Rehabilitation Medicine

Principles and Practice

Third Edition

Rehabilitation Medicine

Principles and Practice

Third Edition

EDITOR-IN-CHIEF

Joel A. DeLisa, M.D., M.S.
Professor and Chairman
Department of Physical Medicine and Rehabilitation
University of Medicine and Dentistry of New Jersey
New Jersey Medical School
Newark, New Jersey; and
President
Kessler Medical Rehabilitation Research and Education Corporation; and
Senior Vice President and Chief Medical Officer
Kessler Rehabilitation Institute
West Orange, New Jersey; and
Chairman
Department of Physical Medicine and Rehabilitation
St. Barnabas Medical Center
Livingston, New Jersey

EDITOR

Bruce M. Gans, M.D., M.S.
Professor and Chairman
Department of Physical Medicine and Rehabilitation
Wayne State University School of Medicine
Senior Vice President
Rehabilitation Institute of Michigan
The Detroit Medical Center
Detroit, Michigan

ASSOCIATE EDITORS

William L. Bockenek, M.D.
Donald M. Currie, M.D.
Steve R. Geiringer, M.D.
Lynn H. Gerber, M.D.
James A. Leonard, Jr., M.D.
Malcolm C. McPhee, M.D.
William S. Pease, M.D.
Nicolas E. Walsh, M.D.

With 169 contributing authors

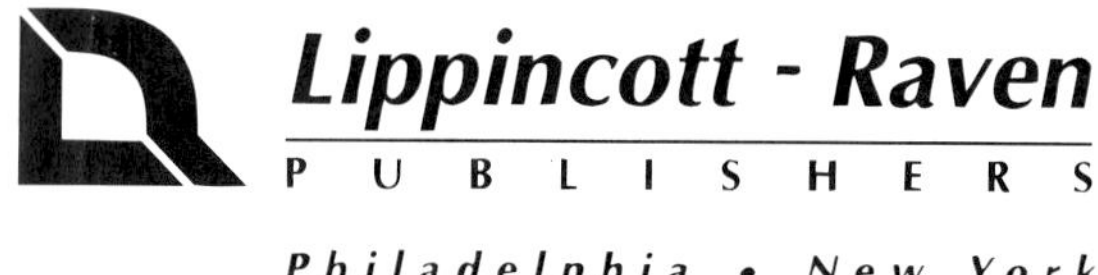

Philadelphia • New York

Acquisitions Editor: Elizabeth Greenspan
Developmental Editor: Emilie M. Linkins and Susan Rhyner
Manufacturing Manager: Dennis Teston
Production Manager: Jodi Borgenicht
Production Editor: Raeann Touhey
Cover Designer: Joseph DePinho
Indexer: Jayne Percy
Compositor: Maryland Composition
Printer: Quebecor Kingsport

Printed in the United States of America

9 8 7 6 5 4 3 2 1

Library of Congress Cataloging-in-Publication Data

Rehabilitation medicine : principles and practice / editors, Joel A. DeLisa, Bruce M. Gans ; section editors, William L. Bockenek ... et al.] ; with 169 contributing authors. — 3rd ed.
p. cm.
Includes bibliographical references and index.
ISBN 0-7817-1015-4
1. Medical rehabilitation. 2. Medicine, Physical. I. DeLisa, Joel A. II. Gans, Bruce M. III. Bockenek, William L.
[DNLM: 1. Rehabilitation. 2. Physical Medicine—methods. WB 320 R3458 1998]
RM930.R364 1998
615.8′2—DC21
DNLM/DLC
for Library of Congress

Care has been taken to confirm the accuracy of the information presented and to describe generally accepted practices. However, the authors, editors, and publisher are not responsible for errors or omissions or for any consequences from application of the information in this book and make no warranty, express or implied, with respect to the contents of the publication.

The authors, editors, and publisher have exerted every effort to ensure that drug selection and dosage set forth in this text are in accordance with current recommendations and practice at the time of publication. However, in view of ongoing research, changes in government regulations, and the constant flow of information relating to drug therapy and drug reactions, the reader is urged to check the package insert for each drug for any change in indications and dosage and for added warnings and precautions. This is particularly important when the recommended agent is a new or infrequently employed drug.

Some drugs and medical devices presented in this publication have Food and Drug Administration (FDA) clearance for limited use in restricted research settings. It is the responsibility of the health care provider to ascertain the FDA status of each drug or device planned for use in their clinical practice.

To our patients,
who challenge us to continually strive to improve their health,
function, and quality of life

To our teachers,
who challenged us to develop a scientific approach to problem-solving and
instilled in us the need for continuous learning

To our students,
who challenge and stimulate us to keep at the cutting edge. They are our
hope for the future

To our families,
who provided the inspiration, support, and patience necessary to
make this text a reality

Contents

Part II. Management Methods

Contributing Authors

Craig Alexander, Ph.D.
Associate Professor
Department of Physical Medicine and Rehabilitation
University of Medicine and Dentistry of New Jersey
New Jersey Medical School
150 Bergen Street
Newark, New Jersey 07103; and
Kessler Institute for Rehabilitation
1199 Pleasant Valley Way
West Orange, New Jersey 07052

Michael Andary, M.D., M.S.
Associate Professor
Department of Physical Medicine and Rehabilitation
Michigan State University
College of Osteopathic Medicine
B401 West Fee Hall
East Lansing, Michigan 48824

Don Anderson, M.A.
Coordinator
Disability Rights and Education
Ann Arbor Center for Independent Living
2568 Packard Road
Ann Arbor, Michigan 48104

John R. Bach, M.D.
Professor and Vice Chairman
Department of Physical Medicine and Rehabilitation
University of Medicine and Dentistry of New Jersey
New Jersey Medical School
150 Bergen Street, Room B403
Newark, New Jersey 07103

Richard D. Ball, M.D., Ph.D.
Attending Physician
Department of Physical Medicine
Munson Medical Center
1221 6th Street, Suite 300
Traverse City, Michigan 49689

Laura L. Barnett, M.C.S.D./C.C.C.-S.L.P.
Speech-Language Pathologist
Department of Rehabilitation Services
University of Utah Hospital
50 North Medical Drive
Salt Lake City, Utah 84132

Jeffrey R. Basford, M.D., Ph.D.
Associate Professor
Mayo Medical School
Consultant
Department of Physical Medicine and Rehabilitation
Mayo Clinic
200 1st Street Southwest
Rochester, Minnesota 55905-0001

John V. Basmajian, O.C., O.Ont., M.D., F.R.C.P.C., F.R.C.P.C. (Glasg), F.A.C.A., F.S.B.M., F.A.B.M.R., F.A.F.R.M.-R.A.C.P. (Australia), Hon Dip (St LC)
Professor Emeritus in Medicine and Anatomy
Department of Medicine
Chedoke Rehabilitation Centre of Hamilton Health Science Corporation
Chedoke, Box 2000
Hamilton, Ontario L8N 3Z5
Canada

Lee A. Beatty, M.D.
Adjunct Clinical Assistant Professor
Department of Family Medicine
University of North Carolina at Chapel Hill
School of Medicine
215 South Main Street
Mount Holly, North Carolina 28120

Bruce E. Becker, M.D.
Associate Professor
Department of Physical Medicine and Rehabilitation
Wayne State University School of Medicine
Rehabilitation Institute of Michigan
261 Mack Boulevard
Detroit, Michigan 48201

Jeanne L. Beer, R.D.
Clinical Dietitian
Department of Nutrition Services
Virginia Mason Medical Center
1100 9th Avenue, X2-DTO
Seattle, Washington 98111

Fadi J. Bejjani, M.D., Ph.D.
Atlantic Occupational Orthopaedic Centers
14 Franklin Street
Belleville, New Jersey 07109

Kathleen R. Bell, M.D.
Assistant Professor
Department of Rehabilitation Medicine
University of Washington Medical Center
1959 Northeast Pacific Street Box 256490
Seattle, Washington 98195

Barbara T. Benevento, M.D.
Assistant Professor
Department of Physical Medicine and Rehabilitation
University of Medicine and Dentistry of New Jersey
New Jersey Medical School
150 Bergen Street
Newark, New Jersey 07103; and
Staff Physiatrist
Kessler Institute for Rehabilitation
1199 Pleasant Valley Way
West Orange, New Jersey 07052

Keith A. Bengtson, M.D.
Instructor
Department of Physical Medicine and Rehabilitation
Mayo Medical Center
200 1st Street Southwest
Rochester, Minnesota 55905

Marla Bernbaum, M.D.
Associate Professor
Department of Internal Medicine
Division of Endocrinology
St. Louis University Health Sciences Center
1402 South Grand Boulevard
St. Louis, Missouri 63104

Champa V. Bid, M.D.
Assistant Professor of Clinical Physical Medicine and Rehabilitation
Department of Physical Medicine and Rehabilitation
University of Medicine and Dentistry of New Jersey
New Jersey Medical School; and
Kessler Institute for Rehabilitation
300 Market Street
Saddle Brook, New Jersey 07663

William L. Bockenek, M.D.
Director
Spinal Cord Injury Program
Residency Training Director
Clinical Assistant Professor
Department of Physical Medicine and Rehabilitation
Charlotte Institute of Rehabilitation
Carolinas Medical Center
1100 Blythe Boulevard
Charlotte, North Carolina 28203

Francis J. Bonner, Jr., M.D.
Clinical Professor of Medicine
Chairman
Department of Physical Medicine and Rehabilitation
Allegheny Graduate Hospital
One Graduate Plaza, Pepper Pavillion 1000
Philadelphia, Pennsylvania 19146

Murray E. Brandstater, M.B.B.S., Ph.D., F.R.C.P.(C)
Professor and Chairman
Department of Physical Medicine and Rehabilitation
Loma Linda University Medical Center
11234 Anderson Street
Loma Linda, California 92354

Brian A. Casazza, M.D.
Assistant Professor
Department of Physical Medicine and Rehabilitation
Director
Division of Spine and Sports Care
University of Virginia Health System
2955 Ivy Road, Suite 311
Charlottesville, Virginia 22903

John Chae, M.D.
Assistant Professor
Center for Physical Medicine and Rehabilitation
Case Western Reserve University
MetroHealth Medical Center
2500 MetroHealth Drive
Cleveland, Ohio 44109

Charles D. Chesnut III, M.D.
Professor
Department of Medicine and Radiology
Adjunct Professor
Department of Orthopaedics
University of Washington Medical Center
218 40th Avenue East
Seattle, Washington 98112

Joseph W. Cheu, R.Ph., D.O.
Instructor
Department of Physical Medicine and Rehabilitation
University of Medicine and Dentistry of New Jersey
New Jersey Medical School
150 Bergen Street
Newark, New Jersey 07103

Naoichi Chino, M.D., M.S. (Phys Med), D.M.Sc.
Professor and Chairman
Department of Rehabilitation Medicine
Keio University School of Medicine
35 Shinano-Machi
Shinjuku-ku, Tokyo 160
Japan

Charles H. Christiansen, Ed.D.
Dean and George T. Bryan Distinguished Professor
School of Allied Health Sciences
University of Texas Medical Branch at Galveston
301 University Boulevard
Galveston, Texas 77555-1028

Robert P. Christopher, B.S., M.D.
Professor and Chief
Division of Rehabilitation Medicine
University of Tennessee College of Medicine
800 Madison Avenue
Memphis, Tennessee 38163

Gary S. Clark, M.D.
Associate Professor of Clinical Rehabilitation Medicine
Head
Department of Rehabilitation Medicine
Buffalo General Hospital
100 High Street
Buffalo, New York 14203-1154

Bruce A. Cohen, M.D.
Associate Professor
Department of Neurology
Northwest University Medical School
645 North Michigan Avenue Suite 1058
Chicago, Illinois 60611

Andrew J. Cole, M.D., F.A.C.S.M.
Puget Sound Sports and Spine Physicians
1600 East Jefferson Street, Suite 401
Seattle, Washington 98122

Jeffrey L. Cole, M.D.
Associate Professor
Department of Physical Medicine and Rehabilitation
The New York Hospital Medical Center of Queens
56-45 Main Street
Flushing, New York 11355

Ann C. Cotter, M.D.
Assistant Professor of Clinical Physical Medicine and Rehabilitation
Department of Physical Medicine and Rehabilitation
University of Medicine and Dentistry of New Jersey
New Jersey Medical School
150 Bergen Street
Newark, New Jersey 07103; and
Staff Physiatrist
Physical Medicine and Rehabilitation Service
Veterans Administration Medical Center
East Orange, New Jersey; and
Consultant
Center for Complementary and Alternative Medicine
Kessler Medical Rehabilitation Research and Education Corporation
1199 Pleasant Valley Way
West Orange, New Jersey 07052

Graham H. Creasey, B.Sc., M.B., Ch.B., F.R.C.S.Ed.
Assistant Professor
Regional Spinal Cord Injury Service
MetroHealth Medical Center
2500 MetroHealth Drive
Cleveland, Ohio 44109

G. Fred Cromes, Jr., Ph.D.
Associate Professor of Rehabilitation Psychology
Department of Physical Medicine and Rehabilitation
The University of Texas—Southwestern Medical Center at Dallas
5323 Harry Hines Boulevard
Dallas, Texas 75235-9055

Donald M. Currie, M.D.
Associate Professor
Department of Rehabilitation Medicine
University of Texas Health Science Center at San Antonio
7703 Floyd Curl Drive
San Antonio, Texas 78284-7798

Gerben DeJong, Ph.D.
Professor
Department of Family Medicine
National Rehabilitation Hospital Research Center
Georgetown University
1016 16th Street, Northwest
Washington, D.C. 20010

Barbara J. de Lateur, M.D., M.S.
Professor
Department of Physical Medicine and Rehabilitation
The Johns Hopkins University School of Medicine
5601 Loch Raven Boulevard-Professional Office Building Room 406
Baltimore, Maryland 21239

Joel A. DeLisa, M.D., M.S.
Professor and Chairman
Department of Physical Medicine and Rehabilitation
University of Medicine and Dentistry of New Jersey
New Jersey Medical School
150 Bergen Street, UH B261
Newark, New Jersey 07103; and
President
Kessler Medical Rehabilitation Research and Education Corporation; and
Senior Vice President and Chief Medical Officer
Kessler Rehabilitation Institute
1199 Pleasant Valley Way
West Orange, New Jersey 07052; and
Chairman
Department of Physical Medicine and Rehabilitation
St. Barnabas Medical Center
Livingston, New Jersey 07039

Bruce J. Diamond, M.Ed., Ph.D.
Assistant Professor
Departments of Physical Medicine and Rehabilitation and Research
University of Medicine and Dentistry of New Jersey
New Jersey Medical School
150 Bergen Street, UH B-261
Newark, New Jersey 07103;
Kessler Medical Rehabilitation and Education Corporation
1199 Pleasant Valley Way
West Orange, New Jersey 07052

Daniel Dumitru, M.D.
Professor and Deputy Chairman
Department of Rehabilitation Medicine
University of Texas Health Science Center at San Antonio
7703 Floyd Curl Drive
San Antonio, Texas 78284-7798

Rolland P. Erickson, M.D.
Consultant and Assistant Professor
Department of Physical Medicine and Rehabilitation
Mayo Clinic-Scottsdale
13400 East Shea Boulevard
Scottsdale, Arizona 85259

Avital Fast, M.D.
Professor
Department of Rehabilitation Medicine
Montefiore Medical Center
Albert Einstein College of Medicine
111 East 210th Street
Bronx, New York 10467

Steven M. Fine, M.D.
Instructor and Fellow
Department of Medicine—Infectious Diseases Unit
University of Rochester School of Medicine and Dentistry
601 Elmwood Avenue, Box 689
Rochester, New York 14642

Steven V. Fisher, M.D., M.S.
Chief and Associate Professor
Department of Physical Medicine and Rehabilitation
University of Minnesota Medical School
Hennepin County Medical Center
701 Park Avenue
Minneapolis, Minnesota 55415

Amy Fitzsimmons, M.D.
Staff Physician
Department of Physical Medicine and Rehabilitation
Graduate Hospital
Philadelphia, Pennsylvania 19146

Angeles M. Flores, M.D.
Clinical Professor
Department of Physical Medicine and Rehabilitation
University of Medicine and Dentistry of New Jersey
New Jersey Medical School
150 Bergen Street
Newark, New Jersey 07103; and
Veterans Administration Medical Center
385 Tremont Avenue
East Orange, New Jersey 07018

Christopher S. Formal, M.D.
Assistant Professor
Department of Rehabilitation Medicine
Thomas Jefferson University Hospital
111 South 11th Street
Philadelphia, Pennsylvania 19102

Gerard E. Francisco, M.D.
Associate Director
Brain Injury Program
The Institute for Rehabilitation and Research
1333 Moursund Avenue
Houston, Texas 77030

Mitchell K. Freedman, D.O.
Instructor
Department of Physical Medicine and Rehabilitation
Magee Rehabilitation Hospital
6 Franklin Plaza
Philadelphia, Pennsylvania 19102

Guy W. Fried, M.D.
Assistant Professor
Department of Rehabilitation Medicine
Thomas Jefferson University Hospital; and
Magee Rehabilitation Hospital
6 Franklin Plaza
Philadelphia, Pennsylvania 19102

Bruce M. Gans, M.D., M.S.
Professor and Chairman
Department of Physical Medicine and Rehabilitation
Wayne State University School of Medicine
Senior Vice President
Rehabilitation Institute of Michigan
The Detroit Medical Center
261 Mack Avenue
Detroit, Michigan 48201-2417

Steve R. Geiringer, M.D.
Professor
Department of Physical Medicine and Rehabilitation
Wayne State University
36301 Warren Road
Detroit, Michigan 48201

Lynn H. Gerber, M.D.
Chief
Department of Rehabilitation Medicine
National Institutes of Health
9000 Rockville Pike
Bethesda, Maryland 20892-1604; and
Professor of Internal Medicine
Department of Rheumatology
Georgetown University Medical Center
4000 River Road, Northwest
Washington, D.C. 20057; and
Associate Professor of Internal Medicine
George Washington University Medical Center
901 23rd Street, Northwest
Washington, D.C. 20037

Carol J. Gill, Ph.D.
Assistant Professor
Department of Disability and Human Development
University of Illinois at Chicago
1640 West Roosevelt Road, Suite 236
Chicago, Illinois 60608

Gunnar Grimby, M.D., Ph.D.
Professor
Department of Rehabilitation Medicine
Göteborg University
Sahlgenska University Hospital
S-41345 Göteborg
Sweden

Michael E. Groher, Ph.D.
Chief
Department of Audiology and Speech Pathology
James A. Haley Veteran's Hospital
13000 Bruce B. Downs Boulevard
Tampa, Florida 33612

Janet F. Haas, M.D.
William Penn Foundation
Two Logan Square, 11th Floor
100 North 18th Street
Philadelphia, Pennsylvania 19103-2757

Eugen M. Halar, M.D.
Professor
Department of Rehabilitation Medicine
University of Washington Medical Center
1959 Northeast Pacific Avenue, Box 358280
Seattle, Washington 98195

Farrukh Hamid, M.D., F.A.A.D.E.P.
Assistant Professor
Department of Physical Medicine and Rehabilitation
The University of Texas—Southwestern Medical Center at Dallas
5323 Harry Hines Boulevard
Dallas, Texas 75235-9055

Margaret C. Hammond, M.D.
Associate Professor
Department of Physical Medicine and Rehabilitation
University of Washington
Box 356490
Seattle, Washington 98195

Karen Hardwick, B.S.O.T., M.Ed., Ph.D.
Director
Department of Habilitation Therapies
Austin State School
2203 West 35th Street
P.O. Box 1269
Austin, Texas 78767

Tessa Hart, Ph.D.
Clinical Neuropsychologist
Drucker Brain Injury Center
Moss Rehabilitation Hospital
1200 West Tabor Road
Philadelphia, Pennsylvania 19141

Robert K. Heinrich, Ph.D.
Clinical Psychologist
McAuley Mental Health Services
St. Joseph Mercy Hospital
Ann Arbor, Michigan 48105

Phala A. Helm, M.D., B.S.
Professor
Department of Physical Medicine and Rehabilitation
University of Texas—Southwestern Medical Center at Dallas
5323 Harry Hines Boulevard
Dallas, Texas 75235-9055

Stanley A. Herring, M.D.
Clinical Associate Professor
Departments of Rehabilitation Medicine and Orthopaedics
University of Washington
1959 Northeast Pacific Avenue
Seattle, Washington 98195; and
Puget Sound Sports and Spine Physicians
1600 East Jefferson Street, Suite 401
Seattle, Washington 98122

Mary L. Heye, R.N., Ph.D.
Assistant Professor
Department of Acute Nursing Care
University of Texas Health Science Center at San Antonio
7703 Floyd Curl Drive
San Antonio, Texas 78284

Jeanne E. Hicks, M.D.
Deputy Chief
Department of Rehabilitation Medicine
National Institutes of Health
9000 Rockville Pike
Bethesda, Maryland 20892-1604; and
Associate Professor
Department of Internal Medicine
George Washington University Medical Center
901 23rd Street, Northwest
Washington, D.C. 20037; and
Associate Professor of Physical Medicine and Rehabilitation
Department of Orthopedic Surgery
Georgetown University Medical Center
4000 River Road, Northwest
Washington, D.C. 20057; and
Assistant Professor of Internal Medicine
Uniformed Armed Services Institutes
4301 Jones Bridge Road
Bethesda, Maryland 20814

Kathleen A. Hinderer, M.S., M.P.T., P.T.
Doctoral Candidate
Center for Human Motor Research
Department of Movement Science
Division of Kinesiology
University of Michigan
401 Washtenaw Avenue, CCRB
Ann Arbor, Michigan 48109-2214; and
Senior Physical Therapist
Rehabiliation Insitute of Michigan
261 Mack Avenue
Detroit, Michigan 48201-2417

Steven R. Hinderer, M.D., M.S., P.T.
Assistant Professor
Department of Physical Medicine and Rehabilitation
Wayne State University School of Medicine
Rehabilitation Institute of Michigan
261 Mack Avenue
Detroit, Michigan 48201-2417

Martin D. Hoffman, M.D.
Associate Professor
Physical Medicine and Rehabilitation
Medical College of Wisconsin
5000 West National Avenue
Milwaukee, Wisconsin 53295

Todd G. Holmes, M.D.
Clinical Assistant Professor
Department of Physical Medicine and Rehabilitation
Michigan State University
College of Osteopathic Medicine
East Lansing, Michigan 48824; and
Staff Physician
Sister Kenny Institute
800 East 28th Street at Chicago
Minneapolis, Minnesota 55407

Barbara Hopkins, M.M.Sc., R.D., L.D.
Instructor
Department of Nutrition
Georgia State University
College of Health and Human Sciences
Atlanta, Georgia 30303

Satiko Tomikawa Imamura, M.D., Ph.D.
Director of Physical Medicine and Rehabilitation
Institute for Orthopaedics and Traumatology
Hospital das Clinicas
University of Sao Paulo Medical School
Sao Paulo
Brazil

Sudesh S. Jain, M.D.
Associate Professor of Clinical Physical Medicine and Rehabilitation
Department of Physical Medicine and Rehabilitation
University of Medicine and Dentistry of New Jersey
New Jersey Medical School
150 Bergen Street, Room B261
Newark, New Jersey 07103;
Department of Clinical Physical Medicine and Rehabilitation
St. Barnabas Medical Center
Suite 309, Old Short Hills Road
Livingston, New Jersey 07039

Mark V. Johnston, Ph.D.
Associate Professor
Department of Physical Medicine and Rehabilitation
University of Medicine and Dentistry of New Jersey
New Jersey Medical School
150 Bergen Street
Newark, New Jersey 07103; and
Director of Outcomes Research
Kessler Medical Rehabilitation Research and Education Corporation
1199 Pleasant Valley Way
West Orange, New Jersey 07052

Susan M. Kaschalk, B.S., P.A.-S.
Exercise Physiologist
St. Joseph Mercy Hospital
888 Woodward Avenue, Suite 304
Pontiac, Michigan 48320

Glenn M. Kaye, M.D.
Department of Otolaryngology—Head and Neck Surgery
McGill University
Montreal, Quebec H3G 1Y6
Canada

D. Casey Kerrigan, M.D., M.S.
Assistant Professor
Department of Physical Medicine and Rehabilitation
Harvard Medical School
Spaulding Rehabilitation Hospital
125 Nashua Street
Boston, Massachusetts 02114

Paul R. Kileny, Ph.D.
Professor of Otolaryngology
Director of Audiology and Electrophysiology
Department of Otolaryngology—Head and Neck Surgery
University of Michigan Medical Center
1500 East Medical Center Drive
Ann Arbor, Michigan 48109

Kevin Kilgore, Ph.D.
Department of Orthopaedics
MetroHealth Medical Center
2500 MetroHealth Drive
Cleveland, Ohio 44109

John C. King, M.D.
Associate Professor
Department of Rehabilitation Medicine
University of Texas Health Science Center at San Antonio
7703 Floyd Curl Drive
San Antonio, Texas 78284

R. Lee Kirby, M.D., F.R.C.P.C.
Professor and Head
Division of Physical Medicine and Rehabilitation
Dalhousie University
1341 Summer Street
Halifax, Nova Scotia B3H 4K4
Canada

Kristi L. Kirschner, M.D.
Assistant Professor
Department of Physical Medicine and Rehabilitation
Rehabilitation Institute of Chicago
Northwestern University Medical School
345 East Superior Street
Chicago, Illinois 60611

Steven C. Kirshblum, M.D.
Assistant Professor and Residency Training Director
Department of Physical Medicine and Rehabilitation
University of Medicine and Dentistry of New Jersey
New Jersey Medical School
150 Bergen Street
Newark, New Jersey 07103; and
Director
Spinal Cord Injury Program
Kessler Institute for Rehabilitation
1199 Pleasant Valley Way
West Orange, New Jersey 07052

Robert Klecz, M.D.
31 Sherwood Court
River Edge, New Jersey 07661

David S. Klein, M.D.
Shenandoah Valley Pain Clinic
109 Mackenly Place
Staunton, Virginia 24461

William J. Kraemer, Ph.D.
Professor
Department of Applied Physiology
Director of Research
Center for Sports Medicine
The Pennsylvania State University
21 REC Building
University Park, Pennsylvania 16802

Andrea Laborde, M.D.
Clinical Assistant Professor
Department of Physical Medicine and Rehabilitation
Temple University School of Medicine
Philadelphia, Pennsylvania 19140; and
Attending Physician
Drucker Brain Injury Center
Moss Rehabilitation Research Institute
1200 West Tabor Road
Philadelphia, Pennsylvania 19141

Indira S. Lanig, M.D.
Assistant Clinical Professor
Department of Physical Medicine and Rehabilitation
University of Colorado Health Science Center
Craig Hospital
3425 South Clarkson
Englewood, Colorado 80110

James A. Leonard, Jr., M.D.
Clinical Professor and Chair
Department of Physical Medicine and Rehabilitation
University of Michigan Medical Center
1500 East Medical Center Drive
Ann Arbor, Michigan 48109-0042

Stephen F. Levinson, M.D., Ph.D.
Assistant Professor
Department of Physical Medicine and Rehabilitation
University of Rochester School of Medicine and Dentistry
601 Elmwood Avenue
Rochester, New York 14642

Robert Lindsay, M.D., Ph.D.
Professor of Clinical Medicine
Department of Medicine
Columbia University
New York, New York 10027; and
Chief of Internal Medicine
Department of Medicine
Helen Hayes Hospital
West Haverstraw, New York 10993

Todd A. Linsenmeyer, M.D.
Associate Professor
Departments of Physical Medicine and Rehabilitation and Surgery (Urology)
University of Medicine and Dentistry of New Jersey
New Jersey School of Medicine
150 Bergen Street
Newark, New Jersey 07103; and
Director
Department of Urology
Kessler Institute for Rehabilitation
1199 Pleasant Valley Way
West Orange, New Jersey 07052

James W. Little, M.D., Ph.D.
Assistant Professor
Department of Rehabilitation Medicine
University of Washington School of Medicine
1959 Northeast Pacific Street, BB-919 HSB RJ-30
Seattle, Washington 98195

E. Patrick Maloney, M.D., M.P.H.
Volunteer Faculty
Department of Physical Medicine and Rehabilitation
University of Arkansas for Medical Sciences
4301 West Markham Street
Little Rock, Arkansas 72205

Miriam Maney, M.A.
Program Evaluation Manager
Kessler Institute for Rehabilitation
1199 Pleasant Valley Way
West Orange, New Jersey 07052

Nancy Mann, M.D.
Assistant Professor and Associate Chair
Department of Physical Medicine and Rehabilitation
Wayne State University School of Medicine
Rehabilitation Institute of Michigan
261 Mack Boulevard
Detroit, Michigan 48201

Rebecca A. Marburger, M.E.B.M.E., O.T.R.
Assistant Director
Department of Occupational Therapy
Austin State School
2203 West 35th Street
Austin, Texas 78703

Gordon M. Martin, M.D., M.S.
Emeritus Professor
Department of Physical Medicine and Rehabilitation
Mayo Medical School and Mayo Graduate School of Medicine; and
Department of Physical Medicine and Rehabilitation
Mayo Clinic
200 1st Street Southwest
Rochester, Minnesota 55905-0001

Teresa L. Massagli, M.D.
Associate Professor
Departments of Rehabilitation Medicine and Pediatrics
University of Washington School of Medicine
1959 Northeast Pacific Street, Box 356490
Seattle, Washington 98195

B. Cairbre McCann, M.D.
Department of Rehabilitation Medicine
Maine Medical Center
22 Brumhall Street
Portland, Maine 04102-3175

Malcolm C. McPhee, M.D.
Associate Professor
Department of Physical Medicine and Rehabilitation
Mayo Clinic-Scottsdale
13400 East Shea Boulevard
Scottsdale, Arizona 85259

Robert H. Meier III, M.D.
Director of Medical Rehabilitation
O'Hara Regional Center for Rehabilitation
1500 Hooker Street
Denver, Colorado 80204

Robert M. Miller, Ph.D.
Chief
Department of Audiology and Speech Pathology
Veterans Administration Puget Sound Health Care System; and
Clinical Associate Professor
Department of Rehabilitation Medicine
University of Washington
1660 South Columbian Way
Seattle, Washington 98108

Carol Adams Mushett, M.Ed., C.T.R.S., M.S.W.
Department of Kinesiology and Health
Georgia State University
College of Education
University Plaza
Atlanta, Georgia 30303

Jodi Weiss Nadler, B.S.
Occupational Therapist
Department of Occupational Therapy
Kessler Institute for Rehabilitation—Welkind Facility
Pleasant Hill Road
Chester, New Jersey 07930

Scott Nadler, D.O.
Assistant Professor
Department of Physical Medicine and Rehabilitation
University of Medicine and Dentistry of New Jersey
New Jersey Medical School
90 Bergen Street
Newark, New Jersey 07103

Sangeetha Nayak, Ph.D.
Research Scientist
Kessler Medical Rehabilitation Research and Education Corporation
1199 Pleasant Valley Way
West Orange, New Jersey 07052

T. Russell Nelson, Ph.D.
Clinical Associate Professor
Department of Rehabilitation Medicine
University of Texas Health Science Center at San Antonio
7703 Floyd Curl Drive
San Antonio, Texas 78284; and
Speech Pathologist
Department of Veterans Affairs
South Texas Health Care System
7400 Merton Minter Boulevard
San Antonio, Texas 78284

Kevin C. O'Connor, M.D.
Assistant Professor
Department of Physical Medical and Rehabilitation
University of Medicine and Dentistry of New Jersey
New Jersey Medical School
150 Bergen Street
Newark, New Jersey 07103; and
Kessler Institute for Rehabilitation
1199 Pleasant Valley Way
West Orange, New Jersey 07052

Kenneth J. Ottenbacher, Ph.D., O.T.R.
Professor and Vice Dean
School of Allied Health Sciences
University of Texas Medical Branch at Galveston
301 University Boulevard
Galveston, Texas 77555-1028

Liina Paasuke, M.A., C.R.C.
Certified Rehabilitation Counselor
Department of Rehabilitation Services
Michigan Jobs Commission
I H 225 University Hospital
1500 East Medical Center Drive
Ann Arbor, Michigan 48109-0050

Jeffrey B. Palmer, M.D.
Associate Professor
Departments of Physical Medicine and Rehabilitation and Otolaryngology
Johns Hopkins University
Good Samaritan Hospital
Baltimore, Maryland 21218

Geetha Pandian, M.D.
Assistant Professor and Residency Program Director
Department of Physical Medicine and Rehabilitation
University of Texas—Southwestern Medical Center at Dallas
5323 Harry Hines Boulevard
Dallas, Texas 75235-9055

Shailesh S. Parikh, M.D.
Assistant Professor of Clinical Medicine and Rehabilitation
Department of Physical Medicine and Rehabilitation
University of Medicine and Dentistry of New Jersey
New Jersey Medical School; and
Kessler Institute for Rehabilitation
300 Market Street
Saddle Brook, New Jersey 07663

Jaywant J.P. Patil, M.B., B.S., F.R.C.P.C.
Assistant Professor of Medicine
Department of Physical Medicine and Rehabilitation
Dalhousie University
1526 Dresden Row, Fourth Floor
Halifax, Nova Scotia B3J 3K3
Canada

William S. Pease, M.D.
Associate Professor and Chairperson
Department of Physical Medicine and Rehabilitation
Medical Director
Dodd Hall Rehabilitation Program
The Ohio State University College of Medicine and Public Health
1018 Dodd Hall
480 West 9th Avenue
Columbus, Ohio 43210

Bonnie Pond, B.S.
Department of Rehabilitation Services
University of Utah Hospital
50 North Medical Drive
Salt Lake City, Utah 84132

Joel M. Press, M.D.
Assistant Professor
Department of Physical Medicine and Rehabilitation
Northwestern University
1030 North Clark Street
Chicago, Illinois 60611

Kent Questad, M.D.
Assistant Professor of Clinical Psychology
Department of Rehabilitation Medicine
University of Washington
124 Harborview Hall
Seattle, Washington 98195

Kristjan T. Ragnarsson, M.D.
Dr. Lucy G. Moses Professor
Department of Rehabilitation Medicine
The Mount Sinai Medical Center
1425 Madison Avenue, Box 1240
New York, New York 10029

Somayaji Ramamurthy, M.D.
Professor
Department of Anesthesiology
University of Texas Health Science Center at San Antonio
7703 Floyd Curl Drive
San Antonio, Texas 78284-7838

Mary E. Schmidt Read, M.S., P.T.
Director
Department of Physical Therapy
Director
Spinal Cord Injury Program
Magee Rehabilitation Hospital
6 Franklin Plaza
Philadelphia, Pennsylvania 19102; and
Adjunct Assistant Professor
Allegheny University of the Health Sciences
Philadelphia, Pennsylvania 19102

James J. Rechtien, D.O., Ph.D.
Professor
Department of Physical Medicine and Rehabilitation
Michigan State University
College of Osteopathic Medicine
A-434 East Fee Hall
East Lansing, Michigan 48824

Thomas S. Rees, Ph.D.
Associate Professor
Department of Otolaryngology—Head and Neck Surgery
University of Washington
1660 South Columbine Way
Seattle, Washington 98108; and
Chief
Department of Audiology
Harborview Medical Center
Audiology Box 359894
325 9th Avenue
Seattle, Washington 98104

Judy Panko Reis, M.A., M.S.
Administrative Director
Health Resource Center for Women with Disabilities
Rehabilitation Institute of Chicago
345 East Superior
Chicago, Illinois 60611

Kenneth J. Richter, D.O.
Clinical Associate Professor
Department of Rehabilitation Medicine
St. Joseph Mercy at Oakland
Michigan State University
888 Woodward Avenue
Pontiac, Michigan 48341

Haim Ring, M.D., M.Sc. PM&R
Professor of Physical Medicine and Rehabilitation
Chairman, Department of Neurological Rehabilitation and Institute for Functional Evaluation
Deputy Director
Loewenstein Hospital Rehabilitation Center
Tel Aviv University Medical School
P.O. Box 3
Raanana 43100
Israel

James P. Robinson, M.D., Ph.D.
Clinical Assistant Professor
Department of Rehabilitation Medicine
University of Washington Hospital
Box 356490
Seattle, Washington 98195; and
University of Washington Pain Center
4245 Roosevelt Way, Northeast
Seattle, Washington 98105

Keith M. Robinson, M.D.
Assistant Professor
Department of Rehabilitation Medicine
University of Pennsylvania Health System
3400 Spruce Street
Philadelphia, Pennsylvania 19104

James N. Rogers, M.D.
Associate Professor
Department of Anesthesiology
University of Texas Health Science Center at San Antonio
7703 Floyd Curl Drive
San Antonio, Texas 78284

Daniel E. Rohe, Ph.D., A.B.P.P.
Associate Professor
Departments of Psychiatry and Psychology
Mayo Clinic and Foundation
200 1st Street Southwest
Rochester, Minnesota 55905

Robert D. Rondinelli, M.D., Ph.D.
Associate Professor and Chairman
Department of Physical Medicine and Rehabilitation
University of Kansas Medical Center
3901 Rainbow Boulevard
Kansas City, Kansas 66160-7306

Mitchell Rosenthal, M.A., Ph.D.
Professor and Associate Chair
Department of Physical Medicine and Rehabilitation
Wayne State University
Rehabilitation Institute of Michigan
261 Mack Avenue
Detroit, Michigan 48201

Sandy Salerno, O.T.R.
Clinical Specialist
Department of Occupational Therapy
St. Francis College
Brooklyn, New York; and
Kean College
Union, New Jersey; and
Kessler Institute for Rehabilitation
1199 Pleasant Valley Way
West Orange, New Jersey 07052

Michael Schaufele, M.D.
Department of Physical Medicine and Rehabilitation Medicine
Harvard Medical School
Spaulding Rehabilitation Hospital
125 Nashua Street
Boston, Massachusetts 02114

Steven J. Scheer, M.D.
Professor and Director
Department of Physical Medicine and Rehabilitation
University of Cincinnati Medical Center
231 Bethesda Avenue
Cincinnati, Ohio 45267-0530

Carson D. Schneck, M.D., Ph.D.
Professor of Anatomy and Diagnostic Imaging
Department of Anatomy and Cell Biology
Temple University School of Medicine
3400 North Broad Street
Philadelphia, Pennsylvania 19140

Andrew A. Schoenberg, Ph.D.
Associate Professor of Medicine and Bioengineering
Department of Physical Medicine and Rehabilitation
University of Utah Hosptial
50 North Medical Drive
Salt Lake City, Utah 84132

Nancy E. Schoenberger, Ph.D.
Assistant Professor
Department of Psychiatry and Physical Medicine and Rehabilitation
University of Medicine and Dentistry of New Jersey
New Jersey Medical School
150 Bergen Street
Newark, New Jersey 07103; and
Assistant Program Director
Kessler Medical Rehabilitation Research and Education Corporation
1199 Pleasant Valley Way
West Orange, New Jersey 07052

Lawrence S. Schoenfeld, Ph.D.
Professor
Department of Psychiatry
University of Texas Health Science Center at San Antonio
7703 Floyd Curl Drive
San Antonio, Texas 78284-7792

Ann H. Schutt, M.D., B.S.
Associate Professor
Department of Physical Medicine and Rehabilitation
Mayo Medical Center
200 1st Street Southwest
Rochester, Minnesota 55905

Lois M. Sheldahl, Ph.D.
Associate Professor
Department of Medicine
Veterans Administration Medical Center
Medical College of Wisconsin
5000 West National Avenue
Milwaukee, Wisconsin 53295

Claudine Sherrill, Ed.D.
Professor of Adapted Physical Activity
Department of Kinesiology
Texas Woman's University at Denton
11168 Windjammer Drive
Denton, Texas 76204

Samuel C. Shiflett, Ph.D.
Assistant Professor
Departments of Psychiatry and Physical Medicine and Rehabilitation
University of Medicine and Dentistry of New Jersey
New Jersey Medical School
150 Bergen Street;
Newark, New Jersey 07103; and
Director, Center for Research in Complementary and Alternative Medicine
Kessler Medical Rehabilitation Research and Education Corporation
1199 Pleasant Valley Way
West Orange, New Jersey 07052

Hilary C. Siebens, M.D.
Associate Director
Department of Physical Medicine and Rehabilitation
Harvard Medical School
Massachusetts General Hospital
55 Fruit Street, V BK 820
Boston, Massachusetts 02114-2696

Eugenia L. Siegler, M.D.
Associate Professor of Clinical Medicine
Department of Medicine
New York University School of Medicine
Brooklyn Hospital Center
121 Dekalb Avenue
Brooklyn, New York 11201

Marca L. Sipski, M.D.
Associate Professor
Department of Physical Medicine and Rehabilitation
University of Medicine and Dentistry of New Jersey
New Jersey Medical School
150 Bergen Street
Newark, New Jersey 07103;
Director of Medical Systems Development
Kessler Rehabilitation Corporation
1199 Pleasant Valley Way
West Orange, New Jersey 07052

James A. Sliwa, D.O.
Associate Professor
Department of Physical Medicine and Rehabilitation
Northwestern University Medical School
Rehabilitation Institute of Chicago
345 East Superior
Chicago, Illinois 60611

Dennis S. Smith, F.R.C.P., F.R.A.C.P.
Professor
Department of Rehabilitation Medicine
Wessex Rehabilitation Centre
University of Southhampton
''Clyro'', Steyne Road, Seaview
Isle of Wight PO345EP
United Kingdom

William E. Staas, Jr., M.D.
Professor
Department of Physical Medicine and Rehabilitation
Thomas Jefferson University
111 South 11th Street
Philadelphia, Pennsylvania 19107; and
President and Medical Director
Magee Rehabilitation Hospital
Six Franklin Plaza
Philadelphia, Pennsylvania 19102

Todd P. Stitik, M.D.
Assistant Professor
Department of Physical Medicine and Rehabilitation
University of Medicine and Dentistry of New Jersey
New Jersey Medical School
150 Bergen Street
Newark, New Jersey 07103; and
Doctors Office Center, Suite 3100
90 Bergen Street
Newark, New Jersey 07103-2499

James M. Stone, M.D., F.A.C.S.
Northern California Surgical Group
2510 Airpark Drive, Suite 301
Redding, California 96001

Joel E. Streim, M.D.
Associate Professor of Psychiatry
Departments of Psychiatry and Rehabilitation Medicine
Hospital of The University of Pennsylvania
Ralston-Penn Center
3615 Chestnut Street
Philadelphia, Pennsylvania 19104-2676

Ingeborg Swanson, M.S., R.D.
Clinical Dietitian
Department of Nutrition Services
Virginia Mason Medical Center
1100 9th Avenue, X2-DTO
Seattle, Washington 98111

James R. Swenson, M.D.
Professor
Department of Physical Medicine and Rehabilitation
University of Utah School of Medicine
50 North Medical Drive
Salt Lake City, Utah 84132

Denise G. Tate, Ph.D.
Associate Professor
Department of Physical Medicine and Rehabilitation
University of Michigan Medical Center
1500 East Medical Center Drive
Ann Arbor, Michigan 48109-0050

Mark Thomas, M.D.
Assistant Professor
Department of Rehabilitation Medicine
Montefiore Medical Center
Albert Einstein College of Medicine
111 East 210th Street
Bronx, New York 10467

Mary Nelle D. Titus, M.A.O.T., M.A.Ed., O.T.R.
Consultant in Medical Rehabilitation
14202 Red Maple Wood
San Antonio, Texas 78249-1859

Ronald J. Triolo, Ph.D.
Assistant Professor
Departments of Orthopaedics and Biomedical Engineering
Case Western Reserve University
MetroHealth Medical Center
2500 MetroHealth Drive
Cleveland, Ohio 44109

Margaret A. Turk, M.D.
Associate Professor
Departments of Physical Medicine and Rehabilitation and Pediatrics
State University of New York Health Science Center at Syracuse
750 East Adams Street
Syracuse, New York 13210

Thomas C. Turturro, M.Div., P.T., O.C.S.
Assistant Professor
Department of Physical Therapy
University of Texas Health Science Center at San Antonio
7703 Floyd Curl Drive
San Antonio, Texas 78284

Mary Vargo, M.D.
Assistant Professor
MetroHealth Medical Center
2500 MetroHealth Drive
Cleveland, Ohio 44109

Stanley F. Wainapel, M.D., M.P.H.
Associate Professor and Clinical Director
Department of Rehabilitation Medicine
Montefiore Hospital
Albert Einstein College of Medicine
111 East 210th Street
Bronx, New York 10467

Nicolas E. Walsh, M.D.
Professor and Chairman
Department of Rehabilitation Medicine
University of Texas Health Science Center at San Antonio
7703 Floyd Curl Drive
San Antonio, Texas 78284-7798

Robert J. Weber, M.D.
Professor and Chairman
Department of Physical Medicine and Rehabilitation
State University of New York Health Science Center at Syracuse
750 East Adams Street
Syracuse, New York 13210

Stuart M. Weinstein, M.D.
Clinical Assistant Professor
Department of Rehabilitation Medicine
University of Washington
1959 Northeast Pacific Avenue
Seattle, Washington 98195; and
Puget Sound Sports and Spine Physicians
1600 East Jefferson Street, Suite 401
Seattle, Washington 98122

Sandra Welner, M.D.
Medical Staff
Department of Obstetrics and Gynecology
Sibley Memorial Hospital
Washington, D.C. 20016

Marco N. Wen, M.D.
Instructor
Department of Physical Medicine and Rehabilitation
Harvard Medical School
Spaulding Rehabilitation Hospital
125 Nashua Street
Boston, Massachusetts 02114

John Whyte, M.D., Ph.D.
Professor
Department of Physical Medicine and Rehabilitation
Temple University School of Medicine
3401 North Broad Street
Philadelphia, Pennsylvania 19140; and
Director
Moss Rehabilitation Research Institute
MossRehab
1200 West Tabor Road
Philadelphia, Pennsylvania 19141

J. Michael Wieting, D.O., M.Ed.
Associate Professor
Department of Physical Medicine and Rehabilitation
Michigan State University
College of Osteopathic Medicine
B401 West Fee Hall
East Lansing, Michigan 48824

Deborah L. Wilkerson, M.A.
Director
Department of Research and Quality Improvement
CARF—The Rehabilitation Accreditation Commission
4891 East Grant Road
Tucson, Arizona 85712

Faren H. Williams, M.D., M.S., R.D.
Assistant Clinical Professor
Department of Rehabilitation Medicine
University of Washington
Box 356490
1959 North East Pacific Street
Seattle, Washington 98195; and
Physiatrist
Virginia Mason Medical Center
1100 9th Avenue, G2-1
Seattle, Washington 98111

Kathryn M. Yorkston, Ph.D.
Professor
Department of Rehabilitation Medicine
University of Washington
Box 356490
Seattle, Washington 98195-6490

Jeffrey L. Young, M.D., M.A.
Associate Professor
Department of Physical Medicine and Rehabilitation
Albert Einstein College of Medicine of Yeshiva University; and
Associate Director
Department of Spine and Sports Rehabilitation
Beth Israel Medical Center
10 Union Square East
New York, New York 10003

Ross O. Zafonte, D.O.
Assistant Professor and Medical Director
Chief, Traumatic Brain Injury Unit
Department of Physical Medicine and Rehabilitation
Wayne State University
Rehabilitation Institute of Michigan
261 Mack Boulevard
Detroit, Michigan 48201

Jerald R. Zimmerman, M.D.
Chief
Department of Rehabilitation Medicine
Englewood Hospital and Medical Center
350 Engle Avenue
Englewood, New Jersey 07631

Lenore R. Zohman, M.D.
Consultant
Cardiac Rehabilitation Service
Department of Physical Medicine and Rehabilitation
Montefiore Medical Center
111 East 210th Street
Bronx, New York 10467

Teresa A. Zwolan, Ph.D.
Assistant Research Scientist
Department of Otolaryngology
University of Michigan
475 Market Place Building 1, Suite A
Ann Arbor, Michigan 48108

Preface

There have been a surprising number of changes in the field of physical medicine and rehabilitation (PM&R) since the publication of the Second Edition of this book. Among these changes are advances in the amelioration of spinal cord and traumatic brain injury, advances in robotics and microelectronics, the explosion of the Internet as a communication channel, and substantial changes in the health care delivery system, with the evolution of managed care heading the list. This edition brings the latest knowledge of these and a myriad of other issues to bear on the core of the practice of PM&R.

All the chapters have been updated and 19 new chapters have been added. We especially want to call attention to the chapters on injection procedures, primary care for persons with disabilities, health issues for women with disabilities, complementary and alternative medicine, rehabilitation of total hip and total knee replacements, and vestibular rehabilitation.

This textbook is organized into four broad sections: (i) overview and principles of evaluation and diagnosis (19 chapters), (ii) management methods (16 chapters), (iii) major rehabilitation problems (12 chapters), and (iv) rehabilitation of specific disorders (24 chapters).

In compiling the book, we stressed the scientific basis of our specialty, but simultaneously strove to have the information be practical and clinically useful. Chapters are multi-authored and the authors were chosen for their expertise in their specific area. There are a total of 169 contributing authors representing all areas of the world.

In an attempt to cover the breadth and scope of the specialty, we have added chapters on the rehabilitation of patients with visual impairments and hearing impairments, as well as primary care for patients with disabilities and international rehabilitation. We hope that you, our readers, will benefit from all of the efforts of our authors and ourselves to provide the best comprehensive source of state-of-the-art knowledge about the field of PM&R.

We welcome your comments and suggestions for future editions.

Joel A. DeLisa, M.D., M.S.
Bruce M. Gans, M.D.
William L. Bockenek, M.D.
Donald M. Currie, M.D.
Steve R. Geiringer, M.D.
Lynn H. Gerber, M.D.
James A. Leonard, Jr., M.D.
Malcolm C. McPhee, M.D.
William S. Pease, M.D.
Nicolas E. Walsh, M.D.

PART I

Overview and Principles of Evaluation and Diagnosis

Rehabilitation Medicine: Principles and Practice, Third Edition,
edited by Joel A. DeLisa and Bruce M. Gans.
Lippincott–Raven Publishers, Philadelphia © 1998.

CHAPTER 1

Rehabilitation Medicine

Past, Present, and Future

Joel A. DeLisa, Donald M. Currie, and Gordon M. Martin

Rehabilitation is the process of helping a person to reach the fullest physical, psychological, social, vocational, avocational, and educational potential consistent with his or her physiologic or anatomic impairment, environmental limitations, and desires and life plans. Patients, their families, and their rehabilitation teams work together to determine realistic goals and to develop and carry out plans to obtain optimal function despite residual disability, even if the impairment is caused by a pathologic process that cannot be reversed (1).

Rehabilitation is a concept that should permeate the entire health-care system. It should be comprehensive and include prevention and early recognition, as well as outpatient, inpatient, and extended care programs. Anticipated patient outcomes of such a comprehensive and integrated rehabilitation program should include increased independence, a shortened length of stay, the most efficient use of evolving health-care systems, and an improved quality of life.

PATIENT CARE TEAMS

Rehabilitation medicine is based on a holistic and comprehensive approach to medical care, using the combined expertise of multiple caregivers. The team approach is critical in solving the complex problems associated with various disabilities. A health-care team is defined as a group of health-care professionals from different disciplines who share common values and objectives (2). Halstead performed a literature review, covering the years 1950 to 1975, on team care in chronic illness and found three major broad categories that he described as "bases." The "opinion base" reflects statements of belief and faith in the team approach to chronic illness. The "descriptive base" contains details and personal testimony of programs using team concepts. The "study base" includes serious research efforts that investigated the effectiveness of the team care approach in various settings. It should be noted that only 10 studies were found in the research category. Halstead concluded that a coordinated team care approach appears to be more effective than fragmented care for patients with long-term illness (2).

Organization

There are many ways to organize a team, and many differences exist with respect to integration, collaboration, hierarchical organization, horizontal and vertical communications, and individual responsibilities. Some teams are organized by body systems, whereas others are organized by practice specialty, concepts of delivery of care, and focus of delivery of care.

Health-care providers may be classified into one of four groups: the medical model (without a formal team), the multidisciplinary model, the interdisciplinay model, and the transdisciplinary model. The reader is referred to Chapter 13 for more thorough discussion of these four models in terms of styles of interaction; application of a multiplicity of caregivers to solve patients problems; communication via referrals, orders, and other methods of interaction; and the

J.A. DeLisa: Department of Physical Medicine and Rehabilitation, University of Medicine and Dentistry of New Jersey, New Jersey Medical School, Newark, New Jersey 07013; and Kessler Medical Rehabilitation Research and Education Corporation; and Kessler Rehabilitation Institute, West Orange, New Jersey 07052; and Department of Physical Medicine and Rehabilitation, St. Barnabas Medical Center, Livingston, New Jersey 07039.

D.M. Currie: Department of Rehabilitation Medicine, University of Texas Health Science Center at San Antonio, San Antonio, Texas 78284-7798.

G.M. Martin: Department of Physical Medicine and Rehabilitation, Mayo Medical School and Mayo Graduate School of Medicine, and Department of Physical Medicine and Rehabilitation, Mayo Clinic, Rochester, Minnesota 55905.

current state of research related to efficacy and advantages and disadvantages of the four models. This chapter focuses on issues that affect team effectiveness regardless of the model used.

Because rehabilitation teams are usually multidisciplinary or interdisciplinary, a few comments about these two models are made here. The multidisciplinary model is analogous to the classic pyramid-shaped model of management, which features vertical communication between supervisor and subordinates. The interdisciplinary model is analogous to matrix organization. The project-orientation of matrix organization is similar to the problem-orientation and function-orientation of medical rehabilitation and meshes well with the concept of diagnostically oriented specialty teams within the broader team (3). Because the interdisciplinary model is designed to facilitate lateral communication, it is theoretically better suited for rehabilitation teams (4–6). The interdisciplinary model has been described as a compromise between the benefits of specialization and the need for continuity and comprehensiveness of care (7).

Team Development and Dynamics

Although the team concept appears to be straightforward, the development and maintenance of an effective team requires time and effort from all the team members. An effective team is efficient in reaching its goals and creates an exciting and stimulating work environment for its members. Douglas McGregor, a founder of neoclassicist organization theory, developed one of the first descriptions of an effective team, noting that it must have the 11 characteristics outlined in Table 1-1 (8).

The focus of the rehabilitation team is the well-being of the patient. A common goal is shared by all the members (8). When a team exhibits McGregor's characteristics, it has a built-in feedback mechanism through which it constantly

TABLE 1-1. *McGregor's characteristics of an effective work team*

1. The atmosphere tends to be informal, comfortable, and relaxed. There are no obvious tensions. It is a working atmosphere in which people are involved and interested. There are no signs of boredom.
2. There is a lot of discussion in which virtually everyone participates, but it remains pertinent to the task of the group. If the discussion gets off the subject, someone will bring it back in short order.
3. The task or the objective of the group is well understood and accepted by the members. There will have been free discussion of the objective at some point, until it was formulated in such a way that the members of the group could commit themselves to it.
4. The members listen to each other! The discussion does not have the quality of jumping from one idea to another unrelated one. Every idea is given a hearing. People do not appear to be afraid of being foolish by putting forth a creative thought even it if seems fairly extreme.
5. There is some disagreement. The group is comfortable with this and shows no signs of having to avoid conflict or to keep everything on a plane of sweetness and light. Disagreements are not suppressed or overridden by premature group action. The reasons are carefully examined, and the group seeks to resolve them rather than to dominate the dissenter. On the other hand, there is no "tyranny of the minority." Members who disagree do not appear to be trying to dominate the group or to express hostility. Their disagreement is an expression of a genuine difference of opinion, and they expect a hearing so that a solution may be found. Sometimes there are basic disagreements that cannot be resolved. The group finds it possible to live with them, accepting them but not permitting them to block its efforts. Under some conditions, action will be deferred to permit further study of an issue between the members. On other occasions, when the disagreement cannot be resolved and action is necessary, it will be taken but with open caution and recognition that the action may be subject to later reconsideration.
6. Most decisions are reached by a consensus, in which it is clear that everybody is in general agreement and willing to go along. However, there is little tendency for members who oppose the action to keep their opposition private and thus let an apparent consensus mask real disagreement. Formal voting is at a minimum; the group does not accept a simple majority as a proper basis for action.
7. Criticism is frequent, frank and relatively comfortable. There is little evidence of personal attack, either openly or in a hidden fashion. The criticism has a constructive flavor in that it is oriented toward removing an obstacle that faces the group and prevents it from getting the job done.
8. Team members are free in expressing their feelings as well as their ideas both on the problem and on the group's operation. There is little pussyfooting, there are few hidden agendas. Everybody appears to know quite well how everybody else feels about any matter under discussion.
9. When action is taken, clear assignment are made and accepted.
10. The chairman of the group does not dominate it, nor does the group defer unduly to him or her. In fact, as one observes the activity, it is clear that the leadership shifts from time to time, depending on the circumstances. Different members, because of their knowledge or experience, are in a position at various times to act as resources for the group. The members use them in this fashion and they occupy leadership roles while they are thus being used. There is little evidence of a power struggle as the group operates. The issue is not who controls but how to get the job done.
11. The group is self-conscious about its own operations. Frequently, it will stop to examine how well it is doing or what may be interfering with its operation. The problem may be a matter of procedure, or it may be a member whose behavior is interfering with the accomplishment of the group's objectives. Whatever it is, it gets open discussion until a solution is found.

Adapted from McGregor D. *The human side of enterprise.* New York: McGraw-Hill, 1960; 232–235.

monitors itself and maintains its effectiveness. When a team is not functioning well, effective function can be developed or restored through the process of team building (8). Team building requires commitments of time and energy, but the rewards of improved patient outcomes and satisfaction of the team members are worth the effort. Team building is discussed briefly in the section on communication in this chapter and in more detail in other sources (8–10).

A newly formed team or a team with several new members faces several major tasks that must be accomplished if the team is to function effectively (8,9). The members must build a working relationship and establish a facilitative climate. They must work out methods for setting goals, solving problems, making decisions, ensuring follow-through on task assignments, developing collaboration of effort, establishing lines of open communication, and ensuring an appropriate support system that will let team members feel accepted yet allow open discussion and disagreement. In a newly formed team it is advisable to designate meetings to share personal expectations and develop working policies.

Conflict and Disagreement

Conflict is a normal, necessary, and not always destructive part of team development (10,11). The potential for conflict is high in health services organizations (12). How it is handled will determine its effect on team objectives and the group process. A good rehabilitation team creates an atmosphere in which members can agree to disagree without making personal accusations or faulting each others' personalities. In this atmosphere, conflict can be used as a vehicle for growth and innovation.

When conflict repeatedly occurs with no resolution, action must be taken to restore the team's effectiveness. An appropriate setting for conflict resolution is a team-building session. The reader is referred to the section on communication for more details about overcoming communication barriers and conflict on a rehabilitation team.

Complacency

Another factor that may be detrimental to the team's effectiveness is complacency (8,11). A complacent team may be recognized by one or more of the following characteristics: the same members seem to be doing the same things the same way year after year despite advances in the field; products prescribed are predictable; new members transfer out of the team because of the lack of challenge; there is a fear of or resistance to risk taking; and the rewards go to team members with average performance. These characteristics are especially detrimental to the rehabilitation team when the external conditions that define the team's direction are always changing. Despite similar diagnoses, each patient presents a unique picture; thus, treatment goals and procedures should vary. Treatment techniques change in response to new research findings; creativity and problem solving are important to the functioning of a rehabilitation team. Steiner has identified the following characteristics of a creative team: it includes unusual types of people, has open channels of communication, encourages contact with outside sources, experiments with new ideas, is not run as a "tight ship," its members have fun, rewards go to people with ideas, and there is a risk-taking ethos (8).

Leadership

The physician leader of a rehabilitation team has broad responsibilities as the director of the combined medical treatment and rehabilitation programs. This physician has primary responsibility for medical and rehabilitative evaluation and treatment and for coordinating and integrating a complex care program with multiple goals and caregivers. Managerial skills, such as the ability to motivate and direct the team, and the willingness to acknowledge and appropriately defer to the opinions of team members are necessary elements. The leadership qualities defined by Lundberg should be cultivated by rehabilitation team leaders approaching this task (Table 1-2) (13).

The physiatrist is especially equipped to direct the team care of rehabilitation patients. Examples of the breadth of training and expertise that make physiatrists suitable for this leadership role include knowledge and skills in the following areas, which are frequently important in the care of patients treated by a rehabilitation team:

Neurophysiology
Exercise physiology
The psychology of disability
Management of a broad array of medical and surgical problems
The functional effects of these problems and associated physical impairments
Familiarity with the knowledge and skills of the various members of the rehabilitation team
Managerial skills necessary to direct teams and lead team meetings

TABLE 1-2. *Some qualities of a leader*

- Knows where he or she is going
- Knows how to get there
- Has courage and persistence
- Can be believed
- Can be trusted not to "sell out" a cause for personal advantage
- Makes the mission seem important, exciting and possible to accomplish
- Makes each person's role in the mission seem important
- Makes each member feel capable of performing his or her role

Modified from Lundborg LB, *The art of being an executive.* Reprinted with the permission of The Free Press, a Division of Macmillan, Inc. © 1981 by Barbara W. Lundborg.

The traditional autocratic model of leadership, in which the physician assumes an authoritarian role and other team members obey, is not effective in the rehabilitation setting (10). In this setting every team member should be encouraged to develop leadership skills and to perform the tasks necessary for meeting the patient goals. A successful interdisciplinary team has an administrative leader or coordinator, but leadership is passed from one member to another during team meetings. There is coordination, cooperation, and open communication among team members who know each other's skills and are willing to share the responsibility for the team's actions. Patients are perceived as comanagers of their rehabilitation and must be taught and are expected to accept more responsibility for their own care as the rehabilitation process goes on.

Managing a Team Meeting

A rehabilitation team's success depends on effective team meetings. A good meeting is productive, stimulating, and goal oriented and involves creativity, problem solving, and interaction. The team leader, usually the physiatrist, has the responsibility of conducting the meeting and maintaining the team's productivity.

The organization of a team meeting can facilitate an effective team process. The simplest and most popular structure for team meetings is for a member from each discipline to give a progress report for each patient. This structure can work well because each member tends to concentrate his or her effort on one problem or a related set of problems. Another approach is the problem-oriented agenda, where the problem list for each patient is the outline for discussion at the meeting. As each problem on the agenda is discussed, any team member may address his or her role in managing the problem. This format tends to promote the synergistic interdisciplinary approach. For example, when discussing a patient's ischial ulcer, the physiatrist may present a physiologically sound overview of the strategy being applied to allow healing and prevent recurrence, the plastic surgeon may discuss surgical considerations, the nurse may describe the effects of the topical dressings, the dietitian may mention the implications of dietary proteins and nutritional support for optimal wound healing, the occupational therapist may describe how the patient's daily activities have been adapted to avoid ischial pressure, and the physical therapist may note the effects of hydrotherapy and the patient's ability and dependability in weight-shifting maneuvers. It may be easier to keep the meeting goal oriented because the problem list inherently defines the objectives for the meeting; however, this model requires more skill on the part of the team leader to keep the meetings efficient.

A special problem with rehabilitation team meetings is the presence of many different disciplines in rehabilitation (14). This issue is discussed further in the section on communication.

Regardless of which model is used, it is the team leader's responsibility to keep the group focused on the task. This involves facilitating discussion, ensuring that ideas are understood, negotiating compromises, and clarifying responsibilities (15). The minutes that document the meeting must include an action summary of the agreed upon responsibilities, assignments, and deadlines. The action summary should be distributed to team members as a form of documentation and reminder (Fig. 1-1).

The physical setting is important for facilitating communication within a team meeting. A specific meeting time must be designated, and team members must be committed to this time.

The meeting room's size, lighting, and temperature may help or hinder effective group process. Seating should allow face-to-face communication among all members. This criterion typically is met by sitting around a table or in a circle. Having adequate physical space and time can prevent communication barriers.

Communication

Communication is the creation or exchange of information and understanding between senders and receivers (16,17).

An effective communicator has the following attributes:

- Accepts differences in perspectives of others
- Functions independently
- Negotiates roles with other team members
- Forms new values, attitudes, and perceptions
- Tolerates constant review and challenge of ideas
- Takes risks
- Possesses personal identity and integrity
- Accepts the team philosophy of care (9)

The maintenance of effective communication requires constant application of all these qualities by all team members.

Decision	Who is to do it	Date of completion	Date to report progress
Train to do safe independent car transfers with a sliding board	Jan Hoover, PT Patient's mother is to bring her car in for use in the training sessions	May 23	May 27 (next scheduled team meeting)

FIG. 1-1. Example of an action summary.

Communication can be studied using management theory (16,17). Classical management theory recognizes five functions of management:

Planning
Organizing
Directing
Coordinating
Controlling

Recently, directing and coordinating have been combined as ''leading'' (18). All these management functions require communication, but it is in leading that communication theory may have its greatest application to health-care teams. Communication networks associated with rehabilitation are complex, and there are many potential barriers to effective communication. Understanding flows of communication and strategies to overcome communication barriers can improve internal communication within the rehabilitation team and health-care organization and thus improve patient care. Communicating well in a rapidly changing health-care market, especially external communication with stakeholders outside the typical rehabilitation facility, also can benefit the health-care organization, providing rehabilitation services in ways that ensure the health, or even survival, of the organization. For example, the rehabilitation organization that communicates well may benefit in terms of being selected as the first-choice provider of rehabilitation services, obtaining contracts with favorable reimbursement levels for services, or helping establish favorable regulatory policies (17).

Another consideration for facilitating communication is the identification and resolution of barriers to communication. Given and Simmons have identified communication barriers that can interfere with the achievement of treatment goals:

- Autonomy
- Individual members' personal characteristics that may contribute to personality conflicts
- Role ambiguity
- Incongruent expectations
- Differing perceptions of authority
- Power and status differentials
- Varying educational preparation of the patient care team members
- Hidden agendas (9)

These barriers stem from interpersonal, interprofessional, and practice issues and are not intrinsic defects of the team concept.

A special barrier to effective communication on rehabilitation teams is the presence of many disciplines in rehabilitation, particularly the different perspectives of professionals with a physical background (e.g., physicians and physical therapists) and a psychosocial background (e.g., psychologists and social workers). The use of a communication instrument to help keep the information communicated comprehensible, relevant, and compact can help improve communication between professionals with different backgrounds (14).

Another barrier is varying definitions and understanding of rehabilitation-related terminology by different members of the rehabilitation team. A recent study provided objective evidence that members of rehabilitation teams have ''a disturbing lack of common understanding for some basic rehabilitation terminology'' and that ''only about half of the personnel providing rehabilitation services are currently sensitive to this issue'' (19). The authors suggested several courses of action for this problem: alert rehabilitation professionals that it exists, adopt a standardized rehabilitation glossary for the team, avoid the use of vague terms, define terms operationally, and express descriptions of patients and their progress objectively using standardized functional assessment instruments (19).

Lack of communication can be detrimental to the rehabilitation process, as well as uncomfortable for team members. Time must be designated to maintain effective team process and overcome communication barriers. When a team is functioning suboptimally owing to conflict, complacency, or poor communication, the problem can be resolved through the team-building process (8).

Dyer cites three prerequisites for conflict negotiation:

1. All parties must agree to come together and work on the problems.
2. Members must agree that there are problems that need to be solved and that solving them is everyone's responsibility.
3. Members accept the position that the end result is that the team will communicate better, thus enhancing the rehabilitation process (8).

Once these prerequisites have been met, the team identifies the conflicts or barriers to communication in need of resolution. It is important that concrete suggestions be made for the resolution of these problems and that the team agree on the solutions. This creates a problem-solving session rather than a detrimental process in which the members attempt to determine fault or place blame. Once solutions are agreed on, each member has the responsibility to follow through according to his or her role.

An outside consultant may be extremely helpful (8). Some symptoms of poor team function are more easily discerned by an outsider. Other symptoms are more easily seen by team members, but an outside consultant can help interpret and resolve these symptoms. The consultant can guide the team away from interpretations of problems that are not likely to lead to resolution, such as erroneously labeling incomplete or inadequate conflict resolution as an inevitable personality conflict (8). They can lead the team toward constructive ways to resolve problems such as the use of the expectation theory, which states that negative reactions can be predicted whenever the behavior of one person violates the expectations of another. A vicious cycle of escalating conflict can result when the negative reaction itself violates the expectations of the first person. However, because this theory focuses on behavior rather than personality, it allows a greater possibility for conflict resolution. If the parties involved, or even one of the parties, can identify the behaviors that violate expectations, then behaviors can be changed, or agreements can be reached, so that team members can reward each other's behaviors rather than negatively reinforce them (8). The consultant can help the team learn to sustain healthy communication by developing its own internal mechanisms for problem identification and diagnosis, planning remediation, implementing changes, and evaluating its own results in a healthy feedback loop. The beneficiaries of healthy communication on the rehabilitation team are the patients and the team members.

The interactionist perspective is a current view toward conflict. According to this view, a certain level of conflict is healthy and leads to a group that is viable, self critical, and innovative. A group can have too little conflict. When it does, it may be viewed as harmonious, cooperative, and tranquil, but the team may become apathetic, noninnovative, and nonresponsive to needs for change and may show low productivity. Team members may leave because they are bored. If this occurs, it becomes the responsibility of team leaders to stir up enough conflict to promote creativity, innovation, and productivity among the team members. The interactionist manager must use great care and skill to not allow conflict to accelerate to the point where it becomes disruptive or chaotic. If conflict is not controlled, cooperation ceases and the quality of patient care decreases (11).

It is especially important that health-care teams and organizations be able to manage a particular type of conflict: the conflict that arises when something goes wrong. Even in the best managed organization, things go wrong. In a health-care organization, the result can be injury, pain, suffering, or even death. In such cases the rehabilitation team and the organization also experience distress. There are always ripple effects that can affect multiple stakeholders inside and outside the organization. Excellent communication skills in this situation can contain the damage and redress the consequences, the most difficult step. Healthy communication when things go wrong can potentially strengthen future relationships with affected stakeholders as well as help prevent recurrences of similar mishaps (17).

To make rehabilitation teams more effective and interdisciplinary, Rothberg believes the following functions must be performed (7):

- Teach team members how to work together and provide sufficient practice time in team work.
- Ensure that all members learn, understand, and respect the knowledge and skills of others.
- Develop clear definitions of the roles and behaviors expected of team participants and lessen ambiguities regarding expectations of others.
- Encourage use of the full potential of each member.
- Direct attention to initiation and maintenance of communication and to the breaking down of remediable barriers to interdisciplinary communications.
- Attend to the maintenance of the teams in the same way that other organizations engage in activities that strengthen their cohesion and offer satisfaction to their personnel.
- Acknowledge that leadership should shift as necessary in terms of the patient's paramount needs.
- Ensure that the person in the leadership role respects the other members, as evidenced by consultation, listening, and involving them in planning.
- Develop an internal system for demonstrating the accountability of each team member to the group and to the institution in which the team practices.
- Develop a process to acknowledge conflict as it arises and to address it in a manner that strengthens the group and its members.

Team Size and Membership

This section describes the disciplines that are most commonly represented on the rehabilitation team. There may be some overlap among team members in their areas of expertise and training.

The Occupational Therapist

Occupational therapists usually focus on functional activities and provide the following services to rehabilitation patients:

- Evaluate and train the patient in self-care activities (e.g., dressing, eating, bathing, and personal hygiene) to maximize independence. Teach the patient how to use orthoses or adaptive equipment, which may be fabricated by the therapist, when necessary. Teach wheelchair transfer techniques for home and community use (e.g., wheelchair to toilet).
- Train the patient in home management skills, presenting simpler modified methods to minimize fatigue and conserve energy.
- Explore vocational skills and avocational interests. Work with the vocational counselor when a change in employment or further education is anticipated.
- Aid in maintaining and improving joint range of motion (ROM), muscle strength, endurance, coordination, and dexterity, particularly in the upper extremities.
- Evaluate and train the patient to compensate for sensory, perceptual, and cognitive deficits as they relate to function.
- Evaluate the home and suggest modifications to provide a barrier-free environment.
- Evaluate the patient's skills within the community and train the patient in modified strategies and the use of equipment when necessary.
- Assess predriving and driving behaviors and abilities and retrain when necessary, using appropriate assistive devices.

Educate the patient's family by demonstrating techniques designed to maintain patient independence and to minimize overprotection.
Train the patient in the functional use of upper extremity prostheses.
Evaluate and train patients in the use of assistive technology systems (e.g., environmental controls and computer systems) and the ability to operate switches to access high technology assistive devices.
Train patients or significant others in the maintenance of equipment.
Evaluate and manage dysphagia in collaboration with speech language pathologists and nurses.

The Physical Therapist

Physical therapists assist the patient in functional restoration, especially for gross motor functions. Tasks may include the following:

Restore and preserve joint ROM through mobilization techniques and exercises.
Evaluate muscle length and perform stretching exercises and soft-tissue mobilization to enhance muscle elasticity.
Perform muscle strength evaluation and quantification.
Evaluate muscle hypotonicity or hypertonicity and provide exercises to normalize motor control.
Evaluate and train sitting and standing balance, transfers, and mobility, including wheelchair use and ambulation. Progressive gait training with or without ambulatory aids may be offered and includes instruction in negotiating barriers and obstacles such as rough ground, ramps, and stairs.
Evaluate and train users of lower extremity orthoses and prostheses to facilitate their gait independence and function.
Evaluate level of dependence during position changes and provide mobility training to enhance function.
Offer exercises to increase strength, endurance, and coordination for specific muscle groups or the entire body.
Assess skin integrity and sensation and provide precautionary instructions for skin care.
Manage edema and musculoskeletal pain by physical measures.
Offer various physical therapy modalities, such as superficial and deep heat and cold, as well as hydrotherapy techniques, electrical stimulation, traction, and massage.
Assess total body posture and provide education and exercises to improve alignment.
Perform auscultation to lung fields and render percussion and vibration, breathing exercises, incentive spirometry, and postural drainage in some settings.
Aid in home evaluations to make the environment barrier free and accessible.
Assess the patient's wheelchair needs, including maintenance, and assist with individualized wheelchair prescriptions.
Teach functional employment skills, including proper lifting techniques, functional strength testing, and ergonomic considerations.

The Certified Therapeutic Recreation Therapist

Recreation therapists use recreational activities for purposive intervention in some physical, social, or emotional behavior to bring about a desired change in that behavior and promote the growth and development of the patient. Therapeutic recreation includes the following measures:

Assess in detail the patient's
- interests
- resources
- level of participation
- social capability
- cognitive functioning
- physical limitations or abilities
- perceived barriers
- emotional functioning
- level of resource awareness

Educate patients in leisure activities, including
- specialized recreation and sports equipment and training in their use
- adapted sports
- increasing awareness of leisure time and alternatives to prior life-styles
- acquiring new leisure skills
- self-initiation at leisure pursuits
- developing or increasing social skills

Actively participate in patient rehabilitation by using recreational and community activities to increase attention span, concentration, or maintenance of physical strength, social skills, and motivation.
Assist in adjustment to disability.
Assist in the family's adjustment to disability.
Decrease atypical behaviors.
Increase independence.
Reinforce other therapies.
Provide community integration.
Further evaluate level of functioning.
Provide recreation activities that are nonstructured and more suited to the patient's wants than needs to facilitate participation in previously acquired leisure interests. This also provides a form of self-expression, a healthy outlet for frustrations, maintenance of health, and a nonthreatening atmosphere for patient-staff interaction or patient social interaction.
Develop program plans specifically suited to the patient's needs that include the preceding.
Integrate the patient into the community through a safe, nonthreatening, and graduated program of recreational outings into the community.

Assist the patient in exploring resources for postdischarge activities such as support groups.

The Prosthetist-Orthotist

The prosthetist-orthotist is responsible for the evaluation, design, and fabrication of orthoses (i.e., braces) or prostheses (i.e., artificial limbs). The prosthetist-orthotist ensures that the device functions and fits properly and that the patient adjusts to its presence. Patient and family instruction in the care and use of the prostheses or orthoses, as well as follow-up maintenance and repair, should be stressed. The prosthetist-orthotist should be certified by the American Board for Certification in Orthotics and Prosthetics.

The Rehabilitation Nurse

Rehabilitation nurses specialize in the direct personal care of physically impaired patients. They evaluate the health status of the patient and help determine short- and long-term goals. The nurse helps educate patients and their families about the physical, social, and behavioral sciences related to their disability. The nurse assesses and addresses the following patient needs:

Hygienic factors
Bowel or bladder programs to promote optimum independence
Specific interventions related to skin integrity
Environmental factors such as heat and noise, control of personal property, sanitation, infection control, and safety
The use of adaptive equipment needed by patients to communicate, eat, move, eliminate, dress, and ambulate
Specific preventive measures to minimize the effects of inactivity
Specific measures to promote optimal independence
Helping patients manage their time, including integrating the various therapies into their daily activities
Medication management

The Speech-Language Pathologist

The speech-language pathologist evaluates and treats patients with neurogenic disorders such as aphasia, dysarthria, apraxia, cognitive-communication impairments secondary to right hemisphere cerebrovascular accident or traumatic brain injury, and dysphagia. The responsibilities of the speech-language pathologist include the following:

Detailed assessment of language processing and remediations of impairments in speech, comprehension, reading, and writing
Evaluation of the swallowing mechanism, including videofluoroscopic swallow study, with subsequent recommendations and implementation of feeding regimens
Assessment of and intervention for pragmatic and cognitively based communicative disorders
Motor-speech assessment and treatment
Evaluation and training of patients requiring augmentative and alternative communication approaches, including use of high-technology devices, talking tracheostomy tubes, and electrolarynxes
Family and patient education and counseling

The Psychologist

The psychologist helps the patient and significant others to prepare psychologically for full participation in rehabilitation. This can involve a number of activities, including the following:

Testing, involving
  personality style (e.g., manipulative, dependent, dogmatic)
  ways of dealing with stress
  problem-solving skills
  psychological status (e.g., neurosis, psychosis)
Incorporation of the test results into the care plan
Counseling in
  adjustment to body changes
  development of problem-solving skills
  secondary problems caused by the disease and its disability
  adjustment to changes in sexual functioning and viable alternatives
  death and dying
Testing of intelligence, memory, and perceptual functioning

The Social Worker

Social workers interact with the patient, family, and rehabilitation team (including insurers) and can assist in the following ways:

Evaluate the patient's total living situation, including lifestyle, family, finances, employment history, and community resources, and assess the impact of the disease or disability on these areas.
Maintain a continuing relationship with the patient and family.
Coordinate funding resources and discuss financial arrangements and concerns. This may include a case management role.
Help the family develop the skills needed to participate actively in treatment procedures in the home.
Provide assistance in locating alternative living situations.
Assess vocational barriers.
Provide emotional support to the patient and family in stressful situations.
Facilitate discharge planning.

The Vocational Counselor

Vocational counselors assist the patient in developing and attaining realistic vocational goals. Major areas of responsibility include the following:

Evaluate vocational interests, aptitudes, and skills.
Counsel patients who must shift to alternate occupations or return to their prior position with adjustments in the work environment.
Organize activities, individual or group, to improve job-related behaviors (e.g., job interview skills, work skills, resume development, employer–employee relationship behaviors).
Act as a liaison between the patient and agencies that provide training or job placement services.
Provide counseling, education, and support to potential employers (e.g., job analysis on worksite).
Mentor

Other Rehabilitation Health-Care Professionals

Allied health-care professionals from several other disciplines may be brought onto the team depending on the patient's needs. The following professionals often are consulted:

Psychiatrist
Enterostomal therapist
Maxillofacial prosthetist
Podiatrist
Dentist
Audiologist
Dietitian
Durable medical equipment vendor
Bioengineer
Hospital-based schoolteacher
Chaplain (see Chapter 13, Fig. 13-1)

Although their roles with rehabilitation patients possess some special features, their areas of responsibility are familiar enough not to require further clarification. Other professionals are less well known and not as readily available but can provide important services to selected patients. Some of these are listed below and in Table 1-3.

The Child Life Specialist

The child life specialist acts as the advocate for a child. Child life specialists usually work with hospitalized children, but also may practice in ambulatory care settings. The philosophy of child life programs is to minimize the interruption and disruption of normal life experiences caused by hospitalization or illness and to make hospitalization a positive growth experience for a child and family. Some of the specialist's activities include the following:

Use play and homelike activities to foster continued development.
Encourage and facilitate continuation of school and family relationships during hospitalization and illness.
Provide developmentally appropriate explanations of health-care procedures to children, sometimes using props such as dolls or puppets.

Child life specialists work closely with other allied health team members. Child life specialists have bachelor's degree academic preparation in fields as varied as nursing, psychology, social work, special education, and occupational therapy.

The Kinesiotherapist

The Kinesiotherapy Association defines kinesiotherapy as the applied science of medically prescribed therapeutic exercise, education, and adapted physical activities to improve the quality of life and health of adults and children by developing physical fitness, increasing functional mobility and independence, and improving psychosocial behavior. The kinesiotherapist seeks a coach–player relationship in which he or she helps the patient reach the goal of becoming an independent, self-sustaining person. The potential overlaps among kinesiotherapy, physical therapy, occupational therapy, and recreational therapy need to be resolved in each setting. Compared with physical therapists, with whom there is probably the most potential overlap, kinesiotherapists put more emphasis on geriatric care, extended care, reconditioning and fitness, and psychiatric care. A large percentage of kinesiotherapists practice in Veterans Administration hospitals and can provide the following programs:

Gross motor and remedial exercise programs
Adapted driver education
Home maintenance programs for fitness for physically disabled children
Fitness as a means of stress management for psychiatric patients
Gait training and fitness programs for amputees
Fitness-promoting therapeutic recreation programs for acute, chronic, and convalescent patients

The Horticultural Therapist

In addition to improving physical capabilities required for gardening, the raising of flowers, vegetables, and other plants is thought to have therapeutic value in building or rebuilding personal confidence and self-esteem. Horticultural therapists offer the following services:

Work with a variety of patients, including those with mental retardation and psychiatric diagnoses as well as physically disabled and hospitalized children and adults, to promote independence, motor skills, and psychological well-being
Help prepare selected patients for vocations involving work with plants, gardening, and grounds keeping

The Music Therapist

Music therapists works with patients with a broad variety of diagnoses and therapeutic goals. The interventions may

TABLE 1-3. *Facts about some rehabilitation team members*

Discipline	Organization	Journal	Certification required
Occupational Therapist	American Occupational Therapy Association 4720 Montgomery Lane P.O. Box 31220 Bethesda, MD 20824-1220 Tel: (301) 652-2682 Fax: (301) 652-7711	*American Journal of Occupational Therapy* (monthly) *OT Weekly* (weekly) *OT Practice* (monthly)	Yes
Physical Therapist	American Physical Therapy Association 1111 North Fairfax Street Alexandria, VA 22314 Tel: 1-800-999-APTA Fax: (703) 706-3169	*Physical Therapy Journal* (monthly)	Yes
Prosthetist/ Orthotist	American Orthotic and Prosthetic Association 1650 King Street Suite 500 Alexandria, VA 22314 Tel: (703) 836-7116 Fax: (703) 836-0838	*The Journal of Prosthetics and Orthotics* (quarterly) *The Almanac* (annually)	Yes
Rehabilitation Nurse	Association of Rehabilitation Nurses 4700 West Lake Avenue Glenview, IL 60025 Tel: (847) 375-4710 Fax: (847) 375-4777	*Rehabilitation Nursing* (bimonthly)	Yes
Speech Pathologist	American Speech-Language-Hearing Association 10801 Rockville Pike Rockville, MD 20852 Tel: (301) 897-5700 Fax: (301) 571-0457	*Journal of Speech and Hearing Research* (bimonthly) *American Journal of Audiology* (3 issues per year)	Yes
Social Worker	National Association of Social Workers 750 First Street Ne Suite 700 Washington, DC 20002 Tel: (202) 408-8600 Fax: (202) 336-8310	*Social Work* (bimonthly) *Health and Social Work* (quarterly) *Social Work Research* (quarterly) *Social Work Abstracts* (quarterly) *Social Work and Education* (quarterly)	Yes
Vocational Counselor	American Association for Counseling and Development 5999 Stevenson Avenue Alexandria, VA 22304 Tel: (703) 823-9800 Fax: (703) 823-0252	*Journal of Counseling and Development* (6 issues per year) *Counseling Today* (monthly newspaper)	Yes
Child Life Therapist	Association for the Care of Children's Health 7910 Woodmont Avenue Suite 300 Bethesda, MD 20814 Tel: (301) 654-6549 Fax: (301) 986-4553	*Journal of the Association for the Care of Children's Health* (quarterly) *Association for the Care of Children's Health Advocate* (two issues per year)	No
Kinesiotherapist (Corrective Therapist)	American Kinesiotherapy Association 4456 Corporation Lane Suite120 Virginia Beach, VA 23462 Tel: (800) 326-0268 Fax: (800) 296-2582	*Clinical Kinesiotherapy* (quarterly)*Journal of the American Kinesiotherapy Association* (quarterly)	Yes
Horticultural Therapist	American Horticulture Therapy Association 362 A Christopher Avenue Gaithersburg, MD 20879 Tel: (301) 948-3010 Fax: (301) 869-2397	*Journal of Therapeutic Horticulture* (annually)	Yes

(continued)

TABLE 1-3. *Continued.*

Discipline	Organization	Journal	Certification required
Music Therapist	National Association of Music Therapists 8455 Colesville Road Suite 930 Silver Spring, MD 20910 Tel: (301) 589-3300 Fax: (301) 589-5175	*Journal of Music Therapy* (quarterly) *Music Therapy Perspective* (two issues yearly)	Yes
Recreation Therapist	National Therapeutic Recreation Society 2775 South Quincy Street Suite 300 Arlington, VA 22206 Tel: (703) 820-4940 Fax: (703) 671-6772	*Therapeutic Recreation Journal* (quarterly)	Yes
	American Therapeutic Recreation Association P.O. Box 15215 Hattiesburg, MS 39404-5215 Tel: (601) 264-3413 Fax: (601) 264-3337	*Annual of Therapeutic Recreation* (annually)	
Dance Therapist	American Dance Therapy Association 2000 Century Plaza Suite 108 Columbia, MD 21044 Tel: (401) 997-4040	*American Journal of Dance Therapy* (semi-annually)	Yes

involve musical performance with instruments, voice, or body movements; listening to music; or attending musical events. Possible goals and treatments include the following:

Help children with cerebral palsy or other paralytic conditions, or adults with paralysis, to improve coordination and develop gross and fine motor skills through playing selected instruments or exercising to music.

Relaxation, sedation, or control of pain or anxiety for therapeutic procedures or control of acute or chronic pain.

Improve speech through articulation training or melodic intonation therapy.

Prepare selected patients for music-related careers (e.g., musicians, visually impaired piano tuners).

Improve socialization skills, self-confidence, and self-esteem through group music activities.

Improve quality of life for patients in palliative or hospice care.

The Dance Therapist

Dance therapists, sometimes called movement therapists, focus on rhythmic body movement as a medium of physical and psychological change. Dance therapy is practiced more often with mental health patients than with physically disabled patients. A master's degree is required by the American Dance Therapy Association to award the credentials Dance Therapist Registered (DTR). Dance therapists can use rhythmic movements and music to help patients in the following ways:

Improve gross motor control

Relieve and improve awareness of tension and stress, and awareness and expression of other emotions, especially when verbal expression is limited

Improve body image and awareness

Classify and describe body movements

TREATMENT STRATEGIES IN CHRONIC DISEASE

The history and physical examination techniques that, when applied to patients with chronic disease, permit the identification of disability problems are described in Chapter 5. The disability associated with chronic disease or severe trauma, such as spinal cord injury, is chronic when the pathologic process is irreversible. In these cases remediation of the disability depends on techniques that are directed not at the pathologic condition but at achieving maximum independence despite the disorder. These techniques and principles are applicable to the rehabilitation of patients with specific disease states or organ system dysfunctions that will appear throughout this textbook.

There are six classes of treatment strategies to help mitigate disability (20). A few examples for each strategy are given to help appreciate this approach to disability.

Prevent or Correct Additional Disability

Medications to prevent congestive heart failure in patients with cardiac disease

Good glucose control in patients with diabetes with the hope of delaying retinopathy, neuropathy, and nephropathy

Regular foot care for patients with peripheral vascular disease to avoid skin lesions and decrease the risk of amputation

High-caloric nutritional supplements in specific patients with swallowing impairment to prevent malnutrition
Passive joint ROM exercises to avoid contractures in paretic limbs
Adequate bladder hygiene for patients with indwelling catheters to avoid bladder calculi formation, ureter reflux, or pyelonephritis
Muscle stretching exercises to correct contractures in spastic limb muscles
Periodic pressure relief over anesthetic bony surfaces to avoid pressure ulcers and loss of skin integrity
Patient education and training in tracheostomy care to prevent formation of mucus plugs and tracheal obstruction

Enhance Systems Unaffected by the Pathologic Condition

Train laryngectomy patients to trap air in the esophagus and release it through the esophageal-pharyngeal junction for voice production
Progressive resistive exercises to the nonparalyzed side of a hemiplegic stroke patient or to upper extremities of paraplegic patients to aid in transfers
Visual feedback for hand function in patients with a sensory deficit
Speech-reading training for patients with severe hearing loss and after cochlear implantation for the patient with total deafness
Develop overarticulation to enhance speech intelligibility for the laryngectomy patient using an electrolarynx

Enhance Functional Capacity of Systems Affected by the Disease

Hearing aids to compensate partially for hearing loss
Graded exercise programs to improve general conditioning for patients who have had a myocardial infarction
Progressive resistive exercises to weakened muscles to enhance their strength
Training dysarthric speakers to reduce their speaking rates for improved intelligibility
Visual written cues (i.e., prosthetic memory) in brain-damaged patients to assist memory function
Serial pumping of lymphedema to improve cosmesis and use of extremity

Use of Adaptive Equipment to Promote Function

Electrolarynx for voice production after laryngectomy
Canes, crutches, or orthoses to achieve ambulation
Augmentative communication devices for patients with unintelligible dysarthric speech
Wheelchair training when walking is not possible
Equipment to extend hand function in dressing (i.e., long shoehorns, stocking pullers, buttonhooks)
Hand controls for the automobile of paraplegic or quadriplegic patients
Shoe modifications to improve standing balance
Prostheses for amputees to achieve walking or upper extremity function
Closed caption television systems for the hearing-impaired patient
Voice activation to direct a computerized robot or animal assistant to perform duties for patients with severe disabilities

Modify Social and Vocational Environment

Move to a one-level home for patients who are unable to climb stairs.
Widen bathroom doorways to allow a wheelchair to pass.
Add rails on stairs to promote stair climbing.
Provide assistance in the home for physical dependency needs.
Shift employment to sedentary activities for patients with reduced ambulation skills.
Redesign work areas for wheelchair users.
Modify diet for certain swallowing problems.
Train family members not to reinforce sick behavior but to reinforce well behavior.

Psychological Techniques to Enhance Patient Performance and Patient Education

Repetition in training patients with memory problems in self-care techniques
Teach new skills by verbal instruction for patients with memory problems
Teach new skills by demonstration (i.e., pantomime) for patients with language deficits
Develop skill in task performance by operant methods (i.e., behavior therapy)
Group therapy for patients with similar disabilities

HISTORICAL PERSPECTIVES ON PHYSICAL MEDICINE AND REHABILITATION

The history of the beginnings and the evolution of the medical specialty of physical medicine and rehabilitation (PM&R) has proven fascinating to a number of historically oriented physicians and writers (21). The roots of physical medicine have been traced back as far as the ancients, who were aware of the beneficial effects of various physical agents. Heliotherapy and hydrotherapy were recognized and operational at the time of the Roman Empire and perhaps even earlier. In the eighteenth and nineteenth centuries, applications of galvanic and faradic currents were prescribed as valuable therapeutic methods. About 1890, high-frequency currents from spark-gap diathermy machines were introduced by d'Arsonval in France for both medical and surgical treatment (22). If this important milestone is singled out as a logical beginning point for the history of the specialty, we now are entering the second century of evolution, growth, and development.

During and after World War I, diathermy, electrical stimulation, heat, massage, and exercise were used increasingly as therapeutic tools in the United States (23–26). Army medical hospitals made extensive use of physical and occupational therapy. Colonel Harry Mock of the Army Medical Corps referred to the importance of these services in the rehabilitation of wounded and other disabled people during World War I (26). Dr. John Coulter, an Army Medical Corps physician, promoted physical therapy and rehabilitation. He later became involved in establishing this discipline at Northwestern University (23). The uses of physical therapy during World War I were followed by more extensive, updated, and sophisticated uses of physical and rehabilitation medicine in military settings during World War II (27).

A medical specialty evolves when a group of physicians recognizes that a special body of knowledge, along with certain procedural skills, should be nurtured and developed so that its benefits can be made available to patients whose needs in that special area are not being met adequately.

A detailed, well-documented account of many highlights in the long and complex history of the specialty appears as the first chapter in Dr. Frank Krusen's pioneering textbook *Physical Medicine,* published in 1941 (22). This classic reference still is recognized as an outstanding source book. Other authors have reviewed various aspects of the evolution of the specialty, particularly the physician-oriented organizations that have played significant roles in the development and evolution of the specialty. In 1969, Dr. Krusen reviewed 40 years of history of interest areas and activities related to the specialty (28).

Special reference also must be made to Dr. Paul Nelson's notable in-depth study of the origins and evolution of a principal publication of the specialty in the *Archives of Physical Medicine and Rehabilitation.* Nelson's 1969 article, recognizing and honoring 50 years of publication of the *Archives,* includes extensive historical data and pictures of the physicians of the decade from 1915 to 1925 who were pioneers in the medical uses of x-ray and electrotherapeutics (29). Nelson's article is a unique data source on the organizations whose activities, interests, and publications served the new specialty effectively. In an article published in 1973, Nelson reviewed the early interrelationships of electrotherapeutics and radiology (30). In addition to the *Archives,* another significant periodical is the *American Journal of Physical Medicine,* which has a distinguished editorial board and was edited by Dr. H.D. Bouman from 1952 through 1987. In 1988, the journal was renamed the *American Journal of Physical Medicine and Rehabilitation.* The *Journal* is sponsored by the Association of Academic Physiatrists (AAP), with Dr. Ernest W. Johnson as editor.

The historical development of the various methods and devices that are used today in PM&R are discussed in the chapters pertaining to these topics (see Chapters 15, 16, and 20–30). The discussion in Chapter 1 focuses on the important organizations that have evolved to represent this specialty, along with some special clinical areas that, although now superseded, were milestones in the development of the specialty.

American Congress of Rehabilitation Medicine

The complexities of the evolving specialty can be appreciated and understood best by an overview of several important organizations and their areas of major interest, functions, expertise, and performance in relation to physical and rehabilitation medicine. Nelson stated that among the early organizations related to the specialty was the American Electrotherapeutic Association, founded in 1890 (30). It consisted of physicians with varied interests who banded together for the study and promotion of electrotherapeutic measures. It included physicians who were particularly involved with irradiation; ear, nose, and throat medicine; general surgery; neurology; and general medicine. In 1929, this organization merged with the Western Association of Physical Therapy, a regional association of physicians interested in physical therapy, whose leaders and organizers were based in Omaha and Des Moines. Another parent organization began in 1923 as the American College of Radiology and Physiotherapy. The name of this organization was changed in 1925 to the American Congress of Physical Therapy. Ten years of its progress were reviewed by Hollander in 1935 (31).

In 1933, the American Physical Therapy Association, an organization of physicians interested in physical treatment, merged with the American Congress of Physical Therapy. The new organization continued to use the term "congress" while undergoing several other name changes. In 1945, it became known as the American Congress of Physical Medicine; in 1952, the American Congress of Physical Medicine and Rehabilitation; and, in 1966, the American Congress of Rehabilitation Medicine (ACRM). Through the years, membership in the ACRM has been open to any physician with an interest in physical medicine or rehabilitation. In addition to physiatrists, it has included family practitioners, internists, orthopedists, neurologists, surgeons, and dermatologists. Since 1975, membership in the ACRM has been extended to include nonphysicians with advanced degrees in allied health or basic science fields pertinent to rehabilitation. This expanded membership includes psychologists, speech-language pathologists, physical therapists, occupational therapists, social workers, vocational rehabilitation specialists, rehabilitation nurses, and others. Those concerned with rehabilitation of hearing- and vision-impaired people also may be included.

The membership of the ACRM reached 3,200 in 1987, with 2,260 physicians and 940 nonphysicians. In 1996 membership had decreased to 1,679, with 949 physician members, and an office separate from the American Academy of Physical Medicine and Rehabilitation was established. The administrative officers of the ACRM and the Academy have included Dr. Walter Zeiter of Cleveland, Dr. Glenn Gullickson, Jr. of Minneapolis, and Creston Herald, Ike Mayeda, Ronald Henrichs, Irene Tesitor, Richard Muir, and Diane Burgher of Chicago.

The ACRM's annual scientific meeting provides opportunities for nonphysician professionals to present papers or poster exhibits on research aspects pertinent to their involvement and interests. Five of the past ten presidents of the ACRM have been nonphysicians.

In addition to scientific involvement, this organization and the Academy are deeply concerned with many aspects of the changing pictures in the economics, organization, and delivery of health care at federal, state, and local levels. The ACRM, Academy, and AAP are represented by Richard E. Verville, an attorney from Washington, DC, who informs the organizations regarding pending and proposed legislation that might affect either recipients or providers of health care and rehabilitation services.

A list of the past presidents of the ACRM indicates the wide geographic base of the top leadership of the organization since early in this century. Each of these leaders and his or her organizational associates have contributed significantly to the evolution and growth of the specialty.

American Registry of Physical Therapists and the American Physiotherapy Association

Dr. Paul Magnuson established a physical therapy department at Wesley Memorial Hospital at Northwestern University in 1919 and developed a teaching course for physical therapy technicians in 1927 (23). Dr. Harry Mock developed a similar program at St. Luke Hospital, Chicago, when he returned from World War I. In 1926, he became the first chairman of the Council on Physical Therapy of the American Medical Association (AMA). In 1944, the AMA trustees changed the name to the Council of Physical Medicine.

The American Registry of Physical Therapists was organized under the auspices of the American Congress of Physical Medicine and the Council on Physical Therapy of the AMA in 1935 to approve training schools, establish educational standards, and provide certification of registered therapists. Physical therapy schools date back to training programs established at Walter Reed Army Hospital during World War I.

The American Physiotherapy Association (APTA) was formed in 1921 and 1922. By 1947 its membership had increased to 4,000 and by 1986 to 37,000. In 1934, the APTA asked the Council on Medical Education and Hospitals of the AMA to assist with the certification of approved training schools. In December 1971, the APTA withdrew from its functionally cooperative status with the AMA and the ACRM and assumed responsibility for approving training programs and certifying therapists, at first in cooperation with the Council on Allied Health Education Accreditation, and later under the auspices of the Council on Postsecondary Accreditation.

Section Council on Physical Medicine and Rehabilitation of the American Medical Association

The AMA Section Council on Physical Medicine and Rehabilitation provides specialty representation at the AMA. Beginning in the early 1940s, the Section Council sponsored scientific sessions and exhibits at the annual conventions until they were discontinued in the late 1970s. The Section Council maintained an active liaison with other specialty section councils on topics of mutual concern. The section councils of the various specialties also have representation in the AMA House of Delegates. Currently, Section Council members participate in the AMA nominations for directorships on the American Board of Physical Medicine and Rehabilitation. Beginning in the 1930s as the Council on Physical Therapy, and extending to 1950, the Section Council was involved with the evaluation, testing, and approval of diagnostic and physical therapy devices.

The American Academy of Physical Medicine and Rehabilitation

The American Academy of Physical Medicine and Rehabilitation (AAPM&R) had its official origin in 1938. Since 1947, Academy membership has comprised board-certified physiatrists. A membership status of "Fellow of the American Academy of Physical Medicine and Rehabilitation" is available only to certified diplomates of the American Board of Physical Medicine and Rehabilitation (ABPM&R). Its roots and precursor organizations were researched by Dr. G.K. Stillwell and described in the 1982 Zeiter lecture (32). Some of these earlier organizations also had overlapped with physician groups that could be considered allied to those of the pre-ACRM era. The first president of the Academy of Physical Medicine and Rehabilitation was Dr. John Coulter of Northwestern University, Chicago (Table 1-4). The organization originally comprised primarily physicians practicing almost full time in physical medicine.

One of the primary aims of the group in the early 1940s was to support the founding and development of a certifying board for the new specialty of physical medicine. This emerging organization (the Academy) provided financial support for the committee that was to be involved in the preliminary planning for the specialty board. The Academy thus became the primary sponsoring organization of the specialty board, which was established in 1947. When the first diplomates were certified, it was decided that membership in the Academy would require board certification in physical medicine. At a later date, the Academy decided that fully qualified members of the Academy would be known as Fellows of the American Academy of Physical Medicine and Rehabilitation. Although the growth of the Academy was relatively slow during the early years, membership has increased appreciably during the past decade. As of 1997, the Academy had 3,428 fellows plus associate, affiliate, corresponding, senior, life, inactive, and honorary members for a total membership of 5,499.

TABLE 1-4. *Past Presidents, American Academy of Physical Medicine and Rehabilitation*

John S. Coulter, 1938–1939, Chicago
F. W. Ewerhardt, 1939–1940, St. Louis
William Bierman, 1940–1941, New York
Frank H. Krusen, 1941–1942, Rochester, MN
K. G. Hasson, 1942–1943, New York
William H. Schmidt, 1943–1944, Philadelphia
Fred B. Moor, 1944–1945, Los Angeles
Fred B. Moor, 1945–1946, Los Angeles
William D. Paul 1946–1947, Iowa City, IA
Earl C. Elkins, 1947–1948, Rochester, MN
Arthur E. White, 1948–1949, Washington, DC
Charles O. Molander, 1949–1950, Chicago
Miland E. Knapp, 1950–1951, Minneapolis
Frances Baker, 1951–1952, San Francisco
Walter S. McClellan, 1952–1953, Saratoga Springs, FL
Donald L. Rose, 1953–1954, Kansas City, KS
Harold Dinken, 1954–1955, Denver
Ben L. Boynton, 1955–1956, Chicago
Murray B. Ferderber, 1956–1957, Pittsburgh
George D. Wilson, 1957–1958, Asheville, NC
Louis B. Newman, 1958–1959, Chicago
Clarence W. Dail, 1959–1960, Los Angeles
Rav Piakoski, 1960–1961, Milwaukee
Robert W. Boyle, 1961–1962, Milwaukee
Max K. Newman, 1962–1963, Detroit
Morton Hoberman, 1963–1964, New York
Herman L. Rudolph, 1964–1965, Reading, PA
A. B. C. Knudson, 1965–1966, Washington, DC
Michael M. Dasco, 1966–1967, New York
Robert C. Darling, 1967–1968, New York
G. Keith Stillwell, 1968–1969, Rochester, MN
Herman J. Bearzy, 1969–1970, Dayton, OH
Glenn Gullickson, Jr., 1970–1971, Minneapolis
Arthur S. Abramson, 1971–1972, New York
Justus F. Lehmann, 1972–1973, Seattle
Leonard F. Bender, 1973–1974, Ann Arbor, MI
Eugene Moskowitz, 1974–1975, New York
Carl V. Granger, 1975–1976, Boston
Ernest W. Johnson, 1976–1977, Columbus, OH
Joseph Goodgold, 1977–1978, New York
Frederick J. Kottke, 1978–1979, Minneapolis
Joseph C. Honet, 1979–1980, Detroit
William M. Fowler, 1980–1981, Los Angeles
John F. Ditunno, Jr, 1981–1982, Philadelphia
Murray M. Freed, 1982–1983, Boston
Arthur E. Grant, 1983–1984, San Antonio, TX
George H. Kraft, 1984–1985, Seattle
Myron M. LaBan, 1985–1986, Detroit
Richard S. Materson, 1986–1987, Houston
Joachim L. Opitz, 1987–1988, Rochester, MN
Barbara deLateur, 1988–1989, Seattle
Erwin G. Gonzalez, 1989–1990, New York
James T. Demopoulos, 1990–1991, Philadelphia
Ian C. MacLean, 1991–1992, Chicago
James T. Demopoulos, 1992–1993, Philadelphia
Leon Reinstein, 1993–1994, Baltimore
Robert P. Christopher, 1994–1995, Memphis
Randall E. Braddom, 1995–1996, Indianapolis
James R. Swenson, 1996–1997, Salt Lake City
Barry S. Smith, 1997–1998, Dallas, TX

The Academy, in collaboration with the ACRM, is involved in the sponsorship, management, and production of the Archives of Physical Medicine and Rehabilitation. The Academy has an 11-member board of governors that includes the current officers, the past president, and five members at large. The list of past presidents of the Academy (Table 1-4) reflects the wide geographic distribution of these officers.

The American Board of Physical Medicine and Rehabilitation

In 1936, Dr. Louis Wilson, then president of the Advisory Board of Medical Specialties, suggested the need for a certifying board in physical medicine. In the late 1930s and early 1940s, plans for the establishment of an accrediting board were developed. Much of the groundwork was laid by Drs. Frank Krusen, John Coulter, and Walter Zeiter. It was believed to be essential to develop a plan of organization of a board of physical medicine that was acceptable to the Advisory Council of Medical Specialties. It also was necessary to seek the support of other, already established boards when the proposal was presented to the Advisory Board. After considerable exchange of views with the existing boards, and much controversy regarding the use of the term "rehabilitation" in the title, the American Board of Physical Medicine was approved by the Advisory Board for Medical Specialties in January 1947. It was authorized to begin certification procedures under the advisory capacity of the American Board of Medicine, the American Board of Orthopaedics, and the American Board of Radiology.

The 11 original members of the American Board of Physical Medicine were Dr. Kristian Hansson of New York, Dr. Richard Kovacs of New York, Dr. Walter Zeiter of Cleveland, from the American Society of Physical Medicine, now the American Academy of Physical Medicine and Rehabilitation; Dr. Frank Krusen of Rochester, Minnesota, and Dr. Arthur Watkins of Boston, from the AMA; Dr. Leonard Huddleston of Los Angeles, Dr. Benjamin Strickland, Jr., of Washington, DC, and Dr. William Schmidt of Philadelphia, from the American Congress of Physical Medicine, now the ACRM; and Dr. Robert Bennett of Warm Springs, Georgia, and Dr. Frank Ewerhardt of St. Louis, from the Section of Physical Medicine of the Southern Medical Association. The Board was incorporated in Illinois on February 27, 1947, and the first meeting was held in Atlantic City, New Jersey, on June 6, 1947. The officers of the Board elected at this meeting were Dr. Krusen, chairman; Dr. Strickland, vice chairman; and Dr. Bennett, secretary-treasurer.

The American Board of Physical Medicine was organized under the auspices of the Advisory Board for Medical Specialties as an affiliated board functioning under the direction of the Committee on Standards and Examinations of the Advisory Board for Medical Specialties and under the auspices of the boards of medicine, orthopaedics, and radiology. After 2 years it became an independent board with full representation on the Advisory Board for Medical Specialties and was approved by the Council on Medical Education and

Hospitals, now known as the Council on Medical Education, of the AMA.

The first certifying examinations of the American Board of Physical Medicine were held in Minneapolis in August 1947, during which 91 diplomates were certified. About half of these individuals were certified on the basis of peer recognition for full-time practice in the field. This was the only time such "grandfathering" was used as a basis for certification. It is interesting to note that a large number of those considered eligible to be grandfathered responded to a request of the Board to take the written examinations to help the Board and the Examinations Committee establish baseline pass-fail performance standards.

In June 1949, the American Board of Physical Medicine became the ABPM&R with the approval of the Advisory Board for Medical Specialties, now known as the American Board of Medical Specialties (ABMS).

The gradual growth of the total number of diplomates certified by the Board from 1947 through 1996 is shown in Figure 1-2; the number certified annually ranged from 17 to

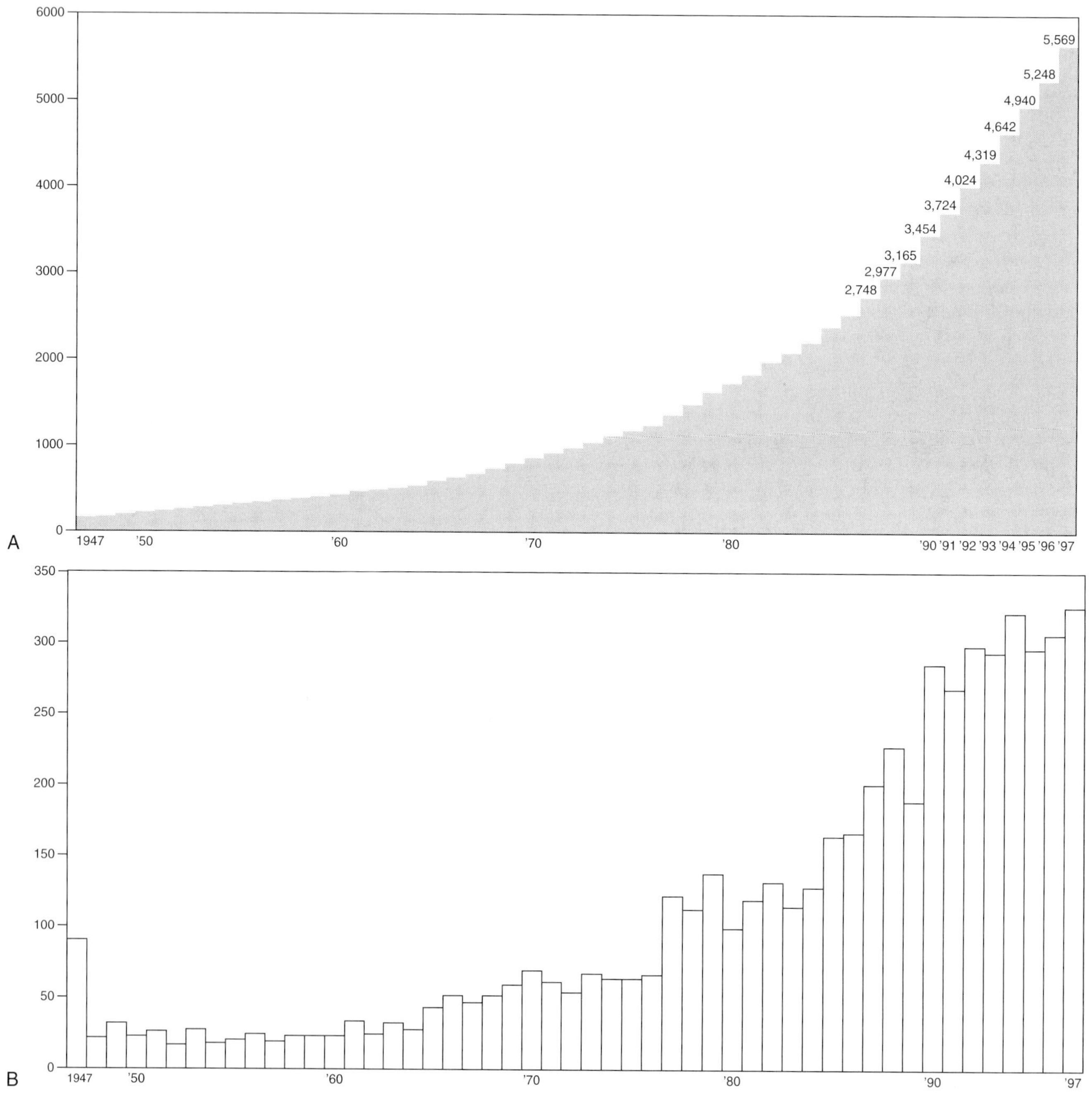

FIG. 1-2. A: Progressive growth of the number of diplomates in physical medicine and rehabilitation occurred from 1947 through 1997. **B:** Total certificates awarded annually ranged from 17 to 300, for a total of 5,569 diplomates; 3,023 have been certifed since 1987.

71 through 1976. Beginning in 1977, the number certified each year increased significantly, ranging from 101 to 323 annually. As of 1997, 5,569 physicians have been certified as diplomates. Each year since 1947 the Board has given a two-part written and oral examination to candidates who have satisfactorily completed a residency program approved by the Residency Review Committee in Physical Medicine and Rehabilitation and accredited by the Accreditation Council on Graduate Medical Education.

Before 1980, candidates applying for admission to the certification process could use an option of submitting documented evidence of 2 years of full-time clinical practice in PM&R as an alternative for 1 year of satisfactorily completed accredited residency training in the specialty. This option was terminated in July 1981.

Written Examination

The Board has given a written examination as part I of the certification process annually since 1947. The written examination committee currently includes three subsections on content: neuromuscular; musculoskeletal issues; and cardiovascular, pulmonary, pain, and other subjects. Each section enlists the assistance of experienced physiatrists as written examination associates. Together, the written examination associates and the Board's written examination committee develop questions relevant to the specialty. A large computerized test bank has been compiled. The Board strives to use new questions for 60% of each written examination. To improve the quality of subsequent examinations, responses to each question are carefully analyzed after the examination. Questions with desirable positive discrimination indices may be used in subsequent examinations.

Oral Examination

The Board has given oral examinations (i.e., part II of the certification examinations) annually since 1947 to candidates who present evidence of a minimum of 1 full year of broadly based clinical practice in PM&R after satisfactory completion of the residency training program, or an acceptable fifth year of advanced residency involvement or other suitable alternative. Before 1977, the clinical practice requirement had been 2 years. Essentially the same format for the oral examinations has been used since the founding of the Board. Each candidate has three 45-minute oral examinations with three separate examiners. Before 1965, all oral examinations were given by members of the Board. As the number of candidates increased, however, it became necessary to invite selected certified diplomates to assist the Board members as guest oral examiners. Since 1965, 400 guest oral examiners have assisted the Board in the evaluation process, and several have become Board directors. The format for the oral examination is specified, and a training manual and training session are provided by the Board so that there is a unified, structured format with minimal duplication of subject matter. Principles of scoring and grading candidates are carefully structured and standardized. The format has worked well for many years, and studies have shown that new examiners grade comparably with the experienced examiners and Board members. At variance with procedures used in some specialty Board oral examinations, specific questions and answers are not prescribed by the Board's examination committee.

During the past 18 years, the Board has conducted an annual survey of all residency training programs to obtain current statistical data on the number of trainees by postgraduate year, plus some demographic aspects of residents in training. These data are shared with the residency training program directors and have proved to be a valuable source of information relating to person-power studies in the specialty.

The progressive growth in the number of residents in training, along with the residency positions available in all accredited training programs, is shown in Figure 1-3. The total number of training programs has remained fairly constant, between 70 and 80, during the past decade. Occasionally, a program loses accreditation or withdraws, and new programs receive provisional approval by the accrediting authority of the Residency Review Committee.

Some demographic aspects of residents in training in recent years in relation to international and American medical graduates are shown in Figure 1-4. Changes in percentages of male and female residents are indicated in Figure 1-5.

The 24 specialty boards that are members of the ABMS provide quality assurance services to the public and medical profession. All of these specialty boards are autonomous, nonprofit corporations maintaining functional liaisons with the AMA and the specialty organizations in their field. Specifically, the purpose of the ABPM&R is to standardize qualifications for specialists in the field and to certify as specialists the physicians who have appeared voluntarily before it for recognition and certification according to its requirements.

The history of the Board was reviewed by Koepke in the Zeiter lecture of 1971 (33). Its further history, including presentation of statistical studies and analysis related to Board certification, was reviewed by Martin, Gullickson, and Gerken in 1980 (34). In 1996 the Board had 14 directors, the majority of whom had been intimately involved with residency training programs in PM&R. New members of the Board of Directors are elected from lists of five nominees submitted by the American Academy of Physical Medicine and Rehabilitation, the AMA, and the AAP. Members usually serve one or two 6-year terms, and broad geographic representation is considered desirable. The directors of the Board and the oral examiners serve without remuneration. The Board's activities in graduate medical education and certification are coordinated and integrated with the activities of the Residency Review Committee, the Accreditation Council on Graduate Medical Education, the residency training programs, and the ABMS. The original 1947 incorporation of the ABPM&R in Illinois was dissolved in 1981, when

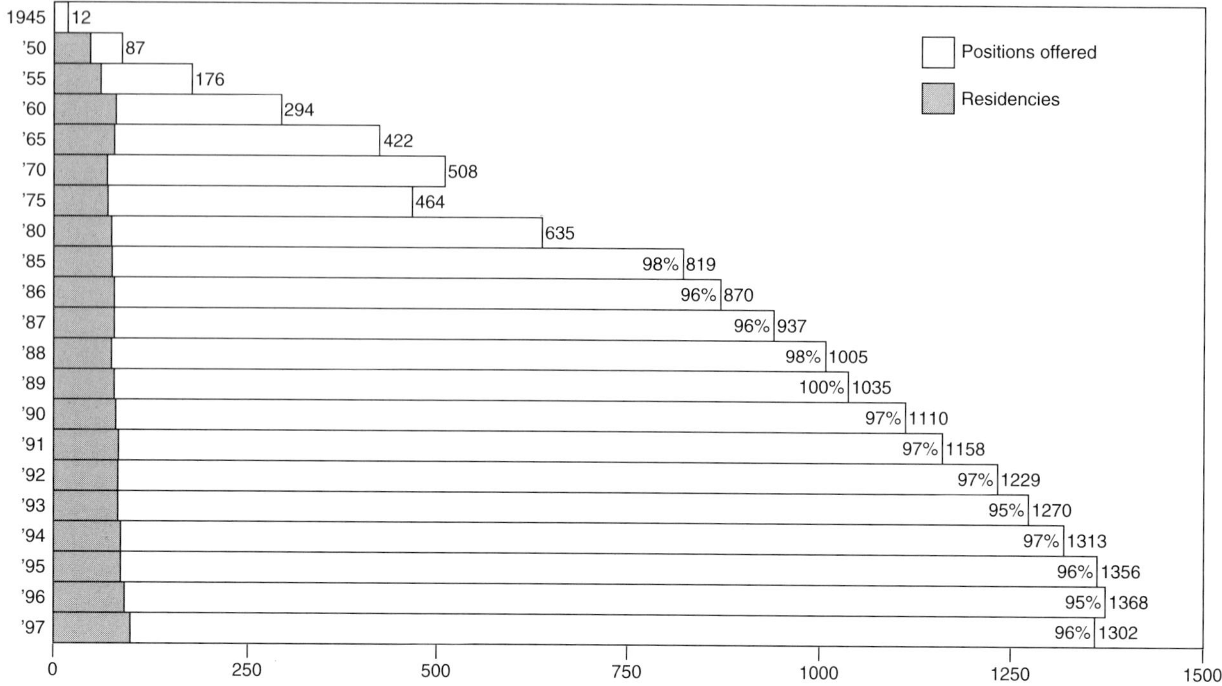

FIG. 1-3. The number of training programs in physical medicine and rehabilitation since 1945 has increased to 73 in 1960 and remains fairly constant. Total residency positions reached 1,302 in 1997.

it was incorporated as an autonomous, nonprofit corporation in the State of Minnesota. The Board celebrated its 50th anniversary in May 1997, and this was marked by a special supplement Board issue in the *Archives of Physical Medicine and Rehabilitation* (35).

In 1995 the ABPM&R was approved to issue a subspecialty certificate in Spinal Cord Injury Medicine. The first examination is tentatively scheduled for October 1998. The requirements of the ABPM&R for proposing the establishment of subspecialty certification was published in 1995 (35).

Time-Limited Certification and Recertification

The ABPM&R issued a letter of intent to begin issuing 10-year time-limited certificates in 1993. This was done in response to demand from the public, government, and third-party payers that physicians show evidence that they have stayed abreast of developments in their particular specialty, The first recertification examination is scheduled for the year 2,000, with examinations thereafter held annually.

The goals of the recertification program are to (a) encourage, stimulate, and support the diplomates in a program of self-directed lifelong learning, through the pursuit of continuing medical education; (b) permit diplomates to demonstrate that they continue to meet the requirements of the Board; and (c) provide evidence to patients and their families, to funding agencies, and to the public that PM&R diplomates are current in their medical knowledge.

The current and past directors of the ABPM&R are listed in Table 1-5.

Residency Review Committee for Physical Medicine and Rehabilitation

Organizational plans for the establishment of a residency review committee in PM&R were undertaken in 1953 following a letter from Dr. Edward Leveroos for the Council on Medical Education of the AMA to the ABPM&R. Before this time, residencies were granted approval for training by the Council of Medical Education of the AMA. A prototype for the function of the specialty Board as a cosponsor of a Residency Review Committee had existed for several years in internal medicine. By 1953, there were 10 other functioning residency review committees, whose methods for the evaluation and approval of residency programs were proving to be effective and efficient. It was proposed that the Residency Review Committee include three representatives of the ABPM&R and three representatives of the Council, two of whom were to be physiatrists. It was stated that the chairman of the committee was to be a Board representative, whereas the secretary was to be a member of the Council. All expenses for the administration and meetings of the committee were to be covered by the Council on Education of the AMA.

The first official meeting of the Residency Review Committee was held in 1954 and included, representing the Board, Drs. Robert L. Bennett, Earl C. Elkins, and Walter M.

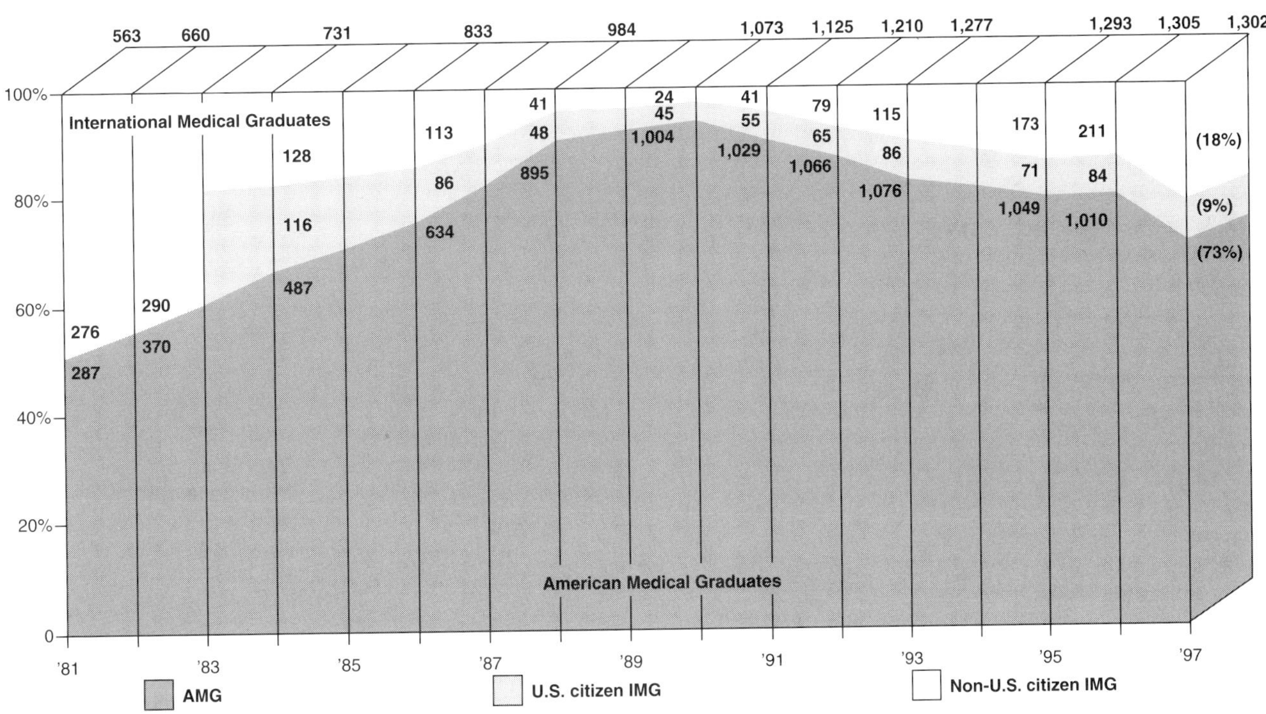

FIG. 1-4. Demographics of residents in physical medicine and rehabilitation indicate increasing numbers and percentages of American medical graduates since 1981. Approximately three quarters currently are American medical graduates. *AMG*, American medical graduates; *IMG*, international medical graduates.

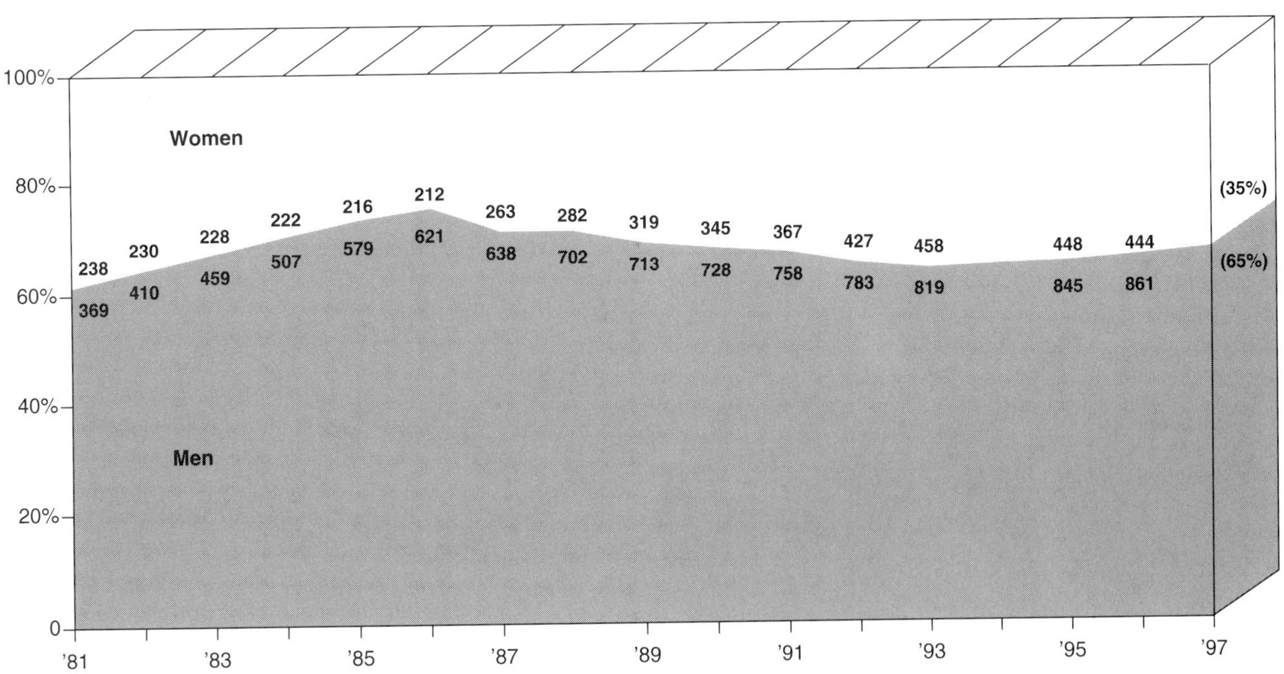

FIG. 1-5. Demographics of male and female residents in physical medicine and rehabilitation from 1981 to 1997 indicate that about one third are women.

TABLE 1-5. *Directors and Past Directors, American Board of Physical Medicine and Rehabilitation*

Chairmen of the Board	
Frank Krusen, M.D.	1947–1949
Walter Zeiter, M.D.	1949–1953
Robert Bennett, M.D.	1953–1963
Frederic Kottke, M.D.	1963–1969
George Koepke, M.D.	1969–1976
Glenn Gullickson, M.D.	1976–1981
John Dittunno, M.D.	1981–1984
B. Stanley Cohen, M.D.	1984–1988
John L. Melvin, M.D.	1988–1993
Joel A. DeLisa, M.D.	1993

Directors of the Board

Johns S. Coulter, M.D., 1947–1949, Chicago, IL
Frank H. Krusen, M.D., 1947–1949, Rochester, MN
Frank Dwerhardt, M.D., 1947–1948, St. Louis, MO
Benjamin A. Strickland, Jr., M.D., 1947–1950, Washington, DC
Richard I. Kovacs, M.D., 1947–1950, New York, NY
Walter J. Zeiter, M.D., 1947–1955, Cleveland, OH
Arthur L. Watkins, M.D., 1947–1958, Boston, MA
Robert L. Bennett, M.D., 1947–1963, Warm Springs, GA
Kristian G. Hansson, M.D., 1947–1960, New York, NY
O. Leonard Huddleston, M.D., 1947–1960, Denver, CO
William H. Schmidt, M.D., 1947–1964, Philadelphia, PA
Earl C. Elkins, M.D., 1949–1977, Rochester, MN
A. B. C. Knudsen, M.D., 1949–1966, Washington, DC
William Bierman, M.D., 1950–1966, New York, NY
Donald A. Covalt, M.D., 1951–1962, New York, NY
Walter M. Solomon, M.D., 1951–1954, Cleveland, OH
Frederick J. Kottke, M.D., 1955–1969, Minneapolis, MN
H. Worley Kendell, M.D., 1956–1965, Peoria, IL
Donald L. Rose, M.D., 1956–1967, Kansas City, KS
Arthur S. Abramson, M.D., 1957–1968, New York, NY
Edward E. Gordon, M.D., 1958–1960, Chicago, IL
Thomas F. Hines, M.D., 1959–1964, New Haven, CT
Justus F. Lehmann, M.D., 1961–1972, Seattle, WA
Edward W. Lowman, M.D., 1962–1972, New York, NY
Joseph G. Benton, M.D., 1965–1976, Brooklyn, NY
George H. Koepke, M.D., 1965–1976, Ann Arbor, MI
Edward M. Krusen, M.D., 1965–1976, Dallas, TX
Alfred Ebel, M.D., 1966–1978, New York, NY
Jerome W. Gersten, M.D., 1966–1977, Denver, CO
Glenn Gullickson, Jr., M.D., 1969–1981, Minneapolis, MN
Thomas C. Hohmann, M.D., 1969–1974, Pittsburgh, PA
Leonard D. Policoff, M.D., 1970–1980, Princeton, NJ
John F. Dittunno, M.D., 1972–1984, Philadelphia, PA
Arthur A. Rodriquez, M.D., 1972–1980, Chicago, IL
Murray M. Freed, M.D., 1974–1987, Boston, MA
B. Stanley Cohen, M.D., 1976–1988, Baltimore, MD
Victor Cummings, M.D., 1976–1988, Toledo, OH
Arthur E. Grant, M.D., 1976–1988, San Antonio, TX
Gordon M. Martin, M.D., 1977–1992, Rochester, MN
John W. B. Redford, M.D., 1977–1989, Kansas City, KS
Catherine N. Hinterbuchner, M.D., 1978–1990, New York, NY
Barbara J. deLateur, M.D., 1980–1992, Seattle, WA
Donald H. See, M.D., 1981–1987, San Francisco, CA
John L. Melvin, MD., 1981–1993, Milwaukee, WI
Phala A. Helm, M.D., 1984–1996, Dallas, TX
James R. Swenson, M.D., 1989–1997, Salt Lake City, UT
Malcolm C. McPhee, M.D., 1987–present, Scottsdale, AZ
Robert P. Christopher, M.D., 1987–present, Memphis, TN
Bruce M. Gans, M.D., 1988–present, Detroit, MI
Joel A. DeLisa, M.D., 1988–present, Newark, NJ
F. Patrick Maloney, MD., 1988–present, N. Little Rock, AR
Joseph C. Honet, M.D., 1990–present, Detroit, MI
Joachim L. Opitz, M.D., 1992–1995, Rochester, MN
Murray E. Brandstater, M.D., 1992–present, Loma Linda, CA
Margaret C. Hammond, M.D., 1993–present, Seattle, WA
Gerald Felsenthal, M.D., 1993–present, Baltimore, MD
Nicolas E. Walsh, M.D., 1993–present, San Antonio, TX
William, E. Staas, Jr., M.D., 1995–present, Philadelphia, PA
Margaret A. Turk, M.D., 1996–present, Syracuse, NY
Stephen F. Noll, M.D., 1996–present, Rochester, MN
Jay V. Subbarao, 1997–present, Maywood, IL

Solomon; representatives of the Council were Drs. Harold Dinken, Donald L. Rose, and Edward Leveroos. Dr. Elkins was elected the first chairman and Dr. Leveroos the first secretary. The members were, and continue to be, elected or appointed for a 3-year term and are eligible to serve two terms. Original appointments were made on a staggered basis.

The Residency Review Committee meets for two full days twice a year to consider applications for accreditation of new residency programs and renewal of accreditation. Residency survey reports prepared by AMA site visitors are reviewed and discussed. Site visitors are trained as analysts, and requests are sent out by the AMA office for review of one or several residency programs at an institution. The members of the Committee are not eligible to serve as site visitors. The site visitors have current information, which is submitted by the program directors, plus a protocol and format to be completed and returned to the Residency Review Committee. The Committee generally is the body that decides when use of a specialist site visitor is indicated. The Residency Review Committee decides on one of several options regarding the status of a residency program. A new program that appears to have potential for success is given provisional approval for 3 years. Full approval usually is granted after 3 years of effective performance under provisional status, and accreditation generally is renewed after surveys made at 3- to 5-year intervals. Probationary status for a program may be in order when significant questions arise regarding faculty, didactic programs, or clinical teaching and experience. Before a decision is made to give a probationary rating or to withdraw approval, the representatives of the program and the supporting institution have the opportunity to respond to concerns and criticisms made by the Residency Review Committee.

The actions of the Residency Review Committee are subject to final approval by the Accreditation Council on Graduate Medical Education, one of its parent bodies. If members of a residency training program, and the sponsoring institution, are dissatisfied with a ruling or action of the Residency Review Committee, they can appeal at the Committee and, if advisable, the Council level.

Usually, 15 to 20 programs are fully or partially considered at a given meeting of the Residency Review Committee. The specialty board works closely with the Committee and maintains an up-to-date listing of the accredited programs, the names of the program directors, the names of physiatrists responsible for the residents in training, and details of the training program. Additionally, information is provided by the Board office, from program or institutional staff, from the residents, or by the record of performance of the residents in the certification process. The Executive Secretary of the Residency Review Committee is on the staff of the Accreditation Council on Graduate Medical Education and the AMA and provides information on the activities of the Committee to the Council on Education of the AMA.

Another important function of the Residency Review Committee is to prepare a statement and detailed description of the program requirements for a residency training program in PM&R, which is published annually by the AMA in the *Directory of Graduate Medical Education Programs* (i.e., "Green Book"). The "program requirements" section is part of the section on "accredited residencies in graduate medical education: institutional and program requirements." The *Directory* includes a complete listing of all accredited residency training programs.

The current and past members of the Residency Review Committee in Physical Medicine and Rehabilitation are listed in Table 1-6.

TABLE 1-6. *Members and past members, Residency Review Committee for Physical Medicine and Rehabilitation*

Current members (1996)	*Past members*
American Academy of Physical Medicine and Rehabilitation	Robert L. Bennett, M.D.[a]
Gerald Felsenthal, M.D. (Chairman)	B. Stanley Cohen, M.D.
Phyllis Page, M.D.	Donald A. Covalt, M.D.
	Victor Cummings, M.D.[a]
American Board of Physical Medicine and Rehabilitation	Harold Dinken, M.D.
Murray E. Brandstater, M.D.	John F. Ditunno, M.D.
Margaret C. Hammond, M.D.	Alfred Ebel, M.D.
Mark Raymond, Ph.D., ex officio	Earl C. Elkins, M.D.
	William J. Erdman, II, M.D.
Council on Medical Education	Murray M. Freed, M.D.
Barry S. Smith, M.D.	Erwin G. Gonazlez, M.D.
Marc E. Duerden, M.D.	Arthur M. Grant, M.D.
	Glenn Gullickson, Jr., M.D.
	Catherine N. Hinterbuchner, M.D.
Resident Representative	Thomas F. Hines, M.D.
Alice Chen, M.D.	Joseph C. Honet, M.D.[a]
	Ernest W. Johnson, M.D.
Staff	Nancy Kester, M.D.
Paul O'Connor, Ph.D. (Executive Secretary)	A. B. C. Knudson, M.D.
Sheila Hart (Accreditation Administrator)	George H. Koepke, M.D.
	Frederic J. Kottke, M.D.
	Edward M. Krusen, M.D.
	Edward Leveroos, M.D.
	Edward W. Lowman, M.D.
	Gordon M. Martin, M.D.
	Richard S. Materson, M.D.
	Malcolm C. McPhee, M.D.[a]
	John L. Melvin, M.D.
	Roger Pesch, M.D.
	Leonard D. Policoff, M.D.
	James W. Rae, M.D.
	Donald L. Rose, M.D.
	Oscar Selke, M.D.
	Walter M. Solomon, M.D.
	Jerome Tobis, M.D.
	Arthur L. Watkins, M.D.
	Walter J. Zieter, M.D.

[a] Representative of the American Board of Physical Medicine and Rehabilitation.

The American Board of Medical Specialties

The concept of a specialty board in medicine was first proposed in 1908 at the meeting of the American Academy of Ophthalmology and Otolaryngology. The first board to be formed was the American Board for Ophthalmic Examinations, which was incorporated in 1917; the name was changed in 1933 to the American Board of Ophthalmology (1). The second specialty board was the American Board of Otolaryngology, founded and incorporated in 1924. The third and fourth boards, the American Board of Obstetrics and Gynecology and the American Board of Dermatology and Syphilology, were established in 1930 and 1932. In 1933, a conference attended by representatives of the four specialty boards, plus the American Hospital Association, the Association of American Medical Colleges (AAMC), the Federation of State Medical Boards, the AMA Council on Education and Hospitals, and the National Board of Medical Examiners, was held, during which the Advisory Board for Medical Specialties was created. Dr. Louis Wilson was elected as the first president.

Since 1934, official recognition of specialty boards in medicine has been under the jurisdiction of the Advisory Board for Medical Specialties and later its successor, the ABMS and the AMA Council on Medical Education (36). This mechanism was formalized through the establishment of a Liaison Committee for Specialty Boards and the publication of the Essentials of Approval of Examining Boards in Medical Specialties (37). This document has undergone several revisions but remains the standard for recognition of new specialty boards. By 1948, 18 specialty boards had received approval and recognition. Between 1949 and 1969, no new boards were approved by the ABMS and the Liaison Committee for Specialty Boards. Between 1969 and 1979, five specialty boards were approved: Allergy and Immunology, Emergency Medicine, Family Practice, Nuclear Medicine, and Thoracic Surgery. The American Board of Medical Genetics was approved in 1991.

The ABMS has continued to grow and to expand its interests and concerns. It also provides a forum for representation of all specialty boards. At semiannual sessions, the ABMS considers policies regarding certification procedures and requirements of various boards, length of residency training, and standards for residency programs.

An extensive program involving publications based on several conferences sponsored by the ABMS on examination procedures, educational concepts, and teaching methods is functioning effectively. A continuing project of the ABMS is the publication of directories of certified specialists in each specialty.

One division of the ABMS is concerned with research on education in specialty fields, examination procedures for certification, and in-service resident evaluation procedures and their potential role in the certification process. Through annual surveys, the ABMS maintains data on residency training and certification in all of the accredited specialties. The ABPM&R, an active member of the ABMS, has three official delegates and three alternates to provide active participation and voting representation at the annual and semiannual meetings.

In addition to its own organizational activities, the ABMS maintains official functional liaison with the Council for Medical Affairs, Accreditation Council for Graduate Medical Education, Accreditation Council for Continuing Medical Education, National Resident Matching Program, National Board of Medical Examiners, Educational Commission for Foreign Medical Graduates, and Liaison Committee for Specialty Boards.

The Association of Academic Physiatrists

An organization with a strong academic orientation and involvement of its members was needed to gain representation for the specialty in the Association of American Medical Colleges (AAMC). The AAP was founded in 1967 to address this need and to stimulate interest in and share expertise related to undergraduate and graduate academic physiatry (38). The AAP was selected to be a member of the AAMC in 1970. It has experienced steady growth to a membership of 1,366, including 301 residents, in 1996. The AAP has achieved recognition both within the specialty and in several other areas of academic medicine.

The AAP has sponsored workshops and sessions for improving curriculum planning and teaching skills, as well as developing and expanding research and grant-writing skills. The AAP provides a forum for the ABPM&R and its residency training program directors and faculties. It encourages increased faculty and resident involvement in high-quality basic and clinical research. The AAP has four councils: resident's council, chairman's council, resident program director's council, and the council of directors and coordinators of research.

The AAP provides advisory services for matching academic positions with potential candidates. It is also one of the nominating organizations for selection of directors for the ABPM&R.

In addition to the *American Journal of Physical Medicine and Rehabilitation,* the AAP publishes a quarterly newsletter with information of interest to those involved in medical school and graduate medical education and for residents with the potential for an academic career. Grant announcements and research opportunities are stressed. It also provides curricular and other academic consultation to medical schools requesting such assistance. In addition, the AAP works with the American Medical Student Association to provide career information. Recently the AAP developed a Web page to provide better communication and more interaction with internet users.

The Executive Director is Carolyn Braddom, Ed.D., and the office is located in Indianapolis, Indiana. AAP presidents have included the following physicians:

William J. Erdman II, M.D., 1967–1968
Henry B. Betts, M.D., 1968–1969
Mieczyslaw Peszcynski, M.D., 1969–1970
Murray M. Freed, M.D., 1970–1971
Nadene Coyne, M.D., 1971–1972
Joseph Goodgold, M.D., 1972–1973
John F. Ditunno, Jr., M.D., 1973–1975
Justus F. Lehmann, M.D., 1975–1977
Ernest W. Johnson, M.D., 1977–1979
George H. Kraft, M.D., 1979–1981
Paul J. Corcoran, M.D., 1981–1983
Martin Grabois, M.D., 1983–1985
John L. Melvin, M.D., 1985–1987
Paul E. Kaplan, M.D., 1987–1989
Randall L. Braddom, M.D., 1989–1991
Joel A. DeLisa, M.D., 1991–1993
Bruce M. Gans, M.D., 1993–1995
Robert Meier, III, M.D., 1995–1997
Nicolas E. Walsh, M.D., 1997–1999

The International Rehabilitation Medicine Association

Since 1940, several international organizations have been formed with various goals and related in many ways to specialty areas related to rehabilitation medicine. The most active of these organizations, and the one with the widest membership, is the International Rehabilitation Medicine Association (IRMA). The IRMA was founded by Dr. Sidney Licht in 1969. Dr. Licht, editor of the 11-volume *Physical Medicine Library* and a Connecticut-based physiatrist, had established many professional and personal contacts with physicians interested in physical and rehabilitation medicine throughout the world.

The IRMA is a society of physicians from all specialties of medicine and surgery who are interested in promoting the art and science of medicine and the improvement of health through the understanding and use of rehabilitation medicine. The IRMA's objectives are based on the recognition that at least 300 million people of all ages require rehabilitation services in the treatment of their disabilities. The goal of IRMA is to educate and encourage governments and societies to recognize the reality of this need and to provide rehabilitation medicine services for the vast number of chronically diseased and disabled people, including the aged, and to promote medical research in this area.

The IRMA offers its members the opportunity to broaden their professional competence through the formation of and participation in activities of scientific sections geared to medical and surgical specialties and to other areas of interest, including education and research. The IRMA sponsors a world congress every 4 years and publishes a quarterly newsletter and periodic scientific monographs.

The IRMA maintains liaison with the International Federation for Physical Medicine and Rehabilitation, Medical Commission of Rehabilitation International, and World Health Organization. The IRMA is governed by a board of directors of eight members, including four officers and four members at large. The presidents of this organization since its founding have included Drs. C. Wynn Perry of Great Britain, Silvano Boccardi of Italy, Luis Ibarra of Mexico, Wilhelm Zinn of Switzerland, Herman Flax of Puerto Rico, Tyrone Reyes of the Philippines, Arturo Arino-Molina of Madrid, Spain, and Dr. Martin Grabois of Houston, Texas.

The Baruch Committee on Physical Medicine and Rehabilitation

In the early 1940s, Bernard Baruch, a renowned financier, philanthropist, and personal advisor to the presidents of the United States from World War I until his death in 1965, became vitally interested in the developing specialty of PM&R. His interest was initiated by admiration for his father, Dr. Simon Baruch, who had been a physician involved with the care of Civil War soldiers and who later practiced in New York City. He had been particularly interested in physical activities and hydrotherapy in the rehabilitation and return of soldiers to active duty. *An Epitome of Hydrotherapy* by Dr. Baruch was published in 1920 and republished in 1950 under Bernard Baruch's auspices in honor of his father (39). As a memorial to his father, he wished to provide significant support to the development of physical medicine as a specialty area. In 1942, he approached Dr. Frank Krusen at the Mayo Clinic, who assembled and organized a committee of physiatrists and noted consultants from several other specialties and from the basic sciences of physiology and physics (24,40). This committee, under the chairmanship of Dr. Ray Lyman Wilbur, and its consultants included approximately 41 enthusiastic and capable scientists who proposed and initiated opportunities and encouragement for training of residents in physical medicine, established model training and research centers, and encouraged and supported pertinent research projects in specialized institutions.

The Baruch Committee was very active for 4 years, during which its basic aims were achieved. Its influence has continued within the specialty. Approximately 50 physicians have received sponsorship and aid with their residency training from the Baruch Committee. The principal research and development centers that were established by this Committee were Columbia University College of Physicians and Surgeons, to establish a model center for basic research and teaching of physical medicine, as well as the University of Minnesota Medical School, Harvard Medical School, University of Southern California, Medical College of Virginia, and New York University College of Medicine. The Massachusetts Institute of Technology was awarded a grant to establish a center on biophysics, electronics, and instrumentation related to medicine.

The Baruch Committee and the Special Exhibit Committee on Physical Medicine of the AMA sponsored and arranged for extensive state-of-the-art scientific exhibits for the AMA conventions and interim meetings in 1948 and 1949. These were described by Krusen and associates (22).

After World War II, there was rapidly increasing interest and development in rehabilitation concepts and services, which had evolved significantly in military medicine. Dr. Howard Rusk was a prime developer and promoter in this area after his involvement in the Air Force medical services (41). His enthusiasm, coupled with his organizational, promotional, and communication abilities, rapidly raised the level of interest of many physicians, hospitals, and medical centers in providing effective medical rehabilitation services and training programs for physicians and other essential rehabilitation personnel.

Dr. Rusk developed the New York University Rehabilitation Center, which became the largest residency training program in the United States. His writing for the *New York Times,* as an associate editor, was an important public relations resource for PM&R. Dr. Rusk is recognized for his efforts in involving many foreign countries and their physicians in rehabilitation medicine. Through the World Rehabilitation Fund, trainees were aided in obtaining training in the United States. In addition, educational and service programs have been organized and implemented in many parts of the world.

Another pioneer in the field of rehabilitation was Dr. Henry H. Kessler. Dr. Kessler served in the Navy during World War II and became the director of the Navy Rehabilitation and Amputation Center at Mare Island, one of the leading centers in the country at the time. After World War II, Dr. Kessler focused his energies on enlarging the scope of postwar rehabilitation to include civilians as well as veterans. He returned to his home state of New Jersey and founded the Kessler Institute, based on his desire to provide care for the entire person rather than merely treating the medical aspects of a disability.

Dr. Kessler took his ideals for rehabilitation of the whole person to an international level and was in the forefront of the development of rehabilitation clinics and increased recognition of the field in Yugoslavia, Indonesia, India, the Philippines, Israel, and many other parts of the world. Dr. Kessler also was pivotal in the refinement of the workers' compensation program and disability determination process to better enable physicians to determine the extent of a disability and have the patient return to the work environment.

In addition to his work in developing rehabilitation on a national and international scale, Dr. Kessler is credited with introducing to the United States the surgical technique of cineplasty for the muscular control of an artificial arm. He also further enhanced its use and applications.

The Impact of Specific Disorders in the Development of Rehabilitation Medicine

Poliomyelitis

In the 1940s there was a revolution in the management of patients with both acute and chronic poliomyelitis. Before the use of new concepts promulgated by the Australian nurse Sister Elizabeth Kenny, patients who had paralytic poliomyelitis were treated for many weeks and months with plaster-shell supports of the extremities, and trunk muscles weakened by the anterior horn cell involvement of poliomyelitis. These long periods of supportive bed rest and splinting generally were followed by efforts at re-establishing ambulation, often involving extensive bracing, crutches, walkers, and wheelchairs.

Sister Kenny, through her observation of the clinical course and management of poliomyelitis patients in Australia and England, had developed concepts of the pathophysiology that were not compatible with the pathologists' descriptions of anterior horn cell inflammation and destruction as the basic lesion. A new term, "mental alienation," was used instead of "paralysis," and daily treatment with hot packs for pain and spasm followed by passive and retraining exercises was prescribed. Sister Kenny and her colleagues used precise, standardized manual muscle testing and grading procedures performed at frequent intervals. A Sister Kenny Institute for treatment of poliomyelitis was established in Minneapolis with a number of affiliated satellite centers, some with support from the National Foundation for Infantile Paralysis.

Dr. Miland Knapp, a pioneer physiatrist in Minneapolis who, with his associates, worked with Sister Kenny for several years in the management of these patients, modified and refined some of her original concepts of the disease and its manifestations. At the same time, he acknowledged the important contributions Sister Kenny had made on the subject of poliomyelitis (42):

1. She emphasized muscle shortening as a cause of deformity, and pointed out that this shortening is not secondary to anterior horn cell damage but is a positive entity that requires positive treatment in the early stages if future deformity is to be minimized.
2. She systematized a technique of muscle re-education, which deserves the name "re-education" and is based on sound physiologic principles and logical reasoning.
3. She emphasized a positive approach to treatment of the disease, stressing those aspects that can be treated with some hope of success such as muscle shortening, reversible paralyses, and incoordination, and relatively ignoring those effects for which no treatment is successful, namely, anterior horn cell degeneration with motor denervation (42).

As Sister Kenny's methods and observations gained the support of physicians at the University of Minnesota and elsewhere, the importance of the new specialty of physical medicine in providing a new style of treatment for poliomyelitis rapidly evolved. Dr. Robert L. Bennett, longtime medical director and physiatrist at the Georgia Warm Springs Foundation, pointed out the importance of the evolution of a sound basis for the practice of physical medicine (43):

> "Polio, more than any other disease, was the workshop and the showcase for demonstration of the physical aspects of medical care. The pathology of polio was never very difficult to understand . . . ."

Even though confined almost entirely to lower motor neurons, polio is never monotonous in its manifestations. Each patient seen is a neuromuscular puzzle with patterns of weakness and paralysis of endless variety. If the puzzle is not solved—and solved quickly—musculoskeletal complications result that create new and intriguing puzzles for us to solve. Probably from no other disease have we learned so much about the pathogenesis of musculoskeletal deformities and their functional significance.

The severe impairment not infrequently caused by polio has had great influence on the development of the concept of realistic functional goals for these patients. Highly refined methods of muscle evaluation and care were developed that we believe keep impairment within the bounds of irreversible pathology. Such evaluation and the subsequent formulation of the prescription for care required a knowledge of functional anatomy and muscle retraining. It was through our experience with polio that this knowledge became one of the cornerstones of physical medicine.

There is no reason to believe that manual muscle testing was devised entirely for evaluation of the patient with poliomyelitis, but certainly the systems of manual muscle testing now used to determine and record voluntary muscle strength were developed and refined from the demands of caring for such patients.

Muscle re-education was, and of course still is, a natural follow-through of thorough muscle testing. It seems unnecessary to state that exercise of weakened muscles without accurate knowledge of their strength and their response to exercise is as illogical as it is dangerous.

Functional training was a natural outgrowth of muscle re-education. Functional achievement for the polio patient required new and different techniques in both physical and occupational therapy, and new and different orthotic devices. Literally hundreds of functional orthotic devices all developed from our experience with polio.

As we learned how to save the lives of patients with severe and extensive damage to the nervous system, knowledge and experience gained from polio were immediately applicable to the care of the paraplegic, the hemiplegic, the quadriplegic, and even the severely brain-damaged patient (42).

> Dr. Bennett continued: "I am convinced that it was through contact with patients who had polio that physiatrists first were established as clinicians with the special interest, essential training and recognized competence in handling those conditions that require carefully prescribed activity" (43).

Changes in the management of poliomyelitis were paralleled by the rapid development of new tools for patients with respiratory impairment and paralysis. Body respirators of several types were introduced, improved, and functionally refined. The large tank-type negative-pressure respirators (i.e., iron lungs) became the standard device and in many instances proved to be life-saving supportive equipment. These devices were stockpiled by the National Foundation for Infantile Paralysis in a number of cities during epidemic years and were made available to hospitals, treatment centers, and patients at home. Other devices included cuirass-type respirators that could be used in wheelchairs and beds, rocking beds, and abdominal pressure belts called pneumobelts. Phrenic nerve stimulators for respiratory paralysis were used successfully in several centers and later were used for selected high-cervical-level traumatic quadriplegic patients.

Spinal Cord Injury and Cerebrovascular Accident

Active interest in the rehabilitation of patients with spinal cord injuries evolved in the 1940s, in both England and the United States. Dr. Ludwig Guttmann founded the Stoke-Mandeville National Spinal Cord Injury Center in 1932 in Aylesbury, England (44). By 1965 there were seven other national centers in Great Britain. In 1946 Guttmann described some of the problems in the management of those patients (45). In the United States, the first large and comprehensive spinal cord injury center was established at the Hines Veterans Administration Hospital in suburban Chicago. Extensive developments and progress in this area are well documented in several standard textbooks and reference articles.

An in-depth analysis of the needs of persons with hemiplegia for expanding rehabilitation services was made in the challenging 1973 Zeiter lecture given by Dr. Kottke (46).

Summary of History

A historical perspective of the specialty of PM&R shows the first glimmers of a new specialty originating in the 1920s. At first, and during the 1930s, a base group of physicians determined the direction for the specialty and began seeking more physician support. During the 1940s, the specialty evolved from a physical treatment base to the larger concept incorporating total rehabilitation. The growth in residency training and certification of specialists has been the most significant thrust since 1947.

Additionally, the specialty has gained increased recognition since 1960 by the medical community and the public owing to a growing awareness of the need for rehabilitation services for the disabled, handicapped, and aging population.

The developments to date indicate growing and active specialty organizations, most notably the following:

American Congress of Rehabilitation Medicine—74 years old with 1,650 members, comprising many medical and allied health professionals

American Academy of Physical Medicine and Rehabilitation—65 years old with 5,499 fellows, associates, and junior members

American Board of Physical Medicine and Rehabilitation—50 years old with 5,569 certified diplomates

Association of Academic Physiatrists—30 years old with 1,366 members
International Rehabilitation Medicine Association—27 years old with 1,801 members.

The scientific programs and exhibits at the annual Academy and ACRM meetings, plus publications in the *Archives of Physical Medicine and Rehabilitation* and the *American Journal of Physical Medicine and Rehabilitation,* reveal increasing research productivity as well as growing involvement in other areas such as sports medicine, pediatric rehabilitation, and geriatrics.

CURRENT ACADEMIC STATUS OF PHYSICAL MEDICINE AND REHABILITATION

The health-care system, including the $27 billion medical rehabilitation industry, is in the process of changing from a provider-driven fee-for-service system to a payer-driven system. It is currently unclear whether it will ultimately be provider, payer, or consumer driven. Nevertheless, it would be an advantage to our specialty to establish an outcomes-driven, market-based approach to the delivery of rehabilitation (47).

The immediate catalyst for change has been the recent proliferation of managed care and its touted advantages of cost effectiveness, case management, medical technology assessment, practice pattern, and continuous quality improvement analysis (48). Managed care penetration has increased in the private insurance market from 26% in 1993 to 38% in 1994 and about 60% in 1996. It is predicted to exceed 85% by the year 2000 (47). Overall managed care also has begun to enter the public sector, which funds Medicare and Medicaid fee-for-service programs. Although in 1994 only 9% of Medicare beneficiaries were enrolled in managed care, DeJong predicts that this will be 70% to 85% by the year 2000 (47). Because Medicare accounts for about 70% of all inpatient rehabilitation revenue, further penetration will have a profound effect on the field.

In addition, the states are moving rapidly to convert their Medicaid programs from traditional fee-for-service programs to managed care programs (49). DeJong predicts that by 1998, 85% of Medicaid participants, exclusive of those in nursing homes, will be in some form of managed care (47).

Individuals with disabilities are most likely to be insured under public programs such as Medicare and Medicaid. They also are more likely to be dependent on their health-care coverage with respect to assistive technology and personal assistance services. The central health-care issue for individuals with disabilities is timely access to appropriate high-quality health care. Individuals with disabilities are likely to need more health care and thus to be more affected by cost constraints on the volume or quality of services.

In markets with high levels of managed care, health-care providers are consolidating into a few competing integrated provider networks that offer a comprehensive continuum of care. Rehabilitation providers are being forced to align themselves with these networks, some of which require exclusive agreements. Because rehabilitation is often a "downstream" provider, it is very much at risk for a guaranteed flow of patients. A better approach may be to try to align with all the major health-care networks in the area. To succeed as nonaligned however, a rehabilitation hospital may need to be reorganized as a center of excellence with a broad national and/or international referral base.

The payer-driven system encourages competition based on costs and financial risks more than prestige, and unfortunately, quality of care is assumed. Many for-profit providers have entered the rehabilitation market. These investor-owned for-profit companies look to Wall Street for financing. Not-for-profit organizations rely on debt financing, which must be covered through billing and revenue. The two largest for-profit organizations in the medical rehabilitation industry in 1997 are HealthSouth and Horizon/Continental Medical Systems. It is estimated that they own about 60% of the free-standing rehabilitation hospitals. Nova Care, Manor Care, and Theratx are three other for-profit companies that are heavily involved in providing subacute rehabilitation. Some believe that many not-for-profit hospitals will convert to for-profit status in order to obtain capital without incurring significant debt.

In order to maintain their market share, rehabilitation programs are diversifying to include subacute beds, ambulatory satellites, home care, durable medical equipment companies and assisted living. They are trying to eliminate excess capacity and to move patients more efficiently to the most cost-effective rehabilitation treatment modalities. The goal is to have patient care delivered in the most cost-efficient, appropriate setting to maximize outcomes and to achieve a high level of patient satisfaction. The driving force is almost exclusively cost. Comprehensive hospital inpatient rehabilitation often costs more than $1,000 a day. It has declined in mature managed care markets, whereas rehabilitation providers are cutting costs and inpatient lengths of stay are decreasing. Subacute inpatient rehabilitation units that are often housed in skilled nursing facilities are expanding. Although they provide services for only $300 to $500 per day, they usually require longer lengths of stay and provide less intensive therapies. Despite the fact that there are no good prospective studies evaluating costs or outcomes of patients, many orthopedic joint replacements and stroke patients are now rehabilitated in subacute units. Many providers are going to a treatment team product model and streamlining their therapy teams as well as developing integrated systems for the full continuum of care. Many systems are also increasing consumer involvement in the care decisions and their implementations.

At-Risk Relationships Between Providers and Insurers

Capitation is a method of caregivers being paid to provide care to a defined number of enrollees for a fixed amount of money per member per month. In a capitated system, revenue is earned up front when contracts are negotiated. Management of costs becomes the provider's challenge. Capitation raises problems because it creates financial interests that conflict with the interest physicians have in maximizing the welfare of their patients. There is little case-rate capitation experience in medical rehabilitation.

Although cost is dominating the system, patient satisfaction surveys are considered important, especially because the consumer usually has the option of at least three plans and the opportunity to change plans annually. However, except for length of stay, infection rates, and mortality rates, most hospital systems lack quality-of-care monitors that truly indicate outcomes. Consumer satisfaction eventually deals with individual health plans as well as individual providers. In some cities, formal health outcomes report cards are being developed and disseminated.

Quality of care needs to remain as important as price. Quality indicators need to be determined for each diagnostic group, and they need to be risk adjusted for age, case mix, severity of illness, and severity of impairment. Although it may require the participation of large multicenter groups to develop meaningful statistics, it is only by quality of care and outcomes analysis that we will be able to educate payers, consumers, and health-care providers on the short- and long-term cost effectiveness of rehabilitation.

The field of PM&R has not had to address the diagnostic related group (DRG) prospective payment system (PPS) that was implemented by Medicare in the acute hospitals in 1983. However, since 1990, Medicare has been reassessing reimbursement models for rehabilitation hospitals and units that are exempt from the PPS. A PPS based on functional-independent measure function-related group (FIM-FRG) is currently being explored by the Health Care Finance Administration (HCFA) that would be the rehabilitation analog to DRGs (50). This system would risk-adjust payment based on patient impairment, function, and age at admission. However, it has been criticized for lack of explicit financial incentive for good outcomes (51).

OPPORTUNITIES IN REHABILITATION

Manpower

With the managed care emphasis on minimizing costs and with gate-keepers limiting access to specialists to underutilize the system, it has been predicted that there will be a significant excess of physicians, especially specialists, by the year 2000 (52). The Council on Graduate Medical Education (COGME) has recommended moving to a system of 50% of physicians practicing general medicine and reducing the total number of first-year residents to 110% of United States Medical Graduates. The AAPM&R, AAP, ABPM&R, and American Physiatric Education Council commissioned Lewin VHI, a private research firm, to conduct a physiatric manpower study. They developed a supply-and-demand model to assess future physiatric needs based on various scenarios (49,53). Their study indicated that PM&R is still a shortage specialty with opportunity for growth. However, this is true only if an aggressive educational campaign about the specialty and its cost-effectiveness is successfully conducted and aimed at managed care organizations and other health-care providers (49,54,55). At this time the south appears to be the region with the greatest growth potential, whereas the northeast and Great Lakes region are more likely to experience a surplus.

Besides quantity, the quality of the trainees produced by physiatry training programs is important. Physiatrists need to do a better job of promoting PM&R to United States medical students to attract the best and the brightest, especially those with good interpersonal and communications skills (55). Currently there are 1,305 residents in training. Eight hundred sixty-one (66%) are male, and 444 (34%) are female, with 1,010 (77%) being American medical graduates. Some are beginning to question whether we are training too many physiatrists (56).

If the specialty were to increase its provision of primary care to the severely disabled (see Chapter 36), the demand for physiatrists would markedly exceed the supply. During admission to inpatient units, a physiatrist serves as the primary care physician, addressing both medical and rehabilitation needs. Once discharged from the hospital, these individuals typically follow up with their regular doctor for medical problems and with the physiatrist for disability-related concerns. However, some patients, such as certain previously healthy persons with a spinal cord injury, and many patients with other severe disabilities have no such regular doctor and rely on the physiatrist to fulfill all their ongoing medical needs.

Disabled individuals now live longer and develop the same chronic health problems (e.g., cardiac disease, hypertension, diabetes mellitus) experienced by the nondisabled population (57). Individuals with disabilities often are vulnerable to secondary conditions that may exacerbate their original disability (58). They are concerned about a lack of appropriate primary care and are apprehensive about the effects of capitated systems on the quality and quantity of care that will be available to them.

Many believe that general medical problems are better handled by the traditional primary care providers, such as internists and family practitioners, or by specialists who have had more formal and extensive training in general medicine than a typical physiatrist. Most primary care physicians, however, are not experienced and comfortable in dealing with the needs of the disabled, particularly the severely affected. Although these individuals with disabilities have tried to educate their primary care providers about the medical complications of their impairment, this has often been unsatisfactory. This has resulted in difficulty for the disabled to access effective primary care. This in turn has led to delays in diagnosis and management and high rehospitalization rates. Thus, there is a need for physicians qualified and willing to provide both medical and rehabilitation services for disabled individuals.

The challenge to our field is considerable: Should we expand skills and encourage practice patterns that would provide full primary care services to disabled individuals? If the specialty chooses to offer primary care for the disabled, there are multiple models that should be considered (59).

1. *Collaboration*. In this model, PM&R specialists would establish collaborative relationships with primary care practitioners, with PM&R providing expertise about long-term care of the disability issues and the primary care practitioner providing the 24-hour coverage for medical problems of a general nature. The collaborative model would involve linking with physicians practicing family medicine or general internal medicine. This model has been described by Gans and colleagues (60) and does not require modification of the present PM&R training requirements.
2. *Individual practice model*. In this arrangement, individual PM&R practitioners would incorporate primary care into their practice. This has already begun in various centers. An analogy might be the use of spinal injections such as epidural steroids for those providing primary spine care. Individual PM&R practitioners are beginning to acquire skills in spinal injections and to incorporate these into their practices. This is not part of regular residency training, nor a traditional part of PM&R practice.
3. *Subspecialty*. This would be either an added or special qualification and would require acceptance by organized medicine: the American Board of Medical Specialties (ABMS) and the Accreditation Council of Graduate Medical Education (ACGME) (61). It would require an additional year of training but would grant specific recognition by organized medicine of the practitioners' skills.
4. *Double boarding*. Dual certification agreements were formalized in 1987 with the American Board of Pediatrics, in 1989 with the American Board of Internal Medicine, and in 1991 with the American Board of Psychiatry and Neurology. Pediatrics/PM&R and internal medicine/PM&R are pathways recognized by organized medicine that have the potential to provide primary care practitioners for persons with disabilities. These double-boarding programs integrate the training required in two specialties, making it possible for a resident to complete both training requirements in 1 year less time than would be required to complete the two individual residencies. However, Medicare has reduced reimbursement for training beyond the initial residency.
5. *Physical medicine and rehabilitation as a primary care specialty*. In this model, all PM&R residents doing their residency training would have sufficient exposure to primary care practice so that they would be able to offer primary care if they chose, once they were in practice. This would represent a major shift in the definition of our field, and in training. It would have to be accomplished without diminishing the present emphasis on both physical medicine and on rehabilitation. Hopefully, it could be accomplished without additional training time. The model would represent an expansion of the discipline of PM&R to include, within its scope of practice, primary care for the disabled along with those other traditional components of PM&R, namely physical medicine, medical rehabilitation, and electrodiagnosis. The obvious parallel to this model is the initiative by obstetrics and gynecology to become a recognized primary care specialty for a defined patient group.

Another priority that the specialty needs to address is teaching rehabilitation to students and residents destined for a career in primary care. We have not, in general, concerned ourselves with the rehabilitation education of non-PM&R trainees. It is our obligation to provide them with the special knowledge and/or accommodations needed by individuals with disabilities, especially, if we do not provide some of the primary care.

Managed care is putting tremendous pressure on the entire academic community, which is struggling to maintain an adequate patient care network for education and research. Quality control and effective teaching, as well as health services and outcomes research, also must be assured. These networks will probably extend beyond the walls of the traditional academic medical center hospital. Some training will have to occur in community-based locations. As the academic medical center tries to reduce costs and shift some clinical responsibilities to network hospitals, careful planning will be needed to maintain high-quality resident/fellow training programs (62). Innovative paradigms will be needed for educating tomorrow's physicians, while at the same time providing high-quality patient care and focusing on investigation-initiated and -targeted research.

The involvement of academic medical centers and their patient care networks will create a degree of tension between health-care sites in the community aligned with competing networks (63). As a result, there may be pressure to limit educational programs to institutions within the patient care network of the academic medical center, regardless of their patient mix, to meet the curricular objectives of the educational program. Thus, training sites may have to be added or eliminated based on patient flow rather than on educational needs (62).

Physical medicine and rehabilitation is presently taught in only 88 of our nation's medical schools, and often it is elective, not a requirement. Thus, many medical students are not exposed to rehabilitation principles and techniques. Physiatry needs to be taught in all medical schools and needs to obtain mandatory as well as elective curriculum time (64). We need to develop a standard curriculum and modify it to match the advances in clinical care. We need to develop national clerkship objectives, as well as a syllabus and a "shelf examination" possibly coordinated by the AAP. If we undertake this, we will need to increase our academic faculty (55).

Generally, the process of choosing a specialty has involved two main areas: analysis of what the specialty has to offer (content, patient problems encountered, intellectual challenge, etc.) and suitability of the specialty for the individual (personality, skills, and abilities). The profile of a physiatrist indicated five factors most important in their career decision. These were sufficient time/flexibility for family obligations; opportunity to make a difference in people's lives; interest in helping people; types of patient problems encountered; and consistency with personality (65).

We need to develop our practice parameters and critical pathways (66). We must demonstrate the cost effectiveness of our specialty and emphasize to the medical students early on the excitement of basic and clinical investigation in our specialty (64).

SUMMARY

Rehabilitation medicine encompasses a special body of knowledge and procedural skills to help patients with acute or chronic disease maximize their level of function and independence. The specialty is relatively young but already has proven its clinical practice value and has the ideal training to produce primary care providers for patients with disabilities. The academic aspects of the specialty need further development, and a core research base with ties to basic science must be established. It is an exciting, growing specialty that emphasizes prevention and treatment. It is not organ based; it can be either hospital or nonhospital based; and it treats all age groups, which allows the practitioner the maximum flexibility to develop a challenging, dynamic practice.

REFERENCES

1. Haas J. Ethical considerations of goal setting for patient care in rehabilitation medicine. *Am J Phys Med Rehabil* 1993; 72:228–232.
2. Halstead LS. Team care in chronic illness: a critical review of literature of past 25 years. *Arch Phys Med Rehabil* 1976; 57:507–511.
3. Gaston EH. Developing a motivating organizational climate for effective team functioning. *Hosp Commun Psychiatry* 1980; 31:407–412.
4. Longest BB. *Management practices for the health professional,* 4th ed. Norwalk, CT: Appleton & Lange, 1990; 100–102.
5. Longest BB. *Health professionals in management.* Stamford, CT: Appleton & Lange, 1996; 166–168.
6. Melvin JL. Interdisciplinary and multidisciplinary activities and the ACRM. *Arch Phys Med Rehabil* 1980; 61:379–380.
7. Rothberg JS. The rehabilitation team: future direction. *Arch Phys Med Rehabil* 1981; 62:407–410.
8. Dyer WG. *Team building: issues and alternatives.* Reading, MA: Addison-Wesley, 1977.
9. Given B, Simmons S. Interdisciplinary health care team: fact or fiction? *Nurs Forum* 1977; 15:165–184.
10. Sharf BF (in consultation with Flaherty JA). *The physician's guide to better communication.* Glenview, IL: Scott, Foresman & Co, 1984; 82–91.
11. Robbins SP. *Organizational behavior: concepts, controversies, and applications,* 4th ed. Englewood Cliffs, NJ: Prentice Hall, 1989; 366–395.
12. Longest BB. *Management practices for the health professional,* 4th ed. Norwalk, CT: Appleton & Lange, 1990; 168–170.
13. Lundberg LB. What is leadership? *J Nurse Admin* 1982; 12:32–33.
14. Jelles F, van Bennekom CAM, Lankhorst GJ. The interdisciplinary team conference in rehabilitation medicine: a commentary. *Am J Phys Med Rehabil* 1995; 74:464–465.
15. Bair J, Gray MS, eds. *The occupational therapy manager.* Rockville, MD: American Occupational Therapy Association, 1985.
16. Longest BB. *Management practices for the health professional,* 4th ed. Norwalk, CT: Appleton & Lange, 1990; 144–155.
17. Longest BB. *Health professionals in management.* Stamford, CT: Appleton & Lange, 1996; 277–305.
18. Longest BB. *Health professionals in management.* Stamford, CT: Appleton & Lange, 1996; 47–49.
19. Wanlass RL, Reutter SL, Kline AE. Communication among rehabilitation staff: "mild," "moderate," or "severe" deficits? *Arch Phys Med Rehabil* 1992; 73:477–481.
20. Stolov EC, Hays RM, Kraft GH. In: Hays RM, Kraft GH, Stolov WC, eds. *Treatment strategies in chronic disease and disability: a contemporary rehabilitation approach to medical practice.* New York: Demos, 1994; 27–31.
21. Stillwell GK. Meeting a need. *Arch Phys Med Rehabil* 1969; 50: 489–494.
22. Krusen FH. *Physical medicine: the employment of physical agents for diagnosis and therapy.* Philadelphia: WB Saunders, 1941; 9–143.
23. Coulter JS. History and development of physical medicine. *Arch Phys Med Rehabil* 1947; 28:600–602.
24. Kovacs R. Progress in physical medicine during the past twenty-five years. *Arch Phys Med Rehabil* 1946; 27:473–477.
25. Krusen FH, Overholser W, Rusk HA, et al. Exhibit on physical medicine: physical therapy, occupational therapy and rehabilitation [committee report]. *Arch Phys Med* 1946; 27:491–498.
26. Mock HE. Rehabilitation. *Arch Phys Med* 1943; 24:676–678 (reprinted *Arch Phys Med Rehabil* 1969; 50:474–475).
27. Strickland BA Jr. Physical medicine in the Army. *Arch Phys Med Rehabil* 1947; 28:229–236.
28. Krusen FH. Historical development in physical medicine and rehabilitation during the last forty years. *Arch Phys Med Rehabil* 1969; 50: 1–5.
29. Nelson PA. History of the archives: a journal of ideas and ideals. *Arch Phys Rehabil* 1969; 50:367–405.
30. Nelson PA. History of the once close relationship between electrotherapeutics and radiology. *Arch Phys Med Rehabil* 1973; 54: 608–640.
31. Hollander AR. The American Congress of Physical Therapy: ten years of progress. *Arch Phys Ther X-ray Rad* 1935; 16:425–528 (reprinted *Arch Phys Med Rehabil* 1969; 50:223–226).
32. Stillwell GK. Whence our academy? *Arch Phys Med Rehabil* 1983; 64:97–100.
33. Koepke GH. The American Board of Physical Medicine and Rehabilitation: past, present and future. *Arch Phys Med Rehabil* 1972; 53: 10–13.
34. Martin GM, Gullickson G Jr, Gerken C. Graduate medical education and certification in physical medicine and rehabilitation. *Arch Phys Med Rehabil* 1980; 61:291–297.
35. American Board of Physcial Medicine and Rehabilitation: the first 50 years. *Arch Phys Med Rehabil Suppl* 1997; 78(suppl 2):1–59.
36. American Board of Physical Medicine and Rehabilitation. Requirements of the American Board of Physical Medicine and Rehabilitation for proposing the establishment of subspecialty certification. *Arch Phys Med Rehabil* 1995; 76:888.
37. American Board of Medical Specialties. *50th Anniversary edition annual report and reference handbook.* Evanston, IL: American Board of Medical Specialties, 1983.
38. Johnson EC. The Association of Academic Physiatrists (personal communication), 1986.
39. Baruch S. *An epitome of hydrotherapy for physicians, architects and nurses.* Philadelphia: WB Saunders, 1920.
40. Krusen FH. And now to carry the torch of Aesculapius [Editorial]. *Arch Phys Med Rehabil* 1969; 50:709–712.
41. Rusk HA. The growth and development of rehabilitation medicine [Editorial]. *Arch Phys Med Rehabil* 1969; 50:463–466.
42. Knapp ME. The contribution of Sister Elizabeth Kenny to the treat-

ment of poliomyelitis. *Arch Phys Med Rehabil* 1969; 50:535–542 (abridged form of 1941 article).
43. Bennett RL. The contribution to physical medicine of our experience with poliomyelitis [Editorial]. *Arch Phys Med Rehabil* 1969; 50: 522–524.
44. Guttmann L. *Spinal cord injuries: comprehensive management and research.* Oxford: Blackwell Scientific Publications, 1973.
45. Guttmann L. Problems of physical therapy for persons with traumatic paraplegia. *Arch Phys Med Rehabil* 1946; 27:750–756.
46. Kottke FJ. Historia obscura hemiplegia. *Arch Phys Med Rehabil* 1974; 55:4–13.
47. DeJong G. Current Status of the Medical Rehabilitation Industry and Prospects for an Outcomes Driven System of Service Delivery and Financing. Presentation: Advances in Accreditation: Focus on Outcomes Sponsored by CARF, July 21, 1996, Tucson, AZ.
48. Hughes EFX. A perspective on the future of american medicine: implications for managed care and its role in the future. In: Hughes EFX, ed. *Health care in the 1990s and beyond—focus on outcomes.* Princeton, NJ: Excerpta Medica, 1991; 1–10.
49. Lewin VHI. *Adapting to a managed care world: the challenge for physical medicine and rehabilitation.* Chicago: American Academy of Physical Medicine and Rehabilitation, 1995; 1–80.
50. Stineman MG, Hamilton BB, Granger CV, Goin JE, Escarce JJ, Williams SV. Four methods for characterizing disability in the formation of function related groups. *Arch Phys Med Rehabil* 1994; 75: 1277–1283.
51. Sutton JP, DeJong G, Wilkerson D. Function-based payment model for inpatient medical rehabilitation: an evaluation. *Arch Phys Med Rehabil* 1996; 77:693–701.
52. Weiner JP. Forecasting the effects of health reform on U.S. physician workforce requirement: evidence from HMO staffing patterns. *JAMA* 1994; 272:222–230.
53. Hogan PF, Dobson A, Haynie B, et al. Physical Medicine and Rehabilitation Workforce Study: the supply of and demand for physiatrists. *Arch Phys Med Rehabil* 1996; 77:95–99.
54. DeLisa JA. Challenges for academic physiatry in the era of health care reform: a commentary. *Am J Phys Med Rehabil* 1995; 74: 159–160.
55. DeLisa JA. Need for academic physiatry in the era of health care reform: a commentary. *Am J Phys Med Rehabil* 1995; 74:234–236.
56. DeLisa JA, Jain SS. Analyzing the national resident match data: are there too many physical medicine and rehabilitation training positions? A commentary. *Am J Phys Med Rehabil* 1996; 75:141–143.
57. DeVivo MJ, Fine PR, Maetz HM, Stover SL. Prevalence of spinal cord injury: a re-estimation of employing life table techniques. *Arch Neurol* 1980; 37:707–708.
58. Burns TJ, Batavia AJ, Smith QW, DeJong G. Primary health care needs of persons with physical disabilities: what are the research and service priorities? *Arch Phys Med Rehabil* 1990; 71:138–143.
59. Brandstater M. Personal correspondence.
60. Gans BM, Mann NR, Becker BE. Delivery of primary care to the physically challenged. *Arch Phys Med Rehabil* 1993; 74(suppl): 515–519.
61. DeLisa JA. Organized specialty medicine with respect to primary care in the severely disabled. *Am J Phys Med Rehabil* 1997; (suppl): S30–S34.
62. DeLisa JA, Jain SS. Managed care and its effect on residency training in physical medicine and rehabilitation: a commentary. *Am J Phys Med Rehabil* 1995; 74:380–382.
63. Maintaining educational quality in the context of health system change: report of the American Medical Association Section on Medical Schools Working Group on Medical Education. December 1994.
64. DeLisa JA. Academic physiatry trends, opportunities and challenges. *Am J Phys Med Rehabil* 1993; 72:113–116.
65. DeLisa JA, Kirshblum S, Jain SS, et al. Practice and career satisfaction among physiatrists: a national survey. *Am J Phys Med Rehabil* 1997; 76:90–101.
66. DeLisa JA, Granger C, LaBan M. Practice parameters for medicine and rehabilitation: a commentary. *Am J Phys Med Rehabil* 1993; 72:398–400.

Rehabilitation Medicine: Principles and Practice, Third Edition,
edited by Joel A. DeLisa and Bruce M. Gans.
Lippincott–Raven Publishers, Philadelphia © 1998.

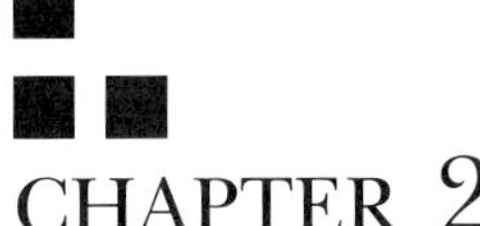

CHAPTER 2

Ethical Issues in Rehabilitation Medicine

Janet F. Haas

A 59-year-old man suffered a left hemispheric cerebrovascular accident. Two weeks later, he was admitted to a rehabilitation unit for treatment of deficits resulting from expressive language impairment and right-sided weakness. He did not agree with the self-care, mobility, and speech goals proposed by the rehabilitation team. Instead, he was anxious to return to his home and work. His wife of 30 years was apprehensive about caring for him at his current level of disability and urged the team to continue therapy.

Patients, family members, and practitioners not uncommonly disagree about the goals, processes, or utility of rehabilitation therapy. Health-care practitioners face difficult dilemmas as they attempt to set a course that all can promote. In this patient's case, they were torn between respecting the patient's desire to be discharged and respecting the concerns and wishes of his wife. They did not want to treat a patient who failed to provide informed consent. On the other hand, the practitioners realized that the patient's wife was not prepared to care for him at home. They knew that training would improve his functional abilities and enhance his eventual return home.

Rehabilitation practitioners confront moral quandaries often during the course of practice. A single moral principle—such as that of autonomy or beneficence—may not outweigh all others, yet choices must be made. Practitioners must attempt to reconcile and assign priority to conflicting moral obligations (1). Decisions of a moral nature are distinguishable from those of the law, technology, religion, and politics. They focus on what is proper rather than on what is possible or legally permissible. Considerations of etiquette, cost, and convenience play an insignificant role in moral decision making.

The terms "moral" and "ethical" are closely related; Cicero apparently used the Latin word *moralis* to translate the Greek *ethikos* (2). Both terms stress manners, customs, and character. Contemporary usage reflects a divergence of meaning, however. "Ethics" refers to theoretical and contemplative descriptions of values. "Morality" describes conduct, that is, whether behaviors are right or wrong.

HISTORICAL DEVELOPMENT

Religious Influences

In the 5th century B.C., Hippocrates described scientific, technological, and ethical facets of medical care (3). The Hippocratic Oath developed from the traditions of a religious sect known as the Pythagoreans. The Oath pertained to a small group of physicians who lived on the Isle of Cos. It required them to vow secrecy and loyalty to their teachers, refuse to give deadly drugs to their patients, and strive to attain virtues of purity and holiness. Physicians were compelled to help patients and forbidden from harming them. They alone were qualified to determine how to benefit sick patients.

Religious traditions influenced the development of medical ethics through the Middle Ages, when monks dominated medical practice, and beyond (4). Since that time, Catholics have integrated principles of medical decision making into their moral theology (3). Protestants have examined specific ethical topics in detail and have incorporated concepts of medical ethics into a larger, systematic theology (3). Orthodox Jews historically have linked Talmudic and rabbinical teachings to the practice of medicine, emphasizing values of preservation and sanctity of life (3).

Secular Influences

During the Enlightenment, the influence of religion on morality in medicine was eclipsed by secular theories of reason and philosophy. Discussion and controversy flourished as scholars studied and debated various viewpoints. A number of works were published and disseminated (3).

J.F. Haas: William Penn Foundation, Philadelphia, Pennsylvania, 19103-2757.

Codes of medical practice developed in time; the first followed an epidemic of typhoid in 1789. Chaos erupted in an English hospital when staff members were required to assume additional, unfamiliar tasks. As tension heightened and some staff members resigned, a retired physician named Thomas Percival sought to restore calm. He designed a code of professional conduct later published in a book entitled *Medical Ethics* (3). The virtues of physicians, "tenderness with steadiness and condescension with authority," were expected to "inspire the minds of their patients with gratitude, respect, and confidence" (5). Percival's very words were included in the first professional code of ethics, published in 1847 by the American Medical Association. Physicians were instructed to address the needs of individual patients rather than those of the larger society (3).

Recent Developments

The nature of medicine has changed dramatically in the past 40 years. Technological advances have established a scientific basis for medical treatment. Many diseases can now be cured. Developments in the biologic sciences and health-care fields have given rise to complex and profound moral dilemmas. The study of ethical problems, a central focus of contemporary medicine, transcends discrete professional boundaries.

Daniel Callahan describes five factors that underlie the development of ethical issues in medicine (6). Technologies such as renal dialysis, organ transplantation, genetic engineering, and embryonal transplantation have expanded our ability to intervene in nature. A strong social commitment to health care coupled with a compelling tendency to apply available technology has made it difficult to restrict technology's use.

Second, medical resources are costly. When medicine could do little to help people, care tended to be cheap. But now that improved neonatal, emergency, and acute care medicine saves many lives, the chronicity and cost of disease have skyrocketed. Americans spent almost 14% of the gross national product on medical care in 1994 (7).

Callahan cites an expanded role of the public as a third factor prompting recognition of ethical issues (6). The solitary and secretive aura of Hippocratic medicine has been supplanted by an environment in which there is more public input. More than 80% of Americans die in hospitals. Taxpayers support medical research and fund health-care entitlement programs. Research on human subjects is regulated by federally mandated Institutional Review Boards. Legal issues are increasingly salient in medicine (8).

The language of rights is another evolving concept. Strong support of individualism in American society and the recognition of rights such as those of racial minorities and women have generated discussion about patients' rights. Medical personnel who respect self-determination and personal dignity acknowledge that patients have a right to make their own decisions (3).

Finally, Callahan cites increasing concern about quality of life. Certainly, many lives are now preserved and extended. We may wonder, however, what kind of life some people will be able to lead (9). At times, the cure clearly is worse than the disease, with its burdens outweighing its benefits (10).

Dramatic change has occurred in the health-care insurance industry as well in recent years. Mechanisms of reimbursement for health care have shifted as systems of managed care, many operating on a for-profit basis, have spread rapidly. Expectations, relationships, and roles of payers, providers, and consumers have been profoundly altered.

What About Rehabilitation?

Until the recent past, little formal attention was directed to the ethical aspects of rehabilitative care. A number of explanations exist (11). As a relatively young field, rehabilitation medicine has concentrated on acquiring recognition and acceptance by the medical community (12). Its chronic care dilemmas may seem to lack the drama of life-and-death decisions. Patients often are treated over an extended period of time by a broad range of professionals, none of whom clearly possess responsibility for addressing ethical issues. Educational and training programs have not always sought to promote student awareness of ethical issues.

As moral problems have been identified in fields of chronic care, however, descriptions of ethical dilemmas inherent to rehabilitative practice also have appeared in the literature (11,13–29). Questions have been raised about duties of professionals, dynamics of professional–patient relationships, roles and expectations of family members, and goals of care. A discussion of fundamental ethical principles furnishes a conceptual framework to study these issues.

Ethical Principles: Beneficence, Autonomy, and Justice

The term "beneficence" connotes kindness, charity, and the doing of good; it refers to a moral obligation to help other people, refrain from harming them, and attempt to balance benefits with harms. In the health-care setting, beneficence entails an obligation to promote the health and well-being of patients and to prevent disease, injury, pain, and suffering (2).

However, the issue of beneficence becomes complicated when patients' values conflict with traditional medical values of healing and care. There can be a difference of opinion among patients, family members, and professionals about what should be considered the best interests of patients or about what constitutes a good quality of life. Balancing many different interests within a moral framework can pose difficulties. Beauchamp and McCullough wrote that "beneficence includes the obligation to balance benefits against harms, benefits against alternative benefits, and harms against alternative harms" (4). It may not be possible to objectify so many conditions, much less to determine whose perspective should serve as the standard.

The principle of autonomy is grounded in the notion of respect for the values and beliefs of other people. Humans are entitled to privacy and to make decisions about their lives. They are seen to possess a right to self-determination that ensures freedom to make personal choices and to resist the intervention of others. The principle of autonomy gives rise to the principle of respect for other people. Within the context of health care, autonomy underlies the medical doctrine of informed consent. There is an obligation to give patients accurate information about their diagnoses and treatment alternatives, as well as to seek their permission before instituting treatment. Decisions are respected, even if they appear to be unwise (2,4).

Many authors describe tension between the principles of beneficence, which requires acting in a patient's best interests, and autonomy, which entails respecting patient choices (2–4,30). Balancing the two principles is a perpetual struggle for health caregivers who deem some patient decisions harmful. When patients refuse to accept information, they may be seen to be acting autonomously or, conversely, they may in fact be shirking autonomy. To Englehardt, "the moral obligation to respect persons will often constrain physicians to acquiesce in patients' choices—choices that most likely will lead to the loss of important goods" (30). In fact, health caregivers may be tempted to act paternalistically to restrict patient freedom to make autonomous choices if these are seen to compromise the patient's best interests.

The principle of justice concerns questions of what is due to whom and how to distribute the burdens and benefits of living in a society. An egalitarian model obliges society to provide all its members with a fair share of health-care resources and to treat people equitably. Scarcity of resources or competition for them can create conflict (2). It may be that people should share social goods equally or that an unequal distribution of goods should benefit those who are favored least.

American society has yet to define the basic medical services required by all people. For example, despite the fact that measles and sexually transmitted diseases are public health hazards, some people receive neither prevention nor treatment efforts. Others, however, can obtain organ transplants or extensive cosmetic surgery. Emergency treatments generally are available, but aftercare and rehabilitation to improve the lives saved often are not funded adequately. Entitlement programs in some states pay for procedures not funded in others. Millions of Americans, many of whom work, do not qualify for publicly funded insurance programs yet cannot afford to buy private health-care insurance. Insurance coverage—which is often provided through employment-related programs—offers differing benefits.

Our emphasis on individual desires and dignity has transcended our concern with society's needs. Daniel Callahan asks what kind of medicine is needed by a good society and what role medicine should play in our mix of education, housing, welfare, and culture (9). If we are to determine how much health care to afford, we must reflect on what we want for the lives we lead within our larger society. Fundamental questions are difficult to frame and to answer; it is not surprising, then, that we have yet to develop and implement a health-care delivery system undergirded by a just social policy.

PATIENT CARE–RELATED REHABILITATION ISSUES

The field of rehabilitation, unlike traditional medicine, does not center around a sick patient whom treatment is expected to cure. Acute care physicians attempt to reverse the course of pathologic processes, relieve symptoms, save lives, and discharge medically stable patients. Rehabilitation practitioners, on the other hand, treat dysfunctions that are chronic, often irreversible, and rarely curable. Residual disability may well persist throughout a person's life.

Medical rehabilitative care addresses impairment caused by pathologic processes that include disease, accident, and congenital abnormality. Disabled persons experience a restricted ability to perform activities in a normal manner. When unable to perform activities important to normal role fulfillment, a person is said to be handicapped (31). Rehabilitation therapy attempts to ameliorate handicap by restoring skills and capabilities through functional retraining and environmental adaptation. Many professionals, including but not limited to physicians, nurses, psychologists, social workers, and educators, as well as physical, speech, occupational, recreational, and vocational therapists, contribute to this effort. They must reach beyond pathologic condition and physiologic function to learn about the unique familial, social, vocational, psychological, and financial characteristics of patients. Otherwise, a set of stairs, an unavailable family member, or limited skin-pressure tolerance may destroy a successful discharge plan.

Relationships integral to rehabilitation are more complicated than those of a more traditional medical dyad, doctor, and patient. An entire community, including family members, concerns itself intimately with each patient's treatment. A triangle with points bearing patient; family, which often includes at least several people; and health-care team, which always includes a number of people, can portray the many relationships involved. People at each point of the triangle share concerns with the others, but have unique considerations as well. Blurred responsibilities and loyalties can cause confusion. Competing rights and obligations of patients, family members, and practitioners can trigger conflict.

Goal Setting Within the Field of Rehabilitation

Goal setting is a central moral issue often disc rehabilitation practitioners. Phrases such as "hi of health," "integration into society," "produc "quality of life" are used to define goals of

(32–36). But such ambiguous and open-ended terms are difficult to apply to patient care. Our society does not instruct us about relating concepts of health and function to cherished personal values such as autonomy and independence. Medical practitioners do not have a special talent for identifying or prescribing notions such as "quality of life."

Balancing Medical and Rehabilitative Needs

Moral quandary may arise as rehabilitation practitioners seek to balance medical and rehabilitative treatments for patients who need both. Providers teach skills to enable patients to adapt to disability and meet environmental demands. They also direct medical resources to maintain and improve the general health of patients. At times, health problems overshadow rehabilitative needs.

The introduction of diagnosis-related groups has encouraged acute care practitioners to transfer patients to rehabilitation settings as soon as possible during recovery from acute disease. Transfer may be sought even before patients are able to participate meaningfully in rehabilitation training. Rehabilitation practitioners may be torn between satisfying the needs of acute care providers for early transfer and initiating treatment at an ideal time for the patient. Sometimes patients who have thrived in a rehabilitation setting may suddenly experience serious medical complications. Although rehabilitation physicians may be qualified to provide appropriate medical care, they may prefer to restrict their interventions to treatments within the purview of their specialized training.

When a patient's ability to participate in treatment is limited, the patient, family members, or even staff personnel may become discouraged. The rehabilitation stay may be prolonged, increasing costs. Yet, even brief transfer to an acute care setting may prove disruptive to patients or relatives. Although rehabilitation practitioners must determine the efficacy of treatments to prescribe, few guidelines exist to specify how to balance medical and rehabilitative needs of patients.

Treatment Practices

Many rehabilitation providers have a strong desire to achieve respect and recognition for the field as a discrete specialty of medicine (37). Distinction has not come readily to a relatively new specialty that lacks the glamour and prestige of other subspecialties (38). Practitioners have sometimes found it difficult to prove their field's worth, perhaps in part because they provide services to disabled people who themselves until recently have had little political appeal.

Empiricism rather than science has undergirded some rehabilitation interventions. Methods to document outcomes of therapy have been developed only relatively recently (39). Prospective epidemiologic studies have been largely unavailable; even retrospective studies of sizable patient populations are few in number. Rehabilitation practitioners must attempt to validate treatments and should inform patients if an intervention is recommended for its theoretical potential rather than demonstrated efficacy. Treatments still to be scientifically validated should be established as part of a research protocol, and informed consent should be sought accordingly.

Reflection on other goals of rehabilitation invites recognition of moral dilemmas. As the field evolves and new technologies become available, rehabilitation practitioners must define criteria to select those to embrace. We must learn to harness sophisticated technologies without allowing technology to become an end in itself. We must decide for whom to provide customized vans, environmental control systems, ramps, respite care, and vocational retraining. We must consider how to respond to the ever-expanding demands of people who want limitless services.

Selection of Patients

Provision of medical care in the United States is based only in part on demonstration of need. More than 40 million Americans lack insurance to reimburse health-care expenses. Many studies have shown that factors such as race and income affect the care given even to patients who are insured by a single plan such as Medicare (40). Persons whose lives have been saved by acute care interventions may not be entitled to reimbursement for rehabilitative care, for supply of rehabilitative care historically has fallen short of demand.

To distribute available resources, rehabilitation practitioners screen potential patients to select those to treat. Practitioners consult with referring and other treating professionals and use information derived from hospital records. Although they may examine patients or interview family members, they generally do not seek input from most team members. They recognize that not all patients will benefit from therapy; some have impairments that cannot be rehabilitated, others are too ill to participate in therapy, and still others have relatively insignificant deficits of functional skills (41).

Medical Factors

Providers consider a variety of medical and nonmedical factors when determining whether to initiate therapy (16). Medical diagnosis and prognosis are paramount. For example, physicians may view people with spinal cord injury, amputation, or stroke as more likely to achieve functional gains than patients with other diagnoses. Secondary diseases, medical complications, and requirements for specialized equipment such as respirators must be manageable in a rehabilitation environment. Impairments in cognitive or sensory capacity must not preclude effective therapy.

Ability to learn and retain information is considered crucial because rehabilitation often requires patients to solve problems by applying new approaches to old skills. Patient age and predicted course of recovery also influence decisions to initiate care. Despite severe dysfunction, patients who are expected to make significant progress are usually viewed as good candidates.

Nonmedical Factors

Practitioners also explore nonmedical parameters. They direct particular attention to whether family members are available geographically and emotionally to support patients because strong social support is known to correlate with positive outcomes (42). Ability to pay is a powerful determinant of access to services, and practitioners may recognize a hierarchy of preferred insurance coverage. They know that comprehensive coverage of services and equipment permits optimal rehabilitation and that gains made during treatment are more likely to be retained in a setting with adequate financial resources.

Features of the rehabilitation unit also influence selection of patients. Some units specialize in treating specific impairments or in addressing priorities of regional or national treatment centers. Those that emphasize training for work require patients to demonstrate vocational potential. Fluctuation in availability of beds or staffing patterns may affect selection; surplus capacity at a given time may prompt admission of patients who would otherwise be rejected (16).

Values

Practitioners are guided in the selection process by values of efficiency, potential to benefit, ability to pay, and the burden that will be placed on staff members who provide patient care. The absence of formal admission criteria that are known to the public gives practitioners significant flexibility to make judgments. Unregulated decision making carries a potential for injustice, however, because bias or subjectivity may influence decisions. Having received little formal training with respect to moral problems, practitioner judgments are likely to reflect personal experience, belief systems, and values that may differ significantly from those of particular patients (16). Practitioners may not recognize the extent to which society's desire to save money while caring for its disabled members may influence their judgments (17).

Practitioners face difficult decisions. Should they treat a patient with great need but a relatively poor prognosis, or one with lesser disability but the promise of a better outcome? Should there be a bias to accept young patients who have a long life span during which to use their training, or those who are older? Should they treat persons who bear responsibility for their disability or who have been noncompliant with past treatment?

Our system of selection seems to favor those already well off. Engelhardt's description of "lotteries" can be applied to rehabilitation. The "natural lottery" describes one's talents and abilities, diseases and illnesses; the "social lottery" refers to social attention, jobs, education, good insurance, and secure finances (43). "Winners" know how to make demands on a complex medical system to help them cope with disease. "Losers" lack sophisticated resources; they may not even know of available services. Already disadvantaged by socioeconomic factors, patients may experience restricted access to rehabilitation for much the same reason. Some may know nothing about procedures for making selection decisions. Lacking an explanation for rejection, they are unable to challenge selection decisions effectively.

Recommendations

An enormous potential for injustice exists in a system that places power in the hands of those who make selection decisions yet fails to provide clear criteria or standards for making those determinations. Although screening is necessary to assure that patients have remediable functional disabilities and are not too sick or unstable to treat, shortcomings of the screening process must be addressed. We should openly describe the process by which candidates are selected for treatment, explain clearly reasons for rejecting patients, and offer to reevaluate patients for future services. A single decision made relatively early in the course of disease should not preclude all future rehabilitative care. A mechanism for patient appeals could provide valuable checks and balances. Broader staff discussions could help practitioners develop more objective selection guidelines that could, in time, be formulated in writing.

Patient–Practitioner Relationships

Relationships between rehabilitation patients and healthcare providers are likely to be of long duration. The nature of the moral rules and principles that determine exchange of information and provision of services bears exploration. Such relationships differ from those of acute care medicine, in which an often solitary provider tries to cure a competent patient (15).

Contractual Model

As patients have been accorded greater rights, a new and more egalitarian relationship has replaced the paternalistic connection between patients and providers (17). This arrangement, known as a contractual model, requires practitioners to tell patients the truth, to present options in an accurate and balanced manner, and to avoid deceiving patients. The duty to act beneficently toward patients is constrained by respect for their autonomy. Physicians supply the medical care that autonomous people making informed decisions desire and permit. Respect for confidentiality and privacy are central to trusting and egalitarian relationships between patients and physicians.

Caplan describes a number of factors that compromise the value of applying the contractual model to rehabilitation (15). The model presumes a relationship between two parties, but in rehabilitation, patients work with many healthcare providers, only some of whom are physicians. Family members often play an integral role in treatment as well. Circumstances under which informed consent should be obtained are not always clear; a general consent for rehabilitation treatment and specific permission for invasive procedures may not be morally sufficient. Perhaps patients should consent to all interventions and should renew their consent periodically over the weeks, months, or even years during which treatment continues.

The competence of patients during the earliest phases of rehabilitative treatment may be questioned (17,22,26,27). People who have experienced sudden, severe impairment need time to adjust to the reality of disability. Many feel anguished by altered function and fear the future. They might not be ready to make decisions for themselves (44). Even those who retain decision-making capacity may know little about disability and how it affects their choices. Similarly, family members may not understand capacities that the patient is likely to have and decisions that will be faced in the future.

Educational Model/Recommendations

Caplan believes that rehabilitation professionals are justified in overriding autonomous wishes of patients who have not yet had sufficient time to adapt to impairment and to appreciate future possibilities (15). He argues that, early in therapy, practitioners are warranted in using persuasion and other means designed to restore patient identity, capacity to cope, and autonomy in the long run. His educational model of rehabilitative care is designed to earn the patient's understanding and cooperation rather than to give orders and is sensitive to the complex and evolving nature of relationships between patients and providers. The model emphasizes instructing patients about disability and encouraging their participation in rehabilitation. It tolerates a greater level of beneficence on the part of providers than is usually accepted in contemporary medicine.

If an educational model for relationships were to be adopted in rehabilitation, periodic assessment of patients' capacities to make autonomous choices would be needed. An independent committee could appraise the evolution of patient autonomy during treatment, for practitioners would need to be mindful that paternalism is appropriate only in a limited sense, and only in the service of restoring autonomous control to patients (17). Patients would be consulted incrementally about the nature of their treatments, and after an opportunity to adjust to the consequences of impairment, they would resume decision making.

Goal-Setting for Individual Patients

Identification of patient needs prior to acceptance for rehabilitation therapy enables goals to be set early in treatment. Many people contribute to this complicated process. Staff members review the history and physical examination and discuss requirements of the postdischarge environment with the patient and family in order to formulate and recommend a plan of treatment. During the course of treatment, goals are periodically reviewed and adjusted to ensure that they are appropriate and realistic.

Several authors have addressed goal-setting during patient care (22,24,25,32,33,36). Trieschman asserts the importance of consulting patients and family members as goals are cast and later refined, and refraining from imposing goals on patients who may reject them in the long run anyway. She cautions caregivers against assuming that skills mastered in the rehabilitation setting will transfer readily to a home environment (45). Becker emphasizes the benefits of sharing individualized written goals with all persons concerned with patient care in order to identify discrepancies in goals and enhance family and staff interaction (32).

Problems of Current Practice

Although rehabilitation practitioners encourage most patients from the moment of treatment to assume an active role in designing their program, patients may have difficulty setting goals. They may feel vulnerable from pain, weakness, fatigue, depression, or anxiety (46). They may not have come to terms with new or exacerbated disability. They may know little about what they will achieve from rehabilitation and may find the rehabilitation unit an unfamiliar and unsettling environment. Behaviors that seemed desirable on the acute care ward—cooperation, passivity, acceptance of frightening or painful interventions—no longer apply. Instead, patients are encouraged to socialize with strangers who may have visible, often distressing bodily scars and dysfunctions. Deprived of most daytime visitors, feeling stranded, insecure, and scared, patients are nonetheless expected to assume responsibility for their actions and decisions and to participate in treatment. Even those who are familiar with disability may experience difficulty clarifying goals during the course of rehabilitation. Many lack knowledge about the demands of their new situation because they have yet to return home to live as disabled people but are instead isolated from the real life experiences that could illuminate their postdischarge needs (25).

Whose Goals?

Goal-setting is complicated. People may not agree about the needs to be met or how to satisfy them and may interpret data about probabilities and outcomes differently. Approaches to information about risks and benefits, pain, cost, health, and disability are strongly influenced by personal values. Patients, family members, health-care teams, and insurers may encounter conflict as they select discrepant or even mutually exclusive goals. Patients may want to make independent decisions, knowing well how exhausted or disheartened they feel and what is meaningful to them. Relatives may believe that their caretaking role should lend their opinions priority. Practitioners who respect professional experience with disability more than the ideas of inexperienced laymen may be tempted to usurp decision-making power rather than to allow patients and families to waste time, money, or effort for an unnecessarily poor outcome.

Recommendations

The principle of autonomy holds self-determination as a fundamental right regardless of whether patients make ill-advised choices. We know that people often lose autonomy just by becoming patients who know less about medicine than do their caregivers. But technical expertise does not imply moral authority; professionals should refrain from imposing their values on patients who know best what is possible for themselves. So often, when finally free to do as they wish, patients discard splints, ignore home exercise programs, or allow themselves to be dressed by caretakers. They refuse tasks that require too much time, patience, or concentration to be satisfying and discard equipment that is ugly, cumbersome, or difficult to repair. Available finances, transportation, or social networks may be insufficient to the support progress they made in the rehabilitation setting (25).

The process of setting goals may unveil tension in patient–provider relationships (25–27). Practitioners should be cognizant of their power in relationships with patients who have experienced a profound, often sudden loss of physical abilities. Persistent beneficence, however well-meaning, may compromise the patient's best interests. Patients should be educated about costs, risks, and effectiveness of treatment alternatives, as well as the medical and functional ramifications of their decisions. Their preferences should be respected unless they are incompetent in relevant aspects of decision making. Time and experience will accustom them to disability and to their evolving capacities and needs.

Professional and Team Issues

Rehabilitation treatment is often delivered by a multidisciplinary group of professionals who work as a team to address patients' functional deficits and psychosocial and vocational needs. Professionals believe that teams provide a coordinated, comprehensive approach not offered by individual caregivers working independently. Teams can render services efficiently as a result of experience, economies of scale, and organization of functions (19,22).

Moral Problems of Teams

Patients and family members may be unaccustomed to health-care teams, however. The locus of authority is often unclear. Patients or family members may tell ''secrets'' to one provider who is instructed not to tell other team members. If such information is important to the patient's rehabilitation, practitioners may be conflicted about whether to honor confidentiality or to act in the patient's apparent best interests. Team members may gather discrepant information from patients and relatives that may be difficult to reconcile without alienating some family members.

Members of a rehabilitation team should recognize the vulnerability of patients to subtle pressure. Exhausted, frightened, or confused patients may be intimidated by experienced professionals who mean well. Purtilo suggests that patients who feel outnumbered by the team may feel compelled to follow recommendations with which they do not agree (19).

Conflicts and Loyalties

Practitioners serve as teachers or guides who enhance individual patient function and assist adjustment to disability. Team members must address the needs of many patients at once in an efficient and cost-effective manner. Activities of patients, including smoking, eating, dressing, following a schedule, and watching television, are often governed by institutional policies. When policies clash with the desires of particular patients, the team must balance the interests of individuals with those of the collective (17).

Controversy about authority and responsibility can arise among team members who recommend discrepant goals for patients or who disagree about how to set priorities among goals. Team members may work with patients in dissimilar or conflicting ways. They may disagree about the arrangement of patients' schedules or about the amount of time patients should spend with each professional. Dissension may be difficult to resolve within a team that functions in an egalitarian manner. Team members who share long and difficult hours of work often develop a sense of loyalty to one another that may deter one team member from questioning another's competency.

Recommendations

Purtilo suggests that a ''common moral language'' is needed to frame ethical decisions and that teams would benefit from exercises to clarify values (19). Teams need administrative mechanisms to identify and resolve conflicts in a timely manner (17). All members must be accountable to the entire team for their actions and must be willing to raise questions about professional behaviors that appear to compromise patient interests. Team members must treat all patients respectfully, particularly those who are noncompliant or difficult to manage. Recognizing that the team itself may inadvertently intimidate patients, its members must strive to listen carefully to patients' wishes at all times.

Professionals should explain to patients and their relatives the shared responsibility and authority of team function (17). They should clarify lines of communication to alleviate patient concerns and anxieties. Practitioners should protect patient privacy and confidentiality, but must emphasize to patients and relatives the need to share information among those concerned with a patient's care. Patients should be informed if confidential information must be divulged and should understand clearly the nature and degree of family involvement in decision making. Conflicts must be resolved promptly to assure effectiveness of patient care.

Termination of Treatment

Many factors contribute to decisions to terminate treatment in the rehabilitation setting (17). Patients are expected to make steady and measurable progress toward attaining their goals. When progress slows significantly or patients appear to have reached a plateau in degree of improvement, members of the treatment team may doubt whether continued therapy is worthwhile. Questions about the efficacy of treatment are typically raised first by professionals who often do not consult patients and relatives who may wish to continue working toward goals that professionals deem insignificant or unrealistic.

Whose Values?

The moral values of team members may greatly influence their decisions. Practitioners must assess rather nebulous concepts such as "benefit" and "functional improvement" as they delineate meaningful and reasonable end-points of treatment. Their subjective judgments about the ability of patients to cope with impairments outside the rehabilitation setting affect their appraisals. Their values concerning acceptable levels of function do likewise, regardless of whether these values differ from those of patients (17).

The progress of some patients undergoing rehabilitation may be examined sooner than that of others. Certain patients—those who may be labeled noncompliant, uncooperative, or poorly motivated—may be so difficult to manage that the team discusses discharge relatively early in the course of treatment. Others have very limited insurance coverage. Pressure to use scarce resources for new patients may prompt caregivers to cease care for longer term patients. A patient's home setting and anticipated level of assistance affect the timing of the decision to curtail care as well.

Recommendations

Caregivers must be morally sensitive and wise to allocate care among patients. Sometimes rehabilitation teams fail to explain the criteria used in decisions to end treatment. For example, nonprofessionals may not fully appreciate the significance of financial restrictions or understand the methods that practitioners use to monitor whether progress is sufficient to allow continued care. Surely patients and their relatives have a right to know the parameters by which patient progress will be measured and the standards that determine whether treatment is continued. Rehabilitation practitioners have a duty to document information about patient progress so that data underlie the decision to stop care. Patients and relatives should be informed about team discussions concerning termination of care. Their opinions should be sought and honored to the extent possible (17).

Duties and Rights of Family Members

Family members often play an extremely important role in the care of disabled people. The presence of interested and committed family may determine whether a patient is admitted for rehabilitation. During treatment, family members meet with the team to discuss goal-setting and postdischarge arrangements.

Obligations

There is an expectation on the part of society that family members will assist one another when needs arise. Family or familylike relationships are considered unique in extensiveness and interdependence (17). Family members often undertake special caretaking duties with the understanding that they can provide emotional support and affection as well as the physical care that patients require (14).

The need for family caretaking has increased (47). Rehabilitation professionals find that early discharge enhances patient autonomy and enables patients to experience a real-life setting to test their skills and the feasibility of their goals. Outpatient or home settings are less expensive than inpatient facilities and are preferred by many patients. Thus, some rehabilitative care has shifted to home settings.

Callahan has noted that many families discover that providing care to their disabled members is mutually satisfying and rewarding (14). Caretakers develop skills and resources that enable them to adapt effectively to new demands. They may take pride in their ability to identify patient needs and to give care in a kind and sensitive way. They may be exceptionally responsive to the patient's situation and offer the care most compatible with it.

Other families experience difficulties, however. Unresolved problems between patients and caregivers may interfere with a satisfactory relationship. The demands of caring for a disabled person may exceed the capacities of family members. Strain may result from limited financial resources or inadequate physical facilities. Family members may feel angry, sad, or depressed about the patient's condition. They may feel ill equipped to deal with a disabled person who has an uncertain prognosis or who faces years of severe disability. Plunged into an unexpected and unchosen situation, they may find their own happiness and welfare threatened.

Limits of Duty

There is no simple formula to determine how much family members ought to give to patients or what the limits of duty may be. Some people may gladly dedicate the remainder of their days to care for a patient; others may view this as unjustified self-sacrifice (14). Commitments are complicated by the fact that families are smaller and more dispersed now than in the past; several people may not be able to share caregiving tasks. Women may feel a special responsibility to act as caretakers, but many work outside the home and are unavailable to perform traditional caretaking roles. Some families are not in a position to provide adequate care despite wishing to do so, whereas others have inadequate financial or emotional resources.

Health-care providers have insufficient knowledge of the lives and relationships of patients and family members to know how to advise them. It may be difficult to identify the nature of trust and intimacy within specific relationships in a family. Practitioners realize that although patients' needs and vulnerabilities may best be addressed by family caregivers who can provide a nurturing and regenerative environment, family members may be unwilling to relinquish plans, hopes, or dreams of their own (14).

Recommendation

Practitioners may not know to what extent to use persuasion as they attempt to convince potential caregivers to commit themselves to patients. When patient needs are minor and family members are expected to sacrifice little, consideration of the patient's best interests may well permit encouraging relatives to fulfill obligations. When disability is severe and great sacrifice will be required, however, strong persuasion does not appear justified. Callahan points out that our society neither rewards nor honors people who transcend their own needs to care for others; such people are more likely to meet with social isolation than with commendation. They are not treated as heroes and should not be expected to act as such (14).

As a society, we have yet to develop mechanisms to reimburse the financial and psychological services that could serve to minimize the burden on caregivers. We need to furnish family members with the tools that would help to sustain them, for example, day care centers, respite care, counseling and self-help groups, and adequate physical facilities (47). Only then can society expect any but the most extraordinary people to embrace an opportunity to care for a seriously disabled relative.

POLICY ISSUES

Allocation of Resources

The number of patients who can benefit from rehabilitation grows steadily. Babies who would have died from complications of prematurity or congenital abnormality only a few years ago now survive, often with significant residual disability. Many injured and sick people recover from life-threatening conditions. Americans live considerably longer than did previous generations; by the year 2040, 23% of the population is expected to be older than 65 years (48). Not surprisingly, chronic disease is increasingly prevalent. Disability affects over 30 million Americans, 75% of whom cannot function normally either at work, school, or in the home. At some point many of these people require rehabilitation services to enhance their functional skills (49).

Costs of Health Care

The costs of all medical care, including rehabilitation, are increasing well above the level of inflation (48). During the period from 1970 to 1994, annual costs increased an average of 11.3% (7). This was an average annual rate of 3% in real terms (50). Between 1989 and 1990, the cost of health-care premiums increased by more than 17% (51). Even average Americans have become worried that they could be excluded from necessary health-care services due to inability to pay (52).

Extrapolation of trends in the early 1990s indicated that health-care costs would reach 20% of our gross domestic product by the end of the twentieth century (53). Medicare is predicted to become bankrupt in 2001 (54). Fee-for-service reimbursement plans and the practice of defensive medicine act as incentives for physicians to render more services (48). Our preoccupation with expensive technology and our generous use of hospital-based services increase costs dramatically. Our desire for perfect health and our willingness to provide medical care for patients who will experience marginal benefit do likewise.

People who in the past would have died of spinal cord or head injury may receive care worth several hundred thousand dollars. Additional costs result from lost wages and needed income and social supports. Increasing numbers of patients and the higher costs associated with treating them augment the demand for rehabilitation resources. Tighter economic times have forced Americans to choose only certain services to fund.

Limited Access

Our unwillingness to afford health care to all who want it has created a system that curtails access to health care. Many poor urban and rural people receive little medical care. Categorical restrictions and income eligibility ceilings in the Medicaid program exclude many working people whose income is below the poverty level (55). Innovations such as diagnosis-related groups, health maintenance organizations, and preferred provider organizations have reduced health care available to underinsured people by precluding practices used in the past to shift costs to insured patients (48). Geographic maldistribution of health-care resources also restricts access to care because insufficient numbers of physicians practice in inner city and rural areas. People who lack medical services are known to have worse health than those who receive services, even if factors such as increased stress and poor hygiene are controlled (56).

Churchill claims that we do ration health care according to ability to pay, although we find the idea morally repugnant

(48). Physicians who determine access to care have little public accountability regarding whom they treat. Care, even if desperately needed, is given sporadically at best to those without financial resources. Many forego basic services such as eyeglasses, hearing aids, and routine dental care. Interest groups compete with one another at the federal and state levels to capture and retain limited amounts of funding.

We have come to emphasize interventions designed to extend life, but not always to enhance its quality. The heroes and personal dramas of rescue medicine prevail over the more mundane preventive medicine. Our fragmented system of private health insurance and publicly funded entitlement programs fails many. We lack a coherent and comprehensive approach that would enable us to address the needs of people of various ages, income levels, and types and degrees of illness. We do not know how to place the needs of one person within a context of others, nor how to weigh priorities when making allocation decisions (9).

Principle of Justice

A system of medical care should be considered morally acceptable only if it encompasses principles of equity and justice. Allotting health care to favor those who are insured, wealthy, and white cannot stand in a just society; rationing is not simply unfortunate, it is unfair. Life within a community incurs social obligations to care for those who are sick. We can respect a community that offers mutual and reciprocal assistance to its members. After all, no one is immune to disease or calamity that can strike at any time. Misfortune can in fact serve to link us to one another (48).

But what services will be offered in a society that cannot afford everything? Principles of utility emphasize the desirability of services that provide the greatest good for the greatest number of people (2). Principles of justice imply that services should be based on need. People define "need" differently, however, and genuine needs may be difficult to distinguish from hopes and preferences (9).

When health care is apportioned, as it must be in an era of limited resources, we should avoid discriminating among individuals. Limits should be established by applying generic guidelines to people with common conditions. Private, personal appeals for specialized services should not be encouraged (48). Quality, not simply length of life, should be stressed. Americans should be assured universal access to basic and primary care services. Access to additional care should depend on its effectiveness and the efficiency with which it can be provided. Costly care of marginal benefit should be discouraged.

It is not easy to define health needs or characteristics such as "quality," "efficiency," and "benefit" (57). Specialties such as rehabilitation will be called on to demonstrate how their treatments promote health, prevent illness and deterioration, and contribute to useful functioning. Services that are demonstrated to be important and effective are most likely to be considered worthy of continued funding.

Managed Care

Despite enjoying the most advanced medical technology in the world, Americans worry that this care may one day be beyond their economic reach. In 1993, cognizant of concern about health-care security, President Clinton assembled a task force to draft a health reform act that would guarantee universal, affordable health care (58). Although legislation failed, the intense focus on the health-care industry catalyzed widespread changes within it.

Managed care played a limited role in health care until the past several years, during which time it has expanded dramatically. It is based on the concept of utilitarianism and predicated on an assumption that payers are more qualified to oversee treatment than are either users or providers. Managed care seeks to enhance access to comprehensive, coordinated care delivered in a cost-effective manner. It has markedly altered medical practice and has affected relationships among payers, providers and patients. It has led to major discordances in the care that patients desire and providers wish to give, and that which payers are willing to reimburse (29). In particular, many managed care plans do not cover significant rehabilitation services.

Administrators of managed care plans have not yet focused on measuring quality of outcome after treatment. Rather, plans compete for customers on the basis of price and results of plan-administered general surveys of consumer satisfaction. Information about quality of care has not been accessible to consumers; it is still an open question whether the health status of enrollees has improved (59).

The many and varied needs of a particularly vulnerable population of patients may be difficult to meet within the resource constraints of managed care organizations. Ethical questions at the confluence of managed care and rehabilitation of severely disabled individuals concern use of research and outcome information, roles and responsibilities of practitioners, respect for individualism, patient privacy and informed consent, and the moral character of a responsible rehabilitation institution (28).

In the past, professionals were expected to provide services, but today they must also delineate probable outcomes of therapy before delivering the services intended to accomplish treatment goals. It is necessary not only to align expectations of patients, families, providers, and payers in regard to outcome, but for payers and providers to negotiate about finances required to implement treatment programs. Knowledge about likely patient outcomes plays an essential role in the struggle to balance ethically appropriate services with fiscally responsible expenditures (60).

Professionals who act as "gatekeepers" to managed care services experience tension between containing medical costs by efficient delivery of services and advocating for additional resources to benefit individual patients. Caplan argues that gatekeeping at the bedside is not an ethical solution to the problem of limited resources but serves to undermine patient ability to trust caregivers. Coverage decisions should rest instead on broad guidelines determined publicly with input from providers, patients, and families (61). National standards are needed to delineate minimal services that must be offered by treatment plans. Appeals processes for patients who find their treatment alternatives unreasonably limited are also important (62).

Managed care has had a significant impact on the integrity of the practice of informed consent. Gag rules may prohibit physicians from describing to patients those services that could be of benefit as well as financial incentives and conflicts of interest that pertain to professionals practicing within the plan. Patients must receive and understand all relevant information to make truly informed decisions (62). The bias to limit treatment inherent to capitated managed care systems may be particularly relevant to rehabilitation, a field whose importance may be unrecognized. It may be tempting to shortchange treatment that appears arduous despite having a potential for benefit.

Moral values that underscore respect for individual rights and freedoms have had a powerful influence on contemporary health care. Values that foster individualism discourage mutual obligations to one another, including to disabled persons who may not be deemed capable of contributing fully to society. Managed care plans compromise quality or duration of treatment for chronic impairment. Yet a just health-care system should seek to remedy the characteristics of disease and disability that lead to social disadvantage (63).

Similarly, "good" rehabilitation institutions function for the benefit of individual patients, especially those who are most vulnerable, as well as for the broader community. Utilitarianism, a principle that compares units of money to units of healing, may fail as a dominant form of moral reasoning in the context of already marginalized patients. A virtuous institution conveys morally sound values as it assures skilled care of patients and families within a fiscally responsible environment (64).

Professional Responsibilities

Research

Professionals in rehabilitation claim that treatment helps patients improve their lives as well as their skills (65). Therapy is thought to diminish the burden of disability on patients and their relatives. Although outcome research has substantiated some claims, many rehabilitation practitioners emphasize the need for further research to enable more practices to be founded on demonstrated facts and knowledge (12).

Rehabilitation practitioners continually seek to increase the prominence of their field in the eyes of those who fund scientific studies. There is more money available now for scientific evaluation of rehabilitation processes than at any time in the past (17). However, Fuhrer cited three factors that inhibit public support of rehabilitation research (66):

1. Insufficient appreciation of the potential of disabled people for self-sufficiency and economic productivity
2. Skepticism on the part of those who fund research about studies directed to palliative efforts rather than to cures for underlying impairments
3. A belief that research will produce technology that is excessively sophisticated and expensive

Fuhrer advises practitioners to seek to increase federal funding of research by creating greater awareness of past research successes and demonstrating the monetary benefit of treating disabled people. To justify claims for additional resources, rehabilitation practitioners must prove the efficacy of treatments and new processes (67). De Lateur suggests that controlled clinical trials and outcome-oriented research will be required to allow a stronger case to be made in the effort to secure additional public funding for medical rehabilitation (12).

Professional Standards

Rehabilitation professionals have a duty to maintain professional standards of competence in their field. Codes of ethics of many of the specialists who participate in treatment fail to address issues that arise when professionals interface with one another (17). Practitioners must develop systems that enable them to question the conduct of co-workers or colleagues in other institutions when necessary. They must decide whether to function in roles that may be required by the team, but that have not been part of their professional training and experience.

Public Policy

Prevention Efforts

Some rehabilitation patients became disabled as a result of accident or choices of life-style. In many situations, altered behavior patterns would have avoided disability altogether. Alcohol use leads to accidents of all kinds. Excessive speed commonly precedes traffic accidents. Road injuries are more serious when seat belts or car seats are not used. Absence of helmets worsens head injuries of motorcyclists and bicyclists. Firearms produce severe and disabling accidental injuries.

The knowledge that so many of their patients have sustained preventable disability should mobilize rehabilitation practitioners to advocate measures such as gun control, stiff penalties against drunk driving, and moderate speed limits. Regardless of their own choices of life-style, it would seem that practitioners have an obligation to influence public policies in order to prevent needless disability; no one can portray more vividly the devastating ramifications of impairments such as spinal cord injury or severe brain injury. Practitioners must work to ensure that legislation such as the 1990 Americans with Disabilities Act is enforced properly.

Human Immunodeficiency Virus Infection

For patients who have human immunodeficiency virus infection or acquired immunodeficiency syndrome and are approaching death, rehabilitative treatment will be too strenuous or of insignificant benefit. But many patients can live for years after diagnosis. Some will be able to benefit significantly from treatment and so are referred for rehabilitation services to address and remediate aspects of daily life at home and work (23).

Principles of justice require practitioners to serve all patients. Persons who entered the medical profession did so of their own accord with the knowledge that exposure to contagious disease is an inherent condition of practice. Professionals thus have a duty to treat patients when there is a limited risk of incurring infection themselves (68). Although high risk of infection would not require them to act heroically, this is unlikely to pertain in a rehabilitation setting. Universal precautions should be used when working with patients.

Pedagogic Issues

Training Programs

In recent years, a number of institutions and professional societies have made significant efforts to include topics of ethics in their educational programs. Concerted efforts have yet to be made in the field of rehabilitation. Very few professional training programs in rehabilitation medicine, nursing, allied health, or social work offer courses in this area. Faculty members have not been encouraged to make ethics a focus of their teaching and research. Relatively few published articles and case materials apply specifically to rehabilitation (17).

If rehabilitation ethics is to be considered important to the education of students, faculty members will have to be supplied the resources and time needed to become familiar with and to teach about ethics. Effective teaching requires competent and committed professionals. As the number of knowledgeable instructors increases, rehabilitation practitioners may wish to add formal certification requirements in ethics for schools and specialty training programs. Some professions (e.g., nursing) and specialties (e.g., family practice, internal medicine) have introduced an ethics requirement into their certification process. Rehabilitation accrediting agencies also could emphasize formal teaching of ethics (17).

Continuing Education

Continuing education in rehabilitation may emphasize study of ethics as well. Some institutions have initiated "ethics grand rounds" for discussing topics in ethics. Some rehabilitation hospitals have developed ethics committees similar to those in many acute care hospitals to explore educational issues and sponsor workshops. Rehabilitation professionals should work closely with these committees to draw attention to ethical problems.

Journal editors could encourage more scholarly writing about policy aspects of rehabilitation and more examination of clinical case studies. Organizers of ethics conferences could solicit symposia and panel discussions of rehabilitation topics. Rehabilitation professionals should work closely with community groups and organizations to enhance discussion about ethical aspects of care. Advocacy groups, institutional trustees, staff, patients, and family members should be educated about the ethical challenges that confront us now, and those that patients and providers will soon encounter in rehabilitation medicine (17).

CONCLUSION

Rehabilitation practitioners will face important moral challenges in the coming years. Certainly, they must strive to ensure excellent patient care undergirded by scientific study, but they also must examine whether patients are treated with compassion and respect in an era dominated by financial competition and technological development. Close attention should be directed to the personal qualities, manners, sensibilities, and everyday practice procedures of practitioners. Whether they tolerate differences and how they listen to and speak with people are more important than ever in view of the complicated, intimidating, and expensive nature of today's treatments. The provision of reassurance and comfort should be emphasized as institutional policies are crafted.

Health-care practitioners also have a duty to recognize and address problems and inequities of our current medical system. Our competitive, free-market structure has prompted development of joint venture investments, for-profit facilities, and commercial insurance. In recent years, increasing numbers of doctors have invested in laboratories, imaging centers, and physical therapy clinics. Charges in these "joint venture" centers exceed those of similar facilities not owned by doctors. A study of doctor-owned physical therapy facilities in Florida reported that they provide a lower quality of care and employ fewer licensed therapists, each of whom is allotted less time with each patient, than is true of facilities not owned by doctors. Scheduling of extra patient visits allows more revenue to be derived from each patient. Access to care for poor people or those who live in rural areas is limited (69).

For-profit facilities, including some rehabilitation facilities, have a negligible commitment to medically indigent people, who are considered highly unprofitable. Many insurers preferentially select persons with good health records to insure. Often others who are expected to require costly treatment—including some who develop chronic disease—are turned away. Some persons have had their policies canceled by commercial insurers.

As rehabilitation practitioners examine the quality and availability of medical resources, they must respond to society's failure to provide millions of Americans with basic medical resources. They should identify conflicts of interest in their practices and set high and exacting standards for professional conduct. Practitioners have a responsibility to ponder the role of medical rehabilitation in an era of limited resources. Conscious of the fact that some medical needs will remain unmet in a society that has other important needs, they must identify and limit care of marginal benefit or excessive cost. They must inform and educate Americans about important medical needs and help society in its attempt to balance needs of individuals with those of the larger society.

REFERENCES

1. Ross WD. *The right and the good.* Oxford: Oxford University Press, 1930.
2. Beauchamp TL, Childress JF. *Principles of biomedical ethics.* New York: Oxford University Press, 1989.
3. Veatch RM. *A theory of medical ethics.* New York: Basic Books, 1981.
4. Beauchamp TL, Mcullough LB. *Medical ethics: the moral responsibilities of physicians.* Englewood Cliffs, NJ: Prentice Hall, 1984.
5. Percival T. *Percival's medical ethics.* [Originally published 1803.] Reprint, Leake CD, ed. Baltimore: Williams & Wilkins, 1927.
6. Callahan D. Personal communication.
7. Pear R. Health care costs are growing more slowly, report says. *New York Times,* p. 13, May 28, 1996.
8. Editors. Legal issues in medicine—a new series. *N Engl J Med* 1991; 325:354–355.
9. Callahan D. *What kind of life: the limits of medical progress.* New York: Simon & Schuster, 1990.
10. Dutton DB. *Worse than the disease: pitfalls of medical progress.* Cambridge: Cambridge University Press, 1988.
11. Haas JF. Ethics in rehabilitation medicine. *Arch Phys Med Rehabil* 1986; 67:270–271.
12. De Lateur BJ. Fostering research in the physiatrist's future. *Arch Phys Med Rehabil* 1990; 71:1–2.
13. Brody BA. Justice in allocation of public resources to disabled citizens. *Arch Phys Med Rehabil* 1988; 69:333–336.
14. Callahan D. Families as care givers: the limits of morality. *Arch Phys Med Rehabil* 1988; 69:323–328.
15. Caplan AL. Informed consent and provider-patient relationships in rehabilitation medicine. *Arch Phys Med Rehabil* 1988; 69:312–317.
16. Haas JF. Admission to rehabilitation centers: selection of patients. *Arch Phys Med Rehabil* 1988; 69:329–332.
17. Caplan AL, Callahan D, Haas J. Ethical and policy issues in rehabilitation medicine. *Hastings Cent Rep* 1987; 17(special suppl):1–20.
18. Jennings B, Callahan D, Caplan AL. Ethical challenges of chronic illness. *Hastings Cent Rep* 1988; 18(special suppl):1–16.
19. Purtilo RB. Ethical issues in teamwork: the context of rehabilitation. *Arch Phys Med Rehabil* 1988; 69:318–322.
20. Haas JF, MacKenzie CA. The role of ethics in rehabilitation medicine. *Am J Phys Med Rehabil* 1993; 72:48–51.
21. Callahan D. Allocating health care resources: the vexing case of rehabilitation. *Am J Phys Med Rehabil* 1993; 72:101–105.
22. Meier RH III, Purtilo RB. Ethical issues and the patient-provider relationship. *Am J Phys Med Rehabil* 1994; 72:365–366.
23. Strax TE. Ethical issues of treating patients with AIDS in a rehabilitation setting. *Am J Phys Med Rehabil* 1994; 73:293–295.
24. Purtilo RB, Meier RH III. Team challenges: regulatory constraints and patient empowerment. *Am J Phys Med Rehabil* 1993; 72:327–330.
25. Haas J. Ethical considerations of goal setting for patient care in rehabilitation medicine. *Am J Phys Med Rehabil* 1993; 72:228–232.
26. Venesy BA. A clinician's guide to decisionmaking capacity and ethically sound medical decisions. *Am J Phys Med Rehabil* 1994; 73: 219–226.
27. Jennings B. Healing the self: the moral meaning of relationships in rehabilitation. *Am J Phys Med Rehabil* 1993; 72:401–404.
28. Haas JF. Ethical issues in physical medicine and rehabilitation: conclusion to a series. *Am J Phys Med Rehabil* 1995; 74(suppl):54–58.
29. Haas JF, Mattson Prince J. Ethics and managed care in rehabilitation medicine. *J Head Trauma Rehabil* 1997; 12:vii–xiii.
30. Englehardt HT Jr. *The foundations of medical ethics.* New York: Oxford University Press, 1986.
31. Acton N. The world's response to disability: evolution of a philosophy. *Arch Phys Med Rehabil* 1982; 63:145–149.
32. Becker MC, Abrams KS, Onder J. Goal setting: joint patient-staff method. *Arch Phys Med Rehabil* 1974; 55:87–89.
33. Kottke FJ. Future focus of rehabilitation medicine. *Arch Phys Med Rehabil* 1980; 61:1–6.
34. Rusk HA. Rehabilitation medicine: knowledge in search of understanding. *Arch Phys Med Rehabil* 1978; 59:156–160.
35. Spencer WA. A new use for the rehabilitation process—introspection. *Arch Phys Med Rehabil* 1970; 51:187–197.
36. Wallace SG, Anderson AD. Imprisonment of patients in the course of rehabilitation. *Arch Phys Med Rehabil* 1978; 59:424–429.
37. Spencer WA. Changes in methods and relationships necessary within rehabilitation. *Arch Phys Med Rehabil* 1969; 50:566–580.
38. Gritzer G, Arluke A. *The making of rehabilitation.* Berkeley: University of California Press, 1985.
39. Granger CV, Hamilton BB, Forer S. Development of a uniform national data system for medical rehabilitation. *Arch Phys Med Rehabil* 1985; 66:538.
40. Gornick M, Eggers P, et al. Effects of race on mortality and use of services among medicare beneficiaries. *N Engl J Med* 1996; 335: 791–799.
41. Kottke FJ, Lehman JF, Stillwell GK. Preface. In: Kottke FJ, Stillwell GK, Lehman JF, eds. *Krusen's handbook of physical medicine and rehabilitation.* 3rd ed. Philadelphia: WB Saunders, 1982; xi–xix.
42. De Vellis RF, Sauter SVH. Recognizing the challenges of prevention in rehabilitation. *Arch Phys Med Rehabil* 1985; 66:52–54.
43. Englehardt HT Jr, Rie MA. Intensive care units, scarce resources, and conflicting principles of justice. *JAMA* 1986; 255:1159–1164.
44. Kerson TA, Kerson LA. *Understanding chronic illness.* New York: Free Press, 1985.
45. Trieschmann RB. Coping with a disability: a sliding scale of goals. *Arch Phys Med Rehabil* 1974; 55:556–560.
46. Anderson TP. Educational frame of reference: an additional model for rehabilitation medicine. *Arch Phys Med Rehabil* 1978; 59:203–206.
47. Lubin IM. *Chronic illness: impact and interventions.* Boston: Jones & Bartlett, 1990; 200–217.
48. Churchill LR. *Rationing health care in America: perceptions and principles of justice.* Notre Dame, IN: University of Notre Dame Press, 1987.
49. Evans RW. Health care technology and the inevitability of resource allocation and rationing decisions. *JAMA* 1983; 249:2047–2053.
50. Fuchs VR. The health sector's share of the GNP. *Science* 1990; 247: 534–538.
51. Freudenheim M. Health care: a growing burden. *New York Times,* p. D1, January 29, 1991.
52. Wine M, Pear R. President finds he has gained even if he lost on health care. *New York Times,* p. 1, July 30, 1996.
53. Hasan M. Let's end the nonprofit charade. *N Engl J Med* 1996; 334: 1055–1057.
54. Zaldivar RA. Crisis is near for Medicare, trustees say. *Philadelphia Inquirer,* p. 1, June 6, 1996.
55. Davis K, Rowland D. Uninsured and underserved: inequities in health care in the US. *Milbank Mem Fund Q* 1983;61:149–152.
56. Bayer R, Caplan A, Daniels N, eds. *In search of equity: health needs and the health care system.* New York: Plenum, 1983.
57. Blumenthal D. Quality of care-what is it? *N Engl J Med* 1996; 335: 891–893.
58. Haas JF. Recent changes in health care insurance. *J Head Trauma Rehabil* 1997; 12:1–9.
59. Prince JM, Haas JF. A vision for the future: an interview with Gerben DeJong, Ph.D. *J Head Trauma Rehabil* 1997; 12:71–86.
60. Schmidt N. Outcome-oriented rehabilitation: response to managed care. *J Head Trauma Rehabil* 1997; 12:44–50.
61. Caplan AL. The ethics of gatekeeping in rehabilitation medicine. *J Head Trauma Rehabil* 1997; 12:29–36.
62. Dougherty C. Managed care and (un)informed consent. *J Head Trauma Rehabil* 1997; 12:21–28.
63. Banja J. Values, function and managed care: an ethical analysis. *J Head Trauma Rehabil* 1997; 12:60–70.
64. Thobaben J. The moral character of rehabilitation institutions. *J Head Trauma Rehabil* 1997; 12:10–20.
65. Rusk HA. World to care for. New York: Random House, 1972.
66. Fuhrer MJ. Issues in the federal funding of rehabilitation research. *Arch Phys Med Rehabil* 1985; 66:661–668.
67. Braddom RL. Why is physiatric research important? *Am J Phys Med Rehabil* 1991; 70(suppl):2–3.
68. Daniels N. Duty to treat or right to refuse? *Hastings Cent Rep* 1991; 21:36–46.
69. Pear R. Study says fees are often higher when doctor has stake in clinic. *New York Times,* p. 1, August 9, 1991.

Rehabilitation Medicine: Principles and Practice, Third Edition,
edited by Joel A. DeLisa and Bruce M. Gans.
Lippincott–Raven Publishers, Philadelphia © 1998.

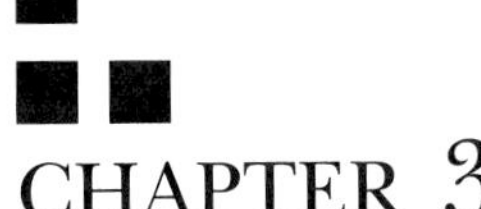

CHAPTER 3

International Issues in Rehabilitation Medicine

Naoichi Chino, Gunnar Grimby, Dennis S. Smith, Haim Ring, and
Satiko Tomikawa Imamura

The demand for rehabilitation medicine services has increased as the world's population has grown older and as the number of disabled persons has increased. The development of rehabilitation medicine has varied in each country and area of the world. It is difficult to survey the status of rehabilitation medicine in every country worldwide. This chapter provides an overview of the development of rehabilitation medicine outside of North America, in Asia, Europe, the Mediterranean, South America, Australia, New Zealand, and the South Pacific.

ASIA

Japan

There is some controversy over the terms "rehabilitation medicine" versus "physical medicine and rehabilitation" (PM&R). In Asian countries the former term is now more prevalent than the latter. This relates to the history of how the specialty has developed.

Dr. F.H. Krusen is recognized as the father of our specialty. In his textbook, Dr. Krusen stated that PM&R consists of two areas: (a) physical medicine, a branch of medicine using physical agents (e.g., light, heat, water, electricity, and mechanical agents) in the management of disease, and (b) rehabilitation, the treatment and training of patients to attain the maximal potential for normal living physically, psychologically, socially, and vocationally (1).

With the passage of time, the term "rehabilitation medicine" has subsumed the concept of physical medicine, and use of the name "rehabilitation medicine" has become dominant in Asian countries.

In Japan, the concept of medical rehabilitation (especially for children) was introduced in the 1920s by the late Professor K. Takagi. An academic organization, the Japanese Association of Rehabilitation Medicine was founded in 1963 under the auspices of the governmental delegates, who had been World Health Organization–sponsored fellows in the United States and Europe.

The 64 founders of the association were from the fields of orthopedics, internal medicine, pediatrics, psychiatry, surgery, ophthalmology, otolaryngology, public health, and speech pathology. At the opening ceremony, the late Professor S. Mizuno declared that this association shall help those persons disabled by ailment and accident to regain their maximal potential and to return to their previous social setting with productive lives (2).

The principal focus of this association was rehabilitation medicine, with little early attention to physical medicine. With a gradual increase in the number of rehabilitation medicine training programs in medical schools and residency programs, more emphasis on physical medicine has occurred.

Membership in the Japanese Association of Rehabilitation Medicine numbered 2,266 in 1983. A specialty certification board examination system sponsored by the Japanese Association of Rehabilitation Medicine was started in 1980. Fifteen members were certified at that time. In 1990, with the proposal for a medical specialty system sponsored by the Japanese Medical Association and the Committee of Japanese Specialty Board, more physicians, including orthopedic surgeons, internists, and neurosurgeons, joined the Japanese

N. Chino: Department of Rehabilitation Medicine, Keio University School of Medicine, Tokyo 160, Japan.

G. Grimby: Department of Rehabilitation Medicine, Göteborg University, Sahlgenska University Hospital, S-41345 Göteborg, Sweden.

D.S. Smith: Department of Rehabilitation Medicine, Wessex Rehabilitation Centre, University of Southhampton, Isle of Wight PO34 5EP, United Kingdom.

H. Ring: Department of Neurological Rehabilitation and Institute for Functional Evaluation; and Loewenstein Hospital Rehabilitation Center, Tel-Aviv University Medical School, Raanana 43100, Israel.

S. Tomikawa Inamura: Institute for Orthopaedics and Traumatology, Hospital das Clinicas, University of São Paulo Medical School, São Paulo, Brazil.

Association of Rehabilitation Medicine and the membership of the Association jumped to 8,639 in 1996. Those who are board-certified members of rehabilitation medicine numbered 5,254, and those who are board-certified physiatrists reached 615. The latter practice primarily rehabilitation medicine.

Since 1996, in order to be board-certified members of rehabilitation medicine, candidates must complete at least 1 year of a rehabilitation residency program during 4 years of postgraduate training and pass a written examination. Board certified physiatrists must fulfill a 3-year rehabilitation training program during a total of 5 training years and pass an oral examination.

Rehabilitation medicine is taught in all Japanese medical schools. However, a 1996 survey indicated that only 10 of 80 Japanese medical schools have independent departments of rehabilitation medicine. About one third of the university hospitals have training programs for rehabilitation medicine. There are 258 training programs in the university-affiliated hospitals, general hospitals, and rehabilitation institutions that are scattered around the country.

On September 2, 1996, the Japanese government adopted the term "rehabilitation medicine" to be used officially and legally as one of the clinical specialties. Before then, only the terms "physical medicine" or "physical therapy" were used.

A registration system for physical therapists and occupational therapists was started in 1965. In 1994, 14,205 physical therapists and 7,028 occupational therapists were registered. Speech therapists are not licensed in Japan, but about 2,000 trained speech therapists work under the supervision of physicians and will be posted for national licensure in the very future.

Rehabilitation medicine has developed in other Asian countries due to their own efforts and the assistance of the United States.

South Korea

In 1953, rehabilitation medicine was introduced by American missionaries and the America-Korea Foundation. The specialty has grown slowly during the past 45 years. In 1972 the Korean Academy of Rehabilitation Medicine was founded, and in 1983 a specialty board examination was initiated. The number of Korean Academy members in 1996 was 507. In this organization 270 are board certified and 237 are resident physicians. Korean medical students are exposed to rehabilitation medicine in 31 of 32 schools. A 4-year residency program is offered in 53 hospitals. Rehabilitation medicine is now a rapidly growing specialty field in Korea.

Indonesia

In Indonesia, rehabilitation medicine started after World War II and the War of Independence. The late Professor Dr. Soeharso, an orthopedic surgeon, set up a rehabilitation service, initially for prosthetic limb fitting. The Government of Indonesia, particularly its Department of Health, realized the necessity for rehabilitation medicine, and in 1979 Dr. A.R. Nastion was appointed as the head of the Rehabilitation Medicine Unit in the teaching hospital for the Faculty of Medicine of the University of Indonesia. In 1987, Dr. Soelarto assumed leadership of the service and organized residency training programs in rehabilitation medicine and education and culture. As of 1992, there were three recognized residency training centers. They have considered the development of neuro-musculo-skeletal, pediatric, cardiac, and geriatric subspecialties (3).

China

The People's Republic of China, with the largest population in the world, has only recently instituted its rehabilitation program. It is estimated that there are 50 million disabled Chinese, 5% of the total population. The national program for the disabled addresses three target areas: blindness, infantile paralysis (or polio), and deafness. Medical social workers are the primary advocates for rehabilitation. So far, 1 million individuals with cataracts and 360,000 cases of infantile paralysis have been treated, and 50,000 deaf children have received language training (4).

Europe

Physical medicine and rehabilitation is a full and complete specialty in 15 member states of the European Union (Austria, Belgium, Denmark, Finland, France, Germany, Greece, Ireland, Italy, Luxembourg, The Netherlands, Portugal, Spain, Sweden, and the United Kingdom) and in the four countries of the European Association of Free Exchanges (Iceland, Lichtenstein, Norway, and Switzerland). Within this European area there is, in principle, free movement for physicians. Medical school examinations and specialist certificates are recognized between the countries. Naturally, there are certain differences in the content and emphasis in the specialty between the different countries. This could explain the different names used for the specialty. In Ireland, Sweden, and the United Kingdom it is called rehabilitation medicine; in The Netherlands, *revaliditie*; and in France and Luxembourg, *reducation et radaptation fonctionnelles.* PM&R in European countries outside this area, mainly the Eastern European and Balkan countries, is not included in this discussion.

The European Union of Medical Specialists has been of great importance for collaboration between the specialist associations in the different countries. Each specialty has its own section. The PM&R section set up the European Board of PM&R in 1991, with the objectives to study, promote, and protect the highest possible uniformity of care given to patients in Europe in the field of rehabilitation medicine. The present Secretary of the Board, Dr. Antoine Macouin from France, has summarized facts and figures about the specialty in Europe in two recent publications (5,6).

There is an uneven distribution of specialists in PM&R among the European countries. According to data published in 1995, the highest number of specialists per 100,000 inhabitants is in Belgium (4.11 PM&R specialists). France, Italy, Portugal, and Spain also have a relatively high number of PM&R specialists. Very few specialists were reported from Greece, Ireland, and the United Kingdom (Tables 3-1 and 3-2).

It should be noted that the specialty in its present form was only recognized in 1990 in England and Wales and in 1992 in Germany. In Denmark, the situation is somewhat special; PM&R had been an independent specialty but is now a part of rheumatology.

With the exception of the smallest European countries, there is ongoing training of new specialists, but with somewhat varying ratios between specialists and trainees. Most countries also have university professors who are responsible for teaching at medical schools and participating in specialist and continuing education. Several journals of rehabilitation medicine are published in Europe.

The European Board of PM&R has worked toward common content and quality of specialist training in Europe by creating a curriculum for studies, by establishing an annual Europe-wide certifying examination, and by recognizing training institutions by peer review visits. A minimum of 4 years training is required, of which 2 years are spent in PM&R units. Many countries require longer specialist training, as in Sweden, where the minimum is 5 years.

One factor that may explain the different structures of PM&R and how it is practiced in different European countries is the differences in the health-care systems. Another factor may be the history of the development of PM&R. In some countries on the continent, the special spa institutions have a strong tradition, whereas this is not the case in northwestern Europe and Scandinavia. As in the United States, the need for rehabilitation of war victims had a strong impact in some countries on the development of PM&R, as did the increasing occurrence of traffic accidents in later years.

There is also a long tradition of special care and rehabilitation programs for certain categories of the disabled, including those with congenital defects, tuberculosis, polio, and blindness and deafness.

Sweden

The first Department of Rehabilitation Medicine in Sweden started in 1958 at the county hospital in Bors in southwestern Sweden. It was followed by departments at other hospitals during the following decade. The first professor of rehabilitation medicine was appointed at Göteborg University in 1966. Rehabilitation medicine was recognized as a specialty in 1969. It is now represented in nearly all major hospitals in each of the 24 counties.

Rehabilitation medicine in Sweden, as in a number of other European countries, can be looked upon as a highly specialized field, with approximately 160 rehabilitation medicine specialists. In all departments rehabilitation is based on multiprofessional teams, including physicians, nurses, occupational therapists, physiotherapists, psychologists, social workers, and speech therapists. The inpatient service treats many stroke and other brain injury patients, whereas the outpatient service treats patients with other types of disabilities, including chronic pain.

TABLE 3-1. *PM&R specialists practicing in Europe*

Country	Specialists per 100,000 inhabitants
Belgium	4.11
Spain	3.71
Italy	3.50
France	3.21
Portugal	3.20
Denmark	2.30
Switzerland	2.20
Finland	2.20
Sweden	1.88
Luxembourg	1.50
The Netherlands	1.31
Austria	1.20
Greece	0.60
The United Kingdom	0.15
Ireland	0.11

Reprinted with permission from Macouin A. Physical medicine and rehabilitation in Europe. *Eur Med Phys* 1995; 31:61–66.

Rehabilitation medicine is an academic discipline represented by full professors at five of the six medical schools in the country. At all universities there is exposure of medical students to rehabilitation medicine, occupational therapy, physiotherapy, and other allied health professions.

Postgraduate courses are offered for specialist training, and there are also courses and scientific meetings in continuing education. Research is conducted in rehabilitation medicine at all universities, and it is possible to receive a Ph.D. in Rehabilitation Medicine in the Faculty of Medicine. A Ph.D. program is also available to specially qualified persons from allied health professions. There is close collaboration with the Colleges of Allied Health in teaching and in research training.

After the Swedish equivalent to internship and certification as a physician, specialist training begins. Training is guided by a number of officially established goals and is a minimum of 5 years. Around 3 years are spent in the Department of Rehabilitation Medicine, including inpatient and outpatient rehabilitation. There is no compulsory examination. The specialist certificate is issued by the National Board of Health and Welfare when the supervisors can state that the goals have been fulfilled. The Swedish Medical Society and the specialist associations have created a voluntary specialist examination, which includes both written and clinical sections.

The Mediterranean

Historically, the Mediterranean basin has been a crossroad where north met south and west met east, each having its

TABLE 3-2. *Ratio of trainees to the number of practicing PM&R specialists*

Country	Trainees/ practicing specialists
Greece	1/1.9
Austria	1/2.1
The United Kingdom	1/2.6
Finland	1/2.7
Switzerland	1/2.8
Portugal	1/3.2
The Netherlands	1/3.3
Belgium	1/5.6
Spain	1/6.0
Italy	1/7.5
Sweden	1/8.0
France	1/11.0
Denmark	1/12.0

Reprinted with permission from Macouin A. Physical medicine and rehabilitation in Europe. *Eur Med Phys* 1995; 31:61–66.

distinct characteristics. This cultural and demographic heterogeneity is reflected in the current status of the rehabilitation discipline in the Mediterranean basin. As in other parts of the world, there is some hesitation in the Mediterranean region whether to use the term ''rehabilitation medicine'' or ''physical medicine and rehabilitation.''

The history of rehabilitation systems in the Mediterranean basin is young compared with that of other regions. Rehabilitation systems first appeared in several countries, including Turkey and Spain, about 60 to 70 years ago, then in Slovenia and Israel in the 1940s. The impetus for their emergence varied from country to country. In Turkey and Israel, it emerged as a result of war. In others, it developed as a result of epidemics (such as polio in Italy) or work accidents (Spain). In France, back pain, scoliosis, and amputees remained the main issues until the World War II. In most countries, decades of informal or isolated activities preceded the installment of university services or drafting of appropriate legislation to legitimately establish rehabilitation among the medical professions.

In looking at the general organization of the systems, it is interesting to see that medical and social systems run parallel in various places such as Spain, Italy, and Israel. Perhaps the fact that most rehabilitation work in the region is performed in the public sector is representative of the stressed importance on the social aspects of rehabilitation in rehabilitation services.

The number of rehabilitation specialists or rehabilitation beds, whether absolute or relative, appears to vary both in terms of the number of medical doctors in any given country and in the way they are defined. With rehabilitation medicine being a very heterogeneous field, ranging from burns to cardiology to pain, and spanning pediatrics to geriatrics, it is often difficult to distinguish between the two specialties. In general, it appears that there is a shortage of mainstream rehabilitation for strokes and spinal cord injuries. Such rehabilitation beds represent 1% to 2% of the total number of beds. The number of PM&R specialists, predominantly in France, Italy, and Spain, is estimated at 5,000.

The scope of clinical rehabilitation work varies from country to country. In Turkey and Spain rheumatology and orthopedics appear to dominate, whereas in Israel and France and to some extent in Italy neurorehabilitation has a very prominent place. Spinal cord injury treatment was pioneered by Sir Ludwig Guttman in the United Kingdom and was emulated by his trainees from Israel, Spain, and other countries. Functional electrical stimulation was almost exclusively developed in the Lubljana Rehabilitation Center in Slovenia. It then rapidly spread to other countries such as Italy and Israel, where technological advancement allowed an integration of this field into the clinical and research work of locomotor disabilities.

In most of the ''active'' countries, a 3- to 5-year curriculum syllabus for becoming a PM&R specialist was developed and approved by the academic authorities. In most of the active places, there is also a well-structured postgraduate PM&R program. Undergraduate rehabilitation teaching is uniformly reported as occurring in the last (fifth or sixth) years of medical school, seldom earlier.

All countries with formal rehabilitation systems have some organs of expression—journals, bulletins, and the like—and several countries have more than one.

Although the style and content of clinical work remain different among the countries, the future direction is one of convergence. The expansion of rehabilitation services from medical centers to be assimilated into the community, active participation in primary care, integration with basic sciences and advanced research, incorporation of high technology in the routine treatments, rehabilitation for new pathologies such as acquired immunodeficiency syndrome, rehabilitation cost-effectiveness studies, and implementation of quality assurance principles all appear to be common to the future agenda of the various systems.

As the 21st century dawns, there is room for some optimism. Although political developments appear remote from the daily clinical work, they do form an integral part of the existence of rehabilitation. Historic events are bringing together rehabilitation experts. In the First Mediterranean Congress of Physical Medicine and Rehabilitation, held in Herzlyia, Israel, May 12 to 16, 1996, under the motto of ''Rehabilitation Without Frontiers,'' over 420 colleagues from 40 different countries in this region and beyond met and discussed common issues and their possible solutions at the scientific sessions, workshops, and other informal activities during the Congress.

Australia, New Zealand, and the South Pacific

Modern rehabilitation in Australia, New Zealand and the South Pacific has its roots in World War II. There was a need in the early 1940s to return skilled and trained airmen of the Royal Australian Air Force (RAAF) to flying duties as soon as possible after injury. The process was developed for rehabilitation by such pioneers as the late Dr. George Burniston during his service in the medical branch of the RAAF. The development of rehabilitation medicine in Australia has progressed to achieve world standards of practice and as a specialized branch of internal medicine.

In the early 1970s, Dr. Burniston, at that time the Director of Rehabilitation Medicine at the University of New South Wales Teaching Hospitals, submitted the paper entitled "The Physically Handicapped—A Comment on Some Aspects of their Care and Welfare Today" to an Australian Senate Committee. This paper remains today a comprehensive and scholarly review of Australian attitudes to the problems of the disabled from a medical viewpoint. Burniston pointed out that voluntary hospitals, created in the latter part of the 18th century in Great Britain, were, unlike their predecessors, largely concerned with the process of healing. They therefore increasingly restricted admissions to patients with short-term, curable ailments. The disabled and chronically sick had to be accommodated elsewhere and were not subjected to funding from the voluntary sector. As a result, it was necessary for the government to set up its own accommodation for the chronically sick.

Teaching hospitals were based on the acute voluntary model and thus, the undergraduate curriculum was also based on this voluntary model of management. In fact, the Flexnerian model, which continues to dominate the design of undergraduate courses of medicine, is concerned with the training of undergraduates in the principles of physics, chemistry, and biological science. The subsequent medical curriculum is also strictly based on the applied consequences of these subjects to the determinate of pathology and its clinical manifestations. Hence, modern hospital services have been slow to recognize the important psychosocial needs of the chronically sick, as well as of people with disabilities. Such needs, among others, have remained the responsibility of the State Community Services, who have largely interpreted their role as custodial and caring in nature. Burniston went on to elaborate that care for the disabled was based on a passive caring model, quite different from the dynamic curative model epitomized by the curriculum and contents of the large teaching hospitals, and that this passive caring model was often inappropriate. Dr. Burniston's postgraduate medical training and subsequent experience in the medical branch of the Royal Australian Air Force accounted for this belief.

According to the "Official Medical Services History of the Second World War,"

> The problem was a shortage of skilled man power, notably pilots, during a period of active war . . . . It was essential to restore these airmen to their previous state of fitness, high morale and motivation as rapidly as possible. They were discharged from hospital(s) as soon as their primary surgical management had been completed . . . . There, away from the hospital, the germ of invalidism could be attacked. The medical officers, after assessing the patients, prescribed a program of activities, including remedial exercises, physiotherapy, and occupational therapy, designed to advance the restoration of fitness, and promote healing of fractures and other injuries. The results were excellent. Out of the first 13,500 airmen, 85% of the aircrew returned to flying duties, 96% of the ground staff returned to duty, and 5% were discharged from the service. These figures compare to a 50% discharge rate before this program.

In 1943, Burniston helped set up the RAAF Rehabilitation Service, which was eventually passed over to the Commonwealths Rehabilitation Services. By 1948, Australia had a number of rehabilitation centers, remote from hospitals, but they were only used for the rehabilitation of invalid pensioners. The success rate, measured by the nominated goal of return to work, was between 5% and 15%, or if you like, an 85% failure rate. Burniston, in his submission to the government in 1970, critically appraised this service. He had become increasingly convinced that the Commonwealth Rehabilitation Service was an anachronism.

The Royal South Sydney Rehabilitation Centre was opened in September 1956, with Dr. Marie Naomi Wing as the Honorary Medical Director. This was originally a 2-year pilot project, and when it opened it had only one patient and one occupational therapist. The latter was a highly trained Australian graduate in Occupational Therapy, Mr. Frank Dargan, who had returned from extensive postgraduate training in the United States under the direction of Dr. Howard Rusk. Dr. Rusk, in world terms, was a giant in the genesis of rehabilitation. He believed that although rehabilitation should be essentially hospital based and should extensively be based on the somewhat limited concepts of physical medicine or physiatry, it should develop as a separate principle specialty, separate from Internal Medicine. It would be true to say that his influence on the pioneers of rehabilitation in Australia was largely responsible for the initial development of rehabilitation as a specialty in its own right.

The third member of this visionary group of doctors was Dr. Bruce Ford, who was appointed to the position of Consultant in Rehabilitation to the Canberra Hospital in 1960. His training was in general practice and public health medicine. His empathy with people with disabilities and his drive were related to his determination not to let his handicap of severe motor cerebral palsy interfere with any significant aspect of his very active life. Over a matter of 10 years in Canberra, Ford created a model service based entirely on his own concepts of what was needed. The service that he created was a tertiary referral service, that is, he only took patients referred to him from other specialists. He told them that he would be happy to take on the rehabilitation management of any patient with a significant problem related to disability. This resulted in the development of a service that would still be looked on as innovative for people with disabilities of any age. Because this assessment-based goal-directed service did not have age as a limitation, it spanned the fields of pediatrics and geriatrics.

In Australia, the process that was to lead to the establishment of a Diploma in Physical Medicine and Rehabilitation in the 1970s and a College of Rehabilitation Medicine in

1980 was given a boost by the introduction of an amendment to the Workers' Compensation Act of New South Wales in December 1970. In Section 10 of the Act, the words "medical rehabilitation and the necessary accompanying services were included by both Houses of the Parliament. This amendment enabled rehabilitation services to be paid for, and was a substantial benefit to both the unit at Royal South Sydney Hospital and the unit run at that time by Dr. Adrian Paul at Prince Alfred Hospital. Also of considerable strategic importance were the "Report of the Federal Senate Committee" in 1971, the Health Services Commission report "A Medical Rehabilitation Program for Australia" in 1973, and in particular, the Meares Woodhouse report "The National Committee of Inquiry into Compensation and Rehabilitation in Australia" in 1974.

Kenneth Jenkins, the Chief Executive of Bedford Industries, South Australia, the largest rehabilitation workshop in Australia, was the president of Rehabilitation International and a proponent of the International Year of the Disabled in 1982. He was largely responsible for creating the Chair of Rehabilitation at Flinders University in South Australia. There are now three such positions currently in existence in Australia.

The specialty of rehabilitation was recognized by the National Specialist Advisory Committee (NSQAC) in 1978. With the support of other colleges, the Australian Association of Physical Medicine and Rehabilitation, under its active president, Dr. Ben Marosseky, in 1977 took initiatives and established the Australian College of Rehabilitation in 1979. Its first president was appropriately Dr. George Burniston.

The professional training programs developed in the College are of a very high standard. Each candidate must have a minimal 3 years general clinical training approved by the Board of Censors before he or she is eligible for taking the entrance examination. The examination consists of two multiple-choice papers of 3 hours' duration, questions of which are selected on the basis of high discriminatory content and relevance. The successful candidates are then examined clinically on a long case and a selection of short cases. Those candidates who pass this part 1 examination enter the 3-year advanced training program. At the end of the 3-year program, the candidate takes the part 2 examination, which consists of a multiple-choice paper, an essay paper, and, if successful, a clinical examination consisting of a long consultation, three or four short cases, and an oral examination. At the end of this 6-year training program, the trainee is awarded his or her Diploma of Fellowship and can register as a Consultant in Rehabilitation Medicine.

South America

In South America, rehabilitation medicine developed after World War II. The poliomyelitis epidemic in the 1950s had a profound impact on the development of rehabilitation medicine in Brazil as opposed to other countries, where rehabilitation medicine was shaped by neurologic and orthopedic trauma suffered during wartime combat. The number of specialists has increased over the past decade in many South American countries, especially Brazil, Argentina, Columbia, and Venezuela. Rehabilitation medicine is becoming recognized among other specialties, with the need increasing for specialists in the field. The scientific and practical concepts of rehabilitation medicine are included in the curricula of many medical schools, even though these are frequently optional.

In Brazil the concept of rehabilitation medicine started in 1854 at Pedro II Hospital in Rio de Janeiro, where patients with mental disorders performed occupational tasks at such places as the shoemaker's, the dressmaker's, and the florist's. In the 19th century, Emperor Pedro II founded the Institute for the Blind, which is considered to be the initial mark of the specialty in this country. In 1878 the first physical therapy service was created in South America at the Santa Casa de Misericórdia General Hospital in Rio de Janeiro. In 1919, after World War I, Raphael Penteado de Barros, Professor of Biological Physics at the University of São Paulo School of Medicine, founded the Department of Medical Electricity at that university. In 1947 physiatrist Waldo Rolim de Moraes created the first service for PM&R at the Hospital das Clinicas of the University of São Paulo School of Medicine. In 1952 the discipline of physical therapy was reborn at the School of Medical Sciences in Rio de Janeiro.

In 1954, rehabilitation medicine was recognized as a medical specialty with the foundation of the Brazilian Society of Physical Medicine and Rehabilitation. The Society affiliated with the Brazilian Medical Association in 1973. In 1956 the first Congress was held in the Institute of Orthopaedics and Traumatology at Hospital das Clinicas, University of São Paulo School of Medicine (7). Since that time, 14 national congresses of the specialty have been held. There are now 13 regional societies in Brazil.

In 1972 the Brazilian Academy of Rehabilitation Medicine was founded. In 1973 the first board examination for PM&R was given with theoretical and practical sections. Since then, the number of specialists and rehabilitation services at the university level has increased. There are 820 physiatrists in Brazil, and 468 have passed the board examination, 50% of whom are in the state of São Paulo. In Chile there are approximately 90 physiatrists, in Argentina 200, Peru 60, Columbia 200, Venezuela 123, and Uruguay 42, most of whom are concentrated in the capital cities (8).

Both graduate and postgraduate levels are involved in the university education of specialists. Graduate courses have a total accreditation of 30 to 60 hours and include the presentation of the specialty, with emphasis on the importance of disability in the various fields of medicine and of preventive rehabilitation procedures. The evaluation of a patient with a physical impairment, functional residual capacities, and the main rehabilitation issues usually are offered in the fourth year of medical school (9). Postgraduate courses include medical residency of 3 years' duration: the first year in internal medicine and 2 years in PM&R. The residency program can be accomplished at a university or at a private hospital. The University of São Paulo, Federal University of São Paulo, Santa Casa School of Medicine, Federal University of Rio de Janeiro, State University of Rio de Janeiro, Federal University of Bahia, and the Federal University of Rio Grande do Sul all have residency programs in rehabilitation medicine. In Chile, the residency program can be completed at one of three different locations, one of which is the University of Chile in Santiago.

A specialty board examination is held every year in Brazil, consisting of 2 days of both theoretical and practical tests. The first board examination took place in Brazil in 1973. In Chile the board examination lasts 1 week and takes place in the year after the completion of a residency program.

In Brazil, the *Medicina de Reabilitao* periodical is published every 4 months and is indexed in the *Latin America Index Medicus.* The first issue was published in 1956.

INTERNATIONAL ORGANIZATIONS

There are several international meetings related to rehabilitation medicine: the International Federation of Physical Medicine and Rehabilitation (IFPMR), the International Rehabilitation Medicine Association (IRMA), and the Medical Commission of Rehabilitation International (RIMC). These international bodies collaborate with the World Health Organization to influence rehabilitation services throughout the world.

International Federation of Physical Medicine and Rehabilitation

The history of the IFPMR dates back to the last decade of the 19th century, when the American Electro-Therapeutic Association (one of the oldest organizations related to physical medicine) had strong ties to England and France. Several international congresses related to electrotherapeutics and radiology were held up until the early decades of 20th century in the European countries (10,11).

In 1952, after World War II, the IFPMR was officially created by the Interim Committee that included Drs. F. Krusen (Chairman, U.S.A.), P. Bauwens (Honorary Secretary, Great Britain); H. Burt (Honorary Treasurer, Great Britain); S. Clemmensen (Denmark); and W. Tegner (Great Britain). The Federation promoted the advancement of all aspects of PM&R for the benefit of mankind by (a) linking on an international level local (national and regional) societies of PM&R; (b) hosting the meeting of International Congresses of PM&R at regular intervals; (c) fostering the collection and exchange of information on matters pertaining to PM&R between members of the Federation; (d) organizing symposia and seminars in subjects proper and related to PM&R; and (e) promoting the advancement of PM&R by any other means that in the opinion of the International Committee shall tend to further the objectives of the Federation.

The first International Federation of Physical Medicine was held in London in 1952. Since that time, the IFPMR has met at 4-year intervals. In 1964, an application to become an affiliated member of the World Health Organization was approved. As the scope of the field has broadened, in 1972 the name of the Congress changed to the IFPMR.

After the first Congress in London in 1952, meetings were held in Copenhagen in 1956, Washington in 1960, Paris in 1964, Montreal in 1968, Barcelona in 1972, Rio de Janeiro in 1976, Stockholm in 1980, Jerusalem in 1984, Toronto in 1988, Dresden in 1992, and Sydney in 1995. At the 12th World Congress in Sydney, the Board, chaired by Dr. E. Conradi, selected Washington, DC, as the site of the 13th World Congress, with Dr. J. Melvin as President of the Congress. He was at the same time named President-Elect of the IFPMR for the term 1995 to 1999. Dr. P. Disler was selected as Secretary and Dr. M. Grabois as Treasurer.

The IFPMR will merge with the International Rehabilitation Medicine Association to become a single organization as explained later in this chapter.

International Rehabilitation Medicine Association

The IRMA was founded by Dr. S. Licht in 1969. The main difference between the IRMA and the IFPMR is that the former consists of member physicians and surgeons individually who are interested in rehabilitation medicine. The latter offers membership to only one established national society.

Since 1969, two major international congresses have been held, as has the meeting of the Medical Commission of Rehabilitation International. Efforts to form a single international rehabilitation medical organization began at the 7th World Congress of IRMA held in Washington, DC, in April 1994. The name of the new organization is expected to be the International Society of Physical and Rehabilitation Medicine (ISPRM). The ISPRM plans to hold a congress every 2 years.

Medical Commission of Rehabilitation International

The RIMC was founded in 1922 as a federation of national and international organizations and agencies working for the prevention of disability, the rehabilitation of disabled people, and the equalization of opportunities within society on behalf of disabled people and their families throughout the world. The RIMC maintains official relations with the United Nations Economic and Social Council, the World Health Organization, the International Labor Office, UNICEF, and other related committees.

REFERENCES

1. Krusen FH. The scope of physical medicine and rehabilitation. In: Krusen FH, Kottke FJ, Ellwood PM, eds. *Handbook of physical medicine and rehabilitation.* Philadelphia: WB Saunders, 1965; 1–11.

2. Mizuno S. Establishment of the Japanese Association of Rehabilitation Medicine [in Japanese]. *Jpn J Rehabil Med* 1964; 1:57–61.
3. Everett JP. Past, present and the future of PM&R in Indonesia. News and views. *IRMA* spring, 1992.
4. Wu CZ. Rehabilitation, education and employment of China disabled. News and views. *IRMA* fall, 1995.
5. Macouin A. The specialty of physical medicine and rehabilitation in Europe; 1993 facts and figures. *J Rehabil Sci* 1993; 6:100–104.
6. Macouin A. Physical medicine and rehabilitation in Europe. *Eur Med Phys* 1995; 31:61–66.
7. Leitao, A. *Clinica de reabilitaco,* 2nd ed [in Portuguese]. Rio de Janeiro: Atheneu Ed., 1995.
8. Organizacion Panamericana de la Salud. Directorlo AMLAR (Associacion Medica Latina Americana de Rehabilitacion), Febrera, 1994. Document OPS/HSS/94.02, Washington, D.C.
9. Lianza S. *Medicina de reabilitaco,* 2nd ed [in Portuguese]. São Paulo, Brazil: Guanabara Koogan, 1995.
10. Nelson P. History of the once close relationship between electrotherapeutics and radiology. *Arch Phys Med Rehabil* 1973; 54:608–640.
11. Jimenez J, ed. *International Federation of Physical Medicine and Rehabilitation—regulations and list of members: 1992–1995.* Toronto: International Federation Physical Medicine and Rehabilitation, 1992; 1–39.

Rehabilitation Medicine: Principles and Practice, Third Edition,
edited by Joel A. DeLisa and Bruce M. Gans.
Lippincott–Raven Publishers, Philadelphia © 1998.

CHAPTER 4

Impairment, Disability, and Handicap

R. Lee Kirby

One might say that such matters are outside the healing art. Why, forsooth, trouble one's mind further about cases which have become incurable? This is far from the right attitude. The investigation of these matters too belongs to the same science; it is impossible to separate them from one another.
Hippocrates, 460–377, B.C.

A physician is obliged to consider more than a diseased organ, more even than the whole man—he must view the man in his world.
Harvey Cushing, 1869–1939

This chapter addresses concepts that are the essence of medical rehabilitation, what makes a physiatrist different from most other physicians. The difference between the clinical evaluation by a physiatrist and that of other physicians is not a mere collection of isolated disagreements on findings, such as about the grading of a knee jerk or whether the pedal pulses are palpable. Rather, the physiatric evaluation at its best provides a clear picture of how illnesses affect peoples' lives—what they can no longer do and how that precludes what is meaningful to them.

More specifically, the purpose of this chapter is to help physicians who are interested in rehabilitation accomplish educational objectives. Each physician should be able to:

- Define, compare, and contrast the terms impairment, disability, and handicap.
- Identify a person's impairments, disabilities, and handicaps in the clinical setting.
- In defining a person's functional capacity, identify the current and required level of function, the severity of the limitation, and the limiting factors.
- In managing a person with disability, assist the person in adapting to the limitation, in minimizing the intrinsic and extrinsic limiting factors, and in changing the nature of the task to render it possible.

R.L. Kirby: Division of Physical Medicine and Rehabilitation, Dalhousie University, Halifax, Nova Scotia B3H 4K4, Canada.

THE WORLD HEALTH ORGANIZATION'S CLASSIFICATION

In 1980, the World Health Organization (WHO) published the International Classification of Impairments, Disabilities and Handicaps (ICIDH) (1). Since then, the ICIDH has been extensively studied and its merits debated—the WHO has a bibliography that lists over 1,000 references to the ICIDH (2–4). Despite consensus on some needed improvements (e.g., clarifying the role of the social and physical environment in the process of handicap, providing a means to indicate severity, and avoiding cultural specificity), the ICIDH concepts have been widely adopted, with the classification available in 13 languages (4). A revision is underway, with a target of 1999 for completion of the second version—details can be found on the WHO web site (http://www.who.ch1).

IMPAIRMENT

Impairment: any loss or abnormality of psychological, physiological, or anatomical structure or function (1).

Any tissue, organ, or system can respond in only a finite number of ways to the seemingly unlimited combinations and permutations of etiologic insults. These responses are the impairments, sometimes called the clinical features or manifestations of the disease or condition. Examples of impairments are weakness, limited range of motion, pain, and confusion. It should be noted that function, as referred to in the ICIDH definition of impairment, is the function of a body part (e.g., the thyroid), not the whole-person function, which will be discussed in the next section.

DISABILITY

Disability: any restriction or lack resulting from an impairment of ability to perform an activity in the manner or within the range considered normal for a human being (1).

Any causal relationship between impairment and disability is a loose and polyfactorial one. Indeed, the relationship

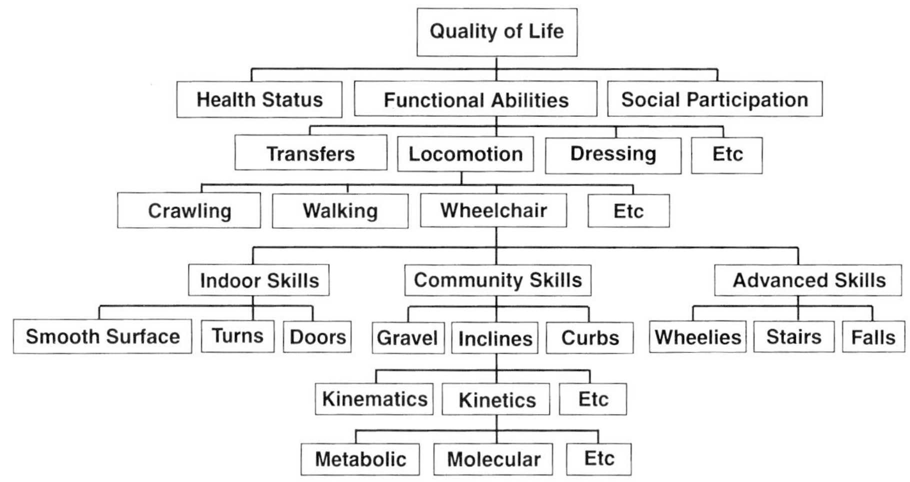

FIG. 4-1. A hierarchy of evaluation measures relevant to rehabilitation.

may be bidirectional (4), for example, the inability to walk (a disability) may lead to muscle weakness and contractures (impairments). Because so many factors (e.g., motivation, emotional state, fatigue, pain) influence final performance, even with the most accurate list of impairments, a physician can make only an educated guess about the functional limitations. Badley and colleagues (5) and Levack and associates (6) found low correlations between ranges of joint motion and functional scores. Similarly, Hagglund and colleagues found that biomedical indicators of arthritis disease activity did not correlate well with functional status (7). Tinetti and Ginter, in a study of elderly people living in the community, found that the conventional neuromuscular examination correlated poorly with functional mobility (8).

Furthermore, deteriorations in functional capacity may occur in a stepwise fashion despite a smooth progressive loss of strength, range, or aerobic capacity (9). For example, a loss of knee flexion range from 90° to 80°, what may seem to be a minor deterioration, can be enough to prevent sitting-to-standing transfers in some patients (10). On the other hand, the simultaneous occurrence of two or more impairments may not produce additional functional difficulties because one impairment may preempt the other. For instance, a person with hemiplegia who requires an amputation on the same side may have his or her overall ambulation function improved by the second impairment, with a passive prosthesis preferable to spastic equinovarus.

Figure 4-1 illustrates where an evaluation tool (like one that assesses wheelchair skills) would fit in the overall hierarchy of evaluations that make up health-related quality of life. The second level of the hierarchy corresponds to the three broad ICIDH categories (impairment, disability. and handicap), but uses the more positive expressions "health status," "functional abilities," and "social participation." The next two levels reflect the usual broad activities of daily living (ADL) categories (Table 4-1) and some subcategories in the locomotion domain. Although a number of global rating scales (e.g., the Functional Independence Measure [FIM]) (11) have been developed for quantitating disability at these levels, and they represent valuable contributions from the perspective of program evaluation (12), they generally lack the specificity needed to manage individual patients. The next two levels illustrate a way in which wheelchair skills can be subdivided into individual tasks. The final two levels relate to progressively more detailed evaluations, such as the task determinants at the biomechanical and subcellular levels.

The specificity needed for a functional diagnosis is at the level of meaningful whole-person tasks, often referred to as ADLs. (Some clinicians refer to the more complex ADLs that involve a number of constituents as instrumental ADLs [IADLs].) ADLs are behaviors in that they are observable and measurable. The terms used are defined by the task (e.g., typing) rather than the region (e.g., hand function) because it is possible to have no arms and to type with one's feet.

TABLE 4-1. *An ADL classification*

Domain	Examples
Locomotion	Walking, wheeling, stairs
Transport	Driving, use of public conveyance
Transfers	Bed mobility, bed-wheelchair, sit-stand
Personal Hygiene	Bathing, shaving, grooming, toileting
Dressing	Clothing, shoes, orthoses or prostheses on and off
Feeding	Ingestion of food, liquid, pills
Environmental Control	Control of lights, temperature, television
Communication	Speaking, writing, typing, telephone use
Recreation	Knitting, cards, sports
Homemaking	Shopping, bed making, vacuuming, kitchen
Work	Lifting, equipment operation

ADL, activities of daily living.

Many classifications of ADL have been described, one of which is shown in Table 4-1. Most classification systems contain unavoidable areas of overlap, such that a given ability (e.g., donning trousers after a bowel movement) might be assigned to more than one category (e.g., dressing and personal hygiene).

As noted earlier, the ICIDH definition of disability focuses on the "ability to perform an activity" (1). The term "disability" is therefore meaningless without a description of what it is the person is unable to do; one may be disabled from the perspective of climbing stairs but be able to play the piano. For any specific task, one can compare a person's functional capacity to that of his or her peers. However, a rigid adherence to this criterion would not allow us to consider a person who began significantly more able than his or her peers as disabled, such as a world-champion swimmer slowed, although not necessarily to the point of losing, by a knee ailment. In such circumstances, the person's performance should be compared with his or her own previous performances. However, this approach fails to accommodate the person with a congenital disability.

This dilemma may be solved by resorting to a form of double definition. The extent of disability may be expressed as the discrepancy between a person's current functional capacity (CFC) and normal functional capacity (NFC), preferably the person's own capacity before the onset of the disabling conditions, but if such information is not available, then that of his or her peers. In the equation that follows, note that the only way that true disability (TD) can be decreased is by increasing CFC, because NFC cannot be changed:

$$TD = (NFC - CFC)/NFC \times 100\%$$

Significant disability (SD) is different; this term represents an important clinical distinction, but not one made in the ICIDH. Significant disability relates to the discrepancy between functional requirements and actual capabilities (13). Normally, functional capacity exceeds requirements, and one is said to possess a functional reserve. If a person needs or wants to perform a task, however, and is incapable of doing so, then he or she is significantly disabled, the extent of which may be expressed by the equation below. Note that SD can be decreased either by increasing CFC (as for TD) or by decreasing the required functional capacity (RFC), such as in a lowering of expectations (Fig. 4-2).

$$SD = (RFC - CFC)/ RFC \times 100\%$$

A severe true disability, such as inability to walk, may be only mildly significant to a person whose interests are aesthetic. Disability may even be an asset in some respects, if there are secondary gains such as freedom from responsibility and financial worries, or if the disability provides a stimulus for an improved outlook on life.

Despite the availability of the equations noted earlier, it is often difficult to quantify disability—few norms are available, the clinician seldom knows exactly what the functional

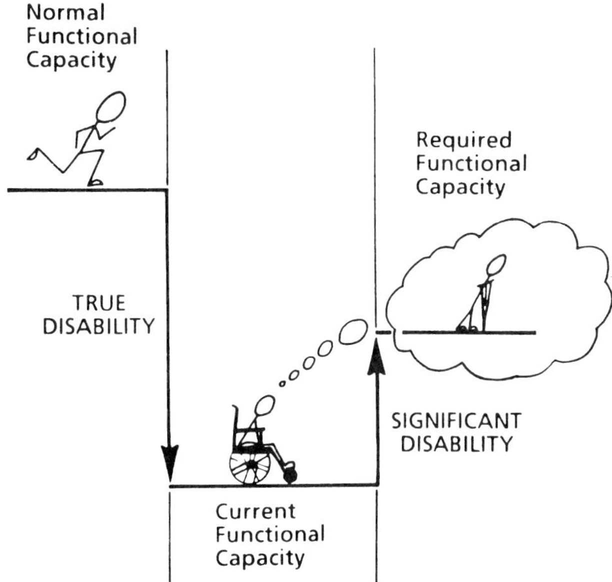

FIG. 4-2. True disability is the discrepancy between current functional capacity and normal capacity. Significant disability is the discrepancy between current functional capacity and what the person needs or wants to do (i.e., the required functional capacity).

capacity was before an injury or illness, and a person's requirements may be difficult to determine precisely. It is therefore customary to describe the person's current functional capacity rather than to attempt to measure disability. This is not only practical, but also preferable on humanistic grounds because it emphasizes the positive residual abilities: what is left, not what has been lost.

HANDICAP

> Handicap: a disadvantage for a given individual resulting from an impairment or a disability that limits or prevents the fulfillment of a role that is normal (depending on the age, sex, and social and cultural factors) for that individual (1).

If an impairment represents the problem at the tissue and organ level, and disability represents the problem at the whole-person level, then handicap represents the problem at the environmental and societal level (Fig. 4-3). For clinical

WHO
DEFINITIONS
LEVELS
Handicap
Society
Disability
Whole Person
Impairment
Organ or Tissue

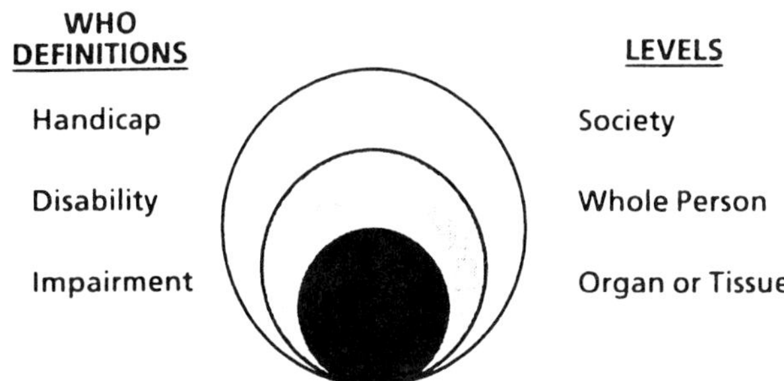

FIG. 4-3. Impairment, disability, and handicap are manifestations of a problem at the tissue or organ, whole person, and societal levels, respectively.

purposes, one may think of a handicap as an extrinsic limiting factor, or a factor in the environment (e.g., accessibility) that limits function. Unlike a work disability, where a person is unable to perform the work activity, a work handicap involves an external limitation (e.g., the unwillingness of an employer to make a necessary architectural modification). It is apparent from this that a person may be handicapped without being disabled; an example would be a person with a Symes amputation (i.e., through the ankle joint) who may be physically capable of driving a truck when wearing a prosthesis, but precluded from doing so by licensing authorities.

CLINICAL EVALUATION OF FUNCTIONAL ABILITIES

Clinical evaluation will be discussed in depth elsewhere in the textbook, but a few points will be useful here to advance the conceptual framework that is the focus of this chapter. If a functional problem in an ADL is suspected (e.g., difficulty with a task such as dressing), it should be explored further through history, physical examination, and investigation until the physician is satisfied that the problem is insignificant or until there is sufficient information to permit management. A clear understanding of the problem in the ADL setting should include three components:

- Determination of the current and required levels of function
- Identification of the severity of the limitation
- Identification of the limiting factors

Current and Required Levels of Function

Within each broad ADL category there are several subtasks. For example, locomotion (getting from one point to another) may occur by a variety of techniques (e.g., walking, crawling, hopping, wheelchair propulsion) and includes locomoting over smooth and rough surfaces, through doors, and ascending and descending inclines, curbs, and stairs. Within a given ADL category, some tasks are consistently more difficult than others. Having determined what the person can do, the physician ordinarily may assume that the person can perform less difficult items but cannot perform more difficult ones. For example, for a person with osteoarthritis of the hips who is able to rise from an armchair, but with difficulty, it may be assumed that he or she can rise easily from a tall stool, but is unlikely to be able to get out of an unmodified bathtub. These assumptions usually are confirmed by evaluating a few more and less difficult tasks. This validation is necessary because the order of difficulty may vary subtly from one disorder to the next; although a person with osteoarthritis may be able to walk but not hop, a person with an amputation may be able to hop but not walk. As noted earlier, a determination of the functional level is academic without an understanding of what the person needs or wants to do. To permit the significance of a disability to be estimated, the person's functional requirements or goals must be addressed.

Severity of the Limitation

For any specific functional limitation, the severity can be quantitated by timing the task and/or numerically expressing the degree of assistance needed (Table 4-2). Assistance to function may take the form of help from an assistive device or from a person (or animal). A person should not be penalized for the use of assistive devices; such a device is not a problem, but rather may be the solution to a person's functional need. In the assisted category of Table 4-2, standby assistance and supervision have been grouped with physical assistance because the commitment of an assistant's time (if not physical effort) is often as great (if not more) when providing supervision rather than physical assistance.

The 3-point scale shown in Table 4-2 has several desirable features: there are few enough categories to be easily remembered; the lowest level is 0 (in some scales, including the widely used FIM, 1 is the lowest level) (11); and the higher score reflects a higher level of function (some scales have 1 as the highest level and 7 as the lowest; they measure disability rather than independence); and the distinctions are clear-cut, which enhances reliability. Although Hamilton and colleagues (14) have reported good interrater reliability for the 7-point FIM scale, most clinicians experience difficulty in estimating the percentage of physical assistance needed. The most valid objection to a condensed scale like the one shown in Table 4-2 is the potential loss of sensitivity and responsiveness in the measure. This limitation can be obviated by evaluating a diversity of tasks and by timing them.

Independence from others may be an appropriate goal for some people with functional limitations, but not for all. Indeed, for a person with severe inflammatory polyarthritis, the demands of independence on inflamed joints may be harmful. In such circumstances, dependence on a visiting homemaker for housework may be preferable to a zealous

TABLE 4-2. *An ordinal scale to quantify functional ability*

Grade	Definition	Explanation
2	Independent	Completes the task without assistance, safely, and in a functional period of time. Aids permitted.
1	Assisted	Requires the physical or supervisory assistance of one or more persons to accomplish the task, safely, and in a functional period of time. However, the person actively participates, physically or otherwise.
0	Dependent	The person is unable to physically or verbally assist in performing the task.

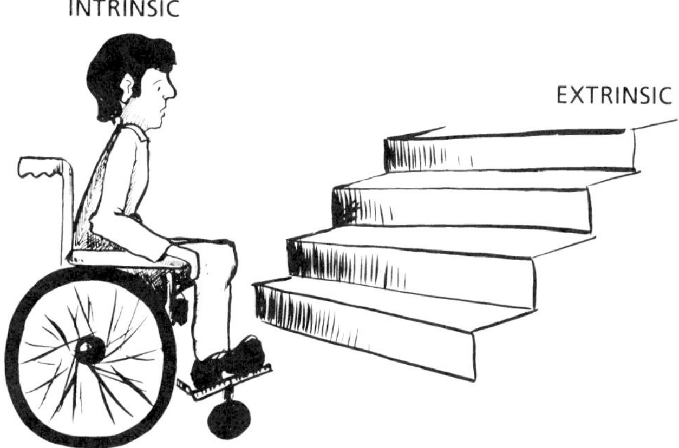

FIG. 4-4. Limiting factors may be intrinsic (e.g., weakness of leg muscles) or extrinsic (e.g., stairs).

drive for complete personal independence. Indeed, the goal may be to help the person accept a higher level of dependence. Although this may seem counterintuitive, remember that most able-bodied people also depend on other people for their standard of living.

Limiting Factors

Limiting factors are those that preclude a higher level of function. Their identification is of paramount importance to the clinician because a major component of the therapeutic strategy is aimed at correcting or bypassing these factors in people with significant disabilities. Limiting factors may be intrinsic or extrinsic (Fig. 4-4). Intrinsic limiting factors are the impairments due to a disease or condition (e.g., muscle weakness, limitation of motion). Extrinsic limiting factors are those in the environment (e.g., a flight of stairs, an employer's attitude) that preclude functioning at the limits of intrinsic capabilities (see section on Handicaps).

A cautionary note: the correction of one limiting factor may uncover others. For example, hip replacement may eliminate hip pain as the limiting factor to stair climbing, but uncover a previously unrecognized limitation, such as knee pain or dyspnea. Attempting to increase functional capacity can sometimes seem like peeling away the layers of an onion.

MANAGEMENT OF DISABILITIES

The specifics of management vary with the disease, the functional limitation, and the person. However, a few general principles will complete the conceptual framework. In choosing a therapeutic strategy to overcome a specific disability, the management can be broken down into four components:

- Ensure that the degree of significance of a disability is appropriate.
- Minimize the intrinsic limiting factors.
- Minimize the extrinsic limiting factors.
- Change the nature of the task.

Ensure that the Degree of Significance of a Disability is Appropriate

The important distinction between true and significant disability was described above. If a person with a bad back has adjusted to the fact that he or she can no longer perform a specific task, and accepts this limitation without any substantial sense of loss, then there is no reason why the clinician should be overly eager to restore this function. Ouslander and Beck (15) found that young health professionals tend to judge others as being in poorer health than do the people themselves.

In a gradually progressive disease such as arthritis or multiple sclerosis, however, the person may have unnecessarily accepted a diminished functional capacity. Although, as noted earlier, it is impossible to estimate accurately the appropriate extent of functional limitation from a knowledge of the physical impairments, some rough estimates are possible. If the person appears to be far more disabled than would have been anticipated, the clinician may be justified in attempting to raise the person's expectations, if satisfied that he or she is not paternalistically imposing goals on the person.

For a more acutely lost ability, when it appears that the precipitating event (e.g., spinal cord injury) is irreversible, then the physician's role may lie in helping the person lower his or her expectations appropriately (Fig. 4-5). The person may go through the stages of grief (e.g., denial, anger, bar-

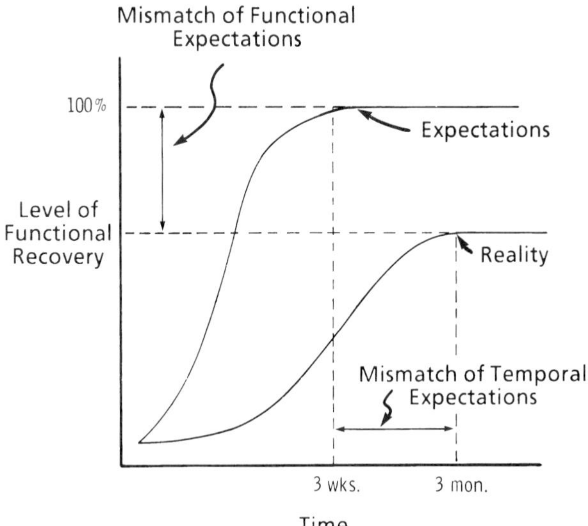

FIG. 4-5. A discrepancy may exist between expectations and reality with respect to the rate and extent of recovery that can be expected.

gaining), just as in the stages of grief leading to the acceptance of death. Whereas acceptance is the target before death, in adjusting to disability, the clinician hopes the person will then go beyond acceptance to adapt and achieve in spite of the loss. In helping a patient establish realistic goals, education and counseling are the tools at hand, and the coordinated efforts of an interdisciplinary team working with the patient and his or her family can be invaluable in this regard.

Minimize the Intrinsic Limiting Factors

Many of the intrinsic limiting factors (i.e., impairments) can be treated by such therapeutic modalities as patient education, behavioral strategies, drugs, physical measures, and surgery. These modalities are presented in detail in other chapters. Although a number of attributes (including an excellent understanding of disability and handicap) distinguish physiatrists from most other physicians, a major role of the physiatrist within the interdisciplinary team is to identify and remediate intrinsic limiting factors (e.g., the urinary tract infection, which is aggravating the spasticity, which is interfering with the seating position, which is preventing the wheelchair user from leaning forward, which prevents him from successfully propelling the wheelchair up an incline).

Minimize the Extrinsic Limiting Factors

As noted earlier, the limiting factors to an activity are often external (i.e., handicaps), including financial limitations, social circumstances, architectural barriers, and the attitudes of others. Some of these factors are amenable to the coordinated efforts of the team, particularly those of the social worker or the vocational counselor, but many reflect the physical environment and the society in which we live (16). Although there have been dramatic changes in these factors in this century, the evolution is far from complete. Notwithstanding the laudable efforts by many health-care professionals and people with disabilities to change the system, the role of members of the health-care team as advocates for an individual patient is to assist the person through the maze of barriers to a realistic endpoint.

Change the Nature of the Task

One of the most feasible and rewarding methods of addressing specific disabilities is to use aids and appliances to improve functional capacity through modification of the task. A patient may not have the endurance to walk up a hill to visit a friend, but a motorized scooter can make the visit possible. Before prescribing aids, however, the clinician should determine that the person is willing to comply with the trial-and-error, fine-tuning, and training that often is necessary and that there are no major external limiting factors (e.g., inability to pay for the device). Prescription of devices should be made with care, with input from appropriate members of the team, and preferably after a supervised trial with the aid.

Many of the aids and appliances that have been developed for people with functional difficulties are equally useful for the able bodied. Good ergonomic design benefits everyone and decreases the stigmatization that may accompany the use of a special device. There is tremendous technological scope for such therapies. Devices range from those as simple and inexpensive as a long handle for a comb to the highly elaborate environmental control systems and robotics available for people with the most severe disabilities.

CONCLUSION

In this chapter, the interrelated concepts of impairment, disability, and handicap have been described from the perspective of the practicing clinician, providing a framework for clinical evaluation and management.

REFERENCES

1. World Health Organization (WHO). *International classification of impairments, disabilities, and handicaps: a manual of classification relating to the consequences of disease*. Geneva, Switzerland: World Health Organization, 1980.
2. Chamie M. The status and use of the International Classification of Impairments, Disabilities and Handicaps (ICIDH). *World Health Stat Qu* 1990; 43:273–279.
3. Brandsma JW, Heerkens YF, van Ravensberg CD. The International Classification of Impairments, Disabilities and Handicaps (ICIDH): a manual of classification relating to the consequences of disease? *J Rehabil Sci* 1995; 8:2–7.
4. World Health Organization. Foreword to the 1993 reprint. *The International Classification of Impairments, Disabilities and Handicaps (ICIDH)*. Geneva, Switzerland: World Health Organization, 1993: 1–6.
5. Badley EM, Wagstaff S, Wood PH. Measures of functional ability (disability) in arthritis in relation to impairment of range of joint movement. *Ann Rheum Dis* 1984; 43:563–569.
6. Levack B, Rassmussen GL, Day S, Freeman MAR. Range of motion poor index of hip function. *Acta Orthop Scand* 1988; 59:14–15.
7. Hagglund KJ, Haley WE, Reveille JD, Alarcon GS. Predicting individual differences in pain and functional impairment among patients with rheumatoid arthritis. *Arthritis Rheum* 1989; 32:851–858.
8. Tinetti ME, Ginter SF. Identifying mobility dysfunctions in elderly patients: standard neuromuscular examination or direct assessment? *JAMA* 1988; 259:1190–1193.
9. Young A. Exercise physiology in geriatric practice. *Acta Med Scand* 1985; 711(suppl):227–232.
10. Fleckenstein SJ, Kirby RL, MacLeod DA. Effect of limited knee-flexion range on peak hip joint moments of force in humans transferring from sitting to standing. *J Biomech* 1988; 21:915–918.
11. Granger CV. A conceptual model for functional assessment. In: Granger CV, Gresham GE, eds. *Functional assessment in rehabilitation*. Baltimore: Williams & Wilkins, 1984; 14–25.
12. Stineman MG, Hamilton BB, Goin JE, Granger CV, Fiedler RC. Functional gain and length of stay for major rehabilitation impairment categories. Patterns revealed by function related groups. *Am J Phys Med Rehabil* 1996; 75:68–78.
13. Mittelsten-Scheid EE. Abilities and requirements profiles: a tool to facilitate reintegration of people with disabilities into employment. *Int J Rehabil* 1985; 7:82–84.
14. Hamilton BB, Laughlin JA, Fiedler R, Granger CV. Interrater reliability of the 7-level Functional Independence Measure (FIM). *Scand J Rehabil Med* 1994; 26:115–119.
15. Ouslander JG, Beck JC. Defining the health problems of the elderly. *Ann Rev Public Health* 1982; 3:55–83.
16. Zola IK. Toward the necessary universalizing of a disability policy. *Milbank Q* 1989; 67(suppl 2):401–428.

Rehabilitation Medicine: Principles and Practice, Third Edition,
edited by Joel A. DeLisa and Bruce M. Gans.
Lippincott–Raven Publishers, Philadelphia © 1998.

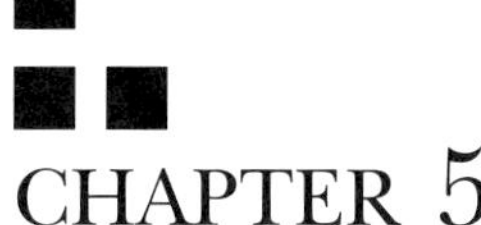

CHAPTER 5

Clinical Evaluation

Rolland P. Erickson and Malcolm C. McPhee

OVERVIEW

As with other branches of medicine, the cornerstone of rehabilitation medicine is a meticulous and germane patient evaluation. Therapeutic intervention must be based on proper patient assessment. The disability cannot be isolated from preexisting and concurrent medical problems. Although the rehabilitation evaluation encompasses all elements of the general medical history and physical examination, its scope is more comprehensive; thus, the rehabilitation evaluation provides a unique perspective.

The Rehabilitation Evaluation Is an Evaluation of Function

Medical diagnosis concentrates on the historical clues and physical findings that lead the examiner to the correct identification of disease. Once the medical diagnosis is established, the rehabilitation physician must then ascertain the functional consequences of disease that constitute the rehabilitation diagnosis. An adept functional assessment requires that the examiner have a clear understanding of the distinctions among disease, impairment, disability, and handicap, as discussed in Chapter 4.

If the disease cannot be challenged directly through medical or surgical means, measures are used to minimize the impairment. For example, a weak muscle can be strengthened or a hearing impairment can be minimized through an electronic aid. With chronic disorders, disease and impairment are not reducible; hence, intervention must address the disability and the handicap. The identification of intact functional capabilities is essential to successful rehabilitation. When intact capabilities can be augmented and adapted to new uses, functional independence can be enhanced.

R. P. Erickson and M. C. McPhee: Department of Physical Medicine and Rehabilitation, Mayo Clinic-Scottsdale, Scottsdale, Arizona 85259.

A.W. had gained much enjoyment and self-esteem as a competitive runner before his spinal cord injury. During and after inpatient rehabilitation, he vigorously pursued a cardiovascular and upper extremity conditioning program. After obtaining an ultra-lightweight sport wheelchair, he resumed competitive athletics as a wheelchair racer, winning several regional races.

Comment: A.W.'s intact capabilities included normal arm strength, a competitive spirit, and self-discipline. Through augmentation and adaptation, he regained enjoyment and self-esteem in his athletic endeavors.

Despite best efforts, the physician is occasionally unable to ascertain the specific disease responsible for a patient's constellation of historical, physical, and laboratory findings. Medical management must then be symptomatic. Although highly desirable, the diagnosis of disease is not a necessary prerequisite to the identification and subsequent management of functional loss. The rehabilitation physician will then attempt to characterize historically the temporal nature of the disease process in an effort to determine expectations of future disease activity based on past activity.

F.Z., a 62-year-old woman, presented with difficulty climbing stairs. Questioning revealed that she and her husband had been in the habit of taking a 30-minute evening walk for many years, but 2 years previously fatigue began to limit her to no more than a few blocks. During the previous year she had had difficulty rising from low seating, and 6 months previously she reluctantly quit taking the walks. During the preceding few weeks she had found that climbing stairs was a burden and had started taking showers because she needed assistance getting out of the bathtub.

F.Z. reported no sensory deficits. Physical examination showed hypotonic muscle stretch reflexes and predominantly proximal muscle weakness. Electrodiagnostic studies and muscle biopsy demonstrated a noninflammatory myopathy; however, further extensive evaluation failed to determine a cause. She was provided with a bath bench, a toilet seat riser, a lightweight folding wheelchair for long-distance mobility, and a cane for short distances. She was instructed in safe ambulation with a cane, operation of the wheelchair, energy conservation techniques, and the proper placement of bathroom safety bars. Safe automobile operation was documented, and she was provided with a parking sticker for handicapped people. The philosophy of rehabilitation medicine concerning her potentially progressive muscle weakness was discussed with her, and she was given supportive counseling.

When F.Z. returned for a follow-up examination 1 month later, muscle testing showed only slight progression of her weakness, and her functional capabilities had not changed. Another follow-up examination was scheduled for 6 weeks later.

Comment: Although a specific diagnosis of disease was not established, rehabilitation intervention specific to F.Z.'s functional losses was accomplished. Such extrapolations are not always accurate; however, serial evaluations performed at regular follow-up intervals allow the rehabilitation physician to identify and minimize future functional loss.

The Rehabilitation Evaluation Is Comprehensive

Unlike some medical specialities, rehabilitation medicine is not limited to a single organ system. Attention to the whole person is a rehabilitation absolute. The goal of a rehabilitation physician is to restore handicapped people to the fullest possible physical, mental, social, and economic independence; therefore, one must analyze a diverse aggregate of information to achieve the stated goal. Consequently, the person must be evaluated in relation to not only the disease but also the way in which the disease affects and is affected by the person's family and social environment, vocational responsibilities and economic state, avocational interests, hopes, and dreams.

C.C., a 63-year-old piano tuner, had a left cerebral infarction manifested only as minimal dominant right hand dysfunction. Despite demonstrating discrete digit function in the involved hand on physical examination, he was psychologically devastated to find that he could no longer accomplish the fine but elegant motor patterns necessary to perform his profession.

B.D., a 63-year-old corporate attorney, had a left cerebral infarction resulting in severe spastic weakness of his nondominant upper extremity. He accomplished some paperwork every day during his inpatient rehabilitation and returned to full-time employment shortly after dismissal.

Comment: For each person, the degree of impairment has little or no relationship to the severity of resultant disabilities and handicaps.

The Rehabilitation Evaluation Is Interdisciplinary

Although most of this chapter addresses the patient history and physical examination as they relate to the rehabilitation evaluation, these are only part of the comprehensive rehabilitation assessment. This statement is not meant to deprecate the usefulness of these traditional physician's tools. The patient interview and physical examination are of critical importance and serve as the basis for further evaluation; yet, by their nature, they are also limited. Speech and language disorders can inhibit communication. Subjective interpretation of the facts by the patient and by the family, when present, can cloud the objective assessment of function. Performance is not optimally assessed by interview.

For example, inquiry about ambulation skills during the interview may identify a potential problem, but they can be objectively and reliably assessed only by having the physician and physical therapist observe the patient during ambulation in various situations. Likewise, the occupational therapist must assess the performance of activities of daily living, and the rehabilitation nurse must assess the safety and judgment of the patient while in the ward. The speech therapist furnishes a measured assessment of language function and, through special communication skills, may obtain information from the patient that was missed during the interview. The rehabilitation psychologist provides a quantified and standardized assessment of cognitive and perceptual function and a skilled assessment of the patient's current psychological state. Through interaction with the patient's family and employer, the social worker can provide useful information that is otherwise unavailable regarding the patient's social support system and economic resources. The concept of the rehabilitation team applies not only to evaluation of the patient but also to the ongoing management of the patient.

SETTING AND PURPOSE

Because of the expanding scope of rehabilitation medicine, the evaluation setting can be diverse. A necessary corollary to the setting is the purpose of the evaluation. Both the setting and the purpose will have an impact on the format and extent of the evaluation. Traditionally, the inpatient rehabilitation unit has been the optimal setting for a comprehensive evaluation by the entire rehabilitation team. However, in these days of increasing medical costs and intervention by the government and other third-party payers, creativity is being used to accomplish comprehensive rehabilitation evaluations in the clinic and elsewhere in the community (Table 5-1).

PATIENT HISTORY

Ordinarily, the patient history is obtained via interview of the patient by the physician. If communication disorders and cognitive deficits are encountered during the rehabilitation evaluation, additional and collaborative information must be obtained from significant others accompanying the patient. The spouse and family members are valuable resources. The physician also may find it necessary to interview other caregivers, such as paid attendants, the public health nurse, and the home health agency aide.

The major components of the history are the chief complaint, history of the present illness, functional history, past medical history, review of systems, patient profile, and family history.

Chief Complaint

In assessing the chief complaint, the intent is to document the patient's primary concern in his or her own words. The complaint often is an impairment in the form of a symptom that implies a certain disease or group of diseases. The com-

TABLE 5-1. *The rehabilitation evaluation: setting and purpose*

Setting	Purpose
Hospital	
Inpatient rehabilitation unit	Comprehensive evaluation by team
Off-service consultation	Assessment by physician of potential for rehabilitation benefit
Clinic	
General rehabilitation clinic	Comprehensive evaluation by team
	Assessment by physician of potential for rehabilitation benefit
	Limited evaluation of specific musculoskeletal disorder
Special clinic	Limited evaluation of specific disease group (e.g., muscular dystrophy, sports injury)
Day rehabilitation program	Comprehensive evaluation by team
Impairment/disability clinic	Evaluation determined by requirement of referring agency (e.g., workers' compensation, Social Security)
Community	
Nursing home	Comprehensive evaluation by team
	Limited assessment by selected members of rehabilitaiton team
	Assessment by physician of potential for rehabilitation benefit
School	Limited evaluation of physical disability
	Limited evaluation for participation in sports
Transitional living facilities	Comprehensive evaluation by team
	Limited assessment of specific problem

plaint of "chest pain when I walk up a flight of stairs" suggests cardiac disease, and a report that "my hands ache and go numb when I drive" hints at carpal tunnel syndrome.

Of equal importance is recognition that the chief complaint, when lost function is expressed, also may be the first implication of a disability or handicap. The homemaker's report that "my balance has been getting worse and I've fallen several times" may be related to disease involving the vestibular system and to the disability created by unsafe ambulation. Similarly, the farmer's declaration that "I can no longer climb up onto my tractor" not only suggests a neuromuscular or orthopedic disease but also conveys to the physician that the disorder has resulted in a handicap by virtue of the inability to accomplish vocational expectations.

History of the Present Illness

The history of the present illness is obtained when the patient tells the story of the medical predicament. It is safe to state that all physicians at some time during their years of medical education have been admonished to "listen to your patients, for they will tell you their diagnosis." Few maxims are more true. When necessary, the patient should be asked to define the specific words he or she uses. It is often surprising to find out what "numbness" or "weakness" really means to some patients. At other times, specific questions relating to a particular symptom may help focus the interview. Using these techniques, the patient is gently guided by the physician to follow a chronologic sequence and to describe fully the symptoms and their consequences. Above all, the patient should be allowed to tell the story. More than one complaint may be elicited during the interview, and the physician should characterize each problem in an orderly fashion (Table 5-2) (1).

A complete list of current medications should be obtained. Polypharmacy is commonly encountered in people with chronic disease, at times with striking adverse effects. Side effects of medications can further impede cognition, psychological state, vascular reflexes, balance, bowel and bladder control, muscle tone, and coordination already impaired by the present illness or injury.

The history of the present illness should include a record of handedness, which is important in many areas of rehabilitation.

Functional History

The rehabilitation evaluation of chronic disease often shows lost function. Through the functional history, the physician must characterize the disabilities that have resulted from disease and identify remaining capabilities. It is considered part of the history of the present illness by some physicians and a separate segment of the patient interview by others. The examiner must know not only the functional status associated with the present illness but also the level

TABLE 5-2. *Analysis of symptoms*

1. Date of onset
2. Character and severity
3. Location and extension
4. Time relationships
5. Associated complaints
6. Aggravating and alleviating factors
7. Previous treatment and effects
8. Progress, noting remissions and exacerbations

From Department of Neurology and Department of Physiology and Biophysics, Mayo Clinic and Mayo Foundation. *Clinical examinations in neurology*, 6th ed. St. Louis: Mosby–Yearbook, 1991. By permission of the Mayo Foundation.

of function at one or more times before the present illness; therefore, we prefer to consider it separately.

Although the specific organization of the activities of daily living is somewhat variable, the following elements of personal independence remain constant: communication, eating, grooming, bathing, toileting, dressing, bed activities, transfers, and mobility.

When obtaining the functional history, the physician may record in a descriptive paragraph the patient's level of independence in each activity. However, functional stability is best communicated, followed over time, and made accessible for study when the physician uses a standard functional assessment scale, as discussed in Chapter 7.

Communication

A major component of rehabilitation is education; thus, communication is critical. The interviewer must assess the patient's communication options. In the clinical situation, this is an aspect of the evaluation in which the distinction between history and physical examination blurs. It is difficult to interact with the patient in a meaningful way without coincidentally examining his or her ability to communicate; significant speech and language deficiencies become obvious. However, for purposes of discussion, certain facets of the assessment relate more specifically to the history and will be discussed here. Additional facets are presented below in the section on the physical examination.

Speech pathology has provided clinicians with numerous classification systems for speech and language disorders (see Chapter 12). From a functional view, the elements of communication hinge on four abilities:

1. Listening
2. Reading
3. Speaking
4. Writing (2)

By assessing these factors, one can determine a patient's communication abilities.

Representative questions include the following:

Do you have difficulty hearing?
Do you use a hearing aid?
Do you have difficulty reading?
Do you need glasses to read?
Do others find it hard to understand what you say?
Do you have problems putting your thoughts into words?
Do you have difficulty finding words?
Can you write?
Can you type?
Do you use any communication aids?

Eating

The abilities to present solid food and liquids to the mouth, to chew, and to swallow are basic skills taken for granted by able-bodied people. However, in individuals with neurologic, orthopedic, or oncologic disorders, these tasks can be formidable. When dysfunctional, eating can be associated with far-reaching consequences, such as malnutrition, aspiration pneumonitis, and depression. As in the assessment of other skills for activities of daily living, inquiries about eating function should be specific and methodical.

Representative questions include the following:

Can you eat without help?
Do you have difficulty opening containers or pouring liquids?
Can you cut meat?
Do you have difficulty handling a fork, knife, or spoon?
Do you have problems bringing food or beverages to your mouth?
Do you have problems chewing?
Do you have difficulty swallowing solids or liquids?
Do you ever choke?
Do you regurgitate food or liquids through your nose?

Patients with nasogastric or gastrostomy tubes should be asked who helps them prepare and administer the feedings. The type, quantity, and schedule of feedings should be recorded.

Grooming

Grooming may not be considered as important as feeding. However, the inability to make oneself attractive and presentable to oneself and others can have injurious effects on one's body image and self-esteem, social sphere, and vocational options. Consequently, grooming skills should be of real concern to the rehabilitation team.

Representative questions include the following:

Can you brush your teeth without help?
Can you remove and replace your dentures without help?
Do you have problems fixing or combing your hair?
Can you apply your makeup independently?
Do you have problems shaving?
Can you apply deodorant without assistance?

Bathing

The ability to maintain cleanliness also has far-reaching psychosocial implications. In addition, deficits in cleaning can result in skin maceration and ulceration, skin and systemic infections, and the spread of disease to others. Independence in bathing should be sought.

Representative questions include the following:

Can you take a tub bath or shower without assistance?
Do you feel safe in the tub or shower?
Do you use a bath bench or shower chair?
Can you accomplish a sponge bath without help?
Are there parts of your body you cannot reach?

For patients with sensory deficits, bathing is also a convenient time for skin inspection, and inquiry about the patient's inspection habits should be made. For patients using a wheelchair, architectural barriers to bathroom entry should be determined.

Toileting

To the cognitively intact person, incontinence of stool or urine can be the most psychologically devastating deficit of personal independence. Ineffective bowel or bladder control has an adverse impact on self-esteem, body image, and sexuality and often prevents the sufferer from employment and social relationships. Dignity may even prohibit the person from venturing from the house for fear of an accident. Soiling of skin and clothing often results in ulceration, infection, and urologic complications. The rehabilitation physician should vigorously pursue toileting dependency with sensitivity.

Representative questions include the following:

Can you use the toilet without assistance?
Do you need help with clothing before or after using the toilet?
Do you need help with cleaning after a bowel movement?

For patients with indwelling urinary catheters, usual management of the catheter and leg bag should be understood. If bladder emptying is accomplished by intermittent catheterization, the examiner should learn who performs the catheterization and have a clear understanding of the technique used. For patients who have had ostomies for urine or feces, the examiner should determine who cares for the ostomy and ask to have the technique described.

Feminine hygiene is generally performed while on or near the toilet, so at this point in the interview it may be convenient to inquire about problems with sanitary napkin and tampon use.

Dressing

We dress to go out into the world—to be employed in the workplace, to dine in a restaurant, to be entertained in a public place, and to visit friends. Even within one's home, convention dictates that we dress to entertain anyone except close friends and family. We dress for protection, warmth, self-esteem, and pleasure. Dependency in dressing obviously results in a severe limitation to personal independence and should be investigated thoroughly during the rehabilitation interview.

Representative questions include the following:

Do you dress daily?
What articles of clothing do you regularly wear?
Do you require assistance putting on or taking off your underwear, shirt, slacks, skirt, dress, coat, stockings, panty hose, shoes, tie, or coat?
Do you need help with buttons, zippers, hooks, snaps, or shoelaces?
Do you use clothing modifications?

Bed Activities

The most basic stage of functional mobility is independence in bed activities. The importance of this functional level should not be underestimated. If a person cannot turn from side to side to redistribute pressure and periodically expose skin to the air, he or she is at high risk to develop pressure sores over bony prominences and skin maceration from heat and occlusion. For the person who cannot stand upright to dress, bridging (lifting the hips off the bed in the supine position) will allow the donning of underwear and slacks. Independence is likewise enhanced by an ability to move between a recumbent and a sitting position. Sitting balance is required to accomplish many other activities of daily living, including transfers.

Representative questions include the following:

Can you turn onto your front, back, and sides without assistance?
Can you lift your hips off the bed when supine?
Do you need help to sit or lie down?
Do you have difficulty maintaining a seated position?
Can you operate the bed controls on an electric hospital bed?

Transfers

The second stage of functional mobility is independence in transfers. Skills to move between a wheelchair and the bed, toilet, bath bench, shower chair, standard seating, or car seat often serve as precursors to independence in other areas. Although a male patient can use a urinal to void without transferring, a female patient cannot be independent in bladder care without the ability to transfer to the toilet and will probably require an indwelling catheter. Travel by airplane or train is difficult without the ability to transfer from the wheelchair to other seating. Bathing or showering is not independent without the ability to move to the bath bench or shower chair. The inability to transfer to a car seat precludes the use of a motor vehicle with standard seating. Also included in this category is the ability to move from a seated position to a standing position. Low seats without arm supports present a much greater problem than straight-backed chairs with arm supports.

Representative questions include the following:

Can you move between the bed, toilet, bath bench, shower chair, standard seating, or car seat and the wheelchair without assistance?
Can you get out of bed without difficulty?
Do you require assistance to stand from low or high seats?
Can you get on and off the toilet without help?

Mobility

Wheelchair Mobility

The next level of mobility to be assessed is operation of a wheelchair. Although wheelchair independence is more prone to inhibition by architectural barriers than is walking, it provides excellent mobility for the nonwalking person. With today's manual wheelchairs of lightweight materials and efficient engineering, the energy expenditure of wheeling on flat ground is only slightly higher than that of walking. With the addition of a motorized drive, battery power, and controls for speed and direction, a person without the upper extremity strength necessary to propel a manual wheelchair can still maintain significant independence in mobility.

Quantification of manual wheelchair skills can be accomplished in several ways. A person may report in feet, yards, meters, or city blocks the distance he or she is able to traverse before resting. Alternatively, the number of minutes one can continuously propel the chair can be specified, or the environment in which one is able to use the chair can be described (e.g., within a single room, around the house, or throughout the community).

Representative questions include the following:

Do you propel a wheelchair?
Do you need help to lock the wheelchair brakes before transfers?
Do you require assistance to cross high-pile carpets, rough ground, or inclines?
How far or how many minutes can you wheel before you must rest?
Can you independently move about your living room, bedroom, and kitchen?
Do you go shopping, to restaurants, and to friends' homes?

With any of these functional levels of wheelchair mobility, the patient should be asked what keeps him or her from going farther and whether help is needed to lift the wheelchair into an automobile.

Ambulation

The final level of mobility is ambulation. In the narrow sense of the word, ambulation is walking, and we have used this definition to simplify the following discussion. However, within the sphere of rehabilitation, ambulation often is any useful means of movement from one place to another. In the view of many rehabilitation professionals, the bilateral above-knee amputee ambulates with a manual wheelchair, the patient with C4 tetraplegia ambulates with a motorized wheelchair, and a polio victim in an underdeveloped country might ambulate by crawling. To some, driving a motor vehicle also is a form of ambulation. Ambulation ability can be quantified in the same ways as wheelchair mobility. A person may report the distance he or she is able to walk, the duration between necessary rest periods, or the scope of the environment within which he or she walks.

Representative questions include the following:

Do you walk unaided?
Do you use a cane, crutches, or a walker to walk?
How far or how many minutes can you walk before you must rest?
What stops you from going farther?
Do you feel unsteady or do you fall?
Can you go upstairs and downstairs unassisted?
Do you go shopping, to restaurants, and to friends' homes?
Can you use public transportation (e.g., bus, subway) without assistance?

Operation of a Motor Vehicle

In the perceptions of many patients, full independence in mobility is not attained until one is able to accomplish independent operation of a motor vehicle. Although driving skills are by no means a necessity to an urban dweller with readily available public transportation, they are of great importance to a person living in a suburban or rural environment. Driving skills should always be assessed in patients of driving age.

Representative questions include the following:

Do you have a valid driver's license?
Do you own a car?
Do you drive your car to go shopping, to restaurants, and to friends' homes?
Do you drive in heavy traffic or over long distances?
Do you use hand controls or other automobile modifications?
Have you experienced any motor vehicle accidents or received any citations for improper operation of a motor vehicle since your illness or injury?

Past Medical History

The past medical history is a record of a patient's significant illness, trauma, and health maintenance during his or her life. The effects of certain past conditions will continue to affect the present level of function. Identification of these conditions affords the rehabilitation physician the opportunity to better characterize the patient's baseline functional level before the present disorder. The examiner must take special care to decipher whether the patient's diagnostic terms accurately represent the true diagnoses. Although many past conditions associated with significant immobilization, deconditioning, and disability are themselves amenable to rehabilitation measures, they will tend to define the goals for future rehabilitation efforts.

P.B., a 66-year-old woman, was referred for rehabilitation after right above-knee amputation due to vascular disease. The past history was significant for a right cerebral infarction 7 years earlier. Despite comprehensive rehabilitation after the stroke, she was able to ambulate only one block with a quadripod cane and ankle-foot orthosis because of spastic left hemiparesis.

Comment: After prosthetic fitting and training, most people in P.B.'s age group with an above-knee amputation regain ambulation skills, although many will require a cane or other gait aid. However, because she had significant ambulation disability due to the left hemiparesis that occurred before amputation, rehabilitation goals included a wheelchair prescription, with consideration of a hemi-chair if she could not accomplish wheeling with the left arm, and training in wheelchair activities. Even though ambulation beyond a few yards was not feasible, a preparatory prosthesis with manual knee lock was provided on a trial basis to determine whether it aided transfers. In this example, ambulation disability was dictated more by previous impairments than by impairments associated with the present illness.

All elements of the standard past medical history should be completed; however, a history of neurologic, cardiopulmonary, or musculoskeletal disease should alert the rehabilitation physician. Psychiatric disorders are also of special interest to the rehabilitation physician and are discussed below in the section on the psychological and psychiatric history.

Neurologic Disorders

Most frequently encountered in older populations but possibly present in any age group, a past history of neurologic disease can have a tremendous impact on the rehabilitation outcome of an unrelated present illness. Whether congenital or acquired, preexisting cognitive impairment places restrictions on educationally oriented rehabilitation intervention. Disorders with sensory manifestations such as loss of touch, pain, or joint position and afflictions characterized by perceptual dysfunction retard the patient's ability to monitor performance during the acquisition of new functional skills. These maladies also render the patient more likely to be unresponsive to soft-tissue injury from prolonged or excessive skin surface pressures during periods of immobility. When they are coupled with pre-existing visual or auditory impairment, function is further encumbered. Likewise, a residual motor deficit can inhibit new motor learning through spasticity, weakness, or decreased endurance. A diligent search for antecedent neurologic disease is a fundamental part of the rehabilitation evaluation.

Cardiopulmonary Disorders

In patients with motor disabilities, activities of daily living are accomplished with higher than normal energy cost. When pre-existing cardiopulmonary disorders limit the capacity to tolerate the greater energy expenditures imposed on the patient by the motor disability, further functional deficits follow. This is also the case with many forms of hematologic, renal, and hepatic dysfunctions. The physician is encouraged to gather as much cardiopulmonary data as needed to estimate cardiac reserve accurately. Only when disease of the cardiopulmonary system is identified can rehabilitation be tailored and medical intervention be initiated to maximize cardiac reserve.

Musculoskeletal Disorders

Weakness, joint ankylosis or instability from previous trauma or arthritis, amputation, and other musculoskeletal dysfunctions can all deleteriously affect functional capacity. A search for such disorders is a necessary prerequisite to a complete rehabilitation evaluation.

Review of Systems

The systems are reviewed to screen for clues to disease not otherwise identified in the history of the present illness and the past medical history. A thorough review should always be completed. Many diseases have potential for adverse effects on rehabilitation outcome. However, as described previously, certain disorders are of special interest to the rehabilitation physician. This part of the evaluation considers constitutional, head and neck, respiratory, cardiovascular, gastrointestinal, genitourinary, neurologic, and musculoskeletal symptoms.

Constitutional Symptoms

Of particular interest to the examiner are suggestions of infection and nutritional deficiency. Fatigue can be a prominent complaint in patients with multiple sclerosis.

Head and Neck Symptoms

Vision, hearing, and swallowing deficits must be identified.

Respiratory Symptoms

Any pulmonary condition that inhibits the delivery of oxygen to the tissues will adversely affect endurance. Symptoms such as the following should be identified: dyspnea, cough, sputum, hemoptysis, wheezing, and pleuritic chest pain.

Cardiovascular Symptoms

The manifestations of heart disease restrict cardiac reserve and endurance. When identified, many can be ameliorated through medical management. Identification of arrhythmias is important for the prevention of recurrent strokes of embolic cause. The presence of the following symptoms should be determined: chest pain, dyspnea, orthopnea, palpitations, and lightheadedness.

Peripheral vascular disease is the leading cause of amputation. The potential for ulceration and gangrene from bed rest, orthoses, pressure garments, and other rehabilitation equipment can be minimized if peripheral disease is recognized. The patient should be asked about claudication, foot ulcers, and varicosities.

Gastrointestinal Symptoms

Almost any form of gastrointestinal disease can result in nutritional deficiency, a particularly insidious condition that limits rehabilitation efforts more frequently than previously realized (3). Bowel control is of special interest in patients with neurologic disorders. The patient should be asked about incontinence, bowel care techniques, and use of laxatives.

Genitourinary Symptoms

Manifestations of neurogenic bladder must be sought. Questions about the following should be asked: specific fluid intake, voiding schedules, specific bladder emptying techniques, urgency, frequency, incontinence, retention and incomplete emptying, sensation of fullness and voiding, dysuria, pyuria, infections, flank pain, hematuria, and renal stones.

For female patients, a menstrual and pregnancy history should be obtained, and inquiries about dyspareunia, vaginal and clitoral sensation, and orgasm should be made. Male patients should be asked about erection, ejaculation, progeny, and pain during intercourse.

Neurologic Symptoms

Because of the high prevalence of neurologic disorders in patients in a rehabilitation program, a methodical neurologic review should always be performed. The following items should be addressed: sense of smell, diplopia, blurred vision, field cuts, imbalance, vertigo, tinnitus, weakness, tremors, involuntary movements, convulsions, depressed level of consciousness, ataxia, loss of touch, pain, temperature, dysesthesias, hyperpathia, and changes in memory and "thinking."

Chewing, swallowing, hearing, reading, and speaking may be addressed in either the functional history or the review of systems. Inquiry about psychological and psychiatric issues can be made either during the review of symptoms or, as we prefer, when obtaining the psychosocial history for the patient profile.

Musculoskeletal Symptoms

The musculoskeletal review also must be extremely thorough because of the high frequency of musculoskeletal dysfunction in patients in a rehabilitation program. Inquiry should be made regarding the following: muscle pain, weakness, fasciculation, atrophy, hypertrophy, skeletal deformities and fractures, limited joint motion, joint stiffness, joint pain, and swelling of soft tissues and joints.

Patient Profile

The patient profile provides the interviewer with information about the patient's present and past psychological state, social milieu, and vocational background.

Personal History

Psychological and Psychiatric History

Any present illness accompanied by functional loss is of itself psychologically challenging. A quiescent major psychiatric disturbance can resurface during such stressful times to hinder or halt rehabilitation efforts. When the examiner is able to identify a history of psychiatric dysfunction, the necessary support systems to lessen the chances of recrudescence can be applied prophylactically during the rehabilitation process. The examiner is encouraged to seek a history of previous psychiatric hospitalization, psychotropic pharmacologic intervention, or psychotherapy. The patient should be screened for past or current anxiety, depression and other mood changes, sleep disturbances, delusions, hallucinations, obsessive and phobic ideas, and past major and minor psychiatric illness. A review of the patient's prior and current responses to stress often helps us to understand and modify behavioral responses to catastrophic illness or trauma. Therefore, it is important to know the patient's emotional responses to previous illness and family troubles and how the stress of the current illness is being addressed. Tests to clarify psychological symptoms or a personality disturbance may be requested from a clinical psychologist if initial screening results suggest abnormality.

Life-Style. Leisure activities can promote both physical and emotional health. The patient's leisure habits should be reviewed to identify special rehabilitation measures that might return independence in these activities. Examples of questions to consider include the following (4):

What sort of interests does the patient have?

Does the patient most enjoy physical endeavors, sports, the outdoors, and mechanical avocations (i.e., motor oriented)?

Is the patient more interested in intellectual pursuits (i.e., symbol oriented)?

Does the patient derive the most pleasure from social interactions, organizations, and group functions (i.e., interpersonally oriented)?

Has the patient been actively pursuing these interests?

The work-oriented person without avocational interests before the present illness will need recreational counseling during rehabilitation.

Diet. Inadequate nutrition may inhibit rehabilitation efforts. In addition, even after initial myocardial and cerebrovascular events due to atherosclerosis, some secondary prevention can be accomplished through dietary manipulation. The patient's ability to prepare meals and snacks, usual dietary habits, and special diets should be determined.

Alcohol and Drugs. Drug, alcohol, and nicotine use must be assessed. Patients with cognitive, perceptual, and motor deficits can be further impaired to a dangerous degree through substance abuse. Drugs and alcohol are frequent factors in the cause of head and spinal cord injury. Identification of abuse and dependency provides the opportunity to

TABLE 5-3. *The CAGE questionnaire*

1. Have you ever felt you ought to ***C***ut down on your drinking?
2. Have people ***A***nnoyed you by criticizing your drinking?
3. Have you ever felt bad or ***G***uilty about your drinking?
4. Have you ever had a drink first thing in the morning to steady your nerves or get rid of a hangover (***E***yeopener)?

Reprinted with permission from Ewing JA. Detecting alcoholism: the CAGE questionnaire. *JAMA* 1984; 252:1905–1907.

modify future behaviors through counseling. The CAGE questionnaire is a brief but useful screening vehicle for the identification of alcohol abuse and dependency (Table 5-3); a single affirmative answer should initiate further investigation (5).

Social History

Family

Catastrophic illness in a family member places enormous stress on the rest of the family. When the family is already facing other problems with interaction, health, or substance abuse, the potential for disintegration of the family unit is greater. This is unfortunate because the availability of a sturdy system of family and friends can be as predictive of disposition as functional outcome. The patient's marriage history and status should be determined. Other family members who live at home and their names and ages should be sought. The established roles of each member should be clearly understood (e.g., who handles the finances, the cooking, the cleaning, the discipline). Determine whether other family members live nearby. For all potential assistants, inquire about their willingness and ability to participate in the care of the family member and about their work or school schedule to ascertain potential availability.

Home

The patient's home design should be reviewed for architectural barriers. Determine whether the patient owns or rents, the location of the home (e.g., urban, suburban, or rural), the distance between the home and rehabilitation services, the number of steps into the home, the presence of or room for entry ramps, and the accessibility of the kitchen, bath, bedroom, and living room.

Vocational History

Education and Training

Although the level of education does not predict intellectual function, the educational level achieved by the patient may suggest intellectual skills upon which the rehabilitation team could draw during the patient's convalescence. In addition, when coupled with the assessment of physical function, the educational background will dictate future educational and training needs. The years of education completed by the patient and whether high school, undergraduate, or graduate degrees were obtained are determined and the patient's performance reviewed. The acquisition of special skills, licenses, and certifications is noted. Future vocational goals are always important to address but are of particular concern with adolescent patients. Discussion of these goals will indicate the need for and type of interest, aptitude, and skills testing and vocational counseling appropriate for the patient.

Work History

An understanding of the patient's work experience can also determine whether further education and training will be necessary. In addition, it provides an idea of the patient's motivation, reliability, and self-discipline. The duration and type of previous jobs and the reason for job changes are recorded. Not only titles but also actual job descriptions must be obtained, and the patient should be asked about architectural barriers at the workplace. These principles apply equally to the patient who is a homeworker. The evaluator must define the specific work expectations relating to meal preparation, shopping, home maintenance, cleaning, child rearing, and discipline. In addition, the patient should be asked where the clothes washing is done and whether architectural barriers prevent the patient from reaching appliances or areas in the home and yard.

Finances

The physician should have a basic understanding of the patient's income, investment, and insurance resources, disability classifications, and debts.

Family History

The family history is used to identify hereditary disease within the family and to assess the health of people within the patient's home support system. Knowledge of the health and fitness of the spouse and other family members may be very important in dismissal planning.

PHYSICAL EXAMINATION

The physical examination performed by the rehabilitation physician shares much with the general medical examination. Of necessity, it is a well-practiced art. Through perceptions gleaned from observation, palpation, percussion, and auscultation, the examining physician seeks physical findings to support and formulate the diagnosis further and to screen for other conditions not suggested by the history.

The physical examination also is different from the general medical examination. After investigating the physical findings that help to establish the medical diagnosis, the rehabilitation physician still has two principal tasks:

1. To scrutinize the patient for physical findings to define the disabilities and handicaps that emanate from the disease.
2. To identify remaining physical, psychological, and intellectual strengths to serve as the base from which to re-establish functional independence.

In this characterization, rehabilitation medicine places special emphasis on the orthopedic and neurologic examinations, and functional assessment becomes an integral part of the examination.

Severe motor, cognitive, and communication impairments make it difficult or impossible for some patients to follow through with directions from the physician and place limitations on certain traditional physical examination maneuvers. Creativity is often required to accomplish the examination. Particularly expert examination skills are necessary in such situations.

We assume that the reader has developed competence in the performance of the general medical examination (6). In the following discussion, priority is placed on the aspects of the physical examination that have special relevance to rehabilitation medicine. The major segments of the physical examination in rehabilitation medicine are the following: vital signs and general appearance, integument and lymphatics, head, eyes, ears, nose, mouth and throat, neck, chest, heart and peripheral vascular system, abdomen, genitourinary system and rectum, musculoskeletal system, neurologic examination, and functional examination.

Vital Signs and General Appearance

The recording of blood pressure, pulse, temperature, weight, and general observations is important. The identification of hypertension may be meaningful to the secondary prevention of stroke and myocardial infarction. Supine, sitting, and standing blood pressures should be obtained to rule out orthostasis in any patient with unexplained falls, lightheadedness, or dizziness. Tachycardia can be the initial manifestation of sepsis in a patient with high-level tetraplegia or can suggest pulmonary embolism in an immobilized patient. Initial weight recordings are invaluable to identify and follow up malnutrition, obesity, and fluid and electrolyte disorders common to various forms of brain injury. A notation is made if patients are hostile, tense, or agitated, or if their behavior is uncooperative, inappropriate, or preoccupied. The gestalt of a patient at initial contact can reveal problems not recognized at close scrutiny.

Integument and Lymphatics

Skin disorders are frequently encountered in rehabilitation medicine. Prolonged pressure in patients with peripheral vascular disease, sensory disorders, immobility, and altered consciousness often results in damage to skin and underlying tissues. Many diseases common to disabled people, and their treatments, render the skin more prone to trauma and infection. Skin problems that are only bothersome to able-bodied people can be devastating to those with disabilities when these problems prevent the use of prostheses, orthoses, and other devices. Workers providing rehabilitation services to patients with cancer often confront lymphedema in the extremities after proximal node excision and irradiation.

The skin is inspected in good light. If the skin is considered as each separate body region is examined, the entire body surface can be studied without total exposure of the patient. In particular, the skin over bony prominences and in contact with prosthetic and orthotic devices is examined for lichenification, erythema, or breakdown. Intertriginous areas are inspected for maceration and ulceration; the distal lower extremities in patients with vascular disease are examined for pigmentation, hair loss, and breakdown; and the hands and feet in insensate patients are observed for unrecognized trauma. All common lymph node sites are palpated for enlargement and tenderness, and areas of edema are palpated for pitting.

Head

The head is inspected for signs of past or present trauma. Gentle palpation is performed for evidence of previous trauma or neurosurgical procedures, shunt pumps, and other craniofacial abnormalities. Auscultation for bruits is done when considering vascular malformations.

Eyes

Unrecognized acuity errors can hamper rehabilitation efforts, especially in patients needing good eyesight to compensate for disorders of other sensory systems. With the patient's usual eyewear in place, far and near vision is tested with the use of standard charts. If charts are not available, the patient's vision is compared with the examiner's vision by object identification and description for far vision and by reading material of several print sizes for near vision. Findings are substantiated with refraction when circumstances permit. A funduscopic examination is performed; if dilatory agents are necessary, one of short duration is used, and notation is made in the patient's chart of the time of administration and the name of the preparation. Evidence of erythema and inflammation of the globe or conjunctiva is sought; aphasic patients and those with altered consciousness may not adequately express the pain of acute glaucoma or the discomfort of conjunctivitis. The eyes of comatose patients are inspected for inadequate lid closure; corneal ulcerations from deficient lubrication should be prevented.

Ears

Unrecognized hearing impairment also may limit rehabilitation efforts. Hearing acuity is checked with the "watch test" or by having the patient repeat words presented with a whispered voice. If a unilateral hearing deficit is identified, Weber and Rinne tests are used to determine whether it is a nerve or conductive loss. Findings are substantiated with an audiogram. An otoscopic examination is performed. If otorrhea is present in head-injured patients, the presence of sugar, which would indicate cerebrospinal fluid, is assessed using Benedict's solution.

Nose

A routine examination of the nose generally suffices. If clear or blood-tinged drainage is noted in head-injured patients, the presence of cerebrospinal fluid is determined.

Mouth and Throat

The oral and pharyngeal mucosa is inspected for poor hygiene and infections (e.g., candidiasis in patients taking corticosteroids and broad-spectrum antibiotics), the teeth for disrepair, and the gums for gingivitis or hypertrophy. Dentures are checked for fit and maintenance needs. In patients with arthritis or trauma, the temporomandibular joints are inspected and palpated for crepitation, tenderness, swelling, or limited motion. Any of these problems can threaten food intake and result in poor nutrition.

Neck

A routine examination of the neck generally suffices. One should be sure to listen for carotid bruits in patients with atherosclerosis and cerebrovascular disorders. In patients with musculoskeletal disorders, range of motion (ROM) is assessed. However, neck motion is not checked in patients with recent trauma or chronic polyarthritides until radiographic studies have ruled out fracture or instability.

Chest

Tolerance to exercise is significantly affected by pulmonary function. For the patient in whom exercise tolerance is already compromised by neurologic or musculoskeletal disease, the examiner must rigorously search for pulmonary dysfunction to minimize the deficit. The standard medical maneuvers are usually sufficient; however, certain aspects of the chest examination merit mention.

The chest wall is inspected to note the rate, amplitude, and rhythm of breathing. The presence of cough, hiccups, labored breathing, accessory muscle activity, and chest wall deformities is noted. Rheumatologic disorders such as the late stages of HLA-B27 arthropathies and scleroderma restrict respiratory excursion and lead to shallow, tachypneic respirations. Likewise, restrictive pulmonary disease with hypoventilation is common in muscular dystrophy and other congenital diseases of the motor unit, severe kyphoscoliosis, and chronic spinal cord injuries. Tachypnea and tachycardia may be the only readily apparent manifestations of pulmonary embolism, pneumonia, or sepsis in patients with high-level spinal cord injuries. The finding of a barrel chest may lead the examiner to document obstructive pulmonary disease so that medical management can minimize its effect on function.

The patient is instructed to cough, and notation is made of the force and efficiency of this action. If the cough is weak, the patient is assisted by exerting manual pressure over the abdomen coincidentally with the cough attempt to observe the effect. The chest wall is palpated for tenderness, deformity, and transmitted sounds. During the acute care of a head-injured patient, rib fractures can be missed. Percussion is performed to document diaphragmatic level and excursion. Auscultation is performed to characterize breath sounds and identify wheezes, rubs, rhonchi, and rales. Pneumonitis can be especially insidious in the immunosuppressed patient.

When pulmonary disease is suggested, it is documented with function tests and determination of blood gas levels. If the patient has a tracheostomy, the skin around the opening is examined, the type of apparatus is recorded, and cuff leaks are noted. Any opportunity to screen for breast malignancy in both men and women should not be wasted.

Heart and Peripheral Vascular System

Like pulmonary disease, cardiovascular dysfunction can adversely affect exercise tolerance already encumbered by neurologic or musculoskeletal disease. When cardiovascular disorders are identified, intervention can relieve or reduce the deleterious effects on exercise tolerance and general health. Secondary prevention of embolic stroke is contingent on the identification of arrhythmias, valvular disease, and congenital anomalies. The general medical cardiac examination will suffice.

In the clinical situation, the peripheral circulation is usually assessed during scrutiny of the extremities. When bracing is contemplated, one should always search for the pallor and cool dystrophic skin of arterial occlusive disease; inappropriate devices may lead to skin breakdown and subsequent amputation. Deep venous thrombosis is a major risk to patients immobilized by other conditions. When venous stasis and incompetency complicate the situation, the risk is greater. A search is made for varicose and incompetent veins. Bedside Doppler studies should be used whenever necessary to help delineate arterial or venous concerns. Evaluation is done to determine the presence of Raynaud's phenomenon.

Abdomen

In many patients, the general medical examination of the abdomen will be all that is necessary to screen for abnormality and assess gastrointestinal complaints. Again, however, special situations warrant mention. In patients with widespread spasticity, such as occurs with multiple sclerosis and myelopathy, inspection and auscultation are done before attempting palpation and percussion. Manipulation of the abdominal wall often results in a wave of increased tone that will temporarily render the remainder of the abdominal examination difficult or impossible to accomplish. Vigorous abdominal palpation in patients with disordered peristalsis from certain central nervous system diseases may initiate regurgitation of stomach contents. Such patients are examined gently when they are in the semireclined position.

Genitourinary System and Rectum

The genitalia should be examined during any comprehensive evaluation. However, a thorough examination of the male and female genitalia is particularly necessary to evaluate patients with disorders of continence, micturition, and sexual function. In the presence of incontinence in either gender and in male patients using an external collecting device such as the condom catheter, maceration and ulceration can result. Examination of the penile skin in male patients, the periurethral mucosa in female patients, and all intertriginous perineal areas for maceration and ulceration is performed. The scrotal contents are palpated for orchitis and epididymitis in male patients with indwelling catheters. Incontinence from neurogenic causes is common in the rehabilitation population; however, the examiner should not miss a cystocele or other remediable structural cause for the incontinence. Patients with chronic indwelling catheters should be checked for external urethral meatal ulceration and male patients for penile fistulas. Whenever urinary retention is suspected, the physical examination should be followed by an in-and-out catheterization to measure the amount of residual urine.

The rehabilitation assessment is not completed without digital examination of the rectum, anus, anal tone, and perineal sensation. In any patient with suspected central nervous system, autonomic, or pelvic disease, the bulbocavernosus reflex is evaluated. This is accomplished by firmly compressing the glans of the penis or clitoris with one hand while inserting the index finger of the other hand into the anus to monitor sphincter tone. Sphincter tone is increased with many upper motor lesions and decreased or absent with neurogenic disease of or peripheral to the sacral cord (S2–S4).

Musculoskeletal System

Disorders of the musculoskeletal system are a major portion of the pathologic conditions addressed by the rehabilitation physician. The examiner must possess expert skills in the evaluation of all musculoskeletal components; while attending to each body region, the bone, joint, cartilage, ligament, tendon, and muscle should be assessed in an orderly fashion. To accomplish this task, full familiarity with surface landmarks and the underlying anatomy is needed.

Assignment of many examination components to the musculoskeletal and neurologic examinations is an arbitrary exercise because neuromusculoskeletal function is so integrated. For discussion, examination of the musculoskeletal system is divided into inspection, palpation, ROM assessment, joint stability assessment, and muscle strength testing.

Inspection

Inspection is done for scoliosis, abnormal kyphosis, and lordosis; joint deformity, amputation, absence and asymmetry of body parts (leg-length discrepancy); soft-tissue swelling, mass, scar, and defect; and muscle fasciculations, atrophy, hypertrophy, and rupture. At times, the dysfunction is subtle and decipherable only through careful observation of the patient. While proceeding with the examination, the physician makes note of any wary and tentative movements of the patient in pain, of the exaggerated and inconsistent conduct of the malingerer, and of the bizarre behavior of the hysterical patient.

Palpation

Localized abnormalities identified through inspection and body regions of concern to the patient should be palpated to ascertain the structural origin of tenderness and deformity. For any such abnormality, it is important to first determine whether the basic consistency is that of soft tissue or bone and whether it is of normal anatomic structure. For soft-tissue abnormalities, an attempt is made to identify them further as pitting or nonpitting edema, synovitis, or a mass.

All skeletal elements near areas of hemorrhage and ecchymosis in patients with altered consciousness are palpated. The elderly patient with traumatic subdural hematoma may have experienced an extremity fracture associated with a fall. During the critical care of a motorcyclist with a head injury, an incidental fracture may have been missed. Likewise, any in-hospital fall by a confused patient warrants a search for occult bony trauma.

Range-of-Motion Assessment

Human joint motion is measured during clinical evaluation by many health-care professionals for various reasons, including initial evaluation, evaluation of treatment procedure, feedback to a patient, assessment of work capacity, or research studies. Of the different methods available, we prefer to regard the anatomic position as the baseline (zero starting point) when identifying a starting point for measuring the ROM of a joint. If rotation is being measured, the midway point between the normal rotation range is chosen as the zero starting point. The technique of measurement was published in detail by Norkin and White (7).

Considerable variation exists among people when ROM measurements are compared. Factors such as age, gender, conditioning, obesity, and genetics can influence the normal ROM. A publication of the American Academy of Orthopaedic Surgeons includes average ranges of joint motion for the joints of the human body (8).

When the patient does not assist the examiner while the joint is taken through a ROM, the measurement is a passive ROM. If the patient performs the ROM without assistance from the examiner, then the range is an active ROM. If comparisons are made between active and passive ROM, the starting position, stabilization, goniometer, alignment, and type of goniometer should be the same.

Different methods of recording the results of the ROM measurements are available. Graphic recordings are often helpful if feedback to the patient or to a third party is needed. Sometimes the lag between the patient's range and a normal range is of special interest to the examiner, such as when the surgeon wants to periodically evaluate finger motion as a guide to recovery after a hand operation.

The goniometer position, starting position, and average ROM of the more commonly measured joints are shown in Figures 5-1 through 5-26.

Joint Stability Assessment

Joint stability is the capacity of the structural elements of a joint to resist forces of inappropriate vector. It is determined by the degree of bony congruity, cartilaginous and capsular integrity, ligament and muscle strength, and the forces required of the joint. For example, the ball-and-socket arrangement of the hip joint is inherently stable because of bony congruity, whereas the glenohumeral joint must rely on musculoligamentous support because of the incongruity of the spherical humeral head in relation to the flat glenoid fossa.

Joint stability is often compromised by disorders common to rehabilitation medicine. Inflammatory synovitis associated with polyarthritis weakens the joint capsule and surrounding ligaments, and the resulting pain inhibits muscle contraction. This inhibition renders the involved joint susceptible to trauma from normal and abnormal forces and leads to joint instability. Instability of extremity and spinal joints is common in traumatic and neurogenic conditions.

Excessive joint motion is often identified during the ROM assessment. However, several specialized physical examination maneuvers (e.g., Larson's test, Lachman's test, pivot-shift test) provide the examiner with tools to assess individual joint integrity. Although a discussion of each of these tests is beyond the scope of this chapter, excellent texts are available (6,9,10).

The stability of each joint is assessed in an orderly fashion. A routine series of individual joint maneuvers is used as part of the general examination, and additional tests are performed as necessary to identify more subtle instability when suggested by the history or general examination.

If joint instability is recognized or suspected by physical examination, radiographic studies are often helpful for quantifying the extent of instability. At times, flexion-extension views of the spine and stressed joint views of extremity joints can be helpful; however, these should never be considered until the physical examination and nonstressed films have determined such maneuvers to be safe.

Muscle Strength Testing

Manual muscle testing provides an important means of assessing strength but also can be viewed as a means of assessing weakness. The examiner needs to keep in mind many factors that can affect the effort that a patient is willing to put into the testing. Such factors are age, gender, pain, fatigue, low motivation, fear, misunderstanding of the test, and the presence of lower or upper motor neuron disease.

Lower motor neuron diseases result in patterns of motor loss that depend on the location of the disease. For example, a peripheral neuropathy shows a pattern of weakness in the muscles supplied by the affected nerve, or the residual weakness in poliomyelitis is often scattered. The flaccid characteristic of a paretic muscle or muscle group in lower motor neuron disease allows the testing procedure to be uncomplicated by the spasticity or rigidity of upper motor neuron disease. Knowledge of the appearance of the muscle surface when a muscle undergoes atrophy from lower motor neuron disease also can be helpful to the clinician. If the joint crossed by the muscle being tested is unstable because of a chronic flaccid state, the grade of weakness may be much more difficult to estimate.

Upper motor neuron diseases frequently result in spastic muscles, which make manual testing challenging. For example, the antagonist muscle may be spastic and resist the action of the muscle being tested, or contractures may have developed, complicating the testing by limiting the available ROM.

For a detailed discussion of the technique of manual muscle testing, the reader is referred to the publications of Kendall and McCreary (11) or Daniels and Worthingham (12). The anatomic basis for manual muscle testing of the major groups of muscles is discussed below (1).

Outline of Anatomic Information Required for Tests of Strength of Specific Muscles

In the following descriptions of the tests, the name of each muscle is followed in parentheses by the corresponding peripheral nerve and spinal segmental supply. There is considerable variability in segmental supply, particularly to certain muscles, as given by different authorities. Furthermore, there is some anatomic variation both in the plexuses and in the peripheral nerves. Therefore, the segments listed cannot be regarded as absolute. The principal and usual supply is underlined. Under the "Action" heading are listed only the principal and important secondary or accessory functions—those particularly useful in testing and those that may cause confusion by substituting for the activity of other muscles. In the description of the test itself, the position and movement given first refer to the patient, unless otherwise clearly stated. In some instances the movement is adequately indicated by the action of the muscle and, hence, is omitted

(text continues on p. 81)

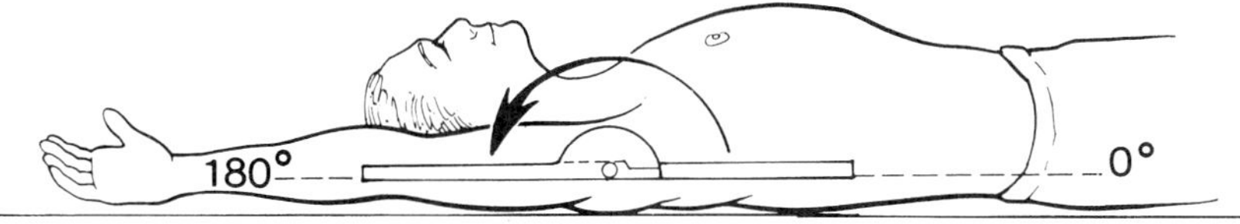

FIG. 5-1. Shoulder flexion (courtesy of J.F. Lehmann, M.D.).

Starting position	Measurement
Supine Arm at side with hand pronated	Sagittal plane Substitution to avoid: Arching back Rotating trunk Goniometer: Axis lateral to joint and just below acromion Shaft parallel to midaxillary line of trunk Shaft parallel to midline of humerus

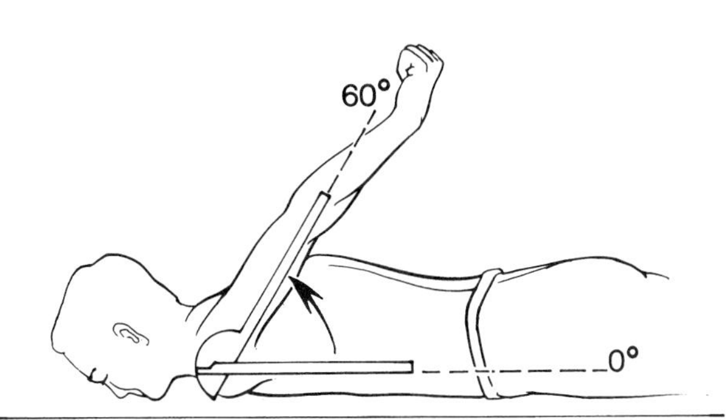

Starting position	Measurement
Prone Arm at side with hand pronated	Sagittal plane Substitution to avoid: Lifting shoulder from table Rotating trunk Goniometer: same as in Figure 5-1

FIG. 5-2. Shoulder hyperextension (courtesy of J.F. Lehmann, M.D.).

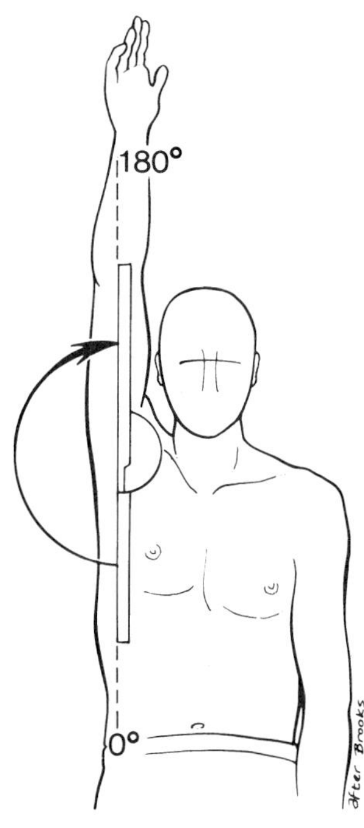

Starting position	Measurement
Supine Arm at side	Frontal plane (must externally rotate shoulder to obtain maximum) Substitution to avoid: Lateral motion of trunk Rotating trunk Goniometer: Axis anterior to joint and in line with acromion Shaft parallel to midline of trunk Shaft parallel to midline of humerus

FIG. 5-3. Shoulder abduction (courtesy of J.F. Lehmann, M.D.).

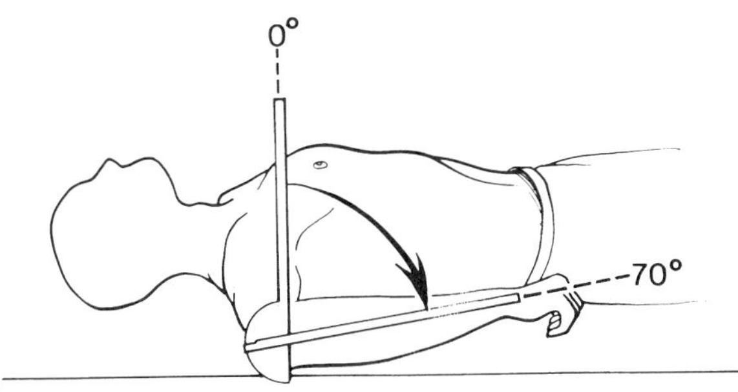

Starting position

Supine
Arm abducted to 90° and elbow off table
Elbow flexed to 90° and hand pronated
Forearm perpendicular to floor

Measurement

Transverse plane
Substitution to avoid:
- Protracting shoulder
- Rotating trunk
- Changing angle at shoulder or elbow

Goniometer:
- Axis through longitudinal axis of humerus
- Shaft perpendicular to floor
- Shaft parallel to midline or forearm

FIG. 5-4. Shoulder internal rotation (courtesy of J.F. Lehmann, M.D.).

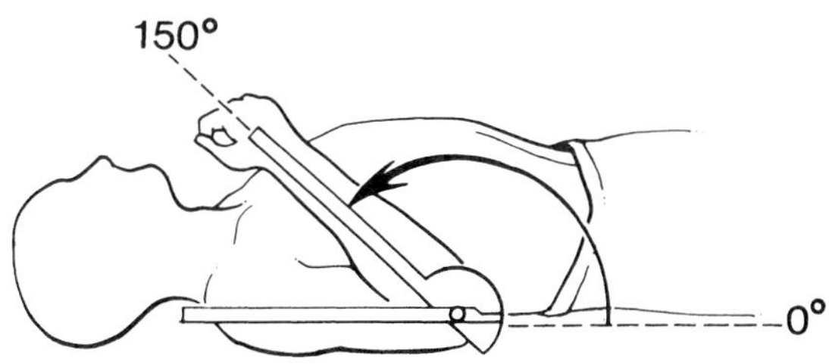

Starting position

Supine
Arm at side with elbow straight

Hand supinated

Measurement

Sagittal plane
Goniometer:
- Axis lateral to joint and through epicondyles of humerus
- Shaft parallel to midline of humerus
- Shaft parallel to midline of forearm

FIG. 5-6. Elbow flexion (courtesy of J.F. Lehmann, M.D.).

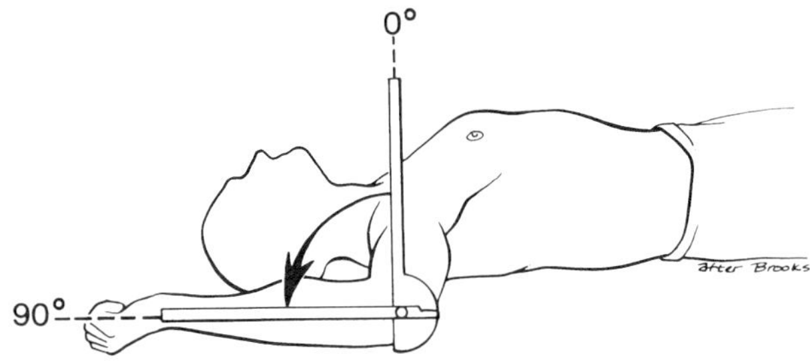

Starting position

Same as in Figure 5-2

Measurement

Transverse plane
Substitution to avoid:
- Arching back
- Rotating trunk
- Changing angle at shoulder or elbow

Goniometer: same as in Figure 5-4

FIG. 5-5. Shoulder external rotation (courtesy of J.F. Lehmann, M.D.).

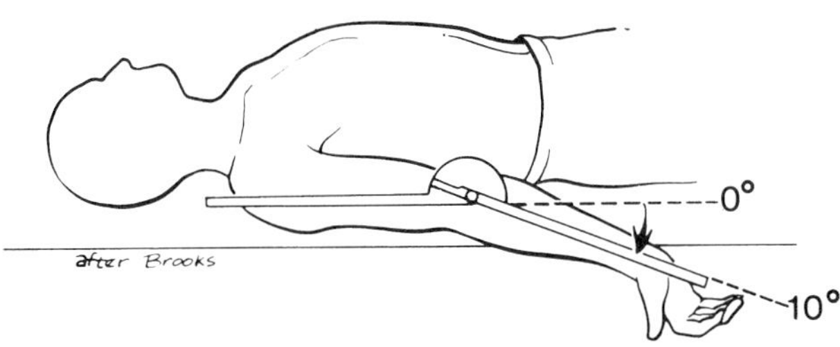

FIG. 5-7. Elbow hyperextension. Demonstration of the method of measuring excessive mobility past the normal starting position (courtesy of J.F. Lehmann, M.D.).

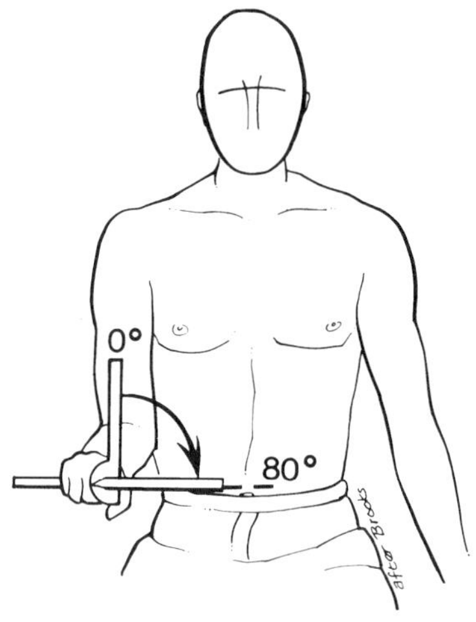

Starting position	Measurement
Sitting (or standing) Arm at side with elbow held close to trunk Elbow bent to 90° Forearm in neutral position between pronation and supination Wrist in neutral position Pencil held securely in midpalmar crease	Transverse plane Substitution to avoid: Rotating trunk Moving arm Changing angle at elbow Angulating wrist Goniometer: Axis through longitudinal axis of forearm Shaft parallel to midline of humerus Shaft parallel to pencil (on thumb side)

FIG. 5-8. Forearm pronation (courtesy of J.F. Lehmann, M.D.).

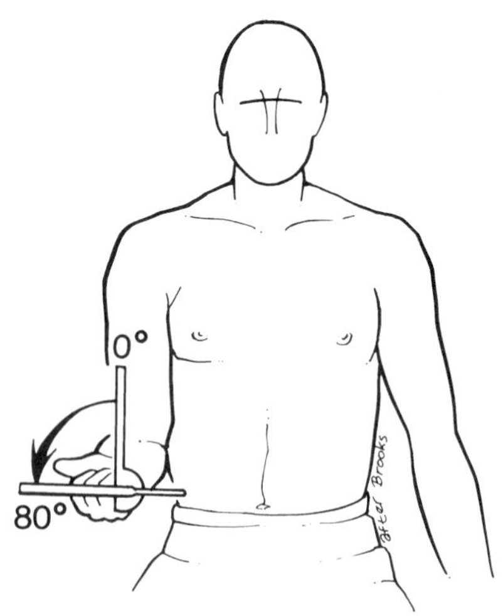

Starting position	Measurement
Same as in Figure 5-8	Same as in Figure 5-8

FIG. 5-9. Forearm supination (courtesy of J.F. Lehmann, M.D.).

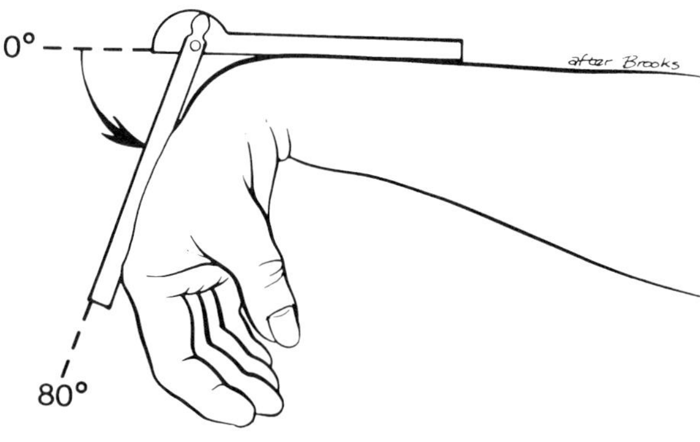

Starting position	Measurement
Elbow bent Forearm and wrist in neutral position	Sagittal plane Goniometer: Axis over dorsum of wrist (in line with third metacarpal bone) Shaft on mid-dorsum of forearm Shaft on mid-dorsum of hand

FIG. 5-10. Wrist flexion (courtesy of J.F. Lehmann, M.D.).

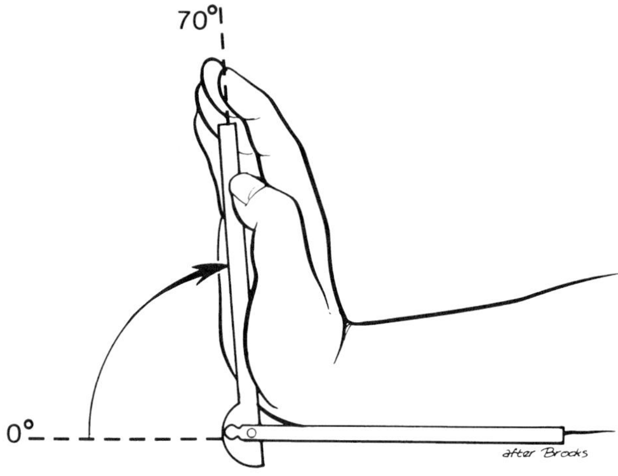

Starting position	Measurement
Same as in Figure 5-10	Sagittal plane Goniometer: Axis on ventral surface of wrist (in line with third metacarpal bone) Shaft on midventral surface of forearm Shaft on midpalmar surface of hand

FIG. 5-11. Wrist extension (courtesy of J.F. Lehmann, M.D.).

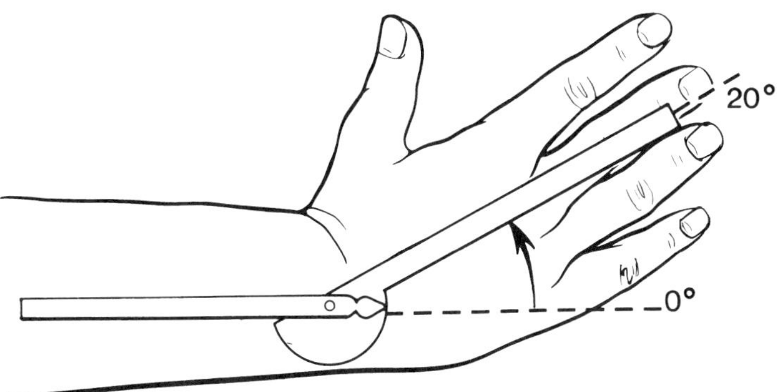

Starting position

Forearm pronated
Wrist in neutral position

Measurement

Frontal plane
Goniometer:
Axis over dorsum of wrist centered at midcarpal bone
Shaft on mid-dorsum of forearm
Shaft on shaft of third metacarpal bone

FIG. 5-12. Wrist radial deviation (courtesy of J.F. Lehmann, M.D.).

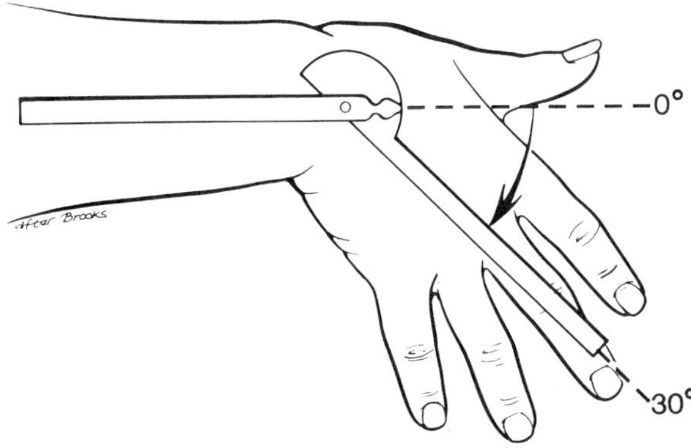

Starting position

Same as in Figure 5-12

Measurement

Same as in Figure 5-12

FIG. 5-13. Wrist ulnar deviation (courtesy of J.F. Lehmann, M.D.).

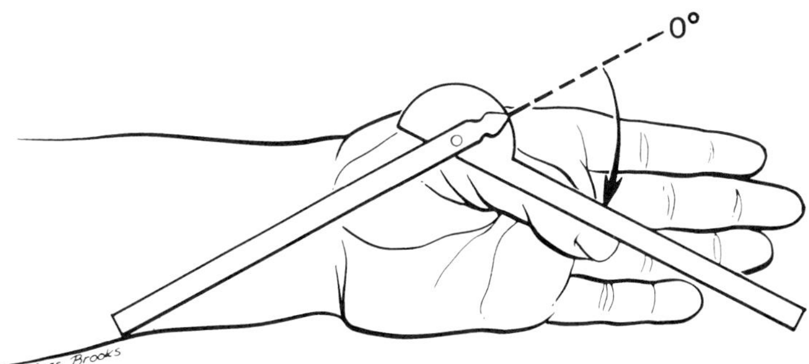

Starting position

Elbow slightly flexed
Hand supinated
Fingers and thumb extended

Measurement

Frontal plane
Goniometer:
Axis on lateral aspect of metacarpophalangeal joint
Shaft parallel to midline of first metacarpal bone
Shaft parallel to midline of proximal phalanx

FIG. 5-14. First metacarpophalangeal flexion (courtesy of J.F. Lehmann, M.D.).

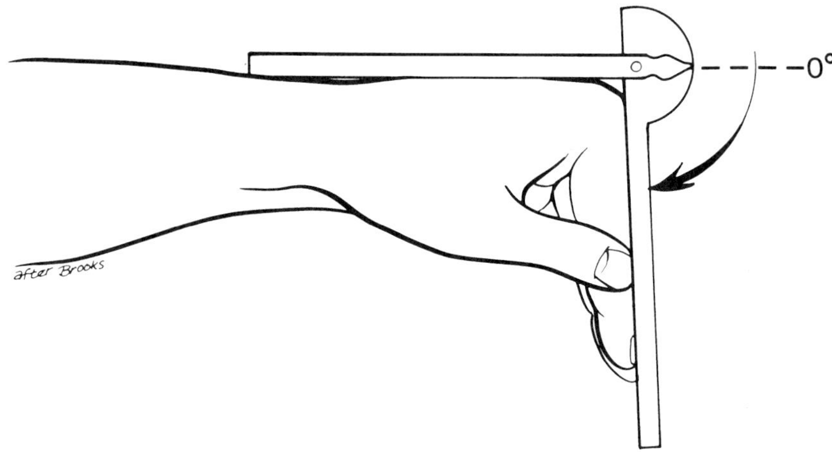

Starting position

Elbow flexed
Hand pronated
Wrist in neutral position

Measurement

Sagittal plane
Goniometer:
Axis on mid-dorsum of joint
Shaft on mid-dorsum of metacarpal bone
Shaft on mid-dorsum of proximal phalanx

FIG. 5-15. Second, third, and fourth metacarpophalangeal flexion (courtesy of J.F. Lehmann, M.D.).

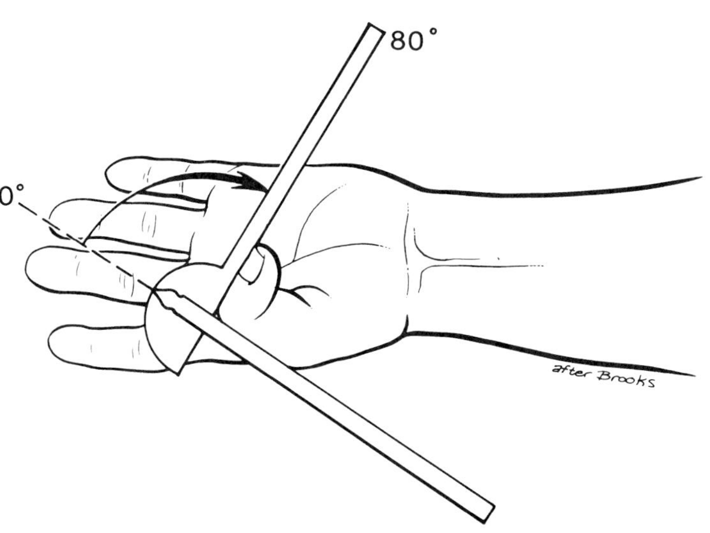

Starting position

Elbow flexed
Forearm supinated
Interphalangeal joint extended

Measurement

Frontal plane
Goniometer:
Axis on lateral aspect of interphalangeal joint
Shaft parallel to midline of proximal phalanx
Shaft parallel to midline of distal phalanx

FIG. 5-16. First interphalangeal flexion (courtesy of J.F. Lehmann, M.D.).

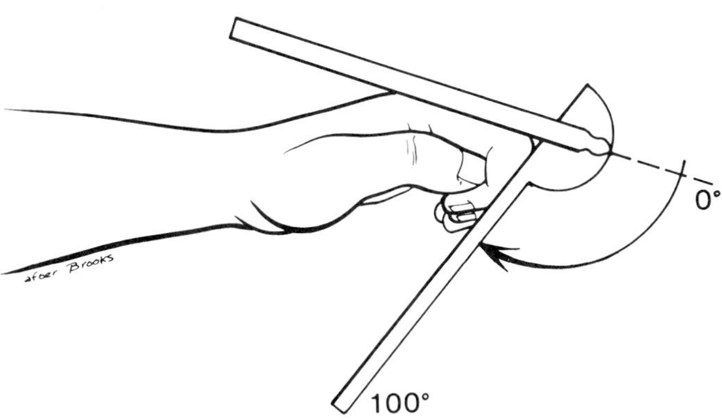

Starting position

Elbow flexed
Forearm pronated
Interphalangeal joint extended

Measurement

Sagittal plane
Goniometer:
- Axis over dorsal aspect of joint
- Shaft over mid-dorsum of proximal phalanx
- Shaft over mid-dorsum of more distal phalanx

FIG. 5-17. Second, third, and fourth interphalangeal flexion (courtesy of J.F. Lehmann, M.D.).

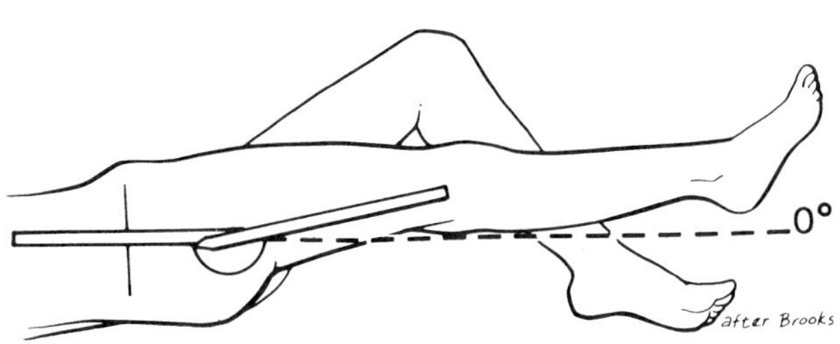

FIG. 5-18. Hip extension. See Fig. 5-19. (Courtesy of J.F. Lehmann, M.D.)

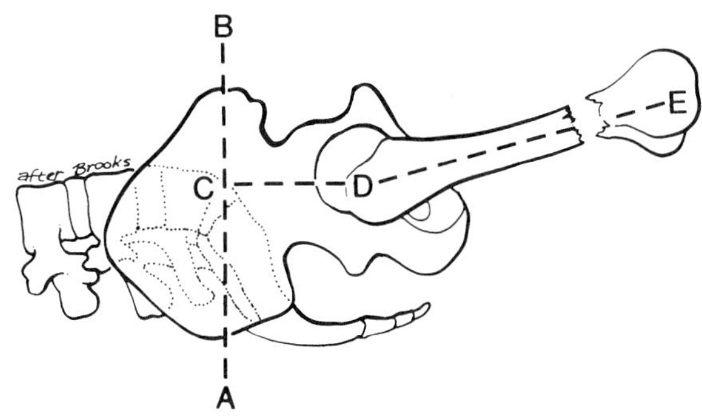

Starting position

Lying on side (or supine)
Lower leg bent for support

Measurement

Sagittal plane
Draw line from anterosuperior to posterosuperior iliac spines (B–A)
Drop a perpendicular to the greater trochanter (C–D)
Center axis of goniometer at greater trochanter (D)
Shaft along perpendicular (C–D)
Shaft along shaft of femur (D–E)

FIG. 5-19. Hip extension (courtesy of J.F. Lehmann, M.D.).

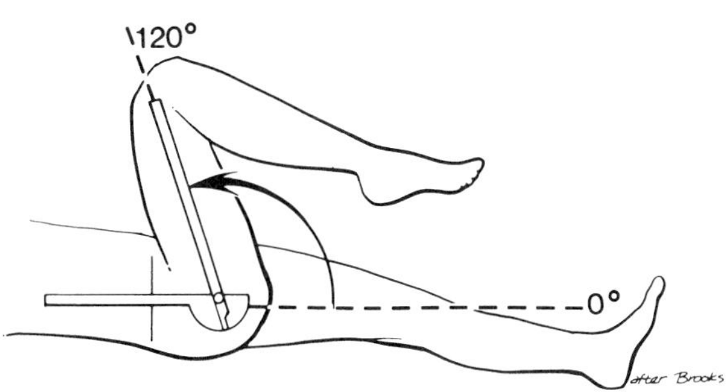

Starting position

Lying on side or supine (may flex lower knee slightly for support)

Measurement

Sagittal plane
Relocate greater trochanter and redraw C–D, as described in Figure 5-19
Goniometer placement is the same as in Figure 5-19

FIG. 5-20. Hip flexion (courtesy of J.F. Lehmann, M.D.).

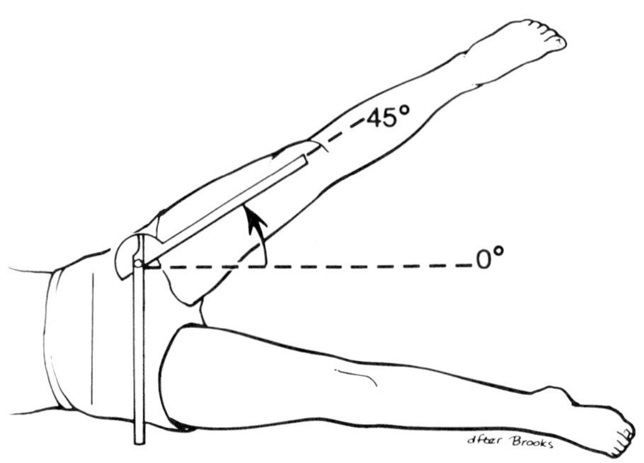

FIG. 5-21. Hip abduction (courtesy of J.F. Lehmann, M.D.).

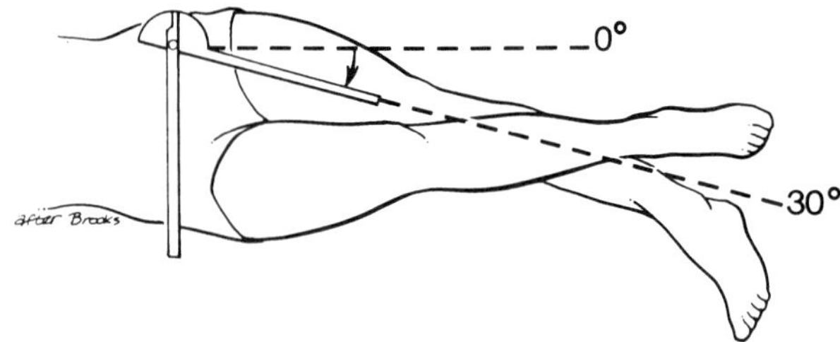

Starting position

Supine
Leg extended and in neutral position

Measurement

Frontal plane
Mark both anterosuperior iliac spines, and draw a line between them
Goniometer:
- Axis over hip joint
- Shaft parallel to line between spines of ilium
- Shaft along shaft of femur

FIG. 5-22. Hip adduction (courtesy of J.F. Lehmann, M.D.).

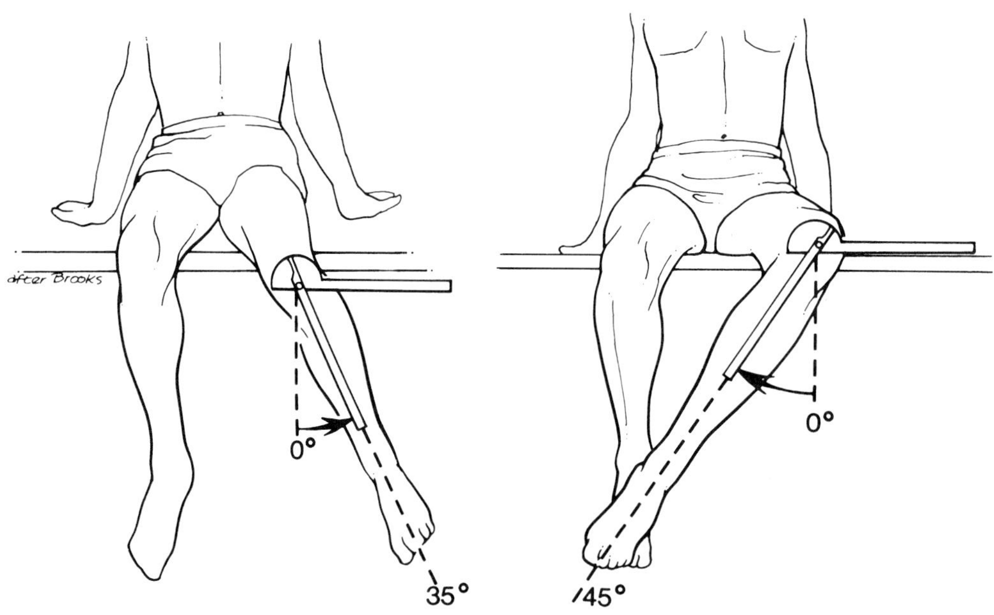

Starting position

Prone, sitting, or supine (indicate position on record)
Knee flexed to 90°

Measurement

Transverse plane
Substitution to avoid:
- Rotating trunk
- Lifting thigh from table

Goniometer:
- Axis through longitudinal axis of femur
- Shaft parallel to table
- Shaft parallel to lower part of leg

FIG. 5-23. Hip internal rotation *(left)* and hip external rotation *(right)* (courtesy of J.F. Lehmann, M.D.).

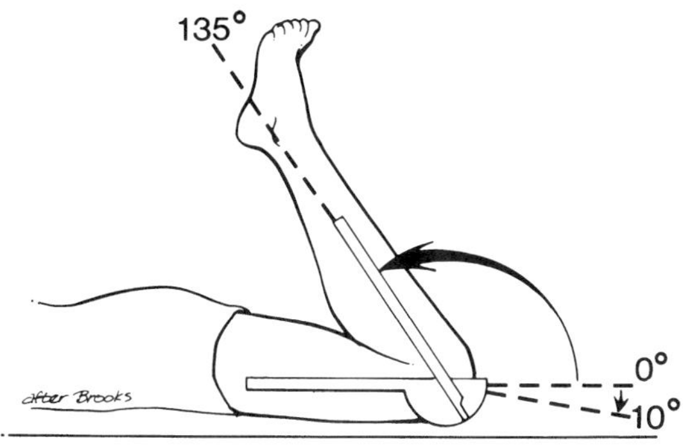

Starting position	Measurement
Prone (or supine with hip flexed if rectus femoris limits motion)	Sagittal plane Goniometer: Axis through knee joint Shaft along midthigh Shaft along fibula

FIG. 5-24. Knee flexion. *Small arrow* indicates hyperextension (courtesy of J.F. Lehmann, M.D.).

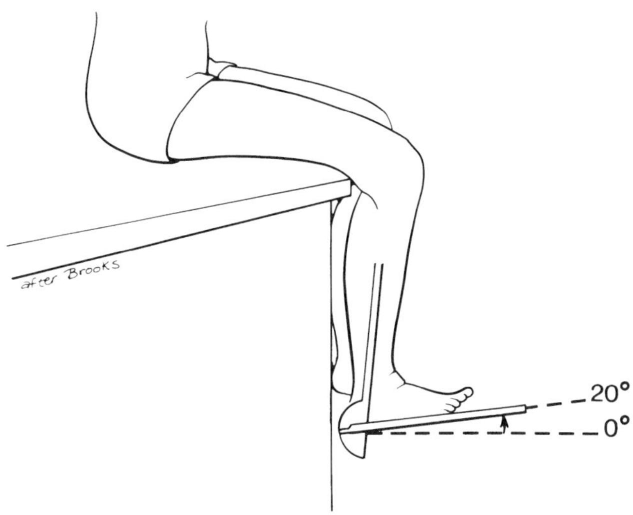

Starting position	Measurement
Sitting Knee flexed to 90° Foot at 90° angle to leg	Sagittal plane Goniometer: Axis on sole of foot Shaft along fibula Shaft along fifth metatarsal bone

FIG. 5-25. Ankle dorsiflexion (courtesy of J.F. Lehmann, M.D.).

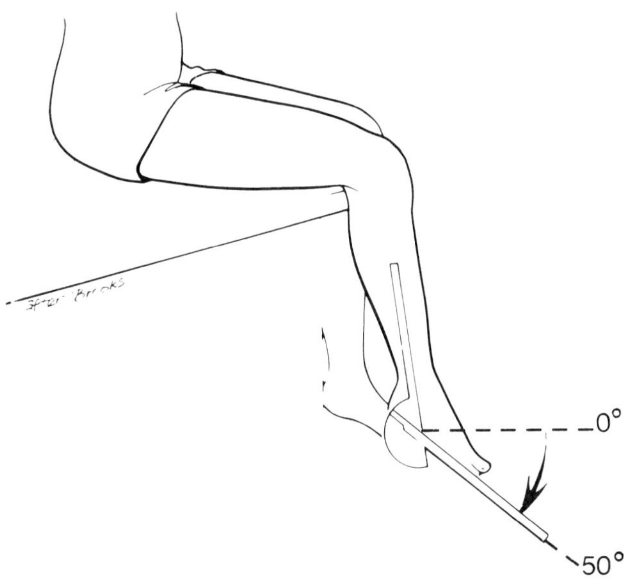

Starting position	Measurement
Same as in Figure 5-25	Same as in Figure 5-25

FIG. 5-26. Ankle plantar flexion (courtesy of J.F. Lehmann, M.D.).

here. The term "resistance," unless otherwise specifically stated, refers to the pressure applied by the examiner, and this is in the direction opposite that of the movement. For brevity and uniformity in description of the tests, the method of testing in which the patient initiates action against the resistance of the examiner is given except when the other method is distinctly more applicable. However, this concession to uniformity and brevity of description is not meant to imply a preference for the method of testing in which the patient initiates action. The location of the belly of the muscle and its tendon is often given to stress the importance of observation and palpation in identifying the function of that particular muscle. Only those participating muscles are listed that have a definite action in the movement being tested and that may substitute at least in part for the muscle being discussed.

The following text is reprinted from *Clinical Examinations in Neurology* with the permission of the editors. We feel it is an excellent summary and appreciate their contributions.

TRAPEZIUS

(Spinal accessory nerve) (Figs. 5-27 and 5-28)

Action

Elevation, retraction (adduction), and rotation (lateral angle upward) of scapula, providing fixation of scapula during many movements of arm.

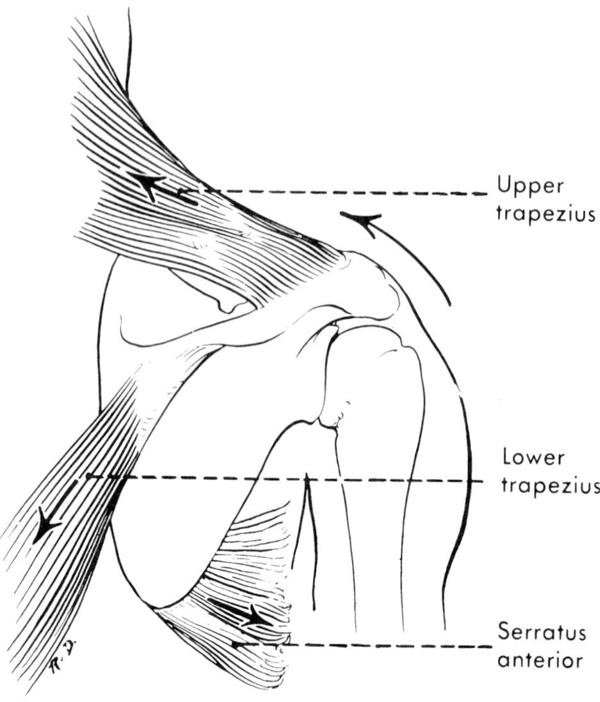

FIG. 5-27. Upward rotators of the scapula. (Reprinted with permission from Hollinshead WH. *Functional anatomy of the limbs and back: a text for students of physical therapy and others interested in the locomotor apparatus,* 3rd ed. Philadelphia: WB Saunders, 1969.)

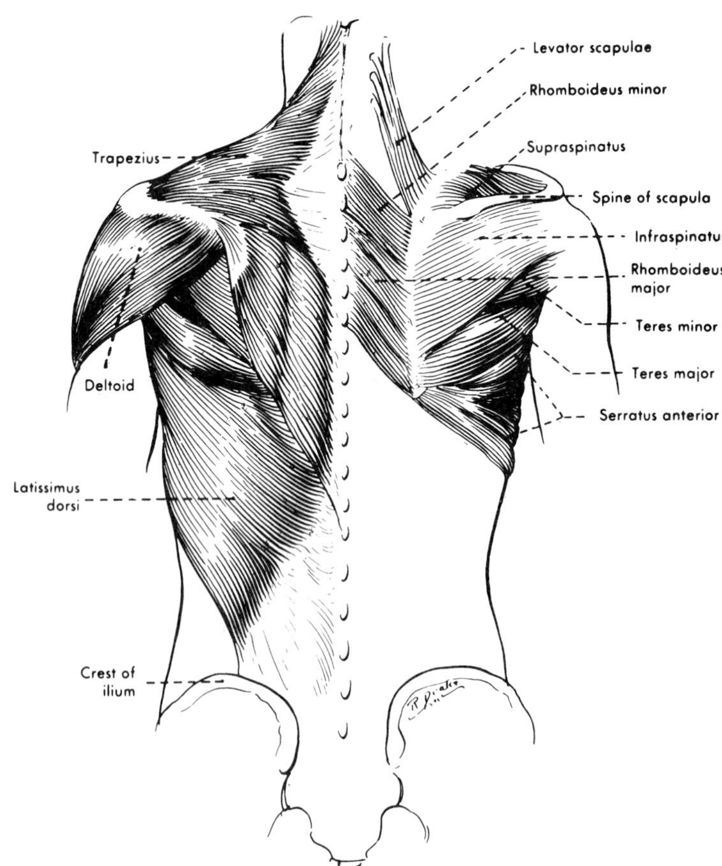

FIG. 5-28. Musculature of the shoulder from behind. (Reprinted with permission from Hollinshead WH. *Functional anatomy of the limbs and back: a text for students of physical therapy and others interested in the locomotor apparatus,* 3rd ed. Philadelphia: WB Saunders, 1969.)

Test

Elevation (shrugging) of shoulder against resistance tests upper portion, which is readily visible.

Bracing shoulder (backward movement and adduction of scapula) tests chiefly middle portion.

Abduction of arm against resistance intensifies winging of scapula.

In isolated trapezius palsy with the shoulder girdle at rest, the scapula is displaced downward and laterally and is rotated so that the superior angle is farther from the spine than the inferior angle. The lateral displacement is due in part to the unopposed action of the serratus anterior. The vertebral border, particularly at the inferior angle, is flared. These changes are accentuated when the arm is abducted from the side against resistance. On flexion (forward elevation) of the arm, however, the flaring of the inferior angle virtually disappears. These features are important in distinguishing trapezius palsy from serratus anterior palsy, which produces an equally characteristic winging of the scapula but in which movement of the arm in these two planes has the opposite effect. Atrophy of the trapezius is evident chiefly in the upper portion.

Participating Muscles

- Elevation: levator scapulae (third and fourth cervical nerves and dorsal scapular nerve, C3–C5).
- Retraction: rhomboids.
- Upward rotation: serratus anterior.

RHOMBOIDS

(Dorsal scapular nerve from anterior ramus, C5) (Fig. 5-28)

Action

Retraction (adduction) of scapula and elevation of its vertebral border.

Test

Hand is on hip; arm is held backward and medially. Examiner attempts to force elbow laterally and forward, observing and palpating muscle bellies medial to scapula.

Participating Muscles

Trapezius; levator scapulae: elevation of medial border of scapula.

SERRATUS ANTERIOR

(Long thoracic nerve from anterior rami, C5–C7) (Fig. 5-27)

Action

Protraction (lateral and forward movement) of scapula, keeping it closely applied to thorax.

Assistance in upward rotation of scapula.

Test

Outstretched arm is thrust forward against wall or against resistance by examiner.

Isolated palsy results in comparatively little change in the appearance of the shoulder girdle at rest. However, there is slight winging of the inferior angle of the scapula and slight shift medially toward the spine. When the outstretched arm is thrust forward, the entire scapula, particularly its inferior angle, shifts backward away from the thorax, producing the characteristic wing effect. Abduction of the arm laterally, however, produces comparatively little winging, demonstrating again an important difference from the manifestations of paralysis of the trapezius.

SUPRASPINATUS

(Suprascapular nerve from upper trunk of brachial plexus, C4, C5, C6) (Fig. 5-29)

Action

Initiation of abduction of arm from side of body.

Test

Above action is tested against resistance.

Atrophy may be detected just above the spine of the scapula, but the trapezius overlies the supraspinatus, and atro-

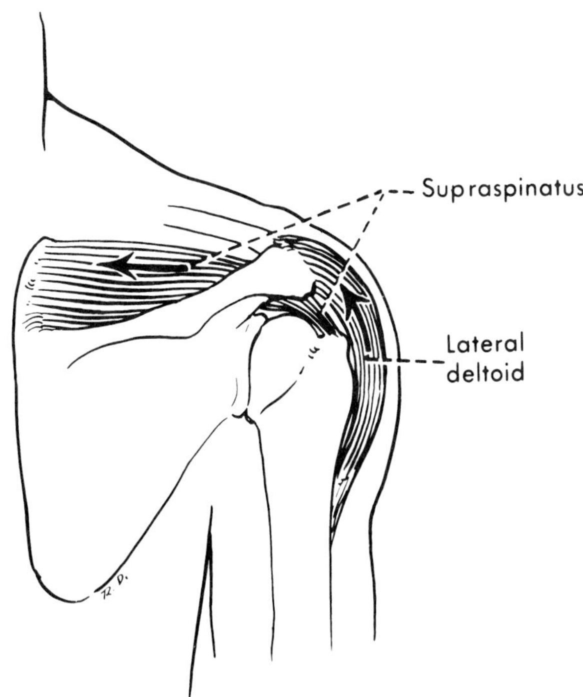

FIG. 5-29. Abductors of the humerus. (Reprinted with permission from Hollinshead WH. *Functional anatomy of the limbs and back: a text for students of physical therapy and others interested in the locomotor apparatus,* 3rd ed. Philadelphia: WB Saunders, 1969.)

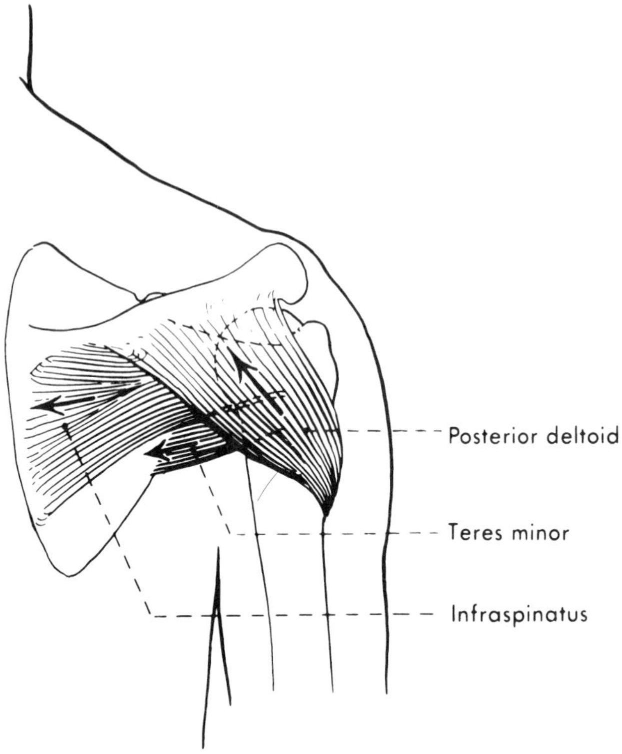

FIG. 5-30. Chief external rotators of the humerus. (Reprinted with permission from Hollinshead WH. *Functional anatomy of the limbs and back: a text for students of physical therapy and others interested in the locomotor apparatus,* 3rd ed. Philadelphia: WB Saunders, 1969.)

phy of either muscle will produce a depression in this area. Scapular fixation is important in this test.

Participating Muscle

Deltoid.

INFRASPINATUS

(Suprascapular nerve from upper trunk of brachial plexus, C4, C5, C6) (Fig. 5-30)

Action

Lateral (external) rotation of arm at shoulder.

Test

Elbow is at side and flexed 90°. Patient resists examiner's attempt to push the hand medially toward the abdomen.

The muscle is palpable, and atrophy may be visible below the spine of the scapula.

Participating Muscles

Teres minor (axillary nerve); deltoid, posterior fibers.

PECTORALIS MAJOR (FIG. 5-31)

Clavicular portion (lateral pectoral nerve from lateral cord of plexus, C5, C6, C7).

Sternal portion (medial pectoral nerve from medial cord of plexus, lateral pectoral nerve, C6, C7, C8, T1).

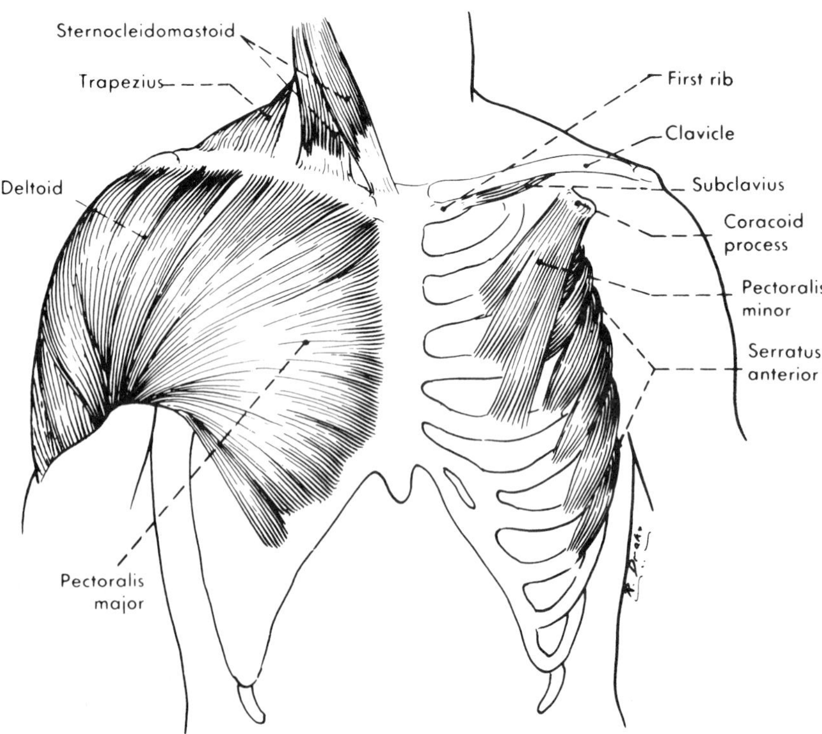

FIG. 5-31. Muscles of the pectoral region. (Reprinted with permission from Hollinshead WH. *Functional anatomy of the limbs and back: a text for students of physical therapy and others interested in the locomotor apparatus,* 3rd ed. Philadelphia: WB Saunders, 1969.)

Action

Adduction and medial rotation of arm. Clavicular portion, assistance in flexion of arm.

Test

Arm is in front of body. Patient resists attempt by examiner to force it laterally.

The two portions of the muscle are visible and palpable.

LATISSIMUS DORSI

(Thoracodorsal nerve from posterior cord of plexus, C6, C7, C8) (Fig. 5-32)

Action

Adduction, extension, and medial rotation of arm.

Test

Arm is in abduction to horizontal position. Downward and backward movement against resistance is applied under elbow.

The muscle should be observed and palpated in and below the posterior axillary fold. When the patient coughs, a brisk contraction of the normal latissimus dorsi can be felt at the inferior angle of the scapula.

TERES MAJOR

(Lower subscapular nerve from posterior cord plexus, C5–C7) (Fig. 5-32*A*)

Action and test are the same as for latissimus dorsi.

The muscle is visible and palpable at the lower lateral border of the scapula.

DELTOID

(Axillary nerve from posterior cord of plexus, C5, C6) (Figs. 5-31 and 5-32*C*)

Action

Abduction of arm.

Flexion (forward movement) and medial rotation of arm, anterior fibers.

Extension (backward movement) and lateral rotation of arm, posterior fibers.

Test

Arm is in abduction almost to horizontal. Patient resists effort of examiner to depress elbow.

Paralysis of the deltoid leads to conspicuous atrophy and serious disability because the other muscles that participate in abduction of the arm (the supraspinatus, trapezius, and

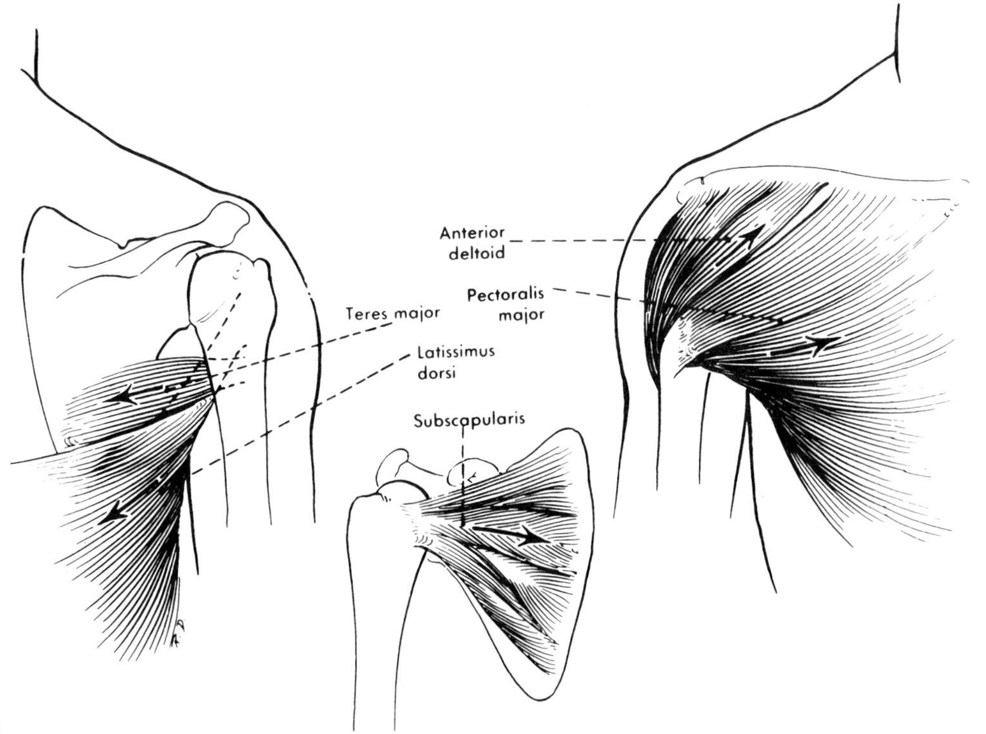

FIG. 5-32. A–C: Chief internal rotation of the humerus. (Reprinted with permission from Hollinshead WH. *Functional anatomy of the limbs and back: a text for students of physical therapy and others interested in the locomotor apparatus,* 3rd ed. Philadelphia: WB Saunders, 1969.)

serratus anterior, the last two by rotating the scapula) cannot compensate for lack of function of the deltoid.

Flexion and extension of the arm are tested against resistance.

Participating Muscles

Abduction: given above.
Flexion: pectoralis major, clavicular portion; biceps.
Extension: latissimus dorsi; teres major.

SUBSCAPULARIS

(Upper and lower subscapular nerves from posterior cord of plexus, C5, C6, C7) (Fig. 5-32*B*)

Action

Medial (internal) rotation of arm at shoulder.

Test

Elbow is at side and flexed 90°. Patient resists examiner's attempt to pull the hand laterally.

Because this muscle is not accessible to observation or palpation, it is necessary to gauge the activity of other muscles that produce this movement. The pectoralis major is the most powerful medial rotator of the arm; hence, paralysis of the subscapularis alone results in relatively little weakness of this movement.

Participating Muscles

Pectoralis major; deltoid, anterior fibers; teres major; latissimus dorsi.

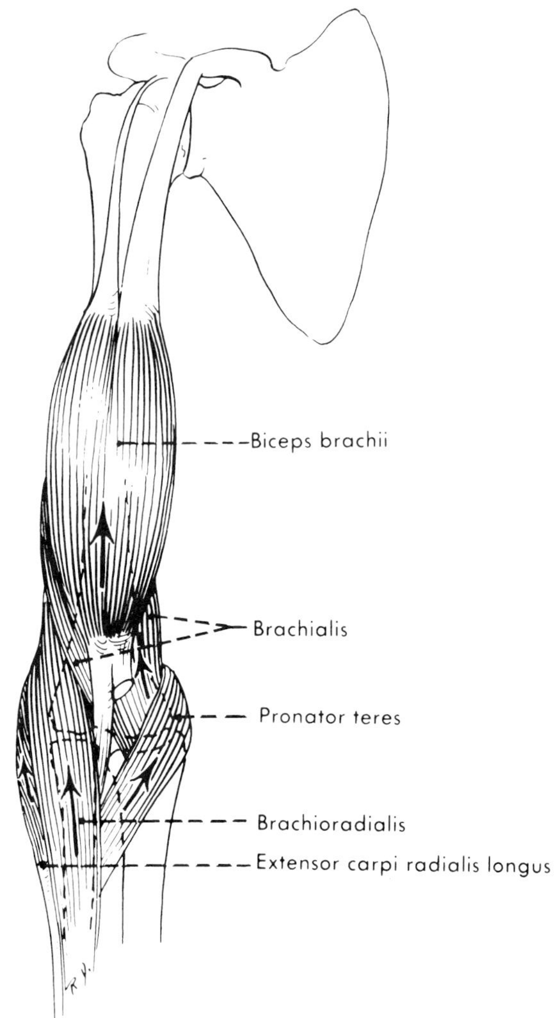

FIG. 5-33. Flexors of the elbow. (Reprinted with permission from Hollinshead WH. *Functional anatomy of the limbs and back: a text for students of physical therapy and others interested in the locomotor apparatus,* 3rd ed. Philadelphia: WB Saunders, 1969.)

BICEPS; BRACHIALIS

(Musculocutaneous nerve from lateral cord of plexus, C5, C6) (Fig. 5-33)

Action

Biceps: flexion and supination of forearm and assistance in flexion of arm at shoulder.

Brachialis: flexion of forearm at elbow.

Test

Flexion of forearm is tested against resistance. Forearm should be in supination to decrease participation of brachioradialis.

TRICEPS

(Radial nerve, which is continuation of posterior cord of plexus, C6, C7, C8) (Fig. 5-34)

Action

Extension of forearm at elbow.

Test

Forearm is in flexion to varying degree. Patient resists effort of examiner to flex forearm farther. Slight weakness is more easily detected when starting with forearm almost completely flexed.

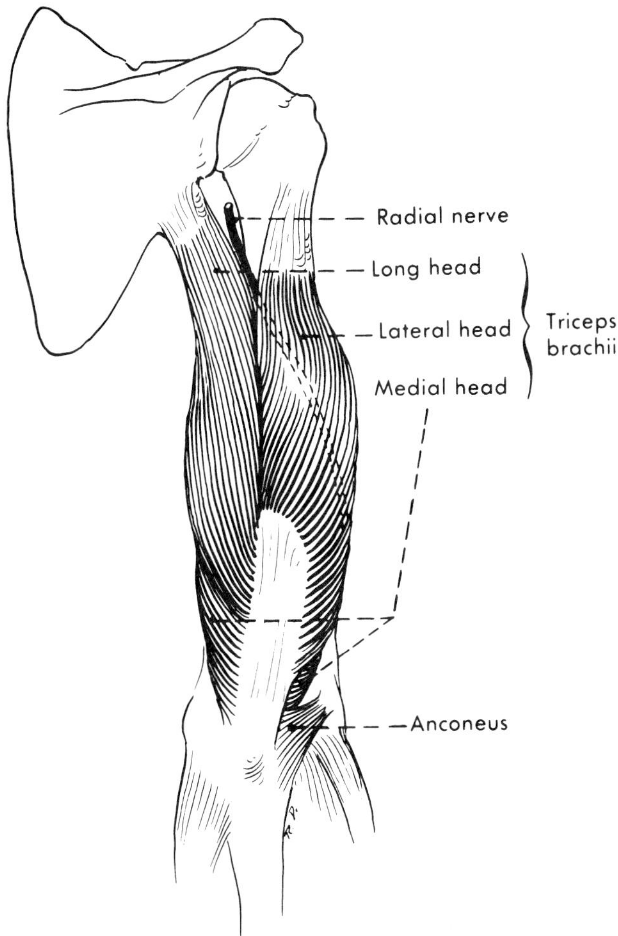

FIG. 5-34. Muscles of the extensor (i.e., posterior) surface of the right arm. (Reprinted with permission from Hollinshead WH. *Functional anatomy of the limbs and back: a text for students of physical therapy and others interested in the locomotor apparatus,* 3rd ed. Philadelphia: WB Saunders, 1969.)

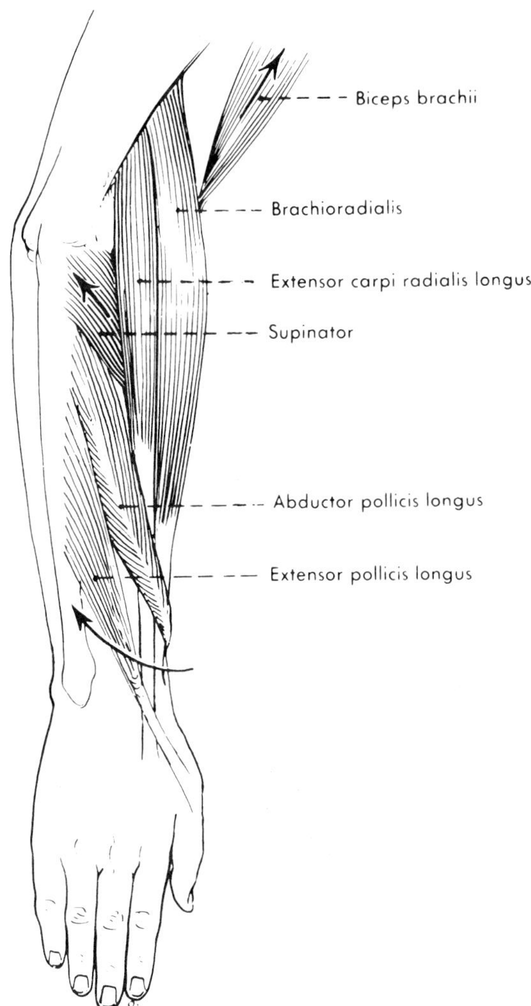

FIG. 5-35. Chief supinators of the forearm. (Adapted Reprinted with permission from Hollinshead WH. *Functional anatomy of the limbs and back: a text for students of physical therapy and others interested in the locomotor apparatus,* 3rd ed. Philadelphia: WB Saunders, 1969.)

BRACHIORADIALIS

(Radial nerve, C5, C6) (Fig. 5-35)

Action

Flexion of forearm at elbow.

Test

Flexion of forearm is tested against resistance with forearm midway between pronation and supination.

The belly of the muscle stands out prominently on the upper surface of the forearm, tending to bridge the angle between the forearm and arm.

Participating Muscles

Biceps; brachialis.

SUPINATOR

(Posterior interosseous nerve from radial nerve, C5–C7) (Fig. 5-35)

Action

Supination of forearm.

Test

Forearm is in full extension and supination. Patient attempts to maintain supination while examiner attempts to pronate forearm and palpates biceps.

Resistance to pronation by the intact supinator can usually be felt before there is appreciable contraction of the biceps.

EXTENSOR CARPI RADIALIS LONGUS

(Radial nerve, C6, C7, C8) (Fig. 5-36)

Action

Extension (dorsiflexion) and radial abduction of hand at wrist.

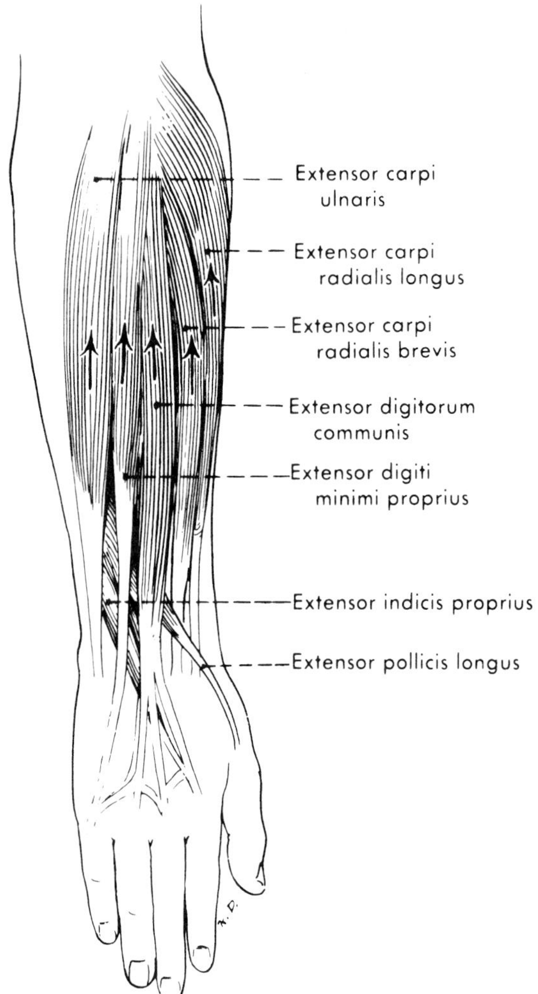

FIG. 5-36. Chief extensors of the wrist. (Reprinted with permission from Hollinshead WH. *Functional anatomy of the limbs and back: a text for students of physical therapy and others interested in the locomotor apparatus,* 3rd ed. Philadelphia: WB Saunders, 1969.)

Test

Forearm is in almost complete pronation. Dorsiflexion of wrist is tested against resistance applied to dorsum of hand downward and toward ulnar side.

The tendon is palpable just above its insertion into the base of the second metacarpal bone. The fingers and thumb should be relaxed and somewhat flexed to minimize participation of the extensors of the digits.

EXTENSOR CARPI RADIALIS BREVIS

(Posterior interosseous nerve from radial nerve, C6, C7, C8) (Fig. 5-36)

Action

Extension (dorsiflexion) of hand at wrist.

Test

Forearm is in complete pronation. Dorsiflexion of wrist is tested against resistance applied to dorsum of hand straight downward.

The tendon is palpable just proximal to the base of the third metacarpal bone. The fingers and thumb should be relaxed and somewhat flexed to minimize participation of the extensors of the digits.

EXTENSOR CARPI ULNARIS

(Posterior interosseous nerve from radial nerve, C7, C8) (Fig. 5-36)

Action

Extension (dorsiflexion) and ulnar deviation of hand at wrist.

Test

Forearm is in pronation. Dorsiflexion and ulnar deviation of wrist are tested against resistance applied to dorsum of hand downward and toward radial side.

The tendon is palpable just below or above the distal end of the ulna. The fingers should be relaxed and somewhat flexed to minimize participation of the extensors of the digits.

EXTENSOR DIGITORUM

(Posterior interosseous nerve from radial nerve, C6, C7, C8) (Fig. 5-36)

Action

Extension of fingers, principally at metacarpophalangeal joints.

Assistance in extension (dorsiflexion) of wrist.

Test

Forearm is in pronation. Wrist is stabilized in straight position. Extension of fingers at metacarpophalangeal joints is tested against resistance applied to proximal phalanges.

The distal portions of the fingers may be somewhat relaxed and in slight flexion. The tendons are visible and palpable over the dorsum of the hand.

Extension at the interphalangeal joints is a function primarily of the interossei (ulnar nerve) and lumbricals (median and ulnar nerves).

The extensor digiti quinti and extensor indicis (posterior interosseous nerve, C7, C8), proper extensors of the little and index fingers, respectively, can be tested individually while the other fingers are in flexion to minimize the action of the common extensor. In a thin person's hand the tendons can usually be identified.

ABDUCTOR POLLICIS LONGUS

(Posterior interosseous nerve from radial nerve, C7, C8) (Fig. 5-35)

Action

Radial abduction of thumb (in same plane as that of palm, in contradistinction to palmar abduction, which is movement perpendicular to plane of palm).

Assistance in radial abduction and flexion of hand at wrist.

Test

Hand is on edge (forearm midway between pronation and supination).

Radial abduction of thumb is tested against resistance applied to metacarpal.

The tendon is palpable just above its insertion into the base of the metacarpal bone and forms the anterior (volar) boundary of the "anatomic snuffbox."

Participating Muscle

Extensor pollicis brevis.

EXTENSOR POLLICIS BREVIS

(Posterior interosseous nerve from radial nerve, C7, C8)

Action

Extension of proximal phalanx of thumb.

Assistance in radial abduction and extension of metacarpal of thumb.

Test

Hand is on edge. Wrist and particularly metacarpal of thumb are stabilized by examiner. Extension of proximal phalanx is tested against resistance applied to that phalanx, whereas distal phalanx is in flexion to minimize action of extensor pollicis longus.

At the wrist the tendon lies just posterior (dorsal) to the tendon of the abductor pollicis longus.

Participating Muscle

Extensor pollicis longus.

EXTENSOR POLLICIS LONGUS

(Posterior interosseous nerve from radial nerve, C7, C8) (Fig. 5-36)

Action

Extension of all parts of the thumb but specifically extension of the distal phalanx.

Assistance in adduction of the thumb.

Test

Hand is on edge. Wrist, metacarpal, and proximal phalanx of the thumb are stabilized by examiner with the thumb close to palm at its radial border. Extension of distal phalanx is tested against resistance.

If the patient is permitted to flex the wrist or abduct the thumb away from the palm, some extension of the phalanges results simply from lengthening the path of the extensor tendon. At the wrist the tendon forms the posterior (dorsal) boundary of the anatomic snuffbox.

The characteristic result of radial nerve palsy is wrist drop. Extension of the fingers at the interphalangeal joints is still possible by virtue of the action of the interossei and lumbricals, but extension of the thumb is lost.

The next group of muscles examined is that supplied by the median nerve, which is formed by the union of its lateral root, from the lateral cord of the brachial plexus, and its medial root, from the medial cord of the plexus. Then the muscles supplied by the ulnar nerve (arising from the medial cord of the brachial plexus) are tested. However, for convenience in order of examination, some of the muscles in the ulnar group are tested with the median group.

PRONATOR TERES

(Median nerve, C6, C7) (Fig. 5-37)

Action

Pronation of forearm.

Test

Elbow is at side of trunk, forearm is in flexion to right angle, and arm is in lateral rotation at shoulder to eliminate effect of gravity, which, in most positions, favors pronation. Pronation of the forearm is tested against resistance, starting from a position of moderate supination.

Participating Muscle

Pronator quadratus (anterior interosseous branch of median nerve, C7, C8, T1)

FLEXOR CARPI RADIALIS

(Median nerve, C6, C7) (Figs. 5-37 and 5-38)

Action

Flexion (palmar flexion) of hand at wrist.

Assistance in radial abduction of hand.

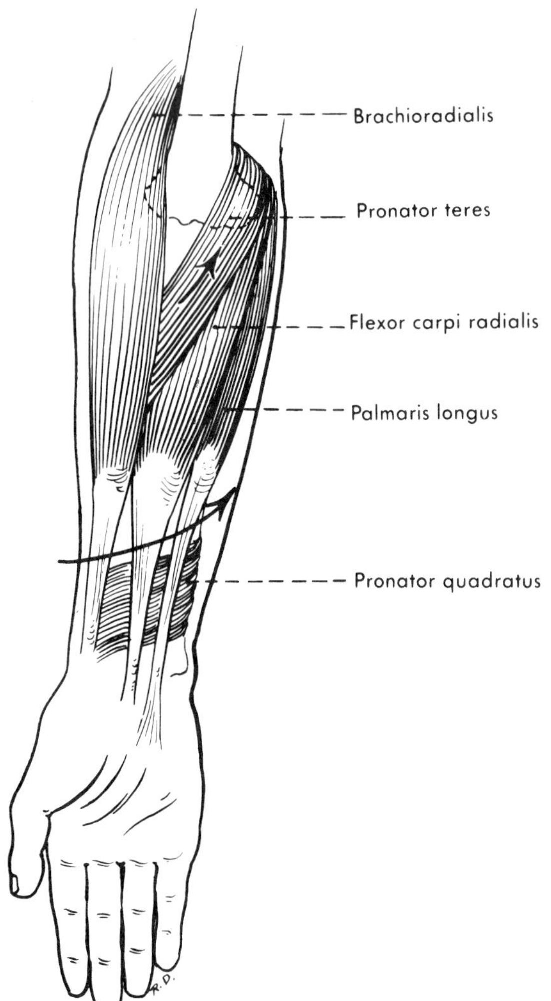

FIG. 5-37. Pronators of the forearm. (Reprinted with permission from Hollinshead WH. *Functional anatomy of the limbs and back: a text for students of physical therapy and others interested in the locomotor apparatus,* 3rd ed. Philadelphia: WB Saunders, 1969.)

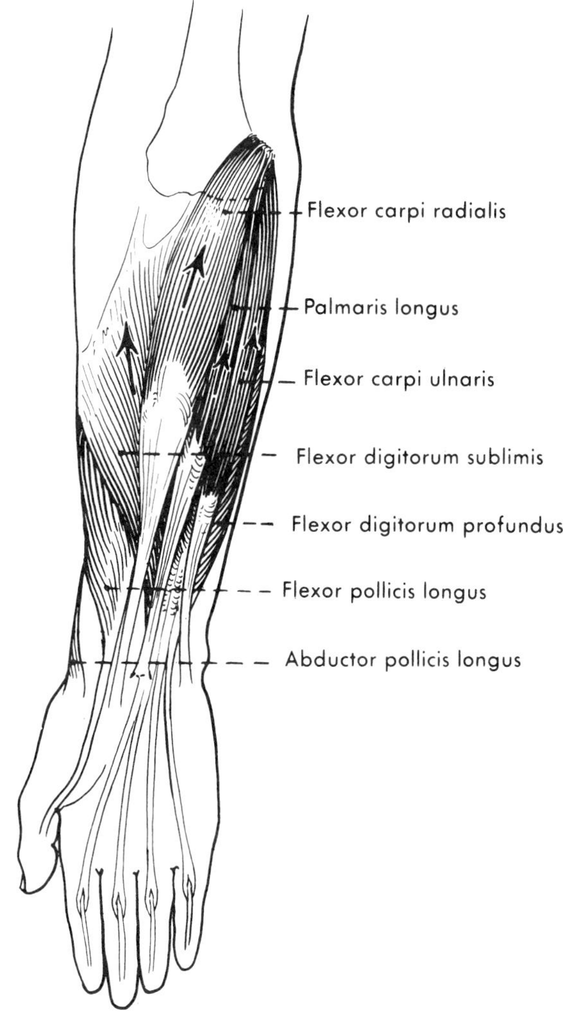

FIG. 5-38. Chief flexors of the wrist. (Reprinted with permission from Hollinshead WH. *Functional anatomy of the limbs and back: a text for students of physical therapy and others interested in the locomotor apparatus,* 3rd ed. Philadelphia: WB Saunders, 1969.)

Test

Flexion of the hand is tested against resistance applied to the palm. Fingers should be relaxed to minimize participation of their flexors.

The tendon is the more lateral (radial) one of the two conspicuous tendons on the volar aspect of the wrist.

In complete median nerve palsy, flexion of the wrist is considerably weakened but can still be performed by the flexor carpi ulnaris (ulnar nerve) assisted to some extent by the abductor pollicis longus (radial nerve). In this event, ulnar deviation of the hand usually accompanies flexion.

PALMARIS LONGUS

(Median nerve, C7, C8, T1) (Figs. 5-37 and 5-38)

Action

Flexion of hand at wrist.

Test

Same as for flexor carpi radialis. The tendon is palpable at the ulnar side of the tendon of the flexor carpi radialis.

FLEXOR CARPI ULNARIS

(Ulnar nerve, C7, C8, T1) (Fig. 5-38)

Action

Flexion and ulnar deviation of hand at wrist.

Fixation of pisiform bone during contraction of abductor digiti quinti.

Test

Flexion and ulnar deviation of the hand are tested against resistance applied to the ulnar side of the palm in the direction of extension and radial abduction. Fingers should be relaxed.

The tendon is palpable proximal to the pisiform bone.

FLEXOR DIGITORUM SUBLIMIS

(Median nerve, C7, C8, T1) (Fig. 5-38)

Action

Flexion of middle phalanges of fingers at first interphalangeal joints primarily; flexion of proximal phalanges at metacarpophalangeal joints secondarily.

Assistance in flexion of hand at wrist.

Test

Wrist is in neutral position; proximal phalanges are stabilized. Flexion of middle phalanx of each finger is tested against resistance applied to that phalanx, with the distal phalanx relaxed.

FLEXOR DIGITORUM PROFUNDUS (FIG. 5-38)

- Radial portion: usually to digits II and III (median nerve and its anterior interosseous branch C7, C8, T1)
- Ulnar portion: usually to digits IV and V (ulnar nerve, C7, C8, T1)

Action

Flexion of distal phalanges of fingers specifically; flexion of other phalanges secondarily.

Assistance in flexion of hand at wrist.

Test

Flexion of distal phalanges is tested against resistance with proximal and middle phalanges stabilized in extension.

With middle and distal phalanges folded over edge of examiner's hand, patient resists attempt by examiner to extend distal phalanges.

FLEXOR POLLICIS LONGUS

(Anterior interosseous branch of median nerve, C7, C8, T1) (Fig. 5-38)

Action

Flexion of thumb, particularly distal phalanx.

Assistance in ulnar adduction of thumb.

Test

Flexion of distal phalanx is tested against resistance with thumb in position of palmar adduction and with stabilization of metacarpal and proximal phalanx.

ABDUCTOR POLLICIS BREVIS

(Median nerve, C8, T1) (Fig. 5-39)

Action

Palmar abduction of thumb (perpendicular to plane of palm).

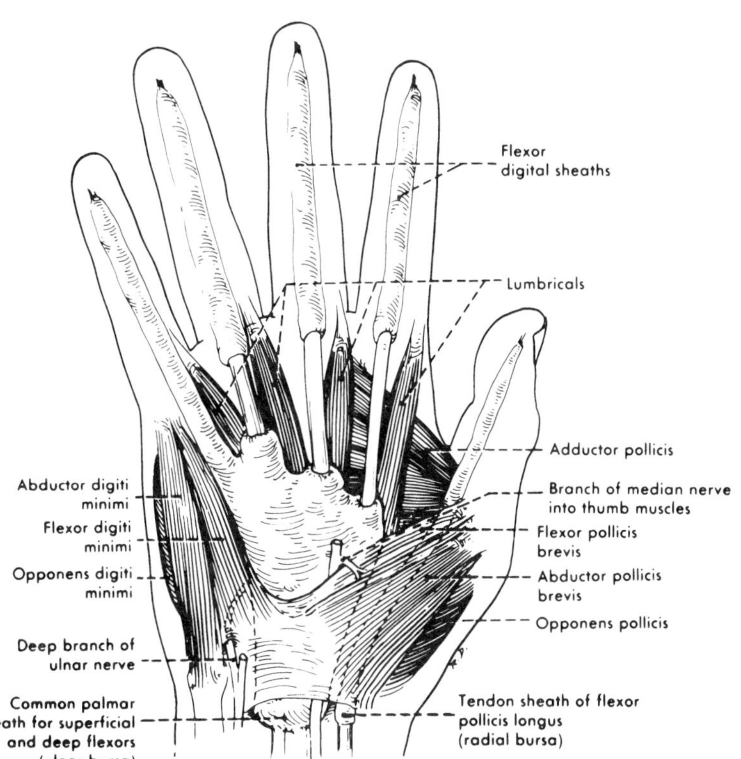

FIG. 5-39. Short muscles of the thumb and little finger. (Reprinted with permission from Hollinshead WH. *Functional anatomy of the limbs and back: a text for students of physical therapy and others interested in the locomotor apparatus,* 3rd ed. Philadelphia: WB Saunders, 1969.)

Assistance in opposition and in flexion of proximal phalanx of thumb.

Test

Palmar abduction of thumb is tested against resistance applied at metacarpophalangeal joint.

The muscle is readily visible and palpable in the thenar eminence.

Participating Muscle

Flexor pollicis brevis (superficial head).

OPPONENS POLLICIS

(Median nerve, C8, T1) (Fig. 5-39)

Action

Movement of first metacarpal across palm, rotating it into opposition.

Test

Thumb is in opposition. Examiner attempts to rotate and draw the thumb back to its usual position.

Participating Muscles

Abductor pollicis brevis; flexor pollicis brevis.

FLEXOR POLLICIS BREVIS

Superficial head (median nerve, C8, T1); deep head (ulnar nerve, C8, T1) (Fig. 5-39)

Action

Flexion of proximal phalanx of the thumb.

Assistance in opposition, ulnar adduction (entire muscle), and palmar abduction (superficial head) of the thumb.

Test

Thumb is in position of palmar adduction with stabilization of metacarpal. Flexion of proximal phalanx is tested against resistance applied to that phalanx while distal phalanx is as relaxed as possible.

Participating Muscles

Flexor pollicis longus; abductor pollicis brevis; adductor pollicis.

Severe median nerve palsy produces the ''simian'' hand, wherein the thumb tends to lie in the same plane as the palm, with the volar surface facing more anteriorly than normal. Atrophy of the muscles of the thenar eminence is usually conspicuous.

Three muscles supplied, at least in part, by the ulnar nerve have already been described: flexor carpi ulnaris, flexor digitorum profundus, and flexor pollicis brevis. The remaining muscles supplied by this nerve follow.

HYPOTHENAR MUSCLES

(Ulnar nerve, C8, T1)

Action

Abductor digiti quinti and flexor digiti quinti: abduction and flexion (proximal phalanx) of little finger.

Opponens digiti quinti: opposition of little finger toward thumb.

All three muscles: palmar elevation of head of fifth metacarpal, helping to cup palm.

Test

Action usually tested is abduction of little finger (against resistance).

The abductor digiti quinti is readily observed and palpated at the ulnar border of the palm. Opposition of the thumb and little finger can be tested together by gauging the force required to separate the tips of the two digits when opposed, or by attempting to withdraw a piece of paper clasped between the tips of the digits.

INTEROSSEI

(Ulnar nerve, C8, T1) (Figs. 5-40 and 5-41)

Action

Dorsal: abduction of index, middle, and ring fingers from middle line of middle finger (double action on middle finger, both radial and ulnar abduction, radial abduction of index finger, ulnar abduction of ring finger).

First dorsal: adduction (especially palmar adduction) of thumb.

Palmar: adduction of index, ring, and little fingers toward middle finger.

Both sets: flexion of metacarpophalangeal joints and simultaneous extension of interphalangeal joints.

Test

Abduction and adduction of individual fingers are tested against resistance with fingers extended. Adduction can be tested by retention of a slip of paper between fingers, and between thumb and index finger, as examiner attempts to withdraw it.

Ability of patient to flex proximal phalanges and simultaneously extend distal phalanges.

Extension of middle phalanges of fingers against resistance while examiner stabilizes proximal phalanges in hyperextension.

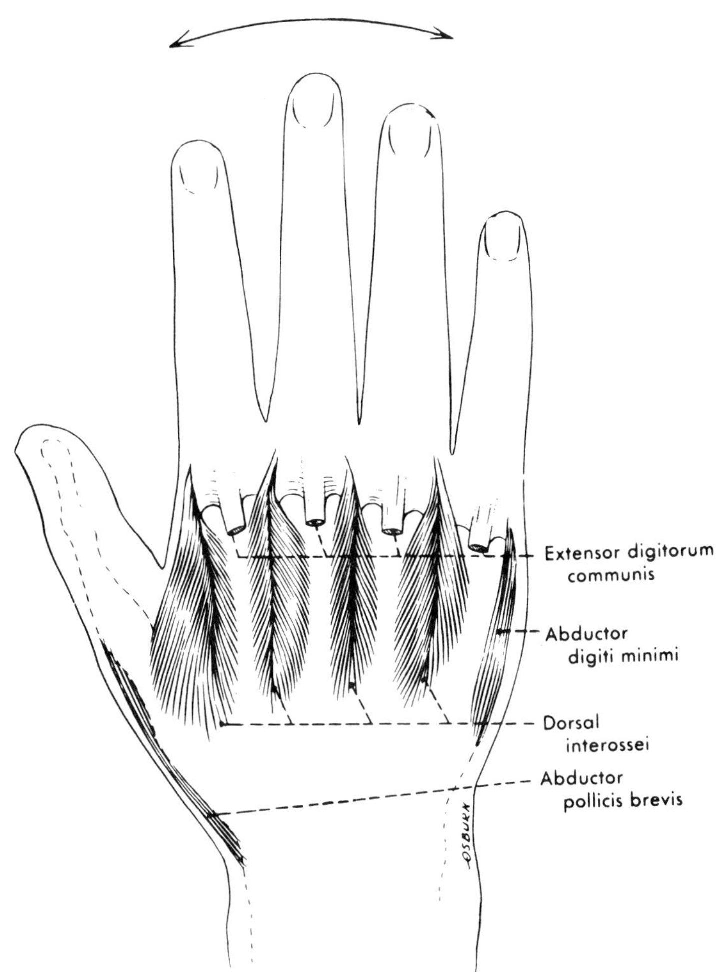

FIG. 5-40. Dorsal view of the chief abductors of the digits. (Reprinted with permission from Hollinshead WH. *Functional anatomy of the limbs and back: a text for students of physical therapy and others interested in the locomotor apparatus,* 3rd ed. Philadelphia: WB Saunders, 1969.)

The long extensors of the fingers (radial nerve) and the lumbrical muscles (median and ulnar nerves) assist in extension of the middle and distal phalanges. The first dorsal interosseous is readily observed and palpated in the space between the index finger and the thumb.

ADDUCTOR POLLICIS

(Ulnar nerve, C8, T1)

Action

Adduction of thumb in both ulnar and palmar directions (in plane of palm and perpendicular to palm, respectively).

Assistance in flexion of proximal phalanx.

Test

Adduction in each plane is tested against resistance by retention of slip of paper between thumb and radial border of hand and between thumb and palm, without flexion of distal phalanx.

It is often possible to palpate the edge of the adductor pollicis just volar to the proximal part of the first dorsal interosseous.

Participating Muscles

Ulnar adduction: first dorsal interosseous; flexor pollicis longus; extensor pollicis longus; flexor pollicis brevis.

Palmar adduction: first dorsal interosseous particularly; extensor pollicis longus.

The muscles of the neck and trunk may be examined in groups in most instances.

FLEXORS OF NECK

(Cervical nerves, C1–C6)

Test

In sitting or supine position, flexion of neck, with chin on chest, is tested against resistance applied to forehead.

EXTENSORS OF NECK

(Cervical nerves, C1)

Test

In sitting or prone position, extension of neck is tested against resistance applied to occiput.

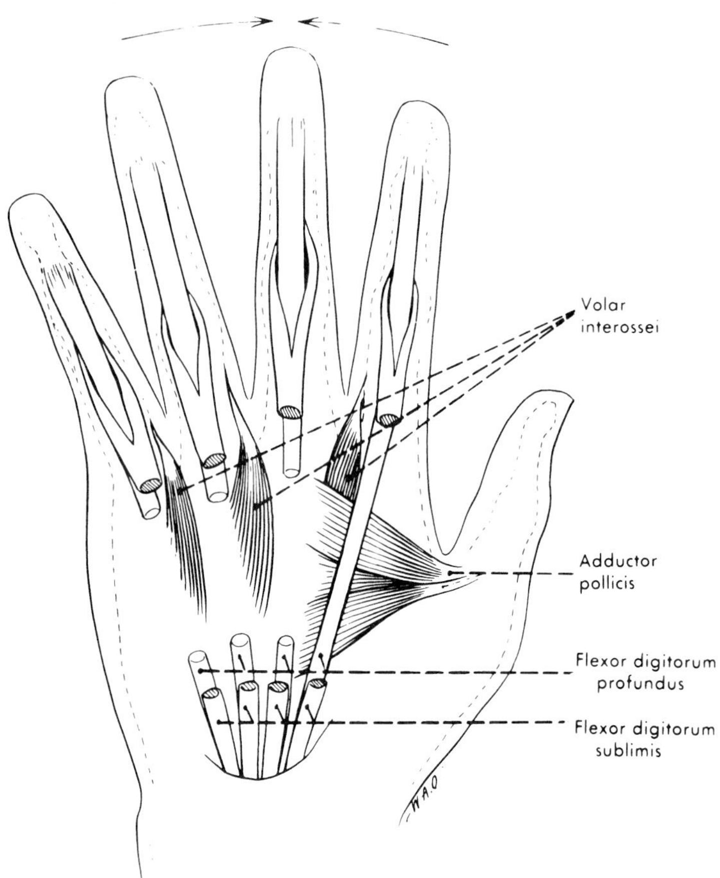

FIG. 5-41. Chief adductors of the digits. (Reprinted with permission from Hollinshead WH. *Functional anatomy of the limbs and back: a text for students of physical therapy and others interested in the locomotor apparatus,* 3rd ed. Philadelphia: WB Saunders, 1969.)

DIAPHRAGM

(Phrenic nerves, C3–C5)

Action

Abdominal respiration (inspiration), as distinguished from thoracic respiration (inspiration), which is produced principally by the intercostal muscles.

Test

Patient is observed for protrusion of upper portion of abdomen during deep inspiration when thoracic cage is splinted.

Patient is observed for ability to sniff.

Litten's sign (successive retraction of lower intercostal spaces during inspiration) is sought.

Diaphragmatic movements are observed fluoroscopically.

Weakness of the diaphragm should be suspected in disease of the spinal cord when the deltoid or biceps is paralyzed, because these muscles are supplied by neurons situated very near those innervating the diaphragm.

INTERCOSTAL MUSCLES

(Intercostal nerves, T1–T11)

Action

Expansion of thorax anteroposteriorly and transversely, producing thoracic inspiration.

Test

Observation and palpation of expansion of thoracic cage during deep inspiration while maintaining pressure against thorax.

Observation for asymmetry of movement of thorax, particularly during deep inspiration.

Other more general tests of function of the respiratory muscles are as follows:

- Observation of patient for rapid shallow respiration, flaring of alae nasi, and use of accessory muscles of respiration
- Ability of patient to repeat three or four numbers without pausing for breath
- Ability of patient to hold breath for 15 seconds

ANTERIOR ABDOMINAL MUSCLES

Upper (T6–T9); lower (T10–L1)

Test

Supine: flexion of neck is tested against resistance applied to forehead by examiner.

Contraction of the abdominal muscles can be observed and palpated. Upward movement of the umbilicus is associated with weakness of the lower abdominal muscles (Beevor's sign).

Supine: hands on occiput. Flexion of trunk by anterior

abdominal muscles followed by flexion of pelvis on thighs by hip flexors (chiefly iliopsoas) to reach sitting position. Examiner holds legs down.

Completion of this test excludes significant weakness of either the abdominal muscles or the flexors of the hips. Weak abdominal muscles, in the presence of strong hip flexors, result in hyperextension of the lumbar spine during attempts to elevate the legs or rise to a sitting position.

EXTENSORS OF BACK

Test

In prone position with hands clasped over buttocks, the head and shoulders are elevated off the table while the examiner holds legs down.

The gluteal and hamstring muscles fix the pelvis on the thigh.

ILIOPSOAS

Psoas major (lumbar plexus, L1, L2, L3, L4); iliacus (femoral nerve, L2, L3, L4) (Fig. 5-42)

Action

Flexion of thigh at hip.

Test

Sitting: flexion of thigh is tested by raising knee against resistance by examiner.

Supine: flexion of thigh is tested by raising extended leg off table and maintaining it against downward pressure by examiner applied just above knee.

Participating Muscles

Rectus femoris and sartorius (both, femoral nerve, L2–L4); tensor fasciae latae (superior gluteal nerve, L4, L5, S1)

ADDUCTOR MAGNUS, LONGUS, BREVIS

(Obturator nerve, L2, L3, L4; part of adductor magnus is supplied by sciatic nerve, L5, and functions with hamstrings) (Fig. 5-42)

Action

Principally adduction of thigh.

Test

Sitting or supine: knees are held together while examiner attempts to separate them.

The two legs also can be tested separately and the muscles palpated.

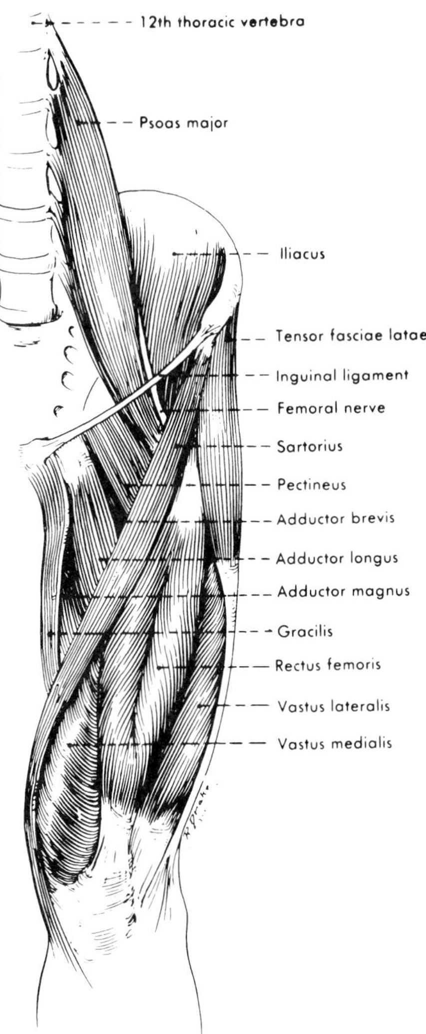

FIG. 5-42. The superficial muscles of the anterior aspect of the thigh. (Reprinted with permission from Hollinshead WH. *Functional anatomy of the limbs and back: a text for students of physical therapy and others interested in the locomotor apparatus,* 3rd ed. Philadelphia: WB Saunders, 1969.)

Participating Muscles

Gluteus maximus; gracilis (obturator nerve, L2–L4)

ABDUCTORS OF THIGH

(Superior gluteal nerve, L4, L5, S1) (Fig. 5-43)

Gluteus medius and gluteus minimus principally.

Tensor fasciae latae to a lesser extent.

Action

Abduction and medial rotation of thigh.

Tensor fasciae latae assists in flexion of thigh at hip.

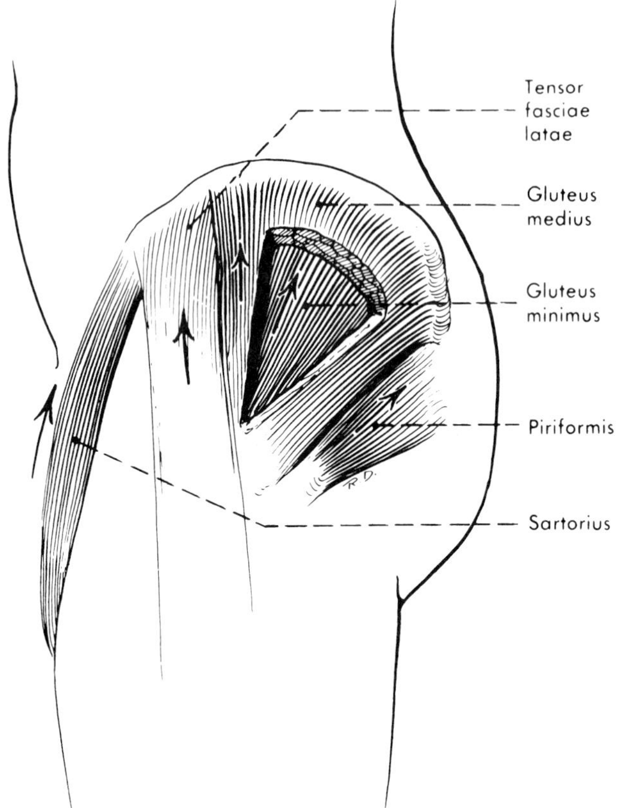

FIG. 5-43. Abductors of the thigh. (Reprinted with permission from Hollinshead WH. *Functional anatomy of the limbs and back: a text for students of physical therapy and others interested in the locomotor apparatus,* 3rd ed. Philadelphia: WB Saunders, 1969.)

Test

Sitting: knees are separated against resistance by examiner.

In this position the gluteus maximus and some of the other lateral rotators of the thigh function as abductors, hence diminishing the accuracy of the test.

Supine: same test as above, but more exact.

Lying on opposite site: hip is abducted (upward movement) while examiner presses downward on lower leg and stabilizes pelvis.

The tensor fasciae latae and to a lesser extent the gluteus medius can be palpated.

MEDIAL ROTATORS OF THIGH

(Same as abductors)

Test

Sitting or prone: knee is flexed to 90°. Medial rotation of thigh is tested against resistance applied by examiner at knee and ankle in an attempt to rotate thigh laterally.

LATERAL ROTATORS OF THIGH

(L4, L5, S1, S2) (Fig. 5-44)

Gluteus maximus (inferior gluteal nerve, L5, S1, S2) chiefly.

Obturator internus and gemellus superior (nerve to obturator internus, L5, S1, S2).

Quadratus femoris and gemellus inferior (nerve to quadratus femoris, L4, L5, S1).

Test

Sitting or prone: knee is flexed to 90°. Lateral rotation of thigh is tested against attempt by examiner to rotate thigh medially.

The gluteus maximus is the muscle principally tested and can be observed and palpated in the prone position.

GLUTEUS MAXIMUS

(Inferior gluteal nerve, L5, S1, S2) (Fig. 5-44)

Action

Extension of thigh at hip.

Lateral rotation of thigh.

Assistance in adduction of thigh.

Test

Sitting or supine: starting with thigh slightly raised, extension (downward movement) of thigh is tested against resistance applied by examiner under distal part of thigh.

This is a rather crude test, and the muscle cannot be observed or readily palpated.

Prone: knee is well flexed to minimize participation of hamstrings. Extension of thigh is tested by raising knee from table against downward pressure applied by examiner to distal part of thigh.

The muscle is accessible to observation and palpation in this position.

QUADRICEPS FEMORIS

(Femoral nerve, L2, L3, L4) (Fig. 5-45)

Action

Extension of leg at knee.

Rectus femoris assists in flexion of thigh at hip.

Test

Sitting or supine: lower leg is in moderate extension. Maintenance of extension is tested against effort of examiner to flex leg at knee.

Atrophy is easily noted.

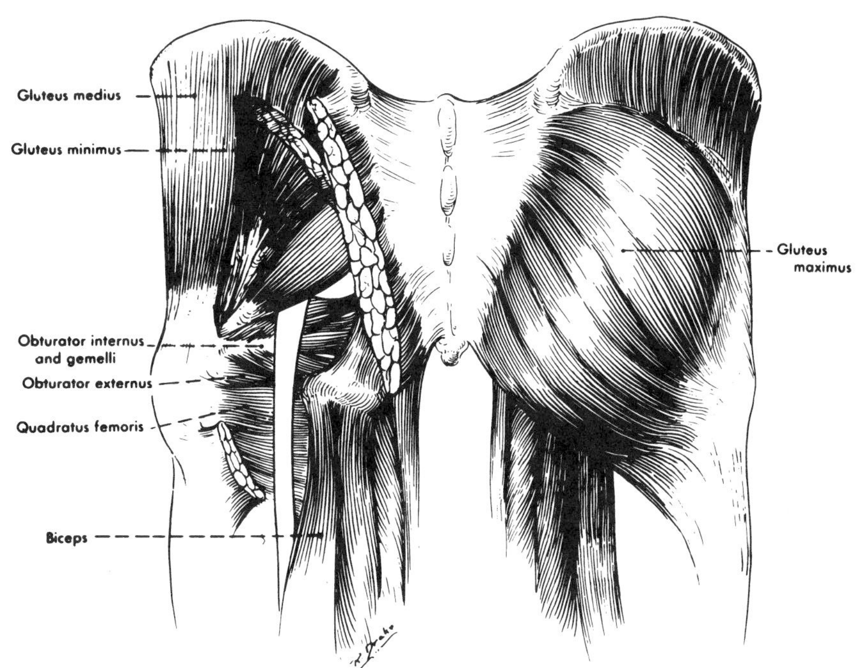

FIG. 5-44. Posteriorly placed external rotators of thigh. (Reprinted with permission from Hollinshead WH. *Functional anatomy of the limbs and back: a text for students of physical therapy and others interested in the locomotor apparatus,* 3rd ed. Philadelphia: WB Saunders, 1969.)

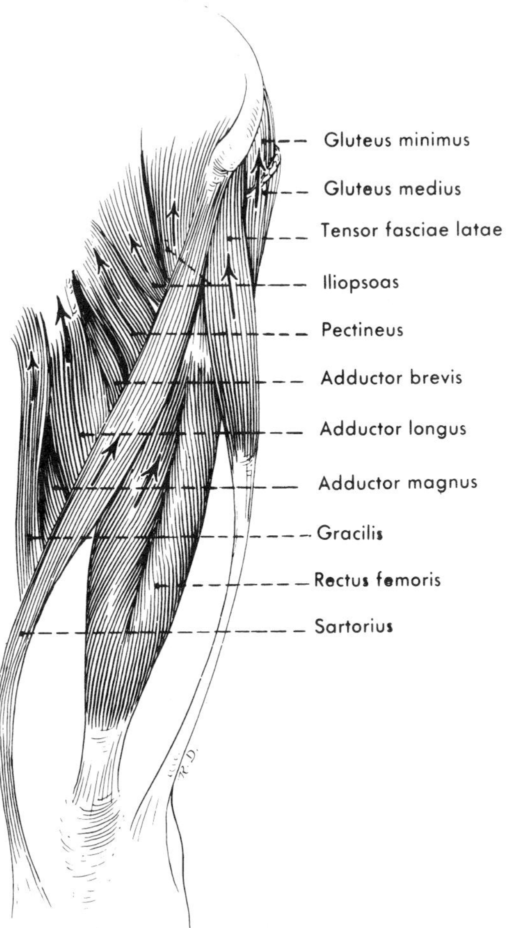

FIG. 5-45. Flexors of the thigh. (Reprinted with permission from Hollinshead WH. *Functional anatomy of the limbs and back: a text for students of physical therapy and others interested in the locomotor apparatus,* 3rd ed. Philadelphia: WB Saunders, 1969.)

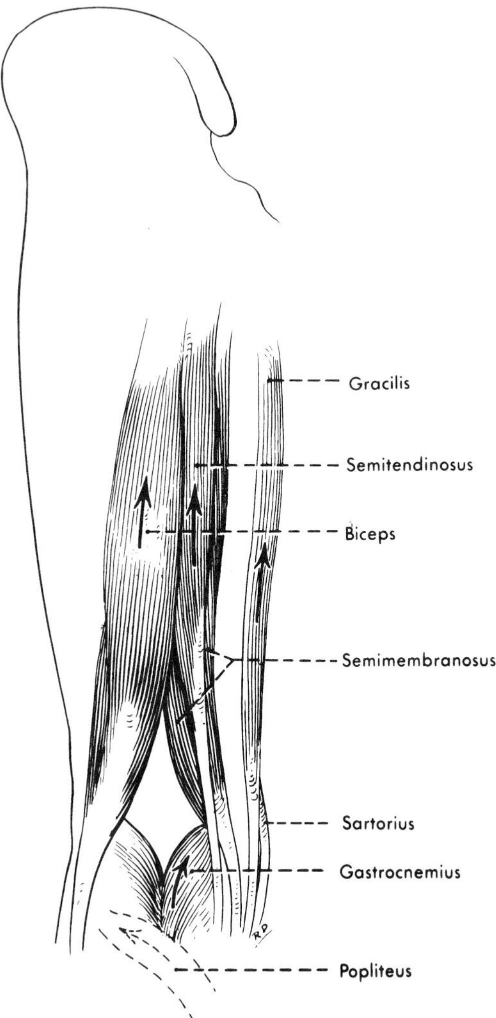

FIG. 5-46. Flexors of the knee. (Reprinted with permission from Hollinshead WH. *Functional anatomy of the limbs and back: a text for students of physical therapy and others interested in the locomotor apparatus,* 3rd ed. Philadelphia: WB Saunders, 1969.)

HAMSTRINGS

(Sciatic nerve, L4, L5, S1, S2) (Fig. 5-46)

Biceps femoris: external hamstring (L5, S1, S2).
Semitendinosus.
Semimembranosus.

Action

Flexion of leg at knee.
All but short head of biceps femoris assist in extension of thigh at hip.

Test

Sitting: flexion of lower leg is tested against resistance.
Prone: knee is partly flexed. Further flexion is tested against resistance. Observation and palpation of the muscles and tendons are important for proper interpretation.

TIBIALIS ANTERIOR

(Deep peroneal nerve, L4, L5, S1) (Figs. 5-47 through 5-49)

Action

Dorsiflexion and inversion (particularly in dorsiflexed position) of foot.

Test

Dorsiflexion of foot is tested against resistance applied to dorsum of foot downward and toward eversion.

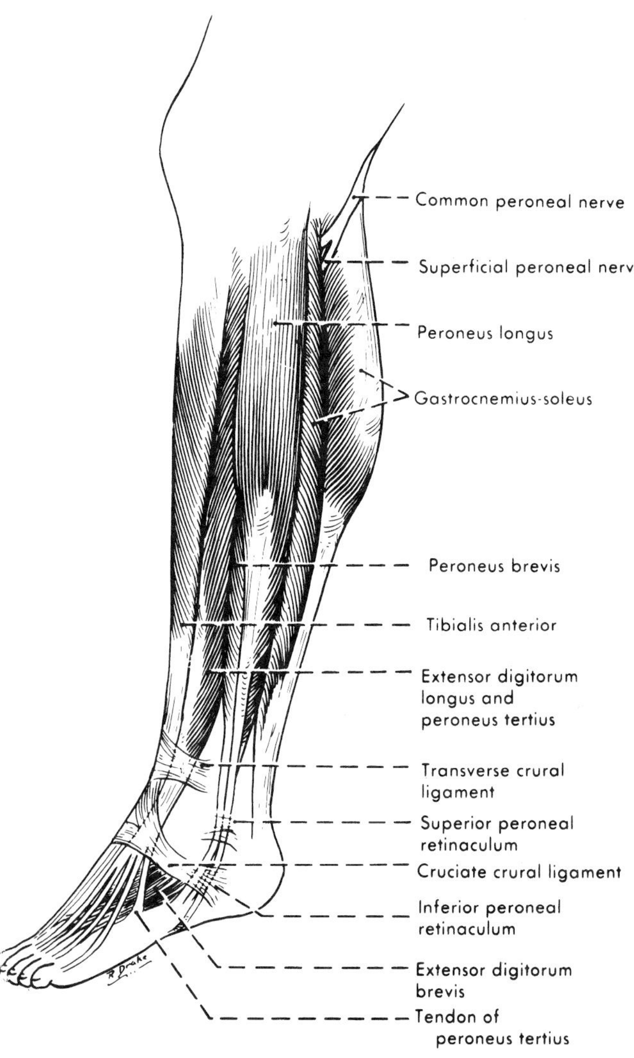

FIG. 5-47. Lateral muscles of the leg. (Reprinted with permission from Hollinshead WH. *Functional anatomy of the limbs and back: a text for students of physical therapy and others interested in the locomotor apparatus,* 3rd ed. Philadelphia: WB Saunders, 1969.)

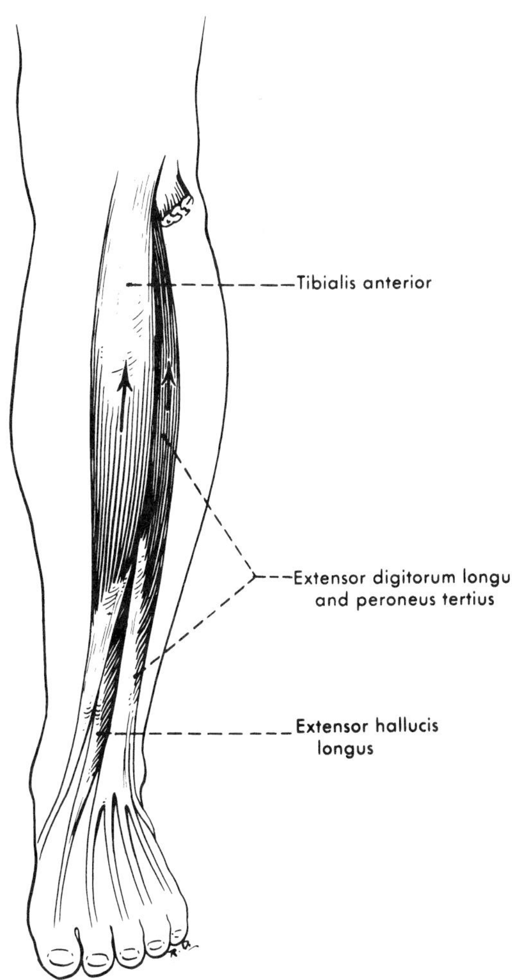

FIG. 5-48. Dorsiflexors of the foot. (Reprinted with permission from Hollinshead WH. *Functional anatomy of the limbs and back: a text for students of physical therapy and others interested in the locomotor apparatus,* 3rd ed. Philadelphia: WB Saunders, 1969.)

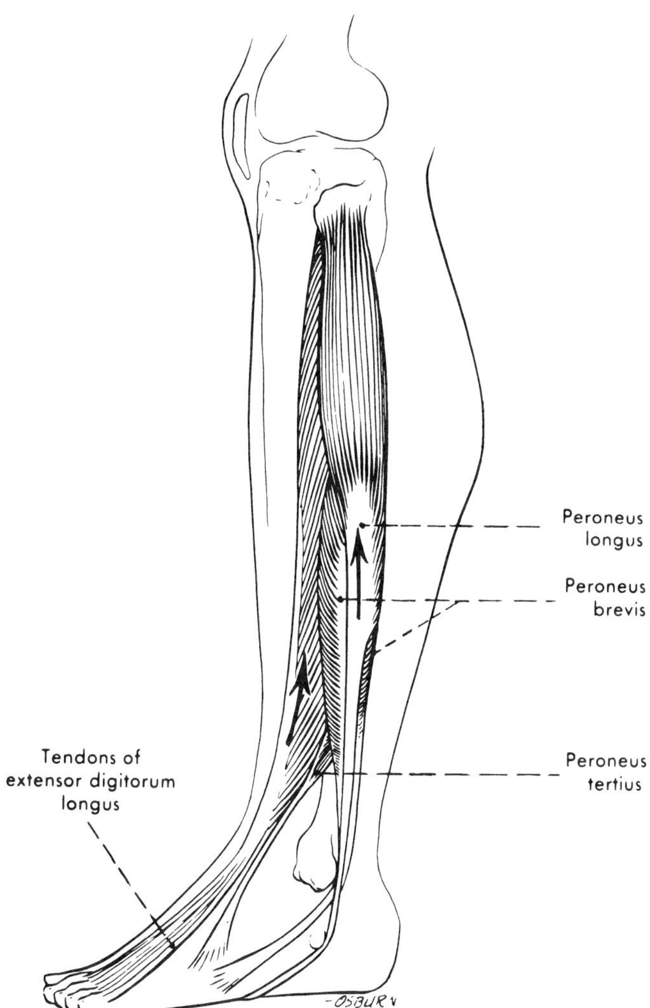

FIG. 5-49. Evertors of the foot. (Reprinted with permission from Hollinshead WH. *Functional anatomy of the limbs and back: a text for students of physical therapy and others interested in the locomotor apparatus,* 3rd ed. Philadelphia: WB Saunders, 1969.)

The belly of the muscle just lateral to the shin and the tendon medially on the dorsal aspect of the ankle should be observed and palpated. Atrophy is conspicuous.

Participating Muscles

Dorsiflexion: extensor hallucis longus; extensor digitorum longus

Inversion: tibialis posterior

EXTENSOR HALLUCIS LONGUS

(Deep peroneal nerve, L4, L5, S1) (Fig. 5-48)

Action

Extension of great toe and dorsiflexion of foot.

Test

Extension of great toe is tested against resistance while foot is stabilized in neutral position.

The tendon is palpable between the tendons of the tibialis anterior and the extensor digitorum longus.

EXTENSOR DIGITORUM LONGUS

(Deep peroneal nerve, L4, L5, S1) (Figs. 5-47 and 5-48)

Action

Extension of lateral four toes and dorsiflexion of foot.

Test

Test is similar to that for action of extensor hallucis longus.

The tendons are visible and palpable on the dorsal aspect of the ankle and foot lateral to the tendon of the extensor hallucis longus.

EXTENSOR DIGITORUM BREVIS

(Deep peroneal nerve, L4, L5, S1) (Fig. 5-47)

Action

Assists in extension of all toes except little toe.

Test

Belly of muscle is observed and palpated on lateral aspect of dorsum of foot.

PERONEUS LONGUS, BREVIS

(Superficial peroneal nerve, L4, L5, S1) (Fig. 5-49)

Action

Eversion of foot.
Assistance in plantar flexion of foot.

Test

Foot is in plantar flexion. Eversion is tested against resistance applied by examiner to lateral border of foot.

The tendons are palpable just above and behind the external malleolus. Atrophy may be visible over the anterolateral aspect of the lower leg.

GASTROCNEMIUS; SOLEUS

(Tibial nerve, L5, S1, S2) (Fig. 5-50)

Action

Plantar flexion of foot.

The gastrocnemius also flexes the knee and cannot act effectively in plantar flexion of the foot when the knee is well flexed.

Test

Knee is extended to test both muscles. Knee is flexed to test principally soleus. Plantar flexion of foot is tested against resistance.

The muscles and tendon should be observed and palpated. Atrophy is readily visible. The gastrocnemius and soleus are very strong muscles, and leverage in testing favors the patient rather than the examiner. For this reason, slight weakness is difficult to detect by resisting flexion of the ankle or by pressing against the flexed foot in the direction of extension. Consequently, it is advisable to test the strength of these muscles against the weight of the patient's body. The patient stands on one foot and flexes the foot so as to lift himself or herself directly and fully upward. Sometimes it is necessary for the examiner to hold the patient steady as this test is performed.

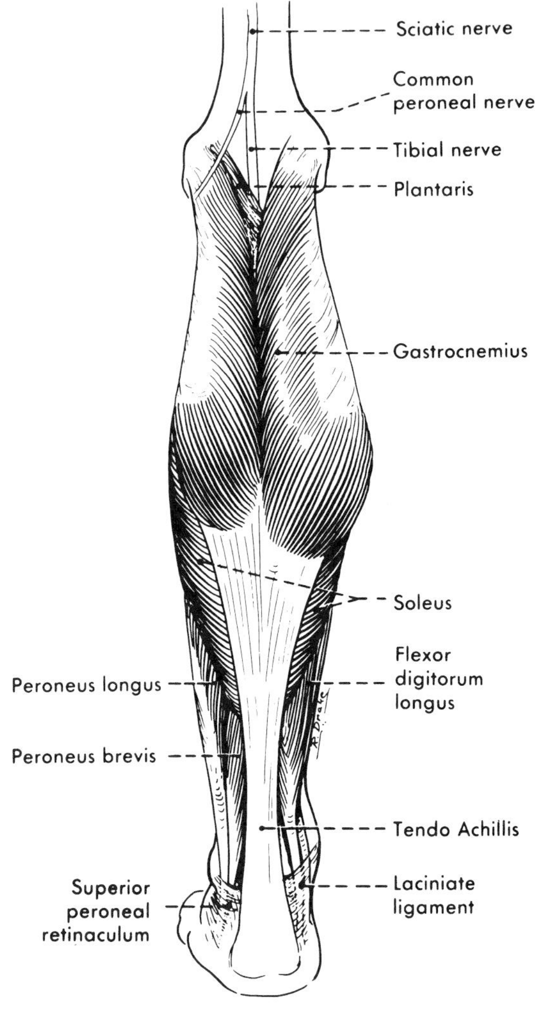

FIG. 5-50. Musculature of the calf of the leg, first layer. (Reprinted with permission from Hollinshead WH. *Functional anatomy of the limbs and back: a text for students of physical therapy and others interested in the locomotor apparatus,* 3rd ed. Philadelphia: WB Saunders, 1969.)

Participating Muscles

Long flexors of toes; tibialis posterior and peroneus longus and brevis (particularly near extreme plantar flexion).

TIBIALIS POSTERIOR

(Posterior tibial nerve, L5, S1) (Fig. 5-51)

Action

Inversion of foot.
Assistance in plantar flexion of foot.

Test

Foot is in complete plantar flexion. Inversion is tested against resistance applied to medial border of foot and directed toward eversion and slightly toward dorsiflexion.

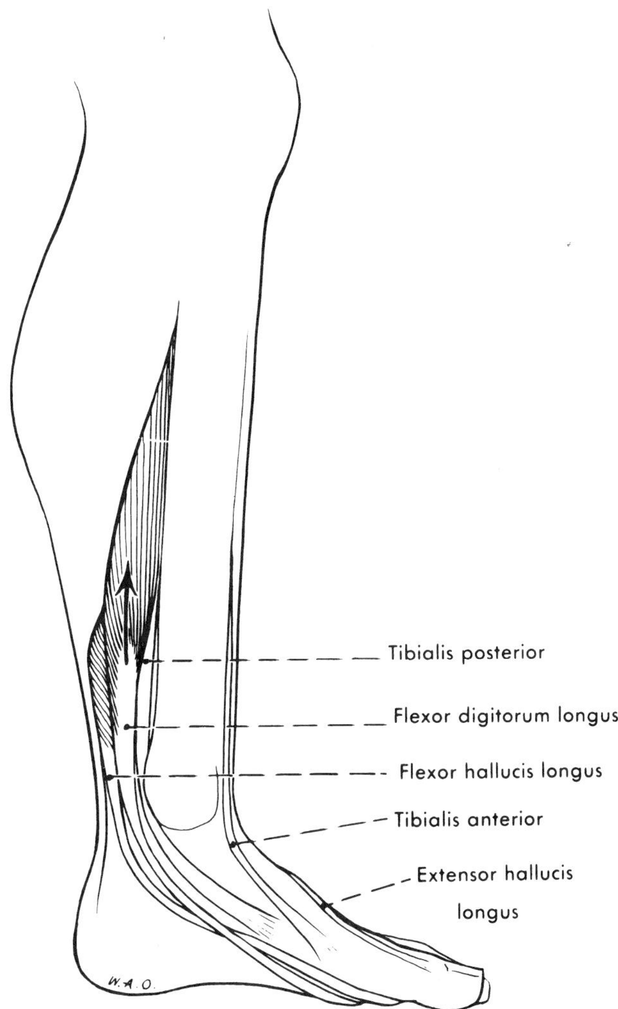

FIG. 5-51. Invertors of the foot. (Reprinted with permission from Hollinshead WH. *Functional anatomy of the limbs and back: a text for students of physical therapy and others interested in the locomotor apparatus,* 3rd ed. Philadelphia: WB Saunders, 1969.)

This maneuver virtually eliminates participation of the tibialis anterior in inversion. The toes should be relaxed to prevent participation of the long flexors of the toes.

LONG FLEXORS OF TOES

(Posterior tibial nerve, L5, S1, S2)

- Flexor digitorum longus.
- Flexor hallucis longus.

Action

Plantar flexion of toes, especially at distal interphalangeal joints.

Assistance in plantar flexion and inversion of foot.

Test

Foot is stabilized in neutral position. Plantar flexion of toes is tested against resistance applied particularly to distal phalanges.

INTRINSIC MUSCLES OF FOOT

These include virtually all muscles except extensor digitorum brevis (medial and lateral plantar nerves from posterior tibial nerve, L5, S1, S2).

Action

Somewhat comparable with that of intrinsic muscles of the hand. Many people have very poor individual function of these muscles.

Test

Cupping sole of foot is adequate test for most clinical purposes.

Neurologic Examination

With the exception of the musculoskeletal examination, no other component of the standard physical examination is more important to the rehabilitation assessment than the neurologic examination. Although often conducted to identify disease, the neurologic examination provides the rehabilitation physician with the opportunity to identify both the neurological impairments to be addressed and the residual abilities to be used in maximizing the functional outcome of the patient.

Although it is customary to record the results of the neurologic examination in a separate portion of the examination report, the examination is rarely performed all at one time. The examiner often finds it convenient to integrate the appropriate portions of the neurologic examination into the assessment of a specific region of the body. For example, cranial nerve assessment is often performed with other components of the head and neck examination because the patient is positioned appropriately for both. For purposes of discussion, the neurologic examination is addressed separately and is divided into assessments of mental status, speech and language function, cranial nerves, reflexes, central motor integration, sensation, and perception. Muscle strength is discussed in the section on examination of the musculoskeletal system. The assessment of complex motor activities is discussed in the section on the functional examination. The reader is referred to *Clinical Examinations in Neurology* for a comprehensive discussion of the neurologic evaluation (1).

Mental Status

Level of Consciousness

Before performing a formal mental status examination, the patient's level of consciousness is determined. Qualita-

TABLE 5-4. *Glasgow coma scale*[a]

Eye Opening	
Spontaneous	E4
To speech	E3
To pain	E2
Nil	E1
Best Motor Response	
Obeys	M6
Localizes	M5
Withdraws	M4
Abnormal flexion	M3
Extensor response	M2
Nil	M1
Verbal Response	
Orientated	V5
Confused conversation	V4
Inappropriate words	V3
Incomprehensible sounds	V2
Nil	V1

[a] Coma score (E + M + V) = 3 to 15.

From Jennett B. Teasdale G. *Management of head injuries.* Philadelphia: FA Davis, 1981.

tive terms such as drowsy, lethargic, and stuporous are useful in a descriptive sense, but they suffer from a lack of precise definition. "Stuporous" to one examiner may be "lethargic" to another. A definitive classification of mental status requires a standardized approach (13–15). In the Glasgow Coma Scale, the examiner classifies the patient's eye, motor, and verbal responses to verbal or physical stimuli according to a numerical scale that is quantifiable and reproducible (Table 5-4) (16). Such a standardized scale is necessary to assess changes over time and to facilitate communication among physicians, nurses, therapists, and family. In patients with traumatic brain injury, other aspects of the neurologic assessment such as pupillary responses, ocular movements, and respiration will provide information about the cause of altered consciousness but do not quantifiably relate in a statistical sense to eventual outcome.

Cognitive Evaluation

With the conscious patient, assessment of mental status begins when the physician enters the room, and it continues throughout the examination. However, as with the assessment of the level of consciousness, a formal approach to the mental status examination is beneficial to identify and quantify specific impairments and residual capacity, to recognize subtle temporal changes, and to facilitate communication among caregivers. Excellent systems have been developed to assess intellectual performance in specific populations (10,16). Although some systems include perceptual testing, speech and language assessment, or an inventory of thought processing, and other systems do not, certain components of the evaluation remain constant.

Orientation. The patient is asked to report his or her name, address, and telephone number and the building (e.g., hospital, clinic), city, state, year, month, and day.

Attention. Attention is assessed with digit repetition; the patient is asked to repeat a series of random numbers. Two numbers are used initially (e.g., "4, 9"); if the patient answers correctly, increase the sequence by one digit until the patient either repeats seven digits correctly or makes a mistake. Note the number of digits repeated correctly.

Recall. Three numbers or three objects are listed, and the patient is asked to remember them because he or she will be asked to repeat them later. A response from the patient is requested in 5 minutes, and the number of correct responses is recorded. If all responses are correct, recall responses are obtained at 10 and 15 minutes.

General Fund of Information. Questions are asked appropriate to the patient's age, cultural interests, and educational background. For example, the names of the past five presidents or other country leaders, the current vice president, and the home-state governor can be requested, or inquiries can be made for information about current events and other nearly universal subjects (e.g., world wars and basic scientific principles).

Calculations. The patient is asked to count by sevens, and the last correct response is recorded. Arithmetic calculations of increasing difficulty are presented.

Proverbs. An explanation of three common proverbs is requested. The patient is assessed as to whether he or she abstracts the principle from the adage or explains it in concrete terms.

Similarities. The patient is requested to describe what is common to an orange and an apple, a desk and a bookcase, and a cup and a fork. The number of correct responses is recorded.

Judgment. The patient is presented with three problems (e.g., smelling smoke in a movie theater, finding a stamped and addressed envelope on the sidewalk, and finding a friend in an unfamiliar city) and asked how to handle the situations.

Speech and Language Function

As with the assessment of mental status, analysis of communicative function occurs throughout the entire examination. The patient should be evaluated for the presence and extent of aphasia, apraxia, and dysarthria, and residual communicative skills should be identified. At times, effort is required to discriminate among the disorders of aphasia, apraxia of speech, and the language dysfunction associated with a more generalized cognitive deficit. Expert assessment of speech production and language processing can be a valuable tool for the diagnosis of neurologic disease (see Chapter 12). However, as described in the preceding section, assessment of the four basic elements of communication provides a practical framework for functional evaluation.

Listening

After first determining that the patient does not have a significant hearing loss, had spoken your language before the onset of disease, and has the requisite motor and visual skills, the physician tests the patient's auditory comprehension, noting his or her ability to follow specific directions without gestures from the examiner. Often, it is useful to characterize the degree of impairment with stepped commands. First, the patient's ability to follow one-step commands is assessed by asking him or her to perform three different single motor activities, such as "take off your glasses," "touch your nose," and "open the book." Each command should be given separately, and a prolonged pause should be allowed to observe the response. These responses are rated and notation made of whether the patient requires pantomime of the activity before performing the task. If two of the three responses are correct, the patient's skill is assessed at following two-step commands, such as "touch your nose, then take off your glasses," "point to the window, then close the book," and "touch my hand, then touch your knee." If the patient can follow two-step commands, then three-step commands are assessed in a similar fashion. A simple object such as a toothbrush is held up and the patient is asked to demonstrate its use. This request is repeated at least two times with different objects. If speech is functional, a short phrase is spoken and the patient is asked to repeat it. The response is observed for perseveration and jargon.

Reading

It is important to be sure the patient had reading skills before onset of the neurologic disorder. The patient is asked to read a short written command and perform the activity; the patient also can try two- and three-step commands. If writing is otherwise functional, the patient is asked to read aloud what he or she has written.

Speaking

If auditory comprehension is adequate, language production is tested in the following ways. An object is indicated and the patient is asked to name it and to state its function; at least three objects are used. The patient is asked to report his or her name, home town, telephone number, or other simple verifiable fact. A picture can be shown and the patient asked to describe it. Tests for phonation and resonance deficits are performed by asking the patient to say a prolonged "aaah" and observing for force and steadiness of pitch and tone. The patient is asked to say "pa-pa-pa" to test lip closure, "ta-ta-ta" to test tongue function, and "ka-ka-ka" to test speed, regulatory, and posterior pharyngeal function. If reading is otherwise functional, the patient is asked to read aloud a short passage with various vowels and consonants to assess articulation further.

Writing

The patient is asked to write his or her name, address, and telephone number and to write a brief paragraph.

Cranial Nerves

Cranial Nerve I (Olfactory)

Olfactory function is evaluated routinely. Deficits are common after head trauma.

Cranial Nerve II (Optic)

Visual field testing of each eye is performed individually, with a temporary patch over the contralateral side. It is best to test each quadrant diagonally to identify quadrantanopias. Although visual double simultaneous stimulation may be more correctly classified under cortical sensation, it is convenient to assess for extinction during visual field testing, once full fields have been ensured. Visual acuity is discussed in the section on eye examination.

Cranial Nerves III (Oculomotor), IV (Trochlear), and VI (Abducens)

Visual pathways are assessed by evaluating pupil size, pupillary reactions, and extraocular movements. Strabismus is evaluated by testing corneal light reflections.

Cranial Nerve V (Trigeminal)

The muscles of mastication and facial sensation are tested.

Cranial Nerve VIII (Vestibular/Auditory)

Nystagmus is sought. Auditory function is discussed in the section on ear examination.

Cranial Nerves VII (Facial), IX (Glossopharyngeal), X (Vagus), and XII (Hypoglossal)

Isolating individual cranial nerve function emanating from the lower part of the brain stem is difficult. Cranial nerves are often grouped by function. Taste (nerves VII, IX, and X), muscles of facial expression (nerve VII) and articulation (nerves VII, IX, X, and XII), and swallowing function (nerves IX, X, and XII) are evaluated.

Cranial Nerve XI (Accessory)

Sternocleidomastoid and trapezius function is frequently assessed during manual muscle testing.

Brain stem and visual-evoked responses, electromyography and other forms of electrodiagnostic testing, and swallowing videofluoroscopy are often necessary for better delineation of dysfunction of cranial nerves and their brain stem interactions.

Reflexes

Muscle Stretch Reflexes

After the patient is relaxed, muscle stretch reflexes are tested. Commonly, the biceps (C5–C6), triceps (C6–C8), brachioradialis (C5–C6), quadriceps (L2–L4), and triceps surae (L5, S1–S2) are tested. The masseter (cranial nerve V), internal hamstring (L4–L5, S1–S2), and external hamstring (L5, S1–S2) reflexes are tested in selected cases. The patient is observed for clonus.

Superficial Reflexes

Segmental reflexes are often helpful for localizing the lesion. The corneal (cranial nerves V and VII), gag (cranial nerves IX and X), anal (S3–S5), and plantar (L5, S1–S2) reflexes are tested. At times, it is useful to include the epigastric (T6–T9), mid-abdominal (T9–T11), hypogastric (T11–T12, L1), and cremasteric (L1–L2) reflexes.

Pathologic Reflexes

Elicitation of the Babinski reflex is attempted. In questionable cases, the confirmatory Chaddock, Oppenheim, and Stransky reflexes are tested.

Central Motor Integration

Muscle Tone

Spasticity, rigidity, and hypotonicity are sought by assessing the patient's resistance to passive movement, pendulousness, and ability to posturally fixate.

Coordination

Coordination in the upper extremities is assessed with the finger-nose, finger-nose-finger, and knee-pat tests. Coordination in the lower extremities is evaluated with the toe-finger and heel-knee-shin test.

Alternate Motion Rate

The tongue-wiggle, finger-wiggle, and foot-pat tests are used to identify subtle spasticity, rigidity, and incoordination.

Involuntary Movements

The patient is observed for tremors, chorea, athetosis, ballismus, dystonia, myoclonus, asterixis, and tics and are described if present.

Apraxia

Apraxia is a failure of motor planning and execution without deficits of strength, coordination, or sensation; however, deficits of strength, coordination, and sensation are often also present because of the extent of the lesion. Automatic motor activities are observed while the patient manipulates a pen or pencil, handles clothing, and moves about the examination room; then the patient's ability to perform some of the same maneuvers on command is assessed. The patient is asked to touch his or her nose, drink from a glass, put a pencil in the glass, strike a match and blow it out, and use scissors. The patient is asked to perform these activities without the objects and with each hand. Inefficient or fumbling movements or failure to accomplish the task is noted. Dressing apraxia is assessed by asking the patient to put on a coat. To assess for more subtle deficits, one sleeve of the coat is first turned inside out. Constructional apraxia is evaluated by asking the patient to copy a geometric design or draw the face of a clock.

Sensation

Superficial Sensation

Light touch is tested with a wisp of cotton, superficial pain with a single-use pin, and temperature with two test tubes, one with hot and the other with cold tap water. Abnormal findings are recorded on a drawing of the human figure and compared with standard charts of spinal dermatomes and peripheral nerves (1).

Deep Sensation

The evaluation of joint position sense is started with distal hand and foot joints and moved proximally until normal sensation is identified. Testing for deep pain in the upper extremities is done by hyperextension of small finger joints and in the lower extremities by firm compression of the calf muscles or Achilles tendon. Vibration sense is often evaluated, but its isolated absence does not result in functional deficit.

Cortical Sensation

If superficial and deep sensations are intact, two-point discrimination, graphesthesia, stereognosis, and double simultaneous stimulation are evaluated.

Perception

Disorders of perception are most common with lesions of the nondominant parietal lobe but also can occur with lesions on the dominant side. Chapter 48 provides an in-depth discussion of perceptual disorders.

Agnosia

Agnosia is a failure to recognize familiar objects despite intact vision, hearing, sensation, and language function (although language is often also deficient because of the extent of the lesion). Pictures of common objects or the objects themselves are shown and the patient is asked to identify them and to describe their components. Agnosia of body parts is assessed by asking the patient to identify his or her or the examiner's arm, finger, or eye. Unilateral environmental neglect assessed by observing ambulation or wheelchair operation for difficulty clearing corners and doorjambs, extinction on double simultaneous stimulation, and failure to scan the complete page width when asked to read a passage or to cross out all the occurrences of the letter "E." Body scheme agnosias are evaluated by searching for denial of obvious physical impairments when the patient is asked to describe them.

Right-Left Disorientation

If agnosia of body parts is not present, the patient is asked to indicate various body parts on the right and left sides.

Other Perceptual Tests

If perceptual deficits are identified with the maneuvers described above, additional deficits are tested for, such as geographic and spatial orientation and figure-ground relationships. Comprehensive, formal, quantitative testing of perception by a psychologist and an occupational therapist is warranted if any deficits are found during the physical examination.

Functional Examination

Once impairments have been identified, the consequences of these impairments on the function of the patient must be appraised. Prediction of functional status should not be attempted from the history and physical examination; instead, function is examined. For a comprehensive assessment, the patient must be evaluated by individual rehabilitation team members in settings where the activities are actually performed. Bathing skills should be observed by the rehabilitation nurse in the bathroom while the patient attempts to bathe; eating skills should be analyzed by the occupational therapist while the patient eats a meal; and car transfer skills should be assessed by the physical therapist with use of the patient's car. Each team member will use unique skills to contribute to a comprehensive determination of functional status. Many functional evaluative processes cannot be accomplished at a single point. Safety and judgment can be assessed only from observation of the patient in varying situations within both the rehabilitation environment and the community.

However, the rehabilitation physician in many instances must glean a basic view of functional status at the time of the initial evaluation. For instance, in the clinic the physician may be consulted to determine a patient's need for rehabilitation services. It is unlikely that the physician will be able to observe the patient during a meal, in the bathroom, or transferring from the car. In such cases, the physician must use creativity to place the patient in situations that are similar to those of daily life. Examples are given below.

Components of the communication assessment were discussed in the sections on the history and physical examination and will not be repeated here.

Eating

The patient is requested to use examining equipment in place of feeding utensils to demonstrate proficiency in bringing food to the mouth. The patient is provided with a glass of water and asked to drink if aspiration has not already been identified.

Grooming

The patient is asked to comb hair and mimic the activities of brushing teeth or putting on makeup.

Bathing

The patient is observed mimicking the activities of bathing. It is important to note if any body parts cannot be reached by the patient, particularly whether the patient can reach the back, scalp, and the axilla and arm contralateral to hemiparesis.

Toileting

The patient must have adequate unsupported sitting balance, must have the requisite wrist and hand motion to reach

TABLE 5-5. *Gait analysis*

Standing Balance
Observe for steadiness of position. Push the patient off balance and note the patient's attempts to regain balanced posture
Individual Body Part Movements During Walking
Observe for fixed or abnormal postures and inadequate, excessive, or asymmetrical movements of body parts.
Head and trunk: listing or tilting, shoulder dipping, elevation, depression, protraction, and retraction
Arm swing: protective positioning or posturing
Pelvis and hip: hip hiking, dropping (Trendelenburg), or lateral thrust
Knee: genu valgum, varum, or recurvatum
Foot and ankle: excessive inversion or eversion
Gait Cycle Factors
Cadence: rate, symmetry, fluidity, and consistency
Stride width: narrow or broad base, knee and ankle clearance
Stride length: shortened, lengthened, or asymmetrical
Stance phase: normal heel-strike, foot flat, push-off; knee stability during all components of stance; coordination of knee and ankle movements
Swing phase: adequate and synchronized knee and ankle dorsiflexion during swing, abduction or circumduction

the perineum adequately, must be able to handle toilet paper, and must be able to rise from low seating.

Dressing

The patient is observed during undressing before the examination and dressing after completion of the examination. It is wise to explain the purpose of the observation and to be accompanied by a nurse or aide.

Bed Activities

During the physical examination, notation is made of whether the patient has difficulty moving between the seated and the supine position, can roll from front to back and back to front, and can raise the pelvis off the examining table while in the supine position.

Transfers

The patient is observed rising from seating with and without armrests and moving between bed and chair.

Wheelchair Mobility

The patient is asked to demonstrate wheeling straight ahead and turning, on both carpeted and noncarpeted floors, if available; locking the brakes; and manipulating the leg rests.

Ambulation

To adequately recognize disturbances of gait, the examiner must be able to view body parts. If the examining room is secluded, the assessment is performed while the patient is wearing underwear. If privacy is not possible, the patient

FUNCTIONAL STATUS

NAME John Doe 3-418-448 — Ⓛ Hemiparesis

ACTIVITY	Independent	Independent with aids	Requires Assistance	Dependent
Listening		aid-Ⓛ ear		
Reading			verbal cues to scan Ⓛ	
Speaking	dysarthria			
Writing	✓			
Eating			set up meal; needs rocker knife; scoopplate	
Grooming			verbal cues for Ⓛ body shave Ⓛ face	
Bathing			verbal cues for Ⓛ body wash Ⓡ trunk	
Toileting		bladder with urinal	1 person assist for transfer to commode	
Dressing			1 person assist lower body; fasteners	
Bed Activities		hospital bed with bed rails		
Transfers			verbal cues; lock brakes protect Ⓛ arm ↓ judgement	
Wheel Chair			verbal cues to scan Ⓛ unlock wc brakes	
Ambulation				✓
Driving				✓

If the activity is Independent or Dependent, mark with a check
If the activity is Independent with Aids, list the aids needed
If the activity Requires Assistance, describe the assistance and list the aids needed

FIG. 5-52. Sample of a functional status record.

should have access to washable or paper shorts. Assuming that the examiner does not already have knowledge of the patient's ambulation skills, it is wise to provide the patient with a safety belt before gait is assessed. If specific gait abnormalities are to be discerned, both the individual components and the composite activity must be studied. The patient is observed from the front, the back, and the sides. If the patient experiences pain during ambulation, the temporal relationship to the gait cycle is noted. The analysis must be approached in an orderly fashion. One routine for gait analysis is outlined in Table 5-5 (4,17). See Chapter 8 for a comprehensive discussion of gait.

Operation of a Motor Vehicle

Driving is best assessed in an automobile. However, the examiner can gain some information about the patient's motor abilities to drive by requesting the patient to demonstrate the motions of operating the pedals and hand controls.

Quantitation of Function

Several scales can be used to document and quantify functional status in activities of daily living. These are extremely useful to assess a patient's rehabilitation progress (see Chapter 15). When validated and standardized, they become essential tools for analysis of rehabilitation outcome for a series of patients participating in a specific intervention program. When these scales are used by multiple rehabilitation centers to share data, significant information can be obtained to advance the state of the art and assess the cost versus benefit of rehabilitation. The reader is encouraged to develop expertise in the use of these valuable tools.

However, the data collection for most validated functional scales requires additional time because of interdisciplinary input; therefore, the initial documentation of functional status by the physician must be practical and complete. One such system is shown in Figure 5-52. Findings from both the history and the physical examination should be used to define functional status.

SUMMARY AND PROBLEM LIST

Once the history is obtained, the physical examination has been performed, and the results recorded, the rehabilitation physician summarizes the findings, constructs a problem list, and formulates a plan.

A summary of findings often has been an inconsistent component of the written record. Often of two or three sentences in length, the summary can provide the reader with a succinct and memory-jogging description of significant findings in the history and examination.

For the management of chronic diseases, rehabilitation medicine must commonly address myriad physical, psychological, social, and vocational problems. Weed's problem-oriented medical record (18) has been applied to the management of patients undergoing rehabilitation (19–22). Although use of the problem list itself is the essential factor, a consensus as to the organization and use of the entire system in the rehabilitation setting has proved challenging. The recommendation of Grabois that medical and rehabilitation problems be separately listed is beneficial (21). In addition, it may be helpful to delineate individual plans for each problem at the conclusion of the workup (Table 5-6).

TABLE 5-6. *Example of summary, problem list, and plan*

Summary

55-year-old male carpenter with left hearing deficit and poorly treated hypertension; 4 days following sudden moderate left-side spastic hemiparesis, moderate sensory deficits, left neglect, nocturnal bladder incontinence, dysarthria. He is alert, oriented, and normotensive; left hip and knee motor function is returning; high serum cholesterol level. He is divorced, lives alone, and has no close family. CT scan of head shows moderate right subcortical infarction. Ischemia is not shown in ECG.

Medical Problems/Plans

1. Right hemisphere infarction with motor, sensory, perceptual, speech deficits: monitor neuromuscular fx, maintain ROM, control spasticity (air splint, positioning, consider meds) motor re-ed, patient ed/risk factors.
2. Hypertension: maintain below 140/90 mm Hg with propranolol, 40 mg quid po
3. Hypercholesterolemia: low-fat diet, patient ed/diet and food preparation
4. Urinary incontinence: check residual urine volume, culture specimens; treat urosepsis. If residual volume is low, offer urinal frequently, +/− nocturnal condom cath. If residual volumes are high, begin 1800-ml fluid intake schedule, q6h cath, urodynamics, bladder retraining.

Rehabilitation Problems/Plans

1. Communication deficits: speech pathologist for evaluation and therapy
2. Left neglect: OT for perceptual testing, retraining, and compensation; verbal clues to scan left, RN and RT to reinforce OT
3. Left sensory deficits: monitor skin, patient ed/insensate skin care
4. Self-care deficits: OT for upper extremity ROM, re-ed, strengthening, ADL retraining, adaptive aids
5. Safety and judgment deficits: 4 bed rails, RN to monitor closely at night, verbal clues, physical spotting
6. Transfer deficits: PT for retraining, left WC brake extension
7. Mobility deficits: PT for lower extremity ROM, re-ed, strengthening, gait retraining, gait aids
8. Driving, dependency: retesting and retraining if improvement
9. Community re-entry/poor support system: assess home for architectural barriers, assess home health services, identify additional social support
10. Reactive depression: psychological support
11. Vocational issues: consider prevocational counseling and testing

+/−, presence or absence; ADL, activities of daily living; cath, catheterization; CT, computed tomography; ECG, electrocardiogram; ed, education; fx, fracture; OT, occupational therapy; PT, physical therapy; RN, registered nurse; ROM, range of motion; WC, wheelchair.

REFERENCES

1. Department of Neurology and Department of Physiology and Biophysics, Mayo Clinic and Mayo Foundation. *Clinical examinations in neurology,* 6th ed. Philadelphia: Mosby-Yearbook, 1991.
2. Darley FL. Treatment of acquired aphasia. *Adv Neurol* 1975; 7: 111–145.
3. Newmark SR, Sublett D, Black J, Geller R. Nutritional assessment in a rehabilitation unit. *Arch Phys Med Rehabil* 1981; 62:279–282.
4. Stolov WE, Hays RM. Evaluation of the patient. In: Kottke FJ, Lehmann JF, eds. *Krusen's handbook of physical medicine and rehabilitation,* 4th ed. Philadelphia: WB Saunders, 1990; 1–19.
5. Ewing JA. Detecting alcoholism: the CAGE questionnaire. *JAMA* 1984; 252:1905–1907.
6. DeGowin EL, DeGowin RL. *Bedside diagnostic examination,* 5th ed. New York: Macmillan, 1987.
7. Norkin CC, White DJ. *Measurement of joint motion: a guide to goniometry.* Philadelphia: FA Davis, 1985.
8. Committee for the Study of Joint Motion, American Academy of Orthopaedic Surgeons. *Joint motion: method of measuring and recording.* Chicago: American Academy of Orthopaedic Surgeons, 1965.
9. D'Ambrosia RD, ed. *Musculoskeletal disorders: regional examination and differential diagnosis,* 2nd ed. Philadelphia: JB Lippincott, 1986.
10. Hoppenfeld S. *Physical examination of the spine and extremities.* New York: Appleton-Century-Crofts, 1976.
11. Kendall FP, McCreary EK. *Muscles: testing and function,* 3rd ed. Baltimore: Williams & Wilkins, 1983.
12. Daniels L, Worthingham C. *Muscle testing: techniques of manual examination,* 5th ed. Philadelphia: WB Saunders, 1986.
13. Folstein MF, Folstein SE, McHugh PR. ''Mini-mental state'': a practical method for grading the cognitive state of patients for the clinician. *J Psychiatr Res* 1975; 12:189–198.
14. Levin HS, O'Donnell VM, Grossman RG. The Galveston orientation and amnesia test: a practical scale to assess cognition after head injury. *J Nerv Ment Dis* 1979; 167:675–684.
15. Strub RL, Black FW. *The mental status examination in neurology,* 2nd ed. Philadelphia: FA Davis, 1985.
16. Jennett B, Teasdale G. *Management of head injuries.* Philadelphia: FA Davis, 1981.
17. Lehmann JF, de Lateur BJ. Gait analysis: diagnosis and management. In: Kottke FJ, Lehmann JF, eds. *Krusen's handbook of physical medicine and rehabilitation,* 4th ed. Philadelphia: WB Saunders, 1990; 108–125.
18. Weed LL. *Medical records, medical education, and patient care: the problem-oriented record as a basic tool.* Cleveland, OH: The Press of Case Western Reserve University, 1971.
19. Dinsdale SM, Gent M, Kline G, Milner R. Problem oriented medical records: their impact on staff communication, attitudes and decision making. *Arch Phys Med Rehabil* 1975; 56:269–274.
20. Dinsdale SM, Mossman PL, Gullickson G Jr, Anderson TP. The problem-oriented medical record in rehabilitation. *Arch Phys Med Rehabil* 1970; 51:488–492.
21. Grabois M. The problem-oriented medical record: modification and simplification for rehabilitation medicine. *South Med J* 1977; 70: 1383–1385.
22. Milhous RL. The problem-oriented medical record in rehabilitation management and training. *Arch Phys Med Rehabil* 1972; 53:182–185.

Rehabilitation Medicine: Principles and Practice, Third Edition,
edited by Joel A. DeLisa and Bruce M. Gans.
Lippincott–Raven Publishers, Philadelphia © 1998.

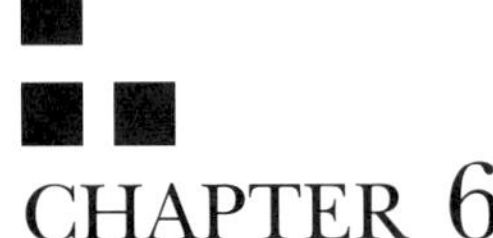

CHAPTER 6

Principles and Applications of Measurement Methods

Steven R. Hinderer and Kathleen A. Hinderer

Objective measurement provides a scientific basis for communication between professionals, documentation of treatment efficacy, and scientific credibility within the medical community. Federal, state, private third-party payer, and consumer organizations increasingly are requiring objective evidence of improvement as an outcome of treatment. Empirical clinical observation is no longer an acceptable method without objective data to support clinical decision making. The lack of reliability of clinicians' unaided measurement capabilities is documented in the literature (1–7), further supporting the importance of objective measures. In addition, comparison of alternative evaluation or treatment methods, where more than one possible choice is available, requires appropriate use of measurement principles (8–11).

Clinicians and clinical researchers use measurements to assess characteristics, functions, or behaviors thought to be present or absent in specific groups of people. The application of objective measures uses structured observations to compare performances or characteristics across individuals (i.e., to discriminate), or within individuals over time (i.e., to evaluate), or for prognostication based on current status (i.e., to predict) (12,13). It is important to understand the principles of measurement and the characteristics of good measures to be an effective user of the tools. Standards for implementation of tests and measures have been established within physical therapy (14,15), psychology (16), and medical rehabilitation (17) to address quality improvement and ethical issues for the use of clinical measures.

The purpose of this chapter is to discuss the basic principles of tests and measurements and to provide the reader with an understanding of the rationale for assessing and selecting measures that will provide the information they require to interpret test results properly. A critical starting point is to define what is to be measured, for what purpose, and at what cost. Standardized measurements meeting these criteria should then be assessed for reliability and validity pertinent to answering the question or questions posed by the user. Rothstein stated that unless "measurements are shown to be valid and reliable they do not yield information, but rather numbers or categories that give a false impression of meaningfulness" (18).

The initial section of this chapter discusses the psychometric parameters used to evaluate tests and measures. Principles of evaluation, testing, and interpretation are detailed in the second section. The third section provides guidelines for objective measurement when a standardized test is not available to measure the behavior, function, or characteristic of interest.

The complexity and diversity of the tests and measures used in rehabilitation medicine clinical practice and research preclude itemized description in a single chapter. Appendix A provides sources of available objective tests and measures and serves as a resource for the reader to seek further information on measures in their domain or domains of interest. (See Appendix A at the end of this chapter.) Reviewing the references provided in Appendix A in conjunction with the principles provided in this chapter will enable the reader to become a more sophisticated user of objective measurement tools. Although there are several good measures listed in Appendix A, there is much developmental work that needs to be completed for many of these tests. A measurement is not objective unless adequate levels of reliability have been demonstrated (18). Therefore, it is imperative that the user be able to recognize the limitations of these tests to avoid inadvertent misuse or misinterpretation of test results.

S. R. Hinderer: Department of Physical Medicine and Rehabilitation, Wayne State University School of Medicine, Rehabilitation Institute of Michigan, Detroit, Michigan 48201-2417.

K. A. Hinderer: Center for Human Motor Research, Department of Movement Science, Division of Kinesiology, University of Michigan, Ann Arbor, Michigan 48109-2214; and Rehabilitation Institute of Michigan, Detroit, Michigan 48201-2417.

PSYCHOMETRIC PARAMETERS USED TO EVALUATE TESTS AND MEASURES

The methods developed primarily in the psychology literature to evaluate objective measures generally are applicable to the standardized tests and instruments used in rehabilitation medicine. The topics discussed in this section are the foundation for all useful measures. Measurement tools must have defined levels of measurements for the trait or traits to be assessed and a purpose for obtaining the measurements. Additionally, tests and measures need to be practical, reliable, and valid.

Levels of Measurement

Tests and measures come in multiple forms because of the variety of parameters measured in clinical practice and research.

Despite the seemingly overwhelming number of measures, there are classified levels of measurement that determine how test results should be analyzed and interpreted (19). The four basic levels of measurement data are nominal, ordinal, interval, and ratio. Nominal and ordinal scales are used to classify discrete measures because the scores produced fall into discrete categories. Interval and ratio scales are used to classify continuous measures because the scores produced can fall anywhere along a continuum within the range of possible scores.

A nominal scale is used to classify data that do not have a rank order. The purpose of a nominal scale is to categorize people or objects into different groups based on a specific variable. An example of nominal data is diagnosis.

Ordinal data are operationally defined to assign individuals to categories that are mutually exclusive and discrete. The categories have a logical hierarchy, but it cannot be assumed that the intervals are equal between each category, even if the scale appears to have equal increments. Ordinal scales are the most commonly used level of measurement in clinical practice. Examples of ordinal scales are the manual muscle test scale (20–22), activities of daily living scales (e.g., Kohlman Evaluation of Living Skills) (23,24), and functional outcome measures (e.g., Functional Independence Measure) (25).

Interval data, unlike nominal and ordinal scales, are continuous. An interval scale has sequential units with numerically equal distances between them. Interval data often are generated from quantitative instrumentation as opposed to clinical observation. An example of an interval measurement is range-of-motion scores reported in degrees.

A ratio scale is an interval scale where the zero point on the scale represents a total absence of the quantity being measured. An example is force scores obtained from a quantitative muscle strength testing device.

Interval and ratio scales are more sophisticated and complex than nominal and ordinal scales. The latter are more common because they are easier to create. However, analysis of nominal and ordinal scales requires special consideration to avoid misinference from test results (26,27). The major controversies surrounding the use of these scales are the problems of unidimensionality and whether scores of items and subtests can be summed to provide an overall score. Continuous scales have a higher sensitivity of measurement and allow more rigorous statistical analyses to be performed.

Purpose of Testing

After the level of the measure has been selected, the purpose of testing must be examined. Tests generally serve one of two purposes: screening or in-depth assessment of specific traits, behaviors, or functions.

Screening Tests

Screening tests have three possible applications:

1. To discriminate between "suspect" and "normal" clients
2. To identify people needing further assessment
3. To assess a number of broad categories superficially

One example of a screening test is the Test of Orientation for Rehabilitation Patients, administered to individuals who are confused or disoriented secondary to traumatic brain injury, cerebrovascular accident, seizure disorder, brain tumor, or other neurologic events (28–31). This test screens for orientation to person and personal situation, place, time, schedule, and temporal continuity. Another well-developed screening test is the Miller Assessment for Preschoolers (MAP) (32). This test screens preschoolers for problems in the following areas: sensory and motor, speech and language, cognition, behaviors, and visual-motor integration.

The advantages of screening tests are that they are brief and sample a broad range of behaviors, traits, or characteristics. They are limited, however, because of an increased frequency of false-positive results due to the small sample of behaviors obtained. Screening tests should be used cautiously for diagnosis, placement, or treatment planning. They are used most effectively to indicate the need for more extensive testing and treatment of specific problem areas identified by the screening assessment.

Assessment Tests

Assessment tests have four possible applications:

1. To evaluate specific behaviors in greater depth
2. To provide information for planning interventions
3. To determine placement into specialized programs
4. To provide measurements to monitor progress

An example of an assessment measure is the Boston Diagnostic Aphasia Examination (33). The advantages of assessment measures are that they have a lower frequency of false-positive results, they assess a representative set of behaviors, they can be used for diagnosis, placement, or treatment planning, and they provide information regarding the functional level of the individual tested. The limitations are that an extended amount of time is needed for testing and they generally require specially trained personnel to administer, score, and interpret the results.

Criterion-Referenced versus Norm-Referenced Tests

Proper interpretation of test results requires comparison with a set of standards or expectations for performance. There are two basic types of standardized measures: criterion-referenced and norm-referenced tests.

Criterion-Referenced Tests

Criterion-referenced tests are those for which the test score is interpreted in terms of performance on the test relative to the continuum of possible scores attainable (18). The focus is on what the person can do or what he or she knows rather than how he or she compares with others (34). Individual performance is compared with a fixed expected standard rather than a reference group. Scores are interpreted based on absolute criteria, for example, the total number of items successfully completed. Criterion-referenced tests are useful to discriminate between successive performances of one person. They are conducted to measure a specific set of behavioral objectives. The Tufts Assessment of Motor Performance (which has recently undergone further validation work and is being renamed the Michigan Modified Performance Assessment) is an example of a criterion-referenced test (35–39). This assessment battery measures a broad range of physical skills in the areas of mobility, activities of daily living, and physical aspects of communication.

Norm-Referenced Tests

Norm-referenced tests use a representative sample of people who are measured relative to a variable of interest. Norm referencing permits comparison of a single person's measurement with those scores expected for the rest of the population. The normal values reported should be obtained from, and reported for, clearly described populations. The normal population should be the same as those for whom the test was designed to detect abnormalities (34). Reports of norm-referenced test results should use scoring procedures that reflect the person's position relative to the normal distribution (e.g., percentiles, standard scores). Measures of central tendency (e.g., mean, median, mode) and variability (e.g., standard deviation, standard error of the mean) also should be reported to provide information on the range of normal scores, assisting with determination of the clinical relevance of test results. An example of a norm-referenced test is the Peabody Developmental Motor Scale (40). This developmental test assesses fine and gross motor domains. Test items are classified into the following categories: grasp, hand use, eye-hand coordination, manual dexterity, reflexes, balance, nonlocomotor, locomotor, and receipt and propulsion of objects.

Practicality

A test or instrument should be practical—easy to use, insensitive to outside influences, inexpensive, and designed to allow efficient administration (41). For example, it is not efficient to begin testing in a supine position, switch to a prone position, then return to supine. Test administration should be organized to complete all testing in one position before switching to another. Instructions for administering the test should be clear and concise, and scoring criteria should be clearly defined. If equipment is required, it must be durable and of good quality. Qualifications of the tester and additional training required to become proficient in test administration should be specified. The time to administer the test should be indicated in the test manual. The duration of the test and level of difficulty need to be appropriate relative to the attention span and perceived capabilities of the client being tested. Finally, the test manual should provide summary statistics and detailed guidelines for appropriate use and interpretation of test scores based on the method of test development.

Reliability and Agreement

A general definition of reliability is the extent to which a measurement provides consistent information (i.e., is free from random error). Granger and associates (42) provide the analogy "it may be thought of as the extent to which the data contain relevant information with a high signal-to-noise ratio vs. irrelevant static confusion." In contrast, agreement is defined as the extent to which identical measurements are made. Reliability and agreement are distinctly different concepts and are estimated using different statistical techniques (43). Unfortunately, these concepts and their respective statistics often are treated synonymously in the literature.

The level of reliability is not necessarily congruent with the degree of agreement. It is possible for ratings to cluster consistently toward the same end of the scale, resulting in high reliability coefficients, and yet these judgments may or may not be equivalent. High reliability does not indicate whether the raters absolutely agree. It can occur concurrently with low agreement when each rater scores clients differently, but the relative differences in the scores are consistent for all clients rated. Conversely, low reliability does not necessarily indicate that raters disagree. Low reliability coefficients can occur with high agreement when the range of scores assigned by the raters is restricted or when the variability of the ratings is small (i.e., in a homogeneous population). In instances where the scores are fairly homogeneous, reliability coefficients lack the power to detect relationships and are often depressed, even though agreement between ratings may be relatively high. The reader is referred to Tinsley and Weiss for examples of these concepts (44). Both reliability and agreement must be established on the target population or populations to which the measure will be applied, using typical examiners. There are five types of reliability and agreement:

1. Interrater
2. Test-retest
3. Intertrial
4. Alternate form
5. Population specific

Each type will be discussed below, along with indications for calculating reliability versus agreement and their respective statistics.

Interrater Reliability and Agreement

Interrater or interobserver agreement is the extent to which independent examiners agree exactly on a client's performance. In contrast, interrater reliability is defined as the degree to which the ratings of different observers are proportional when expressed as deviations from their means; that is, the relationship of one rated person to other rated people is the same, although the absolute numbers used to express the relationship may vary from rater to rater (44). The independence of the examiners in the training they receive and the observations they make is critical in determining interrater agreement and reliability. When examiners have trained together or confer when performing a test, the interrater reliability or agreement coefficient calculated from their observations may be artificially inflated.

An interrater agreement or reliability coefficient provides an estimate of how much measurement error can be expected in scores obtained by two or more examiners who have independently rated the same person. Determining interrater agreement or reliability is particularly important for test scores that largely depend on the examiner's skill or judgment. An acceptable level of interrater reliability or agreement is essential for comparison of test results obtained from different clinical centers. Interrater agreement or reliability is a basic criterion for a measure to be called objective. If multiple examiners consistently obtain the same absolute or relative scores, then it is much more likely that the score is a function of the measure, rather than of the collective subjective bias of the examiners (18).

Pure interrater agreement and reliability are determined by having one examiner administer the test while the other examiner or examiners observe and independently score the person's performance at the same point in time. When assessing some parameters, where the skill of the examiner administering the test plays a vital role (e.g., sensory testing, range of motion testing) or where direct observation of each examiner is required (e.g., strength), it is impossible to assess pure interrater agreement and reliability. In these instances, each examiner must test the individual independently. Consequently, these interrater measures are confounded by factors of time and variation in client performance.

Test-Retest Reliability and Agreement

Test-retest agreement is defined as the extent to which a client receives identical scores during two different test sessions, when rated by the same examiner. In contrast, test-retest reliability assesses the degree of consistency in how a person's score is rank ordered relative to other people tested by the same examiner during different test sessions. Test-retest reliability is the most basic and essential form of reliability. It provides an estimate of the variation in client performance on a different test day, when retested by the same examiner. Some of the error in a test-retest situation also may be attributed to variations in the examiner's performance. It is important to determine the magnitude of day-to-day fluctuations in performance so that true changes in the parameters of interest can be determined. Variability of the test or how it is administered should not be the source of observed changes over time. Additionally, with quantitative measuring instruments the examiner must be knowledgeable in the method of and frequency required for instrument calibration.

The suggested test-retest interval is 1 to 3 days for most physical measures and 7 days for maximal effort tests where muscle fatigue is involved (45). The test-retest interval should not exceed the expected time for change to occur naturally. The purpose of an adequate but relatively short interval is to minimize the effects of memory, practice, and maturation or deterioration on test performance (46).

Intertrial Reliability and Agreement

Intertrial agreement provides an estimate of the stability of repeated scores obtained by one examiner within a test session. Intertrial reliability assesses the consistency of one examiner rank ordering repeated trials obtained from clients within a test session. Intertrial agreement and reliability also are influenced by individual performance factors such as fatigue, motor learning, motivation, and consistency of effort. Intertrial agreement and reliability should not be confused with test-retest agreement and reliability. The latter involves test sessions usually separated by days or weeks as opposed to seconds or minutes for intertrial agreement and reliability. A higher level of association is expected for results obtained from trials within a test session than those from different sessions.

Alternate Form Reliability and Agreement

Alternate form agreement refers to the consistency of scores obtained from two forms of the same test. Equivalent or parallel forms are different test versions intended to measure the same traits at a comparable level of difficulty. Alternate form reliability refers to whether the parallel forms of a test rank order people's scores consistently relative to each other. A high level of alternate form agreement or reliability may be required if a person must be tested more than once and a learning or practice effect is expected. This is particularly important when one form of the test will be used as a pretest and a second as a posttest.

Population-Specific Reliability and Agreement

Population-specific agreement and reliability assess the degree of absolute and relative reproducibility, respectively, that a test has for a specific group being measured. A variation of this type of agreement and reliability refers to the population of examiners administering the test (18).

Interpretation of Reliability and Agreement Statistics

Because measures of reliability and agreement are concerned with the degree of consistency or concordance between two or more independently derived sets of scores, they can be expressed in terms of correlation coefficients (34). The reliability coefficient is usually expressed as a value between 0 and 1, with higher values indicating higher reliability. Agreement statistics can range from -1 to $+1$, with $+1$ indicating perfect agreement, 0 indicating chance agreement, and negative values indicating less than chance agreement. The coefficient of choice varies, depending on the data type analyzed. The reader is referred to Bartko and Carpenter (47), Hartman (48), Hollenback (49), Liebetrau (50), and Tinsley and Weiss (44) for discussions of how to select appropriate measures of reliability and agreement. Table 6-1 provides information on appropriate statistical procedures for calculating interrater and test-retest reliability and agreement for discrete and continuous data types. No definitive standards for minimum acceptable levels of the different types of reliability and agreement statistics have been established; however, guidelines for minimum levels are provided in Table 6-1. The acceptable level varies, depending on the magnitude of the decision being made, the population variance, the sources of error variance, and the measurement technique (e.g., instrumentation versus behavioral assessments). If the population variance is relatively homogeneous, lower estimates of reliability are acceptable. In contrast, if the population variance is heterogeneous, higher estimates of reliability are expected. Critical values of correlation coefficients, based on the desired level of significance and the number of subjects, are provided in tables in measurement textbooks (51,52). It is important to note that a correlation coefficient that is statistically significant does not necessarily indicate that adequate reliability or agreement has been established, since the significance level only provides an indication that the coefficient is significantly different from zero (Table 6-1).

TABLE 6-1. *Interrater reliability, test-retest reliability, and agreement analysis: appropriate statistics and minimum acceptable levels*

	Reliability analysis		Agreement analysis	
Data type	Appropriate statistic	Level	Appropriate statistic	Level
Discrete				
Nominal	ICC or κ_w	>0.75	κ	>0.60
Ordinal	ICC	>0.75	κ_w	>0.60
Continuous				
Interval	ICC	>0.75	χ^2 and T	$P < 0.05$
Ratio	ICC	>0.75	χ^2 and T	$P < 0.05$

References: ICC: discrete (47,55), ordinal (47), continuous (44,47), minimal acceptable level (56); Cohen's κ—κ (44,47,57,58), κ_w (47,59,60), κ_w equivalence with ICC for reliability analysis of minimal data (61–64), minimal acceptable level (65); Lawlis and Lu's χ^2 and T: statical and minimal level (43,44).

ICC, intraclass correlation; κ, kappa; κ_w, weighted kappa; T, T index.

Agreement and reliability both are important for evaluating client ratings. As discussed earlier, these are distinctly different concepts and require separate statistical analysis. Several factors must be considered to determine the relative importance of each. Decisions that carry greater weight or impact for the people being assessed may require more exact agreement. If the primary need is to assess the relative consistency between raters, and exact agreement is less critical, then a reliability measure alone is a satisfactory index. In contrast, whenever the major interest is either the absolute value of the score, or the meaning of the scores as defined by the points on the scale (e.g., criterion-referenced tests), agreement should be reported in addition to the reliability (44). Scores generated from instrumentation are expected to have a higher level of reliability or agreement than scores obtained from behavioral observations.

A test score actually consists of two different components: the true score and the error score (34,53). A person's true score is a hypothetical construct, indicating a test score that is unaffected by chance factors. The error score refers to unwanted variation in the test score (56). All continuous scale measurements have a component of error and no test is completely reliable. Consequently, reliability is a matter of degree. Any reliability coefficient may be interpreted directly in terms of percentage of score variance attributable to different sources (18). A reliability coefficient of 0.85 signifies that 85% of the variance in test scores depends on true variance in the trait measured and 15% depends on error variance.

Specific Reliability and Agreement Statistics

There are several statistical measures for estimating interrater agreement and reliability. Four statistics commonly used to determine agreement are the frequency ratio, point-by-point agreement ratio, kappa (κ) coefficients, and Lawlis and Lu's χ^2 and T-index statistics. For reliability calculations, the most frequently used correlation statistics are the

Pearson product-moment (Pearson r) and intraclass correlation coefficients (ICC). When determining reliability for dichotomous or ordinal data, specific ICC formulas have been developed. These nonparametric ICC statistics have been shown to be the equivalent of the weighted kappa (κ_w) (61–64). Consequently, the κ_w also can be used as an index of reliability for discrete data and the values obtained can be directly compared with equivalent forms of ICCs (62). The method of choice for reliability and agreement analyses partially depends on the assessment strategy used (44,47–50,66). In addition to agreement and reliability statistics, standard errors of measurement (SEM) provide a clinically relevant index of reliability expressed in test score units. Each statistic is described below.

Frequency Ratio

This agreement statistic is indicated for frequency count data (46). A frequency ratio of the two examiners' scores is calculated by dividing the smaller total by the larger total and multiplying by 100. This statistic is appealing because of its computational and interpretive simplicity. There are a variety of limitations, however. It only reflects agreement of the total number of behaviors scored by each observer; there is no way to determine whether there is agreement for individual responses using a frequency ratio. The value of this statistic may be inflated if the observed behavior occurs at high rates (66). There is no meaningful lower bound of acceptability (48).

Point-by-Point Agreement Ratio

This statistic is used to determine if there is agreement on each occurrence of the observed behavior. It is appropriate when there are discrete opportunities for the behavior to occur or for distinct response categories (46,67,68). To calculate this ratio, the number of agreements is totaled by determining the concurrence between observers regarding the presence or absence of observable responses during a given trial, recording interval, or for a particular behavior category. Disagreements are defined as instances where one observer records a response and the other observer does not. The point-by-point agreement percentage is calculated by dividing the number of agreements by the number of agreements plus disagreements, and multiplying by 100 (68). Agreement generally is considered to be acceptable at a level of 0.80 or above (68).

The extent to which observers are found to agree is partially a function of the frequency of occurrence of the target behavior and of whether occurrence and/or nonoccurrence agreements are counted (67). When the rate of the target behavior is either very high or very low, high levels of interobserver agreement are likely for occurrences or nonoccurrences, respectively. Consequently, if the frequency of either occurrences or nonoccurrences is high, a certain level of agreement is expected simply owing to chance. In such cases, it is often recommended that agreements be included in the calculation only if at least one observer recorded the occurrence of the target behavior. In this case, intervals where none of the observers records a response are excluded from the analysis. It is important to identify clearly what constitutes an agreement when reporting point-by-point percentage agreement ratios because the level of reliability is affected by this definition.

Kappa Coefficient

The κ coefficient provides an estimate of agreement between observers, corrected for chance agreement. This statistic is preferred for discrete categorical data because, unlike the two statistics discussed above, it corrects for chance agreements. In addition, percentage agreement ratios often are inflated when there is an unequal distribution of scores between rating categories. This often is the case in rehabilitation medicine, where the frequency of normal characteristics is much higher than abnormal characteristics (69,70). In contrast, κ coefficients provide accurate estimates of agreement, even when scores are unequally distributed between rating categories (70).

Kappa coefficients are used to summarize observer agreement and accuracy, determine rater consistency, and evaluate scaled consistency among raters (66). Three conditions must be met to use κ:

1. The clients must be independent.
2. The raters must independently score the clients.
3. The rating categories must be mutually exclusive and exhaustive (69,70).

The general form of κ is a coefficient of agreement for nominal scales where all disagreements are treated equally (44,47,50,57,58,65,72). The κ_w statistic was developed for ordinal data (47,50,59,60), where some disagreements have greater gravity than others (e.g., the manual muscle testing scale, where the difference between a score of 2 and 5 is of more concern than the difference between a score of 4 and 5). Refer to the references cited above for formulas used to calculate κ and κ_w.

Several other variations of κ have been developed for specific applications. The kappa statistic κ_v provides an overall measure of agreement, as well as separate indices for each subject and rating category (73). This form of κ can be applied in situations where subjects are not all rated by the same set of examiners. The variation of κ described by Fleiss is useful when there are more than two ratings per client (63); a computer program is available to calculate this statistic (69). When multiple examiners rate clients and a measure of overall conjoint agreement is desired, the kappa statistic κ_m is indicated (74). Standard κ statistics treat all raters or units symmetrically (63). When one or more of the ratings is considered to be a standard (e.g., scores from an experienced rater), alternate analysis procedures should be used (74–76).

Lawlis and Lu χ^2 and T Index

These measures of agreement are recommended for continuous data (44). They permit the option of defining seriousness of disagreements among raters. A statistically significant χ^2 indicates that the observed agreement is greater than that expected owing to chance. The T index is used to determine whether agreement is low, moderate, or high. The reader is referred to Tinsley and Weiss (44) for a discussion of the indications for, calculation of, and interpretation of these statistics.

Pearson Product-Moment Correlation Coefficient

Historically, the Pearson r has been used commonly as an index of reliability. It is a parametric statistic intended for use with continuous data. The Pearson r was designed to determine the relationship between two sets of scores, each from a different test. The generally accepted minimum level of this coefficient is 0.80; however, levels above 0.90 often are considered more desirable (34,51). The distribution of these two sets of scores is referred to in statistics texts as bivariate. The repeated measurement of individuals on the same test, as is done to determine reliability, is a univariate variable. It is therefore more appropriate to use a univariate statistic, such as the ICC, for reliability testing (45). Another disadvantage of using the Pearson r instead of an ICC is that the Pearson r provides only an index of the strength of the relationship between scores and is insensitive to consistent differences between scores. Consequently, a linear regression equation must be reported in addition to the Pearson r to indicate the nature of the relationship between the scores (18). In contrast, the ICC is sensitive to score differences, and no additional linear regression analyses are required.

Intraclass Correlation Coefficients

Intraclass correlation coefficients provide an index of variability resulting from comparing rating score error with other sources of true score variability (42,52,54). As indicated above, it is the coefficient of choice for reliability analyses. The ICC is based on the variance components from an analysis of variance (ANOVA), which includes not only the between-subject variance, as does the Pearson r, but also other situation-specific variance components such as alternate test forms, maturation of subjects between ratings, and other sources of true mean differences in the obtained ratings (77). The individual sources of error can be analyzed to determine their percentage contribution to the overall error variance using generalizability analysis (53,56). For further information regarding the use of generalizability theory to distinguish between sources of error, the reader is referred to Brennan (78) and Cronbach and associates (79).

There are six different ICC formulas (56). The correct ICC formula is selected based on three factors:

1. The use of a one-way versus two-way ANOVA
2. The importance of differences between examiners' mean ratings
3. The analysis of an individual rating versus the mean of several ratings (44,56)

Selection of the proper formula is critical and is based on the reliability study design (56,77,80). It is important to report which type of ICC is used to compute reliability because the calculations are not equivalent. Variations of the ICC formulas also exist for calculating ICCs using dichotomous (55) and ordinal (44) nonparametric data. The marginal distributions do not have to be equal, as was originally proposed for nonparametric ICCs (62). These nonparametric ICC formulas have been demonstrated to be equivalent to weighted κ coefficients, provided that the mean difference between raters is included as a component of variability and the rating categories can be ordered (62).

Standard Error of Measurement

It has been suggested that measurement error estimates are the most desirable index of reliability (18,34,54). The SEM is an estimate, in test score units, of the random variation of a person's performance across repeated measures. The SEM is an expression of the margin of error between a person's observed score and his or her true ability (46). The SEM is an important indicator of the sensitivity of the test to detect changes in a person's performance over time.

The formula for the SEM is

$$SD\sqrt{1 - r_{rr}}$$

where SD is the standard deviation of the test scores and r_{rr} is the reliability coefficient for the test scores (34,45,54). Correlating scores from two forms of a test is one of several ways to estimate the reliability coefficient (54) and often is used in psychology when parallel forms of a test are available. In rehabilitation medicine, however, equivalent forms of a test often are not available. The test-retest reliability coefficient therefore is the coefficient of choice for calculating the SEM in most rehabilitation applications because the primary interest is in the variation of subject performance. The SEM is a relatively conservative statistic, requiring larger data samples (approximately 300 to 400 observations) in order to not overestimate the error (15).

It is best to report a test score as a range rather than as an absolute score. The SEM is used to calculate the range of scores (i.e., confidence interval) for a given person; that is, the person's true performance ability is expected to fall within the range of scores defined by the confidence interval. A person's score must fall outside of this range to indicate with confidence that a true change in performance has occurred. Based on a normal distribution, a 95% confidence interval would be approximately equal to the mean ± 2 SEM. A 95% confidence interval is considered best to use when looking for change over time. This rigorous level of confidence minimizes the likelihood of a type I error (i.e., there is only a 5% chance that differences between scores obtained from a given person during different test sessions will not fall within the 95% confidence interval upper and lower values). Consequently, there is less than a 5% chance that differences between scores exceeding the upper end of the confidence interval are due to measurement error (i.e., they have a 95% chance of representing a true change in performance).

Factors Affecting Reliability

There are four sources of measurement error for interrater reliability (18,45):

1. Lack of agreement among scorers
2. Lack of consistent performance by the individual tested
3. Failure of the instrument to measure consistently
4. Failure of the examiner to follow the standardized procedures to administer the test.

Threats to test-retest reliability similarly are caused by four factors:

1. The instrument
2. The examiner
3. The client
4. The testing protocol

Sources and prevention of examiner error will be discussed in the section on Principles of Evaluation, Testing, and Interpretation.

There are several factors conducive to good reliability of a measure (45). These factors are the power to discriminate among ability groups; sufficient time allotted so that each client can show his or her best performance without being penalized for an unrepresentative poor trial; test organization to optimize examinee performance; and test administration and scoring instructions that are clear and precise. Additionally, the testing environment should support good performance and the examiner must be competent in administering the test. For tests designed to be appropriate for a wide age range, reliability should be examined for each age level rather than for the group as a whole (53).

In summary, reliability and agreement are essential components to any objective measurement. Rothstein stated that "measurements that do not have test-retest reliability can be considered so full of error as to be useless because the numbers obtained do not reflect the variable measured" (18). Reliability is an important component of validity, but good reliability or agreement does not guarantee that a measure is valid. A reliable measurement is consistent, but not necessarily correct. However, a measurement that is unreliable cannot be valid.

Validity

Validity is defined as the accuracy with which a test measures that which it is intended to measure. As Rothstein explained, "The concept refers to the appropriateness, meaningfulness, and usefulness of a test for a particular application" (18). Validity is initially investigated while a test or instrument is being developed and confirmed through subsequent use. Four basic aspects of validity will be discussed: content, construct, criterion-related, and face validity.

Content Validity

Content validity is the systematic examination of the test content to determine if it covers a representative sample of the behavior domain to be measured. It should be reported in the test manual as descriptive information on the skills covered by the test, number of items in each category, and rationale for item selection. Content validity generally is evidenced by the opinion of experts that the domain sampled is adequate. There are two primary methods that the developer of a test can use for obtaining professional opinions about the content validity of an instrument (81). The first is to provide a panel of experts with the items from the test and request a determination of what the battery of items is measuring. The second method requires providing not only the test items but also a list of test objectives so that experts can determine the relationship between the two. For statistical analysis of content validity, the reader is referred to Thorn and Deitz (82).

Construct Validity

Construct validity refers to the extent to which a test measures the theoretical construct underlying the test. Construct validity should be obtained whenever a test purports to measure an abstract trait or theoretical characteristics about the nature of human behavior such as intelligence, self-concept, anxiety, school or work readiness, or perceptual organization. The following five areas must be considered with regard to construct validity in test instruments (34,81).

Age Differentiation

Any developmental changes in children or changes in performance due to aging must be addressed as part of the test development.

Factor Analysis

Factor analysis is a statistical procedure that can be performed on data obtained from testing. The purpose of factor analysis is to simplify the description of behavior by reducing an initial multiplicity of variables to a few common underlying factors or traits that may or may not be pertinent to the construct or constructs that the test was originally designed to measure. The reader is referred to Cronbach (54), Wilson (83), Wright and Masters (84), and Wright and Stone (85) for in-depth discussions of factor analysis. The more recent development of confirmatory factor analysis

(86,87) overcomes the relative arbitrariness of traditional factor analysis methods. Confirmatory factor analysis differs from traditional factor analysis in that the investigator specifies, before analysis, the measures that are determined by each factor and which factors are correlated. The specified relationships are then statistically tested for goodness of fit of the proposed model compared with the actual data collected. Confirmatory factor analysis is therefore a more direct assessment of construct validity than is traditional factor analysis.

Internal Consistency

In assessing the attributes of a test, it is helpful to examine the relationship of subscales and individual items to the total score. This is especially important when the test instrument has many components. If a subtest or item has a very low correlation with the total score, the test developer must question the subtest's validity in relation to the total score. This technique is most useful for providing confirmation of the validity of a homogeneous test. A test that measures several constructs would not be expected to have a high degree of internal consistency. For dichotomous data, the Kuder-Richardson statistic is used to calculate internal consistency (34). Cronbach's coefficient alpha (α) is recommended when the measure has more than two levels of response (34). The minimum acceptable level of α generally is set at 0.70 (88).

Convergent and Divergent Validity

Construct validity is evidenced further by high correlations with other tests that purport to measure the same constructs (i.e., convergent validity) and low correlations with measures that are designed to measure different attributes (i.e., divergent validity). It is desirable to obtain moderate levels of convergent validity, indicating that the two measures are not measuring identical constructs. If the new test correlates too highly with another test, it is questionable whether the new test is necessary because either test would suffice to answer the same questions. Moderately high but significant correlations indicate good convergent validity, but with each test still having unique components. Good divergent validity is demonstrated by low and insignificant correlations between two tests that measure theoretically unrelated parameters, such as an activities of daily living assessment and a test of expressive language ability.

Discriminant Validity

If two groups known to have different characteristics can be identified and assessed by the test, and if a significant difference between the performance of the two groups is found, then incisive evidence of discriminant validity is present.

Criterion-Related Validity

Criterion-related validity includes two subclasses of validity: concurrent validity and predictive validity (34,46). The commonality between these subclasses of validity is that they refer to multiple measurement of the same construct. In other words, the measure in question is compared with other variables or measures that are considered to be accurate measures of the characteristics or behaviors being tested. The purpose is to use the second measure as a criterion to validate the first measure.

Criterion-related validity can be assessed statistically, providing clear guidelines as to whether a measure is valid. Frequently, the paired measurements from the tests under comparison have different values. The nature of the relationship is less important than the strength of the relationship (18). Ottenbacher and Tomchek (89) showed that the limits of agreement technique provided the most accurate measurement error when comparing test results, versus other statistics frequently used for such comparisons.

Concurrent Validity

Concurrent validity deals with whether an inference is justifiable at the present time. This is typically done by comparing results of one measure against some criterion (e.g., another measure or related phenomenon). If the correlation is high, the measure is said to have good concurrent validity. Concurrent validity is relevant to tests used for diagnosis of existing status, rather than predicting future outcome.

Predictive Validity

Predictive validity involves a measure's ability to predict or forecast some future criterion. Examples include performance on another measure in the future, prognostic reaction to an intervention program, or performance in some task of daily living. Predictive validity is difficult to establish and often requires collection of data over an extended period of time after the test has been developed. Hence, very few measures used in rehabilitation medicine have established predictive validity. A specific subset of predictive validity that is important to rehabilitation medicine practice is ecological validity. This concept involves the ability to identify impairments, functional limitations, and performance deficits within the context of the person's own environment. Measures with good concurrent validity sometimes are presumed to have good predictive validity, but this may not be a correct assumption. Unless predictive validity information exists for a test, extreme caution should be exercised in interpreting test results as predictors of future behavior or function.

Face Validity

Face validity is not considered to be an essential component of the validity of a test or measure. It reflects only whether a test appears to measure what it is supposed to, based on the personal opinions of those either taking or giving the test (18). A test with high face validity has a greater likelihood of being more rigorously and carefully administered by the examiner, and the person being tested is more likely to give his or her best effort. Although it is not essential, in most instances, face validity is still an important component of test development and selection. Exceptions include personality and interest tests where the purpose of testing is concealed to prevent client responses from being biased.

Summary

The information discussed in this section provides the basis for critically assessing available tests and measures. The scale of the test or instrument should be sufficiently sophisticated to discriminate adequately between different levels of the behavior or function being tested. The purposes for testing must be identified and the test chosen should have been developed for this purpose. The measure selected should be practical from the standpoint of time, efficiency, budget, equipment, and the population being tested. Above all, the measure must have acceptable reliability, agreement, and validity for the specific application it is selected. Reliability, agreement, and validity are important for both clinical and research applications. The power of statistical tests depends on adequate levels of reliability, agreement, and validity of the dependent measures (90). Consequently, it is essential that adequate levels of reliability, agreement, and validity be assessed and reported for dependent measures used in research studies.

For additional information on the test development process, the reader is referred to Miller (91). For information on the principles of tests and measurements, the reader is referred to Anastasi (34), Baumgartner and Jackson (45), Cronbach (54), Safrit (51), Rothstein (18), Rothstein and colleagues (15), and Verducci (52).

Identification of the most appropriate test for a given application, based on the psychometric criteria discussed above, does not guarantee that the desired information will be obtained. Principles of evaluation, testing, and interpretation must be followed to optimize objective data acquisition.

PRINCIPLES OF EVALUATION, TESTING, AND INTERPRETATION

Systematic testing using standardized techniques is essential to quantify a client's status objectively. Standardized testing is defined as using specified test administration and scoring procedures, under the same environmental conditions, with consistent directions (34,46). Standardized testing is essential to permit comparison of test results for a given person over time and to compare test scores between clients (92). In addition, consistent testing techniques facilitate interdisciplinary interpretation of clinical findings among rehabilitation professionals and minimize duplication of evaluation procedures.

Examiner Qualifications

Assessments using objective instrumentation or standardized tests must be conducted by examiners who have appropriate training and qualifications (14,16,17,34,92,93). The necessary training and expertise varies with the type of instrument or test used. The characteristics common to most rehabilitation medicine applications will be discussed. Examiners must be thoroughly familiar with standardized test administration, scoring, and interpretation procedures. Training guidelines specified in the published test manual must be strictly adhered to. A skilled examiner is aware of factors that might affect test performance and takes the necessary steps to ensure that the effects of these factors are minimized. Interrater reliability needs to be attained at acceptable levels with examiners who are experienced in administering the test to ensure consistency of test administration and scoring.

Examiners also must be knowledgeable about the instruments and standardized tests available to assess parameters of interest. They need to be familiar with relevant research literature, test reviews, and the technical merits of the appropriate tests and measures (14,16,17,34). From this information, examiners should be able to discern the advantages, disadvantages, and limitations of using a particular test or device. Based on the purpose of testing and characteristics of the person being assessed, examiners need to be able to select and justify the most appropriate assessment method from the available options.

When interpreting test results, examiners must be sensitive to factors that may have affected test performance (34). Conclusions and recommendations should be based on a synthesis of the person's scores, the expected measurement error, any factors that might have influenced test performance, the characteristics of the given person compared with those of the normative population, and the purpose of testing versus the recommended applications of the test or instrument. Written documentation of test results and interpretation should include comments on any potential influence of the above factors.

Examiner Training

Proper training of examiners is critical to attaining an acceptable level of interrater reliability for test administration and scoring (92). Examiners should be overtrained to minimize later decrements in performance (66). Training methods should be documented carefully so that they can be replicated by future examiners.

Training Procedures

As part of their training, examiners should read the test manual and instructions carefully. Operational definitions and rating criteria need to be memorized verbatim (94). A written examination should be administered to document the examiners' assimilation of test administration and scoring procedures (66). This information should be periodically reviewed to produce close adherence to the standardized protocol. It is helpful for examiners to view a videotape of an experienced examiner conducting the test. If test administration and scoring techniques need to be adjusted for the varying abilities of the target population (e.g., children of different age levels), the experienced examiner should be observed testing a representative sample from the target population to demonstrate the various testing, scoring, and interpretation procedures.

Videotapes also are useful to clarify scoring procedures and establish consistency of scoring between and within raters (66,92). Once scoring procedures have been reviewed adequately, interrater reliability can be established by having trainees view several clients on videotape then compare their scores with those from an experienced examiner. Scoring discrepancies should be discussed and trainees should continue to score videotaped segments until 100% agreement is established with an experienced examiner (94). Intrarater consistency of scoring also can be established by having an individual examiner score the same videotape on multiple occasions. Sufficient time should elapse between multiple viewings so examiners do not recall previous ratings.

For assessments that involve multiple trials (e.g., strength assessments), intertrial reliability can be calculated to provide a measure of the examiner's consistency of administering multiple trials within a given test session. As was mentioned previously, intertrial reliability also is influenced by factors such as fatigue, motor learning, motivation, and the stability of performance over a short period of time. Multiple trials administered during a given session generally are highly correlated; thus, intertrial reliability coefficients are expected to be very high. Although this measure provides feedback on consistency in administering multiple trials, it should not be considered a substitute for establishing other types of reliability during the training phase.

Establishing Procedural Reliability

Procedural reliability is defined as the reliability with which standardized testing and scoring procedures are applied. As part of training, examiners should be observed administering and scoring the test on a variety of people with characteristics similar to those of the target population (92). Procedural reliability should be established by having an experienced examiner observe trainees to determine if the test is being administered and scored according to the standardized protocol. Establishing procedural reliability greatly increases the likelihood that the observed changes in performance reflect true changes in status and not alterations in examiner testing or scoring methods. Unfortunately, this type of reliability often is neglected. According to Billingsley and associates (95), failure to assess procedural reliability poses a threat to both the internal and external validity of assessments.

Procedural reliability is assessed by having an independent observer check off whether each component of an assessment is completed according to the standardized protocol while viewing a live or videotaped assessment. Specific antecedent conditions, commands, timing of execution, and positioning are monitored, and any deviations are noted. Procedural reliability is calculated as a percentage of correct behaviors (95). Checklists should include all essential components of the standardized protocol. An example of a procedural reliability checklist for selected items on the MAP is provided in Figure 6-1 (92). In this example, the checklist varies for each item administered. Another example of procedural reliability is referenced for strength testing using a myometer (96). In this case, the protocol was standardized across muscle groups, including the command sequence, tactile input, myometer placement, start and end positions, and contraction duration.

Deviation from the standardized protocol can be minimized by conducting periodic procedural reliability checks (95). Procedural reliability should be assessed on an ongoing basis at random intervals in clinical or research settings, in addition to the training period. Assessments should be conducted at least once per phase during a research study. Examiners should be informed that procedural reliability checks will occur randomly, and ideally should be unaware of when specific assessments are conducted, to avoid exam-

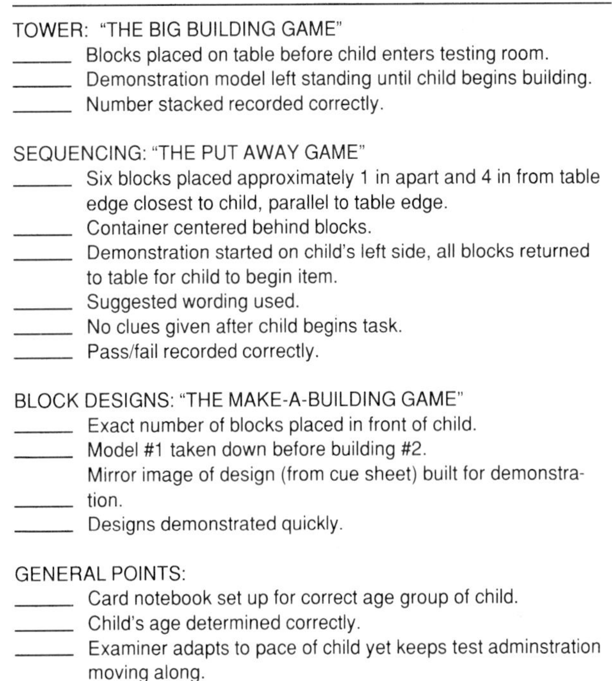
TOWER: "THE BIG BUILDING GAME"
_____ Blocks placed on table before child enters testing room.
_____ Demonstration model left standing until child begins building.
_____ Number stacked recorded correctly.

SEQUENCING: "THE PUT AWAY GAME"
_____ Six blocks placed approximately 1 in apart and 4 in from table edge closest to child, parallel to table edge.
_____ Container centered behind blocks.
_____ Demonstration started on child's left side, all blocks returned to table for child to begin item.
_____ Suggested wording used.
_____ No clues given after child begins task.
_____ Pass/fail recorded correctly.

BLOCK DESIGNS: "THE MAKE-A-BUILDING GAME"
_____ Exact number of blocks placed in front of child.
_____ Model #1 taken down before building #2.
_____ Mirror image of design (from cue sheet) built for demonstration.
_____ Designs demonstrated quickly.

GENERAL POINTS:
_____ Card notebook set up for correct age group of child.
_____ Child's age determined correctly.
_____ Examiner adapts to pace of child yet keeps test adminstration moving along.

FIG. 6-1. Procedural reliability checklist for selected items on the Miller Assessment for Preschoolers. (Reprinted with permission from Gyurke J, Prifitera A. Standardizing an assessment. *Phys Occup Ther Pediatr* 1989; 9:71.)

iner reactivity. A minimum acceptable level of procedural reliability should be established for clinical or research use (generally, 90% to 100%). During the training phase, a 100% level should be attained. Feedback on procedural reliability assessments should be provided to examiners. If an examiner's score decreases below the acceptable level, pertinent sections of the standardized protocol should be reviewed.

Establishing Interrater Reliability and Agreement

Once an examiner has demonstrated consistency in scoring by viewing videotaped assessments and reliability in test administration through procedural reliability checks, then interrater reliability and/or agreement should be established with an experienced examiner (66,92). Both examiners should independently rate people with characteristics similar to the target population. Reliability and agreement assessments should be conducted under conditions similar to those of the actual data collection procedures (67). As with procedural reliability, interrater assessments should be conducted periodically in both clinical and research settings. It is essential to establish interrater reliability and/or agreement at least once per phase in a research study to determine the potential influence of examiner rating differences on the data recorded (66,67). When calculating interrater agreement where the experienced examiner's scores are considered to be a standard, specific statistical procedures are indicated (74–76).

For assessments where the person's performance can be observed directly (e.g., developmental or activities of daily living assessments), it is preferable to establish interrater reliability and agreement with the examiner in training administering the test while the experienced examiner simultaneously observes and independently scores the person, so that pure interrater reliability and agreement can be assessed. When measuring parameters such as range of motion, sensation, or strength, it is imperative that both examiners independently conduct the tests because the measurement error depends to a large extent on the examiner's skill and body mechanics in administering the test. In addition, direct observation of these parameters by each examiner is required. In these instances, interrater reliability and agreement are confounded by factors of time and variation in client performance, as discussed above in the section on Interrater Reliability and Agreement.

If examiners are aware that interrater reliability and/or agreement is being assessed, the situation is potentially reactive (67). Reactivity refers to the possibility that behavior may change if the examiners realize they are being monitored. Examiners demonstrate higher levels of reliability and agreement when they are aware that they are being observed. It is difficult, however, to conduct reliability and agreement assessments without examiner awareness; consequently, during a research study, it might be best to lead examiners to believe that all of their observations are being monitored throughout the investigation (67). It is important to note that levels of reliability and agreement attained when examiners are aware that they are being monitored are potentially inflated compared with examiner performance in a typical clinic setting where monitoring occurs infrequently.

Detecting Examiner Errors

When training examiners in the use of rating scales, interrater reliability and agreement data should be examined to determine if there are any consistent trends indicative of examiner rating errors. These data should be obtained from testing clients who represent a broad-range sample of pertinent characteristics of the population, so that a relatively normal score distribution is expected. In many circumstances, a representative group of clients can be observed efficiently on videotape by multiple examiners. The distribution of examiners' scores across clients is then compared for error trends (52). If only one examiner is using a given rating scale, so that multiple examiners' scores cannot be compared for rating errors, rating errors still can be detected by examining the distribution of one examiner's ratings across multiple clients. Rasch analysis is another useful method for detecting examiner errors on specific items or as an overall trend. Rating errors can be classified into five categories:

1. Error of central tendency
2. Error of standards
3. Halo effect error
4. Logical error
5. Examiner drift error

An indication of an error of central tendency is where one rater's scores are clustered around the center of the scale and the other raters' scores are spread more evenly over the entire scale. Errors of standards occur when one rater awards either all low or all high scores, indicating that his standards are set either too high (i.e., error of severity) or too low (i.e., error of leniency), respectively. Leniency errors are the most common type of rating error (52). Halo effect errors can be detected if several experienced examiners rate a number of people under identical conditions and the score distributions are examined. There should be little variability between well-trained examiners' scores. If one examiner's scores fall outside of this limited range of variability, a halo rating error may have occurred as a result of preset examiner impressions or expectations. A logical error occurs when multiple traits are rated and an examiner awards similar ratings to traits that are not necessarily related.

A fifth type of rating error is examiner drift. Examiner drift refers to the tendency of examiners to alter the manner in which they apply rating criteria over time (67). Examiner drift is not easily detected. Interrater agreement may remain high even though examiners are deviating from the standardized rating criteria (66,67). This occurs when examiners who work together discuss rating criteria to clarify rating definitions. They may inadvertently alter the criteria, diminishing rating accuracy, and yet high levels of interrater agreement are maintained. If examiners alter rating criteria over time, data obtained from serial examinations may not be comparable. Examiner drift can be detected by assessing interrater agreement between examiners who have not worked together, or by comparing ratings from examiners who have been conducting assessments for an extended period of time with scores obtained from a newly trained examiner (67). Presumably, recently trained examiners adhere more closely to the original criteria than examiners who have had the opportunity to drift. Comparing videotaped samples of client performance from selected evaluation sessions with actual examiner ratings obtained over time is another method of detecting examiner drift.

Reducing Examiner Errors

Examiner ratings can be improved in several ways (52,66,67). Operational definitions of the behavior or trait must be clearly stated, and examiners must understand the rating criteria. If examiners periodically review rating criteria, receive feedback on their adherence to the test protocol through procedural reliability checks, and are informed of the accuracy of their observations through interrater agreement checks, examiner drift can be minimized. Examiners should be aware of common rating errors and how these errors may influence their scoring. Adequate time needs to be provided to observe and rate behaviors. If the observation period is too brief for the number of behaviors or people to be observed, rating accuracy is adversely affected. The reliability of ratings also can be improved by averaging ratings from multiple observers because the effects of individual rater biases tend to be balanced. Averaging multiple scores obtained from one rater is not advantageous for reducing rating error, however, because a given rater's errors tend to be relatively constant.

The complexity of observations negatively affects interrater reliability and agreement because observers may have difficulty discriminating between rating criteria (67). With more complex observations, examiners need to attain higher levels of agreement for each behavior during the training phase. These high levels of interrater agreement need to be achieved under the exact conditions that will be used for data collection (67). If multiple behaviors are observed on several clients, it is best to rate all clients on one behavior before rating the next behavior. This practice facilitates more consistent application of operational definitions and rating criteria for the individual behavior. It also tends to reduce the incidence of logical errors.

Another method for improving scoring is to make raters aware of examiner idiosyncrasies or expectations that can affect ratings. According to Verducci (52), there are five client-rater characteristics that may affect scoring:

1. If an examiner knows the person being evaluated, ratings can be either positively or negatively influenced—the longer the prior relationship has existed, the more likely the ratings will be influenced.
2. The rater tends to rate more leniently if the rater is required to disclose ratings directly to the person, or if the person confronts the examiner about the ratings.
3. Examiner gender also can influence ratings. In general, male examiners tend to rate more leniently than female examiners.
4. There is a tendency to rate members of one's gender higher than those of the opposite gender.
5. Knowledge of previous ratings may bias examiners to rate similarly. Consequently, examiners should remain blind to previous scores until current ratings have been assigned.

Other potential sources of rater bias are the examiner's expectations about the client's outcome and feedback received regarding ratings (66,67). If examiners expect improvement, their ratings are more likely to show improvement. This is especially true when examiners are reinforced for client improvement. In a research setting, examiner bias can be minimized if the observers remain blind to the purposes and hypotheses of the study. In a clinical setting, the baseline, intervention, and follow-up sessions often can be videotaped. Blind, independent observers can then rate the behaviors when shown the videotaped sessions in a random order.

Test Administration Strategies

Consistency in test administration is essential to permit comparison of test results from one session to another or between people. Multiple factors that might influence performance must be held constant during testing. These factors include test materials and instrumentation, the testing environment, test procedures and scoring, state of the person being assessed, observers present in the room, and time of day. Examiners must be aware of the potential influence of these factors and document any conditions that might affect test performance. Examiners ideally should remain blind to previous test results until after conducting the evaluation to avoid potential bias.

If more than one method is acceptable for testing, it is important to document which protocol is used so that the same method can be used during future evaluations. If it is necessary to alter the method of measurement as a result of a change in status or the development of an improved measurement technique, measurements should be taken using both the new and old methods so there is overlap of at least one evaluation. This overlap permits comparison with previous and future test results so that trends over time can be monitored.

Multiple trials should be administered when assessing traits, such as muscle strength, which require consistent efforts on the part of the client. An average score of multiple trials is more stable over time than a single effort (96). A measure of central tendency and the range of scores both should be reported.

Standardized test positions always should be used unless a medical condition prevents proper positioning (e.g., joint contractures). In this event, the client should be positioned as closely as possible to the standardized position and the altered position should be documented. It is important to make sure that clients are posturally secure and comfortable during the evaluation. For clients with neurologic involvement, the head should be positioned in neutral to avoid subtle influences of tonic neck reflexes. An exception occurs when testing is conducted in the prone position. In this case, the head should be turned consistently toward the side being tested.

A key to obtaining reliable and valid test results is providing clear directions and demonstrations to the client. Standardized instructions always must be provided verbatim and may not be modified or repeated unless specifically permitted in the test manual. Verbal directions often are enhanced by tactile, kinesthetic, and visual cues, if permitted. If confusion about the task is detected, this should be documented. If the examiner believes that a given client could complete a task successfully with further instructions that are not specified in the standardized protocol, this item can be readministered at the end of the test session. The person's test score should be based solely on performance exhibited when given standardized instructions. Test performance with augmented instructions can be documented in the clinical note but should not be considered when scoring.

When conducting tests that do not have standardized instructions (e.g., strength testing), it is important to use short, simple, consistent commands. If repetitive or sustained efforts are required, the examiner's voice volume needs to be consistent and adequate to heighten the arousal state and motivate clients to give their best effort.

Verbal reinforcement and feedback regarding performance can influence performance levels (97). Consequently, it must be provided consistently, according to the procedures specified in the test manual. For tests where reinforcement and feedback intervals are not specified and are permitted as needed, the frequency and type of feedback provided should be documented.

Test Scoring, Reporting, and Interpretation of Scores

Examiners should be thoroughly familiar with scoring criteria so that scores can be assigned accurately and efficiently during evaluation sessions. It is not appropriate for examiners to look up scoring criteria during or after the evaluation. Uncertainty about the criteria prolongs the evaluation and leads to scoring errors. It is helpful to include abbreviated scoring criteria on the test form to assist the examiner during the evaluation. Test forms should be well organized and clearly written to facilitate efficient and accurate recording of test results. If multiple types of equipment and test positions are required, it is useful if the equipment and position are identified on the score sheet using situation codes for each item. Such a coding system expedites test administration by assisting the examiner in grouping test items with similar positioning and equipment requirements. Examples of well organized test forms that use situation codes are the Bayley Scales of Infant Development (98), the MAP (32), and the revised version of the Peabody Developmental Motor Scales test forms (40).

If the scoring criteria for a test are not well defined, it may be necessary for examiners within a given center or referral region to clarify the criteria. This was the case for many items on the Peabody Developmental Motor Scales. Interrater reliability levels of highly trained examiners were low for several items, so therapists at the Child Development and Mental Retardation Center in Seattle, Washington, clarified the scoring criteria to improve reliability. Examiners in the surrounding referral area were educated about the clarified criteria by means of inservices and videotapes to ensure that all examining centers in the area would be using identical criteria (40). If scoring criteria are augmented to improve reliability, it is imperative to document that the test was administered with altered criteria. Future results are comparable only if administered using identical scoring criteria. Additionally, if scores are compared with normative data, it is important to document that the test scores obtained may not be directly comparable because altered scoring criteria were used.

Raw scores obtained from testing are meaningless in the absence of additional interpretive data. To compare meaningfully a person's current test results to previous scores, the SEM of the test must be known. To determine how a person's performance compares with that of other people, normative data must come from a representative standardized sample of people with similar characteristics. In the latter case, the raw score must be converted into a derived or relative score, to permit direct comparison with the normative group's performance. These concepts are discussed in detail below.

Raw scores may be compared with previous scores obtained from a given person to monitor changes in status. However, the SEM of the test must be known to determine if a change in a score is clinically significant. A change in a test score exceeding the SEM is indicative of a meaningful change in test performance. As was discussed earlier, in the section on reliability and agreement, it is best to report test scores as a range, based on confidence intervals, rather than as an absolute score. This is because a person's score is expected to vary as a result of random fluctuations in performance. It is only when a score changes beyond the range of random fluctuation that we can be confident that a true change in performance has occurred. This true score range usually is based on the 95% confidence interval. This rigorous level of confidence minimizes the likelihood of a type I error (i.e., believing a change occurred when actually there was no change) and is considered the confidence level of choice when looking for improvement in performance, resulting from a specific treatment regimen or improved physical status. A lower level of confidence (e.g., 75%, 50%) may be desirable when monitoring the status of people who are at risk for loss of function over time. For these people, it is important to minimize the likelihood of a type II error (i.e., believing no change occurred when actually there was a change). In such cases, if a person's score falls outside a true score range that is based on a lower level of confidence, it may indicate the need to conduct further diagnostic tests or to monitor the person more closely over time.

If normative data are available for a given test, a person's score can be compared directly to the normative group performance by converting the score into a derived or relative score. Normative scores provide relative rather than absolute information (99). Normative data should not be considered as performance standards but rather as a reflection of how the normative group performed. Derived scores are expressed either as a developmental level or as a relative position within a specified group. Derived scores are calculated by transforming the raw score to another unit of measurement that enables comparison with normative values. Most norm-referenced tests provide conversion tables of derived scores that have been calculated for the raw scores so that hand calculations are not required. However, it is important for examiners to understand the derivation, interrelationship, and interpretation of derived scores. Specific calculation of these scores is beyond the scope of this chapter. For computational details and the practical application of these statistical techniques, the reader is referred to textbooks on psychological or educational statistics and measurement theory (91,92,99).

Selection of the particular type of score to report depends on the purpose of testing, the sophistication of the people reading the reports, and the types of interpretations to be made from the results (99). Table 6-2 summarizes various descriptive and standard scores that are commonly used. Figure 6-2 shows the relationship of these scores to the normal distribution and the interrelationship of these scores. Calculation of standard scores (e.g., z scores, T scores, stanines, developmental motor quotients, deviation IQ) is appropriate only with interval or ratio data. They express where a person's performance is with regard to the mean of the normative group, in terms of the variability of the distribution. These standard scores are advantageous because they have uniform meaning from test to test. Consequently, a person's performance can be compared between different tests.

Written Evaluation

Thorough documentation of testing procedures and results is essential in both clinical and research settings to permit comparison of test results between and within individuals.

TABLE 6-2. *Descriptive and standard scores commonly reported in rehabilitation medicine*

Summary statistic	Definition and interpretation
Descriptive Score	
Raw scores	Expressed as number of correct items, time to complete a task, number of errors, or some other objective measure of performance
Percentage scores	Raw scores expressed as percent correct
Percentile scores	Expressed in terms of the percentage of people in the normative group who scored lower than the client's score (e.g., a client scoring in the 75th percentile on a norm-referenced test has performed better than 75% of the people in the normative group). Often stratified for age, gender, or other pertinent modifying varieties
Age-equivalent score	Average score for a given age group
Grade-equivalent score	Average score for a given grade level
Developmental age	The basal age score, plus credit for all items earned at higher age levels (up to the ceiling level of the test). Also called motor age for tests of motor development. The basal age level is defined as the highest age at and below which all test items are passed.
Scaled score	The client's total score, summed across all sections of the test. Used for comparison to previous and future scores.
Standard Scores	
Z Score	The client's raw score minus the mean score of normative group, divided by the standard deviation of the normative group. The mean of a z score is 0 with a standard deviation of 1. Scores may be plus or minus. Reported to two significant digits.
T Score	Z-score times 10 plus 50. The mean of a T score is 50 with a standard deviation of 10.
Stanine	Standard scores which range from 1 to 9. A stanine of 5 indicates average performance and the standard deviation deviation is 2. Often used to minimize the likelihood of overinterpreting small differences between individual scores.
DMQ	The ratio of the client's actual score on the test (expressed as developmental age) and the client's chronologic age, DMQ = DA/CA. The DMQ equals the z score times 15, plus 100. The mean DMQ is 100, with a standard deviation of 15.
Deviation IQ	A standard score derivative of the ratio between the client's actual score on the test, expressed as a mental age and the client's chronological age. The mean deviation IQ is 100, with a standard deviation of 15, based on the Wechsler deviation IQ distribution.

CA, chronological age; DA, developmental age; DMQ, developmental motor quotient; IQ, intelligence quotient; MA, motor age.

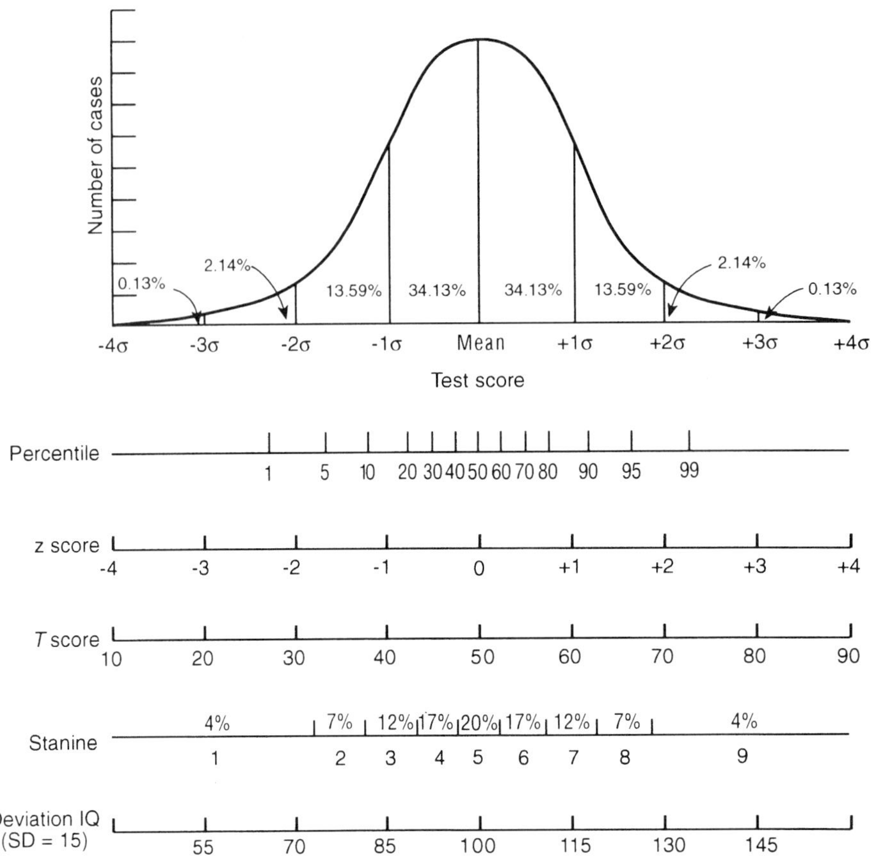

FIG. 6-2. Relationships among standard scores, percentile ranks, and the normal distribution. (Adapted with permission from Anastasi A. *Pschological testing,* 6th ed. New York: Macmillan, 1988; 97.)

The tests administered should be identified clearly. Any deviations from the standardized procedures, such as altered test positions or modified instructions, should be documented (14). If multiple procedural options are available for a given test item (e.g., measuring for a flexion contracture at the hip), the specific method used should be specified in the report. The client's behavior, level of cooperation, alertness, attention, and motivation during the evaluation should be documented. Any potential effect of these factors on test performance should be stated. Other factors that might have influenced the validity of test results also should be noted (e.g., environmental factors, illness, length of test session, activity level before the test session). It should be indicated whether optimal performance was elicited. If a person's performance is compared with normative data, the degree of similarity of the person's characteristics to those of the normative group should be stated. It is imperative to distinguish between facts and inferences in the written report.

The use of a standard written evaluation format facilitates communication between and within disciplines. In addition, computerized data bases provide standardized formats useful for both clinical and research purposes. Serial examinations of a given person can be reviewed easily, and a client's status can be compared directly with that of other people with similar characteristics. Clinical and research applications of computer data bases for documentation in rehabilitation medicine are discussed by Shurtleff (100), Lehmann and associates (101), and Magnuson and Stenehjem (102).

OBJECTIVE MEASUREMENT WHEN A STANDARDIZED TEST IS NOT AVAILABLE

Rationale for Systematically Observing and Recording Behavior

Standardized tests and objective instrumentation are not always available to measure the parameters of clinical and research interest. Consequently, rehabilitation professionals often resort to documentation of subjective impressions (e.g., "head control is improved," "wheelchair transfers are more independent and efficient"). However, functional status and behaviors can be documented objectively by observing behavior using standardized techniques that have been demonstrated to be reliable. Systematically observing and recording behavior provides objective documentation of behavior frequency and duration, identifies the timing and conditions for occurrence of a particular behavior, and identifies small changes in behavior. Several of the procedures for objective documentation described below are based on the principles of single-case research designs. These research designs have been suggested to be the most appropriate method of documentation of treatment-induced clinical change in rehabilitation populations, owing to the wide variability in clinical presentation, even within a given diagnostic category (93,103). In addition, such designs have been recommended to evaluate and compare the effects of two different treatments on individual patients (104). Selected single-case research concepts that specifically pertain to objective documentation for either clinical or research purposes are presented in this chapter. The reader is referred to Barlow and colleagues (105), Barlow and Hersen (66), Bloom and Fisher (46), Kazdin (67), and Ottenbacher (93) for more thorough discussions of documentation using single-case research standardized testing techniques.

Procedures for Objective Observation and Recording of Behavior

Step 1: Identify the Target Behavior to Be Monitored

The target behavior must be identified by specifying the parameters of interest and their associated conditions. The prerequisite conditions required must be defined, such as verbal directions, visual or verbal cues, or physical assistance provided. In addition, environmental conditions must be described because different responses may be observed in the therapy, inpatient ward, or home setting. The duration, frequency, and timing of the observation period also must be specified. Ideally, these conditions should be constant from one observation period to the next for comparison purposes.

Step 2: Operationally Define the Target Behavior

An operational definition is stated in terms of the observable characteristics of the behavior that is being monitored. The definition must describe an observable or measurable action, activity, or movement that reflects the behavior of interest. The beginning and ending of the behavior must be clearly identified. Objective, distinct, and clearly stated terminology should be used (66,93). The definition should be elaborated to point out how the response differs from other responses. Examples of borderline or difficult responses, along with a rationale for inclusion and exclusion, should be provided. An example of an operational definition used to determine success or failure in drawing a circle is provided in Figure 6-3.

Step 3: Identify the Measurement Strategy

There are five methods of sampling behavior: event recording, rate recording, time sampling, duration recording, and discrete categorization (46,66,93). Each of these methods will be described below, along with indications and contraindications for their use.

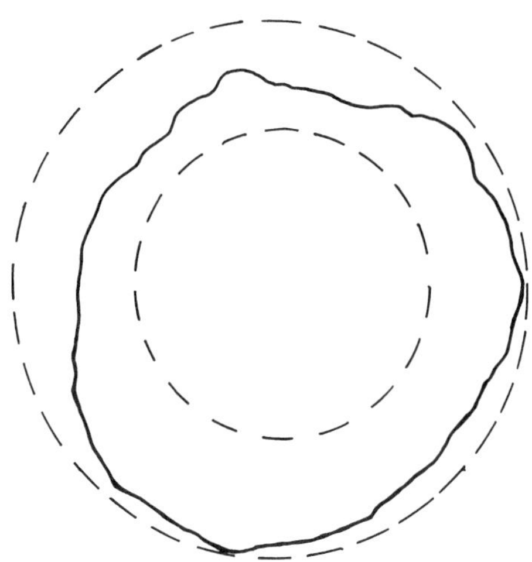

FIG. 6-3. The operational definition of a circle (*dashed lines*, circle path template; *solid line*, client's drawing of a circle). The client is instructed to draw a circle inside the two dashed lines. An adequate circle is one in which the two ends meet, and the line of the circle stays within the circle path template. It can touch the edges of the template but cannot extend beyond the edges.

Event Recording

The number of occurrences of the behavior is tallied in a given period of time or per given velocity, in the case of mobility activities. Indications for event recording include when the target response is discrete, with a definite beginning and end, or when the target response duration is constant. The target behavior frequency should be low to moderate and the behavior duration should be short to moderate. It is best to augment the number of occurrences with real-time information to permit sequential, temporal, and reliability and agreement analyses. Contraindications for using event recording techniques include behaviors that have a high incidence of occurrence, because of the increased probability of error in counting the high-frequency behavior, and behaviors that have an extended duration or that occur infrequently (66,93) (e.g., wheelchair transfers). Duration recording should be used in the latter case. The following is an example of event recording:

A man with hemiplegia successfully fastened five of 10 shirt buttons during a 10-minute period of time using his involved hand to hold his shirt and his uninvolved hand to manipulate the buttons. The number of successes, number of trials, and duration of the observation period were recorded.

Rate Recording

The number of occurrences of the behavior is divided by the duration of the observation period (e.g., the number of occurrences per minute). This method is indicated when the observation period varies from session to session. Rate recording is advantageous because it reflects changes in either the duration or frequency of response and is sensitive for detecting changes or trends because there is no theoretical upper limit. The following is an example of rate recording.

A child with Down syndrome exhibits five occurrences of undesirable tongue thrusting during a 10-minute observation period the first day and eight times during a 20-minute observation period the second day. The observations were made from videotapes recorded immediately after the child's oral motor therapy program. An independent observer, who was blind to the child's intervention program, performed the frequency counts. The rate of responding was 0.5 behaviors per minute (five per 10 minutes) for the first day and 0.4 behaviors per minute (eight per 20 minutes) for the second day.

Time Sampling

This method involves recording the state of a behavior at specific moments or intervals in time. It also has been described in the literature as scan sampling, instantaneous time sampling, discontinuous probe time sampling, and interval sampling. Time sampling is analogous to taking a snapshot and then examining it to see if a particular behavior is occurring. This method often is used in industrial settings to determine exposure to risk factors or compliance with injury prevention techniques.

To monitor behavior using this method, the behavior of interest is observed for a short block of time (e.g., a 5-second observation period) at specified recording intervals (e.g., 5-minute intervals) during a particular activity (e.g., a 30-minute meal period). The recording interval is signaled to the observer by means of a timer, audiotape cue, or a tone generator. The target behavior is scored as either occurring or not occurring during the observation period of each recording period. Fixed (i.e., preset) or random intervals can be used, but it is important to avoid a situation where the signal coincides with any regular cycle of behavior. The sampling should occur at various times throughout the day and in different settings to obtain a representative picture of the behavior frequency. The recording interval length depends on the behavior duration and frequency, as well as on the observer's ability to record and attend to the person. The more frequent the behavior, the shorter the interval. For low to medium response rates, 10-second intervals are recommended. For high response rates, shorter intervals should be used (106). An advantage of this type of recording is that several clients can be observed simultaneously by one rater in a group setting (e.g., during meal times or recreational events), by staggering the recording intervals for each client.

Variations of time sampling include observing the behavior during a single block of time that is divided into short intervals (i.e., interval recording) or during brief intervals that are spread out over an entire day (i.e., time sampling); combining time sampling and event recording, where the number of responses occurring during a given interval are recorded; and combining time sampling and duration recording where the duration of the response during a given interval is recorded. The following are examples of time sampling.

To document a client's ability to maintain his head in an upright position, the nursing staff observed him for 15 seconds at 5-minute intervals during one 30-minute meal period, during one 30-minute self-care/dressing period, and during one 30-minute recreation period.

To estimate compliance of 12 industrial workers with suggestions provided in a back school program, the time individual workers spent in appropriate versus inappropriate postures was recorded for 5 minutes each hour during an 8-hour shift.

Duration Recording

Either the duration of the response or the length of the latency period is recorded. The duration is reported as the total time if the observation period is constant, or as the percentage of time that a behavior occurred during observation periods of varying length. Indications for this method include continuous target responses, behaviors with high or even response rates, and behaviors with varying durations such as a wheelchair transfer, where a frequency count would be less meaningful. The behavior duration is timed with a stopwatch, electromechanical event recorder, or electronic keyboard. Variations of duration recording include timing the response latency (i.e., the time that elapses between a cue and a response; measuring the time required to complete a particular task; or monitoring the time spent performing a particular activity. The following are examples of duration recording:

The amount of time that it takes an adult with a spinal cord injury to dress in the morning.

The length of time that a child is able to stand independently with and without orthotics before losing his or her balance.

Discrete Categorization

With this method of behavior measurement, several different behaviors of interest are listed and checked off as being performed or not performed. This method is useful in determining whether certain behaviors have occurred. It is indicated when behavioral responses can be classified into discrete categories (e.g., correct/incorrect, performed/not performed). An example of this method is a checklist of the different steps for performing a wheelchair transfer, such as positioning the wheelchair, locking the brakes, removing feet from footrests, and so forth. The observer checks off whether each of these steps was performed during a given transfer.

Step 4: Establish Interrater Reliability

There are four reasons for assessing interrater (i.e., interobserver) reliability and agreement.

1. To establish how consistently two observers can measure a given behavior.
2. To minimize individual observer bias by establishing interrater reliability and then retraining observers if the level of reliability is unacceptable.
3. To reduce the chances of an examiner altering or "drifting" from the standard method of rating by implementing periodic interrater reliability or agreement checks to ensure that observers are consistent over time.
4. To examine the adequacy of operational definitions, rating criteria, and scoring procedures. Items that have poor agreement should be revised.

Before the onset of data collection, two people should independently observe and score pilot subjects who have characteristics that are similar to those of the clinical or study population. Behaviors of interest are rated according to predetermined operational definitions. Interrater reliability and agreement are then calculated using an appropriate statistic (see section on Reliability and Agreement). The minimum acceptable level of agreement depends on the type of statistic calculated (see Table 6-1).

If interrater reliability or agreement is below the target level, improvement may occur by discussing operational definitions of the behaviors. If problems with reliability or agreement continue, it may be necessary to redefine behaviors, improve observation and recording conditions, reduce the number of behaviors being recorded, provide additional training, and, if necessary, further standardize the data collection environment (57,84). Interrater reliability or agreement should be re-established once remedial steps have been taken. As stated previously, periodic checks of interrater reliability or agreement should be conducted in the clinic and at least once during each phase of a research study (57,58). Reliability and agreement data should be plotted along with clinical or research data to show the level of consistency in measurements.

Step 5: Report Scores and Graph Data

Baseline, intervention, and follow-up data should be plotted on a graph or chart to provide a pictorial presentation of the results. Graphing strategies include using standard graph paper or a Standard Behavior Chart (i.e., six-cycle graph paper). Advantages of the latter are that it permits systematic, standardized recording using a semilog scale that allows estimation of linear trends. Extremely high and low rates can be recorded on the chart. Behavior rates that range from once per 24 hours to 1,000 per minute can be accommodated; therefore, data are not lost as a result of floor or ceiling effects. In addition, continuous recording of data for up to 20 weeks is permitted. For further information on graphing strategies, the reader is referred to White and Haring (107) and Carr and Williams (108) for use of the Standard Behavior Chart in clinical settings.

The time period of data collection is plotted on the horizontal axis (e.g., hours, days, weeks) and changes in the target behavior on the vertical axis. Appropriate scaling should be used to accommodate the highest expected response frequency and the longest anticipated documentation period duration. The measurement interval on both axes should be large enough to permit visual detection of any changes in behavior. Interrater reliability data from each phase should be plotted on the same graph, along with the study results, as discussed previously.

Considerations When Reporting Scores

The percentage of correct scores often is reported because of the ease of calculation and interpretation. However, usefulness of this summary statistic is limited because it does not provide information on the number of times a client has performed correctly (93). Consequently, it can be misleading if the total number of opportunities varies from day to day. For example, three successes of six trials on day 1 versus three successes out of four trials on day 2 would yield percentages of 50% and 75%, respectively. Based on percentage scores, it would appear that the client's performance was improved, and yet the absolute number of successes has not changed. Additionally, if an odd number of trials is administered on some days and an even number of trials on other days, performance changes may occur based on percentage scores simply because it is not possible to receive half-credit for a trial on days when an odd number of trials are given (e.g., five successes out of 10 trials versus three successes out of five trials).

SUMMARY

Rehabilitation practitioners and researchers in rehabilitation medicine increasingly are using objective tests and measurements as a scientific basis for communication, to establish credibility with other professionals, and to document treatment effectiveness. The increased use of such measures has resulted in greater responsibility of the user for appropriate implementation and interpretation of tests and measures. Rehabilitation professionals must be familiar with the principles of objective measurement to use the tools properly.

The initial section of this chapter described the psychometric parameters used to evaluate the state of development and quality of available objective measures. The four basic levels of measurement—nominal, ordinal, interval, and ratio scales—were defined. The purposes for testing were discussed, including screening tests, in-depth assessment tests, and criterion-referenced tests. Several issues of practicality for selection and use of tests also were identified. The various forms of reliability, agreement, and validity described are of great importance for using the various measurements effectively. A test that does not provide reproducible results, or does not measure what it is purported to measure, is of no value and is potentially harmful, by giving a false implication of meaningfulness. Consequently, caution in the use and interpretation of test results must be exercised when information on reliability or validity of a measure is not available or if their values are below accepted levels.

The second section of this chapter discussed the principles of evaluation, testing, and interpretation that help to ensure that adequate reliability and validity are obtained from test administration. The issues of standardization, interrater reliability, and procedural reliability are of particular importance. Care must be taken during test administration to control for the potential rater errors of central tendency, standards, halo effect, logical errors, and examiner drift.

For many applications in rehabilitation medicine practice and research, standardized measures have not yet been developed. Methods derived from single-subject research paradigms provide guidelines for objective measurement when a standardized test is not available. These guidelines, which are discussed in the third section of this chapter, include identifying the behavior to be monitored; operationally defining the behavior; identifying the measurement strategy (e.g., event recording, rate recording, time sampling); establishing interrater reliability; and properly reporting scores and graphing the data.

Specific tests and objective measurement instruments are not discussed owing to the number and broad spectrum of measures used by rehabilitation professionals. Rather, a detailed table of references (see Appendix A) describing measures is provided, categorizing measures by the domains assessed.

The principles discussed in this chapter provide the framework for the readers critically to assess the measures available for their specific application needs. Such critical analysis will further emphasize the need for ongoing development and improvement of objective measures at the disposal of rehabilitation professionals.

Appendix A. *Measurement scales and test methods used in physical medicine and rehabilitation: critiques and references*

Adaptive equipment assessments for positioning and function
- Biomechanics of wheelchair propulsion as a function of seat position and user-to-chair interface (109)
  - Describes an experimental protocol for determining three-dimensional wheelchair propulsion kinematics with varied hand placements (push-levers versus handrims) and seat positions.
- Development of a clinical measure of postural control for assessment of adaptive seating in children with neuromotor disabilities (110)
  - Reviews the literature on seating assessment, including measures that require complex instrumentation and clinical evaluation scales.
  - Describes the development of a clinical evaluation scale, the Seated Postural Control Measure (SPCM) for use with children requiring adaptive seating systems. The SPCM consists of postural alignment and functional movement items, scored on a four-point scale. A modified version of the Level of Sitting Ability Scale (LSAS) also is described. The LSAS is used to rate sitting ability based on the amount of support required to maintain sitting and the degree of sitting stability. Interrater and test-retest reliability data are reported for both scales.
- Effects of seat-surface inclination on postural stability and function of the upper extremities of children with cerebral palsy (111)
  - Describes methods of evaluating optimal seating surface inclination through postural, center of pressure, and upper extremity function data,
  - Postural data were obtained by means of videotape analysis. Center of pressure data were acquired using a force platform. Upper extremity performance was assessed through six motor control tasks.
- Improvement of functional sitting position for children with cerebral palsy (112)
  - Describes a method of determining the most optimal functional sitting position by using videotapes and photographs. The Sitting Assessment Scale was used to rate head control, trunk control, foot control, arm function, and hand function. Interrater reliability of this scale is reported.
- Pediatric power wheelchairs: evaluation of function in the home and school environments (113)
  - Describes a standardized functional task assessment for use in evaluating indoor function in a wheelchair, both at home and at school. The tasks assessed are classified into three categories: positioning, reaching, and driving.
- Pressure sores: clinical practice and scientific approach (114)
  - Describes pressure distribution measurements, movement studies during sleep, and remote monitoring mechanical force measurements, wound healing measurements, tissue distortion measurements, and compressive loading regimens of wheelchair sitting behavior.
- Prevention of pressure sores: engineering and clinical aspects (115)
  - Describes skin blood flow measurement, seat cushion evaluation techniques, pressure measurement using bladder pressure sensors and conventional pressure sensors, interface pressure distribution visualization, and sheer measurement techniques.

Balance measurement techniques
- Method for the display of balance platform center of pressure data (116)
  - Describes the measurement of center of pressure.
- Assessing the influence of sensory interaction on balance (117)

Appendix A. *Continued.*

Describes procedures for assessing balance under six conditions in the typical clinic setting. Three visual conditions, (i.e., normal, blindfolded, visual-conflict dome) are tested with two surface inputs (i.e., normal, standing on foam). Suggestions of quantifying postural sway under each condition are provided.

Adapting reflexes controlling the human posture (118)

Describes a method of assessing balance using a displacement platform and a visual surround, which is used to assess the influence of various sensory conditions on balance.

Biomechanics and Motor Control Assessment Techniques

Biomechanics and Motor Control of Human Movement (119)

Describes measurement of kinematic data (e.g., by using goniometers, accelerometers, and imaging techniques); anthropometric data (e.g., density, mass, center of mass, moment of inertia, joint centers of rotation, muscle anthropometry); kinetic data (e.g., joint reaction forces, bone-on-bone forces, force transducers, force plate data, muscle force estimates); mechanical work, energy, and power measurements; muscle mechanics; and electromyography.

Methodology for studying motor behavior (120)

Describes methods of measuring movement kinematics, electromyography, movement errors, tracking, balance, coordination, reaction time, movement time, and motor skills.

Techniques of the study of movement (121)

Describes methods of studying movements, including cinematography, stroboscopic photography, cyclography, stereoscopic recording, determining masses and centers of gravity, electrogoniometry, ultrasound, optoelectronics, accelerometry, photogrammetry, rigid-body kinematics, derivative estimation, state-space modeling, force plates, body segment description, kinetic modeling, and data processing. Includes descriptions of historical techniques and compares these to contemporary methods.

Computerized assessment data bases and techniques

Computer data bases for pediatric disability: clinical and research applications (100)

Reviews computer-based medical records and evaluation systems for individuals with disabilities. These systems have applications for clinical and research settings.

Computerized data management as an aid to clinical decision making in rehabilitation (101)

Describes a computerized data base that has been developed for clinical decision making in rehabilitation. Multidisciplinary patient performance data can be stored and accessed by all team members.

Computers in rehabilitative medicine (102)

Describes computerized assessments to monitor behavior (e.g., pressure relief), physiologic parameters, cognition, communication, eye-hand coordination, gait, balance, electrodiagnosis, and functional assessment.

Computerized medical instrument data bases and citation indexes.

Health instruments file data base (122)

A computerized data base that contains information on instruments (e.g., questionnaires, interview protocols, observation checklists, index measure, rating scales, projective techniques, tests) in health, health-related, and behavioral sciences. Designed to identify measures needed for research studies, clinical assessments, and program evaluation. The data base contains information on selected measurement instruments, instruments constructed for a particular study, and modifications of existing instruments.

Medical/health science bibliographies (123)

A computerized data base of annotated test bibliographies. The data base includes tests of personality, sensory-motor function, vocation/occupation, behavior, developmental scales, family interaction, environmental influences, manual dexterity, learning, social skills, and social perception and judgment.

Medical device register: United States and Canada (124)

Cross-references lists of medical instruments and devices.

Science citation index (125)

References that have cited specific instruments are indexed according to the specific name of the instrument.

Elderly assessment instruments

Assessing the elderly (126)

Reviews selected instruments for measuring physical health, physical functioning, activities of daily living, cognitive functioning, affective functioning, general mental health, social interactions and resources, person–environment compatability, and multidimensional measure.

Electrodiagnostic assessment techniques

Electrodiagnostic evaluation of the peripheral nervous system (127)

Describes electrodiagnostic procedures, including sensory nerve conduction studies, motor nerve conduction studies, single-fiber electromyography, needle electrode examination, and findings for specific diagnostic categories.

Manual of nerve conduction velocity and somatosensory evoked potentials (128)

Describes techniques and normal value ranges for nerve conduction studies and somatosensory evoked potentials.

Functional assessment instruments

A critical review of 12 activities of daily living (129)

Discusses parameters measured, type of scoring, scaling of scores, and the advantages and disadvantages of each scale.

A critical review of scales of activities of daily living (130)

Reviews scales of basic self-care according to standard criteria. The evaluation criteria include: purpose, clinical utility, test construction, standardization, reliability, and validity. Specific recommendations are made regarding which activities of daily living scales are most suitable for describing, predicting, or evaluating activities of daily living function.

(continued)

Appendix A. *Continued.*

Functional assessment in rehabilitation (131)
Reviews functional assessments for people with physical disabilities, mental retardation, and psychiatric impairments, functional communication assessments, quantitative muscle function testing, upper extremity functional capabilities, job-related social competence, learning potential for people with mental retardation, environmental influences on behavior, rehabilitation indicators, self-observation and report techniques, and vocational rehabilitation assessments.
Functional assessment in rehabilitation medicine (25)
Reviews functional assessment instruments used in outcome measurement, rehabilitation nursing, and in assessing the elderly, the arthritic patient, and people with mental retardation. Also reviews functional measurement of verbal impairments, assessments of support systems for the elderly, assessment of family functioning, and functional assessments used in primary care.
Measurement of activities of daily living (132)
Reviews the characteristics of several commonly used standardized activities of daily living assessments. The characteristics reviewed include number of test items, target population, parameters assessed, method of administration, and reliability.
Measurement of time in a standardized test of patient mobility (133)
Describes a standardized assessment for evaluating the efficiency of bed mobility, wheelchair activities, transfer activities, and ambulation.
Normative values are provided for 20- to 69-year-old people
Gait assessment techniques
Footprint analysis in gait documentation (134)
Provides instructions for obtaining footprint data in the typical clinic setting. Instructions for measuring velocity, cadence, foot progression angle, base of support, stride length, and step length are provided. Observations of toe drag and symmetry of pressure also are suggested.
Functional community ambulation: what are your criteria (135)
Criteria are provided for evaluating functional community ambulation. Distances required for independent community ambulation at the post office, bank, doctor's office, supermarket, department store, drug store, and to cross intersections are provided. Typical curb heights and crosswalk times also are presented.
Gait analysis: normal and pathological function (136)
Discusses observational gait analysis, oxygen consumption measures, ground reaction force measurements, dynamic electromyography, and gait assessment using motion analysis systems. Normal and pathologic gait patterns are described. Applications of assessment techniques to specific patient populations are discussed.
Interrater reliability of videotaped observational gait analysis assessments (137)
Interrater reliability of 54 therapists observing videotapes of patients exhibiting abnormal gait was determined. The parameters assessed included knee flexion, genu valgum, cadence, step length, stride length, stance time, and step width. The therapists received no special training in preparation for this study, beyond their physical therapy education. The results indicate that observational gait analysis, in the absence of common rater training, has low to moderate interrater reliability.
Reliability of observational kinematic gait analysis (138)
Methods of observational analysis are discussed. Descriptions are provided of the procedures used to develop a reliable observational gait analysis format and the protocol used to train raters. Interrater and test-retest reliability data were obtained by having raters observe gait videotapes. The results indicate that observational kinematic gait analysis is a convenient but only moderately reliable technique.
Strategies for the assessment of pediatric gait in the clinical setting (139)
Describes observational and video gait analysis, measurement of time–distance parameters, electromyography, kinematics, kinetics, and energy expenditure. The pros and cons of each method are discussed, and instrumentation required is described. The use of gait analysis measurements for surgical and orthotic decision making also is presented.
Biomechanics and motor control of human gait (140)
Discusses gait terminology, temporal and stride measures, kinematics, kinetics, electromyography. Selected normal values are provided.
Multifactorial rehabilitation assessment references
Clinical measurements (141)
Reviews measures of isokinetic strength, clinical measures, functional disability, sensorimotor performance, range of motion, developmental parameters, infant movement, postural control and cardiopulmonary function.
Measurement in physical therapy (142)
Reviews measures of strength testing (e.g., manual muscle testing, instrumented muscle performance measures), joint motion, functional assessment, gait assessment, children with central nervous system dysfunction, pulmonary function testing, cardiovascular function, nerve conduction velocity, and electromyographic testing.
Measurement tools with application to brain injury (143)
Reviews measures of coma and global function, disability measures, communicative function, cognitive function, degree of handicap, general outcome measures, environmental measures, preinjury history, and sensory impairments.
Measuring health: a guide to rating scales and questionnaires (144)
Reviews measures of functional disability and handicap, activities of daily living, psychological well-being, social health, quality of life and life satisfaction, pain measurements, and general health measurements.
Quality of life assessments in clinical trials (145)

Appendix A. *Continued.*

Reviews economic scales and tests, quality of life assessments, social interaction tests and scales, psychological tests and scales, and functional disability scales. Applications of these scales in rehabilitation and for specific patient populations are discussed.

Tenth-Mental Measurements Yearbook (146)

Reviews standardized tests in the areas of achievement, aptitude, development, education, intelligence, neuropsychology, personality, sensory-motor, speech and hearing, and vocation. Contains a bibliography and critical test reviews of 396 commercially available tests, new or revised, since the publication of the *Ninth Mental Measurements Yearbook* in 1985. Bibliographies of references for specific tests, related to the construction, validity, or use of the tests in various settings also are included. The tests are indexed by periodical, author, publisher, tests or book title, and tests classification. Reviews, descriptions, and references associated with older tests are contained in previous editions of the *Yearbook.*

Muscle strength assessment techniques

Manual muscle strength assessment methods (20–22)

Describes standard tests positions and grading criteria for manual assessment of strength.

Muscle strength development and assessment in children and adolescents (3)

Reviews the literature pertaining to the reliability and validity of strength testing using manual muscle testing and objective techniques.

Describes principles of strength testing with both traditional manual methods and objective myometry techniques. Suggestions for testing infants, children, and adolescents are provided.

Muscle strength testing: instrument and noninstrumented systems (147)

Discusses strength assessment techniques, including: skeletal muscle strength testing with instrumented and noninstrumented systems, isometric testing with fixed-load cells, dynamic strength testing, trunk strength testing, and grip and pinch strength measurements.

Technical manual: hand strength and dexterity tests (148)

Describes tests of grip strength, pinch strength, and finger–hand coordination, and provides normative values.

Muscle tone assessment techniques

Clinical measures of spasticity: are they reliable? (4)

Intertrial, interrater, and test-retest reliability results of clinical measures of spasticity obtained on a group of people with traumatic spinal cord injuries are reported.

H-reflex and recovery cycle in spastic and normal children (149)

Intraindividual, Interindividual, and Intergroup Comparisons are provided. Describes reflex quantification by means of H-reflex recovery curves.

Microprocessor-based instrument for achilles tendon reflex measurements (150)

Describes quantification of reflex responses by means of tendon tapping with measured forces.

Spasticity: quantitative measurements as a basis for assessing effectiveness of therapeutic intervention (151)

Detailed description of a method for measuring mechanical output from spastic reflex muscle response to sinusoidal ankle motion at varying frequencies of oscillation.

Occupational biomechanics, ergonomics, and work capacity evaluation techniques

Ergonomic design for people at work (152)

Volume 1 discusses design issues for the workplace, equipment, hand tools, and the environment. Volume 2 describes evaluation of job demands, lifting, manual materials handling by means of surveys, timed activity analysis, biomechanical analysis, energy expenditure measurements, and motion analysts techniques.

Occupational Biomechanics (41)

Reviews measurement of anthropometry, joint motion, muscle strength, motion analysis, postural analysis, force platform data, work capacity, vibration exposure, manual materials handling, hand tool analysis, preemployment screening, job analysis, and ergonomic assessments in clerical and industrial settings. Manual work evaluation techniques also are discussed, including motion time measurement methods, physical demands analysis, manual lifting analysis, job static strength analysis, and job postural analysis.

Work hardening (153)

Describes equipment used for work hardening and ergonomic assessments and the evaluation process.

Work hardening: state of the art (154)

Describes work-hardening evaluations and intervention techniques, including equipment and tools required.

Work injury: management and prevention (155)

Describes ergonomic, functional capacity, and work hardening evaluations.

Occupational therapy evaluation techniques

An annotated index of occupational therapy evaluation tools (156)

Reviews the purposes, advantages, and limitations of standardized and nonstandardized tests of activities of daily living, adaptive skills, cognitive skills, developmental skills, oral function, person-environment interactions, play skills, psychosocial, roles and habits, sensory integration, visual-perceptual skills, and vocational skills.

Housing accessibility checklist (157)

Specific criteria are described for determining housing accessibility. Recommended minimum standards are provided for parking areas, walks and ramps, curbs, stairs, doorways, elevators, and interior rooms.

Mental health assessment in occupational therapy (158)

(continued)

Appendix A. *Continued.*

Reviews selected assessments of human function pertaining to mental health, including checklists, interest inventories, assessment of older adults, prevocational assessments, work tolerance screening, research analysis of evaluation tools used to assess mental health clients, and the Milwaukee Daily Living Skills and Kohlman Evaluation of Living Skills assessment scales.

Willard and Spackman's occupational therapy (159)

Reviews tests of manual dexterity, motor function, developmental, sensory integration, intelligence, and psychological tests.

Pediatric assessment instruments

Pediatric functional outcome measures (160)

Reviews the technical and clinical merits of selected functional outcome measures used in pediatric rehabilitation practice.

Review of selected measures in neurodevelopmental rehabilitation

Reviews measures of gross and fine motor function, activities of daily living, general cognitive abilities, speech and language, and child and parent adjustment.

Physical function assessment techniques

Assessment of fitness (161,162)

Discusses methods of objective assessment and interpretation of test results for objective evaluation of flexibility, body composition (e.g., body density, anthropometry, total body water, muscle mass estimation), muscle strength and endurance, anaerobic abilities, aerobic abilities, leisure time and occupational activity, and physiologic fitness (e.g., blood pressure, blood lipids and lipoproteins, glucose intolerance). References for specific tests are provided.

Human muscle function and fatigue (163)

Describes the mechanism of muscle fatigue, distinguishing between central and peripheral factors. Describes tests of contractile function and electromyographic changes with fatigue.

Introduction to measurement in physical education and exercise science (51)

Reviews measures of physical fitness, including body composition (e.g., hydrostatic weighing, skinfold thickness), aerobic fitness tests, performance-based measures, muscle strength and endurance, balance, flexibility, posture, and motor ability.

Measurement for evaluation in physical education and exercise sciences (45)

Reviews measures of physical abilities (e.g., muscle strength, power, endurance, flexibility, balance, kinesthetic perception), youth fitness, aerobic fitness, body composition (e.g., hydrostatic weighing, skinfold thickness), and skill achievement.

Methodology in human fatigue assessment (164)

Describes methods of assessing fatigue, including psychological ratings, the blink method, urinary metabolite measurements, assessment of fatigue at work, direct estimation of circulatory fatigue using bicycle ergometry, determination of muscular work performed with different muscle groups, increasing work loads under different environmental conditions, mental fatigue and stress, and fatigue assessments of specific worker populations.

Patient evaluation methods for the health professional (165)

Describes standardized techniques for measuring limb girth, limb length, limb volume, joint range of motion, muscle length, activities of daily living, motor control, and neurologic parameters.

Quantitative Assessment of Physical Performance (166)

Describes techniques for measuring range of motion, strength and power, endurance and fatigue, sensation, pain algometry, coordination, muscle tone, gait, hand function, functional parameters, and degree of disability.

Psychosocial assessment instruments

A Sourcebook for Mental Health Measures (167)

Contains 1,100 abstracts of mental health-related psychological measures that describe questionnaires, scales, inventories, tests, and other types of measuring devices. The emphasis is on instruments that have been developed for research or clinical purposes and are less well known than commercially published tests. Abstracts are grouped into 45 categories. These categories include alcoholism, cognitive tests, counseling and guidance, crime and juvenile delinquency, differential psychological diagnosis, drugs, educational adjustment, environments, family interaction, generations differences, geriatrics, marriage and divorce, mental health attitudes, mental retardation, mental status and level of psychological functioning, occupational adjustment, parent behavior and viewpoints, personal history and demographic data, personality, physical handicap, racial attitudes, psychiatric rehabilitation, service delivery, sex, social issues, student and teacher attitudes, suicide and death, therapeutic outcomes, therapeutic processes, and vocational tests. A description of each instrument is provided, along with the source. In addition, the sourcebook references several other sources of mental health measures.

Evaluating Practice: Guidelines for the Accountable Professional (46)

Reviews a group of nine instruments that measure generalized contentment, self-esteem, marital satisfaction, sexual satisfaction, parental attitudes, child's attitudes, family relations, and peer relations. Also provides references and briefly discusses reviews of various psychological measures, including mental health measures, psychotherapy change measures, behavioral assessment questionnaires, behavior checklists, psychological assessment, social attitudes, social functioning, adult assessment, rapid assessment instruments for practice, and rating scales which are useful to evaluate client performance using an interview or observation format.

Neuropsychological assessment (168)

Reviews measures of intellectual abilities, verbal functions, perceptual functions, constructional functions, memory functions, conceptual function, executive functions, motor performance, orientation, attention, tests for brain injury, observational methods, rating scales, and inventories, and tests of personal adjustment and functional disorders.

Psychological testing (34)

Appendix A. *Continued.*

Reviews intelligence and developmental tests for the general population and special populations, educational achievement and competency tests, creativity and reasoning tests, projective testing techniques, environmental attitudes tests, vocational aptitude tests, occupational cognitive screening, psychomotor tests, aptitude tests, personality tests, behavioral assessments, measures of interests, values, and personal orientation, and tests for learning disabilities and neuropsychological dysfunctions.

Self-report inventories in behavioral assessment (169)

Reviews instruments that measure fears, anxiety, assertiveness, social skills, and depression.

Range-of-motion and muscle extensibility assessment techniques

Measurement of joint motion (170)

Reviews static and dynamic methods of measuring joint motion.

Measurement of joint motion: a guide to goniometry (171)

Describes standardized procedures for measuring range of motion of the extremities, spine, and temporomandibular joint. Photos show each test position. Normative values are provided for ranges of motion of each joint.

Measurement of trunk motion and flexibility (172–180)

This series of references describe measurement techniques and reliability of trunk lateral flexion (174,177,178,180), forward flexion (172,179), and extension (173,175,176,180).

Speech assessment techniques

Appraisal and diagnosis of speech and language disorders (33)

Reviews measures of articulation, speech-sound discrimination, language, developmental skills, motor skills, nonverbal intelligence, speech production, structural disorders, fluency, and neurologic disorders.

Diagnosis of speech and language disorders (181)

Reviews content areas of tests for language disturbances (e.g., aphasia, apraxia), articulation, language production, language comprehension, speech intelligibility, phonologic processes, auditory abilities and behavior, comprehension, discrimination, memory, language development, language inventories, communicative abilities, learning aptitude, nonverbal communication, stuttering, grammatical comprehension, sound discrimination, and listening accuracy.

Diagnostic Handbook of Speech Pathology (182)

Lists quick screening tests for speech and language, articulation tests, auditory tests, language tests, and tests in related areas (e.g., adaptive behavior, basic concepts, intelligence tests, developmental tests, visual perception, learning aptitude, motor accuracy, performance and attainment scales).

REFERENCES

1. Frese E, Brown M, Norton BJ. Clinical reliability of manual muscle testing: middle trapezius and gluteus medius muscles. *Phys Ther* 1987; 67:1072–1076.
2. Harris SR, Smith LH, Krukowski L. Goniometric reliability for a child with spastic quadriplegia. *J Pediatr Orthop* 1985; 5:348–351.
3. Hinderer KA, Hinderer SR. Muscle strength development and assessment in children and adolescents. In: Harms-Ringdahl K, ed. *Muscle strength series: international perspectives in physical therapy. Muscle strength.* Edinburgh: Churchill-Livingstone, 1993.
4. Hinderer SR, Nanna M, Dijkers MP. The reliability and correlations of clinical and research measures of spasticity [Abstract]. *J Spinal Cord Med* 1996; 19:138.
5. Iddings DM, Smith LK, Spencer WA. Muscle testing. part 2: reliability in clinical use. *Phys Ther Rev* 1961; 41:249–256.
6. Lilienfeld AM, Jacobs M, Willis M. A study of the reproducibility of muscle testing and certain other aspects of muscle scoring. *Phys Ther Rev* 1954; 34:279–289.
7. Sacket DC, Haynes RB, Tugwell P. *A basic science for clinical medicine.* Boston: Little, Brown, 1985.
8. Bartlett MD, Wolf LS, Shurtleff DB, Staheli LT. Hip flexion contractures: a comparison of measurement methods. *Arch Phys Med Rehabil* 1985; 66:620–625.
9. Hinderer KA, Gutierrez T. Myometry measurements of children using isometric and eccentric methods of muscle testing [Abstract]. *Phys Ther* 1988; 68:817.
10. Hinderer KA, Hinderer SR. Stabilized vs. unstabilized myometry strength test positions: a reliability comparison [Abstract]. *Arch Phys Med Rehabil* 1990; 71:771–772.
11. Hinderer KA, Hinderer SR, Deitz JL. *Reliability of manual muscle testing using the hand-held dynamometer and the myometer: a comparison study.* Presented at American Physical Therapy Association Midwinter Sections Meeting, Washington, DC, February 11, 1988.
12. Gowland C, King G, King S, et al. *Review of selected measures in neurodevelopmental rehabilitation: a rational approach for selecting clinical measures.* Research report no. 91-2. Hamilton, Ontario: McMaster University, Neurodevelopmental Clinical Research Unit, 1991.
13. Kirshner B, Guyatt G. A methodological framework for assessing health indices. *J Chronic Dis* 1985; 38:27–36.
14. American Physical Therapy Association. Standards for tests and measurements in physical therapy practice. *Phys Ther* 1991; 71:589–622.
15. Rothstein JM, Echternach JL. *Primer on measurement: an introductory guide to measurement issues.* Alexandria, VA: American Physical Therapy Association, 1993.
16. American Educational Association, American Psychological Association, National Council on Measurement in Education. *Standards for educational and psychological testing.* Washington, DC: American Psychological Association, 1985.
17. Johnston MV, Keith RA, Hinderer SR. Measurement standards for interdisciplinary medical rehabilitation. *Arch Phys Med Rehabil* 1992; 73(suppl 12S):S3–S23.
18. Rothstein JM. Measurement and clinical practice: theory and application. In: Rothstein JM, ed. *Measurement in physical therapy.* New York: Churchill-Livingstone, 1985; 1–46.
19. Krebs DE. Measurement theory. *Phys Ther* 1987; 67:1834–1839.
20. Hislop HJ, Montgomery J. *Daniels and Worthingham's muscle testing: techniques of manual examination,* 6th ed. Philadelphia: WB Saunders, 1995.
21. Janda V. *Muscle function testing.* Boston: Butterworths, 1983.
22. Kendall FP, McCreary EK, Geise PG. *Muscle testing and function.* 4th ed. Baltimore: Williams & Wilkins, 1993.
23. McGourty LK. *Kohlman evaluation of living skills*, 2nd ed. Seattle: KELS Research, 1979.
24. McGourty LK. Kohlman evaluation of living skills (KELS). In: Hemphill BJ, ed. *Mental health assessment in occupational therapy.* Thorofare, NJ: Black Publishers, 1988; 131–146.
25. Granger CV, Gresham GE, eds. *Functional assessment in rehabilitation medicine.* Baltimore: Williams & Wilkins, 1984.
26. Merbitz C, Morris J, Grip JC. Ordinal scales and foundations of misinference. *Arch Phys Med Rehabil* 1989; 70:308–312.

27. Wright BD, Linacre JM. Observations are always ordinal; measurements, however, must be interval. *Arch Phys Med Rehabil* 1989; 70: 857–860.
28. Deitz JC, Beeman C, Thorn DW. *Test of orientation for rehabilitation patients (TORP).* Tucson, AZ: Therapy Skill Builders, 1993.
29. Deitz JC, Tovar VS, Beeman C, Thorn DW, Trevisan M. The test of orientation for rehabilitation patients: test-retest reliability. *Occup Ther J Res* 1992; 12:172–185.
30. Deitz JC, Tovar VS, Thorn DW, Beeman C. The test of orientation for rehabilitation patients: interrater reliability. *Am J Occup Ther* 1990; 44:784–790.
31. Thorn DW, Deitz JC. A content validity study of the Test of Orientation for Rehabilitation Patients. *Occup Ther J Res* 1990; 10:27–40.
32. Miller LJ. *Miller assessment for preschoolers.* San Antonio, TX: Psychological Corporation, 1988.
33. Peterson HA, Marquardt TP. *Appraisal and diagnosis of speech and language disorders.* 3rd ed. Englewood Cliffs, NJ: Prentice-Hall, 1994.
34. Anastasi A. *Psychological testing,* 6th ed. New York: Macmillan, 1988.
35. Gans BM, Haley SM, Hallenborg SC, Mann N, Inacio CA, Faas RM. Description and inter-observer reliability of the Tufts Assessment of Motor Performance. *Am J Phys Med Rehabil* 1988; 67:202–210.
36. Haley SM, Ludlow LH, Gans BM, Faas RM, Inacio CA. Tufts Assessment of Motor Performance: an empirical approach to identifying motor performance categories. *Am J Phys Med Rehabil* 1991; 72: 359–366.
37. Ludlow LH, Haley SM. Polytomous Rasch models for behavioral assessment: the Tufts Assessment of Motor Performance. In: Wilson M, ed. *Objective measurement: theory into practice.* Vol. 1. Norwood, NJ: Ablex Publishing, 1992; 121–137.
38. Haley SM, Ludlow LH. Applicability of the hierarchical scales of the Tufts Assessment of Motor Performance for school-aged children and adults with disabilities. *Phys Ther* 1992; 72:191–206.
39. Ludlow LH, Haley SM, Gans BM. A hierarchical model of functional performance in rehabilitation medicine: the Tufts Assessment of Motor Performance. *Evaluation Health Prof* 1992; 15:59–74.
40. Hinderer KA, Richardson PK, Atwater SW. Clinical implications of the Peabody Developmental Motor Scales: a constructive review. *Phys Occup Ther Pediatr* 1989; 9:81–106.
41. Chaffin DB, Anderson GBJ. *Occupational biomechanics.* 2nd ed. New York: Wiley, 1991.
42. Granger CV, Kelly-Hayes M, Johnston M, Deutsch A, Braun S, Fiedler RC. Quality and outcome measures for medical rehabilitation. In: Braddom RL, ed. *Physical medicine and rehabilitation.* Philadelphia: WB Saunders, 1996; 239–253.
43. Lawlis GF, Lu E. Judgment of counseling process: reliability, agreement, and error. *Phys Occup Ther Pediatr* 1989; 9:81–106.
44. Tinsley HE, Weiss DJ. Interrater reliability and agreement of subjective judgements. *J Counsel Psychol* 1975; 22:358–376.
45. Baumgartner TA, Jackson AS. *Measurement for evaluation in physical education and exercise science,* 4th ed. Dubuque, IA: William C Brown, 1991.
46. Bloom M, Fischer J, Orme JG. *Evaluating practice: guidelines for the accountable professional.* Boston: Allyn & Bacon, 1995.
47. Bartko JJ, Carpenter WT. On the methods and theory of reliability. *J Nerv Ment Dis* 1976; 163:307–317.
48. Hartmann DP. Considerations in the choice of interobserver reliability estimates. *J Appl Behav Anal* 1977; 10:103–116.
49. Hollenbeck AR. Problems of reliability in observational research. In: Sackett GP, ed. *Observing behavior: data collection and analysis methods.* Vol. 2. Baltimore: University Park Press, 1978; 79–98.
50. Liebetrau AM. Measures of association. *Sage University paper series on quantitative applications in the social sciences.* Series no. 07-032. Newbury Park, CA: Sage, 1983.
51. Safrit MJ. *Introduction to measurement in physical education and exercise science,* 2nd ed. St. Louis: Times Mirror/Mosby College Publishing, 1990.
52. Verducci FM. *Measurement concepts in physical education.* St. Louis: CV Mosby, 1980.
53. Deitz JC. Reliability. *Phys Occup Ther Pediatr* 1989; 9:125–147.
54. Cronbach LJ. *Essentials of psychological testing,* 5th ed. New York: Harper & Row, 1990.
55. Fleiss JL. Estimating the accuracy of dichotomous judgments. *Psychometrika* 1965; 30:469–479.
56. Shrout PE, Fleiss JL. Intraclass correlations: uses in assessing rater reliability. *Psychol Bull* 1979; 86:420–428.
57. Cicchetti DV, Aivano SL, Vitale J. Computer programs for assessing rater agreement and rater bias for qualitative data. *Educ Psychol Measure* 1977; 37:195–201.
58. Cohen J. A coefficient of agreement for nominal scales. *Educ Psychol Measure* 1960; 20:37–46.
59. Cicchetti DV, Lee C, Fontana AF, Dowds BN. A computer program for assessing specific category rater agreement and rater bias for qualitative data. *Educ Psychol Measure* 1978; 38:805–813.
60. Cohen J. Weighted kappa: nominal scale agreement with provision for scaled disagreement or partial credit. *Psychol Bull* 1968; 70:213–220.
61. Fleiss JL. Measuring agreement between two judges on the presence or absence of a trait. *Biometrics* 1975; 31:651–659.
62. Fleiss JL, Cohen J. The equivalence of weighted kappa and the intraclass correlation coefficient as measures of reliability. *Educ Psychol Measure* 1973; 33:613–619.
63. Fleiss JL. The measurement of interrater agreement. In: Fleiss JL, ed. *Statistical methods for rates and proportions,* 2nd ed. New York: Wiley, 1981; 212–236.
64. Krippendorff K. Bivariate agreement coefficients for reliability of data. In: Borgatta EF, ed. *Sociological methodology.* San Francisco: Jossey-Bass, 1970; 139–150.
65. Landis JR, Koch GG. The measurement of observer agreement for categorical data. *Biometrics* 1977; 33:159–174.
66. Barlow DH, Hersen M. *Single case experimental designs: strategies for studying behavior change.* 2nd ed. New York: Pergamon, 1984.
67. Kazdin AE. *Single-case research designs.* New York: Oxford University Press, 1982.
68. Harris FC, Lahey BB. A method for combining occurrence and nonoccurrence interobserver agreement scores. *J Appl Behav Anal* 1978; 11:523–527.
69. Haley SM, Osberg JS. Kappa coefficient calculation using multiple ratings per subject: a special communication. *Phys Ther* 1989; 69: 90–94.
70. Plewis I, Bax M. The uses and abuses of reliability measures in developmental medicine. *Dev Med Child Neurol* 1982; 24:388–390.
71. Soeken KL, Prescott PA. Issues in the use of kappa to estimate reliability. *Med Care* 1986; 24:733–741.
72. Hubert L. Kappa revisited. *Psychol Bull* 1977; 84:289–297.
73. Fleiss JL. Measuring nominal scale agreement among many raters. *Psychol Bull* 1971; 76:378–382.
74. Light RJ. Measures of response agreement for qualitative data: some generalizations and alternatives. *Psychol Bull* 1971; 76:365–377.
75. Wackerly DD, McClave JT, Rao PV. Measuring nominal scale agreement between a judge and a known standard. *Psychometrika* 1978; 43:213–223.
76. Williams GW. Comparing the joint agreement of several raters with another rater. *Biometrics* 1976; 32:619–627.
77. Krebs DE. Computer communication. *Phys Ther* 1984; 64: 1581–1589.
78. Brennan RL. *Elements of generalizability theory.* Iowa City, IA: ACT Publications, 1983.
79. Cronbach LJ, Gleser GC, Nanda H, Rajaratnam N. *The dependability of behavioral measurements.* New York: Wiley, 1972.
80. Lahey MA, Downey RG, Saal FE. Intraclass correlations: there's more there than meets the eye. *Psychol Bull* 1983; 93:586–595.
81. Dunn WW. Validity. *Phys Occup Ther Pediatr* 1989; 9:149–168.
82. Thorn DW, Deitz JC. Examining content validity through the use of content experts. *Occup Ther J Res* 1989; 9:334–346.
83. Wilson M, ed. *Objective measurement: theory into practice.* Monterey, CA: Ablex, 1991.
84. Wright BD, Masters GN. *Rating scale analysis.* Chicago: Mesa Press, 1982.
85. Wright BD, Stone MH. *Best test design: Rasch measurement.* Chicago: Mesa Press, 1979.
86. Francis DJ. An introduction to structural equation models. *J Clin Exp Neuropsychol* 1988; 10:623–639.
87. Long JS. Confirmatory factor analysis. *Sage University paper series on quantitative application in the social sciences.* Series no. 07-033. Newbury Park, CA: Sage Publications, 1983.

88. Law M. Measurement in occupational therapy: scientific criteria for evaluation. *Can J Occup Ther* 1987; 54:133–138.
89. Ottenbacher KJ, Tomchek SD. Measurement variation in method comparison studies: an empirical examination. *Arch Phys Med Rehabil* 1994; 75:505–512.
90. Cleary TA, Linn RL, Walster GW. Effect of reliability and validity on power of statistical tests. In: Borgatta EF, ed. *Sociological methodology*. San Francisco: Jossey-Bass, 1970; 130–138.
91. Miller LJ, ed. Developing norm-referenced standardized tests. *Phys Occup Ther Pediatr* 1989; 9:1–205.
92. Gyurke J, Prifitera A. Standardizing an assessment. *Phys Occup Ther Pediatr* 1989; 9:63–90.
93. Ottenbacher KJ. *Evaluating clinical change: strategies for occupational and physical therapists.* Baltimore: Williams & Wilkins, 1986.
94. Paul GL, Lentz RJ. *Psychosocial treatment of chronic mental patients: milieu versus social-learning programs.* Cambridge, MA: Harvard University Press, 1977.
95. Billingsley F, White OR, Munson R. Procedural reliability: a rationale and an example. *Behav Assess* 1980; 2:229–241.
96. Hinderer KA. Reliability of the myometer in muscle testing children and adolescents with myelodysplasia. Unpublished master's thesis, University of Washington, Seattle, WA, 1988.
97. Schmidt RA. Feedback and knowledge of results. In: Schmidt RA, ed. *Motor control and learning,* 2nd ed. Champaign, IL: Human Kinetics Publishers, 1988; 423–455.
98. Bayley NA. The Bayley scales of infant development. New York: The Psychological Corporation, 1969.
99. Cermak S. Norms and scores. *Phys Occup Ther Pediatr* 1989; 9: 91–123.
100. Shurtleff DB. Computer data bases for pediatric disability: clinical and research applications. *Phys Med Rehabil Clin North Am* 1991; 2: 665–687.
101. Lehmann JF, Warren CG, Smith W, Larson J. Computerized data management as an aid to clinical decision making in rehabilitation medicine. *Arch Phys Med Rehabil* 1984; 65:260–262.
102. Magnuson RL, Stenehjem J. Computers in rehabilitative medicine. In: Goodgold J, ed. *Rehabilitation medicine.* St. Louis: CV Mosby, 1988; 879–891.
103. Martin JE, Epstein L. Evaluating treatment of effectiveness in cerebral palsy. *Phys Ther* 1976; 56:285–294.
104. Guyatt G, Sackett D, Taylor W, Chong J, Roberts R, Pugsley S. Determining optimal therapy. *N Engl J Med* 1986; 314:889–892.
105. Barlow DH, Hayes SC, Nelson RO. *The scientist practitioner: research and accountability in clinical and educational settings.* New York: Pergamon, 1984.
106. Repp AC, Roberts DM, Slack DJ, Repp CF, Berkler MS. A comparison of frequency, interval, and time-sample methods of data collection. *J Appl Behav Anal* 1976; 9:501–508.
107. White OR, Haring NG. *Exceptional teaching: a multimedia training package.* Columbus, OH: Charles E Merrill, 1976.
108. Carr BS, Williams M. Analysis of therapeutic techniques through the use of the Standard Behavior Chart. *Phys Ther* 1982; 62:177–183.
109. Hughes CJ, Weimar WH, Sheth PN, Brubaker CE. Biomechanics of wheelchair propulsion as a function of seat position and user-to-chair interface. *Arch Phys Med Rehabil* 1992; 73:263–269.
110. Fife SE, Roxborough LA, Armstrong RW, Harris SR, Gregson JL, Field D. Development of a clinical measure of postural control for assessment of adaptive seating in children with neuromotor disabilities. *Phys Ther* 1991; 71:981–993.
111. McClenaghan BA, Thombs L, Milner M. Effects of seat-surface inclination on postural stability and function of the upper extremities of children with cerebral palsy. *Dev Med Child Neurol* 1992; 34:40–48.
112. Myhr U, von Wendt L. Improvement of functional sitting position for children with cerebral palsy. *Dev Med Child Neurol* 1991; 33: 246–256.
113. Deitz JC, Jaffe KM, Wolf LS, Massagli TL, Anson DK. Pediatric power wheelchairs: evaluation of function in the home and school environments. *Assist Technol* 1991; 3:24–31.
114. Bader DL, ed. *Pressure sores: clinical practice and scientific approach.* London: Macmillan, 1990.
115. Webster JG, ed. *Prevention of pressure sores.* Bristol, England: Adam Hilger Publishers, 1991.
116. Harris GF. A method for the display of balance platform center of pressure data. *J Biomech* 1982; 15:741–745.
117. Shumway-Cook A, Horak FB. Assessing the influence of sensory interaction on balance. *Phys Ther* 1986; 66:1548–1554.
118. Nashner LM. Adapting reflexes controlling the human posture. *Exp Brain Res* 1976; 26:59–72.
119. Winter DA. *Biomechanics and motor control of human movement,* 2nd ed. New York: Wiley, 1990.
120. Schmidt RA. Methodology for studying motor behavior. In: Schmidt RA, ed. *Motor control and learning.* 2nd ed. Champaign, IL: Human Kinetics Publishers, 1988; 45–73.
121. Bernstein N, Wilberg RB, Woltring HJ. The techniques of the study of movement. In: Whiting HTA, ed. *Human motor actions: Bernstein reassessed.* Amsterdam: Elsevier, 1984; 1–73.
122. University of Pittsburgh. *Health instruments file database.* Pittsburgh, PA: University of Pittsburgh, 1992.
123. Educational Testing Service. *Medical/health science bibliographies.* Princeton, NJ: Educational Testing Service, 1992.
124. Medical Device Register, Inc. *Medical device register: United States and Canada.* Stanford, CT: Medical Device Register, Inc., 1990.
125. Institute for Scientific Information, Inc. *Science citation index.* Philadelphia: Institute for Scientific Information, Inc., 1945–present.
126. Siu AL, Reuben DB, Moore AA. Comprehensive geriatrics assessment. In: Hazard WR, Bierman EL, Blass JP, Ettinger WH, Halter JB, eds. *Principles of geriatric medicine and gerontology,* 3rd ed. New York: McGraw-Hill, 1994; 203–211.
127. Dumitru D. *Electrodiagnostic medicine.* Philadelphia: Hanley & Belfus, 1995.
128. Delisa JA, Lee HJ, Baran EM, Lai K, Spielholz N. *Manual of nerve conduction velocity and somatosensory evoked potentials,* 3rd ed. New York: Raven, 1994.
129. Bruett BS, Overs RP. A critical review of 12 ADL scales. *Phys Ther* 1969; 49:857–862.
130. Law M, Letts L. A critical review of scales of activities of daily living. *Am J Occup Ther* 1989; 43:522–528.
131. Halpern AS, Fuhrer MJ, eds. *Functional assessment in rehabilitation.* Baltimore: Paul H Brookes, 1984.
132. Barer D, Nouri F. Measurement of activities of daily living. *Clin Rehabil* 1989; 3:179–187.
133. Jebsen RH, Taylor N, Trieschmann RB, Trotter MH. Measurement of time in a standardized test of patient mobility. *Arch Phys Med Rehabil* 1970; 51:170–175.
134. Shores M. Footprint analysis in gait documentation. *Phys Ther* 1980; 60:1163–1167.
135. Lerner-Frankiel MB, Vargas S, Brown M, Krusell L, Schoneberger W. Functional community ambulation: what are your criteria? *Clin Manage* 1986; 6:12–15.
136. Perry J. *Gait analysis: normal and pathological function.* Thorofare, NJ: Slack, 1992.
137. Eastlack ME, Arvidson J, Synder-Mackler L, Danoff JV, McGarvey CL. Interrater reliability of videotaped observational gait-analysis assessments. *Phys Ther* 1991; 71:465–472.
138. Krebs DE, Edelstein JE, Fishman S. Reliability of observational kinematic gait analysis. *Phys Ther* 1985; 65:1027–1033.
139. Rose SA, Ounpuu S, DeLuca PA. Strategies for the assessment of pediatric gait in the clinical setting. *Phys Ther* 1991; 71:961–980.
140. Winter DA. *The biomechanics and motor control of human gait.* Waterloo, Ontario: University of Waterloo Press, 1987.
141. Lister MJ, Currier DP. Clinical measurement. *Phys Ther* 1987; 67: 1829–1897.
142. Rothstein JM, ed. *Measurement in physical therapy.* New York: Churchill-Livingstone, 1985.
143. Johnston MV, Findley TW, DeLuca J, Katz RT. Research in physical medicine and rehabilitation. XII: measurement tools with application to brain injury. *Am J Phys Med Rehabil* 1991; 70(suppl):114–130.
144. McDowell I, Newell C. *Measuring health: a guide to rating scales and questionnaires,* 2nd ed. New York: Oxford University Press, 1996.
145. Spilker B, ed. *Quality of life assessments in clinical trials.* New York: Raven, 1990.
146. Conoley JC, Kramer JJ. *The mental measurements yearbook,* 10th ed. Vols. 1–2. Lincoln, NE: University of Nebraska, Buros Institute of Mental Measurements, 1989.
147. Amundsen LR, ed. *Muscle strength testing: instrumented and non-instrumented systems.* New York: Churchill-Livingstone, 1990.
148. Kellor M, Kondrasuk R, Iversen I, Frost J, Silberberg N, Hoglund M.

Technical manual: hand strength and dexterity tests. Minneapolis, MN: Sister Kenny Institute, 1977.

149. Tardieu C, Lacert P, Lombard M, Truscelli D, Tardieu G. H-reflex and recovery cycle in spastic and normal children: intra- and inter-individual and inter-group comparisons. *Arch Phys Med Rehabil* 1977; 58:561–567.
150. Frollo I, Kneppo P, Krizik M, Rosik V. Microprocessor-based instrument for Achilles tendon reflex measurements. *Med Biol Eng Comput* 1981; 19:695–700.
151. Lehmann JF, Price R, de Lateur BJ, Hinderer S, Traynor C. Spasticity: quantitative measurements as a basis for assessing effectiveness of therapeutic intervention. *Arch Phys Med Rehabil* 1989; 70:6–15.
152. Rodgers SH. *Ergonomic design for people at work.* Vols. 1 and 2. Rochester, NY: Eastman Kodak, 1983, 1986.
153. Ellexson M. Work hardening. In: Hertfelder S, Gwin C, eds. *Work in progress.* Rockville, MD: American Occupational Therapy Association, 1989.
154. Ogden-Niemeyer L, Jacobs K. *Work hardening: state of the art.* Thorofare, NJ: Slack, 1989.
155. Isernhagen SJ. *Work injury: management and prevention.* Rockville, MD: Aspen Publishers, 1988.
156. Asher IE. *An annotated index of occupational therapy evaluation tools.* Rockville, MD: American Occupational Therapy Association, Inc, 1989.
157. Wittmeyer M, Barrett JE. *Housing accessibility checklist.* Seattle, WA: University of Washington, Health Sciences Learning Resources Center, 1980.
158. Hemphill BJ, ed. *Mental health assessment in occupational therapy.* Thorofare, NJ: Black Publishers, 1988.
159. Hopkins HL, Smith HD. *Willard and Spackman's occupational therapy.* 8th ed. Philadelphia: JB Lippincott, 1993.
160. Haley SM, Coster WJ, Ludlow LH. Pediatric functional outcome measures. *Phys Med Rehabil Clin North Am* 1991; 2:689–723.
161. Gledhill N. Discussion: assessment of fitness. In: Bouchard C, Shephard RJ, Stephens T, Sutton JR, McPherson BD, eds. *Exercise, fitness, and health.* Champaign, IL: Human Kinetics Books, 1991; 121–126.
162. Skinner JS, Baldini FD, Gardner AW. Assessment of fitness. In: Bouchard C, Shephard RJ, Stephens T, Sutton JR, McPherson BD, eds. *Exercise, fitness, and health.* Champaign, IL: Human Kinetics Books, 1990; 109–119.
163. Edwards RHT. Human muscle function and fatigue. In: *Ciba Foundation symposium 82 on human muscle fatigue: physiological mechanisms.* London: Pitman Medical, 1981:1–18.
164. Hashimoto K, Kogi K, Grandjean E. *Methodology in human fatigue assessment.* London: Taylor & Francis, 1971.
165. Minor MAD, Minor SD. *Patient evaluation methods for the health professional.* Reston, VA: Reston, 1985.
166. Barry DT. Quantitative assessment of physical performance. In: Kottke FJ, Lehmann JF, eds. *Krusen's handbook of physical medicine and rehabilitation,* 4th ed, Philadelphia: WB Saunders, 1990:61–71.
167. Comrey AL, Backer TE, Glaser EM. *A sourcebook for mental health measures.* Los Angeles: Human Interaction Research Institute, 1973.
168. Lezak MD. *Neuropsychological assessment.* 3rd ed. New York: Oxford University Press, 1995.
169. Bellack AS, Hersen M. *Behavioral assessment: a practical handbook,* 3rd ed. New York: Pergamon, 1988.
170. Nicol AC. Measurement of joint motion. *Clin Rehabil* 1989; 3:1–9.
171. Norkin CC, White DJ. *Measurement of joint motion: a guide to goniometry,* 2nd ed. Philadelphia: FA Davis, 1995.
172. Batti MC, Bigos SJ, Fisher LD, et al. The role of spinal flexibility in back pain complaints within industry. *Spine* 1990; 15:768–773.
173. Burton, AK. Regional lumbar sagittal mobility: measurement by flexicurves. *Clin Biomech* 1986; 1:20–26.
174. Domjan L, Nemes T, Balint GP, Toth Z, Gomor B. A simple method for measuring lateral flexion of the dorsolumbar spine. *J Rheumatol* 1990; 17:663–665.
175. Hart DL, Rose SJ. Reliability of a noninvasive method for measuring the lumbar curve. *J Orthop Sports Phys Ther* 1986; 8:180–184.
176. Lovell FW, Rothstein JM, Personius WJ. Reliability of clinical measurements of lumbar lordosis taken with a flexible rule. *Phys Ther* 1989; 69:96–105.
177. Mellin GP. Physical therapy for chronic low back pain: correlations between spinal mobility and treatment outcome. *Scand J Rehabil Med* 1985; 17:163–166.
178. Mellin GP. Accuracy of measuring lateral flexion of the spine with a tape. *Clin Biomech* 1986; 1:85–89.
179. Merrit JL, McLean TJ, Erickson RP, Ojford KP. Measurement of trunk flexibility in normal subjects: reproducibility of three clinical methods. *Mayo Clin Proc* 1986; 61:192–197.
180. Rose MJ. The statistical analysis of the intra-observer repeatability of four clinical measurement techniques. *Physiotherapy* 1991; 77: 89–91.
181. Nation JE, Aram DM. *Diagnosis of speech and language disorders,* 2nd ed. Boston: College-Hill Publication, 1984.
182. Hutchinson B, Hanson M, Mechan M. *Diagnostic handbook of speech pathology.* Baltimore: Williams & Wilkins, 1979.

Rehabilitation Medicine: Principles and Practice, Third Edition,
edited by Joel A. DeLisa and Bruce M. Gans.
Lippincott–Raven Publishers, Philadelphia © 1998.

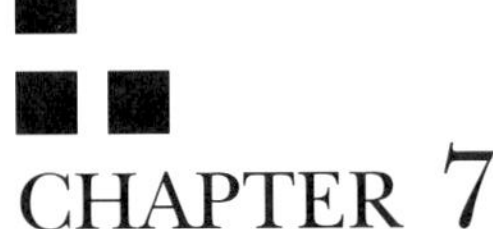

CHAPTER 7

Evaluation and Management of Daily Self-Care Requirements

Charles H. Christiansen and Kenneth J. Ottenbacher

SELF CARE: DEFINITION AND SIGNIFICANCE

Enabling the accomplishment of daily self-care tasks may be one of the most significant goals undertaken by the rehabilitation team. Although most self-care tasks are performed routinely by able-bodied persons, they can become extraordinary challenges for persons with cognitive, motor, or sensory impairments and disability. They often assume symbolic meaning for the individual in a rehabilitation program because independent eating, dressing, and toileting are milestones during the early stages of typical development, and because grooming and dressing are instrumental to the presentation of self so necessary for living in a social world (1).

Reference to self-care tasks typically refers to dressing, eating, bathing, grooming, use of the toilet, and mobility within the home. These are customary tasks included within the general rubric of activities of daily living (ADL). Other important activities in this general category are those that Lawton described as instrumental activities of daily living (IADL) (2). These include food preparation, laundry, housekeeping, shopping, the ability to use the telephone, use of transportation, medication use, and financial management. Child care also is an important responsibility in the daily routine of many people.

About 30% of a typical person's waking hours are spent performing self-maintenance activities, including basic self care and IADL (3). In fact, self care is such a critical part of everyday activity that the ability to perform self-care tasks is a critical factor in discharge decisions after rehabilitation. Research has shown that over 70% of the variance in discharge decisions after stroke rehabilitation is determined by the ability to function independently in the performance of self-care tasks necessary for bathing, toileting, social interaction, dressing, and eating (4).

Overall functional status encompasses physical, mental, emotional, and social dimensions of performance, and this is also true for self care. Meeting self-care needs is vital to success in adapting to the social environment because appropriate dress, personal appearance, hygiene, and other expectations influence perceptions of the self and others (5). Self-esteem, or the value accorded oneself, is determined by how well self-evaluation matches the values perceived as being important in the social environment (6). Self-esteem is influenced by social acceptance and through one's success in achieving a desired social identity (7). Because the ability to perform self-care tasks contributes to both acceptance and identity, it can have a direct effect on self-esteem. In fact, social factors have been shown to explain life satisfaction and perceived well-being to a greater extent than functional limitations for persons who must adjust to the consequences of aging (8), injury (9), or disease (10).

The importance of independence in self-care is obvious at a very young age. As a child becomes independent in self-care tasks, such as in using eating utensils, it is an indication that the child can participate in wider social arenas with the accompanying personal and social privileges of those situations. Once self-care skills are mastered and become part of the daily routine, however, their perceived importance diminishes and other social, educational, and vocational activities replace them in significance (11). Independence in daily living skills allows for freedom to perform the work and leisure tasks that become meaningful to the person. Nevertheless, the ability to accomplish these skills is a requirement for perceived success in most social environments.

Usually, self-care activities are taken for granted by the person and society unless successful performance is con-

C. H. Christiansen and K. J. Ottenbacher: School of Allied Health Sciences, University of Texas Medical Branch at Galveston, Galveston, Texas 77555-1028.

strained. Difficulty in performing self-care tasks and dependency on others for their completion can have a devastating effect on a person's psychological, social, and financial well-being. Depression, diminished self-confidence, and lack of motivation can result from the inability of the individual to perform these tasks, whereas successful performance can lead to increased self-concept (12–14).

A study of the self-concept of 71 persons who had spinal cord injuries showed that the subjects who believed they were as physically independent as possible had a more positive self-concept than did subjects who felt less independent than their capability (15). Another study of persons with spinal cord injury found that the perception of control over life decisions was strongly associated with feelings of well-being. These two studies indicate that an important goal of rehabilitation should be to help patients learn to take control of decisions about daily living because this may contribute positively to their sense of well-being (16).

FAMILY AND SOCIAL ISSUES INFLUENCING SELF CARE

Disability affects families. When a member of the family is no longer able to perform expected activities and roles, the daily routine may be upset, creating stress and conflict (17,18). The family must adjust their expectations of the member who is disabled as well as adjusting to changes in the total family dynamics.

Families are systems, and they have life cycles with stages and time periods, each with characteristic issues that affect family dynamics. Important issues related to self-care and caregiving needs must be considered in light of these stages, with recognition that needs will change over time (19). The most significant change affecting caregiving is the number of family members who are available to provide support as a family life cycle matures.

Necessary adjustments made by families or caretakers confronted with rehabilitation challenges often include a reassignment of homemaking tasks or changes in priorities and may impose additional financial or social burdens due to the need to hire outside assistance or rely on volunteers. Jones and Vetter found that the curtailment of the caretaker's social life as a result of the time needed to provide self-care assistance was more stressful than the actual tasks they performed (20). Their study and others (21,22) showed that levels of depression, anxiety, and somatic complaints are higher among caretakers and family members of disabled people living in the home environment than the general population.

A stable and supportive family unit can be of great assistance during the rehabilitation process, whereas families that are functioning poorly can impede rehabilitation (23,24). Poor outcomes can be traced to a lack of family involvement, whereas too much support can encourage dependency (25). The family should be involved in all aspects of rehabilitation, including evaluation and the setting of rehabilitation goals and treatment strategies before and after discharge.

A primary source of adjustment difficulties for people with physical disabilities comes from societal treatment of them as socially inferior. The common belief that strength, independence, and appearance are important aspects of self-worth is damaging to people with disabilities. Being included as a significant member of a social group often depends on the ability to perform at the group's expected level (26,27).

Kielhofner contends that society expects adults to be independent in self care, yet devalues self-care tasks because their accomplishment does not directly contribute a meaningful commodity to the societal group (28). Self-care tasks are not publicly valued in the same manner as gainful employment. Ironically, they assume importance principally when one's inability to perform them leads to a label of "handicapped." Bartels suggests that when a person is independent in living skills, society's view of what it means to be disabled is drastically changed (29). Independence in ADL helps to refute the idea that a person with a disability may be a financial or social burden to society. Bartels notes that a concept basic to the independent living philosophy is that a disability becomes a barrier to achievement only when it is perceived to be one by others or the environment makes it so.

SELF-CARE AND FUNCTIONAL PERFORMANCE

Traditionally, intervention for people who have difficulty performing self-care tasks has begun with training in the hospital or rehabilitation center environment. Typically, such intervention has started with instruction in procedures to regain dressing, grooming, hygiene, and eating skills (30). More recently, the use of adaptive devices and training in homemaking skills have been recognized as important goals. In pursuit of these goals, rehabilitation sessions have been conducted within the patient's hospital room or in simulated ADL settings within occupational therapy clinics so that compensatory strategies can be performed at home after discharge.

ADL training in a rehabilitation setting does not guarantee skill generalization to the discharge location (31). DiJoseph notes that patients may perform well in an occupational therapy clinic but that such learned adaptive behavior may not even transfer to the individual's bedside environment, much less the normal living setting (32). Environmental and psychosocial factors that directly influence task performance may be too varied between settings for the person receiving rehabilitation to generalize the learned skills. The individual may become dependent on the staff for self-care performance or lack the opportunity to perform new skills on a regular basis. Performance after discharge may reflect a lack of confidence or motivation.

COMMUNITY FOCUS

During the 1970s in the United States, the emphasis on the location of rehabilitation services was expanded to focus on the needs of the patient in the home and community. A concern for disabled persons' rights and abilities in the community became an issue, as reflected in legislation on education, housing, and vocational and medical needs, as well as in a more active consumer advocacy movement (33). Intervention in the community allowed the medical professions to reach more patients who might not be able to get to the hospital (34). Environmental factors began to be viewed as important in determining degrees of independence for people with disabilities (35). The focus of evaluation and treatment expanded to include the needs of individuals in their home, work, and community. Community skills such as banking, shopping, and going to restaurants began to be addressed by health-care professionals (36). In the United States, passage of the Americans with Disabilities Act has provided additional impetus toward recognition of full inclusion of persons with disability and the importance of eliminating barriers to access in communities (37).

Sometimes intervention in the home environment allows the rehabilitation team to confront each problem with greater insight and sensitivity, and problems can be solved more rapidly than in the hospital or rehabilitation facility setting (38). The environment can be evaluated in terms of architectural, transportation, and communication barriers and how these affect the individual's daily living skills. Colvin and Korn described a major city program in which architectural barriers were removed from the homes of people with disabilities (39). It was proposed that if these barriers were removed and the individual was provided with environmental control devices, greater benefit could be derived from home care programs and individuals would be able to participate more fully in self-care and home activities. The participants in this project contended that the environmental modifications made an improvement in their personal and family lives and that they felt safer and more independent.

In addition to expansion into the home and community, the use of high-technology assistive devices has greatly influenced the field of rehabilitation. These developments have the potential to assist the patient to gain environmental control for self care and vocational and recreational pursuits. With the aid of computers and environmental control devices, some patients who previously required institutional care now have the potential to live in community settings (40,41).

MANAGEMENT OF OPTIONS OF SELF-CARE TASKS

The patient's bill of rights adopted by the American Hospital Association in the 1970s set the stage for a management approach toward self care that fully informs and involves the individual receiving rehabilitation services. At the root of this document was the goal to provide information for patients with the objective of investing the patient in decision making and therefore increasing involvement with the process and satisfaction with outcomes (42). Building on this model, the approach to self-care deficits and independent living skills has broadened in the past decade, principally owing to the inclusion of patient participation criteria in accreditation standards (43,44), improved rehabilitation procedures and assistive technologies, increased attention to the rights of persons with disabilities, and increased emphasis on care of individuals in their environmental settings. Despite the broad appeal of this philosophy, the goals of intervention are determined too frequently without significant input from the person receiving care and his or her social support system. A study of the extent to which occupational therapists practicing in adult physical rehabilitation settings met 23 patient and family involvement criteria showed that although involvement occurred, much potential for collaborative planning was unrealized (45). An interesting study of housing decisions after discharge of persons recovering from stroke showed that in 86% of the cases, the affected family member was not included in the meetings of providers and family members in which discharge-related decisions were made (46).

When goals are set in collaboration with the individual receiving care, the motivation to learn and maintain a skill is better than if the goals are determined by rehabilitation professionals or caregivers. Burke notes that motivation comes from self-initiated and self-guided behavior (47). Each self-care behavior should be evaluated to see if the individual is motivated to learn and maintain it. In a study by Chiou and Burnett, stroke patients' views of the importance of self-care skills were compared with the views of their occupational therapists and physical therapists. The results showed that the patients and therapists viewed the importance of specific self-care items differently (48). This suggests that rehabilitation goals and procedures should be individualized, and assumptions about functional outcomes avoided.

Choice and perceived control over the environment are important to life satisfaction and general well-being (49). Decker and Schultz contend that an important aspect of occupational therapy should be to help improve the patient's perception of self-control over his or her physical and psychological environment. Their study of middle-aged persons with spinal cord injuries showed that subjects with a high level of life satisfaction tended to perceive themselves as in control of their lives. However, some research has shown that the degree to which perceived control results in positive psychological outcomes depends on the patient's personality, with those having an internal locus of control affected most adversely by perceived lack of control (50).

The role of the rehabilitation professional must change from one who dictates the treatment goals for the patient to one who can inform the patient about the rehabilitation options available to attain the desired degree of self-care functioning. The professional's role is to provide the necessary information to enable patients to make successful choices about their independence in self-care activities, because these relate to their total social and physical environment. Through a wide range of intervention options, the professional can be available to participate in the attainment of patients' individualized goals and can explain these options so that a choice about how to accomplish tasks at the desired degree of independence can be made.

One of the first options the professional and person receiving rehabilitation should explore concerning the performance of any self-care task is whether the task is necessary or desired. There may be self-care tasks that were performed premorbidly that the individual may no longer desire to perform. For example, a woman with hemiplegia who formerly rolled her hair on rollers on a daily basis may decide to have it cut in an easier-to-manage style rather than learn to use rollers with one hand. This type of decision should be based on individual preferences.

In some instances, training procedures can be used to regain a desired skill. After a cerebrovascular accident (CVA), for example, the therapist may be able to retrain the person to perform the task as it was performed premorbidly if there is sufficient return of voluntary movement. In some instances, the individual may no longer have the perceptual or physical capability to perform a task as before; however, he or she may be able to learn to accomplish the task using different movement patterns or with different body parts.

Environmental changes represent an additional array of intervention options that can be explored by the individual and his or her rehabilitation team as a means of gaining independence in self care. In some instances simply rearranging the physical environment may allow the disabled person to perform tasks independently. For example, moving dishes to lower shelves so that the patient can reach them from a wheelchair would represent a modification of the environment requiring only simple rearrangement. Structural changes in the physical environment also may be necessary. These can include major changes such as the architectural modification of rooms to accommodate wheelchair movement or less extensive improvements such as replacing round doorknobs with lever handles for a person who has weak grasp, or installing bathroom rails and grab bars for persons with unsteady gait or balance difficulties.

Bates and others (51,52) have recommended that physical space also be considered from the standpoint of its negotiability, which suggests that in addition to being accessible, the environment must support its successful use with adaptive aids in a manner acceptable to the individual. For example, it does not matter that the doors to a food vending area at a workplace are wide enough for a wheelchair if the machines themselves cannot be used by disabled persons.

Assistive technology can be used to aid in the satisfactory performance of a desired task. Adaptive equipment and devices can range from simple, inexpensive articles, such as bathtub seats, to the use of expensive equipment such as computers for environmental control and communication. Many labor-saving devices are now widely available in catalogs and retail outlets catering to the general population. A line of fashionable apparel designed for easy dressing and maintenance is now available for persons with disability. The rehabilitation professional's role is to inform the patient of the existence and cost of these devices and to train the individual and caregiver in their use and maintenance.

Finally, assistance from other people for the partial or total completion of a desired task is another option available to the individual receiving care. Assistance may come from spouses, friends, or paid personal care attendants. The role of the professional in this case must be to instruct the individual and/or their care attendant on optimal approaches to working together for the completion of identified self-care tasks.

Collectively, the personal and environmental intervention options described in this section form the basis for collaborative decision making and treatment planning. Neither diagnosis alone nor the extent of impairment can serve as an adequate basis for planning self-care intervention. Together, the rehabilitation team and the individual receiving care must determine those interventions that represent the most realistic and achievable goals based on the abilities, values, and social circumstances of the person. Only in this way will optimal results be achieved after discharge (Fig. 7-1).

ASSESSMENT OF SELF-CARE INDEPENDENCE

Functional assessment has been defined by Granger (53) as a method for describing abilities and limitations and to measure an individual's use of the variety of skills included in performing tasks necessary to daily living, leisure activities, vocational pursuits, social interactions, and other required behaviors. Assessment must take place within a conceptual framework, and the most often cited model for this purpose is that of the World Health Organization's International Classification for Impairment, Disability and Handicap (ICIDH) (54). Despite the controversy over use of the term "handicap," the ICIDH model provides a useful conceptual framework for assessing functional performance (55,56). Under this model, an impairment (such as loss of sensation) may or may not yield a deficit in the ability to perform tasks of living such as dressing or grooming (disability), which in turn may compromise role performance (such as being unable to function as a homemaker or worker outside the home) (57,58).

Assessment at any level has as its ultimate purpose the ability to make informed decisions. Scales and instruments designed to assess the ability of the individual to perform self-care tasks may assist in intervention or discharge planning by describing or documenting current abilities or monitoring changes in functional status. More global scales, which may include self-care components, are used to provide information on the effectiveness of rehabilitation programs, thus playing an important role in program evaluation.

Lawton has noted that formalized assessment of the pa-

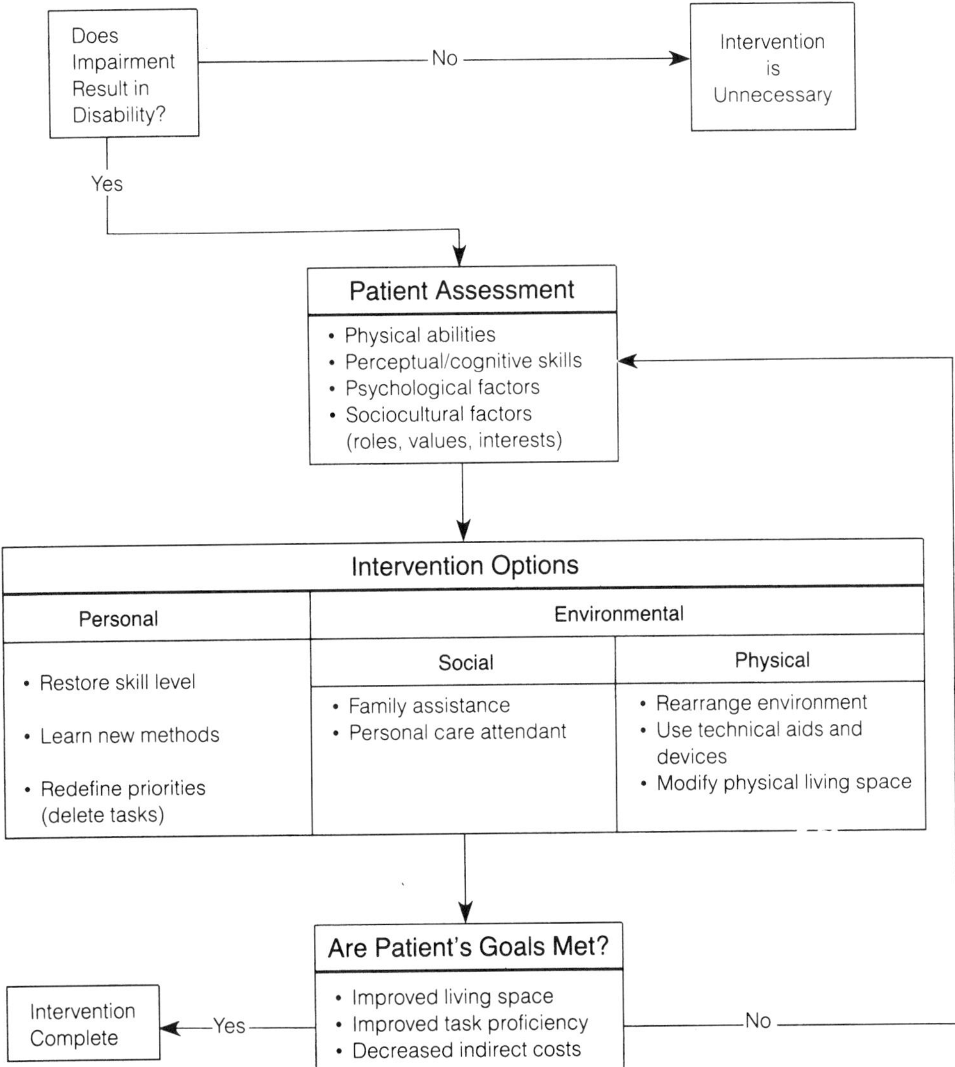

FIG. 7-1. Decision-making algorithm for self-care intervention.

tient's functioning yields a comprehensive picture of the strengths as well as the weaknesses of a patient and can provide objective evidence of clinical impressions (2). By providing a documented baseline of the individual's level of functioning, the formalized assessment facilitates communication with other members of the rehabilitation team.

Vash has suggested that because decisions made on the basis of assessment have the greatest ultimate impact on the individual receiving care, results of assessments should be shared with them (59). In this way, individuals receiving care enter into the decision-making process and become consultants. Such involvement in decision making is viewed as an important collaborative dimension of the rehabilitation process.

History and Development of Self-Care Assessment Tools

Assessment of the individual's ability to function independently has been conducted in medical rehabilitation for nearly 50 years. In an early review of the problems of measurement and evaluation in rehabilitation published in 1962, Kelman and Willner found that poorly conceptualized outcome criteria, lack of standardization, disagreement about methods, multidimensional scales, and the influence of the setting on performance were barriers to effective management (60).

Law and Letts reviewed several scales from the standpoint of clinical utility, scale construction, standardization, reliability, and validity (61). They concluded that the development of new scales should be curtailed, with greater effort devoted to the refinement and validation of existing scales. Currently, although there has been increased agreement about which abilities to measure, many of the problems noted above remain (62–65).

Capability versus Characteristic Behavior

It was noted earlier that function cannot be considered in isolation from its environmental context. This is made especially clear by the distinction between capability and actual behavior. Alexander and Fuhrer have noted this distinction as it pertains to measures of functional ability (66). Measures of capability represent what the patient can do, whereas measures of actual behavior indicate what the patient does do.

Most self-care assessments in use during the past 30 years have been designed to measure what the patient is capable of doing within the rehabilitation environment. An assessment of actual behavior, however, must take place in the daily living environment in which the person performs the tasks. This helps to explain why some studies have shown an apparent decline in patient function after discharge from the rehabilitation setting. Awareness of the distinction between capability and actual behavior and their relationship to the patient's environment has had an important impact on the development of new approaches to the assessment of self-care abilities.

Skills Versus Task Completion

A related issue is the need to distinguish between the measurement of isolated abilities and skills rather than task completion. In her paper on the concept of function, Unsworth noted that reviews of assessments have tended to emphasize technical issues such as reliability and validity rather than design and structural concerns related to the concept of function (67). She notes that some scales combine the measurement of tasks or activities with the measurement of skills and abilities, as though the two fit naturally together. Although there is no question that cognitive and motor skills are necessary for task performance, it has been shown that measurement at this level does not adequately predict task performance. Therefore, if measurement of function is to describe the extent of disability or social disadvantage, then measures of task performance are necessary for an appropriate representation of function in these classifications.

The Criterion Problem in Functional Outcome

Frey (68) and Keith (69) have noted that increased emphasis on accountability and the need for determining the benefit-cost ratios of rehabilitation have shown ambiguities within the definition of rehabilitation success. For example, gains in self-care ability, although important to the patient, may not be perceived as beneficial within a system that perceives employability as the sole criterion of success. This has created additional pressure for the development of assessment devices that consider postdischarge function.

Fortunately, the increased attention to these issues has resulted in increased research, which has encouraged the refinement or development and validation of several scales that assess self-care performance. Some of these scales possess characteristics suitable for program evaluation and research as well as clinical decision making. However, the need remains for greater awareness of the problems associated with functional assessment and the importance of using instruments that possess necessary measurement characteristics.

Standards

Influenced by the well-known standards developed by the American Psychological Association and the American Educational Research Association (70), the American Physical Therapy Association published measurement standards in 1991 (71). Similarly, the American Congress of Rehabilitation Medicine developed the Measurement Standards for Interdisciplinary Medical Rehabilitation in 1992 (72). Each of these standards provide important guidelines for the appropriate use and interpretation of measures, including self-care scales. They also provide definitions of important terms relevant to test development and refer to technical problems which should be avoided by developers and users. Although both practical and technical problems related to the assessment process have thus far precluded the development of an ideal self-care assessment tool, characteristics such an instrument should possess are described in the following section.

Desirable Attributes of Self-Care Assessment Scales

Standardization

To be standardized, a scale must have explicitly stated procedures for administration and scoring, as well as performance data from a normal population, preferably of varying ages; information on the measurement properties of the scale (e.g., its computed reliability); and a statement of the necessary qualifications of the examiner. Very few self-care scales now in use meet these guidelines for standardization. It probably is not possible to develop standardized scales that are useful both as measures of capability as well as of actual functioning because the environmental context so important to patient functioning will not be comparable in the administration across the different settings.

Scalability

Scaling procedures serve to quantify a person's responses to a defined set of tasks so that they are distributed along a continuum of performance. For an assessment device to be considered a true scale, it must be established that the tasks performed will cumulatively yield a score or descriptor that represents increasing capability or independence. A commonly reported index of scalability is Guttman's scalogram analysis (73).

Reliability

An acceptable scale should provide a reliable measure of the patient's level of performance. Reliability refers to a scale's consistency in providing information, regardless of the time, setting, or person performing the assessment. Scales that have carefully defined methods and scoring criteria are likely to be more sensitive and consistent and present a more accurate picture of the patient than those that do not.

Validity

A scale cannot be valid if it is not reliable. Validity is related to theoretical as well as methodological issues and therefore depends on a number of factors. These include the extent to which the scores on the assessment are related to some external criterion, the degree to which the instrument contains items or tasks that represent the domain of interest, and the relationship of the instrument to other measures that collectively support various theoretical assumptions. To the extent that observations of a scale's relationship with other measures and its corroboration with clinical expectations are demonstrated, the scale can be said to demonstrate evidence of validity. Kaufert notes that a number of factors make it difficult to establish the validity of functional ability indices. Specifically, he asserts that the impact of aids, adaptations, and helpers must be considered in measuring functional independence. Moreover, such factors as situational conditions, the patient's level of motivation, the professional perspective of the rater, and the role expectations of the patient can compromise efforts at establishing the validity of these scales. Because there is no standard index for indicating validity, the clinician and researcher should consider these factors in determining the overall merit of a particular scale.

Comprehensive

Self-care assessments are more useful if they determine performance levels for all basic ADL skills and are applicable to every diagnosis. Because patients have the universal need to perform or have performed for them basic self-care tasks, broad applicability is appropriate and facilitates comparison of research findings among differing patient groups. Including instrumental ADL measures makes a scale more useful as a measure of independence in postdischarge settings.

Performance Based

This characteristic eliminates measurement error due to selected observations or inaccurate memory, which can mitigate against scales that are based on patient interviews or reports of professional caregivers. Although self-care abilities have been assessed using scales that are self-administered and through interviews, the validity of such approaches is controversial (74). McGinnis and colleagues compared therapists' ratings with patients' self-reports on the Barthel Index and found that the self-report scores were significantly lower (75). Klein-Parris and colleagues found that interviews were more accurate when clients were high functioning and the items were less complex (76). Performance-based scales should not emphasize speed because speed is irrelevant if a patient cannot perform the task. Moreover, therapeutic intervention frequently is aimed at improving the quality of movement demonstrated by patients with central nervous system dysfunction. In these cases, performance often is improved if tasks are accomplished more slowly or deliberately (77). Time is an issue in performance, however, because it becomes impractical to perform some tasks independently if the amount of time required for completion is disproportionate to the value of the activity as perceived by the patient or significant other.

Practical

The extent to which a scale is designed to facilitate decision making and research is an important consideration in instrument selection. The number of items should be sufficient to permit reliability while requiring a reasonable length of time (i.e., 30 to 45 minutes) for administration. To the extent possible, items should not require equipment that would unduly limit locations where the scale could be administered. Scoring sheets should contain clear explanations of criteria and should be designed to permit accurate recording as well as coding for data processing. Terminology should be readily understandable, with abilities expressed using everyday language. Finally, the meaning of obtained scores should clearly convey a patient's level of functional independence to caregivers as well as to members of the patient's family.

Resolving Measurement Problems in Functional Assessment

A topic of considerable importance in the area of functional assessment is that of how numbers are assigned to performance observations and later interpreted. Most self-care scales use ordinal rankings to assign numbers to patient performance on selected items. Merbitz and colleagues have identified the limitations of such rankings, based on the characteristics of ordinal measurement scales (78). They point out that the properties of ordinal scales do not permit valid conclusions to be drawn on the summed or averaged scores obtained from them and that their misuse in this way is misleading and subject to invalid inferences. Furthermore, because they are given equal weight in scoring, the implied assumption of most scales of functional ability is that the items being measured are equally important, either to the professional or to the individual being measured. This is clearly an invalid assumption.

Using techniques developed by Rasch and others (79,80), however, observations of functional ability (from items and persons) can be translated into linear measures. The logit unit of measurement produced by the Rasch model is the natural log of the odds of a correct response. This transformation allows the researcher to interpret the person and item information using the same units of measure. Once the scores for the persons and items have been transformed using Rasch scaling, other information about the persons and items can be obtained using a variety of statistical methods. These transformed scales possess the properties necessary for valid inferences (81). In effect, these statistical transformations lead to scores that are corrected for differences in items or raters. Such techniques are increasingly being applied to existing scales (82,83).

Widely Used Self-Care Scales

Although dozens of instruments designed to assess self-care performance have been reported in the literature, consensus has not been achieved for use of a single scale. The past decade has shown a remarkable growth in the use of the Functional Independence Measure (FIM), largely due to a growing body of research demonstrating its validity, as well as the creation of a database (the Uniform Data System for Medical Rehabilitation [UDSMR]), which includes a large number of rehabilitation cases whose progress and outcomes have been documented using the FIM (84).

Besides the FIM, a handful of scales have demonstrated sufficient validity and frequency in the literature to warrant their review here. In the following paragraphs, we review the composition, measurement properties, and scoring of several scales and summarize the literature on their use with varying patient populations and evidence of validity. The scales to be reviewed in this section are the PULSES Profile (85), the Katz Index of Independence in ADL (86), the Barthel Index, and the FIM (87). These scales are reviewed here in the order of their development and appearance in the literature.

The PULSES Profile

The PULSES Profile, published by Moskowitz and McCann in 1957, has been described as the first major formalized functional assessment instrument to be widely used in U.S. medical rehabilitation settings (88,89). The instrument evolved out of a perceived need for a more structured approach to functional assessment and represented an adaptation of a military classification system used by U.S. and Canadian armed forces in the 1940s to classify the overall physical status of military personnel. PULSES is an acronym formed of initials representing the subsections comprising the overall instrument, which is of the global variety. These subsections are designed to measure: *P*hysical condition, performance using the *U*pper extremities, mobility as permitted by the *L*ower extremity function, communication and *S*ensory performance, bowel and bladder or *E*xcretory performance, and psychosocial *S*tatus.

Within each section, numerical grades ranging from 1 (i.e., no abnormalities) to 4 (i.e., severe abnormalities limiting independence) are assigned based on the patient's functional ability as assessed by an examining physician.

The original PULSES Profile had notable weaknesses, including a lack of specifically defined criteria and an underlying assumption that impairment equates with disability. The profile was modified by Granger and associates in 1975 to include a scoring system and improved rating criteria (90). Studies since that time have added to evidence of its utility in classifying independent status in a wide variety of patient samples (91–93). Research suggests that the PULSES Profile appears to be more useful in detecting change before discharge and is most effective in those situations in which substantial changes in functional status are likely to occur, such as in a patient with CVA or spinal cord injury.

The Katz Index of Independence in Activities of Daily Living

The Katz Index of Independence in ADL was developed to study results of treatment and prognosis in the elderly and chronically ill (94). Development of the index was based on observations of a large number of activities performed by a group of patients with fracture of the hip.

The index is based on an evaluation of the functional independence of patients in bathing, dressing, toileting, transfers, continence, and feeding. Using three descriptors for rating independence in each of six subscales, the rater is able to derive an overall grade of independence with the aid of specific rating criteria. Depending on the determined level of independence, a patient is graded as A, B, C, D, E, F, G, or other. According to the scale, a patient graded as A would be functioning independently in all six functions, whereas a patient graded as G would be dependent in all rated functions. Patients graded as "other" are dependent in at least two functions but not classifiable as C, D, E, or F. Through observations over a definite period of time, the observer determines whether the patient is assisted or whether the patient functions on his or her own when performing the six activities. Assistance is classified as active personal assistance, directive assistance, or supervision.

In studies of the Katz Index involving over 1,000 patients, the scale was found to result in an ordered pattern, so that a person able to perform a given activity independently also would be able to perform all activities performed by people graded at lower levels. This hierarchical structure correctly classifies the functional ability of patients 86% of the time and is the characteristic that makes this index a true Guttman scale.

The Katz Index of Independence in ADL has been used as a tool to accumulate information about recovery after CVA (95,96), the need for care among patients with rheumatoid arthritis, and as an instrument to study information about the dynamics of disability in the aging process. Brorsson and Asberg used the scale in a study of internal medicine patients in a general hospital in Sweden (97). Their study found a high degree of interrater reliability as well as high coefficients of scalability, which was interpreted as an index of its construct validity.

TABLE 7-1. *Barthel Index items and scoring weights*

	With help	Independent
1. Feeding (If food needs to be cut up = help)	5	10
2. Moving from wheelchair to bed and return (includes sitting up in bed)	5–10	15
3. Personal toilet (wash face, comb hair, shave, clean teeth)	0	5
4. Getting on and off toilet (handling clothes, wipe, flush)	5	10
5. Bathing self	0	5
6. Walking on level surface (or, if unable to walk, propel wheelchair)	10 0[a]	15 5[a]
7. Ascend and descend stairs	5	10
8. Dressing (includes tying shoes, fastening fasteners)	5	10
9. Controlling bowels	5	10
10. Controlling bladder	5	10

[a] Score only if unable to walk.

A patient scoring 100 BI is cotinent, feeds himself, dresses himself, gets up out of bed and chairs, bathes himself, walks at least a block, and can ascend and descend stairs. This does not mean that he is able to live alone; he may not be able to cook, keep house, and meet the public, but he able to get along without attendant care.

From Mahoney FI, Barthel DW. Functional evaluation: the Barthel index. *Maryland State Med* 1965; 14:61–65.

The Barthel Index

In 1965, Mahoney and Barthel published a weighted scale for measuring basic ADL with chronically disabled patients (Table 7-1) (98). Described as "a simple index of independence to score the ability of a patient with a neuromuscular or musculoskeletal disorder to care for himself," the Barthel Index included 10 items, including feeding, transfers, personal grooming and hygiene, bathing, toileting, walking, negotiating stairs, and controlling bowel and bladder. Items are scored differentially according to a weighted scoring system that assigns points based on independent or assisted performance. For example, a person who needs human assistance in eating would receive 5 points, whereas independence in eating would be awarded 10 points. A patient with a maximum score of 100 points is defined as continent, able to feed and dress himself or herself, walk at least a block, and climb and descend stairs. The authors were careful to note that a maximum score did not necessarily signify independence because instrumental ADL such as cooking, housekeeping, and socialization are not assessed. The stability (i.e., test-retest reliability) of the original Barthel Index has been reported by Granger and colleagues as 0.89, whereas interrater reliability coefficients were above 0.95.

The Barthel Index is one of the most widely studied of published self-care assessments. Several studies have shown that the scale is sensitive to change over time, that it is a significant predictor of rehabilitation outcome, and that it relates significantly with other measures of patient status.

For example, Wade and colleagues found that scores on the Barthel Index were positively correlated with functional status 6 months later in a sample of 83 patients with CVA. Similarly, the initial Barthel Index score was found to be the most reliable predictor of final rehabilitation outcome in a 31-month study of 41 stroke patients conducted by Hertanu and colleagues (99). That study concluded that the Barthel Index was a more reliable predictor of rehabilitation outcome than estimates based on computed tomography showing the extent of the lesion after CVA. The Barthel Index also has been found to correlate significantly with type of discharge and shorter length of stay for patients with CVA (100,101), as well as independent living outcome for patients with spinal cord injury (102).

In a study of 307 randomly selected severely disabled patients at 10 comprehensive medical rehabilitation centers, the Barthel Index and the PULSES Profile were used to determine functional changes over time. The investigators found that scores for the two instruments were highly correlated, with coefficients ranging from 0.74 to 0.80 for point of measurement and 0.61 to 0.74 for difference scores (90). A more recent study of patients with dysvascular amputations also has shown a correspondence between scores on the Barthel Index and the PULSES Profile (103).

There are at least five versions (including the original) of the Barthel Index that have been used in the literature, reflecting various modifications of levels (104,105), scoring (106), and sensitivity (107). Because of this, it is important for researchers to indicate the precise version when reporting studies involving use of the instrument.

The Functional Independence Measure

The FIM evolved from a Task Force of the American Congress of Rehabilitation Medicine and the American Academy of Physical Medicine and Rehabilitation, which met to develop a reliable and valid instrument that could be used to document the severity of disability as well as the outcomes of rehabilitation treatment as part of a uniform data system (108). The FIM consists of 18 items organized under six categories, including self care (e.g., eating, grooming, bathing, upper body dressing, lower body dressing, and toileting); sphincter control (i.e., bowel and bladder management); mobility (e.g., transfers for toilet, tub, or shower, as well as bed, chair, and wheelchair); locomotion (e.g., walking, wheelchair, and stairs); communication, including comprehension and expression; and social cognition (e.g., social interaction, problem solving, and memory). Using the FIM, patients are assessed on each item with a 7-point scale, ranging from complete independence (value = 7) to complete dependence (total assistance required = 1; Fig. 7-2).

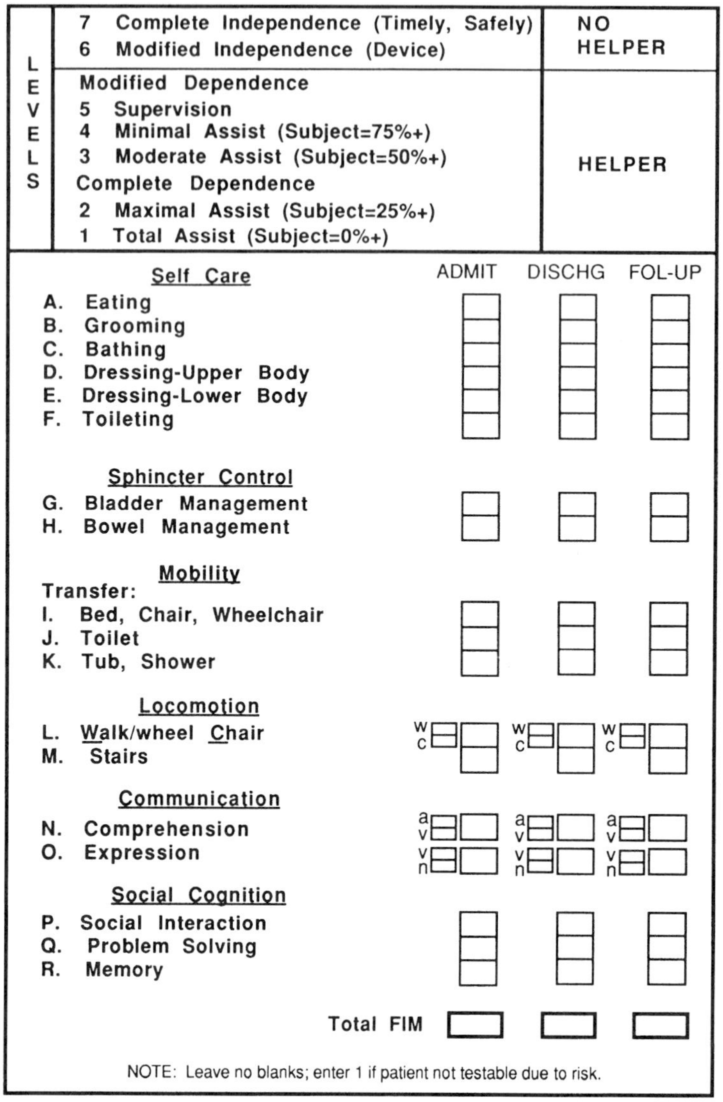

L E V E L S		
	7 Complete Independence (Timely, Safely) 6 Modified Independence (Device)	NO HELPER
	Modified Dependence 5 Supervision 4 Minimal Assist (Subject=75%+) 3 Moderate Assist (Subject=50%+) Complete Dependence 2 Maximal Assist (Subject=25%+) 1 Total Assist (Subject=0%+)	HELPER

	ADMIT	DISCHG	FOL-UP
Self Care			
A. Eating			
B. Grooming			
C. Bathing			
D. Dressing-Upper Body			
E. Dressing-Lower Body			
F. Toileting			
Sphincter Control			
G. Bladder Management			
H. Bowel Management			
Mobility			
Transfer:			
I. Bed, Chair, Wheelchair			
J. Toilet			
K. Tub, Shower			
Locomotion			
L. Walk/wheel Chair	w / c	w / c	w / c
M. Stairs			
Communication			
N. Comprehension	a / v	a / v	a / v
O. Expression	v / n	v / n	v / n
Social Cognition			
P. Social Interaction			
Q. Problem Solving			
R. Memory			
Total FIM			

NOTE: Leave no blanks; enter 1 if patient not testable due to risk.

FIG. 7-2. Functional Independence Measure. (Copyright 1990 by the Research Foundation of the State University of New York. Reprinted with permission.)

Since 1983, the FIM has been studied extensively, with pilot and trial studies designed to refine the instrument's items and determine reliability, validity, and precision. During trial studies using an earlier version of the scale, data were collected on 250 patients at 25 facilities throughout the United States. Nearly 900 assessments were performed at admission, discharge, and, where feasible, follow-up. Based on that study, interrater reliability for the FIM was estimated at 0.86 for assessments performed on admission to 0.88 on discharge. Studies with the current (i.e., revised) version of the scale (18 items and seven levels) have shown an interrater reliability of 0.95 for the total scale. The intraclass correlation coefficients (ICC) for individual elements were 0.96 motor, 0.96 cognitive, and 0.94 self care. Kappa coefficients ranged from 0.53 (memory) to 0.66 (stair climbing) (109). Other studies have confirmed satisfactory interrater reliability of the revised FIM (110–112).

In a study to determine the equivalence of the scales sections, Bunch and colleagues assessed the perceived importance of areas on the FIM as viewed by therapists and rehabilitation nurses in four of six sections (113). The study showed that communication skill was valued most, followed by continence, mobility, and self care. Despite these findings, differences between categories were not large enough statistically to compromise treating category scores as equal intervals.

Granger and colleagues found that the FIM, the Incapacity Status Scale, the Environmental Status Scale, and the modified Barthel Index had high intercorrelations with each other (114). The FIM was found to be the most useful in predicting the physical care needs of subjects with multiple sclerosis. In combination with the Brief Symptom Inventory and the Environmental Status Scale, the FIM contributed to predicting the patient's general satisfaction as well.

A comprehensive analysis of the FIM reported in 1990 found that the burden of care for a person with a disability is a two-dimensional concept, reflecting both motor and cognitive dimensions (115). Consequently, the FIM was found to have acceptable scalability only when broken down into two parts that treat the 13 motor and five cognitive items as separate subscales. Scaled measures derived from this treatment demonstrated statistically and clinically significant increases in motor and cognitive function from admission to discharge across all impairment groups studied. Regression analyses supported the predictive validity of the FIM, although the success in predicting outcome varied across impairment groups.

Muecke and colleagues studied the FIM as a predictor of rehabilitation outcome in lower limb amputees (116). The FIM did not predict outcome of lower functioning patients (bottom quartile) at admission, but predicted rehabilitation success well in higher functioning patients.

A large number of validity studies have been reported since the inception of the FIM, which have demonstrated that the scale has concurrent (117–122), predictive (123–125), and construct validity (126–129). These results also have been demonstrated with foreign versions of the scale (130–132).

Comparisons Among Self-Care Scales

A comparison of the self-care scales reviewed in this section shows that each focuses on basic ADL, each is based on professional observation and judgment, each derives an interpretable score that can be used in studies of prediction, and each has some evidence of reliability and predictive validity. Only the Katz Index of Independence in ADL and, to a lesser extent, the FIM derive scores that are readily interpretable in terms of the specific tasks a patient is able to perform independently. A graphic comparison of the important characteristics of each of these self-care scales is provided in Table 7-2.

Several studies have reported concurrent use of various combinations of the PULSES Profile, Barthel Index, and Katz Index of Independence in ADL. In general, the scales have correlated significantly with one another, providing evidence of their concurrent validity.

Unfortunately, most of these scales possess shortcomings that can be addressed only incompletely here. Their value

TABLE 7-2. *Self-care scale comparison*

PULSES (Moskowitz and McCann, 1957)	Katz Index of Independence in ADL (Katz et al., 1963)	Barthel Index (Mahoney and Barthel, 1965)	Functional Independence Measure (Hamilton et al., 1987)
Domain/tasks assessed			
Physical condition Upper extremity Lower extremity Sensory components Excretory (bowel and bladder) Status of patient (mental and physical)	Bathing Dressing Going to toilet Transfer Continence Feeding	Feeding Wheelchair transfer Grooming Toilet transfer Bathing Level walking Stairs Dressing Bowel control Bladder control	Self-care (feeding, grooming, bathing, upper and lower extremity dressing, toileting) Sphincter control Mobility Locomotion Communication Social cognition
Scoring			
Numerical 4-point scale. Range 0–24. Adapted version relates upper and lower extremity function to ADL tasks and mobility.	Ordinal ranking A–G based on descending levels of independence.	Adapted version is based on weighted numerical scale yielding mobility and self-care score. Range 0–100.	Items scored 1–7 from total assist to complete independence. Overall score derived from rating 18 items comprising total scale.
Reliability validity			
Reported coefficients: test-retest reliability = 0.87, interrater reliability = >0.95. Evidence of predictive and concurrent validity.	Coefficient of scalability = 0.89. Some evidence of predictive and concurrent validity.	Reported test-retest reliability = 0.89, interrater reliability = >0.95. Evidence of predictive and concurrent validity.	Interrater reliability of 0.95 (i.e., intraclass correlation of total FIM Scores has been reported on 18-item, 7-level version. Some evidence of concurrent and predictive validity has been reported.
Strengths/limitations			
Widely used among varying patient populations. Lacks subscore detail in discrete ADL variables.	Derived score yields specific information about patient's functional independence.	Comprehensive and widely used in U.S. Adapted versions permit distinction between levels of independence.	Using the Uniform Data System, several hundred facilities throughout North America have provided assessment data from versions of the FIM

ADL, acitivities of daily living; FIM, Functional Independence Measure.

as reliable assessment instruments hinges on careful adherence to rating criteria by informed raters, and they do not readily serve as precise guides to treatment planning. Moreover, in most scales, the scope of assessed functioning is limited to basic ADL, including mobility and communication, that collectively represent a limited, albeit important, portion of the overall domain of independent living tasks. Perhaps most importantly, the scales were designed to assess capability rather than actual performance in the discharge environment, thus limiting their relevance as tools for measuring rehabilitation outcomes.

Approaches to Comprehensive Functional Assessment

During the past two decades, much effort has been devoted to developing innovative systems for gathering and reporting the functional status of patients, both within and outside the rehabilitation facility. Four notable examples are described in this section: the Rehabilitation Indicators Project, the Patient Evaluation and Conference System (PECS), the Assessment of Motor and Process Skills (AMPS), and the Canadian Occupational Performance Measure (COPM).

Rehabilitation Indicators Project

Between 1974 and 1982, a federally funded project at New York University's Institute of Rehabilitation Medicine sought to develop instruments that would sensitively describe the impact of rehabilitation on client functioning and provide a detailed and systematic view of the benefits of rehabilitation. The instruments that were developed under the aegis of this project are collectively referred to as rehabilitation indicator (RI) instruments (133). The RI instruments have the common characteristic of generating moderately to highly detailed functional assessment data that provide descriptive profiles of client functioning. The instruments are designed so that detailed data can be collapsed into broad indicators for predictive and diagnostic purposes.

Compared with other measures of functional assessment, the RI instruments have the capability of providing detail for professionals desiring more exact pictures of the needs of clients, while also permitting information on a broader scale. The terminology used in the assessments incorporates lay language as much as possible to facilitate communication.

One of the strongest characteristics of the RI assessment tools is overall flexibility. By incorporating levels of measurement ranging from individual skills as reflected in skill indicators to activity clusters referred to as activity pattern indicators, the instruments can be used to serve a wide range of purposes, ranging from clinical management to outcome evaluation. Additionally, client data can be gathered in different ways, ranging from direct observation to self- or professional staff report. Because the instruments evolved from a model in which rehabilitation is viewed as a process dependent on the service system, the person receiving care, and the characteristics of the environment, their design reflects these factors and their inherent complexities.

The flexibility of the RI instruments, although increasing their use as tools for different purposes and settings, restricts attempts to determine their reliability under varying types of administration. This characteristic also precludes any attempt to standardize the various scales, especially the self-care items assessed through the activity pattern indicators. Despite these limitations, the authors believe that the practical benefits derived from having a flexible instrument are more important than the lack of comparability incurred through lack of standardization.

Patient Evaluation and Conference System (PECS)

The PECS was developed in 1979 for the purpose of structuring team conferences in clinical settings (134). The purposes of the system are to record the patient's progress and define treatment goals. The PECS is a broadly ranging instrument originally comprising 115 items divided into 16 different disciplinary sections. Each section is completed by the discipline that is primarily responsible for the specific aspect of the care. The 16 sections include medical, nursing, physical mobility, ADL, communication, medications, nutrition, assistive devices, psychology, neuropsychology, social issues, vocational and educational activity, therapeutic recreation, pain, pulmonary rehabilitation, and pastoral care.

A 7-point ordinal scale is used for most items, with 1 representing most dependent and 7 indicating full independence. The use of assistive devices to complete items lowers the score. The 7-point scale makes the instrument sensitive to minor changes in functional level. Factor analysis and Rasch analysis of the PECS has revealed four unidimensional interval scales underlying the PECS (135). These four subscales and the items comprising them are shown in Table 7-3.

The PECS has been used to predict the level of care needed after discharge from a treatment facility (134). The clinical validity also has been estimated by determining the relationships between the predictive value of a computed tomography scan and the PECS score (136). The results showed a high correlation. The interrater reliability for different sections of the PECS ranges from intraclass correlation coefficient (ICC) = 0.68 to 0.80 (137). Silverstein and colleagues have conducted factor analyses of the PECS to determine its underlying structure and relationship to existing constructs of disability (80). A computerized graphic profile has been developed based on this research and is used to display the client's progress and goals using the information in the PECS sections. This profile is designed to facilitate team conferences and can be used in research to predict which individuals will be most successful in reaching goals associated with independent function (138).

A factor analysis of the PECS performed at the Marianjoy Rehabilitation Center showed eight PECS factors that collec-

TABLE 7-3. *PECS items and subscales*

Impairment severity
Motor loss
Spasticity/involuntary movement
Joint limitations
Autonomic disturbance
Sensory deficiency
Associated medical problems
Postural deviations
Applied self-care
Performance of bowel program
Performance of urinary program
Performance of skin program
Responsibility for self-care
Performance in assigned interdisciplinary activities
Patient education
Resocialization
Safety awareness
Knowledge of medication
Motoric competence
Performance of transfers
Performance of ambulation
Performance of wheelchair mobility
Ability to handle environmental barriers
Performance of car transfers
Responsibility for mobility
Position changes
Endurance
Balance
Performance in feeding
Performance in hygiene/grooming
Performance in dressing
Mobility in the home environment
Bathroom transfers
Cognition
Impairment in short-term memory
Impairment in long-term memory
Impairment in verbal linguistic processes
Impairment in visual spatial processes
Impairment in basic intellectual skills
Orientation
Alertness/coma state
Ability to comprehend spoken language
Ability to produce spoken language
Ability to comprehend written language
Ability to produce written language
Perceptual and cognitive deficiency
Ability to problem-solve and utilize resources

Adapted from Kilgore KM, Fisher WP Jr, Silverstein B, Harley JP, Harvey RF. Application of Rasch analysis to the patient evaluation and conference system. *Phys Med Rehab Clin North Am* 1993; 4: 493–516.

tively accounted for 60% of the item variance. These factors were cognition, motor competence, applied self care, communication skills, impairment severity, assistive devices, social/recreational involvement, and family support. The motor competence factor was defined by physical mobility and ADL items (139). This and additional studies, including Rasch analysis, suggest that the PECS has the potential for reliable and valid measurement; however, concern remains about adding individual item scores to obtain a global functional performance score (139).

Assessment of Motor and Process Skills (AMPS)

The Assessment of Motor and Process Skills is an observational evaluation that is used to simultaneously examine both the ability to perform IADL and the underlying motor and process capacities necessary for successful performance (140). The AMPS is an assessment system that requires a clinician to observe a person performing IADL as he or she would normally perform them. The individual to be measured selects two or three familiar tasks from among more than 50 possibilities described in the AMPS manual. These include such options as sweeping the floor, folding laundry, making a bed, washing clothes, potting a plant, or ironing clothes. After the observation, the clinician rates the person's performance in two skill areas: IADL motor and IADL process. The motor and process areas are listed in Table 7-4. Motor skills are observable actions that are thought to be related to underlying abilities, including postural control, mobility, coordination, and strength. The AMPS motor items represent an observable taxonomy of actions used to move the body and objects during actual performance. Process skills reflect the organization and execution of a series of actions over time in order to complete a specified task. Thus, process skills are thought to be related to a person's underlying attentional, conceptual, organizational, and adaptive capabilities. Like the AMPS motor skill items, the AMPS pro-

TABLE 7-4. *AMPS motor and process skill items by group*

Motor skill groups and items	Process skill groups and items
Posture	Using knowledge
Stabilizes	Chooses
Aligns	Uses
Positions	Handles
Mobility	Heeds
Walks	Inquires
Reaches	Notices
Bends	Temporal organization
Coordination	Initiates
Coordinates	Continues
Manipulates	Sequences
Flows	Terminates
Strength and effort	Space and objects
Moves	Searches
Transports	Gathers
Lifts	Organizes
Calibrates	Restores
Grips	Adaptation
Energy	Accommodates
Endures	Adjusts
Paces	Navigates
	Benefits
	Energy
	Paces
	Attends

Adapted from Fisher WP, Fisher AG. Applications of Rasch analysis to studies in occupational therapy. *Phys Med Rehab Clin North Am* 1993; 4:493–516.

cess skill items represent a universal taxonomy of actions that can be observed during any task performance.

During each IADL task performed for the assessment, and for each of the 16 motor and 20 process skills (Table 7-4), the person is rated on a 4-point scale: 1 = deficit, 2 = ineffective, 3 = questionable, and 4 = competent. The raw ordinal scores are analyzed using many-faceted Rasch analysis. This approach rests on a mathematical model of likelihood that the person will receive a given score on each of the motor and process skill items. The observed counts of the raw scores of IADL motor and process skill items constitute ordinal (ranked) data. These counts are converted by logistic transformation into additive, linear measures. Once the raw scores are computer analyzed, the derived person ability measures (motor and process) become estimates of the person's position on the two AMPS scales. That is, the AMPS motor and process scales represent continua of increasing IADL motor or process skill ability, and the person's estimated position on the AMPS motor and process scales, expressed in logits, represents his or her IADL motor and process skill ability (141).

The many-faceted Rasch analysis used in the AMPS allows simultaneous calibration of three aspects of performance: item easiness, task simplicity, and rater leniency. Each of these item characteristics is determined by using a probabilistic model. The ability measure produced by the Rasch analysis is the estimated person ability plotted on a linear scale and is defined by a skill's item easiness and task simplicity but adjusted for the rater who scored the task performance (80).

Because the person ability measures on the AMPS are adjusted for task simplicity, a clinician can use the ability measure to predict whether a person possesses the motor and process skills necessary to perform tasks that are more difficult than those the person was observed performing. Also, because the AMPS includes a large number of possible IADL tasks (n = 50) and each person is observed performing only two or three, the number of possible alternative task combinations is large. Regardless of how many different tasks the individual performs, however, the ability measure will always be adjusted to account for the easiness and simplicity of those particular tasks, so direct comparisons can be made among persons even though they performed completely different tasks.

Fisher and colleagues have conducted a series of investigations using the AMPS with persons who have psychiatric, orthopedic, neurologic, cognitive, and developmental disabilities (141–144). Studies also have been conducted using the AMPS with older adults living in the community (134). These investigations have established the preliminary reliability and validity of the AMPS. The AMPS is a new instrument and approaches the assessment of functional performance in a nontraditional manner, that is, using many-faceted Rasch analysis. This approach has advantages, but it also has disadvantages. The logic of the Rasch approach is not familiar to many rehabilitation providers, and the mathematical modeling used to the develop the scoring system is complex. For these reasons, its widespread use may be impractical. However, the AMPS and other Rasch-based instruments are alternatives to traditional assessment approaches and represent an important new dimension in the evolution of functional assessment.

Canadian Occupational Performance Measurement

The COPM is a criterion measure developed in consultation with the Department of National Health and Welfare and the Canadian Association of Occupational Therapists (145–147). The COPM reflects a client-centered practice philosophy of measurement and incorporates roles and role expectations within the client's own environment. The descriptor "client-centered" means that the assessment incorporates roles and role expectations from within the client's living environment using a semi-structured, individualized interview approach (148).

The COPM encompasses the areas of self-care, productivity and leisure as the primary outcomes being measured but can also include an assessment of performance components in order to gain an understanding of why the client may be having difficulty in a particular functional area. The COPM was designed to help therapists establish functional performance goals based on client perceptions of need and to measure change objectively in defined problem areas.

The COPM measures the client's identified problem areas in daily functioning. In those instances where a client is unable to identify problem areas (e.g., a young child, an individual with dementia) a caregiver may respond to the measure. The COPM considers the importance, to the person, of the occupational performance areas as well as the client's satisfaction with present performance. The instrument takes into account client roles and role expectations and, in focusing on the client's own environments and priorities, ensures the relevance of identified areas in the assessment process.

The COPM can be used to measure a client outcome with different objectives for treatment, whether it is developmental, maintenance, restoration of function, or prevention of future disability. Because it is generic (not diagnosis specific) and can be used across different age groups, it has wide applicability. The instrument is administered in a five-step process using a semi-structured interview conducted by the therapist together with the client and/or caregiver. The five steps in the process include problem identification/definition, initial assessment, occupational therapy intervention, reassessment and calculation of change scores. The original version included a procedure whereby rated importance was used as a weighting factor in calculating performance and satisfaction scores. However, this has been eliminated in the second edition based on findings from pilot studies that indicated the equivalence of scores, whether or not importance weights are included (145).

First, problems are defined jointly with the client and appropriate caregivers. Then the client is asked to rate the importance of each activity on a scale of 1 to 10. The client (or caregiver) is also required to rate his or her ability to perform the specified activities and his or her satisfaction with performance on the same scale of 1 to 10. These scores are then compared across time. There are two scores: one for performance and one for satisfaction. Administration time averages about 30 to 40 minutes.

The authors reported findings on an extensive pilot study of the COPM that involved administration of the instrument to 256 clients in many facilities across Canada and in other countries, including New Zealand, Greece, and Great Britain (148). Data gathered during this multi-phase study included feedback from therapists and clients about the clinical utility of the COPM, data on the sensitivity of the instrument to change, and descriptive statistics on identified problems and client scores. The findings indicated that the average change scores for performance and satisfaction were approximately 1.5 times the standard deviation of the scores, indicating sensitivity of the instrument to perceived changes in occupational performance by clients. Comments by therapists involved in the pilot studies were generally favorable regarding the clinical utility of the measure. Because the assessment involves an interview with clients who are often unaccustomed to participating in the identification of their own problems, some awkwardness with administration has been reported by therapists during their initial attempts at administration. Also, due to its reliance on client participation in the assessment process, it is viewed as unsuitable for use with clients having significant cognitive impairment. The perceived clinical utility of the COPM relates to its flexibility, the use of client-centered approaches in practice, and support by administrators who value the philosophy underlying the instrument (149).

Research continues on the COPM, with particular attention to its validity as a bona fide measure of real changes in occupational performance. Although it is a new instrument, the COPM has the potential to provide useful and important information regarding self-care performance. One unique feature of the COPM is the quantitative emphasis on client satisfaction.

Important Factors in Informal Assessment

The above sections provide a historical and conceptual review of structured approaches to measuring functional independence in self care. However, a complete analysis of patient assessment in this area must address other factors that may have an important relationship to the degree of functional independence achieved after rehabilitation. These factors have not been included in traditional assessment instruments and, with few exceptions, may be given insufficient attention in a consideration of the patient's rehabilitation program. These factors include the patient's ability to manage devices that extend independence through environmental control; the family resources available to the patient in the environment to which he or she is to be discharged; the amount of time or energy required to perform tasks independently; and the degree of safety with which patients are able to perform tasks.

Developments in high technology for independent living have made it possible and important to assess people with severe disability in terms of their available movements and physical resources for controlling switches to activate environmental control units. Paradoxically, these devices are more likely to extend the patient's ability to perform instrumental ADL more proficiently than self-care tasks.

The inability to perform self-care tasks independently, of course, does not dictate discharge to institutional care if human resources are available in an alternative environment. Frequently the patient can rely extensively on the assistance of the spouse, other family members, or friends to assist with self-care tasks. It can be argued that the presence of these resources, although commonly determined by the social worker in planning discharge, should be given early consideration in planning rehabilitation intervention.

Additional considerations include the amount of time and energy required to perform the task independently versus the value of the task as perceived by the patient. It cannot be assumed, given competing requirements for time and energy, that all patients assign the independent performance of all self-care tasks the same degree of importance. Thus, the motivation to complete the task independently after discharge is likely to be a function of the alternatives available for task completion, the importance of the task to the patient, and the amount of time and energy required to perform the task independently in the face of competing demands.

Weingarden and Martin reported a study of 10 postdischarge spinal cord–injured patients to determine if time was a factor in the decision to retain, modify, or completely delegate dressing activities (150). Although all 10 patients were capable of dressing independently at home, none did so routinely. The authors concluded that the person's concept of appropriate time and energy expenditure are important considerations in postdischarge decisions on the use of functional skills.

The degree of safety with which a task is performed may be of more obvious importance to the practitioner than to the patient or those caregivers in the environment who may be providing assistance with self-care tasks. It is therefore important that training in self-care assistance be provided as a part of the rehabilitation effort and that the ability of helpers to render this assistance in a safe and effective manner be assessed before the patient is discharged.

Significance to the Patient as a Consideration in Assessment

No discussion of self-care assessment is complete without a consideration of the values that may be reflected in the process. Although assessment is a judgmental process, it should not be unnecessarily value laden. In fact, the rehabilitation goal of independent functioning itself reflects a societal value not shared to the same extent by all cultures. Patients with profound differences in cultural heritages and life experiences may bring differing sets of values about independence and self care to the rehabilitation setting. Effective management of the patient requires an appreciation of these differences and an appreciation that interdependence may be more typical than independence. It may therefore be important for assessment to include methods for determining premorbid activity patterns and leisure interests as well as values and attitudes toward assistance. Characteristic methods for performing basic and instrumental ADL and characteristic aspects of the environment in which these have been performed may be important information in planning successful intervention strategies for management of self-care and other ADL.

Self-Care Assessment in Children: Special Considerations

Information presented to this point has been based on self-care assessment as it pertains to adults. Self-care assessment of the pediatric patient requires a number of special considerations. These pertain to incorporating developmental milestones into the structure of the assessment, interacting with the child during the assessment process, and reporting information to parents. Although little has been published in this area, the reader is referred to work accomplished at the Children's Hospital at Stanford University for more specific information (151).

Functional Independence Measure for Children

In 1987, the FIM was adapted to meet the need for a reliable and valid functional assessment tool that would be useful in measuring the severity of disability in children. The resulting Functional Independence Measure for Children (WeeFIM) (152) was designed to measure functional ability in a developmental context. Each of the 18 items is considered in relation to chronologic age, developmental norms, and realistic expectations for children from 6 months to 7 years of age. Rather than replacing assessment tools that analyze individual component skills of ADL, the WeeFIM is meant to give clinicians an overall view of the child's actual daily performance in six areas, including self care, mobility, locomotion, sphincter control, communication, and social cognition. The WeeFIM uses the same 7-point ordinal scale to assess level of function as does its parent, the FIM.

Studies of the WeeFIM have shown a strong correlation between the scale and age. Increased variability in scoring was noted for children above 4 years of age, with the most variability occurring in the locomotion category. Data showed that tasks on the WeeFIM demonstrate a developmental sequence, with an observed positive relationship between the complexity of tasks and the age at which children achieve independence in their performance (153). Additional studies have shown that the WeeFIM demonstrates acceptable reliability (154) and validity in tracking the impact of developmental disability in children of preschool and middle childhood (155,156), and in documenting the outcomes of rehabilitation in children after intervention for primary brain tumors (157), and after traumatic brain injury (158).

Pediatric Evaluation of Disability Inventory

The Pediatric Evaluation of Disability Inventory (PEDI) was developed to provide functional assessment of children 6 months to 7.5 years of age (159,160). The instrument is designed to assess functional status and change along three dimensions: functional skill level, caregiver assistance, and modifications of adaptive equipment used. It has 197 functional skill items and 20 complex functional items for which caregiver assistance and modification are assessed across three content domains, including self care, mobility, and social function. An overview of the content is provided in Table 7-5.

The scale is intended to be used as a discriminative device to identify functional deficits as well as an evaluative instrument to monitor progress in rehabilitation programs. The PEDI has been standardized on a normative regional (New England) sample of 412 nondisabled children.

Several reliability and validity studies have been conducted since the scale's inception. Feldman and colleagues found evidence of concurrent validity between the PEDI and the Batelle Developmental Inventory Screening Test (161). The scale has been used successfully in studies to document outcomes after interventions for cerebral palsy (dorsal rhizotomy) (162,163) and traumatic brain injury (164).

MANAGEMENT OF SELF-CARE SKILLS

The assessment process characterizes the strengths and weaknesses of each patient in relation to self-care skills. The management process uses this description to develop options that will enable the patient to become more independent in self-care activities. Experience has shown that patients offered a number of options become active and responsible participants in their own rehabilitation. Medical management of self care can be viewed as an information management process. The practitioner attempts to develop a comprehensive listing of training methods, devices, environmental modifications, and human resources. From these a subset is selected to maximize patient functioning within the constraints of limited time, money, and patient potential for improvement. Most, if not all, of such options fall into one of three goal categories: to improve living space, to minimize indirect costs of self-care independence, and to decrease the time or energy required to perform self-care tasks. A study of self care and aging by Norburn and associates (165) identified three types of self-care coping strategies. These were use of equipment or devices, changes in behavior, and modi-

TABLE 7-5. *Content of the Pediatric Evaluation of Disability Inventory*

	Self-care domain	Mobility domain	Social function domain
Function skills scales	Types of food textures Use of utensils Use of drinking containers Toothbrushing Hairbrushing Nose care Handwashing Washing body and face Pullover/front-opening garments Fasteners Pants Shoes/socks Toileting tasks Management of bladder Management of bowel	Toilet transfers Chair/wheelchair transfers Car transfers Bed mobility/transfers Tub transfers Method of indoor locomotion Distance/speed indoors Pulls/carries objects Method of outdoor locomotion Distance/speed outdoors Outdoor surfaces Upstairs Downstairs	Comprehension of word meanings Comprehension of sentence complexity Functional use of expressive communication Complexity of expressive communication Problem resolution Social interactive play Peer interactions Self-information Time orientation Household chores Self-protection Community function
Complex activities assessed with caregiver assistance and modifications scales	Eating Grooming Bathing Dressing upper body Dressing lower body Toileting Bladder management Bowel management	Chair/toilet transfers Car transfers Bed mobility/transfers Tub transfers Indoor locomotion Outdoor locomotion Stairs	Functional comprehension Functional expression Joint problem solving Peer play Safety

fications of environment. The study also found that receiving assistance may supplement self-care coping strategies.

Improve Living Space

People with disabilities usually want the same freedom they enjoyed before their illness or accident. They wish to select their own living conditions and companions. Rehabilitation professionals should respect the choices of patients and recognize their needs rather than to opt for safe, secure, inexpensive, or convenient options when discharge is being considered. The growth of the independent living movement among the disabled in the United States has been described by De Jong (166) and Neistadt and Marques (167). Self-care training must be structured toward maximizing the potential of patients to live where they choose and with whom they choose. Neistadt and Marques (145) described a program in which independent living skills are taught in addition to traditional self-care skills to institutionalized mentally handicapped adults. They suggest that such programs should not focus narrowly on the patient's strengths and weaknesses but should focus on a larger community in which the patient desires to live. Adaptive community skills such as banking, budgeting, consumer advocacy, personal health care, and attendant management are important training areas often neglected by traditional therapy programs. In addition to conceptualizing self-care goals in the context of community, Levine urges therapists to "enter the patient's world" and to "adapt treatment to suit the patient's needs" (168). Cultural and ethnic considerations of life-style should provide a framework in which the patient defines preferences and needs.

Minimize Indirect Costs

Physicians and therapists who rely on hospital billing departments and social workers to handle financial arrangements may not be aware of economic constraints on a patient. All too often the self-care options presented to a patient are based on the availability of equipment and not on the ability of the patient to afford such items. To plan self-care remediation strategies realistically, there must be some attempt to gather data on available resources and to use these to determine which options are feasible for the patient. The philosophy that should guide selection should be the least expensive and simplest to effect the largest conservation of resources with the least modification/adaptation of performance or tools that still can permit independent self care.

Decrease Time Required for Performance

Time is precious. It is perhaps the most neglected of resources for the physically disabled. Rehabilitation professionals may train patients to perform self-care tasks without considering whether it is worth the patient's time to do so. Few people would spend 20 minutes each morning just to put on their shoes and socks, yet patients may be asked to consider this despite its obvious temporal demand. The conservation of time should be a goal of all self-care training. As Shillam and associates reported in their study of the role of occupational therapy in bathing independence for the disabled, decreasing the time it takes to perform routine self-care is important not only to the patient but also to family members and other caregivers (169).

Frank has written that,

> "In medicine and in the allied health fields such as occupational therapy, despite the probabilities that might bear on a given case, the goal of rehabilitation is to achieve a result that is actual, against an indeterminate field of possibility" (170).

In our experience, results do not emerge from a field of indeterminate possibility but rather from defined listings of options that have been considered with respect to given self-care goals as well as with respect to living space, costs, and the time required for performance.

AN OVERVIEW OF INTERVENTION APPROACHES

The context of self-care rehabilitation is one in which options are tailored to the economic, social, and time requirements of the patient. These options can include a variety of training approaches, assistive technologies, environmental modifications, or personal attendants.

Training

Self-care rehabilitation is a learning process by which patients must adapt to the effects of illness, accident, or birth defect because they affect the demands of everyday life. The initial acquisition of skills by those who are developmentally or congenitally disabled is a markedly different learning process from the reacquisition of self-care skills by those who have been independent at such tasks before becoming disabled. When the goals of training are to develop skills in a person with a congenital condition, the training process is termed habilitation. When the therapist seeks to restore normal function for a person with an acquired disability, the training process is called restorative. In those instances in which there is either a poor prognosis for development of self-care skills or the patient has failed to benefit from habilitation or restorative training, the approach is known as compensatory training.

Developmental or Habilitation Training

Practice is an important aspect of all motor training (171). Mere repetition of activity is not therapeutic training. The rehabilitation provider or other self-care trainer must provide task structuring, strategic prompts, and suggestions for improvement of performance. The patient or learner must learn to monitor and correct performance errors. Over time, desirable behaviors must be systematically rewarded and undesirable behaviors ignored or extinguished (172).

Children normally learn self-care tasks over extended periods of time. Most often, operant conditioning is provided in which successive approximations toward each goal (e.g., feeding, bowel and bladder control, grooming, dressing, bathing) are rewarded. Four stages of learning are described by Snell, including acquisition, maintenance, fluency, and generalization (173). This incremental learning process, moving from initial instruction to mastery with graded assistance, is often termed scaffolding. Practice usually occurs only at the time or times each day that a task is appropriate. Learners are encouraged to do what they can to help—sometimes starting a task that the therapist will need to finish and sometimes completing a task that the therapist initiates.

During the initial or acquisition stages of instruction, therapists can promote generalization and mastery by teaching under natural conditions, using real equipment rather than simulated tools, involving multiple teaching conditions (locations, instructors, materials), and selecting the instructional examples carefully, with attention to those that best sample the range of variation likely to be encountered in task performance (174,175).

Trombly has reported that there is a demonstrated sequence of self-care independence that is supported by child development and anthropologic observations (176). Feeding, grooming, continence, transfers, undressing, dressing, and bathing usually occur in order. Even such limited information as this may be useful in habilitation training. Using a distributed practice schedule (i.e., teaching self-care activities only during those times they would normally be performed) is critical for the person unfamiliar with the concept of the task. Part of self-care training is learning the appropriate times and natural sequences of daily activities. The patient who is relearning a task often retains an appreciation of when it is to be performed, but the patient being habilitated needs to learn not only the skills but also the context appropriate to each task. Jarman and colleagues have demonstrated that this approach can be effective in training multiply handicapped children to perform their morning care routines (177). Walker and Vogelsburg similarly demonstrated the effectiveness of structured practice with a nonambulatory, severely handicapped woman who was taught to be mobility independent (178). Habilitation in self care not only teaches specific tasks but also fosters the attitudes and values that sustain motivation to do these tasks independently. The assumption that all patients should be trained to perform similar tasks using the same practice schedules, reinforcement schedules, and task structuring is one that should be challenged (179). Learning and relearning may be related phenomena, but they are different. Failure to appreciate this may lead to inappropriate selection of activities for self-care training.

Restorative Training

The literature on stroke rehabilitation shows that gains in organ/physiologic (impairment) skills do not automatically result in improved functional performance (180,181). The results of several studies in which correlations between motor impairment and ADL were aggregated have been reported by Trombly (182). Her findings indicate that the amount of variance in ADL accounted for by motor impairment was 31%. The majority (approximately 69%) of the variance associated with ADL performance was derived from other factors.

For the patient with an acquired disability, relearning self-care independence is a distinctly different process than for the habilitation patient. First, there is a loss of self-esteem and sense of failure and frustration when one is unable to perform those tasks that often are taken for granted by the persons without disability. Initial learning usually is motivated by intrinsic rewards of increased competency at self-care tasks (183), as well as by the positive social reinforcement of parents and other caregivers. In learning a task, negative reinforcement (i.e., avoiding unpleasant experiences or consequences), such as avoiding embarrassment over having to ask for assistance for feeding or toileting, may be far more effective than positive social reinforcement. The therapist who tries to use social praise to reinforce practice of toileting skills will find that it is not effective. In fact, it probably will be viewed as demeaning to praise an adult in a situation reminiscent of a childhood experience.

For the person who has not been previously adept at self-care, the context and timing of practice are more important than for the adult seeking to regain skills. Simulation may be effective as a training method, using partial-task practice on just those components of activity that are deficient. This may be a better choice than whole-task distributed practice. Using partial-task training and moderately massed practice, skill components can be retrained. In restoration of skills, a patient may make considerable contributions to the therapy process based on his or her previous knowledge and understanding of how the task was performed.

Such patients can monitor their own errors and often use appropriate strategies to minimize deficits. In this case the treatment session is used to develop a practice strategy, and the patient practices self care at each opportunity whether or not the therapist is present. Problems occurring between treatments are discussed, and possible solutions can be practiced during the next treatment session.

There is one category of patient that clearly does not benefit from this approach. This category includes patients with closed head injury or CVA who also have significant cognitive or perceptual deficits. As Bjornby and Reinvang have pointed out, such conditions as apraxia may significantly influence the effects of self-care training and may need to be remediated before or in conjunction with remediation of self-care dependency (184). For such patients and those for whom other approaches have failed to produce results, compensatory training should be considered.

Compensatory Training

When habilitation or relearning fails or is inappropriate, other options remain available. Often a skill the patient would like to perform in a normal manner can be accomplished successfully some other way. The person with bilateral above-elbow amputations may not do well at feeding using prostheses but may perhaps develop superior toe prehension and use the feet rather than the hands to eat, write, and manipulate tools. Adaptive equipment may substitute for lost or impaired abilities that limit function. The use of such devices will be discussed in the next section. Regardless of how compensatory training is approached, the philosophical principle that should guide therapy is that there are many approaches to accomplishing the same task. Creative alterations in task performance may allow people to do something for themselves that under other circumstances they would be dependent on another to perform. It is characteristic of compensatory training that it is the end result of patient activity, whether it is clean teeth or tied shoelaces, and not the method used to perform the task that is important.

Assistive Technology

In the past 20 years there has been an unprecedented increase in the numbers and kinds of devices available to assist the disabled person. It has become impossible for rehabilitation professionals to be aware of, or have access to, information on all such devices. Research suggests that there are nearly 2,000 sources of such equipment worldwide, offering an estimated 25,000 to 30,000 products for sale. The typical occupational or physical therapist, speech pathologist, or physician may have 20 to 50 catalogs readily available for finding devices but remains unaware of vast numbers of other specific items that could benefit patients. One solution to this problem is to use computerized listings or data bases of such devices, catalogued according to their areas of application. ABLEDATA is a technology data base that describes over 15,000 commercially available rehabilitation products, providing equipment descriptions, information about manufacturers, and other comments (185). This data base is now available on the internet. A second data base, REHABDATA, is supplied by the National Rehabilitation Information Center (under contract with the National Institute on Disability and Rehabilitation Research). Assistive technology information is but one aspect of that service, which also includes publications, reports, and journal entries related to rehabilitation. REHABDATA is also available on the internet.

Taylor and associates have described a growing specialty of occupational therapy in which therapists become evaluators and providers of increasingly numerous and complex aids to independence (186). Their call for an expanded role of rehabilitation therapists in providing technical aids to independence was issued at approximately the same time that Newrick and Langton-Hewer published findings that over two thirds of a group of 42 patients with motor neuron disease could have benefited from aids to independence that had never been prescribed (187).

Systems and Devices for Persons with Disability

To determine which systems or devices each person needs, an array of equipment must be available. A compre-

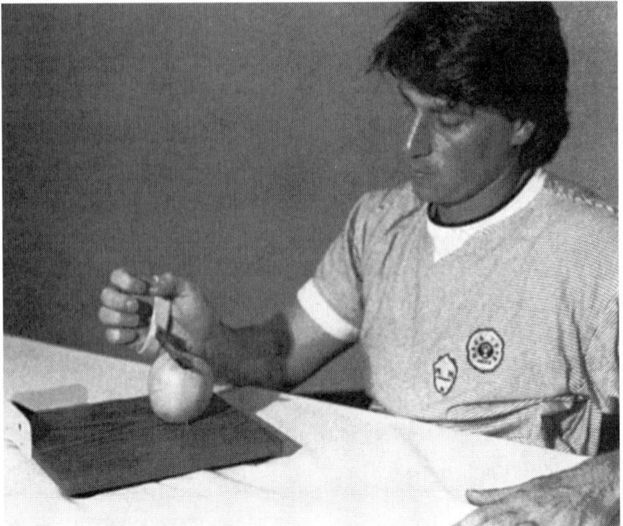

FIG. 7-3. Adapted knife and cutting board.

hensive team evaluation leads to a list of possible solutions for each identified problem, providing ample information for the patient to make the ultimate decision in the selection of equipment. In every instance, the goal of assessment is to find the simplest, least expensive device that best meets the needs of the patient (Figs. 7-3 through 7-6)

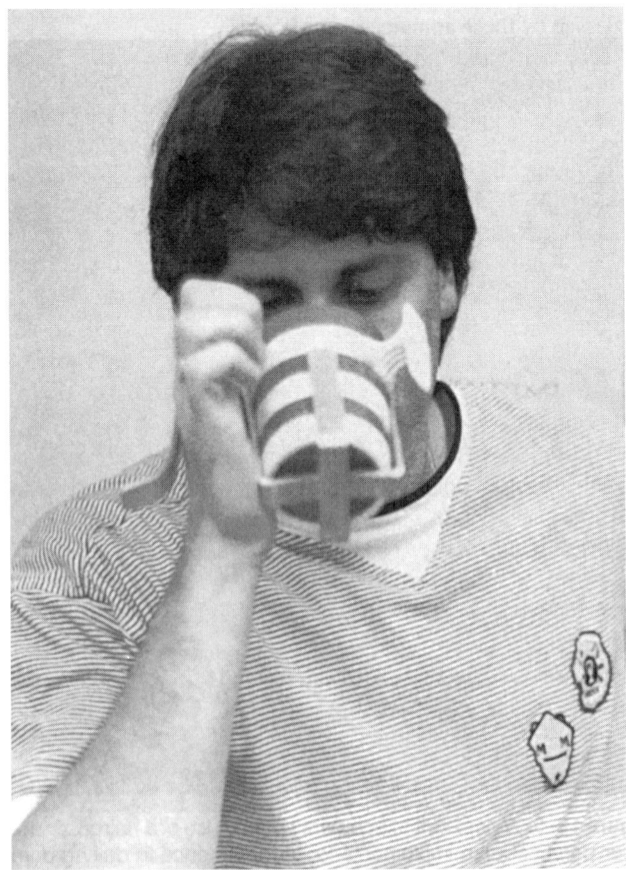

FIG. 7-4. Adapted cup holder.

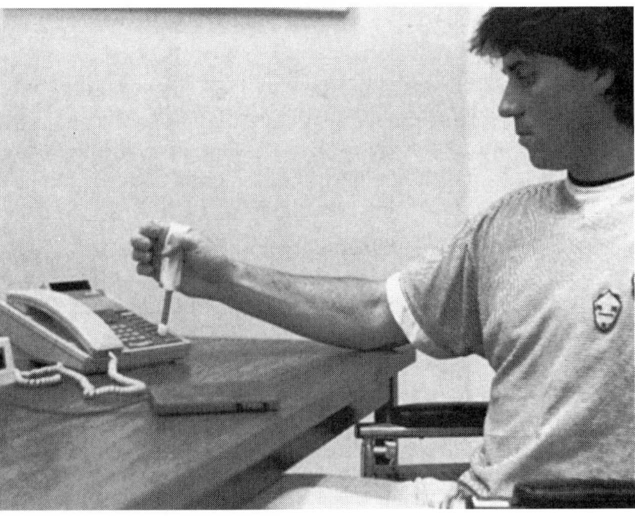

FIG. 7-5. An environmental control device with a large-pad pressure switch allows control of electrical devices in the kitchen and throughout the home. Also, a speaker phone with automatic dialing functions is activated through use of a cuff-mounted pointer stick.

A special case of the use of devices or adaptive equipment is the application of technology to increase the disabled person's independence. High-technology devices and systems are characterized by sophisticated electronic components. These include computers, robots, speech synthesizers, and environmental control systems. Symington has provided an excellent review of the role of environmental control devices in fostering independent living (188).

Low-technology items are simple mechanical aids, such as built-up handles for an arthritic person or shoelaces that can be tied with one hand. Such low-technology items are far more numerous than high-technology devices, yet they are less well known to many disabled people. The technol-

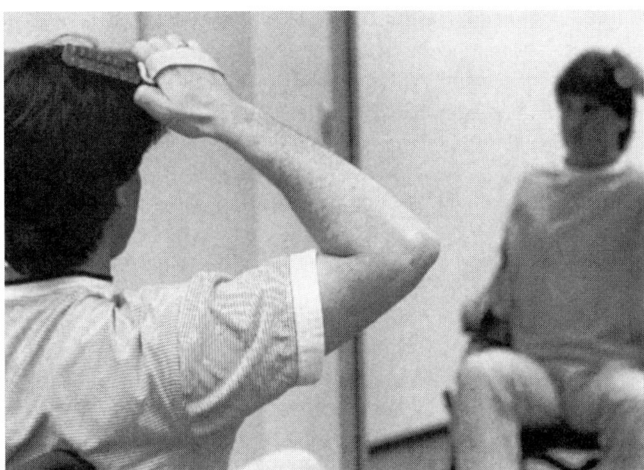

FIG. 7-6. Velcro cuff attachments permit use of a hairbrush and other personal care implements for independence in daily grooming.

ogy of remote control has become increasingly available in our society. For a person unable to reach a light switch, radio, television, thermostat, door lock, or curtain cord, an environmental control system can provide an important new degree of independence. Ultrasonic or infrared signals, sent from a command center, may allow a disabled person to use a variety of electronically activated appliances.

In recent years, the development of robotic devices has continued, including those aimed at serving as independent living assistants. In general, progress with these specialized assistive devices has not proceeded with the degree of success predicted in the 1980s (189). However, some promise has been realized for limited applications (such as retrieval and manipulative functions) in home settings (190).

The use and acceptance of assistive technology for self care is not always related to function or independence. Stein and Walley reported that 60% of the upper extremity amputees fitted with myoelectric versus conventional prostheses preferred the myoelectric ones even though they wore them fewer hours per day and were twice as slow at tasks as with the conventional prostheses (191). Presumably, cosmesis was a major consideration unrelated to self-care independence that influenced the choice of device by these amputees.

Smith has observed that patients often are provided with technological aids they do not need because of the widespread perception that technologic advancements equate with improved function (192). He notes that the best solution to a functional problem often is found with less sophisticated devices or through approaches that require no technology at all. Devices are not always a solution reserved for cases that have failed to respond to other measures. Often assistive technology is needed during one stage of recovery and later can be replaced by more normal tools or approaches. Haworth studied the use of devices and aids to independence by 163 patients with total hip replacement and clearly showed that patients used devices for ambulation, safety, dressing, and toileting and stopped using them when they were able to manage without such aids (193). Mann and colleagues studied assistive device use by older persons with cognitive and physical impairments living in their homes and found that impairment category was associated with the number of devices used and the satisfaction with assistive devices. Overall, however, subjects used 79% of the devices they owned and were satisfied with 72% of those devices (194).

Rogers and Figone assessed the extent of use of self-care skills learned during rehabilitation as well as the orthotic devices provided to support function in 35 patients with traumatic cervical cord injury 1 to 4 years after discharge from a rehabilitation unit (195). They found that the level of self-care achieved during rehabilitation was maintained by the majority of patients at follow-up. Both improvement as well as regression in function occurred variably among the rehabilitants, reflecting a reordering of time and energy based on personal priorities and other situational factors. The authors suggested that disuse of skills, caused by mobility barriers to important places where skills normally are performed (such as bathrooms), might help explain some regression in function. Moreover, the authors questioned whether rehabilitation training goals of dressing independence for those with spinal cord injury at level C6–C7 were realistic, given the impracticality of such activities for rehabilitants in community living. In other studies of assistive device use, Gitlin and colleagues (196) found that devices for older adults with mixed disabilities were seldom used, concluding that instruction within the home setting was frequently inadequate.

Environmental Modifications

Both training and devices for self-care independence must be appropriate to the living space of the patient. Modifications of living spaces and the architectural barriers they often impose may greatly enhance independent function in ADL. Such modifications may range from minimal in the case of rearrangement of furniture, to extensive when apartments or homes must be specially designed for the disabled. Intermediate to these extremes are the cases in which modifications or additions to existing space and equipment may be used to enhance function. In a study of 545 patients with rheumatoid arthritis and 170 patients with ankylosing spondylitis, Ur-b'anek and colleagues found that environmental conditions such as narrow apartment space negatively influenced the activity of the rheumatoid disease process itself (197). Liang and colleagues have pointed out the inadequacies of the U.S. health care system in meeting the needs of the estimated one million homebound patients in the United States (198). They described how many of them could be helped by modifications of their home environment or occupational and physical therapy. This was confirmed in a study by the National Center for Health Statistics, which reported that nearly one quarter of adults over age 65 require some type of assistive device or accessibility modification in the home, with this percentage steadily increasing as the age bracket increases (199).

Rearrange Existing Living Space

Many simple modifications that can improve self-care can be suggested by the occupational therapist or the practitioner during the course of a predischarge home visit. When upper extremity range of motion is limited, pots, pans, cosmetics, canned goods, and other essential daily living items can be stored on counters rather than in their traditional places, which often are difficult or impossible to reach. For the patient with a visual field deficit such as homonymous hemianopia, moving the bed and furniture into the patient's intact visual field when viewed from the doorway may make it easier and safer to move around the room. Of course, the view and placement of objects relative to the bed also must be strategically considered for the same reasons. Removal of throw rugs and other common obstacles for the mobility impaired person may make a nighttime trip to the bathroom considerably safer.

Modify Existing Living Space

The range of possibilities for modification of living space to meet the needs of disabled people is extensive. Examples of common modifications include widening doorways, adding ramps, converting a den or family room into a wheelchair-accessible bedroom, and adding tub rails, toilet rails, and other safety equipment in the bathroom. Several extensive studies have focused solely on the design and modification of bathrooms with respect to both disabled and nondisabled people (200,201). Lowman and Klinger have presented many ideas for environmental adaptations catalogued by self-care skill category and by patient deficits (202). Resources such as the American National Standards Institute's Specifications for Making Buildings and Facilities Accessible to and Usable by Physically Handicapped People give explicit guidelines for many common problems (203). Unfortunately, lack of information usually is not what prevents patients and caregivers from effecting changes in living space. Expense and, for those who rent, ownership often are barriers to change. Lack of support by third-party payers in the reimbursement of environmental modifications is particularly frustrating. Some health-care providers have attacked these problems directly by developing partnerships between governmental and community agencies to fund programs designed to eliminate architectural barriers within the home. Colvin and Korn have described one such partnership in New York City between United Cerebral Palsy of New York, Inc., the Mayor's Office for the Handicapped, and the Department of Housing Preservation and Development. This project was found to be both cost effective and to improve the quality of life for those served by it.

Design New Components in Living Space

The most extensive and expensive of options is to redesign or renovate existing living space. However, for many of the most severely disabled people, the only alternative to making such modifications is institutionalization. Everett and Colignon have discussed the architectural and self-care needs for independent living by severely disabled people (204). They suggest that such needs are part of a complex set of interrelated problems for disabled people and that public policy must be developed to support programs that will provide extensive architectural intervention for these patients. Architectural renovations alone, however, may not solve the problem. To renovate an apartment for a person with high-level quadriplegia by adding a roll-in shower stall, rerouting pipes to allow wheelchair access to sinks, and performing other changes may not make the person more independent if he or she lacks transportation, has no job, or is unable to communicate. Major modifications of living space must be subject to cost-benefit analysis and justified with respect to the overall level of functioning they permit. Such considerations include, but extend beyond, independence in self-care.

Use of Personal Care Attendants

There is no combination of training, devices, or environmental modifications that will enable some severely disabled persons to function independently in self-care. For such people to live independently outside an institution they must depend on family members (informal support) or personal care attendants (formal support) to assist them. Part of the rehabilitation process for people who are going to require attendant care is that they learn to recruit, hire, supervise, and, if necessary, terminate personal care attendants.

Recruitment of Personal Care Attendants

There are a number of excellent manuals and guides to attendant care (205,206); however, the availability and quality of personal care attendants vary greatly from one community to the next. One source of attendants is through home health-care agencies, many of which provide pre-employment screening and placement for a fee. Nurse placement services and agencies specializing in unskilled or temporary help also are possible sources of attendants. Classified advertising in local newspapers and announcements strategically placed on bulletin boards at colleges, religious institutions, and supermarkets also can be effective. Often the most difficult task for the patient is that of defining the tasks that require assistance, the degree of assistance that is desired, and the hours of the day when these tasks need to be performed. Because hours, pay, and working schedules (i.e., often attendants are needed seven days per week) often are not competitive with other types of employment, turnover among attendants is high. The occupational therapist or other appropriately trained health-care professional often can assist the patient in writing the job description for a personal care attendant and in some cases may work with the patient to be an effective supervisor. Baum and Levesser note that selection and recruitment can be facilitated through the use of carefully defined tasks (207). The use of checklists with required tasks and procedures can serve as a specification for interviews, training, and performance appraisal (208).

Guidelines for the Appropriate Use of Care Attendants

An important and difficult aspect of working with a care attendant is to be able to define all of the self-care and daily living activities that will require assistance. Many tasks, such as brushing one's teeth, dressing, and grooming, are performed daily. Other tasks such as washing one's hair or having a bowel movement may be performed less frequently but still quite regularly. Still other tasks such as doing the laundry or changing the bed are even less frequent but still are performed regularly. Finally, there will be tasks such as mending torn clothing or washing windows that are infrequent and not performed on a regular basis. This listing must then be categorized into three distinct classes of activities: those that the patient can perform alone, those that the patient can perform with some assistance, and those that must be performed by the personal care attendant.

The attendant who wants to care totally for the patient or is too impatient to wait for the patient to assist with a task is as harmful as the attendant who neglects the patient. When rehabilitation personnel assist the patient in achieving a realistic and comprehensive understanding of his or her self-care strengths and limitations, more effective use of care attendants is possible.

In 1991, the World Personal Assistance Services Symposium was sponsored by the World Institute on Disability, resulting in a resolution on strategies for the development of a personal assistance services system. The resolution recognized the United Nations World Program of Action, which holds that member states should encourage the provision of support services to enable disabled people to live as independently as possible in the community and in so doing should ensure that persons with a disability have the opportunity to develop and manage these services for themselves (209). The document also includes various principles that collectively advocate the need for governmental assistance in the provision of personal assistance services and expresses the importance with which access and management issues related to personal assistance for persons with disabilities are viewed.

Major Self-Care Considerations by Functional Limitation

A most important concept in self-care rehabilitation is that neither the type nor severity of the disability can be used to predict how independent a given patient will be. Pressures from new Medicare reimbursement guidelines and the accompanying need for medical care cost containment tend to foster the notion that with controlled studies the factors that predict rehabilitation outcomes can be identified. The intent of such efforts is to shift resources toward those patients believed to have better chances at independence and away from those with less likelihood of functioning independently. That this is a misguided approach is supported by studies such as those by Neill and associates who studied 100 men with coronary disease (210). They found that there was little or no relationship between physical limitations and the activities performed by those patients. Patient perceptions and not cardiac symptoms accounted for the patterns of independence/dependence in household and social activities. Limited capacity for exertion, which is used by many occupational and physical therapists to recommend appropriate activities, is in fact not a determinant of the activities those cardiac patients performed as part of their daily routine. Is it useful then, to discuss self-care considerations by functional limitations? If the goal is to become aware of special problems or issues unique to a particular disability and not to predict outcomes, then the answer clearly is affirmative.

Cognitive-Perceptual Deficits and Self-Care

There are a number of principles that can be applied to the patient with cognitive or perceptual deficits. Right-sided brain damage is associated with visual perceptual and visual search disorders that make self-care training more difficult. Anstine and Isaacs found that problems with dressing were more common in subjects with right hemispheric damage (211). Gordon and colleagues investigated 78 patients with right-sided brain damage and showed that patients given a comprehensive perceptual remediation program did better at such tasks on discharge than the controls not given this program (212). After discharge, the controls tended to show improvement, whereas the experimental group had reached a plateau. This suggests that rehabilitation training may accelerate recovery of perceptual abilities but is not a *sine qua non* for improvements. Dudgeon and colleagues found that among patients with right-sided brain damage, those with defective optokinetic nystagmus (OKN) reflexes showed less improvement in upper extremity dressing than did those with normal OKN, but that both groups showed improvement over time (213). The OKN deficit group had an average 40% longer hospitalization and a higher incidence of nursing home placement at discharge.

Panikoff described the course of functional recovery from head injury over a 2-year period for 80 head-injured adults (214). That study found that the longer the period of coma, the greater the disability and dependency at 1 year and 2 years after injury. However, the majority of patients continued to show improvement in ADL and other skills over the 2-year period. Goldkamp studied 53 patients with cerebral palsy for periods of 6 to 25 years and found that the only variable that appeared to influence ADL independence directly was intelligence (215). Bjornby and Reinvang investigated the relationship of apraxia to ADL skills in 120 people with right-sided hemiplegia after left-sided CVA (184). They found that apraxia variables were significant predictors of dependency and that even less severely involved patients who showed progress in the hospital setting regressed in ADL function after returning home. Their conclusion was that these patients have difficulty in transferring skills learned in the clinic to the home environment and that such patients might best be treated in their own homes.

These results are consistent with a study of 25 stroke patients in which a clear relationship between apraxia and ADL skills was shown (216). Similarly, Bernsprang and colleagues found that perceptual motor abilities were significant predictors of self-care and ADL in stroke patients (217). However, deficits in visual perception did not correlate significantly with ADL performance, suggesting that abilities that require organization and action are the most essential to competent performance of self-care activities. It appears that cognitive-perceptual limitations may make self-care rehabilitation training more difficult. Patients with such limitations can and do make progress, albeit more slowly than similar patients without such deficits.

Upper Extremity Impairment

Patients with unilateral upper extremity impairment most often compensate by using the uninvolved extremity. When disability affects the preferred hand, there will be a need to transfer skill to the other hand. This may or may not require coordination and dexterity training. Bilateral upper extremity weakness, loss of motion, and amputations are more serious threats to self-care independence. For such people, orthotic and prosthetic devices often are useful. In some cases teeth are used for prehension privately, whereas the prosthesis may be used publicly. Cosmesis often is as much or more a consideration than function in the selection of a prosthesis (218).

Lower Extremity Impairment

Mobility and transfer limitations are the most significant self-care problems for lower extremity disabled people, including those with hip fractures, amputations, arthritis, and paraplegia. Often wheelchairs or other ambulation aids are needed for independent mobility. Bathroom safety equipment, dressing aids such as extended handle shoehorns, and raised seats may be used either temporarily or permanently. Rearrangement of living space to permit wheelchair access or access using other mobility aids often is necessary. Ramps, chairlifts, and additional railings may be needed if stairs are present. For the person dependent on a wheelchair, it also may be helpful to consider rearrangement of shelves, drawers, and closet space to permit items that are used frequently to be reached from the wheelchair. Narang and associates reported that of 500 lower extremity amputees they studied, 55% were totally independent in all self-care, 40% required only additional aids to independence for self-care, and 5% were confined to wheelchairs or not totally independent (219). Haworth investigated the patterns of use of aids to independence in 163 patients after total hip replacement (220). Findings suggested that aids were used only as long as needed for bathroom safety, dressing, and toileting and that patients discarded them when they could manage independently.

Upper and Lower Extremity Impairment

People with quadriparesis or quadriplegia from traumatic spinal cord injury, brain disorders, muscular dystrophy, multiple sclerosis, or amyotrophic lateral sclerosis must rely on a wide range of options for self-care independence. In most cases there will be a need for attendant care, assistive devices, and modifications of living space. Such people often require high-technology devices such as environmental controls, augmentative communications, and other microprocessor-based systems to be fully independent in their own home. DeJong and colleagues have reported that independence for patients with spinal cord injury is a complex and interdependent process in which severity of injury, transportation, education, marital status, and economic disincentives all play a role (221). A concerted effort to address such issues, including a broader definition of self-care training, appears to be needed to enable such patients to live more productively and in less restrictive environments.

Hemiparesis

Considerations of cognitive and perceptual deficits have been discussed earlier. Perhaps the most important finding that has been emerging is that the side of the lesion may predict a pattern of problems but does not predict self-care outcomes. Mills and DeGenio compared 50 right-hemispheric CVA patients with 52 left-hemispheric CVA patients and found that there was no significant difference in ADL independence between the two groups (222). Wade and colleagues studied 42 consecutive acute CVAs and found that neither gender nor side of weakness influenced functional recovery *per se* but that patients with left-hemispheric CVA attended rehabilitation therapies longer so that they appeared to have made better functional gains at discharge (223).

The differences between left- and right-side brain damage do not affect prognosis for self-care independence directly. Instead, it appears that patients with left-sided brain damage are easier to train, receive more training, and progress more rapidly. Patients with right-sided damage tend to be more difficult to train, take longer to train, and tend to receive less training. The suggestion that cannot be ignored is that the attitudes and skills of therapists and the economics of medical rehabilitation may be biased toward those with left-sided brain damage. As Dudgeon and colleagues have suggested, the availability of more sensitive tests to predict the patterns of self-care difficulties that may be encountered is needed. Therapists and physicians need to be aware of the implications of their decisions about intensity and duration of training for right- versus left-sided brain-damaged patients. remembering that both groups show gains over time in self-care and that the hospital discharge prognosis for ADL independence is not necessarily the long-term self-care prognosis (180).

Limitations in Joint Range of Motion

Problems of limited range of motion that result in difficulty reaching common ADL items are best addressed by rearrangement of living space. Urb'anek and associates have shown that the home environment, both in its physical dimensions and with respect to support of the family, is significantly related to independence (197). An occupational therapist or other health-care provider making a home visit can suggest safety equipment for the bathroom, removal of obstacles that could contribute to falls, and other adaptive devices that are needed. With respect to training, an emphasis on compensatory training regarding work simplification and energy conservation techniques is needed.

SUMMARY

Assessment and management strategies for promoting independence in self care represent, from the patient's standpoint, one of the most practical and important aspects of medical rehabilitation. As a rehabilitation goal, independence in self care has been approached all too frequently from the narrow perspective of the professional and the rehabilitation setting. In this chapter, we have presented a decision process for managing options in which the patient and the professional collaborate in determining goals and methods for managing these important life tasks after discharge. In this decision-making process, the patient's preferences, experiences, and postdischarge living environment assume at least as much importance as the diagnosis or physical limitations. Moreover, such factors as costs of time and energy must enter into decisions about the value of various options for independence.

Options include determining if the task is feasible, if retraining or new training is desirable, if the environment needs to be altered, if assistance needs to be provided through other people, or if adaptive equipment and devices, including high technology, may be useful.

Technological developments to permit independent function will continue to offer promise for the future. In the meantime, however, we are confident that the participation of the patient in determining self-care goals ultimately will represent an equally important achievement in independent living.

ACKNOWLEDGMENTS

The work of Richard Schwartz and Karin Barnes was instrumental to the development of earlier versions of this chapter and is acknowledged with appreciation. We also thank Ralph Cheeseman, Shaffiq Rahemtulla, and Gary Bowman for their help in preparing photographs of assistive devices, as well as Will Shaller and Kristin Tate for assistance in locating important reference materials.

REFERENCES

1. Christiansen C. A social framework for understanding self-care performance. In: Christiansen C, ed. *Ways of living: self care strategies for special needs.* Bethesda: American Occupational Therapy Association. 1994; 1–26.
2. Lawton MP. The functional assessment of elderly people. *J Am Geriatr Soc* 1971; 14:465–481.
3. Christiansen C. Three perspectives on balance in occupation. In: Zemke R, Clark F, eds. *Occupational science: the evolving discipline.* Philadelphia: FA Davis, 1996; 431–451.
4. Mauthe RW, Haaf DC, Hayn P, Krall JM. Predicting discharge destination of stroke patients using a mathematical model based on six items from the Functional Independence Measure. *Arch Phys Med Rehabil* 1996; 77:10–3.
5. Parsons T. Definitions of health and illness in the light of American values and social structure. In: Jaco EG, ed. *Patients, physicians and illness.* Glencoe, IL: Free Press, 1958; 165–187.
6. Christiansen CH. Assessing occupational performance. In: Christiansen CH, Baum C, eds. *Occupational therapy: overcoming human performance deficits.* Thorofare, NJ: Slack, 1991; 375–426.
7. Hogan R. A socioanalytic theory of personality. *Nebraska Symp Motivation* 1982; 30:55–89.
8. Bowling AP, Edelmann RJ. Loneliness, mobility, well-being and social support in a sample of over 85 year olds. *Personality Individual Differences* 1989; 10:1189–1192.
9. Rintala D, Young ME. Social suport and the well being of persons with spinal cord injury living in the community. *Rehabil Psychol* 1992; 37:155–163.
10. Affleck G, Pfeiffer CA. Social support and psychosocial adjustment to rheumatoid arthritis: quantitative and qualitative findings. *Arthritis Care Res* 1988; 1:71–77.
11. Rohrer K, Adelman B, Puckett J. Rehabilitation in spinal cord injury: use of a patient-family group. *Arch Phys Med Rehabil* 1980; 61: 225–229.
12. Rice FP. *The adolescent: development, relationships and culture,* 2nd ed. Boston: Allyn & Bacon, 1978.
13. Aitken MJ. Self-concept and functional independence in the hospitalized elderly. *Am J Occup Ther* 1982; 36:243–250.
14. Malick MH, Almasy B. Assessment and evaluation: life work tasks. In: Hopkins HL, Smith HD, eds. *Willard and Spackman's occupational therapy,* 7th ed. Philadelphia: JB Lippincott, 1982.
15. Green BC, Pratt CC, Grigsby TE. Self-concept among persons with long-term spinal cord injury. *Arch Phys Med Rehabil* 1984; 65: 751–754.
16. Decker SD, Schulz R. Correlates of life satisfaction and depression in middle-aged and elderly spinal-injured persons. *Am J Occup Ther* 1985; 39:740–745.
17. Leathem J, Health E, Woolley C. Relatives perceptions of role change, social support and stress after traumatic brain injury. *Brain Injury* 1996; 10:27–38.
18. Deutsch CP, Goldston JA. Family factors in home adjustment of the severely disabled. *J Marriage Family* 1960; 21:312–316.
19. Barber PA, Turnbull AP, Behr SK, Kerns GM. A family systems perspective on early childhood special education. In: Odom SL, Karnes MB, eds. *Early intervention for infants and children with handicaps: an empirical base.* Baltimore: Paul H Brookes, 1989; 179–197.
20. Jones DA, Vetter NJ. A survey of those who care for the elderly and home: their problems and their needs. *Soc Sci Med* 1984; 19:511–514.
21. Evans RL, Bishop DS, Ousley RT. Providing care to persons with physical disability. Effect on family caregivers. *Am J Phys Med Rehabil* 1992; 71:140–144.
22. Wilcox VL, Kasl, SV, Berkman, LF. Social support and disability in older people after hospitalization: a prospective study. *Health Psychol* 1994; 13:170–179.
23. Zisserman L. The modern family and rehabilitation of the handicapped: a macrosociological view. *Am J Occup Ther* 1981; 35:14–20.
24. Bishop DS, Epstein NB. Family problems and disability. In: Bishop DS, ed. *Behavioral problems and the disabled.* Baltimore: Williams & Wilkins, 1980; 337–364.
25. Wilcox VL, Kasl SV, Berkman LF. Social support and physical disability in older people after hospitalization: a prospective study. *Health Psychol* 1994; 13:170–179.
26. Weinberg N. Physically disabled people assess the quality of their lives. *Rehabil Lit* 1984; 45:12–15.
27. Hogan R. A socioanalytic theory of personality. *Nebraska Symp Motivation* 1982; 30:55–89.
28. Kielhofner G. Occupation. In: Hopkins HL, Smith DH, eds. *Willard and Spackman's occupational therapy,* 7th ed. Philadelphia: JB Lippincott, 1988; 84–92.
29. Bartels EC. A contemporary framework for independent living rehabilitation. *Rehabil Lit* 1985; 46:325–327.
30. Malick M. Activities of daily living and homemaking. In: Willard HS, Spackman CS, eds. *Occupational therapy,* 7th ed. Philadelphia: JB Lippincott, 1988; 258–271.
31. Haworth RJ, Hollings EM. Are hospital assessments of daily living activities valid? *Int Rehabil Med* 1979; 1:59–62.
32. DiJoseph LM. Independence through activity: mind, body, and environment interaction in therapy. *Am J Occup Ther* 1982; 36:740–744.
33. Wade DT, Wood VA, Hewer RL. Recovery after stroke: the first 3 months. *J Neurosurg Psychiatry* 1985; 48:7–13.

34. Newrick PG, Langton-Hewer R. Motor neuron disease: can we do better? A study of 42 patients. *Br Med J [Clin Res]* 1984; 289: 539–542.
35. Wiemer RB, West WL. Occupational therapy in community health care. *Am J Occup Ther* 1970; 24:323–328.
36. Williams GH. The movement for independent living: an evaluation and critique. *Soc Sci Med* 1983; 17:1003–1010.
37. Batavia A, Dejong G, Eckenhoff EA, Materson RS. After the Americans with disabilities act: the role of the rehabilitation community. *Arch Phys Med Rehabil* 1990; 71:1014–1015.
38. Neistadt ME, Marques K. An independent living skills training program. *Am J Occup Ther* 1984; 38:671–676.
39. Colvin ME, Korn TL. Eliminating barriers to the disabled. *Am J Occup Ther* 1984; 38:748–753.
40. Seplowitz C. Technology and occupational therapy in the rehabilitation of the bedridden quadriplegic. *Am J Occup Ther* 1984; 38: 743–747.
41. Smith RO. Technological approaches to performance enhancement. In: Christiansen C, Baum C, eds. *Occupational therapy: overcoming human performance deficits.* Thorofare, NJ: Slack, 1991; 747–788.
42. Countryman KM, Gekas AB. Development and implementation of a patient s bill of rights in hospitals. Chicago: American Hospital Association, 1980.
43. Commission on Accreditation of Rehabilitation Facilities. *The standards manual for organizations serving people with disabilities.* Tucson: Commission on Accreditation of Rehabilitation Facilities, 1992.
44. Joint Commission on Accreditation of Healthcare Organizations. *The 1993 joint commission accreditation manual for hospitals.* Vol. 1. Standards. Chicago: Joint Commission on Accreditation of Rehabilitation Facilities, 1992.
45. Northen JG, Rust DM, Nelson CE, Watts JH. Involvement of adult rehabilitation patients in setting occupational therapy goals. *Am J Occup Ther* 1995; 49:214–220.
46. Unsworth C. Clients perceptions of discharge housing decisions after stroke rehabilitation. *Am J Occup Ther* 1996; 50:207–216.
47. Burke JP. A clinical perspective on motivation: pawn versus origin. *Am J Occup Ther* 1977; 31:254–258.
48. Chiou IL, Burnett CN. Values of activities of daily living: a survey of stroke patients and their home therapists. *Phys Ther* 1985; 65: 901–906.
49. Rodin J, Langer E. Aging labels: the decline of control and the fall of self esteem. *J Social Issues* 1980; 36:12–29.
50. Coulton CJ, Dunkle RE, Haug M, Chow JC, Vielhaber DP. Locus of control and decision-making for post hospital care. *Gerontologist* 1989; 28:627–631.
51. Bates PS. The self care environment: issues of space and furnishing. In: Christiansen C, ed. *Ways of living: self care strategies for special needs.* Bethesda, MD: American Occupational Therapy Association, 1994; 423–452.
52. Norris-Baker C, Willems EP. Environmental negotiability as a direct measurement of behavior-environment relationships: some implications for theory and practice. In: Seidel AD, Danford S, eds. *Proceedings of the 10th Annual Conference of the Environmental Design Research Association.* Houston: Environmental Design Research Association, 1978; 209–214.
53. Granger CV. A conceptual model for functional assessment. In: Grangerand CV, Gresham GE, eds. *Functional assessment in rehabilitation medicine.* Baltimore, MD: Williams & Wilkins, 1984; 14–25.
54. Wood PHN. Appreciating the consequences of disease—the classification of impairments, disabilities and handicaps. *WHO Chron* 1980; 34:376–380.
55. Mather JH. The problem of functional assessment: political and economic perspectives. *Am J Occup Ther* 1993; 47:240–246.
56. Towsend E, Ryan B, Law M. Using the World Health Organization's International Classification of Impairments, Disabilities, and Handicaps in occupational therapy. *Can J Occup Ther* 1990; 57:16–25.
57. Christiansen C. Occupational therapy: intervention for life performance. In: Christiansen C, Baum C, eds. *Occupational therapy: overcoming human performance deficits.* Thorofare, NJ: Slack, 1991; 1–47.
58. Ottenbacher K, Christiansen C. Functional performance assessment. In: Christiansen C, Baum C, eds. *Occupational therapy: enabling functional performance and well being.* Thorofare, NJ: Slack, 1997.
59. Vash CL. Evaluation from the client's point of view. In: Halpern AS, Fuhrer MJ, eds. *Functional assessment in rehabilitation.* Baltimore: Paul H Brookes, 1984; 253–268.
60. Kelman HR, Willner A. Problems in measurement and evaluation of rehabilitation. *Arch Phys Med Rehabil* 1962; 43:172–181.
61. Law M, Letts L. A critical review of scales of activities of daily living. *Am J Occup Ther* 1989; 43:522–527.
62. Jette AM. Health status indicators: their utility in chronic-disease evaluation research. *J Chronic Dis* 1979; 33:567–579.
63. Kaufert JM. Functional ability indices: measurement problems in assessing their validity. *Arch Phys Med Rehabil* 1983; 64:260–267.
64. Keith RA. Functional assessment measures in medical rehabilitation: current status. *Arch Phys Med Rehabil* 1984; 65:74–78.
65. Christiansen C. Continuing challenges in functional assessment. *Am J Occup Ther* 1993; 48:258–259.
66. Alexander JL, Fuhrer MJ. Functional assessment of individuals with physical impairments. In: Halpern AS, Fuhrer MJ, eds. *Functional assessment in rehabilitation.* Baltimore: Paul H Brookes, 1984; 45–60.
67. Unsworth CA. The concept of function. *Br J Occup Ther* 1993; 56: 287–292.
68. Frey WD. Functional assessment in the 80s: a conceptual enigma, a technical challenge. In: Halpern AS, Fuhrer, MJ, eds. *Functional assessment in rehabilitation.* Baltimore: Paul H Brookes, 1984; 11–44.
69. Keith RA. Functional assessment in program evaluation for rehabilitation medicine. In: Granger CV, Gresham GE, eds. *Functional assessment in rehabilitation medicine.* Baltimore: Williams & Wilkins, 1984.
70. American Educational Research Association, American Psychological Association, National Council on Research in Education. *Standards for educational and psychological testing.* Washington, DC: American Psychological Assocation, 1985.
71. American Physical Therapy Association. Standards for tests and measurements in physical therapy practice. *Phys Ther* 1991; 71:589–621.
72. Johnston MV, Keith RA, Hinderer SR. Measurement standards for interdisciplinary medical rehabilitation. *Arch Phys Med Rehabil* 1992; 73:S3–S23.
73. Guttman L. The basis of scalogram analysis. In: Stouffer SA, Guttman L, Suchman EA, Lazarsteld PF, Star SA, Clausen JA, eds. *Measurement and prediction: studies in social psychology—World War II.* Princeton, NJ: Princeton University Press, 1950.
74. Guccione AA. Physical therapy diagnosis and the relationship between impairment and function. *Phys Ther* 1991; 71:499–504.
75. McGinnis GE, Seward M, DeJong G, Osberg JS. Program evaluation of physical medicine and rehabilitation departments using self-report Barthel. *Arch Phys Med Rehabil* 1986; 67:123–125.
76. Klein-Parris C, Clermont MT, O'Neill J. Effectiveness and efficiency of criterion testing versus interviewing for collecting functional assessment information. *Am J Occup Ther* 1986; 40:486–491.
77. Klein RM, Bell B. Self-care skills: behavioral measurement with Klein-Bell ADL scale. *Arch Phys Med Rehabil* 1982; 63:335–338.
78. Merbitz C, Morris J, Grip JC. Ordinal scales and foundations of misinference. *Arch Phys Med Rehabil* 1989; 70:308–312.
79. Rasch G. *Probabilistic models for some intelligence and attainment tests.* Copenhagen: Danmarks Paedogogistic Institut, 1960. [Reprinted with foreword and afterword by Wright BD. Chicago: University of Chicago Press, 1980.]
80. Silverstein B, Kilgore KM, Fisher WP, Harley JP, Harvey RF. Applying psychometric criteria to functional assessment in medical rehabilitation: I. Exploring unidimensionality. *Arch Phys Med Rehabil* 1991; 72:631–637.
81. Wright B, Linacre JM. Observations are always ordinal: measurements, however, must be interval. *Arch Phys Med Rehabil* 1989; 70: 857–860.
82. Silverstein B, Kilgore K, Fisher W. *Implementing patient tracking systems and using functional assessment scales.* Wheaton, IL: Marianjoy Rehabilitation Center, 1989.
83. Heinemann AW, Linacre JM, Wright BD, Hamilton BB, Granger C. Prediction of rehabilitation outcomes with disability measures. *Arch Phys Med Rehabil* 1994; 75:133–143.
84. Hamilton BB, Granger CV. Disability outcomes following inpatient rehabilitation for stroke. *Phys Ther* 1994; 74:494–503.
85. Moskowitz E, Fuhn ER, Peters ME. Aged infirm residents in a custodial institution. *JAMA* 1959; 169:2009–2012.

86. Katz S, Downs T, Cash H, Grotz R. Progress in development of the index of ADL. *Gerontologist* 1970; 10:20–30.
87. Granger CV, Hamilton BB, Sherwin FS. *Guide for use of the uniform data set for medical rehabilitation.* Buffalo, NY: Uniform Data System for Medical Rehabilitation, 1986.
88. Gresham GE, Labi MLC. Functional assessment instruments currently available for documenting outcomes in rehabilitation medicine. In: Granger CV, Gresham GE, eds. *Functional assessment in rehabilitation medicine.* Baltimore: Williams & Wilkins, 1984.
89. Moskowitz E, McCann CB. Classification of disability in the chronically ill and aging. *J Chronic Dis* 1957; 5:342–346.
90. Granger CV, Albrecht GL, Hamilton BB. Outcome of comprehensive medical rehabilitation: measurement by Pulses Profile and the Barthel Index. *Arch Phys Med Rehabil* 1979; 60:145–154.
91. Granger CV, Dewis LS, Peters NC, Sherwood CC, Barrett BA. Stroke rehabilitation: analysis of repeated Barthel Index measures. *Arch Phys Med Rehabil* 1979; 60:14–17.
92. Kelly CR, Rose DL. Grading the rehabilitation effort. *J Kansas Med Soc* 1971; 72:154–156.
93. Moskowitz E, Lightbody FEH, Freitag NS. Long term follow-up of the post stroke patient. *Arch Phys Med Rehabil* 1972; 53:167–172.
94. Katz S, Ford AB, Moskowitz RW. Studies of illness in the aged: the Index of ADL: a standardized measure of biological and psychosocial function. *JAMA* 1963; 185:914–919.
95. Anderson TP, Boureston N, Greenberg FR, Hilyard VG. Predictive factors in stroke rehabilitation. *Arch Phys Med Rehabil* 1974; 55: 545–553.
96. Gibson CJ. Epidemiology and patterns of care of stroke patients. *Arch Phys Med Rehabil* 1974; 55:398–403.
97. Brorsson B, Asberg KH. Katz index of independence in ADL: reliability and validity in short-term care. *Scand J Rehabil Med* 1984; 16: 125–132.
98. Mahoney F, Barthel DW. Functional evaluation: the Barthel Index. *Maryland State Med J* 1965; 14:61–65.
99. Hertanu JS, Demopoulos JT, Yang WC, Calhoun WF, Fenigstein HA. Stroke rehabilitation: correlation and prognostic value of computerized tomography and sequential functional assessments. *Arch Phys Med Rehabil* 1984; 65:505–508.
100. Granger CV, Hamilton BB, Gresham GE, Kramer AA. The stroke rehabilitation outcome study: Part II: relative merits of the total Barthel Index score and a four-item subscore in predicting patient outcomes. *Arch Phys Med Rehabil* 1989; 70:100–103.
101. Wylie CM, White BK. A measure of disability. *Arch Environ Health* 1964; 8:834–839.
102. DeJong G, Branch LG, Corcoran PJ. Independent living outcomes in spinal cord injury: multivariate analyses. *Arch Phys Med Rehabil* 1984; 65:66–73.
103. O'Toole DMK, Goldberg RT, Ryan B. Functional changes in vascular amputee patients: evaluation by Barthel Index, Pulses Profile and Escrow Scale. *Arch Phys Med Rehabil* 1985; 66:508–511.
104. Granger CV, Albrecht GL, Hamilton BB. Outcome of comprehensive medical rehabilitation: measurement by pulses profile and the barthel index. *Arch Phys Med Rehabil* 1979; 60:145–154.
105. Fortinsky MA, Granger CV, Seltzer GB. The use of functional assessment in understanding home care needs. *Med Care* 1981; 19:489–497.
106. Collin C, Wade DT, Davies S, Horne V. The Berthel ADL Index: a reliability study. *Int Disability Studies* 1988; 11:40–44.
107. Shah S, Vanclay F, Cooper B. Efficiency, effectiveness and duration of stroke rehabiltitaion. *Stroke* 1990; 21:241–246.
108. Deutsch A, Braun S, Granger CV. The Functional Independence Measure and the Functional Independence Measure for Children: ten years of development. *Crit Rev Phys Med Rehab* 1996; 8:267–281.
109. Hamilton BB, Granger CV, Sherwin FS, Zielezny M, Tashman MJ. A uniform national data system for medical rehabilitation. In: Fuhrer MJ, ed. *Rehabilitation outcomes: analysis and measurement.* Baltimore: Paul H Brookes, 1987; 137–147.
110. Fricke J, Unsworth C, Worrell D. Reliability of the functional independence measure with occupational therapists. *Aust Occup Ther J* 1993; 40:7–15.
111. Chau N, Daler S, Andre JM, Patris A. Inter-rater agreement of two functional independence scales: the Functional Independence Measure and a subjective uniform continuous scale. *Disability Rehabilitation* 1994; 16:63–71.
112. Hamilton BB, Laughlin JA, Fiedler RC, Granger CV. Interrater reliability of the 7-level functional independence measure (FIM). *Scand J Rehabil Med* 1994; 26:115–119.
113. Bunch WH, Dvonch VM. The value of functional independence measure scores. *Am J Phys Med Rehabil* 1994;73:40–43.
114. Granger CV, Cotter AC, Hamilton BB, Fiedler RC, Hens MM. Functional assessment scales: study of persons with multiple sclerosis. *Arch Phys Med Rehabil* 1990; 71:870–875.
115. Heinemann AW, Hamilton BB, Betts HB, Aguda B, Mamott BD. *Rating scale analysis of functional assessment measures.* Chicago, IL: Rehabilitation Institute of Chicago, 1991.
116. Muecke L, Shekar S, Dwyer D, Israel E, Flynn JP. Functional screening of lower limb amputees: a role in predicting rehabilitation outcome? *Arch Phys Med Rehabil* 1992; 73:851–858.
117. Kidd D, Stewart G, Baldry J, et al. The Functional Independence Measure: a comparative validity and reliability study. *Disability Rehabil* 1995; 17:10–14.
118. Fisher WP Jr, Harvey RF, Taylor P, Kilgore KM, Kelly CK. Rehabits: a common language of functional assessment. *Arch Phys Med Rehabil* 1995; 76:113–122.
119. Ottenbacher KJ, Mann WC, Granger CV, Tomita M, Hurren D, Charvat B. Inter-rater agreement and stability of functional assessment in the community-based elderly. *Arch Phys Med Rehabil* 1994; 75: 1297–1301.
120. Segal ME, Schall RR. Determining functional health status and its relation to disability in stroke survivors. *Stroke* 1994; 25:2391–2397.
121. Kaplan CP, Corrigan JD. The relationship between cognition and functional independence in adults with traumatic brain injury. *Arch Phys Med Rehabil* 1994; 75:643–647.
122. Segal ME, Gillard M, Schall R. Telephone and in person proxy agreement between stroke patients and caregivers for the functional independence measure. *Am J Phys Med Rehabil* 1996; 75:208–212.
123. Cowen CD, Meythaler JM, DeVivo MJ, Ivie CS, Lebow J, Novack TA. Influence of early variables In traumatic brain injury on functional independence measure scores and rehabilitation length of stay and charges. *Arch Phys Med Rehabil* 1995; 76:797–803.
124. Granger CV, Divan N, Fiedler RC. Functional assessment scales. A study of persons after traumatic brain injury. *Am J Phys Med Rehabil* 1995; 74:107–113.
125. Granger CV, Divan N, Fiedler RC. Functional assessment scales. A study of persons with multiple sclerosis. *Arch Phys Med Rehabil* 1990; 71:870–875.
126. Segal ME, Schall RR. Determining functional health status and its relation to disability in stroke survivors. *Stroke* 1994; 25:2391–2397.
127. Segal ME, Ditunno JF, Staas WE. Interinstitutional agreement of individual functional independence measure (FIM) items measured at two sites on one sample of SCI patients. *Paraplegia* 1993; 31:622–631.
128. Heinemann AW, Linacre JM, Wright BD, Hamilton BB, Granger C. Relationships between impairment and physical disability as measured by the functional independence measure. *Arch Phys Med Rehabil* 1993; 74:566–573.
129. Granger CV, Cotter AC, Hamilton BB, Fiedler RC. Functional assessment scales: a study of persons after stroke. *Arch Phys Med Rehabil* 1993; 74:133–138.
130. Weh L, Ramb JF. Functional independence measure as a predictor of expected rehabilitation outcome in patients with total endoprosthesis replacement and after apoplectic infarct [in German]. *Z Orthop* 1992; 130:333–338.
131. Tsuji T, Sonoda S, Domen K, Saitoh E, Liu M, Chino N. ADL structure for stroke patients in Japan based on the functional independence measure. *Am J Phys Med Rehabil* 1995; 74:432–438.
132. Turkalj Z, Colja-Matic S, Vlah N, Topoljak D, Pokos L, Zadravec S. [Results of rehabilitation after ischemic cerebrovascular stroke]. *Lijecnicki Vjesnik* 1995; 117:268–271.
133. Brown M, Gordon WA, Diller L. Rehabilitation indicators. In: Halpern AS, Fuhrer MJ. *Functional assessment in rehabilitation.* Baltimore: Paul H Brookes, 1984; 187–204.
134. Harvey RF, Jellinek HM. Patient profiles: utilization in functional performance assessment. *Arch Phys Med Rehabil* 1983; 64:268–271.
135. Harvey RF, Silverstein B, Venzon MM, et al. Applying psychometric criteria to functional assessment in medical rehabilitation: III. Construct validity and predicting level of care. *Arch Phys Med Rehabil* 1992; 73:887–892.
136. Chaudhuri G, Harvey RF, Sulton LD, Lambert R. Computerized to-

mography head scans as predictors of functional outcome of stroke patients. *Arch Phys Med Rehabil* 1988; 69:496–498.
137. Jellinek HM, Torkelson RM, Harvey RF. Functional abilities and distress levels in brain injured patients at long-term follow-up. *Arch Phys Med Rehabil* 1982; 63:160–162.
138. Harvey RF, Jellinek HM. Functional performance assessment: a program approach. *Arch Phys Med Rehabil* 1981; 62:456–461.
139. Silverstein B, Fisher WP, Kilgore KM, Harley JP, Harvey RF. Applying psychometric criteria to functional assessment in medical rehabilitation. II. Defining interval measures. *Arch Phys Med Rehabil* 1992; 73:507–518.
140. Fisher AG. *Assessment of motor and process skills* (Research ed. 7.0). Fort Collins, CO: Department of Occupational Therapy, Colorado State University, 1994.
141. Fisher AG. The assessment of IADL motor skill: an application of the many-faceted Rasch analysis. *Am J Occup Ther* 1993; 47:319–329.
142. Fisher AG, Liu Y, Velozo CA, Pan A. Cross-cultural assessment of process skills. *Am J Occup Ther* 1992; 46:876–885.
143. Nygard L, Bernspang B, Fisher AG, Winbald B. Comparing motor and process ability of persons with suspected dementia in home and clinical settings. *Am J Occup Ther* 1994; 48:689–696.
144. Park S, Fisher AG, Velozo CA. Using the Assessment of Motor and Process Skills to compare occupational performance between clinic and home settings. *Am J Occup Ther* 1994; 48:697–709.
145. Law M, Baptiste S, McColl MA, Carswell-Opzoomer A, Polotajko H, Pollock N. The Canadian Occupational Performance Measure: an outcome measure for occupational therapy. *Can J Occup Ther* 1994; 57:82–87.
146. Pollock N. Client-centered assessment. *Am J Occup Ther* 1993; 47: 298–301.
147. Pollock N, Baptiste S, Law M, McColl MA, Opzoomer A, Polatajko H. Occupational performance measures: a review of based on the guidelines for the client-centered practice of occupational therapy. *Can J Occup Ther* 1990; 57:77–81.
148. Law M, Polotajko H, Pollock N, McColl M, Carswell A, Baptiste S. Pilot testing of the Canadian Occupational Performance Measure: clinical and measurement issues. *Can J Occup Ther* 1994; 61: 191–197.
149. Toomey M, Nicholson D, Carswell A. The clinical utility of the Canadian Occupational Performance Measure. *Can J Occup Ther* 1995; 62:242–249.
150. Weingarden SI, Martin C. Independent dressing after spinal cord injury: a functional time evaluation. *Arch Phys Med Rehabil* 1989; 70: 518–519.
151. Coley IL. *Pediatric assessment of self-care activities.* St. Louis: CV Mosby, 1978.
152. Uniform Data System for Medical Rehabilitation. *Guide for the use of the pediatric functional independence measure.* Buffalo, NY: Research Foundation-State University of New York, 1990.
153. Braun SL, Granger CV. A practical approach to functional assessment in pediatrics. *Occup Ther Pract* 1991; 2:46–51.
154. Ottenbacher KJ, Taylor ET, Msall ME, et al. The stability and equivalence reliability of the functional independence measure for children. *Dev Med Child Neurol* 1996; 38:907–916.
155. Msall ME, DiGaudio KM, Rogers BT, et al. The Functional Independence Measure for Children (WeeFIM). Conceptual basis and pilot use in children with developmental disabilities. *Clin Pediatr* 1994; 33: 421–430.
156. Msall ME, DiGaudio, KM, Duffy, LC. Use of functional assessment in children with developmental disabilities. *Phys Med Rehabil Clin North Am* 1993; 4:517–527.
157. Philip PA, Ayyangar R, Vanderbilt J, Gaebler-Spira DJ. Rehabilitation outcome in children after treatment of primary brain tumor. *Arch Phys Med Rehabil* 1994; 75:36–39.
158. DiScala C, Grant CC, Brooke MM, Gans BM. Functional outcome in children with traumatic brain injury. Agreement between clinical judgment and the functional independence measure. *Am J Phys Med Rehabil* 1992; 71:145–148.
159. Haley SM, Coster WJ, Ludlow LH. *Pediatric evaluation of disability Inventory: development, standardization and administration manual.* Boston: PEDI Research Group, New England Medical Center Hospitals.
160. Haley SM, Ludlow LH, Coster WJ. Pediatric evaluation of disability inventory. *Phys Med Rehabil Clin North Am* 1993; 4:529–540.
161. Feldman AB, Haley SM, Coryell J. Concurrent and construct validity of the Pediatric Evaluation of Disability Inventory. *Phys Ther* 1990; 70:602–610.
162. Bloom KK, Nazar GB. Functional assessment following selective posterior rhizotomy in spastic cerebral palsy. *Childs Nervous System* 1994; 10:84–86.
163. Dudgeon BJ, Libby AK, McLaughlin JF, Hays RM, Bjornson KF, Roberts TS. Prospective measurement of functional changes after selective dorsal rhizotomy. *Arch Phys Med Rehabil* 1994; 75:46–53.
164. Coster WJ, Haley SM, Baryza MJ. Functional performance of young children after traumatic brain injury: a six month follow-up study. *Am J Occup Ther* 1994; 48:211–218.
165. Norburn JE, Bernard SL, Konrad TR, et al. Self care and assistance from others in coping with functional status limitations among a national sample of older adults. *J Gerontol* 1995; 50(suppl):101–109.
166. DeJong G. *Meeting the personal care needs of severely disabled citizens in Massachusetts: report number two.* Waltham, MA: Brandeis University Levinson Policy Distribution, 1977; 239.
167. Neistadt ME, Marques K. An independent living skills training program. *Am J Occup Ther* 1984; 38:671–676.
168. Levine RE. The cultural aspects of home care delivery. *Am J Occup Ther* 1984; 38:734–738.
169. Shillam LL, Beeman C, Loshin PM. Effects of occupational therapy intervention on bathing independence of disabled persons. *Am J Occup Ther* 1983; 37:744–748.
170. Frank G. Life history model of adaptation to disability: the case of a congenital amputee. *Soc Sci Med* 1984; 19:639–645.
171. Cross KW. Role of practice in perceptual-motor learning. *Am J Phys Med* 1967; 46:487–510.
172. Schoening HA, Iversen IA. Numerical scoring of self-care status: a study of the Kenny self-care evaluation. *Arch Phys Med Rehabil* 1968; 49:221–229.
173. Snell ME. Principles for teaching self-care skills. In: Christiansen C, ed. *Ways of living: self care strategies for special needs.* Bethesda, MD: American Occupational Therapy Association, 1994; 77–100.
174. Cross KW. Role of practice in perceptual-motor learning. *Am J Phys Med* 1967; 46:487–510.
175. Snell ME. *Instruction of students with severe disabilities.* New York: Macmillan, 1993.
176. Trombly CA. Activities of daily living. In: Trombly CA, ed. *Occupational therapy for physical dysfunction,* 2nd ed. Baltimore: William & Wilkins, 1984.
177. Jarman PH, Iwata BA, Lorentzson AM. Development of morning self-care routines in multiply handicapped persons. *Appl Res Mental Retardation* 1983;4:113–122.
178. Walker RI, Vogelsberg RT. Increasing independent mobility skills for a woman who was severely handicapped and nonambulatory. *Appl Res Mental Retardation* 1985; 6:173–183.
179. Schwartz RK. *Therapy as learning.* Dubuque, IA: Kendall-Hunt, 1985.
180. Wagenaar RC, Meijer OG. Effects of stroke rehabilitation: a critical review of the literature. *J Rehabil Sci* 1991; 4:61–73.
181. Wagenaar RC, Meijer OG. Effects of stroke rehabilitation: a critical review of the literature. *J Rehabil Sci* 1991; 4:97–109.
182. Trombly CA. Occupation: purposefulness and meaningfulness as therapeutic mechanisms. 1995 Eleanor Clarke Slagle Lecture. *Am J Occup Ther* 1995; 49:960–972.
183. White RW. Motivation reconsidered: the concept of competence. *Psychol Rev* 1959; 66:297–333.
184. Bjornby ER, Reinvang IR. Acquiring and maintaining self-care skills after stroke: the predictive value of apraxia. *Scand J Rehabil Med* 1985; 17:75–80.
185. *ABLEDATA.* Newington, CT: Trace Research and Development Center and Newington Children's Hospital, 1989.
186. Taylor SJ, Trefler E, Nwaobi O. Occupational therapy and rehabilitation engineering: delivering technology to the severely physically disabled. *Occup Ther Health Care* 1984; 1:143–154.
187. Newrick PG, Langton-Hewer R. Motor neuron disease: can we do better? A study of 42 patients. *Br Med J [Clin Res]* 1984; 289: 539–542.
188. Symington DC, Batelaan J, O'Shea BJ, White DA. *Independence through environmental control systems.* Canada: Canadian Rehabilitation Council for the Disabled, 1980.
189. Lees D, Lepage P. Will robots ever replace attendants? Exploring the

current capabilities and future potential of robots in education and rehabilitation. *Int J Rehabil Res* 1994; 17:285–304.

190. Regalbuto MA, Krouskop, TA, Cheatham JB. Toward a practical mobile robotic aid system for people with severe physical disabilities. *J Rehabil Res Dev* 1992; 29:19–26.
191. Stein RB, Walley M. Functional comparison of upper extremity amputees using myoelectric and conventional prostheses. *Arch Phys Med Rehabil* 1983; 64:2443–2448.
192. Smith RO. Technological approaches to performance enhancement. In: Christiansen C, Baum C, eds. *Occupational therapy: overcoming human performance deficits.* Thorofare, NJ: Slack 1991; 747–786.
193. Haworth RJ. Use of aids during the first three months after total hip replacement. *Br J Rheumatol* 1983; 22:29–35.
194. Mann WC, Hurren D, Tomita M. Comparison of assistive device use and needs of home based older persons with different impairments. *Am J Occup Ther* 1993; 47:980–987.
195. Rogers JC, Figone JJ. Traumatic quadriplegia: follow-up study of self-care skills. *Arch Phys Med Rehabil* 1980; 61:316–321.
196. Gitlin LN, Levine R, Geiger C. Adaptive device use by older adults with mixed disabilities. *Arch Phys Med Rehabil* 1993; 74:149–152.
197. Urb'anek T, Si'tajov'a H, Hud'akov'a G. Problems of rheumatoid arthritis and ankylosing spondylitis patients in their labor and life environments. *Czech Med* 1984; 7:78–89.
198. Liang MH, Gell V, Partridge A, Eaton H. Management of functional disability in homebound patients. *J Fam Pract* 1983; 17:429–435.
199. LaPlante MP, Hendershot GE, Moss AJ. *Assistive technology devices and home accessibility features: prevalence, payment, need and trends.* Hyattsville, MD: USDHHS, National Center for Health Statistics. Advance Data from Vital and Health Statistics, 1992; n217.
200. Malassigne PM. *Design of bathrooms, bedroom fixtures and controls for the able bodied and disabled: annual report.* Blacksburg, VA: Virginia Polytechnic Institute and State University College of Architecture and Urban Studies, 1977.
201. Malassigne PM. *Design of bathrooms, bathroom fixtures and controls for the able bodied and disabled: final report.* Blacksburg, VA: Virginia Polytechnic Institute and State University College of Architecture and Urban Studies, 1980.
202. Lowman E, Klinger JL. *Aids to independent living.* New York: McGraw-Hill, 1969.
203. American National Standards Institute (ANSI). *Specifications for making buildings and facilities accessible to and usable by physically handicapped people.* New York: ANSI, 1980.
204. Everett TH, Collignon FC. *Cost and policy considerations in improving the capacity for independent living of the most severely handicapped.* Berkeley, CA: Berkeley Planning Associates, 1975.
205. Larson MR, Snobl DE. *Attendant care manual.* Marshall, MN: Southwest Minnesota State University, 1977.
206. Roberts S, Sydow N. *Consumer's guide to attendant care.* Madison, WI: Access for Independence, 1981.
207. Baum CM, Levesser P. Caregiver assistance: using family members and attendants. In: Christiansen C, ed. *Ways of living: self care strategies for special needs.* Bethesda, MD: American Occupational Therapy Association, 1994; 453–482.
208. Ulicny G, Jones ML. Enhancing the attendant management skills of persons with disabilities. *Am Rehabil* 1985; 2:18–20.
209. World Institute on Disability. *Resolution on personal assistance services.* Passed at the International Personal Assistance Symposium Oakland, CA, September 29 to October 1, 1991.
210. Neill WA, Branch LG, DeJong G. Cardiac disability: the impact of coronary heart disease on patients' daily activities. *Arch Intern Med* 1985; 145:1642–1647.
211. Anstine LA, Isaacs LI. *Diagnostic, predictive and operational significance of self-care (dressing) problems in hemiplegia rehabilitation.* Boston: Boston University Medical Center University Hospital, 1971.
212. Gordon WA, Hibbard MR, Egelko S, et al. Perceptual remediation in patients with right brain damage: a comprehensive program. *Arch Phys Med Rehabil* 1985; 66:353–359.
213. Dudgeon BJ, DeLisa JA, Miller RM. Optokinetic nystagmus and upper extremity dressing independence after stroke. *Arch Phys Med Rehabil* 1985; 66:164–167.
214. Panikoff LB. Recovery trends of functional skills in the head-injured adult. *Am J Occup Ther* 1983; 37:735–743.
215. Goldkamp O. Treatment effectiveness in cerebral palsy. *Arch Phys Med Rehabil* 1984; 65:232–234.
216. Titus M, Gall N, Yerxa EJ, Roberson TA, Mack W. Correlation of perceptual performance and activities of daily living. *Am J Occup Ther* 1991; 45:410–418.
217. Bernsprang B, Asplund K, Erriksson S, Fugl-Meyer A. Motor and perceptual impairments in acute stroke patients: effects on self-care ability. *Stroke* 1987; 18:1081–1086.
218. Stein RB, Wally M. Functional comparison of upper extremity amputees using myoelectric and conventional prosteheses. *Arch Phys Med Rehabil* 1983; 64:2443–2448.
219. Narang IC, Mathur BP, Singh P, Jape VS. Functional capabilities of lower limb amputees. *Prosthet Orthot Int* 1984; 8:43–51.
220. Haworth RJ, Hollings EM. Are hospital assessments of daily living activities valid? *Int Rehabil Med* 1979; 1:59–62.
221. DeJong G, Branch LG, Corcoran PJ. Independent living outcomes in spinal cord injury: multivariate analyses. *Arch Phys Med Rehabil* 1984; 65:66–73.
222. Mills VM, DiGenio M. Functional differences in patients with left or right cerebrovascular accidents. *Phys Ther* 1983; 63:481–488.
223. Wade DT, Hewer RL, Wood VA. Stroke: influence of patient's sex and side of weakness on outcome. *Arch Phys Med Rehabil* 1984; 65: 513–516.

Rehabilitation Medicine: Principles and Practice, Third Edition,
edited by Joel A. DeLisa and Bruce M. Gans.
Lippincott–Raven Publishers, Philadelphia © 1998.

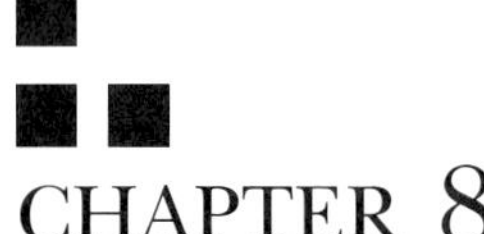

CHAPTER 8

Gait Analysis

D. Casey Kerrigan, Michael Schaufele, and Marco N. Wen

Gait, referring in humans to walking and running, is one of the most fundamental actions in life. Rehabilitation clinicians can especially appreciate the complexity of gait in the face of impairment or functional limitation. Often, an individual has difficulty walking, and for some, gait may be functionally impossible. It is the physiatrist's task to determine the specific causes of why a person cannot walk well, not only at the pathophysiology level, but also at the impairment and functional limitation levels as well. The effectiveness of any physiatric treatment relies heavily on the ability to accurately determine these causes.

NOMENCLATURE

An understanding of gait analysis first requires familiarization with the currently accepted terminology. Because gait is habitual in nature, we often focus our analysis on the functional unit of gait, called the gait cycle, or stride. Various temporal and functional parameters within the gait cycle, presented by Perry and colleagues (1) (Fig. 8-1), form a frame of reference to discuss both nondisabled and disabled gait. This standard classification divides the gait cycle into the stance and swing periods. Similarly, the gait cycle is divided into three basic functional tasks. Weight acceptance and single limb support are the functional tasks occurring during stance, whereas limb advancement is the functional task primarily occurring during swing. These functional tasks are further broken down into eight phases during the gait cycle. The phases of initial contact and loading response comprise the functional task of weight acceptance. The phases of mid-stance and terminal stance comprise single limb support. Limb advancement begins in the final phase of stance (preswing) and then continues through the three phases of swing (initial swing, midswing, and terminal swing). The terms "heel strike" and "toe-off," corresponding to initial contact and preswing, respectively, may be inappropriate and inaccurate in many atypical gait patterns.

Gait velocity refers simply to the speed of gait. Stride time is defined from the time of initial contact of one limb to the next initial contact of the same limb. Step time is defined from the time of initial contact of one limb to the time of initial contact of the contralateral limb. Stride length and step length are the distances covered during their respective time frames. The cadence of gait can be expressed in either strides per minute or steps per minute. At an average walking velocity, the stance period comprises about 60% of the gait cycle, whereas the swing period comprises 40%. In walking, at least one foot is on the ground at all times. During the stance period, there are two time intervals when both feet are on the ground, termed double limb support. One of these time intervals occurs from initial contact into loading response and the other during preswing. Single limb support refers to the time interval in stance when the opposite limb is in swing. At an average walking speed, each double limb support time comprises approximately 10% of the gait cycle, whereas single limb support comprises about 40%. Typical values (1) for temporal gait parameters in adult nondisabled subjects, walking comfortably on a level surface, are summarized in Table 8-1. At slower walking velocities, the double limb support times are greater. Conversely, with increasing walking speeds, the double limb support time intervals decrease. Walking becomes running when there is no longer an interval of time in which both limbs are in contact on the ground.

ENERGY CONSERVATION AND THE DETERMINANTS OF GAIT

To the casual observer, nondisabled walking is a smooth and almost effortless task of locomotion. This efficiency is made possible by minimizing the displacement of the body's center of mass (COM) during walking (2,3). The COM, de-

D. C. Kerrigan, M. Schaufele, and M. N. Wen: Department of Physical Medicine and Rehabilitation, Harvard Medical School; and Spaulding Rehabilitation Hospital, Boston, Massachusetts 02114.

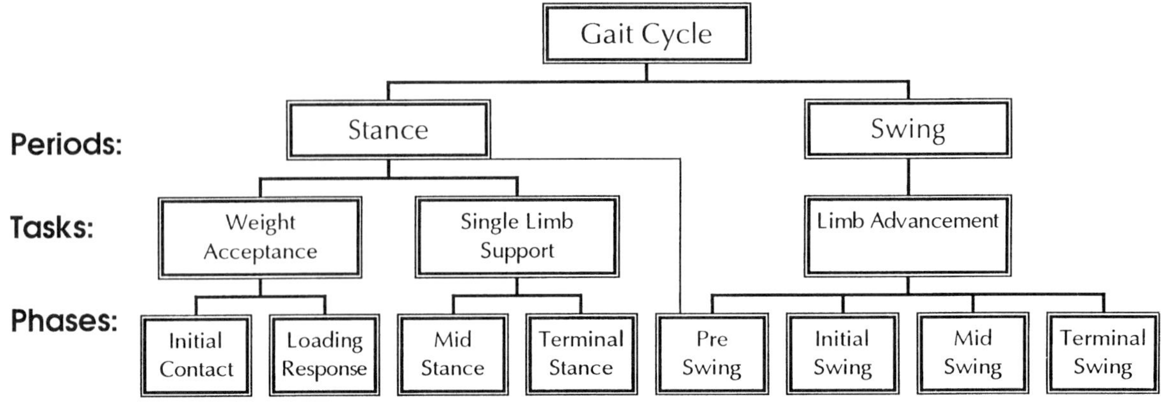

FIG. 8-1. Periods of the gait cycle. The gait cycle is separated into two distinct periods of stance and swing. Functional tasks include weight acceptance and single limb support during stance and limb advancement during swing. The stance period of the gait cycle includes initial contact, loading response, midstance, terminal stance, and preswing. The swing period includes initial swing, midswing, and terminal swing.

fined as the hypothetical point at which all mass can be considered to be concentrated, is located just anterior to the second sacral vertebrae in the average human lying in the anatomic position (4). During walking, the COM normally travels along a sinusoidal up-and-down and side-to-side path with each step. It reaches its highest point during single limb support and its lowest point during double limb support. With regard to efficiency of walking, the vertical displacement of the COM is far more relevant than the lateral displacement (5). The major mechanisms by which the body minimizes the displacement of the COM during walking are via a series of maneuvers described as the determinants of gait by Saunders and colleagues (6):

- Pelvic rotation in the transverse plane
- Pelvic obliquity in the coronal plane
- Lateral displacement in the coronal plane
- Interchange between knee, ankle, and foot motion

The subsequent figures serve as simple models to illustrate how each determinant contributes to reducing the COM displacement. Figure 8-2 demonstrates a hypothetical "compass" that assumes what walking would be like without any of these determinants (6). The legs are represented as rigid levers without foot, ankle, or knee components, and articulations only at the hip joints. Normally, pelvic rotation in the transverse plane reduces the drop in the COM during double limb support (Fig. 8-3). A slight amount of pelvic obliquity (i.e., Trendelenburg) reduces the peak of the COM during single limb support (Fig. 8-4). Diminution of the lateral displacement of the pelvis are influenced by two factors. One, the body is shifted toward the side of the stance limb during loading. Two, the natural valgus between the femur and tibia allow the feet to be closer together during forward progression (Fig. 8-5).

TABLE 8-1. *Typical temporal gait parameters for comfortable walking on level surfaces in adult subjects*[a]

Temporal gait parameter	Average value
Velocity (m/min)	~80
Cadence (steps/min)	113
Stride length (m)	1.41
Stance (percent of gait cycle)	~60
Swing (percent of gait cycle)	~40
Double support (percent per leg per gait cycle)	~10

[a] From Perry J. *Gait analysis: normal and pathological function.* Thorofare, NJ: Slack, 1992.

The interchange between knee, ankle, and foot motion is a mechanism that further reduces the vertical displacement of the COM during walking and helps alter the pattern of COM motion from a series of arcs as in the hypothetical compass gait situation to the actual characteristic smooth sinusoidal appearance (Fig. 8-6). These joint motions are described in detail in a later section. Relevant to this discussion, the ankle moves into controlled plantarflexion from initial contact into loading, and the knee flexes slightly to reduce the peak of COM displacement in single limb support. Also during single limb support, there is progressive ankle dorsiflexion that similarly effectively reduces the peak of COM displacement. The ankle plantarflexes again in double limb support, which effectively raises the COM's lowest point. All of these actions occur gradually and in rhythm so as to also smooth the curve of COM motion during gait.

If it were not for the combined action of the determinants of gait, the average total vertical displacement of COM would be about twice the value that it actually is (7,8). Many impairments and functional limitations can interfere with one or more of these determinants and thus increase the COM displacement and energy cost of walking.

ENERGY COST OF GAIT

At an average comfortable walking velocity of 80 m/min in nondisabled subjects, the energy expenditure is about four times the basal metabolic rate (5). Interestingly, the velocity

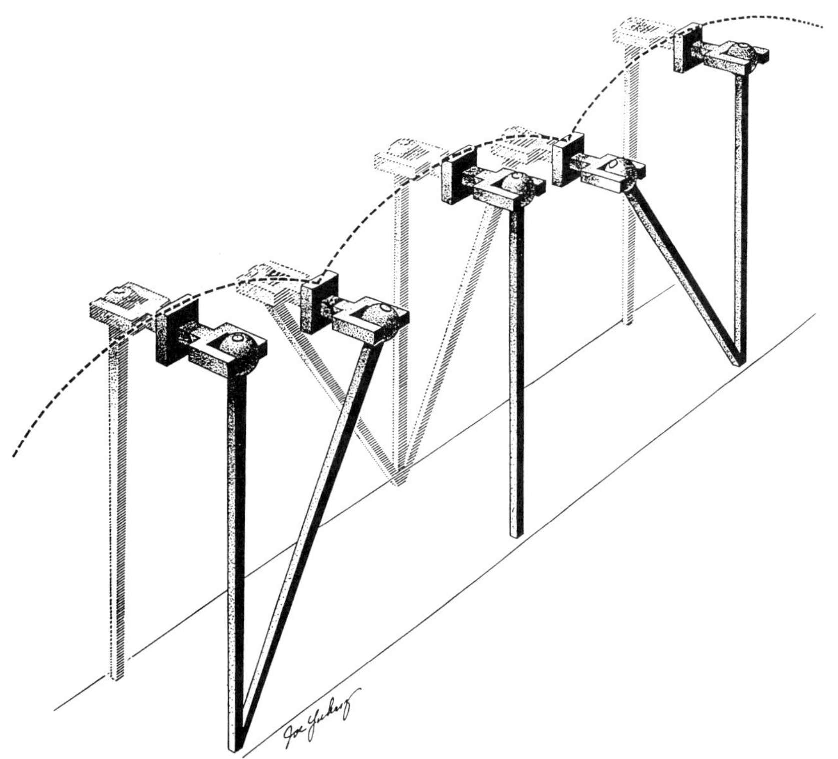

FIG. 8-2. Hypothetical "compass" gait. The pelvis is represented by a single bar with a small cuboid representing the body's COM. The legs are rigid bars articulating only at the hip. No foot, ankle, or knee joints are present. The pathway of the COM is a series of interconnecting arcs. (Reprinted from Rose J, Gamble JG. *Human walking,* 2nd ed. Baltimore: Williams & Wilkins, 1994, with permission.)

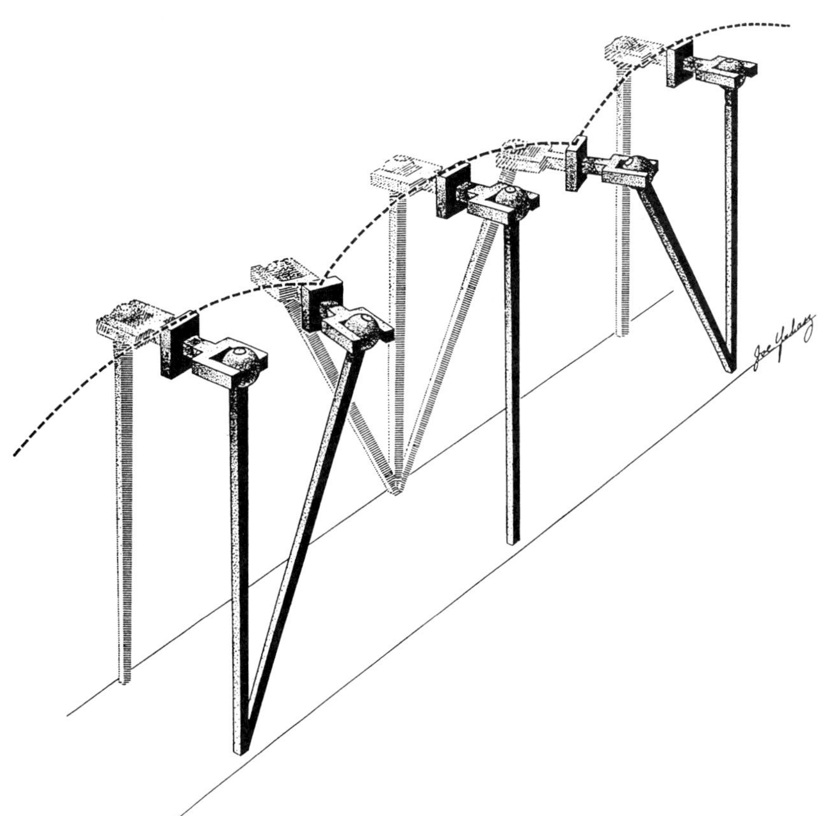

FIG. 8-3. Effect of pelvic rotation in the tranverse plane. The slight rotation of the pelvis in the transverse plane during double-limb support reduces the elevation needed by the COM when passing over the weight-bearing leg during midstance. (Reprinted from Rose J, Gamble JG. *Human walking,* 2nd ed. Baltimore: Williams & Wilkins, 1994, with permission.)

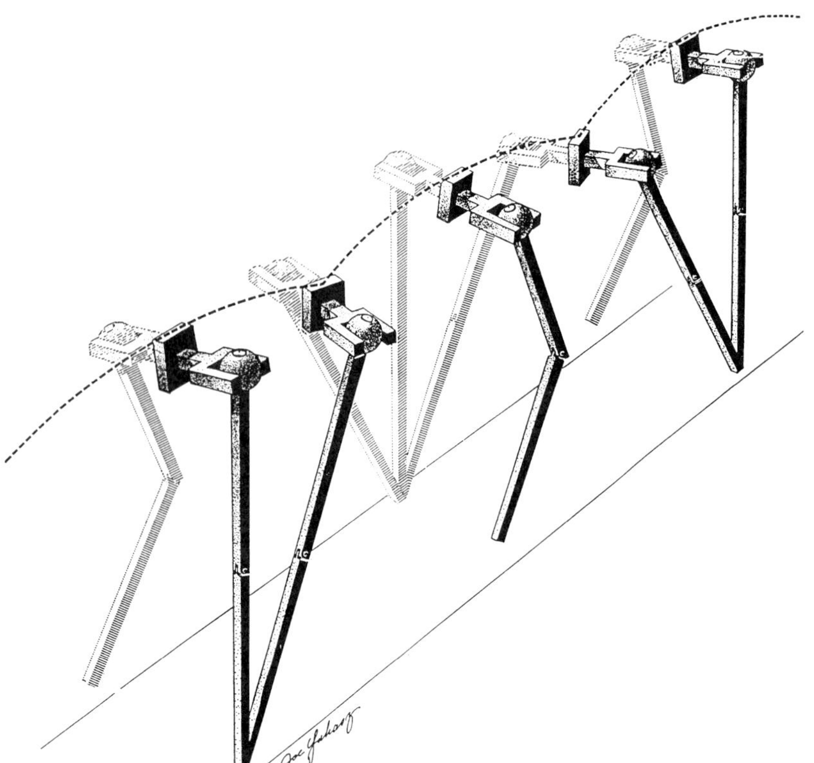

FIG. 8-4. Pelvic obliquity during single-limb support. A drop in the pelvis on the non–weight-bearing side allows for a reduction in the peak height of the COM during mid-stance. (Reprinted from Rose J, Gamble JG. *Human walking,* 2nd ed. Baltimore: Williams & Wilkins, 1994, with permission.)

that subjects choose as their comfortable speed is also the velocity that requires the least energy per unit distance (9). Walking faster or running usually requires anaerobic metabolism. On the other hand, walking slower requires extra energy, probably for balance support, rather than for propelling the body forward (10). Importantly, the rate of energy expended during comfortable walking is consistent across the nondisabled and disabled gait populations (5). A person with a gait disability tends to walk slower than a person without a gait disability (11). Thus, although the energy expenditure per unit time is consistent in subjects with gait disability, increases in energy expenditure per unit distance are common. For instance, patients with hemiplegia affecting their gait spend the same amount of energy per time during comfortable walking as subjects without gait disability, but they walk slower and spend 37% (12) to 62% (13) more energy per unit distance.

An important aim of improving gait disability may be to reduce the energy required to walk. To this end, the effectiveness of a particular type of rehabilitation treatment can be assessed by evaluating the energy expended during walking. The most direct method to evaluate energy expended is via measuring the oxygen that is consumed during walking. This involves having the subject breathe into a mask that is linked to a gas analyzer. The analyzer determines how much oxygen is being used, and from this, a calculation of energy expenditure is given, based on the knowledge that about 4.83 kcal of energy is expended for every liter of oxygen consumed (5). Alternatively, an estimate of energy expended can be obtained by measuring heart rate before and during walking because the change in heart rate that occurs with walking is linearly correlated with oxygen consumption measurements (14). An easier, although more indirect, method to evaluate the energy required to walk is to measure the comfortable walking speed. This can be performed using a stopwatch and a designated walking distance. This simple measure rests on the fact noted above that subjects with gait disability tend to walk at a consistent energy rate, just slower. Thus, comfortable walking speed relates indirectly to the energy required to walk. Unfortunately, all of these measures, including oxygen consumption, heart rate, and comfortable walking speed, relate not only to biomechanical aspects of walking, but to cardiopulmonary conditioning and psychological factors including mood as well. Quantitative gait measures described in a later section, although useful in determining the mechanisms of the gait impairment, are insufficient in evaluating the efficiency of walking. A so-called biomechanical efficiency quotient was proposed (8,15) based on the concept of minimizing the COM displacement through the determinants of gait. This measure was introduced as a means to specifically evaluate biomechanical walking efficiency in subjects with gait disability, independent of cardiopulmonary conditioning and psychological factors. The quotient is the measured vertical displacement of the COM divided by the predicted vertical displacement, the latter being a function of the subject's average stride length and height of the pelvis from the ground. Patients with gait disability tend to have higher biomechanical

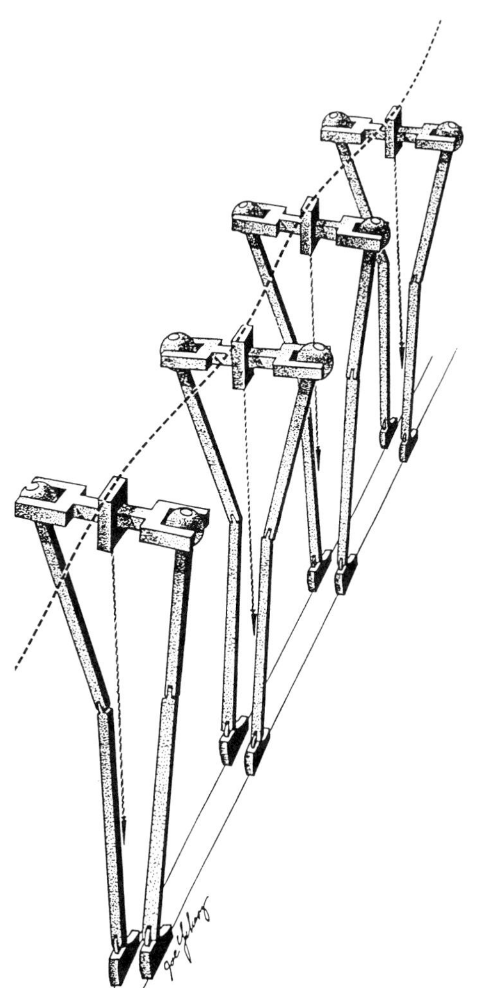

FIG. 8-5. Effect of narrowing the walking base. A shift in the position of the body over the stance limb, combined with the natural valgus between the femur and tibia allow for a reduction in the lateral displacement of the pelvis. Reduction in the width of the gait cycle reduces the displacement of the COM. (Reprinted from Rose J, Gamble JG. *Human walking,* 2nd ed. Baltimore: Williams & Wilkins, 1994, with permission.)

efficiency quotients than subjects without gait disability and treatments such as an ankle-foot-orthosis tend to reduce the biomechanical efficiency quotient (15).

CONCEPTS FOR UNDERSTANDING GAIT EVENTS

Inasmuch as the determinants of gait result in a more efficient method of human locomotion, they make human walking a rather complex concept to understand. In order to evaluate the mechanisms of a gait disability and therefore to identify individualized therapeutic interventions, a basic knowledge of the events during a normal gait cycle is necessary. Kinematics describe the spatial motions of joints and limb segments. Quantitative gait analysis, described in a later section, can be used to quantitate normal kinematics during the gait cycle (16,17). However, observational gait analysis also can provide important qualitative kinematic information. Kinetics describe the moments or torques and forces that cause joint and limb motion, and these are not intuitive from observational gait analysis. Only quantitative gait analysis can provide kinetic information. Similarly, the firing patterns of muscles can be determined only with the aid of dynamic electromyographic (EMG) measurement used in quantitative gait analysis.

Broadly speaking, the study of kinetics includes the study of muscular activity as well as the study of forces, calculated using physics, and provides insight about the causes of the observed kinematics. In quantitative gait analysis, we are often interested in computing the net moments acting on muscles, tendons, and ligaments. A moment about a joint occurs when a force is acting at a distance from the joint through a lever, causing acceleration of the joint angle. For instance, an externally applied extensor moment about the elbow is produced when a weight is placed in the hand. In this case, the lever is the forearm and the elbow will tend to accelerate uncontrollably into extension. The external moment can be mathematically calculated as the product of the weight of the object and the length of the forearm. In order that a joint angle remains stable, all the moments acting about the joint must sum to zero. An internal force from the biceps humerus acting through its forearm lever can provide a resisting internal flexor moment such that the elbow joint is stabilized. Depending on the magnitude of the force through the biceps, the elbow joint angle will extend in a controlled fashion (eccentric contraction), stay the same (isometric contraction), or flex (concentric contraction). These concepts are applied repeatedly in gait analysis. At each point in the gait cycle, the hip, knee, and ankle joints are stabilized, such that all the moments about a particular joint are in a state of equilibrium. The externally applied moments from gravity, inertia, and the ground are countered by internal joint moments generated by muscle activity and/or soft tissue. During the swing period of the gait cycle, most of the external moments occurring about the lower limb joints are a result of gravitational and inertial forces from the individual limb segments. For instance, during swing, both the weight of the foot and the inertial force from the swinging lower leg will generate an external plantarflexor moment that needs to be restrained by an internal dorsiflexion moment provided by the ankle dorsiflexors in order to prevent foot drop.

During the stance period of the gait cycle, most of the external moments occurring about the hip, knee, and ankle joints are produced from the ground reaction force (GRF). In quiet standing, the body weight pushes against the ground. The ground reacts with an equal and opposite GRF, the vector of which passes through the base of support (the feet) up toward the COM of the body. When we walk, the GRF is essentially a result of both the weight of the body and the body's accelerations and decelerations as our COM moves up and down. Knowing where the line of the GRF lies with

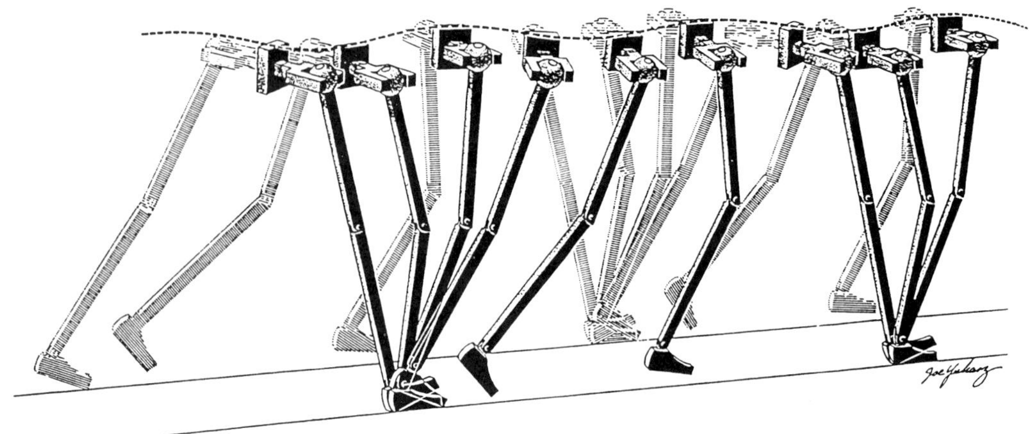

FIG. 8-6. Sinusoidal pathway of the COM. The combined interaction of the knee, ankle, and foot allows for the reduction and smoothing out of the displacement of the COM. (Reprinted from Rose J, Gamble JG. *Human walking,* 2nd ed. Baltimore: Williams & Wilkins, 1994, with permission.)

respect to the hip, knee, and ankle joints gives us a reasonable approximation of the external moments occurring about each of these joints. The GRF can be directly measured with a force plate, described later in the quantitative gait analysis section. A more exact estimation of the external moments during the stance period, which includes the additional effects of gravitational and inertial forces, is ordinarily performed with quantitative gait analysis. These additional gravitational and inertial forces are small during stance at slow and normal walking speeds and thus can be ignored for now in understanding normal gait function (18). Visualizing where the GRF lies with respect to a joint provides a means to understand what internal moments must be generated in order to stabilize that joint. For instance, if the GRF line lies posterior to the knee, an external knee flexor moment is produced that is the product of the GRF multiplied by the distance of the GRF line from the knee joint. In order to maintain stability so that the knee does not collapse uncontrollably into flexion, an internal knee extensor moment must occur. This moment, provided by the knee extensors, is equal in magnitude to the external flexor moment.

The concept of joint stabilization and the importance of knowing where the GRF lies in relation to the joints are best exemplified during quiet standing. In quiet standing, the GRF extends from the ground through the mid-foot, passing anterior to the ankle and knee joints and posterior to the hip joints (Fig. 8-7). At the hip, the external extensor moment is countered passively by the iliofemoral ligaments. Similarly, at the knee, the external knee extensor moment is countered passively by the posterior capsule and ligaments at the knee. At the ankle, the external dorsiflexion moment can be countered with an internal ankle plantarflexor moment provided by the ankle plantarflexors (or alternatively with an ankle-foot-orthosis with a dorsiflexion stop equivalent). Thus, the only lower extremity muscles that need to be con-

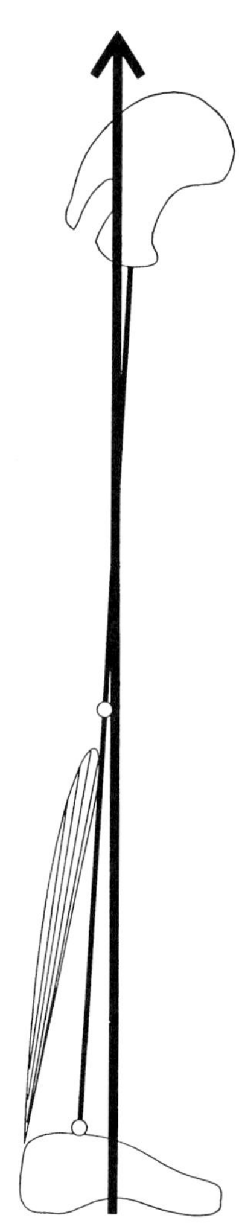

FIG. 8-7. Quiet standing. The GRF, represented by the *solid line* with an *arrow,* is located anterior to the knee and ankle and posterior to the hip. The soleus muscle is active to stabilize the lower limb.

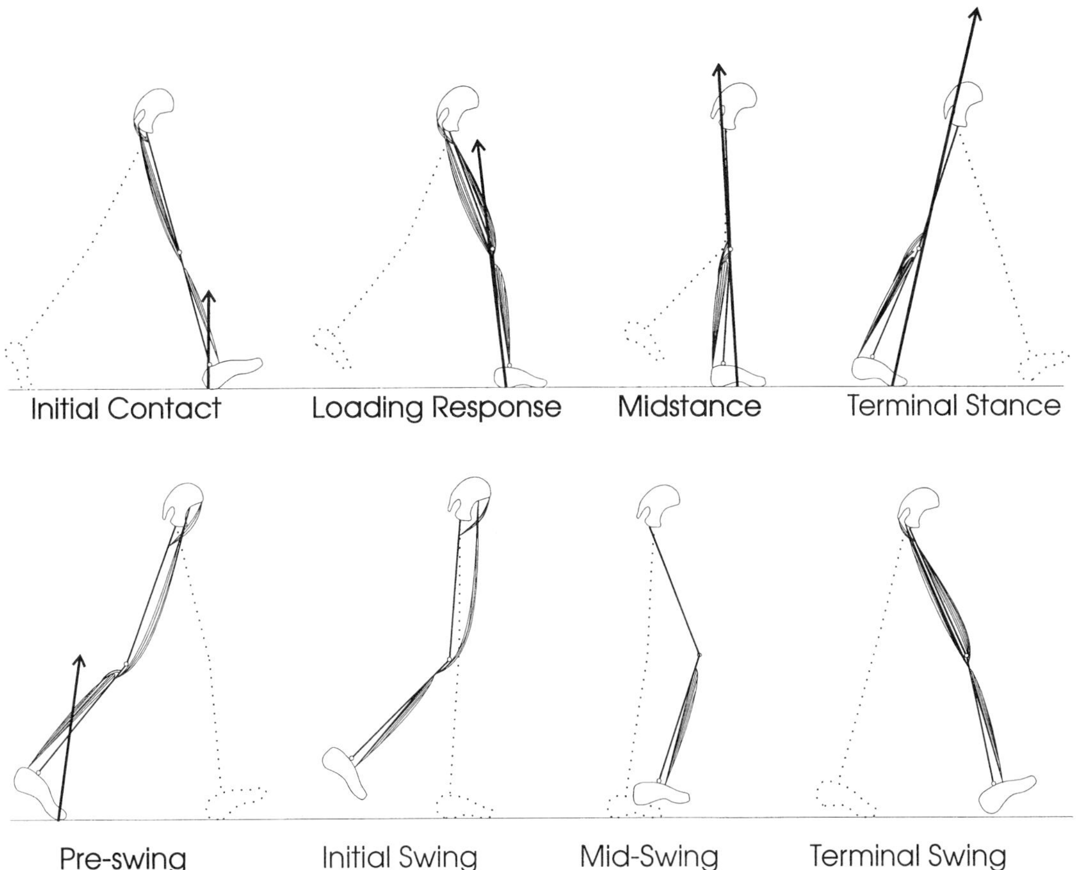

FIG. 8-8. The eight phases of the gait cycle include initial contact, loading response, midstance, terminal stance, preswing, initial swing, midswing, and terminal swing. The GRF vector is represented by a *solid line* with an *arrow*. The active muscles are shown during each phase of the gait cycle. The uninvolved limb is shown as a *dotted line*.

sistently active during quiet standing are the ankle plantarflexors.

During walking, the GRF line moves in a posterior-anterior direction as the body progresses forward (Fig. 8-8). During loading response, the vector is anterior to the hip and posterior to the knee and ankle. In mid-stance, the vector passes through the hip and knee joints and is anterior to the ankle. During terminal stance, the vector moves posterior to the hip, anterior to the knee joint, and maximally anterior to the ankle. With these dynamics in mind, normal gait function is easier to interpret. The muscles fire in response to the need for joint stability. Furthermore, whether the muscle is firing concentrically or eccentrically depends on the corresponding joint motion at that time. In quantitative gait analysis, whether a muscle group is firing concentrically or eccentrically can be determined by measuring the joint power that is mathematically the product of the joint moment and the joint angular velocity. A positive joint power implies that the muscle group is firing concentrically, whereas a negative joint power implies that the muscle group is firing eccentrically. Interestingly, most of the muscle activity that occurs in walking is eccentric. Also, it is interesting to note that each muscle group undergoes a phase of stretching and or eccentric contraction before each concentric contraction.

NORMAL KINEMATICS, KINETICS, AND MUSCLE FUNCTION

The following descriptions of normal kinematics, kinetics, and muscle activity are based on data collected from the Spaulding Rehabilitation Hospital Gait Laboratory and are similar to those reported elsewhere. The following general patterns of movement are fairly representative in nondisabled subjects across most ages after the age of 3 years (19,20).

Sagittal Plane Motion

For each phase, the kinematics, kinetics, and muscle activities are described. Figure 8-8 illustrates the chief actions occurring in each phase with a visual representation of the limb and joint positions, the GRF line, and the muscles that are active during that phase. It also may be useful to refer to Figure 8-12, later in this chapter, which graphically demonstrate the joint motion, moments, and powers throughout the gait cycle.

Initial Contact

Initial contact with the ground typically occurs with the heel in nondisabled gait. The hip is maximally flexed at 30°, the knee is fully extended, and the ankle is in a neutral position. Because the GRF is anterior to the hip, the hip extensors (gluteus maximus and hamstrings) are firing to maintain hip stability. At the knee, the GRF creates an extensor moment, which is countered by hamstring activity. The foot is supported in a neutral position by the ankle dorsiflexors.

Loading Response

The primary purpose of loading response is to provide weight acceptance and shock absorption while maintaining forward progression. The hip extends and will continue to extend into the terminal stance phase. Because the GRF is anterior to the hip, the hip extensors must be active to resist uncontrolled hip flexion. This hip extension implies that the hip extensors are concentrically active. With the location of the GRF now posterior to the knee joint, an external flexor moment is created. This external moment is resisted by an eccentric contraction of the quadriceps allowing knee flexion to approximately 20°. Because the GRF is posterior to the ankle, an external plantarflexion moment occurs that rapidly lowers the foot into 10° of plantarflexion. This action is controlled by an eccentric contraction of the ankle dorsiflexors. At the end of loading response, the foot is in full contact with the ground.

Midstance

During midstance, the limb supports the full body weight as the contralateral limb swings forward. The GRF vector passes through the hip joint, eliminating the need for hip extensor activity. At the knee, the GRF moves from a posterior to an anterior position, similarly eliminating the need for quadriceps activity. Knee extension occurs and is restrained passively by the knee's posterior capsule and ligaments and is possibly actively restrained as well by eccentric popliteus and gastrocnemius action. At the ankle, the GRF is anterior to the ankle, thus producing an external ankle dorsiflexion moment. This moment is countered by the ankle plantarflexors, which eccentrically limit the dorsiflexion occurring during this phase.

Terminal Stance

In terminal stance the body's mass continues to progress over the limb as the trunk falls forward. The GRF at the hip is now posterior, creating an extensor moment that is countered passively by the iliofemoral ligaments. The hip is now maximally extended at 10°. At the knee, the GRF moves from an anterior to a slightly posterior position. As the heel rises from the ground, the GRF becomes increasingly anterior to the ankle joint, and this dorsiflexion moment continues to be stabilized by ankle plantarflexor activity. During this phase, the ankle is plantarflexing; thus, the action of the ankle plantarflexors has switched from eccentric to concentric.

Preswing

The purpose of preswing is to begin propelling the limb forward into swing. This second interval of double limb support is occurring as the contralateral limb now advances through initial contact and loading response. From maximal hip extension, the hip now begins flexing and will continue flexing throughout the swing period. The hip flexors (combined activation of the iliopsoas, hip adductors, and rectus femoris) are concentrically active. The knee swiftly flexes into 40° of flexion as the GRF progresses rapidly posterior to the knee. Knee flexion may be controlled by rectus femoris activity. Thus, the rectus femoris is simultaneously acting concentrically at the hip and eccentrically at the knee. The ankle continues plantarflexing to approximately 20° with continued concentric activity of the ankle plantarflexors.

Initial Swing

The purpose of initial swing is to continue propelling the limb forward. Hip flexion occurs because of the hip flexion momentum initiated in preswing and the continued concentric activity of the hip flexors. During initial swing, the limb accelerates mainly as a result of concentric hip flexor activity. The knee continues to flex to approximately 65°. This knee flexion occurs passively as a combined result of hip flexion and the momentum generated from preswing. The ankle dorsiflexors are concentrically active as the ankle dorsiflexes.

Midswing

In midswing the limb continues to advance forward, primarily as a pendulum from inertial forces generated in pre- and initial swing. The hip continues to flex, now passively, as a result of the momentum generated in initial swing. The knee begins to extend passively as a result of gravity. The ankle remains in a neutral position with the continued activity of the ankle dorsiflexors.

Terminal Swing

At terminal swing the previously generated momentum has to be controlled to maintain sufficient stability before the upcoming weight acceptance phase. At the hip and knee joint, strong eccentric contraction of the hamstrings decelerate hip flexion and control knee extension. The ankle dorsiflexors remain active to ensure a neutral ankle position at initial contact.

Coronal and Transverse Plane Motion

Most lower extremity motion during gait occurs in the sagittal planes. The joint motions and kinetics about the hip in the transverse plane and about the knee and ankle in both the coronal and transverse planes are normally quite small. Although significant motion and associated moments occur in these planes in various gait disabilities, it is difficult to reliably measure these parameters with current quantitative gait analysis techniques. However, significant coronal plane motion and kinetics do occur about the hip (and pelvis) normally and can be accurately evaluated with quantitative analysis. At initial contact both the pelvis and hip are in neutral positions in the coronal plane. During loading response, GRF passes medially to the hip joint center as the opposite limb is unloading. This medial GRF causes an external adductor moment, which tends to allow the contralateral side of the pelvis to drop slightly (the slight Trendelenburg noted previously as one of the determinants of gait). This motion is controlled by eccentric contraction of the hip abductors. During mid-stance and terminal stance, the GRF is still medial to the hip; however, now the contralateral side of the pelvis is lifted concentrically by the hip abductors. During preswing, unloading of the limb causes the ipsilateral side of the pelvis to drop again.

GENERAL APPROACH TO EVALUATING A PATIENT WITH AN ATYPICAL GAIT PATTERN

Although a number of atypical gait patterns have been described, each patient has a unique set of impairments, functional limitations, and associated compensations causing these patterns. Examples of atypical gait patterns associated with distinct diagnoses are described in the following sections. Especially in the case of upper motor neuron (UMN) pathology, a stereotypical description of the gait pattern may be sufficient for an initial classification but is too imprecise for determining the mechanisms in an individual patient. It is important to determine these mechanisms in individual patients because they are the basis for directing optimal rehabilitation treatment.

It should be noted that an atypical gait pattern may or may not be functionally significant and thus may or may not be considered a true gait disability. Thus, the atypical gait pattern first should be evaluated with respect to each of the following:

- Energy requirement
- Risk of falling
- Biomechanical injury
- Cosmesis

Treatment to change the gait pattern should be prescribed if the pattern is functionally significant with respect to these four criteria. For instance, the pattern of knee recurvatum (or hyperextension) can be functionally significant if it increases the energy required to walk by not allowing the peak of the COM to be minimized during single limb support. Alternatively, knee recurvatum may or may not be associated with increased forces across the posterior capsule and ligaments of the knee (21), which would predispose to biomechanical injury. Another example is equinus during the swing period, which may or may not predispose to falling depending on the associated compensations. To this end, the associated compensatory gait patterns also need to be evaluated with respect to these four criteria. In the case of equinus in swing, a compensation at the pelvis such as hip hiking would interfere with the pelvic obliquity determinant and thus increase the energy required to walk. Finally, an atypical gait pattern should be evaluated with respect to cosmesis. For this assessment, the patient's own perceptions are far more important than the clinician's perceptions.

From the examples above, it is clear that a detailed evaluation of the patient is required. The summary of the patient's history and musculoskeletal examination, observational gait analysis, and information from a quantitative gait analysis assist in determining the functional significance of the gait patterns and help identify specific causes for each pattern. Based on these results, a detailed treatment plan can be prescribed.

STATIC EVALUATION

History

The initial part of a comprehensive gait evaluation should include a focused history and physical examination. Based on this evaluation, the underlying diagnosis (or diagnoses) can be classified as a UMN pathology, lower motor neuron (LMN) pathology, orthopedic disorder, amputation (the evaluation of which is described in another chapter), cerebellar or basal ganglia related disorder, or psychogenic cause, to name a few. It is helpful to anticipate certain gait patterns associated with these diagnoses as well as to anticipate the need for various components of a quantitative gait analysis. For example, the use of dynamic EMG is particularly useful in detecting inappropriate firing patterns in patients with UMN pathology but may not be necessary for every patient with one of the other mentioned diagnostic categories. The reason for referral should be identified, and the patient's chief complaint with regard to walking should be considered. Any previous medications, neurolytic procedures, or surgeries affecting the lower extremities should be noted. Also, a detailed history of strengthening and stretching exercises previously and currently being performed should be ascertained. Finally, the use of assistive devices and/or orthotics should be recorded.

Physical Examination

The physical examination should focus on the neurologic and musculoskeletal system and include a static evaluation of the patient's strength, joint range of motion, tone, and proprioception. Although static evaluation is a routine part of a gait consultation and should be included in the assessment of every patient with an atypical gait pattern, it is generally agreed upon that, especially in the case of an UMN pathology, the static evaluation has limited usefulness in determining the underlying mechanisms responsible for the atypical gait pattern (22–24). Thus, often the results from the static evaluation need to be combined with those obtained from quantitative gait analysis to provide dynamically relevant information on which to base treatment.

Strength

Classic evaluation of strength involves quantitative manual muscle testing about each joint. It requires the ability of the patient to cooperate with resistive movement of the examiner (25), which often is difficult in patients presenting with a UMN pathology. The patient with a UMN pathology has impaired voluntary muscle control in the affected limbs so that selectively activating an agonist while simultaneously relaxing the antagonist may be impossible. Thus, the result is a limited relationship between static strength performance and dynamic strength associated with gait. For example, a patient with hemiplegia affecting his or her gait may not be able to dorsiflex the foot during static examination, yet when walking may be able to actively dorsiflex during the swing period of the gait cycle (26,27), presumably under the control of primitive reflexes. Conversely, a patient with normal dorsiflexion strength of the ankle during static evaluation may demonstrate an equinus gait during the swing period of gait.

Range of Motion

Determining the passive range of motion at each joint is the traditional method to assess soft tissue contracture and should be performed in at least the lower extremities in all patients presenting with a gait disability. However, it is important to note that this static testing is somewhat limited, particularly in the case of UMN pathology. Differentiating between contracture of a one-joint and a two-joint muscle is difficult in patients with a UMN pathology, undoubtedly because of impaired selective control of these muscles. Furthermore, there seems to be a limited relationship between static range of motion observed with passive ranging and the dynamic range of motion that occurs during gait.

Three clinical tests are commonly performed in patients with UMN pathology to screen for contractures of a two-joint muscle. The Duncan-Ely-test differentiates between a rectus femoris and a iliopsoas contracture given that the rectus femoris is both a hip flexor and knee extensor. In this test, the patient is placed in a prone position and the knee is rapidly flexed. With a contracture of the rectus femoris, the hips will flex and the buttocks will rise off the table. Although this test is somewhat useful, EMG studies have demonstrated that this test induces activity not only in the rectus femoris, but also in the iliopsoas in some patients with cerebral palsy affecting their gait (28). The Silverskiold test is used to differentiate between a contracture of the soleus and the gastrocnemius muscle. Whereas the soleus is a one-joint muscle, the gastrocnemius is both a knee flexor and ankle plantarflexor. With the patient in the sitting position, the knee is flexed at 90° and the foot is brought to maximal dorsiflexion. With a gastrocnemius contracture, some of the ankle dorsiflexion will be lost when the knee is extended. It has been shown that this test is not always clinically reliable (29). The Phelps test differentiates a contracture of the gracilis from the other hip abductors, given that the gracilis is the only hip adductor that crosses the hip and the knee. With the patient in a prone position, the knees are flexed and the hips are brought into an abducted position. A gracilis contracture is present when the hip adducts when one knee is extended.

Structural deformities also may contribute to reduced range of motion and gait. If indicated, further clinical tests and x-rays are helpful to document common problems such as femoral anteversion, knee valgus and varus, tibial torsion, and foot abnormalities. These structural problems are sometimes associated with other underlying diagnoses and impairments and can have significant impact on the patient's walking.

Tone

Tone in all muscle groups should be assessed in each patient presenting with a gait disability. Clinical examination of tone involves testing for resistance by passively moving a joint through its range of motion. This assessment is fairly subjective and is dependent on time of day, temperature, and limb position. Thus, as in the other static tests, there is often a limited association between what is observed statically and what actually occurs during gait.

Proprioception

Joint sense position should be evaluated in all patients in whom a neurologic diagnosis is suspected. If this is impaired, it is important to also evaluate the degree of impairment by evaluating joint position sense not only at the great toe, but at the ankle, knee, and hip as well.

OBSERVATIONAL GAIT ANALYSIS

Observational gait analysis is common practice for physiatrists. The observer describes the gait after watching the patient walk without the aid of any electronic devices. However, it is often difficult to appreciate all limb segment and joint motions throughout the different phases of gait because of the difficulty in concurrently observing the multiple body segments and joint motion (30). Videotaping can be an important part of observational gait analysis because it allows repeated viewing of the patient's gait pattern without causing undue patient fatigue. The patient should be observed from the side and from behind. Stride and step length, width, and symmetry should be noted. By concentrating on one joint at a time, including hip, knee, and ankle, atypical motions may be easier to identify. Having the patient walk at faster speed sometimes exaggerates an atypical motion. Observational gait analysis can identify obvious atypical gait patterns, such as excessive ankle plantarflexion or reduced knee flexion in swing. However, in certain cases this approach may not show all atypical patterns. For example, an increased lumbar lordosis or anterior pelvic tilt due to a hip flexion contracture may be apparent only via quantitative analysis. Moreover, quantitative gait analysis can be quite helpful in delineating the specific causes for each atypical pattern and thus help direct the appropriate treatment.

A number of terms are commonly used to characterize various atypical gait patterns that are obvious from observational assessment alone. For instance, antalgic gait has been described as a pattern common to patients with pain in one lower extremity. In this pattern, gait is modified to reduce weight bearing on the involved side. The uninvolved limb is rapidly advanced to shorten stance on the affected side. Gait is often slow and steps are short in order to limit the weight-bearing period. Steppage gait is a compensatory gait pattern used to describe excessive hip and knee flexion to assist a ''functionally long'' lower leg to clear the ground in swing. Festinating gait have been described as a characteristic pattern of Parkinson's disease, in which there is a tendency to take short accelerating steps. Shuffling gait is also common in Parkinson's disease and refers to the feet shuffling during swing. Ataxic gait, associated with cerebellar pathologies, peripheral neuropathies, and dorsal column pathologies, is a broad term used to describe a pattern of apparent poor balance, a wide base of support, and variable motions from stride to stride.

Various gait patterns associated with the use of assistive gait devices are easily noted with observational analysis. The specific indications and use of each of these type of devices are described in detail in another chapter. A cane essentially increases the base of support by providing an additional point of contact with the ground. When pathology, impairment, and functional limitation involve bilateral extremities, two canes or crutches are occasionally used. In this situation, an alternating two-point gait is commonly used in which one cane and opposite lower limb are in contact with the ground alternating with the opposite cane and lower limb in each successive step. In three-point gait, contact with one limb that fully bears weight onto the ground alternates with full weight-bearing through two crutches that make simultaneous contact with the ground. In four-point gait, which provides maximal stability and base of support (at the cost of reduced speed of locomotion), there is always three points of support on the ground at all times. It is initiated by forward movement by an upper extremity crutch, followed by forward movement of the contralateral lower limb, then forward movement of the other crutch followed by forward movement of the other lower limb.

QUANTITATIVE GAIT EVALUATION

Modern-day quantitative gait analysis systems typically include measurement of three primary components: kinematics, kinetics, and muscle activity. Quantitative gait analysis also can include other components such as footswitches and oxygen consumption monitoring to measure overall energy expenditure. To measure these various components, a variety of equipment is used, including optoelectronic motion analysis systems to measure kinematics, force plates to help measure kinetics, and a multi-channel dynamic EMG apparatus to measure electrical muscle activity in multiple muscles during gait. Given the previously described limitations of static evaluations and of observational gait analysis, quantitative gait analysis can be a particularly useful clinical tool for developing a treatment plan.

Modern quantitative gait analysis is clearly recognized as useful in outlining an effective orthopedic surgical treatment plan in patients with spastic paretic gait from cerebral palsy (23,31–33). Children with cerebral palsy often undergo tendon lengthening or transfer procedures to improve range of motion in the lower extremities in an effort to improve gait disability. The results from a detailed quantitative gait analysis can help determine the best surgical plan (i.e., which tendons should be lengthened or transferred) to provide the most optimal gait. In the same way that quantitative gait analysis is helpful in orthopedic decision making in patients with UMN pathology, it should be similarly useful in directing these patients' rehabilitation management. Many physiatric treatments, as described in other chapters, include intramuscular neurolytic techniques, strengthening, bracing, functional electrical stimulation, stretching, modalities, and many other management techniques aimed at (a) strengthening or compensating for weakness, (b) stretching a contracture, and/or (c) reducing tone in a spastic muscle. The outcome of these treatments ultimately rely on the proper determination of the specific underlying impairment or functional limitation causing the gait disability. In some instances, rehabilitation treatments are aimed at improving motor control through, for example, EMG biofeedback or neuromuscular re-education. In these instances, quantitative gait analysis is especially helpful in determining which specific muscle groups are firing at inappropriate times.

Unfortunately, skepticism still persists about the value of quantitative gait analysis in defining a physiatric therapeutic plan because there have been few reports about the value of quantitative gait analysis as a useful evaluation tool in rehabilitation. Human gait is complex. Quantitative analysis offers a clinical tool to better understand these complexities and thus prescribe an optimal rehabilitation treatment program (34). Some of the reluctance in using quantitative gait analysis may be due to the heavy time commitment necessary to understand and interpret the data and the necessity for teamwork between many disciplines, including medicine and engineering. The cost for gait analysis systems is declining, and the technology required for acquiring and analyzing the data is continually improving. A rapid expansion of computer and optoelectronic technology has brought dramatic changes in image-based motion analysis in the past 10 years. It is anticipated that quantitative gait analysis will soon become a routine clinical evaluation, much like electrodiagnosis has become a routine clinical extension of our physiatric examination. Formal training in quantitative gait analysis, which is already a mandatory part of our physiatric residency curriculum, is likely to become the norm.

Systems to Evaluate Temporal Parameters of Gait

Common temporal parameters such as velocity, cadence, and stride length can be measured to monitor a patient's progress outside of a sophisticated gait laboratory. As noted previously, velocity can be measured simply with a stopwatch as a patient traverses a designated distance. Similarly, step and stride length can be measured without sophisticated equipment if the walkway is sprinkled with talcum powder. Computerized stride analyzers may provide this same information in a more automated fashion (35,36). They usually consist of instrumented insoles with footswitches (i.e., pressure sensitive transducers), typically attached to the heel, toe, and occasionally the metatarsal region. They are connected to data boxes worn by the patient either around the waist or the ankle. These sensors measure the duration of floor contact via opening and closing switches. After acquisition, data transfer and analysis are typically performed using a personal computer.

Footswitches are also commonly used in gait laboratories to help determine the beginning and end of the stance period, allowing calculation of temporal gait parameters such as the duration of the stance and swing periods, single and double support time, and cadence. These parameters are useful in interpreting the temporal relationships of kinematic, kinetic, and particularly dynamic EMG data. Although this same information can be obtained directly from force plate data, footswitches are particularly helpful in the gait laboratory when force plate data cannot be obtained.

Foot Pressure Systems

Foot pressure systems are electronic instruments to measure pressure distributions in the soles of the feet. The systems work via a large number of capacitive or force sensitive sensors in foot insoles or platforms and are linked to a computer by either cable or radiowave telemetry. Several commercial systems are available and used clinically and for research. These systems may help direct appropriate shoe wear and orthotic prescriptions by providing information about abnormal pressure distributions, particularly in patients with structural foot deformities or in patients at risk for developing skin ulcerations in the feet because of diabetes mellitus or other underlying vascular and peripheral neuropathy disorders.

Kinematics

Electrogoniometers

Electrogoniometers are computerized versions of simple goniometers, which are commonly used in clinical practice to assess joint range of motion. An electrogoniometer consists of one or more potentiometers placed between two bars, with one bar strapped to the proximal limb segment and the other strapped to the distal limb segment (Fig. 8-9). The potentiometer, which is placed over the joint, provides a varying electrical impulse, depending on the instantaneous angle between the two limb segments. This electrical impulse information is then interfaced to an analog-to-digital converter in a personal computer to plot joint angle information over time. A combination of three potentiometers allows for measuring three rotations between limb segments (37). A major disadvantage of current electrogoniometers is relatively poor accuracy because they are difficult to apply, particularly about the hip and ankle. Unfortunately, even in the case of good accuracy, the results obtained from electrogoniometers provide only relative joint angle information, not absolute positions of the joints of limb segments. Because of these limitations, electrogoniometers cannot be used in conjunction with force plate data to evaluate joint kinetic data.

Cinematography

Historically, gait analysis was performed using sequential photographs or motion pictures. Markers placed over various anatomic landmarks can be used to help identify the location of limb segments and joints. The location of markers can

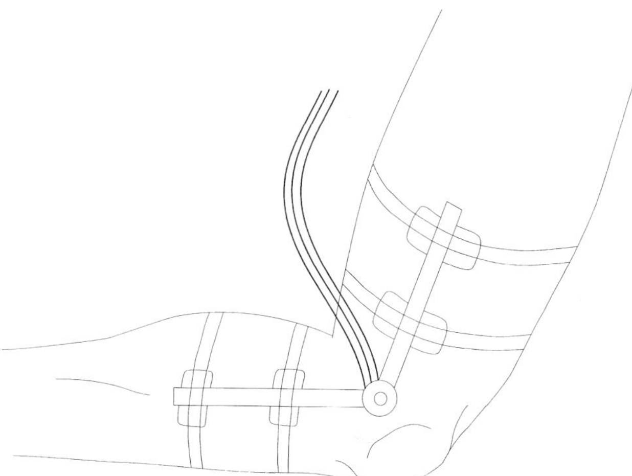

FIG. 8-9. Electrogoniometer. A potentiometer placed at the joint center records varying electrical impulses depending on the relative position of the proximal and distal segments.

then be manually digitized, frame by frame, so that the marker position in two dimensions can be determined. In both cinematographic and optoelectronic systems, a single camera provides two-dimensional information. By using two cameras, triangulation can be performed to determine the three-dimensional position of each marker. Although the cinematographic system is theoretically as accurate as what can be obtained with modern-day optoelectronic systems, the time necessary to manually digitize and process the data is of such great magnitude that it makes this procedure unfeasible for routine clinical evaluation.

Optoelectronic Motion Analysis

Modern-day quantitative gait analysis typically involves a sophisticated computerized video camera apparatus, referred to as an optoelectronic motion analysis system. These systems measure the three-dimensional location of an individual marker in a manner similar to that in cinematography, but with far greater ease and speed. The system automatically digitizes the position of each marker from each video camera and then automatically triangulates the information to provide a three-dimensional position of each marker at each frame. A layout of a typical laboratory space that includes an optoelectronic motion analysis system is illustrated in Figure 8-10. Typically, an optoelectronic system can detect the true three-dimensional position of a marker within a few millimeters in each of the three axes. The specific type of camera or lenses that are used, the algorithms used to digitize or identify markers, the size of the markers, and the laboratory environment are all factors that determine the specific accuracy of any given system. Marker position is typically determined at every 1/50, 1/100, or 1/200 of a second, depending on the speed of the cameras used. Multiple

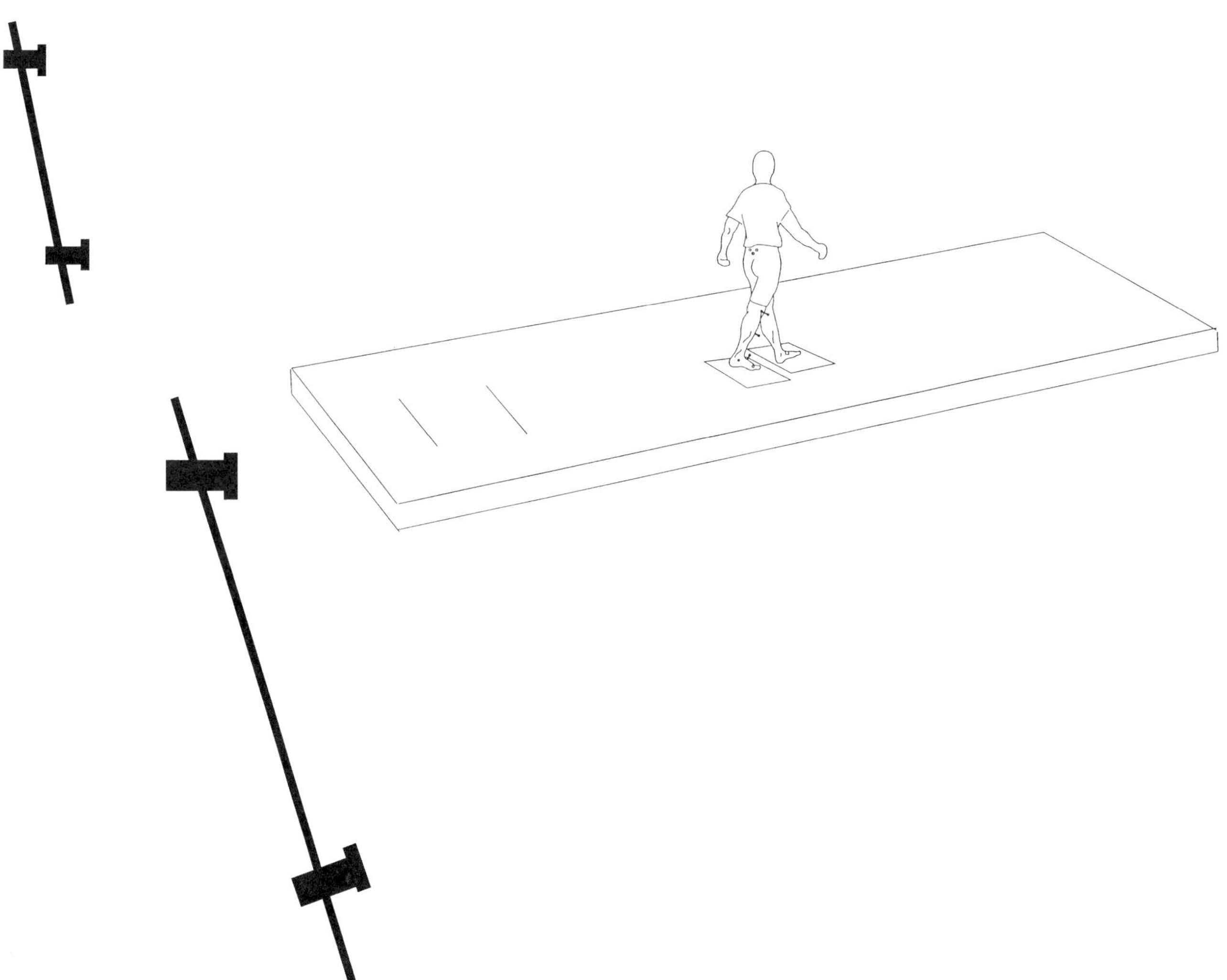

FIG. 8-10. Optoelectronic motion analysis system. Patient walks along a walkway with reflective markers attached to specific anatomic reference points. Camera pairs record the three-dimensional locations of the reflective markers. Force plates located in the center of the walkway record GRFs. Computer programs combine three-dimensional coordinates and GRFs to calculate joint kinetics and kinematics.

markers are affixed to the skin of the pelvis and the lower extremities in relationship to bony landmarks. Similar to the cinematographic method, two cameras are necessary to visualize each marker to obtain its three-dimensional position. Often a camera cannot visualize a marker during a particular part of a movement because of limb rotation or because another limb segment gets in the way. For this reason, sometimes a laboratory uses more than two cameras to ensure that at every given frame of movement, at least two cameras can visualize each of the markers. In the case where three or more cameras visualize a marker, an algorithm must be used to determine the true position of the marker because there is invariably some error such that not all cameras converge on the identical three-dimensional position. Other laboratories strategically position the markers so that the same two cameras can visualize a particular marker throughout the movement.

Currently, there are two different types of optoelectronic systems used for quantitative gait evaluation: (a) active marker systems, where the markers are actively illuminated by a computer, and (b) passive marker systems. A built-in advantage of an active marker system is that the computer knows in advance which marker it is illuminating at any given frame so that the markers are automatically identified as the lateral femoral epicondyle marker, the lateral malleolus marker, etc. The main disadvantage of current active marker systems, however, is that the illuminators require power; thus, multiple wires connected to a power source need to be attached to the patient, which tend to encumber the patient's gait. In contrast, passive marker systems require only that a small infrared reflective piece of material be placed over each anatomic landmark. Although passive markers do not encumber the patient, they do require some additional type of system to determine which marker is which. Fortunately, sophisticated computer software programs have been developed that automate this procedure. Thus, passive marker optoelectronic systems have become the preferred systems for routine clinical practice and are readily commercially available with all necessary software programs.

In order to obtain estimates of joint motion, the optoelectronic system is coupled to a biomechanical or mathematical model that defines where on the body the markers are optimally placed (Fig. 8-11). A simple model to measure knee motion might involve placement of one marker over the greater trochanter, one marker over the lateral femoral epicondyle, and one over the lateral malleolus. The angle formed between the line connecting the greater trochanter with the lateral femoral epicondyle and the line connecting the lateral femoral epicondyle and the lateral malleolus would represent knee flexion. However, this model would be too simplistic in that knee varus or valgus could easily be misread as true knee flexion. To accurately define sagittal motions such as knee flexion, geometry dictates that three

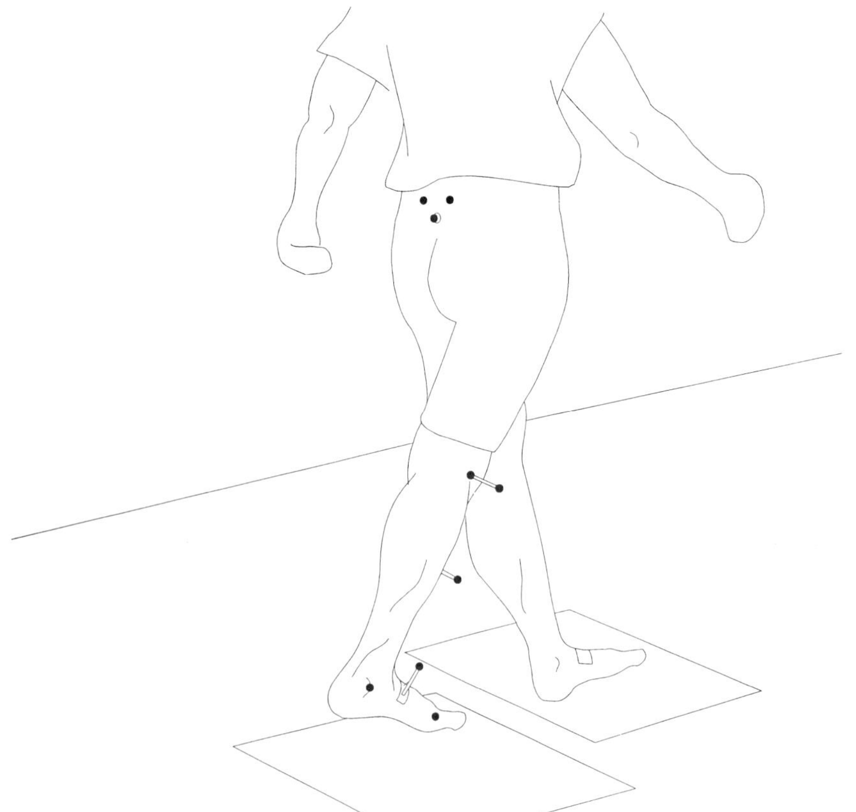

FIG. 8-11. An example of marker arrangement. Markers are placed on a variety of anatomic landmarks allowing for the collection of three markers or marker equivalents per rigid body segment.

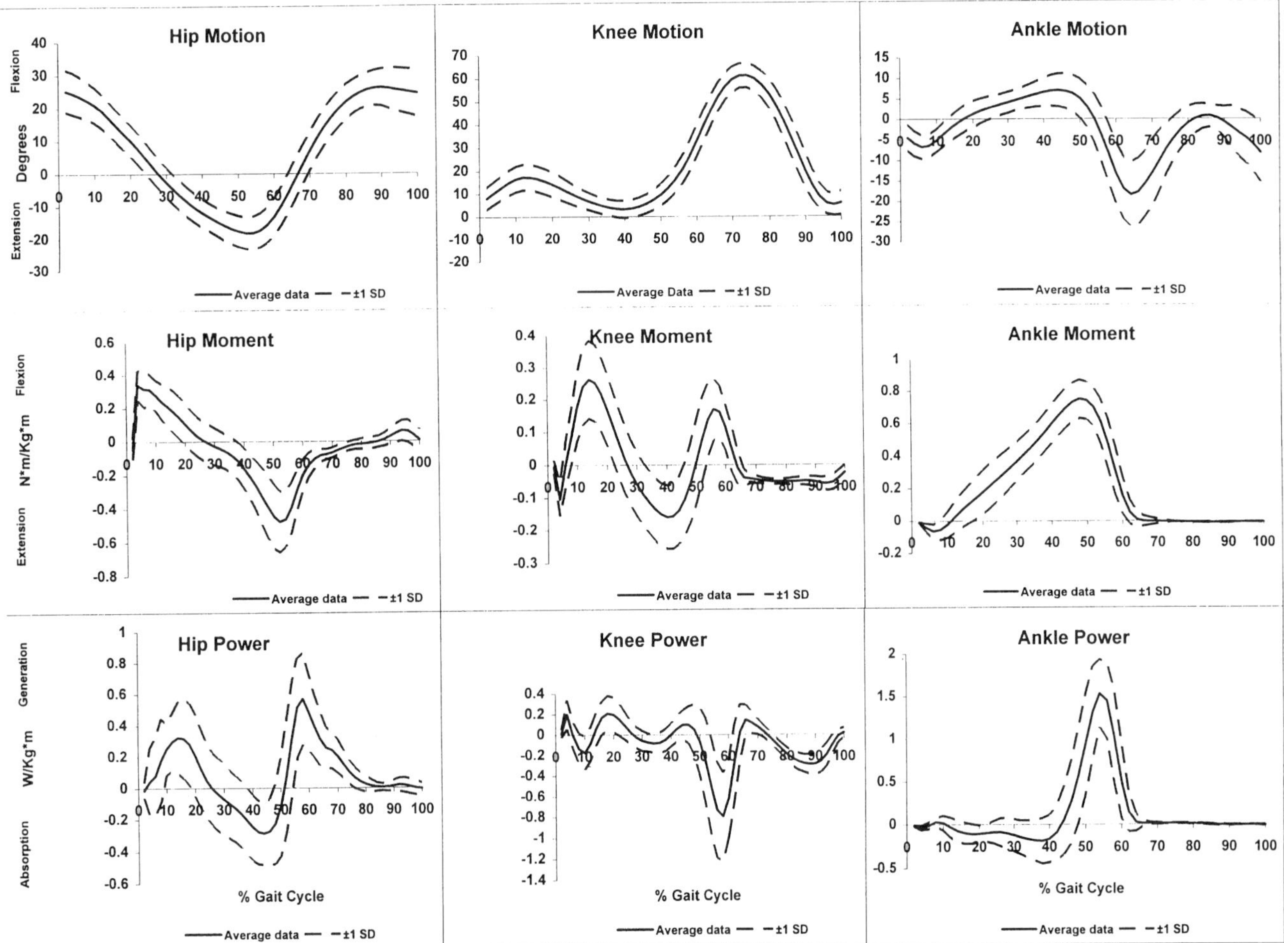

FIG. 8-12. Kinetics and kinematics at the hip, knee, and ankle. Sagittal joint motion, moments, and powers are shown.

markers (or marker equivalents) be placed on each limb segment, assumed to be rigid, to define the three-dimensional coordinate system for that segment (Fig. 8-12). A marker equivalent could be some imaginary anatomic point calculated on the basis of the position of real markers. For instance, three markers could be used to define a plane in the pelvis. From this and the known geometry of the pelvis, the location of the hip joint center can be calculated. The hip joint center then becomes an imaginary marker equivalent and can be used in defining the thigh segment coordinate system. Marker locations are often chosen in order to facilitate estimating joint centers as well as to ensure that the markers can be visualized by the camera system.

Typically, markers are placed over bony landmarks to ensure consistent applications as well as to reduce skin movement artifact. With three markers or marker equivalents for each body segment, the segment can be represented in the form of a local coordinate system whose orientation is determined with respect to a global coordinate system. The local coordinate system is defined by three mutually perpendicular vectors. Joint angle information then can be ascertained from the proximal and distal limb segment local coordinate systems. Several methods exist for determining joint angle information. Commonly, one axis is chosen to be parallel to the proximal segment local coordinate system axis, and a second axis is chosen to be parallel to the distal segment local coordinate system axis (38). In this way, a medial/lateral axis is selected from the proximal segment local coordinate system and is considered to be the axis about which joint flexion/extension occurs. A longitudinal axis chosen from the distal segment local coordinate system represents the axis about which internal/external rotation occurs. Finally, an axis formed mutually perpendicular to these two axes is considered the axis about which abduction/adduction occurs (Fig. 8-13).

Kinetics

Joint moments and power are commonly measured with quantitative gait analysis. The concept of a joint moment has already been described. A joint power, also referred to previously, represents the net rate of generating or absorbing

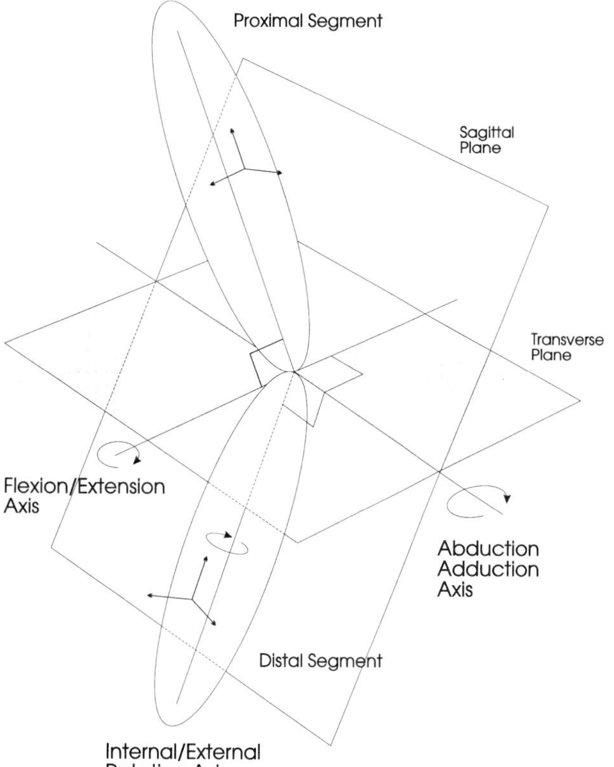

FIG. 8-13. Determination of axes of rotation. Flexion/extension, abduction/adduction, and internal/external rotation axes are determined based on the proximal and distal segments' local coordinate systems.

energy and is the mathematical product of the joint moment and joint angular velocity. A positive joint power implies that the muscle contraction is concentric because the joint angular velocity and moments are in the same direction. A negative power implies that the muscle contraction is eccentric because angular velocity and joint moments are in opposite directions. Joint kinetics are calculated in part using inverse dynamic techniques according to Newton's second law of motion, which essentially calculate the joint moments based on the motion and mass characteristics of the limb segments. Although theoretically the kinetics could be calculated from the kinematic data alone, these calculations would be extremely complicated and prone to error. Kinetics are therefore typically calculated using a combination of GRF data along with inverse dynamic techniques. Thus, kinetic calculations are usually based on (a) knowledge of the position of the joint in relationship to the GRF, (b) estimates of body segment masses and moments of inertia, and (c) knowledge of the body segment positions, velocities, and acceleration.

GRFs are measured using force plates that are comprised of piezoelectric or strain-gauge transducers. One or more force plates are imbedded in the ground of the walkway (see Fig. 8-10). As the patient walks, he or she steps on the force plate. To obtain useful GRF data, only one foot must strike the plate without interference from the other foot or an assistive device. Also, to feasibly assess joint kinetics, kinematic measurements must be collected synchronously with force plate data. The locations of the force plates are predetermined within a calibrated volume where the kinematic data are measured. A combination of various measurements taken on the patient are used in conjunction with look-up tables, based on cadaver data, to estimate body segment masses and moments of inertia (4,39). Clinical gait laboratories report joint moments as either external or internal. An external moment refers to the net external load applied to the joint measured via inverse dynamic techniques. The internal moment, which is equal and opposite in sign to the external moment is the presumed moment due to the muscle activity and/or soft tissues to fulfill the requirement that the joint is in equilibrium. For example, an external dorsiflexion moment about the ankle during the stance period of a gait cycle implies that an equal and opposite internal moment provided by the ankle plantarflexors or heel cord is present to maintain joint stability. Similarly, an external flexor moment about the hip during the stance implies that the hip extensors must be active in order to maintain stability. The typical kinetics and kinematics at the hip, knee, and ankle are shown in Figure 8-12. This type of graphic format is typically used for reporting quantitative kinetic and kinematic gait information in the clinical setting.

Dynamic Electromyography

Quantitative gait analysis also includes measurements of muscle activity during walking obtained using dynamic EMG measurement. When combined with kinematic and kinetic data, dynamic EMG provides useful information about whether a muscle is firing appropriately and if not, how this nonphasic activity impacts on gait, particularly in patients with spastic paretic gait. Because muscle activity does not linearly relate to the magnitude of force generated, quantifying the amplitude of activity is not practical in patients. However, relative normalization to the peak level activity over the gait cycle or the peak level activity, whether it occurs during strength testing or during walking, improves the clinical usefulness of the EMG data (1).

Muscle activity is measured using either surface electrodes affixed to the skin or fine-wire electrodes inserted in the muscles. Surface electrodes are adequate in studying activity in large superficial muscle groups. In addition to the fact that surface electrodes are less invasive than fine-wire electrodes, a major advantage of surface electrodes is that the data obtained are more easily replicated. This latter advantage is undoubtedly due to the fact that surface electrodes, as compared with fine-wire electrodes, sample data from an inordinately greater number of muscle fibers, representing a far greater number of motor units. Because of this same fact, fine-wire electrodes are not as prone as superficial electrodes to interference or "cross-talk" from nearby muscles. Surface electrodes are commonly used for many large superficial muscles in the lower extremity. Fine-wire electrodes are necessary for analyzing activity from smaller, deeper muscles, such as the iliopsoas and posterior tibialis. In addition, fine-wire electrodes are useful for differentiating activity from overlapping muscles such as the rectus femoris and vastus intermedius.

Surface EMG is typically recorded using disposable, gelled electrodes attached to the patient's skin overlying the muscle to be sampled. Usually, bipolar electrodes are used and the signal recorded is the potential difference between the two electrodes. Fine-wire EMG is often recorded using a wire bipolar electrode consisting of two thin, insulated wires with bared tips. The wires are placed through the shaft of a 25-gauge needle with the two ends bent over the needle and the bared tips staggered so as to avoid contact between them. The needle is inserted through the skin into the muscle, and then quickly removed, leaving the fine-wire in place. When in place, the bend in the wires provides a means for the electrodes to "catch" on the muscle fascicles. Again, the signal recorded is the potential difference between the two electrode ends. At the end of the study, the wires are removed with a gentle pull.

Preamplified EMG signals, either from fine-wire electrodes or surface electrodes, can be transmitted by cable or radiowave telemetry to a receiver that is connected to a computer system. The EMG signals are usually filtered to remove artifacts created by the mechanical movement. The signals are displayed and the gait cycle events identified. Some laboratories report raw EMG signals, whereas others report rectified and smooth EMG activity as well. The timing of the activity is typically what is important in the assessment. The normal timings of activity of major muscle groups are summarized in Figure 8-14. Muscle timing errors in patients with UMN pathology traditionally are classified into seven categories: premature onset, delayed onset, curtailed period, prolonged, absent, out of phase, or continuous (40). Although these categorizations are useful in describing activity in each muscle, it is important to note that they do not necessarily imply pathology about that particular muscle. In some instances, muscle activity differs from that of a nondisabled subject because of compensatory actions. As an example, prolongation of quadriceps activity into the mid- and terminal stance phases would be compensatory in a patient with an excessive external knee flexor moment. Thus, muscle firing patterns are optimally assessed in conjunction with the kinetics to help dissociate impairment from compensatory action.

Overall Gait Analysis

The overall gait laboratory analysis procedures takes approximately 2 hours for data acquisition and an additional 2 hours for analysis and interpretation. The majority of the acquisition time is spent applying and confirming placement of the multiple markers and EMG electrodes. The patient is typically evaluated under several conditions, i.e., barefoot, with shoes, and with and without an orthosis or assistive device.

EXAMPLES OF EVALUATION APPROACH TO SPECIFIC ATYPICAL GAIT PATTERNS

Gait Patterns Associated with UMN Pathology

A number of atypical gait patterns can be observed in patients with hemiparetic, paraparetic or diplegic impairments affecting their gait, regardless of the underlying UMN pathology (41–45). These atypical patterns include but are

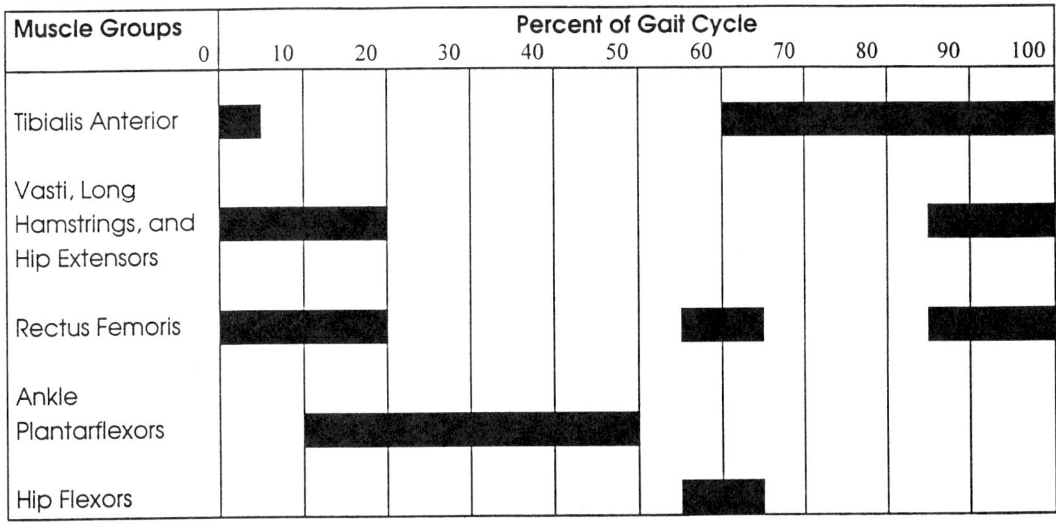

FIG. 8-14. General muscle group activity as a percentage of the gait cycle.

not limited to reduced knee flexion in swing, also referred to as stiff-legged gait, excessive knee flexion in stance referred to as crouched gait, equinus or excessive ankle plantarflexion occurring during one or more phases in either stance and/or swing, and knee hyperextension or recurvatum occurring in one or more phases of stance. Also common are presumably compensatory atypical gait patterns, including hip hiking, circumduction, and steppage gait. The important point to remember is that the causes of each of these atypical gait patterns are not necessarily the same from individual to individual and thus often necessitate a detailed evaluation including quantitative gait analysis.

Spastic Paretic Stiff-Legged Gait

Spastic paretic stiff-legged is a classic atypical gait pattern observed in patients with UMN pathology. Stiff-legged gait can be functionally significant from several views. From an energy standpoint, a lack of knee flexion in swing creates a large moment of inertia that significantly increases the energy required to initiate the swing period of the gait cycle. Additionally, associated compensatory actions to clear the stiff limb such as vaulting on the unaffected side and excessive pelvic motion can increase the vertical COM displacement, thereby increasing energy expenditure. From a biomechanical standpoint, these same compensatory actions could place the unaffected knee at risk for posterior capsule damage or the lower back to injury. Finally, lack of knee flexion may cause toe drag during swing, which could increase the risk of falling.

One cause of stiff-legged gait is inappropriate activity in one or more heads of the quadriceps during the pre- and/or initial swing phases of gait (46–49). Reduced knee flexion also may be caused by weak hip flexors, inappropriate hamstring activity, and/or insufficient ankle plantarflexor muscle action (49). For many patients with spastic paretic stiff-legged gait who undergo a quantitative gait analysis, the cause of the stiff-legged gait is not at all obvious from the static or observational gait evaluations. For instance, patients with increased knee extensor tone often can be found to have quiescent quadriceps EMG activity during preswing and initial swing. Conversely, a patient with normal knee extensor tone can have inappropriate activity during these phases in one or more heads of the quadriceps. In the latter case, if the inappropriate activity is limited to just one head, an intramuscular neurolytic procedure would be a reasonable treatment to improve the gait pattern. On the other hand, quantitative gait analysis may point to dynamically significant weak hip flexors, indicated by slow progression into hip flexion and poor hip power generation in preswing. These findings commonly are not correlated with hip flexion strength evaluated by static testing. In this case, hip flexion strengthening would be the optimal prescription. In another scenario, a reduced external ankle dorsiflexion moment during stance would imply insufficient ankle plantarflexor muscle action, in which case an ankle-foot-orthosis with a dorsiflexion stop might be the most appropriate treatment. A quantitative gait analysis also can help provide information about the functional significance of the atypical gait pattern. For instance, the risk for injury to the posterior capsule and ligaments of the unaffected knee can be assessed by measuring the extensor moment during that limb's stance period. Finally, a follow-up quantitative gait assessment may be useful in quantifying the improvement in knee flexion as well as ascertaining that the treatment itself did not cause any new problems.

Dynamic Knee Recurvatum

Hyperextension of the knee during the stance period, referred to as dynamic knee recurvatum, is a common observation in patients with UMN pathology. This atypical gait pattern may be caused by one or more of the following impairments: quadriceps weakness or spasticity, ankle plantarflexor weakness or spasticity, dorsiflexor weakness, and heel cord contracture (1,50). A primary functional concern for patients with dynamic knee recurvatum is that the hyperextension may produce an abnormal external extensor moment across the knee, placing the capsular and ligamentous structures of the posterior aspect of the knee at risk for injury. Injury to these issues may cause pain, ligamentous laxity, or bony deformity. Not all patients have an abnormal knee external moment, however, in which case the risk for injury is probably less (21). Knee recurvatum is also important from the standpoint of energy expenditure. The lack of knee flexion can cause a greater displacement of the COM because of the lack of knee flexion during the stance period.

Although multiple factors may contribute to knee recurvatum, it is useful to determine the primary cause in each patient so as to prescribe an optimal treatment plan. In some cases, dynamic recurvatum may be advantageous by providing a control mechanism for an otherwise unstable limb during the stance period of the gait cycle. If the associated knee extensor moment is small, then attempts to improve this atypical pattern may not be the appropriate treatment plan. Thus, quantitative gait analysis provides information that can help assess the functional significance of the atypical gait pattern as well as information that can help delineate the pattern's underlying impairment(s).

Diplegic-Crouched Gait

Crouched gait is defined as excessive knee flexion during the stance period of the gait cycle and is most commonly described in diplegic gait specific to cerebral palsy (51–53). Associated gait patterns are adduction and internal rotation at the hips, as well as equinus and forefoot abduction during stance. Reduced knee flexion in swing is also common. Dynamically, hamstring spasticity has been implicated as the principal cause of excessive knee flexion in stance (51–53). However, clinical experience suggests that dynamically tight hip flexors, plantarflexor weakness, and heel cord contracture also may be causative. These potential causes are best evaluated using the combined information obtained from static evaluation and observational and quantitative gait analysis.

Equinus Gait

Excessive ankle plantarflexion or equinus occurring in either stance or swing is common in patients with neurologic lesions. The differential cause for this pattern is inappropriate soleus, gastrocnemius or posterior tibialis activity, heel cord contracture, or weakness of the ankle dorsiflexors. As in the other atypical gait patterns described, the functional significance of the pattern needs to be determined. For instance, excessive plantarflexion during stance may inhibit tibial advancement, thereby interfering with forward progression necessary for efficient ambulation. During swing, excessive plantarflexion may place the patient at increased risk for tripping and falls. Dynamic EMG is useful in identifying the presence of inappropriate soleus, gastrocnemius, or posterior tibialis activity as a cause of the excessive plantarflexion. For equinus in swing, the lack of ankle plantarflexor activity suggests either a heel cord contracture or weak ankle dorsiflexors as a cause. Each patient also should be evaluated for functionally significant compensatory mechanisms as well as increased hip flexion and hip hiking in swing. Finally, it is important to consider the possibility that the excessive ankle plantarflexion itself is a compensatory response for some other impairment or functional limitation such as weakness. This scenario has been reported to occur in muscular dystrophy (54) and is likely to also occur in patients with weakness from UMN. Thus, a reduction in the peak knee flexor moment in a particular patient with excessive ankle plantarflexion during stance may indicate that the ankle plantarflexion is occurring as a compensation for weak knee extensors. Again, because of the complexities of gait, these possibilities are best assessed using quantitative gait analysis including kinetics.

Gait Patterns Associated with LMN and Orthopedic Disorders

Unlike in most patients with UMN pathology, the atypical gait patterns associated with specific peripheral nerve injuries cause discrete patterns of muscle weakness and associated characteristic atypical gait patterns. The following examples illustrate atypical gait patterns that arise from weakness of one specific functional muscle group. Unlike in patients with UMN pathology, in order to determine the underlying impairment and functional limitation responsible for the atypical gait pattern, static evaluation and observational analysis are usually adequate. Kinetic assessment is often useful, however, in helping to determine the functional significance of an atypical gait pattern.

Gait Associated with Femoral Neuropathy

Selected quadriceps weakness, which can occur in femoral neuropathy in diabetes, femoral nerve entrapment, or poliomyelitis, impairs weight-bearing stability during stance. The quadriceps eccentrically contract to control the rate of knee flexion during the loading response of the limb. With weakness, the knee would tend to ''buckle.'' The effective compensatory action is to position the lower extremity such that the GRF lies anterior to the knee joint, imparting an extension moment during stance phases. This is first achieved during initial contact by plantarflexing the ankle. Contraction of the hip extensors also can help to hold the knee in hyperextension. As noted previously, quantitative gait analysis may be useful in evaluating the associated knee extensor moment, which, if excessive, could place the posterior capsule and ligamentous structures at risk for injury.

Atypical Gait Patterns Associated with Weak Ankle Dorsiflexion

Dorsiflexion weakness also has a characteristic gait pattern. Clinical conditions in which this is seen is peroneal nerve palsy occurring as a result of entrapment at the fibular head or more proximally as an injury to a branch of the sciatic nerve, or in an L5 radiculopathy. If the ankle dorsiflexors have a grade of 3 or 4/5, the characteristic clinical sign is ''foot slap'' occurring soon after initial contact, due to the inability of the ankle dorsiflexors to eccentrically control the rate of plantarflexion after normal heel contact. If the ankle dorsiflexors have less than 3/5 strength, toe drag and/or a steppage gait pattern with excessive hip flexion in swing is likely. The cause of these patterns can usually be determined with a careful history, physical examination, and standard electrodiagnostic procedures (as opposed to a dynamic EMG assessment).

Atypical Gait Patterns Associated with Generalized LMN Lesions

More generalized LMN lesions commonly involve variable weakness patterns and thus often have unpredictable and often complex associated gait patterns. Poliomyelitis and Guillain-Barré syndrome are examples. For these diagnoses, kinetic assessment can be particularly useful in determining excessive joint moments, implying excessive soft-tissue strain or the need for increased compensatory muscle action in another muscle group.

Trendelenburg Gait

Trendelenburg gait (gluteus medius gait), describes a pattern of either excessive pelvic obliquity during the stance period of the affected side (so-called uncompensated Trendelenburg gait) and/or excessive lateral truncal lean during the stance period of the affected side (so-called compensated Trendelenburg gait). Weakness or reluctance to use the gluteus medius can cause this atypical gait pattern. The most common cause of Trendelenburg gait is osteoarthritis of the hip. In this case, the gait pattern (regardless of whether it is compensated or uncompensated) occurs as a compensatory response to reduce the overall forces across the hip during stance. This can be seen as a reduction in the external hip adductor moment, which ordinarily occurs in the stance period.

Atypical Gait Patterns Associated with Orthopedic Conditions

In cases of specific orthopedic conditions, the atypical gait pattern is fairly predictable and the cause directly relates to the structural abnormality. For instance, the cause of absent knee flexion during gait may simply be the result of a knee fusion. Studies about the diagnostic use of quantitative gait analysis in structural abnormalities are scant. Nevertheless, quantitative analysis may be useful in evaluating complex orthopedic conditions involving multiple joints and in evaluating the functional relevance of associated gait patterns. For instance, one study demonstrated that kinematic and kinetic measurements were helpful in directing and documenting the effects of gait training in patients with symptomatic knee hyperextension due to posterolateral ligament complex injury (55). Other studies have reported the usefulness of quantitative gait assessments to identify abnormal joint forces in patients with anterior cruciate ligament–deficient knees and osteoarthritis of the knee, which may help to identify patients with risk of further deterioration (56,57).

ACKNOWLEDGMENT

We thank Mary K. Todd and Thomas A. Ribaudo for their assistance in preparing figures for this chapter. The work in this chapter was supported in part by National Institutes of Health Grant HD01071-03 from the Public Health Service and by the Ellison Foundation.

REFERENCES

1. Perry J. *Gait analysis: normal and pathological function.* Thorofare, NJ: Slack, 1992.
2. Inman VT. Conservation of energy in ambulation. *Arch Phys Med Rehabil* 1967; 47:484–488.
3. Klopsteg PE, Wilson PD, eds. *Human limbs and their substitutes.* New York: McGraw-Hill, 1954.
4. Dempster WT. *Space requirements of the seated operator.* Ann Arbor, MI: University of Michigan, 1955.
5. Gonzalez EG, Corcoran PJ. Energy expenditure during ambulation. In: Downey JA, Myers SJ, Gonzalez EG, et al., eds. *The physiological basis of rehabilitation medicine.* Stoneham, MA: Butterworth-Heinemann, 1994; 413–446.
6. Saunders JBD, Inman VT, Eberhart HD. The major determinants in normal and pathological gait. *J Bone Joint Surg [Am]* 1953; 35: 543–558.
7. Inman VT, Ralston HJ, Todd F. Human Locomotion. In: Rose J, Gamble JG, eds. *Human walking.* Baltimore: Williams & Wilkins, 1994; 3–22.
8. Kerrigan DC, Viramontes BE, Corcoran PJ, et al. Measured versus predicted vertical displacement of the sacrum during gait as a tool to measure biomechanical gait performance. *Am J Phys Med Rehabil* 1995; 74:3–8.
9. McDonald I. Statistical studies of recorded energy expenditure of man. Part II: Expenditure on walking related to weight, sex, height, speed, and gradient. *Nutr Abstr Rev* 1961; 31:739–762.
10. Duff-Raffaele M, Kerrigan DC, Corcoran PJ, et al. The proportional work of lifting the center of mass during walking. *Am J Phys Med Rehabil* 1996; 75:375–379.
11. Corcoran PJ. Energy expenditure during ambulation. In: Downey JA, Darling RD, eds. *Physiological basis of rehabilitation medicine.* Philadelphia: WB Saunders, 1971; 185–198.
12. Bard B. Energy expenditure of hemiplegic subjects during walking. *Arch Phys Med Rehabil* 1963; 44:368–370.
13. Corcoran PJ, Jebsen RH, Brengelmann GL. Effects of plastic and metal leg braces on speed and energy cost of hemiparetic ambulation. *Arch Phys Med Rehabil* 1970; 51:69–77.
14. Astrand PO, Rodahl K. *Textbook on work physiology.* New York: McGraw-Hill, 1970.
15. Kerrigan DC, Thirunarayan MA, Sheffler LR, et al. A tool to assess biomechanical gait efficiency: a preliminary clinical study. *Am J Phys Med Rehabil* 1996; 75:3–8.
16. Murray MP, Drought AB, Kory RC. Walking patterns of normal men. *J Bone Joint Surg [Am]* 1964; 46:335–360.
17. Kadaba MP, Ramakrishnan HK, Wootten ME. Measurement of lower extremity kinematics during level walking. *J Orthop Res* 1990; 8: 383–392.
18. Wells RP. The projection of the ground reaction force as a predictor of internal joint moments. *Bull Prosthet Res* 1981; 18:15–19.
19. Sutherland DH, Olshen RA, Biden EN, et al. *The development of mature walking.* Philadelphia, Mac Keith Press, 1988.
20. Murray MP, Kory RC, Clarkson BH. Walking patterns in healthy old men. *J Gerontol* 1969; 24:169–178.
21. Kerrigan DC, Deming LC, Holden MK. Knee recurvatum in gait: a study of associated knee biomechanics. *Arch Phys Med Rehabil* 1996; 77:645–650.
22. Gage JR. *Gait analysis in cerebral palsy.* Philadelphia: Mac Keith Press, 1991.
23. Lee EH, Nather A, Goh J, et al. Gait analysis in cerebral palsy. *Ann Acad Med Singapore* 1985; 14:37–43.
24. DeLuca PA. Gait analysis in the treatment of the ambulatory child with cerebral palsy. *Clin Orthop* 1991; 264:65–75.
25. Brain Editorial Committee for the Guarantors of Brain. *Aids to the examination of the peripheral nervous system.* Oxford, England: Alden, 1986.
26. Perry J, Giovan P, Harris LJ, et al. The determinants of muscle action in the hemiparetic lower extremity (and their effect on the examination procedure). *Clin Orthop* 1978; 131:71–89.
27. Perry J, Mulroy SJ, Renwick SE. The relationship of lower extremity strength and gait parameters in patients with post-polio syndrome. *Arch Phys Med Rehabil* 1993; 74:165–169.
28. Perry J, Hoffer MM, Antonelli D, et al. Electromyography before and after surgery for hip deformity in children with cerebral palsy. A comparison of clinical and electromyographic findings. *J Bone Joint Surg [Am]* 1976; 58:201–208.
29. Perry J, Hoffer MM, Giovan P, et al. Gait analysis of the triceps surae in cerebral palsy. A preoperative and postoperative clinical and electromyographic study. *J Bone Joint Surg [Am]* 1974; 56:511–520.
30. Saleh M, Murdoch G. In defence of gait analysis. Observation and measurement in gait assessment. *J Bone Joint Surgery [Br]* 1985; 67: 237–241.
31. Gage JR. Gait analysis for decision-making in cerebral palsy. *Bull Hosp Joint Dis Orthop Inst* 1983; 43:147–163.
32. Gage JR. Gait analysis: an essential tool in the treatment of cerebral palsy. *Clin Orthop* 1993; 288:126–134.
33. Lee EH, Goh JC, Bose K. Value of gait analysis in the assessment of surgery in cerebral palsy. *Arch Phys Med Rehabil* 1992; 73:642–646.
34. Kerrigan DC, Glenn MB. An illustration of clinical gait laboratory use to improve rehabilitation management. *Am J Phys Med Rehabil* 1994; 73:421–427.
35. Turnbull GI, Wall JC. The development of a system for the clinical assessment of gait following a stroke. *Physiotherapy* 1985; 71: 294–298.
36. Hausdorff JM, Ladin Z, Wei JY. Footswitch system for measurement of the temporal parameters of gait. *J Biomech* 1995; 28:347–351.
37. Chao EYS. Justification of triaxial goniometer for the measurement of joint rotation. *J Biomech* 1980; 13:989–1006.
38. Grood ES, Suntay WJ. A joint coordinate system for the clinical de-

scription of three-dimensional motions: applications to the knee. *J Biomech Eng* 1983; 105:136–144.

39. Zatsiorsky VM, Seluyanov VN. The mass and inertia characteristics of the main segments of the human body. In: Matsui H, Kobayashi K, eds. *Human kinetics.* Champaign, IL: 1983; 1152–1159.
40. Bekey GA, Chang CJP, et al. Pattern recognition of multiple EMG signals applied to the description of human gait. *Proc IEEE* 1977; 65: 674–691.
41. Hirschberg GG, Nathanson M. Electromyographic recordings of muscular activity in normal and spastic gaits. *Arch Phys Med Rehabil* 1947; 33:217–224.
42. Peat M, Dubo HI, Winter DA, et al. Electromyographic temporal analysis of gait: hemiplegic locomotion. *Arch Phys Med Rehabil* 1976; 57: 421–425.
43. Knutsson E, Richards C. Different types of disturbed motor control in gait of hemiparetic patients. *Brain* 1979; 102:405–430.
44. Shiavi R, Bugle HJ, Limbird T. Electromyographic gait assessment. Part 2: Preliminary assessment of hemiparetic synergy patterns. *J Rehabil Res Dev* 1987; 24:24–30.
45. Winters TF Jr, Gage JR, Hicks R. Gait patterns in spastic hemiplegia in children and young adults. *J Bone Joint Surg [Am]* 1987; 69:437–441.
46. Waters RL, Garland DE, Perry J, et al. Stiff-legged gait in hemiplegia: surgical correction. *J Bone Joint Surg [Am]* 1979; 61:927–933.
47. Treanor WJ. The role of physical medicine treatment in stroke rehabilitation. *Clin Orthop* 1969; 63:14–22.
48. Sutherland DH, Santi M, Abel MF. Treatment of stiff-knee gait in cerebral palsy: a comparison by gait analysis of distal rectus femoris transfer versus proximal rectus release. *J Pediatr Orthop* 1990; 10: 433–441.
49. Kerrigan DC, Gronley J, Perry J. Stiff-legged gait in spastic paresis: a study of quadriceps and hamstrings muscle activity. *Am J Phys Med Rehabil* 1991; 70:294–300.
50. Simon SR, Deutsch SD, Nuzzo RM, et al. Genu recurvatum in spastic cerebral palsy. Report on findings by gait analysis. *J Bone Joint Surg [Am]* 1978; 60:882–894.
51. Gage JR, Perry J, Hicks RR, et al. Rectus femoris transfer to improve knee function of children with cerebral palsy. *Dev Med Child Neurol* 1987; 29:159–166.
52. Sutherland DH, Cooper L. The pathomechanics of progressive crouch gait in spastic diplegia. *Orthop Clin North Am* 1978; 9:143–154.
53. Thometz J, Simon S, Rosenthal R. The effect on gait of lengthening of the medial hamstrings in cerebral palsy. *J Bone Joint Surg [Am]* 1989; 71:345–353.
54. Johnson EW, Walter J. Zeiter lecture: pathokinesiology of Duchenne muscular dystrophy: implications for management. *Arch Phys Med Rehabil* 1977; 58:4–7.
55. Noyes F, Dunworth L, Andriacchi T, et al. Knee hyperextension; gait abnormalities in unstable knees. *Am J Sports Med* 1996; 24:35–45.
56. Noyes FR, Schipplein OD, Andriacchi TP, et al. The anterior cruciate ligament-deficient knee with varus alignment: an analysis of gait adaptations and dynamic joint loadings. *Am J Sports Med* 1992; 20: 707–716.
57. Goh JCH, Bose K, Khoo BCC. Gait analysis study on patients with varus osteoarthrosis of the knee. *Clin Orthop* 1993; 294:223–231.

Rehabilitation Medicine: Principles and Practice, Third Edition,
edited by Joel A. DeLisa and Bruce M. Gans.
Lippincott–Raven Publishers, Philadelphia © 1998.

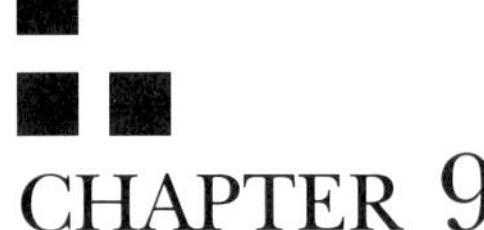

CHAPTER 9

Psychological Aspects of Rehabilitation

Daniel E. Rohe

This chapter begins by reviewing the history and current status of rehabilitation psychology. This is followed by a description of the direct and indirect services typically provided by rehabilitation psychologists. Frequently encountered psychological measures are described, and their importance for rehabilitation planning is stressed. The final section examines theories of adjustment to disability.

REHABILITATION PSYCHOLOGY: HISTORY AND CURRENT STATUS

History

The field of rehabilitation psychology received initial impetus from the rehabilitation needs of veterans returning from the two world wars in the first half of this century. After World War II, the Veterans Administration focused on the psychological needs of the physically disabled, which led to acceptance of psychologists as providers of mental health services. During this same time period, Howard A. Rusk developed the first comprehensive rehabilitation center, which led, with the assistance and leadership of others, to the development and acceptance of physical medicine and rehabilitation as a specialty and enhanced the development of physical and occupational therapy. Thus, the birth and maturation of the disciplines comprising the rehabilitation team have overlapping histories (1,2).

As the number of psychologists working in rehabilitation settings grew, the need for a professional forum arose. In 1949, a special-interest group within the American Psychological Association (APA) was created and, in 1958, was granted division status. The Division of Rehabilitation Psychology of the APA provides leadership in formulating federal legislation among various other professional and lay organizations. The Rehabilitation Act of 1973 and the Education for All Handicapped Children Act of 1975 provided mandates for the participation of rehabilitation psychologists in services to the disabled (3). Rehabilitation psychologists supported the passage of the Americans with Disabilities Act of 1990 and its ongoing implementation (4).

D. E. Rohe: Departments of Psychiatry and Psychology, Mayo Clinic and Foundation, Rochester, Minnesota 55905.

Current Status

Rehabilitation psychologists have struggled with an identity problem since the field's inception. Shontz and Wright argued for the distinctiveness of rehabilitation psychology, and others proposed a continuum within the related fields of medical psychology, health psychology, and behavioral medicine (5–7). Part of the identity problem stems from the fact that rehabilitation psychologists typically have doctoral degrees in clinical or counseling psychology and enter the field through internship training. Their professional identity is molded by their degree program rather than through didactic exposure to rehabilitation theories, principles, literature, and research. Historically, there have been only a handful of doctoral programs in rehabilitation psychology. Consequently, some practitioners lack theoretical models of rehabilitation on which to base clinical decisions.

The training and practice of rehabilitation psychologists are changing for several reasons. First, the APA has evolved a new model of education in which the graduate-level curriculum will be generic, with specialization occurring through postdoctoral training. To this end, the Division of Rehabilitation Psychology, in conjunction with the American Congress of Rehabilitation Medicine, developed and in 1995 disseminated guidelines for postdoctoral training in rehabilitation psychology (8). These guidelines provide consensus documentation of what constitutes valid postdoctoral training of rehabilitation psychologists. Currently, there are roughly 25 postdoctoral training programs in the United States. Second, the American Board of Rehabilitation Psychology (ABRP) was established in 1995, with the first diplomate in rehabilitation psychology awarded in 1996. The ABRP provided a comprehensive rationale for specialty definition and practice standards. Those awarded the diplomate have typically completed postdoctoral training plus 5 years of clinical service in rehabilitation psychology. The ABRP is part of the American Association of Professional Psychology, a larger umbrella organization of psychologists that accredits subspecialties much as the American Board of Medical Specialties does for medical specialties.

The goal of the Division of Rehabilitation Psychology is to expand knowledge and seek solutions to problems related to disability and the rehabilitation process. The mission of the organization states:

> By the year 2000, the Division of Rehabilitation Psychology will: a) be APA's voice for the science and practice of psychology as it relates to changes in abilities and social roles arising from illness and disability; b) be recognized by constituents internal and external to APA for the redefinition of "rehabilitation psychology" as an expanded spectrum of community and clinical services including prevention, rehabilitation, and postacute health care within the context of quality of life across the life-span; and c) influence the healthcare marketplace such that rehabilitation psychology services are widely available and accessible and that the quality of life perspective counterbalances both the economic and the medical/curative approaches (9).

Finally, the delivery of rehabilitation psychology services is changing with changes in the health care marketplace. Rehabilitation psychologists are shifting their venues from hospitals to less expensive settings such as subacute and outpatient rehabilitation facilities. The shift in provider systems to health maintenance and preferred provider organizations presents an evolving challenge to the delivery of cost-effective, quality rehabilitation psychology services. Despite the consolidation of health care payer and delivery systems, consumers continue to demand quality and value. Rehabilitation psychology's long-standing emphasis on the psychological and social adjustment to disability remains a vital component of quality rehabilitation services. The value of rehabilitation psychology services is acknowledged by the Commission on the Accreditation of Rehabilitation Facilities through their mandated provision for the presence of the rehabilitation psychologist as part of the rehabilitation team in both acute and subacute rehabilitation facilities. Rehabilitation psychology's focus on enhancing the quality of life for those with chronic illness and disability remains a central goal despite changes in health care.

DIRECT SERVICES

Assessment

Nonstandardized Assessment: The Clinical Interview

The psychologist's first contact with a patient is often pivotal in the development of a therapeutic relationship and may occur before transfer to a rehabilitation unit. The psychologist may visit the patient before the initial interview and explain his or her role. The patient's expectations of meeting with the psychologist are frequently determined by previous exposure to mental health professionals, communications from other team members including the physician, and preliminary explanations from the psychologist. The patient's willingness to interact meaningfully with the psychologist can be strongly influenced by the physician. Physiatrists who view rehabilitation as predominantly a process of "applied physical medicine" are less likely to communicate the importance of working with the psychologist. At the introduction, the psychologist will state that comprehensive rehabilitation includes help with problematic thoughts and feelings occasioned by the disability. Frequently, patients are relieved to discover that contact with the psychologist is a routine part of comprehensive rehabilitation.

The initial interview may last an hour or more. Patients with cognitive impairment may be seen only long enough for a general determination of their information-processing capacity and emotional state. Further assessment will await improvement in their cognitive status or contact with an informed family member. The length of the initial interview with patients not cognitively impaired depends on the complexity of the medical or social issues. There are two major goals for the initial interview. First, a comprehensive history of the patient's social background is obtained. Frequently asked biographical questions are listed in Table 9-1. These data provide insight into previous learning experiences that may affect rehabilitation-related attitudes and behaviors. Second, the psychologist attempts to understand the disability as the patient sees it. The foundation for a meaningful therapeutic relationship is laid in part by taking sufficient time to elicit the patient's perspective. The patient often faces a medical situation that he or she does not fully comprehend. Anxiety and fear often block the reception and communication of information between the patient and rehabilitation team members, especially physicians. The opportunity to have one's perspective, including cognitive and emotional aspects, aired in a supportive and clarifying manner is often therapeutic in itself.

The psychologist occupies an unusually difficult position vis-à-vis other team members. Although a team member, the psychologist also has the professional responsibility of maintaining the confidentiality of the therapeutic relationship. The patient may confide information that is personally sensitive and inappropriate to share with other team members. If directly asked by other team members about such information, the psychologist may have to explain that the information is confidential. Usually the patient is informed that any information considered sensitive by the psychologist or so indicated by the patient will not be communicated to others. General information of a less sensitive nature is dictated and typed in the form of an initial interview note. Subsequent therapeutic contacts are recorded in the hospital chart or summarized periodically. The frequency of these contacts depends on such factors as the goals established during the initial interview, the current degree of psychological distress, the potential for behavioral decompensation, and overall staffing levels.

TABLE 9-1. *Psychosocial information sought during initial interview*

Data on Family of Origin
- Names, ages, occupations, marital status, and residence of parents and siblings
- Religious training
- Stability of family during early development
- History of major mental disorder in immediate and extended family, including a history of sexual abuse, chemical dependency, suicide, or psychiatric hospitalization

Relevant Patient Information
- Educational background and school achievement
- Occupation and vocational history
- Avocational activities
- History of adjustment to structured environments, such as school, work and military service
- Social adjustment, including any previous arrests, chemical dependency treatment, or psychiatric diagnosis
- Prior association with hospitals and health care
- Preinjuiry stresses at the time of injury
- Most difficult loss the patient has had to adjust to previously; success in that task
- Former associations with people having disabilities

Family Structure
- Names, ages, and quality of relationship with spouse and children
- Background of dating and sexual relationship with current spouse
- Marital adjustment

Understanding the Patient's Perspective
- The patient's understanding of the cause and probable course of the disability
- The patient's initial thoughts at the onset of the disability (if traumatic)
- The patient's most pressing immediate concern
- How well the patient thinks he or she is coping with the situation
- The patient's perception of how the disability will change lifestyle, including relationships, vocational future, and self-concept
- The patient's understanding of the behavioral expectations in the rehabilitation unit compared with those in the acute care unit of the hospital
- The degree to which the patient's sense of self-esteem related to physique or physical skills
- The patient's comfort in meeting with a psychologist
- Techniques the patient has used successfully in the past to cope with stressful events
- Techniques the patient uses to get and maintain a sense of control over the environment

Standardized Assessment

Because of the time-consuming and subjective nature of clinical interviews, rehabilitation psychologists use standardized tests to speed assessment and enhance interventions (10,11). This section describes a number of helpful or frequently used instruments. Standardized measures of personality, intellectual ability, and academic achievement are briefly discussed. The domains of neuropsychological and chemical use assessment are covered in more detail because of their particular relevance in rehabilitation settings.

Personality

A personality test conventionally refers to a measure of personal characteristics, such as emotional status, interpersonal relations, motivation, interests, and attitudes. Currently, there are several hundred personality tests. Personality inventory development has generally involved one or more methods, including content validation, empirical criterion keying, factor analysis, and personality theory. Frequently, a measure uses several of the above-mentioned techniques. Personality measurement has generated controversy over two issues. The first concerns the stability of personality traits across situations as opposed to the situational specificity of behavior (12). The second issue is the degree to which a given personality characteristic reflects a mere transitory state rather than a stable underlying trait. Anastasi provided a thorough overview of these issues and of other psychological measurement concepts, including norms, item analysis, reliability, and validity (13). Elliott and Umlauf caution that the inappropriate and insensitive use of personality measures with individuals who have medical symptoms or limited physical abilities can produce erroneous and misleading results (14). The most frequently used personality inventory designed to measure psychopathology is the Minnesota Multiphasic Personality Inventory (MMPI). Two personality measures of nonpathologic or ''normal'' personality relevant to rehabilitation are the Revised NEO Personality Inventory (NEO-PI-R) and the Strong Interest Inventory. Space limitations preclude discussion of the measurement of mood in persons with physical disability. Eliott and Frank reviewed the literature on depression and spinal cord injury (15). Rohe discussed the differentiation of grief from depression after onset of disability (16).

Minnesota Multiphasic Personality Inventory

The MMPI is the most widely used and thoroughly researched objective measure of personality (17–19). The inventory is composed of statements describing thoughts, feelings, ideas, attitudes, physical and emotional symptoms, and previous life experiences. In general, the material included on the MMPI is usually covered in a clinical interview; however, factors of privacy, time savings, and the clinical relevance of the items have ensured its acceptance in health care settings.

The MMPI was originally designed to yield information about personality factors related to the major psychiatric syndromes. The 550 true–false questions are grouped into ten clinical scales (Table 9-2) that continue to reflect important aspects of personality despite their obsolete psychiatric titles. The items composing each scale were determined statistically. An item was included only if a carefully diagnosed group of patients (e.g., those hospitalized for depression) answered that question in a manner statistically different from that of other carefully diagnosed groups of patients (e.g., schizophrenics) and from a normal control group. This

TABLE 9-2. *Brief description of the Minnesota Multiple Personality Inventory validity and clinical scales*

Scale		Number of items	Elevated scores suggest
Number	Name		
Q	Cannot say	550	That a large number of items have not been answered, a possible indication that the patient is resentful or is uncomfortable with ambiguity
L	L scale	15	An effort to create the impression of being a person with high moral, social, and ethical values
F	F scale	64	That the whole questionnaire has been invalidated by some factor, such as lack of comprehension, poor reading ability, mental confusion, a deliberate desire to fake psychiatric difficulty, random marking of responses, or scoring errors
K	K Scale	30	A self-view of being well adjusted, capable, and confident, which, at higher scale elevations, is likely to be a denial of the true state of affairs
1	Hypochondriasis	33	Undue concern with bodily states and preoccupation with possible symptoms of physical illness
2	Depression	60	Depression, sadness, pessimism, guilt, passivity, and tendency to give up hope easily
3	Hysteria	60	Psychological immaturity, self-centeredness, superficial relationships, and frequent use of denial in everyday life
4	Psychopathic deviate	50	Assertiveness and nonconformity at moderate elevations; angry rebelliousness and noncompliance with social mores at extreme levels
5	Masculinity–femininity	60	The degree of identification with roles traditionally assigned to the sex opposite that of the respondent
6	Paranoia	40	Interpersonal oversensitivity and irritability about motives or behavior of others, and at extreme elevations, suspicious thinking similar to that of people with paranoid personality traits
7	Psychasthenia	48	General feelings of anxiety, with excessive rumination about personal inadequacies
8	Schizophrenia	78	Feelings of detachment from the social realm, extending to frank mental confusion and interpersonal aversiveness
9	Hypomania	46	Talkativeness, distractability, physical restlessness, and, at times, impatience, irritability, or rapid mood swings
0	Social introversin	20	Social introversion and a lack of desire to be with others

system of item selection (i.e., empirical criterion keying) led to the inclusion of subtle items that make the MMPI less easily faked than other personality measures. The empirical nature of the inventory has permitted construction of special scales. For example, there are scales to help predict rehabilitation motivation, headache proneness, and tendencies toward the development of alcoholism. Additionally, there are extensive MMPI norms on persons with specific diagnoses such as multiple sclerosis and spinal cord injury (20,21).

The ten clinical scales are interpreted with the aid of four validity scales (see Table 9-2). These scales provide information on the client's response style, such as literacy, cooperation, tendency toward malingering, comprehension, and use of denial or defensiveness. Norms are reported as standard scores with a mean of 50 and a standard deviation of 10. A score of 70 or greater is traditionally considered suggestive of a pathologic level of the trait in question.

The MMPI requires a sixth-grade reading level and is not suitable for children. The test requires between 1.5 and 2 hours for completion. Although many computerized scoring services are available, this does not obviate the need for interpretation by an experienced psychologist. A variety of factors, including race, socioeconomic status, unique family circumstances, ethnic background, and physical disability may distort the MMPI profile (22).

In 1989, a new version of the MMPI, the MMPI-2, was published (23). The MMPI-2 retains the same validity and clinical scales of the original test and adds 15 new content scales. The MMPI-2 provides larger, nationally representative norms and updated item content. The standardization sample consisted of 2,600 persons from seven states chosen to reflect several national census parameters, including minority group status. Unfortunately, the sample's mean level of education and occupational status was higher than national averages. When compared to the MMPI, the MMPI-2 requires a higher reading level (eighth grade versus sixth grade) and is to be used only with adults 18 years of age or older. A version of the MMPI entitled the MMPI-A was recently developed for use with adolescents (24). Colligan and Offord published contemporary norms for 1,315 normal adolescents aged 13 through 17 using the original MMPI (25).

The first goal of the MMPI-2 update was to improve the normative sample. Although the MMPI-2 successfully addressed the problem of the outdated and nonrepresentative original norming sample, that problem was already mitigated by Colligan and colleagues, who established new norms for the MMPI (26). Their large random sample of 1,408 normal subjects, subdivided by gender and age, excluded individuals with a history of major medical or psychiatric illness. Their data showed that the scores of contemporary normal individuals are only slightly different from those of the original normative sample. The changes average less than one-half standard deviation (5 *T* points) per scale; these small changes in profile elevation would have little impact on clinical interpretation. A complementary study examined scale changes in four code types for psychiatric samples over 40 years and found remarkable stability over this period of time (27).

Two additional goals of the MMPI-2 were to revise the outdated item content and wording while simultaneously preserving sufficient item continuity to allow for the generalizability of the voluminous MMPI research literature to the MMPI-2. Unfortunately, although the first goal was achieved, the second was not. Humphrey and Dahlstrom reported that profiles generated by the MMPI and the MMPI-2 on the same subjects are too frequently at variance for the two instruments to be considered interchangeable (28). Hence, it would be an error to assume that the MMPI clinical research literature can be generalized to the MMPI-2 for all patients. In short, the MMPI-2 represents a new instrument whose acceptance will be determined by clinical utility and research evidence. There are sufficient weaknesses in the new version to preclude unquestioned acceptance from clinicians who are expert on the original MMPI. Moreover, many of the criticisms of the MMPI remain problematic for the MMPI-2 (29).

The NEO-PI-R

The NEO-PI-R reflects the culmination of decades of personality research that concluded that personality traits can be summarized in terms of the so-called "five-factor model" (30,31). The NEO-PI-R is designed to measure the five major dimensions, or domains, thought to be central to normal adult personality (32). These dimensions are entitled Neuroticism (N), Extraversion (E), Openness (O), Agreeableness (A), and Conscientiousness (C). Each domain scale has six facet scales, resulting in a total of thirty-five scales on the inventory. Neuroticism refers to a general tendency to experience negative affect, self-consciousness, poor coping, irrational ideas, feelings of vulnerability, and difficulties controlling cravings and urges. Extraversion relates to interpersonal warmth, gregariousness, assertiveness, activity, excitement-seeking, and the tendency to experience positive emotions. Openness pertains to depth of imagination, esthetic sensitivity, intensity of feelings, preference for variety, intellectual curiosity, and independence of judgment. Agreeableness includes the characteristics of trust, straightforwardness, altruism, manner of handling interpersonal conflict, humbleness, and sympathy for others. Finally, conscientiousness encompasses the characteristics of competence, organization, reliability, achievement striving, self-discipline, and deliberation before acting.

NEO-PI-R item construction was based on rational-theoretical considerations. Item selection was based on internal consistency and factor-analytic data. The scale's 240 items are rated on a 5-point continuum from strongly disagree to strongly agree. The inventory is designed for adults aged 17 or older. The inventory requires a sixth-grade reading level and about 45 minutes for completion. There are separate norms for those aged more than 21 and less than 21. The NEO-PI-R has both a self report (Form S) and an observer rating form (Form R). This dual-form feature is unique among personality measures and is especially relevant to rehabilitation research. Also noteworthy, the NEO-PI-R items do not contain references to physical abilities or sensations that might distort a physically disabled subject's responses.

The NEO-PI-R is a reliable and valid measure. The internal consistency values for the domain scales range from 0.86 to 0.95. The initial version of the instrument demonstrated 6-year test–retest reliabilities of 0.86 to 0.91 for the domain scales and 0.66 to 0.92 for the facet scales. Validity has been established through numerous studies that correlate the NEO-PI-R with other measures of personality. All of these correlations have been in accord with theory and expectation (32). There are two limitations to the NEO-PI-R. The NEO-PI-R assumes an honest respondent, and no subtle items or validity scales are provided. In addition, it remains unclear how much the subject's current mood (state) may impact on the response to test items that describe long-standing personality characteristics (trait).

The NEO-PI-R has not been systematically studied with rehabilitation subjects. In one study, Rohe and Krause administered the initial version of the NEO-PI-R to men with traumatic spinal cord injurt 16 years after injury (33). The subjects scored lower on the scales of conscientiousness, assertiveness, and activity and higher on the scales of excitement seeking and fantasy than did the adult male normative sample. Scales reflective of negative affect were not elevated. The reduced conscientiousness and nonelevated neuroticism scale scores have negative implications for adherence to rehabilitation regimens and positive implications for long-term coping abilities.

The Strong Interest Inventory

The Strong Interest Inventory (SII) is traditionally considered a measure of vocational interests; however, research has supported its use as a valid non-pathology-oriented measure of personality (34). The 1994 version of the Strong Vocational Interest Blank (SVIB) includes numerous improvements such as larger normative samples and a greater number of skilled trade and technical occupations. First published in 1927, it is one of the most thoroughly researched, highly respected, and frequently used psychological tests. The SII asks the respondent to indicate liking, indifference, or dislike for occupations, school subjects, activities, leisure activities, and types of people. Two subsections ask for preferences between two occupational activities and between pairs of work dimensions. Finally, one section asks the respondent to rate his or her possession of 13 personal characteristics. The test contains 317 items, requires 35 to 40 minutes to complete, and is written at an eighth- to ninth-grade reading level (35).

The General Occupational Themes, one of the three types of scales on the SII, are based on trait theory as derived by John Holland (36). Holland drew on factor-analytic studies of personality and Guilford's factor analysis of human interests to produce a typology of six basic personality types. These types are titled Realistic, Investigative, Artistic, Social, Enterprising, and Conventional. Rohe and Athelstan administered the SII to a national sample of persons with spinal cord injury (SCI) (37). Contrary to previous research, they found unique personality characteristics associated with persons having SCI of traumatic onset. These characteristics included an interest in activities requiring physical interaction with things, such as machinery, and a disinterest in activities that require intense or complex interaction with either data or people. Malec used the Eysenck Personality Inventory with persons having SCI of traumatic onset and discovered a pattern of personality characteristics congruent with that found in Rohe and Athelstan's study (38). Rohe's review of the literature suggested that when a disability is of traumatic onset and secondary to the individual's behavior, earlier statements in the literature about the lack of relationship between disability and personality characteristics appear to be inaccurate (39). He noted that the previous literature either used pathology-oriented measures (e.g., MMPI) or studied individuals whose disability was not the result of trauma associated with their behavior. An additional study sought to determine if those personality characteristics associated with persons having SCI would change after years of living with the disability. The data indicated that overall personality characteristics remained constant over an average of 10 years (40). Rohe and Krause conducted a follow-up study to the aforementioned personality stability study. They found that men with traumatic SCI displayed marked consistency in personality characteristics over an 11-year follow-up period (41).

The MMPI, NEO-PI-R, and SII represent three measures of personality relevant to clinical rehabilitation settings. These measures can help answer pressing diagnostic and management questions. For example, the MMPI has been used successfully to diagnose the presence of psychopathology expressed in the form of physical disability—the so-called conversion disorders. Additionally, a patient's unwillingness to comply with requested medical interventions or the structure imposed by the hospital environment can be discerned with the use of personality measures. Knowledge of such personality characteristics can help prevent ill-advised interventions and can create a treatment environment to maximize patient compliance.

Intellectual Ability

Intellectual ability tests characteristically provide a summary score that serves as a global index of a person's general problem-solving ability. The score generated from the intellectual ability test is usually validated against a broad criterion, such as scholastic achievement or occupational success. Although such tests are ordinarily constructed of a number of subtests that sample facets of intellectual functioning, they are usually weighted towards tasks requiring verbal ability. The degree to which general problem-solving ability is present may have a significant impact on the type and complexity of medical and vocational rehabilitation goals established. The intellectual ability test also serves as the cornerstone of neuropsychological assessment. The most frequently encountered measure of intellectual ability is the Wechsler Adult Intelligence Scale, Revised (WAIS-R) (42). The revised version of the WAIS-R, entitled the WAIS-III, will become available in 1997. This discussion provides preliminary information available on the WAIS-III supplemented by comparisons with the WAIS-R (43).

The WAIS-III is the second revision of the Wechsler Adult Intelligence Scale, originally published in 1955. The WAIS-III was standardized on a normative sample of 2,450 "normal adults" from ages 16 to 89. They were carefully chosen to be representative of the United tates population as determined by the 1993 census update. The sample was further stratified by gender, educational level, ethnicity, and region of the country. The new form alters or eliminates test items that have become obsolete because of societal changes or found to be biased against individuals of African-American or Hispanic ethnicity. The WAIS-III must be administered by a trained examiner and requires 75 to 90 minutes for completion.

The subtest structure of the WAIS-III will closely resemble the WAIS-R, which has 11 subtests. On the WAIS-R, six subtests are used in the computation of the so-called verbal IQ, and five subtests determine the performance IQ. These subtests and what they purport to measure are included in Table 9-3 and are numbered in their order of administration. The subject's score on some subtests is based on both accuracy and speed. These timed subtests are arithmetic, picture arrangement, block design, object assembly, and digit-symbol. All WAIS-R subtest scores are corrected for age and standardized with a mean of 10 and a standard deviation of 3. The full-scale IQ is determined by averaging scores obtained from the verbal and performance IQs.

Cohen and subsequent investigators have consistently found three factors that account for most of the WAIS-R test variance (44). A subset of WAIS-R subtests constitute these factors and are sometimes administered to reduce testing time. The factor scores and the subtests used to compute them are verbal comprehension (i.e., information, vocabulary, comprehension, similarities), freedom from distractibility (i.e., digit span, arithmetic), and perceptual organization (i.e., block design, object assembly). As with the traditional IQ scores, factor scores have a mean of 100 and a standard deviation of 15. They are sometimes reported in lieu of the traditional IQ scores. The WAIS-III contains two additional subtests entitled "Cancellation" and "Letter-Number Se-

TABLE 9-3. *The eleven subtests of the Wechsler Adult Intelligence Scale, Revised*

Test Number	Test Title	Number of items	Task	Measures
Verbal Scale				
1	Information	29	Answer oral questions about diverse information acquired through living in the United States	Retention of long-term general knowledge
3	Digit span		Listen to and orally repeat increasingly long lists of numbers, with separate lists presented in forward and reverse directions	Ability to attend; immediate auditory recall
5	Vocabulary	35	Define the meaning of words presented both orally and visually	Verbal and general mental ability
7	Arithmetic	14	Solve arithmetic problems presented in a story format without using pencil or paper	Concentration and freedom from distractibility
9	Comprehension	16	Explain what should be done under certain circumstances and why certain social conventions are followed; interpret proverbs	Common sense, abstract reasoning, and social judgment
11	Similarities	14	Explain the way in which two things are alike	Verbal concept formation
Performance Scale				
2	Picture completion	20	Determine which part is missing from a picture of an object or scene	Visual recognition, remote memory, and general information
4	Picture arrangement	10	Arrange sets of cards containing cartoonlike drawings so that they tell a story	Social judgement, sequential thinking, foresight and planning
6	Block design	9	Reproduce a two-dimensional design on a card by using 1-inch blocks whose sides are red, white, or red and white	Visuospatial organizing ability
8	Object assemby	4	Properly arrange four cut-up cardboard figures of familiar objects	Visual concept formation and visuospatial reasoning
10	Digit symbol		In a timed code substitution task, pair nine symbols with nine digits	Concentration and psychomotor speed

quencing.'' The latter subtest is designed to measure a proposed fourth factor entitled ''speed of information processing,'' as suggested by the work of Malec and colleagues (45).

Because of the emotional significance of IQ scores, psychologists usually convert both IQ scores and discussions about them into either percentiles or classifications (Table 9-4). When a physician is confronted with questions about test results from patients, the use of either percentiles or classifications is recommended. Measures of intellectual ability help the physiatrist set appropriate expectations about the rate and complexity of learning legitimately expected from the patient. They also serve as the cornerstone for determining the presence of organic brain dysfunction and provide guidance for postdismissal vocational planning.

TABLE 9-4. *IQ scores, percentile ranges, and classifications for the Wechsler Adult Intelligence Scale, Revised*

IQ score	Percentile range	Classification
130 and above	98 or greater	Very superior
120–129	91 to 97	Superior
110–119	74 to 89	High average
90–109	25 to 73	Average
80–89	9 to 23	Low average
70–79	2 to 8	Borderline
60–69	<2	Mild mental retardation
35–49	<1	Moderate mental retardation
20–34	<1	Severe mental retardation
Below 20	<1	Profound mental retardation

Academic Achievement

A frequently overlooked but nonetheless important factor within rehabilitation settings is academic achievement. Reading and mathematics achievement are of particular concern not only during inpatient rehabilitation but also for longer-range educational and vocational planning. The patient's reading level is a potential limiting factor in tasks ranging from filling out hospital menus to incorporating ideas presented in patient education materials. The average reading level in the United States is roughly that of the sixth grade. Patient education materials, however, often reflect the reading levels of the professionals who devise them. As the patient's reading level falls below the national average, progressively greater reliance on oral instruction and audiovisual materials becomes necessary. Patients are often expected to use mathematics when recording fluid intake and taking correct dosages of medications. Two frequently used measures of reading and mathematical achievement are the

Wide-Range Achievement Test-3 and the Woodcock–Johnson Psycho-Educational Battery-Revised.

Wide-Range Achievement Test 3 (WRAT-3)

The WRAT-3 is the current edition of the Wide Range Achievement Test (46). The test provides assessment of three types of academic achievement: reading, spelling, and arithmetic. The test is to be used for individuals from ages 5 through 75. There are alternate forms, entitled ''Tan''and ''Blue.''The reading subtest requires the subject to recognize and name letters and correctly pronounce individual words ranging from ''see''to ''synecdoche.'' The reading test is not a measure of reading comprehension. The spelling test requires correct spelling of words presented by the examiner separately and in the context of a sentence. The level of difficulty ranges from ''in''to ''vicissitude.'' Finally, the mathematics test ranges in difficulty from simple counting to performing advanced algebra problems and has a time limit of 15 minutes. The entire test can be completed in roughly 30 minutes, and results are presented in the form of standard scores, percentiles, and grade equivalents. The WRAT-3 is reliable, and the national stratified sample of 5,000 individuals is a significant improvement over the older version of the test. Critics highlight that the correct pronunciation of individual words represents a limited index of reading comprehension.

Woodcock–Johnson Psycho-Educational Battery—Revised (WJ-R)

The WJ-R contains 35 subtests subdivided into two parts: cognitive ability (21 subtests) and academic achievement (14 subtests). The original test received critical acclaim for ease of administration, reliability, validity, and normative sampling procedures (47,48). The authors improved the original test by expanding the number of subtests, increasing the national normative sample, extending the age range from 2 to 95 years, and providing parallel achievement test forms (49).

The academic achievement subtests are grouped into five clusters: reading, mathematics, written language, knowledge, and skills. Reading achievement is determined by averaging four subtests requiring a total of 20 minutes to complete. These four subtests assess letter-word identification, phonetic analysis, passage comprehension, and reading vocabulary. Thus, the resulting score reflects diverse aspects of reading, not just correct word pronunciation. Achievement scores are reported in age- and grade-normed percentiles, and reading ranges from easy to difficult. Mathematics achievement is based on two subtests consisting of story problems and calculations that require about 20 minutes to complete. The three remaining achievement clusters are of less relevance to inpatient rehabilitation but may be of use in postdismissal planning.

Both the WRAT-3 and the WJ-R provide insight into the patient's current level of academic achievement. This information aids in determining the most appropriate manner of instructing the newly disabled. Those with low reading and math achievement levels may require special care when being provided patient education. This information is invaluable at the time of postdismissal educational and vocational planning.

Neuropsychological Assessment

People with cognitive dysfunction form one of the largest groups receiving rehabilitation services. For many, the deficits are transient, and for some, cognitive deficits are permanent and not only will complicate the learning of independent living skills but also will determine future living arrangements, social interactions, and vocational prospects. In both situations, the psychologist is frequently asked to clarify the nature and type of cognitive deficits. This section provides information on two helpful screening tests of cognitive status. Both tests can readily be used by the physician to determine the need or readiness for more extensive neuropsychological assessment. Next, two approaches to neuropsychological assessment, the quantitative approach as exemplified by the Halstead–Reitan Neuropsychological Battery and the qualitative approach as exemplified by the Boston Process Approach, are described. As noted by Lezak, the use of fixed neuropsychological test batteries is waning in favor of a flexible choice of tests (50). The test battery typically chosen will consist of instruments that assess those cognitive functions most frequently impacted by the specific neurological disorder under investigation. This approach is critical in rehabilitation because of the presence of sensory and motor impairments, which make administration of some tests difficult or impossible. A recent report by the American Academy of Neurology confirmed the efficacy of neuropsychological assessment (51).

Screening Measures of Cognitive Status

The physician frequently encounters patients of doubtful potential for a rehabilitation program. A question that often arises is whether the patient shows evidence of organic brain dysfunction. More than a dozen scales designed to assess the presence of dementia are available (52). Although each has particular strengths, many do not offer the diversity of content or wide applicability needed for use with a general rehabilitation population. Mental status scales can be divided into three groups: lengthy scales with multiple content, abbreviated scales with one or two items per cognitive area, and short scales of ten or fewer items. Lengthy scales often require 1 hour to administer and may not provide enough information to warrant the time required. Short scales tend to focus on orientation questions, ignoring the diversity of cognitive abilities. Kokmen and colleagues devised the Short Test of Mental Status to address the above-mentioned limitations (53).

The Short Test of Mental Status has diverse content, is easily learned, and requires only 5 minutes to administer. Content includes orientation, attention, learning, calculation, abstraction, information, construction, and delayed recall. The test was normed by comparing 93 consecutive neurologic outpatients without dementia to 87 outpatients with dementia. The maximum possible score is 38. A cut score of 29 or less resulted in a sensitivity of 92% and a specificity of 91% for the diagnosis of dementia. When this test was compared with standardized tests of cognitive function, a high degree of correlation was demonstrated (54).

Although the Short Test of Mental Status is useful for answering the question of whether to refer for neuropsychological assessment, the physician must decide when to refer for testing. This is particularly true for individuals with a closed head injury or slowly resolving coma. The Glasgow Coma Scale is useful for assessment of wakefulness during the acute stage of head injury but is not designed to guide the timing of psychological assessment (55).

The Galveston Orientation and Amnesia Test (GOAT), developed by Levin and colleagues, assesses amnesia and disorientation after head injury (56). The scale consists of ten questions that focus on temporal orientation, recall of biographical data, and memory of recent events. The patient can obtain a maximum of 100 points; the final score is computed by subtraction of the number of error points. The GOAT was standardized on a group of 50 young adults (median age, 23) who had recovered from mild closed head injury, usually consisting of a momentary loss of consciousness. Scores below those received by all members of the control group (<65) are designated impaired, scores between 66 and 75 are designated borderline, and those above 75 are considered normal. The greatest scoring difficulty would appear to occur when points are assigned for the patient's accuracy in recalling events before trauma. Posttraumatic amnesia is defined as the time during which the GOAT score is 75 or less. Validity data were generated by a comparison of the length of the posttraumatic amnesia with the variables of initial neurologic impairment and scores on the Glasgow Outcome Scale. In both cases, the GOAT score readily discriminated according to the severity of head injury. Scaling recovery of cognitive function in the noncomatose patient permits meaningful discussion with the family and rehabilitation team members. Most important, attempts at more involved neuropsychological assessment usually prove nonproductive until the patient consistently obtains scores of 70 or greater. Once a score of 70 is achieved, neuropsychological test data usually are reliable for further rehabilitation and postdismissal planning. Further detail on the GOAT is provided in Chapter 49.

Goals of Neuropsychological Assessment

The field of neuropsychological assessment has come full circle since 1935, when Ward Halstead established his laboratory (57) Halstead observed the behavior of patients with brain damage and then developed psychological tests to measure the characteristics that he observed. Thus, the initial goal of assessment was a better understanding of brain–behavior relationships, particularly in patients with brain impairments. Halstead's assessment methods quickly proved their worth, when used by experienced clinicians, by reliably and validly diagnosing brain damage and localizing malfunctioning regions of the brain. Their use as a neurodiagnostic instrument gained prominence and is now routine. Their diagnostic validity has been shown to be equal to that of neurodiagnostic techniques in use before the introduction of computed tomography and magnetic resonance imaging (58). As brain imaging technology has improved, however, the importance of neuropsychological assessment has begun to return to the original goal of describing brain–behavior relationships.

The next and final stage in the field of neuropsychological assessment will be the development of new methods for assessing rehabilitation potential, functional competence, and valid cognitive remediation procedures for patients with brain damage (59–63). Unfortunately, most neuropsychological tests were designed with diagnosis, not prediction or remediation, as their major goal. The tests were not constructed to provide crisp discriminations about which combinations of cognitive abilities are minimally necessary for survival in complex environments. Heaton and Pendleton, in a comprehensive review of the neuropsychological literature, lament that prediction of everyday functioning is a largely ignored topic of research in a field still dominated by diagnostic issues (64).

Ultimately, new neuropsychological measures will have to be constructed. The normative comparison groups will include cognitively impaired individuals who demonstrate appropriate adaptational skills in their home and work environments. If the brain-injured subject could score sufficiently high on combinations of these measures, one could then have faith that the subject would be able to function adequately outside of a sheltered environment. Traditionally, measurement has focused on the patients and not the unique environment to which they will return. There has been increased recognition of the inherent limits of neuropsychological assessment. Optimal prediction about the satisfactory matching of persons with environments will require new approaches to the measurement of environments (65).

Halstead–Reitan Neuropsychological Battery (HRNB)

The HRNB consists of three batteries (i.e., child, intermediate, and adult) (66). The focus here is on the adult version, which consists of Halstead's original five tests of seven variables selected for their ability to distinguish people who have frontal lobe dysfunction. Halstead's first graduate student, Ralph Reitan, established his own laboratory and added measures of aphasia, sensory-perceptual integrity, grip strength, and sequential visual scanning, collectively entitled "Allied Procedures."In addition to the HRNB, a complete battery usually includes the WAIS-R and a measure of personality (e.g., the MMPI).

The results of the HRNB can be presented as the Halstead Impairment Index, a summary value computed by dividing the number of test scores in the impaired range by 7. Boll provided a thorough description of the HRNB and stressed that the impairment index is not by itself a meaningful indicator of brain damage (57). Rather, the index should be seen as a summary score and should be placed in the context of other test data analyzed by inferential methods. Reitan described these inferential methods as follows (67):

- Level of performance. The individual's score is compared with that of a criterion group, and the normality or abnormality of the score is determined. In addition, statements describing the amount or degree of a specific attribute can be provided.
- Pattern of performance. Variations of scores within and between tests within the battery can be analyzed for specific strengths and weaknesses.
- Specific behavioral deficits or pathognomonic signs. Behaviors occurring only with brain damage (e.g., anomia, hemianopsia, and hemiplegia) can be detected.
- Comparison of performance of the right and left sides of the body. Measures of motor, sensory, and sensory-perceptual functions from one side of the body are compared with those of the opposite side. Significant discrepancies are likely to reflect brain dysfunction and can help rule out competing explanations of poor performance on more complex neuropsychological tests.

In rehabilitation, as opposed to general medicine, the issue of diagnosing brain damage is of reduced importance. Brain damage is frequently the criterion for entry to a rehabilitation unit. Rehabilitation team members are more concerned with the degree to which the patient will be able to understand and profit from rehabilitation services. A lengthy test battery may not be physically possible because of recent onset of impairment. In these cases, the neuropsychologist attempts to administer portions of the standard HRNB flexibly or to use tests that place fewer demands on the patient. Before dismissal from the hospital or immediately thereafter, a more complete battery of neuropsychological tests may be administered to assess more fully current cognitive function and to provide guidance on the need for supervision or the ability to return to work.

Although the HRNB can validly and reliably diagnose the presence and type of brain dysfunction, it is not without its limitations and critics. For example, Halstead's original cutting scores were based on the performance of young patients, with age-graded norms becoming available only recently (68). Patients with minimal education may spuriously score in the impaired range. Finally, the battery's ability to consistently localize lesions and discriminate psychiatric from organically impaired patients remains problematic (50).

The Boston Process Approach to Neuropsychological Assessment (BPA)

The BPA is the designation given to neuropsychological assessment that focuses on the manner in which the patient produced the response rather than concentrating solely on test norms and patterns of scores. The three goals of the BPA are to (a) understand the qualitative nature of the behavior being assessed, (b) reconcile descriptive richness with the reliability and validity of quantitative tests, and (c) relate the behavior assessed to neuropsychological theory (69).

The BPA began with the efforts of Edith Kaplan to utilize developmental psychology's distinction between "process and achievement" to understand the disintegration of function in patients with brain damage. Kaplan and her colleagues, known collectively as "the Boston group," employed tests with proven validity in identifying patients with brain damage and then systematically observed the problem-solving strategies used by these patients. This method allowed both a quantitative assessment and a dynamic description of the information processing style of each patient.

The BPA uses a core set of tests with supplementary tests to clarify problem areas and confirm clinical hypotheses. The core set consists primarily of frequently used tests that assess functions in six cognitive domains, including intellectual and conceptual, memory, language, visuoperceptual, academic achievement, self-control, and motor control (69). Although standardized test instructions are generally adhered to, some modifications were made to facilitate data collection on the patient's cognitive strategies. These modifications typically do not interfere with the standard administration of the tests. The BPA emphasizes "testing the limits," which refers to asking the patient to respond to test items beyond the standard cutoff scores or time limits for test discontinuation. Other modifications include adding new components to established tests (70).

The BPA is concerned with the extent to which the patient gives priority to processing low-level detail or "featural" information versus higher-level "configural" or "contextual" information. Patients who show impairment in contextual processing are often found to have difficulties organizing and directing their behavior. The BPA is as valid for the detection and localization of cortical lesion as quantitative methods.

Both the quantitative and qualitative approaches to neuropsychological assessment have proponents. The process approach is perhaps more compatible with the rehabilitation emphasis on practical and functional improvements. Given its focus on qualitative observation, the process approach provides potential insights regarding the most effective cognitive rehabilitation methods to use for remediation of cognitive deficits. The effectiveness of cognitive rehabilitation remains controversial and is reviewed in Chapter 49.

Chemical Use Assessment

Background

In the early 1970s, rehabilitation discovered its failure to assess and intervene in the domain of sexuality. In the mid-1980s, Rohe and DePompolo reviewed the literature on chemical abuse and physical disability (71). They found a similar failure to assess and intervene in the domain of chemical health among those with disabilities. They noted that physicians seldom receive training in chemical abuse assessment and intervention. Throughout this section, alcohol and drug abuse are considered jointly. The focus of discussion, however, is on alcohol, the more frequently abused drug.

The importance of alcohol screening is related to both the drug's impact on bodily functions and the associated behavioral aberrations occasioned by its excessive use. Eckardt and colleagues reviewed the detrimental effect of alcohol on most organs, especially the liver, pancreas, and heart (72). Alcohol ingestion may potentiate the action of prescribed medications, most notably central nervous system (CNS) depressants. This potentiation of action is of particular importance for rehabilitation patients. For example, medications that control blood clot formation and reduce spasticity are frequently used with rehabilitation patients. Alcohol may decrease blood clotting activity and act in an additive manner with muscle relaxants such as diazepam (Valium [Roche Products, Manati, Puerto Rico]) and baclofen (Cliorsel [CIBA Geneva, CIBA Geigy, Summit, NJ]). In addition, altered consciousness may result in less vigilance in health-compromising situations. If alcohol is ingested in the form of beer, the large fluid volume could seriously compromise a bladder-retraining program (73).

The cognitive and behavioral aberrations associated with drug intoxication often result in the onset of a disability. Rohe and DePompolo cite evidence that vehicular crashes and falls, especially while the individual is under the influence of alcohol, account for a large proportion of admissions to rehabilitation units (71). Retrospective chart reviews of persons with CNS trauma often show alcohol present at the time of injury. Fullerton and colleagues found that 50% of their spinal cord-injured patients admitted to drinking before their injury (74). Heinemann and associates found that 39% of their spinal cord-injured patients admitted to being intoxicated at the time of injury (75). Corrigan's review of the literature found that nearly two-thirds of head-injured patients may have a history of substance abuse that preceded their injury. These studies revealed alcohol intoxication present in one-third to one-half of hospitalizations (76). Heinemann, Schmidt, and Semik found that drinking patterns before and after spinal cord injury are strongly related (77). In a study of long-term spinal cord-injured patients, problems resulting from substance abuse were reported by more than one-half of the patients sampled (78). In a prospective study, Rimel found that 72% of 1330 consecutive CNS trauma admissions had a positive blood alcohol level (79). Fifty-five percent were legally intoxicated, with blood alcohol levels of 1,000 μg/ml or higher. The above-mentioned data suggest that individuals admitted to rehabilitation units with traumatic CNS injuries are not a random sample of the drinking public. Failure to assess and intervene with this population represents a missed opportunity to reduce future medical, social, and personal costs. Corrigan argues that rehabilitation professionals, under scrutiny from third-party payers, cannot afford to have a significant proportion of their patients display poor long-term outcomes secondary to failure to address substance abuse (76).

The screening for chemical health of all rehabilitation patients must become standard practice. For this to occur, the administration of rehabilitation facilities will have to require that drug screening be standard policy and that rehabilitation professionals, especially physiatrists, have necessary screening skills. Unfortunately, although most representatives of physical medicine and rehabilitation training programs indicated concern about alcohol or drug abuse problems in their patients, only 22% reported that staff were provided education on the issue (71). Little has changed since Rohe and DePompolo's call for improved staff training, screening, and treatment of chemical health issues. For example, Schmidt and Gavin found that only 4% of persons receiving initial traumatic brain injury rehabilitation were screened for substance abuse (80). In this study, an in-service training program resulted in improved frequency of chemical health assessment and referral, but this only occurred for patients who were obviously intoxicated at injury onset. The authors found that proactive attention to substance abuse prevention after onset of disability was not evident (81). Obtaining accessible substance abuse treatment for persons with physical disabilities remains difficult (82). Screening and intervention for nicotine dependence has yet to be systematically addressed by rehabilitation providers.

Screening for Chemical Dependency

Individual attitudes about alcohol use, like attitudes about sexuality, are diverse and strongly held and determine the perception of another person's use. Unless one first examines personally held attitudes and values about alcohol use, perceptions of another's use may be highly biased. A training program developed by the Center for Substance Abuse Prevention stresses the importance of attitudes in prevention programs (83). The two most frequent problems encountered during screening are viewing alcohol as a moral problem and judging the deviance of the patient's drinking through comparison with the interviewer's personal pattern of use. Weinberg stated that the most important aspects of interviewing about alcohol use are:

- Getting a detailed history
- Demonstrating nonjudgmental acceptance
- Asking direct, specific, and factual questions
- Maintaining persistence

- Never discussing alibis
- Titrating hostility (84)

Two measures useful in assessing alcohol use are the CAGE Questionnaire and the Self-Administered Alcoholism Screening Test (SAAST).

The CAGE Questionnaire was originally developed on 130 randomly selected medical and surgical inpatients at North Carolina Memorial Hospital. The goal was to find the least number of questions that would reliably identify those suffering from alcoholism. The four CAGE questions are:

1. Have you ever felt you ought to ***C***ut down on your drinking?
2. Have people ***A***nnoyed you by criticizing your drinking?
3. Have you ever felt bad or ***G***uilty about your drinking?
4. Have you ever had a drink first thing in the morning to steady your nerves or to get rid of a hangover (i.e., an ***E***ye opener)?

Ewing summarized the scale's development and data on four normative samples (85). One positive response to any of the questions raises the suspicion that alcohol dependence is present. Two positive responses identified 97% of his alcoholic sample correctly and only 4% of his nonalcoholic sample incorrectly. Three or more responses are clearly symptomatic of alcohol dependence.

One measure designed to aid in the process of accurate and reliable assessment of alcohol use is the SAAST. Developed by Swenson and Morse (86), it is a modified version of the Michigan Alcoholism Screening Test (87). The SAAST comprises 35 items presented in a yes/no format. A score of 7 to 9 suggests possible alcohol dependence. A score of 10 or greater suggests probable dependence. An advantage of the SAAST is its ability to be administered in a structured interview or independently. Hurt and colleagues reported SAAST data on more than 1,000 consecutive patients receiving general medical examinations (88). The study concluded that the SAAST is an effective tool for the detection of alcohol dependence in a general medical setting.

The field of rehabilitation has yet to fulfill its responsibility in the screening and treatment of chemical abuse and dependency. Research data suggest that patients with traumatic CNS injuries have a high probability of chemical use. Physiatrists have a responsibility for learning the skills needed for systematic screening of their patients. This intervention, early in the rehabilitation process, is a crucial aspect of prevention of future medical complications.

PSYCHOTHERAPEUTIC INTERVENTIONS

Individual Psychotherapy

Psychotherapy is a generic term denoting psychological interventions that ameliorate a wide variety of emotional and behavioral difficulties. Psychotherapy can be broadly defined as an interpersonal process whose goal is modification of problematic affect, behavior, or cognition (89). Of the more than 130 varieties of psychotherapy, research has yet to demonstrate that any specific variety shows clear superiority. Instead, effectiveness seems related to a therapist's degree of training in and enthusiasm for the theory and methods espoused by the particular therapy. Data suggest that psychotherapy does produce measurable change in patients. This change, however, can be negative as well as positive. The important principle of "above all, do no harm" is as important in psychotherapy as it is in medicine. Inadequately trained therapists are thus a source of concern in a field lacking firm boundaries.

The three basic assumptions underlying psychotherapy are as follows:

1. The person seeking services desires change.
2. The dysfunctional affect, behavior, or cognition is understood and amenable to change.
3. The process is a collaborative endeavor that assumes active client participation.

Psychotherapeutic intervention is thus contraindicated in patients on whom it must be forced or in those with significant communication or learning impediments. Additionally, if the difficulties result from factors solely in the patient's environment (e.g., long hospitalization, unpleasant medical interventions, prejudice, nonunderstanding staff), the focus of the psychotherapist's intervention may shift from the patient to the environment.

The qualities of effective therapists have been studied and delineated. Therapeutic effectiveness initially depends on good assessment skills. Knowing when and how to intervene and, conversely, when to do nothing is fundamental to the process. Effective therapists are able to instill trust, confidence, and hope in their clients. Irrespective of the type of therapy practiced, effective therapists have been shown to communicate the specific attitudinal qualities of genuineness, unconditional positive regard, and empathy. As opposed to mere friendship, the therapist provides an atmosphere of acceptance, respect, understanding, warmth, and help in conjunction with deliberate efforts to avoid criticizing, judging, or reacting emotionally with the patient. The creation of this atmosphere results in a framework unmatched by any other human relationship, one conducive to therapeutic change.

Most people living in rehabilitation units are faced with discovering and coping with permanent physical, cognitive, and social losses. This discovery is often accompanied by significant levels of anger, anxiety, dysphoria, grief, and fear. Clinical experience suggests that the patient population can be divided into thirds according to the severity of their reactions. One-third of the patients cope extremely well through use of previously established skills and the support of significant others. Another one-third have greater difficulties but, through rather minimal psychotherapeutic intervention, are able to successfully manage the crisis. The final one-third have significant difficulties in coping. They frequently have histories of difficulties in adjustment, such as chemical abuse, major mental disorder, and inability to tolerate structured living environments. This group is of paramount concern to the rehabilitation psychologist and consumes large amounts of professional time.

Because of the pressing practical problems faced by rehabilitation inpatients and the increasingly short period of hospitalization, rehabilitation psychologists tend to use time-limited forms of therapy, also known as brief therapy (90). Brief therapy is a general term denoting therapies with a small number of sessions (i.e., six to ten) and limited, focused, and readily attainable goals. These goals often include amelioration of the most disabling symptoms, reestablishment of previous levels of functioning, and development of enhanced coping skills. The sessions are focused on concrete content and the "here and now." Rehabilitation psychologists frequently apply techniques termed cognitive–behavioral. This concept has been summarized by Turk and associates (91).

Even though cognitive–behavioral techniques are implemented in diverse ways, some common elements can be identified. Interventions are usually active, time-limited, and fairly structured, with the underlying assumption that affect and behavior are largely determined by the way in which the individual construes the world. Therapy is designed to help the patient identify, reality-test, and correct maladaptive, distorted conceptualizations and dysfunctional beliefs. The patient is assisted in recognizing the connections among cognition, affect, and behavior, together with their joint consequences, and is encouraged to become aware of and monitor the role that negative thoughts and images play in the maintenance of maladaptive behavior.

Behavioral Management and Operant Conditioning Techniques

Medical rehabilitation involves a coordinated effort to slow, stop, or reverse the loss of a person's functional abilities. The ultimate criterion of success is the degree to which the patient is able to maintain or improve functional performance. Thus, in medical rehabilitation, in contrast to other areas of medicine, there is a strong and systematic interaction between the medical and the behavioral sciences. Although the physiatrist would not be expected to devise or implement a detailed behavioral modification program, knowledge of the laws of behavior is essential when problems are conceptualized.

This section discusses the three types of learning:

1. Observational learning
2. Classic or respondent conditioning
3. Operant conditioning or behavior modification

Because of their relevance to rehabilitation, the principles underlying behavior modification are discussed in detail. Included are the topics of token economies, behavioral contracting, and misconceptions about behavior modification. The following material is drawn from the writings of Martin and Pear (92), Reynolds (93), Kazdin (94), and Brockway and Fordyce (95).

Three Types of Learning

Observational Learning

Observational learning, also known as modeling, occurs when a person observes a model's behavior but makes no overt response and receives no direct consequences. The behavior is learned through watching a model without actually performing the behavior. In modeling, a critical distinction is made between learning and performance. The only requirement for learning by modeling is observation of the model. Performance of the learned response, however, depends on the response consequences or incentives connected with the response. Thus, although rehabilitation professionals can effectively use observational learning when instructing patients about desired responses, the principles of behavior modification operate to determine if the observed behavior is actually performed. The likelihood of spontaneously emulating a model depends on a variety of factors, including whether the model is rewarded after the behavior, the similarity of the model to the observer, and the prestige, status, and expertise of the model.

Classic Conditioning

Classic, or respondent, conditioning is the process of repeatedly pairing a neutral stimulus with stimuli that automatically elicit respondent behavior. Some examples of respondents are salivation in response to food in the mouth, muscle flexion in response to pain, and accelerated heart rate in response to loud, unexpected noise. Thus, respondents are responses associated with the organism's glands, reflexes, and smooth muscle. Respondent conditioning does not involve the learning of new behavior but rather involves the capacity of a previously neutral stimulus to elicit a respondent. Respondent behavior is innate, part of the inherited structure of the organism. In respondent conditioning, stimuli that precede the behavior elicit the response. The resulting behavior is stereotyped and rather invariant across species, whereas in operant conditioning, behavior is emitted without any apparent prior stimulus.

The principles of respondent conditioning are used in the treatment of phobias and compulsions. For example, the relatively well-known therapeutic procedure of systematic desensitization involves pairing subjective states of deep muscle relaxation with graded approximations of the stimuli identified as eliciting the pathologic anxiety or fear response. Respondent conditioning techniques have been applied to enuresis, excessive eating, smoking, drinking, and deviant sexual behavior.

Operant Conditioning

Operant conditioning is a process by which the frequency of a bit of behavior is modified by the consequences of the behavior. Such behaviors are termed operants because they are emitted responses that operate on the environment. Operants are behaviors involving the striated muscles. Most behaviors occurring in everyday life, including those in rehabilitation units, are operants. When an operant is followed by a positive consequence (i.e., reinforcer), its frequency increases. Behavior that results in the termination of an aversive stimulus (e.g., turning off an alarm clock) is said to be negatively reinforced. When an operant is followed by a negative consequence (i.e., punisher), its frequency decreases. Operants no longer followed by reinforcers decrease in frequency and eventually disappear, a process known as extinction. An additional method of decreasing an undesirable behavior is to reinforce an alternative behavior, one that is incompatible with undesirable behavior. In simple terms, rehabilitation is the process of reinforcing disability-appropriate behaviors and extinguishing or punishing disability-inappropriate behaviors.

Environmental events that regularly precede and accompany operants are said to "set the occasion" on which the operant has been reinforced. These environmental stimuli, also known as discriminative stimuli, signal the availability of reinforcement should the previously reinforced behavior occur. Examples of such stimuli are a doorbell ringing, a traffic light turning green, and an "open" sign on the front door of a business. Discriminative stimuli are important because their presence increases the likelihood that a previously reinforced behavior will be emitted.

The speed, amount, and schedule of reinforcement are major determinants of the effectiveness of reinforcement. If possible, the reinforcer should be delivered immediately after the response to maximize the effect of reinforcement. The greater the amount of the reinforcer, the more frequent the response. Schedules of reinforcement have a major impact on the rate of emission of a behavior; they are succinctly described by Reynolds (73). When one is increasing a low-frequency behavior, it is best to reinforce each occurrence of the behavior. Once the behavior is established, the frequency can be maintained with less frequent (i.e., intermittent) reinforcement. The steps for setting up a behavioral modification program are presented in Table 9-5.

TABLE 9-5. *Steps in setting up a behavior modification program*

1. Define the behavior to be increased or decreased.
2. Define units of that behavior that can be readily measured, such as the beginning or end of a movement cycle.
3. Record the rate of occurrence of the behavior (i.e., movement cycle or time).
4. Identify potentially effective and readily controlled reinforcers.
5. Determine a schedule of reinforcement.
6. Implement and modify the program on the basis of outcome obtained.

Types of Reinforcers

There are three types of reinforcers. Primary or unconditioned reinforcers are present at birth. They include food, water, sexual stimulation, rest after activity and activity after rest, a band of temperatures, air, and cessation of aversive stimuli. Conditioned reinforcers are stimuli that have been repeatedly paired with primary reinforcers. They are idiosyncratic and are based on the learning history of the person. Generalized reinforcers are stimuli that have been paired with two or more conditioned reinforcers. The prime example of a generalized reinforcer is money; however, verbal responses such as "thank you," "correct," and "great" also are in this category. In addition to the three types of reinforcers, there is an important principle, the Premack principle, which states that any high-frequency behavior can be used to reinforce a low-frequency behavior. For example, a high-frequency behavior such as watching television can be made contingent on performing a low-frequency behavior such as stretching exercises.

Token Economies

A token economy refers to a reinforcement system based on tokens. The tokens, frequently poker chips, function as generalized reinforcers and can be exchanged at agreed-on rates for back-up reinforcers, such as food, activities, and privileges. The behaviors to be changed (i.e., target behaviors) are specified along with the number of tokens earned for their performance. The stipulations of the economy are usually written in the form of a contract; a "reinforcement menu," which indicates exchange rates and back-up reinforcers, is displayed in a prominent place. Token economies have been used extensively in special education and psychiatric settings. They can be useful with troublesome rehabilitation patients for such behaviors as arriving at therapy sessions late, lack of compliance with fluid schedules, and failure to perform activities of daily living. As with behavioral contracts, ethical considerations and the success of the program mandate full involvement of the patient in the initial design of the program.

Behavioral Contracts

Behavioral contracts, also known as contingency contracts, are written agreements between people who desire a change in behavior (i.e., rehabilitation team members) and those whose behavior is to be changed (i.e., patients). The contract precisely indicates the relationship between behaviors and their consequences. The contract serves four important functions. First, it ensures that the rehabilitation team and the patient agree on goals and procedures. Second, because the goals are specified behaviorally, evidence is readily available regarding fulfillment of the contract. Third, the patient has a clear picture of what behaviors are expected if he or she is to remain in the rehabilitation program. Fourth, the signing of a document functions as a powerful indicator of commitment and helps ensure compliance with the agreement.

Common Misconceptions About Behavior Modification

Behavior modification has aroused the ire of some people, usually because of a misunderstanding of its underlying principles. Kazdin presented a succinct overview of common objections, two of which are iterated here (94). A frequent objection is that use of tangible reinforcers is the same as bribery. Bribery can be differentiated from reinforcement, because bribery is used to increase behavior that is considered illegal or immoral and usually involves delivery of the payoff before performance of the behavior, not, as in behavior modification, afterward. Bribery and reinforcement share the similarity of being ways of influencing behavior, but that is where the similarity ends.

A second objection is that behavior modification is "coercive." Although behavior modification is inherently controlling and designed to alter behavior, multiple safeguards prevent its misapplication. These safeguards include involving the patient when contingencies are negotiated, constructing programs that rely on positive reinforcement rather than negative reinforcement or punishment, and making response requirements for reinforcement lenient at the beginning of the program (96). The use of behavioral modification in rehabilitation units requires careful training of staff. A limiting factor in many inpatient rehabilitation units is the lack of stability in team membership, especially where shifts in nursing personnel occur frequently.

Social Skills Training

Changes in Social Interaction After Disability

Although only a limited number of the recently disabled may profit from psychotherapy, most can benefit from social skills training. Research on the social psychology of disability is plentiful and underscores the social disadvantages encountered by the disabled, especially the recently disabled (97–108). Richardson summarized the literature and found consistently negative public attitudes toward the disabled (104). He noted that on first encountering a disabled person, the nondisabled experience heightened emotional arousal, anxiety, and feelings of ambivalence. These learned but somewhat involuntary reactions usually result in distorted social interactions.

Often, the nondisabled focus solely on the disability and ignore personal characteristics normally used to evaluate people and establish relationships. The disabled also suffer from the societal norm to be kind to the disabled, which results in a dearth of honest feedback and decreased accuracy in social perception by the disabled person (109). Consequently, the physically disabled often learn to discount praise and pay close attention to criticism. The factors mentioned above suggest that social interactions between the disabled and the nondisabled are complex, ambiguous, and unpredictable. Interventions that ameliorate difficulties with social interaction might help reduce emotional distress, speed the slow process of community reintegration (110), and reduce the risk of future medical problems (111).

Social Skills: Types and Methods of Assessment

Social skills is an inexact term used to describe a wide range of behavior thought necessary for effective social functioning (112,113). Dunn and Herman listed three types of social skills: general, general disability-related, and specific disability-related (Table 9-6) (114). Patients with onset of disability before adolescence may require intensive remedial help with the development of general social skills. Patients with onset of disability after adolescence enter the social arena with various competencies in general social skills. However, those with onset after adolescence experience social situations for which they have no previous socialization experiences; hence the importance for training to handle these situations. General social skills can be assessed through a variety of means, including paper-and-pencil tests, behavioral assessment, and observational techniques.

A social skill frequently identified as a problem is assertiveness; hence, it is used here to illustrate three assessment

TABLE 9-6. *General, general disability, and disability-specific social skills*

General Social Skills
Listening
Positive and negative assertion
Self-disclosure
Receiving compliments
Confrontation
Touching
Conversation
Maximizing physical attractiveness
Meeting new people
Use of humor
Heterosocial skills
General Disability-Related Social Skills
Acknowledgment of the disability
Asking for help
Acknowledgment of unstated attitudes (making the implicit explicit)
Refusing undesired help
Managing unwelcome social advances
Dealing with staring
Handling unwanted questions
Disability-Specific Social Skills
Facilitating communication
Overcoming early deficits in socialization
Managing bowel and bladder problems
Handling reactions to deformity and disfigurement
Disclosing nonvisible disabilities
Dealing with reactions to prostheses

From Dunn ME. Social skills and rehabilitation. In: Caplan B, ed. *Rehabilitation psychology desk reference.* Rockville, MD: Aspen Publishers, 1987; 345–381, by permission of the publisher.

methods. A well-known paper-and-pencil measure of assertiveness is the Gambrill Assertion Inventory (115). The Gambrill Assertion Inventory presents the subject with 40 situations described by a short phrase, for example, "turn off a talkative friend." The subject then rates his or her degree of discomfort for each situation on a five-point scale ranging from "none" to "very much." Next, the subject rates his or her response probability for each situation on a five-point scale ranging from "always do it" to "never do it." Normative data allow comparisons with the general population and with those having assertiveness difficulties. A measure of assertiveness more relevant to disability is the Spinal Cord Injury Assertion Questionnaire (116). The format of this questionnaire is similar to that of the Gambrill Assertion Inventory, but social situations that are potential problems for wheelchair users are described.

Behavioral measures help clarify the frequently found discrepancy between what people say they do and what they actually do. Behavioral measures offer direct and quantifiable data on both verbal and nonverbal aspects of social interactions. Such measures might include checklists or rating scales that permit counting responses, measuring length of time spent interacting, and so on. For example, studies using behavioral measures have shown that disabled people receive offers of help from strangers less frequently than do the nondisabled. However, if help is offered to the disabled, it tends to be overly solicitous (117,118). Hastorf and associates found that strangers were more willing to work on a cooperative project if the disabled partner assertively acknowledged the handicap at the beginning of the interaction (109). Finally, behavioral measures have been used during evaluation of the efficacy of assertion training with disabled people (119–122).

Observational techniques can be used by the person, significant others, or staff members. Generally, this type of assessment is less objective than that provided by behavioral measures. Nonetheless, reduced precision is counterbalanced by the opportunity to observe qualitative aspects of the social skill in a natural setting. Several research projects (e.g., Longitudinal Functional Assessment System and Rehabilitation Indicators Project) use observational techniques in the form of diaries, self-reports, and environmental surveys. Thorough descriptions of methods of assessing social skills can be found in a variety of publications (119,123,124). The reader is encouraged to consult relevant social skills training manuals for intervention techniques (125,126). Social skills training programs for wheelchair users are described by Hobart (unpublished data) and Dunn and Herman (114); a program for the traumatic brain injured is described by Brotherton and colleagues (127).

INDIRECT SERVICES

The rehabilitation psychologist's overall aim is to enhance the quality of rehabilitation outcomes for patients. Indirect services in the form of maximizing team interaction skills, staff development, administration, and research provide avenues for enhancing patient outcomes that are as important as those of direct patient services.

The rehabilitation team is a unique structure in the delivery of health care resources (128). Nowhere else are so many professionals with diverse backgrounds of training expected to communicate in a clear, timely, and comprehensive manner. This communication may become tenuous because of different professional terminologies, overlap in roles, and more recently pressures of productivity in a competitive health care environment with decreased lengths of inpatient hospitalizations (129). The psychologist can enhance patient outcomes by facilitating cohesion of the rehabilitation team (130). This task can be accomplished through a variety of methods, including chairing committees to improve interdisciplinary cooperation and leading staff meetings to clarify overlap in professional roles (131). The rehabilitation psychologist's knowledge of normal and abnormal behavior is frequently called on for staff in-service training. Although some in-service topics focus on patient variables, such as practical management suggestions and brain–behavior relationships, other topics include personal concerns of the staff, such as job stress and communication skills. The psychologist's interpersonal skills often lead to selection for administrative positions.

Rehabilitation psychologists trained at the doctoral level are usually the only team members with specific expertise in research design and statistical methods. As such, they are often consulted by other team members interested in conducting research. They frequently coordinate research or direct research committees. The research expertise of psychologists is used through their presence on editorial boards of numerous rehabilitation-related publications. They are also found in local, state, and national organizations whose function is to promote quality rehabilitation or social justice for the physically disabled.

PSYCHOLOGICAL ADJUSTMENT TO DISABILITY

This section is divided into two parts. The first part provides a brief overview of theories of adjustment to disability. The second part describes three models of adjustment to disability. The stage model emphasizes internal cognitions; the behavioral model emphasizes external events; and the coping skills model emphasizes both internal cognition and external events in the adjustment to disability.

Overview of Theories of Adjustment to Disability

Theories of adjustment to disability can be grouped along an internal-to-external continuum (132). On one end are theories that emphasize internal cognitive events, termed mentalistic theories, and on the other end are theories that emphasize events external to the individual, termed social theories or behavioral theories. The middle of the continuum contains integrative theories that attempt to meld the internal (i.e., mentalistic) aspects with the external (i.e., social and environmental) determinants.

Before formal theorizing about adjustment to disability, most people believed that the primary source of suffering connected with disability was the disability itself. Hence, removal or amelioration of the disability would presumably reduce distress. However, practice demonstrated that after removal of a disability, some people continued to remain incapacitated. The search for explanations shifted to the then-contemporary principles of dynamic psychology and focused on internal events such as motivation. Patients' difficulties in adjusting to disability were conceptualized in psychodynamic terms, and their incapacitation was transformed into problems of mental health (133).

As time progressed, it became increasingly clear that dynamic psychology models, especially the classic psychoanalytic model with its emphasis on disease, provided insufficient explanatory power. Professionals came to recognize that physical and social barriers, barriers external to the patient, produce the major source of adjustment problems. Emphasis on sociologic concepts such as "sick role" (134) and "illness behavior" (135) ensued. These sociologic theories added to the understanding of adjustment to disability on a societal level (136). When individual behavior is of concern, however, the emphasis of learning theory on the sensitivity of behavior to its consequences provides significant explanatory power. The behavioral model of adjustment to disability is described more fully in a later section.

Theories that attempt to take into account the internal events of the person and the external demands of the environment are called "integrative field theories" (132). Integrative field theories grew out of Lewin's concept of "life space" (137). These theories state that behavior is a joint function of the person and his environment: $B = f(P,E)$. Myerson, Trieschmann, and Wright applied Lewin's basic formulation to problems encountered by the physically disabled (138–140). For example, Trieschmann discussed the "educational model of rehabilitation," in which behavior is the joint function of personal, organic, and environmental variables, designated by the formula $B = f(P \times O \times E)$. Her acknowledgment of organic variables highlights the concept that behavior is fundamentally dependent on and limited by the physical capacities of the person.

Models of Adjustment to Disability

Stage Model

Stage theory states that people undergoing a life crisis follow a predictable, orderly path of emotional response. Shontz is the major contributor to the application of stage theory to adjustment to disability (141,142). Stage theory appears both explicitly and implicitly in a wide variety of rehabilitation-related literature, including that on cancer (143), hemodialysis (144,145), spinal cord injury (146–149), and amputation (150). Additional writers who make implicit or explicit reference to a stage model of adjustment to disability are Dembo and associates, Siller, and Gunther (99,105,151). Unfortunately, these studies are merely descriptive and are based on interview data or anecdotal reports.

Most stage theories set up a series of three to five steps beginning with shock and ending with some form of adaptation. Three commonly held assumptions appear to underlie stage theory formulations applied to the disabled. First, people respond to the onset of disability in specific and predictable ways. Second, they go through a series of stages over time. Finally, they eventually accept or resolve their emotional crises. The following discussion draws on the work of Silver and Wortman (152) and Trieschmann (139).

Are There Universal Responses to Disability Onset?

Both Gunther (151) and Shontz (141,142) indicated that once the crisis of disability is realized, virtually all people experience shock. Unfortunately, the vast majority of studies report retrospective accounts of initial feelings and behavior. In one such study, Parkes interviewed widows and amputees after their losses (150). Initial feelings of shock and numbness were reported by roughly 50% of the sample. Tyhurst observed disaster victims and described three types of reactions (153). One group reacted with classic signs of shock, another group appeared cool and collected during the acute situation, and a third group responded with reactions of paralyzing anxiety and hysterical crying. Shock was a predominant but far from universal reaction. Silver and Wortman's literature review concluded that there is little evidence supporting the belief that people react in specific and predictable ways to undesirable life events (152). Although some patterns are evident, individual variation is inevitably present.

Do Emotional Responses Follow a Pattern After Injury?

The concept that people follow a predictable pattern of emotional response after the onset of a disability is widely held. References to stage models of emotional response occur in the professional literature of nurses (154,155), social workers (156), clergy (157), health care professionals (158), and psychologists (105,141,142,151).

Silver and Wortman were unable to discover any studies specifically testing stage theory by measurement of affective states over time (152). Four related studies, all conducted on patients with spinal cord injury, failed to support state theory. Dunn studied seven psychological variables during three phases of rehabilitation (159). He was unable to discover a pattern of change in nor variability among the patients was the norm. McDaniel and Sexton assessed psychological status over four points in time from ratings by rehabilitation team members (156). Ratings of negative mood states remained relatively constant over the length of the study and were independent of staff ratings of the patient's degree of acceptance of loss. Dinardo, in a cross-sectional study, found that the degree of depression experienced by his subjects was independent of the time that had elapsed since their injury (160). Finally, Lawson, in a longitudinal study, used a variety of methods to assess the presence of depression (161). He found no period of at least a week when any of his patients scored consistently in the depressive range on any of the measures. His results suggest that patients with spinal cord injury do not experience a stage of depression during initial rehabilitation.

Although there is much popular and professional literature attesting to the veracity of stages of adjustment to disability, the empirical data do not support such a contention. Silver and Wortman summarized the available data by stating: "Perhaps the most striking feature of available research, considered as a whole, is the variability in the nature and sequence of people's emotional reactions and coping mechanisms as they attempt to resolve their crises" (152). Wright noted: "The process of acceptance of loss is not accomplished once and for all, nor does it march through fixed stages to ultimate acceptance" (140).

Is a Final Stage of Resolution Reached?

Do people who have suffered a major undesirable life event eventually reach a final stage of resolution or acceptance of their disability? The findings across studies suggest that a large minority of people continue to suffer years after a traumatic life event. The unquestioned expectation of resolution or acceptance appears unwarranted for such traumatic life events as severe burns, spinal cord injury, cancer, death of a spouse, and rape (152). For example, Shadish and associates studied a cross-sectional sample of patients with spinal cord injury (162). They found that those who had been disabled for as long as 38 years continued to think about and miss physically impossible activities.

Given the lack of support for three common assumptions underlying stage theory, one must look to alternative explanations of why such beliefs permeate clinical folklore and descriptive writing in the area. Although numerous hypotheses could be considered, two come readily to mind. First, professionals working with the recently disabled often encounter unpredictable and emotionally charged situations. One way to help neutralize fears occasioned by such situations is to label the patient as being in a particular stage. This may help transform potentially threatening and seemingly unpredictable behavior into meaningful and predictable categories. A negative outcome of such conceptualizing may be the well-documented tendency for rehabilitation personnel to overdiagnose psychopathological conditions in patients (163). This interpretation of behavior may also result in the staff inappropriately distancing themselves from the patient by negating the necessity for careful listening. A second reason for the popularity of stage theory may be the enticing belief that all patients eventually resolve the negative effect occasioned by their disability and achieve a final stage of adjustment or resolution. Such a belief has intrinsic appeal to health care professionals, who strive to maximize functional abilities and enhance quality of life.

Behavioral Model

The behavioral model of disability adjustment emphasizes the importance of external factors in determining a person's adjustment. In this model there is reduced interest in the patient's cognitions and a primary focus on observable behaviors. The most frequently cited proponent of this model is Fordyce, and much of what follows is culled from his writings (95,164). Additional applications of the behavioral model to rehabilitation problems can be found in the works of Ince (165,166) and Berni and Fordyce (167). In the behavioral model of adjustment to disability, the newly disabled face four tasks. The patient must remain in the rehabilitation environment, eliminate disability-incongruent behaviors, acquire disability-congruent behaviors, and maintain the output of disability-congruent behaviors.

The onset of physical disability and entry into the rehabilitation environment represent punishment to most people. In learning theory, punishment is defined as the loss of access to positive reinforcers or the response-contingent onset of aversive stimuli. Thus, the newly disabled find themselves initially operating under a pattern of punishment. Two types of behavior follow the onset of aversive stimuli. The first is escape or avoidance, and the second is aggression. Escape or avoidance behavior is frequently seen in the rehabilitation setting in the form of daydreaming, verbal disclaimers of disability, unauthorized forays off the medical unit, and refusal to participate in scheduled treatments. Aggressive behaviors may consist of either rebellious and capricious behavior or verbal and sometimes physical attack. If avoidant or aggressive behaviors are not understood and dealt with therapeutically, rehabilitation may either never begin or end prematurely.

The intervention strategy for these problems involves the discovery and, if possible, reduction of aversive aspects of the rehabilitation environment. This is accompanied by reinforcement of approximations to active participation in the rehabilitation program. Selecting and systematically graphing a mutually agreed on indicator of rehabilitation progress can help the patient focus on tangible improvements. Patient reactions of hostility are common and should be tolerated within limits. These reactions should never be dealt with through counterhostility, which only increases the probability that the environment, including the treatment staff, will become conditioned aversive stimuli. Systematically ignoring unwanted behavior and establishing therapeutic rapport enhance the probability that the patient will remain in the rehabilitation environment.

The reduction of disability-inappropriate behaviors and the acquisition of disability-congruent behaviors are synonymous with the concept of "adjustment to disability." Disability-inappropriate behaviors are decreased by withdrawal of reinforcers after their occurrence, a process known as extinction. Paradoxically, the laws of behavior demonstrate that withdrawal of reinforcers initially results in a temporary increase in the rate of behavior. This is true for both verbal and performance behaviors.

The patient's verbal behavior is likely to change more slowly than performance behavior. Statements indicating a belief in the eventual return of physical function may require years to extinguish; the staff should neither reinforce nor punish unrealistic verbalizations. Rather, a verbal response suggesting the need to maintain hope tempered with a focus on the present is least likely to offend the patient. These statements of patients are more frequent at the onset of rehabilitation and possibly reflect the beginning of extinction. Detailed explanations of anticipated recovery of functional abilities help decrease unrealistic patient or family verbalizations and keep everyone focused on achievable functional goals. This is especially important for family members, who may erroneously believe that the proper way to help the disabled family member cope is through agreeing with unrealistic fantasies about eventual recovery of function.

Difficulties in the acquisition of disability-congruent behaviors are usually considered to be problems in motivation. Learning theory rejects this formulation because it relies on an inference about the internal state of the person. Usually, this label is applied to people who have failed to reach expected levels of performance set by the rehabilitation staff. In learning theory, the problem is that of adjusting contingencies to increase the rate of desired behavior or reduce the rate of behaviors competing with the desired behavior. Unfortunately, most disability-congruent behaviors are initially of low frequency, strength, and value. The steps in changing this situation include establishing reinforcing relationships with the treatment staff, enhancing long-term reinforcers for disability-congruent behaviors, and introducing contingency management interventions that promote the acquisition of disability-congruent behaviors.

Maintaining the output of disability-appropriate behaviors is the final and most important step in adjustment to disability. Rehabilitation is unsuccessful if the behaviors learned in the rehabilitation unit cannot be transferred to the patient's home environment (168). Although the patient may demonstrate the ability to perform a task, the probability of its occurrence depends on contingencies operating in the home environment. Disability-congruent behaviors, such as propelling a wheelchair, maintaining a fluid schedule, and using gait aids, are unlikely to be reinforcing in themselves.

Two strategies for improving generalization are bringing disability-congruent behaviors under the control of reinforcers occurring naturally in the environment and reprogramming the patient's home environment to deliver appropriate reinforcement contingently. The first strategy is promoted through interventions designed to re-engage the patient in meaningful vocational and avocational activities after dismissal. Therefore, vocational counseling and therapeutic recreation are important as part of inpatient rehabilitation. Gradual and systematic rehearsal of newly learned skills in the home environment during weekend visits is an additional method encouraging generalization. The second strategy is promoted through such interventions as home modifications, assigning a family member to monitor and reinforce home therapy programs, and contracting with the patient for continued compliance. Unfortunately, powerful contingencies may be operating to prevent generalization. For example, the patient may receive reinforcers in the form of increased attention or financial rewards from litigation, a condition also known as secondary gain. Inability to control sources of secondary gain may prevent generalization of disability-congruent behaviors to the home environment. Family interventions are critical to prevent these problems.

Coping Skills Model

The coping skills model (169), which emphasizes both cognitive and behavioral factors, is based on the crisis theory originally formulated by Lindemann (170). Crisis theory asserts that people require a sense of social and psychological equilibrium. After a traumatic event, a state of crisis and disorganization occurs. At the time of the crisis, a person's characteristic patterns of behavior are ineffectual in establishing equilibrium. This state of disequilibrium is always temporary, and a new balance is achieved within days to weeks. The coping skills model comprises seven major adaptive tasks and seven major coping skills. The coping skills are elaborated below.

Denying or Minimizing the Seriousness of a Crisis

This coping skill may be directed at the illness or at its significance and helps to reduce negative emotions to manageable levels. This reduction enhances the mental clarity needed for quick and effective action in emergency situations. The likelihood of implementing a greater range of coping responses is also increased.

Seeking Relevant Information

Often, emotional distress is occasioned by a misunderstanding of medical diagnoses and procedures. Understanding often reduces anxiety and provides predictability and a sense of control. The act of gathering information gives the patient and family a concrete task and the accompanying feeling of purposefulness. One longitudinal study of people with chronic illness showed that information-seeking has salubrious effects on adjustment (171).

Requesting Reassurance and Emotional Support

The literature shows that perceived social support, adjustment during a crisis, and improved health outcomes are interrelated (172–174). Component parts of social support are perceiving that one is cared for, being encouraged to openly express beliefs and feelings, and being provided material aid. Social support may enhance coping by reducing counter-productive emotional states, building self-esteem, and increasing receptivity to new information. Cobb suggested that social support enhances health outcome either directly through neuroendocrine pathways or indirectly through increased patient compliance (175,176). He cited evidence showing that patients who receive social support are more likely to stay in treatment and follow their physicians' recommendations. Turner found a reliable association between social support and psychological well-being, especially during stressful circumstances (177).

Learning Specific Illness-Related Procedures

This skill reaffirms personal competence and enhances self-esteem, which is often undermined by physical disability. Bulman and Wortman asked social workers and nurses on a rehabilitation unit to define good and poor coping in patients with spinal cord injury (178). Both groups agreed that good coping included the willingness to learn physical skills that would minimize disability. Conversely, the definition of poor coping included an unwillingness to improve the condition or attend physical therapy.

Setting Concrete Limited Goals

Limited goal-setting breaks a large task into small and more readily mastered components. as each component is mastered, self-reinforcement accrues and sets the stage for further learning. Limited goal setting decreases feelings of being overwhelmed and enhances the opportunity to achieve something considered meaningful.

Rehearsing Alternative Outcomes

Activities such as mental rehearsal, anticipation, discussions with significant others, and incorporation of medical information are involved in this skill. Here, the patient considers possible outcomes and determines the most fruitful manner of handling each. Recalling previous periods of stress and how these were successfully managed is an example of this coping skill. The patient engages in behaviors that alleviate feelings of anxiety, tension, fear, and uncertainty. A cognitive road map is delineated to provide guidance on how any of a variety of possible future stressors will be minimized.

Finding a General Purpose or Pattern of Meaning in the Course of Events

Physical disability is a crisis that can destroy a person's belief that the world is a predictable, meaningful, and understandable place. There appears to be a compelling psychological need to believe that the world is just (179) and to make sense out of a crisis experience. Some theorists claim that the search for meaning is a basic human motivation (180). Bulman and Wortman studied 29 subjects with spinal cord injury and concluded that "the ability to perceive an orderly relationship between one's behaviors and one's outcomes is important for effective coping" (178). Krause, in a 15-year prospective study of persons with spinal cord injury, found that survival was directly related to higher activity levels and being employed (181).

SUMMARY

This chapter began with a review of the history and current status of rehabilitation psychology. This was followed by an overview of services offered by the rehabilitation psychologist and theories of adjustment to disability. Although the rehabilitation psychologist provides a wide variety of direct and indirect services, certain skills are particularly relevant to rehabilitation. These are training in the standardized measurement of human attributes, behavior modification, and research. Rehabilitation environments represent settings in which people under physical and emotional distress are asked to learn. Many of these people not only are emotionally upset but also have brain injuries that further impair learning efficiency. Standardized measurement of personality, intellectual ability, academic achievement, neuropsychological integrity, and chemical health provide a valid and reliable base on which to set rehabilitation goals.

Rehabilitation is specifically concerned with the behavior and functional performance of a person. Rehabilitation team members provide diverse interventions to ensure that the person can physically perform specific activities. Whether this person will actually do so is determined by contingencies in the rehabilitation unit and, more important, in the home environment. The rehabilitation psychologist's behavioral modification skills permit the careful assessment and harnessing of these contingencies in the service of the patient.

Progress in any scientific activity depends on research of high quality. Such research is of particular concern for rehabilitation because outcomes are determined by an unusually large and complex set of physical and social variables. Doctoral-level psychologists are usually the only rehabilitation team members with training in research. Traditionally, this training follows the clinician-researcher model, which stresses the asking of practical research questions relevant to clinical problems. These clinical problems may consist of the evaluation of entire rehabilitation service delivery systems.

Theories of adjustment to disability are numerous and can be grouped along a continuum stressing internal cognitive events on the one end and external social and behavioral events on the other. Stage theory is a widely held but largely unsubstantiated model that stresses internal events. Alternative models worth considering are the behavioral model and the coping skills model.

REFERENCES

1. Eisenberg MG, Jansen MA. Rehabilitation psychology: state of the art. *Annu Rev Rehabil* 1983; 3:1–31.
2. Fraser RT. An introduction to rehabilitation psychology. In: Golden CJ, ed. *Current topics in rehabilitation psychology.* Orlando, FL: Grune & Stratton, 1984; 1–15.
3. DeLeon PH, Forsythe P, VandenBos GR. Federal recognition of psychology in rehabilitation programs. *Rehabil Psychol* 1986; 31:47–56.
4. Bruyere SM, ed. Special issue on the implications of the Americans with Disabilities Act of 1990 for psychologists. *Rehabil Psychol* 1993; 38:71–148.
5. Shontz FC, Wright BA. The distinctiveness of rehabilitation psychology. *Prof Psychol* 1980; 11:919–924.
6. Grzesiak RC. Psychological services in rehabilitation medicine; clinical aspects of rehabilitation psychology. *Prof Psychol* 1979; 10: 511–520.
7. Elliott TR, Gramling SE. Psychologists and rehabilitation: new roles and old training models. *Am Psychol* 1990; 45:762–765.
8. Patterson DR, Hanson SL. Joint Division 22 and ACRM guidelines for postdoctoral training in rehabilitation psychology. *Rehabil Psychol* 1995; 40:299–310.
9. Caplan B. Statement of vision and mission: APA division 22. *Rehabil Psychol News* 1996; 23:14.
10. Cushman LA, Scherer MJ, eds. *Psychological assessment in medical rehabilitation.* Washington, DC, American Psychological Association, 1995.
11. Kramer JJ, Conoley JC, eds. *The 11th mental measurements yearbook.* Lincoln: The University of Nebraska Press, 1992.
12. Epstein S, O'Brien EJ. The person–situation debate in historical and current perspective. *Psychol Bull* 1985; 98:513–537.
13. Anastasi A. *Psychological testing, 6th ed.* New York: Macmillan, 1988.
14. Elliott TR, Umlauf RL. Measurement of personality and psychopathology following acquired physical disability. In: Cushman LA, Scherer MJ, eds. *Psychological assessment in medical rehabilitation.* Washington, DC: American Psychological Association, 1995; 325–358.
15. Elliott TR, Frank RG. Depression following spinal cord injury. *Arch Phys Med Rehabil* 1996; 77:816–823.
16. Rohe DE. Loss, grief and depression in persons with laryngectomy. In: Keith RL, Darley FL, eds. *Laryngectomee rehabilitation, 3rd ed.* Austin, TX: Pro-Ed Publications, Inc., 1993; 487–514.
17. Dahlstrom WG, Welsh GS, Dahlstrom LE, eds. *An MMPI handbook, Vol. 1. Clinical interpretation, rev. ed.* Minneapolis: University of Minnesota Press, 1972.
18. Dahlstrom WG, Welsh GS, Dahlstrom LE, eds. *An MMPI handbook, Vol. 2. Research applications, rev. ed.* Minneapolis: University of Minnesota Press, 1975.
19. Greene RL, ed. *The MMPI-2: an interpretive manual, 2nd ed.* Boston: Allyn & Bacon, 1991.
20. Swenson WM, Pearson JS, Osborne D. *An MMPI source book: basic item, scale, and pattern data on 50,000 medical patients.* Minneapolis: University of Minnesota Press, 1973.
21. Levitt EE, Gotts EE. *The clinical applications of the MMPI special scales, 2nd ed.* Hillsdale, NJ: Lawrence Erlbaum Associates, 1995.
22. Rodevich MA, Wanlass RL. The moderating effect of spinal cord injury on MMPI-2 profiles: a clinically derived T score correction procedure. *Rehabil Psychol* 1995; 40:181–190.
23. Butcher JN, Dahlstrom WG, Graham JR, Tellegen A, Kaemmer B. *MMPI-2, manual for administration and scoring.* Minneapolis: University of Minnesota Press, 1989.
24. Butcher JN, Williams CL, Graham JR, Archer RP, Tellegen A, Ben-Porath YS, Kaemmer B. *Minnesota multiphasic personality inventory—adolescent, manual for administration, scoring and interpretation.* Minneapolis: University of Minnesota Press, 1992.
25. Colligan RC, Offord KP. Adolescents, the MMPI, and the issue of K correction: a contemporary normative study. *J Clin Psychol* 1991; 47:607–631.
26. Colligan RC, Osborne D, Swenson WM, Offord KP, eds. *The MMPI: a contemporary normative study of adults, 2nd ed.* Odessa, FL: Psychological Assessment Resources, 1989.
27. Greene RL. Stability of MMPI scale scores within four codetypes across forty years. *J Pers Assess* 1990; 55:1–6.
28. Humphrey DH, Dahlstrom WG. The impact of changing from the MMPI to the MMPI-2 on profile configurations. *J Pers Assess* 1995; 64:428–439.
29. Helmes E, Reddon JR. A perspective on developments in assessing psychopathology: a critical review of the MMPI and MMPI-2. *Psych Bull* 1993; 113:453–471.
30. Digman JM. Personality structure: emergence of the five-factor model. In: Rosenzweig MR, Porter LW, eds. *Annual review of psychology*, vol. 41. Palo Alto, CA: Annual Reviews, 1990; 417–440.
31. Goldberg LR. The structure of phenotypic personality traits. *Am Psychol* 1993; 48:26–34.
32. Costa PT Jr., McRae RR. *NEO-PI-R professional manual.* Odessa, FL: Psychological Assessment Resources, 1992.
33. Rohe DE, Krause JS. *The five factor model of personality: findings among males with spinal cord injury.* Paper presented at 101st Annual Meeting, American Psychological Association, Toronto, August 22, 1993.
34. Costa PT Jr, McCrae RR, Holland JL. Personality and vocational interests in an adult sample. *J Appl Psychol* 1984; 69:390–400.
35. Harmon LW, Hansen JC, Borgen FH, Hammer AL. *Strong interest inventory: applications and technical guide.* Palo Alto: Consulting Psychologists Press, 1994.
36. Holland JL. *Making vocational choices: a theory of personalities and work environments, 2nd ed.* Englewood Cliffs, NJ: Prentice-Hall, 1985.
37. Rohe DE, Athelstan GT. Vocational interests of persons with spinal cord injury. *J Couns Psychol* 1982; 29:283–291.
38. Malec J. Personality factors associated with severe traumatic disability. *Rehabil Psychol* 1985; 30:165–172.
39. Rohe DE. Personality and spinal cord injury. *Top Spinal Cord Inj Rehabil* 1996; 2(9):1–10.
40. Rohe DE, Athelstan GT. Change in vocational interests after spinal cord injury. *Rehabil Psychol* 1985; 30:131–143.
41. Rohe DE, Krause JS. Stability of interests after severe physical disability: an 11-year longitudinal study. *J Voc Behav* 1998; 52 (in press).
42. Wechsler D. *The Wechsler Adult Intelligence Test: revised manual.* New York: Psychological Corporation, 1983.
43. Tulsky DS, Zhu J, Prifitera A. *An introduction to the Wechsler Adult Intelligence Scale, 3rd ed.* Paper presented at 104th Annual Meeting, American Psychological Association, Toronto, August 17, 1996.
44. Cohen J. A factor-analytically based rationale for the Wechsler Adult Intelligence Scale. *J Consult Psychol* 1957; 21:451–457.
45. Malec JF, Ivnik RJ, Smith GE, Tangalos EG, Petersen RC, Kokmen E, Kurland LT. Mayo's older adult normative studies: utility of corrections for age and education for the WAIS-R. *Clin Neuropsychol* 1992; 6(Suppl):31–47.
46. Wilkinson GS. *Wide-Range Achievement Test administration manual.* Wilmington, DE: Wide Range, Inc., 1993.
47. Cummings JA. Review of Woodcock–Johnson Psycho-Educational Battery. In: Mitchell JV Jr, ed. *The ninth mental measurements yearbook, Vols. 1 and 2.* Lincoln, NE: University of Nebraska Press, 1985; 1759–1762.
48. Kaufman AS. Review of Woodcock–Johnson Psycho-Educational Battery. In: Mitchell JV Jr, ed. *The ninth mental measurements yearbook, Vols. 1 and 2.* Lincoln, NE: University of Nebraska Press, 1985; 1762–1765.
49. Woodcock RW, Johnson MB. *Woodcock–Johnson PsychoEducational Battery—revised.* Allen, TX: DLM Teaching Resources, 1989.
50. Lezak MD, ed. *Neuropsychological assessment, 3rd ed.* New York: Oxford University Press, 1995.
51. Therapeutics and Technology Assessment Subcommittee of the American Academy of Neurology. Assessment: neuropsychological testing of adults. *Neurology* 1996; 47:592–599.
52. Kochansky GE. Psychiatric rating scales for assessing psychopathology in the elderly: a critical review. In: Raskin A, Jarvik LF, eds. *Psychiatric symptoms and cognitive loss in the elderly: evaluation and assessment techniques.* Washington, DC: Hemisphere Publishing Company, 1979.
53. Kokmen E, Naessens JM, Offord KP. A short test of mental status: description and preliminary results. *Mayo Clin Proc* 1987; 62: 281–288.
54. Kokmen E, Smith GE, Petersen RC, Tangalos E, Ivnik RC. The short test of mental status: correlations with standardized psychometric testing. *Arch Neurol* 1991; 48:725–728.

55. Teasdale G, Jennett B. Assessment of coma and impaired consciousness: a practical scale. *Lancet* 1974; 2:81–84.
56. Levin HS, O'Donnell VM, Grossman RG. The Galveston Orientation and Amnesia Test: a practical scale to assess cognition after head injury. *J Nerv Ment Dis* 1979; 167:675–683.
57. Boll TJ. The Halstead–Reitan Neuropsychology Battery. In: Filskov SB, Boll TJ, eds. *Handbook of clinical neuropsychology.* New York: John Wiley & Sons, 1981: 577–607.
58. Filskov SB, Goldstein SG. Diagnostic validity of the Halstead–Reitan Neuropsychological Battery. *J Consult Clin Psychol* 1974; 42: 382–388.
59. Caplan B. Neuropsychology in rehabilitation: its role in evaluation and intervention. *Arch Phys Med Rehabil* 1982; 63:362–366.
60. Dunn EJ, Searight HR, Grisso T, Margolis RB, Gibbons JL. The relation of the Halstead–Reitan Neuropsychological Battery to functional daily living skills in geriatric patients. *Arch Clin Neuropsychol* 1990; 5:103–117.
61. Heinrichs RW. Current and emergent applications of neuropsychological assessment: problems of validity and utility. *Prof Psychol Res Pract* 1990; 21:171–176.
62. Meier MJ, Benton AL, Diller L, eds. *Neuropsychological rehabilitation.* New York: Guilford Press, 1987.
63. Satz P, Fletcher JM. Emergent trends in neuropsychology: an overview. *J Consult Clin Psychol* 1981; 49:851–865.
64. Heaton RK, Pendleton MG. Use of neuropsychological tests to predict adult patients' everyday functioning. *J Consult Clin Psychol* 1981; 49:807–821.
65. Wicker AW. Nature and assessment of behavior settings: recent contributions from the ecological perspective. In: McReynolds P, ed. *Advances in psychological assessment, Vol. 2.* San Francisco: Josey-Bass, 1981.
66. Reitan RM. Theoretical and methodological bases of the Halstead–Reitan Neuropsychological Test Battery. In: Grant I, Adams KM, eds. *Neuropsychological assessment of neuropsychiatric disorders.* New York: Oxford University Press, 1986; 3–30.
67. Reitan RM. A research program on the psychological effects of brain lesions in human beings. In: Ellis NR, ed. *International review of research in mental retardation, Vol. 1.* New York: Academic Press, 1966; 153–218.
68. Heaton RK, Grant I, Matthews CG. *Comprehensive norms for an expanded Halstead–Reitan battery.* Odessa, FL: Psychological Assessment Resources, 1991.
69. Milberg WP, Hebben N, Kaplan E. The Boston process approach to neuropsychological assessment. In: Grant I, Adams KM. eds. *Neuropsychological assessment of neuropsychiatric disorders.* New York: Oxford University Press, 1986; 65–86.
70. Kaplan E, Fein D, Morris R, Delis D. *WAIS-R as a neuropsychological instrument.* San Antonio: The Psychological Corporation, 1991.
71. Rohe DE, DePompolo RW. Substance abuse policies in rehabilitation medicine departments. *Arch Phys Med Rehabil* 1985; 66:701–703.
72. Eckardt MJ, Harford TC, Kaelber CT, et al. Health hazards associated with alcohol consumption. *JAMA* 1981; 246:648–666.
73. Cameron JS, Halla-Poe D. *Alcohol and spinal cord injury.* Minneapolis: Brad Thompson, 1985.
74. Fullerton DT, Harvey RF, Klein MH, Howell T. Psychiatric disorders in patients with spinal cord injuries. *Arch Gen Psychiatry* 1981; 38: 1369–1371.
75. Heinemann AW, Mamott BD, Schnoll S. Substance use by persons with recent spinal cord injuries. *Rehabil Psychol* 1990; 35:217–228.
76. Corrigan JD. Substance abuse as a mediating factor in outcome from traumatic brain injury. *Arch Phys Med Rehabil* 1996; 76:302–309.
77. Heinemann AW, Schmidt MF, Semik P. Drinking patterns, drinking expectancies, and coping after spinal cord injury. *Rehabil Counsel Bull* 1994; 38:135–153.
78. Heinemann AW, Doll MD, Armstrong KJ, Schnoll S, Yarkony GM. Substance use and receipt of treatment by persons with long-term spinal cord injuries. *Arch Phys Med Rehabil* 1991; 72:482–487.
79. Rimel RW. A prospective study of patients with central nervous system trauma. *J Neurosurg Nurs* 1981; 13:132–141.
80. Schmidt MF, Garvin LJ. *Substance abuse prevention for people with traumatic brain injury.* Paper presented at the 12th annual conference of the National Head Injury Foundation, Chicago, November 10, 1994.
81. Schmidt MF, Heinemann AW, Semik P. The efficacy of inservice training on substance abuse and spinal cord injury issues. *Top Spinal Cord Inj Rehabil* 1996; 2:11–20.
82. Cherry L. *Summary report. Alcohol, drugs, and disability II: second national policy and leadership development symposium.* San Mateo, CA: Institute on Alcohol, Drugs and Disability, 1994.
83. Center for Substance Abuse Prevention. *Rehabilitation Specialists Prevention Training System.* Rockville, MD: Center for Substance Abuse Prevention, United States Department of Health and Human Services, 1994.
84. Weinberg JR. Interview techniques for diagnosing alcoholism. *Am Fam Physician* 1974; 9:107–115.
85. Ewing JA. Detecting alcoholism: the CAGE questionnaire. *JAMA* 1984;252:1905–1907.
86. Swenson WM, Morse RM. The use of a Self-Administered Alcoholism Screening Test (SAAST) in a medical center. *Mayo Clin Proc* 1975; 50:204–208.
87. Selzer ML. The Michigan Alcoholism Screening Test: the quest for a new diagnostic instrument. *Am J Psychiatry* 1971; 127:1653–1658.
88. Hurt RD, Morse RM, Swenson WM. Diagnosis of alcoholism with a Self-Administered Alcoholism Screening Test: results with 1,002 consecutive patients receiving general examinations. *Mayo Clin Proc* 1980; 55:365–370.
89. Strupp HH. Psychotherapy research and practice: an overview. In: Garfield SL, Bergin AE, eds. *Handbook of psychotherapy and behavior change: an empirical analysis, 2nd ed.* New York: John Wiley & Sons, 1978; 3–22.
90. Butcher JN, Koss MP. Research on brief and crisis-oriented therapies. In: Garfield SL, Bergin AE, eds. *Handbook of psychotherapy and behavior change: an empirical analysis, 2nd ed.* New York: John Wiley & Sons, 1978; 725–767.
91. Turk DC, Meichenbaum D, Genest M. *Pain and behavioral medicine: a cognitive–behavioral perspective.* New York: Guilford Press, 1983.
92. Martin G, Pear J. *Behavior modification: what it is and how to do it, 2nd ed.* Englewood Cliffs, NJ: Prentice-Hall, 1983.
93. Reynolds GS: *A primer of operant conditioning, revised edition.* Glenview: Scott, Foresman and Company, 1975.
94. Kazdin AE. *Behavior modification in applied settings, 5th ed.* Pacific Grove, CA: Brooks Cole, 1994.
95. Brockway JA, Fordyce WE. Psychological assessment and management. In: Kottke FJ, Lehmann JF, eds. *Krusen's handbook of physical medicine and rehabilitation, 4th ed.* Philadelphia: WB Saunders, 1990; 153–170.
96. Malec JF, Lemsky C. Behavioral assessment in medical rehabilitation: traditional and consensual approaches. In: Cushman LA, Scherer MJ, eds. *Psychological assessment in medical rehabilitation.* Washington, DC: American Psychological Association, 1995; 199–236.
97. Asch A. The experience of disability: a challenge for psychology. *Am Psychol* 1984; 39:529–536.
98. Davis F. Deviance disavowal: the management of strained interaction by the visibly handicapped. *Soc Problems* 1961; 9:120–132.
99. Dembo T, Leviton GL, Wright BA. Adjustment to misfortune: a problem of social-psychological rehabilitation. *Rehabil Psychol* 1975; 22: 1–100.
100. Goffman E. *Stigma: notes on the management of spoiled identity.* Englewood Cliffs, NJ: Prentice-Hall, 1963.
101. Hanks M, Poplin DE. The sociology of physical disability: a review of literature and some conceptual perspectives. *Dev Behav* 1981; 2: 309–328.
102. Meyerson L. The social psychology of physical disability: 1948 and 1988. *J Soc Issues* 1988; 44:173–188.
103. Nagler M, ed. *Perspectives on disability, 2nd ed.* Palo Alto, CA: Health Markets Research, 1993.
104. Richardson SA. Attitudes and behavior toward the physically handicapped. *Birth Defects* 1976; 12(4):15–34.
105. Siller J. Psychological situation of the disabled with spinal cord injuries. *Rehabil Lit* 1969; 30:290–296.
106. Tajfel H. Social psychology of intergroup relations. *Annu Rev Psychol* 1982; 33:1–39.
107. Yuker HE, ed. *Attitudes toward persons with disabilities.* New York: Springer, 1988.
108. Dunn DS, ed. Psychosocial perspectives on disability. *J Soc Behav Pers* 1994; 9:1–424.
109. Hastorf AH, Northcraft GB, Picciotto SR. Helping the handicapped:

how realistic is the performance feedback received by the physically handicapped? *Pers Soc Psychol Bull* 1979; 5:373–376.
110. Cogswell BE. Self-socialization: readjustment of paraplegics in the community. *J Rehabil* 1968; 34:11–40.
111. Norris-Baker C. Behavioral discriminators of health outcomes in spinal cord injury (abstract). *Arch Phys Med Rehabil* 1982; 63: 503.
112. Conger JC, Farrell AD. Behavioral components of heterosocial skills. *Behav Ther* 1981; 12:41–55.
113. Curran JP. Skills training as an approach to the treatment of heterosexual–social anxiety: a review. *Psychol Bull* 1977; 84:140–157.
114. Dunn M, Herman SH. Social skills and rehabilitation. In: Caplan B, ed. *Rehabilitation psychology desk reference.* Rockville, MD: Aspen Publishers, 1987; 345–364.
115. Gambrill ED, Richey CA. An assertion inventory for use in assessment and research. *Behav Ther* 1975; 6:550–561.
116. Dunn M. Social discomfort in the patient with spinal cord injury. *Arch Phys Med Rehabil* 1977; 58:257–260.
117. Piliavin IM, Piliavin JA, Rodin J. Costs, diffusion, and the stigmatized victim. *J Pers Soc Psychol* 1975; 32:429–438.
118. Soble SL, Strickland LH. Physical stigma, interaction, and compliance. *Bull Psychon Soc* 1974; 4:130–132.
119. Dunn M, Van Horn E, Herman SH. Social skills and spinal cord injury: a comparison of three training procedures. *Behav Ther* 1981; 12:153–164.
120. Ginsburg ML. Assertion with the wheelchair-bound: measurement and training. *Diss Abstr Int B* 1979; 39:5552-B.
121. Mischel MH. Assertion training with handicapped persons. *J Couns Psychol* 1978; 25:238–241.
122. Morgan B, Leung P. Effects of assertion training on acceptance of disability by physically disabled university students. *J Couns Psychol* 1980; 27:209–212.
123. Curran JP, Monti PM, eds. *Social skills training: a practical handbook for assessment and treatment.* New York: Guilford Press, 1982.
124. Hersen M, Bellack AS. Assessment of social skills. In: Ciminero AR, Calhoun KS, Adams HE, eds. *Handbook of behavioral assessment.* New York: John Wiley & Sons, 1977.
125. Bellack AS, Hersen M. *Introduction to clinical psychology.* New York: Oxford University Press, 1980.
126. Wilkinson J, Canter S. *Social skills training manual.* New York: John Wiley & Sons, 1982.
127. Brotherton FA, Thomas LL, Wisotzek IE, Milan MA. Social skills training in rehabilitation of patients with traumatic closed head injury. *Arch Phys Med Rehabil* 1988; 69:827–832.
128. Keith RA. The comprehensive treatment team in rehabilitation. *Arch Phys Med Rehabil* 1991; 72:269–274.
129. Rothberg JS. The rehabilitation team: future direction. *Arch Phys Med Rehabil* 1981; 62:407–410.
130. Diller L. Fostering the interdisciplinary team, fostering research in a society in transition. *Arch Phys Med Rehabil* 1990; 71:275–278.
131. Ackermann L, Campbell D, Hall J, Hawkins H. Role clarification: a procedure for enhancing interdisciplinary collaboration on the rehab team (abstract). *Arch Phys Med Rehabil* 1983; 64:514.
132. Shontz FC. Psychological adjustment to physical disability: trends in theories. *Arch Phys Med Rehabil* 1978; 59:251–254.
133. Kahana RJ, Bibring GL. Personality types in medical management. In: Zinberg NE, ed. *Psychiatry and medical practice in a general hospital.* New York: International Universities Press, 1964; 108–123.
134. Parsons T. Definitions of health and illness in the light of American values and social structure. In: Jaco EG, ed. *Patients, physicians and illness: a sourcebook in behavioral science and health, 2nd ed.* New York: Free Press, 1972; 99–117.
135. Mechanic D. The concept of illness behavior. *J Chron Dis* 1962;15: 189–194.
136. Kutner B. The social psychology of disability. In: Neff WS, ed. *Rehabilitation Psychology.* Washington, DC: American Psychological Association, 1971; 143–67.
137. Lewin K. *Principles of topological psychology*, translated by F Heider, G Heider. New York: McGraw-Hill, 1936.
138. Myerson L. Somatopsychology of physical disability. In: Cruickshank WM, ed. *Psychology of exceptional children and youth, 2nd ed.* Englewood Cliffs, NJ: Prentice-Hall, 1963; 1–52.
139. Trieschmann RB. *Spinal cord injuries: psychological, social, and vocational rehabilitation, 2nd ed.* New York: Demos Publications, 1988.
140. Wright BA. *Physical disability, a psychosocial approach, 2nd ed.* New York: Harper & Row, 1983.
141. Shontz FC. Reactions to crisis. *Volta Rev* 1965; 67:364–370.
142. Shontz FC. *The psychological aspects of physical illness and disability.* New York: Macmillan, 1975.
143. Gullo SV, Cherico DJ, Shadick R. Cited in Garber J, Seligman MEP, eds. *Human helplessness: theory and applications.* New York: Academic Press, 1980.
144. Beard BH. Fear of death and fear of life: the dilemma in chronic renal failure, hemodialysis, and kidney transplantation. *Arch Gen Psychiatry* 1969; 21:373–380.
145. Reichsman F, Levy NB. Problems in adaptation to maintenance hemodialysis: a four-year study of 25 patients. *Arch Intern Med* 1972; 130: 859–865.
146. Bray GP. Rehabilitation of spinal cord injured: a family approach. *J Appl Rehabil Couns* 1978; 9:70–78.
147. Cohn N. Understanding the process of adjustment to disability. *J Rehabil* 1961; 27(6):16–18.
148. Weller DJ, Miller PM. Emotional reactions of patient, family, and staff in acute-care period of spinal cord injury: Part I. *Soc Work Health Care* 1977; 2:369–377.
149. Weller DJ, Miller PM. Emotional reactions of patient, family, and staff in acute-care period of spinal cord injury: Part II. *Soc Work Health Care* 1977; 3:7–17.
150. Parkes CM. Components of the reaction to loss of a limb, spouse or home. *J Psychosom Res* 1972; 16:343–349.
151. Gunther MS. Emotional aspects. In: Ruge D, ed. *Spinal cord injuries.* Springfield, IL: Charles C Thomas, 1979; 93–108.
152. Silver RL, Wortman CB. Coping with undesirable life events. In: Garber J, Seligman MEP, eds. *Human helplessness: theory and applications.* New York: Academic Press, 1980; 279–340.
153. Tyhurst JS. Individual reactions to community disaster: the natural history of psychiatric phenomena. *Am J Psychiatry* 1951; 107: 764–769.
154. Engel GL. Grief and grieving. *Am J Nurs* 1964; 64:93–98.
155. Zahourek R, Jensen JS. Grieving and the loss of the newborn. *Am J Nurs* 1973; 73:836–839.
156. McDaniel JW, Sexton AW. Psychoendocrine studies of patients with spinal cord lesions. *J Abnorm Psychol* 1970; 76:117–122.
157. Nighswonger CA. Ministry to the dying as a learning encounter. *J Thanatol* 1971; 1:101–108.
158. Bernstein L, Bernstein RS, Dana RH. *Interviewing: a guide for health professionals, 4th ed.* Norwalk, CT: Appleton-Century-Crofts, 1985.
159. Dunn D. Cited in Trieschmann RB. *Spinal cord injuries: psychological, social, and vocational rehabilitation, 2nd ed.* New York: Demos Publications, 1988.
160. Dinardo QE. Psychological adjustment to spinal cord injury. *Diss Abstr Int B* 1972; 32:4206-B.
161. Lawson NC. Depression after spinal cord injury: a multimeasure longitudinal study. *Diss Abstr Int B* 1976; 37:1439-B.
162. Shadish WR Jr, Hickman D, Arrick MC. Psychological problems of spinal cord injury patients: emotional distress as a function of time and locus of control. *J Consult Clin Psychol* 1981; 49:297.
163. Gans JS. Depression diagnosis in a rehabilitation hospital. *Arch Phys Med Rehabil* 1981; 62:386–389.
164. Fordyce WE, ed. *Behavioral methods for chronic pain and illness.* St Louis: CV Mosby, 1976.
165. Ince LP, ed. *Behavior modification in rehabilitation medicine.* Springfield, IL: Charles C Thomas, 1976.
166. Ince LP, ed. *Behavioral psychology in rehabilitation medicine: clinical applications.* Baltimore: Williams & Wilkins, 1980.
167. Berni R, Fordyce WE, eds. *Behavior modification and the nursing process, 2nd ed.* St Louis: CV Mosby, 1977.
168. Davidoff G, Schultz JS, Lieb T, et al. Rehospitalization after initial rehabilitation for acute spinal cord injury: incidence and risk factors. *Arch Phys Med Rehabil* 1990; 71:121–124.
169. Moos RH, Tsu VD, eds. *Coping with physical illness.* New York: Plenum Medical, 1977; 3–21.
170. Lindemann E. Symptomatology and management of acute grief. *Am J Psychiatry* 1944; 101:141–148.
171. Felton BJ, Revenson TA. Coping with chronic illness: a study of

illness controllability and the influence of coping strategies on psychological adjustment. *J Consult Clin Psychol* 1984; 52:343–353.

172. Cutrona C, Russell D, Rose J. Social support and adaptation to stress by the elderly. *Psychol Aging* 1986; 1:47–54.
173. Gottlieb BH. Social support as a focus for integrative research in psychology. *Am Psychol* 1983; 38:278–287.
174. Schaefer C, Coyne JC, Lazarus RS. The health-related functions of social support. *J Behav Med* 1981; 4:381–406.
175. Cobb S. Social support as a moderator of life stress. *Psychosom Med* 1976; 38:300–314.
176. Cobb S. Cited in Garber J, Seligman MEP, eds. *Human helplessness: theory and applications.* New York: Academic Press, 1980.
177. Turner RJ. Social support as a contingency in psychological well-being. *J Health Soc Behav* 1981; 22:357–367.
178. Bulman RJ, Wortman CB. Attributions of blame and coping in the ''real world:'' severe accident victims react to their lot. *J Pers Soc Psychol* 1977; 35:351–363.
179. Lerner MJ. *The belief in a just world: a fundamental delusion.* New York: Plenum Press, 1980.
180. Frankl VE. *Man's search for meaning: an introduction to logotherapy, rev. ed.*, translated by I Lasch. Boston: Beacon Press, 1963.
181. Krause J. Survival following spinal cord injury: a fifteen-year prospective study. *Rehabil Psychol* 1991; 36:89–98.

Rehabilitation Medicine: Principles and Practice, Third Edition, edited by Joel A. DeLisa and Bruce M. Gans.
Lippincott–Raven Publishers, Philadelphia © 1998.

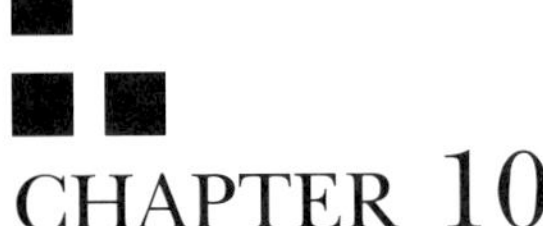

CHAPTER 10

Occupational Rehabilitation and Disability Determination

Robert D. Rondinelli, James P. Robinson, Steven J. Scheer, and Stuart M. Weinstein

Within the field of physical medicine and rehabilitation (PM&R), occupational rehabilitation includes those injuries and illnesses arising in the workplace, which are compensable and generally treatable under workers' compensation. It is essential that the physiatrist managing such cases be able to recognize and adeptly manage an array of conditions that are particularly prone to the development of chronicity and prolonged work disability. One should become familiar with expected patterns of recovery from musculoskeletal injuries while recognizing the potential negative influence of the claims process and litigation on outcomes in certain cases. The rules and statutory requirements of the workers' compensation system must be followed in order to maintain professional credibility and minimize compliance frustrations. The physician must develop fair and equitable impairment ratings and make safe, valid, and reliable return-to-work determinations on a routine basis. Furthermore, one may be expected to serve as an independent medical examiner empowered by a medicolegal system whose moral and ethical imperatives extend well beyond the confines of the traditional patient–physician relationship.

The scope and purpose of this chapter are threefold: first, to familiarize the reader with the unique features of occupational rehabilitation that qualify it as a subspecialty area; second, to illustrate the comprehensive evaluation and treatment approach to acute, subacute, and chronic work injury through a focus on occupational low back pain (LBP); and third, to provide an overview of impairment ratings, work disability determinations, and the independent medical evaluation through an approach that is based on the AMA Guides (1) and is consistent with workers' compensation law and the Americans with Disabilities Act (ADA). The special case of cumulative trauma disorders, an occupational illness, is dealt with exclusively in Chapter 65 and is not discussed in detail here.

R. D. Rondinelli: Department of Physical Medicine and Rehabilitation, University of Kansas Medical Center, Kansas City, Kansas 66160-7306.

J. P. Robinson: Department of Rehabilitation Medicine, University of Washington Hospital, Seattle, Washington 98195; and University of Washington Pain Center, Seattle, Washington 98105.

S. J. Scheer: Department of Physical Medicine and Rehabilitation, University of Cincinnati, Cincinnati, Ohio 45267-0530.

S. M. Weinstein: Department of Rehabilitation Medicine, University of Washington, Seattle, Washington 98195; and Puget Sound Sports and Spine Physicians, Seattle, Washington 98122.

OCCUPATIONAL REHABILITATION AS A SUBSPECIALTY AREA

Natural History of Work-Related Injury

Epidemiology

Overall Statistics

The Bureau of Labor Statistics (2) reported a total of approximately 6.8 million occupational injuries and illnesses for 1992, a rate of 8.9 per 100 workers. Of these, over 92% were injuries, and the remainder illnesses. The total cost of workers' compensation to business in 1992 was estimated at $55 billion. Of this total, $18.3 billion (33%) was directed toward medical treatment, and $26.4 billion (48%) toward survivor benefits and disability payment, with the remaining costs attributed to administration of all industrial compensation systems (3). Such costs appear even more staggering if one considers the likelihood of significant underreporting of industrial problems in general and illnesses in particular (4). Furthermore, of the problems that are reported, not all are accepted as being valid industrial injuries or illnesses. Ap-

TABLE 10-1. *1988 Washington State injury profile by nature of injury*

Nature of injury	All claims	Percent of claims that produce time loss >120 days	Number of claims with time loss >120 days
Contusions, bruises, cuts, lacerations, punctures, scratches, abrasions	74,713 (47.6%)	0.8%	644 (9.6%)
Sprains, strains	59,729 (37.6%)	7.5%	4,456 (66.1%)
Fractures	7,424 (4.7%)	11.9%	882 (13.1%)
Burns	5,777 (3.6%)	0.6%	38 (0.6%)
Multiple injuries	2,689 (1.7%)	10.2%	273 (4.0%)
Dislocations	1,483 (0.9%)	19.0%	282 (4.2%)
Amputations	237 (0.1%)	18.1%	43 (0.6%)
Other	5,918 (3.7%)	2.1%	123 (1.8%)
Totals	158,970 (100%)	—	6,741 (100%)

From Washington State Department of Labor and Industries (unpublished).

proximately 18% of industrial illness claims and 4% of industrial injury claims are rejected (5).

Common Work Injuries and Illnesses

A breakdown of injuries that occurred among workers in Washington State in 1988 is presented by type of injury in Table 10-1 and by body part affected in Table 10-2. The largest proportion of injuries comprises contusions, bruises and lacerations (47.6%), followed by sprains and strains (37.6%). Whereas hand or finger injuries are the single most commonly affected body part (17.7%), injuries to the back (16.2%) or back and neck (5%), when viewed collectively, are even more common. Approximately 90% of back injuries are attributable to sprains or strains.

Among occupational illnesses, it is striking that approximately 60% involve repetitive trauma, usually of the upper extremity (carpal tunnel syndrome is a subset of upper extremity illnesses which may be caused by repetitive trauma). The next most frequently reported illnesses are skin disorders (14%) and respiratory conditions associated with toxic agents (5%) (2, p. 7). The most frequent types of repetitive activities associated with occupational illnesses are repetitive grasping or moving objects (other than tools) and repetitive use of tools (2, p. 135). As might be expected, the overwhelming majority of repetitive injuries occur in manufacturing jobs, and the 25 industries with the highest rates of repetitive trauma are all manufacturers (2, p. 7), with meat packing and motor vehicle assembly plants leading the way. Keyboarding is also a significant cause of repetitive trauma-induced occupational illness but is less important than repetitive grasping or repetitive use of tools (2, p. 135).

Conditions Associated with Prolonged Work Disability

Not all reported work injuries and illnesses are disabling. Of the 6.8 million claims filed in 1992, 2.8 million involved at least one additional day off work (beyond the day of injury), and 4.5 million did not involve time loss from work (2, p. 1). Many of the latter are effectively treated in emergent or urgent care facilities, if at all, and these may variably be referred to the physiatrist. Among disabling conditions, it is important to distinguish those associated with brief periods off work from those associated with prolonged time loss. Although any injured worker who reports inability to work should be handled with concern, the majority of injuries involving time loss from work end uneventfully with the worker returning to the job after a short time off. For example, the median time off work because of back injury in 1992 was 7 days (2, p. 180).

The physiatrist is most likely to be consulted for conditions associated with prolonged disability (time off work

TABLE 10-2. *1988 Washington State injury and illness profile by body part*

Body part	All claims	Percent of claims that produce time loss >120 days	Number of claims with time loss >120 days
Finger	29,721 (17.7%)	0.7%	207 (2.8%)
Back	27,196 (16.2%)	9.6%	2,598 (34.6%)
Eyes	17,981 (10.7%)	0.1%	19 (0.2%)
Hand/wrist	17,444 (10.4%)	3.7%	643 (8.5%)
Back and neck	8,427 (5.0%)	8.7%	734 (9.8%)
Knee	7,478 (4.4%)	8.1%	609 (8.1%)
Foot	6,611 (3.9%)	2.6%	173 (2.3%)
Multiple	5,583 (3.3%)	10.2%	571 (7.6%)
Other	47,616 (28.3%)	4.1%	1,945 (25.9%)
Totals	168,057 (100%)	—	7,499 (100%)

From Washington State Department of Labor and Industries (unpublished).

exceeding 120 days). Of those conditions listed in Table 10-1, dislocations and amputations are highly prone, and fractures, multiple trauma, and sprains and strains are moderately prone, to result in prolonged time loss from work. Because sprains and strains are relatively common among claims overall, workers experiencing these conditions account for 66% of cases with extended time loss. Similarly, and according to affected body part (Table 10-2), 9.6% of patients with back disorders remain off work more than 120 days. However, because back problems occur frequently, 34.6% of claims associated with prolonged time loss for injury or illness are attributable to them.

Biological Factors

The data presented above indicate that conditions commonly treated by physiatrists, particularly LBP and carpal tunnel syndrome (CTS), are associated with protracted disability. Several factors that may be predictive of chronic disability include:

1. Severity of injury. An expected relationship between severity of injury and duration of disability has been shown in extreme cases where ''catastrophic injury'' (requiring hospitalization within 28 days of injury) results in 2.5-fold increase in duration of work disability relative to noncatastrophic injury (6). However, only a small portion (6%) of cases are catastrophic and a predictive model for the noncatastrophic group is lacking.
2. Diagnosis. Risk of prolonged disability varies by diagnosis, and within a diagnostic category some prediction is also possible. For example, studies have shown that prolonged disability is more likely in LBP when sciatica is present (7). Injured workers given a specific diagnosis within 1 week of injury (i.e., sciatica, disk injury, or facet joint syndrome) are also more likely to demonstrate prolonged disability than those with nonspecific diagnoses such as ''lumbar strain'' (8,9). However, the percentage of patients receiving specific diagnoses is small (8) and not useful for predicting variability in chronicity for the nonspecific group.
3. Age. Although older workers appear less likely to sustain work-related injuries than younger ones, they are at greater risk of experiencing chronic disability when such injuries occur (2,6,10).

Skewed Recovery Curves

Most occupational back injuries appear to be self-limited, with an estimated 40% to 50% of workers returning to work within 2 weeks, 70% to 80% back by 4 weeks, and fewer than 10% remaining out of work at 3 to 6 months after injury (6,7,11,12). However, those remaining out of work are at progressive risk of chronic disability (13). The Clinical Standards Advisory Group's estimated long-term recovery curve for LBP indicates that the probability of ever returning to work is only 25% for an injured worker who has been off work for 1 year and 10% after 2 years (12). Up to one-third of those returning to work may continue to experience ongoing symptoms and functional compromise beyond a 6-month healing period (14,15).

The skewed recovery curves noted above are by no means uniquely descriptive of back pain. Similar skewed curves have been noted for carpal tunnel syndrome, fractures, and other unspecified industrial injuries (Fig. 10-1) (6). Furthermore, costs of care associated with skewed claims can be staggering. To illustrate, in Washington State, fewer than 5% of total reported injuries result in prolonged time loss from work (exceeding 120 days), yet this subgroup accounts

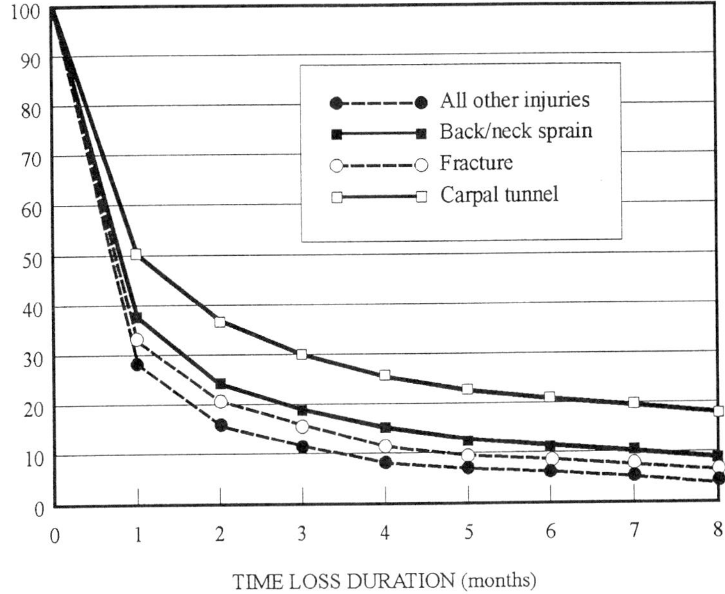

FIG. 10-1. Skewed recovery curves among workers disables by various conditions. (From Cheadle A, Franklin G, Wolfhagen C, et al. Factors influencing the duration of work-related disability: A population-based study of Washington State Workers' Compensation. *Am J Public Health* 1994; 84(2):194.)

for 84% of total disability payments reported for the entire group (16, p.3). The percentage of annualized costs associated with occupational LBP and directly attributed to disability payments has been estimated as high as 66% (17, vol. 40(9), p. 7); however, the percentage of costs associated with medical care is rising gradually, and as of 1993, an estimated 58% of the annualized costs were for disability payments (18).

Industrial Claims: Potential Effects on Outcome

Role of the Workplace

A number of work-related risk factors for back injury have been identified and may include heavy physical demands of the job, task repetition, static and dynamic postures during physical work, frequent bending or twisting activity, and forceful movement of lifting, carrying, pushing, and pulling (19). Certain occupations (e.g., material handling) have been shown to be ''high risk'' in terms of associated rates of LBP (19–22).

Long-term outcomes analysis for industrial injuries has shown that an injured worker who is temporarily disabled is more likely to return to work if the return is to the same employer where the injury occurred (23). If this is not feasible, significant barriers to reemployment may exist. For example, new employers may be reluctant to hire an individual who has been out of the workplace because of an industrial injury and whose claim has been settled (24, p. 954).

Intensity of Treatment

A comparison of costs and duration of medical treatment for injuries associated with industrial compensation claims versus comparable injuries treated through private insurance companies such as Blue Cross and Blue Shield (25) reveals the following: the industrially based treatment group is characterized by a more invasive, high-intensity, and short-duration treatment, whereas the private insurance group is typified by a less invasive and more conservative lengthy approach. Other research confirms these observations (26). It is understandable that both injured workers and their physicians want to use available technologies to promote rapid recovery, especially if an injury has caused the worker to go on disability. However, there is good evidence that injured workers are less likely to benefit from medical or surgical treatment for a variety of conditions than their counterparts with noncompensable injuries (27–32). A paradox thus arises whereby injured workers may receive more intensive treatment that is less likely to be beneficial. This raises a possibility that iatrogenic factors associated with aggressive or invasive interventions may contribute negatively to outcomes in industrially related claims, particularly as they apply to ''failed back syndrome'' (33,34).

Socioeconomic Determinants

Employment opportunities at the community level may have an impact on frequency and severity of work-related claims. In communities where the unemployment rate is high, workers tend to file claims more frequently and experience more protracted disability (6,35). Under the rules of Workers' Compensation, it appears reasonable to expect that the injured worker will continue to report physical incapacity until he or she is successfully able to reintegrate into the work force. If local socioeconomic pressure impedes effective reintegration, disability may become a ''path of least resistance.''

Workers' Compensation provides time-loss benefits during the period of treatment in which the claimant is medically determined to be unable to work. Such payment may serve as a disincentive for workers to return to work, even after a sufficient recovery period. As the wage replacement ratio (the ratio between an injured worker's time-loss payment and preinjury wage level) increases, there are corresponding increases in both frequency and duration of claims (36). Paradoxically, the system rewards failure at multiple levels. Failure to respond favorably to medical treatment is typically rewarded by extending treatment and time-loss benefits. Failure to reintegrate at the workplace may be rewarded by vocational retraining, and failure of vocational rehabilitation may be rewarded by pensioning. Many of the policies designed to ease suffering or hardship associated with industrial injury may, in effect, serve as incentives for delayed recovery and prolonged disability.

Psychological Determinants

There is a general consensus that psychological variables contribute significantly to chronic pain and disability, with a range of contributing factors having been identified. These include history of childhood physical, sexual, or psychological abuse, history of substance abuse, recent life stressors, family dysfunction, and concomitant psychiatric disorders including depression or anxiety (37). Associations have also been drawn between cognitive factors and chronic pain, including patient belief systems and coping strategies. It appears plausible that a worker facing the adaptive demands of work injury and who may have been subjected to an abusive childhood, or who experiences a concomitant psychiatric disorder or maintains a dysfunctional belief system, may lack the resilience and coping skills needed to meet such demands and is thereby prone to an outcome of chronic disability.

''Compensation neurosis'' is one of several terms used to describe the conscious or unconscious tendency of certain patients to magnify symptoms when there is the potential for financial gain. Compensation neurosis has been described as '' . . . . .a state of mind, born out of fear, kept alive by avarice, stimulated by lawyers, and cured by a verdict'' (38, p. 20). The essential feature of a compensation neurosis is that the claimant describes an incapacity in terms of physical limitations and symptoms, while observers suspect underlying motivational factors and secondary gain. The concept of compensation neurosis has been criticized as a diagnosis that is, by nature, inferential, subjective, and pejorative. Patients so labeled may have little in common except for their compensation claim (39). The central tenet that a verdict is somehow curative lacks empirical validation, and, in fact, many claimants out of work at the time a verdict is rendered remain symptomatic and disabled beyond case closure. Despite the above caveats, most clinicians who treat injured workers believe that some of them report symptoms that are not explained biologically but, rather, reflect influences of the disability system as filtered by psychological tendencies within the patients. The term "chronic disability syndrome" (40) is sometimes used to describe these patients, rather than the more pejorative "compensation neurosis." Whether clinicians use "compensation neurosis," "chronic disability syndrome," or some other descriptive label for injured workers who appear to be "stuck" in the disability system, they need to be observant for "symptom magnification" when evaluating such patients. Symptom magnification is a useful clinical descriptor that conveys the observable discrepancy between pain behavior and objectifiable underlying pathology, without implying deception or malintent.

Workers' Compensation System

Historical Development

Before the 1880s a worker who was injured on the job could only seek redress against his or her employer by bringing suit for negligence under Common Law. The employer's oft-successful defense rested upon grounds of employee contributory negligence, assumption of risk, and the "Fellow Servant Doctrine" implicating co-worker contributory negligence. Winning meant a large lump-sum payment for damages, whereas losing meant no reimbursement for medical expenses or time loss compensation. The first workers' compensation system was introduced by Germany in 1884 (41, p. 1), and the first U.S. industrial compensation system was established in Wisconsin in 1911. Other states rapidly followed suit, and, as a result, Workers' Compensation now exists in all 50 states as well as the District of Columbia (41, p. 43). Between 1911 and 1972, Workers' Compensation expanded its coverage both in terms of work categories and benefits. By 1970 the Occupational Safety and Health Act (OSHA) was passed which included establishing a U.S. National Commission on State Workmen's Compensation Laws. Initially, the Commission provided impetus to correct inconsistencies and inadequacies among state compensation systems through expansion of services and the creation of new programs. More recently, state compensation systems have focused on cost containment strategies (42).

Workers' compensation in the United States is decentralized. Each state has its own compensation system, and there are significant differences from one system to another. In general, though, compensation systems share the following common features:

1. The system is no-fault, and the employer assumes liability for all claims arising as a result of injury or illness directly attributable to the workplace. In return, the worker gives up the right to bring suit against the employer for separate damages.
2. Benefits are provided only for work-related conditions which are medically determined to arise directly out of and during the course of employment.
3. A distinction is made between "industrial injury" where there is a clear history of a precipitating event, and "occupational illness" in which the condition arises from activity/exposure over a period of time. (In reality, the legal distinction may blur, and conditions such as occupational LBP are typically regarded as injuries when research has shown that symptoms frequently begin without a precipitating event.)
4. The course of recovery is assumed to follow a predictable pattern whereby a plateau is reached. At this point, the condition is judged to be "fixed and stable" or to have reached "maximum medical improvement" (MMI, see below) (Fig. 10-2). At this juncture compensation law dictates termination of treatment and development of a vocational plan or provision of a pension, and an additional cash settlement award for damages suffered according to permanent medical physical impairment.
5. There is no cap on the dollar amount payable for treatment until MMI is achieved.
6. Compensation is provided for time lost due to temporary incapacitation throughout the course of treatment and until MMI is achieved.

The types of conditions regarded as treatable under Workers' Compensation have evolved to include subtle injuries or illnesses attributable to repetitive motion strain, including upper extremity cumulative trauma disorders (CTD) and LBP. Causality for such conditions is often difficult to establish (43), and their association with prolonged disability in some cases makes them quite costly. Furthermore, perceived disability due to these conditions may be largely subjective, and consequently, there is often reluctance on the part of the insurer to provide coverage.

Particulars of the Patient–Physician Relationship

The Patient as Claimant

When a patient has an active or pending claim for compensable injury, additional factors may impact upon the traditional patient-physician relationship and affect patient outcomes and physician expectations. If a claim is industrially-based, the physician is typically asked to make judgments concerning causality of illness or injury due to occupational

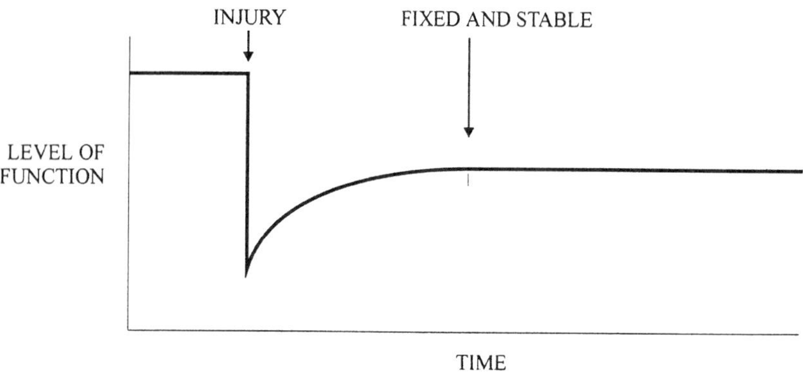

FIG. 10-2. Hypothetical recovery curve following work injury.

exposure, and must also determine the patient's ongoing fitness for duty. Such concerns are generally irrelevant in private insurance claims. Furthermore, the employer may play a decisive role in determining whether or not the employee files a claim, and participates in an adversarial or cooperative manner with the physician and other health care providers. Longitudinal studies have shown that workers are more likely to file claims if they are dissatisfied with their jobs (44). Once a claim has been filed, a sympathetic employer can facilitate recovery by taking an active interest in the injured employee's condition and cooperating with options for transitional return to work (45).

Typically, there are multiple parties to complex industrial claims beyond the treating physician. They may include the employer, a claims manager, physician consultant specialists, therapists, a vocational counselor, and, often, an attorney. The communication channels are manifold with multiple opportunities for confused or mixed messages to arise, which can fuel patient fears or suspicions. This may hasten attorney involvement which, in turn, may be associated with less successful rehabilitation (46) and more costly claims (47). In many states the injured worker retains the right to choose a treating physician regardless of said physician's expertise and familiarity with the industrial compensation system or the special needs of injured workers. Conflicts may arise between claimant and employer concerning necessity and appropriateness of treatment, which frequently must be mediated by an independent medical examiner (see following).

The Physician as Patient and System Advocate

The industrial rehabilitation physician must broaden the sphere of concern beyond patient advocacy to actively include the interests of the employer and insurance carrier alike. Pressure may be applied to terminate treatments that are primarily palliative in nature, to hasten the injured worker's return to work or objectify reasons for not doing so, and to render objective opinions on medical impairment rating and permanent work disability. The ethical dilemmas posed are not unlike those arising in the context of rapid growth and expansion of managed care, where contracted physicians may face financial incentives to limit or withhold treatment. Such complex decision making becomes a matter of routine and should be rendered within the context of a sound understanding of the functional implications of a particular industrial illness or injury, and a firm commitment to fostering and maintaining the highest functional outcome possible in every case.

PATIENT EVALUATION

History and Physical Examination

Patient History

The history provided by the injured worker is perhaps the single most useful indicator of diagnosis, prognosis for return-to-work, and management strategies likely to be beneficial in a given case (48–50). If the worker seeks immediate medical attention following acute injury, prognosis is more favorable than when the presenting complaint is delayed (17). A careful history should include a precise description of the precipitating event as well as the type and frequency of physical tasks with which the worker is typically involved. Pain complaints should be characterized according to nature, location, duration and severity, and any palliative or aggravating factors should be identified. History of prior work-related injuries should be documented and their associated outcomes noted with respect to time to recovery and any residual impairment. The worker's own perception of their functional disability should also be noted in light of potential modified duty options available from the employer (49–53).

Patients experiencing LBP may develop sciatica—pain that radiates from the low back into a lower limb (usually below the knee). Such symptoms may appear acutely, or more gradually over a period of days, weeks or even months following onset of back symptoms (54). Sciatica is thought to result from nerve root displacement by disk material or from the gradual development of chemically-mediated radiculitis (55). Leg pain may arise on referral from nonneurogenic structures (56); however, the presence of sciatica is strongly suggestive (specificity = 88%, specificity = 95%) of nerve root impingement at the L4–L5 and L5–S1 disk levels (57). Additional history should include inquiry about lower extremity weakness or sensory changes, bladder or bowel incontinence or erectile dysfunction (suggests cauda equina syndrome), or exacerbation of pain with valsalva maneuver.

Additional important elements of the history should focus upon the work environment, job tasks and physical requirements, and employer flexibility with respect to modified duty options (53), in order to address feasibility of return to work during the recovery period.

Physical Examination

In the evaluation of acute occupational LBP the examining physician should focus on the following three issues: 1) ruling out a specific (i.e. nonmechanical) cause of back pain; 2) assessing indications for surgical intervention (i.e. severe and/or progressive neurological deficit, bladder or bowel dysfunction); and 3) identifying key findings likely to affect specific aspects of treatment (57).

Physical examination should include attention to symmetry and integrity of dermatomal sensory levels, muscle stretch reflexes and muscle strength at the lumbar and sacral root levels (58). The examiner should perform the classical "straight leg raise" test (SLR) as well as check for root tension signs in order to verify possible root irritation (59,60). In the presence of nerve root tension, the SLR is provocative of pain radiating posteriorly into the leg, when the hip is flexed 30° to 60° with the knee extended. The SLR is 80 % sensitive (negative SLR rules out nerve root impingement)(60,61); however, central disk herniation may be present with a negative SLR. Root tension signs include evoking hip flexion in the supine position with cervical flexion, hip internal rotation and ankle dorsiflexion maneuvers (59,62). The crossed SLR (provocation of sciatica on the affected side with contralateral SLR) is highly specific of L4–L5 or L5–S1 disk herniation (specificity = 90%) but is not sensitive (54,61).

Confirmation of lumbar root irritation at more proximal levels (L3,L4) through physical examination requires use of the "femoral stretch test" (provocation of pain radiating into the anterior thigh by flexing the knee while the patient is prone (58). Muscle weakness at the quadriceps or gastrocnemius muscle is specific for L3/L4 or S1 root irritation, respectively (61), but the reliability of these and other findings remains questionable (63,64).

A common presentation is the patient lacking neurological symptoms or radicular findings (reflex changes, weakness, hypesthesia, or decreased sphincter tone) on physical examination. In such cases the SLR may often be equivocal or positive (20) and probably represents disk injury without nerve root tension.

Risk Factors for Delayed Recovery

"Delayed recovery" refers to the lack of favorable response to appropriate medical and rehabilitative care during an adequate time period for healing to occur following an industrial injury (65). During the history and physical examination, the physiatrist should routinely screen for potential enablers and confounders of recovery as listed in Table 10-3 (53,65). Patients at high risk of delayed recovery may require formal psychological evaluation to identify potential psychological and psychosocial barriers to recovery and to develop strategies for neutralizing any such barriers. Treatment should focus away from a passive and palliative approach and toward active strategies as much as possible (see following).

Nonorganic Versus Organic Findings

The initial and ongoing assessment of the injured worker should seek to validate medical impairment in terms of plausibility and reproducibility of findings and degree and consistency of effort put forward. Waddell's signs may aid in

TABLE 10-3. *Enabling and confounding factors affecting return to work following occupational injury*

	Medical	Psycho-social	Course of treatment	Employer	Occupational	Insurance carrier	Attorney
Enablers	Mild pathology Timely assessment Competent and compassionate care	Strong work ethic	Expedited care Active exercise emphasized Work directed	Concerned Advocating Flexible	Adaptable Limited duty or transitional work options available High job satisfaction	Facilitating	Job discrimination averted
Confounders	Severe pathology Prior history of injury Excessive diagnostic and treatment efforts Delays in evaluating or initiating treatment	Poor English Proficiency Family history of disability Substance abuse history Dysfunctional family history	Delayed initiation of treatment Passive interventions emphasized Job functions not addressed	Aloof or indifferent Lack of flexibility	No limited duty or transitional work options available Low job satisfaction with supervisor conflicts	Barriers to treatment authorization and start up	Litigation

From Scheer SJ. The role of the physician in disability management. In: Shrey DE, Lacerte M, eds. *Principles and practices of disability management in industry.* Winter Park: GR Press, 1995; 189; and Deerbery VJ, Tullis WH. Delayed recovery in the patient with a work compensible injury. *J Occup Med* 1983; 25:829–835.

the identification of physiological inconsistency or incongruity on examination (66), and meticulous documentation of initial and subsequent observations allows determination of inconsistencies over time. Symptom magnification is frequently encountered in patients with compensable injury (67,68). Displays of exaggerated pain behavior and physiological inconsistency need to be identified, documented, and appropriately weighed without necessarily invoking malingering or other pejorative connotations (see above). Isokinetic ergometers have been used to determine consistency of effort in testing patients with LBP (69) and upper extremity conditions (70,71). The "coefficient of variability" (standard deviation divided by the performance mean) has been determined for such equipment for healthy, unimpaired individuals and can be expected to increase in the presence of skewed performance or other abnormalities (71). However, the application of such normative data to injured workers experiencing pain or possible symptom magnification has been critically reviewed (72), and such equipment may be no more effective than traditional means of assessing and managing this complex patient group (73).

Diagnostic Testing

If a history of severe trauma or other risk factors for vertebral fracture is obtained, plain lumbar radiographs or nuclear imaging are appropriate initial studies (74,75). Otherwise, radiographic imaging of the spine is generally not indicated within the first 6 weeks of the presenting complaint (57,74,76).

In cases in which uncomplicated radiculopathy is suspected, the clinician may justifiably defer additional diagnostic imaging in favor of nonsurgical treatment for at least 6 to 8 weeks (75,77). In effect, favorable clinical response to nonoperative care obviates the need for confirmatory imaging at that point.

In refractory patients who fail to show the expected improvement or who worsen clinically, in cases where additional motivation of the anxious patient is needed, and in situations where surgical intervention is indicated, further confirmation of the cause and location of the lesion is needed. Each of the preferred imaging methods for viewing the lumbar spine—myelography, computerized axial tomography (CAT), and magnetic resonance imaging (MRI)—has a low false-negative rate for significant disk disruption but a high false-positive rate for detection of asymptomatic disk herniation or spinal stenosis (78–80). Sequestered disk fragments are exceedingly rare in asymptomatic patients (81) and are best visualized using MRI, where 85% accuracy has been reported (82).

Alternative imaging options have appropriate selected indications. In cases of suspected neoplasm or spinal fracture, plain films or bone scan imaging may be indicated, and potential segmental instability is perhaps best visualized using flexion–extension films (74,75). Although controversial, discography allows clarification of the nature and extent of intervertebral disk derangement and is considered useful by some (83).

Electrodiagnostic examination may be considered a useful extension of the clinical examination with a low rate of false-positive studies in acute radiculopathy (84,85). However, the rate of false negatives may be as high as 30%.

In most cases of occupational LBP, a firm objective diagnosis cannot be achieved with certainty (57,58,86), even with advanced imaging techniques (58). The differential diagnosis is broad and may include muscle and ligamentous strain and sprain, annular tear, disk herniation or degeneration, vertebral endplate fracture, facet joint inflammation, sacroiliac dysfunction, or, more generally, "lumbar strain or sprain" (50,58). Ascertaining an exact diagnosis is often unnecessary in view of the self-limited course and generally favorable outcome in most cases (57,58).

Functional Capacity Evaluation

Functional capacity evaluation (FCE) is a systematic method of measuring a worker's ability to perform meaningful job-related tasks safely and dependably (87). The purposes for FCE include:

Matching the worker's functional capacity to particular job demands.
Designing individualized programs of incremental exercise/activity to improve work tolerance and objectify progress.
Identifying presence and degree of work disability.

Basic components of the FCE include the assessment of strength, flexibility, endurance, lifting and carrying capacity, pushing and pulling capacity, balance and climbing activity, finger and hand dexterity, movement accuracy and skill. The FCEs can assist the physician examiner in the process of assessing medical impairment, job disability, and return-to-work feasibility following work injury. They are typically administered by a trained physical or occupational therapist and, if used appropriately, can enable a more reliable prediction of work capacity than can typically be arrived at through the physician's office examination (50). Because the scope and content (and costs) of FCE testing can vary considerably depending on the targeted purpose and assessment process in question, the choice of measures should be directed by considerations of safety, feasibility, reliability, validity, and relevance in each case. Because most tests have the potential to cause harm, procedural rules with exclusionary and performance guidelines must be followed. The evaluator is urged to obtain signed and informed consent before carrying out the FCE.

Psychological Evaluation

As noted earlier, there is a consensus that a wide range of psychosocial factors can adversely influence the recovery of an injured worker. Some of these factors are considered psychiatric disorders. In fact, according to the *Diagnostic and Statistical Manual of Mental Disorders,* fourth edition (American Psychiatric Association, 1994) there are at least eight psychiatric diagnoses recognized as associated with chronic pain and disability, including somatization disorder, undifferentiated somatoform disorder, conversion disorder, pain disorder associated with psychiatric disorders, hypochondriasis, factitious disorder, malingering, and substance dependence and abuse (88). In addition, anxiety and depression are the most common psychiatric comorbidities of acute and chronic pain conditions, respectively, and both conditions frequently accompany chronic pain of more than 6 months' duration (89).

However, some of the processes that may adversely influence injured workers are subtle and cannot easily be related to a psychiatric diagnosis. Examples include poor stress management skills and suboptimal motivation to return to work. A rehabilitation psychologist can often identify these subtle barriers to recovery as well as identify psychiatric disorders in injured workers. The psychologist may use a number of standardized and objective assessment tools to facilitate evaluation (90). These include the Minnesota Multiphasic Personality Inventory (MMPI), McGill Pain Questionnaire, Beck Anxiety Scale, Beck and Zung Depression Indices, and the Westhaven–Yale Multidimensional Pain Inventory (WHYMPI). The psychologist may offer counseling services to assist the worker with coping and complying with treatment during the recovery phase. Finally, the psychologist may ultimately assist with rendering a statement of psychiatric or psychological impairment at case closure (see below).

TREATMENT OPTIONS

Acute Strategies

In the majority of acute cases of industrial-related LBP, recovery in terms of return to work can be expected within the first few weeks. Lengthy rest periods are generally unnecessary and should be discouraged. At least one randomized control study has shown that two days of rest is preferable to seven days in expediting return to work (48). A recent study also suggests that a gradual and judicious return to functional activity is more efficacious than either enforced bed rest or a regimented exercise approach (91). A detailed set of physician recommendations regarding return to function seems intuitively appealing; however, the one randomized control study examining the use of specific advice in this regard was no more efficacious than a vague "let pain be your guide" approach (92). Nonsteroidal anti-inflammatory agents or acetaminophen, icing and advice concerning activities and posture to minimize stress may improve comfort, whereas opioid analgesics and muscle relaxants have not been proven to be of additional benefit (93).

The benefits of "back school" in acute LBP have been questioned. Whereas one randomized control study demonstrated favorable return-to-work outcomes when back school was added (94), there have been three comparable studies that failed to show added benefit from this approach (95).

Exercise has not been shown to expedite return to work in randomized control studies (95) during the first few weeks following acute low back injury. However, most such studies comparing exercise groups to controls utilized a single exercise approach across all subjects in the exercise groups; consequently, the potential benefits of an individualized exercise approach have not been adequately assessed (96).

Spinal manipulation has been recommended during the first 2 weeks following back injury according to the Agency for Health Care Policy and Research practice guidelines (92). This remains controversial among allopathic physicians, and available literature ranges from neutral to supportive of benefits from manipulation (97,98). It is also unclear which patients are likely to derive consistent benefit from this procedure, or whether manipulation *per se* or the facilitating approach of the chiropractor is of greater value.

Finally, there is evidence that, in addition to specific treatment modalities, the messages given by health care providers about return to work are important. Specifically, workers are more likely to return to their jobs when an unrestricted return to work is recommended (99).

Subacute Strategies

In situations where radicular pain fails to centralize or respond to initial management, continued nonoperative care might include a trial of epidural corticosteroids (100,101). A recent meta-analysis suggests that adding epidural steroid injections can produce a modest additional benefit beyond what can be provided by other nonoperative measures (102).

Various physical approaches and options such as the McKenzie (103), dynamic lumbar stabilization (104), and traction have been advocated for the treatment of discogenic back pain with radicular symptoms. Dynamic lumbar stabilization has been shown in a retrospective uncontrolled study to enable a rapid return to work in most such cases (104). Another study has retrospectively examined cost effectiveness and long-term outcomes for discectomy after 3 months of refractory radicular pain versus continued nonsurgical care (105). Overall, costs and return-to-work rates were similar; however, the surgically treated group showed significantly fewer missed days after return to work. A prospective randomized comparison of operative versus nonoperative care for nonemergent disk herniation and radicular symptoms revealed significant improvement in the latter group within the first 3 months (106); substantial crossover from the nonsurgical to the surgical treatment group also occurred. In general, surgical management for nonemergent disk herniation is not recommended during the first 3 months following onset. However, in mitigating circumstances (e.g., free disk fragment unresponsive to epidural steroids and other interventions after 4 weeks), an earlier surgical consultation appears warranted.

Work Hardening and Transitional Return-to-Work Programs

Work hardening is a concept designed to rehabilitate injured workers by incorporating job-oriented functional activities into a physical restorative program (107). Such programs are typically carried out off-site in a refurbished warehouse or satellite health facility and are generally directed toward patients with chronicity and delayed recovery. Although such programs may be poorly understood and viewed as costly by employers, they have several advantages over more traditional approaches: They adopt an active as opposed to passive therapy focus, and espouse a philosophy of enablement on the part of the injured worker. One particular benefit is requiring the ''temporarily totally disabled'' individual to participate in a regularly occurring, structured routine that mimics their ordinary job and minimizes the reinforcement and incentives for illness behavior.

Transitional return-to-work programs provide the injured worker with on-site opportunities to engage in supervised work activity of incremental complexity and physical demand. This progression continues until there is sufficient capacity to perform at full duty without exacerbation of symptoms or undue risk of reinjury. Such programs are both physically therapeutic and psychologically gratifying and allow maximum transferability of functional gains during treatment to an actual job setting. They also ensure employer ''buy-in'' and active participation in the potentially more favorable recovery process (108).

Vocational Assessment

Job and Workplace Evaluation

The ideal vocational outcome after time loss from an industrial injury is return of the injured worker to the same job or to a modified job at the same company. An FCE may be helpful to characterize the work task abilities of the returning worker as described above, and particularly if used in conjunction with an accurate job site and work task analysis. Any limitations of the worker thus identified may become the focus for further rehabilitation if significant improvement is expected. Possibilities for ergonomic improvement can also be explored to lessen the physical stresses associated with the job and to facilitate return to work.

Ergonomic Modifications

Ergonomics is the study of fitting the job to the worker and the worker to the job. The primary goal of ergonomic interventions is the improvement of workers' performance and safety through the study and development of principles to guide the interaction of workers within their working environments (52). Administrative ergonomic controls may include those interventions relating to worker schedules, job task rotation, lightening of workload burdens, and employee training in back protection techniques. Engineering controls may consist of job site changes, use of load-bearing equipment, tool changes or modifications in design, and other environmental improvements that lessen the physical and emotional stress of work (109).

Injury Prevention Strategies

The discussion of ergonomic improvements that lessen the burden of work is best undertaken preventively, such that job tasks predisposing to work-related injury are minimized (primary ergonomic prevention). Secondary ergonomic prevention efforts are undertaken after a high-risk job has been identified by repeated occurrence of work injury. Often, job changes that have a favorable ergonomic impact are much less expensive than might otherwise be expected. For example, in 1995, job accommodations were recommended to over 500 employers by the Job Accommodation Network in West Virginia, and these cost less than $500 in approximately two-thirds of the cases; the median cost of accommodation was only $200 (110).

MEDICAL IMPAIRMENT RATING

Purpose and Derivation of the *AMA Guides*

The *American Medical Association Guides to the Evaluation of Permanent Impairment,* fourth edition *(AMA Guides)* (1) has been developed as a standard reference to assist the physician in evaluating and reporting medical impairment of any human organ system. The estimates derived according to the *AMA Guides* are generally applicable to disability claims evaluations under Workers' Compensation, Social Security Administration, and other claim systems. Under Workers' Compensation law, physician involvement is mandatory in order to determine causality or association of illness or injury with the workplace; to coordinate and direct medical care; to determine MMI; to provide a medical impairment rating; and to render determination of work capacity and restrictions if applicable. In 1956, the AMA created an ad hoc committee to address physician concerns and provide guidelines concerning these reporting requirements. The committee published 13 separate articles over the period from 1958 to 1970 and subsequently compiled them into the first *AMA Guides* in 1971. The *AMA Guides* have undergone four subsequent revisions to their currently accepted form.

Use of the *AMA Guides* is currently mandatory or recommended by law under Workers' Compensation in approximately 55% of its 53 existing jurisdictions; it is frequently used in another 21% and not mandated, recommended, or frequently used in 24% of jurisdictions (1). Readers are encouraged to become familiar with the laws and requirements of the particular state or jurisdiction in which they practice and to comply fully with prescribed guidelines and reference materials available pertaining to impairment rating practices.

Using the *AMA Guides*

The Musculoskeletal System

Space limitations preclude a fully detailed review of the impairment rating process and guidelines for each organ system. Because the physiatrist typically deals with impairment and disability directly pertaining to the musculoskeletal system, certain details and key points related to musculoskeletal impairment rating are highlighted here. The reader is referred to an excellent companion volume to the *AMA Guides* (111) for more detailed and expanded discussions of other organ systems, in particular, the cardiopulmonary and respiratory systems.

Impairments affecting the musculoskeletal system are generally viewed in terms of three regional units (i.e., the hand and upper extremity, the lower extremity, and the spine). Medical impairment is assessed independently for each of these units. The hand and upper extremity are further divided into regional subunits of thumb, finger, wrist, elbow and shoulder. The lower extremity is divided into five subunits to include the toes, foot, ankle, knee, and hip. The spine is divided into cervical, thoracic, lumbar, and sacral subunits. Within each regional unit, impairment is calculated for the smallest applicable subunit. Separate impairments within a subunit are combined before impairments among subunits are combined within a region. Similarly, individual impairments within a regional unit are combined before impairments among regions. When two impairment values are combined within or between regional units or subunits, the smaller value *(B)* is combined with the larger value *(A)* by the formula:

$$C\ (\%) = A\ (\%) - B\ (\%)\ [100 - A\ (\%)]$$

This adjustment is necessary in order that the cumulative impairment for a regional unit or subunit does not exceed 100%. A reference table of "combined values" is provided to facilitate these conversions (1, pp. 322–324). Impairment to the upper extremity regional unit can be converted to a "whole person" estimate by multiplying by 0.6, or to the lower extremity by multiplying by 0.4. Impairment to the spine regional unit is always determined to the "whole person."

Medical impairments may be derived using qualitative descriptors for such conditions as amputation, joint ankylosis, or bone/joint deformity secondary to arthritis or similar disorders. They may be quantitatively derived, based on estimated loss of motion at specific joints (see following), or they may be diagnosis-based, in which case a clear history of injury pertaining to the rated diagnosis is emphasized (see following).

The "Range-of-Motion" Model

The "range-of-motion" model enables a determination of impairment according to loss of motion from the neutral position of a joint, with reference to the cardinal planes of motion and normative range of motion for that particular joint. Reference tables are provided to determine the amount of impairment corresponding to degrees of motion lost for each joint within each regional unit. For the spine regional unit, a categorical listing of impairments according to specific disorders (e.g., fractures, intervertebral disk lesions, spondylolysis or spondylolisthesis, or spinal stenosis) is also provided (1, p. 113). Each category has its own determinants of severity, and the resulting impairment figures can be combined with estimates derived for loss of spinal motion.

The "Diagnosis-Related Estimates" Model

In cases involving the spinal regional unit, the *AMA Guides* (1) recognize a separate "injury model" based on a "diagnosis-related estimates" (DRE) model of impairment. Application of DREs is predicated on obtaining a history of an injury that, with medical probability, caused specific and associated impairment to the spine. Under the DRE model, the spine is composed of three regional subunits (cervicothoracic, thoracolumbar, and lumbosacral). For each subunit, seven common, objective differentiators of severity are listed, resulting in eight categories of impairment, respectively. Impairment estimates derived according to the DRE model and from the range-of-motion model are mutually exclusive and should not be combined.

Limitations of the *AMA Guides*

A number of limitations pertaining to the theoretical underpinnings and practical implications of the *AMA Guides* deserve mention. To begin with, the impairment percentages listed according to the *AMA Guides* are intended to represent an "informed estimate of the degree to which an individual's capacity to carry out daily activity has been diminished" (1). In effect, such determinations have been rendered by consensus and are in no way supported by the rigorously collected, behaviorally based observations that are necessary for scientific validation.

The reliability of commonly accepted impairment measurement techniques is also questionable and has been debated in the literature with particular reference to surface inclinometry techniques for determining spinal flexibility (112,113). Subjectivity on the part of claimant and/or examiner, as well as consistency of effort put forth by the claimant, may further skew or otherwise affect the reliability of impairment measurements obtained. The physician examiner can frequently expect to encounter elements of symptom magnification, particularly in the presence of chronicity and pain. Exaggerated displays of pain behavior and related inconsistencies should be noted and documented; when properly accounted for, they should not result in inflated impairment ratings nor inappropriate penalizing of the claimant who exhibits them.

The conceptual issues surrounding the definition of pain and measurement of pain behavior are well documented (114). Detailed discussions of the relationships between pain and suffering (115) and pain and disability (116) are presented elsewhere (see Chapter 56). For purposes of the impairment rating process, the experience of pain is not directly and objectively measurable. The relationship between pain and suffering is entirely subjective, and consequently, pain behavior should not serve as the sole basis for an impairment rating in the absence of objective corroborative findings.

The *AMA Guides* (1) assert that impairment is determined by ''medical means'' and disability by ''nonmedical means.'' However, the relative emphasis placed on structural versus functional criteria to derive the impairment rating varies by organ system, and some ratings are largely determined by functional criteria pertaining to imputed disability (117). Furthermore, the normative foundations for weighting impairment have been challenged in terms of an existing gender bias (117).

Deviating from the *AMA Guides*

The *AMA Guides* are intended to be just that—guides to aid the physician in analyzing and reporting data concerning medical impairment. However, in some cases (e.g., pain), objective and reliable data are lacking; in others, adequate normative data concerning function are unavailable. In such cases, the judgment and consensus represented by the *AMA Guides* is not intended to supersede that of the individual rating physician, who is expected to exercise independent judgment and go beyond the boundaries and limits specified by the *AMA Guides* when the situation warrants.

WORK DISABILITY DETERMINATION AND THE ADA

Medical impairment may affect ''employability,'' the capacity to meet the demands and conditions of employment set forth by an employer. Employability requires the physical capacity to travel to and from the job site, to be present at the job site for a sustained period of time, and to be able to perform a predetermined array of tasks and duties in exchange for wages. Knowledge of medical impairment *per se* may not be a necessary nor sufficient criterion for determining employability, and the physiatrist making such determinations must also be aware of and consider criteria and perspectives offered by the ADA.

Under Title I of the ADA, individuals with disabilities are afforded protection against discrimination in the workplace for businesses that employ 25 or more persons. Accordingly, employability for a specific job can be viewed as the ability to perform the essential functions of that job—the fundamental duties of the employment position—which can be identified according to physical demands and are typically listed in a job description. Accommodation involves modification of a job description or workplace to enable an employee with an impairment or disability to meet the essential functions. The ADA requires the availability to the disabled of reasonable accommodation—accommodation that can be carried out without posing undue hardship on the employer (in terms of added costs or logistic difficulties) or a direct threat to the health and safety of the disabled employee or any co-workers (118).

At present the ADA concepts and mandates have not been fully integrated into workers' compensation law and rather represent a separate and parallel system. However, the physiatrist may render an ADA-compatible return-to-work determination for an impaired worker that specifically addresses essential functions and employer willingness or ability to accommodate in each case. In essence, work disability can be operationally dealt with in relation to medical impairment, essential functions, and reasonable accommodation as the following scenarios and Table 10-4 illustrate.

Assume an injured worker suffers permanent impairment as a result of partial amputation of the dominant hand. The impact of this defined impairment on disability has a wide range depending on whether the employee is, for example, a construction worker, police officer, concert musician, or surgeon. If the job requires the safe operation of heavy equipment at a construction site, and the worker can perform the essential functions without accommodation, therefore, no work disability is present. If the job requires the ability to safely and reliably handle small firearms, accommodation may be required and may necessitate reassignment to a dis-

TABLE 10-4. *Examples of medical impairment and work disability relative to reasonable accommodation and the ADA*

Impairment	Job category	Sample essential functions	Essential functions performed	Accommodation needed	Reasonable accommodation afforded	Work disability present
Partial hand amputee (dominant)	Construction worker	Operates heavy equipment	+	–	Not applicable	–
	Policeman	Proficiency with handgun	+	+ + +	+ (reassign as dispatcher)	–
	Concert musician	Live concert appearances	±	+ + +	+ (provide synthesizer for studio performance)	±
	Surgeon	Operates on chest	–	+ + +	– (physician extender not feasible)	+

ADA, Americans with Disabilities Act.

patching operation. With that accommodation, no work disability is present. If the job involves live concert performances, the individual may not be able to meet the essential functions but may still be able to compose and deliver studio performances through the use of an electronic synthesizer or other suitable equipment. In this case, some degree of work disability is present in spite of reasonable accommodation. If the job requires a high degree of manual dexterity, such as surgery, accommodation might involve use of a surgical assistant or physician extender to provide intraoperative manual assistance. However, medicolegal and financial considerations might pose sufficient logistic barriers to preclude such accommodation (even if available), and consequently, work disability is present.

Determination of "fitness for duty" involves the evaluation of the worker's ability to safely and dependably meet or exceed the job task demands (87,119). The physiatrist is encouraged to obtain a functional capacity evaluation and valid job description on which to base medical opinions concerning fitness for duty and the match between worker abilities and the essential function task demands. Figure 10-3 illustrates an integrated approach to job analysis and functional capacity evaluation, allowing the therapist and vocational analyst to compare and report worker fitness relative to a variety of job-specific task demands. Such information is valid when good performance effort is given, is highly relevant to the question of job-specific work disability, and can be invaluable to the physiatrist seeking to minimize risk yet endorse maximum work ability. In the event that a mismatch between job task demands and worker ability is identified, the physiatrist should determine valid restrictions to minimize direct threat or personal risk. The employer is responsible for reasonable accommodation and may be assisted by the coordinated efforts of the therapist, ergonomist, and vocational analyst as the situation warrants. It is not the responsibility of the physiatrist to determine the essential functions of the job, to devise accommodation, or to determine reasonableness of any proposed accommodation (119).

TREATING, RATING, AND TERMINATION ISSUES

Treating Versus Rating Physician

The conflicts inherent to the roles of treating versus rating physician have been well documented (120) and are summarized briefly as follows: The treating physician acts primarily as a patient advocate and seeks to diagnose and treat in order to minimize suffering. In treating the injured worker, the physician may prioritize symptom alleviation and functional recovery ahead of return-to-work considerations. Case termination becomes an objective only after medical impairment is minimized and return to work, when feasible, has been achieved. By contrast, a rating physician may face an inverse set of priorities, whereby endpoints of impairment rating and work disability determination are the primary objectives. Case termination is of paramount importance in order to enable a rating to occur (see MMI determination), and return-to-work considerations are a priority objective to enable case closure. Satisfactory diagnostic and therapeutic results are of interest in promoting successful return to work. The physiatrist as treating or rating physician can potentially bridge this conflict and perform both roles equally by maintaining a priority focus on functional improvement. Diagnostic evaluations and medical and rehabilitative treatment remain viable objectives as long as functional improvement during treatment is demonstrated. When functional improvement is no longer tenable, case termination is warranted, and an impairment rating and work disability determination can be made. If further care of a "nonrestorative" nature appears indicated beyond case closure, the physiatrist may advocate for treatment outside the Workers' Compensation system through alternative legal and administrative channels. It is thereby possible for the injured worker and physiatrist to maintain a functionally based therapeutic alliance throughout their course of interactions.

Determination of Maximum Medical Improvement

Maximum medical improvement (MMI) is the point when a medical impairment becomes stable such that additional diagnostic and/or therapeutic interventions are not reasonably expected to produce further improvement. The MMI is felt to have occurred when a "sufficient "healing period has elapsed (the *AMA Guides* previously recognized 6 months as a sufficient healing period; the fourth edition no longer specifies the duration of "sufficient" healing); when the medical condition has resolved; or when there is no reasonable ongoing or anticipated progress toward resolution of the condition (1). From a physiatric perspective, this endpoint is reached when functional improvement is no longer tenable, and MMI determination should be based primarily on lack of demonstrable progress according to measurable functional gains rather than symptom reduction.

Sometimes a patient meets criteria for MMI in the sense that the condition in question is no longer improving but is of a type that is expected to deteriorate over time. An example would be a fracture into a joint. In this situation, the physiatrist can still declare the patient to have reached MMI. The issue of long-term deterioration is handled in either of two ways, depending on the patient's compensation system. One method requires the physiatrist to provide an estimate of the patient's future medical needs regarding the condition. The other is to identify that the patient has reached MMI and is ready for claim closure but to note that a reopening of the claim might be necessary and appropriate at a future date.

Role of the Independent Medical Examination

In cases of industrial injury where a legal claim dispute arises, the claimant or insurer or a neutral party (often an administrative law judge) may engage the services of an

Job Title: Name of individual:

Who/how information obtained:

Key: **N=never** **O=Occasionally** (0-2.5 hrs/day) **F=Frequently** (2.5-5.5 hrs/day) **C=Constantly** (5.5+ hrs/day)

	JOB	**EMPLOYEE STATUS**	**COMMENTS**
Strength			
Sedentary	N____ O____ F____ C____	N____ O____ F____ C____	______
Light	N____ O____ F____ C____	N____ O____ F____ C____	______
Medium	N____ O____ F____ C____	N____ O____ F____ C____	______
Heavy	N____ O____ F____ C____	N____ O____ F____ C____	______
Very Heavy	N____ O____ F____ C____	N____ O____ F____ C____	______
Functions (list weights/distance):			
Walking	N____ O____ F____ C____	N____ O____ F____ C____	______
Standing	N____ O____ F____ C____	N____ O____ F____ C____	______
Sitting	N____ O____ F____ C____	N____ O____ F____ C____	______
Lifting	N____ O____ F____ C____	N____ O____ F____ C____	______
Carrying	N____ O____ F____ C____	N____ O____ F____ C____	______
Pushing	N____ O____ F____ C____	N____ O____ F____ C____	______
Pulling	N____ O____ F____ C____	N____ O____ F____ C____	______
Twisting	N____ O____ F____ C____	N____ O____ F____ C____	______
Reaching (list weights):			
Below knees	N____ O____ F____ C____	N____ O____ F____ C____	______
Knee/Waist	N____ O____ F____ C____	N____ O____ F____ C____	______
Waist/Chest	N____ O____ F____ C____	N____ O____ F____ C____	______
Chest/Shoulder	N____ O____ F____ C____	N____ O____ F____ C____	______
Above Shoulder	N____ O____ F____ C____	N____ O____ F____ C____	______
Climbing:			
Stairs	N____ O____ F____ C____	N____ O____ F____ C____	______
Ladders	N____ O____ F____ C____	N____ O____ F____ C____	______
Scaffolds	N____ O____ F____ C____	N____ O____ F____ C____	______
Balancing:			
Narrow	N____ O____ F____ C____	N____ O____ F____ C____	______
Slippery	N____ O____ F____ C____	N____ O____ F____ C____	______
Moving	N____ O____ F____ C____	N____ O____ F____ C____	______
Stooping:	N____ O____ F____ C____	N____ O____ F____ C____	______
Kneeling:	N____ O____ F____ C____	N____ O____ F____ C____	______
Squatting:	N____ O____ F____ C____	N____ O____ F____ C____	______
Crawling:	N____ O____ F____ C____	N____ O____ F____ C____	______
Handling/Fingering (list weights when applicable):			
Simple Grasping	N____ O____ F____ C____	N____ O____ F____ C____	______
Power Grasping	N____ O____ F____ C____	N____ O____ F____ C____	______
Pushing/Pulling	N____ O____ F____ C____	N____ O____ F____ C____	______
Wrist Twisting	N____ O____ F____ C____	N____ O____ F____ C____	______
Fine Motor	N____ O____ F____ C____	N____ O____ F____ C____	______

Comments, Concerns, Recommendations:

____

____

____

____

____

____

____

____

____

____

Job Analyzer:______________________ **Date**______________

Therapist:______________________ **Date**______________

FIG. 10-3. Job analysis and physical demand comparison.

impartial physician to render an "independent medical evaluation" (IME). The IME physiatrist must not have prior familiarity with or direct involvement in the case at time of referral. The independent physician is expected to fairly and impartially represent the interests of all parties to the dispute and, therefore, cannot be the treating physician of record.

The independent medical examiner can typically be expected to address the following nine questions in the evaluation and report (53, p. 194):

1. What is the diagnosis and extent of severity of the condition in question? The IME physiatrist must review available treatment records and perform an appropriate history and physical exam pursuant to the presenting complaint(s). Additional diagnostic tests or procedures may be requested and authorized in order to render a diagnostic impression and by themselves do not denote a treating relationship.
2. What is the cause of the condition? Causality refers to the medical probability of association between a causal event and its purported effect. Medical probability is the physician's estimate that something is more likely than not (probability exceeds 50%), as opposed to medical possibility (probability is equal to or less than 50%). Causality requires determination that a causal event took place that could give rise to the condition in question, that the claimant experiencing the event has the condition in question, and that it is medically probable that the event gave rise to the condition. Judgments regarding causality are typically not difficult when a previously healthy worker experiences a clear-cut injury with obvious clinical findings. However, they can be quite challenging when a worker has a prior history of problems in the currently affected area or when the alleged cause of symptoms is cumulative trauma rather than a single event (121).
3. Have the necessary tests been performed? The IME physiatrist should ensure that a sufficient diagnostic workup has been provided.
4. Has appropriate treatment been rendered? The IME physiatrist should determine if necessary and appropriate therapies and treatment have been provided.
5. What additional diagnostic or therapeutic recommendations might improve outcome and hasten recovery? The IME physiatrist may recommend additional tests and treatments but should avoid contributing to the development of an "illness conviction" mindset through an endorsement of excessive diagnostic inquiries or inappropriate and perhaps futile treatment efforts. Only those treatments directed at reducing the objective impairment should be endorsed.
6. Has MMI been reached? The IME physiatrist can typically expect to address issues of MMI determination and present or future medical needs to maintain MMI, as discussed above.
7. What is the permanent impairment rating? The permanent total or partial physical impairment associated with the condition should be determined according to methods and procedures summarized above (1), where permitted by law. Jurisdictional rules and reference systems may vary, and the IME physiatrist must comply with local requirements or risk impeachment of the medical opinions and conclusions otherwise rendered.
8. Can the injured worker return to the former job and, if so, how soon? Job analysis and functional capacity evaluation can assist the physiatrist in determining fitness for duty following work injury, as detailed previously. In cases where valid performance measurements are available, those data should guide the physiatrist's estimate of ability of an injured worker to perform the essential functions of the job safely and effectively. In cases where performance is invalid because of inconsistencies and submaximal effort, the physiatrist's assessment becomes increasingly subjective and conjectural in nature.
9. What activity is permitted, and what work restrictions are recommended? As previously mentioned, the physiatrist should rely on valid, empirically based performance data where available and match restrictions to essential functions of a specific job whenever possible.

Legal and Ethical Considerations

Medicolegal aspects of rehabilitation medicine are discussed in detail in Chapter 11. It is important to note that medicolegal accountability of physicians continues to increase for their opinions rendered with respect to workers' compensation disability and independent medical evaluations. The industrial rehabilitation physician can frequently expect to be deposed or offer courtroom testimony regarding his or her findings and opinions and may be held accountable for details recorded months or even years previously. Consequently, data collection, organization, and reporting should be carried out in a thorough, systematic, and sufficiently detailed manner to facilitate retrieval of specific information at any future time.

Several of the ethical dilemmas confronting the physician as treater versus rater and at case termination have been highlighted above. Additional concerns include the potential that the physiatrist acting as a "double agent" might exploit patient candor and trust or inappropriately apply medical skills and authority to nonmedical agendas under workers' compensation law. The very process of MMI determination and work disability determination is potentially countertherapeutic insofar as it conveys a message that treatment is ended and future recovery is not anticipated. The physiatrist facing these ethical challenges should recognize that compensable injuries have potential inherent disincentives towards recovery that tend to promote disability. Furthermore, physician actions (regardless of intent) that enable excessive or inappropriate diagnostic and therapeutic efforts, or result in prolongation of claims, may help to confirm a "disability conviction'' on the part of the patient, further impeding functional recovery. The difficult questions concerning terminating treatment, rating impairment, and determining work disability must be handled with finesse and dexterity and, above all, with the fairness, objectivity, and consistency that a functionally-oriented focus can provide.

REFERENCES

1. American Medical Association. *Guides to the evaluation of permanent impairment,* 4th ed. Milwaukee: American Medical Association, 1993.
2. US Department of Labor, Bureau of Labor Statistics. *Occupational injuries and illnesses: Counts, rates, and characteristics, 1992.* Washington, DC: US Government Printing Office, 1995.
3. Schmulowitz J. Workers' compensation: Coverage, benefits and costs, 1992–93. *Soc Sec Bull* 1995; 58(2):51–57.
4. McCurdy SA, Schenker MB, Samuels SJ. Reporting occupational injury and illness in the semiconductor manufacturing industry. *Am J Public Health* 1991; 81:85–89.
5. Blessman JE. Differential treatment of occupational disease v occupational injury by workers' compensation in Washington State. *J Occup Med* 1991; 33:121–126.
6. Cheadle A, Franklin G, Wolfhagen C, et al. Factors influencing the duration of work-related disability: A population-based study of Washington State Workers' Compensation. *Am J Public Health* 1994; 84(2):190–196.
7. Andersson GB, Svensson O, Oden A. The intensity of work recovery in low back pain. *Spine* 1983; 8:880–884.
8. Abenhaim L, Rossignol M, Gobeille D, et al. The prognostic consequences in the making of the initial medical diagnosis of work-related back injuries. *Spine* 1995; 20:791–795.
9. Franklin GM, Haug J, Heyer NJ, McKeffrey SP, Picciano JF. Outcome of lumbar fusion in Washington State workers' compensation. *Spine* 1994; 19:1897–1904.
10. Rossignol M, Suissa S, Abenhaim L. Working disability due to occupational back pain: three-year follow-up of 2,300 compensated workers in Quebec. *J Occup Med* 1988; 30:502–505.
11. Magora A, Taustein I. An investigation of the problem of sick-leave in the patient suffering from low back pain. *Ind Med Surg* 1969; 38: 398–408.
12. Waddell G. *Epidemiology review: the epidemiology and cost of back pain.* London: Her Majesty's Stationery Office, 1994.
13. McGill CM. Industrial back problems: A control program. *J Occup Med* 1968; 10:174–178.
14. Von Korff M. Studying the natural history of back pain. *Spine* 1994; 19(18S):2041S–2046S.
15. Carey TS, Garrett J, Jackman A, et al. The outcomes and costs of care for acute low back pain among patients seen by primary care practitioners, chiropractors, and orthopedic surgeons. *N Engl J Med* 1995; 333:913–917.
16. Washington State Department of Labor and Industries. Long-term disability prevention pilots. *Annual Report to the Legislature, 1994.* Olympia, WA: Department of Labor and Industries, 1994.
17. Leavitt SS, Johnston TL, Beyer RD. The process of recovery: Patterns in industrial back injury, Parts 1–4. *Ind Med* 1971–1972; 40(8): 7–14,40(9):7–15,41(1):7–11,41(2):5–9.
18. Burton JF. Workers' compensation benefits and costs: significant developments in the early 1990s. In: Burton JF, ed. *1996 Workers' Compensation year book.* Horsham, PA: LRP Publications, 1995.
19. Andersson GB. Epidemiologic aspects of low back pain in industry. *Spine* 1981; 6:53–60.
20. Magora A. Investigation of the relation between low back pain and occupation. *Scand J Rehabil Med* 1975; 7:146–151.
21. Kelsey JL, White AA. Epidemiology and impact of low back pain. *Spine* 1980; 5:133–142.
22. Riihimaki H, Tola S, Videman T, Hanninen K. Low back pain and occupation: a cross-sectional questionnaire study of men in machine operating, dynamic physical work, and sedentary work. *Spine* 1989; 14:204–209.
23. Butler RJ, Johnson WG, Baldwin ML. Managing work disability: Why first return to work is not a measure of success. *Ind Lab Relat Rev* 1995; 48(3):452–469.
24. Greenough CG, Fraser RD. The effects of compensation on recovery from low-back injury. *Spine* 1989; 14:947–955.
25. Parry T. *Medical benefit delivery-group medical versus workers' compensation in California.* San Francisco, CA: California Workers' Compensation Institute, 1994.
26. Abeln SH. ''Rehabilitating'' Workers' Comp: Factors in selecting and contracting with rehab providers. *J Care Manage* 1995; 1(2):39ff.
27. Rohling ML, Binder LM, Langhinrichsen-Rohling J. Money matters: A meta-analytic review of the association between financial compensation and the experience and treatment of chronic pain. *Health Psychol* 1995; 14(6):537–547.
28. Catts PF, Aroney M, Indyk JS. Laparoscopic repair of inguinal hernia. *Med J Aust* 1994; 161(4):242–245.
29. Davis RA. A long-term outcome analysis of 984 surgically treated herniated lumbar discs. *J Neurosurg* 1994; 80(3):415–421.
30. Greenough CG, Taylor LJ, Fraser RD. Anterior lumbar fusion. A comparison of noncompensation patients with compensation patients. *Clin Orthop* 1994; 300:30–37.
31. Myerson MS, McGarvey WC, Henderson MR, et al. Morbidity after crush injuries to the foot. *J Orthop Trauma* 1994; 8(4):343–349.
32. Roth JH, Richards RS, MacLeod MD. Endoscopic carpal tunnel release. *Can J Surg* 1994; 37(3):189–193.
33. Lau LS. Lumbar facet joint block: a simplified technique. *Aust Radiol* 1986; 30:251.
34. Norton WL. Chemonucleolysis versus surgical discectomy. *Spine* 1986; 11:440–443.
35. Volinn E, VanKoevering D, Loeser JD. Back sprain in industry: the role of socioeconomic factors in chronicity. *Spine* 1991; 16:542–548.
36. Loeser JD, Henderlite SE, Conrad DE. Incentive effects of workers' compensation benefits: a literature synthesis. *Med Care Res Rev* 1995; 52(1):34–59.
37. Weiser S, Cedraschi C. Psychosocial issues in the prevention of chronic low back pain—a literature review. *Baillier's Clin Rheum* 1992; 6(3):657–684.
38. Kennedy F. The mind of the injured worker. *Comp Med* 1946; 1(6–7): 19–24.
39. Mendelson G. *Psychiatric aspect of personal injury claims.* Springfield, IL: Thomas, 1988.
40. Strang PJ. The chronic disability syndrome. In: Aronoff GM, ed. *Evaluation and treatment of chronic pain.* Baltimore: Urban & Schwarzenberg, 1985.
41. Williams CA. *An international comparison of Workers' Compensation.* Boston: Kluwer Academic Publishers, 1991.
42. Grannemann TG. *Review, regulate or reform? What works to control workers' compensation medical costs.* : Workers' Compensation Research Institute, 1994.
43. Bigos SJ, Spengler DM, Martin NA, et al. Back injuries in industry: a retrospective study. II. Injury factors. *Spine* 1986; 11:246–251.
44. Bigos SJ, Battie MC, Spengler DM, et al. A prospective study of work perceptions and psychosocial factors affecting the report of back injury. *Spine* 1991; 16(1):1–6.
45. Habeck R, Leahy M, Hunt H, et al. Employer factors related to workers' compensation claims and disability management. *Rehab Counsel Bull* 1991; 34; 210–236.
46. Dichraff RM. When the injured worker retains an attorney. *AAOHN J* 1993; 41(10):491–498.
47. Kramer O, Briffault R. *Workers' Compensation.* New York: Insurance Information Institute Press, 1991.
48. Deyo RA, Diehl A, Rosenthal M. How many days of bed rest for acute low back pain? A randomized clinical trial. *N Engl J Med* 1986; 315:1064–1070.
49. Scheer SJ. Commonalities of measuring capacity to work. In: Scheer SJ, ed. *Multidisciplinary perspectives in vocational assessment of impaired workers.* Gaithersburg: Aspen Publications, 1990; 19–29.
50. Scheer SJ, Wickstrom RJ. Vocational capacity with low back pain impairment. In: Scheer SJ, ed. *Medical perspectives in vocational assessment of impaired workers.* Gaithersburg: Aspen Publications, 1991; 19–63.
51. Yelin EH, Henke CJ, Epstein WV. Work disability among persons with musculoskeletal conditions. *Arthritis Rheum* 1986; 29:1322-33.
52. Chaffin D, Andersson GB. Worker selection. In: Chaffin D, Anders-

son GB, eds. *Occupational biomechanics*. New York: John Wiley & Sons, 1984; 399–410.

53. Scheer SJ. The role of the physician in disability management. In: Shrey DE, Lacerte M, eds. *Principles and practices of disability management in industry*. Winter Park: GR Press, 1995; 175–205.
54. Spangfort EV. Lumbar disc herniation: a computer aided analysis of 2504 operations. *Acta Orthop Scand [Suppl]* 1972; 142:1–93.
55. Olmarker K, Rydevik B, Nordborg C. Autologous nucleus pulposus induces neurophysiologic and histologic changes in porcine cauda equina nerve roots. *Spine* 1993; 18:1425–1432.
56. Robinson JP, Brown PB, Fisk JD. Pathophysiology of lumbar radiculopathies and the pharmacology of epidural corticosteroids and local anesthetics. *Phys Med Rehabil Clin North Am* 1995; 6(4):671–690.
57. Deyo RA, Rainville J, Kent DL. What can the history and physical examination tell us about low back pain? *JAMA* 1992; 268:760–765.
58. Frymoyer J, Andersson GB. Clinical classification. In: Pope MH, Andersson GB, Frymoyer JW, et al, eds. *Occupational low back pain*. New York: Praeger, 1991; 44–70.
59. Troup JD, Martin JW, Lloyd DC. Back pain in industry: a prospective study. *Spine* 1981; 6:61–69.
60. Kosteljantez M, Espersen JO, Halaburt H, et al. Predictive value of clinical and surgical findings in patients with lumbago-sciatica: a prospective study (part 1). *Acta Neurochir* 1984; 73:67–76.
61. Hakelius A, Hindmarsh J. The comparative reliability of preoperative diagnostic methods in lumbar disc surgery. *Acta Orthop Scand* 1972; 43:234–238.
62. Brieg A, Troup JD. Biomechanical considerations in the straight-leg raising test: cadaveric and clinical studies of medial hip rotation. *Spine* 1979; 4:242–250.
63. Nelson M, Allen P, Clamp S, et al. Reliability and reproducibility of clinical findings in low-back pain. *Spine* 1979; 4:97–101.
64. McCombe PF, Fairbank JC, Cockersole BS, et al. Reproducibility of physical signs in low-back pain. *Spine* 1989; 14:908–918.
65. Deerbery VJ, Tullis WH. Delayed recovery in the patient with a work compensible injury. *J Occup Med* 1983; 25:829–835.
66. Waddell G, McCulloch J, Kummel E, et al. Non-organic physical signs in low-back pain. *Spine* 1980; 5:117–125.
67. Smith WC. *Principles of disability evaluation*. Philadelphia: JB Lippincott, 1959; 15–19.
68. Matheson LN. Symptom magnification syndrome structured interview: rationale and procedure. *J Occup Rehabil* 1991; 1:43–56.
69. Hazard RG, Reid S, Fenwick J, et al. Isokinetic trunk and lifting strength measurements: variability as an indicator of effort. *Spine* 1988; 13(1):54–57.
70. Stokes H. The seriously uninjured hand: weakness of grip. *J Occup Med* 1983; 25:683–684.
71. Chengalur SN, Smith GA, Nelson RC, et al. Assessing sincerity of effort in maximal grip strength tests. *Am J Phys Med Rehabil* 1990; 69(3):148–153.
72. Newton M, Waddell G. Trunk strength testing with iso-machines. Part 1. Review of a decade of scientific evidence. *Spine* 1993; 18:801–811.
73. Timm KE. A randomized-control study of active and passive treatments for chronic low back pain following L5 laminectomy. *J Orthop Sports Phys Ther* 1994; 20:276–286.
74. Boden SD, Wiesel SW. Errors in decision making following radiographic investigations of the spine. *Semin Spine Surg* 1993; 5:90–100.
75. Simmons ED, Guyer RD, Graham-Smith A, et al. Contemporary concepts in spine care: radiographic assessment for patients with low back pain. *Spine* 1995; 20:1839–1841.
76. US Department of Health and Human Services, Agency for Health Care Policy and Research. *Acute low back problems in adults. Clinical practice guideline number 14*. AHCPR Publication No. 95-0643, 1994.
77. Herzog RJ, Guyer RD, Graham-Smith A, et al. Contemporary concepts in spine care. Magnetic resonance imaging: use in patients with low back or radicular pain. *Spine* 1995; 20:1834–1838.
78. Hitselberger WE, Witten RM. Abnormal myelograms in asymptomatic patients. *J Neurosurg* 1968; 28:204–206
79. Wiesel SW, Bell GR, Feffer HL, et al. A study of computer-assisted tomography: I. The incidence of positive CAT scans in an asymptomatic group of patients. *Spine* 1984; 9:549–551.
80. Boden SD, Davis DO, Dina TS, et al. Abnormal magnetic resonance scans of the lumbar spine in asymptomatic subjects: a prospective investigation. *J Bone Joint Surg (Am)* 1990; 72:403–408.
81. Jensen MS, Brant-Zawadski N, Obuchowksi N, et al. Magnetic resonance imaging of the lumbar spine in people without back pain. *N Engl J Med* 1994; 331:69–73.
82. Masaryk TJ, Ross JS, Modic MT, et al. High-resolution MR imaging of sequestered lumbar intervertebral disks. *Am J Roentgenol* 1988; 150:1155–1162.
83. Executive Committee of the North American Spine Society. Position statement on discography. *Spine* 1988; 13:1343.
84. Haldeman S. The electrodiagnostic evaluation of nerve root function. *Spine* 1984; 9(1):42–48.
85. Partanen J, Partanen K, Oikarinem H, et al. Preoperative electroneuromyography and myelography in cervical root compression. *Electromyogr Clin Neurophysiol* 1991; 31:21–26.
86. White AA, Gordon SL. Synopsis: workshop on idiopathic low-back pain. *Spine* 1982; 7:141–149.
87. Matheson LN. Functional capacity evaluation. In: Demeter SL, Anderson GB, Smith GM, eds. *Disability evaluation*. St. Louis: Mosby/AMA, 1996; 168–188.
88. Katz RT. The difficult patient. In: *Disability evaluation*. Chicago, IL: American Association for Physical Medicine and Rehabilitation Certificate Program Syllabus, 1996.
89. Eisendrath SJ. Psychiatric aspects of chronic pain. *Neurology* 1995; 45(Suppl 9):S26–S34.
90. Tait RC. Psychological factors in the assessment of disability among patients with chronic pain. *J Back Musculoskel Rehabil* 1993; 3(1): 20–47.
91. Malmivaara A, Hakkinen U, Aro T, et al. The treatement of acute low back pain—bed rest, exercises, or ordinary activity? *N Engl J Med* 1995; 332:351–355.
92. Fordyce WE, Brockaway J, Bergman J, et al. Acute back pain: a control-group comparison of behavioral vs. traditional management methods. *J Behav Med* 1985; 9:127–140.
93. Bigos SJ, Bower OR, Braen GR, et al. *Acute low back problems in adults. Clinical practice guideline no. 14*. Rockville, MD: Agency for Health Care Policy and Research, Public Health Service, US Department of Health and Human Services, AHCPR Publication No. 95-0642, 1994.
94. Bergquist-Ullman M, Larsson U. Acute LBP in industry. *Acta Orthop Scand* 1977; 170(Suppl):1–113.
95. Scheer SJ, Radack KL, O'Brien DR. Randomized controlled trials in industrial low back pain relating to return to work. Part 1. Acute interventions. *Arch Phys Med Rehabil* 1995; 76:966–973.
96. Mooney V. Letter to the editor. *Spine* 1994; 19:1101–1104.
97. Shekelle PG, Adams AH, Chassin MR, et al. Spinal manipulation for low-back pain. *Ann Intern Med* 1992; 117:590–598.
98. Assendelft WJ, Koes BW, Van Der Heijden G, et al. The efficacy of chiropractic manipulation for back pain: blinded review of relevant randomized clinical trials. *J Manip Physiol Ther* 1992; 15:487–494.
99. Hall H, McIntosh G, Melles T, et al. Effect of discharge recommendations on outcome. *Spine* 1994; 19(18):2033–2037.
100. Weinstein SM, Herring SA, Derby R. Contemporary concepts in spine care. Epidural steroid injections. *Spine* 1995; 20:1842–1846.
101. Spaccarelli KC. Lumbar and caudal epidural corticosteroid injections. *Mayo Clin Proc* 1996; 71:169–178.
102. Rapp SE, Haselkorn JK, Elam JK, et al. Epidural steroid injection in the treatment of low back pain: a meta-analysis (abstract). *Anesthesiology* 1994; 81:923.
103. McKenzie R. *The lumbar spine: mechanical diagnosis and therapy*. Weikane, New Zealand: Spinal Publications, 1981.
104. Saal JA. Intervertebral disc herniation: advances in nonoperative treatment. *Phys Med Rehabil State Art Rev* 1990; (4):175–190.
105. Shvartzman L, Weingarten E, Sherry M, et al. Cost-effectiveness analysis of extended conservative therapy versus surgical intervention in the management of herniated lumbar intervertebral disc. *Spine* 1992; 17:176–182.
106. Weber H. Lumbar disc herniation. A controlled, prospective study with ten years of observation. *Spine* 1983; 8:131–140.
107. Matheson LN, Ogden LD, Violette K, et al. Work hardening: occupational therapy in industrial rehabilitation. *Am J Occup Ther* 1985; 39: 314–321.
108. Shrey DE, Olsheski JA. Disability management and industry-based work return transition programs. *Phys Med Rehabil State Art Rev* 1992; 6(2):303–314.

109. Scheer SJ. Ergonomics. *Phys Med Rehabil Clin North Am* 1992; 3(3): 599–614.
110. *Job Accomodation Network U.S. quarterly report.* Morgantown, WV, April–June, 1995.
111. Demeter SL, Andersson GB, Smith GM, eds. *Disability evaluation.* St. Louis: Mosby/AMA, 1996.
112. Keely J, Mayer T, Cox R, et al. Quantification of lumbar function: Part 5. Reliability of range of motion measures in the sagittal plane and an *in vivo* torso rotation measurement technique. *Spine* 1986; 11: 31–35.
113. Rondinelli R, Murphy J, Esler A, et al. Estimation of normal lumbar flexion with surface inclinometry: a comparison of three methods. *Am J Phys Med Rehabil* 1992; 71:219–224.
114. Fordyce WE. *Behavioral methods for chronic pain and illness.* St. Louis: Mosby, 1976.
115. Fordyce WE. *Back pain in the workplace.* Seattle: ISAP Press, 1995.
116. Osterweis M, Kleinman A, Mechanic D, eds. *Pain and disability: clinical, behavioral, and public policy perspectives.* Washington, DC: National Academy Press, 1987.
117. Pryor ES. Flawed promises. A critical evaluation of the American Medical Association Guides to the Evaluation of Permanent Impairment. *Harvard Law Rev* 1990; 103:964–976.
118. Bell C. Overview of the Americans with Disabilities Act and the Family and Medical Leave Act. In: Demeter SL, Andersson GB, Smith GM, eds. *Disability evaluation.* St. Louis: Mosby/AMA, 1996; 582–591.
119. Johns RE, Elegante JM, Teynor PD, et al. Fitness for duty. In: Demeter SL, Andersson GB, Smith GM, eds. *Disability evaluation.* St. Louis: Mosby/AMA, 1996; 592–604.
120. Sullivan MD, Loeser JD. The diagnosis of disability. Treating and rating disability in a pain clinic. *Arch Intern Med* 1992; 152: 1829–1835.
121. Kramer MS, Lane DA. Causal propositions in clinical research and practice. *J Clin Epidemiol* 1992; 45(6):639–649.

Rehabilitation Medicine: Principles and Practice, Third Edition,
edited by Joel A. DeLisa and Bruce M. Gans.
Lippincott–Raven Publishers, Philadelphia © 1998.

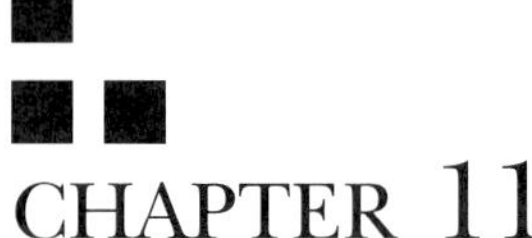

CHAPTER 11

Interactions with the Medicolegal System

Steve R. Geiringer

Most clinicians who evaluate or treat patients with rehabilitation-related problems will eventually interact with the legal system. For some practitioners these interactions may occur daily, for others, a few times yearly, and still others may interact with the legal system once or twice a month. Medicolegal horror stories abound, many starting with, "The worst deposition I ever sat through . . . . " Although few relish this aspect of the musculoskeletal or rehabilitation practice, it need not be that onerous. One goal of this chapter is to remove some negative feelings about this type of work, not necessarily by casting it in a favorable light but rather by desensationalizing the process through familiarization and preparation.

There are many types of medicolegal interactions, with the most common being depositions, expert witness reviews, independent medical evaluations (IMEs), and malpractice complaints.

Giving a deposition is quite commonplace and is a medicolegal interaction most of us will encounter throughout our careers. A main theme of this chapter is, therefore, a detailed review of the process of giving a deposition. Physiatrists are often asked to perform IMEs, and that process is also detailed below. Even though there may or may not be an attorney involved with an IME, being available for and performing them frequently leads to a subsequent deposition. Expert witness reviews are less common, and a brief discussion appears at the end of the chapter, along with miscellaneous considerations. Optimistically, malpractice complaints will not be experienced often, if ever, and are mostly beyond the scope of this chapter.

Many medical professionals dislike anything related to medicolegal proceedings and consequently carry negative feelings about being forced to deal with them. Some even avoid the type of clinical work that more likely leads to depositions, and others feel there is no such thing as a truly "impartial" medical evaluation. Much of this dislike and mistrust arises from unfamiliarity and misunderstanding of the processes involved; the experience should be no worse than neutral if a clear awareness of the details is present ahead of time.

S. R. Geiringer: Department of Physical Medicine and Rehabilitation, Wayne State University, Detroit, Michigan 48201.

STANDARDS OF CLINICAL PRACTICE RELATED TO MEDICOLEGAL WORK

Medicolegal issues should be considered during, but not be the driving force behind, the development of sound standards of clinical practice, including principles of history taking, physical examination, and report generation and storage. Adherence to some common-sense guidelines will make life infinitely easier when later reviewing a chart for medicolegal reasons. On the other hand, one should not prepare reports as if their primary purpose is an eventual deposition. Most importantly, your routine clinical decision making should never be shaped solely by legal considerations.

Reviewing Outside Records

Especially in the case of an IME, a packet of outside medical records will often accompany the patient or will have been sent ahead of time. A few narrative reports can be read at the time of the examination, but a voluminous file should be reviewed earlier, then quickly scanned again just before the history and physical examination. Radiographs should be studied if made available. It is not necessary to examine or document records that are not pertinent to your examination of the patient. For example, although you may note underlying cardiovascular disease, there is no need to review innumerable diagnostic studies, laboratory results, and the like. Your opinions in those areas will not be legally admissible anyway, other than how they directly affect physical medicine and rehabilitation. Never discard any records forwarded to you, even if they are peripheral to your assessment. An attorney may want to review everything that was ever sent to you; suspicions may be raised, if files are missing, that they were deliberately discarded for some less than noble reason.

Taking the History

As with all cases, it is crucial to be thorough while not allowing the process to become engulfed in superfluous detail. The proper degree of completeness allows for full reproduction of the history months or even years later, when direct recall of the patient is likely nil. One should use common language to define any jargon or terms specific to the case. A chronological sequencing of events will simplify future review. The line of questioning should be orderly, starting with the onset of the problem, prior and current symptoms, diagnostic studies, the patient's understanding of test results, prior and current treatment efforts, and pertinent past medical history. An occupational or functional summary is often critical, including the relationship of symptoms or job status to intercurrent events. Your report might be the only place where such crucial information appears. A patient might have had a work-related injury, and during treatment been involved in a motor vehicle accident. Separate the effects of these as much as possible within the history. Either throughout the history or in summary form at its end, provide a detailed description of the effect of the patient's problem on impairment related to physical, psychological, social, and vocational issues.

The Physical Examination

Naturally, a thorough physical examination is mandatory. If any aspect of the physical relies purely on a subjective response from the patient, this should be clearly noted in the report. Third-party payers often balk at a diagnosis based solely on reports from the patient without objective abnormalities. Whenever possible, generate as objective a set of observations as possible to counter future attempts by an attorney to dismiss all subjective reporting as unreliable. A common example in the pain practice is the distribution of trigger points in a patient with myofascial pain syndrome. In these cases, it is extremely helpful years later to have documentation in the chart that the tender points were at reproducible, characteristic locations described in textbooks (upper trapezius fibers, insertion of levator scapula into the superior medial border of the scapula, lateral epicondyle, etc.). On the other hand, if the patient has pain with minimal pressure over every spot examined, that is atypical for known myofascial disorders, and one should describe it as such. This type of reporting lends a warranted objective dimension to what is inherently a subjective topic. Similarly, it will be more helpful to document reduced range of motion at any joint in terms of percentage lacking or absolute degrees rather than by using such modifiers as "mildly" or "moderately" reduced. However, do not think that endless goniometric joint motion or computerized strength measurements will lend additional credence to your report. A medical report is useful because of the clear logic and objective reasoning used in reaching the conclusion, not because of an overabundance of data.

Whenever any aspect of the physical examination is described as "positive," it is important to detail for what symptom or sign it is positive. To illustrate, if the straight leg raise test is "positive for pain," be sure to distinguish pain radiating from the back down the posterior thigh into the foot at 45° from a pull or stretching discomfort isolated to the hamstring muscles at 80°. When you review a chart years later, this type of differentiation will be critical. The same holds true for the Spurling maneuver, Tinel's sign, and many others.

The Report

Mention who referred the patient to the clinic, whether it is another practitioner, a third party payer, a nurse manager hired by an insurance company, or if the patient was self-referred (not possible for an IME). In the case of IMEs, dictate a standard line noting that no doctor–patient relationship was established.

Your report should acknowledge any outside medical records by stating who sent them to you and what they contain. The type of report, its date, conclusions reached, and other pertinent findings should be catalogued, either chronologically or by type of report (medical, radiographic, electrodiagnostic, etc.). It is sufficient to summarize these as "medical reports from Drs. Smith and Jones" or "handwritten physical therapy progress notes that are largely illegible," etc. It is not necessary to paraphrase every such note as to date, content, or conclusion. If you refer to an outside record in your dictated report, the appropriate amount of detail can be added at that point. If you studied radiographs, your report must also note if you read the formal radiology interpretation. This does not mean that you should avoid reaching your own conclusion about such films, but keep in mind that an attorney will be quick to point out during deposition that you are not formally qualified to do so. There is no need to vary from your own standard of practice.

Months to years later, clinic visit reports may be the only documentation of evaluation and treatment efforts. It is imperative that no important point in the history or physical examination is left to memory, as even the best memory will eventually fail to recall what prove to be critical details. It is inadequate to keep the final chart report in handwritten form; all reports and communications should be done with word processing, generated with a laser printer. This allows for legibility even when reports have been telefaxed, photocopied, and faxed again. Exceptions include brief handwritten notes documenting a telephone call, prescription refill, or similar matters. It is sound practice, though, to dictate a note concerning any direct communication with the patient. If one takes handwritten notes during a clinic visit, they are to be kept in the permanent record. An attorney will often ask if such notes are taken. If they are as a routine but are not available at the time of the deposition, the suspicion can be raised that they were destroyed just recently for some sinister reason. It is preferable to modify the clinic schedule to allow for dictation time immediately following each patient encounter, to eliminate the need for handwritten notes. If dictated in this fashion, the content of the notes may be less suspect than if all reports from a day are dictated at a later time.

The history, physical examination, and conclusions must be summarized objectively. As the impressions are expressed, one should not resort to judgmental or pejorative terms. For example, it is impossible to detect that a patient is "exaggerating" symptoms or blowing them out of proportion. There is no method of determining whether a patient is "enhancing" reports of pain. Similarly, never report that the patient does not appear "legitimate." The use of such terms is counterproductive, and one can easily challenge their basis. Preferably, report that the examination can or can not explain the patient's symptoms. One conclusion might be, "The impairment found on today's examination, combined with review of diagnostic testing, includes mild tightness of the left upper trapezius muscle. This does not explain the chronic symptoms of low back and neck pain, bilateral arm numbness, or the 9 months Mr. X has been disabled from work." It is of course equally germane to outline those impairments that do account for signs and symptoms. For example, "C7 nerve root abnormality on the right is documented on today's examination, with reduced triceps reflex and strength, and a positive Spurling maneuver. This corresponds to the MRI scan showing a disc herniation in the low cervical spine on the right and to the recent EMG showing a C7 radiculopathy." Thinking and reporting in this manner will simplify the process of chart review and of participating in a deposition at a later date.

For most situations involving treatment, it helps to conclude the report with a summary of what was said to the patient, including specific instructions for follow-up visits or testing. (This does not pertain to IMEs, because there is no doctor–patient relationship established.) There should also be a designated form in the chart for the office staff to document telephone calls, prescription refills, and no-show, rescheduled, or canceled appointments.

INDEPENDENT MEDICAL EVALUATION

Definition

An IME is arranged when a party desires to obtain a medical opinion from a practitioner who has never before examined the patient. That opinion is typically requested as a step toward resolving a conflict between the patient and a third party, often an employer or an agent of the employer. The request may originate from a company physician, the insurance company backing an employer's workers compensation program, a case manager hired by that insurance company, or an attorney for either the patient or the employer.

An IME may be sought because of medical expertise in a particular area, but performing one does not constitute the establishment of a doctor–patient relationship. An attorney therefore cannot introduce into the legal record the results of that IME. That point of jurisprudence, combined with the nature of the evaluations being carried out, means that more IMEs will likely lead to depositions in typical clinic practice.

As a point of explanation, a patient who initiates legal action of this sort is a plaintiff. Although there is no accusation of criminal action, the party the patient is acting against is the defendant. The representing attorneys are named correspondingly.

Ethics of Independent Medical Evaluation

The requisite condition of an underlying conflict, as mentioned above, is the genesis of much of the controversy surrounding IMEs. For example, a case manager is typically hired by an insurance company that underwrites an employer's workers' compensation program or by an automobile insurance firm that is being asked to provide benefits to one of its insured. One might reasonably infer that, for that case manager to remain in good standing with her employer, she would try to reduce the amount of money paid out in a claim. Understandably, the case manager would develop a list of physicians who reliably determine, via an IME, that there is no impairment present, or at least that the impairment is not as severe, long-lasting, or expensive as the patient's own physician believes. The converse also applies to plaintiff-oriented attorneys, who know which specialists will routinely determine that a severe and long-lasting disability is present, even when objective impairment is minimal, if present at all. Thus, the "impartial" in IME is often compromised. Some physicians have built a particular reputation hand in hand with a lucrative practice, fueled by referrals from either the defense side (companies, company physicians, case managers, defense attorneys) or from the plaintiff side (most prominently plaintiff attorneys). Therefore, you may be asked during deposition what percentage of your medicolegal work originates from the plaintiff and/or defense sides. A physician who performs IMEs predominantly or exclusively for only one side may be considered less than fully credible.

It may now be more apparent why some believe that the medicolegal world of IMEs and depositions is one to avoid. Fortunately, there is reason for optimism. Judges, administrative law clerks, and mediators now tend to recognize a "boilerplate" IME and their authors, and will discount or even ignore their conclusions. Case managers, company attorneys, insurers, and even the employers themselves eventually come to the understanding that these one-sided opinions do not hold up under scrutiny and may cost more time and money over the long run, as challenges and appeals drag out. Most importantly, one can hope that physicians will become less willing to be tempted into one camp or another.

The simple, underlying principle in the world of IMEs (as with the rest of medical practice) is to keep in mind what is in the best interest of the patient. That would seem to be an obvious thought, without the need to repeat it or even state it in the first place. It may also seem to sway physicians toward the plaintiff side of most proceedings, and, after all, we should be patient advocates. In reality, an ethical physician, who as a matter of course takes into account the best interest of the patient, will not be labeled as belonging to either the plaintiff or defense camp. That attests to a high level of objectivity. Some examples will illustrate this principle.

A young adult sustains a C6 complete spinal cord injury in a motor vehicle accident. After the acute medical stage has passed, the insurance company wishes to settle its financial responsibility via a lump-sum payment. The patient's attorney does not feel that sum is nearly adequate, even if invested wisely, to cover lifetime expenses. As a specialist in spinal injury, your IME opinion in this case only secondarily concerns the diagnosis. You agree that the long-term expenses would be more likely met by rejecting the lump sum and opting for an ongoing responsility on the part of the insurance company. That is in the best interest of the patient.

Now consider the case of a middle aged assembly-line worker who sustains a back injury. A friend has recommended a physician who determines that the patient is totally disabled indefinitely, perhaps permanently. Treatment includes three times weekly hot packs in that physician's office. Your IME, along with directed diagnostic testing, finds the only impairment to be mild lumbar muscle tightness. It is clearly not in the best interest of the employer or its insurance company to have the patient disabled, but most importantly, it is certainly not in the best interest of the patient (or his family, or for that matter society) to recommend ongoing disability when gainful employment would be a simple matter to achieve.

Impartiality is not difficult to conceptualize or attain. Each case is judged on its own merits, with emphasis on objective data. These can include physical examination findings, diagnostic test results, laboratory study results, or even a surveillance videotape recording showing the plaintiff moving heavy furniture into his mother's house. If you are successful in this regard, you will develop a reputation that your reports do not automatically favor either party. Some companies or attorneys might not refer IMEs to you because of that, but that is business you are wise to do without.

The IME Without Treatment

This is the most common mode of referral. Your service is sought for a one-time evaluation, with the outcome that you will provide an expert answer to one or several questions. This may be as deceivingly simple as: "Did this patient sustain a mild closed head injury?" In the musculoskeletal area, numerous questions are usually asked:

- What is the impairment?
- Is there a causal relationship between the injury/accident and the current impairment?
- What is the disability arising from the objective impairment?
- Has the treatment to date been effective?
- What further treatment is recommended?
- Has the patient reached maximal medical improvement (MMI)? In other words, do you believe that further formal medical treatment will improve the impairment (not necessarily just provide symptomatic relief)?
- Is the patient able to return to work? With restrictions? How long should the restrictions last?
- In some states, you may also be asked to calculate that patient's percentage of permanent impairment (*Guidelines to the evaluation of permanent impairment, 4th ed.* American Medical Association, 1990.).

There may be other questions as well, depending on the specifics of the case at hand.

Serial IMEs

By definition, the initial IME does not allow the physician to assume the role of prescribing or overseeing treatment. It can become quite frustrating to witness inadequate, insufficient, or improper care without the opportunity to rectify the situation. Some third parties will ask for follow-up IMEs, which is an intermediate step along the spectrum of opinion only versus treatment. You might determine that an injured worker cannot return to the assembly line for 3 months, while the original impairment is treated. After that interval the worker is returned to your clinic for a follow-up IME, for you to ascertain whether your suggestions were followed and for an updated opinion on work status. Some patients are returned for serial IMEs up to six or eight times over a span of up to several years.

DEPOSITION

Definition

A deposition is the process of taking your testimony, under oath, as part of a formal legal record. This information is for subsequent use, either in trial before a jury or at an arbitration hearing before a lay or expert panel, and takes the place of your personal testimony in court. Keep in mind that whatever you say at the time of your deposition carries all the weight and responsibility of courtroom testimony, and you should handle it with equal respect. In these cases, you have either evaluated or both evaluated and treated a patient. This could have been a single visit for your opinion, IME, or an ongoing treating relationship. The results of the practitioner–client interactions have been documented in the notes generated at the times of office visits, but a deposition allows for expansion and clarification. A critical point to remember is that the medical professional may offer *opinion,* not just reiteration of what is already written. The lay person can only testify as to *facts,* with no interpretation thereof.

A deposition is "called" when a case involving one of your patients has progressed (or degenerated) to the point of legal action. This is typically a civil case involving compensation or insurance benefits (automobile, worker's compensation, disability) or other payback carrying a perceived value to both parties. The fact that you receive a subpoena for a deposition implies that a disagreement exists between the sides, one that has not been rectified during initial attempts at negotiation, compromise, and mediation.

An interesting question to ponder is, if testimony is needed for court proceedings, why are medical practitioners not simply given a subpoena to appear in court? The answer, based in years of tradition, is that the attorney who wants your opinion does not want to inconvenience you. If you were required to schedule time away from your clinic, or were subjected to repeated cancellations because of the quirks of the court system, you might turn into a "hostile witness." The one thing feared most by an attorney is that what you say during testimony will be a surprise to them. Depositions are therefore typically scheduled in your office, at times convenient for you, provided both attorneys agree. The conventions and standard practices in this regard vary widely among states and counties.

Scheduling the Deposition

After you have participated in your first deposition, you might understand that it is a good idea to delineate specific criteria for the future scheduling process. This is because attorneys will often use the presence of an upcoming deposition to "encourage" the opposing party to settle the case out of court. There are several reasons lawyers are more willing to settle (rather than litigate) cases than the practitioners or organizations they represent. One is financial, as a settlement ensures at least some remuneration to the attorney, whereas a trial verdict may not. Depositions are therefore often canceled at the last minute, without regard to the havoc wrought on your clinic schedule.

Take the time to thoughtfully draft a form letter that your office staff will transmit to an attorney whenever deposition time is requested. The letter should include your office protocol, including at least:

1. The fee. Typically this includes the hourly rate, with a 1-hour minimum charge. If your practice leads to many short depositions of 30 minutes or less, you may consider a minimum rate based on the shorter time. As well, there is often a slightly discounted fee for half-day or full-day blocks of time. Your calculated time should include review of the file as well as any additional preparation time (videotape review, discussions with the attorney, etc.).
2. Prepayment procedure. To avoid frequently being left with a large hole in the clinic schedule because of deposition cancellations, consider the following: The deposition is not scheduled until the prepayment of 1 hour's fee has been received, has been deposited, and has cleared payment at the bank. This guideline may seem harsh, but remembering why depositions are often scheduled in the first place makes it more reasonable and understandable.
3. Time allotment. It makes sense to schedule depositions for the end of the day, as it is impossible to predict with any accuracy the duration of a given deposition. Generally, 45 to 90 minutes is the amount of time needed. One can decide either to displace the last clinic patient slot or two or simply add the deposition to the end of the daily schedule. However, be prepared to be flexible in your time allotment. Depositions on cases in which the clinician interaction has consisted of only one evaluation or IME may take 2 hours, yet in some seemingly complex cases, the testimony may be over in 20 minutes. Finally, make sure your office staff confirms the deposition that morning, just to be certain it has not been canceled without your having been notified.
4. Cancellation policy. The letter needs to be very clear about the negative consequences of waiting until the last minute for notification that the deposition has been called off. To carry any weight, the consequences need to be financial. The percentage of the prepayment your office will reimburse in case of cancellation depends on how many days of notice are given and on the ability of the office staff to fill the void. A typical schedule might be 100% reimbursement if your office receives notice five or more business days ahead of time, 50% reimbursement for two or three days' notice, and no refund if less notice is given.

You should not feel guilty or defensive about your fee or cancellation policies; keep in mind that the large block of time set aside for the deposition displaces revenue-generating activity. Although it is theoretically possible for an attorney to become so upset about these preliminary details that the court mandates your presence, the likelihood is small.

The Day of the Deposition

In the morning your office should routinely verify that the deposition will still be taken, as last-minute cancellations are common, often without notice to the physician. Your clinic schedule should end at least 15 minutes before the designated time to allow for chart review (if the file is small) and a brief meeting with the attorney who was responsible for arranging the deposition. If the chart is at all sizable, meaning you saw the patient more than two or three times, you will need additional time that day for review. It is perfectly legitimate to charge for your preparation time before the deposition.

It is generally not necessary to review any chart content other than what you are directly responsible for. Results of tests you ordered should be flagged, as should reports from other practitioners who saw the patient on your referral. Physical therapy progress notes, from treatment you ordered, should be reviewed as well. Attorneys will typically not question you about reports from other clinicians, which are legally "hearsay" to you.

All reports, test results, and other documents you have generated or were otherwise responsible for are open for detailed questioning during the deposition. It is to your distinct advantage to spend adequate time in preparation, using a highlighter, underlining, or marking key passages. The crucial information should be nearby during questioning. In the initial encounter report, highlight important aspects of the history and key positive and negative physical examination findings. Later reports should document test results, treatment efforts, and the patient's response to treatment, including pertinent changes in symptoms or physical examination.

Immediately before the deposition starts, it is customary for the attorney responsible for arranging it to meet briefly with you in private. This meeting is not to be used to form strategy, as clinicians should never think of the deposition as an "us versus them" situation. Rather, the attorney can review the process, then try to ascertain what the general tone of your responses will be. I have always thought it would be wise for a lawyer to contact me before considering taking my deposition, in case my opinion is inconsistent with the one sought. You should inquire about diagnostic test results or clinical impressions generated after you saw the patient, so that you will not be surprised if these are raised by the other attorney during the proceedings.

It is possible that the attorney may cancel a deposition after this "preconference" if it becomes evident that testimony would be harmful to the case. Assuming the preconference does take place, the lawyer who was not there may later ask if you and the initiating attorney discussed details of the case or planned what you would say during the deposition. It is wise to understand ahead of time that you should not reach that level of detail in a predeposition conference.

The typical deposition involves four people: the clinician, two attorneys, and a legal reporter, who will be typing on a shorthand machine during the entire proceeding. Occasionally, there may be more than one lawyer representing one side, or one from another interested party, such as the state worker's compensation fund. The patient is rarely present; in those cases, it would be natural to formulate answers in a more circumspect fashion than customary.

Most depositions are taken in the above manner; sometimes the proceeding is video recorded. You will sit across from the camera, which will likely be focused on you no matter who is speaking. A video technician becomes an additional party present, and the court reporter may or may not be typing as usual.

A deposition is a legal proceeding, and the attorneys act just as they would in a courtroom, except of course there is no judge or jury present. You are a sworn witness, and the first line of business is to be sworn in by the court reporter. If you normally speak rapidly, learn to slow down. Talk in measured, clear sentences, making sure the reporter can see and hear you. The attorney who called the deposition will first make introductions. You will then be asked to state your full name, and there will likely be questions about your curriculum vitae, one copy of which you will have to provide. The point is to establish your educational credentials and academic or clinical qualifications, not to cover every line; the entire C.V. might be typed into the record or included as an attachment. This background establishes you as qualified to act as an *expert witness,* one who can provide opinion, and not a witness who can only testify about facts. You might also be asked to provide a summary of what your field of medical specialty entails. Be brief and use lay terms. Those individuals deciding the outcome of the case may not have heard of a neuropsychologist, or how that differs from a psychologist involved with a chronic pain management program. They almost certainly have never heard of a physiatrist. Remember that the jury's educational level may range from no formal education to extensive graduate-level training.

The main point of the deposition follows. The attorney who called the deposition will put you through the *direct examination.* You will probably be asked how this patient happened to be referred to you, in what location you performed the examinations, and if you made records of these visits. The preliminary questioning will vary in time from case to case. Finally, you will be questioned directly about your care of the patient, what points of history and physical examination you found and recorded, and what your conclusions and treatment plans were. Do not hesitate to use the chart reports for reference; no one expects you to remember details of an old case. If the records have been reviewed and organized just prior to the deposition, it will be a minor task to answer questions quickly, accurately, and with confidence. The answers to questions should reflect what is written in the records; inconsistencies will become apparent. If a question is unclear, ask the attorney to repeat it. If a topic is out of your realm of expertise, say so. You may still be asked to provide a response, as long as it is clear that your knowledge is that of any other medical practitioner, or even a lay person, on that topic.

A cardinal point during depositions has to do with the frame of mind taken by the clinician with respect to the questioning from either attorney. The physician is there to represent a professional opinion, not as an advocate for the attorney, the opposing attorney, the employer, or an insurance company. Although the lawyers are in fact in opposition, the physician is not on anyone's "side." The principal distinguishing feature of expert medical testimony, when compared to testimony from a lay person, is that you may *give opinion,* not simply recall what occurred. An attorney might at times perceive an opinion as counter to the interests of his or her client, and verbally dance around these topics. A response to this may be to creatively fashion your answers to have the record reflect your opinions.

As previously mentioned, this meeting holds all the legal weight of a court appearance, and as such, the same legal procedures can and are used. After one attorney poses a question, the other might object, giving the reasons for the objection. Following this exchange, the questioning attorney will instruct you to answer the question anyway. Whether the jury eventually hears the question or the response to it depends on how the judge later rules on that particular point.

Direct examination usually concludes when all reports have been covered, and medical impressions and conclusions from the last patient visit have been stated. Next is the *cross examination.* The other attorney has the chance to ask you about anything broached by the first. Again, interruptions in the form of objections may occur. The line of questioning can alternate between the direct, cross, redirect, recross, and so on, indefinitely, though in reality there are rarely more than two such cycles before the entire deposition concludes.

Either of the attorneys might ask you to consider a hypothetical situation, which will markedly resemble the particulars of this case. They raise hypotheticals to elicit your general opinion regarding the case, e.g., whether in these circumstances it is reasonable to conclude that ongoing pain or disability might or might not result. Hypothetical questions raised by one side are universally challenged by the other, citing lack of foundation. As before, simply listen until it is time to answer, then do so. It is natural to feel defensive at times during a deposition, most often during cross examination. The second attorney might ask why certain aspects of the physical examination were or were not performed, or if important information might have been gained by ordering a diagnostic test that was not done, and so on.

It is vital to keep a cool head during the entire episode, as the physician is a witness, not the defendant. These are tried-and-true tactics to put you off guard and perhaps to lead you away from an opinion not favored by one attorney. All the tricks of the trade are just that, and you should not take them personally. One can fully understand this after witnessing two lawyers go for each other's throats like worst enemies and then, once the deposition is concluded, discuss where to have lunch. Only occasionally is true and palpable animosity apparent in the air. Your goal should be to accurately represent what you believe to be the truth, at least in those areas where you are considered an expert; leave the legal maneuvering to the lawyers. It is not necessary to be apprised about the outcome of the litigation, although there is no legal reason to prevent your inquiry.

EXPERT WITNESS REVIEWS

At some point in your career, you might be asked if you are interested in reviewing a chart to provide your expert opinion about a particular issue. More often than not, these are medical malpractice cases in which an attorney is looking for a physician to support the side of the client he or she is representing. Your name might be familiar to the lawyer from prior depositions you have given or might have been suggested by the physician being sued. Medical practitioners typically review charts on the side of the defendant, that is, the person being sued, with the goal in mind of showing there was no malpractice committed. On the other hand, some clinicians are well known for always providing an opinion favoring the plaintiff. An ''expert'' who always reaches a conclusion favorable to one side is more a mercenary than an expert.

There are several points to consider before accepting an expert review. The foremost point is whether you really want to get involved in this type of work; some view it as beneath their dignity, given the cast of characters sometimes associated. Next is the time required for a helpful review. The attorney will rely on your opinion, and it is incumbent on you to scour the records thoroughly and thoughtfully for scraps that have so far eluded others. This can take several hours, particularly if there are handwritten reports to decipher. Finally, you must be painfully honest with the attorney, especially if your opinion is damaging to the case of the client that attorney represents. It is extremely harmful to the client if the case proceeds to trial because of an opinion that was not thoughtfully produced and that later proves to be unsupported by expert testimony. If the practitioner being sued truly did not meet the standards of practice as you interpret them, say so.

Before accepting a case for review, become familiar with its framework. It may not reside within your realm of expertise. Once the case is accepted, the attorney will provide a copy of the entire record, and a time frame will be set for completion. Most often, there will be no requirement for a written summary or a face-to-face meeting; the pertinent information can be relayed by telephone. The attorney will use your opinion to help decide if and how to proceed with the case. You may be called on to provide testimony at deposition, although it is less likely you will be subpoenaed as an expert witness in a trial setting. This is primarily because most malpractice cases never come to trial; they are either dismissed or settled before then.

REMUNERATION FOR MEDICOLEGAL WORK

Medicolegal work can be lucrative. It is not uncommon for physicians to charge at least several hundred dollars hourly for deposition or expert review time. Where should the money go? The answer will depend on the particulars of each situation, although some guidelines are generally accepted. Above all, be certain to have the monetary issues clearly delineated prospectively to avoid disputes after the fact.

For the clinician who is self-employed, there is no controversy about where the medicolegal fees go. In a group private practice, though, the practice plan should have this spelled out. There are two obvious alternatives: the funds go to the individual or to the practice as a whole. The same dichotomy is often true in the academic world, and the rules should be clear. Typically, if depositions arise within the usual course of seeing patients in a practice, the fees go into the practice coffers. Expert reviews do not by nature originate from the practice itself, as they involve outside cases. The fees for expert reviews therefore often go directly to the reviewer if the review is done outside work hours. Naturally, if you cancel clinic time to accomplish a chart review, you should not expect to keep the review fees. The exception might be in the academic setting, if there is time allotted each month for outside work, typically consulting. Each center has rules about such work, which probably include the department chairperson approving the activity for nonconflict of interest with department affairs. Funds derived from expert witness reviews might seem tainted to some; a possible solution is to donate the funds to some aspect of your department or field or to a charity.

MISCELLANEOUS CONSIDERATIONS

Malpractice Complaints

Statistics point out that most physicians will be served with malpractice complaints more than once during their careers. Reading such a complaint, even on cases that are quickly dismissed, makes it sound as if your entire medical career is an abomination, and the hospital or clinic at which you practice would be better off razed. It is easy, and indeed natural, to become outraged at the language and accusations found in such documents. There is never a more important time to keep in mind that one should not take this personally. A plaintiff attorney is acting in the best interest of the client, given the ground rules now present in our system. Never attempt to respond to the plaintiff attorney, or the complaining patient, yourself. Your practice or your hospital will arrange for its representative, a defense attorney, to review and respond legally to the complaint and direct the actions thereafter.

It is important to understand ahead of time if your legal defense firm generally believes strongly in proceeding with litigation, rather than agreeing to negotiated settlements. Plaintiff attorneys typically do not realize reimbursement unless there is a payoff; that is, their getting paid is ''contingent'' on the outcome of the case. They are not usually paid hourly, as are defense lawyers. A plaintiff attorney's interest may well be in spending the least amount of time on the case, with the most lucrative payment. That often means avoiding a trial. Although ''settling'' may also be a more conservative approach to the defense side (some payout now versus the chance of a large one later), all such outcomes appear as negative for the physician, regardless of the particulars of the cases. Put another way, it may be tempting from pure financial terms for even the defense side to settle, even though the facts point to no wrongdoing on your part. Hence, it is necessary to know the philosophy of a defense legal firm. Further discussion regarding medical malpractice complaints are beyond the scope of this chapter.

Threats of Harm

Patients encountered during the practice of medicine might be upset with their employer, fellow employees, themselves, other health practitioners, or you. On occasion that anger is voiced to the point of a threat of harm that the patient might inflict on others. A general rule is that, if specific names have been stated of people whom the patient threatens, it is your obligation to notify law enforcement agencies accordingly. Because these guidelines vary locally and regionally, one should always check with a hospital attorney or other expert before proceeding.

ADDITIONAL READINGS

American Medical Association. *Guides to the evaluation of permanent impairment,* 4th ed. Chicago: American Medical Association, 1990.

Bascom R. A medicolegal primer for physicians. *Phys Med Rehabil Clin North Am* 1992; 3:325–339.

Bonfiglio RP, Bonfiglio RL. Medical testimony in workers' compensation matters. *Phys Med Rehabil Clin North Am* 1992; 3:665–676.

Deutsch PM. *Rehabilitation testimony: Maintaining a professional perspective.* Albany: Matthew Bender and Co., 1985.

Geiringer SR. Clinician interactions with the medicolegal system. *Adv Med Psychother* (in press).

Johnston W. Importance of communication between physician and attorney. *Phys Med Rehabil Clin North Am* 1992; 3:677–695.

Rondinelli RD, Robinson JP, Scheer SJ, Weinstein SM. Occupational rehabilitation and disability determination. Delisa DA, Gans BM, eds. *Rehabilitation medicine: principles and practice, 3rd ed.* Philadelphia: Lippincott–Raven Publishers, 1998; 213–230.

Rehabilitation Medicine: Principles and Practice, Third Edition,
edited by Joel A. DeLisa and Bruce M. Gans.
Lippincott–Raven Publishers, Philadelphia © 1998.

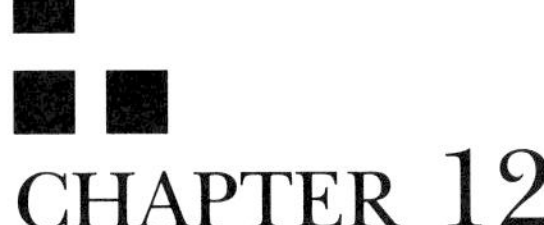

CHAPTER 12

Speech, Language, Swallowing, and Auditory Rehabilitation

Robert M. Miller, Michael E. Groher, Kathryn M. Yorkston, Thomas S. Rees, and Jeffrey B. Palmer

Speech and language are dynamic, multidimensional behaviors that constantly are influenced by physiological, psychological, and environmental factors. Speech uses anatomic structures and physiological reflexes that are common to both respiration and swallowing. Language is intimately related to cognition and the integration of sensory modalities, most commonly the auditory sense. Because of the complexity of human communication, a number of specialists are involved in studying and treating components of these communication behaviors and the disease states that impair their function.

An introduction to the processes of human communication, a description of disorders that are recognized at each level of the process, and a rationale for the evaluation and rehabilitation procedures that are used for each condition are presented in this chapter. Because of the complexity of these behaviors, the discussion is limited to the major areas of acquired dysfunction found in an adult population. The major divisions include normal processes for human speech and language, motor speech disorders, laryngectomee rehabilitation, language and intellectual disorders, swallowing evaluation and management, and auditory evaluation and the management of hearing loss.

R. M. Miller: Department of Audiology and Speech Pathology, Veterans Administration Puget Sound Health Care System; and Department of Rehabilitation Medicine, University of Washington, Seattle, Washington 98108.

M. E. Groher: Department of Audiology and Speech Pathology, James A. Haley Veteren's Hospital, Tampa, Florida 33612.

K. M. Yorkston: Department of Rehabilitation Medicine, University of Washington, Seattle, Washington 98108-6490.

T. S. Rees: Department of Otolaryngology—Head and Neck Surgery, University of Washington, Seattle, Washington 98108; and Department of Audiology, Harborview Medical Center, Seattle, Washington 98104.

J. B. Palmer: Departments of Physical Medicine and Rehabilitation and Otolaryngology, Johns Hopkins University, and Good Samaritan Hospital, Baltimore, Maryand 21218.

NORMAL PROCESSES

The process of human speech is accomplished through the systems of cerebration, respiration, phonation, and articulation. Neural organization by the brain programs and sequences the physical processes. The resonating cavities of the pharynx, mouth, and nose influence the acoustic product.

Respiration

Two forms of respiration are recognized: chemical and mechanical. Chemical respiration is concerned with the exchange of oxygen and carbon dioxide to and from the blood, whereas mechanical respiration is concerned with the movement of tidal air in and out of the lungs. The expiration of air through the vocal mechanism, the larynx, is the power plant for audible speech. Inhalation is an active process that is accomplished by the contraction of the diaphragm, which increases the vertical diameter of the thorax. The decrease in pressure within the thoracic cavity allows air to flow into the lungs. Other notable muscles of inhalation are the costal elevators, serratus muscles, and certain muscles of the neck and back that elevate the ribs.

Unlike inhalation, exhalation is more passive. Tissue elasticity and gravity contribute to this act as the diaphragm returns to its relaxed position. The abdominal and intercostal muscles can provide force to exhalation or help to control prolonged exhalation for speech.

Phonation

Energy, in the form of exhaled air, passes from the lungs into the subglottic region where the vocal cords are capable of modifying the air stream. Complete closure can result in a Valsalva effect, whereas close approximation increases subglottic pressure and creates a vibratory separation–apposition cycle that results in audible sound energy or voice production. Vocal intensity is increased by raising the level of subglottic pressure. Higher pitch is achieved primarily by increasing the length and tension of the vocal cords and by increasing subglottic air pressure and elevating the larynx. A normal voice is therefore the product of a controlled exhalation of air, steady maintenance of subglottic air pressures, and delicately balanced vocal cords capable of producing regular air pulsations.

Resonation

The raw vocal tone is modified and amplified by resonance within the pharyngeal, oral, and nasal cavities, which are referred to collectively as the vocal tract. The shape of the vocal tract is altered by changing the tension of the pharyngeal walls, by raising or depressing the larynx, by modifying the position of the jaw, tongue, and lips, and by occluding or lowering the soft palate. The innumerable configurations of the shape of the vocal tract provide the human voice with a tremendous variety of potential qualities.

Articulation

The physical event that lends meaning to the resonating voice is articulation. The coordinated action of the tongue, lips, jaw, and soft palate produces the meaningful sounds of speech called phonemes. These structures may shape the vocal tract to produce vowels or voiced consonants, or they may relax, compress, or momentarily stop the air stream as it passes through the oral cavity to produce unvoiced consonants.

Cerebration

Thought transformed into symbols and communicated by speech, writing, or gestural sign is considered language. A broad area of associational cortex in the left hemisphere of the brain is responsible for converting thoughts into symbols and then into words or language. The words are organized into a meaningful arrangement using rules of grammar and are eventually transmitted either through the physical efforts previously described for speech or by gesture or writing. The brain, more specifically the left frontal cortex, is responsible for organizing and patterning the muscle actions of respiration, phonation, and articulation to produce recognizable speech.

COMMUNICATION PATHOLOGY

A pathologic condition that affects any organ involved in the process of speech or language influences the final product *en masse.* At times the pathologic condition is limited to a single speech or language organ, and the dysfunction can be detected in only one component of the process (e.g., an isolated voice or articulation impairment). More commonly, however, the pathologic condition of a single organ influences other elements of the communication process in ways that are predictable, considering the integrated nature of speech and language. For example, severe obstructive pulmonary disease does not just impair the respiratory support for speech but results in alterations in vocal pitch, vocal intensity, and phrasing modifications through compensations for an impaired ability to sustain air flow. Certain disease states, involving organs that are not directly involved in speech or language, can affect the final communication product in a more diffuse manner. Some endocrine disorders, such as hypothyroidism, can influence voice quality as an isolated component of speech and also lead to language confusion and impaired memory. Because of the complexity and interactive nature of the speech and language processes, whenever one evaluates or treats a patient with a communication disorder, some considerations must be given to overall human physiology as well as to the dynamic speech and language systems.

Dysarthria

Definitions and Differential Diagnosis

The dysarthrias are a group of motor speech disorders characterized by slow, weak, imprecise, or uncoordinated movements of speech musculature. Rather than a single neurologic disorder, the dysarthrias vary along a number of dimensions. The neuroanatomic site of lesion can be either the central or peripheral nervous system or both, including the cerebrum, cerebellum, brainstem, and cranial nerves. One or a combination of pathophysiological processes may be involved, including spasticity, flaccidity, ataxia, tremor, rigidity, and chorea (1). A number of diagnoses may be associated with dysarthria, including cerebral palsy, parkinsonism, multiple sclerosis, amyotrophic lateral sclerosis, brainstem stroke, bilateral cortical strokes, and traumatic brain injury. All or several speech subsystems may be involved to varying degrees, including the respiratory, phonatory, velopharyngeal, and oral articulatory subsystems.

As a first step, differential diagnosis involves distinguishing the dysarthrias from other neurogenic communication disorders. The dysarthrias are distinct from aphasia in that language function (i.e., word retrieval, comprehension of both verbal and written language) is preserved in dysarthria but impaired in aphasia. Although both apraxia and dysarthria are considered motor speech disorders, they can be distinguished on the basis of several clinical features. In apraxia, automatic (i.e., nonspeech) movements are intact, whereas in dysarthria they are not. Highly consistent articulatory errors are characteristic of dysarthria, whereas inconsistent errors are a hallmark of apraxia. Finally, in most dysarthrias, all speech subsystems, including respiration and phonation, are involved; in apraxia, respiratory or phonatory involvement is rare. It should be recognized that patients

TABLE 12-1. *Summary of the etiologies, neuropathologies, and neuromuscular deficits characteristic of the common dysarthrias*

Type	Example	Location of neuropathology	Neuromuscular deficit
Flaccid	Bulbar palsy	Lower motor neuron	Muscular weakness; hypotonia
Spastic	Pseudobulbar palsy	Upper motor neuron	Reduced range, force, speed; hypertonia
Ataxic	Cerebellar ataxia	Cerebellum (or tracts)	Hypotnia; reduced speed; inaccurate range, timing, direction
Hypokinetic	Parkinsonism	Extrapyramidal system	Markedly reduced range; variable speed of repetitive movements; movement arrests; rigidity
Hyperkinetic			
Quick	Chorea Myclonus Gilles de la Tourette syndrome	Extrapyramidal system	Quick, unsustained, random, involuntary movements
Slow	Athetosis Dyskinesias Dystonia	Extrapyramidal system	Sustained, distorted movements and postures; slowness; variable hypertonus
Tremors	Organic voice tremor	Extrapyramidal system	Involuntary, rhythmic, purposeless, oscillatory movements
Mixed	Amyotrophic lateral sclerosis Multiple sclerosis Wilson disease	Multiple motor systems	Muscular weakness, limited range and speed

Adapted from Rosenbek JC, LaPointe LL. The dysarthrias: description, diagnosis and treatment. In: Johns DF, ed. *Clinical management of neurogenic communication disorders.* Austin, TX: ProEd, 1985; 97–152.

can have elements of both dysarthria and apraxia, particularly those with bilateral brain damage.

Differential diagnosis among the dysarthrias is an area that has received more systematic attention than any other aspect of the disorder. Information related to the various dysarthrias is summarized in Table 12-1 (2). In studies carried out at the Mayo Clinic, the perceptual features of the speech of seven groups of dysarthric patients were examined (3,4). These groups contained patients who were unequivocally diagnosed as having one of the following conditions: pseudobulbar palsy, bulbar palsy, amyotrophic lateral sclerosis, cerebellar lesions, parkinsonism, dystonia, and choreoathetosis. Speech samples were rated along 38 dimensions, which described pitch characteristics, loudness, vocal quality, respiration, prosody, articulation, and general impression dimensions. Results of this study indicated that each of the seven neurologic disorders could be characterized by a unique set of clusters of deviant speech dimensions and that no two disorders had the same set of clusters. Thus, differential diagnosis among the dysarthrias can be made in part on the basis that one type of dysarthria sounds different from others. Single features, however, such as imprecise consonants or nasal emission, may not be sufficient to distinguish one type of dysarthria from another. Instead, differential diagnosis is made on the basis of clusters of features reflecting underlying pathophysiology and the examination of the musculature. The following are perceptual descriptions of the unique features of selected types of dysarthria (5).

Pseudobulbar Palsy

Speech is slow and labored, and the articulation is rather consistently imprecise, especially on more complicated groups of consonant sounds. Pitch is low and monotonous. Voice quality is harsh and often strained or strangled.

Bulbar Palsy

Hypernasality is associated with nasal emission of air during speech. Inhalation often is audible and exhalation breathy. Air wastage is manifest by short phrases. Articulation often is imprecise because consonants may be weak through failure to impound sufficient intraoral breath pressure owing to velopharyngeal incompetence, or there may be immobility of tongue and lips due to impairment of the hypoglossal and facial nerves, which prevents normal production of vowels and consonants.

Amyotrophic Lateral Sclerosis

The combined spastic and flaccid dysarthria in this disorder causes progressive deterioration of speech. In an earlier stage, either spastic or flaccid speech and nonspeech signs predominate; in an advanced stage, both sets of features described above are present. Slow rate, low pitch, hoarse and strained–strangled quality, highly defective articulation, marked hypernasality, and nasal emission combine to make the speaker struggle to produce short, barely intelligible phrases.

Parkinsonism

In hypokinetic dysarthria, vocal emphasis, peaks and valleys of pitch, and variations of loudness are flattened, resulting in monotony. Short rushes of speech are separated by illogically placed pauses, the rate being variable and often accelerated. Consonant articulation in contextual speech and syllable repetition is blurred as muscles fail to go through their complete excursion. Difficulty initiating articulation is shown by repetition of initial sounds and inappropriate silences. The voice often is breathy, and loudness is reduced, at times to inaudibility.

Dystonia

Involuntary body and facial movements cause unpredictable voice stoppages, disintegration of articulation, excessive variations of loudness, and distortion of vowels. Perhaps in anticipation of these interruptions, normal prosody is altered by slowing of rate, reduction in variations of pitch and loudness, prolongation of interword intervals, and interposition of inappropriate silences.

Choreoathetosis

The involuntary movements that alter the normal breathing cycle result in sudden exhalatory gusts of breath, bursts of loudness, elevations of pitch, and disintegration of articulation. The overall loudness level may be increased. Anticipated breakdowns are managed by varying the rate, introducing and prolonging pauses, and equalizing stress on all syllables and words.

Assessment

The model of chronic disease has been applied to the area of dysarthria (6,7). Impairment refers to "any loss or abnormality of psychological, physiological, or anatomical structure or function." Functional limitation, on the other hand, refers to "any restriction or lack (resulting from impairment) of the ability to perform any activity in the manner or within the range considered normal for the human being."

In a dysarthric speaker, the impairment would include the movement deficits seen in the respiratory, phonatory, velopharyngeal, and oral articulatory subsystems. The functional limitation resulting from the motor speech impairment is characterized by reduced speech intelligibility, rate, and naturalness. In the assessment of a dysarthric speaker, both the impairment and the functional limitation must be considered (8).

Assessing the Impairment

During the assessment of the impairment, focus is placed on the speech production process. The clinician seeks to understand how the weakness, slowness, discoordination, or abnormal tone of the speech musculature has influenced points or places along the speech mechanism, including respiratory, phonatory, velopharyngeal, or oral articulatory subsystems (9). A number of perceptual or instrumental tools are available for measuring speech performance (10,11). The perceptual tools are those that rely on the trained eyes and ears of the clinician, whereas instrumental approaches to assessment include devices that provide information about the acoustic, aerodynamic movement, or myoelectric aspects of speech. Before we proceed with a more detailed description of the assessment of the various speech subsystems, a word of caution is warranted. Viewing speech as a series of isolated points or components would seriously oversimplify a complex process. In dysarthria, the impairment almost never is restricted to a single dimension. Rather, impairments of varying levels of severity may occur at numerous points, all of which are interdependent. For example, consider the function of the muscles and structures of respiration as a pump to provide breath support for speech. The adequacy of respiratory support may be influenced by the efficiency of all the "upstream" valves. For example, inadequate laryngeal, velopharyngeal, or oral articulatory valving interacts with poor respiratory support to create a cumulative negative effect.

Assessment of the respiratory subsystem begins with perceptual measures, including ratings of the number of words produced per breath and the loudness of samples of connected speech or visual observations of the presence of clavicular breathing. Instrumental approaches to the measurement of respiratory function may include acoustic measures of vocal intensity and utterance durations. Aerodynamically, respiratory performance may be assessed by estimating the subglottal air pressure generated by the speaker (12,13). Respiratory inductive plethysmography, commercially available as the Respitrace, is an instrumental means of obtaining information about the movements of the rib cage and abdomen during breathing and speech.

Assessment of the phonatory or laryngeal subsystem typically begins with perceptual ratings of pitch characteristics (e.g., pitch level, pitch breaks, monopitch, voice tremor), loudness (e.g., monoloudness, excess loudness, variation of volume), and voice quality (e.g., harsh voice, hoarseness, wet voice, breathiness, strained–strangled voice). Acoustically, vocal fundamental frequency and intensity can be measured in the clinical setting (14,15). Aerodynamically, measures of laryngeal resistance can be obtained (16).

Assessment of the velopharyngeal mechanism can be made with perceptual judgments of hypernasality or occurrence of nasal air emission. Nasalization also can be measured acoustically. Precise inferences can be made about the timing of velopharyngeal closure by obtaining simultaneous aerodynamic measures of air pressure and air flow during selected speech samples (17,18). Movement of the velopharyngeal mechanism can be observed through cineradiographic techniques.

Assessment of oral articulation can be made perceptually by rating consonant and vowel precision. Although movements also can be inferred using cineradiographic technique and myoelectric activity with electromyographic recordings, these techniques are not used in routine clinical practice.

Assessing the Functional Limitation

The overall speech disability observed in dysarthric speakers may be characterized by abnormalities in speech intelligibility, rate, and naturalness. Of these measures of disability, intelligibility has received the most attention in the clinical literature for a number of reasons. First, measures of speech intelligibility, when accompanied by measures of speaking rate, provide a useful index of the severity of the disorder. Second, reduced speech intelligibility and speaking rate is a nearly universal characteristic of dysarthria, regardless of the underlying neuromotor impairment (19). Finally, intelligibility appears to be closely related to other aspects of the impairment, including measures of information conveyed (20), movement rates, sounds produced recognizably, and judgments of speech disability (21,22).

Despite the importance of intelligibility, care must be taken in clinically measuring this aspect of dysarthria (23). Research literature contains numerous examples of how intelligibility scores can be changed depending on the speakers' task, the transmission system, and the judges' task (19,24). Standard tools are available for measuring sentence and single-word intelligibility and speaking rate using reading or imitation tasks (19). These measures are used clinically as an index of severity of the disability to monitor change over time, and as a measure of the effectiveness of specific intervention techniques such as rate control or palatal lift fitting.

Treatment Considerations

Decisions about the management of dysarthric speakers are twofold. The first level involves the most general decisions about goals of treatment, and the second involves the selection of specific treatment approaches to achieve those goals. General goals of treatment vary with the severity of the disability and with the natural course of the disorder (8).

For severely involved speakers, whose intelligibility is so poor that they are unable to communicate verbally in some or all situations, the general goal of treatment involves establishing a functional means of communication using augmentative approaches. The term "communication augmentation" refers to any device designed to augment, supplement, or replace verbal communication for someone who is not an independent verbal communicator. Systems range from communication boards and books to computer-based speech synthesis systems (25–27). The selection of an appropriate augmentation system necessitates a thorough evaluation of the person's communication needs. These needs may vary considerably; some people need a system for survival communication, whereas others manage basic communication well but need assistance in education or vocational communication. Concurrent with the needs assessment, physical and cognitive capabilities are assessed. This assessment tests cognition, language, memory, physical control, vision, and hearing. Because of the person's limited response options, these tests must be carefully selected or modified for the individual. Once the capabilities have been ascertained, system components can be selected, and an appropriate system developed.

For those moderately involved speakers who are able to use speech as their sole means of communication but who are not completely intelligible, the general goal of treatment involves maximizing intelligibility. The term "compensated intelligibility" aptly describes the goal of this phase of intervention (1). Achieving compensated intelligibility may take a variety of forms depending on the speaker and the nature of the underlying impairment. For some severely dysarthric people, use of an alphabet supplementation system, in which they point to the first letter of each word as they say the word, assists in the transition to intelligible speech (26). For other dysarthric people, treatment involves an attempt to decrease the impairment by exercises that will improve performance on selected aspects of speech production. For example, exercises may involve developing more adequate respiratory support for speech (28). For still others, treatment may include training to establish an appropriate speech rate (29). It also may involve prosthetically managing a severely impaired velopharyngeal mechanism through the use of a palatal lift (30,31), which is a dental retainer with a shelf attached to elevate the soft palate to the height necessary to reduce hypernasality and nasal air emission. An appropriately fitted palatal lift will allow certain dysarthric speakers to better produce speech sounds that require the buildup of oral air pressure, such as \p\, \t\, and \d\. In other cases, maximizing intelligibility involves teaching dysarthric speakers to emphasize speech sounds in the final position of words, to control the number of words per breath, and to stress important words in a sentence.

For the mildly involved dysarthric speaker whose speech is characterized as intelligible but less efficient and less natural than normal, treatment planning must first determine whether there is a handicap. For some speakers, these mild reductions in speech efficiency pose no problems. For other mildly involved speakers, however, treatment is warranted. The general goals of treatment for dysarthric people with mild disabilities include maximizing communication efficiency while maintaining intelligibility and maximizing speech naturalness. Maximizing naturalness is accomplished by teaching appropriate phrasing, stressing patterning, and intonation (32).

Treatment approaches for patients with progressive disorders such as parkinsonism, multiple sclerosis, and amyotrophic lateral sclerosis are different from those used with the recovering dysarthric speaker (33). Initially, the patients are encouraged to maximize the functional communication level by paying specific attention to the clarity and precision of their speech. At some point, the patients will need to modify their speaking patterns by controlling rate and consonant emphasis and reducing the number of words per breath. Some patients with progressive dysarthria make the adjustments in their speech pattern without specific treatment; others may need to practice these modifications with a speech pathologist or trained family member until the changes become habitual. In severe cases, a communication augmentation system may be considered. These systems usually are chosen or designed to accommodate the life style of the patient while serving his or her communication needs over the longest period of time.

Laryngectomee Rehabilitation

Cancer of the larynx may be treated by a single treatment modality or a combination of modalities. Surgery, irradiation, and chemotherapy all are used to treat this condition, and the decision may be made on the basis of the extent of the tumor, the presence of diseased lymph nodes, and the general health of the patient, including vitality of specific organs and physiological systems. There are several surgical options. In general terms, some tumors that are limited to the region above the glottis may be treated by supraglottic laryngectomy, lesions lateralized to one side may be treated with hemilaryngectomy, and tumors that involve the glottic area with one mobile arytenoid may be dealt with by a subtotal laryngectomy. In each of these conservation operations, the patient's laryngeal tumor is removed, yet voice is maintained. Postoperative rehabilitation usually centers more on training compensations for swallowing than voice restoration.

Total laryngectomy remains a common procedure for the treatment of laryngeal cancer. In addition to the obvious need for speech rehabilitation, these patients require education for tracheostoma care and adjustment to tracheostoma breathing. For example, the patient must adjust to the relatively dry air entering the lungs without benefit of mucosal humidification from the nose, mouth, and pharynx. Humidifiers and moist stomal covers often are required to prevent crusting and the formation of mucus plugs, especially in the first few postoperative months. Shower bibs, neck wear, and stoma filters may be obtained to assist the patient in adjusting to neck breathing and the changes in appearance.

Speech Options

There are several options available to patients for speaking. External prosthetic devices, specifically electrolarynxes and pneumatic external reeds, offer most patients an opportunity to speak within days after surgery. A tracheal–esophageal puncture (TEP) with insertion of a small one-way valved prosthesis enables some laryngectomees to produce an esophageal vibratory voice. A third option, which is effective for a small percentage of patients, is learned esophageal speech.

Electrolarynx

Commercially available electrolarynxes are designed to introduce vibratory sound either directly into the oral cavity through a catheter or indirectly through the neck tissues. In each case, the tone resonates within the oral and pharyngeal cavities and is modified by the dynamic process of articulation to form audible, intelligible words. Often, an intraoral electrolarynx can be used within 2 or 3 days after surgery and provides the patient with a means of communication. Speech therapy that is begun early can prevent the problem of trismus that is so common in head and neck surgical patients who do not use their jaw muscles in speech or mastication for almost 2 weeks after surgery. Intraoral devices can be used long term for patients with necks that are unsuitable for sound transmission, usually because of pain, edema, or scar tissue. Experience suggests that good speech is slower to develop using an intraoral device; therefore, care must be taken to help the patient avoid early frustration associated with not being understood immediately. Although most electrolarynxes designed for neck placement easily can be converted for intraoral use, they are intended to transmit the vibration through the submandibular or neck tissue into the oral and pharyngeal cavities. Patients usually can begin to use the neck-held instruments when they are allowed to take nutrition by mouth. In patients with a suitable neck, intelligible speech can be achieved after one or two practice sessions.

Pneumatic Reeds

Another type of external voice prosthesis is the pneumatic reed. This device is placed over the tracheostoma to allow exhaled air to pass across a reed to produce a tone that is carried into the mouth, much like an intraoral electrolarynx. Although these devices are inexpensive and capable of producing a pleasant quality of voice, they are somewhat cumbersome and conspicuous to use and have not gained wide popularity.

Tracheal–Esophageal Puncture

Tracheal–esophageal puncture procedures have been used since 1980 as a relatively simple means of voice restoration (34). The TEP can be performed either as a primary procedure at laryngectomy (35) or almost any time during the postoperative period. A small one-way valved voice prosthesis is inserted through the TEP (Fig. 12-1) to allow the patient to shunt pulmonary air into the esophagus without having esophageal contents enter the TEP. Air passing through the prosthesis and up the esophagus vibrates the pharyngoesophageal segment to produce an esophageal voice. The prosthesis is not the source of the voice, but the speech outcome depends on the size and the design of the prosthesis chosen for the patient. Prostheses may be chosen which require weekly cleaning and replacement or indwelling devices that remain in place for five to eight months (36). Early speech success following TEP and voice prosthesis fitting has been reported at almost 90% (37,38). Reports of long-term success are between 93% for patients given primary TEP and 83% for those given secondary pro-

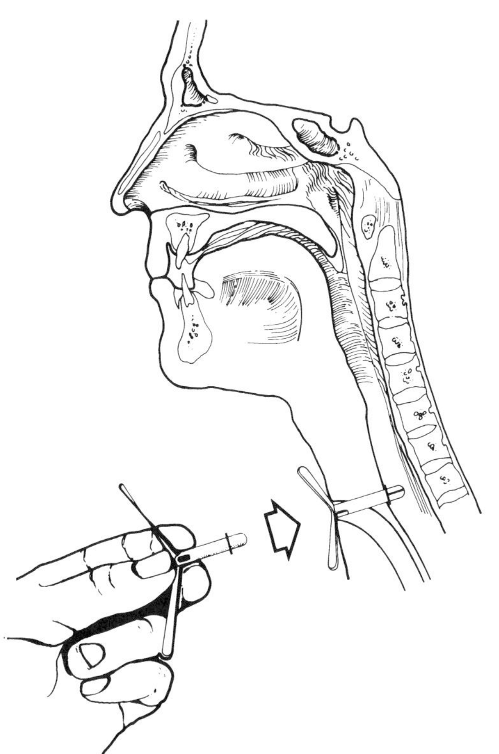

FIG. 12-1. A one-way valved voice prosthesis can be placed in a surgically created tracheal–esophageal fistula to allow pulmonary air to be shunted into the esophagus for esophageal voice production.

cedures (39). Success largely depends on patient selection, and in some cases success can be enhanced by surgical techniques such as pharyngeal plexus neurectomy or cricopharyngeal myotomy performed to prevent a pharyngoesophageal segment spasm (40). Other factors to consider in patient selection are motivation, intellect, dexterity, eyesight, stoma size and sensitivity, hand hygiene, surgical risk, and cost.

Esophageal Speech

Esophageal speech is accomplished by training the patient to move air from the oral and pharyngeal cavities into the esophagus by injection or suction methods, to hold the air in this esophageal reservoir, and then to release it in a controlled manner through the pharyngoesophageal segment. This method of voice production uses the same anatomic vibratory site as the TEP technique but is accomplished without the necessity of occluding the tracheostoma. Because the volume of air maintained in the esophagus is much less than the pulmonary capacity used by the TEP speaker, the reservoir must be replenished constantly. Accomplished esophageal speakers can speak clearly and effortlessly; however, many laryngectomy patients are unable to learn this technique. Failure may represent insufficient or excessive pharyngoesophageal segment tone, scarring, nerve damage, or learning disorders.

LANGUAGE DISTURBANCE

An understanding of the mechanisms responsible for the processing and formulation of language is critical to good rehabilitation practice. Success in rehabilitation depends on a patient learning a new skill. Learning this new skill depends on how well the clinician and patient communicate. The success of this interaction is crucial to the speed, efficiency, and retention of newly learned behavioral patterns. Loss or disruption of available learning (i.e., communication) input and output modalities can impede this process unless compensations are made. The necessary compensations are achieved with an understanding of how to assess the patient's language strengths and weaknesses and how these modalities compare with nonlanguage learning modalities. A description of the learning strengths and limitations of patients with those language disorders frequently associated with cortical and subcortical disease, both focal and diffuse, is presented in this section.

Aphasia

Aphasia is a disorder of both the expression and reception of propositional language secondary to cortical or subcortical disease, usually in the left hemisphere. It interferes with the ability to manipulate the meaning (i.e., semantics) or order (i.e., syntax) of words and gestures. There are three important points to emphasize in this definition.

First, the term aphasia implies impairment in both receptive and expressive language modalities. Expression may be more severely involved than reception, whereas reception appears grossly intact. If the testing instrument is sensitive to subtle change in language behavior, however, pathology can be identified in the more intact modality. Second, aphasia, by itself, is consistent only with focal disease, usually of the left hemisphere. Aphasic symptoms may be part of a diffuse pathologic condition; however, these patients evidence more than disruptions in their ability to manipulate linguistic symbols, such as disorientation. Prognosis and recovery for this group is markedly different from those who evidence aphasia alone. And finally, although it is well known that aphasic disturbances primarily are a consequence of cortical disease, identification and classification of more atypical aphasic syndromes are associated now with subcortical infarction and hemorrhage (41).

Language Characteristics

Comprehension impairment of spoken language includes deficits of auditory perception and auditory retention. Auditory misperceptions are characterized by a tendency to confuse words that are similar in either meaning or sound. These confusions create a distorted message resulting in errors of comprehension. Most aphasics will experience more errors in comprehension as the length of the auditory input increases. In general, the speed of auditory input, combined with increased length, leads to errors in auditory retention. In addition, increased sentence length often presupposes a more difficult syntax and vocabulary, combining to make comprehension more liable to error. It has been demonstrated that some aphasics retain more information from the beginning of an utterance, whereas others retain information from the end (42). Evaluation of this aspect of the patient's auditory capacity is especially important if rehabilitation is to succeed. Comprehension of graphic material (i.e., reading) also is impaired. The severity of this impairment often is greater than that of the linguistic deficits in other modalities.

Expressively, patients might evidence anomia, agrammatism, paragrammatism, or paraphasias, or they may produce jargon, stereotypic, or echolalic language patterns. Although most aphasics display an overall reduction in word classes available for production, they show particular deficits in the retrieval of nouns (i.e., anomia). Because nouns carry a large part of the meaning during an intended message, the language of the anomic patient is described as ''empty'' because sentences often lack a subject or referent. In their attempts to retrieve words, aphasics make ''paraphasic'' language errors. When the substitution for the intended word is from the same word class, such as ''chair'' for ''table,'' it is a semantic paraphasia. The substitution of like sounds or syllables, such as ''flair'' for ''chair'' is classified as a phonemic paraphasia. A final class of paraphasic error is the neologism. These productions are words that are attempts at the target but bear no phonemic or semantic relationship to that target, such as ''I want to brush my ploker.'' Patients who find word retrieval difficult but who do not produce paraphasic language errors in their search for the intended word often circumlocute or talk around the intended noun, such as saying ''I wear it on my wrist'' instead of ''watch.''

Agrammatism is a form of expressive deficit characterized by reliance on nouns and verbs (i.e., content words) to the exclusion of articles, verb auxiliaries, pronouns, and prepositions (i.e., function words). Agrammatic productions often are described as telegraphic. Paragrammatic language is characterized by a misuse, rather than an omission, of grammatical elements.

Patients whose expressive output is largely incomprehensible, even though the utterance is well articulated and excessive (i.e., press for speech), display a form of expressive deficit called jargon. Concentrations of neologisms are called neologistic jargon and may be associated with stereotypes such as ''blam, blam, blam'' substituted for all attempts at verbalization. A preponderance of unrelated semantic paraphasias is semantic jargon. Finally, some patients evidence echolalia, typified by the patient echoing in response the same utterance he or she has just heard.

Expressive graphic output usually is impaired in aphasia, as is the ability to use gestures as a substitute form of expression (43). A summary of the terminology used to describe expressive language deficits in aphasia is presented in Table 12-2.

TABLE 12-2. *Summary of the terminology used to describe expressive disorders of aphasia*

Term	Definition
Agrammatism	The absence of recognized grammatical elements during speech attempts
Anomia	Difficulty producing nouns
Circumlocution	Attempts at word retrieval end in descriptions or associations related to the word
Echolalia	An accurate repetition of a preceding utterance when repetition is not required
Empty speech	A fluent utterance that lacks substantive parts of language, such as nouns and verbs
Jargon	Mostly incomprehensible, but well-articulated language
Neologistic jargon	Mostly incomprehensible, some words are partially recognizable, others are contrived or "new"
Paragrammatism	Misuse of grammatical elements, usually during fluent utterances
Phonemic paraphasia	"Flair" for "chair," also called literal paraphasia
Press for speech	Excessively lengthy, often incomprehensible, well-articulated language
Semantic jargon	A combination of unrelated semantic and phonemic paraphasia, together with recognizable words
Semantic paraphasia	"Table" for "chair," also called nominal paraphasia
Stereotypes	Nonsensical repetition of similar syllables for all communicative attempts, such as "dee, dee, dee"
Telegraphic speech	Language similar to a telegram, mostly nouns and verbs

Classification of Aphasic Syndromes

Historically, there have been many attempts to place pathologic language symptoms into homogeneous groups permitting reference to specific aphasic subtypes. The Boston classification system standardizes terminology beginning with a broad classification of disorders into those in which expressive skills are predominantly fluent and those in which they are predominantly nonfluent (44). Although such a distinction might be useful clinically, it often can be difficult to make, as in the case of a conduction aphasic (i.e., fluent aphasia) who may have long pauses and expressive struggle (i.e., nonfluency) during speech. The eight major types of aphasia in the Boston system are the more common forms of Broca aphasia and Wernicke aphasia, anomia, conduction, and global and the less frequent transcortical types (Table 12-3). Each of these syndromes is correlated with a specific localized cortical lesion, some with subcortical extension.

Improvements in brain imaging have made it possible to

TABLE 12-3. *Summary of the Boston classification system of aphasia*

Type	Language characteristics
Nonfluent	
Broca	Telegraphic, agrammatic expression often associated with apraxia; good comprehension except on more abstract tasks
Transcortical motor	Limited language output; fair naming; intact repetition; fair comprehension
Global	Severe expressive and receptive reduction in language
Mixed transcortical	Severe reduction in expression and reception; repetition intact
Fluent	
Anomia	Word-finding difficulty without other serious linguistic deficits
Conduction	Phonemic paraphasic errors; good comprehension; fluency in bursts; deficits in repetition of low probability phrases
Wernicke	Phonemic and semantic paraphasias; poor comprehension
Transcortical sensory	Fluent neologistic language; poor comprehension; intact repetition

correlate disturbances in language with lesions in the corpus striatum and thalamus. The data are still incomplete, but most of the syndromes described differ from those associated with confirmed cortical disease. Although some characteristics show patterns consistent with site, not every investigator describes the same speech and language deficits from identical lesions.

Preliminary evidence suggests that the speech and language disorders are confined to left hemispheric subcortical structures (45). There is suggestion that the causative factor, infarct versus hemorrhage, at the same site may produce differential effects. Lesion size also may be important. Lesions involving the putamen and caudate with anterosuperior extension into the capsule reportedly have produced more dysarthric (i.e., reduced vocal volume) and labored speech (46,47). Grammar and comprehension were unaffected. Paraphasia and poor comprehension were associated most with a posterior extension of the lesion. A combination of anterior and posterior capsular lesions resulted in global aphasia. Patients with anterior capsular lesions have been found to have articulation disturbances consistent with buccofacial apraxia plus disturbances of comprehension (48).

Linguistic deficits secondary to thalamic hemorrhage also have been reported (49,50). A great deal of variation is observed in language performance, with some patients having almost normal language performance and others demonstrating marked paraphasia and periods of fluctuating unconsciousness (50). These fluctuations may be related more to the role of the thalamus in arousal and selective attention as prerequisites to communication than to actual deficits of language (49).

Although most studies confirm the notion that the symptoms associated with subcortical disease may be transitory, patients seen in our clinic who evidence attentional and arousal deficits beyond the acute stage of illness have not been able to learn compensations for their communication failures in spite of comprehension skills that approach normality.

Differentiation from Other Disorders

Aphasia, particularly in the acute stages, may be difficult to differentiate from other disorders that compromise communication. Accurate differentiation is necessary because each communication disorder requires separate treatment and management approaches. It should be noted that aphasia may occur in conjunction with other syndromes. A comparison of linguistic and nonlinguistic behaviors among disorders that commonly interfere with communication is provided in Table 12-4.

Agnosia

Agnosia is the inability to interpret or recognize information when the end organ is intact. For example, a patient with auditory agnosia would have normal hearing thresholds but cannot interpret speech signals at the cortical level; hence, auditory comprehension will be severely compromised. Patients with agnosia can be differentiated from those with aphasia because they will be impaired in only one modality—the patient with auditory agnosia who has severe comprehension deficits will be able to read the same words through the intact visual modality.

Apraxia

In its pure form, oral apraxia is the motor counterpart of agnosia. Lesions in the premotor cortex are a frequent finding (51). Apraxia of speech is characterized by labored and dysprosodic productions resulting in errors of omission, substitution, and repetition. There is debate as to whether apraxia is a pure motor or linguistic (i.e., phonemic) disturbance (43,52,53). Patients have difficulty programming the positioning of the speech musculature and sequencing the movements necessary for speech. Apraxia occurs in the absence of significant weakness and incoordination of muscles, with automatic and reflexive movements undisturbed. It is seen by some as a distinct condition that often coexists and complicates aphasia, whereas others regard the characteristics as part of the nonfluent Broca aphasia. Apraxia of speech carries a negative prognosis for recovery if there is a moderate to severe aphasia in tandem. When it occurs without the concomitant language disturbance, therapy can focus on retraining the patients's ability to program sound patterns,

TABLE 12-4. *Aphasia differentiated from other cortical and subcortical speech and language disorders*

Characteristic	Agnosia	Aphasia	Apraxia	Confusion	Dementia	Dysarthria	Subcortical aphasia
Auditory comprension	+/−	+/−	+	+/−	+/−	+/−	+/−
Auditory memory	+	+/−	+	−	−	+	+/−
Visual memory	+	+	+	−	−	+	+/−
Naming	+	+/−	+	+/−	−	+	+/−
Reading/writing	+/−	−	+	−	−	+	+/−
Generalized cognitive deficits	+	+	+	−	−	+	+/−
Inappropriate behaviors	+	+	+	−	−	+	+/−
Disturbance of attention	+	+	+	−	−	+	−
Learn well	+	+	+	+/−	−	+	+/−
Disorder confined to one input/output modality	−	+	−	+	+/−	+	+
Regular errors of speech output	+	+	+	+	+	−	+/−
Irregular errors of speech output	+	+	−	+	+	+	+/−

In acute stages: +, usually unimpaired; −, usually impaired; +/−, patient dependent.

to shift from one sound to another, and to use preserved melodic and rhythmic patterns to facilitate speech.

Dementia

Dementia is a syndrome of progressive cognitive deterioration that adversely affects the ability to communicate (54). Although specific expressive and receptive language disturbances can present as part of a dementing process, the aphasic patient may not evidence cognitive deficits in such areas as orientation, judgment, self-care, and visual-perceptual skills. The distinction between those patients with language deficits secondary to aphasia and those with diffuse disease is particularly relevant in rehabilitation because the prognosis for retraining specific skills and developing independence is more favorable for the aphasic.

Confusion

Confused language is characterized by reduced recognition, reduced understanding of and responsiveness to the environment, faulty memory, unclear thinking, and disorientation (54). It often is associated with head trauma. It is differentiated, in part, from the language disorders of dementia because the prognosis for recovery after traumatic injury is more favorable and the course is not progressive.

Tests for Aphasia

Tests for aphasia measure the patient's receptive and expressive language capacities by sampling different types of language skills through systematically controlled channels. For example, an examination of the visual input system (i.e., reception) might begin with a concrete task such as copying or matching and proceed to more difficult tasks such as the reading of sentences for comprehension. Tests of expression might range from simple repetition, to naming, to providing definitions. Most test batteries currently in use attempt to provide a representative sample from which inferences can be made about performance in similar linguistic situations. Although most tests of aphasia do sample linguistic competencies, they are not equipped to measure the least and most severe disorders. Therefore, in selected cases, the examination will have to be supplemented by other specialized formal and nonformal measures.

The Minnesota Test for Differential Diagnosis of Aphasia

The Minnesota Test for Differential Diagnosis of Aphasia is the most comprehensive test battery, taking an average of 3 hours to administer (55). The test has 47 subtests and is particularly useful for recognizing and classifying deficits of auditory comprehension. Means and standard deviations are available for each subtest, and patients can be rated from 0 to 6 in each major area of performance (i.e., comprehension, reading, expression, writing). Because of the length of the test, it must be given in multiple sessions. Scoring is cumbersome, and subtest instructions for the examiner are not always clear. Patients can be classified into groups by aphasia type, on which a prognosis for recovery is based.

The Boston Diagnostic Aphasia Examination

The Boston Diagnostic Aphasia Examination (BDAE) provides the examiner with 27 subtests and an additional group of non-language-based subtests as part of a battery to evaluate parietal lobe dysfunction (44). It is particularly valuable as a classification tool because it assesses deficiencies in language consistent with the Boston schema of aphasia classification. The examiner rates the patient's conversational speech and auditory comprehension on a seven-point scale. This scale is used for patient classification and is tied to lesion site. Test scores are summarized by modality and are presented as percentiles compared with a large sample of patients.

The Western Aphasia Battery

The Western Aphasia Battery is a modification and expansion of the BDAE (56). Subtest scores provide the information used in classification. Auditory and expressive modality scores yield an aphasia quotient (AQ) that is calculated taking spontaneous recovery into account. An AQ score below 93 (8) is consistent with aphasia. The patient is assigned a performance quotient (PQ) on the basis of tests of reading, writing, drawing, calculation, block design, and portions of the Raven's Progressive Matrices. A summary of cognitive function combines the PQ and AQ scores. This summary score is useful in assessing patients with cognitive deficits after traumatic injury.

The Porch Index of Communicative Ability

The Porch Index of Communicative Ability contains 18 subtests and uses ten common objects to elicit patient responses (57). Examiners must be trained a minimum of 40 hours and then meet reliability criteria before using the test. The uniqueness of this battery is its 16-point scoring scale. Every response on each subtest is scored from 1 to 16 based on the completeness, accuracy, promptness, responsiveness, and efficiency of the patient's response. Percentile scores by modality can be compared with scores of patients with bilateral and left hemisphere damage. Modality or overall test scores can be used to predict recovery. The test is particularly useful in planning programmed treatment and research. It is not particularly sensitive to patients with mild or severe linguistic deficits because it assesses a narrow range of verbal functions.

The Token Test

The Token Test is designed to detect subtle auditory comprehension disorders and often is administered to patients who reach ceiling levels on standardized aphasia batteries (58). The patient is given 20 tokens with two shapes, two sizes, and five colors and is asked through nonredundant language to manipulate them. The five sections, comprised of 62 total items, increase in difficulty by length and linguistic complexity. Normative data do not come with the test but must be obtained from the literature (59,60). Test interpretation can be difficult because patients can make errors owing to pure linguistic auditory comprehension problems or auditory memory deficits. A more standardized version (i.e., The Revised Token Test) also is available (61). A version in which the examiner moves the tokens and the patient describes what he or she has seen is the Reporter's Test (62).

The Reading Comprehension Battery

The Reading Comprehension Battery comprises ten subtests that are used to assess reading skills in greater detail than most standardized aphasia batteries (63). Subtests include comprehension of morphosyntactic structure, functional reading, synonym recognition, and sentence and paragraph comprehension.

Approaches to Treatment

Aphasia treatment should be patient dependent, maximizing communicative strengths in actual interactive situations. Aphasics, even those with similar types of lesions, represent a heterogeneous group. Because of this, attempts to evalvate outcomes of treatment are often unpredictable. In addition to building on the patient's communicative strengths, remediation should be directed toward helping the patient, family, and friends accept the person's liabilities.

Traditionally, the focus of aphasia remediation has been on the stimulation–facilitation approach, in which the patient and clinician interact within a stimulus–response framework on tasks that are thought to be related to communication (64,65). Although this approach may be most beneficial for the more severely impaired, its relevance in helping the patient solve everyday communicative needs remains questionable. The notion that the clinician's role should be guided toward helping the patient adjust to his or her own particular environment presupposes that family, friends, and employers will receive as much remediation as the patient because they will have to learn how to enhance the patient's communicative competencies. To accomplish this, the speech pathologist must analyze the patient's communicative strengths and weaknesses and then objectify and teach the pragmatics of communication to the language-impaired person and his or her significant others.

In general, patients who evidence diffuse cortical signs in addition to their linguistic deficits, those with unilateral multilobe disease, especially secondary to hemorrhage, and those with a severe reduction of test scores after the first month will not be candidates for direct daily speech and language remediation. Monthly reassessment of these patients with either standardized or nonformal testing instruments is necessary to identify any emerging communicative strengths so that they may be further enhanced with treatment. This reassessment should continue until 6 months after the insult and then in 2-month intervals up to 1 year. Treatment with globally involved patients should focus on their ability to learn a new task in a prescribed amount of time. Such tasks usually do not require a great deal of complex processing, such as matching picture to object, object to object, or word to object. Data should be kept on the patient's accuracy and processing time as measures of change. Learning success provides prognostic information for further daily remediation in using direct approaches to treatment.

Training in communicative interaction must focus on the following:

- Appropriate rates of auditory presentation and the importance of pause times
- Differences between concrete and abstract language

- Use of redundancy to improve comprehension
- Ways to carry the load of a conversation while still involving the patient
- Utilization of contextual cues to comprehend what the patient may be communicating
- Ways to verify messages from the patient
- Ways to combine gesture and oral language to facilitate communication
- Allowing the appropriate amount of time for a patient to formulate a response before restimulation (i.e., questioning or repeating)

The training modules should be divided into four parts: direct work with the patient and clinician, demonstrations of pragmatics with the family, patient–family interactions critiqued by the clinician, and environmental control training.

Environmental controls are similar to environmental language stimulation described by Lubinski (66). The patient's environment should be evaluated to determine how it might be manipulated to enhance communicative skills and compensate for deficits. These manipulations should focus on ways to control for distractions, to provide favorable seating and lighting when possible, to control the number of speakers, to suggest the time of day when the patient's performance is best, to control daily situations so that the patient has a need to communicate, and to provide adequate reinforcement for communication. Other environmental controls that enhance communication because they allow for linguistic predictability include the design of a daily regimented schedule and keeping items in the environment such as chairs, utensils, and food items in familiar places. Although these controls may be needed to maximize communicative effectiveness, patients who react favorably to such controls should have them removed at prescribed times, forcing them to use their language in reaction to less predictable situations. These encounters, if positive, can lead to significant improvement in communication.

Communication Impairment After Right Hemisphere Damage

It is well known that the right hemisphere plays a major role in initiating planned action, making judgments based on visual perception, and remembering information that must be visually coded. In some, neglect or denial of the environment makes these deficits more pronounced and harder to manage. It is easy to overlook these deficits because of the patient's stronger communication skills. Typically, the verbal performance is so strong that the reasons for the poor visual motor skills might be questioned (Fig. 12-2). Evidence suggests that even though the patient with right hemisphere damage may suffer more from visual than linguistic deficits, there is also affective and extraverbal communication impairment.

The right hemisphere's role in affective aspects of communication is continuing to be explored. Affective aspects, such as the lack of facial expression while speaking, failure to maintain eye contact, failure to use gesture, and a lack of vocal inflection, all have been described in the patient with right hemisphere damage (67). Loss of inflectional patterns that signal anger or frustration is not surprising given the role the right hemisphere plays in decoding and recalling melodies. It is important that the clinician recognize the possibility of such a pathologic process because loss of these affective cues often is mistaken for the functional states of rudeness or unconcern for another's feelings.

Additional problems with extraverbal aspects of communication also help explain the ''difficult-to-get-along-with'' personality of the patient with right hemisphere damage. Extraverbal skills include behaviors such as appreciation of humor and figurative language and the use of pragmatics such as the ability to maintain a conversational topic and turn-taking during conversation. These patients have difficulty in organizing information and they fail to make use of contextual cues. Failure to recognize these cues results in many conversational irrelevancies and poor monitoring of rate and amount of expressive language as they stray from, or completely lose, the thread of the conversation. Failure to recognize humor and metaphoric language structures may be translated behaviorally into a noncaring, depressed personality. Problems in interpreting incoming visual and auditory information, long known to be a right hemisphere function, make it difficult for these patients to get the point of discourse, leading to further frustration on the sender's part.

Assessment

Before the Clinical Management of Right Hemisphere Dysfunction (68), no formal assessment tool was available for the systematic evaluation of the communication skills of the patient with right hemisphere damage. The test offers a scoring system for assessment of the use of pragmatics, nonverbal skills such as eye contact and facial gestures, interpretation of metaphoric language, memory skills, writing, visual scanning and tracking, and an analysis of conversation, including topic maintenance, verbosity, and reference. Approaches to treatment based on the analysis are presented.

Informal assessment tools are described by West and colleagues (69). Their battery includes a screening of basic language skills, an analysis of single-word responses to part–whole tasks, oral opposites, written opposites, oral analogies, and printed analogies. Other sections include interpretation of idioms and proverbs, effects of imagery, and evaluation of the patient's ability to appreciate humor.

Treatment

Treatment should concentrate on three broad areas. First, the clinician should use the patient's stronger language capabilities to compensate for poor visuomotor skills. Unable to learn new motor patterns by demonstration, some patients

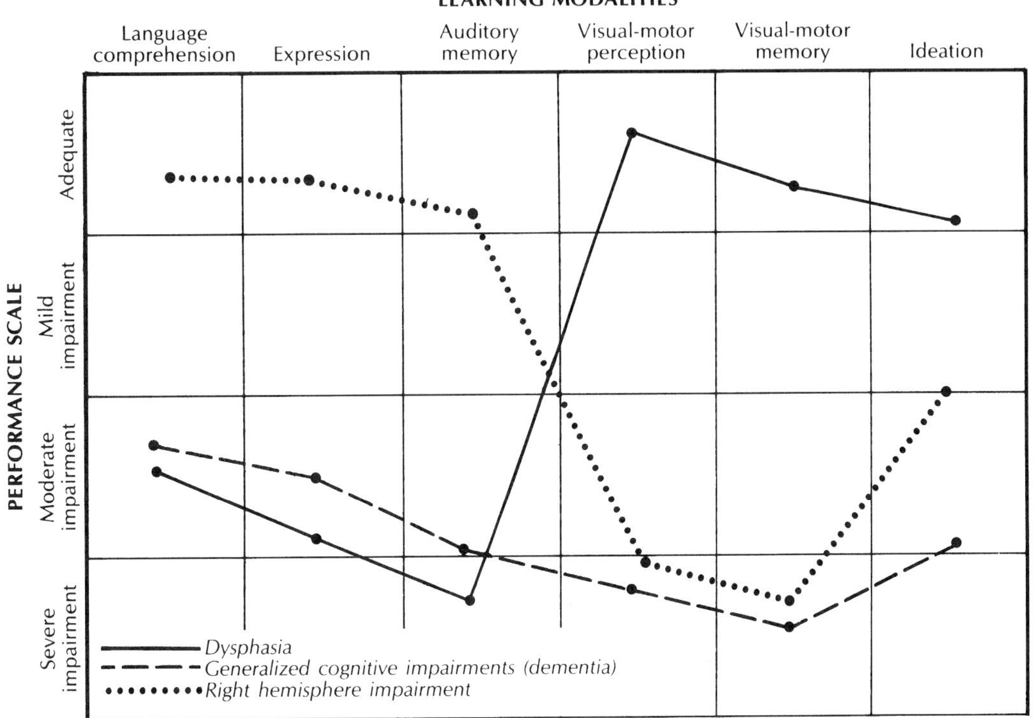

FIG. 12-2. Comparison of learning strengths and weaknesses of patients with right and left hemisphere pathology and dementia. (From DeLisa JA, Miller RM, Melnick RR, Mikulie MA. Stroke rehabilitation. Part I. Cognitive deficits and prediction of outcome. *Am Fam Physician* 1982; xx:208, with permission.)

with right hemisphere damage can be taught through intact auditory or graphic channels. Second, the communication specialist should develop tasks that help the patient attend to contextual cues in an effort to reduce verbosity and improve topic maintenance, retell stories in a fashion that highlights the main points, and produce language that follows a logical sequence. Although these tasks appear related to the impairment, there are no data supporting success or failure using such strategies. Third, counseling the patient's family on how the loss of pragmatic and affective language can affect their perception of the patient's personality must not be underestimated. Rehabilitation successes in other areas will be diminished or lost if the patient's family does not make the adjustment to a new personality and the reasons it is manifest.

Communication Impairment After Traumatic Injury

Patients with language impairment caused by traumatic injury may display a combination of disorientation, aphasia, and memory deficits (70). Acutely, disorders of perception and behavior mask the severity of deficits, and chronically they may interfere with rehabilitation. These patients' specific difficulty with attention and arousal, lack of insight, and failure to self-correct make rehabilitation challenging. The combination of these disturbances has become known as ''generalized deficits of cognition,'' and the treatment offered is thus labeled ''cognitive rehabilitation.'' This designation highlights the importance of recognizing the significance of their diffuse disease manifested by both right (i.e., perceptual) and left (i.e., linguistic) pathologic conditions as well as deficits in memory, problem solving, and other behaviors that depend on bilateral cooperation. In this way, the language of confusion that often is associated with diffuse traumatic brain injury differs from that in aphasia and focal disease.

Typically, these patients are young, and recovery of linguistic deficits as measured by standardized aphasia batteries is good. Higher-level language difficulties not assessed by traditional means may persist, however. Recovery of concrete language skills generally precedes return of orientation and memory independent of length of coma (71). It is difficult to separate communicative recovery from cognitive recovery. The return of communication is hierarchic and occurs in the following order:

1. Prelinguistic skills of internal and external attention
2. Discrimination
3. Seriation
4. Recovery of memory
5. Categorization
6. Association
7. Analysis and synthesis (72)

Specific linguistic deficits in diffuse traumatic brain injury include the following:

- Problems retrieving auditory and visual information
- Anomia
- Decreased auditory comprehension, especially for longer and syntactically more complex utterances
- Reduced reading comprehension
- Difficulty integrating, analyzing, and synthesizing through all modalities

Expressive language in these patients lacks relevance and is marked by verbosity, confabulation, and circumlocution. At 6 months after the insult, many patients are able to make their needs known but continue to have ideational perseverations, incomplete thought content in expression, and poor verbal reasoning capacities. These cognitive deficits were categorized by Hagen and associates based on recovery through eight stages (73). Stage 1 represents patients who are unaware of any external input; stage 4 (i.e., confused-agitated) represents patients who respond primarily to internal confusion with inappropriate verbalizations and confabulation; and stage 8 (i.e., purposeful and appropriate) is reached when the patient can communicate more efficiently by integrating past, present, and future. Social, emotional, and intellectual capabilities remain impaired for more complex language manipulations.

Assessment

Because these patients often show deficits of language, perception, and memory, all of these modalities should be evaluated with available measures. Because linguistic skills recover quickly, most standardized aphasia batteries are insensitive to change after 6 months, and the clinician must develop methods of analyzing expressive and receptive discourse, such as those described by Coelho and colleagues (74). Such measures should include an analysis of relevance, auditory analysis and synthesis, expressive integration, serial discrimination and expression, and problem-solving skills that rely on linguistic processing. There is no test capable of assessing each of these skills, forcing the clinician to rely on subtests from both standard and nonstandardized measures. Most of the available testing resources do not provide normative data for the head-injured population. Therefore, their interpretation is done best by comparing test results with premorbid educational levels and by single-subject performance comparisons on serial testing. Halper and colleagues review those portions of test batteries in use, together with suggestions for which severity level each subtest is most appropriate (75).

Treatment

The traumatically brain injured usually are under 30 years of age, display generalized cognitive deficits, recover language at a fast rate, improve for a longer period of time, and often have a chance to return to the work force (76). These circumstances suggest that treatment strategies for this population may differ from those for patients with impairment from vascular etiologies. Although the patient may benefit from more traditional rehabilitative techniques, especially in the acute stages, he or she will need additional concentration on tasks that improve orientation and memory, help in developing selective attention and discrimination, and eventually must be involved in receptive and expressive language tasks that emphasize analysis and synthesis. Remediation should be directed toward helping the patient retain specific pieces of information gathered from progressively longer utterances. The patient should practice shifting topics without significant delay. Success in job performance and psychosocial adjustment depends on how well the patient can perform on these more abstract linguistic tasks.

Because loss of memory, with its consequences for learning and orientation, is a significant finding in this group, tasks must be designed to compensate for memory deficits. Of critical importance to this is the structuring of the patient's environment so that predictability will reinforce recall and retention. Mnemonic training aids, together with the patient's written or auditory recording of daily events, will help solidify this aspect of rehabilitation.

Disturbances of attention, memory, and nonlanguage problem solving lend themselves to computerized remediation applications. Computer programs are particularly useful in treatment of the head-injured patient because of the computer's ability to control stimuli in a repeatable format, helping to focus attention on selected linguistic parameters. Furthermore, the ease of response makes the computer nonthreatening and reinforcing. There are a number of computer-based programs that highlight the skills important in cognitive training. Some, like those designed by Hartley Courseware, focus on aspects of vigilance and attention needed as prerequisites to learning. Other, more generic software not specifically designed for this population but easily adapted includes offerings from Developmental Learning Materials and Psychological Software Service. These materials are designed to improve problem-solving skills through linguistic and nonlinguistic manipulations. A series of more linguistically based programs that can be adapted for the high-level patient are available from Aspen Publishers.

Language Deficits and Dementia

Patients with dementia present with a generalized intellectual impairment that compromises communication efficiency (54). The severity of the dementia will correlate with the degree of communication impairment. Wertz characterized the linguistic performance of these patients as a deterioration of capacities in all communication modalities consistent with the deterioration of all other mental functions (77). Because dementia usually results from a progressive, diffuse pathologic process, patients rarely improve, and it is difficult to identify any learning strengths. The learning strengths and weaknesses of patients with dementia compared with those with right and left cortical disease are presented in Figure 12-2.

There is now evidence to show that language may be a barometer of change in charting the deterioration in dementia (78). Knowledge of these changes may be useful in family counseling and subsequent management of the communication disorder.

The inability of a demented patient to communicate a message that is relevant, timely, and completely understood by the listener often will depend on the severity of the disruption of those cognitive constructs that subserve language, such as general orientation, attention, memory, and visual-perceptive integration. Although some patients in the early stages of dementia may complain of an inability to produce nouns as their major communication deficit, this is not a consistent finding in all patients. Most sensitive to linguistic compromise is the patient's ability to name items in a category of either semantically or letter-related items (79). Progressive deterioration of memory skills is particularly coincident with interruptions in normal communicative discourse. Inability to monitor (i.e., identify, sort, remember, integrate) auditory/visual messages and verbal and graphic output may result in a paucity of information, problems in topic cohesion (i.e., relevance), indefinite phrases, and perseveration of words and ideas. Such disability will interfere with communicative exchanges. As the severity of dementia progresses, both syntax and phonology are preserved remarkably until the final stages. Discourse is characteristically neologistic and echolalic at this stage, but repetition without comprehension may be spared. In the most severe cases, meaningful communication is absent, and the patient may be mute.

Assessment

Assessment of linguistic skills usually is informal but should be accomplished at regular intervals to chart progression. Obler suggests the following categories for evaluation: orientation, naming (i.e., confrontation and responsive), analysis of discourse, comprehension, repetition, verbal fluency, idioms and proverbs, sentence construction, number facts, automatic speech, and reading and writing (80). Tests that assess memory, because of its close relationship to linguistic ability, also need to be administered at regular intervals. The impact of memory on linguistic communication can be measured by the Arizona Battery for Communication Disorders of Dementia (81). The test is comprised of 16 subtests, four of which (i.e., Story Retelling, Delayed; Word Learning, Free Recall; Word Learning, Total Recall; Word Learning, Recognition) can be used as a screening device to help differentiate the linguistic communicative deficits of patients with Alzheimer disease from those with normal skills.

Treatment

Treatment for patients with communication disorders secondary to dementia should be supportive. Treatment goals should include environmental controls, capitalization on preserved procedural memory, and family education. Environmental structure provides orientation and reinforces memory that, in turn, will improve the accuracy of linguistic attempts. Interactions with the patient should be structured to reduce any demands beyond the limits of the cognitive system as established by psychometric evaluation. Frequent measures of linguistic function are part of the treatment and are necessary so that family and friends can be informed about how much to expect receptively and expressively from the patient. This knowledge will reduce frustration for both the patient and family. Some patients retain skills longer than others, and knowledge of the best input and expected output modalities is useful in management. Because dementia often results in diminution of all linguistic modalities, performance may be strengthened through multiple channels such as the combination of gestural, written, and verbal language. This strategy is a process that needs to be demonstrated and taught to family members.

Although the evidence that certain medications facilitate memory in patients with dementia remains controversial, there are no data to support the notion that these facilitative drugs enhance language.

SWALLOWING IMPAIRMENT

Swallowing is an essential organismic function that begins *in utero* and continues throughout life. It is necessary to survival both because it is the source of hydration and alimentation and because it has a crucial role in maintaining airway integrity by clearing residue from the oral cavity and pharyngeal tract. Abnormal swallowing (dysphagia) may lead to dehydration, starvation, aspiration pneumonia, or airway obstruction. Dysphagia is frequently associated with cerebrovascular disease, traumatic brain injury, head and neck cancer, and a variety of other conditions common in rehabilitation patients. In many cases, swallowing impairments are amenable to a rehabilitation approach.

Physiology of Swallowing

Swallowing is coordinated with other patterned behaviors, including respiration and mastication; each is controlled by a central pattern generator in the brainstem. For convenience, swallowing is typically divided into three phases based on the anatomic location of the bolus (23,82). These phases may overlap in their timing and coordination.

Oral Phase

The oral phase begins with the oral preparation of the bolus, which precedes the swallow *per se.* The manner in which the bolus is prepared for swallowing varies depending on the consistency of the material. When liquid is ingested, there is no need for mastication. Liquids may be held between the tongue and palate or in the lingual sulcus but generally pass through the oral cavity in a continuous process. Soft foods may be held immediately between the tongue and anterior hard palate or lateralized for mastication before resuming a midline position for swallowing.

The process of preparation for solid food entails several distinct but overlapping processes (84). Ingestion is passage of food through the lips and into the mouth by biting or manual placement. This is followed immediately by stage I transport, propulsion of food from the anterior to the middle or posterior oral cavity. If food particles are still too large or coarse for swallowing, they remain in the mouth. During mastication, food is softened, and food particles are reduced in size by chewing (incising, crushing, and grinding) and mixing with saliva. Food in the mouth stimulates mechanoreceptors for the fifth cranial nerve located in the periodontal membrane and palate. Stimulation of these receptors activiates the central pattern generator for mastication, producing sequential contraction and relaxation of the elevator and depressor muscles of the mandible and resulting in cyclic opening and closing of the mouth. This cyclic grinding motion of the jaws is coordinated with rotation of the tongue, which pushes the food between the upper and lower teeth. Saliva is milked from the salivary glands, helping to break down the food and stimulate the taste buds. The physical consistency of the food is monitored continuously by oral mechanoreceptors. Once a small portion of the food is fully prepared (triturated), a cycle of stage II transport is initiated. The tongue pushes upward and forward in the mouth, contacting the anterior portion of the hard palate. The area of tongue–palate contact expands backward, propelling the small portion of the triturated food through the faucial arches and into the oropharynx. This small portion of food may remain in the oropharynx while chewing continues for several more jaw cycles, and additional small portions of triturated food may be propelled into the oropharynx. When a large enough bolus has been prepared, a swallow is initiated. A large bolus of food in the oral cavity is propelled through the faucial pillars, joining the small portion of triturated food already in the oropharynx. The pharyngeal phase of swallowing follows immediately.

Pharyngeal Phase

When appropriate sensory input reaches the medullary swallowing center (central pattern generator for swallowing), a complex motor sequence is elicited to propel a bolus through the pharynx, around the larynx, through the pharyngoesophageal (PE) sphincter, and into the esophagus. The events of the pharyngeal phase occur almost simultaneously, having a duration of about 1 second. Respiration ceases, and the palatopharyngeal isthmus closes, sealing off the nasopharynx. The tongue pushes back into the pharynx like a plunger, pushing the bolus downward. The epiglottis inverts, deflecting the bolus around the larynx and away from the airway. The larynx closes via contraction of the vocal folds and sealing of the laryngeal vestibule. The PE sphincter opens, allowing the bolus to pass into the esophagus. Opening of the PE sphincter is a complex process: the cricopharyngeus muscle relaxes, allowing the sphincter to open; the submandibular muscles pull the hyoid bone, the larynx, and the attached anterior wall of the pharynx upward and forward (away from the posterior pharyngeal wall), and the pressure of the descending bolus helps push the PE sphincter open (85). The pharyngeal constrictors contract sequentially with a peristaltic-like wave from top to bottom, clearing the pharynx of residue.

Esophageal Phase

The pharyngeal constricting wave that cleared the bolus into the esophagus continues throughout the esophagus as a primary peristaltic wave that strips the bolus through the gastroesophageal sphincter (GES) and into the stomach (82). Esophageal clearance is assisted by gravity but requires relaxation of the GES. Reflux of stomach contents is prevented by tonic contraction of the GES and reflex esophageal swallowing that is triggered by esophageal distension (secondary peristalsis).

Evaluation of Swallowing

When dysphagia is recognized, or a complaint about swallowing is registered, a special evaluation is required (83,86,87). Such an evaluation should consist of a complete medical history, a detailed description of the complaint, and a physical examination of the peripheral deglutitory motor and sensory system, including trial swallows under observation. Diagnostic studies, including videofluorography, manometry, electromyography, and fiberoptic endoscopy, are indicated in selected cases.

History

Data should be compiled from a review of the patient's general health history. Special attention should be paid to the neurologic history, which might suggest contributing factors such as stroke, head trauma, Parkinsonism, or central demyelinating disease, each of which may cause dysphagia. All prior operations should be noted, especially those involving the head and neck. All current prescription and nonprescription medications should be listed. Those that have side effects of sedation, muscle weakness, drying of mucous membranes, disorientation, or dyskinesia may contribute to dysphagia. Anticholinergic and psychoactive medications are specially noted.

Psychosocial factors may have a significant impact on swallowing, especially for elderly individuals. An individual living alone may be unable to obtain supervision during meals. For a nursing home resident, prescribing a special diet may be unrealistic. Swallowing must be considered in the context of feeding. Feeding dependency is an enormous problem for the elderly. Problems with feeding may be difficult to differentiate from impairments of swallowing *per se* (88).

Description of the Complaint

In many instances the subjective description of the problem gives the examiner clues to the cause of the swallowing problem. Critical data include a sensation of food sticking in the throat or chest, difficulty initiating swallowing, occurrence of coughing or choking spells associated with eating, drooling or difficulty clearing oral secretions, weight loss, change in diet or eating habits, episodes of aspiration pneumonia, and symptoms referable to gastroesophageal reflux. Difficulties swallowing solids and liquids should be contrasted and compared.

With liquids, patients may complain of coughing or choking during drinking. These symptoms are suggestive of aspiration (misdirection of food through the larynx and into the trachea) and are common in patients with neurogenic swallowing impairment. A complaint of food sticking in the throat or chest is common with solid food and raises the possibility of foodway obstruction. It may have many causes, however, including bulbar palsy, pharyngoesophageal diverticula, tumor, stricture, or esophageal dysmotility. The sensation of food sticking in the chest (thoracic dysphagia) is usually associated with disease of the esophagus or GES. Pharyngeal dysphagia, however, has poor localizing value and may be caused by dysfunction of the pharynx, PE sphincter, esophagus, or GES. Nasal regurgitation is associated with weakness or incompetence of the palatopharyngeal mechanism. Oral malodor may suggest a pharyngoesophageal diverticulum but may also be associated with mastication problems, poor oral hygiene, pharyngeal retention of food, tumor, or infection. Pain on swallowing (odynophagia) is a worrisome symptom, often associated with cancer of the esophagus. Heartburn, acid or sour regurgitation, and regurgitation of digested food suggest GE reflux disease. Reflux of stomach contents, especially at night, can lead to severe aspiration pneumonia. Instances of aspiration pneumonia should be recorded as a measure of severity. Because the anatomic and neuromuscular systems used for speech and swallowing are common, any speech or voice changes should be carefully noted and described. Weight loss or change in eating habits often reflect an underlying problem with swallowing.

Clinical Examination

A general physical examination is essential to look for evidence of cardiopulmonary, gastrointestinal, or neurologic disease that may impair swallowing. The exam includes assessment of mental status and the patient's ability to cooperate. A screening of language functions (e.g., following spoken commands, expressing thoughts), memory, and visual–motor–perceptual function is helpful (89). Cranial nerves should be assessed carefully. The respiratory system is examined for signs of obstruction or restriction such as tachypnea, stridor, use of accessory muscles, paradoxic motion of the chest wall, or labored breathing. Speech is examined for evidence of dysarthria or dysphonia.

The head and neck are inspected and palpated for structural lesions. The hyoid bone and laryngeal cartilages are palpated carefully and gently mobilized. Facial sensation is checked bilaterally. The muscles of the face, mouth, and neck are examined beginning with the muscles of facial expression. The examination should compare movement of the two sides of the face for signs of weakness. The masseter and temporalis can be palpated as the patient bites and chews. Movements of the lower jaw are assessed in three dimensions.

The examination proceeds to inspection of the intraoral mucosa. Careful attention should be paid to the presence of lesions, oral debris, abnormal movement, and dryness. Palpation with gloved hand on the floor of the mouth, gum lines, tonsillar fossa, and tongue serves to help rule out neoplastic growth. Atrophy, weakness, and fasciculations of the tongue should be noted. Tongue strength can be assessed by placing fingers against the outer cheek and resisting the patient's tongue as it is pushed into the inner cheek. The palate is inspected for symmetry at rest and during phonation. Each side of the palate is stimulated, and gag reflexes are observed; the soft palate and pharyngeal walls should contract briskly and symmetrically, but gag reflexes may be difficult to elicit in some normal individuals. The presence of primitive reflexes associated with chewing and swallowing (such as the sucking, biting, or snout reflexes) should be noted. These pathologic reflexes are often found in patients with bilateral hemispheric or frontal lobe damage and may indicate impairments of oral motor control.

The comprehensive examination includes observing the patient eating and drinking (87). Trial swallows are an essential portion of the examination but carry a small risk of aspiration. It is advisable initially to use a substance that is relatively safe if aspirated and to ensure that the patient is able to cough to protect the airway; a sip of water is relatively innocuous. The examiner observes for the promptness of the swallow and palpates the anterior neck to assess the adequacy of laryngeal elevation. Behaviors that should be noted include drooling, slow rate of eating, residual food in the mouth after swallowing, frequent throat clearing, change in voice quality, and posturing of the head and neck with swallowing. A spoonful of crushed ice may elicit chewing because of its texture and temperature. The examiner can observe the chewing action and feel for the laryngeal elevation to indicate that a swallow has occurred. Once it has been determined that the patient adequately elevates the larynx and that there is an adequate protective cough, other substances with varying textures and consistencies can be tried. Soft solid foods will also elicit chewing and allow the examiner to feel for laryngeal elevation. The mouth is inspected for retention after swallowing.

The purposes of the history and physical examination are

to assess components of the swallowing mechanism, to characterize the nature and severity of the swallowing deficit, to assess the patient's ability to perform compensatory maneuvers, and to determine whether further diagnostic studies are necessary. The physical examination is neither sensitive nor specific for identifying aspiration and cannot prove or disprove that a patient aspirates (90).

Diagnostic Studies

The videofluorographic swallowing study (VFSS) is the *sine qua non* of diagnostic tests for dysphagia. The rehabilitation approach to videofluorography is to have the patient eat various radio-opacified foods, using appropriate modifications, toward the goal of establishing a safe and efficient method of eating. An empirical approach is used to identify variables associated with safe and unsafe swallowing such as physical consistency of food, posture of the patient (especially position of the head and neck), and the means for presenting the food. These variables are altered systematically during the VFSS, and the effects on swallowing are observed (91–93).

Indications for a VFSS include frequent choking episodes, difficulty managing secretions, wet-hoarse voice quality, respiratory complications, and unexplained weight loss. Relative contraindications include inability to cooperate with the examination and severe respiratory dysfunction. Although static x-ray films may be valuable to detect morphologic changes in the pharynx or esophagus, they are not useful in studying the dynamics of swallowing. A complete examination should be conducted beginning with a small amount of liquid barium. Both lateral and anteroposterior views should be obtained with the patient in an upright posture. The oral and pharyngeal stages of swallowing should be studied with the camera focused superiorly on the hard palate and inferiorly on the cervical esophagus. Many clinicians recommend using a variety of textures (e.g., thin and thick liquid barium, puree, and cookie). Because simultaneous disorders of the pharynx and esophagus are frequent, the examination should include a study of the esophagus whenever possible. The esophagus and GE junction are best visualized with the patient in a prone position.

A protocol for fiberoptic endoscopic examination of swallowing (FEES) has been described by Langmore and colleagues (94) as a means to detect aspiration in patients for whom radiographic studies are difficult. A FEES carries the added benefit of directly visualizing the pharynx and larynx, to inspect for mucosal lesions or motion impairment of the vocal folds. Esophagoscopy is essential for detecting a variety of esophageal and GES disorders and provides the opportunity for diagnostic biopsy. Electrodiagnostic studies may be helpful for detecting motor unit dysfunction of the larynx, pharynx, and oral musculature but can not substitute for VFSS (95).

Management of Swallowing Impairment

Once the patient's swallowing has been described, the impairment identified, and the compensatory strengths recognized, a recommendation is made to feed the patient by mouth or to manage nutrition by an alternative route such as feeding tube. When oral feeding is recommended, a plan is needed that will maintain optimum calorie and fluid intake while minimizing the patient's risk for aspiration. Each plan must be individualized and based on what is known about the normal physiology of swallowing, the specific physiological abnormality, the cause of the disorder, and the prognosis for recovery (96). Table 12-5 lists some of the therapeutic and compensatory techniques that can be employed for patients with oral–pharyngeal forms of dysphagia.

Mechanical Disorders

Disruptions in the transmission of food and beverage from the anterior oral cavity into the pharynx and esophagus caused by structural abnormalities such as mucosal inflammation, trauma, tumor, or surgical alteration (in the mouth, pharynx, or larynx) may be described as mechanical disturbances of swallowing (97).

One type of mechanical disorder is found in the patient with partial or total glossectomy. If pharyngeal sensation and motor function are preserved, a special feeding spoon with a plunger to propel food into the posterior oral cavity can be used. A cohesive bolus of soft food can be pushed toward the back of the tongue. Liquids can be placed directly

TABLE 12-5. *Some therapeutic and compensatory techniques for managing patients with dysphagia*

Technique	Desired Effect
Flex neck	Reduce aspiration
Turn head to one side	Direct bolus to the ipsilateral side (away from side of weakness)
Hold breath before swallowing	Seal larynx, reduce aspiration
Thicken liquids (avoid thin)	Reduce aspiration, improve bolus control
Thin liquids (avoid thick)	Reduce pharyngeal retention
Slow rate of eating	Improve oral bolus control, avoid overloading pharynx
Mendelsohn maneuver	Prolong PE sphincter opening, improve pharyngeal clearance
Glottic adduction exercises	Improve airway protection, reduce aspiration
Use glossectomy spoon	Bypass anterior mouth, place food directly into posterior oral cavity
Stimulate soft palate with cold	Increase sensitivity for eliciting swallow
Feeding gastrostomy	Bypass oral cavity and pharynx

PE, pharyngoesophageal.

into the posterior oral cavity or oropharynx by using a syringe and length of tubing that will reach the faucial pillars.

Complications to swallowing for many surgical head and neck cancer patients are caused by radiation therapy. Xerostomia, or dry mouth, results from destruction of the salivary glands and other moisture-producing cells in the mucous lining. Artificial saliva may be used just before meals to provide moisture. Lemon-glycerin swabs, used to clean out oral debris, can be helpful for some patients, although others complain they increase dryness. The diet of these patients should emphasize foods lubricated with sauces, gravies, and butter. Mucosal pain associated with irradiation can be managed in part by the use of topical anesthetics; however, patients with impaired pharyngeal swallowing will have a greater aspiration risk because of the reduction of sensation.

Patients who have undergone a supraglottic laryngectomy are at risk for aspiration because of the loss of the epiglottis and altered sensation. Aspiration can be minimized by training the patient to inhale and hold breath before swallowing, to swallow, to cough gently while exhaling, and to reswallow. This procedure ensures that the patient has an adequate amount of air in the lungs to cough out debris that has penetrated the unprotected laryngeal region.

Disorders of the Motor Unit

Diseases that affect the lower motor neuron, neuromuscular junction, or muscle may result in weakness or paralysis of the swallowing musculature. These include brainstem stroke or tumor (particularly lateral medullary syndrome), motor neuron disease, myasthenia gravis, botulism, and inflammatory muscle disease. If the condition is progressive, and examination indicates that oral intake is reasonably safe, management centers on minimizing aspiration risks and preventing the secondary complications of dehydration and malnutrition (87,98). The posture should be adjusted to keep the patient upright with the neck flexed and chin down toward the chest. This posture typically helps to reduce aspiration. In lateral medullary syndrome, there is unilateral weakness of pharyngeal constrictor muscles. Turning the head toward the side of weakness directs the bolus to the stronger side of the pharynx, improving pharyngeal clearance (99). Some can be trained either in the breath-holding technique described for the patient with supraglottic laryngectomy or to prolong laryngeal elevation while swallowing repeatedly (the Mendelsohn maneuver). Care providers should be taught assistive coughing techniques but also should be instructed to recognize that the patient must be allowed every opportunity to clear material with an unassisted cough. The diet should be adjusted to provide foods that hold together as cohesive boluses. Dry and sticky foods should be avoided.

In those patients with potentially improving conditions, the same principles of management apply; however, exercise may hasten recovery of some motor functions. Vocal cord adduction may be strengthened by performing Valsalva maneuvers for exercise.

Some patients with specific muscle weakness can be assisted in swallowing and airway protection by surgical intervention. For example, laryngeal surgical procedures can be used to improve glottic function in some patients with vocal cord paralysis. Cricopharyngeal myotomy, a surgical procedure to slit the cricopharyngeal muscle and facilitate its opening during the swallow, may be beneficial to patients with demonstrated impairment of sphincter opening (85). In the event of persistent aspiration, surgical closure of the glottis with tracheostomy can be considered. Some techniques are potentially reversible should the patient recover function, whereas others, including total laryngectomy, are permanent (100). An alternative form of communication becomes the primary consideration.

Supranuclear Impairments

Supranuclear or pseudobulbar swallowing impairments result from neurological lesions above the level of the somatic motor nuclei in the brainstem. These include hemispheric stroke, brain tumor, and Parkinsonsim. In supranuclear impairments, there may be cognitive, sensory, and upper motor neuron dysfunction. The active swallowing muscles may be spastic or poorly coordinated, with diminished speed and delayed initiation of motion. Unlike patients with paralysis of swallowing, the patients with pseudobulbar impairment generally retain reflexes associated with airway protection, such as the gag and cough. The voluntary initiation of swallowing and coughing may be impaired, but each can be elicited by sensory stimulation.

Cognitive deficits can mimic or exascerbate supranuclear swallowing difficulties. Perceptual-motor impairments, judgment deficits, and language disorders are common in these patients, and may complicate the feeding process (89). Behavioral manifestations include failure to chew and swallow owing to impaired awareness or distractibility; taking excessively large bites or eating quickly owing to impaired judgment or motor planning (causing oral and pharyngeal overload); retaining food in the mouth between bites and ignoring food on the one side of the tray owing to sensory neglect; and failure to appreciate the importance of eating, which may be attributed mistakenly to depression or lack of motivation in patients with various forms of attention deficits.

Management is similar in many respects to the principles described for the patient with paralysis of swallowing (98). Placing patients in an upright posture with the neck flexed, providing foods that maintain a cohesive bolus, and ensuring that patients are in an optimal state of nutrition and hydration are very important considerations. Maintenance of good oral hygiene is a necessity. Additional attention should be paid to selecting foods that stimulate receptors associated with swallowing. Temperature, texture, volume, and taste may all help elicit a swallow. Foods should be pleasant in appearance and aroma. Items that are sticky, dry, tough to chew, or fall apart in the mouth are avoided.

Each patient with supranuclear swallowing difficulty must be evaluated individually to determine the nature and extent of cognitive impairment. The dysphagia treatment plan must be adapted to compensate for intellectual deficits. For example, the patient with distractability or language deficits may require an environment for eating that is free of distracting conversation. Patients with motor planning deficits may need verbal cues to begin eating and to maintain the process. Patients with impaired perception, judgment, or neglect require close, quiet supervision and monitoring. Most patients with supranuclear swallowing problems function best in a quiet setting with simple verbal instructions.

AUDITORY REHABILITATION

Two million people in the United States are either totally deaf or lack sufficient hearing to understand speech. Another 12 million have a serious hearing impairment. Some degree of hearing loss is present in 20 million Americans, or nearly one in ten. With increasing life expectancy as well as increasing noise exposure, the number of Americans who will suffer the effects of hearing loss will become even greater. The effect of hearing impairment on a person's life may be critical because of the communication problems it may cause or exacerbate.

Psychosocial Implications of Hearing Impairment

Although hearing impairment is not life-threatening, nor does it directly restrict physical activity, it is disabling because it interferes with quality of life. The psychosocial impact of a hearing loss is poorly understood and appreciated. The many ways in which we depend on our hearing simply are not recognized until hearing loss is experienced directly or unless a very close acquaintance has impaired hearing. There are few aspects of daily living that are not, in some way, affected by a hearing loss.

The primary impact of a hearing loss is on communication and, most notably, free and easy communication. Because of the interference with communication caused by hearing loss, a sense of isolation is imposed that can hinder opportunities for education, work, recreation, worship, and entertainment. A further sense of isolation can result from the inability to relate to the variety of sounds that keep us in contact with our environment, such as the sounds of nature, civilization, warning, or danger, as well as the many sounds that provide important everyday information.

Unfortunately, there is built into our cultural heritage misunderstanding, mistrust, and lack of sympathy for the hearing impaired, in a way certainly quite different from our perceptions and treatment of visual impairments. Often the symptoms of hearing loss (e.g., not answering when spoken to, answering inappropriately, requiring repetition) encourage others to talk and treat the hearing impaired as if their cognitive abilities also were diminished. This attitude is especially pertinent with the elderly hearing impaired, because associations with senility also are construed.

The two most commonly reported consequences of hearing loss are depression and social isolation. In addition, hearing loss can produce or aggravate embarrassment, fatigue, irritability, tension, and avoidance. A relationship of hearing loss with symptoms of paranoia has been suggested. Because hearing loss typically is very gradual in onset and progression, the affected person and friends may not be aware of the deficit. Not being able to hear can create frustration, suspiciousness, and anger that others are whispering and perhaps talking about the hearing-impaired person. Over time, social relationships may deteriorate, resulting in isolation and diminished quality of life. At the least, the psychosocial ramifications of hearing loss indicate the social need for an understanding of the deficit and efforts toward early identification and rehabilitation by the health care providers.

Assessment of Auditory Function

Basic Hearing Evaluation

The tests used in routine assessment of hearing include air and bone conduction and pure-tone and speech audiometry. The measurement of hearing sensitivity involves obtaining thresholds for both pure-tone and speech stimuli. The graph used to record hearing test results is called an audiogram (Fig. 12-3). The frequency (i.e., pitch) scale along the abscissa is measured in hertz (Hz). Even though young normal adults can hear frequencies as low as 20 Hz to as high as 20,000 Hz, the frequencies used in clinical hearing measurement include only those from 250 Hz up to 8,000 Hz. The most critical frequencies for the reception and understanding of speech are 500, 1,000, 2,000, and 3,000 Hz. The intensity scale on the ordinate of the audiogram is measured in decibels (dB) and encompasses a range from a very faint sound of 10 dB hearing level (HL) up to a very intense sound of 110 dB. The 0 dB HL for each frequency represents the average hearing sensitivity for a young normal adult.

Pure-tone air conduction audiometry provides information on the degree of hearing impairment as well as the configuration of the hearing loss. Sensitivity thresholds are obtained for the various audiometric frequencies for each ear separately using earphones. Air conduction evaluation thus measures the responsiveness of the entire auditory system from the external auditory canal through the middle ear mechanism to the cochlea, and associated neural pathways to the brain. Therefore, a hearing impairment shown by pure-tone air conduction measurement may result from a disorder anywhere in the auditory system.

Pure-tone bone conduction audiometry assists in defining the general anatomic location of the hearing disorder. A small vibrator placed on the mastoid process behind the ear to be tested conducts sound vibrations directly to the cochlea, and thresholds can be obtained for the frequencies 250 through 4,000 Hz. Because sound transmission by bone con-

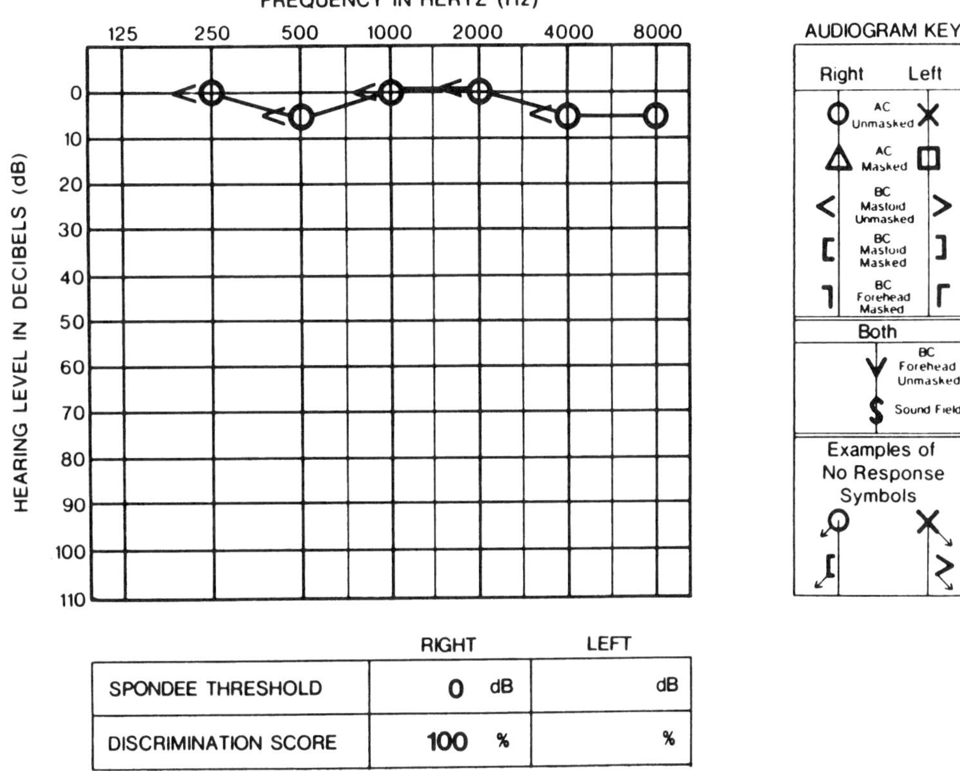

FIG. 12-3. Audiogram of a normal ear.

duction bypasses the outer and middle ear, bone conduction results reflect the sensitivity of the sensorineural system only. The use of a masking noise in the nontest ear often is necessary to ensure that the bone conduction responses are not being perceived in the nontest ear.

In addition to pure-tone threshold measurements, the basic audiologic evaluation includes the measurement of threshold sensitivity for speech and the determination of speech recognition (i.e., understanding) abilities. The Speech Reception Threshold (SRT) test serves primarily as a reliability check on the pure-tone threshold levels. Familiar two-syllable words (e.g., airplane, sidewalk, playground) are presented to each ear separately through earphones, and the softest intensity level at which 50% of the words are correctly repeated is defined as the SRT. The SRT should agree within + 10 dB of the pure-tone average (PTA) threshold levels at 500, 1,000, and 2,000 Hz. If not, exaggerated hearing loss must be suspected.

A hearing impairment may be reflected not only in a sensitivity loss but also in an impairment in the ability to understand speech even when speech is sufficiently loud. The assessment of speech discrimination analyzes the ability to understand speech when presented at comfortably loud levels; it is not a threshold or sensitivity test. Standardized word lists of 25 or 50 phonetically balanced single-syllable words (e.g., darn, art, chief) are presented to each ear separately at comfortably loud intensity levels. These words are repeated back by the patient and the percentage of correct responses is the speech discrimination score. The speech discrimination score may range from 0% to 100%, and scores of 90% to 100% are considered normal.

Audiometric Test Interpretation

Degree of Hearing Loss

The threshold results obtained using pure-tone air conduction assessment provide quantitative information about the amount of hearing loss present. Classification systems have been devised in an effort to relate the amount of air conduction hearing loss to the expected degree of handicap imposed by a hearing loss. Such systems typically use the PTA to estimate various hearing loss categories and the expected effects of the loss on speech understanding. An example of such a classification system is as follows:

The American Medical Association uses a percentage hearing loss system, and a formula is used to calculate hearing loss percentage based on the frequencies from 500 Hz to 3,000 Hz. Any type of audiometric classification system, however, must be interpreted with caution because most are based on pure-tone air conduction thresholds alone and do not incorporate the effects of speech discrimination difficulties, etiologic factors, or hearing loss configuration. In addition, people with similar amounts of pure-tone hearing loss may be affected in far different ways, depending on their life styles, hearing demands, and other psychosocial factors.

Location of Auditory Impairment

The general anatomic location of a hearing impairment can be determined by comparing the air conduction and bone conduction thresholds. A conductive hearing loss is present when air conduction results demonstrate a hearing loss but bone conduction results are within normal range (Fig. 12-4). The difference between the air and bone conduction thresholds reflects the amount of conductive involvement and is called the air–bone gap. A conductive hearing loss could be caused by any obstruction in the sound-conducting mechanism of the ear, from the external auditory canal (e.g., cerumen impaction, foreign body) through the middle ear (e.g., middle ear effusion, otosclerosis). On the basis of the audiometric results alone, the specific etiology or location cannot be predicted. Although otoscopic evidence of a cerumen impaction, tympanic membrane perforation, or serous otitis could account for a conductive hearing loss, there are conductive pathologies that present with normal otoscopic examinations, such as otosclerosis or ossicular discontinuity.

Patients with pure conductive hearing loss demonstrate normal speech discrimination scores (90% to 100%) because the sensorineural system is intact. Speech needs only to be presented at louder levels than normal to compensate for the conductive deficit.

When a hearing loss is present by air conduction and similarly by bone conduction, the impairment is called a sensorineural loss (Fig. 12-5). The hearing disorder could be located in the cochlea, the associated neural pathways, or in both. The specific etiology of the sensorineural hearing loss cannot be determined by the audiometric results alone. Although the audiogram can provide diagnostic cues to the etiology of the impairment, the patient's history and other tests need to be reviewed to provide a diagnosis.

Speech discrimination results in sensorineural hearing loss often provide important diagnostic and rehabilitative signs. In general, cochlear involvements demonstrate speech discrimination scores compatible with the degree of hearing loss. The greater the hearing loss in cochlear disorders, the poorer the speech discrimination. On the other hand, neural auditory disorders often yield speech discrimination scores disproportionately poorer than would be expected from the pure-tone thresholds. That is, a 40 dB HL sensorineural hearing loss with a 72% speech discrimination score would be consistent with cochlear involvement, whereas a similar amount of hearing loss with only 10% speech discrimination would suggest the possibility of eighth-cranial-nerve involvement. From a rehabilitative standpoint, the higher the speech discrimination score, the better the prognosis for hearing aid success because there is less distortion in the auditory system.

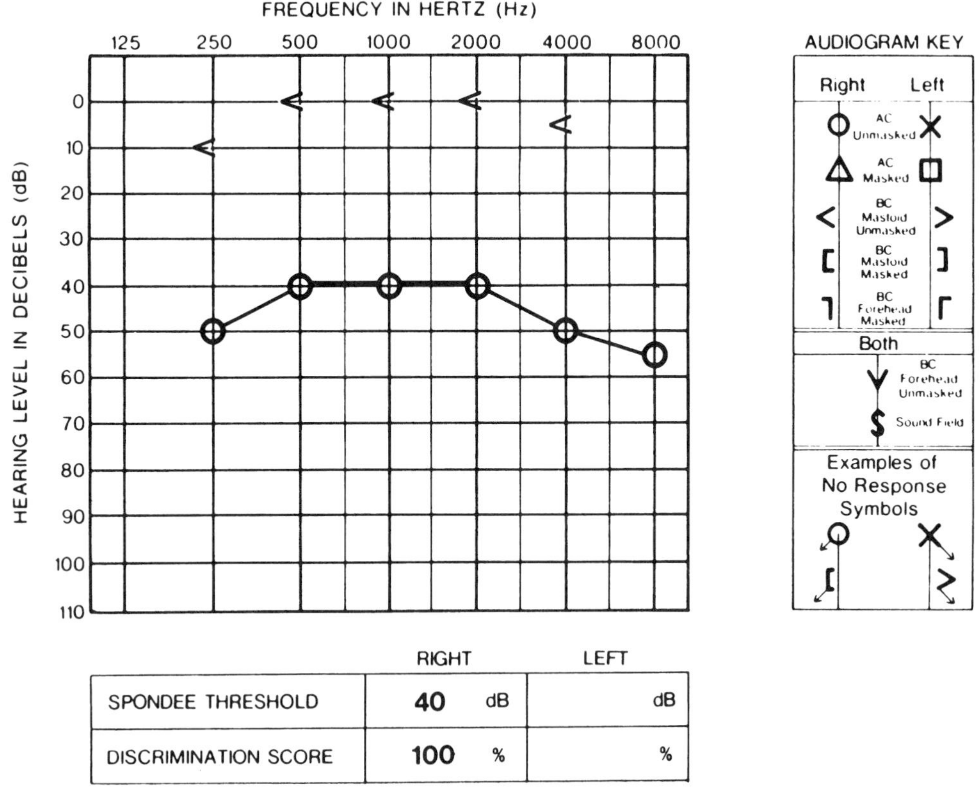

FIG. 12-4. This audiogram shows that the patient has a mild conductive hearing loss. Note that the air conduction thresholds reveal a hearing impairment of 40 dB, but the bone conduction responses are within the normal range. Therefore, an air–bone gap of 35 dB is present. Speech discrimination is normal because no sensorineural involvement is present.

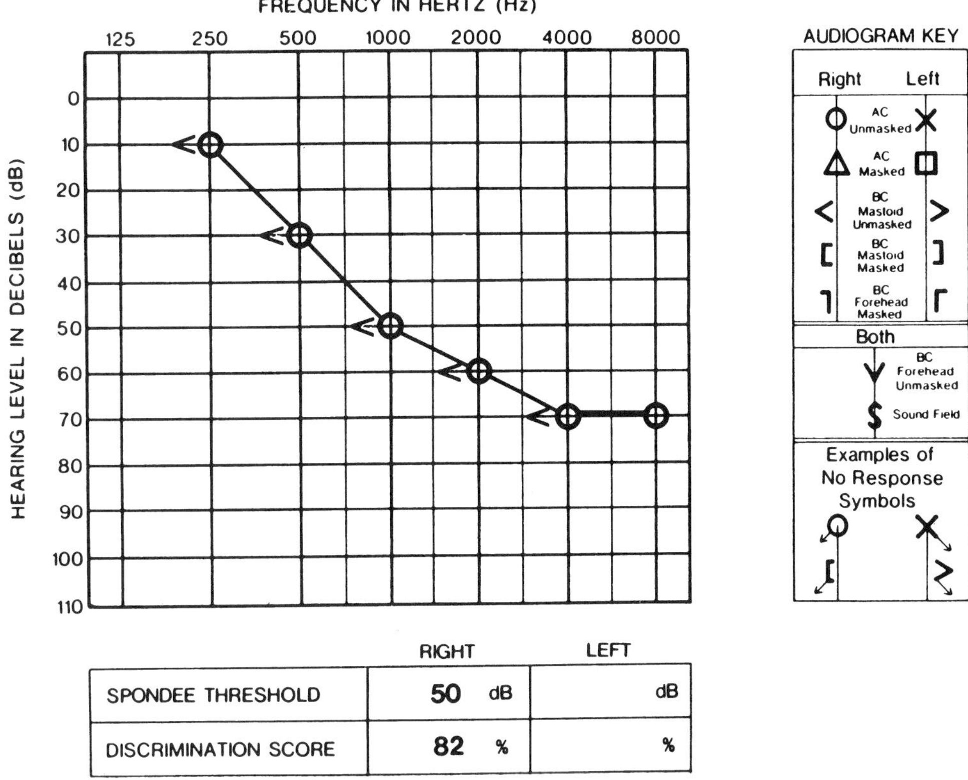

FIG. 12-5. This audiogram shows that the patient has a sensorineural hearing loss—both the air conduction and the bone conduction thresholds are similarly depressed. Speech discrimination at a comfortable level is relatively good in this illustration (82%) but is reduced from normal performance.

A loss in hearing sensitivity for bone conduction with a greater loss for air conduction represents a mixed hearing loss (Fig. 12-6). A sensorineural hearing loss is present, as reflected by the reduced bone conduction levels, and conductive loss also is present, as reflected by the air–bone gaps. Speech discrimination performance reflects the amount and etiology of the sensorineural involvement. Correction of the conductive component by medical or surgical treatment should result in a sensorineural loss alone, as reflected by the bone conduction levels.

Site-of-Lesion Evaluation

The basic audiologic test battery of pure-tone air conduction, bone conduction, SRT, and speech discrimination assessment represents the minimum audiologic protocol for evaluating patients with hearing impairment. In the case of an asymmetric sensorineural deficit or clinical suspicion of eighth-nerve or central auditory involvement, special audiologic procedures to define the site of impairment are available. The audiologic site-of-lesion battery includes tests to determine the presence of loudness recruitment, which is a cochlear sign; abnormal auditory adaptation, which is a neural sign; and speech discrimination rollover, which is also a neural sign. The evaluation of the integrity of the stapedius (i.e., acoustic) reflex by immittance measurement is a helpful test in differentiating between cochlear and eighth-nerve involvement. Abnormalities in the stapedius reflex (e.g., elevated reflexes, absent reflexes, reflex decay) often are related to an eighth-nerve tumor. The electrophysiological analysis of brainstem auditory evoked potentials (BAEPs) provides a sensitive procedure for the diagnosis of acoustic tumors. Electrocochleography also is available for measuring the electrophysiological activity originating with the cochlea and can supplement information provided by BAEP audiometry.

Measures for Special Populations

If a patient cannot respond appropriately to conventional tests, as in the case of the neonate, infant, or mentally handicapped patient, other audiologic techniques are indicated. The field of pediatric audiology has many behavioral approaches available to assess the auditory capabilities of these special populations. Reliable and valid measures of hearing sensitivity can be obtained using innovative audiologic methods in infants as young as 6 months, and the presence or absence of significant hearing impairment can be determined in neonates by behavioral observation audiometry. When behavioral measures prove unsuccessful, or when additional documentation is needed, the use of BAEP audiometry is indicated.

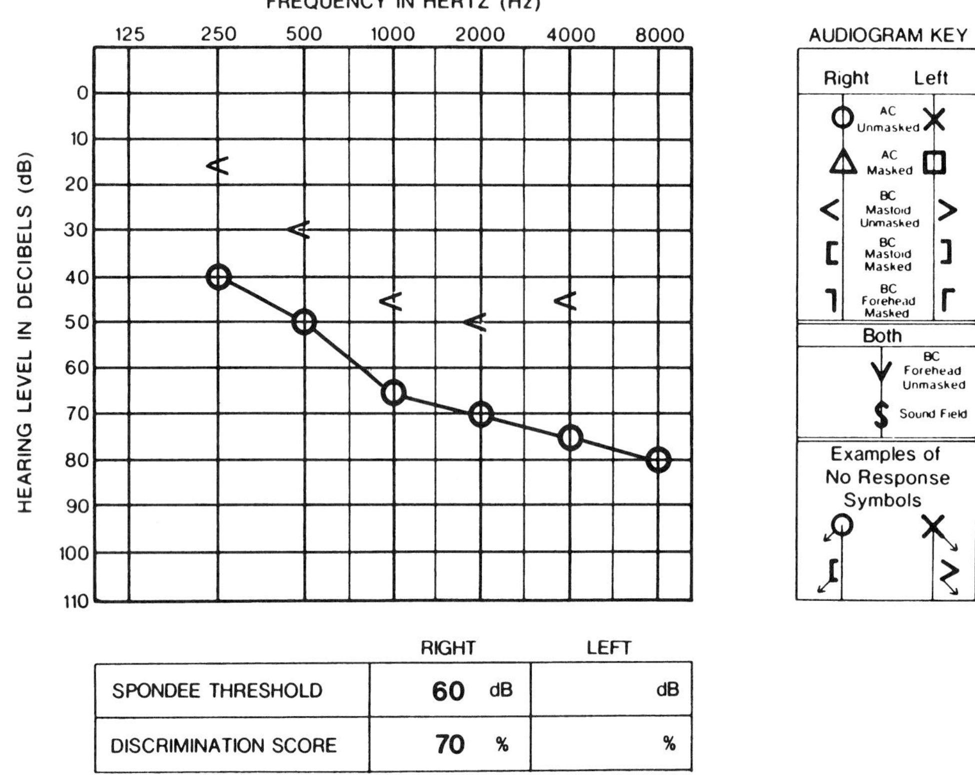

FIG. 12-6. This audiogram shows that the patient has a mixed hearing loss. Although both the air conduction and the bone conduction thresholds are reduced, a greater impairment is evident for air conduction. Speech discrimination is reduced (70%), reflecting the sensorineural component of the loss.

The assessment of the patient suspected of manifesting functional (i.e., exaggerated) hearing loss requires the use of special audiologic test procedures developed specifically for this purpose.

Management of Hearing Impairment

The management of the person with hearing loss should begin with a complete otologic evaluation. Although hearing loss most often occurs alone, it may be one manifestation of a syndrome or part of a more generalized disease process. As with any symptom or clinical finding, treatment should be based on the underlying pathophysiological condition. A specific diagnosis should be sought with the objective of reversal of the hearing loss or prevention of additional impairment.

A thorough otologic history should be obtained, including questions about the time of onset, whether the loss was sudden or gradual, and if associated symptoms are present (e.g., tinnitus, vertigo, discharge, aural fullness, pain). In addition, questioning should review family history of hearing loss, loud noise exposure, head trauma, and ototoxic drug use. After the history, physical examination with special attention to the head and neck region is completed. The otoscopic examination should include otomicroscopic evaluation and pneumo-otoscopy to assess tympanic membrane mobility. Some practitioners may use tympanometry, a measurement of the compliance of the tympanic membrane and middle ear system. The standard audiologic evaluation is then administered, and any special audiologic tests are recommended. The use of associated neurologic, laboratory, and radiologic studies also may be helpful. Only after the assessment has been completed and a diagnosis has been established should rehabilitation of the hearing loss be initiated. All too frequently, patients with hearing loss are approached for rehabilitation without antecedent medical evaluation. Many hearing-impaired patients are fit with hearing aids without medical evaluation of their hearing loss. Neither hearing aid dispensers nor audiologists have the appropriate training to diagnose the etiology of hearing loss.

Medical–Surgical Rehabilitation

Medical or surgical treatment of hearing loss most often is available for people with impairments of the conductive auditory system. When hearing loss originates in the external auditory canal, it usually is related to a mechanical obstruction in the form of cerumen or foreign body; cerumen impaction is the most common cause of conductive hearing loss. Removal of the obstruction will improve or restore hearing. Infections of the lining of the external canal (i.e., otitis externa) can be treated with topical antibiotics. Hearing impairment originating in the middle ear system may be treated with otologic surgery. Surgical procedures such as myringoplasty (i.e., repair of tympanic membrane perforation), tympanoplasty (i.e., ossicular reconstruction), stapedectomy for otosclerosis, and myringotomy with placement of ventilating tubes for middle ear effusion often can correct the conductive hearing loss. The otologist bases a surgical recommendation on the amount of conductive involvement and the possibility that closure of the air–bone gaps would improve hearing significantly. Even in cases of mixed hearing loss, surgical correction of the conductive component may enable the patient to use a less powerful hearing aid or require an aid only on a limited basis.

Otologic surgery sometimes is required for treatment of life-threatening disease and not for hearing improvement. Pathologic conditions such as cholesteatoma, glomus tumor, or chronic middle ear disease necessitate surgery. In addition, otoneurosurgery is necessary for sensorineural impairment caused by eighth-nerve tumors. Although hearing preservation is possible in some patients, the primary goal is the removal of the neoplasm.

Otologic treatment of congenital or hereditary sensorineural hearing loss, noise-induced hearing loss, presbycusis, and most other types of sensorineural impairment is not possible at this time. Perhaps the greatest advance in the surgical rehabilitation of sensorineural impairments is now available with the development of the cochlear implant for profound hearing loss.

Hearing Aid Amplification

The most common rehabilitative therapy for hearing impairment is the hearing aid. Appropriate amplification improves receptive communicative functioning for people with untreatable auditory disorders. A hearing aid is a miniature amplifier of sound, designed to increase the intensity of sound and to deliver it to the hearing-impaired ear. Although the physical appearance of hearing aids may vary considerably, all electroacoustic hearing aids have the following basic components: an input microphone to convert airborne sound to electrical energy; an amplifier to increase the strength of the electrical signal; an output receiver to convert the amplified signal back to acoustic energy; a battery to provide power for the aid; and a volume control to permit the user to adjust the loudness of the sound. The various types of hearing aid are as follows (Fig. 12-7).

Body Hearing Aid

The body or pocket hearing aid houses the microphone and amplifier in a case worn at chest level, with a cord connected to an external receiver fit into an earmold. This aid is considerably larger than other hearing aids and is regarded as the most powerful, durable, and least cosmetic. Body aids fulfill a need only for people with severe or profound hearing loss as well as those who cannot manipulate the smaller aids because of dexterity problems or other physical limitations.

Behind-the-Ear Aid

The components of the behind-the-ear (BTE) aid are fit into a curved case that rests behind the ear. Sound is amplified and then delivered through a short length of plastic tubing to an earmold fit into the ear canal. These aids generally have replaced body aids for those with severe hearing losses, as they now have the power equivalent to many body aids. They also are helpful for mild and moderate hearing loss patients, especially those who need tone controls and other features not available in smaller hearing aids.

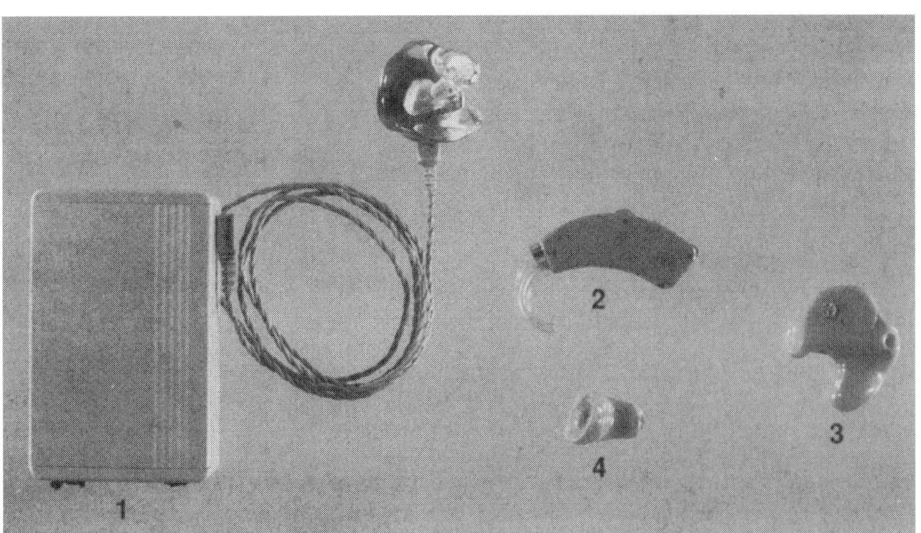

FIG. 12-7. Various types of hearing aids: *(1)* body, *(2)* behind-the-ear, *(3)* in-the-ear, and *(4)* in-the-canal.

Eyeglass Hearing Aid

The components of the eyeglass hearing aid all fit within the temple bow of an eyeglass frame. Eyeglass aids are seldom fit today because of the difficulties in the adjustment of these aids with eyeglass frames, and part-time eyeglass or hearing aid wearers are annoyed when both are in the same unit.

In-the-Ear Hearing Aid

The in-the-ear (ITE) aid is a self-contained hearing aid that fits entirely into the concha of the external ear. These aids have the advantages of cosmetic appeal and ease of insertion and adjustment compared with BTE hearing aids. The ITE aid is custom-fit to the wearer's ear as well as to the specific amplification requirements of the hearing loss.

In-the-Canal and Completely-in-the-Canal Hearing Aids

The in-the-canal (ITC) and completely-in-the-canal (CIC) hearing aids are the smallest and most "cosmetic" of all hearing aids, as they are molded to fit entirely within the ear canal. They incorporate suitable amplification for mild and moderate degrees of hearing loss. Their major drawback relates to the lack of space available for inclusion of sophisticated circuitry and telephone coils. In addition, those persons with poor finger dexterity have considerable difficulty in insertion and adjustment of these small devices. The cost of these aids is usually quite high ($1,000 to $1,800 each), although it is surprising how many persons forego financial considerations in order to wear "the smallest aid possible."

Programmable Hearing Aids

These hearing aids offer the most advanced technology in amplification. They are individually computer programmed and provide advanced signal-processing circuitry. Multiple-program aids offer the user the choice of several situation-specific programs for use in a variety of listening situations (i.e., quiet, small groups, large groups, telephone, etc.). They are operated with a user-operated remote control. Some aids have no volume controls, as the aids automatically adjust the volume to incoming sounds. As expected these instruments are the most expensive ($1,500 to $2,500 each).

Contralateral Routing of Signals Hearing-Aid System

The contralateral routing of signals (CROS) hearing aid system was developed to assist those people with a unilateral unaidable ear, such as a severe/profound unilateral deafness with normal hearing in the good ear. An aid containing a microphone is placed on the unaidable ear side and sound is transmitted to any aid on the better ear using radio transmission. The aid on the poor ear acts as a radio transmitter to send the sound to the receiver aid on the better ear side. This permits the wearer to hear people speaking to their severe hearing loss ear simply by sending sounds to the good hearing ear. A modification of the CROS system is the BI-CROS aid, which is intended for patients with bilateral hearing loss whose poorer ear is not suitable for amplification. In addition to the CROS side pick-up, sound also is amplified to the better hearing ear.

Special Features

Special features serve to increase the fitting flexibility of many aids and provide options for specific hearing loss requirements or personal needs. Telephone circuits (i.e., T coil) are available in all hearing aid types, with the exception of the ITC aid. A magnetic induction coil inside the aid picks up sounds directly from the receiver of the telephone, bypassing the external microphone. The volume control of the hearing aid can increase the loudness of the telephone voice without amplifying background noise. Although some newer telephones do not generate an adequate magnetic field for T coil use, a special device is available to connect to the telephone to restore efficient use of the T coil. Telephone circuits also can be used in auditoriums and classrooms where induction loop amplification systems are installed.

Many hearing aids incorporate controls for dispenser adjustment of the aid's power, tone, and other acoustic variables. These internal adjustments increase the fitting applications, as a particular aid can be made suitable for a wide range of hearing loss requirements and configurations. Some hearing aids also have user-operated tone controls, which permit the user to change the tone response. This is helpful in situations with background noise, as the adjustment of the tone control can reduce the low-frequency amplification of the aid, decreasing noise interference.

Hearing aid technology has not yet achieved computerization; hearing aids are analog devices. Although digitally programmable hearing aids are now being introduced, there still is no fully digital hearing aid available for consumers. Digitally programmable aids enable the dispenser and wearer to digitally program several different responses into a single hearing aid. This permits the user to select the acoustic response in his or her hearing aid that is most helpful for a particular listening environment by means of a remote control selector. The hearing aid user can select a different response for a quiet versus a noisy environment, thus enhancing speech understanding. These devices also cost considerably more than conventional hearing aids. When fully digital hearing aids are made available, hearing aid costs will increase dramatically. Hearing aid costs are most often paid by the person, since they are not covered under Medicare or the majority of insurance policies.

Determination of Hearing Aid Candidacy

There are no accepted rules or criteria as to who should be considered to be a hearing aid candidate. Although hearing loss greater than 40 dB HL certainly warrants consideration for the fitting of amplification, there are those with even moderate to severe hearing impairment who reject such advice. Psychological attitudes such as denial of a hearing loss, putting the blame of hearing difficulties on others (e.g., people just don't speak clearly), and fear that a hearing loss reflects aging results in some people being poor hearing aid candidates and rejecting hearing aid use. The most important criteria for successful hearing aid use relate to the person's self-perceived hearing difficulties, acceptance of the hearing loss, and motivation to use amplification. Any person who expresses hearing difficulties that handicap daily social or professional activities should be considered a prospective hearing aid candidate. This recommendation for possible hearing aid use should be accompanied by a very positive and uplifting approach by the practitioner. The practitioner should never discourage a hearing aid trial, nor should one suggest that the hearing-impaired person can get by without amplification. Discouraging a hearing aid trial for a person with hearing difficulties and a potentially remediable hearing loss serves only to invite isolation and frustration.

The prospective candidate should receive a hearing aid evaluation performed by a certified clinical audiologist. Although some hearing aid dealers are relatively skilled in the fitting of hearing aids, others possess only minimal training and are more oriented to sales. Many states, in fact, require that a hearing aid dealer meet only minimal requirements, and educational criteria typically are not required. The clinical audiologist, on the other hand, holds at least a master's degree in the evaluation and rehabilitation of hearing impairment. During the hearing aid evaluation, the patient may be evaluated with several electroacoustically appropriate hearing aids. Tests are administered through a loudspeaker in a sound-treated room to determine which hearing aid or aids best suit the patient's acoustic and psychological needs. Whether regulated by state law or local dispensing practices, most hearing aids are fit on at least a 30-day trial-rental period before purchase. Critical to successful hearing aid prognosis are factors unrelated to the audiologic assessment. Lack of motivation, negative attitudes, family pressure, denial of hearing difficulties, and other psychological factors often result in unsuccessful hearing aid fitting.

The rehabilitation of hearing loss with a hearing aid does not cure the hearing impairment, nor does it restore normal hearing. Hearing aid amplification does represent the best treatment available, however, and will improve the ability to communicate effectively and reduce the handicapping consequences of hearing loss for most hearing-impaired people.

Speech Reading and Auditory Training

Speech reading is the use of visual cues in the recognition of speech and incorporates the interpretation of facial expressions, body movements, and gestures. Everyone uses speech reading to some extent, although usually we are not conscious of the importance of visual input in helping us to recognize what is being said. Many hearing-impaired people, particularly those with a gradually progressive hearing loss, develop this skill through necessity.

The use of speech reading alone cannot be the sole rehabilitative approach in providing the hearing-impaired patient with complete understanding of speech. Although a considerable amount of the speech signal can be perceived visually, only about one-third of English speech sounds are clearly visible. Certain sounds (e.g., \f\ and \th\) are relatively easy to see on the lips, others (e.g., \k\ and \g\) are not visible, and some (e.g., \p\ and \b\) are indistinguishable.

Speech reading usually is taught in conjunction with a program of auditory training. Auditory training teaches the patient to make the most effective use of the minimal auditory cues imposed by the hearing loss. The combination of visual input and auditory input is superior to either one alone in understanding speech. Aural rehabilitation strategies also try to teach the hearing-impaired person to become a more assertive listener. Those who quietly accept not hearing and understanding merely invite continued social isolation. The hearing-impaired listener needs to inform others as to the most effective means of communication. Self-help groups are available, most notably the Self Help for Hard of Hearing People organization, which offers local groups as well as an active national organization and journals.

Assistive Listening Devices

Despite the substantial improvements in hearing aid design and application, few hearing-impaired people can achieve normal auditory receptive functioning with hearing aid use alone. The levels of noise and background interference found in many public places often renders speech recognition of the desired message unintelligible to the hearing-impaired person. The amplification of unwanted sounds (e.g., other talkers in a crowd, ventilation hum, background music) to an ear with sensorineural hearing loss often interferes with the reception and comprehension of the desired message.

The use of assistive listening devices (ALDs) can make the difference between satisfactory and unsatisfactory communication in adverse listening situations. The primary difference between ALDs and hearing aids is that ALDs are designed to help only in selected listening environments. Many ALDs use a microphone placed close to the desired sound source (e.g., television, theater stage, speaker's podium), and sound is transmitted directly to the hearing-impaired listener. Transmission methods include infrared, audio loop, FM radio, or direct audio input to a hearing aid. The direct transmission of the sound to the listener's hearing aid or receiver unit improves the signal-to-noise ratio; that is, the desired message is enhanced while competing extraneous noises are decreased. The key to success is the direct electronic coupling reaching from the microphone at the desired sound source to the ear of the listener. Some churches, theaters, and classrooms are now equipped with ALDs.

Amplified telephones, low-frequency doorbells and telephone ringers, and closed-captioned TV decoders are just a few examples of a number of devices available for situation-specific assistance for the hearing impaired. Flashing alarm clocks, alarm bed vibrators, and flashing smoke detectors help to alert the deaf person. Telephone communication for severely hearing-impaired people is possible with the use of telephone devices for the deaf. These systems use a typed message for transmission and a written read-out either to a LED display or printer.

Cochlear Implant (see Chapter 70)

The cochlear implant is an auditory prosthesis designed to provide hearing for the profoundly deaf by electrically stimulating residual eighth-nerve neurons in the cochlea. Prospective implant candidates require an extensive audiologic evaluation to document that powerful hearing aids would not be of help. The implant operation involves placing an electrode wire or electrode array into the cochlea and connecting it to an internal coil placed under the skin behind the ear, aligned with an external coil placed behind the ear. After the healing period, the patient is fit with a microphone and stimulator/signal processor unit. The microphone, usually worn at ear level, picks up sound and transmits the sound to a signal processor unit that resembles a body-type hearing aid. The processor converts the sound to electrical signals that are transmitted to the external coil, through the skin to the internal coil, and to the electrodes in the cochlea. Current flows between the active electrodes and a ground electrode placed in the eustachian tube, stimulating remaining nerve fibers and producing a sensation of sound.

The cochlear implant, unlike a hearing aid, does not change the electrical impulses back into amplified sounds. Rather, sound is changed into electrical impulses that are delivered directly to the cochlea. Sounds perceived with a cochlear implant are entirely different from sounds heard with a hearing aid. Implanted patients have described the sounds they hear as buzzes, whistles, or metallic sounds; only rarely are sounds described as speech-like. Although the implant does allow the profoundly deaf person to detect speech, this does not imply the ability to discriminate (i.e., understand) speech. Electrical stimulation does provide considerable loudness and timing information to the patient, aiding in speech reading. In addition, the implant can help to provide the user with an awareness of environmental sounds.

Tactile Aids

For those profoundly deaf patients who are not candidates for cochlear implants and who receive no help from hearing aids, tactile devices are available. These devices convert sound into vibrations to provide the patient with awareness of sound.

REFERENCES

1. Duffy JR. *Motor speech disorders: Substrates, differential diagnosis and management.* St. Louis: CV Mosby, 1995.
2. Rosenbek JC, LaPoint LL. The dysarthrias: description, diagnosis and treatment. In: Johns DF, ed. *Clinical management of neurogenic communication disorders.* Austin, TX: ProEd, 1985; 97–152.
3. Darley FL, Aronson AE, Brown JE. Differential diagnostic patterns of dysarthria. *J Speech Hear Res* 1969; 12:246–269.
4. Darley FL, Aronson AE, Brown JE. Clusters of deviant speech dimensions in the dysarthrias. *J Speech Hear Res* 1969; 12:462–496.
5. Darley FL, Aronson AE, Brown JE. Motor speech signs in neurologic disease. *Med Clin North Am* 1968; 52:835–844.
6. Yorkston KM, Strand EA, Kennedy MRT. Comprehensibility of dysarthric speech: implications for assessment and treatment planning. *Am J Speech-Lang Pathol* 1996; 5:55–66.
7. Pope AM, Tarlov AR, eds. *Disability in America: toward a national agenda for prevention.* Washington, DC: National Academy Press, 1991.
8. Yorkston KM, Beukelman DR, Bell KR. *Clinical management of dysarthric speakers.* Austin, TX: ProEd, 1988.
9. Netsell R. Speech physiology. In: Minifie FD, Hixon TJ, Williams F, eds. *Normal aspects of speech, hearing, and language.* Englewood Cliffs, NJ: Prentice-Hall, 1973.
10. Gerratt BR, Till JA, Rosenbek JC, Wertz RT, Boysen AE. Use and perceived value of perceptual and instrumental measures in dysarthria management. In: Moore CA, Yorkston KM, Beukelman DR, eds. *Dysarthria and apraxia of speech: perspectives on management.* Baltimore: Paul H. Brookes, 1991; 77–94.
11. Netsell R, Lotz WK, Barlow SM. A speech physiology examination for individuals with dysarthria. In: Yorkston KM, Beukelman DR, eds. *Recent advances in clinical dysarthria.* Austin, TX: ProEd, 1989; 3–38.
12. Hixon TJ. Respiratory function in speech. In: Minifie FD, Hixon TJ, Williams F, eds. *Normal aspects of speech, hearing, and language.* Englewood Cliffs, NJ: Prentice-Hall, 1973; 75–125.
13. Netsell R, Hixon TJ. A noninvasive method of clinically estimating subglottal air pressure. *J Speech Hear Disord* 1978; 43:326–350.
14. Keller E, Vigneuz P, Lafamboise M. Acoustic analysis of neurologically impaired speech. *Br J Disord Commun* 1991; 26:75–94.
15. Ramig LA, Scherer RC, Tize IR, Ringel S. Acoustic analysis of voices of patients with neurologic disease: rationale and preliminary data. *Ann Otol Rhinol Laryngol* 1988; 97:164–172.
16. Smitheran J, Hixon TJ. A clinical method for estimating laryngeal airway resistance during vowel production. *J Speech Hear Disord* 1981; 46:138–146.
17. Barlow SM. High-speed data acquisition for clinical speech physiology. In: Yorkston KM, Beukelman DR, eds. *Recent advances in dysarthria.* Boston: College-Hill Press, 1989; 39–52.
18. Hardy JC, Netsell R, Schweiger JW, Morris HL. Management of velopharyngeal dysfunction in cerebral palsy. *J Speech Hear Disord* 1969; 34:123–137.
19. Yorkston KM, Beukelman DR, Traynor CD. *Computerized assessment of intelligibility of dysarthric speech.* Tigard, OR: CC Publications, 1984.
20. Beukelman DR, Yorkston KM. The relationship between information transfer and speech intelligibility of dysarthric speakers. *J Commun Disord* 1979; 12:189–196.
21. Platt LJ, Andrews G, Young M, Neilson PD. The measurement of speech impairment of adults with cerebral palsy. *Fol Phoniatr* 1978; 30:30–58.
22. Platt LJ, Andrews G, Young M, Quinn P. Dysarthria of adult cerebral palsy: intelligibility and articulatory impairment. *J Speech Hear Res* 1980; 23:28–40.
23. Yorkston KM, Dowden PA, Beukelman DR. Intelligibility as a tool in the clinical management of dysarthric speakers. In: Kent RD, ed. *Intelligibility in speech disorders: theory, measurement and management.* Amsterdam: John Benjamins, 1992; 265–286.
24. Yorkston KM, Beukelman DR. *Assessment of intelligibility of dysarthric speech.* Tigard, OR: CC Publications, 1981.
25. Brandenburg S, Vanderheiden G. *Communication, control and computer access for disabled and elderly individuals: communication aids.* Austin, TX: ProEd, 1987.
26. Yorkston KM, Beukelman DR. Motor speech disorders. In: Beukel-

man DR, Yorkston KM, eds. *Communication disorders following traumatic brain injury: management of cognitive, language, and motor impairment.* Austin, TX: ProEd, 1991; 251–316.
27. Beukelman DR, Mirenda P. *Augmentative and alternative communication: management of severe communication disorders in children and adults.* Baltimore: Paul H. Brookes, 1992.
28. Netsell R, Daniel B. Dysarthria in adults: physiologic approach to rehabilitation. *Arch Phys Med Rehabil* 1979; 60:502–508.
29. Yorkston KM, Hammen VL, Beukelman DR, Traynor CD. The effect of rate control on the intelligibility and naturalness of dysarthric speech. *J Speech Hear Disord* 1990; 55:550–561.
30. Gonzalez J, Aronson A. Palatal lift prosthesis for treatment of anatomic and neurologic palatopharyngeal insufficiency. *Cleft Palate J* 1970; 7:91–104.
31. Yorkston KM, Honsinger MJ, Beukelman DR, Taylor T. The effects of palatal lift fitting on the perceived articulatory adequacy of dysarthric speakers. In: Yorkston KM, Beukelman DR, eds. *Recent advances in clinical dysarthria.* Austin, TX: ProEd, 1989; 85–98.
32. Bellaire K, Yorkston KM, Beukelman DR. Modification of breath patterning to increase naturalness of a mildly dysarthric speaker. *J Commun Disord* 1986; 19:271–280.
33. Yorkston KM, Miller RM, Strand EA. *Management of speech and swallowing disorders in degenerative disease.* Tucson: Communication Skill Builders, 1995.
34. Singer MI, Blom ED. An endoscopic technique for restoration of voice after laryngectomy. *Ann Otol Rhinol Laryngol* 1980; 89:529–533.
35. Hamaker RC, Singer MI, Blom ED, Daniels HA. Primary voice restoration at laryngectomy. *Arch Otolaryngol* 1985; 111:182–186.
36. Hilgers FJM, Balm AJM. Long-term results of vocal rehabilitation after total laryngectomy with the low-resistance, indwelling Provox™ voice prosthesis system. *Clin Otolaryngol* 1993; 18:517–523.
37. Singer MI, Blom ED, Hamaker RC. Further experience with voice restoration after total laryngectomy. *Ann Otol Rhinol Laryngol* 1981; 90:498–502.
38. Wetmore SJ, Johns ME, Baker SR. The Singer-Blom voice restoration procedure. *Arch Otolaryngol* 1981; 107:674–676.
39. Kao WW, Rose MM, Kimmel CA, Getch C, Silverman C. The outcome and techniuques of primary and secondary tracheoesophageal puncture. *Arch Otolaryngol Head Neck Surg* 1994; 120:301–307.
40. Singer MI, Blom ED, Hamaker RC. Pharyngeal plexus neurectomy for alaryngeal speech rehabilitation. *Laryngoscope* 1986; 96:50–54.
41. Robin DA, Schienberg S. Subcortical lesions and aphasia. *J Speech Hear Disord* 1990; 55:90–100.
42. Brookshire RH. Recognition of auditory sequences by aphasic, right hemisphere damaged and non-brain damaged subjects. *J Commun Disord* 1975; 8:51–59.
43. Duffy RJ, Duffy JR, Pearson KL. Pantomime recognition in aphasics. *J Speech Hear Res* 1975; 18:115–132.
44. Goodglass H, Kaplan E. *The assessment of aphasia and related disorders.* Philadelphia: Lea & Febiger, 1983.
45. Wallesch G, Kornhuber H, Brunner R, Kinz T, Hollerbach B, Sugar G. Lesions of the basal ganglia, thalamus, and deep white matter: differential effects on language functions. *Brain Lang* 1983; 20: 286–304.
46. Naeser MA. CT scan lesion size and lesion locus in cortical and subcortical aphasias. In: Kertesz A, ed. *Localization in neuropsychology.* New York: Academic Press, 1983; 63–120.
47. Naeser MA, Alexander MP, Helm-Estrabrooks N, Levine N, Laughlin SA, Geschwind NA. Aphasia with predominantly subcortical lesion sites: description of 3 capsular/putaminal aphasia syndromes. *Arch Neurol* 1982; 39:2–14.
48. Damasio A, Damasio H, Rizzo, Varney N, Gersch F. Aphasia with non-hemorrhagic lesions in the basal ganglia and internal capsule. *Arch Neurol* 1982; 39:15–20.
49. Alexander MP, LoVerme SR. Aphasia after left hemisphere intracerebral hemorrhage. *Neurology* 1980; 30:1193–1202.
50. Mohr JP, Watters WC, Duncan GW. Thalamic hemorrhage and aphasia. *Brain Lang* 1975; 2:3–17.
51. Darley FL. *Aphasia.* Philadelphia: WB Saunders, 1982.
52. Buckingham HW. Explanation in apraxia with consequences for the concept of apraxia of speech. *Brain Lang* 1979; 8:202–226.
53. Martin AD. Some objections to the term apraxia of speech. *J Speech Hear Disord* 1974; 39:53–64.
54. Bayles KA, Kaszniak AW. *Communication and cognition in normal aging and dementia.* Austin, TX: ProEd, 1987.
55. Schuell H. *The Minnesota test for the differential diagnosis of aphasia.* Minneapolis, MN: University of Minnesota Press, 1965.
56. Kertesz A. *The Western aphasia battery.* New York: Grune & Stratton, 1982.
57. Porch BE. *The Porch index of communicative ability.* Palo Alto, CA: Consulting Psychology Press, 1967.
58. DeRenzi E, Vignolo LA. The token test: a sensitive test to detect receptive disturbances in aphasia. *Brain* 1962; 85:665–678.
59. Noll JD, Randolph SR. Auditory semantic, syntactic, and retention errors made by aphasic subjects on the token test. *J Commun Disord* 1978; 11:543–553.
60. Swisher LP, Sarno MT. Token test scores of three matched patient groups: left brain damaged with aphasia; right brain damaged without aphasia; non-brain damaged. *Cortex* 1969; 5:264–273.
61. McNeil MR, Prescott TE. *Revised token test.* Baltimore: University Park Press, 1978.
62. DeRenzi E, Ferrai C. The reporter's test: a sensitive test to detect expressive disturbances in aphasics. *Cortex* 1978; 14:279–293.
63. LaPoint LL, Horner J. *Reading comprehension battery.* Tigard, OR: CC Publications, 1979.
64. Albert ML, Helm-Estabrooks N. Diagnosis and treatment of aphasia. Part I. *JAMA* 1988; 259:1043–1047.
65. Albert ML, Helm-Estabrooks N. Diagnosis and treatment of aphasia. Part II. *JAMA* 1988; 259:1205–1210.
66. Lubinski R. Environmental language intervention. In: Chapey R, ed. *Language intervention strategies in adult aphasia.* Baltimore: Williams & Wilkins, 1981; 223–245.
67. Simmons N. Interaction between communication and neurologic disorders. In: Darby JK, ed. *Speech and language evaluation in neurology: adult disorders.* Orlando, FL: Grune & Stratton, 1985; 3–28.
68. Burns MS, Halper AS, Mogil SI. *Clinical management of right hemisphere dysfunction.* Rockville, MD: Aspen Systems Corporation, 1985.
69. West JF, Leader BJ, Costagliola C. *Screening battery assessing cognition in patients with right cerebrovascular accidents.* Paper presented at New York State Speech and Hearing Association meeting, 1982.
70. Beukelman DR, Yorkston KM, eds. *Communication disorders following traumatic brain injury: management of cognitive, language, and motor impairments.* Austin, TX: Pro-Ed, 1991.
71. Groher M. Language and memory disorders following closed head trauma. *J Speech Hear Disord* 1977; 20:212–220.
72. Hagen C, Malkmus D, Burditt G. *Intervention strategies for language disorders secondary to head trauma.* Paper presented at short course, American Speech and Hearing Association convention, Atlanta, 1979.
73. Hagen C, Malkmus D, Durham E. Levels of cognitive functioning. In: *Rehabilitation of the head injured adult.* Downey, CA: Professional Staff Association, 1979.
74. Coelho CA, Liles BZ, Duffy RJ. Analysis of conversational discourse in head-injured adults. *J Head Trauma Rehabil* 1991; 6(2):92–99.
75. Halper AS, Cherney LR, Miller TK. *Clinical management of communication problems in adults with traumatic brain injury.* Gaithersburg, MD: Aspen Publishers, 1991.
76. Groher M. Communication disorders in adults. In: Rosenthal M, Griffith ER, Bond MR, Miller JD, eds. *Rehabilitation of the adult and child with traumatic brain injury.* Philadelphia: FA Davis, 1990; 148–162.
77. Wertz RT. Neuropathologies of speech and language: an introduction to patient management. In: Johns DF, ed. *Clinical management of neurogenic communication disorders.* Boston: Little, Brown, 1991; 1–96.
78. Bayles K. Language function in senile dementia. *Brain Lang* 1982; 16:265–280.
79. Bayles KA, Salmon DP, Tomoeda CK, et al. Semantic and letter category naming in Alzheimer's patients: a predictable difference. *Dev Neuropsychol* 1989; 5:335–347.
80. Obler L. *Language in age and dementia. Short course abstract.* Washington, DC: American Speech, Language, and Hearing Association, 1985.
81. Bayles KA, Tomoeda C. *Arizona battery for communication disorders of dementia.* Tucson, AZ: Canyonland, 1991.
82. Gelfand DW, Richter JE. *Dysphagia: diagnosis and treatment.* New York: Igaku-Shoin, 1989.

83. Logemann J. *Evaluation and treatment of swallowing disorders.* San Diego: College-Hill Press, 1983.
84. Palmer JB, Rubin NJ, Lara G, Crompton AW. Coordination of mastication and swallowing. *Dysphagia* 1992; 7:187–200.
85. Goyal RK. Disorders of the cricopharyngeus muscle. *Otolaryngol Clin North Am* 1984; 17:115–130.
86. Miller RM. Evaluation of swallowing disorders. In: Groher M, ed. *Dysphagia: diagnosis and management.* Boston: Butterworths, 1984; 85–110.
87. Palmer JB, DuChane AS. Rehabilitation of swallowing disorders in the elderly. In: Felsenthal G, Garrison SJ, Steinberg FU, eds. *Rehabilitation of the aging and older patient.* Baltimore: Williams & Wilkins, 1994; 275–287.
88. Siebens H, Trupe E, Siebens A, et al. Correlates and consequences of eating dependency in institutionalized elderly. *J Am Geriatr Soc* 1986; 34:192–198.
89. Martin BJW, Corlew MM. The incidence of communications disorders in dysphagic patients. *J Speech Hear Disord* 1990; 55:28–32.
90. Horner J, Massey EW. Silent aspiration following stroke. *Neurology* 1988; 38:317–319.
91. Palmer JB, DuChane AS, Donner MW. The role of radiology in the rehabilitation of swallowing. In: Jones B, Donner MW, eds. *Normal and abnormal swallowing: imaging in diagnosis and therapy.* New York: Springer-Verlag, 1991; 215–225.
92. Palmer JB, Kuhlemeier KV, Tippett DC, Lynch C. A protocol for the videofluorographic swallowing study. *Dysphagia* 1993; 8:209–214.
93. Logemann JA. *Manual for the videofluorographic study of swallowing.* Boston: College-Hill, 1986.
94. Langmore SE, Schatz K, Olsen N. Fiberoptic endoscopic examination of swallowing safety: a new procedure. *Dysphagia* 1988; 2:216–219.
95. Palmer JB, Holloway AM, Tanaka E. Detecting lower motor neuron dysfunction of the pharynx and larynx with electromyography. *Arch Phys Med Rehabil* 1991; 72:237–242.
96. Miller RM, Groher M. General treatment of swallowing disorders. In: Groher M, ed. *Dysphagia: diagnosis and management.* Boston: Butterworths, 1984; 113–132.
97. Fleming SM. Treatment of mechanical swallowing disorders. In: Groher M, ed. *Dysphagia: diagnosis and management.* Boston: Butterworths, 1984; 157–172.
98. Palmer JB, DuChane AS. Rehabilitation of swallowing disorders due to stroke. *Phys Med Rehabil Clin North Am* 1991; 2:529–546.
99. Logemann JA, Kahrilas PJ, Kobara M, et al. The benefit of head rotation on pharyngoesophageal dysphagia. *Arch Phys Med Rehabil* 1989; 70:767–771.
100. Lindemann RC. Diverting the paralyzed larynx: a reversible procedure for intractable aspiration. *Laryngoscope* 1975; 85:157–180.

Rehabilitation Medicine: Principles and Practice, Third Edition,
edited by Joel A. DeLisa and Bruce M. Gans.
Lippincott–Raven Publishers, Philadelphia © 1998.

CHAPTER 13

Prescriptions, Referrals, Order Writing, and the Rehabilitation Team Function

John C. King, T. Russell Nelson, Mary L. Heye, Thomas C. Turturro, and Mary Nelle D. Titus

Comprehensive rehabilitation patients require the services of multiple health care providers who possess unique skills and training that may be necessary for the full restoration of these patients' function. The competent physiatrist must be able to communicate in an optimal fashion to all these providers to meet all the needs and services required by the patient. Prescriptions, referrals, and orders are basic tools by which the physiatrist may communicate the desired involvement of other rehabilitation or medical specialties in assessment, treatment planning, treatment delivery, provision of equipment, and fitting of adaptive devices. Medical specialties that are commonly involved with the rehabilitation patient may include neurosurgery, neurology, geriatrics, primary care, family practice, internal medicine, and pediatrics, psychiatry, and orthopedics. Other specialties are consulted as needed. Assessment, treatment planning, and therapy are often provided by rehabilitation clinicians specializing in occupational therapy, physical therapy, kinesiotherapy, psychology and neuropsychology, recreational therapy, speech–language pathology, rehabilitation nursing, social work, dietary science, and case management (see Chapter 1 and Fig. 13-1) (1). Which professions are involved with a particular patient and the extent of those involvements are largely determined by the nature of the patient's deficits and the structure of the setting in which rehabilitation is being conducted. As indicated by assessment, the physiatrist requests the participation of other rehabilitation specialists in determination of appropriateness for rehabilitation, planning, conduct, and monitoring of treatment, discharge planning, and patient/family education.

Writing physical medicine and rehabilitation (PM&R) therapy referrals, equipment prescriptions, and coordinating care requires the skills of a comprehensive clinician adept in both therapist and patient interactions. Deficits in knowledge base or team and patient interaction skills lead to suboptimal treatment plans. The well-trained rehabilitation medicine specialist is able to develop comprehensive PM&R treatment plans of substantial detail if warranted. The degree of documentation and specification required depends on the mode of team interaction and treatment adopted by the professionals involved. Effective participation in treatment planning nevertheless requires the ability both to generate and support the rationale behind multiple interventions. These interventions must be appreciated in terms of their impact on function as well as on pathophysiological processes.

Treatment plans are generated from goals that arise from the problem list developed during evaluation. The evaluation (see Chapters 4 through 12) results in a set of identified problems that can be variously classified, often as medical, rehabilitation, and social problems. A set of goals or desired treatment outcomes is generated, along with an estimate of the duration of therapy necessary to accomplish each. Such goals form the heart of a comprehensive treatment plan. This plan is a tool that patients, families, and therapists or other treating professionals examine for prognosis and expectations. It forms the basis from which all team members may suggest additions or deletions. The treatment plan is not a

J. C. King: Department of Rehabilitation Medicine, University of Texas Health Science Center at San Antonio, San Antonio, Texas 78284.

T. R. Nelson: Department of Rehabilitation Medicine, University of Texas Health Science Center at San Antonio, San Antonio, Texas 78284; and Department of Veterans Affairs, South Texas Veterans Health Care System, San Antonio, Texas 78284.

M. L. Heye: Department of Acute Nursing Care, University of Texas Health Science Center at San Antonio, San Antonio, Texas 78284.

T. C. Turturro: Department of Physical Therapy, University of Texas Health Science Center at San Antonio, San Antonio, Texas 78284.

M. N. D. Titus: Medical Rehabilitation, San Antonio, Texas 78249–1859.

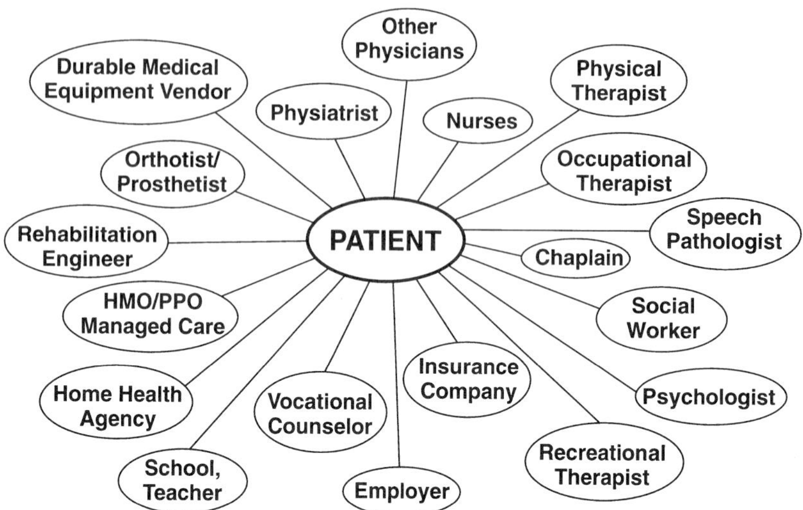

FIG. 13-1. Multiple caregivers may be required in comprehensive rehabilitation.

static document but remains dynamic as goals are accomplished, new goals are identified and added, or some goals become irrelevant or unachievable and are deleted.

Treatment strategies are developed to accomplish the identified goals. The specific strategies can be physician-directed, therapist-directed, or, most ideally, mutually derived by the patient and team through the interdisciplinary process. The rehabilitation medicine specialist should be knowledgeable about all pertinent therapies to apply and the specific interventions available to each therapy specialty that might help accomplish the desired goals (see Chapter 1). The availability, benefits, and risks of adaptive equipment and their use to facilitate independence in activities of daily living (ADL), improve mobility, communication, and leisure activities, or decrease pain must be well understood to be prescribed appropriately. A knowledge of expected effects and potential side effects, as well as a pathophysiological and pharmacologic knowledge base, allow therapeutic interventions to be made with the least possible morbidity. This occurs when treatment is supervised by a physiatrist who can offer appropriate precautions and monitoring of referrals and prescriptions. The comprehensive treatment plan is initiated by referrals, prescriptions, and direct physician interventions. Factors that influence the form and details of the written therapy referral or equipment prescription include team communication needs, styles of interaction, and the need for quality control.

TEAM COMMUNICATION

Comprehensive medical rehabilitation requires the interactions of multiple caregivers to provide the breadth of services needed by people with physical and cognitive impairments (2–4). Patient needs range from acute and chronic medical problems to physical impairments, their complex interactions, and the impact each has on the patient's psychological, vocational, and social integration. The primary goal of interactions between care providers is communication of the patient's needs and coordination of their efforts in a synergistic manner (5). Physician-initiated prescriptions, referrals, or orders are written communications that intend to provide for patient needs by requesting the services provided by multiple caregivers. The form such written communications take depends in part on the style of interaction adopted by involved professionals. Redundant, uncoordinated, or incomplete care can occur when patients' desires and needs are addressed from multiple vantage points without communication or coordination among the different caregiver professionals. Despite the widespread perception that a coordinated team effort enhances the effectiveness of such complex patients' care, definitive studies are lacking, and results depend on the variables examined in the few studies that have been reported (2,6,7).

Accrediting agencies such as the Commission on Accreditation for Rehabilitation Facilities (CARF) and, more recently, the Joint Commission on the Accreditation of Healthcare Organizations (JCAHO) as well as federal regulations in certain instances require "interdisciplinary teams" (6,8–10), yet many styles of interaction exist that are influenced in part by the practice environment (11). Four general styles of interaction between physicians and other professional caregivers are discussed: the traditional *medical model* without a formal team; the *multidisciplinary team,* which some call the traditional medical model of team interaction; the *interdisciplinary* model; and the *transdisciplinary* model. Each model's advantages and disadvantages are outlined, and their impact on prescriptions, orders, referrals, and treatment plan writing is discussed. These four models of interaction are described in pure form, though features of each are often combined to take the greatest advantage of the benefits each model may offer for a particular practice setting. Effective team dynamics and communication are always important, but especially for successful implementation of the interdisciplinary and transdisciplinary models. The reader is referred to the sections on team development and dynamics, conflict and disagreement, and communication in Chapter 1 for a more thorough discussion of these issues.

STYLES OF INTERACTIONS

Medical Model

Traditional medical care results in a model in which a physician attends to the patient's needs. If services of another discipline are desired, that professional is consulted and given either specific or general requests for assistance to meet the needs of the patient as perceived by the attending physician. The quality of the service rendered and thus future consultations depend on meeting those perceived needs. The consultant would usually discuss any additional identified needs first with the attending physician before proceeding with additional treatment, in recognition of the fact that the attending physician may have additional information and insight not available to the consultant. This traditional system results in a clear chain of responsibility that continues to be well respected medicolegally. Multiple consultations may result in many professionals doing multiple tasks. Coordination of these efforts by the attending physician or among the involved professionals can be difficult or incomplete, resulting in less efficient patient care. This is one of the major disadvantages to the medical model of patient care (3,5,12).

Multidisciplinary Team Model

The multidisciplinary team model provides a means for multiple professionals who require frequent interactions to meet and coordinate efforts on a consistent basis. It typically remains an attending-physician-controlled team in which most interactions are between consultants and the primary attending. Discussion between consulting professionals is held to a minimum or, at best, directed by the attending physician when necessary. This emphasis on vertical communication (Fig. 13-2) evolved from the medical model attending physician's role and relationship with consultants (11).

Team conferences can be conducted efficiently with such clear lines of authority and control, but lateral communication (see Fig. 13-2) may suffer (12,13). This tendency to impede the free flow of communication horizontally between the team members is recognized as an obstacle to the optimal use of each participant's specific expertise and problem-solving skills. This may negate the possible group synergism, which can create a product greater than the sum of its parts or, in clinical terms, a care plan better than any one participant could have developed alone (11,14). The interdisciplinary team model attempts to improve communication and enhance group synergism, thus fostering a sense of mutual authority and responsibility (4,13,14).

Interdisciplinary Team Model

Interdisciplinary teams benefit from lateral communication flow that occurs as easily as vertical communication in the multidisciplinary team. This is because the expected norm is group decision making and group responsibility for developing optimal care planning (13). The problem orientation and ease of flow of lateral communication in the interdisciplinary team processes are similar in function to the project orientation and communication patterns of matrix organization (16,17). The patient is considered part of this planning group and has a central role in the team's considerations (Fig. 13-1) (5,18,19). With the emphasis on mutual communication and responsibility, the patient care-coordinating conferences may be led by any team member (Fig. 13-4) (12,20). One objective of this model is to allow a freer exchange of ideas and thereby benefit from the group synergy concept (5,21). Disadvantages can include considerably less time effectiveness in completing patient care conferences; in theory, this is offset somewhat by improved communication and better problem solving. Such teams also require considerable training in the team process, generally not received during the years of formal training in the individual disciplines (13). Team communication and conflict resolution are discussed further in Chapter 1. This non-patient-care training is expensive and does not ensure success (4,13,22). The commitments and personality traits found in

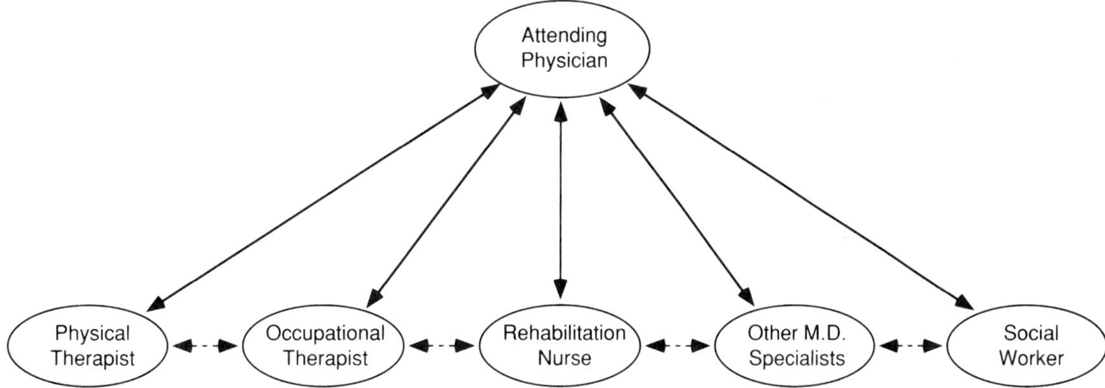

FIG. 13-2. Multidisciplinary team conference structure. Vertical communication *(solid lines)* may serve to limit horizontal communication *(dotted lines)* between team care providers.

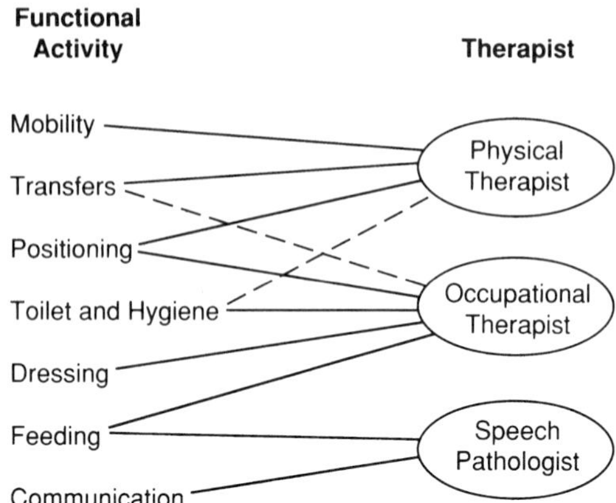

FIG. 13-3. The appropriate therapy specialties must be chosen for the patient's specific deficiencies. Examples from physical therapy, occupational therapy, and speech pathology are shown. Team coordination is required to prevent duplication of services and avoid gaps in services needed.

the members of a successful interdisciplinary team are similar to those that engender good referral patterns between physicians (Table 13-1) (12,22). The physician may be uncomfortable with the team decision-making process because the physician is the one who must usually assume the greatest medicolegal responsibility for the team's actions and plans. There may be difficulty in having the physician complete the appropriate prescription for such team-generated plans, especially if the plans seem to be different from what the physician recalled or desired. Such conflicts are ideally resolved in team meetings, but delays in completion of the paperwork can jeopardize the anticipated optimal patient care.

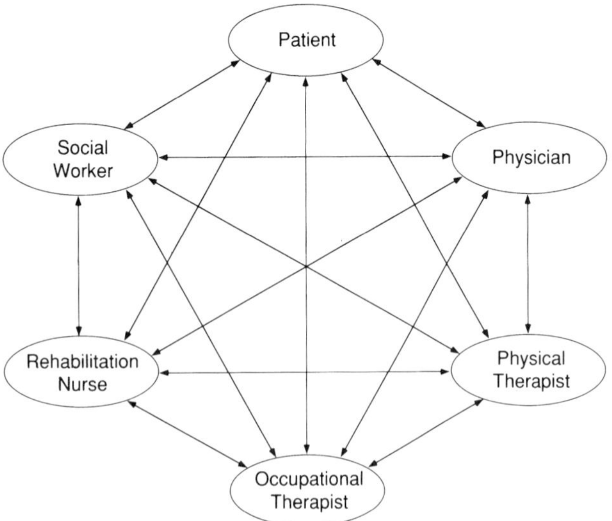

FIG. 13-4. In an interdisciplinary team, communication and decision-making mutualism are encouraged. One team member usually acts as the patient care coordinator, but lack of role dominance allows any team member to be eligible for this role.

TABLE 13-1. *Personal characteristics of successful interdisciplinary team participants*

1. Accept differences and perspectives of others
2. Function interdependently
3. Negotiate role with other team members
4. Form new values, attitudes, and perceptions
5. Tolerate constant review and challenge of ideas
6. Take risks
7. Possess personal identity and integrity
8. Accept team philosophy of care

Adapted from Given B, Simmons S. The interdisciplinary health-care team: fact or fiction? *Nurs Forum* 1977; 16: 165–183, with permission.

Transdisciplinary Team Model

Transdisciplinary teams, a more recent development, encourage not only communication but cross-treatment between disciplines. These have developed largely out of educational models (3,11,24,25) and have been justified on the basis of economic market forces and inadequate numbers of therapy professionals (4,26–28). Cross-training, or multiskilling, of available teachers and aides is reported to be very helpful in providing the needed services. Such programs, when self-rated against no integration of the disciplines, are rated very favorably (23,24,27). The transdisciplinary team has also found favor with traumatic brain injury teams (11,27). Consistency of information exchange, with the patient intrinsic to cotreatment, is cited as an advantage (24,25,27). Furthermore, the exchange of information between disciplines is highly valued, with therapists or teachers noting expansion of their own professional expertise. A future corps of rehabilitation generalists as the main therapy providers has been prognosticated and advocated (26,28). Whether such informally shared professional knowledge and cotreatment leads to competent therapists in each other's fields is doubtful. The issues of technically competent care, state licensure, and qualifications may limit the development of truly transdisciplinary rehabilitation generalist therapists (6,28). This approach nevertheless is highly valued in certain settings.

Research is lacking to determine which of the previous models is most effective. The usefulness of such studies almost certainly will depend on which parameters are examined (i.e., team and patient satisfaction versus outcome). It may be that different models are more effective in different practice environments. The medical care, multidisciplinary team, interdisciplinary team, and transdisciplinary team models can be found in various settings in rehabilitation. In a free-standing office practice or in inpatient consultations in an acute care hospital, the medical care model often is used. This becomes especially true when referrals are made to therapists who are geographically distant or with whom frequent interaction may be difficult. Standing hospital programs that often include nonphysiatric physicians, such as cardiac rehabilitation, pulmonary rehabilitation, geriatrics, prosthetics clinic, myelomeningocele clinic, and the like, may use the multidisciplinary model with a primary physician in charge. Interdisciplinary teams generally consist of a stable population of health caregivers that often can be found in association with specialized units in a comprehensive rehabilitation hospital, unit, or service. Transdisciplinary teams are more common when a stable population of professionals is to provide long-term care for a patient, and cognitive-educational needs are more prominent than intense physical needs.

These models of interaction are meant to enhance communication and thereby coordination of care. The practicing physiatrist may prefer one style over the others but often finds it necessary to communicate with patients and multiple care providers in all of these models, or some combination, depending on practice setting. Specificity of orders and the methods in which treatment plans are developed vary with the treatment and communication models adopted.

MULTIPLICITY OF CARE PROVIDERS

Comprehensive rehabilitation of people with physical and/or cognitive impairments can be an enormously complex task. The desired goals are not disorder-specific. The patient's psychological, religious, vocational, social, and personal needs, desires, and priorities are used to establish and prioritize rehabilitation goals. As an integrated member of the treatment team, the patient is expected to make a transition from the passive observer role common during the acute treatment phase of an injury or debilitating disease to an active participatory role. This shift in roles requires some patient orientation and education about the team process of evaluating and establishing goals. Patient autonomy should be supported and encouraged. Not only are patients' medical needs addressed, but the psychological, social, religious, and vocational impacts of their disabling disorder require attention. Planning and facilitating all desired interventions can be accomplished best by multiple disciplines evaluating issues with the patient from their unique points of expertise. This knowledge must then be shared and formulated into a cohesive plan of treatment.

Professional healthcare givers in the many disciplines common to rehabilitation (see Fig. 13-1) spend many years acquiring specific skills necessary to effectively assess patient problems that fall within their professional expertise. This often includes the use of test instruments standardized for specific disorders. They learn to formulate and communicate their discipline-specific treatment plans and goals; educate patients, family, and other professionals; apply discipline-specific interventions; and monitor progress. From their unique vantage points, they often uncover problems or issues not apparent to others. Although physiatrists have the most wide-based training among physician specialties in the issues involved in physical impairments, disabilities, and handicaps, their perspective generally will not be as specific in any one area as that of a therapist who focuses exclusively in that area. Because the interventions required are more than any one provider can reasonably give, the expertise of many professionals is used to divide up needs according to areas of treatment or intervention expertise. To avoid fracturing or neglecting needs and goals that cross disciplines, team communication is used to formulate comprehensive treatment plans (4). Descriptions and roles of the various healthcare providers commonly found on the rehabilitation team are outlined in Chapter 1. The competent rehabilitation medicine physician will appreciate those skills listed and develop an extensive knowledge base of the capabilities these specialists possess.

Through the medical model, the patient often first encounters a physiatrist, a specialist in PM&R, by referral. With rehabilitation as the first goal, the physiatrist also will address associated medical problems unique to disabling disorders such as dysfunctional spasticity or optimal pharmacologic bladder management in the spinal-cord-injured patient. The physiatrist often initiates the referrals to the remaining rehabilitation professionals. In the inpatient comprehensive rehabilitation setting, the physiatrist may be the sole physician involved.

A physiatrist is knowledgeable in the medical care issues of physically debilitating diseases and trauma and also has the broadest knowledge of the expertise available from each of the various team professionals (see Fig. 13-1). Identifying the areas of patient need addressed by each of these professionals will ensure that appropriate resources are used; examples are shown in Figure 13-3. The physician who specializes in medical rehabilitation must be aware of techniques and therapeutic interventions available from each discipline that could have positive impact on the care of their patients as well as which interventions are specifically contraindicated.

The appropriate consulted professionals, the patient, and family form the rehabilitation team. The multiplicity of potential needs—medical, physical, psychological, vocational, educational, social, or spiritual—require multiple health care professionals to whom referrals, orders, or prescriptions may be sent. The combined input of the team members should form the basis for a coordinated, comprehensive treatment plan including methods, goals, and estimates of length of time for completion of each. The treatment plan is dynamic and will require frequent modifications, updates, and revisions as the patient progresses.

THERAPY REFERRALS AND ORDER WRITING

Therapy referrals and order writing are based on the initial evaluation (see Chapters 4 through 12). This may or may not include team evaluation input or consensus toward the treatment plan. In the medical model and multidisciplinary team model, orders and treatment plans usually are developed initially by the physiatrist, although they may be modified later as input is received from consultants. In the interdisciplinary team model, a period of evaluation by appropriate disciplines occurs before group development and consensus on the comprehensive treatment plan. Depending on frequency of team meetings, this may introduce a delay before coordinated team interventions begin. In the transdisciplinary model, transdisciplinary evaluations are the rule, frequently allowing team treatment plans to be developed during the same evaluation and treatment session. Although time efficient, the transdisciplinary team may have less time available for deliberation or complex problem solving, given the concurrent patient treatment occurring.

Once the problems and treatment goals have been delineated, the process of referrals and order writing can proceed. Often this can be facilitated by organizing problems into functional areas of concern. One organizational scheme is to list problems that are primarily medical in nature first, followed by functional limitations or rehabilitation problems, and then associated social-environmental problems. This allows orders to be broken down into medical, therapy, and psychosocial issues, though overlap of problems between these categories is common. Problem-based medical management of medical issues is now commonplace and integrates well into this scheme.

Interacting with the professionals providing rehabilitation of the complex problems requires the physiatrist to possess a diverse professional knowledge and highly developed communication skills. The resources available should be applied optimally to obtain the best results for the patient. Through correct identification of the suitable providers, appropriate referrals or orders communicate in as complete a fashion as possible without limiting creative problem solving or the reciprocal feedback that helps take full advantage of the available expertise. The format of these orders and referrals depends on the practice setting and the model of communication customary in that setting.

Medical Model Referrals and Orders

In the outpatient setting, the practice may involve a well-integrated cohesive team, but more often the rehabilitation medicine specialist is a sole practitioner using community-wide resources. The former type is discussed below under the appropriate team model section. The latter outpatient practice is similar to inpatient physiatric consultations in an acute care hospital where individual therapy departments may exist without organized teams to coordinate the activities of multiple providers. In such settings, referrals and orders need to be more specific because frequent verbal feedback and clarification is not as readily available. Charting helps with inpatient coordination and communication but is less available in the outpatient setting. Written prescriptions help avoid ambiguity and ensure that the patient is being treated as desired (see Written Prescriptions, Orders, and Referrals).

Although treatment recommendations ideally are based on clear physiological rationales and clinically proven efficacy, such a literature base often is lacking or incomplete. Practitioners tend to be strongly influenced by their own personal successes and failures, applying lessons learned from past patients to future patients. If the physiatrist does not know which approach to treatment a consulted discipline is taking, then it is unlikely any specific learning will occur from that interaction to benefit the rehabilitation physician's future management of similar patients. Thus, knowing the particular interventions to be used will help enhance the clinical acumen of the referring physiatrist. Indeed, knowledge of how to prescribe in as much detail as is necessary is one measure the American Board of Physical Medicine and Rehabilitation examiners use to determine competence.

Another unique advantage the physiatrist holds is the understanding of how therapeutic interventions affect the pathophysiological process of disease states. This knowledge may serve as a safety check for his or her patients. The physical medicine aspect of physiatry demands that the physics, biophysics, physiology, and pathophysiology of all prescribed physical modalities be well appreciated. This allows rational prescription of intensity, application methods, sites, duration, frequency, and precautions as warranted for such treatments. The physiatrist must both prescribe appropriate interventions and proscribe inappropriate interventions. It is from such patient safety concerns that legal requirements for physician prescriptions were mandated. Without specific understanding and concurrence in the treatment strategies used, this safety net of supervision is lost.

The major disadvantage in an extremely precise prescription format is that it may be taken as a signal by the consultant not to think or be creative in addressing the patient's problems but, rather, merely to perform the services of a technician. This may occur even though an order to evaluate the patient has been included—this often is legally required by state rules whether prescribed or not. To minimize this potential negative impact on professional creativity and problem-solving expertise, requests for feedback should be specifically included. It often is helpful to request phone consultation with therapists after their evaluation but before they begin treatment to explore additional options or to convey significant yet sensitive information. If a phone consultation is requested, priority must be given to receiving such calls, or this form of feedback and collaboration will not be sufficiently reinforced to be maintained. Phone consultations may allow a more optimal treatment approach to be pursued through modifications to orders by phone while providing the attending rehabilitation physician with the knowledge to adequately coordinate the specific interventions being applied. This will also help provide the order specifics often necessary for reimbursement of therapist-provided services.

Occasionally, team members are found who are unwilling to follow specific treatment orders and who proceed on a treatment plan based on their impression of what is in the patient's best interests, without consulting the prescribing physician. This violates the trust placed in the consultant and rules by which one should engender referrals from physicians (see Table 13-2) (29). Such practices also expose the therapist and patient to medically unsupervised care. If this situation cannot be corrected, the patient, for his or her safety

TABLE 13-2. *Personal practices that engender referrals from other physicians*

1. Never say anything bad about another physician, especially in front of a patient.
2. Send a typed note to the referring physician every time you see the patient as an outpatient.
3. Tell the referring physician in person or by phone of major changes in a patient's condition or treatment plan.
4. Never discharge another physician's patient from a hospital without informing that physician.
5. Do not provide care to referred patients that is in the area of expertise of the referring physicians, unless they have asked you to do so.
6. Regardless of your opinion on providing free care, do not refuse to see a patient who cannot pay or who has poor insurance if referred by a physician who also sends you many paying patients.
7. Do not communicate with the referring physician directly in hospital chart notes, particularly about an item of disagreement. Remember that the chart is a legal document. A lawyer may ask you to read your chart notes in court.
8. Get to know your referring physicians and their individual ways of handling patients. Avoid violating personal habits and biases.
9. Never send a patient who has been referred to you to another specialist unless the referring physician concurs.
10. Never leave a referring physician uninformed about the disposition of his or her patient. Physicians usually stop sending you patients if they know they will never see them again.
11. Answer consultations promptly.
12. Keep up your competence. Your referring physicians expect you to be on the cutting edge of your field.
13. Give the referring physician some suggestions or leads if you cannot definitively help him or her with a referred patient.
14. Let physicians' calls come through to you, but take a number and call back other persons.
15. Use a tickler file to keep up with patient needs.
16. Have a method for handling angry patients. Let them get all their emotion out—do not interrupt. Lower your voice and talk slowly. Never argue with their feelings, only with the facts of the case.

From Braddom RL. Practice issues in the hospital-based rehabilitation unit. In: Melvin JL, Odderson IR, eds. Clinical rehabilitation and physiatric practice. *Phys Med Rehabil Clin North Am* 1996; 7:31–41, with permission.

and optimal care, should be redirected to more cooperative therapy professionals. General orders requesting "evaluate and treat," sometimes because of lack of better knowledge, tend to promote such practices. Although this takes advantage of the therapist's creativity and expertise, it may restrict the physician's ability to supervise or coordinate patient care and tends to reduce the advantage of multiple professionals' synergism. Habitual poor physician support has, in part, encouraged some therapy groups to seek independent practices, also called direct access, wherein no medical supervision is required (30). The relationship between a physiatrist and consulted professionals should be a collegial, mutually supportive one because a domineering, rigid posture serves only to dampen creativity and problem solving between professionals and thus may diminish the quality of patient care (23). Managed care may restrict access to only certain providers. This adds weight to the value of being able to generate rapport, collegiality and a sense of teamwork with many different rehabilitation professionals in many different settings.

A physiatrist may evaluate patients in the outpatient setting, in which no other professional consultations are required. In this situation, instructions to the patient about medications, side effects, therapeutic exercise home programs, or simple modalities (e.g., heating pads, ice packs, home traction) are the important communications. Informational brochures and pictographic flyers frequently are available from national advocacy groups (see Table 13-3), or can be devised to help reinforce patient comprehension and therefore compliance with the prescribed home program. Without the benefit of a therapist who interacts frequently with the patient and reports problems regularly, more frequent reevaluations may be necessary to ensure both compliance and progress. Increasingly case management nurses may become involved and may serve as valuable coordination resources and advocates for the patient with third party payors.

When formal therapy is ordered, treatment referrals should specify any patient education or instruction desired. This includes requesting home programs and follow-up to verify compliance as necessary. Home health care services often terminate treatment because of funding constraints before all goals have been accomplished. Using therapy time before such terminations to provide patient and family training in home programs may significantly extend gains.

Multidisciplinary Team Referrals and Orders

In the multidisciplinary team setting, the physiatrist may be a team member, a consultant, or more often act as the

TABLE 13-3. *Patient education resources*

Scriptographic Booklets
Channing L. Bete Co., Inc.
South Deerfield, MA 01373

Krames Communication
1100 Grundy Lane
San Bruno, CA 94066-3030

The Source Book of Patient Education Materials for Physical Medicine and Rehabilitation, extremely complete resource for patient education materials for people with any disability; over 700 pages. New edition is due in 1997.
The Center for Disability and Rehabilitation
Comanche County Memorial Hospital
P.O. Box 129
Lawton, OK 73502
(405)355-8620, ext. 3271

primary attending physician. In such a group, the same specificity of orders often is required to initiate therapy, but is modified more readily after input from consultants at regularly scheduled patient care team conferences. Priorities of goals and treatments also are more easily discussed verbally than in the written form. This allows some of the subtleties of comprehensive management to be more effectively conveyed and coordinated. Some degree of coordination between consultants also occurs at multidisciplinary conferences, but not as free a flow of problem-solving creativity as allowed at interdisciplinary team conferences. Format usually consists of consultants giving their reports (i.e., initial evaluations or progress since last conference) and recommendations. Other members ideally monitor the input, but the primary consultant determines the solution to any perceived problems and organizes all the input into a modified problem list and treatment plan. Many treatment modifications are made by verbal orders, with feedback guaranteed by regular meetings. In this setting, it is not necessary to include the time until next physician follow-up or desired frequency and mechanism of follow-up therapy reports on the original orders.

Interdisciplinary Team Referrals and Orders

The format of initial orders to consultants who comprise an interdisciplinary team often is based on requesting a general evaluation, with specific evaluation instruments and the comprehensive treatment plans to be discussed and mutually derived. Occasionally, to avoid delays in initiating therapy, broad categories of intervention also are requested (e.g., "ADL training"). The specifics, however, should be discussed and integrated by the team into a comprehensive individualized patient treatment plan. If the patient's treatment plan is not specified but consists only of general orders for initial evaluations and general treatment, or treatment ordered according to a protocol (e.g., "quadriplegic protocol"), then the shortcomings of a setting with no dynamic, creative problem-solving interactions may persist. Also, a generalized order format implies little attention to the patient's specific and unique needs. It may be countered that therapists adapt the program to this patient's unique needs, but professionalism still functions in isolation, which defeats the advantage of the interdisciplinary team process. Although the mutualism of the interdisciplinary team implies no dominant specialty, it does not exclude any member from the responsibility to be interdependent of the creative input from other members in establishing his or her own specific treatment interventions. This means the physician should consider input from the physical therapist and therapeutic recreation specialist as well as from a consulting psychiatrist before starting antidepressant medications. Territory is both relinquished by all and embraced by all, although, in the end, specific needs and interventions are assigned by the group to those individual team members who have the greatest expertise in that area, as determined by team consensus.

Because the comprehensive treatment plan is not developed solely by the admitting physician, and specific interventions are decided by mutual consensus among all team members, the actual specifics of treatment can be cryptic for the PM&R resident physician in training. This is especially true if the medicolegally required orders remain generalized or if the specific treatment plans are signed much later by the attending physician without the resident necessarily being in the loop. This may occur because only the attending signature is required to meet hospital and third-party payer rules. Much of resident training is funded by inpatient rehabilitation hospitals or units in which the interdisciplinary team process is most often used. It is necessary not only that generalized order formats be appreciated but that the specifics of therapy interventions and efficacy be prescribed for other less-integrated settings. If the specifics are not discussed in team meetings, then the full benefit of the interdisciplinary team process is not being realized. Many times, multidisciplinary teams with good mutual interactive skills will be labeled interdisciplinary, but each professional maintains full control of his or her specialty's area, with little cross-disciplinary discussion of methods and approaches. Such teams remain multidisciplinary despite labels to the contrary. In this setting, general orders may become accepted but may be counterproductive to the educational process of the physician, the medical supervision of the patient, and the collective group synergism that can enhance creative problem solving. Becoming interdisciplinary is threatening, challenging, and time consuming but satisfying in increasing collegial relationships and in deriving optimal treatment plans. A marginal professional cannot hide, but the team process attempts to compensate for such members (6). Professional growth is challenged, and many are not comfortable in such an exposed position (see Table 13-1).

Transdisciplinary Team Referrals and Orders

All members are involved collaboratively in treatments in the transdisciplinary team approach. Doing is an excellent method for learning, especially when the information shared among the treating professionals is pertinent and applicable to the moment. Having another professional depend on your input as you are cotreating is both rewarding and self-affirming. The importance of each member's beliefs can be emphasized and appreciated in a very practical hands-on experience. The team member does not have to wonder whether a communication about a belief's importance was received adequately when it becomes essential to the treatment approach integrated between professionals during a cotreatment. Many reports on the transdisciplinary approach emphasize the high ratings such approaches received by the treating disciplines (24,25,27). Collaboration and coordination of effort certainly are optimized because the disciplines have the opportunity to communicate throughout both the evaluation and treatment of patients. This sometimes leads to no formal team meetings aside from patient care except perhaps to provide regulation or third-party payer-necessitated documentation. If all the disciplines in comprehensive rehabilitation could be integrated sufficiently that each felt comfortable treating any patient's problem, regardless of usual discipline specificity, then a rehabilitation therapy generalist could be envisioned (26). Such a corps of professionals would certainly appreciate problems from a broader perspective and, in an era of shortage, allow for a certain ease of cross-coverage. The greatest impediment to such a development is the necessity by certification laws and ethical considerations of providing skilled, competent professional care (4,6). Billing also can be an ethical dilemma. Should a single patient treated for 1 hour by three cotreating professionals be billed for 1 hour of therapy or 3? Should the therapy time be billed on the schedule of the best-paying specialty present or equally divided among the therapy disciplines treating? It remains an open question as to whether cotreatment results in each professional becoming more competent or simply exposes the patient to subprofessional care in areas in which the cotreating caregiver lacks certified expertise.

The advantage of fluid treatment plans that adapt to the patients' changing status can be a disadvantage when such plans must be developed on the spot. This allows little time for deliberation or consideration of alternatives because treatment must be given promptly. Written plans may not keep up with the current flow of treatment, causing difficulties when a patient must make the transition to other care providers. Indeed, written treatment plans often are generated as a retrospective report of the patient's past treatments and progress.

If the physician team member is a part of the treatment team, then any concerns about medical safety and medical treatment coordination can be addressed as treatment progresses. This, however, is unusual, with the rehabilitation physician often referring patients to such teams in which the physician will not act as a cotherapist. In such a setting, the more generalized order format may not allow adequate communication of the physician's concerns and treatment goals, especially because formal team conferences may not be frequent. Because the treating professionals may be addressing areas outside their specific expertise, the comprehensiveness with which all specific therapy issues are addressed may be of concern. In such a setting, it may be to the patient's advantage for the physician to write more specific and detailed orders to ensure that the breadth of patient issues identified by the physician will be addressed. Some mechanism to allow flexibility in approaches while maintaining direction toward the desired goals is important. Thus, treatment orders or referrals are written in a very goal-directed way, giving suggestions for treatment methods or models to consider. A mechanism for feedback on the approaches taken also is important to enhance the prescribing physician's supervision and learning experience. Without such interaction, prolonged ineffectiveness or perhaps even contraindicated approaches may result without the benefit of a physiatrist's professional expertise. Because of the possible professional "dilution" in the transdisciplinary approach, even closer reevaluation of care by the prescribing professional may be indicated.

WRITTEN PROTOCOLS, PRESCRIPTIONS, ORDERS, AND REFERRALS

Communication

The purpose of physician-generated protocols, prescriptions, orders, and referrals is to communicate patient needs adequately and to request services from another professional. In the case of medications, this applies to the prescription sent to the pharmacist. In rehabilitation, it applies to the services requested from the various professionals described above. The rehabilitation medicine specialist must use his or her expertise first to decide what the patient's needs are. The physiatrist's broad knowledge of the capabilities of various rehabilitation professionals allows selection of the appropriate professionals to be consulted (see Figs. 13-1 and 13-3). Each selected professional is then sent a referral or orders, depending on the setting. The content depends on the team process in effect in that setting. Referrals in the medical model or multidisciplinary team model should include all elements listed in the first part of Table 13-4 to provide adequate communication (4). The referral should include a mechanism for feedback and possibly an invitation for pretreatment discussion should there exist some doubt as to the most efficacious plan of treatment. If such an approach is taken, priority must be given to responding to therapist-initiated phone consultations, similar to the courtesy that should be offered to referring physicians (see Table 13-2) (29). Referrals to interdisciplinary team members often are requests for evaluation, with the specifics of treatment to be discussed and agreed on at the next team conference, wherein a written treatment plan and orders will be developed. Referrals that are to be addressed by a transdisciplinary team can be performed in a way similar to the interdisciplinary team, if a postevaluation conference can be planned, but otherwise are best left in the detailed format of the medical model. Protocols may be established by the collective consensus of a treatment team, especially for commonly seen disorders, that require little variation in approach. These should be concurred on by all treating professionals before their implementation and often require significant development time. A protocol must not become an excuse not to think or customize the treatment approach according to the patient's unique needs and circumstances. All formats for orders should provide a mechanism for feedback and subsequent discussion should changes in treatment needs be perceived by the treating team as the patient progresses.

Quality Control

Without follow-up, the efficacy of any intervention cannot be evaluated or documented. Referrals for therapy as well

TABLE 13-4. *Seven requirements for therapy referrals*

Required of *All* Referrals

1. Discipline of therapist to whom referral is directed: may include referral to a specific team
2. Diagnosis for which treatment is being requested
3. Request for evaluation
4. Goals of treatment with expected duration
5. Intensity, frequency, and initial duration of treatment desired: may be modified after consultation with therapy professional according to patient's rate of progress
6. Precautions: includes other diagnoses or problems that could impede or contraindicate certain interventions, and necessary patient monitoring during therapy with recommended limitations to maintain patient's safety
7. Mechanism for feedback, date, and signature: date when physician is to reevaluate patient, request for phone consultation or progress reports, or implied team staffing if referred to an established team

Specifics *Possibly* Needed in Therapy Referrals

1. a. If a specific therapist is desired may be listed as *"Discipline*/Attention: *Therapist's Name"*
   b. If to a specific team, may include each therapy discipline desired or left to be defined, implying referrals will be generated to all disciplines for an initial evaluation; specific therapy orders would then be determined at team conference
2. a. Onset of diagnosis or associated problem
   b. Include both physical problem and relevant medical diagnosis and onset
   c. May include multiple relevant problems and respective underlying diagnoses
   d. Associated psychosocial problems that may affect goals or outcome
3. a. Specify desired testing and reporting mechanisms
   b. Specify intervals between any retesting or reevaluation desired
4. a. Detailed short- and long-term goals usually based on problems listed above, or
   b. Detailed component tasks to be accomplished and sequence desired
   c. Estimated length of time expected to accomplish each of the above goals
5. a. Location of therapy desired (e.g., bedside, department or gym, inpatient, outpatient)
   b. Desired duration of each treatment session
   c. Specific therapeutic modalities desired, with intensity, duration, frequency, and timing with other therapeutic interventions described (see Chapters 17 through 29)
   d. Endpoints or decision points and criteria for increasing or decreasing therapy in general, or specific interventions' frequency
   e. Specific education for patient and mechanism to evaluate effectiveness of this teaching
   f. Home program training desired, including timing or criteria for such transition
   g. Nature of home program to be taught: frequency, duration, and intensity of modalities, therapeutic exercise, or other interventions
   h. Handout materials specifically desired
   i. Anticipated or desired home equipment training or trials
   j. Duration until therapist follow-up if any desired, to reverify or enhance compliance with home program and maintenance of gains
6. a. Specifics of monitoring desired: type, frequency, timing during therapeutic interventions, and criteria to discontinue or specifically modify intervention
   b. Criteria for immediate physician notification
   c. Specific precautions to ensure therapist safety (e.g., infectious, patient behavior, or violence risks)
   d. Specific modality precautions given the patient's diagnoses
   e. Complete list of patient problems or complete diagnosis list
   f. May include physician's evaluation report
7. a. Next physician follow-up date
   b. Anticipated physician follow-up frequency
   c. Possibly desired phone consultation before initiating therapy
   d. Desired frequency of follow-up reports and mechanism (written or phone)
   e. Details desired in follow-up reports
   f. Third-party reporting required or desired
   g. Criteria to discontinue or duration to continue therapy should physician follow-up not be obtained
   h. Date or week desired first to discuss this patient at team conference
   i. Frequency of team conferencing desired, especially if different than team's norm
   j. Desired emergency health system to be activated should patient decompensate
   k. Provision of phone, address, and paging numbers to contact the referring physician; mechanism for emergency contact provided

as any prescribed equipment or medication require follow-up. Often what was desired and presumably well communicated by written prescription or referral is not what occurred. Feedback enhances the accuracy of conveying the correct messages and should be encouraged (14). Receiving feedback helps the rehabilitation physician obtain a broader and more complete perspective on the patient's required needs and provides information necessary to evaluate progress. A certain degree of feedback is built into the multidisciplinary and interdisciplinary models as well as the transdisciplinary model if the physician is a cotherapist. Otherwise, mechanisms to ensure feedback are essential to good written referrals and orders. Quality control requires not only feedback and follow-up but appropriate corrective actions (Fig. 13-5).

In the medical model, the attending physician alone bears the responsibility for ensuring feedback, appropriate follow-up, and initiating additional contacts as problems arise. The physician's judgment determines whether outcomes are adequate and whether treatment is brought to closure. Examples of referrals and orders that arise from this model are shown in Table 13-5.

In the multidisciplinary team, the members give input as to whether goals are being achieved and, if not, why. Prob-

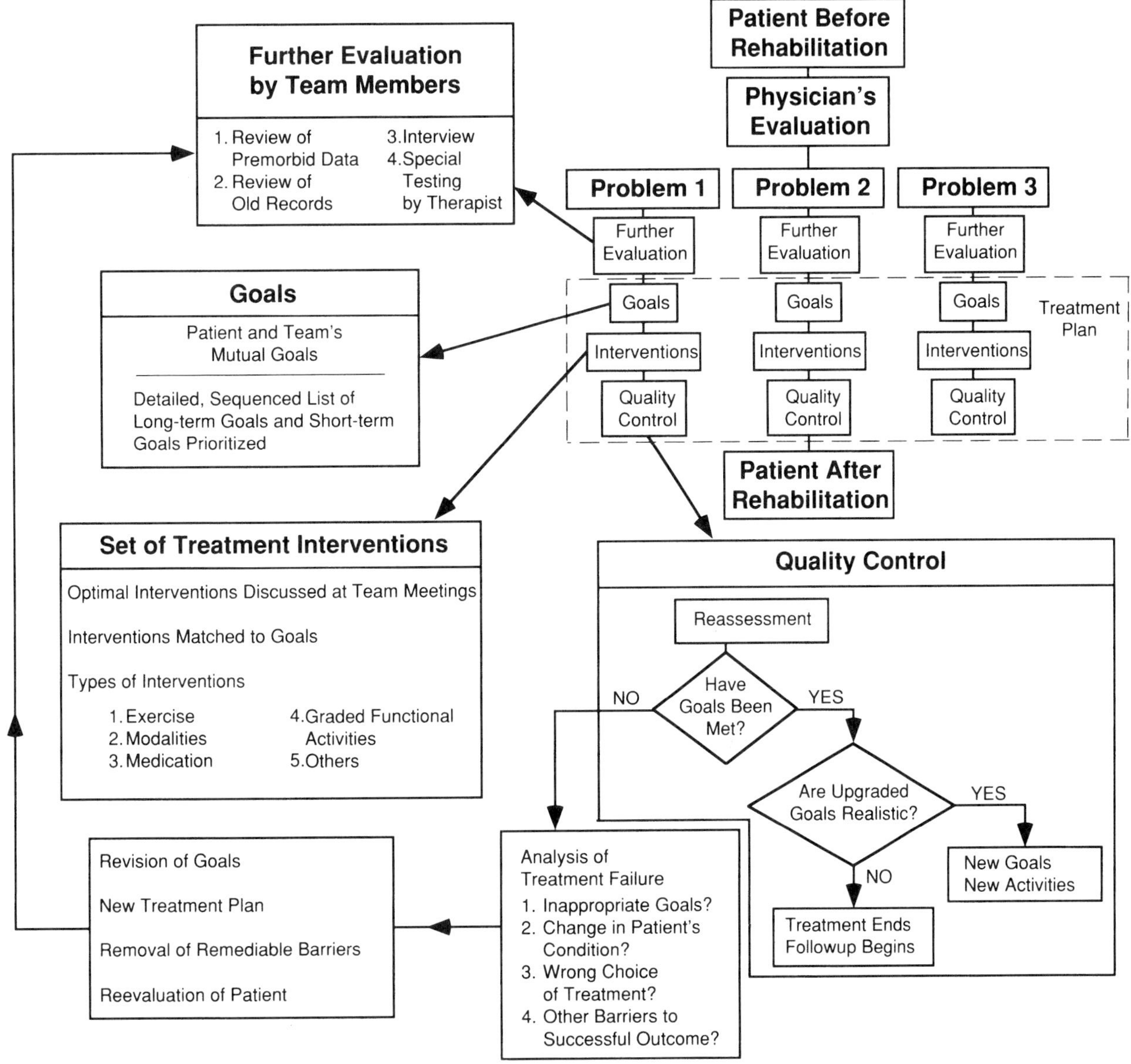

FIG. 13-5. Treatment-planning algorithm.

lems with progress also can be discussed in team conferences, with solutions derived between the consultants and the primary team-leading physician. Identification of problems and necessary corrective actions becomes a more joint effort as the consultants collectively discuss a single patient's care.

In the interdisciplinary team, a sense of mutual responsibility demands rapid identification and problem solving by the team for any problem perceived by a member. Solutions are achieved by interactive discussions, brainstorming, and finally by mutual consensus over the optimum course to be taken. Problem identification and corrective actions are a team process. It is this process that forms the strength of the interdisciplinary team and occupies the greatest time in patient care team conferences.

In the transdisciplinary team, problems are agreed on so rapidly during treatment that larger-scale or longer-term problems may be ignored or not formally considered. If such a problem currently is affecting treatment, it will be solved by mutual discussion and problem solving. Feedback, discussion, and problem solving occur so fluidly and rapidly that the physician member, if not a cotherapist, may be left out until after a solution has been decided and enacted. This diminishes the value of the physician's expertise to the team and can create conflicts should the physician subsequently believe alternative approaches are indicated. Even if by mutual consent the treating therapist and patient concur, doubts may be generated in the patient as to the treatment team's and physician's expertise. More likely, the physician's opinion will be viewed as obtrusive given the relative paucity of time he or she has been involved in the patient's team care. Thus, determining corrective action can be a disjointed

TABLE 13-5. *Examples of detailed prescription for durable medical equipment (DME) and therapy generated from problem list leading to goals which leads to interventions*

Problems ⇓	Peroneal palsy, likely recovery within 6 months	Left shoulder adhesive capsulitis
Goals ⇓	Eliminate toe catching with ambulation	Improve shoulder external rotation and then abduction, while avoiding impingement, to functional and if possibly normal range
Interventions	DME prescription: Please fit with off-the-shelf polypropylene ankle-foot orthosis set at 90°; and provide single cane adjusted to patient. Diagnosis: Foot drop secondary to peroneal palsy; needed for more than 6 months; medically necessary to provide safe gait. Date. Therapy referral: Date: P.T. ×1 visit Dx: Peroneal palsy with footdrop. Goals: Improved gait safety/efficiency and eliminate toe catching during gait; prevent heel cord contracture Precautions: Mildly decreased sensation on foot dorsum, gait instability, chronic intermittent hepatitis B fluid and secretion precautions Please evaluate and train in the use of AFO including donning, doffing and skin checks. Teach home program for gastroc. stretching. Also teach proper gait, including stairs and rough terrain, with cane to be used until patient becomes comfortable with balance. I will follow up pt in 2 weeks; please send report.	DME: Please issue yellow, red, and green theraband exercise elastic cords. Diagnosis: Deficient rotator cuff on left; medically needed over 6 months for proper shoulder function. Date. Therapy referral: Date: P.T. Maximum 12 visits over 4 weeks Dx: Left shoulder adhesive capsulitis Goals: Improve external rotation by 20° and shoulder abduction by 30° by 4 weeks Precautions: Patient S/P rotator cuff repair 12 weeks ago with weak rotator cuff muscles and increased impingement risk; pulleys are contraindicated. Please evaluate and manually stretch left shoulder, avoidng impingement, while applying ultrasound to anterior, then posterior joint to start at 1.5 watts/cm^2 and adjust to highest level comfortable for 10 minutes at each site. If stretch is poorly tolerated may add TENS during sessions. Teach home program for self stretching of external rotation only (abduction to be added later), and rotator cuff muscle strengthening with progressive therabands. Pt will be reevaluated in 4 weeks. Please send progress report, including shoulder active and passive range of motion measurements each 2 weeks. Please call 123-4567 for any questions. Thank you.

process in the transdisciplinary model unless the physician is an integral cotherapist.

Diagnostically related groups (DRGs), implemented in 1983 to cap Medicare expense growth, created incentives for improved efficiency in terms of hospital costs. This prompted the development of care paths in an attempt to optimize hospital resource utilization. Now a prospective payment system (PPS) for rehabilitation based on functional independence measure–function-related groups (FIM-FRG) is being explored by the Health Care Finance Administration (28). Besides increasing the efficiency of cost containment, managed care desires to document maintenance of quality. The ability to measure quality requires some degree of uniformity of approach across institutions for comparisons. Care paths, or protocols for patient treatment, help establish a greater degree of uniformity of patient care. Care paths are ideally targeted for populations for whom 75% are expected to follow a typical course. More customization is typically required in rehabilitation than for other medical care. Care paths are most easily developed for postsurgical patients in whom few complications are expected such as elective orthopedic cases. In acute care settings, 20% to 60% shorter lengths of stay have been obtained by implementing such protocols. Few studies have been done in rehabilitation settings, but one study showed no impact on cost or length of stay when a care path was used versus the usual interdisciplinary team approach. The high level of coordinated care that already exists in comprehensive rehabilitation settings may explain this result (31).

The Uniform Data System (UDS) allows rehabilitation hospitals and units to compare their efficiencies, which may become more and more used in a competitive fashion by managed care companies. Managed care is expected to dominate 60% of the market by the year 2000 (32). This competition and the quality improvement management techniques fostered by the JCAHO and CARF promote the development and implementation of care paths even in rehabilitation, where their value has yet to be firmly established (8,9,31). Care paths or treatment protocols have many labels including critical paths, practice guidelines/parameters, clinical guidelines, clinical pathways, care maps, flow charts, anticipated recovery plans, or case management (31,33). Care paths for inpatient comprehensive rehabilitation units will become more common as managed care increases. The development of such paths always needs to be customized to each particular setting, ideally by an interdisciplinary team. It is hoped that such protocols will improve efficiency without sacrificing the customization of care required by most complex rehabilitation inpatients.

EQUIPMENT PRESCRIPTIONS

Prescriptions can involve not only needed therapies but necessary adaptive equipment as well. The use of adaptive equipment is an important component of the rehabilitation of the physically disabled (34,35). Frequently, appropriate adaptive equipment may represent the difference between being functionally independent and requiring the assistance of a caregiver to perform necessary tasks required for self-care and daily living. The ultimate goal in rehabilitation is for the patient to achieve the highest level of independence possible. This requires the effective integration of adaptive equipment into the patient's individualized treatment as necessary (36). Effective prescription writing to obtain appropriate equipment is discussed.

The importance of adaptive equipment and devices is illustrated by the diversity of items available to enhance mobility or perform ADL (37). Adaptive devices and equipment are categorized according to the functional skills they are devised to facilitate; these include ADL, mobility (e.g., gait aids, positioning and transfer equipment, wheelchairs), communication, environmental management (e.g., adaptations, controls), and leisure and recreation.

Concomitant with the availability of an increasing array of adaptive aids is the inconsistent evaluation of the efficacy of these devices (38). Development and research are variable, as are printed information resources. Changes in patients' functional status through the rehabilitative process introduce another aspect of consideration in adaptive equipment use and length of need. Improved function through time could mean decreased need for adaptive equipment. The goal would be the attainment of the highest level of independence with the least adaptive equipment. All of these factors are part of the process for the selection of adaptive equipment.

Devices and equipment can be very costly. Costs can be minimized by using rentals or 30-day trial usage when utility is uncertain. The production of items for a small percentage of the population tends to be expensive. Some of this cost may be decreasing, however, because some adaptive devices are being used by a normative aging population to facilitate their self-care and functional performance. An example is the use of a reacher rather than standing on a step stool to reach items in the closet or pantry; another is a long-handled shoe horn that makes it unnecessary to bend over when putting on shoes.

Frequently, commercial devices must be adapted to the patient to provide for appropriate, individualized fit. Training also is required for the patient to achieve proper and optimum use of the equipment. In addition, the items of adaptive equipment on the market do not remain static; there are ongoing additions to the available repertoire. These changes can represent refinements on current items, new adaptations, or equipment using new technology.

Types of Adaptive Equipment and Devices

Self-Care/Activities of Daily Living Equipment

This category encompasses a large variety of items designed to make the everyday tasks of self-care easier. These adaptive devices generally contribute to the patient's independence in performing these activities. The assessed ADL dysfunction dictates the type of adaptation needed. For example, a stroke patient may be able to perform only onehanded activities owing to residual upper extremity hemiparesis. To facilitate eating, a plate guard and adaptive eating utensils (e.g., a rocker knife) may be appropriate. The use of the equipment would serve two purposes: to provide the patient independence in eating a meal and to release the caretaker from the supervisory or assistive task during the eating process. Other examples for this patient might include a suction-based hand brush to assist in hygiene and a dressing stick to help in performing dressing activities independently.

The diagnosis and residual function of the patient indicate the types and extent of equipment (39,40). A general rule of thumb is that the more disabled the patient may be in performing ADL, the more adaptive equipment may be needed for that person; also, the more extensive will be the collaboration among occupational therapists, physical therapists, and speech-language pathologists to provide adequately for the patient. Rehabilitation engineers also can be helpful members, particularly when the equipment adaptations are extensive or complex. Common vendor sources are listed in Table 13-6, data bases in Table 13-7, and consumer sources in Table 13-8. Many consumer advocacy groups and their available patient information materials can now be accessed through the internet. A few of these internet addresses are listed in these tables.

Mobility

There are several categories of equipment for mobility. Much emphasis is given to ambulation, and there are varied types of items devised to assist in the process. Canes and walkers are frequently used items. Each offers a method of facilitating ambulation as well as a measure of safety for the person. Prostheses or orthoses also are designed to assist in ambulation and mobility.

Positioning adaptations and seating systems can range from the very simple to the intricate. Proper positioning provides the preliminary and necessary basis of posture for the teaching and development of skills. Good body support and head control are essential prerequisites. Positioning can be simple, such as the placement of a wedge or bolster. It also can involve elaborate seating configurations that require training for proper measurements and construction. The

TABLE 13-6. *Major sources of ADL devices*

AliMed
297 High St.
Dedham, MA 02026
(800)225-2610

Concepts ADL Inc.
P.O. Box 339
Benton, IL 62812-0339
(800)626-3153

Independent Living Aids, Inc.
27 East Mall
Plainview, NY 11803-4404
(800)537-2118

Don Johnson Incorporated
P.O. Box 639
1000 N. Rand Road, Building 115
Wauconda, IL 60084
(800)999-4660

Lumex
100 Spence Street
Bay Shore, NY 11706
(800)645-5272

Maddak, Inc.
Pequannock, NJ 07440-1993
(800)443-4926

North Coast Medical, Inc.
187 Stauffer Boulevard
San Jose, CA 95125-1042
(800)821-9319

Sammons Preston Inc.
P.O. Box 5071
Bolingbrook, IL 60440-5071
(800)323-5547

Smith & Nephew Rehabilitation Division
One Quality Drive, P.O. Box 1005
Germantown, WI 53022-8205
(800)558-8633

ADL, activities of daily living

maintenance of skin integrity is another aspect of seating and positioning equipment that must be considered. As with adaptive devices, the more involved the seating requirements are, the more important it is to have representatives from occupational therapy and physical therapy with the physiatrist to formulate the seating requirements.

Transfer equipment to facilitate a patient's movement from one place to another will depend on the amount of assistance required by the patient for the transfer. A transfer board is the simplest item of equipment for transfer. This is used to facilitate movement of the patient from a wheelchair to a bed or a chair or to an automobile. The less able the patient is to assist in the transfer process, the more elaborate or complex is the equipment needed. Transfer equipment can be manually or electronically operated and may require little or no exertion by the person being transferred or the person assisting in the transfer.

Wheelchairs are another category of mobility equipment and may be manually or electronically operated. Wheel-

TABLE 13-7. *Databases and resources for rehabilitation*

ABLEDATA
Listings of assistive technology products and devices for people with disabilities. The database includes architectural elements, communication, computers, controls, education management, homemanagement, orthotics, personal care, prosthetics, recreation, seating, sensory disabilities, therapeutic aids, transportation, vocational management, walking and wheeled mobility.
ABLEDATA
8455 Colesville Road-Suite 935
Silver Spring, MD 20910
(800)227-0216 (V/TT)
http://www.abledata.com

Accent on Living
Information on rehabilitation aids and devices, disability service organizations, and publications; buyers' guide biannually.
Accent on Information
P.O. Box 700
Bloomington, IL 61702
(800)787-8444
http://www.blvd.com/accent

CTG (Closing the Gap) Solutions
Focuses on computer services and applications for the disabled.
Closing the Gap
P.O. Box 68
Henderson, MN 56044
(507)248-3294
http://www.closingthegap.com

National Health Information Center
This health information referral service was established by the Office of Disease Prevention and Health Promotion (ODPHP) within the Public Health Service. The objectives are to identify health information resources, channel requests for information to these resources, and to develop publications in print and electronic form on health-related topics of interest to health professionals, health-related media, and the public.
National Health Information Center
P.O. Box 1133
Washington, DC 20013-1133
(800)336-4797
http://nhic-nt.health.org(NHIC)

National Rehabilitation Information Center (NARIC)
This is a library and information center on disability and rehabilitation funded by the National Institute on Disability and Rehabilitation Research (NIDDR). The collection includes commercially published books, journal articles and audiovisuals, as well as federally funded research projects. Documents cover all aspects of disability and rehabilitation, including physical disabilities, independent living, employment, mental retardation, medical rehabilitation, assistive technology, psychiatric disabilities, special education, and law and public policy. REHABDATA is the bibliographic database that contains citations and abstracts of the materials in the collection.
REHABDATA
8455 Colesville Road-Suite 935
Silver Spring, MD 20910-3319
(800)346-2742(V/TT)
http://www.naric.com/naric

TABLE 13-8. *Sources for direct consumer adaptive aids*

Adapt Ability
P.O. Box 515
Colchester, CT 06415-0515
(800)937-3482

Aviano USA
1199-K Avenida Acaso
Camarillo, CA 93012

Bruce Medical Supply
411 Waverly Oaks Road
P.O. Box 9166
Waltham, MA 02254-9166
(800)225-8446

Enrichments
P.O. Box 5050
Bolingbrook, IL 60440
(800)323-5547

Independent Living Aids, Inc.
27 East Mall
Plainview, NY 11803-4404
(800)537-2118

North Coast Medical, Inc.
North Coast After Therapy Catalog
187 Stauffer Boulevard
San Jose, CA 95125-1042
(800)821-9319

chairs are discussed further in Chapter 30. The selection of the type of mobility aid will depend on the person's residual motor power to facilitate the process. Car and van adaptations for driving are another aspect of mobility. This, as well as community mobility in general, is discussed in Chapter 29.

Communication

Adaptations and augmentative devices for communication represent an ever-increasing area for consideration. The various devices to enhance communication are becoming increasingly more involved and more readily available. The physiatrist should work with a speech-language pathologist and occupational therapist to select a device. The speech-language pathologist would assist in the selection of the most appropriate device for communication; the occupational therapist would assist in the selection of the most appropriate motorically operative devices or switches for the patient.

Environmental Management

There are various adaptive devices available to provide assistance in the home (41). Most of the devices are engineered for use in the kitchen. These can include one-handed cutting boards, one-handed sandwich holders, stove overhead mirrors for wheelchair-mobile people to see the top of the stove, and other items. Adaptations also are available for washer and dryer operation. Numerous devices are available for the bathroom to assist in independence and safety. Environmental controls for home management are another example of assistive devices. Environmental control systems can have a few simple devices, such as for turning on and off a light or television, or more elaborate systems that manage many of the electric functions in a home.

Adaptations can be made in the work environment to facilitate use by those requiring modifications. Frequently this is done on an individualized basis. If necessary, site visits are made to determine the needs for either adaptations or equipment. Considerations such as space needed for a wheelchair to turn or go through a door and alterations of table position or height to a comfortable work level are examples of work adaptations.

Leisure and Recreation

People may want to pursue old hobbies or develop new leisure and recreational activities. Because of dysfunction, adaptations of equipment required for an activity may be indicated. Just as with other previously described devices, coordination would be indicated for equipment provision. The therapeutic recreation specialist may assist in the identification of the leisure or recreational activity that a patient wants to pursue. The occupational therapist or orthotist may assist in the provision and fitting of the appropriate adaptation or splint needed to perform tasks involved in the activity of interest.

Resources

Many adaptive devices and equipment are readily available through commercial vendors (42). Most items can be used as purchased. Others, however, will need adaptations that customize the devices for the person. At other times, equipment will have to be designed and constructed to meet patient needs. These are done on an individual basis, often by bioengineering or orthotics, with professional input from occupational or physical therapy, or others.

There is wide variance in the cost of equipment, the requirements for documentation for procurement of equipment, and the availability of equipment for patient evaluation trials for efficacy. Some items, such as wheelchairs and environmental control systems, can be very costly to procure. Ideally, there would be a range of items within each category (e.g., ADL, mobility, communication) available to use for patient assessment or training, but this essentially is not economically feasible. Vendors sometimes can provide equipment for patient assessment and use. Equipment pools are another resource. For example, equipment no longer needed by people or equipment shared among several facilities in an area could be used to assist in the evaluative and training process.

Prescriptions for Devices

Any device, be it a simple plate guard for eating to the most elaborately configured electric wheelchair, requires a physician prescription. Those items that are considered durable medical equipment (DME) require specific information. Not all items are DME. To avoid confusion, however, it would be useful to provide a comprehensive equipment prescription for all devices.

The patient's name and diagnosis are included in the information part of the prescription. Then, the initial part of the prescription is the name of the item, the stock number or other identifiers, and, when appropriate, the source of the item. All parts, sizes, adaptations, colors, and the like, are included, as applicable. The justification and rationale for the item are included, as well as the estimated duration of use. A permanent need is documented as "greater than 12 months" for Medicare prescriptions. When expensive devices are being requested, it usually is necessary to receive approval from the third-party payer before ordering such equipment.

Quality Control

Regardless of what adaptive equipment or device is ordered for a patient, there is a responsibility to ensure that the patient receives training in its use. Also, there are those items (e.g., wheelchairs) that require fitting. It is the responsibility of the physician and therapist requesting the equipment to assure that the equipment fits the patient and that the equipment received is operational. This is especially true in managed care settings in which negotiated durable medical equipment contracts may exist and determine what equipment is available. Timely follow-up is indicated for reassessment of the patient's use of the equipment and to ensure that the items serve the purpose for which they initially were intended and ordered.

SUMMARY

The ability to comprehensively define the rehabilitation needs of the patient and to request specific, appropriate therapeutic interventions distinguishes the physiatrist from all other medical specialties. To successfully identify and accomplish the goals of rehabilitation, the physical medicine and rehabilitation physician works closely with the allied health rehabilitation disciplines and other medical specialties. Referrals, orders, and equipment prescriptions are basic mechanisms by which the physiatrist requests the participation of the other professions in assessment, planning, and delivery of patient care. The necessary elements and specificity of detail included in the referrals or orders are largely determined by the mode of professional interaction and style of communication developed among the members of the rehabilitation team. A cohesive team with well-developed mechanisms for clear communication among its members can result in an approach to rehabilitation strategy that exceeds the sum of its parts. Nevertheless, the rehabilitation medicine physician must be knowledgeable about the treatment strategies used and their potential interactions with the patient's medical problems. Providing appropriate therapy precautions is a particular responsibility of physiatrists. Effectively written referrals, orders and equipment prescriptions will fully communicate patient needs, desired interventions, appropriate precautions, expectations and provide adequate mechanisms for feedback and quality control.

REFERENCES

1. Greshan GE, Duncan PW, Stason WB, et al. *Post-stroke rehabilitation, clinical practice guideline, no. 16.* Rockville, MD: U.S. Department of Health and Human Services, Public Health Service, Agency for Health Care Policy and Research, AHCPR Publication No. 95-0662, May 1995.
2. Keith RA. The comprehensive treatment team in rehabilitation. *Arch Phys Med Rehabil* 1991; 72:269–274.
3. Nevlud GN. The team approach: current trends and issues in rehabilitation. *Texas J Audiol Speech Pathol* 1990; 16:21–23.
4. Spencer WA. Changes in methods and relationships necessary within rehabilitation. *Arch Phys Med Rehabil* 1969; 50:566–580.
5. Schulz IL, Texidor MS. The interdisciplinary approach: an exercise in futility or a song of praise? *Med Psychother* 1991; 4:1–8.
6. Portilo RB. Ethical issues in teamwork: the content of rehabilitation. *Arch Phys Med Rehabil* 1988; 69:318–322.
7. Halstead LS. Team care in chronic illness: critical review of literature of past 25 years. *Arch Phys Med Rehabil* 1976; 57:507–511.
8. Joint Commission on Accreditation of Healthcare Organizations. *1996 Accreditation Manual for Hospitals.* Oakbrook Terrace, IL: Author, 1995.
9. Commission on Accreditation for Rehabilitation Facilities. *1996 Standards Manual and Interpretive Guidelines for Medical Rehabilitation.* Tucson, AZ: Rehabilitation Accrediting Commission (CARF), 1996.
10. Melvin JL. Status report on interdisciplinary medical rehabilitation. *Arch Phys Med Rehabil* 1989; 70:273–276.
11. Deutsch PM, Fralish KB. *Innovations in head injury rehabilitation.* New York: Mathew Bender, 1989.
12. Rothberg JS. The rehabilitation team: future directions. *Arch Phys Med Rehabil* 1981; 62:407–410.
13. Given B, Simmons S. The interdisciplinary health-care team: fact or fiction? *Nurs Forum* 1977; 16:165–183.
14. Walton RE, Dutton JM. The management of interdepartmental conflict: a model and review. *Admin Sci Q* 1969; 14:73–84.
15. Melvin JL. Interdisciplinary and multi-disciplinary activities and the ACRM. *Arch Phys Med Rehabil* 1980; 61:379–380.
16. Gaston EH. Developing a motivating organizational climate for effective team functioning. *Hosp Commun Psychiatry* 1980; 31:407–417.
17. Longest BB. *Management practices for the health professional*, 4th ed. Norwalk, CT: Appleton & Lange, 1990.
18. Anderson TP. An alternative frame of reference for rehabilitation: the helping process versus the medical model. *Arch Phys Med Rehabil* 1975; 56:101–104.
19. Becker MC, Abrams KS, Onder J. Goal setting: a joint patient-staff method. *Arch Phys Med Rehabil* 1974; 55:87–89.
20. Halstead LS, Rintala DH, Kanellos M, et al. The innovative rehabilitation team: an experiment in team building. *Arch Phys Med Rehabil* 1986; 67:357–361.
21. Tollison CD. Preface. In: Tollison CD, ed. *Handbook of chronic pain management.* Baltimore: Williams & Wilkins, 1989; ix–x.
22. Mazur H, Beeston JJ, Yerxa EJ. Clinical interdisciplinary health team care: an educational experiment. *J Med Educ* 1979; 54:703–713.
23. Darling LA, Ogg HL. Basic requirements for initiating an interdisciplinary process. *Phys Ther* 1984; 64:1684–1686.
24. Lyon S, Lyon G. Team functioning and staff development: a role release approach to providing educational services for severely handicapped students. *J Assoc Severe Handicap* 1980; 5:250–263.
25. Gast DL, Wolery M. Severe developmental disabilities. In: Berdine

WH, Edward AE, eds. *An introduction to special education,* 2nd ed. Boston: Little, Brown, 1985; 469–729.
26. Melvin JL. Rehabilitation in the year 2000. *Am J Phys Med Rehabil* 1988; 67:197–201.
27. Hoffman LP. Transdisciplinary team model: an alternative for speech-language pathologists. *Texas J Audiol Speech Pathol* 1990; 16:3–6.
28. Tresolini CP, Bailit HL, Conway-Welch C, et al. *Health professions education and managed care: challenges and necessary responses.* San Francisco: Pew Health Professions Commission, 1995.
29. Braddom RL. Practice issues in the hospital-based rehabilitation unit. In: Melvin JL, Odderson IR, eds. Clinical rehabilitation and physiatric practice. *Phys Med Rehabil Clin North Am* 1996; 7:31–41.
30. Colachis SC. New directions in health care. *Arch Phys Med Rehabil* 1984; 65:291–294.
31. Odderson IR. Pathways to quality care at lower cost. In: Melvin JL, Odderson IR, eds. Clinical rehabilitation and physiatric practice. *Phys Med Rehabil Clin North Am* 1996; 7:147–165.
32. Odderson IR, Melvin JL. Overview of the spectrum of rehabilitation services. In: Melvin JL, Odderson IR eds. Clinical rehabilitation and physiatric practice. *Phys Med Rehabil Clin North Am* 1996; 7:1–4.
33. Lumsdon K, Hagland M. Mapping care. *Hosp Health Netw* 1993; 20: 3440.
34. Hall M. Unlocking information technology. *Am J Occup Ther* 1987; 41:722–725.
35. Vanderheiden GC. Service delivery mechanisms in rehabilitation technology. *Am J Occup Ther* 1987; 41:703–710.
36. Smith R. Quality assurance in equipment ordering for the spinal cord-injured client. *Am J Occup Ther* 1988; 42:36–39.
37. Enders A, ed. *Technology for independent living sourcebook.* Washington, DC: Association for the Advancement of Rehabilitation Technology, 1984.
38. American Occupational Therapy Association. *Technology review '89: perspectives on occupational therapy practice.* Rockville, MD: Author, 1989.
39. Hopkins H, Smith H, eds. *Willard and Spackman's occupational therapy,* 7th ed. Philadelphia: JB Lippincott, 1989.
40. Trombly C, ed. *Occupational therapy for physical dysfunction,* 3rd ed. Baltimore: Williams & Wilkins, 1989.
41. Dickey R, Shealey, SH. Using technology to control the environment. *Am J Occup Ther* 1987; 41:717–721.
42. American Occupational Therapy Association. *Technology review '90: perspectives on occupational therapy practice.* Rockville, MD: Author, 1990.

Rehabilitation Medicine: Principles and Practice, Third Edition,
edited by Joel A. DeLisa and Bruce M. Gans.
Lippincott–Raven Publishers, Philadelphia © 1998.

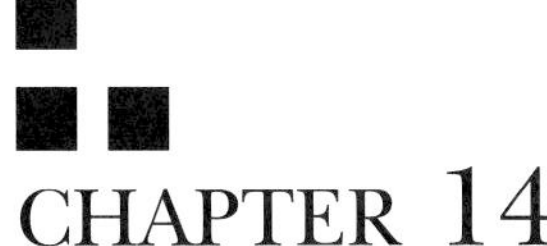

CHAPTER 14

Systematically Assuring and Improving the Quality and Outcomes of Medical Rehabilitation Programs

Mark V. Johnston, Miriam Maney, and Deborah L. Wilkerson

It was once commonly said that the quality of medical care could not be defined but could be recognized when seen. Like beauty, quality was in the eye of the beholder. Adherents of this view are still with us, but the dominance of the notion of implicit quality has waned. Progress has been made in development of outcome norms for medical rehabilitation programs. The most common important features of quality in health care are now convincingly articulated in many publications. Quality in medical care is now understood to be connected to knowledge of the likely benefits and risks, that is, to treatment effectiveness and outcomes. Promising models of outcomes-oriented quality assurance and quality improvement are now available from areas of health care related to medical rehabilitation. Rehabilitation programs are changing in response to new market pressures. ''Outcomes management'' is affecting the practice of rehabilitation, changing treatment and administrative processes with untested impact on patient welfare. Quality and its improvement in actual programs is now understood as complex, requiring several different generic strategies and with local variations so numerous that quality improvement cannot be expected without the involvement of every clinical professional and staff in the relevant care process. New strategies of quality improvement (QI) and outcomes management, although they still need considerable development for medical rehabilitation, are more action-oriented and promising than older methods of program evaluation and quality assurance (QA), which form the basis for the new strategies.

Medical rehabilitation is complex and multifaceted. Quality improvement efforts draw from all of the knowledge in this thick textbook, and more. Methods of assuring and improving the quality and outcomes of medical rehabilitation are correspondingly multifaceted. The broad thesis of this chapter is that multiple strategies and systems are useful for assuring and improving the effectiveness of medical rehabilitation in practice. Both process-focused and outcomes-focused methods are needed, and the two strategies need to be connected. This chapter is designed to be a guide and reference work for physicians, administrators, QI specialists, and any other professionals concerned with quality and patient outcomes in medical rehabilitation.

M. V. Johnston: Department of Physical Medicine and Rehabilitation, University of Medicine and Dentistry of New Jersey—New Jersey Medical School, Newark, New Jersey 07103; and Kessler Medical Rehabilitation Research and Education Corporation, West Orange, New Jersey 07052.

M. Maney: Kessler Institute for Rehabilitation, West Orange, New Jersey 07052.

D. L. Wilkerson: Department of Research and Quality Improvement, CARF—The Rehabilitation Accreditation Commission, Tucson, Arizona 85712.

MOTIVATIONS AND BACKGROUND

Quality and Outcomes Improvement Systems

The need for adequate quality and outcomes monitoring has never been greater. As in medical care as a whole, demands for accountability, quality, and improved outcomes have grown in rehabilitation. Government scrutiny of rehabilitation continues. Managed care organizations have especially pressured rehabilitation facilities to lower their cost or do not refer to rehabilitation hospitals at all. As fee-for-service passes, the need to assure quality and patient outcomes grows sharper.

At a more basic level, the most careful of studies have shown that there are problems in the quality of medical care. For instance, the Harvard Medical Practice Study documented serious errors or problems in 4% of hospitalizations, 14% of which were fatal (1). This is the equivalent of three jumbo jets crashing every 2 days. There are no reliable figures for avoidable disablement, but errors or insufficiencies of funding for interventions designed to improve the health, function, and affective quality of life of patients with disabilities surely occur. The number of physically disabled persons in our population is increasing, and the quality of their lives remains unsatisfactory (2,3).

The primary motivation for quality and outcomes improvement systems in rehabilitation is not avoidance of outright bad care and patient injury. Although these certainly occur, they are in our experience not common in rehabilitation. Medical rehabilitation facilities are caring environments. It is clear that the great majority of patients in inpatient rehabilitation hospitals improve in function (4). The usual motivation is—or should be—to pursue excellence and to improve the lives of persons with disabilities.

Health care professionals should be concerned that:

> in their zeal to document and improve the technical quality of care, health care plans and purchasers may use approaches that are conceptually flawed or based on inaccurate data. An example is the Health Care Financing Administration's program for measuring and publishing hospital mortality rates among Medicare patients. After many years of publishing such statistics, the agency came to the conclusion that without a better method to adjust for the severity of illness, the data were too inaccurate to be useful, and the program was abandoned. (5)

To paraphrase Blumenthal, rehabilitation professionals owe it to themselves and their patients to master the substantive issues that underlie current discussions about the quality and outcomes of rehabilitative care.

Nature and Goals of Medical Rehabilitation

The goals of medical rehabilitation are broad. The aim of rehabilitative interventions is to provide sustained, practical improvement in patient function (6–10). The typical objective is to minimize functional limitations, typically in situations where underlying major impairments cannot be reversed. It is also said that the general goal of rehabilitation is to improve patients' lives or to decrease handicap (7,9–12). Clinical goals are also individually tailored, ideally with the involvement of the person with the disability. The significance of different aspects of function varies among individuals, and individual patient choices need to be elicited (13,14).

Such formulations are ideal—humanistic, holistic, caring. The combination of almost universalist goals with individualization for the particular person presents great complexities for empirical quality and outcomes measurement, which require a specific focus. In general, we emphasize the following: *the basic criterion for evaluation of rehabilitation outcomes is the degree to which the program produces sustained improvements in the everyday life of persons served.* The most typical outcome in medical rehabilitation is a measure of practical improvements or reduced functional limitations in everyday life.

Sustaining function after discharge is critical. Measurement of function after discharge is the hallmark of program evaluation, but it is also essential to the judgment of the real quality and outcomes of a rehabilitative intervention. If a functional performance does not transfer to the person's life after discharge, of what real value is it? The improved function should be practical in the sense of helping the person in everyday life or decreasing stress to caregivers. The improved function should enable the person to sustain desired independent living arrangements and productive activity (9–12). Relevant outcomes are those experienced by persons served, who may have a value perspective different from that of professionals.

Safety, stabilization of medical problems, and personal considerate care are also important—even essential—as medical rehabilitation outcomes. Survival times and mortality rates also are relevant, but more as background or minimal measures than as primary measures. The key measures are measures of functional performance, primarily at the level of disability (see Chapter 4). Efficiency, cost, profit, and marketing are also essential, but in this chapter they are not emphasized, for they are not the central goal of rehabilitation.

Clinical Rehabilitation Goals and Objectives

The clinical care process involves assessing (diagnosis and fact finding), planning (and deciding), treating, checking (measuring the result), and then assessing again whether to alter, continue, or discontinue the treatment, leading to another treatment process or ultimately to patient discharge (Fig. 14-1). Clinical practice involves all of these steps, including some check of the success of preceding diagnostic–planning–treatment sequence. In this sense, clinical outcomes measurement is intrinsic and essential to clinical practice. The relevant clinical measures may be indicators of short-term responsiveness to treatment, such as a serum level, an oral response from the patient, or slightly increased strength or normalization of gait. Efforts to improve the quality and outcomes of rehabilitation must understand and improve all elements of this basic cycle.

Monitoring of relevant longer-term outcomes at discharge or follow-up has long been considered to be important to understanding rehabilitation outcomes. The distinction between *short-term objectives* and *long-term goals* is conventional and useful. Short-term objectives are specific points on the way to broader, more significant long-term objectives. Examples of short-term treatment objectives might include increase range of motion (ROM), complete educational workbook, teach four items important in wheelchair management, teach sterile self-catheterization, ambulate on parallel bars 12 feet, or change a serum level. Shorter-term and intermediate measures are valuable in identifying recovery processes associated with rehabilitation and distinguishing them from events due to exogenous factors (15,16).

A useful distinction is that between *treatment objectives*

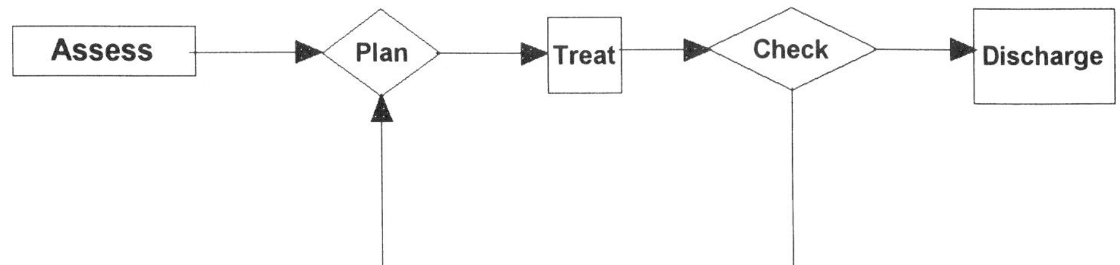

FIG. 14-1. The clinical care process.

and *rehabilitation outcome goals* (9,10,17). Treatment objectives need to have a scientific or at least highly logical relation to the interventions provided. We define treatment objectives as projections of sustained increase in the person's function in the community, after discharge or termination of treatments. Treatment objectives are usually operationalized in terms of a description of the patient's function at discharge. Examples of long-term treatment objectives would include independence in self-care activities of daily living (ADLs) or mobility without accidents, a decrease in the frequency of disruptive verbal behavior to less than once per week, or making the bladder infection free (e.g., urine colony count less than 100,000 without symptoms). Discharge is a key practical terminus of rehabilitation planning, for the person is usually projected to live independently, with defined or implicit continuing supports, and to continue with his or her life activities thereafter.

Rehabilitation outcome goals have been defined at the broader, less specific, but more meaningful level of improvements in the person's life at the level of handicap or role restoration (9–12). Rehabilitation outcome goals are measured after termination of services, when patient function has stabilized to some degree. Existing implementations of this model measure rehabilitation outcomes in terms of productive activity (e.g., paid work, schooling, housework, or other uses of time considered normal for such a person) and independent living (e.g., noninstitutional living arrangement and total support requirements) (9,10,12,18,19).

Rehabilitation Accreditation

Medical rehabilitation is both medical and rehabilitative. It deals with both reduction of neurophysiological impairments (i.e., medical problems) and attainment of disability-reduction goals. Its interventions are a pragmatic combination of medical interventions designed to reduce impairments and therapies involving practice and learning. Reflecting this duality, two independent accrediting bodies have developed in the United States—the Joint Commission on Accreditation of Healthcare Organizations (JCAHO) and the Commission on Accreditation of Rehabilitation Facilities (CARF).

Accreditation by the Joint Commission on Accreditation of Health Organizations is usually essential for hospital licensure and reimbursement in the United States. The JCAHO requires that accredited facilities adhere to standards of patient care, staff education, and organizational performance. Continuous efforts to maintain and improve quality are to be made; QI should be embedded throughout the organization. JCAHO's Agenda for Change in the 1980s increased the emphasis on outcomes. The JCAHO has supported the development of objective indicators of clinical events and mostly short-term outcomes. Publications of JCAHO understandably continue to define quality of care primarily in terms connected to processes and clinical outcomes rather than long-term outcomes.

It has long been recognized that rehabilitation of a person with a disability requires more than medical interventions, in the narrow sense of the term. Generalization of learning and attaining a significant impact on real-world outcomes is integral to quality rehabilitation. As part of the broader rehabilitation movement, medical rehabilitation facilities voluntarily apply for accreditation by CARF to attest to their commitment to maximize the rehabilitation of disabled persons. The standards of CARF are pragmatic, detailed, and optimized for pure rehabilitation, and they emphasize outcomes after discharge (6).

CARF has long specified characteristics of rehabilitation organizations believed to indicate quality and has required that rehabilitation programs eventually establish outcomes-oriented program evaluation systems. Requirements for program evaluation were modified in the mid-1990s. Program evaluation is now subsumed under the rubric ''outcomes measurement and management'' (6).

Dual CARF–JCAHO accreditation has been an expense, but both have been important. During the late 1990s, the two accrediting bodies began work on a collaborative process to streamline rehabilitation accreditation and minimize duplication of effort. Whatever happens to accreditation in the future, medical rehabilitation will continue to deal with both medical problems and broad issues of patients' quality of life.

Continuous Quality Improvement and Total Quality Management

There has been a movement toward *continuous quality improvement* (CQI) (20–23) and *total quality management* (TQM) throughout American health care (24,25). Inspired by the work of Deming (21), Juran (25), Ishikawa, and others on quality control in business and manufacturing (23,26), this movement has worked profound changes in traditional approaches to program evaluation and QA, influencing JCAHO's Agenda for Change, CARF, and current standards of both organizations. Its influence is still strong and perhaps growing. The movement expresses a paradigm shift—a shift in fundamental ways of understanding and acting.

Both CQI and TQM focus on improvement of whole systems or subsystems rather than relying on measurement of either processes or outcomes in isolation (21,22). They emphasize knowledge of processes and involvement of the staff directly involved in any process. They involve fact finding, emphasize prevention of problems, and use measures of processes or of shorter- or longer-term results, depending on the problem. The emphasis, however, is not on measurement but on understanding of the total system and involvement of everyone to diagnose, plan, and fix problems.

Quality and effectiveness depend on the routine system of care much more than on random errors or outliers. A basic assumption, based in experience, is that the root causes of problems are more commonly at the level of the system or of sequences of processes than at the level of individuals or even single departments. The causes of error or undesirable variation in the sequence of activities must be identified and rooted out. The aim is to improve systems, not to blame individuals. Improved protocols for activities and processes need to be developed and implemented as a key element of QI (24,27). Global organizational commitment is a dominant factor in quality of care (21,24,25). The philosophy has moved the field toward integrating outcomes-measurement and process-oriented methods of assuring and improving health care.

Continuous QI emphasizes detailed, expert understanding of what is really happening in the organization and of the processes involved in producing a product. This is rooted in Deming's insight that "profound knowledge" of an organization requires more than knowledge of "general variation" (i.e., statistics and scientific measures): it requires generalized knowledge of "special variation," based on deeper knowledge of the specific processes involved, the organization as a system, "a theory of knowledge" (how people in the organization come to believe they know something), and knowledge of psychology (21,22,28).

Although there is much to learn from CQI and TQM, we believe that approaches to quality and outcomes improvement from manufacturing or provision of hotel services need profound modifications to be optimally applied to medical rehabilitation. Patients cannot be treated as a uniform input, as material inputs to manufacturing can. The response of patients to treatments is not nearly as predictable as the response of physical material to manufacturing processes. *Patient responses must be tested subsequent to treatment rather than assumed.* Idiosyncratic patient desires need to be assessed in rehabilitation, and comorbid conditions commonly alter ordinary treatment patterns. The effect of "context" on therapy is fundamental (29). The principle of reducing variance in treatment processes might need to be redefined in terms involving the tailoring of treatments to the priority needs of the individual. Treatment guidelines or protocols may need to be developed so that we can evaluate the quality of this individualization process.

Sentinel Events

In practice, action to maintain quality of care frequently depends on *sentinel events* (30)—single occurrences that are highly problematic or socially unacceptable. Litigation following patient injury, staff quitting over unacceptable quality or ethical issues, and cockroaches on the walls are not definitive evidence of severe quality problems, but they surely should motivate a detailed review. The premise of this work is that we need to go beyond the level of sentinel events and avoiding scandal. Systematic and continual efforts by professionals are needed to monitor and improve the quality and effectiveness of care.

TERMS AND CONCEPTS

Basic Quality and Outcomes Terms

This section explains basic terms related to quality and outcomes-related systems in medical rehabilitation programs.

One of the most important premises of all systematic approaches to improving quality and outcomes is *the need for objective comparison data as a basis for evaluation.* The necessity for data and preestablished standards of quality and outcome is asserted by JCAHO, CARF, government agencies, and virtually all experts in quality and outcomes monitoring and improvement. JCAHO quite explicitly requires that facilities compare their processes and/or outcomes with those known to be attainable elsewhere (31). CARF publications speak of "benchmarks" (6). Even CQI philosophy assumes a scoreboard in the form of process or general outcome measures (20–22,25).

Quality of care is impossible to define in a few simple words. Quality is always positive, connoting activities that benefit the person served in the short or long term. We connect quality primarily with the concept of effectiveness: quality medical rehabilitation should engender sustained improvement in the function, health, and/or quality of life of patients beyond any improvements that would have occurred with nonprofessional care. Although duration of life is relevant, functional abilities and quality of life are the main issues in medical rehabilitation.

The Institute of Medicine defines quality as the "degree to which health services for individuals and populations increase the likelihood of desired health outcomes and are consistent with current professional knowledge" (32,33). A first approximation to measurement of quality in rehabilitation involves measurement of the degree to which the objectives of care are met.

If quality of care is real, at least approximate standards or objective criteria must exist, although they may usually be implicit, and their specification may be difficult. Explication, validation, implementation, and improvement of guidelines for care are basic to efforts to assure and improve the quality (effectiveness) of care.

Quality care involves at least three components (5,13,34):

1. Choosing to do the right thing, or appropriateness of care. Diagnosis, planning, and decision making are involved, as is the match between treatments chosen and patient conditions and the balancing of likely health benefits against harm and costs.
2. Doing the right thing. The technical competence with which procedures are carried out involves skill, judgment, timeliness, and sustained effort. Both the skill of the individual and the coordination of the individuals on the team are involved.
3. Patient dignity and involvement. The quality of interactions between health care professionals and patients (and family) is also important. Communication, concern, empathy, honesty, sensitivity, and responsiveness to individuals are essential to quality care (35). Patients not only want to be informed about what is going on but also want to be involved in selection of treatment goals. The disability rights movement insists on empowerment of persons with disabilities. Rehabilitation accreditation requires patient involvement in decisions about care and placement (6).

In rehabilitation of patients with complex problems and differing personal circumstances, quality of care surely involves a degree of tailoring of the rehabilitative plan to the individual. Depending on patient response to initial interventions, the treatment approach may need to be adjusted. The durability of outcomes—whether functional gains are sustained—is a major and recurring issue in rehabilitation motivating accreditation requirements for patient follow-up.

We retain the term *quality assurance* (QA). QA means activities to ensure that implicit or explicit standards of care are met. We do not associate the term with reliance on external policing of clinicians, peer review, or other dated techniques. Assuring the quality or at least outcomes of care are critical issues when managed care firms slash the budget for rehabilitative services or when economic incentives exist to provide less care.

Outcomes

Outcomes need to be connected to care processes. The classic method of connecting outcomes to processes involves routine assessment of diagnostic and therapeutic outcomes; related process variables are assessed if outcomes do not meet accepted standards (36).

The term ''outcome'' is commonly used in three overlapping but very different ways: what might be called *life outcomes*—in the sense of role restoration and quality of life generally; *health-related quality of life*—those aspects of life or experience or function that are logically related to physical health or recognized mental disorders; and the *outcomes of care.* ''Rehabilitation outcomes'' implies a causal relationship to treatments provided. Although rehabilitation improves aspects of the quality of patients' lives, it would not be honest to suggest that medical rehabilitation can routinely produce or assume responsibility for massive, global improvements in patients' lives. Although we are concerned with the persons's quality of life as a whole (large circle in Fig. 14-2), medical rehabilitation is primarily directed at health-related quality of life (smaller oval). As medical rehabilitation professionals, we are primarily and directly responsible for those aspects of patients' lives that we can and do affect, namely, treatment outcomes (the small triangle in Fig. 14-2). Distinguishing between life outcomes and treatment outcomes is essential to coherent communication regarding rehabilitation outcomes.

The term *outcome of care* implies a connection to preceding treatments as well as impact on patient functioning or well-being. An *outcome of rehabilitation* is an aspect of function or life related to rehabilitative treatments, beyond effects of natural healing and adaptation (or deterioration) that would occur in the absence in professional rehabilitative care. Outcomes in the absence of intensive specialized rehabilitation cannot be directly measured in QI and outcomes monitoring systems but must be projected or estimated. Although this projection may be implicit, an explicit statistical projection is more precise and definite. Strictly speaking, a *rehabilitation outcome* is a measured deviation from a statistical projection. Evaluations of treatment quality are also either judgmental or extrapolated on the basis of often-limited evidence.

Severity adjustment is basic to outcome evaluation in rehabilitation. Common determinants of case severity within a diagnostic impairment group include disability (i.e., functional dependence) at and before admission, comorbidities, measures of impairment severity such as American Spinal Injury Association (ASIA) motor scores for patients with spinal cord injury (SCI) or Glasgow Coma Scale for trau-

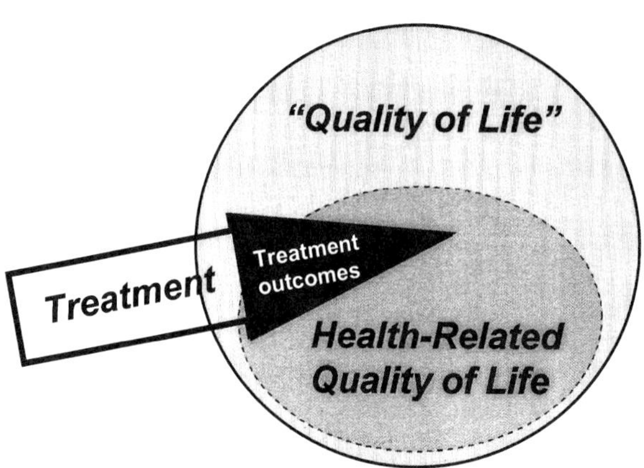

FIG. 14-2. Life, health, and rehabilitation outcomes.

matic brain injury (TBI), extreme age or youth, and many other factors (17). Measurement of baseline stability is essential (37). Severity adjustment factors are identified in longitudinal prognostic research. They are used as covariates when analyzing outcomes and quality measures.

Treatment and long-term continuation of therapeutic activities depend on the cooperation of patients and families. Rehabilitation professionals are responsible for skillfully and sensitively educating patients and families, but their responsibility for outcomes should take patient/family compliance into account.

Similarly, a *risk factor* for a particular functional or health outcome is a characteristic of patients or of their environment that influences the likelihood of occurrence of the health outcome.

Outcomes management and outcomes-focused methods of quality improvement involve attributing outcomes to antecedent events, particularly to antecedent care. Because outcomes typically reflect many factors, the effects of which cannot be precisely separated, statistical control and projection methods are almost universally necessary. Additional technical terms are defined in later sections.

Efficiency and Economic Constraints

Assuring the quality of care would be trivial if money were free. As economic constraints increasingly affect medical care, assuring the quality of care becomes an increasingly sharp and challenging issue.

Efficiency refers to cost-related considerations. Straight cost considerations must be distinguished from cost-effectiveness, which implies balancing improved patient function against the cost of producing that improvement. Measures of effort (e.g., length of stay, number of treatments) are often useful surrogates for detailed measures of cost. Efficiency is always relevant to QI and outcomes evaluation, for resources are always limited. In a managed care environment, we especially need to know whether the imposed limitations have not only cut the traditional quality or intensity of care but also diminished patient outcomes. In a capitated environment, if one spends too much on one patient, there will be fewer resources available for others: information systems need to sketch where the optimum lies.

Treatment Effectiveness

Treatment effectiveness is the concept that ties together processes and outcomes. *Effectiveness* may be defined as the sustained improvement in patient function produced by rehabilitative care beyond those improvements that occur with the natural healing and adjustment that occurs even with less intensive, unspecialized care. Rehabilitation is not worthwhile if the improvement would have occurred even if the person simply stayed home and refused entrance to health care professionals. Effectiveness is assumed by use of the term "rehabilitation outcomes" and is the chief attribute of quality of medical rehabilitation care. Effectiveness encompasses appropriateness of care, the technical competence with which procedures are carried out, risks, and unintended as well as intended consequences.

In simple terms, the primary product of rehabilitation is improved patient function. The aim of both QI and outcomes-monitoring systems is then to increase the degree to which rehabilitative programs routinely improve and sustain patient function.

Both QI and outcomes-monitoring systems are based on already-established knowledge or beliefs regarding effective treatment. Operational clinical data systems are valuable research tools, but prospective, controlled research is needed to reliably establish the efficacy of treatment (37–39).

Both QI and outcomes-monitoring systems also address quality of routine nursing care, hotel services, and patient satisfaction—matters that are both important and more easily measurable than rehabilitation effectiveness (24,40,41).

Validated indicators of causal processes. Ideally, QI and outcomes-monitoring systems evaluate sets of process and outcome measures demonstrated to indicate the effectiveness of interventions. It is technically possible to validate a set of measures indicating effective treatment interventions in a program. Causation is a construct, and studies to establish causal relationships involve construct validation methodologies (17,42,43), including convergent validity studies to ensure that variables correlate as theory would lead one to expect, and discriminant validity studies to distinguish true relationships from confounders. A great deal of research is needed to develop a manageable set of input, process, and outcome measures that validly indicates degree of intervention effectiveness. Such research will employ control groups or stable own-control baseline designs to establish norms and implicit comparison groups. Unfortunately, there is a shortage of well-controlled studies to quantify the effectiveness of interventions in both rehabilitation and medical care as a whole (13,38).

Practical surrogates for effectiveness. In practice, program evaluation and outcomes management in rehabilitation are commonly based on implicit beliefs and practical but flawed surrogate estimates of effectiveness. In program evaluation, the term "effectiveness" is usually used to mean how successful a program is in accomplishing its goals. Improvement in function is also used as an rough proxy indicator of effectiveness. Degree of functional improvement distinguishes rehabilitation programs from chronic disease programs, nursing facilities, and hospices (44). Some QI publications have defined effectiveness as "the degree to which the care is provided in the correct manner, given the current state of the art" (16,45).

Effectiveness is then adherence to normatively based standards and methods of care. This bases practical QI on adherence to practices generally thought to be best. This is a good and reasonable definition. Studies in acute hospitals, for instance, have clearly demonstrated that better adherence to the best practices would improve patient outcomes (13,46–48).

Levels of Measurement

Understanding levels of measurement of health and function is necessary to understanding how to choose and interpret measures in medical rehabilitation. In this chapter, we primarily use the World Health Organization's terminology (49), with a number of modifications and qualifications to adapt the scheme from its original purpose—population epidemiology—to the more detailed requirements of study of the effectiveness of medical rehabilitation. Chapter 4 should be consulted for a full treatment of levels of function. In brief:

- An *impairment* is a ''loss or abnormality of psychological, physiological or anatomical structure or function'' at the level of the organ or organ system (49).
- A *disability* is ''any restriction or lack (resulting from an impairment) of ability to perform an activity in the manner or within the range considered normal for a human being (49).'' Disabilities are composite behaviors or capabilities in everyday life. Disability is commonly measured in terms of assistance requirements in activities of daily living (ADLs), although it can also be measured in terms of qualitative difficulties in performance or the frequency of problems such as noncompletion of a task. Recent measures also attempt to quantify cognitively based problems in daily life and communicative disability (50). Disabilities are determined not only by impairments but also by the extent of compensating functional strengths. Disability measures can have a loose connection to handicap or life satisfaction (17).
- A *handicap* is ''a disadvantage for a given individual, resulting from an impairment or a disability, that limits or prevents the fulfillment of a role that is normal . . . for that individual'' (49). Handicap then implies the interaction of general disabilities with the patient's physical and social environment. Handicap is not a characteristic solely of the person but is equally a characteristic of the environment. Handicap results from role expectations, discrimination, physical barriers, and other features of the environment. Handicap measures include global role performance, employment, general independence of physical assistance, global mobility, income, and economic independence.

Additional Terms

Measures of *pathology*—dysfunction at the cellular or biochemical level—and disease are often essential in medical rehabilitation. *Structural impairments* (e.g., type of spinal cord injury as measured by Frankel grade, ventricular size, presence of large ischemic stroke, leg length discrepancies, or many categoric diagnostic descriptors) may be distinguished from *functional impairments,* which are very specific dysfunctions related to particular organ systems (e.g., electromyograph readings, degree of paralysis as measured by ASIA motor scores in SCI or Fugl-Meyer Scores in stroke) (17).

We use the term *functional limitation* as a near-synonym for disability but more specifically to denote very specific limitations or disabilities of the person, as measured in a controlled environment (3,7).

Social disadvantage is a good near-synonym for handicap (51). *Community integration* is another useful related term.

Measures of patient satisfaction with care are highly practical and are discussed at the end of this major section.

Health status measures. Medical rehabilitation outcome measures have been considered to be a subcategory of health status indicators or quality-of-life measures. Whole books summarizing different measures of health status and quality of life are now available (17,52–54). Perhaps the most commonly used measures of general health are the Sickness Impact Profile (SIP) (55) and the Medical Outcomes Study Short-Form 36 (SF-36) (56). Some of the subscales within these instruments appear to be too broad or are otherwise mistargeted for medical rehabilitation, but many dimensions—such as pain relief, general feelings of health and well-being, and physical function—are at least generically relevant. The sensitivity and applicability of many conventional measures of health status to medical rehabilitation at this point require further verification. An advantage to these scales is that they are well developed. Large-sample norms are available, and they do assess a wider scope of outcomes than do popular medical rehabilitation outcome measures such as the Functional Independence Measure (FIM) or the Barthel.

Quality of Life and Subjective Well-Being

Unqualified ''*quality of life*'' is here used to denote the whole immeasurably complex universe that constitutes the human experience of patients (Fig. 14-2). Although rehabilitation certainly aims to improve patients' quality of life, the concept of ''quality of life'' is also vastly complex and changing. Without qualification, quality of life is too nebulous to serve as a rehabilitation outcome measure. To create a QI or outcomes management system, one needs to specify those aspects of patients' lives that are most likely to be affected by the rehabilitative interventions in question.

Patients' *subjective well-being, life satisfaction,* or *subjective quality of life* are important and deserve assessment, even though they are not part of the current World Health Organization scheme. Although this dimension may not be precisely measured, it can be communicated and roughly indexed. Subjective well-being and related constructs have been increasingly studied for use as ultimate rehabilitation outcomes measures (57). Subjective well-being is statistically associated with health and a loving and satisfying social life, but the weakness and inconsistency of these associations demonstrate that subjective well-being cannot be reduced to indicators of objective health and circumstance. At this point, indices of subjective well-being are well enough understood to be used to begin to understand the value of systems of interventions but are too unreliable and subjective for outcome evaluation to rest on them alone.

Criteria for Choice of Measures

Criteria for choice of measures for process and outcomes improvement projects include (a) psychometric or biometric soundness (reliability and validity or accuracy); (b) logical relatedness to the rehabilitative interventions in the program, that is, to one's treatment theory and the expected results of treatment (15,43); and (c) sensitivity to patient gain (a practical proxy for the preceding). In practice, ease of administration, expense, and budget are of commanding importance. Chapter 6 presents additional clinical criteria for choice of measures.

Psychometric and Biometric Criteria

Rehabilitation professionals need to understand concepts of reliability and validity rather than rely on intuitive notions of "hard" versus "soft" measures, because hard measures can be unreliable and may well be demonstrably invalid for the quality or outcomes measurement purpose (cf. Chapter 6).

Accuracy is the relevant criterion to evaluate the validity of an measure when an extremely accurate, objective "gold standard" is available. Knowledge of sensitivity and specificity are of course basic to assessment of diagnostic tests and other categorical tests, including quality assessments (58). There is reason to believe that many existing assessments of the appropriateness of medical care have a substantial false-positive rate; that is, they tend to overstate the frequency of inappropriate care because the methods are so error-prone (59).

Measurement Standards for Interdisciplinary Medical Rehabilitation are now available to guide clinicians, quality professionals, and researchers in choice and development of measures in domains of human performance, function, or health in which physical gold standards do not exist (58). In brief, we need to know the *reliability*—that is, the stability, agreement, and reproduceability—of measures used for QI or outcomes monitoring. Without this information, results are more subject to error and charges of subjectivity. Unreliability constrains the degree of validity attainable (42).

Validity is a concept associated with utility. Validity is always validity *for some defined purpose* and is always limited. Validity may be seen as the sum of the inferences that one can make from a measure in defined circumstances. The validity of a measure develops with its use in research and in practice, as one learns its meaning and its limitations.

Predictive or criterion-oriented validity information is particularly important: a useful measure should be able to predict some important future event. For instance, a valid measure of general disability should be shown to correlate with total nursing and supervision hours, as the FIM does (60).

Technical criteria. Disability is usually measured by gross rating or, more precisely, by adding together a number of different items. How do we know that the items can really be added together (additivity)? How do we know that they constitute something rather than many things (homogeneity and dimensionality)? When adding things together or applying techniques that assume that intervals between points are of equal magnitude (parametric statistics), they should have equal-interval properties (42,61,62).

Finally, item difficulty also needs to be understood, given the wide range of human performance dealt with in medical rehabilitation, which treats patients who range in ability from complete paralysis and coma to individuals attempting community integration to those attempting to return to demanding occupations that require speed, endurance, and high levels of performance. The field needs measures sensitive to improvement for all of these individuals. Many existing measures are sensitive to the typical range of improvement seen in medical rehabilitation hospitals (7,8,52,61,63) but still have ceiling or floor problems; that is, they may be insensitive to very real improvements that occur in some patient groups (64).

Rasch analysis is applied to determine whether a scale based on adding ordinal raw scores in fact has equal-interval characteristics in terms of difficulty level (i.e., the logit-transformed probabilities of passing items) (42,61,65). If the scale does not have equal-interval characteristics, the numbers representing scale steps can be adjusted to create an equal-interval scale. If some items are nonadditive or do not "fit," they should be treated as representing some other dimension. Rasch analysis has an additional benefit: It produces "person fit" lists that tell one what types of patients the measure works with—and what types it does not. This is a great advantage too, as it is not plausible to believe that the difficulty-level order of functional tasks should be the same across diagnoses. Walking, for instance, may be easy for a person with severely disabling brain injury but is impossible for persons with paraparesis (without impractical functional electrical stimulation). The difficulty structure of memory and complex planning tasks would also be altered across the groups.

Uses of Different Levels of Measures

Measures of pathology, impairment, disability, handicap, and subjective well-being are all needed to understand and evaluate the quality and outcomes of medical rehabilitation programs. It is essential to choose measures of the right type and level, as rehabilitative interventions can be shown to be effective at one level of function but not at another.

Uses of disability measures. Measures of disability or functional limitations are of central importance to medical rehabilitation. Therapeutic interventions involving practice, such as those in physical therapy (PT), occupational therapy (OT), and speech-language pathology (SLP), may be effective at the level of disability but ineffective at the level of basic disease or impairment, as they involve learning of adaptive and compensatory abilities. For instance, practical communication improves in response to speech therapy, but aphasia scores may be unchanged (17), and the underlying brain damage remains. Disability measures may improve even though ASIA motor scores or other measures of functional impairment do not significantly improve (7,17). Measures of practical functional abilities tell us whether an intervention aiming at alleviation of pathology or impairment produced a meaningful, practical improvement in function to the person. Rehabilitation has long focused on ''function'' or functional gain as the first step to begin assessment of the effectiveness of rehabilitative interventions. There are sound reasons for measures of functional gain or reduced functional gain to continue to serve as the core of medical rehabilitation outcomes measurement.

However, measurement should not stop with disability measures. Disability measures are difficult to interpret except in a context that includes consideration of the physiological basis of the disability. The effects of the physical and especially social environment also need to be considered. The significance of the same disability can vary among patients (12–14,52). Improved ability to cook or to climb stairs, for instance, may be critical to one person but irrelevant to another. Life satisfaction, handicap, or individualized needs should be assessed to understand the significance of functional outcomes for individuals.

Uses of impairment measures. Measures of impairment and pathology are so numerous and important to clinical processes that we focus on their role in longer-term outcomes evaluation. Interventions to ameliorate medical pathologies can be extraordinarily powerful, but rehabilitation physicians have largely chosen to care for patients whose problems cannot be cured. The effectiveness of impairment-related interventions in rehabilitation is therefore commonly more limited in rehabilitation than in acute care.

Both QI and outcomes-monitoring systems in medical rehabilitation must at least group patients by their primary etiology or impairment group. Impairment and diagnosis are obviously essential to understanding of appropriateness of treatment planning. They are also needed to set expectations for improvement (10), and for assessment of case severity (e.g., Glasgow Coma Scale, ASIA motor scores) (17).

If an impairment is used as an outcome measure, there should be evidence—not merely an assumption—that the impairment is significantly related to functional outcomes or quality or duration of life. Any number of medical and nursing conditions treated in medical rehabilitation—infection control, reduction of decubitus ulcers, control of blood pressure, prevention and treatment of DVT, diabetes management, pain relief—meet this criterion in principle. Even in these cases, special circumstances could alter their choice or interpretation as treatment objectives. In many circumstances in rehabilitation, however, a pathology or impairment can be treated and technically reduced without alteration of the primary disease or the functional status of the patient (66). Range of motion and even spasticity reduction, for instance, are poorly correlated with functional outcomes (67), probably because they are not the primary barriers to improved function for many patients who have these impairments. Although improved ROM may be a useful intermediate or secondary treatment objective, it does not serve well as a long-term primary treatment objective in rehabilitation. Discriminating more worthwhile from less worthwhile but still technically effective interventions is a challenge for physiatrists and others who plan rehabilitative interventions.

Uses of handicap measures. Reduction of handicap (social disadvantage) can be described as the ultimate goal of rehabilitation, as handicap measures are most relevant to the overall life of persons with disabilities and reflect valued outcomes in the community (9–12,17). Handicap is the most complete outcome measure because it incorporates disability, the environment, disadvantage to the person, and social norms. Reduction of handicap is an appropriate goal for comprehensive, intensive rehabilitation programs and is particularly relevant to later phases of rehabilitation (e.g., outpatient or comprehensive postacute programs when the person is already living in the community) (17–19).

Handicap can be diminished by laws prohibiting discrimination against persons with disability, improving the quality of routine attendant and nursing care, or by simply giving the patient money. The worth of medical rehabilitation programs can be assessed by noting how much they diminish handicap compared to alternatives, even if the alternatives apply very different treatment strategies, provided the patient population is similar.

The breadth of handicap is also its limitation. Handicap is affected by family support, ethnicity, poverty, prior employment history, environmental barriers, and social attitudes. Although medical rehabilitation programs can occasionally influence aspects of these wider social and environmental factors, these factors are primarily beyond its control. Medical rehabilitation aims at decreasing handicap by improving patient function. Handicap measures are not yet as well developed as are measures of disability or impairment (7,17,18,52). Narrower measures more proximal to interventions applied (e.g., functional limitations most characteristic of the diagnostic group) are often a wiser choice for routine outcome monitoring for medical rehabilitation programs.

Sensitivity and Logical Relatedness to Treatment

The minimum simple criterion for choice of outcome measures for quality and outcomes monitoring is demonstrated change in association with treatment. A measure of function or impairment that does not typically change during rehabilitation is not a candidate for an outcome measure.

Many works in medical rehabilitation have for decades interpreted change *per se* as indicating causation or effectiveness. Although the temptation to do this is natural and understandable, and improved function is certainly a crucial indicator in rehabilitation, causation cannot be reliably inferred from measures of functional improvement alone. Causation is inferred from a pattern of improvement highly associated with treatment but not associated with case severity or other exogenous (i.e., nontreatment) factors (37). Controlled research is necessary to infer causation or treatment effectiveness.

More broadly, inference of treatment effectiveness depends on our total knowledge of healing and adaptive rehabilitative processes. A well-validated, sensible theoretical basis is needed to make results credible and to suggest how results can be generalized to practice (68). The essential points of this theoretical basis need to be explicated (15); even a "small" or simple explication of why, how, and when a treatment should work is valuable (43). If the treatment theory deals with pathologic processes (e.g., infections), then indicators of that process should be chosen as central measures (e.g., colony count, organism type). If motor and/or concept learning are core processes, the functional performances the person practices should be measured.

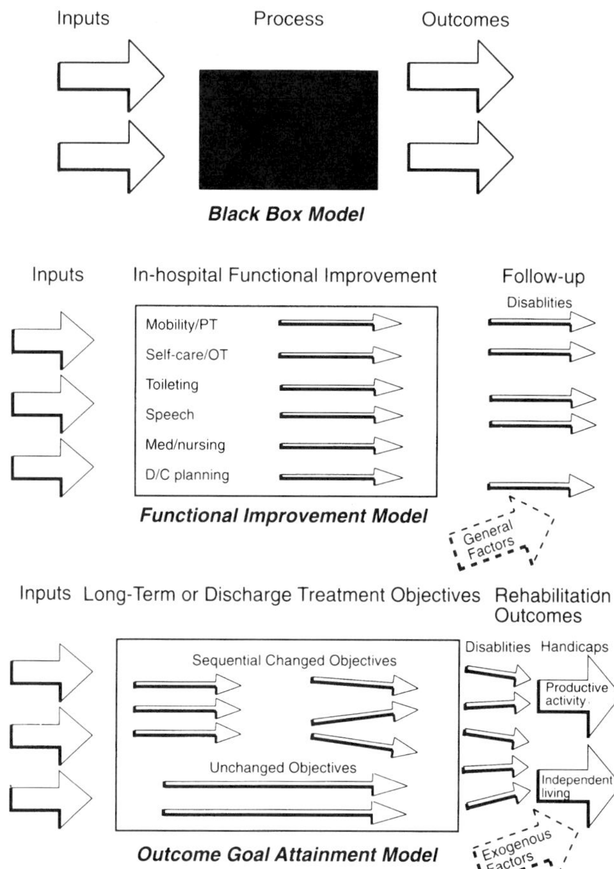

FIG. 14-3. Three simplified schemata for rehabilitation program evaluation and outcomes management.

Causal Models for Monitoring Systems

In general, well-designed quality- and outcomes-monitoring systems involve measures of three types—inputs, processes, and outcomes. Figure 14-3 shows three increasingly sophisticated but still simplified schemata for outcome monitoring systems.

In traditional program evaluation systems in medical rehabilitation, the emphasis has been on outcomes, and the process box is sparse. Commonly, there are virtually no process measures and no explicit theory of effective treatment. Treatment is virtually a black box (top of Fig. 14-3). The approach was useful in the past as a first attempt to understand outcomes of whole comprehensive medical rehabilitation programs, where processes were so complex and numerous that explication of processes and specific treatment objectives has seemed to be an intractable task.

However, limitations of the black box model are increasingly recognized (15,39,43,69,70). When the processes are not measured, one can hardly begin to identify what can be done to improve outcomes. Although the black box model protects caring holistic rehabilitation programs, it also protects disorganized programs and provides virtually nothing that would prohibit cuts of needed care to increase short-term profits.

Although rehabilitation is complex, it is not the case that medical rehabilitation cannot explicate important treatment processes and associated outcomes for commonly encountered, important patient problems. In the last 5 years, many clinical guidelines (listed later in process section) have begun to be written to explicate what is involved in medical rehabilitation.

The middle schema of Figure 14-3 depicts the Functional Improvement Model found in many program evaluation systems. Improvement in specific disabilities associated with primary disciplines within the rehabilitation facility is measured (as represented by arrows). There is some ability to analyze the effect of general factors such as intensity of treatment, primary impairments, payer, and demographic factors.

More sophisticated data systems—tied to the actual rehabilitation planning process for individuals—have been attempted (9,10,71). As displayed at the bottom of Figure 14-3, functional goals and progress are represented by arrows. Evaluation can be based on long-term (i.e., discharge) treatment objectives set by the team for individuals rather than on common goals across patients. Long-term objectives change occasionally during rehabilitation. Short-term daily or weekly objectives are recorded in clinical notes in the record. Functional goals are not treated as parallel and equal but are targeted by the individualized rehabilitation plan at reduction of handicap (as shown by *arrows* pointing to productive activity and independent living after discharge). Follow-up interviews determine whether productive-activity and independent-living outcome goals have been attained and, if not, why. Past publications have called monitoring systems like this *Client-Centered Program Evaluation* (71). When patient goals or objectives are based on actual rehabilitation plans for patients, rather than on typical goals for a broad class, we will refer to it as a true *clinical outcomes management data system.*

Explicating process-outcomes relations requires a knowledge basis. Ultimately, the desire to make quality-outcomes monitoring systems work will require the development and continual updating of detailed, scientifically based, authoritative clinical practice guidelines or clinical paths. Although complexity will defeat attempts to define appropriate clinical interventions for every patient, it is likely that workable guidelines with objective indicators of relevant processes and clinical outcomes can be created for many, perhaps most, common patient problems treated in rehabilitation. One would imagine that such systems would work best if a certain frequency of exceptions and modifications to the guideline are not only allowed but considered optimal.

Patient Satisfaction

Patient satisfaction measures deserve to be part of any clinical data system, because: (a) patient satisfaction is quite measurable at a modest cost (40); (b) a facility's reputation is enhanced by satisfied clients; (c) at the same time, honest patient satisfaction measures can identify significant dissatisfaction and problematic processes; (d) dissatisfaction rates are much higher in facilities that misrepresent the services they offer; and (e) patient satisfaction is important in part because patient valuation of outcomes is different from that of professionals (13,14,40,72,73).

Patient satisfaction measures have limitations and need to be presented to staff in a positive light. Patients tend to express high satisfaction with medical rehabilitation services. ''The most consistent finding is that the characteristics of providers or organizations that result in more 'personal' care are associated with higher levels of satisfaction'' in medical settings (40). Patient satisfaction is poorly related to technical effectiveness or professional standards (40). Satisfaction measures often elicit comments about food, temperature, billing hassles, and other hotel and personal services. Patient satisfaction questionnaires have been published for general medical settings (74) and for inpatient (75) and outpatient (76) rehabilitation programs (22). Many large group health organizations have adopted standard formats for assessment of patient satisfaction based on Ware's research (77).

PROGRAM EVALUATION AND OUTCOMES MANAGEMENT

This section treats systems of measurement or monitoring, interpretation, planning, and action oriented to the outcomes attained by patients after rehabilitative care. Terminology is in flux, and interrelated terms such as program evaluation, outcomes management, outcomes monitoring, outcomes evaluation, and planning are used.

Outcomes Management

The term ''outcomes management'' has become popular. The term is loosely associated with outcomes measurement, program evaluation, case management, and managed care (78). CARF has begun to create standards for ''outcomes measurement and management'' but, reflecting uncertainty in the field, has not yet specified details apart from program evaluation requirements (6). How ''outcomes management'' and ''case management'' relate to the long-established and more basic functions of rehabilitation teams and physicians is often not specified. We will attempt to provide at least some clarification of the terms.

Although the term has come to be used in many ways, Paul Ellwood provided the original and most persuasive conceptualization of ''outcomes management . . . a technology of patient experience designed to help patients, payers, and providers make rational medical care-related choices based on better insight into the effect of these choices on the patient's life'' (79 p. 1551). Outcomes management is based on the increasingly scientific basis of medical care, including the increasing ability to predict outcomes and on advances in health status assessment that permit useful measurement of health and function at the level of patient experience rather than at the level of mortality or disease rates.

Ellwood's concept of outcomes management is based on data sets similar to those long used in program evaluation but expanded to a much wider, population basis. Professional analyses of such huge data bases would, according to Ellwood, provide estimates of the effectiveness and efficiency of medical services in practice. Because rather general outcomes measures are to be used, implications are primarily at the aggregate level—the level of integrated health care systems or programs rather than of management of individual patients.

Outcomes management involves four key techniques:

1. The use of treatment guidelines (or standards) to help clinical professionals to choose appropriate treatments.
2. Routine and systematic measurement of disease-specific outcomes and patients' general health, function, and/or well-being.
3. Combining data on processes and outcomes into extremely large data bases to permit scientific analyses.
4. Dissemination of results in forms appropriate for use by different parties to the health care process.

Although U.S. health care as a whole is far from operationalizing Ellwood's grand plan for outcomes management, each of these is being done on a piecemeal basis as integrated health organizations create their own quality-related data bases and smaller organizations voluntarily join health outcome data bases. Rehabilitation, with its long experience with outcomes-oriented program evaluation systems, should be particularly ready to operationalize outcomes management.

Outcomes management is also used to refer to systems that manage individual patients. We define a *clinical outcomes management system* as a system that involves routine monitoring of outcomes (as well as relevant inputs and processes) and goals or objectives of treatment as defined by the team, case manager, or rehabilitation physician as appropriate for the individual. Clinical outcomes management, as defined here, differs from traditional program evaluation in that standard goals are not routinely applied routinely across a broad and rather diverse diagnostic-functional groups such as stroke, TBI, or SCI without consideration of whether they fit patient or treatment priorities. It may often be most efficient to define certain routine goals or objectives for common clinical presentations (e.g., most knee-replacement or post-elective-arthroplasty patients without complications), but even then a professional familiar with the individual should note whether typical objectives fit or not. As defined here, clinical outcomes management is essentially a structured forms of actual case management or rehabilitation planning for patients, utilizing objective measures for high-frequency or important outcomes. Clinical outcomes management as defined here requires the physician, rehabilitation team, or case manager who knows the patient well to select appropriate treatment objectives. The outcomes management information system provides feedback on results.

''Outcomes management'' is sometimes used to imply regulation of outcomes with a degree of control that is not possible. Quality rehabilitation enhances a patient's likely recovery and adaptation, but the exact level of outcomes to be achieved usually cannot be commanded, engineered, or even predicted with precision. The terms *outcomes planning* and *outcomes evaluation* may be somewhat more realistic than outcomes management. *Outcomes improvement* implies that we do not want to manage outcomes but to do our best to improve them.

Program Evaluation

Program evaluation refers to a variety of information-gathering activities designed to aid in program development or functioning (i.e., formative evaluation) or to decide whether a program as a whole is worthwhile (i.e., summative evaluation) (39). Many approaches evaluation of health service programs have been tested in the last three decades (39). Evaluations of clinical programs typically concentrate on issues of effectiveness and efficiency. Accountability to the public is an outstanding purpose of program evaluation systems. These system also have multiple uses, including marketing, profitability, program planning and development, research, prognosis, utilization review, and improved clinical planning and treatment.

In medical rehabilitation, CARF has defined program evaluation or outcomes-oriented evaluation as ''a systematic procedure for determining the effectiveness and efficiency with which results are achieved by persons served following services'' (6). These results are collected on a regular or continuous basis'' for all patients or for a systematic sample of patients (6,80). Program evaluation in rehabilitation has been oriented toward patient outcomes in the community. An accredited medical rehabilitation program should demonstrate that persons served are making measurable progress toward accomplishment of their functional goals (2, pp. 70–74).

Although CARF has traditionally emphasized functional outcomes, CARF's most recent standards have at last formalized the need to routinely assess medical or physiological outcomes (6). Medical outcomes are especially emphasized when these may effect functional or general health outcomes.

Program evaluation and outcomes management involve setting goals and expectancies (78). If goals are not attained, action should be taken to determine why. In its usual form, program evaluation does not provide answers to specific problem areas but merely identifies that a problem or strength exists. Answers are identified through more in-depth investigations involving further analyses of data, chart review, examination of QI measures (i.e., monitors), and discussions with the knowledgeable staff (20,81–84). Program evaluation systems are used to help make decisions and improve program operations. CARF states that the program evaluation system needs to report the percentage of patients who achieved their discharge goals (7).

History of Program Evaluation

In the 1960s and 1970s, accreditation agencies, payers, and even providers' tracking systems were preoccupied with inputs and processes such as staffing levels, licensure, and authority relationships. Outcomes to patients were typically unknown. Beginning in the 1970s, leaders in rehabilitation realized that the field needed to demonstrate its benefits to the public. Providing a forum and focus for this realization, CARF assumed leadership and developed standards that required well-established rehabilitation facilities to eventually develop program evaluation systems that measure outcomes. In the mid- to late 1970s and 1980s, workable prototype program evaluation designs and guides (85) were tested and developed along with outcome-oriented standards. Accredited programs across the land began to develop program evaluation systems. Many programs, realizing the need for objective comparative data, joined mass data systems, although this was not required by CARF.

Experience with program evaluation systems resulted in a shift of emphasis away from choice of measures and formal design of the program evaluation system beginning with 1982 standards (80–82). Utilization of program evaluation information, regardless of program evaluation system design, became the key point. Program evaluation requirements were incorporated into sections on evaluation, management information systems, and administrative record keeping. Program evaluation was to be integrated into program operations. CARF kept a ''Special Policy'' requiring a program evaluation system that regularly produced useful reports. Beginning in 1995, CARF began to refer to ''outcomes measurement and management,'' and the special policy on program evaluation became ''Policy on Outcomes'' (2, p. 8). The glossary uses the terms program evaluation and outcomes management interchangeably.

In 1996, CARF instituted a ''strategic outcomes initiative'' to respond to increasing demands from consumers, payers as well as providers, for more uniform, meaningful outcome and program quality data. Standards relating to outcome measurement and management were to be reviewed during 1997 for inclusion in 1998 standards. CARF continues its emphasis on outcome-orientation in accreditation, though not to the exclusion of process standards (6).

Although the early enthusiasm for program evaluation has waned, concern about outcomes remains acute. Managed care plans buy rehabilitation services primarily on the basis of cost, but concern about the quality of care and its effects on patients has been heightened. Articles on the quality of health care plans appear recurrently in newspapers and magazines. The need to demonstrate the quality and outcomes of care provided remains pressing. Through program evaluation, medical rehabilitation has two decades of experience with the uses and limitation of outcomes measurement, as much and perhaps more experience than any other sector of the medical care industry.

The Standard Rehabilitation Program Evaluation Model

Over the last three decades or so, medical rehabilitation facilities have developed their own tradition in program evaluation (86). These program evaluation systems are designed to provide an overview of program outcomes. In effect, they are designed to assure outcomes to the public, that is, to be summative evaluation systems. In operation, however, these systems function as formative evaluation systems (82). Information on outcomes is given primarily to program staff, who constitute the main audience for reports. Improved program operations is a primary expectation and an issue in assessing the worth of past program evaluation efforts.

Standard program evaluation systems in rehabilitation have three components: design, goals and objectives, and reports. The standard model sketched here is based on the work of Robert Walker, a chief CARF consultant in the 1970s. Although this basic model is still widely used, considerable updating is occurring as part of CARF's strategic outcomes initiative. In addition to its annual standards manuals, CARF has published monographs on program evaluation help guide programs (80). The current program evaluation materials are in the process of revision, and updated versions may not be available until 1998. Anyone developing, implementing, or using a program evaluation or QI system in rehabilitation should consult these materials as well as the CARF standards manual (6). Readers should call CARF in Tucson or contact their web site (http://www.carf.org) to obtain the most recent information.

Program purpose and description. The program evaluation design is based on a mission statement describing whom the organization serves, what services it provides, and what goals it expects to accomplish. The programs that constitute the organization are then described (e.g., stroke program, brain injury, spinal injury, pain program, general inpatient rehabilitation, transitional living center). Key influencers are listed to ground the statement in reality. These are external agencies that constrain and direct the rehabilitation program, such as the rehabilitation market and clients, referral sources, patients, staff, Medicare, third-party payers, and key government agencies.

Each program within an organization is to be described in terms that should be well-known:

1. General program objectives. These are anticipated results to the primary clients., mission statement for the program. (Here the term ''objectives'' is used for what we call more general ''goals.'')
2. Admission criteria. Both inclusionary (e.g., cerebrovascular accident [CVA]) and exclusionary (e.g., free from communicable disease, over 18, noncomatose, dependent in ADL and ambulation, medically stable for 3 hours/day of therapy, likely to survive at least 6 months) criteria are defined.
3. Persons served, defined by diagnosis and functional problems.
4. Services provided or readily available to the patient, such as routine physiatry, PT, OT, SLP, psychology, social services, and rehabilitation nursing.

General program objectives. CARF publications have defined several objectives that need to occur and be monitored in program evaluation for global program objectives to be attained.

First are *outcome objectives* defined in terms of benefits received by patients or, secondarily, families or caregivers. (We use the term long-term goals or rehabilitation outcome goals for these.) Outcomes are usually measured at admission, discharge, and follow-up, which takes place usually

3 months after discharge but often at 1, 6, or 12 months later.

Also needed are progress objectives in terms of patient improvement in the clinical setting toward outcomes and measures of patient progress in attaining independence of patients in activities such as mobility, self-care and communication. (These are similar to but less specific than our concept of treatment objectives.)

Efficiency objectives are also needed. Resources consumed such as staff time, length of stay, number of treatment sessions, and dollars should be monitored.

Program evaluation and outcomes monitoring measures. The FIM of the Uniform Data System for Medical Rehabilitation is the most commonly used functional outcomes measure in medical rehabilitation. Over 500 facilities contribute data to this data base. The FIM is an 18-item scale that rates each item along a scale ranging from 1 (i.e., total assist) to 7 (i.e., completely independent). The FIM consists of two overall factors (i.e., motor function and cognition), and recent reports indicate acceptable-to-good reliability (65,87).

Typical constituents of a rehabilitation inpatient hospital program evaluation system are shown in Figure 14-4. The sparseness of measures (italicized) in the process box and the larger set of admission (i.e., input) and outcome (i.e., discharge and follow-up) measures show the emphasis of conventional program evaluation systems. Disability measures (e.g., FIM) constitute the primary input (e.g., admission, baseline) and output (e.g., discharge,follow-up) measures. Cost and length of stay are classified here as process measures because they indicate the degree of effort the rehabilitation team chooses to devote to the patient.

Supplementary measures. Program evaluation systems usually have measures used for general descriptive or comparative purposes (cf. Fig. 14-4). Demographic variables (e.g., age, gender, race) are often considered to be input variables. They are listed here as supplemental measures because they may not be very good measures of case severity. Data and reasons for death are essential supplementary measures in program evaluation and QI. Inpatient medical rehabilitation programs frequently deal with aged, infirm, and chronically ill patients. Research has shown that medical rehabilitation programs can increase survival (88). At the same time, rehabilitation does not aim simply to save or extend life. Death rate is not a suitable primary outcome or quality measure for typical medical rehabilitation programs.

The Classic Program Evaluation Model

For almost 20 years, conventional rehabilitation program evaluation systems in rehabilitation involved the following (6,86):

- Program objectives, such as improved function in self-care, mobility, continence, and communication, target length of stay, and patient satisfaction.
- The operational measure, such as the FIM.
- To whom measures apply. In the conventional program evaluation model, program objectives are applied to all patients in the program.

INPUTS		PROCESSES		OUTCOMES
• Function/disability at admission in: *self-care ADLs, mobility, bowel & bladder management, general communicative & cognitive function*, etc. • Demographics (*eg. age, sex, race*) • Marketing data (e.g. referral sources) • *Primary diagnosis, other diagnoses* Key functional impairment measures • Acute hospital function, prior history, *date of onset*, many others.	➡	• Type and amount of therapy • Key tests and measures, and other key services/interventions • Treatment objectives and interrim progress measures. • Complications/problems • Indices of cost/effort (e.g. *charges, length of stay*)	➡	• Function/disability in: *self-care ADLs, mobility, bowel & bladder management, general communicative & cognition function*, etc. at discharge and follow-up. • *Community living arrangement* (vs. nursing home or hospital). • Vocational status (e.g. *full v. part-time employment*) • Many others (e.g. social activities, unpaid activities, disability support costs, preventable complications)

SUPPLEMENTARY MEASURES
• *Payment source*, region of country, and many other descriptors • Date and cause of death

FIG. 14-4. Basic conventional framework for evaluation of rehabilitation programs. Examples from the Uniform Data System are shown in *italics*. From the standpoint of cost–benefit research, cost and length of stay are input variables, but they are classified here as process measures because they are indices of the degree of effort the rehabilitation team chooses to devote to the patient. Demographic variables are usually considered input variables, although often they may not be the relevant index of case severity and therefore should be classified as a supplemental measure. (*ADLs*, activities of daily living.)

- When measures are applied. Most programs measure function at admission and discharge. Assessment of function 1 to 6 months after discharge gives a more valuable picture of patient outcomes.
- Who does the measurement.
- A specific expectancy for each objective. Expectancies are specific statements of the expected level or range of results.
- The relative importance of objectives. Weighs were to be chosen so that multiplying outcomes by these numbers would give an overall goal-attainment percentage for the entire program. All program outcomes were to be summarized into a single number in which optimal attainment of all expectancies was signified by 100.

Comparison of actual outcomes to expectancies was the basis for evaluation of the program in the classic program evaluation model. Realistically, there is a range of tolerable performance. The classic model rather wisely recommended that a range of performance expectancies be defined—minimal, optimal, and maximal. Outcomes were not to fall below the minimum. If outcomes did fall below this level, action was to be taken. The optimal or maximal level is the best that the program feels could be achieved under ideal circumstances (80,85). In these older program evaluation models, expectancies were created by program staff on the basis of local experience and ideas rather than on the basis of normative or published comparison data on what is attainable for patients.

When expectancies were not met, a common response was simply to change the expectancy. Even though accreditation standards allowed completely local measures and standards, the flimsiness of completely local, subjective expectancies has long been recognized. Recognizing this, rehabilitation programs beginning in the 1970s voluntarily created regional and national outcomes data systems, such as the HUP and more recently the Uniform Data System and Formations. Although the evaluation and action component of the classic program evaluation model was weak, the process did at least teach program personnel what realistic outcome expectations were.

Program evaluation systems have been based on straight outcome scores, simple gain scores (i.e., outcome minus admission score), or both (78,83,84). The use of raw outcome scores suffers from the fact that functional outcomes depend strongly on function at admission (7,44,61,89,90). Raw outcome scores need to be adjusted for severity. The correct statistical use of gain scores, like statistical adjustment for case severity, can be tricky (91).

Program Evaluation Reports

Management reports are the routine product of program evaluation and outcomes management information systems. Data are synthesized into periodic (e.g., quarterly or semiannual) management reports on patient progress, outcomes and goal attainment, efficiency, trends in these and in case load, and so on. Reports go to administrative and clinical managers, the governing board, and staff. Data on patient progress or outcomes may also be formatted for release to purchasers of services and the public (6,81,82).

Statistical reports detail program outcomes compared to expected levels of achievement and describe client populations and trends over time. Narrative interpretations are essential for program evaluation or QI data to be meaningful and useful. Reporting and interpretation are so essential that a whole section is devoted to it below.

Shared Data Systems

Because of the need for objective comparison data, most inpatient medical rehabilitation hospitals and many units have joined nationwide or regional data systems.

The largest data system in medical rehabilitation is the Uniform Data System for Medical Rehabilitation. This data set consists of 119 items: 63 FIM, 39 other inpatient variables, and 17 additional follow-up items (92). The central outcome measure is the FIM, a seven-level rating of degree of independence in self-care, mobility, continence, communication, social cognition, and psychosocial function. Every facility subscribing to the service assesses functional progress between admission and discharge; facilities can also assess maintenance of function at follow-up. The Uniform Data System was explicitly designed to be a *minimum data set* to give an overview of practical patient outcomes.

The simplicity of the Uniform Data System explains its practicality and its popularity. It also explains the recurrent criticism that it is incomplete and insufficiently detailed to understand many clinical outcomes and the effectiveness of associated clinical care. The same commentary applies to other outcomes-monitoring systems: there is a trade-off between clinical adequacy and simplicity.

The Program Evaluation Conference System (PECS) developed by Richard Harvey and colleagues at Marianjoy Hospital has been used by dozens of rehabilitation programs across the United States for a decade (61,93). Designed to be clinically useful, the PECS is used to organize communication and set goals in the rehabilitation team conference as well as to evaluate the rehabilitation program and ensure and improve quality of services (93).

It is more complete—and therefore more complex—than the UDS. Excellent psychometric scaling information (61,62) and benchmark comparative data are available. The system produces admirable team conference reports and graphics (cf. Fig. 14-6).

Formations in Health Care offers the Medical Outcome System (94) for respiratory, pain, and wound patients in mostly subacute rehabilitation settings. Patient functional progress is now monitored in term of the FIM. A ''case manager'' is offered that roughly predicts outcomes on the basis of the patient's admission level, increasing the utility of the system.

Formations also offers RESTORE for comprehensive outpatient rehabilitation programs (95). RESTORE measures both functional limitations and general health (using the SF-36). A consortium of outpatient rehabilitation providers, working with university researchers, have developed Focus on Therapeutic Outcomes (FOTO) for back, neck, knee, arthritis, pain, and orthopedic problems seen by physical therapists (PTs) and others in outpatient clinics (96). FOTO uses both measures specific to the problem and the SF-36.

Many other data systems of relevance to some forms of rehabilitation are available (70,78). Certain states and regions have their own data systems, and large rehabilitation corporations have their own proprietary systems. JCAHO continues to develop its indicator measurement and management system, which eventually should come to have elements that apply to medical rehabilitation.

Reports from large data systems reveal that some rehabilitation facilities have high rates of patient progress, whereas others appear to have substantially less. At present, virtually no research identifies reasons for these variations.

Program Evaluation Models for Different Populations

Program evaluation systems in medical rehabilitation are best tailored to diagnostic and functional groups. References are available on how to tailor a program evaluation system for the following situations:

- General inpatient medical rehabilitation, including stroke (7,39,63,80,97)
- SCI (7,63,98)
- TBI (9,10,12,17,99)
- Chronic pain management programs (99)
- Outpatient rehabilitation clinics (76,78,85,90)
- Postacute community reentry (12,18,63) and vocational programs (12,63,100)
- Other chronic diseases (63,101) and fields of health care (39)

CARF is updating its materials on program evaluation to reflect "outcomes management," and readers should contact CARF to obtain the most recent materials. At the time of writing, Forer's *Outcomes Management and Program Evaluation* has up-to-date information on the topic (78).

Because inpatient rehabilitation programs must contend with numerous mixed-diagnosis cases, comorbidities, and rare diagnoses, mixed-diagnosis evaluation systems are a necessity if outcomes (and processes) are to be monitored for all patients. Functional improvement is a meaningful if imperfect way of quantifying the benefits in mixed-diagnosis groups. Mixed-diagnosis systems that focus on functional and handicap-level outcomes appear to be relatively successful for later stages of rehabilitation, including transitional living, community integration, vocational rehabilitation, and long-term nursing home care. Both function and diagnosis are critical in evaluation of processes and outcomes of inpatient, outpatient, and at-home medical rehabilitation programs.

Design Issues in Outcomes Monitoring Systems

This section discusses issues of design of outcomes-monitoring systems that go beyond the standard program evaluation design sketched above.

Generality of measures. Program evaluation and outcomes management measures are usually chosen at a level more general than that used for clinical treatment objectives. Program evaluation goals have typically been designed to credit the program with the larger benefits it produces, such as general independence from assistance (80).

Appeal to a broad audience. Long-term outcome measures can be more valuable for marketing, policy, and accountability to the public if they appeal to a broad audience (81,82). Data on how a program has reduced the frequency with which patients are institutionalized in nursing homes and hospitals after discharge, for instance, are meaningful and even influential with boards of directors, government officials, insurers, families, and referral sources.

Timing of outcome measurement. Outcomes for persons served are best measured following discharge. Although assessing outcomes only at discharge is useful and practical, these outcomes are less informative, as clinical staff tend already to be aware of patient function at discharge. Their concern is about how their patients fared afterwards. Determinants of continued gain versus deterioration after rehabilitation discharge need to be better understood.

CARF's publications (80) state that the achievement of objectives should be assessed "at a point following discharge when results can be considered stable." On the other hand, the achievement of objectives should be assessed "at a time when the information obtained will reflect the impact of services recently provided" (80). The longer one waits, the more results may reflect uncontrollable events after discharge or services provided by other programs after discharge. The status of chronically ill and disabled persons changes. There is no perfect time for follow-up, but rough optima can be defined to avoid follow-up that is too brief or too long. Sometimes short-term follow-up is valuable to assess whether patients have encountered unexpected problems shortly after discharge (e.g., 1 to 2 weeks).

Need for repeated measures and especially intermediate outcomes measures. Rehabilitation involves enhancing healing and adaptation processes, so recovery processes should ideally be measured repeatedly over time. This ideal will remain too expensive for many operational monitoring systems until records are fully automated. Repeated testing can be necessary to ensure a reasonably stable measure of average outcome for both impairments and functional performances that are highly variable (e.g., blood pressure, active ROM, social behavior skills).

We have emphasized the need to measure treatment objectives in a case management or rehabilitation planning context. Other experts in quality and clinical outcomes research also affirm the need to measure *intermediate outcomes* to connect long-term outcomes to clinical care (102).

Performance versus ability. Primary outcomes should be measured in terms of actual patient performance rather than in terms of capability or other terms (63,78,80). Actual performance is usually a more reliable and valid measure than judged ability. Frequently used skills tend to provide greater benefit than rarely used skills. Exceptions to this may exist when dealing with instrumental or extended ADLs, such as cooking, household skills, and community mobility, where skills may be needed even if used on an irregular basis. Weighting or judging need for such skills is an issue here.

Follow-up methods. Outcomes at follow-up are usually assessed by structured telephone calls or clinic visits.

Program evaluation systems have often used structured telephone follow-up calls. Experience and survey research studies have shown that this method can provide a good balance of reliability, low rate of missing data, and modest to moderate costs. Very specific, simple questions need to be asked by skilled, *trained* interviewers using a structured questionnaire. Mail follow-up, though inexpensive, usually suffers from high missing data, although meticulously designed processes can, with extraordinary attention, do much better than this. When 40% to 50% of data are lost to follow-up, a data set can provide suggestions but is useless in characterizing the level of program outcomes.

In-clinic follow-up methods are need to objectively assess medical conditions and impairments. Clinical professionals commonly trust face-to-face in-clinic data more because of familiarity than because of proven validity. Missing data can be a problem with in-clinic follow-up if patients do not return. Observations of patient performance in the outpatient clinic are valuable but are not necessarily the most revealing indicators of patient performance or problems in real life.

Statistical and Metric Considerations

A number of statistical and measurement issues need to be understood by whoever is designing and interpreting a data system. Although phrased in terms of outcomes, these considerations frequently apply to process-monitoring systems as well.

Additive scales. For the sum of set of functional items to make sense, they need to be related both in content and empirically. Empirically, one should know the degree to which the items are unidimensional (42,61,62). If one totals items that are unrelated to each other, the sum may be uninterpretable. Special research techniques such as factor analysis or Rasch analysis are used to study the empirical dimensionality of items (61,62). The FIM, for instance, consists of at least two dimensions, motor ADLs and cognitive–psychosocial function (103). The PECS has eight orthogonal dimensions: cognition/emotional adjustment, motoric competence, applied self-care, communication skills, impairment severity, assistive devices, social/recreational involvement, and family support/discharge preparation (61,62). These are all important dimensions in medical rehabilitation.

Statistical analysis of gain scores. The obvious way to compute gain scores is to subtract the pretest from the posttest score. When the measure is a highly reliable one, pretest scores are highly related to posttest scores, and relationships are linear, simple gain scores can be highly justifiable (104). This is probably the case when computing patient gain using such highly (but hardly perfectly) reliable measures as the FIM, Barthel, or PECS. Potentially important statistical issues remain, including regression artifacts (39,42,61,62): if patients tend to be admitted to rehabilitation for transient crises or exacerbations of unstable problems, there will be a tendency for improvement as they "regress" to a higher mean (average) level. A robust and widely recommended method of adjusting raw outcome scores is by regressing pretest scores on them (i.e., to calculate regressed change scores) (104). The underlying idea is that, to the degree that posttest outcome scores are highly correlated with pretest scores, there is empirical reason to adjust the outcome scores. Many statistical packages—from SAS to SPSS—will do this. Change scores are a complex issue that depends ultimately on one's theory or model of recovery curves (91) or stages (105).

Other Points

Here are some additional points for design of outcome-monitoring systems:

- Patient populations need to be divided into major groups, usually by etiology and functional severity.
- Cases that stay only a few days are not comparable to full-stay cases and need to be looked at as a separate group. The rate of short-term evaluation cases is a characteristic of program function.
- Outcomes-monitoring systems center on episodes of illness rather than on administratively convenient units such as a stay in rehabilitation. Readmissions need to be collapsed or analyzed separately. Efficiency cannot really be achieved by cycling difficult cases back and forth between facilities.
- Some rehabilitation programs distinguish between cases admitted for different reasons. Some patients, for instance, are admitted largely for care of a prominent medical problem (e.g., skin care, urinary tract infections, weaning a patient from a vent), even though the problem may not be seen in most patients in the program. Incorporating measures relevant to the primary reasons for admission or

rehabilitative treatment enhances the meaningfulness of outcomes-monitoring reports.

Analysis and reporting. Routine outcomes reports give rise to hypotheses about problems in the program or reasons outcomes are or are not attained. In-depth analysis and study are needed to discover *reasons* why outcomes are higher or lower than expected. The system for statistical analysis, interpretation, and reporting is as important as the size of the sample or the number of measures.

Critique of the Standard Program Evaluation Model

The standard program evaluation model has a number of strengths. It provides an overview of primary patient outcomes, progress, and cost. If used with a shared national or regional data system, standard program evaluation systems provide an index or benchmark of the effectiveness of the program in improving patient function and placing patients in community settings. Efficiency, or at least an operational utilization review system, is demonstrated if the facility shows a direct correlation between cost or length of stay and improvement (44,89) and if improvement/day rates are similar to those in other rehabilitation facilities for similar diagnostic-functional groups. Program evaluation data have numerous administrative and clinical uses (78). Program evaluation systems have begun to tell us whether rehabilitation programs attain an outcome for their patients.

Dissatisfaction with the traditional program evaluation model has grown over time. CARF is now in the process of reformulating its program evaluation standards toward a currently vague concept of "outcomes management." The main problem has been that program evaluation systems have not provided staff with the specific information they need to improve program operations or outcomes within budgetary constraints. The tie between functional improvement, typically reported in program evaluation, and the real effectiveness of treatment has remained weak. The necessary construct validation work to develop ties between a set of measures and inferences of effective rehabilitative interventions has not been done. Controlled studies are really needed for that.

In addition, when "expectancies" for outcome gain in program evaluation systems are not met, the usual response has been to change the expectancy rather than take action to improve the system of care. Although such changes in expectations are undoubtedly self-serving and convenient, they are not unreasonable. Admission of more severe patients is probably the most common reason for declines in outcomes. Since these patients probably also needed care, action implications have been unclear.

A lesser but still significant problem has been inadequate development of measures. The field has reached agreement on basic domains (e.g., mobility, ADL) (4,58,92), but uniform measures of other critical domains have still to be developed or agreed on (e.g., handicap, extended or instrumental ADLs, ecologically valid measures of communicative and cognitive outcomes, affective quality of life, family and environmental factors) (17,50,53,58). Indices of case severity on admission, including comorbidities, have been poorly developed.

There has been a contradiction between the design of most program evaluation systems in medical rehabilitation and the audience they have had. Conventional program evaluation systems are designed to give an overview of program outcomes. They provide data that, if pooled and analyzed at a nationwide level, could be valuable for identifying systems and strategies of care that best help persons with disabilities. The basic measure set constitutes a useful summative evaluation system for many patient groups. The audience for most program evaluation systems, however, has been internal clinical staff, who already know roughly what is happening to their patients and need more detailed measures and insightful analyses to help them give better care within realistic constraints. Program evaluation systems in medical rehabilitation are often not used because they are designed for public accountability, yet the public and even researchers usually do not have access to the data.

Solutions to the problem will involve methods for access to data by researchers and research to do the needed in-depth analyses and to develop methods of connecting processes with intermediate- and long-term outcomes. Such "second-stage screens" (102) and treatment guidelines, with objective review criteria, are discussed as a New Direction in the last section of this chapter.

Alternative Outcomes–Monitoring Models

The conventional program evaluation model used in rehabilitation is only one of several alternatives. Other fields of health care have used other models (39,106).

Goal Attainment Scaling

Developed in community mental settings, goal attainment scaling (GAS) has been applied in many health-related settings. It has been used in rehabilitation and is reported to be a viable means of documenting therapeutic change and clinical accountability (107). In GAS, the professional defines the goal in by verbally describing levels of desired but attainable future states for each individual client (107,108). Goals are rated on a five-point ordinal scale, anchored on the "expected level of treatment success," ideally in objective terms (107,108). The GAS measures are of unknown and indeterminant reliability and validity, as they are ideographic. In the hands of a skilled professional (e.g., a behavioral psychologist), GAS goals and measures can be highly objective and sensitive to individual needs and possibilities. Although relative optimism or accuracy can be compared across programs, objective results cannot. Elsewhere in this chapter, we discuss "client-centered program evaluation," which is similar to GAS in that goals and/or treatment objectives are chosen by clients and clinicians rather than being preestablished but differs from GAS in that goals and/or treatment objectives are chosen from a preestablished menu.

QUALITY ASSURANCE AND IMPROVEMENT

History

To ensure quality in medical care, it should meet standards that are in some sense predefined (31,109,110). Although efforts to systematically ensure quality in medical care go back to the first quarter of the 20th century, pressure for accountability has increased in recent decades, driven by explosive growth of costs, the health rights movement, and by higher expectations of medical care (109). The federal government and the JCAHO have been major institutional forces behind hospital-care QA in general. CARF also defines structural and process standards for different types of rehabilitation programs (6).

Quality-related efforts of the JCAHO have evolved over the decades. Structural and process indicators of quality were first propounded: care had to be provided by licensed practioners, with certain staffing patterns and authority relationships; extensive record keeping, facility, and equipment standards were prescribed. In the late 1950s and 1960s, peer review of medical records was propounded as a method of quality assurance.

In the 1970s, JCAHO required a system of diagnosis-related chart audits for QA to be done at least quarterly. The peer-review audit method came to face increasing criticism that it did not actually assure or improve the quality of care, although it did improve medical records.

The idea that quality of care could and should be indicated by objective indicators gained currency. The Joint Commission began to recommend use of objective *monitors* or *indicators* of care processes or outcomes in 1981. While the emphasis during the 1970s was on whether the organization had the capacity to provide quality medical care, JCAHO began to revamp its approach to QA in the early 1980s. It introduced a multistage QA program emphasizing measures of important medical care practices and problems and evaluation of whether they met preestablished criteria and standards (69). This became policy in the 1985 Accreditation Manual for Hospitals (AMH). The emphasis was and remains on the quality of the care actually provided to patients, not just capacity.

In 1987, JCAHO initiated its Agenda for Change (109,111). This new approach was partially motivated by the repeated difficulty that clinicians were having in identifying and monitoring critical elements of medical care. Leaving the process of measure and data system development to a busy local committee or QA clerk plainly did not work. The Agenda focused on development and use of a standardized set of severity-adjusted clinical indicators to identify and monitor the quality of clinical practices. Priority is given to *high-volume, high-risk, or problematic clinical practices.* Emphasis on at least short-term clinical outcomes, rather than structure and processes *per se,* increased (109).

The Agenda for Change initiated a multiyear research and development project so that key variables—indicators—related to quality of care can be developed to a professionally respectable level. Health care organizations will be required to send QA results to JCAHO or an approved organization on a continuing basis. With this Agenda, JCAHO has begun to ask whether the organization actually provides high-quality, effective care. The Agenda has stimulated a surge of articles on quality patient care within healthcare organizations.

In 1992, ''quality assessment and improvement'' replaced ''quality assurance'' in the AMH (31). At that time, standards were organized around departments and services, referred to both processes and outcomes, and specified many responsibilities for the leadership of the organization (87). JCAHO standards have evolved with experience, becoming increasingly congruent with CQI and TQM ideas.

Continuous Quality Improvement

The insights of CQI (21,22) introduced as a philosophy near the beginning of this chapter continue to influence quality methods and activities throughout health care. This section will explain several more definite findings or assumptions of CQI.

The need to study the problem and systems in which it is embedded deserves further explication. QI emphasizes review of systems and sequences rather than discrete inspections (20). One must acquire as much knowledge as possible about the system, not just identify errors or outliers as in traditional QA. When variation outside normally observed limits occurs, knowledge of the system explains the cause so that problems are rooted out.

The QI advocates believe, with some basis, that improving routine processes is much more effective than simply trying to eliminate the worst problems or the worst performers. Figure 14-5 displays this in a conventional but revealing way. Assuming that measured quality or results are distributed normally, an approach aimed at eliminating unacceptably poor care would, if successful, eliminate poor care for only a small fraction of patients (the small left tail of the distribution). An approach aimed at improving the process of care and eliminating inappropriate variations in the process (bottom of Fig. 14-5) would lessen variations and improve results for almost all patients. As a byproduct, the fraction of results or care that is clearly below the old threshold is also greatly diminished.

Another basic insight or premise of CQI deserves explanation: most problems are caused by faulty systems rather than the incompetence of particular individuals. The majority of problems, especially remediable ones, in the medical setting are also most likely problems with systems or procedures rather than individuals. Malpractice claims data, for instance, have been used as a basis for an investigation that identified

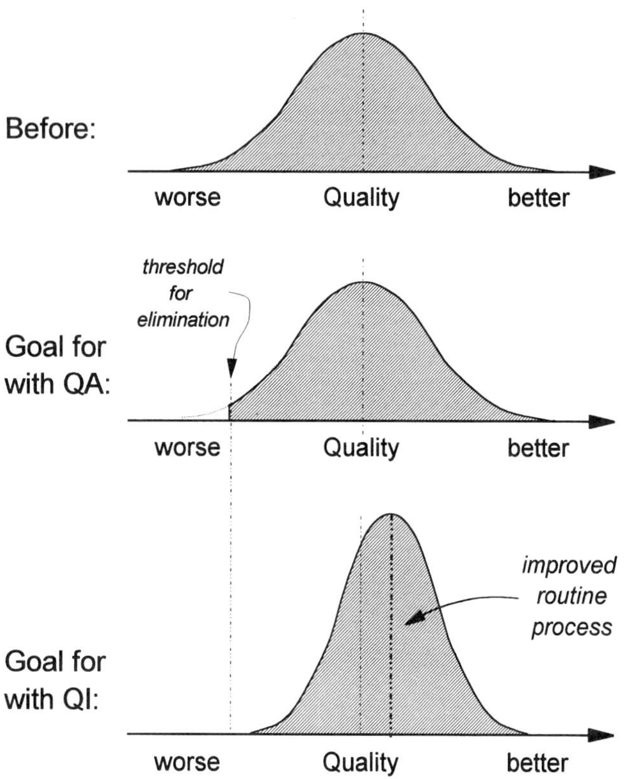

FIG. 14-5. Traditional quality assurance versus quality improvement.

problem-prone clinical processes and suggested improvements to reduce the likelihood of negligence (112). The claims history of individual physicians, however, only weakly predicts claims proneness, so use of such data to target individual physicians is empirically problematic (113). Many articles give examples of systems problems (e.g., in nursing care or the hospital pharmacy) (20,114).

Another insight is that QA systems that depend on mass inspection of discrepancies in outcomes are often ineffective or inefficient (20,24). If QA simply counts errors and points them out to staff, QA will be perceived as an unpleasant policing activity, and the substantial effort to detect outcome anomalies may not be paralleled by efforts to improve production or treatment processes. Deming emphasizes process measures to correct defects as they occur, but outcome measures are also used to monitor quality and verify improvements (22). Multiple statistical measures are needed. Deming's approach integrates knowledge, process, at least short-term outcomes, and action to improve them.

Professional QA and QI Terms

A few basic terms assist in professional QA and QI (109,115). *Norms* are measures of actual clinical practice. Examples are average length of stay, average improvement in FIM scores, and average hours of PT. Norms are most clinically useful when they are specific to a patient diagnosis or otherwise graded to patient characteristics. A similar term—*benchmark*—is popular in rehabilitation. Rehabilitation professionals need to have benchmarks against which to compare their staffing, education, costs, other processes, patient satisfaction, health, functional outcomes, and other outcomes. Norms and benchmarks have greater authority when they are based on large samples or when they tell us what is achievable by the "best" or at least better programs.

Criteria are statements that define appropriate or correct clinical care (109,116). Criteria are typically developed on the basis of professional experience and scientific literature. Some distinguish between a criterion and a *standard* (117), using the former as the more general dimension and the latter as the specific numeric cut-point. We will not rigidly distinguish the two, because a general dimension separate from the quantitative decision point is of little use (109). For instance, the statement that "stroke patients will have a blood level of coumadin in the therapeutic range" is useless without specification of what the range is (e.g., prothrombin time of 1.2 to 1.5 times control). Another example of a criterion or standard is the assertion that inpatients in medical rehabilitation should receive 3 hours per day of PT, OT, and SLP treatment combined. Criteria and standards may describe structure, process, or outcome and in practice involve all three.

An *indicator condition* is a frequent, treatable clinical situation (69,82). The JCAHO defines an *indicator* as an instrument to measure an aspect of care to guide the assessment of performance. Clinical indicators point to clinical processes or procedures that need further analysis to determine if improvements can be made. Improved clinical procedures should lead to improved outcomes.

A *threshold* indicates a preestablished point in an *indicator* that should trigger more in-depth investigation to determine whether a problem or opportunity to improve care exists (69). Action should follow to actually improve the system of care. As a fictitious but clear example, a threshold of 10% might be set for rehabilitation patients discharged back to acute care or to a nursing home. In the past, thresholds have been either rather arbitrary or set by expert judgment; some have suggested statistical criteria (45,69,78,79). The JCAHO has had difficult in setting and implementing thresholds. The concept of threshold is at least more defined that of "benchmarking" in the sense that it at least begins to define action implications.

There are situations where a 0% or 100% threshold is needed (80). For sentinel events such as death or suicide within rehabilitation or within 7 days of discharge, a threshold of 0% would be justifiable: every case needs to be individually investigated. In general, however, a threshold of 100% success or 0% problems can be unrealistic. Setting thresholds at less-than-perfect levels avoids disproportionate use of time to evaluate a few discrepant cases that will probably be found to be clinically justified (69,81). Quality improvement in rehabilitation usually requires discrimination and amelioration of frequently occurring or significant problems, not undiscriminating compulsiveness.

The term "monitor" is popularly used to describe any routinely collected measure on a group of patients. Staff engaged in activities to improve or oversee care monitor aspects of care processes or outcomes. "Monitor" is often used where "indicator" would be more appropriate. Because indicators have yet to be developed, QI efforts for rehabilitation must be undertaken with the use of *ad hoc* monitors. The JCAHO has been testing clinical indicators for anesthesia, obstetrics and gynecology, trauma, cardiovascular disease, and oncology (118). The second generation of indicator development is addressing two key hospital-wide processes—medication use and infection control. The indicator project will ultimately enable accreditation decisions to be based more directly on the actual performance of the health care organization.

Clinical Practice Guidelines

Clinical practice guidelines—also called *care protocols, practice parameters,* or *clinical paths*—are explicit descriptions of how patients should be evaluated and treated. They include enough detail to specify ordinarily appropriate decisions and processes. Care protocols typically involve a sequence of initial measures, alternative clinical processes, and subsequent measures. The terms clinical practice guidelines and standards are also used to describe "standardized specifications for care developed by a formal process that incorporates the best scientific evidence of effectiveness with expert opinion" (119). Initially led by the National Institute of Medicine and the Agency for Health Care Policy and Research, work to develop clinical practice guidelines and similar clinical paths and practice parameters has spread throughout the health care industry (27,120). Medical rehabilitation too has begun to develop guidelines.

There is continuing concern about the legal implications of guidelines and whether clinicians have to follow them. While guidelines are admissible in court, a guideline is a tool to assist clinicians in decision making rather than a standard of care which must be implemented (78).

The explicit purpose of guidelines is to improve the quality of care and to assure it by reducing variation in care provided (27). They are extremely relevant to quality assurance and improvement, for they essentially define the technical quality of care, or at least they define process and outcome indicators that tell a great deal about whether a program is providing standard quality care. When guidelines are based on controlled research on the efficacy of treatment, they link processes and patient outcomes. Guidelines for treatment of functional limitations in rehabilitation have incorporated diagnosis, impairments, and expected improvements in patient function. Outcomes in the clinic are part of these guidelines.

Critical paths may be distinguished from clinical guidelines, paths, or protocols in that the former are simpler and more administratively oriented. A critical path, for instance, might specify that a swallowing evaluation for stroke patients and a PT evaluation occur no later than the second day after admission. A clinical guideline or path should go further and specify the nature of the evaluation, how different interventions depend on differing patient characteristics, and how patient responses (clinical outcomes) are to be measured and evaluated.

Developing clinical guidelines capable of assuring and improving quality involves both sifting the literature and selecting the most reliable of consultants to provide advice that truly improves clinical decision-making and treatment. Formal methods of synthesizing expert judgment and information from varied research studies, such as metaanalysis, may be used. "When systematic assessment of the data is combined with a formal process or consensus to marshall expert clinical judgment, authoritative and reliable practice guidelines can result that give clinicians greater confidence in making treatment decisions" (121, p. 1061).

Over 1,500 practice guidelines, parameters, and similar materials have already been published by government and professional associations (120,122). Among the most relevant high-quality guidelines are those published by the Agency for Health Care Policy and Research for:

- Poststroke rehabilitation (123)
- Treatment of pressure ulcers (124) and their prediction and prevention (125)
- Acute and chronic management of urinary incontinence (126)
- Cardiac rehabilitation (127)

Guidelines for acute low back problems, depression, and acute pain may also be of interest; these and others are available over the Internet (http://www.ahcpr.gov or http://text nlm.nih.gov). Many other efforts are under way to develop guidelines or at least critical paths and forms to structure processes in medical rehabilitation (128). The feasibility of explicating rules or guidelines for treatment of commonly encountered, important problems in rehabilitation has been established.

Research to determine the impact of guidelines on clinical practice, patient outcomes, and costs is ongoing at this point. There have been preliminary reports that detailed clinical paths can improve patient care and outcomes in acute medical care (e.g., stroke patients). Researchers have documented 30% reduction in adverse events from antibiotics, a 27% decline in mortality, and decreased costs when using computer programs that help physicians choose antibiotic treatment (129). A detailed treatment protocol for mechanical ventilation can reduce unwarranted variations from good practice and substantially improve survival (130). Randomized trials have shown that, when combined with feedback on performance and education by respected peers, practice guidelines can improve medical care processes and outcomes (121). Although research on the impact of guidelines is still new, it is already clear that quality care can be "measured" and evaluated.

Clinical guidelines and paths assist in the coordination of multidisciplinary teams by defining procedures more clearly (131). Key clinical process and expected results can be tracked in a check list to be addressed by members of the team. Successful clinical paths should enable teams to provide quality of care more reliably and efficiently, with discussion focusing on a minority of exceptions from the usual path rather than the normal process. For new team members, the path should be educational. Requirements for documentation ideally could also be reduced without loss of meaning.

Rigidity, proliferation of forms, and inapplicability remain as concerns. The only randomized clinical trial of a critical path in medical rehabilitation showed that they did not save money but did decrease patient and staff satisfaction (132). Rehabilitation is so complex that one might expect that only sophisticated guidelines, not simple administrative paths, will actually improve practice. Clinical guidelines and paths in rehabilitation need empirical testing to determine their impact on practice and outcomes. They are likely to need further development and are certain to need recurrent revision.

JCAHO Quality Standards Today

The Agenda for Change is now completed, and JCAHO standards have been revamped. No longer is there a departmental focus, nor a separate chapter discussing quality. The standards relate to patient functions: Patient Rights and Organizational Ethics, Assessment of Patients, Care of Patients, Education and Continuum of Care. Organizational functions include: Improving Organizational Performance, Leadership, Management of the Environment of Care, and Management of Human Resource. The third main category is structures with functions, such as Governance, Management, Medical Staff and Nursing.

The standard "Improving Organizational Performance" expresses much of the philosophy of CQI and TQM, without losing sight of the ultimate purpose of improving patient outcomes. This section discusses quality improvement using a five-step approach (31):

- *Plan.* Planning involves but goes beyond single departments or treatments.
- *Design.* New processes need to be designed well and clinically soundly.
- *Measure.* "Measurement—that is data collection—is the foundation of all performance-improvement activities" (31, p. 250). To measure performance, a hospital collects data on processes and outcomes; outcomes; a comprehensive set of performance measures (indicators); high-risk, high-volume, and problem-prone processes; and other sensors of performance.
- *Assess.* Assessment is defined as transforming data into information by analyzing it (31, p. 261). The significance of measures is assessed or evaluated by comparison with: internal comparison over time (trends); comparison to up-to-date sources of information such as accreditation standards, practice guidelines or practice parameters; similar processes and outcomes in other hospitals, including use of reference data bases; and legal and regulatory requirements (31, p. 242). Appropriate statistical quality control techniques are to be used.
- *Improve.* The hospital is to systematically improve its performance.

It is worth emphasizing that, to JCAHO, thresholds and standards particular to a program are not enough. JCAHO standards state that "Comparative performance data and information are defined, collected, analyzed, transmitted, reported, and used" (31, p. 411). Valuable information may come by comparison to published data or other sources, but there is an explicit requirement that "The hospital uses external reference data bases for comparative purposes" (31, p. 411).

Development of objective indicators has proven to be complex and is still unfolding. Numerous indicators of clinical performance have been developed. Some trial indicators have proven to be expensive to implement, but progress has been made. JCAHO has defined what indicator measurement systems should be and continues to support the development of indicators based on objective data. Ultimately, hospitals will be able to subscribe to the vendor of their choice which the JCAHO has approved. Data on the indicators will then be submitted to JCAHO on a regular basis.

JCAHO makes it clear that extremely relevant comparative knowledge is also to obtained from the published research literature and other sources. "Management of Information" is a responsibility of leadership, according to JCAHO, and important types of information include patient-specific records, aggregate data, and expert knowledge, as well as comparative performance data.

Comprehensive rehabilitation is required, at minimum, to meet the most frequently encountered physical and psychosocial needs of the patient. The services of physical rehabilitation encompass PT, OT, rehabilitation medicine, rehabilitation nursing, social work, and SLP. The JCAHO publications have given examples of quality improvement processes for nursing, psychology, PT, and speech.

QI Methods

In the early 1990s, the JCAHO defined a ten-step process for monitoring and evaluating health care services (133). Although no longer emphasized by JCAHO, the process still describes important steps in QI activities. To emphasize only the gist of the pattern, QI activities (a) begin with the chief or at least requires their support; (b) the scope of care and types of patients to be served must be understood; (c) one should attempt to high-volume, high-risk, or problem-prone care or aspects of care (although it can be just as important and productive to identify care processes that can be improved); (d) one should attempt to identify objective indicators of appropriateness of patient selection, diagnosis, and/or quality or effectiveness of care, or needed resources; (e) one should also attempt to identify some objective threshold or indicator of need (or opportunity) for more in-depth study; (f) one collects data, continuously monitoring important aspects of care. The decision to evaluate care in-depth may in fact involve more than comparison to a single numeric threshold, but it is important (g) to study one's care processes and alternatives in depth when a problem occurs, when outcomes appear to be below expectation, or new strategies or treatments promise a means of improving care and its outcomes. Study leads to development of a plan, and (h) action to solve problems or improve care is needed. The success (i) of efforts to improve care needs to be assessed, and (j) results communicated widely. While the scheme is too abstract to guide specific quality improvement activities, systematic QI involves many of these steps.

Technical Issues in Quality Monitoring

Most the technical and statistical issues discussed previously under outcomes-oriented monitoring systems are also relevant to more process-oriented system. Statistical control principles are highly relevant to quality monitoring. For instance, the patient groups for which an indicator is intended needs to be well defined. Sample size needs to be specified to set a threshold in QI or an expectancy in outcomes monitoring systems. A 50% error rate with two patients is utterly different from the same rate with 100 patients.

Indicators. Many indicators have been developed and are in the process of validation for acute medical care. JCAHO's *National Library of Healthcare Indicators* describes over 200 measures of clinical conditions, functional health status, or satisfaction in a standard format (118). Similarly, the Agency for Health Care Policy and Research distributes a data base ("CONQUEST") in Microsoft Access that describes 53 established clinical performance measures for 52 clinical conditions (134).

There are currently no indicators specific to rehabilitation, although methods for infection control and medication monitoring are also appropriate to medical rehabilitation (135,136). The JCAHO publications have discussed monitoring and evaluation for physical rehabilitation services, including patient goals (133). Possible "monitors" for different departments have included:

- For OT, increase in self-care ADL skills
- For PT, improvement in mobility or other physical dysfunctions or reduction in pain associated with movement
- For prosthetic and orthotic services, patient satisfaction with fit and functioning
- For psychology, cognitive and emotional adaptation of the patient and family to disability
- For recreation therapy, use of leisure time and acquisition of socialization skills
- For social work, whether basic sustenance, shelter, transportation, and comfort needs are met
- For SLP, the effectiveness of actions taken to improve communication skills
- For vocational services, the achievement of work skills
- For rehabilitation medicine, achievement of rehabilitation goals, health maintenance, and prevention of complications common with the disease category

These QI goals and indicators bear more than a passing resemblance to objectives and goals in many extant program evaluation systems in medical rehabilitation. Program evaluation goals, however, have typically been goals for the entire program rather than for any single department. Although discipline-related monitors are understandable, interdisciplinary patient-based monitors are desirable. Patient needs and goals transcend any single department.

The Agenda for Change addressed the fact that problems of system coordination are common in hospitals, which are complex organizations with numerous departments. For example, a departmental laboratory might monitor results of all cultures, and pharmacy staff may monitor timely dispensing of prescriptions. Differences in timing of processes across departments, however, might cause information on sensitivities or even the current prescription to be unavailable at certain times. Errors and costs in one department can easily be decreased, increasing burdens and errors in another department. System costs and errors cannot be identified or fixed without a total systems approach.

IMPLEMENTATION OF QUALITY AND OUTCOMES MONITORING SYSTEMS

The implementation of quality and outcomes monitoring systems is as important as their purpose and measurement factors. A few key points deserve mention.

Costs

Cost is a primary barrier facing any system to continuously monitor processes or outcomes of care. One must keep within the budget. Awareness of budget constraints is especially critical at the point of system design. Realizing that rehabilitation is complex, clinicians often ask that measures be added to account for every factor. Consensus is achieved at the cost of a data system that is too expensive to implement or, if implemented, has so much missing data that it is invalid. At best, data are collected, but there is no time do analyses to clarify the source of problems or for task forces to study problems in sufficient depth to plan actions. Measures need to be ranked by importance, deleting less frequently important items, to construct a data system useful for assessing commonly seen, important patient problems. There should be a plan for analysis and interpretation of every data element included in routine monitoring systems.

Starting With an Existing System

Readers are advised to buy into a shared, already-developed clinical monitoring system rather than to develop their own, whenever possible. You will save a lot of work, and comparative data make results far more interpretable and useful (see Shared Data Systems above). Tailor the system to address your own beliefs and concerns by adding measures. Developing your own system from scratch is more work than you think, and the comparative data provided by shared systems will be informative.

Interpersonal Factors

Organizational climate and political and personal factors are important in development and use of quality and outcomes management systems. Implementation and use of QI and outcomes monitoring systems are most highly associated with support from top management. Broad participation of staff is prudent to improve the technical quality and necessary for implementation of monitoring systems. Staff need to understand the uses of the QI or outcomes system. Provision of meaningful information to staff is the very product of the clinical monitoring information system.

Automation

Quality and outcomes monitoring systems benefit greatly from the use of computers. Simple spreadsheets (Excel, Lotus 1-2-3, Quattro Pro) are useful for *ad hoc* studies. Specialized statistical programs (e.g., SPSS, SAS) have been associated with high levels of user satisfaction in program evaluation data systems. They provide excellent reports and the ability to do the in-depth analyses that lead to reliable understanding and utilization. However, they require some training to master, and an expert statistical consultant may be needed.

Special software programs have been developed for quality and outcomes monitoring, including FIMWare, the Easter Seal System ''Rehabilitation Manager,'' the PECS, R/COM, and others (70,78).

External data systems provide valuable normative comparison data for paying users (e.g., 4). These systems provide routine reports that serve as a first-stage screen, although the reports do not usually identify specific reasons for problems or clues regarding how to go about improving care.

Integrating Information Systems

It is common for hospitals and other complex organizations to have multiple, poorly integrated information systems. The financial information systems is commonly quite from the clinical information system. Routine quality and outcomes monitoring data are commonly abstracted manually from handwritten medical records or entered into a separate computer system, duplicating information in the clinical record.

Integration with the team conference or case management system is particularly important for enhancing the meaningfulness of outcomes monitoring systems in rehabilitation. Outcomes monitoring systems are more meaningful if they relate to the clinical process, including serial assessments of patient function and discharge goals (9,10,41). Integrating the outcomes monitoring system with clinical processes involves more effort than traditional program evaluation, but it reduces duplication of effort and makes the system much more meaningful (101). The process underlies the transformation of traditional program evaluation systems into real clinical outcomes management systems.

Integration of clinical, financial, quality, and outcomes data systems is a goal to be pursued (90). Ultimately a completely integrated clinical–financial information system can be accessed for physicians' orders, pharmacy, current charting, team conference, outcomes management, utilization review, QI, profitability analyses, program planning, marketing reports, reports to third-party payers, referral sources, and regulatory agencies, research, and all levels of staff, consistent with security procedures.

REPORTING AND UTILIZATION

Systems for reporting and utilization are as important as measurement. Many data systems have collected vast quantities of data that are underused because of lack of understanding regarding best use of data and conflicts and fears regarding interpretation. Limitations to inferences from routine reports need to be explicated to avoid misuse of data. This section outlines factors affecting the utility of quality and outcomes reports.

Multiple Uses of Clinical Monitoring Systems

Data can be used for many purposes. Information systems are much more valuable if they are multiuse.

Clinical Uses

Process and outcomes-monitoring data systems have multiple uses in clinical outcomes management. They monitor patient functional status and improvement, which are key indicators in utilization review and assessment of readiness for discharge. Although current standardized measures of disability are somewhat rough tools, they do bracket a range of readiness for discharge (7). Functional status monitoring systems have certainly been widely used in utilization review (e.g., 93) Teams function in an interdisciplinary fashion when they discuss patient function in terms of needed abilities for everyday life.

Clinical data systems can produce displays of individual patient progress used in team conference, case management, and reports to referral sources or payers. Figure 14-6 shows

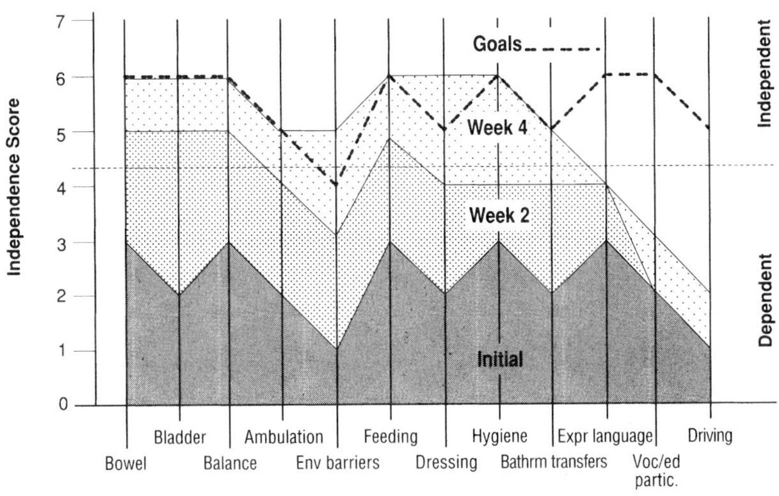

FIG. 14-6. Status and goal profile of a possible discharge candidate. (From Silverstein B, Kilgore KM, Fisher WP. Implementing patient tracking systems and using functional assessment scales, Vol. 1. In Harvey RF, ed. *Center for Rehabilitation Outcome Analysis monograph series on issues and methods in outcome analysis.* Wheaton, IL: Marianjoy Rehabilitation Center, 1989, with permission.)

a graphic report of patient progress from the PECS (61,93). Functional tasks are ordered by difficulty; patients tend first to achieve mobility in tasks to the left. The case displayed is a possible discharge candidate.

Administrative Uses

Program evaluation and QI systems provide data that administrators use in understanding and managing rehabilitation programs. Uses include marketing (83,137), refined profitability analyses, planning, and accreditation (9,10, 12,41,83,84). Another clinical–administrative use is estimation of acuity of patients for staffing. Many hospitals already use nursing acuity rating systems to determine daily nursing rates and daily nursing staffing requirements. These systems incorporate ratings very similar to those in program evaluation and QI systems, along with additional impairment information. Rating scales like the FIM have been shown to be related to hours of care needed (60).

Interpreting Data

Practical QI and outcomes monitoring systems are based on known or at least assumed knowledge of effective treatment. Although elaborate controlled research is needed to establish causal processes, when an intervention has been established as effective, it should be possible to monitor effectiveness using a simpler set of input, process, and outcomes measures. Interventions are typically reassessed, depending on patient response (Fig. 14-1). Patient diagnosis, specific problems and presenting functional level, treatment objectives,treatments implemented, short-term and longer-term patient response would ordinarily be assessed.

Quality and outcomes evaluation systems in practice are looser than scientific research. They do not provide unambiguous answers but strengthen some ideas about intervention effectiveness and weaken others. These systems are, however, essential because only real-world data can tell us whether a program is or is not skillfully implementing treatment methods to patients who are most likely to benefit from them and whether desired results are in fact attained.

There are several common, avoidable traps in interpretation of clinical process-outcomes data. First is the common tendency to assume a massive effect of treatments. Medical rehabilitation, like much and perhaps even most of medical care, is not a simple cure, although it helps—sometimes a little, sometimes a lot. A second major error is assuming that improvement results entirely from rehabilitation. Improvement can also result from case severity, natural recovery, and social and environmental factors.

Although unrealistic beliefs that rehabilitation can produce wonders is flattering and good for marketing, its implication—complete responsibility for outcomes—produces apprehension in rehabilitation professionals. It is unrealistic and incorrect to evaluate rehabilitation programs on the basis of outcomes, improvement, or improvement per day or per dollar, without a good deal more information.

Interpreting Cost-Effectiveness Data

Improvement per day or per dollar is often labeled as a measure of "efficiency" or cost-effectiveness. Such labeling is incorrect and misleading, as patient improvement, length of stay, and costs (usually indexed by charges) are driven by many factors that are at least as powerful as the actual effectiveness and efficiency of administration and clinical care processes. Important exogenous factors include natural healing, case severity, referral processes, base reimbursement rates, cost-charge ratios, the adequacy of postdischarge support and rehabilitation systems, family support, and others. Improvement-per-day figures are not meaningless, but their interpretation is tricky (89). These ratios are at best a heuristic or first-stage screen, meaningful only if further study is done. Other works will help readers to understand cost, cost-benefit, and cost-effectiveness analyses in rehabilitation (38,138).

Understanding basic facts or relationships helps one to interpret cost-effectiveness or improvement-per-day data. More severe cases tend to receive and require longer care (44,61). Outcomes per se often have little relation to effort (or length of stay) (44,61). Improvement in medical rehabilitation hospitals is and should be clearly related to length of stay (44,61). Patients who cease to respond to treatment or to improve should tend to be discharged.

Comparing Outcomes

Conventional program evaluation systems distinguish between types of programs (e.g., between chronic care facilities, skilled nursing facilities, and other facilities marketed but not actually organized as comprehensive, intensive rehabilitation programs). Treatment effects, however, are difficult to distinguish from utilization review procedures that discharge slow-to-respond patients (19,44).

There are several considerations in comparing outcomes or improvement scores for an impairment group in one program to those in others. One must examine alternative plausible explanations for the differences in outcomes observed, including:

1. Functional severity at admission. Improvement may not be equally likely or meaningful across all levels of an admission measure. Some studies have reported curvilinear relationships, that is, greater improvement among patients admitted at intermediate levels of severity (44).
2. Chronicity (i.e., onset–admission interval). After the acute phase of many severe injuries, there is a period of relatively rapid recovery, followed by increasingly slow improvement and eventual asymptote, at least on a group basis. Control for natural history recovery curves is extremely useful.
3. Length of stay. Improvement in rehabilitation tends to be correlated with length of stay.
4. Differences in case mix, comorbidities, and severity of illness or injury (17). Differences in improvement across facilities is frequently a function of selection differences (e.g., differences in case mix and case severity. Differences in effectiveness of treatment and selection–treatment interactions are also possible, of course. Observed differences can best be explained if there is knowledge about the relative patient mixes. For example, a facility with a high proportion of tetraplegic patients, or one that serves ventilator-dependent patients with SCI, would be expected to show lower discharge functional levels on ADL measures, longer length of stay, and higher charges within the SCI impairment group.

Function-related groups (FRGs) have been developed to adjust inpatient medical rehabilitation caseload for case severity in the sense of effort (length of stay) required (139). They predict about 31% of the variance of length of stay in rehabilitation, which is similar to the performance of DRGs for acute hospital length of stay. Patients are categorized on the basis of functional status (FIM) at admission, age, and primary diagnosis. FRGs may also have some applications for quality monitoring (140). FRGs provide a basis for classifying rehabilitation patients into groups which are more clinically homogeneous and interpretable than groupings by primary diagnosis alone. When objective comparison data on functional gain and length of stay for each FRG are available, they should provide a valuable benchmark or first stage screen for evaluation of rehabilitation programs.

There are several additional methods of case mix or severity adjustment for medical rehabilitation (141), based on factors such as functional independence, diagnosis, age, and chronicity (onset-admission days). All these methods of risk or severity adjustment are approximate and typically predict a minority of the variance of length of stay or functional gain. Methods of case mix adjustment to predict mortality in acute hospitals are also approximate; although there is substantial (78% to 95%) agreement, disgreement in ranking of severity is signficant (142).

Conflicting Documentation Requirements

Perhaps the major structural problem with the health care information systems is the presence of multiple, differing, and sometimes even conflicting documentation requirements from different regulatory, payer, accreditation, professional, and business sources. When the uncoordinated demands of each are added, the burden of documentation is extreme (143). What are needed are common standards and definitions so that clinical staff can document once in one place and data can subsequently be reformatted and sent to other parties by computer without burdening clinical staff.

TRENDS AND NEW DIRECTIONS

Driven by increasing demands for accountability and the decreasing cost of computerized information systems, process and outcomes monitoring systems will grow, albeit slowly and perhaps haltingly.

Changes in the Health Care Industry: Cost-Control, Risk Sharing, and Managed Care

Cost control—especially managed care and risk-sharing arrangements and incentives to providers to restrict care—has heightened concern about the quality of care. Although reports on the quality of care have not always shown that managed care firms provide worse care to persons with disabilities and chronic conditions, these firms have incentives to do so, as these patients cost much more to care for than average amounts (144). In 1986, data from the Rand Health Insurance experiment indicated that poor patients with chronic conditions had worse outcomes under even well-regarded health maintenance organizations compared to fee-for-service arrangements (145). Nonetheless, commercial, Medicare, and Medicaid managed care schemes have grown rapidly.

Perhaps no sector of health care is more vulnerable than rehabilitation, which is a relatively high cost service for individuals who cannot for the most part be cured and who would probably survive even without rehabilitation. Severely disabled individuals also tend to be poor and limited in mobility, and some cannot communicate articulately. Rehabilitation specialists are a very small proportion of the whole health care labor force.

Managed care and capitated care systems have the potential to improve care (5,146). Freed from constraints of itemized payment, they provide opportunities for innovation and integration of currently fragmented care systems. Quality and outcomes improvement systems can in principle be implemented with a beneficial wider, long-term perspective. Concern for quality must take into account the needs of health plan enrollees as a group, including individuals who do not receive care. Capitation provides an incentive for prevention and health maintenance. Several studies have reported similar processes and outcomes in capitated systems and fee-for-service, with most studies showing direct costs to be less under capitated system; a number of capitated systems have delivered preventive services more reliably than fee-for-service (146,147). When resources are limited, overall quality of care may be improved by limiting access to more expensive or less effective care so that all members of the group receive certain highly effective services. Evidence for effectiveness of rehabilitative care varies across diagnostic groups and types of rehabilitation (68,148).

Although current evidence is limited, cause for concern remains. Disabled and chronically ill individuals are money losers under capitation, so there is an incentive not to enroll such individuals, to treat them as cheaply as possible, and to hope that limited services will induce them to sign up for alternatives. The most severely disabled of individuals loose their private insurance and shift to Medicaid or Medicare. Because profits can be increased by minimizing care, firms with less concern about quality have a competitive advantage and are less likely to participate in studies of quality and outcomes. There is even reason to question whether costs to the system or even to Medicare have been saved by current managed care firms (149). Administrative costs are high in managed care firms, and much depends on whether long-term costs to society as a whole are included in cost estimates. ''Managed care may be a vehicle for change, but it will require external forces to assure that it moves in the desired direction'' (154).

Managed Care and Case Management Data Bases

Difficulties in utilization of traditional routine clinical monitoring data systems are not primarily due to technical deficiencies, although these exist. When there is a concrete motive (e.g., a financial motive), clinical data systems are used. Managed care organizations have developed their own data bases to track the appropriateness of medical care, including medical rehabilitation. These data bases concentrate on financial factors but increasingly include detailed clinical data. These clinical information systems are certainly used. If the case management agency does not like the outcomes associated with patients sent to a rehabilitation provider, it does not send new cases to that provider. Only a minority of expensive cases are managed with the use of such data bases, but for this minority the external party's data system is essentially the operational program evaluation and utilization review data base. These case management systems are typically proprietary, but their adequacy, criteria, and the associated patient outcomes are of public interest.

Report Cards and NCQA's HEDIS

In response to concerns of the public and of employers regarding the quality of care provided by managed care firms, ''report cards'' have been devised that allow consumers in many regions of the country to compare hospitals and health care systems (150). The National Committee on Quality Assurance (NCQA) has developed the most widely used system for assessing the performance of health plans, the Health Plan Employer Data and Information Set (HEDIS). The current version of HEDIS (2.5) contains nine indicators of quality, seven of which are process indicators, five of these relating to preventive care. NCQA is planning to expand the scope of coverage of HEDIS. NCQA standards for health plan performance now include health outcomes measures. Draft versions of HEDIS 3.0 contain 75 measures that accredited health plans are to use, including measures from the Medical Outcomes Study such as the SF-36 or SF-12 (151).

The validity of report cards on whole systems of care is problematic. More than administrative or structural measures are needed to assess quality and effectiveness of care. One would expect selected processes and associated outcomes would need to be monitored for specific conditions, clinicians, and sites to screen for quality and effectiveness problems or opportunities; detailed clinical measures would be needed to evaluate the actual quality and effectiveness of care. On the other hand, purchasers must have some feasible basis to judge the quality of the health services they purchase.

None of the current HEDIS measures relates to rehabilitation or care of chronic conditions. Efforts to address this deficiency are being made. The issue of public report cards on rehabilitation cuts two ways: We would like systems that provide high quality rehabilitation to have higher scores, but what if these scores induce individuals with chronic conditions to join such a plan, leading to financial losses for such systems?

Prospective Payment and Bundling

The federal government has for many years expressed interest in developing a prospective payment for medical rehabilitation to parallel the diagnosis-related group (DRG) system for acute hospitals. Function-related groups—patient groups defined by FIM at admission, primary impairment group, and age with similar lengths of stay or costs—have been developed as a possible basis for prospective payment for medical rehabilitation hospitals (139,141). Although the proposed FRG system is imperfect, it is surely fairer than the current TEFRA system, which provides cost-based payment for expensive new facilities but squeezes well-established facilities with a low historical cost basis. An FRG system could provide ''rehabilitation carve out'' that would shield rehabilitation from major financial incentives to provide inadequate care.

An alternative, favoring the continued rapid expansion of outpatient and at-home services, is the bundling of rehabilitation with other forms of posthospital care. Another alternative for Medicare and Medicaid is further expansion of riskbearing managed care contracts. The latter choice merely shifts apparent responsibility for providing quality rehabilitation. Surely the responsibility to provide adequate rehabilitation remains. Regardless of financial manipulations, systems to monitor and improve the quality and outcomes of care are needed.

Automation

The advance of automation is an engine for growth of process and outcomes data systems. The expense of data collection has been a limiting factor. As more and more of the clinical record is stored in computers, this expense declines. Nationwide and regional data bases for monitoring of quality and outcomes have grown rapidly, and continued growth may be expected.

Progress in development of clinical information systems has been limited by lack of agreement on measurement of function outside the domain of basic ADLs, by lack of thought given to structure of the clinical recording system, and by incompatibility between requirements of various payors, regulatory agencies, and clinical needs. Clinical knowledge—not mere statistical knowledge—needs to be built into data systems.

Prediction of Outcomes and Expert Systems

The ability to predict rehabilitative outcomes has substantially improved over the years (e.g., following stroke rehabilitation) (152). Although accuracy is limited, computerized outcome prediction systems based on program evaluation and other clinical data are available (90). The incremental cost of predicting outcomes is small once the data are entered into a computer. Current systems are at least capable of distinguishing outliers or problematic cases and bracketing a range of realistic expectations.

Knowledge-based systems—systems that use the computer to ''think'' about data by modeling the thought processes of experts—will continue to multiply over the years, proving themselves in one niche after another (153). Knowledge-based expert systems will over the years greatly increase the routine utility of automated clinical data sets using validated measures.

Future Rehabilitation Information Systems

The long-term future is clear: quality and outcomes management data systems will be part of completely automated total information systems that incorporate financial management, the plan for care of the patient, routine clinical notes, short-term processes, utilization review, QI, and hopefully both short-term patient response and longer term outcomes. Automation is proceeding rapidly, but we still have a long ways to go.

Incorporating Wider Considerations into Accountability

Medical rehabilitation has a history of concern for the lives of persons with disabilities, including long-term care and advocacy for policies to alleviate handicapping social and environmental conditions. Although this chapter has emphasized the effectiveness of rehabilitative care, a wider view—toward the ultimate goals of improving patients' lives—is needed in a public policy, advocacy, and cost-effectiveness analysis.

The monitoring of quality of services provided can beg the question of whether the best type of services are being provided to patients. Services are frequently considered ''appropriate'' even if they do not address other important patient needs and even if somewhat more effective interventions strategies may exist. Similarly, the usual standard in traditional program evaluation is that a program is held accountable ''only for those objectives which are achievable by the services which that program provides'' (86). Although monitoring of processes is appropriate, clinical monitoring systems become more powerful if they consider rehabilitative interventions known to be effective, regardless of whether they are currently offered by the program. Such data document the need for restructuring of the program. For example, one study based on program evaluation data found that TBI patients frequently developed unanticipated behavioral problems after discharge (19). This suggests the need for increased psychological interventions, training for generalization, and definite follow-up of discharged clients.

In QI, the same principle of assessing errors of omission holds. The Harvard study of the quality in acute care hospitals, for instance, found that errors of omission (e.g., a physician not detecting an major diagnostic problem leading to suffering, disability, or death) were more common than errors of commission (not providing the correct treatment for the diagnosis) (47).

The Need for Patient Follow-up

Follow-up and follow-along of patients have long been considered to be important to quality rehabilitation and have long been incorporated in rehabilitation accreditation requirements (6). The problems of rehabilitation patients are commonly long-enduring rather than acute or self-limiting. Short-term in-clinic measures are therefore less satisfactory in rehabilitation than in medical care dealing with time-limited problems, from which most patients fully recover. Not infrequently, patients' most important needs become evident only after they return to the community and attempt to resume their lives. The quality of postdischarge care for rehabilitation patients is variable. With shortening lengths of stay, reliance on outpatient and home health services has increased. While financial pressure can make them difficult, follow-up and follow-along are more important than ever. Outcomes-focused quality strategies are needed to tell us whether changes in the rehabilitative treatment system designed to lessen costs have done so without compromising patient recovery.

New Quality and Outcomes Management Models

Conventional program evaluation and QI systems are only one of many possible approaches (24). The field will do well to learn from program evaluation, CQI, and TQM efforts in health care more generally, including acute medical care, psychiatric care, geriatric medicine, home health care, and long-term care (102,110,154,155). The emerging challenge is integrating different strategies--both process-oriented and outcomes-oriented—and defining which strategy or technique is most valuable in which circumstance.

Conceptualizing Rehabilitation Objectives

Both QI and outcomes management in rehabilitation benefit from distinguishing clinical treatment objectives, usually at the level of specific functional limitations or important impairments, from longer-term outcome goals, measured in broader terms such as handicap reduction or general quality of life (9,10,12). Handicaps are fairly generic across impairment groups and give an overview of patients' lives. Applicable across diagnostic groups, they are useful for assessing comprehensive programs and systems of care. At the level of rehabilitation planning for individuals, handicap-reduction goals help to prioritize more specific treatment objectives and can coordinate multidisciplinary teams toward the achievement of a transdisciplinary outcome.

Client-Centered Outcomes Management Information Systems

Clinical monitoring systems have been developed that focus on the independent living and productive activity goals planned by the team for the person served, rather than being defined in advance (9,10,12). Independent living is defined in terms of the specific living arrangement and supports required for the individual; productive activities, in terms of paid work, school work, parenting, contributions to one's family and household, or healthy leisure activities. Specific treatment objectives are defined to achieve these. Treatment objectives are things that have to be accomplished for the general outcome goal to be attained. They are usually defined in terms of reduced functional limitations, environmental modifications, caregiver training, and reduction of key impairments.

In these experimental systems, the team or case manager selects outcome goals from a list of previously developed and validated measures. Although superficially similar to Goal Attainment Scaling, the procedure is much more objective, as objective outcomes can be measured in ways that are comparable across patients.

A criticism of such a procedure has been that clinicians will choose goals that are easy to attain so they will have good goal attainment rates. Although this can surely occur, there is, in practice, a great deal of pressure from families and payers to set optimistic goals; overly optimistic goals are common in practice (19). In any case, if objective outcomes are assessed, it is possible to compare treatment programs on an objective basis. One can determine whether clinicians who set high goals tend to have better objective outcomes than those who set lower goals. For results to be completely objective, precise means need to be developed to decide when a certain objective applies to an individual. This is difficult, but it is important to begin to explicate how to tailor treatment objectives to the individual patient.

Systems such as these have been called ''client-centered program evaluation'' (71). A more current term is clinical case management information systems or clinical outcomes management. Regardless of rubric, the idea is to base the system on the actual clinical rehabilitation plan for individuals. A key point is incorporating decisions about patients into the outcomes-information system. Monitoring systems that completely standardize monitoring of processes and outcomes in the name of eliminating subjectivity can also make the system irrelevant to clinical decision making, which commonly rests on judgment. In other words, process and outcomes monitoring systems can be of increased value if they are rooted the actual clinical rehabilitation planning process.

Outcomes-Focused Quality Improvement: A Missing Link

The missing link in clinical monitoring and improvement systems is a valid method to connect processes to outcomes. One can do this by starting with treatments that are known to have a reliable connection to an defined outcome—or by monitoring outcomes and investigating processes when there is a discrepancy between measured outcomes and achievable expectancies. Given the lack of evidence for a single best way to deliver rehabilitative care, it makes sense to monitor patient outcomes—as well as key processes—giving programs a degree of leeway in the way that they produce these outcomes (154).

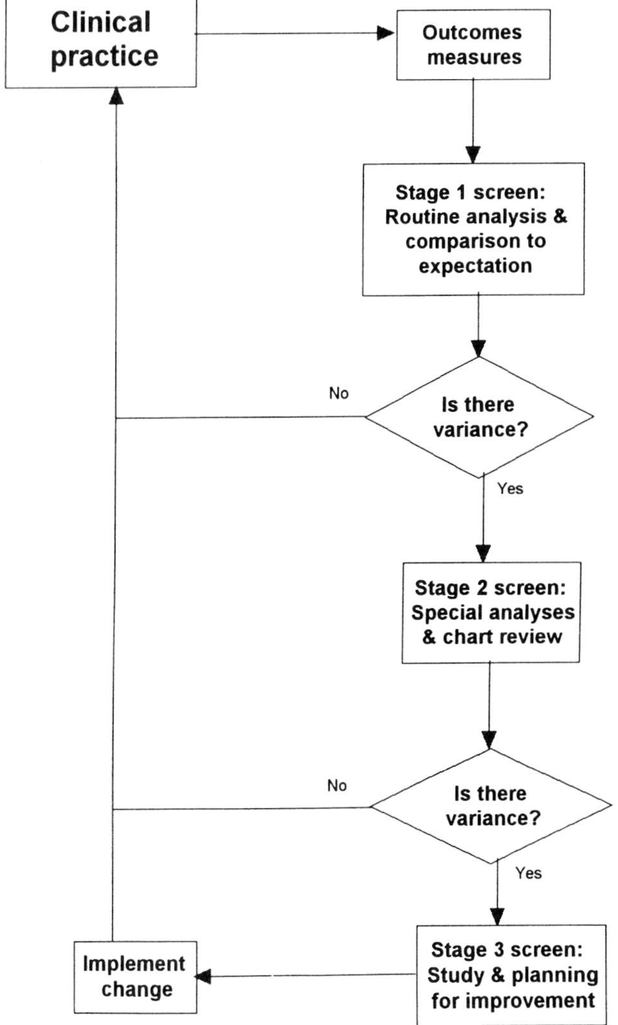

FIG. 14-7. The outcomes-focused quality improvement cycle.

Such outcomes-focused approaches have frequently been misunderstood. In general, *when a program or patient group has higher or lower outcomes than projected, this by itself does not constitute evidence for high or low quality or effectiveness of care.* (There are exceptions to this rule if outcomes are terrible, but in the experience of the authors they are infrequent.) Outcomes are due to many factors beyond the reach of even quality rehabilitative care, and current methods of statistical projection to determine "expected" outcomes typically predicts only a minority of the variance of functional gain or other outcomes. As a consequence, *a discrepancy between measured outcome and a normative expectation is primarily an indicator that second stage of analysis and study is needed.* As a rule then, connecting an outcome to treatment processes is a multi-stage process.

Figure 14-7 depicts the outcomes-focused quality improvement cycle in terms of three stages. Discrepancies from expected outcomes are validly useable only as *first-stage screens*—indicators of a possible problem or opportunity to improve operations, but hardly proof. Many empirical studies show that appropriate use of outcomes data to improve clinical processes "virtually always requires detailed clinical data" (110, p. 868). Discrepancies between actual and expected outcomes are at least as likely to reflect unmeasured patient or environmental factors rather than quality of care. Much more information is needed to infer likely reasons for discrepancies.

Second stage screens or *investigation tools* are needed to guide local staff in their efforts to identify most-likely problems in care processes (or opportunities to improve the effectiveness and efficiency of care). In-depth analyses are commonly needed to confirm a routine report that a statistically stable discrepancy in outcomes actually exists. Clinical guidelines provide a systematic basis for study of program processes. A chart review based on preestablished review criteria would make the process objective and systematic. Objective review criteria are feasible and have begun to be developed for home health services (102). The chart review could focus on patients whose outcomes are particularly discrepant. Alternatively, one could identity patients who experienced variances in care processes and determine if their severity-adjusted outcomes were in fact below expectation. When and if a problem with care processes is identified, the task force should direct its efforts to solving the problem. In this third stage, study, detailed practical planning, and action should actually improve care processes. Continued monitoring will reveal the impact on outcomes.

Perhaps the greatest technical problem with outcomes-focused approaches to quality improvement is that second-stage screens and other systematic tools have not been formally developed to connect variances in measured outcomes to specific antecedents. Instead, the difficult process of determining reasons for sub-optimal outcomes has usually been left to harried local QI committees, part-time program evaluation staff, or peer reviewers without validated tools to focus their efforts. It should not be surprising if they cannot achieve in a few meetings or chart reviews a level of insight into how rehabilitative processes affect patient outcomes that researchers are often unable to achieve even after years of effort. For that matter, review criteria and guidelines for process-focused approaches to quality assurance and improvement in medical rehabilitation have also been inadequately developed and validated against key patient outcomes at the level of independent living or productive activities.

CONCLUSIONS

Quality improvements and outcomes management systems—and cruder report cards on systems of care—should be a major concern to medical rehabilitation professionals, as they are critical to the justification of the field in the eye of payors and the public.

Both QI and outcomes management rest on knowledge of which interventions are highly effective, which are less effective, and which are likely to be ineffective, for well-defined patient groups or problems. This implies that more research is needed. Yet more research is not all that is needed. What we already know needs to be synthesized and distinguished from what we do not know. Although knowledge of the effectiveness of rehabilitation is limited, evidence including a few randomized experiments and a larger number of less controlled research does exist (148). Moreover, rehabilitation involves processes that in some sense are known to be efficacious. Interventions based on learning and physical conditioning surely ''work,'' as do many environmental modifications, prostheses, orthoses, nursing interventions, and pharmaceutical interventions from general medical care (68). Synthesizing the results of many research studies is basic to constructing sound clinical strategies and to systematic QI and outcomes management. Review articles and textbooks provide a useful basis for defining quality of care and understanding outcomes. Formal clinical guidelines—developed on the basis of thorough reviews of the literature, formal meta-analyses, and the consensus of experienced experts—can produce higher quality, more complete, and authoritative bases for monitoring and improvement of treatment quality (13,27,110).

Clinical practice guidelines are critical to systematic efforts to improve the quality of care. If guidelines are based on controlled research and incorporate measures of clinical responsiveness to treatment, they should also improve patient outcomes. There are, however, caveats. Guidelines without adequate scientific basis may merely codify custom and inhibit innovation (154). Guidelines can be rigid, based on the assumption that one single method of care is best even when evidence and experience supports several alternative approaches. Most existing guidelines focus on medical/nursing pathologies rather than functional gain, the core goal of medical rehabilitation. Guidelines need to be developed to the point that detailed criteria enable one to objectively evaluate the degree to which a patient group has received quality care. Guidelines also need to be validated: we need evidence that programs that adhere more closely to guidelines have better severity-adjusted outcomes.

Systematic efforts to assure and improve the quality and outcomes of medical rehabilitation should utilize a toolkit with a variety of methods. Both process-oriented and outcomes-oriented methods are needed. In practice most efforts to assure and improve care justifiably focus on processes and clinically relevant indicators of patient response, that is, on relatively short-term outcomes. There are, however, circumstances where a short-term focus is insufficient. Rehabilitation patients commonly experience long-term problems, and long-term benefits to patients often cannot be reliably projected on the basis of care processes or short-term clinical responses. The routine monitoring of key long-term outcome indicators remains valuable. Measuring whether improvements in patient function are sustained in everyday life after discharge remains a necessary first step in gauging the value of rehabilitative interventions. Regardless of the point in the causal chain one chooses to measure, validated inferential systems are needed to connect care processes, moderate-term clinical outcomes, and longer-term outcomes in the community. The adaptive and healing processes engendered by rehabilitative care also needs to be distinguished from other factors affecting patients.

Both process-focused and outcomes-focused methods are limited by uncertainties in knowledge of the connection between care processes and outcomes, that is, by our currently vague knowledge of the effectiveness of alternative rehabilitative treatments. More definite, quantitative knowledge of which rehabilitative interventions are most effective, and for whom, will increase the utility of QI and outcomes management in medical rehabilitation and thereby advance the field and improve the lives of persons served.

Acknowledgment

We express special thanks to Steven Forer, M.A., M.B.A., for his timely, expert critique of this chapter.

REFERENCES

1. Leape LL. Error in medicine. *JAMA* 1994; 272:1851–1857.
2. DeJong G, Batavia AI, Griss R. America's neglected health minority: working-age persons with disabilities. *Milbank Q* 1988; 67:311–351.
3. Institute of Medicine. *Disability in America.* Washington, D.C.: National Academy of Sciences, 1991.
4. Fiedler RC, Granger CV, Ottenbacher KJ. The Uniform Data System for Medical Rehabilitation: report of first admissions for 1994. *Am J Phys Med Rehabil* 1996; 75(2):125–129.
5. Blumenthal D. Quality of health care: Part 1: Quality of care—What is it? *N Engl J Med* 1996; 335(12):891–894.
6. Commission on Accreditation of Rehabilitation Facilities. *1996 Standards manual and interpretative guidelines for medical rehabilitation.* Tucson: Author, 1996.
7. Granger CV, Gresham G, eds. *Functional assessment in rehabilitation medicine.* Baltimore: Williams & Wilkins, 1984.
8. Keith RA. Functional assessment measures in medical rehabilitation: current status. *Arch Phys Med Rehabil* 1984; 65:74–78.
9. Haffey WJ, Johnston MV. An information system to assess the effectiveness of brain injury rehabilitation. In: Wood R, Eames P, eds. *Models of brain injury rehabilitation.* London: Chapman Hall, 1989; 205–233.
10. Haffey WJ, Johnston MV. A functional assessment system for real world rehabilitation outcomes. In: Tupper D, Cicerone K, eds. *The neuropsychology of everyday life.* Boston: Martinus Nijhoff, 1989; 99–124.
11. DeJong G, Hughes J. Independent living: methodology for measuring long-term outcomes. *Arch Phys Med Rehabil* 1982; 63:68–73.
12. Haffey WJ, Lewis FD. Programming for occupational outcomes following traumatic brain injury. *Rehabil Psychol* 1989; 34:147–158.
13. Brook RH. Quality of care: do we care? *Ann Intern Med* 1991; 115: 486–490.
14. McNeil BJ, Pauker SG, Sox HC Jr, Tversky A. On the elicitation of preferences for alternative therapies. *N Engl J Med* 1982; 306: 1259–1262.
15. Glueckauf RL. Program evaluation guidelines for the rehabilitation professional. *Adv Clin Rehabil* 1990; 3:250–266.
16. Joint Commission on Accreditation of Healthcare Organizations. Characteristics of clinical indicators. *Qual Rev Bull* 1989; 15: 330–339.
17. Whiteneck GG, Charlifue SW, Gerhart KA, Overholser JD, Richardson GN. Quantifying handicap: a new measure of long-term rehabilitation outcomes. *Arch Phys Med Rehabil* 1992; 73:519–526.
18. Johnston MV, Lewis FD. The outcomes of community re-entry pro-

grams for brain injury survivors. Part 1: Independent living and productive activities. *Brain Inj* 1991; 5:141–154.
19. Johnston MV. The outcome of community re-entry programs for brain injury survivors. Part 2: Further investigations. *Brain Inj* 1991; 5: 155–168.
20. Kritchevsky SB, Simmons BP. Continuous quality improvement. *JAMA* 1991; 266(13):1817–1823.
21. Deming WE. *Out of the crisis.* Cambridge, MA: Massachusetts Institute of Technology Center for Advanced Engineering Study, 1986.
22. Lubeck RC, Davis PK. W.E. Deming's 14 points for quality: can they be applied to rehabilitation? *J Rehabil Admin* 1991; 15:216–222.
23. Thompson R. Some practical applications of Deming's fourteen points. *J Qual Assur* 1990; 12(Sept/Oct):22–23.
24. Casalou RF. Total quality management in health care. *Hosp Health Serv Admin* 1991; 36(1):134–176.
25. Juran J. *Quality control handbook*, 4th ed. New York: McGraw-Hill, 1988.
26. Fainter J. Quality assurance quality improvement. *J Qual Assur* 1991; 13:8–9.
27. Committee to Advise the Public Health Service on Clinical Practice Guidelines; Field MJ, Lohr KN, eds. *Clinical practice guidelines.* Washington, D.C.: National Academy Press, 1990.
28. Marder R. Relationship of clinical indicators and practice guidelines. *Qual Rev Bull* 1990; 16:60–61.
29. Haley SM, Costner WJ, Binda-Sundberg K. Measuring physical disablement: the contextual challenge. *Phys Ther* 1994; 74(5):443–451.
30. Rutstein DD, Berenberg W, Chalmers TC, Child CGI, Fishman AP, Perrin EB. Measuring the quality of medical care: a clinical method. *N Engl J Med* 1976; 194;582–588.
31. Joint Commission on the Accreditation of Healthcare Organizations. *1996 Comprehensive accreditation manual for hospitals.* Chicago: Author, 1995.
32. Lohr KN, Donaldson MS, Harris-Wehling J. Medicare: a strategy for quality assurance. Quality of care in a changing health care environment. *Qual Rev Bull* 1992; 18:120–126.
33. Lohr KN, ed. *Medicare: a strategy for quality assurance.* Washington, D.C.: National Academy Press, 1990.
34. Brook RH. Quality of care: do we care? *Ann Intern Med* 1991; 115: 486–490.
35. Donabedian A, Palmer RH. Considerations in defining quality of health care. In: Palmer RH, Donabedian A., Povar GJ, eds. *Striving for quality in health care.* Ann Arbor: Health Administration Press, 1991; 1–53.
36. Williamson JW. Evaluation quality of patient care: a strategy relating outcome and process assessment. *JAMA* 1971; 218(4):564–569.
37. Johnston MV, Ottenbacher K, Reichardt K. Strong quasi-experimental designs for research on the effectiveness of rehabilitation. *Am J Phys Med Rehabil* 1995; 74(5):383–392.
38. Johnston MV, Keith RA. The cost benefits of medical rehabilitation: review and critique. *Arch Phys Med Rehabil* 1983; 64:147–154.
39. Posavac EJ, Carey RG. *Program evaluation: Methods and case studies,* 4th ed. Englewood Cliffs, NJ: Prentice Hall, 1992.
40. Cleary PD, McNeil BJ. Patient satisfaction as an indicator of quality care. *Inquiry* 1988; 25:25–36.
41. Gray CS, Swope MG. Integrated program evaluation and quality assurance processes. In: England B, Glass RM, Patterson CH, eds. *Quality rehabilitation: results-oriented patient care.* Chicago: American Hospital Publishing, 1989; 53–59.
42. Allen MJ, Yen WM. *Introduction to measurement theory.* Monterey, CA: Brooks/Cole, 1979.
43. Lipsey M. Theory as method: small theories of treatments. In: Sechrest L, Perrin E, Bunker J, eds. *Research methodology: strengthening causal interpretations of nonexperimental data (PHS 90-3454).* Rockville, MD: DHHS, PHS, AHCPR, 1990; 33–52.
44. Carey RG, Seibert JH, Posavac EJ. Who makes the most progress in inpatient rehabilitation? An analysis of functional gain. *Arch Phys Med Rehabil* 1988; 69:337–343.
45. Joint Commission on Accreditation of Hospitals. *Primer on clinical indicator development and application.* Chicago: Author, 1990.
46. Donabedian A. *Explorations in quality assessment and monitoring, Vol. 3: Methods and findings of quality assessment and monitoring.* Ann Arbor, MI: Health Administration Press, 1985.
47. Brennan TA, Leape LL, Laird NM, Hebert L, Localio AR, Lawthers AG, Newhouse JP, Weiler PC, Hiatt HH. Incidence of adverse events and negligence in hospitalized patients. Results of the Harvard medical practice study I. *N Engl J Med* 1991; 324:370–376.
48. Kravitz RL, Rolph JE, McGuigan K. Malpractice claims data as a quality improvement tool. I. Epidemiology of error in four specialties. *JAMA* 1991;266:2087–2092.
49. World Health Organization. International classification of impairments, disabilities, and handicaps. Geneva: Author, 1980.
50. Johnston MV, Hall K, Carnevale G, Boake C. Functional assessment and outcome evaluation in TBI rehabilitation. In: Horn LJ, Zasler ND, eds. *Medical rehabilitation of traumatic brain injury.* Philadelphia: Hanley and Belfus, 1996;197–226.
51. National Center for Medical Rehabilitation Research. *Research Plan for the National Center for Medical Rehabilitation Research. NIH Publication No. 93-3509.* Washington, D.C.: US Department of Health and Human Services, Public Health Services, National Institute of Child Health and Human Development, 1993.
52. Spiker B, ed. *Quality of life assessments in clinical trials.* New York: Raven Press, 1990.
53. Wade DT: *Measurement in neurological rehabilitation.* New York, Oxford University Press, 1992.
54. McDowell I, Newell C. *Measuring health: A guide to rating scales and questionnaires,* 2nd ed. New York, Oxford University Press, 1996.
55. Bergner M, Bobbit RA, Carter WB, et al. The Sickness Impact Profile: development and final revision of a health status measure. *Med Care* 1981; 19:787–805.
56. Stewart AL, Ware JE Jr, eds. *Measuring functioning and well-being.* Durham, NC: Duke University Press, 1992.
57. Fuhrer MJ. Subjective well-being: implications for medical rehabilitation outcomes and models of disablement. *Am J Phys Med Rehabil* 1994; 73(5):358–364.
58. Johnston MV, Keith RA, Hinderer S. Measurement standards for interdisciplinary medical rehabilitation. *Arch Phys Med Rehabil* 1992; 73(Suppl 12):S6–S23.
59. Phelps CE. The methodologic foundations of the appropriateness of medical care. *N Engl J Med* 1996; 329(17):1241–1245.
60. Granger CV, Cotter AC, Hamilton BB, Fiedler RC, Hens MM. Functional assessment scales: a study of persons with multiple sclerosis. *Arch Phys Med Rehabil* 1990; 71:870–875.
61. Silverstein B, Kilgore KM, Fisher WP. Implementing patient tracking systems and using functional assessment scales, Vol. 1. In Harvey RF, ed. *Center for Rehabilitation Outcome Analysis monograph series on issues and methods in outcome analysis.* Wheaton, IL: Marianjoy Rehabilitation Center, 1989.
62. Silverstein B, Kilgore KM, Fisher WP, Harley P, Harvey RF. Applying psychometric criteria to functional assessment in medical rehabilitation: I. Exploring unidimensionality. *Arch Phys Med Rehabil* 1991; 72:631–637.
63. Fuhrer MJ, ed. *Rehabilitation outcomes: Analysis and measurement.* Baltimore: Paul Brookes, 1987.
64. Hall KM, Mann N, High WM Jr, Wright J, Kreutzer JS, Wood D. Functional measures after traumatic brain injury: ceiling effects of FIM, FIM-FAM, DRS, and CIQ. *J Head Trauma Rehabil* 1966; 11(5): 27–39.
65. Heinemann AW, Linacre JM, Wright BD, Hamilton BB, Granger C. Relationships between impairment and physical disability as measured by the Functional Independence Measure. *Arch Phys Med Rehabil* 1993; 4(6):566–573.
66. Whyte J. Towards a methodology for rehabilitation research. *Am J Phys Med Rehabil* 1994; 73(6):428–435.
67. Hinderer SR, Gupta S. Functional outcome measures to assess interventions for spasticity. *Arch Phys Med Rehabil* 1996; 77(10): 1083–1089.
68. Johnston MV, Stineman M, Velozo CA. Foundations from the past and directions for the future. In: Fuhrer M, ed. *Assessing medical rehabilitation practices: the promise of outcomes research.* Baltimore: Paul H Brookes, 1997; 1–41.
69. McAuliffe WE. Measuring the quality of medical care: process versus outcome. *Milbank Mem Fund Q* 1979; 57:118–152.
70. Wilkerson DL, Johnston MV. Outcomes research and clinical program monitoring systems: current capability and future directions. In: Fuhrer M, ed. *Medical rehabilitation outcomes research.* Baltimore: Paul H Brookes, 1997; 275–305.
71. Johnston MV, Wilkerson DL. Program evaluation and quality im-

provement systems in brain injury rehabilitation. *J Head Trauma Rehabil* 1993; 7(4)[illegible]–82.

72. Caradoc-Davies TH, Dixon GS, Campbell AJ. Benefit from admission to a geriatric assessment and rehabilitation unit. Discrepancy between health professional and client perception of improvement. *J Am Geriatr Soc* 1989; 37:25–28.
73. Linn LS, DiMatteo MR, Chang BL, Cope DW. Consumer values and subsequent satisfaction ratings of physician behavior. *Med Care* 1984; 22(9):804–812.
74. Ware JE. Research methodology: how to survey patient satisfaction. *Drug Intell Clin Pharm* 1981; 15:892–899.
75. Courts NF. A patient satisfaction survey for a rehabilitation unit. *Rehabil Nurs* 1988; 13:79–81.
76. Davis D, Hobbs G. Measuring outpatient satisfaction with rehabilitation services. *Qual Rev Bull* 1989; 15:192–197.
77. Ware JE Jr, Hays RD. Methods for measuring patient satisfaction with specific medical encounters. *Med Care* 1988; 26(4):393–402.
78. Forer S. *Outcomes management and program evaluation made easy: a toolkit for occupational therapy practioners.* Bethesda, MD: American Occupational Therapy Association, 1996.
79. Ellwood P. Outcomes management: a technology of patient experience. *N Engl J Med* 1988; 318:1549–1556.
80. Commission on Accreditation of Rehabilitation Facilities. *Program evaluation in inpatient medical rehabilitation programs.* Tucson: Author, 1988.
81. Commission on Accreditation of Rehabilitation Facilities. *Program evaluation: a guide to utilization.* Tucson: Author, 1989.
82. Commission on Accreditation of Rehabilitation Facilities. *Program evaluation: utilization and assessment principles.* Tucson: Author, 1989.
83. Forer SK. Outcome analysis for program service management. In: Fuhrer MJ, ed. *Rehabilitation outcomes: analysis and measurement.* Baltimore: Paul Brooks, 1987; 115–136.
84. Forer SK, Magnuson RI. Feedback reporting. In: Granger C, Gresham G, eds. *Functional assessment in rehabilitation medicine.* Baltimore: Williams & Wilkins, 1984; 171–193.
85. Commission on Accreditation of Rehabilitation Facilities. *Program evaluation in outpatient medical rehabilitation programs.* Tucson: Author, 1980.
86. Commission on Accreditation of Rehabilitation Facilities. *Program evaluation in inpatient medical rehabilitation programs.* Tucson: Author, 1988.
87. Commission on Accreditation of Rehabilitation Facilities. *Program evaluation for vocational and employment programs.* Tucson: Author, 1990.
88. Rubenstein LZ, Josephson KR, Wieland GD, English PA, Sayre JA, Kane RL. Effectiveness of a geriatric evaluation unit: a randomized clinical trial. *N Engl J Med* 1984; 311:1664–1670.
89. Johnston MV. *The costs and effectiveness of stroke rehabilitation: measurement and prediction* [Dissertation]. Claremont, CA: Claremont Graduate University, 1983.
90. Carey RG. Integrating case management, program evaluation, and marketing for inpatient and outpatient rehabilitation programs. In: Eisenberg MG, Grzesiak RC, eds. *Advances in clinical rehabilitation,* Vol 3. New York: Springer, 1990;149–219.
91. Collins LM, Horn JL, eds. *Best methods for the analysis of change.* Washington, D.C.: American Psychological Association, 1991.
92. Data Management Service of the Uniform Data System for Medical Rehabilitation. *Guide for use of the uniform data set for medical rehabilitation.* Buffalo: Research Foundation, State University of New York, 1993.
93. Harvey RF, Jellinek HM. Patient profiles: utilization in functional performance assessment. *Arch Phys Med Rehabil* 1983; 64:268–271.
94. Formations in Healthcare. *Medical outcomes system.* Chicago: Formations in Healthcare, 1994.
95. Formations in Healthcare. *Restore outcome system.* Chicago: Formations in Healthcare, 1992.
96. Focus on Therapeutic Outcomes (FOTO). Knoxville, TN; Author, 1993.
97. Gonnella C. Program evaluation. In: Fletcher GF, Banja JD, Jann BB, Wolf SL, eds. *Rehabilitation medicine: contemporary clinical perspectives.* Philadelphia: Lea & Febinger, 1992; 243–268.
98. Commission on Accreditation of Rehabilitation Facilities. *Program evaluation in spinal cord injury programs.* Tucson: Author, 1987.
99. Commission on Accreditation of Rehabilitation Facilities. *Program evaluation in chronic pain management programs.* Tucson: Author, 1987.
100. Commission on Accreditation of Rehabilitation Facilities. *Program evaluation for vocational and employment programs.* Tucson: Author, 1990.
101. Fraser RT, Clemmons D, Trejo W, Temkin R. Program evaluation in epilepsy rehabilitation. *Epilepsia* 1983; 24:734–746.
102. Shaughnessy PW, Crisler KS, Schlenker RE, Arnold AG, Kramer AM, Powell MC, Hittle DF. Measuring and assuring the quality of home health care. *Health Care Financ Rev* 1994(Fall); 16(1):35–67.
103. Linacre JM, Heinemann AW, Wright BD, Granger CV, Hamilton BB. The structure and stability of the Functional Independence Measure. *Arch Phys Med Rehabil* 1994; 75(2):127–132.
104. Cohen J, Cohen P. *Applied multiple regression/correlation analysis for the behavioral sciences,* 2nd ed. Hillsdale, NJ: Lawrence Erlbaum, 1983.
105. Collins LM, Johnston MV. Analysis of stage-sequential change in rehabilitation research. *Am J Phys Med Rehabil* 1995; 74:163–170.
106. Glueckauf RL. Use and misuse of assessment in rehabilitation: getting back to the basics. In: Glueckauf RL, Secrest LB, Bond GR, McDonel EC, eds. *Improving assessment in rehabilitation and health.* Newbury Park, CA: Sage Publications, 1993; 135–155.
107. Ottenbacher KJ, Cusick A. Goal attainment scaling as a method of clinical service evaluation. *Am J Occup Ther* 1990; 44:519–525.
108. Kiresuk TJ, Lund SH. Goal attainment scaling. In: Attkisson CC, Hargreaves WA, Horowitz MJ, Sorensen JE, eds. *Evaluation of human service programs.* New York: Academic Press, 1978; 15–23.
109. Fauman MA. Quality assurance monitoring in psychiatry. *Am J Psychiatry* 1989; 146:1121–1129.
110. Brook RH, McGlynn EA, Cleary PD. Quality of health care: Part 2: Measuring quality of care. *N Engl J Med* 1996; 335(13):966–970.
111. Joint Commission on Accreditation of Hospitals. *Agenda for change update,* Vol 2, no. 1. Chicago: Author, 1988.
112. Kravitz RL, Rolph JE, McGuigan K. Malpractice claims data as a quality improvement tool. I. Epidemiology of error in four specialties. *JAMA* 1991; 266:2087–2092.
113. Kravitz RL, Rolph JE, McGuigan K. Malpractice claims data as a quality improvement tool. II. Is targeting effective? *JAMA* 1991; 266: 2093–2097.
114. Kleefield S, Churchill W, Laffel G. Quality improvement in a hospital pharmacy department. *Qual Rev Bull* 1991; 17:138–143.
115. Batalden P. Building knowledge for quality improvement in healthcare: an introductory glossary. *J Qual Assur* 1991; 13:8–12.
116. Donabedian A. *Explorations in quality assessment and monitoring,* Vol 2. Ann Arbor, MI: Health Administration Press, 1982.
117. Donabedian A. Criteria and standards for quality assessment and monitoring. *Qual Rev Bull* 1986; 12:99–108.
118. Joint Commission on Accreditation of Healthcare Organizations. *National Library of Healthcare Indicators.* Chicago: Author, 1997.
119. Leape L. Practice guidelines and standards: an overview. *Qual Rev Bull* 1990; 16:42–49.
120. *1997 Medical Outcomes & Guidelines Sourcebook.* New York: Faulkner and Gray, 1997.
121. Chassin MR. Quality of health care. Part 3: Improving the quality of care. *N Engl J Med* 1996; 335(14):1060–1063.
122. InterQual, Inc. *A guide for physician reviewers.* North Hampton, NH: Author, 1995.
123. Post-stroke Rehabilitation Guideline Panel. *Post-stroke rehabilitation. Clinical practice guideline number 16. AHCPR publication no. 95-0662.* Rockille MD: US Department of Health and Human Services, Public Health Service, Agency for Health Care Policy and Research, 1995.
124. Bergstrom N, Bennett MA, Carlson CE, et al (Guideline Panel). *Treatment of pressure ulcers. Clinical practice guideline number 15. AHCPR publication no. 95-0652.* Rockville, MD: US Department of Health and Human Services, Public Health Service, Agency for Health Care Policy and Research, 1994.
125. Bergstrom N, Allman RM, Carlson CE, et al (Guideline Panel). *Pressure ulcers in adults: prediction and prevention. Clinical practice guideline number 3. AHCPR publication number 92-0047.* Rockville, MD: US Department of Health and Human Services, Public Health Service, Agency for Health Care Policy and Research, 1992.
126. Fantl JA, Newman DK (chairs), et al (Guideline Update Panel). *Uri-*

nary incontinence in adults: Acute and chronic management. Clinical practice guideline number 2, 1966 Update. AHCPR publication no. 96-0682. Rockville, MD: US Department of Health and Human Services, Public Health Service, Agency for Health Care Policy and Research, 1996.

127. Wenger NK, Froelicher ES, et al (Guideline Panel). *Cardiac rehabilitation. Clinical guideline number 17. AHCPR publication no. 96-0672.* Rockville, MD: Department of Health and Human Services, Public Health Service, Agency for Health Care Policy and Research, 1996.
128. Aspen Reference Group. *Medical rehabilitation services: forms, checklists, & guidelines.* Frederick, MD: Aspen, 1996.
129. Pestotnik SL, Classen DC, Evans RS, Burke JP. Implementing antibiotic practice guidelines through computer-assisted decision support: clinical outcomes and financial outcomes. *Ann Intern Med* 1966; 124; 884–890.
130. James BC. Implementing practice guidelines through clinical quality improvement. *Front Health Serv Manage* 1993; 10(1);3–37.
131. Angstman G. Getting physician and organization buy-in. In: Kaegi L, ed. Practice guidelines: From paper to practice to point of care. *J Qual Improve* 1996; 22(8):551–555.
132. Falconer JA, Roth EJ, Sutin JA, Strasser DC, Chang RW. The critical path method in stroke rehabilitation: lessons from an experiment in cost containment and outcome improvement. *Qual Rev Bull* 1994; 19(1):8–16.
133. Gray CS, Upton BM, Berman S. *Monitoring and evaluation: Physical rehabilitation services.* Chicago: Joint Commission on Accreditation of Healthcare Organizations, 1988.
134. Agency for Health Care Policy and Research. *CONQUEST 1.0: A computerized needs-oriented quality measurement evaluation system. Publication no. 96-N009.* Rockville, MD: US Department of Health and Human Services, Public Health Service, AHCPR Clearinghouse, 1996. Downloadable from www.ahcpr.gov/research/CONQUEST.htm
135. Mayhall CG. *Hospital epidemiology and infection control.* Philadephia; Williams & Wilkins, 1966.
136. Association of Practioners in Infection Control (APIC). *Infection control and applied epidemiology: Principles and practice.* St Louis: Mosby, 1966.
137. Widmer TG, Matthews CB, Gray LW, Everett J, Forer S. Marketing program quality. In: England B, Glass RM, Patterson CA, eds. *Quality rehabilitation: Results-oriented patient care.* Chicago: American Hospital Publishing, 1989; 69–101.
138. Johnston MV. Cost–benefit methodologies in rehabilitation. In: Fuhrer M, ed. *Rehabilitation outcomes: analysis and measurement.* Baltimore: Paul Brooks, 1987; 99–114.
139. Stineman MG, Escarce JJ, Goin JE, Hamilton BB, Granger CV, Williams SV. A case-mix classification system for medical rehabilitation. *Med Care* 1994; 32(4):366–379.
140. Stineman MG, Goin JE, Hamilton BB, Granger CV. Efficiency pattern analysis for medical rehabilitation. *Am J Med Qual* 1995; 10(4): 190–198.
141. Stineman MG. Case-mix measurement in medical rehabilitation. *Arch Phys Med Rehabil* 1995; 76(12):1163–1170.
142. Iezzoni LI, Ash AS, Shwartz M, Daley J, Hughes JS, Mackiernan YD. Predicting who dies depends on how severity is measured: implications for evaluating patient outcomes. *Ann Intern Med* 1995; 123(10):763–770.
143. Himmelstein D, Woolhandler S. Cost without benefit: administrative waste in U.S. health care. *N Engl J Med* 1986; 314(7):441–445.
144. DeJong G, Sutton JP. Rehab 2000: the evolution of medical rehabilitation in American health care. In: Landrum-Kitchell P, Schmidt ND, McLean A Jr, eds. *Outcome-oriented rehabilitation.* Gaithersburg, MD: Aspen, 1995; 3–42.
145. Ware JE Jr, Brook RH, Rogers WH, et al. Comparison of health outcomes at a health maintenance organization with those of fee-for-service care. *Lancet* 1986; 1:1017–1022.
146. Berwick DM. Quality of health care: Part 5: Payment by capitation and the quality of care. *N Engl J Med* 1996; 335(16):1227–1231.
147. Miller RH, Luft HS. Managed care plan performance since 1980: a literature analysis. *JAMA* 1994; 271:1512–1519.
148. Birch and Davis Associates, National Rehabilitation Hospital Research Center. *The state-of-the-science in medical rehabilitation. Volume II. Report submitted to Office of the Civilian Health and Medical Program for the Uniformed Services, Department of Defense.* Falls Church, VA: Birch and Davis Associates, 1996.
149. Brown RS, Bergeron JW, Clement DG, Hill JW, Retchin SM. *Does managed care work for Medicare? An evaluation of the Medicare risk program for HMOs.* Princeton, NJ: Mathematica Policy Research, 1993.
150. Faulkner and Gray. *1997 Comparative performance data sourcebook.* New York: Faulkner and Gray, 1996.
151. Medical Outcomes Trust. National performance standards now include health outcomes. *Med Outcomes Trust Bull* 1996; 4(5):1.
152. Johnston MV, Kirshblum S, Zorowitz R, Shiflett SC. Prediction of outcomes following rehabilitation of stroke patients. *NeuroRehabilitation* 1992; 2(4):71–96.
153. McLean A Jr. Knowledge-based systems in rehabilitation. In: Landrum PK, Schmidt ND, McLean A Jr, eds. *Outcome-oriented rehabilitation.* Gaithersburg, MD: Aspen, 1995; 118–303.
154. Kane RL. Improving the quality of long-term care. *JAMA* 1995; 273(17):1376–1380.
155. Wilson L, Goldschmidt P. *Quality management in health care.* New York: McGraw-Hill, 1995.

Rehabilitation Medicine: Principles and Practice, Third Edition,
edited by Joel A. DeLisa and Bruce M. Gans.
Lippincott–Raven Publishers, Philadelphia © 1998.

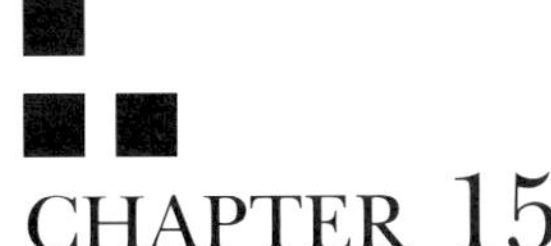

CHAPTER 15

Electrodiagnostic Evaluation of the Peripheral Nervous System

Richard D. Ball

Electrodiagnostic testing of the peripheral nervous system is an adjunct to the history, physical examination, and other laboratory studies in the overall evaluation of neuromuscular disease. Neuromuscular disorders may involve the motor unit (i.e., anterior horn cell body/axon, neuromuscular junction, associated muscle cells), sensory neurons, and related cells (e.g., the Schwann cells). Although the nature of neurologic dysfunction in a specific disease process may be suggested by symptoms or signs obtained during the physical examination, electrodiagnostic studies frequently provide additional information that can be obtained in no other manner. The widespread use of electrodiagnostic testing is based on several facts:

- When used appropriately, it can result in markedly improved diagnostic accuracy.
- It can provide quantitative/semiquantitative data on the severity or prognosis of a disease process.
- It is a relatively objective measure of neurologic function.

The process of performing electrodiagnostic studies consists of the following basic steps:

1. Evaluate the patient by taking a history and performing a physical examination, and arrive at a preliminary differential diagnosis.
2. Use this differential diagnosis to select the proper electrodiagnostic tests to perform.
3. Perform the selected tests in a technically competent manner.
4. Properly interpret the results obtained so as to identify the most likely diagnoses and exclude unlikely diagnoses.

Although these steps seem simple at first glance, the ability to perform them rests on a thorough understanding of a large and complex body of information about the underlying clinical, physiological, and electrical phenomena. Principles and concepts of a general nature are emphasized here rather than specific information that may relate to only a small part of the overall process. The information in this chapter refers exclusively to the peripheral nervous system; electrodiagnostic testing of the central nervous system (CNS) is discussed in Chapter 16.

Although the functional status of the peripheral motor or sensory systems usually can be determined from the history and physical examination, the underlying cause of sensorimotor dysfunction frequently cannot be established in this manner. For example, it may be difficult to decide whether proximal muscle weakness is caused by dysfunction of the neuromuscular junction or by myopathy. Because rational management requires specific diagnoses, the clinician needs information not only on a patient's overall neuromuscular function but also on the specific status of the various physiological and anatomic components of the peripheral nervous system, including the following:

- Motor neurons
- Neuromuscular junction
- Sensory neurons
- Schwann cells (i.e., myelin sheath)
- Muscle cell (i.e., myocyte)

The task of the electrodiagnostician is therefore to determine the isolated electrical properties of these physiological and anatomic components and correlate abnormal electrical properties with the pathologic processes present in specific disease categories; that is, determine whether the electrodiagnostic abnormalities are consistent with the following:

- Anterior horn cell disease
- Polyneuropathy (axonal versus demyelinating; sensory, motor, or sensorimotor)
- Mononeuropathy

R. D. Ball: Department of Physical Medicine, Munson Medical Center, Traverse City, Michigan 49689.

- Mononeuropathy multiplex syndrome
- Plexopathy
- Radiculopathy or polyradiculopathy
- Polyradiculoneuropathy (e.g., Guillain-Barré syndrome)
- Multifocal motor neuropathy
- Neuromuscular junction disorder
- Myopathic process

To perform electrodiagnostic testing accurately and efficiently, a structured approach is necessary. The number of electrodiagnostic tests that could be performed on any one patient is large, the time required may be considerable, and the patient frequently experiences discomfort during the examination. For this reason, the electrodiagnostician must make an effort to obtain the correct answer with a minimum number of individual tests. Most clinicians approach problems by taking a history, performing a physical examination, obtaining results of laboratory studies, and then analyzing the results according to the following questions with respect to involvement of the peripheral nervous system:

- Does the disorder appear to involve the anterior horn cells, sensory neurons, nerve roots, peripheral nerve, neuromuscular junction, or muscle?
- What is the distribution of abnormalities likely to be? Is the problem diffuse and generalized (e.g., myopathy or toxic polyneuropathy), multifocal (e.g., mononeuritis multiplex syndrome), or localized to the distribution of specific roots, plexuses, or peripheral nerves?
- What is the temporal course of the disorder? Is it acute, subacute, chronic, stable, improving, fluctuating, or progressing? How long have the symptoms been present?

The differential diagnoses synthesized from the answers to these questions allow the electrodiagnostician to decide which tests are most likely to lead directly to the most proba-

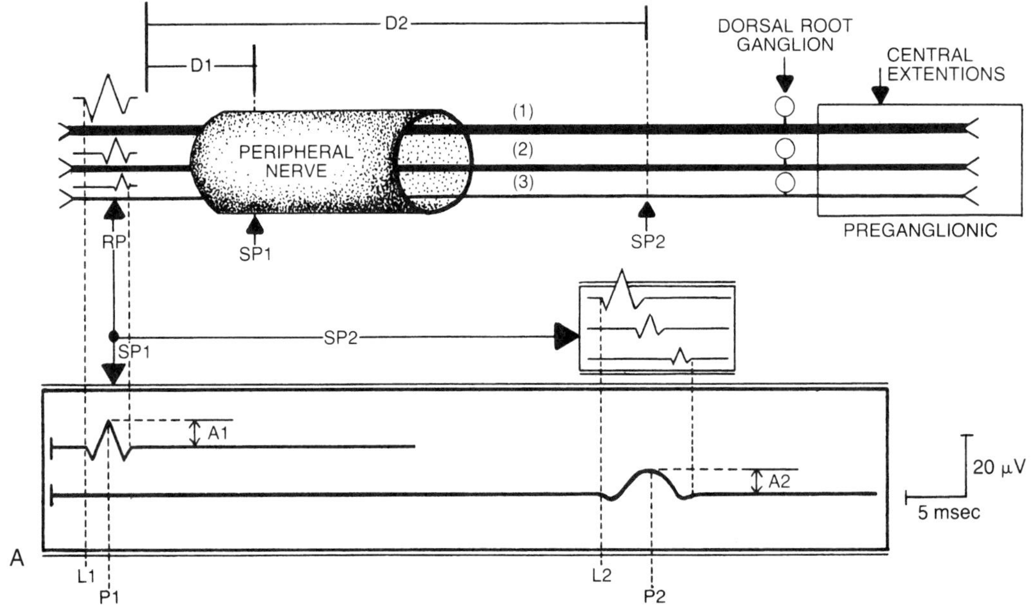

FIG. 15-1. Determination of latencies, nerve conduction velocities, and evoked response amplitudes. **A:** Sensory nerves. The latencies are a function of the length of nerve and the average action potential conduction velocity between the stimulation and recording sites. The distal latency is the latency obtained from the most distal point of stimulation of the nerve. In an analogous fashion, the proximal latency is the latency obtained with the proximal stimulation point. The average conduction velocity of the nerve segment between the stimulation point is calculated as follows: *Conduction Velocity* = $(Distance_2 - Distance_1)/(Latency_2 - Latency_1)$. In general, the latencies used to calculate sensory and motor nerve conduction velocities are measured from the time of the stimulus to the earliest part of the evoked response. Note that this technique measures only the responses of the most rapidly conducting nerve axons. When the sensory nerve action potential (SNAP) distal latency is used in isolation, the distal sensory latency is taken as the time from the stimulus to the peak of the negative deflection of the potential (P_1), not the leading edge of the response (L_1). Latencies are determined in this fashion because the peak of the sensory potential is generally more easily and reproducibly determined than the onset latency. The peak latency is therefore more desirable in general. However, the onset latencies must be used for determining the conduction velocities because this is the only portion of the evoked response that represents the same population of fibers (the fastest) with both distal and proximal stimulation. The action potentials from large *(1)*, medium *(2)*, and small *(3)* myelinated axons are shown. These are intended to represent populations of axons with these size characteristics. Note the change in the SNAP shape and amplitude due to temporal dispersion as the distance over which the action potentials are conducted increases. *(continued)*

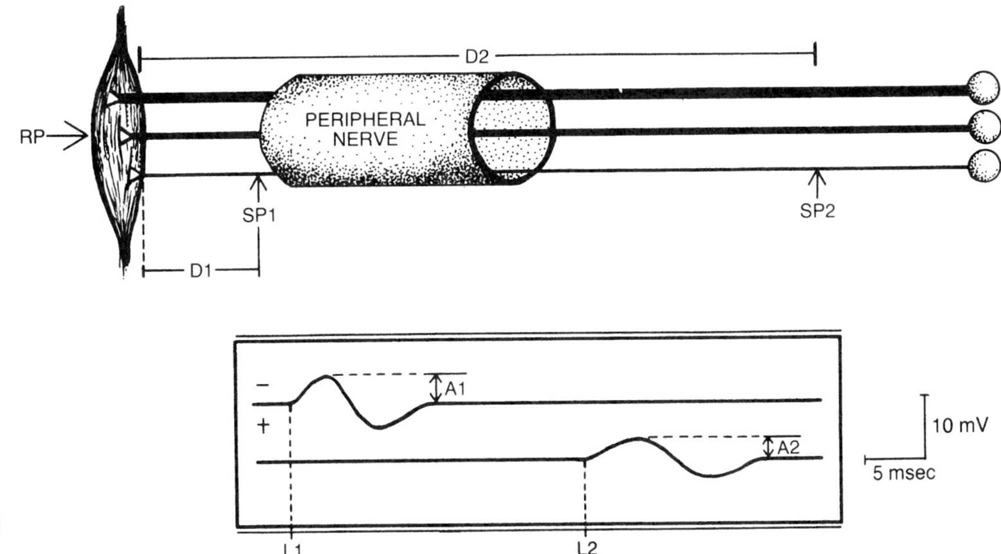

FIG. 15-1. *Continued.* **B:** Motor nerves. Note that the compound muscle action potential (CMAP) is recorded from muscle, not nerve. Three motor units are shown in the diagram, representing motor neurons with large *(1)*, medium *(2)*, and small *(3)* myelinated axons. Temporal dispersion is illustrated in a manner analogous to that for sensory nerves. A_1, amplitude of SNAP **(A)** or CMAP **(B)** obtained with stimulation at SP_1; A_2, amplitude of SNAP **(A)** or CMAP **(B)** obtained with stimulation at SP_2; D_1, distance from SP_1 to *RP*; D_2, distance from SP_2 to RP; L_1, latency 1, time required for fastest conducting fibers to travel distance D_1; L_2, latency 2, the time required for fastest conducting fibers to travel distance D_2; P_1, peak latency of SNAP obtained with stimulation at SP_1; P_2, peak latency of SNAP obtained with stimulation at SP_2; *RP*, recording point; SP_1, stimulus point 1; SP_2, stimulus point 2.

ble diagnosis. *Guidelines in Electrodiagnostic Medicine* (1), published by the American Association of Electrodiagnostic Medicine, should be reviewed for assistance in the design of appropriate electrodiagnostic studies (1). The recent review by Dyck et al. (2) provides an excellent demonstration of these principles applied to the evaluation of peripheral neuropathy.

OVERVIEW OF BASIC ELECTRODIAGNOSTIC TESTS

A discussion of specific electrodiagnostic tests is provided later in this chapter, but first an overview is provided of the most commonly used techniques and the general properties of the peripheral nervous system that are evaluated by these tests. Detailed descriptions of electronic theory and the relevant electronic equipment have been well covered in standard electronic and electromyography (EMG) texts (3–6). A basic understanding of nerve and muscle physiology is assumed. The reader also should become familiar with the statistical aspects of normal values in electrodiagnostic studies (7–9).

Sensory Nerve Conduction Studies

Standard sensory nerve conduction studies are performed by supramaximal stimulation of a nerve at one point and measuring the whole-nerve action potential at some other point (Fig. 15-1*A*). A supramaximal stimulation is defined as having an intensity high enough to initiate an action potential in all axons belonging to the nerve being stimulated. Because the whole-nerve action potential is simply the sum of the action potentials from all axons in the nerve, we are concerned with how the integrity of the peripheral sensory axon action potential is affected by various disease processes. From this standpoint, the anatomic characteristics of peripheral sensory neurons make it useful to divide clinical sensory dysfunction into preganglionic and postganglionic categories, based on whether failure of sensory function is the result of a pathologic process distal or proximal to the sensory neuron cell body. Preganglionic disorders (e.g., radiculopathies, cauda equina lesions, posterior column disease) do not significantly damage the sensory cell body in the dorsal root ganglion and leave the distal axon intact. Sensory electrodiagnostic studies in these disorders are normal even though clinical sensory function may be markedly abnormal. Postganglionic disorders are those disorders that damage the sensory cell body/axon or the associated Schwann cell and result either directly or indirectly in axonal dysfunction. Sensory electrical studies in these disorders may be abnormal if the damage is severe enough.

Information obtained from sensory nerve conduction studies includes the sensory nerve action potential (SNAP) conduction velocity along various segments of the sensory nerve and the amplitude and shape of the SNAP. Analysis of the SNAP amplitude, shape, distal latency, and conduction velocity can provide specific information about the number, type, and state of myelination of sensory axons functioning in various segments of the nerve (10).

Motor Nerve Conduction Studies

Motor nerve conduction studies are performed by stimulating motor nerves and recording the resulting compound muscle action potential (CMAP) from the muscle (Fig. 15-1*B*). The results of motor nerve conduction studies may be affected by any process that damages the anterior horn cell body or axon, associated Schwann cells, the neuromuscular junction, or the muscle cell. In contrast to the sensory neurons, where peripheral lesions could be preganglionic or postganglionic, all peripheral lesions of motor axons occur distal to the cell body, thereby possibly affecting axonal function. This anatomic difference between sensory and motor neurons is sometimes helpful to the electromyographer in differentiating lesions that clinically cause both motor and sensory dysfunction because lesions proximal to the dorsal root ganglion (e.g., radiculopathies) frequently produce abnormal motor studies with concomitantly normal sensory studies, whereas lesions distal to the dorsal root ganglion can affect both motor and sensory electrical function.

As in sensory nerve conduction studies, the major results obtained are the nerve conduction velocity in various nerve segments and the amplitude and shape of the CMAP. Although the interpretation of the motor nerve conduction velocity and CMAP shape is similar to that of sensory nerves, the interpretation of CMAP amplitude is markedly different. The SNAP amplitude of a sensory nerve depends primarily on the number of functioning large myelinated axons present. The CMAP amplitude, on the other hand, depends primarily on the number and density of innervated muscle fibers, not the number of axons innervating them. These two parameters do not always correlate highly with one another. Abnormal neuromuscular junction or muscle cell function, never a factor in sensory studies, also may produce abnormalities in the CMAP amplitude.

Information obtained from motor nerve conduction studies includes the motor nerve action potential conduction velocity along various segments of the motor axons and the amplitude and shape of the CMAP. Analysis of the CMAP amplitude and shape, distal latency, and motor nerve conduction velocity can provide specific information about the state of myelination of motor axons functioning in various segments of the nerve, the number of innervated and functioning muscle fibers, and the function of the neuromuscular junction.

Late Responses

Standard sensory and motor nerve conduction studies usually are performed on distal segments of the nerves, that is, those portions physically located in the extremities. It is difficult to evaluate nerve conduction velocity in extremely proximal segments of peripheral nerve (i.e., the proximal plexuses and roots) because of technical problems associated with selectively stimulating nerves and nerve roots close to the spine. When there is a need to examine these portions of the peripheral nerves, a class of nerve conduction studies known as late responses usually is used. These studies, so called because the response occurs much later after the stimulus than the direct muscle response, include the H reflex and the F_response (Fig. 15-2). For the time being, these nerve conduction studies can be categorized by the fact that they are the result of a distally initiated nerve action potential (i.e., sensory axon for H reflex, motor axon for F_response) that travels proximally, initiating a motor neuron action potential at the level of the spinal cord, which in turn is conducted distally and recorded through the muscle response. The major value of these studies is that they involve conduction over proximal portions of the nerve that are difficult to study with standard techniques. Conduction in proximal nerves also can be studied by the use of direct stimulation of the nerve root or proximal plexus using monopolar stimulation electrodes, although these techniques are somewhat more difficult and uncomfortable for the patient (11).

Repetitive Stimulation

Standard motor nerve conduction studies involve single stimuli delivered to the nerve at a relatively low frequency (i.e., once every several seconds). This does not functionally stress the neuromuscular junction unless severe abnormalities are present. On the other hand, repetitive stimulation of a motor nerve at higher frequencies (2 to 50 Hz) can unmask mild to moderate neuromuscular junction dysfunction. When disorders of the neuromuscular junction such as myasthenia gravis, Eaton–Lambert myasthenic syndrome (ELMS), and others are suspected, repetitive stimulation of motor nerves must be included in the evaluation. Repetitive stimulation also may be used to evaluate other disorders (e.g., myocyte disorders such as myotonic dystrophy) or disorders in which neuromuscular junction transmission may be secondarily abnormal (e.g., rapidly progressive motor neuron disease with extensive denervation and reinnervation).

Needle Electrode Examination

The needle examination is performed by inserting a small recording electrode into skeletal muscle and recording the electrical activity present at rest and during voluntary activation of the muscle. The recording surface of the electrode is small (150 to 600 μm in diameter, depending on electrode type), and as a result, a very small volume of muscle is examined. The action potentials and other electrical phenomena related to individual muscle fibers and motor units are identifiable during these recordings. Specifically, the needle electrode examination evaluates the following muscle characteristics:

1. Insertional activity: electrical activity present as the electrode is passed through muscle cells

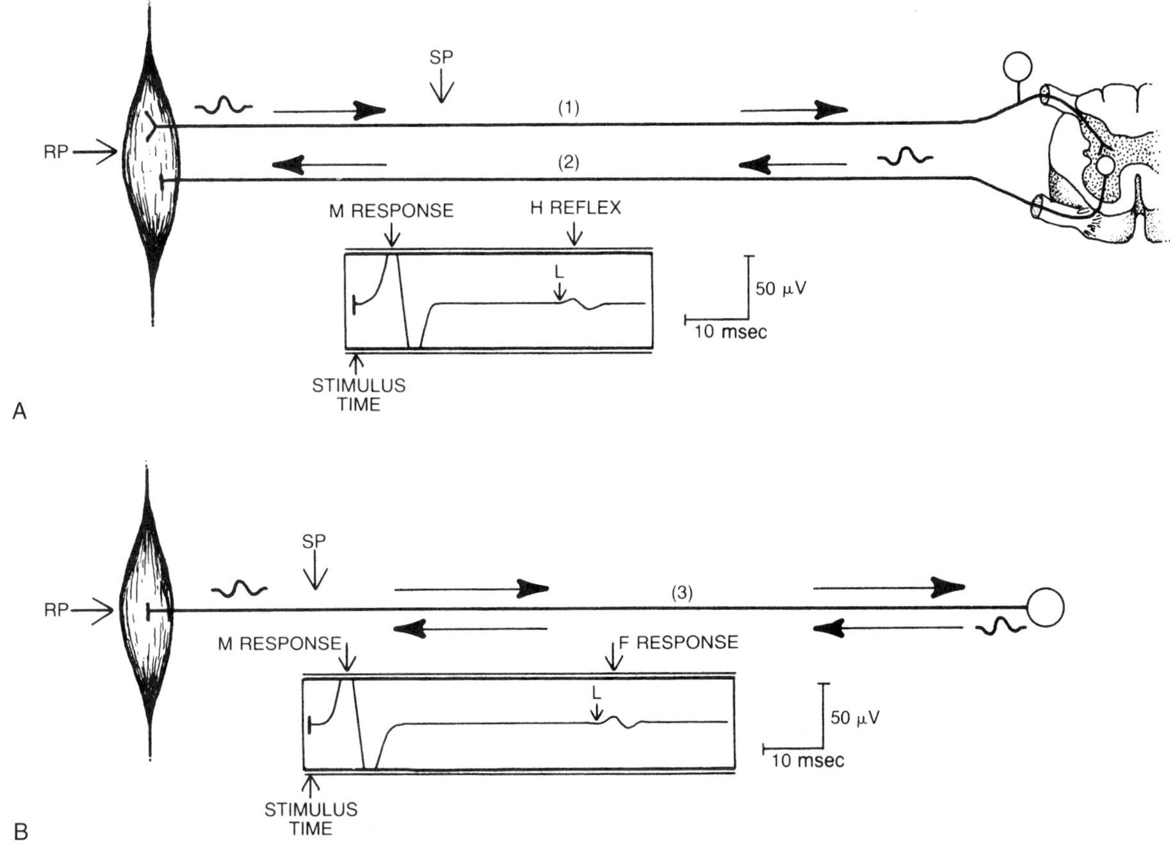

FIG. 15-2. Late responses. **A:** H reflex. A distal stimulus-initiated action potential travels orthodromically along in an Ia afferent sensory axon *(1)* involved in the monosynaptic stretch reflex. On reaching the synapse in the spinal cord, the afferent discharge results in firing of the associated motor neuron *(2)* and a subsequent evoked response in the muscle fibers innervated by that motor neuron. **B:** F_response. A distal stimulus-initiated action potential travels antidromically along the motor axon *(3)* to the motor neuron cell body, where a recurrent discharge is initiated in the same cell. This action potential travels orthodromically and results in an evoked response in the muscle fibers innervated by that motor neuron. *L,* latency; *RP*, recording point; *SP*, stimulus point.

2. Spontaneous activity: electrical activity present when the muscle is at rest and the electrode is not being moved
3. Motor unit action potential (MUAP) shape and amplitude
4. Motor unit recruitment patterns

The needle electrode examination of these items provides close-range evaluation of the electrical characteristics of individual muscle fibers and motor units and can provide information on the state of innervation and integrity of individual muscle fibers and the anatomic organization of motor units (e.g., the number and density of muscle fibers in a motor unit). Analysis of motor unit recruitment patterns provides information on the number and functional status of the anterior horn cells innervating a muscle.

Most of the information provided by the needle electrode examination is complementary to that provided by motor nerve conduction studies. Compound muscle action potential amplitudes obtained during motor nerve conduction studies are a function of the number and functional status of innervated muscle fibers present. As such, the CMAP amplitude is a gross property of the muscle and is insensitive to processes that affect only a small percentage of the total muscle fibers; for example, a process that denervates 5% of the muscle fibers probably will not produce a detectable change in the CMAP even though abnormalities may be present on needle electrode examination. In addition, CMAP amplitude measurements do not provide any information on how the muscle fibers are innervated, only that they are innervated. All other factors being equal, a muscle with 100 normal motor units might have essentially the same CMAP amplitude as a muscle that has lost 80% of its motor neurons and now has 20 markedly abnormal motor units possessing five times the normal number of muscle fibers. Finally, needle electrode examination may identify abnormal electrical events that for one reason or another may not be detected during routine motor nerve conduction studies.

Single-Fiber Electromyography

Certain electrodiagnostic techniques, although not in widespread use, may be of substantial value is some situations. One of the most important of these techniques is that of single-fiber electromyography (SFEMG), a technique for evaluating the performance of the neuromuscular junction. Single-fiber electromyography is much more sensitive than motor nerve repetitive stimulation in detecting the abnormalities that occur in primary disorders of the neuromuscular junction (e.g., myasthenia gravis, ELMS). In situations in which a primary disorder of the neuromuscular junction is suspected, and repetitive stimulation studies are normal, SFEMG will confirm the diagnosis in many cases (12–17).

Neuromuscular junction transmission also may be abnormal where immature neuromuscular junctions are present as a result of ongoing denervation and reinnervation (e.g., in motor neuron disease [MND]). Single-fiber electromyography may provide diagnostically and prognostically useful information in these settings by documenting abnormal neuromuscular junction function consistent with denervation and reinnervation when routine studies are equivocal. Single-fiber electromyography also may be used to estimate motor unit muscle fiber density, another measurement that may be abnormal in myopathies and neuropathies when the results of routine electrodiagnosis are equivocal (13,17). The major drawbacks to the routine use of SFEMG are the time required as well as the need for special equipment and expertise.

Computer-Based Quantitative EMG Techniques

The meaning of the term *quantitative EMG* has changed somewhat in the last few years. Classically, this referred primarily to MUAP analysis using triggered averaging techniques to analyze the first one or two motor units recruited (18). This provides more accurate data regarding MUAP amplitude, duration, and polyphasia than is possible with visual observation of a single occurrence of a MUAP. The major drawback to this form of quantitative EMG is that it is a time-consuming manual technique and is applicable to only the first one or two motor units recruited. In the last several years, however, some advanced EMG machines have provided the capability to perform what has also been labeled as "quantitative EMG." These techniques are computer-based algorithms that allow the electromyographer to analyze certain aspects of the MUAP and of voluntary motor recruitment in a manner that is not possible with purely visual/auditory analysis of the EMG signal or with simple triggered averaging. These include the *turns analysis* technique of Willison, semiautomatic analysis of single MUAPs, and complex template decomposition techniques for analyzing both the MUAP (19) and recruitment characteristics of as many as the first eight motor units recruited. These techniques do not convert an inexperienced electromyographer into an expert but should be considered as an adjunct tool for the experienced electromyographer. With selected patients, computer-based quantitative EMG can be of value in combination with standard electromyographic techniques. Quantitative EMG is still time-consuming and can be viewed somewhat like single-fiber electromyography in that it is generally applied only after the standard electromyographic examination has been performed and the standard techniques have not completely resolved the situation. From a practical standpoint, the techniques are primarily a research tool but should have periodic applications in routine clinical practice. Computer-based quantitative EMG will probably come into increased general use as EMG machines capable of performing these techniques become faster and more widely available, and additional research refines the techniques.

The electrodiagnostic tests described above form the basis for almost all routinely performed electrodiagnostic studies. The reader should understand this section well before proceeding to more advanced sections of this chapter.

NERVE CONDUCTION STUDIES

Basic Techniques and Terminology

Sensory and motor nerve conduction studies involve the analysis of the properties listed below. Discussion of these properties will be organized on the basis of whether the principles underlying that respective property of motor and sensory nerve conduction studies are similar or different. Dumitru provides an excellent discussion of volume conduction in electrodiagnostic phenomena (20).

- *Conduction velocity:* determined primarily by axonal diameter and the state of axonal myelination; the factors underlying normal and abnormal nerve conduction velocities are essentially identical for both motor and sensory nerves and are discussed together.
- *Distal latency* (see Fig. 15-1): an index of conduction velocity in the most distal portion of the nerve.
- *Temporal dispersion* (Fig. 15-3*A*): similar for both motor and sensory nerve conduction studies.
- *Conduction block* (Fig. 15-3*B*): similar for both motor and sensory nerve conduction studies
- *Evoked response amplitude:* physiological factors underlying SNAP and CMAP evoked response amplitudes differ significantly and will be discussed separately for motor and sensory nerve conduction studies.

Nerve Conduction Velocities

Interpreting nerve conduction velocity studies requires knowledge of several facts about axonal action potential propagation. This discussion is restricted to myelinated axons because these are the axons that determine the conduction velocity of motor and sensory nerves. The same physiological principles determine motor and sensory nerve conduction velocities, since it is the conduction velocity of the nerve axon that determines this property in both cases. These properties may be listed as follows:

1. Axonal action potential conduction velocity is related to axonal diameter in roughly a linear fashion, although

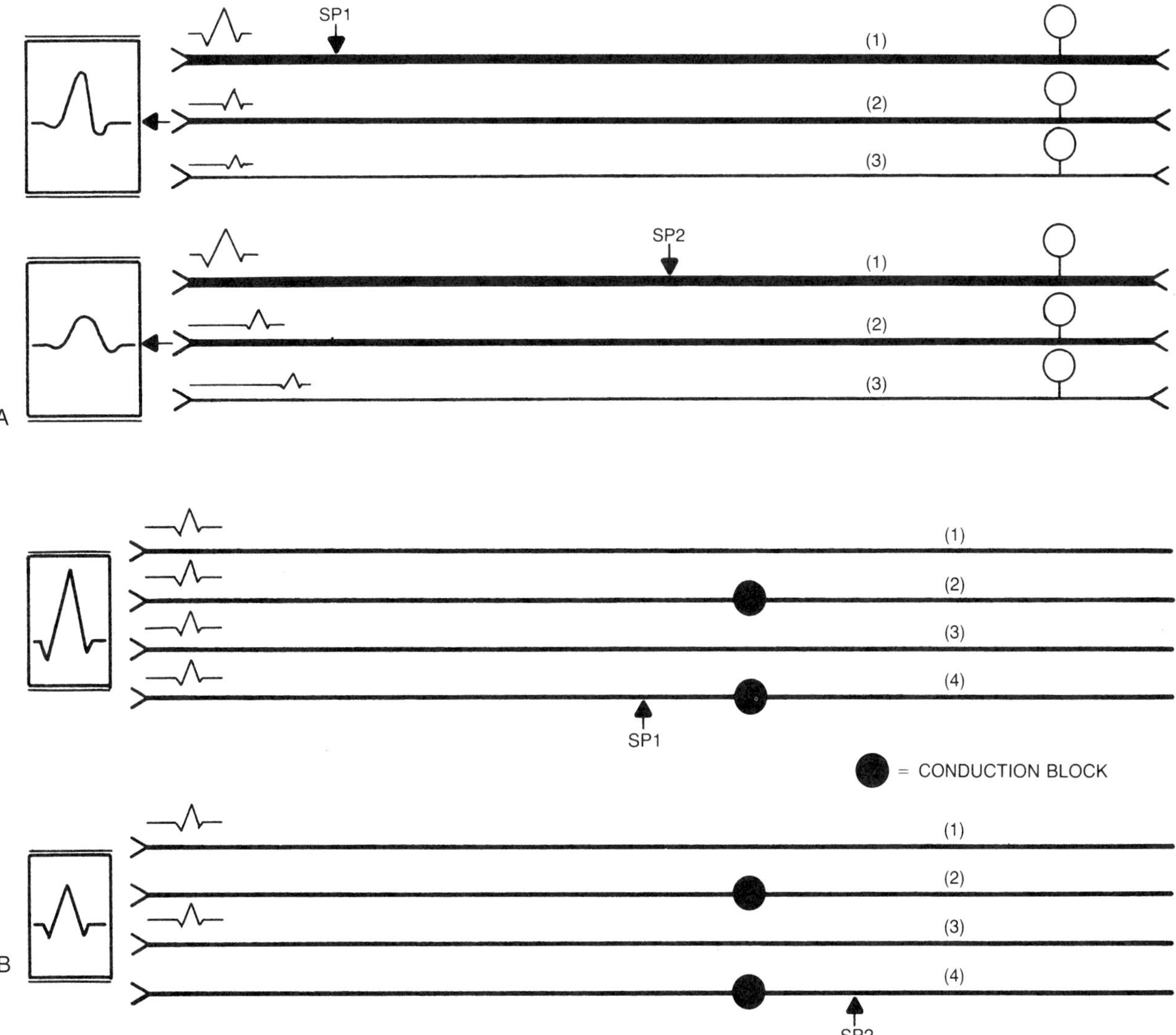

FIG. 15-3. Temporal dispersion and conduction block. **A:** Temporal dispersion. Three myelinated sensory axons with fast *(1)*, medium *(2)*, and slow *(3)* action potential conduction velocities are shown, representing populations of axons with these characteristics. These fast-, medium-, and slow-conducting action potential populations form the leading edge, midportion, and trailing edge of the evoked response. When action potentials are initiated simultaneously in all three axons close to the recording electrode, the time difference between arrival of the fast- and slow-conducting action potentials is minimal, and the evoked response has a relatively short duration and high amplitude. When action potentials are initiated simultaneously in all three axons far from the recording electrode, the time difference between arrival of the fast- and slow-conducting action potentials is exaggerated, and the evoked response has a longer duration and lower amplitude. Temporal dispersion in motor nerves is similar to that in sensory nerves. **B:** Conduction block. Conduction block is the result of any process (e.g., focal demyelination) that prevents an action potential from propagating past a given point while relatively normal distal axonal function permits the distal axon to conduct relatively normally. This excludes the situation occurring immediately following axonal transection, where the distal axon may conduct an action potential for several days before degeneration occurs. Axons 2 and 4 have conduction block at the point indicated. When the nerve is stimulated between the point of conduction block and the recording electrode (SP_1), all axons conduct, and the evoked response amplitude is maximal. If the stimulus is moved proximally on the nerve such that the point of conduction block lies between the stimulus and the recording electrodes (SP_2), the contributions of axons with conduction block will be eliminated, and the resultant evoked response will have a diminished amplitude relative to the evoked response obtained with distal stimulation.

this relationship is complex when comparing a wide range of axonal diameters (21,22).

2. Nerve conduction studies are performed in a manner such that the fastest conducting axons determine the conduction velocity (see Fig. 15-1*A*). There are no easily performed clinical techniques for measuring conduction velocities in slower-conducting axons, although there are some research techniques for this (23).
3. Evaluation of certain autonomic nervous system functions such as the sudomotor responses provides an indirect means of evaluating what is primarily type-C unmyelinated fiber based function (24,25).
4. Conduction velocities may be abnormally low as a result of processes that:
   - Directly affect the conduction velocities of large myelinated fibers (e.g., demyelination). Demyelinating processes may result in conduction velocities ranging from low normal (40 to 50 m/sec) to as low as 5 to 10 m/sec, depending on the severity and nature of the underlying process.
   - Result in a loss of the majority of large myelinated fibers, leaving the smaller, slower-conducting axons to determine the conduction velocity. Loss of faster conducting axons does not result in markedly decreased conduction velocities because conduction velocities usually cannot be determined reliably with routine techniques for technical reasons when all medium and large myelinated fibers are lost. The loss of faster-conducting axons can explain decreases in conduction velocity down to approximately 80% of the lower limit of normal (LLN: 40 to 50 m/sec, depending on the nerve). The relationship of evoked response amplitude to conduction velocity with the loss of large myelinated axons is important and will be discussed subsequently.
   - Interfere with the function of axonal potassium and sodium channels, resulting in reduced conduction velocities in the absence of demyelination or loss of large myelinated axons. Decreases in conduction velocities can be relatively marked. This phenomenon is a recently recognized source of peripheral nerve dysfunction but demonstrates that decreased conduction velocities should no longer be reflexely attributed to demyelination or loss of large myelinated axons. These conditions have been designated as axonal channelopathies resulting from the blockade of sodium and potassium channels by toxins, antibodies, and probable metabolic factors as well (26).
5. The conduction velocity of peripheral nerve tends to decrease in a proximodistal manner (27). This phenomenon is small and not of major importance until the last few centimeters of terminal nerve are reached. The nerve conduction velocity of the terminal nerve branches decreases, probably to as low as 5 to 10 m/sec, owing in part to marked decreases in the diameter of terminal axons. Because nerve conduction velocities along a nerve are heterogeneous, average nerve conduction velocities over specific segments of the nerve are calculated, rather than determining the exact conduction velocity at specific points. For nerve segments proximal to the last 5 to 10 cm of a nerve, the average conduction velocity (i.e., distance traveled divided by time required) is a reasonably accurate estimate of the range of conduction velocities present (see Fig. 15-1). This is not true for the distal few centimeters of a nerve, in which the conduction velocity drops progressively and rapidly as the action potential propagates more distally. Normal conduction velocity behavior of distal nerve is therefore best characterized by determining the time required for an action potential to travel a standardized distance. This is termed a distal latency, with values ranging from 2.5 to 6.5 msec. These data usually are not converted into a conduction velocity because they have less meaning in this form. In the case of motor nerves, the time delay at the neuromuscular junction also is included in the distal latency, introducing a small, but additional error if an action potential conduction velocity is calculated by dividing distance traveled by time required.
6. The conduction velocity of nerve decreases significantly with decreased temperature, and distal latencies become correspondingly prolonged. Most laboratories use a surface temperature of 32°C as standard for determining normal values. Because nerve temperature in the deep tissues of normal limbs is relatively well maintained, conduction velocities in proximal nerve usually are affected only when ambient temperatures are extremely low or when limbs are markedly atrophic. Distal limb temperatures (e.g., finger temperature) are markedly affected by low environmental temperatures and patients must frequently be warmed to 32°C before accurate studies can be performed (28). In addition, more superficial nerves are affected more than deeper nerves—median sensory distal latencies may increase more than ulnar sensory distal latencies with low hand/wrist temperatures. This may create errors when comparing the distal latencies as a means of diagnosing disorders such as the carpal tunnel syndrome. As an approximation, conduction velocities drop by 1.5 to 2.5 m/sec/°C and distal latencies become prolonged by 0.1 to 0.3 m/sec/°C. Nerve evoked response amplitudes tend to increase with decreased temperature, primarily owing to decreased temporal dispersion (29–32).
7. Conduction velocities in newborns are approximately one-half of those in mature adults and are even lower in premature infants. Conduction velocities reach approximately 80% of adult values at 1 year of age and reach adult values at 3 to 5 years of age (32,33).
8. Conduction velocities tend to decrease slightly after 30 to 40 years of age, with the maximum decrement being approximately 10 m/sec at 60 to 80 years of age (29,34).
9. Metabolic abnormalities of the axon have been postulated to be capable of reducing conduction velocities in

the absence of demyelination or loss of large myelinated axons (35). As noted earlier, there are now clear cut examples of this in the form of axonal channelopathies resulting from the blockade of sodium and potassium channels by toxins, antibodies, and probable metabolic factors (26). This must now be included in the differential diagnosis of decreased conduction velocities, and the rigorous determination of demyelination will need to rely on combined electrophysiological and histopathologic criteria, not electrophysiological criteria alone.

10. Nerve conduction velocities are estimated either by calculating an average conduction velocity over a specific nerve segment or by determining the time (i.e., latency) required for the nerve action potential to travel a specified distance. Decreased nerve conduction velocities or increased latencies may indicate demyelination, loss of large, rapidly conducting myelinated axons, an axonal channelopathy, or substandard nerve temperatures.

There are no known pathologic conditions in which conduction velocities are increased. When this appears to occur, it generally is due to technical error or an anatomic anomaly.

Temporal Dispersion

All peripheral nerves contain myelinated axons with heterogeneous sizes and conduction velocities. When a nerve is stimulated supramaximally, an axonal action potential is simultaneously initiated in each axon. If the recording electrode is near the point of stimulation, action potentials from rapidly and slowly conducting axons arrive at the electrode nearly simultaneously and the recorded nerve action potential has a relatively high amplitude and short duration. If the recording electrode is moved farther from the point of stimulation, the time difference between arrival of the action potentials from the faster-conducting axons and the action potentials from slowly conducting axons increases (see Fig. 15-3*A*). The nerve action potential recorded at the longer distance therefore will have a relatively lower amplitude and longer duration than the nerve action potential recorded closer to the stimulus. This phenomenon is referred to as temporal dispersion.

When temporal dispersion is present, phase cancellation secondary to asynchronous arrival of potentials at the recording site also contributes to the decreased evoked response amplitude (36). Phase cancellation is minimal when there is no significant temporal dispersion. In the absence of significant temporal dispersion, action potentials from individual axons, in the case of the SNAP, or muscle fibers in the case of the CMAP, arrive at the recording electrode nearly simultaneously. In this case, positive and negative current flows from individual contributors reinforce each other, and the recorded amplitude is maximal. Phase cancellation results when the asynchronous arrival of the action potentials results in the positive current flow of one generator opposing the negative current flow of others, lowering the net current flow and resultant evoked response amplitude. Phase cancellation due to temporal dispersion is much more prominent with short-duration potentials such as sensory evoked responses as opposed to longer-duration potentials such as motor evoked responses.

Temporal dispersion in both sensory and motor nerves is the result of heterogeneity of axonal conduction velocities. Some temporal dispersion is normal, but it is markedly increased in disease processes causing multifocal demyelination (e.g., Guillain-Barré syndrome). Under these circumstances, axons are demyelinated in an uneven manner, with some axons relatively spared and some heavily involved, resulting in a wide range of conduction velocities. Processes that cause diffuse demyelination (e.g., Charcot-Marie-Tooth disease) affect most axons to approximately the same extent, causing much smaller increases in temporal dispersion than multifocal processes, even though the conduction velocity may be comparably decreased. As a generalization, short-duration, acquired processes such as Guillain-Barré syndrome produce multifocal demyelination, whereas chronic or inherited disorders such as Charcot-Marie-Tooth disease result in diffuse demyelination (37–39). This leads to the generalization that marked temporal dispersion of sensory or motor evoked responses suggests an acquired, relatively short-duration, multifocal process, although Dejerine-Sottas disease (i.e., hereditary sensorimotor neuropathy, HSMN, type III) appears to be an exception to this rule (40) The extremely low nerve conduction velocities (e.g., 4 to 6 m/sec) seen with Dejerine-Sottas disease, however, are less common with other disorders and strongly suggest this diagnosis.

Conduction Block

As a result of saltatory conduction along the nodes of Ranvier, myelinated nerve has a relative high conduction velocity (40 to 80 m/sec) as compared with unmyelinated nerve (1 to 5 m/sec). Damage to Schwann cells and secondary demyelination therefore can cause a significant reduction in the conduction velocity in the affected nerve. If Schwann cell/axonal damage is severe enough, action potentials in individual axons may not propagate past the damaged region, a condition known as conduction block (see Fig. 15-3*B*) (41). Action potential conduction distal to the conduction block frequently is normal, especially when the block is caused by focal damage (e.g., an ulnar pressure neuropathy at the elbow). The presence of conduction block is suggested when the amplitude of a motor or sensory evoked response drops abnormally when the stimulus site is moved more proximally on the nerve, that is, when the test is performed in a manner that requires axonal conduction across the damaged region.

The amplitude of a sensory or motor evoked response may be affected by either temporal dispersion or by conduction block. It would be of value to be able to distinguish absolutely between the two phenomena, and many attempts to do this have been made. Perhaps the most common approach to this problem has been to make use of the fact that the area of an evoked response (i.e., integration of the area under the curve) is affected much less by temporal dispersion than is the amplitude or duration. This has led to the generalization that temporal dispersion does not decrease the area of an evoked response, whereas conduction block does, and the two phenomena can be distinguished in this manner. This is only partially true because phase cancellation secondary to asynchronous arrival of potentials at the recording site also contributes to decreased evoked response amplitudes and areas as well (36,42). Low degrees of conduction block therefore are difficult to identify in the presence of abnormal temporal dispersion. Conduction block is best identified when the ratio of the proximal evoked response amplitudes to the distal evoked response amplitudes in forearm or leg segments drops significantly (<0.7 to 0.8) without significant changes in the ratio of proximal to distal evoked response durations (<1.2) (41,43–48). Additional techniques for detecting focal conduction block include short-segment stimulation in which the stimulating electrode is moved proximally by small increments (e.g., 10 to 15 mm at a time). Any significant drop in amplitude (>10% to 15%) between stimulation sites usually represents conduction block because temporal dispersion is unlikely to be a major factor over a distance this short. Finally, in cases where marked weakness is present and the recruitment pattern is markedly reduced, only a few motor units may be identifiable with voluntary recruitment. Under these circumstances, an individual motor unit may be identified with a needle electrode by submaximal distal stimulation (e.g., at the wrist). Conduction block is assumed when a single motor unit identified in this fashion cannot be activated by maximal volitional activation (45). This technique is difficult, applicable to only a few patients, and not easily applied in routine clinical practice. Cornblath and colleagues have provided a critical analysis of the pitfalls in identifying conduction block by the above techniques (36). In most cases, the absolute distinction between conduction block and temporal dispersion with associated phase cancellation is not of major importance because they are both signs of demyelination and usually carry the same diagnostic or therapeutic significance.

In some situations, conduction block may be reasonably inferred in the presence of decreased motor unit recruitment. A specific case of this phenomenon is discussed in the section on the electrodiagnostic findings associated with multifocal motor neuropathy.

In the presence of conduction block, nerve conduction velocities tend to be underestimated because larger, faster-conducting axons usually are more susceptible. The distal latency obtained by stimulation distal to the block is determined by the faster-conducting axons, whereas the proximal latency obtained by stimulation proximal to the block is determined by slower-conducting fibers. The calculated conduction velocity is then somewhat lower than the true conduction velocity of the slower-conducting axons.

Conduction block may be seen with focal neuropathy (e.g., carpal tunnel syndrome), diffuse disorders (e.g., Guillain-Barré syndrome), or with mononeuropathy multiplex (i.e., multifocal lesions). Other causes of altered proximal-to-distal evoked response amplitude ratios such as anomalous innervation must be excluded. Although the median, ulnar, and peroneal nerves generally follow the criteria for conduction block discussed above, it should be noted that the tibial nerve recorded from the abductor hallicus is not a good nerve to analyze for conduction block because it has a complex motor point arrangement (49), is subject to phase cancellation, and the proximal/distal amplitude ratio is frequently low by the above criteria in the absence of pathology.

Conduction block, when unequivocally present, documents either focal or multifocal demyelination of the nerve in question. Conduction block may be the predominant abnormality in some demyelinating conditions.

Temporal Course of Nerve Conduction Velocity Abnormalities

Demyelinating neurologic lesions and all other types should be analyzed with respect to their stage:

- *Acute:* days to weeks in duration
- *Subacute:* weeks to months in duration
- *Chronic:* months to years in duration, active
- *Old:* months to years since onset, inactive

Several situations may exist in demyelinating processes, depending on the stage and type of disease process. If a demyelinating process is diffuse (e.g., all axons are involved to a similar extent), then the predominant finding will be that of slowed conduction velocity with relatively minimal to moderate temporal dispersion of the evoked response. This diffuse involvement tends to indicate a chronic or old process. On the other hand, a multifocal demyelinating process, which can occur in early Guillain-Barré syndrome, may leave some axons in the nerve relatively uninvolved while others are severely involved. This may result in several different electrodiagnostic pictures with time. If all axons are involved but still conducting action potentials, conduction velocities generally will be reduced with significant temporal dispersion of the evoked response. If a significant number of the large, myelinated fibers are minimally affected, however, the conduction velocity may be normal or near normal, with the dominant abnormality being temporal dispersion or conduction block. Nerve conduction studies may be essentially normal in the presence of significant clinical sensory or motor dysfunction if the majority of conduction block is occurring proximally at the root level. If most of the large myelinated fibers are heavily involved, conduction velocities will be markedly reduced. When evaluating an evolving process, the examiner should be prepared to find any of the above patterns.

Decreased conduction velocities do not necessarily correlate with clinical motor function because nonfunctioning axons have no effect on measured whole nerve conduction velocity, and axonal conduction velocity *per se* has no effect on the force of muscle contraction. Even if conduction velocities are markedly reduced, significant motor dysfunction may not be present if all axons in a nerve are conducting. Sensory function (e.g., vibration or light touch sense) may be abnormal under the same circumstances. Conversely, a patient may present with severe weakness and sensory dysfunction secondary to conduction block in a high percentage of axons. The remaining axons may be minimally demyelinated, resulting in only moderately decreased conduction velocities. As time goes on, the relatively unaffected axons may become more involved while conduction block in severely involved axons begins to resolve. Whole-nerve conduction velocities therefore actually may decrease while the patient's clinical function is improving as a result of resolution of conduction block in axons that initially were nonconducting. Motor nerve evoked response amplitudes may be normal in the presence of severe weakness, with or without slowing of conduction velocity, if the dominant abnormality is conduction block in proximal locations.

Sensory Nerve Conduction Studies

Physiological Factors Determining Sensory Nerve Action Potential Amplitude and Conduction Velocity

The SNAP measured in routine electrodiagnostic studies is a complex function of the sum of the longitudinal currents produced by action potentials of individual sensory nerve axons within the nerve and normally ranges from 2 to 100 μV, depending on the nerve (50). The nerve axon evoked response can be modeled as shown in Figure 15-4. The amplitude of the recorded action potential is proportional to the total current that the underlying nerve action potential longitudinal currents can drive through the tissues separating the recording electrodes. This current is a complex function of the nerve axon diameter, the metabolic condition of these cells, cell density (cells/mm^2), phase cancellation, and the electrical properties of surrounding tissue. In most cases, abnormally low SNAPs result from a loss of functioning axons and subsequent decrease in functioning axonal density or from temporal dispersion and phase cancellation. Abnormal metabolic states, e.g., channelopathies, can diminish the

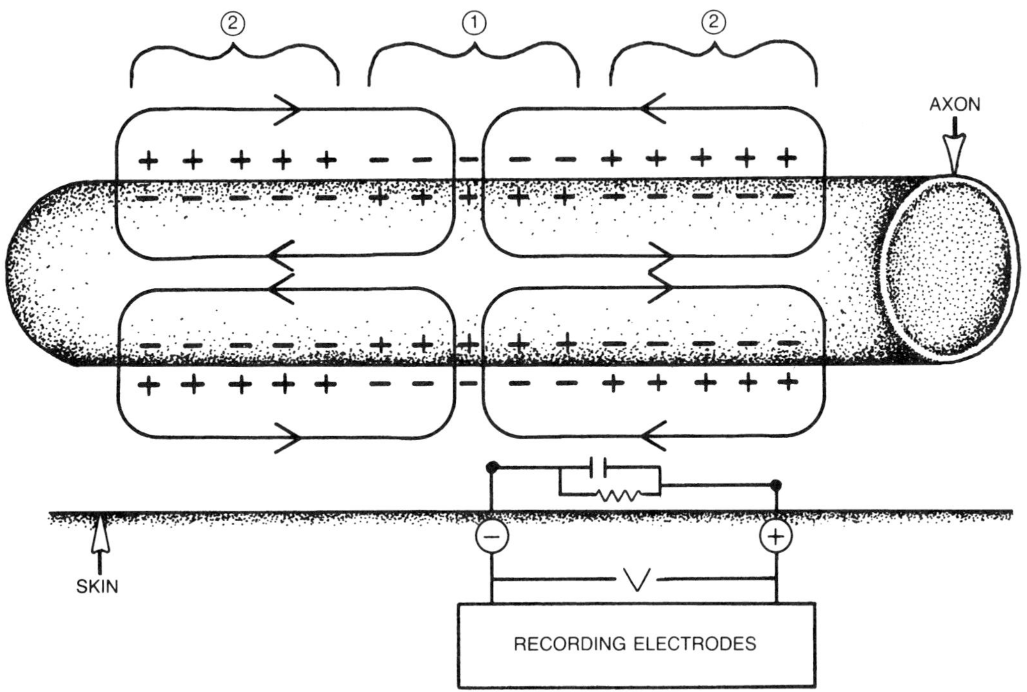

FIG. 15-4. Longitudinal current. The extracellular surface region of an axon that is conducting an action potential *(1)* is electrically negative with respect to other portions of the surface of the axon *(2)*. Likewise, the active intracellular interior of the axon is positive relative to areas of the axon cytoplasm that are not conducting an action potential. The net effect of this situation is that a positive (i.e., conventional) longitudinal current loop is set up on both sides of the active region of the axon in which intracellular current flows away from the active region and extracellular current flow is toward the active region. Conventional electrodiagnostic studies detect the voltage *(V)* produced by this extracellular current loop roughly according to Ohm's law, $V = IZ$, where I is the current/cm^2 conducted through and Z is the impedance (resistance − 1/capacitance) of the tissue separating the recording electrodes. All other factors being equal, the total current, and therefore amplitude of the recorded evoked response, is proportional to the density of axons or muscle cells within the pickup radius of the recording electrodes. The compound motor evoked response can be analyzed in an analogous fashion.

currents produced by the axons and result in decreased SNAP amplitudes, despite normal fiber density. A detailed discussion of the relationship between the action potential and axonal population of the sensory nerve is presented by Lambert and Dyck (21).

At this point, a review of several properties of nerve axons is in order:

1. Axonal conduction velocity is roughly linearly related to axonal diameter.
2. The longitudinal current and the amplitude of the axonal action potential is approximately proportional to the square of the fiber diameter.
3. The evoked response amplitude recorded from a whole nerve is proportional to the density and type of axons present, all other factors being equal.

A myelinated axon with a diameter of 10 μm would therefore have an action potential approximately four times larger and would conduct at a velocity roughly two times faster than a myelinated fiber with a diameter of 5 μm. In normal sensory nerve, there are approximately three times as many unmyelinated as myelinated axons present, with unmyelinated axons ranging from 0.3 to 1.5 μm in diameter. Approximately 30% of the myelinated axons have diameters greater than 8 μm, with a range of 2 to 22 μm. From these data, it can therefore be concluded that both the SNAP amplitude and the conduction velocity are determined primarily by the large-diameter myelinated axons, and that small-diameter myelinated and unmyelinated nerve fibers make a minimal contribution to the SNAP amplitude and temporal dispersion and essentially no contribution to SNAP conduction velocity. A process such as amyloidosis that involves primarily small unmyelinated fibers could completely eliminate the action potentials of these fibers without producing abnormal results in conventional sensory nerve conduction studies.

Temporal Course of Sensory Nerve Conduction Abnormalities

The specific electrodiagnostic findings in a disease may depend highly on the stage of the disease process. Major interpretive errors can be made if this is not taken into account. For this reason, the sensory nerve conduction changes that occur at different times after axonal transection are reviewed. The stages of demyelinating lesions have been reviewed previously.

After a sensory axon has been transected, the segment of nerve distal to the transection point will initially conduct in a normal fashion, with normal conduction velocity and evoked response amplitude. Individual axons within the nerve will cease to conduct action potentials over the next 5 to 10 days, resulting in a progressive loss in SNAP amplitude over time as fewer and fewer axons are functioning. The SNAP amplitude would diminish after 2 to 4 days, and no SNAP would be present after 7 to 11 days (51).

The presence of a SNAP generally is taken to indicate that at least some sensory axons are intact and functioning in a given nerve. If the time interval between axonal injury and subsequent testing is less than 7 to 11 days, a detectable SNAP with distal stimulation does not prove axonal continuity; that is, no clear-cut distinction between conduction block and axonal transection can be made in the first few days after injury.

Normal and Abnormal Sensory Nerve Conduction Studies

Conventional sensory nerve conduction studies provide an evoked response amplitude proportional to diameter, number, density, and metabolic state of functioning axons; a distal latency, which is a function of average distal nerve conduction velocity; segmental conduction velocities, which are a function of axonal diameter and state of myelination/ion channel function; and SNAP conformation, which is a function of temporal dispersion and conduction block. Abnormalities may occur in any one of these measurements, either in isolation or combination.

Prolonged Distal Latency

Prolonged distal latency may occur with the following five conditions (35,41):

1. Low distal limb temperatures
2. Generalized or focal/multifocal processes resulting in demyelination in the distal segment of the nerve
3. Generalized or focal/multifocal processes causing a loss of large, myelinated fibers
4. Processes causing a severe reduction in axonal diameters.
5. Channelopathies or other metabolic dysfunction of the axon.

Examples of generalized, multifocal processes would include Guillain-Barré syndrome and other polyneuropathies, whereas focal processes would include the carpal tunnel syndrome. When a loss of large, myelinated fibers or severe axonal stenosis is the underlying basis for a prolonged distal latency, a decreased evoked response amplitude is seen as well. Because it is the large, myelinated, rapidly conducting fibers that also produce most of the evoked response amplitude, loss of these axons must necessarily result in a low SNAP amplitude in conjunction with the prolonged distal latency. Axonal stenosis, frequently seen in distal polyneuropathies, produces decreased SNAP amplitudes directly and is frequently associated with loss of axons, further decreasing the SNAP amplitude (35). Distal axonal stenosis may be the earliest manifestation of a generalized process.

Decreased Conduction Velocity

Decreased conduction velocity may be seen with the following:

- Diffuse demyelination
- Loss of large, myelinated fibers
- Focal or multifocal demyelination
- Marked axonal stenosis
- Channelopathies or other metabolic dysfunction of the axon.

From an etiologic standpoint, it is important to determine how much conduction velocity decreases and whether it is associated with temporal dispersion or conduction block. Conduction velocities may be mildly decreased secondary to loss of the faster-conducting axons without any significant demyelination occurring. It generally is held that this can be responsible for conduction velocities down to, but not lower than, approximately 80% of the lower limit of normal (35). This explanation for decreased conduction velocities is valid only when the SNAP amplitude is markedly diminished as well (10% to 30% of the lower limit of normal). As discussed previously, it is the large, myelinated, rapidly conducting fibers that also produce most of the evoked response amplitude (35). If the majority of these axons are lost, both the SNAP amplitude and conduction velocity must necessarily decrease. If the SNAP amplitude is not markedly reduced, and temperature is not a factor, conduction velocities less than the lower limit of normal are most consistent with minimal demyelination or other axonal dysfunction. The interpretation of reduced conduction velocities therefore depends on the associated SNAP amplitude. When the SNAP is not markedly reduced, mild demyelination and other axonal dysfunction can produce conduction velocities ranging from 80% to 100% of the lower limit of normal (35).This type of demyelination is present in many conditions and is relatively nonspecific (41). Markedly decreased conduction velocities (e.g., 20% to 80% of the lower limit of normal) are seen in conditions in which demyelination is the predominant feature of the disease and suggest a relatively small group of disorders: Guillain-Barré syndrome (52), Charcot-Marie-Tooth disease (HSMN type I), Dejerine-Sottas disease (40) (HSMN type III), chronic inflammatory demyelinating polyneuropathy (CIDP), diphtheria, metachromatic leukodystrophy, and some dysimmune neuropathies such as those associated with paraproteinemias (53), lymphomas, systemic lupus erythematosus, and Castleman's disease.

For technical reasons, it frequently is impossible to determine sensory nerve conduction velocities when the above abnormalities are present, forcing the electrodiagnostician to rely on analysis of motor nerve conduction studies to evaluate the presence or absence of demyelination. Motor nerves demonstrate essentially the same relationships between CMAP amplitude, loss of large IA myelinated axons, and axonal conduction velocity as do sensory nerves, although for slightly different underlying reasons.

Decreased Sensory Nerve Action Potential Amplitude

Decreased SNAP amplitude may be seen with:

- Temporal dispersion
- Conduction block
- Severe axonal stenosis
- Significant loss of large, myelinated axons

or be caused by technical factors such as poor electrode placement, significant swelling of soft tissue surrounding the nerve, or submaximal stimulation.

When the decreased evoked response amplitude is secondary to severe axonal stenosis, loss of large myelinated axons, or temporal dispersion without conduction block, the distal latency will probably be prolonged as well. Increased distal latencies also may be associated with conduction block because processes causing conduction block also may cause loss of large myelinated axons and focal demyelination, as in the carpal tunnel syndrome.

Increased Temporal Dispersion

Increased temporal dispersion is noted primarily in multifocal disorders in which some axons within a nerve may have only minimal demyelination and demonstrate only mild decreases in conduction velocity, whereas other axons are more significantly involved and conduction velocities are much slower. This is a feature of certain phases of acquired disorders such as acute inflammatory demyelinating polyneuropathy (acute inflammatory demyelinating polyneuropathies [AIDP]; Guillain-Barré syndrome), early CIDP, and other polyneuropathies (52). Long-standing disorders, such as Charcot-Marie-Tooth disease (HSMN type I) or long-standing CIDP, will generally involve all axons within a nerve to a similar degree, producing marked slowing of the nerve conduction velocity but much less temporal dispersion (37–39).

Motor Nerve Conduction Studies

The underlying determinants of motor nerve conduction studies are very similar to those for sensory nerve conduction studies, with the important difference that it is the CMAP that is being measured after motor nerve stimulation, not the nerve action potential. The neuromuscular junction also is involved in producing the evoked response, thereby making motor nerve conduction studies a simultaneous test of nerve, neuromuscular junction, and muscle cell function. One can apply all the logic developed for sensory nerve conduction studies when analyzing conduction velocity, distal latency, temporal dispersion, and conduction block, but different principles must be used to analyze CMAP amplitude. Normal CMAP amplitudes for commonly studied muscles range from 2 to 25 mV depending on the muscle. Miller provides an excellent discussion of the events following injury of peripheral motor nerves (54).

Physical Factors Affecting Compound Muscle Action Potential Amplitude

One difference between sensory and motor nerve conduction studies is related to the physical size of the electrically active tissues. Because of the relatively small size of nerves, surface electrodes used in standard sensory conduction studies record action potentials from essentially all axons in the nerve. This is not always the case with CMAPs because many muscle fibers may be too far from the recording electrode for their longitudinal currents and resultant action potentials to be significant (see Fig. 15-4). In the case of small muscles, such as those of the hands and feet that are used in most routine nerve conduction studies, the electrical activity of most of the muscle fibers in the muscle will be recorded by the electrode. For a large muscle such as the quadriceps, most of the muscle fibers in the muscle are too far from the recording electrode to make a significant contribution to the recorded potential, and the recording electrode therefore measures only action potentials from a small fraction of the total number of muscle fibers. The resultant CMAP therefore is proportional to the longitudinal current produced by the muscle fibers within the pickup range of the electrode, not the total number of fibers in the muscle. All other factors being identical, this longitudinal current is primarily a function of the muscle fiber density (fibers/cm^2). The CMAP amplitude changes observed with pathologic processes that affect the number of innervated muscle fibers (e.g., denervation or segmental necrosis of muscle fibers) will therefore be minimal unless the density of innervated muscle fibers within the recording range of the electrode is altered (21).

Motor Neuron Numbers and Compound Muscle Action Potential Amplitude

The amplitude of the potential is a function of the number and density of innervated muscle fibers, not the number of axons innervating them. In an old lesion, such as might be seen with old poliomyelitis, relatively few axons might survive, but the motor evoked response amplitude may be normal if all the originally denervated muscle fibers are reinnervated. In an acute lesion in which reinnervation has not had time to occur, the evoked response amplitude is roughly proportional to the number of functioning axons.

Disuse Atrophy and Compound Muscle Action Potential Amplitude

The longitudinal current and resulting action potential amplitude of a muscle fiber, as is the case for nerve axons, is proportional to the square of the diameter of the fiber; that is, larger muscle cells produce larger action potentials. Muscle atrophy, with the concomitant reduction in fiber diameters, does not generally produce major reductions in CMAP amplitude because atrophy is offset to a large degree by an increase in fiber density. Although good studies of this problem are lacking, it is generally believed that disuse atrophy cannot easily explain CMAP amplitude decreases below 70% to 80% of the lower limit of normal. This situation is most common with disuse atrophy of the small muscles of the hands, e.g., secondary to severe degenerative hand joint disease.

Metabolic Impairment and Compound Muscle Action Potential Amplitude

If a muscle cell is metabolically impaired, as may occur in some myopathies (e.g., hypokalemic and hyperkalemic periodic paralysis), transmembrane and longitudinal currents and the resulting action potential and CMAP may be diminished or even absent.

Anomalous Innervation and Compound Muscle Action Potential Amplitude

Because the ratio of proximal to distal CMAP amplitudes is of major importance (see sections on conduction block, temporal dispersion), other phenomena that affect CMAP proximal-to-distal amplitude ratios must be discussed. One of these phenomena is the presence of anomalous motor innervation (e.g., an accessory peroneal nerve or the Martin-Gruber anastomosis). When an accessory peroneal nerve is present, it passes behind the lateral malleolus and may innervate some or all of the extensor digitorum brevis. It is not stimulated when peroneal nerve conduction studies are carried out in standard fashion, where the distal stimulation point is over the deep peroneal nerve on the anterior ankle. The amplitude of the CMAP obtained by distal stimulation will be lower than the CMAP obtained with proximal stimulation. The presence of this anomaly may be detected by stimulating behind the lateral malleolus and recording from the extensor digitorum brevis. This usually is not confused with pathologic processes because the proximal-to-distal amplitude ratios are the opposite of those seen with conduction block or temporal dispersion.

The Martin-Gruber anastomosis (Fig. 15-5) occurs when motor axons innervating normally ulnar-innervated intrinsic hand muscles pass in the proximal median nerve and cross over to the ulnar nerve in the forearm. When ulnar nerve conduction studies are performed, the CMAP obtained with distal stimulation is larger than the CMAP obtained with proximal stimulation because the axons that cross over in the forearm are stimulated at the wrist but not at the elbow. This may be mistakenly interpreted as indicating conduction block in the forearm if the Martin-Gruber anastomosis is not detected. The reverse may occur when studying the median nerve; that is, higher median CMAP amplitudes are obtained when stimulating at the elbow because ulnar-bound axons involved in the crossover and innervating muscles of the thenar eminence will be stimulated at the elbow but not at the wrist. The median-to-ulnar crossover should be suspected when the above pattern of median and ulnar proximalto-distal CMAP amplitude ratios is obtained. The anastomosis usually can be confirmed by stimulating the median nerve at the elbow and recording from normally ulnar-innervated intrinsic hand muscles. Combined simultaneous stimu-

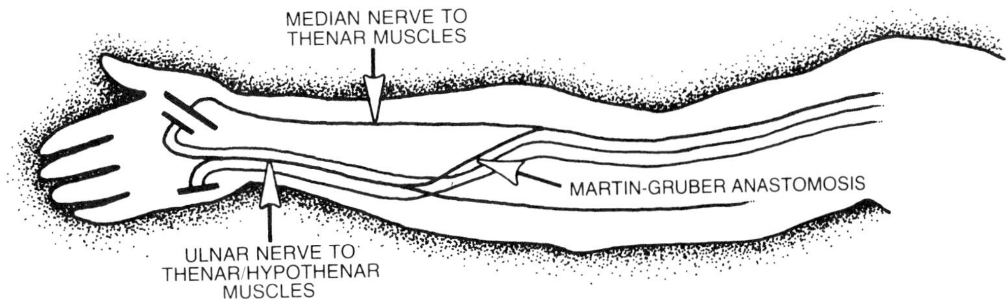

FIG. 15-5. The Martin-Gruber anastomosis is present when motor axons that normally enter the ulnar nerve in the brachial plexus travel instead in the median nerve until the level of the forearm, where they then cross over into the ulnar nerve. This creates a situation in which these fibers are stimulated in the median nerve at the elbow but in the ulnar nerve at the wrist. Ulnar nerve compound muscle action potential (CMAP) amplitudes therefore may appear to drop with stimulation at the elbow relative to the wrist because more axons are stimulated at the wrist. This can mimic conduction block and cause confusion if not identified. The median CMAP amplitude usually is higher with stimulation at the elbow than at the wrist if the crossover involves thenar muscles. Stimulation of the median nerve at the elbow while recording from the abductor digiti quinti muscle usually demonstrates a significant evoked response, and combined simultaneous stimulation of the ulnar and median nerves at the elbow usually reconstitutes a significant portion of the ulnar motor evoked response amplitude observed with ulnar stimulation at the wrist. The amplitude may not be completely reconstituted by combined median/ulnar stimulation at the elbow, presumably secondary to phase cancellation.

lation of the median and ulnar nerves at the elbow while recording over the hypothenar eminence may reconstitute a significant percentage of the amplitude observed with ulnar stimulation at the wrist. Details on variations of the Martin-Gruber crossover are provided by Gutmann and colleagues (55) and Stevens (56).

As previously noted, the tibial nerve, recorded from the abductor hallicus, may give abnormal results, by the criteria used for median/ulnar motor nerves, for proximal/distal evoked response amplitude ratios as a result of a complex motor point anatomy and phase cancellation (49).

Normal and Abnormal Findings in Motor Nerve Conduction Studies

Prolonged Distal Latencies

Distal motor latencies may be interpreted in essentially the same fashion as distal sensory latencies. The relationship between prolonged distal latencies and evoked response amplitude remains the same, although for slightly different reasons.

Decreased Amplitude

Decreased CMAP amplitudes may be seen primarily with the following:

1. Disorders that decrease the density of functionally innervated muscle fibers within the pickup radius of the electrode (e.g., anterior horn cell disease, neuropathies, neuromuscular junction disorders, muscle fiber segmental necrosis)
2. Disorders that affect the action potential current-generating capacity of the muscle fiber (e.g., myopathies)
3. Temporal dispersion
4. Conduction block
5. Anomalous innervation
6. Technical factors such as poor electrode placement, massive soft tissue swelling at the electrode site, or submaximal stimulation

The number of motor axons innervating a muscle may be markedly reduced, but the CMAP can be normal if all muscle fibers have been reinnervated (e.g., as can occur in old poliomyelitis). Compound muscle action potential amplitudes therefore are more likely to be decreased in acute neurogenic lesions in which reinnervation has not had time to occur, as opposed to old or chronic lesions in which enough motor axons have survived to carry out full reinnervation of denervated muscle fibers.

Decreased Conduction Velocities

Decreased conduction velocities in motor nerves can be interpreted according to the same principles as can conduction velocities in sensory nerves.

Increased Temporal Dispersion

Increased temporal dispersion may be interpreted in the same manner as for sensory conduction studies. In the absence of crossovers or conduction block, which might alter the ratio of distal to proximal amplitudes, a proximal-to-distal CMAP amplitude ratio of approximately 0.7 or lower together with a proximal-to-distal CMAP duration ratio greater than approximately 1.2 can be taken as presumptive evidence of temporal dispersion from demyelination (57). If crossovers or conduction block is present, then the proximal-to-distal CMAP amplitude ratio may be of little value, and the identification of temporal dispersion must be made on the basis of the proximal-to-distal CMAP duration ratio alone. Proximal-to-distal CMAP area ratios may be of value in distinguishing temporal dispersion from conduction block, as discussed previously.

Repetitive Firing

Repetitive firing is an infrequently seen phenomenon in which a single stimulus to a motor nerve results in a second peak in addition to the primary response. The second peak usually is superimposed on the trailing edge of the primary peak and usually is of significantly lower amplitude. Repetitive firing is seen with antiacetylcholinesterase toxicity (58,59), and in an extremely rare disorder of the neuromuscular junction, hereditary acetylcholinesterase deficiency (60). It should be specifically sought when myasthenics on large doses of antiacetylcholinesterase medications are being evaluated for an acute exacerbation and it is unclear whether the correct diagnosis is myasthenic crisis or cholinergic crisis.

Temporal Course of Compound Muscle Action Potential Amplitude Abnormalities

Temporal evolution of abnormalities in motor nerve conduction studies may be analyzed according to the same principles as sensory nerve conduction studies, with one exception. When a motor axon is transected, neuromuscular transmission fails well before failure of axonal action potential propagation. As an approximation, complete neuromuscular junction transmission failure occurs by 3 to 7 days, whereas axonal conduction may persist for an additional 3 to 7 days. Because it is the axon potential that is recorded directly in sensory conduction studies, the SNAP can be recorded for 1 to 3 days after CMAPs become unobtainable secondary to failure of neuromuscular transmission.

Late Responses

H Reflex

The H reflex or H response appears to represent the electrical analog of the muscle stretch reflex minus the involvement of the muscle spindle. This reflex is obtained by distal stimulation of IA afferent fibers from muscle spindles, which in turn conduct into the spinal cord, initiating the monosynaptic stretch reflex and evoking a motor response in the muscle involved (see Fig. 15-2*A*). Although it occurs normally in a few other muscles (61), the only H reflex widely used for clinical purposes is that involved in the ankle jerk reflex and recorded from the gastrocnemius and soleus muscles. The widespread presence of the H reflex in muscles in which it does not frequently occur suggests hyperreflexia as a result of an upper motor neuron pathologic process.

In most applications involving the peripheral nervous system, only the latency of the H reflex is generally used since the factors influencing the amplitude are complex, not easily interpreted, and are probably related more to CNS excitability than peripheral nervous system function. While the amplitude of the H reflex is highly variable, the latency is relatively constant (62). The H reflex, as it is commonly used, therefore provides information related to conduction velocity and differs from standard nerve conduction studies in that it involves the proximal portions of the plexuses and roots that are difficult to study directly. This fact allows the H reflex to detect decreased conduction velocities when the pathologic process is limited to the proximal portions of the nerves and roots, a situation in which the results of standard conduction studies usually will be normal. This situation frequently is encountered in evaluating patients with Guillain-Barré syndrome. The H reflex also may prove useful for evaluating focal radicular disease at the S1 level (63,64). It is not a sensitive index of focal radiculopathies at other levels or of lesions such as plexopathies unless they heavily involve S1 axons. Kimura (65) and Dumitru (24) have provided detailed discussions of the H reflex.

The H reflex latency correlates highly with both limb length and age. Braddom and Johnson have published a nomogram that predicts the normal H reflex latency as a function of limb length and age (63,66). The mean H reflex latency in a normal population is 29.8 $\pm$ 2.74 msec with a normal side-to-side difference of 1.0 to 2.0 msec depending on the sensitivity criteria used. Where an S1 radiculopathy is the major consideration, a side-to-side difference exceeding 1.5 to 2.0 msec is felt to be supportive of this diagnosis.

When the H reflex latency is affected by an S1 radiculopathy, the latency is usually either prolonged by no more than 2 to 4 msec or is unobtainable. This probably reflects the fact that slowing of the response occurs over a short segment of nerve root, e.g., 2 to 3 cm on each of the afferent and efferent limbs. For example, if a total of 5 cm of nerve is affected (2.5 cm afferent and efferent), the normal time required for the action potential to traverse this segment would be 1.0 msec at a conduction velocity of 50 m/sec. If the entire increase in the H reflex latency results from slowing across 5 cm of proximal nerve, i.e., the entire delay in the latency can be attributed to peripheral slowing, not changes in central reflex latency at the level of the spinal cord, then the conduction velocity in this segment must drop from 50 m/sec to approximately 17 m/sec to add 2.0 msec to the H reflex latency. To add 4.0 msec to the latency under these circumstances, the conduction velocity must decrease to 10 m/sec. This magnitude of decrease in conduction velocities certainly occurs in other focal compressive nerve lesions such as severe carpal tunnel syndromes. More severe compression, i.e., further root injury and additional slowing of the conduction velocity in the affected segment, is probably associated with substantial temporal dispersion/conduction block and results in loss of the H reflex.

When the H reflex latency is affected by diffuse processes such as an acute inflammatory demyelinating polyneuropathy, the resultant decrease in conduction velocities may affect relatively long segments of nerve, in contrast to the situation with mechanical nerve root compression. If 50 cm (25 cm afferent, 25 cm efferent) of nerve are affected, and the conduction velocity drops from 50 m/sec to 40 m/sec, the time required for the action potential to traverse this segment increases from 10.0 msec to 12.5 msec, increasing the H reflex latency by 2.5 msec. If the involved nerve segment is longer, or the drop in conduction velocity is greater, correspondingly greater increases in H reflex latency will be observed. The H reflex may be prolonged by 10 to 20 msec or more in some cases of acute inflammatory demyelinating polyneuropathy.

F_Response

The F_response or F wave is produced by a stimulus-initiated action potential traveling proximally along the motor axon to the body of the anterior horn cell, triggering a secondary discharge of the same anterior horn cell (see Fig. 15-2*B*). This produces an action potential that travels distally and evokes a muscle action potential (67). The F_response, like the H reflex, is useful primarily as a long-pathway nerve conduction study that examines proximal segments of the nerve, plexuses, and roots. It differs from the H reflex in that it can be elicited from almost all muscles and is therefore of more general applicability. The ease with which F_responses can be elicited does depend on the excitability of the anterior horn cell, which is affected by CNS influences. It is a multi-root-level response and requires that only a small percentage of the axons be intact. It therefore is not sensitive to processes affecting a single root level or plexus branch and has relatively little applicability in the study of focal radiculopathies or plexopathies. Although the F_response may be abnormal with severe radiculopathies or plexopathies, it usually provides little additional information because there are almost always many other electrodiagnostic abnormalities in this setting (68).

The amplitude of the F_response is highly variable and has not proved highly useful clinically. Only the latency is routinely examined. The F_response latency is a highly variable phenomenon; i.e., if one performs multiple stimulations of the nerve at the same sitting, the shortest and longest F_response latencies obtained in a given muscle may vary as much as 3 to 6 msec, depending on the muscle (69). This contrasts with the H reflex latency, which varies much less from trial to trial. The determination of the F_response latency therefore requires some type of statistical approach, i.e., as many as ten to 100 stimulations to obtain valid data, depending on the technique. Largely because of this variability, many different approaches to analyzing F_response latency data have been developed, e.g., minimum latency, mean latency, range of latencies (F chronodispersion), and others. Regardless of the statistical treatment of the data, the F_response is primarily a measure of the average conduction velocity of the involved anterior horn cell axon. The reader is referred to Dumitru (24) for a comprehensive discussion of the F_response and to Fisher (69) for a detailed discussion of the statistical aspects of analyzing F_response latencies.

There is more variability in the normal range of mean side-to-side differences in F_response latency as compared to the H reflex. Normal side-to-side differences for the F_response latencies are approximately 2 msec in the upper extremities and 4 msec in the lower extremities, roughly twice that expected for the H reflex. The F_response is subject to the same influences as the H reflex in investigations of focal lesions affecting only a few centimeters of nerve versus diffuse lesions affecting long segments (see previous). The relatively large variability of the F_response latency makes it insensitive to the 1- to 4-msec increases in latencies predicted for focal lesions such as radiculopathies. For practical purposes, the F_response should be thought of primarily as a test for diffuse moderate slowing over relatively long segments of nerve.

Neither the H reflex nor the F_response is highly useful in precise localization because all they document is that there is a conduction delay somewhere along the path of the action potential. These responses can be evoked with both distal and proximal stimulation, and the contribution of the distal nerve subtracted out mathematically, but all this allows the electromyographer to do is to localize the pathology distally or proximally. It does not allow precise localization within the proximal nerve structures.

Applications of the Late Responses

The late responses are always part of a larger clinical and electrodiagnostic picture and the electromyographer should rely heavily on them only in situations where they actually add substantially and unequivocally to the clinical situation. Their use should be associated with a very low rate of false positivity. Abnormal late response results are usually of minor importance when there are significant abnormalities on the standard nerve conduction studies and/or the needle electrode examination. The following discussion applies primarily to situations where there are minimal or no abnormalities on standard nerve conduction studies and/or the needle electrode examination, i.e., the electromyographer is relying heavily on the results of late response studies for his or her conclusions.

1. When are normal or abnormal late responses clearly of significant value in establishing a specific diagnosis and guiding management decisions?
   A. AIDP, where involvement is primarily proximal and the results of standard distal peripheral nerve conduction studies are normal or equivocal. Substantially prolonged F_response and H reflex latencies strongly support the diagnosis of a demyelinating

process in this situation. Absent late responses in this setting are not nearly as helpful in establishing a rigid diagnosis of AIDP as are markedly prolonged latencies because absence of the response is more nonspecific than marked prolongation.

B. In a setting of acute paralysis, the differential diagnosis includes, among other things, AIDP, acute myelopathies, and malingering/hysteria. The presence of late responses in this situation documents intact peripheral nerve function from the periphery to the spinal cord, thereby disfavoring AIDP or other peripheral nerve lesions and favoring either a central cord lesion or malingering/hysteria. This applies primarily to paralysis or extreme weakness, and when weakness is only mild to moderate, the presence or absence of late responses is much less helpful. Note that the converse does not necessarily apply; e.g., F_responses can be absent in spinal shock, transverse myelitis, etc., so that their absence does not document a peripheral disorder (70). Their absence in some settings can be an important clue to the existence of some type of organic pathology, e.g., the teenager with early transverse myelitis who has weak lower extremities and detectable reflexes who is suspected of malingering/hysterical weakness. F_responses should be readily obtained in a patient such as this, and their absence is highly suspicious.

2. When are normal or abnormal late responses of occasional value in establishing a specific diagnosis and guiding management decisions when taken in the context of other electrodiagnostic, metabolic, and imaging studies?

   A. The H reflex can help influence management decisions regarding S1 radiculopathies when the results of standard electrodiagnostic studies are normal and imaging studies of the lumbosacral spine are equivocal for a surgically significant structural lesion. An abnormal H reflex that correlates with an equivocal structural abnormality and/or clinical finding can help influence a decision to operate or take other aggressive action based on that diagnosis. An abnormal H reflex latency in association with normal structural studies of the lumbosacral spine and otherwise normal electrodiagnostic studies is for the most part of unknown clinical significance and not particularly helpful in clinical management, e.g., one is unlikely to take any aggressive action on the basis of an abnormal H reflex study unless there are other corroborating signs, symptoms, and other abnormal diagnostic tests. It should be remembered that, like the ankle jerk, the H reflex can remain permanently absent or delayed following a previous root injury, e.g., previous S1 radiculopathy.

   B. Nonstructural, e.g., metabolic or vasculitic proximal plexus/root pathology where relatively large portions of the neural structures are involved. External compressive lesions of major nerve trunks usually fall in this category as well, e.g., a sciatic neuropathy related to prolonged pressure during a drug-induced coma, etc. This contrasts specifically with focal, space-occupying lesions discussed below (69).

3. When are normal or abnormal late responses usually of limited value in establishing a specific diagnosis and/or guiding management decisions?

   A. This situation arises most often when focal, space-occupying, compressive lesions, e.g., neoplasms that produce neurologically incomplete radiculopathies, plexopathies, or proximal mononeuropathies are suspected and the results of standard nerve conduction studies and needle electromyography are equivocal or normal. This also includes partial compressive lesions such as a putative piriformis syndrome.

The H reflex has already been discussed with respect to S1 radiculopathies, and it has been pointed out that it is of little value at other root levels. It is of at least theoretical interest with respect to plexopathies or tibial neuropathies affecting plexus/peripheral nerve segments containing significant S1 contributions. However, since the H reflex is based on the latency resulting from the fastest conducting axons, one would predict that if a percentage of the axons carrying S1 axons are intact and undamaged, then the H reflex latency may well be normal; i.e., the H reflex is insensitive to partial lesions. As H reflex studies are usually performed, utilizing tibial nerve stimulation, it is most sensitive when the lesion is large enough to involve all S1-containing segments of the root, plexus, or peripheral nerve. Outside of the nerve root level, where all S1 axons can easily be compressed by a single lesion or major compressive lesions of the tibial nerve, this probably does not occur frequently unless the lesion is quite large and probably well seen on imaging studies. The F_response is subject to the same logic with the qualification that the axons involved are probably even more diffusely localized in the neural structures, and an even more diffuse/larger lesion would be required to produce abnormalities. An abnormal late response latency in this situation would certainly be an indication for imaging studies of the proximal neural structures, e.g., plexus. However, if a mass lesion is a realistic possibility, imaging studies should probably be performed regardless of the results of electrodiagnostic studies. This is due to a significant false negative rate for electrodiagnostic studies in this setting. Contemporary magnetic resonance imaging (MRI) and computed tomography (CT) scanning of the proximal shoulder girdle and pelvis are generally better ways to examine the proximal peripheral nervous system for space occupying structural lesions than are late responses (71) 1944, particularly those lesions for which any specific treatment is available. It should be noted that much of the interest in late responses began in the years before CT and MRI scanning were available, and the late responses were essentially the only techniques, albeit insensitive, with which a clinician could infer the functional state of proximal nerve structures.

It should be emphasized that standard needle electromyography can be quite sensitive in detecting proximal lesions if there has been axonal interruption and spontaneous activity is present. The needle electrode examination, by means of spontaneous activity, can frequently detect abnormalities caused by malignant invasion of a proximal nerve structure at a time when many routine imaging studies are unremarkable. Exhaustive detailed imaging techniques or invasive biopsies, performed primarily because of the results of the electrodiagnostic studies may subsequently demonstrate the lesion. Note, however, that many of these lesions do occur without any significant axonal interruption, at least initially, and they may therefore have a normal needle electrode examination. It should be recognized that MRI, CT scanning, CT directed biopsy, and electrodiagnostic studies are complementary, not exclusive, technologies.

B. Mild prolongation of the late responses in cases of suspected polyneuropathy, in the absence of other electrodiagnostic abnormalities, privides supportive evidence for a very minimal peripheral neuropathy. The late responses are not particularly helpful in this situation in that essentially all management decisions will be made on the basis of the history, physical examination, laboratory results, and the standard electrodiagnostic studies, not the results of the late responses.

EVALUATION OF THE NEUROMUSCULAR JUNCTION

Motor nerve conduction studies analyze the behavior of nerve, neuromuscular junction, and muscle fiber. With the exception of myotonic disorders and the periodic paralyses, the ability of the nerve axon and the muscle fiber to produce normal action potentials is not stressed with short bursts of repetitive stimulation at frequencies below 50 Hz. Fifty hertz is chosen here because it represents a common practical upper limit for stimulation frequencies in electrodiagnostic studies, not because it represents any intrinsic property of nerve or muscle. Repetitive stimulation of motor nerves at frequencies ranging from 2 to 50 Hz may produce clear-cut abnormalities when dysfunction of the neuromuscular junction exists, however, even when the results of standard motor nerve conduction studies are normal (12,14, 16,72–74). For this reason, repetitive stimulation of motor nerves should be included in any electrodiagnostic evaluation in which a disorder of the neuromuscular junction may exist, such as in myasthenia gravis, ELMS, botulism (75), or drug toxicity (76).

Neuromuscular transmission also may be abnormal in immature neuromuscular junctions present as a result of denervation and reinnervation. Although this usually is a nonspecific finding, it may be useful for prognosticating in neuropathic conditions such as MND, in which the presence of abnormal results with repetitive stimulation suggests large amounts of denervation and reinnervation, which implies a poorer prognosis than if the results of repetitive stimulation were normal. Abnormal neuromuscular transmission may rarely be seen as a nonspecific finding with direct muscle cell damage, as can be seen with inflammatory myopathies.

Basic Mechanisms and Pharmacology of Acetylcholine Synthesis, Storage, and Release in the Normal Functioning of Motor Neurons

Acetylcholine is synthesized within the nerve terminal from choline and acetyl-CoA by the enzyme choline-O-acetyltransferase. It is then transported into synaptic vesicles. Current information indicates that the acetylcholine in the nerve terminal can be grossly divided into two major functional pools. The first of these pools is commonly referred to as the immediately available pool and constitutes a small percentage of the total acetylcholine in the nerve terminal. This is the acetylcholine that is biologically available for immediate release into the synaptic cleft during synaptic transmission. The majority of acetylcholine is in the reserve pool and must be transported first into the immediately available pool before it can be used. This phenomenon of transfer to the immediately available pool is referred to as mobilization. When a resting nerve terminal begins to fire repetitively, the size of the immediately available pool decreases transiently until mobilization from the reserve pool occurs.

When an action potential invades the presynaptic nerve terminal, the membrane permeability to calcium increases, leading to markedly increased intracellular calcium concentrations. The increased intracellular calcium concentrations trigger, in some as yet poorly understood manner, the release of acetylcholine from the nerve terminal into the synaptic cleft. The major facts about acetylcholine release are summarized as follows:

1. Acetylcholine release depends on the fourth power of the extracellular calcium concentration.
2. Acetylcholine release is antagonized by hypocalcemia or hypermagnesemia.
3. Acetylcholine is released in discrete quanta, which appear to correspond to the contents of the synaptic vesicles.
4. The number of acetylcholine quanta (M) released by a single nerve action potential can be modeled with the following equation (77):

$$M = P \times N$$

where N is the number of acetylcholine quanta in the immediately available pool, and P is the probability of release. The probability of release is directly related to the intracellular calcium concentration and other factors such as magnesium concentrations, presence of certain antibiotics, and other molecules that are known to affect acetylcholine release.

Acetylcholine diffuses across the synaptic cleft to bind to the postsynaptic acetylcholine receptors, resulting in an increased sodium influx into the muscle cell. This generates the miniature end-plate potentials (MEPP), which sum with other MEPPs to yield the net end-plate potential (EPP). The EPP will initiate a muscle cell action potential if it is suprathreshold. All other things being equal, the amplitude of the muscle cell EPP is proportional to the amount of acetylcholine released by the presynaptic nerve terminal and the number of functional postsynaptic acetylcholine receptors. Decreases in either the amount of acetylcholine released or in the number of functional postsynaptic acetylcholine receptors will decrease the probability of the resultant EPP being suprathreshold. Acetylcholine bound to postsynaptic acetylcholine receptors is in rapid equilibrium with free acetylcholine and is rapidly hydrolyzed to choline and acetic acid by the acetylcholinesterase enzyme bound to the postsynaptic membrane. Free choline is then taken up by the nerve terminal to complete the cycle.

Effects of Repetitive Stimulation on Acetylcholine Release by the Presynaptic Nerve Terminal

The immediately available pool of acetylcholine in the nerve terminal is relatively small and must be replenished by mobilization from the reserve pool during repetitive firing of the nerve terminal. When a resting nerve terminal is stimulated repetitively at 2 to 5 Hz, the rate of mobilization initially lags behind the rate of release of acetylcholine from the immediately available pool, resulting in a transient decrease in the size of the immediately available pool. Since the number of acetylcholine quanta released per nerve stimulus is proportional to the size of the immediately available pool, this means that the actual number of acetylcholine quanta released by a single nerve impulse will decrease progressively with 2- to 5-Hz repetitive stimulation until mobilization can restore the initial size of the immediately available pool. This increased rate of mobilization from the reserve pool takes 500 to 2,000 msec to occur. The net result of this phenomenon is that when a nerve is repetitively stimulated at 2 to 3 Hz, the amount of acetylcholine released drops successively during the first three to five stimuli before returning to baseline. This usually is of no significance to the normal person, in that two to three times as much acetylcholine is released as is necessary to result in a suprathreshold postsynaptic end-plate potential. If, for whatever reason, the amount of acetylcholine initially released is barely sufficient to result in suprathreshold EPPs, this transient drop in the amount of acetylcholine released actually may result in subthreshold EPPs during the initial three to five stimuli at 2 to 3 Hz. When observed at the single-fiber level, an all-or-none phenomenon would be seen (i.e., a normal muscle cell action potential or no potential at all). During the simultaneous observation of a large number of muscle fibers in a muscle, as is done with standard motor nerve conduction studies, a certain percentage of muscle fibers fail to fire. This will manifest itself as a decrement in the CMAP amplitude recorded during several of the initial stimuli at 2 to 5 Hz (Fig. 15-6). The majority of the decrement will occur between the first and second stimuli. This decrement serves as the basis for electrodiagnostic testing of the neuromuscular junction by this technique. Normal subjects demonstrate less than a 5% decrement with repetitive stimulation when technical artifacts such as electrode or stimulator movement are eliminated.

Acetylcholine release is facilitated (i.e., there is an increased probability of release) by high rates of stimulation (e.g., 20 to 50 Hz) or by the functional equivalent, maximal exercise. This phenomenon may outweigh the decrease in the amount of acetylcholine release caused by a decrease in the immediately available pool size. It is then possible that no failure of neuromuscular transmission may be observed at 20 to 50 Hz, whereas clear failure may occur at 2 to 3 Hz. It is for this reason that repetitive stimulation testing at 2 to 3 Hz is included in the evaluation of diseases of the neuromuscular junction such as myasthenia gravis. Stimulation frequencies of 20 to 50 Hz are still used in eliciting facilitation and in the evaluation of ELMS and botulism (78,79).

Facilitation by relatively high stimulation frequencies is

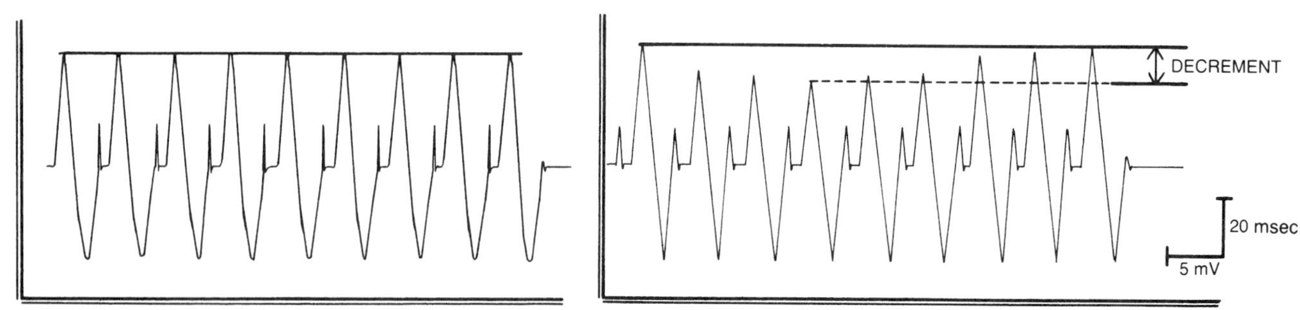

FIG. 15-6. Stimulation of a motor nerve at 2 Hz. **A:** In the normal person, the amplitude of the compound motor evoked response shows no significant decrement (<5%). **B:** When impaired neuromuscular transmission is present, a decrement greater than approximately 5% may be seen during the first one to four stimuli.

believed to occur because higher intracellular calcium concentrations, which result in increased acetylcholine release, can be achieved with high frequencies (20 to 50 Hz) than with frequencies in the 2- to 3-Hz range. This also is the explanation for why a decrement observed on repetitive stimulation in myasthenia gravis will be diminished (i.e., repaired) by having the patient exercise vigorously for 5 to 10 seconds before repetitive stimulation.

In the myasthenic syndrome (i.e., ELMS), a presynaptic defect of neuromuscular transmission results in failure of neuromuscular transmission in rested neuromuscular junctions. This is evidenced in standard nerve conduction studies by a reduced CMAP amplitude. If low CMAP amplitudes are secondary to ELMS, a marked increment (>100%) in the CMAP amplitude will be seen with high-frequency stimulation (20 to 50 Hz) or after maximal exercise. This increment also is believed to be related to increased presynaptic nerve terminal calcium concentrations. The ELMS is probably frequently missed in clinical practice because of omission of the proper tests. Because repetitive stimulation at high frequencies is usually poorly tolerated by patients, equivalent results can be achieved by single stimulations done after approximately 10 seconds of voluntary maximal exercise. This is well tolerated and should be done any time the electromyographer encounters multiple low motor evoked response amplitudes.

Temperature has a significant effect on the NMJ. Low temperatures are protective and high temperatures exacerbate the electrodiagnostic abnormalities associated with MG and ELMS. Electrodiagnostic testing for NMJ dysfunction should therefore take place after warming of the limb.

It should be noted that a significant percentage of patients with a mild to moderate defect in neuromuscular transmission, e.g., myasthenia gravis, will have normal or equivocal results on repetitive stimulation, and SFEMG must be used to document an abnormality.

Single-Fiber Electromyography

Single-fiber electromyography is an extremely powerful tool for the evaluation of the neuromuscular junction (13,14,17). It is performed by positioning an electrode with a very small recording surface (25-μm diameter) such that it simultaneously records the single-fiber action potentials (SFAPs) from two or more muscle fibers within the same motor unit. The interpotential interval between these two SFAPs is then measured and analyzed (Fig. 15-7). It has been well established that the duration of this interpotential interval (1 to 4 msec) is not constant from one firing of the motor unit to the next but has a variation averaging 10 to 60 μsec. This variability occurs primarily in the time required for neuromuscular transmission to occur and is related to the time at which the muscle cell EPP reaches threshold value (see Fig. 15-7). If the EPP amplitude is high, the muscle fiber threshold is reached early in the EPP, and the time of threshold occurrence relative to the arrival of the action potential at the nerve terminal does not vary much from one firing to the next. If the EPP amplitude is low and variable, as is the case in many disorders of the neuromuscular junction, then threshold values are reached near the peak of the EPP, where the time of occurrence relative to the arrival of the nerve action potential may vary widely. This variability is known as the neuromuscular jitter. If the EPP is barely threshold, failure may intermittently occur, a phenomenon known as blocking. If an abnormal decrement of the CMAP amplitude is observed on repetitive stimulation, blocking must be present on SFEMG. Jitter, however, may be markedly increased even when there is no overt failure of neuromuscular transmission. The SFEMG therefore is a much more sensitive, albeit more difficult, technique for diagnosing disorders of the neuromuscular junction than is repetitive stimulation. Patients who have normal standard repetitive stimulation studies but who are strongly suspected of having a disorder of neuromuscular junction function should have SFEMG studies.

Single-fiber electromyography also has the ability to provide an indirect estimate of motor unit fiber density (i.e., the number of muscle fibers per unit cross-sectional area belonging to a single motor unit). This is done by randomly inserting the SFEMG electrode next to a single muscle fiber, triggering on that fiber, and counting the number of additional SFAPs from the same MU that can be recorded in that location. Normal values range from 1.3 to 1.7, depending on the muscle. This parameter frequently will be abnormal in many disease processes that result in anatomic reorganization of the motor unit (e.g., MND, some myopathies).

NEEDLE ELECTRODE EXAMINATION

The needle electrode examination comprises the remaining major component of the electrodiagnostic evaluation. Although nerve conduction studies provide information primarily on the numbers and physiological state of functioning nerve axons and muscle fibers, the needle electrode examination provides additional information on the physiological state of individual muscle fibers, the anatomic organization of the motor unit, motor unit recruitment properties, and other motor unit phenomena (e.g., fasciculations). The monograph by Daube should be considered mandatory reading (80).

Basic Physiology and Pathophysiology

Before we discuss pathophysiology, we review some basic definitions and concepts. Subsequent sections discuss individual topics in more detail.

Insertional Activity

As the needle electrode is passed through muscle fibers, the tip is alternately exposed to and detects the extracellular

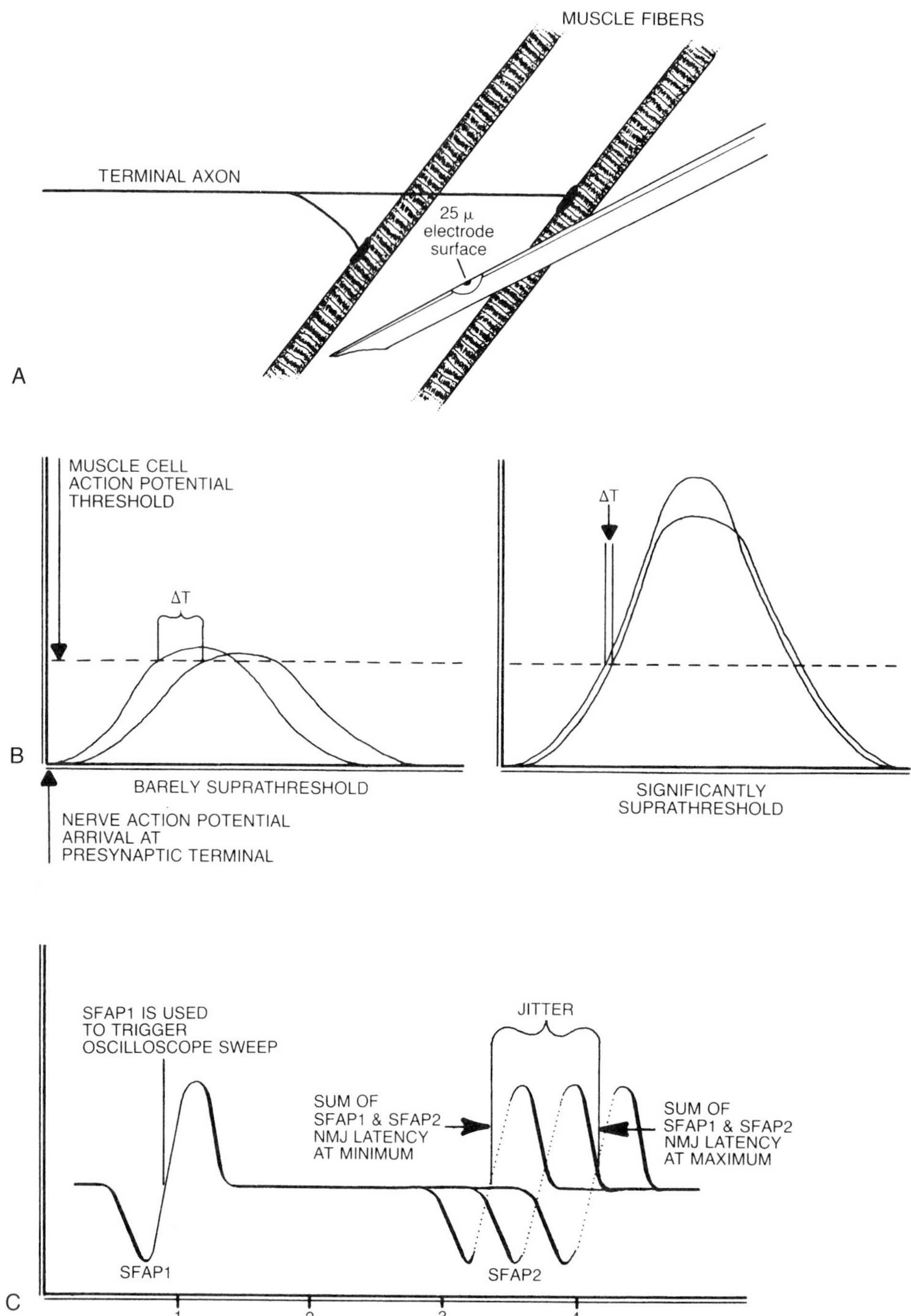

FIG. 15-7. Jitter. **A:** Fiber/electrode position. The recording electrode is positioned such that the single-fiber action potentials *(SFAPs)* from two or more single muscle fibers from the same motor unit are recorded simultaneously. **B:** Muscle cell end-plate potential (EPP). Two barely suprathreshold and two significantly suprathreshold EPPs are shown. The neuromuscular junction *(NMJ)* latency is defined as the elapsed time from the arrival of the nerve action potential at the synaptic terminal to the time that the postsynaptic EPP reaches the threshold for an action potential. Note that the neuromuscular junction latency is relatively independent of EPP amplitude when the EPP is well above the threshold value, whereas the neuromuscular junction latency varies significantly when the EPP is barely suprathreshold. **C:** Jitter. The interpotential interval (IPI) is the difference in time between the arrival of the first and second SFAPs at the recording electrode site. The variability in the IPI has been shown to be caused primarily by variability in the neuromuscular latency of the two fibers involved, which in turn is affected by the factors outlined in **B**. The variability in the IPI is called jitter and is increased when neuromuscular function is abnormal.

potential (approximately 0 mV) and the intracellular potential (approximately −70 mV). Although the standard needle electrodes (diameter approximately 200 μm) are much larger than muscle fibers (diameter 40 to 100 μm), the tip of the electrode is small enough to transiently penetrate muscle fibers. The intracellular potential therefore contributes to the net voltage measured by the electrode during passage through the muscle fiber. Additionally, the muscle cell transmembrane potential may be destabilized enough by the passage of the electrode to generate a muscle membrane action potential, adding to the electrical activity detected by the electrode. Because insertional activity usually is evaluated at an amplifier gain setting of 50 to 100 μV per division (500 to 1,000 μV from the top to the bottom of the screen on most EMG machines), the potential changes encountered by the needle electrode (10,000 to 50,000 μV) are sufficient to cause the trace on the oscilloscope to deflect off of the screen. Depending on the low-frequency response of the amplifier, this insertional activity should return to baseline in 500 to 1,000 msec or less. In normal muscle, there should be near electrical silence after electrode movement ceases. The primary value of insertional activity is that it tells the electromyographer when the needle electrode actually is in muscle tissue. Markedly decreased insertional activity, such as that seen when minimal electric potential changes are detected as the electrode is moved, indicates that either the electrode is not in muscle or that the muscle has undergone severe atrophy and replacement by electrically inactive tissues such as fat or connective tissue. This finding is common in the intrinsic muscles of the feet in the presence of a severe polyneuropathy or in any muscle after long-standing, severe denervation.

Spontaneous Activity

Normal muscle should be virtually electrically silent when the patient is relaxed and the electrode is not being moved. Persistent electrical activity after the needle electrode has stopped moving may be related to the following:

1. Voluntary motor unit activity secondary to poor relaxation
2. Normal electrical events (e.g., motor end-plate noise or nerve potentials, detected because of fortuitous placement of the electrode)
3. Motor unit states associated with abnormal nerve or muscle membrane stability
   A. *Abnormal muscle fiber states:* The most common form of this type of spontaneous activity is the presence of positive sharp waves or fibrillation potentials (Fig. 15-8). Although muscle fiber spontaneous activity may be seen with other conditions (e.g., acid maltase deficiency), the most common etiology is the marked membrane electrical instability that results when a muscle fiber or segment of a fiber loses its innervation. A large amount of electrophysiological data suggest that fibrillation potentials are relatively normal SFAPs recorded remote from the point of generation of the action potential. Positive sharp waves (see Fig. 15-8) also are believed to represent SFAPs. Positive sharp waves are thought to occur when the electrode is in contact with the damaged muscle fiber and the action potential is blocked at this site or the repolarization phase of the action potential is markedly slowed. Fibrillation potentials, on the other hand, are believed to represent a normally conducted action potential recorded at a distance from the muscle fiber. The length of time required for positive sharp waves and fibrillation potentials to appear in a denervated muscle is proportional to the length of nerve remaining in continuity with the muscle. For example, if a nerve root is severed at the spinal foramen, spontaneous activity may appear in the paraspinous muscles 1 to 2 weeks before it appears in distal muscles of the extremities. Likewise, if the median nerve is cut at the wrist, spontaneous activity will appear in the thenar muscles earlier than if the lesion is located in the axilla. It generally is believed that spontaneous activity may take as long as 6 weeks to appear in distal muscles when the lesion is proximal at the root level. These factors should be considered when examining an evolving lesion. The presence of spontaneous activity is related to the stage of a pathologic process. It may take weeks to begin after an insult and may then resolve completely if all of the muscle fibers are reinnervated. This should be considered when attempting to decide whether the absence of spontaneous activity mitigates against a particular diagno-

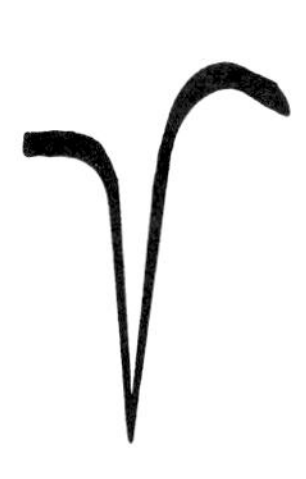

POSITIVE WAVE

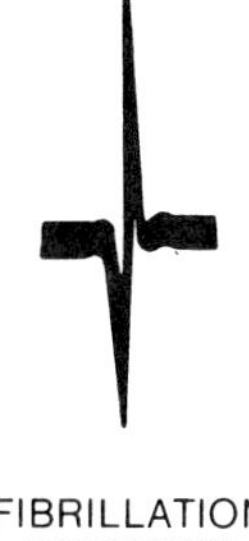

FIBRILLATION POTENTIAL

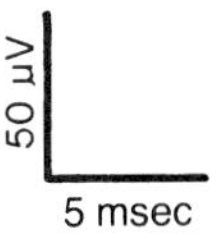

FIG. 15-8. Spontaneous activity.

sis (e.g., the electrodiagnostic examination may have been performed either before or after spontaneous activity was present).

B. *Fasciculations:* Spontaneous, repetitive single discharges of individual motor units. Fasciculations may be seen in MND, polyneuropathies, radiculopathies, and benign idiopathic conditions (81).

C. *Complex repetitive discharges* (CRDs), also known as high-frequency discharges or iterative discharges: A relatively nonspecific abnormality noted in a wide range of disorders such as polyneuropathies, radiculopathies, and inflammatory myopathies; CRDs usually are associated with chronic disorders.

D. *Myotonic discharges:* Associated with myotonic disorders (82), myotonic dystrophy, myotonia congenita, paramyotonia congenita (83), and hyperkalemic periodic paralysis.

E. *Myokymia:* Grouped repetitive discharges most often associated with postirradiation nerve damage, old neurogenic lesions, and multiple sclerosis (84).

F. *Neuromyotonia:* Associated with continuous motor unit activity syndromes.

A more detailed discussion of the characteristics and significance of the types of spontaneous activity is beyond the scope of this section (57,85–87).

Motor Unit Action Potential Configuration

The MUAP represents the summation of SFAPs from the muscle fibers in a given motor unit. Because the origin of the MUAP is complex, an extensive discussion will be devoted to analyzing it. Many types of motor unit pathologic processes will produce characteristic changes in the duration, amplitude, polyphasia, and variability of amplitude of the MUAP (Fig. 15-9).

Recruitment

Recruitment refers to the pattern in which motor units are activated. The force produced by a muscle can be controlled by changing either the number of active motor units, the firing frequency of individual motor units, or both (88). As the motor unit discharge frequency increases, muscle fibers develop increasing force up to a plateau known as the maximum tetanic tension (P_0) (89). In humans, motor units are capable of discharging from a minimum of 2 to 3 Hz up to 30 to 60 Hz (or even as high as 100 Hz and above under special circumstances). The general scheme used by spinal cord mechanisms is to recruit low-threshold motor units and increase force output by increasing their discharge frequency slightly, while simultaneously recruiting additional motor units with slightly higher thresholds. The frequency at which a motor unit starts firing is referred to as its onset frequency, and the frequency at which the next motor unit is recruited is referred to as the recruitment frequency of the preceding unit (90). In conditions in which there is substantial axonal loss, as in a severe radiculopathy or polyneuropathy, onset and recruitment frequencies of the initial motor unit pool are increased. This situation, however, is referred to as decreased recruitment because a given level of force is produced by fewer MUAPs firing at higher average rates relative to the normal situation.

When a myopathy is suspected, the other recruitment abnormality that must be considered is rapid recruitment. To refer to this condition as an abnormality of recruitment is misleading, however, because the pattern of recruitment of individual MUAPs is essentially normal. The abnormality noted in a myopathy is that a larger number of motor units must be recruited or activated to produce a given force output. Evaluating rapid recruitment, therefore, requires knowledge of the force produced in addition to the recruitment information obtained from the needle electrode in the muscle. This is not true in the case of decreased recruitment,

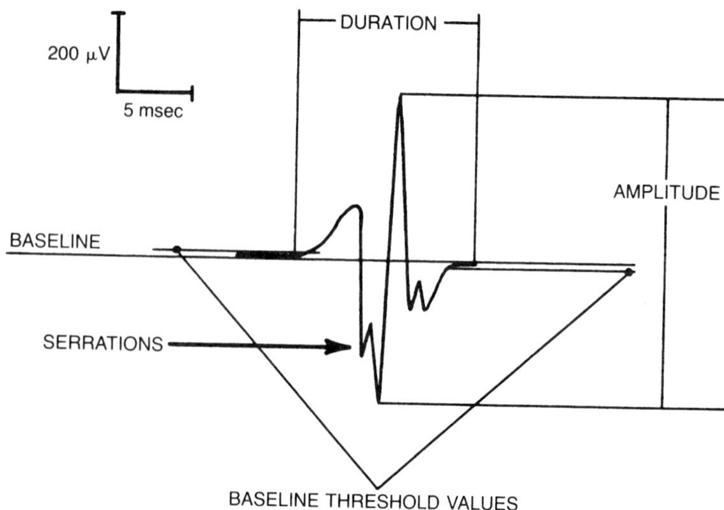

FIG. 15-9. Schematic motor unit action potential (MUAP) characteristics are labeled. This MUAP has four major phases (i.e., three baseline crossings plus one). Note that both of the major positive (i.e., downward) deflections are serrated. Familiarity with the basic definitions and anatomy of skeletal muscle motor units is assumed. Details on normal values for MUAP duration, polyphasia, and amplitude are presented in other sources (78–82).

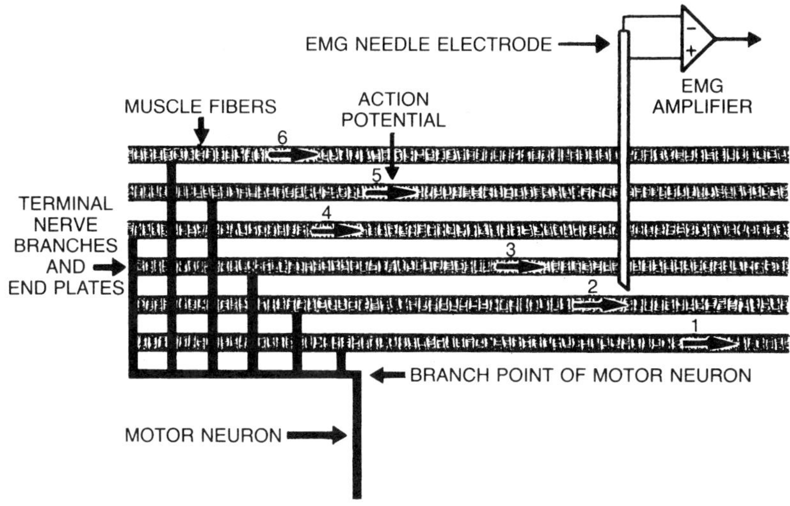

FIG. 15-10. Schematic representation of motor unit action potential generation and recording by concentric needle electrode. The neuronal action potential diverges at the branch point of the motor neurons to asynchronously initiate muscle fiber action potentials. The muscle fiber action potentials then travel toward the electrode position at approximately 4 m/sec. Locations of the respective muscle fiber action potentials at a single time are shown by the *numbered arrows.*

which can be identified using only the information present on the screen of the EMG machine.

Analysis of Motor Unit Action Potential Electrophysiology

The motor unit electrophysiology necessary for an in-depth understanding of the EMG needle electrode examination is discussed in the following section. A mechanistic approach is taken using relatively simple models. Thus, a few comments on biological models are in order. In all cases involving modeling of biological phenomena, there is a trade-off between accuracy and simplicity; that is, the more accurate a model of a given phenomenon, the more complex and less easily understood it is. Simplicity, as opposed to complexity, is emphasized in the following discussion. More detailed descriptions are provided elsewhere (91–95).

Modeling of Motor Unit Action Potential

The motor unit can be considered to consist of approximately 150 infinitely long, parallel muscle fibers arranged in a cylindrical fashion (Fig. 15-10). Between these muscle fibers are fibers belonging to other motor units. The number of muscle fibers per unit cross-sectional area is defined as the fiber density. Do not confuse this with the fiber density as determined by SFEMG. They are different, although they both measure the same motor unit characteristic. An innervation zone is then selected for the fibers where the anterior horn cell divides to provide innervation to each individual muscle fiber. Finally, the electrode is positioned a significant distance away from the innervation zone. The term *significant distance* refers to a point where motor end-plate events related to the initiation of the muscle SFAP are not detected by the electrode; all that the electrode detects is the muscle fiber action potential moving toward it. This arrangement represents the majority of electrode positions used by the clinical electromyographer.

The anterior horn cell action potential travels down the axon to the point where the axon branches to supply all the individual muscle fibers (see Fig. 15-10). At this point, the individual action potentials of the terminal nerve branches are synchronized. Because the lengths of the terminal nerve branches to the individual muscle fibers are not identical, and because the conduction velocities probably are not identical in each terminal nerve branch, all muscle fibers in the motor unit are not activated simultaneously. The action potentials of fibers closest to the branch point of the motor nerve will be initiated before those of the muscle fibers that are farthest away from the motor neuron branch point. Because of the anatomic spread of motor end plates, not all muscle fiber action potentials start exactly in the same location. The action potentials of some muscle fibers therefore have a head start in reaching the electrode. After each individual muscle fiber is activated, their action potentials travel down the muscle fibers at 2 to 4 m/sec toward the electrode position. In addition, because the conduction velocities of individual muscle fibers are not identical, by the time the group of SFAPs reaches the electrode position there will be a difference of approximately 4 msec or less between the time of arrival of the earliest and latest SFAP in a given area of a normal motor unit (17). What the EMG machine displays is the net sum of these individual SFAPs passing by the recording electrode.

It has previously been stated that the MUAP is the summation of the SFAPs in that motor unit, and it has been shown how a group of SFAPs pass the electrode position in a spread-out (i.e., temporally dispersed) fashion. The relative position of the electrode and a given muscle fiber has a major effect on the contribution of that SFAP to the overall MUAP as well.

The potential represented in Figure 15-11*A* is an approximation of the SFAP under the recording conditions used by the clinical electromyographer. An in-depth discussion of this potential is provided by Sanders and Howard (17), and Rosenfalck (96).

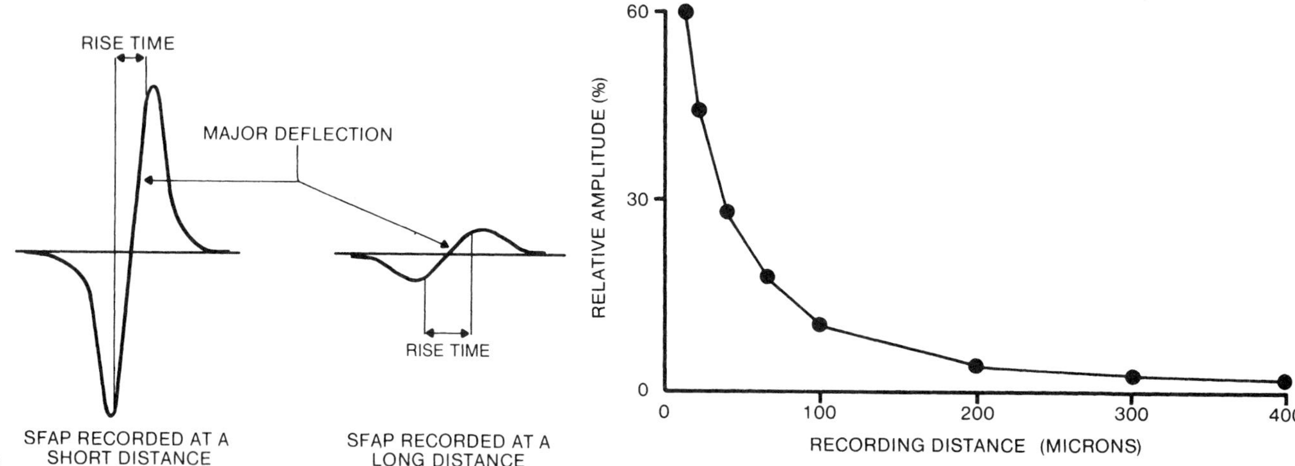

FIG. 15-11. Single-fiber action potential *(SFAP)* characteristics. Examples of SFAPs recorded near and far away from the single fiber show that **A:** the rise time progressively increases and **B:** the peak-to-peak amplitude falls exponentially as the distance from the muscle fiber to the recording electrode increases. This occurs over a relatively short distance. The rise time usually is defined as the time required for a potential to change from 10% to 90% of its maximum value.

The action potential consists of an initial positive deflection and a terminal negative deflection. The positive and negative deflections usually are of approximately equal amplitude and duration, depending on the exact electrode position.

The middle portion of the potential, extending from the positive peak to the negative peak, is the major deflection of the potential, and its slope is related to what is called the rise time of the potential. The higher the slope of the major deflection, the shorter the rise time of the potential. This is a function of the distance from the electrode to the single fiber.

The absolute amplitude of the SFAP is approximately proportional to the square of the diameter of the muscle fiber. For a given electrode position, a 100-μm diameter muscle fiber will produce an action potential roughly four times larger that a 50-μm fiber.

Several major points are revealed in the examination of the effect of electrode distance on the SFAP configuration (see Fig. 15-11*B*):

1. The peak-to-peak amplitude of the action potential decreases exponentially as the distance from the electrode to the single fiber increases.
2. The amplitude of the leading and trailing edges of the SFAP falls off much less rapidly than the peak-to-peak amplitudes as the electrode–fiber distance increases.
3. The slope of the major deflection decreases markedly (i.e., the rise time increases considerably) as the electrode–fiber distance increases.

From these observations, the following conclusions can be made about the effects of fiber-electrode distance on the contribution of individual single fibers to the observed MUAP:

1. The appearance of the MUAP will be dominated by those fibers very close to the electrode because of exponential fall-off of single-fiber peak-to-peak action potential amplitude with increasing distance from the electrode. Extremely high amplitudes can be obtained by being very close to a single fiber. In this situation, however, the high amplitude will be associated with a very short rise time of the major deflection of the potential, and the amplitude observed will be critically dependent on the electrode position (e.g., minor adjustments in electrode position will cause major changes in the peak-to-peak amplitude of the MUAP). This is the major reason why it is difficult clinically to quantitate MUAP amplitude: variable fiber–electrode distances produce marked variations in the observed peak-to-peak amplitude. A wide range of MUAP amplitudes can therefore be obtained from a given motor unit simply by altering electrode position.
2. Fibers that are remote from the electrode will contribute significantly more to the duration than they do to the peak-to-peak amplitude, primarily because of the manner in which duration is determined (see Fig. 15-9). Although one to ten close fibers may dominate MUAP amplitude, there are many more muscle fibers (i.e., 150 to 1,500) that are remote from the electrode, making low-amplitude contributions ($<$10 to 50 μV) to the initial, middle, and trailing edges of the MUAP. Because average MUAP peak-to-peak amplitudes will be in the range of 400 to 2,000 μV for most electrode types, these low-amplitude contributions to overall peak-to-peak amplitude will not be significant. The low-amplitude contribution to the measured MUAP duration does, however, make a significant difference. Because MUAP duration is defined as the difference in time between the

initial deviation from baseline by a threshold amount (e.g., 5 to 10 μV) and the time where it falls below the threshold value in returning to the baseline, small contributions to the amplitude in the leading and trailing regions of the MUAP will increase the measured duration.

Factors Influencing Motor Unit Action Potential Duration, Polyphasia, and Amplitude

Using the above information on the anatomic and physiological factors that determine the MUAP configuration, we refine our understanding as follows.

Duration

The duration of the MUAP is determined by several factors:

1. The difference in arrival time between the earliest and latest SFAPs. Early and late SFAPs from muscle fibers close to the electrode have a major influence on duration.
2. The absolute number of muscle fibers in a motor unit. This is directly correlated with duration because even distant early- and late-arriving muscle fibers will contribute a few microvolts to the leading and trailing edges of the MUAP, respectively, keeping the MUAP amplitude above the threshold values for determining duration.
3. Increased fiber density. All other parameters being equal, this will increase the measured MUAP duration because the SFAPs from more muscle fibers at the leading and trailing edges of the MUAP make a detectable contribution to the potential detected by the electrode.

Amplitude

The amplitude of the MUAP is determined by the number of muscle fibers very close to the electrode. This in turn is a function of muscle fiber density and electrode position. When MUAP amplitude is dominated by a single fiber, the rise time of the major deflection is extremely short, and the MUAP amplitude changes drastically with minor changes in electrode position.

Motor Unit Action Potential Polyphasia

Motor unit action potential polyphasia is a difficult concept to define rigorously, and, in fact, there is no completely satisfactory method of measuring polyphasia. One definition of polyphasia states that the number of MUAP phases is equal to the number of baseline zero crossings plus one, with MUAPs having more than four phases being considered polyphasic (see Fig. 15-9). Although simple and convenient, this definition also is inadequate. The other definition of polyphasia is based on the number of slope reversals, known as serrations, in the MUAP. The serration definition, which is a more general index of polyphasia, is preferable because pathologic processes of interest may produce serrations without crossing the baseline.

Using the model developed so far, one can consider the MUAP that results if all SFAPs reach the electrode simultaneously. The resultant MUAP will resemble a large SFAP, and there will be no polyphasia.

The other extreme of polyphasia can be illustrated by considering a motor unit with ten muscle fibers located equidistant from the electrode. The arrival time of each SFAP will be chosen so that sequential SFAPs reach the electrode as the previous SFAP has almost passed by; ten SFAPs will line up head to tail. The resultant MUAP will have 20 phases, as determined by baseline crossings, plus one with no serrations. Sometimes, an SFAP will arrive so late that it is completely separated from the main MUAP. This is referred to as a satellite potential or linked potential and usually suggests reinnervation with immature, slowly conducting terminal nerve branches. If the arrival times of the SFAPs are moved closer together, the resultant MUAP becomes serrated with fewer baseline crossings but remains highly polyphasic. From these illustrations, it can be concluded that MUAP polyphasia is produced primarily by temporal dispersion of SFAPs from muscle fibers close to the electrode when there is enough temporal separation between SFAPs that they retain their individual identities.

Interference Pattern Analysis

The above discussion covers aspects of the MUAP that are easily analyzed only when individual MUAPs can be identified on the EMG machine screen—that is, only the first few motor units recruited can be studied in this fashion. When the number of motor units recruited is high enough that the discrete features of individual motor units can no longer be discerned, the electrical activity is referred to as the interference pattern. Several techniques for analyzing the interference pattern have been developed, most of them relying on computerized analysis. One useful characteristic of the interference pattern that can be estimated easily by eye during routine EMG is the amplitude of the envelope (i.e., the peak-to-peak amplitude of the interference pattern), which correlates well with the amplitudes of the larger MUAPs (97).

Motor Unit Recruitment

As discussed previously, the spinal cord modulates the force developed by a muscle by controlling both the number of motor units firing and the rate at which the motor units are firing. Excellent discussions of motor unit recruitment (MUR) can be found elsewhere (88,98–100). Now consider the case of a ramp contraction when the force developed by a muscle is gradually and slowly increased from zero up to a

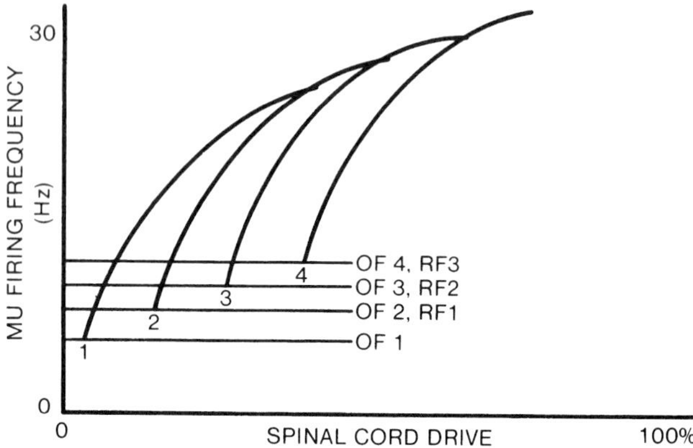

FIG. 15-12. Recruitment. Schematic representation of the discharge characteristics of the first four motor units recruited as the strength of the contraction increases. The electromyographer generally is focusing on the onset and recruitment frequencies of the first few motor units. In this model of recruitment, if motor unit *2* is lost for some reason, the onset frequency of unit *2* and the recruitment frequency of unit *1* are replaced by the onset frequency of unit 3 and the recruitment frequency of unit *2*. The average firing frequency of all motor units will be increased for the number of motor units that have been recruited. *OF*, onset frequency; *RF*, recruitment frequency.

moderate level. This may be 10% to 20% of a maximum voluntary contraction (MVC) for a normal muscle and up to 100% of an MVC in a weak muscle. This is the only type of contraction that is routinely of interest to the electromyographer performing the needle electrode examination. In a ramp contraction, motor units are recruited at their onset frequency and their rate of firing is increased (i.e., rate modulation) until the recruitment frequency is reached and an additional motor unit is recruited. Different muscles use recruitment and rate modulation to varying degrees (88). Disregarding the effects of inhibitory reflexes and other influences not covered here, recruitment will be discussed using the model in Figure 15-12. Detailed discussions of recruitment are provided by Burke (98,99), Henneman (100), and De Luca (88).

Motor unit action potential unit recruitment and modulation of firing rates are done by spinal cord-level mechanisms that receive their input from the corticospinal tracts as well as other neuronal systems. The intensity of this input signal is referred to as spinal cord drive; that is, a weak contraction has a low drive to the spinal cord mechanisms controlling a given muscle, whereas a strong contraction has a high drive.

Each motor neuron belonging to a given muscle pool possesses properties that determine the probability of firing at any given level of spinal cord drive. For example, the first unit recruited has a probability of firing at almost any nonzero spinal cord motor drive level, whereas the last motor unit recruited responds only to the maximum drive level. Low-threshold units are generally type I, fatigue-resistant units, whereas high-threshold units tend to be type II, rapidly fatigable motor units (98,99,101).

Increased spinal cord motor drive will first cause a motor unit to start discharging at its onset frequency when its recruitment threshold is reached. The discharge rate will continue to increase with increasing motor drive until a plateau value is reached.

Decreased Recruitment

Now consider the first six motor units normally recruited in a muscle and assume damage to the motor neurons belonging to motor units 2, 4, and 6 without affecting units 1, 3, and 5. Assume that this does not alter the recruitment properties of units 1, 3, and 5. When spinal cord drive increases to the level attained when the first six motor units were recruited, only units 1, 3, and 5 will be firing and less force will be developed, because the contributions of units 2, 4, and 6 will be missing. As the spinal cord drive is increased from zero, unit 1 is recruited normally, but the recruitment frequency for unit 1 is now the frequency at which unit 3 is recruited, not unit 2 as was the case previously; that is, unit 1 is firing more rapidly than normal when the next unit is recruited. A similar situation occurs for subsequent motor units recruited. Finally, to achieve the previous force levels, spinal cord drive must increase to produce a higher percentage of MVC, resulting in higher overall firing frequencies for each motor unit and perhaps the recruitment of additional motor units. Muscles with both normal and subnormal strength may demonstrate decreased motor unit recruitment. There may be a significant decrease in the number of functioning anterior horn cells innervating a muscle, producing decreased motor unit recruitment, but if all of the muscle fibers are reinnervated by functional axons, strength may be normal. This is frequently seen in old poliomyelitis. The presence of decreased recruitment therefore indicates that a significant percentage of the motor neurons or their axons originally innervating a muscle are nonfunctional. This may derive from irreversible causes (e.g., motor neuron death) or reversible causes (e.g., demyelination and conduction block of the axon). Decreased recruitment may therefore be reversible.

In summary, the major features of decreased recruitment are as follows:

- Elevated recruitment and onset frequencies
- Higher average firing rates of individual motor units for the number of motor units recruited.

This latter condition is the condition most often recognized in clinical practice because recruitment and onset frequencies usually are elevated by very small amounts that must be evaluated on a statistical basis unless axonal loss is extremely severe. It is most easily appreciated because motor units will be observed firing at high rates that would normally be obscured by the concomitant firing of other motor units. No knowledge of force production is necessary to identify the above conditions.

Unless the decrease in numbers of motor units is so severe

that the majority of units are recruited under the conditions used, this technique of examining recruitment involves only the first few motor units recruited, thereby ignoring a large part of the motor unit pool. Much effort has gone into examining late motor unit recruitment, but these techniques have limitations and are not routinely used. Note that the model assumes that axonal loss is randomly distributed over all types of motor units (i.e., early and late recruited units).

One feature of this recruitment model is that for decreased recruitment to occur, a large number of motor neurons must be nonfunctional, meaning that a loss of 5% to 20% of motor units or possibly even more probably will not be detectable. Recruitment analysis is a relatively insensitive indicator of the extent of neuronal damage and demonstrates unequivocal abnormalities only when a large percentage of motor neurons is nonfunctional. Unless highly quantitative research techniques are used, published studies generally show decreased motor unit recruitment only with fairly marked neurogenic lesions (102–105).

Semiquantitative techniques for analyzing decreased MUR during routine electromyography have met with limited success. Because of the statistical nature of MUR, there is little value in measuring the onset and recruitment frequencies of only a few motor units since changes in average firing rates are small unless the abnormalities are severe. This requires that a relatively large number of discharges be analyzed for the results to be statistically valid. It should also be noted that the firing rates of individual motor units are not normally constant, but fluctuate substantially from second to second (106). One method of estimating motor unit firing rates is to capture two or more sequential firings of a single motor unit on the EMG machine screen, and then measure the interpotential interval between these discharges, converting interpotential interval into firing rates. Unfortunately, a relatively wide range of firing rates may be obtained by this approach, depending on whether the motor unit was discharging at the maximum or minimum point of its firing range when the trace was captured. True quantitative analysis of MUR firing rates is therefore quite time consuming and not practical for routine clinical electromyographic studies. However, there are some rough rules of thumb that can be helpful when MUR is decreased near the threshold of detection. One observation is that when the firing frequency of the fastest firing motor unit on the EMG screen is divided by the number of active units, the ratio is approximately five, e.g., if the fastest unit is firing at 20 Hz and there are four active MU s, the ratio is five. In the author s experience, it is frequently difficult to separate out individual motor units and determine their firing rates until MUR is decreased, i.e., if you can easily identify four MUs on the screen and reliably determine that the fastest unit is firing at 20 Hz, MUR is very likely decreased.

Another very rough rule of thumb is that an onset frequency for the first MU of over 15 Hz is most likely indicative of decreased MUR. This is a very crude index and probably results in significant numbers of false negatives.

Newer computer-based decomposition algorithms are the best candidates for quantitative techniques to examine MUR. These techniques allow as many as the first eight motor units in a given region to be analyzed for firing rates in a relatively quantitative and statistical fashion. They will probably be significantly more sensitive in detecting decreased MUR than observational or semi-quantitative analysis. While they are not in widespread clinical use at this time, they hold significant promise for the future. More basic research and normative data is needed prior to their widespread application. As noted earlier, these techniques will be somewhat time consuming and probably not of routine use in every muscle. The electromyographer will still need to rely on observational analysis for the bulk of their work.

Muscle Strength and Recruitment Abnormalities

Recruitment abnormalities are related to muscle strength in most cases, and the electromyographer should learn when, as well as when not to expect recruitment abnormalities based on the results of clinical manual muscle testing (MMT; see Chapter 5). The following discussion refers to qualitative MMT and qualitative analysis of motor unit recruitment as performed during routine clinical studies. Some minor exceptions to the statements made below may exist when highly quantitative research techniques are used.

The observed maximum isometric force generated during any joint movement depends on multiple factors, including:

1. The specific maximum tetanic tension (P_0) of the muscle per cross-sectional area (Newtons/cm^2)
2. The effective muscle cross-sectional area, related to internal muscle architecture (e.g., angle of pennation)
3. The biomechanics of the joint-muscle complex (e.g., effective instantaneous lever arms).

Although much work is being done in this area, it is not yet possible practically to determine all of these parameters for each joint or movement of clinical interest, and the clinician must therefore rely on clinical intuition and experience to estimate what can be called predicted strength for observed muscle bulk and joint condition under test conditions. Unless weakness of a particular movement is so marked that is allows identification on absolute grounds, weakness usually is identified as an asymmetry of strength from side to side.

Several points must be made regarding MMT:

1. The maximum strength of a given movement has not been adequately tested unless the muscles producing that movement have been overpowered during a true maximal contraction and forced into an eccentric (i.e., lengthening) contraction. As an example, a patient may have weakness of elbow flexion with 50 pound-feet of torque on the normal side and 25 pound-feet on the involved side. If the applied test torque is only 20 pound-feet, neither side will be overpowered and will appear

identical (i.e., no weakness will be identified). If the test torque is increased to 40 pound-feet, the weak, but not the normal, side will be overpowered and the weakness will be clearly identified but not quantitated. If the test torque is increased to more than 50 pound-feet, both sides will be overcome and the actual degree of weakness can be estimated.
2. An ideal MMT protocol will therefore overcome every tested movement by use of optimal examiner-patient positioning, leverage, and the like. The ability to do this is a function of technique as well as the relative strength of the examiner and the patient. Additionally, some movers such as ankle plantarflexors or hip extensors are so strong that regardless of the strength of the examiner, they are impossible to test adequately in many patients unless marked weakness is present.
3. Unless the examiner has overcome all muscle groups tested, the results of MMT should be described as unremarkable, not normal, so as to avoid reinforcing the thought that the MMT was adequate.

For the prime movers of any particular joint movement, clinical weakness will be present if:

1. The specific tetanic tension of the prime movers is below normal, as can occur with many myopathies.
2. The functional cross-sectional area of the prime movers is low (e.g., secondary to atrophy of any etiology).
3. Motor units are incompletely activated and their firing rate does not reach the tetanic frequency (e.g., poor volition or upper motor neuron lesions).
4. Motor units or muscle fibers are not activated (e.g., secondary to conduction block, axonotmesis, or other failure of the anterior horn cell/axon).

Only the last condition is of interest with respect to recruitment because no true abnormalities of recruitment will be present with conditions 1 through 3. This effectively restricts the following discussion to neurogenic lesions. For purposes of discussion, the following will refer only to compressive neurogenic lesions, although there is no evidence to suggest that the rationale applied does not generalize to other types of neurogenic lesions as well.

The relationship between abnormalities of muscle strength and motor unit recruitment are as follows:

1. In a previously normal muscle, weakness from an acute compressive lesion is the result of a certain percentage of muscle fibers not being activated as a result of conduction block or interruption of their motor axons. Because this is the same mechanism by which recruitment abnormalities are produced, there will be a direct link between weakness and abnormal recruitment in this situation. Loss of functioning motor units must produce some weakness since the muscle fibers belonging to the inactivated motor units are no longer contributing to force generation. High quality manual muscle testing should be able to detect weakness in the range of 10% with side-to-side comparison. Note that MUAP characteristics will initially be normal in this setting.
2. If there has been a previous permanent loss of motor neurons supplying a muscle (e.g., old polio, compressive radiculopathy) and all muscle fibers have subsequently been reinnervated, maximal strength will be normal. Motor unit recruitment abnormalities related to loss of functioning anterior horn cells may be present if the extent of permanent loss was sufficient, but in this case, the acquisition of additional muscle fibers by remaining motor units will result in increases in MUAP amplitude, duration, and polyphasia.
3. We may therefore conclude that, for practical purposes in a clinical setting, motor unit recruitment abnormalities will not be observed in an adequately tested muscle that demonstrates normal strength, except under condition 2 above. Stated another way, if a muscle demonstrates normal strength with adequate testing and the MUAPs are essentially normal, recruitment almost certainly will be normal. This statement needs to be qualified to recognize that some movements are complex and involve many muscles (e.g., wrist flexion–extension). In this situation, significant weakness in one muscle might be masked by strong function in the remaining movers of that joint. Recruitment abnormalities might then be seen in the weak muscle in the face of what appears to be essentially normal strength of that movement.

It is also hypothesized that the AHC/axons to motor units in a small region of the muscle may be damaged, leaving the majority of axons to the muscle intact. Note that this is really a special, intramuscular, variant of the situation discussed immediately above. It is theoretically possible under these circumstances that abnormalities of MUR could be observed in a small portion of the muscle, but not the entire muscle. This might occur in the absence of detectable weakness. This explanation for possible decreased MUR should be used with caution when the examiner thinks he or she is observing decreased MUR restricted to a small portion of the muscle, but it may well occur. The author is not aware of any published literature specifically addressing this issue.

From the above, the following generalizations can be made:

- If the electromyographer has tested a muscle's strength adequately, finds it to be normal, finds normal MUAPs, and thinks that decreased MUR is present, he or she is probably making either a technical error or error in interpretation in one or more of these phenomena, or the muscle has not been adequately tested. A less likely possibility is that one of the exceptions noted above is being observed.
- Manual muscle testing frequently is more sensitive in identifying conduction block or axonotmesis than is recruitment analysis, unless the muscle cannot be adequately tested manually (e.g., a low examiner-to-patient strength

ratio for that particular movement or the muscle is part of a complex movement using many muscles where most of the other muscles are functioning well). In the author's experience, a Medical Research Council (MRC) level of approximately 4 − /5 to 4/5 is the minimum level of weakness at which one expects to find decreased motor unit recruitment in a muscle with normal motor units.

To summarize, the electromyographer should think of detection of decreased motor unit recruitment as being a situation where one can see the holes in the interference pattern, not the active motor units. This is analogous to leaves falling off a tree in autumn. It is easy to look at the ground and estimate the number of leaves that have fallen, but the tree must lose a large percentage of its leaves before an observer can begin to see through the tree to the other side. The loss of a few leaves will not be detected simply by observation of the tree itself because the remaining leaves are still sufficient to block the sight path through the tree. Recruitment analysis looks at the tree, not the leaves on the ground.

It should be obvious to the reader that, in the presence of upper motor neuron lesions, pain inhibition or poor volition, manual muscle testing is no longer a valid test of motor unit function. It is only when manual muscle testing actually reflects true maximal strength that the above relationships will hold.

In summary, MUR abnormalities should be expected with:

1. Acute/recent lower motor neuron (LMN) lesions associated with weakness below approximately the 4 − /5 to 4/5 level (MRC scale). Decreased MUR may be very valuable in these situations in that its presence reliably differentiates between organically based peripheral neuromuscular dysfunction and problems such as upper motor neuron (UMN) lesions, neuromuscular junction disorders, myopathic processes, malingering, hysteria, pain inhibition, and poor volition. Also note that decreased MUR is present as soon as the AHC ceases to function. This makes its presence particularly valuable in acute processes, since the electromyographer need not wait for the abnormality to develop. This is in contrast to other electrodiagnostic abnormalities such as spontaneous activity, MUAP abnormalities, etc., all of which require days, weeks, or months to develop. This can be extremely valuable in acute situations, e.g., where the electromyographer might need to differentiate between acute Guillain-Barré syndrome and upper motor lesions such as some cases of transverse myelitis, etc.. The unequivocal presence of decreased MUR in this setting essentially documents a lower motor neuron etiology.
2. Old/chronic lesions that have resulted in loss of a significant percentage of the AHC previously present in that muscle. This may be associated with either normal strength or weakness, depending on whether the efficiency of reinnervation was close to 100%. Motor unit action potential amplitude, duration, and/or polyphasia will be unequivocally increased in this situation. Increases in these MUAP parameters can more easily be detected than can decreased MUR, so that as these lesions evolve, increases in MUAP parameters will be noted before the appearance of decreased MUR. In general, the more marked the MUAP increases, the more MUR is decreased.
3. Acute/recent lesions not associated with weakness if the MMT was inadequate.

Times not to expect MUR abnormalities:

1. Acute/recent lesions not associated with weakness if the MMT was adequate.
2. Old/chronic lesions not associated with a loss of a significant percentage of the AHC previously present in that muscle. MUAP parameters are no more than mildly increased in this setting.
3. Disorders/problems such as UMN lesions, neuromuscular junction disorders, myopathic processes, malingering, hysteria, pain inhibition, and poor volition. To the experienced examiner, it is usually, although not always, clear when these conditions are present. MUR analysis usually differentiates reliably between weakness secondary these etiologies and weakness on the basis of peripheral neuromuscular dysfunction if weakness exceeds approximately the 4 − /5 range (MRC scale). MUR probably does not reliably differentiate between these entities when weakness is less marked than this.

Abnormalities Detected by Needle Electrode Examination

The motor unit changes described in subsequent paragraphs are artificially separated according to the underlying mechanism. Many real-life situations will have several of these mechanisms operating simultaneously, producing abnormalities that are the sum of the individual phenomena. Partial loss refers to the loss of a percentage of the motor neurons innervating a given muscle. The reader should review Stalberg for additional information (107).

Significant Partial and Permanent Axonal or Motor Neuron Loss, Discrete Insult, No Continuing Axonal Loss, With Surviving Axons

Partial and permanent axonal or motor neuron loss may be seen in partial nerve transection (i.e., axonotmetic lesion), acute poliomyelitis, some cases of Guillain-Barré syndrome, radiculopathy, plexopathy, and other lesions producing partial axonal disruption. The common factor in each of these situations is that a significant number of muscle fibers is denervated and the remaining motor unit axons are capable of sprouting to reinnervate these muscle fibers. The findings here may be arbitrarily classified according to time course.

Initial Findings

Decreased recruitment will be present immediately when axonal loss occurs, but the axonal loss must be extensive for decreased recruitment to be detected. After an appropriate time interval (1 to 3 weeks) has elapsed, spontaneous activity will be present in the form of positive sharp waves and fibrillations. Spontaneous activity may be present even if only a small percentage of axons are lost (e.g., 2% to 3%).

Intermediate Findings

Remaining motor units pick up additional muscle fibers by axonal sprouting, producing increased fiber density and increased MUAP amplitude, duration, and polyphasia. In addition, conduction velocities in immature nerve terminals are slow, resulting in increased temporal dispersion and leading to increased duration, polyphasia, and possibly satellite or linked potentials. The magnitude of the motor unit abnormalities will increase as more and more muscle fibers are added to each motor unit. Spontaneous activity may disappear if all muscle fibers are reinnervated.

Late Findings

As the previous processes advance, it is hypothesized that maturation of terminal nerves and subsequent increases in conduction velocity will partially offset the increases in duration and polyphasia caused by increased fiber density, whereas the addition of more muscle fibers to the motor unit and increased conduction velocity of maturing new terminal nerve branches both contribute to increased MUAP amplitude (e.g., more SFAPs arriving at the electrode position in a more synchronous manner). This may explain why in cases of old, recovered motor neuron lesions, as seen in old poliomyelitis, increased MUAP amplitude is the dominant abnormality, whereas increased polyphasia is less prominent. Remodeling of motor units also may contribute to this process; for example, a single muscle fiber contributing to increased MUAP polyphasia and duration as a result of being innervated by a long, slowly conducting terminal nerve branch may be transiently denervated and become part of another motor unit where it does not contribute significantly to increased duration or polyphasia.

The extent of the changes seen will be proportional to the number of motor units denervated. As the percentage of motor units denervated increases, more muscle fibers will have to be picked up by fewer remaining functional motor units and the average percent increase in the number of muscle fibers per motor unit will be larger. Spontaneous activity may or may not be present, depending on whether all muscle fibers have been reinnervated.

Discussion

If it is hypothesized that a motor unit must increase its number of muscle fibers by 5% to 20% before MUAP changes can be detected (possibly an underestimate); then spontaneous activity should be seen at some point after injury since that many muscle fibers probably cannot be acutely denervated without spontaneous activity being present at some time. Spontaneous activity will resolve if all denervated fibers are reinnervated. Minor injuries (i.e., approximately 5% of fibers denervated) probably will not be detectable through MUAP configuration changes, although spontaneous activity should be present at some time.

Although quantitative data in all clinical situations are lacking, it generally is believed that depending on the nature and extent of the pathologic insult, a minimum of approximately 4 weeks is required for enough reinnervation to occur to produce detectable MUAP changes (107,108). If the electromyographer finds unequivocal MUAP changes 1 day after an acute partial nerve transection, these cannot be caused by the lesion in question; they must be the result of some previous lesion.

Severe or Complete Neuronal Loss with Reinnervation

If the majority of axons innervating a muscle are disrupted, and enough time has passed to allow some reinnervation to occur, a different picture is obtained. In this case, the majority of MUAPs will be newly created by neurons regrowing into the denervated muscle, rather than by modification of preexisting motor units. The MUAP will have few muscle fibers initially and will subsequently add more muscle fibers until large numbers belong to each motor unit. Because of the low number of muscle fibers present in early motor units formed in this manner, as well as the temporal dispersion produced by slow conduction velocities in immature nerve sprouts, the resultant MUAPs typically have a long duration and low amplitude and are very polyphasic. This type of motor unit is known in the older literature as a nascent motor unit. There also will be a short period in which the motor unit has so few fibers that the duration may be short. As additional muscle fibers are added, these MUAPs eventually will evolve into the long-duration, high-amplitude polyphasic MUAPs characteristic of neurogenic injuries that will evolve as described in the previous section. Profuse spontaneous activity should be present within 1 to 3 weeks after the injury and should persist for long periods of time.

Partial Axonal Loss with Surviving Axons, With or Without Discrete Injury, with Ongoing Axonal Loss and Reinnervation

Partial axonal loss with surviving axons is seen in most axonal neuropathies, MND, and some radiculopathies, plexopathies, and compressive neuropathies. The electrodiagnostic findings relative to MUAP configuration changes here are similar to those discussed previously, except that the number of denervated muscle fibers at any one time may be small, and these few fibers may be reinnervated before they develop detectable spontaneous activity. Therefore, MUAP changes can be seen without evidence of spontaneous activity. In these cases, SFEMG may demonstrate the increased jitter of immature neuromuscular junctions associated with denervation and subsequent reinnervation. With very slowly progressive lesions, as seen in some cases of MND, markedly increased amplitude with less prominent polyphasia may be the predominant feature for the same reasons postulated in previous paragraphs.

It can be hypothesized that as axons are lost in the above manner, decreased motor unit recruitment should accompany the development of MUAP changes. Motor unit action potential changes probably are more easily detected than decreased recruitment, so that the detection of the former is not invariably linked to the unequivocal detection of the latter early in the course of this type of process.

Demyelination of Terminal Nerve Branches

Demyelination of terminal nerve branches is seen in acute demyelinating neuropathic processes, such as Guillain-Barré syndrome, CIDPs, and neuropathies such as HSMN I, III, and IV. It is frequently accompanied by axonal loss.

This phenomenon will increase MUAP duration and polyphasia while possibly decreasing MUAP amplitude if no axonal loss and reinnervation are involved. That is, arrival time differences at the electrode between first and last fibers increase, producing increased polyphasia and duration while the decreased synchrony of SFAP arrival actually decreases MUAP amplitude. Conduction block in terminal nerve sprouts also may contribute to decreased MUAP amplitude. If there is accompanying axonal loss, which is frequently seen, and enough time has elapsed for reinnervation to occur, MUAP amplitude will increase, producing the classic finding associated with neurogenic lesions as described previously.

Processes Producing Severe Atrophy of Muscle Fibers Without Segmental Necrosis of Muscle Fibers

Processes producing severe muscle fiber atrophy are seen in myopathies (e.g., corticosteroid myopathies) in which relatively little actual necrosis of muscle fibers occurs. The predominant underlying process is a decrease in muscle fiber diameter, as well as possible metabolic dysfunction, resulting in a decrease in the SFAP amplitude. This leads to decreased MUAP duration and amplitude with no or minimal increases in polyphasia. Spontaneous activity usually is not seen in these conditions.

Acute Processes Involving Random Segmental Necrosis and Atrophy of Muscle Fibers or Random Denervation of Individual Muscle Fibers

Segmental necrosis may be seen in inflammatory and other myopathies. Because muscle fibers are innervated only at one location, any lesion that anatomically interrupts the muscle fibers produces for all practical purposes two muscle fibers, one that is innervated and one that is not. If the segmental necrosis is extensive and some segments of the muscle fiber are far away from the innervation zone, these muscle segments may never be reinnervated. The result will be chronic spontaneous activity. Some myopathic processes, such as polymyositis, also damage terminal nerve branches and may produce a completely denervated muscle fiber (109). Extensive damage to the neuromuscular junction by botulism toxin may produce similar results. Spontaneous activity therefore is common at some stage of these disorders.

The MUAP lesions seen in this type of process are similar to those described in the previous section, except that the actual loss of muscle fibers results in even greater decreases in MUAP duration and amplitude in the acute setting, whereas the presence of reinnervation can increase MUAP polyphasia or duration later on. Fiber splitting, seen in some myopathies, also may contribute to polyphasia.

Chronic or Old Myopathies with Segmental Necrosis

Reinnervation of denervated muscle segments and fibers may occur, producing changes similar to those discussed for various neuropathic processes. Additionally, if many muscle fibers are not reinnervated and atrophy or degenerate, it is hypothesized that the interfiber distances between muscle fibers belonging to a given motor unit may decrease, resulting in higher muscle fiber density. These factors may produce long-duration, moderately high-amplitude, polyphasic MUAPs in chronic myopathies. A mix of long-duration and short-duration MUAPs may be seen in these situations as well. In some cases, this may produce confusion in the attempt to differentiate chronic neuropathic from chronic myopathic processes.

Abnormal Neuromuscular Transmission of the Type Seen in Myasthenia Gravis

By the criteria and techniques applied in routine clinical examinations, the MUAP seen with myasthenia-gravis-type neuromuscular junction dysfunction has an essentially normal configuration except for moment-to-moment variability in amplitude (110). This variability in amplitude is secondary to the intermittent failure of neuromuscular transmission in individual muscle fibers and therefore can be seen in any disorder in which neuromuscular transmission is abnormal. When examining moment-to-moment variability, the electrodiagnostician must make sure that superimposition of other MUAPs is excluded and that electrode position is absolutely constant. If these precautions are observed, normal MUAPs will have almost no variability in amplitude ($<1\%$) (111).

If the defect in neuromuscular transmission is so severe that transmission is continuously failing in a large percentage of the neuromuscular junctions in each motor unit, short-duration, low-amplitude, polyphasic MUAPs may result.

TABLE 15-1. *Typical effects of repetitive stimulation on motor evoked response amplitudes in several commonly encountered neuromuscular disorders*

Disorder	Single response (normal range 5 to 20 mV)	2-Hz stimulation, rested muscle (normal: decrement <5% to 8%)	20- to 50-Hz stimulation or 2-Hz stimulation immediately postexercise (normal: may increment <20% to 50%)	2-Hz stimulation 2 to 4 min. postexercise (normal: decrement <5% to 8%)
Myasthenia gravis	Normal or low Usually >80% Lower limit of normal	Normal, mild, or marked decrement 0 to 60%	Decrement partially or completely repaired	Decrement may increase or appear (decrement may be present only under these conditions)
Myasthenic syndrome	Low 5% to 90% Lower limit of normal	>5% to 8% decrement	Marked increment 100% to 2000% of baseline response	Decrement may increase
Botulism	Normal or low	Normal or >5% to 8% decrement	No change (severe cases) or increment (mild cases)	Facilitation may persist

This should not be interpreted as suggesting a superimposed myopathic process.

The above phenomena depend on the presence of large amounts of neuromuscular junction blocking, and are not likely to be present if the results of repetitive stimulation studies are not significantly abnormal.

Increased jitter may be observed in MUAPs at fast sweep speeds (e.g., <5- to 10-msec total sweep duration) but not at settings normally used for routine MUAP analysis (e.g., 100-msec total sweep duration).

Abnormal Neuromuscular Transmission of the Type Seen in the Eaton–Lambert Myasthenic Syndrome

As in myasthenia gravis, the MUAP seen in ELMS has significant moment-to-moment variability in amplitude. The characteristic feature of MUAPs in ELMS is that the amplitude is relatively low at low firing frequencies and increases to near normal levels as the motor unit firing rate increases. Increased jitter and blocking seen in ELMS also is rate dependent, improving with higher firing rates (112).

Short-duration, low-amplitude, polyphasic MUAPs may be seen in ELMS for the same reasons given above for myasthenia gravis and should be interpreted in a similar manner. The MUAP abnormalities in ELMS, observed at low firing rates, will generally be more marked than for MG since the neuromuscular junction in ELS is failing at rest, not after use. Single fiber EMG jitter is extremely abnormal in ELMS.

ELECTRODIAGNOSTIC FINDINGS IN NEUROMUSCULAR DISORDERS

The basic electrodiagnostic abnormalities observed in various neuromuscular disorders are summarized in this section. The text by Brown and Boulton is highly recommended and should be considered a major reference for this information (2). Summaries of typical electrodiagnostic findings in neuromuscular diseases are listed in Tables 15-1 through 15-4.

TABLE 15-2. *Typical electrodiagnostic results of motor nerve conduction studies in commonly encountered neuromuscular disorders*

Disorder	Distal latency	Conduction velocity	Evoked response amplitude	Temporal dispersion	Conduction block	Late responses
Motor neuron disease						
Mild	Usually normal	Usually normal	Usually normal	Usually normal	None	Usually normal
Advanced	Normal or slightly prolonged	Normal or slightly decreased	Usually decreased	Usually normal	None	Normal or mildly prolonged
Entrapment neuropathy						
Mild	Prolonged if across lesion	Slow across lesion	Usually normal	Usually normal	Normal to mild	Normal
Severe	Prolonged if across lesion	Slow across lesion	Usually decreased	Normal or slightly increased	Mild to marked	May be mildly prolonged if lesion is proximal to stimulus site
Radiculopathy	Normal	Usually normal	Normal unless severe	Normal	None (distally)	May be slightly prolonged if severe
Neuromuscular junction disorders	Normal	Normal	Normal or decreased	Normal	None	Normal
Myopathies	Normal	Normal	Normal or decreased	Normal	None	Normal

TABLE 15-3. *Typical electrodiagnostic results of motor nerve conduction studies in polyneuropathies*

Disorder	Distal latency	Conduction velocity	Evoked response amplitude	Temporal dispersion	Conduction block	Late responses
Axonal polyneuropathy						
Mild	Normal or slightly prolonged	Normal or slightly decreased	Usually normal	Usually normal	Usually none	Normal or slightly prolonged
Severe	Normal or prolonged	Usually slightly decreased	Usually decreased (may be marked)	Normal or slightly increased	None to minimal	May be mildly prolonged or absent
Demyelinating polyneuropathy						
Mild	Usually prolonged	Usually decreased	Normal or decreased	Normal to marked[a]	None to mild	Normal to aprolonged or absent
Severe	Usually prolonged (may be marked)	Usually decreased (may be marked)	Usually decreased	Normal to marked[a]	Mild to marked	Usually prolonged or absent

[a] Temporal dispersion may be prominent in acquired demyelinating polyneuropathies, whereas it is less marked in hereditary polyneuropathies.

Motor Neuron Disease

The reader is referred to the references by Daube for a comprehensive discussion of the electrodiagnostic abnormalities in generalized MND (113–115). The reader should appreciate that MND describes a group of diseases, and that MND is not necessarily synonymous with amyotrophic lateral sclerosis (ALS). Focal and monomelic forms of MND (i.e., Sobuye's disease) are also described (116–119).

Sensory Nerve Conduction Studies

Sensory nerve conduction studies generally are normal, although minor abnormalities may be seen (120,121). The presence of significant electrodiagnostic sensory abnormalities suggests either a different or additional diagnosis.

Late Responses

F_response and H reflex latencies generally are normal.

Repetitive Stimulation

A small decrement may be present if extensive denervation–reinnervation is occurring. The presence of a decrement is a negative prognostic factor, signifying relatively rapid motor neuron loss. In addition to denervation–reinnervation, there is recent evidence suggesting that neuromuscular junction function may be primarily affected in ALS as well (122).

Motor Nerve Conduction Studies

The results of motor nerve conduction studies are either normal or demonstrate low evoked response amplitudes. Sig-

TABLE 15-4. *Typical electrodiagnostic results of sensory nerve conduction studies in commonly encountered neuromuscular disorders*

Disorder	Distal latency	Conduction velocity	Evoked response amplitude	Temporal dispersion	Conduction block
Motor neuron disease					
Mild	Normal	Normal	Normal	Normal	None
Advanced	Normal	Normal	Normal	Normal	None
Polyneuropathy					
Axonal					
Mild	Normal or prolonged	Normal or slightly low	Normal or decreased	Normal or slightly increased	None to slight
Severe	Usually prolonged	Usually slightly low	Decreased or absent	Normal or slightly increased	None to slight
Demyelinating					
Mild	Usually prolonged	Usually decreased	Normal or decreased	Usually increased	None to moderate
Severe	Prolonged (may be marked)	Decreased (may be marked)	Decreased or absent	Usually increased (may be marked)	None to marked
Entrapment neuropathy					
Mild	Prolonged if across lesion	Slow across lesion	Normal or low	Usually normal to mildly increased	Normal or slight
Severe	Prolonged if across lesion	Slow across lesion	Low or absent	Normal to moderately increased	Slight to marked
Radiculopathy	Normal	Normal	Normal	Normal	None
Neuromuscular junction disorders	Normal	Normal	Normal	Normal	None
Myopathies	Normal	Normal	Normal	Normal	None

nificant conduction block or temporal dispersion generally is not present, although evoked responses may appear dispersed as an artifact of markedly reduced amplitudes. Conduction velocities may be mildly decreased if the evoked response amplitude is very low. Low motor-evoked response amplitudes are associated with a poor overall prognosis. In some cases, multifocal motor neuropathy may mimic MND, and the presence of proximal conduction block specifically should be sought in these cases (123–125).

Needle Electrode Examination

Spontaneous activity may be present and is a negative prognostic factor in that it signifies either a very rapid axonal loss or loss of a large percentage of the original motor neurons (114,115). The MUAP abnormalities noted are those associated with progressive chronic motor neuron loss. The dominant abnormality is the presence of MUAPs with moderately to markedly increased amplitude and lesser degrees of increased polyphasia and duration. Late in the disease process, low-amplitude, short-duration, polyphasic MUAPs may occur along with the larger MUAPs as individual motor units degenerate and possess only a few muscle fibers.

Discussion

The electrodiagnostic abnormalities of advanced MND usually are marked and widespread, involving all four extremities and possibly bulbar muscles. Early MND, however, can present in a radicular or much less commonly, a peripheral nerve distribution, making it difficult in some cases to differentiate MND from other neurologic disorders, such as syringomyelia, radiculopathy, polyradiculopathy, or neuropathies when sensory abnormalities are not prominent (e.g., multifocal motor neuropathies). Previous neurologic disease resulting in the loss of significant numbers of motor neurons (e.g., old poliomyelitis) also may mimic MND electrodiagnostically. Electrodiagnostic studies generally should not be considered as strongly supporting the diagnosis of MND unless abnormalities are present in three or more extremities or bulbar muscles, and previous neurologic disease resulting in the loss of anterior horn cells has been ruled out. Even with these criteria, old poliomyelitis or multiple radiculopathies secondary to bony spine disease involving both cervical and lumbosacral regions may be difficult to differentiate electrodiagnostically from MND. The diagnosis of MND must therefore be based on both clinical and electrodiagnostic criteria (126).

In the evaluation of possible MND in the childhood and adolescent years (e.g., Werdnig-Hoffmann disease, Kugelberg-Welander disease), the differential diagnosis discussed above is much less of a factor, because superimposed diseases are present less frequently.

Multifocal Motor Neuropathies

It has been recognized in recent years that multifocal motor neuropathy (MMN) is a condition that can mimic true MND. This applies primarily to lower motor neuron presentations of MND, not MND variants such as ALS, which have a significant component of upper motor signs. Multifocal motor neuropathy is not associated with upper motor neuron signs and symptoms. Although MMN is relatively rare, differentiating MMN from MND has become important because of the therapeutic implications; i.e., MMN is a potentially treatable condition, whereas true motor neuron disease is for the most part untreatable. The MMN probably represents a predominantly motor variant of a chronic inflammatory demyelinating polyneuropathy (127). The AAEM minimonograph by Parry (127) is an excellent summary of the clinical and electrodiagnostic features of MMN. A key feature of MMN versus MND is that abnormalities in MMN tend to occur in the distribution of peripheral nerves, trunks, etc., whereas the most common pattern in MND is that of spinal segmental involvement. In performing electrodiagnostic studies, care must be taken to study involved distributions because uninvolved nerves may demonstrate normal electrodiagnostic studies. This frequently means performing special motor nerve conduction studies, e.g., radial, axillary, musculocutaneous nerve conduction studies in addition to the more commonly studied nerves, e.g., median, ulnar.

Sensory Nerve Conduction Studies

Distal sensory nerve conduction studies generally are normal, although mild abnormalities are not uncommon (127–129). The primary feature of MMN is that motor abnormalties are far out of proportion to the sensory abnormalities noted, not the fact that it is an absolutely pure motor syndrome. Sensory conduction may occur normally in a segment of nerve where profound motor nerve conduction abnormalities are present.

Late Responses

F_response and H reflex latencies may be prolonged in involved nerves.

Repetitive Stimulation

A small decrement may be present if extensive denervation–reinnervation is occurring.

Motor Nerve Conduction Studies

The hallmark of MMN is motor conduction block in focal segments of involved nerves. This is frequently severe by the time that most patients present for study and can be as high as 80% to 100%. These abnormalities are presumably less marked in patients who are diagnosed early. Nerve conduction velocities in the involved focal segments are usually markedly reduced, but may be essentially normal or only minimally abnormal in uninvolved segments of an affected nerve or in uninvolved nerves. Amplitudes of distal responses are frequently reduced, reflecting a component of axonal involvement. The distal amplitude can be a clue to the diagnosis in that a normal or only mildly reduced motor evoked response amplitude in a profoundly weak muscle strongly suggests the possibility of conduction block in proximal sites.

Needle Electrode Examination

The needle electrode examination is generally abnormal and usually demonstrates spontaneous activity such as positive waves and fibrillations, reflecting an axonal component to the process. Myokymia may also be seen, a rare finding in true motor neuron disease. At the time of diagnosis, motor unit action potentials are usually increased in duration, polyphasia, and amplitude, reflecting an element of denervation and reinnervation over the usual long duration of the disease prior to diagnosis. Presumably, these changes are less prominent in those atypical cases where the diagnosis is made relatively early. Motor unit recruitment in weak muscles is usually markedly decreased.

The following pattern of abnormalities in the needle electrode examination has been of use to the author in identifying presumed conduction block in special cases, supporting a diagnosis of MMN when this could not clearly be demonstrated on the basis of nerve conduction studies alone. One patient, whose long-term clinical course has been consistent with MMN, presented initially with a 6- to 12-month history of progressive weakness in multiple extremities without significant clinical or electrodiagnostic sensory findings, and could not be shown to demonstrate classic conduction block on any standard motor nerve conduction studies. On needle electrode exam, the patient was noted to have essentially normal MUAPs with the exception of mildly increased polyphasia. Very little spontaneous activity was present. Motor unit recruitment was dramatically decreased in muscles that were clinically weak. These findings persisted without significant change over several months.

The near normal MUAP characteristics suggested that there had been very little permanent cumulative axonal loss over the previous 6 to 12 months. The markedly decreased motor unit recruitment suggested that a large percentage of the motor axons were nonfunctional because of either conduction block or axonal interruption. If the decreased MUR were secondary to axonal interruption, one would postulate that large amounts of spontaneous activity such as positive waves and fibrillations should have been present at some point in time. The minimal nature of the spontaneous activity observed suggested that the predominant etiology of the decreased MUR was either large amounts of conduction block in the motor axon, or, less likely, large amounts of very recent axonal damage where spontaneous activity had not had time to develop. Large amounts of spontaneous activity did not develop in the next several months, disfavoring the later possibility. The electrodiagnostic observation of near-normal MUAPs, markedly decreased MUR, and minimal spontaneous activity over weeks to months of observation, therefore suggests that conduction block is the basis for the patient's decrease MUR and clinical weakness, not axonal interruption. It is unlikely that this situation would develop in classical motor neuron disease, and these findings strongly support the diagnosis of MMN.

Polyneuropathies

There are many different hereditary and acquired etiologies of peripheral nerve dysfunction that affect distal and proximal, and motor and sensory components of the peripheral nervous system in a differential fashion, with or without significant demyelination. Different disease processes also may vary widely in their temporal course. Consequently, many different motor, sensory, axonal, demyelinating, anatomic, and temporal patterns of electrodiagnostic abnormalities can be seen, although more severe involvement usually occurs in distal locations and lower extremities (130). The specifics of individual disease processes are discussed elsewhere (39,130–136).

Sensory Nerve Conduction Studies

Electrodiagnostic sensory abnormalities may include prolonged distal latencies, abnormal conduction velocities, conduction block, temporal dispersion, and decreased evoked response amplitudes. Significant temporal dispersion suggests an acquired multifocal demyelinating polyneuropathy (see Table 15-4).

F_Response

The F_response, if obtainable, usually is moderately to markedly prolonged in neuropathies in which demyelination is prominent and is normal to mildly prolonged in other neuropathies. It frequently is unobtainable when the neuropathy is severe, regardless of the underlying mechanism.

H Reflex

The H reflex follows a pattern similar to that observed for the F_response.

Repetitive Stimulation

A small decrement may be present if large amounts of denervation and reinnervation are present.

Motor Nerve Conduction Studies

As in sensory nerve conduction studies, electrodiagnostic motor nerve conduction study abnormalities may include prolonged distal latencies, abnormal conduction velocities, conduction block, temporal dispersion, and decreased evoked response amplitudes (see Table 15-3). Significant temporal dispersion suggests an acquired multifocal demyelinating polyneuropathy (37–39). In many neuropathies, temporal dispersion and conduction block must be determined solely from motor nerve conduction studies because the proximal sensory response may not be detectable.

Needle Electrode Examination

Spontaneous Activity

If axonal loss is occurring at a significant rate and sufficient time has elapsed, spontaneous activity usually will be present. If the rate of axonal loss is low and reinnervation is occurring rapidly, significant axonal loss may occur without detectable spontaneous activity.

Motor Unit Action Potentials

If a substantial percentage of the axons supplying a muscle has been lost and the denervated muscle fibers have been added to remaining motor units, MUAP amplitude, duration, and polyphasia will increase in proportion to the number of muscle fibers added to the average motor unit.

Motor Unit Recruitment

Motor unit recruitment will be decreased if a substantial percentage of the motor axons is lost. For technical reasons, MUAP conformation changes probably will be detectable before recruitment abnormalities are unequivocally present.

Entrapment Neuropathies

The most common entrapment neuropathies are those of the median nerve at the wrist (56,137,138), the ulnar nerve at the elbow (139,140), the peroneal nerve at the fibular head (51), and the tarsal tunnel syndrome (141,142), although many other variants occur (143–146). Hallett (147) and Wilbourn (51) have provided excellent discussion of the general pathophysiology underlying entrapment neuropathies. Additional major references include Dawson and colleagues (148) and Pecina and associates (149).

Sensory Nerve Conduction Studies

Abnormalities noted on sensory nerve conduction studies include slowing of the SNAP across the lesion, mild temporal dispersion, and decreased evoked response amplitudes secondary to either temporal dispersion, conduction block, or axonotmesis.

F_Response

F_response latencies may be prolonged in cases where severe focal compression is present. They will be most sensitive if the stimulus is applied distal to the lesion since the action potential must cross the lesion twice in this situation. F_response latencies usually are very insensitive in detecting entrapment neuropathies owing to the long length of normal nerve included in the conduction pathway. They are not highly valuable in the detection of uncomplicated entrapment neuropathies.

Motor Nerve Conduction Studies

As is the case for sensory nerve, abnormalities noted include slowing of the nerve action potential across the lesion, mild temporal dispersion, and decreased evoked response amplitudes secondary to either conduction block or axonotmesis.

Needle Electrode Examination

If axonotmesis has occurred and sufficient time has elapsed, spontaneous activity may be detected on needle electrode examination. If a large percentage of axons are nonconducting for any reason, motor unit recruitment may be decreased. If significant permanent axonal loss has occurred with subsequent reinnervation, increases in MUAP duration, polyphasia, and amplitude will be observed.

Mononeuropathy Multiplex Syndromes and Plexopathies

Mononeuropathy multiplex syndromes are characterized by multifocal lesions of peripheral nerves and are associated with systemic disorders such as diabetes, vasculitis, amyloidosis, direct tumor involvement, and paraneoplastic syndromes (150,151). Aside from the anatomic distribution of abnormalities, plexopathies share the same electrodiagnostic features as the mononeuropathy multiplex syndromes in that they are both lesions of peripheral nerves that result in primarily axonal damage of both motor and sensory fibers. Mononeuropathy multiplex syndromes can be distributed bilaterally distally and proximally throughout the body and have a predilection for associated entrapment neuropathies, whereas plexopathies tend to be localized to the proximal portions of the peripheral nerve structures innervating the limbs and trunk. A plexopathy may, in fact, be part of a mononeuropathy multiplex syndrome, and the differential diagnosis is similar (see Tables 15-2 through 15-4). Diabetic amyotrophy (152) and the so-called acute brachial neuropathy/neuralgic amyotrophy (153,154) also may be included in this category. The thoracic outlet syndrome (TOS) deserves special mention because of the high frequency with which it appears in the differential diagnosis of upper extremity pain or numbness, although electrodiagnostic tests are rarely positive. Electrodiagnostic testing in suspected TOS is primarily of value in evaluating other alternative or coexisting diagnoses such as carpal tunnel syndrome or cervical radiculopathy and very, very, rarely in providing a positive diagnosis of TOS (8,151,155,156). The TOS is generally a clinical, not a laboratory diagnosis (157).

Sensory Nerve Conduction Studies

The lesion or lesions in these disease categories are distal to both the motor and sensory cell bodies and result in either axonal disruption or abnormal axonal conduction. A major distinguishing point between radiculopathies and plexopathies is that sensory studies usually are normal in the former and frequently abnormal in the latter. This distinction may be important clinically and is subject to the following qualifications. Sensory nerve conduction studies will be abnormal in the presence of axonal disruption if the sensory axons of the nerve being studied pass through the involved area and are interrupted. The appropriate sensory nerve must therefore be studied (158). If an L4 radiculopathy or plexopathy is suspected on the basis of electrodiagnostic and clinical evidence, the sural nerve, involving predominantly the S1 level, cannot be used to distinguish an L4 radiculopathy from a plexopathy involving primarily L4 muscles.

Sensory nerve conduction studies will be abnormal only if a large enough percentage of the sensory axons is damaged. A lesion that eliminates conduction in 10% of the sensory axons will produce a loss of SNAP amplitude that may not be unequivocally detectable. Axonotmesis in that many motor axons will probably produce easily detectable spontaneous activity after an appropriate time interval. The presence of a normal sensory response may therefore be seen in a plexopathy in which spontaneous activity is present, even when the appropriate sensory nerve is studied.

Late Responses

Late response latencies may be prolonged or absent.

Repetitive Stimulation

A small decrement may be present if significant denervation–reinnervation is present.

Motor Nerve Conduction Studies

Motor nerve conduction abnormalities are similar to those seen in axonal polyneuropathies and entrapment neuropathies with the exception of the anatomic distribution.

Needle Electrode Examination

Abnormalities noted on needle electrode examination are those associated with axonal dysfunction as listed for radiculopathies and neuropathies.

Discussion

The electrodiagnosis of plexopathies and mononeuropathy multiplex syndromes is subject to many pitfalls. These have been reviewed by Ball (8). In general, diagnosis rests on a careful history, physical exam, and comprehensive electrodiagnostic studies with proper emphasis being given to each of the electrodiagnostic abnormalities identified.

Radiculopathy and Polyradiculopathy

A radiculopathy may occur with extensive bony spine disease, intervertebral disc injury, carcinomatous–lymphomatous meningitis, other mass lesions, and some metabolic or inflammatory disorders (159,160). Cord-level lesions (e.g., syringomyelia, intramedullary mass lesions) that damage anterior horn cells are difficult to distinguish electrodiagnostically from radiculopathies and always should be considered if clinically appropriate. One of the primary features of radiculopathies and polyradiculopathies is that damage to the nerve root usually occurs proximal to the sensory neuronal cell body. Electrodiagnostic abnormalities therefore are restricted to the motor unit unless a secondary process (e.g., a sensorimotor polyneuropathy) is present. Typical findings in radiculopathies and polyradiculopathies are discussed both in terms of severity of neuronal damage and chronology of electrodiagnostic abnormalities. Wilbourn also provides an excellent discussion of the electrodiagnostic findings in radiculopathies (161).

Sensory Nerve Conduction Studies

Sensory nerve conduction studies almost always are normal. In rare cases, the dorsal root ganglia may be damaged, producing sensory abnormalities.

F Wave

F wave latencies usually are normal unless the radiculopathy is severe or multilevel. The F wave usually provides little additional information because there generally are significant abnormalities on the needle electrode examination or motor nerve conduction studies by the time the F wave latencies become abnormal (68).

H Reflex

The H reflex may be abnormally prolonged in S1 radiculopathies and may assist in making the diagnosis under some circumstances (64,159). Prolongation or absence of the H reflex correlates well with a diminished or absent ankle reflex in radicular disease, although not necessarily in polyneuropathy.

Repetitive Stimulation

A small decrement may be present if extensive denervation and reinnervation is present.

Motor Nerve Conduction Studies

Motor nerve conduction studies usually are normal in radiculopathies unless a large percentage of the axons innervating the muscle being tested has been anatomically interrupted (i.e., axonotmesis). When this occurs under acute conditions, the amplitude of the motor evoked response is normal initially and decreases to its nadir 3 to 7 days after injury. Motor nerve conduction velocities and temporal dispersion usually are normal unless the motor evoked response amplitude is markedly decreased. If the lesion is chronic or old, and the majority of the originally denervated muscle fibers has been reinnervated by surviving axons, the motor-evoked response amplitude may be normal in spite of significant permanent axonal loss. High-amplitude, long-duration, polyphasic MUAPs should be present on needle electrode examination in this situation. If axonal loss is severe and permanent, CMAP amplitudes may remain low, in which case spontaneous activity should persist for long periods of time, or even permanently. Lesions of the nerve root producing only conduction block (i.e., neurapraxia) do not affect the results of standard nerve conduction studies because the nerve is stimulated distal to the conduction block.

Needle Electrode Examination

Spontaneous Activity

In acute or short-duration radiculopathy (i.e., 1 to 3 months), abnormalities in needle electrode examination results are caused primarily by (a) the presence of spontaneous activity if axonotmesis has occurred and sufficient time has elapsed, or (b) decreased motor unit recruitment if a large enough percentage of the axons are not conducting action potentials.

Spontaneous activity will be the most sensitive indicator of neuronal damage if axonal interruption occurs, because a small percentage of motor axonal loss (2% to 3%) probably will be detectable.

Spontaneous activity may require 1 to 2 weeks to appear in the proximal muscles (i.e., paraspinal muscles) and 2 to 6 weeks to appear in distal muscles. Spontaneous activity therefore is not routinely of significant value in evaluating radiculopathies in the acute setting in which symptoms have been present only a few days. Clear-cut spontaneous activity present only days after a clinical insult is probably the result of an injury antedating the event in question. This may have some applicability in a medicolegal setting.

Spontaneous activity may resolve earlier in proximal muscles than in distal muscles. The electrodiagnostician therefore may observe a pattern in which spontaneous activity may be present only in proximal muscles, present in both proximal and distal muscles, or present in distal muscles only, depending on the timing of the examination with respect to the injury. No spontaneous activity may be detected at any time if anatomic axonal interruption does not occur or if reinnervation is rapid.

The presence of spontaneous activity in a muscle often is taken to indicate ongoing denervation, a conclusion that is incorrect in many cases. It is known that spontaneous activity can persist for many years when major axonal loss has left a muscle with relatively few functioning axons. This usually occurs in the setting of severe old poliomyelitis, near-complete peripheral nerve lesions, and the like, and probably reflects the inability of the remaining motor neurons to reinnervate the denervated muscle fibers. The situation is much less clear in settings in which only a small percentage of the axons have been damaged, as is the case with most radiculopathies. In most cases involving spontaneous activity, the following conditions are present:

1. The patient has no superimposed neurologic disease that would affect the ability of motor neurons to sprout and reinnervate denervated muscle fibers.
2. The majority of the original motor neurons are intact and functioning. The number of muscle fibers per motor unit therefore will not be excessively large and the ability of the motor neuron to innervate additional muscle fibers is not impaired.
3. The mechanism underlying spontaneous activity is denervation.

In this setting, it is unlikely that significant numbers of muscle fibers could remain denervated for long periods of time in the absence of recent injury. The presence of spontaneous activity under these conditions strongly favors the conclusion that denervation has occurred within the past several weeks or months. This logical framework is useful when analyzing the significance of spontaneous activity in the muscles of patients who present with symptoms of short duration (i.e., weeks to a few months) and a history of neurologic injury in the remote past. This logic does not assist in deciding whether denervation actually is occurring at the moment of the electrodiagnostic examination.

It often is difficult to determine the significance of spontaneous activity in the paraspinal muscles after laminectomies. Spontaneous activity in this setting may be the result of direct surgical damage to muscle fibers or intramuscular nerve branches, or it may be secondary to axonotmesis produced by a new radiculopathy. Although it has been proposed that spontaneous activity located more that 3 cm from the scar usually is not the result of surgical trauma (64), this assumption should be made with reservation since the location and size of the surface wound does not always identify the location and extent of the surgical trauma. Damage to nerves innervating the paraspinal muscles also may result in spontaneous activity remote from the surgical scar. This discussion may be qualified by considering the surgeon and surgical technique. In the hands of a careful surgeon, a one-level microdiscectomy using an operating microscope is unlikely to produce major damage to paraspinal muscles or muscular nerve branches compared with a wide laminectomy and fusion involving multiple levels and extensive periosteal stripping. It is not unusual for there to be no residual spontaneous activity several months after a one-level microdiscectomy through a small (e.g., 3-cm) incision.

Spontaneous activity in the paraspinal muscles after laminectomy should be analyzed as follows:

1. When examining a postlaminectomy patient for the first time, or if no accurate records on previous studies after laminectomy are available, spontaneous activity in the paraspinal muscles should probably be attributed to surgical trauma, particularly if low amplitude. This assumption may be modified by considering the surgeon and surgical technique.
2. When performing electrodiagnostic studies on a postlaminectomy patient, the posterior myotomes should be searched carefully and the spontaneous activity present described accurately. If needed, an evaluation for initial documentation should take place no sooner than 1 to 2 months after surgery.
3. Subsequent studies should attempt to document an interval increase in the distribution or amount of spontaneous activity present in the paraspinal muscles before deciding that abnormalities are relevant to the current clinical complaints.

It should be noted that spontaneous activity in the cervical paraspinal muscles is exceedingly rare after an uncomplicated anterior cervical discectomy.

Please see Prognosis and Progression in the final section of this chapter for suggestions regarding describing these various situations in the conclusion of the electrodiagnostic report.

Motor Unit Recruitment

Decreased motor unit recruitment will be present immediately on injury if the percentage of nonconducting axons innervating that muscle is large enough. Abnormalities of motor unit recruitment may resolve completely if secondary to conduction block or may be permanent if axonotmesis occurs and the axons are permanently lost.

Motor Unit Action Potential Configuration

If a significant percentage of the motor axons supplying a muscle are permanently lost, and enough time has elapsed (i.e., 1 to 3 months) so that the muscle fibers originally innervated by those axons are added to other motor units, the amplitude, duration, and polyphasia of the remaining motor units will increase. This may occur with either old (i.e., inactive) or chronic (i.e., active) lesions and depends primarily on the total percentage of axons lost.

Anatomic Distribution of Abnormalities

Many tables exist that list the predominant root level supply of commonly studied muscles of the trunk and limbs (64,162,163). A large amount of variability exists, and the electromyographer should be cautious when relating specific electrodiagnostic abnormalities to spinal root levels (164). Because the axons supplying a given muscle are topographically localized in the nerve root, damage may occur to the axons innervating any or all of the muscles supplied by that root. On this basis alone, electrodiagnostic abnormalities may be present in only one or a few of the muscles supplied by a given nerve root and, in fact, may not even involve the entire muscle (165). Finally, reinnervation is significantly more efficient in proximal muscles, with the result that persistent abnormalities may be noted only in distal muscles innervated by that root (165). When these phenomena are combined with the time course of abnormalities discussed previously, it should be clear that marked variations in the pattern of electrodiagnostic abnormalities may occur with radiculopathies (166). It is only in the severe radiculopathy that a majority of the axons in the nerve root are damaged, producing unequivocal, long-standing abnormalities in multiple anterior and posterior myotome muscles predominantly innervated by that root. Electrodiagnostic abnormalities in a single muscle are sufficient for a probable diagnosis of radiculopathy in the appropriate clinical setting. The often heard criterion that a radiculopathy should have electrodiagnostic abnormalities in two to three muscles or more is probably too restrictive in most cases. Granted, the reliability of the diagnosis improves as abnormalities are identified in a larger number of muscles with a common predominant root level supply of a single root, particularly when they are innervated by different peripheral nerves and plexus structures. However, when the electromyographer considers the history and physical examination in most cases of suspected radiculopathy, there is usually no other likely explanation for abnormalities in a single muscle other than a mild radiculopathy.

Normal Electrodiagnostic Studies in Compressive Radiculopathy

When a radiculopathy is strongly suspected, but the electrodiagnostic studies are normal, the author usually includes the following phrase in the discussion of the results: "Negative electrodiagnostic studies in this setting signify that if a compressive radiculopathy is present, there has been no significant nerve root damage either now or in the past, or if there has, it is recent and minor." This statement signifies that no matter how long the process has been going on, there has been no significant cumulative axonal loss (as evidenced by the lack of MUAP changes) and also covers the situation where spontaneous activity associated with recent axonotmesis has not yet had time to develop. This assists the referring physician who may not understand some of the subtleties of the electrodiagnostic examination with respect to radiculopathies.

Polyradiculoneuropathy

The term polyradiculoneuropathy generally designates a disease process that affects peripheral nerve but, in contrast to generalized polyneuropathies, demonstrates an additional predilection for the nerve roots themselves. Many of these disorders appear to be immunologic, vasculitic, or toxic in origin, and this particular anatomic distribution is believed to reflect the relative permeability of the blood-nerve barrier at the point where the nerve roots enter the subarachnoid space, providing access to injurious agents. Polyradiculopathies due to structural etiologies with superimposed polyneuropathies should be considered as a separate entity where the electrodiagnostic abnormalities present are essentially the sum of the abnormalities seen with each individual disease process. Acutely presenting polyradiculoneuropathies usually are considered to fall under the differential diagnosis of the Guillain-Barré syndrome. The majority, although not all, of these acute disorders have demyelination as a predominant feature and therefore are classified as AIDP.

Classification of chronic polyradiculoneuropathies is poorly defined, and for this discussion will be taken to refer to CIDP. The references by Albers and colleagues provides an excellent discussion of the clinical and electrodiagnostic features of the inflammatory demyelinating polyradiculoneuropathies (45,52,167).

Before discussing the details of electrodiagnostic studies in AIDP and CIDP, it should be pointed out that electrodiagnostic findings may vary widely depending on the individual patient and the time course of the disease (168). It is not unusual for early abnormalities in AIDP to be restricted entirely to the level of the nerve roots, consisting of either conduction block or axonotmesis. In this situation, the results of peripheral nerve conduction studies will be entirely normal with the exception of F_responses and H reflexes, which frequently are absent if weakness is marked. The only other abnormality seen in this situation will be decreased motor unit recruitment. The electromyographer should not rely only on slowing of nerve conduction velocities and temporal dispersion to make a diagnosis of AIDP. Although significantly less common, there are what appear to be primarily axonal forms of Guillain-Barré syndrome in which significant electrodiagnostic abnormalities suggestive of demyelination are minimal or lacking (169). Guillain-Barré syndrome and AIDP therefore are not always technically synonymous. Prior to diagnosis an axonal form of GBS, the electromyographer should consider the possibility of distal demyelination and conduction block producing low or absent motor evoked response amplitudes without evidence of slowing or temporal dispersion in the proximal nerve (170). This pattern may mimic the electrodiagnostic findings on motor nerve conduction studies associated with axonal damage, but the prognosis is much better for a demyelinating lesion. If appropriate, acute myopathies associated with loss of muscle electrical excitability should also be considered when no motor evoked response can be obtained (171).

Sensory Nerve Conduction Studies

Electrodiagnostic sensory abnormalities may include prolonged distal latencies, abnormal conduction velocities, conduction block, temporal dispersion, and decreased evoked response amplitudes. One peculiarity of these disorders is the frequent relative preservation of the sural sensory evoked response whereas median and sometimes ulnar sensory evoked responses are significantly abnormal (52). Extreme prolongation of distal latencies and slowing of nerve conduction velocities may be present. It frequently is impossible to determine sensory conduction velocities because temporal dispersion and conduction block make the proximal, and sometimes the distal, sensory response undetectable (see Table 15-4).

F_Response

The F_response, if obtainable, may be moderately to markedly prolonged when demyelination is prominent. It may be one of the most important studies in cases where acute inflammatory demyelinating polyneuropathy is suspected because all nerve involvement may be proximal e.g., at the root level, resulting in normal distal peripheral nerve conduction studies. F_response latencies may be markedly prolonged under these conditions, when other portions of the electrodiagnostic studies are within normal limits. The F_response latency may be normal in Guillain-Barré syndrome if conduction block is the dominant abnormality and those axons that are conducting the F_response are conducting relatively normally. The F_response usually is unobtainable when the neuropathy is severe.

H Reflex

The H reflex follows a pattern similar to that observed for the F_response.

Repetitive Stimulation

A small decrement may be present if large amounts of denervation-reinnervation are present. While repetitive simulation is not usually useful in establishing the diagnosis of GBS itself, it should always be performed in patients with acute weakness to evaluate the possibility of a rapid onset neuromuscular junction disorder.

Motor Nerve Conduction Studies

Electrodiagnostic motor abnormalities may include prolonged distal latencies, abnormal conduction velocities, conduction block, temporal dispersion, and decreased evoked response amplitudes as is seen with sensory nerves. Abnormalities may be marked, with distal latencies two to three times the upper limit of normal and nerve conduction velocities of 20% to 30% of the lower limit of normal. Motor nerve conduction studies usually are the only way that conduction block and temporal dispersion can be identified because it is common for the proximal sensory response to be undetectable. Conduction block and temporal dispersion may occur in the presence of normal conduction velocities. Low nerve conduction velocities are not necessarily a negative prognostic factor, since the prognosis for demyelinating lesions is much better than that for lesions involving axonal loss. Distal CMAP amplitudes determined after the disease has stabilized correlate directly with prognosis (see Table 15-3).

Needle Electrode Examination

Spontaneous Activity

If significant axonal loss has occurred and sufficient time has elapsed, spontaneous activity usually will be present. In the case of an acute presentation, spontaneous activity will not be present at the time of the initial diagnostic evaluation. If the rate of axonal loss is low and reinnervation is occurring rapidly, axonal loss may occur without detectable spontaneous activity. All other factors being equal, the presence of significant amounts of spontaneous activity is a negative prognostic factor because it signifies axonal loss.

Motor Unit Action Potentials

If a substantial percentage of the axons supplying a muscle have been lost and the denervated muscle fibers have been added to remaining motor units, MUAP amplitude, duration, and polyphasia will increase in proportion to the number of muscle fibers added to the average motor unit. Again, in the acute presentation, MUAPs usually will be normal unless some antecedent neurologic insult has occurred in the remote past. Mild increases in polyphasia and duration may be present early if demyelination affects the terminal nerve branches.

Motor Unit Recruitment

Motor unit recruitment will be decreased if a substantial percentage of the motor axons are nonconducting. In an acute presentation, decreased motor unit recruitment may be the only abnormality noted during the electrodiagnostic examination if the lesions are predominantly those of conduction block at the nerve root level. When patients are seen very early in the course of their acute weakness, it is frequently difficult to rule out an acute myelopathy or other upper motor neuron lesion. Severe weakness should always be associated with decreased motor unit recruitment, and when normal motor unit recruitment is observed in the presence of severe weakness, an upper motor neuron lesion is likely.

Discussion

When patients with AIDP are seen in the first few days post-onset, weakness may be mild, and it is the presence of prominent sensory complaints that raises the possibility of AIDP. Under these circumstances, the results of electrodiagnostic studies may be minimally or equivocally abnormal, and laboratory studies (e.g., cerebrospinal fluid protein levels) may be normal. The clinician then may need to make a provisional diagnosis of AIDP based on clinical criteria so as to avoid a delay in appropriate treatment.

Neuromuscular Junction Disorders

The electrodiagnostic abnormalities noted in disorders of the neuromuscular junction are described in Tables 15-1 through 15-4 and in selected texts (2,13,14,16,75).

Sensory Nerve Conduction Studies

These are normal.

F_Response

These are normal.

H Reflex

These are normal.

Repetitive Stimulation

See the section on evaluation of the neuromuscular junction and Table 15-1.

Motor Nerve Conduction Studies

See Table 15-2.

Needle Electrode Examination

See section on abnormalities detected by needle electrode examination.

Critical Illness Syndromes

The electromyographer is frequently called to the intensive care unit to evaluate patients with severe generalized weakness. These patients can be those just admitted to the intensive care unit (ICU) with severe weakness and impending respiratory failure, or they can be patients who were admitted to the ICU for some other reason, e.g., sepsis, acute reactive airway disease, and who subsequently fail to wean from mechanical ventilation. In the case of those patients admitted with weakness, the differential diagnosis is broad and includes CNS etiologies, acute polyradiculoneuropathies/neuropathies, acute defects in neuromuscular transmission, and acute myopathies. When a patient fails to wean from mechanical ventilation, all of these diagnoses must still be considered, in that, on occasion, primary neuromuscular disease was not recognized on admission, or subsequently developed during the course of the hospitalization. In addition, several relatively distinct syndromes have been recognized that are more or less unique to the ICU setting. These are broad categories of disorders known as critical illness polyneuropathy and critical illness myopathy. They are discussed in the same section here because of their common clinical setting, and the fact that they frequently need to be distinguished from one another.

Critical illness polyneuropathy is frequently associated with sepsis and multisystem organ failure, usually lasting in excess of 2 to 4 weeks. Risk factors for critical illness myopathy include these same risk factors, as well as treatment with nondepolarizing neuromuscular blocking agents and/or high dose corticosteroids. Patients with critical illness myopathy usually have two or more of these risk factors. Further complicating matters, both critical illness polyneuropathy and myopathy may coexist in the same patient.

Critical illness polyneuropathy is primarily an axonal sensorimotor polyneuropathy that may range from mild to severe. In those cases where it is the explanation for problems such as failure to wean from mechanical ventilation, it is generally severe. The dominant electrodiagnostic features are either absent or markedly reduced sensory/motor evoked responses. Conduction velocities are usually reduced only to the extent that would be expected in association with low evoked response amplitudes. Conduction block and/or temporal dispersion is not a prominent feature, and there is usually no significant decrement to repetitive stimulation. Needle electrode examination demonstrates the findings discussed previously for axonal polyneuropathies. If the patient survives the critical illness, prognosis is usually good once the underlying factors have been corrected, although poor outcomes may be associated with severe neuropathies.

The electrodiagnostic findings in critical illness myopathy are somewhat complex. Sensory nerve conduction studies are generally normal unless there is superimposed acute/chronic polyneuropathy (not uncommon). The dominant electrodiagnostic abnormalities are those of low/absent motor-evoked response amplitudes and an abnormal response to repetitive stimulation in some cases. Critical illness myopathy appears to have two variants (172). The first is that of profound weakness that lasts for hours to as long as approximately 1 week following the discontinuation of nondepolarizing neuromuscular blocking agents. This variant appears most likely to reflect the persistence of the neuromuscular blocking agent and its metabolites and is frequently linked to renal failure. A decrement is frequently present on repetitive stimulation. The second variant produces severe weakness or paralysis for weeks to months and appears to be a true myopathy with multiple etiologies (171–173). A decrement is frequently absent on repetitive stimulation with this variant. In some cases of acute myopathic quadriparesis, muscle may be electrically inexcitable and the lack of a motor evoked response may be erroneously attributed to a severe axonal polyneuropathy. One should keep this in mind when interpreting markedly low or absent motor evoked responses in this setting. Direct stimulation of skeletal muscle may be of value in identifying this situation (171). The presence of abnormalities on sensory nerve conduction studies cannot be used to make an absolute distinction between neuropathic and myopathic etiologies for severely reduced/absent motor evoked response amplitudes since sensory abnormalities may only reflect a mild to moderate sensorimotor polyneuropathy superimposed on a severe myopathy. The key feature here is that in most uncomplicated axonal sensorimotor polyneuropathies, sensory abnormalities are more marked than motor abnormalities, e.g., it is unusual for sensory evoked responses to be present if the motor amplitudes are severely reduced. The presence of only mild to moderate sensory amplitude electrodiagnostic abnormalities in conjunction with severe motor amplitude abnormalities should alert the electromyographer to the possibility of an underlying severe myopathy. Needle electrode examination frequently demonstrates decreased insertional activity, mild to marked positive waves and fibrillations, and rapid recruitment of small polyphasic MUAPs although patients may be unable to voluntarily activate any motor units in severely involved muscles, precluding any analysis of MUAPs and motor unit recruitment. The unusual combination of low-amplitude, polyphasic, short-duration MUAPs and decreased motor unit recruitment may be seen if both a severe myopathy and neuropathy coexist.

Primary Muscle Disorders

Attempting to discuss general abnormalities in myopathies is difficult because the term represents a large group of diseases. As might be expected, the clinical and electrodiagnostic characteristics of these disorders vary widely (85,174–178). These disorders include acquired diseases such as metabolic/endocrine disorders, infections with a variety of different agents, inflammatory processes and toxic etiologies, as well as inherited/congenital problems such as the various muscular dystrophies, myotonic disorders, periodic paralysis, mitochrondrial myopathies, and metabolic myopathies. When faced with these problems clinically, the electromyographer must review the specifics of each specific diagnosis under consideration. A detailed discussion of each disorder is beyond the scope of this chapter (179). The following discussion focuses on general features of this class of muscle disorders.

Sensory Nerve Conduction Studies

Sensory nerve conduction studies are generally normal in myopathic processes. However, in situations such as severe metabolic/endocrine disorders, e.g., severe hypothyroidism or fulminant vasculitic processes, both muscle and nerve function may be abnormal electrodiagnostically, each target organ responding to a systemic insult in its own characteristic manner.

Late Responses

F_response and H reflex latencies generally are normal, subject to the qualification noted above for sensory nerve conduction studies.

Repetitive Stimulation

The results of repetitive stimulation usually are normal. A mild decrement may be present if neuromuscular junctions are abnormal as a result of primary muscle cell dysfunction. Decrements also may be present in myotonic disorders as a result of abnormal muscle fiber membrane function and the resulting inability to repetitively generate normal muscle cell action potentials (180).

Motor Nerve Conduction Studies

The results of motor nerve conduction studies usually are normal with the exception of the evoked response amplitude, which may be decreased.

Needle Electrode Examination

The abnormalities noted on the needle electrode examination in primary muscle diseases depend highly on the disease process and as such are discussed by group.

Muscular Dystrophies

The muscular dystrophies include a large number of disorders with widely varying characteristics. Abnormalities on needle electrode examination may be distal, proximal, craniopharyngeal, or a combination of these; spontaneous activity may or may not be present; and MUAP changes may vary widely, ranging from near normal to short-duration, low-amplitude MUAPs to moderately high-duration, normal- to high-amplitude MUAPs, depending on the disease and its stage. A mixed picture with some MUAPs having increased duration and others having decreased duration also may be seen. Although MUAP polyphasia usually is increased, it may not be prominent. Details are provided in the works of Daube (85) and Buchtal (181).

Acquired Inflammatory Myopathies

The untreated, acquired inflammatory myopathies are characterized classically by the presence of spontaneous activity, decreased MUAP amplitude and duration with increased polyphasia, and rapid motor unit recruitment (182–185). Treatment with steroids or other immunosuppressant drugs may suppress spontaneous activity. In contrast, the MUAPs in chronic acquired inflammatory myopathies may evolve into moderately high-amplitude, long-duration, polyphasic MUAPs. Electrodiagnostic findings in inflammatory myopathies therefore may be confusing and clinical correlation with the stage of the disease is essential (182,186,187).

Endocrine Myopathies

Endocrine myopathies (e.g., steroid, hypothyroid, hyperthyroid, hyperparathyroid) generally show MUAPs that either are normal or demonstrate minimally decreased amplitude and duration. Motor unit recruitment usually is rapid in proportion to clinical weakness. Fibrillations and positive waves are not generally a feature of these disorders, although increased insertional activity, short myotonic discharges, doublets, fasciculations, and other poorly defined irregular spontaneous discharges may be seen in disorders such as hypothyroidism and hyperparathyroidism.

Toxic Myopathies

Toxic myopathies, such as those seen with alcoholic myopathy (188), lovastatin and gemfibrozil, or lovastatin alone, may present with findings similar to those seen with inflammatory myopathies if muscle fiber damage is severe enough. Many toxic myopathies (e.g., those seen with chloroquine and clofibrate) are significantly milder and present as electrodiagnostic abnormalities similar to those observed in endocrine myopathies. Pentazocine and other injected drugs may produce focal myopathies after repeated use.

Inherited Myopathies

Inherited myopathies generally demonstrate decreased MUAP amplitude and duration, increased polyphasia, and rapid motor unit recruitment although abnormalities may be minimal or nonexistent. Electrodiagnostic abnormalities are usually associated with those diseases where there are structural abnormalities of the muscle fiber on histologic examination, e.g., central core disease, nemaline myopathy, etc. Disorders consisting primarily of abnormal fiber type distributions or muscle fibers size without other abnormalities usually have minimal or no electrodiagnostic abnormalities. Spontaneous activity may be profuse (e.g., acid maltase deficiency) or absent (e.g., fiber type disproportion).

Periodic Paralysis

The characteristic feature of periodic paralysis is the impaired ability of the muscle cell membrane to generate a normal action potential (157). This results in electrical silence with paralytic attacks, during which insertional activity is decreased, voluntary MUAPs are absent, and no CMAP can be elicited by stimulation of the motor nerve. Lesser degrees of abnormalities are noted during milder attacks, which produce weakness, not paralysis. Depending on the degree of impairment of muscle fiber action potential generation, MUAPs may range from normal to low amplitude and short duration. In hyperkalemic periodic paralysis, fibrillations and myotonic discharges may be seen between attacks, although they disappear during an attack. Hypokalemic periodic paralysis does not demonstrate spontaneous activity but may demonstrate an abnormal drop (>50%) in the CMAP amplitude after exercise or in response to intra-arterial injection of epinephrine (189).

Myotonic Disorders

The myotonic disorders include myotonic dystrophy, myotonia congenita, and paramyotonia congenita (190–192). The hallmark of these disorders is the myotonic discharge (193), a repetitive discharge of single muscle fibers that varies widely in frequency and amplitude, giving rise to what is usually described as a dive-bomber sound. Firing rates vary from 2 to 100 Hz. Myotonic discharges are not absolutely specific for the myotonic disorders and also can be seen in hyperkalemic periodic paralysis, acid maltase deficiency, hypothyroid myopathy, myotubular myopathy, and inflammatory myopathies.

INTERPRETATION OF ELECTRODIAGNOSTIC RESULTS

Analysis of results obtained during the electrodiagnostic evaluation is one of the most challenging aspects of the overall process. The following scheme is one approach to this problem. As presented, it assumes that no technical errors have been made (e.g., low distal limb temperatures resulting in prolonged distal latencies). The raw data obtained during the examination should be reviewed and their major features summarized.

Nerve Conduction Study Analysis

A summary of the typical nerve conduction study abnormalities found in commonly encountered neuromuscular disorders is provided in Tables 15-1 through 15-4. The following questions should be asked when reviewing the collected data:

1. Were all of the necessary tests performed? A negative examination frequently is the result of neglecting a key test. Review the initial differential diagnosis as well as any abnormal results obtained during the examination to decide this. Ask yourself this question while you are still in the room with the patient.
2. If nerve conduction studies are abnormal, determine the distribution of abnormalities. Are abnormalities symmetrical or asymmetrical, focal or diffuse/multifocal, distal or proximal?
3. Are abnormalities sensory, motor, or both?
4. If CMAP amplitudes are generally low, was the patient tested for a defect in neuromuscular transmission?
5. If obtained, were F_response or H reflex latencies disproportionately prolonged relative to distal nerve conduction velocities, suggesting proximal demyelination?
6. Is abnormal temporal dispersion present in evoked responses following proximal and distal stimulation, suggesting multifocal demyelination?
7. Is there evidence of conduction block in any nerve tested, suggesting a focal lesion in between the stimulus sites?
8. If clinical and electrodiagnostic findings are predominantly motor, was proximal stimulation (e.g., at the axilla, Erb's point) carried out to test for proximal conduction block?
9. Is there evidence of significant demyelination as evidenced by markedly reduced conduction velocities?

Needle Electrode Results Analysis

The following questions should be asked when insertional activity, spontaneous activity, MUAP abnormalities, or recruitment abnormalities are analyzed:

1. Were the appropriate muscles examined?
2. Are abnormalities symmetrical or asymmetrical, focal or diffuse/multifocal, distal or proximal? Do they follow the distribution of a specific peripheral nerve, plexus, or root?
3. What type and stage of disease process is suggested by the abnormalities?
4. Can abnormalities noted on motor nerve conduction studies be verified on needle electrode examination? Processes of pathologic significance that produce a true abnormality in CMAP amplitude usually produce abnormalities on needle electrode examination, although this is not necessarily true for those processes resulting in only motor nerve conduction velocity abnormalities.
5. Do the results of MMT, MUAP analysis, and motor unit recruitment analysis correlate with one another?

Conclusion

Final Diagnosis

The results of this analysis should allow identification of the most likely underlying pathologic process, such as sensory, motor, or sensorimotor polyneuropathy, mononeuropathy, multiple mononeuropathies (i.e., mononeuropathy multiplex), polyradiculoneuropathy such as that seen with Guillain-Barré syndrome, MND, MMN, polyradiculopathy, radiculopathy, plexopathy, disordered neuromuscular transmission, or myopathic processes. In some cases it is necessary to invoke multiple diagnoses to explain all electrodiagnostic abnormalities. Examples of this might include a polyneuropathy with superimposed entrapment neuropathies (e.g., carpal tunnel syndrome).

Etiologies

The summary should guide the referring clinician in further evaluation of the patient by including a differential diagnosis of etiologies that could produce the electrodiagnostic findings noted on the examination.

Relationship to Clinical Complaints

When electrodiagnostic abnormalities are present, but the electrodiagnostician does not believe that they are likely to be the basis of the patient's clinical complaint, some statement should be made to this effect. This can avoid confusion in the nonelectromyographer who reads the report.

Dating of Pathologic Processes

When possible, the electrodiagnostic findings should be classified as being consistent with acute, subacute, chronic, or old pathologic processes. This information frequently is of value in interpreting the electrodiagnostic results when the duration of clinical symptoms and the estimated age of the electrodiagnostic abnormalities do not correlate well with one another (e.g., the presence of marked increase in MUAP duration, polyphasia, and amplitude is not consistent with a process of 1 week's duration). In this particular case, the significance of electrodiagnostic abnormalities would be diminished in explaining the major clinical complaint, or the differential diagnosis might be considerably shortened.

Progression and Prognosis

When the diagnosis is relatively certain, some statement should be made regarding prognosis and progression of the disease, if possible. Considerable confusion often occurs in this area, and considerable attention is therefore devoted to this topic.

Electrodiagnostic data may be used in certain conditions to estimate the prognosis for recovery of neurologic function or for estimating the rate of progression of a disease. This must be done on a disease-by-disease basis. Diseases for which this may be done include MND, peripheral nerve injury, acquired polyneuropathies, myasthenia gravis, inflammatory myopathies, inflammatory demyelinating polyneuropathies, and others.

When using electrodiagnostic findings in isolation, progressive or ongoing processes can be evaluated only by demonstrating an interval change between two serial electrodiagnostic studies. Even under these circumstances, the only conclusion that can be drawn is that the event responsible for the interval change occurred shortly before the first examination or between the two examinations, not that progression is occurring at the time of the second examination. As an example, the presence of spontaneous activity often is interpreted as being diagnostic of ongoing denervation. This is incorrect because under certain conditions spontaneous activity may persist for years after the responsible insult. An example of this would be a complete and rapid transection of the median nerve at the wrist. An electrodiagnostic study performed 1 hour after nerve transection will not demonstrate spontaneous activity, whereas repeat studies 1 month later will demonstrate marked spontaneous activity. Although denervation occurred only transiently, spontaneous activity will be recorded from distal median innervated muscles for months to years; that is, profuse spontaneous activity will be present even though there is no ongoing denervation. Under the proper circumstances (see discussion of radiculopathy in previous section), the presence of spontaneous activity suggests that a recent neurologic insult has occurred, although it still is not possible to state that injury is occurring at the time of the electrodiagnostic examination. Similar analysis can be made of most types of electrodiagnostic abnormalities, including demyelination, increased neuromuscular jitter, abnormal decrements on repetitive stimulation, low motor/sensory evoked response amplitudes, pathologic MUAP changes, and motor unit recruitment abnormalities.

Fibrillation potential amplitude may be useful as an indicator of the age of a lesion (194,195). The presence of large numbers of very low-amplitude fibrillation potentials (5 to 25 μV), as occurs when denervated muscle fibers undergo severe atrophy with time, signifies an event that occurred in the remote past. Large-amplitude fibrillation potentials (100 to 200 μV) suggest a recent or ongoing event.

These limitations of the electrodiagnostic examination must be kept in mind when making a statement as to whether a disease process is ongoing. The electromyographer must learn to integrate historical, clinical, and electrodiagnostic data to estimate the probability that a disorder is ongoing at the time of evaluation. To do this, the electrodiagnostician must have a thorough understanding of the clinical presentation and course and electrodiagnostic abnormalities associated with the disease under consideration (e.g., the presence of spontaneous activity may be useful in determining the recent course of an inflammatory myopathy and may assist in evaluating the effectiveness of recent therapy, whereas the same findings may be of no value in deciding whether a radiculopathy of recent onset is currently active). Statements about ongoing progression of a disease process may have considerable practical significance for medical or surgical management and should be made with care.

The author generally uses the following phraseology to guide the referring physician as to the significance of the presence/absence of positive sharp waves and fibrillations.

1. If positive sharp waves and fibrillations are present and of high amplitude, the phrase "The electrodiagnostic findings on this examination are consistent with denervation due to a recent, but resolved process, or an active/currently ongoing process," is used.
2. If positive sharp waves and fibrillations are present, but of low amplitude, the statement "The electrodiagnostic findings are most consistent with denervation in the remote past, favoring an old, probably inactive, process, but not absolutely excluding an ongoing process," is used.

3. If there are no positive sharp waves and fibrillations present, but other abnormalities such as MUAP changes are present, the phrase "The electrodiagnostic findings on this examination are consistent with either an old, inactive (resolved) process, or an ongoing, active process," is used. This phrase covers both the situation where the process in truly old and resolved, as well as the situation where denervation/reinnervation may be occurring, but it is occurring at such a slow rate that denervated muscle fibers are reinnervated before they display detectable spontaneous activity.

Improbable Diagnoses

Finally, a statement should be made about diagnoses that are virtually excluded by the electrodiagnostic results. In many cases, it is a simple task to eliminate a particular diagnosis by electrodiagnostic criteria when it is impossible to do so on the basis of clinical or other laboratory data.

REFERENCES

1. American Association of Electrodiagnostic Medicine. Guidelines in electrodiagnostic medicine. *Muscle Nerve* 1992; 15:229–253.
2. Dyck PJ. Dyck JB, Grant IA, Fealey RD. Ten steps in characterizing and diagnosing patients with peripheral neuropathy. *Neurology* 1996; 47:10–17.
3. Brown WF, Boulton CF. *Clinical electromyography.* Boston: Butterworth, 1984.
4. Malmstadt HV, Enke CG, Crouch SR. *Electronics and instrumentation for scientists.* Reading, MA: Benjamin/Cummings, 1981.
5. Gitter AJ, Stolov WC. AAEM minimonograph 16: Instrumentation and measurement in electrodiagnostic medicine—Part I. *Muscle Nerve* 1995; 18:799–811.
6. Gitter AJ, Stolov WC. AAEM minimonograph 16: Instrumentation and measurement in electrodiagnostic medicine—Part II. *Muscle Nerve* 1995; 18:812–824
7. Robinson LR, Temkin, MR, Fujimoto WY, Stolov WC. Effect of statistical methodology on normal limits in nerve conduction studies. *Muscle Nerve* 1991; 14:1084–1090.
8. Ball RD. Plexopathies. Electrodiagnosis. *State Art Rev Phys Med Rehabil* 1989; 3:725–740.
9. Rivner MH. Statistical errors and their effect on electrodiagnostic medicine. *Muscle Nerve* 1994; 17:811–814.
10. Shefner JM, Dawson MD. The use of sensory action potentials in the diagnosis of peripheral nerve disease. *Arch Neurol* 1990; 47:341–348.
11. Berger AR, Busis NA, Logigian EL, et al. Cervical root stimulation in the diagnosis of radiculopathy. *Neurology* 1987; 37:329–332.
12. Brown WF. *The physiological and technical basis of electromyography.* Boston: Butterworth, 1984; 369–428.
13. Jablecki CK. Electrodiagnostic evaluation of patients with myasthenia gravis and related disorders. *Neurol Clin* 1985; 3:557–572.
14. Kimura J. Techniques of repetitve stimulation. In: Kimura J, ed. *Electrodiagnosis in diseases of nerve and muscle: principles and practice,* 2nd ed. Philadelphia: FA Davis, 1989; 184–198.
15. Kimura J. Single-fiber and macro electromyography. In: Kimura J, ed. *Electrodiagnosis in diseases of nerve and muscle: principles and practice,* 2nd ed. Philadelphia: FA Davis, 1989; 288–304.
16. Sanders DB. Acquired myasthenia gravis. In: Brumback RA, Gerst J, eds. *The neuromuscular junction.* Mount Kisco, NY: Futura, 1984; 257–294.
17. Sanders DB, Howard JF. AAEM minimonograph 25: single fiber electromyography in myasthenia gravis. *Muscle Nerve* 1986; 9:809–819.
18. Dumitru D. Special needle electromyographic techniques. In: Dumitru D, ed. *Electrodiagnostic medicine.* Philadelphia: Hanley and Belfus, 1995; 249–280.
19. Bischoff C, Stalberg E, Falck B, Eeg-Olofsson KE. Reference values of motor unit action potentials obtained with multi-MUAP analysis. *Muscle Nerve* 1994; 17:842–851.
20. Dumitru D, DeLisa JA. AAEM minimonograph 10: volume conduction. *Muscle Nerve* 1991; 14:605–624.
21. Lambert EH, Dyck PJ. Compound action potentials of sural nerve *in vitro* in peripheral neuropathy. In: Dyck PJ, Thomas PK, Lambert EH, Bunge R, eds. *Peripheral neuropathy,* 2nd ed. Philadelphia: WB Saunders, 1984; 1030–1044.
22. Waxman SG. Determinants of conduction velocity in myelinated nerve fibers. *Muscle Nerve* 1980; 3:141–150.
23. Kakigi R, Endo C, Neshige R, Kuroda Y, Shibasaki H. Estimation of conduction velocity of A fibers in humans. *Muscle Nerve* 1991; 14:1193–1196.
24. Dumitru D. Special nerve conduction techniques. In: Dumitru D, ed. *Electrodiagnostic medicine.* Philadelphia: Hanley and Belfus, 1995; 177–210.
25. Ravits J, Hallett M, Nilsson J, Polinsky R, Dambrosia J. Electrophysiological tests of autonomic function in patients with idiopathic autonomic failure syndromes. *Muscle Nerve* 1996; 19:758–763.
26. Gutmann L, Gutmann L. Axonal channelopathies: An evolving concept in the pathogenesis of peripheral nerve disorders. *Neurology* 1996; 47:18–20.
27. Zwartz MJ, Guechev A. The relation between conduction velocity and axonal length. *Muscle Nerve* 1995; 18:1244–1249.
28. Franssen H, Wieneke GH. Nerve conduction and temperature: Necessary warming time. *Muscle Nerve* 1994; 17:336–344.
29. Brown WF. *The physiological and technical basis of electromyography.* Boston: Butterworth, 1984; 95–168.
30. Kimura J. Principles of nerve conduction studies. In: Kimura J, ed. *Electrodiagnosis in diseases of nerve and muscle: principles and practice,* 2nd ed. Philadelphia: FA Davis, 1989; 78–102.
31. Kimura J. Nerve conduction studies and electromyography. In: Dyck PJ, Thomas PK, Lambert EH, eds. *Peripheral neuropathy,* 2nd ed. Philadelphia: WB Saunders, 1984; 919–966.
32. Denys EH. AAEM minimonograph 14: the influence of temperature in clinical neurophysiology. *Muscle Nerve* 1991; 14:795–811.
33. Kimura J. Anatomy and physiology of the peripheral nerve. In: Kimura J, ed. *Electrodiagnosis in diseases of nerve and muscle: principles and practice,* 2nd ed. Philadelphia: FA Davis, 1989; 55–77.
34. Wagman IH, Lesse H. Maximum conduction velocities of motor fibers of ulnar nerve in human subjects of various ages and sizes. *J Neurophysiol* 1952; 15:235–244.
35. Buchthal F, Rosenfalck A, Behse F. Sensory potentials of normal and diseased nerves. In: Dyck PJ, Thomas PK, Lambert EH, Bunge R, eds. *Peripheral neuropathy,* 2nd ed. Philadelphia: WB Saunders, 1985; 981–1015.
36. Cornblath DR, Sumner AJ, Daube J, et al. Conduction block in clinical practice. *Muscle Nerve* 1991; 14:869–871.
37. Lewis RA, Sumner AJ. Electrodiagnostic distinctions between chronic acquired and familial demyelinating neuropathies. *Neurology* 1982; 32:592–596.
38. Miller RG. Hereditary and acquired neuropathies: electrophysiologic aspects. *Neurol Clin* 1985; 3:543–556.
39. Miller RG, Gutmann L, Lewis TA, Sumner A. Acquired versus familial demyelinative neuropathies in children. *Muscle Nerve* 1985; 8: 205–210.
40. Benstead TJ, Kuntz NL, Miller RG, Daube JR. The electrophysiologic profile of Dejerine-Sottas disease (HMSN III). *Muscle Nerve* 1990; 13:586–592.
41. Brown WF. *The physiological and technical basis of electromyography.* Boston: Butterworth, 1984; 37–94.
42. Shin LJ, Kim DE, Kuruoglu HR. What is the best diagnostic index of conduction block and temporal dispersion? *Muscle Nerve* 1994; 17:489–493.
43. Olney RK, Miller RG. Conduction block in compression neuropathy: recognition and quantification. *Muscle Nerve* 1984; 7:662–667.
44. Brown WF. Electrophysiologic features of Guillain-Barré syndrome. In: *American Association of Electrodiagnostic Medicine annual course B: demyelinating neuropathies and the electrophysiology of conduction block.* Rochester, MN: American Association of Electrodiagnostic Medicine, 1991; 21–31.
45. Albers JW. Electrophysiologic features of chronic demyelinating neuropathies. In: *American Association of Electrodiagnostic Medicine annual course B: demyelinating neuropathies and the electrophysiol-*

ogy of conduction block. Rochester, MN: American Association of Electrodiagnostic Medicine, 1991; 32–47.

46. Brown WF, Feasby FE. Conduction block and denervation in Guillain-Barré polyneuropathy. *Brain* 1984; 107:219–239.
47. Kelly JJ. Differential diagnosis of demyelinative polyneuropathies. In: *American Academy of Neurology annual course 146: clinical electromyography.* Minneapolis, MN: American Academy of Neurology, 1989; 107–124.
48. Olney RK, Budiingen HJ, Miller RG. The effect of temporal dispersion on compound action potential area in human peripheral nerve. *Muscle Nerve* 1987; 10:728–733.
49. Del Toro DR, Park TA. Abductor hallicus false motor points: Electrophysiologic mapping and cadaveric dissection. *Muscle Nerve* 1996; 19:1138–1143
50. Junge D. *Nerve and muscle excitation,* 2nd ed. Sunderland, MA: Sinauer Associates, 1981; 1–16.
51. Wilbourn AJ. Common peroneal mononeuropathy at the fibular head. *Muscle Nerve* 1986; 9:825–836.
52. Albers JW. Inflammatory demyelinating polyradiculoneuropathy. In: Brown WF, Boulton CF, eds. *Clinical electromyography.* Wolbourn, MA: Butterworth, 1987; 209–244.
53. Kelly JJ. The electrodiagnostic findings in peripheral neuropathy associated with monoclonal gammopathy. *Muscle Nerve* 1983; 6: 504–509.
54. Miller RG. AAEM minimonograph 28: injury to peripheral motor nerves. *Muscle Nerve* 1987; 10:698–710.
55. Gutmann L, Gutierrez A, Ruggs JE. The contribution of median–ulnar communications in diagnosis of mild carpal tunnel syndrome. *Muscle Nerve* 1986; 9:319–321.
56. Stevens JC. The electrodiagnosis of carpal tunnel syndrome. *Muscle Nerve* 1987; 10:99–113.
57. Albers JW, Donofrio PD, McGonagle TK, et al. Sequential electrodiagnostic abnormalities in acute inflammatory demyelinating polyradiculoneuropathy. *Muscle Nerve* 1985; 8:528–539.
58. Maselli RA, Soliven BC. Analysis of the organophosphate-induced electromyographic response to repetitive nerve stimulation: paradoxical response to edrophonium and D-tubocurarine. *Muscle Nerve* 1991; 14:1182–1188.
59. Besser R, Vogt T, Gutmann L, Wessler I. High pancuronium sensitivity of axonal nicotinic-acetylcholine receptors in humans during organophosphate intoxication. *Muscle Nerve* 1991; 14:1197–1201.
60. Engle AG, Lambert EH, Gomez MR. A new myasthenic syndrome with end-plate acetylcholinesterase deficiency, small nerve terminals, and reduced acetylcholine release. *Ann Neurol* 1977; 1:315–330.
61. Jabre JF, Stalberg EV. Single-fiber EMG study of the flexor carpi radialis H reflex. *Muscle Nerve* 1989; 12:523–527.
62. Jabre JF, Rainville J, Salzaieder SM, Smuts J, Linke J. Correlates of motor unit size, recruitment threshold, and H reflex jitter. *Muscle Nerve* 1995; 18:1300–1305.
63. Braddom R, Johnson EW. Standardization of "H" reflex and diagnostic use in S1 radiculopathy. *Arch Phys Med Rehabil* 1974; 55: 161–166.
64. Clairmont AC, Johnson EW. Evaluation of the patient with possible radiculopathy. In: Johnson EW, Pease WS, eds. *Practical electromyography,* 3rd ed. Baltimore: Williams & Wilkins, 1996; 115–130.
65. Kimura J. H, T, masseter, and other reflexes. In: Kimura J, ed. *Electrodiagnosis in diseases of nerve and muscle: principles and practice,* 2nd ed. Philadelphia: FA Davis, 1989; 356–374.
66. Braddom RL, Johnson EW. H reflex: review and classification with suggested clinical uses. *Arch Phys Med Rehabil* 1974; 55:412–417.
67. Kimura J. The F wave. In: Kimura J, ed. *Electrodiagnosis in diseases of nerve and muscle: principles and practice,* 2nd ed. Philadelphia: FA Davis, 1989; 332–355.
68. Aminoff MF, Goodin DS, Parry GJ, et al. Electrophysiologic evaluation of lumbosacral radiculopathies: electromyography: late responses, and somatosensory evoked potentials. *Neurology* 1985; 35: 1514–1518.
69. Fisher MA, Hoffen B, Hultman C. Normative F wave values and the number of recorded F waves. *Muscle Nerve* 1994; 17:1185–1189.
70. Dumitru D. Special nerve conduction techniques. In: Dumitru D, ed. *Electrodiagnostic medicine.* Philadelphia: Hanley and Belfus, 1995; 177–210.
71. Syme JA, Kelly JJ. Absent F waves early in a case of transverse myelitis. *Muscle Nerve* 1994; 17:462–465.
72. Chu-Andrews J, Johnson RJ. *Electrodiagnosis: an anatomical and clinical approach.* Philadelphia: JB Lippincott, 1986; 258–263.
73. Clinchot D, Levy C. Generalized weakness. In: Johnson EW, Pease WS, eds. *Practical electromyography,* 3rd ed. Baltimore: Williams & Wilkins, 1996; 339–350.
74. Pickett JB. Neuromuscular transmission. In: Sumner AJ, ed. *The physiology of peripheral nerve disease.* Philadelphia: WB Saunders, 1980; 239–264.
75. Pickett JB. AAEM case report 16: botulism. *Muscle Nerve* 1987; 10: 1201–1205.
76. Keesey JC. AAEM minimonograph 33: electrodiagnostic approach to defects of neuromuscular transmission. *Muscle Nerve* 1989; 12: 613–626.
77. McArdle JJ. Overview of the physiology of the neuromuscular junction. In: Brumback RA, Gerst J, eds. *The neuromuscular junction.* Mount Kisco, NY: Futura, 1984; 65–120.
78. Cornblath DR, Sfladky JT, Sumner AJ. Clinical electrophysiology of infantile botulism. *Muscle Nerve* 1983; 6:448–452.
79. Cornblath DR. Disorders of neuromuscular transmission in infants and children. *Muscle Nerve* 1986; 9:606–611.
80. Daube JR. AAEM minimonograph 11: needle examination in clinical electromyography. *Muscle Nerve* 1991; 14:685–700.
81. Layzer RB. The origin of muscle fasciculations and cramps. *Muscle Nerve* 1994; 17:1243–1249.
82. Streib EW. AAEM minimonograph 27: differential diagnosis of myotonic syndromes. *Muscle Nerve* 1987; 10:603–615.
83. Subramony SH, Malhotra CP, Mishra SK. Distinguishing paramyotonia congenita and myotonia congenita by electromyography. *Muscle Nerve* 1983; 6:374–379.
84. Gutmann L. AAEM minimonograph 37: facial and limb myokymia. *Muscle Nerve* 1991; 14:1043–1049.
85. Daube JR. Electrodiagnosis of muscle disorders. In: Engle AG, Baker BQ, eds. *Myology,* Vol 1. New York: McGraw-Hill, 1986; 1081–1121.
86. Kimura J. Neuromuscular diseases characterized by abnormal muscle activity. In: Kimura J, ed. *Electrodiagnosis in diseases of nerve and muscle: principles and practice,* 2nd ed. Philadelphia: FA Davis, 1989; 558–578.
87. Dumitru D. Needle electromyography. In: Dumitru D, ed. Kimura J, ed. *Electrodiagnostic medicine.* Philadelphia: Hanley and Belfus, 1995; 211–248.
88. DeLuca CJ. Control properties of motor units. In: Basmajian JV, De Luca CJ, eds. *Muscles alive: their functions revealed by electromyography.* Baltimore: Williams & Wilkins, 1985; 125–167.
89. Podolsky RJ, Schoenberg M. Force generation and shortening in skeletal muscle. In: Peachey L, ed. *Handbook of physiology: section 10, skeletal muscle.* Baltimore: Williams & Wilkins, 1983; 173–187.
90. Petajan JH. Motor unit frequency control in normal man. In: Desmedt JE, ed. *Motor unit types, recruitment and plasticity in health and disease.* Basel: S Karger, 1981; 184–200.
91. Boyd DC, Lawrence PD, Bratty PJA. On modeling the single motor unit action potential. *IEEE Trans Biomed Eng* 1978; 25:236–243.
92. Griep PAM, Boon, KL, Stegeman DF. A study of the motor unit action potentials by means of computer simulation. *Biol Cybern* 1978; 30:221–230.
93. Andreassen S. Methods for computer-aided measurement of motor unit parameters. In: Ellingson RJ, Murray NFM, Halliday AM, eds. *The London symposia (EEG supplement 39).* Amsterdam: Elsevier, 1987; 13–20.
94. Nandedkar SD, Sanders DB, Stalberg EV, Andreassen S. Simulation of concentric needle EMG motor unit action potentials. *Muscle Nerve* 1988; 11:151–159.
95. Nandedkar SD, Sanders DB. Simulation of myopathic motor unit action potentials. *Muscle Nerve* 1989; 12:197–202.
96. Rosenfalck P. Intra- and extracellular potential fields of active nerve and muscle fibers. *Acta Physiol Scand [Suppl]* 1969; 321:1–168.
97. Nandedkar SD, Sanders DB. Measurement of the amplitude of the EMG envelope. *Muscle Nerve* 1990; 13:933–938.
98. Burke RE. Motor units in mammalian muscle. In: Sumner AJ, ed. *The physiology of peripheral nerve disease.* Philadelphia: WB Saunders, 1980; 133–194.
99. Burke RE. Motor units: anatomy, physiology, and functional organization. In: Brookhart JM, Mountcastle VB, eds. *Handbook of physiology: section 1, the nervous system. vol. II: Motor control, part 1.* Baltimore: Williams & Wilkins, 1981; 345–422.

100. Henneman E, Mendell LM. Functional organization of the motoneuron pool and its inputs. In: Brookhart JM, Mountcastle VB, eds. *Handbook of physiology: Section 1, the nervous system. vol. II: Motor control, part 1*. Baltimore: Williams & Wilkins, 1981; 423–507.
101. Jabre JJ, Spellman NT. The demonstration of the size principle in humans using macro electromyography and precision decomposition. *Muscle Nerve* 1996; 19:338–341.
102. Miller RG, Sherratt M. Firing rates of human motor units in partially denervated muscle. *Neurology* 1978; 28:1241–1248.
103. Rodriquez AA, Agre JC, Black PO, Franke TM. Motor unit firing rates in postpolio and control subjects during submaximal contraction. *Am J Phys Med Rehabil* 1991; 70:191–194.
104. Herdmann J, Reiners K, Freund H-J. Motor unit recruitment order in neuropathic disease. *Electromyogr Clin Neurophysiol* 1988; 28: 53–60.
105. Reiners K, Herdmann J, Freund H-J. Altered mechanisms of muscular force generation in lower motor neuron disease. *Muscle Nerve* 1989; 12:647–659.
106. Sogaard K. Motor unit recruitment pattern during low-level static and dynamic contractions. *Muscle Nerve* 1995; 18:292–300.
107. Stalberg E. Invited review: electrodiagnostic assessment and monitoring of motor unit changes in disease. *Muscle Nerve* 1991; 14:293–303.
108. So YT, Olney RK. AAEM case report 23: acute paralytic poliomyelitis. *Muscle Nerve* 1991; 14:1159–1164.
109. Robinson LR. AAEM case report 22: polymyositis. *Muscle Nerve* 1991; 14:310–315.
110. Jablecki CK. AAEM case report 3: myasthenia gravis. *Muscle Nerve* 1991; 14:391–397.
111. Stalberg EV, Sonoo M. Assessment of variability in the shape of the motor unit action potential, the jiggle, at consecutive discharges. *Muscle Nerve* 1994; 17:1135–1144.
112. Chaudhry V, Watson DF, Bird SJ, Cornblath DR. Stimulated single-fiber electromyography in Lambert-Eaton myasthenic syndrome. *Muscle Nerve* 1991; 14:1227–1230.
113. Daube JR. AAEM minimonograph 11: needle examination in clinical electromyography. *Muscle Nerve* 1991; 14:685–700.
114. Daube JR. *AAEM minimonograph 18: EMG in motor neuron diseases.* Rochester, MN: American Association of Electrodiagnostic Medicine, 1982.
115. Daube JR. Electrophysiologic studies in the diagnosis and prognosis of motor neuron disease. *Neurol Clin* 1985; 3:473–494.
116. Sobuye I, Saito N, Iida M, Ando K. Juvenile type of distal and segmental muscular atrophy of upper extremities. *Ann Neurol* 1978; 3: 429–432.
117. Oryema J, Ashby P, Spiegel S. Monomelic atrophy. *Can J Neurol Sci* 1990; 17:124–130.
118. Biondi A, Dormont D, Weitzner I, Bouche P, Chaine P, Bories J. MR imaging of the cervical cord in juvenile amyotrophy of distal upper extremity. *Am J Neuroradiol* 1989; 10:263–268.
119. Donofrio PD. AAEM Case report 28:Monomelic amyotrophy. *Muscle Nerve* 1994; 17:1129–1134.
120. Behnia M, Kelly JJ. Role of electromyography in amyotrophic lateral sclerosis. *Muscle Nerve* 1991; 14:1236–1241.
121. Shefner JM, Tyler HR, Krarup C. Abnormalities in the sensory action potential in patients with amyotrophic lateral sclerosis. *Muscle Nerve* 1991; 14:1242–1246.
122. Killian JM, Wilfong AA, Bernett L, Appel SH, Boland D. Decremental motor responses to repetitive nerve stimulation in ALS. *Muscle Nerve* 1994; 17:747–754.
123. Parry GJ, Clarke S. Multifocal acquired demyelinating neuropathy masquerading as a motor neuron disease. *Muscle Nerve* 1988; 11: 103–107.
124. Pestronk A. Invited review: motor neuropathies, motor neuron disorders, and antiglycolipid antibodies. *Muscle Nerve* 1991; 14:927–936.
125. Pestronk A, Chaudhry V, Feldman EL, et al. Lower motor neuron syndromes defined by patterns of weakness, nerve conduction abnormalities, and high titers of antiglycolipid antibodies. *Ann Neurol* 1990; 27:316–326.
126. Denys EH. AAEM case report 5: Amyotrophic lateral sclerosis. *Muscle Nerve* 1994; 17:263–268.
127. Parry GJ. AAEM case report 30: multifocal motor neuropathy. *Muscle Nerve* 1996; 19:269–276.
128. Chaudry V, Corse AM, Cornblath DR, Kuncl RW, Freimer ML, Griffin JW. Multifocal motor neuropathy: Electrodiagnostic features. *Muscle Nerve* 1994; 17:198–205.
129. Oh SJ, Claussen GC, Odabasi Z, Palmer CP. Multifocal demyelinating motor neuropathy: Pathologic evidence of inflammatory demyelinating polyradiculopathy. *Neurology* 1995; 45:1828–1832.
130. Donofrio PD, Albers JW. AAEM minimonograph 34: polyneuropathy: classification by nerve conduction studies and electromyography. *Muscle Nerve* 1990; 13:889–903.
131. Dyck PJ, Lambert EH, Thomas PK, Bunge R, eds. *Peripheral neuropathy.* Philadelphia: WB Saunders, 1984.
132. Dyck PJ, Thomas PK, Asbury AK, et al. *Diabetic neuropathy.* Philadelphia: WB Saunders, 1987.
133. McLeod JG, Evans WA. Peripheral neuropathy in spinocerebellar degenerations. *Muscle Nerve* 1981; 4:51–61.
134. Schaumberg HH, Spencer PS, Thomas PK. *Disorders of peripheral nerves.* Philadelphia: FA Davis, 1983.
135. Shields RW. Alcoholic polyneuropathy. *Muscle Nerve* 1985; 8: 183–187.
136. Kelly JJ. The electrodiagnostic findings in polyneuropathies associated with IgM monoclonal gammopathies. *Muscle Nerve* 1990; 13: 1113–1117.
137. Chang CW, Lien IN. Comparison of sensory nerve conduction in the palmar cutaneous branch and first digital branch of the median nerve: a new diagnostic method for carpal tunnel syndrome. *Muscle Nerve* 1991; 14:1173–1176.
138. Stevens JC. AAEM minimonograph 26: the electrodiagnosis of carpal tunnel syndrome. *Muscle Nerve* 1987; 10:99–113.
139. Miller RG. AAEM case report 1: ulnar neuropathy at the elbow. *Muscle Nerve* 1991; 14:97–101.
140. Kincaid JC, Phillips LH, Daube JR. The evaluation of suspected ulnar neuropathy at the elbow. *Arch Neurol* 1986; 43:44–47.
141. Felsenthal G, Butler DH, Shear MS. Across tarsal tunnel motor nerve conduction technique. *Arch Phys Med Rehabil* 1992; 73:64–69.
142. DeLisa JA, Saeed MA. The tarsal tunnel syndrome. *Muscle Nerve* 1983; 6:664–670.
143. Omer GE, Spinner M, eds. *Management of peripheral nerve problems.* Philadelphia: WB Saunders, 1980.
144. Spinner M. *Injuries to the major branches of peripheral nerves in the forearm.* Philadelphia: WB Saunders, 1978.
145. Sunderland S. *Nerves and nerve injuries.* Edinburgh: Churchill-Livingstone, 1978.
146. Mumenthaler M, Schliack H, eds. *Peripheral nerve lesions.* Stuttgart: Georg Thieme Verlag, 1991.
147. Hallett M. Electrophysiologic approaches to the diagnosis of entrapment neuropathies. *Neurol Clin* 1985; 3:531–542.
148. Dawson DM, Hallett M, Millender LH. *Entrapment neuropathies.* Boston: Little, Brown, 1990.
149. Pecina MM, Krmpotic-Nemanic J, Markiewitz AD. *Tunnel syndromes.* Boca Raton, FL: CRC Press, 1991.
150. Parry GJG. AAEM case report 11: mononeuropathy multiplex. *Muscle Nerve* 1985; 8:493–498.
151. Wilbourn AJ. Electrodiagnosis of plexopathies. *Neurol Clin* 1985; 3: 511–531.
152. Chokroverty S. AAEM case report 13: diabetic amyotrophy. *Muscle Nerve* 1987; 10:679–684.
153. Brown WF. *The physiological and technical basis of electromyography.* Boston: Butterworth, 1984; 37–94.
154. Subramony SH. AAEM case report 14: neuralgic amyotrophy (acute brachial neuropathy). *Muscle Nerve* 1988; 11:39–44.
155. Roos DB. The thoracic outlet syndrome is underrated. *Arch Neurol* 1990; 47:327–328.
156. Wilbourn AJ. The thoracic outlet syndrome is over diagnosed. *Arch Neurol* 1990; 47:328–330.
157. Lindgren KA, Manninen H, Rytkonen H. Thoracic outlet syndrome—a functional disturbance of the thoracic upper aperture? *Muscle Nerve* 1995; 18:526–530.
158. Ferrante MA, Wilbourn AJ. The utility of various sensory nerve conduction responses in assessing brachial plexopathies. *Muscle Nerve* 1995; 18:879–889.
159. Eisen A. Electrodiagnosis of radiculopathies. *Neurol Clin* 1985; 3: 494–510.
160. Wilbourn AJ. The value and limitations of electromyographic examination in the diagnosis of lumbosacral radiculopathy. In: Hardy RW, ed. *Lumbar disc disease.* New York: Raven Press, 1982; 65–109.

161. Wilbourn AJ. AAEM minimonograph 32: the electrodiagnostic examination in patients with radiculopathies. *Muscle Nerve* 1988; 11: 1099–1114.
162. Chu-Andrews J, Johnson RJ. Kimura J, ed. *Electrodiagnosis: an anatomical and clinical approach.* Philadelphia: JB Lippincott, 1986; 253–254.
163. Kimura J. Anatomic basis for localization. In: Kimura J, ed. *Electrodiagnosis in diseases of nerve and muscle: principles and practice,* 2nd ed. Philadelphia: FA Davis, 1989; 3–24.
164. Phillips LH, Park TS. Electrophysiologic mapping of the segmental anatomy of the muscles of the lower extremity. *Muscle Nerve* 1991; 14:1213–1218.
165. Chamely A, Husid M, Wilbourn AJ. The intramyotomal distribution of abnormalities with L5 and S1/S2 radiculopathies. *Muscle Nerve* 1987; 10:654.
166. Levin KH, Maggiano HJ, Wilbourn AJ. Cervical radiculopathies: Comparison of surgical and EMG localization of single root lesions. *Neurology* 1996; 46:1022–1025.
167. Albers JW, Kelly JJ. Acquired inflammatory demyelinating polyneuropathies: Clinical and electrodiagnostic features. *Muscle Nerve* 12: 435–451,1898.
168. Albers JW. AAEM case report 4: Guillain-Barré syndrome. *Muscle Nerve* 1989; 12:705–711.
169. Feasby TE. Axonal Guillain-Barré Syndrome. *Muscle Nerve* 1994; 17:678–679.
170. Cros DC, Triggs WJ. There are no neurophysiologic features characteristic of axonal Guillain-Barré syndrome. *Muscle Nerve* 1994; 17: 675–677.
171. Rich MM, Teener JW, Raps EC, Schotland DL. Muscle is electrically inexcitable in acute quadriplegic myopathy. *Neurology* 1996; 46: 731–736.
172. Gooch JL. AAEM case report 29: Prolonged paralysis after neuromuscular blockade. *Muscle Nerve* 1995; 18:937–942.
173. Ruff RL. Acute illness myopathy. *Neurology* 1996; 46:600–601.
174. Gutmann L, Blumenthal D, Gutmann L, Schochet SS. Acute type II myofiber atrophy in critical illness. *Neurology* 1996; 46:819–821.
175. Brooke MH. *A clinician's guide to muscle diseases*, 2nd ed. Baltimore: Williams & Wilkins, 1986.
176. Engle AG, Baker BQ, eds. *Myology.* New York: McGraw-Hill, 1986.
177. Layzer RB. *Neuromuscular manifestations of neuromuscular disease.* Philadelphia: FA Davis, 1985.
178. Walton JN. *Disorders of voluntary muscle,* 4th ed. London: Churchill-Livingstone, 1981.
179. Bodensteiner JB. Congenital myopathies. *Muscle Nerve* 1994; 17: 131–144.
180. Miller RH, Buchthal F. Autosomal recessive myotonia congenita: Marked muscle weakness in a 16 year old boy. *Muscle Nerve* 1992; 15:111–113.
181. Buchthal F. Electromyography in the diagnosis of muscle disease. *Neurol Clin* 1985; 3:573–598.
182. Trojaborg W. Quantitative electromyography in polymyositis: a reappraisal. *Muscle Nerve* 1990; 13:964–971.
183. Trojaborg W. Motor unit disorders and myopathies. In: Halliday AM, Butler S, Paul R, eds. *A textbook of clinical neurophysiology.* New York: John Wiley & Sons, 1987; 417–428.
184. Joy JL, Oh SJ, Baysal AI. Electrophysiological spectrum of inclusion body myositis. *Muscle Nerve* 1990; 13:949–951.
185. Trojaborg W. EMG in myositis. *Electroencephalogr Clin Neurophysiol* 1987; 66(Suppl):105–106.
186. Barkhaus PE, Nandedkar SD, Sanders DB. Quantitative EMG in inflammatory myopathy. *Muscle Nerve* 1990; 13:247–253.
187. Uncini A, Lange DJ, Lovelace RE, Solomon M, Hays AP. Long-duration polyphasic motor unit potentials in myopathies: a quantitative study with pathological correlation. *Muscle Nerve* 1990; 13:263–267.
188. Haller RG. Experimental acute alcoholic myopathy: a histochemical study. *Muscle Nerve* 1985; 8:195–203.
189. Engel AG, Lambert EH, Rosevear JW, Tauxe WN. Clinical and electromyographic studies in a patient with primary hypokalemic periodic paralysis. *Am J Med* 1965; 38:626–640.
190. Ricker R, Rudel R, Lehmann-Horn F, Kither G. Muscle stiffness and electrical activity in paramyotonia congenita. *Muscle Nerve* 1986; 9: 299–305.
191. Streib EW. Paramyotonia congenita: successful treatment with tocainide: clinical and electrophysiologic findings in seven patients. *Muscle Nerve* 1987; 10:155–162.
192. Streib EW. AAEM minimonograph 27: differential diagnosis of myotonic syndromes. *Muscle Nerve* 1987; 10:603–615.
193. Brown WF. Normal and abnormal spontaneous activity in muscle. In: The physiological and technical basis of electromyography. Boston: Butterworth, 1984; 339–368.
194. Dumitru D. Single muscle fiber discharges (Insertion activity, end-plate potentials, positive sharp waves, and fibrillation potentials): A unifying proposal. *Muscle Nerve* 1996; 19:221–226,229–230.
195. Kraft GH. Issues and Opinions. Single muscle fiber discharges (insertion activity, end-plate potentials, positive sharp waves, and fibrillation potentials): A unifying proposal. Rebuttal. *Muscle Nerve* 1996; 19:227–228.

Rehabilitation Medicine: Principles and Practice, Third Edition, edited by Joel A. DeLisa and Bruce M. Gans. Lippincott–Raven Publishers, Philadelphia © 1998.

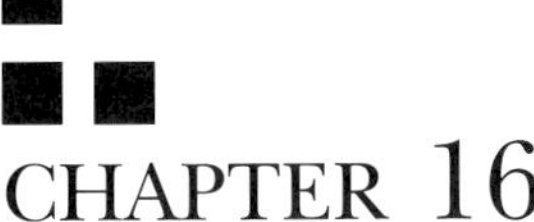

CHAPTER 16

Central Nervous System Electrophysiology

Jeffrey L. Cole

Physiatric applications of central nervous system (CNS) electrodiagnostic examinations include stimulus-specific studies that allow functional correlations to be made about losses and residual capabilities after any individual disease process or injury. These tools yield information that is often quantifiable for almost any type of stimulus-specific response, including all sensory pathways. Additionally, the initiation of peripheral motor responses or efferent neurogram activity can be examined using event-related cortical potentials and by direct motor cortex or spinal cord stimulation. The information from these tests can be related to physiological function, transmission, and processing of information in addition to anatomy changes or gross loss of tissue. This information, therefore, can be complementary to that gathered by imaging studies, which only define the local anatomic changes. The imaging studies and the electrodiagnostic studies should never be considered mutually exclusive. These electrophysiological studies can produce functional and prognostic information, define acute intraoperative changes, or stand alone as unique diagnostic data.

The first observations of the nature of electrical activity on the brain were by Canton in 1875, when he reported detection of electrical currents from electrodes placed on the skull or exposed brains of animals (1). The first reported use of photographic averaging by trace superimposition was by Dawson in 1947, to improve his ability to see synchronized responses to a particular event (2,3).The giant myoclonic somatosensory evoked potentials (SEP) that he observed serendipitously were the first event-related cerebral responses to a peripheral nerve stimulation and opened an entire area of electrodiagnostics (3). Later, he designed and built the first electromechanical averager to increase the signal-to-noise (S/N) ratio and improve his ability to see these potentials, which are extremely small relative to the ongoing electroencephalograph (EEG) and amplifier noises.

J. L. Cole: Department of Physical Medicine and Rehabilitation, The New York Hospital Medical Center of Queens, Flushing, New York 11355.

More widespread interest in evoked potential (EP) studies occurred approximately 20 years later, when available electronic averaging equipment and amplifier noise levels improved the effective S/N ratios and became available to more clinically oriented researchers. The final phase of their application on a routine clinical level was the development and the availability, at a reasonable cost, of integrated circuits so that all electrophysiological equipment could be supplied with electronic averaging capabilities, putting EP studies within the realm of every clinician's office. Despite this, it remains a poorly understood diagnostic tool, for although there is a large data base of normal values and gross correlation with a variety of pathologic conditions, there is little understanding of the generator sources. It generally is accepted that the scalp potentials recorded are the sum of multiple neuronal tracts, nuclei, and processes that are conducted to the scalp through different tissues.

These procedure results should never be used with rote pattern recognition or in isolation to establish a specific diagnosis. The physician performing these studies must review the relevant history and physical examination before planning the neurophysiological studies. The interpretation of the results must address the specific clinical questions that prompted the referral, and the results must be correlated with other available laboratory and radiologic information. Some of the basic science, applications, interpretation, and technical pitfalls of the different studies are presented as a starting point from which to build clinical experience. This brief overview is an initial exposure that should lead interested clinicians to further reading and training before they practice EP techniques.

ROUTINE ELECTRODIAGNOSIS IN CENTRAL NERVOUS SYSTEM DISEASE

It should be noted that abnormal needle electromyography (EMG) findings frequently are seen in muscles weakened by CNS disease, especially during the acute injury phase

(4,5). Awareness of this finding will prevent overdiagnosis of the peripheral nerve injuries that can occur in association with the CNS problem. In general, spontaneous potentials and increased insertional activity are seen in muscle during the flaccid period after acute injury, and they diminish as spasticity or voluntary movement develops (6,7).

In spinal cord injury (SCI), serial studies have confirmed that fibrillation potentials are seen in most patients with recent complete injury in the 3^+ to 4^+ grade range (5,7,8). The abnormalities diminish over time in the proximal muscles more than in the distal muscles (5,7). All nine subjects seen by Campbell and Herbison had persistence of spontaneous potentials below the knee when seen 3 years or more after the injury (5). Motor and sensory nerve conduction velocities were normal in seven of the nine subjects and only mildly abnormal in the two others. Hemiplegia secondary to stroke can result in similar abnormalities (4,6). Johnson demonstrated in serial studies of 16 patients with acute stroke that positive sharp waves and fibrillation potentials develop during the second week after injury (6). The abnormalities tend to resolve within 6 to 12 months, usually as tone returns to the muscles (4,6). Motor unit potentials, when active, remain normal in configuration.

During the acute phase of hemiplegia after stroke, the F-wave response is diminished in amplitude and persistence in direct proportion to the severity of weakness (9). Chronic spastic hemiparesis results in an increase in the F-wave amplitude when compared with the contralateral limb (10), whereas the M and H responses remain symmetric. The blink reflex also commonly is abnormal after cortical and subcortical stroke (11,12). The R2 component on the hemiplegic side is most likely abnormal and in proportion to the degree of paresis and can show significantly prolonged duration as reorganization occurs. Brainstem studies have been reported more commonly as producing abnormal blink reflexes (12). In coma, a persistent blink reflex suggests a good prognosis.

NEUROPHYSIOLOGY OF THE POTENTIAL GENERATOR

Before we discuss correlation of stimulus-contingent information on a clinical level, we would like to attempt to understand the relationship between the recorded waveforms and their underlying generators. These information-processing areas of the brain that produce the electrical response can be thought of as a localized receptor field. For clinical studies at this time, there is only gross anatomic localization to brain regions. Clearly, the most efficacious applications and ultimate correlation of CNS electrodiagnostic studies will be with identification of the peripheral afferent pathways utilized and the CNS anatomic structures, neuroelectrical activity, and processes involved.

Whenever neuron and glial cell membranes depolarize, there is an inward flow of current, and a potential difference is created between different locations in the extracellular space (Fig. 16-1). These ionic movements usually are related to transient changes in membrane-embedded ionic channel proteins. Such transient flows may be produced by voltage-sensitive transitions in membrane conductance, as in sodium channel activation supporting the axonal conduction of an action potential or from chemically mediated changes in postsynaptic membrane conductance produced through the presynaptic release of a neurotransmitter. Transmembrane ionic currents can be defined precisely in basic cellular studies by using intracellular microelectrodes and recording the transmembrane voltages directly. The ionic flow potential differences can be recorded by placing a pair of electrodes into the extracellular space. With one electrode fixed in place, it is possible to move the other electrode around throughout the extracellular space and define the spatial distribution of these electric potentials in the potential field. Thus, the primary event is the ionic current flow across a cellular membrane that generates a potential field that distributes throughout the volume conductor of the extracellular space. The cells giving rise to the transmembrane current flows, the source or field generator, produce the volume-conducted extracellular potential fields that can be recorded at large distances or from the skin overlying the actual source. The resultant surface potential represents the linear summation of the individual cellular generators, their temporal synchronization of activation, their spatial orientation to each other, and the geometry of the volume conductor.

Based on this electric field theory, the recorded scalp potentials result from the superposition of the brain's electrostatic fields. Because the total net electrical charge of the brain generators is zero, only pairs of separated positive and negative charges can give rise to potential fields. This separated pair of electric charges, called a dipole (see Fig. 16-1), is represented by a vector whose magnitude is given by the product of the separated amount of charge multiplied by the distance of separation and whose direction along an imaginary line drawn between the separated point charges is determined by the orientation. The field generator activity is modeled electrically as either a sheet or point dipole whose orientation relative to the recording electrodes will determine the general configuration of the potential distribution. A radially oriented dipole will be maximal overlying the dipole location, regardless of polarity, and its amplitude will fall off as the electrode moves away from the source in any direction. It is this dipole type that most effectively generates a positive scalp potential. A tangentially oriented dipole gives rise to a polarity reversal in the surface distribution with a positive peak on one end and a negative peak on the other. Obliquely oriented dipoles give rise to distributions that are effectively hybrids of these two types of field. From the scalp, it is not possible to identify the specific cellular areas giving rise to the signal, or even whether the response(s) reflect excitatory or inhibitory processes.

When activity is recorded without the application of specific stimuli, this is referred to as spontaneous or background activity, the usual mode for recording the EEG. When seg-

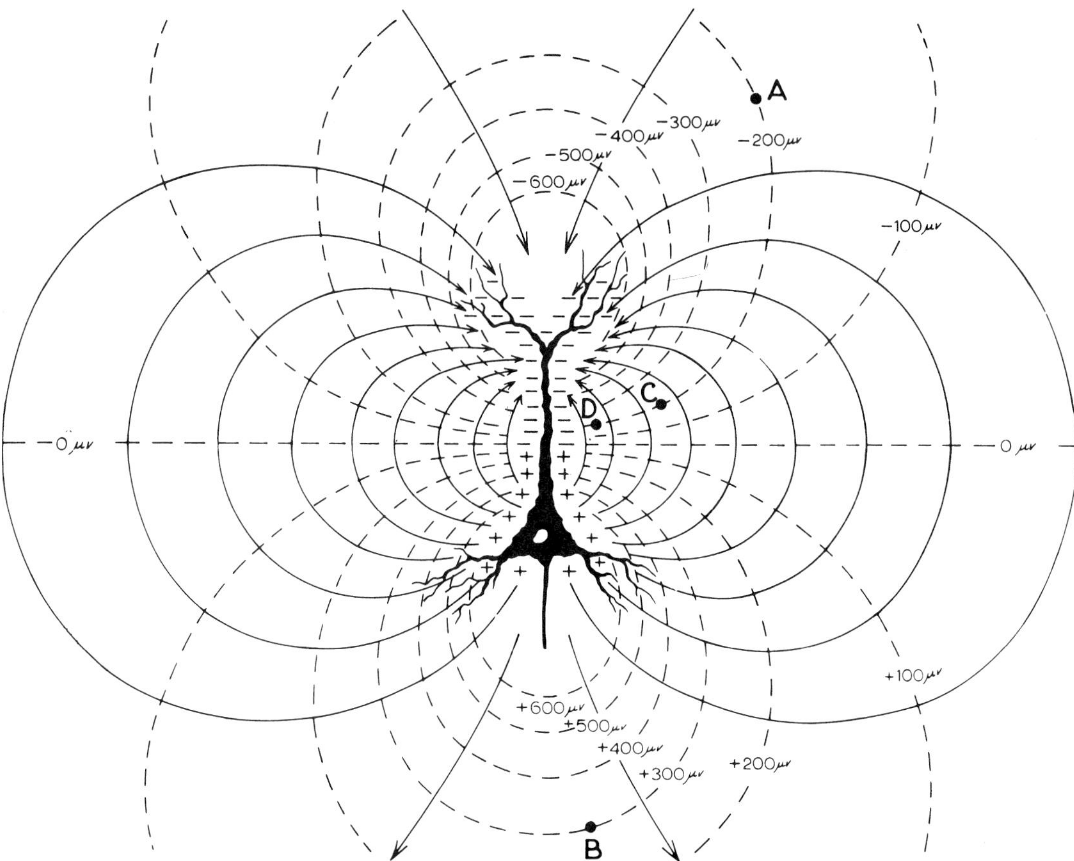

FIG. 16-1. Dipole modeling of generators. The fundamental dipole of the cortex is the pyramidal cell. A dipolar field is generated when the cellular membrane receives synaptic input to the dendritic tree. This creates a net relative negativity or positivity superficially in the apical dendrites that generates a potential difference between the cell body and basal dendrites and the apical dendrites. For example, superficial excitatory input, as illustrated here, causes a relative negativity of the apical dendrites and positivity in the cell body and basal dendrites. The transient dipolar field causes a current to flow through the volume conductor, and this is recorded as a voltage on the scalp. This resultant surface potential *(dashed lines)* represents the linear summation of the individual cellular generators and will depend on synchronization of generator activation as well as on the geometry of both the generators and the volume conductor. Current flows are shown as *solid lines.* (From Gloor P. Neuronal generators and the problem of localization in electroencephalography: application of volume conductor theory to electroencephalography. *J Clin Neurophysiol* 1985; 2:327–345.)

ments of the data are recorded after application of a discrete stimulus, this is referred to as evoked activity or sensory EPs. Depending on the stimulation rate, the EP responses may be either transient or steady-state. With transient EP, the rate of stimulation is slow enough that the response to one stimulus is completed before the next stimulus is applied. With steady-state EP, the stimulus rate is high enough that one response appears to interact with the next response of the series. Depending on the stimulation rate, responses can overlap and may reduce or augment the resultant response. Because the processes underlying the EP generally are nonlinear, the transient and steady-state EP can provide complementary information about the underlying generative processes. In clinical applications, at this time, only transient stimuli are used.

When extracellular activity is recorded close to the generator site, as from electrodes placed on the surface of the exposed primary sensory cortex, the EP after application of a peripheral stimulus can be recognized with a single trial. This technique has been used with intraoperative recording in epileptic patients to map regions of the somatosensory cortex. When the evoked activity is recorded on the scalp at some distance from the source, signal averaging usually must be used to enable extraction of the recorded activity that correlates consistently with the application of the evoking stimulus. With the assumption that background noise has a random nature, the S/N ratio shows improvement in proportion to the square root of the number of averaged sweeps.

A percutaneous peripheral nerve stimulation, which produces a clear motor action potential, also will produce an afferent traveling wave of neural extracellular negativity called a somatosensory afferent neurogram. To be able to record a distinct response, the conducting nerves must be congruous, for with loss of coherency, the spatial and temporal field summation contributed by each axon is reduced, and the recorded potential becomes lower in amplitude, wider in duration, or more complex in morphology. The response would be referred to as being dispersed. Dispersion usually is encountered in peripheral nerve conduction studies, but when CNS recording activity is being generated, the activity is generated primarily by synchronous postsynaptic potential activation and apparently can appear dispersed by other mechanisms.

The nerve cell population's geometry is important in determining the field generator's recordable activity. The parallel-oriented nerve tracts produce an open conduction pattern as would be seen in peripheral nerve conduction studies (Fig. 16-2). The radially oriented nuclei set up a closed potential field presentation that, by its complex spherical alignment, tends effectively to cancel out the distantly recorded neural activity, yielding a zero net electrical domain. Depending on whether the internal structure is spatially regular or randomly oriented, the activity may or may not be clearly evident in a distant extracellular recordings. If the brain cells in a responding population are synchronously activated, and, in addition, they all are oriented in the same direction (e.g., cortical pyramidal cells), then the potentials associated with each cell in the group also will have the same orientation, and their fields will spatially sum for a large net potential. A spatially regular neural population in which the geometry of the cells aligns gives rise to an open field generator. In an open field, the extracellular activity produced by the neural population can be recorded at a distance from the generator. Spatial cancellation results if the cells are not all oriented in the same direction, and thus structures such as deep nuclei may make relatively little contribution to the extracellular potential field outside the immediate vicinity of the source. Penetrating intracranial electrodes must be inserted to detect their activity. This situation is referred to as the closed field generator. Thus, source geometry is critical in determining the spatial distribution of the extracellular activity that can be recorded remotely from the source population.

When the source of the activity is relatively close to the recording electrode sites, this is referred to as near-field recording (Fig. 16-3), as when a scalp electrode is recording activity directly over a cortical generator. Near-field recordings are characterized by large spatial gradients in the potential field because there is less spread of the extracellular activity through the volume conductor between the site of generation and the site of recording. Near-field recordings can be done with electrodes that are relatively close together on the surface and in the region of the spatial gradient, as a bipolar recording, or they can be recorded with one electrode placed close to the source with the other electrode at a relatively inactive and distant reference site, as a monopolar recording. It must be recognized that this differentiation is only a relative one that can be misleading because, in fact, there is no ideal reference site. All electrode locations on the skin, including the ground electrode, will have some significant activity so that all surface recording systems are really bipolar. When a recorded potential deflection is seen, it is important to recognize that both the active and reference electrodes are contributing to the recorded potential. On the other hand, far-field recordings are produced when the generator site is much further from the accessible surface, as would be the case of the brainstem generating auditory evoked responses. As in this case, the amplitudes usually are low, and a great deal more averaging is needed. From the recording surface, far-field potential field spatial gradients are low, and the extracellular distribution spread is broad. Therefore, these potentials must necessarily be recorded with electrodes that are fairly widely separated to detect and sample the spatial gradient.

The volume conductor's geometry (e.g., the arm tissue being stimulated during an upper extremity SEP study) also can have an important effect on the EP waveform components' identification and interpretation. Kimura and col-

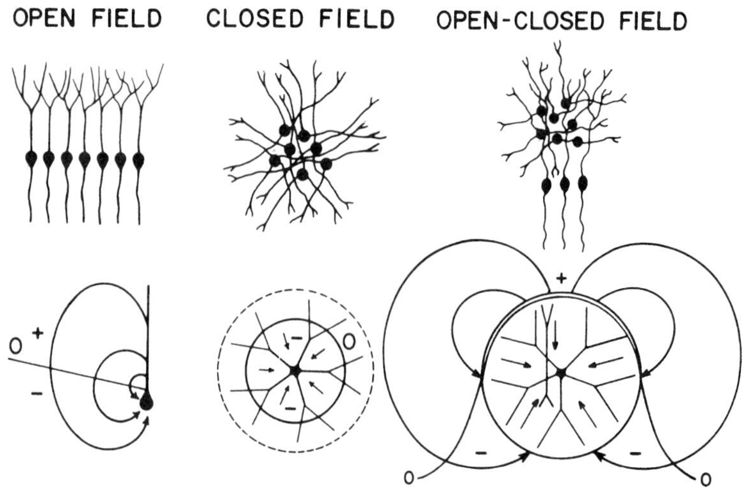

FIG. 16-2. The effect of source geometry on field potential recording. Current flow and potential field produced by synchronous depolarization of the cell bodies of a row of neurons with parallel orientation *(open field)*, with the cell bodies clustered and dendrites spreading radially *(closed field)*, and with a combination of radial and parallel elements *(open–closed field)*. (From Allison T, Wood CC, McCarthy G. The central nervous system. In: Coles MGH, Donchin E, Porges SW, eds. *Psychophysiology: systems, processes and applications.* New York: Guilford Press, 1986; 5–25. Adapted from Lorente de No R. Action potential of the motor neurons of the hypoglossus nucleus. *J Cell Comp Physiol* 1947; 29:207–287.)

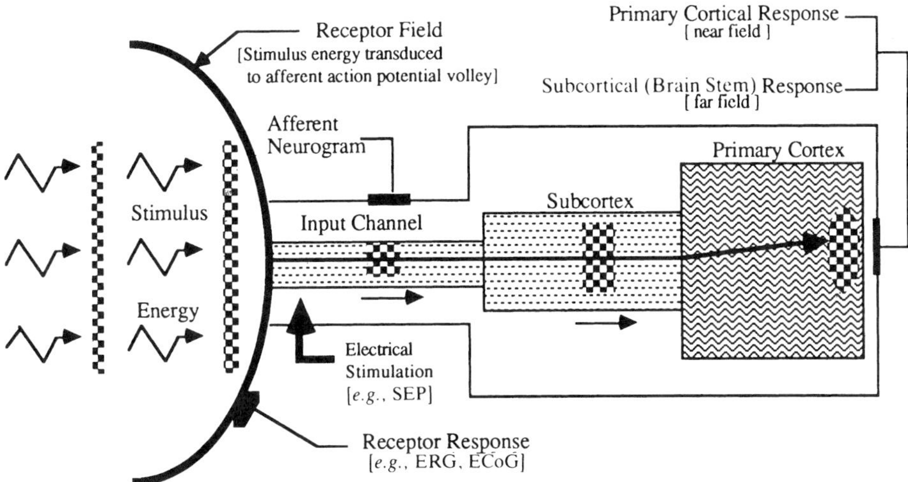

FIG. 16-3. Recording paradigm common to all evoked potentials. Discrete, repeating stimuli are applied to a receptor field or peripheral nerve of the relevant part of the nervous system being studied to give rise to an electrophysiological signal. This series of synchronous afferent volleys traverses the chosen input pathway to its primary cortical region to be recorded as a somatosensory evoked potential *(SEP)*. Signals theoretically can be recorded from the receptors themselves (e.g., as an electroretinogram, *ERG*, or electrocochleogram, *ECoG*) or along its peripheral or subcortical course as well while a particular sensory stimulus or the start of a motor response recurs.

leagues demonstrated that some far-field EP components may be contributed to or be the result of the transmitted volley's activity passing across a discontinuous junction, at which point the volume conductor geometry changes significantly (13). Some of these phenomena reflect the distant recording of the change in current density produced as the propagating electrical field being confined (and therefore concentrated) or expanded (diluting the recordable power) as it flows away from the stimulus. The elbow is such a junction, as the transmission moves from the lower to upper arm. This phenomenon, in which stationary components are generated, has been modeled using basic field theory and computer simulations of volume conduction through structures of various geometries (13,14). Extreme caution must be exercised in assigning relevance to early and middle far-field components without concurrent tracking of the afferent volley's timing, particularly when the moving current may be crossing a boundary where the volume conductor geometry changes, because the principle of generator algebraic superposition is always at play. That means that at any given time, the activity from spatially distinct generators is volume conducted, and their simultaneous activity overlaps. Thus, scalp potential field summations can produce either masking, truncation, or enhancement of the individual components. The individual SEP cortical peaks have been attributed to responses from (a) parallel conducted peripheral information and/or from (b) sequentially produced cerebral processing. This is reviewed further under Clinical Correlation.

To discuss CNS electrophysiology processes accurately and to have the capability to interpret clinical studies, it is necessary to achieve a broad familiarity with seemingly diverse topics, including anatomic and neurophysiological factors, electric field theory, the technical aspects of instrumentation, and recording techniques for specific procedures being applied. It generally is accepted that the scalp potentials recorded are the sum of multiple neuronal tracts and nuclei that are then conducted up to the scalp through different tissues. Because of these factors and observed differences in the responses under different recording conditions, there have been cycles of condemnation and acceptance throughout the growth and adoption of CNS electrodiagnostics. The actual bioelectrical phenomenon that is evoked in response to a given stimulation has not changed since Dawson first recorded the scalp information with his photo-averaging technique (2), but what has changed is how we envision and record the EPs and our ability to refine and correlate these data with clinical information. When rigorous recording criteria are used, it is an excellent diagnostic tool whose full potential has yet to be realized. Beyond current concepts of recording EPs are many new applications of this information for the rehabilitation process that have not yet been developed.

RECORDED EVOKED POTENTIALS

An EP represents the algebraic sum of the electrical activity seen across the scalp at a given time related to a stimulus delivered through a predetermined sensory pathway. Scalp potentials recorded today commonly measure the voltage changes at a point on the scalp plotted against time following a stimulus. The recorded scalp potential therefore is the sum of some or all of the stimulus-evoked, event-related, and bioelectrical potentials from, depending on the area being studied, the peripheral nerve, retina, or cochlear mechanism;

from the spinal cord or central conduction pathways; and from cortical and subcortical cerebral structures.

Even assuming that the applied stimulus is adequate to produce these potentials and the recording electrodes are applied properly, recording is an enterprise fraught with difficulties and contaminating signals and noises (15,16). Among these are the bioelectric signals such as cardiac and skeletal muscle potentials, ongoing EEG and spinal cord activity, ocular movement and corneoretinal potentials, and cerebrospinal fluid volume-conducted potentials. In addition, there are electromagnetic noises and artifacts from the electronic circuit components plus the random interference from the environment. Sixty-cycle interference from line current, fluorescent lights, and unshielded and motor-driven devices that are in close proximity or plugged into the same power line are especially troublesome. A plugged-in, unshielded extension cord with nothing plugged into it or inadequate equipment and patient grounding can generate sufficient interference to prevent signal acquisition when an averager voltage input limiter is used, as is common in most averaging devices. These voltage input limiters are routinely set to prevent the input of any signal that is too large (90% of maximal display presentation) relative to the amplifier gain setting for the test. Another phenomenon that can be troublesome is called ringing, which is manifested by time-locked baseline oscillations within filter networks.

Although EP studies are being used routinely as a clinical tool for diagnostic and therapeutic determinants in patient care, this is still a developing science. The growing wealth of literature attests that there are varied methodologies and poorly standardized ways of recording the various studies. Many think that this is desirable because standardization would tend to inhibit the clinicians who experiment with new technical approaches.

In the sections that follow, recording parameters and electrode montage guides are the most commonly used recommendations. In no way do we imply that these are the only recognized recording techniques, and continued experimentation is highly desirable once the individual practitioner has developed sufficient experience to understand the impact that each change will have on the recorded information.

The most frequent recording paradigm for looking at the scalp EP is from electrode pairs with voltage plotted against time. The more powerful computer-based equipment being produced enables us to look at more dynamic and varied brain information. Spectral analyses are being reapplied to the EP in attempts to improve component sensitivity and ability to detect pathologic processes (17). The calculated second derivative (i.e., the rate of change of the rate of change) of the scalp potential is a particularly powerful tool known as the scalp current density that gives information on the local current flow from the resultant dipole source. This gives better information on biogenerator localization, improved correlation with known pathologic conditions and neural transmission, and will be more widely available in the near future (18–21,23,24). The graphic technique of brain electrical activity mapping (BEAM) is the representation of electrical potential differences across the entire recorded scalp surface at a fixed time after the triggered stimulus. The interpolated map produced uses a scale of colors to represent the voltage gradients based on the electrode array of at least 32 channels. Wide clinical application has been slow because its best application is with longer-latency cognitive studies that require a large, well-controlled data base to be used clinically, and arbitrary color scales can camouflage pathologic processes or encourage excessive false positives with all but the most experienced practitioners. Three-dimensional vector analysis techniques are finding application in the analysis of scalp far-field potentials in auditory brainstem responses (ABR, formerly called brainstem auditory evoked responses [BAER]), with the main conceptual difference in data representation being the plotting of voltage versus voltage sequentially instead of against time to give a pattern of loops much like an electrocardiogram vector analysis (25,26). The data analysis adaptation and representation simplicity are based on the credulous assumption that the vector can be shown as a single, generator-dependent instantaneous dipole.

Result reporting should include the relevant aspects of the history and physical examination and the reason for the referral. The traces used for the data analysis and interpretation must be recorded from at least two clearly reproduced runs to demonstrate reliability and must be printed with the report, including the electrode montage and recording amplitude and time-base calibrations. The stimulus and equipment recording parameters used for the test should be included with the data as well as a brief description of the technique used. Interpretation of latency, amplitude, and waveform morphology always should be based on appropriate statistical analysis.

THE INTERNATIONAL 10–20 SYSTEM

The first prominent conference to standardize EEG electrode placements and their nomenclature was in 1947, which resulted in the 1958 proposal of what we now refer to as the International 10–20 System for technique, scalp electrode placements, and standardized labeling of electrode sites that is identical in all languages (27). This well-planned scheme for scalp coverage, using a limited number of electrode sites whose locations could be reproduced easily and accurately, was necessary to permit good serial comparison and the exchange of comparative EEG data. Although these needs are common to EP work, we are looking at very different types of electrophysiological information and therefore need additional flexibility. The reader should learn proper electrode site placements before looking at the occasional deviations and their generally recognized nomenclature.

The 10–20 system allows for uniform positioning relative to fixed landmarks that would then give uniformly proportionate electrode placements no matter what the subject's skull size. There are anatomically proven correlates for each electrode site (Fig. 16-4) that are consistent from patient to

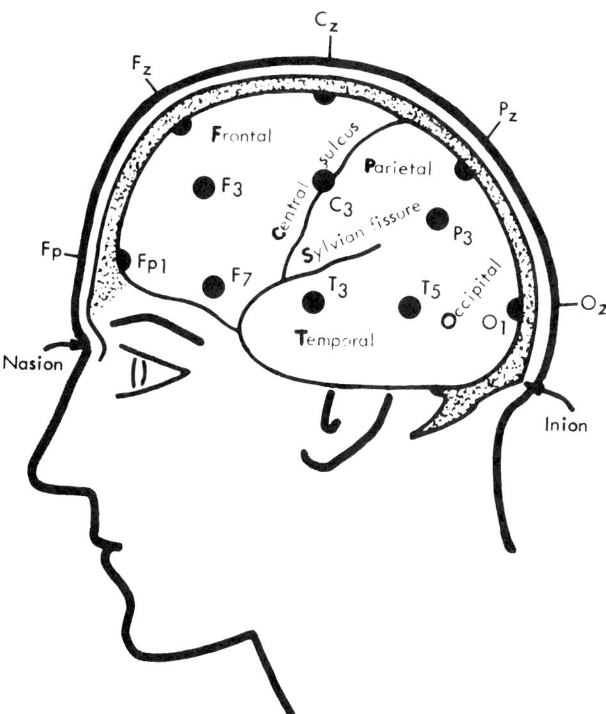

FIG. 16-4. Anatomic correlations between the midline electrode positions and the brain lobes, central sulcus, and Sylvian fissure.

patient, and a large enough area of scalp is included to provide adequate brain coverage for all areas of cortical representation.

The first measurement made is the nasion to inion distance in centimeters. This distance is then subdivided into 10% and 20% increments (Fig. 16-5) for the first Fp, Fz, Cz, Pz, and O site locations. The sites are marked with a wax pencil or marker on the scalp; for example, the central zero or vertex (Cz) anterior-to-posterior mark is located at the midpoint (50%) of the total measurement from nasion to inion. There are 21 regularly used scalp electrode sites: two nonscalp sets at the earlobes (i.e., A_1, A_2) and nasopharyngeal region (i.e., Pg_1, Pg_2); and two for cerebellar activity (i.e., Cb_1, Cb_2) that are rarely used because it is thought that they do not accurately reflect local activity from the cerebellum.

When one is recording from an infant's or newborn's head, it is not necessary or desirable to use a full complement of electrodes because of the larger variation between the skull landmarks and the underlying cortical structures (28). The nine generally used recording electrodes and two auricular locations (see Figs. 16-4 and 16-5) are derived in the same manner and using the same relative percentages as outlined above for adults. After 6 months of age, a full electrode complement usually can be applied. When the shape of the head is distorted or deformed, electrode application should proceed as normally as possible, with the reference points and Cz location based on the most normal-appearing (i.e., least deformed) side proportions or by maintaining symmetry and routine percentages for the electrode locations if the deformity is diffuse.

The 10–20 system was developed to answer the needs of EEG. The site label nomenclature was borrowed for use in EP studies; however, its rigidity demanded certain modifications during their evolution. A fairly common practice in cortical SEP studies is to place an electrode behind a designated site and use a prime mark (′) for each 1-cm distance away. This evolved in SEP work because these subtle shifts of the electrodes were found to maximize the averaged evoked amplitude or improve the separation or identification of certain peaks. An example of this would be placement of an electrode 2 cm behind the Cz site, toward the inion, to be designated Cz″. Also, when other than scalp recording sites are used, the area should be designated precisely with clear anatomic references. The "O" site is sometimes labeled "Oz" when used in SEP and visual evoked potential (VEP) studies. We must stress that although these necessary adaptations are frequent practices and appear in the literature for EP studies, they are common uses and abuses of the nomenclature and are not permitted in the 10–20 system for EEG recordings.

EQUIPMENT

Suppose that we were summoned to the Coronary Care Unit because readings on the monitor indicated that a patient

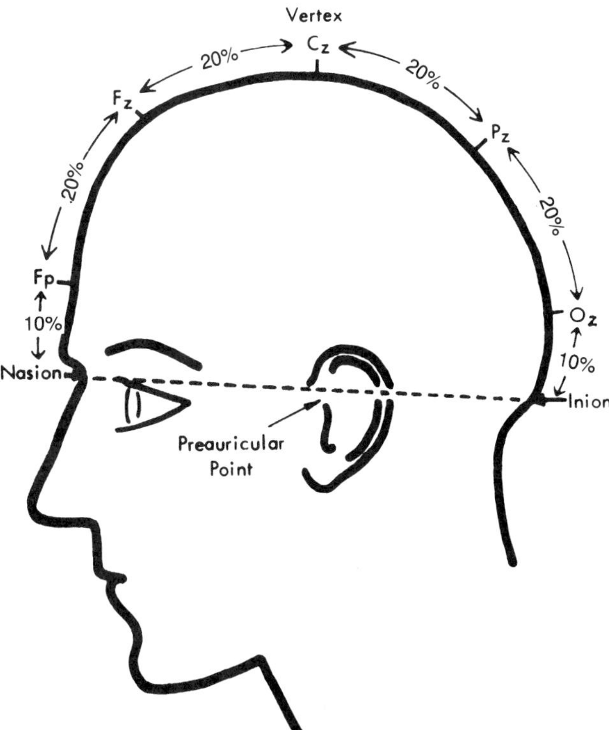

FIG. 16-5. Reference point landmarks on the skull, including the *nasion*, right and left *preauricular points*, and *inion*, from the left lateral view. The percentages of distance between electrode sites are shown along the midline measurement from nasion to inion.

to which it was attached had essentially no cardiac output and we found that the patient was sitting comfortably in bed without clinically evident cardiopulmonary compromise. The lines would be checked for placement and patency, and the medical decision might be to disconnect the monitor because it appeared to have malfunctioned. In such a situation, we could easily examine the patient's pulse and lung sounds for confirmatory diagnostic information and accept that the equipment could be at fault. Unfortunately, because of the nature of CNS electrophysiological testing, we are much more dependent on the machine's output.

If we are generally intimidated by the equipment and do not recognize when we are faced with a technical error or malfunction, we can be misled. Unlike peripheral neuromuscular studies, direct clinical data correlation is more obfuscated, and because the information sought is of very low amplitude, is embedded in electronic and bioelectrical noise, and often is surrounded by larger contaminating bioelectric signals, information processing is necessary. This puts the tester in a passive role during the data collection process but does not obviate the need for physician interaction, examination, and development of an appropriate game plan.

Electrodes

For the skin–electrode interface, the scalp should be scrubbed with a lightly abrasive solution for surface recording or cleaned for needle insertion. An electrode is applied where needed and fixed in place with collodium or elasticized tape to minimize movement during testing. The interface so formed, at the electrode contact point, has characteristics that vary significantly with the type of electrode (e.g., cup, disc, intradermal, pin, Ag/AgCl, surface clip) applied. This is because the interface formed behaves electrically as a resistor and capacitor wired in parallel so that alternating current (AC) and direct current (DC) signals can cross this interface (15,29,30). The absolute values of the resistance and capacitance vary with the skin location being used, the type of electrode and electrolyte solution or gel selected, and the skin preparation technique. The relative values of the resistance and capacitance, combined as impedance, vary with the frequency and voltage of the biological signals. At low frequencies the impedance approaches the resistance of the coupling electrolyte, and at the higher frequencies it is inversely proportional to the signal's current density. It is desirable to test the electrodes with an impedance meter whose AC frequency is at the lower end of the frequency of the biological signal that is to be recorded. Most commercial impedance meters use 30- to 60-Hz generators and give fairly representative values. The resultant impedance should be between 2,000 and 5,000 Ω with a properly applied surface electrode. Intradermal pin- or clip-type surface electrodes have inherently higher impedances that cannot be reduced because of the nature and size of the skin–electrode interface (31), which can theoretically contribute to greater stimulus artifact (32). Electrode testing with a DC ohmmeter cannot determine the actual impedance reading and generates an electrical charge at the skin–electrode interface.

When multichannel recordings are used, we recommend that individual electrodes for each channel input be placed at each site to be used instead of using jumper wires to split the electrode for input into more than one channel. Not only can jumpers affect the signal quality, they can inadvertently cause shunting of the signal or effectively short out a preamplifier input. This shorting can occur because the majority of systems use a common-mode rejection design that requires a single ground connected to all amplifiers.

For the most precise recordings, the patients are advised to wash their scalp and hair the morning of the test and not to apply anything to the hair. Deceptively low impedance readings can be attained because the salts in sweat and a variety of hair conditioning agents can produce bridging between the electrodes. If the electrodes are shorted out in this manner, no clinically significant recording can be obtained.

Among the differences between peripheral and central electrophysiological studies is the effect the ground electrode placement may have on the EP waveform. Theoretically, it should eliminate signals by common-mode rejection, but with small-amplitude responses, it can produce a signal by common-mode amplification because it is sending information to two amplifiers that are never perfectly matched. The ground site can be on the extremity being stimulated, located proximal to the stimulation site or at a relatively indifferent site near the active and reference electrodes. In either case, the electrode should be similar to those used in the remainder of the study, and the site similarly prepared. In addition, because of the potential for disease transmission, pin or needle electrodes and surface electrodes used in the genital areas should be soaked in bleach or equivalent disinfectant and then processed by regular gas or high-vacuum sterilization (33).

Filters and Filtering

The information of interest for recording has its electrical energy within a specific limited frequency range. One way to improve measurement of this desired signal would be to diminish those signals whose frequencies are above or below that range with a frequency discrimination device. This is called an electronic wave filter, or simply a filter. If a heterogeneous signal (i.e., white noise) is input through such a frequency-selective device, certain parts of the signal (i.e., output voltage) will be passed through unaltered, and the electrical energy at certain frequencies will be dispersed or blocked out. The cutoff or break frequency of a filter is defined as the frequency at which the gain (i.e., the ratio of output voltage to input voltage) drops to a fixed level, typically between 70% and 50% of the input amplitude in a typical filter. This definition leaves out all consideration of the signal's dropoff rate, which is discussed later.

A low-pass filter passes the signals with little attenuation up to the cutoff frequency. Those signal components with higher frequencies are attenuated, and the lower frequencies are passed through. This device will determine the upper frequency setting of the bandwidth being examined. A high-pass filter will attenuate the frequencies between zero and the determined cutoff and allow the majority of signals above the cutoff frequency to pass. Because frequencies are permitted to pass above the cutoff but are attenuated below, this device will determine the bandwidth's lower frequency setting being examined. Equipment manufactured with bandpass filters pass a selected group of frequencies with little attenuation between the two determined cutoff frequencies. The difference between the two preselected numbers is the bandwidth permitted through for analysis. These devices limit the ability to adjust the machine adequately. In a band-reject filter (with its frequency response opposite that of the bandpass filter), the frequencies below the lower cutoff and above the higher cutoff are passed with little attenuation while the signal whose frequencies lie between the lower and higher cutoff levels are attenuated appreciably. If the attenuated frequency range is very narrow, it is called a notch filter. During EEG recording, the notch filter can be used to eliminate 60-Hz interference, but EP signals, except in brainstem studies, contain much information through that range, and so notch filters should not be used. Additionally, notch filters can produce a transient ringing or oscillations of the baseline that can obliterate data acquisition or cause misinterpretation of results. Ringing occurs when the signal being analyzed has significant energy in the frequencies being processed out by the filters. If this effect is suspected, the notch filter should be turned off and the filter settings separated so more signal passes unimpeded. Filtering should be used to reduce unwanted noises but not distort the desired signal. Body tissues themselves also produce changes in the amplitude, frequency, and waveform morphology depending on their thickness, conductance, geometry, and the resultant vectors of the pathways being studied relative to the recording electrodes chosen. In general, higher-frequency signals are reduced because they are conducted from deep-lying generators.

Let us go back to the filter's dropoff rate. The power output dropoff (i.e., slope) around the cutoff frequency and, therefore, the signal allowed through on either side of the setting is slightly different from one piece of equipment to another. In some, the dropoff is sharper, and in some, it tapers off more gradually. As an example, consider a low-pass filter with a cutoff frequency of 1,000 Hz in a machine with a more gradual signal attenuation. We are recording a signal that has energy components at 900 to 1,000 Hz. If we switch to equipment that has a filter with sharper attenuation characteristics (remember, both devices will be designated as 1,000-Hz filters) the first filter will block part of the desired information, so a low-pass (i.e., upper) filter setting of 1,200 Hz would have to be used to obtain the same waveforms. This is why it is important not to be rigid in using recommended settings and to experiment with one's own equipment. Equipment that has a broad range of both high and low filters gives more flexibility and better control of the information entering each channel. There is no single correct procedure or standardized way of recording this information. It is necessary to be consistent and to become well versed in the effect each change will have on recorded data. Proper use of filters is a necessity to attain efficient EP acquisition. The application of new filtering techniques allows speed analysis of single-sweep EP recordings as well as rapid looks at stimulus-to-stimulus changes (e.g., during surgery) or changes from multiple variables or stimuli.

The Averaging Process

An averager improves the S/N ratio so that stimulus-time-locked information can be extracted from the background noise through a mathematical process by which one sweep or waveform is synchronously added to the next to bring the stimulus-related events out of the surrounding noise. A natural bioelectrical signal resulting from a biochemical event is a continuously varying voltage, called an analog signal. To amplify or display this type of information is not a problem, but to average it is cumbersome. To facilitate averaging, the analog signal must be digitized; that is, the waveform is separated into discrete levels of voltage and small time intervals. The total amplitude scale of the digitizer is divided into a set of discrete (vertical) levels that represent the voltage variation. The final readings cannot be made in finer divisions than the difference between the discrete averager points. The amplifier gain should be set to the highest sensitivity that will allow data acquisition. The number of time data points along the sweep length is the time sampling rate. This number determines the horizontal resolution. To have good signal analysis, in theory, the time sampling rate must be at least twice the highest frequency of the EP signal that is to be recorded. For accurate clinical reconstruction of the waveform, however, the sampling rate should be three to five times the highest desired frequency or three times the upper (i.e., low-pass) filter setting for that study. To assure faithful signal reproduction, skin–electrode resistance should be minimized, maximal amplifier gain as opposed to the averager's augmentation should be used, the shortest time interval as required should be averaged, and a system with a larger digitizer size and faster sampling rate should be selected. If excessive baseline shift or high-frequency noise is present, the filter settings should be kept as close as possible to the signal's expected power spectrum, which is derived by frequency analysis, while avoiding distortion or dispersion of the derived signal. One should be aware that events that are not directly triggered by the stimulus but that are repeated or time-locked signals also can be averaged in and be misleading. These include line-current noise, regular brain wave rhythms, stimulus-induced filter and amplifier ringing, and myogenic synchronous movements in the extremities from the stimulus. When possible, a stimulation rate that is asynchronous with 60 Hz (e.g., 1.27 Hz instead of 3 or 10 Hz), or an irregular stimulus rhythm, should be used.

The improvement in S/N ratio from use of this averaging process is related directly to the number of sweeps averaged and is approximately equal to the square root of the total number of sweeps counted. If we look at this relationship, and for clinical purposes use a minimal S/N ratio of 3, we can obtain a relatively simple way of knowing when to stop averaging, because overaveraging can increase the relative contribution of the stimulus-dependent noises and can reduce the recorded EP amplitude. Measuring the envelope of noise at a slow sweep speed with an appropriate amplitude setting allows the total noise on that channel to be visualized. By knowing the EP signal amplitude (e.g., based on literature, prior personal data), the measured noise with everything in place and ready to record, and the formula in Figure 16-6, we can estimate the number of sweeps required to obtain the response. For example, if 25 sweeps are averaged, the remaining mean noise amplitude will be reduced by a factor of 5 compared with each single sweep used for the averaging. If 100 sweeps are averaged, the remaining noise should be reduced by a factor of 10. If excess noise still is present, a larger number of sweeps can be averaged together

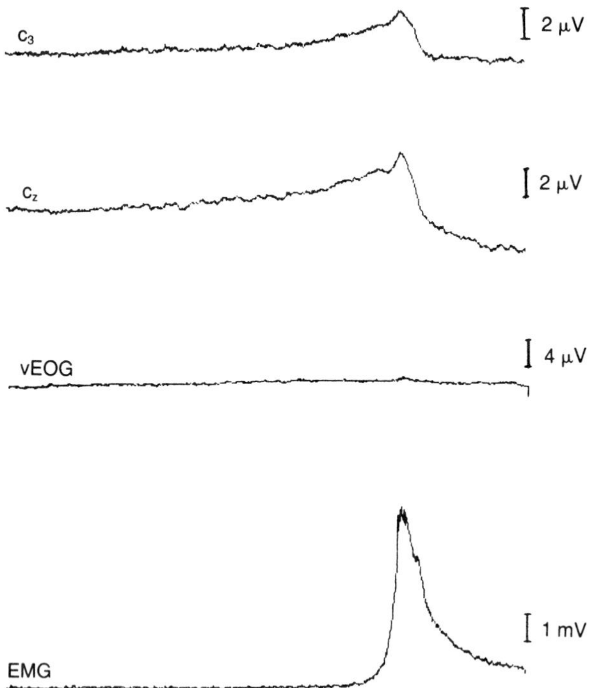

FIG. 16-6. Normal movement-related cortical potential (MRCP). An average is formed from 500 sweeps made 3 seconds before movement and 1 second after rapid flexion of interphalangeal joint of the right thumb (band pass, 0.01 to 100 Hz; gain, 20,000). Channel 1: averaged electroencephalogram recorded from the C_3 electrode. Channel 2: MRCP recorded at C_2 overlying the supplementary motor area. Channel 3: vertical electrooculogram *(vEOG)*. Channel 4: rectified surface electromyogram *(EMG)* recorded from electrodes placed over the motor point of the flexor pollicis longus.

in each run, or more individual runs can be recorded and superimposed, but this should never be a substitute for adequate skin-electrode preparation or for changes in stimulation or recording parameters between runs. If reproducible and superimposable responses are not obtained at that point, all technical reasons must be ruled out and the test rerun before their absence can be interpreted clinically.

Recording Guidelines

Table 16-1 gives routine recording parameters for a variety of CNS electrodiagnostic studies. Newer equipment relies less on dedicated hardware and more on firmware (i.e., programs stored permanently in read-only memory) and software (i.e., enterable programs) to control adjustable parameters. These systems lend themselves to automated recording parameter groupings, real-time manipulation of the recording parameters, and storage of the raw or processed data for reexamination or manipulation at a later time. Special filtering programs, Fourier analysis, spectral density analysis, and varied graphic representation of the data are now available with little if any additional hardware. The flexibility and power of software signal processing programs will allow new areas of clinical application while carrying with it the burden of understanding the impact of the new technology on data representation.

AUDITORY BRAINSTEM RESPONSES AND OTOACOUSTIC EMISSIONS

The ABR components as defined by Picton and Hillyard generally occur within the first 8 msec after an auditory stimulus is delivered (34). These potentials are the smallest of the EP responses customarily recorded in clinical practice, and their amplitude usually is no more than 600 nV. Before Picton's description and classification in 1974, all auditory EP before 60 msec were referred to as early (34). After Jewett's (35) and Picton's (34) work, the early auditory responses were defined as occurring before 10 msec, middle components were looked for in the 10- to 60-msec area, and late potentials beyond that. The late potentials include the cognitive evoked potential (CEP), the cognitive negative variation, and vertex potentials. In 1978, Kemp (36) described the dynamic acoustic signals produced by the inner ear, the otoacoustic emissions (OAE) (37). These are the minuscule but discrete sounds that are produced by the cochlear outer hair cells vigorous motility, which generates its own vibrational energy. This mechanical energy is transmitted from the cochlea, spreading outward via the middle ear and tympanic membrane. The motility energy spectra can be measured in the external ear canal as a frequency specific OAE response (38). These tests have great correlation with the maturation of the peripheral auditory organs in preterm infants and other difficult-to-test patients and can help differentiate between nerve deafness and cochlear hair cell deafness because it analyzes the responses that antecede the first

TABLE 16-1. *Evoked potential recording parameters: general guidelines for select studies*

	Auditory evoked potentials	Visual evoked potentials	Upper extremity SSEP	Lower extremity and pudendal SSEP	ESG	Cognitive evoked potentials
Amplifier						
Sensitivity	0.5–2.0 μV/div	5–10 μV/div	2.0–5.0 μV/div	5–10 μV/div	0.5–5.0 μV/div	2.0–5.0 μV/div
Sweep speed	1 msec/div	20–40 msec/div	5 msec/div	10 sec/div (120 msec/div intraoperatively)	5–10 msec/div	50–100 msec/div
Filters						
Low (high pass)	80–160 Hz	0.8–1.0 Hz	2–20 Hz (noncephalic reference or 16–32 Hz cephalic reference)	8–16 Hz (16–64 Hz intraoperatively)	20 or 200 Hz	0.1–0.3 Hz
High (low pass)	2500–3600 Hz	80–100 Hz	1600–2000 Hz	1000–2000 Hz	1000–3000 Hz	70–100 Hz
Stimulator						
Repetition rate	10 pps	2 reversals/sec	3–8pps	1–3 pps	1–4 pps	0.5–1.0 stim/sec
Duration	0.1 msec (100 Hz–8 kHz)		0.05–0.2 msec	0.05–0.2 msec	(0.3 intraoperatively)	0.05–0.2 msec
Stimulus intensity	60–65 above hearing threshold; noise 38 dB below click level	Constant lumens output; maximum (100%) contrast	5 mA above minimal thumb abduction twitch	5mA above minimal hallux abductor/flexor (maximum stimulator voltage intraoperatively) Pudendal stimulation at three times threshold level	10 mA above minimal toe flexion	Variable; may be used as a "target" parameter
Averager						
Number of sweeps for good S/N	1000	100	500–1000	100–500	100–1000	100–500
Electrode Placements (see Fig. 16-4)	C_z—active, A_1/M_1 or A_2/M_2 reference; opposite ear ground stimulus	O_z (occasionally O_1 or O_2)—C_z or F_z; midline ground	C_3/C_3' or C_4/C_3' to contralateral noncephalic reference or F_z (and Erb's point marker)	C_z–F_z (use ESG as proof of entry and marker)	L1–T11 vertebral level (midline at interspinous ligament)	C_z—active; joined A_1—A_2 or M_1–M_2 reference; midline ground

ESG, electrospinogram; SSEP, somatosensory evoked potentials; S/N, signal to noise ratio.
Adapted from Cole JL. Equipment parameter determinants in evoked potential studies. *Bull Am Soc Clin Evoked Potentials* 1984; 3(1):3–9, with permission.

peak of the ABR. The test can be used for superior screening of early hearing problems in infants (39), for early detection of hearing loss from ototoxic drugs (40), and as part of an assessment battery for children with auditory processing deficits, as both peripheral and central auditory problems can be present that would impact rehabilitation strategies (41). Additionally, because OAE is site specific for the outer cochlear hair cells, it can assist in evaluating cochlear damage from noise exposure and when tinnitus is part of the presenting complaint.

The ABR's wide application has come from its reproducibility from subject to subject, anatomic specificity and correlation to brainstem nuclei activity, and resistance to change under a wide variety of physiological and drug-induced stresses. Its role in clinical use remains primarily diagnostic because it generally does not correlate well with subtle changes in clinical course or responses to specific treatments (42,43).

Anatomy of the Auditory Pathways

Short-latency ABR interpretation is better correlated with its anatomic substrate than any other EP study; therefore, understanding the anatomic pathway is essential to its application. The vibrating eardrum transmits its energy through the auditory ossicles to the basilar membrane of the cochlea. The sensory organ in the hearing mechanism is the organ of Corti, which lies in the membranous cochlea contained in the bony cochlea of the petrous temporal bone. An osseous spiral lamina projects from the modiolus into the cochlea.

The modiolus is traversed by many small and one large canal, which run lengthwise in the center and communicate with the canals in the spiral lamina. The afferent fibers of the auditory nerve pierce the small canals of the spiral lamina that connect with the spiral canal containing the spiral ganglion, which in turn contains the bipolar cells. The spiral ganglion axons constitute the cochlear nerve, and the dendrites of the cells arborize with the sensory hair cells. These sensory hair cells are arranged in a single row of inner hair cells and three rows of outer hair cells. The inner hair cells are bulbous-shaped and contain approximately 40 hairs arranged in two rows like an "11." The outer hair cells contain approximately 115 hairs that are embedded in the tectorial membrane.

Two types of nerve endings make contact with these hair cells: type I endings are small, sparsely granulated afferent fibers, and type II endings are larger, more densely granulated efferent fibers from the olivocochlear bundle, which originates from the contralateral brainstem. The acoustic or auditory nerve originates from the axons of the spiral ganglion cells, which are first-order neurons that enter the brainstem in the groove between the pons and medulla. The auditory or cochlear nerve then divides and distributes itself to the dorsal and ventral cochlear nuclei. The tonotopic organization in the organ of Corti, in which high frequencies are represented in the basal area and lower frequencies in the apical areas, is preserved with the high-frequency information distributed ventrolaterally. The nerve fibers then synapse with multiple neurons so that no first-order neurons pass beyond the cochlear nuclei. The fibers leaving the cochlear nuclei then pass by three main routes to the contralateral brainstem and continue as the lateral lemniscus. Some of the fibers continue up to the inferior colliculus, which is another relay nucleus. It is the highest level where auditory fibers cross from one side to another and where tonotopic organization is still preserved. The majority of the fibers leaving the lateral lemniscus go to the superior olivary complex. The lateral superior olivary complex afferents generally come from the ipsilateral ventral cochlear nucleus, and its efferents distribute to the lateral lemnisci on both sides. The signal then passes through the medial geniculate body with the majority of the fibers being fourth order, although some are still third order, at this level. The only obligatory nuclei along the auditory pathway are the spiral ganglion, cochlear nucleus, and medial geniculate body. All other nuclei are variably traversed. The auditory cortex is located on the superior temporal gyrus in area 41, deep in the Sylvian fissure, which corresponds to the primary auditory area. Areas of the parietal and frontal lobes also are believed to be involved as secondary auditory areas.

In the auditory pathway, as in other sensory systems, there is a progressive increase in the number of neurons activated as the afferent signal progresses. As the signal traverses each synapse, the resultant electrical potential is larger in amplitude.

Indications

Adults

In adults the ABR has found utility in a variety of audiologic problems, including unexplained central losses on auditory tests and in the differential diagnosis of sudden-onset unilateral deafness or severe hearing loss. The test has excellent sensitivity in detecting multiple sclerosis (MS), other demyelinating processes, and acoustic neuromas; in intraoperative monitoring; and in monitoring brainstem function during barbiturate coma or in those who appear brain dead.

Children

Audiometry recording the ABR (i.e., objective audiometry) and OAE can be used in infants and newborns to detect the presence of hearing loss. Although ABR studies are still the benchmark, OAE offer the potential of identification earlier and in milder cases when it results from sensory (cochlear) hearing loss. These studies should be considered in infants of 6 months of age or less who are suspected of hearing loss, and in children up to 2 years of age who appear to have hearing or behavioral problems. Detection of hearing loss at an early stage is important because aural rehabilitation can be more successful if therapy is begun early. A follow-up examination usually is necessary to confirm any perceived abnormality. The ABR has been of value for therapeutic consideration in young, physically challenged children who have delayed language development or behavioral difficulties, and for prognostic considerations following hypoxic encephalopathies. In older children, it is of diagnostic value in suspected white matter degenerative disorders, demyelinating disorders, and brainstem tumors.

Procedures and Test Parameters

Any blockage of the external auditory canal should be removed before the studies are performed. The test room should be relatively free of extraneous noises and distractions. The patient should be placed in a supine position with a firm foam pillow under the head or in a high-back or reclining chair so that the head can be supported and the neck muscles relaxed; Cz is marked. The patients are instructed to relax their jaws, close their eyes or look straight ahead, and listen to the clicks on the headset.

We must first orient ourselves, which for ABR, like EEG, implies a positive upward recording, and Cz is the active electrode. Because most electrodiagnostic equipment is configured for positive down, the Cz electrode should be inserted into the anode jack (red) so that the correct polarity will be displayed. If the equipment is software driven, the manual must be checked. The reference electrode is placed on the ear lobe at A1 or A2, or behind the ear on the mastoids, which sometimes are designated M1 on the left and M2 on the right. For each test, the reference electrode is ipsilateral to the stimulus. The ear contralateral to the side of stimulation can be used as the ground site. When the electrodes and earphones are in place, the interelectrode impedances are checked.

The common method of stimulation is a click delivered to an individual ear. The opposite ear usually is masked with white noise so that it does not process any ambient noises or the bone- or air-conducted stimulus from the opposite ear. The hearing threshold for each ear is determined individually by having the subject signal when he or she first hears the click as the intensity is increased, and when he or she loses it as it is decreased. The click polarity is based on a mechanical phenomenon within the stimulating headset. Rarefaction designates that the earphone diaphragm's initial movement is away from the tympanic membrane; condensation is when the earphone diaphragm moves toward the tympanic membrane during its initial movement. The diaphragm of the earphones is obligated to move in both directions to ultimately produce the clicking sound wave, but there is a small latency difference from the stimulus polarity. Rarefaction generally produces a shorter-latency peak than does condensation when all other recording parameters are the same. There is still considerable disagreement as to which is the correct stimulation technique. It generally is accepted that only one polarity should be used during any series of trials; with most machines, there is a tendency to have a baseline shift in one direction or another from the summating (i.e., mechanical shock artifact) auditory stimulation by the headset. This baseline shift produces noise when the averaged response is enlarged for marking the response peaks. Alternate rarefaction and condensation stabilizes the baseline; however, because of the peak shifts, a blurred, smaller-amplitude response is obtained, making peak identification slightly more difficult.

Clinical Interpretation

Jewett and Williston concluded in 1971 that the response (i.e., peak I) originated in the auditory nerve (Fig. 16-7) (35). The second wave appears to be generated in the cochlear nucleus at the pontomedullary junction area and usually is designated peak II, although its presence is variable. The third wave (i.e., peak III) appears to be generated at or near the superior olivary complex in the caudal pons. Peak IV is generated by synchronized conduction through the lateral lemniscus in the pons and also can be inconsistent. The fifth wave, peak V, is generated in the inferior colliculus in the midbrain and represents the most important wave for comparison to earlier potentials as well as for its absolute latency. The sixth wave (VI) appears to be generated in the medial geniculate body of the thalamus, and peak VII is believed to be the response over the auditory radiations of the thalamocortical tract. These latter two waves are inconsistent in normal control studies and have not been found to provide good correlation in pathologic conditions. Table 16-2 gives a set of normal adult values ($N = 63$) for the absolute peak and interpeak latencies using 10 click/sec rarefaction stimuli at 60 to 65 dB above hearing threshold with white noise masking of the contralateral ear at 30 dB below the stimulus level, a filter range of 100 to 3,000 Hz, and 1,000 sweeps averaged per run. Normal values should be established for each laboratory using similar baseline criteria (44). Runs always should be at least duplicated to be certain that interatrial latency differences do not exceed 0.25 msec.

TABLE 16-2. *Normal ABR adult values for the absolute peak and interpeak latencies using 10 click/sec rarefaction stimuli at 60 to 65 dB above hearing threshold, with contralateral masking noise at 30 dB below the stimulus level* [a]

Jewett Peak Latencies	Interpeak Latency Differences
I. = 1.35 → 2.08 msec.	I–III = 1.93 → 2.30 msec.
II. = 2.54 → 3.22 msec.	I–IV/V = 3.60 → 4.20 msec.
III. = 3.58 → 4.30 msec.	I–V = 3.75 → 4.38 msec.
IV. = 5.00 → 5.60 msec.	III–IV/V = 1.50 → 2.10 msec.
IV/V. = 5.25 → 6.00 msec.	III–V = 1.74 → 2.18 msec.
V. = 5.32 → 6.16 msec.	
VI. = 7.05 → 7.78 msec.	
VII. = 8.70 → 9.45 msec.	

[a] See Figure 16-7 for far-field responses and their anatomic correlates.
ABR, auditory brainstem response.

The I–III interpeak latency difference has shown excellent correlation with documented lesions in the peripheral auditory mechanism, auditory nerve, and lower pons level lesions. The I–V interpeak latency difference has had application in brainstem, thalamic, and cortical structure injuries when the I–III interpeak latency is normal (45). In addition, there can be diffuse involvement in both the I–III and III–V interpeak central conduction times with MS and other demyelinating processes. Hearing losses are suggested by large latency shifts of wave I peak latency from stimulus intensity changes.

The individual waves sometimes are difficult to record, and so a variety of filtering techniques, electrode placements, and stimulation parameters are used to better define individual components. For example, using the ipsilateral ear as active electrode and the contralateral ear as reference (i.e., a horizontal montage) increases the amplitudes of waves I and III while reducing wave V. Often the IV and V peaks partially or completely overlap when recorded Cz to ipsilateral ear, but they may separate when recorded from Cz to the contralateral ear. Slowing down the stimulus repetition rate may better define the IV–V complex by giving a better relative amplitude to peak V. Slowing the rate can augment the I and III waves. Augmentation of these early waves sometimes can be improved by increasing the stimulation decibel level. Reducing the stimulus intensity can reduce their amplitude and shift the entire ABR complex. When peak identification is difficult, these tricks help in a few studies but cannot correct for a noisy environment, poorly applied electrodes, or inconsistent interatrial recording criteria.

In an audiologic setting, the ABR can be used as a range

of stimulus intensity series levels for those patients who cannot be tested by conventional audiometric methods. The ABR amplitudes are directly proportional, and the latencies are inversely proportional, to the stimulus intensities used. The I–V or I–IV/V interpeak latency difference generally remains stable except when marked hearing losses or disrupted central conduction are present. Similar ABR values should be obtained using air-conducted stimuli by subtracting 30 dB of stimulus intensity from bone-conducted tests. These types of testing protocols are done most commonly in conjunction with routine audiometric testing.

SOMATOSENSORY EVOKED POTENTIALS

Many disabling neuromuscular conditions are associated with significant sensory impairments as well as loss of motor function; hence, the ability to open a physiological window on such functions provides the physiatrist with important information for planning rehabilitation programs. In a recent patient with paraplegia caused by a conversion reaction, the SEP studies were found to be entirely normal. The results of the study were explained to her, and a confident prediction that her impairment would improve was made. She subsequently made a rapid and complete recovery with physical therapy and supportive counseling (46). This case demonstrates that testing can be used to obtain objective evidence that either confirms or conflicts with subjective examination findings. These studies are particularly useful in subjects in whom a clinical sensory examination is either unreliable or not possible. They also help to quantify the degree of somatosensory pathway damage and characterize and localize the impairment to some extent.

Scalp potentials elicited by electrical stimulation of the ulnar nerve were first recorded by Dawson in a patient with progressive myoclonic epilepsy, a condition associated with very large-amplitude SEPs (3). With the proliferation of microcomputer-based systems for signal processing, the ability to record these potentials has become widespread, and their application to clinical situations common. Problems remain in defining appropriate applications, interpretation standardization, and localization of generators associated with the individual components. However, there appears to be consistent evidence that the cortically referenced far-field early response (first onset to peak) is generated in the subthalamic to thalamic regions.

The SEP can be viewed in a simplistic but useful sense as the central equivalent of the peripheral sensory nerve action potential study. With the SEP technique, the electrodiagnostician traces the afferent impulses produced by electrical stimulation of a peripheral nerve along their proximal route through to the spinal cord and from there to the brainstem and cerebrum. Because the SEP pathways can involve the longest axons in the body with the greatest span of the CNS, the SEP tends to be more useful than visual and auditory studies for detecting impairment at various anatomic levels traversed by these fibers. The somatosensory route also includes proximal peripheral nerve, plexus, root, and spinal cord, which, when injured, can affect study results.

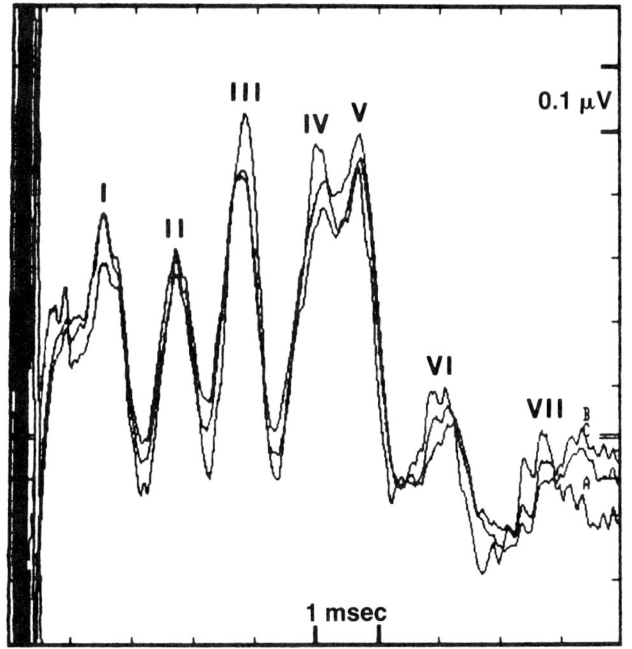

FIG. 16-7A, B. The normal auditory brainstem response (ABR) typically contains seven waves, which are designated as peaks I through VII. *(continued)*

Anatomy of the Somatosensory Pathway

Whereas in the visual and auditory modalities, the commonly used techniques involve natural stimulation of the receptors, in SEP the peripheral receptors in the skin commonly are bypassed, and electrical stimulation of the peripheral (i.e., mixed) nerve axons is used, producing a highly unphysiological afferent volley. It is possible to demonstrate a SEP with mechanical tapping of the skin and muscle stretch, but the advantages of using electrical stimulation include the fact that it permits the synchronous activation of a large proportion of the low-threshold, large-diameter fibers, which produces a highly coherent transmission. When a mixed nerve such as the median or tibial nerve is stimulated, this coherent volley of action potentials is conducted along the peripheral processes of the large-diameter, high-speed epicritic sensory system and continues along the central processes of these cells to travel rostral in the ipsilateral dorsal column of the spinal cord to synapse at the cervicomedullary junction in the dorsal column nuclei. Lumbar and sacral root fibers ascend medially as the fasciculus gracilis, and cervical root fibers ascend laterally as the fasciculus cuneatus to reach their respective nuclei. Axon branches also enter the dorsal horn gray matter at the segmental level and contact cells in the nucleus proprius and other areas of the spinal gray matter. Second-order cells in the dorsal column nuclei give rise to fibers that continue to propagate rostrally,

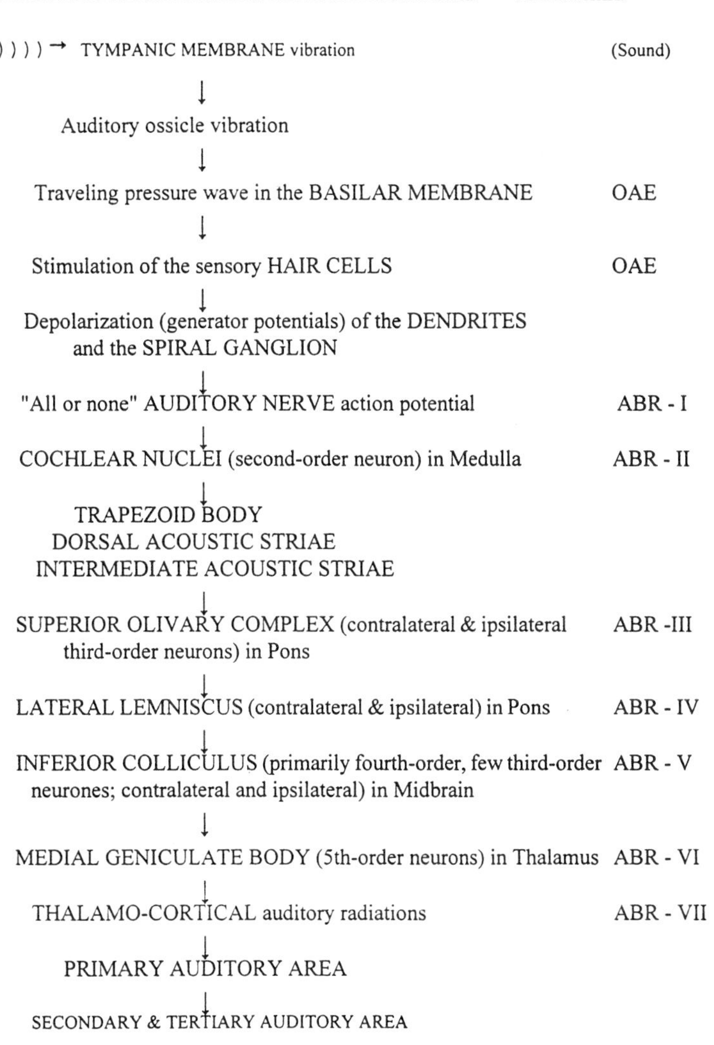

FIG. 16-7A, B. *Continued.* The OAE **(B)** is the recordable response from the coclear mechanism's outer hair cell. The ABR is recorded as a series of high-frequency vertex (Cz)-positive far-field potentials **(A)** during the first 10 msec after a discrete stimulus (see Table 16-2).

crossing the internal arcuate fibers in the lower medulla and continuing to the ventral, posterolateral thalamus by way of the medial lemniscus. From the thalamus, third-order fibers continue transmission to the region of the primary somatosensory cortex. Thus, tibial nerve stimulation at the ankle activates medial regions of the contralateral hemisphere, receiving input from the leg and foot regions and producing a focus of activation that usually is of highest amplitude just posterior to the scalp vertex, whereas median nerve stimulation at the wrist produces a focus of activation located over the central parietal convexity contralateral to the side being stimulated, as the cortical homunculus would predict.

Testing Procedures

As mentioned earlier, establishing a rapport with the patient is important to ensure a good working relationship with a cooperative subject, just as positioning and muscle relaxation are critical for reducing EMG artifact. In an unusually anxious adult, a mild sedative (e.g., chloral hydrate or diazepam) may be used. In children or cognitively impaired patients who are unable to cooperate, sedation is commonly used to ensure technically adequate studies. Both upper and lower limb studies are usually recorded with the patient supine, resting comfortably with the head and neck supported on an examination table or reclining chair. Lower limb (LL) studies with spinal recordings are performed prone, with a pillow under the trunk to relax the lumbosacral paraspinal muscles. After positioning and skin preparations are complete, all recording, ground, and stimulation electrodes should be attached to their respective inputs.

Bipolar near-field recordings sometimes are preferred to non-cephalic-referenced far-field because the potentials are larger and more easily recorded with less contamination noises (48). The main disadvantage of cephalic-referenced bipolar recordings is their cancellation of the earlier, small-amplitude, far-field potentials.

The electrode site selections are directed to answer the particular clinical problem being studied, the sites are marked, and the electrodes are firmly attached. The skin over the stimulation and ground sites should be similarly prepared and checked. The ground electrode may be a large plate or band electrode when placed proximally on the limb being stimulated; however, it should be similar to the recording electrodes (e.g., cup, needle) when used in their vicinity.

The stimulating electrodes are secured longitudinally over the nerve with the cathode proximal, or with the cathode over the nerve and a larger anode on the limb's opposite side. The stimulus duration should be adequate to excite group Ia muscle and group II cutaneous afferents (49). Stimulating current is adjusted to the sensory threshold and is then slowly raised until it is two and one-half to three times the threshold level, or until there is a moderate but brisk distal muscle contraction. The patient is allowed to accommodate to the stimulation before data acquisition is actually begun. Instruct the patient to open his or her mouth loosely to allow jaw and temple muscles to relax, and to try to refrain from swallowing, yawning, talking, or moving about while the signals are being recorded. Alternating left and right side stimulation can improve the ability to compare between sides (50,51).

Usually the active and reference electrodes are placed on the scalp; however, if cortical and subcortical information is desired in the same recording channel, then a noncephalic reference electrode site should be used. This latter technique is most useful for upper extremity studies. As the electrodes' separation is increased, more noise will be allowed into the system and the potentials' amplitude will be more variable. For all lower extremity and pelvic area nerves, whether mixed or pure sensory, the active electrode should be between Cz and Cz'', referenced to Fz for primary clinical interpretation. Likewise, for all upper extremity studies, one channel must record from the hemisphere's central site (typically C3 to C3'' or C4 to C4'') contralateral to the stimulus and referenced to the Fz or an inactive noncephalic site (e.g., the acromioclavicular joint opposite the stimulus). Averaging begins with the stimulation rate between 0.5 and 4 stimuli/sec. Averages usually are collected up to a total of 500 sweeps, and one or more retests are performed for validation of the data.

Once all the data have been recorded and deemed acceptable, the electrodes may be removed. Component latencies and amplitudes are measured and distances between recording electrodes recorded so that peripheral and central conduction velocities can be computed. Data sensitivity can be improved by using interpeak latencies and by comparing values from one side to the other (i.e., neutralizing height effects). Sensitivity also can be improved if subject variables, such as age and height, are regressed out using standard linear regression methods, because component latencies and amplitude ratios generally are assumed to be normally distributed. Depending on how conservative the clinician wishes to be in the judgment of abnormality, the upper limits of normal range can be set at two and one-half or three standard deviations beyond the mean values. Alternatively, the result can be reported in terms of the number of standard deviations beyond the mean to indicate the probability that the obtained reading is abnormal.

Various peripheral nerves can be selected to look at different root levels or to investigate proximal peripheral nerve lesions (e.g., meralgia paresthetica [52], plexopathy). Lower extremity nerve studies give access to transmission through the lumbar and thoracic spine segments whereas stimulation of upper extremity nerves can be used to focus on transmission through the brachial plexus and cervical spinal cord. Mixed nerves contain large populations of muscle afferents that contribute to the recorded information in addition to its somatic sensation. The tibial nerve at the popliteal fossa or medial malleolus level, or the peroneal nerve at the fibular neck level usually are stimulated transcutaneously. Alternatively, percutaneous stimulation can be done using dermal wire or monopolar needle electrodes that are inserted to lie adjacent to the nerve, requiring much less current and reaching deep nerves.

There is no mandatory minimum number of channels required to record clinical SEP studies. A single-channel, noncephalic-referenced upper extremity study can contain all the needed data, or serial studies of different levels or paradigms can be obtained. The advantage of multichannel systems includes more data acquisition per stimulus and per time, as well as better documentation of signal entry and transmission along the studied pathway. Simultaneous recordings can be obtained from electrodes placed over the peripheral nerve (i.e., afferent neurogram), over different spinal levels (i.e., electrospinographic [ESG] potential), or over relevant regions of the scalp (i.e., cortical evoked potential). An example of a four-channel tibial nerve SEP is shown in Figure 16-8, from stimulation just below the medial malleolus. Stimulation of the median nerve at the wrist (Fig. 16-9) demonstrates proximal progression of the afferent volley from peripheral arm stimulation to the primary somatosensory cortex. Notice that the Erb's point potential must be referenced to a noncephalic site.

Clinical Correlation

The generators for the various components of the cervical, upper extremity cortical SEP have not been clearly defined and some controversy remains. The N9 component is thought to be generated by the cervical roots and by transmission of the dorsal columns, (54) whereas the P/N13 may be a postsynaptic potential generated locally by a focal stationary source in the spinal cord interneurons with a horizontally oriented anteroposterior dipole (53). The dorsal column nuclei also may be contributing to this P/N13 component. The later upper extremity negativity may be of thalamic or thalamocortical radiation origin (54), or from cortical sources (55). Some investigators contend that there is a single tangentially oriented dipole in the posterior central sulcus (i.e., Brodmann's area 3b) dominating the response and explaining the polarity reversal in the N20 and P20 components

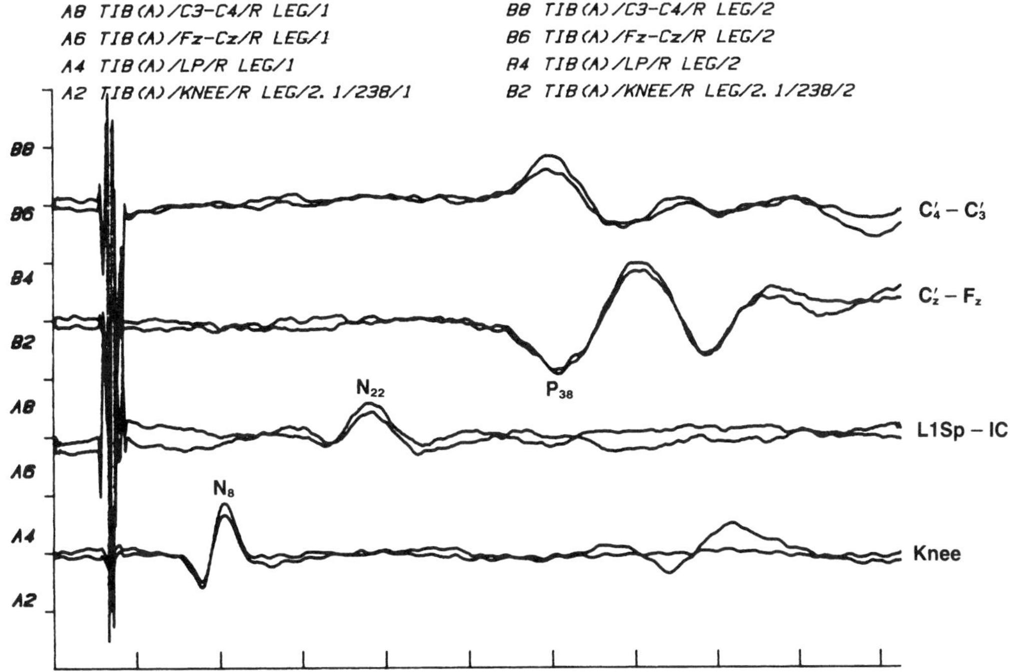

FIG. 16-8. Normal four-channel posterior tibial nerve somatosensory evoked potential study. The traces shown each represent an average of 1,000 sweeps with two averages superimposed. The time base is 5.5 msec/division Channel 1 **(bottom)**: afferent neurogram recorded over the ipsilateral popliteal fossa; scale, 5 μV/division. Channel 2 shows lumbar potential (i.e., electrospinogram) recorded at the level of the L1 vertebral body as monopolar response referenced to the contralateral iliac crest; scale, 2 μV/division. Channel 3 shows standard lower extremity midline recording from active electrode at C''_2 (negative grid 2 cm dorsal to vertex) referenced to F_2 (positive grid) site; scale, 1.5 mV/division. Channel 4 **(top)** shows active recording from C'_4 referenced to C'_3; scale, 3 μV/division.

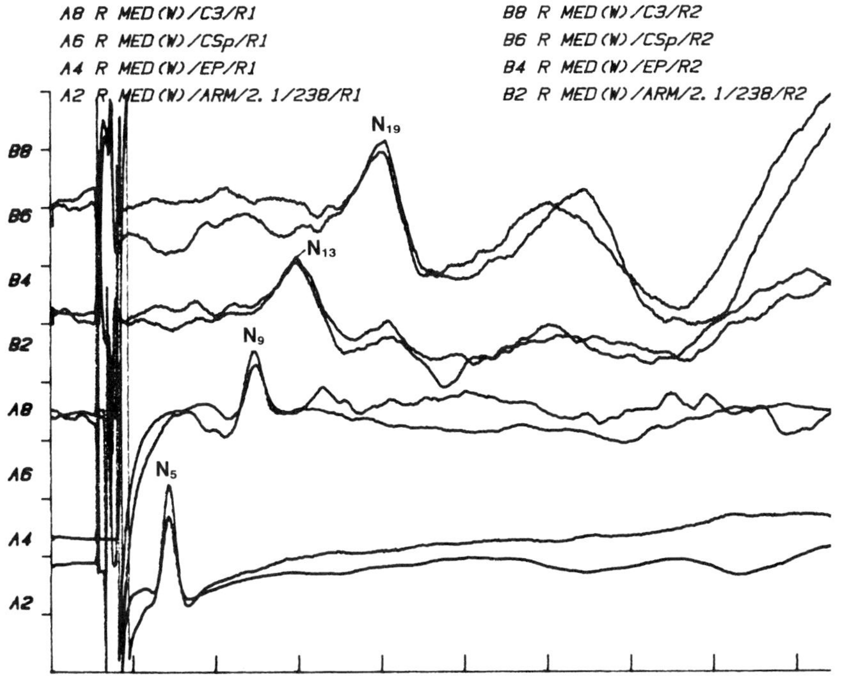

FIG. 16-9. Normal median nerve somatosensory evoked potential study demonstrating the normal components of the afferent volley with a four-channel system. The traces shown each represent an average of 500 sweeps with two averages superimposed. The time base is 5.5 msec/division. Channel 1 **(bottom)** shows afferent neurogram recorded over the ipsilateral median nerve at the elbow level; scale, 10 μV/division. Channel 2 shows an afferent neurogram from the shoulder level recorded over the ipsilateral clavicle (i.e., Erb's point) area and referenced to the contralateral midclavicle; scale, 5 μV/division. Channel 3 shows cervical spinal level potentials recorded over C2 vertebral spinous process, referenced to a midfrontal (Fz site) electrode; scale, 2 mV/division. Channel 4 **(top)** shows C'_3 or C'_4 responses from the contralateral hemisphere central (relative to the side of stimulation) to a cephalic reference at the Fz site; scale, 1 μV/division.

observed between parietal and frontal recording sites, respectively (56–59). Others suggest a separate frontal generator in the primary precentral motor and supplementary motor cortex (60–62). which is supported by the observation of a variable latency delay between the parietal N19 and the frontal P22 peaks as well as the observation that patients with cerebral lesions can have disassociated loss of these components. Electrocorticographic recordings have been reported to support this latter idea (63), and there appears to be retention of a precentral SEP component following complete removal of the postcentral gyrus (64). A third element of the frontal response may be related to the P25 component recorded from the postcentral region, which does not have a clear frontal counterpart. Allison and colleagues have suggested that the P25 and the following negativity (N35) may relate to the response of a second somatosensory receiving area, in Brodmann's area 1 of the postcentral gyrus (57).

The cortical response tends to be dominated by the fast-conducting, large afferent fiber population conducted primarily through the dorsal columns (65). Animal studies on lower extremity nerves indicate that the large-diameter peripheral nerve fibers and dorsal columns contribute primarily to waveform components seen under 40 msec, whereas the small-diameter peripheral nerve fibers and anterolateral columns contribute to the components observed at 70 msec or later (66). The waveform between 40 and 70 msec is produced with contributions from the large and small diameters and the dorsal and anterolateral columns. Patients with dissociated sensory loss show abnormal SEP components on the side with proprioceptive impairment, whereas little change, if any, occurs in association with loss of pain and temperature sensation alone (67,68). Namerow reported that the SEP was unchanged following section of the spinothalamic tracts (69), and Cusick and associates showed that the SEP cortical components were abolished with complete lesions of the dorsal columns (70).

Applications and Interpretation

The general strategy for near-field recording interpretation is to look for the major components of the SEP at each level in the pathway and to evaluate the conduction times between these major peaks. In far-field or combined near-field and far-field recordings, the absolute and interpeak latencies from a single channel's traces may be compared to standardized data or compared to an uninvolved contralateral equivalent study. These approaches can be used to localize a problem that produces either a block of conduction to more proximal sites, giving a dropout or loss of the proximal components, or a significant delay in conduction in a segment of the pathway, as evidenced by abnormal delay between components that still are recordable. Abnormality thus can be related to loss of expected components, prolonged central conduction times within one trace or between traces of serial levels, abnormal latency differences between sides, or abnormal amplitude ratios. Peripheral conduction velocity also can be measured and, when slow, cause delay or dispersion of the central responses. Therefore, a SEP study must never be labeled abnormal without knowing the state of the peripheral components. Upper extremity values generally are more dependent than trunk dermatomal, pudendal nerve, and lower extremity values on the specific paradigm and electrode montage used and require individual normal data.

Many other useful SEP paradigms can be employed using similar techniques by stimulating different nerves or dermatomes or by looking at alternative electrode configurations to examine different structures. Pudendal nerve (PN) (71–73), trigeminal nerve (74), nerve root dermatomes (75–77), and other specific sensory nerves also may be used. Because of the growing and diverse applications of SEP studies, a detailed consideration of all areas cannot be attempted, and the reader is referred to other sources for this information (78–80).

In addition to their well-documented utility for establishing diagnoses and uncovering unsuspected subclinical lesions, the SEP offers an opportunity to the physiatrist to open a physiological window onto sensory function that may help to quantify sensory impairment associated with various forms of disability. This ultimately may lead to the development of rational observation-based criteria for the selection of different forms of rehabilitation therapy for individual patients. Furthermore, the SEP is useful in documenting sensory impairment in infants and patients in coma or persistent vegetative state who could not be evaluated objectively in any other fashion. These studies also may prove extremely useful in the process of developing prognoses and rehabilitation goals. As a powerful clinical research tool, SEP may be applied to obtain important insights into the processes of adaptation and recovery of function following brain damage.

Electrospinograms

In the adult of average height, the T12—L1 interspinous ligament represents the spinal cord entry level for the roots of the tibial nerve. The simplest technique of ESG recording uses a 25-mm monopolar EMG needle inserted vertically or slightly rostrally into the T12-L1 interspinous ligament, maintaining an adequate clearance dorsal to the ligamentum flavum. The reference electrode is placed in the midline, 5 cm or two intervertebral spaces rostral to the active needle electrode. This bipolar recording configuration yields an open, high-frequency, near-field potential with a narrow waveform morphology as a somatosensory afferent neurogram for which latency is predictable from the person's height. The reference electrode should be a second needle rather than a surface electrode. The stimulation rate is about 1 Hz.

Normal Data and Interpretation

The ESG latency in normal subjects has an excellent linear relationship to height. Left-to-right differences in the normal population range up to 1.1 msec (mean 0.08 msec; standard deviation 0.34 msec), making this a sensitive indicator of pathologic processes. Abnormal left-to-right differences, not absolute latency prolongations, appear to be the most sensitive indicator of unilateral radicular pathologic condition. The mean amplitude is just under 2 μV, but because of the large standard deviation observed, it generally is held that any good and clearly reproducible response is acceptable.

Application of the ESG as an entry marker can delineate the peripheral nervous system from the CNS and evaluate central conduction times during SEP. When used with more rostral SEP studies from the LL, it can improve the diagnostic yield by reducing the errors seen at the extremes of height. The technique outlined above can easily be used for any LL peripheral nerve. From multiple vertebral level ESG data, segmental conduction velocities along the spinal column can be calculated to evaluate the impact of local lesions of the spinal cord, such as tumors or stenotic lesions. It can be applied in early MS, neuropathic conditions, or other processes that produce conduction disruptions in the CNS to correlate with clinical findings. In cases of multiple disc herniations, ligamentum flavum hypertrophies, or other conditions in which anatomic imaging studies show diffuse involvement, the ESG can show the level of primary physiological disruption. In addition, in sacral root sensory radiculopathies, an asymmetric ESG, by itself or in conjunction with abnormal H reflex studies, has been the only indicator of pathologic process.

Pudendal Nerve Somatosensory Evoked Potential Studies

Pudendal nerve cortical SEP studies became a welcome addition in 1982 to the diagnostic evaluation of pelvic problems; it is an easy and reliable methodology (71–73,81,82). The PN is involved in the functions of ejaculation, penile erection, sexual responsiveness, and urinary and bowel voiding and continence. The nerve is derived from the second, third, and fourth sacral nerve roots and from the pelvic sympathetic plexuses. Its parasympathetic fibers leave the spinal cord with the anterior spinal nerve roots, and after passing through the sacral foramen, these nervi erigentes enter the pelvic nerve plexus. The sympathetic fibers are derived from the 12th thoracic and upper lumbar cord segments, which descend through the abdomen to the presacral aortic bifurcation area, where they join the hypogastric plexus. These sympathetic nerves from the hypogastric plexus go to the prostate and seminal vesicles, giving motor and ejaculation function.

In men, the penile nerve supply is derived from the PN and the pelvic autonomic plexus. It innervates the bulbocavernosus (BC) and ischiocavernosus muscles, the urogenital diaphragm, and the external urethral sphincter. Its sensory branches receive information from the skin of the penis (i.e., the dorsal nerves), from the perineum, and from the posterior scrotum.

In women, the PN divides into three branches. The inferior hemorrhoidal nerve supplies the external anal sphincter and perianal skin; the perineal nerve supplies the external anal sphincter and levator ani muscles, the superficial and deep perineal muscles, the ischiocavernosus and BC muscles, and the labia; and the mixed motor and sensory dorsal nerve goes to the glans of the clitoris and from the clitoris and medial and lateral labia. Cutaneous innervation in this area from other nerves includes the anterior labial branches of the ilioinguinal nerve to the mons pubis and upper portion of the labium.

Genitourinary and sexual dysfunction can accompany lumbosacral lesions, neuromuscular diseases, metabolic problems, or depression, the latter of which often is seen with chronic pain. Improved understanding of the etiologies and more willingness to discuss these problems has led to better therapeutic choices (81–83). Problems that can be evaluated by PN SEP include symptomatic patient with reduced rectal manometric pressure with no obvious explanation (''idiopathic'' rectal and/or urinary incontinence); abnormal rectal sphincter manometric or cystometric workup without rectal, bladder, or pelvic floor anatomic explanation; severe distal lower extremity pain or muscle spasms (algodystrophy) associated with any bowel or bladder complaints; unexplained perineal numbness or pain; localizing the site of peripheral sacral level nervous system dysfunction; diabetic peripheral polyneuropathy, other metabolic or toxic (poly)-neuropathic conditions, or autonomic neuropathies associated with bowel, bladder, or sexual dysfunction; sacral level radiculopathy or radiculomyelopathy; central nervous system causes of anorectal dysfunction such as myelopathy (spinal stenosis) or radiculomyelopathy, spinal cord injury, amyotrophic lateral sclerosis, Shy–Drager syndrome, multiple sclerosis (upper and lower motor neuron damage) when it presents with detrusor/sphincter dyssynergia, urinary incontinence, or other neurogenic bladder problems; impotence or orgasmic and gynecologic disturbances; impaired pyramidal tract function (detrusor–sphincter dyssynergia syndrome), Parkinson's disease and other motor control problems, cauda equina and conus medullaris syndromes, spina bifida occulta, cerebrovascular accidents, or traumatic brain injury; inadequately localized and characterized neuromyopathic and myopathic dysfunction or diseases affecting continence; acute rectal sphincter trauma (with the possibility of concurrent pudendal nerve or pathway injury); traumatic injury to rectum and/or surrounding area or a history of prior anorectal surgery associated with the subsequent development of rectal sphincter problems; occult or protracted (traumatic) injury to the anorectal sphincter and pelvic floor neuromuscular structures; rectocele with or without failure to relax the sphincter skeletal muscle during attempted defecation (anismus), pelvic floor (muscular) dysfunction, nerve injury from excessive traction and stretching during perineal descent as the proximal part of the pudendal nerve is bound or ''entrapped'' in connective tissue as it angulates around the ischial spine (73).

Among the more common etiologies of recurrent/chronic

traction (partial) injuries to the pudendal or perineal nerve distal motor branches (that innervate the perineum and anus) are prolapse, anorectal dyschezia, multiparity, forceps delivery, increased duration of the second stage of labor, a third-degree perineal tear, high-birth-weight children, prior pelvic surgery, chronic ''straining'' from constipation, and/or when such problems appear to be an anomalous accompaniment of aging. Fecal incontinence in any woman who had forceps deliveries or progressive incontinence with aging (even 20 years or more following the first delivery) should be evaluated, as both conservative and surgical therapeutic intervention, when guided by these diagnostic tests, has proven beneficial in a majority of cases. Additionally, PN SEP studies can be performed as intraoperative monitoring in addition to routine studies for cases in which there are suspected sacral nerve root problems or injuries or when os sacralis or pelvic ring fractures are being corrected.

Normal Values and Interpretation

The waveform shows an initial positive deflection that commences in the range from between 30 and 42 msec (see Table 16-3). This shift point from the baseline usually is referred to as the P1 (onset) but also has been designated as the N0. The waveform then reaches its first positive apex, P1 (peak), ranging between 37 and 47 msec. This is followed by a negative deflection, N1, which peaks between 48 and 60 msec. This initial ''W'' pattern is followed by a series of more variable, longer-latency, alternating positive and negative waves. In men, the P1 to N1, or N1 to P2 peak-to-peak amplitudes are 1.25 to 5 μV. The amplitude usually is lower in women, using the individual right and left nerves (0.5 to 3 μV). The averaged SEP waveform configuration for the peroneal nerve, tibial nerve, and PN all are similar. The P1 (onset) latency of the PN SEP is generally 6 to 10 msec longer than that from the peroneal nerve response from knee-level stimulation and generally is in the same range as the P1 (onset) for the posterior tibial nerve SEP from ankle-level stimulation.

Because the PN SEP has less distance to travel, why then does it appear to take relatively longer to enter the lumbosacral spinal levels? The principal reason is related to the fact that the PN originates from the S2–S5 root levels, whereas the peroneal nerve is primarily supplied by the L4 and L5 spinal roots, and the posterior tibial nerve by the L5 and S1 roots. Another reason is the difference in nerve types being compared. The PN fibers stimulated are purely exteroceptive compared with the mixed fibers of the leg peripheral nerves, which include rapidly conducting muscle afferents, and it has been shown that there is little or no cutaneous contribution to the earlier EP peak components (65).

Pudendal nerve SEPs are easily recorded neurophysiological information that can add to our understanding of a patient's genitourinary or sacral area problems, and more clinical indications are being described. Normal PN SEP results should not be thought to exclude true or organic disease or problems but rather be considered an integral part of a workup for a complex functional system.

VISUAL EVOKED POTENTIALS

Anatomy

When light stimulates the retinal photoreceptors (i.e., the rods and cones), a signal is transmitted to the bipolar cells and then to the ganglion cells of the inner retina. These ganglion cell axons of the retina exit through the sclera as the optic nerve. The optic nerves transmit the signal intracranially through the chiasm forming the optic tracts so that the right visual field transmissions from both eyes are carried in the left optic tract and vice versa. Each optic tract's fibers synapse in the lateral geniculate body located at the lateral dorsum of each thalamus. The neurons in the lateral genicu-

TABLE 16-3. *Normal latency data (in msec) for pudendal nerve somatosensory evoked potential by height in 25 men and women*

Height (inches)	P1 (onset)	P1 (peak)	N1	P2	N2	P3
60	28.36	35.40	45.65	58.32	73.40	91.16
61	28.88	35.97	46.20	58.80	73.84	91.89
62	29.39	36.55	46.77	59.27	74.28	92.63
63	29.90	37.12	47.33	59.74	74.71	93.36
64	30.42	37.70	47.89	60.22	75.15	94.09
65	30.93	38.28	48.45	60.69	75.59	94.82
66	31.44	38.85	49.00	61.16	76.03	95.55
67	31.95	39.43	49.57	61.64	76.46	96.28
68	32.47	40.00	50.13	62.11	76.90	97.00
69	32.98	40.58	50.69	62.59	77.33	98.47
70	33.50	41.16	51.25	63.06	77.77	98.47
71	34.01	41.73	51.81	63.54	78.21	99.20
72	34.52	42.31	52.37	64.01	78.65	99.93
73	35.04	42.89	52.93	64.50	79.09	100.66
Group mean (standard deviation)	31.15 (2.73)	38.25 (2.72)	48.68 (2.97)	60.89 (3.58)	75.77 (5.14)	95.12 (7.91)

N1, first negative peak; N2, second negative peak; P1, first positive peak; P2, second positive peak; P3, third positive peak.

late body, like those of the retina, respond strongly to sharp, contrasting borders, opponent colors, and spots of light. Each geniculate cell responds to one eye but not both. The signals are relayed through the optic radiation to the primary visual cortex (i.e., area 17) in the calcarine fissure. Binocular convergence occurs at the visual cortex. The primary visual cortex passes the information to areas 18 and 19, where integration and visual perception occur. The central visual field function of the macula is represented 35 times more than the periphery, and so the VEP primarily reflects the 3° to 6° of central vision. These few degrees of macular activity are sent to the occipital lobe surface, whereas the more peripheral retina projects to more deeply situated areas in the calcarine fissure.

Procedure

Corrective lenses, preferably the reading glasses if more than one prescription is used, must be brought for the test. Mydriatic agents should be avoided for 12 hours before testing. The visual fields must be checked because their deficits necessitate laterally placed (i.e., O_1 and O_2) recordings in addition to a standard midline electrode montage. When a field defect or hemianopsia is present, hemifield stimulation should be used with the additional electrodes placed at O_1 and O_2 and referenced to Fz.

The most commonly used site is at Oz with reference at Cz and ground at Fz. There is wide occipital VEP representation, and a few subjects demonstrate larger potentials when recording is done from Pz, but Pz should never be a sole recording site. An Oz-to-Cz arrangement can yield the maximal available P100 amplitude by summation of potentials of opposite polarity through differential amplification, but because of the anatomic and field gradient variations discussed previously, there can be wide differences in the normal population, making interpretation of pathologic conditions difficult.

The equipment is set to analyze a 200- to 400-msec sweep with a gain of 5 to 10 μV/division. A filter bandwidth from 0.8 to 100 Hz and an average of 100 to 500 pattern reversal responses are programmed. The stimulus luminance must be bright (40 to 100 cd/m^2), the room darkened, and the pattern's contrast at the maximum allowed (50% saturation level) by the monitor. The test usually is conducted with the head supported to relax the neck muscles, with the eyes straight ahead. The stimulus criteria are determined by retinal area to be activated and the level of cooperation possible. Patterned (e.g., checkerboard) or unpatterned (e.g., flashing strobe) stimuli routinely are used (86). The visual cortex is arranged to transform images into information that is specifically oriented in bar or line segments, not primarily by light spot or luminance, as in the retina, although these also are processed. The most commonly used pattern stimulus is a monitor or light-emitting diode (LED) array shift or reversal display that gives constant luminance because the checks are visible at all times. This display eliminates the flash-stimulus problem, reduces certain acuity and astigmatism variables, and gives more easily standardized responses. A checkerboard's element (i.e., one light or dark box) size can be equated to the degrees of retinal visual arc stimulated by that element. To obtain the visual arc from a measured check size, the following formula should be used: the angle in minutes = 3.438 times the check size in millimeters. Larger checks produce VEP responses that are similar to those obtained with flash stimulation. The usual distance is 70 to 100 cm with a check size <30 minutes of arc (0.5°) to reduce the likelihood of pattern defocusing. The VEP amplitude normally is inversely proportional to check size, so multiple check sizes can be used during a test series to improve detection of CNS pathology (84). Flash or goggle stimulators can be used on children, with patients who are not able to maintain steady focusing as a result of behavioral or neuromuscular difficulties, during operations, with sedation or unconsciousness, or where visual acuity precludes shorter distance or larger check-patterned stimulus testing. The eyes are first tested together with the pattern reversing twice per second, with the subject's attention on a focusing aid (e.g., colored dot, LED) in the middle of the pattern. Each eye should be tested individually, and the results of each trial are duplicated.

Normal Values

The most important VEP criterion is latency (85). The wave usually has three peaks (Fig. 16-10) that are labeled by their polarity and position (e.g., N1, P1, N2) or their polarity and latency (i.e., N75, P100, N140) (78). The N75 has a normal range from 65 to 90 msec, the P100 will range from 88 to 114 msec, and the N2 (N140) up to 151 msec in normal subjects. Visual acuity losses, even with the use of corrective lenses, may attenuate the P100 amplitude but should have little effect on the latency. In addition, there is a general correlation of visual acuity with the check size used so that a good P100 response at 10 minutes of arc stimulation implies 20/25 acuity, 20 minutes of arc implies 20/50 acuity, 30 minutes of arc implies 20/100 acuity, and 45 minutes of arc implies 20/200 acuity. The P100 latencies shorten during the first year of life, reach a plateau by 6 or 7 years of age, and then increase gradually with age after 60 years. Women tend to have slightly shorter latencies. Low stimulus luminance and pattern contrast can delay the latency and reduce the response amplitude.

When hemifield stimulation is used to evaluate a unilateral occipital cortex lesion, a paradoxical response can be observed with lateral occipital (i.e., O_1 and O_2) lobe electrodes. In a left occipital cerebrovascular accident (CVA) example, a left nasal retinal response crosses the chiasm and joins the right temporal retinal response. The postchiasm tract transmits the signal to the medial surface of the normal right occipital lobe, giving a normal, large VEP on the left and a smaller, normal VEP on the right. The right hemifield stimulation will produce a small response on the right and

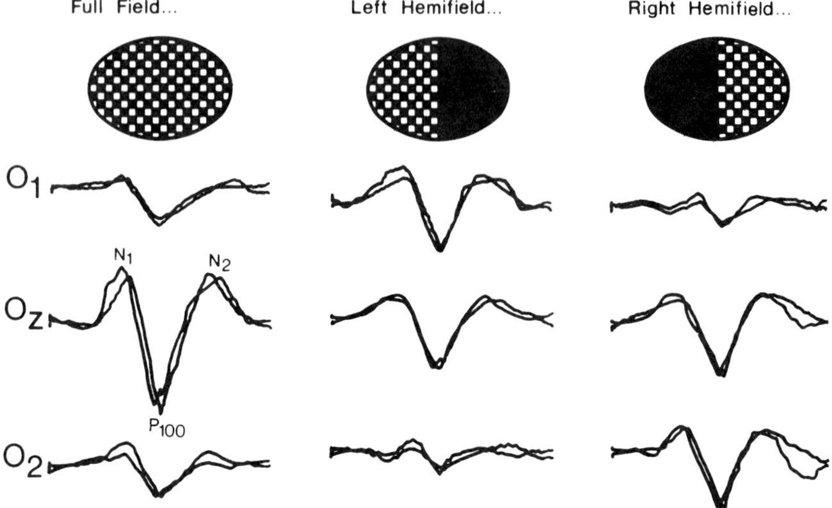

FIG. 16-10. Normal visual-evoked potentials recorded at the O_1, O_z, and O_2 electrode sites in response to *full-field, left-hemifield,* and *right-hemifield* pattern-reversal stimuli to both eyes. The full-field response from O_z is labeled to show typical peak nomenclatures.

an even smaller, less defined response at O_1. The paradoxical response is observed because the larger potential in this example, recorded over the left occipital (i.e., O_1) lobe from left hemifield stimulation, is believed to be the result of the P100 vector being directed contralaterally as it approached the medial surface of the primary visual cortex.

Indications and Interpretation

The VEP is particularly useful in complementing the neuroophthalmologic examination when clinical problems are associated with mild or even subclinical visual dysfunction. Conditions that affect central retinal or macular function can cause alterations in the VEP amplitude or waveform, rather than the latency, and require that a small check pattern be used (87). In fact, larger check patterns may fail to demonstrate several CNS pathologic conditions. Peripheral retinal diseases will not significantly alter the VEP until the macula is involved, and central retinal artery occlusion may not produce any VEP abnormality, whereas ischemic or compressive optic neuropathies can cause waveform and amplitude abnormalities that are out of proportion to the latency delays (88,89). Papilledema, in the absence of secondary ischemic atrophy, may not give any VEP abnormalities. Cortical blindness usually abolishes the VEP, so this test can be of some value in differentiating conversion symptoms from organic lesions. The greatest utility of the VEP is for patients with optic nerve diseases (e.g., optic neuritis) or MS and other demyelinating diseases giving latency prolongations up to the 250-msec range. Toxic or nutritional amblyopias, which are considered demyelinating, usually are not associated with significant VEP alteration.

Chiasmal lesions, which usually are space-occupying masses (e.g., pituitary adenoma, craniopharyngioma, meningioma), generally alter the VEP bilaterally. The resulting waveform distortion and amplitude losses usually are disproportional to the modest latency delays of up to 25 msec. Postchiasmal focal lesions (e.g., tumors, CVA) are best defined with partial or hemifield stimulation, but it must be remembered that the comparatively larger paradoxical response usually is found over the involved hemisphere in occipital cortex lesions. A normal VEP is consistent with an intact pathway through the primary visual cortex, but lesions beyond area 17 require imaging studies for detection.

COGNITIVE EVOKED POTENTIALS

A second category of EP is the so-called endogenous EP. Unlike SEP and VEP, endogenous EPs are stimulus nonspecific, do not require specific receptors, and do require that subjects actively participate in the procedure by carefully attending to a sequence of stimuli and making a decision about them according to certain preset rules to obtain a maximal response.

The CEP, also known as the event-related potential (ERP), is a vertex positivity generated when the subject recognizes a change (i.e., the target) interspersed in an ongoing stimulus pattern (Fig. 16-11). The ERP, however, is stimulus nonspecific because it does not matter what the actual stimulus is. For example, it can be auditory, visual, or somatosensory, or even be the absence of an expected stimulus.

Because the CEP is generated when the brain "decides" that a specific change has occurred, it is also called a decision potential. More common terms are P3 or P300, (typical latency 300 msec). The CEP is not generated by receptors or specific pathways except, of course, those that convey the stimulus to the brain. Because the CEP occurs after the stimulus has been received and then processed by the brain, the latency of the CEP is considerably longer than the exogenous EP latency.

The three factors that have been shown to affect the peak latency of the P300 are the ease with which the target and nontarget stimuli can be discriminated, the age of the subject, and dementia.

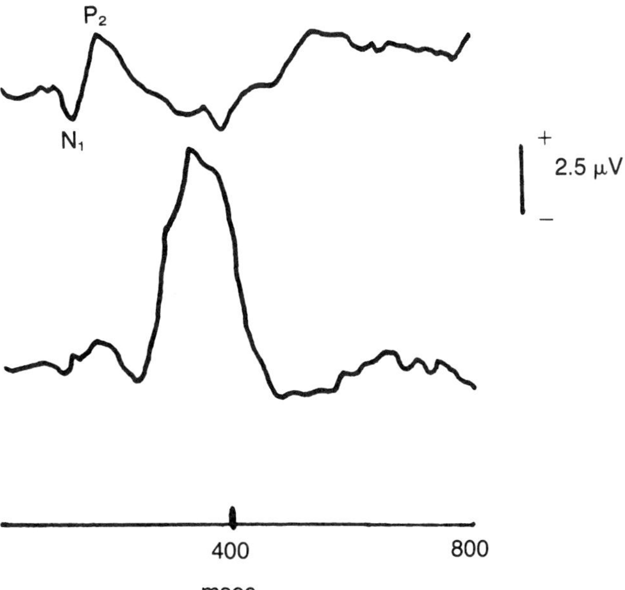

FIG. 16-11. Vertex event-related potentials recorded from a normal 55-year-old subject. Averaged response to frequent 1,000-Hz tones showing typical N_1–P_2 complex or auditory potential **(top)**. Response to 2,000-Hz rare tones after subtracting the averaged response to the frequent tones **(bottom).** This difference potential accentuates the P300 by reducing components that were common to both, including N_1 and P_2.

The easier it is to discriminate between target and nontarget, the shorter the latency of the P300. For example, whereas it is fairly easy to discriminate pitches of 2,000 Hz from those of 1,000 Hz, it is somewhat more difficult to distinguish 1,100 Hz from 1,000 Hz. When the pitches are more similar, it takes longer for the brain to ''decide'' that it has heard the target tone, and this in turn would be reflected in a longer average latency compared with the easier discrimination task.

For a given discrimination task, such as between 1,000- and 2,000-Hz tones, the P300 latency increases with age. Indeed, latencies may approach 400 msec at age 80. The regression line of latency versus age was found to be linear, 1.7 msec/year (89) to 2.8 msec/year in subjects over the age of 15 (90).

Dementing illnesses, even when age corrected, are associated with marked increases in P300 latency. However, false negatives, normal P300 latencies in demented patients, do occasionally occur (91), and prolonged P300 latencies, by themselves, do not differentiate between different causes of dementia (92).

As with latency, there also are a number of factors that appear to influence or correlate with the ERP amplitude. The more expected the stimulus or the greater the probability of its occurrence, the lower will be the P300 amplitude (93). As stated earlier, the ERP requires that the subject generally attend to the ongoing stimulus train and pick out the targets from the nontargets. If the difference between the frequents and rares is great enough, however, subjects who purposefully are not attending to the stimulus still generate P3OOs, although they are smaller in amplitude and of longer latency than under active concentration (94,95). The P300 cannot be completely suppressed voluntarily when an unpredictable stimulus is perceived or appreciated by an intact sensory pathway. In situations where malingering or hysteria is present, as when a subject intentionally blurs or defocuses a VEP pattern stimulus, the P300 can be detected. For example, if a bar pattern is rarely presented during a routine checkerboard VEP trial, when a normal subject defocuses on the monitor, the VEP P100 will be attenuated, but the P300 will come through in response to the different display. In our later years, the P300 amplitude can decreases at a rate of up to 0.2 μV per year (89,90).

MOTOR EVOKED POTENTIALS

Motor evoked potentials (MEP) are the heterogeneous group of responses that have in common their use of one or more neural components that include the efferent spinal motor conduction pathway. Studies of MEPs can provide documentation of neural transmission through the efferent anterior spinal cord pathways as a complement to the afferent dorsal column and anterolateral tract information derived from SEP studies. The MEP response can be elicited from either magnetic or electrical stimulation of the cerebral motor cortex or spinal cord neurons and can be recorded over a relatively superficial motor or mixed peripheral nerve as an efferent neurogram or directly in a targeted peripheral muscle. Magnetic stimulators are stand-alone devices that externally trigger the epoch. In general, the cortical and spinal magnetic stimulators are used in clinical laboratory settings while the cortical and spinal cord electrical stimuli are used during an intraoperative procedure when the subject is under anesthesia. Magnetically stimulated transcranial MEPs can utilize different stimulator shapes and positions to trigger assorted motor cortex patterns, which could then select individual peripheral motor areas. With proper stimulator angular position, some selected subcortical sites can be provoked. Magnetic cortical stimulation has not been widely applied because of the potential for activating seizures. Electric cortical stimulation can be performed using either cortical–cortical or cortical–palatine electrodes and spinal cord stimulation via several approaches. Stimulus site specificity and a lower potential for seizure disorder arousal are among the advantages of electric over magnetic cortical stimulation; however, the stimulus intensity required practically limits its use only to intraoperative applications. To maximize the magnetic MEP responses, on the other hand, they should be performed on awake, cooperative subjects who can voluntarily contract the ''target'' muscles to obtain better information. The transcranial magnetic stimulus delivered during voluntary activity produces a prolonged postexcitatory volitional activity inhibition called the ''silent period.'' Intervertebral space magnetic stimulation, like electrospirograms

TABLE 16-4. *Physiological presentations and diagnostic clinical correlations of magnetic transcranial MEPs*

Conditions	Motor evoked potential		Poststimulation silent period
	Latency	Amplitude	
Physiological factors			
Normal aging	Linear increase	No change to a mild linear increase	Slightly decreased
Increased stimulus intensity	Decreases	Increases	Increases
With volition	Decreases	Increases	Unchanged
Spinal cord lesions			
Cervical myelopathy	Normal or increased	Normal	Decreases (despite volitional contraction of target muscle)
Extramedullary cervical lesion	Increase in 60%	—	—
Intramedullary cervical lesion	Increase in 30%	—	—
Syringomyelia	Prolonged	Decreased or absent	—
Lumbosacral myelopathy	Increased	Normal	—
Various diseases			
Amyotrophic lateral sclerosis	Minimally increased	Decreased	—
Hemiparetic lesions	Normal	Decreases	Very increased
Huntington's disease	Normal	Normal	—
Peripheral neuropathy	Increased	Decreases	Unchanged
Friedreich's ataxia	Increased[a]	Decreases[a]	—
Hereditary spastic paraplegia	UE—Normal	—	—
	LE—NL or increased	—	—
Multiple sclerosis	Very increased	Decreased	Increased
Myotonic dystrophy	Normal	Slight decrease	Unchanged
Parkinsonism	Decreases	Increases	Decreases

[a]Change proportional to disease duration.

(ESG), can derive relatively short spinal segment information or can establish the peripheral motor latency (PML). The central motor latency (CML) or conduction time is the difference between the cortically evoked and the spinal or peripheral nerve latencies (CML − MEP latency = PML). Magnetic transcranial MEPs have been correlated with several physiological factors and clinical conditions (Table 16-4).

Intraoperatively, electrical cortical and/or spinal cord stimulation offers several advantages over magnetic stimuli, as it can be delivered at a higher rate, permitting more rapid data acquisition, and can be obtained in the presence of neuromuscular blockage agents and other medications typically used during surgery. The cranial and (usually cervical) vertebral (or any site rostral to the surgery) stimulating electrodes are more easily placed and physically and electromagnetically are less troublesome for the anesthesiologist and surgeon. The most direct and efficient, especially in terms of being able to utilize conventional electrophysiological equipment, is the placement of laminal depth stimulating monopolar needle electrodes to trigger the spinal cord. Electrical tissue burns from the stimulating electrodes are a potential problem that can be minimized by increasing the electrode–tissue interface area, which reduces the effective current density. However, R-on-T phenomena and potentially dangerous ground loops can occur from the electrodiagnostic apparatus or any concurrently used equipment if a failure occurs.

MOVEMENT-RELATED POTENTIALS

Central Motor-Evoked Potentials

Merton and colleagues stimulated the precentral motor cortex and the spinal cord with surface electrodes placed on the scalp and over the spine to generate compound muscle action potentials (CMAP) in extremity muscles (96). This can be accomplished using 50-μsec high-voltage (i.e., up to 2,000 volts) stimuli. Alternative techniques include using unipolar electric (97) or high-current magnetic field stimulation (98). Although it is gaining broader use, transcranial cortical stimulation still is undergoing clinical trials to evaluate patient safety and has not yet been approved for general application.

By using induced cerebral motor cortex excitation, the corticospinal tract can be made to generate efferent impulses to evoke a CMAP (Fig. 16-12) in the peripheral muscles, and its latency or propagation time can be measured. By comparing the transcranial stimulation latencies with latencies obtained by cervical spinal cord transcutaneous stimulation, it is possible to measure and compute a central efferent conduction time.

The central stimulation technique complements the SEP examination in that it can provide important information about the functional integrity of the descending motor pathways that produce movement. These muscle contractions are entirely involuntary. From the perspective of the electromyographer, studying the brain and spinal cord efferent pathways with central motor evoked potentials is a logical extension of peripheral motor nerve conduction study.

Readiness Potentials and Back Averaging

This approach involves capturing the EEG signal before, as well as after, a self-generated voluntary movement is produced. The technique used is called back averaging. Back averaging is accomplished with concurrent collection in a circular buffer memory of EEG and peripheral muscle action potential data. The CMAP triggers an averager so that its analysis window time-locks events that precede and follow the triggering. Using the buffered data, the EEG signals are then averaged together. A slow negative drift of the scalp potential can be identified (see Fig. 16-6), particularly in the central regions, beginning up to 1 second before the CMAP onset occurs (99–101). This readiness potential (RP) or Bereitschaft potential presumably is involved in the cortical processes of preparing, initiating, and executing a voluntary motor activity. It can be recorded in advance of speech and saccadic eye movements as well as movements of the hands and feet. The RP and cognitive negative variation may be applied to the examination of how voluntary action and anticipatory learning are normally organized by brain structures and how these critical processes are affected by different disabling conditions.

CLINICAL USES OF EVOKED POTENTIALS

Cerebrovascular Accidents

Evoked potential studies have been used for more than 20 years to evaluate patients with cerebrovascular lesions. Among the early pioneers in this field was Liberson, who, in 1966, studied aphasics using SEP and noted that preservation of a normal SEP was most frequently accompanied by a significant clinical improvement (102). In the last decade, EP studies were used to study various aspects of stroke from both the diagnostic (103–106) and prognostic (104,107–111) perspectives.

Brainstem auditory evoked response studies are of value primarily in brainstem and related area infarctions and massive hemispheric infarctions. In capsular, parietal, and temporal lobe infarctions, the ABR usually is normal (105). The clinically uninvolved side, as in normal subjects (see Fig. 16-7), generally should yield normal wave I through V latencies. However, possibly because of edema producing bilateral

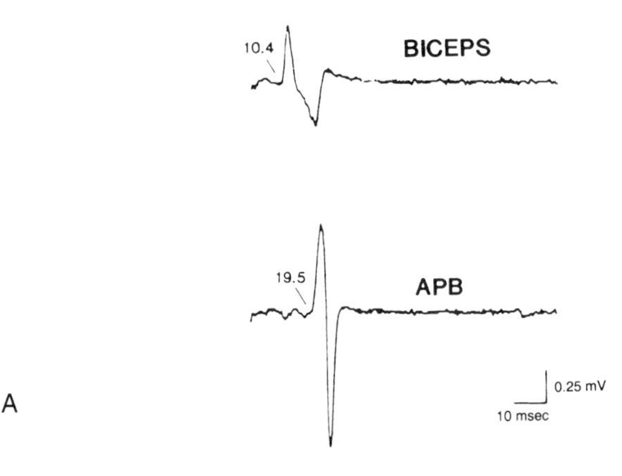

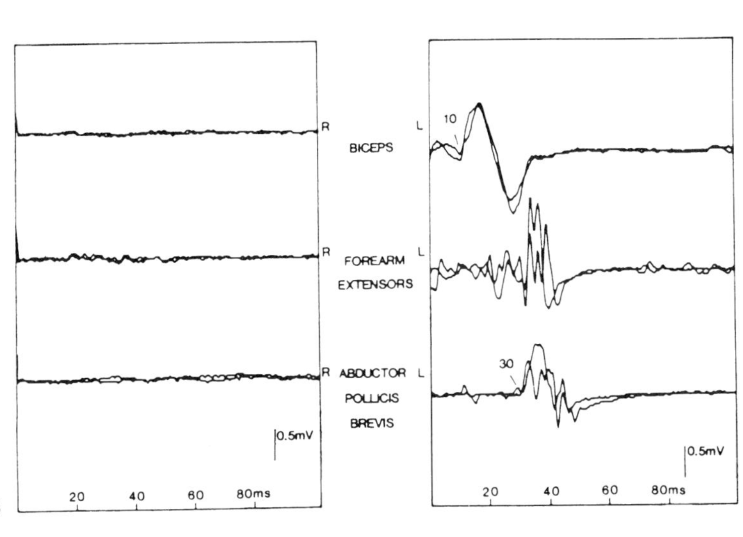

FIG. 16-12. Compound muscle action potential recorded from biceps and thenar eminence after transcranial cortical stimulation. **A:** Surface electromyogram responses recorded at the *biceps* and abductor pollicis brevis *(APB)* after stimulation of contralateral motor cortex by a transcranial current produced by a brief, high-current stimulus. **B:** Compound muscle action potentials produced by transcranial cortical stimulation in a patient who sustained a C3–C4 fracture-dislocation and cervical spinal cord injury. Clinically, the patient improved on the left but had a residual paralysis of the right arm and leg. These studies show absent responses from the right arm with left motor cortex stimulation and delayed motor responses in the left APB following right motor cortex stimulation. (Data from Thompson PD, Dick JP, Asselman P, et al. Examination of motor function in lesions of the spinal cord by stimulation of the motor cortex. *Ann Neurol* 1987; 21:389–396.)

compromise or accentuation of the physiological effects in the usually older age group involved, the normal-side peak V latency in CVA patients is slightly longer than that in the general population, with an acceptable range (mean ± 3 SD) up to 6.49 msec.

A strobe light can be used for VEP, but, in most instances, a checkerboard pattern, usually black and white, on a monitor or through goggles is used. Full-field stimulation is normal in the majority of CVA patients, so hemifield stimulation frequently is used to better define retrochiasmatic lesions, such as unilateral occipital infarctions and homonymous hemianopsia (78,85,109,112). The visual stimuli are delivered to each eye in turn, then both eyes, and the recordings are compared.

The VEP amplitude of the P100 wave is quite variable in CVA studies, and it can vary significantly from one subject to another or from one test to another carried out on the same person. The normal variation in amplitude from one eye to another is large, and some authors consider amplitude comparisons unreliable; however, it is the author's consensus that in a carefully controlled study, amplitude variations greater than 50% usually are significant (113).

Following a CVA, the ability to record a MEP from cortical stimulation within an involved area suggests a better short-term prognosis than when the response is unrecordable (105). The rate of magnetically stimulated MEP abnormality was higher in patients with hemorrhage than in those with infarction, and the degree of weakness appears to correlate with the severity of cortical MEP findings (114).

The quest for a good CVA outcome predictor has challenged the imagination of a myriad of researchers. The possible relationship between EP studies and stroke outcome has been explored by a number of these. Liberson, in 1966, noted a correlation between SEP and the outcome of aphasia in 15 patients with stroke (102). Vredevelt reported on 97 hemiplegic patients, and found that absence of the N19/20 peak was accompanied by a poor functional recovery (111). Patients in whom N19/20 was present, even if attenuated, had a higher percentage of better functional recovery. La Joie and associates, in 1982, studied the correlation of median nerve SEP and right arm return of function in 68 right hemiplegic patients (108). Of 42 patients with absent SEP, only one showed some functional gain in the upper extremity, whereas more than 36% of the patients with normal or diminished SEP studies showed some functional gain on discharge. Despland and colleagues studied the SEP N19/20 peak and recovery of sensory deficits in hemispheric infarction in 50 patients and noted a significant correlation between the two (115). Ignacio and colleagues (107), in 1982, reported on the relationship between SEP and functional outcome in 130 patients following an acute CVA using the method of bilateral median nerve stimulation with simultaneous C3 and C4 recordings (106), with the studies carried out within 2 weeks of CVA onset and with ongoing correlations through the recovery phase. A very good correlation was found between the CNS electrodiagnostic abnormality and the degree of functional recovery. Patients with low-grade changes showed return of function in the affected hand and were able to carry out self-care activities independently or with minimal assistance and to ambulate independently. Severely affected patients, on the other hand, did uniformly poorly. None of them regained any useful function in the affected hand, none regained independence in self-care activities or functional ambulation, and 50% of them had to be placed in nursing homes.

Spinal Cord Injury

One of the challenges in caring for SCI patients has been in predicting outcome. When recovery does occur, it indicates that the lesion did not progress beyond the stage of neurapraxia, whereas permanent involvement indicates that long tracts have degenerated. Experience has shown that two types of patients frequently demonstrate at least some return of function. The first group consists of those with clinically incomplete lesions, and the second are patients who show early partial return during the first 48 hours. Interestingly, and germane to the major purpose of this section, preservation of even partial sensory function alone often has been followed by return of voluntary motion (see Chapter 51).

Working within the realities of human SCI, Nuomoto and associates reported a fairly good correlation between the SEP and motor function return (116). Subsequent animal studies confirmed that early return of the SEP was usually, though not always, a harbinger of motor recovery (117). Other investigations correlated the presence or absence of the SEP with the anatomic changes found in impacted spinal cords (118), in compressed spinal cords (119), and with motor evoked potentials after graded compression of the spinal cord (120).

Within 24 to 48 hours after a SCI in humans, the presence of a SEP, even one with altered morphology, from either peroneal or posterior tibial nerve stimulation usually was associated with some degree of clinical improvement in the legs (121–124). At least some improvement in upper limb function was reported when a median nerve SEP was obtained after cervical cord trauma (125). All patients who had an SEP from lower extremity stimulation also were diagnosed as having incomplete lesions based on neurologic examination, whereas patients with clinically complete lesions had no SEP from below the level of the lesion, and their recovery usually was nil or minimal at best. Spielholz and colleagues, however, found that the SEP could not be obtained in about 15% of clinically incomplete patients, yet these patients did just as well as other clinically incomplete patients in whom the SEP was present (124). It would appear, then, in the awake, cooperative patient, as opposed to the unconscious one, a routine SEP study does not substitute for a thorough clinical examination, which still appears to be the best prognostic tool.

Intraoperative Monitoring

Spine Surgery

Up to 1% of patients who undergo Harrington or C-D rodding (fusion) instrumentation for treatment of scoliosis develop varying degrees of spinal cord dysfunction (126), and more than 10% of pedicle screw placement surgeries are associated with some postoperative complication or neurologic deficit. However, this is not the typical complication rate observed by most. Early distraction lesions usually are reversible, and removal of the rods or fixation within 6 hours usually resolves the problem. Direct neural tissue trauma from a misguided pedical screw or drill bit is less likely to fully or rapidly reverse. Regardless of the etiology of the SEP or MEP response degradation, the earliest recognition still will afford the patient the greatest chances for return to normal or preoperative function through a systematic review of the current operative activity, the monitoring equipment, and the patient's vital signs. The first intraoperative monitor, still in use today in certain quarters, is the wake-up test. Subsequently, electrophysiological methods were developed, including the following:

- Epidural stimulation with epidural recording (127)
- Peripheral nerve stimulation with epidural recording (128)
- Real-time/ongoing EMG from a paraspinal muscle or peripheral extremity muscle can be used in cases that involve cauda-equina-level surgeries (if no neuromuscular blockage agent was administered except for intubation purposes)
- Peripheral nerve stimulation with ESG recording by means of needles inserted into the exposed spinous process or adjacent ligament (51) or percutaneously in the interspinous ligament above or below the operative site (129)
- Peripheral nerve stimulation with ESG recording by means of Steinmann pins in spinous processes of vertebrae (130)
- Peripheral nerve stimulation with scalp SEP recording (131)
- Using a magnetic cortical or spinal level stimulation with the evoked motor potential recorded from an extremity muscle,
- Cortical–cortical or palatine–cortical electrical MEP with a targeted peripheral extremity muscle or efferent peripheral nerve (neurogram)
- Spinal cord (bilateral monopolar laminal level stimulating electrodes) electrical stimulation with the recording site in a peripheral muscle or over a relatively superficial nerve as an efferent neurogram.

Of these methods, the ESG recorded from the interspinous ligament or vertebrae and the SEP are most widely practiced. The SEP is usually of larger amplitude than the ESG and theoretically requires less averaging. The SEP, however, has a much greater sensitivity than the ESG to anesthetic agents, producing a dose-related amplitude decrease and latency prolongation. As these effects (enflurane more than isoflurane, and least with halothane) (131,132) are a likely confounding variable in studies where a 40% amplitude reduction can make a critical difference in the surgical decision, their use should be avoided. Other anesthetic agents and physiological factors that affect the IOM/EP studies include narcotics (fentanyl, for example, significantly reduces, while naloxone increased, the later peak amplitudes of SEP and ABRs) and other anesthetic medication (133,134), blood pressure, oxygen carrying capacity of the blood, and/or significant changes in hematocrit, hypothermia, and P_{CO_2} (135). Because of these factors, SEP alterations must be analyzed carefully for other contributing reasons before spinal cord compromise can be ascertained. These tests have advantages and disadvantages, but both share a common shortcoming in that neither measures conduction in motor pathways. It is possible for either of them to remain unaltered during surgery and yet for the patient to wake up paralyzed or with bladder or bowel impairment.

What then are the criteria for alerting the surgeon to a possible problem? Different institutions have different requirements, but the following has been a reliable protocol for many years (134):

- All peaks of the SEP or the MEP response (after repeat studies confirm a change) either disappear entirely or become markedly smaller, or significant latency prolongation occurs relative to postanesthesia predistraction data.
- The peaks remain in the above state for a number of repeat trials over the next 5 minutes or more.
- Checking with the anesthesiologist fails to reveal an anesthetic (e.g., recent bolus of narcotic, change in inhalation agents) or other systemic reason (e.g., drop in blood pressure, significant drop in hematocrit, increase in P_{CO_2}).
- Checking the stimulating circuit and recording inputs does not reveal any malfunction along the pathway being studied, and confirmation of the equipments continued operating is established through a normal study utilizing a nonoperative site.

It is important to remember that loss of the intraoperative SEP during spinal surgery or instrumentation distraction forces does not require immediate action because the rod can be removed several hours later and recovery will still occur. This time latitude is not always available when the changes result from anoxic/ischemic impairment. However, it is imperative that the surgeon and anesthesiologist be immediately and clearly notified and that all of the data and circumstances of the surgical procedure be correlated as well as can be annotated.

Aortic Surgery

Paraplegia is a recognized possible complication of surgery on the aorta. Its incidence is estimated at 0.5% for coarctation of the aorta to as high as 15% for thoracoabdominal aneurysms (136). A number of reports describe the use of SEP to determine whether spinal cord or cerebral blood flow remains adequate during cross-clamping of the aorta or whether a bypass or shunt is required to maintain adequate spinal cord perfusion (136,137).

In dogs and humans, spinal cord ischemia produces detectable changes in the SEP starting after 3 minutes, with total loss of all peaks after about 9 minutes. An important difference here from monitoring for spinal cord distraction is the time limit to identify and correct problems. In vascular cases, the physician should sample recordings more frequently and attempt to use a case-to-case standardized minimum number of sweeps per recording to rapidly recognize changes during the procedure. Maneuvers designed to increase both distal spinal cord blood flow and perfusion have resulted in SEP reappearance without postoperative neurologic deficits.

Carotid Endarterectomy

Intraoperative SEP monitoring during carotid endarterectomy surgery accurately identifies cerebral ischemia secondary to carotid clamping; however, controversy still exists over the value of intraoperative monitoring if a shunt is to be performed electively, such as with contralateral carotid occlusion or previous stroke (138). A number of reports have appeared attesting to the SEP's ability to detect early cerebral ischemia and, thus, presumably identify patients in whom a bypass shunt is required (139,140). Nonshunting of patients in whom the SEP or EEG (followed as an open running channel) disappeared during clamping has been followed by neurologic deficits, whereas shunting that restored the deteriorated SEP was followed by an uneventful outcome (141). Most equipment available today has the capacity to simultaneously record an averaged signal (SEP) while displaying the real-time input information (EEG). The intraoperative SEP technique most often used is to stimulate the posterior tibial nerves, or the median nerve contralateral to the side being operated on. Disappearance or marked SEP attenuation during the clamping time is an indication that the shunt is needed to maximize the patient's outcome (142). Rapid reestablishment of circulation frequently is associated with the SEP return to its preclamping levels.

The pathophysiological process that presumably underlies the SEP changes in patients who require a shunt during carotid artery clamping is the inability of the brain to maintain appropriate electric capabilities as it becomes ischemic. Studies have shown, in both humans and baboons, that when regional cerebral blood flow is greater than about 20 ml/100 g per minute, electrical activity, whether monitored by EEG or SEP, is normal. In the range, approximately, of 16 to 18 ml/100 g per minute, the SEP latency begins to lengthen, and changes start occurring in the EEG. At about 10 ml/100 g per minute, both electric indices are essentially flat (143,144).

Multiple Sclerosis

About a decade ago, it was noted that VEP were abnormal in patients with optic neuritis (145,146). Because it is one of the frequent and early manifestations of MS, VEP soon proved to be a very useful adjunct in diagnosis. As more EP studies were done in this new diagnostic field, it was soon discovered that short-latency ABR and SEP studies also are abnormal in a high percentage of patients (see Chapter 50).

The VEP abnormalities associated with MS are related most often to optic neuritis. They may encompass a single eye or both eyes, with one usually affected more than the other. The principal VEP changes associated with MS are the following:

- Prolonged P100 latency
- Interocular latency differences
- Relative amplitude diminution
- Dispersion or change in duration of the P100 potential
- Other waveform morphology changes

In a large series of MS cases, the mean for P100 was 10 to 30 msec greater than that of normal subjects (139); however, the most sensitive indicator of optic nerve dysfunction is the interocular latency difference. In many MS patients, especially in the early stages, only one eye is involved, and this is reflected by an increase in the interocular latency difference; latency abnormalities usually precede amplitude changes. With the full-field stimulation technique, a total amplitude less than 3 mV should be considered suspicious, and a side-to-side amplitude difference greater than 50% may be considered abnormal (146).

The P100 shape often is abnormal in MS patients, especially if they have visual symptoms. The characteristic V-shaped peak is at times converted to a bifid or "W," or at times, the concavity of the "V" is greatly increased, skewed, or dispersed. The P100 is a far-field potential, and thus, the latency should best be marked by visualizing the peak's overall middle or by extrapolation from the peak's sides, and not at the first positive component of the waveform's peak.

In early MS, abnormalities frequently are present when the patient has no visual symptoms or other objective findings. The pattern-shift VEP sensitivity in uncovering optic tract demyelinating lesions has been documented in a number of studies (140,145). Halliday studied MS patients with pattern-shift VEP at intervals over several years and noted latency prolongation with relapses associated with visual impairment. Pavot and colleagues found similar results and found no other relationship between the VEP and nonvisual status. Brooks and Chiappa reported on 198 MS patients who had various neuroophthalmologic tests (147). In their report, when the pattern-shift VEP was normal, there was never an abnormality found on clinical examination. Even when the pattern-shift VEP was abnormal, various clinical examinations remained normal; however, when optic neuritis was clearly present, more than 95% of patients had VEP abnormalities. When there was no clinical evidence of optic nerve involvement, the incidence of VEP abnormalities was 51%. Varying the check sizes (87) and hyperthermia (148) increase the test's sensitivity.

The ABR in MS also has been extensively studied throughout the world for its distinct value in the diagnosis and possible management of this condition. The ABR has been found to be abnormal in 30% of possible MS, 41% of probable MS, and 67% of definite MS patients (135). The principal abnormalities noted fall into the following categories:

- Absence of waves, especially peak V
- Marked diminution of amplitude of the waves
- Increased interpeak latency differences
- Reversal of I/V amplitude ratio

Any of the waves, or combination of them, may be prolonged, attenuated, or abolished; the most commonly involved is peak V, then, less frequently, peak III (45,149). Exacerbations in clinical course do not correlate with the ABR, however. Side-to-side comparisons are of better value because the findings frequently are more pronounced on one side.

Interpeak latency prolongation is one of the frequent findings in MS, with the III–V difference generally more frequently involved than the I–III. Occasionally, an abnormally prolonged III–V latency may be encountered in the presence of a normal peak V latency or normal I–V interval, but, most frequently, wave V prolongation is present. If the calculated I/V amplitude ratio (i.e., the ratio of wave I/wave V amplitudes) exceeds normal values, it is suggestive of a conduction defect rostral to lower pons. Amplitude criteria, however, remain a precarious basis for establishing a diagnosis because a few normal patients may show a reversal of the ratio.

Upper and lower extremity SEP studies in MS patients are more frequently abnormal than ABR or VEP (149–151). Chiappa reported that in a group of 114 MS patients, 54% had abnormal upper limb SEP, and 64% abnormal lower limb SEP findings (149). The abnormalities demonstrated include the following:

- Peak latency prolongation
- Prolongation of interpotential latency
- Diminution of amplitude
- Absence of component peaks
- Change in the morphology (150)

Prolongation of the absolute peak or interpeak latencies is among the most commonly found abnormalities. Because MS or its sequelae may affect peripheral nerves, the spinal cord, or the CNS, SEP will show various combination of abnormalities. A marked diminution of amplitude typically affecting several rather than a single potential is a common finding in MS. The amplitude will be diminished at times to the point where the potential is almost imperceptible or appears to be absent. This disappearance of one, or at times several, potentials is not uncommon with clinically advanced MS (151).

The overall incidence of abnormal SEP studies is approximately 58% for all clinical MS classifications. The abnormality rate was 77% in patients with definite MS, 67% in probable MS, and 49% in possible MS. A larger percentage of SEP abnormalities are present from the lower extremities (64%) than from the upper extremities (54%).

Comparison of the relative diagnostic value of SEP, VEP, and ABR studies suggests that the SEP is abnormal in over 40% of cases, whereas the ABR is abnormal in fewer than 25%, and the VEP is abnormal in approximately 37% of those referred for study. This appears to be primarily a function of the tract's length or the white matter pathway being tested and, second, the individual system's susceptibility to demyelination.

Motor cortex electrical or magnetic stimulation for the study of central and peripheral conduction in normal subjects and MS patients showed the cord-to-axilla conduction to be normal in both groups, whereas central conduction (e.g., cord-to-cord conduction) was markedly slowed in MS patients (152).

The arrival of magnetic resonance imaging (MRI) revolutionized the diagnosis of MS by its ability to detect small demyelinating lesions in both brain and spinal cord. In these circumstances, it often is superior to EP studies in the probable MS category (153). In brainstem lesions, however, the ABR is more sensitive than MRI. Also, in optic neuritis secondary to MS, the MRI usually has been normal, whereas pattern-shift VEPs are abnormal in approximately 95% of patients. Giesser and associates showed that of 23 "possible MS" patients studied with trimodal EPs and MRI, the EP studies were abnormal in 18, whereas the MRI showed changes in only 15 patients (154).

Head Injury

In head injuries (HI), the magnitude and degree of impairment vary greatly from one case to another, and numerous attempts to predict long-term outcome have been made. Multimodality-evoked potentials (MmEP) can be used for diagnostic localization of lesions (155,156) as well as to gather information for prognostic value. Multimodality-evoked potential studies in large HI patient populations using long-window (i.e., 150 to 300 msec) SEP, ABR, and VEP have a distinct advantage in patients with altered levels of consciousness or who are confused or uncooperative (156). In addition, these tests serve as a method of assessing brain function during barbiturate coma treatment for specific HI patients. Evoked potential testing appears to have less value in mild closed HI (158) and in predicting outcome (as compared to clinical assessment scales) (159–161) than they do in CVA.

Greenberg studied short, intermediate, and long-latency potentials and devised a four-level classification based on the degree of complexity of the EP responses and the presence or absence of potentials (155). Grade I was essentially normal responses. In grade II, there was absence of long- and preservation of short- and intermediate-latency potentials. Absence of long and intermediate potentials defined grade III, and in grade IV, only some with short latency were identified. In this study, grade I had a good prognosis and recovered within 3 months (155). The chances for a good functional outcome diminished in grade II and were even less in grade III. Patients classified as grade IV either died or ended up in a vegetative state. Involvement of only one system generally carried a better prognosis than involvement of two or three systems. Comparison of the MmEP with other clinical indices such as neurologic examination, computed tomography scan, Glasgow outcome scale, and the like revealed that MmEP provided a 91% accuracy of predicting outcome, which is the best prediction obtained by any single indicant (156). In the SEP studies, the contralateral–ipsilateral amplitude difference may be a better marker of extent and severity of injury than the differences in latency and may also be helpful in localizing site of injury, particularly if it is an interhemispheric or corpus callosal injury (157). Furthermore, addition of MmEP results to those of other measures improved the accuracy and the confidence limits of prediction (158), as patients with no SEP activity beyond 50 msec in either hemisphere either have a high probability of dying or will probably remain in a vegetative state.

Rappaport and colleagues also reported on MmEP studies carried out in comatose patients (159,160). They found that correlation between the degree of abnormality of the EP patterns and the severity of patients' disability increased from 0.55 when one sensory modality was used to 0.98 when three modalities (i.e., ABR, VEP, and SEP) were used. Correlation of diagnostic/outcome scales, such as the Coma/Near-Coma (CNC) scale, which is designed to measure small clinical changes in patients with severe traumatic and nontraumatic brain injuries, shows a significant correlations with MmEP abnormality scores (161–164). They found that ABR generally were less correlated with disability than cortical responses, at least among long-term survivors of traumatic brain injury. Rappaport has shown that EP results obtained up to 1 year after a severe insult to the CNS can provide useful information on the status and ultimate outcome for individual patients. The MmEP studies carried out within 1 month after trauma (162), when graded with the same system described previously for CVA patients, showed a high degree of correlation between the EP grade and the outcome.

Identification of reliable prognostic indicators for patients with severe HI is important to provide objective information for appropriate allocation of rehabilitation services, family counseling, and for clinical investigation and assessment of our therapeutic approaches. Multimodality evoked potential studies have been shown to be such a tool for assessing the degree of disability and in predicting long-term functional outcome in patients with HI.

Brain Death

The definition of brain death most often is based on a serial or duplicated clinical determinations; however, there are circumstances under which an unimpeachable documentation is required. Evoked potential recording, intracranial pressure measurement, serial EEG recording, cerebral blood flow measurement, apnea testing, and ultrasound techniques have all been used as monitoring methods. EEG findings do not correlate well with the diagnosis of brain death as the EEG is essentially a test of cortical function and brain death is better correlated with the irreversible loss of brainstem function. Absence of a cortical SEP with preservation of the ABR correlated with loss of cortical function and preservation of brainstem function in hypoxic insults who developed a chronic vegetative state. An absent or abnormal SEP may help to identify the sensory pathway loss, but it does not indicate its location, therefore, it is essential that entry markers, that is Erb s point responses for the upper extremities and ESG or afferent neurograms form the lower extremities, be recorded to confirm the peripheral nerve stimulation and the equipment s operation. In upper extremity SEP studies, the presence of the thalamic components (P13 through P17 peak latencies) suggests continuing brainstem activity (162). Evoked potential studies can be a reliable diagnostic and prognostic predictor of outcome (163,164,166).

In brain death, the ABR typically has no identifiable waves or only isolated unilateral or bilateral wave I can be recorded. Only rarely is wave II present. When the first wave is recordable its latency can range from normal to significantly delayed (163). Over the observable clinical course, the wave I can show further delay and/or disappear due to progressive hypoxic-ischemic dysfunction of the cochlea and the eighth nerve. The ABR recordings in decerebration and bulbar syndromes, in contrast to the stabile latencies of healthy subjects, show considerable instability and an increase in the wave latencies. In decerebrate patients the wave I latency and the interpeak latencies for the medullo-pontine and ponto-mesencephalic segments as well as the central conduction time are typically increased and marked peak III and V amplitude reductions. This is presumed to be due to the mesencephalic and pontine functional disturbance during decerebration (164). In the diagnosis of multiple sclerosis, as in the diagnosis of brain death, MmEP testing has been shown to be more effective than any one EP test used alone (165). In head trauma, MmEP testing potentially offer a means of localization and prognostication (165).

NEUROPLASTICITY AND THE ADAPTIVE PROCESS

Physiology is an important basic science and, specifically in this context, clinical neurophysiology is an important investigative tool of rehabilitation medicine. These disciplines involve the study of dynamic processes associated with adaptation. It is within the context of these considerations that the role of clinical neurophysiology takes on special importance as a means of investigating the functional mechanism in normal subjects and disabled patients. It becomes a part of the functional examination, permitting a careful operational analysis of clinical recovery, in addition to providing clues to an understanding of the basic mechanisms associated with adaptation and functional recovery. The following are some of the current and potential applications of clinical neurophysiology in physical medicine and rehabilitation:

- Guiding the development of individualized programs and assisting in decision making about the design of such programs
- Assessing prognosis for recovery or the stage to which recovery has progressed
- Evaluation of the therapy's impact and detecting clinically unsuspected malfunction of the neural system
- Assessing function in patients difficult to evaluate clinically (e.g., children, comatose or aphasic patients)
- Monitoring objective changes in physiological status, recognizing that the tests are essentially noninjurious and thus can be repeated to evaluate longitudinal change without additional risk to the patient
- Detecting principles of physiological change associated with recovery of function and predicting responsiveness to therapies
- Helping to guide and assist the development of new rehabilitation methods and to evaluate their effectiveness
- Early detection of dysfunction in the physically challenged child to permit the earliest corrective technological intervention where possible and institution of a rehabilitation program.

In the rehabilitation management of the patient with peripheral nerve damage, EMG provides a vista of the disability to correlate with the clinically observed muscle weakness. The clinician is able to assess, in an objective and quantitative manner, the extent to which the recovery processes of sprouting, axonal regrowth, and reinnervation have progressed. Such information helps evaluate treatments, such as surgical release or repair, and aids management decisions, such as splinting and exercise programs. Our goal is to achieve a similar understanding of the role of clinical neurophysiology in the rehabilitation management of disability arising from CNS impairment. Although we are just beginning to understand the basic neurophysiological processes involved in recovery of function following CNS lesions such as CVA and HI (165,166), clinical neurophysiology can be applied for the assessment of CNS function in a manner analogous to peripheral nerve dysfunction. It must be understood that there still remains a great deal of basic and applied research to be done to fully appreciate the potential research and clinical value of these powerful tests in physical medicine and rehabilitation, and the authors hope that this chapter serves as a catalyst to that process.

REFERENCES

1. Canton R. The electrical currents of the brain. *Br Med J* 1985; 2:278.
2. Dawson GD. Cerebral responses to electrical stimulation of peripheral nerve in man. *J Neurol Neurosurg Psychiatry* 1947; 10:134–140.
3. Dawson GD. Investigations on patient subject to myoclonic seizures after sensory stimulation. *J Neurol Neurosurg Psychiatry* 1947; 10: 141–149.
4. Benecke R, Berthold A, Conrad B. Denervation activity in the EMG of patients with upper motor neuron lesions: time course, local distribution and pathogenic aspects. *J Neurol* 1983; 230:143–151.
5. Campbell JW, Herbison GJ, Chen YT, Jahweed MM, Gussner CG. Spontaneous electromyographic potentials in chronic spinal cord injured patients: relation to spasticity and length of nerve. *Arch Phys Med Rehabil* 1991; 72:23–27.
6. Johnson EW, Denny ST, Kelly JP. Sequence of electromyographic abnormalities in stroke syndrome. *Arch Phys Med Rehabil* 1975; 56: 468–473.
7. Spielholz N, Sell GH, Goodgold J, Rusk HA, Greene SK. Electrophysiological studies in patients with spinal cord lesions. *Arch Phys Med Rehabil* 1972; 53:558–562.
8. Taylor RG, Kewelramani LS, Fowler WM. Electromyographic findings in lower extremities of patients with high spinal cord injury. *Arch Phys Med Rehabil* 1974; 55:16–23.
9. Fisher MA, Shahani BT, Young RR. Assessing segmental excitability after acute rostral lesions: I. The F response. *Neurology* 1978; 28: 1265–1271.
10. Liberson WT, Chen LY, Fok SK, Patel KK, Yu G, Fried P. ''H'' reflexes and ''F'' waves in hemiplegics. *Electromyogr Clin Neurophysiol* 1977; 17:247–264.
11. Colombo A, Guerzoni MC, Bortolotti P, Schoenhuber R. Blink reflex in unilateral hemiplegic cerebrovascular lesions. *Electromyogr Clin Neurophysiol* 1986; 26:735–741.
12. Cole JL. Facial muscle electrodiagnostic and electrophysiological assessment of functional strength after injury. In: Rubin LR, ed. *The paralyzed face*. St. Louis: Mosby-Yearbook, 1991; 30–39.
13. Kimura J, Nitsudome A, Yamada T, Dickins QS. Stationary peaks from a moving source in far-field recording. *Electroencephalogr Clin Neurophysiol* 1984; 58:351–361.
14. Cunningham K, Halliday AM, Jones SJ. Simulation of ''stationary'' SAP and SEP phenomena by two-dimensional potential field modelling. *Electroencephalogr Clin Neurophysiol* 1986; 65:416–428.
15. Cole JL. Equipment parameter determinants in evoked potential studies. *Bull Am Soc Clin Evok Potentials* 1984; 3:3–9.
16. Gopalan L, Parker PA, Scott RN. Microprocessor-based system for monitoring spinal evoked potentials during surgery. *IEEE Trans Biomed Eng* 1986; 33:982–985.
17. Roberts KB, Lawrence PD, Eisen A. Dispersion of the somatosensory evoked potential (SEP) in multiple sclerosis. *IEEE Trans Biomed Eng* 1983; 30:360–364.
18. Ary UP, Klein SA, Fender DH. Localization of sources of evoked scalp potentials: corrections for skull and scalp thickness. *IEEE Trans Biomed Eng* 1981; 28:447–452.
19. Gevins AS. Analysis of the electromagnetic signals of the human brain: milestones, obstacles, and goals. *IEEE Trans Biomed Eng* 1984; 31:833–850.
20. McKay DM. On line source density computation with a minimum of electrodes. *Electroencephalogr Clin Neurophysiol* 1983; 56:696–698.
21. Perrin F, Bertrand O, Pernier J. Scalp current density mapping: value and estimation from potential data. *IEEE Trans Biomed Eng* 1987; 34:283–288.
22. Srebro R. Localization of visually evoked cortical activity in humans. *J Physiol* 1985; 360:233–246.
23. Srebro R, Sokol B, Wright W. The power spectra of visually evoked potentials to pseudorandom contrast reversals of gratings. *Electroencephalogr Clin Neurophysiol* 1981; 51:63–68.
24. Wood CC. Application of dipole localization methods to source identification of human evoked potentials. *Ann NY Acad Sci* 1982; 388: 139–155.
25. Martin WH, Pratt H, Bleich N. Three-channel Lissajous' trajectory of human auditory brainstem evoked potentials: II. Effects of click intensity. *Electroencephalogr Clin Neurophysiol* 1986; 63:54–61.
26. Paqueroau J, Marillaud A, Ingrand P, Kremer-Merere C. Three-dimensional curves: main parameters of brainstem auditory evoked responses in the normal subject. *Audiology* 1986; 25:107–115.
27. Jasper HH. The ten-twenty electrode system of the International Federation. *Electroencephalogr Clin Neurophysiol* 1958; 10:371–375.
28. Blume WT, Buza RC, Okazaki H. Anatomic correlates of the

ten–twenty electrode placement system in infants. *Electroencephalogr Clin Neurophysiol* 1974; 36:303–307.
29. Geddes LA. Electrodes: what we know and don't know about them. In: *Proceedings of the Seventh Annual Conference of the IEEE Engineering in Medicine and Biology Society.* Chicago: IEEE-EMBS, 1985; 1:154–158.
30. Geddes LA. *Electrodes and the measurement of bioelectric events.* New York: John Wiley & Sons, 1972.
31. Copland JG, Davies CT. A simple clinical skin electrode. *Lancet* 1964; 1:416.
32. McLean L Scott RN, Parker PA. Stimulus artifact reduction in evoked potential measurements. *Arch Phys Med Rehabil* 1996; 77: 1286–1292.
33. Karam DB. AIDS and the electromyographer. *Arch Phys Med Rehabil* 1986; 67:491.
34. Picton T, Hillyard S. Human auditory evoked potentials: II. effects of ttention. *Electroencephalogr Clin Neurophysiol* 1974; 36:191–199.
35. Jewett DL, Williston JS. Auditory evoked far-fields averaged from the scalp in humans. *Brain* 1971; 94:681–696.
36. Kemp DT. Stimulated acoustic emissions from within the human auditory system. *J Acoust Soc Am* 1978; 64:1386–1391.
37. Ravazzani P, Grandori F. Evoked otoacoustic emissions: nonlinearities and response interpertation. *IEEE Trans Biomed Eng* 1993; 40(5): 500–504.
38. Hall JW, Chase P. Answers to 10 common clinical questions about otoacoustic emissions today. *Hearing J* 1993; 46(10):29–32.
39. White KR, Vohr BR, Behrens TR. Universal newborn hearing screening using transient evoked otoacoustic emissions: Results of the Rhode Island Hearing Assessment Project. *Semin Hearing* 1993; 14:18–29.
40. Norton SJ. Application of transient evoked otoacoustic emissions to pediatric populations. *Ear Hearing* 1993; 14(1):64–73.
41. National Institute of Health Consensus Development Conference: *Early identification of hearing impairment in infants and young children.* Washington, DC: Author, 1993.
42. Aminoff MJ, Davis SL, Panitch HS. Serial evoked potential studies in patients with definite multiple sclerosis. *Arch Neurol* 1984; 41: 1197–1202.
43. Walsh JC, Garrick R, Cameron J, McLeod JG. Evoked potential changes in clinically definite multiple sclerosis: a two year follow-up study. *J Neurol Neurosurg Psychiatry* 1982; 45:494–500.
44. Rowe MJ. Normal variability of the brainstem auditory evoked response in young and old adult subjects. *Electroencephalogr Clin Neurophysiol* 1982; 53:73–77.
45. Picton TW. Abnormal brainstem auditory evoked potentials: a tentative classification. In: Cracco RQ, Bodis-Wollner I, eds. *Evoked potentials.* New York: Alan R. Liss, 1986; 373–378.
46. Howard JE, Dorfman LJ. Evoked potentials in hysteria and malingering. *J Clin Neurophysiol* 1986; 3:39–49.
47. Aminoff MJ. *The clinical role of somatosensory evoked studies: a critical appraisal. AAEM minimonograph 21.* Rochester, MN: American Association of Electrodiagnostic Medicine, 1984.
48. Kimura J, Kimura A, Machida M, Yamada T, Mitsudome A. A model for far-field recordings of SEP. In: Cracco RQ, Bodis-Wollner I, eds. *Evoked potentials.* New York: Alan R. Liss, 1986; 246–261.
49. Veale JL, Mark RF, Refs S. Differential sensitivity of motor and sensory fibers in human ulnar nerve. *J Neurol Neurosurg Psychiatry* 1973; 36:75–86.
50. Goldberg G, Schmier N. Alternating lateralized stimulation technique for recording somatosensory evoked potentials. *Muscle Nerve* 1986; 9:663.
51. Yamada T, Dickins QS, Machida M, Oishi M, Kimura J. Somatosensory evoked potentials to simultaneous median nerve stimulation in man: method and clinical application. In: Cracco RQ, Bodis-Wollner I, eds. *Evoked potentials.* New York: Alan R. Liss, 1986; 45–47.
52. Po HL, Mei SN. Meralgia paresthetica: the diagnostic value of somatosensory evoked potentials. *Arch Phys Med Rehabil* 1992; 73:70–72.
53. Desmedt JE, Oheron G. Prevertebral (esophageal) recording of subcortical somatosensory evoked potentials in man: the spinal P13 component and the dual nature of the spinal generators. *Electroencephalogr Clin Neurophysiol* 1981; 52:257–275.
54. Goldie WD, Chiappa KH, Young RR, Brooks EB. Brainstem auditory and short-latency somatosensory evoked responses in brain death. *Neurology* 1981; 31:248–256.
55. Mauguiere F, Desmedt JE, Courjon J. Neural generators of N18 and P14 far-field somatosensory evoked potentials studied in patients with lesions of thalamus or thalamo-cortical radiations. *Electroencephalogr Clin Neurophysiol* 1983; 56:283–292.
56. Allison T. Scalp and cortical recordings of initial somatosensory cortex activity to median nerve stimulation in man. *Ann NY Acad Sci* 1982; 388:671–678.
57. Allison T, Goff WR, Williamson PD, Van Gilder JC. On the neural origin of early components of the human somatosensory evoked potential. *Prog Clin Neurophysiol* 1980; 7:51–68.
58. Lueders H, Andrich J, Gurd A, Weiker G, Klem G. Origin of far-field subcortical potentials evoked by stimulation of the posterior tibial nerve. *Electroencephalogr Clin Neurophysiol* 1981; 52:336–344.
59. Wood CC, Cohen D, Cuffin BN, Yarita M, Allison T. Electrical sources in human somatosensory cortex: identification by combined magnetic and potential recordings. *Science* 1985; 227:1051–1053.
60. Desmedt JE. Generator sources of SEP in man. In: Cracco RQ, Bodis-Wollner I, eds. *Evoked potentials.* New York: Alan R. Liss, 1986; 246–261.
61. Desmedt JE, Bourguet M. Color imaging of parietal and frontal somatosensory potential fields evoked by stimulation of median or posterior tibial nerve in man. *Electroencephalogr Clin Neurophysiol* 1985; 62:1–17.
62. Nauguiere F, Desmedt JE, Courjon J. Astereognosis and dissociated loss of frontal or parietal components of somatosensory evoked potentials in hemispheric lesions. *Brain* 1983; 106:271–311.
63. Papakostopoulos D, Crow HJ. Direct recording of the somatosensory evoked potentials from the cerebral cortex of man and the difference between precentral and postcentral potentials. *Clin Neurophysiol* 1980; 7:15–26.
64. Slimp JC, Tamas LB, Stolov WC, Wyler AR. Somatosensory evoked potentials after removal of somatosensory cortex in man. *Electroencephalogr Clin Neurophysiol* 1986; 65:111–117.
65. Burke D, Skuse NF, Lethlean AK. Cutaneous and muscle afferent components of the cerebral potential evoked by electrical stimulation of human peripheral nerve. *Electroencephalogr Clin Neurophysiol* 1981; 51:579–588.
66. Simpson RK, Blackburn JG, Martin HF, Katz S. Peripheral nerve fiber and spinal cord pathway contributions to the somatosensory evoked potential. *Exp Neurol* 1981; 73:700–715.
67. Giblin DR. Somatosensory evoked potentials in healthy subjects and in patients with lesions of the nervous system. *Ann NY Acad Sci* 1964; 112:93–142.
68. Halliday AM, Wakefield GS. Cerebral evoked potentials in patients with dissociated sensory loss. *J Neurol Neurosurg Psychiatry* 1961; 26:211–219.
69. Namerow NS. Somatosensory evoked responses following cervical cordotomy. *Bull LA Neurol Soc* 1969; 34:184–188.
70. Cusick JF, Myklebust JB, Larson EJ, Sances A. Spinal cord evaluation by cortical evoked responses. *Arch Neurol* 1979; 39:140–143.
71. Haldeman S. Pudendal nerve evoked spinal, cortical, and bulbo-cavernosus reflex responses: methods and application. In: Cracco RQ, Bodis-Wollner I, eds. *Evoked potentials.* New York: Alan R. Liss, 1986; 68–75.
72. Haldeman S, Bradley WB, Bhatia NN, Johnson BK. Cortical evoked potentials on stimulation of pudendal nerve in women. *Urology* 1983; 21:590–593.
73. Cole JL, Gottesman L. Anal electrophysiology and pudendal nerve evoked potentials. In: Smith, LE, ed. *Practical guide to anorectal testing*, 2nd ed. New York: Igaku-Shoin, 1995; 207–220.
74. Bennett MH, Jannetta PJ. Evoked potentials in trigeminal neuralgia. *Neurosurgery* 1983; 13:242–247.
75. Aminoff MJ, Goodin DS, Parry GJ, Barbaro NM, Weinstein PR, Rosenblum ML. Electrophysiologic evaluation of lumbosacral radiculopathies: electromyography, late responses and somatosensory evoked potentials. *Neurology* 1985; 35:1514–1518.
76. Katifi HA, Sedgwick EM. Somatosensory evoked potentials from posterior tibial nerve and lumbosacral dermatomes. *Electroencephalogr Clin Neurophysiol* 1986; 65:249–259.
77. Slimp JC, Rubner DE, Snowden ML, Stolov WC. Dermatomal somatosensory evoked potentials: cervical, thoracic, and lumbosacral levels. *Electroencephalogr Clin Neurophysiol* 1992; 84:55–70.
78. Chiappa KH. *Evoked potentials in clinical medicine.* New York: Raven Press, 1983.

79. Nodar RH, Barber C, eds. *Evoked potentials II.* Boston: Butterworth, 1984.
80. Spehlmann R. *Evoked potential primer.* Boston: Butterworth, 1985.
81. Ertekin C, Akyurekli D, Burses RN, Turgut H. The value of somatosensory evoked potentials and bulbocavernosus reflex on patients with impotence. *Acta Neurol Scand* 1985; 71:48–53.
82. Haldeman S, Bradley WB, Bhatia N. Evoked responses from the pudendal nerve. *J Urol* 1982; 128:974–980.
83. Haldeman S, Bradley WB, Bhatia NN, Johnson BK. Pudendal evoked responses. *Arch Neurol* 1982; 39:280–223.
84. Neima D, Regan D. Pattern visual evoked potentials and spatial vision in retrobulbar neuritis and multiple sclerosis. *Arch Neurol* 1984; 41: 198–201.
85. Halliday AM, Barret G, Carroll WM, Kris A. Problems in defining the normal limits of the visual evoked potentials. In: Courjon J, Mauguiere F, Revol M, eds. *Clinical applications of evoked potentials in neurology.* New York: Raven Press, 1982; 1–9.
86. Erwin CW. Pattern reversal evoked potentials. *Am J Electroencephalogr Technol* 1981; 20:161–184.
87. Sokol S, Moskowitz A, Toule VL. Age related changes in the latency of the visual evoked potential: influence of check size. *Electroencephalogr Clin Neurophysiol* 1981; 51:559.
88. Wilson WB. Visual-evoked response differentiation of ischemic optic neuritis from optic neuritis of multiple sclerosis. *Am J Ophthalmol* 1978; 86:530–535.
89. Syndulko K, Hansch EC, Cohen SN, et al. Long-latency event related potentials in normal aging and dementia. In: Courjon J, Maugiere F, Revol M, eds. *Clinical applications of evoked potentials in neurology.* New York: Raven Press, 1982; 279–285.
90. Goodin D, Squires K, Henderson B, Starr A. Age-related variation in evoked potentials to auditory stimuli in normal human subjects. *Electroencephalogr Clin Neurophysiol* 1978; 44:447–458.
91. Brown WS, Marsh J, LaRue A. Event-related potentials in psychiatry: differentiating depression and dementia in the elderly. *Bull LA Neurol Soc* 1982; 47:91–107.
92. Polich J, Ehler CL, Otis S, Mandell AJ, Bloom FE. P300 latency reflects the degree of cognitive decline in dementing illness. *Electroencephalogr Clin Neurophysiol* 1986; 63:133–148.
93. Squires KC, Donchin E, Herning RI, McCarthy G. On the influence of task relevance and stimulus probability components. *Electroencephalogr Clin Neurophysiol* 1977; 42:1–14.
94. Polich J. Attention, probability and task demands as determinants of P300 latency from auditory stimuli. *Electroencephalogr Clin Neurophysiol* 1986; 63:251–259.
95. Squires N, Ollo C. Human evoked potential techniques: possible applications to neuropsychology. In: Hannay J, ed. *Experimental techniques in human neuropsychology.* Oxford: Oxford University Press, 1985.
96. Merton PA, Morton HB, Hill DK, Marsden CD. Scope of a technique for electrical stimulation of human brain, spinal cord and muscle. *Lancet* 1982; 2:597–600.
97. Rossini PN, DiStefano E, Stanzione P. Nerve impulse propagation along central and peripheral fast conducting motor and sensory pathways in man. *Electroencephalogr Clin Neurophysiol* 1985; 60: 320–334.
98. Barker AT, Jalinous R, Freeston IL. Non-invasive magnetic stimulation of the human motor cortex. *Lancet* 1985; 1:1106–1107.
99. Deecke L, Grozinger B, Kornhuher HH. Voluntary finger movements in man: cerebral potentials and theory. *Biol Cybern* 1976; 23:99–119.
100. Deecke L, Boschert J, Weinberg H, Brickett P. Magnetic fields of the human brain (Bereitschaftsmagnetfeld) preceding voluntary foot and toe movements. *Exp Brain Res* 1983; 52:81–86.
101. Tamas LB, Shibasaki H. Cortical potentials associated with movement: a review. *J Clin Neurophysiol* 1985; 2:157–171.
102. Liberson WT. Study of evoked potentials in aphasics. *Am J Phys Med* 1966; 45:135–142.
103. Ignacio DR, Lightfoote WE, Pavot AP. Somatosensory cerebral evoked potentials, electroencephalogram and C.T. scan in acute stroke. *Arch Phys Med Rehabil* 1982; 63:536.
104. Pavot AP, Ignacio DR, Lightfoote W. Diagnostic and prognostic value of somatosensory evoked potentials in cerebrovascular accidents. *Electroencephalogr Clin Neurophysiol* 1983; 56:149.
105. Pavot AP, Ignacio DR, Lightfoote W. Correlation of somatosensory evoked potentials study with the site of lesion in acute cerebrovascular accident. *Arch Phys Med Rehabil* 1984; 65:628.
106. Yamada T, Graff-Radford N, Kimura J, Stokes-Dickens Q, Adams HP. Topographic analysis of somatosensory evoked potentials in patients with well-localized thalamic infarctions. *J Neurol Sci* 1985; 68: 31–46.
107. Ignacio DR, Pavot AP, Kuntavanish A. Somatosensory evoked potentials: their prognostic value in the management of stroke. *Arch Phys Med Rehabil* 1982; 63:537.
108. La Joie WJ, Reddy NM, Melvin JL. Somatosensory evoked potentials: their predictive value in right hemiplegia. *Arch Phys Med Rehabil* 1982; 63:223–226.
109. Pavot AP, Ignacio DR, Kuntavanish A, Lightfoote W. The prognostic value of somatosensory evoked potentials in cerebrovascular accidents. *Electromyogr Clin Neurophysiol* 1986; 26:333–340.
110. Pavot AP, Kuntavanish A, Ignacio D. Somatosensory evoked potentials as a predictor of long-term functional outcome in stroke. *Arch Phys Med Rehabil* 1986; 67:617.
111. Vredeveld JW. Predictive somatosensory evoked potentials. *Electroencephalogr Clin Neurophysiol* 1983; 52:340.
112. Haimovic IC, Pedley TA. Hemifield pattern reversal visual evoked potentials: II. lesions of the chiasm and posterior visual pathways. *Electroencephalogr Clin Neurophysiol* 1982; 54:121–131.
113. Ignacio DR, Lightfoote WE, Pavot AP. Visual evoked potentials in acute cerebrovascular disorders. *Arch Phys Med Rehabil* 1984; 65: 667.
114. Misra UK. Kalita J. Motor evoked potential changes in ischaemic stroke depend on stroke location. *J Neurol Sci* 1995; 134(1–2):67–72.
115. Despland PA, Regli F. Clinical usefulness of early somatosensory evoked potentials in 50 patients with unilateral cerebral vascular lesions. In: *Proceedings of the third European conference of electroencephalography and clinical neurophysiology, Basel, Switzerland.* Amsterdam: Elsevier, 1983; 12–14.
116. Nuomoto M, Flanagan ME, Wallman LJ, Donaghy RMP. Prognostic significance of sensory evoked potential and H-reflex in spinal cord injury. In: *Proceedings of the 18th Spinal Cord Injury Conference of the VA.* Washington, DC: Department of Veterans Affairs, 1971; 227–230.
117. Campbell JB, DeCrescito V, Tomasula JJ, Demopoulas HG, Flamm ES, Ransohoff J. Experimental treatment of spinal cord contusion in the cat. *Surg Neurol* 1973; 1:102–106.
118. D'Angelo CM, Van Gilder JC, Taub A. Evoked cortical potentials in experimental spinal cord trauma. *J Neurosurg* 1973; 38:332–336.
119. Schramm J, Hasizume K, Fukushima T, Takahashi H. Experimental spinal cord injury produced by slow, graded compression. *J Neurosurg* 1979; 50:48–57.
120. Croft TJ, Brodsky JS, Nulson FE. Reversible spinal cord trauma: a model for electrical monitoring of spinal cord function. *J Neurosurg* 1972; 36:402–406.
121. Perot PL, Vera CL. Scalp-recorded somatosensory evoked potentials to stimulation of nerves in the lower extremities and evaluation of patients with spinal cord trauma. *Ann NY Acad Sci* 1982; 388: 359–368.
122. Rowed DW. Value of somatosensory evoked potentials for prognosis in partial cord injuries. In: Tator CH, ed. *Early management of acute spinal cord injury.* New York: Raven Press, 1982; 167–180.
123. Simpson RK, Blackburn JG, Martin HF, Katz S. The effects of spinal cord injury on somatosensory evoked potentials produced by interactions between afferent pathways. *Neurol Res* 1983; 5:39–56.
124. Spielholz NI, Benjamin MV, Engler GL, Ransohoff J. Somatosensory evoked potentials and clinical outcome in spinal cord injury. In: Popp AJ, ed. *Neurologic trauma.* New York: Raven Press, 1979; 217–229.
125. Perot PL. The clinical use of somatosensory evoked potentials in spinal cord injury. *Clin Neurosurg* 1973; 20:367–381.
126. MacEwen GD, Bunnel WP, Sriran K. Acute neurological complications in the treatment of scoliosis: a report of the Scoliosis Research Society. *J Bone Joint Surg [Am]* 1975; 57:404–408.
127. Tamaki T, Noguchi T, Tokano H, et al. Spinal cord monitoring as a clinical utilization of the spinal evoked potential. *Clin Orthop* 1984; 184:58–64.
128. Shimoji K, Higashi H, Kano T. Epidural recording of spinal electrogram in man. *Electroencephalogr Clin Neurophysiol* 1971; 30: 236–239.
129. Cole JL, Ducommun EJ. Electrospinograms: evolution and applica-

tion as a clinical tool. *Bull Am Soc Clin Evoked Potentials* 1987; 5: 21–26.

130. Maccabbee PJ, Levine DB, Pinkhasov EI, Cracco RQ, Tsairas P. Evoked potentials recorded from scalp and spinous processes during spinal column surgery. *Electroencephalogr Clin Neurophysiol* 1983; 56:569–582.
131. Engler GL, Spielholz NI, Bernhard WN, Danziger F, Merkin H, Wolff T. Somatosensory evoked potentials during Harrington instrumentation for scoliosis. *J Bone Joint Surg [Am]* 1978; 60:528–532.
132. Peterson DO, Drummond JC, Todd MM. Effects of halothane, enflurane, isoflurane, and nitrous oxide on somatosensory evoked potentials in humans. *Anesthesiology* 1986; 65(1):35–40.
133. Parthak KS, Brown RH, Cascorbi HF, Nash CL. Effects of fentanyl and morphine on intraoperative somatosensory cortical evoked potentials. *Anesth Analg* 1984; 63:833–837.
134. Spielholz NI, Engler GL, Merkin H. Spinal cord monitoring during Harrington instrumentation. *Bull Am Soc Clin Evoked Potentials* 1986; 4:12–16.
135. Grundy BL, Nash CL, Brown RH. Deliberate hypotension for spinal fusion: prospective randomized study with evoked potential monitoring. *Can Anaesth Soc J* 1982; 29:452–462.
136. Cunningham JN, Laschinger JC, Merkin JH, et al. Measurement of spinal cord ischemia during operations upon the thoracic aorta: initial clinical experience. *Ann Surg* 1982; 196:285–296.
137. Laschinger JC, Cunningham JN, Nathan IM, Knopp EA, Cooper MM, Spencer FC. Experimental and clinical assessment of the adequacy of partial bypass in maintenance of spinal cord blood flow during operations on the thoracic aorta. *Ann Thorac Surg* 1983; 36:417–426.
138. Schwartz ML, Panetta TF, Kaplan BJ, Legatt AD, Suggs WD, Wengerter KR, Marin ML, Veith FJ. Somatosensory evoked potential monitoring during carotid surgery. *Cardiovasc Surg* 1996; 4(1):77–80.
139. Cant BR, Hume AL, Shaw NA. Effects of luminance on the pattern visual evoked potential in multiple sclerosis. *Electroencephalogr Clin Neurophysiol* 1978; 45:496–504.
140. Moorthy SS, Narkand ON, Dilley RS, McCammon RL, Warren CH. Somatosensory evoked responses during carotid endarterectomy. *Anesth Analg* 1982; 61:879–883.
141. Russ W, Fraedich G, Hehrlein FW, Hampelmann G. Intraoperative somatosensory evoked potentials as a prognostic factor of neurologic state after carotid endarterectomy. *Thorac Cardiovasc Surg* 1985; 33: 392–396.
142. Schwartz ML, PanettaTF, Kkaplan BJ, Legatt AD, Suggs WD, Wengerter KR, Marin ML, Veith FJ. Somatosensory evoked potential monitoring during carotid surgery. *Cardiovasc Surg* 1996; 4(1):77–80.
143. Branston NM, Symon L, Crockard HA, Pasztor E. Relationship between the cortical evoked potential and local cortical blood flow following acute middle cerebral artery occlusion in the baboon. *Exp Neurol* 1974; 45:195–208.
144. Hagardine JR, Branston NH, Symon L. Central conduction time in primate brain ischemia: a study in baboons. *Stroke* 1980; 11:637–642.
145. Halliday AM, McDonald WI, Mushin J. Visual evoked responses in the diagnosis of multiple sclerosis. *Br Med J* 1973; 4:661–664.
146. Shahrokhi F, Chiappa KH, Young RR. Pattern shift visual evoked responses: two hundred patients with optic neuritis and/or multiple sclerosis. *Arch Neurol* 1978; 35:65–71.
147. Brooks EB, Chiappa KH. A comparison of clinical neuroophthalmological findings and pattern shift visual evoked potentials in multiple sclerosis. In: Courjon JJ, ed. *Neurology*. New York: Raven Press, 1982; 435–437.
148. Phillips KR, Potvin AR, Syndulko K, Cohen SN, Tourtellotte WW, Potvin JH. Multimodality evoked potentials and neurophysiological tests in multiple sclerosis: effect of hyperthermia on test results. *Arch Neurol* 1983; 40:159–164.
149. Chiappa KH. Pattern shift visual, somatosensory evoked potentials in multiple sclerosis. *Neurology* 1980; 30:110–123.
150. Eisen A, Odusote K. Central and peripheral conduction times in multiple sclerosis. *Electroencephalogr Clin Neurophysiol* 1980; 48: 253–265.
151. Matthews WB, Small DG. Serial recording of visual and somatosensory evoked potentials in multiple sclerosis. *J Neurol Sci* 1979; 40: 11–21.
152. Mills KR, Murray NMF. Corticospinal tract conduction time in multiple sclerosis. *Ann Neurol* 1985; 18:601–605.
153. Pavot AP, Lightfoote WF, Wener L, Ignacio D. The use of magnetic resonance imaging in the diagnosis of multiple sclerosis. *Arch Phys Med Rehabil* 1986; 67:679.
154. Giesser BS, Kurtzbereg D, Vaughan HG, et al. Trimodal evoked potentials compared with magnetic resonance imaging in the diagnosis of multiple sclerosis. *Arch Neurol* 1987; 44:281–284.
155. Greenberg RP, Becker DP, Miller JD, Mayer DJ. Evaluation of brain function in severe human head trauma with multimodality evoked potentials: Part 2. localization of brain dysfunction and correlation with posttraumatic neurological condition. *J Neurosurg* 1977; 47: 163–167.
156. Newlon PG, Greenberg RR. Assessment of brain function with multimodality evoked potentials. In: Rosenthal M, ed. *Rehabilitation of the head injured adult*. Philadelphia: FA Davis, 1983; 75–96.
157. Rappaport M, Leonard J, Ruiz Portillo S. Somatosensory evoked potential peak latencies and amplitudes in contralateral and ipsilateral hemispheres in normal and severely traumatized brain-injured subjects. *Brain Injury* 1993; 7(1):3–13.
158. Werner RA, Vanderzant CW. Multimodality evoked potential testing in acute mild closed head injury. *Arch Phys Med Rehabil* 1991; 72: 31–34.
159. Johnston MV, Hall KM. Outcomes evaluation in TBI rehabilitation. Part I: Overview and system principles. *Arch Phys Med Rehabil* 1994; 75(12 Spec No.):SC1–SC9, discussion SC27–SC28.
160. Nativ A, Lazarus JA, Nativ J, Joseph J. Potentials associated with the go/no-go paradigm in traumatic brain injury. *Arch Phys Med Rehabil* 1994; 75(12):1322–1326.
161. Boake C. Supervision rating scale: a measure of functional outcome from brain injury. *Arch Phys Med Rehabil* 1996; 77(8):765–772.
162. Rappaport M. Brain evoked potentials in coma and the vegetative state. *J Head Trauma Rehabil* 1986; 1:15–29.
163. Rappaport M, Hopkins HK, Hall K, Bellexa T. Evoked potentials and head injury: 2. Clinical applications. *Clin Electroencephalogr* 1981; 12:167–176.
164. Rappaport M, Dougherty AM, Kelting DL. Evaluation of coma and vegetative states. *Arch Phys Med Rehabil* 1992; 73(7):628–634.
165. Machado C, Valdes P, Garcia-Tigera J, Virues T, Biscay R, Miranda J, Contin P, Roman J, Garcia O. Brain-stem auditory evoked potentials and brain death. *Electroencephalogr Clin Neurophysiol* 1991; 80(5): 392–398.
166. Jenkins WM, Merzenick NM. Reorganization of neocortical representations after brain injury: a neurophysiological model of the bases of recovery from stroke. *Prog Brain Res* 1987; 71:249–266.

Rehabilitation Medicine: Principles and Practice, Third Edition,
edited by Joel A. DeLisa and Bruce M. Gans.
Lippincott–Raven Publishers, Philadelphia © 1998.

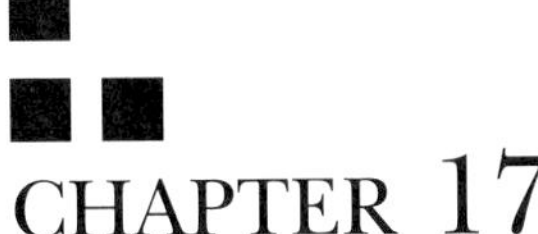

CHAPTER 17

Research in Physical Medicine and Rehabilitation

Barbara J. de Lateur and Kent Questad

GENERAL CONSIDERATIONS

Asking the Research Question

The importance of asking the research question cannot be overstated. Whether or not explicitly stated, obtaining the answer to the research question must be the primary objective of any study. It has occasionally happened that a large data base has been collected without a clear statement (in advance of the data collection) of the question(s) to be answered. This runs the risk of needless expenditure of time and other resources for collection of data not used, while simultaneously failing to collect data essential to answering the questions that were subsequently asked.

Deciding upon the Appropriate Type of Study

One might be interested in characterizing the biomechanical and functional consequences of osteoarthritis (OA) of the knee and comparing the characteristics with those of OA of the hip. This is a descriptive study—a highly technical and detailed study to be sure—but a descriptive study nevertheless. Whether or not a funding agency, governmental or private philanthropic, will consider such research a priority for funding will depend on a number of factors (some of them political). Two major factors are the importance of the condition (seriousness and prevalence) and the state of knowledge concerning the topic. The study group reviewing the proposal might think that OA of the hip and knee have already been sufficiently characterized and that the money might be better spent on evaluating a novel intervention. In that case, the randomized, controlled, double-blind trial will be the "gold standard" of intervention. In contrast to a descriptive study, the research intervenes in the process, to determine if the course of the disease and/or its consequences can be altered.

B. J. de Lateur: Department of Physical Medicine and Rehabilitation, The Johns Hopkins University School of Medicine, Baltimore, Maryland 21239.
K. Questad: Department of Rehabilitation Medicine, University of Washington, Seattle, Washington 98195.

Selecting Dependent Variables or Outcome Measures

The measures selected must have reliability and validity. The reliability is equivalent to reproducibility, that is, how closely a repeated test will approximate the value of the first test if nothing has changed. For example, a hematocrit taken 5 minutes after a first hematocrit would be almost identical to the first, if the patient is not actively bleeding; thus, a hematocrit is considered to be a highly reliable test. A hematocrit would also be considered a valid measure of the red cell mass in the body; it would not be considered a valid measure of acute infection or even of chronic infection, even though chronic infection may contribute to anemia, as reflected in a lowered hematocrit. The linkage is too loose. Another way of defining validity would be the extent to which the test faithfully represents or reflects the variable being measured. One of the most famous controversies is the extent to which intelligent quotient (IQ) tests measure intelligence (or, are all IQ tests hopelessly culturally biased and reflective of educational achievement rather than true "native" intelligence?). Many would say that these tests are not valid, even while conceding that the tests are reliable.

Statistical Significance versus Practical Significance

Large data bases and powerful computing techniques currently available allow detection of statistical relationships that may not be meaningful or practical. A statistical relationship has been found between the number of bathtubs per capita and coronary artery disease. The idea of causal relationship between the two is preposterous. This is an epiphenomenon and no doubt reflects the fact that, in general, those who have more bathtubs have better socioeconomic conditions, with greater and more regular access to calories and fat. Another study might show that purchase and use of a very expensive set of machines costing $30,000 to build would save only $5.00 per car. If the variability were low and the statistical power to detect differences were high, one could easily establish that this difference was statistically significant, but there would probably not be a practical difference (benefit) because the company would have to sell far more cars that it could ever expect to do in order to recover the costs.

CASE STUDIES

The late B.F. Skinner noted that very few, if any, great scientific discoveries were initially the result of well-controlled, multiple group experiments and statistical analysis. His point was that most truths worth knowing are obvious if the right data are gathered systematically. Data from one subject, if they are gathered so that it is possible to replicate the experiment, can be as useful as data from thousands.

Most contemporary studies of medical treatments have a provision for discontinuing random assignment if one treatment is obviously superior to the others. This is done out of the concern for subjects who would be denied a more effective treatment needlessly. Thus, there is an ethical imperative that researchers have some means of evaluating the results of data from small numbers of subjects.

Finally, there are other pragmatic reasons for conducting case-controlled studies. It is often difficult to plan a clinical study without some initial or pilot experience. Single subject research designs provide methods for gathering pilot data. In addition, the best planned studies can fall victim to unforeseen changes. Data can be gathered to permit single subject analysis that can be folded into a repeated-measures, group experimental design. The following is an example of how this can be accomplished.

Brooke and colleagues (1) reported the results of a descriptive study of incidence and prevalence of agitated behavior after traumatic brain injury. The next phase of the project was to test treatments for agitation.

Their initial data from the descriptive study suggested that it might be difficult to enroll enough subjects for a between-groups experimental design. Although the incidence of the behavior they labeled as restlessness (general restless movement) was high, the incidence of agitation (focused aggressive behavior) was low, approximately 10%. It was also of short duration; most subjects who were agitated, were agitated for 1 week or less.

In addition, for the primary drug to be studied, propranolol, the best method of setting the dose was to increase it slowly until the patient's behavior changed, the maximum dose was reached, or undesirable side effects occurred. Thus, the study design must include a treatment period of up to 3 weeks to reach the optimum dose.

Although these circumstances presented a number of challenges, they also seemed ideal for a case-controlled approach. Adjusting the dose of propranolol (or placebo) required daily monitoring of subjects' medical status and behavior. If we used a single subject design, we would know quickly if the drug were clearly more effective than the placebo. Finally, even if it proved impossible to enroll enough subjects for a group analysis, we would be sure to have meaningful data regarding the effectiveness of propranolol.

They considered two common single-subject designs. The first was a multiple baseline design. Any case-controlled study requires a means of comparing the individual to himself or herself under different conditions. In a multiple baseline design, two or more attributes of the individual are tracked simultaneously. After a baseline period, a treatment is introduced that, hypothetically, will influence only one of the attributes. Then another treatment is added to influence another attribute and so on until all the tracked variables are under treatment. If the targeted attribute changes after the treatment is introduced and the others do not, then the hypothesis is confirmed.

In this case, they considered using agitation and restlessness in a multiple baseline design. They hypothesized that propranolol would reduce agitation and not restlessness. On the other hand, they expected an antianxiety agent, such as Ativan, to reduce restlessness. The effectiveness of propranolol could be tested by collected daily data on agitation and restless while treating the patient with Ativan and propranolol, for equal periods of time, in a random double-blinded fashion. Although this would have been a valid approach, it was rejected because of practical difficulties of using two drugs.

They chose to use a simple reversal design instead. This design included two equal periods in which the subject was treated with a placebo and active drug in a double-blind reversal. Data from the first few subjects suggested that there was a real, but not dramatic, difference between the two conditions. This disappeared entirely by the reversal phase.

The experience with these subjects helped us to estimate the number of subjects we needed to perform a group analysis with adequate statistical power. They also learned quickly that an effective dose of propranolol was often much greater than that typically used at the time. The final analysis compared subjects in the propranolol (first) group to the subjects in the placebo (first) group in a repeated-measures analysis (2).

In this example the use of a single subject design allowed the investigators to (a) evaluate quickly whether the treatment under study was clearly superior, (b) design a better group study of the treatment, and (c) treat each subject with the best dose of the treatment drug. It illustrates how case-controlled techniques can form a nexus between good clinical practice and valid clinical research.

REASONABLE USE OF STATISTICS

Figure 17-1 shows the temperature distribution in six human thighs at the completion of 20 minutes of exposure to shortwave diathermy applied with the monode applicator with 3 mm of terry cloth inserted between applicator and skin (3). Each series of dots connected by a line represents the temperatures on the skin or at various depths of the thigh of a single subject. Note that there is no overlap of the "before treatment" group of lines and the "after treatment" group. The distance between the groups is greatest at the surface, but even at the greatest depth of the muscle measured, there is no overlap of the temperature curves. One could apply statistical analysis, perhaps a form of the analysis of variance (ANOVA) known as trend analysis, but this is not necessary. The clear separation of the two groups of curves that consist of multiple measures is sufficient to conclude that the diathermy produced a definite temperature increase on and in the tissues. The curves are different because of the multiple measures. If there were only four per line, they could look different by chance. Whether this temperature increase produced, in turn, a therapeutic effect would have to be determined by other data. However, one may obtain some clue to this possibility by further inspection

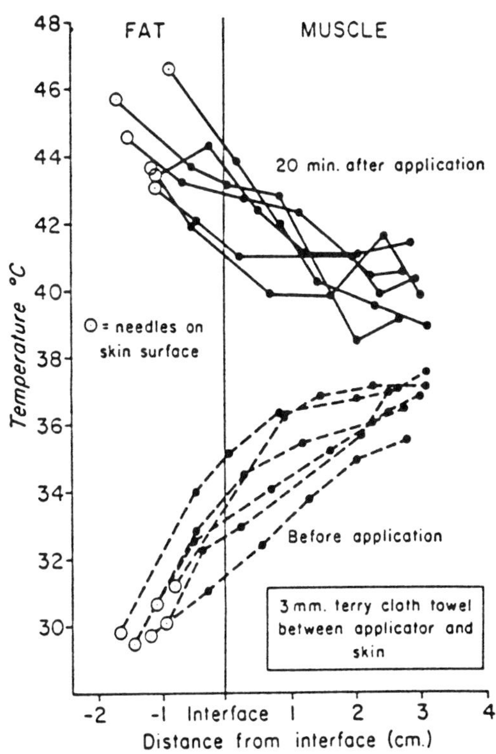

FIG. 17-1. Temperature distribution in the human thigh at the completion of 20 minutes of exposure to short wave (27.12 MHz) applied with the monode with 3 mm of terry cloth inserted between applicator and skin. (Reprinted with permission from Lehmann JF, de Lateur BJ, Stonebridge JB. Selective heating by short wave diathermy with a helical coil. *Arch Phys Med Rehabil* 1969; 50:117–123.)

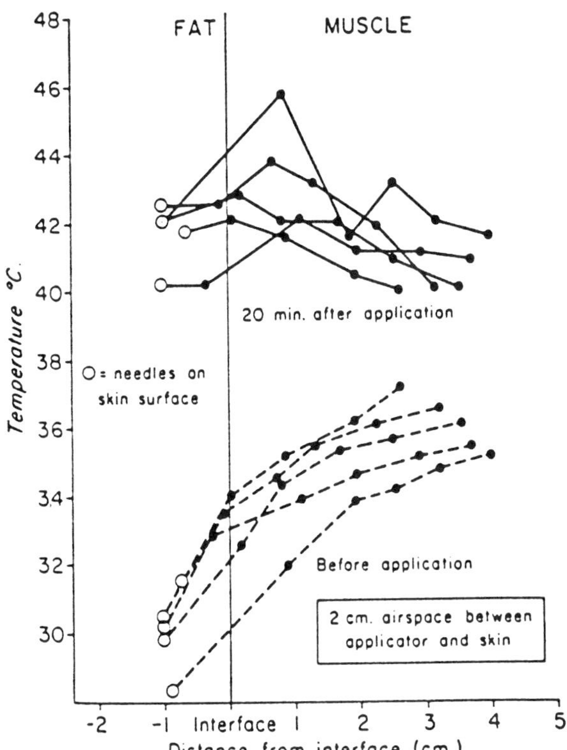

FIG. 17-2. Temperature distribution in the human thigh at the completion of 20 minutes of exposure to short wave (27.12 MHz) applied with the monode with 2 cm of air space between applicator and skin. (Reprinted with permission from Lehmann JF, de Lateur BJ, Stonebridge JB. Selective heating by short wave diathermy with a helical coil. *Arch Phys Med Rehabil* 1969; 50:117–123.)

of the "after" treatment curves and recalling that the therapeutic temperature range is generally considered to be from 40 to 45°C. Note that two of the surface thermisters register temperatures higher than 45°C, whereas the thermisters in the greatest depth of the muscle register temperatures from 39 to 41°C, i.e., just below or in the lower portion of the therapeutic range. Clearly, the vigor of the effect on and in the muscle is limited by the much higher temperatures on the surface (3).

Figure 17-2 shows the same types of measurements made in five different volunteers before and after 20 minutes of shortwave diathermy, also with a monode applicator, but with a different technique of application (3). Rather than 3 mm of terry cloth, 2 cm airspace separates applicator and skin. One can readily see that there is much more uniform heating of the thigh, from skin to muscle. One might wish to apply trend analysis to the "after" group to ascertain that there is not a significant trend from surface to depth, but, here again, visual inspection of the graphically displayed data is sufficient.

In contrast to the ease of detection of the temperature increase produced in the human thigh by the application of shortwave diathermy with a helical coil, consider the diffi-

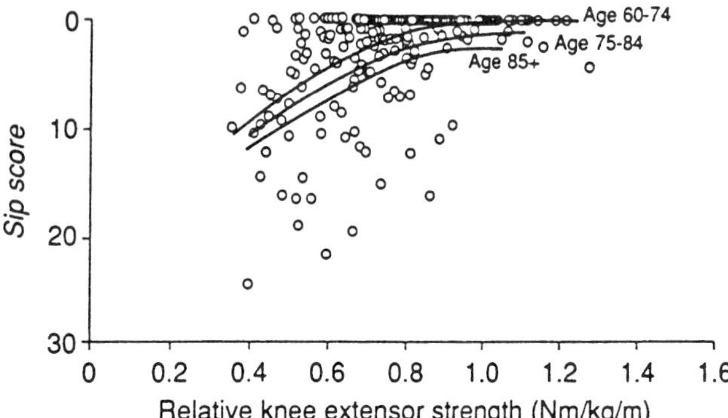

FIG. 17-3. Relative knee extensor strength versus SIP physical dimension score. Data from n = 434 adults ≥60 years of age with only every other point plotted. SIP scale is oriented so that higher scores, which reflect poorer function, are at the bottom. Curves derived from polynomial regression. (Reprinted with permission from Buchner DM, de Lateur BJ. The importance of skeletal muscle strength to physical function in older adults. *Ann Behav Med* 1991; 13:91–98.)

culty researchers have had in their attempts to relate strength to function, or, conversely, to relate weakness to dysfunction or disability. Based on extensive experience, clinicians have long suspected such a relationship, and in the case of frank paralysis, such a relationship is quite apparent. However, among persons without such paralysis, this relationship has not been easy to establish. Perhaps this is because many researchers were looking for a linear relationship between strength and function. Another "dead end" has been the search for a relationship between "absolute" strength as opposed to "relative" strength. Let us begin by defining these terms. Absolute strength is the maximum torque produced by a muscle. Typical units in current use are newton-meters, or, in the older literature, foot-pounds. Absolute strength says nothing about the daily demands placed on the muscle by the weight of the person using that muscle. In contrast, relative strength relates the torque produced to the body weight of the person. For example, the relative strength of the quadriceps might be expressed as maximum or peak torque in newton-meters, divided by the person's weight in kilograms. One can improve the predictive ability slightly by considering the length of the levers, which are proportionate to the height. The final units for relative strength in that case would be torque in newton-meters/weight in kilograms/height in meters. Figure 17-3 shows the relationship between relative strength of the quadriceps and self-reported difficulty performing various usual activities (4). The data were taken from a large population of older persons, members of the Group Health Cooperative of Puget Sound. The instrument used for self-reported impairment was the Sickness Impact Profile (SIP), a well-tested instrument, the reliability and validity of which have been established in a variety of settings. Because higher numbers represent greater self-reported difficulty, the numbers on the ordinate are reversed, i.e., proceed from higher to lower as one ascends the ordinate. If one were to inspect the data points without benefit of mathematical analysis, one would not readily intuit the curves that the authors derived. The "best fit" is not obtained by any single curve, certainly not a single straight line. The mathematical formula shows a curvilinear rather than a linear relationship. The fit can be further improved by drawing three curves, based on age, rather than a single curve, grouping all older persons. These curves show that there is a threshold of relative strength, below which persons are likely to describe themselves as having difficulty with certain ordinary activities, and that threshold is lower with advancing age. Although sophisticated analysis was necessary to establish this relationship, once pointed out, it certainly withstands the scrutiny of common sense. A heavier person may well have more difficulty climbing stairs and getting out of a bathtub, even if somewhat stronger, in absolute terms, than a lighter person (4).

In the process of establishing the reliability and normative values of a physiologic test, statistical methods are of the essence. This is particularly true when the variations in response are subtle. Shehab and Butinar studied the pronator teres reflex, a reflex found useful in evaluating the C6 and C7 roots but also a reflex without normative values and not widely known (5). A standard procedure for eliciting (mechanical/physiologic) and recording (electrophysiologic) the pronator teres reflex was used to study the right and left sides of 25 healthy subjects, 11 female and 14 male (it would have been better to have equal numbers of the sexes, but this approximation is adequate because the norms and confidence intervals [CIs] were reported separately). Figure 17-4 shows the type of reproducible response that was obtained from both right and left sides of all subjects (5). The next important step was to obtain the test-retest reliability. Figure 17-5 is a graphic display of the linear relationship of the latency of the first test with the latency of the retest in the 25 subjects (5). The statistical significance of the linearity was confirmed by using Pearson's correlation coefficient, which yielded a correlation coefficient (r) value of 0.827, with $p < 0.001$. Another way of stating this result, in ordinary parlance, would be to say that the chances are fewer than one in a thousand that the test-retest values are poorly related and that the correlation coefficient of 0.827 occurred purely by chance. The next step was to display the actual values of these latencies. As expected, these values varied from one subject to another, from side to side, and from male to female. One problem is how to describe these values in a way that permits assignment of future subjects, with symptoms suggestive of a C6 radiculopathy, to the "normal" or "abnormal" category. The first descriptive statistic given is a measure of central tendency, usually the arithmetic average or mean. If a future patient's values fall right on the mean, there is no problem assigning this result to the normal study category. However, many values will be longer (or shorter, but our concern here is with the longer latencies) than the mean; how do we decide whether or not these values

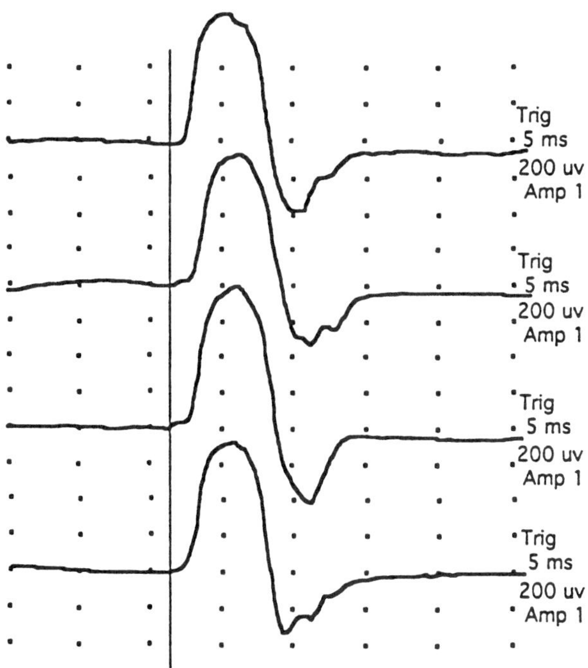

FIG. 17-4. The pronator teres reflex, electromyographic response. A reproducible diphasic response with an initial negative deflection is found in all tested individuals. All recordings were made over the pronator teres muscles.

Basic statistics for the 25 individuals in the study

	Mean	SD	Range	Minimum	Maximum
Female	11 (44%)				
Male	14 (56%)				
Age (yr)	35.8	6.7	26.0	24	50
Arm (cm)	70.7	3.7	18.0	62	80
Right latency (ms)	16.8	1.5	6.4	13.4	19.8
Left latency (ms)	16.9	1.7	6.3	13.4	19.7

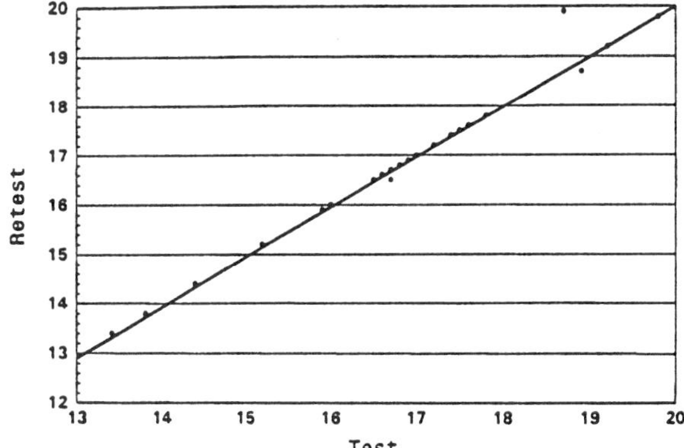

FIG. 17-5. Relationship between the latency of test and retest. Significant relationship is found between the latency of the pronator teres reflex for the test and retest for the 25 individuals (r = 0.827; $p < 0.001$).

are normal? We thus have to look at measures of dispersion. We could simply look at the range of values found in these healthy subjects, and in fact, Shehab and Butinar (5) do give us the range. However, if we had only the range, and decided to call only those subjects who fell outside the range abnormal, we would almost certainly fail to detect some subjects who had early or subtle effects of a C6 radiculopathy. So we need some other measures of dispersion, and Shehab and Butinar (5) give us two very good ones, the standard deviation and the 95% CI, shown in Table 17-1 (Table 2 from the article).

For normally distributed variables (the distribution follows a bell-shaped curve), the mean ± 3 standard deviations (SD) will include more than 99% of the values. Any latency longer than the mean + 3 SD is clearly statistically abnormal. Here again, calling only those values abnormal that are more than 3 SD longer than the mean will likely miss some subtle abnormalities, especially because the normative group was relatively small. (Because the formula for determining the SD has the sample size (n) in the denominator, larger samples will have smaller SDs, other things being equal.) Thus, Shehab and Butinar (5) also give us the 95% CI; if a value falls within that interval, the chances are 95 out of 100 that it is a (statistically) normal value. Finally, one should note that the study took place in a country other than the United States (Kuwait). Can one simply take these values to one's own laboratory and begin using them as norms? Probably not. If one determines normal values for one's own laboratory, these values may turn out precisely the same as those reported in this study, but one cannot assume that, at least not until several workers around the country have made those determinations in their laboratories.

EPIDEMIOLOGIC RESEARCH

Health policy and health-care financing are, or ought to be, solidly based on epidemiologic research, and few would deny that such policy and financing affects the daily practices of each of us and prompt vigilance, not sleep. The following study, reported in the *Journal of American Medical Association*, illustrates the point that one avoids such information at one's own (and the nation's) peril.

Hoffman and colleagues (6) analyzed the 1987 National Medical Expenditure Survey, the 1990 National Health Interview Survey, and *Vital Statistics of the United States* for their report on "Persons with Chronic Conditions: Their Prevalence and Costs." Their approach to the data was conservative; for example, whenever treatment was sought for a condition that could be acute or chronic, such as bronchitis, the condition was considered acute (if there was no way of ascertaining which it actually was). This conservative approach means that if there was a reporting error, it was in

TABLE 17-1. *Mean and 95% confidence interval (CI) of the latency (MS) for right and left in males and females*

	Right		Left	
	Female	Male	Female	Male
Mean	15.9 (±1.3)	17.4 (±1.4)	15.9 (±1.6)	17.9 (±1.2)
95% CI	15.1–16.8	16.6–18.2	14.8–17.0	17.1–18.7

Relationship between arm length and latency. Significant correlation between arm length and latency of pronator teres, tested individuals with 95% CI ($r = 0.497$; $p = 0.012$).

the direction of under-reporting the prevalence and costs of chronic conditions. Figure 17-6 graphically displays one of the more striking findings of the study. Persons with one or more chronic conditions represented 46% of the population, but their care (not counting institutional services) required 76% of the expenditures. As Hoffman et al. (6) noted, this occurs at a time when our health-care system is still firmly rooted in (and oriented toward) acute and episodic care. This study points up the need for health policy and financing changes that truly support continuity of care and health maintenance for persons with chronic conditions rather than attempting to control costs by reducing services and expenditures per acute episode of illness or acute exacerbation of chronic illness (6).

RANDOMIZED CONTROLLED TRIALS

In this type of interventional study, subjects are randomly assigned, with a table of random numbers or other such device, to the various treatment groups or to the treatment versus the control group. Why not match the groups, rather than randomly assigning subjects? Sometimes matched groups of subjects are used, but this approach assumes that the investigator knows (all) the important variables for which

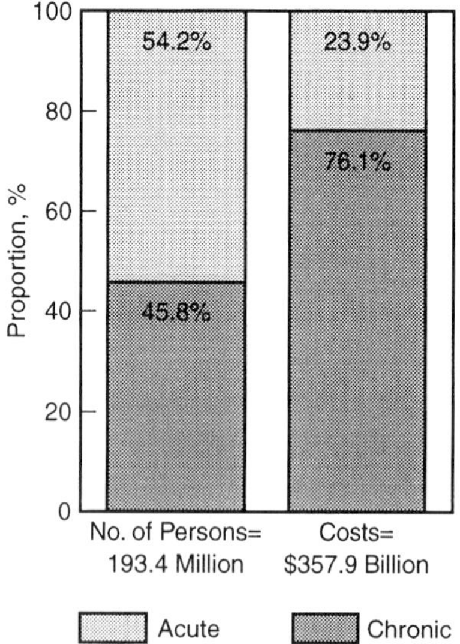

FIG. 17-6. Proportion of persons versus health care expenditures, by conditions, 1987 (total health care expenditures do not include institutional services in this figure). (From Hoffman C, Rice D, Sung H. Persons with chronic conditions, their prevalence and costs. *JAMA* 1996; 276:1477.)

to match the subjects. Failure to match the groups for even one of the important variables could result in a systematic error in either direction, either failing to detect a significant treatment effect that occurred, or claiming a treatment effect when no such effect existed.

Randomization, on the other hand, will likely result in more or less equal numbers of the important variables landing in each of the groups, provided that the study sample is large enough or uniform enough. Even then, checking randomization by testing for statistical differences across key descriptive variables is a good precaution. It is important to conduct a power analysis to be sure that one has enough subjects to detect, with a high degree of probability, a significant effect. The number of subjects needed depends on the size of the treatment effect (realistically) anticipated, the variability of the groups, the power of detection desired (preferably 0.9, i.e., the chances are 9 of 10 that a "real" effect of anticipated size will be found statistically significant), and the value of alpha selected, in advance. It is not appropriate, for example, to select an alpha (p value) of 0.01, and then, after the results are in and fail to reach significance at the 0.01 level, change the alpha to 0.05. When we say that the results are significant at the 0.05 level, we mean that either a rare thing has happened (fewer than five chances in a hundred) or that the treatment effects were "real," i.e., did not occur by chance. Intellectual honesty requires that one decide in advance the p value that one will consider a rare event. Changing it after examining the data is trying to force the data to prove something rather than looking to see what they prove.

The term "controlled" means that, insofar as possible, all things are kept the same between (or among) the groups except for the intervention. One of the early controlled studies in the field of physical medicine was conducted by Lehmann and coworkers (7) in the 1950s. They compared the effects of ultrasonic diathermy with those of microwave diathermy, each combined with massage and standard exercise therapy, on the range of motion of subjects with periarthritis of the shoulder. It was ascertained that the subjects were statistically comparable with respect to age, duration of symptoms, and pretreatment range of motion, as shown in Figures 17-7, 17-8, and 17-9. Results are shown in Table 17-2. Ultrasound treatment resulted in significantly greater increase in range of motion than did microwaves. It should be emphasized that both groups received standard exercise programs. Had neither group received the exercise, it would have been easy to conclude, erroneously, that neither treat-

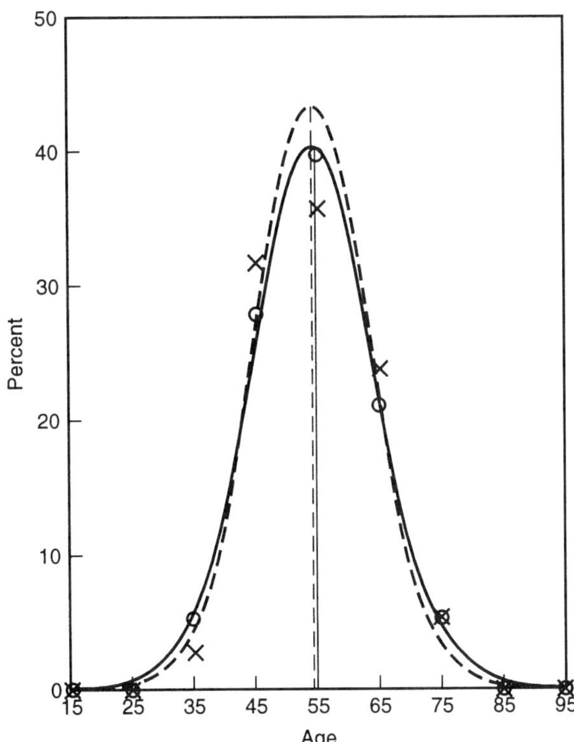

FIG. 17-7. Calculated distribution of age within the group of patients treated with ultrasound *(solid line)* and with microwave *(broken line)*. Data from ultrasound observations indicated by *circles*; data from microwave observations shown by *crosses*. (Reprinted with permission from Lehmann JF, Erikson DJ, Martin GM, Krusen FH. Comparison of ultrasonic and microwave diathermy in the physical treatment of periarthritis of the shoulder. *Arch Phys Med Rehabil* 1954; 35:627–634.)

ment did any good, because neither form of heat can increase range of motion without range of motion exercise (7).

OUTCOMES RESEARCH OR COHORTS/CASE-CONTROLLED STUDIES

There are many situations in rehabilitation, especially comprehensive rehabilitation, as opposed to specific physical medicine interventions, in which a randomized, controlled trial is not feasible, for any of a number of reasons, including societal expectations, ethical considerations, and legal or regulatory constraints. In those situations, outcomes studies are often appropriate and useful, although one must use caution in attempting to ascribe the benefits obtained to any one aspect of the program because it might be the program as a whole yielding the benefit; conversely, one should use caution in claiming that the entire program is necessary to obtain the benefit because a single therapy may be responsible for the specific benefit obtained. Thus, compared with randomized, controlled trials, outcomes studies may be conducted where the former are not feasible; however, the conclusions must be more circumspect.

Goodie and colleagues (8) conducted an outcome study on the change in gait velocity during rehabilitation after stroke. Clearly, there was no ethical possibility of randomization. The first step was to establish the deficit, and this was achieved by comparing the gait velocity of the stroke patients with that of a similar number (44 patients and 42 controls) of age- and sex-matched healthy subjects, because age and sex are known to affect gait velocity. The controls were community dwelling, as were the study subjects, before their strokes. Gait velocity was determined shortly after admission to rehabilitation and again 8 weeks later, regardless of the duration of the inpatient rehabilitation admission. Several analyses of the results were made; Figure 17-10 is very informative and gives the reader great confidence in the results and conclusion. This figure is a frequency distribution of change scores. Of particular interest in the demarcation of the 95% CI for error of measuring change. This shows that 18 of the patients (42.8%) only made changes in gait velocity that were within the limits of accuracy of measuring change. It likewise shows that the 23 (54.8%) who improved beyond the 95% CI made ''real'' improvements, and that only one patient actually deteriorated in gait velocity. Goodie and colleagues pointed out that because the patients only made up about one fourth of the initial velocity deficit, there is no ''ceiling effect'' to this measure, in contrast to certain functional measures, where all patients received a maximum score on ambulation. Finally, one should note the circumspectness of the authors' conclusions: ''Gait velocity discriminated the effect of stroke and the change during rehabilitation'' (8).

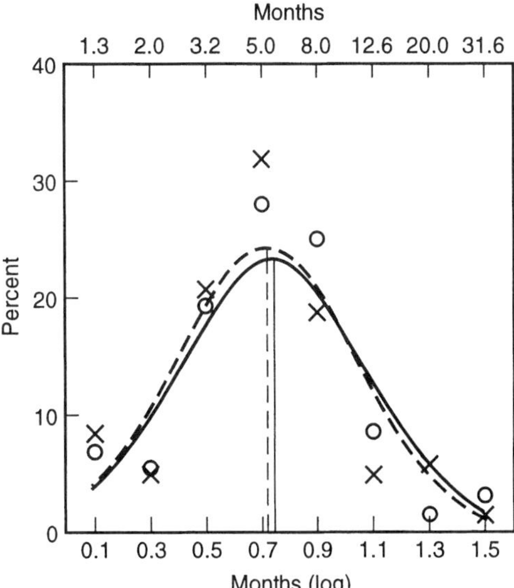

FIG. 17-8. Calculated distribution of the duration of symptoms before first visit in patients treated with ultrasound *(solid line)* and with microwave *(broken line)*. Data observed in ultrasound group indicated by *circles*; data from microwave group indicated by *crosses*. (From Lehmann JF, Erikson DJ, Martin GM, Krusen FH. Comparison of ultrasonic and microwave diathermy in the physical treatment of periarthritis of the shoulder. *Arch Phys Med Rehabil* 1954; 35:627–634.)

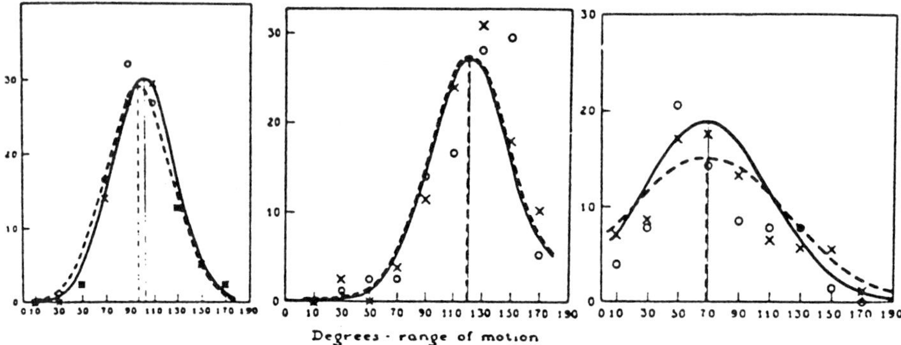

FIG. 17-9. Calculated distribution of range of motion before treatment in group of patients later treated with ultrasound *(solid lines)* and with microwave *(broken lines)*. Data observed after ultrasound indicated by *circles*; after microwave by *crosses*. *Left*, range of abduction; *center*, range of forward flexion; *right*, range of rotation. (Reprinted with permission from Lehmann JF, Erikson DJ, Martin GM, Krusen FH. Comparison of ultrasonic and microwave diathermy in the physical treatment of periarthritis of the shoulder. *Arch Phys Med Rehabil* 1954; 35:627–634.)

TABLE 17-2. *Gain in range of motion after ultrasonic and microwave treatment*

	After treatment with	
	Ultrasound	Microwaves
Forward flexion	27.4° ± 2.3°[a]	16.1° ± 1.5°
Abduction	32.6° ± 2.5°	21.2° ± 2.1°
Rotation	45.4° ± 2.8°	17.3° ± 4.0°

[a] Standard error of the mean.

Reprinted with permission from Lehmann JF, Erickson DJ, Martin GM, Krusen FH: Comparison of ultrasonic and microwave diathermy in the physical treatment of periarthritis of the shoulder. *Arch Phys Med Rehabil* 1954; 36:627–634.

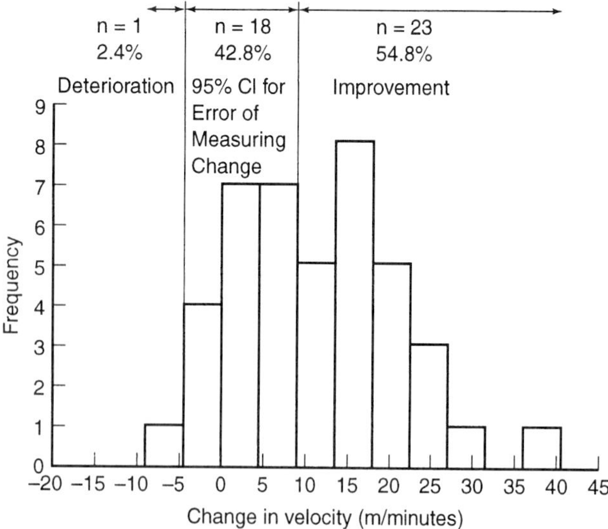

FIG. 17-10. Frequency distribution of change scores for gait velocity with 95% CI for error of measuring change in gait velocity superimposed (−4.54 to 9.3 m/min). (From Goldie PA, Matyas TA, Evans OM. Deficit and change in gait velocity during rehabilitation after stroke. *Arch Phys Med Rehabil* 1996; 77:1078.)

REPORTING OF RESEARCH

The most current guideline for reporting of research results in scientific and biomedical journals is the "Special Report" of the International Committee of Medical Journal Editors: Uniform Requirements for Manuscripts Submitted to Biomedical Journals (9), and the Manuscript Evaluation Guidelines and Glossary of Methodologic Terms (10).

SUMMARY

Research, properly named, is data based. The type of study should be appropriate to the questions asked and to the physical, social, ethical, legal, and financial circumstances. Data analysis may range from simple graphic display to sophisticated statistics but should promote intellectual honesty and clarity of understanding. Research rarely consists just of data, with no further implications; research adds to a body of knowledge, either in terms of describing a previously unknown syndrome, a new treatment approach, verifying or disputing another study or by explaining how an organ or system works.

REFERENCES

1. Brooke M, Questad K, Patterson D, Bashak K. Agitation and restlessness after closed head injury. *Arch Phys Med Rehabil* 1992; 73: 320–323.
2. Brooke M, Questad K, Patterson D, Farrell-Roberts L, Cardenas D. The treatment of agitation during hospitalization after traumatic brain injury. *Arch Phys Med Rehabil* 1992; 73:917–921.
3. Kottke FJ, Lehmann JF, eds. *Krusen's handbook of physical medicine and rehabilitation*, 4th ed. Philadelphia, WB Saunders, 1990 [reprinted from Lehmann JF, de Lateur BJ, Stonebridge JB. Selective heating by short wave diathermy with a helical coil. *Arch Phys Med Rehabil* 1969; 50:117–123].
4. Buchner DM, de Lateur BJ. The importance of skeletal muscle strength to physical function in older adults. *Ann Behav Med* 1991; 13:91–98.
5. Shehab D, Butinar D. Pronator teres reflex: reliability and normal value. *Am J Phys Med Rehabil* 1996; 75:328–331.
6. Hoffman C, Rice D, Sung H. Persons with chronic conditions, their prevalence and costs. *JAMA* 1996; 276:1473–1479.

7. Lehmann JF, Erickson DJ, Martin GM, Krusen FH. Comparison of ultrasonic and microwave diathermy in the physical treatment of periarthritis of the shoulder. *Arch Phys Med Rehabil* 1954; 35:627–634, 1954 [quoted in Lehmann JF, ed. *Therapeutic heat and cold,* 4th ed. Baltimore: Williams & Wilkins, 1990; 550–553].
8. Goldie PA, Matyas TA, Evans OM. Deficit and change in gait velocity during rehabilitation after stroke. *Arch Phys Med Rehabil* 1996; 77: 1074–1082.
9. International Committee of Medical Journal Editors. Special report: uniform requirements for manuscripts submitted to biomedical journals. *N Engl J Med* 1997; 336:309–315.
10. Information for Authors. *Arch Phys Med Rehabil* 1997; 78:i–xiv.

ADDITIONAL READINGS

Finley T, Buchner DM, Davis AM, et al. Physiatric research: a hands-on approach. *Am J Phys Med Rehabit* 1991; 70(Suppl 1):S1–S171.

Moher D, Dulberg CS, Wells GA. Statistical power, sample size, and their reporting in randomized controlled trials. *JAMA* 1994; 272:122–124.

The standards of reporting trial group: a proposal for structured reporting of randomized controlled trials. *JAMA* 1994; 272:1926–1931.

Wen SW, Hernandez R, Naylor CD. Pitfalls in nonrandomized outcomes studies. *JAMA* 1995; 274:1687–1691.

Rehabilitation Medicine: Principles and Practice, Third Edition,
edited by Joel A. DeLisa and Bruce M. Gans.
Lippincott–Raven Publishers, Philadelphia © 1998.

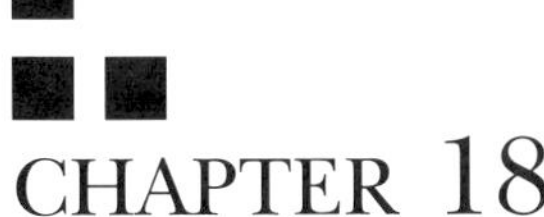

CHAPTER 18

Administration and Management in Physical Medicine and Rehabilitation

F. Patrick Maloney

Physicians' involvement in management is increasing as hospital administrations, practice managers, and health-care organizations realize that physician input is essential for the achievement of success in modern health-care delivery. Although rehabilitation physicians are trained in team efforts for their patients and spend more time than the average physician in patient care and program development meetings, the broader scope of management from an institutional or governmental perspective may be new and strange territory.

Clinicians approach things differently than administrators. The importance of this fact should not be overlooked when clinicians are placed in interactive situations with administrators. In order to become more effective in a managerial sense, physicians need to become acquainted with some terms and processes that are common in the world of managers. This chapter will cover some fundamental concepts and theory and provide examples of medical administration functions.

A satisfactory definition of management is illusive because the term is applied to several types of activities and levels of responsibility. In terms of medical management, the manager's roles have been expanding with the advent of cost containment and managed care organizations (MCOs). Perhaps an effective way to define this subject is to look at what a manager does. Mintzberg (1) listed 10 basic roles common to all managers (Table 18-1). Kurtz (2) amplified eight roles for medical managers (Table 18-2). These roles can be expanded upon to a variety of tasks involved in hospital functions, institutional committees, and various boards (3) (Table 18-3).

STYLES OF MANAGEMENT

The foregoing was concerned with what a manager does. However, effective management is dependent on a knowledge of the corporate culture and the individual's management style, the "how" of management. During the past century management theory has evolved from a purely autocratic approach to various degrees of participation. Each change in underlying philosophy led to modifications in management practice. These have been described as schools of management theory and have developed as follows:

1. Scientific management school. This method relied on hypothesis formation, testing, and analysis of data. Human relations were not factors. Instead, an assumption was made that economic forces drove the company and that people were simply extensions or parts of the machinery of the corporation.
2. Administrative management school. This method used a more intuitive or common sense approach. It attempted to establish useful, fundamental principles based on what was perceived to work.
3. Human relations school. This school recognized that productivity was directly related to employee factors. Psychology and cultural factors became important. Although this school focused attention on the worker as an individual and social being and noted that attention to these factors increased productivity, it did not have the complete desired effect. The missing ingredient was analysis of these interactions.
4. Behavioral science school. This school extends the human relations area to more emphasis on morale and job satisfaction.
5. Management science. Management science, also known as systems management, is an analytic approach to management. It attempts to describe the overall parts of an operation and how these function together to produce whatever the company or corporation intends to produce. It involves participation from a variety of people, including the workers, and builds on using a scientific approach to management including employee and consumer factors.

F. P. Maloney: Department of Physical Medicine and Rehabilitation, University of Arkansas for Medical Sciences, Little Rock, Arkansas 72205.

TABLE 18-1. *The basic managerial roles*

Leadership Roles	
The figurehead role	Performance of ceremonial duties
The leader role	Direct involvement to approve decisions and choose a management team
The liaison role	Dealing with outside people
Informational Roles	
The monitor role	Receiving and sending information for control purposes
The dissemination role	Sharing of information, collected as monitor, with subordinate
The spokesman role	Speaks for department
Decisional Roles	
The entrepreneur role	Involvement with constant addition or deletion of new projects
The disturbance handler role	Attention to problems arising out of strikes, bankruptcies, and interference
The resource allocator role	Allocation of budgets, time, and information
The negotiator role	Ranges from negotiation of an argument to negotiation of a labor contract

Reprinted with permission from Mintzberg H. The manager's job: folklore and fact. *Harvard Bus Rev* 1975; 53: 49–61.

The managed care era and the constraints placed by efforts toward cost containment have fostered attempts at further extending and evolving the basic schools of management. The reorganizations and downsizing that are occurring tend to stress the management systems that are being used. The "management by objectives" used in the past emphasized managerial outcomes rather than costs. At the present time cost reduction appears to be the objective all too often. The suggestion by Paul Elwood (4) for health care to move toward outcome management seems to be catching hold. Unfortunately, the emphasis currently appears to be on cost rather than quality. Nevertheless, the physician profiling that is being conducted by third parties to place and keep physicians on their managed care panels appears to be a variation of outcome management.

TABLE 18-2. *The eight basic role tasks of medical directors*

1. Determining/improving medical practices used in patient care
2. Dealing with problems or differences between physicians
3. Evaluating physician care provided in the organization
4. Advising, counseling, and/or otherwise motivating physicians
5. Recruiting physicians to the organizations
6. Improving the quality of patient care
7. Dealing with medical organizations and societies outside the organization
8. Improving own professional knowledge and skills

Reprinted with permission from Kurtz ME. Role of the physician as manager. *Phys Med Rehabil State Art Rev* 1987; 1:185–196.

TABLE 18-3. *Results of a survey of 750 hospitals conducted by Witt Associates, Inc.*

Percentage of medical directors performing hospital function	
Medical staff affairs	90.3
Quality assurance review	78.5
JCAH compliance	77.4
Credentialing	78.8
Utilization review	62.4
Medical education	60.2
Physician recruitment	55.9
PRO	53.8
Medical manpower planning	49.5
Institutional liaison work	49.5
Disciplinary action	39.8
Housestaff coordination	36.6
Risk management	26.9
Recruitment of other personnel	26.9
Salary negotiations	15.1
Marketing	12.9
Research	11.8
Laboratory	8.6
Radiology	8.6
Physical therapy	7.5
Health services agency	7.5
Pharmacy	4.3
Nursing services	1.1
Percentage of medical directors serving on institutional committees	
Executive	87.1
Credentials	79.6
Medical education	65.6
Bylaws	64.5
Patient care	53.8
Medical records	50.5
Infection control	48.4
Library	47.3
Information systems	31.2
New technologies	24.7
Percentage of medical directors serving on board committees	
Medical staff	50.5
Long-range planning	50.5
Quality assurance	49.5
Executive	29.0
Utilization review	24.7
Finance/budget	18.3
Education	10.8
Bylaws	9.7
Building/grounds	9.7
Audit	9.7

Reprinted with permission from Lloyd J: Growth in medical director numbers continue. *Physician Executive* 1986; 12:10. © American Academy of Medical Directors (now American College of Physician Executives), with permission.

MOTIVATIONAL THEORIES

Theories X, Y, and Z have been described as ways to look at how management has considered the work force in the past and present.

Theory X purports an autocratic approach to management. The philosophy is that the worker dislikes work and, therefore, management is suspicious of workers. External controls of behavior are implemented through a variety of rules and control mechanisms with the assumption that people will avoid responsibility. Theory Y is more people oriented and proposes that people under certain circumstances enjoy working and will be productive as long as their work is rewarded. The reward comes through self-satisfaction rather than purely monetarily. Theory Z was promoted in the 1980s in Japan. This involved high worker participation through the use of quality circles and had job security through long-term employment. Although this system gained popularity in the United States, it became evident that the culture and employee attitudes were significantly different in the two countries, and theory Z as practiced in Japan needed to be modified to a great extent in the United States. However, small group participation is fairly common in many areas and certainly is a mainstay in rehabilitation.

The recognition that productivity is related to employee motivational factors led to a theoretical construct that became known as Maslow's hierarchy of needs. This hierarchy begins with basic needs of people and proceeds through stages to self-actualization (Fig. 18-1). This pyramid of needs shows a breakdown between what is called hygiene factors and motivational factors. The basic premise is that each level of the pyramid, beginning with the base to the peak, must be satisfied in more or less that order. It means that the basic environment of work, safety, and a feeling of belonging must be present to permit motivational factors to come into play. These hygiene factors, by themselves, are not motivators. If they are absent, however, they are demotivators. An interesting factor pertains to the need of a level of income sufficient to have comfortable living. Once this level is reached, the need for income is no longer a motivator.

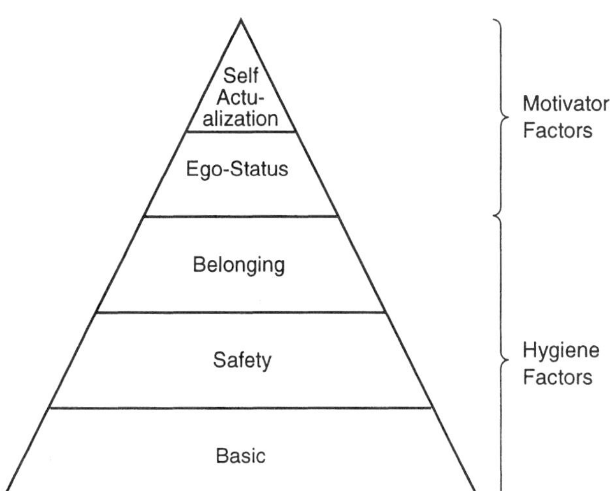

FIG. 18-1. Maslow's hierarchy of needs. (Reprinted with permission from Kurtz ME. Leadership styles. *Phys Med Rehabil State Art Rev* 1987; 1:203.)

TABLE 18-4. *Differences between clinicians and managers*

Clinicians	Managers
Doers	Planners, designers
1:1 Interactions	1:N Interactions
Reactive personalities	Proactive personalities
Require immediate gratification	Accept delayed gratification
Deciders	Delegators
Value autonomy	Value collaboration
Independent	Participative
Patient advocate	Organization advocate
Identify with profession	Identify with organization
Independent	Interdependent

Reprinted with permission from Kurtz ME. Role of a physician as manager. *Phys Med Rehabil State Art Rev* 1987; 1:190.

The stronger needs are for ego status and self-actualization. Two ego status needs were posited by Kurtz (5):

1. Self esteem: needs for self confidence, independence, achievement, competence, and knowledge.
2. Reputation: need for status, recognition, appreciation, and the deserved respect of one's fellows.

LEADERSHIP STYLES

Clinicians view situations differently from managers. The importance of recognizing these differences cannot be overestimated. These contrasts are particularly evident in times of crisis or when rapid decision making seems indicated. Table 18-4 lists these differences. Clinicians are educated to make rapid decisions based on the information at hand. Managers, on the other hand, tend to want input from a variety of sources before important decisions are made. Clinicians tend to think of meetings as a waste of time and time away from patient care, whereas managers seek consensus and at times of crises tend to call meetings to discuss options. Therein lies a potential point of conflict between management and a physician in a management or leadership role. An understanding of these differences will enhance the physician's ability to function in a managerial role. However, there is no expectation that the physician or clinician will change his or her philosophy.

MODELS OF LEADERSHIP STYLES

It is important that the clinician recognize that there are a variety of leadership styles. Although an individual manager tends to use one of these styles as a usual way of managing, other styles may be used depending on the situation at hand. Figure 18-2 indicates a continuum of styles from an autocratic to what can be called an abdicratic method. Extremes of the continuum are generally not viable ways of handling situations. Note that as the style changes to one of more participation and decision making that the involvement of

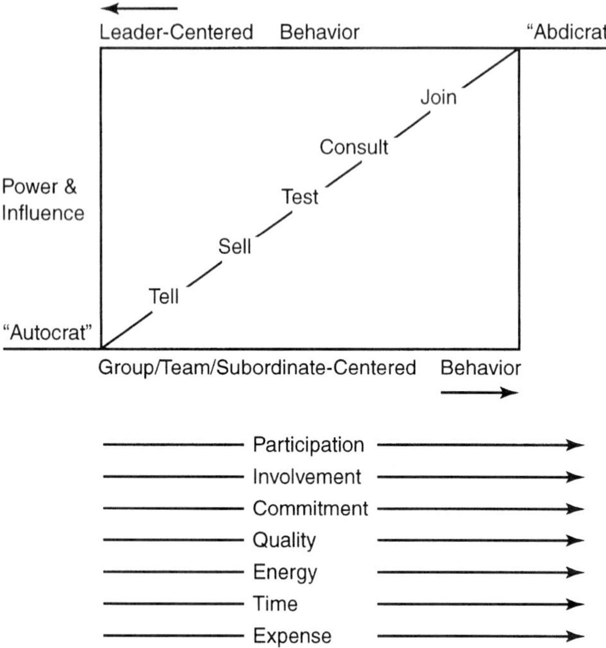

FIG. 18-2. The seven outcomes listed below the model increase as the leadership style moves from authoritarian *(left)* to shared responsibility *(right)*. (Reprinted with permission from Kurtz ME. Organizational behavior. In: Schenke R, ed. *The physician in management.* Tampa, FL: American College of Physician Executives, 1980.)

more people increases, commitment that people have toward the outcome increases, and the quality of the decisions tends to be better. However, the energy required in terms of number of people and the time and expense of these methods are greater. Thus, for major changes or shifts in facility operations and program development, the participatory methods are usually worth the time, expense, and energy involved. However, there are several situations that involve simple matters that would be very inefficient and unwise to make anything other than a fairly autocratic decision. The latter is helped to a great extent by having specific ground rules of when these various methods will be used. Another way of depicting a management style is using a managerial grid. Figure 18-3 shows this grid. This method of analyzing management style shows the relative importance of concern for people and concern for purpose. The descriptions in the figure are self-explanatory. In the present environment where downsizing and costs have become the most important factors, the shift toward high purpose and low concern for people may become evident. It can be very problematic for organizations that have had a high concern for people when they shift to a greater concern for purpose.

TIME MANAGEMENT

Although it has always been important for physicians to know how best to manage their day, it has become much more important recently to account for their time from the standpoint of productivity. It is therefore important for the

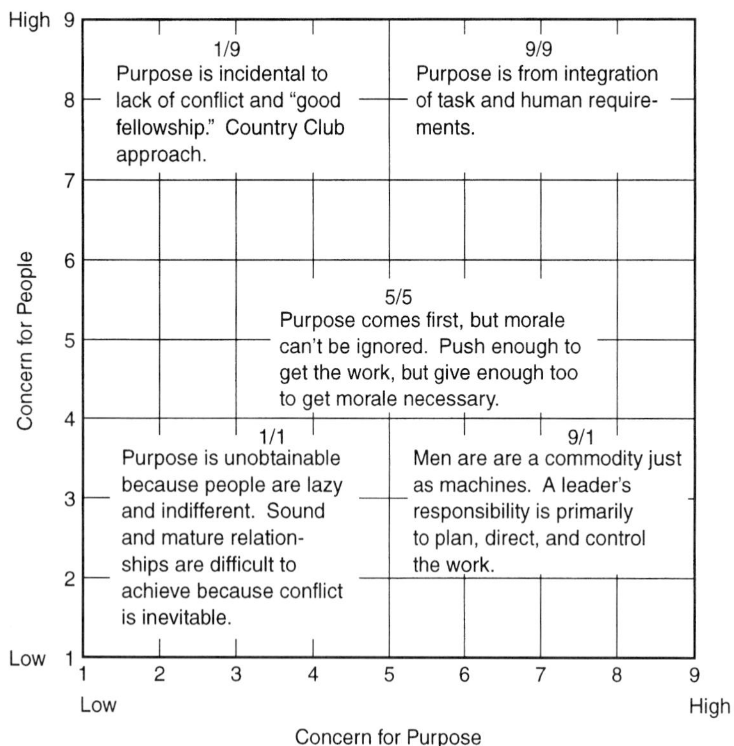

FIG. 18-3. The leadership grid model for assessing leadership practices is based on four factors present in all organizations: purpose, people, power, and philosophy. Each style of leadership reflects a different interplay among these four factors. (Reprinted with permission from the Styles of Leadership Survey. The Woodlands, TX: Teleometrics International, 1968.)

physician manager to establish an order of priorities, some of which will have direct financial implications and others that will only have these indirectly. Furthermore, if the manager is responsible for other physicians, the same must be considered. Finally, the costs of the managers' activities to the institutions in which they function must be factored into the issue of time management.

As indicated in Figure 18-2, participation in group activities toward setting goals, program development, facility reorganization, and various patient care meetings is costly not only from the standpoint of whether the physician can bill for these activities, but also because of the salary cost of the time involved by a variety of professionals. Therefore, it is important that the number of meetings be limited to what is essential. The leader or manager should plan meetings in advance to maximize their productivity and efficiency. It is worthwhile to periodically review the purpose and effectiveness of all meetings in an organization. Frequently, weekly meetings may be reduced to every other week, and some meetings that have lost their usefulness may be discontinued.

Therefore, the manager must be cognizant of managing his or her own time and that of his or her subordinates and colleagues. It is valuable to not only establish a balance between patient care activities and managerial activities, but to also establish a relative cost for these. The manager should be compensated for his or her time as a manager, and the clinical activity should rely on establishing a certain income per scheduled time.

PRODUCTIVITY

Physician profiling is, or will be, used by the federal government, corporations, MCOs, hospitals, and group practices. Nationally, the Healthplan Employee Data and Information Set (HEDIS) scores groups of physicians on performance and outcomes. HEDIS intends to focus on individual physicians in the future. Dr. Richard W. Besdine, Director of Health Standards and Quality Bureau of the Health Care Finance Administration (HCFA), in his keynote address at the 1996 American Board of Physical Medicine and Rehabilitation Annual Conference pointed out that although the HCFA has data on MCOs now, in the future this will be expanded to fee for service (FFS) with emphasis on outcome measurements. Interest in monitoring outcomes and making decisions about payment based on this will make the HCFA a purchaser of health care rather than an insurer. The *American Medical Association News* has reported that some corporations are moving forward with their own measures of physician performance and are willing to ''overlook some of the scientific, validity and sample-size questions to get outcomes and results'' (6). MCOs are profiling physicians. Some of the areas of data collection are listed as follows:

1. Retrospective utilization management
2. Physician quality management
3. Analysis of variations between providers
4. Identification of best practices/providers
5. Quality index scoring
6. Differential payment

Various factors are taken into consideration to develop an index score, including case mix and complexity. Payment is then geared to the index score, with lower scores paid less than higher scores. Counseling for low scores is attempted, and if scores do not increase, the physician is dropped from the provider panel.

Physician profiling can be used as part of time management to feed back to the manager and the individual physician a comparison of how time is used across physicians with the same case mix. Hospitals that employ physicians may use profiles to estimate employment needs. Multispecialty groups can use profiles to recommend or deny the addition of physicians. For example, the average length of stay for five physicians with the same case mix is about the same, but one physician's hospital charges an average $3,000 more than the other four. The profile shows an increase in laboratory, x-ray, and drug charges plus an admission functional independence measure (FIM) (7) average that is less than that of the other physicians. The manager's role may be to look into the reasons for this difference. The physician could be admitting patients too quickly from acute care, necessitating more medical workups that delay the rehabilitation program from being fully implemented, may have patients prone to be transferred back to acute care, or may be admitting more severely involved patients at lower functional levels. Should this be the case, these facts would be discussed with the physician and changes suggested and consequences specified. If changes did not occur, the consequence could be a referral to the Utilization Review Committee for disposition. Physicians who are employed by hospitals or groups may find that their contracts may not be renewed. Similar profiling can lead to nonreappointment in academic departments.

Another example could concern an academic department at a university whose clinicians have formed a group practice. This department wishes to hire an additional faculty member to develop a procedure-oriented approach to pain management. In the past, all that was required was to look at the financial situation of the department and discuss the addition with the dean. However, now the chairperson of the department must justify this addition to the executive committee of the group practice. In this environment, several questions arise and must be addressed. For example:

1. Does the school need this addition? (as opposed to, Does the department need this addition?)
2. Is there too much overlap with existing faculty in other departments?
3. Are the procedures this new faculty member will perform part of the scope of physiatric practice?
4. What are the income projections for the addition and how were the figures generated?

5. Can the educational needs of the department be met by cooperation with other departments that are performing the requested procedures?

It is becoming common for physicians to work part time either combining private practice and employment, cutting back, or taking time to raise a family. The manager must be aware of how many equivalents of full-time physicians are needed for the department or facility. The terms used are "full-time equivalent" (FTE) or "full-time equivalent employee" (FTEE). Advantages of a part-time FTE are that benefits are usually not paid to persons working less than half time, and there is flexibility in having a diverse group of physicians. The disadvantages can be that part-time people may not be able to cover some services (such as large inpatient services), may not be available for call coverage, and could have conflicts of interest. The manager must weigh the pros and cons of employing part-time people and use income projections to justify the complement of physicians.

The foregoing relates to situations where physicians are either employed or are involved in a hospital with a closed staff. In an open staff environment, hospital privileges cannot be denied to a qualified physician. This means additional physicians can affect the income of the other physicians by competing for the same patients unless new sources of patients are developed. Creating new programs, consulting at additional hospitals, and outreach to other geographic areas are examples of finding new sources.

There are other items that can be factored into the costs of time spent by a medical manager, such as the ability of the manager to influence the case mix for the hospital or medical group to influence the medical staff in maintaining acceptable lengths of inpatient stay and their reduction of ancillary charges. Assistance with discharge planners in acute care hospitals to properly triage difficult cases, and establishment of protocols and care paths, are also useful and documentable functions.

ORGANIZATIONAL STRUCTURE

Frequently, the clinician is satisfied to see patients and to attend the minimum number of meetings necessary to maintain hospital privileges. The underlying hospital organization and structure of the medical staff is not a matter of interest. However, when the clinician assumes a managerial role, these matters become important. Hospitals have a specific hierarchical structure, and the medical staff, likewise, has a structure. The two are separate organizationally but report to a single board of trustees. The structure of the hospital and medical staff varies according to whether it is in the private, state, or federal system.

Five types of organizational structures have been described (8):

1. Simple structure. The simple structure is one with few people. The new office or department that starts with a few physicians and few office staff would be an example. The simple structure has the advantage of being very flexible. It can change quickly and respond to change with minimal difficulty because communication occurs freely among the group and middle management does not exist. The disadvantage is that there are usually limited or no formal policies and procedures.

2. Machine bureaucracy. Larger organizations require some centralization and usually develop layers of middle management. A chain of command is common, and delegation of authority is limited. Protocols, policies, and procedures are needed. The disadvantage is that the layers of management makes this fairly inflexible. Many large corporations are examples of this type.

3. Professional bureaucracy. This form also has layers of middle management, but skills are obtained through the process of hiring rather than developed in the organization as occurs in the machine bureaucracy. Medical schools function as a professional bureaucracy with fairly autonomous units. Only large decisions are completely centralized.

4. Divisional bureaucracy. The divisional form has a centralized decision-making body but allows for autonomous divisions. The divisions can be either machine or professional bureaucracies depending on their mission. This type has heavy administrative numbers of personnel and has the advantages and disadvantages of whatever type of structures are used as mentioned above. It has the additional benefit of providing diversity.

5. Adhocracy. The adhocracy is a team approach to management. It combines persons from a variety of disciplines and establishes a project director who has authority over the project and, therefore, the people involved as they relate to the project. However, the individuals are still assigned to and employed by their base department. The NASA moon project is usually used as the example of this structure, in which a project director had people from a variety of organizations brought together for a defined goal. A rehabilitation team could also be considered an adhocracy when dealing with each individual patient, the physician being the project director. Hospital task forces and committees also may function in this way. This structure allows flexibility within a larger organization.

Other terms that have been used to describe structure are vertical, horizontal, and matrix. A staff conference would be an example of a matrix structure that is a combination of a vertical and horizontal structure. An example of the verticality is that the therapists and nurses administratively report to a chain of command in the hospital hierarchy, but for purposes of patient care combine an adhocracy in a horizontal fashion across disciplines to treat the patient.

Problems arise in situations that are not clearly part of the patient care adhocracy. For example, the physician (project director) wants to prescribe a piece of equipment such as a wheelchair and the therapists agree from the standpoint of patient need. However, a hospital policy known to all physicians states that if the wheelchair is obtained during hospitalization, it may be considered as part of the set amount of total payment a third party will pay for the patient's entire hospital stay. This additional cost may cause a loss to the hospital and therefore as a usual policy the wheelchair should be obtained after the patient is discharged (usually the same day). The therapists then are caught between the vertical hospital structure and the horizontal adhocracy of the matrix. The outcomes are usually negotiated and require compromise on a case-by-case need.

HOSPITAL ORGANIZATION

As indicated before, the medical staff organization is usually separate from the hospital organization, so differences in patient care issues can be approached through both hierarchies. The medical staff has a chief of staff, committees, and sections, whereas the hospital has directors, chief executive, and chief operating officers. Most medical staff and hospital administration disputes are settled amicably when both sides have the opportunity to fully discuss the issue. In those rare instances in which a difference cannot be settled, it is taken to the Joint Conference Committee for resolution. This Committee is conducted monthly by the Board of Trustees. Both the medical staff (physicians' organization) and the hospital administration (hospital organization) report to the Joint Conference Committee, whose decision is final.

The manager needs to be aware of the types of authority possible in situations. Line authority is direct authority from a manager to other people. For example, the Chief of Service at the Veterans Administration has line authority for physical, occupational, and kinesiotherapists. In other words, the Chief of Service can direct the staff to develop certain programs or procedures. Staff authority is authority by influence, suggestion, and persuasion. The medical directors of private hospitals usually have no direct line authority to the therapists and certainly do not have this authority regarding the medical staff of an open staffed hospital. Program development and other managerial changes are achieved through persuasion and suggestion.

The authority and responsibility of a medical director can vary according to the structure of the institution in which he or she functions. In the Veterans Administration, the Chief of Service has direct authority for the physicians in the Physical Medicine and Rehabilitation Service. The chief of service also reports through the chief of staff to the director or chief executive officer (CEO) of the hospital. An equivalent role can be found in some closed staff environments where a CEO or medical director of a physician group contracts with a hospital for medical services. The same individual may function as the medical director of the hospital, thus providing the dual role.

In many private settings the medical director functions only in a direct hierarchical line from hospital administration and on a dotted line to the medical staff. Figure 18-4 is an example of this structure. This is a bridging function, but it clearly remains that the physician in that role is an employee of the hospital and not of the medical staff. Figure 18-5 shows another example of a hospital in a multihospital system after the implementation of a patient focused care reorganization establishing program directors instead of therapy and nursing supervisors.

In some instances in an open staff environment the medical director may be one of a group of physicians but not the sole group that have active privileges at that hospital. Thus, for their own group, a medical director has the dual function as indicated above but only has staff authority when it comes to the rest of the medical staff. In many instances the authority for the entire medical staff is derived through the medical staff's delegation of authority to the medical director for purposes of monitoring various medical functions through utilization review, quality assurance, and other defined mechanisms.

In the official structure of an organization it is important to recognize that there is also an informal structure or "grapevine." Everyone is aware that some individuals have more influence on the workings of an organization or department than their official designation would indicate. These are the persons whom others consult to find out information or to work around the system. Because in most instances medical managers are not in a direct line of authority, it is very important that they be aware of this informal structure and how it works.

ACCREDITING BODIES

Managers participate in preparation for various accrediting organizations and surveys and are expected to participate in the site visits that occur. The Joint Commission on Accreditation of Health Care Organizations (JCAHO), the Commission on Accreditation of Rehabilitation Facilities (CARF), state health departments, residency review committees, and various internal reviews are common periodic surveys. Although overlap exists as far as the data needed for all these reviews, the thrust of each is different. JCAHO and CARF are implementing a joint survey that may save time and expense for facilities. Although each of these surveys has value, the staff and physician time and expense consumed in preparation for them is considerable.

It is common practice to engage an experienced surveyor to perform a site visit several months before JCAHO and CARF surveys to identify areas that need additional preparatory work. The medical manager usually has the responsibility of assuring that aspects related to the medical staff are in order and well documented.

Two areas that have particular emphasis for physicians are the organizational function of leadership and the standards involving the function of the medical staff. The manager should become familiar with these standards and the scoring guidelines for the specific standards. In the JCAHO 1996

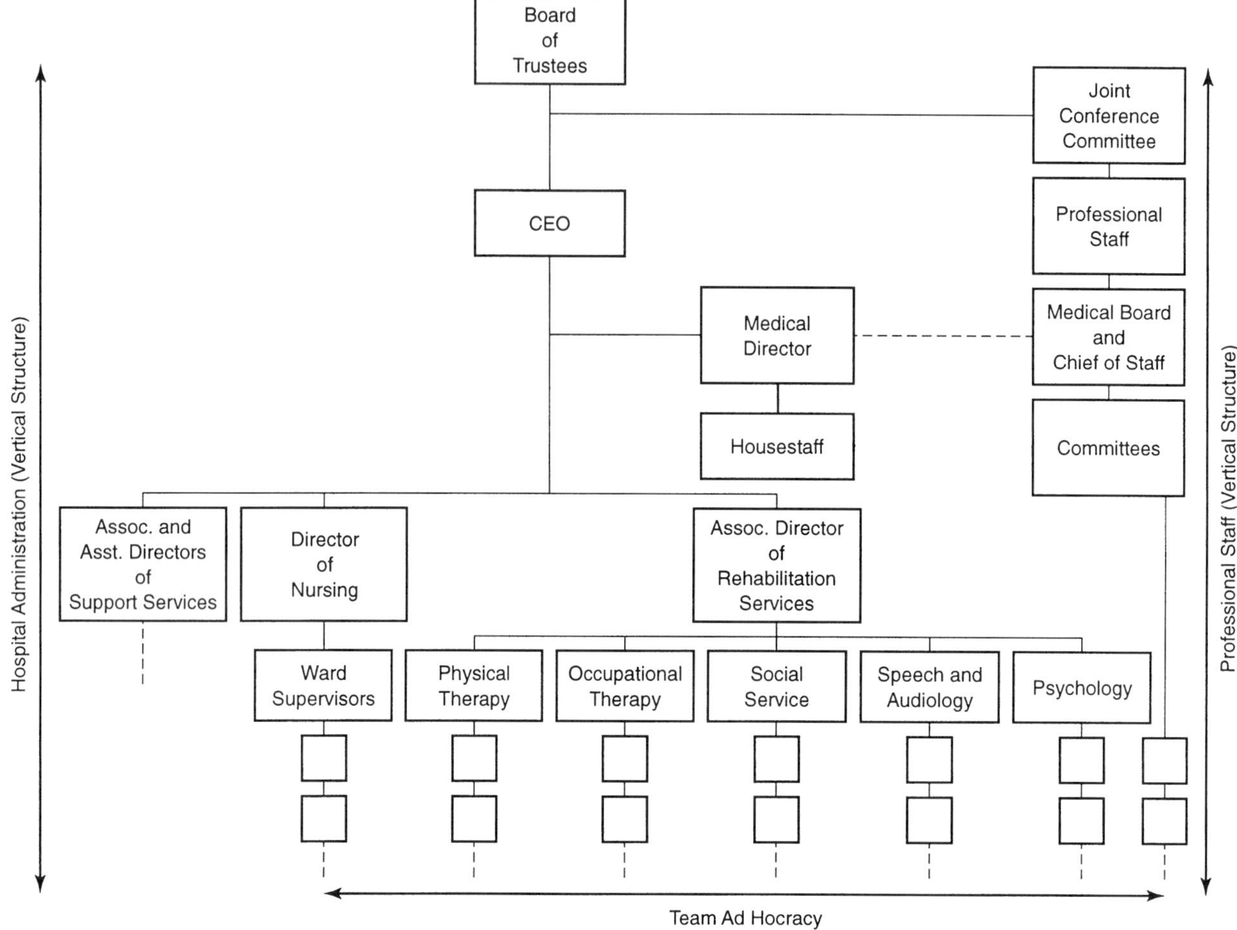

FIG. 18-4. Matrix. Medical director with staff authority. In this configuration the medical director is an advisor. The *solid line* represents direct responsibility to the CEO. The *broken line* indicates the relationship to the medical staff. (Reprinted with permission from Maloney FP, ed. *A primer on management for rehabilitation medicine.* Philadelphia: Hanley & Belfus, 1987.)

Comprehensive Accreditation Manual for Hospitals (9), the list of leadership functions involves the following general areas:

Planning and designing services
Directing services
Integrating and coordinating services
Improving performance

A common aphorism for surveys is, "If it isn't written, it wasn't done." This means that a great deal of attention is placed on how the medical chart documents patient care. Policies and procedures and medical staff rules and regulations are reviewed for content. Chart reviews and interviews with staff are conducted to see if the facility and staff follow the accreditor's standards and the facility's own policies and rules. The accrediting standard may provide a general guideline for what is needed, but the facility policy spells out the details for the institution. Careful thought should be given to writing these policies. The medical manager needs to be especially familiar with those aspects relating to medical care and able to match the accreditation standards to internal policies and their documentation.

For example, a JCAHO standard indicates that a physician's quality of care should be considered at the time of reappointment to the medical staff. It is the medical staff's responsibility to establish the details as to how this is done. The surveyor would then look over this process to see that there is a procedure for the standard and if documentation of adherence to one's own policy exists.

The JCAHO of late is emphasizing the facility staff's understanding of a variety of processes. More time is being spent by surveyors on the wards, reviewing active charts and asking questions to not only caregivers, but also the support staff. Eventually, ongoing information will be sent to JCAHO for a continuous review mechanism.

THIRD PARTIES

A variety of third parties purchase health care. Although each physician has responsibility for his or her own adher-

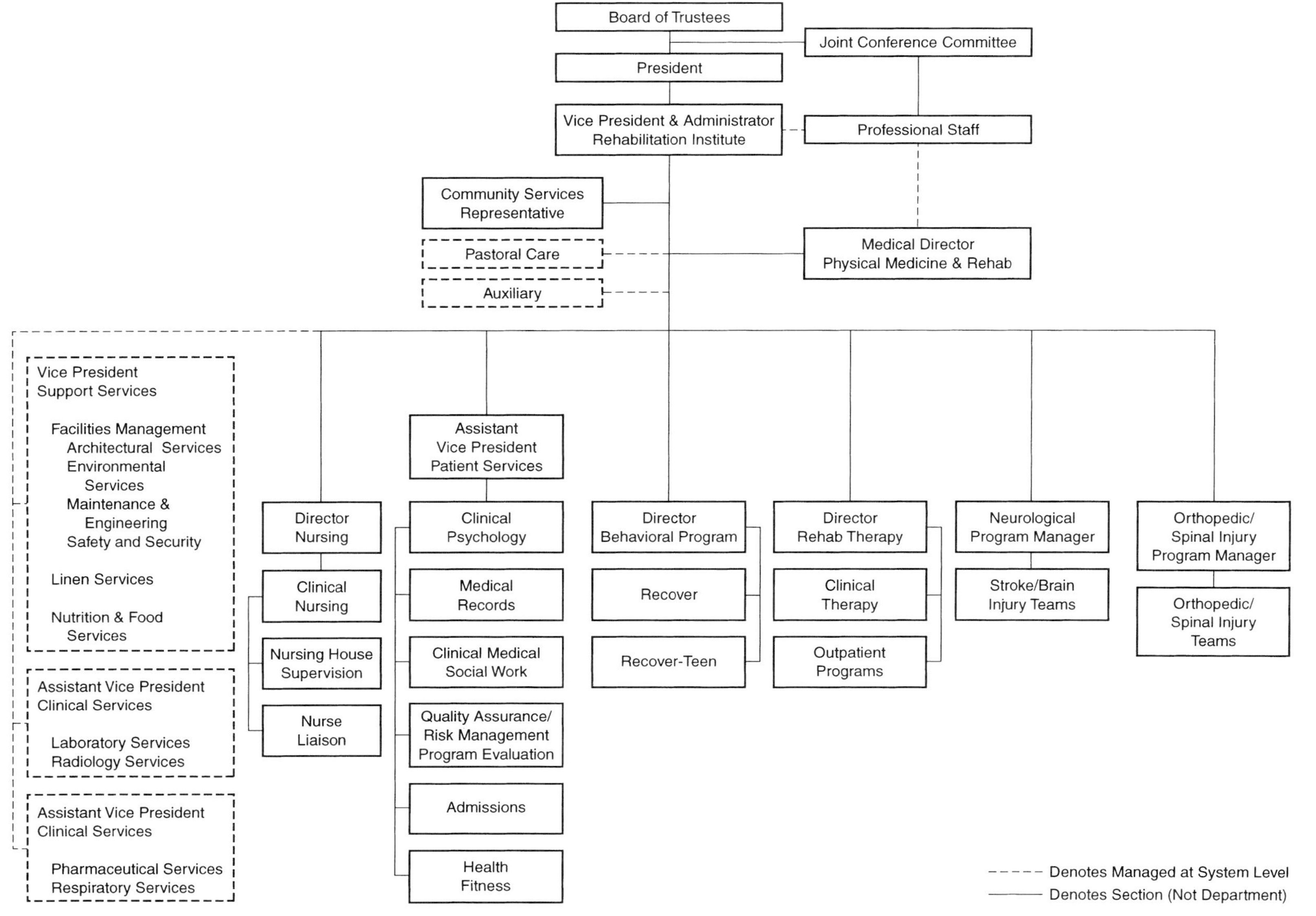

FIG. 18-5. Matrix structure in a multihospital system after patient focused care has reorganized middle management and the institution into teams with program directors. *Dotted lines* represent system functions except as they relate to the professional staff. *Dotted lines from the professional staff* indicate the indirect relationship of the hospital CEO and the medical director.

ence to the third party's guidelines, the medical manager is frequently involved in assisting the facility in responses to denials of payment and justifications for admission, length of stay, and equipment.

MEDICARE

Medicare's peer review organizations (PROs) have extensive guidelines. Frequently the physician will be paid even though the hospital is denied payment for all or part of an admission. The incentive for the physician to challenge the denial, however, is to prevent a negative PRO profile. Every inpatient and outpatient denial should be challenged unless there has been a very obvious failure to meet a guideline. The proportion of Medicare outpatient charges in acute care settings may be small in comparison to rehabilitation facilities. The PRO may experience few challenges from facilities that have small numbers of Medicare cases because the facility may not have a systematic way of dealing with, or believe that it is not cost effective to challenge, such a low volume of charges. Therefore, denials of payment that could legitimately be appealed are written off. This may lead the PRO to incorrectly believe that their decisions were valid. This represents a significant educational problem for rehabilitation facilities. Direct contact with the PRO's medical director and administration is extremely important so that the PRO has a clear understanding of rehabilitation goals and treatments. It is worthwhile to exchange visits. Mutual respect and understanding go a long way to keep denials of payment to a minimum.

The medical manager must keep abreast of changes in the way that Medicare reimburses in the future. The future intent for Medicare is probably to provide a capitated fee for services. The current way that Medicare reimburses rehabilitation facilities should be considered interim, although the method has been in place since 1983. The Tax Equity and Fiscal and Responsibility Act of 1982 (TEFRA) established a fixed Medicare payment for each rehabilitation hospital admission. In acute care, the prospective payment system (PPS) is based on diagnostic related groups. Diagnosis alone does not account for differences between the costs of rehabilitation cases. However, recent indications are that a reimbursement system based on functional related groups may be used to determine case-specific payment for Medicare admissions. This system combines diagnosis and patient function on admission. Managers must be aware of this potential development so that data can be collected and decisions made (10).

Bundling of costs is another possible future method of payment. Bundling all facility and postfacility charges into one payment has been suggested. One method would be to attach all post–acute care costs (rehabilitation, skilled nursing, home health) to the acute care facility. Although subacute rehabilitation has not been recognized by the HCFA, it would be included in this bundle. The other method of bundling is to combine all post–acute care separately from acute care so that the acute care facility does not have the incentive to bypass needed acute rehabilitation. The American Academy of Physical Medicine and Rehabilitation has published a position paper on post–acute care payments (11). Their position is as follows:

1. The payment is focused only on the disabled and on post–acute care so that underservice risks are minimized.
2. Payments are sufficient in amount to meet the needs of all patients included in the program and are, optimally, risk adjusted.
3. A team of rehabilitation professional assesses the need for care and develops a plan of care with full participation by the patient.
4. Payments consider appropriate intensity of service relative to patients' needs and ability to progress with treatment.
5. Payments are made to a post–acute care entity (either a full-service network or coalition of rehabilitation providers) that has the appropriate accreditations and the capability of integrating and accessing services among the full spectrum of post–acute care settings (not to the discharging acute care hospital).
6. Case management is provided by physicians specializing in physical medicine and rehabilitation or other physicians with expertise in the management of post–acute care and the condition involved.

Medicare regulations are continually changing either in content or in interpretation. Interpretations may vary by region. The manager should be familiar with these regulations to assure compliance. The HCFA's proposed Medicare regulations are published in the *Federal Register* to give an opportunity for comment before implementation (12).

A rehabilitation unit that is exempt from the Medicare PPS must have at least 75% of its discharge diagnoses be from the following:

1. Stroke
2. Spinal cord injury
3. Congenital deformity
4. Amputation
5. Major multiple trauma
6. Fracture of femur (hip fracture)
7. Brain injury
8. Polyarthritis, including rheumatoid arthritis
9. Neurological disorders, including multiple sclerosis, motor neuron disease, polyneuropathy, muscular dystrophy, and Parkinson's disease
10. Burns

Efforts to add other diagnoses such as pain management and certain cardiac and pulmonary problems have been proposed.

Among aspects that need to be followed to comply with

TABLE 18-5. *Exemptions from Medicare PPS*

1. Evidence of a preadmission screening process
2. Documented admission criteria to determine if a prospective patient is reasonably likely to benefit from admission
3. Units must be a separate cost center to avoid co-mingling of patients and having multipurpose beds
4. The accounting system most properly allocates costs
5. A provision for medical supervision availability 24 hours per day
6. A written plan of treatment
7. Team conferences at least every two weeks; a team is at a minimum, a physician, rehabilitation nurse, and therapist.
8. A director of rehabilitation who is a doctor of medicine or osteopathy.
   a) For units within hospitals 20 hours per week is the guideline
   b) For rehab hospitals 35 hours per week is the guideline
9. Although the patient must have a reasonable expectation of improvement, for some patients a 3- to 10-day evaluation period is permitted. This period should be designated as an evaluation period and should not be used frequently.
10. The intensity of service should be such as to require inpatient rehabilitation. This has been defined as a need for a minimum of three hours of therapy and 5.5 hours of rehabilitation nursing

the conditions of participation for Medicare PPS, exemptions are found in Table 18-5.

OTHER INSURERS

Some insurers have case managers who control the delivery of care for individual cases. MCOs establish contracts with facilities and physicians for their payment. To decide whether to contract with the MCO, the manager must have data and systems available to judge what discounts can reasonably be offered to an MCO. Factors to consider include volume and exclusivity. A different rate could be negotiated with an MCO that will provide great numbers of patients or give the physician or facility exclusive referrals. Some third parties are seeking the equivalent of a capitated fee. Capitation is a method of compensation that provides a predetermined payment for all care that is delivered. This means that physician charges are combined with the facility charges. The physician must therefore be aware of what amount is reasonable for an entire admission. Insurers are seeking to share risk. If an admission costs less than anticipated, the physician and facility will profit. However, if the costs are greater than anticipated, the physician and facility must absorb the loss. Miscalculation of capitation fees for a high-volume admission such as stroke could be very costly for the provider. Accurate information is essential.

MARKETING

The first point that should be made is that advertising is only a part of marketing. The two terms are not synonymous. Advertising is a strategy by which a service or product gains market recognition by the population at large or a focused group such as other specialties or third-party payers. Some hospitals and rehabilitation programs have successfully used this method by creating a demand for the service that they offer. In this way the consumer will seek from their primary provider the desired service. This has been called a pull strategy. Alternatively, there is a push strategy that attempts to influence intermediaries directly to use a service or product. This method is used by facilities that send representatives to present information at physicians' offices, small medical staff meetings, discharge planners, and various third-party payers. The physician may be called upon to participate in these endeavors. The push strategies are more specific and therefore focused but more expensive and time consuming. These may also be more effective. The pull strategies tend to be more sensitive in that they cover a wide number of people with possibly a poor result in terms of use. Most people who hear or see an advertisement do not need the service or product at the time it is advertised.

An important factor in marketing is the natural history or life cycle of a product. For any new product, an introductory phase may last for considerable time while consumer awareness develops. This phase is followed by a growth phase wherein rapid advancement and use takes place. Sometime during this phase competition develops. This is where large corporations may buy out or overwhelm the smaller initiators of a product with discounts on expanded service. This growth will level out in a mature phase where demand generally equals production. Eventually the demand lessens during a decline phase. Usually the decline occurs because of changes in the marketplace or in demographics. The occupancy rate in hospitals is an example of this decline, whereas outpatient programs have not yet developed a mature phase. The development of MCOs is in a growth phase.

It is important to recognize the phase various programs are in or approaching so that appropriate strategies can be planned. Inpatient rehabilitation is approaching a mature phase in many communities. This has already occurred for acute care facilities, many of which have closed, merged, or been subsumed by national chains. The manager must analyze the situation and decide on prudent courses of action. These may include development of new programs (such as sports medicine or contracting with subacute rehabilitation facilities) or expansion of existing programs (such as development of procedures that are underserved in the community).

Whether or not marketing consultants are used, a marketing plan should be developed together with a budget. For each established goal that is listed, the needed steps should have a budgeted amount, together with timelines and the methods or tools to be used. Some types of measurement of success are useful. They might include increases in numbers of phone contacts, referrals from targeted sources, and so forth.

COMPUTER APPLICATIONS

The electronic era necessitates that managers have at least a rudimentary familiarity with computer use and potential. In the future even this fundamental knowledge will not be sufficient to function in a managerial role.

Hospitals are moving toward the electronic chart (computer-based patient record). JCAHO will implement electronic transfers of ongoing data. Electronic billing direct from offices to billing agencies is available, and E-mail is becoming a preferred way to transmit information rather than by hard copy.

User-friendly programs are readily available. Relational data bases (Access, Paradox, etc.) make analyses of hospital and practice management possible at the desktop rather than waiting months to obtain sufficient priority to have new programs devised by a central computer programming group. A user can query this system about a variety of issues and receive information back in minutes, limited only by the data available and the familiarity of the managers with the system.

ACCOUNTING AND FINANCE

Space permits addressing only a few basic concepts of accounting and finance. The reader is referred to other texts available on this subject (13–15).

The terms ''accounting'' and ''finance'' must be differentiated. Accounting or financial accounting tells us the financial situation of an organization at a point in time. By the time a formal accounting is reported, several months are likely to have transpired. The financial accounting is therefore a historic document and tells the reader about the financial situation of a department or organization at a former point in time. Annual reports and year-end hospital and department reports are examples. Managerial accounting, however, provides some prospective information that is to be used to make decisions about the future. The managerial accountant therefore is providing information that will be used to project or analyze what will be done in the future and is used primarily for budgeting. Finance also involves the analysis of fiscal performance projections.

Cost accounting in a strict sense allocates costs of equipment and services. For example, the cost of an outpatient visit includes small parts of a number of salaries (receptionist, transcriptionist, nurse), plus the cost of lights, copying, files, etc. In a large organization, the personnel not involved in direct patient care, such as housekeeping and administration, must be considered so that the cost of services is also apportioned to the income-producing areas.

The way this is done varies from facility to facility by using formulas in a cascading stepwise manner. It is useful to become somewhat familiar with the methodology that is used. For example, a common item in the first step may be space, such as cost per square foot. Subsequent steps are add-ons and multipliers of each other. If the area charged to the department is larger than is actually used, the allocated cost may be thousands of dollars too high. For example, in one hospital the several areas used for therapies within a physical medicine and rehabilitation department had been reallocated to other services because of changes in priorities and division of services. The accountants did not make this change. When the error was discovered several years later, it made the difference between the department being profitable or not.

There are several terms for which a degree of familiarity is useful.

Fixed Costs

These are costs that do not vary from month to month. Regular employee salaries are fixed costs. This means that when a census is low in a hospital or when an office practice has fewer patient visits than usual, the expense of these salaries remains the same. Fixed costs are always problematic for fiscal viability in a contracting environment when census is low.

Variable Costs

These costs can change monthly, weekly, or daily. The use of nursing pools and hourly transcription services are examples. Also, consumables and medications can be variable.

In this regard, there are some costs that depend on the fiscal soundness of an organization. For example, travel expenses for educational meetings are technically a variable expense but can be allocated in a department budget at $3,000 per person. This would appear to the recipient as being a usual fixed expense. However, if revenues are less than expected, this can be reduced, changing it from a fixed to a variable cost.

Figure 18-6 shows a simplified example of the differences

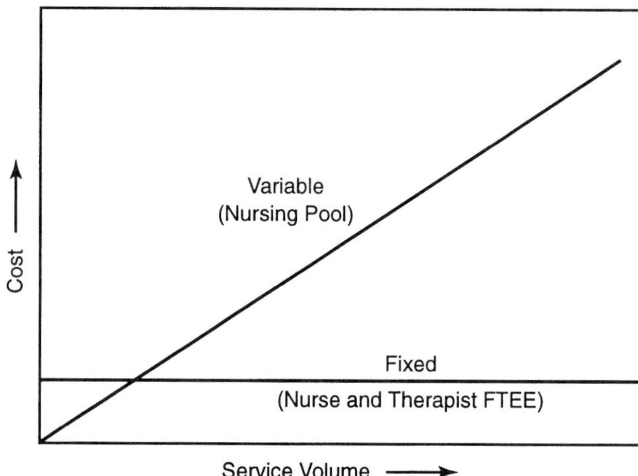

FIG. 18-6. Costs versus service volume. Fixed costs are the same regardless of volume. Therefore, the cost per unit of service decreases as the volume increases. Variable cost increases proportionally with volume.

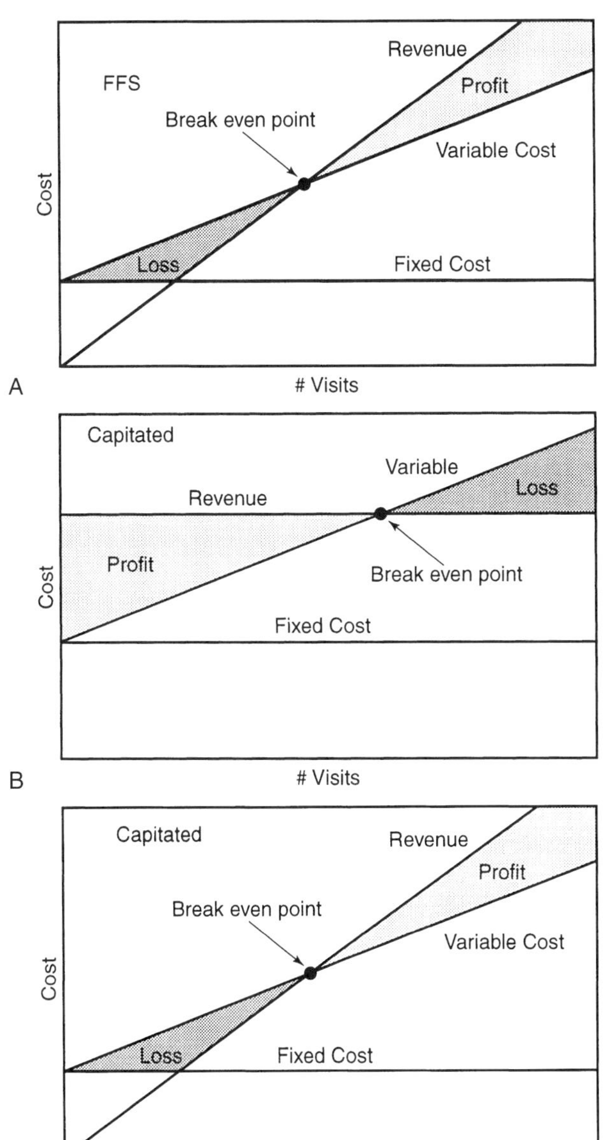

FIG. 18-7. FFS versus capitated costs. **A:** FFS profit occurs with stable fixed costs and an increase in volume. **B:** Capitated. Initial revenue is high, but profitability decreases as volume increases. **C:** Capitated. Profitability increases with the addition of covered lives.

between fixed and variable costs. As volume of a service increases, the fixed cost per unit becomes less, and vice versa. Nursing and therapy salary costs for FTEEs become proportionally less when the census is up. On the other hand, the variable costs per unit of service remain the same and are based on volume.

An expansion of the consideration of fixed and variable costs is applicable to the difference between FFS and capitated situations. Figure 18-7*A* shows that for FFS as the number of visits increases, the billing increases and the profitability increases. This is because the fixed cost per unit of service decreases with an increase in volume. The variable cost slope is less than the revenue slope. Figure 18-7*B*, on the other hand, shows that although the revenue is initially higher, it is constant, so the profitability decreases with an increase in the number of visits and increase in variable costs. Another way to look at a capitated delivery of care is that profitability increases as the number of people covered increases (Fig. 18-7*C*). Thus the MCO's common reference to number of covered lives.

Accrual Accounting

This accountant's tool assigns a value to a service as it occurs. Revenue is the amount of money entered by the accountant at a point in time. It may or may not represent actual cash. It is not collections. Thus, an FFS patient designated as self pay is credited with the amount billed even though it is very possible that collections will be minimal. The same applies to the expense of providing this service. It is recorded at the time of the service. Depreciation of capital expenses comes into play here as an exception. All of the costs of a piece of equipment are not charged at the time of acquisition. For example, it may be assumed the useful life of a piece of equipment, such as diagnostic equipment, is 5 years. It is unfair to expense it all in the first year because the cost of using the equipment may be spread out over its useful life.

Generally Accepted Accounting Principles

The Financial Accounting Standards Board is the policy-setting organization for the accounting profession. In concert with the Securities and Exchange Commission, the generally accepted accounting principles (GAAPs) define the methods of auditing and fiscal reporting. Audits should not be accepted unless they are stated to conform to GAAPs.

Financial Statements

The common financial statements for an organization are the income statement (or statement of performance or profit and loss sheet), the balance statement or balance sheet, and the cash flow statement.

The income statement lists revenues and expenses and provides a net positive or negative total. Table 18-6 is a simplified example for an individual physician.

The balance sheet depicts the situation of an organization at a specific time. It lists assets, liabilities, and equity. The formula that is used is

$$\text{Assets} = \text{liabilities} + \text{owner's equity}$$

Equity is the owner's interest in an endeavor. The elements used for assets are as follows:

Current assets, including cash, net accounts receivable, and supply inventory
Marketable securities

TABLE 18-6. *Dr. Jones's income statement for January, 1995.*

Revenue	
Payments from inpatients	10,500
Payments from Outpatient Site 1	2,000
Payments from Outpatient Site 2	1,500
	14,000
Expenses	
Rent (including utilities)	2,500
Salaries	2,500
Phone	300
Office supplies	200
Travel	1,000
Miscellaneous	500
	7,000
Net Income	7,000

Property, including land, building, and equipment less depreciation

Other assets

All factors may not be present at a department or office situation, but will certainly be there for hospitals. Table 18-7 is a simple example of a balance sheet.

In this example Dr. Jones invests $20,000 of his own money (equity) and borrows $3,000 to buy equipment (accounts payable). The cash is the difference between the physician's equity and the new expenses (asset) of the examination table. More elaborate balance sheets contain lists of assets and liabilities, but the concept is the same.

An important line on reports summarizes the status of revenues compared with expenses and provides a measure of the relationship of revenues/expenses. This figure is not a ratio but simply shows revenues minus expenses. A positive figure indicates that revenues exceed expenses and a negative indicates a loss. These figures are usually reported for the month and year to date. Another figure is the fund balance, which is the carryover of revenue from prior months. Therefore, this figure indicates the reserve amount available. A substantial fund balance makes it more possible to try new ventures that can show losses (revenue/expense) for a time.

Although the income statement shows revenues and expenses, it focuses on the costs of operation, whereas the cash flow statement focuses on the details of cash input and outgo. The cash flow statement provides information about the liquidity or viability of an organization and is a required audit statement. A typical cash flow statement for an institution would categorize operating activities, investing activities, and financing activities. Operating activities include net income and various adjustments to this income that can increase or decrease this net. Common adjustments that add value are reductions in accounts receivable, salaries, and increases in accounts payable. Decreases can occur with a decrease in accounts payable. Investing activities include the purchase of new equipment. Financing activities include mortgages and payment of dividends. These statements are summarized by a net increase/decrease in cash and a comparison of cash at the beginning and end of a year.

A number of ratios are commonly used to describe financial situations. The common ratios that may be useful to an organization relate to liquidity, efficiency, and profitability. The most common liquidity ratio is the current ratio: current ratio = current assets ÷ current liabilities. This relates to whether an organization can meet its obligations. If it is high, then perhaps the enterprise can afford to incur additional debt to give the business higher yield. A low ratio is a red flag for potential default on existing obligations

Efficiency Ratios

How efficiently does an institution manage resources? The common efficiency ratios used in rehabilitation relate to change in FIM divided by cost.

Profitability Ratios

Profit margin = net income ÷ total revenue. Useful ratios of the return on investment are return on assets = net income ÷ total assets, as well as return on net assets = net income ÷ stockholders equity.

None of these ratios by themselves should be used to make decisions. Factors can intervene that make a ratio an incorrect picture of an organization. These are included here so the medical manager is aware of the terms and understands their general use.

BUDGETING

A budget is a plan of expenses, usually for a year. The expenses are matched to an expected income. These projec-

TABLE 18-7. *Balance sheet for physician A as of January 31, 1992*

Assets		=	Liabilities	+	Owner's Equity
Cash	$14,000		Accounts payable $3,000		Physician A Capital $20,000
Office equipment	3,000				
Exam table	6,000				
TOTAL	$23,000	=	$3,000		$20,000

$14,000 = 20,000 − 6,000 paid for examination table

Modified with permission from Weeks D. *Phys Med Rehabil State Art Rev* 1993; 7:258.

tions are educated guesses about the future. Once established, every effort should be given to stay within the budget. Trouble occurs with having no budget, having exaggerated projections of revenue, or encountering unanticipated expenses. For example, with the advent of increased MCO activity in a community, a history of yearly increases of revenues by 10% may be expected to decrease to a lower percentage for the following year. At the same time, shortages of nurses or therapists may require a mid-year upward adjustment in salaries. The combination of these factors can cause shortfalls of considerable amounts.

ORGANIZATIONAL CHANGE

One of the common ways that these factors are being addressed is by reorganization and downsizing. Usually these changes involve eliminating middle management positions, converting professional positions to paraprofessionals, and contracting out services at lower cost. For example, therapy heads and head nurses may be subsumed into a program director designation that combines several functions (Fig. 18-5). Medical managers should participate in such reorganization plans to advise on medical care needs so that downsizing does not have detrimental effects on patient care.

SUMMARY

This chapter provides a management overview beginning with basic concepts and outlining a few applications. The reader is referred to other references for expansion of this information. The books and periodicals listed are a good starting point. The *Primer on Management and Management for Rehabilitation Medicine* (13,14) includes expanded overviews. As mentioned earlier, *Finance and Accounting for Non-Financial Managers* (15) is a bridge between overviews and in-depth accounting and finance texts.

The American Academy of Physical Medicine and Rehabilitation has developed a *Practice Management Manual* (16) that may prove useful for a variety of areas, including marketing and promotion. The other sections covered in this manual are ''Managing Personnel,'' which includes details on equal opportunity employment; ''Hiring and Compensation,'' plus some legal issues; ''Finances and Operations''; ''Managed Care''; and, ''Risk.''

The American College of Physician Executives hold several courses each year geared to physician managers at varying levels of sophistication. They also have several publications that are helpful. Their address is 4890 W. Kennedy Boulevard, Suite 200, Tampa, Florida 33009-9944. They also publish a monthly journal, *Physician Executive,* which contains useful articles.

REFERENCES

1. Mintzberg H. The manager's job: folklore and fact. *Harvard Bus Rev* 1975; 53:45–61.
2. Kurtz ME. Role of a physician as manager. *Phys Med Rehabil State Art Rev* 1987; 1:185–196.
3. Lloyd J. Growth in medical director numbers continue. Witt Associates Inc. Results of a survey of 750 hospitals. American Academy of Medical Directors (now American College of Physician Executives). *Physician Executive* 1986; 12:10.
4. Ellwood P. Shattack lecture: outcomes management. A technology of patient experience. *N Engl J Med* 1988; 318:1549–1556.
5. Kurtz ME. Leadership styles. *Phys Med Rehabil State Art Rev* 1987; 1:197–212.
6. American Medical News. American Medical Association, August 5, 1997.
7. *Guide for Uniform Data Set for Medical Rehabilitation (Adult FIM^SM)*, Version 4.0, 1993. State University of New York, Buffalo, NY 14214.
8. Mintzberg H. Structure in 5's: a synthesis of the research on organization design. *Management Sci* 1980; 26:322–339.
9. *JCAHO 1996 Comprehensive Accreditation Manual for Hospitals.* JCAHO: Oakbrook Terrace, IL, 1995.
10. Fleming JW. Current issues in rehabilitation: the view from ProPac. American Rehabilitation Association Medical Rehab Report, May 1996.
11. Position Paper on Bundling of Post Acute Care Payments. American Academy of Physical Medicine and Rehabilitation. Chicago, August 1996.
12. Medicare Coverage of Inpatient Rehabilitation Services. Federal Register 50:31040–31042, July 31, 1985, Provided by transmittal 1293, September 12, 1986.
13. Maloney FP, ed. *A primer on management for rehabilitation medicine.* Philadelphia: Hanley & Belfus, 1987.
14. Maloney FP, Gray RP, eds. *Management for rehabilitation medicine II.* Philadelphia: Hanley & Belfus, 1993.
15. Finkler SA. *Accounting and finance for non-financial managers.* Englewood Cliffs, NJ: Prentice Hall, 1992.
16. American Academy of Physical Medicine and Rehabilitation. *Practice management manual.* Chicago: American Academy of Physical Medicine and Rehabilitation, 1997.

Rehabilitation Medicine: Principles and Practice, Third Edition,
edited by Joel A. DeLisa and Bruce M. Gans.
Lippincott–Raven Publishers, Philadelphia © 1998.

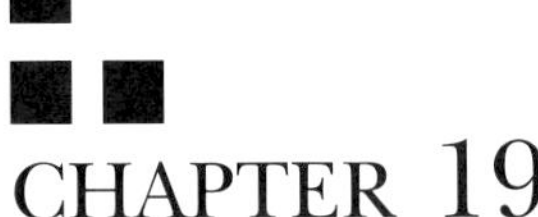

CHAPTER 19

Imaging Techniques Relative to Rehabilitation

Carson D. Schneck

A brief presentation of imaging techniques that are of interest to the physiatrist must necessarily be selective. Because the diagnosis and initial treatment of fractures is the responsibility of the orthopedic surgeon, with the rehabilitation professional typically involved only later in the course, a full discussion of fractures is not presented in this chapter. Only those fractures that bring patients under the long-term care of the physiatrist are included (e.g., vertebral fractures with the potential to damage the spinal cord). Similarly, tumors and infectious processes are de-emphasized. Rather, emphasis is placed on imaging degenerative musculoskeletal processes, spine and head trauma, stroke, and degenerative central nervous system (CNS) diseases commonly seen by the physiatrist.

In the past two decades, computed tomography (CT) and magnetic resonance imaging (MRI) have become the most sophisticated imaging modalities for evaluating the musculoskeletal system and the CNS. Therefore, this chapter focuses mainly on the recent applications of CT and MRI in the imaging of musculoskeletal and neural pathology of interest to the physiatrist.

MUSCULOSKELETAL IMAGING

CT images may be displayed with various windows suitable to resolve different structures. Bone window images provide the highest resolution of compact and cancellous bone. Soft-tissue window CT offers moderate resolution of muscle, tendon, ligament, fat, cartilage, and neural structures. CT imaging is typically performed in the axial (i.e., transverse) plane, with the option to reconstruct the data in any other plane. Some body parts can be inserted into the CT gantry in a manner in which direct imaging in sagittal or coronal planes could be achieved.

The good resolution and enhanced contrast of MRI for soft-tissue structures, together with its direct multiplanar imaging capability, make it a superb modality for evaluating all of the principal constituents of the musculoskeletal system. Although a technical discussion of the physics of MRI is beyond the scope of this chapter, the physiatrist should know the normal and abnormal MRI appearance of various tissues to be able to look at an MR image with confidence and explain the findings to a patient. The MRI signal intensity of any tissue primarily reflects its proton density, its T1 relaxation time, and its T2 relaxation time. Various techniques, including manipulating the repetition time (TR) between the application of radiofrequency pulses or the echo time (TE) between the radiofrequency pulse and the recording of a signal (i.e., echo) produced by the tissue, can emphasize the proton density, T1 relaxation time, or T2 relaxation time features of any tissue (1). The TR and TE are expressed in milliseconds. The most commonly used technique is spin echo, in which short TR and TE will emphasize the T1 relaxation time of a tissue, the so-called T1-weighted image. In general, an image is said to be T1 weighted if TR is less than 1,000 milliseconds and TE is less than 30 milliseconds (e.g., TR = 500 milliseconds, TE = 20 milliseconds). A T2-weighted image generally is accomplished with a TR longer than 1,500 milliseconds and a TE greater than 60 milliseconds (e.g., TR = 2,000 milliseconds, TE = 85 milliseconds). Proton density images are obtained with a long TR and a short TE (e.g., TR = 2,000 milliseconds, TE = 20 milliseconds).

Most normal tissues demonstrate similar signal intensities on both T1- and T2-weighted images. Compact bone, fibrocartilage, ligament, tendon, and the rapidly flowing blood within the blood vessel typically produce very low signal intensity, referred to as a signal void, and appear black (Fig. 19-1). Muscle demonstrates a moderately low signal intensity and appears dark gray. Peripheral nerves demonstrate a slightly higher signal intensity than muscle because of the fat content of their myelinated fibers. Hyaline cartilage produces moderate signal intensity and appears light gray. Fat

C. D. Schneck: Department of Anatomy and Cell Biology, Temple University School of Medicine, Philadelphia, Pennsylvania 19140.

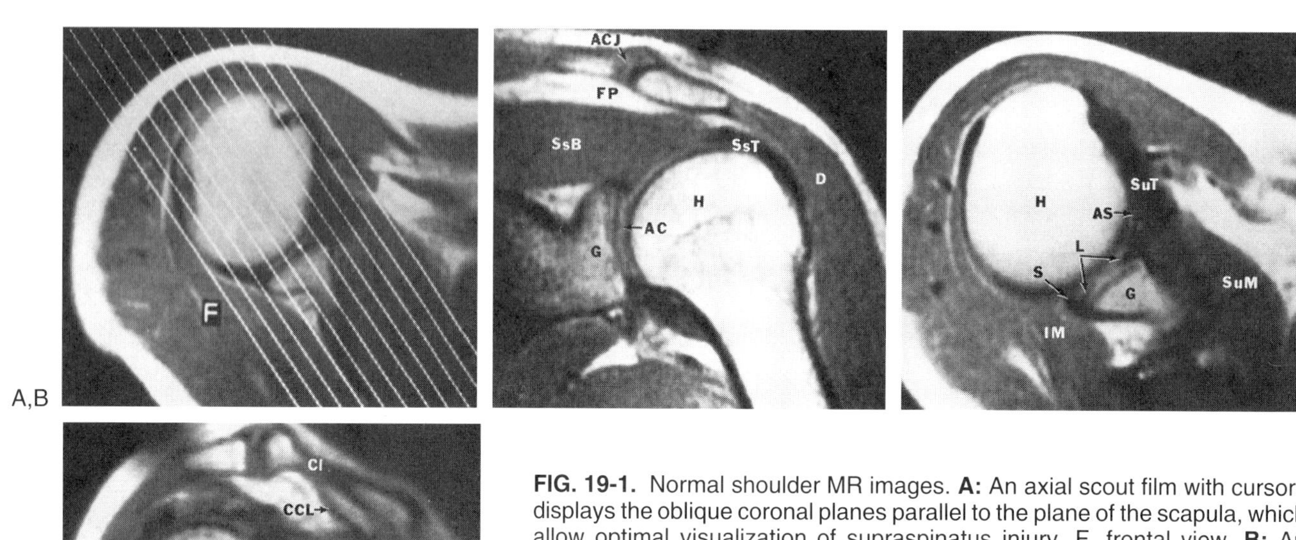

FIG. 19-1. Normal shoulder MR images. **A:** An axial scout film with cursors displays the oblique coronal planes parallel to the plane of the scapula, which allow optimal visualization of supraspinatus injury. F, frontal view. **B:** An oblique coronal image demonstrates the supraspinatus muscle belly *(SsB)*, supraspinatus tendon *(SsT)*, subacromial-subdeltoid fat plane *(FP)*, acromioclavicular joint *(ACJ)*, deltoid muscle *(D)*, articular cartilage of humeral head and glenoid *(AC)*, glenoid *(G)*, and humeral head *(H)*. **C:** An axial image displays humeral head *(H)*, glenoid *(G)*, glenoid labrum *(L)*, anterior shoulder capsule *(AS)*, posterior shoulder capsule *(PS)*, subscapsularis muscle *(SuM)*, subscapularis tendon *(SuT)*, and infraspinatus muscle *(IM)*. **D:** A coronal section demonstrates good resolution of the coracoclavicular ligament *(CCL)* extending from the coracoid process *(CP)* to the clavicle *(Cl)*.

produces very high signal intensity and appears white. Because fat is frequently situated adjacent to ligaments and tendons, it can provide a high contrast interface for evaluating the integrity of these structures. Adult bone marrow also shows high signal intensity because of its high fat content. Most normal body fluids that are not flowing show low signal intensity on T1-weighted images and high signal intensity on T2-weighted images.

Pathologic processes such as tumor, infection, and abnormal fluids (e.g., edema, joint effusion) show an intermediate signal intensity on T1-weighted images and become very hyperintense on T2-weighted images. Pathologic calcifications demonstrate very low signal intensity on both T1- and T2-weighted images.

The direct multiplanar imaging capability of MRI is particularly useful in evaluating obliquely oriented musculoskeletal structures such as the supraspinatus tendon, the cruciate ligaments, and the lateral collateral ligaments of the ankle.

MRI has proved useful in evaluating traumatic, degenerative, inflammatory, and neoplastic pathology of the limbs and spine. It is useful in detecting acute or chronic traumatic injuries and degenerative conditions involving bones, muscles, tendons, ligaments, fibrocartilage, and nerves. Bone pathology particularly well detected by MRI includes contusions, osteochondral injuries, stress fractures, and ischemic necrosis. Muscle lesions that MRI is especially sensitive at identifying include strain or contusion, complete rupture, compartment syndrome, myopathies, and atrophy (2). Tendon conditions well depicted by MRI include partial and complete tear, tendinitis, and tenosynovitis. MRI is also very sensitive for detecting partial or complete ligament tears. Fibrocartilaginous injuries or diseases well delineated by MRI include pathology of the menisci, the glenoid labrum, the triangular fibrocartilage of the wrist, and the intervertebral disc. Nerve entrapments well visualized by MRI include spinal nerve encroachment by disc disease or spinal stenosis and carpal tunnel syndrome (CTS) or other entrapment syndromes.

Osteomyelitis causes a reduction in bone marrow signal intensity on T1-weighted images because of the replacement of normal fatty marrow by inflammatory exudate. In T2-weighted images, these areas of active infection become hyperintense.

MRI has particular value in evaluating both bony and soft-tissue neoplasms. Most of them demonstrate moderately low signal intensity on T1-weighted images and very high signal intensity on T2-weighted images.

Emphasis will now be directed to the application of imaging modalities to common regional pathologic conditions of the musculoskeletal system. Particular focus will be given to MRI because of its superb soft-tissue imaging capabilities and its rapidly expanding diagnostic applications.

Shoulder

MRI has become valuable in evaluating a host of shoulder abnormalities very familiar to the physiatrist. These include impingement syndrome, other rotator cuff abnormalities, instability syndrome, and bicipital tendon abnormalities. It is also useful in demonstrating arthritic changes, occult fractures, ischemic necrosis, and intra-articular bodies. MRI shows particular promise in replacing invasive procedures such as conventional and CT arthrography for evaluating rotator cuff and labral pathology. The use of MRI for shoulder evaluation avoids radiation exposure to the nearby thyroid gland, which can occur with CT examinations. The excellent visualization of marrow by MRI permits early diagnosis of ischemic necrosis, infection, and primary or metastatic tumors.

Because of the oblique orientation of the scapula on the chest wall and the consequent anterolateral facing direction of the glenoid, the direct multiplanar imaging capability of MRI provides optimal visualization of all the important shoulder structures. Oblique coronal images parallel to the plane of the scapula provide full-length views of the rotator cuff musculature, especially the supraspinatus (Fig. 19-1*A* and *B*). Oblique sagittal imaging planes parallel to the glenoid provide cross-sectional views of the rotator cuff apparatus. Axial imaging planes provide good visualization of the anterior and posterior capsular apparatus, glenoid labrum, bony glenoid rim, and humeral head (Fig. 19-1*C*). Straight coronal images provide optimum views of the major stabilizer of the acromioclavicular joint, the coracoclavicular ligament (Fig. 19-1*D*).

Shoulder Impingement Syndrome and Supraspinatus Injury

The MRI findings of shoulder impingement syndrome and its associated supraspinatus injury are best seen on oblique coronal MR images that visualize the full length of the supraspinatus muscle belly and tendon (Fig. 19-1*B*). The normal muscle belly displays moderately low signal intensity. The tendon is visualized as a very low signal intensity structure that blends with the low signal intensity of the superior capsule as it courses to its insertion on the greater tubercle of the humerus. The inferior aspect of the tendon is delimited below by the moderate signal intensity of the hyaline cartilage on the superior aspect of the humeral head. The superior aspects of both the muscle belly and tendon are delimited by a high signal intensity subacromial and subdeltoid fat plane. The normal subacromial–subdeltoid bursa is not specifically visualized because its walls are separated only by monomolecular layers of a synovial-type fluid, but it is situated between the supraspinatus tendon and the fat plane. Above the fat plane, the clavicle, acromioclavicular joint, acromion, and deltoid muscle are demonstrated on different oblique coronal sections.

Neer stated that 95% of rotator cuff tears are associated with chronic impingement syndrome (3) and described three stages in the progression of rotator cuff injury. These can be visualized by MRI (4–6). Stage 1 is characterized by edema and hemorrhage within the supraspinatus tendon characteristic of an early tendinitis. On MRI, this appears as a diffuse moderate increase in signal intensity within the

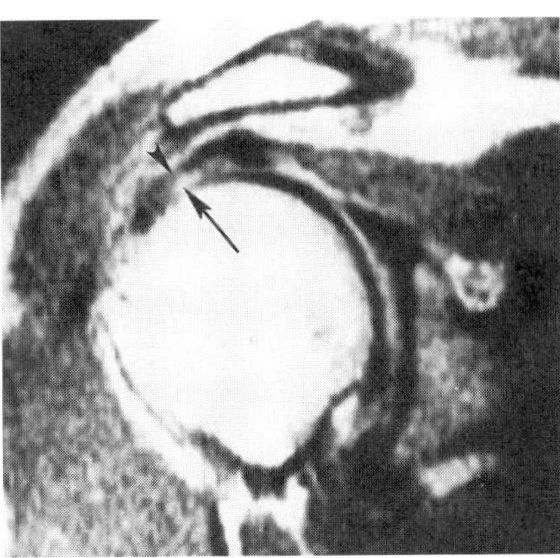

FIG. 19-2. T2-weighted MRI of a stage 2 partial supraspinatus injury demonstrates an area of high signal intensity within the critical zone of the tendon *(arrow)* and thinning and irregularity of the tendon *(arrowhead).*

tendon. In stage 2, Neer described both inflammation and fibrosis within the tendon; MRI shows this as thinning and irregularity of the tendon (Fig. 19-2). Stage 3 is a frank tear of the supraspinatus tendon. On MRI, complete tears are noted by a discontinuity of the tendon with a well-defined focus of high signal intensity on T2-weighted images (Fig. 19-3). The most susceptible area is the critical zone of hypovascularity, located about 1 cm from the insertion (7). With small or partial tears there is no retraction of the muscle–tendon junction, the subacromial–subdeltoid fat plane is commonly obliterated, and fluid may accumulate in the subacromial–subdeltoid bursa, which becomes hyperintense on T2-weighted images. There also may be effusion of the shoulder joint, which may extend inferiorly along the tendon sheath about the long head of the biceps. With a complete supraspinatus tendon tear, the muscle belly may retract medially, and atrophy may occur as the tear becomes chronic (Fig. 19-4). Muscle atrophy appears as areas of high signal intensity because of fatty replacement within the muscle belly and decreased muscle mass. Finally, the acromiohumeral interval narrows as the humeral head migrates superiorly, because of the loss of supraspinatus restraint to the deltoid's tendency to sublux the humerus superiorly during abduction.

Shoulder Instability and Disruption of the Anterior Capsular Mechanism

Axial MR images provide the best visualization of the anterior and posterior glenoid labra, capsule, and lower rotator cuff muscles (Fig. 19-1*C*). Anteriorly, the moderate signal intensity subscapularis muscle belly and its low signal intensity tendon are visualized. The tendon fuses with the low signal intensity anterior capsule as it courses to its insertion on the lesser tubercle. The fibrocartilaginous anterior and posterior labra appear as low signal intensity triangular or rounded areas attached to the glenoid rim. The higher signal intensity opposed hyaline cartilage surfaces of the

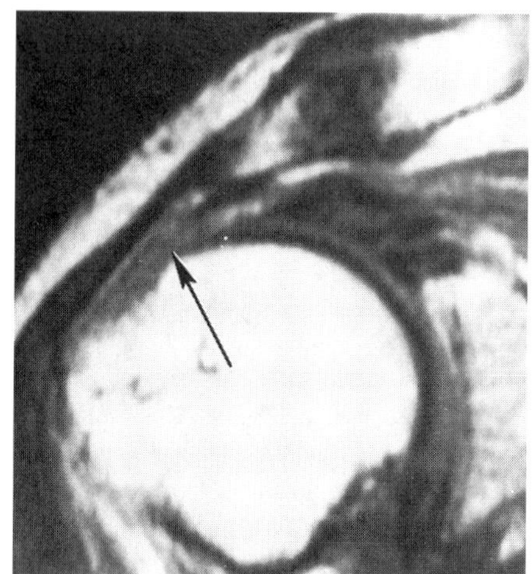
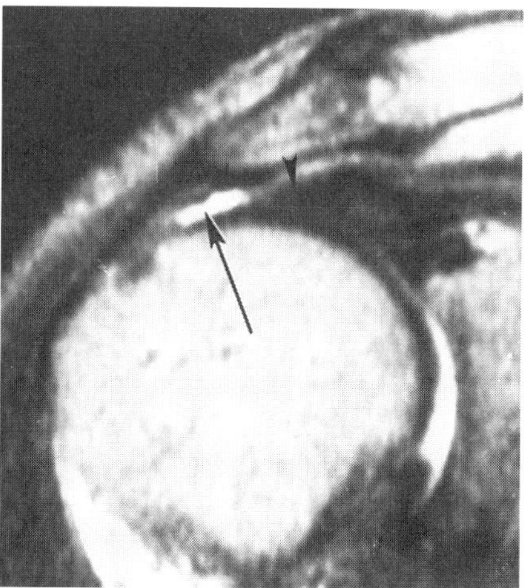

A,B

FIG. 19-3. Acute complete rupture of the supraspinatus tendon is seen in **(A)** a T1-weighted and **(B)** T2-weighted MRI. The T1-weighted image demonstrates a moderate signal intensity *(arrow)* where the signal void of the tendon should insert into the greater tubercle. This moderate intensity becomes hyperintense on the T2-weighted image *(arrow)*, indicating that it is an area of edema or subacute hemorrhage. The signal void of the tendon *(arrowhead)* has retracted medially. The humeral head is superiorly subluxed, and the subdeltoid fat plane is attenuated. A hyperintense joint effusion occupies the glenohumeral joint interval.

glenoid and humeral head separate the low signal intensity subarticular bone of the glenoid and humeral head, which is bounded deeply by high signal intensity marrow. The posterior capsule is visualized as a low-intensity area blending with the deep surface of infraspinatus and teres minor muscles as they extend to their insertions on the greater tubercle of the humerus. The long tendon of the biceps is demonstrated as a round, low signal intensity area within the intertubercular sulcus.

Shoulder instability and the associated disruption of the anterior capsular mechanism can cause chronic shoulder pain and disability. The instability may be caused by an acute traumatic episode or can occur with no history of a traumatic event. Both recurrent traumatic subluxation and nontraumatic instability are typically associated with disruption of the anterior capsular mechanism. Anteriorly, where most instability occurs, this mechanism includes the subscapularis muscle and tendon, the anterior joint capsule, three underlying glenohumeral ligaments, the synovial lining, and the anterior labrum. With instability, the labrum shows tears, separation from the glenoid rim, or degeneration (8). Also frequently present are medial stripping of the capsule from its normal attachment to the labrum and glenoid rim, an enlarged fluid-filled subscapular bursa secondary to joint effusion, attenuation of the glenohumeral ligaments, and injury or laxity of the subscapularis muscle or tendon.

By MRI, labral tears may be visualized as discrete linear areas of increased signal intensity within the normal signal void of the labrum (Fig. 19-5). These areas show moderate intensity on T1-weighted images and high intensity on T2-weighted images. With recurrent dislocation or subluxation, the labrum can become fragmented or attenuated.

Capsular detachment from the scapula (i.e., stripping) is visualized by T2-weighted MRI as an area of high signal intensity fluid dissecting medially from the glenoid rim (Fig. 19-5). With trauma to the subscapularis tendon there can be medial retraction of the muscle–tendon junction when the tendon is completely ruptured. Chronic atrophy of the subscapularis muscle belly is identified by high signal intensity fatty replacement. The glenoid marrow underlying a labral

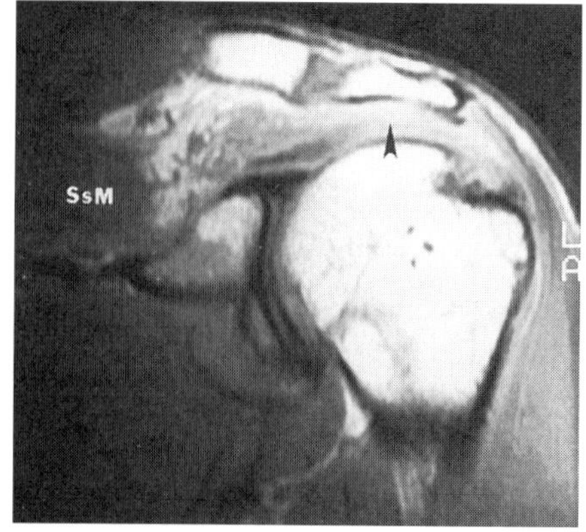

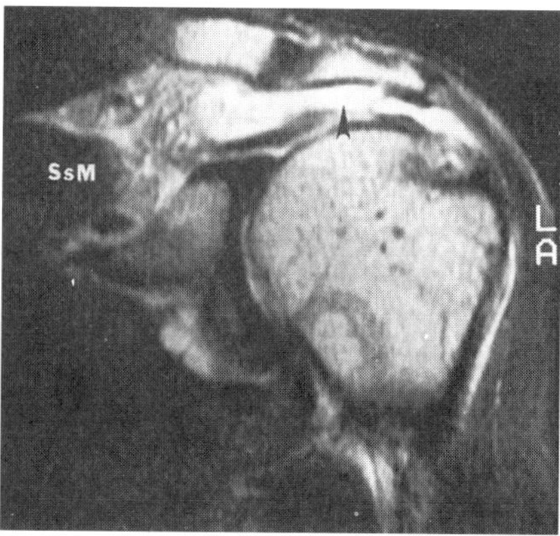

A,B

FIG. 19-4. Chronic complete rupture of the supraspinatus tendon is seen in **(A)** a T1-weighted MRI and **(B)** a T2-weighted MRI. The supraspinatus muscle *(SsM)* has totally retracted medially. On the T1-weighted image, the subacromial region normally occupied by the distal muscle and tendon shows a large area of moderate signal intensity *(arrowhead)* that becomes hyperintense on the T2-weighted image, indicating edema. The subacromial-subdeltoid fat plane is totally obliterated, and the humeral head is subluxed superiorly.

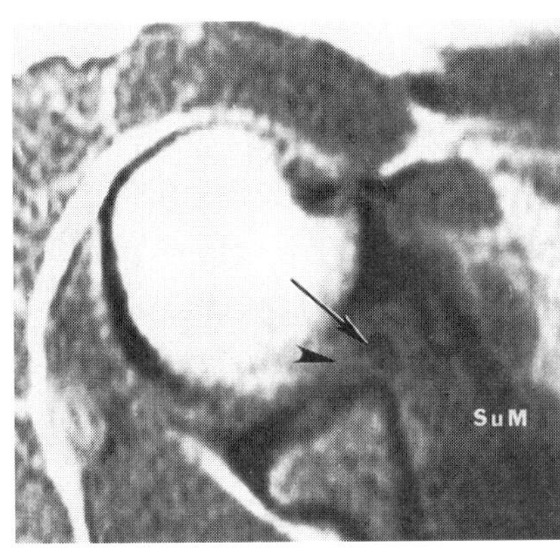

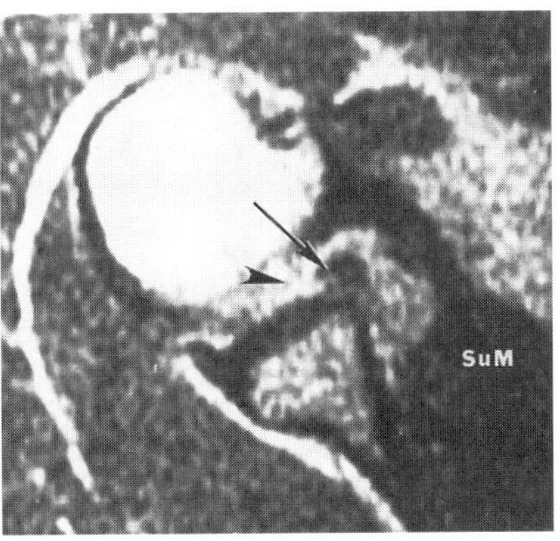

A,B

FIG. 19-5. Anterior labral detachment is seen in **(A)** a T1-weighted MRI and **(B)** a T2-weighted MRI. The anterior labrum *(arrow)* has been completely detached from the glenoid rim. The labral fragment is surrounded by moderate-intensity fluid *(arrowhead)* on the T1-weighted image; this fluid becomes hyperintense on the T2-weighted image. Because the fluid extends into the shoulder joint interval, it is joint effusion. The anterior capsule has been disrupted and the subscapularis muscle *(SuM)* elevated by extension of the effusion into the subscapular bursa.

detachment may show pathologically decreased signal intensity even before the plain film radiograph shows an osseous Bankart lesion. MRI and CT can be used to visualize Bankart fractures of the anterior glenoid and the Hill-Sachs compression deformity of the posterolateral humeral head (9,10). Patients with the rarer posterior instability show similar posterior labral, capsular, and muscular defects.

Tendinitis or Rupture of Other Shoulder Muscles

Tendinitis and rupture also can involve the subscapularis, infraspinatus, and teres minor or biceps tendons, although far less commonly than the supraspinatus. Early tendinitis involves an increased signal intensity area within the tendon. This can proceed to calcification, which is demonstrated by a signal void, sometimes with a surrounding high signal intensity rim of edema on T2-weighted images, as seen in subscapularis tendinitis (Fig. 19-6). This can progress to frank rupture of the tendon with a high signal intensity area at the site of the tear on T2-weighted images and may be associated with joint effusion. A complete tear will eventually cause muscle retraction and later atrophy.

Increased high-intensity fluid about the biceps tendon on T2-weighted MR images can be produced by either a biceps tenosynovitis or a shoulder joint effusion because the tendon sheath normally communicates with the shoulder. Rupture of the biceps tendon is demonstrated by absence of the biceps tendon within the intertubercular sulcus and by distal retraction of the muscle, which is seen on imaging the arm (11). Dislocation of the biceps tendon is identified by medial displacement of the biceps tendon out of the intertubercular sulcus.

Ischemic Necrosis of the Humeral Head

As in other joints, ischemic necrosis of the humeral head is depicted as an area of decreased signal intensity within the subarticular bone marrow in T1-weighted images (Fig. 19-7). On T2-weighted images, adjacent bright bands may

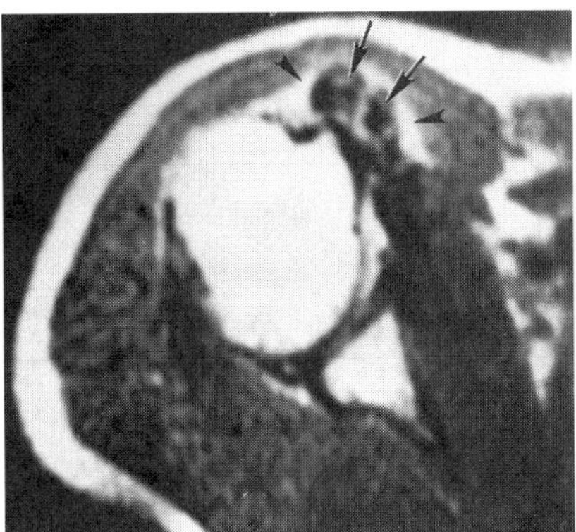

FIG. 19-6. Chronic subscapularis tendonitis with calcification. This T2-weighted MRI demonstrates two hypointense masses *(arrows)* protruding forward into the overlying deltoid muscle. The hypointensity and irregularity of the masses are compatible with calcification. The masses are surrounded with a hyperintense rim of edema *(arrowheads).*

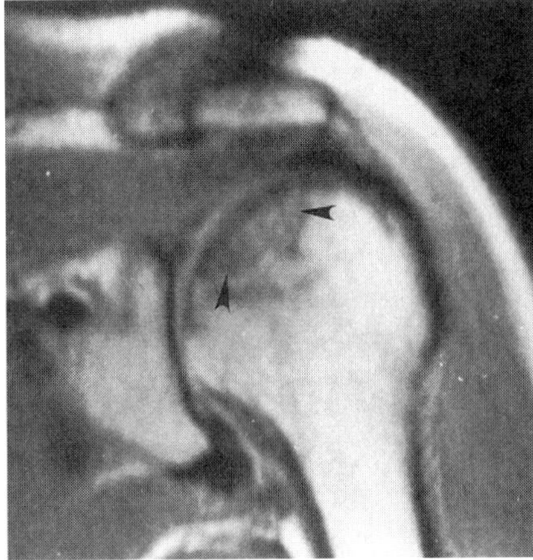

FIG. 19-7. Ischemic necrosis of the humeral head. On this T1-weighted MRI, the area of ischemic necrosis appears as a hypodense region *(arrowheads)* surrounded by a slightly darker band that indicates fibrosis of healing sclerotic bone.

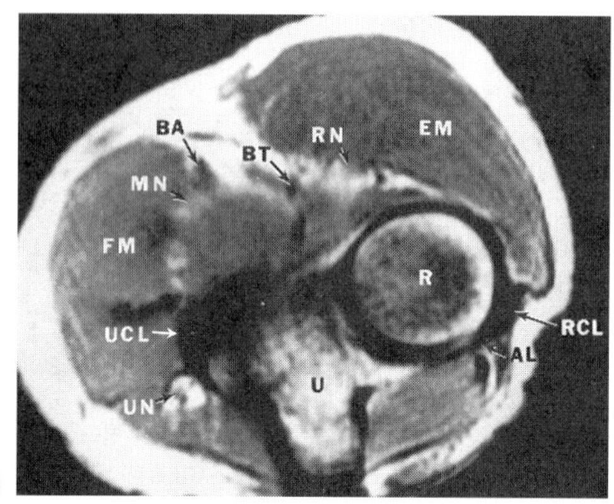

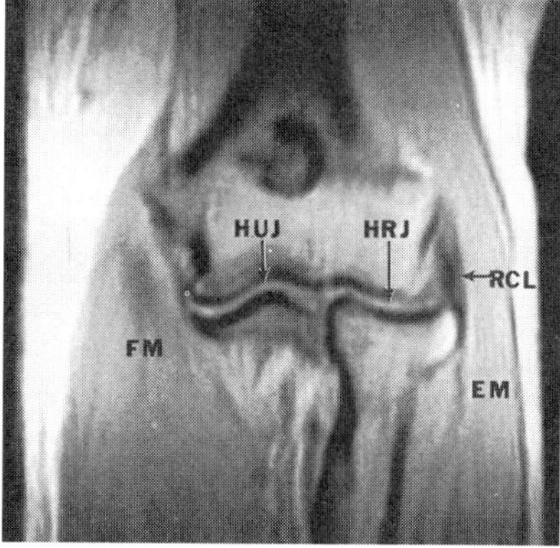

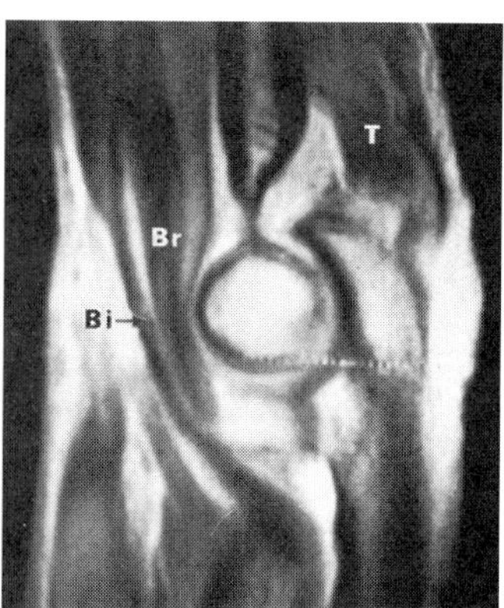

A,B C

FIG. 19-8. Normal elbow as seen on T1-weighted MR images. **A:** The axial MRI displays the ulna *(U)*, radius *(R)*, anular ligament *(AL)*, radial collateral ligament *(RCL)*, ulnar collateral ligament *(UCL)*, brachial artery *(BA)*, biceps tendon *(BT)*, forearm flexor muscles *(FM)*, forearm extensor muscles *(EM)*, median nerve *(MN)*, ulnar nerve *(UN)*, and radial nerve *(RN)*. **B:** The coronal MRI displays the humeroulnar joint *(HUJ)*, humeroradial joint *(HRJ)*, radial collateral ligament *(RCL)*, forearm flexor muscles *(FM)*, and forearm extensor muscles *(EM)*. **C:** The sagittal MRI through the humeroulnar joint demonstrates the biceps *(Bi)*, brachialis *(Br)*, and triceps *(T)*.

indicate edema, and adjacent darker bands may represent fibrosis or healing sclerotic bone. Ischemic necrosis is more fully described with the hip, where its incidence is higher.

Elbow

MRI has not been applied to the evaluation of elbow pathology as extensively as it has to other large joints, but its ability to visualize all of the bony, ligamentous, muscular, neural, and vascular structures around the elbow offers great promise for the detection of elbow lesions (12).

Axial MRI views of the elbow region permit good visualization of the biceps, brachialis, triceps, and all of the extensor and flexor muscles of the forearm (Fig. 19-8*A*). High signal intensity fat planes and low signal intensity intermuscular septa permit clear delineation of each muscle and their tendons of insertion or origin. Axial images clearly depict brachial, ulnar, and radial arteries and all of the subcutaneous and deep veins. They also allow identification of the ulnar nerve within the cubital tunnel and the radial nerve in the brachioradialis–brachialis interval and under the supinator muscle's arcade of Frohse, where it is commonly entrapped. The median nerve is visualized at all of its common elbow entrapment sites, including under the bicipital aponeurosis, between the heads of the pronator teres, and under the fibrous arch of the flexor digitorum superficialis.

The humeroulnar, humeroradial, and proximal radioulnar joint spaces and articular cartilages are well visualized on both coronal and sagittal MR images (Fig. 19-8*B* and *C*). The low signal intensity ulnar collateral, radial collateral, and anular ligaments are depicted on both axial and coronal MR images. Sagittal images delineate the anterior and posterior subsynovial fat pads.

MRI has the capability of directly visualizing traumatic rupture of the anular and the radial and ulnar collateral ligaments. These appear as discontinuities of the low signal intensity ligament. The T2-weighted images disclose hyperintense edema and hemorrhage between the torn ends of the ligament and extending into the joint interval and adjacent soft tissues (Fig. 19-9).

MRI also provides good visualization of the sites of muscle injury about the elbow (13). Figure 19-10 shows a case of direct forearm trauma causing hemorrhage and edema

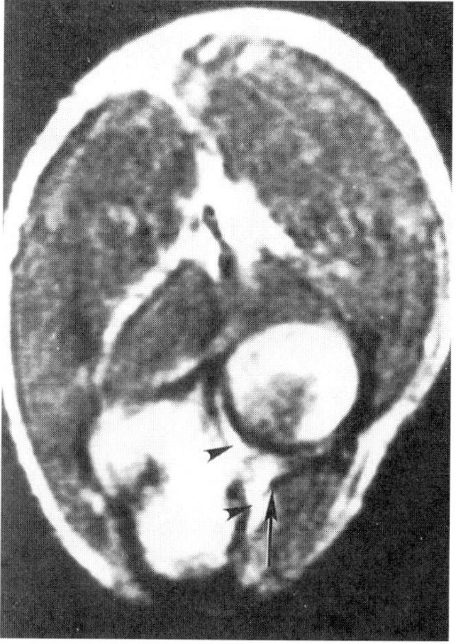

FIG. 19-9. Football-induced rupture of the anular ligament. This T2-weighted MRI shows the disruption of the posterior attachment of the anular ligament to the ulna *(arrow)*. The hyperintense area between the torn end of the ligament and the ulna, which extends deeply into the proximal radioulnar joint interval and superficially into the overlying anconeus muscle, is edema and hemorrhage *(arrowheads)*.

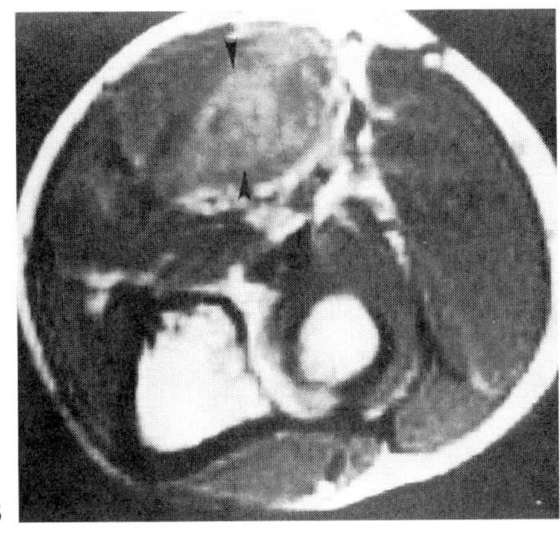
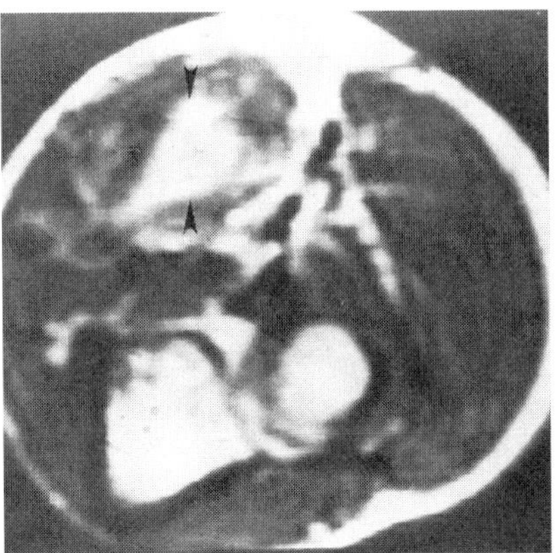

A,B

FIG. 19-10. Pronator teres injury with median nerve entrapment neuropathy is seen on **(A)** a T1-weighted MRI and **(B)** a T2-weighted MRI. The pronator teres displays an abnormal, moderately intense signal *(between arrowheads)* on the T1-weighted image that becomes hyperintense on the T2-weighted image, indicating the presence of edema and hemorrhage secondary to direct trauma. Because the median nerve typically penetrates the pronator teres at this level (see Fig. 19-8*A*), this is the likely entrapment site of the median nerve.

largely confined to the pronator teres muscle in a patient who also demonstrated distal median nerve signs and symptoms. The T1-weighted image shows a slight increase in signal intensity in this muscle, which becomes very hyperintense on the T2-weighted image, especially within the pronator teres. Because the median nerve traverses the pronator teres, this is a likely etiologic site for the clinical median nerve findings, although a forearm flexor compartment syndrome is also a possibility. Figure 19-11 depicts a case of muscle strain produced by a weight-lifting injury that caused pain and swelling of the anterior forearm. Only the T1-weighted image was available, and it demonstrates increased signal intensity in the muscle belly of the pronator teres, flexor carpi radialis, and flexor digitorum superficialis, which extended well down the forearm.

MRI also has the potential to demonstrate tendinitis involving the common extensor and flexor tendon origins from the lateral and medial aspects of the humerus with findings similar to those described in tendinitis about the shoulder. It also can display degenerative joint disorders about the elbow.

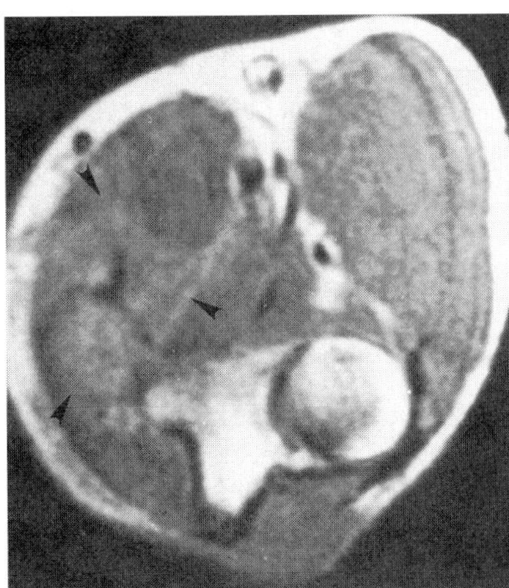

FIG. 19-11. Weight lifting-induced muscle strain. The T1-weighted MRI shows moderately increased signal intensity *(between arrowheads)* involving the deep part of the pronator teres, flexor carpi radialis, and flexor digitorum superficialis compatible with intramuscular hemorrhage and edema.

Wrist

Plain film radiography and CT provide good visualization of the bony structures of the wrist, and arthrography and CT arthrography provide information about ligamentous disorders of the wrist. The ability of MRI to visualize soft-tissue pathology already has been shown to be of great value in assessing CTS and may prove useful in imaging cases of unexplained wrist pain (14–17).

Axial MR images through the wrist from the distal radioulnar joint to the metacarpals provide excellent visualization of all of the bones, joints, ligaments, muscles, tendons, nerves, and vessels in the wrist area (Fig. 19-12). They also clearly display all of the boundaries and contents of the carpal tunnel and Guyon's canal.

Carpal Tunnel Syndrome

MRI can serve as an adjunct diagnostic tool for CTS when the clinical or neurophysiologic findings are equivocal. There are four universal findings of CTS visible by MRI regardless of etiology:

1. Swelling of the median nerve (i.e., pseudoganglion) in the proximal part of the carpal tunnel at the level of the pisiform
2. Increased signal intensity of the edematous median nerve on T2-weighted images
3. Palmar bowing of the flexor retinaculum
4. Flattening of the median nerve in the distal carpal tunnel at the level of the hamate (Fig. 19-13)

MRI also has the potential to establish the cause of CTS. Some of the etiologies visualized by MRI include traumatic tenosynovitis (Fig. 19-14), rheumatoid tenosynovitis (Fig. 19-15), a ganglion cyst of a carpal joint, excessive fat within

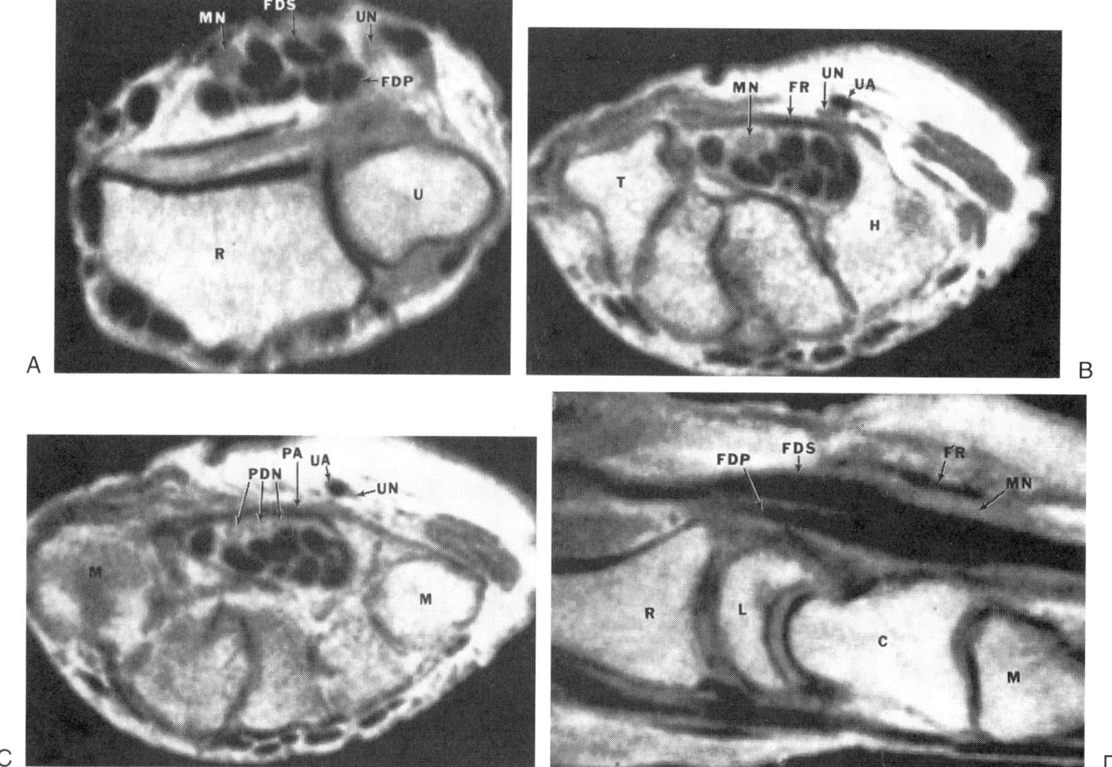

FIG. 19-12. Normal wrist as seen on T1-weighted MR images. Axial MR images are at the levels **(A)** of the distal radioulnar joint, **(B)** the distal carpal tunnel, and **(C)** just distal to the carpal tunnel. Longitudinal MRI **(D)** through the median nerve within the carpal tunnel. *C*, capitate; *FDP*, flexor digitorum profundus; *FDS*, flexor digitorum superficialis; *FR*, flexor retinaculum; *H*, hamate; *L*, lunate; *M*, metacarpals; *MN*, median nerve; *PDN*, palmar digital branches of the median nerve; *R*, radius; *T*, trapezium; *U*, ulna; *UA*, ulnar artery; *UN*, ulnar nerve.

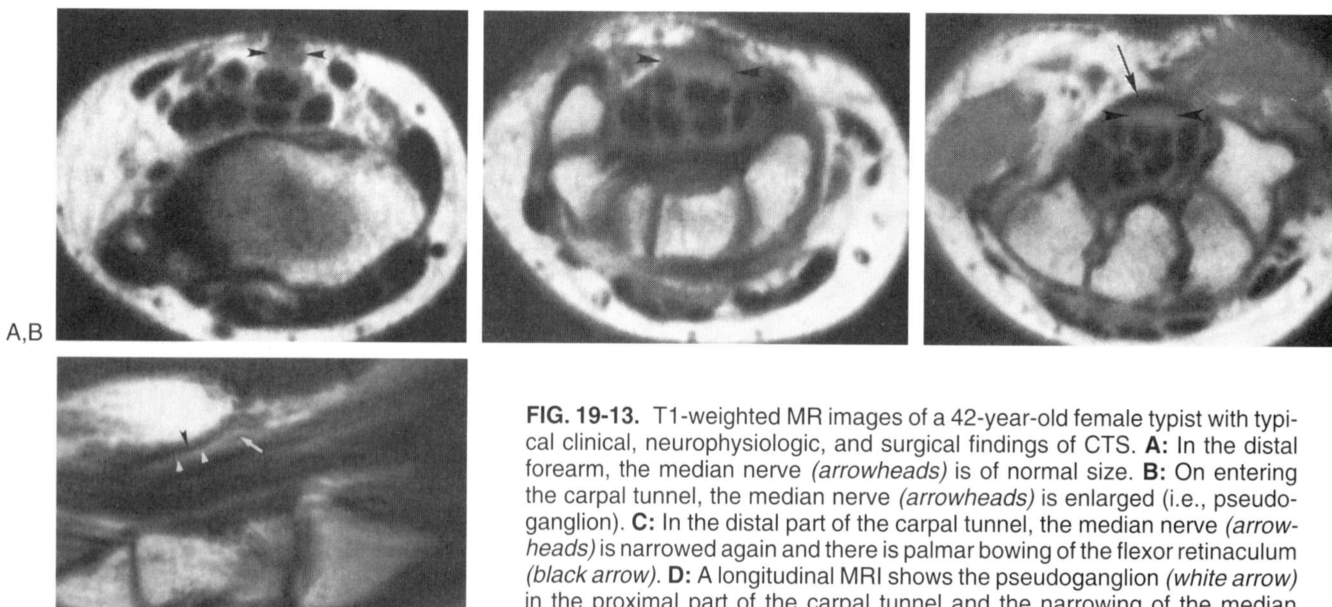

FIG. 19-13. T1-weighted MR images of a 42-year-old female typist with typical clinical, neurophysiologic, and surgical findings of CTS. **A:** In the distal forearm, the median nerve *(arrowheads)* is of normal size. **B:** On entering the carpal tunnel, the median nerve *(arrowheads)* is enlarged (i.e., pseudoganglion). **C:** In the distal part of the carpal tunnel, the median nerve *(arrowheads)* is narrowed again and there is palmar bowing of the flexor retinaculum *(black arrow)*. **D:** A longitudinal MRI shows the pseudoganglion *(white arrow)* in the proximal part of the carpal tunnel and the narrowing of the median nerve *(white arrowheads)* in the distal carpal tunnel where it lies deep to the flexor retinaculum *(black arrowhead)*.

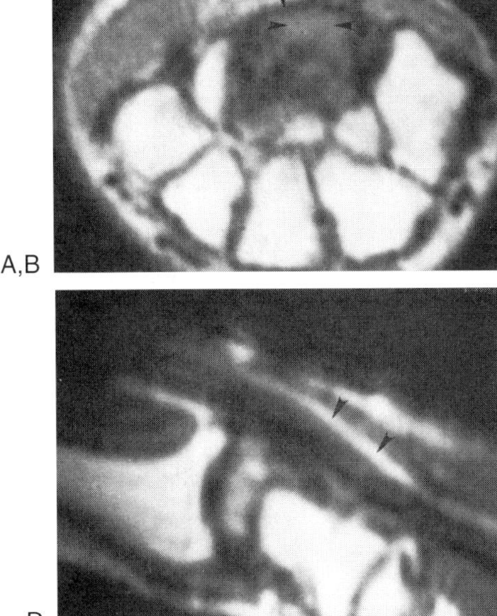

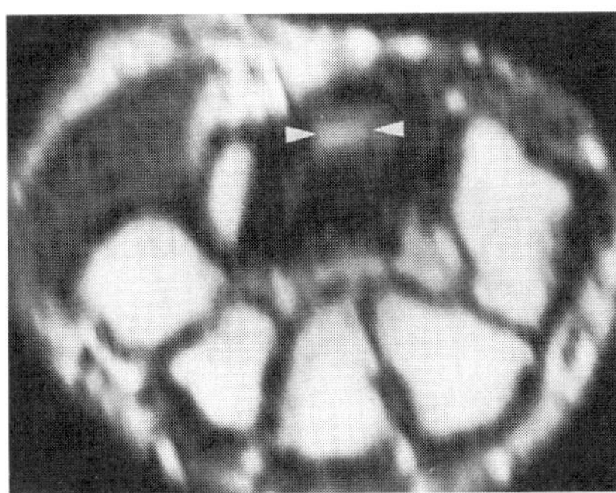

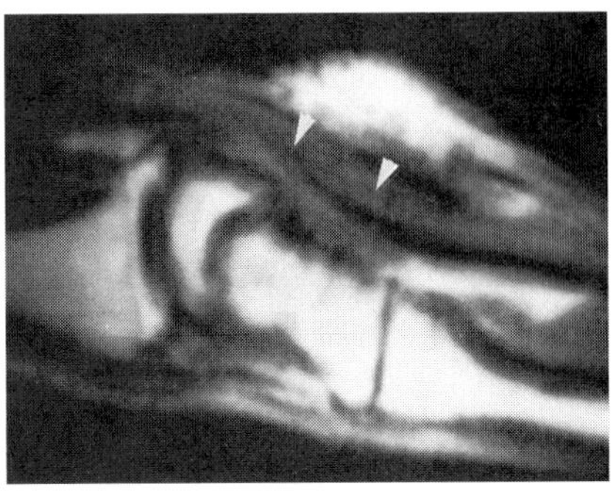

FIG. 19-14. A 33-year-old man with CTS caused by a traumatic tenosynovitis that was relieved by corticosteroid injection. **A:** A T1-weighted axial MRI demonstrates poor definition of the tendons under the flexor retinaculum because of the tenosynovitis. The median nerve *(arrowheads)* is poorly defined beneath the palmarly bowed flexor retinaculum *(arrow)*. **B:** A T2-weighted axial MRI shows increased signal intensity within the edematous median nerve *(arrowheads)*. A comparison of **(C)** T1-weighted and **(D)** T2-weighted sagittal MR images demonstrates that the moderate signal intensity of the median nerve *(arrowheads)* on the T1-weighted image becomes hyperintense *(arrowheads)* on the T2-weighted image.

the carpal tunnel, a hypertrophied adductor pollicis muscle in the floor of the carpal tunnel, and a persistent median artery (15).

MRI also provides a means of postoperative evaluation of those patients in whom the symptoms persist, to ensure that the flexor retinaculum has been completely incised and that there are no other complicating postoperative factors producing continuing discomfort. When the flexor retinaculum has been completely incised, the incision site is well documented by MRI and the contents of the carpal tunnel are typically displaced forward (Fig. 19-16*A*). If the distal part of the flexor retinaculum has been incompletely incised, this can be demonstrated by MRI, and the preoperative MRI findings of CTS will persist (Fig. 19-16*B* and *C*).

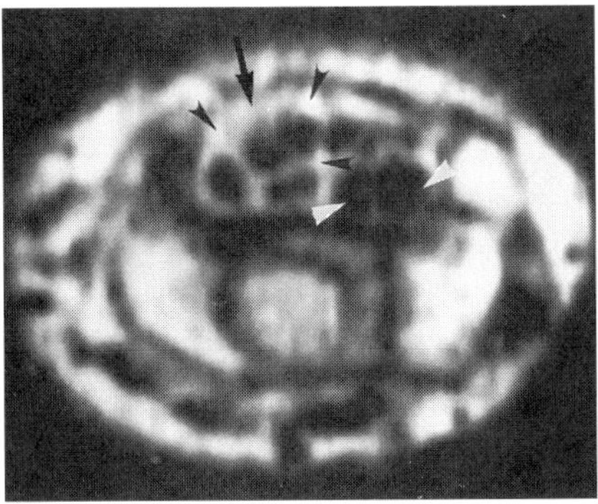

FIG. 19-15. A T2-weighted image of a 53-year-old woman with CTS caused by rheumatoid tenosynovitis. There is a high signal intensity edema *(black arrowheads)* surrounding the median nerve *(black arrow)* and the more radial tendons in the carpal tunnel. The more ulnarly situated flexor digitorum tendons are matted together into a low signal intensity mass characteristic of chronic fibrosis *(white arrowheads)*.

Other Wrist Abnormalities

MRI can visualize postincisional neuromas as lobulated masses in the typical location of the palmar cutaneous branches of the median nerve, which lie between the long digital flexor tendons and superficial to the lumbrical muscles (Fig. 19-17). It can also demonstrate tenosynovitis involving any of the tendons crossing the wrist (Fig. 19-18). MRI also displays marrow abnormalities such as replacement by tumor or ischemic necrosis of the proximal fragment of a scaphoid fracture where the marrow shows reduced signal intensity (18). The ability of MRI to visualize the carpal collateral ligaments, all of the palmar, dorsal, and intercarpal ligaments, and the triangular fibrocartilage also offers promise of visualizing the ligamentous disruptions responsible for carpal instabilities (19).

Hip

MRI of the hip is usually performed in standard axial, coronal, and sagittal planes. The normal marrow of the femoral head epiphysis and the greater trochanter displays very high signal intensity and is surrounded by a thin layer of compact bone that appears as a signal void. However, in children and young adults the marrow of the femoral neck and shaft normally shows a lower signal intensity, because it contains some residual hematopoietic marrow. The acetabulum has imaging characteristics similar to those of the femoral neck. The periphery of the hip joint interval displays the moderate signal intensity of the apposed hyaline cartilage surfaces of the femoral head and acetabulum, whereas the centrally situated acetabular notch contains high signal intensity fat. The thick, very low signal intensity hip joint capsule blends with the acetabular labrum proximally and

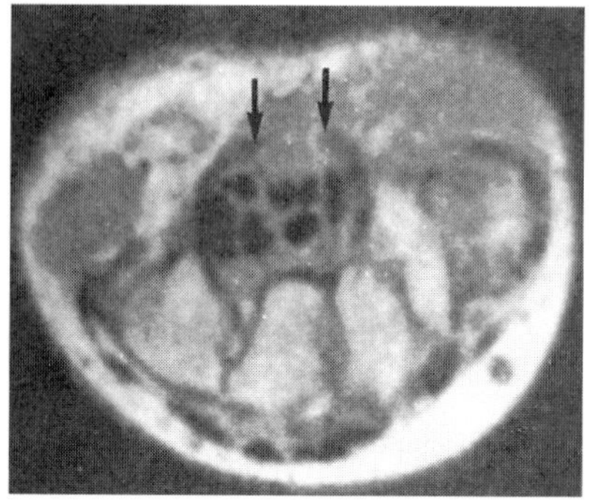
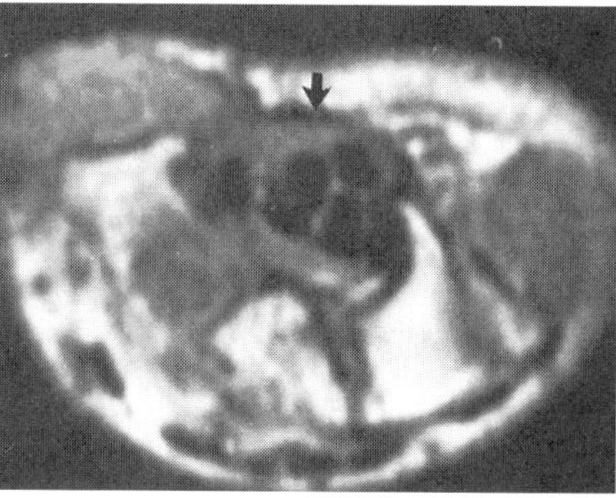
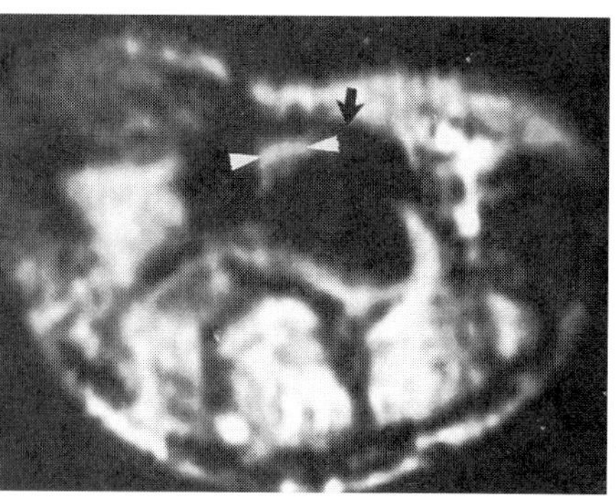
A,B C

FIG. 19-16. MRI evaluation of the postoperative CTS patient. **A:** A satisfactory surgical incision of the flexor retinaculum was obtained in the patient seen in Figure 19-13. The incised ends of the flexor retinaculum *(black arrows)* are displaced palmarward, as are the median nerve and tendon contents of the carpal tunnel. T1-weighted **(B)** and T2-weighted **(C)** images of a patient whose CTS symptoms persisted after surgery. The proximal flexor retinaculum had been cut, but both of these images display an intact palmarly bowed distal flexor retinaculum *(black arrows)*. The median nerve *(white arrowheads)* is still hyperintense on the T2-weighted image, indicating its continued inflammation.

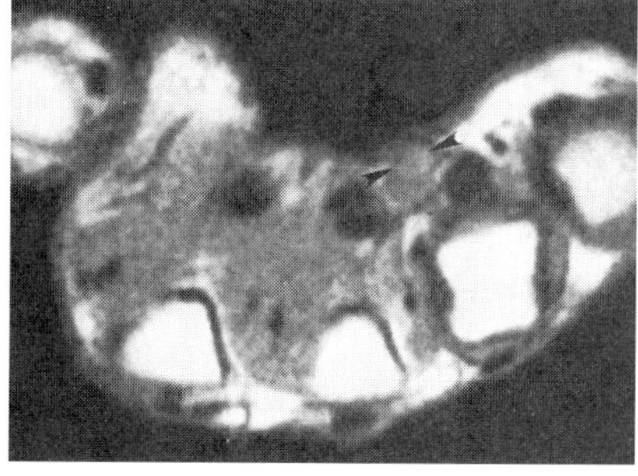

FIG. 19-17. A T1-weighted MRI of a patient with multiple traumatic neuromas that produced pain in the distribution of the median nerve. One of these lobulated masses *(arrowheads)* is lying in the position of a palmar digital branch of the median nerve anterior to the lumbrical muscle in the interval between the long flexor tendons of the digits.

the cortex of the femoral neck distally. All of the muscles, nerves, and blood vessels crossing the hip are well visualized.

Ischemic Necrosis

One of the common indications for MRI of the hip is to determine the presence of ischemic necrosis. This is bone death produced by a compromised blood supply. It also has been called avascular necrosis, osteonecrosis, or aseptic necrosis. Predisposing factors that should raise the physician's index of suspicion include corticosteroid therapy, alcoholism, known hip trauma, chronic pancreatitis, Gaucher's disease, sickle cell disease, exposure to hypobaric conditions, subcapital fractures, childhood septic arthritis or osteomyelitis of the hip, and congenital hip dislocation (20). If undetected early, the disease can progress and finally undergo irreversible collapse of the femoral head. MRI has been dem-

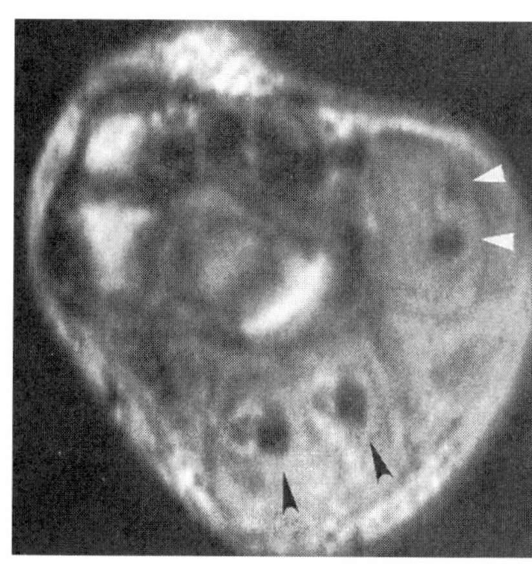
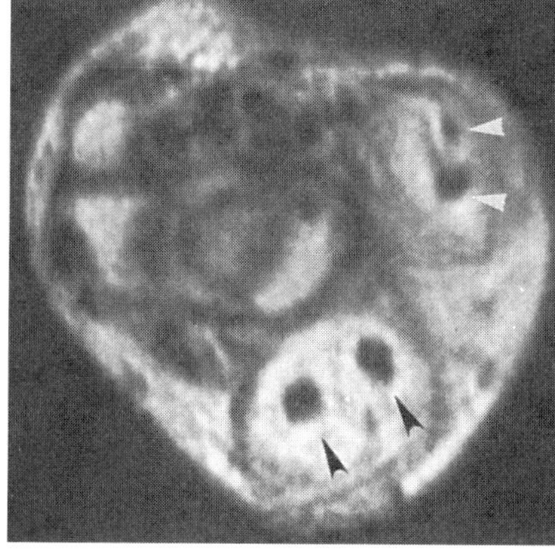
A,B

FIG. 19-18. Tuberculous tenosynovitis of the tendon sheaths around the abductor pollicis longus and extensor pollicis brevis *(white arrowheads)* and the extensor carpi radialis longus and brevis *(black arrowheads)*. **A:** The T1-weighted MRI displays the edema as moderate signal intensity. **B:** The T2-weighted MRI depicts the edema as hyperintense.

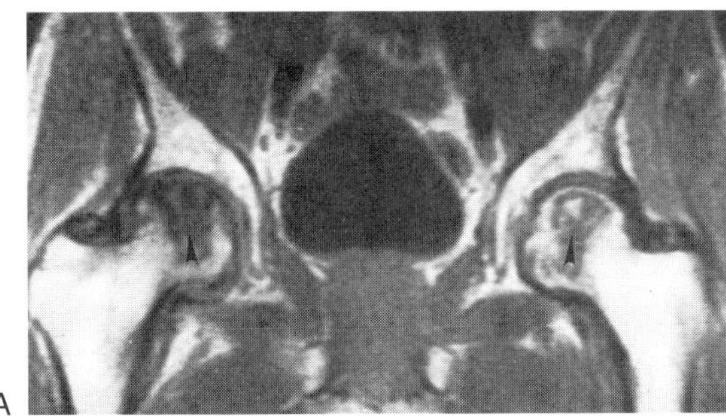

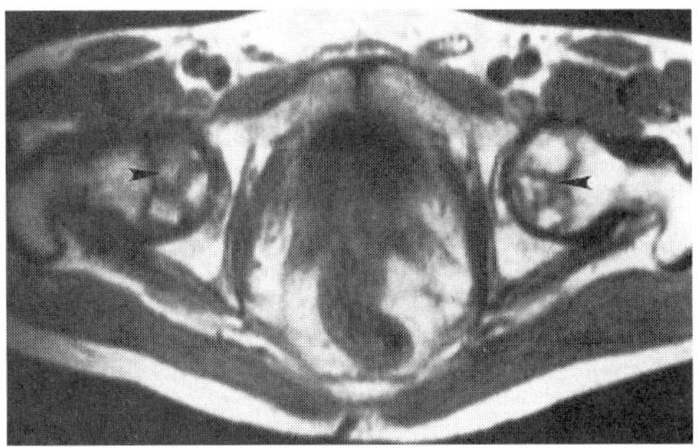

FIG. 19-19. Bilateral ischemic necrosis of the femoral head is seen in **(A)** a coronal T1-weighted MRI and **(B)** an axial T1-weighted MRI. The ischemic necrosis is visualized as relatively well-delimited marrow regions of reduced signal intensity fibrosis *(arrowheads)* with a margin of even lower intensity sclerotic bone.

onstrated to be even more sensitive and specific than bone scintigraphy for the early diagnosis of ischemic necrosis of the femoral head (21–24).

On T1-weighted MRI, the foci of ischemic necrosis of the femoral head appear as homogeneous or inhomogeneous well-delimited or diffuse areas of decreased signal intensity in the shape of rings, bands, wedges, or crescents, or in an irregular configuration (Fig. 19-19) (25,26). The low signal intensity is caused by death of marrow fat and replacement of the marrow by a fibrous connective tissue. Some cases show a lower signal band surrounding the lesion, and this has been attributed to healing sclerotic bone at the interface between normal and necrotic bone. On T2-weighted images, many cases show a double-line sign with a high signal intensity zone just inside of a low signal intensity margin. This is thought to be produced by granulation tissue surrounded by sclerotic bone (24–26).

Other Hip Abnormalities

Transient regional osteoporosis presents with a low signal intensity lesion on T1-weighted images that is similar to ischemic necrosis, but it typically involves both femoral head and neck and becomes hyperintense on T2-weighted images, suggesting the presence of edema. MRI demonstrates osteoarthritic subchondral sclerosis as low signal intensity zones in the subchondral marrow of both the femoral head and acetabulum. MRI also has been found to be very useful for identifying stress or occult fractures. These appear as low signal intensity areas containing an oblique or wavy line of still lower signal intensity, representing the actual fracture site. On T2-weighted images these areas become hyperintense, suggesting that they are edema. MRI also can identify many types of soft-tissue abnormalities about the hip. Figure 19-20 demonstrates a giant synovial cyst extending along the iliopsoas muscle up into the pelvic inlet region.

Another hip region imaging application of potential interest to physiatrists involves the use of technetium bone scanning to evaluate recently described "thigh splints" caused by exaggerated stride length by short female basic trainees in the unisex-oriented military (27). Seven cases of thigh pain in female recruits at one military base were imaged after administration of technetium 99, with the expectation of finding stress fractures. Instead, the scans showed longitudinal linear accentuation sites in the upper or mid-femur that were consistent with periosteal elevation and corresponded with the sites of insertion of one or more of the adductor muscles (Fig. 19-21). The reason these findings occur only

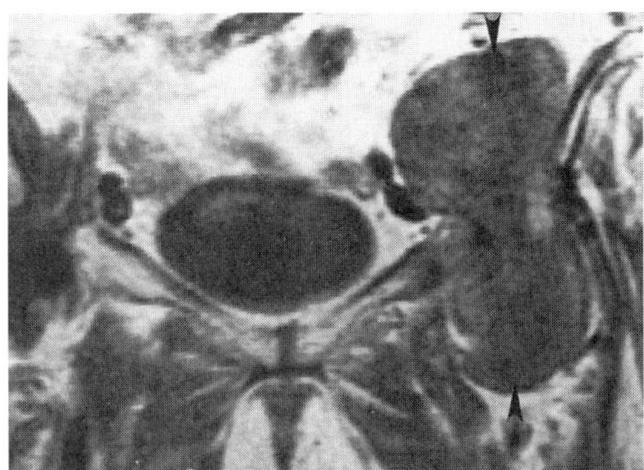

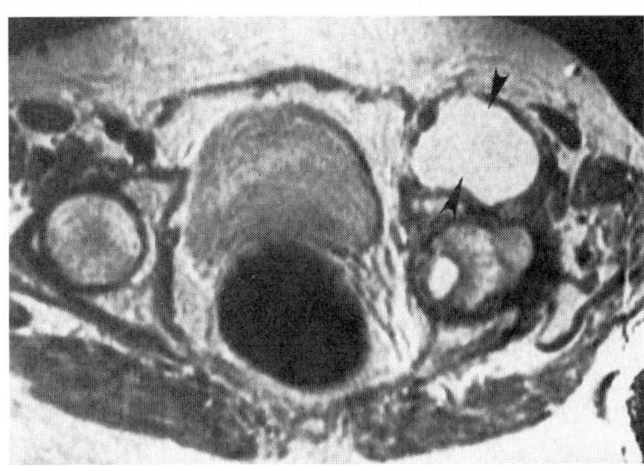

FIG. 19-20. Giant synovial cyst secondary to rheumatoid arthritis of the hip. **A:** A T1-weighted coronal MRI displays a hypointense giant synovial cyst *(arrowheads)* extending from the thigh to the pelvis. **B:** A T2-weighted axial MRI shows the synovial cyst as hyperintense *(arrowheads).* The inflammatory rheumatoid changes in the left femoral heads are also hyperintense.

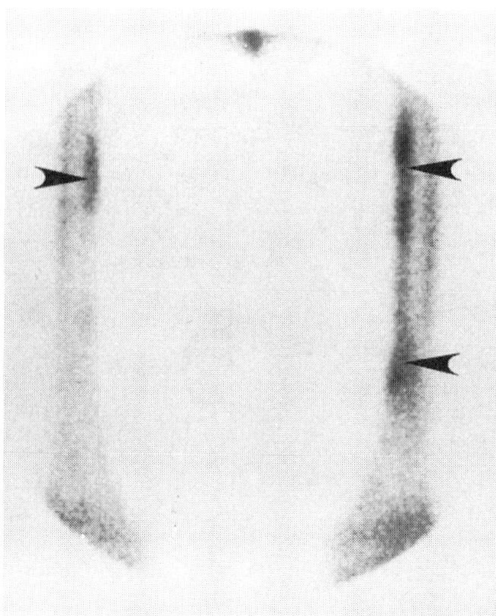

FIG. 19-21. Thigh splint sites demonstrated by technetium 99 scintigraphy. The accentuation sites *(arrowheads)* correspond to the insertions of the adductor longus and magnus muscles.

in female trainees is explained by a Saunders and colleagues' classic description of pelvic rotation as the first of their six determinants of gait (28). Because the shorter female recruits had to march with taller males, their stride had to be lengthened to maintain straight lines of march, and exaggerating the normal pelvic rotation lengthens stride. The adductor muscles are important pelvic rotators, and their overuse apparently produced avulsion and elevation of the periosteum adjacent to their femoral insertions.

Knee

The use of MRI in the evaluation of bony and soft-tissue derangements of the knee has increased substantially in recent years. MRI of the knee is the most commonly performed non-neurologic MRI study. At most institutions it has completely replaced knee arthrography as a diagnostic tool (29).

Meniscal Injuries

All parts of both menisci are well visualized by MRI. Sagittal MR images provide good views of the anterior and posterior horns and a fair view of the body of both menisci. In more central sections, both horns of the menisci appear as wedge-shaped signal voids contrasted on their superior and inferior surfaces by the moderate signal intensity of the hyaline cartilage on the articular surfaces of the femur and tibia (Fig. 19-22*A*). In more peripheral sections, where the images are tangential to the circumference of the menisci, they appear bow tie shaped (Fig. 19-22*B*). Coronal MR images provide the best visualization of the bodies of both menisci.

There are three types of meniscal findings visualized by MRI (11,30,31). One is the presence of small globular or irregular high signal intensity foci confined to the interior of the meniscus. This is considered to be an early type of mucoid degeneration. A second type of meniscal MRI finding is the presence of a linear region of increased signal intensity within the meniscus that does not extend to either the femoral or tibial articular surface of the meniscus but may extend to the meniscocapsular junction. Histologically, this represents fragmentation and separation of the fibrocartilage and is considered by many to be an intrameniscal tear. The significance of the globular or linear signals that do not extend to either articular surface of the meniscus is not fully agreed upon (32). Frank meniscal tears are demonstrated by MRI as linear or irregular areas of signal intensity that extend to one or both articular surfaces of the meniscus (Fig. 19-23*A*). The high signal intensity is produced by synovial fluid in the crevices within the meniscus. These meniscal tears can be horizontal, vertical, or complex. Bucket-handle tears are vertical tears where the inner meniscal fragment is displaced toward the intercondylar notch (Fig. 19-23*B*). At times, repeated trauma or chronic degeneration may cause a gross distortion of meniscal shape, and the meniscus may then appear to have a truncated apex or to be grossly small with a free fragment (Fig. 19-23*C*).

Other meniscal abnormalities well visualized by MRI in-

A,B

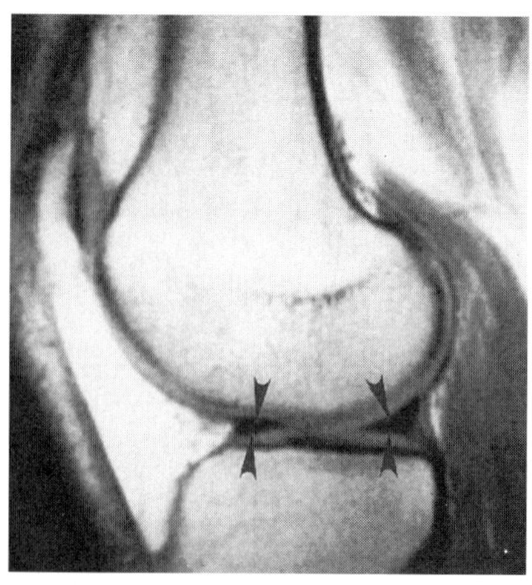

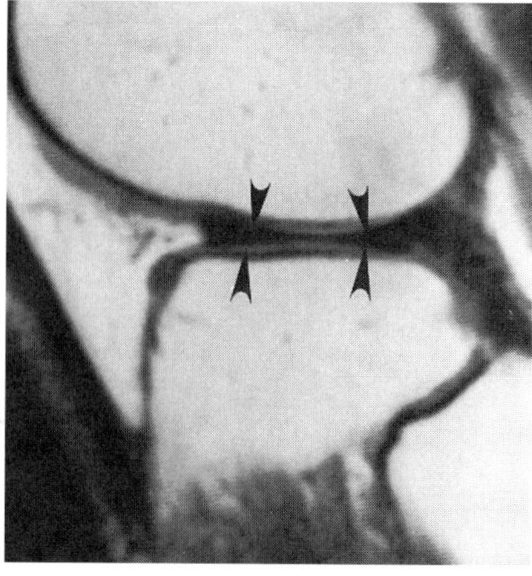

FIG. 19-22. Sagittal MR images through normal menisci. **A:** More central section through the anterior and posterior horns of the lateral menisci where they appear wedge-shaped *(arrowheads)*. **B:** More peripheral cut through the body of the lateral meniscus where it appears bowtie shaped *(arrowheads)*.

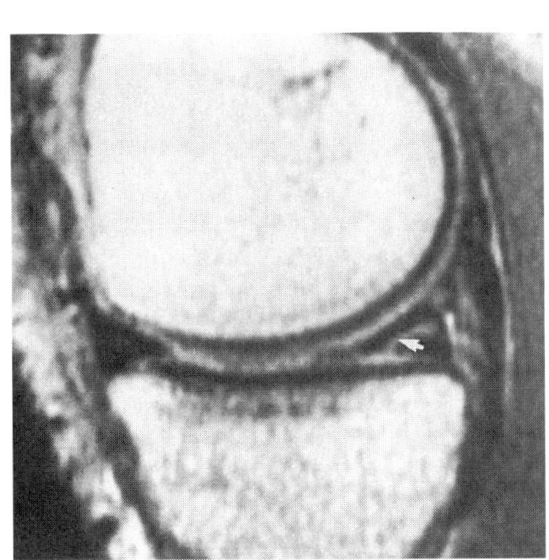
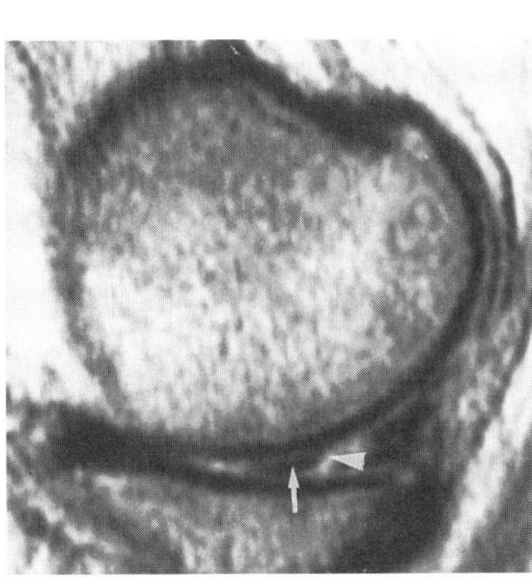
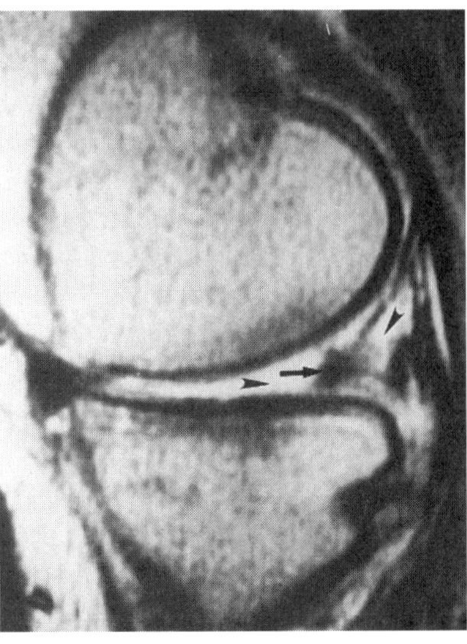

A,B C

FIG. 19-23. Meniscal injuries. **A:** T1-weighted MRI of a frank tear *(arrow)* of the posterior horn of the medial meniscus that extends to its tibial articular surface. **B:** T2-weighted bucket-handle tear *(arrowhead)* of the posterior horn of the medial meniscus with the inner fragment *(white arrow)* displaced centrally. **C:** T2-weighted MRI of a distorted chronically degnerated posterior horn *(black arrow)* of the medial meniscus surrounded by a chronic joint effusion *(black arrowheads)*.

clude discoid meniscus, meniscal cysts, and abnormalities involving the postoperative meniscus. In discoid meniscus, typically involving the lateral meniscus, there is a continuous bridge of meniscal tissue between the anterior and posterior horns in the central part of the joint. Meniscal cysts are usually associated with underlying horizontal meniscal tears through which synovial fluid collects at the meniscocapsular junction (29). They show high signal intensity on T2-weighted images. MRI also can be used to evaluate the post-meniscectomy patient with continuing or recurrent symptomatology (30). It can detect an incompletely excised meniscal tear, retained meniscal fragments, or a tear developing within the residual part of the meniscus.

Cruciate Ligament Injuries

The cruciate ligaments are best visualized by sagittal or oblique sagittal MR images that display the full length of the ligaments (Fig. 19-24). On straight sagittal images, the slender nature of the anterior cruciate ligament and its oblique course cause a volume-averaging effect that averages fat signal intensity about the ligaments with the normal low signal intensity of the ligament so that the anterior cruciate ligament frequently does not appear as a complete signal void (Fig. 19-24*A*). Furthermore, straight sagittal images typically fail to demonstrate the anterior cruciate ligament's femoral attachment because of its oblique orientation in both sagittal and coronal planes. Oblique sagittal images that par-

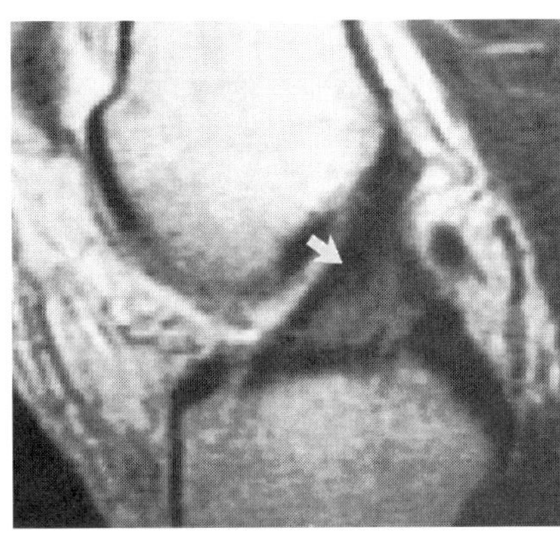
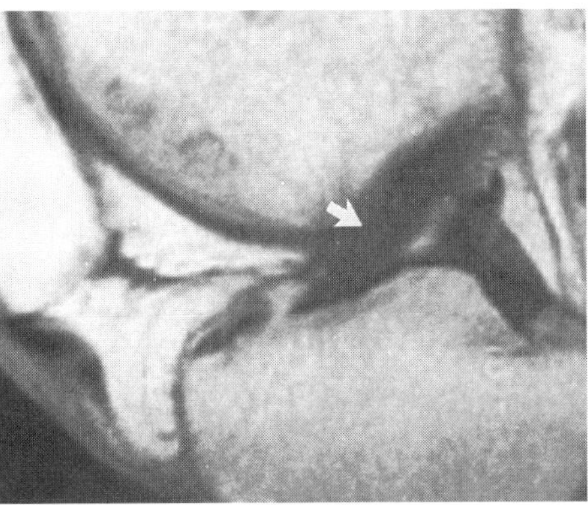
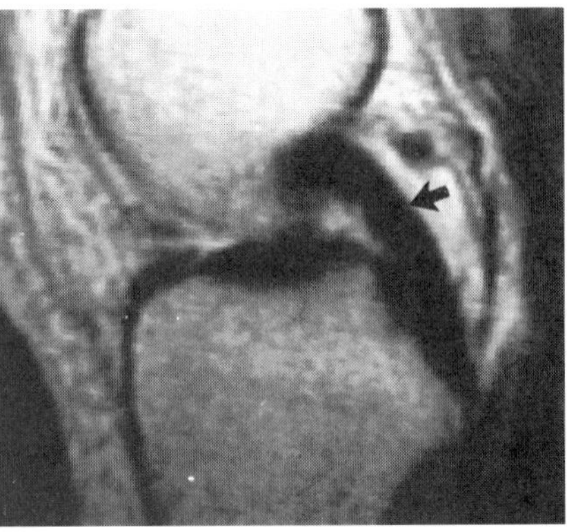

A,B C

FIG. 19-24. Normal cruciate ligaments. **A:** A straight sagittal T1-weighted MRI provides partial visualization of the anterior cruciate ligament *(arrow)*. **B:** An oblique sagittal MRI parallel to the anterior cruciate ligament demonstrates excellent visualization of all borders and attachments of the anterior cruciate ligament *(arrow)*. **C:** A T2-weighted MRI of the posterior cruciate ligament *(arrow)*, which is normally posteriorly bowed when the knee is extended.

allel the ligament show the full thickness and length of the anterior cruciate ligament without subjecting it to partial volume averaging (Fig. 19-24*B*) (33). In the extended position of the knee, which is typically used for MR images, the anterior cruciate ligament is normally taut. The posterior cruciate ligament is a thicker ligament, and is therefore well visualized on straight sagittal MR images (Fig. 19-24*C*). It can be visualized as a signal void structure from its attachment to the posterior tibial intercondylar area to its attachment on the medial femoral condyle. With the knee extended, the posterior cruciate ligament is visualized as thick and posteriorly bowed. It straightens with knee flexion.

The MRI appearance of an anterior cruciate ligament injury depends on the site and degree of disruption, as well as on the age of the tear. A complete tear may be visualized as a discontinuity of the ligament (Fig. 19-25*A* and *B*). In the acute complete tear, the interval between the torn ends of the ligament is often occupied by a mass of intermediate signal intensity on T1-weighted images that becomes hyperintense on T2-weighted images (34). At other times, the torn ligament may present as a fusiform or irregular soft-tissue mass of intermediate signal intensity on T1-weighted images that becomes hyperintense on T2-weighted images. These fluid masses are usually a combination of edema and hemorrhage, and there may be an associated joint effusion. In partial tears there is no complete discontinuity, but the ligament

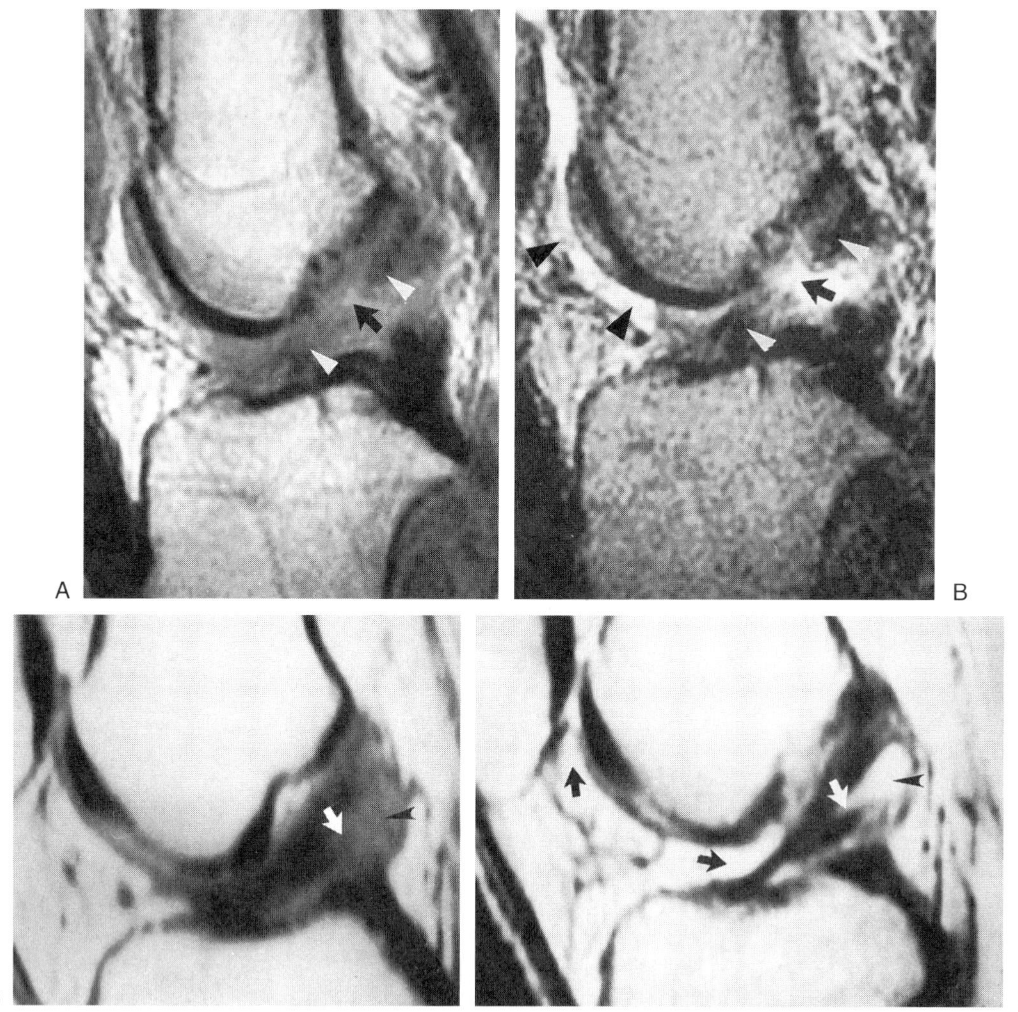

FIG. 19-25. Anterior cruciate ligament injuries. T1-weighted **(A)** and T2-weighted **(B)** MR images of a complete tear of the mid-portion of the anterior cruciate ligament. The T1-weighted image shows only the tibial and femoral ends of the ligament *(white arrowheads)* separated by a moderate signal intensity mass *(black arrows)* that becomes hyperintense on the T2-weighted image, indicating edema, hemorrhage, or both. There is also a joint effusion *(black arrowheads)*. T1-weighted **(C)** and T2-weighted **(D)** MR images of a partial tear of the posterior aspect of the anterior cruciate ligament *(white arrow)*. The T1-weighted image shows a moderate-intensity edema–hemorrhage mass at the site of the tear that becomes hyperintense on the T2-weighted image *(black arrowheads)*. Joint effusion anterior to the anterior cruciate ligament and behind the patella becomes hyperintense on the T2-weighted image *(black arrows)*.

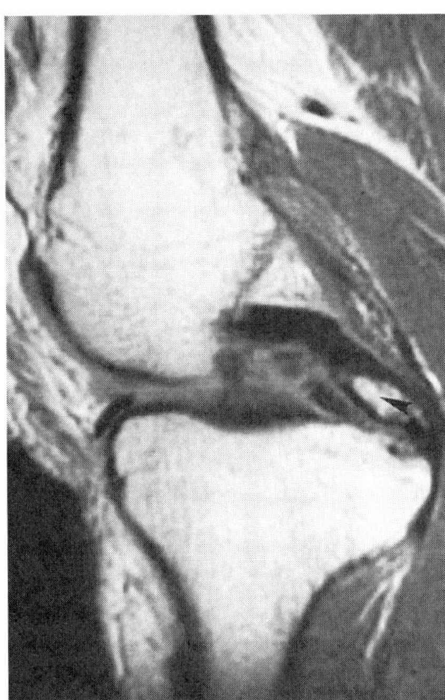

FIG. 19-26. Complete tear of the posterior cruciate ligament. This T2-weighted image shown an avulsion of the tibial attachment of the posterior cruciate ligament with hyperintense edema and hemorrhage *(arrowhead)* within the ligament at the site of the injury.

that appears intact on a T1-weighted image may show a hyperintense signal on T2-weighted images, or the ligament may display an interrupted or concave anterior or posterior margin when the knee is extended (Fig. 19-25*C* and *D*) (29). In chronic anterior cruciate ligament deficiency there may be a complete absence of the ligament or there may be only remnants remaining in its usual location. Some secondary signs of anterior cruciate ligament injury may be present. These include a forward shift of the tibia and an anterior bowing or buckling of the posterior cruciate ligament caused by the position of the knee within the coil, which duplicates the knee position of an anterior drawer or Lachman test (30).

On T1-weighted MR images, partial tears of the posterior cruciate ligament typically appear as foci of increased signal intensity within the normal black signal void of the ligament. These become hyperintense on T2-weighted images. With complete tears, a frank discontinuity is visualized with an intervening fluid mass that becomes hyperintense on T2-weighted images (Fig. 19-26). The gap between the ends of a completely torn posterior cruciate ligament can be exaggerated by imaging the knee in flexion, which tenses the posterior cruciate ligament.

Collateral Ligament Injuries

The collateral ligaments are best visualized by coronal MR images (Fig. 19-27*A*). The medial collateral ligament appears as a narrow low signal intensity band extending from the medial epicondyle of the femur to an attachment on the anteromedial aspect of the tibia 5 to 6 cm below the joint line. It is overlaid at its tibial attachment by the tendons of the pes anserinus, which are separated from it by an intervening anserine bursa that is not visualized unless it is inflamed. Deep to the tibial collateral ligament, the medial capsular ligament, sometimes called the deep portion of the tibial collateral ligament, has femoral and tibial attachments close to the joint interval and deep attachments to the medial meniscus, referred to as the meniscofemoral and meniscotibial or coronary ligaments. Valgus and rotary stresses can injure the medial capsular ligament or the tibial collateral ligament, usually in that order (30). In a complete rupture (i.e., grade III injury), MRI can show discontinuity, serpiginous ligamentous borders, and edema within adjacent connective tissues (Fig. 19-27*B*). In a partial tear (i.e., grade II injury), or in the case of microtears confined to the ligament substance (i.e., grade I injury), the ligament may show no discontinuity, but the overlying subcutaneous fat typically demonstrates

A

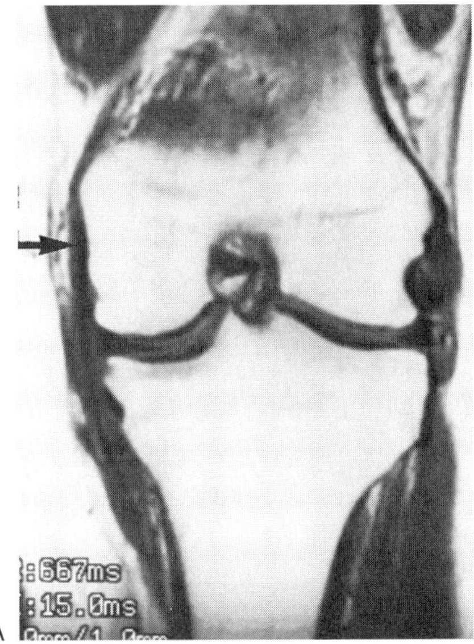

B

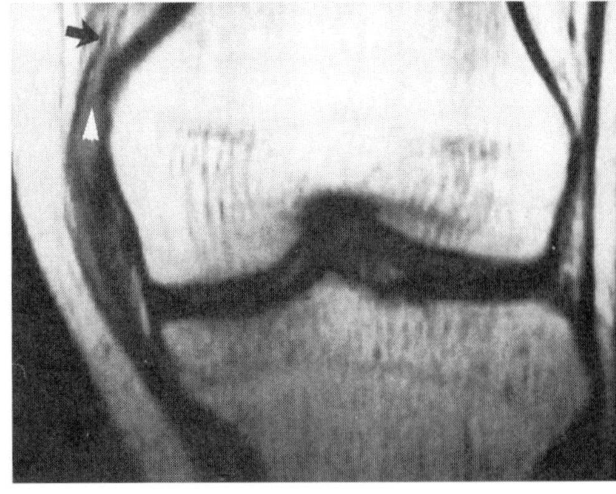

FIG. 19-27. Tibial collateral ligament injury. **A:** Normal tibial collateral ligament *(arrow)*. **B:** A T1-weighted image shows a complete rupture of the medial collateral ligament from its femoral attachment *(arrow)*. The more deeply lying, moderately intense mass is edema and hemorrhage *(arrowhead)*.

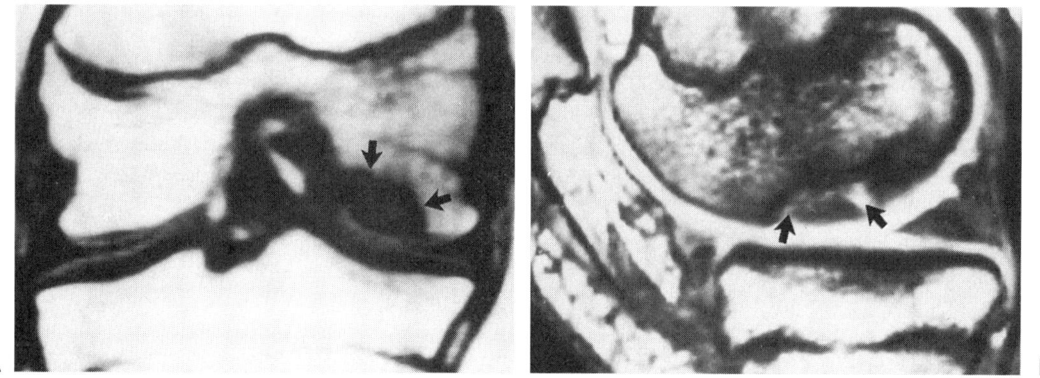

FIG. 19-28. T1-weighted MR images of osteochondritis dissecans. **A:** A coronal view shows an area of hypointensity on the intercondylar aspect of the medial femoral condyle *(black arrows)*. **B:** A sagittal view of the medial femoral condyle demonstrates a completely separated osteochondral fragment *(black arrows)*.

edema and hemorrhage, which is indicated by moderate signal intensity on T1-weighted images and high signal intensity on T2-weighted images. Injury to the tibial collateral ligament is commonly associated with injuries to the anterior cruciate ligament and medial meniscus.

The lateral collateral ligament is seen on coronal MR images as a low signal intensity band extending somewhat obliquely from the lateral femoral epicondyle to the fibular head. It is usually injured by varus and rotary stresses to the knee, although its frequency of injury is less than that of the tibial collateral ligament. The MRI findings of the injured fibular collateral ligament are similar to those for the tibial collateral ligament.

Other Knee Abnormalities

Patellar tendinitis (jumper's knee) is demonstrated by MRI as an area of edema within the patellar ligament (i.e., tendon) at its patellar or tibial tuberosity attachment. There is also associated edema in the adjacent subcutaneous fat or the infrapatellar fat pad.

Ischemic necrosis about the knee most commonly involves the weight-bearing surface of the medial femoral condyle, and its MRI findings are as described for the hip.

Osteochondritis dissecans occurs mainly in adolescents and involves a partial or total separation of a segment of articular cartilage and subchondral bone from the underlying bone (30). It commonly involves the intercondylar portion of the medial femoral condyle's articular surface. It is visualized on T1-weighted MR images as a low signal intensity region in the subchondral bone with or without disruption of the overlying articular cartilage (Fig. 19-28). If the involved osteochondral segment becomes completely separated from the underlying bone, it becomes an intra-articular loose body. The role of MRI in osteochondritis dissecans is mainly to determine the stability of the fragment because the treatment hinges on that.

Chondromalacia patella can be diagnosed and graded noninvasively by MRI (31). In stage I, the posterior patellar articular cartilage demonstrates local areas of cartilage swelling with decreased signal intensity on both T1- and T2-weighted images. Stage II is characterized by irregularity of the patellar articular cartilage with areas of thinning. Stage III demonstrates complete absence of the articular cartilage with synovial fluid extending through this cartilaginous ulcer to the subchondral bone (Fig. 19-29).

Popliteal (i.e., Baker's) cysts and other synovial cysts about the knee appear hyperintense on T2-weighted images (Fig. 19-30). They can be visualized on axial, sagittal, or coronal images. Popliteal cysts are usually an enlargement of the semimembranosus-gastrocnemius bursa, which is located between the tendon of insertion of the semimembranosus and the tendon of origin of the medial head of the gastrocnemius. Popliteal cysts may communicate with the knee joint

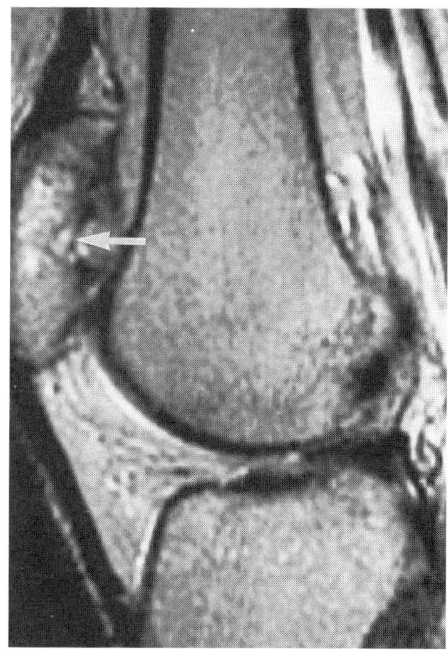

FIG. 19-29. Grade III chondromalacia patella. A T2-weighted MRI demonstrates a cartilaginous ulcer extending to the subchondral bone *(arrow)*.

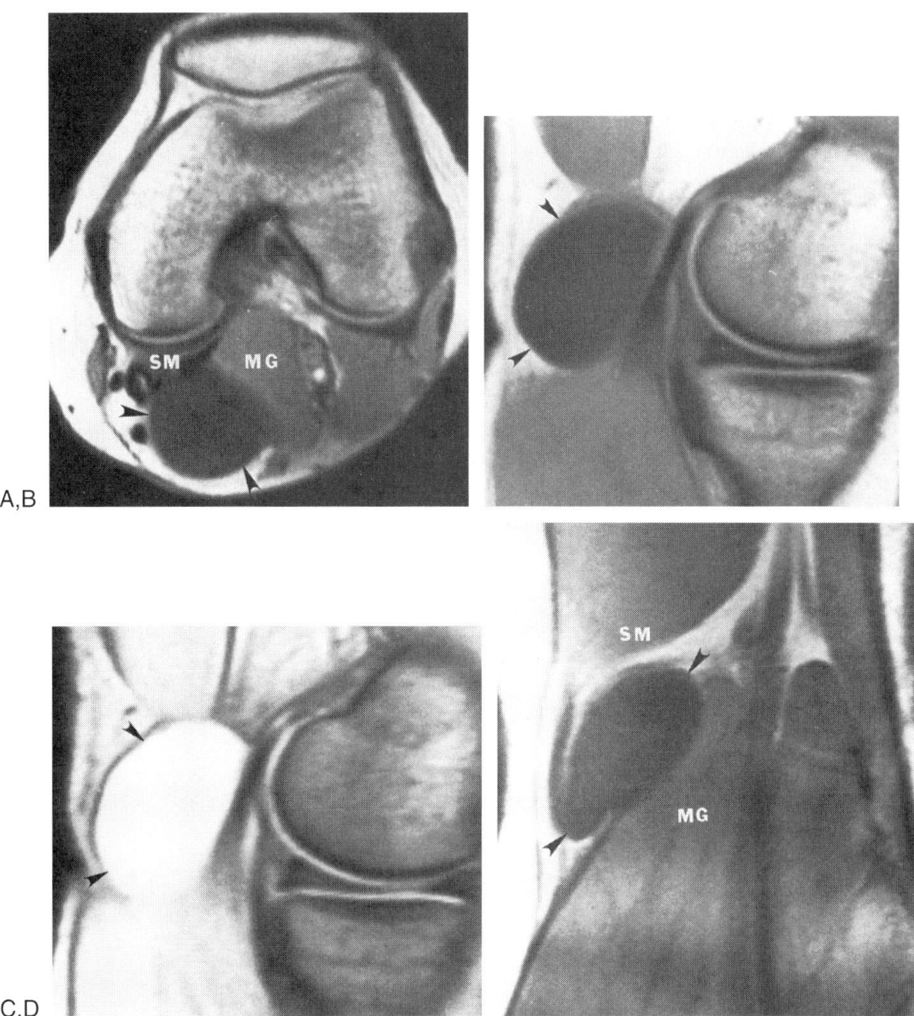

FIG. 19-30. Baker's cyst. **A:** A T1-weighted axial MRI demonstrates a hypointense Baker's cyst *(arrowheads)* in the interval between the semimembranosus *(SM)* and the medial head of the gastrocnemius *(MG)*. T1-weighted **(B)** and T2-weighted **(C)** sagittal MR images through the Baker's cyst *(arrowheads)*. Note that the hypointense fluid in the cyst in the T1-weighted image becomes hyperintense on the T2-weighted image. **D:** A coronal T1-weighted image locates the cyst between the *SM* and the *MG*.

and therefore may be caused by chronic knee joint pathology that produces effusion. A previously undescribed bursa is now known to be consistently present between the tibial collateral ligament and a major slip of the semimembranosus tendon that extends beneath it, and may serve to clarify many cases of previously unexplained medial knee pain (35). Inflammation of this bursa is well demonstrated by MRI (Fig. 19-31).

Ankle

MRI is valuable as a screening modality for assessing a variety of painful ankle disorders (36–40).

Ligament Injuries

Previously, arthrography and tenography were the primary means of imaging ankle ligament injuries. They had the limitations of being invasive, providing only an indirect depiction of ankle ligament disruption, and yielding potentially false-negative results. MRI provides a noninvasive means of directly imaging all of the ligaments in the vicinity of the ankle as well as all of the other bony and soft tissues.

Axial MR images provide good visualization of the tibiofibular ligaments of the tibiofibular mortise. However, all of the lateral collateral ligaments of the ankle have an oblique orientation, and to image these ligaments in full length, either an oblique imaging plane that parallels their length must be chosen, or the foot must be placed in sufficient dorsiflexion or plantar flexion to bring the ligaments into one of the standard imaging planes. With the imaging plane parallel to the anterior talofibular ligament, it is displayed as a low signal intensity band extending anteromedially from the lateral malleolus to gain attachment to the talus just anterior to its fibular articular surface (Fig. 19-32*A*) (39). The calcaneofibular ligament is visualized as a low signal intensity structure extending from the lateral malleolus to the calcaneus, with the peroneus longus and brevis tendons situated superficial to its fibular end (Fig. 19-32*B*). The posterior talofibular ligament is visualized as a wide low signal inten-

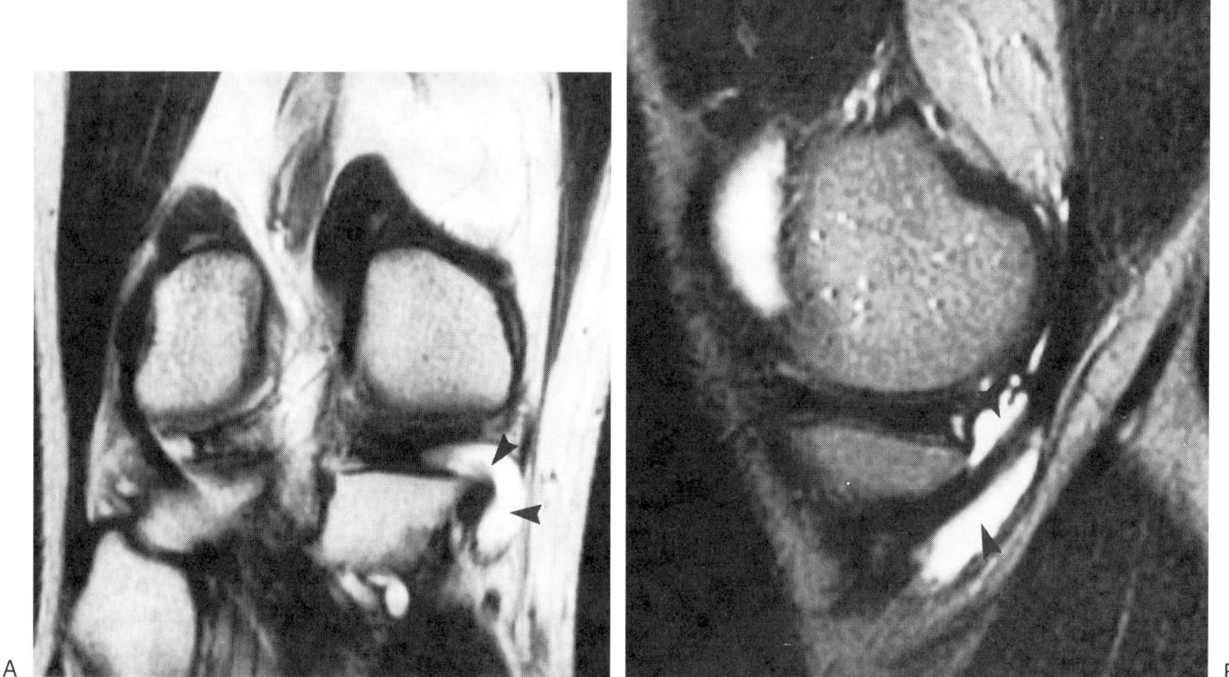

FIG. 19-31. A coronal T2-weighted MRI **(A)** and a sagittal T2-weighted MRI of a 42-year-old man who sustained a twisting injury to the medial side of the knee that produced a bursitis of the semimembranosus–tibial collateral bursa. This is visualized as a high signal intensity area *(black arrowheads)* partially surrounding the semimembranosus tendon *(S)* **(A)** and a high signal intensity *(black arrowheads)* area above and below the semimembranosus tendon *(S)* **(B)**.

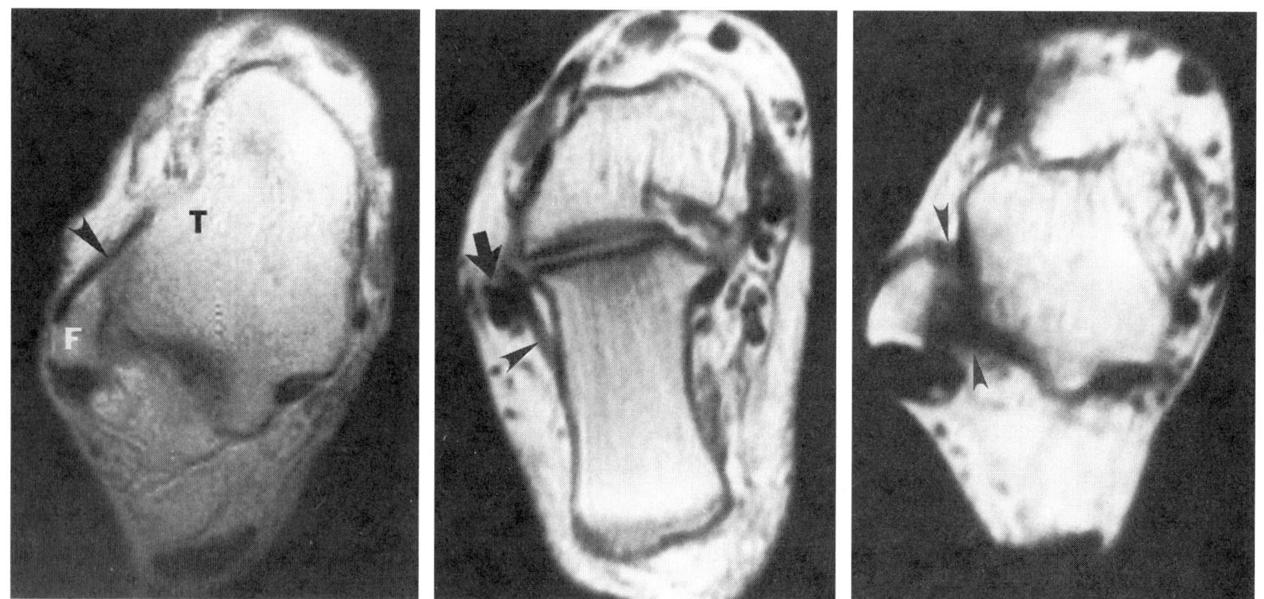

FIG. 19-32. T1-weighted MR images of the normal collateral ligaments of the ankle. **A:** The anterior talofibular ligament *(arrowhead)* extends from the fibular malleolus *(F)* to the talus *(T)*. **B:** The calcaneofibular ligament *(arrowhead)* attaches to the calcaneus and is overlaid by the peroneus tendons *(arrow)*. **C:** The broad posterior talofibular ligament *(between arrowheads)*.

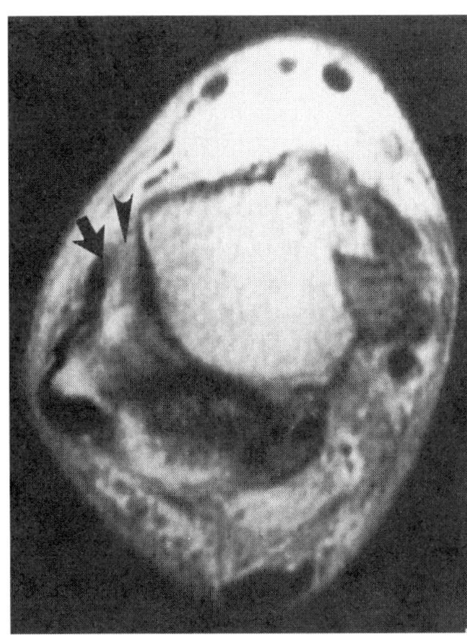
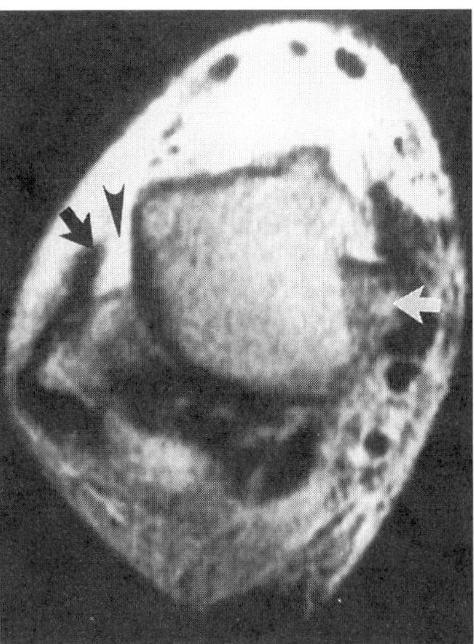

A,B

FIG. 19-33. Complete rupture (grade III sprain) of the anterior talofibular ligament. **A:** A T1-weighted MRI demonstrates the ruptured anterior end of the anterior talofibular ligament *(arrow)*, which is separated from the talus by moderate-intensity hemorrhage and edema *(arrowhead)*. **B:** T2-weighted MRI showing that the hemorrhage–edema about the ruptured end of the anterior talofibular ligament *(black arrow)* has become hyperintense *(arrowhead)*. The T2-weighted image also shows a minute area of increased signal intensity within the substance of the posterior tibiotalar portion of the deltoid ligament *(white arrow)* that was moderately intense on the T2-weighted image. This is compatible with the intraligamentous hemorrhage and edema of an accompanying grade 1 sprain of the deltoid ligament.

sity structure extending from the deep surface of the lateral malleolus to a broad attachment on the talus from its fibular articular surface to its posterior process (Fig. 19-32*C*).

MRI of ankle ligament injuries offers promise for the noninvasive evaluation of the site and severity of both acute ankle ligament injuries and chronic ankle instability (40).

The mechanism of injury of the lateral collateral ligaments typically involves plantar flexion and inversion, and they are usually injured in a predictable sequence from anterior to posterior. The anterior talofibular ligament is the most commonly injured, followed in sequence by injury to the calcanofibular and posterior talofibular ligaments. The major MRI finding in a complete rupture (i.e., grade III sprain) of the anterior talofibular ligament is a complete discontinuity of the ligament visualized at all imaging levels (Fig. 19-33). This is accompanied by periarticular edema or hemorrhage and joint effusion because this ligament is a thickening of the ankle joint capsule. The edema and effusion are visualized with moderate signal intensity on T1-weighted MR images and hyperintensity on T2-weighted images. A partial tear (i.e., grade II sprain) of the anterior talofibular ligament is visualized on MRI as a discontinuity of the upper part of the ligament, with the lower portion remaining intact (Fig. 19-34). Again, there is periarticular edema, hemorrhage, and

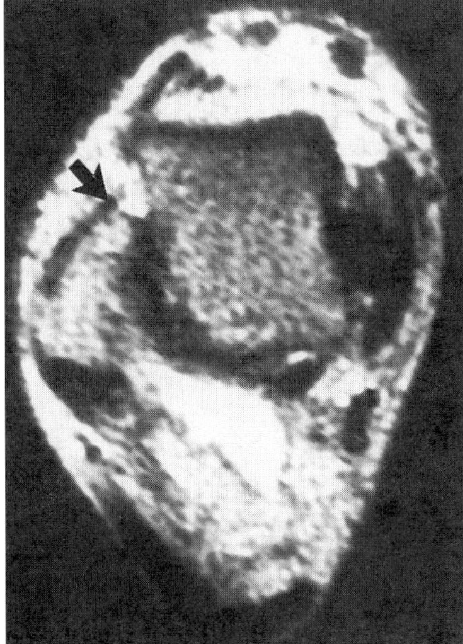
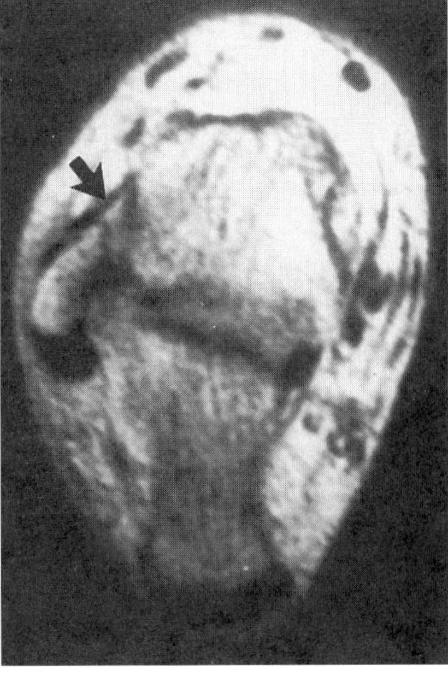

A,B

FIG. 19-34. Partial tear (grade II sprain) of the anterior talofibular ligament. **A:** A T2-weighted MRI shows an interruption of the upper portion of the anterior talofibular ligament *(arrow)*. **B:** The lower portion of the ligament is still intact *(arrow)*.

joint effusion. Grade II sprains of the calcaneofibular ligament may appear as a longitudinal splitting or waviness of the ligament with fluid accumulation within the tendon sheath of the overlying peroneal tendons (Fig. 19-35).

In contrast to the three discrete lateral collateral ligaments, the medial collateral or deltoid ligament is a continuous ligamentous sheet with an apical attachment to the tibial malleolus, and a broad base attaching below to the navicular, talar neck, spring ligament, sustentaculum tali of the calcaneus, and posterior talus. The posterior tibiotalar part of the deltoid ligament is its thickest and strongest (41). The deltoid ligament can be visualized by either axial or coronal MRI. Axial images allow simultaneous visualization of all parts of the deltoid ligament, the overlying flexor retinaculum, and the walls and contents of the tarsal tunnel (Fig. 19-36*A*). The contents of the four compartments under the flexor retinaculum include, from anterior to posterior, the tibialis posterior tendon, flexor digitorum longus tendon, posterior tibial artery, tibial nerve, and flexor hallucis longus tendon. Coronal MR images through the deltoid ligament display the proximal and distal attachments of each part of the deltoid ligament (Fig. 19-36*B*).

MRI appears to have the potential to visualize even grade I sprains, which are microtears confined to the interior of the ligament. The minute foci of edema and hemorrhage accompanying such tears become hyperintense on T2-weighted images. Findings compatible with such grade I tears have been identified in the posterior tibiotalar portion of the deltoid ligament (Fig. 19-33*B*). They are frequently accompanied by fluid within the tendon sheath of the overlying tibialis posterior.

In chronic ankle instability, MR images show thinned, lengthened, wavy ligaments in some locations and thickened scarred ligaments in others (Fig. 19-37).

Other Ankle Abnormalities

Technetium 99 scintigraphy is valuable for detecting stress fractures of metatarsal and tarsal bones, and CT has high accuracy for detecting osteochondral fracture. In foot pain of undetermined etiology, however, MRI is an excellent screening modality because it permits direct evaluation of all bony and soft-tissue structures.

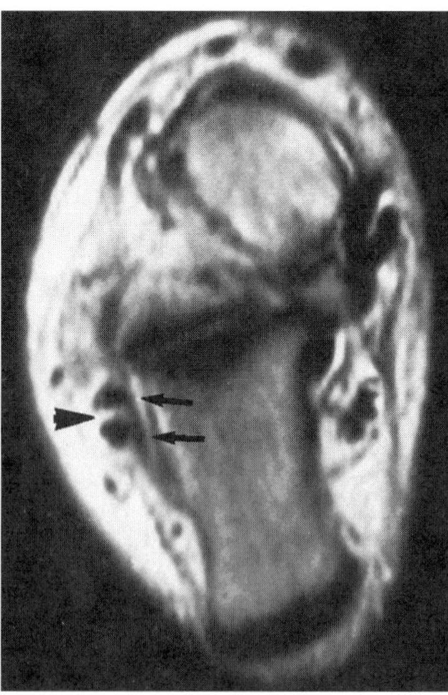

FIG. 19-35. Partial tear (grade II sprain) of the calcaneofibular ligament appears on this T2-weighted MRI as a longitudinal split of the ligament *(arrows)* with hyperintense edema–hemorrhage within the overlying peroneus tendon sheath *(arrowhead).*

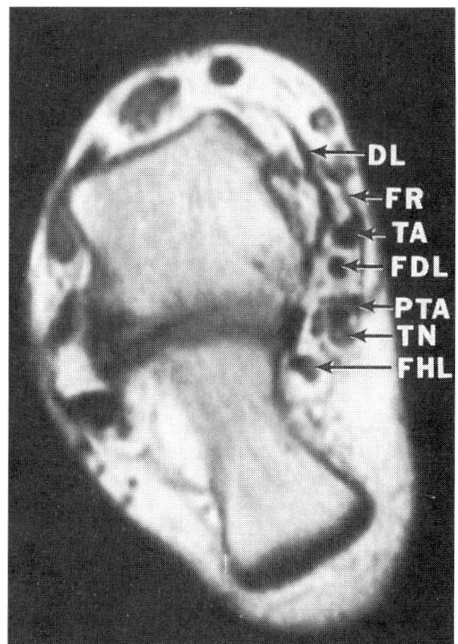

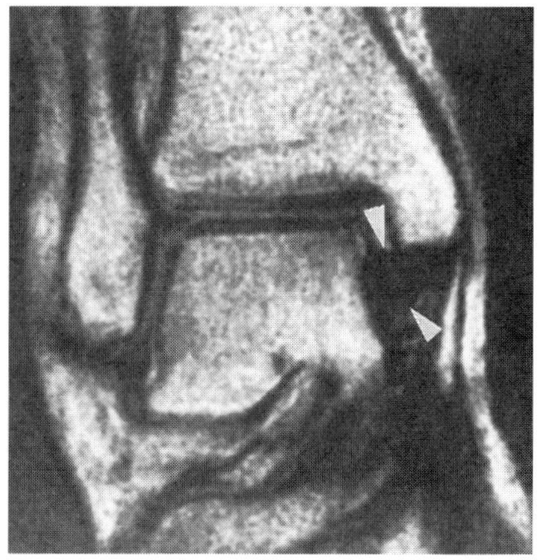

FIG. 19-36. Normal tibial collateral (i.e., deltoid) ligament and tarsal tunnel. **A:** A T1-weighted axial MRI demonstrates the deltoid ligament *(DL)*, the overlying flexor retinaculum *(FR)*, and the contents of the tarsal tunnel: tibialis anterior *(TA)*, flexor digitorum longus *(FDL)*, posterior tibial artery *(PTA)*, tibial nerve *(TN)*, and flexor hallucis longus *(FHL)*. **B:** Coronal T1-weighted MRI through the thick posterior tibotalar part of the deltoid ligament *(between arrowheads).*

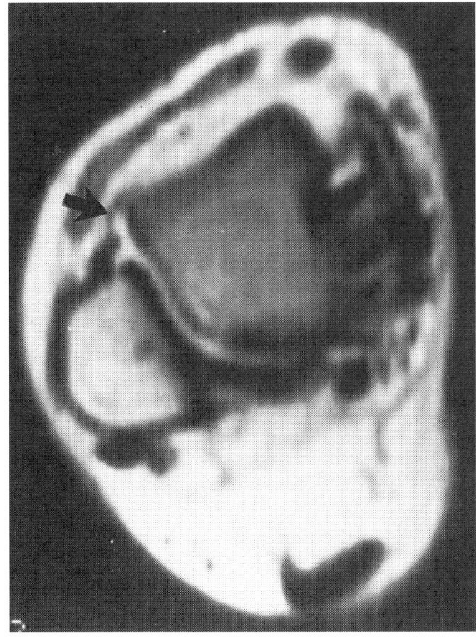

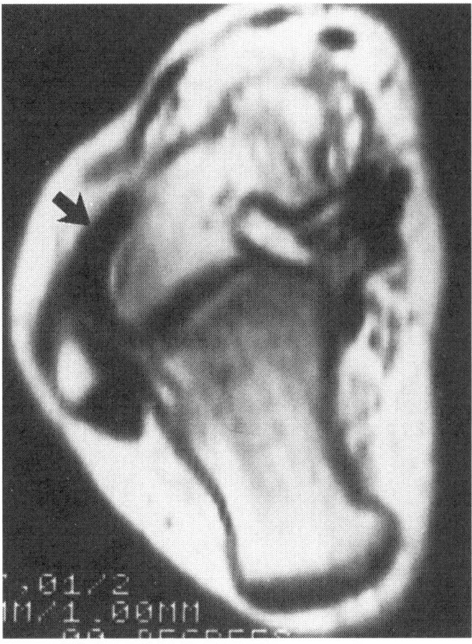

FIG. 19-37. Chronically unstable ankle. High-level **(A)** and low-level **(B)** axial sections, respectively, through the anterior talofibular ligament of a patient with a chronically unstable ankle. The upper portion of the ligament displays an anterior portion that is thinned and wavy *(arrow)*, implying weakening and lengthening of the ligament as the result of repeated trauma. The lower portion of the ligament is considerably thickened and hypointense *(arrow)*, indicating the presence of chronic scar tissue.

MRI is superior to any other modality in displaying tendon pathology (36,37). In tenosynovitis, MRI detects fluid within the tendon sheath as having moderate signal intensity on T1-weighted images and as hyperintense on T2-weighted images. Tendinitis is commonly observed in the Achilles, tibialis posterior, flexor hallucis longus, tibialis anterior, and peroneal tendons. Tendinitis is visualized as a focal or diffuse thickening of the tendon that may show areas of increased signal intensity on T2-weighted images. Plantar fasciitis shows similar changes within the plantar aponeurosis. With a complete tendon rupture, axial MR images show absence of the tendon and its replacement by edema. Sagittal and coronal MR images display the site of discontinuity, with edema occupying the gap and surrounding the torn ends of the tendon.

Stress fractures of the tarsal or metatarsal bones appear on MRI as linear areas of decreased marrow signal intensity. There are adjacent areas of marrow edema that are hypointense relative to marrow fat on T1-weighted images and hyperintense on T2-weighted images (36). By MRI, osteochondral fractures (e.g., of the talar dome) have an appearance similar to that of osteochondritis dissecans of the knee. The primary task of MRI is to determine the stability of the fragment by demonstrating the integrity of the articular cartilage and the absence of fluid between the osteochondral fragment and the parent bone. Synovial cysts of intertarsal joint origin demonstrate moderate signal intensity on T1-weighted images and high signal intensity on T2-weighted images (Fig. 19-38).

Some Common Arthritides

The usual mode for diagnosing the arthritides is plain film radiography. Only the findings of the more common arthropathies will be described.

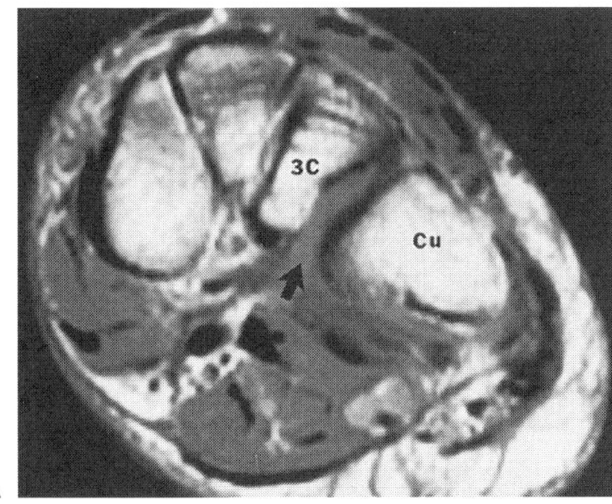

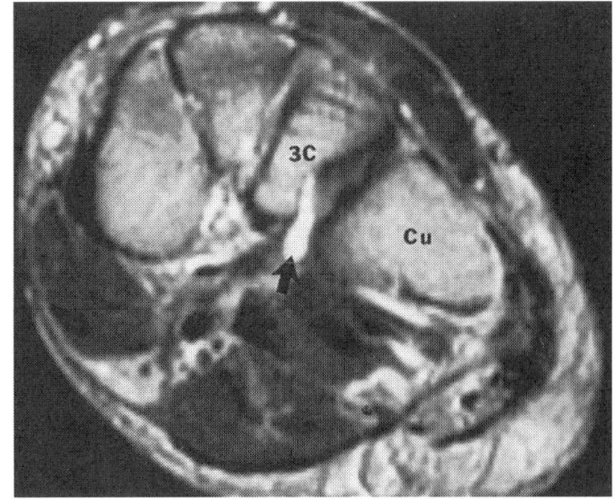

FIG. 19-38. Intertarsal synovial cyst in a patient presenting clinically with foot pain of undetermined etiology is seen in **(A)** T1-weighted and **(B)** T2-weighted axial MR images. On the T1-weighted image, there is a moderately intense (i.e., gray) mass *(arrow)* between the third cuneiform *(3C)* and the cuboid *(Cu)*, which on the T2-weighted image becomes hyperintense *(arrow)* and is seen to bulge into the plantar soft tissues.

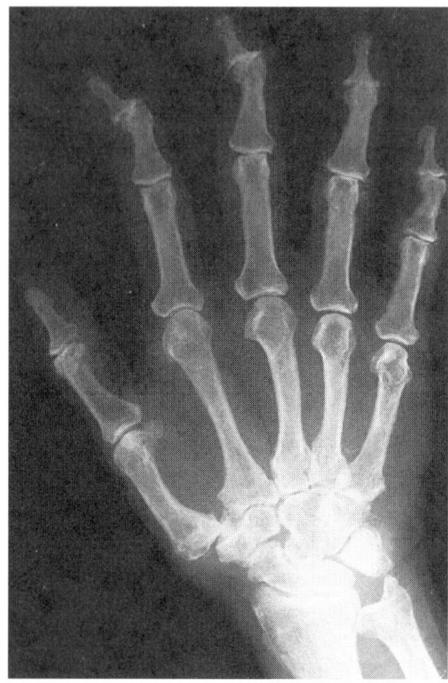
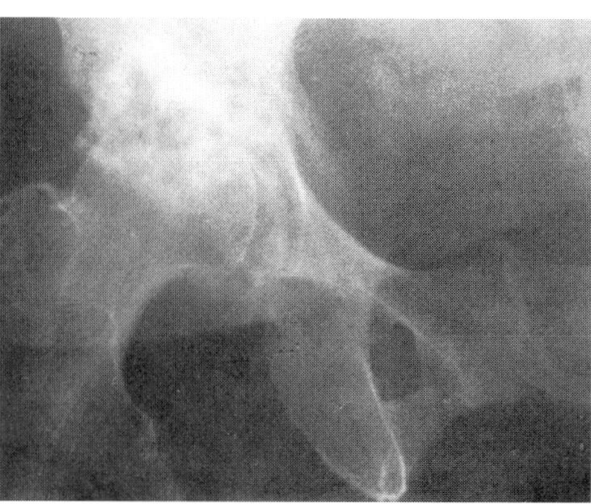

A,B

FIG. 19-39. Osteoarthritis. **A:** Osteoarthritic changes predominantly involving the distal interphalangeal joints. **B:** Osteoarthritis of the hip. Both show joint space narrowing and subchondral sclerosis.

Osteoarthritis

Osteoarthritis is an asymmetric, usually bilateral mechanical degenerative process that involves joints significantly involved in weight bearing, such as the hip, knee, and spine, and those involved in frequent repetitive mechanical trauma, such as the distal interphalangeal joints of the fingers, trapezium–first metacarpal joint, trapezium–scaphoid joint, and metatarsophalangeal joint of the great toe. The most common radiographic findings include the following:

1. A nonuniform loss of joint space caused by cartilage degeneration in high load areas (e.g., the superior aspect of the hip and medial knee)
2. Sclerosis of the subchondral bone
3. Osteophyte formation at the margins of the articular surfaces
4. Cystlike rarefactions in the subchondral bone that may collapse to produce marked joint deformities
5. Adjacent soft-tissue swelling (e.g., that which occurs with Heberden's nodes of the distal interphalangeal joints of the fingers) (Fig. 19-39) (42)

Rheumatoid Arthritis

Rheumatoid arthritis is a bilaterally symmetric inflammatory degenerative disease that involves the following joints in order of decreasing frequency:

1. Small joints of the hands and feet, with the exception of the distal interphalangeal joints
2. Knees
3. Hips
4. Cervical spine
5. Shoulders
6. Elbows

The major radiographic findings include the following:

1. Symmetric periarticular soft-tissue swelling
2. Juxta-articular osteoporosis proceeding to diffuse osteoporosis
3. Erosions of the intracapsular portions of the articulating bones not covered by cartilage, which can proceed to severe subchondral bone erosion
4. Uniform loss of joint space
5. Synovial cysts (e.g., Baker's cysts behind the knee)
6. Subluxations (e.g., boutonniere or swan-neck deformities of the fingers, and palmar and ulnar subluxation of the proximal phalanges on the metacarpal heads) (Fig. 19-40) (43)

Gout

Gout most commonly involves the feet, especially the first metatarsophalangeal joint, as well as the ankles, knees, hands, and elbows in asymmetric fashion. It is produced by a deposition of monosodium urate crystals in tissues with a poor blood supply, such as cartilage, tendon sheaths, and bursae. The radiographic features of gout typically do not appear until after years of episodic arthritis. Radiographic features characteristic of gout include the following:

1. Tophi or periarticular soft-tissue masses created by the deposition of urate crystals that may contain calcium
2. Tophi-induced periarticular or intra-articular bone erosion
3. Prominent cortical edges overhanging the tophi and bone erosions (Fig. 19-41) (43)

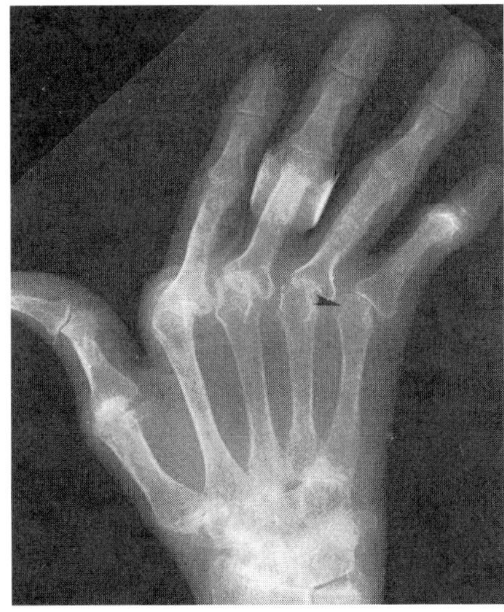

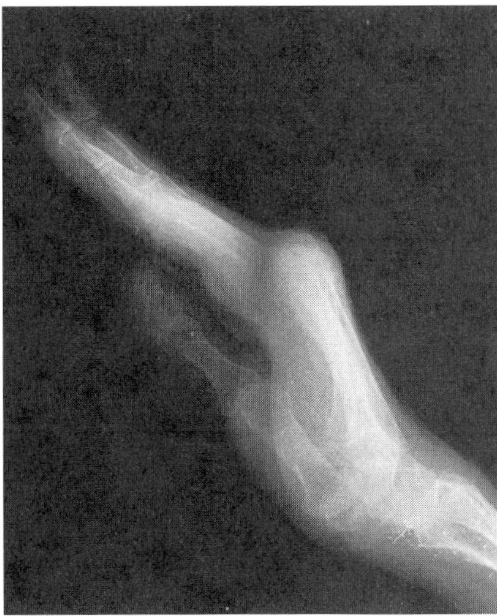

A,B

FIG. 19-40. Rheumatoid arthritis. Posteroanterior **(A)** and lateral **(B)** hand radiographs demonstrate ulnar and palmar subluxations of the proximal phalanges, periarticular soft-tissue swelling, juxta-articular osteoporosis, and erosion of non–cartilage-covered intra-articular bone sufaces *(arrowhead)*.

Diffuse Idiopathic Skeletal Hyperostosis

Diffuse idiopathic skeletal hyperostosis (DISH) is not really an arthropathy because it spares synovium, articular cartilage, and articular bony surfaces. It is an ossification process involving ligamentous and tendinous attachments to bones and occurs in 12% of the elderly (44). It most commonly affects the spine but also may involve the pelvis, foot, knee, and elbow. It can involve ossification of all of the ligaments surrounding the vertebral bodies, particularly the anterior longitudinal ligament. By definition, DISH must involve a flowing ossification of at least four contiguous vertebral bodies (Fig. 19-42). There must be normal disc spaces and facet joints.

SPINE AND SPINAL CORD IMAGING

Although plain radiographs remain valuable for detecting many types of spine fractures and degenerative changes, the high resolution of bony and soft-tissue structures provided by CT and MRI has made these modalities invaluable for the diagnosis of degenerative, traumatic, neoplastic, and infectious diseases of the spinal column and spinal cord.

Degenerative Spine Disorders

CT and MRI provide complementary information about degenerative diseases of the spine. CT offers better distinction between bony spurs and disc herniation or other soft-tissue masses protruding into the spinal canal and the neural foramina. MRI permits noninvasive visualization of the spinal cord and subarachnoid space within the spinal canal and the nerve roots within the neural foramina. Discrimination of these structures by CT requires injection of intrathecal contrast agents. MRI has a superior ability to evaluate intramedullary abnormalities. It also offers direct multiplanar imaging without the usual degradation of image quality that occurs with CT reformation.

Axial CT images of the normal spine provide good visualization of all bony elements, including the facet joints and Luschka's joints (Fig. 19-43*A*). Soft-tissue windows typically permit visualization of the moderate radiodensity of the soft-tissue structures, such as the intervertebral disc, ligamenta flava, transverse atlantal ligament, and thecal sac (Fig. 19-43*B*). Contributing to the radiodensity of the thecal sac are the dura, the cerebrospinal fluid (CSF), the spinal cord, and the intradural course of the nerve roots. Its periphery is delimited at many spinal levels by radiolucent epidural fat. The epidural fat contains the internal vertebral venous

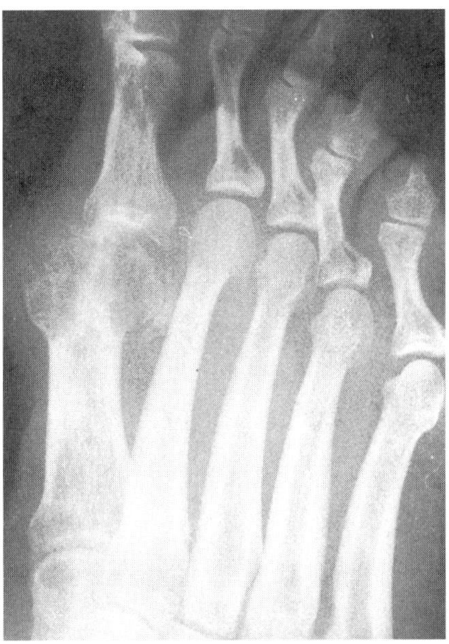

FIG. 19-41. Gout involving the first metatarsophalangeal joint with tophi-induced bone erosions surrounded by cortical bone.

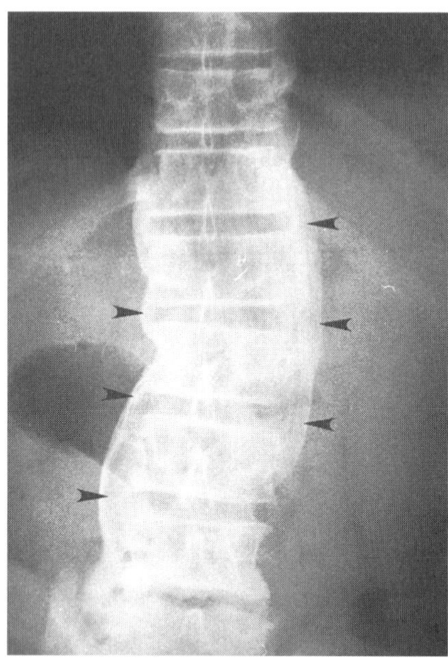
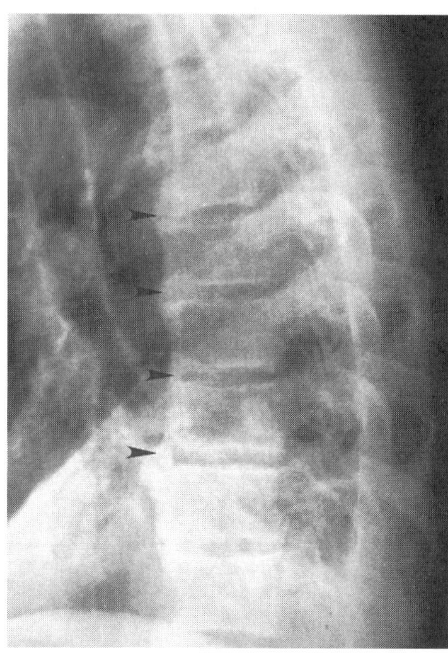

A,B

FIG. 19-42. Diffuse idiopathic skeletal hyperostosis. Anteroposterior **(A)** and lateral **(B)** spine radiographs show lateral lumbar and anterior thoracic ossification of the anterior longitudinal ligament *(arrowheads)*.

plexus, which can be enhanced by a circulating bolus of contrast material to improve visualization of soft-tissue encroachments into the spinal canal, such as herniated discs. Introduction of contrast material into the subarachnoid space (i.e., CT myelography) delimits the contained spinal cord and nerve roots (Fig. 19-43*C*).

Sagittal T1-weighted MR images of the cervical, thoracic, or lumbar spine provide excellent noninvasive survey images to evaluate patients with suspected regional spinal pathology. Mid-sagittal T1-weighted images display the high signal intensity marrow of the vertebrae bounded by low signal intensity cortical bone. Structures displaying very low signal intensity include the peripheral part of the anulus fibrosus of the intervertebral disc, all ligaments, the dura, and the CSF, and these are usually indistinguishable from each other (Fig. 19-44*A* and *B*). The nucleus pulposus, and probably the inner portion of the anulus fibrosus, shows a moderate signal intensity. The spinal cord and nerve roots display moderate signal intensity, which is well contrasted against the low signal intensity CSF. Collections of epidural fat, which are largest at lumbar levels, produce high signal intensity. On T2-weighted MR images, CSF and the normal well-hydrated nucleus pulposus assume a high signal intensity (Fig. 19-44*C*).

Atlantoaxial Instability

Atlantoaxial instability can be produced by softening, laxity, or rupture of the transverse atlantal, alar, and apical ligaments of the dens (i.e., odontoid). These ligaments hold the odontoid in its proper position against the anterior arch of the atlas and below the level of the foramen magnum. Such ligamentous changes can be produced by rheumatoid arthritis, Down syndrome, or traumatic rupture. Rheumatoid

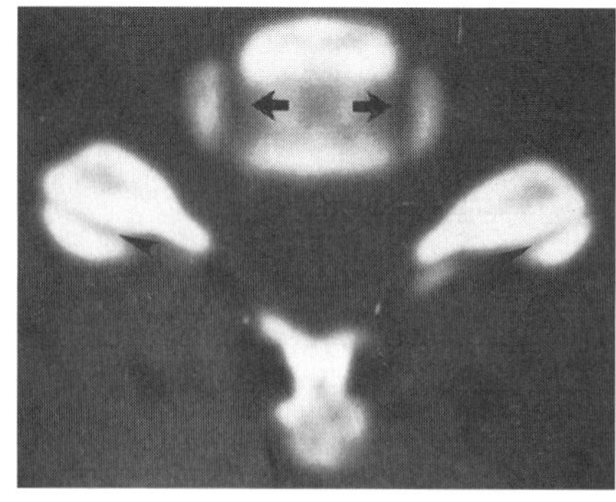
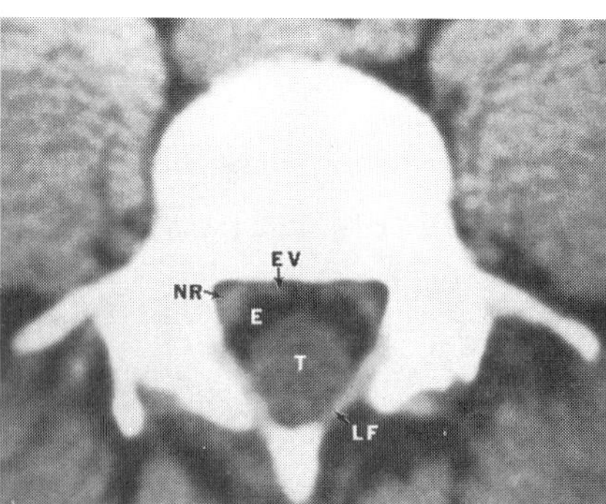

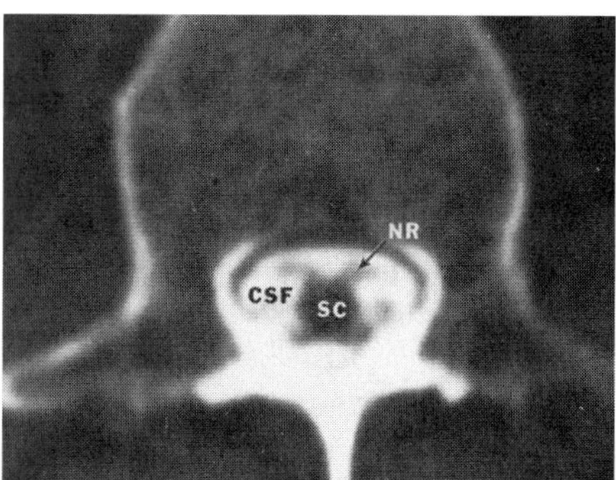

A,B C

FIG. 19-43. CT of the normal spine and spinal cord. **A:** Bone window CT of the cervical spine displays normal facet joints *(arrowheads)* and Luschka's joints *(arrows)*. **B:** Soft-tissue window CT of L5 demonstrating thecal sac *(T)*, nerve roots *(NR)* within the lateral recess, epidural fat *(E)*, epidural veins *(EV)*, and ligamentum flavum *(LF)*. **C:** Metrizamide CT myelogram at L1 level delimiting the spinal cord *(SC)*, nerve roots *(NR)* arising from the cord, and the contrast-enhanced CSF.

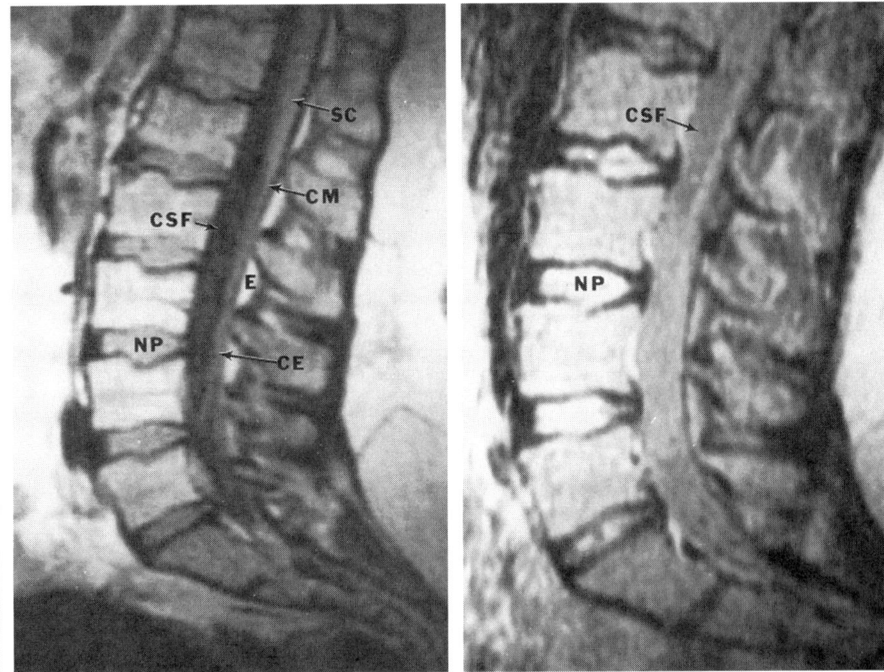

FIG. 19-44. MRI of the normal spine and spinal cord. **A:** A T1-weighted axial MRI of L5 shows the thecal sac *(T)* as an area of low signal intensity, the nerve roots *(NR)* within their lateral recesses as areas of moderate signal intensity, and the epidural fat *(E)* as hyperintense. **B:** T1-weighted mid-sagittal MRI of the lumbosacral spine displays the nucleus pulposus *(NP)* of the intervertebral discs, spinal cord *(SC)*, conus medullaris *(CM)*, and nerve roots of the cauda equina *(CE)* as areas of moderate signal intensity. CSF is of low signal intensity, and epidural fat *(E)* is hyperintense. **C:** T2-weighted mid-sagittal MRI of the lumbosacral spine demonstrates the increased intensity of the nucleus pulposus *(NP)* and CSF.

changes that destroy the articular cartilage and bone of the atlantoaxial joints can further increase the instability. Atlantoaxial instability also can be caused by odontoid abnormalities, such as an unfused apical portion of the odontoid (i.e., os odontoideum), or by odontoid fractures. Normally, the cartilaginous radiolucent interval between the anterior arch of the atlas and the dens does not exceed 3 mm in the adult. With ligamentous abnormalities, lateral radiographs of the flexed cervical spine may show a posterior subluxation of the odontoid into the spinal canal that increases the atlas–dens interval to more than 3 mm. When posterior subluxation of the odontoid exceeds 9 mm, it is likely to compromise the spinal cord and produce neurologic abnormalities (45). There also can be a superior subluxation of the odontoid above the level of the foramen magnum that can cause death by impingement upon the medulla or the vertebral arteries. These subluxations are well visualized by CT and MRI. MRI also can directly evaluate the ligaments. CT myelography and MR images in the axial or sagittal planes can assess the involvement of the spinal cord or medulla by the subluxation.

Cervical Disc Herniation

Disc herniation is typically preceded by degenerative changes in the mucopolysaccharides of the nucleus pulposus, which produce fibrillation of the collagen (46). This eventually causes dehydration and loss of disc volume. As a result, the nucleus pulposus no longer serves as a normal load-dispersing mechanism, and excessive stress is borne by the anulus fibrosus. This produces anular fissuring and tears that can culminate in herniation of the nucleus pulposus. The loss of the load-diffusing function of the normal disc also causes marginal osteophytosis of the vertebral body ends, and the facet joints degenerate by virtue of the increased loads these joints must bear.

Cervical disc herniation occurs with less frequency than lumbar disc herniation. About 90% of cervical disc herniations occur, in order of decreasing frequency, at C5–C6, C6–C7, and C4–C5 (47,48). Plain film myelography shows loss of disc height and indentation of the thecal sac. On CT examination, a herniated cervical disc appears as a dense soft-tissue mass protruding from the disc space centrally or paracentrally into the spinal canal or posterolaterally into the neural foramen (Fig. 19-45). With intrathecal contrast, compression of the thecal sac and spinal cord compression or rotation are well visualized by CT.

On T1-weighted MR images, the herniated cervical disc appears as a posterior extension of the moderate signal intensity of the disc into the low signal intensity region of the thecal sac (Fig. 19-46). Because the spinal cord appears as a relatively high signal intensity structure outlined by the

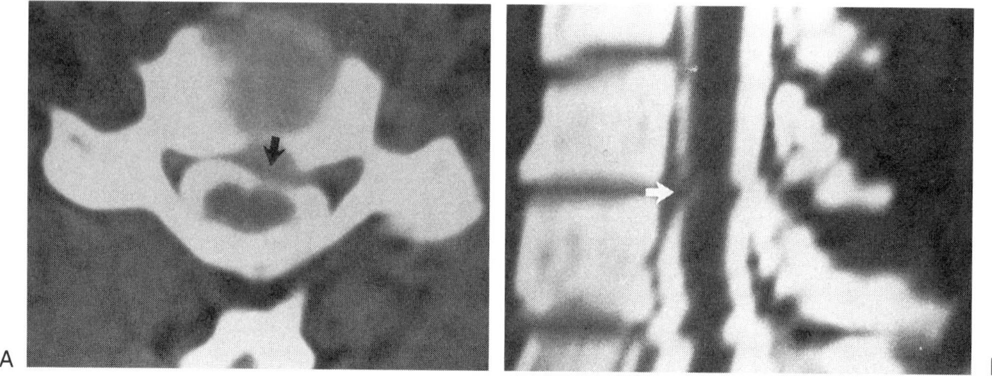

FIG. 19-45. CT evaluation of a herniated C5–C6 nucleus pulposus. **A:** An axial CT myelogram shows a radiodense protrusion of the C5–C6 disc *(arrow)* that distorts the left anterior aspect of both the thecal sac and the spinal cord. **B:** Sagittal reconstruction shows the herniated C5–C6 nucleus pulposus *(arrow)* indenting both the radiodense thecal sac and the radiolucent spinal cord.

low signal intensity cerebral spinal fluid (CSF), the relationship of the herniated disc to the spinal cord can be visualized directly by MRI. On T2-weighted MR images, the degenerated disc appears as a narrowed disc interval. The disc herniation appears as a moderate to low signal intensity impingement on the now high signal intensity CSF. The posterior margin of the herniated disc may have a very low signal intensity margin interfacing with the CSF. This may be a posterior longitudinal ligament elevated by the herniated disc, or it may be fragments of the posterior part of the anulus fibrosus (47). T2-weighted images also permit evaluation of the relationship of the herniated disc to the spinal cord to determine its probability of causing a patient's myelopathic findings. It is sometimes difficult to differentiate lateral herniations of the disc into the neural foramen from osteophytic encroachments by MRI because they may both demonstrate

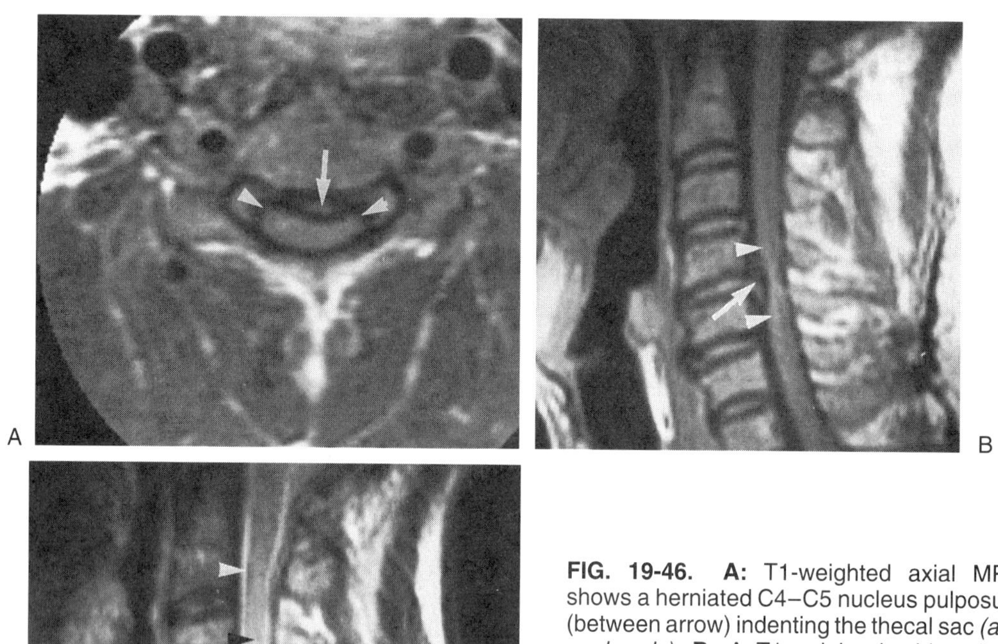

FIG. 19-46. A: T1-weighted axial MRI shows a herniated C4–C5 nucleus pulposus (between arrow) indenting the thecal sac *(arrowheads)*. **B:** A T1-weighted mid-sagittal MRI shows the herniated C4–C5 disc *(arrow)* impinging on the moderately low signal intensity thecal sac *(arrowheads)*. **C:** A T2-weighted mid-sagittal MRI demonstrates that the herniated C4–C5 disc *(arrow)* is compressing not only the high signal intensity dural sac *(white arrowhead)* but also the moderate signal intensity spinal cord *(black arrowhead)*.

low signal intensity. In these circumstances, CT provides good differentiation between bone and soft-tissue density.

Cervical Spinal Stenosis and Foraminal Stenosis

Cervical spinal stenosis can be congenital or acquired. In the less common congenital stenosis, a small spinal canal is produced by short pedicles and thick laminae (48). It commonly remains asymptomatic until degenerative changes are superimposed on the congenital stenosis later in life.

Acquired stenosis can be produced by a host of hypertrophic degenerative changes often collectively referred to as cervical spondylosis. These include osteophytic lipping of the posterior margins of the vertebral body ends bounding the disc, hypertrophic degenerative changes involving Luschka's joints or the facet joints, buckling or hypertrophy of the ligamenta flava, and ossification of the posterior longitudinal ligament. All of these structures bound the spinal canal; therefore, hypertrophic degenerative changes can produce spinal canal stenosis. Because Luschka's joints, the facet joints, and the ligamenta flava also bound the neural foramen, their involvement by degenerative processes can produce foraminal stenosis.

Although hypertrophic degenerative changes of any of the structures bounding the spinal canal or neural foramen can occur in isolation, they are commonly precipitated by intervertebral disc degeneration. As the disc degenerates and loses its normal load-dispersing ability, loads tend to become concentrated on the vertebral body margin toward which the spine is bent. This excessive loading can produce marginal osteophytes around the entire circumference of the vertebral body ends. Those osteophytes developing on the posterior margin can encroach the spinal canal to produce spinal stenosis (Fig. 19-47). Luschka's (i.e., uncovertebral) joints are situated between the uncinate processes that protrude from the lateral or posterolateral margins of the upper surface of the vertebral bodies and a reciprocal convexity on the lateral aspect of the inferior surface of the next higher vertebral body. Recent evidence indicates that they are not true joints (49). Rather, they are degenerative clefts within the lateral part of the intervertebral disc that begin in the second decade of life. The increased loading of Luschka's joints produced by these degenerative changes produces bony spurs that can extend posteriorly into the lateral part of the spinal canal or posterolaterally into the neural foramen (Fig. 19-48).

Because disc degeneration is accompanied by dehydration and loss of disc height, as the vertebral bodies approximate, facet joint loads are increased. The resultant facet joint degeneration involves cartilage erosion with joint space narrowing, subchondral bone sclerosis, and osteophyte forma-

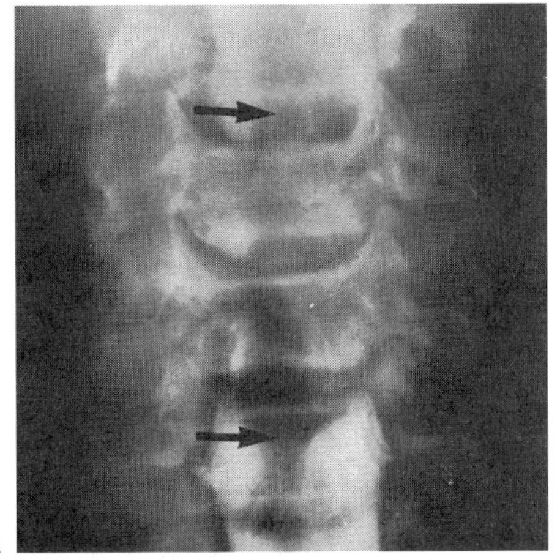
A

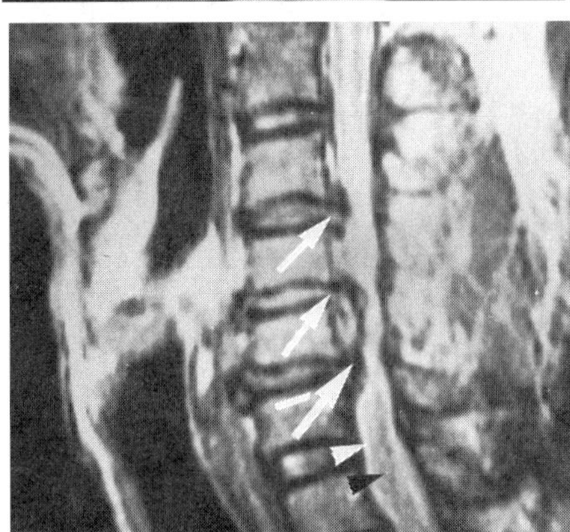
B

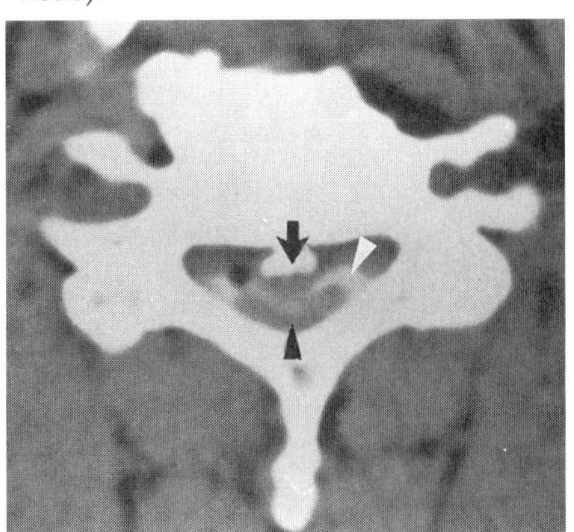
C

FIG. 19-47. Cervical spinal stenosis. Degeneration of C3–C4, C4–C5, and C5–C6 intervertebral discs with posterior body osteophytes and an ossified posterior longitudinal ligament producing complete myelographic block and cord compression. **A:** An anteroposterior myelogram shows a complete block (between arrows) of the contrast column at the C3–C4, C4–C5, and C5–C6 levels. **B:** A T2-weighted mid-sagittal MRI demonstrates degenerated discs *(arrows)* at these levels that impinge on both the high-intensity thecal sac *(white arrowheads)* and the moderate-intensity spinal cord *(black arrowheads)*. **C:** A CT myelogram shows an associated ossification of the posterior longitudinal ligament *(arrow)* that also encroaches on the thecal sac *(white arrowhead)* and compresses the spinal cord *(black arrowhead)*.

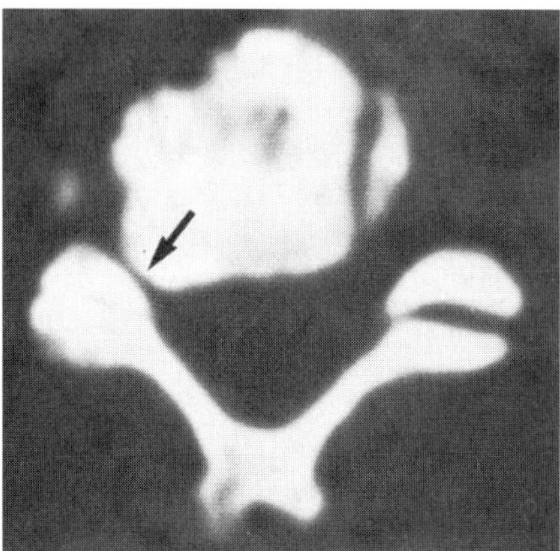

FIG. 19-48. CT of hypertrophic degenerative changes involving Luschka's joint. These changes cause osteophytic encroachment *(arrow)* upon the right C3–C4 intervertebral foramen.

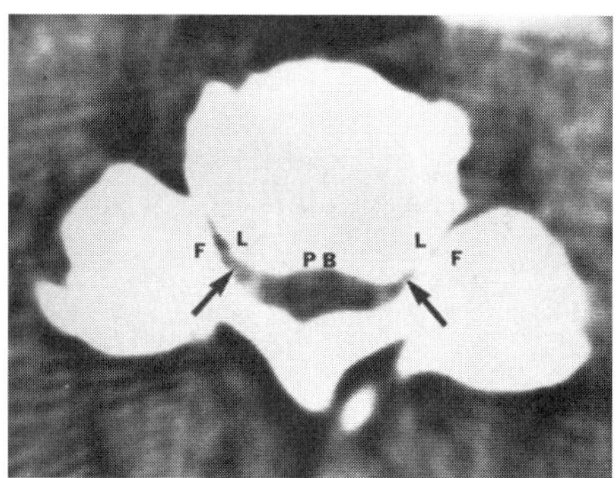

FIG. 19-49. CT of central cervical stenosis and foraminal stenosis. Hypertrophic degenerative changes involving Luschka's joints *(L)*, facet joints *(F)*, and posterior vertebral body margins *(PB)* have caused severe narrowing of the anteroposterior dimension of the cervical spinal canal and bilateral foraminal stenosis *(arrows)*.

tion. The osteophytes may encroach upon the spinal canal or neural foramen.

Loss of disc height can cause the laminae to approximate, and this in turn causes the ligamenta flava to buckle and bulge into the spinal canal, contributing to the spinal stenosis. Because the ligamenta flava continue laterally into the facet joint capsule, buckling of this part of the ligamenta flava can cause foraminal stenosis.

Ossification of the posterior longitudinal ligament occurs more commonly at cervical than at other vertebral levels. It is best visualized via CT, where it appears as an ossification extending over several vertebral levels, separated from the posterior margin of the vertebral bodies by a thin radiolucent interval (Fig. 19-47*C*).

When any of these potential causes of cervical stenosis sufficiently narrow the spinal canal, cord compression can produce myelopathic signs and symptoms. Spinal stenosis most frequently narrows the anteroposterior (AP) dimension of the spinal canal (Fig. 19-49). Although the cross-sectional area of the spinal canal is smallest at the C4 and C7 levels, the smallest AP diameter is usually at the C3 through C5 levels (48). It has been stated that all spinal stenosis that reduces the AP dimension to less than 10 mm will produce quadriplegia (50).

Although the uppermost cervical cord segments are nearly round, at most cervical levels the cord has an elliptical outline with its major axis transversely oriented. With encroachment of the cord by spinal stenosis, it is usually first flattened anteriorly by an encroaching osteophyte (Fig. 19-50*A*). With progression, the anterior median fissure becomes indented and widened until the cord assumes a kidney bean shape (Fig. 19-50*B*) (48). The lateral funiculi may become tapered anterolaterally because of tension on the denticulate ligaments. The cord may become notched dorsally because of posterior white column atrophy. It has been estimated that a 30% reduction in cord cross-sectional area may be required

A

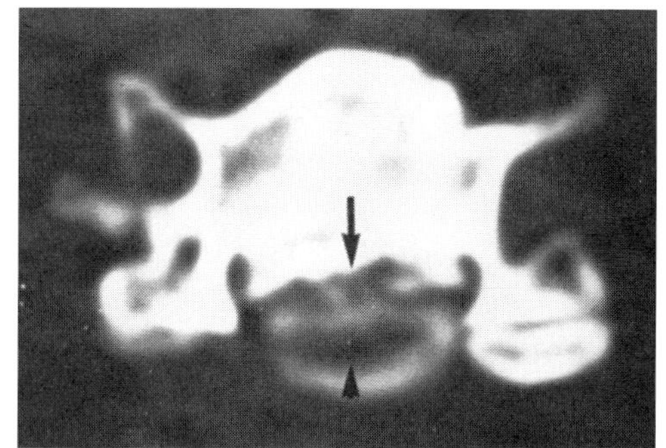

B

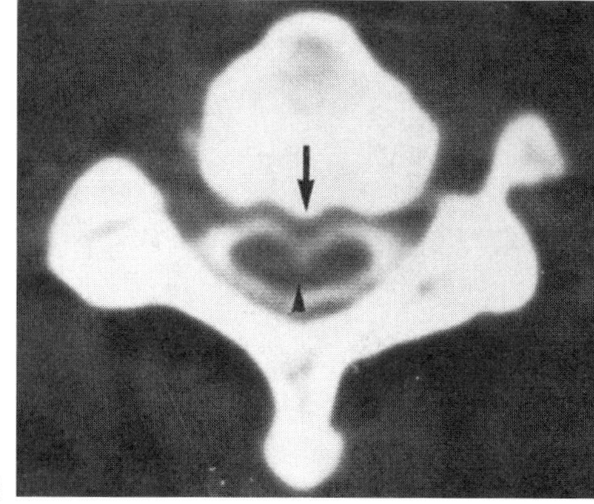

FIG. 19-50. Cord compression by cervical stenosis. **A:** CT myelogram of a patient with prior C3–C6 laminectomies who demonstrated progressive quadriparesis because of marked spondylosis of the C5–C6 and C6–C7 vertebral body margins *(arrow)*. The cord shows anteroposterior compression *(arrowhead)*. **B:** A CT myelogram of another patient showing a midline C3–C4 osteophyte *(arrow)* indenting the anterior aspect of the spinal cord *(arrowhead)*.

to produce signs of ascending and descending tract degeneration (51).

Thoracic Spine Abnormalities

Both thoracic disc herniation and thoracic spinal stenosis are rare compared with cervical and lumbar level disease. When thoracic disc herniation does occur, it most frequently involves discs below T8 (52). The CT findings are similar to those of cervical levels, except that calcification of the disc protrusion is more common at thoracic levels. The causes and CT and MRI findings of thoracic spinal stenosis are similar to those at cervical levels.

Lumbar Disc Herniation

The correlation of lumbar disc herniation with a patient's complaints of low back pain or sciatica is not always clearly established. It has been estimated that as many as 20% of patients with disc herniation are asymptomatic (53). Furthermore, when disc herniation occurs in symptomatic patients, other findings are often present that also could explain the clinical findings.

Lumbar disc herniations most frequently occur posterolaterally because the anulus is thinnest posteriorly but reinforced in the midline by the posterior longitudinal ligament. Also, the most prevalent lumbar spine motion—flexion—places greatest stress on the posterior part of the disc. When the disc herniates posterolaterally, it frequently does not impinge on the spinal nerve roots emerging from the neural foramen to which the disc is related, because the nerve roots occupy the upper portion of the foramen whereas the disc is situated in the anterior wall of the lower part of the foramen. Therefore, when the L5–S1 disc herniates posterolaterally, it frequently spares the L5 nerve roots exiting through the upper portion of the L5–S1 neural foramen. Instead, it more commonly involves the S1 nerve roots that descend across the posterolateral aspect of the L5–S1 disc before their exit from the S1 sacral foramina. Less common lumbar disc herniations are placed centrally or far laterally. Central herniations can involve any or all of the rootlets of the cauda equina. The infrequent far lateral herniations occur outside of the neural foramina. When present, they usually impinge on the ventral ramus that has just emerged from that foramen.

By plain film myelography, the herniated lumbar disc appears as an indentation into the thecal sac contrast column or as a cutoff of the nerve root sleeves (Fig. 19-51*A* and *B*). Visualization of posterolateral herniations is usually optimized by oblique views that place the herniation in profile (Fig. 19-51*B* and *C*).

Noncontrast CT has been described as being as accurate as standard myelography in diagnosing disc herniations. On CT examination, the herniated disc appears as a focal protrusion of the disc that displaces the epidural fat (Fig. 19-52*A*).

A,B
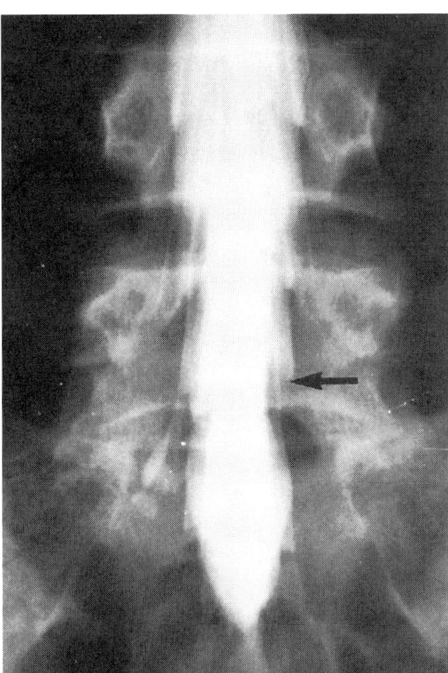
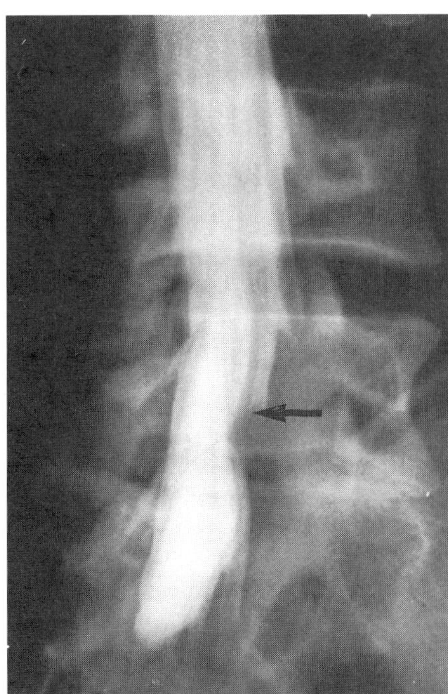
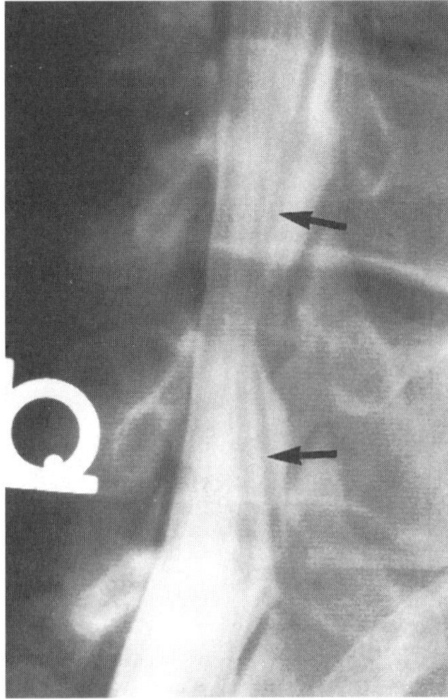
C

FIG. 19-51. Anteroposterior **(A)** and oblique myelograms **(B)** show an L5–S1 herniated disc cutting off the left S1 nerve root sleeve *(arrow)*. The oblique film better displays the indentation of the thecal sac by the herniated disc. Right anterior oblique view **(C)** shows an L3–L4 herniated disc encroaching the L4 nerve roots *(arrows)* while they are still within the thecal sac.

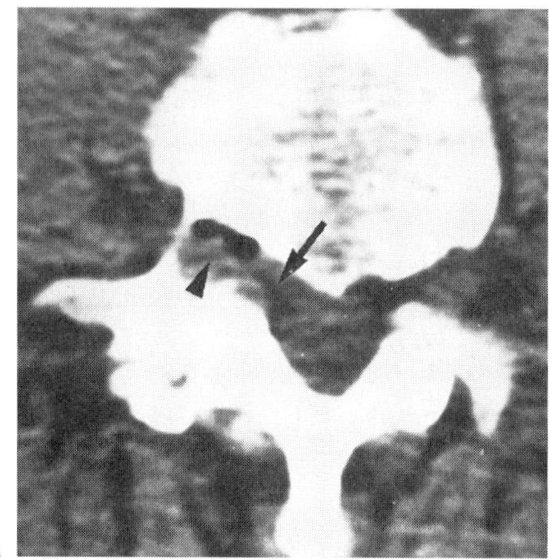

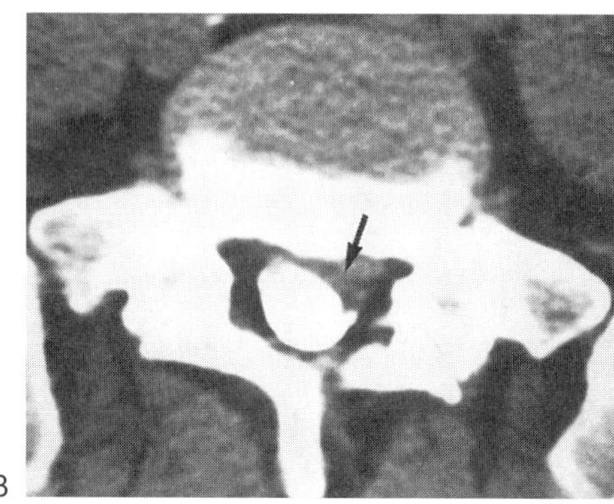

FIG. 19-52. CT evaluation of herniated lumbar discs. **A:** A noncontrast CT image at the L4–L5 level shows a dense mass *(arrow)* containing gas that displaces the right epidural fat and effaces the right L4 nerve roots within their neural foramen *(arrowhead)*. Note the normal epidural fat on the left and the normal fat outlining the left L4 nerve roots. **B:** A CT myelogram showing a left posterolateral herniation of the L5–S1 disc *(arrow)* encroaching upon the left anterior aspect of the contrast-enhanced thecal sac.

The herniated disc material is typically hyperdense relative to the non–contrast-enhanced dural sac and its adjacent nerve roots. With or without intrathecal contrast, the dural sac or adjacent nerve roots may be seen to be indented, displaced, or compressed (Fig. 19-52*B*). In more lateral herniations, the soft-tissue material of the disc can encroach upon the neural foramen or the extraforaminal soft tissues, where it also displaces fat, and here it may encroach upon the dorsal root ganglion, spinal nerve, or its ventral ramus. Herniated lumbar discs may calcify or contain gas. Extruded disc fragments can become separated from the disc and are thus able to migrate superiorly, inferiorly, or laterally. A herniated disc should be distinguished from a bulging anulus. A bulging anulus is produced by dehydration and volume loss within the nucleus pulposus. In contrast to the focal protrusion of a herniated disc, the bulging anulus typically has a symmetrical smooth contour bulging beyond all margins of the vertebral body.

On T1-weighted sagittal and axial MR images, the herniated lumbar disc appears as a moderate signal intensity intrusion into the high signal intensity epidural fat or upon the moderate to low signal intensity thecal sac or the lumbar nerve roots within their dural sleeves (Fig. 19-53). Similarly, disc herniation into the neural foramen is visualized by a moderate signal intensity mass displacing the foraminal fat and encroaching upon the dorsal root ganglion or nerve roots.

On T2-weighted sagittal MR images, the low signal intensity of a degenerated disc contrasts sharply with the high signal intensity of the nucleus pulposus of adjacent well-hydrated discs (Fig. 19-53*B* and *D*). Any intrusion of the low signal intensity disc herniation on the thecal sac is well seen because of the high signal intensity myelographic effect of the CSF on T2-weighted images.

Discography remains a controversial diagnostic imaging modality. It appears that its major diagnostic value lies in the reproduction of the patient's specific pain on contrast injection of a given disc, with controls demonstrating that injection of adjacent discs produces either no pain or foreign pain. Discography, especially when combined with CT, may provide information about degeneration and the extent of fissures and rupture (Fig. 19-54).

Lumbar Spinal Stenosis and Foraminal Stenosis

Like cervical stenosis, lumbar spinal stenosis is frequently precipitated by disc degeneration with subsequent marginal osteophytosis of the vertebral body ends, hypertrophic degeneration of the facet joints, and bulging of the ligamenta flava. Lumbar stenosis may be lateral, central, or combined. The lower lumbar vertebrae normally have shorter pedicles that cause the superior articular processes to intrude into the spinal canal to cut off narrow lateral recesses (Fig. 19-44*A*). The lateral recesses are bounded by the pedicles laterally, the vertebral body anteriorly, and, most important, the superior articular processes posteriorly. The lateral recesses are occupied by the nerve roots of the next spinal nerve to exit as they descend within their dural sleeve. Osteophytes that develop on the anteromedial margin of the superior articular processes of the next lower vertebra are most likely to encroach upon the lateral recess to produce lateral stenosis. Because the inferior articular processes of the next higher vertebra are situated posteromedial to the superior articular processes, osteophytes developing on their anterior margin are more likely to produce central stenosis. In central stenosis, any or all of the rootlets of the cauda equina can be encroached upon. Vertebral body margin osteophytes and buckling of the ligamenta flava can contribute to lumbar spinal stenosis.

Hypertrophic degenerative changes involving the facet joints can also encroach upon the posterior aspect of the neural foramen and produce foraminal stenosis with compression of the nerve roots exiting that foramen. Therefore, hypertrophic degenerative changes involving a single superior articular process can involve the roots of two closely adjacent nerves, with the possibility of producing both fo-

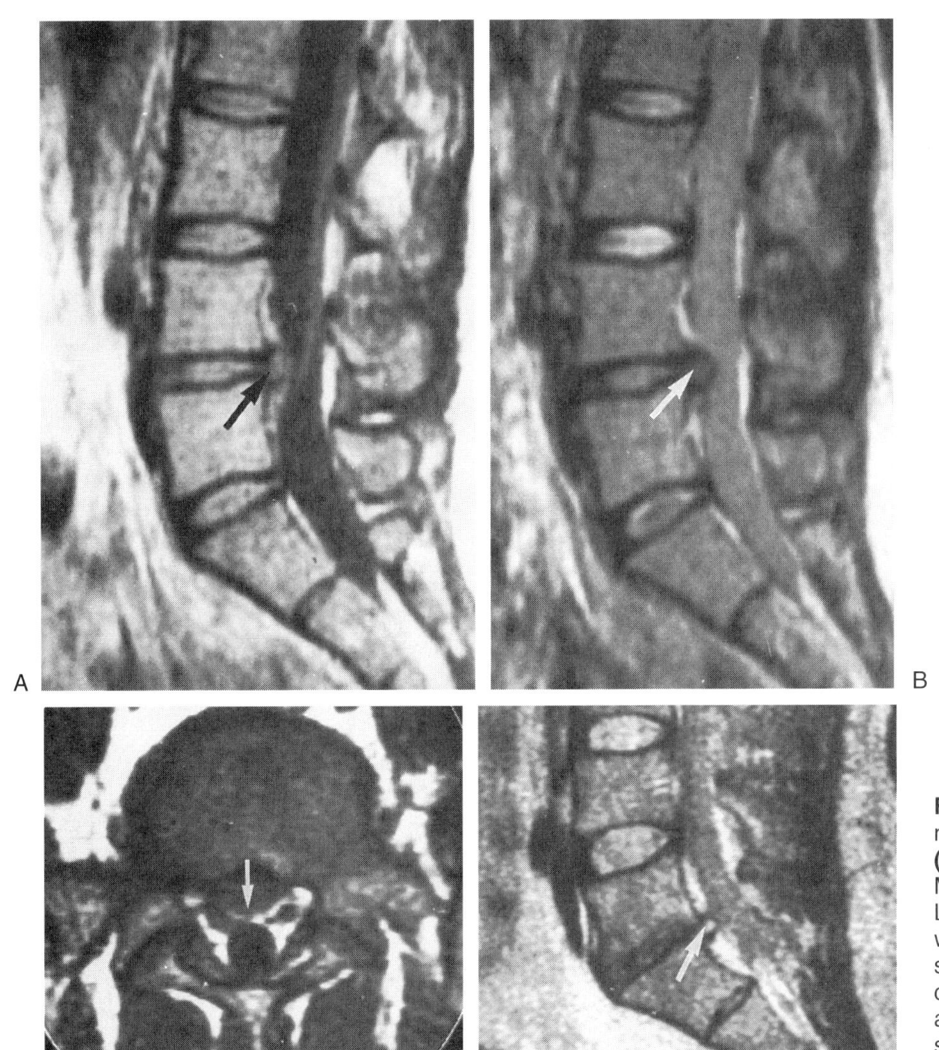

FIG. 19-53. MRI evaluation of herniated lumbar discs. T1-weighted **(A)** and T2-weighted **(B)** sagittal MR images show a herniated L4–L5 disc *(arrows)*. On the T2-weighted image, note the loss of signal intensity from the L4–L5 nucleus pulposus. A T1-weighted axial MRI **(C)** and a T2-weighted sagittal MRI **(D)** show a herniated L5–S1 disc *(arrows)*.

raminal and lateral spinal stenosis. With disc degeneration and loss of disc height, the neural foramen can be further compromised by the upward and forward displacement of the superior articular process into the upper part of the neural foramen where the nerve roots are situated. In addition, because of the obliquity of the facet joint, the accompanying downward displacement of the inferior articular process of the next higher vertebra can produce retrolisthesis (i.e., backward displacement) of its vertebral body into the upper portion of the neural foramen.

By standard myelography, the protruding disc anteriorly and the bulging ligamenta flava posteriorly can produce an hourglass appearance of the thecal sac (Fig. 19-55). By CT, all osteophytes are clearly visualized, and measurements of the AP dimension of lateral recesses that are less than 3 mm are strongly suggestive of lateral stenosis (Fig. 19-56) (54). The hypertrophic changes producing central and foraminal stenosis are also well visualized. Sagittal reformations are especially helpful in evaluating foraminal stenosis.

Facet anatomy is well seen by MRI, with subchondral bone appearing as a signal void. On T1-weighted images, articular cartilage is visualized as a moderate signal intensity interval between the subchondral bone of the two articular processes. This becomes more signal intense on T2-weighted images. Facet joint degeneration appears as an irregularity or reduction in the thickness of the articular cartilage. Osteophytes are usually displayed as signal voids encroaching into the foramen, lateral recess, or spinal canal. Occasionally, osteophytes show a high signal intensity interior, indicating the presence of marrow.

Spondylolysis and Spondylolisthesis

Spondylolysis is a defect in the pars interarticularis, commonly involving the L5 and occasionally the L4 vertebrae. Most spondylolysis is thought to be produced by repetitive stress. The gravitational and muscular loads acting across the steep incline of the upper surface of the sacrum can be resolved into a shearing component, which tends to displace the L5 vertebral body forward on S1, and a compressive component at right angles to the superior surface of S1 (Fig. 19-57). In accordance with Newton's third law, S1 will exert an equal and opposite force against the inferior aspect of the L5 vertebral body. The tendency of L5 to be displaced forward on S1 is largely resisted by the impaction of the inferior articular processes of L5 upon the superior articular processes of S1. Again, Newton's third law dictates that there will be an equal and opposite force exerted against the inferior articular process of L5. The upward and forward force of the sacral body upon the L5 body and the upward and backward force of the superior articular process of the sacrum upon the inferior articular process of L5 cause shearing stresses to be concentrated on the pars interarticularis, and this can produce a stress fracture.

Spondylolisthesis is an anterior subluxation of one vertebral body upon another. It can occur at any vertebral level, but the mechanics of the lumbosacral junction cause a higher incidence at this level. The most common cause at this level is spondylolysis, where the impaction of the inferior articular process of L5 or L4 will no longer be able to resist forward displacement of the vertebral body. Whether or not a spondylolisthesis follows a spondylolysis is largely determined by the resistance of the other supporting structures of the lumbosacral junction, which include the intervertebral disc, the anterior longitudinal ligament, and the iliolumbar ligaments. When they fail, the lysis becomes a listhesis.

Other causes of spondylolisthesis include degenerative changes in the facet joints and disc that produce joint insta-

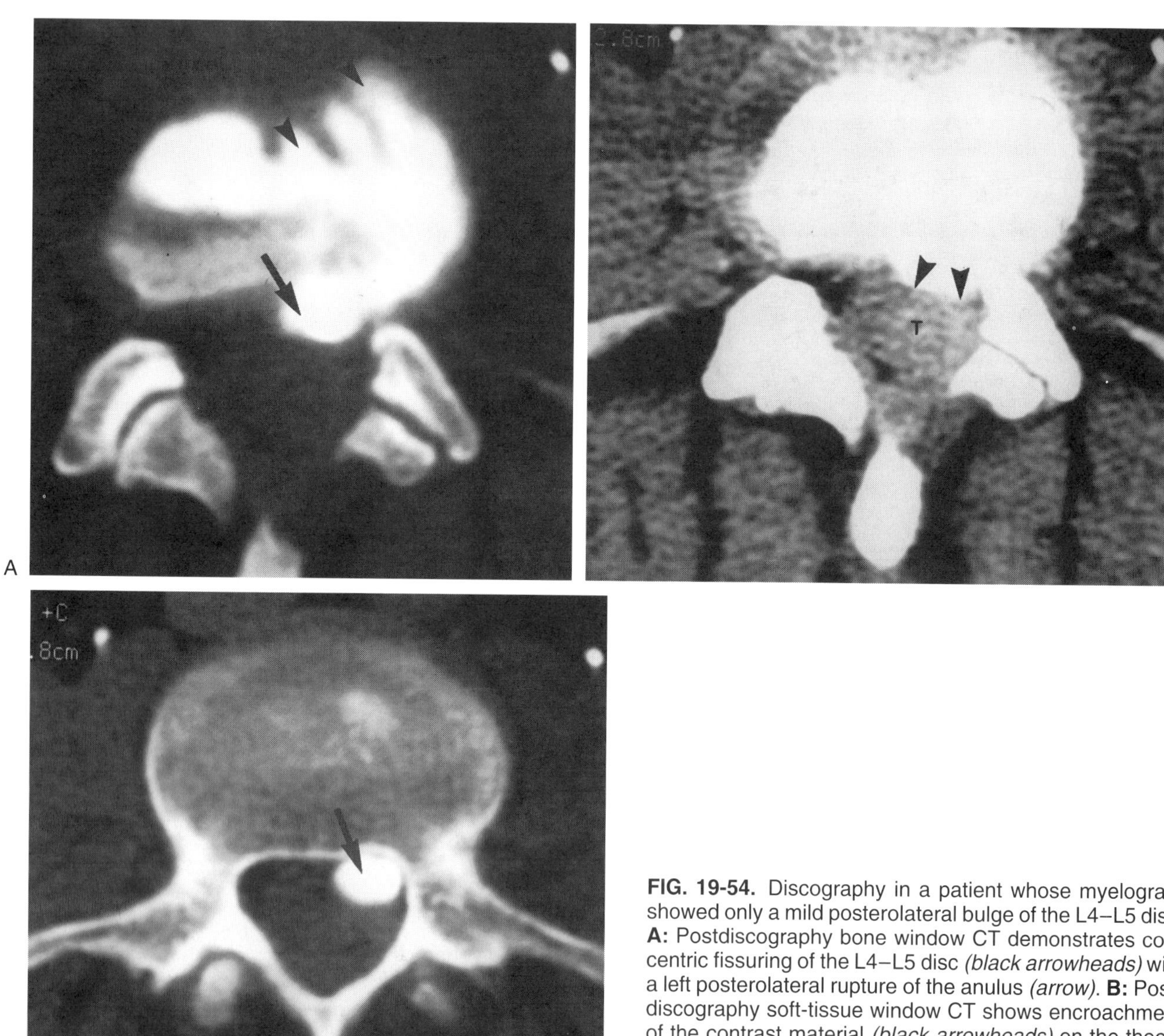

FIG. 19-54. Discography in a patient whose myelogram showed only a mild posterolateral bulge of the L4–L5 disc. **A:** Postdiscography bone window CT demonstrates concentric fissuring of the L4–L5 disc *(black arrowheads)* with a left posterolateral rupture of the anulus *(arrow)*. **B:** Postdiscography soft-tissue window CT shows encroachment of the contrast material *(black arrowheads)* on the thecal sac *(T)*. **C:** Postdiscography bone window CT through L4 demonstrates a cranial migration of the contrast material into the left lateral recess of L4 *(arrow)*.

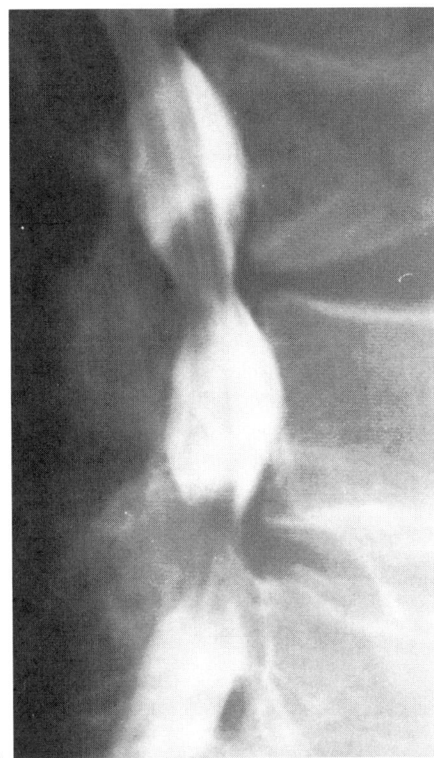

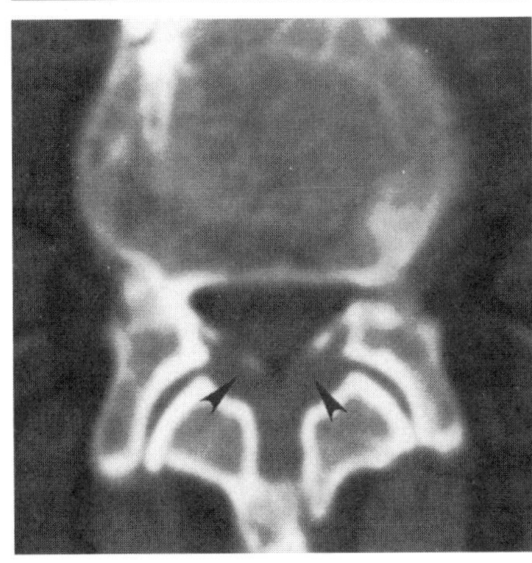

FIG. 19-55. Lumbar spinal stenosis caused by both protruding discs and bulging ligamenta flava. **A:** Lateral myelogram showing the hourglass appearance of the thecal sac. **B:** Axial CT shows the thickened ligamenta flava *(arrowheads)*.

bility, fractures, dysplasia of the upper sacrum or the neural arch of L5, generalized pathology such as Paget's disease, or iatrogenically induced laminectomy or facetectomy (48).

On oblique plain films, spondylolysis is visualized as a break in the neck of the ''Scotty-dog'' outline, which is produced by the ipsilateral transverse process forming a nose, the ipsilateral pedicle an eye, the pars interarticularis a neck, the ipsilateral inferior articular process a forelimb, the lamina a body, the contralateral inferior articular process a hindlimb, and the spinous process a tail (Fig. 19-58*A*).

Spondylolisthesis is graded by the amount of subluxation, with grade I being a forward displacement of less than 25%, grade II a forward displacement of 25% to 50%, grade III 50% to 75%, and grade IV a displacement greater than 75%. Grading the spondylolisthesis is usually accomplished by lateral plain films (Fig. 19-58*B* and *C*).

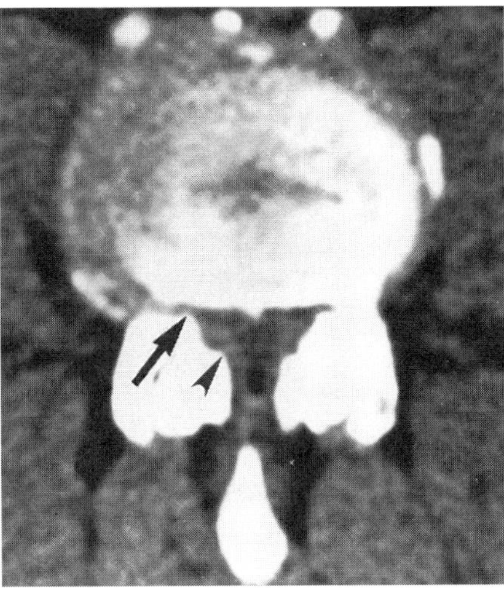

FIG. 19-56. CT at the L4–L5 level shows hypertrophic degenerative changes of the L5 superior articular process *(black arrow)*, which produce lateral stenosis, and hypertrophic changes of the L4 inferior articular process *(black arrowhead)*, which cause central stenosis.

On CT, the defect of spondylolysis is differentiated from the facet joint interval by its location at the axial level of the pedicles rather than at the level of the neural foramen, as well as by the defect's irregular margins and adjacent

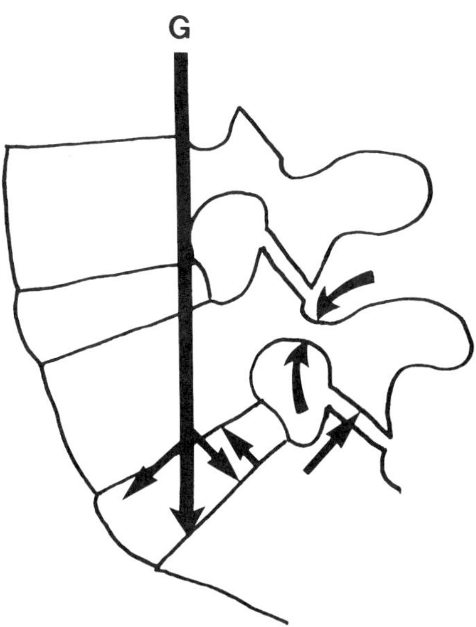

FIG. 19-57. The gravitational load *(G)* is applied across the lumbosacral junction. The equal and opposite forces acting on the inferior aspect of the L5 body and the anterior aspect of the inferior articular process of L5 cause shearing stresses to be concentrated on the pars interarticularis of L5 *(curved arrows)*. This produces the stress fracture of spondylolysis.

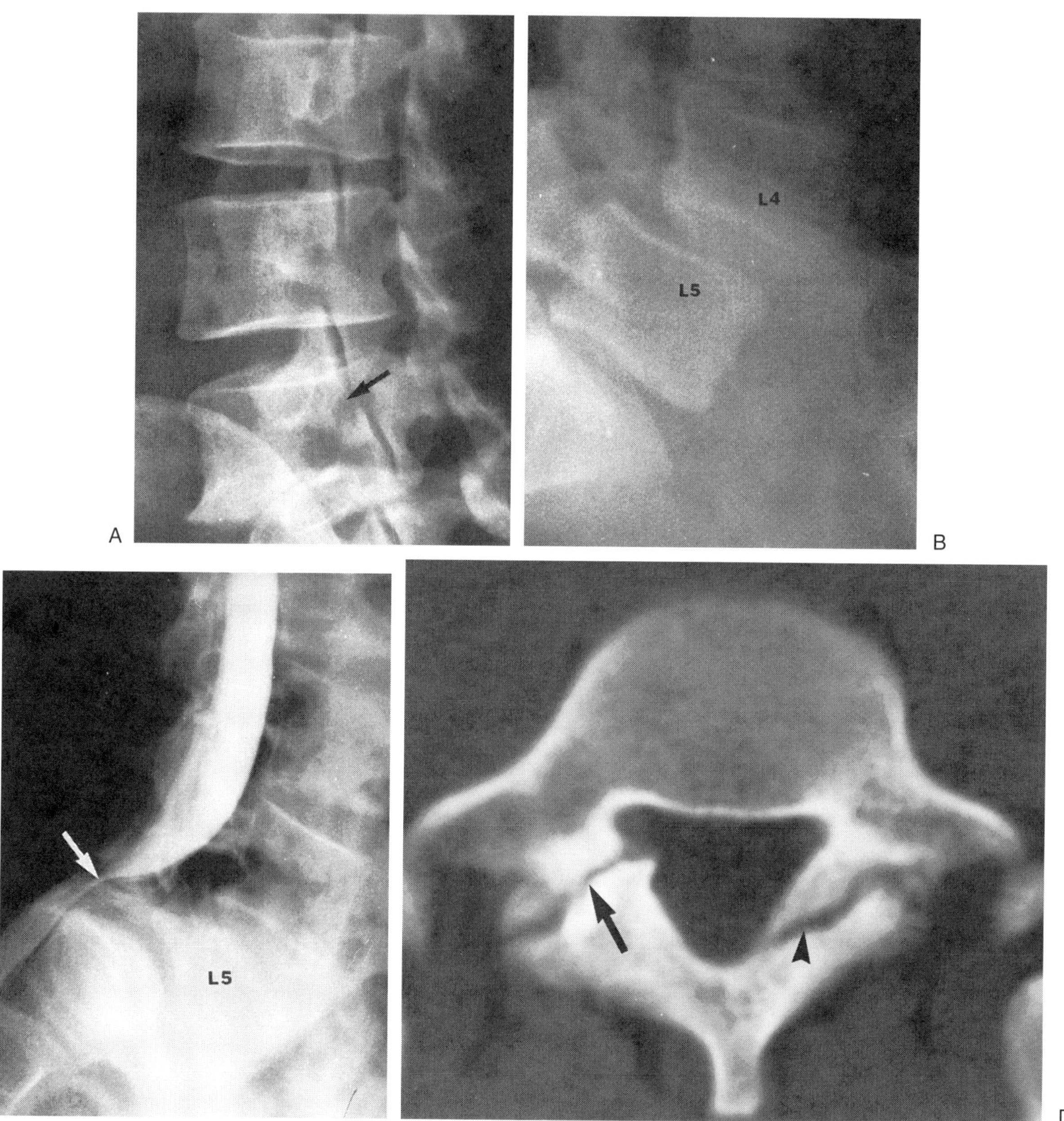

FIG. 19-58. Spondylolysis and spondylolisthesis. **A:** An oblique radiograph demonstrates a spondylolytic defect in the pars interarticularis of L4 *(arrow).* Note the intact neck in the "Scotty dog" outline in the L3 vertebra. **B:** A lateral radiograph shows that there is a grade II spondylolisthesis of L4 on L5. **C:** A lateral myelogram of another patient with a grade III spondylolisthesis of L5 on S1 causing impingement of the thecal sac *(arrow)* by the lamina of L5. **D:** CT demonstrates bilateral L5 spondylolysis with an old nonunited spondylolysis on the right showing irregular margins and adjacent slerosis *(arrow)* and an acute fracture on the left *(arrowhead).*

sclerosis (Fig. 19-58*D*). By MRI, the defect in the pars is visualized as a low signal intensity zone within the high signal intensity marrow of the pars.

Spinal Trauma

Although much spinal trauma is well visualized on plain films or conventional tomography, CT has a number of advantages over these modalities. These include the demonstration of fractures not seen in plain films, an accurate determination of the amount of spinal canal encroachment by fracture fragments (Fig. 19-59*A*), the identification of neural foramen impingement by fractures involving its boundaries, and a more precise evaluation of facet disruption.

CT myelography also can display impingement upon the dural sac or the spinal cord by bone fragments, as well as any resultant cord atrophy (Fig. 19-59*B*). It can demonstrate acute cord enlargement as a sign of cord edema or hemor-

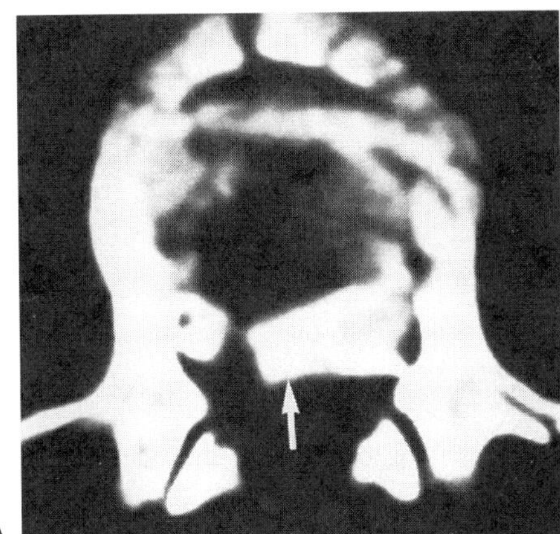

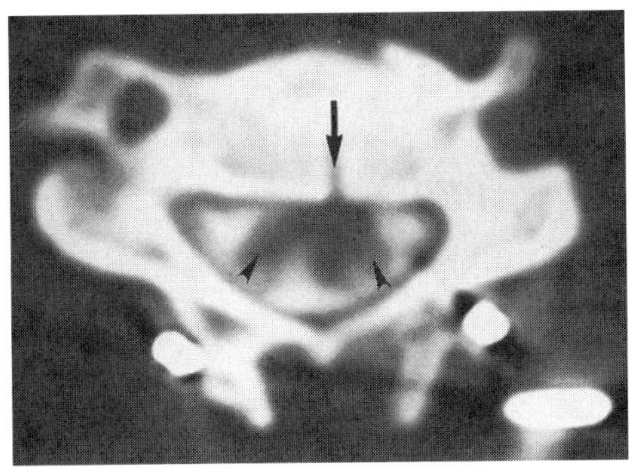

FIG. 19-59. CT visualization of spinal trauma. **A:** CT of a burst fracture of L2 shows displacement of a fracture fragment into the spinal canal *(arrow)*. **B:** A CT myelogram of a sagittal fracture of C5 *(arrow)* 6 months after surgical stabilization shows the irregular outline of an atrophic spinal cord *(arrowheads)* in a quadriparetic patient with some residual upper limb function.

rhage. CT myelography can be used to diagnose posttraumatic cystic myelopathy because the cyst will take up the contrast and be displayed as a well-marginated, homogenous, high-density region within the cord.

CT also can augment the interpretation of the signs of vertebral instability seen on plain radiographs (Fig. 19-60) (56). These signs include the following:

1. Vertebral displacements involving the whole vertebra or fracture fragments
2. Widening of the interspinous interval, which implies injury to the posterior spinal ligaments secondary to hyperflexion injury
3. Increased dimensions of the vertebral canal in the sagittal or coronal plane often evaluated by an increased interpedicle distance, which implies a complete disruption of the vertebral body in the sagittal plane
4. Widening of the facet joint interval, which implies ligamentous disruption
5. Disruption of the alignment of the posterior aspect of the vertebral bodies, such as occurs in burst fractures or lap seat belt fractures

T1-weighted sagittal and axial MR images provide the best evaluation of vertebral alignment and the bony and ligamentous boundaries of the spinal canal. They also allow the best delineation of the low signal intensity of a traumatic syringomyelia against the higher signal intensity of the surrounding spinal cord. T2-weighted sagittal MR images that produce a high signal intensity CSF provide the best estimate of the degree of encroachment of a bony fragment upon the thecal sac or the spinal cord.

MRI has a number of advantages over other modalities for imaging spinal trauma. First, it permits evaluation of vertebral alignment at the cervicothoracic junction of the spine, which is relatively inaccessible by other modalities. Second, it provides a means to evaluate adjacent soft-tissue damage (Fig. 19-60*D*). For example, hemorrhage in the prevertebral space that can occur with hyperextension injuries is identified on T2-weighted images as a high signal intensity area. MRI also identifies high signal intensity hemorrhage in the posterior paravertebral muscles that can occur secondary to hyperflexion injuries. Of importance is the fact that MRI provides a noninvasive means of evaluating the relationship of retropulsed vertebral body fragments or anteriorly displaced neural arch fragments to the spinal cord. In some centers, MRI has replaced myelography as the procedure of choice for evaluating the effects of vertebral trauma on the spinal cord. Most important, MRI can evaluate the extent and type of spinal cord injury (56,57).

An acutely injured spinal cord tends to enlarge, thereby filling the spinal canal and displacing the epidural fat. This can be visualized by both CT and MRI. However, MRI provides the best means of evaluating the type of spinal cord trauma and its evolution. MRI is valuable in the early stages of spinal cord injury in determining the type of spinal cord injury and the prognosis for recovery. It can identify the level and completeness of cord transection by direct visualization of the transection site (Fig. 19-61). In the nontransected cord it can discriminate cord hemorrhage from cord contusion with edema. Spinal cord contusion with edema causes high signal intensity on T2-weighted images within the first 24 hours of injury. Acute hemorrhage of less than 24 hours' duration appears as a low signal intensity area on T2-weighted images. Within a few days of the trauma the subacute hemorrhage site becomes hyperintense on T2-weighted images as a result of the accumulation of paramagnetic methemoglobin (Fig. 19-60*D*). Kulkarni and colleagues found that the type of injury visualized by MRI correlated with the patient's recovery of neurologic function (58). Those patients with cord contusion and edema exhibited significant functional recovery, whereas those with hemorrhage made little functional progress. Therefore, the MRI characteristics of the injury may provide the clinician with important prognostic data.

MRI is also invaluable for identifying late sequelae of spinal cord trauma, including myelomalacia and posttraumatic spinal cord cysts or syringomyelia. Myelomalacia is thought to develop within an injured segment of the spinal cord as a result of ischemia or the release of enzymes from damaged spinal cord tissues, or both (59). The myelomalacic

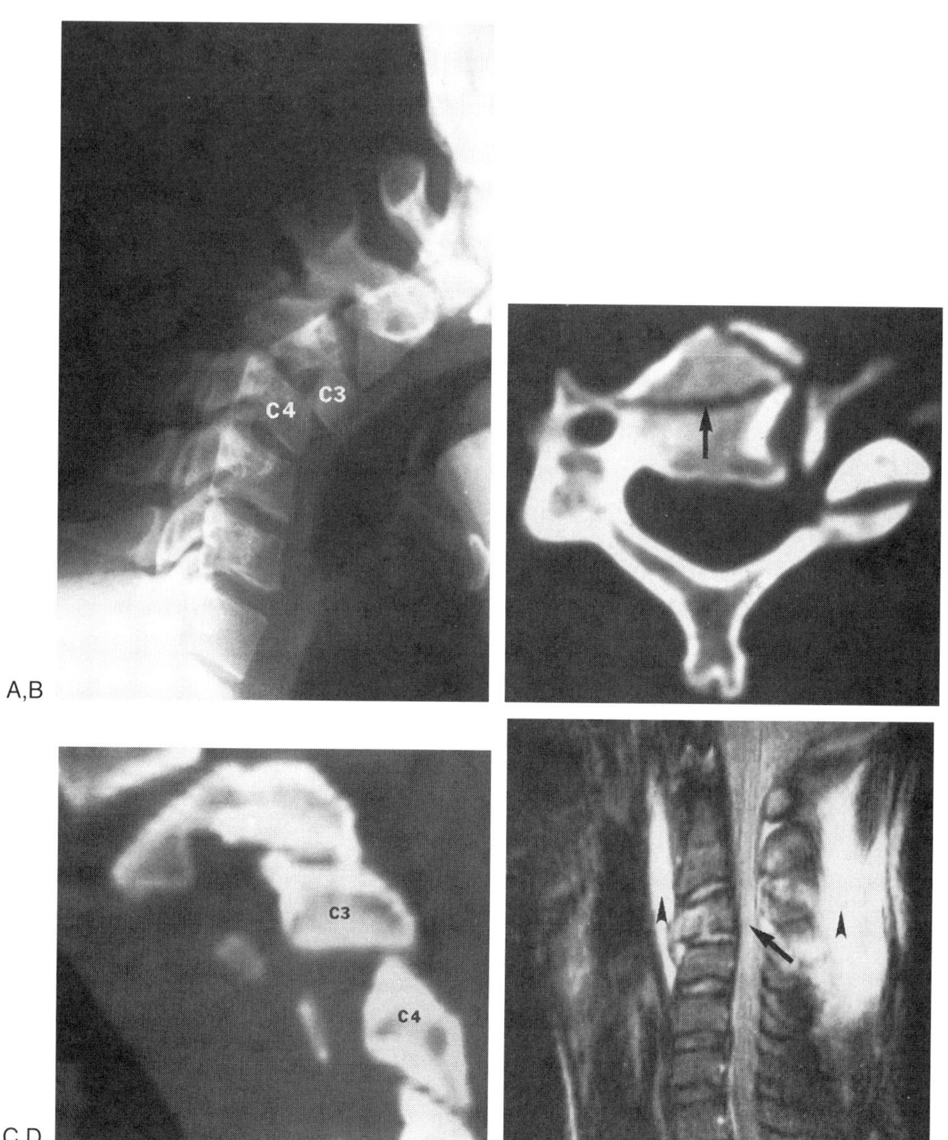

FIG. 19-60. Fracture–dislocation of C3. **A:** A lateral radiograph demonstrates the dislocation of C3 on C4. **B:** Axial CT demonstrates the fracture of the C3 vertebral body *(arrow)*. **C:** A sagittal reconstruction of the CT axial images through the articular pillars demonstrates the anterior dislocation of the C3 inferior articular process on C4. **D:** A T2-weighted mid-sagittal MRI displays hyperintense spinal cord hemorrhage *(arrow)* and hemorrhage within the prevertebral space and posterior paravertebral muscles *(arrowheads)*.

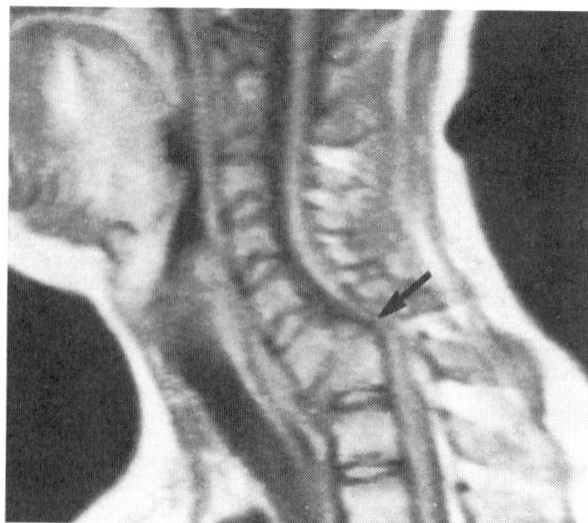

FIG. 19-61. Fracture–dislocation of C6–C7 with cord compression *(arrow)* as seen on a T1-weighted mid-sagittal MRI.

area is made up of the products of neuronal degeneration, scar tissue, and microcysts. It is thought that the myelomalacic areas become larger intramedullary cysts because the scar tissue about the injured cord tethers the cord to the dura so that the episodic changes in CSF pressure that occur during daily activities tend to be concentrated on the injured cord segment as stretching forces. It is hypothesized that these stresses cause coalescence of the myelomalacic microcysts into a progressively enlarging gross cyst. CSF is theorized to enter the cyst along enlarged perivascular Virchow-Robin spaces that connect the subarachnoid space to the cyst.

On T1-weighted images, myelomalacia appears within the segment of the spinal cord near the area of injury as a region of lower signal intensity than the spinal cord but higher signal intensity than the CSF. It has indistinct margins with the surrounding spinal cord. In contrast, intramedullary cysts have signal intensity approximating that of CSF and sharply marginated borders with the surrounding spinal cord or an adjacent area of myelomalacia. The development of an intramedullary cyst in a spinal cord patient whose clinical picture had previously stabilized may cause the patient to develop progressive sensory and motor deficits. Although myelomalacia has no definitive treatment mode, a spinal cord cyst can be surgically decompressed with a shunt to achieve improvement or at least an arrest of the patient's neurologic deterioration. Therefore, the MRI distinction between cysts and myelomalacia is important. MRI can also be used in postoperative follow-up to ensure that the cyst has been fully decompressed and that the catheter is continuing to function to prevent reaccumulation of fluid within the cyst.

BRAIN IMAGING

In this survey of brain imaging relevant to rehabilitation, emphasis is placed on the imaging of ischemic and hemorrhagic strokes, head trauma, and the common degenerative diseases. The imaging of brain neoplasms and infections is not described.

Stroke

The term ''stroke'' typically applies to a sudden neurologic affliction of nontraumatic vascular etiology. An early diagnostic concern is to differentiate between the ischemic and hemorrhagic categories of stroke to determine if anticoagulant therapy is contraindicated. CT continues to be the initial imaging modality for most acute stroke patients for three reasons. First, CT detects intracerebral hemorrhage with great specificity and sensitivity because freshly extravasated blood is more radiodense than either gray or white matter. Second, MRI is unable to detect the oxyhemoglobin that predominates in the hemorrhage in the early hours after a stroke because it is a nonparamagnetic substance. Third, the uncooperativeness of many acute stroke patients during the long MRI scan times and the incompatibility of critical monitoring equipment with the strong magnetic fields often preclude early MRI examination.

Ischemic Stroke

Cerebral ischemia can be produced by thrombosis of large extracranial or small intracerebral vessels, emboli originating from atherosclerotic plaques or thrombi within more proximal vessels or the heart, or decreased perfusion of systemic origin, such as shock, decreased cardiac output, or respiratory failure.

Transient ischemic attacks, in which the neurologic deficits clear completely within 24 hours and frequently within a few minutes or hours, typically produce no findings by either CT or MRI because they are thought to produce no significant cerebral infarction.

When ischemia produces infarction, the first pathologic change is edema. It is this accumulation of water within the involved gray and white matter that produces the earliest CT and MRI findings. Although CT rarely detects infarction in the first few hours, by 18 to 24 hours there are often minor findings on non–contrast-enhanced CT scans. These include a slight hypodensity of the affected area, loss of some of the distinction between gray and white matter, and a subtle mass effect that may be indicated only by effacement of overlying cortical sulci (Fig. 19-62*A*) (60). Edema reaches its peak at 3 to 5 days, and by this time non–contrast-enhanced CT typically demonstrates a well-defined hypodense area that usually corresponds to the vascular territory of one of the cerebral arteries or its branches (Fig. 19-62*B*). With large infarctions, the brain swelling can cause large midline shifts, herniation of the brain under the falx cerebri or through the tentorium, and ventricular enlargement secondary to obstruction of the cerebral aqueduct (Fig. 19-63). With subse-

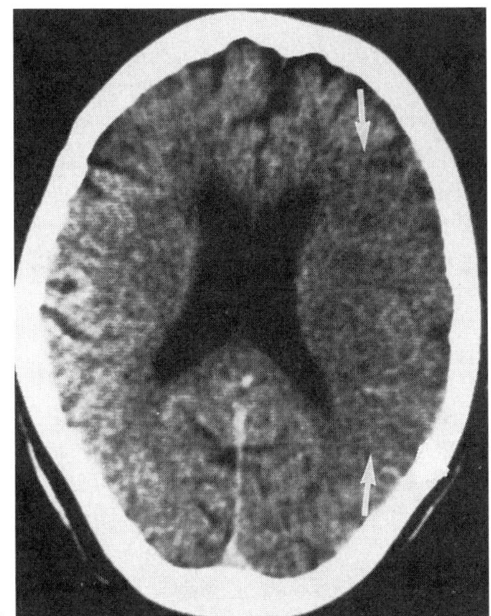
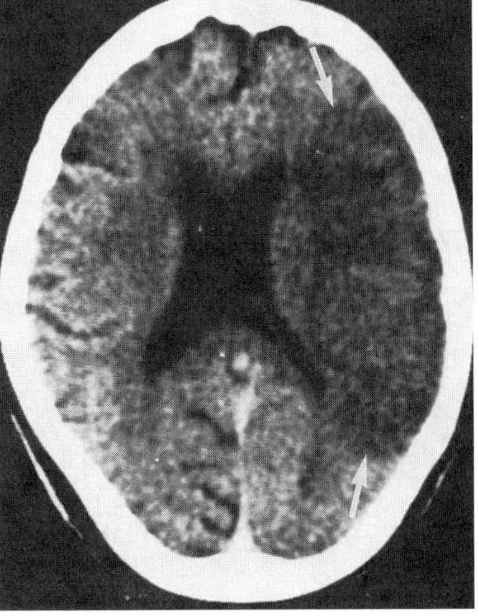

A,B

FIG. 19-62. Early CT changes of left middle cerebral artery infarction. **A:** Within 12 hours, the only CT changes are a slight hypodensity, loss of normal gray-white matter differentiation, and effacement of overlying cortical sulci in the region between the arrows. **B:** By 5 days, postinjury edema has peaked and the infarcted area is shown as a distinct hypodensity conforming to the territory of the middle cerebral artery *(between arrows).*

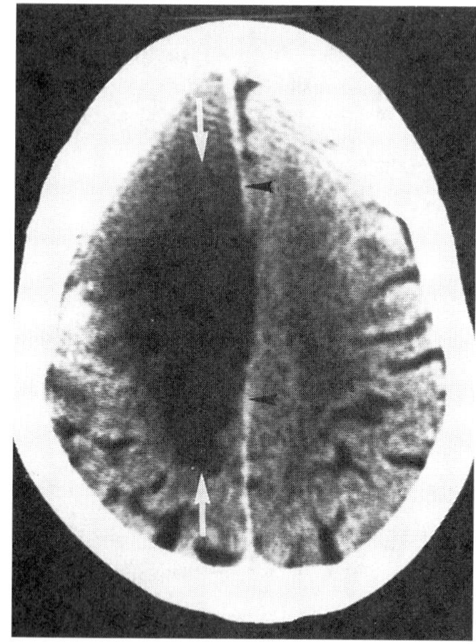

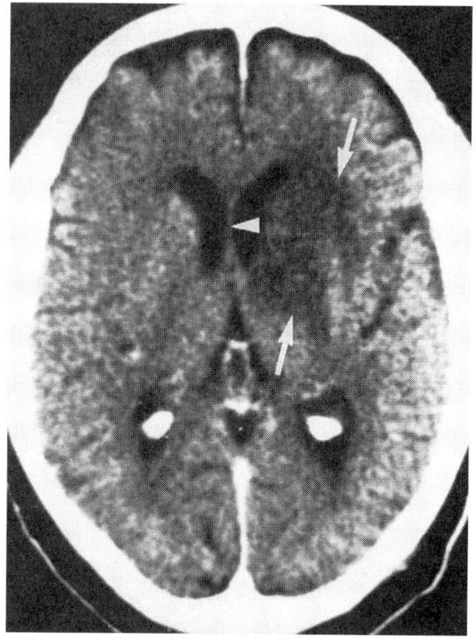

A,B

FIG. 19-63. CT evaluation of large infarctions that cause midline brain shifts and herniations. **A:** The hypodensity of a right anterior cerebral artery infarction *(between arrows)* caused a herniation of the right hemisphere under the falx cerebri *(arrowheads)*. **B:** The hypodensity of an infarction involving the left caudate, lenticular nucleus, thalamus, and internal capsule *(between arrows)* displaced the midline septum pellucidum *(arrowhead)* to the right.

quent degeneration and phagocytosis of the infarcted brain tissue there is volume loss that causes an increase in size of the overlying cortical sulci and underlying ventricles (61). When the infarction is caused by a systemically induced general reduction in brain perfusion, the infarcted areas correspond to the border zones between the territories of the major cerebral arteries because perfusion is most tenuous here (Fig. 19-64). Emboli can at times be directly visualized by noncontrast CT as hyperdensities within arteries. Hemorrhage can occur within an infarcted area, where it will appear as a hyperdense mass within the hypodense edema of the infarct.

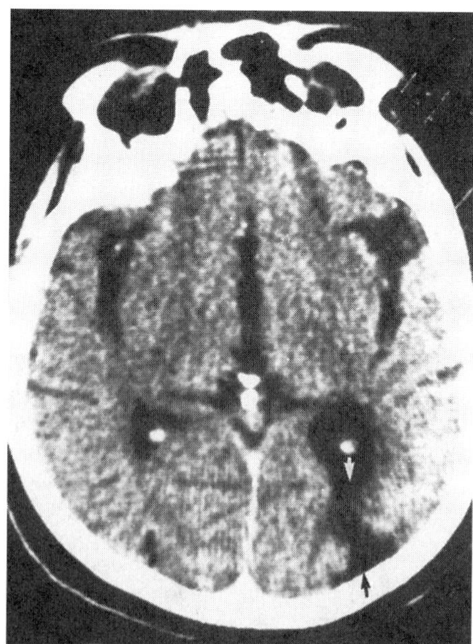

FIG. 19-64. A border zone infarct is seen on CT as a hypodense region *(between arrows)* between the territories of the middle and posterior cerebral arteries.

Injection of intravenous contrast provides no brain enhancement in the first day or two after a stroke. Contrast enhancement must await sufficient damage to the blood–brain barrier. It reaches its peak at 1 to 2 weeks and usually ceases to occur after 2 or 3 months (62). The greatest vascular damage to intact vessels is at the periphery of the infarct. Therefore, contrast-enhanced CT frequently visualizes a contrast-enhanced ring about the infarcted area or in the immediately adjacent cortical gyri (Fig. 19-65).

By MRI, the edema of the early infarct is imaged as a low-intensity area on T1-weighted images and a high-intensity area on T2-weighted images (Fig. 19-66). This can be visualized by MRI sooner than by CT, typically within a few hours of the onset of the infarct. With the administration of intravenous gadolinium-DTPA, a damaged blood–brain barrier is often visualized as a hyperintense area on T1-weighted images. MRI is more sensitive than CT at detecting lacunar infarcts. Lacunar infarcts are small infarcts, less that 1.5 cm in major dimension (61). They are typically situated in the basal ganglia, in periventricular areas, and at brain stem levels (Fig. 19-67). They are most commonly caused by hypertension or diabetes-induced arteriolar occlusive disease of the deeply penetrating arteries, such as the lenticulostriate branches of the middle cerebral arteries. MRI also demonstrates ischemic infarcts of the posterior cranial fossa better than CT because MR images are not degraded by bone artifacts.

MRI can visualize normal and abnormal vessels without the introduction of contrast. Normal vessels are depicted as a flow void. Intra-arterial thrombus is seen as an area of increased signal intensity. An internal carotid artery dissection is depicted as a high signal intensity perivascular thrombus.

Cerebral venous thrombosis can cause infarction and has characteristic imaging features. Whether the thrombosis in-

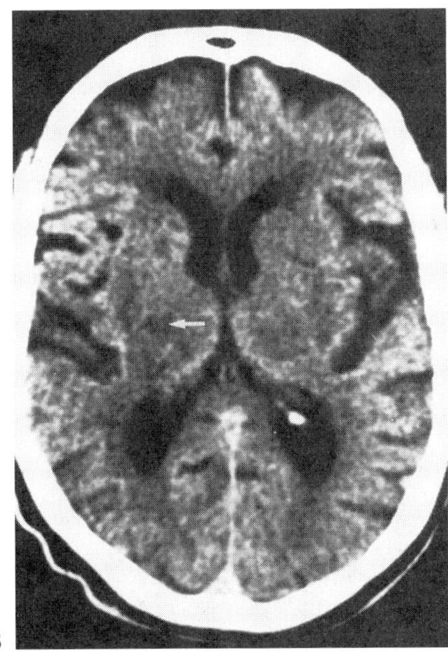
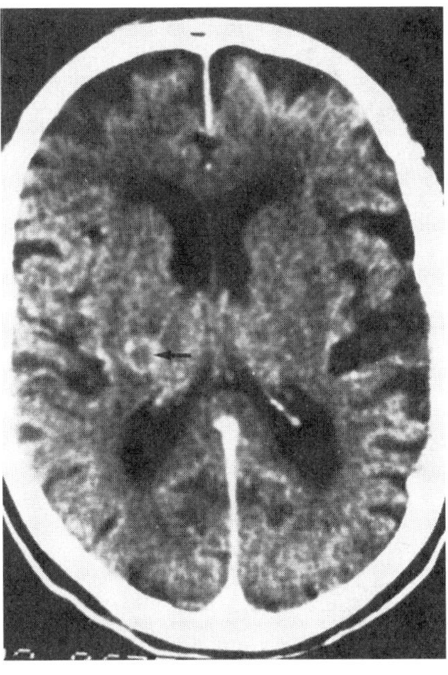

A,B

FIG. 19-65. A: A small lacunar infarct within the posterior limb of the internal capsule shows up as a barely perceptible hypodensity *(arrow)* on noncontrast CT. **B:** With contrast injection, a contrast-enhanced ring appears around the hypodense region *(arrow).*

volves a cerebral vein or one of the dural venous sinuses, the thrombus can be detected on a noncontrast CT as a hyperdensity within the vein (63). The hyperdensity may have a hypodense center, implying a residual lumen. In a contrast-enhanced CT, tortuous dilated collateral venous channels may be demonstrated around the thrombosed vein. By MRI, while the thrombus is still in the oxyhemoglobin stage, which is isodense to brain tissue, it can be suspected by the absence of the normal flow void in that vessel. In the deoxyhemoglobin stage, the thrombus is hypointense, and in the later methemoglobin stage it becomes hyperintense. The venous thrombus typically does not proceed to the hemosiderin phase because it usually lyses spontaneously and flow is re-established.

Hemorrhagic Stroke

Hypertension is the most common cause of intraparenchymal hemorrhage, but it also can be caused by ruptured aneurysm or arteriovenous malformation and, more rarely, by infarction, neoplasms, blood coagulation defects, and cerebral arteritis (63). Common hemorrhage sites include the putamen and thalamus, which receive their major blood supply from the lenticulostriate and thalamogeniculate arteries, respectively.

Because freshly extravasated blood is more radiodense than gray or white matter, an acute hemorrhagic stroke is well visualized by CT as a hyperdense region usually conforming to an arterial distribution (Fig. 19-68). The radiodensity of the clot increases over 3 days because of clot retraction, serum extrusion, and hemoglobin concentration. The extruded serum may form a hypodense rim around the hyperdense clot (Fig. 19-68*C*). As edema develops over 3 to 5 days, the hypodense rim may increase. The hyperdensity of the clot gradually fades and usually disappears by 2 months, leaving only a narrow hypodense slit to mark the site of the hemorrhage (Fig. 19-68*D*).

The appearance of hemorrhage by MRI depends on the state of the hemoglobin in the hemorrhage (63). The oxyhemoglobin present in the fresh hemorrhage is nonparamagnetic; therefore, very early hemorrhage is not detected by MRI. Within a few hours, the oxyhemoglobin will be converted to deoxyhemoglobin, which is a paramagnetic substance. Intracellular deoxyhemoglobin will cause acute hemorrhage to appear very hypointense on T2-weighted images and slightly hypointense or isointense on T1-weighted images (Fig. 19-69*A*). By 3 to 7 days, intracellular deoxyhemoglobin is oxidized to methemoglobin as the clot enters the subacute phase. Although the subacute hemorrhage has several subphases in which the signal intensity of methemoglobin varies, in general the methemoglobin appears hyperintense on both T1- and T2-weighted images (Fig. 19-69*B*). Because the conversion to methemoglobin begins at the periphery of the clot, early in the subacute phase the hemorrhage can have a hyperintense margin and a central hypointense region still containing deoxyhemoglobin. Eventually the entire region of subacute hemorrhage becomes hyperintense. Over several months, the methemoglobin is gradually resorbed and the clot develops a rim of hemosiderin-containing macrophages. Hemosiderin is hypointense on both T1- and T2-weighted images. Therefore, a chronic hemorrhage of several months duration often has a hyperintense methemoglobin center and a hypointense hemosiderin rim. Because the hemosiderin deposits remain indefinitely, an old hemorrhage of several years duration shows up as a totally hypointense area. So although CT provides the very earliest information about hemorrhage, MRI provides the best evaluation of the locus of old hemorrhages.

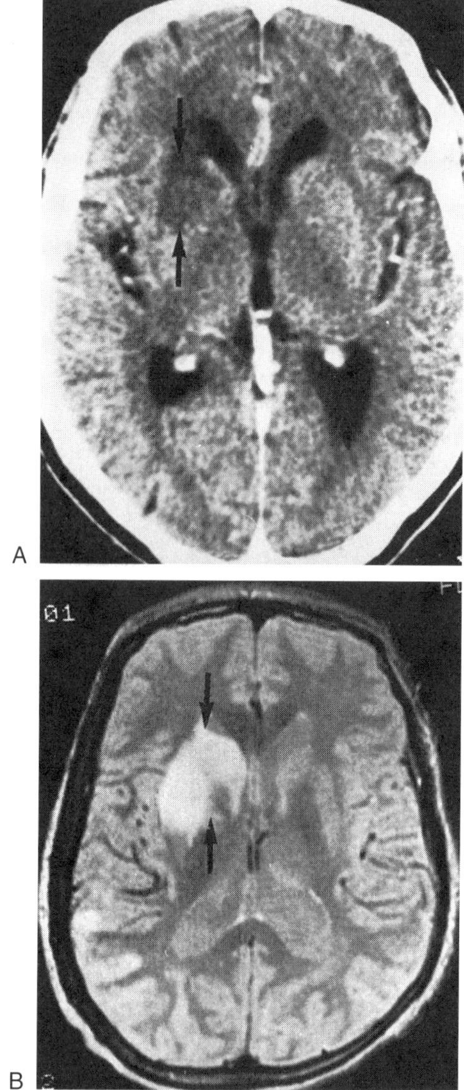

FIG. 19-66. Comparison of CT and MRI evaluation of an early deep infarction. **A:** By CT, the infarction is visualized as a hypodense area *(between arrows)* involving the caudate, lenticular nucleus, and anterior limb of the internal capsule. **B:** MRI shows the same early infarcted area as hyperintense on a T2-weighted image *(arrows)*.

Subarachnoid and Intraventricular Hemorrhage

Because subarachnoid and intraventricular hemorrhage can be spontaneous, as in the case of a bleeding aneurysm or arteriovenous malformation, or secondary to trauma, it can be included under the heading of stroke or head trauma. CT is the imaging modality of choice for evaluating these types of hemorrhages because it detects the hemorrhage from its onset as a hyperdensity. However, subarachnoid hemorrhage is not as radiodense as epidural or subdural hemorrhage because the blood will be diluted by CSF. Unless blood replaces at least 70% of the CSF, the subarachnoid hemorrhage remains isodense to adjacent gray matter (64). When the volume of blood is sufficient to make the hemorrhage hyperdense, it accumulates in the extensions and expansions of the subarachnoid space. Therefore, it appears as linear radiodensities within the sulci or fissures or as larger aggregations in the basal cisterns (Fig. 19-70). MRI will not visualize a very early hemorrhage when oxyhemoglobin, a nonparamagnetic substance, is the primary constituent. Subarachnoid and intraventricular hemorrhage can cause a communicating hydrocephalus by virtue of red blood cells blocking the arachnoid granulations, the CSF resorption site.

Aneurysms and arteriovenous malformations can be de-

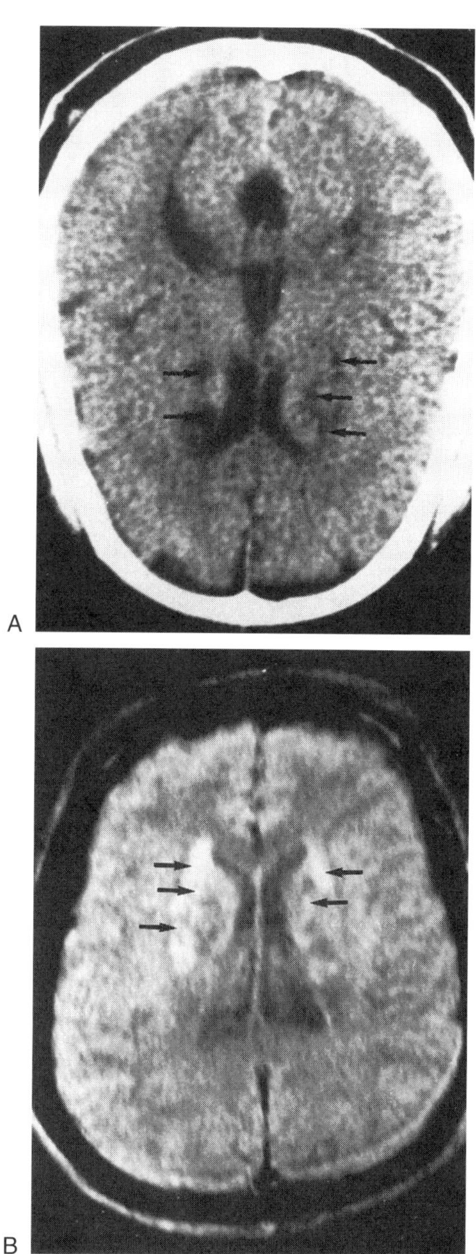

FIG. 19-67. Lacunar infarcts. **A:** CT shows multiple bilateral lacunar infarcts as small hypodense areas *(arrows)*. **B:** By MRI these infarcts are shown as multiple hyperintense areas *(arrows)*.

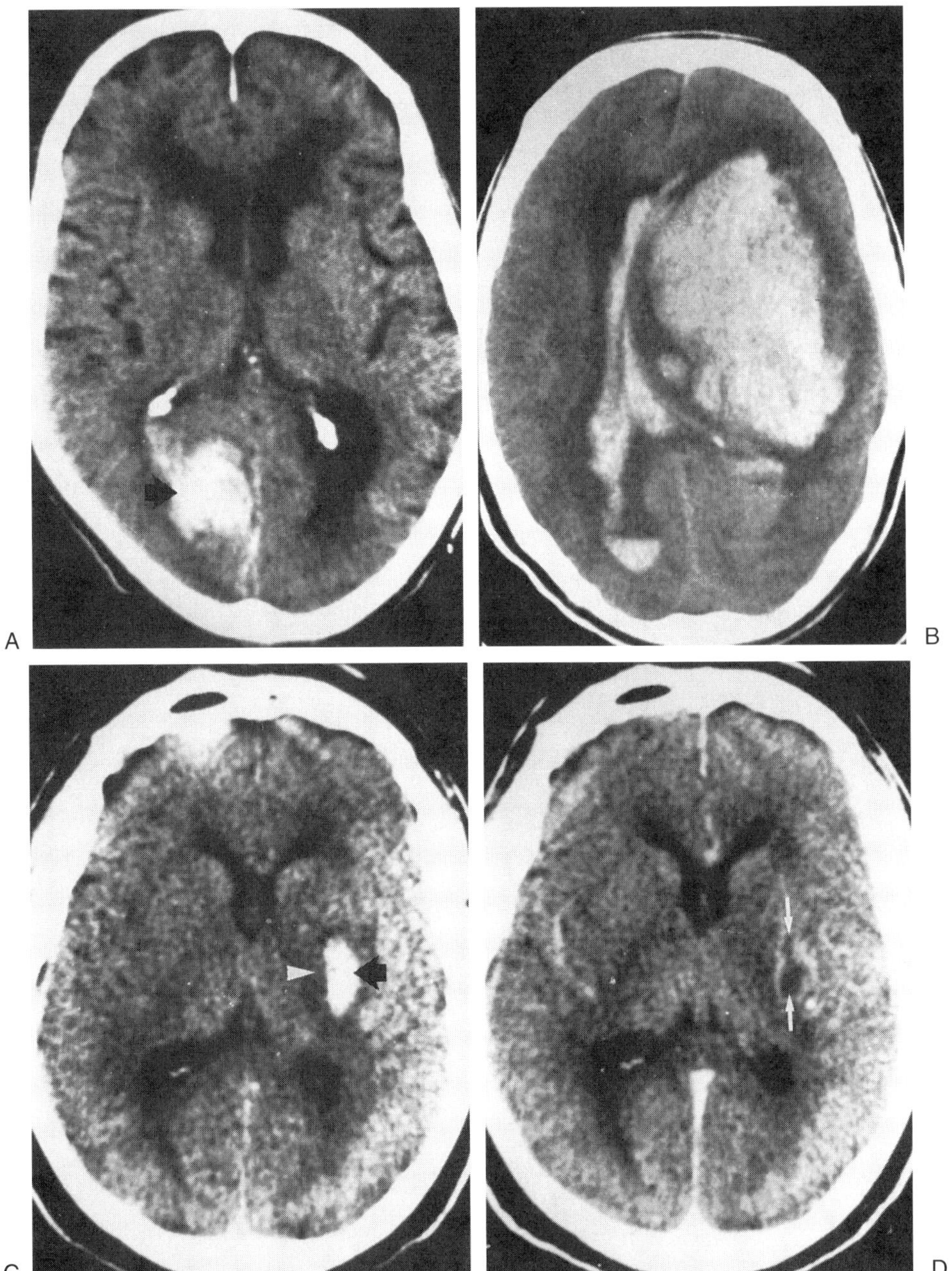

FIG. 19-68. CT evaluation of early and evolving hemorrhagic strokes. **A:** Recent hemorrhagic stroke has occurred in the distribution of the right posterior cerebral artery, which appears hyperdense *(arrow)*. **B:** A massive hypertensive hemorrhage involving most of the interior of the left cerebral hemisphere with intraventricular hemorrhage, midline shift to the right, and herniation of the left hemisphere under the falx cerebri. **C:** A 5-day old hemorrhagic stroke involving the lenticular nucleus shows a hyperdense hemorrhagic center *(arrow)* and a hypodense edematous rim *(arrowhead)*. **D:** The same stroke patient displays replacement of the hyperdense hemorrhage with a narrow hypodense interval *(arrows)* several months later.

tected directly by contrast-enhanced CT and by their flow void characteristics on MR images (Fig. 19-71).

Head Injuries

Head injury can be produced by direct contact or impact loading, where impacts either set a resting head in motion or stop a moving head, or it can be produced by impulse or inertial loading, where the head is suddenly placed in motion or suddenly stopped without impact (65). Fractures and epidural hematomas are produced only by impact loading, but other types of head injury can be produced by either type of loading. Head injury is typically categorized as focal or diffuse. Focal injuries include extracerebral hemorrhages such as epidural or subdural hematomas, intraparenchymal hematomas, cerebral contusion or laceration, and fractures. Diffuse brain injuries include diffuse axonal injury, diffuse cerebral swelling, and edema.

CT is typically the imaging modality of choice for the patients immediately posttrauma. This is because it is very accurate at detecting the depressed fractures and acute hematomas that require emergency surgery. Its other advantages include rapid scanning and continuation of close monitoring and support devices for the critically injured patient. MRI has the disadvantages of longer scans, high susceptibility to motion artifacts by an uncooperative patient, inability to detect very recent hemorrhage, and difficulty evaluating fractures because of the signal void characteristics of cortical bone.

Epidural Hematoma

Epidural hematoma is caused by tears of the middle meningeal artery or vein, or of a dural venous sinus. The blood accumulates in the interval between the inner table of the calvarium and the dura by gradually stripping the dura from its bony attachment. CT visualizes the epidural hematoma as a well-localized biconvex radiodense mass (65). It is commonly, though not invariably, associated with a skull fracture. It causes a mass effect on the adjacent brain with effacement of the underlying sulci, preservation of the gray-white junction, compression of the brain and ventricles, and possible midline shift. When there is a question about whether the mass might be intraparenchymal, contrast injection enhances the dura, establishing the epidural position of the clot. As the clot lyses over the next few weeks, it shrinks and changes to isodense and then hypodense relative to the brain. The inner aspect of the clot vascularizes, and this may produce a thicker rim of enhancement on late contrast studies. The overlying dura may calcify. Epidural hematoma may be associated with subdural, subarachnoid, or intraparenchymal hemorrhage.

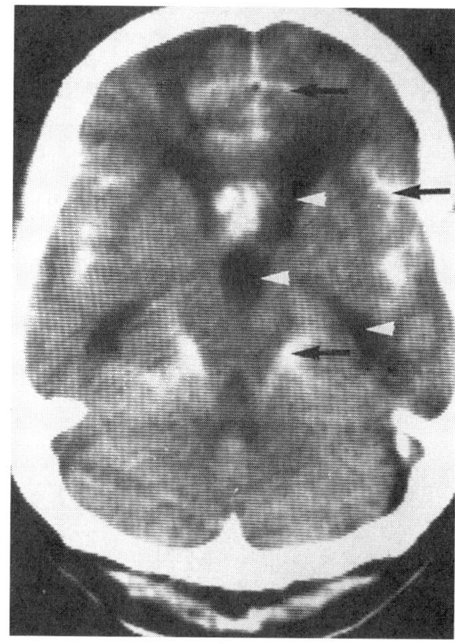

FIG. 19-70. Subarachnoid hemorrhage secondary to an anterior cerebral artery aneurysm. CT shows this condition as hemorrhagic radiodensities within sulci and cisterns *(arrows)*. There is ventricular dilatation *(arrowheads)* secondary to the obstruction of CSF resorption by the hemorrhage.

A

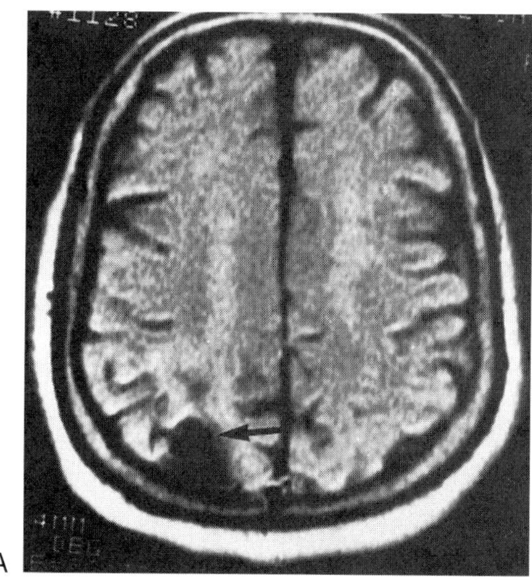

B

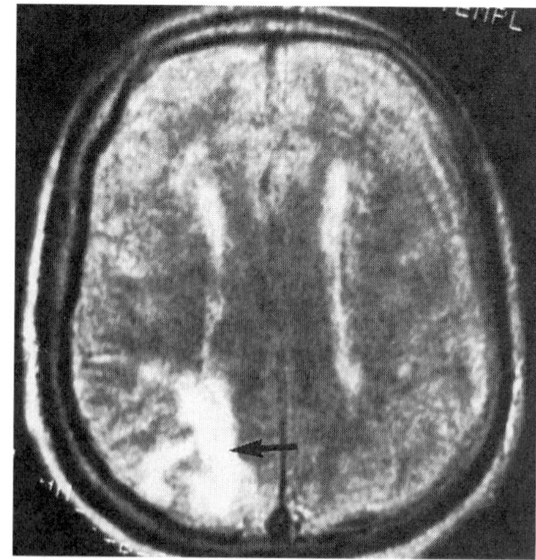

FIG. 19-69. MRI evaluation of hemorrhagic stroke. **A:** An acute hemorrhagic stroke involving the occipital lobe appears hypointense *(arrow)*. **B:** In the subacute phase, the same area appears hyperintense *(arrow)*.

Subdural Hematoma

Subdural hematoma is most commonly caused by acceleration or deceleration shearing stresses that rupture the bridging veins that extend from the movable brain to the fixed dural venous sinuses. The blood accumulates in a pre-existing but essentially volumeless subdural space. Normally, the pressure of the CSF holds the arachnoid in contact with the dura, thereby creating a real interval that is without significant volume. Because the subdural space is a real space surrounding all external surfaces of the brain, subdural hem-

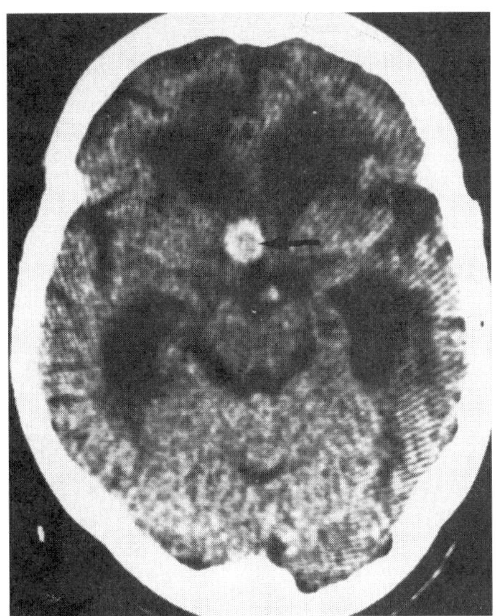
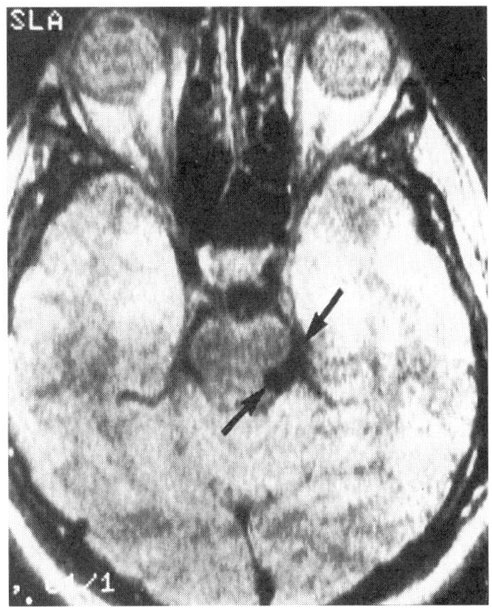

A,B

FIG. 19-71. **A:** CT of an anterior cerebral artery aneurysm *(arrow)* that produced a subarachnoid hemorrhage with secondary hydrocephalus. **B:** MRI demonstrates the flow void of an arteriovenous malformation along the left side of the mid-brain *(between arrows).*

orrhage tends to spread extensively over many aspects of the brain surface.

On CT examination, the typical acute subdural hematoma appears as a diffuse crescent-shaped radiodensity that may extend onto many surfaces of the brain, including the cerebral convexity, skull base, interhemispheric fissure, upper or lower surface of the tentorium, and around the brain stem (Fig. 19-72). There are two ways of classifying subdural hematomas based on their changing radiographic appearance over time (65). One scheme divides them into acute (i.e., more radiodense than adjacent gray matter), subacute (i.e., isodense to gray matter), and chronic (i.e., hypodense to gray matter). Another scheme simply lumps the subacute and chronic into the chronic category. The subdural hematoma typically effaces the adjacent gyri, produces inward displacement of the gray–white matter junction, and may compress

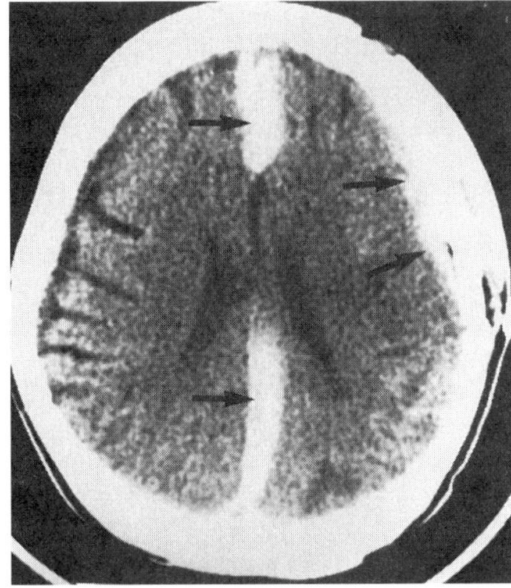

FIG. 19-72. An acute subdural hematoma *(arrows)* overlies the left frontal lobe and extends into the interhemispheric fissure along the falx cerebri.

the ventricle or cause brain herniation under the falx or through the tentorium.

As the subdural hematoma ages, the hemoglobin protein producing its radiodensity is broken down and removed and a vascular granulation tissue develops along its inner surface. Over a few weeks, the subdural hematoma usually becomes isodense or hypodense to gray matter (66). Because of volume loss, the chronic subdural hematoma may lose its concave inner border and become more focal, and even at times assume a biconvex outline. Isodense subdural hematomas are less easy to discriminate. Their presence can be implied indirectly by their mass effects on the underlying brain. An injection of contrast material will enhance both the vascular membrane and the displaced cortical vessels, allowing discrimination of the hematoma from the adjacent cortex.

Patients who present first with a chronic subdural hematoma may have no recollection of any antecedent trauma because the traumatic episode may have been so slight that it was forgotten. Chronic hematomas commonly involve the elderly, where loss of cerebral volume puts the bridging veins under increased stress and makes them more susceptible to rupture by minor trauma.

MRI has valuable unique imaging properties that make it very sensitive to the detection of some extracerebral hemorrhages. First, the high signal intensity that subacute hematomas display on T1- and T2-weighted images makes MRI more sensitive than CT for detecting hematomas that are isodense by CT (58). Even chronic subdural hematomas remain hyperintense to CSF and gray matter for several months, which is long after they have become isodense or hypodense on CT. Also, the ability of MRI to discern the displaced signal voids of cortical or dural vessels facilitates the identification of small extracerebral hemorrhages. In addition, when the hematoma collects around the obliquely placed tentorium, axial CT images may average it into adjacent tissues. Here, the multiplanar imaging properties of

MRI can be very valuable. Also, small hematomas next to the calvarium can be better seen by MRI because they are contrasted against the bony signal void.

Contusions and Intraparenchymal Hemorrhage

Focal parenchymal injuries such as contusions and intraparenchymal hemorrhage usually develop as a result of contact of the brain with the bony walls of the cranial cavity. The coup-type injuries occur at the point of contact, and the contrecoup injuries occur on the opposite side of the brain. Contusions often occur in areas where the walls of the cranial cavity are irregular, such as the anterior and middle cranial fossae. Therefore, frontal and temporal lobe contusions are common because of the sliding displacements of the brain along these irregularities (67).

Cerebral contusions are heterogeneous lesions containing edema, hemorrhage, and necrosis, with any element predominating. When blood makes a major contribution, the contusion appears on CT as a poorly delimited irregular area of hyperdensity (Fig. 19-73). Contusion with edema or necrosis predominating may not be detectable immediately, but after a few days it appears as a hypodense region. Where there is a general admixture of elements, contusions may have a heterogeneous density. Old contusions appear as hypodense areas. By MRI, the edematous and necrotic areas appear as low signal intensity areas on T1-weighted images and become hyperintense on T2-weighted images. MRI is more sensitive than CT in identifying these nonhemorrhagic contusions. The areas of hemorrhage in a contusion older than a few days will be hyperintense on both T1- and T2-weighted images.

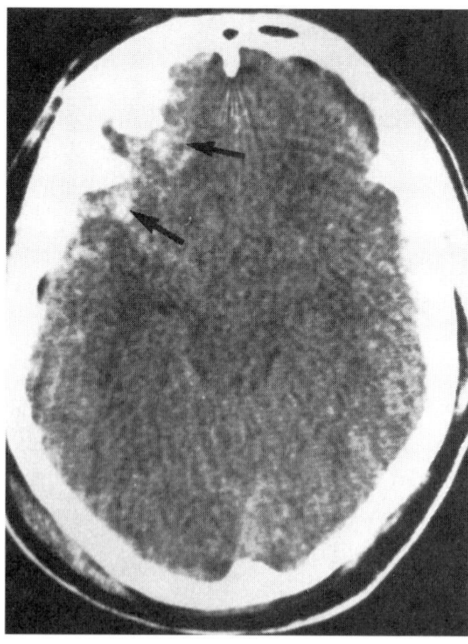

FIG. 19-73. CT of a trauma-induced contusion of the right frontal lobe *(arrows)* and generalized brain edema. Note the loss of all cortical sulci and the perimesencephalic cisterns by the edematous hypointense hemispheres.

Intraparenchymal hemorrhage differs from contusions by having better demarcated areas of more homogeneous hemorrhage. The CT and MRI characteristics of acute and evolving intraparenchymal hemorrhage are the same as for hemorrhagic stroke.

Diffuse Brain Injuries

Diffuse brain injuries include diffuse axonal injury, diffuse cerebral swelling, and edema. Diffuse axonal injury is produced by high shearing stresses that occur between different parts of the brain and at gray matter–white matter interfaces. These disruptions of axonal continuity commonly involve the corpus callosum, anterior commissure, and upper brain stem. Vessels may or may not be disrupted. When vessels are uninterrupted, the scattered small areas of edema are best demonstrated by T1-weighted MR images as slightly hypointense or isointense regions that become hyperintense on T2-weighted images. When vessel disruption produces hemorrhages, they appear early on CT as multiple sites of hyperdensity.

Diffuse cerebral swelling occurs with many types of head injury. It is thought to be produced by a rapidly increased volume of circulating blood. By MRI and CT, the general brain enlargement is visualized by an obliteration or encroachment of the normal CSF spaces: the cortical sulci, the perimesencephalic and basal cisterns, and the ventricles (67). By CT, the enlarged brain may show slightly increased density.

In generalized cerebral edema, the enlarged brain also encroaches upon the CSF spaces, but by CT the edema produces a generalized hypodensity that usually takes longer to develop than diffuse cerebral swelling (Fig. 19-73). The edema may obscure gray matter–white matter boundaries.

Penetrating Trauma

Bullets and other types of penetrating objects will cause brain laceration by both the penetrating objects and the fragments of subcutaneous tissues, bone, and dura driven into the brain. The imbedded fragments of the foreign object and bone are well visualized by CT, as are the accompanying cerebral edema and various types of intracerebral or extracerebral hemorrhage.

Complications of Brain Injury

Brain injury may be accompanied by a number of late or long-term complications. Cerebral herniation may occur under the falx cerebri or through the tentorium. This can cause compression of adjacent brain substance or vessels, with the production of secondary signs and symptoms. Penetrating injuries or fractures can injure nearby large or small vessels, producing thrombosis, embolism, traumatic aneurysm, or internal carotid–cavernous sinus fistula. Basal skull fractures involving the dura and arachnoid can cause CSF leaks that show up as CSF rhinorrhea or otorrhea. Local or diffuse brain enlargement can compress the cerebral aqueduct or fourth ventricle, producing obstructive hydrocephalus. Subarachnoid hemorrhage may obstruct CSF resorption and cause a late-developing communicating hydrocephalus. Focal cerebral atrophy can occur at sites of infarction, hemorrhage, or trauma. Generalized atrophy can follow diffuse injuries and can be demonstrated by an increased size of sulci, fissures, cisterns, and ventricles.

Degenerative Diseases of the Central Nervous System

Degenerative diseases of the CNS can include white and gray matter diseases and the general degenerative changes of aging or the dementias.

White Matter Diseases

White matter diseases can be divided into demyelinating diseases, in which the white matter is normally formed and then pathologically destroyed, and dysmyelinating diseases, in which there is usually a genetically determined enzymatic disorder that interferes with the normal production or maintenance of myelin (68). The enzymatic disturbances are relatively rare; therefore, their imaging characteristics will not be described.

The most common of the demyelinating disorders is multiple sclerosis (MS). The demyelinating plaques of MS are better visualized by MRI than by CT. In fact, MRI has become the primary complementary test to confirm a clinical diagnosis of MS. It also provides a quantitative means of evaluating the present state of a patient's disease and a mode of following its progress (69). Although the T1-weighted MR images are usually normal, the T2-weighted images demonstrate MS plaques as high signal intensity areas. These are most frequently seen in the periventricular white matter, especially around the atrium and the tips of the anterior and posterior horns of the lateral ventricles (Fig. 19-74). The high signal intensity plaques also can be seen in other white matter areas of the cerebral hemispheres, the brain stem, and even the upper spinal cord. When these lesions are seen in patients younger than 40 years of age, they tend to be relatively specific for MS (68). In patients over 50 years of age, the MRI findings of MS are similar to findings in some aging brains, and correlation with the clinical findings helps establish the diagnosis. Recent MS plaques that involve damage to the blood–brain barrier frequently enhance with the use of intravenous gadolinium-DTPA as a paramagnetic substance.

CT demonstrates MS plaques with less reliability than does MRI. They appear as areas of hypodensity. Recent plaques in the acute phase of an exacerbation of the disease will have damage to the blood–brain barrier, and intravenous contrast will then enhance the periphery of the lesion. In the chronic plaque, no contrast enhancement occurs. Other demyelinating diseases, although numerous, are of relatively low incidence and therefore are not described.

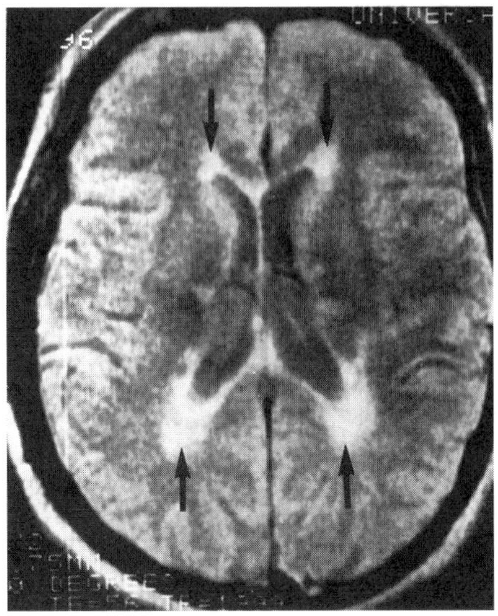

FIG. 19-74. T2-weighted MRI demonstrates the periventricular demyelinating plaques of multiple sclerosis as hyperintense areas *(arrows)* adjacent to the anterior horns and atria of the lateral ventricles.

Gray Matter Diseases

Although imaging of gray matter disorders has not become widely used clinically, there are some early reports that MRI may be able to discriminate a number of movement disorders that are characterized by changes in the size or iron content of a number of deep nuclei (70). Normal nuclei that contain high iron levels, such as the globus pallidus, reticular part of the substantia nigra, red nucleus, and dentate nucleus of the cerebellum, appear hypointense on T2-weighted images. In Parkinson's disease, T2-weighted MRI shows a hypointensity in the putamen that may exceed the normal hypointensity of the globus pallidus. In Huntington's chorea, MRI consistently shows atrophy of the head of the caudate with dilation of the adjacent frontal horn of the lateral ventricle. Some patients with Huntington's chorea also show a hypointensity of the caudate or putamen on T2-weighted images and atrophy predominating in the frontal lobe. Some forms of secondary dystonia show increased signal intensity of the putamen and caudate in T2-weighted images.

Age-Related Changes and Dementing Disorders

The aging brain is characterized on CT or MRI as demonstrating volume increases in both cortical sulci and ventricles (Fig. 19-75). T2-weighted MR images also frequently display small areas of hyperintense signal along the anterolateral margins of the anterior horns of the lateral ventricles.

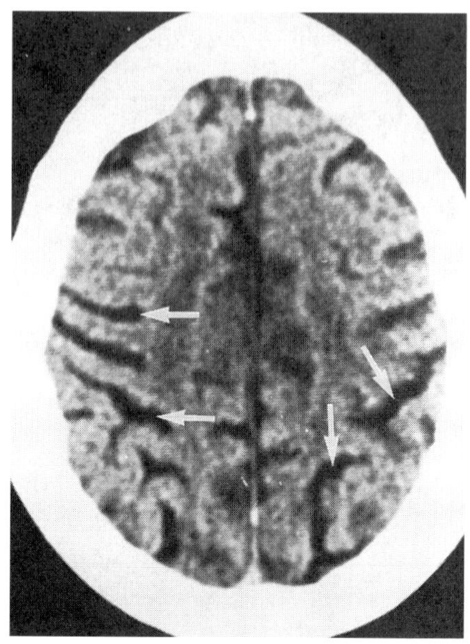

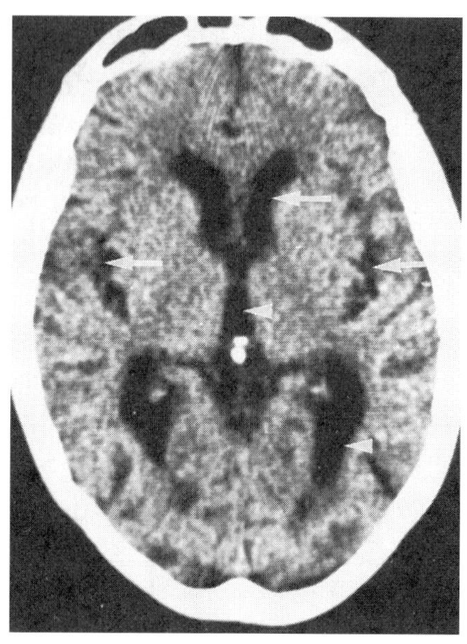

A,B

FIG. 19-75. Two cases of mild cortical atrophy of aging as seen by CT. **A:** Enlargement of cortical sulci *(arrows).* **B:** Enlargement of the sylvian fissure *(arrows)* and ventricular dilatation *(arrowheads).*

These changes may or may not be associated with neurologic findings.

Patients with Alzheimer's disease (AD) and other dementing disorders consistently show these age changes, but because many normal elderly do also, these changes cannot be used to diagnose AD. However, the absence of these findings typically excludes AD. Findings more specifically related to AD are those involving the temporal lobe. The earliest findings in AD involve atrophy of the temporal lobe with dilation of the inferior (i.e,. temporal) horn of the lateral ventricle and a dilation of the choroidal and hippocampal fissures caused by atrophy of the hippocampus, subiculum, and parahippocampal gyrus (71).

CONCLUSIONS

MRI and CT are assuming an expanding role in the diagnosis and follow-up of pathology of the musculoskeletal and nervous systems. MRI, in particular, is experiencing a plethora of technological enhancements that will further expand its role from the diagnosis of pathologic anatomy to the realm of evaluating the physiology and pathophysiology of tissues and organs. The rehabilitation professional must keep abreast of the current and likely future applications of these imaging modalities to ensure that the rehabilitation patient will maximally benefit from the new technology.

REFERENCES

1. Seeger LL, Lufkin RB. Physical principles of MRI. In: Bassett LW, Gold RH, Seeger LL, eds. *MRI atlas of the musculoskeletal system.* London: Martin Dunitz, 1989; 11–24.
2. Deutsch AL, Mink JH. Magnetic resonance imaging of musculoskeletal injuries. *Radiol Clin North Am* 1989; 27:983–1002.
3. Neer CS. Impingement lesions. *Clin Orthop* 1983; 173:70–77.
4. Tsai JC, Zlatkin MB. Magnetic resonance imaging of the shoulder. *Radiol Clin North Am* 1990; 28:279–291.
5. Zlatkin MB, Reicher MA, Kellerhouse LE, McDade W, Vetter L, Resnick D. The painful shoulder: MR imaging of the glenohumeral joint. *J Comput Assist Tomogr* 1988; 12:995–1001.
6. Seeger LL. The shoulder. In: Bassett LW, Gold RH, Seeger LL, eds. *MRI atlas of the musculoskeletal system.* London: Martin Dunitz, 1989; 95–128.
7. Berquist TH. Shoulder and arm. In: Berquist TH, ed. *MRI of the musculoskeletal system.* Philadelphia: Lippincott-Raven, 1996; 517–607.
8. McCauley TR, Pope CF, Jokl P. Normal and abnormal glenoid labrum: assessment with multiplanar gradient-echo MR imaging. *Radiology* 1992; 183:35–37.
9. Workman TL, Burkhard TK, Resnick D. Hill Sachs lesion, comparison of detection with MR imaging, radiography and arthroscopy. *Radiology* 1992; 185:847–852.
10. Rafii M. Magnetic resonance imaging of the shoulder joint. In: Beltran J, ed. *Current review of MRI.* Philadelphia: Current Medicine, 1995; 203–214.
11. Resnick D. Internal derangements of joints. In: Resnick D, ed. *Bone and joint imaging.* Philadelphia: WB Saunders, 1996; 819–883.
12. Bunnell DH, Bassett LW. The elbow. In: Bassett LW, Gold RH, Seeger LL, eds. *MRI atlas of the musculoskeletal system.* London: Martin Dunitz, 1989; 129–138.
13. Mesgarzadeh M, Schneck C, Ross G, Bonakdarpour A. MR imaging of the most commonly injured and diseased structures of the elbow and ankle. *Radiology* 1987; 165(suppl):377.
14. Mesgarzadeh M, Schneck CD, Bonakdarpour A. Carpal tunnel: MR imaging, Part I. Normal anatomy. *Radiology* 1989; 171:743–749.
15. Mesgarzadeh M, Schneck CD, Bonakdarpour A, Mitra A, Conaway D. Carpal tunnel: MR imaging, Part II. Carpal tunnel syndrome. *Radiology* 1989; 171:749–754.
16. Mesgarzadeh M, Schneck CD, Bonakdarpour A. The wrist and hand. In: Bassett LW, Gold RH, Seeger LL, eds. *MRI atlas of the musculoskeletal system.* London: Martin Dunitz, 1989; 139–174.
17. Mesgarzadeh M, Triola J, Schneck CD. Carpal tunnel syndrome: MR imaging diagnosis. *MRI Clin North Am* 1995; 3:249–264.
18. Quinn SF, Belsole RJ, Greene TL, Rayhack JM. Advanced imaging of the wrist. *Radiographics* 1988; 9:229–246.
19. Schoenberg N, Rosenberg ZS. Magnetic resonance imaging of the elbow, wrist and hand. In: Beltran J, ed. *Current review of MRI.* Philadelphia: Current Medicine, 1995;2 15–228.
20. Ficat RP, Arlet J. Bone necrosis of known etiology. In: Hungerford D, ed. *Ischemia and necrosis of bone.* Baltimore: Williams & Wilkins, 1980; 111–130.
21. McGlade CT, Bassett LH. The hip. In: Bassett LW, Gold RH, Seeger LL, eds. *MRI atlas of the musculoskeletal system.* London: Martin Dunitz, 1989; 175–214.
22. Coleman BG, Kressel HY, Dalinka MK, Sheibler ML, Burk DL, Cohen

RK. Radiographically negative avascular necrosis: detection with MR imaging. *Radiology* 1988; 168:525–528.

23. Tervonen O, Mueller DM, Matterson EL, Velosa JA, Ginsburg WW, Ehman RL. Clinically occult avascular necrosis of the hip. Prevalence in an asymptomatic population at risk. *Radiology* 1992; 182:845–847.
24. Resnick D, Sweet DE, Madowell JE. Osteonecrosis and osteochondrosis. In: Resnick D, ed. *Bone and joint imaging*. Philadelphia: WB Saunders, 1996; 941–977.
25. Totty WG, Murphy WA, Ganz WI, Kumar B, Daum WJ, Siegel BH. Magnetic resonance imaging of the normal and ischemic femoral head. *AJR* 1984; 143:1273–1280.
26. Mitchell DG, Rao VM, Dalinka MK, et al. Femoral head avascular necrosis: correlation of MR imaging, radiographic staging, radionuclide imaging and clinical findings. *Radiology* 1987; 162:709–715.
27. Charkes ND, Siddhivarn N, Schneck CD. Bone scanning in the adductor insertion avulsion syndrome (thigh splints). *Nucl Med* 1987; 28: 1835–1838.
28. Saunders JBM, Inman VT, Eberhardt HD. The major determinants in normal and pathological gait. *J Bone Joint Surg [Am]* 1953; 35: 543–558.
29. Burk DL, Mitchell DG, Rifkin MD, Vinitski S. Recent advances in magnetic imaging of the knee. *Radiol Clin North Am* 1990; 28: 379–393.
30. Langer JE, Meyer SJF, Dalinka MK. Imaging of the knee. *Radiol Clin North Am* 1990; 28:975–990.
31. Hartzman S, Gold RH. The knee. In: Bassett LW, Gold RH, Seeger LL, eds. *MRI atlas of the musculoskeletal system*. London: Martin Dunitz, 1989; 215–65.
32. Dillon EH, Pope CF, Jokl P, Lynch JK. Follow-up of grade 2 meniscal abnormalities in the stable knee. *Radiology* 1991; 181:849–852.
33. Mesgarzadeh M, Schneck CD, Bonakdarpour A. Magnetic resonance imaging of the knee: correlation with normal anatomy. *Radiographics* 1988; 8:707–733.
34. Vahey TN, Broome DR, Kayes KJ, Shelbourne KP. Acute and chronic tears of the anterior cruciate ligament: differential features of MR imaging. *Radiology* 1991; 181:251–253.
35. Hennigan SP, Schneck CD, Mesgarzadeh M, Clancy M. The Semimembranosus-tibial collateral ligament bursa. *J Bone Joint Surg [Am]* 1994; 76:1322–1327.
36. Kier R, McCarthy S, Dietz MJ, Rudicel S. MR appearance of painful conditions of the ankle. *Radiographics* 1991;11:401–414.
37. Cheung Y, Rosenberg ZS, Magee T, Chinitz L. Normal anatomy and pathologic conditions of ankle tendons: current imaging techniques. *Radiographics* 1992; 12:429–444.
38. Forrester DM, Kerr R. Trauma to the foot. *Radiol Clin North Am* 1990; 28:423–433.
39. Schneck CD, Mesgarzadeh M, Bonakdarpour A, Ross GJ. MR imaging of the most commonly injured ankle ligaments. Part I. Normal anatomy. *Radiology* 1992; 184:499–506.
40. Schneck CD, Mesgarzadeh M, Bonakdarpour A. MR imaging of the most commonly injured ankle ligaments. Part II. Ligament injuries. *Radiology* 1992; 184:507–512.
41. Siegler S, Block J, Schneck C. The mechanical characteristics of the collateral ligaments of the human ankle joint. *Foot Ankle* 1988; 8: 234–242.
42. Brower AC. *Arthritis in black and white*. Philadelphia: WB Saunders, 1988; 213–30.
43. Schumacher EH. *Primer on the rheumatic diseases*. Atlanta: Arthritis Foundation, 1988; 60–76.
44. Brower AC. *Arthritis in black and white*. Philadelphia: WB Saunders, 1988; 243–256.
45. Weissman BNW, Aliabadi P, Weinfeld MS, Thomas WH, Sosman JL. Prognostic features of atlanto-axial subluxation in rheumatoid arthritis patients. *Radiology* 1982; 144:745–751.
46. Naylor A. The biophysical and biochemical aspects of intervertebral disc herniation and degeneration. *Ann R Coll Surg Engl* 1962; 31: 91–114.
47. Jahnke RW, Hart BL. Cervical stenosis, spondylosis and herniated disc disease. *Radiol Clin North Am* 1991; 29:777–791.
48. Kemp SS, Rogg JM. CT of degenerative and nonneoplastic spine disorders. In: Latchaw RE, ed. *MR and CT imaging of the head, neck and spine*. St. Louis: Mosby-Year Book, 1991; 1109–1157.
49. Sherk HH, Parke WW. Developmental anatomy. In: *The cervical spine*. Philadelphia: JB Lippincott, 1983; 1–8.
50. Stanley JH, Schabel SI, Frey GD, Hungerford GD. Quantitative analysis of the cervical spinal canal by computed tomography. *Neuroradiology* 1986; 28:139–143.
51. Penning L, Wilmink JT, VanWorden HH, Knol E. CT myelographic findings in degenerative disorders of the cervical spine: clinical significance. *AJR* 1986; 146:793–801.
52. McAllister VL, Sage MR. The radiology of thoracic disc protrusion. *Clin Radiol* 1976; 27:291–299.
53. Wiesel SW, Tsourmas N, Feffer HL. A study of computer assisted tomography. 1. The incidence of positive CAT scans in an asymptomatic group of patients. *Spine* 1984; 9:549–551.
54. Ciric L, Mikhael MA, Tarkington JA, Vick NA. The lateral recess syndrome: a variant of spinal stenosis. *J Neurosurg* 1980; 53:433–443.
55. Bogduk N, Aprill C, Derby R. Discography. In: White AH, Schofferman JA, eds. *Spine care*. St. Louis: CV Mosby, 1995; 219–238.
56. Daffner RH, Rothfus WE. Spinal trauma. In: Latchaw RE, ed. *MR and CT imaging of the head, neck and spine*. St. Louis: Mosby-Year Book, 1991; 1225–1255.
57. Kulkarni MV, Bondurant FJ, Rose SL, Narayana PA. 1.5 tesla magnetic resonance imaging of acute spinal trauma. *Radiographics* 1988; 8: 1059–1082.
58. Kulkarni MV, McArdle CB, Kopanicky D, et al. Acute spinal cord injury: MR imaging at 1.5 T. *Radiology* 1987; 164:837–843.
59. Quencer RM. Post-traumatic spinal cord cysts: characterization with CT, MRI and sonography. In: Latchaw RE, ed. *MR and CT imaging of the head, neck and spine*. St. Louis: Mosby-Year Book, 1991; 1257–1267.
60. Wall SD, Brant-Zawadski M, Jeffrey RB, Barnes B. High frequency CT findings within 24 hours after cerebral infarction. *AJNR* 1981; 2: 553–557.
61. Hecht ST, Eelkema EA, Latchaw RE. Cerebral ischemia and infarction. In: Latchaw RE, ed. *MR and CT imaging of the head, neck and spine*. St. Louis: Mosby-Year Book, 1991; 145–169.
62. Inoue Y, Takemoto K, Miyamoto T, et al. Sequential computed tomography scans in acute cerebral infarction. *Radiology* 1980; 135:655–662.
63. Grossman RI. Intracranial hemorrhage. In: Latchaw RE, ed. *MR and CT imaging of the head, neck and spine*. St. Louis: Mosby-Year Book, 1991; 171–202.
64. Chakeres DW, Bryan RN. Acute subarachnoid hemorrhage. In vitro comparison of magnetic resonance and computed tomography. *AJNR* 1986; 7:223–228.
65. Eelkema EA, Hecht ST, Horton JA. Head trauma. In: Latchaw RE, ed. *MR and CT imaging of the head, neck and spine*. St. Louis: Mosby-Year Book, 1991; 203–265.
66. Bergstrom M, Ericson K, Levander B, Svendsen P, Larsson S. Variations with time of the attenuation values of intracranial hematomas. *J Comput Assist Tomogr* 1977; 1:57–63.
67. Zimmerman RA, Bilaniuk LT, Bruce D, Dolinskas C, Obrist W, Kuhl D. Computed tomography of pediatric head trauma: acute general cerebral swelling. *Radiology* 1978; 128:403–408.
68. Weinstein MA, Chuang S. Diseases of the white matter. In: Latchaw RE, ed. *MR and CT imaging of the head, neck and spine*. St. Louis: Mosby-Year Book, 1991; 347–395.
69. Gebarski SS. The passionate man plays his part: neuroimaging and multiple sclerosis. *Radiology* 1988; 169:275–276.
70. Drayer BP. Brain iron and movement disorders. In: Latchaw RE, ed. *MR and CT imaging of the head, neck and spine*. St. Louis: Mosby-Year Book, 1991; 399–412.
71. George AE, DeLeon MJ. Computed tomography, magnetic resonance imaging and positron emission tomography in aging and dementing disorders. In: Latchaw RE, ed. *MR and CT imaging of the head, neck and spine*. St. Louis: Mosby-Year Book, 1991; 413–442.

PART II

Management Methods

Rehabilitation Medicine: Principles and Practice, Third Edition,
edited by Joel A. DeLisa and Bruce M. Gans.
Lippincott–Raven Publishers, Philadelphia © 1998.

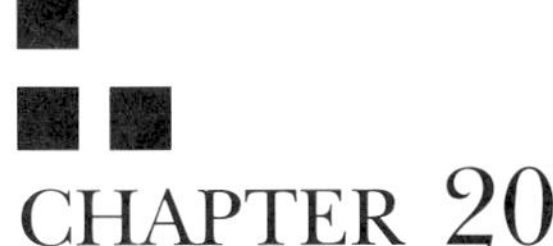

CHAPTER 20

Physical Agents

Jeffrey R. Basford

This chapter reviews the physical agents with an emphasis on their clinical use, scientific basis, and effectiveness. Although the properties of many agents overlap, discussion will first emphasize superficial heat and cold. The diathermies, hydrotherapy, and electrical therapies will then be examined. The chapter will conclude with an analysis of some of the less established modalities, such as pulsed fields, vibration, and low-intensity electrical stimulation.

HEAT AND COLD

Heat and cold have potent effects on tissue. For example, temperatures above 45°C are uncomfortable and, with prolonged exposure, may cause injury (1). Temperatures below 13°C are also uncomfortable, and if systemic temperatures fall below 28°C, death is possible (1). In addition, metabolism and enzymatic processes are temperature dependent: an increase of 3°C increases collagenase activity severalfold (2). Heating the hands to 45°C reduces metacarpophalangeal joint stiffness 20%, whereas cooling them to 18°C increases stiffness by a similar amount (3). Temperature changes of a few degrees alter nerve conduction, and changes of 5°C to 7°C alter blood flow (4–6) and collagen extensibility (7). In practice, most heat treatments attempt to warm deep tissues to between 40°C and 45°C.

Although the heating modalities differ in many ways, they all gain their effects by producing analgesia, hyperemia, local or systemic hyperthermia, and reduced muscle tone. As a result, they share many of the indications (Table 20-1) and contraindications (Table 20-2) of heat in general. Cold's main effects are analgesia and tone reduction. As a result, cold has indications (Table 20-3) and contraindications (Table 20-4) that are often surprisingly similar to heat.

J. R. Basford: Mayo Medical School; and Department of Physical Medicine and Rehabilitation, Mayo Clinic, Rochester, Minnesota 55905-0001.

Superficial Heat

There are only three ways to heat or cool tissue: conduction, convection, and conversion. Among the superficial agents, hot packs exemplify conduction, hydrotherapy emphasizes convection, and heat lamps employ conversion (i.e., convert radiant energy to heat).

The physical properties of superficial modalities differ, but none is able to overcome the combination of skin tolerance, tissue thermal conductivity, and the body's responses to produce localized temperature changes of more than a few degrees at depths of a few centimeters (8). The following sections review the characteristics of the most common superficial agents.

Hot Packs

Hot packs (e.g., Hydrocollator packs) typically consist of segmented canvas sacks filled with a silicon dioxide that when exposed to moisture absorbs many times its own weight of water. These packs are available in various sizes and are suspended on racks in 70°C to 80°C water. When needed, the packs are removed from the baths and, once excess water has been drained off, wrapped in an insulating cover or toweling (Fig. 20-1). Packs cool slowly and maintain therapeutic temperatures for 30 minutes.

Hot pack advantages include low cost, minimal maintenance, long life (i.e., packs last as long as 5 years; reservoirs up to 30 years), good patient acceptance, and ease of use. Self-treatment is possible, and some packs can be heated in a microwave oven.

Hot packs have few risks that are not outlined in Table 20-2. To avoid scalding, however, excess water should be drained before use, the insulating pad checked for excessive dampness, and the pack placed on, not under, the patient.

Kenny Packs

Kenny packs are wool cloths that are soaked in 60°C water and spun dry before use. After spinning, the cloths contain

TABLE 20-1. *General indications for therapeutic heat*

Pain
Muscle spasm
Contracture
Tension myalgia
Production of hyperemia
Acceleration of metabolic processes
Hematoma resolution
Bursitis
Tenosynovitis
Fibrositis
Fibromyalgia
Superficial thrombophlebitis
Induction of reflex vasodilation
Collagen vascular diseases

little water and cool rapidly. As a result, they are replaced during treatment at 5- to 10-minute intervals. Kenny packs, thus, produce a cyclic heating pattern and were once considered particularly effective for the muscle pain and spasms of polio myelitis. These packs are now rarely used due to high equipment and labor requirements.

Electric heating pads, hot water bottles, and circulating water heating pads are alternatives to hot packs. Many of these do not cool spontaneously. Burns are possible and for many devices exposure should be limited to 20 minutes.

Heat Lamps

Radiant heat is an inexpensive, versatile, and easy way to warm superficial tissue. Specialized infrared sources are often used due to their convenience and durability. However, inexpensive incandescent lights release most of their energy as heat, and clamp lamps or incubator lights using these bulbs can be used both at home and in the clinic.

Skin temperatures are controlled by adjusting the distance between the heat source and the patient. Point sources such as light bulbs heat according to the inverse distance squared law. Elongated sources such as quartz lamps and those with specialized reflectors may follow an inverse distance relationship. In practice, heat sources are usually placed about 40 to 50 cm from the patient.

TABLE 20-2. *General contraindications and precautions for therapeutic heat*

Acute inflammation, trauma, or hemorrhage
Bleeding disorders
Insensitivity
Inability to communicate or respond to pain
Poor thermal regulation (e.g., from neuroleptics)
Malignancy
Edema
Ischemia
Atrophic skin
Scar tissue

TABLE 20-3. *General indications for therapeutic cold*

Acute musculoskeletal trauma
Edema
Hemorrhage
Analgesia
Pain
Muscle spasm
Spasticity
Adjunct in muscle reeduation
Reduction of local and systemic metabolic activity

Choice

The physiologic effects of dry heat from a heat lamp differ little from those of moist heat of a hot pack. As a result, agent choice depends on the situation. If the patient is in bed or cannot tolerate pressure, radiant heat is the better option. Similarly, if a patient feels that radiant heat dries their skin or prefers moist heat, the choice is also easy. Many times, ease of use and preference dictate the choice. Some find that the cleanliness, convenience, and reduced laundry costs of heat lamps outweigh most advantages of hot packs.

Safety

The precautions in Table 20-2 apply to the superficial heating agents. In addition, these modalities can burn the patient, produce erythema (erythema ab igne) and, with chronic use, cause a permanent brown skin mottling.

Hydrotherapy

Hydrotherapy uses a fluid medium to transfer thermal and mechanical forces to tissue. Whirlpool baths (Fig. 20-2) and Hubbard tanks (Fig. 20-3) use agitated water to produce convective heating, cooling, massage, and gentle debridement. Agitation is not essential. For example, sitz baths, paraffin baths, and contrast baths all use a stationary medium. This section discusses these therapies as well as alternatives such as balneotherapy and water exercise.

Whirlpool Baths and Hubbard Tanks

Tanks vary in size from small portable whirlpools designed to treat a single extremity to Hubbard tanks contain-

TABLE 20-4. *General precautions and contraindications for therapeutic cold*

Ischemia
Cold intolerance
Raynaud's phenomenon and disease
Severe cold pressor responses
Cold allergy
Insensitivity

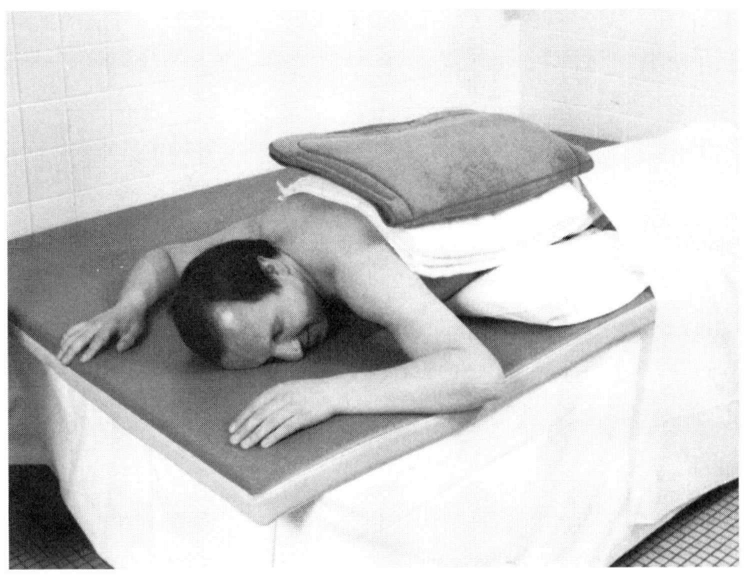

FIG. 20-1. Hot pack treatment of the low back. The pack is covered with an insulated wrapper and separated from the patient with several layers of toweling. Note that the patient must be positioned carefully and be able to tolerate the weight of the pack.

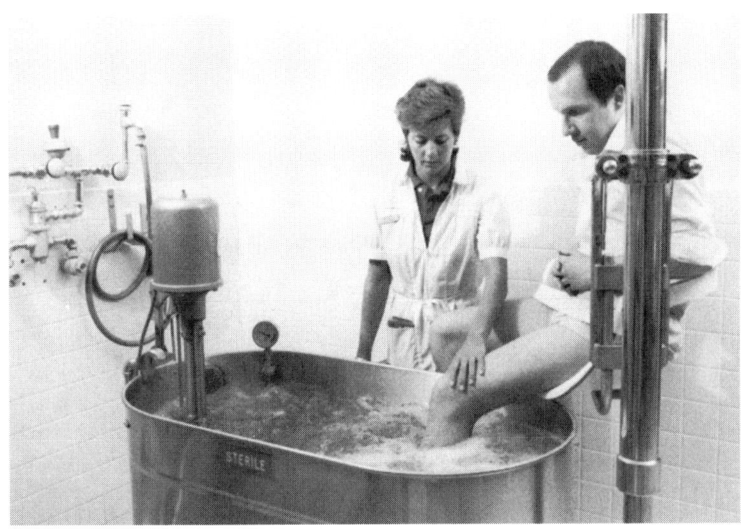

FIG. 20-2. Whirlpool treatment of the lower extremity. Water temperatures may range from 11 to 43°C depending on the patient's condition and the amount of surface area treated. Positioning as well as entering and leaving the bath is made less difficult with a hydraulic chair.

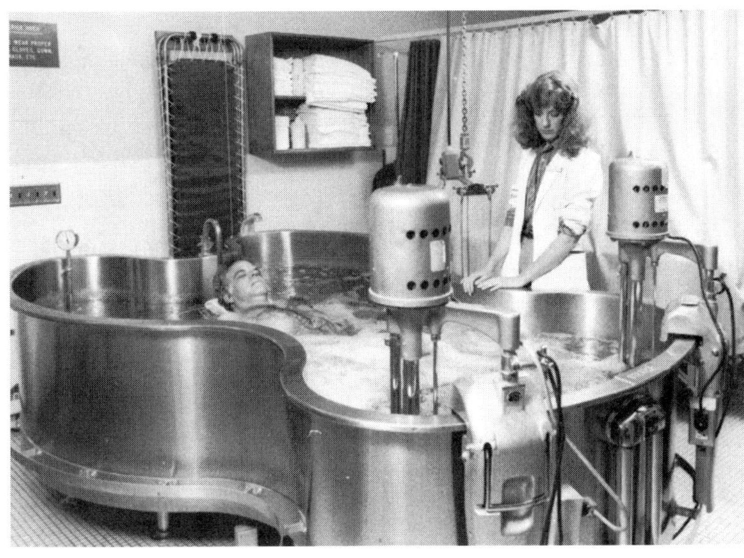

FIG. 20-3. Hubbard tank treatment. These tanks are large, expensive to operate, and occupy large amounts of floor space. Nevertheless, they are necessary for the cleaning of large wounds and helpful in treating patients with conditions involving multiple joints.

ing several thousand liters. Pools and tanks are not essential; hand-held shower heads and small water jets are often used for vigorous local treatment such as the irrigation and debridement of deep wounds and burns.

Water temperature choice depends on the amount of the body immersed, treatment goals, and the patient's medical condition. Neutral temperatures of 33°C to 36°C are usually well tolerated on limited portions of the body, although for a healthy patient, temperatures of 43°C to as much as 45°C or 46°C are possible. Full body immersion can alter systemic temperatures, and Hubbard tank temperatures are usually limited to 39°C. Temperature selection should take into account the fact that turbulent water heats and cools more vigorously than stationary water of the same temperature.

Whirl pools and Hubbard tanks are well suited for wound and burn treatment in which gentle agitation, heat, and solvent action are needed. Neutral temperatures (to somewhat warmer as more of the body is immersed) are chosen and, after the patient is immersed, agitation is increased to provide gentle debridement and aid in dressing removal. Sterile tanks should be specified for burns and wounds. Although true sterility is not possible, a sufficient approximation is possible to make disease transmission unlikely. If wounds are large, or if there is a significant exposure of internal tissue, sodium chloride may be added to the water (5 kg or more for a Hubbard tank) to improve comfort and lessen the risks of hemolysis and electrolyte imbalance. Additional agents such as potassium permanganate and gentle detergents may be added as desired.

Hydrotherapy is also a common adjunct to the treatment of rheumatoid arthritis, diffuse tension myalgia, muscle spasm, and joint mobilization after cast removal. Immobilized patients and those with wounds often find hydrotherapy frightening. Treatment should be reviewed before the first session with emphasis on its comfort, transfers, and any use of plinths and hoists.

Hydrotherapy is resource intensive, expensive, and consumes large amounts of hot water. To save space and money, therapy departments substitute small specialized units for large units as much as possible.

Contrast Baths

Contrast baths use two baths, one at 43°C and the other at 16°C, to produce reflex hyperemia and neurologic desensitization. Effectiveness is thought to be due to alternating exposure to heat and cold. Treatments typically begin with an initial soaking of the hands or feet in the warm bath for about 10 minutes and then proceed to four cycles of alternate 1- to 4-minute cold soaks and 4- to 6-minute warm soaks (9).

Contrast baths are frequently used in treatment programs for rheumatoid arthritis and sympathetically mediated pain (reflex sympathetic dystrophy). Rheumatoid arthritics often benefit but may find simple warm water soaks as effective and simpler. Patients with sympathetically mediated pain often prefer to begin with less extreme bath temperatures. These latter patients also seem to benefit, but this improvement is difficult to separate from the effects of other desensitization and activity programs.

Sitz Baths

Warm sitz baths are enshrined in the treatment of hemorrhoids and anorectal pain. Research supports this practice. For example, sitting in water between 40° and 50°C (with warmer temperatures perhaps more effective) lessens sphincter activity and anal pressures in normal subjects as well as those with hemorrhoids and anorectal fistulas (10).

Edema

The ancient Greeks and 18th century physicians treated edema with water immersion, a practice mimicked today with pneumatic sleeves. Research supports this intuitively reasonable treatment: immersion increases renal water and salt loss in normal subjects as well as those with the nephrotic syndrome and cirrhosis (11). Because warmth produces a reactive vasodilation, neutral temperatures would seem to be the most effective.

Water-Based Exercise

Although patients with rheumatoid and osteoarthritis often like water and pool-based exercise, benefits may not be as clear as they might seem. For example, a comparison of land- and water-based postsurgical anterior cruciate rehabilitation programs found that the water-based program produced less knee pain and swelling, but that land exercises increased knee strength more rapidly (12). In addition, home hip osteoarthritis exercise programs may be as effective as the same programs supplemented with twice-a-week pool exercise (13).

Balneotherapy

Balneotherapy (spa) therapy was once popular in North America but today is little more than a curiosity. In Europe, however, acceptance remains stronger, and visits to spas are still supported by some governments and insurance companies.

Balneotherapy is based on the belief that specific waters containing dissolved gases (such as nitrogen, carbon dioxide, methane), elements (calcium, magnesium, zinc, cobalt, etc.), and compounds (e.g., hydrogen sulfide) (14,15) have therapeutic effects. Although intact skin is relatively impervious to these substances, that of patients with an impaired skin barrier (such as psoriatics in which blood concentration of bromine and rubidium are increased after bathing in the Dead Sea) (16), allows some penetration.

The inflammatory and degenerative arthridities are common indications for balneotherapy. Although most U.S. physicians are skeptical, some controlled investigations support its use. For example, rheumatoid arthritics treated with mineral-rich hot packs improved more in terms of comfort and grip strength than did similar patients treated with identical packs whose mineral concentrations had been depleted 100-fold by repeated rinsing (17). Another controlled study compared the effects of balneotherapy, water jets, and underwater traction on low back pain (18). This study found that all three groups improved, but it could not isolate specific balneotherapy benefits. Other, less rigorously controlled and blinded studies also support the benefits of balneotherapy for rheumatoid arthritis (19) and chronic back pain (20,21).

Fluidotherapy

Hydrotherapy usually uses water as the heat-exchanging medium, but substances such as pulverized corn cobs and small beads "fluidized" by hot air jets may be substituted. Although these devices have been available since the 1970s (22,23), the benefits of this high-temperature, low heat capacity approach remain controversial.

Safety

The general precautions of heat (Table 20-2) apply to hydrotherapy. Drowning, cardiac disease, systemic hyperthermia, and disease transmission are also concerns, but they may be overemphasized.

Cardiac disease is often a contraindication to hyperthermia. Nevertheless, Finnish heart attack survivors return to sauna bathing without apparent increased risk (24,25), and 15-minute soaks in 40°C hot tubs do not create ischemic electrocardiogram changes or alter systolic and diastolic blood pressures more than cardiac rehabilitation stationary bicycle exercises (26).

Hydrotherapy-associated infections seem to be rare. However, there may be some reproductive consequences. Neural tube defects may be increased (relative risk 2.6 to 2.9) in the children of women who sauna bathe during early pregnancy (27), and sperm counts may be lowered after isolated or repeated sauna sessions (28).

Paraffin Baths

Paraffin baths are thermostatically controlled reservoirs filled with a 1:7 mixture of mineral oil and paraffin. Bath temperatures (52°C to 54°C) are higher than in most hydrotherapy, but are well tolerated due to the low heat capacity of the mixture and the tendency for an insulating layer of wax to build up on the surface of the treated area.

Two paraffin treatment approaches predominate. Dipping is the most common and consists of the patient submerging the treated extremity in the bath 10 times, with pauses between dips to permit a layer of paraffin to solidify. The treated area is then covered with a plastic sheet and placed in an insulating cover for about 20 minutes (Figs. 20-4 and 20-5). The paraffin is then stripped off and returned to the container.

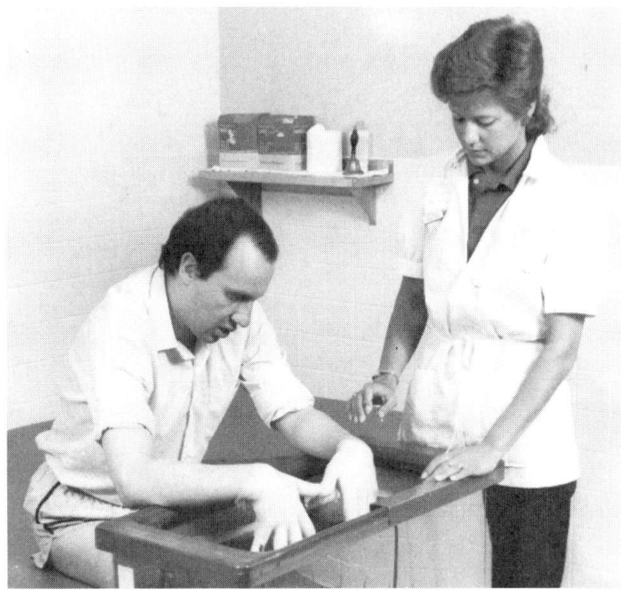

FIG. 20-4. Paraffin bath treatment. Two approaches are common. In the dipping technique, the extremity is immersed in the bath, removed briefly to allow the wax to solidify, and redipped for a total of 10 repetitions. After the dipping, the extremity is wrapped in an insulating cover for about 20 minutes before the wax is removed. The immersion technique provides a more vigorous heating and is similar to the dipping approach except that after a few dips, the extremity is kept immersed in the paraffin.

Dipping initially increases skin temperatures to about 47°C, but by the end of a 30-minute session, skin temperatures fall to within a few degrees of baseline. Deeper tissues respond to a lesser extent: subcutaneous temperatures may increase by 3°C and intramuscular temperatures by 1°C (29).

Continuous immersion is an alternative approach in which the treated extremity is dipped once or twice in the paraffin and then kept immersed for 20 to 30 minutes. Heating is more intense with this method but is still well tolerated because a layer of insulating solidified paraffin forms on the skin. Immersion produces the same initial maximum skin temperature as dipping. However, temperatures decrease less rapidly. At the end of a session, skin temperatures are about 41.5°C, with subcutaneous and intramuscular temperature increases (about 5°C and 3°C, respectively) higher and more persistent than from dipping (29).

Paraffin baths are often used to treat the hand contractures associated with rheumatoid arthritis, scleroderma, burns, and injury. Dipping or immersion is most common, but paraffin at times will be brushed on sensitive or difficult-to-treat areas. Reports in the literature are scant, but these messy treatments seem frequently helpful.

Safety

A thermometer should be kept in the reservoir and paraffin temperature checked before use to avoid burns. (A film of

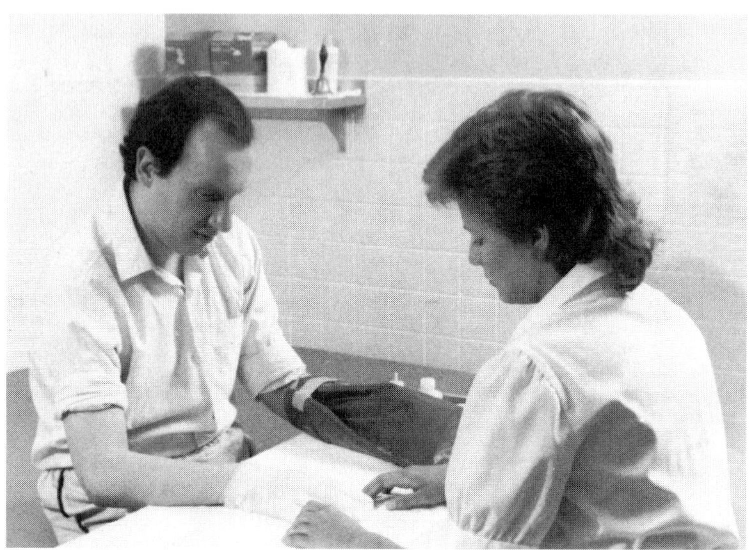

FIG. 20-5. Paraffin dipping technique. After completion of the dipping, the extremity is placed in a plastic-coated, insulated bag to slow cooling. As an alternative, the hand may be wrapped in a plastic sheet and toweling.

solidified wax around the margins of a reservoir is a sign that the temperature is too high.) Some patients use paraffin at home. Although paraffin–oil mixtures can be heated in a double boiler on a stove, small commercial units are convenient and safer. The feet have poor circulation, and a few insulating layers of paraffin may be painted on them before they are dipped or immersed (30).

Most clinicians do not heat acutely inflamed joints and tissues vigorously. However, even a few degrees temperature elevation such as may occur with paraffin baths or hot soaks increases intra-articular enzymatic activity (2). Although there has been controversy about whether or not superficial heat and cold have paradoxical effects (31–35), warmth clearly improves comfort, and most clinicians use superficial heat in the subacute situation.

Diathermy

There are three diathermy (i.e., through-heating) agents: ultrasound (US), shortwave diathermy (SWD) and microwave diathermy (MWD). US and SWD are the most common and are discussed in detail. MWD is now rare but is reviewed because of its continued specialized use.

Ultrasound

US is sound that occurs above the 17,000- to 20,000-Hz limit of human hearing. As such, it shares the characteristics of sound in general: its waves consist of alternating compressions and rarefactions; it requires a medium for transmission; it transmits energy; and it can be focused, refracted, and reflected. Although arguments are made for a variety of frequencies, most therapeutic US occurs between 0.8 and 1 MHz due to the practical considerations of focusing, penetration, and standardization.

Biophysics

US has both thermal and nonthermal effects. Heat production is the best known, but nonthermal processes, including cavitation, streaming, standing waves, mechanical deformation, and shock waves, also may be important. The first of these, cavitation, occurs when high intensity US passes through a liquid and produces small bubbles. Once produced, these bubbles may either rhythmically oscillate in size (stable cavitation) or may grow and abruptly collapse (unstable cavitation). In either case, localized large temperature and pressure changes are created (36). Although unstable cavitation seems most capable of damaging tissue, each produces mechanical distortion, localized motion, and destruction. Pressure asymmetries produced by sound can generate media movement (streaming), which may damage tissue and accelerate metabolic processes (37). Standing waves are generated from the resonant superposition of sound waves and produce fixed regions of high and low pressure at one-half–wavelength intervals (which for 1 MHz US [tissue velocity 1,500 m/sec] is about 0.75 mm) (38). Graphic effects are possible; US exposure produces repetitive bands of red blood cells in chick embryo vessels (39).

US penetration into tissue depends on a number of factors. In particular, penetration decreases by a factor of 6 as the frequency increases from 0.3 to 3.3 MHz (38). Orientation is also important. For example, about 50% of a 0.87-MHz US beam penetrates 7 cm in a direction parallel to muscle fibers, but the same beam penetrates only 2 cm in a direction perpendicular to the fibers (38). Tissue type is also important. Fifty percent of an US beam penetrates several centimeters in muscle, only a few tenths of a millimeter in bone, and 7 to 8 cm in fat (38,40).

Sound absorption discontinuities produce localized heating. Large absorption changes are present at bone–soft tissue interfaces and may generate 5°C temperature elevations

(40,41). Heat is lost from tissue as the result of conduction and cooling effects of the local blood flow.

Equipment

US machines use ceramics or piezoelectric crystals to convert electrical energy into sound. Each machine has a timer, indicates when the applicator is energized, and, when appropriate, indicates the waveform and frequency. Additional options, such as concurrent electrical stimulation, are also available.

US frequencies are relatively stable and usually remain within 5% of the manufacturer's specifications (42). Output powers and intensities (power output divided by the active area of the applicator), on the other hand, may vary by 20% or more during a session and as a unit ages (42–44). Machines should be routinely calibrated.

Technique

There are two philosophies of US therapy. The most widely held is that ultrasound's benefits are due to heat. This approach typically uses an unmodulated, continuous-wave (CW) US beam with intensities limited to 0.5 to 2.5 W/cm^2 by tissue tolerance. The second approach emphasizes ultrasound's nonthermal properties. In this case the beam is modulated to deliver brief pulses of high-intensity US separated by longer pauses of no power. Thus, ultrasound's nonthermal effects are emphasized, but the average power delivered is the same as, or less than, that of the CW US.

US is usually delivered by moving the applicator (Fig. 20-6) over the treated area in slow (1 to 2 cm/sec) overlapping strokes. Treatments cover areas of about 100 cm^2 and last 5 to 10 minutes. Indirect US is less common and is used to treat irregular surfaces (such as the foot and ankle), where it is difficult to keep the applicator in contact with the skin. In these situations, the body part is placed in a container filled with water. The applicator is held a short distance away and moved without touching the skin. Power intensities may need to be higher owing to absorption in the water.

Coupling between the applicator and the skin is not a trivial issue. The treatment area should be cleansed before treatment, and a coupling agent is necessary. Degassed water (water that has been allowed to sit for several hours) is used for indirect US because the dissolved gases in water fresh from the tap form bubbles during treatment and attenuate the beam. Little practical difference exists between degassed water, commercial gels, and mineral oil for direct applications. Glycerin is somewhat less efficient, but is acceptable (45–47).

Phonophoresis is a variant of US in which biologically active substances are combined with the coupling medium, in the hope that the US will force the active material into tissue. Neither effectiveness, penetration depth, nor the amount of material lost to the subcutaneous circulation is well established. Phonophoresis does introduce detectable concentrations of lidocaine into rabbit muscle (48). Although claims of increased cortisol concentrations at depths of several centimeters after corticosteroid phonophoresis are made (49), our own research as well that of others (50) finds limited evidence for deep penetration. One clinical study compared the effectiveness of lidocaine and corticosteroid phonophoresis with similar US treatment using an inert coupling agent (51). Although the US groups fared better than control patients receiving sham treatment, the difference between the them was not statistically significant. Other clinical studies report successful phonophoresis with phonophoretic carbocaine anesthesia during fracture reduction (52) and with phenylbutazone and chymotrypsin (53).

Indications

Tendinitis and Bursitis

The research supporting this common indication is surprisingly mixed. For example, a study of 50 patients with

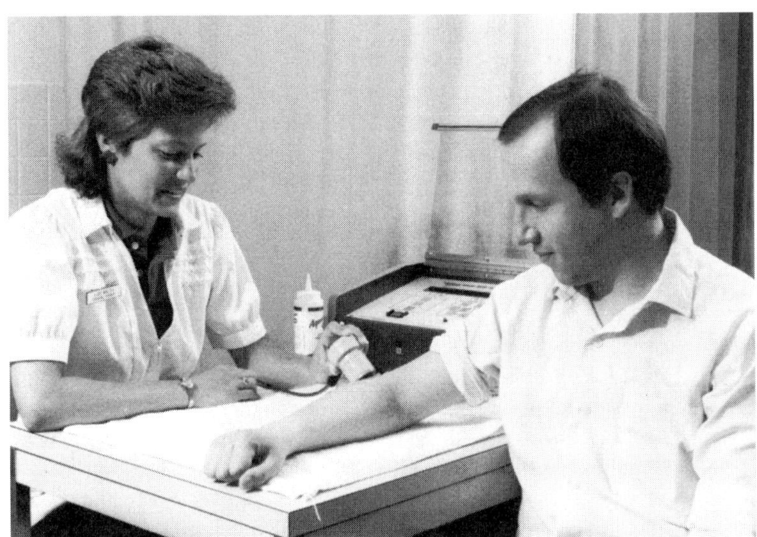

FIG. 20-6. Direct-contact US treatment of the knee. Note the use of a folded towel to comfortably support the patient. Although not shown in the picture, a coupling agent is needed to acoustically couple the applicator and the skin.

bursitis and bicipital tendinitis treated 3 to 5 days a week with 1.2 to 1.8 W/cm^2 of 1 MHz US found good to fair improvement in pain and motion in more than 85% of the patients (54). Two uncontrolled studies found 80% to 90% of 223 patients treated with corticosteroid injections in conjunction with daily or alternate day 1 MHz US (up to 3 W/cm^2) had excellent or moderate improvement (55,56). Whether these subjects would have improved spontaneously is unknown. Although US may delay the onset of postexercise pain (57) and may be more beneficial than corticosteroid injection in the treatment of shoulder pain, some studies find it no more effective than placebo or anti-inflammatories for subacromial bursitis or myofascial face pain (58–61). Although these studies raise legitimate issues, most physicians and therapists remain convinced that US is useful for the treatment of at least some musculoskeletal pain.

Degenerative Arthritis

US is used in addition to exercise, joint protection, and education in the hopes that it will lessen pain and speed recovery from spinal and peripheral osteoarthritis. Treatments are restricted to circumscribed areas and usually involve 5- to 10-minute sessions at intensities of 0.5 to 2 W/cm^2. Studies may report significant (frequently 70% to 80%) improvement with treatment but are limited by subjectivity and poor controls (62).

Contractures

US is effective in increasing the range of motion of periarthritic shoulders and contracted hips (63,64). In fact, it is the only agent that can significantly heat (by 8°C to 10°C) the hip joint (65,66). Hand and Dupuytren (67) contractures also may benefit from US (57). However, these contractures often have a superficial component, and one small burn study (which applied stretching after US) did not find treatment beneficial (68). Collagen and tendon extensibility increases and decreases as temperatures increase or decrease (7). As a result, stretching should begin during heating and should continue as the tissue cools and "sets."

Soft-Tissue Wounds and Inflammation

US treatment of wounds and inflammation is based on the belief that either heating (by increasing blood flow, metabolic or enzymatic activity) or nonthermal effects (perhaps by changing cell wall permeability) accelerates healing. Results of laboratory work offer some support (69). Human studies are more mixed. One study, for example, found pulsed, low intensity 3.28 MHz ineffective in the treatment of nursing home patients with decubitus ulcers (70), whereas another using a similar regimen along with ultraviolet (UV-C) light (71) found treatment helpful. Other poorly controlled studies may find healing improved and pain reduced by US (72). Studies of lower extremity stasis ulcers show both positive and negative results (73–75).

Some feel that inflammation and swelling are indications for US. Others believe that the heating and membrane permeability changes associated with US are contraindications. Studies, including some of the jaw (76), perineum (77), and rat (78) show little clear benefit.

Trauma

Although US may aggravate tissue damage and swelling if used too soon after an injury, injection indurations (79), subacute hematomas (80), and postpartum perineal pain (81) may improve more rapidly with treatment. In addition, US is reported to be more effective than radiant heat, SWD, or paraffin baths in helping patients with a variety of soft-tissue injuries to return to work (82). The benefits of US in addition to an otherwise adequate therapy program are often unclear (83).

Fractures

Ultrasound's ability to improve the healing of boney injuries was established in the 1980s (84). Treatment intensities are remarkably low. For example, a recent study found 30 mW/cm^2 pulsed 1.5 MHz US accelerated the healing of closed and open grade 1 fractures (85). Because US has been approved by the U.S. Food and Drug Administration (FDA) for the treatment of some fractures, and 5% to 10% of fractures heal slowly (84), there may be a wide applicability for this treatment in the future.

Other Indications

Posttherpetic neuralgia is resistant to conventional treatment. Treatment with pulsed and continuous 1 to 1.5 MHz US also has been evaluated. Studies have been poorly controlled and the results are unclear: some investigators have found improvement (86,87), whereas others have not (88). Because US has thermal, and possibly nonthermal, effects on nerve conduction (89–91), further evaluation seems appropriate. Plantar warts treaatment is also unsuccessful. US has also been evaluated here. Study quality has been limited and the results conflicting: benefit at conventional doses (e.g., 0.5 W/cm^2 at 0.8 or 1 Mhz) may (92,93) or may not (94) occur. Scars and keloids respond inconsistently to injection, surgery, and radiation. US is also used for their treatment, but at least one small study found no improvement from a course of 0.5 to 0.8 W/cm^2 treatments (95).

Precautions and Contraindications

US produces intense heating and nonthermal effects such as shockwaves, cavitation, and media motion. The precautions in Table 20- 2 should be heeded. In addition, fluid-filled cavities such as the eyes and gravid uterus are avoided due to the risks of cavitation and heat damage. The heart, brain, cervical ganglia, tumors, acute hemorrhage sites, ischemic areas, pacemakers, and infection sites should not be treated for obvious heat, neurophysiologic, and mechanical reasons. The spine should not be exposed to high intensities, and laminectomy sites, in particular, should be skirted. US is not used over immature or acutely inflamed joints because intra-articular temperature elevation increases enzymatic activity and may harm immature growth plates (96–98).

It is often reported that US treatment over metal in muscle or next to bone elevates temperature tissue temperatures more than would occur in its absence (99–101). These studies investigated a limited number of objects and geometries, it seems possible that other conformations might produce localized heating.

Short-Wave Diathermy

SWD heats tissue with a combination of induced electrical currents and the vibration it imposes on the molecules of a tissue. The shortwaves of SWD are radiowaves and can cause electrical interference. The U.S. Federal Communications Commission (FCC) has therefore restricted the industrial, scientific, and medical (ISM) use of SWD to 27.12-, 13.56-, and 40.68-MHz (wavelengths of 11, 22, and 7 m), respectively. Most SWD machines in the United States operate at 27.12 MHz.

Biophysics

Radiowaves attenuate as they pass through tissue, but actual penetration depths depend on the specifics of tissue as well as the frequency and characteristics of the applicator. Inductive applicators generate magnetically induced eddy currents in tissue and, as a rule, produce the highest temperatures in water-rich, highly conductive tissues such as muscle. Capacitively coupled applicators, on the other hand, emphasize electric field heating. Maximum temperatures tend to occur in water-poor substances such as fat (102), and significant heating is possible. SWD can increase subcutaneous fat temperatures by 15°C and 4- to 5-cm deep muscle temperatures by 4°C to 6°C (103).

SWD machines may produce pulsed as well as CW output. CW SWD is used when the treatment goal is heating. Pulsed SWD, in contrast, alternates brief periods of high power with longer periods of no power output. The average output power may be the same in both approaches, but the pulsed approach emphasizes nonthermal effects. (Some investigators, for example, feel that certain pulse frequencies, even at low intensities, have resonant effects on cell function.) Although nonthermal SWD phenomena (e.g., pearl chains) have been known for more than 40 years (104), their clinical benefits remain elusive.

Technique

An SWD machine is essentially a radio transmitter that is tuned in the same way that any transmitter is tuned. The patient is in the machine's field and is protected from injury by tuning the circuit (automatically in modern SWD machines) for maximum coupling. Once coupling is maximized, movement can only reduce heating.

There are a variety of inductive applicators (Fig. 20-7*A*). Drum applicators consist of coils encased in rigid containers, a number of which may be connected by hinges to allow placement around regions such as the shoulder. Pad applicators are commercially available, semiflexible mats containing a coil that is connected to an SWD machine and placed against the patient. Pads may have dimensions of 0.5 × 0.75 m and typically are used on the low back. Cable applicators consist of rubber-coated cables that were wrapped around an extremity or laid over the body. Cables were once common, but due to safety concerns and the need for careful placement, they have been replaced by drums and pads.

In the most common capacitive arrangement, the patient is placed between two platelike electrodes (Fig. 20-7*B*). Rectal and vaginal applicators are capacitive probes that were used for pelvic heating. The probes were inserted carefully—the vaginal probe under the cervix in the posterior fornix—and an external pad used to complete the circuit. These probes were resisted by patients and are now seldom used despite past use for pelvic inflammatory disease, chronic prostatitis (85), and pelvic floor myalgia. Today, external SWD over the sacrum and pelvic floor is often substituted.

Microwave Diathermy

Electromagnetic radiation can be well focused when the wavelength of the radiation is comparable with the dimensions of the antenna. The FCC-approved ISM frequencies for MWD are 915 and 2,456 MHz (33-cm and 12-cm wavelengths, respectively). Clinical applicators have dimensions between 15 and 30 cm. Thus, MWD satisfies the wavelength-antenna requirements and, unlike shortwaves, can be relatively easily focused.

Biophysics

Microwaves do not penetrate tissue as deeply as SWD and US. In addition, penetration decreases as frequency increases, and deeper heating occurs at 434 MHz than at 915 MHz or 2,450 MHz (102,105,106). Leakage and focusing become more difficult problems with longer wavelengths.

Microwave radiation is absorbed selectively by water and should preferentially heat muscle. However, fat usually overlies muscle and absorbs a significant portion of the beam. As an example, at 915 MHz subcutaneous fat temperatures may increase by 10°C to 12°C, whereas 3- to 4-cm deep muscles will be heated only 3°C to 4°C (107).

Technique

Microwave diathermy was used to heat superficial muscles and joints such as the shoulder. Other uses, such as

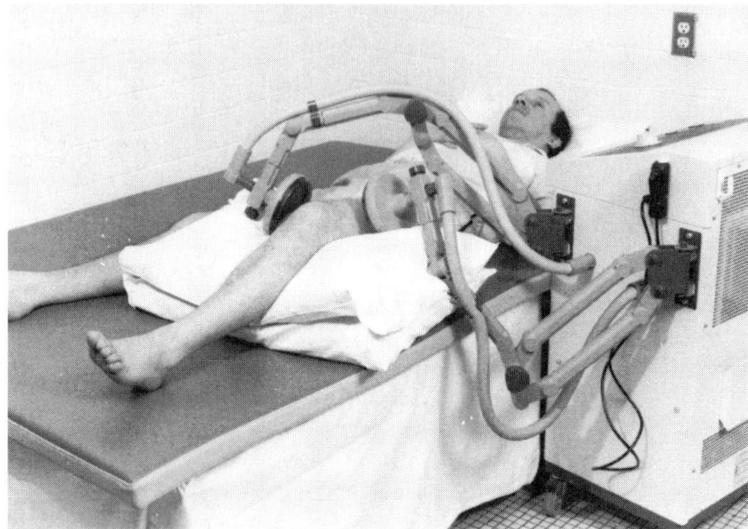

A

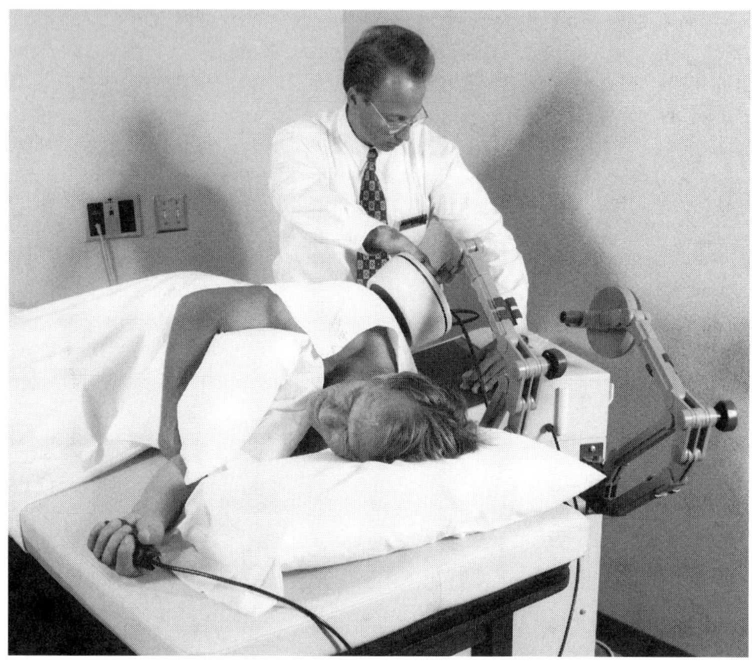

B

FIG. 20-7. A: Short-wave diathermy treatment using a capacitive plate arrangement. Careful positioning is necessary. The patient should wear no jewelry and lie on a nonconductive table. **B:** Short-wave diathermy treatment using an inductive applicator. Note the capacitive plate to the side and the emergency cut-off switch in the patient's hand. Again, metal is avoided and the patient is carefully positioned on a nonconducting surface.

speeding hematoma resolution (108), were also common. Today MWD is used to potentiate the effects of chemotherapy and radiation (109) but has otherwise been replaced with SWD and US.

Precautions and Contraindications

The general contraindications listed in Table 20-2 apply to SWD and MWD. Additional restrictions stem from their electromagnetic nature. For example, perspiration is conductive and, if present in a field, heats the skin. Metal produces localized heating in a field; patients should not wear jewelry, and treatment is given on a nonconductive table. Pacemakers, stimulators, surgical implants, contact lenses, metallic intrauterine devices, and the menstruating or pregnant uterus should not be exposed SWD or MWD. Many feel that small, metallic surgical clips do not produce significant localized temperature elevations. This may be correct, but at least one study found that 1-cm wires positioned to mimic a surgical site, produced temperature elevations 3 to 4°C greater than occurred in their absence during 90-MHz diathermy (109). Many investigators follow a rule of ''no metal'' when using diathermy. Newborns have been exposed to MWD without complications (110), but the effects of diathermy on the immature skeleton is not well established. Microwaves selectively heat water, and MWD of edematous tissue, moist skin, fluid-filled cavities, and blisters can produce unacceptable temperature elevations (111). Microwaves can produce cataracts (112) if protective eye wear is not worn.

Inductive SWD applicators have higher magnetic leakages than capacitive electrodes, which have higher electrical leakages. Leakage varies between applicators, but at dis-

TABLE 20-5. *American National Standards Institute guidelines for radio frequency protection*

Frequency (MHz)	Intensity (mW/cm^2)
0.3–3	100
3–30	900/(MHz)^2
30–300	1
300–500	(MHz)/300
1500–100,000	5

tances of 50 to 60 cm is usually less than 10 mW/cm^2 (102, 113). The American National Standards Institute (ANSI) guidelines (Table 20-5) are frequency dependent (114) and for SWD at 27.12 MHz are about 1 mW/cm^2. MWD leakage depends on a variety of parameters, including the applicator, wave mode, shielding, and spacing (102,106), but also decreases to <10 mW/cm^2 50 to 60 cm from the applicators (102,115). ANSI MWD exposures (Table 20-5) are 3 mW/cm^2 at 915 MHz and 5 mW/cm^2 at 2,450 MHz. These standards are time averaged over the workday. Because therapists work only intermittently with SWD or MWD, their exposures seem to fall well within these guidelines.

Using any diathermy on an acutely inflamed joint is controversial. Patients have reported that treatment improves comfort (97,98), and some investigators feel that synovial temperature elevations to 42°C or more denature enzymes and produce a thermal synovectomy (97,98). However, most clinicians remain skeptical and avoid diathermy in this situation. (As noted above, similar, but less marked, controversy also surrounds the use of superficial heating for the inflammatory arthridites.)

Epidemiologic studies seem to support the workplace safety of SWD and MWD. One study did report that miscarriage rates were increased in women therapists exposed to MWD (116), but other investigations found no alterations in miscarriage rates, sex ratios of offspring, or congenital malformations in the children of therapists working with SWD or MWD (116–118).

Cold (Cryotherapy)

Chilling a limited portion of the body produces local and distant physiologic effects. If the cooling agent is ice, skin temperature initially decreases rapidly and then more slowly approaches an equilibrium of about 12° to 13°C in 10 minutes. Subcutaneous temperatures decline more slowly and decrease by 3°C to 5°C at 10 minutes. Deeper, intramuscular temperatures decrease the least and after 10 minutes have dropped a degree or less (119). Chilling for longer periods generates more pronounced cooling with intramuscular forearm temperature decreases of 6°C to 16°C after 20 minutes to 3 hours of cooling (4,35,96,120). Hollander and Horvath (32–34) reported 50 years ago that superficial heat and cold had paradoxic effects: superficial cold increased joint temperatures and superficial warmth decreased them. More recent work seems to support the more intuitive expectation: intra-articular knee temperatures decrease 6°C over a 3-hour period of cooling with ice chips (35).

Cooling produces an initial period of vasoconstriction that may (121) or may not be followed by a reactive vasodilation that occurs as cold paralyzed vascular smooth muscle relaxes at about 15°C (121–123). Vasoconstriction becomes evident within 5 minutes of cooling, and after 25 minutes of packing a knee in ice, soft tissue and bone blood flow is decreased by 30% and 20%, respectively (35). Superficial cold also decreases metabolic activity, lessens muscle tone, inhibits spasticity (120,124,125), increases gastrointestinal motility (126), slows nerve conduction (4), and produces analgesia (6).

Technique

Ice packs, iced compression wraps, and slushes have high heat capacities and cool treated areas rapidly. Treatments tend to last 20 to 30 minutes. Techniques are straightforward, but if ice packs are used, the skin is often coated with a thin film of mineral oil and a towel is placed around the pack.

Iced whirlpools cool vigorously and usually are used for 20- to 30-minute periods. Although an athlete may be motivated to tolerate them, the average patient finds temperatures below 13°C or 15°C uncomfortable. If the feet or hands are exposed to a cold bath, neoprene booties or gloves may increase tolerance.

Ice massage consists of rubbing a piece of ice (e.g., an ice cube or water frozen in a small cup) over the painful area. Analgesia can be achieved in 7 to 10 minutes, with most patients reporting successive sensations of cold, burning, aching, and numbness. Although chemical and refrigerated agents may have temperatures below 0°C and can produce frostbite, ice treatments of healthy people for periods of less than 30 minutes do not seem to cause injury (120,127).

Vapocoolant and liquid nitrogen sprays can abruptly reduce skin temperature by 20°C (35) and are used for local skin analgesia and the "spray and stretch" techniques of Travell (128). Prepackaged chemical ice packs may consist of two compartments (e.g., one filled with water, the other with ammonium nitrate), which, when broken and the contents mixed, produce a cooling, endothermic reaction. Although these packs are convenient and pliable, they are small, expensive, and tend to cool poorly. Alternatives such as refrigerated and pressurized water pressure cuffs (Fig. 20-8) are also available. Twelve-ounce frozen orange juice containers and plastic packages of frozen peas, which conform to the body when struck on a hard surface, are effective for home use.

Indications

Trauma

Many studies find chilling limits hypoxic damage, lessens edema, speeds recovery, and reduces compartmental pres-

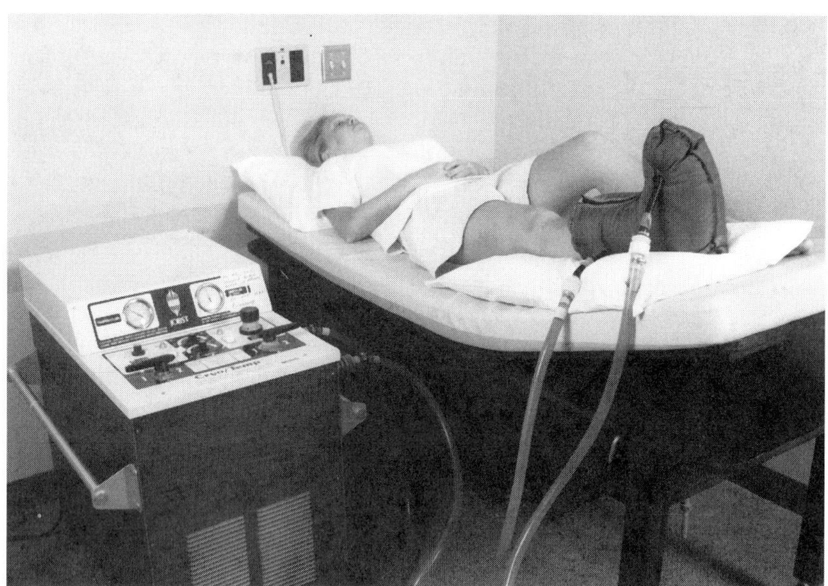

FIG. 20-8. Ice is the mainstay of cryotherapy. Nevertheless, more sophisticated approaches are possible. This machine uses a chilled, inflated cuff to apply pressure and cooling to a knee injury.

sures after injury (129–132). Although there are concerns that cooling does not reduce posttraumatic swelling (133), it does lessen metabolism and blood flow (122). Cooling may slow the deterioration and improve neovasularization of surgical grafts (134).

Rest, ice, compression, and elevation are the initial steps in treating many musculoskeletal injuries. Ice for 20 minutes per half hour to 30 minutes per 2 hours is, for the first 6 to 24 hours, a common ankle sprain regimen (135,136). Early intervention appears important, and acute sprains, fractures, and other trauma should be cooled (and elevated) during the initial evaluation (137). Although ice is the mainstay of acute soft-tissue injury treatment (127), it is interesting that clinical studies of the postsurgical knee (138,139) and cesarean section (140) may not find cryotherapy helpful.

After the first 48 hours, the choice between cryotherapy and heat is a matter of preference and experience. Some prefer cooling and believe that a combination of icing for 10 to 20 minutes to reduce pain and active exercising is the most effective way to speed recovery. In any event, heat and cold are only adjuncts to a mobilization and strengthening program.

Chronic Pain

Patients with chronic musculoskeletal pain occasionally find ice extraordinarily effective. Some research supports their reports. For example, one study of 117 patients hospitalized with low back pain showed that an exercise program with either hot packs or ice massage produced equally effective results, but that there was a nonsignificant tendency for the patients with chronic pain to respond more favorably to the ice regimen (141). Other investigators have found transcutaneous electrical nerve stimulation (TENS) and ice massage equally effective in patients with chronic low back pain (142).

Spasticity

Ten to twenty minutes of vigorous cooling reduces the tone of spastic muscle and may improve the isolation of voluntary function (120,125). Although cooling muscles before therapy might be helpful, its utility must be balanced against the time required.

Precautions and Contraindications

The precautions of Table 20-4 should be heeded. Pressor responses aggravating cardiovascular disease should be considered, as should the effects of direct and consensual vasoconstriction on ischemic limbs and those with Raynaud's phenomenon. Cold hypersensitivity and urticaria are possible; insensate areas and unresponsive patients should be avoided. Cryotherapy is uncomfortable, and it is important to explain its rationale before beginning treatment.

ULTRAVIOLET THERAPY

The UV spectrum is defined in a number of ways. The nonmedical literature divides it into two portions: near (i.e., nearest the visible spectrum, 0.4 to 0.29 μm) and far (less than 0.29 μm) UV. The biomedical literature uses a three-part classification: UV-A (0.315 to 0.4 μm), UV-B (0.29 to 0.315 μm), and UV-C (0.2 to 0.29 μm). This latter division tends to reflect biologic properties. UV-A penetrates deeply (it is the portion of the UV spectrum closest to visible light) but has little biologic activity. UV-B produces sunburn and skin erythema at rates orders of magnitude greater than UV-A. UV-C (the most energetic form of UV) is bactericidal.

Treatment

Broad-spectrum hot quartz lamps were once common but have been replaced with smaller, more convenient, hand-held "cold quartz" lamps that operate at low temperatures and contain mercury at low pressure in a quartz tube. In contrast to the broad spectrums of hot quartz lamps, cold sources produce a narrow band of UV-C light at 0.2537 μm (143). Black light sources (e.g., a Wood's lamp) are simply UV sources filtered to eliminate visible radiation.

UV exposure is limited by the nature of the tissue treated, source intensity, and separation. In practice, exposures are quantified in terms of the time required to produce a minimal erythema (i.e., a minimal erythemal dose [MED]). One MED (usually requiring 5 to 30 seconds) is established by exposing the volar forearm to a source and determining the time required to produce a minimal erythema several hours later. For reference, 2.5 MEDs cause reddening and pain that persist for a few days; five MEDs produce local edema, pain, and desquamation; and 10 MEDs result in blistering (143). Source strength changes with age, and the MED should be redetermined several times a year.

In general, UV treatments begin with one or two MEDs and are kept to less than five MEDs to avoid tissue damage (143). Open wounds are treated directly with a lamp. Specially designed orificial probes may be used for fistulas, undermined wounds, or the oral cavity.

UV was once a common skin ulcer treatment. There is support for this practice in that UV-C kills motile bacteria (spore-forming bacteria are resistant during the spore stage) and may increase wound margin vascularization. There are reports of UV-accelerated wound healing (71,143), but other studies may find alternatives such as occlusive dressings more effective (144). UV is now a rare physical therapy treatment but still has a place in dermatology and neonatology.

Precautions and Contraindications

Sunburn and eye injury are the most plausible concerns. As a result, only the treated area is exposed to UV, and the patient and the therapist should wear protective eye wear. Individuals using photosensitizing medication (e.g., tetracycline, green soap) or cosmetics, or who have a fair complexion, scars, or atrophic skin will be unusually sensitive to UV. In these cases, treatment may be deferred, dosages reduced, and progression to higher exposures slowed.

ELECTROTHERAPY

The ancient Greeks knew that amber rubbed with wool attracted light objects (*elektron* is the Greek word for amber) and that electric eels, rays, and catfish could produce numbness (145,146). This knowledge had little practical benefit. In the 18th and 19th centuries, the invention of electrostatic generators and storage devices was followed by an explosive growth in the understanding of electricity and electromagnetism: Ohm's law was established by 1827, and Maxwell's electromagnetic field equations were known by the late 1860s. This knowledge was accompanied by a growing interest in the medical aspects of electricity. Early "medicinal" electricity applications were enthusiastic and haphazard (146,147). Electrostatic air baths, spark treatments, and galvanically induced limb movement all had momentary popularity. Unfortunately, their utility was minimal, and public as well as scientific interest in therapeutic electricity waned until this century.

Today, high-intensity electrical stimulation is used to strengthen muscles and to move paralyzed limbs. Less intense stimulation produces analgesia and delivers medications percutaneously. Stimulation at still lower intensities has gained FDA approval for fracture healing. Soft-tissue wounds, osteoporosis, and musculoskeletal pain represent additional potentially important, but still investigational, electrical stimulation applications. This section discusses these agents.

Transcutaneous Electrical Nerve Stimulation

The gate theory postulated in 1965 that cells in the substantia gelatinosa are stimulated by both nociceptive and sensory signals and serve as gates by inhibiting the passage of nociceptive information to the brain if sensory afferent signals are present (149). TENS provided sensory afferent signals and, after some successful trials, became widely accepted.

The TENS mechanism of action remains controversial. Thus, although research shows that stimulation reduces dorsal horn cell activity (150), the gate theory does not explain phenomena such as painless sensory neuropathy, analgesia persisting after stimulation, and delayed onset of analgesia. As a result, other explanations, such as those involving frequency-dependent effects and central nervous system endorphins, have been advanced.

TENS units consist of a rechargeable battery, one or more signal generators, and a set of electrodes. Units are small, frequently programmable, and generate a variety of stimuli with currents of less than 100 mA, pulse rates ranging from a few to 200 Hz, and pulse widths from 10 to a few hundred microseconds. Asymmetric, biphasic waveforms are favored to improve comfort and to avoid the electrolytic and iontophoretic effects associated with unidirectional currents. Additional features such as "burst" modes and wave-train modulation are common but of unclear benefit.

Electrode positioning is more art than science. Placement over the painful area is usually the first choice, but locations over afferent nerves, nerve roots, acupuncture and trigger points, and auricular sites, as well as contralateral to the pain, are also possible. Although carbon-impregnated rubber electrodes are inexpensive, more expensive self-adhesive electrodes are far more convenient.

Stimulus parameter choice is also subjective. Many prefer to begin with low-amplitude, 40- to 80-Hz conventional TENS settings and try the less comfortable high-intensity 4- to 8-Hz, low TENS alternative if the first trials are unsuccessful. Response is difficult to predict, and parameter selection is ultimately based on trial and error.

Evaluation is not easy. Ideally, initial benefit is established in a few therapy sessions and an overnight trial. If TENS appears effective, the patient should rent an identical unit for a month or more. Because these devices are expensive (many $700 or more) and benefits often wane with time, purchase should be considered only if benefits persist for at least a few months.

Indications

TENS studies range in quality from well-designed, prospective, randomized, controlled trials, to case reports. Success rates vary from placebo levels to 95% and may be affected by the stimulating parameters (151), electrode placement, conditions treated, chronicity, previous treatment, experimental design, and length of follow-up. Even when studies are controlled, it is not clear whether the controls should be dummy TENS or an alternative treatment.

Many studies, especially in the late 1970s and 1980s, found that TENS reduced postoperative and first-stage labor pain by about 80%, decreased narcotic use, shortened intensive care unit stays, improved respiratory status, lessened ileus, and improved mobility (152). Acute pain and trauma studies tended to find TENS as successful as limited amounts of analgesics and narcotics, whereas chronic pain studies found success rates varying from placebo levels to about 85% with success decreasing as the duration of follow-up increased (152). More recent research supports these findings but tends to put a harsher light on them. Again, evaluation is difficult due to varying study designs, incomplete parameter descriptions, and varying lengths of follow-up. Conflicts persist, but negative results seem more pronounced than a decade or two ago. For example, recent studies found no benefit on respiratory function after surgery (153), but reported a reduction in posthysterectomy vomiting (154), reduced pain with arthrography (155), and a lessened need for postsurgical analgesia (156). Studies of more chronic conditions also often find limited benefit. Thus, a study comparing TENS to other modalities such as chiropractic manipulation, corsets, and massage in the treatment of low back pain found no benefit of one approach over the others (157). Two other studies found TENS ineffective or adding nothing to an exercise program for patients with low back pain (158,159), whereas a third found high-intensity TENS more effective than placebo (160). Studies of knee osteoarthritis found TENS and naproxen equally effective in reducing knee pain (161) and both capable of reducing the pain of dysmenorrhea (interestingly, with only naprosyn reducing the strength of uterine contractions) (162). A temporomandibular joint pain study found 24-hour-a-day occlusal splint use more effective than TENS (163).

Only a limited proportion of patients who try TENS benefit (164). Some clinicians feel that less than half the patients with chronic musculoskeletal conditions find TENS helpful initially and that benefits persist more than a month in less than half of these. However, some patients conclude that TENS is beneficial enough to justify continued use despite its inconvenience. Studies of these long-term users find that about 75% of individuals who have purchased (or had purchased for them) a unit may be still using it after 6 months to a year (165,166) but that use continues to decline to about 30% at 3 years (167). The best results in these chronic users seem to occur in musculoskeletal pain, neurogenic pain, and angina, with psychogenic pain, central pain, autonomic dysfunction, and social distress responding far less well (167).

Vasodilation is another contentious area. TENS seems to have no effects on normal subjects (168) but is reported to improve cutaneous perfusion, increase distal skin temperatures, and lessen pain in people with scleroderma and diabetic neuropathy (169). Spasticity reduction is reported for both stroke and spinal cord–injured patients, but effects may (170) or may not be significant (171). TENS is reported to reduce cardiac ischemia, perhaps by lessening sympathetic tone, and cardiac blood flow is reported to increase after treatment (172).

Precautions and Contraindications

TENS has few safety issues other than contact dermatitis and skin irritation, which usually respond to changes in electrode type and placement. High current densities, either due to the setting of the unit or a partially detached electrode, are uncomfortable but are easily corrected. Cardiac pacemakers seem resistant to TENS, but prudence dictates avoidance in patients with pacemakers, electrical implants, and dysrhythmias (173,174). Treatment near the carotid sinus and epiglottis and over the low backs, abdomens, and proximal lower extremities of pregnant women is avoided. TENS is used for an amazing variety of conditions (Table 20-6) and often with limited, rigorous evaluation. This should be kept in mind when prescribing. Psychogenic pain is particularly resistant to TENS, and use in this setting should be judicious. These precautions err on the side of caution; there is little documentation to support their validity.

Iontophoresis

Iontophoresis uses electrical fields to force electrically charged or polarized atoms and molecules into tissue. Speed of movement is related to voltage and field strength, whereas the amount of material driven into the tissue is proportional to the current. Penetration depends on the substance and may be particularly intense at sweat glands and areas of skin breakdown (175–177).

An iontophoretic unit is simple and may be contained within a skin patch. In general, it consists of a direct-current power source, two electrodes, and a pad moistened with a dilute (often 1%) solution of the desired (charged or polar) substance placed under the electrode of the same polarity. Currents are determined by multiplying the area of the active

TABLE 20-6. *Surgical and obstetric transcutaneous electrical nerve stimulation*

Etiology of pain	Experimental design	Results
General Surgery		
Abdominal surgery (164–168)	Randomized, controlled	Placebo levels to 77% of patients reporting "good or excellent" relief; 50%–67% reporting reduction in medication use
Abdominal and thoracic surgery (168,170)	Randomized	TENS groups tend to have less pain, less atelectasis, less ileus, and shorter ICU stays
Mixed surgery and trauma (171)	Uncontrolled; patients with prolonged postoperative and post-traumatic ileus	80% were relieved of protracted ileus within 24 hours
Orthopaedic Surgery		
Total hip replacement (172)	Randomized	Reduced medication use in TENS group
Knee surgery (173)	Consecutive patients; no controls	Increased ROM; 75%–100% reduction of narcotics
Low back surgery (174)	Randomized, controlled	TENS group reduced narcotic consumption 57%
Podiatric surgery (143)	Controlled	TENS groups required fewer narcotics; 75% with TENS noted excellent pain relief compared with 17% of controls
Hand wounds	Randomized, controlled	TENS group displayed improved mobility and less analgesic use
Obstetrics		
Labor and delivery (145–147,176)	Uncontrolled	78%–88% reported some relief; best relief in first stage; 70% required pudendal or epidural blocks

ICU, intensive care unit; ROM, range of motion; TENS, transcutaneous electrical nerve stimulation.

electrode by 0.1 to 0.5 mA/cm^2. The size of the inactive electrode is immaterial but is kept as large as convenient for patient comfort.

Indications

Tap water iontophoresis is successful in 90% of patients with hyperhidrosis, and benefits may persist 4 to 5 weeks or more (177–179). The hands or feet may be placed in a container with both the anode and cathode, or one extremity and one electrode may be positioned in each of two containers. Currents vary with the approach but are about 10 to 30 mA. The mechanism of action is unclear but may result from the preferential flow of ions along the sweat ducts.

Sodium fluoride iontophoresis is reported to reduce tooth hypersensitivity (180,181). Ionotophoresis also facilitates delivery of gentamicin, penicillin, and cefoxitin into the poorly vascularized tissues of the eye, burns, middle ear, and cartilage (182–185).

Case reports and uncontrolled studies report successful iontophoresis of salicylates for postsurgical pain, iodine for reduction of scar tissue and tendon adhesions (186,187), zinc to speed ischemic ulcer healing (188), lidocaine for myringotomy pain, and idoxuridine for aphthous ulcers (189). Although there is controversy over its effectiveness, corticosteroid iontophoresis has been recommended for Peyronie's disease and facial pain (190,191).

Electric and Low-Intensity Electromagnetic Fields

Although brief high-intensity fields (perhaps 100 + kV/m) produce electroporation and transiently increase cell wall permeability (192,193), it is also known that bone and soft-tissue injuries produce electrical fields and currents that can alter cell orientation, activity, proliferation, calcium concentrations, and mobility (194,195). These latter fields are much smaller than those of the cells themselves: approximately 1 V/m rather than the 70,000 V/m (70 mV/μm) associated with membrane potentials. The mechanism of action of these low-power fields is elusive but may include a switch effect that alters cell permeability.

Interest in electrically stimulated wound healing extends back to late 1960s and early 1970s reports that low-intensity direct current (LIDC) accelerated the healing of ischemic wounds in humans (196,197). These studies were marred by poor controls and unusual protocols. LIDC was not widely accepted, but interest never disappeared. Today protocols remarkably similar to the original LIDC trials use low-frequency (10 to 200 Hz) and low-intensity (10 μA/cm^2) electric currents and electromagnetic field (EMF) fields to treat poorly healing wounds. Benefits are still difficult to judge, but there is experimental support. For example, TENS stimulation may lessen pain, improve healing, and elevate distal limb temperatures in patients with diabetic neuropathy and scleroderma (198,199). In addition, many studies find bone growth stimulated in these fields (200,201) and other studies of varying quality show that low and high voltage stimulation accelerates healing of chronic skin ulcers and pressure sores (202–204). Musculoskeletal pain studies are also intriguing but less than convincing. For example, controlled studies found that low-intensity pulsed SWD (27.12 MHz, 1.5 mW/cm^2) produced clinically and statistically significant improvements in neck pain or ankle sprain (205,206). Ultimate acceptance of electrical and EMF stimulation as a treatment option for slowly healing wounds will depend on FDA approval, cost, comfort, convenience, and effectiveness greater than alternatives such as occlusive dressings.

Interferential Current

TENS units and muscle simulators are limited at times by the discomfort that strong stimulation at low (e.g., less than 80 Hz) frequencies produce at the skin. However, skin impedance decreases with frequency, and higher frequency waves penetrate through the skin without discomfort. Interferential current (IFC) devices (Fig. 20-9) take advantage of this fact by having two 2,000- to 4,000-Hz sine waves differing by 20 to 100 Hz overlap each other in tissue. Beat frequencies equal to the sum and difference of the sine waves are produced in the tissue with the difference in frequency within the therapeutic 20- to 80-Hz range. IFC appears useful when a TENS or muscle-stimulating effect is desired, but clear demonstration of superiority over other devices is lacking.

Safety

These devices operate at low powers and are used for limited periods of time. Not surprisingly, all appear safe, and the only precautions necessary seem to be those outlined for TENS. Epidemiologic studies have at times associated prolonged exposure to low-intensity EMF fields (such as those occurring in homes near power lines and with handheld electrical equipment such as hair dryers) with increased rates of leukemia, miscarriage, and brain tumors. These studies, whether or not showing increased risk, all have methodologic shortcomings, and a 1996 National Research Council review panel concluded that there is no conclusive or consistent evidence that low-intensity EMF fields increase the frequency of cancer, neurobehavioral problems, or reproductive dysfunction (207). This question will never disappear, but at this point risks seem minimal, and if present, subtle.

Alternative Therapies

Vibration

Vibration and tapping are used to facilitate muscle function and re-education in neuromuscular rehabilitation. Although tapping is often effective, vibration is easier to sustain. A variety of vibrators are available, but some clinicians believe that frequencies of about 150 Hz and amplitudes of 1.5 mm are particularly effective (208–210).

Uncontrolled studies find that vibration between 100 and 200 Hz has analgesic effects as effective as TENS or aspirin in 70% of those with musculoskeletal pain or sinusitis (211–213). Vibration also may improve wound healing: mice treated three times a day over a 6-month period with vibration had significantly less edema, fewer adhesions, and improved lymphatic and venous repair than did untreated controls (214).

Low-Intensity Laser Therapy

Low-power lasers have been used for 30 years to lessen pain and speed healing. Initially, treatment involved short exposures to a variety of <1- to 5-mW lasers. With time, therapy practices have coalesced, and now most treatments are performed with approximately 30- to 90-mW infrared

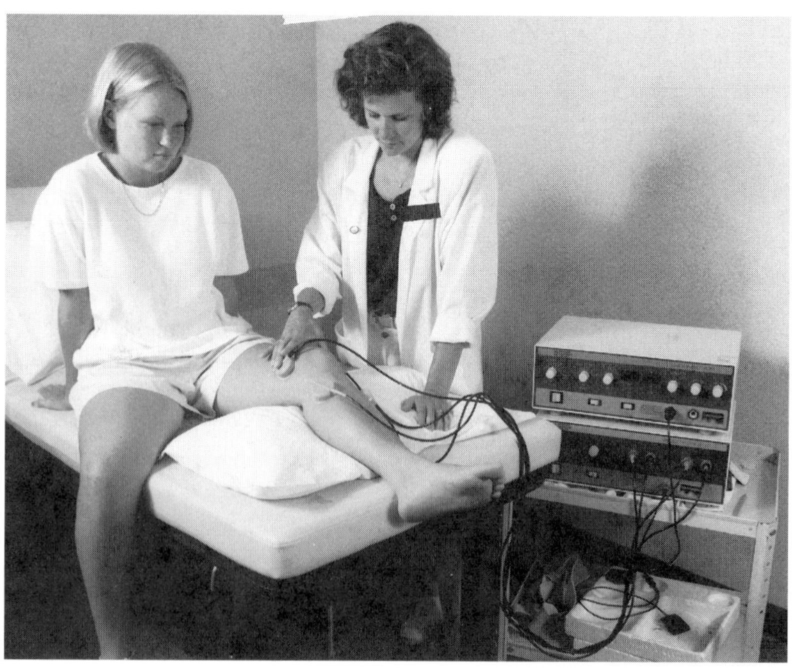

FIG. 20-9. Interferential current treatment. This treatment uses the interference pattern of two higher frequency sine waves to apply electrical stimulation. Although only three electrodes can be seen in the picture, four are required (two for each wave train).

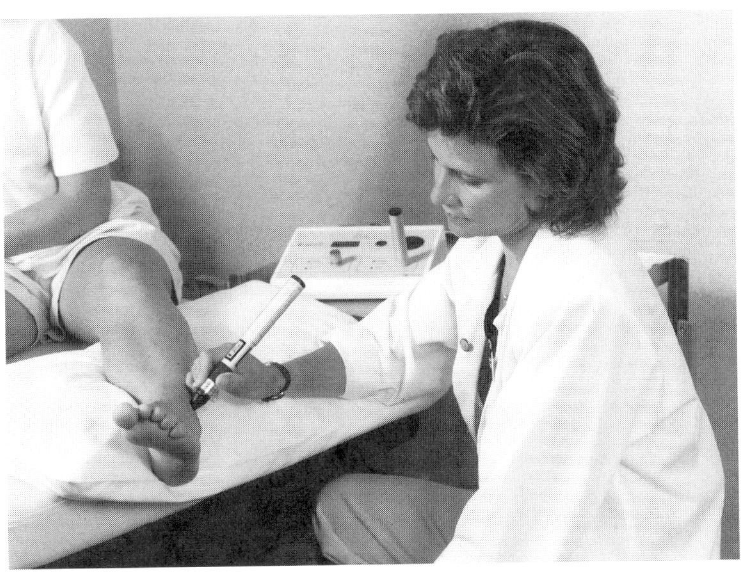

FIG. 20-10. Laser therapy. In this case a hand-held 30-mW IR diode laser is being used to treat an ankle sprain. This therapy is available in many parts of the world, but has yet to gain U.S. FDA approval for any indication.

(IR) laser diodes (Fig. 20-10). Even though treatments do not elevate tissue temperatures more than a few tenths of a degree, laboratory studies find irradiation stimulates collagen production, alters DNA synthesis, and improves the function of damaged neurologic tissue. Unfortunately, extension of these effects to humans is far less convincing. Although this laser therapy is available in many parts of the world, it has yet to receive FDA approval for any indication (215).

MODALITY CHOICE AND PRESCRIPTION

The physical agents are typically prescribed as part of a program that also includes massage, exercise, and education (Table 20-7). As this table shows, a well-written prescription involves the same elements of who (the patient), what (agent), why (the diagnosis), where (treatment area), when (frequency and duration), and how (other treatment, exercise, education) common to good writing. The specifics of the treatment intensities and durations depend on the modality used. A recheck plan should be outlined. Explicit therapy goals were once rare but are becoming more common as documentation requirements become stricter.

TABLE 20-7. *Physical therapy prescription*

Patient
Diagnosis
Modality
Treatment area
Treatment parameters (intensity, power, frequency, duty cycle)
Treatment frequency and duration
Additional treatments (e.g., massage)
Exercise
Patient education
Recheck schedule
Treatment goals

Modality choice depends on a balancing of the diagnosis, the characteristics of the agents, concurrent issues (e.g., level of cooperation, anticoagulation, preference, etc.), and treatment goals. General rules introduce some order into the situation. For example, acute (less than 24 to 48 hours) musculoskeletal conditions are usually treated with cooling. Hot packs, cool packs, hydrotherapy, shortwave diathermy, and some of the electrical therapies are commonly used to treat broad areas such as the low back. More intense agents such as US and ice massage are more common if smaller areas are to be treated. The diathermies are frequently favored for deeper tissues, but the reflex and comfort-inducing effects of superficial agents may be as beneficial. In the end, choice involves blending a physiologic understanding of the agents, experience, preference, and equipment availability. As research continues, our knowledge will grow. Choices common today will seem quaint in the future.

REFERENCES

1. Franchimont P, Juchmes J, Lecomite J. Hydrotherapy: mechanisms and indications. *Pharmacol Ther* 1983; 20:79–93.
2. Harris ED, McCroskery PA. The influence of temperature and fibril stability on degradation of cartilage collagen by rheumatoid synovial collagenase. *N Engl J Med* 1974; 290:1–6.
3. Wright V, Johns RJ. Quantitative and qualitative analysis of joint stiffness in normal subjects and in patients with connective tissue diseases. *Ann Rheum Dis* 1961; 20:36–46.
4. Denys EH. AAEM minimonograph #14: the influence of temperature in clinical neurophysiology. *Muscle Nerve* 1991; 14:795–811.
5. Guyton AC. *Textbook of medical physiology*, 7th ed. Philadelphia: WB Saunders, 1986; 336–346.
6. Knight KL. *Cryotherapy: theory, technique and physiology*, 1st ed. Chattanooga, TN: Chattanooga Corporation, 1985; 83–100.
7. Lehmann JF, Masock AJ, Warren CG, Koblanski JN. Effect of therapeutic temperatures on tendon extensibility. *Arch Phys Med Rehabil* 1970; 51:481–487.
8. Lehmann JF, Silverman DR, Baum BR, et al. Temperature distributions in the human thigh, produced by infrared, hot pack and microwave applications. *Arch Phys Med Rehabil* 1966; 47:291–299.
9. Woodmansey A, Collins DH, Ernst MM. Vascular reactions to the

contrast bath in health and in rheumatoid arthritis. *Lancet* 1938; 2: 1350–1353.

10. Pinho M, Correa JCO, Furtado A, Ramos JR. Do hot baths promote anal sphincter relaxation? *Dis Colon Rectum* 1993; 36:273–274.
11. Adler AJ. Water immersion: lessons from antiquity to modern times. *Contrib Nephrol* 1993; 102:171–186.
12. Tovin BJ, Wolf SL, Greenfield BH, Crouse J, Woodfin BA. Comparison of the effects of exercise in water and on land on the rehabilitation of patients with intra-articular anterior cruciate ligament reconstructions. *Phys Ther* 1994; 74:710–719.
13. Green J, McKenna F, Redfern EJ, Chamberlain MA. Home exercises are as effective as outpatient hydrotherapy for osteoarthritis of the hip. *Br J Rheumatol* 1993; 32:812–815.
14. Forster MM. Mineral springs and miracles. *Can Fam Physician* 1994; 40:729–737.
15. Rishler M, Brostovski Y, Yaron M. Effect of spa therapy in tiberias on patients with ankylosing spondylitis. *Clin Rheumatol* 1995; 14: 21–25.
16. Sukenik S, Giryes H, Halevy S, Neumann L, Flusser D, Buskila D. Treatment of psoriatic arthritis at the dead sea. *J Rheumatol* 1994; 21:1305–1309.
17. Sukenik S, Buskila D, Neumann L, Kleiner-Baungarten A. Mud pack therapy in rheumatoid arthritis. *Clin Rheumatol* 1992; 11:243–247.
18. Konrad K, Tatrai T, Hunka A, Vereckei E, Korondi I. Controlled trial of balneotherapy in treatment of low back pain. *Ann Rheum Dis* 1992; 51:820–822.
19. Sukenik S, Neumann L, Flusser D, Kleiner-Baumgarten A. Balneotherapy for rheumatoid arthritis at the Dead Sea. *Isr J Med Sci* 1995; 31:210–214.
20. Constant F, Coloin JF, Guillemin F, Boulange M. Effectiveness of spa therapy in chronic low back pain: a randomized clinical trial. *J Rheumatol* 1995; 22:1315–1320.
21. Guillemin F, Constant F, Collin JE, Boulange M. Short and long-term effect of spa therapy in chronic low back pain. *Br J Rheumatol* 1994; 33:148–151.
22. Alcorn R, Dowser B, Henley EJ, Holloway V. Fluidotherapy and exercise in the management of sickle cell anemia. *Phys Ther* 1984; 64:1520–1522.
23. Borrell RM, Parker R, Henley EJ, et al. Comparison of in vivo temperatures produced by hydrotherapy, paraffin wax treatment and fluidotherapy. *Phys Ther* 1980; 60:1273–1276.
24. Luurila OJ. Cardiac arrhythmias, sudden death and the Finnish sauna bath. *Adv Cardiol* 1978; 25:73–81.
25. Romo J. Factors related to sudden death in acute ischemic heart disease: a community study in Helsinki. *Acta Med Scand (Suppl)* 1972; 547:1–92.
26. Allison TG, Miller TD, Squires RW, Gau GT. Cardiovascular responses to immersion in a hot tub in comparison with exercise in male subjects with coronary artery disease. *Mayo Clin Proc* 1993; 68:19–25.
27. Pleet H, Graham JM Jr, Smith DW. Central nervous system and facial defects associated with maternal hyperthermia at four to 14 weeks' gestation. *Pediatrics* 1981; 67:785–789.
28. Kauppinen K, Vuori I. Man in the sauna. *Ann Clin Res* 1986; 4: 173–185.
29. Abramson DI, Tuck S, Chu LSW, Agustin C. Effect of paraffin bath and hot fomentations on local tissue temperatures. *Arch Phys Med Rehabil* 1964; 45:87–94.
30. Helfand AE, Bruno J. Therapeutic modalities and procedures: part 1. Cold and heat. *Clin Podiatr* 1984; 1:301–313.
31. Weinberger A, Fadilah R, Lev A, Pinkhas J. Intra-articular temperature measurements after superficial heating. *Scand J Rehabil Med* 1989; 21:55–57.
32. Hollander JL, Horvath SM. The influence of physical therapy procedures on the intra-articular temperature of normal and arthritis subjects. *Am J Med Sci* 1949; 218:543–548.
33. Horvath SM, Hollander JL. Intra-articular temperature as a measure of joint reaction. *J Clin Invest* 1949; 28:469–473.
34. Hollander JL, Horvath SM. Changes in temperature produced by diseases and by physical therapy (preliminary report). *Arch Phys Med* 1949; 30:437–440.
35. Oosterveld FGJ, Rasker JJ. Effects of local heat and cold treatment of surface and articular temperature of arthritic knees. *Arthritis Rheum* 1994; 37:1578–1582.
36. Flint EB, Suslick KS. The temperature of cavitation. *Science* 1991; 253:1397.
37. Dyson M. Non-thermal cellular effects of ultrasound. *Br J Cancer* 1982; 45:165–171.
38. Goldman DE, Heuter TF. Tabular data of the velocity and absorption of high-frequency sound in mammalian tissues. *J Acoust Soc Am* 1956; 28:35–37.
39. Dyson M, Pond JB, Woodward B, Broadbent J. The production of blood cell stasis and endothelial damage in the blood vessels of chick embryos treated with ultrasound in a stationary wave field. *Ultrasound Med Biol* 1974; 1:133–148
40. Lehmann JF, deLateur BJ, Stonebridge JB, Warren CG. Therapeutic temperature distribution produced by ultrasound as modified by dosage and volume of tissue exposed. *Arch Phys Med Rehabil* 1967; 48: 662–666.
41. Lehmann JF, deLateur BJ, Warren CG, Stonebridge JB. Heating of joint structures by ultrasound. *Arch Phys Med Rehabil* 1968; 49: 28–30.
42. Stewart HF, Harris GR, Herman BA, et al. Survey of use and performance of ultrasonic therapy equipment in Pinellas County, Florida. *Phys Ther* 1974; 54:707–714.
43. Coakley WT. Biophysical effects of ultrasound at therapeutic intensities. *Physiotherapy* 1978; 64:166–169.
44. Allen KGR, Battye CK. Performance of ultrasonic therapy instruments. *Physiotherapy* 1978; 64:174–179.
45. Balmaseda MT, Fatehi MT, Koozekanani SH, Lee AL. Ultrasound therapy: a comparative study of different coupling media. *Arch Phys Med Rehabil* 1986; 67:149–152.
46. Reid DC, Cummings GE. Efficiency of ultrasound coupling agents. *Physiotherapy* 1977; 63:255–257.
47. Warren CG, Koblanski JN, Sigelmann RA. Ultrasound coupling media: their relative transmissivity. *Arch Phys Med Rehabil* 1976; 57: 218–222.
48. Novak EJ. Experimental transmission of lidocaine through intact skin by ultrasound. *Arch Phys Med Rehabil* 1964; 45:231–232.
49. Griffin JE, Touchstone JC, Liu A. Ultrasonic movement of cortisol into pig tissue: II. movement into paravertebral nerve. *Am J Phys Med* 1965; 44:20–25.
50. Bare AC, McAnawa MB, Pritchard AE, et al. Phonophoretic delivery of 10% hydrocortisone through the epidermis of humans as dtermined by serum cortisol concentrations. *Phys Ther* 1996; 76:738–749.
51. Moll MJ. A new approach to pain: lidocaine and decadron with ultrasound. *USAF Medical Service Digest* 1977; 30:8–11.
52. Cameroy BM. Ultrasound enhanced local anesthesia. *Am J Orthop* 1966; 8:47.
53. Wanet G, Dehon N. Etude clinique de l'ultrasonophorese avec un topique associant phenylbutazone, et alpha-chymotrypsine. *J Belge Rhumatol Med Physique* 1976; 31:49–58.
54. Echternach JL. Ultrasound: an adjunct treatment for shoulder disabilities. *Phys Ther* 1965; 45:865–869.
55. Coodley EL. Bursitis and post-traumatic lesions: management with combined use of ultrasound and intra-articular hydrocortisone. *Am Practitioner* 1960; 11:181–188.
56. Newman MK, Kill M, Frampton G. Effects of ultrasound alone and combined with hydrocortisone injections by needle or hypospray. *Am J Phys Med* 1958; 37:206–209.
57. Hasson S, Mundorf R, Barnes W, Williams J, Fugii M. Effect of pulsed ultrasound versus placebo on muscle soreness perception and muscular performance. *Scand J Rehabil Med* 1990; 22:199–205.
58. Downing DS, Weinstein A. Ultrasound therapy of subacromial bursitis: a double blind trial. *Phys Ther* 1986; 66:194–199.
59. Dijs H, Mortier G, Driessens M, De Ridder A, Willems J, De Vroey T. A retrospective study of the conservative treatment of tennis-elbow. *Acta Belg Med Phys* 1990; 13:73–77.
60. Lundeberg T, Abrahamsson P, Haker E. A comparative study of continuous ultrasound and rest in epicondylalgia. *Scand J Rehabil Med* 1988; 20:99–101.
61. Taube S, Ylipaavaliniemi P, Kononen M, Sunden B. The effect of pulsed ultrasound on myofacial pain: a placebo controlled study. *Proc Finn Dent Soc* 1988; 84:241–246.
62. Aldes JH, Jadeson WJ. Ultrasonic therapy in the treatment of hypertrophic arthritis in elderly patients. *Ann West Med Surg* 1952; 6:545–550.
63. Lehmann JF, Erickson DJ, Martin GM, Krusen FH. Comparison of

ultrasonic and microwave diathermy in the physical treatment of periarthritis of the shoulder. *Arch Phys Med Rehabil* 1954; 35:627–634.
64. Lehmann JF, Fordyce WE, Rathbun LA, et al. Clinical evaluation of a new approach in the treatment of contracture associated with hip fracture after internal fixation. *Arch Phys Med Rehabil* 1961; 42:95.
65. Lehmann JF, deLateur BJ, Warren CG, Stonebridge JB. Heating of joint structures by ultrasound. *Arch Phys Med Rehabil* 1968; 49: 28–30.
66. Lehmann JF, McMillan JA, Brunner GD, Blumberg JB. Comparative study of the efficiency of short-wave, microwave and ultrasonic diathermy in heating the hip joint. *Arch Phys Med Rehabil* 1959; 40: 510–512.
67. Markham DE, Wood MR. Ultrasound for Dupuytren's contracture. *Physiotherapy* 1980; 66:55–58.
68. Ward RS, Hayes-Lundy C, Reddy R, Brockway C, Mills P, Saffle JR. Evaluation of topical therapeutic ultrasound to improve response to physical therapy and lessen scar contracture after brain injury. *J Burn Care Rehabil* 1994; 15:74–79.
69. Young S, Dyson M. Effect of therapeutic ultrasound on the healing of full-thickness excised skin lesions. *Ultrasonics* 1990; 28:175–180.
70. ter Riet G, Kessels AGH, Knipschild P. Randomized clinical trial of ultrasound treatment for pressure ulcers. *Br Med J* 1995; 310: 1040–1041.
71. Nussbaum EL, Biemann I, Mustard B. Comparison of ultrasound/ultraviolet-C and laser for treatment of pressure ulcers in patients with spinal cord injury. *Phys Ther* 1994; 74:812–823.
72. Paul BJ, Lafratta CW, Dawson AR, et al. Use of ultrasound in the treatment of pressure sores in patients with spinal cord injury. *Arch Phys Med Rehabil* 1960; 41:438–440.
73. Rozsivalova V, Nozickova M, Jelinkova R, Cernochova Z. Management of painful leg ulcers by ultrasound therapy. *Sb Ved Pr Lek Fak Univ Karlovy* 1987; 30:325–329.
74. Dyson M, Frank C, Suckling J. Stimulation of healing of varicose ulcers by ultrasound. *Ultrasonics* 1976; 14:232–236.
75. Callam M, Harper D, Dale J, et al. A controlled trial of weekly ultrasound therapy in chronic leg ulceration. *Lancet* 1987; 25:204–206.
76. Hashishi I, Hai HK, Harvey W, Feinmann C, Harris M. Reduction of postoperative pain and swelling by ultrasound treatment: a placebo effect. *Pain* 1988; 33:303–311.
77. Grant A, Sleep J, McIntosh J, Ashurst H. Ultrasound and pulsed electromagnetic energy treatment for perineal trauma: a randomized placebo-controlled trial. *Br J Obstet Gynaecol* 1989; 96:434–439.
78. Goddard DJ, Revell PA, Cason J, Gallagher S, Currey HLF. Ultrasound has no anti-inflammatory effect. *Ann Rheum Dis* 1983; 42: 582–584.
79. Mune O, Thoseth K. Ultrasonic treatment of subcutaneous infiltrations after injections. *Acta Orthop Scand* 1963; 33:347–349.
80. Oakley EM. Evidence for effectiveness of ultrasound treatment in physical medicine. *Br J Cancer* 1982; 45:233–237.
81. Foulkes J, Yeo B. The application of therapeutic pulsed ultrasound to the traumatised perineum. *Br J Clin Pract* 1980; 34:114–117.
82. Middlemost S, Chatterjee DS. Comparison of ultrasound and thermotherapy for soft tissue injuries. *Physiotherapy* 1978; 64:331–332.
83. Williamson JB, George TK, Simpson DC, Hannah B, Bradbury E. Ultrasound in the treatment of ankle sprains. *Injury* 1986; 17:176–178.
84. Einhorn TA. Current concepts review enhancement of fracture-healing. *J Bone Joint Surg [Am]* 1995; 77:940–956.
85. Heckman JD, Ryaby JP, McCabe J, Frey JJ, Kilcoyne RF. Acceleration of tibial fracture-healing by non-invasive, low intensity pulsed ultrasound. *J Bone Joint Surg [Am]* 1994; 76:26–34.
86. Garrett AS, Garrett M. Ultrasound therapy for herpes zoster pain. *J R Coll Gen Pract* 1982; 32:709–710.
87. Jones RJ. Treatment of acute herpes zoster using ultrasonic therapy: report on a series of twelve patients. *Physiotherapy* 1984; 70:94–95.
88. Payne C. Ultrasound for post-herpetic neuralgia: a study to investigate the results of treatment. *Physiotherapy* 1984; 70:96–97.
89. Currier DP, Greathouse D, Swift T. Sensory nerve conduction: effect of ultrasound. *Arch Phys Med Rehabil* 1978; 59:181–185.
90. Farmer WC. Effect of intensity of ultrasound on conduction of motor axons. *Phys Ther* 1968; 48:1233–1237.
91. Gersten JW. Non-thermal neuromuscular effects of ultrasound. *Am J Phys Med* 1958; 37:235–237.
92. Cherup N, Urben J, Bender LF. The treatment of plantar warts with ultrasound. *Arch Phys Med Rehabil* 1963; 44:602–604.
93. Vaughn DT. Direct method versus underwater method in the treatment of plantar warts with ultrasound: a comparative study. *Phys Ther* 1973; 53:396–397.
94. Braatz JH, McAlistar BR, Broaddus MD. Ultrasound and plan tar warts: a double blind study. *Milit Med* 1974; 139:199–201.
95. Wright ET, Haase KH. Keloids and ultrasound. *Arch Phys Med Rehabil* 1971; 52:280–281.
96. Dussick CT, Fritch DJ, Kyraizidan M, Sear RS. Measurement of articular tissues with ultrasound. *Am J Phys Med* 1958; 37:160–165.
97. Weinberger A, Fadilah R, Lev A, Levi A, Pinkhas J. Deep heat in the treatment of inflammatory joint disease. *Med Hypotheses* 1988; 25:231–233.
98. Weinberger A, Fadilah R, Lev A, Shohami E, Pinkhas J. Treatment of articular effusions with local deep microwave hyperthermia. *Clin Rheumatol* 1989; 8:461–466.
99. Brunner GD, Lehmann JF, McMillan JA, et al. Can ultrasound be used in the presence of surgical metal implants: an experimental approach. *Phys Ther* 1958; 38:823–824.
100. Gersten JW. Effect of metallic objects on temperature rises produced in tissue by ultrasound. *Am J Phys Med* 1958; 37:75–82.
101. Skoubo-Kristensen E, Sommer J. Ultrasound influence on internal fixation with a rigid plate in dogs. *Arch Phys Med Rehabil* 1982; 63: 371–373.
102. Kantor G. Evaluation and survey of microwave and radiofrequency applicators. *J Microw Power Electromagn Energy* 1981; 16:135–150.
103. Lehmann JF, deLateur BJ, Stonebridge JB. Selective heating by shortwave diathermy with a helical coil. *Arch Phys Med Rehabil* 1969; 50:117–123.
104. Wildervanck A, Wakim KG, Herrick JF, Krusen FH. Certain experimental observations on a pulsed diathermy machine. *Arch Phys Med Rehabil* 1959; 40:45–55.
105. Dutreix J, Cosset JM, Salama A, et al. Experimental studies of various heating procedures for clinical application of localized hyperthermia. *Prog Clin Biol Res* 1982; 107:585–596.
106. Witters DM, Kantor G. An evaluation of microwave diathermy applicators using free space electric field mapping. *Phys Med Biol* 1981; 26:1099–1114.
107. DeLateur BJ, Lehmann JF, Stonebridge JB, et al. Muscle heating in human subjects with 915 MHz: microwave contact applicator. *Arch Phys Med Rehabil* 1970; 51:147–151.
108. Lehmann JF, Dundore DE, Esselman PC. Microwave diathermy: effects on experimental muscle hematoma resolution. *Arch Phys Med Rehabil* 1983; 64:127–129.
109. Lee ER, Sullivan DM, Kapp DS. Potential hazards of radiative electromagnetic hyperthermia in the presence of multiple metallic surgical clips. *Int J Hyperthermia* 1992; 8:809–817.
110. Rubin A, Erdman WJ. Microwave exposure of the human female pelvis during early pregnancy and prior to conception. *Am J Phys Med* 1959; 38:219–220.
111. Worden RE, Herrick JF, Wakim KG, Krusen FH. The heating effects of microwaves with and without ischemia. *Arch Phys Med Rehabil* 1948; 29:751–758.
112. Richardson AW, Duane TD, Hines HM. Experimental lenticular opacities produced by microwave irradiations. *Arch Phys Med Rehabil* 1948; 29:763–769.
113. Stuchly MA, Repacholi MH, Lecuyer DW, Mann RD. Exposure to the operator and patient during short wave diathermy treatments. *Health Phys* 1982; 42:341–366.
114. American National Standards Institute, Inc. *Safety levels with respect to human exposure to radio frequency electromagnetic fields, 300 kHz to 100 GHz.* Washington, DC: American National Standards Institute, 1982.
115. Moseley H, Davison M. Exposure of physiotherapists to microwave radiation during microwave diathermy treatment. *Clin Phys Physiol Meas* 1981; 2:217–221.
116. Ouellet-Hellstrom R, Stewart WF. Miscarriages among female physical therapists who report using radio- and microwave-frequency electromagnetic radiation. *Am J Epidemiol* 1993; 138:775–786.
117. Larsen AI. Congenital malformations and exposure to high-frequency electromagnetic radiation among Danish physiotherapists. *Scand J Work Environ Health* 1991; 17:318–323.
118. Guberane E, Campana A, Faval P, et al. Gender ratio of offspring and exposure to short-wave radiation among female physiotherapists. *Scand J Work Environ Health* 1994; 20:345–348.

119. Lehmann JF, de Lateur BJ. Diathermy and superficial heat and cold therapy. In: Kottke FJ, Stillwell GK, Lehmann JF, eds. *Krusen's handbook of physical medicine and rehabilitation,* 3rd ed. Philadelphia: WB Saunders, 1982; 275–350.
120. Hartviksen K. Ice therapy in spasticity. *Acta Neurol Scand* 1962; 38: 79–84.
121. Guyton AC, Hall JE. Body temperature, temperature regulation and fever. In: *Textbook of medical physiology,* 9th ed. Philadelphia: WB Saunders, 1996; 911–922.
122. Ho SSW, Illgen RL, Meyer RW, Torok PJ, Cooper MD, Reider B. Comparison of various icing times in decreasing bone metabolism and blood flow in the knee. *Am J Sports Med* 1995; 23:74–76.
123. Taber C, Contryman K, Fahrenbruch J, Lacount K, Cornwell MW. Measurement of reactaive vasodilation during cold gel pack application to nontraumatized ankles. *Phys Ther* 1992; 72:294–299.
124. Knutsson E, Mattsson E. Effects of local cooling on monosynaptic reflexes in man. *Scand J Rehabil Med* 1969; 1:126–132.
125. Miglietta O. Action of cold on spasticity. *Am J Phys Med* 1973; 52: 198–205.
126. Bisgard JD, Nye D. The influence of hot and cold application upon gastric and intestinal motor activity. *Surg Gynecol Obstet* 1940; 71: 172–180.
127. Knight KL. *Cryotherapy: theory, technique and physiology,* 1st ed. Chattanooga, TN: Chattanooga Corporation, 1985; 15–26.
128. Travell J. Ethyl chloride spray for painful muscle spasm. *Arch Phys Med Rehabil* 1952; 33:291–298.
129. Basur RL, Shephard E, Mouzas GL. A cooling method in the treatment of ankle sprains. *Practitioner* 1976; 216:708–711.
130. Moore CD, Cardea JA. Vascular changes in leg trauma. *South Med J* 1977; 70:1285–1286.
131. Schaubel HJ. The local use of ice after orthopedic procedures. *Am J Surg* 1946; 72:711–714.
132. Bert JM, Stark JG, Maschka K, Chock C. The effect of cold therapy on morbidity subsequent to arthroscopic lateral retinacular release. *Orthop Rev* 1991; 20:755–758.
133. Matsen FA, Questad K, Matsen AL. The effect of local cooling on postfracture swelling: a controlled study. *Clin Orthop* 1975; 109: 201–206.
134. Hirase Y. Postoperative cooling enhances composite graft survival in nasal-alar and finger tip reconstruction. *Br J Plast Surg* 1993; 46: 707–711.
135. Knight KL. Ice, compression and elevation for initial injury care. In: *Cryotherapy: theory, technique and physiology,* 1st ed. Chattanooga, TN: Chattanooga Corporation, 1985; 53–54.
136. Sloan JP, Hain R, Pownall R. Clinical benefits of early cold therapy in accident and emergency following ankle sprain. *Arch Emerg Med* 1989; 6:1–6.
137. Hocutt JE, Jaffe R, Rylander R, Beebe JK. Cryotherapy in ankle sprain. *Am J Sports Med* 1982; 10:316–319.
138. Whitelaw GP, DeMuth KA, Demos HA, Schepsis A, Jacques E. The use of the cryo/cuff versus ice and elastic wrap in the postoperative care of knee arthroscopy patients. *Am J Knee Surg* 1995; 8:28–30.
139. Daniel DM, Stone ML, Arendt DL. The effect of cold therapy on pain, swelling, and range of motion after anterior cruciate ligament reconstructive surgery. *Arthroscopy* 1994; 10:530–533.
140. Amin-Hanjani S, Corcoran J, Chatwani A. Cold therapy in the management of postoperative cesarean section pain. *J Obstet Gynecol* 1992; 167:108–109.
141. Landon BR. Heat or cold for the relief of low back pain. *Phys Ther* 1967; 47:1126–1128.
142. Melzack R, Jeans ME, Stratford JG, Monks RC. Ice massage and transcutaneous electrical stimulation: comparison of treatment for low back pain. *Pain* 1980; 9:209–217.
143. Stillwell GK. Ultraviolet therapy. In: Krusen FH, Kottke FJ, Elwood PM, eds. *Handbook of physical medicine and rehabilitation,* 2nd ed. Philadelphia: WB Saunders, 1971; 363–373.
144. Basford JR, Hallman HO, Sheffield CG, Mackey GL. Comparison of cold quartz ultraviolet, low-energy laser, and occlusion in wound healing in a swine model. *Arch Phys Med Rehabil* 1986; 67:151–154.
145. Sears FW, Zemanski MW. *Coulomb's law in college physics.* Reading, MA: Addison-Wesley, 1960; 449–467.
146. Kane K, Taub A. A history of local electrical analgesia. *Pain* 1975; 1:125–128.
147. Geddes LA. A short history of the electrical stimulation of excitable tissue including electrotherapeutic applications. *Physiologist* 1984; 27(suppl):515–547.
148. Melzack R, Wall PD. Pain mechanisms: a new theory. *Science* 1965; 150:971–979.
149. Melzack R, Stillwell DM, Fox EJ. Trigger points and acupuncture points for pain: correlations and implications. *Pain* 1977; 3:3–23.
150. Garrison DW, Foreman RD. Effects of transcutaneous electrical nerve stimulation (TENS) on spontaneous and noxiously evoked dorsal horn cell activity in cats with transected spinal cords. *Neurosci Lett* 1996; 216:125–128.
151. Walsh DM, Liggett C, Baxter D, Allen JM. A double-blind investigation of the hypoalgesic effects of transcutaneous electrical nerve stimulation upon experimentally induced ischaemic pain. *Pain* 1995; 61: 39–45.
152. Basford JR. Physical agents. In: DeLisa JA, Gans BM, Currie DM, et al., eds. *Rehabilitation medicine: principles and practice,* 2nd ed. Philadelphia: JB Lippincott, 1993; 404–424.
153. Forster EL, Kramer JF, Lucy SD, Scudds RA, Novick RJ. Effect of TENS on pain, medications, and pulmonary function following coronary artery bypass graft surgery. *Chest* 1994; 106:1343–1348.
154. Fassoulaki A, Papilas K, Sarantogpoulos C, Zotou M. Transcutaneous electrical nerve stimulation reduces the incidence of vomiting after hysterectomy. *Anesth Analg* 1993; 76:1012–1014.
155. Morgan B, Jones AR, Mulcahy KA, Finlay DB, Collett B. Transcutaneous electric nerve stimulation (TENS) during distension shoulder arthrography—a controlled trial. *Pain* 1996; 64:265–267.
156. Rainov NG, Heidecke V, Albertz C, Burkert W. Transcutaneous electrical nerve stimulation (TENS) for acute postoperative pain after spinal surgery. *Eur J Pain* 1994; 15:44–49.
157. Pope MH, Phillips RB, Haugh LD, Hsieh CY, MacDonald L, Haldeman S. A prospective randomized three-week trial of spinal manipulation, transcutaneous muscle stimulation, massage and corset in the treatment of subacute low back pain. *Spine* 1994; 19:2571–2577.
158. Deyo RA, Walsh NE, Martin DC, Schoenfeld LS, Ramamurthy S. A controlled trial of transcutaneous electrical nerve stimulation (TENS) and exercise for chronic low back pain. *N Engl J Med* 1990; 322: 1627–1634.
159. Herman E, Williams R, Stratford P, Fargas-Babjak A, Trott M. A randomized controlled trial of transcutaneous electrical nerve stimulation (CEDETRON) to determine its benefits in a rehabilitation program for acute occupational low back pain. *Spine* 1994; 19:561–568.
160. Marchand S, Charest J, Li J, Chenard JR, Lavignolle B, Laurencelle L. Is TENS purely a placebo effect? A controlled study on chronic low back pain. *Pain* 1993; 54:99–106.
161. Lewis B, Lewis D, Cumming G. The comparative analgesic efficacy of transcutaneous electrical nerve stimulation and a non-steroidal anti-inflammatory drug for painful osteoarthritis. *Br J Rheumatol* 1994; 33:455–460.
162. Milsom I, Hedner N, Mannheimer C. A comparative study of the effect of high-intensity transcutaneous nerve stimulation and oral naproxen on intrauterine pressure and menstrual pain in patients with primary dysmenorrhea. *Am J Obstet Gynecol* 1994; 170:123–129.
163. Linde C, Isacsson G, Jonsson BG. Outcome of 6-week treatment with transcutaneous electric nerve stimulation compared with splint on symptomatic temporomandibular joint disk displacement without reduction. *Acta Odontol Scand* 1995; 53:92–98.
164. Reeve J, Menon D, Corabian P. Transcutaneous electrical nerve stimulation (TENS): a technology assessment [Review]. *Int J Technol Assess Health Care* 1996; 12:299–324.
165. Fishbain DA, Chabal C, Abbott A, Heinle LW, Cutler R. Transcutaneous electrical nerve stimulation (TENS) treatment outcome in long-term users. *Clin J Pain* 1996; 12:201–214.
166. Verdouw BC, Zuurmond WWA, De Lange JJ, Metz CGH, Wagemans MFM. Long-term use and effectiveness of transcutaneous electrical nerve stimulation in treatment of chronic pain patients. *Pain Clin* 1995; 8:341–346.
167. Meyler WJ, de Jongste MJ, Rolf CA. Clinical evaluation of pain treatment with electrostimulation: a study on TENS in patients with different pain syndromes. *Clin J Pain* 1994:10:22–27.
168. Nolan MF, Hartsfield JK Jr, Witters DM, Wason PJ. Failure of transcutaneous electrical nerve stimulation in the conventional and burst modes to alter digital skin temperature. *Arch Phys Med Rehabil* 1993; 74:182–187.
169. Kaada B, Helle KB. In search of mediators of skin vasodilation in-

duced by transcutaneous nerve stimulation: IV. In vitro bioassay of the vasoinhibitory activity of sera from patients suffering from peripheral ischaemia. *Gen Pharmacol* 1984; 15:115–122.

170. Goulet C, Arsenault AB, Bourbonnais D, Laramee MT, Lepage Y. Effects of transcutaneous electrical nerve stimulation on h-reflex and spinal spasticity. *Scand J Rehabil Med* 1996; 28:169–176.
171. Levin MF, Hui-Chan CW. Relief of hemiparetic spasticity by TENS is associated with improvement in reflex and voluntary motor functions. *Electroencephalog Clin Neurophysiol* 1992; 85:131–142.
172. Chauhan A, Mullins PA, Thuraisingham SI, Taylor G, Petch MC, Schofield PM. Effect of transcutaneous electrical nerve stimulation on coronary blood flow. *Circulation* 1994; 89:694–702.
173. Eriksson M, Schuller H, Sjolund B. Hazard from transcutaneous nerve stimulation in patients with pacemakers. *Lancet* 1978; 1:1319.
174. Chen D, Philip M, Phillip PA, Monga TN. Cardiac pacemaker inhibition by transcutaneous electrical nerve stimulation. *Arch Phys Med Rehabil* 1990; 71:27–30 [erratum *Arch Phys Med Rehabil* 1990; 71: 3881].
175. Chantraine A, Ludy JP, Berger D. Is cortisone iontophoresis possible? *Arch Phys Med Rehabil* 1986; 67:38–40.
176. O'Malley EP, Oester YT. Influence of some physical chemical factors on iontophoresis using radio isotopes. *Arch Phys Med Rehabil* 1955; 36:310–316.
177. Hill AC, Baker GF, Jansen GT. Mechanisms of actin of iontophoresis in the treatment of palmar hyperhidrosis. *Cutis* 1981; 28:69–70,72.
178. Peterson JL, Read SI, Rodman OG. A new device in the treatment of hyperhidrosis by iontophoresis. *Cutis* 1982; 29:82–83,87–89.
179. Shrivastava SN, Singh G. Tap water iontophoresis in palmoplantar hyperhidrosis. *Br J Dermatol* 1977; 96:189–195.
180. Holman DJ. Desensitization of dentin by iontophoresis: a review. *Gen Dent* 1982; 30:481–483.
181. Lutins ND, Grecot GW, McFall WT. Effectiveness of sodium fluoride on tooth hypersensitivity with and without iontophoresis. *J Periodontol* 1984; 55:285–288.
182. Fishman PH, Jay WM, Rissing JP, et al. Iontophoresis of gentamicin into aphakic rabbit eyes. Sustained vitreal levels. *Invest Ophthalmol Vis Sci* 1984; 25:343–345.
183. Greminger RF, Elliott RA, Rapperport A. Antibiotic iontophoresis for the management of burned ear chondritis. *Plast Reconstr Surg* 1980; 66:356–360.
184. Passali D, Bellussi L, Masieri S. Transtympanic iontophoresis: personal experience. *Laryngoscope* 1984; 94:802–806.
185. LaForest NT, Cofrancesco C. Antibiotic iontophoresis in the treatment of ear chondritis. *Phys Ther* 1978; 58:32–34.
186. Langley PL. Iontophoresis to aid in releasing tendon adhesions: suggestions from the field. *Phys Ther* 1984; 64:1395.
187. Tannebaum M. Iodine iontophoresis in reducing scar tissue. *Phys Ther* 1980; 60:792.
188. Cornwall MW. Zinc iontophoresis to treat ischemic skin ulcers. *Phys Ther* 1981; 61:359–360.
189. Lekas MD. Iontophoresis treatment. *Otolaryngol Head Neck Surg* 1979; 87:292–298.
190. Kahn J. Use of iontophoresis in Peyronie's disease: a case report. *Phys Ther* 1982; 62:995–996.
191. Kahn J. Iontophoresis and ultrasound for post-surgical temporomandibular trismus and paresthesia. *Phys Ther* 1980; 60:307–308.
192. Marcer M, Musatti G, Bassett CAL. Results of pulsed electromagnetic fields (PEMEFs) in ununited fractures after external skeletal fixation. *Clin Orthop* 1984; 190:260–265.
193. Albanese R, Blaschak J, Medina R, Penn J. Ultrashort electromagnetic signals: biophysical questions, safety issues, and medical opportunities. *Aviat Space Environ Med* 1994; 65(suppl):A116–A120.
194. Cheng N, Van Hoof H, Bockx E, et al. The effects of electric currents on ATP generation, protein synthesis and membrane transport in rat skin. *Clin Orthop* 1982; 171:264–271.
195. Robinson KR. The responses of cells to electrical fields: a review. *J Cell Biol* 1985; 101:2023–2027.
196. Wolcott LE, Wheeler PC, Hardwicke HM, Rowley BA. Accelerated healing of skin ulcers by electrotherapy: preliminary clinical results. *South Med J* 1969; 62:795–801.
197. Gault WR, Gatens PF Jr. Use of low intensity direct current in management of ischemic skin ulcers. *Phys Ther* 1976; 56:265–268.
198. Vodovnik L, Karba R. Treatment of chronic wounds by means of electric and electromagnetic fields. Part 1 literature review. *Med Biol Eng Comput* 1992; 30:257–266.
199. Kaada B. Vasodilatation induced by transcutaneous nerve stimulation in peripheral ischemia (Raynaud's phenomenon and diabetic neuropathy). *Eur Heart J* 1982; 3:303–341.
200. Brighton CT. Treatment of nonunion of the tibia with constant direct current (1980 Fitts Lecture, AAST). *J Trauma* 1981; 21:189–195.
201. Mammi GI, Rocchi R, Cadossi R, Massari L, Traina GC. The electrical stimulation of tibial osteotomies. *Clin Orthop* 1993; 288:246–253.
202. Kloth LC, Feedar JA, Gentzkow GD. Pulsed electrical stimulation accelerates healing of chronic dermal ulcers. In: Transactions XI: Bioelectrical Repair and Growth Society, 11th annual meeting, September 29–October 2, 1991.
203. Gentzkow GD, Miller KH, Kause JD. Dermapulse for the treatment of decubitus ulcers: a baseline controlled trial. In: Transactions XI: Bioelectrical Repair and Growth Society, 11th annual meeting, September 29–October 2, 1991.
204. Barron JJ, Jacobson WE, Tidd G. Treatment of decubitus ulcers: a new approach. *Minn Med* 1985; 68:103–106.
205. Foley-Nolan D, Barry C, Coughlan RJ, O'Connor P, Roden D. Pulsed high frequency (27MHz) electromagnetic therapy for persistent neck pain. A double blind, placebo controlled study of 20 patients. *Orthopedics* 1990; 13:445–451.
206. Binder A, Hazelmann B, Pang P, Fitton-Jackson D. Pulsed electromagnetic field therapy on rotator cuff tendinitis. A double blind controlled assessment. *Lancet* 1984; 1:695–698.
207. Kaiser J. Panel finds EMFs post no threat. *Science* 1996; 274:910.
208. Bishop B. Vibratory stimulation: Part I. Neurophysiology of motor responses evoked by vibratory stimulation. *Phys Ther* 1974; 54: 1273–1282.
209. Bishop B. Vibratory stimulation: Part II. Vibratory stimulation as an evaluation tool. *Phys Ther* 1975; 55:28–34.
210. Bishop B. Vibratory stimulation: Part III. Possible applications of vibration in treatment of motor dysfunctions. *Phys Ther* 1975; 55: 139–143.
211. Lundeberg T, Ekblom A, Hannsson P. Relief of sinus pain by vibratory stimulation. *Ear Nose Throat J* 1985; 64:163–167.
212. Lundeberg T, Nodemar R, Ottoson D. Pain alleviation by vibratory stimulation. *Pain* 1984; 20:25–44.
213. Lundeberg T. The pain suppressive effect of vibratory stimulation and transcutaneous electrical nerve stimulation (TENS) as compared to aspirin. *Brain Res* 1984; 294:201–209.
214. Leduc A, Lievens P, Dewald J. The influence of multi-directional vibrations on wound healing and on regeneration of blood and lymph vessels. *Lymphology* 1981; 14:179–185.
215. Basford JR. Low intensity laser therapy: still not an established clinical tool. *Lasers Surg Med* 1995; 16:331–342.

Rehabilitation Medicine: Principles and Practice, Third Edition,
edited by Joel A. DeLisa and Bruce M. Gans.
Lippincott–Raven Publishers, Philadelphia © 1998.

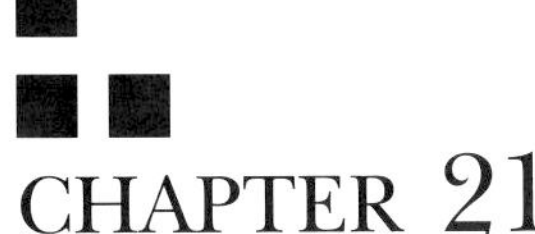

CHAPTER 21

Biofeedback in Physical Medicine and Rehabilitation

John V. Basmajian

Biofeedback (BF) as a clinical tool became recognized in the 1960s. At that time, three main scientific sources flowed together to form the broad stream that is modern BF: electromyography (EMG), electroencephalography (EEG), and cardiovascular research by psychophysiologists. Although the second and third sources are important, their influence on rehabilitation has been limited. The rehabilitation applications of the first arose from diagnostic and research work in EMG. For one half of a century, clinical electromyographers were quite aware of the considerable help they derived from the instant feedback of the myoelectric signals. Even in the adolescent period of EMG, in the 1940s, I often used the sound of motor unit potentials to grade the desired strength of contractions and often recruited the help of the patient.

In the more mature 1950s and early 1960s, my team was using feedback signals to train exquisite controls in normal muscles of handicapped persons to substitute for lost limbs and to augment the strength of weakened parts of the body (1–3). Our concerns were twofold: to determine and define the normal mechanisms of motor control in all parts of the body, and to develop methods and improve devices for treating neurologically and orthopedically handicapped patients. In the midst of these studies, I found that when our subjects were provided with instant visual and acoustic feedback from the EMG, they could learn to perform elaborate tricks with the tiniest units of muscle: the motor units. Throughout the 1960s, 1970s, and 1980s, many investigations of motor unit control of a highly technical nature were reported around the world, giving electromyographic biofeedback (EMGBF) a solid foundation (4).

Clinical EMGBF, the most widely used form of this modality, was an outgrowth of diagnostic EMG and research on the fine control of motor units. In rehabilitation, EMGBF has gained a firm place in the treatment of upper motor neuron lesions, particularly in retraining muscles and inducing relaxation of spastic muscles of stroke patients. In cerebral palsy and musculoskeletal disturbances, additional feedback transducers (e.g., electrogoniometers, pressure-sensitive and position-sensing devices) are gaining wider use. Spasmodic torticollis has proved to be particularly suitable for behavioral methods of treatment, including EMG feedback.

J. V. Basmajian: Department of Medicine, Chedoke Rehabilitation Centre of Hamilton Health Science Corporation, Hamilton, Ontario L8N 3Z5, Canada.

BIOFEEDBACK

In general, the field of BF may be defined as the technique of using equipment—usually electronic—to reveal to human beings some of their internal physiologic events, normal and abnormal, in the form of visual and auditory signals to teach them to manipulate these otherwise involuntary or unfelt events by manipulating the displayed signals. This technique inserts a person's volition into the gap of an open feedback loop—hence the artificial name "biofeedback," a term that some scientists and clinicians abhor for linguistic and other reasons. Unlike conditioned responses, the animal involved—here, necessarily, a human being—must want to voluntarily change the signals to meet a goal.

Teaching patients to control a wide range of physiologic processes occasionally has amazing therapeutic results, but legitimate clinical use of BF as described in this book must be differentiated from the fad that caught the popular imagination in the late 1960s. Although many self-serving promoters of general BF are still at work, true clinical BF has quietly taken a place as a genuine treatment for a growing number of neurologic and psychosomatic ailments. Both scientific and practical studies provide us with sufficient concrete evidence that objective neurologic signs and symptoms can be altered, particularly in patients with upper motor neuron paralysis and spasticity due to brain damage. The easiest form of do-it-yourself BF—alpha brain wave BF—is still not understood scientifically. Alpha feedback is still a mystery, and it is not a definitive treatment method. Other forms of EEG feedback have shown considerable promise in the experimental situation, but they will not be covered in this chapter (5).

Electromyographic Biofeedback

In rehabilitation, the most useful feedback has been myoelectric, or EMG. ''Electromyographic'' is probably not a good adjective to apply to this form of BF, because the patient and the clinician do not directly view electromyograms or an electromyograph. Instead, the myoelectric signals from the muscle are translated into simple acoustic and visual signals that are very easy to understand (e.g., lights and buzzing sounds) or graphic computer displays.

Position Biofeedback

This technique is indicated when the goal of training is the regulation of movement, provided the patient is able to voluntarily recruit and relax the appropriate muscle groups. Position or movement feedback is used to train the appropriate timing and coordination needed to control a movement. Examples of the application of position feedback in neural rehabilitation include the following:

Training for head position control (6)
Coordination and control of hand movements in ataxia and after hand surgery (7)
Training for knee joint position in children with cerebral palsy (8), adults with hemiplegia (9,10), and prosthesis wearers (11)

In addition, position feedback may be used in stroke rehabilitation when the muscle that must be monitored is inaccessible or difficult to isolate (e.g., in training pronation and supination of the forearm).

Pressure or Force Biofeedback

Force monitoring may be indicated when information concerning the amount of force being transmitted through a body segment or assistive device is desired. For example, for training of symmetrical standing or gait, the Krusen limb load monitor (LLM), developed at the Krusen Research Center of the Moss Rehabilitation Center in Philadelphia, may be used with hemiplegic adults (12) and children (13) to monitor the force transmitted through an extremity. Similarly, the use of a feedback cane can help train hemiplegic patients to monitor the amount of force being borne on an assistive device. In addition, the LLM is potentially an inexpensive evaluative tool to analyze gait (14). Other successful postural BF techniques have been described (15–17).

Temperature and Peripheral Blood Flow Biofeedback

Temperature or peripheral blood flow control of the extremities has become one of the major tools of clinical psychologists and their scientific associates. Considerable controversy continues as to whether direct blood flow measurements, photoplethysmography, or skin temperature–sensing devices are preferable. These matters are discussed elsewhere in books and journals devoted to BF (5).

Blood Pressure Biofeedback

Blood pressure BF usually uses regular plethysmography. Patients are trained to modify its outputs with the added support of relaxation training with EMGBF and temperature control of the extremities (5).

Sphincteral Control Training

By using perineal EMGBF with pressure transducers in the anal canal or vagina, incontinent patients are provided with electronic monitoring coupled with a modified form of operant conditioning. Usually considered to be the province of urologists, gynecologists, proctologists, psychologists, and gerontologists, this type of training should be of increasing interest to the interdisciplinary rehabilitation team and will be discussed later in this chapter.

Respiratory Biofeedback

Application of research findings remains uncommon for conditions that would seem ideal for the use of electronic monitoring for BF training (e.g., asthma, high-level spinal cord injuries [SCIs]). Pulmonologists and therapists appear to be overlooking a ''sure bet'' for aiding their patients.

Miscellaneous Techniques

Almost all physiologic functions, from eye blinking to gastric and bowel activity, are under investigation with appropriate sensors (e.g., microphones, chemical probes, gas pressure balloons). None of these studies would seem to have a direct application to rehabilitation medicine today, but they may be useful in the future after additional research (5).

APPLIED FIELDS

Psychotherapy

Unquestionably, the largest application of BF is in clinical psychotherapy. Thousands of research papers on the whole gamut of BF therapies have been written and are being put to practical use. One of the early sources was the work done by Jacobson in the 1920s and 1930s (18). He developed and became an enthusiastic proponent of relaxation therapy, in which he used rather primitive EMG equipment to monitor the level of tension in the muscles of his patients. Limited by the apparatus available at that time, Jacobson developed methods of electrical measurement of the muscular status of tension, and with these measurements he facilitated progressive somatic relaxation for a variety of psychoneurotic syndromes. Meanwhile, in Germany, Shultz (19) developed his related technique, autogenic training, which was widely popularized in Canada by his pupil Luthe (20). Although autogenic training used no specific EMG equipment, it was one of the early sources of much of today's BF application to the treatment of psychosomatic and neurotic symptoms.

Although medical specialists and psychologists who knew of these relaxation techniques kept them alive and growing, the field of diagnostic EMG was spreading slowly. Only a scattering of research papers kept alive the flow of data regarding myoelectric BF. Thus, in 1934, Olive Smith (21), and soon after, Lindsley (22), emphasized that at rest "subjects can relax a muscle so completely that . . . no active units are found." Relaxation sometimes requires conscious effort, and in some cases special training.

Lindsley found that complete relaxation was not difficult in any of his normal subjects. This finding has since been confirmed by thousands of investigators using modern electrical apparatus. Gilson and Mills (23), Harrison and Mortensen (24), and I (1,25) have continued this type of work. Using fine-wire electrodes that I had recently developed for other purposes, I was able to train normal subjects to activate many separate motor units and to activate them consciously. This was a form of single spinal motor neuron training. Then, a long series of studies with my students and colleagues led progressively toward a confluence with the other branches that were to form modern BF.

The fields of myoelectric control and muscle relaxation joined in the mid-1960s. After my publication on single motor unit controls (1,2), Budzynski and colleagues (26) developed a technique for relief of tension headaches. This type of application of myoelectric feedback has grown to dominate the entire field. Although medical rehabilitation groups emphasize targeted relaxation or targeted retraining of semiparetic muscles, clinical psychologists and specialists in psychosomatic medicine almost limit their clinical work to general deep relaxation, often combining jacobsonian techniques and autogenic training along with instrumental relaxation.

Other applications became apparent in the mid-1960s. One of these was the increasing use of operant conditioning in animal psychological research. Thus, the cardiovascular conditioning by Miller and his colleagues (27–29) caught the imagination of many scientists and clinicians (5). At the same time, experts in EEG began to report interesting correlations between the state of emotional set and consciousness, and the amount of alpha waves generated by the subject. By the end of the 1960s, all of the various branches of modern BF research were integrated.

In the 1970s, the shape of BF changed dramatically. The most dominant form, alpha feedback, which received the greatest publicity in the late 1960s, virtually dried up as a scientifically defensible clinical tool. Where it is still used by serious clinicians, it is combined with other techniques to achieve relaxation. However, it has also returned to the research laboratory from which it probably should not have emerged prematurely. Through the next generation of scientific investigation, it may return as a useful applied technique, possibly in rehabilitation.

In psychotherapy today, EMGBF has taken over the dominant role, and, either alone or in combination with thermal feedback and adjuncts (e.g., meditation, exercises), it is the primary tool of psychotherapists who daily use BF. Somewhat ironically, much of the benefits their patients derive ought to be more easily transferable to patients in rehabilitation facilities. Only where psychologists have a significant presence in rehabilitation centers have these beneficial transfers occurred to provide relief of various symptoms of stress. Tension headache, chronic back problems, and anxiety are prime targets, and the literature on their management with BF relaxation is expanding rapidly.

Deep relaxation strikes directly at the cause (i.e., muscle tension). There are other ways in which relaxation can be taught effectively, but BF gadgets are useful in accelerating the treatment, and good psychotherapists quickly wean their patients from the gadgets. They teach their patients self-control as part of their long-term treatment. General or total body relaxation also has proved to be very useful in the rehabilitation clinic, along with targeted relaxation of specific muscles in spasm. Thus, in patients with dyskinesias (e.g., spasmodic torticollis) and cerebral palsy, and for patients who have suffered stroke and have spasticity, relaxation therapy enhances their subsequent training of improved motor performance.

Branches of Clinical Medicine

Acknowledging the importance of embracing the benefits of behavioral medicine noted above, there are many other practical uses of BF technology in clinical medicine. For the purpose of this book, rehabilitation medicine is pre-eminent among the branches and will be considered separately and fully later in this chapter. Most closely related—almost inseparably—are neurology, geriatrics, and orthopedics; their rehabilitative concerns are integrated into that later discussion. Perhaps the same may be said about chronic pain management and sphincter control management because they figure so prominently in rehabilitation centers. However, because of certain unique features, they will be considered now. Also considered are Raynaud's disease, incontinence, sports medicine, and psychoimmunology.

Chronic Pain Management

Although the treatment of frequent tension headaches with EMGBF (5) and vascular headaches (i.e., migraine) with peripheral temperature control training (2) is well established in clinical psychology, in clinical medicine the treatment of chronic pain in the back and extremities is the main target of BF therapy. Most of the cases treated are managed in back pain clinics and related rehabilitation facilities.

As Johnson and Hockersmith point out, patients with chronic low back pain are characteristically found to be chronically depressed with strong feelings of helplessness, anger, and resistance to most proposed treatment (30). Therefore, EMGBF is an effective nonthreatening way to regain the lost confidence in clinicians by increasing self-awareness and self-esteem. Because they are given low initial goals, the patients usually find success with the equipment and a sense of accomplishment. Usually this success has been rare for them in the therapeutic milieu, where passively receiving treatment from others has been the mode.

Some disagreement exists as to which muscle groups should be trained to relax. The obvious target of the paravertebral muscles is not universally accepted. Psychotherapists generally prefer the easily accessible forehead or neck muscles. The whole-body musculature is advocated by Johnson and Hockersmith (30). Other EMGBF sources have their defenders as well. The end results, however, are similar: a statistically and clinically useful therapy in the total management of low back pain (5).

Raynaud's Disease

Behavioral techniques emphasizing self-regulation, especially with BF in the training sessions, permit 80% of patients with primary Raynaud's disease to self-regulate the symptoms caused by the idiopathic vasospasms in the hands (31). A program combining EMG and skin temperature feedback with autogenic training is generally advised. Subsequent reinforcement sessions are sometimes necessary. Unfortunately, similar treatment of secondary Raynaud's phenomenon has been found to be considerably less successful.

Urinary and Fecal Incontinence

First there was the early demonstration by Schuster of the effectiveness of operant conditioning with the use of a series of rectal and anal balloons to train the anal sphincter to respond appropriately (32,33). This quite effective technique has been accepted by colorectal surgeons more readily than by other clinicians, for obvious reasons. Most rehabilitation and psychotherapy practitioners prefer local EMGBF for BF training of the pelvic floor for incontinence of the bladder, the rectum, or both. Bladder incontinence is a distressingly common symptom even in normal healthy young women, 51% of whom occasionally experience stress incontinence as a result of laughing or sneezing (34). Up to 50% of institutionalized patients are incontinent (34).

In recent years, a generalized training of the pelvic floor muscles with a modified EMGBF device such as the Kegel perineometer (PerryMeter Systems, Stratford, PA) (34) has gained increasing acceptance. With or without the device, perineal exercises are an effective method to reachieve continence, but the use of both is twice as effective (91% successful subjects) as the exercises alone (55% successful subjects) (34).

Biofeedback in Paraclinical Fields

Sports Medicine

Increasingly, trainers are using EMGBF both for relaxation training and for muscle strengthening and coordination of skilled movement. The theoretical basis for both approaches is obvious, but the general enthusiasm has not resulted in valid research results. Perhaps it is possible to measure results in an unbiased fashion, but a true double-blind test appears to be difficult or even impossible.

Psychoimmunology

An enormous new application of BF has emerged through the discovery that immune systems can be influenced by stress management achieved through BF and visualized imagery. Visualization "tells our body what to do and BF tells us how well the body carries out our instructions" (35). There is a large body of literature relating the immune system to stress and to specific conditions such as depression, schizophrenia, Huntington's disease, and multiple sclerosis. Obviously, clinicians are exploring ways to influence the immune system with psychotherapy of stress (36).

REHABILITATION MEDICINE AND THERAPY

Interdisciplinary Factors in Biofeedback

In the introduction of any novel treatment, the interdisciplinary team often is suspicious and skeptical. In time, if one or more of the partners in the group becomes knowledgeable and convinced of the value of the new approach and finds some evidence of its worth, resistance declines and may be replaced by silent acceptance. If results are clearly manifest to all members of the team, particularly to the patient and family, the new therapy becomes a regular feature.

Such has been the process in the case of BF's introduction into rehabilitation practice. If even one member of the team has absolutely no enthusiasm for it, then its use declines or may never occur. Where it is used persistently, it becomes a regular part of the team's expectations.

Physicians

Generally, few physiatrists perform BF personally; instead they rely on other members of the health-care team. However, through the overt and covert signals they emit—especially if they are the team leader and cost-containment is a problem—they greatly influence the adoption of methods by their colleagues. On the other hand, physicians have taken a leading role in research and advocacy in EMGBF.

Rehabilitation Therapists

Throughout the world, the largest user group for EMGBF outside of psychotherapy has been physical therapy (PT). For motor retraining, spasticity reduction, and general relaxation training, physical therapists have molded EMGBF into their practice to varying degrees from low to very high. Many occupational therapists use EMGBF for manual skill retraining and for relaxation therapy. The treatment of communications disorders by speech therapists has been augmented by EMGBF of laryngeal functions or of respiratory functions (37).

The psychologist member of the team often is the most enthusiastic about applying EMGBF techniques carried over from general psychotherapy and general relaxation therapy. On the other hand, nursing, the largest and most important group in rehabilitation teams, has had only a superficial opportunity to us the technology of BF. In those centers where nurses have been involved in the mystique, they are making significant contributions to relaxation therapy in pain clinics and outpatient classes for arthritis, postcardiac, and other patients.

Environmental Factors

Most types of guided learning of skills require an environment that fosters that process. Therefore, ideal BF in its various forms requires (and sometimes demands) special surroundings. These are not prohibitive in cost, although in some busy departments they may be difficult to achieve: small, quiet, simply furnished rooms, peaceful corners of therapy gymnasiums, and gait laboratories. Some learning, especially at the later stages of transfer of skills to the everyday environment, can and should be performed against a background of distracting influences. A skill learned in a vacuum is of limited use; it must be carried over to the activities of daily living, one half of which are not a private affair.

Equipment Factors

Basic Electronics

The practitioner who uses any of the BF tools must have a relationship with the devices that is based on a familiarity with the fundamentals and terminology of medical electronics. To be unfamiliar with Ohm's law ($E = IR$) and the power equations ($P = I^2R$ and $P = E^2R$ or $P = EI$) suggests that the physician or therapist is locked into the eighteenth or nineteenth century. An appreciation of current flow and root mean square values of parameters that determine specifications of medical electronic equipment is essential. Electrical factors rule the specifications of all electrical equipment used. These factors may include the following:

Voltage–current relationships
Resistance
Inductance
Capacitance
Impedance
Rectification
Integration
Filters
Differential amplifiers
Circuit block diagrams

Figure 21-1 summarizes the basic circuitry of an EMGBF device (5).

Most EMGBF devices on the market today were designed for psychotherapy. Nevertheless, they are practical in most rehabilitation settings, and because they are cheaper than several excellent special computerized devices, they may continue to dominate the field. Generally, they cost about $1,000 and have one- or two-channel inputs, bipolar surface electrodes for each channel, excellent differential amplifiers, and some form of semi-integration of the signals. Thus, the raw EMG signal is processed to give an increasing and decreasing voltage, usually with variable time bases provided. This voltage then acts on simple visual and acoustic output devices rather than on the type of outputs (e.g., cathode ray oscilloscopes) familiar to the diagnostic clinician. These include microvoltage meters, digital displays, threshold setters, banks of lights, and sound transducers that produce

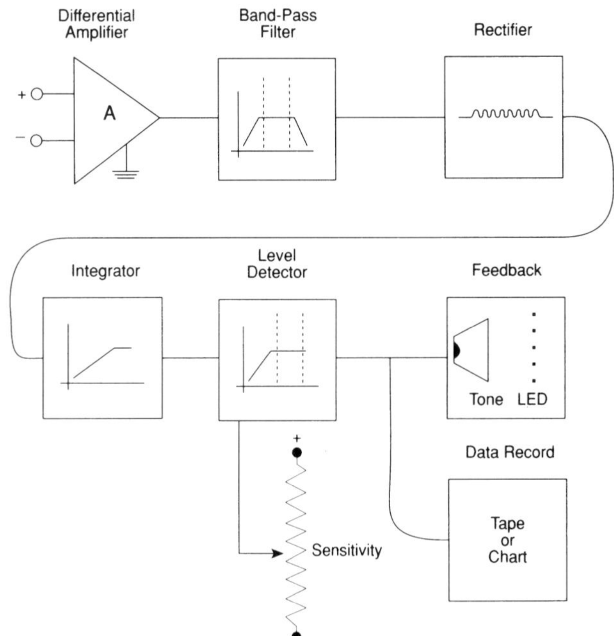

FIG. 21-1. Basic block diagram of an EMGBF device. LED, light-emitting diode. (Reprinted with permission from Basmajian JV, ed. *Biofeedback: principles and practice for clinicians,* 3rd ed. Baltimore: Williams & Wilkins, 1989.)

noises such as clicks, warbles, and buzzes. Patients require very little training to understand the signals produced. These audio signals can be presented in a variety of ways to help shape patient responses. Also, the outputs can be fed into auxiliary devices for further functions, including computation.

Auditory Feedback

Some devices emit clicks that increase in frequency proportional to increases in EMG voltage, and others give short tones or beeps. A beep is heard when the integrated EMG increases; the device emits no sound during relaxation. This approach encourages the patient to work harder for another beep. The opposite is possible with a different mode setting: as the EMG activity decreases, the beep is heard. Silence occurring during periods of increased muscle activity is useful for teaching relaxation of spastic muscle. It can be a positive reinforcement because the patient must try to repeat within a specified period of time whatever it was that caused the beep to occur. Many devices have variable time constants that determine when a feedback tone or visual change is provided to the patient.

Use of a short time constant results in a shorter delay between a change in integrated EMG and the feedback; this is useful during training that requires dynamic muscle contraction. Selection of longer time constants is often advisable when training for general relaxation in the absence of dynamic activity.

In some threshold devices, a monotone buzzer is heard only when the patient achieves a specific level of muscle activity preset by the therapist. A low-threshold setting may be used in training for recruitment of activity above a given level in a weak or paretic muscle. Once the patient reliably exceeds this level, the threshold is raised progressively. This is often referred to as shaping. The reverse shaping strategy to reduce integrated EMG levels (i.e., reduction of resting hypertonus) also may be used.

Visual Feedback

Displays in EMG feedback devices include oscilloscopes, banks of lights, or activated meters with increasing levels of integrated EMG activity. The threshold level for the visual feedback can be set by either the therapist or the patient. In either case, a meter deflection helps maintain continuity and gives both therapist and patient a more precise measure of activity. The meter also can be an excellent source of motivation. Increasingly, sophisticated (and more expensive) computerized devices are coming into vogue (Fig. 21-2).

An oscilloscope tracing can be helpful to the clinician who is familiar with EMG. Local and extraneous EMG as well as artifacts can be distinguished. The therapist also can optimize electrode placements, combining EMG displayed on an oscilloscope with integrated EMG on the audio. Visual feedback is particularly valuable to detect possible artifact or interference that could provide erroneous information. Patients usually prefer to watch a meter rather than an oscilloscope because it gives them a clearer measure.

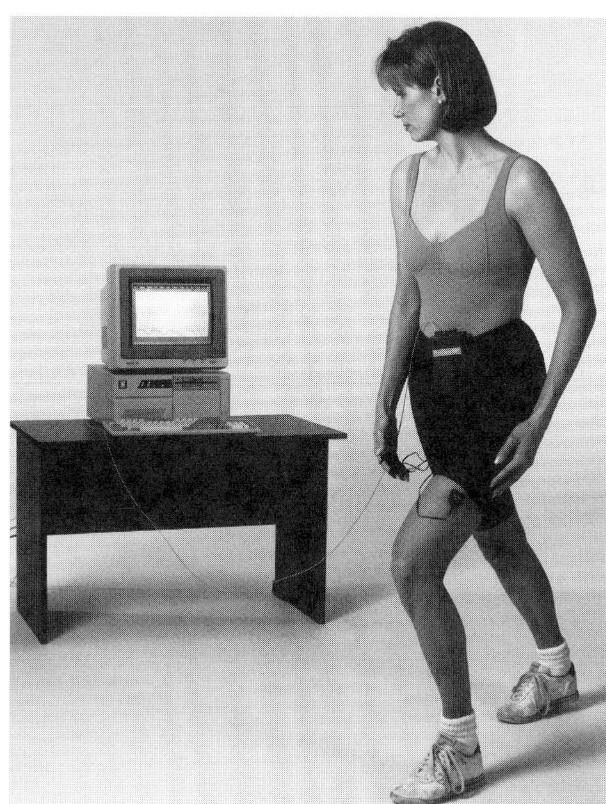

FIG. 21-2. Computerized EMGBF equipment for rehabilitation clinical use (this example is made by Thought Technology Ltd, Montreal, Canada).

If the electrodes are properly applied, it is theoretically possible to obtain accurate readings of activity as low as 1 μV, but such low integrated levels are important only during generalized relaxation training. Retraining patients with musculoskeletal weakness (e.g., the quadriceps after meniscectomy) requires a feedback device with comparatively low sensitivity settings because such patients often learn to generate several hundred microvolts of integrated EMG during isometric or isokinetic contractions.

Electronic interfaces are available to allow simultaneous use of both the BF device and an external oscilloscope. They must incorporate isolation of the battery-run BF equipment from the alternating current needed to drive the oscilloscope to ensure patient safety against possible current leaks.

The most elaborate and expensive equipment is not necessarily the best. It must be suited for the specific clinic. The equipment should be versatile enough to be meaningful to as many patients as possible. If the therapist works primarily with old people, large visual feedback is advisable. On the other hand, the size of visual feedback may not be as significant a consideration with children as is the variety of feedback alternatives needed to capture and maintain interest and motivation.

Electrodes

Skin or surface electrodes predominate in EMGBF. Although indwelling electrodes permit large-amplitude and localized, well-defined pick-up of muscle potentials, they must be inserted percutaneously and so are not practical for BF training in most clinics, except for muscles that are not easily isolated by surface electrodes. Sometimes needle electrodes can be used in cases where no signs of activity could be elicited. A clinical EMG should determine if any viable motor units have survived.

Surface electrodes are round disks, having silver chloride or gold recording surfaces that are recessed within a plastic cup. The surface diameters vary in size up to 12.5 mm. Commercial miniature electrodes (e.g., Beckman, The Electrode Store, Yucca Valley, CA; 4 mm in diameter) are used for monitoring small areas or muscles such as hand muscles. Disposable electrodes are also available; they are usually quite large and made for electrocardiographic recordings.

Electrode placement for re-education of weak muscles requires precision. The electrodes should be placed over target muscles in an area of relative anatomic isolation from the surrounding musculature. Wide spacing of electrodes causes cross-talk (e.g., over the tibialis anterior, they will pick up signals from a spastic gastrocnemius). Consistent electrode placement is essential from session to session, giving validity to the meter reading as an indication of general progress.

Problems

Most equipment-related problems have easy solutions for the electronically sophisticated clinician or an electronics associate. Artifacts can arise from undesired sources nearby (e.g., electrode movements, antagonist muscles, electrocardiographic signals, electrode artifacts, poor grounding) or from more distant environmental sources (e.g., an electrically noisy elevator or radiology department nearby). Most can be eliminated in a few moments. While visiting groups who were having serious problems with their equipment, I have occasionally found that the battery was run down and required recharging.

Cautions

Almost all commercially available BF devices are self-contained and battery operated, and they are completely safe. However, makeshift connections to recording and computer devices that are operated on 110 or 220 V and are faulty introduce a risk to both the patient and the clinician. Only a qualified electrical engineer or technologist can ensure the safety of such equipment linkages (5).

Training Strategies

These have been presented in detail elsewhere (5). Experienced clinicians will complement their present strategies with the careful melding of the influence of the BF of different types.

Placebo Factors

In another article, I addressed placebo factors extensively in all therapies, including BF (38). It is a potent factor that accounts for more than one third of all cures. Therefore, it needs to be understood, used wisely, and not sneered at. It must not be used as deception.

Resistance to Novelty

The history of health care almost always shows that every innovation begins with a tiny group of passionate advocates who are opposed overwhelmingly by antagonists who want to thwart change. This generally has not been the case for BF in psychotherapy, where it was warmly accepted from the earliest days. However, it was true in medical rehabilitation. Fortunately, a solid base of advance and concurrent research was and is available, and the transition to comfortable acceptance is occurring. One hindrance for some physical therapists is the mind set that condemns them to do things to patients rather than helping patients to learn for themselves. An enormous revolution is in progress as therapists recognize their greater role as teachers and trainers rather than modern bone-setters.

NEUROLOGIC BASIS OF ELECTROMYOGRAPHIC BIOFEEDBACK

Wolf and Binder-MacLeod have asked, ''How do patients process feedback information? What factors account for the patient's ability to gradually become less dependent upon artificially induced information signals . . . after failing to achieve significant gains using conventional rehabilitation procedures?'' (39).

As is well known, the central nervous system employs a multitude of internal modulatory networks (39) The role of the somatosensory areas, other subcortical areas, and the basal ganglia should not be underemphasized. They make voluntary movements meaningful. Cutaneous receptors, proprioceptors, and auditory and visual inputs are harmonized into the controls, as is the cerebellum. Therefore, a damaging external or internal trauma to area 4 of the cerebral cortex may spare pathways that are primarily conditioned for skilled movements, or they may spare redundant pathways that EMGBF training can bring into play.

Plasticity and relearning by the brain should be thought of as a more complex phenomenon than the taking over of the mature role of specialized areas by the neighboring cortex. It also may involve an activation of pathways that had not been trained previously by the natural selection of the best pathways. Along with this idea, some investigators invoke the possibility of dendritic sprouting occurring in the relearning stages to account for the reacquisition of skills. The jury is still out regarding these intriguing questions.

CLINICAL APPLICATIONS IN REHABILITATION

Electromyographic and Force Biofeedback for Stroke Patients

Undoubtedly, stroke rehabilitation is a major application of EMGBF in rehabilitation hospitals and outpatient clinics.

Wolf and colleagues investigated patient characteristics that may affect the outcome of EMGBF training of hemiplegic patients (40,41). Age, gender, hemiparetic side, duration of stroke, previous rehabilitation, and number of training sessions did not have a significant effect. The presence of proprioceptive loss appeared to diminish the probability of making functional gains in the upper limb. In general, patients showed greater functional improvement with lower limb training than with upper limb training.

It is now known that there is no clear relationship between successful retraining and age or duration of hemiparesis (5), and patients should not be excluded from feedback training based solely on either age or length of time since their stroke. However, the optimal time for introducing BF appears to be the same as for any rehabilitation efforts—fairly early.

The effectiveness of force feedback on symmetrical standing in chronic hemiplegic patients is also related to the ability to successfully use the feedback information during the first training session, less severe disturbances in standing asymmetry, and a right hemiparesis. However, many questions still exist as to the best candidates for feedback training. Some of the more significant factors are listed as follows:

1. Potential for voluntary control must exist before feedback training is begun.
2. Motivation and cooperation are essential. Fortunately, the introduction of the feedback frequently serves to motivate patient and therapist alike.
3. Inability to follow commands and receptive aphasia make BF training practically impossible.
4. Severe proprioceptive loss, marked spasticity, and the inability to voluntarily initiate exploratory (i.e., reaching) movements of an extremity all appear to correlate to diminished functional improvements.

Lower Limb

Targeted training of the lower limb is simpler than that of the upper limb and so is discussed first. The primary functional goals are improved ambulation and development of the relatively limited number of stereotyped patterns used during ambulation. Training of the lower limb need not follow the proximal-to-distal progression for the upper limb. Instead, it builds in complexity, involving the training of several limb segments simultaneously in specific movement patterns. BF can fit nicely into many traditional exercise approaches designed to train the lower limb.

Hip and Knee Extension

This combination is an important component of the stance phase of gait. General weakness of these muscles is most commonly observed during the early stages of recovery before the appearance of a strong extensor synergy. EMGBF can be incorporated into many exercises that individually train the gluteus maximus.

Similarly, EMGBF can be used to encourage recruitment of the quadriceps or relaxation of the hamstrings, or both. Relaxation of the hamstrings may need to be practiced at rest and after static and dynamic stretches. Dual-channel monitoring may be used to facilitate contraction of the quadriceps and relaxation of the hamstrings. Prompt relaxation of the quadriceps at the termination of the range, and even the reversal of activity back into flexion, should be practiced early in training because of the frequent development of spasticity in the quadriceps.

Finally, EMGBF can be used to train combined hip and knee extension. Patterned movements can be practiced against manual or mechanical resistance while feedback is provided from a weak prime mover or from overactive synergistic or antagonistic muscles. Feedback can be used along with an isometric, isotonic, or isokinetic contraction, although the therapist should be aware of the differences in the EMG interference patterns associated with each type of contraction (42). Combining functional electrical stimulation (FES) with either EMGBF or positional BF has shown promising added effectiveness in multiple studies (43–46).

Hip Flexion with Knee Extension

The combination of hip flexion and knee extension occurs during the terminal phase of the swing phase of gait. Only accessory muscles of hip flexion (i.e., rectus femoris, sartorius) can be monitored with surface electrodes. For most patients, hip flexion is strongest when combined with knee flexion, and knee extension is strongest as part of a total extensor pattern of the lower extremity. If weak, these muscles may first need to be trained within the synergy pattern, and then out of that pattern. The combined movement of hip flexion and knee extension may next be practiced when up in a weight-bearing position.

Hip Extension with Knee Flexion

This is difficult for many stroke patients. Mat exercises begin with active flexing of the knee while not increasing the hip flexor activity. The quadriceps and hip flexors must both be trained to relax while the patient recruits the hamstrings. Next, the patient is brought to a standing position where knee flexion with hip extension can be practiced.

Hip Abduction

Weakness in the gluteus medius occurs in many hemiplegic patients during the stance phase of gait. The hip adductors, if spastic, may require relaxation before training the abductors. Reflex contraction of the abductors can be evoked in most patients by a strong isometric contraction of the abductors on the normal side (i.e., Raimiste's phenomenon) (47). The patient then uses the EMG feedback to volitionally augment the reflex response. Gradually, the reflex facilitation is reduced and the patient performs the contraction voluntarily. If necessary, the hip adductors can be simultaneously monitored to enhance their relaxation.

Ankle Dorsiflexion

One of the first areas of BF training was for the treatment of footdrop (5) caused by paralysis of the ankle dorsiflexors and spasticity of the plantar flexors, which are easy muscles to monitor with surface electrodes. Training may begin with either relaxation of the gastrocnemius or recruitment of the dorsiflexors. Recruitment of the dorsiflexors during relaxation of the gastrocnemius also may need to be trained. Training for dorsiflexion is begun with the patient seated and the ankle again resting unsupported in plantar flexion. Dual-channel monitoring is used, if available. Primarily auditory feedback is used as the patient is encouraged to watch the foot avoid marked inversion.

As control of the dorsiflexors improves and the patient learns to dorsiflex the ankle without apparent hip and knee flexion, the patient begins exercising with greater knee extension. The next task is to attempt to recruit the dorsiflexors and relax the plantar flexors while the knee is passively held in progressively more extension.

If the patient has appreciable active dorsiflexion, the therapist may combine position feedback with EMG feedback from plantar flexors with a relatively simple electrogoniometer (9). When position feedback is combined with EMG feedback of the plantar flexors, it is possible for the dorsiflexion to trigger the feedback signal while maintaining an appropriate level of relaxation of the plantar flexors.

Ambulation Training

Electromyographic and position feedback are used along with force feedback to train specific muscles or movements necessary for ambulation. Each of the practiced exercises and other necessary movements are trained and then integrated into the walking pattern. Many repetitions make any learned movement automatic.

BF training when the patient is up and standing or walking can be divided into exercises to improve either the stance phase or swing phase of gait.

Stance Phase

Equal weight distribution onto both lower extremities may be facilitated by force feedback used from the very early stages of treatment while learning to rise from a chair, stand, and return to sitting. A useful feedback device is the Krusen LLM. Quantification of the analog voltage output of the LLM can be obtained with an oscilloscope or strip chart recorder.

The force feedback is used to train the force and temporal components of weight shifting during the stance phase of gait with either the LLM (14) or a feedback cane (48). By varying the threshold of either device, the peak force borne on the involved lower extremity can be shaped. For the training of the temporal component (i.e., the duration of stance), the LLM along with a time delay modification developed at Emory University (49) can be used to shape a more symmetric gait.

Swing Phase

Feedback is used while rehearsing many of the previously practiced movements and for the integration of these movements into a functional gait pattern. Position feedback from the ankle joint may be combined with EMGBF feedback from the necessary ankle, knee, or hip muscles. The strategies are similar to those used during mat activities and those used in training for the relaxation of hip adductors during active flexion of the hip to avoid scissoring of the extremity. Training generally begins in the parallel bars and progresses to ambulation with assistive devices.

Upper Limb

BF has been used in the treatment of hemiplegia of the arm since the 1960s (50). Most of the early reports were case studies or clinical reports. Only a few systematically controlled experiments that purported to demonstrate the benefits of EMGBF in rehabilitation of muscle function were reported (50). Flaws in methodology limited the validity of conclusions that had been generally very favorable.

Controlled Studies and Meta-Analyses

Meta-analyses by three separate study groups have given conflicting conclusions ranging from "effective tool for neuromuscular re-education in the hemiplegic stroke patient" (51) to "not conclusively indicate superiority" (52) and "do not support the efficacy of BF in restoring the range of motion of hemiparetic joints" (53), with a caution that a type II error may be masking "an important clinical benefit." Combining upper limb results (generally very dismal with all treatments) with lower limb results (excellent with EMGBF) has been a confounding factor.

In a formal preliminary study, we treated the hemiplegic upper limb in 37 patients with a wide range of severity and duration after stroke (54). They were randomly assigned to either a 5-week, 15-session program of integrated EMGBF plus PT or a standard exercise therapy program with the same time elements and intensity. In both groups, tested independently, some cases showed improved useful function. Patients' conditions were classified as early-mild, early-severe, late-mild, and late-severe. All patients in the early-mild group had substantial improvement, whereas those in the late-severe group did not improve. It became imperative to investigate the other two groups—early-severe and late-mild.

Meanwhile, reports of other independent controlled studies by Wolf and Binder-MacLeod (55) and Inglis and associates (56) appeared; EMGBF plus PT had been tested against PT alone. Both studies found that in chronic stroke patients, EMGBF, when used as an adjunct to PT, resulted in improvement in upper limb range of motion and muscle strength. Although positive, these investigators were more restrained in their enthusiasm for BF for the upper limb than were authors of earlier uncontrolled clinical reports. Nevertheless, they brought new insights into the effects of both standard and BF-behavioral approaches to the hemiparetic upper limb. They also emphasized that EMGBF is an adjunctive and not a total therapy.

At the start of our formal second study, we were impressed by the apparent importance of the elapsed time before therapy and severity of the functional loss (57). In addition, the possible influence of behavioral factors in both groups appeared to require more careful attention. Therefore, the study was fashioned as a comparison of "integrated behavioral-physical therapy versus a traditional physical therapy program " (57).

The primary objective was to demonstrate a clinically and statistically significant difference in upper limb function between the two groups at the end of therapy and at 9-month follow-up. Specifically, the objective was to show that a greater number of patients in one treatment group improved at least 10 points on the Carroll Upper Extremity Function Test (UEFT), shown in the pilot study (54) to be a valid indicator by correlating well with activity-of-daily-living functions and being quantitative, valid, and reliable. The UEFT shows the amount of change needed to demonstrate significant clinical improvement or regression and is the most useful tool in predicting functional outcome. A second measure of physical ability, the finger oscillation test, measured speed of movement.

Our extended study suggested that the functional recovery after a formal behavioral approach (e.g., BF and cognitive therapy) is equal to, but not superior to, a matched program of Bobath-based PT. Both approaches were clinically effective, and significantly so. These results do not tell us to advocate dropping one form of therapy in favor of the other. Instead, they dramatize that, in a substantial but still poorly defined proportion of stroke patients with hemiplegic upper limbs, clinically useful improvement is achievable and worth the effort. However, the specific patients who would benefit most from one or the other of these two approaches are still not clarified, and further study is essential, along with further study to establish the physiologic basis of the functional changes.

A study by our group (58) casts new light on the underlying neural deficit in the hemiplegic limb. The poor motor responses were long held to be due to inhibition of the desired movement by antagonist activity, as taught by the Bobaths (59). We found the opposite to be true: the lack or absence of movement is simply due to a poverty of motor unit recruitment in the prime movers. Physical therapists must revise their systematic approach to upper limb retraining.

Motivation enhancement is obviously needed in both approaches, and in this study the behavioral approach was not more successful than the PT approach in altering locus of control, mood, affect, and so forth. Thus, we cannot document superior psychological changes as having come from the psychological approach. This behavioral technique by physical therapists (e.g., EMGBF and cognitive therapy) rivals traditional neurophysiologic hands-on PT; both bring about clinically worthwhile and lasting improvement in substantial numbers of patients. The time, costs, and required training for EMGBF are modest, and the treatments can be performed on an outpatient basis. Of particular interest is the effectiveness of EMGBF on shoulder subluxation with or without a recovery of functional use of the hand. The latter presents a major problem compared with the relatively straightforward biomechanical principles, procedures, and good outcome of EMGBF for subluxation.

Shoulder Subluxation

This is a common problem among flaccid hemiplegic patients. Since our earliest clinical experience at Emory University, my colleagues and I have had excellent results in decreasing shoulder subluxation by remobilizing the shoulder. By gaining control and strength in the upper trapezius and anterior deltoid, the patient not only tends to reduce subluxation but also improves the active range of motion. We have found that feedback from the scapular muscles can be confusing to the patient and not as satisfactory as the indirect approach of feedback from the anterior deltoid.

The upper trapezius is a good muscle to start training. Initiating activity in the upper trapezius can be learned easily by most patients. With electrodes over the muscle belly, the patient may be first asked to shrug either the involved or both shoulders, with feedback provided from the involved muscle. A mirror is also used to provide visual feedback of the movement performed. Targeted levels of motor unit recruitment followed by prompt relaxation should be encouraged early in the retraining process because overactivity of the upper trapezius often appears. Although movement may not be seen initially, increasing the targeted level of recruitment will show overt movement eventually. With increasing control of the shoulder elevators, restoration of normal scapular posture should result in the reduction of subluxation (5).

Therapists' Strategies for Upper Limb Training

The following section is based on Stuart Binder-MacLeod's broader description of strategies in my book *Biofeedback: Principles and Practice for Clinicians* (60).

Shoulder

Shoulder flexion is often the most difficult shoulder movement for stroke patients to perform because it brings on the flexion synergy pattern that includes scapular elevation and shoulder abduction. The therapist may need to introduce dual-channel monitoring to break up this synergistic movement pattern. The patient can be trained to reduce the upper trapezius or the middle deltoid activity while recruiting the anterior deltoid. All muscles are easily monitored, but the anterior and middle deltoid activity is difficult to isolate except with extremely close spacing and a posterolateral placement of the electrodes over the middle deltoid.

If the patient is primarily having problems with abduction, instead of elevation, start with the middle and anterior deltoid muscles, usually with the patient reclined. The therapist can begin with the involved shoulder passively flexed to 90°, with neutral shoulder rotation and the elbow fully flexed. The patient's task is to first maintain shoulder flexion without moving into abduction. The patient attempts to recruit activity from the anterior deltoid while staying below threshold for the middle deltoid. The next step may be to work on eccentric contraction of the anterior deltoid. Starting at 90°, the patient lowers his or her arm slowly. When the patient is able to show control over the complete range, we progress to training concentric contractions until the patient displays control over the full range of shoulder flexion and extension. Similarly, exercises may be performed while monitoring the upper trapezius, if shoulder elevation is also a problem.

Training next progresses to more functional activities with specific exercises, depending on the individual patient's needs and problems.

BF may be used for relaxation training of a spastic pectoralis major. The patient is first trained to relax the pectoralis major at rest and then during distraction (e.g., during conversation), during movement of the normal limbs, and while the muscle is placed and maintained in progressively increasing lengthened positions, within the patient's pain-free range of motion (ROM). Next, relaxation of the pectoralis major may be combined with feedback training for various active movements of the shoulder.

Elbow and Forearm

Problems include insufficient recruitment or relaxation of the elbow flexors or extensors to produce complete active ROM. The flexors generally have the greatest problem relaxing during passive stretch, whereas all muscles may require training during active movement. Relaxation training begins with the muscles to be trained positioned in a shortened position, the forearm well supported, and the patient comfortably seated. The previously described steps of training at rest, during distraction, and during static and dynamic stretching are then followed.

Dual-channel monitoring may be used to train for reciprocal relaxation and recruitment between the elbow flexors and extensors. Movements through small and relatively easy segments of the range are practiced—first one way and then the other. The patient recruits the agonist while maintaining relaxation of the antagonist, silencing the agonist activity each time before attempting the reversal of activity. A skateboard during the initial stages of movement training to reduce friction, as well as various supplementary techniques, can be used to facilitate a poorly recruited muscle (e.g., vibration, quick stretching, tapping, resistance) (60).

After training of isolated elbow flexion and extension, these movements are then combined with shoulder flexion. The patient slides a bean bag to a predetermined place on the table, and the task is made more difficult by increasing the distance or height of the object.

During all stages of training, an attempt is made to wean the patient from the feedback. If the performance deteriorates, or if we progress to a more difficult task, the feedback is reintroduced.

Position feedback is used during training of pronation and supination of the forearm because EMG activity from the pronators and supinators is difficult to isolate from other EMG activity present in the forearm. EMGBF may be combined with position feedback in cases of severe spasticity or flaccidity.

Combined Limb Movements

Finally, the patient must learn to combine dynamic control of the whole limb with perhaps only auditory EMG feedback from one elbow or shoulder muscle. For instance, the patient may be training to relax his biceps and maintain his forearm in a neutral or supinated position while reaching for an object. Threshold feedback from the forearm, reminding the patient to avoid pronation, may be combined with EMG feedback from the biceps to encourage relaxation. If the patient pronates the forearm or tenses the biceps, the respective feedback signals are triggered. The patient can then use this feedback to help shape the appropriate response (60).

Wrist and Fingers

Targeted training usually starts with relaxation of the frequently spastic wrist and finger flexors, which are monitored with one pair of electrodes placed over the center of the forearm flexor muscles.

First, the limb should be positioned so as to quiet the flexors. EMGBF, along with any other desired technique, can then be used to help train relaxation. Next, the patient attempts to maintain this relaxation of the forearm flexors during diversionary conversation and contralateral limb movements and as the wrist flexors are placed and maintained in progressively increased lengthened positions. The wrist and finger flexors are then stretched simultaneously.

Dynamic stretches are next introduced, first slow and then faster stretches of the wrist. Next, the fingers are stretched with the wrist in progressively increasing extension. This teaches a method of targeted relaxation of the forearm flexors, which can be practiced at home even without EMGBF to maintain or increase the passive ROM of the wrist and finger flexors. Next, relaxation of the forearm flexors may be combined with active wrist extension (60).

An isometric contraction against resistance appears to facilitate recruitment of the extensors. Targeted levels of EMG recruitment from the extensors are practiced while the patient maintains minimal levels of activity in the flexors. Facilitation techniques, such as tapping, quick stretches, or heavy resistance, may be observed, and feedback as well as changes in the limb position can be used to help reduce these synergistic patterns.

Initiating finger extension is often difficult for many patients. In chronic stroke patients (i.e., after 1 year), active finger extension is seldom attained in the absence of some active extension. In those who have some active finger extension, the results are encouraging. Marked improvements in movement and function have been noted with treatment. Training starts with the wrist and fingers flexed and progresses by increasing the amount of wrist extension. As with the wrist, various limb positions and facilitation techniques can be used in conjunction with the BF to train isolated finger extension (60).

The patient next progresses to controlling the proximal limb segments while training the wrist and fingers. Feedback from a proximal segment can be used while training the wrist and fingers. This may be followed by a combination of movements of the proximal and distal segments during functional activities.

Fine manipulative movements of the thumb are not only difficult to regain but are difficult to monitor for feedback training.

BIOFEEDBACK IN OTHER CONDITIONS

Spinal Cord Injuries

Except for the work of Wolf and various colleagues (61–66), reports of EMGBF for patients with SCIs are rather brief or limited to single-subject designs, but they are quite promising. Newton and Coolbaugh demonstrated substantial increases in active ROM and EMG output in the triceps brachii of a 25-year-old man with a fracture of the sixth cervical level (67). During feedback training, there was generalization to the flexor carpi radialis bilaterally. Dunn and colleagues demonstrated that muscle feedback was beneficial for three quadriplegic patients who gained control over the amplitude of their spasms when feedback was introduced (68). Inevitably, the presentation of a feedback signal resulted in voluntary reduction of integrated EMG. Unfortunately, removal of the feedback signal resulted in increased levels of EMG.

Rehabilitation researchers at Emory University have developed their own approach to treatment of SCI patients with EMG feedback (62). The principles embodied in the following discussion represent only one approach to interfacing patients with a modality. They are designed for patients with both acute and chronic SCI at virtually any level of the spinal cord who have demonstrable voluntary activity in muscles innervated by motor neurons below (i.e., caudal to) the site of injury. Feedback may be beneficial for these patients because the modality may be easily incorporated into exercise programs with immobilized patients during the acute phase of injury; it provides immediate information to the patient concerning the level of voluntary muscle activity; and, by so doing, this modality may help patients obtain spatial and temporal summation of muscle potentials leading toward increased contractility, and therefore preparing the patient for a more vigorous therapy program.

The primary goals for interfacing the SCI patient with EMG feedback are much the same as those outlined previously for stroke patients. First, attempts are made to reduce hypermotor responses to induced length changes in spastic muscles. Such hyperactive behavior of spastic muscles may occur during spontaneous episodes of clonus or during induced clonic seizures when the lower or upper extremity responds to various tactile stimuli.

Once the patient is able to reduce such responses in supine, sitting, and ultimately standing postures, efforts are directed toward recruitment of weak muscles. In treating patients with paraplegia, attempts are made to reduce activity in the adductors of the thigh and the gastrocnemius–soleus complex.

In partial lumbar SCI patients, feedback training at Emory University enabled many to increase the speed at which they ambulate and to reduce the number of required assistive devices. For quadriparetic patients with obvious voluntary movement, feedback combined with an exercise program facilitated active ROM and improved upper extremity function. However, in cases where little activity could be observed among chronic SCI patients, feedback provided little or no significant benefit toward restoration of function (61).

Cerebral Palsy and Traumatic Head Injuries

The clinical appearance of spastic patients and their difficulties with daily living are really due less to spasticity itself than to the related deficits in strength and control (69).

Holt argued that abnormal EMG activity of spastic muscles in children with cerebral palsy often cannot be reasonably attributed to exaggerated stretch reflex activity (70). Bobath maintains that abnormal muscle tone in individual muscles should not be the focus of treatment efforts (71). He has stressed the importance of overall postural and movement patterns in controlling the distribution of muscle tone and criticized the ''peripheral'' view of cerebral palsy, which explains overall abnormality as a summation of abnormal responses of individual muscles. Historically, neuromuscular re-education by physical therapists has moved steadily away from training of individual muscles to an increasing emphasis on patterns of posture and movement (72).

Harrison and Connolly trained four diplegic spastic subjects to discretely control very low amplitude spikes in spastic forearm muscles while inhibiting other EMG activity (73). They were uncertain that the spikes were single motor units because of limitations in the recording equipment.

Harrison later provided a particularly interesting series of experiments on the nature and limitations of control of spastic musculature and the effect of EMG feedback training (74). The spastic subjects are not described, but we can infer that they were adults with cerebral palsy. In Great Britain, the term "spastic" is often used to denote cerebral palsy. The spastic forearm flexor muscles were studied, and the same five spastic subjects were compared with normal subjects or with themselves after successive training interventions. These studies are too lengthy to detail here, except to indicate how EMGBF was used and what changes ensued.

Harrison compared normal and spastic subjects first on their ability to repeat muscular tension levels and then on scaling of muscular tension between minimum and maximum levels. Spastic subjects were significantly inferior on both tasks. Spastic subjects then repeated the muscular tension level repetition task, using a meter display of integrated EMG to guide their efforts; some improvement in accuracy of reproduction was noted. They then repeated the scaling study without feedback; the brief exposure to EMGBF produced a marked improvement in ranking and scaling of muscular tension efforts in some subjects.

Harrison then put all five spastic subjects through a training program to learn to produce three levels of integrated forearm EMG with stringent accuracy. The subjects did not receive concurrent feedback but were told by the experimenter immediately after each training trial whether the effort was too high, too low, or correct. Training continued until subjects could respond correctly for several successive trials. After this training, the spastic patients were retested without any feedback on the scaling task. All five subjects now did quite well at ranking and scaling their efforts.

Harrison also compared the amount of time required by normal and spastic subjects to relax the spastic forearm muscles thoroughly after tensing to various specified levels. Spastic subjects took significantly longer to achieve complete relaxation. All subjects quickly relaxed to just above baseline and spent most of their time eliminating the low level of remaining activity. The experiment was repeated for the five spastic subjects with use of a meter to provide EMG feedback. They halved their relaxation times but were still more then twice as slow as normal subjects working without feedback.

The five spastic subjects and five normal subjects were then tested on their forearm activity for 10 seconds without feedback. Normal subjects could maintain various levels accurately with little deviation. Spastic subjects deviated more and failed to check a gradual reduction in EMG activity during the 10-second period. The spastic subjects repeated this experiment using EMGBF from a meter. There was a significant improvement in their accuracy, although their efforts still tended to fall away from the target levels during the 10-second period.

Special devices for head position monitoring and control of drooling also have been used with children who have cerebral palsy, but formal studies are sparse.

Multiple Sclerosis

Ladd and colleagues applied the EMGBF technique to patients with spastic paraparesis from MS (75). The soleus muscle was used for training because it was the most spastic. Before administration of an antispasticity drug (Dantrium, Proctor & Gamble Pharmaceuticals, Cincinnati, OH), four of the eight subjects were able to isolate a single motor unit; with Dantrium, seven of the eight patients could do so. Reviewing results from all four tests, the authors concluded that the ability of patients to establish voluntary control over fine neuromuscular activity in the spastic soleus was considerably inferior to that of normal subjects, but this ability was significantly improved to near that of normals by Dantrium.

My own experience with many inpatients and outpatients with MS has persuaded me that the abnormal fatigue induced by any form of training reduces the usefulness of EMGBF for motor retraining. However, in selected patients it may be useful in training muscle relaxation of mild spasticity and of general tenseness. For moderate and marked spasticity, I do not advocate EMGBF, preferring one or another of the specific antispasticity drugs.

Dystonias and Dyskinesias

Ignoring the many conflicting theories of etiology that provide no clear guides to therapy, we briefly discuss here a number of movement disorders that have responded well to behavioral therapy featuring EMGBF. They present themselves mainly in isolated muscle groups; spasmodic torticollis is the best example, but also included are the rarer blepharospasm, hemifacial spasm, oromandibular dystonia, writer's cramp, and severe torsional dystonias of the torso (i.e., malignant dystonia musculorum deformans). Many brief case studies have been reported. The most thorough studies of many patients successfully treated with EMGBF combined with other behavioral techniques were reported by Brudny and colleagues (76) and by Cleeland (77). Cleeland's thorough summary (78) is recommended. Cleeland also has reported some success with the symptoms of Parkinsonism. One of my very serious cases, a young woman with dystonia musculorum deformans, responded with a complete "cure" after a lengthy program of EMGBF training in the early 1980s. This case study was documented with videotapes but never formally reported in the literature.

Peripheral Nerve Denervation

Booker and colleagues (79) and our group at Emory University (80) described patients with paralysis resulting from a facial nerve lesion in whom a portion of the 11th or 12th cranial nerve was anastomosed to the distal segment of the facial nerve. After EMGBF training, there was substantial improvement in facial symmetry and voluntary functions.

This form of neuromuscular re-education allows the patient to process visual and auditory signals representing continuous covert physiologic events of which he would normally be unaware. The procedure permits the patient to gain functional control of a muscle or muscle groups by monitoring motor unit activity. With available feedback alternatives, each patient can first learn to activate a few motor units and subsequently produce a partial movement.

Pain Management and Biofeedback

Elsewhere in this book the comprehensive treatment management of chronic pain (see Chapter 56) and of spinal pain (see Chapter 57) are covered. In this chapter, it is appropriate to note that related disciplines, especially psychotherapy and pain clinics, widely use EMGBF for relaxation—both general and specific (5). In addition, skin temperature feedback training is used for treating pain conditions normally not seen by rehabilitation clinicians (e.g., migraine) with generally good results (5). The present level of confidence in the outcomes remains controversial.

Acute and chronic back pain treatment with targeted EMGBF remains controversial. More recently, there has been widespread interest among clinical psychologists and chiropractors in treating back pain with surface EMG training of back muscles (which are believed to be in asymmetrical states of contraction). In view of the widespread interest at this writing, a group of which I am co-director is currently conducting a large randomized controlled study of two opposite forms of lumbar EMG and an untreated control group of patients. Results are not expected until after the publication date of this book.

Orthopedic Rehabilitation

Feedback Goniometers

These devices have been successfully used in retraining of hand function after reparative surgery (81–83) of traumatized fingers and their motor nerves. Active ROM exercises and related activities are an important means of applying progressive stress to induce remodeling of various tissues that restrict ROM in the hand and wrist. Supplying joint-angle feedback to patients as they exercise can help them more consistently reach the therapist. To accomplish this aim, feedback goniometers have been developed that are worn on the hand during exercise and therapeutic activities. These devices supply a threshold feedback signal when a predetermined joint angle is attained. Clinical trials indicate that many patients in a comprehensive hand rehabilitation program after injuries or corrective surgery will improve somewhat more in active ROM if they use feedback goniometers while exercising.

Other portions of the musculoskeletal system are also targets for EMGBF. For example, Draper and Ballard showed in a controlled study that BF alone is more effective than electrical stimulation alone in the recovery of the peak torque or force of extension of the knee after anterior cruciate ligament surgery (84). However, they conceded that an aggressive rehabilitation program coupled with EMGBF would be preferable to the experimental situation.

SUMMARY AND CONCLUSIONS

Clinical BF, particularly EMGBF, is finally melding into the practice of physicians, psychotherapists, and therapists in rehabilitation medicine. The major application undoubtedly is in retraining motor skills and inhibiting spasticity arising from brain injuries of all types and at all ages. A wide variety of other conditions usually considered resistant to therapy are also improved by feedback training of various kinds. These are based on pick-up from electronic sensors of physiologic functions ranging from skin temperature to pressure and joint-angle changes. No longer a novelty, BF is an important adjunct to the tools of the rehabilitation team. Unlike almost all of the rehabilitation therapies, it has had intensive scientific scrutiny with controlled studies from its very beginnings, and ineffective procedures are being weeded out. As with all rehabilitation (85), many more randomized controlled studies are needed for all applications of BF in rehabilitation.

REFERENCES

1. Basmajian JV. Control and training of individual motor units. *Science* 1963; 141:440–441.
2. Basmajian JV. *Muscles alive: their functions revealed by electromyography,* 1st ed. Baltimore: Williams & Wilkins, 1962.
3. Basmajian JV, Kukulka CG, Narayan MG, Takebe K. Biofeedback treatment of foot-drop after stroke compared with standard rehabilitation technique: effects on voluntary control and strength. *Arch Phys Med Rehabil* 1975; 56:231–236.
4. Basmajian JV, DeLuca CJ. *Muscles alive,* 5th ed. Baltimore: Williams & Wilkins, 1985.
5. Basmajian JV, ed. *Biofeedback: principles and practice for clinicians,* 3rd ed. Baltimore: Williams & Wilkins, 1989.
6. Leiper CI, Miller A, Lang J, Herman R. Sensory feedback for head control in cerebral palsy. *Phys Ther* 1981; 61:512–518.
7. Brown DM, DeBacher GA, Basmajian JV. Feedback goniometers for hand rehabilitation. *Am J Occup Ther* 1979; 33:456–463.
8. Wooldridge CP, Leiper C, Ogston DG. Biofeedback training of knee joint position of the cerebral palsied child. *Physiother Can* 1976; 28: 138–143.
9. Koheil R, Mandel AR. Joint position biofeedback facilitation of physical therapy in gait training. *Am J Phys Med* 1980; 59:288–297.
10. Mandel AR, Nymark JR, Balmer SJ, et al. Electromyographic versus rhythmic positional biofeedback in computerized gait retraining with stroke patients. *Arch Phys Med Rehabil* 1990; 71:649–654.
11. Fernie G, Holden J, Soto M. Biofeedback training of knee control in the above-knee amputee. *Am J Phys Med* 1978; 57:161–166.
12. Wannstedt GT, Herman R. Use of augmented sensory feedback to achieve symmetrical standing. *Phys Ther* 1978; 58:553–559.
13. Seeger BR, Caudrey DJ, Scholes JR. Biofeedback therapy to achieve symmetrical gait in hemiplegic cerebral palsied children. *Arch Phys Med Rehabil* 1981; 62:364–368.
14. Wolf SL, Binder-MacLeod SA. Use of the Krusen Limb Load Monitor

to quantify temporal and loading measurements of gait. *Phys Ther* 1982; 61:976–982.
15. Shumway-Cook A, Anson D, Haller S. Postural sway biofeedback: its effect on re-establishing stancestability in hemiplegic patients. *Arch Phys Med Rehabil* 1988; 69:395–400.
16. Hocherman S, Dickstein R, Pillar T. Platform training and postural stability in hemiplegia. *Arch Phys Med Rehabil* 1984; 65:588–592.
17. Winstein CJ, Gardner ER, McNeal DR, et al. Standing balance training: effect on balance and locomotion in hemiparetic adults. *Arch Phys Med Rehabil* 1988; 70:755–762.
18. Jacobson E. Electrical measurements concerning muscular contraction (tonus) and the cultivation of relaxation in man. *Am J Physiol* 1933; 1207:230–248.
19. Schultz JH, Luthe W. *Autogenic training.* New York: Grune & Stratton, 1959.
20. Luthe W. *Autogenic therapies.* Vols. 1–6. New York: Grune & Stratton, 1969.
21. Smith OC. Action potentials from single motor units in voluntary contraction. *Am J Physiol* 1934; 108:629–638.
22. Lindsley DB. Electrical activity of human motor units during voluntary contraction. *Am J Physiol* 1935; 114:90–99.
23. Gilson AS, Mills WB. Activities of single motor units in men during slight voluntary efforts. *Am J Physiol* 1941; 133:658–669.
24. Harrison VF, Mortensen OA. Identification and voluntary control of single motor unit activity in the tibialis anterior muscle. *Anat Rec* 1962; 144:109–116.
25. Basmajian JV. New views on muscular tone and relaxation. *Can Med Assoc J* 1957; 77:203–205.
26. Budzynski TH, Stoyva JM, Adler CS, Mullaney DJ. EMG biofeedback and tension headache: a controlled outcome study. *Psychosom Med* 1973; 35:484–496.
27. Miller NE, Bunuazizi A. Instrumental learning by curarized rates of a specific visceral response, intestinal or cardiac. *J Comp Psychol* 1968; 65:1–7.
28. Miller NE. Biofeedback and visceral learning. *Annu Rev Psychol* 1978; 29:373–404.
29. Miller NE. Biomedical foundation for biofeedback as a part of behavioral medicine. In: Basmajian JV, ed. *Biofeedback: principles and practice for clinicians,* 3rd ed. Baltimore: Williams & Wilkins, 1989; 5–16.
30. Johnson HE, Hockersmith V. Therapeutic electromyography in chronic back pain. In: Basmajian JV, ed. *Biofeedback: principles and practice for clinicians,* 3rd ed. Baltimore: Williams & Wilkins, 1989; 311–316.
31. Sedlacek K. Biofeedback treatment of primary Raynaud's disease. In: Basmajian JV, ed. *Biofeedback: principles and practice for clinicians,* 3rd ed. Baltimore: Williams & Wilkins, 1989; 317–322.
32. Schuster MM. Operant conditioning in gastrointestinal dysfunction. *Hosp Pract* 1974; 9:135.
33. Schuster MM. Biofeedback control of gastrointestinal motility. In: Basmajian JV, ed. *Biofeedback: principles and practice for clinicians,* 3rd ed. Baltimore: Williams & Wilkins, 1989; 273–280.
34. Campbell D. Biofeedback training of the pelvic floor and incontinence. In: Basmajian JV, ed. *Biofeedback: principles and practice for clinicians,* 3rd ed. Baltimore: Williams & Wilkins, 1989; 281–286.
35. Norris PA. Clinical psychoimmunology: strategies for self-regulation of immune system responding. In: Basmajian JV, ed. *Biofeedback: principles and practice for clinicians,* 3rd ed. Baltimore: Williams & Wilkins, 1989; 57–66.
36. Smith GR Jr. Intentional psychological modulation of the immune system. In: Basmajian JV, ed. *Biofeedback: principles and practice for clinicians,* 3rd ed. Baltimore: Williams & Wilkins, 1989; 49–56.
37. Carman BG, Ryan G. Electromyographic biofeedback and the treatment of communication disorders. In: Basmajian JV, ed. *Biofeedback: principles and practice for clinicians,* 3rd ed. Baltimore: Williams & Wilkins, 1989; 287–296.
38. Basmajian JV. The problem of the placebo in rehabilitation. *Physiother Can* 1978; 30:246–248.
39. Wolf SL, Binder-MacLeod SA. Neurophysiologic factors in electromyographic feedback for neuromotor disturbances. In: Basmajian JV, ed. *Biofeedback: principles and practice for clinicians,* 3rd ed. Baltimore: Williams & Wilkins, 1989; 17–36.
40. Wolf SL, Baker MP, Kelly JL. EMG biofeedback in stroke: effect of patient characteristics. *Arch Phys Med Rehabil* 1979; 60:96–103.
41. Wolf SL, Baker MP, Kelly JL. EMG biofeedback in stroke: a one-year follow-up of the effect on patient characteristics. *Arch Phys Med Rehabil* 1980; 61:351–355.
42. Heckathorne CW, Childress DS. Relationships of the surface EMG to the force, length, velocity, and contraction rate of the cineplastic human biceps. *Am J Phys Med* 1981; 60:1–17.
43. Bowman BR, Baker LL, Waters RL. Positional biofeedback and electrical stimulation: an automated treatment for the hemiplegic wrist. *Arch Phys Med Rehabil* 1979; 60:497–502.
44. Winchester P, Montgomery J, Bowman B, Hislop H. Effects of feedback stimulation training and cyclical electrical stimulation in knee extension in hemiplegic patients. *Phys Ther* 1983; 63:1096–1103.
45. Cozean CD, Pease WS, Hubbell SL. Biofeedback and functional electrical stimulation in stroke rehabilitation. *Arch Phys Med Rehabil* 1988; 69:401–405.
46. Krafft GH, Fitts SS, Hammond MC. Techniques to improve function of the arm in chronic hemiplegics. *Arch Phys Med Rehabil* 1992; 73: 220–227.
47. Brunnstrom S. *Movement therapy in hemiplegia: a neurophysiological approach.* New York: Harper & Row, 1970.
48. Baker MP, Hudson JE, Wolf SL. A "feedback" cane to improve the hemiplegic patient's gait. *Phys Ther* 1979; 59:170–171.
49. Wolf SL, Hudson JE. Feedback signal based upon force and time delay. *Phys Ther* 1980; 60:1289–1290.
50. Basmajian JV. Biofeedback in rehabilitation: review of principles and practices. *Arch Phys Med Rehabil* 1981; 62:469–475.
51. Schleenbaker RE, Mainous AG III. Electromyographic biofeedback for neuromuscular re-education in the hemiplegic stroke patient: a meta-analysis. *Arch Phys Med Rehabil* 1993; 74:1301–1304.
52. Moreland J, Thompson MA. Efficacy of electromyographic biofeedback compared with conventional physical therapy for upper-extremity function in patients following stroke: a research overview and meta-analysis. *Phys Ther* 1994; 74:534–547.
53. Glanz M, Klawansky S, Stason W, Berkey C, Shah N, Phan H, Chalmbers TC. Biofeedback therapy in post-stroke rehabilitation: a meta-analysis of the randomized controlled trials. *Arch Phys Med Rehabil* 1995; 76:508–515.
54. Basmajian JV, Gowland C, Brandstater ME, Swanson L, Trotter J. EMG feedback treatment of upper limb in hemiplegic stroke patients: pilot study. *Arch Phys Med Rehabil* 1982; 63:613–616.
55. Wolf SL, Binder-MacLeod SA. Electromyographic biofeedback applications to hemiplegic patient: changes in upper extremity neuromuscular and functional status. *Phys Ther* 1983; 63:1404–1413.
56. Inglis J, Donald MW, Monga TN, Sproule M, Young MJ. Electromyographic biofeedback and physical therapy of hemiplegic upper limb. *Arch Phys Med Rehabil* 1984; 65:755–759.
57. Basmajian JV, Gowland CA, Finlayson AJ, et al. Stroke treatment: comparison of integrated behavioral-physical therapy vs traditional physical therapy programs. *Arch Phys Med Rehabil* 1987; 68:267–272.
58. Gowland C, deBruin H, Basmajian JV, Plews N, Burcea I. Agonist and antagonist activity during voluntary upper-limb movement in patients with stroke. *Phys Ther* 1992; 72:624–633.
59. Bobath B. *Adult hemiplegia: evaluation and treatment.* London: William Heinemann Medical, 1978.
60. Binder-MacLeod SA. Biofeedback in stroke rehabilitation. In: Basmajian JV, ed. *Biofeedback: principles and practice for clinicians,* 2nd ed. Baltimore: Williams & Wilkins, 1983; 73–89.
61. Nacht MB, Wolf SL, Coogler CE. Use of electromyographic biofeedback during the acute phase of spinal cord injury. *Phys Ther* 1982; 62: 290–294.
62. Wolf SL. Electromyographic feedback for spinal cord injured patients: a realistic perspective. In: Basmajian JV, ed. *Biofeedback: principles and practice for clinicians,* 2nd ed. Baltimore: Williams & Wilkins, 1983; 130–134.
63. Wolf SL, Catlin PA, Blanton S, Edelman J, Lehrer N, Schroeder D. Overcoming limitations in elbow movement in the presence of antagonist hyperactivity. *Phys Ther* 1994; 74:35–44.
64. Segal RL, Wolf SL. Operant conditioning of spinal stretch reflexes in patients with spinal cord injuries. *Exp Neurol* 1994; 130:202–213.
65. Wolf SL, Segal RL, Heter ND, Catlin PA. Contralateral and long latency effects of human biceps brachii stretch reflex conditioning. *Exp Brain Res* 1995; 197:96–102.
66. Wolf SL, Segal RL. Downtraining human biceps-brachii spinal stretch reflexes. *J Neurophysiol* 1996; 75:1637–1645.
67. Newton FA, Coolbaugh CF. Bilateral EMG biofeedback training of

the triceps brachii and generalization effects in a quadriplegic. *Biofeedback Self Regul* 1981; 6:434–435.

68. Dunn M, Davis J, Webster T. Voluntary control of muscle spasticity with EMG biofeedback in three spinal cord injured quadriplegics. *Proceedings of the Ninth Annual Meeting of the Biofeedback Society of America*. Albuquerque, NM, 1970; 122.
69. DeBacher G. Biofeedback in spasticity control. In: Basmajian JV, ed. *Biofeedback: principles and practice for clinicians,* 2nd ed. Baltimore: Williams & Wilkins, 1983; 141–151.
70. Holt KS. Facts and fallacies about neuromuscular function in cerebral palsy as revealed by electromyography. *Dev Med Child Neurol* 1966; 8:255–268.
71. Bobath K. The motor deficit in patients with cerebral palsy. In: *Clinics in Developmental Medicine No. 23: Spastics Society Medical Education and Information Units.* London: Heinemann, 1966.
72. Basmajian JV. Neuromuscular facilitation technique. *Arch Phys Med Rehabil* 1971; 52:40–42.
73. Harrison A, Connolly K. The conscious control of fine levels of neuromuscular firing in spastic and normal subjects. *Dev Med Child Neurol* 1972; 13:762–771.
74. Harrison A. Studies of neuromuscular control in normal and spastic individuals, and training spastic individuals to achieve better neuromuscular control using electromyographic feedback. *Clin Dev Med* 1975; 55:51–101.
75. Ladd H, Oist C, Jonsson B. The effect of Dantrium on spasticity in multiple sclerosis. *Acta Neurol Scand* 1974; 50:397–408.
76. Brudny J, Korein J, Grynbaum BB, et al. EMG feedback therapy: review of treatment of 114 patients. *Arch Phys Med Rehabil* 1976; 57: 55–61.
77. Cleeland CS. Behavioral technics in the modification of spasmodic torticollis. *Neurology* 1973; 23:1241–1247.
78. Cleeland CS. Biofeedback and other behavioral techniques in the treatment of disorders of voluntary movement. In: Basmajian JV, ed. *Biofeedback: principles and practice for clinicians,* 2nd ed. Baltimore: Williams & Wilkins, 1983; 135–148.
79. Booker HE, Robow RT, Coleman PJ. Simplified feedback in neuromuscular retraining in automated approach using electromyographic signals. *Arch Phys Med Rehabil* 1969; 50:621–625.
80. Brown DM, Nahai F, Wolf S, Basmajian JV. Electromyographic feedback in the re-education of facial palsy. *Am J Phys Med* 1978; 57:183.
81. Brown DM, DeBacher GA, Basmajian JV. Feedback goniometers for hand rehabilitation. *Am J Occup Ther* 1979; 30:458–463.
82. Brown DM, Nahai F. Biofeedback strategies of the occupational therapist in total hand rehabilitation. In: Basmajian JV, ed. *Biofeedback: principles and practice for clinicians,* 2nd ed. Baltimore: Williams & Wilkins, 1983; 90–106.
83. DeBacher G. Feedback goniometers for rehabilitation. In: Basmajian JV, ed. *Biofeedback: principles and practice for clinicians,* 2nd ed. Baltimore: Williams & Wilkins, 1983; 352–362.
84. Draper V, Ballard L. Electrical stimulation versus electromyographic biofeedback in the recovery of quadriceps femoris muscle function following anterior cruciate ligament surgery. *Phys Ther* 1991; 71: 455–464.
85. Basmajian JV, Banerjee SN. *Clinical decision making in rehabilitation: efficacy and outcomes.* New York: Churchill Livingstone, 1996.

Rehabilitation Medicine: Principles and Practice, Third Edition,
edited by Joel A. DeLisa and Bruce M. Gans.
Lippincott–Raven Publishers, Philadelphia © 1998.

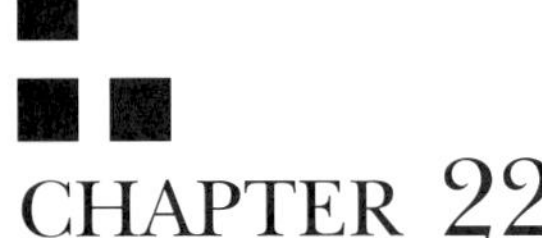

CHAPTER 22

Manipulation, Massage, and Traction

James J. Rechtien, Michael Andary, Todd G. Holmes, and J. Michael Wieting

The treatment modalities discussed in this chapter have been used for several thousand years. Each has been used in various forms throughout the world, having arisen independently in one civilization after another. Traction, manipulation, and massage are all treatments for the relief of painful conditions—sometimes with noticeable immediate effects—that are sought after by an ever-increasing number of people. Despite these favorable factors, complete acceptance within the medical community has not been forthcoming.

At best, the medical community does not uniformly accept the efficacy of these modalities. A discussion of manipulation, for example, rarely fails to evoke strong feelings. Proponents note that over 90 million manipulations are performed yearly in the United States alone (1), that patients generally feel better after a series of manipulations, and that complications rarely arise, and only then because of an unqualified practitioner performing an inappropriate maneuver. Opponents argue that patients who improve with manipulation would have done so anyway; that complications, although rare, are often grievous and sometimes fatal; that treatments are aimed at the pocketbook and not the pain; and that claims of success, especially concerning visceral, nonmuscloskeletal disorders, are totally unproven (2). The recent Agency for Health Care Policy Research (AHCPR) (3) recommendations that include manipulation as an option in acute low back pain management have done little to resolve these differences (4).

What has led to the apparently dichotomous thinking among some physiatrists who dismiss manipulation but accept other treatments such as transcutaneous electrical nerve stimulation (TENS), when neither has been proven scientifically to be efficacious? One reason may be that the traditional, allopathic medical community looks askance at any modality of treatment not developed by its own members. Traction, manipulation, and massage, described centuries to millennia ago, fit into that category. In addition, they are treatments that can be performed by nonphysicians, particularly manipulation and massage. A treatment appears less scientific and perhaps less efficacious if it can be obtained from nonphysician, even nonlicensed, practitioners. A more acceptable rationale for rejecting these treatments may be the lack of scientific proof of benefit. The principles of traction are the most well established of the three modalities, and are based on objective experimental data. Not surprisingly, use of traction among allopathic physicians is less controversial than use of manipulation.

The use of any treatment should be limited to those conditions that can reasonably be expected to improve with the physiologic effects of that treatment. The macroscopic effects of traction and massage have been well elucidated and offer reliable guidance regarding indications. This is not yet true for manipulation, and empirical findings and speculation are largely responsible for shaping the clinician's opinion.

MANIPULATION

Although spinal manipulation has been practiced in almost all countries of the world since at least the time of Hippocrates (5), the subject rarely fails to evoke strong emotional responses among health care professionals, particularly in the United States and Great Britain. Since the 1890s, when manipulation became a cornerstone of the therapeutic approach of the Osteopathic and Chiropractic Schools of Medicine, the subject has polarized physicians to the point where dialogue has often been impossible. Proponents note the rapid and continuing growth of the use of manual care and the ever-increasing public constituency that seeks it, whereas opponents point to the relative lack of proof of efficacy and the rare, but occasionally catastrophic, complica-

J. J. Rechtien, M. Andary and J. M. Wieting: Department of Physical Medicine and Rehabilitation, Michigan State University, College of Osteopathic Medicine, East Lansing, Michigan 48824.
T. G. Holmes: Department of Physical Medicine and Rehabilitation, Michigan State University, College of Osteopathic Medicine, East Lansing, Michigan 48824; and Sister Kenny Institute, Minneapolis, Minnesota 55407.

tion. Medical common sense ensures that a middle ground exists between ''it cures nothing'' and ''it cures everything,'' but few data exist to help establish this.

Some of this divergence of viewpoint can be explained by the fact that each group purports to treat the other's failures. The fact that manipulation requires skills significantly different from those acquired in most allopathic medical schools serves to separate practitioners who possess those skills from those who do not. In continental Europe, professional conflict has been relatively absent; the discussion of manipulation (6), although not uniformly welcomed, has developed in an anger-free, knowledge-seeking environment.

Osteopathic and chiropractic physicians perform spinal manipulation for a number of different reasons (7). The facts pertinent to physiatry are provided as follows.

> Most of the 90 million annual chiropractic manipulations performed in the United States (1), and probably most manipulations by practitioners of other disciplines, are for complaints of musculoskeletal pain in the back and neck. Spinal manipulation is neither chiropractic nor osteopathic *per se*, but is an application of forces to the muscles, tendons, ligaments, joints and capsules, bones, and cartilage of the vertebral column or related tissues, which has as a major goal the restoration of normal spinal motion and the elimination of pain secondary to disturbed biomechanics.

Most physiatrists see patients who present with problems potentially treatable by spinal manipulation. In fact, many patients treated by physiatrists have had or soon will undergo manipulation. At the very least, therefore, all physiatrists should know the types of manipulation their patients might encounter, along with associated contraindications. Only some physiatrists will actively refer patients, usually those who fail to improve with initial therapeutic interventions, to practitioners of manipulation, and fewer still will incorporate manipulation into their own practice of physiatry.

This section will provide some of the information the practitioner needs to rationally select one of the above relationships to spinal manipulative therapy. After proposing a definition, three major factors involved in the choice will be discussed.

1. Perceived risk-to-benefit ratio
2. Perceived need
3. The availability of manipulation to patients.

Definition

The definition of manipulation is controversial, but a consensus definition is that it is ''the use of the hands in a patient's management process using instructions and maneuvers to achieve maximal painless movement of the musculoskeletal system and postural balance'' (8). That definition is too broad for the purposes of this chapter, where the following definition will be used. Spinal manipulation is ''a passive mechanical treatment applied to a specific vertebra or vertebral region, including the sacroiliac region and the rib cage, by a physician or therapist with the primary goal of restoration of lost vertebral motion.'' Nonthrust techniques, (''mobilization'' to a physical therapist) are encompassed by this definition. Active exercise, self-applied forces, or self-induced motion, although occasionally effective in the restoration of vertebral hypomobility, and nonspinal articulation techniques are not included. Massage, which is applied only to soft tissue, and traction, which is nonspecific to a vertebral region, are excluded by this definition, although the reader will recognize that some overlap among manipulation, traction, and massage occurs. The interested reader will find a detailed history of manipulation in a number of sources (5,9,10,11).

Choosing Manipulation

Risks and Benefits

Few risks are involved in spinal manipulative therapy. Complications resulting from isometric or articulatory treatment have not been reported. There are reports of complications of thrust manipulation, but the number of reported problems, which is in the hundreds (12), is actually quite small considering that at least 90 million manipulations are performed annually in the United States alone. In addition, as will be discussed, most of these complications probably are avoidable.

Osteopathic and chiropractic proponents of spinal manipulative therapy believe in distant visceral benefits, beyond the systemic benefits produced by good structural and biomechanical efficiency and relief of pain (7). However, distant visceral complications temporally related to manipulation have been documented only twice in the last 100 years (13,14); therefore, the physiatrist may safely evaluate the benefits or detriments of manipulation solely on musculoskeletal results.

Benefits of manipulation have not been definitively proven. Proponents anecdotally report excellent results in treating acute musculoskeletal problems, and good results in treating chronic conditions. Empirically, these outcomes are comparable with those achieved with ''conventional'' modalities, which also often carry no proof of efficacy. If nothing else, the growing number of patients obtaining manipulative therapy indicates a perceived benefit.

Applicability to a Physiatrist's Practice

A physiatrist who accepts the basic premises of manipulative therapy will be able to identify, via a focused examination, that subpopulation of patients most likely to benefit from a manipulative approach. Although some manipulative techniques may have hospital applicability, for example, rib mobilization in patients receiving respiratory therapy, most patients with conditions appropriate for manipulation are in the outpatient setting. This group includes people with structural problems such as pelvic asymmetries and vertebral rotations, and others whose diagnosis relies on palpatory expertise. Patients with chronic back pain might be referred for a course of manipulation in conjunction with epidural injections, TENS, psychological counseling, and other interventions.

Patient Selection

A general physiatric examination should be performed on every new patient. Any underlying impairment must be identified and treated, including fractures, disc herniations with neurologic signs and symptoms, and major sprains, strains, tears, hematomas, and joint injuries. Considerations of imaging and electromyography would be no different for the physician using forms of manipulation therapy than any other type of therapy intervention. For thrusting and articulatory manipulation there are specific contraindications that must be considered, discussed later in this chapter.

Next, the physiatrist contemplating manipulative intervention performs a focused, detailed vertebral structural examination in areas suggested by symptoms or by the general examination with the goal of finding treatable "manipulable lesions." This evaluation involves both careful observation and active gross spinal motion assessment as well as a palpatory and passive segmental vertebral motion examination. Subsequent success with manipulative therapy will depend on an accurate diagnosis of lost vertebral motion. The findings of palpation and segmental autonomic changes constitute the most important components of structural diagnosis.

The factors generally sought on the vertebral or segmental levels are asymmetry of bony structures, restriction of vertebral motion relative to adjacent vertebrae in any of the three planes (flexion, extension, side-bending, or rotation), and tissue texture changes (thought to be mediated by segmental autonomic reflexes). Local tenderness on palpation or induced motion is a component identified by many authors as important or even essential (15).

Tenderness elicited by pressure over vertebral processes or by induced vertebral motion is noted (16). Passive vertebral motion is evaluated for range, symmetry, and the force needed to achieve full range (17). The latter is discussed in the literature as the quality or feel of motion (1,18). Combinations of vertebral motions, such as flexion and rotation, are examined. Springing of the vertebra (1) and tenderness elicited by local pressure on the interspinous ligament (19) are useful clues to dysfunctional conditions and loss of joint play. Subcutaneous tissue texture changes (e.g., edema, fibrosis) (1), noted by palpation and skin rolling (20), are signs of dysfunction, and some manipulators look carefully for segmental autonomic changes such as perspiration (21) and hyperemic response to a light scratch. The ribs, occiput, and pelvis often need to be included in this part of the examination. Vertebrae identified by positive findings in this type of examination are considered dysfunctional and, if the result is relative hypomobility, are candidates for manipulation unless contraindications exist.

Hypermobile vertebral segments are themselves not amenable to manipulative therapy (9) but may signal the presence of hypomobile segments elsewhere in the spine. Hypermobile vertebrae should, therefore, prompt a search for reduced motion elsewhere. If nontender hypomobile segments are found, successful manipulation there could conceivably resolve a distant hypermobility. This interconnectedness of the vertebrae is one of the features that makes dysfunctions of the spine difficult yet fascinating to study.

A structural examination of this type will add 5 to 10 minutes to an initial visit and less than 5 minutes to subsequent examinations. The physiatrist choosing to do manipulation will of course need to do this evaluation with a relatively high degree of acumen and skill. Physiatrists referring a patient to another physician or a therapist for manipulation can probably stop with identification of a hypomobile and/or tender segment and leave some of the detailed motion analysis to the person providing the manipulation. However, enough of the examination must be accomplished to identify the vertebral segment needing attention and to establish an endpoint of therapy that the physiatrist can verify.

Modes of Practice

Availability of spinal manipulative therapy depends on which mode of practice is chosen. Physiatrists who wish to use spinal manipulative therapy but not practice it themselves have two alternatives.

Referral to a Physician

The referral of the patient for concurrent manipulative care to another practitioner works well in some instances (22), but potential problems exist. Among these, other practitioners may consider themselves competent to care for the patient, so control of the patient can become an issue. This impediment may be addressed via a specific referral that states its exact nature and the scope of treatment requested, that encourages discussion with the referring physician, and that makes clear the intent of the physiatrist to resume the remainder of care. Furthermore, the physiatrist may not be able to assess the manipulator's competence, and, moreover, some patients may resent a referral to another practitioner.

Referral to a Licensed Nonphysician

The second option is for the physiatrist to diagnose the problem and write a prescription for manipulation to be performed by a licensed nonphysician, typically a physical therapist (16). As more nonphysicians acquire training in spinal manipulation, this becomes a viable option. In the United States, physical therapists traditionally have been limited to providing isometric and articulatory techniques, although strain–counterstrain and myofascial release techniques are becoming more popular. The manipulation can be provided as part of a comprehensive physical therapy program. Even with such a referral pattern, however, the physician must at least acquire basic palpatory diagnostic skills. This allows one to write a detailed prescription for an anatomic area to be treated and motion to be restored, along with the technique to be used, and frequency and length of treatment. The physician can then monitor progress of the therapy objectively and determine the endpoint and possible side effects or failure of the manipulation. Sequential monitoring of each manipulative intervention can be left to the therapist; this is acceptable, given the time course and safety of isometric and articulatory techniques. The acquisition of minimal diagnostic palpatory skills may take 1 to 2 weeks. However, the physiatrist probably will use these skills frequently and maintain them easily. The time commitment and economic investment are far less for this option than in the provision of manipulative therapy itself.

Most manipulators believe that restoration of the vertebral joint's normal passive and active ranges of motion and resting equilibrium position is the endpoint of treatment (17,23). In this view, spinal manipulative therapy is analogous to peripheral passive range of motion and end stretching. It is a natural extension of the physical therapy that physiatrists already prescribe for spine problems, as it simply addresses individual joints rather than the spine as a whole. The differences from the approach taken with peripheral joints are as follows:

1. Most patients cannot actively range specific vertebral joints, so passive ranging is necessary.
2. The vertebral bones have short lever arms and small normal ranges of motion, so loss of mobility is hard to detect compared to limbs.
3. Other vertebrae usually compensate for the loss of a single joint's mobility, so gross spinal motion often remains normal or nearly so.
4. Forceful thrusting maneuvers have been traditionally used in spinal manipulative therapy to restore range of motion, but this is less commonly done on the larger peripheral joints.

The practice of physician referral of patients to physical therapists for manipulative treatment is likely to become more common in the United States and to bring the benefits of spinal manipulative therapy to those patients who have chosen the traditional physiatric approach to health care for musculoskeletal problems. In some localities, referral to other licensed nonphysicians such as skilled athletic trainers may be appropriate.

Acquiring Manipulation Skills

There are three obstacles to the physiatrist performing manipulation:

1. Acquiring initial skills
2. Maintenance of skills
3. Economics of manipulation

Thrusting types of manipulation, because of significant forces involved and potential for harm, are best learned on volunteers, not patients, under the close direction of a skilled operator. Estimates of the minimum initial learning time required vary from 3 to 12 months (6,15). Even the lower estimates place this type of training out of the reach of most physiatrists. Because of their inherent safety, isometric/muscle energy and articulatory techniques sufficient for therapy initiation can be acquired by most in 1 to 2 weeks of formal course work. The training time for isometrics is shorter because an inappropriate or nonindicated isometric technique, unless repeated very frequently or over a prolonged period, rarely causes detrimental effects. Thus, the operator may begin working with patients early in training and develop improved techniques with time.

Postdoctoral programs such as those approved by the American Academy of Physical Medicine and Rehabilitation can provide a mechanism for the physiatrist to become acquainted with the skills necessary to begin manipulation. There are numerous other courses available which may also be of use to the physiatrist, but would have to be investigated individually. There is interest among physiatric residents in acquiring this type of training (24), which may lead to expanded training possibilities in the future.

Maintenance of skills is relatively easy for a full-time manipulator, but may be problematic for the physiatrist whose practice is general in nature or heavily hospital oriented. Manipulative skills are not comparable with those involved, for example, in riding a bicycle—infrequent use tends to decrease competence. The actual minimum frequency of use needed to maintain competence or excellence varies considerably from person to person. Clearly, however, the potential user should consider maintenance of skills before investing time and money in the acquisition of these skills. Closely tied to the frequency of use is the economics of performing this service. Manipulation, if done well, can be time consuming and reimbursement rates are extremely variable.

Although manipulation techniques can be studied by any physician, skillful manipulation is demanding, and not all physicians will derive satisfaction from providing it. Anecdotally, at least, manipulators who do not enjoy performing manipulation may not do it well.

Indications for Spinal Manipulative Therapy

Spinal manipulative therapy is applicable in all musculoskeletal pain problems of the back, pelvis, and neck in which loss of vertebral function or localized tenderness on induced motion may be a contributing factor, if there are no contraindications. Some recent injuries (fractures, tears, sprains, strains, disc herniations with neurologic signs, tumors, anomalies, joint disease, inflammation, stenosis) will not respond to manipulation because of the resultant hypermobility, or because local conditions constitute contraindications. Again, all visceral or systemic pathologic conditions must be excluded, or at least under concurrent care. As noted earlier, nontender vertebrae may be treated, but there is substantial controversy regarding this issue (25).

Another issue is manipulation for prophylaxis. Osteopathic and chiropractic physicians tend to treat vertebral motion restrictions in asymptomatic patients for these reasons: future stress in the form of mechanical use, systemic illness, psychogenic problems, or a loss of compensatory motion in an aging mechanical system will eventually cause problems in the restricted area; structural normality lessens metabolic demands; there may be visceral effects; and restrictions become fixed by fibrosis or a type of neurologic set (i.e., engram) if untreated. The individual physiatrist must decide how much of this philosophy to accept, and weigh this against the potential obstacles, e.g., third-party payors, time.

Side Effects

There are a number of reported side effects of spinal manipulative therapy (12). The most common is a transient increase in discomfort for 6 to 72 hours after therapy (26). This should resolve to a level less than that of the pretreatment pain and should be less of a problem with each successive treatment. Minor autonomic effects, such as increased perspiration and early or increased menses, have been reported (27).

Duration of Therapy

Thrusting has an immediate effect, and improvement should be seen within 1 week of initiation of therapy (20). Isometrics take longer and are often applied concurrently with physical therapy. However, lack of improvement in objective findings after 2 to 4 weeks would suggest the need to re-evaluate the diagnosis or therapeutic plan. Some problems do not resolve despite accurate diagnosis and treatment, but long-term therapy does appear to have some subjective value. Duration of therapy is decided on an individual basis.

Contraindications

Spinal manipulative techniques differ as to their degree of invasiveness. Because of the higher forces involved, thrust is considered the most invasive, whereas articulation, isometrics, and functional approaches are considered less invasive. The more invasive the approach, the more likely it is to be contraindicated. The literature concerning contraindications for thrusting techniques has been reviewed comprehensively by Kleynhans (12); contraindications to articulation are discussed by several investigators (18,28–31).

Absolute contraindications for manipulation, especially nonthrusting techniques, are rare, and relative contraindications are few in number. Clearly, manipulation should only be performed for a hypomobile vertebral segment that might respond to manipulation; therefore, accurate diagnosis is important. Inadequate skill of the practitioner is a major contraindication for all types of manipulation.

Articulation is contraindicated in the following:

- Vertebral malignancy
- Infection or inflammation
- Cauda equina syndrome
- Myelopathy or spondylosis
- Multiple adjacent radiculopathies
- Vertebral bone diseases
- Vertebral bony joint instability (e.g., fractures, dislocations)
- Rheumatoid disease in the cervical region

Thrust is clearly contraindicated in these cases, plus the following:

- Presence of spinal deformity and most anomalies
- Systemic anticoagulation, either disease-related or pharmacologic
- Severe diabetes
- Atherosclerosis
- Severe degenerative joint disease
- Vertigo or symptoms and signs of vertebral basilar disease or insufficiency (cervical region)
- Spondyloarthropathies (e.g., psoriatic, ankylosing spondylitis, Reiter's syndrome)
- Inactive rheumatoid disease
- Ligamentous joint instability or congenital joint laxity and syndromes such as Marfan, Ehlers-Danlos, and Down syndrome
- Aseptic necrosis
- Local aneurysm
- Osteomalacia
- Osteoporosis
- Acute disc herniation

Spondylolisthesis does not contraindicate manipulation localized to neighboring vertebrae. Excessive range of motion in a vertebral joint (i.e., hypermobility) of any cause is a contraindication to further manipulation of that joint (31,32).

Certain patients with a tendency toward obsessional neurosis and fixation on painful anatomic areas probably are poor candidates for thrust (18). In addition, some investigators consider the absence of any pain-free direction of vertebral motion a contraindication to thrust. Pregnancy with known threat of miscarriage is an absolute contraindication to manipulation. The normal low-risk pregnancy is discussed by Grieve (18), who avoids compressive and rotational thrusting techniques but performs very conservative mobilization techniques up to the eight month. Because the disturbed biomechanics and hormonal ligamentous interactions of pregnancy are frequently implicated in back pain of pregnancy, this subject continues to stimulate discussion in the literature (33–36).

Objective radicular signs are a contraindication to articulation or thrust. The question of manipulation for clearly defined root pain without objective neurologic findings is controversial (37), with some investigators avoiding rotational thrust in a side-lying position and others avoiding any forceful intervention at all. Isometrics in a nonlateral position appear to be safe, but there is no conclusive literature on this or any other contraindication to isometrics. Vertebral isometric techniques should not be used if the lesion would preclude passive range of motion, gentle stretching, or isometrics in a peripheral joint with the same condition. Catastrophic results do not occur in isometric techniques; some of the absolute contraindications to thrust and articulation, specifically osteoporosis, severe diabetes, rheumatoid disease distant from the cervical area, degenerative joint disease, and joint laxity, may become relative contraindications, and patients with these problems probably can be cautiously treated with isometrics. Concurrent active myositis may contraindicate isometrics because of the patient's active muscular contraction; however, functional techniques or counterstain could be safely applied in this condition. No contraindications for functional and counterstain techniques have been documented, but it would seem reasonable to assume these may parallel restrictions against massage, discussed later in the chapter.

Complications

Complications generally arise from performance of contraindicated procedures. There are no documented or anecdotal reports of complications arising from articular, isometric, counterstain, functional, soft-tissue, or myofascial release. The situation with craniosacral manipulation is best discussed with the description of that technique. Most reported complications, particularly the major disasters occurring after manipulation, often involve thrust techniques in the cervical region. In almost all cases, the neck was extended during the procedure and the complication was a vascular insult to the basilar system or the spinal cord (17,38–40). These extremely serious consequences of thrust manipulation, albeit disturbing, still appear to occur with a relatively low frequency, estimated by Powell et al. to be one case per 1 to 1.5 million manipulations (41). Recently Carlini has stated ". . . as to whether or not healthy patients should be concerned with the risk of cervical manipulation . . . I can only answer that the risk appears to be quite small" (42).

No cases of permanent problems after isometric cervical manipulation have been reported. It seems prudent, however, to exclude all patients with objective signs or symptoms referable either to the vertebrobasilar artery system, cervical spondylosis or instability from forceful cervical spinal manipulative therapy. Whether patients without signs or symptoms should receive provocative examinations such as those described by Bourdillon (17) and Maigne (26) is debatable, and is thoroughly discussed by Maigne (15). It should be remembered, though, that it is difficult to predict vertebrobasilar problems in the elderly even with provocative tests. Even if isometric techniques are used, excessive neck extension should be avoided.

Even if less invasive techniques are used in the cervical spine, risk to the patient is minimized by adhering to the following:

1. Proper positioning of the patient with avoidance of extremes of cervical flexion, extension, side-bending and rotation
2. Careful evaluation and treatment of patients with or suspected to have osteoporosis or spinal stenosis
3. The patient should be appropriately dressed, relaxed, able to breathe deeply, and able to experience unrestricted motion during the manipulation

Severe complications in lumbosacral manipulation are very rare and have been limited to thrust manipulation (43–45). Coincidental development of a disc syndrome during a course of manipulation has occurred, but has not been documented definitively in the literature. However, such a possibility emphasizes the need for the physiatrist to examine and document the vertebral dysfunction before and during the performance of spinal manipulative therapy. New incidents or complications appear in the literature sporadically (46), and have been reviewed elsewhere (40,47–49).

Techniques of Spinal Manipulative Therapy

In the following introductions to the most common techniques of spinal manipulation used in the United States, discussion is limited to those that the physiatrist is most likely to encounter early in the investigation of manipulative therapy.

Thrust

Other terms for thrust techniques (23,50–52) include impulse, which is of European origin (8), high velocity/low amplitude, adjustment, and spinal manipulative therapy (SMT), which are of chiropractic origin. In most approaches, the operator diagnoses the dysfunctional vertebral segment by identification of position or motion abnormalities or by related tissue changes, including tenderness to palpation or induced motion. He or she then rotates, side-bends, and flexes or extends the vertebral segments below it, thereby "locking" the facets so that further motion is limited to the vertebra in question. This vertebra is then passively moved to its limit of motion (i.e., its barrier) to remove all slack motion. A small force, localized to the joint in question and in the direction of the restricted motion, is applied to hold this position. Finally, a brief (53) controlled thrust is applied to the involved vertebra in the direction perceived as limited, and a small motion in the desired direction, either flexion, extension, rotation, or side-bending, occurs as the vertebra traverses the barrier (Fig. 22-1). Often an audible "pop" (54) or "click" (55) is produced. The source of this sound has been attributed to cavitation (56) and nitrogen release in the synovial facet joint. Its presence infers a mechanical process has occurred over a much shorter time than for inaudible events, e.g., reflex muscle contraction. This further

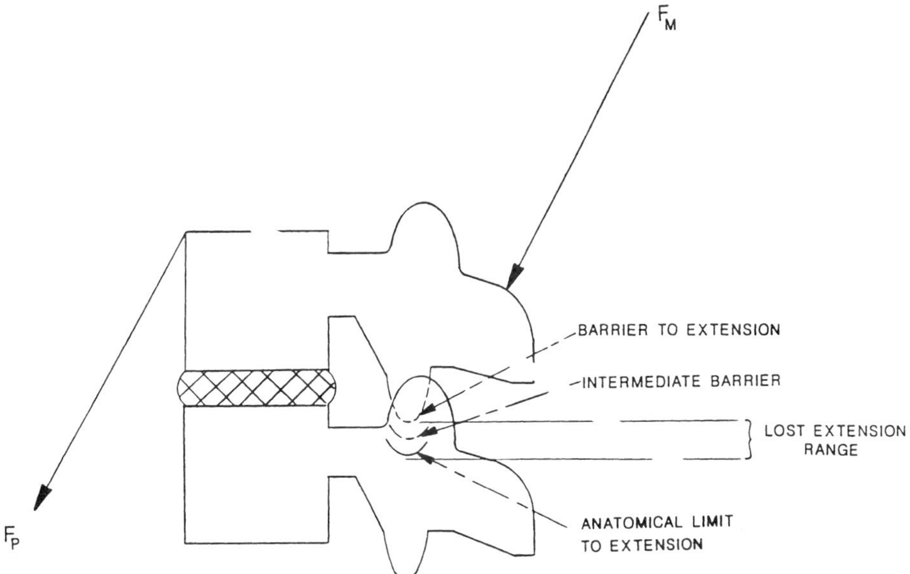

FIG. 22-1. In the thrust technique, the patient is relaxed and is not applying force *(Fp)*. The manipulator applies a quick force *(Fm)* in the direction shown, to extend the upper vertebrae to the anatomic limit in one motion. In the muscle energy technique, the manipulator applies force *(Fm)* and the patient contracts muscles with net force *(Fp)* in the directions shown so that no torque exists around the center of flexion–extension rotation. After 5 seconds patient and doctor relax, and a new extension barrier to passive range of motion nearer to the anatomic limit is found. Repeated manipulations will bring succeeding barriers closer to the normal passive anatomic limit.

suggests that audible thrusting procedures have a different mechanisms of action and possibly different efficacy of action compared with other manipulative procedures. It is arguable as to whether there is clinical relevance to this sound (15,36). The acceleration, forces, and durations of actions (57), and some displacement values (58) in thrusting techniques have been measured recently. The forces appear to peak in the range of 100–400 Newtons (59), occurring on a time scale of about 150 milliseconds.

If the force is applied over a spinous or transverse process, the procedure is known as a short-lever technique. If the force is applied distant from the vertebra through the locked vertebral column, the procedure is called a long-lever technique. All thrust techniques can do harm if the forces are misdirected or not well localized to the vertebra or vertebral region involved.

Some manipulators take up slack and apply thrust in a direction opposite the restriction (19,26). This type of approach, away from the restriction, is called an indirect technique. The success of this approach probably implies a facet-locking mechanism as opposed to a soft-tissue restriction source of dysfunction. Other manipulators work with less specificity, but may add traction and direct the thrust at relocating a bulging disc (60).

Articulatory

The articulatory technique (9,61,62), also called mobilization in Europe and low velocity/high amplitude in the United States, is very similar to oscillatory (28) techniques performed in Australia. The vertebral joint is passively moved within the reduced range defined by its resting position and the dysfunctional limit of motion. The extent of motion and its endpoint are varied according to a grading scheme, but ultimately the endpoint and dysfunctional barrier become the same, and the barrier is teased with repeated motion. Ideally, the quality or feel of the induced motion, as well as the quantity of force and excursion, are normalized by this procedure. Occasionally, a small amount of additional force takes the vertebra through its barrier or restriction, and this technique blends into thrust. Other variables include frequency of repetition, duration of "hold time" at the extremes, and velocity of motion. Oscillatory techniques are similar in that there are various magnitudes of pressure applied, but in these techniques, the pressure is applied and removed at a rate of 120 or more times a minute, for 15 to 20 seconds (54).

Positional Techniques

The underlying principle in counterstain and functional techniques is that the somatic dysfunction or hypomobility is caused by an inappropriately firing muscle, that is, active tissue, rather than a shortened passive tissue such as capsule, myofascia, or ligament. Thrust, articulation, and muscle energy techniques all employ forces that might be expected to lengthen shortened passive tissues, whereas the positioning techniques attempt to change an inappropriate engram of vertebral muscle behavior, similar to what is done in rehabilitation of head injury and tendon transplants.

Counterstrain

Counterstrain (9,63–66) is an indirect myofascial technique developed by Jones (67), that shares with functional technique (discussed elsewhere in this chapter) the emphasis on relative positioning of a joint or body part as an essential component of the actual therapy. Treatment involves placing the joint or body part into its position of maximal ease or comfort, relaxing myofascial or ligamentous soft tissues. This allows inappropriately shortened muscles (causing the somatic dysfunction) to "reset" their spindles, which then normalize their proprioceptive input to the spinal cord. Generally, the restricting muscle is overly shortened by this positioning (counterstain) and its antagonist muscle is gently over-stretched (strained) in the process. The treatment position is found by minimizing the pain associated with palpatory pressure over a "tender point" and once the position of maximum comfort is found, it is held for some 90 to 120 seconds with concurrent monitoring of the tender point (36). During this time the tenderness underneath the palpating hand should fade to at least 20% to 30% of its initial value. On occasion, small "fine tuning" passive repositioning movements with feedback from the patient may be needed. Because tenderness is a part of this feedback system, the patient must respond to the questions of the practitioner. The patient is then slowly returned to the neutral position, usually in one plane of motion at a time, to prevent resumption of the inappropriate muscle firing. Structural reassessment is then repeated.

Counterstain is considered indirect because, like functional technique, the positioning is always in a direction away from the restricted motion. If multiple tender points are present, the most tender is treated first, then the next most tender, etc.; areas of highest accumulation of tender points, proximally then distally, should then be treated (67).

The "tender points" essential to the treatment are found beneath the skin by palpatory examination over the shortened and restricted posterior muscles or over related anterior anatomic structures such as a muscle, tendon, and ligament. They do not coincide with the trigger points of Travell (68) or the similarly named tender points associated with fibromyalgia. The tender points of counterstain are usually small, discrete, fibrotic areas thought to be manifestations of distant somatic dysfunction; they are neither paired nor associated with the other signs of fibromyalgia such as stiffness, fatigue, and sleep disorders. They are widely distributed in reproducible locations depending on the nature and location of the associated somatic dysfunction. These associations are not based on known neurophysiologic or neuroanatomic referral patterns; in this way they are similar to the mapping characteristics of the Eastern variants of massage noted later in the chapter. They are similar to those found in fibromyalgia in that they cause pain locally when palpated rather than in a distant referral pattern.

Counterstain is considered to be gentle, safe, effective, and atraumatic. Because of its gentleness, it is said to be useful (as is functional technique) for elderly or hospitalized patients, for children, and for patients with fear of pain. This technique is easy to perform and relatively forgiving. It is easily incorporated into a home exercise program as well. Practitioner time may be problematic because tender point release often requires a significant time outlay, especially when there are multiple areas of dysfunction; on the other hand, significant training and experience are not considered nearly as important in this technique as in other functional or indirect techniques. Additionally, treating only a few of tender points in one session decreases the incidence of post-traumatic "flare" of nearby muscle aches.

Functional Techniques

These techniques (9,69–72) developed in the 1940s and 1950s, share with counterstrain a methodology oriented to resetting inappropriate afferent impulses from nociceptors and mechanoreceptors (and the resultant efferent alpha motor activity to the skeletal muscle) by placing the joint or body part into a position of maximum ease (9). Unlike counterstain, the position is found and monitored by the hand of the practitioner sensing either increased resistance to trials of small induced motions, or increased tissue tension of the nearby tissues when motion is induced. The most relaxed position is held in this "balanced" state. Practitioners feel that inherent body motions, such as respiration, then allow the firing pattern of the aberrant muscles to reset such that they are normalized in a neutral position. This approach, unlike counterstrain, does not make use of tender points and is, in principle, more objective because only the practitioner's palpation determines the positions of balance. The patient is put through a sequence of these positions, hopefully progressing toward anatomic neutral as the position of maximum ease or balance.

Proponents of functional techniques and counterstrain often state that the forces involved are negligible, but the patient is often treated in the seated position. Internal muscle forces to overcome gravity, particularly in positions away from anatomic neutral, are asymmetric and potentially substantial. Nonetheless, functional techniques (nontraumatic and repeatable) are useful in both acute and chronic conditions. The focus of this treatment is in the quality, (i.e., the force it takes to move the vertebra) rather than on the quantity of the motion of the vertebra, with restoration of normal function implying normal quality and range of motion. Functional techniques require significant experience on the part of the practitioner.

Muscle Energy

This nonthrusting technique (31,63,73–75) is also called isometrics and, by some Europeans, mobilization; it bears a strong relationship to proprioceptive neuromuscular facilitation (76). The muscle energy technique requires the operator to position the patient and remove slack as in thrust procedures. The operator prevents active motion of the affected vertebra away from its barrier. The patient then exerts small to moderate force against the resistance offered by the operator, for 5 to 10 seconds, and then relaxes. After this isometric maneuver, the operator finds that the barrier has been displaced and the affected vertebra now moves beyond the original barrier. The procedure is repeated two to three times, with diminishing gains in range being achieved. Although generally painless, muscle energy often needs to be repeated and generally requires accompanying physical therapy to maintain the corrections so obtained. The time scale for treatment, normally every other day to every third day, fits in coincidentally with the usual physical therapy prescription for spine pain. Muscle energy techniques also have been used in an indirect approach.

Soft-Tissue Techniques

This approach uses mechanical stretch of the skin, muscle, and fascia to increase their motion. Lateral stretch (or ''bowstringing''), linear stretch, and deep inhibitory pressure are the most common procedures. This approach is useful in virtually all patients, often as a first step in treatment involving multiple manipulative approaches. Encouraging overall circulation and enhancing venous and lymphatic flow are central to these techniques (9). The overall purpose of soft-tissue technique is to relieve superficial muscle and fascial tension. These techniques are easy to learn in a short time and can be incorporated into outpatient clinical practice without difficulty.

Myofascial Release

This approach (9,77–80) to manipulation overlaps somewhat with massage and, conceivably, with traction. It can be directed at hypomobility of a vertebra, of a vertebral segment (as in spinal manipulation) or of the entire body, in which case it resembles some massage techniques. It can be indirect, whereby a restricted area is placed into a position of little resistance until relaxation occurs, or direct, in which case the affected area is placed against the restriction barrier with constant force until a fascial release occurs. Conceptually, in this approach, all the myofascia in the body are interconnected, and when one area is tight or restricted, diminished movement results locally and in related areas.

Successful practitioners continually palpate to assess tissue response, and adjust the applied forces of stretch, traction, pressure, or twist they are using, until the affected tissues are felt to change toward normal. This often happens over a short time scale and is called a ''release.'' The actual forces are combinations of those used in massage, soft-tissue, muscle energy, and possibly craniosacral techniques. The mechanism of the release of the ''tightness'' can be biomechanical (such as viscoelastic strain), or neuroreflexive, but, when accomplished, fascial resistance to forces applied should be symmetric and the tissues should be relatively mobile, that is, responsive to the force. In practice, the operator appears to be performing a type of massage, although the application of forces and the actual motions do not systematically coincide with classical massage.

Myofascial release combines the mechanical approach of thrust, articulation, and muscle energy techniques with the neuroreflexive approach of counterstrain, functional, soft-tissue, and craniosacral techniques. This technique requires considerable palpatory skill and experience and rigorous training on the part of the practitioner, and demands concentration on this task for relatively long periods of time. These relative impediments need to be appreciated before this type of therapy is employed.

Craniosacral Therapy

Craniosacral manipulative therapy (9,81,82) is an approach based on the concept of a primary respiratory mechanism, said to be a cyclic, palpable, rhythmic wave of inherent motion, most easily appreciated in the cranial and sacral areas. Proponents believe that this wave represents a continuous state of flux of the cerebrospinal fluid (36). It is not clear whether this wave is related to low frequency waves noted in CSF monitoring (83). This primary mechanism is felt to entail the inherent mobility of the central nervous system (CNS), cerebrospinal fluid fluctuation, the articular mobility of the cranial bones, involuntary motion between the ilia and sacrum, and the mobility of intercranial and interspinal membranes (81,84).

The practitioner palpates the head and/or the sacrum to feel pulsations of the postulated wave motion in the 8 to 12 per minute range, and for symmetry, amplitude, regularity and frequency of the wave. In infants and those with head injury, it is easy to accept the concept of motion, but in the normal adult, motion at the cranial sutures must be quite small, animal studies notwithstanding (85). Whether elastic distortions could give rise to these motions or to palpable changes in elastic compliance (86) is unclear. In any event, when abnormalities are found, the practitioner uses gentle pressure on the skull and sacral areas to restore the wave to its normal symmetry, rhythm, and amplitude.

This type of therapy is related to the previously discussed types of manipulation only because many conventional practitioners and therapists incorporate it into their practices. There is no credible scientific explanation for the positive effects reported anecdotally; this technique, therefore, remains controversial even among practitioners in manipulation. However, its largest subset of potential patients, infants with birth defects and the head-injured, intersects strongly with the patient base of many physiatrists, and its recent growth in popularity demands inclusion in any current discussion of manipulation. Importantly, there is some indication that in the head injury population, craniosacral manipulation can produce undesirable results (87).

Hypotheses of Etiology of the Dysfunction

Manipulation is basically a mechanical intervention, and it is not surprising that most hypotheses offered in explanation of the underlying dysfunction or the cure, involve position and motion of the vertebral body and its accompanying soft tissues. Generally, demonstrable pathology such as fractures, sprains, strains, tears, avulsions, tumors, and joint inflammation are excluded from consideration because it is recognized that manipulation rarely would be considered as a primary therapy for those conditions. Fibrotic contractures may be exceptions, because these may be amenable to manipulation, particularly thrust. Most hypotheses, though, invoke some pattern of neuromuscular behavior that results in localized vertebral hypomobility in the early stage. Pain and edema may cause immobility that leads to contracture or an abnormal neuromuscular pattern. Thus, the precipitating pathology may be largely resolved by the time the dysfunctional condition is diagnosed. However, pain also may arise from the dysfunction, and can therefore be incorporated into these hypotheses as a cause or effect, both, or neither, and has an inconsistent role in explanations offered to date.

All hypotheses are at least somewhat empirical; none has become a theory in the scientific sense. They differ as to whether efficacy is evaluated by measures of pain or palpable findings. It is helpful to recognize that various terms refer to the same entity. For instance, minor intervertebral derangement, osteopathic lesion, chiropractic subluxation, manipulable lesion, joint blockage, segmental dysfunction, somatic dysfunction, and painful minor intervertebral dysfunction all describe the same entity (9,15,19,26,88).

Barrier models have been suggested by several investigators to explain palpable findings (32,89,90) (Fig. 22-2). Normal joints possess an active range of motion and a larger passive range of motion. A barrier or motion restriction, produced by abnormal muscle contraction, capsular or ligamentous shortening, forms in one or more directions between the neutral position and the normal limit, so that the patient cannot achieve normal range; the manipulator needs additional force to achieve the normal passive range. Asymmetry of the applied force may lead to a new resting position for the vertebra, away from anatomic neutral. A variant of this approach considers strain of soft tissue as the basic

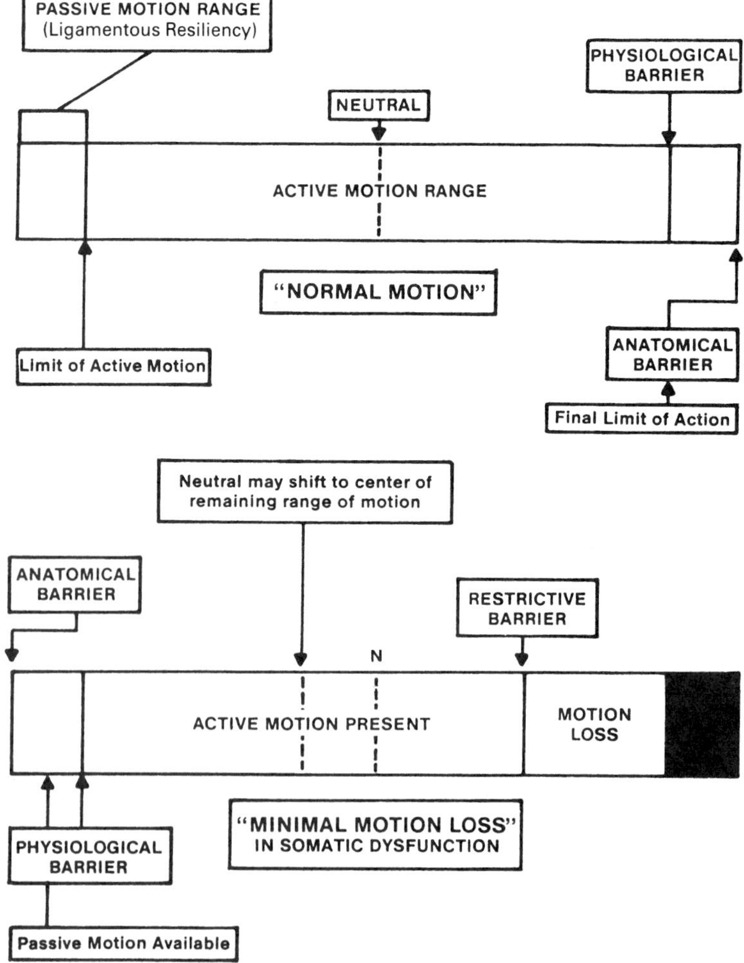

FIG. 22-2. A model of barrier motion restriction. The motion represented may be rotation, side bending, or flexion–extension. The anatomic barrier consists of cartilage and bony elements, whereas the restrictive and physiologic barriers are made up of muscular and ligamentous elements. (Modified with permission from Kimberly PE. Formulating a prescription for osteopathic manipulative treatment. *J Am Osteopath Assoc* 1980; 79:506–513.)

pathologic conditions (91); the resulting inflammation and edema then start a local vicious cycle resulting in pain and spasm. With time, edematous thickening leads to barrier formation.

The facilitated segment model assumes that a vertebral body, chronically malpositioned by contracture or overly active muscle, floods the segmentally related area of the spinal cord with inappropriate nonfatiguing proprioceptive impulses. These in turn spill over and facilitate outgoing motor neurons and autonomics in the same vertebral segment of the cord (92). Thus, pathways are present for interaction between soma and viscera at related segments, and palpatory diagnosis of visceral disease and manipulative influence on the viscera are possible. This also allows abnormal segmental areas that were asymptomatic to develop symptoms from general illness, emotional stress, or distant disease. Physiatrists familiar with reflex bladders and autonomic hyperreflexia will probably accept the concepts of somatovisceral reflexes and segmental spillover, but the magnitude and importance of these effects in the spinal-intact human is unclear (93–96).

Modern extrapolations of this postulate accept the fact that the gamma input is only one of many to the spinal cord, which must therefore respond to a pattern of afferent impulses (92). Spinal cord ''vertigo'' can result from conflicting proprioceptive and gamma afferent input information (97). The possibility of chronic problems caused by spinal cord learning, similar to cortical engram formation (98), also has been proposed. This hypothesis has been criticized on the basis of the plurisegmental nature of proprioceptive afferent and the complexity and suprasegmental nature of known viscerosomatic pain reflexes (21). Consideration of these phenomena has led to a model, almost directly opposed to that of the facilitated segment, suggesting that manipulation functions by *increasing* proprioceptive input to the dorsal root. This input competitively prevents pain input from cephalad transmission (i.e., the gate of the gate theory). Here, manipulation acts like mechanical TENS. The tendency of afferent input from a joint at its end range of motion to be attenuated, at least temporarily, by passive excursion beyond that endrange (99), also may contribute to the increased range of motion and reduced pain (100) often noted after manipulation.

Distinct from the various neurophysiologic hypotheses is the primarily mechanical model of altered ''joint play'' or accessory movements (101). All normal voluntary joint motion is accompanied by ''wiggle'' in a direction perpendicular or, possibly, tangential to the plane of that motion (20,102,103). This joint play exists because joint surfaces are not perfectly congruent. This play conceptually differs from coupling (104), which is obligate related *voluntary* motions, e.g. rotation and side-bending. Loss of play due to soft-tissue restriction may inhibit voluntary motion because the *involuntary* component is absent. Passive intervention is needed to normalize function, because the lost play is in an involuntary direction. Pain is not addressed directly by this model, but it arises from poor mechanical function.

A bulging disc or dislodged disc fragment pressing on the posterior longitudinal ligament can cause pain (25). One model suggests that manipulation, often accompanied by manual traction, acts to replace the fragment or reduce the bulge, with subsequent pain relief. A modification of this approach (19,26) suggests that the effect of the bulge is to create asymmetry and locking or wedging in the facet joints so that motion is lost as a consequence. Further voluntary motion would accentuate the problem, and passive intervention is needed. The possibility of asymptomatic dysfunctional joints creating symptoms under stress is part of this model, although the author of this theory (15) now requires pain to be present, distinguishing this approach from the primary hypomobility hypothesis.

McKenzie defines three classes of abnormality (25):

1. A postural syndrome with intermittent pain from postural stress
2. A dysfunctional syndrome with pain and lost vertebral motion similar to the barrier picture (see Fig. 22-1)
3. A derangement syndrome involving disc abnormalities

Numerous hypotheses have been offered by the chiropractic profession to explain the relationships between altered structure and resultant pathologic conditions. These are adequately reviewed by Janse (105). The deleterious neurophysiologic effects that result from nerve compression caused by vertebral derangement have been conjectured to be a major cause of both somatic and visceral complaints; this viewpoint, which has been prominent since the earliest foundations of chiropractic, is perhaps the one most associated with chiropractic by other professionals. However, other concepts, including neurodystrophic effects, viscerosomatic reflexes, and a proprioceptive insult phenomenon similar to the segmental facilitation model discussed earlier, also appear. Some European authors believe that there is soft material in the vertebral joint spaces (i.e., a meniscoid), which can become trapped between the cartilage surfaces and block smooth joint motion until moved by manipulative gapping or repeated mobilization (6).

Soft-tissue pain and palpatory findings, although related to vertebral dysfunction, do not always follow obvious segmental patterns (17). An attempt to incorporate these findings (myotendinosis) into the classical picture has coined the term ''spondylogenic reflex'' to describe the suprasegmental organizing process (106). There have been other efforts to unify the various hypotheses (107), but they have had limited success to date.

Hypotheses of Action of Manipulation

The mechanism by which spinal manipulative techniques relieve pain is unknown (100,108,109). A simple categorization separates treatments into those that mechanically lengthen tight soft tissues from those that alter the firing pattern of an inappropriately shortened muscle to achieve relaxation. Either of these will eliminate hypomobility of the offending segment if the soft tissue is lengthened or the muscle is relaxed. Functional, muscle energy, most myofascial release, and strain/counterstrain techniques, using small forces, probably can work only on the neuroreflexive alteration of muscle activity. This is the spinal segmental equivalent of re-educating an inappropriate primitive engram, similar to CNS rehabilitation. Thrust and articulatory techniques involve larger forces and presumably can stretch and elongate tissue; these might work purely in the mechanical mode. Pain, though, is not typically addressed, other than to suppose it is lessened by reducing hypomobility. Given the importance of pain relief in a physiatric practice, this approach is disappointing. The hypotheses focus on different specific actions of the therapy:

- Restoration of vertebral range of motion
- Restoration of symmetry at the disc and/or facet levels
- Production of an afferent signal to the cord, evoking the gate effect
- Release of endorphins, increase pain threshold or decrease severity
- Placebo effect

1. Restricted motion arises from muscle contraction and shortened or stiffened soft tissues. All forms of manipulation are thought to interfere with abnormal muscular contraction, either by production of afferent stimuli that attenuate a hyperexcitable gamma system, or by elimination of proprioceptive input that stimulates the gamma system. In addition, thrust and possibly articulatory and isometric techniques can stimulate Golgi tendon organ input (110). Articulatory and isometric techniques may elicit permanent lengthening of collagenous tissue by inducing a permanent set with repeated stretching in the viscoelastic range (111). Alternatively, repeated deformation of soft tissue may normalize its mechanical response to load, that is, soften the material so that deformation occurs at lower load (112). This functional lengthening of the tissue can be a passive phenomenon, but the time scale of isometric and articulatory treatment (i.e., days) might allow metabolic response of the tissue to occur. Thrust techniques result in high stress levels and probably very high strain rates in the soft tissues over a very short time. It seems reasonable to speculate that a nonuniform distribution of strain will result, which may lead to very localized tissue injury and subsequent healing with permanent elongation. The net result is that the vertebra will regain normal play of motion, and the forces needed to produce motion will be normalized. Pain is reduced secondary to return of function.

2. Facet malposition or malfunction can be directly influenced by passive motion of the joint (19), or a malpositioned meniscoid can be relocated (6). A bulging disc (60) is envisioned as being reduced or normalized by manipulation with accompanying traction. This relieves compressive stresses on the disc, creates suction, and, via the stretched posterior longitudinal ligament, replaces the bulge anteriorly.

3. The change in proprioceptive input to the spinal cord is theorized to close the gate on pain or to remove an abnormal facilitating proprioceptive input. A "hysteresis" induced loss of afferent input at the joint's endpoint of motion also might be a factor in pain modulation (99,100).

4. Despite one report that thrust may have an effect on circulating cells or the immune system (113), there are only contradictory data regarding the possibility of manipulation induced endorphin release (114–118).

5. The placebo effect, which may always be present to some extent, seems to favor manual medicine techniques over less "hands-on" approaches (119).

It should be clear that manipulation success is reported in many, if not most, patients, using widely varying techniques and operating under very different assumptions as to the cause of the problem and action of therapy. It would seem that any procedure that induces muscular relaxation or vertebral motion has some chance of success. Because most of the postulated actions of manipulation are accomplished by most techniques, success itself provides little feedback as to validity of the model. There is as yet too much "joint play" in our knowledge to discern the pathway to a definitive understanding either of technique or of back pain. All, or possibly none, of the hypotheses presented may ultimately be found valid. The placebo effect, which may be diminished or enhanced when the manipulation is relegated to nonphysicians, is impossible to gauge or compare with the various approaches.

Physiatric Use of Manipulation

The goals of spinal manipulation are the restoration and maintenance of optimal biomechanical function by improving vertebral motion, thereby facilitating spinal mobility, minimizing spinal and other pain, and increasing the patient's level of wellness.

Scientific evidence for efficacy of manipulation for the treatment of acute spinal pain (3) has been mounting, with gradual acceptance by the physiatric community. Similar scientific evidence regarding chronic spinal pain is not as yet generally accepted (120,121). These studies (122) are much more difficult to perform because total eradication of chronic pain is rare regardless of the techniques employed. Manipulation therapy in these cases should be directed at the restoration of normal spinal segmental motion, thereby reducing pain, with the hope that overall physical activity may increase (123). The somatic dysfunction(s) may have been the original source of pain, but what this means in terms of the effect of manipulation on the patient is not obvious given our present lack of understanding of the relationship of pain to either the dysfunction or chronic pain syndrome.

Prescribing Manipulation

The referral of a patient for manipulation requires a prescription. This can be, and perhaps is best done, via conversation with the provider, implying the physician has chosen a practitioner with appropriate credentials and training. The manipulative care will usually be included as part of a general ranging, strengthening, and educational program. What will be added to the prescription is the specific vertebral region to be manipulated, the suggested technique to be used, and any specific side effects or medical issues the provider must be aware of. For example, a patient with low back pain, for whom demonstrable pathology has been ruled out, with the palpable finding of hypomobility of T12 relative to L1 would have a prescription as follows:

Patient age: ______
Precautions: Avoid thrusting techniques
Diagnosis: Unresolved mechanical low back pain without radiographic or neurologic findings. Somatic dysfunction T12
Rx: Back stabilization program
Back education program
Muscle energy procedures to T12 to restore normal T12 mobility relative to L1
Home program
Frequency: 3 times per week
Duration: 3 weeks or until T12 motion is normalized
Options: May use soft-tissue massage before manipulation, may use superficial hot–cold modalities to supplement above. Please call to discuss other treatment options if indicated.
Other: Notify physician if patient complains of increased pain lasting more than 8 hours after last session. Notify physician if mobility in T12 relative to L1 is normalized.

If known, the actual hypomobility restrictions could be added (e.g., T12 is restricted in flexion, left side-bending and left rotation relative to L1), but this takes a higher diagnostic acumen than that needed to detect hypomobility of T12. However, the more specific and localized the treatment, the more likely it is to correct the specific localized dysfunction.

Follow-up patient examination, in this case to confirm the restoration of T12 mobility, occurs as with any other physical therapy program. If treatment was unsuccessful, reformulation of the diagnosis or of therapy would follow. The next step might be escalating the invasiveness of the manipulation to articulatory or thrusting techniques, if no contraindications exist. Conversely, if manipulation is producing discomfort lasting greater than 8 hours, consider switching to the less invasive counterstrain or functional techniques.

The manipulation technique utilized will be determined by the time course of the problem, the patient's age, general physical condition, presence of any contraindications, and the expertise of the practitioner. The former considerations explain the need for a careful history, physical examination, segmental structural examination, and functional diagnosis, while the latter justifies the choice of a particular practitioner for a problem. The provider should be allowed some input to the technique or approach, with agreement reached before therapy is initiated. A manipulable lesion must be identified for manipulation to be effective for any patient; this is particularly important for the subacute or chronic population that the physiatrist frequently encounters. Patients cannot localize muscular forces to a particular segment or joint in the spine, so self mobilization of the vertebra is not feasible. The manipulative process will therefore always need to be performed by a provider (operator). Also, there is rarely complete eradication of pain in these patients. These factors lead to the possibility of dependence on manipulation, and the physiatrist should be aware of this possibility. Having well defined biomechanical endpoints, i.e. normal range of motion and tissue compliance, will help objectify the endpoint to manual treatment. If pain relief alone is used as an endpoint, treatment may continue indefinitely. There is no well established literature on this point, but experience with chronic pain patients suggests that manipulation, with accompanying physical therapy, should be directed at obtaining an optimal biomechanical condition as quickly as possible, and thereafter used only infrequently to "tune up" the mechanics as needed. There is no evidence that prolonging care is in the patient's best interest.

An additional benefit of manipulative therapy may come to those physiatrists providing the manipulation themselves. The application of "hands on" treatment facilitates trust in the practitioner; this can only help the in doctor–patient relationship. Physical therapists routinely experience this phenomenon.

Research Relevant to Manipulation

There probably is no other medical modality that has had so many practitioners (50,000 doctors of osteopathy and chiropractic in the United States), consumers (90,000,000 chiropractic manipulations alone are performed annually in the U.S.), and critics (a significant but decreasing proportion of the allopathic medical profession), with so little hard data to support or refute it.

Efficacy Studies

Forty-six clinical trials of spinal manipulative therapy have been summarized by Brunarski (124). More detailed reviews and critiques of selected trials have been published by Evans (125), Haldeman (1), Tobis and Hoehler (126), Curtis (127), and Abenhaim and Bergeron (128); it has been the subject of two international meetings (129,130). Recent trials have attempted to improve our knowledge by comparing thrust to nonthrust techniques (131) and joint-specific to non–joint-specific manual therapy (132), by using more frequent and intense interventions (133), and comparing different types of joint specific manipulation (134). The conclusions of the various studies are difficult to compare (135). For example, Coxhead and colleagues reported no significant differences using manipulation as compared with traction, corset, or exercises (136), whereas Rasmussen reported that 11 of 12 manipulative patients reported pain relief, compared to 3 of 12 patients receiving placebo short-wave diathermy (137). However, to truly understand these conflicting data, one needs to know that Rasmussen eliminated chronic back pain patients from the study, used rotational manipulation in the pain-free direction, studied the effects at 2 weeks after starting therapy, and had favorable, but somewhat different, results when using the modified Schober test for his criteria for improvement. Coxhead and colleagues studied patients with sciatic pain with or without back pain, used Maitland's technique of manipulation (28), and evaluated improvement at 4 weeks and 4 months after therapy initiation. Thus, criteria for inclusion were different, manipulative techniques were different, criteria for improvement were partially different, and time of the evaluation was different. These differences are representative, and it is therefore not surprising that the results of these studies are equivocal. The wide variations among studies have even frustrated attempts at blinded reviews and meta-analysis (138,139,140).

In general, studies vary regarding the entry or improvement criterion (pain or motion), duration of the problem, time of evaluation, nature of the placebo or control, type and specificity of technique used, and method of statistical analysis used. With rare exceptions (141), the studies address a chief complaint of pain without regard to objective findings. Given the spectrum of pathologic conditions that cause back pain, the perplexity of the results is understandable. The situation is analogous to studying whether surgery is a more efficacious therapy than bed rest for a complaint of abdominal pain when neither the etiology of the abdominal pain nor the surgical procedure used is defined. In addition, designers of studies who are denied the double-blind techniques of drug research are confronted with the strong emotional bias of those who must do the manipulation and are sure it works, and of those who must evaluate the results and are often sure it does not. The development of appropriate statistical methods may help (142), but the solution to this dilemma is not obvious.

Physics and Anatomy of Manipulation

The basic physics of manipulation have been discussed and explored theoretically in recent years (143–147), and an experimental attempt has been made to look at changed spinal mobility resulting from manipulation (148). The alterations to the anatomy of the dysfunctional joint are poorly understood despite numerous efforts to delineate them (149), and this constitutes a major area needing elucidation.

In recent years there has been significant advancement in our knowledge of the biomechanics of thrust manipulation. The external mechanical forces involved (57), the duration of application of these forces (59), and some gross anterior/posterior displacements have been measured in human subjects (58), and relative displacements have been measured in cadavers (150). These measurements represent the first steps toward understanding the relevant biomechanics. Study of the internal forces and relative displacements of vertebral bodies resulting from these applied forces still needs to be done. The cavitation phenomenon (56) also has recently been reviewed and is to a large measure understood. Some research has been conducted regarding the neurologic (151) and the neuromuscular responses (59) to the thrust procedure, but these are also the first steps. Little has been done to elucidate the other types of manipulative therapy in terms of either biomechanical parameters or physiologic responses to them.

On a more positive note, much has been learned in the last 20 years about pain and mechanoreceptors (152,153), spinal cord physiology (92,93), and normal spinal biomechanics (154). Application of this information toward an understanding of manual medicine dysfunction and treatment is ongoing (96). Knowledge about small tissue strains (as opposed to the injury level large deformations familiar to orthopedic surgery) is now being accumulated and assimilated into manual medicine thinking (155). The potential visceral effects of manipulative intervention, or lack thereof, are undergoing continuing investigation (96). Notwithstanding these advances, the interrelationships among therapy, patient, and dysfunction remain elusive, and the design of more credible clinical efficacy trials is still a formidable problem.

There are two areas of research development that are strikingly absent. One involves the lack of any firm association of somatic dysfunction to pain. Although somatic dysfunction is the entity treated by manipulation, the nearly universal reason for treatment is pain relief. However, the relationship between these two basic concepts is ignored even in the hypothesis stage of most models. The second area involves the absence of any instrument or device that can objectively measure a somatic dysfunction in a patient. Whether one's hands are sensitive to lost vertebral motion, quality of motion, end feel, or any other palpatory cue, it should be possible to objectively validate with today's technology. This would move the investigation of manipulation from the province of those few providers with the requisite skills to detect subtle palpatory changes into the mainstream of medical research. Almost all medical development has progressed slowly from clinical practice to scientific validation, usually by development of new technology over periods of years to decades. Manipulation in the United States is now over 100 years old; and it would seem that appropriate research could be generated regarding its use. Certainly, the ongoing concern about health-care cost containment will demand answers to the questions of mechanism and efficacy raised in this section. However, this objective validation is a daunting prospect, given our present level of knowledge; while much of medical practice is indeed not based on objective findings, efforts should continue to maximize current objective data. Until such time as these questions are resolved, the physiatrist will be forced to evaluate manipulation based on incomplete information and the similarity or dissimilarity between manipulation and other relatively unproved techniques of physical medicine.

MASSAGE

Massage is one of the oldest treatment modalities in medicine (156,157). Throughout history it has been woven into the cultural context of medicine. In this sense, it may be viewed as an essential component of traditional medicine, with the word ''traditional'' implying an old and/or very common usage. Massage may be classified, admittedly with significant overlap, into western and eastern variants. In the west, mentioned as early as the time of Hippocrates (157), its practice and popularity has waxed and waned over the centuries. The interested reader can find detailed accounts of the history in various sources (157–163). In recent years a prior decline in its popularity, probably related to technologic developments in medicine, has been reversed by a resurgence of interest in alternative therapies (160). Some claims for massage by the proponents may sound implausible, but there can be little doubt that it is efficacious for certain conditions. However, it is safe to say that there is a dramatic need for additional research regarding mechanisms and efficacy.

Definition/Relation to Other Mechanical Therapies

Massage is defined as the therapeutic manipulation of the soft tissues of the body with a goal of normalization of those tissues. It is also defined as ''hand motion practiced on the surface of the living body with a therapeutic goal,'' (164) or, ''a group of procedures which are usually done with the hands, such as friction, kneading, rolling, and percussion of the external tissues of the body in a variety of ways, either with a curative, palliative, or hygienic object in view'' (165).

Manipulation and massage both involve similar hand positions and movements, and some techniques overlap significantly. Soft-tissue manipulation, performed to loosen and relax tissues before vertebral manipulation, is partially composed of the various massage techniques. Myofascial release (77) uses stretching forces similar to those used in massage, albeit in myofascial release the object of the stretch is a poorly functioning vertebral region rather than the soft tissue *per se*. Myofascial release and craniosacral manipulation, discussed in the manipulation section of this chapter, are often available from massage therapists and massage can easily be a preliminary treatment to manipulation. Regardless of the similarities, however, massage clearly targets the health of the soft tissues while spinal manipulation targets vertebral motion; soft-tissue health is optimized only secondarily with manipulation.

The difference between massage and traction is easier to delineate. Massage consists mostly of hand movements, some of which may be traction based. Traction as a therapy usually involves machinery, but also can be applied manually, but the latter would not use other massage movements. In addition, traction tends to effect changes in the spinal column *per se* with soft tissues only secondarily modified. Like traction, however, massage effects tend to be nonspecific.

Massage can have mechanical, reflexive, neurologic, and psychological effects, and can be used to reduce pain or adhesions, promote sedation, mobilize fluids, increase muscular relaxation, and cause vasodilation (166,167).

Basic Western Massage Procedures

There is probably no area of manual medicine where there is more confusion in terminology than massage. Much of the basic terminology for western massage was introduced by Pare (168) but there is a tendency for textbooks and practitioners to use idiosyncratic variants and readers must be vigilant to this. The essence of massage is the use of the hands to apply mechanical forces to the skeletal muscles and skin, although the intent may be to influence either more superficial or deeper tissues. The types of massage prevalent in the western hemisphere are derived from the Swedish system. They are categorized by whether (a) the focus of pressure is moved by the hands gliding over the skin; (b) soft tissue is compressed between the hands or the fingers; (c) the skin and muscle are impacted with repetitive compressive blows by the hands; or (d) shearing stresses are created at tissue interfaces below the skin. The three former techniques retain their classic French names, *effleurage*, *petrissage*, and *tapotement*, whereas the fourth is called deep friction massage.

Effleurage or Stroking Massage

The operator's hands glide across the skin overlying the skeletal muscle being treated (158,159,161–163,166,169). Often oil or powder is incorporated to reduce the friction between the hands and the skin. Any part of the hand can be used but many applications require the palm to be in good contact with the skin. In all stroking techniques, hand-to-skin contact should be maintained throughout the stroke. If the compressive force on the muscle is kept relatively light, this is called superficial stroke massage; if it is relatively heavy, it is called deep stroke massage. Presumably, a light stroke energizes cutaneous receptors and acts by some neuroreflexive mechanism or possibly vascular reflexive mechanism, whereas a deep stroke is more capable of mechanically mobilizing fluids in the tissues beneath it, including the muscle, in the direction of the stroke. Therefore, deep stroking should be in the direction of venous or lymphatic flow, whereas light stroking can be in any direction.

Effleurage tends to be a technique common to all massage therapy because it is used to gain initial relaxation and patient confidence, to diagnose regions of spasm and tightness, and most importantly, to get the operator's hands from one problem area to another, where other techniques may be employed. Effleurage has as its main mechanical effect the application of sequential pressure over contiguous soft tissues with the result that fluids will be displaced ahead of the hands as the tissue is compressed.

Petrissage or Kneading Massage

This more invasive form of massage involves compression of the underlying skin and muscle either between the fingers and thumb of one hand or between the two hands of the masseur/masseuse. The entrapped tissue is squeezed gently as the hands move in a circular motion perpendicular to the direction of compression (158,159,161,162). Some investigators call this "kneading" the tissue whereas others separate "kneading" from petrissage, depending on the direction of the compression and force of the motion. The pressure is such that the skin can move over the underlying tissue, but practitioners disagree on whether the operator's hand should slip relative to the skin. Mobilization of fluid would be a result with this type of treatment, but petrissage has as its main mechanical effect the compression and subsequent release of soft tissues, reactive blood flow, and neuroreflexive response to the flow.

Tapotement or Percussion Massage

This consists of the operator striking the soft tissue with repetitive blows using both hands (158,159,161,162). It is done rhythmically, gently, and rapidly. There is no rigid frequency requirement, but typically these motions occur about three times per second (163). There are numerous variants defined by the part of the hands that make the impact; using the back of the medial fingers is called hacking; the volar surface of all the fingers is called slapping; the hypothenar eminence is called beating; the pads of the fingers or the tips of the fingers is called tapping. If the thumb and index finger do a light pinch on contact, it is called pincement. A form more familiar to physicians occurs when the cupped palm of the hand is used to make the impact. This tends to make a clapping noise on each impact. The therapeutic effect is hypothesized to result from a compression of the trapped air that occurs on impact. Because the frequency of sound is low, the waves can penetrate to deep structures, but whether this is the therapeutic effect is not clear. If done over the upper back, the lung tissue may absorb the waves; a variant of this technique called clappatage is used by respiratory therapists to loosen bronchial secretions.

The effect of tapotement is thought to be stimulatory. It tends to be used more often on healthy people by nonmedical practitioners in a nontherapeutic milieu. Nonetheless, it also is part of the armamentarium of medically trained practitioners.

Friction or Deep Friction Massage

Pressure of varying intensities is applied with the ball of the thumb or fingers to the skin and muscle of the patient. With constant pressure, the digit is moved in small circular motions for several cycles before the pressure is released and the application performed in a new location (158,159,161,162,170). There is no gliding as in effleurage and no compression between the fingers as in petrissage. The main mechanical effect of friction massage is probably the application of shear stresses to the underlying tissue, particularly at the interface between two types of tissue, for example, dermis–fascia, fascia–muscle, muscle–bone, scar tissue–bone, etc. It is probably impossible to affect abnormalities within one tissue, e.g. muscle. The effect of the pressure is to keep the superficial tissues under the thumb from shearing so that the shear and force are directed to a deeper interface. The higher the applied pressure, the thicker the level of nongliding tissue and the deeper the level that shear takes effect. Various techniques have the motion across fibers, parallel to fibers, or random. Friction massage is, perhaps, the primary method of preventing or treating adhesions of scar tissue to bone and deeper structures. For this reason, physiatrists involved in amputee rehabilitation may encounter this application more often than other techniques.

All of these techniques have variants, and each has its proponents. A variant of tapotement called vibration differs by the fact that the hands do not lift off the skin at the end of each cycle. Variants of petrissage depend on the forces applied to the tissue trapped between the fingers or hands. The technique, called picking-up, requires the tissue to be first compressed against deep structures, then pinched, then released for advancement of the hands to a new area for treatment. Wringing requires one hand or finger of the practitioner to push the trapped tissue while the other hand pulls, perhaps shearing even deep tissue planes between them. Rolling, which often is done just to the skin in diagnosis of manipulative lesions, allows the tissue to roll between the fingers and thumb, often combined with gliding of the digits over the skin. In shaking, the entrapped tissue is shaken by the operator's hand as it glides down the length of tissue.

Each of these variants arises by changing the dominant force used, then adding a new sequence of shear, compression, and glide that basic techniques provide. For a given patient, the correct combination of these forces may be more important than the sequence of their application.

Eastern Massage

Eastern massage systems have evolved over many centuries and are integrated within the culture of the country where they are practiced. The systems for evaluation, diagnosis, and treatment are, for the most part, not based on known western neurophysiology. It is unlikely that western physiatrists will need detailed knowledge of these systems, but it seems probable that western massage will incorporate some of the more valuable eastern concepts as time goes on. Many of these techniques resemble variants of classical western massage, although they are often used for visceral complaints. There are many more gradations of technique, as many as 24 in one Chinese system (171), varying from simple pressure application to stretching reminiscent of muscle energy or proprioceptive neuromuscular facilitation (PNF) approaches. Often further subdivision is done with regard to which body part of the operator is applying the corrective forces. Some systems have developed followings of such size that separate names have been attached to them.

Acupressure

This system applies massage forces, largely digital pressure, to the same points treated with the better known acupuncture needles, and for the same reasons (158,160). Energy or *Chi* is said to circulate in the body along 12 meridians or pathways unrelated to the neuroreferral patterns known to western medicine. Imbalances of energy found along the meridians are felt to cause disease and can be rectified by localized finger pressure accompanied by circular movements similar to deep friction.

The pressure is generally increased until it is relatively heavy and then held constant. The similar Japanese form is called Shiatsu.

Reflexology and Auriculotherapy

The meridian concept is a part of these systems also (158,159). The meridians are felt to have whole-body representation like a homunculus on the extremities, particularly, the feet (reflexology) and the ear (auriculotherapy). All parts of the body and its organs are mapped to points on the foot or ear, and massage of a point is felt to produce change in the organ or structure mapped to that point.

Massage Variables

There are certain variables of massage that will need to be controlled by the operator (158,159). The physiatrist may wish to specify these if ordering massage although often they are left to the provider.

Milieu

The massage should be performed in a warm, (to the partially undressed patient) quiet area, where neither the patient nor the operator need be concerned about interruptions. Draping of untreated areas must be loose so that no constrictions limit the potential flow of fluids mobilized from the massage itself. The operator's hands should be clean, warm, and well manicured, and any liquid medium applied also should be warm to the touch. The patient must be comfortable, in a position chosen to enhance the goals of the massage. For example, if percussion is being used to mobilize bronchial secretions, the patient should be positioned so that gravity will assist the flow of secretions away from the segment being treated. The practitioner also must be comfortable, e.g. the height of the treatment table must be compatible with the height of the therapist. Unlike manipulation, where the course of treatment may range from seconds to minutes, massage treatments often last 15 to 45 minutes so that the practitioner's comfort is essential for effective treatment. The use of pillows, rolls, pads, etc. can be used to cushion the patient against the firm compressive forces often required for massage.

Treatment Variables

Friction-Reducing Medium

In effleurage, the hands of the therapist move relative to the patient's skin, so a medium to reduce friction between them may be advisable, particularly when significant pressure is to be applied to the skin surface. Powders are sometimes used to minimize friction and have the advantage that they also eliminate moisture on the practitioner's hands so that abrasion of the patient's skin does not occur. Talcum or boric acid powder (159) have been used, as have oils and solid-oily lubricants (159) to soften the skin as well as keep it smooth and slippery. Mineral oil, glycerin, and coconut oil are among the liquids mentioned in the literature, and cold creams and cocoa butter have been suggested as solid lubricants. Deep friction treatments do not generally require lubricants because the procedure requires the thumb and patient's tissues to move in unison. Opponents of the use of lubricants state that sensitivity is lost by their use, and this is probably true. Unless there is a particular medium that would be contraindicated for the patient, the use of and choice of lubricants is probably best negotiated between the practitioner and the patient.

Rhythm

Any massage stroke should be regular and cyclic. Scientific support for this is lacking, but it seems reasonable when one considers that relaxation is one of the desirable outcomes of the treatment.

Rate

The rate of application of the massage force varies with the type of technique used. Tapotement or percussion is generally given several times per second (163). Other strokes are much slower, perhaps 15 per minute or in essence at the patient's respiratory rate. One author (159) recommends a velocity of 7 inches per second for the hand speed during effleurage which is probably congruent with the 15 per minute rate noted above.

Pressure

The amount of pressure used is strongly dependent on the technique and desired result of the treatment. Light pressure is said to produce sedation and relaxation and may decrease spasm, while breakdown of adhesions may require heavy pressure. The treatment of edema and the stretching of connective tissue typically require an intermediate pressure, although some new techniques for lymphedema use very low pressures. There are no good data to define light, moderate, and heavy, so to a certain extent this will vary among providers.

Direction

The direction of effleurage generally has been centripetal because one of the desired effects is to mobilize fluids, best done by having them flow towards the heart. The sequence of tissues treated is also often centripetal. When muscle is treated, motions are usually parallel to the muscle fibers, the exception occurring in deep friction techniques. To reduce adhesions, the shearing motion is either circular to cover all directions, or at least includes cross fiber components.

Area to be Treated

This depends on the condition to be treated. Unlike manipulation addressing dysfunctional tissue, massage is used for pathologic tissue, e.g., affected by fibrosis or contracture. The area can thus be circumscribed in many cases, although contiguous areas might also need to be treated because physiology there also could be disturbed. Unlike recreational massage, whole body treatment is seldom appropriate for musculoskeletal conditions.

Duration of Individual Treatments

This will depend on patient tolerance and, once again, on the area being treated. There is wide variation of duration and the operator has to be guided by the tissue changes occurring during the actual procedure. In addition, if massage is done prior to other treatments, e.g. range of motion or strengthening, the duration may be determined by the result needed for optimization of the next treatment. It is safe to say that the patient, practitioner, and physiatrist must be in agreement on this point, and some negotiation among the three is desirable.

Frequency

There are also no scientific guidelines here. Daily treatments might be appropriate in some cases, but weekly or bi-weekly treatments are more common. Because massage is expensive and may not be included in insurance packages, the physiatrist should negotiate duration and frequency with the patient, provider, and, in select cases, third-party carriers.

Duration of the Program

This can range anywhere from a week to months, and will depend on the verifiable goals of the massage. Often these goals will be encompassed in a general therapy program for which massage serves as a first step. Patients need to be re-examined after a time interval commensurate with the diagnosis and the general therapy goals.

Physiological Effects

Mechanical Effects

Vascular changes are recognized as a clear mechanical effect of massage. Mechanical pressure on soft tissue will displace any fluids that are not chemically bound by the tissue or physically bound by compartmentalization. The fluid can move in a low-resistance direction under the static hand force, but a moving locus of pressure will create a gradient of pressure. Assuming no significant resistance, pressure is lower ahead of (usually proximal to) the advancing hand. Once the mobilized fluid leaves the cells or interstitium, it can enter the venous or lymphatic low pressure systems, with valvular mechanisms that help prevent fluid return. Areas are typically worked distal to proximal, centripetally, to keep the fluid movement toward the heart, which along with the kidneys will be required to handle an additional load. The amount of fluid mobilized in any one treatment is probably quite small, and major effects to the heart have not been noted. Nonetheless, the physiatrist needs be aware of this physiologic effect in the cardiovascular or renal compromised patient. Proponents of the "complex physical therapy" approach to lymphedema, espousing gently applied massage, tend to massage the proximal lymph area first, then move distally. The belief is that proximal blockage areas in the lymph channels must be opened first, perhaps reflexively, to allow subsequent distal mobilization of the fluid and protein (172,173). Scientific evidence for a distal-to-proximal approach or the converse is lacking.

Kneading and stroking massage both decrease edema, and compression will convert nonpitting to pitting edema (174). Friction massage is probably not effective in this regard. In addition to that strictly mechanical effect, it is thought that histamine is released by the massage, causing superficial vasodilation to assist in the washing out of metabolic waste products (166,167). Venous return is thereby increased, and in healthy patients, stroke volume will increase (175). There is contradictory evidence that massage to one limb will increase the blood flow contralaterally (176,177). If this is true, the mechanism is uncertain. Effleurage may be more effective than either diathermy or ultrasound in increasing blood flow (178). Clearly, these effects on the mobilization of fluids will be more important in the flaccid or mechanically inactivated limb, because the normal compression supplied by skeletal muscle contraction is absent in those cases.

Recent findings suggest that massage may decrease blood viscosity and hematocrit and increase circulating fibrinolytic compounds (179,180). Although these are preliminary data it would help to explain the apparent success of massage in decreasing instances of deep vein thrombosis (181). Massage nonetheless is still contraindicated in the presence of existing thrombosis. Other blood compounds thought to be increased by massage include myoglobin, glutamic oxaloacetic transaminase, creatine kinase, and lactic dehydrogenase (182,183). One suspects that these transient increases represent local muscle cell leakage from the applied pressure. Lactate does decrease in massaged muscle cells (184). Massage is said to decrease muscle spasm and increase force of contraction and endurance of skeletal muscle (185,186). One can rationalize the decrease of spasm and the increase of endurance as occurring secondary to washout of metabolic waste products by the mobilization of fluids and increased blood flow. The enhanced contractual force though, is based on remote publications and needs new validation and elucidation, particularly because the mechanism is not obvious. The decrease in muscle soreness that many patients relate is probably also from the wash out of metabolites, and the cycle may be broken permanently if the spasm was responsible for the original build-up of the metabolites and immobility of the muscle.

The shearing forces of deep friction massage have not been studied adequately, but it is accepted that they can break down or prevent adhesions and increase fascial mobility (162,163,170,187,188). Limited local tissue damage, with hyperemia and mild inflammation, may occur when adhesions are reduced.

A special case of the mechanical effects of massage on the lymphatic system is the ''lymphatic pump'' often used as part of manipulation techniques for patients with respiratory compromise (9). This is a type of petrissage done to the chest and rib cage that is hypothesized to draw lymph into the patient's thoracic duct and hence to the venous circulation because of the alternating increase and release of pressure on the chest cavity.

Similar to manipulation, endogenous endorphins have also been postulated to be released by massage (166,189). Here, too, there is little supportive evidence for this, and further studies will be needed to establish this effect either way.

Reflexive Changes

Massage can stimulate cutaneous receptors and possibly the spindle receptors in superficial skeletal muscles (167). These produce impulses that reach the spinal cord, which once there, conceivably can produce myriad effects (166,167,190). One such effect would be moderation of the so-called ''facilitated segment,'' (92) discussed in more detail in the manipulation section. Somatovisceral reflex changes to the viscera are possible in this model, although evidence for this is lacking. Our knowledge of somatovisceral and viscerosomatic reflexes is rudimentary enough to allow almost any effect, but allowing for such a system, massage could have distant visceral effects. Others might include input to the ''gate'' of the dorsal column of the spinal cord, thereby reducing pain like a mechanical TENS unit (190). Possibly the increased afferent input can influence the activity of the cord itself. Some of the vascular effects noted above could be secondary to reflexive vasodilation, although one might justifiably question why vasoconstriction does not also occur. It does seem safe to acknowledge that reflexive effects occur in massage, with further details awaiting scientific validation. One method of massage that depends heavily on reflex mechanisms, and which may be encountered by the physiatrist, is the German *Bindegewebmassage,* or connective tissue massage (158,191,192). This is based on the concept that autonomic vascular, rather than somatic, nerves are the channels for reflex systems that give rise to skin symptoms or palpatory changes, not necessarily along accepted dermatomes. The skin massage here is done very lightly, presumably in areas related to the viscera, to influence the connective tissue, trigger reflex mechanisms, and ultimately to modify the target viscera. Studies of its effects are contradictory (193–196). Some of the Eastern approaches to massage noted earlier, (reflexology and auriculotherapy) are also dependent on reflexive mechanisms, most of which have little or no basis in conventional Western neurophysiology and neuroanatomy.

These types of hypothetical postulates, which are difficult to prove and even more difficult to disprove, form the basis of massage and manipulation practitioners' efforts to treat visceral diseases with these methods. Physiatrists need not enter this controversy, yet can rest assured that, as in manipulation, there are few if any complications of massage that cannot be explained on purely mechanical or well-established physiologic grounds. A recent discussion of the ability of somatic problems to mimic visceral pathology may be the first step in understanding some of these approaches (197).

Psychological Effects

Most people experiencing any form of massage will attest to the feeling of relaxation and well being that it produces. Whether this is a placebo effect or the result of some hitherto undiscovered reflex is unknown, but this has stimulated interest in the use of massage for acute and chronic pain conditions as well as in anxiety states (157,194,197–199). Some practitioners incorporate a variety of other psychological techniques, such as guided imagery, into the massage treatment. Yet another massage approach incorporates psychosomatic integration. This is called ''rolfing''® (after the originator) or ''structural integration'' (200). Rolfing® incorporates sometimes uncomfortable deep friction massage aimed at realigning and balancing the patient's body relative to the gravitational field, with predetermined sequences of treatments unrelated to individual symptomatology. The rebalancing is thought to optimize both the psychological and physical states of the patient.

Therapeutic Goals of and Indications for Massage Therapy

Massage will be utilized either as a therapeutic intervention alone or more commonly as an adjunct to other modalities. It will be indicated by a need for one of its physiologic, reflexive, or psychological effects as noted above. Thus, it might be ordered to mobilize interstitial fluids, to reduce or modify edema (201–208), to increase local blood flow, to decrease muscle soreness or stiffness, to moderate pain, to prevent or eliminate adhesions, or to facilitate relaxation.

In a physiatric practice, these indications may be considered in patients with sprains, strains, fractures, mechanical back pain, contractures, myofascial pain syndromes with accompanying tightness, myoedema, and spasms, flaccid or immobilized limbs, amputations and sympathetic dystrophy (209). In these patients, massage may be used to alter the pathophysiology of the primary condition (e.g., contracture) or to prevent or modify the negative ramifications of the primary treatment modality (i.e., nonobstructive limb edema from immobilization). The physiatrist will most frequently be involved with the chronic sequelae of these impairments and massage is, perhaps, more useful in chronic rather than acute conditions. In almost all cases, however, massage is secondary to and less important than the primary treatment therapies (i.e., immobilization, ranging, strengthening) and must be utilized in such a way that it acts synergistically with and not antagonistically to them. The sedative effect may be of complementary use in any of a large number of painful or anxiety stimulating conditions.

Contraindications

Massage is contraindicated when it would cause worsening of a condition, unwanted destruction of tissue, or spread of the condition (158). Malignancy, thrombi, atherosclerotic plaques, and infected tissue could be spread by massage, and their presence is felt to be an absolute contraindication to massage. Relative contraindications include: the treatment of scar tissue that is not fully healed; patients who are anticoagulated, either therapeutically or by disease; calcified soft tissues; skin grafts; inflamed tissue; atrophic skin; and tissue that is susceptible to further edema if circulation is increased by the massage technique.

Although not rigidly a contraindication, chronic pain situations must be approached cautiously by the physiatrist if massage is going to be used. Because it has a hands-on nature and potentially strong psychological effects, the risk of dependency of the patient is always present. Patient satisfaction, of course, may increase with this type of approach, but objective improvement in the impairment may not occur. To use massage for chronic pain, endpoints must be established before institution of the treatment, and treatment terminated when they are reached.

Practical Problems in Physiatric Application of Massage

Four practical issues may confront the physiatrist. The first, patients entering the physiatric milieu for the first time with a massage history already in place, will require some action on the part of even those physicians not interested in the utilization of massage. Many of these patients will have received massage directed at relaxation, sometimes ordered by physicians as a therapy for stress relief, but more often entered into by the patient by self-referral. While this type of therapy is seldom directed primarily at musculoskeletal problems, the practitioners often have varying degrees of experience in athletic training or other such vocations, and thus may address musculoskeletal issues in the course of the massage. An accurate history of the patient's experience is relevant and the physiatrist may wish to consider including the massage therapist in the overall care plan. At the very least, intervention when contraindications are present may become the responsibility of the physician.

The second practical issue facing the physiatrist committed to the use of the massage is the choice of a therapist. Competent practitioners in a therapeutic milieu may be nurses, physical therapists, occupational therapists, athletic trainers, or respiratory therapists. When the massage is to be used as an adjunct, the choice is usually dictated by the concomitant therapy. Thus, the type of provider chosen often will depend on skills other than massage skills. Most physical therapists and many occupational therapists receive massage training during their professional education. Massage involves as much art as science, though, and different providers might obtain markedly different results with what appear to be identical techniques. Thus, trial and error and local reputation are probably the most useful criteria involved in the choice of a specific practitioner.

A third issue is the cost and insurance coverage of the massage treatment. Massage alone is rarely reimbursed, and generally it will need to be bundled into the overall therapy plan to be viable for most patients. This aspect usually acts to the patient's benefit for two reasons. The accompanying therapies will tend to prevent dependency on massage, particularly in chronic pain conditions. Secondly, the other therapies involved usually have well established functional endpoints which can be utilized to justify the overall program and validate its composite efficacy, an issue of some importance with massage alone. In those few cases where function is not the desired outcome (the cosmetic result of lymphedema reduction, for example) the physician will have more difficulty establishing the usefulness of massage.

Lastly, a massage prescription may need to be generated, particularly if a long term program is anticipated. Such a prescription should include the relevant diagnoses, precautions, the area to be treated, and the specific massage variables discussed earlier. Some of these variables cannot be determined by the physician *a priori* since tissue feedback often guides the provider, but limits can be delineated by the physician. Verifiable goals of the overall treatment plan should be included in the prescription.

Efficacy

Long-term efficacy of massage has not been validated in almost any of the conditions noted above. Most applications of interest to the physiatrist involve a limited course of therapy directed at permanent improvement of a condition. The situation is analogous to the use of an antibiotic to cure an infection as opposed to an anti-hypertensive medication designed to be used indefinitely. Long-term effects are therefore of paramount interest, but have not been investigated. One issue is that the underlying physiology of the tissues is not well understood so that it becomes difficult to understand how massage would affect that physiology. At this time, the therapeutic use of massage must be undertaken with the understanding that its value lies either in demonstrable short-term improvements (such as decreased edema, soreness, sensitivity) or in longer term verifiable outcomes of the accompanying therapies that it facilitates.

Given the increasing use of massage in the face of tightening health care expenditures, it is important that the long-term efficacy of this modality be established scientifically, including accurate outcome measures. In addition, entry criteria to identify the subset of patients most likely to benefit from massage would be useful. Massage continues to provide a valuable modality for physical medicine practitioners. It is user friendly, low risk, and does not rely on high technology. As a result, it is available world wide, and should continue to provide valuable health benefits in the future.

TRACTION

Traction is the act of drawing or pulling, or a pulling force. In medicine, forces are applied to the body generally to stretch a given part or separate two or more parts. Traction continues to be effectively used in the treatment of fractures of the extremities and the spine. In physiatry, traction is usually limited to the cervical or lumbar spine with the hope of relieving pain in, or originating from, those areas, and this section will address only spine traction.

Since the days of Hippocrates, attempts at correction of scoliosis have frequently involved traction in one form or another. Treatment of long bone fractures led to the development of many traction techniques in the 1800s (210). More recent attempts at spinal traction have included: applying the pulling force manually (211), with free weights and a pulley (212), with the patient supplying the pull with his hands or feet (213), with motorized equipment (214), by inversion and gravity supplying the pull (215), and an overhead harness in conjunction with treadmill walking (216).

Physiological Effects

Cervical Spine

The most reproducible result of traction to the cervical spine is elongation. Cyriax has reported that applying a force of 300 pounds manually results in a 1-cm increase in cumulative interspace distance (211). A study to determine optimal weight for cervical traction concluded that the minimum weight to accomplish any vertebral separation is 25 pounds (217). Greater forces (218), and in some cases much greater forces (219), have been used, but most studies have concluded that elongation of 2 to 20 mm of the cervical spine is achievable with 25 or more pounds of tractive force. In another investigation, the anterior and posterior intervertebral spaces (IVS) and the facet joint space at neck positions of 30° of flexion, neutral, and 15° of extension were quantified under 30 pounds of intermittent traction (8 seconds of traction followed by 6 seconds of rest) after a total traction time of 20 minutes. The anterior IVS was increased most in 30° of flexion, ranging from 18% to 21% with the largest IVS at C6–C7. The effect of traction on the facet joint was, in all three positions, not statistically significant. Traction in neck extension was noted by many subjects in the study to be painful, and the posterior IVS actually decreased in some instances. The investigators, citing these reasons, in addition to the increased risk of complications from vertebral basilar insufficiency and the possibility of spinal instability, did not recommend the use of traction in extension (220). The vertebral separation accomplished after traction has been reported as temporary, with return to normal height the morning after traction (218). The effect of traction on paraspinal muscles is not well known. Cyriax has postulated traction leads to fatigue and then relaxation (211). However, another study found greater muscle relaxation in the cervical traction group with a 2-pound placebo traction than in a group with 6 to 12 pounds of traction (221,222).

Lumbar Spine

Once friction is overcome with either adequate force of pull (223) or a split table (224), the major physiologic effect of traction of the lumbar spine is elongation. Investigators who report widening of the lumbar interspaces used between 70 and 300 pounds of pull to obtain this widening. The widening, when apparent, averages up to slightly more than 3 mm at one intervertebral foramen (225–228). The length of time that this separation persists remains indeterminate, with one study unable to document residual distraction 30 minutes posttreatment (227) and another demonstrating residual separation at least 10 minutes posttreatment, which was the extent of the observations (229).

Data have been generated on the dimensional and pressure changes caused by traction in lumbar discs, both in the normal spine and after herniation. A decrease in the intradiscal pressure of patients treated with 50 to 100 pounds of traction on a split table has been documented (224), but there is evidence that some such applications actually cause an increase in intradiscal pressure that, in principle, would exacerbate nerve compression from a herniated component of the disc (230). Discograms performed during both compression and distractive traction showed large variations (greater than 10%) of the radiologic disc area in patients with "disc syndrome," but failed to demonstrate area changes in normal subjects (231). Reduction of prolapsed discs during lumbar traction has been noted by epidural contrast (232) and computed tomography scanning techniques (233). The latter study was marred by lack of blinding and long-term follow-up. Thus, the evidence is inconclusive, with considerable information favoring at least temporary reduction of the herniated component of an abnormal lumbar disc under the influence of traction.

The issue of whether the disc changes size is really not identical to pressure relief on the nerve root or reversal of abnormal physiology in radiculopathy. This much more clinically relevant question has received surprisingly little attention in the literature to date. However, a study by Knutsson and colleagues demonstrated an improvement in lower extremity voluntary muscle strength and normalization of bilateral somatosensory evoked potentials and skin temperature (via thermography) after autotraction in patients with lumbar and sacral radiculopathies (234). Unfortunately, the investigators were not blinded, and controls and long-term follow-up evaluations were not included. Nonetheless, this research breaks ground in the area of inquiry that is of most interest to physiatry. It should be noted that there is a tendency for some physicians to use lumbar traction as a means of enforcing bed rest (235,236). The benefits of strict bedrest for low back pain are questionable, and physiologic effects in these are discussed in the chapter on Immobilization.

Outcome

There are few scientifically rigorous studies in the literature that allow the effect of traction to be distinguished from the natural history of the pathology (usually radiculopathy) being treated. Deyo has suggested criteria that would allow the true effects of traction to be delineated in the face of confounding variables. Studies meeting these criteria should use (a) randomized, controlled trials; (b) blinded outcomes assessment; (c) equivalent cointerventions; (d) monitored compliance; (e) minimal attrition; (f) minimal contamination; (g) adequate statistical power; (h) adequate description of study design, patients, and interventions; and (i) relevant, functional outcomes (237). No traction outcome study has achieved all these criteria to date. Despite this, there are randomized, controlled trials that meet many of these and give clinicians some insight into the efficacy of traction.

Lumbar Traction

The AHCPR recently reviewed the literature on traction and made recommendations as part of the clinical practice guideline on acute low back problems in adults. Thirty-one articles were examined, of which six randomized, controlled trials met criteria for their review. Additionally, the panel did a meta-analysis of traction. The AHCPR conclusion was that "spinal traction is not recommended in the treatment of acute low back problems" (3). This is a strong, negative recommendation that does not appear to be refuted by other randomized, controlled trials using good methodology.

The studies that claim improvement after traction report modest, short-term improvements with limited or no improvement in functional outcome and have study design flaws. Some examples of specific studies that report improved outcome after traction illustrate the lack of convincing evidence for traction efficacy. Eighty-two patients with acute sciatica and positive straight leg-raising signs were assigned randomly to either corset and bed rest (not timed controlled placebo) or autotraction (238). Evaluation was performed at one and three weeks posttreatment by a blinded observer and at 3 months by questionnaire. Traction subjects were treated either as outpatients, who were usually driven home by ambulance, or as inpatients. Placebo controls did not have the time intensive ambulance rides or overnight hospital stays. While no outcome differences between those treated with traction and those treated as controls was apparent at 3 months during follow-up, the traction-treated group reported modest pain relief without documented functional improvement at both 1 and 3 weeks posttreatment.

Pain relief has been reported in patients who were treated with traction for 6 days for a chief complaint of back pain and sciatica (239). This improvement was limited to a subgroup of women under age 45, follow-up was only 2 weeks, and functional outcomes were not measured. Another investigation showed that patients with sciatica treated with traction and exercise had more favorable pain improvement than a cohort treated with hot packs, massage, and spinal mobilizing and strengthening exercises. The actual control group in this study received a placebo therapy of hot packs and rest and had similar improvement to the traction group. Nonetheless, these similar results were interpreted as a "significant priority" for those treated with pelvic traction (240). Other controlled trials evaluating primarily patients with sciatica do not report clear benefit for traction (241–245). Of course the "absence of proof is not the proof of absence." It is entirely possible that a subgroup of patients (e.g. lateral herniated discs with radiculopathy) will benefit from a particular type of traction for either short-term or long-term improvement in functional outcome. At this stage, the literature does not clearly delineate these subgroups.

Cervical Traction

There are few randomized, controlled trials to address patient outcome after cervical traction. Methodology problems are similar to those noted previously regarding lumbar traction. A review of the randomized, controlled trials available will give clinicians an idea of the potential efficacy and limitations of cervical traction.

Perhaps the most ambitious trial was conducted by the British Association of Physical Medicine and published in 1966. A total of 466 neck and arm pain patients were randomly assigned into one of five groups: (a) traction; (b) placebo traction (positioning); (c) instruction in posture and cervical collar; (d) placebo as untuned shortwave diathermy; and (e) placebo tablets. A blinded assessment was performed at 2 and 4 weeks with letter follow-up at 6 months. Outcome measures included range of motion, pain, and function. There was no statistical difference between the groups and no noticeable trends in subgroups. The authors suggest that none of these treatments alters the natural history of the problem. The major potential criticism of this study is that the traction treatment was not completely standardized. The investigators reported that the traction was "given every chance to succeed" and thus the therapist had latitude to customize the traction (246).

Three randomized trials have reported improvements in patients treated with cervical traction. Goldie and Landquist reported on the results of a randomized, controlled trial in 73 neck and arm pain patients who were placed into one of three groups: (a) traction; (b) isometric exercises; and (c) instruction only (no time-controlled placebo). There was slight improvement in both of the treatment groups over no treatment, with patient report, blinded physician report, and range of motion measurement used as outcome measures. Of note, there was no difference in "sick leave," although there was a trend for less time off work in the instruction only group (247). Zylbergold and Piper reported on a controlled trial of 100 patients randomized into one of four groups: (a) static traction; (b) intermittent traction; (c) manual traction; and (d) nontraction treatment (hot packs, exercise, and range of motion not strictly time controlled with other traction groups). Blinded observers noted that the intermittent traction caused improvement over the other three treatments in range of motion (neck flexion and rotation) (248). Klaber-Moffett et al. reported a statistically significant improvement in neck range of motion in patients receiving continuous traction. Although *statistically* significant findings were reported in these studies, the actual *clinical* significance of 5° to 10° of neck movement is unclear. Measures of pain, sleep disturbance, social dysfunction, and activities of daily living did not show statistically significant improvement in the traction group (221–222).

Techniques of Applying Traction

Manual

Cyriax has written most extensively about manual application of spinal traction primarily as an adjunct or precursor to spinal manipulation (211,249).

Cervical

Traction generally is transmitted to the spine by a free weight and pulley system or an electrical motorized device. Adequate pull for the cervical spine is achievable by using a head or chin sling attached to a system that can provide pull in a cephalad direction. The motorized devices have the advantage of allowing easy application of intermittent traction but require the patient to be in the clinic. Free weight and pulley systems have been developed for home use. Many units for home traction consist of a bag filled with 20 or more pounds of water or sand, and a pulley system attached to a door. If a tractive force of only 20 pounds is possible, then the system probably will fail to achieve therapeutic results because one half of that weight counterbalances the head in the sitting position (250), and only a suboptimal 10 pounds of traction remains. This limitation has led to the development of supine cervical traction units that sacrifice only a few pounds of pull to overcome friction. Cervical traction should not be attempted at home alone because if patients get into uncomfortable positions, they may need help extricating themselves. Additionally, most of these systems are difficult for the patient to set up without assistance. Home cervical traction can cause an increase in pain or fail to produce significant pain relief unless it is professionally monitored periodically. Improper head and neck position and inadequate tractive force lead to ineffectual therapy. At the initiation of home traction, the patient should demonstrate proper use of the equipment to the satisfaction of the therapist. This demonstration should be repeated at intervals, starting at 1 week and gradually progressing up to 2 to 4 weeks.

Lumbar

Adequate pull with weights and pulleys or motorized device (233) to achieve vertebral distraction also can be attained in the lumbar spine with the proper apparatus. A harness is usually attached around the pelvis (to deliver the caudal pull), and the upper body is stabilized by a chest harness or voluntary arm force (for cephalad pull). Motorized units have the relative advantage of allowing intermittent traction with less therapist supervision. If the goal of traction is distraction of lumbar vertebrae, then 70 to 150 pounds of pull is generally employed (236). The friction between the treatment table and body usually requires a traction force of 26% of the total body weight before there is any effective traction to the lumbar spine (223). Thus, if lumbar traction is applied to a 200-pound patient, the first 50 pounds of traction would not be therapeutic to the lumbar spine. Many traction devices use a "split table" that essentially eliminates the lower body segment friction (251). There are very few practical home lumbar traction units.

Gravity

Theoretically, body weight provides sufficient pull to distract lumbar vertebrae and eliminates much of the necessary mechanical apparatus. Gravity traction is used almost exclusively for lumbar traction. Inversion traction is accomplished by patients hanging upside down with their feet strapped in special boots. After 10 minutes of inversion traction, there has been documented increased intervertebral foraminal separation (228). However, reported side effects have included increase in blood pressure, periorbital and pharyngeal petechiae, persistent headaches, persistent blurred vision, musculoskeletal pain, and contact lens discomfort (252). The use of inversion therapy has greatly decreased in recent years, and many clinicians feel the risks outweigh the benefits. Other gravitational lumbar traction systems involve corsetlike vests worn around the ribcage, causing the patient's feet to be lifted from the ground with the weight of the legs and pelvis supplying the traction force to the lumbar spine (227,252). Recently this type of suspension has been combined with a treadmill to allow exercise and normal activity during traction (216).

Autotraction

Autotraction devices allow the patient to provide tractive forces by pulling with their arms on a specially designed table (213,228,253,254). One randomized treatment trial with nonblinded observers suggested that autotraction was more efficacious than passive traction (255).

Parameters

As with many other areas of physiatric therapeutics, little has been proven about the exact parameters of traction and their relationship to the efficacy of traction. Preferences of specific parameter settings (e.g., sitting versus supine, continuous versus intermittent) depend more on the practitioner's empirical observation than on objective data. Individual physicians should, within limits dictated by common sense and the experiences of others, develop personal guidelines regarding the amount of weight, duration of traction, and other parameters. Above all, the patient should be comfortable during traction therapy; monitoring by the physical therapist is essential to ensure that the traction applied is not ineffective or aggravating a painful condition.

Positioning

Cervical

In cervical traction, the choice of sitting versus supine positioning should be based on patient comfort and ability to relax. Crue was the first to suggest the importance of neck position in cervical traction (256,257). This may be related to widening of the intervertebral foramina and/or intervertebral spaces. The maximal effect of distraction seems to occur between 20° and 30° of flexion with no rotation or sidebending components (220,258). Nearly all studies report difficulties with the cervical spine in extension; thus, neck extension during traction should be avoided (220).

Lumbar

Lumbar traction can be accomplished in the upright body suspension, but chest discomfort from the harness is often a limiting factor (227), so the supine position is most commonly chosen. Hip flexion (15° to 70°) is routinely incorporated to cause relative lumbar spine flexion, theoretically leading to optimal vertebral separation. Reliable studies comparing different positions of lumbar traction are lacking.

Continuous Versus Intermittent Traction

Cervical

A larger improvement in range of motion with less accompanying pain was noted in patients subjected to intermittent traction of 25 pounds peak (10 seconds on, 10 seconds off, total duration of 15 minutes), than in cohorts subjected either to 15 minutes of manual traction or 15 minutes of static traction of 25 pounds. All three groups were treated with the cervical spine flexed at 25° (248). Data show that a constant cervical distraction force of 30 pounds effects maximum vertebral separation in 7 seconds or less, and that no more is gained by applications of 30 or 60 seconds (229). If so, then strictly skeletal effects require no longer application times in order to be optimized but, of course, accompanying musculoligamentous relaxations (211) may require much longer times of application. These studies, in conjunction with the fact that patients may prefer the improved comfort of intermittent pull, suggest some advantage to an intermittent over continuous protocol (217,248,259).

Lumbar

There is limited information on this topic for lumbar traction. Cyriax has reported that continuous traction is necessary to fatigue the muscles and allow strain to fall on the joints (211). Despite this claim, no statistical difference in x-rays was noted for normal subjects treated with either continuous traction of 100 pounds for 5 minutes or intermittent traction of 100 pounds peak for 15 minutes (10 seconds traction, 5 seconds rest) (212). Similarly, the data seem conclusive for the skeletal effects, but it is conceivable that some of the benefits of traction occur in the soft tissues, which may respond much differently in terms of sensitivity to time. Again, improved patient tolerance seems to favor the use of intermittent traction (214).

Weight

Cervical

If cervical traction is performed with the patient in the sitting position, about 10 pounds are required to counterbalance the patient's head (250). Amounts less than this may be used initially to condition the patient to the feel of the halter and pull. In the literature there is a great deal of variation, with the amount of force reported varying from 6 to 440 pounds of traction (260). Colachis and Strohm have shown that 30 pounds of traction to a neck flexed to 24° can cause vertebral separation, particularly posteriorly, but an increase of force to 50 pounds produced no clear-cut additional separation (258). This correlates with the earlier finding that a minimum of 25 pounds was needed before the vertebrae separated (217). An initial "test dose" of 5 or 10 pounds of traction followed by a gradual increase in weight to 45 or 50 pounds has been advocated (217).

Lumbar

Friction becomes an important consideration in the lumbar spine. In a widely quoted article, Judovich reported that a pull equal to about one half the weight of a body part is needed to overcome friction: for the lower body, this becomes 26% of total body weight (223). Either this amount of force needs to be applied before true traction on the spine is accomplished or a split table must be used (223,251,261). Regardless of whether the effect of friction is overpowered or by-passed, another 25% or more of body weight is then needed to cause vertebral separation. For example, Colachis and Strohm used 50 and 100 pounds of lumbar traction with a split table and measured statistically significant vertebral separation with both weights (212). Posterior vertebral separation predominated at 50 pounds; anterior and posterior widening occurred at 100 pounds. The usual range of traction is between 70 and 150 pounds, averaging 100 pounds (236,262). With tractive forces above 100 pounds, the counterforce, in the form of a chest or axillary harness, causes pain and is the limiting factor for many patients.

Duration

Cervical

The exact and optimal duration of traction has not been clearly shown. Recommendations have varied from 2 minutes to 24 hours for each session (248). Intermittent traction with the neck in flexion for a total traction time of 15 minutes (248), or 20 minutes (220), or 25 minutes (226) has produced physiologic effects. A duration of 15 to 25 minutes, if tolerated by patients, is commonly prescribed. There is also significant variability in the frequency of application and duration of program parameters ranging from daily for 2 months to two or three times per year. Traction is most commonly prescribed at a frequency of daily for the first week, then every other day (or 3 times per week) for a total treatment time of 3 or 4 weeks. Most reported trials use 10 to 15 sessions over a 3 to 4 week period (246,247,248,260).

Lumbar

The information pertinent to duration of force application is limited and does not allow definitive judgments to be made. In cadavers, 85% of lumbar elongation retraction occurred immediately (263). Others have applied traction for 5 minutes to 8 hours (218,227,228). Lumbar traction with minimum weight often has been used for many days to enforce bed rest without the expectation of the physiologic effect of the traction itself. Treatment recommendations are usually recommended in the 8 to 40 minute range per session (236).

Recommendations for frequency are similar to those for cervical traction, i.e., daily for the first week then every other day (or 3 times per week) for a total treatment time of 3 or 4 weeks. Most reported trials use 10 to 15 sessions over a 3- to 4-week period (236,246–248,260,262).

For both cervical and lumbar traction, goals of treatment should dictate the time course and determine the endpoint of treatment. Potential endpoints of treatment include (a) pain relief; (b) normal range of motion; (c) return to work or appropriate activity; (d) exacerbation of symptoms during treatment; (e) inability or unwillingness of patient to schedule traction; (f) lack of improvement in symptoms and/or activity any time after four to six sessions of traction; and (g) 3 or 4 weeks of traction. Any of these can be used for individual rehabilitation programs depending on the role of traction in the overall program.

Indications for Traction

The literature does not give clear indications for what type of neck or low back pain can benefit from traction. In fact, the preponderance of studies strongly suggest that traction does not significantly influence the long-term outcomes of neck or low back pain (264). Thus, defining indications in the face of poor scientific evidence of efficacy is very difficult. Physicians who prefer sound scientific evidence for the efficacy of treatment probably will rarely use traction for spinal pain. Without additional scientifically valid outcome studies, it is possible that spinal traction as a treatment for neck and back pain will gradually decrease. For clinicians who are willing to recommend empirical treatments, the indications for traction are outlined below.

Theoretically, if traction can separate vertebrae and decrease the size of herniated discs, then patients with this problem and radiculopathy would be the most likely to benefit. Indeed, most studies attempt to target this population, with little demonstrated efficacy. There is considerable disagreement among investigators. Weinberger has suggested that traction is "irrational, counterproductive, nonphysiologic and traumatic" (265). Yates has stated that there is no reason to suggest traction will be any more useful to treat degenerative spondylosis of the cervical spine than traction to a hip or knee with osteoarthritis (266).

Cervical

Cervical traction has been used for a wide spectrum of painful conditions based on its physiologic effects of vertebral separation, widening of the intervertebral nerve root foramina, and possible reduction of herniated disc material and muscle relaxation. Neck and arm pain have been historically used as the indications (246).

Lumbar

Low back pain caused by herniated nucleus pulposus, lumbar radiculopathy, or muscle spasm might improve with appropriately applied traction of adequate force (249). Additionally, some clinicians use lumbar traction as an enforcement of bed rest in the treatment of acute low back pain. There are no data to suggest that nonpainful radiculopathy with clear neurologic deficit will benefit from traction.

Contraindications

There are few anecdotal reports and no scientific reports that clearly delineate the contraindications of traction. Thus, clinicians must rely on empirical information and opinion to guide them. Old age is a relative contraindication, given the likelihood that at least one of the described conditions is more likely to be present in the elderly. Should a practitioner wish to prescribe traction for an elderly person, a careful screening process should be used.

In general, the following are considered contraindications to cervical or lumbar traction: ligamentous instability; osteomyelitis; discitis; primary or metastatic bone tumor (267); spinal cord tumor; severe osteoporosis; untreated hypertension; severe anxiety; clinical signs of myelopathy; or inadequate expertise.

Cervical traction requires additional considerations. Patients with vertebral basilar artery insufficiency could theoretically experience a stroke due to traction, particularly with the neck in extension. In the elderly it is difficult to confidently eliminate the diagnosis of vertebral basilar insufficiency. Thus, patients with a history at all suggestive of vertebral basilar insufficiency should not have cervical traction. Additionally, patients with rheumatoid arthritis and other connective tissue disorders are at high risk for atlantoaxial instability. This also may be difficult to diagnose, and thus patients with rheumatoid arthritis should undergo cervical traction with extreme caution, if at all. Patients with midline herniated nucleus pulposus and/or acute torticollis should not have cervical traction (217).

Lumbar traction has fewer factors that require special consideration. However, patients with restrictive lung disease or other breathing disorders should not be subjected to the pull of a chest harness. Additionally, the presence of the following have been listed as contraindications without supporting evidence: pregnancy, active peptic ulcers, hiatal hernia, other hernias, aortic aneurysm, gross hemorrhoids, and evidence for cauda equina compromise (260). After evaluation of the patient, if there is any question of spine instability, imaging studies, especially flexion–extension x-rays of the spine, should be considered.

Writing the Referral

The practitioner can no more write ''cervical traction, please'' as a treatment prescription than to ask for ''physical therapy for back pain'' or ''medications for infection.'' One is obliged to write a detailed parameter-specific prescription for cervical or lumbar traction. As with other physical therapy referrals, the following patient information is included: age, gender, diagnosis, underlying medical conditions, precautions to be taken, patient symptoms that would signal a need to discontinue the traction, and recommended medical follow-up.

Cervical or lumbar traction should not be used as a single modality but rather as one aspect of an overall rehabilitation program. Traction as a modality to improve activity, mobility, and function (e.g., return to work) is probably most effective. If patients are required to miss 2 to 3 hours of work per day to undergo traction and physical therapy, one could argue this is ineffective treatment and may actually be counterproductive to the patient's overall recovery and well-being.

The patient's interests are not served by writing a prescription for a home cervical traction unit and expecting a pharmacy clerk to explain its use, nor is lumbar traction reliably self-applied by the patient at home. The therapist's input therefore becomes critical to the successful and safe use of traction. If traction, for any reason, exacerbates symptoms, it should be discontinued and the efficacy and rationale of continued traction should be closely examined. There is no evidence to date to suggest that the patient should ''endure the side effects'' of traction in order to enjoy its therapeutic effect.

The following specific parameters should be outlined in all traction referrals.

Position
- Body position: sitting, supine, standing, or walking on treadmill.
- Neck position (cervical traction): between neutral and 30° of neck flexion.
- Hip/Knee position (Pelvic traction): full extension to 90° of flexion can be used.

Mode of application
- Continuous or intermittent: Intermittent is preferred for patient comfort. Variable times have been used, e.g., 7 to 15 seconds of traction with 5 to 10 seconds rest or 30 to 60 seconds of force with 10 to 20 seconds of rest. Some equipment allows adjustment of the speed that each cycle allows to reach maximum force (rise time).

Weight
- A range is necessary to allow patient acclimatization. Usually a small amount of traction is used at the beginning with additional weight added later.
- Cervical: 5 to 45 pounds (starting low and gradually increasing/decreasing each session or over a number of sessions).
- Lumbar: 50 to 150 pounds.

Other modalities: superficial heat for relaxation before or during traction may be used.

Time: in most instances, 10 to 30 minutes.

Frequency and duration: 3 to 5 times per week for 3 to 6 weeks.

Physician re-evaluation: 2 to 14 days

Guidelines for discontinuation: if symptoms become worse or new symptoms develop (e.g., pain, dizziness, weakness, autonomic symptoms) traction should be discontinued.

Goals and endpoint: delineating endpoints that the physiatrist can identify is helpful. Some of these are discussed above in the duration session. Working on protocols with therapists can be useful.

Home traction: If a supervised trial of cervical traction is successful, a home unit can be prescribed with the contingency that the therapist check the patient for correct head and neck positioning and for the use of adequate weight initially and at intervals. The monitoring interval may vary depending on the patient but will likely increase over time.

The Future of Traction

Traction has a long history of clinical acceptance based on surprisingly little understanding of its mechanism of action or suggestions, let alone proof, of efficacy. Although it seems natural to associate separation of the vertebrae with relief of pressure on the spinal nerves in situations where herniated discs are present in the lateral recesses, little or no evidence exists for this mechanism. Even if it does occur in this manner, the question arises as to whether the pressure relief is permanent and, if not, is it reasonable to believe that a neuropathic process will reverse itself in the short time the separation is present. If not, then might not some of the perceived benefits result from changes in the musculoligamentous system via relaxation, vasodilation, neurologic reflexes, or any other of numerous mechanisms that might occur? Twenty years ago these questions were unanswerable, but modern and future imaging and physiologic instruments are able to evaluate neurologic, muscular, and soft-tissue structures also. Unlike manipulation, which deals with normal but dysfunctional tissue (i.e., no clear neurologic damage), traction generally has been studied in patients with apparent abnormal structure. Perhaps traction really only addresses the soft tissues, and the wrong subset of patients (neck or back pain secondary to radiculopathy) has been evaluated.

It seems difficult if not impossible to document the actual prevalence of the use of traction in clinical practice today; based on anecdotal discussions and the paucity of fresh literature on the subject, it appears its use has diminished significantly over the past few years. It would be unfortunate if traction were to fall out of favor because no one has used modern technology to study it. This is particularly true at a time when spine pain is a growing societal burden, and no other highly effective treatments appear on the horizon.

REFERENCES

1. Haldeman S. Spinal manipulative therapy in the management of low back pain. In: Finneson BE, ed. *Low back pain,* 2nd ed. Philadelphia: JB Lippincott, 1980; 245–275.
2. Stillwell GK, deLateur BJ, Geiringer SR, Keen M, Kevorkian CG, Steinberg F. *Self-directed medical knowledge program in physical medicine and rehabilitation, syllabus,* 2nd ed. Chicago: American Academy of Physical Medicine and Rehabilitation, 1986; 1–22.
3. U.S. Department of Health and Human Services. *Acute low back problems in adults.* (AHCPR Publication no. 95-0642). Washington, DC: U.S. Government Printing Office, 1994.
4. *PM&R in Practice.* 1996; 4(3):4.
5. Schiotz EH, Cyriax J. *Manipulation past and present.* London: William Heinemann, 1975.
6. Lewitt K. *Manipulative therapy in rehabilitation of the motor system.* London: Butterworths, 1985.
7. Miller WD. Treatment of visceral disorders by manipulative therapy. In: Goldstein M, ed. *The research status of spinal manipulative therapy.* DHEW publication no. (NIH) 76-998. Bethesda, MD: National Institutes of Health, 1975; 295–301.
8. Dvorak J, Dvorak V, Schneider W, eds. *Manual medicine.* Berlin: Springer-Verlag, 1984.
9. Greenman PE. *Principles of manual medicine,* 2nd ed. Baltimore: Williams & Wilkins, 1996.
10. Harris JD. History and development of manipulation and mobilization. In: Basmajian JV, Nyberg R, eds. *Rational manual therapies.* Baltimore, MD: Williams & Wilkins, 1993; 7–19.
11. Cyriax J, Russel G. *Textbook of orthopaedic medicine.* Vol. 2: Treatment by manipulation, massage, and injection. London: Bailliere Tindall, 1980.
12. Kleynhans AM. Complications and contraindications to spinal manipulative therapy. In: Haldeman S, ed. *Modern developments in the principles and practice of chiropractic.* Norwalk, CT: Appleton-Century-Crofts, 1980; 359–384.
13. Gorman RF. Cardiac arrest after cervical mobilization. *Med J Aust* 1978; 2:169.
14. Rettig H. Observation of an acute Basedow's syndrome after chiropractic treatment of the cervical spine. *Med Klin* 1955; 26:1528.
15. Maigne R. *Diagnosis and treatment of pain of vertebral orgin.* Baltimore: Williams & Wilkins, 1996.
16. Nyberg R. Role of therapists in spinal manipulation. In: Basmajian JV, ed. *Manipulation, traction and massage,* 3rd ed. Baltimore: Williams & Wilkins, 1985; 22–46.
17. Bourdillon JF. *Spinal manipulation,* 3rd ed. New York: Appleton-Century-Crofts, 1983.
18. Grieve GP. *Mobilization of the spine,* 3rd ed. Edinburgh, Scotland: Churchill-Livingstone, 1979.
19. Maigne R. Manipulation of the spine. In: Basmajian JV, ed. *Manipulation, traction and massage,* 3rd ed. Baltimore: Williams & Wilkins, 1985.
20. Mennell JM. *Back pain.* Boston: Little, Brown, 1960.
21. Paterson JK, Burn L. *An introduction to medical manipulation.* Lancaster: MTP Press, 1985.
22. Cassidy JD, Kirkaldy-Willis WH, McGregor M. Spinal manipulation of chronic low back and leg pain: an observational study. In: Buerger AA, Greenman PE, eds. *Validation of spinal manipulation.* Springfield, IL: Charles C Thomas, 1985; 119–148.
23. Stoddard A. *Manual of osteopathic practice*, 2nd ed. New York: Harper & Row, 1969.
24. Atchison JW; Newman RL, Klim GV. Interest in manual medicine among residents in physical medicine and rehabilitation. The need for increased instruction. *Am J Phys Med Rehabil* 1995; 74:439–443.
25. Mckenzie RA. *The lumbar spine.* Walkanae, New Zealand: Spinal Publications, 1981.
26. Maigne R. *Orthopedic medicine.* Springfield, IL: Charles C Thomas, 1972.
27. Haldeman S, Rubinstein SM. The precipitation for aggravation of musculoskeletal pain in patients receiving spinal manipulative therapy. *J Manipulative Physiol Ther* 1993; 16:47–50.
28. Maitland GD. *Vertebral manipulation,* 5th ed. London: Butterworths, 1986.
29. Reid DC, Robinson BE. Contraindications and precautions to spinal joint manipulation: a review. Part I: specific spinal conditions. *Can J Rehabil* 1988; 2:19–30.
30. Reid DC, Robinson BE. Contraindications and precautions to spinal joint manipulation: a review. Part II: selected patient groups and special conditions. *Can J Rehabil* 1988; 2:71–78.

31. Goodridge JP. Muscle energy technique: definition, explanation, methods of procedure. *J Am Osteopath Assoc* 1981; 81:249–252.
32. Kappler RE. Direct action techniques. *J Am Osteopath Assoc* 1981; 81:239–243.
33. Diakow PR, Gadsby TA, Gadsby JB, Gleddie JG, Leprich DJ, Scales AM. Back pain during pregnancy and labor. *J Manipulative Physiol Ther* 1991; 14:116–118.
34. Daly JM, Frame PS, Rapoza PA. Sacroiliac subluxation: a common, treatable cause of low back pain in pregnancy. *Fam Pract Res J* 1991; 11:149–159.
35. Parson C. Back care in pregnancy. *Mod Midwife* 1994; 4:16–19.
36. DiGiovanna EL, Schiowitz S. *An osteopathic approach to diagnosis and treatment.* Philadelphia: JB Lippincott, 1991; 3–8.
37. Quon JA, Cassidy JD, O'Connor SM, Kirkaldy-Willis WH. Lumbar intervertebral disc herniation: treatment by rotational manipulation. *J Manipulative Physiol Ther* 1989; 12:220–227.
38. Krueger BR, Okazaki H. Vertebral-basilar distribution infarction following chiropractic cervical manipulation. *Mayo Clin Proc* 1980; 55: 322–332.
39. Sherman DG, Hart RG, Easton JD. Abrupt change in head position and cerebral infarction. *Stroke* 1981; 12:2–6.
40. Terrett AG, Kleynhans AM. Cerebrovascular complications of manipulation. In: Haldeman S, ed. *Principles and practice of chiropractic,* 2nd ed. Norwalk, CT: Appleton & Lange, 1992; 579–598.
41. Powell FC, Hanigan WC, Oliero WC. A risk/benefit analysis of spinal manipulation therapy for relief of lumbar or cervical pain. *Neurosurgery* 1993; 33:73–79.
42. Wiesel SW, ed. Complications of cervical manipulation are rare but may include stroke and spinal cord injury. *The Back Letter.* 1995; 10(6):61–72.
43. Hooper J. Low back pain and manipulation paraparesis after treatment of low back pain by physical methods. *Med J Aust* 1973; 1:549–551.
44. Kornberg E. Lumbar artery aneurysm with acute aortic occlusion resulting from chiropractic manipulation: a case report. *Surgery* 1988; 103:122–124.
45. Richard J. Disk rupture with cauda equina syndrome after chiropractic adjustment. *NY State J Med* 1967; 67:2496–2498.
46. Haldeman S, Rubinstein SM. Cauda equina syndrome in patients undergoing manipulation of the lumbar spine. *Spine* 1992; 17: 1469–1473.
47. Vick DA, McKay C, Zengerle CR. The safety of manipulative treatment: review of the literature from 1925 to 1993. *J Am Osteopath Assoc* 1996; 96:113–115.
48. Lee KP, Carlini WG, McCormick GF, Albers GW. Neurologic complications following chiropractic manipulation: a survey of California neurologists. *Neurology* 1995; 45:1213–1215.
49. Dvorak J, Kranzlin P, Muhlemaunn D, Walchi B. Musculoskeletal complications. In: Haldeman S, ed. *Principles and practice of chiropractic,* 2nd ed. Norwalk, CT: Appleton & Lange, 1992; 549–577.
50. Blackman J, Prip K. *Mobilization techniques.* Edinburgh, Scotland: Churchill-Livingstone, 1988.
51. Fisk JW. *Medical treatment of neck and back pain.* Springfield, IL: Charles C Thomas, 1987.
52. Gitelman R. A chiropractic approach to biomechanical disorders of the lumbar spine and pelvis. In: Haldeman S, ed. *Modern developments in the principles and practice of chiropractic.* Norwalk, CT: Appleton-Century-Crofts, 1984; 297–330.
53. Tobis JS, Hoekler F. *Musculoskeletal manipulation: evaluation of scientific evidence.* Springfield, IL: Charles C Thomas, Springfield, 1986.
54. Nwuga VCB. *Manual treatment of back pain.* Malabar, FL: RE Krieger, 1986.
55. Kirkaldy-Willis WH. *Manipulation.* In: Kirkaldy-Willis WH, ed. *Managing low back pain.* New York: Churchill-Livingstone, 1983.
56. Brodeur R. The audible release associted with joint manipulation. *J Manipulative Physiol Ther* 1995; 18:155–164.
57. Herzog W. Biomechanical studies of spinal manipulative therapy. *J Can Chiropract Assoc* 1991; 35:156–164.
58. Lee R, Evans J. Load-displacemnt time characteristics of the spine under posteroanterior mobilization. *Aust J Physiother* 1992; 38: 115–123.
59. Herzog W. Mechanical and physiological responses to spinal manipulative treatments. *J Neuromusc Systems* 1995; 3:1–9.
60. Cyriax J. *Textbook of orthopaedic medicine.* Vol. 2, 2nd ed. London: Balliere Tindall, 1984.
61. Grieve GP. *Common vertebral joint problems,* 2nd ed. Edinburgh, Scotland: Churchill-Livingstone, 1988.
62. Trott PH, Grant R, Maitland GD. Manipulative therapy for the low lumbar spine: technique selection and application to some syndromes. In: Twomey LT, Taylor JR, eds. *Physical therapy of the low back.* New York: Churchill-Livingstone, 1987; 199–224.
63. Sydenham RW. Manual therapy techniques for the thoracolumbar spine. In: Donatelli R, Wooden MJ, eds. *Orthopaedic physical therapy.* London: Churchill-Livingstone, 1989; 359–401.
64. Brandt B, Jones LH. Some methods of applying counterstrain. *J Am Osteopath Assoc* 1976; 75:786–789.
65. Kusunose RS. Strain and counterstrain. In: Basmajian JV, Nyberg R, eds. *Rational manual therapies.* Baltimore: Williams & Wilkins, 1993; 323–333.
66. Yates HA, Glover JC. *Counterstrain a handbook of osteopathic technique.* Tulsa, OK: Yknot, 1995.
67. Jones LH. Strain and counterstrain. Boise: Jones Strain-Counterstrain Inc., 1995; 92.
68. Travell JG, Simons DG. *Myofascial pain and dysfunction, the trigger point manual.* Baltimore: Williams & Wilkins, 1983.
69. Johnston WL, Friedman HD. *Functional methods.* Indianapolis: American Academy of Osteopath, 1994.
70. Bowles CH. Functional technique: a modern perspective. *J Am Osteopath Assoc* 1981; 80:326–331.
71. Neumann HD. *Introduction to manual medicine.* Berlin: Springer-Verlag, 1989.
72. Tehan PJ. Functional technique: a different perspective in manipulative therapy. In: Glasgow EF, Twomey LT, Scull ER, Kleynhans AM, eds. *Aspects of manipulative therapy.* London: Churchill-Livingstone, 1980; 94–96.
73. Mitchell FL, Mitchell PK. *The muscle energy manual.* Vol. 1. East Lansing, MI: MET Press, 1995.
74. Fowler C. Muscle energy techniques for pelvic dysfunction. In: Grieve GP, ed. *Modern manual therapy of the vertebral column.* New York: Churchill-Livingstone, 1986; 805–814.
75. Mitchell FL, Moran PS, Pruzzo NA. *Evaluation and treatment manual of osteopathic muscle energy technique.* Valley Park, MO: Moran & Pruzzo, 1979.
76. Tanigawa MC. Comparison of the hold relax procedure in passive mobilization on increasing muscle length. *Phys Ther* 1972; 32: 725–735.
77. Ward RC. Myofascial release concepts. In: Basmajain JV, Nyberg R, eds. *Rational manual therapies.* Baltimore: Williams & Wilkins, 1993; 223–240.
78. Hanten WP. Effects of myofascial release leg pull and sagittal plane isometric contract-relax techniques on passive straight-leg raise angle. *J Orthop Sports Phys Ther* 1994; 20:138–144.
79. Murphy T. Myofascial techniques. In: DiGiovanna EL, Schiowitz S, eds. *An osteopathic approach to diagnosis and treatment.* Philadelphia: JB Lippincott, 1991; 81–84.
80. Ward RC. *Myofascial release: concepts and treatment.* East Lansing, MI: Michigan State University Press, 1985.
81. Upledger JE, Vredevoogd JD. *Craniosacral therapy.* Seattle: Eastland Press, 1983.
82. Upledger JE. *Craniosacral therapy II.* Seattle: Eastland Press, 1987.
83. Urayama K. Origin of lumbar cerebrospinal fluid pulse wave. *Spine* 1994; 19:441–445.
84. Sutherland Cranial Teaching Foundation of the Cranial Academy: Osteopathy in the Cranial Field. Kirksville, MO: Journal Printing, 1976.
85. Adams T, Heisey RS, Smith MC, Briner BJ. Parietal bone mobility in the anesthetized cat. *J Am Osteopath Assoc* 1992; 92:599–622.
86. Heisey RS, Adams T. Role of cranial bone mobility in cranial compliance. *Neurosurgery* 1993; 33:869–877.
87. Greenman PE, McPartland JM. Cranial findings and iatrogenesis from craniosacral manipulation in patients with traumaatic brain syndrome. *J Am Osteopath Assoc* 1995; 95:182–188; 191–192.
88. Kenna C, Murtagh J. *Back pain and spinal manipulation.* Sydney: Butterworths, 1989.
89. Grice AS. A biomechanical approach to cervical and dorsal adjusting. In: Haldeman S, ed. *Modern developments in the principles and prac-*

tice of chiropractic. Norwalk, CT: Appleton-Century-Crofts, 1984; 331–358.

90. Kimberly PE. Formulating a prescription for osteopathic manipulative treatment. *J Am Osteopath Assoc* 1980; 79:506–513.
91. Brodin H, Bang J, Bechgarrd P, Kaltenborn F, Schiote E, eds. *Manipulation av ryggraden,* as reported by Nwuga VC. *Manipulation of the spine.* Baltimore: Williams & Wilkins, 1974.
92. Korr IM. Neural basis of the osteopathic lesion. *J Am Osteopath Assoc* 1947; 47:191–198.
93. Coote JH. Somatic sources of afferent input as factors in aberrant autonomic, sensory and motor function. In: Korr IM, ed. *Neurobiologic mechanisms in manipulative therapy.* New York: Plenum, 1978; 91–111.
94. Sato A. Physiological studies of the somato autonomic reflexes. In: Haldeman S, ed. *Modern developments in the principles and practice of chiropractic.* Norwalk, CT: Appleton-Century-Crofts, 1985; 91–105.
95. Sato A, Schmidt RF. The modulation of visceral functions by somatic afferent activity. *Jpn J Physiol* 1987; 37:1–16.
96. Slosberg M. Effects of altered afferent articular input on sensation, proprioception, muscle tone and sympathetic reflex responses. *J Manipulative Physiol Ther* 1988; 11:400–408.
97. Korr IM. Somatic dysfunction, osteopathic manipulative treatment, and the nervous system: a few facts, some theories, many questions. *J Am Osteopath Assoc* 1986; 86:109–114.
98. Patterson MM. Louisa Burns Memorial Lecture 1980. The spinal cord: active processor not passive transmitter. *J Am Osteopath Assoc* 1980; 80:210–216.
99. Grigg P, Greenspan BJ. Response of primate joint afferent neurons to mechanical stimulation of the knee joint. *J Neurophysiol* 1977; 40: 1–8.
100. Zusman M. Spinal manipulative therapy: review of some proposed mechanisms, and a new hypothesis. *Aust J Physiother* 1986; 32: 89–99.
101. Magee DJ. *Orthopedic physical assessment,* 2nd ed. Philadelphia, PA: WB Saunders, 1992.
102. Kaltenborn FM. *Mobilization of the extremity joints,* 3rd ed. Oslo, Norway: Olaf Norlis, 1980.
103. Wolff HD. The theory of joint play. In: Greenman P, ed. *Concepts and mechanisms of neuromuscular functions.* Berlin: Springer-Verlag, 1984; 108–110.
104. White AA, Panjabi MM. *Clinical biomechanics of the spine.* Philadelphia: JB Lippincott, 1990.
105. Janse J. History of the development of chiropractic concepts: chiropractic terminology. In: Goldstein M, ed. *The research status of spinal manipulative therapy.* DHEW publication no. (NIH) 76-998. Bethesda, MD: National Institutes of Health, 1975; 25–42.
106. Dvorak J. Neurological and biomechanical aspects of back pain. In: Buerger AA, Greenman PE, eds. *Validation of spinal manipulation.* Springfield, IL: Charles C Thomas, 1985; 241–266.
107. Neuman HD. A concept of manual medicine. In: Buerger AA, Greenman PE, eds. *Validation of spinal manipulation.* Springfield, IL: Charles C Thomas, 1985; 267–272.
108. Haldeman S. Manipulation and massage for the relief of pain. In: Wall PD, Melzack R, eds. *Textbook of pain.* Edinburgh: Churchill-Livingstone, 1989; 942–951.
109. Raftis KL. Manipulation for back pain. In: Warfield CA, ed. *Manual of pain management.* Philadelphia: JB Lippincott, 1991; 291–297.
110. Korr IM. Proprioceptors and somatic dysfunction. *J Am Osteopath Assoc* 1985; 74:638–650.
111. Viidik A. Biomechanical behavior of soft connective tissues. In: Akkas N, ed. *Progress in biomechanics.* The Netherlands: Sijthoff & Noordhoff, 1979; 75–113.
112. Hubbard RP, Chun KJ. Repeated extensions of collagenous tissue: measured responses and medical implications. In: Orphanoudakis SC, ed. *Proceedings of the Twelfth Annual Northeast Bioengineering Conference.* New Haven, CT: Institute of Electrical and Electronic Engineers, 1986; 157–160.
113. Brennan PC, Triano JJ, McGregor M, Kokjohn K, Hondras MA, Brennan DC. Enhanced neutrophil respiratory burst as a biological marker for manipulation forces: duration of the effect and association with substance P and tumor necrosis factor. *J Manipulative Physiol Ther* 1992; 15:83–89.
114. Christian GF, Stanton GJ, Sissons P, et al. Immunoreactive ACTH, beta-endorphin, and cortisol levels in plasma following spinal manipulative therapy. *Spine* 1988; 13:1411–1417.
115. Payson SM, Holloway HS. Possible complications of using naloxone as an internal opiate antagonist in the investigation of the role of endorphins in osteopathic manipulative treatment. *J Am Osteopath Assoc* 1984; 84(suppl):152–156.
116. Sanders GE, Reinert O, Tepe R, Maloney P. Chiropractic adjustive manipulation on subjects with acute low back pain: visual analog pain scores and plasma beta endorphin levels. *J Manipulative Physiol Ther* 1990; 13:391–395.
117. Vernon H. Exploring the effect of a spinal manipulation on plasma beta-endorphin levels in normal men. *Spine* 1989; 14:1272–1273.
118. Vernon HT, Dhami MS, Howley TP, Annett R. Spinal manipulation and beta-endorphin: a controlled study of the effect of a spinal manipulation on plasma beta-endorphin levels in normal males. *J Manipulative Physiol Ther* 1986; 9:115–123.
119. Cherkin DC, MacCornack FA. Patient evaluations of low back pain care from family physicians and chiropractors. *West J Med* 1989; 150: 351–355.
120. Laban MM, Taylor RS. Manipulation: an objective analysis of the literature. *Orthop Clin North Am* 1992; 23:451–459.
121. Winkel D. *Diagnosis and treatment of the spine.* Gaithersburg, MD: Aspen, 1996.
122. Koes BW, Bouter LM, van Mameren H, Essers AH, Verstegen GM, Hofhuizen DM, Houben JP, Knipschild PG. Randomised clinical trial of manipulative therapy and physiotherapy for persistent back and neck complaints: results of one year follow-up. *Br Med J* 1992; 304: 601–605.
123. Stanton DF, Wieting JM. The use of manipulation in the treatment of chronic pain syndrome. *Adv Med Psychother* 1997–1998; 9:119–127.
124. Brunarski DJ. Clinical trials of spinal manipulation: a critical appraisal and review of the literature. *J Manipulative Physiol Ther* 1984; 7: 243–249.
125. Evans DP. The design and results of clinical trials of lumbar manipulation: a review. In: Buerger AA, Greenman PE, eds. *Validation of spinal manipulation.* Springfield, IL: Charles C Thomas, 1985; 228–238.
126. Tobis JS, Hoehler F. *Musculoskeletal manipulation.* Springfield, IL: Charles C Thomas, 1986.
127. Curtis P. Spinal manipulation: does it work? *Spine State Art Rev* 1987; 2:31–44.
128. Abenhaim L, Bergeron AM. Twenty years of randomized clnical trials of manipulative therapy for back pain: a review. *Clin Invest Med* 1992; 15:527–535.
129. Buerger AA, Greenman PE, eds. *Validation of spinal manipulation.* Springfield, IL: Charles C Thomas, 1985.
130. Buerger AA, Tobis JS. *Approaches to the validation of manipulation therapy.* Springfield, IL: Charles C Thomas, 1977.
131. Hadler NM, Curtis P, Gillings DB, Stinnett S. A benefit of spinal manipulation as adjunctive therapy for acute low back pain: a stratified controlled trial. *Spine* 1987; 12:702–706.
132. Kinalski R, Kuwik W, Pietrzak D. The comparison of manual therapy versus physiotherapy methods used in the treatment of patients with low back pain syndromes. *J Manipulative Med* 1989; 4:44–46.
133. MacDonald RS, Bell CM. An open controlled assessment of osteopathic manipulation in nonspecific low-back pain. *Spine* 1990; 15: 364–370.
134. Meade TW, Dyer S, Browne W, Townsend J, Frank AO. Low back pain of mechanical origin: randomised comparison of chiropractic and hospital outpatient treatment. *Br Med J* 1990; 300:1431–1437.
135. Koes BW, Bouter LM, van der Heijden GJ. Methodological quality of randomized clinical trials on treatment efficacy in low back pain. *Spine* 1995; 20:228–235.
136. Coxhead CE, Inskip H, Meade PW, North WRS, Troup JDG. Multicenter trial of physiotherapy in the management of sciatic symptoms. *Lancet* 1981; 1:1065–1068.
137. Rasmussen GG. Manipulation in treatment of low back pain (a randomized clinical trial). *Manuelle Medizin* 1978; 1:8–10.
138. Koes BW, Assendelft WJ, van-der-Heijden GJ, Bouter LM, Knipschild PG. Spinal manipulation and mobilisation for back and neck pain: a blinded review. *Br Med J* 1991; 303:1298–1303.
139. Shekelle PG, Adams AH, Chassin MR, Hurqitz EL, Brook RH. Spinal manipulation for low-back pain. *Ann Intern Med* 1992; 117:590–598.
140. Anderson R, Meeker WC, Wireich BE, Mootz RD, Kirk DH, Adams

A. A meta-analysis of clinical trials of spinal manipulation. *J Manipulative Physiol Ther* 1992; 15:181–194.
141. Godfrey CM, Morgan PP, Schatzken J. A randomized trial of manipulation for low back pain in a medical setting. *Spine* 1984; 9:301–304.
142. Hoehler FK, Tobis JS. Appropriate statistical methods for clinical trials of spinal manipulation. *Spine* 1987; 12:409–411.
143. Haas M. The physics of spinal manipulation: part I. The myth of F = ma. *J Manipulative Physiol Ther* 1990; 13:204–206.
144. Haas M. The physics of spinal manipulation: part II. A theoretical consideration of the adjustive force. *J Manipulative Physiol Ther* 1990; 13:253–256.
145. Haas M. The physics of spinal manipulation: part III. Some characteristics of adjusting that facilitate joint distraction. *J Manipulative Physiol Ther* 1990; 13:305–308.
146. Haas M. The physics of spinal manipulation: part IV. A theoretical consideration of the physician impact force and energy requirements needed to produce synovial joint cavitation. *J Manipulative Physiol Ther* 1990; 13:378–383.
147. Lee M. Mechanics of spinal joint manipulation in the thoracic and lumbar spine: a theoretical study of posteroanterior force techniques. *Clin Biomechanics* 1989; 4:249–251.
148. Burton AK, Tillotson KM, Edwards VA, Sykes DA. Lumbar sagittal mobility and low back symptoms in patients treated with manipulation. *J Spinal Disorders* 1990; 3:262–268.
149. Rahlmann JF. Mechanisms of intervertebral joint fixation: a literature review. *J Manipulative Physiol Ther* 1987; 10:177–187.
150. Gal JM, Herzog W, Kawchuk GN, Conway PJ, Zhang YT. Forces and relative vertebral movements during SMT to unembalmed post-rigor human cadavers: peculiarities associated with joint cavitation. *J Manipulative Physiol Ther* 1995; 18:4–9.
151. Murphy BA, Dawson NJ, Slack JR. Sacroiliac joint manipulation decreases the H-reflex. *Electromyogr Clin Neurophysiol* 1995; 35: 87–94.
152. Haldeman S. The neurophysiology of spinal pain syndromes. In: Haldeman S, ed. *Modern developments in the principles and practice of chiropractic.* Norwalk, CT: Appleton-Century-Crofts, 1980; 119–142.
153. Wyke B. The neurology of low back pain. In: Jayson MIV, ed. *Lumbar spine and back pain,* 2nd ed. Kent, England: Pitman Medical, 1980; 265–340.
154. Goel VK, Weinstein JN. Role of mechanics in lumbar spine disease. In: Goel VK, Weinstein JN, eds. *Biomechanics of the spine.* Boca Raton, FL: CRC Press, 1990; 1–7.
155. Hubbard RP. Mechanical behavior of connective tissue. In: Greenman PE, ed. *Neuromuscular functions.* Berlin: Springer-Verlag, 1984; 47–54.
156. Huang Ti. *The yellow emperor's classic of internal medicine* [translated by Veith I]. Baltimore: Williams & Wilkins, 1949.
157. Kanemetz HL. History of massage. In: Basmajian JV, ed. *Manipulation, traction and massage,* 3rd ed. Baltimore: Williams & Wilkins, 1985.
158. Tappan FM. *Healing massage techniques: holistic, classic, and emerging methods,* 2nd ed. Norwalk, CT: Appleton & Lange, 1988.
159. Wood EC, Becker PD. *Beard's massage,* 3rd ed. Philadelphia: WB Saunders, 1981.
160. Rubik B, et al. *Manual healing methods in alternative medicine: expanding medical horizons. A report to the National Institutes of Health on Alternative Medical Systems and Practices in the United States.* Washington, DC: US Government Printing Office, 1994.
161. Goats GC. Massage—the scientific basis of an ancient art: part 1. The techniques. *Br J Sp Med* 1994; 28:149–152.
162. Geringer SR, Kincaid CB, Rechtien JR. Traction, manipulation, and massage. In: Delisa JA, ed. *Rehabilitation medicine: principles and practice,* 2nd ed. Philadelphia: JB Lippincott, 1993.
163. Atchison JW, Stoll ST, Gilliar WG. Manipulation, traction, and massage. In: Braddom RL, ed. *Physical medicine and rehabilitation.* Philadelphia: WB Saunders, 1996.
164. Borgey MAJ. *Manel de massage.* Paris: Masson, 1950.
165. Graham D. *Practical treatise on massage.* New York: Wm Wood, 1884.
166. Goats GC. Massage—the scientific basis of an ancient art: part 2. Physiological and therapeutic effects. *Br J Sp Med* 1994; 28:153–156.
167. Wakim KG. Physiologic effects of massage. In: Basmajian JV, ed. *Manipulation, traction and massage,* 3rd ed. Baltimore: Williams & Wilkins, 1985.
168. Pare A. *Oeuvres completes.* Paris: JB Balliere, 1941.
169. Basmajian JV, ed. *Manipulation, traction and massage,* 3rd ed. Baltimore: Williams & Wilkins, 1985.
170. Cyriax JH. Clinical applications of massage. In: Basmajian JV, ed. *Manipulation, traction and massage,* 3rd ed. Baltimore: Williams & Wilkins, 1985.
171. Lee HM, Whincup G, translators. *Chinese massage therapy.* Boulder, CO: Shambhala, 1983.
172. Brennan MJ. Focused review; post mastectomy lymphedema. Arch *Phys Med Rehabil* 1996; 77(suppl):74–80.
173. Foldi E, Foldi M, Clodius L. The lymphedema chaos: a lancet. *Ann Plast Surg* 1989; 22:505–515.
174. Pflug JJ. Intermittent compression; a new principle in treatment of wounds. *Lancet* 1974; 2:355–356.
175. Carrier EB. Studies on the physiology of capillaries. V. The reaction of the human skin capillaries to drugs and other stimuli. *Am J Physiol* 1922; 61:528–547.
176. Severini V, Venerando A. The physiological effects of massage on the cardiovascular system. *Eur Medicophys* 1967; 3:165–183.
177. Wakim KG, Martin GM, Terrier JC, Elkins EC, Krusen FH. The effects of massage on the circulation on normal and paralyzed extremities. *Arch Phys Med Rehabil* 1949; 30:134–144.
178. Hansen TI, Kristensen JH. Effect of massage, shortwave diathermy and ultrasound upon 133 Xe disappearance rate from muscle and subcutaneous tissue in the human calf. *Scand J Rehabil Med* 1973; 5:179–182.
179. Ernst E, Matrai A, Magyarosy I, Liebermeister RGA, Eck M, Breu MC. Massages cause changes in blood fluidity. *Physiotherapy* 1987; 73:43–45.
180. Allenby F, Boardman L, Pflug JJ, Calnan JS. Effects of external pneumatic intermittent compression of fibrinolysis in man. *Lancet* 1973; 2:1412–1414.
181. Knight MTN, Dawson R. Effect of intermittent compression of the arms on deep venous thrombosis in the legs. *Lancet* 1976; 2: 1265–1267.
182. Danneskiold-Samsoe B, Christiansen E, Lund B, Andersen RB. Regional muscle tension and pain (fibrositis): effect of massage on myoglobin in plasma. *Scand J Rehabil Med* 1983; 15:17–20.
183. Bork K, Korting GW, Faust G. ACtion of serum enzymes following whole body muscle massage: contribution to the problem of physical therapy in dermatomyosis. *Arch Dermatol Forsch* 1971; 240: 342–348.
184. Bale P, James H. Massage, warm-down and rest as recuperative measures after short term intense exercise. *Physiother Sport* 1991; 13: 4–7.
185. Suskind MI, Hajek NM, Hines HM. Effects of massage on denervated skeletal muscle. *Arch Phys Med* 1946; 27:133–135.
186. Wood EC, Kosman AJ, Osborne SL. Effects of massage in delaying atrophy in denervated skeletal muscle of the dog. *Phys Ther Rev* 1948; 28:284–285.
187. Chamberlain GJ. Cyriax's friction massage: a review. *J Orthop Sports Phys Ther* 1982; 4:16–22.
188. Hunter SC, Poole RM. The chronically inflamed tendon. *Clin Sports Med* 1987; 6:371–388.
189. Kaada B, Torsteinbo O. Increase of plasma beta-endorphins in connective tissue massage. *Gen Pharmacol* 1989; 20:487–489.
190. Melzack R, Wall PD. Pain mechanisms: a new theory. *Science* 1965; 150:971–979.
191. Ebner M. *Connective tissue manipulation: theory and therapeutic application,* 3rd ed. Malabar, FL: RE Krieger, 1975.
192. Dicke E. *Meine Bindegewebsmassage.* Stuttgart: Hippokrates-Verlag, 1956.
193. Reed B, Held J. Effects of sequential connective tissue massage on autonomic nervous system of middle-aged and healthy adults. *Phys Ther* 1988; 68:1231–1234.
194. McKechnie AA, Wilson F, Watson N, Scott D. Anxiety states: a preliminary report on the value of connective tissue massage. *J Psychosom Res* 1983; 27:125–129.
195. Frazer F. Persistent post sympathetic pain treated by connective tissue massage. *Physiotherapy* 1978; 64:211–212.
196. Robertson A, Gilmore K, Frith PA, Antic R. Effects of connective tissue massage in subacute asthma. *Med J Aust* 1984; 140:52–53.

197. Nansel D, Szlazak M. Somatic dysfunction and the phenomenon of visceral disease simulation: a probable explanation for the apparent effectiveness of somatic therapy in true visceral disease. *J Manipulative Physiol Ther* 1995; 18:379–397.
198. Longsworth JCD. Psychophysiological effects of slow stroke back massage in normotensive females. *Adv Nurs Sci* 1982; July:44–61.
199. Valentine KE. Massage in psychological medicine—modern use of an ancient art. *N Z J Physiother* 1984; 12:15–16.
200. Cantu RL, Grodin AJ. *Myofascial manipulation: theory and clinical application.* Gaithersburg, MD: Aspen, 1992.
201. Mason M. The treatment of lymphoedema by complex physical therapy. *Aust Physiother* 1993; 39:41–45.
202. Lerner R. The ideal treatment for lymphedema. *Massage Ther J* 1992; winter:37–39.
203. Swedborg I. Effectiveness of combined methods of physiotherapy for post-mastectomy lymphoedema. *Scand J Rehabil Med* 1980; 12: 77–85.
204. Casley-Smith JR, Casley-Smith JR. Modern treatment of lymphoedema I. Complex physical therapy: the first 200 Australian limbs. *Aust J Dermatol* 1992; 33:61–68.
205. Gillham L. Lymphoedema and physiotherapists: control not cure. *Physiotherapy* 1994; 80:835–843.
206. Zanolla R, Monzeglio C, Balzarini A, Martino G. Evaluation of the results of three different methods of postmastectomy lymphedema treatment. *J Surg Oncol* 1984; 26:210–213.
207. Boris M, Weindorf S, Lasinski B, Boris G. Lymphedema reduction by noninvasive complex lymphedema therapy. *Oncology* 1994; 9: 95–106.
208. Morgan RG, Casley-Smith JR, Mason MR, Casley-Smith JR. Complex physical therapy for the lymphoedematous arm. *J Hand Surg [Br]* 1992; 17:437–441.
209. Dietz FR, Mathews KD, Montgomery WJ. Reflex sympathetic dystrophy in children. *Clin Orthop* 1990; 258:225–231.
210. Peltier LF. A brief history of traction. *J Bone Joint Surg [Am]* 1968; 50:1603–1617.
211. Cyriax JH. *Textbook or orthopaedic medicine: diagnosis of soft tissue lesions,* 8th ed. London: Balliere Tindall, 1982.
212. Colachis SC, Strohm BR. Effects of intermittent traction on separation of lumbar vertebrae. *Arch Phys Med Rehabil* 1969; 50:251–258.
213. Tesio L, Luccarelli G, Formari M. Natchev's auto-traction for lumbago-sciatica: effectiveness in lumbar disc herniation. *Arch Phys Med Rehabil* 1989; 70:831–834.
214. Rogoff JB. Motorized intermittent traction. In: Basmajian JV, ed. *Manipulation, traction and massage,* 3rd ed. Baltimore: Williams & Wilkins, 1985; 201–207.
215. Mara JR. Gravity inversion. *Aches Pains* 1983; 4:6–12.
216. Ducommun JR. Personal communication.
217. Judovich BD. Herniated cervical disk: a new form of traction therapy. *Am J Surg* 1952; 84:646–656.
218. Lawson GA, Godfrey CM. A report on studies of spinal traction. *Med Services J Can* 1958; 14:762–771.
219. DeSeze S, Levernieux J. Les tractions vertebrales. Premieres etudes experimentales et results therapeutiques d'apres une experience d'une quatre annees. *Semin Hop Paris* 1951; 27:2085–2104.
220. Wong AM, Leong CP, Chen CM. The traction angle and cervical intervertebral separation. *Spine* 1992; 17:136–138.
221. Klaber-Moffett JA, Hughes GI, Griffith P. An investigation of the effects of cervical traction. Part 1. Clinical effectiveness. *Clin Rehabil* 1990; 4:205.
222. Klaber-Moffett JA, Hughes GI, Griffith P. An investigation of the effects of cervical traction. Part 2. The effects on the neck musculature. *Clin Rehabil* 1990; 4:287.
223. Judovich BD. Lumbar traction therapy: elimination of physical factors that prevent lumbar stretch. *JAMA* 1955; 159:549–550.
224. Ramos G, Martin W. Effects of vertebral axial decompression on intradiscal pressure. *J Neurosurg* 1994; 81:350–353.
225. Bridger RS, Ossey S, Fourie G. Effect of lumbar traction on stature. *Spine* 1990; 15:522–524
226. Colachis, SC, Strohm BR, Effect of duration of intermittent cervical traction on vertebral separation. *Arch Phys Med Rehabil* 1966; 47: 353–359.
227. Lehmann JF, Brunner GD. A device for application of heavy lumbar traction: its mechanical effects. *Arch Phys Med Rehabil* 1958; 39: 696–700.
228. Kane MD, Karl RD, Swain JH. Effects of gravity-facilitated traction on intervertebral dimensions of the lumbar spine. *J Orthop Sports Phys Ther* 1985; 6:281–288.
229. Colachis SC, Strohm BR. Relationship of time to varied tractive force with constant angle of pull. *Arch Phys Med Rehabil* 1965; 46: 815–819.
230. Andersson GBJ, Schultz AB, Nachemson AL. Intervertebral disc pressures during traction. *Scand J Rehabil Med* 1983; 9:88–91.
231. Masturzo A. Vertebral traction for the treatment of sciatica. *Rheumatism* 1955; 1:62.
232. Mathews JA. Dynamic discography; a study of lumbar traction. *Ann Phys Med* 1968; 9:275.
233. Onel D, Tuzlaci M, Sari H, Demir K, Computed tomographic investigation of the effect of traction on lumbar disc herniations. *Spine* 1989; 14:82–90.
234. Knutsson E, Skoglund CR, Natchev E. Changes in voluntary muscle strength, somatosensory transmission, and skin temperature concomitant with pain relief during autotraction in patients with lumbar and sacral root lesions. *Pain* 1988; 33:173–179.
235. Cheatle MD, Esterhai JL. Pelvic traction as treatment for acute back pain. *Spine* 1991; 16:1379–1381.
236. Pellecchia G. Lumbar traction: a review of the literature. *J Orthop Sports Phys Ther* 1994; 20:262–266.
237. Deyo R. Conservative therapy for low back pain. Distinguishing useful from useless therapy. *JAMA* 1983; 250:1057–1062.
238. Larson U, Choler U, Lidstrom A, et al. Autotraction for treatment of lumbago-sciatica. *Acta Orthop Scand* 1980; 51:791–798.
239. Mathews J, Mills S, Jenkins V, et al. Back pain and sciatica controlled trials of manipulation, traction, sclerosant and epidural injections. *Br J Rheumatol* 1987; 26:416–423.
240. Lidstrom A, Zachrisson M. Physical therapy on low back pain and sciatica. An attempt at evaluation. *Scand J Rehabil Med* 1970; 2: 37–42.
241. Coxhead C, Meade T, Inskip H, et al. Multicentre trial of physiotherapy in the management of sciatic symptoms. *Lancet* 1981; 1: 1065–1068.
242. Christie BGB. Discussion on the treatment of backache by traction. *Proc R Soc Mod* 1955; 48:811.
243. Mathews J, Hickling J. Lumbar traction; a double blinded control study for sciatica. *Rheum Rehabil* 1975; 14:222–225.
244. Weber H, Ljunggren A, Walker L. Traction therapy in patients with herniated discs. *J Oslo City Hosp* 1984; 34:61–70.
245. Pal B, Mangion P, Hossain M, Diffey B. A controlled trial of continuous lumbar traction in the treatment of low back pain and sciatica. *Br J Rheumatol* 1986; 25:181–183.
246. British Association of Physical Medicine. Pain in the neck and arm: a multicentre trial of the effects of physiotherapy. *Br Med J* 1966; 1: 253.
247. Goldie I, Lundquist A. Evaluation of the effects of different forms of physiotherapy in cervical pain. *Scand J Rehabil Med* 1970; 117:2–3.
248. Zylbergold RS, Piper MC. Cervical spine disorders, a comparison of three types of traction. *Spine* 1985; 10:867–870.
249. Cyriax JH. Conservative treatment of lumbar disc lesions. *Physiotherapy* 1964; 50:300–303.
250. Jackson R. *The cervical syndrome,* 2nd ed. Springfield, IL: Charles C Thomas, 1958.
251. Goldish GD. A study of the mechanical efficiency of split-table traction. *Spine* 1989; 15:218–219.
252. Gianakopoulos G, Waylonis GW, Grant PA, Tottle DO, Blazek JV. Inversion devices: their role in producing lumbar distraction. *Arch Phys Med Rehabil* 1985; 66:100–102.
253. Lind GAM. Auto-traction treatment of low back pain and sciatica [Thesis]. Linkoping, Sweden: University of Linkoping, 1974.
254. Natchev E, Valentino V. Low back pain and disc hernia observation during auto-traction treatment. *Manual Med* 1984; 1:39–42.
255. Tesio L, Merlo A. Autotraction versus passive traction: an open controlled study in lumbar disc herniation. *Arch Phys Med Rehabil* 1993; 74:871–876.
256. Crue BL. Importance of flexion in cervical traction for radiculitis. *US Air Force Med J* 1957; 8:374–380.
257. Crue BL, Importance of flexion in cervical halter traction. *Bull Los Angeles Neurol Soc* 1965; 30:95–98.
258. Colachis SC, Strohm BR. A study of tractive forces and angle of pull

on vertebral interspaces in the cervical spine. *Arch Phys Med Rehabil* 1965; 46:820–830.
259. Caillet R. Neck and arm pain. Philadelphia: FA Davis, 1972; 79–83.
260. Hinterbuchner C. Traction. Basmajian JV, ed. *Manipulation, traction and massage,* 3rd ed. Baltimore: Williams & Wilkins, 1985; 173–201.
261. Judovich BD, Nobel GR. Traction therapy; a study of resistance forces. *Am J Surg* 1957; 93:108.
262. Hickling J. Spinal traction technique. *Physiotherapy* 1972; 58:58.
263. Twomey LT. Sustained lumbar traction: an experimental study of long spine segments. *Spine* 1985; 10:146–149.
264. Spitzer W, Le Blanc F, Dupuis M, et al. Scientific approach to the assessment and management of activity related spinal disorders; a monograph for clinicians. Report of the Quebec Task Force on Spinal Disorders. *Spine* 1987; 12(suppl):1–57.
265. Weinberger LM. Trauma or treatment? The role of intermittent traction in the treatment of cervical soft tissue injuries. *J Trauma* 1976; 16:377–382.
266. Yates DAH. Indications and contra-indications for spinal traction. *Physiotherapy* 1972; 54:55.
267. Laban MM, Meerschaert JR. Quadriplegia following cervical traction in patients with occult epidural prostatic metastasis. *Arch Phys Med Rehabil* 1975; 56:455–458.

Rehabilitation Medicine: Principles and Practice, Third Edition, edited by Joel A. DeLisa and Bruce M. Gans. Lippincott–Raven Publishers, Philadelphia © 1998.

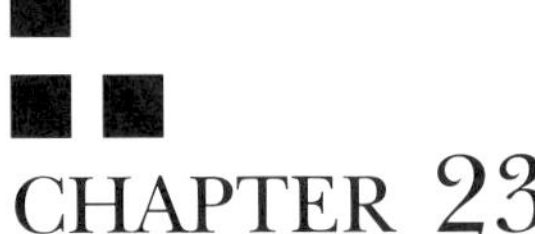

CHAPTER 23

Injection Procedures

Nicolas E. Walsh, James N. Rogers, and Jaywant J.P. Patil

Injection of the nerves, muscles, and skeletal structures (bursae, joints, and tendons) provides an important intervention in the management of pain and dysfunction. Injection techniques constitute both diagnostic and therapeutic modalities in many settings. As in all patient care, the origin of pain and/or dysfunction involves careful history taking and a complete physical examination. The details of these techniques are generally addressed in Chapter 5 with a specific focus in Chapters 56 and 57.

HISTORICAL

Since antiquity, sharp objects have been used to inject various concoctions into the body as remedies for pain and dysfunction (1,2). The tools of modern-day injection procedures include the hollow needle developed by Rynd in 1845 (3) and the syringe developed by Pravaz (4) (1853) and Wood (5) (1855). Medications to inject for anesthesia were developed in the late 1800s, with extensive use of cocaine as a local analgesic (6) and as an injected analgesic (7). The application of these tools to achieve local anesthesia for relief of pain was described by Corning (8) in 1894. Historical information on neural blockade has been reviewed in detail by Fink (2).

Since the early 1900s, procaine had been injected into the synovium of inflamed joints for temporary relief of pain. Hench in 1949 (9) introduced systemic corticosteroids to suppress the inflammatory changes in rheumatoid arthritis. However, large doses of corticosteroids given systemically resulted in complications. In 1951, Hollander (10) introduced and reported on low-dose local (intra-articular and periarticular) injections of hydrocortisone acetate to control pain and inflammation caused by trauma and inflammatory joint disease. Historical information on intra-articular injection has been reviewed in detail by Hollander (11).

Tender points in the muscle were identified in the 1800s by multiple investigators (12,13). Kraus (14) (in 1937) and Travell (15) (in 1942) introduced the treatment of myofascial pain by direct trigger point injection and use of vapocoolant spray and emphasized the importance of exercise in the treatment of patients with pain due to trigger points. Historical information on myofascial pain has been reviewed in detail by Simons (12).

GENERAL

The general principles for utilization of neural blockade were described in detail by Bonica in 1953 (16). Injections of local anesthetic agents has been shown to be effective in managing patients with acute and chronic pain. The mechanism of action is the blockade of nociceptive input along the pathway of transmission (17). Intra-articular and periarticular injections of corticosteroids have been shown to reduce inflammation and pain, as well as to facilitate mobility and function (18). Unfortunately, injection of medication is often used in isolation for the management of many pain problems. It is important to use injections as one component in a vast armamentarium of interventional techniques that are often best used in concert with each other. An injection unaccompanied by appropriate therapy, exercise, and other treatment is often incomplete in alleviating pain or restoring function. This is best demonstrated by the "block clinics," highly popular in the 1930s and 1940s but which have since been superseded by multidisciplinary pain clinics. Injection procedures should be performed within the context of total patient rehabilitation. It is common for noninvasive treatments (e.g., modalities, medication, exercise) to be used before injection.

N. E. Walsh: Department of Rehabilitation Medicine, University of Texas Health Science Center at San Antonio, San Antonio, Texas 78284-7798.

J. N. Rogers: Department of Anesthesiology, University of Texas Health Science Center at San Antonio, San Antonio, Texas 78284.

J. J. P. Patil: Department of Physical Medicine and Rehabilitation, Dalhousie University, Halifax, Nova Scotia B3J 3K3, Canada.

Knowledge and Training

The physician using injection procedures must have the requisite knowledge to understand the diagnosis and treatment of pain syndromes. The practitioner should understand the limitations, complications, advantages, and disadvantages of each procedure and alternative treatments in order to decide the best therapy or combination of therapies. The physician must be highly skilled in injection techniques based on education, training, and experience. This requires a thorough knowledge of the anatomic basis of the procedure and the characteristics of the injectable medication, including expected side effects of the procedure, as well as unexpected complications and their prevention and prompt treatment (17).

Communication

Communication with the patient is essential in all activities, including injection. Providing the patient with a complete explanation of the procedure will result in the individual having increased confidence and reduced anxiety. During the procedure the physician should continually inform and ensure the patient as to the progress of the procedure.

Informed Consent

Although state laws vary in terms of the documentation required, informed consent involves providing the patient with enough information about the injection procedure so that consent is given with an understanding of the entire procedure. This involves a thorough discussion of the procedure with the patient, including the possible benefits, alternative treatments, common side effects, and risks. The patient should be given the opportunity to ask questions about details of the injection. It is recommended that the patient receive no medications that will significantly impair responses before the consent is given. Depending on the state, the patient may or may not be required to sign an informed consent form. The common side effects of injection procedures are provided in Table 23-1.

TABLE 23-1. *Common complications*

Systemic toxic reaction
Other systemic reactions
Epinephrine reaction
Vasovagal reaction
Allergic reaction
Accidental spinal block
Concurrent medical episode
Infection
Pneumothorax
Nerve Injury
Other complications
Hypotension
Hematoma

Universal Precautions

Universal precautions are required for all injection techniques to reduce the incidence of transmission of infectious agents. These include the use of gloves and protective eye wear. Possible transmission of blood-borne pathogens during medical procedures is a common concern among patients and health-care workers due to its potentially devastating consequences. Although this concern has largely focused on the human immunodeficiency virus (HIV), other agents, particularly hepatitis B, C, and G viruses, are of significantly greater risk. The data show that the risk to health-care workers from patients is far greater than the risk to patients from health-care workers (19). It is important to maintain proper sharps disposal containers in all areas where needles are used. Needlesticks pose the greatest risk of occupational transmission, with studies following health-care workers after such exposures finding the following seroconversion rates: hepatitis B, 5% to 37%; hepatitis C, 3% to 10%; and HIV, 0.2% to 0.8% (20–24). Research shows that recapping a needle increases the risk of needle stick, so needles should either be laid down in the sterile field or disposed uncapped in an appropriate container.

Positioning

Optimal results of any injection depends on proper positioning before, during, and after the injection procedure. The proper position should facilitate access to the injection site with the patient as comfortable as possible. Bony prominences should be cushioned where needed to avoid discomfort from pressure. When possible, the recumbent position is used because it is usually the most comfortable for the patient and minimizes the incidence of orthostatic hypotension caused by vasovagal reaction during the procedure. Positioning to avoid ergonomic stress on the patient and physician is essential.

Skin Preparation

Strict aseptic technique is required in all injection procedures. The injection site is prepared by scrubbing with an antiseptic to reduce cutaneous micro-organisms to the lowest level. Commonly used agents include chlorhexidine (Hibiclens, Zeneca Pharmaceuticals, Wilmington, DE), iodophors (Betadine, Purdue Frederick, Norwalk, CT), and alcohol (25). It is important to wait approximately 2 minutes after the application of any of the above antiseptics to obtain maximal reduction in cutaneous bacteria. It is rarely justified to remove hair from the skin for an injection procedure (26).

Needle Insertion

To reduce pain of the initial needle insertion, the skin may be stretched while rapidly piercing the skin. Once the skin is pierced, the tension is released and the needle is advanced slowly. Rapid infusion of medication may result in tissue distention, causing pain. Other methods of reducing pain with initial needle insertion include the use of topical anesthetics and vapocoolant sprays.

Conscious Sedation

The procedures described in this chapter rarely require conscious sedation. In circumstances where conscious sedation is used, appropriate airway protection and monitoring equipment must be used. Resuscitation equipment and personnel must be readily available.

SIDE EFFECTS AND COMPLICATIONS

The injection procedures described here are associated with various side effects, although the risk of significant complications is very low. The physician who performs injection procedures should have the training and education to recognize and treat a wide range of potential complications (Table 23-2). Advanced life support (ACLS) protocols are used in airway management and cardiorespiratory resuscitation (27).

Systemic Toxic Reaction

Various toxic reactions have been reported after use of local anesthetics, but with very low incidence. Local anesthetic agents are relatively lipid-soluble, low molecular weight compounds that readily cross the blood–brain barrier. As toxic levels are reached, disturbances of central nervous system (CNS) function are observed initially, producing signs of CNS excitation. Early symptoms of overdose include headache, ringing in the ears, numbness in the tongue and mouth, twitching of facial muscles, and restlessness. As blood levels increase, generalized convulsions of a tonic–clonic nature occur. If sufficiently high blood levels are reached, the initial excitation is followed by generalized CNS depression. Respiratory depression and ultimately respiratory arrest may occur secondary to the toxic effect of the local anesthetic agent on the respiratory center in the medulla. Occasionally, the excitatory phase may not occur, and toxicity presents as CNS depression.

Cardiovascular system (CVS) effects either result indirectly from inhibition of autonomic pathways during regional anesthesia (as in high spinal or epidural) or are directly due to depressant actions on the CVS. The CVS is generally more resistant than the CNS to toxicity. The CVS/CNS toxicity ratio is lower for bupivacaine and etidocaine than for lidocaine. Convulsive activity may initially be associated with an increase in heart rate, blood pressure, and cardiac output. As the blood concentration of a local anesthetic agent further increases, CVS depression occurs, resulting in a decrease in blood pressure secondary to myocardial depression, impaired cardiac conduction, and eventual peripheral vasodilation. Ultimately, circulatory collapse and cardiac arrest may result. In addition, certain agents such as bupivacaine may cause ventricular arrhythmias and fatal ventricular fibrillation. The onset of CVS depression with bupivacaine may occur relatively early and be resistant to

TABLE 23-2. *Differential diagnosis of local anesthetic reactions*

Etiology	Major clinical feature	Comments
Systemic toxic reaction		
Intravascular injection	Immediate convulsion and/or cardiac toxicity	Injection into vertebral or a carotid artery may cause convulsion and administration of small dose
Relative overdose	Onset in 5 to 15 minutes with irritability, progressing to convulsions	
Epinephrine reaction	Tachycardia, hypertension, headache, apprehension	May vary with vasopressor used
Vasovagal reaction	Rapid onset Bradycardia Hypotension Pallor, faintness	Rapidly reversible with elevation of legs
Allergy		Allergy to amides extremely rare
Immediate	Anaphylaxis (↓blood pressure, bronchospasm, edema)	Cross-allergy, e.g., with preservatives in local anesthetics and food
Delayed	Urticaria	
High spinal or epidural	Gradual onset Bradycardia[a] Hypotension Possible respiratory arrest	May lose consciousness with total spinal block and onset of cardiorespiratory effects more rapid than with high epidural or with subdural block
Concurrent medical episode (e.g., asthma attack, myocardial infarct)	May mimic local anesthetic reaction	Medical history important

[a] Sympathetic block above T4 adds cardioaccelerator nerve blockade to the vasodilatation seen with blockade below T4; total spinal block may have rapid onset.

Reprinted with permission from Covino BG: Clinical pharmacology of local anesthetic agents. In: Cousins MJ, Bridenbaugh PO, eds. *Neural blockade in clinical anesthesia and management of pain,* 2nd ed. Philadelphia: JB Lippincott, 1988; 134.

usual therapeutic modalities. The pregnant patient is more sensitive to the cardiotoxic effects of bupivacaine.

Systemic toxicity may be due to unintentional intravascular injection or drug overdose. Intravascular injection produces signs of toxicity (usually seizures) during the injection itself. A relative overdose results in toxic reactions when peak blood levels are reached, approximately 20 to 30 minutes after the injection. Factors that affect the blood concentration (site of injection, drug, dosage, addition of vasoconstrictor, speed of injection) influence the potential for systemic toxic reactions to develop.

To minimize systemic reactions to local anesthetic agents, avoid intravascular injection, the most common cause of seizures. Use careful, intermittent aspiration before injecting large quantities of local anesthetic agents. Patient complaints of metallic taste, numbness around the mouth, or ringing in the ears is suggestive of intravascular needle placement. Patients may be premedicated with midazolam or diazepam to raise the seizure threshold if necessary.

Systemic toxicity is treated with general supportive measures. If early signs of toxicity occur, maintain constant verbal contact, administer oxygen, encourage breathing, and monitor CVS function. If seizure activity occurs, maintain a clear airway and administer oxygen by assisted or controlled ventilation. If seizures continue, administer thiopental (50 to 100 mg) or diazepam (2.5 to 5.0 mg) intravenously (IV), but avoid large doses of thiopental, which may produce additional CVS or CNS depression. If airway maintenance is jeopardized, use succinylcholine to facilitate endotracheal intubation. Muscular convulsive activity is terminated with succinylcholine, but the seizure activity in the brain is not affected. If CVS depression occurs, treat hypotension by increasing IV fluids, proper positioning (elevate the legs), and vasopressors such as ephedrine (Table 23-3).

TABLE 23-3. *Treatment of acute local anesthetic toxicity*

Airway
Establish clear airway; suction, if required
Breathing
Oxygen with face mask
Encourage adequate ventilation (prevent cycle of acidosis, increased uptake of local anesthetic into CNS, and lowered seizure threshold)
Artificial ventilation, if required
Circulation
Elevate legs
Increase IV fluids if ↓ blood pressure
CVS support drug if ↓ blood pressure persists (see below) or ↓ heart rate
Cardioversion if ventricular arrhythmias occur
Drugs
CNS depressant
Diazepam 5–10 mg, IV
Thiopental 50 mg, IV, incremental doses until seizures cease
Muscle relaxant
Succinylcholine 1 mg/kg, if inadequate control of ventilation with above measures (requires artificial ventilation and may necessitate intubation)
CVS support
Atropine 0.6 mg, IV, if ↓ heart rate
Ephedrine, 12.5–25 mg, IV, to restore adequate blood pressure
Epinephrine for profound cardiovascular collapse

CNS, central nervous system; CVS, cardiovascular system; IV, intravenous.

Reprinted from Covino BG: Clinical pharmacology of local anesthetic agents. In: Cousins MJ, Bridenbaugh PO, eds. *Neural blockade in clinical anesthesia and management of pain,* 2nd ed. Philadelphia: JB Lippincott, 1988; 135.

Epinephrine Reaction

Reaction to epinephrine may sometimes be confused with local anesthetic overdose. Systemic absorption of epinephrine produces palpitations and restlessness approximately 1 to 2 minutes after completion of the injection. Consider avoiding epinephrine in patients who are sensitivity prone (e.g., hypertensive, or hyperthyroid, arrhythmic patients). Do not use epinephrine for blocks of the fingers, toes, or penis due to the possibility of localized vasoconstriction. An epinephrine reaction is treated with a small dose of fast-acting barbiturate to reduce blood pressure to within normal limits. If hypertension persists, a vasodilator may be required.

Vasovagal Reaction

Vasovagal reaction is a frequent response to injection procedures that is attributable to physiologic and psychological factors. This response may result in bradycardia and hypotension, often accompanied by loss of consciousness. This usually occurs in the initial portion of the procedure before any medication is injected. Vasovagal reaction is often mislabeled as an allergic reaction to the medication. This response is often preceded by dizziness, faintness, sweating, and pallor. Vasovagal reaction is rapidly reversible by placing the patient in the Trendelenburg position and removal of painful stimuli. If this fails to relieve the symptoms, then treatment with general supportive measures is indicated, including airway maintenance, oxygen, IV fluids, and vasopressors such as ephedrine (Table 23-3).

Allergic Reaction

An allergic response to local anesthetic agents rarely occurs and in some instances may be confused with a vasovagal reaction or a reaction to epinephrine. Ester anesthetic agents (e.g., procaine, tetracaine), are more frequently associated with allergic reactions than amide anesthetic agents (e.g. lidocaine, ropicaine) because esters are derivatives of para-aminobenzoic acid (PABA). However, the use of amides from multiple-dose vials may result in an allergic reaction secondary to the preservative methylparaben. Allergic reaction is treated with general supportive measures and the administration of antihistamine or epinephrine. The patient should be closely monitored for a clear airway.

Although this is a rare event, if there is a question of

patient hypersensitivity to anesthetic agents, intradermal skin tests (injection with diluted [1 : 1,000] followed by undiluted local anesthetic) can be used successfully to diagnose adverse responses. However, false-positive results may occur. Anaphylactic shock is treated as systemic toxic reaction with attention to maintaining cardiovascular and ventilatory function (Table 23-3).

Accidental Spinal Block

Inadvertent subarachnoid or epidural blockade can occur with any injection that is performed close to the spine. These include intercostal nerve blocks, sympathetic blocks, and nerve root injections. Proper equipment and staff should always be available to treat any possible complication. This includes the ability to administer fluids if the patient develops hypotension from sympathetic blockade, and to maintain ventilation with oxygen if the patient has impaired respiratory function.

Concurrent Medical Episode

Concurrent medical problems may be exacerbated by injection procedures. Hypotension will reduce myocardial profusion and may be a major factor for reinfarction in patients with ischemic heart disease. Patients with chronic renal failure are more susceptible to toxicity from local anesthetics. Diabetic patients have an increased sensitivity to the effects of corticosteroid injection. Patients with liver disease may have reduced metabolism of local anesthetic medications resulting in an increased possibility of toxicity at standard doses. Other medical illnesses may decompensate clinically due to mild toxicity and changes in fluid and electrolyte balance. These risks are minimized with appropriate monitoring and optimal medication regimes. Patients should be medically stable before undergoing elective injection procedures.

Infection

Although infectious complications rarely occur, cutaneous and joint infection, epidural abscess, bacterial meningitis, and adhesive arachnoiditis have been associated with injection procedures. Preparation of the injection site in a standard aseptic fashion and use of sterile technique throughout the procedure minimize these risks. The majority of injection techniques described in this chapter do not require surgical draping; however, the phrase "sterile technique is used throughout the procedure" indicates an increased risk for major infectious complications, including epidural abscess, meningitis, and adhesive arachnoiditis. Epidural abscess usually arises indigenously from hematogenous spread of an infectious process located elsewhere in the body. The abcess may cause spinal cord compression. Signs and symptoms of epidural abscess are severe back pain, localized tenderness, fever, leukocytosis, cervical rigidity, increased protein and leukocytes in the cerebral spinal fluid, and abnormal imaging studies of the spine. Early diagnosis and prompt treatment are essential to avoid catastrophic complications. Meningitis and adhesive arachnoiditis are the result of the introduction of bacterial or irritating contaminants into the spinal fluid as well as trauma during the procedure.

Pneumothorax

Injections into the thoracic region have the potential to cause a pneumothorax. In procedures that put the patient at risk for needle penetration of the lung, fewer than 1% develop a pneumothorax. Most of these patients can be easily treated with administration of supplemental oxygen, close monitoring (e.g., O_2 saturation, vital signs) of the patient, and, when necessary, needle aspiration of air. Only those pneumothoraces that result in significant dyspnea or those under tension require chest tube thoracostomy and vacuum drainage.

Nerve Injury

Three major factors contribute to nerve injury during injections: trauma, toxicity, and ischemia, with all three contributing to most nerve injuries. Nerve blocks are the result of infiltration of anesthetic agents around the nerve, not directly into the neural tissue. Intraneural injections directly injure nerve fibers, as well as cause a breakdown in the blood–nerve barrier. The use of short beveled needles has significantly reduced nerve injuries from injections. Intense pain in the nerve distribution on injection is often the result of intraneural needle placement and necessitates immediate cessation of the injection and repositioning of the needle.

Other Complications

Local anesthetic agents used in recommended clinical concentrations have minimal irritating effects on the nerves, skin, and fat. Complete recovery of function occurs after regional blocks. The administration of large doses of prilocaine may lead to methemoglobinemia owing to the accumulation of a metabolite (OH-toluidine), which can convert hemoglobin to methemoglobin. It may be treated by IV methylene blue.

Hypotension may result from sympathetic blockade. This commonly occurs in patients who are hypvolemic and receive a spinal or epidural block involving a large portion of the body. Hypotension is treated with general supportive measures, including administration of IV fluids, proper positioning (elevate the legs), and vasopressors such as epinephrine to maintain blood pressure within normal limits.

Bleeding at the site of injection occurs commonly at the surface. Hematoma at the site of injection is a possibility but usually not clinically significant. If arterial puncture occurs, prolonged direct pressure is usually adequate to prevent the development of a hematoma.

MEDICATIONS

Injection procedures use three primary classes of medication: local anesthetic agents, neurolytic agents, and corticosteroids. All of these medications have multiple clinical applications and are documented to be safe and effective when used appropriately.

It is incumbent on the practitioner to understand the efficacy, complications, and common side effects of these agents.

Anesthetic Agents

The mechanism of local anesthetic action is likely a reversible block of ion flux through the axon's sodium channels. By blocking transmission from the peripheral nerves, no input is detected at the central nervous system. The degree of neural blockade depends on the properties, absorption, amount, location, and other characteristics of the drug injected (28,29) (Table 23-4).

Neurolytic Agents

Neurolytic nerve blocks were popular in the early 1900s. However, improved use of analgesics, as well as the use of radiofrequency and cryoablative techniques, have replaced their use in most instances. Alcohol and phenol are the most widely used neurolytic agents in the United States. These agents indiscriminately affect motor and sensory nerves.

Phenol can be used intrathecally, epidurally, as well as for peripheral nerve and motor point blocks. It is poorly soluble in water and is often added to glycerine to achieve concentrations higher than 7%. It also can be added to radiographic contrast to allow fluoroscopic visualization of the spread during injection. Phenol has a local anesthetic effect, resulting in less pain after the injection. Because of this, long-term effects of the block cannot be evaluated for 24 to 48 hours after the effects of the local anesthetic dissipate. Doses greater than 100 mg can result in serious toxicity (30).

Alcohol is used primarily intrathecally for nerve roots and locally for sympathetic blockade. Because alcohol is hypobaric in cerebrospinal fluid (CSF), positioning with intrathecal use is extremely important. It is readily soluble in body tissues and produces intense burning on injection. It requires 12 to 24 hours before block effects can be determined.

Corticosteroids

Glucocorticosteroids are used in the injection treatment of inflammatory processes (31) (Table 23-5). Some of the commonly used forms of corticosteroid available for intra-articular injections are listed as follows:

- Betamethasone sodium phosphate and acetate (Celestone Soluspan, Schering), 6 mg/ml
- Methylprednisolone acetate (Depo-medrol, Upjohn), 40 and 80 mg/ml
- Prednisolone sodium phosphate (Hydeltrasol, Merck), 20 mg/ml
- Prednisolone terbutate (Hydeltra-TBA, Merck), 20 mg/ml
- Triamcinolone acetonide (Kenalog, Squibb), 40 mg/ml
- Triamcinolone hexacetonide (Aristospan, Lederle), 20 mg/ml

The above corticosteroids vary in strength, concentration, duration, and side effects. All of the above corticosteroid preparations are effective. Triamcinolone hexacetonide has the longest duration of suppression of inflammatory activity.

TABLE 23-4. *Anesthetic Agents*

Characteristics	Procaine (Novocaine)	Lidocaine (Xylocaine)	Prilocaine (Citanest)	Mepivacaine (Carbocaine)	Bupivacaine (Marcaine)	Tetracaine (Pontocaine)	Etidocaine (Duranest)	Ropivocaine (Naropin)
Physicochemical								
Relative Potency[a]	1	3	3	3	15	15	15	15
Relative Toxicity[a]	1	1.5	1.5	2.0	10	12	10	10
pH of solution	5–6.5	6.5	4.5	4.5	4.5–6	4.5–6.5	4.5	7.4
Clinical								
Onset	Moderate	Fast	Fast	Fast	Moderate	Very Slow	Fast	Slow
Dispersion	Moderate	Marked	Marked	Marked	Moderate	Poor	Moderate	Moderate
Duration of Action	Short	Intermediate	Intermediate	Intermediate	Long	Long	Long	Long
Relative Duration[a]	1	1.5–2	1.75–2	2–2.5	6–8	6–8	5–8	6–8
Concentration of Solution (%)	1–2	1–2	1–2	1–2	0.25–0.5	0.1–0.25	0.5–1	0.25–0.5
Maximum Recommended Dose (mg/kg, adult)	10–14	6–10	6	6–10	2–3	2	4–5	3–4
Total Dose (mg, adult)	500	300	—	400	150	—	300	200
Toxic Blood Levels (μg/ml)								
CNS	—	18–21	20	22	4.5–5.5	—	4.3	4.3
CVS	—	35–50	—	—	6–10	—	—	—

[a] Procaine = 1
CNS, central nervous system; CVS, cerebrovascular system.

TABLE 23-5. *Corticosteroids*

Characteristics	Hydro-cortisone (Cortisol)	Prednisolone (Hydeltra)	Methyl-prednisolone (Depo-Medrol)	Triamcinolone (Aristospan, Kenalog)	Beta-methasone (Celestone)
Physiochemical					
Relative Anti-Inflammatory Potency[a]	1	4	5	5	25
Relative Mineralcorticoid Potency[a]	1	0.8	0	0	0
pH of Solution	5.0–7.0	6.0–8.0		4.5–6.5	6.8–7.2
Clinical					
Onset	Fast	Fast	Slow	Moderate	Fast
Dispersion	Moderate	Poor	Poor	Moderate	
Duration of Action	Short	Intermediate	Intermediate	Intermediate	Long
Salt Retension	2+	1+	0	0	0
Plasma Half-Life (Min)	90	200	180	300	100–300
Concentration Mg/ml	50	20	40–80	20	6
Range of Usual Dose (mg)	25–100	10–40	10–40	5–20	1.5–6

[a] Relative to hydrocortisone.

Fluorinated corticosteroids are rarely chosen for soft-tissue injection (e.g., triamcinolone) because they are more likely to cause tissue atrophy. Prednisolone terbutate and methylprednisolone acetate are often used for soft-tissue injections due to efficacy and cost.

Contraindications

Injection procedures encompass a wide variety of techniques, including epidural, caudal, nerve, motor point, joint, and muscle. Although relative advantages and disadvantages exist, certain conditions comprise contraindications to performing any injection technique. Certain medical conditions also may preclude an injection. For example, a patient with severe lung disease should not have a rib block with its attendant risk of pneumothorax.

Absolute Contraindications

Absolute contraindications to injection procedures include patient refusal, localized infection, dermatologic conditions that preclude adequate skin preparation, existence of a tumor at the injection site, history of allergy to local anesthetic agents, the presence of severe hypovolemia, gross coagulation defects, increased intracranial pressure (for epidural procedures), and septicemia.

Relative Contraindications

Relative contraindications include lack of education, training, and skill on the physician's part, and minor coagulation abnormalities, including the use of mini-dose heparin. Diabetes is a relative contraindication for injections with corticosteroids due to the possibility of hyperglycemia, glycosuria, electrolyte imbalance, as well as increased risk of infection.

COMMON NERVE BLOCK TECHNIQUES

After informed consent is obtained from the patient, the injection site is prepared in a standard aseptic fashion and draped appropriately. All medications, syringes, needles, and other equipment should be readily available. Syringe volume may vary from 3 to 12 ml. Needles commonly vary from as small as half an inch, 25 gauge to 3 1/2 inch, 21 gauge. For convenience, an 18-gauge needle should be available to draw medications from the vial. All caregivers participating in the injection procedure should be gloved with universal precautions applying to all.

General

The placement of local anesthetics at various sites along the neural axis is an important tool in the diagnosis and treatment of a variety of pain disorders, such as reflex sympathetic dystrophy and postherpetic neuralgia, among others. Peripheral nerve blocks also can provide muscle relaxation and pain relief to facilitate an active physical therapy program.

When the point of injection has been determined, it is best marked with the tip of a retracted ball point pen or a needle hub by pressing the skin to produce a temporary indentation to mark the point of entry. The skin is then prepared in a standard sterile fashion and sterile technique used throughout the procedure. The skin and subcutaneous tissue at the injection site may be anesthetized by injecting 1% lidocaine with no epinephrine using a 25- to 30-gauge needle. Alternatively, a vapocoolant spray applied to the skin surface may be used to provide adequate anesthesia.

Before injecting the medication, always attempt to aspirate to avoid accidental intravascular injection. After ensuring that the needle is in the joint space, the medication should be injected in a slow steady fashion.

Indications for Nerve Blocks

Neural blockade may be used for the diagnosis, prognosis, and treatment of pain. Selective nerve blocks are indicated to determine the etiology of pain by isolation of specific anatomic structure(s). Selected nerve blockade is used to determine specific nociceptive pathways and other mechanisms involved in pain generation. Diagnostic blocks assist in narrowing the differential diagnosis of the site and cause of pain. Prognostic neural blockade is used to evaluate the possible outcome from neurolytic procedures. Therapeutic nerve blocks are indicated to decrease morbidity in acute postoperative pain, posttraumatic pain, and pain resulting from self-limiting conditions. Nerve blockade may provide rapid relief of pain and facilitate the patient's participation in a comprehensive rehabilitation program. Therapeutic nerve blocks may interrupt the pain cycle sufficiently to provide prolonged pain relief.

Contraindications for Nerve Blocks

Absolute contraindications to regional anesthesia include localized infection, a skin condition that prevents adequate skin preparation, the existence of a tumor at the injection site, a history of allergy to local anesthetics, the presence of severe hypovolemia (for blocks that could result in significant sympathetic blockade), gross coagulation defects, septicemia, and increased intracranial pressure (spinal, caudal, and epidural).

Prilocaine should not be used in doses greater than 600 mg because significant methemoglobinemia may result. The use of corticosteroids with preservatives is contraindicated in epidural and subarachnoid techniques as the preservative may result in seizures and permanent central nervous system damage.

Relative contraindications include general medical conditions that would put the patient at increased risk. These include aortic stenosis, severe lung disease, sickle cell anemia, and pre-existing neurologic diseases such as multiple sclerosis or amyotrophic lateral sclerosis, which could be worsened during regional anesthesia.

Complications

Complications common to nerve blocks include hypotension from sympathetic blockade. This usually occurs in patients who are hypovolemic and receive a block covering a large portion of the body, such as a spinal or epidural blockade. Local anesthetic overdose or intravascular injection can result in CNS toxicity and, in some cases, pulmonary and cardiac arrest. Nerve injury from contact with the needle may occur, but is rare, especially when a short beveled needle is

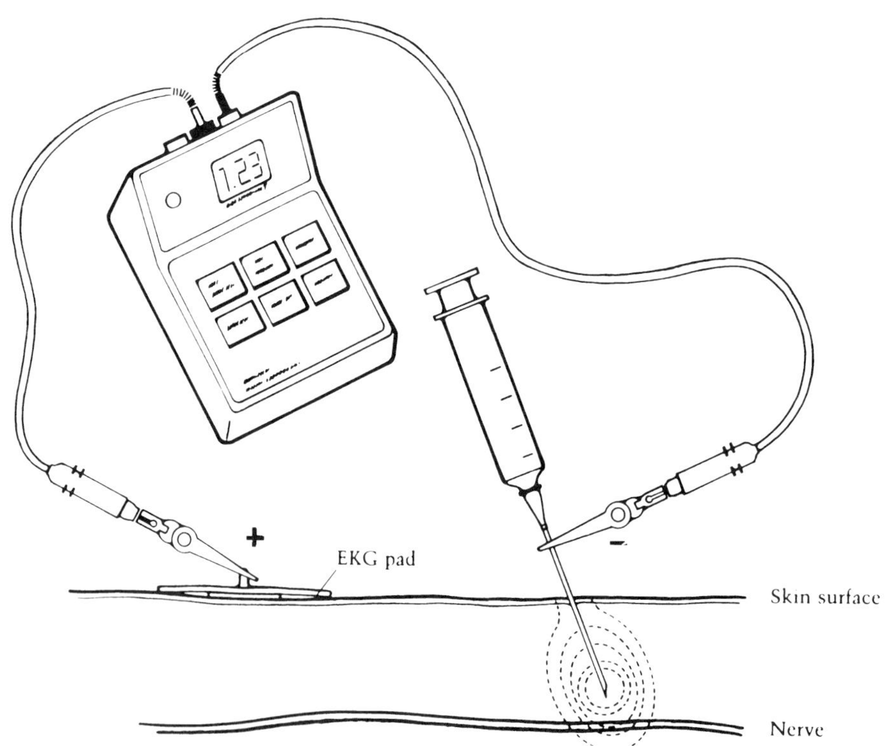

FIG. 23-1. Nerve stimulator attached to regional block nerve. The negative (black) lead is attached to the exploring needle, whereas the positive (red) lead is connected to the reference EKG pad used as the ground reference. Note the current distribution pattern for this uninsulated needle. (Reprinted with permission from Mulroy MF. *Regional anesthesia—an illustrated procedural guide.* Boston: Little, Brown, 1989; 63.)

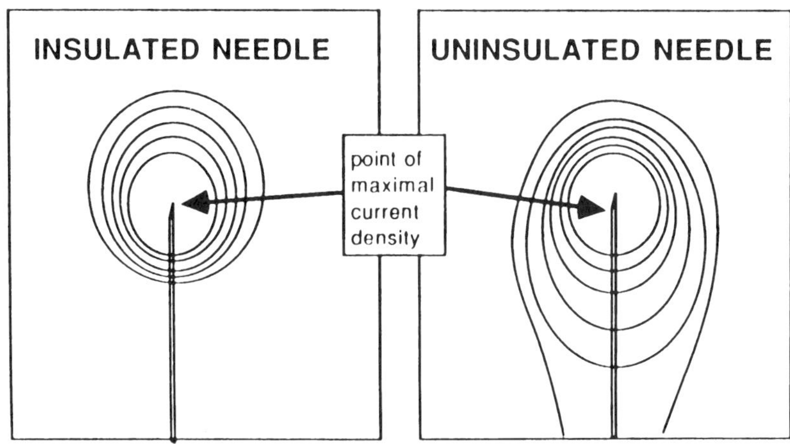

FIG. 23-2. Current density pattern for insulated and uninsulated needles. (Reprinted with permission from Brown RE. Monitoring and equipment for regional anesthesia. In: Raj PP, ed. *Clinical practice for regional anesthesia.* New York: Churchill-Livingstone, 1991; 43.)

used. Other complications are dependent on the location of the block and will be discussed separately.

Techniques

Before the injection, locate and mark the appropriate landmarks. Scrub the skin and allow the antiseptic to dry for 2 minutes. The wearing of sterile gloves is required so that the bony landmarks in the sterile field may be palpated throughout the procedure. Standard sterile technique is required to minimize risk of a septic joint. It is preferable to use single-dose vials of the local anesthetic because this further reduces the risk of infection. A 25- to 27-gauge needle is used with approximately 1% lidocaine with no epinephrine to raise a small skin wheal for skin anesthesia. Routinely a 1 1/2 inch (4 cm) 21- to 25-gauge needle transverses the skin, joint capsule, and synovial lining, sliding smoothly into the joint cavity.

Aspirate to ensure no intravascular penetration. If this occurs, the needle should be repositioned and aspirated to ensure that blood vessels have been avoided, and then the medication slowly injected. After the medication has been injected, the needle should be cleared with a new syringe containing a small amount of lidocaine or saline. The needle is then withdrawn with pressure applied to minimize bleeding.

Nerve Stimulator

Peripheral nerves may be localized with a nerve stimulator using a small adjustable amount of electrical current to depolarize neural tissue in proximity to the needle. The cathode (negative) terminal is connected to the needle, and the anode (positive) terminal is connected to a service electrode. The stimulator initially is set to deliver 10 to 20 mA of current to detect the general area of the nerve. The current is then reduced to further localize the nerve. The needle is positioned to produce the maximal twitch at the lowest stimulus. The needle is usually adjacent to the nerve when 0.5 to 0.1 mA produce motor stimulation with an insulated needle and 1 mA with an uninsulated needle (Fig. 23-1).

Nerve stimulators do not substitute for a knowledge of anatomy and proper needle placement. Insulated needles increase the point of maximal current density at the needle tip and are used for precise localization of specific nerves. Uninsulated needles are often accurate enough for many nerve blocks; however, both the tip and shaft of the needle have sufficient current density to stimulate a nerve. Local muscle twitches from the shaft of the uninsulated needle should not be confused with the response from the nerve to be blocked (Fig. 23-2).

SPECIFIC NERVE BLOCKS

Occipital Nerve Block

Indication

The occipital nerve blockade is used both diagnostically and therapeutically in the treatment of occipital neuralgia.

Techniques

After informed consent is obtained, the patient is placed in the sitting position with the head flexed forward. The occipital nerve is located at the mid-point between the mastoid process and the greater occipital protuberance at the superior nuchal line. The patient is prepared in a standard aseptic fashion and a 1 inch (2.5 cm) 21- to 25-gauge needle is inserted perpendicular to the superior nuchal line. Before reaching the periosteum of the skull, paresthesias in the occipital nerve distribution may be elicited. If not, the periosteum is contacted and the needle withdrawn slightly. After negative aspiration, 3 to 5 ml of local anesthetic is injected to block the occipital nerve (Fig. 23-3).

Comments

Localization of the nerve may be accomplished by palpation of the occipital artery just lateral to the nuchal ridge. The

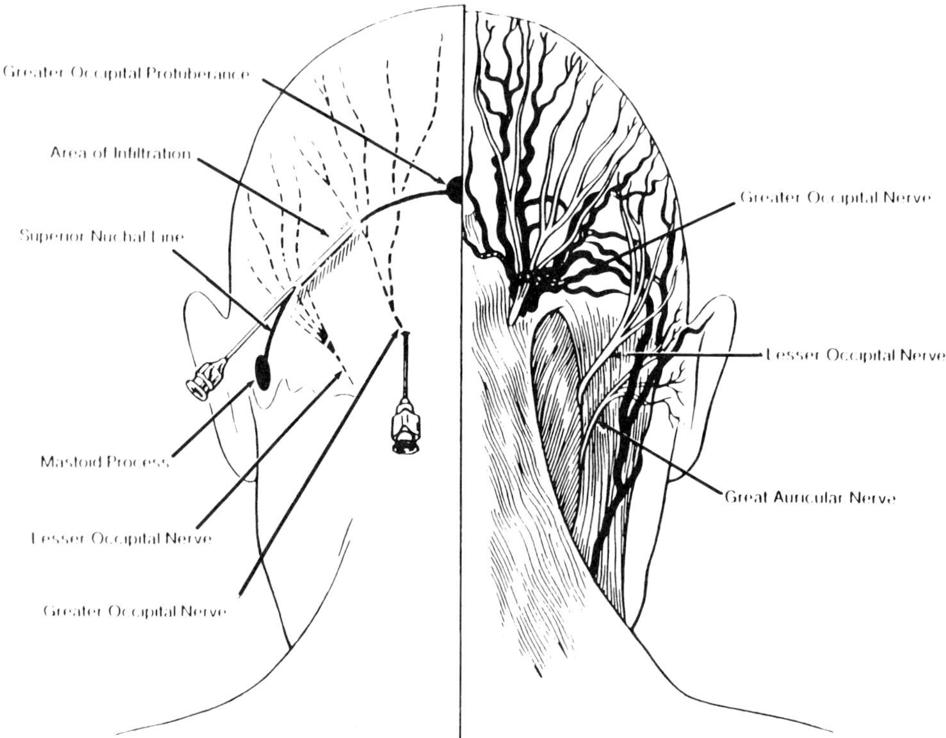

FIG. 23-3. Occipital nerve block. Approach for occipital nerve block and neural blockade. (Reprinted with permission from Murphy TM. Somatic blockade of the head and neck. In: Cousins MJ, Bridenbaugh PO, eds. *Neural blockade in clinical anesthesia and management of pain.* Philadelphia: JB Lippincott, 1988; 552.)

nerve runs with the occipital artery, innervating the posterior portion of the skull. A nerve stimulator may be used for precise needle placement. An alternate approach may be used with the patient positioned as above with anatomic landmarks identified. A 2 inch (4 cm) 21- to 25-gauge needle is inserted subcutaneously along the middle third of the superior nuchal line. After negative aspiration, 5 ml of local anesthetic is injected to block the greater and lesser occipital nerve (Fig. 23-3).

Complications

Intravascular injection can occur, resulting in systemic toxicity and seizures, especially if larger volumes are used. Bleeding due to vascular injury also may occur. Nerve injury secondary to injection into the nerve may result in persistent numbness over the posterior portion of the scalp.

Stellate Ganglion Block

Indication

Stellate ganglion blockade is useful for diagnosing and treating pain of sympathetic origin. This includes pain involving the face, head, neck, and upper extremities secondary to causalgia, reflex sympathetic dystrophy, acute herpes zoster, and phantom limb pain.

Techniques

After informed consent is obtained, the patient is placed in the supine position with a pillow under the shoulders and the neck extended. The patient is prepared in a standard aseptic fashion, and sterile technique is used throughout the procedure. The transverse process of the C6 vertebral body is palpated between the cricoid cartilage and the carotid artery. A 1 1/2 inch (4 cm) 22-gauge needle is inserted vertically and advanced to touch the periosteum of the C6 transverse process. The needle is withdrawn slightly, and after negative aspiration a 1-ml test dose of local anesthetic is injected. After unremarkable test dose and repeated aspiration, 9 ml of local anesthetic is injected, in divided doses with continuous monitoring, to block the stellate ganglion (Fig. 23-4).

Comments

This technique is commonly used for differential diagnosis and is the preferred treatment of sympathetic mediated pain involving the upper extremity. The stellate ganglion is located between the anterior lateral surface of the seventh cervical vertebral body. It is formed by the inferior cervical ganglion and first thoracic sympathetic ganglion. Autonomic mediated pain does not usually correspond to segmental or peripheral nerve distribution.

This procedure requires full monitoring capability to include blood pressure, heart rate, level of consciousness, and pulse oximeter. Temperature should be monitored and recorded for each hand before, during, and after the procedure. The patient is continuously monitored for change and level of consciousness or for adverse reaction. Stellate ganglion blockade is confirmed by elevated temperature on the block side as well as evidence of a Horner's syndrome (miosis, ptosis, anhydrosis, and enophthalmos). Nasal congestion and hoarseness may occur with this injection. It is recommended that IV access be available before the block in the event of intravascular injection and resulting seizure activity (32). Rarely are ablative nerve procedures (neurolysis) required in the management of sympathetic mediated pain.

Complications

Performance of this procedure outside of a fully monitored environment is not recommended. Resuscitation equipment and personnel must be readily available. While appearing technically simple, this block has multiple potential hazards due to the proximity of the common carotid artery, vagus nerve, jugular vein, vertebral artery, trachea, esophagus, lung, and dura. Intra-arterial and intradural injection of local anesthetic may result in death, seizure, respiratory arrest, cardiac arrest, cerebral damage with multiple sequelae, and other lesser complications. The risk of intervascular injection may be reduced if a test dose is given, the total dose is injected incrementally, and aspiration is performed before each injection.

Cervical Epidural Steroid Injection

Indications

Cervical epidural injection is primarily used to treat pain arising from cervical herniated discs or spinal stenosis.

Techniques

After informed consent is obtained, the patient is placed in either the lateral decubitus position or sitting position with the neck flexed. The sitting position, with the head resting on the examination table, provides better stabilization of the neck during the procedure but may be a problem if the patient is prone to lightheadedness. The patient is prepared in a standard aseptic fashion, and strict sterile technique is used throughout the procedure. Local skin anesthesia is provided with 1% to 2% lidocaine at the C7–T1 interspace. A Tuohy epidural needle is advanced in a midline horizontal fashion until well seated in the posterior ligaments. A winged needle is preferred because it allows two-handed control of the needle as it is directed toward the epidural space. A midline approach is used to avoid the large epidural veins that lie laterally. The stylet is then removed and a "loss-of-resistance" syringe is attached to the hub of the needle. Either 2 to 3 ml of air or normal saline should be in the syringe. The needle is slowly advanced 1 to 2 mm at a time with constant checking for loss of resistance by tapping on the plunger of the syringe. Once a distinct loss of resistance is obtained, the needle is halted and an attempt is made to aspirate blood or CSF. After negative aspiration, 80 mg of methylprednisolone acetate or equivalent is injected. Care

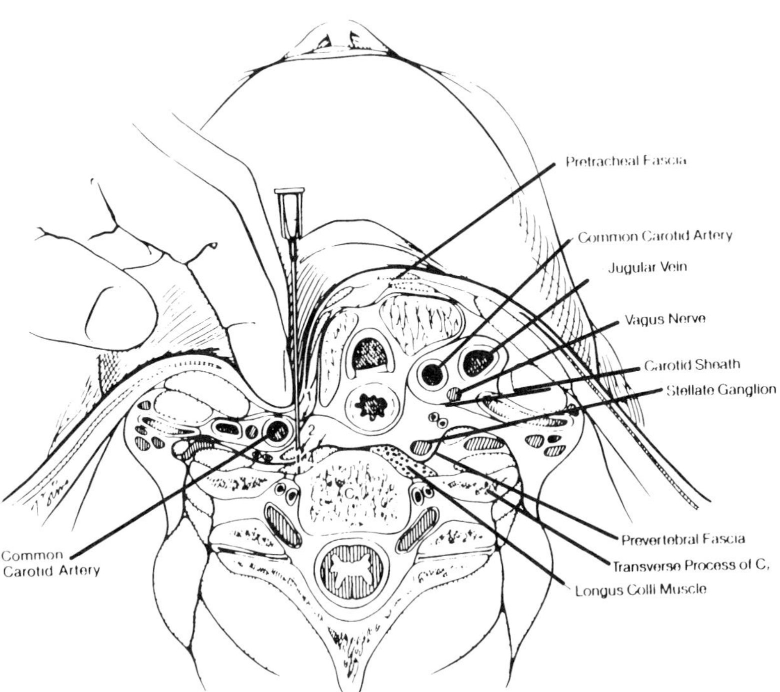

FIG. 23-4. Stellate ganglion block. Approach for stellate ganglion injection and neural blockade. Cross section at C6. (Reprinted with permission from Raj PP. Chronic pain. In: Raj PP, ed. *Clinical practice of regional anesthesia.* New York: Churchill-Livingstone, 1991; 495.)

should be made to flush the needle with normal saline and to replace the stylet before the needle is removed to avoid depositing steroid in the needle track to the skin.

Comments

Cervical epidural injections are similar in technique to lumbar epidural injections. The cervical spinous processes at C7 and T1 are oriented almost horizontally, as in the lumbar region. Of note, caution must be taken because the cervical ligamentum flavum is thinner in this region than at any other spinal level, and the width of the epidural space is only 3 to 4 mm.

Complications

The most frequent complication of a cervical epidural injection is subarachnoid penetration (wet tap), due to the thinner ligamentum flavum and the reduced width of the cervical epidural space. Cervical epidural injections should only be attempted by those physicians with a great deal of experience with lumbar epidural techniques because the spinal cord lies in close proximity to the epidural space. Injection of local anesthetics into the cervical epidural space can result in respiratory depression, particularly if the phrenic nerve roots are blocked (C3–C5).

Infection or bleeding into the closed epidural space also can result in significant neurologic deficits, including quadriplegia. Any complaint of increasing pain or neurologic changes should be investigated immediately. Early recognition can prevent permanent injury.

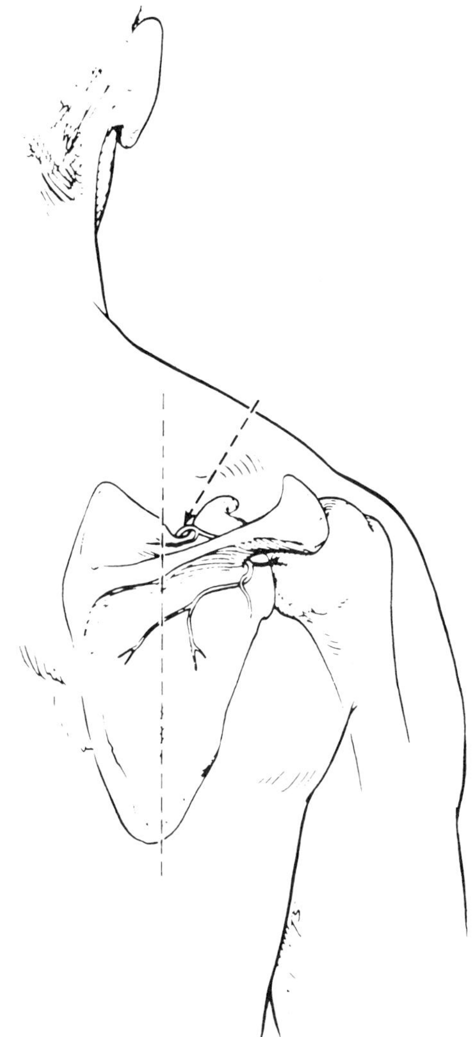

FIG. 23-5. Suprascapular nerve block. Approach for suprascapular nerve injection and neural blockade. (Reprinted with permission from Murphy TM, Raj PP, Stanton-Hicks M. Techniques of nerve blocks—spinal nerves. In: Raj PP, ed. *Practical management of pain.* Chicago: Yearbook Medical, 1986; 621.)

Suprascapular Nerve Block

Indication

The suprascapular nerve blockade is useful as a therapeutic procedure in patients for pain in the shoulder region. This block is used as an adjuvant to physical therapy for patients with limited range of motion secondary to arthritic shoulder pain, shoulder hand syndrome, and shoulder pain.

Techniques

After informed consent is obtained, the patient is placed in the sitting position. The spine of the scapula is divided by a line formed by the bisection of the scapular angle. The upper outer quadrant formed from the spine of the scapula and the vertical line bisecting the angle of the scapula is bisected and a point is marked 2 cm along this line for needle insertion. The patient is prepared in a standard aseptic fashion, and a 3 inch (8 cm) 23- to 25-gauge needle is inserted perpendicular to the skin and, using a nerve stimulator, advanced until needle placement is confirmed by movements of the supraspinatus and infraspinatus muscles. After negative aspiration, 5 ml of local anesthetic is injected (Fig. 23-5).

Comments

The suprascapular nerve is a branch from the trunk of the brachial plexus, which enters the scapular region through the suprascapular notch on the cephalic border of the scapula. Confirmation of the block is determined when abduction of the arm is diminished over the first 15°. If a nerve stimulator is not available, the same technique is used with the needle being advanced to the dorsal surface of the scapula. The needle is then walked along the edge of the scapula to the suprascapular notch.

Complications

Intraneural injection may result in nerve damage. Severe pain on injection suggests the possibility of an intraneural injection, and the needle should be repositioned immediately. Hematoma and intravascular injection are possible due to the close proximity of the suprascapular vessels. Pneumothorax is possible if the needle is advanced beyond the scapula and into the pleura. Most pneumothoraces can be treated easily with administration of supplemental oxygen and close observation and, when necessary, needle aspiration of air. Only those pneumothoraces that result in significant dyspnea or those under tension require chest tube thoracotomy and vacuum drainage.

Intercostal Nerve Block

Indications

Intercostal blockade is used to treat pain from herpes zoster, rib fractures, and intercostal neuropathies. It is also used to diagnose unusual abdominal or chest wall pain.

Techniques

After informed consent is obtained, the patient is placed in either the prone or lateral position. In the lateral position, the injection site is along the mid-axillary line, which may result in incomplete blockade of the lateral cutaneous branch of the intercostal nerve. In the prone position, the injection site is along the angle of the rib posteriorly. Mark the ribs to be injected at the angle of the rib or along the mid-axillary line. If the ribs are not easily palpated, an alternative injection technique such as an epidural or root block may be considered. The patient is prepared in a standard aseptic fashion, and strict sterile technique is used throughout the procedure. The index finger of the nondominant hand is used to palpate the rib and identify the intercostal space. The tip of the finger is placed in the intercostal space and the skin slid over the superior rib. A 5/8 inch (1.5 cm) 25-gauge needle is inserted directly over the rib until contact is made with the rib. The long axis of the needle and syringe should have a slight cephalad tilt and be perpendicular to the long axis of the rib. The needle is then moved to the inferior edge of the rib by walking (i.e., repeatedly slightly withdrawing) the needle in the subcutaneous tissue and allowing the skin to slowly move back to its original position. The needle should retain its slight cephalad tilt. As the needle slips off the inferior ridge of the rib, advance the tip approximately 3 mm and aspirate. If aspiration is positive for blood or air, reposition needle; otherwise, 2 to 5 ml of local anesthetic is injected to block the intercostal nerve (Fig. 23-6).

Comments

A new needle should be used for each nerve blocked. Intercostal blocks are a simple and effective method of providing analgesia for painful disorders of the chest and abdominal walls. Due to the wide distribution of intercostal nerve innervation, the intercostal nerves above and below the level of pain must be blocked to gain optimal pain relief.

Complications

Intercostal blockade is often underutilized because of an exaggerated fear of pneumothorax. In actuality, less than 1% of all patients having an intercostal block develop a pneumothorax. Most can be easily treated with administration of supplemental oxygen and close observation, and when necessary, needle aspiration of air. Only those pneumothoraces that result in significant dyspnea or those under tension require chest tube thoracotomy and vacuum drainage. Local anesthetic toxicity can occur because of the rapid absorption after intercostal injection. Toxicity can easily be avoided by limiting the total amount injected to a known, safe level (Table 23-2).

Spinal Nerve Root Block

Indications

Nerve root blockade is useful in diagnosing and treating pain present in a dermatomal distribution.

Techniques

After informed consent is obtained, the patient is placed in the prone position and a line perpendicular to the axis of the spine is drawn across the top of the spinous process. In the lumbar region, a line drawn along the inferior edges of the two transverse processes will intersect the spinous process of the same vertebra at its most cephalad point. In the thoracic region, this line can extend as much as two vertebral levels caudally, particularly in the mid-thoracic region. The patient is prepared in a standard aseptic fashion, and strict sterile technique is used. A 4 inch (10 cm) 22-gauge needle is inserted 3 to 5 cm lateral from the midline, which should overlie the transverse process. The needle is advanced perpendicular to the skin until contact is made with the transverse process. The depth is noted at this point. The needle is pulled back to skin level and redirected to pass below the transverse process. Appropriate response with a nerve stimulator or paresthesia indicates correct placement. After negative aspiration, 2 to 5 ml of local anesthetic is injected to block the spinal nerve root (Fig. 23-7).

Comments

The technique of nerve root blockade is similar to that of the intercostal block. The transverse process serves as the depth marker for nerve roots. A sound knowledge of the relationship of the transverse process and the spinous processes is necessary to precisely locate the selected nerve

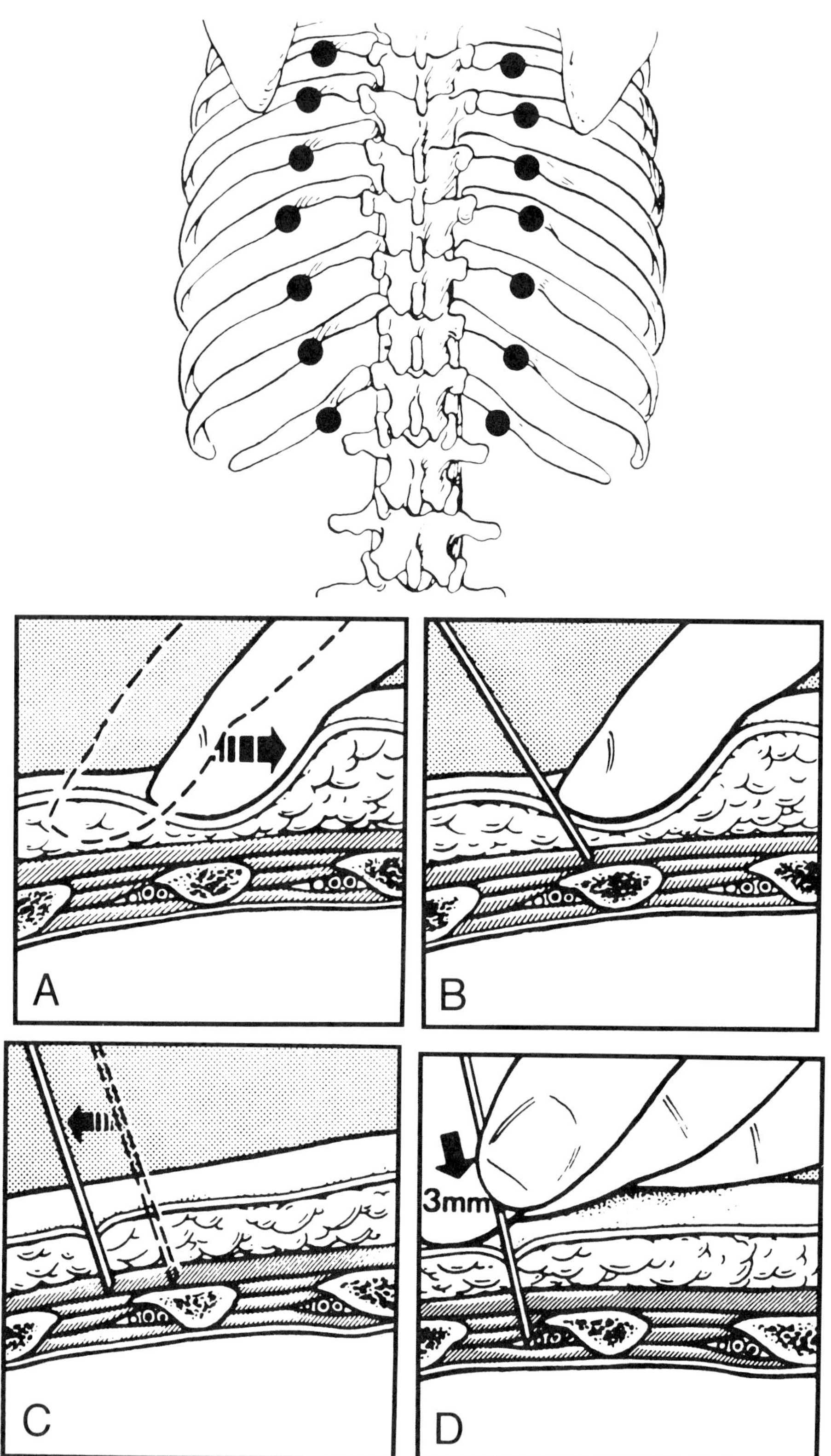

FIG. 23-6. Intercostal nerve block. Approach for intercostal nerve injection and neural blockade with injection sites marked at the angle of the rib. **A:** The tip of the finger is placed in the intercostal space and the skin slid over the superior rib. **B:** The needle is inserted directly over the rib until contact is made. **C:** The needle is walked to the inferior edge of the rib while maintaining a slight cephalad tilt. **D:** As the needle slips off the inferior edge of the rib, advance the needle approximately 3 mm, where it is adjacent to the intercostal nerve. (Reprinted with permission from Thompson GE, Moore DC. Celiac plexus, intercostal, and minor peripheral blockage. In: Cousins MJ, Bridenbaugh PO, eds. *Neural blockade in clinical anesthesia and management of pain,* 2nd ed. Philadelphia: JB Lippincott, 1988; 513.)

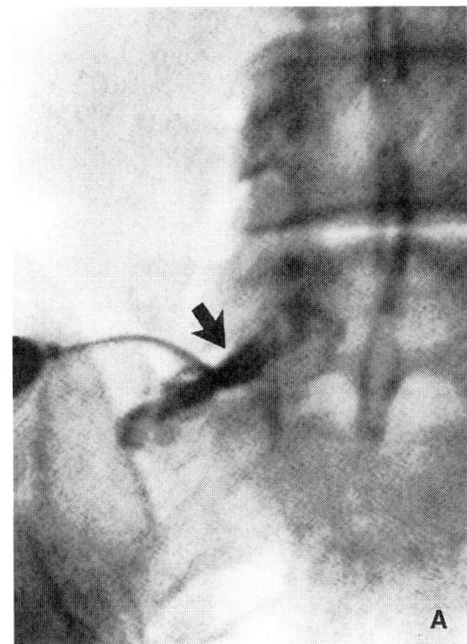

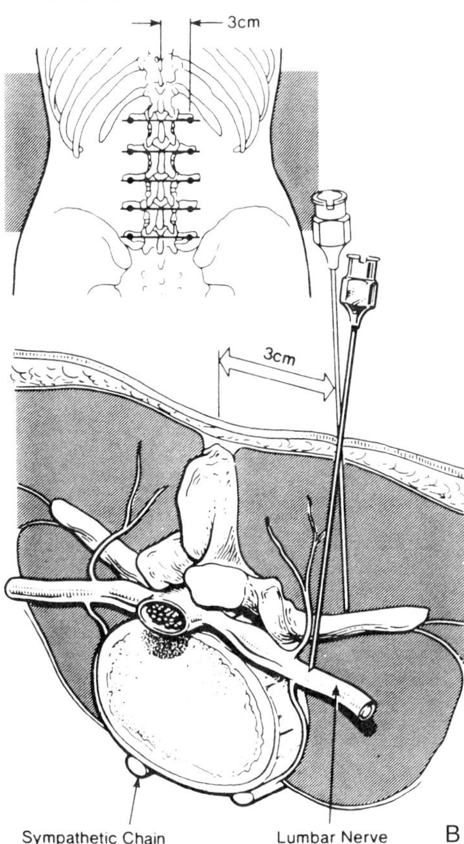

FIG. 23-7. Spinal nerve root block. **A:** Fluoroscopic view for L5 nerve root block *(arrow)*. **B:** Approach for spinal nerve root injection and neural blockade. (Reprinted with permission from Cousins MJ, Bridenbaugh PO, eds. *Neural blockade in clinical anesthesia and management of pain,* 2nd ed. Philadelphia: JB Lippincott, 1988; 420.)

root. Any disorder that responds to intercostal blockade also should respond to selective nerve root blockade.

Complications

Complications usually occur from injection of local anesthetic agents into areas adjacent to the paravertebral space such as the epidural or subarachnoid space. Puncture of retroperitoneal organs and bleed also can occur if care is not taken to fully consider the anatomy.

Celiac Plexus Block

Indications

Celiac plexus blockade is useful for diagnosing and treating pain of sympathetic origin. This includes pain involving the viscera, abdomen, and pelvis secondary to causalgia, reflex sympathetic dystrophy, and vasospastic disorders.

Techniques

After informed consent is obtained, the patient is placed in the prone position with a pillow under the abdomen. The inferior edge of the spinous process of the first lumbar vertebra and the lower border of each 12th rib at 7 cm from the spinous process of the first lumbar vertebra is identified and marked. The patient is prepared in a standard aseptic fashion, and a 6 inch (15 cm) 22-gauge needle is inserted at the mark on the 12th rib toward the spinous process of L1 at 60° from perpendicular. The needle is advanced until it contacts the lateral side of the L1 vertebra. The depth is noted at this point. The needle is pulled back to subcutaneous level and reinserted at 45° toward the spinous process of L1 and slightly cephalad until it slips off the edge of the vertebra. This is approximately 2 to 3 cm deeper than the original depth. After negative aspiration, 20 ml of local anesthetic is injected (Fig. 23-8).

Comments

This technique is commonly used for differential diagnosis and is the preferred treatment of sympathetic mediated pain involving the viscera and pelvis. The celiac plexus is located in the prevertebral region at the level of the L1 vertebral body. It is formed by the right and left celiac, superior mesenteric, and aorticorenal ganglia. Autonomic mediated pain does not usually correspond to segmental or peripheral nerve distribution. Lateral and anteroposterior fluoroscopic views are recommended to ensure that the needle is properly positioned. It is recommended that IV access be available before the block in the event of intravascular injection and resulting seizure activity. It is necessary to perform this procedure bilaterally for a complete celiac plexus block. Rarely are ablative nerve procedures (neurolysis) required in the management of sympathetic mediated pain.

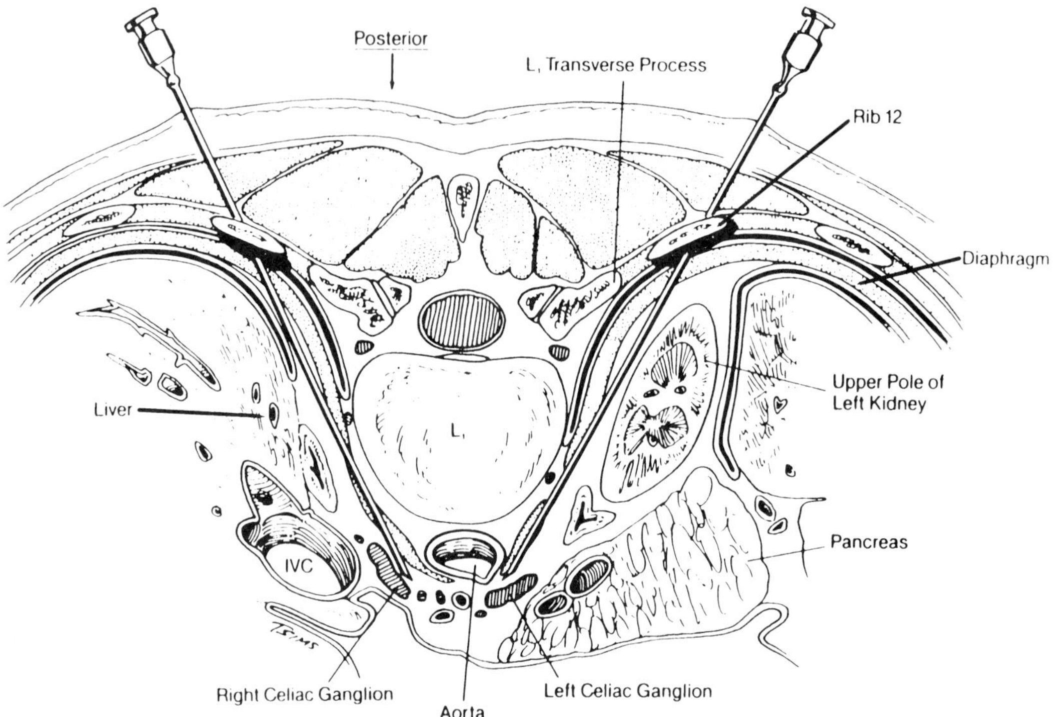

FIG. 23-8. Celiac plexus block. Approach for celiac plexus injection and neural blockade. (Reprinted with permission from Raj PP, Pai U, Rawal N. Techniques of regional anesthesia in adults. In: Raj PP, ed. *Clinical practice of regional anesthesia.* New York: Churchill-Livingstone, 1991; 496.)

Complications

Performance of this procedure out of a fully monitored environment is not recommended. Resuscitation equipment and personnel must be readily available. While appearing technically simple, this block has multiple hazards due to the proximity of the aorta, kidney, pancreas, diaphragm, thoracic duct, and other vascular structures. Intra-arterial or intradural injection of local anesthetic may result in death, seizure, respiratory arrest, cardiac arrest, cerebral damage with multiple sequelae, and other lesser complications. The risk of intravascular injection may be reduced if a test dose is given, the total dose is injected incrementally, and aspiration is performed before each injection.

Lumbar Epidural Steroid Injection

Indications

Epidural steroid injection (ESI) is most effective for lumbosacral radiculopathy associated with intervertebral disc herniation, bulging, or degeneration. The main criterion for success is the presence of nerve root inflammation that can be relieved by the steroid. ESI also has been used to treat pain from degenerative joint disease, scoliosis, spondylolysis, spondylolisthesis, postlaminectomy syndrome, facet abnormalities, herpes zoster, and postherpetic neuralgia.

Techniques

After informed consent is obtained, the patient is placed either in the lateral decubitus position or sitting with the back, hips, and knees flexed. The injection should be performed as close as possible to the bony level of the nerve root irritation. The patient is prepared in a standard aseptic fashion with strict sterile technique used throughout the procedure. Local skin anesthesia is provided with 1% to 2% lidocaine. A Tuohy epidural needle is then advanced between the spinous processes in a midline approach until the needle is well seated in the posterior ligaments. The stylet is then removed and a loss-of-resistance syringe is attached to the hub of the needle. Either 2 to 3 ml of air or normal saline should be in the syringe. The needle is slowly advanced 1 to 2 mm at a time with constant checking for loss of resistance by tapping on the plunger of the syringe. Once a distinct loss of resistance is obtained, the needle is halted and an attempt is made to aspirate blood or CSF. After negative aspiration, either 80 to 120 mg of methylprednisolone acetate or 50 mg of triamcinolone diacetate is injected. The steroids can be injected as is or diluted in 5 to 10 ml of preservative-free normal saline. If multiple levels are involved, dilution will ensure better spread of the steroid. The needle should be flushed with normal saline and the stylet replaced before it is removed from the skin to avoid tracking steroid to the skin. If on aspiration blood is obtained, reposition the needle. If CSF is obtained on aspiration, continue with the procedure, but a spinal headache may result from dural puncture (Fig. 23-9).

Comments

A complete evaluation of the pain should be undertaken before ESI to rule out serious neurologic dysfunction or malignancy. Local infection, sepsis, coagulation abnormalities, or patient refusal are contraindications to ESI. Success is higher if the patient has had no previous back surgeries and the pain has been present less than 6 to 12 months. Methylprednisolone acetate is best used for localized nerve root irritation. Triamcinolone diacetate is water soluble and results in optimal outcome in generalized nerve root irritation such as arachnoiditis.

The paraspinous approach may be used if difficulty is encountered with the midline approach. A Tuohy epidural needle is inserted alongside the caudal edge of the inferior spinous process to the bony level of nerve root irritation. The needle is inserted with a 45° angulation to the long axis of the spine below and a 10° offset from midline and advanced between the spinous processes until it is well seated in the posterior ligaments.

Complications

Inadvertent dural puncture may result in a postdural puncture headache. Intrathecal injection of steroid may result in aseptic meningitis, adhesive arachnoiditis, or conus medullaris syndrome. Each milliliter of methylprednisolone acetate contains approximately 30 mg of polyethylene glycol, which has been associated with nerve damage in experimental models (33). Epidural steroids can suppress plasma cortisol levels for approximately 3 to 5 weeks. Iatrogenic Cushing's syndrome, fluid retention, and elevated serum glucose levels also can occur (34).

Infection or bleeding into the closed epidural space also can result in significant neurologic deficits, including quadriplegia. Any complaint of increasing pain or neurologic changes should be investigated immediately. Early recognition can prevent permanent injury.

Lumbar Sympathetic Block

Indications

Lumbar sympathetic blockade is useful for diagnosing and treating pain of sympathetic origin. This includes pain involving the pelvis and lower extremity secondary to causalgia, reflex sympathetic dystrophy, vasospastic disorders, and phantom pain.

Techniques

The spinous process of the second or third lumbar vertebra is palpated and a point 4 cm lateral to the middle of the spinous process is marked. The patient is prepared in a standard aseptic fashion and sterile technique is used. A 4 inch (10 cm) 22-gauge needle is inserted and advanced cephalad until contact is made with the transverse process. The needle is pulled back to skin level and redirected to pass between the transverse processes and alongside the anterolateral aspect of the vertebral body. After negative aspiration, 20 ml of local anesthetic is injected (Fig. 23-10).

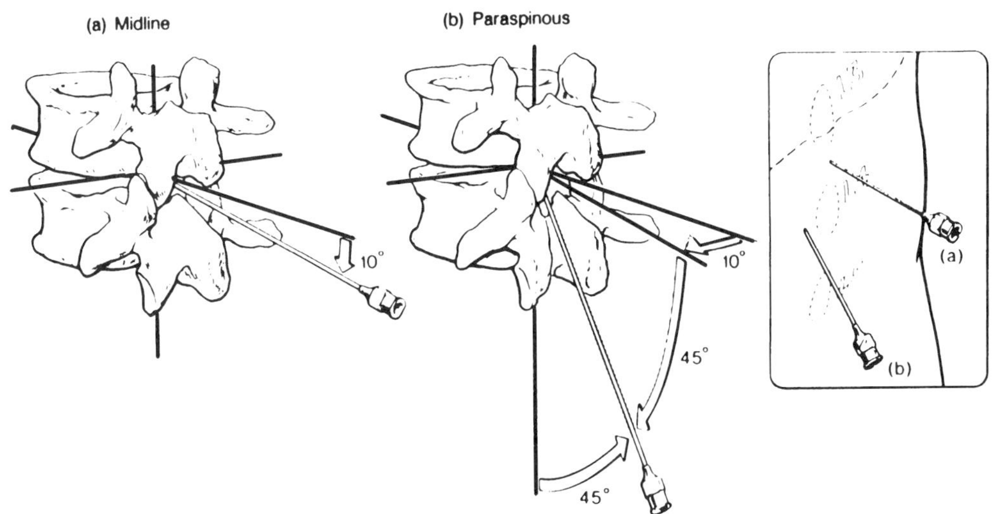

FIG. 23-9. Lumbar epidural steroid injection. Approach for lumbar epidural steroid injection. **a:** Midline. Note insertion is closer to the superior spinous process and with a slight upward angulation. **b:** Paraspinous (paramedian). Note insertion alongside caudal edge of "inferior" spinous process with 45° angulation to long axis of spine below. (Reprinted with permission from Cousins MJ, Bridenbaugh PO, eds. *Neural blockade in clinical anesthesia and management of pain,* 2nd ed. Philadelphia: JB Lippincott, 1988; 323.)

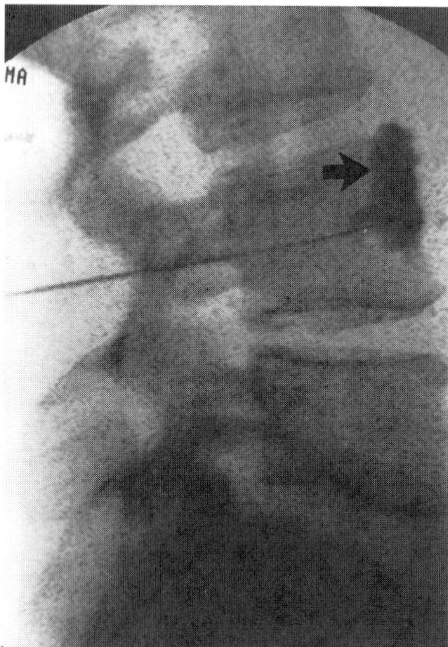

FIG. 23-10. Lumbar sympathetic approach. Fluoroscopic approach for lumbar sympathetic injection and neural blockade *(arrow)*.

Comments

This technique is commonly used for differential diagnosis and is the preferred treatment of sympathetic mediated pain involving the upper extremity. The lumbar sympathetic ganglion is located along the anterior lateral surface of the lumbar vertebral bodies and anteromedial to the psoas muscle. Autonomic mediated pain does not usually correspond to segmental or peripheral nerve distribution. Lateral and anteroposterior fluoroscopic views are recommended to ensure that the needle is properly positioned. It is recommended that IV access be available before the block in the event of intravascular injection and resulting seizure activity. Rarely are ablative nerve procedures (neurolysis) required in the management of sympathetic mediated pain.

Complications

Performance of this procedure outside of a fully monitored environment is not recommended. Resuscitation equipment and personnel must be readily available. While appearing technically simple, this block has multiple hazards due to the proximity to the aorta, inferior venacava, kidney, pancreas, and intestines. Intra-arterial or intradural injection of local anesthetic may result in death, seizure, respiratory arrest, cardiac arrest, cerebral damage with multiple sequelae, and other lesser complications. The risk of intravascular injection may be reduced if a test dose is given, the total dose is injected incrementally, and aspiration is performed before each injection.

Caudal Injection

Indications

The caudal approach to the epidural space is used to treat pain in the lower back and pelvis.

Techniques

After informed consent is obtained, the patient may be placed in a variety of positions, with patient comfort probably the prime concern. The preferred position is the lateral Sim's position with the left side down for right-handed clinicians. With the upper leg flexed, the buttocks are separated, allowing easy access to the sacral–coccygeal junction. The patient is prepared in a standard aseptic fashion over a large area to allow palpation of landmarks. The midline is identified by palpating the tip of the coccyx with a finger and moving cephalad about 4 to 5 cm in an adult, until the fingertip lies over the sacral hiatus with the sacral cornua palpable on each side. The palpating hand is kept in position, and a 2 inch (5 cm) 18-gauge short beveled needle is inserted. The initial angle of insertion is about 120° to the coccyx. A "pop" is felt as the sacrococcygeal ligament is penetrated. The needle is then depressed to align with the long axis of the canal and inserted 1 cm. Once the caudal space has been entered, the position is confirmed by aspiration of CSF, then 80 to 120 mg methylprednisolone acetate or 50 mg of triamcinolone diacetate is injected. The steroids can be injected as is or diluted in 5 to 10 ml of preservative-free normal saline (Fig. 23-11).

Comments

Epiduroscopy, a technique used to visualize the lumbar epidural space, depends on this approach because the fiberoptic catheter cannot tolerate bending. Advantages of this approach include minimal risk of inadvertent dural puncture. Continuous catheter techniques can be used, but maintenance of site cleanliness is more difficult when compared with the lumbar approach to the epidural space. A Tuohy needle is not used for catheter placement because it will direct the catheter against the wall of the caudal canal and make catheter advancement difficult. Methylprednisolone acetate is best used for localized nerve root irritation. Triamcinolone diacetate is water soluble and results in optimal outcome in generalized nerve root irritation such as arachnoiditis.

Complications

Improper needle placement can result in inadequate or absent block. This is due to variability in anatomy and inexperience. Rapid injection of large volumes of fluid is not recommended because this may result in large increases in CSF pressures, with the risk of cerebral hemorrhage, visual disturbances, headache, or compromised spinal cord blood

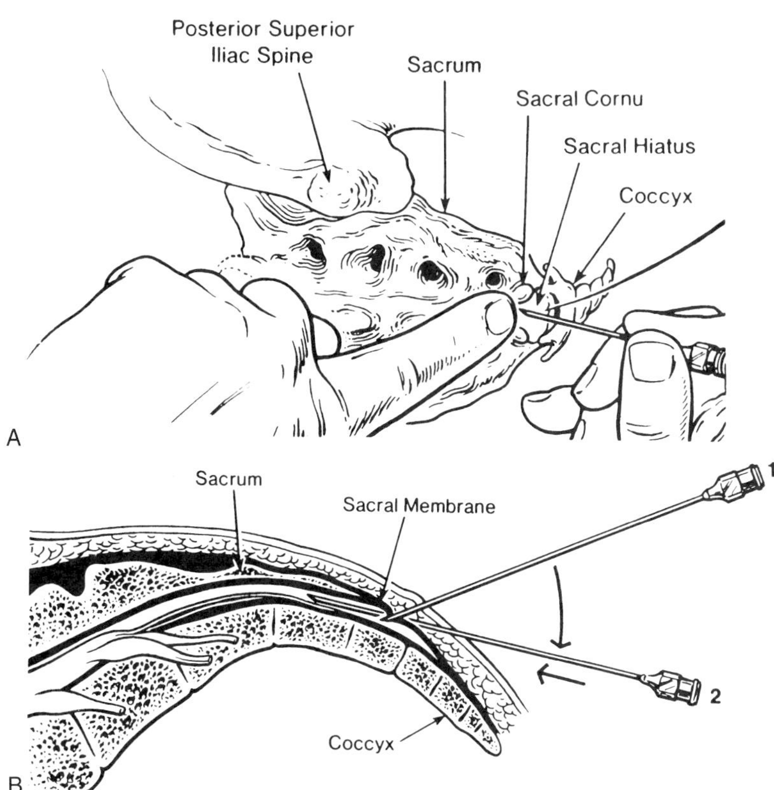

FIG. 23-11. Caudal injection. **A:** Landmarks and approach for needle insertion. **B:** Needle insertion through sacral-coccygeal membrane for injection. (Reprinted with permission from Willis RJ. Caudal epidural blockade. In: Cousins MJ, Bridenbaugh PO, eds. *Neural blockade in clinical anesthesia and management of pain,* 2nd ed. Philadelphia: JB Lippincott, 1988; 373.)

flow. Pain at the injection site is a common complaint. Urinary retention can result from local anesthetic injection and should last only as long as the block.

Lateral Femoral Cutaneous Nerve Block

Indications

Lateral femoral cutaneous nerve blockade is useful for diagnosing and treating pain in the lateral thigh, thought to be from irritation of this nerve.

Techniques

After informed consent is obtained, the patient is placed in a supine position and the anterior superior iliac spine is palpated. The patient is prepared in a standard aseptic fashion, and a 1 1/2 inch (4 cm) 21- to 23-gauge needle is inserted 1 cm medial and below the anterior superior iliac spine. The needle is advanced deep into the fascia lata toward the shelving of the iliac crest. After negative aspiration, 5 ml of local anesthetic is injected in a fanwise manner (Fig. 23-12).

This nerve can be blocked via an alternative approach by directing the needle superiorly beneath the inguinal ligament into the fascial compartment containing the nerve above the level of the inguinal ligament. This fascial compartment can be identified by directing a short bevel needle medial to the anterior superior iliac spine and advancing through the

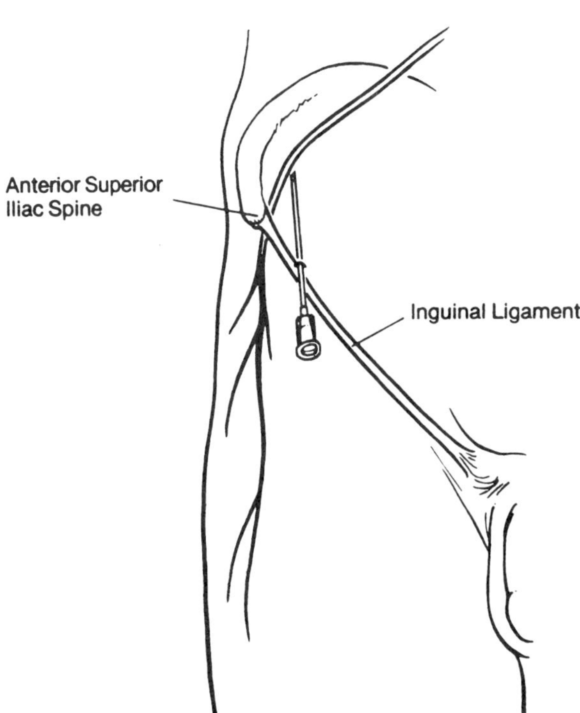

FIG. 23-12. Lateral femoral cutaneous nerve block. Approach for lateral femoral cutaneous nerve injection and neural blockade. (Reprinted with permission from Raj PP, Pai U, Rawal N. Techniques of regional anesthesia in adults. In: Raj PP, ed. *Clinical practice of regional anesthesia.* New York: Churchill-Livingstone, 1991; 496.)

external oblique aponeurosis, the internal oblique muscle, and through the fascia iliaca. The short bevel needle allows the physician to feel a distinct loss of resistance or characteristic pop as the two fascial layers are penetrated. After negative aspiration, 5 ml of local anesthetic is injected to block the lateral femoral cutaneous nerve.

Comments

The lateral femoral cutaneous nerve emerges along the lateral border of the psoas muscle below the ilioinguinal nerve. It runs obliquely under the iliac fascia across the iliacus muscle and enters the thigh by passing posterior to the inguinal ligament, just medial to the anterior superior iliac spine. It provides cutaneous innervation to the lateral aspect of the thigh to the knee. A large area over the lateral aspect of the thigh can be easily blocked with this technique.

Complications

The lateral femoral cutaneous nerve block has no significant complications, with the rare exception of a dysesthesia if the nerve is injured during the injection. Severe pain on injection suggests the possibility of an intraneural injection, and the needle should be immediately repositioned. It is possible to inadvertently block the femoral nerve when large amounts of local anesthetic are injected, resulting in a temporary weakness of knee extension and impaired ambulation. This occurs secondary to medial spread of local anesthetic beneath the fascia iliaca.

Femoral Nerve Block

Indications

Femoral nerve blockade is useful in conjunction with other lower extremity blocks in treating reflex sympathetic dystrophy and as an aid to decrease knee and ankle pain during physical therapy.

Techniques

After informed consent is obtained, the patient is placed in the supine position and the femoral artery is located. After the patient is prepared in a standard aseptic fashion, the femoral artery is palpated below the inguinal ligament. A 1 1/2 inch (4 cm) 22-gauge needle is inserted 1 to 2 cm below the inguinal ligament and lateral to the femoral artery. The needle is advanced in a lateral and posterior direction just distal to the inguinal ligament. A characteristic pop, when using a short beveled needle, can be used to identify penetration of the fascia lata and the fascia iliaca, remembering that the femoral nerve lies deep to both. When a nerve stimulator is used, contraction of the quadriceps muscle confirms correct placement of the needle. After negative aspiration, 10 ml of local anesthetic is injected to block the femoral nerve (Fig. 23-13).

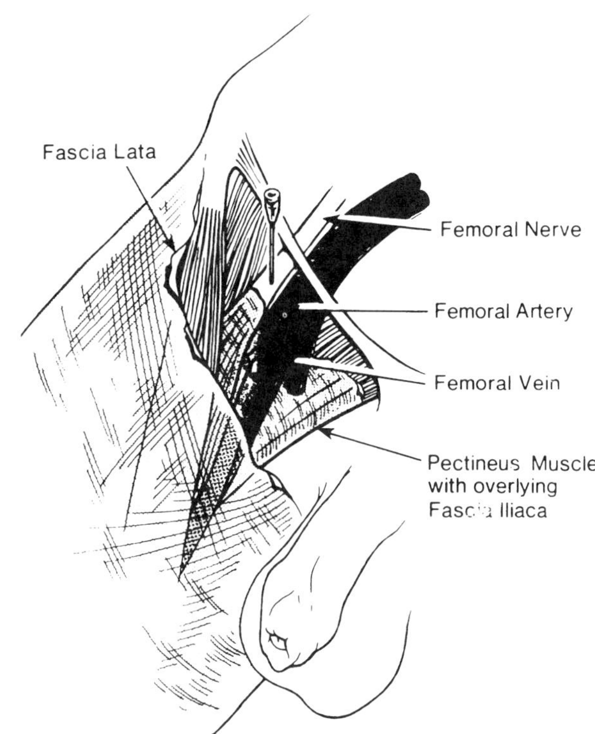

FIG. 23-13. Femoral nerve block. Approach for femoral nerve injection and neural blockade. (Reprinted with permission from Bridenbaugh PO. The lower extremity: somatic block. In: Cousins MJ, Bridenbaugh PO, eds. *Neural blockade in clinical anesthesia and management of pain,* 2nd ed. Philadelphia: JB Lippincott, 1988; 421.)

Comments

At the level of the inguinal ligament, the femoral nerve lies anterior to the iliopsoas muscle and slightly lateral to the femoral artery. It does not lie within the femoral sheath. The nerve lies underneath the fascia lata and fascia iliaca within its own sheath. At the level of the inguinal ligament, the femoral nerve divides into anterior (superficial) and posterior (deep) bundles. The anterior bundle provides cutaneous innervation of the skin overlying the anterior surface of the thigh as well as providing motor innervation to the sartorius muscle. The posterior bundle provides innervation to the quadriceps muscles and the knee joint. It also gives off the saphenous nerve, which supplies cutaneous innervation to the medial aspect of the calf to the level of the medial malleolus. A catheter also can be placed within the femoral nerve sheath for continuous infusion of local anesthetics.

It is important to remember that the upper portion of the anterior thigh is innervated by the ilioinguinal and genitofemoral nerves and is not blocked when performing a femoral nerve block.

Complications

Significant complications associated with femoral nerve blockade are uncommon. Dysesthesia may result if the nerve is injured during the injection. Hematoma at the site is a possibility but is usually not clinically significant. If an arterial puncture occurs, prolonged direct pressure is usually adequate to prevent the development of a hematoma. The presence of a femoral artery vascular graft is a relative contraindication to femoral nerve blockade.

Obturator Nerve Block

Indications

Obturator nerve blockade is extremely useful as a diagnostic, prognostic, or therapeutic procedure in patients with adductor spasm that interferes with rehabilitation or personal hygiene.

Techniques

After informed consent is obtained, the patient is placed in the supine position with the leg to be blocked placed in slight abduction. It is not necessary to shave the pubic area. The patient is prepared in a standard aseptic fashion, and a 3 inch (8 cm) 22-gauge needle is inserted perpendicular to the skin at a point 1.5 cm lateral and inferior to the pubic tubercle. The needle is advanced until the inferior ramus of the pubis is contacted. The needle depth at which the bone is contacted should be noted. The needle is withdrawn to skin level and redirected in a lateral and slightly superior direction, parallel to the superior ramus of the pubis. The needle is advanced 2 to 3 cm beyond the previously noted depth until a paresthesia is elicited. A nerve stimulator makes it relatively easy to identify the obturator nerve by adductor muscle contraction. After negative aspiration for blood, 10 ml of local anesthetic is injected to block the obturator nerve. This traditional approach was first described by Labat (35) (Fig. 23-14).

Using the above techniques, Wassef has described an alternative approach using the femoral artery and adductor longus tendon as landmarks (36). A mark is made on the skin 1 to 2 cm medial to the femoral artery just below the inguinal ligament. This mark is used to indicate the direction of the needle toward the obturator canal. The adductor longus tendon is then identified near its insertion site at the pubis. A 3 inch (8 cm) 22-gauge insulated needle is introduced behind the adductor longus tendon and directed laterally, with a slight posterior and superior inclination toward the skin mark. The needle is advanced until adductor muscle contraction is elicited with a nerve stimulator (37).

Comments

The obturator nerve is formed by the union of the ventral branches of the anterior primary rami of L2, L3, and L4 within the substance of the psoas muscle. It emerges from the medial border of the psoas muscle at the brim of the pelvis. The nerve runs caudad and anteriorly along the lateral wall of the pelvis along the obturator vessels to the obturator foramen. There it enters the thigh, supplying the adductor muscles and providing innervation to the hip and knee joints.

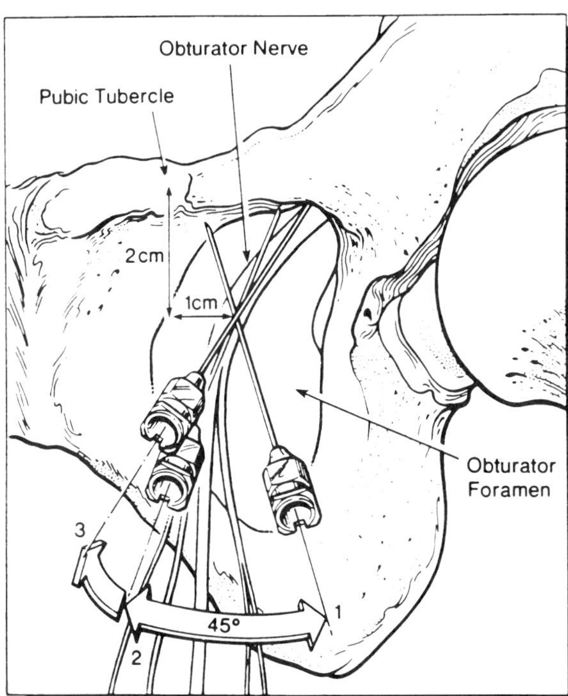

FIG. 23-14. Obturator nerve block. Approach for obturator nerve injection and neural blockade. (Reprinted with permission from Bridenbaugh PO. The lower extremity: somatic block. In: Cousins MJ, Bridenbaugh PO, eds. *Neural blockade in clinical anesthesia and management of pain,* 2nd ed. Philadelphia: JB Lippincott, 1988; 432.)

As the nerve passes through the obturator canal, it divides into anterior and posterior branches. The anterior branch supplies the hip joint, the anterior adductor muscles, and cutaneous branches to the medial aspect of the thigh. The cutaneous innervation of the obturator nerve can be extremely variable and can be nonexistent in some people. The posterior branch supplies the deep adductor muscles and frequently sends a branch to the knee joint.

This procedure is often performed on rehabilitation patients with spasticity and/or contractures that result in positioning difficulty. Confirmation of a successful obturator nerve block is demonstrated by paresis of the adductor muscles because the cutaneous contribution of the obturator nerve is inconsistent. An alternative to this procedure is selective root blockade at levels L2, L3, and L4 using a nerve stimulator to establish muscle innervation.

Complications

Hematoma and intravascular injection are possible due to the close proximity of the obturator vessels. If an arterial puncture occurs, prolonged direct pressure is usually adequate to prevent the development of a hematoma.

Sciatic Nerve Block

Indications

Sciatic nerve blockade is typically used to treat painful conditions of the lower leg such as reflex sympathetic dystrophy and to facilitate physical therapy by decreasing pain in the lower extremity.

Techniques

A regional block of the sciatic nerve can be achieved anywhere along the course of the nerve. Most of the approaches have been developed mainly to avoid positioning problems that may be present in trauma patients or in the elderly. The nerve can be blocked at the sciatic notch, at the level of the ischial tuberosity, greater trochanter, or superior aspect of the popliteal fossa.

Classic Approach

The classic technique described by Labat (35) blocks the nerve at the level of the greater sciatic notch, using the piriformis muscle as a landmark. After informed consent is obtained, the patient is placed in the lateral Sims position with the side to be blocked uppermost. The upper knee is flexed and the patient's back rotated slightly forward. Some patients may find this position uncomfortable, particularly those with orthopedic problems.

The landmarks are the cephalad portion of the greater trochanter and the posterior superior iliac spine. A line is drawn connecting these two points, corresponding to the superior border of the piriformis muscle and the upper border of the sciatic notch. A perpendicular line is drawn distally from the mid-point of the first line. The point of injection is 3 to 5 cm distal on the perpendicular line. Verification of the insertion point can be made by drawing a third line connecting the cephalad portion of the greater trochanter and the sacrococcygeal joint. This third line is used to compensate for the height of the patient. The intersection of lines 2 and 3 is the point of needle insertion (Fig. 23-15).

The patient is prepared in a standard aseptic fashion, and a 4 to 5 inch (10 to 12 cm) 22-gauge spinal needle is introduced at right angles to the skin and advanced to a depth of 6 to 10 cm until a paresthesia is reported in the distribution of the sciatic nerve, preferably involving the foot. If periosteum is contacted, the needle is then redirected medially or superiorly. Touching the periosteum may produce a local paresthesia, which could be mistaken for a true sciatic nerve paresthesia. A nerve stimulator is extremely helpful in locating the nerve (37).

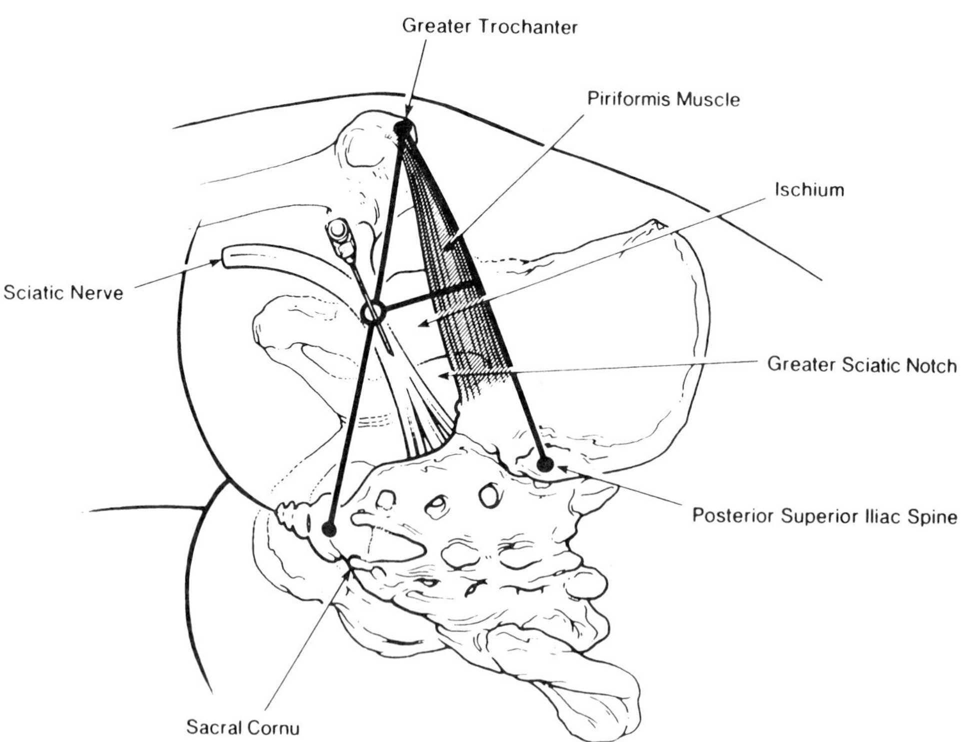

FIG. 23-15. Sciatic nerve block—classic approach. Classic approach for sciatic nerve injection and neural blockade. (Reprinted with permission from Bridenbaugh PO. The lower extremity: somatic block. In: Cousins MJ, Bridenbaugh PO, eds. *Neural blockade in clinical anesthesia and management of pain,* 2nd ed. Philadelphia: JB Lippincott, 1988; 424.)

Doppler ultrasound also can be used to locate the dominant arterial structure within the sciatic notch (38). The needle is then advanced in the same orientation as the probe until a paresthesia is obtained. Successful blockade has been reported after one or two attempts in 70% of patients. After negative aspiration for blood, 20 to 30 ml of local anesthetic is injected to block the sciatic nerve.

A continuous sciatic nerve block can be performed by using a standard 16-gauge IV infusion cannula attached to a nerve stimulator. After obtaining muscle contraction in the lower leg, preferably dorsal or plantar flexion of the foot, an epidural catheter is advanced about 6 cm into the neurovascular space. Continuous infusion of a local anesthetic using an infusion pump can then be used to provide continuous analgesia (39). With the classical approach, both the posterior femoral cutaneous and pudendal nerves are usually blocked with the sciatic nerve.

Posterior Approach

An alternate approach may be used, with the patient positioned as above or prone. The ischial tuberosity and the greater trochanter are identified and a line drawn connecting these two points. The patient is prepared in a standard aseptic fashion, and a 3 to 4 inch (8 to 10 cm) 22-gauge spinal needle is inserted at the mid-point of the line until a paresthesia is elicited in the lower leg. After negative aspiration, 20 to 30 ml of local anesthetic is injected to block the sural nerve. The posterior femoral cutaneous nerve is often blocked at this level, but the pudendal nerve is frequently spared.

Anterior Approach

The anterior approach allows the sciatic nerve to be blocked without moving the patient, enabling the patient to remain in the supine position (35,40). This approach is especially helpful in trauma patients with a painful leg but is quite painful, with sedation often necessary. The nerve is very deep at this point and can be difficult to locate. In adults, the sciatic neurovascular compartment is usually 4.5 to 6 cm below the surface of the femur. In children, however, the distance varies according to age and size of the child (41). The use of a nerve stimulator is advised in identifying the nerve. The posterior cutaneous nerve of the thigh may not be blocked with this approach, resulting in tourniquet pain if a thigh tourniquet is applied (Fig. 23-16).

The patient is placed in the supine position with the leg in a neutral position. The anterior superior iliac spine and the pubic tubercle are identified and marked. A line is then drawn connecting these two points, overlying the inguinal ligament, and trisected into equal parts. A perpendicular line is drawn distally from the junction of the medial and middle thirds. A third line is drawn parallel to the first starting from the cephalad aspect of the greater trochanter. The point of

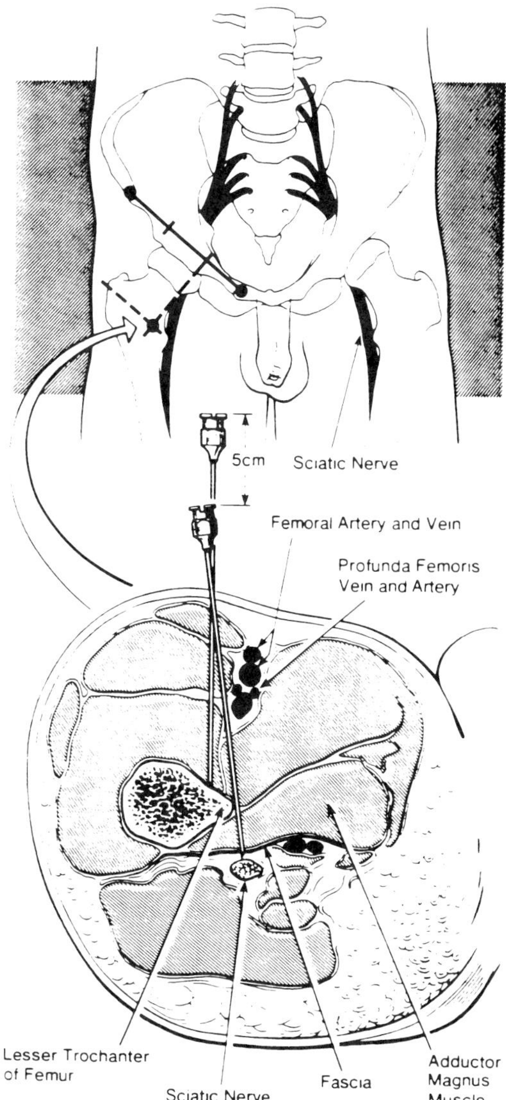

FIG. 23-16. Sciatic nerve block—anterior approach. Anterior approach for sciatic nerve injection and neural blockade. Cross-section of the leg at the level of the lesser trochanter to show the relationship between the sciatic nerve and femur, and the fascia separating it from the adductor magnus. (Reprinted with permission from Bridenbaugh PO. The lower extremity: somatic block. In: Cousins MJ, Bridenbaugh PO, eds. *Neural blockade in clinical anesthesia and management of pain,* 2nd ed. Philadelphia: JB Lippincott, 1988; 426.)

intersection of this third line and the perpendicular line is the insertion point of the needle.

The patient is prepared in a standard aseptic fashion, and a 6 inch (15 cm) 22-gauge spinal needle is inserted and directed slightly laterally from a plane perpendicular to the skin. The needle is advanced until periosteum is contacted (usually the lesser trochanter). The needle is partially withdrawn and redirected medially and posteriorly to pass approximately 5 cm beyond the femur until a paresthesia is elicited. After negative aspiration, 20 to 25 ml of local anesthetic agent is injected to block the sural nerve.

Lateral Approach

The lateral approach, initially described by Ichiyanaghi (42), was found to be very difficult and never became popular. A new lateral approach described by Guardini et al. (43) is easier. It blocks the sciatic nerve just posterior to the quadratus femoris muscle in the subgluteal space.

The greater trochanter is identified, and the patient is prepared in a standard sterile fashion. A 5 to 6 inch (12 to 15 cm), 22 gauge spinal needle is advanced 3 cm distal to the maximum lateral prominence of the trochanter, close to its posterior margin. The needle is inserted until the periosteum is contacted. The needle is then partially withdrawn and redirected posteriorly and medially to slide beneath the femoral shaft until a paresthesia, or contraction of the calf or the anterior compartment muscles, occurs with the use of a nerve stimulator. After negative aspiration, 20 to 30 ml of local anesthetic is injected to block the sural nerve.

The main advantage of this technique is that the patient can remain in the supine position and the leg need not be manipulated. When using a nerve stimulator, it is important to make sure the muscle contractions occur in the calf muscles or in the muscles of the anterior compartment. It is possible with this technique to inadvertently stimulate the nerve branch supplying the two heads of the biceps femoris muscle, producing thigh muscle contraction and misplacement of the local anesthetic.

Comments

The sciatic nerve is the largest in the body. It arises from both the lumbar and sacral plexuses. Anatomically, the sciatic nerve consists of two major nerve trunks: the tibial and common peroneal components. The tibial nerve is derived from the anterior rami of L4–S3 nerve roots. The common peroneal nerve is derived from the dorsal branches of the anterior rami of the same roots.

It leaves the pelvis along with the posterior cutaneous nerve of the thigh through the sciatic foramen beneath the inferior margin of the piriformis muscle. It passes halfway between the greater trochanter and the ischial tuberosity. It becomes superficial at the inferior border of the gluteus maximus muscle and travels down the posterior aspect of the thigh. At the superior aspect of the popliteal fossa, the sciatic nerve physically separates into the tibial and common peroneal nerves.

In the past, the sciatic nerve block was considered unreliable, technically difficult, and uncomfortable for the patient. Sedation was often required, and this interfered with the patient's ability to provide accurate verbal feedback. This was especially the case if a paresthesia was used to identify the nerve. Reported rates of success ranged between 33% and 95% using various techniques. Today's insulated needles and nerve stimulators have made it easier to perform this block safely in sedated or even anesthetized patients with a higher rate of success.

Complications

Although the sciatic nerve is composed of mostly somatic nerves, it has a sympathetic component. The resulting sympathetic block may allow some mild venous pooling, but this is usually insufficient to cause clinically significant hypotension. Residual dysesthesias have been reported but usually improve in 1 to 3 days. This may be the result of nerve injury from the use of long beveled needles. Using short beveled needles for regional blocks may decrease the incidence of nerve injury.

NERVE BLOCKS AT THE KNEE

Nerve blockade at the knee is primarily used to treat pain disorders in specific nerve distributions. Diagnostic tibial nerve blocks also can be helpful in evaluating patients with spastic hemiparesis or myotonic disorders (44). Many early textbooks of regional blockade discouraged individual nerve blocks at the knee because they were thought to be difficult to perform and there was a possibility of a postanesthetic neuritis (45). Recently, studies have shown these nerve blocks can be safely and successfully performed at the knee, even in children (46,47).

The common peroneal and tibial nerves are extensions of the sciatic nerve. The sciatic nerve bifurcates at the superior aspect of the popliteal fossa, bordered by the biceps femoris muscle laterally and the semimembranosus and semitendinosus muscles medially. The two heads of the gastrocnemius muscle border the lower half of the popliteal fossa. Techniques have been described in which the tibial and common peroneal nerves are blocked with one injection, but it is possible to miss one of the branches (48). Identifying the two nerves separately and performing individual nerve blocks increases the likelihood of success.

Tibial Nerve Block

Indications

Tibial nerve blockade is useful as a diagnostic, prognostic, or therapeutic procedure in painful disorders involving the ankle and foot.

Techniques

After informed consent is obtained, the patient is placed in the prone position. The knee is flexed to allow palpation of the superior popliteal fossa borders and identification of the skin crease behind the knee joint. The patient is prepared in a standard aseptic fashion, and a 1 1/2 inch (3 to 4 cm) 21- to 23-gauge needle is inserted just above the crease line in the middle of the popliteal fossa. A nerve stimulator is used to identify the tibial nerve by eliciting plantar flexion of the foot. The average depth from skin to nerve in adults is 1.5 to 2.0 cm. After negative aspiration, 5 ml of local anesthetic is injected to block the tibial nerve (Fig. 23-17).

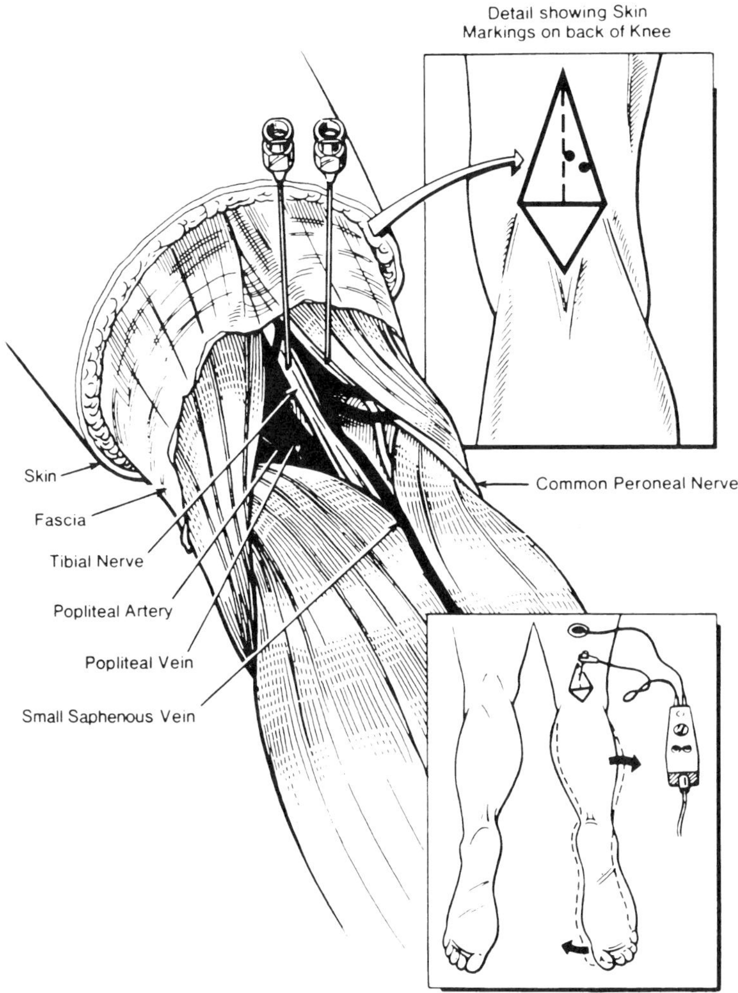

FIG. 23-17. Tibial and common peroneal nerve block at the knee. Approach for tibial and common peroneal nerve injection and neural blockade at the knee. Tibial and common peroneal (lateral popliteal) nerve. (Reprinted with permission from Bridenbaugh PO. The lower extremity: somatic block. In: Cousins MJ, Bridenbaugh PO, eds. *Neural blockade in clinical anesthesia and management of pain,* 2nd ed. Philadelphia: JB Lippincott, 1988; 433.)

Comments

The tibial nerve is the larger of the two branches of the sciatic nerve and supplies motor innervation to the flexor muscles at the back of the knee joint and calf. The cutaneous innervation supplies the skin overlying the popliteal fossa and down the back of the leg to the ankle. It travels through the center of the popliteal fossa as it proceeds distally down the leg.

Complications

Hematoma and intravascular injection are possible due to the close proximity of the popliteal vessels. If an arterial puncture occurs, prolonged direct pressure is usually adequate to prevent the development of a hematoma.

Common Peroneal Nerve Block

Indications

Common peroneal nerve blockade is useful as a diagnostic, prognostic, or therapeutic procedure in painful disorders involving the ankle and foot.

Techniques

After informed consent is obtained, the patient is placed in the supine or lateral position. The common peroneal nerve can be easily palpated as it crosses the neck of the fibula. The patient is prepared in a standard aseptic fashion, and a 1 inch (2.5 cm) 25-gauge needle is inserted next to the nerve and advanced to contact the periosteum, taking care to avoid an intraneural injection. A sudden, intense pain on injection suggests intraneural injection. If this occurs, reposition the needle and proceed. A nerve stimulator may be used to identify the nerve by eliciting contraction of the anterior compartment muscles. The needle is withdrawn slightly, and after negative aspiration, 5 ml of local anesthetic is injected to block the peroneal nerve (Fig. 23-17).

Comments

The common peroneal nerve is about half the size of the tibial nerve and contains articular branches to the knee joint and provides motor innervation to the extensor muscles of the foot and cutaneous nerves to the lateral aspect of the leg, heel, and ankle. It separates from the tibial nerve at the superior aspect of the popliteal fossa and courses laterally around the fibular head where it divides into the deep and superficial peroneal nerves.

Complications

Complications from the common peroneal nerve block are rare, especially when care is taken to avoid an intraneural injection. Severe pain on injection suggests the possibility of an intraneural injection, and the needle should be immediately repositioned.

Saphenous Nerve Block

Indications

Saphenous nerve blockade is useful as a diagnostic, prognostic, or therapeutic procedure in painful disorders involving the ankle and foot.

Techniques

After informed consent is obtained, the patient is placed in the supine or lateral position. The saphenous nerve is located at the medial surface of the medial condyle of the femur at approximately the same level as the apex of the patella. The patient is prepared in a standard aseptic fashion, and a 1 1/2 inch (4 cm) 25-gauge needle is inserted perpendicular to the skin just below the medial surface of the tibial condyle. After negative aspiration, 5 to 10 ml of local anesthetic is injected subcutaneously to block the saphenous nerve (Fig. 23-18).

Comments

The saphenous nerve is the terminal branch of the femoral nerve. It provides cutaneous innervation to the skin overlying the medial, anteromedial, and posteromedial aspects of the leg from just above the knee to the level of the medial malleolus and in some patients to the medial aspect at the base of the great toe. There is no motor component.

Complications

The saphenous vein may accompany the saphenous nerve and the patient should be made aware of the possibility of a hematoma from venous puncture. Other complications from the saphenous nerve block are rare, especially when care is taken to avoid an intraneural injection. Severe pain on injection suggests the possibility of an intraneural injection, and the needle should be repositioned immediately.

NERVE BLOCKS AT THE ANKLE

Nerve blockade at the ankle is primarily used to treat pain disorders in specific nerve distributions. There are five terminal branches of the tibial, common peroneal, and femoral nerves that supply the ankle and foot: posterior tibial, sural, superficial peroneal, deep peroneal, and saphenous nerves. These nerves are relatively easy to block at the level of the ankle.

In general, five nerve blocks form a ring of infiltration around the ankle at the level of the malleolus. It is important to remember that large volumes of local anesthetic, especially those containing epinephrine, may cause vascular occlusion. Otherwise, neural blockade at the ankle is safe and highly successful.

Tibial Nerve Block

Indications

Tibial nerve blockade is used to treat pain disorders in the tibial nerve distribution of the foot.

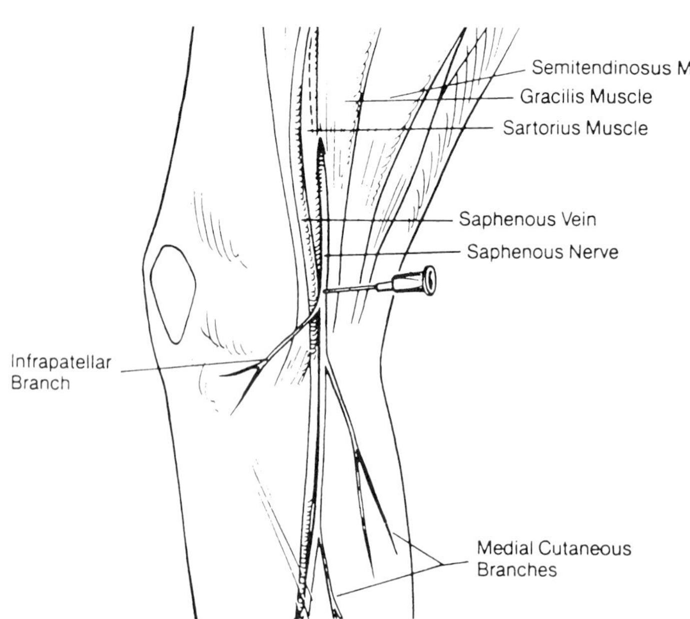

FIG. 23-18. Saphenous nerve block at the knee. Approach for saphenous injection and neural blockade at the knee. (Reprinted with permission from Raj PP, Pai U, Rawal N. Techniques of regional anesthesia in adults. In: Raj PP, ed. *Clinical practice of regional anesthesia.* New York: Churchill-Livingstone, 1991; 321.)

Techniques

After informed consent is obtained, the patient is placed in the prone position with the foot supported by a pillow. The patient is prepared in a standard aseptic fashion, and a skin wheal is raised along the medial aspect of the Achilles tendon at the level of the superior border of the medial malleolus. A 1 inch (2.5 cm) 25-gauge needle is advanced through the wheal toward the posterior aspect of the tibia, behind the posterior tibial artery. If a paresthesia is elicited after negative aspiration, 3 to 5 ml of local anesthetic is injected after negative aspiration. If a paresthesia is not elicited, the needle is advanced until the tibial periosteum is contacted. The needle is withdrawn 0.5 cm, and after negative aspiration, 5 to 7 ml of local anesthetic is injected to block the posterior tibial nerve. A nerve stimulator may be used to identify the posterior tibial nerve by eliciting contraction of muscles in the sole of the foot (Fig. 23-19).

Comments

The posterior tibial nerve is located along the medial aspect of the Achilles tendon, lying just behind the posterior tibial artery. The nerve gives off a medial calcaneal branch to the medial aspect of the heel, then divides behind the medial malleolus into the medial and lateral plantar nerves. The medial plantar nerve supplies the medial two thirds of the sole of the foot as well as the plantar portion of the medial three and one half toes. The lateral plantar nerve supplies the lateral one third of the sole and the plantar portion of the lateral one and one half toes.

Complications

Intraneural injection may result in nerve damage. Severe pain on injection suggests the possibility of an intraneural injection, and the needle should be repositioned immediately. Hematoma and intravascular injection are possible due to the close proximity of the posterior tibial vessels. If an arterial puncture occurs, prolonged direct pressure is usually adequate to prevent the development of a hematoma.

Sural Nerve Block

Indications

Sural nerve blockade is used to diagnose and treat pain disorders in the sural nerve distribution.

Techniques

After informed consent is obtained, the patient is placed in a prone position with the foot supported by a pillow. The patient is prepared in a standard aseptic fashion, and a skin wheal is raised lateral to the Achilles tendon at the level of the lateral malleolus. A 1 inch (2.5 cm) 25-gauge needle is inserted to a depth of 1 cm directed toward the lateral border of the fibula. If a paresthesia is elicited, 2 to 3 ml of a local

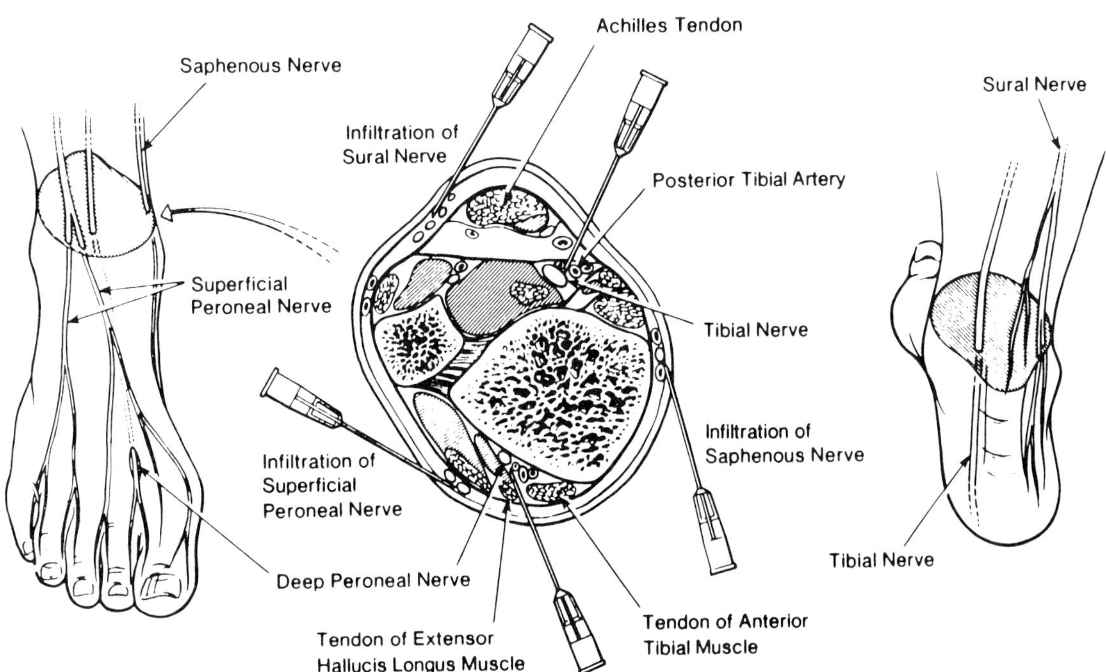

FIG. 23-19. Nerve blocks at the ankle. Approach for nerve injection and neural blockade at the ankle. (Reprinted with permission from Bridenbaugh PO. The lower extremity: somatic block. In: Cousins MJ, Bridenbaugh PO, eds. *Neural blockade in clinical anesthesia and management of pain,* 2nd ed. Philadelphia: JB Lippincott, 1988; 435.)

anesthetic is injected after negative aspiration. If a paresthesia cannot be elicited, after negative aspiration, 3 to 5 ml of local anesthetic is injected subcutaneously in a fan distribution from the lateral border of the Achilles tendon to the lateral border of the fibula to block the sural nerve (Fig. 23-19).

Comments

The sural nerve is a cutaneous nerve that contains fibers from both the tibial and common peroneal nerves. It lies subcutaneous somewhat distal to the middle of the leg and travels with the short saphenous vein behind and below the lateral malleolus. It supplies the posterolateral surface of the leg, the lateral side of the foot, and the lateral aspect of the fifth toe.

Complications

Intraneural injection may result in nerve damage. Severe pain on injection suggests the possibility of an intraneural injection, and the needle should be immediately repositioned. Hematoma and intravascular injection are possible due to the close proximity of the sural vessels. If an arterial puncture occurs, prolonged direct pressure is usually adequate to prevent the development of a hematoma.

Superficial Peroneal Nerve Block

Indications

Superficial peroneal nerve blockade is used to diagnose and treat pain disorders of the superficial peroneal nerve distribution in the foot.

Techniques

After informed consent is obtained, the patient is placed in a supine position with the foot elevated on a pillow. The patient is prepared in a standard aseptic fashion, and a 1 inch (2.5 cm) 25-gauge needle is inserted just lateral to the anterior border of the tibia at the proximal level of the lateral malleolus. The needle is carefully advanced to the superior aspect of the lateral malleolus. After negative aspiration, 5 ml of local anesthetic is injected over the course of the needle to block all the branches of the superficial peroneal nerve (Fig. 23-19).

Comments

The superficial peroneal nerve exits the deep fascia of the leg at the anterior aspect of the distal two thirds of the leg. From that point, the superficial peroneal nerve runs subcutaneously to supply the dorsum of the foot and toes, with the exception of the contiguous surfaces of the great and second toes.

Complications

Complications are rare with the superficial peroneal nerve block.

Deep Peroneal Nerve Block

Indications

Deep peroneal nerve blockade is used to diagnose and treat pain disorders in the deep peroneal nerve distribution of the foot.

Techniques

After informed consent is obtained, the patient is placed in a supine position with the foot elevated on a pillow. The patient is prepared in a standard aseptic fashion, and a 1 inch (2.5 cm) 25-gauge needle is inserted between the extensor hallucis longus tendon and the anterior tibial tendon just superior to the level of the malleoli. The extensor hallucis longus tendon can easily be identified by having the patient extend the great toe. If the artery can be palpated, the needle is placed just lateral to the artery. The needle is advanced toward the tibia, and after negative aspiration, 3 to 5 ml of local anesthetic is injected deep to the fascia to block the deep peroneal nerve (Fig. 23-19).

Comments

The deep peroneal nerve travels down the anterior portion of the interosseus membrane of the leg and extends midway between the malleoli onto the dorsum of the foot. At this point, the nerve lies lateral to the extensor hallucis longus tendon and the anterior tibial artery. It supplies motor innervation to the short extensors of the toes and cutaneous innervation to adjacent areas of the first and second toes.

Complications

Hematoma and intravascular injection are possible due to the close proximity of the anterior tibial vessels. If an arterial puncture occurs, prolonged direct pressure is usually adequate to prevent the development of a hematoma.

Saphenous Nerve Block

Indications

Saphenous nerve blockade is used to diagnose and treat pain disorders of the saphenous nerve distribution in the foot.

Techniques

After informed consent is obtained, the patient is placed in a prone position with the foot elevated on a pillow. The patient is prepared in a standard aseptic fashion, and a 1 inch

(2.5 cm) 25-gauge needle is inserted immediately above and anterior to the medial malleolus and advanced to the anterior border of the tibia. After negative aspiration, 3 to 5 ml of local anesthetic is injected over the course of the needle to block the saphenous nerve (Fig. 23-19).

Comments

The saphenous nerve is the terminal branch of the femoral nerve. It becomes cutaneous at the lateral aspect of the knee joint and follows the great saphenous vein to the medial malleolus. It supplies cutaneous innervation to the medial aspect of the lower leg anterior to the medial malleolus and the medial aspect of the foot and may extend as far forward as the metatarsophalangeal joint.

Complications

Hematoma and intravascular injection are possible due to the close proximity of the great saphenous vessels. If an arterial puncture occurs, prolonged direct pressure is usually adequate to prevent the development of a hematoma.

Intramuscular Nerve (Motor Point) Block

Indications

Intramuscular nerve blockade is used for diagnostic, prognostic, and therapeutic treatment of non–velocity-dependent muscle tone, flexor spasm, and dystonia.

Techniques

After informed consent is obtained, the patient is positioned comfortably to allow optimal access to the muscle(s) involved. The patient is prepared in a standard aseptic fashion, and a skin wheal is raised over the main muscle bulk of the muscle(s) to be injected. A 1 1/2 to 4 inch (2.5 to 10 cm) insulated needle is advanced through the wheel with a nerve stimulator used to localize the motor nerve branches or motor points. The current is reduced until the minimum current is required to elicit muscle contraction. When the needle tip is within 1 mm of the motor nerve and after negative aspiration, 1 to 2 ml of 4% to 6% phenol is injected for neurolysis (Fig. 23-1).

Comments

Intramuscular nerve or motor point blockade are reported to have a duration of effect from 1 to 36 months (median = 11.5 months). No dose-response or dose–duration of effects relationship has been demonstrated for motor point blocks (49–51). The needle is positioned to produce the maximal twitch at the lowest stimulus. The needle is usually adjacent to the nerve when 0.5 to 0.1 mA produces motor stimulation with a insulated needle and 1 mA with an uninsulated needle. The motor points of each muscle cluster at the mid-point of the muscle fibers.

Complications

Significant complications are rare with intramuscular nerve injections, and transitory side effects include pain of mild intensity, tenderness and swelling at injection sites, and dysesthesia. Inadvertent neurolysis of a mixed nerve results in painful paresthesia in approximately 11% of the patients.

COMMON MUSCLE INJECTION TECHNIQUES

Informed consent should be obtained from the patient, the injection site prepared in a standard aseptic fashion, and draped appropriately. All medications, syringes, needles, and other equipment should be readily available. Syringes may vary from 3 to 12 ml. Needles may vary from as small as 1/2 inch (1 cm) 25-gauge needles to 3 1/2 inch (9 cm) 21-gauge spinal needles. For convenience, an 18-gauge needle should be available to draw medications from the vial. All caregivers participating in the injection procedure should be gloved with universal precautions applying to all.

General

Trigger points may occur in any muscle or muscle group of the body. They are commonly found in muscle groups that are routinely overstressed or those that do not undergo full contraction and relaxation cycles. Many trigger points are characterized by pain originating from small circumscribed areas of local hyperirritability involving myofascial structures resulting in local and referred pain. Pain is aggravated by stretching, cooling, and compression of the affected area, which often gives rise to a characteristic pattern of referred pain (12,13).

Trigger points are best localized by deep palpation of the affected muscle, which reproduces the patient's pain complaint both locally and in the referred zone. Trigger points are usually a sharply circumscribed spot of exquisite tenderness when they are present, passive, or active stretching of the affected muscle routinely increases the pain. When compared with equivalent palpation pressure in normal muscle, the trigger point region displays isolated bands, increased tenderness, and referred pain. The muscle in the immediate vicinity of the trigger point is often described as ropey, tense, or a palpable band. The trigger point is injected after palpation of the affected muscle, and the point of maximal tenderness reproducing the pain complaint is identified. When the point of injection has been determined, it is best marked with the tip of a retracted ballpoint pen or needle hub by pressing the skin to reproduce temporary indentation to mark the point of entry. The skin is then prepared in a standard aseptic fashion, and sterile technique is used throughout the procedure. The skin and subcutaneous tissue at the injection site are usually not anesthetized.

A 1 1/2 to 2 inch (4 to 5 cm) 22- to 25-gauge needle is advanced into the muscle at the point of maximum tenderness. Before injecting the medication, always attempt to aspirate to avoid accidental or intravascular injection. Verification that the needle is at the trigger point may be established by the jump sign or reproduction of the pain complaint. Medication should be injected in a fanwise manner in the area of the trigger point.

Indications for Trigger Point Injections

Trigger point injections may be used to determine the source of pain and to provide maximum pain relief from myofascial pain and to facilitate physical therapy for the stretching of trigger points.

Contraindications for Trigger Point Injections

Absolute contraindications to trigger point injection include localized infection, a skin condition that prevents adequate skin preparation, the existence of a tumor at the injection site, history of allergy to local anesthetics, gross coagulation defects, septicemia, or an uncooperative patient.

Complications

The complications associated with trigger point injections include infection, increased pain, local anesthetic overdose, or intravascular injection that can result in CNS toxicity, and in some cases pulmonary and cardiac arrest. Intraneural injection may result in nerve damage. Severe pain on injection suggests the possibility of an intraneural injection, and the needle should be immediately repositioned. Other complications depend on location of the trigger point injection and will be discussed separately.

Techniques

Before the injection, palpate the affected muscle, and locate and mark the trigger points. Scrub the skin and allow the antiseptic to dry for 2 minutes. The wearing of sterile gloves is required so that muscle in the sterile field may be palpated throughout the procedure. Before the injection, repalpate the trigger point and stabilize between fingers for injection (Fig. 23-20). Routinely a 1 1/2 inch (4 cm) 21- to 25-gauge needle transverses the skin subcutaneous tissue and is advanced smoothly into the area of the trigger point.

Aspirate to ensure no intravascular penetration. If this occurs, the needle should be repositioned and aspirated to ensure that blood vessels have been avoided, and then the medication is injected. A fanwise manner of injection often results in the longest pain relief due to increased distribution of local anesthetic (Fig. 23-21). The needle is then withdrawn with pressure applied to minimize bleeding.

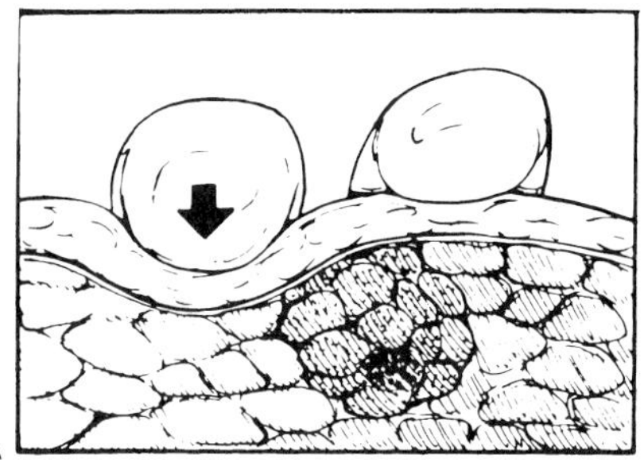

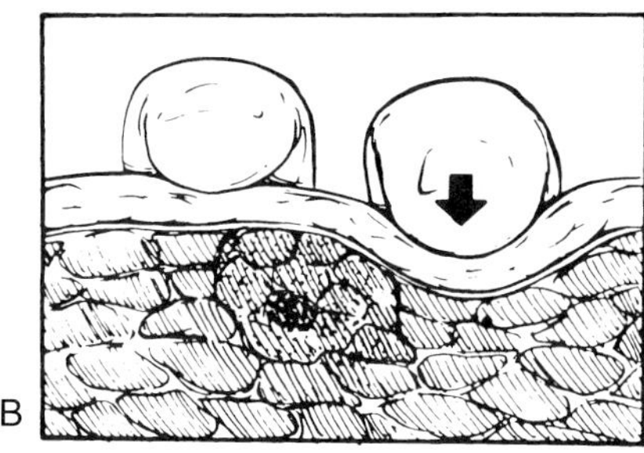

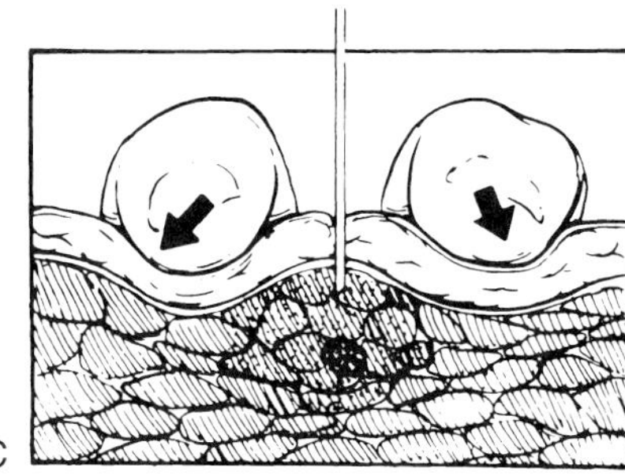

FIG. 23-20. Trigger point palpation. **A** and **B:** Palpation and localization of trigger point. **C:** Stabilization of trigger point for injection. (Reprinted with permission from Raj PP. Chronic pain. In: Raj PP, ed. *Clinical practice of regional anesthesia.* New York: Churchill-Livingstone, 1991; 491.)

SPECIFIC TRIGGER POINT INJECTIONS

Trapezius

Indications

Trigger point injection of the trapezius muscle is used to treat myofascial pain.

Techniques

After informed consent is obtained, the patient is placed in the sitting or prone position. The trapezius muscle is palpated. The injection sites are identified as points of maximal tenderness to deep palpation reproducing the patient's pain complaint. This may or may not result in referred pain. The patient is prepared in a standard aseptic fashion. A 1 1/2 inch (4 cm) 21- to 25-gauge needle is inserted at the point of maximal tenderness and advanced to the area of the trigger point. After negative aspiration, inject the trigger point area with 4 ml of local anesthetic (Fig. 23-22).

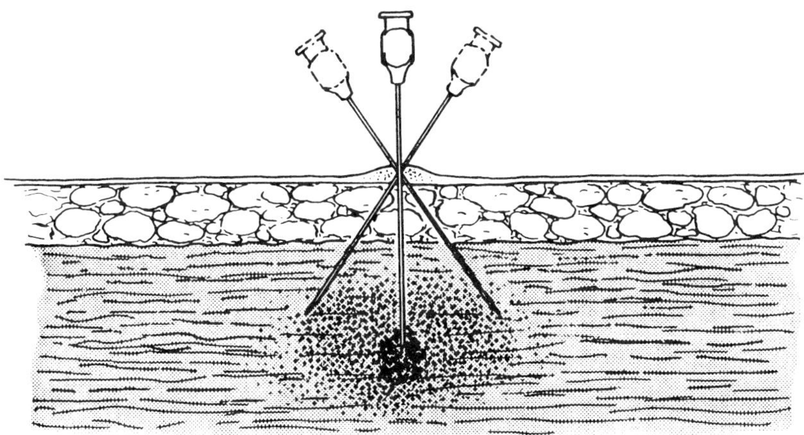

FIG. 23-21. Fanwise injection technique for trigger point. (Reprinted with permission from Raj PP. Chronic pain. In: Raj PP, ed. *Clinical practice of regional anesthesia.* New York: Churchill-Livingstone, 1991; 491.)

Comments

The referred pain pattern for the upper trapezius is often along the posterior lateral aspect of the neck, as well as periarticular and temporal regions. The referred pain pattern for the mid-trapezius often involves the shoulder and paraspinal region. The referred pain pattern for the lower trapezius usually involves the paraspinal region. The patient should be fully familiar with the stretching program for the trapezius muscle and be instructed in a home program. Failure to include a home stretching program usually results in short-term relief.

Complications

Significant complications are uncommon with trapezius trigger point injections.

Levator Scapulae

Indications

Levator scapulae trigger point injection is a useful diagnostic and therapeutic procedure for myofascial pain.

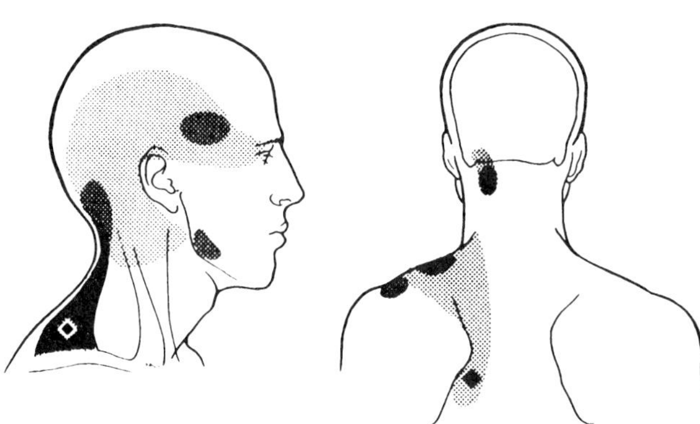

FIG. 23-22. Trapezius. Trigger points and referred pain patterns.

Techniques

After informed consent is obtained, the patient is placed in a sitting or prone position. The levator scapulae muscle is palpated along the attachment at the C1–C4 vertebrae and the superior angle of the scapulae. The injection sites are identified as points of maximal tenderness to deep palpation reproducing the patient's pain complaint. This may or may not result in referred pain. The patient is prepared in a standard aseptic fashion. A 1 1/2 inch (4 cm) 21- to 25-gauge needle, is inserted at the point of maximal tenderness and advanced to the area of the trigger point. After negative aspiration, inject the trigger point area with 4 ml of local anesthetic (Fig. 23-23).

Comment

Palpate the entire body of the levator scapulae muscle from origin to insertion and inject all trigger points. Total injection should not exceed maximum safe dosage. The referred pain pattern for the levator scapular muscle often in-

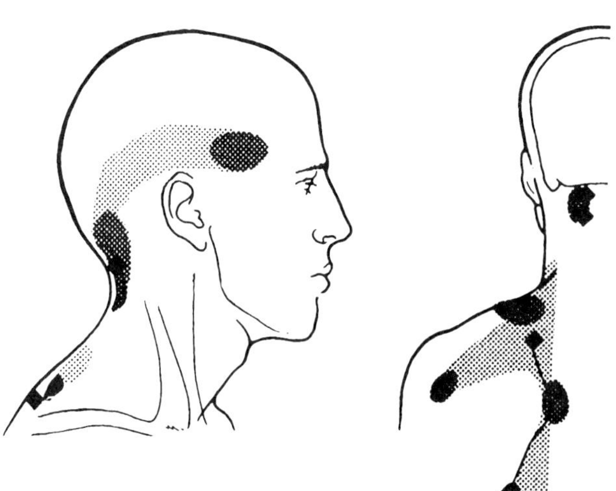

FIG. 23-23. Levator scapulae. Trigger points and referred pain patterns.

cludes a posterior lateral neck and occipital and temporal regions. The patient should be fully familiar with the stretching program for the levator scapulae muscle and be instructed in a home program. Failure to include a home stretching program usually results in short-term relief.

Complications

Nerve root blockade may result from improper needle placement or injection of large quantities of local anesthetic in the vertebral region and may result in nerve root block. Intraneural injection may result in nerve damage. Severe pain on injection suggests the possibility of an intraneural injection, and the needle should be repositioned immediately.

Supraspinatus

Indications

Supraspinatus injection is a useful diagnostic and therapeutic procedure with myofascial pain.

Techniques

After informed consent is obtained, the patient is placed in a sitting or prone position. The supraspinatus muscle is palpated for trigger points from the supraspinous fossa to the humerus. The injection sites are identified as points of maximal tenderness to deep palpation reproducing the patient's pain complaint. This may or may not result in referred pain. The patient is prepared in a standard aseptic fashion. A 1 1/2 inch (4 cm) 21- to 25-gauge needle, is inserted at the point of maximal tenderness and advanced to the area of the trigger point. After negative aspiration, inject the trigger point area with 4 ml of local anesthetic (Fig. 23-24).

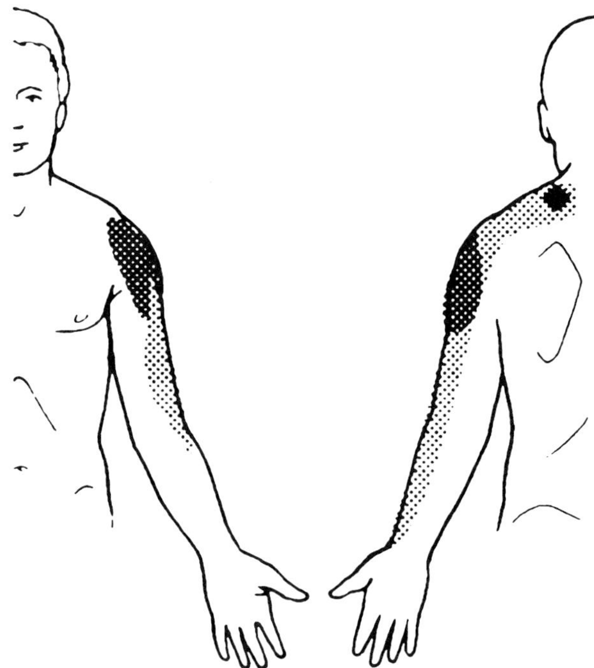

FIG. 23-24. Supraspinatus. Trigger points and referred pain patterns.

Comment

The referred pain pattern for the supraspinatus muscle often involves the posterior lateral aspect of the shoulder and upper extremity. The patient should be fully familiar with the stretching program for the supraspinatus muscle and be instructed in a home program. Failure to include a home stretching program usually results in short-term relief.

Complications

Significant complications are uncommon with supraspinatus trigger point injections.

Infraspinatus

Indications

Infraspinatus injection is a useful diagnostic and therapeutic procedure for myofascial pain.

Techniques

After informed consent is obtained, the patient is placed in the sitting or prone position. The infraspinatus muscle is palpated from the infraspinous fossa of the scapula to the humerus. Trigger points are most often located below the spine of the scapulae. The injection sites are identified as points of maximal tenderness to deep palpation reproducing the patient's pain complaint. This may or may not result in referred pain. The patient is prepared in a standard aseptic fashion. A 1 1/2 inch (4 cm) 21- to 25-gauge needle is inserted at the point of maximal tenderness and advanced to the area of the trigger point. After negative aspiration, inject the trigger point area with 4 ml of local anesthetic (Fig. 23-25).

Comment

The referred pain pattern for the infraspinatus often involves the deltoid muscle, as well as the area over the lateral shoulder and proximal upper extremity. Pain also may be referred in the infrascapular region. The patient should be fully familiar with the stretching program for the infraspinatus muscle and be instructed in a home program. Failure to include a home stretching program usually results in short-term relief.

Complications

Significant complications are uncommon with infraspinatus trigger point injections.

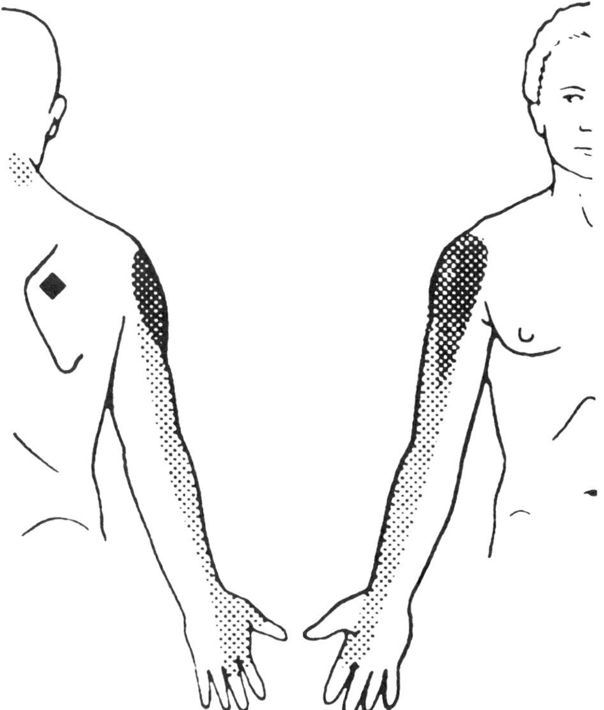

FIG. 23-25. Infraspinatus. Trigger points and referred pain patterns.

Pectoralis

Indications

Pectoralis muscle injection is a useful diagnostic and therapeutic procedure for myofascial pain.

Techniques

After informed consent is obtained, the patient is placed in the supine position. The pectoralis muscles are palpated. The injection sites are identified as points of maximal tenderness to deep palpation reproducing the patient's pain complaints. This may or may not result in referred pain. The patient is prepared in a standard aseptic fashion. A 1 1/2 inch (4 cm) 21- to 25-gauge needle is inserted at the point of maximal tenderness and advanced to the area of the trigger point. After negative aspiration, inject the trigger point area with 4 ml of local anesthetic (Fig. 23-26).

Comment

The referred pain pattern for the pectoralis muscles usually involves the anterior chest wall and breast regions. The patient should be fully familiar with the stretching program for the pectoralis muscle and be instructed in the home program. Failure to include a home stretching program usually results in short-term relief.

Complications

Significant complications are uncommon with pectoralis trigger point injections; however, the anatomy of the region, including the close proximity of the thoracic cavity, must be carefully considered. The risk of pneumothorax is reduced by approaching the trigger point with the needle tangential to the thoracic wall.

Deltoid

Indications

Deltoid muscle injection is a useful diagnostic and therapeutic procedure for myofascial pain.

Techniques

After informed consent is obtained, the patient is placed in the sitting position. The anterior, middle, and posterior components of the deltoid muscle are palpated. The injection sites are identified as points of maximal tenderness to deep palpation reproducing the patient's pain complaint. This may or may not result in referred pain. The patient is prepared in a standard aseptic fashion. A 1 1/2 inch (4 cm) 21- to 25-gauge needle is inserted at the point of maximal tenderness and advanced to the area of the trigger point. After negative aspiration, inject the trigger point area with 4 ml of local anesthetic (Fig. 23-27).

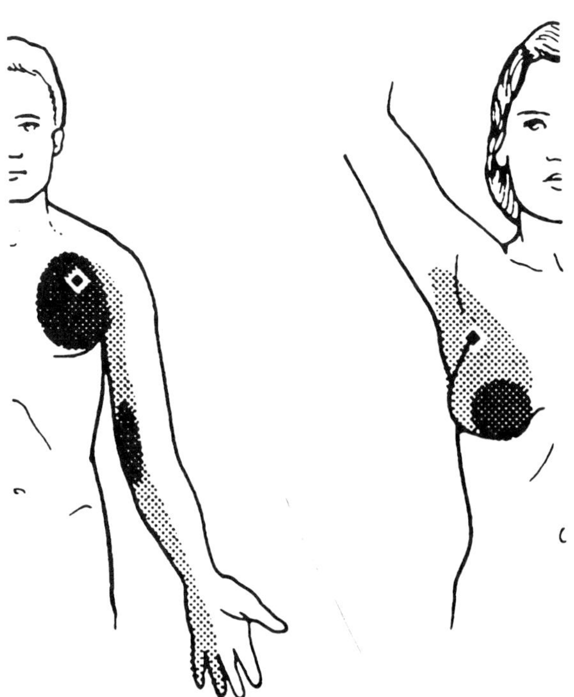

FIG. 23-26. Pectoralis. Trigger points and referred pain patterns.

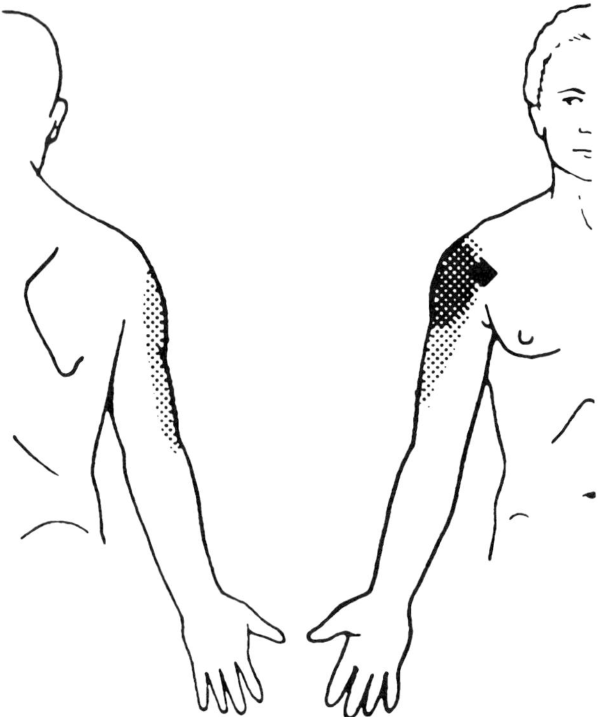

FIG. 23-27. Deltoid. Trigger points and referred pain patterns.

Comment

The referred pain pattern for the deltoid muscle usually involves the shoulder and proximal upper extremity. The patient should be fully familiar with the stretching program for the deltoid muscle and be instructed in a home program. Failure to include a home stretching program usually results in short-term relief.

Complications

Significant complications are uncommon with deltoid trigger point injections.

Quadratus Lumborum

Indications

Quadratus lumborum injection is a useful diagnostic and therapeutic procedure for myofascial pain.

Techniques

After informed consent is obtained, the patient is placed in a prone position. The quadratus lumborum muscle is palpated from the 12th rib to the iliac crest and from vertebral attachments L1–L4 to its lateral border. The injection sites are identified as points of maximal tenderness to deep palpation reproducing the patient's pain complaint. This may or may not result in referred pain. The patient is prepared in a standard aseptic fashion. A 1 1/2 inch (4 cm) 21- to 25-gauge needle is inserted at the point of maximal tenderness and advanced to the area of the trigger point. After negative aspiration, inject the trigger point area with 4 ml of local anesthetic (Fig. 23-28).

Comment

The referred pain pattern for the quadratus lumborum muscle usually involves the iliac crest, hip, and buttock. The patient should be fully familiar with the stretching program for the quadratus lumborum muscle and be instructed in a home program. Failure to include a home stretching program usually results in short-term relief.

Complications

Significant complications are uncommon with quadratus lumborum trigger point injections.

Paraspinal Musculature

Indications

The paraspinal muscle injection is a useful diagnostic and therapeutic procedure for myofascial pain.

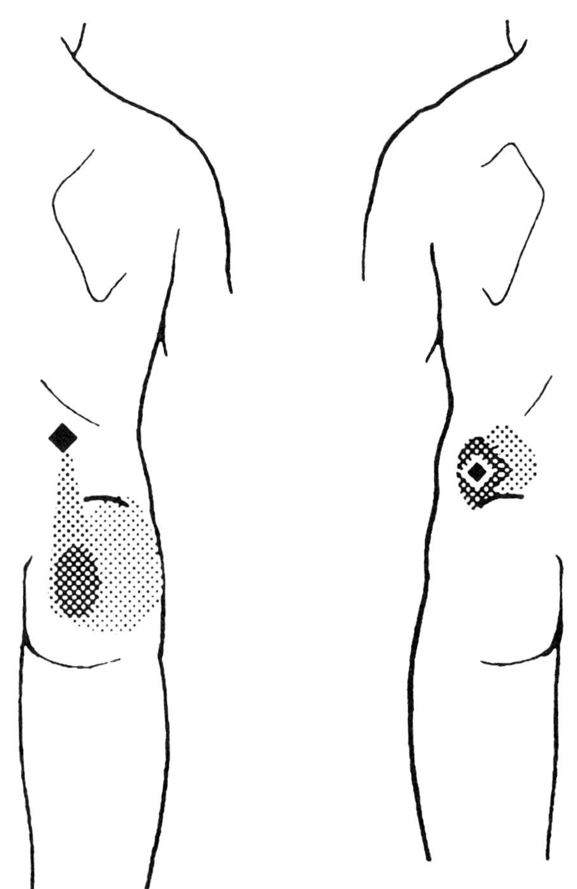

FIG. 23-28. Quadratus lumborum. Trigger points and referred pain patterns.

Techniques

After informed consent is obtained, the patient is placed in the prone position. The appropriate thoracic and/or lumbar regions are palpated. The injection sites are identified as points of maximal tenderness to deep palpation reproducing the patient's pain complaint. This may or may not result in referred pain. The patient is prepared in a standard aseptic fashion. A 1 1/2 inch (4 cm) 21- to 25-gauge needle is inserted at the point of maximal tenderness and advanced to the area of the trigger point. After negative aspiration, inject the trigger point area with 4 ml of local anesthetic (Fig. 23-29).

Comment

The referred pain pattern for the thoracic paraspinal muscles often involves the scapular and chest wall region as well as the lower thoracic paraspinal muscles and abdomen region. The referred pain pattern for the lumbar paraspinal muscles often involves the buttock, iliac crest, and sacroiliac joint region. These muscles involve the erector spinae, semispinalis cervicis, longissimus capitis, longissimus cervicis, longissimus iliocostalis thoracis, iliocostalis lumborum, and semispinalis multifidus. The patient should be fully familiar with the stretching program for the affected paraspinal muscle and be instructed in a home program. Failure to include a home stretching program usually results in short-term relief.

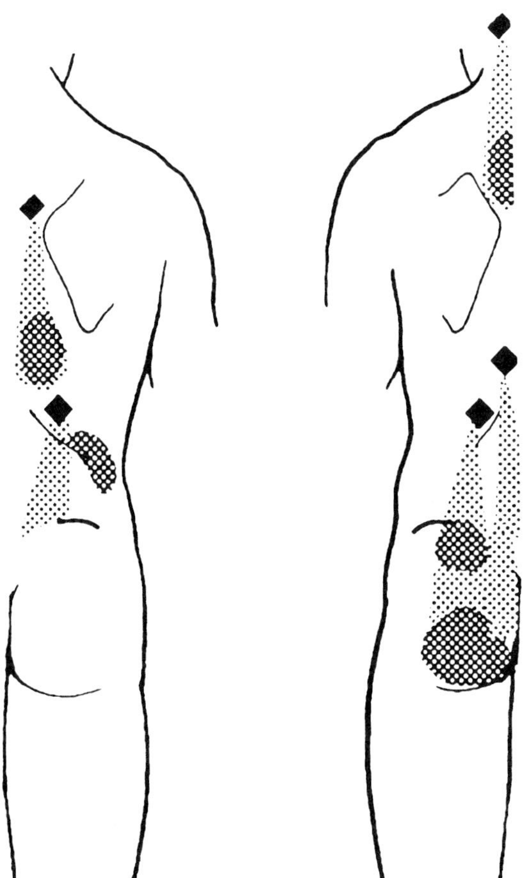

FIG. 23-29. Paraspinal musculature. Trigger points and referred pain patterns.

Complications

Significant complications are uncommon with paraspinal trigger point injections.

Gluteal

Indications

Gluteal muscle injection is a useful diagnostic and therapeutic procedure for myofascial pain.

Techniques

After informed consent is obtained, the patient is placed in the lateral position with the unaffected side down, or in the prone position. The gluteus maximus, minimus, and medius muscles are palpated. The injection sites are identified as points of maximal tenderness to deep palpation reproducing the patient's pain complaint. This may or may not result in referred pain. The patient is prepared in a standard aseptic fashion. A 1 1/2 inch (4 cm) 21- to 25-gauge needle is inserted at the point of maximal tenderness and advanced to the area of the trigger point. After negative aspiration, inject the trigger point area with 4 ml of local anesthetic (Fig. 23-30).

Comment

The referred pain pattern for the gluteus maximus usually involves the sacroiliac joint, hip, and buttock. The referred pain pattern for the gluteus medius often involves the iliac crest, sacroiliac joint, and buttock. The referred pain pattern for the gluteus minimus muscle usually involves the buttock and lateral aspect of the lower extremity. The patient should be fully familiar with the stretching program for the gluteal muscle and be instructed in a home program. Failure to include a home stretching program usually results in short-term relief.

Complications

Significant complications are uncommon with gluteal trigger point injections; however, the anatomy of the region, including the sciatic nerve, must be carefully considered with these injections. Intraneural injection may result in nerve damage. Severe pain on injection suggests the possibility of an intraneural injection, and the needle should be immediately repositioned.

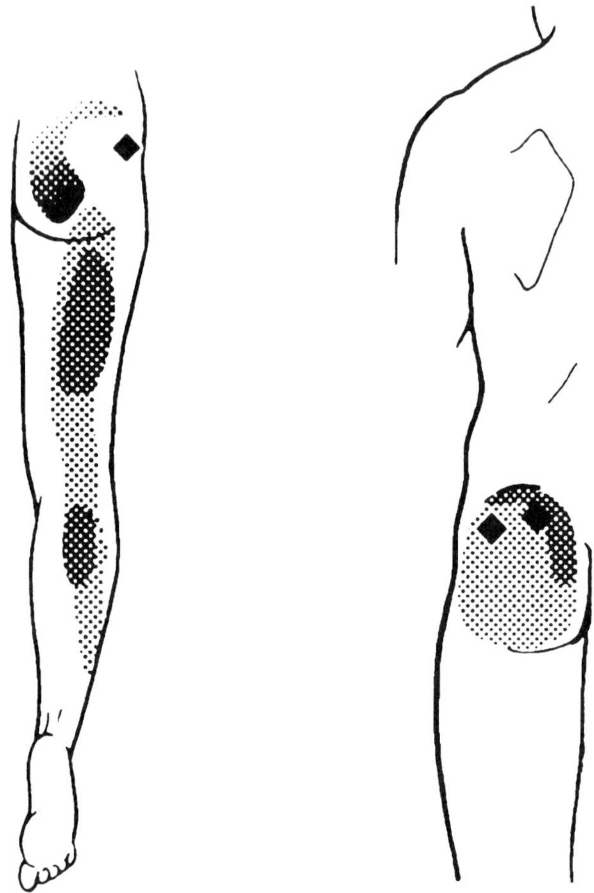

FIG. 23-30. Gluteal trigger points and referred pain patterns.

Piriformis

Indications

Piriformis muscle injection is a useful diagnostic and therapeutic procedure for myofascial pain.

Techniques

After informed consent is obtained, the patient is placed in the lateral Sims' position. The piriformis muscle is palpated from the sacrum toward the hip. The injection sites are identified as points of maximal tenderness to deep palpation reproducing the patient's pain complaint. This may or may not result in referred pain. The patient is prepared in a standard aseptic fashion. A 1 1/2 inch (4 cm) 21- to 25-gauge needle is inserted at the point of maximal tenderness and advanced to the area of the trigger point. After negative aspiration, inject the trigger point area with 4 ml of local anesthetic (Fig. 23-31).

Comments

The referred pain pattern for the piriformis muscle often involves the buttocks, iliosacral region, and posterior hip. The patient should be familiar with the stretching program for the piriformis muscle and be instructed in a home program. Failure to include a home stretching program usually results in short-term relief.

Complications

Attention to the anatomy of the sciatic nerve in this region will prevent intraneural injection; otherwise, significant complications are uncommon with trigger point injections. Severe pain on injection suggests the possibility of an intraneural injection, and the needle should be repositioned immediately.

Hip Adductor

Indications

Hip adductor muscle injection is a useful diagnostic and therapeutic procedure for myofascial pain.

Techniques

After informed consent is obtained, the patient is placed in the supine position and the affected limb flexed, adducted, and externally rotated. The adductor longus, adductor brevis, and adductor magnus are palpated along the medial aspect

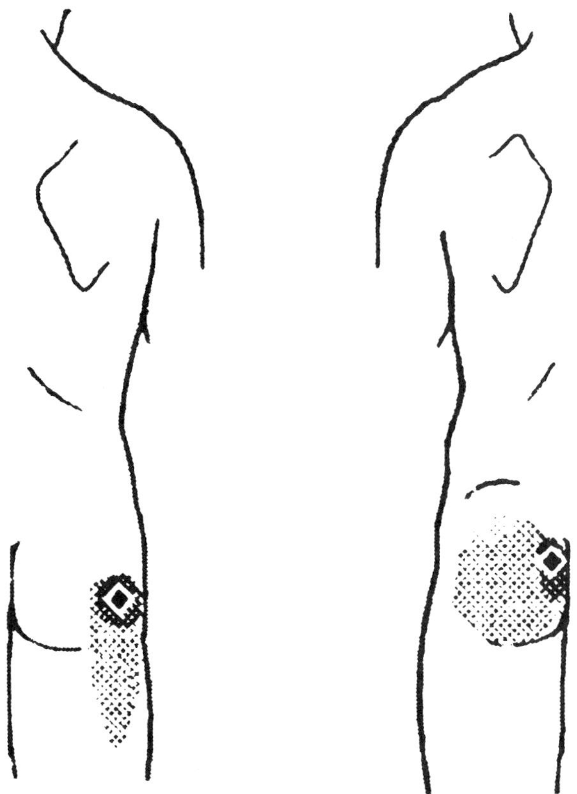

FIG. 23-31. Piriformis trigger points and referred pain patterns.

of the humerus and thigh. The injection sites are identified as points of maximal tenderness to deep palpation reproducing the patient's pain complaint. This may or may not result in referred pain. The patient is prepared in a standard aseptic fashion. A 1 1/2 inch (4 cm) 21- to 25-gauge needle is inserted at the point of maximal tenderness and advanced to the area of the trigger point. After negative aspiration, inject the trigger point area with 4 ml of local anesthetic (Fig. 23-32).

Comment

The referred pain pattern for the adductor muscles of the hip often involves the proximal hip, medial thigh, anterior thigh, and knee. The patient should be fully familiar with the stretching program for the adductor muscle and be instructed in a home program. Failure to include a home stretching program usually results in short-term relief.

Complications

Significant complications are uncommon with trigger point injections.

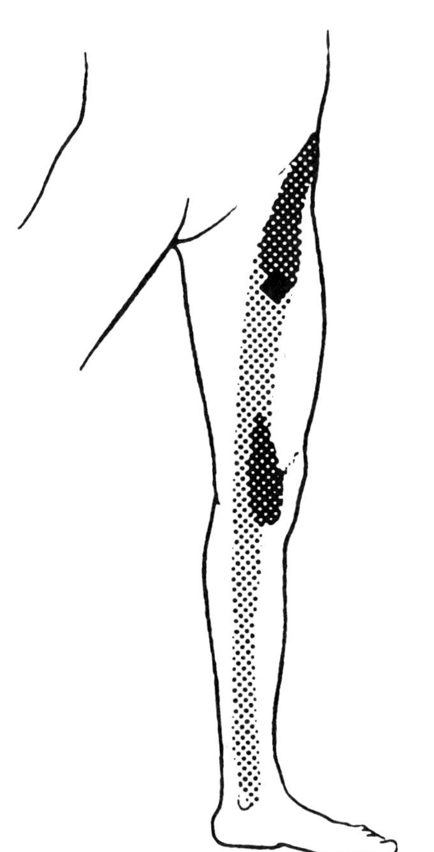

FIG. 23-32. Hip adductor trigger points and referred pain patterns.

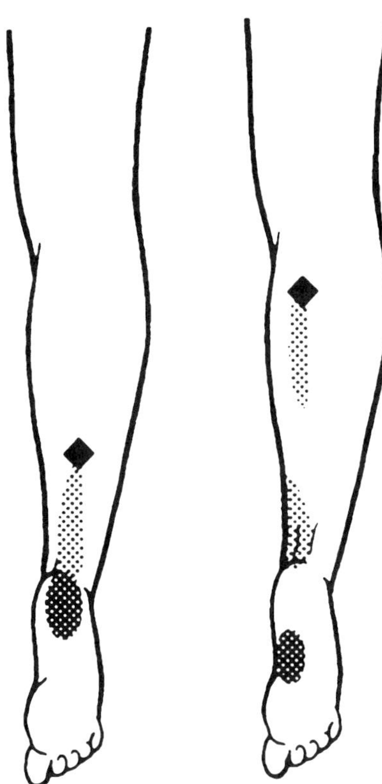

FIG. 23-33. Gastocnemius and solius trigger points and referred pain patterns.

Gastrocnemius

Indications

Gastrocnemius injection is a useful diagnostic and therapeutic procedure for myofascial pain.

Techniques

After informed consent is obtained, the patient is placed in a supine position. The gastrocnemius and soleus muscles are palpated from the knee to the ankle for areas of maximal tenderness reproducing the patient's pain complaint. The injection sites are identified as points of maximal tenderness to deep palpation reproducing the patient's pain complaint. This may or may not result in referred pain. The patient is prepared in a standard aseptic fashion. A 1 1/2 inch (4 cm) 21- to 25-gauge needle, is inserted at the point of maximal tenderness and advanced to the area of the trigger point. After negative aspiration, inject the trigger point area with 4 ml of local anesthetic (Fig. 23-33).

Comment

The patient should be fully familiar with the stretching program for the gastrocnemius muscle and be instructed in a home program. Failure to include a home stretching program usually results in short-term relief. The referred pain pattern for the gastrocnemius and soleus muscles often involve the posterior knee, calf, heel, and plantar aspect of the foot.

Complications

Significant complications are uncommon with trigger point injections.

COMMON JOINT INJECTION TECHNIQUES

After informed consent is obtained from the patient, the injection site is prepared in a standard aseptic fashion and draped appropriately. All medications, syringes, needles, and other equipment should be readily available. Syringes may vary from 3 to 12 ml. Needles may vary from as small as 1/2 inch (1 cm) 25-gauge needles to 3 1/2 inch (9 cm) 21-gauge epidural needles. For convenience, an 18-gauge needle should be available to draw medications from the vial. All caregivers participating in the injection procedure should be gloved, with universal precautions applying to all.

General

The joint is usually injected from the extensor surface at a point where the synovium is closest to the skin. This site minimizes the interference from major arteries, veins, and nerves. When the point of injection has been determined it is best marked with the tip of a retracted ballpoint pen or a needle hub by pressing the skin to produce a temporary indentation to mark the point of entry. The skin is then prepared in a standard aseptic fashion, and sterile technique is used throughout the procedure. The skin and subcutaneous tissue at the injection site may be anesthetized by injecting 1% lidocaine with no epinephrine using a 25- to 30-gauge needle. Alternatively, a vapocoolant spray or 5% lidocaine-prilocaine cream applied to the skin surface may be used to provide adequate anesthesia (52).

A 1 1/2 to 2 inch (4 to 5 cm) 22- to 25-gauge needle is then pushed gently into the joint. Before injecting the medication, always attempt to aspirate to avoid accidental intravascular injection. After ensuring that the needle is in the joint space, the medication should be injected in a slow steady fashion.

Indications for Intra-articular Injection

Intra-articular injections may be used to determine the source of pain as articular or extra-articular and to provide maximal control of inflammation in joints when nonsteroidal anti-inflammatory drug (NSAID) therapy has failed or is contraindicated. Intra-articular injections are indicated to decrease morbidity in self-limited sterile inflammatory conditions. Intra-articular injections provide rapid relief of inflammatory pain and facilitate physical therapy of an inflamed joint. Poorly controlled inflammation in more than three joints requires reconsideration of systemic corticosteroids.

The intra-articular injection of hyaluronan for osteoarthritis is a relatively new technique. The viscosupplement acts like synovial fluid to maintain lubrication of the joint. This may be used in early osteoarthritis but does not appear to be an efficacious treatment in advanced osteoarthritis (53).

Contraindications for Intra-articular Injection

Contraindications must be considered before the injection of any joint. Contraindications to intra-articular injection include overlying soft-tissue sepsis, bacteremia, anatomic inaccessibility, an uncooperative patient, articular instability, septic arthritis, avascular necrosis, osteonecrosis, and neurotrophic joints.

Steroid injection into Charcot joint is contraindicated because local steroids will not provide significant long-term relief of the symptoms. Avascular necrosis in Charcot joints has been correlated to corticosteroid injections. Another specific contraindication is injection of an unstable joint unless the instability is appropriately corrected by bracing or surgery. Traumatic arthritis secondary to fracture through the joint is another contraindication for steroid injection because the beneficial effects of the steroid injections are not long lasting. Severe osteoporosis in areas around the joint is also a contraindication for injecting steroids.

Injection of joints with surgical implants is relatively contraindicated because these joints are more prone to infection than intact joints and are usually inflamed secondary to infection rather than synovitis. Injection of corticosteroids into a nondiarthrodial joint is rarely of value because there is no synovial sac in which to decrease inflammation.

Complications

The few complications associated with corticosteroid injections include infection, postinjection inflammation, and tissue atrophy. The occurrence of joint infection is extremely rare with the use of appropriate sterile techniques. Hollander described an incidence of 14 cases in over 100,000 consecutive intra-articular injections (11). Gatter reported an infection incidence of 0.005% in 400,000 injections (18).

Postinjection inflammation is often secondary to corticosteroid crystal–induced synovitis. This normally lasts 4 to 12 hours and is treated with NSAIDs and local application of ice. If this persists beyond 24 hours, the patient should be re-evaluated to rule out infection. The incidence of postinjection flares has been estimated at 1% to 2%. Repeated intraligamentous injections may result in calcification and rupture of the ligaments. Penetration of the articular cartilage will result in damage. Traumatic injection is prevented by never injecting against resistance.

Inflamed weight-bearing joints should not be injected more frequently than every 3 to 4 months to minimize damage to the cartilage or supporting ligaments. Large joints should not be injected more than three or four times per year or 10 times cumulatively. Small joints should be injected not more than two to three times per year or four times cumulatively (18).

Tissue atrophy in the area of injection occurs when corticosteroid is placed outside the joint space or leaks from the joint space. If a portion of the injected intra-articular corticosteroid is absorbed into the systemic circulation, the result may be an elevation of blood sugar, hormonal suppression, and brief generalized improvement in all inflamed joints.

Corticosteroid injections are not recommended immediately after an acute injury or immediately before an athletic event. A patient should have a period of joint immobilization, rest, and protection from further injury after injection (54).

Techniques

Before the injection, locate and mark the appropriate landmarks. Scrub the skin and allow the antiseptic to dry for 2 minutes. The wearing of sterile gloves is required so that the bony landmarks in the sterile field may be palpated throughout the procedure. Standard sterile technique is required to minimize risk of a septic joint. It is preferable to use single-dose vials of the steroid preparation and local anesthetic agent because this further reduces the risk of infection. A 25- to 27-gauge needle is used with approximately 1% lidocaine with no epinephrine to raise a small skin wheal for skin anesthesia. Routinely a 1 1/2 inch (4 cm) 21- to 25-gauge needle traverses the skin, joint capsule, and synovial lining, sliding smoothly into the joint cavity. One must avoid the periosteum of the bone as well as the articular cartilage during this procedure. Aspirate to ensure no intravascular penetration. The return of synovial fluid ensures the position of the needle in the joint space; however, often there is minimal to no aspirated fluid. If there is an effusion, the fluid is removed in a slow steady fashion until all possible joint fluid is aspirated. If the fluid is yellow colored and clear, the likelihood of infection is minimal, and the corticosteroid may be injected. If the fluid appears turbid, it should be sent for synovial analysis including culture and sensitivity testing for microorganisms. If infection is suspected, the steroid injection into the joint should be postponed until the culture and sensitivity reports are completed. In addition to examining the color of the fluid, the viscosity of the fluid may be determined by putting a couple of drops of the fluid between the gloved thumb and index finger and stretching it. Normal synovial fluid has a good viscosity and is usually able to stretch for 2 to 2.5 cm. However, if there is an inflammatory process occurring in the joint, the viscosity of the fluid will be significantly decreased with a hazy or cloudy presentation (Table 23-6). The synovial fluid analysis completed in the laboratory may include rheumatoid factor, albumin, complements, protein electrophoresis, glucose level, and cell count with differential. A high white cell count may indicate an inflammatory process. The fluid for culture and sensitivity should be sent immediately to the laboratory because infections caused by fastidious gonococcal organisms do not survive long in the test tube. Corticosteroids should not be injected into a joint until infection, including that caused by mycobacteria or fungi, has been excluded.

Aspiration from the joint may be impeded by synovial tissue over the end of the needle, intra-articular debris, and excessive joint fluid viscosity. It also may be difficult to aspirate if the tip of the needle is against or imbedded in the articular cartilage or if the needle is not in the joint cavity. It is important to ensure that the entire needle is withdrawn intact because there have been reports of the separation of the needle from the hub and of needle fracture in articular injections.

The ease with which medication can be injected into the joint provides an indication as to the appropriate placement of the needle. No resistance should be encountered during the injection. If this occurs, the needle should be repositioned and aspirated to ensure that blood vessels have been avoided and then the medication slowly injected. After the medica-

TABLE 23-6. *Characteristics of synovial fluid*

			Inflammatory		
Characteristics	Normal	Noninflammatory (e.g., osteoarthrosis, traumatic arthritis, osteochondritis dissecans, aseptic necrosis)	Group I Rheumatoid arthritis (e.g., seropositive and seronegative spondarthritides)	Group II Septic arthritis (e.g. bacterial infection tuberculosis)	Group III Crystal synovitis (gout and pseudo-gout)
Clarity	Transparent	Transparent	Transparent to opaque, slightly cloudy	Opaque, cloudy	Clear with flakes of fibrin
Color	Pale yellow	Yellow or straw	Yellow	Brown/green/yellow/grey	Yellow
Viscosity	High	High	Low	Very low (may be high with coagulase-positive *staphylococcus*)	Low
WBC/mm^3	<150	$<3,000$	3–50,000	50–300,000	3–50,000
Predominant cell	Mononuclear ($<25\%$ PMN)	Mononuclear ($<25\%$ PMN)	Neutrophil ($>70\%$ PMN)	Neutrophil (70–100% PMN)	Neutrophil ($>70\%$ PMN)
Crystal	No	No	No	No	Yes
Culture	Negative	Negative	Negative	Often Positive	Negative

tion has been injected, the needle should be cleared with a new syringe containing a small amount of lidocaine or saline. The needle is then withdrawn with pressure applied to minimize bleeding. Joint injections are used primarily to deliver corticosteroids and anesthetic agents to treat inflamed synovium, bursa, and tendon.

Long-acting steroid preparations may induce a crystal synovitis 24 hours after the injection that resolves spontaneously. The patient should be cautioned about possible short-term aggravation of symptoms in the affected joint. It is recommended to infiltrate the subcutaneous tissues and the joint capsule with 2 to 4 ml of 1% lidocaine without epinephrine. When long-acting anesthetic agents are injected into the joint, it is important to advise the patient to limit usage during the first 24 hours after injection to prevent injury.

INJECTION OF SPECIFIC SKELETAL STRUCTURES

Cervical Zygapophyseal Joint

Indications

The cervical zygapophyseal joints have been shown to be a potential source of pain from the cranium to the mid-thoracic spine (55). Cervical facet injections can provide diagnostic as well as therapeutic benefits for patients with a wide variety of head and neck pains.

Techniques

After informed consent is obtained, the patient is placed in the prone position with the neck flexed and head turned to the opposite side to open the facet joint. A cushion is placed under the chest to allow neck flexion. The skin entry site lies approximately two vertebral segments below the target joint. The patient is prepared in a standard aseptic fashion, and a 3 inch (8 cm) 22-gauge spinal needle is advanced superiorly to the inferior margin of the joint. While advancing at a 45° angle, care is taken to ensure the needle is directed over the articular pillars and not allowed to stray medially toward the interlaminar space or excessively lateral. The needle is advanced until contact is made with the articular pillar either above or below the targeted joint and then redirected into the joint capsule. Lateral and anteroposterior fluoroscopic views are necessary to ensure that the needle is advanced to the joint mid-point. Injection of contrast media can be used to confirm proper placement in the joint. After negative aspiration, inject the joint with a 1-ml or less mixture of 10 mg triamcinolone hexacetonide (or equivalent) and local anesthetic (Fig. 23-34).

Comments

Total injected volume should not exceed 1 ml because the joint volume is usually 1 ml or less. Anterior needle placement should be avoided because the neural foramen, epidural space, and vertebral artery are in close proximity to the anterior surface of the cervical joint.

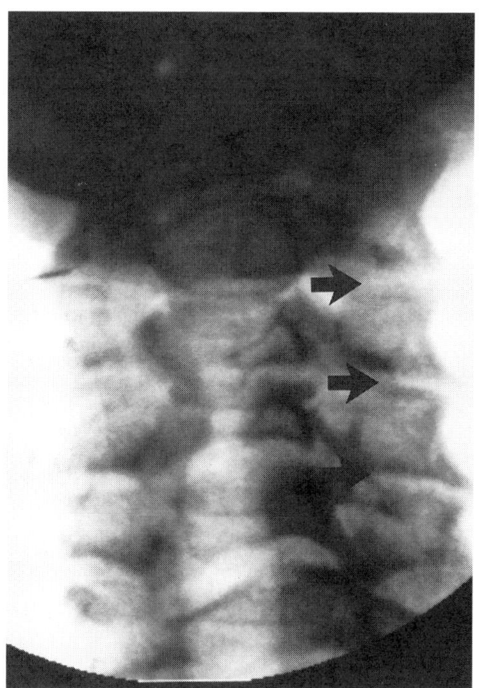

FIG. 23-34. Cervical zagapophyseal joint injection. Fluoroscopic approach for injection *(arrows)*.

Complications

Serious complications from cervical zygapophyseal joint injections are uncommon when meticulous care is given to ensure proper needle placement before injection. Local postinjection pain and lightheadedness may occur. Ataxia and dizziness may occur if local anesthetics are used at the more proximal segments, secondary to loss of postural tonic-neck reflexes and proprioceptive input to the cervical muscles. The type of local anesthetic used will determine the duration of these effects. Vertebral artery injection of even small amounts of local anesthetic can cause a seizure. Epidural or spinal blockade can occur if the needle placement is medial, resulting in regional blockade, respiratory compromise, and hypotension.

Costochondral Junction

Indications

Costochondral junction injection can be very useful as a diagnostic or therapeutic procedure in patients with costochondritis and Tietze's syndrome.

Techniques

After informed consent is obtained, the patient is positioned in the supine position. The involved costochondral joints are palpated for local tenderness and replication of pain complaint. The patient is prepared in a standard aseptic fashion, and a 1 inch (2.5 cm) 25-gauge needle is inserted at the point of maximum tenderness to the level of costochondral cartilage and withdrawn 1 mm. After negative aspiration, inject a 2 ml mixture of 20 mg methylprednisolone acetate or equivalent and local anesthetic into each involved costochondral junction.

Comments

It is not necessary to advance the needle into the costochondral joint. Infiltration of the superficial tissue over the interosseous groove of the joint at the point of maximal tenderness is usually adequate. Tenderness with costochondritis is often present over more than a single costochondral joint. Tenderness and swelling of a single costochondral joint is found with Tietze's syndrome. The presence of chest wall pain does not exclude underlying heart or lung disease. Similar injection techniques are used for the costoclavicular junction (Fig. 23-35).

Complications

Serious complications are uncommon with appropriate needle placement. Pneumothorax is possible with inadvertent penetration of the thorax. Most pneumothoraces can be easily treated with administration of supplemental oxygen and close observation, and when necessary, needle aspiration of air. Only those pneumothoraces that result in significant dyspnea or those under tension require chest tube thoracotomy and vacuum drainage.

Glenohumeral Joint

Indications

Intra-articular injection of the glenohumeral joint can be used to treat rheumatoid arthritis, inflammatory arthropathy, or adhesive capsulitis.

Techniques

After informed consent is obtained, the patient is placed in the sitting position, with the shoulder internally rotated. The glenohumeral joint is palpated by placing the fingers between the coracoid process and humeral head. The joint space can be felt as a groove just lateral to the coracoid process. The patient is prepared in a standard aseptic fashion and a 1 1/2 inch (4 cm) 21- to 23-gauge needle is inserted one fingerbreadth inferior and lateral to the tip of the coracoid process. The needle is directed in the anterior/posterior plane just lateral to the coracoid process and is advanced into the groove. The needle is very gently manipulated through the joint capsule into the synovial cavity. Aspiration is attempted until the needle has entered the synovial space. If there is an effusion of the joint, complete the aspiration. After negative aspiration, or if the aspirated fluid is noninflammatory (clear and viscous), a 2- to 3-ml mixture of triamcinolone hexacetonide (or equivalent) and local anesthetic should be administered (Fig. 23-36).

Comments

Care is required not to direct the needle medially into the neurovascular structures in the axilla.

Complications

Hematoma and intravascular injection are possible due to the close proximity of the axillary vessels. If an arterial puncture occurs, prolonged direct pressure is usually adequate to prevent the development of a hematoma. Do not inject with corticosteroid if there is any suspicion that the joint is infected. If the fluid appears infected, then send it for culture and sensitivity and treat the patient appropriately for the infection.

Acromioclavicular Joint

Indications

Intra-articular injection of the acromioclavicular joint is used to treat an inflamed or painful joint, as well as pain secondary to acromioclavicular joint separation.

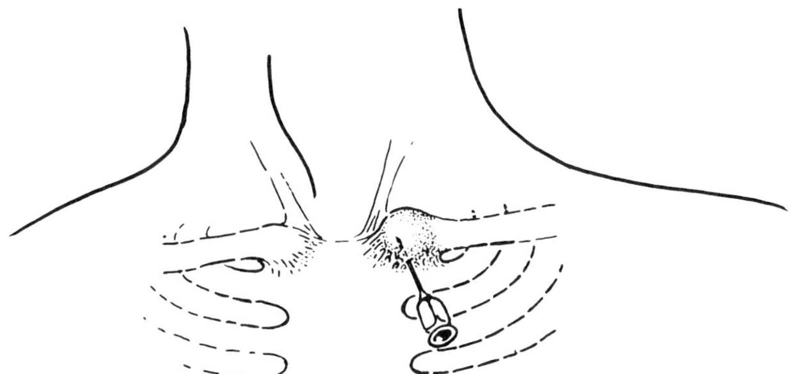

FIG. 23-35. Costochondral and costoclavicular junction injection. Approach for costochondral and costoclavicular junction aspiration and injection. (Reprinted with permission from Steinbrocker O, Neustadt DH. *Aspiration and injection therapy in arthritis and musculoskeletal disorders.* Hagerstown, MD: Harper & Row, 1972; 42.)

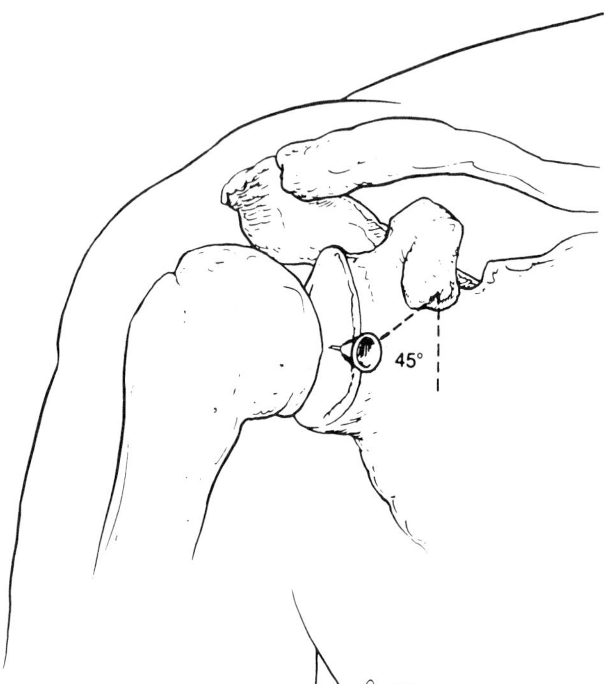

FIG. 23-36. Glenohumeral joint injection aspiration and injection. (Reprinted with permission from Gatter RA. Arthrocentesis technique and intrasynovial therapy. In: Koopman WJ, ed. *Arthritis and allied conditions—a textbook of rheumatology,* 13th ed. Baltimore: Williams & Wilkins, 1997; 753.)

Techniques

After informed consent is obtained, the patient is placed in the sitting position. The acromioclavicular joint is palpated by placing the fingers at the tip of the distal clavicle and medial to the tip of the acromion. The patient is prepared in a standard aseptic fashion, and a 5/8 inch (2 cm), 25-gauge needle is inserted at the joint and advanced to the proximal margin of the joint surface. After negative aspiration, inject the periarticular area with 2 ml of 1% lidocaine for diagnostic purposes. If the local anesthetic provides significant pain relief, inject the periarticular area with a 2-ml mixture of 10 mg methylprednisolone (or equivalent) and local anesthetic (Fig. 23-37A).

Comments

It is not necessary to advance the needle into the acromioclavicular joint. Infiltration of the superficial tissue over the interosseous groove of the joint at the point of maximal tenderness is usually adequate.

Complications

Serious complications are uncommon with injection of the acromioclavicular joint.

Rotator Cuff Tendon/Subacromial Bursa

Indications

Corticosteroid injection procedures are used to diagnose and treat rotator cuff tendonitis or subacromial bursitis. These conditions are often due to nonspecific irritation of the subacromial bursa, lesions of the rotator cuff, calcific tendonitis, or rheumatoid arthritis.

Techniques

After informed consent is obtained, the patient is placed in a sitting position with the arm in the lap. The lateral aspect of the shoulder is palpated for the point of maximal tenderness, usually 1 to 2 cm inferior and 1 to 2 cm anterior to the angle of the acromion. The patient is prepared in a standard aseptic fashion and a 1 1/2 inch (4 cm) 21-gauge needle is inserted below the acromion at the point of maximal tenderness. The needle is gently manipulated under the acromion. Aspiration is attempted until the needle has entered the synovial space. The subacromial bursa is approximately 1 to 2 cm below the skin between the tip of the acromion process and the head of the humerus. If there is an effusion of the bursa, complete the aspiration. After negative aspiration or if the aspirated fluid is noninflammatory (clear and viscous), inject a 5-ml mixture of 20 mg triamcinolone hexacetonide (or equivalent) and local anesthetic. Inject half the mixture under the acromion in the bursa. Withdraw the needle

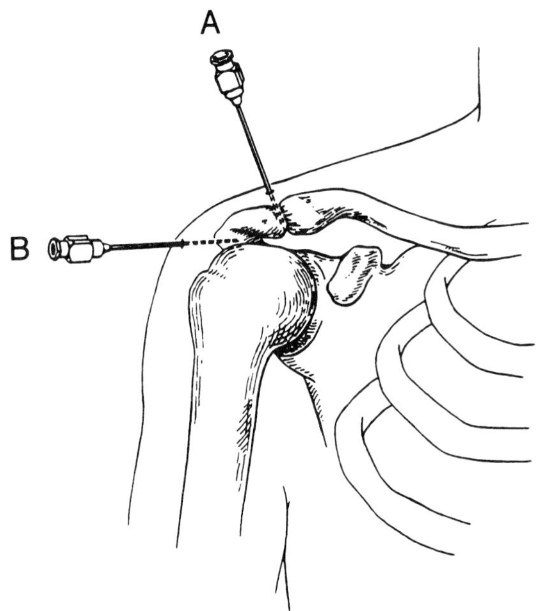

FIG. 23-37. Shoulder joint injections. **A:** Approach for shoulder joint aspiration and injection. Acromioclavicular joint injection. **B:** Approach for shoulder joint aspiration and injection. Rotator cuff tendon/subacromial bursa injection. (Reprinted with permission from Steinbrocker O, Neustadt DH. *Aspiration and injection therapy in arthritis and musculoskeletal disorders.* Hagerstown, MD: Harper & Row, 1972; 42.)

slightly, redirect it toward the anterior part of the rotator cuff, and infiltrate the remainder of the mixture (Fig. 23-37*B*).

Comments

Shoulder x-rays may show the locations of calcific deposits. If noted, a 1 1/2 inch (4 cm) 16- to 18-gauge needle is directed to this area and aspiration attempted. Inject 3 ml of the mixture at this location. Withdraw the needle slightly, redirect it toward the anterior part of the rotator cuff, and infiltrate the remainder of the mixture. This type of injection is usually uncomfortable, and premedication with codeine or oxycodone should be considered.

Complications

Do not inject with corticosteroid if there is any suspicion that the bursa is infected. If the fluid appears infected, then send it for culture and sensitivity and treat the patient appropriately for the infection.

Bicipital Tendon

Indications

Peritendinous injection of the bicipital tendon is a useful diagnostic and therapeutic procedure with bicipital tenosynovitis.

Techniques

After informed consent is obtained, the patient is placed in the seated position with arm externally rotated, lateral to the medial edge of the humeral head. Locate the bicipital groove and palpate the bicipital tendon for the area of marked tenderness. The patient is prepared in a standard aseptic fashion, and a 1 1/2 inch (4 cm) 21- to 23-gauge needle is inserted along the border of the bicipital tendon. A 6-ml mixture of 20 mg triamcinolone hexacetonide (or equivalent) and anesthetic agent is injected 2 ml at a time at the point of maximal tenderness and 1 inch above and below this point along the border of the bicipital tendon sheath (Fig. 23-38).

Comments

There should be no significant resistance encountered when injecting the tenosynovium. Resistance suggests that the tip of the needle is within the body of the tendon. Steroid injection into the tendon should be avoided.

Complications

Injecting directly into the tendon rather than the peritendinous region may result in damage to the bicipital tendon.

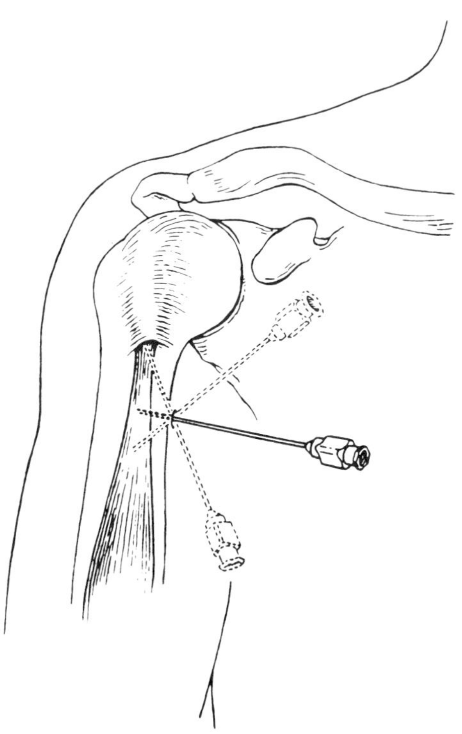

FIG. 23-38. Bicipital peritendonous injection. Approach for bicipital peritendonous aspiration and injection. (Reprinted with permission from Steinbrocker O, Neustadt DH. *Aspiration and injection therapy in arthritis and musculoskeletal disorders.* Hagerstown, MD: Harper & Row, 1972; 46.)

Lateral Epicondyle of the Elbow

Indications

Lateral epicondyle injection is a useful diagnostic and therapeutic procedure for lateral epicondylitis of the elbow (tennis elbow). The condition is usually secondary to occupational or sports-related trauma or recurrent trauma.

Techniques

After informed consent is obtained, the patient is placed in the sitting position, with the arm resting on the examination table, palm down, and the elbow flexed to 45°. The elbow is palpated at the junction of the forearm extensor group at its attachment to the bone near the lateral epicondyle for the point of maximal tenderness. The patient is prepared in a standard aseptic fashion, and a 1 1/2 inch (4 cm) 23-gauge needle is inserted at the point of maximal tenderness. After negative aspiration, inject at the point of maximal tenderness with a 5-ml mixture of 10 mg methylprednisolone acetate (or equivalent) and anesthetic agent (Fig. 23-39).

Comments

The point of maximal tenderness is usually just medial and distal to the lateral epicondyle over the common tendon of the forearm extensor group at its attachment to the bone.

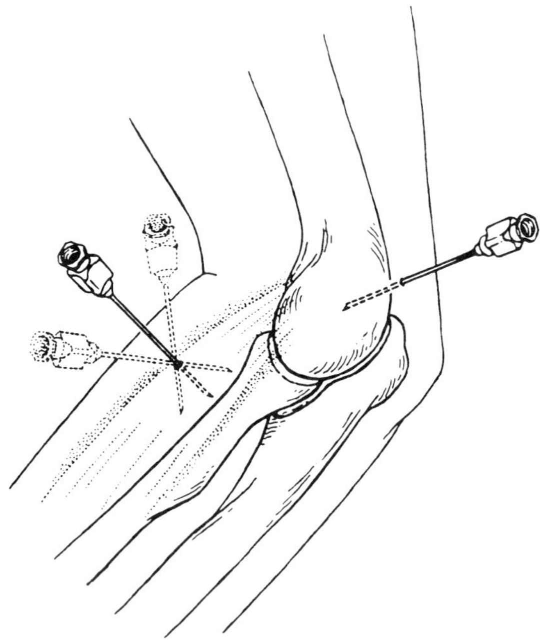

FIG. 23-39. Lateral epicondyle injection. Approach for lateral epicondyle aspiration and injection. (Reprinted with permission from Steinbrocker O, Neustadt DH. *Aspiration and injection therapy in arthritis and musculoskeletal disorders.* Hagerstown, MD: Harper & Row, 1972; 55.)

Complications

Serious complications are uncommon with injection of the lateral epicondyle of the elbow.

Medial Epicondyle of the Elbow

Indications

Medial epicondyle injection is a useful diagnostic and therapeutic procedure with medial epicondylitis (golfer's elbow or tortilla elbow).

Techniques

After informed consent is obtained, the patient is placed in the sitting position, with the arm resting on the examination table, palm up, and the elbow flexed to 45°. The elbow is palpated at the junction of the forearm extensor group at its attachment to the bone at the lateral epicondyle for the point of maximal tenderness. The patient is prepared in a standard aseptic fashion, and a 1 1/2 inch (4 cm) 23-gauge needle is inserted at the point of maximal tenderness. After negative aspiration, inject at the point of maximal tenderness with a 5-ml mixture of 10 mg methylprednisolone acetate (or equivalent) and anesthetic agent.

Comments

The point of maximal tenderness is usually just lateral and distal to the medial epicondyle over the common tendon of the forearm flexor group at its attachment to the bone.

Complications

Avoid injecting the ulnar nerve in the groove just behind the medial epicondyle.

Olecranon Bursa of the Elbow

Indications

Olecranon bursa injection is a useful diagnostic and therapeutic procedure with olecranon bursitis. This condition is usually secondary to trauma or rheumatoid arthritis.

Techniques

After informed consent is obtained, the patient is placed in the sitting position with hand in lap. The olecranon process of the ulna is palpated for swollen bursa. The point of maximum swelling is marked. The patient is prepared in a standard aseptic fashion, and a 1 1/2 inch (4 cm) 21-gauge needle is inserted at the most prominent part of the olecranon bursa. Aspiration is attempted until the needle has entered the synovial space. If there is an effusion of the bursa, complete the aspiration. After negative aspiration or if the aspirated fluid is noninflammatory (clear and viscous), inject the bursa with a 3-ml mixture of 10 mg triamcinolone hexacetonide (or equivalent) and local anesthetic (Fig. 23-40).

Comments

This procedure may require an 18-gauge needle to aspirate the bursa with highly viscous fluid.

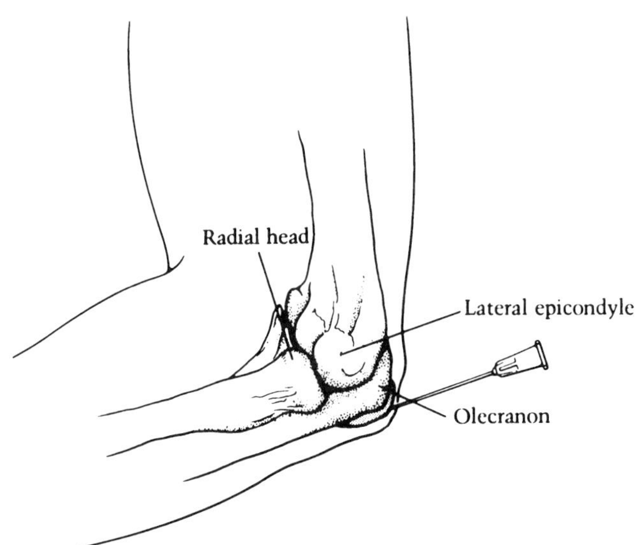

FIG. 23-40. Olecranon injection. Approach for olecranon aspiration and injection. (Reprinted with permission from Akins CM. Aspiration and injection of joints, bursae, and tendons. In: Vander Salm TJ, Cutler BS, Brownell Wheeler H, eds. *Atlas of bedside procedures.* Boston: Little, Brown, 1979; 357.)

Complications

Do not inject with corticosteroid if there is any suspicion that the bursa is infected. If the fluid appears infected, then send it for culture and sensitivity and treat the patient appropriately for the infection.

Radiohumeral Joint (True Elbow Joint)

Indications

Radiohumeral joint injection is used to diagnose and treat the painful and swollen elbow due to rheumatoid arthritis or nonspecific inflammatory arthritides.

Techniques

After informed consent is obtained, the patient is placed in the sitting position with the elbow flexed to 90°. The lateral epicondyle and posterior olecranon are palpated. The patient is prepared in a standard aseptic fashion, and a 1 1/2 inch (4 cm) 21- to 23-gauge needle is inserted into the groove just above and lateral to the olecranon process, just below the lateral humeral epicondyle, and posterior to the head of the radius. The needle is gently manipulated into the joint. Aspiration is attempted until the needle has entered the synovial space. If there is an effusion of the joint, complete the aspiration. After negative aspiration or if the aspirated fluid is noninflammatory (clear and viscous), inject the joint with a 5-ml mixture of 10 mg triamcinolone hexacetonide (or equivalent) and local anesthetic (Fig. 23-41).

Comments

The connective tissue surrounding the elbow joint should be evaluated as a possible source of pain before injection of the radiohumeral joint.

Complications

Do not inject with corticosteroid if there is any suspicion that the bursa is infected. If the fluid appears infected, then send it for culture and sensitivity and treat the patient appropriately for the infection.

Carpal Tunnel

Indications

Injection of the carpal tunnel is used to treat inflammation of the tissue of the tunnel resulting in median nerve entrapment.

Techniques

After informed consent is obtained, the patient is placed in the sitting position with the arm resting on the examination table. The wrist is positioned with the hand dorsiflexed over a towel. The injection site is on the volar wrist surface just proximal to the distal wrist crease between the palmaris longus and flexor carpi radialis tendons. The patient is prepared in a standard aseptic fashion, and a 1 1/2 inch (4 cm) 23- to 25-gauge needle is directed distally at an angle of 60° to the skin and gently manipulated through the flexor retinaculum ligament into the carpal tunnel. The tunnel is approximately 1 to 2 cm from the skin in this position. After negative aspiration, inject the carpal tunnel with a 1-ml mixture of 10 mg methylprenisolone acetate (or equivalent) and local anesthetic (Fig. 23-42).

Comments

Anesthesia in the distribution of the median nerve verifies injection in the carpal tunnel. These paresthesias may last for 1 to 2 weeks.

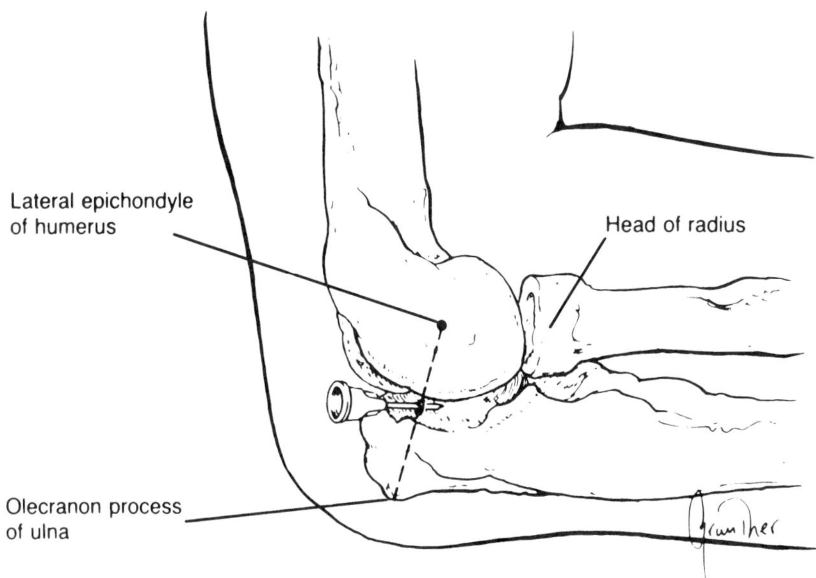

FIG. 23-41. Radiohumeral joint injection. Approach for radiohumeral joint aspiration and injection. (Reprinted with permission from Gatter RA. Arthrosyntesis therapy and intrasynovial injection. In: Koopman WJ, ed. *Arthritis and allied conditions—a textbook of rheumatology,* 13th ed. Baltimore: Williams & Wilkins, 1997; 714.)

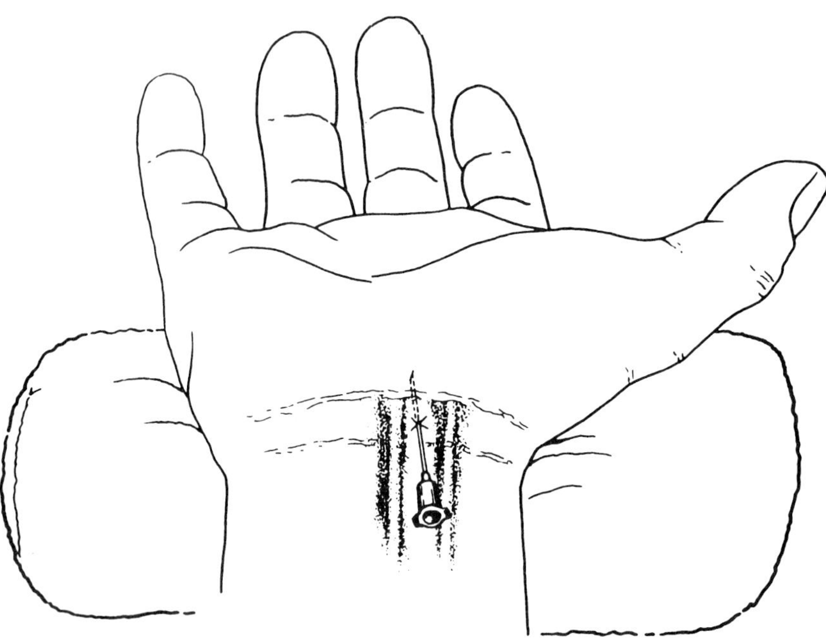

FIG. 23-42. Carpal tunnel injection. Approach for carpal tunnel aspiration and injection. (Reprinted with permission from Steinbrocker O, Neustadt DH. *Aspiration and injection therapy in arthritis and musculoskeletal disorders.* Hagerstown, MD: Harper & Row, 1972; 59.)

Complications

Do not inject the median nerve. The patient will normally report sharp electrical sensation when the needle tip is against the median nerve and excruciating pain if the needle tip pierces the median nerve. If either of the above occurs, withdraw slightly and continue the procedure. The volume injected into the carpal tunnel should be kept to a minimum to reduce postinjection discomfort.

Wrist Joint

Indications

Wrist joint injection is a useful diagnostic and therapeutic procedure for inflammation due to rheumatoid arthritis and other inflammatory arthritides.

Techniques

After informed consent is obtained, the patient is placed in the sitting position with the arm resting on the examination table. The hand is placed palm down with the wrist positioned over a rolled towel. The wrist joint is approached from the dorsal aspect. The patient is prepared in a standard aseptic fashion and a 1 1/2 inch (4 cm) 23-gauge needle is inserted between the distal radius and ulna on the ulnar side of the extensor pollicis longus tendon. The needle is gently manipulated into the joint cavity to a depth of about 1 to 2 cm. Aspiration is attempted until the needle has entered the synovial space. If there is an effusion of the joint, complete the aspiration. After negative aspiration or if the aspirated fluid is noninflammatory (clear and viscous), inject the joint with a 2- to 3-ml mixture of 20 to 40 mg methylprednisolone acetone (or equivalent) and local anesthetic (Fig. 23-43).

Comments

Many of the synovial joints of the wrists are interconnected. No significant resistance should be encountered. If

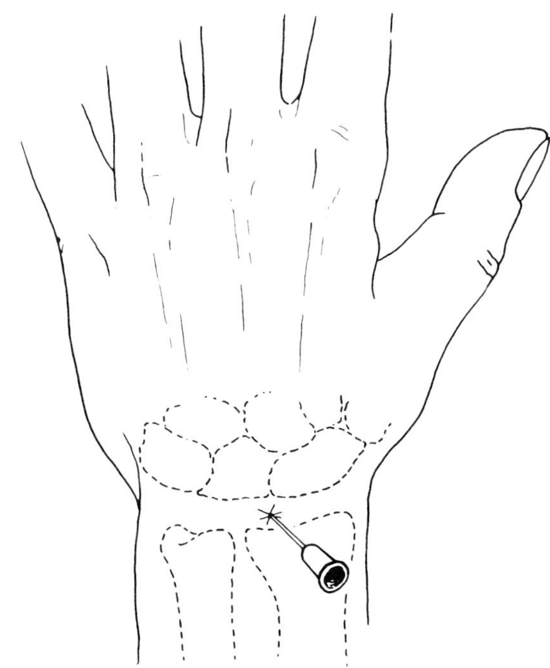

FIG. 23-43. Wrist joint injection. Approach for wrist joint aspiration and injection. (Reprinted with permission from Steinbrocker O, Neustadt DH. *Aspiration and injection therapy in arthritis and musculoskeletal disorders.* Hagerstown, MD: Harper & Row, 1972; 61.)

resistance is encountered, the needle may not be in the joint cavity. Consider scapholunate dislocation, carpal instability, avascular necrosis, or other etiology of chronic conditions before injection. Elastic bandage or splint immobilization for 24 hours after injection may decrease discomfort.

Complications

Intraneural injection may result in nerve damage. Hematoma and intravascular injection are possible due to the close proximity of the vessels. If an arterial puncture occurs, prolonged direct pressure is usually adequate to prevent the development of a hematoma. Do not inject with corticosteroid if there is any suspicion that the joint is infected. If the fluid appears infected, then send it for culture and sensitivity and treat the patient appropriately for the infection.

Abductor Tendon of the Thumb

Indications

Abductor tendon of the thumb injection is a useful therapeutic procedure for tenosynovitis of extensor pollicis brevis and abductor hallicus longus (de Quervain's syndrome) usually associated with repetitive trauma disorder. This procedure involves injection of common tendon sheath of the long abductor and short extensor tendons of the thumb.

Techniques

After informed consent is obtained, the patient is placed in the sitting position with the arm resting on the examination table. The forearm is placed on the ulnar side midway between supination and pronation, with the wrist held in ulnar deviation over a rolled towel stretching the tendons over the radial styloid. Palpate tendons for point of maximal tenderness. The patient is prepared in a standard aseptic fashion, and a 1 1/2 inch (3 cm) 23-gauge needle is inserted in a proximal direction, parallel to the tendon at a tangential angle, aiming for the point of maximal tenderness. Once the needle is in the tenosynovium, 0.25 to 0.5 ml of local anesthetic can be injected with a tuberculin syringe without significant resistance. This results in a small sausage-shaped swelling along the length of the tendons. At this point the syringe containing only local anesthetic is disconnected and another syringe is used to inject the peritendinous area with a 2-ml mixture of 5 mg triamcinolone hexacetonide (or equivalent) and local anesthetic (Fig. 23-44).

Comments

There should be no significant resistance encountered in the tenosynovium. There will be resistance encountered by the plunger of the syringe if the needle is in the tendon. Steroid injection into the tendon should be avoided.

Complications

Injecting directly into the tendon rather than peritendinous region can result in damage to the abductor tendon of the thumb.

First Metacarpal Joint

Indications

First metacarpal joint injection is used to treat pain and inflammation secondary to osteoarthritis.

Techniques

After informed consent is obtained, the patient is placed in a sitting position with the arm resting on the examination table. The forearm is placed on the ulnar side midway between supination and pronation with the thumb adducted and held in flexion with the palm. Palpate the first metacarpal along the dorsal aspect to the groove at its proximal end. The patient is prepared in a standard aseptic fashion, and a 1 inch (2.5 cm) needle is inserted at the point of maximal tenderness. The needle is advanced into the joint space. Aspi-

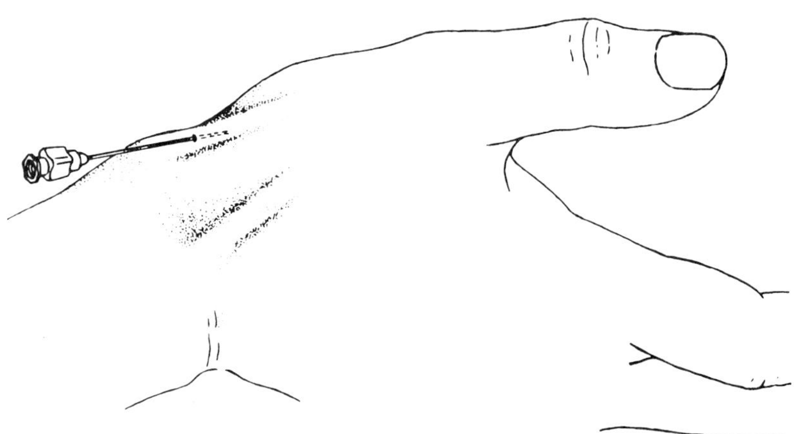

FIG. 23-44. Abductor tendon sheath thumb injection. Approach for abductor tendon sheath of the thumb aspiration and injection. (Reprinted with permission from Steinbrocker O, Neustadt DH. *Aspiration and injection therapy in arthritis and musculoskeletal disorders.* Hagerstown, MD: Harper & Row, 1972; 58.)

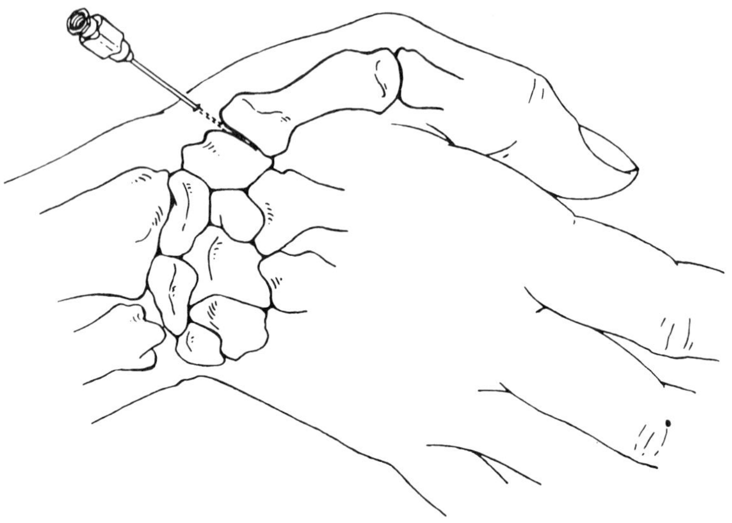

FIG. 23-45. First metacarpal joint injection. Approach for first metacarpal joint aspiration and injection. (Reprinted with permission from Steinbrocker O, Neustadt DH. *Aspiration and injection therapy in arthritis and musculoskeletal disorders.* Hagerstown, MD: Harper & Row, 1972; 63.)

ration is attempted until the needle has entered the synovial space. After negative aspiration or if there is an effusion of the joint, complete the aspiration. If negative aspiration or if the aspirated fluid is noninflammatory (clear and viscous), inject the joint with a 1- to 3-ml mixture of triamcinolone hexacetonide (or equivalent) and local anesthetic (Fig. 23-45).

Comments

Avoid piercing the radial artery and extensor pollicis tendon.

Complications

Radial artery injury, extensor pollicis tendon injury, and increased pain for 1 to 3 days are uncommon but may result from this injection. Hematoma and intravascular injection are possible due to the close proximity of the axillary vessels. If an arterial puncture occurs, prolonged direct pressure is usually adequate to prevent the development of a hematoma. Do not inject with corticosteroid if there is any suspicion that the joint is infected. If the fluid appears infected, then send it for culture and sensitivity and treat the patient appropriately for the infection.

Interphalangeal Joint

Indications

Interphalangeal joint injection is used as a therapeutic procedure to treat inflammation of the metacarpal phalangeal and interphalangeal joints due to rheumatoid arthritis and other inflammatory arthritides.

Techniques

After informed consent is obtained, the patient is placed in the sitting position with the arm resting on the examination table. The hand is placed with the joint extended for approach from the lateral or medial aspect with slight traction applied to the finger. The patient is prepared in a standard aseptic fashion, and a 1 inch (2.5 cm) 25- to 27-gauge needle is inserted at the borders of the joint and advanced gently to the joint capsule. Pericapsular injection without attempting to enter the joint is appropriate. Inject the pericapsular area with a 1-ml mixture of 10 mg methylprednisolone acetate (or equivalent) and local anesthetic (Fig. 23-46).

Comments

No effort should be made to aspirate fluid unless infection is suspected.

Complications

Serious complications are uncommon with appropriate needle placement.

Lumbar Facet Joint

Indications

The lumbar facet joints have been shown to be a potential source of pain involving the low back and buttocks. Facet joint injections can provide diagnostic as well as therapeutic benefits for patients with low back pain.

Techniques

After informed consent is obtained, the patient is placed in the prone position with a pillow under the pelvis to flatten the lumbar curve. The lumbar spine is palpated for point of

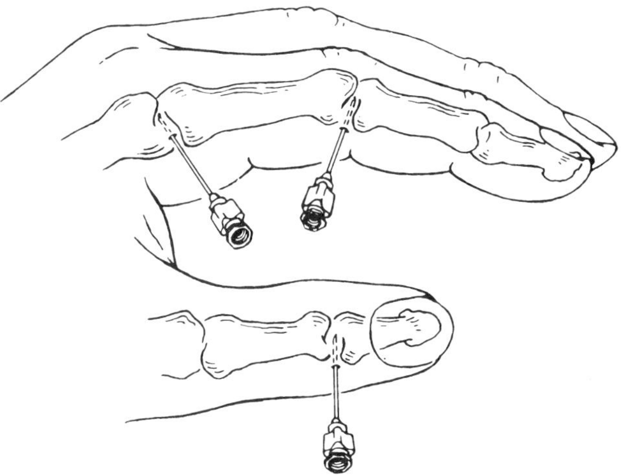

FIG. 23-46. Interphalangeal joint injection. Approach for first metacarpal joint aspiration and injection. (Reprinted with permission from Steinbrocker O, Neustadt DH. *Aspiration and injection therapy in arthritis and musculoskeletal disorders.* Hagerstown, MD: Harper & Row, 1972; 64.)

maximum tenderness. The patient is prepared in a standard aseptic fashion, and a 3 inch (8 cm) 22-gauge needle is inserted at the point of maximum tenderness. The needle is advanced to the joint, with care taken to ensure the needle is directed over the articular pillars and not allowed to stray medially toward the interlaminar space or excessively laterally. The needle is advanced until contact is made with the articular pillar, either above or below the targeted joint and then redirected into the joint capsule. Lateral and anteroposterior fluoroscopy views are necessary to ensure that the needle is advanced to the joint mid-point. Injection of contrast medium may be used to confirm proper placement in the joint. After negative aspiration, inject the joint with a 1-ml or less mixture of 10 mg triamcinolone hexacetonide (or equivalent) and local anesthetic (Fig. 23-47).

Comments

Total injected volume should not exceed 1 ml because joint volume is usually 1 ml or less. Anterior needle placement should be avoided because the dural sleeve, spinal cord, and epidural space are in close proximity to the anterior surface of the cervical joint.

Complications

Serious complications from lumbar zygapophyseal joint injections are uncommon when meticulous care is given to ensure proper needle placement before injection. Local post-injection pain may occur. Intravascular injection of local anesthetic may cause a seizure. Epidural or spinal blockade can occur if the needle placement is medial, resulting in regional blockade, respiratory compromise, and hypotension.

Sacroiliac Joint

Indications

Sacroiliac joint injection is used to treat inflammation of the sacroiliac joints secondary to trauma, rheumatoid arthritis, degenerative joint disease, or stress secondary to mechanical changes in posture or gait.

Techniques

After informed consent is obtained, the patient is placed in the prone position. The patient is prepared in a standard aseptic fashion, and a 6 inch (16 cm) 22-gauge needle is inserted. The needle is advanced under fluoroscopy to the joint. After negative aspiration, joint penetration is confirmed with 1 ml diatrizoate megluimine injection USP 60% (Renografin-60 [Squibb]). After needle location is confirmed, inject with a 10-ml mixture of 40 mg methylprednisolone acetate (or equivalent) and local anesthetic (Fig. 23-48).

Comments

The sacroiliac joint is difficult to aspirate due to the depth and bony structures. Fluoroscopic guidance with the use of contrast media is recommended. It is rare to aspirate fluid from this joint.

Complications

Serious complications are uncommon with appropriate needle placement.

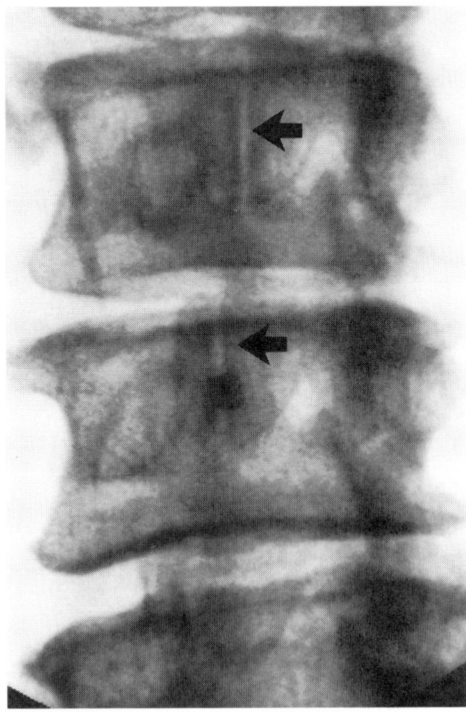

FIG. 23-47. Lumbar facet joint injection. Fluoroscopic approach for lumbar facet joint injection *(arrows).*

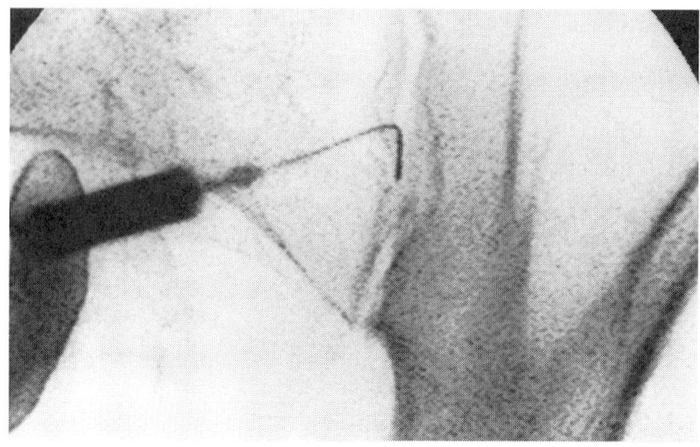

A

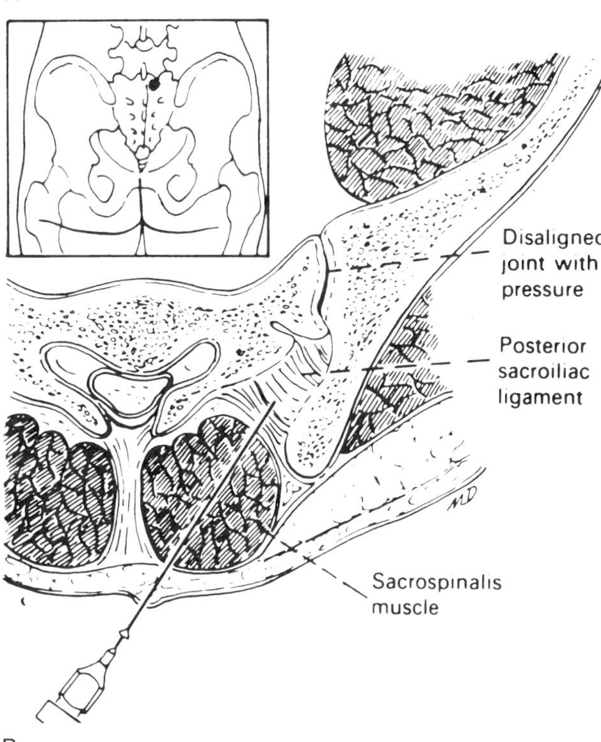

B

FIG. 23-48. Sacroiliac joint injection. **A:** Fluoroscopic approach for right sacroiliac joint. **B:** Approach for sacroiliac joint injection. (Reprinted with permission from Bonica JJ, Buckley FP. Regional analgesia with local anesthetics. In: Bonica JJ, ed. *The management of pain,* 2nd ed. Philadelphia: Lea & Febiger, 1990; 1897.)

Coccygeal Junction

Indication

Infiltration of the coccyx region can be useful as a therapeutic procedure in coccydynia after exclusion of infection or other significant pathology.

Techniques

After informed consent is obtained, the patient is position in the lateral Sims' position with the left side down for right-handed clinicians. With the upper leg flexed, the buttocks are separated, allowing easy access to the sacrococcygeal junction. The patient is prepared in a standard aseptic fashion over a large area to allow palpation of landmarks. The area of tenderness is localized by palpating from the tip of the coccyx to the sacrococcygeal junction. The palpating hand is kept in position, and a 1 1/2 inch (4 cm) 21-gauge needle is inserted at the point of maximal tenderness perpendicular to the skin. After negative aspiration, inject a 3-ml mixture of 20 mg methylprednisolone acetate or equivalent and local anesthetic into the tender area using a fan pattern (Fig. 23-49).

Comments

It is not necessary to advance the needle into the sacrococcygeal junction. Infiltration of the superficial tissue at the point of maximal tenderness is usually adequate.

Complications

Perianal numbness may be noted for 24 hours after injection. Serious complications are uncommon with appropriate needle placement.

Hip Joint

Indications

Hip joint intra-articular injection is used to treat inflammation of the hip secondary to rheumatoid arthritis or osteoarthritis.

Techniques

After informed consent is obtained, the patient is placed in the supine position with the leg straight and externally rotated. A point is marked at 2 cm below the anterior superior spine of the ilium and 3 cm lateral to the palpated femoral pulse at the level of the superior edge of the greater trochanter. The patient is prepared in a standard aseptic fashion, and a 3.5 inch (9 cm) 21-gauge needle is inserted at the mark in the posterior medial direction at an angle 60° to the skin. The needle is advanced through the tough capsular ligaments to the bone and slightly withdrawn. Under fluoroscopy, contrast medium is injected to confirm appropriate needle placement. Aspiration is attempted until the needle has entered the synovial space. If there is an effusion of the joint, complete the aspiration. After negative aspiration or if the aspirated fluid is noninflammatory (clear and viscous), inject the joint with a 2- to 4-ml mixture of 20 mg triamcinolone hexacetonide (or equivalent) and local anesthetic (Fig. 23-50).

Comments

The hip joint is difficult to aspirate or inject due to the depth and limited landmarks. Fluoroscopic guidance with the use of contrast media is recommended. It is rare to aspirate fluid from this joint.

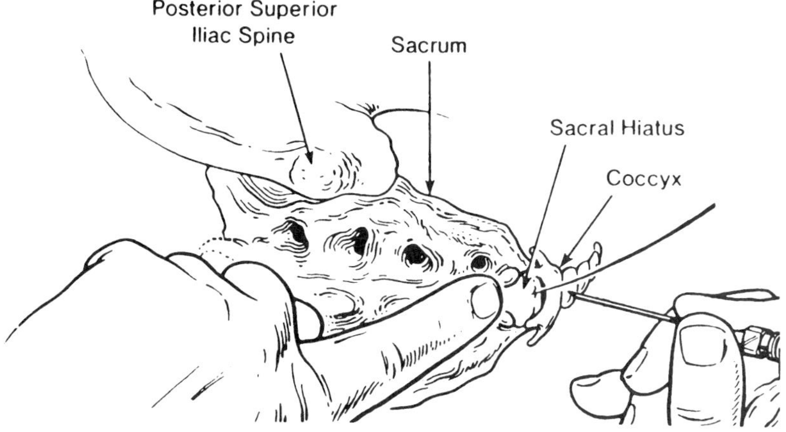

FIG. 23-49. Coccygeal junction injection. Approach for coccygeal junction injection. (Reprinted with permission from Willis RJ. Caudal epidural blockade. In: Cousins MJ, Bridenbaugh PO, eds. *Neural blockade in clinical anesthesia and management of pain,* 2nd ed. Philadelphia: JB Lippincott, 1988; 373.)

Complications

Avascular necrosis of the hip has been reported due to repeated intra-articular injection of corticosteroids. Hematoma and intravascular injection are possible due to the close proximity of the femoral vessels. If an arterial puncture occurs, prolonged direct pressure is usually adequate to prevent the development of a hematoma. Do not inject with corticosteroid if there is any suspicion that the joint is infected. If the fluid appears infected, then send it for culture and sensitivity and treat the patient appropriately for the infection.

Trochanteric Bursa

Indications

Trochanteric bursa injection is used to diagnose and treat bursitis of the hip. This often presents as pain in the lateral thigh during ambulation. Pain may be elicited by placing the hip in external rotation and abduction.

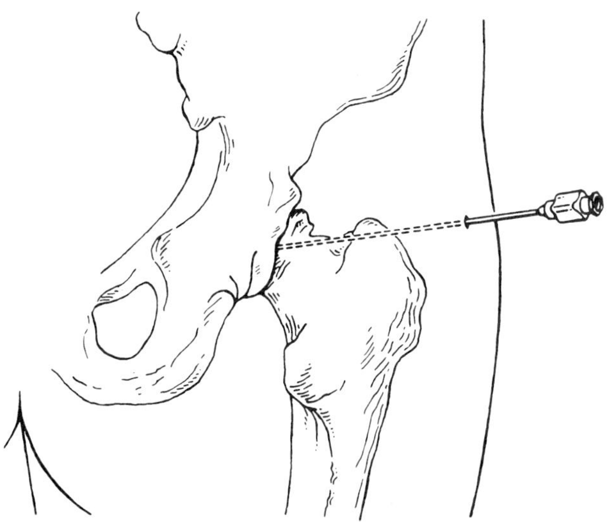

FIG. 23-50. Hip joint injection. Approach for hip joint aspiration and injection. Lateral approach. (Reprinted with permission from Steinbrocker O, Neustadt DH. *Aspiration and injection therapy in arthritis and musculoskeletal disorders.* Hagerstown, MD: Harper & Row, 1972; 83.)

Techniques

After obtaining informed consent, position the patient lying on their side and facing the clinician with the painful hip exposed. The hips and knees are flexed and the affected hip adducted. The protuberance of greater trochanter on the lateral aspect of the thigh is palpated for the point of maximal tenderness. This is usually two fingerbreadths below the tip of the trochanter. The patient is prepared in a standard aseptic fashion, and a 3 inch (8 cm) 21-gauge needle is inserted perpendicular to the skin at the point of maximal tenderness. The needle is advanced with aspiration attempted until the needle has entered the synovial space. If there is an effusion of the joint, complete the aspiration. If the aspirated fluid is noninflammatory (clear and viscous), inject the bursa with a 3-ml mixture of 20 to 40 mg methylprednisolone acetate (or equivalent) and local anesthetic. If unable to enter the synovial space, the needle is advanced to the bone and then withdrawn 2 mm. After negative aspiration, inject with a 3 ml mixture of 20 to 40 mg methylprednisolone acetate (or equivalent) and local anesthetic (Fig. 23-51).

Comments

The clinician should consider other causes of pain if the problem persists after bursa injection and appropriate rehabilitation.

Complications

Do not inject with corticosteroid if there is any suspicion that the bursa is infected. If the fluid appears infected, then send it for culture and sensitivity and treat the patient appropriately for the infection.

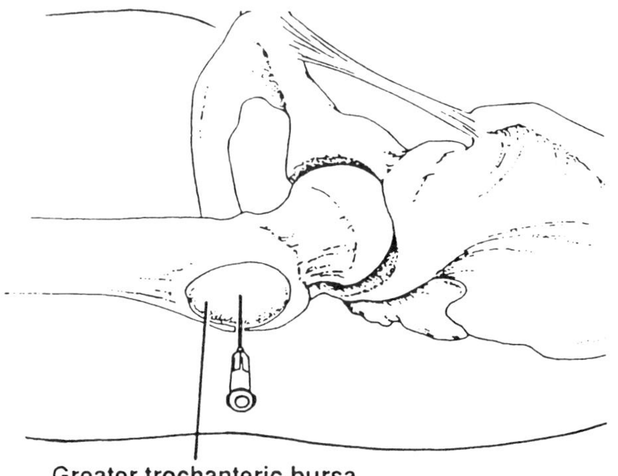

FIG. 23-51. Trochanteric bursa injection. (Reprinted with permission from Akins CM. Aspiration of joints, bursae, and tendons. In: Vander Salm TJ, Cutler BS, Brownell Wheeler H, eds. *Atlas of bedside procedures.* Boston: Little, Brown, 1988; 359.)

Abductor Tendon of the Hip

Indications

Injection of the abductor tendon is a useful diagnostic and therapeutic procedure with tendonitis at the insertion of the gluteal musculature into the greater trochanter.

Techniques

After informed consent is obtained, position the patient lying on their side facing the clinician with the painful hip exposed. The hips and knees are flexed and the affected hip adducted. The hip is palpated above the tip of the trochanter for the point of maximal tenderness. A 3.5 inch (9 cm) 21-gauge needle is inserted at the point of maximal tenderness and directed toward the tip of the greater trochanter, approximating the insertion of the gluteal fasciae. The needle is advanced vertically to a depth that would reach the hip abductor tendon. This depth would vary from patient to patient, which is estimated by palpation of the hip abductor tendon. In obese patients, one would have to use a lumbar puncture needle to reach the tendon area. After negative aspiration, inject the area of maximal tenderness with a 10-ml mixture of 40 mg methylprednisolone acetate (or equivalent) and local anesthetic.

Comments

The injection is not into the tendon but peritendinous. Wide infiltration with a corticosteroid/local anesthetic mixture is recommended. Tender points in the vicinity of the hip joint are often associated with osteoarthritis of the hip. Injection of these sites may provide significant pain relief.

Complications

Injecting directly into the tendon rather than the peritendinous region may result in damage to the abductor tendon of the hip.

Knee Joint

Indications

Intra-articular corticosteroid injection of the knee joint is used to treat noninfective inflammatory joint disease secondary to rheumatoid arthritis, seronegative spondylarthritides, or the chondrocalcinosis inflammatory phase of osteoarthritis.

Techniques

After informed consent is obtained, the patient is placed in the sitting position with the knee flexed to 90°. The patellar tendon is palpated and the middle of the patellar tendon is marked. The patient is prepared in a standard aseptic fashion. A 1 1/2 inch (4 cm) 21-gauge needle is inserted horizontally and advanced to the intercondylar notch. Aspiration is attempted until the needle has entered the synovial space. If there is an effusion of the joint, complete the aspiration. After negative aspiration or if the aspirated fluid is noninflammatory (clear and viscous), inject the joint with a 2-ml mixture of 10 mg of triamcinolone hexacetonide (or equivalent) and local anesthetic (Fig. 23-52).

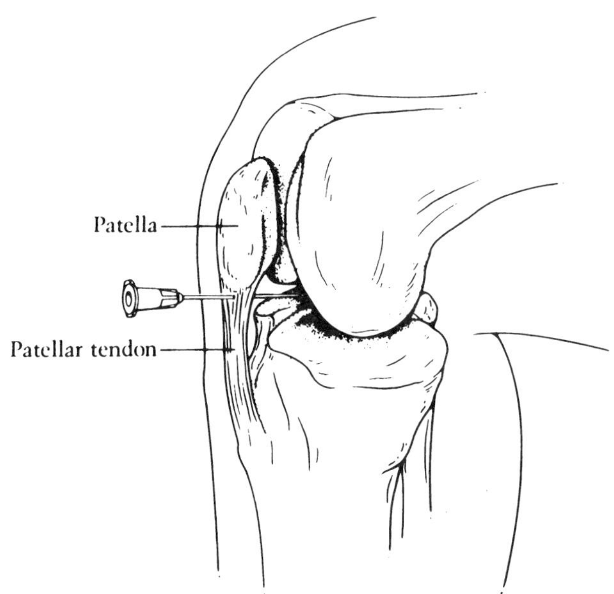

FIG. 23-52. Knee joint injection. Approach for knee joint aspiration and injection. Anterior approach. (Reprinted with permission from Akins CM. Aspiration and injection of joints, bursae, and tendons. In: Vander Salm TJ, Cutler BS, Brownell Wheeler H, eds. *Atlas of bedside procedures.* Boston: Little, Brown, 1979; 363.)

Comments

An alternate approach may be used to access the suprapatellar pouch, which is continuous with the synovial space of the knee. The patient is placed in the supine position with leg fully extended. The patient is prepared in standard aseptic fashion and throughout the procedure the patella should be grasped between the examiner's thumb and forefinger and be able to be moved from side to side to ensure that the quadriceps muscle is relaxed. A 1 1/2 inch (4 cm) 21-gauge needle is inserted horizontally into the suprapatellar pouch at a point lateral and posterior to the patella at the level of its cephalad edge. A small amount of pressure is placed on the patella, pushing it to the side of needle insertion. This improves the ability to direct the needle during advancement (Fig. 23-53). Advise patients to minimize walking activity for 24 hours after injection to minimize dispersion of the corticosteroid from the joint. If fluid is exceptionally viscous, a 1 1/2 inch 18-gauge needle may be required to aspirate the joint.

Complications

Do not inject with corticosteroid if there is any suspicion that the joint is infected. If the fluid appears infected, then send it for culture and sensitivity and treat the patient appropriately for the infection. It is contraindicated to inject this joint in a person with hemophilia unless the risk of intra-articular bleed has been minimized. Corticosteroid injection into the knee joint may impair epiphyseal growth in children, resulting in a significant leg length discrepancy.

Anserine Bursa of the Knee

Indications

Anserine bursa injection is a useful diagnostic and therapeutic procedure in bursitis resulting from osteoarthritis or direct trauma. Pain is noted inferior to the anterior medial surface of the knee when climbing stairs. Pain is reproduced with the knee in flexion extension while internally rotating the leg.

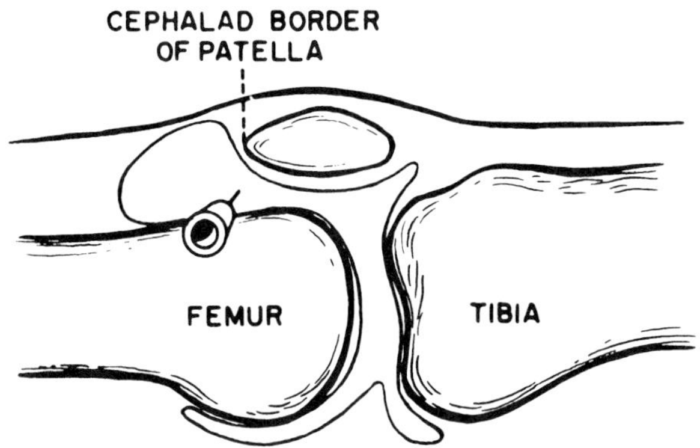

FIG. 23-53. Knee joint injection. Medial approach to suprapatellar pouch for knee joint aspiration and injection. Note connection between suprapatellar pouch and main synovial cavity. (Reprinted with permission from Gatter RA. Arthrocentesis technique and intrasynovial therapy. In: Koopman WJ, ed. *Arthritis and allied conditions—a textbook of rheumatology,* 13th ed. Baltimore: Williams & Wilkins, 1997; 752.)

Techniques

After informed consent is obtained, the patient is placed in the supine position with the knee in extension. The knee is palpated for the point of maximal tenderness over the medial tibial flare. The patient is prepared in a standard aseptic fashion, and a 1 1/2 inch (4 cm) 21-gauge needle is inserted perpendicular to the skin and at the point of maximal tenderness. The needle is advanced to the periosteum and withdrawn slightly. After negative aspiration, a 4-ml mixture of 2 mg methylprednisolone (or equivalent) and local anesthetic is injected (Fig. 23-54).

Comments

The anserine bursa is one of the most common bursa to become inflamed in the lower extremity. Knee pads are recommended for athletes with anserine bursitis secondary to trauma.

Complications

Serious complications are uncommon with injection of the anserine bursa.

Tibiotalar Joint

Indications

Tibiotalar joint injection is a useful therapeutic procedure with inflammation secondary to osteoarthritis, rheumatoid arthritis, or chronic pain from instability. Pain most often occurs with ankle extension and flexion with weight bearing.

Techniques

After informed consent is obtained, the patient is placed in the supine position with the leg extended and the ankle extended over the end of the examination table. Palpate and place a mark just anterior to the medial malleolus at the articulation of the tibia and the talus. The patient is prepared in standard aseptic fashion, and a 1 1/2 inch (4 cm) 21-gauge needle is inserted at the mark perpendicular to the skin. The needle is advanced slightly laterally, penetrating the capsule of the joint. The needle is directed into the tibiotalar joint to a depth of approximately 2 to 3 cm. Aspiration is attempted until the needle has entered the synovial space. If there is an effusion of the joint, complete the aspiration. After negative aspiration or if the aspirated fluid is noninflammatory (clear and viscous), inject the joint with a 2-ml

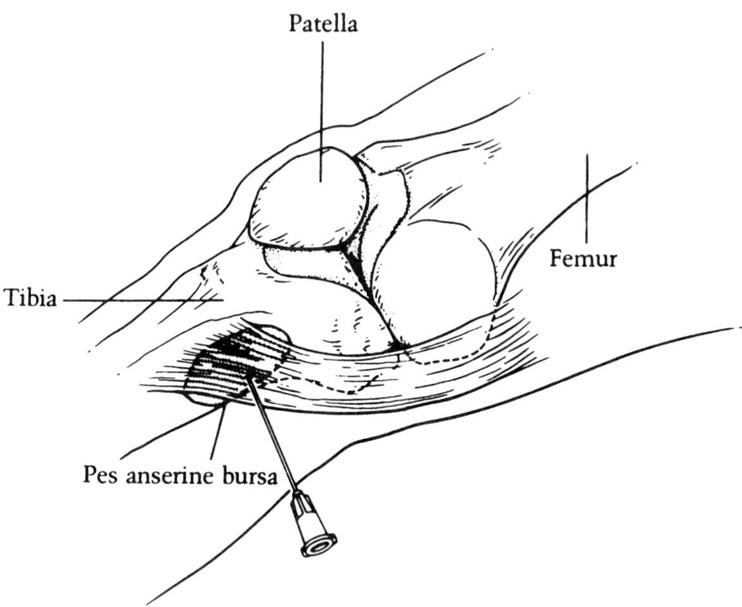

FIG. 23-54. Anserine bursa injection. Approach for anserine bursa aspiration and injection. (Reprinted with permission from Akins CM. Aspiration of joints, bursae, and tendons. In: Vander Salm TJ, Cutler BS, Brownell Wheeler H, eds. *Atlas of bedside procedures.* Boston: Little, Brown, 1988; 361.)

mixture of 10 mg triamcinolone hexacetonide (or equivalent) and local anesthetic (Fig. 23-55).

Comments

Injection of this joint is usually secondary to osteoarthritis resulting from trauma or from repetitive overuse injury such as from ballet dancing. If the swelling and tendonitis is around the lateral aspect of the joint, entry is accomplished just below the lateral malleolus. Gout is not an indication for injecting this joint.

Complications

Do not inject the corticosteroid if there is any suspicion that the joint is infected. If the fluid appears infected, then send if for culture and sensitivity and treat the patient appropriately for the infection.

Subtalar (Talocalcaneal) Joint

Indications

Subtalar joint injection is used to treat inflammation secondary to rheumatoid arthritis and other inflammatory arthritides.

Techniques

After informed consent is obtained, the patient is placed in the prone position with feet extending over the end of the examination table and the foot flexed to approximately 90°. Palpate and mark the location of the subtalar joint, approximately 1 to 2 cm distal to the tip of the lateral malleolus and posterior to the sinus tarsus. The patient is prepared in a standard aseptic fashion, and a 1 1/2 inch (4 cm) 21-gauge needle is inserted perpendicular to the skin at the mark and advanced medially into the subtalar joint. Aspiration is attempted until the needle has entered the synovial space. If there is an effusion of the joint, complete the aspiration. If

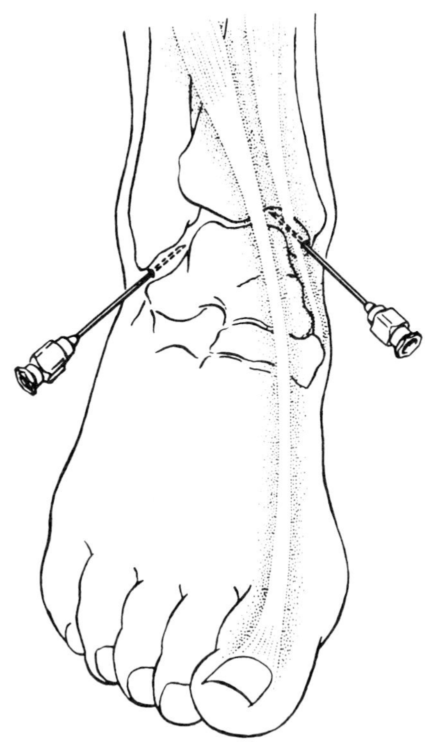

FIG. 23-55. Tibiotalar joint injection. Approach for tibiotalar joint aspiration and injection. (Reprinted with permission from Steinbrocker O, Neustadt DH. *Aspiration and injection therapy in arthritis and musculoskeletal disorders.* Hagerstown, MD: Harper & Row, 1972; 89.)

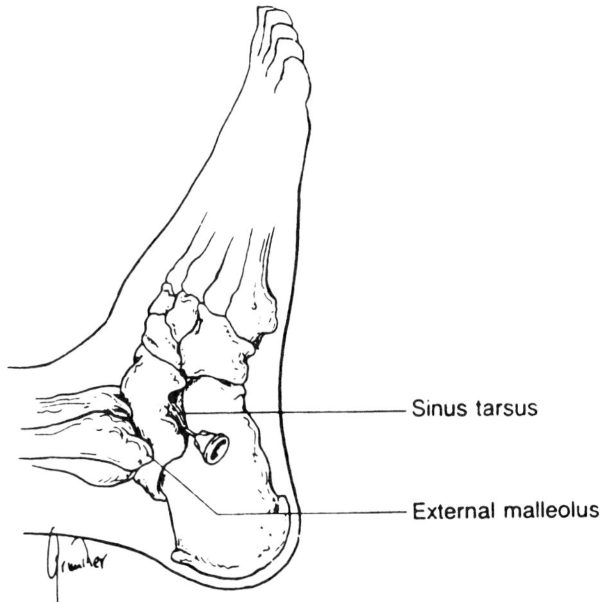

FIG. 23-56. Subtalar (talocalcaneal) joint injection. Approach for subtalar (talocalcaneal) joint aspiration and injection. (Reprinted with permission from Gatter RA. Arthrocentesis technique and intrasynovial therapy. In: Koopman WJ, ed. *Arthritis and allied conditions—a textbook of rheumatology,* 13th ed. Baltimore: Williams & Wilkins, 1997; 752.)

the aspirated fluid is noninflammatory (clear and viscous), inject the joint with a 2-ml mixture of 10 mg triamcinolone hexacetonide (or equivalent) and local anesthetic (Fig. 23-56).

Comments

Injection of this joint is usually secondary to osteoarthritis resulting from trauma or from repetitive overuse injury such as from ballet dancing. Gout is not an indication for injecting this joint.

Complications

Do not inject the corticosteroid if there is any suspicion that the joint is infected. If the fluid appears infected, then send if for culture and sensitivity and treat the patient appropriately for the infection.

Retrocalcaneal Bursa

Indications

Retrocalcaneal bursa injection is a useful therapeutic procedure with bursitis secondary to repetitive overuse disorder or rheumatoid arthritis.

Techniques

After informed consent is obtained, the patient is positioned side lying. The lateral malleolus and the Achilles tendon are palpated. The patient is prepared in a standard aseptic fashion, and a 1 1/2 inch (4 cm) 23- to 25-gauge needle is inserted between the lateral malleolus and the Achilles tendon perpendicular to the skin. The needle is advanced slowly to approximately half the thickness of the width of the Achilles tendon. After negative aspiration, inject a 2-ml mixture of 20 mg methylprednisolone acetate (or equivalent) and local anesthetic (Fig. 23-57).

Comments

This disorder may be seen in runners as they increase mileage early in the season or from an improperly fitting running shoe.

Complications

Do not inject with corticosteroid if there is any suspicion that the bursa is infected. If the fluid appears infected, then send it for culture and sensitivity and treat the patient appropriately for the infection.

Plantar Heel Fascia

Indications

Plantar heel fascia injection is used to treat inflammation at the insertion of the long plantar ligament at the anterior

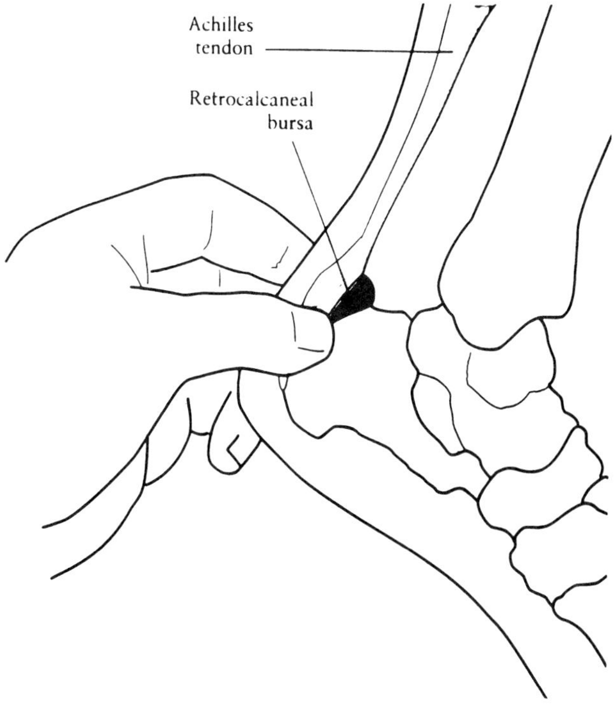

FIG. 23-57. Retrocalcaneal bursa injection. Approach for retrocalcaneal bursa aspiration and injection. (Reprinted with permission from Gross J, Fetto J, Rosen E. *Musculoskeletal examination—the ankle and foot.* Cambridge, MA: Blackwell Science, 1996; 393.)

aspect of the calcaneus secondary to chronic overuse disorder or spondylarthritides.

Techniques

After informed consent is obtained, the patient is placed in the prone position with feet extending over the end of the examination table. The plantar aspect of the heel is palpated in the area of the attachment of the plantar fascia to the calcaneus for the point of maximal tenderness. The patient is prepared in a standard aseptic fashion, and a 1 1/2 inch (4 cm) 23- to 25-gauge needle is inserted at point of maximum tenderness on the plantar surface of the heel, perpendicular to the skin. The needle is gently advanced until the tip touches underlying bone and then is withdrawn 2 mm. After negative aspiration, inject a 2-ml mixture of 20 to 40 mg of methylprednisolone (or equivalent) and local anesthetic. If proper palpation of the point of maximal tenderness is difficult, inject one half the mixture of local anesthetic and corticosteroid in the region of maximal tenderness and the remainder in a fanwise manner around the plantar fascia attachment (Fig. 23-58*A*).

Comments

This is a significantly painful procedure with or without cutaneous anesthesia. After injection, the patient is discouraged from excessive walking until the local anesthetic wears off, and is encouraged to wear a heel cushion inside the shoe.

Complications

Serious complications are uncommon with appropriate needle placement.

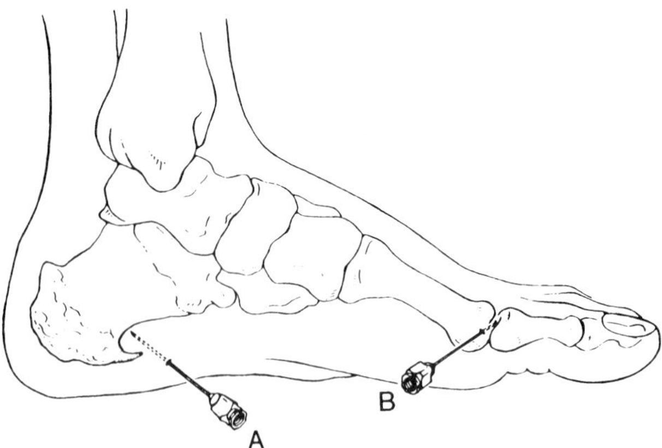

FIG. 23-58. Foot injections. **A:** Approach for plantar fasciitis or calcaneal bursitis injection. **B:** Approach from aspiration and injection of metatarsophalangeal joint. (Reprinted with permission from Steinbrocker O, Neustadt DH. *Aspiration and injection therapy in arthritis and musculoskeletal disorders.* Hagerstown, MD: Harper & Row, 1972; 89.)

Metatarsophalangeal Joint

Indications

Metatarsophalangeal joint injection is a useful procedure in the treatment of joint inflammation secondary to rheumatoid arthritis.

Techniques

After obtaining informed consent, the patient is positioned for optimal access to the dorsal surface of the foot. The metatarsophangeal joints are palpated for swelling and point tenderness. The patient is prepared in a standard aseptic fashion, and light traction is applied to the toe of the joint to be injected. A 1/2 inch to 1 inch (1.5 to 2.5 cm) 25-gauge needle is inserted perpendicular to the skin, directly into the joint space. Aspiration is attempted until the needle has entered the synovial space. If there is an effusion of the joint, complete the aspiration. After negative aspiration or the aspirated fluid is noninflammatory (clear and viscous), inject the joint with 0.5-ml mixture of 5 mg triamcinolone acetate (or equivalent) and local anesthetic (Fig. 23-58*B*).

Comments

These joints are often limited to 0.5 ml of solution. The first metatarsophalangeal joint may be approached from the medial side with the needle advanced tangentially under the extensor tendon.

Complications

Do not inject with corticosteroid if there is any suspicion that the joint is infected. If the fluid appears infected, then send if for culture and sensitivity and treat the patient appropriately for the infection.

Metatarsal Joint

Indications

This injection procedure is used to diagnose and treat Morton's metatarsalgia and Morton's neuroma.

Techniques

After informed consent is obtained, the patient is positioned for optimal access to the dorsal aspect of the foot. The metatarsal joint interspaces are palpated for swelling and tenderness. The patient is prepared in a standard aseptic fashion and a 5/8 inch (2 cm) 25-gauge needle is inserted at the point of maximal tenderness, perpendicular to the skin, and advanced approximately 1 cm. After negative aspiration,

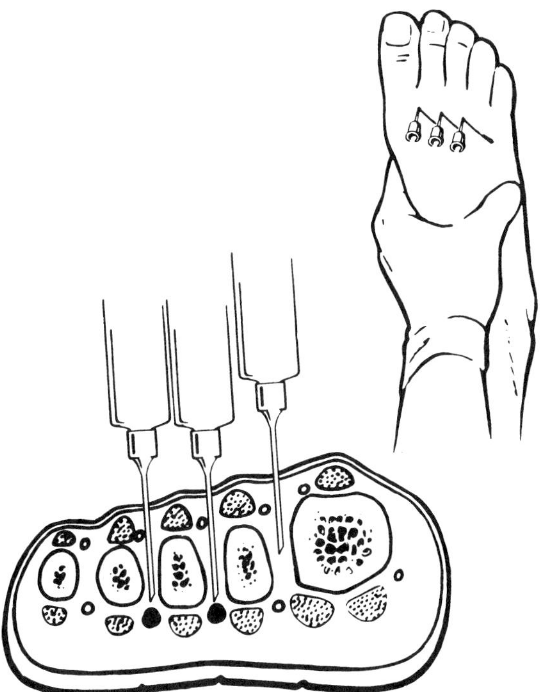

FIG. 23-59. Metatarsal joint injection. Approach for metatarsal joint aspiration and injection. (Reprinted with permission from Katz J. *Atlas of regional anesthesia.* Norwalk, CT: Appleton & Lange, 1994; 93.)

inject with a 2-ml mixture of 20 mg methylprednisolone acetate (or equivalent) and local anesthetic (Fig. 23-59).

Comments

Morton's metatarsalgia often involves the first and second interdigital spaces. Morton's neuroma is neuritis of the plantar digital nerves located between the third and fourth metatarsal heads and occasionally in the nerve between the second and third metatarsal heads. This procedure is used to treat postoperative scar pain often present after surgical removal of a Morton's neuroma.

Complications

Serious complications are uncommon with appropriate needle placement.

CONCLUSION

The injection procedures outlined in this chapter are appropriately used in conjunction with other aspects of rehabilitation to reduce pain and increase function. Aseptic technique and knowledge of anatomic relationships are required.

Aspiration is performed before injecting and repeated as necessary throughout administration of medication to prevent intravascular injection. For optimal results and safety with injection techniques, the practitioner needs the necessary skill, training, and education to perform the procedures. Haste and failure to observe the necessary precautions increase risks for any procedure. Knowledge of the anatomy pertaining to each injection procedure is a requirement for safe and successful outcomes in even the simplest injection.

ACKNOWLEDGMENT

We thank C. Farias, Department of Radiology, University of Texas Health Science Center at San Antonio, for the photographic productions.

REFERENCES

1. Macht DI. The history of opium and some of its preparations and alkaloids. *JAMA* 1915; 64:477–481.
2. Fink BR. History of neural blockade. In: Cousins MJ, Bridenbaugh PO, eds. *Neural blockade in clinical anesthesia and management of pain,* 2nd ed. Philadelphia, PA: JB Lippincott, 1988; 3–21.
3. Rynd F. *Neuralgia—introduction of fluid into the nerve.* Dublin: Dublin Medical Press, 1845; 167.
4. Pravaz CG. Sur un nouveau moyen d ópérer la coagulation du sang dans les artier, applicable à la quérison des anéurismes. *C R Acad Sci (Paris)* 1853; 36:88.
5. Wood A. New method of treating neuralgia by the direct application of opiates to the painful points. *Edinb Med Surg J* 1855; 82:265.
6. Koller C. On the use of cocaine for producing anaesthesia on the eye. *Lancet* 1884; 2:990–992 (translation).
7. Halstead WS. Practical comments on the use and abuse of cocaine; suggested by its invariably successful employment in more than a thousand minor surgical operations. *N Y Med J* 1885; 42:294–295.
8. Corning JL. *Local anaesthesia in general medicine and surgery.* New York: Appleton, 1886.
9. Hench PS, Kendall EC, Slocumb CH, Polley HF. Effect of hormone adrenal cortex (17-hydroxy-11-dehydrocorticosterone; compound E) and of pituitary adrenocorticotrophic hormone on rheumatoid arthritis; preliminary report. *Proc Staff Meet Mayo Clin* 1949; April 13, 24: 181–197.
10. Hollander JL, Brown EM, Jessar RA, Brown CY. Hydrocortisone and cortisone injected into arthritic joints. *JAMA* 1951; 147:1629–1635.
11. Hollander JL, Jessar RA, Brown EM. Intra-synovial corticosteroid therapy: a decade of use. *Bull Rheum Dis* 1961; 11:23–240.
12. Travell JG, Simons DG. *Myofascial pain and dysfunction.* Vol. 1. Baltimore: Williams & Wilkins, 1983.
13. Travell JG, Simons DG. *Myofascial pain and dysfunction.* Vol. 2. Baltimore: Williams & Wilkins, 1992.
14. Kraus H. Another use of surface anesthesia for the treatment of painful motion. *JAMA* 1941; 116:2582–2587.
15. Travell J, Rinzler S, Herman M. Pain and disability of the shoulder and arm: treatment by intramuscular infiltration with procaine hydrochloride. *JAMA* 1942; 120:417–422.
16. Bonica JJ. *The management of pain.* Philadelphia: Lea & Febiger, 1953.
17. Bonica JJ, Buckley FP. Regional analgesia with local anesthetics. In: Bonica JJ, ed. *The management of pain,* 2nd ed. Philadelphia: Lea & Febiger, 1990; 1883–1979.
18. Gatter RA. Arthrocentis technique and intrasynovial therapy. In: Koopman WJ, ed. *Arthritis and allied conditions—a textbook of rheumatology,* 13th ed. Philadelphia: Lea & Febiger, 1997; 751–775.
19. Rhodes RS. Human immunodeficiency virus transmission and surgeons: Update. Department of Surgery, University of Mississippi Medical Center. *South Med J* 1995; 88:251–255.
20. Alter MJ. Epidemiology of hepatitis C in the west. *Semin Liver Dis* 1995; 15:5–14.
21. Hernandez ME, Bruguera M, Puyuelo T, et al. Risk of needlestick injuries in the transmission of hepatitis C virus in hospital personnel. *Hepatology* 1992; 16:56–58.
22. Mitsui T, Iwano K, Masuko K, et al. Hepatitis C virus infection in medical personnel after needlestick accident. *Hepatology* 1992; 16: 1109–1114.

23. Kozoil DE, Henderson DK. Nosocomial viral hepatitis in health care workers. In: Mayhall CG, ed. *Hospital epidemiology and infection control*. Baltimore: Williams & Wilkins, 1996; 825–837.
24. Lo B, Steinbrook R. Health care workers infected with the human immunodeficiency virus. *JAMA* 1992; 267:1100–1105.
25. Ritter MA, French MLV, Eitzen HE, Gior TJ. The antimicrobial effctiveness of operative-site palparative agents. *J Bone Joint Surg [Am]* 1980; 62:826–828.
26. Alexander JW, Fischer JE, Boyajian M, Palmquist J, Morris MJ. The influence of hair removal methods on wound infections. *Arch Surg* 1983;118: 347–352.
27. Emergency Cardiac Care Committee and Subcommittee, American Heart Association: Guidelines for Cardiopulmonary Resuscitration and Emergency Cardiac Care. *JAMA* 1992; 268:2171–2302.
28. Tucker GT, Mather LE. Properties, absorption, disposition of local anesthetic agents. In: Cousins MJ, Bridenbaugh PO, eds. *Neural blockade in clinical anesthesia and management of pain,* 2nd ed. Philadelphia: JB Lippincott, 1988; 47–110.
29. Catterall W, Mackie K. Local anesthetics. In: Hardman JG, Gilman AG, Limbird LE, eds. *The therapeutic basis of therapeutics,* 9th ed. New York: McGraw Hill 1996; 331–347.
30. Swerdlow M. Medicolegal aspects of complications following pain relieving block. *Pain* 1982; 13:321–331.
31. Schimmer BP, Parker KL. Adrenocorticotrapic hormore. In: Hardman JG, Gilman AG, Limbird LE, eds. *The therapeutic basis of therapeutics,* 9th ed. New York: McGraw Hill, 1996; 1459–1485.
32. Brown RE. Monitoring and equipment for regional anesthesia. In: Raj PP, ed. *Clinical practice of regional anesthesiology*. New York: Churchill-Livingstone, 1991; 43–65.
33. Nelson DA. Dangers from methylprednisolone acetate therapy by intraspinal injection. *Arch Neurol* 1988; 45:805–806.
34. Tuel SM, Meythaler JM, Cross LL. Cushing's syndrome from epidural methylprednisolone. *Pain* 1990; 40:81–84.
35. Labat G. *Regional anesthesia: its technic and clinical application.* Philadelphia: WB Saunders, 1924.
36. Wassef MR. Interadductor approach to obturator nerve blockade for spastic conditions of adductor thigh muscles. *Regional Anesthesia* 1993; 18:13–17.
37. Pither CE, Raj PP, Ford DJ. The use of peripheral nerve stimulators for regional anesthesia: a review of experimental characteristics, techniques, and clinical applications. *Regional Anesthesia* 1985; 10:49–58.
38. Hullander M, Spillane W, Leivers D, Balasara Z. The use of Doppler ultrasound to assist with sciatic nerve blocks. *Regional Anesthesia* 1991; 16:282–284.
39. Smith BE, Fischer HBJ, Scott PV. Continuous sciatic nerve block. *Anaesthesia* 1984; 39:155–157.
40. Beck GP. Anterior approach to sciatic nerve block. *Anesthesiology* 1963; 24:222–224.
41. McNicol LR. Anterior approach to sciatic nerve block in children: Loss of resistance or nerve stimulator for identifying the neurovascular compartment. *Anesth Analg* 1987; 66:1199–1200.
42. Ichiyanagi K. Sciatic nerve block: lateral approach with patient supine. *Anesthesiology* 1959; 20:601–604.
43. Guardini R, Waldron BA, Wallace WA. Sciatic nerve block: a new lateral approach. *Acta Anaesthesiol Scand* 1985; 29:515–519.
44. Arendzen JH, van Duijn H, Beckmann MKF, Harlaar J, Vogelaar TW, Prevo AJH. Diagnostic blocks of the tibial nerve in spastic hemiparesis. *Scand J Rehabil Med* 1992; 24:75–81.
45. Lofstrom B. Block at the knee-joint. *Illustrated handbook in local anaesthesia.* Chicago: Year Book Medical, 1969.
46. Kofoed H. Peripheral nerve blocks at the knee and ankle in operations for common foot disorders. *Clin Orthop* 1982; 168:97–101.
47. Kempthorne PM, Brown TCK. Nerve blocks around the knee in children. *Anaesth Intens Care* 1984; 12:14–17.
48. Rorie DK, Byer DE, Nelson DO, Sittipong R, Johnon KA. Assessment of block of sciatic nerve in the popliteal fossa. *Anesth Analg* 1980; 59: 371–376.
49. Khalili AA. Physiatric management of spasticity by phenol nerve and motor point block. In: Ruskin AP, ed. *Current therapy in physiatry.* Philadelphia: WB Saunders, 1984.
50. Bekerman H, Lankhorst GJ, Verbeek ALM, Becher J. The effects of phenol nerve and muscle blocks in treating spasticity: review of the literature. *Crit Rev Phys Med Rehabil* 1996; 8:111–124.
51. Glenn NB. Nerve blocks. In: Glenn NB, Whyte J, eds. *The practical management of spasticity in children and adults.* Philadelphia: Lea & Febiger, 1990; 227–258.
52. Taddio A, Stevens B, Craig K, et al. Efficacy and safety of Lidocaine-Prilocaine cream for pain during circumcision. *N Engl J Med* 1997; 336:1197–1201.
53. Adams ME, ed. Viscosupplementation: a treatment of osteoarthritis. An International Symposium, Ottawa, ON. *J Rheumatol* 1993; 20.
54. Buckwalter JA, Woo Sly. Tissue effects of medications in sports injuries. In: DeLee JC, Drez D, eds. *Orthopaedic sports medicine: principles and practice.* Philadelphia: WB Saunders, 1994; 73–81.
55. Dwyer A, Aprill C, Bogduk N. Cervical zygapophyseal joint pain patterns 1: a study in normal volunteers. *Spine* 1990; 15:453–457.

ADDITIONAL READINGS

Cousins MJ, Bridenbaugh PO, eds. *Neural blockade in clinical anesthesia and management of pain,* 2nd ed. Philadelphia: JB Lippincott, 1988.

Gatter RA. Arthrocentesis technique and intrasynovial therapy. In: Koopman WJ, ed. *Arthritis and allied conditions—a textbook of rheumatology,* 13th ed. Baltimore: Williams & Wilkins, 1997; 751–775.

Lennard TA. *Physiatric injections.* Philadelphia: Hanley & Belfus, 1995; 14–27.

Raj PP, ed. *Clinical practice of regional anesthesiology.* New York: Churchill-Livingstone, 1991.

Steinbrocker O, Neustadt DH. *Aspiration and injection therapy in arthritis and musculoskeletal disorders—a handbook on technique and management.* Hagerstown, MD: Harper & Row, 1972.

Travell JG, Simons DG. *Myofascial pain and dysfunction.* Vol. 1. Baltimore: Williams & Wilkins, 1983.

Travell JG, Simons DG. *Myofascial pain and dysfunction.* Vol. 2. Baltimore: Williams & Wilkins, 1992.

Rehabilitation Medicine: Principles and Practice, Third Edition,
edited by Joel A. DeLisa and Bruce M. Gans.
Lippincott–Raven Publishers, Philadelphia © 1998.

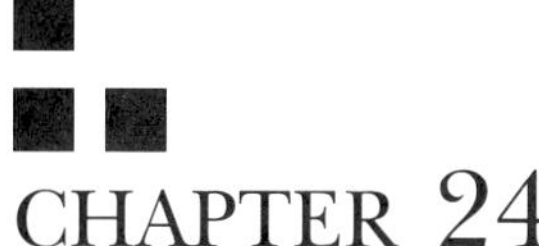

CHAPTER 24

Functional Neuromuscular Stimulation

John Chae, Ronald J. Triolo, Kevin Kilgore, and Graham H. Creasey

The prevention of complications of immobility, implementation of compensatory strategies, and facilitation of psychosocial adjustment to disability and community reintegration are central to the rehabilitation management of persons with hemiplegia, paraplegia, and tetraplegia. The devastating effects of persistent neurologic impairment on disability, handicap, and quality of life are still all too common for many with upper motor neuron paralysis. The challenge before the medical rehabilitation community is to break the glass ceiling on rehabilitation outcome imposed by this persistent neurologic impairment. With recent advances in clinical medicine and biomedical engineering, functional neuromuscular stimulation (FNS) can now be added to the physiatric armamentarium to decrease the debilitating effects of upper motor neuron paralysis. Physiatrists must have an understanding of how the various stimulation systems function, as well as of their strengths, limitations and risks, and indications and contraindications. This information must be conveyed appropriately and accurately to patients so that they may have a clear understanding of how these devices may impact their quality of life.

Neuromuscular stimulation can be broadly categorized as therapeutic or functional. Therapeutic neuromuscular stimulation is defined as the use of repetitive stimulation of paralyzed muscles to minimize specific impairments such as limited range of motion, motor weakness, spasticity, and cardiovascular deconditioning. Although therapeutic neuromuscular stimulation may, and hopefully will, lead to functional improvements, the electrical stimulation does not directly provide function. FNS is defined as the use of electrical stimulation to activate paralyzed muscles in a precise sequence to assist in the performance of activities of daily living. Devices or systems that provide FNS are also appropriately called neuroprostheses.

This chapter will focus on the application of FNS in tetraplegia and paraplegia secondary to traumatic spinal cord injury, and to a lesser degree hemiplegia due to cerebral dysfunction such as stroke or traumatic brain injury. The physiology of neuromuscular stimulation will be reviewed. The components of FNS systems and their evolution in design will be presented. The clinical implementation of FNS will be discussed with respect to upper extremity, lower extremity, and bladder applications. Finally, perspectives on the future developments and directions will be presented.

PHYSIOLOGY OF FUNCTIONAL NEUROMUSCULAR STIMULATION

Excitation of Nervous Tissue by Electrical Stimulation

A short pulse of electrical current applied to the membrane of a neuron can cause the generation of an action potential in that neuron. The action potential produced by electrical stimulation in this manner is identical to the action potential that would be generated by natural physiologic means, and it has the same ''all-or-none'' property. The action potential propagates in both directions along the axon. An action potential is initiated in a neuron by any stimulus pulse that delivers a sufficient charge, i.e., the appropriate combination of pulse duration and current amplitude. The lowest level of charge that will generate an action potential is defined as the stimulus threshold.

The stimulus threshold of any neuron is inversely proportional to the diameter of the neuron. Therefore, large-diameter neurons, such as alpha motor neurons, have the lowest thresholds for stimulation (1,2). Small-diameter neurons, such as C pain fibers, have the highest thresholds for stimula-

J. Chae: Center for Physical Medicine and Rehabilitation, Case Western Reserve University, MetroHealth Medical Center, Cleveland, Ohio 44109.

R. J. Triolo: Departments of Orthopaedics and Biomedical Engineering, Case Western Reserve University, MetroHealth Medical Center, Cleveland, Ohio 44109.

K. Kilgore: Department of Orthopaedics, MetroHealth Medical Center, Cleveland, Ohio 44109.

G. H. Creasey: Regional Spinal Cord Injury Service, MetroHealth Medical Center, Cleveland, Ohio 44109.

tion. As a result, stimulation applied near a nerve will preferentially stimulate larger diameter fibers at lower levels of stimulation. As the stimulus level is increased, smaller diameter fibers will be stimulated. This property of electrical stimulation is referred to as reverse recruitment order. Note that this is the reverse of the physiologic size principle (3), which states that smaller muscle fibers are recruited initially, followed by larger fibers.

The stimulus current diminishes as a function of the distance from the stimulating source (electrode) (2,4). Therefore, neurons that are farther away from an electrode are less likely to receive stimulation at a level above threshold. For example, stimulation applied by surface electrodes placed on the skin are more likely to stimulate the sensory and pain fibers in the skin than the deeper motor neurons because of their proximity to the electrode, even though the motor neurons are much larger.

The threshold for direct muscle fiber excitation is about 100 to 1,000 times higher than the threshold for nerve stimulation (2). Therefore, it is unlikely that direct muscle stimulation occurs as a result of any of the electrical stimulation paradigms described in this chapter. Although FNS systems are often described as involving stimulation of a muscle, technically they are referring to stimulation of the nerves innervating the muscle, resulting in muscle contraction.

Muscle Response to Nerve Stimulation

Muscle Alterations Induced by Electrical Activation

Muscle fibers are divided into three or four groups relating to their contractile properties. At one end of the spectrum are muscle fibers that have fast twitch responses, generate high levels of force, and fatigue fairly quickly. These fibers are referred to as fast-twitch glycolytic (FG) fibers, or type II (4,5) because they have a high capacity for glycolytic metabolism. These muscle fibers are generally larger and are innervated by larger neurons. At the other end of the spectrum are the slow-twitch oxidative (SO) fibers, or type I (4), which have a high capacity for oxidative metabolism. Although they have slow-twitch response and lower force levels, they are fatigue resistant. These fibers tend to be innervated by smaller diameter neurons. Muscle fiber types between these two extremes have also been identified, and they exhibit some of the properties of both types (4,5).

Fatigue resistance is probably the most desirable muscle quality for most electrical stimulation applications involving stimulation of skeletal muscle. Activities such as standing, walking, grasping, and reaching do not necessarily have to be achieved quickly, just consistently. Therefore, recruitment of slow-twitch, slow-fatiguing (SO) muscle fibers is most desirable for FNS. However, there are two conditions that impede this goal. First, as described previously, large fibers have lower thresholds for stimulation. Therefore, the large fast-fatiguing fibers are recruited preferentially. Secondly, in the case of paralyzed muscle, disuse atrophy tends to convert muscle fibers to the fast-twitch, fast-fatiguing type (6). In addition, these atrophied muscles also generate low levels of force.

Fortunately, this muscle atrophy can be reversed using chronic electrical stimulation. Peckham et al. (7) demonstrated that chronic stimulation of 8 to 24 hours per day resulted in changes in the metabolic makeup of muscle fibers in cats. It was then demonstrated that chronic stimulation in paralyzed humans could achieve the same results. Marsolais and Kobetic (8) studied percutaneous stimulation of the paralyzed quadriceps muscle. Stimulation was applied for up to 3 hours per day, and in at least one case there was a 10-fold increase in knee torque after 10 weeks. Recently, Kagaya et al. (9) used percutaneous stimulation in five spinal cord–injured patients for 6 months. They found increases in knee torque from 1.7 to 5.8 times with a corresponding increase in muscle bulk. These studies demonstrated the feasibility of functional use of electrically stimulated muscle. All current FNS applications use some form of muscle conditioning patterned after these studies.

Upper and Lower Motor Neuron Damage

Successful stimulation of muscle for functional purposes requires that the lower (alpha) motor neuron (LMN) be intact. In cases of spinal cord injury, there is frequently some damage to the LMN pool at the level of injury (10). If most or all of the LMNs to a particular muscle are damaged, then it will not be possible to obtain functional levels of force from the muscle with electrical stimulation. Electrical exercise will not reverse atrophy in fibers if the LMN has been damaged. Extensive LMN damage is therefore a contraindication for FNS, and diseases or traumas that involve peripheral nerve damage (such as amyotrophic lateral sclerosis or brachial plexus injury) are not likely to benefit from FNS.

Modulation of Muscle Force

The muscle force generated by electrical stimulation can be modulated by altering the stimulation parameters. There are three stimulus parameters that are controlled in FNS systems: (a) stimulus pulse duration, (b) current amplitude (or voltage amplitude), and (c) frequency. At least one of these three parameters can be changed on a pulse-by-pulse basis by any FNS system. In addition to these three parameters, the shape of the stimulus waveform (rectangular biphasic, exponentially decaying, triangular monophasic, etc.) also can affect the stimulated response, although waveform shape is typically constant in any single system.

When a single stimulus pulse is delivered to a neuron resulting in the generation of an action potential, the motor unit will respond with a twitch contraction of the muscle. For a single motor unit, the magnitude of the twitch will depend on the size of the stimulus pulse and the size of the motor unit. The rate of increase and decrease of the twitch depends on the muscle fiber type. A single muscle twitch reaches peak force in 10 to 50 milliseconds and returns to baseline force within 40 to 100 milliseconds. When repeated stimulus pulses are delivered to a nerve, the muscle twitch response will begin before the previous twitch is complete. As a result, the muscle force begins to summate so that the peak force at each twitch is progressively higher and higher. At low pulse rates (less than 10 Hz), the individual pulses can be seen in the force output as a sinusoidal ripple. This ripple will eventually disappear at higher frequencies, and the contraction will be fused (tetany). However, muscle fibers fatigue faster at higher rates of stimulation. In practical FNS systems, there is a trade-off between obtaining a smooth contraction of the muscle and keeping the fatigue rate low. The ideal frequencies vary depending on the type of function and the type of muscle. For the upper extremity, this frequency is typically 12 to 16 Hz. For lower extremity systems, frequencies are typically 25 Hz.

As the duration or amplitude of a stimulus pulse is increased, the stimulus threshold will be reached for neurons farther from the electrode. Therefore, more neurons will generate action potentials, resulting in a stronger muscle contraction. This is known as spatial summation. It is the primary method used for modulation of muscle force in FNS systems. The mechanisms of force modulation are the same regardless of whether pulse duration or amplitude is used as the controlled stimulus parameter. Crago et al. (11) demonstrated that modulation of pulse duration required less charge transfer per stimulus pulse at any given force level. However, the decision whether to modulate duration or amplitude is usually determined by stimulator circuitry design considerations rather than to the physiologic response.

Although force can be modulated by adjusting the stimulation parameters, the force output is also dependent on several electrode–nerve geometry-dependent properties. For example, muscle length–dependent properties have significant effect on the moments generated at a given joint for several reasons. First, and most important for electrical stimulation, the contraction or passive stretch of a muscle can result in a change in the electrode position relative to the neurons being recruited. This movement can substantially change the recruitment curve characteristics (12,13). The recruitment curve describes the relationship between the stimulus level and the generated force and is almost always nonlinear (11) because the threshold for any neuron is dependent on both the size of the neuron and the distance between the neuron and the stimulating electrode. Secondly, muscles have an inherent length–tension property, so that even at a constant level of recruitment, there will be changes in the force generated by the muscle contractile elements. Finally, changes in tendon moment arm as a function of joint angle affects the moment generated about the joint even if the tension in the tendon is constant. Another electrode–nerve geometry-dependent phenomenon is that the stimulus field that emanates from a single electrode is not affected by anatomically defined muscle boundaries. Therefore, a single electrode is likely to recruit motor units from more than one muscle. The degree to which this happens will depend on the relative location of the muscle innervation to the electrode and the excitability of the nerves to the different muscles. In most functional applications, it is usually desirable to isolate the recruitment to single muscles or muscle groups.

Safe Stimulation of Living Tissue

Effect of Stimulation on Electrode Materials

The parameters for safe stimulation and materials for safe electrodes have been experimentally established (2). Improper stimulation can result in electrochemical changes in the electrode material, leading to corrosion or dissolution of metal ions. Strong negative charge on the electrode can result in hydrogen formation at the electrode. In addition, reactions at the electrode can cause changes in pH that can result in possible tissue necrosis. Despite the potential detrimental reactions that can occur with current levels of stimulation, safe stimulation can be achieved at current levels that are sufficient to stimulate muscles at functionally useful levels.

Tissue damage is related to the charge per unit area of stimulation. It is not related to the voltage of the stimulus. The critical factors for safe stimulation are the current amplitude and the electrode–tissue contact area. It is therefore safer to use constant-current stimulation for electrodes within muscle or nerve tissue because it provides control of the charge density delivered to the tissue, assuming that the contact area of the electrode remains constant. When constant voltage stimulation is used, the current densities are uncontrolled and can become very high if the resistance of the electrode–tissue interface becomes high. Therefore, stimulus current should always be regulated for electrodes located within living tissue.

There are other factors to consider when surface electrodes are used. The electrode–tissue contact area is generally not constant. If the electrode pulls away from the skin, the contact area can become very small. When constant-current stimulation is used, the same amount of current will be driven through a very small contact area, resulting in high current densities. This can result in burning of the tissue. However, when using constant voltage stimulation in this same situation, the increased resistance will result in decreased current delivered to the tissue. Although this may be safer, it results in variations in the stimulation delivered to the muscle, changing the force output. No matter what type of stimulation is used, it is important to maintain good contact between the electrode and skin.

Balanced biphasic stimulation should always be used. The balancing pulse (typically an anodic pulse) balances the charge injected into the tissue and greatly reduces the potential for damage. There is never a reason to use monophasic stimulation for functional intramuscular electrical stimulation.

Effect of Stimulation on Living Tissue

Stimulation of muscles with electrodes applied on the skin surface may result in warming and reddening of the skin and, in certain conditions, burning of the tissue. The warming and reddening of the skin are due to the increase in circulation and are generally benign. However, if the current densities are too high, burning of the tissue can occur. In clinical use, surface stimulation parameters can vary considerably. Typical parameters include amplitudes of up to 100 mA, pulse durations of up to 400 milliseconds and frequencies that range from 15 to 50 Hz. Surface stimulation should be used with caution and with frequent examination of the skin when applied to patients with impaired sensation and cognition.

The risk for muscle damage is more significant with intramuscular stimulation. Safe stimulus levels for balanced biphasic stimulation have been established at 0.4 μC/mm^2 (2). Therefore, the maximum stimulus levels depend on the stimulating surface area of the electrode. The percutaneous electrodes used for many neuromuscular applications have surface areas of approximately 10 mm^2 (2). Safe stimulation levels with this type of electrode are biphasic pulses with an amplitude of 20 mA and a pulse duration of 200 milliseconds. Frequencies are typically in the range of 10 to 50 Hz, although frequency is not a factor in adverse tissue response to stimulation. Intramuscular stimulation using these parameters has been applied for human use for over 15 years without any evidence of significant muscle damage (14).

Most direct nerve stimulation is accomplished using a nerve cuff electrode that encompasses the nerve trunk. Nerve tissue damage can occur through the same electrochemical mechanism as muscle tissue damage, but it also can occur through mechanical movement of the cuff relative to the nerve. In addition, tissue growth around nerve cuff electrodes can result in compression of the nerve and, therefore, secondary damage (15). Despite these potential problems, nerve cuffs have been used safely in many applications (16–18). Stimulation of nerves typically requires about one tenth of the current necessary for intramuscular stimulation.

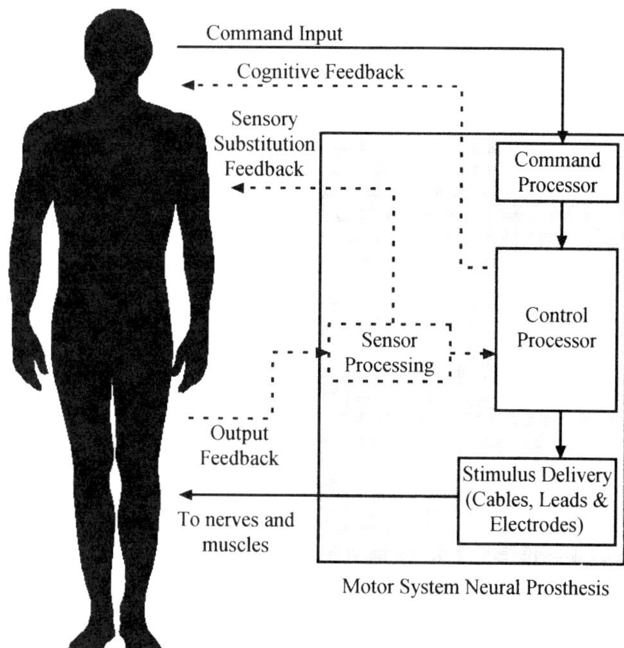

FIG. 24-1. Schematic representation of a basic motor system neuroprosthesis. *Dotted lines* indicate optional components for advanced control. Components of such systems can be implanted if communication channels are maintained with external components via RF links.

SYSTEM COMPONENTS AND EVOLUTION IN DESIGN

System-Level Overview of FNS Technology

All FNS systems intended to provide motor function share several common elements. The fundamental components of a neuroprosthesis for motor function are represented schematically as solid lines in Figure 24-1. First, the user of an FNS system must have a way to communicate his or her intent to the device in order to control the resulting limb movement. This command input can take any number of forms, from simple switch closures and timer settings to more complicated sequences of EMG activity from muscles still under volitional control (8,19–23). Once the command is delivered, the device must process the input, which could be interpreted differently depending on the prior history of stimulation, the current state of the device, or the status of the limb. After the command processor unambiguously recognizes the intent of the user, the neuroprosthesis must take action. The control processor selects the appropriate channels (corresponding to the nerves or muscles required to effect the intended motion) as well as the relative timing, intensity, and frequency of stimulation. These parameters are then used by the stimulus delivery subsystem to create the stimulation waveforms and deliver current to the neural structures. These components of the system include cables, leads, and electrodes that interface with the biologic system. Optional features of a motor prosthesis are indicated by the dotted lines in Figure 24-1. The user can be made aware of what the system is doing through cognitive feedback of the state of the device via displays, warning lights, or audio tones. The majority of clinically applied FNS systems operate open loop; that is, they are unresponsive to the environment and do not automatically correct for errors that arise between the intended and actual motions of the limbs. Sensors have been used experimentally to feed the state of the biologic system (joint angles, contact forces, etc.) back to the controller. Such closed-loop systems require sensors to provide output feedback and a sensor processor to monitor the actions of the limbs and allow the control processor to adjust stimulus levels automatically without conscious input from the user. Finally, the user can be informed of the orientation and state of his own body (rather than the state of the device) through substitute sensory feedback. In this scheme, the closed-loop sensor signals are used to modulate tactile stimulation to sensate areas, or provide other indications of the status of the limbs and joints and their interaction with the environment (24,25).

Various portions of the neuroprosthesis depicted in the shaded region of Figure 24-1 can be made implantable. FNS systems can be completely external, in which case no foreign material is introduced into the body and only the stimulating current crosses the skin boundary. When subsystems are implanted (e.g., the electrodes and/or stimulus delivery circuitry), communication must be maintained with those parts of the system remaining outside of the body. This can be achieved via direct percutaneous connection or radiofrequency (RF) transmission. In the latter case, nothing crosses the skin except electromagnetic energy, reducing the likelihood of infection present with percutaneous connections and improving the convenience of donning and doffing over completely external systems. Implanting components of the system requires additional circuitry (RF transmitters and receivers) to complete the communication pathways indicated by the arrows in Figure 24-1, and may increase the complexity of the design. Despite the required surgery, implantable systems offer the advantages of placing the stimulating electrodes in close proximity to neural structures, greatly increasing the selectivity and efficiency of activation while simultaneously reducing the current required.

Interfacing with the Nervous System: Electrode and Lead Technology

Electrodes for FNS applications are classified according to the location of their stimulating surfaces. They are usually designed to activate nerves in the periphery, and fall into three broad classes: surface electrodes applied to the skin, muscle-based electrodes, and nerve-based electrodes. Alternatively, lead wires connecting the electrodes to the stimulus generating circuitry are described by the course they take and the tissues through which they pass. Electrode leads can be classified as external, percutaneous, or implanted. All surface electrodes will use external leads, whereas muscle- and nerve-based electrodes will be connected to either percutaneous or implanted lead wires.

Surface electrodes deliver charge to the motor nerve transcutaneously. They are affixed to the surface of the skin over the motorpoint, the location exhibiting the largest mechanical response from the target muscle at the lowest levels of stimulation. Transcutaneous stimulation with surface electrodes offers several distinct advantages: (a) The electrodes are generally easy to apply and remove; (b) the stimulation technique is noninvasive and therefore reversible; (c) the use of surface electrodes can be easily learned and applied in the clinic; and (d) neuromuscular stimulators and surface electrodes are relatively inexpensive, readily available, and produced by numerous manufacturers. Stimulation with surface electrodes is the most widely used technique for therapeutic applications.

Despite their apparent convenience when applied individually in small numbers, surface electrodes for transcutaneous stimulation also have several disadvantages: (a) They tend to activate any neural structure lying beneath them, making it difficult to selectively stimulate the motor neuron for a single isolated muscle; (b) daily doffing and donning can complicate use, especially if electrode positions vary slightly from day to day, producing different stimulated responses; and (c) multiple electrode systems rapidly become impractical as the number of muscles (and stimulus channels) required to perform a specific task increases to six or more (26). In this situation, donning, doffing and connecting multiple electrodes can become cumbersome.

In addition, the skin offers substantial resistance to the flow of current. Removing oils, hair, or dead skin cells by cleaning or shaving the skin can reduce the skin resistance and improve current delivery to the deeper neural tissues. Precautions also need to be taken to ensure intimate contact of the electrode with the skin through some highly conductive medium or electrolytic gel. As noted earlier, loss of skin contact will create an area of high charge density, which increases the risk for burning. Large currents may be required to drive sufficient charge through the skin and intervening tissues between the electrode and the peripheral nerve, decreasing the efficiency of surface stimulation. In many cases, cutaneous pain receptors are excited as current passes through these tissues, and patients with preserved or heightened sensation may find it difficult to tolerate surface stimulation at the levels required to produce a motor response. They also have been reported to cause skin irritations in certain individuals (27).

Muscle-based electrodes bypass the high resistance of the skin and cutaneous sensory fibers. They provide a means to produce contractions more efficiently (with small currents) and more selectively than surface electrodes. Stimulation can also be more comfortable as more of the muscle can be recruited without eliciting the sensation of pain from the cutaneous fibers. For these reasons, muscle-based electrodes are preferable for many functional applications of FNS that require discrete and independent control of several isolated muscles. The stimulating tips of intramuscular electrodes reside in the muscle tissue itself and generally include a barbing mechanism to snare the tissue and provide a degree of immediate fixation and resistance to movement until encapsulation occurs. Depending on their intended application, intramuscular electrodes have been designed to be introduced either percutaneously (28–30) or in an open surgical procedure (31). In addition to their selectivity, low current requirements, and ease of implantation, intramuscular electrodes allow access to deep neural structures that are difficult to approach surgically. When used with percutaneous leads, they also can be removed easily and provide a means for producing high-quality contractions on either an acute or longer term basis. Early movement away from the target nerve branch within the first 6 weeks postimplantation (before encapsulation is complete) can result in altered stimulated responses and is the most frequently observed failure mode of these devices (29,30). Epimysial electrodes are sutured directly to the epimysium or fascia to eliminate this early movement and provide immediate and permanent fixation. Because they require a surgical installation, they are used almost exclusively with implantable leads and stimulators (32).

Nerve-based electrodes have a more intimate contact with the peripheral nerve and therefore require even less current than muscle-based electrodes to produce a contraction. They take the form of epineural electrodes, which are sutured to the connective tissue on either side of a motor nerve; cuff electrodes, which envelope the nerve; and intrafascicular or intraneural electrodes, which are still laboratory-based investigational tools. Epineural and nerve cuff designs have both been used as stimulating electrodes in FNS systems to restore motor function in spinal cord injury and stroke (33–36). Cuff electrodes also have been configured to record from afferent nerves in attempts to use the natural sensors in the body to provide feedback signals to control and adjust the stimulation (37).

Electrodes are connected to stimulating or recording circuitry through lead wires. Percutaneous leads have been designed to interface chronically indwelling intramuscular and epimysial electrodes to circuitry external to the body while maintaining a barrier to infection. These devices take the form of multiple strands of stainless steel insulated in Teflon that are helically wound to form a thin, flexible cable of small enough diameter for the tissue to heal around as it exits the skin. The helical configuration converts bending motions to torsional stresses in the coils of the lead, providing mechanical resistance to fracture due to metal fatigue. Alternately, the leads can be coiled around a central core of suture material or wound a second time to form a compound helix to offer additional flexibility near the critical stimulating tip (30). The open coils also promote ingrowth and assist with fixation. A thin layer of endothelial cells proliferates around the coils near the skin surface at sufficient depth to provide a barrier to infection. Because of their small diameter, helically coiled percutaneous leads from multiple electrodes can exit the skin in relatively high densities. These electrodes are then connected to an external stimulator.

Although they facilitate donning and doffing of neuroprosthesis by eliminating the need to apply individual electrodes and simplifying connecting to other electronic components, percutaneous interfaces require continual attention from the user. They must be cleaned, dressed, and properly inspected and maintained. These leads are subject to breakage at areas of high shear stress, such as where they cross fascial planes. Although they can remain functional for years without infection or complication, percutaneous leads are usually reserved for acute applications and are generally considered to be ill-suited for long-term clinical use.

Implanted leads can assume larger dimensions than percutaneous lead wires because they need to be more robust and resistant to failure, and are not required to cross the skin. One popular configuration consists of two Teflon-insulated stranded stainless-steel cables wound in tandem with each other (38). The redundant conductor assembly is then enclosed in an elastomer sheath to prevent ingrowth, provide mechanical stability, and allow the leads to slide through the tissues between the electrode and the implanted stimulating circuitry. To promote serviceability and allow repair or revision of implanted FNS systems, provisions have been made in several designs to isolate system subcomponents from each other via high reliability implantable connectors (39). In-line connectors permit the surgical removal and repositioning of individual electrodes with minimal dissection and without extensive exposure of larger implanted circuit packages. These designs reduce the risk of infection and minimize the likelihood of damage to other implanted components during maintenance procedures. Implantable electronic components also can be designed as passive devices that derive their power from the RF signals providing the communication channels to external command or control processors. Systems using this configuration eliminate the need for additional surgery to replace internal batteries.

UPPER EXTREMITY APPLICATIONS

Objectives of Upper Extremity FNS Systems

FNS has been used to provide grasp and release for individuals with a spinal cord injury at the cervical level (40–70). The objectives of these systems are to reduce the need for individuals to rely on assistance from others, reduce the need for adaptive equipment, reduce the need to wear braces or other orthotic devices, and reduce the time it takes to perform tasks. Neuroprostheses make use of the patient's own paralyzed musculature to provide the power for grasp and the patient's voluntary musculature to control the grasp. These systems are now available clinically and, although they do not provide normal grasp function, they do enable patients to perform tasks more independently. Typically, patients use the neuroprosthesis for such tasks as eating, personal hygiene, writing, and office tasks.

Candidate Selection

The most clinically advanced upper extremity FNS systems have been applied to individuals with C5 and C6 motor level complete spinal cord injury. These patients have fairly good control of shoulder motion and have good elbow flexion. They also may have good wrist extension. Their function enables them to move their arm in space and bring their hand to their face, but they do not have the ability to grasp and hold utensils. For these patients, the provision of grasp opening and closing using FNS provides a distinct functional benefit. For injuries at the C4 level, control of elbow flexion must be provided by stimulation of the biceps and/or brachialis, or by a mechanical or surgical means. FNS has been applied to a limited extent to these individuals, but there are no clinically deployed systems for this population to date. For individuals with strong C6 or C7 level function, there are other surgical options such as tendon transfers to provide function, and FNS is usually not indicated at the present time.

Electrical stimulation is applied to intact motor neurons, as described earlier. With any spinal cord injury, there is some peripheral nerve damage, typically occurring in the nerves just below the level of functional preservation. For the C5 and C6 spinal cord injuries, the muscles most likely to sustain LMN damage are the wrist extensors. Peckham and Keith (71) found that 80% to 100% of the muscles necessary for grasp had sufficient innervation intact to generate functional levels of force. In many cases, other paralyzed muscles can be used to substitute for the function that is not available, although this may require surgical intervention (54).

Neurologic stability is necessary for implanted systems; therefore, implant surgery is not performed until at least 1 year after injury. Joint contractures must be corrected or the grasp functions will be limited. Spasticity must be under control. For implant systems, problems such as persistent urinary tract infections or other chronic infections are contraindications. Neither age nor time postinjury appears to be a major factor when considering neuroprosthetic applications.

Individuals who are motivated and desire greater independence are the best candidates for FNS. In addition, most current FNS systems still require assistance in donning the device, so it is necessary for the individual to have good attendant support.

Operating Principles of Upper Extremity Systems

Grasp Patterns

Two basic grasp patterns are generally provided for functional activities: lateral pinch and palmar prehension, as shown in Figure 24-2 (64). The choice of these two grasp patterns was based on the work of Keller et al. (71), who showed that these two grasp patterns accounted for about 90% of the acquiring and manipulating of objects encountered in everyday activities. Other grasp patterns have been described for use in FNS, including a pinch grip between the index and thumb (72), as well as parallel extension grasp with finger extension and thumb abduction (47).

The lateral pinch is used for holding small utensils such as a fork, spoon, or pencil. In the open phase of this grasp, the fingers and thumb are extended. The fingers are then fully flexed at all joints while the thumb remains extended. The thumb is then flexed against the lateral aspect of the index finger to produce pinch. Strong pinch forces can be achieved, typically up to 30 newtons. Palmar prehension is used for acquiring large objects. The fingers are extended and the thumb is posted in full abduction. The fingers then flex against the thumb, ideally resulting in contact between the tip of the thumb and the tips of the index and long fingers. Thumb flexion can be added to increase grasp force if needed. The pinch grip is a modification of the palmar grasp, where the index finger and thumb make contact, whereas the other fingers remain extended. This grasp is used for picking up and manipulating small objects. The parallel extension grasp involves extension of the fingers and adduction of the thumb. Typically this can be accomplished with stimulation of the ulnar nerve at the wrist, recruiting thumb adductor and finger intrinsic muscles. This grasp is used for holding things in the hand, such as playing cards. Stimulated control of the wrist is sometimes incorporated into the grasp patterns, although most systems use braces to fix the wrist if the patient does not have voluntary control of wrist extension. Without stabilization, stimulation of the finger flexors generates a strong flexion moment about the wrist.

Muscles Stimulated

Essentially every muscle in the forearm and hand has been used in upper extremity FNS systems. However, at least five

A 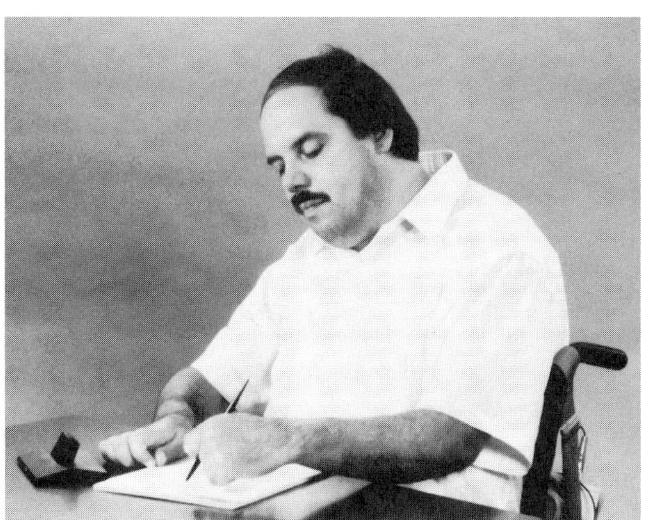

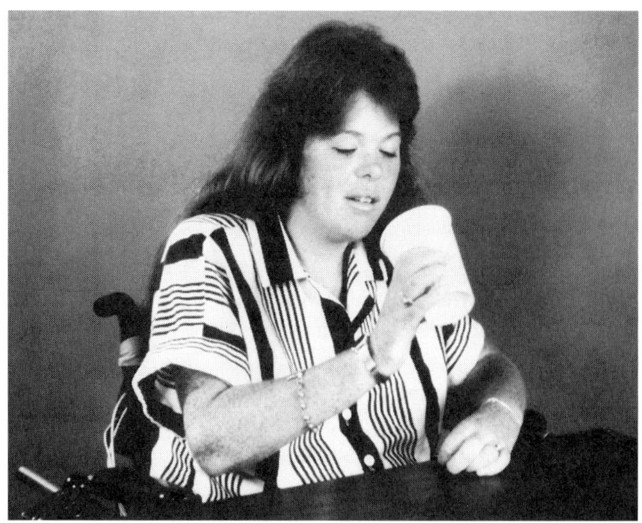 B

FIG. 24-2. Patients using lateral **(A)** and palmar **(B)** grasp patterns to perform activities. (Courtesy of the Cleveland FES Center.)

muscles are necessary to provide a palmar and lateral grasp. The most frequently used muscles are the adductor pollicis (AdP), extensor pollicis longus (EPL), abductor pollicis brevis (AbPB), extensor digitorum communis (EDC), and flexor digitorum superficialis (FDS). Typically, more force is required in flexion, so a second thumb and finger flexor are utilized, usually the flexor digitorum profundus (FDP) and flexor pollicis longus (FPL). Wrist extensors, forearm pronators, and even the finger intrinsic muscles also have been used.

Electrodes

There are three major categories of electrodes used in upper extremity clinical FNS systems: surface, percutaneous, and implanted, as previously described. Surface electrodes are obviously the least invasive but also provide the poorest recruitment properties and require the most time to don and doff. Percutaneous electrodes provide good recruitment properties, but risks for skin infection exist. Implanted electrodes are used in conjunction with implanted stimulator units. They typically provide the best recruitment properties but require surgical exposure for placement (73,74).

Controller/Stimulator

Every neuroprosthesis has an electronic controller/stimulator unit that is typically driven by microprocessor circuitry. The controller/stimulator can be divided into three or four units: (a) a stimulation output stage, (b) a control signal conditioning stage, (c) circuitry to convert the control signal to the necessary stimulus levels, and (d) power supply and regulation. In some cases the stimulator is implanted, but in all applications to date, there is an external control unit. This unit contains the power and intelligence for the system. Grasp patterns are stored in lookup tables in these units. Stimulation is applied through as many as 30 electrodes in the different muscles of the forearm and hand. Stimulus output parameters and waveforms vary considerably among different applications.

Control Methods

Identifying a method of control is probably the biggest challenge in upper extremity neuroprosthetics. Because of their extensive paralysis, quadriplegic individuals have few voluntary movements that can be used as command sources. Ideally, the control source will have the following characteristics (68,75). The control method must not interfere with the other functional movements or activities. It must be discrete, cosmetically acceptable, and should not draw attention to disability. The computational delay must be small. The method should be repeatable, that is, the same input always gives the same output. The method should also be reliable, that is, it distinguishes between user issued commands and background noise or other commands. The control should be natural, easy to learn, and to some degree subconscious (i.e., requires little attention from the user). The system must be durable, and, if necessary, donning and doffing should be easy. Finally, the system should be reasonably priced. None of the control methods developed to date meet all of these characteristics, although each control method excels in a few. The ultimate choice of the control method for a neuroprosthesis depends on the user's goals and physical abilities.

Signals issued by the user are used in one of two ways to control grasp: (a) as a proportional command signal or (b) as a state or logic command. For a proportional command, the magnitude of the system response is graded according to the magnitude of the command signal. State command is typically an on/off or yes/no command, initiating a change in the mode of operation of the system. Many FNS systems use a proportional control for grasp opening and closing and use one or more state commands to switch between different grasp patterns or perform other features.

The simplest form of control is to use switches mounted on the wheelchair or some other location within reach of the patient. They are simple to use and understand, and they provide a reliable and repeatable signal. The major disadvantage of switches is that they require the user to occupy their opposite arm to control their instrumented arm. This usually means that tasks have to be performed one handed. This disadvantage is especially relevant for application to upper extremity hemiplegia. It also can be difficult to locate switches where they are always accessible to the patient.

Movement of the contralateral shoulder to control grasp opening and closing has been a popular choice for proportional control of neuroprostheses (41,45,75–78). Specifically, movement of the sternoclavicular joint is used as a proportional control source for grasp opening and closing. The sternoclavicular angle is determined using a joystick transducer or resistive tube that is taped to the chest. This type of control allows both hands to be free to perform tasks, although there is some interference with two-handed movements (75). The use of shoulder control generally requires that the system has a lock feature because it is too difficult to maintain the shoulder in one position in order to hold the grasp closed for a long period of time such as for writing or eating. The lock enables the user to disconnect the grasp from the proportional control source so that the grasp remains at a constant level regardless of shoulder position (75).

The use of wrist extension/flexion to control grasp opening and closing has been another popular choice (67,79,80). Control of grasp by wrist motion works in coordination with the tenodesis grasp that patients are already trained to use. Wrist extension closes the grasp, and wrist flexion (by gravity) opens the grasp. If a lock is necessary, it is usually provided by a switch. Wrist control is much more amenable to bilateral control than shoulder control because the control is derived from the instrumented hand.

There are fewer options for higher level spinal cord–injured patients. Head movement or orientation also has been used as both a proportional and logic command (45,63,70). Respiration control such as siff/puff has been used for higher level injuries (49). One major disadvantage is that it is difficult to use while eating, which is one of the tasks for which the neuroprosthesis is frequently used.

Voice control is a potentially appealing control method because of the potential to obtain a wide variety of control signals. However, there are two major problems with the implementation of voice control in a neuroprosthesis. First, as with respiration control, it is difficult to use while eating or drinking. Secondly, this method does not meet the criterion of being discreet, and patients consider it to be socially unacceptable to talk to their hand to make it work. It is also more difficult to implement a proportional control using voice commands. Nevertheless, some systems have been developed using voice commands (44,45,60) and have met with some success.

The use of myoelectric signals (MES) from muscles under voluntary control by the patient provides a great variety of potential signal sources. MES were used in the earliest implementation of FNS to the upper extremity (81). There are two major difficulties that have to be overcome to use MES control. First, suitable control muscles have to be found. Potential control muscles include those synergistic to the grasp movement, such as wrist extensors and, to a lesser extent, brachioradialis, as well as nonsynergists such as sternocleidomastoid and auricularis posterior. Secondly, the MES must be obtained in the presence of stimulus artifacts that are huge in comparison with the signal and tend to saturate the amplifiers. These difficulties have been overcome to various degrees in different implementations (63,80,82,83).

Feedback Mechanisms

Feedback in neuroprosthetic systems has been provided in three sensory modalities. First, all clinically deployed systems use visual feedback between the user and his or her hand. Second, audio feedback is frequently used to provide simple system state information (on/off etc.). Finally, electrotactile feedback can be provided by stimulating the skin surface. This can be provided comfortably, and patients describe the sensation as a buzzing or tapping. Both the stimulus frequency and intensity can be used to encode different types of information.

Clinically Evaluated Applications

There are four separate FNS neuroprosthetic systems designed to provide upper extremity function that are currently undergoing multicenter trials and have been transferred out of the research setting and into industry. Table 24-1 shows a comparison of the different features of these four applications.

Two surface stimulation systems are undergoing multicenter clinical trials. Nathan (60,61), from Beersheba, Israel, has developed a splint that incorporates surface electrodes for grasp. The brace fixes the wrist in neutral, making it applicable primarily to C5 level tetraplegic individuals who do not have a tenodesis grasp. Multicenter trials are now underway in the United States, Europe, and Israel. A second surface stimulation system has been developed by Prochazka (67), in Edmonton, Canada. The device uses self-adhesive electrodes over which a neoprene glove is placed to initiate electrode contact with the skin. Wrist motion is used to activate hand opening and closing, making it applicable to individuals with C6 tetraplegia with good wrist control. The device is currently undergoing multicenter study in Canada, the United States, Australia, and Switzerland.

Percutaneous systems were developed to address the problems of specificity and repeatability encountered with surface stimulation systems. The implantation is minimally invasive, requiring needle insertion only, with no surgical exposure. The Cleveland percutaneous clinical system was the first upper extremity neuroprosthesis system to undergo multicenter clinical trials (41,52,65). The system used up to 16 electrodes to provide palmar and lateral grasp for both C5 and C6 completed spinal cord–injured individuals. Hand grasp was controlled using a shoulder position transducer. The clinical trials demonstrated significant improvements in both laboratory and home-based impairment and disability assessments (84–89). This study has now progressed to utilization of an implanted stimulator unit, which is described below. The only commercially available upper extremity percutaneous system was developed by Handa and colleagues (43–50), of Sendai, Japan. The system uses up to 30 percutaneous electrodes to provide palmar, lateral, and parallel extension grasp controlled by a switch operated by the opposite arm or by respiration using a siff/puff type of control.

TABLE 24-1. *Comparison of clinical upper extremity neuroprosthesis systems*

Originating location	Product name	Electrodes	Patient population	Number of channels	Grasp pattern	Control method	Feedback
BeerSheva, Israel	Handmaster	Surface	C5	2–4	Lateral, Palmar, Tip	Switch	Visual
Edmonton, Canada	Bionic Arm	Surface	C6	2–4	Palmar	Wrist angle, Switch	Visual
Sendai, Japan	FESMate 1000	Percutaneous	C5/C6	30	Lateral, Palmar, Extension	Shoulder angle, Switch	Visual
Cleveland	Freehand System	Implant	C5/C6	8	Lateral, Palmar	Shoulder/wrist angel, Switch	Visual, Electrotactile

An implanted upper extremity neuroprosthesis offers several advantages over percutaneous systems. The implanted system obviates the need for constant surveillance for infections and broken electrodes at the percutaneous interface (76–90). Cosmesis is significantly improved as external cabling is minimized. Surgical augmentation of the hand and arm can result in improved hand function both with and without the neuroprosthesis. The implant stimulator and electrodes can be placed in the same surgery, eliminating the need for a second surgical procedure (53,54). The Cleveland percutaneous system has now evolved into an implanted stimulator neuroprosthesis (53–56,65,69,83), shown in Figure 24-3. The eight-channel system provides lateral and palmar grasp to persons with C5 and C6 tetraplegia. The electrodes and the implant receiver-stimulator are fully implanted (69). A radiofrequency-inductive link provides the communication and power to the implant receiver-stimulator. The proportional control of grasp opening and closing is achieved using either shoulder or wrist motion. Outcome studies have demonstrated significant improvements in impairment (86,88) and disability (85,87,89) measures. The system is currently undergoing multicenter trials in the United States, Europe, and Australia.

The Cleveland implanted system appears to be mechanically durable. Of the first 146 electrodes that have been implanted longer than 2 years, three (2%) have failed. There have not been cases of implant failure, although the first implant was replaced after two years due to increased power consumption (53) with no further incident. The replacement device has now been operating for over 8 years. Medical complications associated with the implantable neuroprosthesis have been few. There have been no postoperative infections. One device was explanted after infection secondary to a pressure sore around the leads at the elbow that occurred 1 year after implant. This device was removed after 16 months to ensure that the infection did not track up the leads to the implant. In addition, two devices rotated in situ; and there were two localized infections. In both cases of implant rotation, the implant was surgically exposed, unwound, and resutured in place. Both devices remain functional. For the localized electrode infections, the distal lead of the electrode was cut, and the area was allowed to heal without further incident. In one case the electrode was later replaced. These incidents were minor and did not cause compromise to the patient.

Future Directions for Upper Extremity Neuroprostheses

Future work in upper extremity neuroprostheses will focus on the technologic development of implantable neuroprostheses, control of proximal joints, feedback control systems, and application to other impairment groups with central nervous system injuries. Technologic advancements will include implanted control transducers (91), new electrode technology (92,93), and use of devices that minimize surgical invasiveness (94). Proximal joint control will be implemented to allow triceps extension (60,95) and improve shoulder control (96). Closed-loop systems will improve performance by correcting the output based on knowledge of

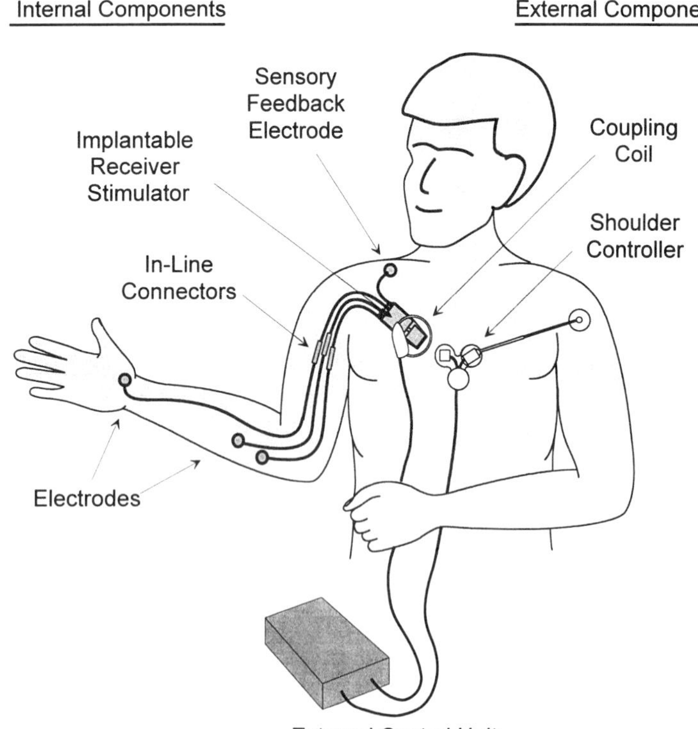

FIG. 24-3. FES hand grasp system. Diagram of implanted neuroprosthesis. The implanted components are the electrodes, leads, and stimulator unit. The external components of the system are the coil, shoulder control device, and an external control unit. The external control unit is battery operated and is placed behind or under the patient's wheelchair. (Courtesy of the Cleveland FES Center.)

the output (82,93,97–99). Finally, upper extremity FNS will be applicable to individuals with head injury (56), stroke (100–102), cerebral palsy (83), and multiple sclerosis (84).

LOWER EXTREMITY APPLICATIONS

Overview and Background

Many clinicians and researchers have pursued lower extremity applications of FNS to restore or improve standing and walking ability in adults with complete or partial paralysis due to spinal cord injury (SCI), head injury, or stroke (8,19–23,33–36,103–109). FNS systems for these applications have ranged from simple single-channel devices to reduce or eliminate footdrop, to complex multichannel microprocessor-controlled devices (35,36,103,110). Stimulation in such systems has been delivered to the nerve transcutaneously from surface electrodes (20–22,103), percutaneously via muscle-based electrodes (8,26,109), or by nerve and muscle-based electrodes connected to completely implantable stimulation systems (33–36,111). Systems using surface stimulation for exercise of the lower extremities or as aids in gait training are commercially available. Representative samples of all these lower extremity FNS systems are presented in the following sections. The discussions are arranged by target patient population and applicable technology.

Lower Extremity Neuromuscular Stimulation in Hemiplegia

FNS can be used to correct a number of gait deficits after stroke. During the swing phase of gait, diminished ankle dorsiflexion, knee flexion, and/or hip flexion can result in inability to clear the floor with the affected limb. In that case, one or more of several compensatory strategies can be adopted, including circumducting the affected limb, dragging the affected limb, and vaulting over the unaffected limb in order to clear the floor with the affected limb. FNS can be used to stimulate insufficiently or inappropriately active limb flexor musculature so that a more normal-appearing swing phase results. Likewise, diminished control of weight-bearing muscles can result in gait deficits during the stance phase of gait. Gait deficits can include stance phase knee hyperextension, hyperflexion of the knee during stance, and deficient weight shifting to the affected limb. FNS can be used to retrain weight-bearing muscles and improve stance phase limb control.

One of the earliest and most successful applications of neuromuscular electrical stimulation for individuals with hemiparesis resulting from a stroke was as a motor neuroprosthesis rather than an exercise or training tool. Stanic et al. studied the use of multiple channels of surface stimulation timed with the gait cycle according to the electromyographic activity observed during normal walking (103). These systems automatically adjusted the stimulation sequences to the preferred cadence of each individual based on the timing of foot–floor contact patterns measured by insole-mounted switches. Significant improvements in the kinematics of gait were observed during walking trials in the laboratory. Simpler applications of FNS in this population focused on the loss of ankle dorsiflexion. Appropriately placed surface electrodes have been used to generate contractions of the tibialis anterior, peroneals, and other muscles that, when appropriately timed to the gait cycle, actively dorsiflex the ankle and allow the foot to clear the floor during swing. Timing in this application can be controlled by simple heel switches or automatic timers that can initiate stimulation at heel rise, and continue stimulation to maintain dorsiflexion until heel contact at the end of swing, or shortly thereafter to resist the rapid acceleration of the foot into plantarflexion.

In the 1970s and early 1980s a single-channel implantable system to correct footdrop was tested and marketed (35,36). The system used a passive receiver-stimulator located in the abdominal region linked by a single cable directly to a cuff electrode in the popliteal area. Stimulated inversion and eversion were balanced intraoperatively at the time of implantation by adding or removing motor branches of the common peroneal nerve to the contact area of the cuff. External components consisted of a heelswitch and small telemetry unit that communicated foot–floor contact information to a belt-worn controller. The unit then produced the RF signals required to control the implanted device through a coupling coil place on the skin over the implanted receiver-stimulator.

The system successfully provided users with active dorsiflexion, and long-term results were generally good. However, the reliability of early versions of the technology, particularly the external heelswitch and foot–floor contact transmitter, proved to be a barrier to use. Other shortcomings were a result of choices made in the design of the system. Because it relied on a single channel of stimulation, it was impossible to actively balance inversion and eversion of the ankle as the stimulated responses changed with time after the system was implanted. The lack of an in-line connector required the removal and replacement of the implanted system in its entirety in the event of an electrode, lead, or receiver problem. In many cases, similar clinical results could be obtained with a simple and inexpensive flexible molded ankle–foot orthosis (AFO).

More recent approaches to lower extremity rehabilitation in stroke have used neuromuscular stimulation as a training tool to facilitate motor relearning after stroke. During the acute poststroke period, Bogataj et al. reported that surface FNS treatment resulted in more rapid gains in limb coordination and walking velocity than did other rehabilitation methods (104,105). Temporary FNS systems using intramuscular electrodes with percutaneous leads are currently being used to eliminate the adverse sensation experienced during surface stimulation. For chronic stroke survivors, researchers have reported that the use of intramuscular electrodes resulted in significantly greater gains compared with the use of surface electrodes and other rehabilitation techniques (106,107). This form of treatment resulted in more improved swing phase limb flexion and improved stance phase limb control. It remains to be determined conclusively whether or not FNS accelerates the relearning of coordination sequences and significantly improve gait patterns when compared with conventional physical therapy.

Lower Extremity Neuromuscular Stimulation in Spinal Cord Injury

Exercise Cycling

Lower extremity FNS can be an effective exercise modality for persons otherwise paralyzed by SCI. Progressive resistance knee extension exercise using dynamic contractions of the quadriceps with electrical stimulation can reverse or prevent disuse atrophy, improve strength, endurance, and appearance, and promote circulation (112). The mechanisms of these changes appear to be peripheral rather than central adaptations and include fiber type conversion (fast to slow twitch), increased concentration of metabolic enzymes, hypertrophy, and higher capillary density (113–115).

FNS protocols similar to voluntary high-resistance weight training are effective in strengthening the paralyzed muscles of individuals with spinal cord injuries (116–119). FNS protocols similar to voluntary high-resistance weight training can strengthen paralyzed muscles. However, such training protocols will not elicit significant central cardiopulmonary responses (119). Stationary bicycle ergometers were developed to address this need and promote cardiovascular fitness in persons with spinal cord injuries. Sophisticated leg cycle ergometers using computer-controlled surface stimulation to the quadriceps, hamstrings, and gluteal groups are commercially available for use in the home or clinic environments and can be prescribed by a physician. An example of one such system (Therapeutic Alliances, Inc. Fairborn, OH) is depicted in Figure 24-4.

Much of the work in the physiologic responses to lower extremity cycling exercise with FNS has been conducted at the Institute for Rehabilitation Research and Medicine at Wright State University in Dayton, Ohio. FNS cycling exercises induce aerobic metabolic and cardiopulmonary responses, as well as favorable central and peripheral hemodynamic responses (120,121). Chronic cycling in this manner has been shown to produce significant physiological and psychological benefits, including increased dimension and thickness of cardiac muscle (122), elevated high-density lipoprotein levels (suggesting reduced risks of coronary heart disease), enhanced immunoreactivity (123), improved scores on depression, self-image, and mood indices (124), and reduced incidence of pressure sores and kidney and bladder infections. These effects may take months to years of regular exercise to manifest themselves.

Cardiovascular fitness training can be further enhanced by adding voluntary arm cranking to the FNS-generated leg cycling exercise program (112,125). Recent studies at Wright State suggest that combining lower extremity FNS and voluntary exercise can provide superior cardiopulmonary training than either mode alone. This may be due to the larger muscle mass used by exercising both upper and lower extremities simultaneously, as well as the enhanced venous return provided by the cyclic contractions of the limbs.

Surface Stimulation for Standing and Walking

Pioneering work in the application of surface stimulation to the restoration of standing and walking function to individuals with complete and incomplete spinal cord injuries

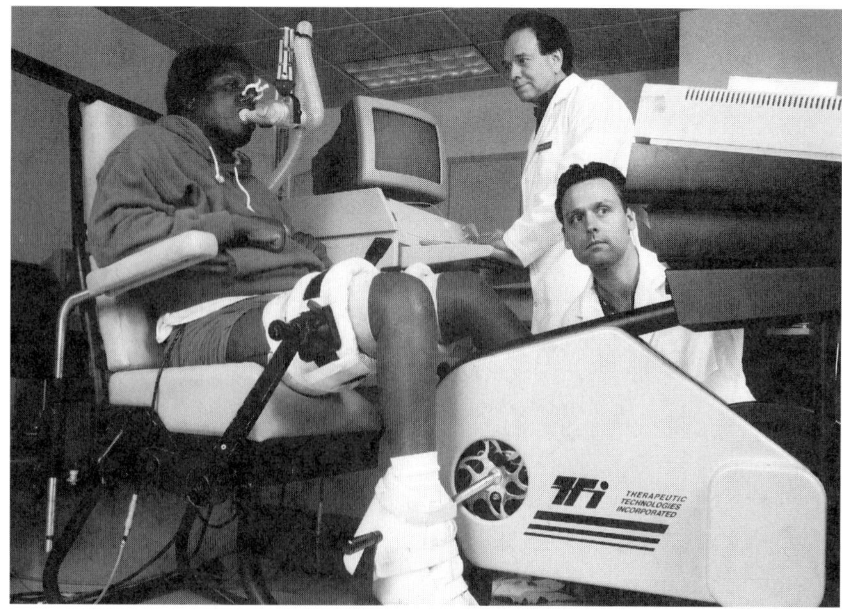

FIG. 24-4. Bicycle ergometer from Therapeutic Associates, Inc., in use at Wright State University. (Courtesy of the Institute for Rehabilitation Research and Medicine, Wright State University, Scott A. Kissel, photographer.)

was conducted in the 1970s and 1980s in Lublijana, Slovenia. The techniques developed by Kralj, Bajd, and others (20–22,126) continue to be used in many laboratories and clinics around the world. Using as few as two surface stimulation channels per leg, standing and reciprocal walking is produced through a combination of direct activation of the quadriceps muscles and the triggering of a flexion withdrawal reflex. Standing is achieved by simultaneously activating the quadriceps bilaterally in response to a command input, such as the simultaneous depression of switches on the handles of a rolling walker or crutches. A stride is produced by maintaining activation to the quadriceps of the stance limb while initiating a flexion withdrawal in the contralateral limb via afferent stimulation of the swing limb side. To complete the reaching phase of the stride, activation of the knee extensors on the swinging limb is initiated while the reflex is still active and flexing the hip. The stimulus producing the flexion reflex is then removed, leaving the user in double-limb support once again with bilateral quadriceps stimulation. The user then moves the walker or other supporting aid and repeats the procedure for the opposite limb. Trunk extension is usually achieved passively by adopting a C-curve posture or by activating the gluteal muscles to extend the hips.

This type of a system has a number of limitations. Active flexion forces at the hip are generated by the rectus femoris when the quadriceps are stimulated with surface electrodes, which compromises standing stability. Not all patients exhibit a flexion withdrawal reflex that is strong or repeatable enough to be used for stepping. Although reflex stepping can be effective in well-selected individuals, it tends to be jerky and inconsistent. The reflex also habituates with repeated activation, limiting the number of steps that can be taken at one time.

The Slovenian group has fit systems of this type to over 50 patients with several years of follow-up and has developed extensive prescriptive criteria for individuals with various neurologic deficits (20). Patients with incomplete injuries are first evaluated for conventional orthoses alone before adding FNS. Individuals with high-level injuries are considered for combinations or orthoses and stimulation, and persons with mid- to low-level paraplegia are candidates for the surface FNS system without orthoses. These systems and implementation procedures have been successfully transferred to clinical practice. Figure 24-5 depicts a commercially available surface stimulation system for standing and stepping that recently was approved by the U.S. Food and Drug Administration (127). Operation of the Parastep system (Sigmedics, Inc. Northfield, IL) is similar to the Slovenian systems just described.

Concentrating exclusively on standing function, rather than walking, allows the command and control structure of these systems to be greatly simplified. Jaeger and colleagues (108,128–130) adopted this approach and used techniques similar to those originally developed in Slovenia. Two channels of surface stimulation were applied to the quadriceps bilaterally, and operation consisted of manipulation of a single switch on the stimulator housing. Stimulation for standing was initiated or deactivated by a single switch depression. When activated, the standing system issued an initial audio tone. A time delay enabled the subject to prepare to stand by repositioning the hands and body immediately before the onset of the stimulation. A second depression of the control switch reversed the sequence and lowered the user back into the wheelchair. Protocols for implementing these systems clinically also have been developed and published along with results from small-scale clinical trials (130).

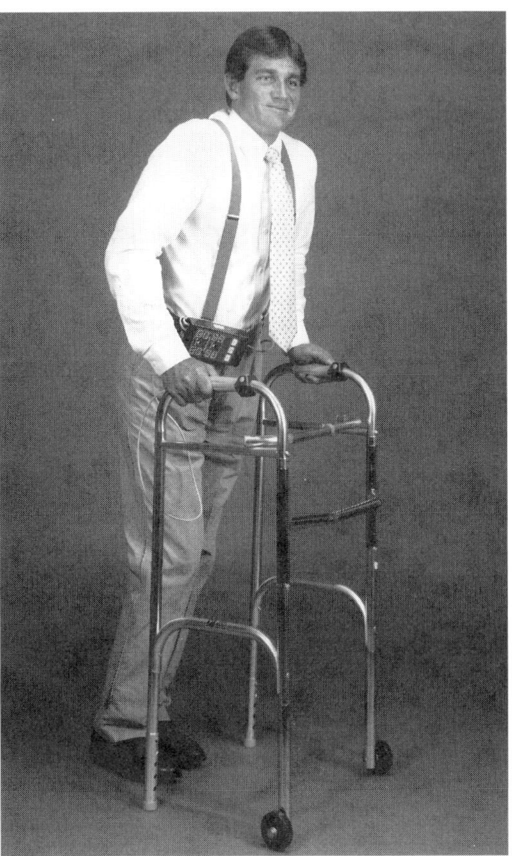

FIG. 24-5. The Parastep System, a four-channel surface stimulation system for standing and walking. (Courtesy of Sigmedics, Inc., Northfield IL.)

Hybrid Systems for Standing and Walking

One method to overcome the disadvantages of standing and walking systems that rely exclusively on surface stimulation involves combining FNS with conventional bracing (131–135). The advantages of orthoses lie primarily in their ability to constrain the motions of the joints, reduce the degrees of freedom of movement, and provide mechanical stability. Standing with FNS alone requires continuous activation of the antigravity muscles, leading to rapid fatigue. Fine control of posture and balance is currently unattainable with the present level of FNS technology. As previously noted, activation of the flexion withdrawal reflex and quadriceps with surface stimulation introduce additional complicating factors. However, walking with hip–knee–ankle–foot orthoses (HKAFOs) alone can also be prohibitively difficult because of the demands placed on the upper extremities. Combining FNS and bracing in a hybrid orthosis offers an opportunity to take advantage of the positive aspects of each technology and minimize the potential shortcomings.

One method of effectively combining the advantages of orthoses and FNS is under investigation at Louisiana State University (LSU). Solomonow and colleagues have been developing a practical hybrid system that uses an LSU reciprocating gait orthosis (RGO) and a custom-designed surface stimulator (133–136). The LSU RGO is a passive mechanical HKAFO consisting of solid custom-molded polypropylene ankle-foot component joined by lateral uprights to lockable knee and hip joints and terminating in a thoracic strap positioned below the axilla. The most important feature of the LSU RGO is the coupling between the hip joints. Two stainless-steel cables inside a low-friction conduit join the hip mechanisms to transmit extension movements on one side to flexion movements on the contralateral side. This reciprocating mechanism engages automatically when the hips are fully extended upon standing up and can be disengaged voluntarily to allow the user to return to the seated position. Individuals with complete paraplegia can walk by shifting their weight onto the stance limb, pushing up on a walker with their arms, and letting the swing limb advance as the stance limb extends.

The FNS component of the system consists of a four-channel surface stimulator and a flexible copolymer electrode cuff that locates and maintains the surface electrodes over the rectus femoris and hamstrings. Stimulating the hamstrings with the knees locked will extend the hip and flex the contralateral limb through the action of the reciprocating mechanism. Conversely, the rectus femoris is used to flex the hip actively, rather than to extend the knee, and to assist with contralateral hip extension via the reciprocating mechanism. Rectus femoris and contralateral hamstrings are activated simultaneously to initiate a step upon the depression of a walker-mounted switch. The hybrid system has been fitted to approximately 50 patients to date with complete or incomplete thoracic or low-level cervical injuries at LSU and collaborating centers (136). Similar systems using a hip-guidance orthosis or alternative reciprocating mechanism have been devised and tested in various centers in North America and Europe (137).

Multichannel Systems with Implanted Electrodes

Clinicians and researchers at the Cleveland Veterans Affairs Medical Center (VAMC) and Case Western Reserve University (CWRU) have been developing systems that use implanted electrodes for personal mobility functions such as standing, one-handed reaching, forward, side, and back stepping, and stair ascent and descent. The approach to lower extremity FNS at the Cleveland VAMC has involved individual activation of many muscles via implanted muscle-based electrodes (intramuscular and epimysial), rather than the use of synergistic patterns such as the flexion withdrawal reflex, or extensive bracing. Intramuscular electrodes afforded access to deep structures or anatomically adjacent nerves that were difficult to isolate and activate separately from the surface. Marsolais and colleagues have synthesized complex lower extremity motions by activating up to 48 separate muscles (via a combination of 40 chronically indwelling intramuscular electrodes with percutaneous leads plus eight surface electrodes) under the control of a programmable microprocessor-based external stimulator (114). Access to deep muscles minimized the need for bracing with the system. Only a freely articulated AFO is used to protect the ligaments and structure of the foot and ankle because all other motions were either created or resisted internally by FNS-activated muscular contractions. All components of the system are worn by the user, freeing him or her from cabling to a walker, wheelchair, or other assistive device that might interfere with transfers or other daily function.

This sophisticated system allowed independent control of stimulus timing, pulse duration, and frequency for each channel. Although synthesizing the stimulus patterns for large complements of electrodes quickly became a difficult task, a general approach to specifying and adjusting stimulation for standing and walking was developed (138). Preprogrammed packages of stimulation were created on a personal computer and transferred to the portable external control unit for clinical use. Users select one of a series of movement patterns by scrolling through a menu of options presented on a liquid-crystal display. Switches on a command ring worn on the index finger are used to activate and deactivate the stimulation patterns. Successive depressions of the switch with the thumb initiated the next step, or insole-mounted pressure sensors can be used to sense foot–floor contact and trigger steps automatically. Figure 24-6 shows one subject with a complete thoracic spinal cord injury using a multichannel percutaneous FNS system for standing and functional reach.

Some well-trained subjects can walk 300 m repeatedly at 0.5 m/sec with this system. By triggering the steps with insole pressure sensors, walking speed can increase to 0.73 m/sec with a cadence of 65 steps/min. Double support and swing times can average close to the nominal values of 15% and 40% of the gait cycle, respectively (139). The quality of the motions produced by FNS with this system depends on the availability, strength, and endurance of paralyzed muscles, the ability of the therapist or engineer to specify patterns of stimulation for ambulation, and the subject's experience with the device (26,139).

Despite these accomplishments, installing and maintaining systems consisting of large numbers of percutaneous intramuscular electrodes becomes impractical or impossible in the clinical setting. For this reason, the Cleveland group is pursuing clinical trials of completely implantable lower

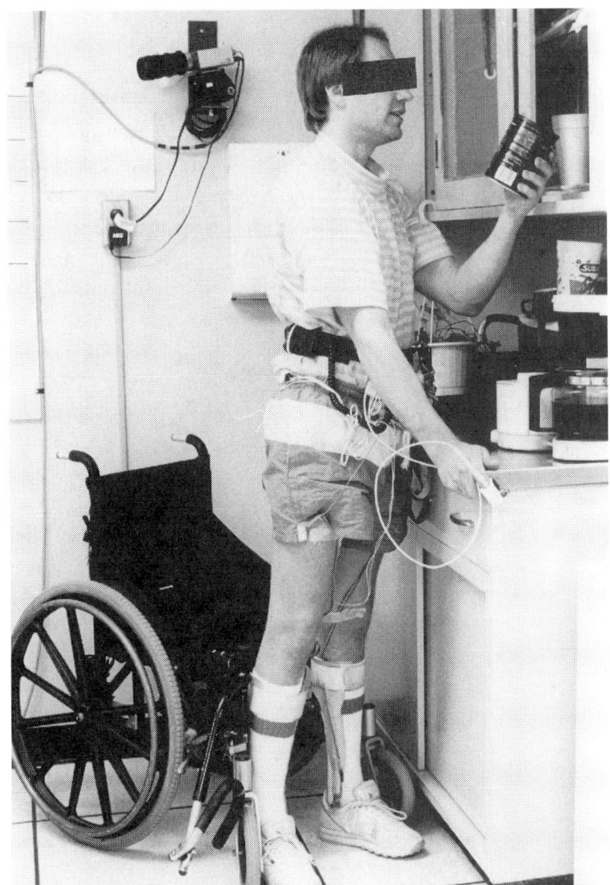

FIG. 24-6. Functional standing with a percutaneous intramuscular FNS system. Stimulation is provided to the individual heads of the quadriceps, hamstrings, posterior portion of the adductor magnus, gluteus maximus, and lumbar erector spinae. (Courtesy of the Motion Study Laboratory at the Cleveland Veterans Affairs Medical Center.)

extremity systems. An eight-channel implantable receiver-stimulator developed at CWRU and the Cleveland Veterans Affairs (VA) Medical Center is being used as the platform for clinical trials of systems to facilitate standing and transfers in persons with neurologically complete or incomplete injuries at the C6–T4 levels (111). Figure 24-7 shows the CWRU/VA standing transfer system. The implantable components of the CWRU/VA implantable receiver-stimulator are pictured in Figure 24-7*A*. The passive electronics package receives control signals and power via an RF link to an external control unit and delivers stimulation to implanted epimysial or implanted intramuscular electrodes via separate implanted leads and in-line connectors. A schematic representation of the clinical system is presented in Figure 24-7*B*. The entire system can be implanted in a single surgical procedure, and Figure 24-7*C* shows an x-ray of such a system installed in one volunteer with incomplete tetraplegia (115).

Standing and stepping can be achieved without braces for persons with complete paraplegia with 16 channels of stimulation. Clinical trials of implanted systems for walking are being planned that will rely on implanting two eight-channel CWRU/VA devices into volunteers with thoracic level injuries. This system is depicted schematically in Figure 24-8*A*. New rechargeable external control units have been developed to coordinate the actions of both implants simultaneously. A prototype of this small, wearable, energy-efficient device is pictured in Figure 24-8*B*.

FNS for Functional Ambulation

The potential for FNS in providing functional ambulation is dependent on the resolution of the significant differences between FNS-induced and normal gait. The best FNS walking systems to date have been successful in advancing the swing limb through stimulation of the hip flexors and knee extensors, preventing collapse with stimulation to the knee and hip extensors, and injecting propulsive forces through stimulation of the hip extensors and ankle plantarflexors. However, consistent foot placement has been difficult to produce without orthoses. Forward progression of the trunk and weight transfer from the trailing to leading limb usually requires significant upper extremity exertion. Automatic postural corrections are not provided, and balance must be maintained with assistive devices. The joint angles of the hip, knee, and ankle during walking with FNS differ from those typical of able-bodied gait at slow or natural cadences (140,141). There are also some differences in the ground reaction forces produced in normal and FNS-generated gait (26,139). Instead of the normal two-peak vertical force associated with weight acceptance and push-off, a more variable three-peak force is observed during stance (139).

Differences in energy consumption also impede the use of FNS for functional ambulation. Major differences in energy consumption become evident as individuals walk with different FNS systems. Hybrid systems have been reported to require less energy to operate than do braces alone. Energy expenditure increases with velocity when walking with either a reciprocating gait orthosis or a hybrid system consisting of a reciprocator and FNS. At slow to moderate speeds, energy consumption for both modes of walking is still significantly less than with FNS alone, which can require as much as seven times the resting metabolic rate (142). However, energy consumption for FNS walking decreases as walking speed increases, suggesting that as velocities approach normal, the differences between walking modalities will be minimized or reversed (with brace walking requiring more energy than FNS).

At present, FNS walking appears to be a promising form of exercise rather than an alternative to wheelchair locomotion. The metabolic energy currently required by any FNS system, hybrid or otherwise, is still too high to make walking with FNS a practical alternative to the wheelchair for long distance transportation over level surfaces. The true value of lower extremity FNS systems in their current forms may lie primarily in their ability to facilitate or provide options for

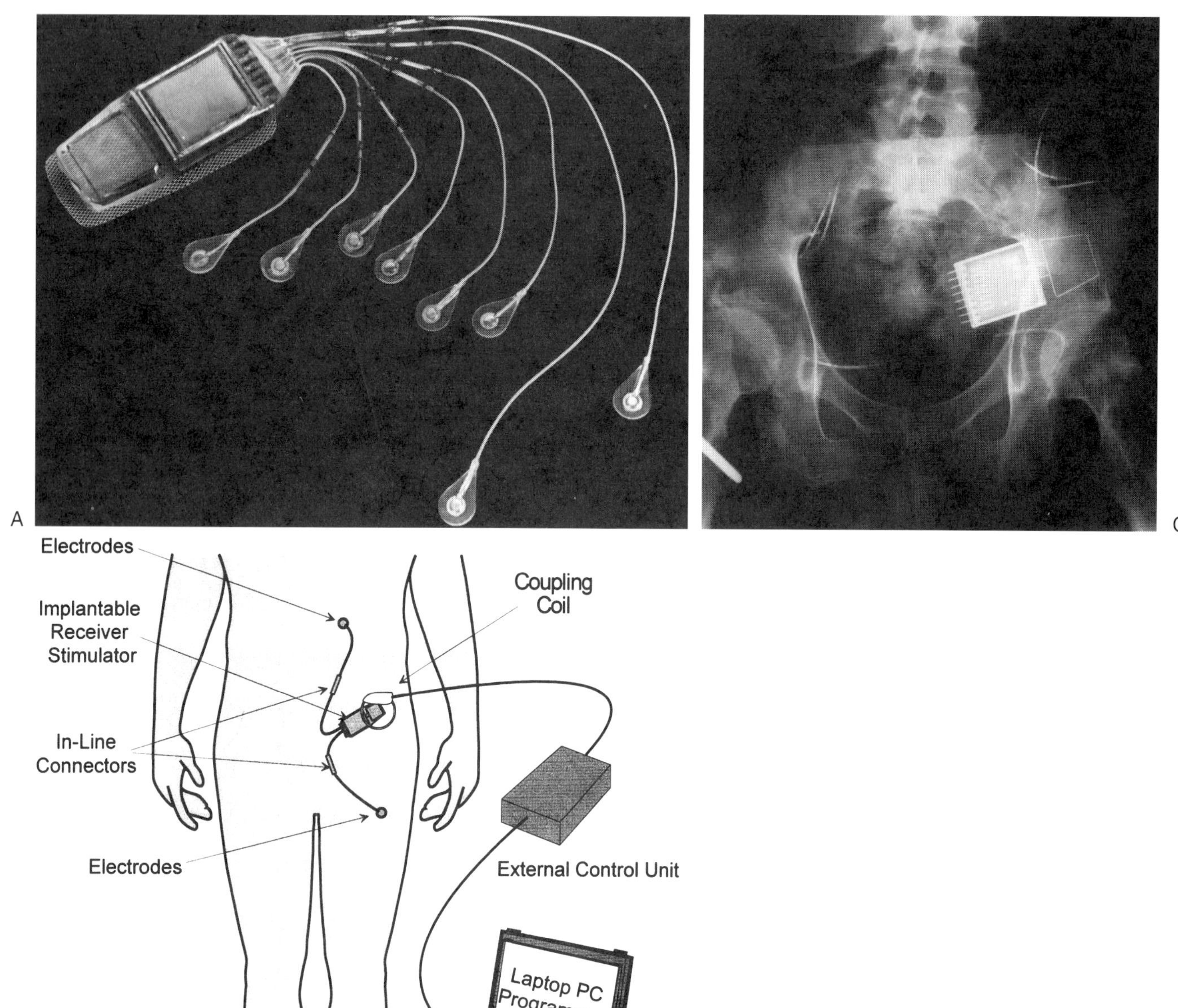

FIG. 24-7. The eight-channel CWRU/VA implantable receiver/stimulator and the standing/transfer system. Implantable components of the system include the stimulator/receiver, in-lead connectors, and epimysial electrodes **(A)**. A schematic representation of the clinical system is given in **(B)** along with an x-ray of the implant installed in a tetraplegic volunteer **(C)**. (Courtesy of the Cleveland Veterans Affairs Medical Center Motion Study Laboratory and the Cleveland FES Center).

short-duration mobility-related tasks, such as overcoming physical obstacles or architectural barriers in the vicinity of the wheelchair.

Clinical Considerations

Not all individuals with SCI may be well suited for lower extremity FNS due to clinical presentations that contraindicate the application of electrical currents, joint mobilization, or weight bearing. However, several precautions can be taken to prevent interfering complications from developing, and several other clinical interventions can be identified to address pre-existing medical contraindications in preparation for standing or walking with FNS. Several medical conditions need to be identified early when screening potential candidates for lower extremity FNS programs. The major physical barriers to application of FNS are summarized below.

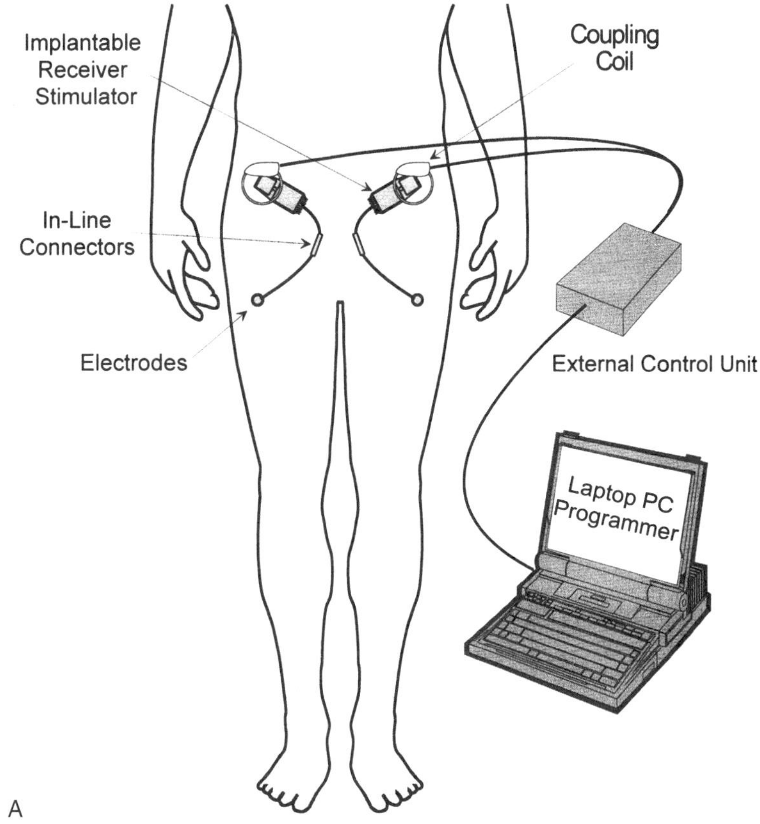

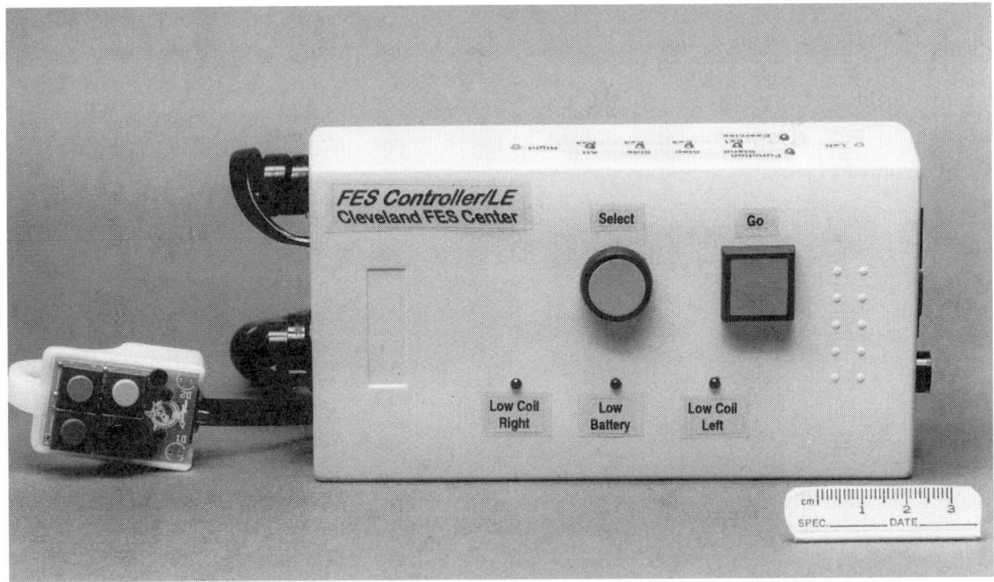

FIG. 24-8. Schematic representation of a dual-implant walking system consisting of two CWRU/VA implanted stimulator/receivers **(A)** and external control unit capable of communicating, powering, and coordinating both implants simultaneously **(B)**. (Courtesy of the Cleveland Veterans Affairs Medical Center Motion Study Laboratory and the Cleveland FES Center.)

Range of motion limitations and soft-tissue contractures significantly limit FNS standing and walking and should be aggressively prevented and treated. Spasticity can be troublesome for the patient trying to stand and walk with FNS. Exercise with FNS appears to result in stronger, but less frequent, involuntary spasms. Medication is recommended for controlling spasticity that may interfere with function. However, neuromuscular blocking agents that may adversely affect the excitability of the peripheral nerve or muscle contractility should be avoided. High grade-pressure sores that may require surgery can be contraindications to the application of FNS. Certain muscles that might be used for standard surgical repairs may be critical for standing or walking with FNS. Joint Instability appears to be a common problem at the hip among spinal cord–injured individuals (143,144). Soft-tissue stretching of the adductors and flexors, control of spasticity, and prophylactic abduction bracing will help prevent the contractions and deforming forces that may contribute to subluxation. Should subluxation occur, surgical procedures such as soft-tissue releases and bony supplementation are possible. Early surgical intervention is strongly recommended for established instabilities (143,144). Spinal deformities occur in many patients with spinal cord injury (145) and may compromise standing posture, requiring excessive use of the arms for stability during lower extremity FNS application. Early prophylactic bracing should be considered for FNS. Once the curve progresses past 40°, a spinal fusion is indicated (145). Caution is advised after spinal fusion because long-term use of FNS for standing and walking will place extra demands on the lumbosacral spine (26). Finally, peripheral denervation is the most common contraindication for FNS application (32). Without an intact and excitable peripheral nerve, high stimulating currents or long-duration stimulating pulses are required to activate the muscle tissue directly. In the lower extremity, the highest incidence of denervation occurs in individuals with T12–L3 level injuries.

Safety Precautions

The application of neuromuscular stimulation for functional use or exercise of the lower extremities presents potential risks, as well as benefits, to the individual with SCI. The dangers include orthopedic injury (fracture, damage of insensate joints), exercise or orthostatic hypotension, autonomic dysreflexia, burn, pressure sores (from orthotic components), and inappropriate thermoregulatory responses. Health-care professionals prescribing lower extremity neuromuscular stimulation systems need to be aware of these risks and take the necessary precautions to minimize them, including informing and educating users to the potential dangers. Patients considering a lower extremity neuromuscular stimulation program should have a thorough physical examination, including radiographs of the lower extremities, magnetic resonance imaging of the ankles, knees, and hips, neurologic evaluation, cardiopulmonary examination, and psychosocial evaluation. Consumer and professional alike need to be actively involved in conscientious monitoring and long-term follow-up of use of neuromuscular stimulation systems in unsupervised settings.

BLADDER APPLICATION

Normal function of the lower urinary tract requires alternation between micturition and continence; micturition requires contraction of the detrusor with relaxation of the sphincter mechanism, whereas continence requires relaxation of the detrusor and maintenance of muscle tone, with occasional strong contraction of the sphincters. Producing these alternating functions with electrical stimulation has been a challenge for many years, but it is now achievable in some conditions, particularly in patients with spinal cord injury.

Continence

Improvement of continence may depend on reduction of unwanted bladder contraction or improvement in sphincter tone and contraction, or both. Electrical stimulation of sacral afferent nerves has frequently been shown to reduce incontinence in selected patients, whether applied via electrodes in the anus or vagina, on the sacral dermatomes, on the pudendal nerves, epidurally, or on the sacral nerves in the spinal canal (146–148). This stimulation reduces hyperactivity of the bladder in some patients, although the mechanism is not well understood. This technique is sometimes called neuromodulation (149) and is probably related to the reduction of spasticity in skeletal muscle, which can sometimes be produced by afferent stimulation. Because the mechanism is incompletely understood, it is difficult to predict which patients will benefit. Patients are typically offered the use of a stimulator with electrodes in the form of an anal plug, vaginal pessary, or adhesive skin patches and instructed to use it several hours a day for a period of some weeks while maintaining a continence diary to evaluate its effects. Some patients report improvement in continence during and even after the use of the device, but many find the electrodes and wires troublesome (150).

In order to reduce the inconvenience of externally applied electrodes, fully implantable stimulators have been developed with electrodes that can be placed in contact with the nerve roots in the sacral foramina. In order to predict which patients will benefit, it is usually necessary to test stimulation by connecting percutaneous electrodes in these foramina to an external stimulator for a period of several days before implanting a stimulator permanently (151).

Stimulation of sacral afferent nerves can produce reflex activation of the efferent nerves to the sphincter, but this reflex is likely to accommodate too rapidly to provide lasting contraction. The external urethral sphincter also can be made to contract by electrical stimulation of efferent fibers in the pudendal nerve via electrodes in the anus or vagina, or by stimulation of sacral nerves or roots via implanted electrodes (152). However, fatigue is likely to reduce the pressure generated in the urethra to a level that can be overcome by a strong bladder contraction. In addition, many patients with stress incontinence have been shown to have damage to the peripheral nerves serving the sphincters and pelvic floor, possibly resulting from obstetric injury, pelvic surgery, or prolonged constipation, and this further limits the contraction that can be obtained from stimulation of these structures.

Improvement in continence associated with electrical stimulation probably has been primarily due to the reduction of unwanted bladder contraction and has mainly been applied in multiple sclerosis and in patients with irritable bladders but without major neurologic disease.

Micturation

Contraction of the detrusor can be produced by electrical activation of the parasympathetic efferent neurons whose cell bodies are in the sacral segments of the spinal cord and whose axons usually travel in the S3 and sometimes S4 or S2 anterior roots and nerves. However, these axons are closely accompanied for most of their course by somatic efferent axons to the external sphincter and pelvic floor. The latter axons, being of larger diameter than the parasympathetic axons, have a lower threshold for electrical activation, and it has therefore been difficult to produce contraction of the detrusor without contraction of the external sphincter. Attempts have been made to reduce sphincter contraction by cutting the pudendal nerves, the levator ani, or the external sphincter itself, but these techniques are not always successful and sometimes produce incontinence. The most successful micturition has been produced by the technique of poststimulus voiding, which uses the fact that the detrusor muscle of the bladder relaxes more slowly than the striated muscle of the external sphincter. Bladder pressure can be built up by a series of bursts of electrical stimulation, each lasting a few seconds, and is maintained between the bursts; the external sphincter contracts strongly during bursts but relaxes rapidly for a few seconds between bursts, allowing urine to flow. It was initially thought that the intermittent contraction of the sphincter during voiding might produce harmful pressures in the bladder leading to ureteric reflux or hydronephrosis, but these fears have not been borne out in practice. The technique usually has been combined with rhizotomy of the posterior sacral nerve roots, which abolishes unwanted bladder contractions and urge incontinence and has been shown to lead to a reduction in ureteric reflux and hydronephrosis in these patients.

Selection of Patients

The technique has mainly been applied to patients with suprasacral spinal cord lesions because it requires intact parasympathetic efferent neurons to the detrusor. The function of these neurons can be demonstrated by the presence of reflex detrusor contractions when performing a cystometrogram; it is desirable to show a pressure increase of at least 35 cm water in a woman and 50 cm water in a man. Other sacral reflexes such as ankle tendon reflexes, the bulbocavernosus reflex, anal skin reflex, and reflex erection are confirmatory. Frequent urinary infection and problems with catheters or anticholinergic medication are further indications.

A hyperactive detrusor causing high storage pressures and endangering the upper tracts or producing incontinence is an indication for concurrent posterior rhizotomy. A posterior rhizotomy offers several advantages. Uninhibited reflex bladder contraction can be abolished, thereby increasing bladder capacity and abolishing reflex incontinence. Normal bladder compliance can be restored, thereby protecting the upper tracts. The abolition of reflex contraction of the sphincter reduces detrusor–sphincter dyssynergia. Finally, autonomic dysreflexia triggered from the bladder or rectum will be abolished. However, posterior rhizotomies also have the following disadvantages. There will be a loss of reflex erection and ejaculation. Erection is commonly produced by the implant and even more effectively by injection of papaverine into the corpora cavernosa. Seminal emission can now be produced from a high proportion of spinal cord–injured men by rectal probe electrostimulation. The micturition produced by the implant is more effective than reflex micturition, but if the implant is not used for any reason, a patient will usually have to resort to intermittent catheterization. Finally, there will be a loss of peripheral sensation if present.

A decision about posterior rhizotomy should therefore be made in each case. Paraplegic and low quadriplegic subjects who can transfer to a toilet seat independently have more to gain from continence and the ability to dispense with a urine collection bag than quadriplegic men who may choose to continue to wear a condom collection device. Female paraplegics with reflex incontinence have more to gain from posterior rhizotomy than do men because of the lack of satisfactory urine collecting devices for females and the fact that they have less to lose from the rhizotomy. Men with poor or absent reflex erection have more to gain and less to lose than do those whose reflex erections already suffice for coitus. However, it is now the usual practice in both genders for the implantation to be accompanied by posterior rhizotomy.

Technique

Electrodes may be placed either intradurally on the sacral anterior nerve roots in the cauda equina or extradurally on the mixed sacral nerves in the sacral canal. The intradural approach has the advantage of avoiding stimulation of afferent neurons, but because these neurons are commonly subjected to rhizotomy, there is a trend toward extradural electrodes, which have less risk of cerebrospinal fluid leakage. Leads from the electrodes are tunneled subcutaneously to a radio receiver-stimulator placed under the skin of the abdomen or chest and powered and controlled by a radio transmitter operated by the patient. The posterior rhizotomy is best done intradurally, where the sensory and motor roots can be more easily separated, particularly where they enter the conus medullaris.

Surgery

Intradural implantation and rhizotomy are performed through a lower lumbar laminectomy and opening of the dura. Extradural electrodes can be placed in the sacral canal via a laminectomy of S1–S3, usually combined with a laminectomy of T12–L1 for intradural division of S2–S5 posterior roots. Intraoperative electrical stimulation and recording of bladder pressure is used to confirm the identity of the nerves supplying the bladder.

Postoperatively, urodynamic studies are used to guide the setting of stimulus parameters to give an acceptable voiding pressure and rate and pattern of flow. The patient usually can be discharged within a week of surgery with a working device. The stimulus program should be checked 1 to 3 months after the operation because the response of the bladder may change with repeated use; thereafter, review is recommended at least annually, monitoring lower and upper urinary tract function.

Results

Micturition

Micturition using this technique was first produced successfully in humans in Britain in 1978, and it is now in use by over 1,000 patients in 20 countries (153–157). Results have been reviewed by several clinicians (158–160). The majority of subjects with an implanted bladder stimulator use it routinely for producing micturition at home four to six times per day. Residual volume in the bladder after implant-driven micturition is usually less than 60 ml and often less than 30 ml (159). A substantial decrease in symptomatic urine infection with or without pyrexia has been reported by many groups after use of the implant (154,159,161,162).

Continence of Urine

In multicenter data, continence is reported to have been achieved in over 85% of patients. This is probably largely attributable to the abolition of detrusor hyperreflexia and increase in bladder compliance which follow posterior sacral rhizotomy and which appear to be long term provided the rhizotomy is complete from S2 caudally. A decrease in residual urine, as a result of stimulated voiding, also allows a patient a longer period of bladder filling before reaching capacity. Reduction of infection also should improve the compliance of the bladder and reduce the likelihood of contraction in response to spinal or nonspinal reflexes.

Urodynamic Studies

Several authors (163,164) have reported the results of urodynamic investigation showing increases in bladder capacity and compliance, which are probably mainly due to posterior rhizotomy.

Concern was initially expressed that the cocontraction of bladder and external sphincter would lead to dangerously high bladder pressures, resulting in trabeculation of the bladder, ureteric reflux, and hydronephrosis. When the sphincter is closed, the pressure in the bladder depends on the stimulus parameters applied to the parasympathetic efferent fibers, and these parameters can be varied to control the detrusor pressure. Detrusor pressure has been recorded during stimulation and voiding by several groups (153,154,161,164,165), and although voiding pressure is sometimes greater than in non–spinal cord injured subjects, it is usually less than in reflex micturition. Several investigators (154,159) have reported on long-term follow-up, particularly of the upper tracts. These reports indicate that trabeculation, ureteric reflux, and hydronephrosis have tended to decrease in patients who have undergone implantation and posterior rhizotomy. It appears likely in these patients that any harmful effects from transient high pressure during micturition are outweighed by the beneficial effects of low pressure during storage of urine.

Autonomic Dysreflexia

In some patients autonomic dysreflexia present before operation has improved with the control of infection and autonomic dysreflexia as triggered by afferents from the bladder, lower bowel, or perineum is usually abolished by posterior sacral rhizotomy. This outcome is particularly beneficial to tetraplegic males formerly dependent on an indwelling catheter prone to blockage from frequent infection. In one multicenter survey, autonomic dysreflexia was reported to be a problem in 26 of 184 patients before operation but in only 10 postoperatively; no patient in this survey developed autonomic dysreflexia following the surgery (159).

Complications

Infection of these implants has been rare, particularly because a technique of coating them with antibiotics was introduced in 1982. Rushton et al. (166) reported that one of 104 coated implants had become infected, and in this case infection appeared to have been introduced at a subsequent operation to close a leak of cerebrospinal fluid. Among early implants not coated with antibiotic, two of 40 became infected. The infection rate for a variety of neural prosthetic implants was shown to be significantly reduced by the antibiotic coating but not by systemic perioperative antibiotics.

Technical faults in the implanted equipment have been uncommon and have been analyzed as occurring on average once every 19.6 implant-years (167). The most common site for faults has been in cables, which are sometimes mechanically damaged by compression against a rib. Repair or replacement of the implanted device has been possible in all cases where this has been attempted, and no fault is known to have led to permanent discontinuation of use of the implant.

Summary

Electrical stimulation can now produce micturition reliably in selected patients with suprasacral spinal cord lesions. Some patients with urge incontinence benefit from stimulation of sacral afferent nerves to reduce hyperactivity of the detrusor, although prediction of which patients will benefit often requires a period of test stimulation. The use of electrical stimulation for treating stress incontinence has been limited by the fact that many patients have damage to the nerves or muscles required for continence, and this limits the effects that can be produced by electrical activation of those nerves or muscles.

SUMMARY AND FUTURE DEVELOPMENTS

The principal goal of the rehabilitation management of persons with upper motor neuron paralysis is to maximize quality of life. Although quality of life is clearly influenced by a wide range of variables, including social, emotional, psychological, vocational, and educational factors, the persistent neurologic impairment after injury to the central motor system remains a powerful reminder and determinant of one's physical disability and handicap. FNS systems bypass the injured central circuitry to activate neural tissue and contract muscles to provide function to what is otherwise a nonfunctioning limb or structure. Recent advances in clinical medicine and biomedical engineering have made the clinical implementation of FNS systems to enhance the mobility and function of paralyzed person more feasible. Hand neuroprosthesis systems can significantly enhance the upper extremity activities of daily living of persons with tetraplegia. A variety of lower extremity systems with and without bracing are being investigated for the purpose of ambulation, transfers, and standing for persons with paraplegia. Bladder FNS system can provide catheter-free micturation for persons with either paraplegia or tetraplegia.

After decades of development, the clinical utility of FNS systems is finally becoming a reality. However, in view of the dynamic nature of the present health-care environment, the future of FNS technology is still difficult to predict. By necessity, scientists and clinicians must continue to explore new ideas and improve upon the present systems. Components will be smaller, more durable, and more reliable. The issues of cosmesis and ease of donning and doffing will require systems to be fully implantable. Control issues will remain central, and the implementation of cortical control will dictate the nature of future generations of FNS systems. Future developments will be directed by consumers. In the present health-care environment, where cost has become an overwhelming factor in the development and implementation of new technology, the consumer will become one of technology's greatest advocates. The usual drive toward greater complexity will be tempered by the practical issues of clinical implementation, where patient acceptance is often a function of a tenuous balance between the burden or cost associated with using a system and the system's impact on the user's life. Finally, FNS will be become available to those with paralysis secondary to cerebral dysfunction such as stroke, cerebral palsy, traumatic brain injury, and multiple sclerosis.

ACKNOWLEDGMENTS

This work was supported in part by grants form the National Institute for Child Health and Human Development, National Institute for Neurological Diseases and Stroke, and the Department of Veterans Affairs.

REFERENCES

1. McNeal R. Analysis of a model for excitation of myelinated nerve. *IEEE Trans Biomed Eng* 1976; 23:329–337.
2. Mortimer JT. Motor Prostheses. In: Brookhart JM, Mountcastle VB, eds. *Handbook of physiology—the nervous system II.* Bethesda, MD: American Physiological Society, 1981; 155–187.
3. Henneman E. Relation between size of neurons and their susceptibility to discharge. *Science* 1957; 126:1345–1347.
4. Burke RE. Motor units: anatomy, physiology, and functional organization. In: Brookhart JM, Mountcastle VB, eds. *Handbook of physiology—the nervous system II.* Bethesda, MD: American Physiological Society, 1981; 345–422.
5. Sweeney JD. Skeletal muscle response to electrical stimulation. In: Reilly JP, ed. *Electrical stimulation and electropathology.* New York: Cambridge University Press, 1992; 283–310.
6. Riley DA, Allin EF. The effects of inactivity, programmed stimulation, and denervation of the histochemistry of skeletal muscle fiber types. *Exp Neurol* 1973; 40:391–398.
7. Peckham PH, Mortimer JT, Marsolais EB. Alteration in the force and fatigability of skeletal muscle in quadriplegic humans following exercise induced by chronic electrical stimulation. *Clin Orthop* 1976; 114:326–334.
8. Marsolais EB, Kobetic R. Functional walking in paralyzed patients by means of electrical stimulation. *Clin Orthop* 1983; 175:30–36.
9. Kagaya H, Shimada Y, Sato K, Sato M. Changes in muscle force following therapeutic electrical stimulation in patients with complete paraplegia. *Paraplegia* 1996; 34:24–29.
10. Peckham PH, Mortimer JT, Marsolais EB. Upper and lower motor neuron lesions in the upper extremity muscles of tetraplegics. *Paraplegia* 1976; 14:115–121.
11. Crago PE, Peckham PH, Thrope GB. Modulation of muscle force by recruitment during intramuscular stimulation. *IEEE Trans Biomed Eng* 1980; 27:679–684.
12. Grandjean PA, Mortimer JT. Recruitment properties of monopolar and bipolar epimysial electrodes. *Ann Biomed Eng* 1986; 14:53–66.
13. Kilgore KL, Peckham PH, Keith MW, Thrope GB. Electrode characterization for functional application to upper extremity FNS. *IEEE Trans Biomed Eng* 1990; 37:12–22.
14. Keith MW, Peckham PH, Thrope GB, et al. Implantable FES in the tetraplegic hand. *J Hand Surg [Am]* 1989; 14:524–530.
15. Naples GG, Mortimer JT, Scheiner A, Sweeney JD. A spiral nerve cuff electrode for peripheral nerve stimulation. *IEEE Trans Biomed Eng* 1988; 35:905–916.
16. Glenn WWL, Phelps ML. Diaphragm pacing by electrical stimulation of the phrenic nerve. *Neurosurgery* 1985; 14:53–66.
17. Kim JH, Manuelidis EE, Glenn WWL, Kaneyuki T. Histopathological changes in the phrenic nerve following long-term electrical stimulation. *J Thoracic Cardiovasc Surg* 1976; 72:602–608.
18. Waters RL, McNeal DR, Faloon W, Clifford B. Functional electrical stimulation of the peroneal nerve for hemiplegia: long-term clinical follow-up. *J Bone Joint Surg [Am]* 1985; 67:792–793.
19. Peckham PH. Functional electrical stimulation: current status and future prospects of applications to the neuromuscular system in spinal cord injury. *Paraplegia* 1987; 25:279–285.
20. Bajd T, Kralj A, Turk R, Benko H, Sega J. The use of a four channel electrical stimulator as an ambulatory aid for paraplegic patients. *Phys Ther* 1983; 63:1116–1120.
21. Kralj A, Bajd T, Turk R, Benko H. Gait restoration in paraplegic patients: a feasibility demonstration using multichannel surface electrode FES. *J Rehab Res Dev* 1983; 20:3–20.
22. Kralj A, Bajd T. *Functional electrical stimulation: standing and walking after spinal cord injury.* Boca Raton, FL: CRC Press, 1989.
23. Graupe D. EMG pattern analysis for patient-responsive control of FES in paraplegics for walker-supported walking. *IEEE Trans Biomed Eng* 1989; 36:711–719.
24. Chizeck HJ, Kobetic R, Marsolais EB, Abbas JJ, Donner IH, Simon

E. Control of functional neuromuscular stimulation systems for standing and locomotion in paraplegics. *Proc IEEE* 1988; 76:1155–1165.
25. Crago PE, Chizeck HJ, Neuman M, Hambrecht FT. Sensors for use with functional neuromuscular stimulation. *IEEE Trans Biomed Eng* 1986; 33:256–268.
26. Triolo RJ, Kobetic R, Betz RR. Standing and walking with FNS: technical and clinical challenges. In: Harris GF, Smith PA, eds. *Human motion analysis: current applications and future directions.* New York: IEEE Press, 1996; 318–350.
27. Benton LA, Baker LL, Bowman BR, Waters RL. *Functional electrical stimulation: a practical clinical guide,* 2nd ed. Downey, CA: Rancho Los Amigos Medical Center, 1981.
28. Marsolais EB, Kobetic R. Implantation techniques and experience with percutaneous intramuscular electrodes in the lower extremities. *J Rehabil Res Dev* 1986; 23:1–8.
29. Memberg WD, Peckham PH, Thrope GB, Keith MW, Kicher TP. An analysis of the reliability of percutaneous intramuscular electrodes in upper extremity FNS applications. *IEEE Trans Rehabil Eng* 1993; 1: 126–132.
30. Scheiner A, Polando G, Marsolais EB. Design and clinical application of a double helix electrode for functional electrical stimulation. *IEEE Trans Biomed Eng* 1984; 41:425–431.
31. Memberg W, Peckham PH, Keith MW. A surgically implanted intramuscular electrode for an implantable neuromuscular stimulation system. *IEEE Trans Rehabil Eng* 1994; 2:80–91.
32. Gradjean PA, Mortimer JT. Recruitment properties of monopolar and bipolar epimysial electrodes. *Ann Biomed Eng* 1986; 14:53–66.
33. Thoma H, Frey M, Holle J, Kern H, Mayr W, Schwanda G, Stoehr H. Functional neurostimulation to substitute locomotion in paraplegia patients. In: Andrade JD, ed. *Artificial organs.* New York: VCH Publishers, 1987; 515–529.
34. Davis R, MacFarland WC, Emmons SE. Initial results of the Nucleus FES-22-implanted system for limb movement in paraplegia. *Stereotactic Func Neurosurg* 1994; 63:192–197.
35. Waters R, McNeal D, Perry J. Experimental correction of footdrop by electrical stimulation of the peroneal nerve. *J Bone Joint Surg [Am]* 1975; 57:1047–1054.
36. Waters R, McNeal D, Faloon W, Clifford B. Functional electrical stimulation of peroneal nerve for hemiplegia. *J Bone Joint Surg* 1985; 67:792–793.
37. Sinkjaer T, Haugland M, Haase J. Natural neural sensing and artificial muscle control in man. *Exp Brain Res* 1994; 98:542–545.
38. Smith B, Peckham PH, Roscoe DD, Keith MW, Marsolais EB. An externally powered, multichannel implantable stimulator for versatile control of paralyzed muscle. *IEEE Trans Biomed Eng* 1987; 34: 499–508.
39. Letechepia JE, Peckham PH, Gazdik M, Smith B. In-line lead connector for use with implanted neuroprostheses. *IEEE Trans Biomed Eng* 1991; 38:707–709.
40. Akazawa K, Makikawa M, Kawamura J, Aoki H. Functional electrical stimulation system using an implantable hydroxyapatite connector and a microprocessor-based portable stimulator. *IEEE Trans Biomed Eng* 1989; 36:746–752.
41. Buckett JR, Peckham PH, Thrope GB, Braswell SD, Keith MW. A flexible, portable system for FNS in the paralyzed upper extremity. *IEEE Trans Biomed Eng* 1988; 35:897–904.
42. Girbardt R. Restoration of the grasp movement of a tetraplegic with the help of functional electric stimulation. In: *International Series on Biomechanics.* Vol. 3A. Dubrovnik. Baltimore: University Park Press, 1981; 301–306.
43. Handa Y, Shimada Y, Komatso S, et al. Electrically induced hand movements and their application for daily living. *Proceedings of the Eighth International Symposium on ECHE,* Dubrovnik, 1984; 169–180.
44. Handa Y, Handa T, Nakatsuchi Y, Yagi R, Hoshimiya N. A voice controlled functional electrical stimulation system for the paralyzed hand. *Jpn J Med Electronics Biol Eng* 1985; 23:292–298.
45. Handa Y, Hoshimiya N. Functional electrical stimulation for the control of the upper extremities. *Med Prog Technol* 1987; 12:51–63.
46. Handa Y, Ohkubo K, Hoshimiya N. A portable multi-channel FNS system for restoration of motor function of the paralyzed extremities. *Automedica* 1989; 11:221–231.
47. Handa Y, Handa T, Ichie M, et al. Functional electrical stimulation (FES) systems for restoration of motor function of paralyzed muscles—versatile systems and a portable system. *Frontiers Med Biol Eng* 1992; 4:214–255.
48. Handa Y, Kameyama J, Hoshimiya N. FNS-control of shoulder motion in hemiplegic and quadriplegic patients. *Proceedings of the Vienna International Workshop on Functional Electrostimulation.* 1992; 127–129.
49. Hoshimiya N, Naito A, Yajima M, Handa Y. A multichannel FES system for the restoration of motor functions in high spinal cord injury patients: a respiration-controlled system for multijoint upper extremity. *IEEE Trans Biomed Eng* 1989; 36:754–760.
50. Hoshimiya N, Handa Y. A master-slave type multichannel functional electrical stimulation (FES) system for the control of the paralyzed upper extremities. *Automedica* 1989; 11:209–220.
51. Kawamura J, Matsuya M, Fukui N, Nishihara K, Sueda O, Tominaga A. Clinical experiences of functional electrical stimulation in Japan. *Proceedings of the Eighth International Symposium on ECHE,* Dubrovnik, 1984; 89–100.
52. Keith MW, Peckham PH, Thrope GB, Buckett JR, Stroh KC, Menger V. Functional FNS neuroprostheses for the tetraplegic hand. *Clin Orthop Rel Res* 1988; 233:25–33.
53. Keith MW, Peckham PH, Thrope GB, et al. Implantable functional FNS in the tetraplegic hand. *J Hand Surg [Am]* 1989; 14:524–530.
54. Keith MW, Kilgore KL, Peckham PH, Wuolle KS, Creasey G, Lemay M. Tendon transfers and functional electrical stimulation for restoration of hand function in spinal cord injury. *J Hand Surg [Am]* 1996; 21:89–99.
55. Kilgore KL, Peckham PH, Keith MW. An implanted upper extremity neuroprosthesis: a twenty patient follow-up [Abstract]. *J Spinal Cord Med* 1995; 18:147.
56. Kilgore KL, Peckham PH, Keith MW, et al. An implanted upper-extremity neuroprosthesis: follow-up of five patients. *J Bone Joint Surg Am* 1997; 79:533–541.
57. Kiwerski J, Pasniczek R. An apparatus making possible restoration of simple functions of the tetraplegic hand. *Paraplegia* 1984; 22: 316–319.
58. Long C, Masciarelli V. An electrophysiologic splint for the hand. *Arch Phys Med* 1963; 44:499–503.
59. Nathan RH. Functional electrical stimulation of the upper limb: charting the forearm surface. *Med Biol Eng Comput* 1979; 17:729–736.
60. Nathan RH, Ohry A. Upper limb functions regained in quadriplegia: a hybrid computerized FNS system. *Arch Phys Med Rehabil* 1990; 71:415–442.
61. Peckham PH, Mortimer JT. Restoration of hand function in the quadriplegic through electrical stimulation. In: Reswick JB, Hambrecht FT, eds. *Functional electrical stimulation: applications in neural prosthesis.* New York: Marcel Dekker, 1977; 83–95.
62. Peckham PH, Marsolais EB, Mortimer JT. Restoration of key grip and release in the C6 tetraplegic patient through functional electrical stimulation. *J Hand Surg* 1980; 5:462–469.
63. Peckham PH, Mortimer JT, Marsolais EB. Controlled prehension and release in the C5 quadriplegic elicited by functional electrical stimulation of the paralyzed forearm musculature. *Ann Biomed Eng* 1980; 8: 369–388.
64. Peckham PH, Thrope GB, Buckett JR, Freehafer AA, Keith MW. Coordinated two mode grasp in the quadriplegic initiated by functional FNS. In: Cambell RM, ed. *IFAC control aspects of prosthetics and orthotics.* Oxford, England: Pergamon, 1983; 29–32.
65. Peckham PH, Keith MW. Motor prostheses for restoration of upper extremity function. In: Stein RB, Peckham PH, Popovic DB, eds. *Neural prostheses: replacing motor function after disease or disability.* New York: Oxford University Press, 1992; 162–190.
66. Perkins TA, Brindley GS, Donaldson NN, Polkey CE, Rushton DN. Implant provision of key, pinch and power grips in a C6 tetraplegic. *Med Biol Eng Comp* 1994; 32:367–372.
67. Prochazka A, Wieler M, Gauthier M. The bionic glove. *Proceedings of the First Annual Conference of the International Functional Electrical Stimulation Society*, Cleveland, OH, May 1996; 13.
68. Scott TRD, Peckham PH, Keith MW. Upper extremity neuroprostheses using functional electrical stimulation. In: Brindley GS, Rushton DN, eds. *Bailliere's clinical neurology.* London: Bailliere Tindall, 1995; 57–75.
69. Smith B, Buckett JR, Peckham PH, Keith MW, Roscoe DD. An externally powered, multichannel, implantable stimulator for versatile control of paralyzed muscle. *IEEE Trans Biomed Eng* 1987; 34:499–508.
70. Weiss M, Kiwerski J, Pasniczek R. An electronic hybrid device for the control of hand functions by electrical stimulation methods. *Proceedings of the 7th International Congress in Biomechanics.* Baltimore: University Park Press, 1981; 397–404.

71. Keller AD, Taylor CL, Zahm V. Studies to determine the functional requirements for hand and arm prosthesis. *Final Report National Academy of Science Contract No. Vam-21223.* New York: Veterans Administration, 1947.
72. Nathan RH. Control strategies in FNS systems for the upper extremities. *Crit Rev Biomed Eng* 1993; 21:485–568.
73. Kilgore KL, Peckham PH, Keith MW, Thrope GB. Electrode characterization for functional application to upper extremity FNS. *IEEE Trans Biomed Eng* 1990; 37:12–21.
74. Smith BT, Betz RR, Mulcahey MJ, Triolo RJ. Reliability of percutaneous intramuscular electrodes for upper extremity functional electrical stimulation in adolescents with C5 tetraplegia. *Arch Phys Med Rehabil* 1994; 75:939–945.
75. Johnson MW, Peckham PH. Evaluation of shoulder movement as a command control source. *IEEE Trans Biomed Eng* 1990; 37:876–885.
76. Betz RR, Mulcahey MJ, Smith BT, et al. Bipolar latissimus dorsi transposition and functional electrical stimulation to restore elbow flexion in an individual with C4 quadriplegia and C5 denervation. *J Am Paraplegia Soc* 1992; 15:220–228.
77. Mortimer JT, Bayer DM, Lord RH, Swanker JW. Shoulder position transduction for proportional two axis control of orthotic/prosthetic systems. In: Heberts P, Kadefors R, Magnusson R, Petersen I, eds. *The control of upper-extremity prostheses and orthoses.* Springfield, IL: Charles C Thomas, 1974; 131–145.
78. Smith BT, Mulcahey MJ, Triolo RJ, Betz RR. The application of a modified neuroprosthetic hand system in a child with a C7 spinal cord injury, case report. *Paraplegia* 1992; 30:598–606.
79. Kilgore KL, Hart RL, Peckham PH. Wrist control of an upper extremity neuroprosthesis. *American Paraplegia Society 42nd Annual Conference.* Las Vegas, NV, 1996; 13.
80. Saxena A, Nikolic S, Popovic D. An EMG-controlled grasping system for tetraplegics. *J Rehabil Res Dev* 1995; 32:17–24.
81. Vodovnik L, Long C, Reswick JB, Lippay A, Starbuck D. Myo-electric control of paralyzed muscles. *IEEE Trans Biomed Eng* 1965; 12: 169–172.
82. Solomonow M, Baratta R, Shoji H, D'Ambrosia RD. The myoelectric signal of electrically stimulated muscle during recruitment: an inherent feedback parameter for a closed-loop control scheme. *IEEE Trans Biomed Eng* 1986; 33:735–745.
83. Triolo R, Nathan R, Handa Y, Keith M, Betz R, Carroll S, Kantor C. Challenges to clinical deployment of upper limb neuroprostheses. *J Rehabil Res Dev* 1996; 33:111–122.
84. Teeter JO, Kantor C, Brown DL. *Functional electrical stimulation (FES) resource guide for persons with spinal cord injury or multiple sclerosis.* Cleveland: FES Information Center, 1995.
85. Mulcahey MJ, Smith BT, Betz RR, Triolo RJ, Peckham PH. Functional FES: outcomes in young people with tetraplegia. *J Am Paraplegia Soc* 1994; 17:20–35.
86. Smith BT, Mulcahey MJ, Betz RR. Quantitative comparison of grasp and release abilities with and without functional electrical stimulation in adolescents with tetraplegia. *Paraplegia* 1996; 34:16–23.
87. Stroh KC, Van Doren CL, Thrope GB, Wijman CAC. Common object test: a functional assessment for quadriplegic patients using an FNS hand system. *Proceedings of the RESNA 12th Annual Conference,* New Orleans, LA, 1989; 387–388.
88. Wuolle KS, Van Doren CL, Thrope GB, Keith MW, Peckham PH. Development of a quantitative hand grasp and release test for patients with tetraplegia using a hand neuroprosthesis. *J Hand Surg [Am]* 1994; 19:209–218.
89. Wijman CA. Stroh KC, Van Doren CL, Thrope GB, Peckham PH, Keith MW. Functional evaluation of quadriplegic patients using a hand neuroprosthesis. *Arch Phys Med Rehabil* 1990; 71:1053–1057.
90. Memberg WD, Peckham PH, Thrope GB, Keith MW, Kicher TP. An analysis of the reliability of percutaneous intramuscular electrodes in upper extremity FNS applications. *IEEE Trans Rehabil Eng* 1993; 1: 126–132.
91. Tang Z, Smith B, Schild JH, Peckham PH. Data transmission from an implantable biotelemeter by load-shift keying using circuit configuration modulator. *IEEE Trans Biomed Eng* 1995; 42:525–528.
92. Grill WM, Mortimer JT. Quantification of recruitment properties of multiple contact cuff electrodes. *IEEE Trans Rehabil Eng* 1996; 4: 49–62.
93. Haugland MK, Hoffer JA, Sinkjaer T. Skin contact force information in sensory nerve signals recorded by implanted cuff electrodes. *IEEE Trans Rehabil Eng* 1994; 2:18–28.
94. Loeb GE, Zamin CJ, Schulman JH, Troyk PR. Indictable microstimulator for functional electrical stimulation. *Med Biol Eng Comput* 1991; 29:NS13–NS19.
95. Miller LJ, Peckham PH, Keith MW. Elbow extension in the C5 quadriplegic using functional FNS. *IEEE Trans Biomed Eng* 1989; 36: 771—780.
96. Kameyama J, Handa Y, Ichie M, Hoshimiya N, Sakurai M. Control of shoulder movement by FNS. *Proceedings of the Annual International Conference of the IEEE Engineering in Medicine and Biology Society,* San Diego, CA, 1993;1342–1343.
97. Crago PE, Nakai RJ, Chizeck HJ. Feedback regulation of hand grasp opening and contact force during stimulation of paralyzed muscle. *IEEE Trans Biomed Eng* 1991; 38:17–28.
98. Riso RR, Ignagni AR, Keith MW. Cognitive feedback for use with FNS upper extremity neuroprostheses. *IEEE Trans Biomed Eng* 1991; 38:29–38.
99. Van Doren CL, Menia LL. Representing the surface texture of grooved plates using single-channel electrocutaneous stimulation. In: Verrillo RT, ed. *Sensory research multimodal perspectives.* Hillsdale, NJ: Lawrence Erlbaum, 1993; 177–197.
100. Hines AE, Crago PE, Billian C. Hand opening by electrical stimulation in patients with spastic hemiplegia. *IEEE Trans Rehabil Eng* 1995; 3:193–205.
101. Merletti R, Acimovic R, Grobelnik S, Cvilak G. Electrophysiological orthosis for the upper extremity in hemiplegia: feasibility study. *Arch Phys Med Rehabil* 1975; 56:507–513.
102. Rebersek S, Vodovnik L. Proportionally controlled functional electrical stimulation of hand. *Arch Phys Med Rehabil* 1973; 54:378–382.
103. Stanic U, Acimovic-Janezic R, Gros N, Trnkocsy A, Bajd T, Kljajic M. Multichannel electrical stimulation for correction of hemiplegic gait. *Scand J Rehabil Med* 1977; 10:175–192.
104. Bogataj U, Gros N, Malezic M, Kelij B, Kljajic M, Acimovic R. Restoration of gait during two of three weeks of therapy with multichannel electrical stimulation. *Phys Ther* 1989; 69:319–326.
105. Bogatgj U, Gros N, Kljajic M, Acimovic R, Malezic M. The rehabilitation of gait in patients with hemiplegia: a comparison between conventional therapy and multichannel functional electrical stimulation therapy. *Phys Ther* 1995; 75:38–52.
106. Daly JJ, Barnickle K, Kobetic R, Marsolai EB. Electrically induced gait changes post stroke, using an FNS system with intramuscular electrodes and multiple channels. *J Neurol Rehabil* 1993; 7:17–25.
107. Daly JJ, Marsolais EB, Mendell LM, Rymer WZ, Stefanovska A, Wolpaw JR, Kanton C. Therapeutic neural effects of electrical stimulation. *IEEE Trans Rehabil Eng* 1996; 4:218–230.
108. Cybulski GR, Penn RD, Jaeger R. Lower extremity functional neuromuscular stimulation in cases of spinal cord injury. *Neurosurgery* 1985; 15:132–146.
109. Marsolais EB, Kobetic R. Functional electrical stimulation for walking in paraplegia. *J Bone Joint Surg [Am]* 1987; 69:728–733.
110. Borges G, Ferguson K, Kobetic R. Development and operation of portable and laboratory electrical stimulation systems for walking in paraplegic subjects. *IEEE Trans Biomed Eng* 1989; 36:798–800.
111. Marsolais EB, Scheiner A, Miller PC, Kobetic R, Daly J. Augmentation of transfers for a quadriplegic patient using an implanted FNS system. Case report. *Paraplegia* 1994; 32:573–579.
112. Glaser RM. Functional neuromuscular stimulation: exercise conditioning of spinal cord injured patients. *Int J Sports Med* 1994; 15: 142–148.
113. Glaser RM. Physiologic aspects of spinal cord injury and functional neuromuscular stimulation. *Cent Nerv Syst Trauma* 1986; 3:49–62.
114. Glaser RM. Physiology of functional electrical stimulation-induced exercise: basic science perspective. *J Neurol Rehabil* 1991; 5:49–61.
115. Martin TP, Stein RB, Hoeppner PH, Reid DC. Influence of electrical stimulation on the morphological and metabolic properties of paralyzed muscle. *J Appl Physiol* 1992; 72:1401–1406.
116. Faghri PD, Glaser RM, Figoni SF, Miles DS. Feasibility of using two FNS exercise modes for spinal cord injured patients. *Clin Kinesiol* 1989; 43:62–64.
117. Gruner JA, Glaser RM, Feinberg SD, Collins SR, Nussbaum NS. A system for evaluation and exercise conditioning of paralyzed leg muscles. *J Rehabil Res Dev* 1983; 20:21–30.
118. Rodgers MM, Glaser RM, Figoni SF, et al. Musculoskeletal responses of spinal cord injured individuals to functional neuromuscular stimulation-induced knee extension exercise training. *J Rehabil Res Dev* 1991; 28:19–26.
119. Figoni SF, Glaser RM, Rodgers MM, et al. Acute hemodynamic responses of spinal cord injured individuals to functional neuromuscular

stimulation-induced knee extension exercise. *J Rehabil Res Dev* 1991; 28:9–18.

120. Ragnarsson KT, O'Daniel W, Edgar R, Pollack S, Petrofsky J, Nash MS. Clinical evaluation of computerized functional electrical stimulation after spinal cord injury: a multicenter pilot study. *Arch Phys Med Rehabil* 1988; 69:672–677.
121. Pollack SF, Axen K, Spielholz N, Levin N, Haas F, Ragnarsson KT. Aerobic training effects of electrically induced lower extremity exercises in spinal cord injured people. *Arch Phys Med Rehabil* 1989; 70: 214–219.
122. Nash MS, Bilsker S, Arcillo AE, et al. Reversal of adaptive left ventricular atrophy following electrically-stimulated exercise training in human tetraplegics. *Paraplegia* 1991; 29:590–599.
123. Twist DJ, Culpepper-Morgan JA, Ragnarsson KT, Petrillo C, Kreck MJ. Neuroendocrine changes during functional electrical stimulation. *Am J Phys Med Rehabil* 1992; 71:156–163.
124. Sipski ML, Delisa JA, Schweer S. Functional electrical stimulation bicycle ergometry: patient perceptions. *Am J Phys Med Rehabil* 1989; 68:147–149.
125. Hooker SP, Figoni SF, Rodgers MM, et al. Metabolic and hemodynamic responses to concurrent voluntary arm crank and electrical stimulation leg cycle exercise in quadriplegics. *J Rehabil Res Dev* 1992; 29:1–11.
126. Bajd T, Kralj A, Turk R. Standing up of a healthy subject and a paraplegic patient. *J Biomech* 1982; 15:1–10.
127. Graupe D, Kohn K. *Functional electrical stimulation for ambulation by paraplegics.* Malabar, FL: Krieger Publishing, 1994.
128. Jaeger RJ, Yarkony GM, Roth EJ. Rehabilitation technology for standing and walking after spinal cord injury. *Am J Phys Med Rehabil* 1989; 68:128–133.
129. Yarkony GM, Jaeger R, Roth E, Kralj A, Quintern J. Functional neuromuscular stimulation for standing after spinal cord injury. *Arch Phys Med Rehabil* 1990; 70:201–206.
130. Jaeger R, Yarkony G, Smith R. Standing the spinal cord injured patient by electrical stimulation: refinement of a protocol for clinical use. *IEEE Trans Biomed Eng* 1989; 36:720–728.
131. Andrews B, Baxendale R. A hybrid orthosis incorporating artificial reflexes for spinal cord damaged patients. *J Physiol (Lond)* 1986; 380: 19P.
132. Marsolais EB, Kobetic R, Chizeck HJ, Jacobs JL. Orthoses and electrical stimulation for walking in complete paraplegia. *J Neurol Rehabil* 1991; 5:13–22.
133. Solomonow M, Baratta RV, Hirokawa S. The RGO generation II:-muscle stimulation powered orthosis as a practical walking system for paraplegics. *Orthopaedics* 1989; 12:1309–1315.
134. Solomonow M. Biomechanics and physiology of a practical functional neuromuscular stimulation powered walking orthosis for paraplegics. In: Stein RB, Peckham PH, Popovic DP, eds. *Neural prostheses: replacing motor function after disease or disability.* New York: Oxford University Press, 1992; 202–232.
135. D Ambrosia R, Solomonow M, Baratta RV. Current status of walking orthoses for thoracic paraplegics. *Iowa Orthop J* 1995; 15:174–181.
136. Kantor C, Andrews BJ, Marsolais EB, Solomonow M, Lew RD, Ragnarsson KT. Report on a conference on motor prostheses for workplace mobility of paraplegic patients in North America. *Paraplegia* 1993; 31:439–456.
137. McClelland M, Andrews BJ, Patrick JH, Freeman PA. Augmentation of the Oswestry Parawalker orthosis by means of surface electrical stimulation: gait analysis of three patients. *Paraplegia* 1987; 25: 32–38.
138. Kobetic R, Marsolais EB. Synthesis of paraplegic gait with multichannel functional neuromuscular stimulation. *IEEE Trans Rehabil Eng* 1994; 2:66–79.
139. Kobetic R, Marsolais EB, Samame P, Borges G. The next step: artificial walking. In: Rose J, Gamble JG, eds. *Human walking,* 2nd ed. Baltimore, MD: Williams & Wilkins, 1994; 225–252.
140. Edwards BG, Marsolais EB. Metabolic responses to arm ergometry and functional neuromuscular stimulation. *J Rehabil Res Dev* 1990; 27:107–114.
141. Inman VT, Ralston HJ, Todd F. *Human walking.* Baltimore: Williams & Wilkins, 1981; 45–46.
142. Winter DA. *Biomechanics and motor control of human movement,* 2nd ed. New York: Wiley, 1990.
143. Betz R, Boden B, Triolo R, Mesgarzadeh M, Gardner E, Fife R. Effects of functional neuromuscular stimulation on the joints of adolescents with spinal cord injury. *Paraplegia* 1996; 34:127–136.
144. Betz RR, Mulcahey M, Smith B, Triolo RJ. Hip dislocation following standing and ambulation with functional electrical stimulation: a case report. (Submitted for publication).
145. Dearolf WW, Betz RR, Vogel LC, Levin J, Clancy M, Steel H. Scoliosis in spinal injured patients. *J Pediatr Orthop* 1990; 10:214–218.
146. Alexander S, Rowan D. Electronic control of urinary incontinence: a clinical appraisal. *Br J Surg* 1970; 57:766–768.
147. Hopkinson BR. Electrical treatment of incontinence. *Ann R Coll Surg Engl* 1992; 50:92–111.
148. Smith JJ. Intravaginal stimulation randomised trial. *J Urol* 1966; 155: 127–130.
149. Thon WF, Baskin LS, Jonas U, Tanagho EA, Schmidt RA. Neuromodulation of voiding dysfunction and pelvic pain. *World J Urol* 1991; 9:138–141.
150. Edwards L, Malvern J. Electronic control of continence: a critical review of the present situation. *Br J Urol* 1992; 44:467–472.
151. Bosch JL, Groen J. Sacral (S3) segmental nerve stimulation as a treatment for urge incontinence in patients with detrusor instability: results of chronic electrical stimulation using an implantable neural prosthesis. *J Urol* 1995; 154:504–507.
152. Ishigooka M, Hashimoto T, Sasagawa I, Nakada T, Handa Y. Electric pelvic floor stimulation by percutaneous implantable electrode. *Br J Urol* 1994; 74:191–194.
153. Arnold EP, Gowland SP, MacFarlane MR, Bean AR, Utley WLF. Sacral anterior root stimulation of the bladder in paraplegics. *Aust N Z J Surg* 1986; 56:319–324.
154. Brindley GS, Polkey CE, Rushton DN, Cardozo L. Sacral anterior root stimulators for bladder control in paraplegia: the first 50 cases. *J Neurol Neurosurg Psychiatry* 1986; 49:1104–1114.
155. Robinson LQ, Grant A, Weston P, Stephenson TP, Lucas M, Thomas DG. Experience with the Brindley anterior sacral root stimulator. *Br J Urol* 1988; 62:553–557.
156. Brindley GS, Rushton DN. Long-term follow-up of patients with sacral anterior root stimulator implants. *Paraplegia* 1990; 28:469–475.
157. Madersbacher H, Fisher J. Sacral anterior root stimulation: prerequisites and indications. *Neurourol Urodyn* 1993; 12:489–494.
158. Creasey GH. Electrical stimulation of sacral roots for micturition after spinal cord injury. *Urol Clin North Am* 1993; 20:505–515.
159. Van Kerrebroeck PEV, Kolewijn EL, Debruyne FMJ. Worldwide experience with the Finetech-Brindley sacral anterior root stimulator. *Neurourol Urodyn* 1993; 12:497–503.
160. Brindley G. The first 500 patients with sacral anterior root stimulator implants: general description. *Paraplegia* 1994; 32:795–805.
161. Madersbacher H, Fischer J, Ebner A. Anterior sacral root stimulator (Brindley): experiences especially in women with neurogenic urinary incontinence. *Neurourol Urodyn* 1988; 7:593–601.
162. Colombel P, Egon G. Electrostimulation of the anterior sacral nerve roots. An International Congress, Le Mans, November 24–25, 1989. *Ann Urol Paris* 1991; 25:48–52.
163. MacDonagh RP, Forster DM, Thomas DG. Urinary continence in spinal injury patients following complete sacral posterior rhizotomy. *Br J Urol* 1990; 66:618–622.
164. Van Kerrebroeck PEV, Kolewijn EL, Wijkstra H, Debruyne FMJ. Urodynamic evaluation before and after intradural posterior sacral rhizotomies and implantation of the Finetech-Brindley anterior sacral root stimulator. *Urodinamica* 1992; 1:7–16.
165. Cardozo L, Krishnan KR, Polkey CE, Rushton DN, Brindley GS. Urodynamic observations on patients with sacral anterior root stimulators. *Paraplegia* 1984; 22:201–209.
166. Rushton DN, Brindley GS, Poldey CD, Browning GV. Implant infections and antibiotic-impregnated silicone rubber coating. *J Neurol Neurosurg Psychiatry* 1989; 52:223–229.
167. Brindley G. The first 500 sacral anterior root stimulators: implant failures and their repair. *Paraplegia* 1995; 33:5–9.

Rehabilitation Medicine: Principles and Practice, Third Edition,
edited by Joel A. DeLisa and Bruce M. Gans.
Lippincott–Raven Publishers, Philadelphia © 1998.

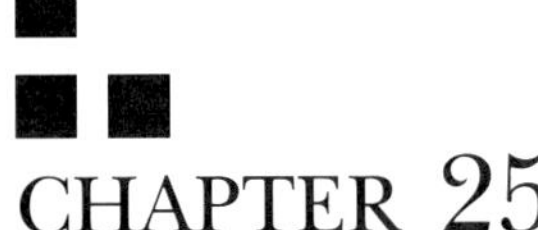

CHAPTER 25

Spinal and Upper Extremity Orthotics

Steven C. Kirshblum, Kevin C. O'Connor, Barbara T. Benevento, and Sandy Salerno

An orthosis is an orthopedic appliance or apparatus used to support, align, prevent, or correct deformities or to improve the function of movable parts of the body (1). Descriptions of orthotic use dates back to ancient times. Although the concepts and goals of orthoses are not new, advances in materials, surgical methods and medical treatments, and modern technology have expanded their use and applications.

There have been a number of different classifications and many names for orthoses. Although many orthoses have specific eponyms based on their founder or location where they were developed, standard orthoses are now described by the joints they encompass and the mechanical motion the orthosis provides (2,3). There are many potential benefits of spinal and upper extremity orthoses, including protection of painful areas, stabilization of body parts, immobilization, and improving function. These will be discussed in further detail. There are also a number of drawbacks, including the difficulty of donning and doffing, skin breakdown, nerve compression, muscle atrophy with long-term use, restriction of the thoracic or abdominal cavity if these orthoses are used, and difficulty swallowing from a cervical orthosis. A major difficulty with all orthoses is the compliance of the patient. The more effective the orthosis as an immobilizer, usually the more uncomfortable. This is especially a problem with removable orthoses that the patient can don and doff at will (4). Unless the patient recognizes the improvements the orthoses offer, they will most often discard them rather than tolerate the discomfort. The nonphysiologic negative effects of some orthoses, especially temporary spinal orthoses, are the cosmetic and psychological aspects, including altered appearance, dependence, and embarrassment.

Orthotics require external compression on the skin molded to the body contours. In order to achieve fixation, skin and body habitus are important factors to consider. Overweight patients may be difficult to fit. Patients with insensate or fragile skin secondary to disease processes are prone to breakdown. These factors must be taken into account when prescribing the orthosic design and fabrication material.

S. C. Kirshblum: Department of Physical Medicine and Rehabilitation, University of Medicine and Dentistry of New Jersey, New Jersey Medical School, Newark, New Jersey 07103; and Spinal Cord Injury Program, Kessler Institute for Rehabilitation, West Orange, New Jersey 07052.

K. C. O'Connor and B. T. Benevento: Department of Physical Medicine and Rehabilitation, University of Medicine and Dentistry of New Jersey, New Jersey Medical School, Newark, New Jersey 07103; and Kessler Institute for Rehabilitation, West Orange, New Jersey 07052.

S. Salerno: Departmemt of Occupational Therapy, St. Francis College, Brooklyn, New York; and Kean College, Union, New Jersey; and Kessler Institute for Rehabilitation, West Orange, New Jersey 07052.

SPINAL ORTHOSES

There are many different spinal orthoses available. The success of spinal bracing depends on the goals to be achieved (Table 25-1) and the ability of the brace to serve these goals. A knowledge of the general principles as well as a clear understanding of the indications and limitations of each specific brace is critical for prescribing the proper orthosis.

The spine for orthotic purposes can be divided into six subgroups: the upper cervical (C1–C2), mid-cervical (C3–T1), thoracic (T2–T10), thoracolumbar (T11–L1), lumbar (L1–L4) and lumbosacral (L4–S1). The most cephalad (upper cervical) and caudal (lumbosacral) areas of the spine are the most difficult to immobilize. Negative effects of spinal orthotics can include skin irritation (5), osteopenia (6,7), muscle atrophy (5), and psychological problems including emotional dependency (8). Other complications are discussed under the specific braces. Neck and trunk exercises within the orthosis can help decrease the degree of decondi-

TABLE 25-1. *Specific functions that spinal orthoses may offer*

Correct deformity
Warmth for pain relief
Stabilize the spine
Psychologic benefits
Limit spinal motion
Mechanical unloading

tioning and atrophy. Spinal orthoses are temporary devices and should be discarded when the goals have been reached. Spine orthoses are indicated in treating many disorders and injuries to the neck, from minor muscle spasm to instability. They can be categorized by the joints they encompass and include:

1. Cervical orthoses (CO)
2. Head cervical orthoses (HCO)
3. Cervical thoracic orthoses (CTO)
4. Cervical thoracic lumbar sacral orthoses (CTLSO)
5. Thoracolumbosacral orthoses (TLSO)
6. Lumbosacral orthoses (LSO)

CERVICAL SPINE: ANATOMIC CONSIDERATIONS

The cervical spine is composed of seven vertebrae and moves in three planes: flexion–extension, lateral bending, and rotation. The occiput-C1 articulation offers a great degree of flexion and extension with limited lateral bending and rotation. The C1–C2 (atlantoaxial) joint is more complex, with rotation as its primary motion with less flexion–extension. Movements between C1 and C2 can occur independently of movements below C2. The cervical segments (C3–C6) are more mobile than C7 and thoracic vertebrae. Total flexion of the cervical spine is approximately 70°. Most flexion–extension occurs between C5 and C6, followed by C6–C7 and C4–C5. The occipito-atlanto-axial complex allows a great amount of flexion, mostly at the occiput-C1 articulation. Full rotation is approximately 75° to 90°, with half to three quarters occurring at C1–C2. Each disc allows only a few degrees of rotation. Lateral bending occurs in the middle portion of the cervical spine (C2–C6).

The type of cervical orthosis recommended depends on the amount of limitation of range of motion (ROM) desired (Table 25-2). No spinal brace provides complete immobilization; however, the more encompassing and the harder the material used, the greater the limitation of range. The cervical spine is the most mobile and has the smallest skin surface area of all segments of the spine. Vital structures contained within this small area include the trachea, larynx, and major vessels. These structures, along with the limited skin surface area upon which to place the pressure from an orthosis, make it difficult to offer adequate immobilization with comfort and safety.

A number of investigators have studied the limitations of motion of cervical orthoses by different techniques (9–13). Most investigators agree that the soft cervical collar offers

TABLE 25-2. *Effects of cervical orthoses on cervical motion (occiput to C7) (%) of mean normal motion allowed*

	Flexion/Extension	Lateral bending	Rotation	Reference
Normal	100	100.0	100.0	
Soft collar	74.2	92.3	82.6	Johnson (11)
	90/95	90/95	100	
	70/73	87	78	
Hard collar	25	25	25–50	Hartman (10)
Philadelphia collar	28.9	66.7	43.7	Johnson (11)
	58/53	66.7	43.7	Lunsford (4)
	26/41	71	51	Ducker (76)
Miami J	52/62	52	24	Lunsford (4)
	15/25	37		Ducker (76)
Malibu	47/43	—	39	Lunsford (4)
SOMI	27.7	65.6	33.6	Johnson (77)
	20–25%	15%	40	Hartman (10)
4 Poster brace	20.6	45.9	27.1	Johnson (11)
	15–20	15–20	40	Hartman (10)
Yale brace	13.3	39.5	25.4	Johnson (77)
Rigid cervicothoracic brace	12.8	50.5	18.2	Hartman (10)
				Drucker (76)
Halo	4.0	4.0	1.0	Johnson (11)
	11.7	8.4	2.4	Lysell (13)
	5–10%	5	0	Hartman (10)
	31%	—	—	Koch (12)
	70%	—	—	Lind (21)
Minerva body jacket	14.0	15.5	0	Maiman (31)

little restriction of cervical spine mobility, with halo-vest fixation the most effective. However, even the halo-vest allows a fair amount of motion in the lower part of the cervical spine and seems to be most dependent on the snugness of the vest to the sternum/chest. Except for the halo device, cervical spine orthoses are indicated only for stable spinal injuries.

CERVICAL ORTHOSES

Cervical orthoses provide no support from the head or thorax. Because of this lack of support, their limitation of cervical motion is minimal. Cervical orthoses include soft and hard collars. A soft cervical collar is made of polyurethane foam rubber with a stockinette cover that attaches with a Velcro closure. The degree of limitation of motion provided by the soft collar has varied in different studies, generally between 3% restriction of flexion and 26.6% restriction of extension (14) and limiting normal rotation by 17% (11). Carter et al. (15) reported that soft collars can limit motion up to 11%; however, the amount of motion was dependent on the collar position. When the Velcro closure of the collar was located posteriorly, extension was more significantly limited; with the closure anterior, flexion was more limited. However, Hartman et al. (10) did not find any difference when the closure was anterior or posterior. Although the soft cervical collar provides little mechanical support, it does provide warmth and physiologic comfort, is well tolerated, acts as a reminder to patients to limit certain movements and supports the head during the acute stages of pain.

The hard cervical collar (e.g., Thomas collar) is made of a rigid polyethylene band with padding that also uses Velcro closures. With optional occipital and mandibular supports added, the hard collar restricts all planes of movement more than the soft cervical collar, but not as much as an HCO, and it causes more discomfort. Hartman et al. (10), in a small study of five healthy subjects, found that the Thomas collar restricted up to 75% of movement in the sagittal plane but offered less control of lateral bending or rotation.

In general, cervical orthoses (soft and hard) may be indicated for patients with uncomplicated neck pain but should not be used in cases where restriction of cervical spine motion is required. Care should be taken not to prescribe these for too long a period, so as to avoid cervical muscle atrophy, which complicates discontinuation of the brace.

Head Cervical Orthoses

This group of orthoses incorporates the head (occiput and chin) to provide additional support to further restrict cervical motion. Examples include the Philadelphia, Miami J, California Stifneck immobilizing, Malibu, and Newport collars. The Philadelphia collar (Westville, NJ) is made of two pieces of plastizote foam with anterior and posterior plastic reinforcements secured by Velcro straps. It is available in a number of sizes according to the circumference and height of the neck, and with or without an opening for a tracheostomy. It has mandibular and occipital supports and extends distally onto the upper thorax. It is more effective in restricting motion of the upper cervical spine. Johnson (11) found that the Philadelphia collar offered 71% restriction of flexion–extension, 66% restriction of rotation, but only 34% restriction of lateral bending. The California Stifneck immobilizing collar (California Medical Products, Long Beach, CA) is a one-piece collar made of polyethylene with a foam cushion and can be used as a prehospital immobilization orthosis (16,17). HCOs are usually indicated for stable mid-cervical bony or ligamentous injuries, sprains, and strains, as well as for postoperative control after spine stabilization. In a small comparison study, the Malibu collar had slightly more restriction of cervical motion in all three planes relative to the Philadelphia, Miami J, and Newport collars (4).

Cervical Thoracic Orthoses

A number of variations of CTOs provide substantial restriction of motion in the middle to lower cervical region. The two-poster brace has anterior and posterior thoracic plates that are connected to chin and occipital supports. The four-poster CTO has padded, molded mandibular and occipital supports with adjustable struts attaching to the thoracic plates. Struts connect the mandibular and occipital supports as well as the anterior and posterior thoracic pads.

The sternal-occipital-mandibular-immobilizer (SOMI) is named for its points of attachment. The detachable chin and occipital supports are attached by adjustable aluminum bars (two from the occipital and one from the mandibular support) to the sternal chest plate anteriorly. The rigid chest plate extends to the xiphoid and has straps that go over the shoulders. A head band that encircles the forehead can be used if the chin piece needs to be removed (i.e., during eating). The SOMI limits normal flexion–extension of the cervical spine by 72% (11), lateral bending by 34.4%, and rotation by 66.4%. An advantage of the SOMI is the lack of posterior rods, making it easier to use in a bedridden patient. The SOMI support is somewhat more restricting than the four-poster brace (9,11). However, if improperly adjusted, the SOMI provides little to no restriction.

The Yale orthosis is essentially an extended Philadelphia collar, continuing down the thorax anteriorly and posteriorly, with a strap under the arms and a higher occipital support. These extensions (cephalad and caudal) increase the restriction of cervical flexion–extension and rotation, but with less effect on lateral bending.

Halo

The halo device is the most restrictive of all cervical orthoses. Although it provides the greatest orthotic restriction of motion of the cervical spine, it does not guarantee the maintenance of alignment nor ultimate bone fusion. It was first described in 1959 (18), and although the design has been modified, the concept of providing rigid fixation of the neck by immobilizing the head relative to the trunk has remained. The halo is the most frequently used brace for treating acute cervical fractures and dislocations. It is made of a rigid lightweight metal or graphite ring that is compatible for use with magnetic resonance imaging and is attached with fixation pins into the outer table of the skull, two in the frontal region and two in the parieto-occipital region. The preferred placement of the pins is anterolaterally above the orbital rim and posterolaterally below the greatest diameter of the skull (19). These positions avoid the thinner frontal sinuses and temporal fossa, prevent piercing of the temporalis muscle, and avoid injury to major sensory nerves. The halo ring has posts extending down most commonly onto a rigid polyethylene vest lined with sheepskin or a soft fabric that extends to the umbilicus. A plaster cast vest also can be used. If more contact area is needed, a body cast that extends to the pelvis can be made; but this extension does not improve the restriction of neck motion in radiologic studies. However, loosening of the pins was more common in patients with the halo cast, and patient acceptance and comfort was greater with the plastic jackets (20). The cast is also more time consuming to fabricate, and skin hygiene may be more difficult. Although the halo offers the most restriction of movement, it does not completely immobilize the spine. Lysell (13) found that the halo restricted 88.3% of normal flexion–extension motion, 91.6% of lateral bending, and 97.6% of rotation. Johnson (11) reported that the halo restricted 96% of flexion–extension and lateral bending and 99% of rotation. Koch and Nichol (12) found a restriction of only 69% of normal spine motion between supine and upright positions. Investigators also have described a ''snaking phenomenon'' during halo immobilization (12,21), which is movement between individual spine segments without significant movement of the head in relation to the thoracic spine. The correct fit of the vest is a major determinant in stability. Rehabilitation exercise does not seem to cause any greater motion to the spine than does daily motion and activity (21); however, shoulder shrugging and abduction greater than 90° should be avoided because this can push up on the shoulder straps of the vest and alter the load on the cervical spine (12). Wang (22) studied the stability of the halo based on the length of the vest and found that upper cervical spine lesions can be treated effectively with a half vest (extending to the level of the nipples), although lesions below the fourth cervical vertebrae required a vest to below the 12th rib for proper stability.

Numerous investigators have detailed the proper applications and maintenance of the halo orthosis. Botte et al. (23) found that pin loosening decreased from 36% to 7% and pin tract infections from 20% to 2% when the pins in the halo were applied using 0.90 newton-meters (8 inches-pounds) of torque rather than 0.68 newton-meters (6 inches-pounds). However, Rizzolo et al. (24) concluded that there was no difference between the two torques. Pins are initially tightened at 24 to 48 hours after placement. The pins can be retightened if loosening occurs as long as resistance (proper torque) is felt; otherwise, pins should be moved to another site. Superficial pin infections are treated with local wound care and oral antibiotics. The routine use of povidine-iodine, hydrogen peroxide, hypochlorite solution, and chlorhexidine is discouraged because all of these have been associated with increased infection, disruption of the healing process, or disruption of the normal flora of the skin (25). The use of ointments blocks the drainage of fluid at the pin site and increases the risk of infection (26). Saline or soap and water are the most beneficial cleansing agents for pin care using cotton-tipped applicators, and this cleaning should be performed twice per day. Complications of the halo apparatus include (in decreasing order of occurrence) pin loosening, infection, pin discomfort, ring migration, pressure sores, and unacceptable scars (19). Infrequent complications include nerve injury, dysphagia, perforation of the skull, brain abscess, degenerative changes of facets from immobilization, avascular necrosis of the dens, limitation of self-care activities and social activities, vascular compression of the duodenum, and a reduction of pulmonary vital capacity (27–29). Suggestions to reduce or monitor complications associated with halos are use of a proper protocol for pin placement and care, a full evaluation for post-halo headaches, monitoring at least daily for decubiti (particularly in the elderly and in patients with impaired sensation), and being attentive to abdominal pain or vomiting so as to recognize superior mesenteric artery syndrome from compression of the vest. Wetzel et al. (30) found that patients experienced a significantly higher incidence of halo associated pain with open versus closed ring halos. However, this study was limited, and further prospective studies are needed. The original Minerva brace was an example of an HCO. However, the newer designs with a thermoplastic body jacket that extends caudally to a level similar to the halo vest and with a circumferential forehead piece proximally, offer excellent restriction of motion and comfort without the need of the invasive pin insertions. This thermoplastic Minerva body jacket (TMBJ) has been studied and found to be comparable with the halo in the degree of restriction of cervical spine movement below C3 (31–34). The TMBJ is the only true noninvasive orthosis that offers the support of the halo for below C2. However, the halo still is better at controlling motion at the occiput to C2 levels (32,34). Gaskill (35) recommended its use in preschool children because of its advantages of noninvasiveness, lightness, and comfort.

THORACIC AND LUMBOSACRAL SPINE

Many of the thoracic braces incorporate the lumbar and sacral spine as well. This section will discuss these areas of the spine in conjuntion with the available orthoses. The control systems for most of these orthoses include three-point pressure (which offers trunk support and restricts motion) and anterior abdominal compression. The abdominal compression tends to straighten lumbar lordosis, decreases intervertebral joint motion, and elevates intracavity pressure to decrease the load on the vertebrae and discs. Restriction of motion from thoracic and lumbosacral orthoses have not been studied as extensively as that of cervical orthoses.

The orthotics will be described from the least to most restrictive. The more firm the material and the more segments of the spine they encompass, the greater stabilization they offer. Thoracic and lumbar orthoses can be described by the plane of movement they limit, including flexion, extension, and lateral control. All of these orthotics may impact function by increasing energy consumption, decreasing respiratory function, and decreasing the patient's cadence or stride length in ambulation. This should be taken into account when prescribing the braces because patients with certain medical conditions (e.g., neuromuscular disease, severe deconditioning) may not be able to tolerate them. As with cervical orthoses, the effectiveness of those orthotics is directly dependent on the proper fit and alignment of its components.

Trochanteric Belt

The trochanteric belt encircles the pelvis between the greater trochanter and the iliac crest and is fastened in the front. It can be made of a variety of materials such as canvas or leather and is usually 2 to 3 inches wide. It is used to support healing pelvic fractures and for management of pain in the sacroiliac region.

Sacral Belt

This is a prefabricated orthosis of heavy cotton or cloth, 4 to 6 inches wide, occasionally reinforced with light-weight plastic or metal stays. Its borders are the iliac crest and pubic symphysis anteriorly, and the posterior border extends to the gluteal fold. Perineal straps can prevent the orthosis from shifting upward. A sacral pad applies pressure over the sacrum. This orthosis helps stabilize the sacroiliac joint and is used in patients who are postpartum and have traumatic sacroiliac separations.

Corsets

A number of different types of corsets are available: sacroiliac, lumbar, lumbosacral, and thoracolumbar. They are the most frequently prescribed orthotic for low back pain.

Sacroiliac Corset

The sacroiliac corset is similar to the sacroiliac belt in that its borders are the iliac crest, pubic symphysis, and gluteal fold. It is also prefabricated and can be adjusted with laces that can be placed at the back, side, or front, and therefore will give a variable amount of pressure to the abdomen. They are made from several different fabrics; with stretching, some loss of support can occur. These orthoses do not restrict motion very well, but they increase abdominal pressure and may help stabilize the pelvic joints. They may be useful for postpartum and posttraumatic stabilization of pelvic joints (sacroiliac and pubic symphysis).

Lumbar (Abdominal) Binder

A lumbar (abdominal) binder is made of an elastic fabric with Velcro closure. It offers some trunk support through elevation of intra-abdominal pressure. It also serves as a reminder to the patient to maintain proper posture. A thermoplastic insert can be molded to the patient's back and inserted in a posterior pocket.

Lumbar and Lumbosacral Corsets

Lumbar corsets are made of cotton, nylon, or rayon and usually close in the front with Velcro. Lumbosacral corsets can be either custom made or prefabricated. They surround both the torso and hips, and they border the xiphoid process or lower ribs, pubic symphysis, inferior angle of the scapula, and gluteal fold. They can be secured by laces, hooks, or Velcro either in the front or back. Because they encompass more of the body, they exert increased intra-abdominal pressure and therefore are thought to decrease the load on the vertebrae and discs. The corset can reduce spinal motion by as much as two thirds (36,37). Metal or plastic stays can be added, which mainly cause painful stimuli if the patient moves against them rather than providing additional rigid support. Corsets overall are most effective in acting as a reminder for the patient to limit motion. However, they also support the abdomen, reduce the load on the lumbosacral spine, provide some restriction of the spine, and reduce excessive lumbar lordosis to provide a straighter and more comfortable low back (38,39). A lumbosacral corset has been shown to restrict lateral bending by 29% (37).

For the treatment of low back pain, these braces are effective in decreasing pain. For additional support and pain relief, a custom thermomolded plastic pad for the patient's low back and sacrum can be inserted into a posterior pocket in the LSO controlling the lumbosacral joint (Warm'N'Form, Thermomold Products, Mt. Laurel, NJ). A disadvantage of these and more encompassing spinal orthoses is that they may result in weakening of the muscles that support the trunk. Patients should therefore be instructed in proper exercises to prevent such muscle atrophy.

Thoracolumbar Corset

The thoracolumbar corset is similar to the lumbosacral corset with a thoracic extension. It extends over the scapula, and shoulder straps are added that help maintain the thoracic extension. This brace stabilizes the trunk, decreases the load on the vertebrae, and reminds the patient to restrict movement.

The shorter corsets (those that encompass less surface area

of the spine) are used for disorders such as low back pain due to sprain, strain, osteoarthritis, or osteoporosis. The longer, full-length corsets are helpful in controlling pain in generalized arthritis, metastatic malignancy, myeloma, and osteoarthritis of the thoracic spine. All of these corsets can be reinforced with plastic or metal paraspinal stays, which adds to the rigidity of the corset and somewhat improves the restriction of spinal motion. The posterior stays should be shaped to flatten, not maintain, lumbar lordosis.

When spinal stability is a concern, a more rigid orthosis must be used. Fortunately, the rib cage provides relative stability and minimizes displacement of a fracture in the upper thoracic spine because this part of the spine is otherwise difficult to immobilize. The more rigid orthoses use three-point fixation to limit flexion and extension. This is accomplished by applying forces both proximally and distally to the segment that is to be immobilized. A third force is applied in the opposite direction between these points, and this provides three-point control. A flexion moment is created if the central counterforce is anterior to the spine with the cranial and caudal forces posterior.

Lumbosacral Orthoses

Lumbosacral Flexion–Extension Control and Lateral Control Orthoses

The chairback brace is an example of a lumbosacral flexion–extension control orthosis. It is a rigid LSO made of metal and covered in fabric, but it also can be made of plastic. This brace has a thoracic band that is placed below the scapula and a pelvic band at the sacrococcygeal junction, which are attached posteriorly by two lumbosacral paraspinal uprights. The abdominal support is fastened to the uprights by straps. The thoracic and pelvic bands provide anteriorly directed forces, and the abdominal support a posteriorly directed force, which together act to limit extension and flexion of the lumbar spine. If the pelvic and thoracic bands are rigid, they provide medially directed forces that can control lateral motion, making this brace a flexion–extension lateral (F-E-L) control brace. This brace has been shown to restrict lateral bending by 45% (37). It helps to unload the intervertebral discs and transmit pressure to the surrounding soft tissue and is used for patients with low back pain but has limited value for fracture management. If the forces are great enough, the brace also can act to decrease lordosis.

The Knight brace is an example of a lumbosacral (F-E-L) control orthosis. This brace is similar to the chairback brace with added lateral bars. This offers lateral control and then only requires an anterior corset panel instead of a full corset. It is mainly used for the treatment of low back pain and disc herniation.

These motion-restricting braces can be a useful prognostic aid for patients who may be candidates for spinal fusion. If symptoms are controlled when in the orthosis and not without, even after a proper exercise program, surgical stabilization may be a reasonable option.

Lumbosacral/Extension–Lateral Control Orthosis

The lumbosacral extension–lateral control orthosis or Williams brace is a short spinal orthosis and is unique in that it is dynamic. It contains an anterior elastic panel to allow for forward flexion. Lateral uprights attach to a thoracic band, and a pelvic band is attached to the lateral upright by oblique bars. The abdominal support is laced to the lateral uprights. The three-point force system limits extension of the trunk and lateral trunk movement. Lumbosacral flexion is maintained and therefore of benefit in patients with spondylosis and spondylolisthesis, but not recommended for use in patients with compression fractures.

Thoracolumbosacral Orthoses

Thoracolumbosacral Flexion–Extension Control Orthosis

Taylor, in 1863, designed a brace that was originally used for the treatment of Pott's disease (40). The Taylor brace is a thoracolumbosacral flexion–extension control orthosis, which has a wide pelvic band that attaches to two posterior paraspinal uprights. These uprights extend to the shoulder and are joined by a mid-thoracic transverse bar. Straps pass from the uprights over the shoulder and under the axilla and then reattach to the transverse bar. The axillary loops reduce dorsal kyphosis. There is also an abdominal apron that is attached by straps and buckles that increase intracavitary pressure. The interscapular band decreases thoracic kyphosis by providing an anteriorly directed force. This brace restricts flexion and extension but limits thoracic motion only if the axillary straps are tightened to the point of discomfort (41). The orthosis is ineffective if the straps are loose and therefore should not be used if strict immobilization is required. It is therefore mainly used for kyphosis due to stable pathologic fractures such as osteoporosis.

Thoracolumbosacral Flexion–Extension Lateral Control Orthosis

The Knight-Taylor brace is a combination of the Knight and Taylor braces with both thoracic and pelvic bands, lateral bars, and posterior uprights offering F-E-L control. It is usually made of aluminum and provides thoracolumbar spine control in the saggital and coronal planes. The thoracic band is placed below the inferior angle of the scapula, and the pelvic band is fitted at the sacrococcygeal junction. Axillary straps are attached to an interscapular band. Either a full corset or an anterior panel provides intracavitary pressure and is laced to lateral uprights. Flexion and extension as well as lateral motion are limited. It can be used for stable or postsurgical stable thoracolumbar fractures or pain due to severe muscle strain (40).

Thoracolumbosacral Flexion Control Orthosis (Anterior Hyperextension Brace)

The Jewett brace is one of the oldest of the TLSOs. It employs a three-point system using anterior pads at the upper sternum and at the pubic symphysis that are opposed posteriorly by a thoracolumbar pad. These forces act to extend the thoracolumbar region (42). It is prefabricated, light weight, and easily adjusted; however, because the forces are concentrated over small areas, the brace may cause discomfort. This brace is unique in that it does not have an abdominal apron and therefore does not offer any abdominal support. The pads control the movement, so the brace frame should not contact the patient. When seated, the sternal pads should be a half an inch inferior to the sternal notch and the suprapubic pad half an inch superior to the pubic symphysis. It is used mainly to prevent flexion and to immobilize the lower thoracic and upper lumbar spine after surgical stabilization of a fracture. It is not recommended for compression fractures secondary to osteoporosis because it can place excessive hyperextension forces on the lower lumbar vertebrae and induce fracture of the posterior elements (41). The brace limits motion only in flexion, does not control rotation, and therefore is not to be used in spinal instability.

The cruciform anterior spinal hyperextension (CASH) brace is another hyperextension orthosis that is shaped like a cross with anterior sternal and pubic pads. The forces from the two anterior pads are opposed by a posterior strap that wraps around the thoracolumbar region. The CASH brace has been used to decrease kyphosis in patients with osteoporosis with questionable success. It is also used in acute low thoracic and upper lumbar vertebral body fractures. The brace is light and easy to don, but is hard to adjust. In unstable fractures or when maximum immobility is needed, a molded spinal orthosis is required that will limit flexion, extension, and rotation at the thoracolumbar and lumbosacral area.

Molded Spinal Orthoses

These orthoses are usually made from plaster of Paris, leather, or plastic and, depending on the material used, provide differing amounts of support. They are either custom fabricated or fitted from prefabricated shells. The Boston overlap modular TLSO is a premolded polyethylene orthosis that is stocked in modules of preformed sizes that can be custom assembled for the patient. Body jackets maintain total contact with the patient and distribute forces over a large area by compression of soft tissues and relief of bony prominences and therefore act to maintain spinal alignment. It maintains flexion, extension, lateral motion, and rotation by having a three-point system for each. Depending on the level of injury and the amount of instability of the fracture, a CTLSO, TLSO, or LSO can be prescribed. A properly fitting TLSO should encompass the sternal notch to the pubis anteriorly, and spine or inferior angle of the scapula to the sacrococcygeal junction posteriorly. For better control of motion, the gluteal mass should be contained and the axilla and the trochanter free (40). They can be washed, modified, and hidden under loose-fitting clothing. A proper fit is imperative in patients with a lack of sensation to avoid skin breakdown with adequate reliefs at bony prominences. This brace is prescribed for maximum restriction of movement in all planes. If spinal stability is not an issue, patients tolerate TLS corsets with stays much better than body jackets.

Use of Thoracic and Lumbosacral Orthoses

Thoracolumbar Fractures

No orthosis will totally immobilize the thoracolumbar spine. Activity restrictions to ensure protection of the spine should be instructed in association with the brace. There are a number of options in orthotic prescription, depending on the level of the fracture. For high-level fractures (T1–T6), there is no consensus. Some believe that a CTLSO—a cervical extension added to a TLSO (hyperextension orthosis, Knight-Taylor brace, or body jacket)—is required (43,44). However, other braces without cervical extensions have been used (45). Lower level fractures of the thoracic and thoracolumbar spine can be treated using body jackets, body casts, and hyperextension orthoses (46,47). For vertebral body compression fractures without neurologic impairment, the use of a thoracoabdominal support to control pain is usually sufficient. Once the pain level allows the patient to assume the upright position (7 to 10 days) a lumbosacral corset may be enough. Even a rigid orthosis will not prevent occasional instances of pain. Transverse process fractures are essentially a soft-tissue injury that heals quickly and is treated with an orthosis that will control the pain. Fractures with posterior element involvement require immobilization to permit skeletal healing. A body jacket is preferable. For spine metastasis without instability or neurologic deficits, a TLSO corset with rigid stays may be sufficient. If there is instability or neurologic deficits, a body jacket is recommended.

The use of a brace after surgery depends on the type of fracture and the surgical procedure/stabilization performed. After Harrington rod instrumentation without sublaminar wiring, bracing (usually a body jacket) for 6 months is recommended. The use of Luque or Contrel-Dubousset instrumentation may or may not require postoperative bracing depending on surgical techniques. In all patients, avoidance of excessive bending and heavy lifting should continue for 3 months, but the patient can participate in a rehabilitation program that can include training in transfer, ambulation, and activities of daily living (ADL).

Orthotic Management of Low Back Pain

Although orthotic prescription for LBP is common, justification for its use is limited. The use of an LSO for a short period of time for acute low back pain may reduce pain and increase activity. Bracing can be used for longer periods for pain relief in patients with compression fractures from osteoporosis or degenerative joint disease (DJD). Braces may work by restricting motion (mechanically and by reminding the patient), employing heat and/or massagelike effect, and providing trunk support (by increasing intra-abdominal pressure); they may also be effective from a psychological aspect. A lumbar binder with a Velcro closure is useful, but a lumbosacral corset may be needed in the obese or elderly for increased support.

Examination of all spinal orthotics is extremely important, to ascertain that the prescription has been followed and that the orthosis meets the needs of the patient. One should check the patient in the seated as well as standing position if possible. After removal of the orthosis, one needs to check for signs of irritation. If redness disappears within 10 minutes, there is usually no cause for concern. Also, make sure that the patient considers the orthosis satisfactory as to weight, comfort, function, and appearance. This will help in maintaining compliance. The use of these braces has been shown to be effective in manual workers in the workplace in reducing back injuries (48). Molded supports can be added to further assist the patient in pain relief.

Certain braces not covered include scoliosis bracing (see Chapter 37) and bracing specific for osteoporosis (Chapter 58).

UPPER LIMB ORTHOTICS

Optimal upper extremity function may be achieved by maintaining or increasing joint mobility, muscle strength, and coordination, as well as by using adaptive equipment or an orthosis. Upper extremity orthotics are often used as an adjunct to facilitate or maintain treatment gains, as well as to encourage hand function for self-care tasks, vocational skills, and recreational activities. They can substitute for decreased or absent muscle strength, support segments that require positioning or immobilization, provide traction, enforce specific directional control, and allow for the attachment of adaptive devices.

Types of Orthoses

The two basic types of upper extremity orthotics are static and dynamic (49). Static orthotics, which have no moving parts, are used to rigidly support or rest the splinted part. Static splints also are used to stretch joint contractures and to align specific joints, nerves, and tendons after surgical procedures to allow optimal healing. A static orthosis should not be used longer than physiologically required and should never include joints other than those being treated because immobilization causes unwanted effects such as contracture and atrophy (50). A dynamic orthotic has moving parts that allow controlled movement for function (50,51). The movement in dynamic splints may be intrinsically powered by another body part or through electrical stimulation of the patient's muscle. Intrinsic power can be provided by elastic pulley traction systems (52,53), springs, pneumatic devices, and motors (49).

Orthotics for Specific Problems

Arthritis

In arthritis, with altered joint mechanics as well as the destruction of articular surfaces, there is instability and ineffective movement of the joints. As a result of this joint degeneration, the normal arches of the hand are disturbed. A progressive deformity is caused by abnormal stresses arising from muscle imbalances and attempts of the hand to adapt despite the degenerative and inflammatory changes. Orthotics can be effective in preserving joint integrity by providing external support to the joint's surrounding structures, and by stabilizing some joints while permitting other joints to move with more freedom and strength. Splints also can be used as an adjunct to, as well as an alternative to, surgery (54,55). The following are some splints which may be used in osteoarthritis and rheumatoid arthritis.

Resting Hand Splint

The resting hand splint is a static wrist–hand orthosis used to immobilize the wrist, fingers, and thumb. It is applied volarly and extends from the fingertips to the proximal third of the forearm. The hand is positioned for function at 20° to 30° of wrist extension, 5° to 10° of ulnar deviation, thumb opposition with abduction, and slight flexion of the fingers (55). The resting hand splint is used primarily to provide rest and pain relief at these joints during periods of acute inflammation in an effort to reduce the inflammation. Because the structures in and around these involved joints become distended, they often assume abnormal postures. Therefore, the resting hand splint not only rests these inflamed joints but also ensures that they rest in functional alignment.

The resting hand splint also can be used in the arthritic hand that is beginning to develop contractures (54). To prevent ulnar deviation in the resting position, an ulnar border is incorporated into the hand portion of the splint. Generally this splint is worn at night, but it may be worn during the day for additional rest, especially during acute inflammation.

Wrist Cock-up Splint

This is a static functional splint that immobilizes the wrist but allows full metacarpophalangeal (MCP) flexion and thumb opposition. It is applied volar, positioned proximal to the distal palmar crease, and extends to the proximal third of the forearm. It also may be applied dorsal, providing the patient with the added advantage of sensory input through the wrist and palm. The indications for this splint in arthritis include the presence of severe, chronic wrist inflammation and pain. At the same time that it provides support to the wrist, it also protects the extensor tendons, which may be weakened by the inflammatory process. This prevents the tendons from becoming overstretched or ruptured during wrist motion or hand use. The support of the splint improves hand function and grip and reduces the possibility that pain would cause the wrist to give way during use. The wrist cock-up splint also may be used after flexor tenosynovectomy to stabilize the wrist in a fixed position with tension on the tendons while encouraging the action of finger flexion (56). This splint may be combined with an MCP support that maintains the MCP joints in normal alignment. This addition is of particular value to the arthritic hand affected with MCP synovitis with or without mild or moderate ulnar deviation.

Tri-point Finger Splint

Deformities commonly seen in the rheumatoid hand are swan-neck and boutonniere deformities. The tri-point finger splint or ring splint, may be used to prevent these deformities from becoming fixed and to improve hand function. This splint applies pressure at three points on the finger: proximal and distal to the dorsal surface of the proximal interphalangeal (PIP) joint and central to the volar aspect of that joint. It prevents PIP hyperextension and allows active PIP flexion (55). If a swan-neck deformity is surgically repaired, the splint may be used postoperatively in an effort to prevent the return of the deformity (55,57). In the boutonniere deformity, the splint is applied with volar pressure applied proximal and distal to the PIP joint and dorsal pressure at the PIP joint to inhibit PIP flexion contractures (55,58,59).

Thumb Splints

The thumb carpometacarpal (CMC) stabilization (thumb spica) splint is a static, functional splint that immobilizes the wrist and CMC joint of the thumb. It is applied volarly and extends from the area proximal to the distal palmar crease to the proximal third of the forearm with built-in support around the first metacarpal, restricting motion at the CMC joint while allowing MCP and interphalangeal (IP) notion. The splint is used for the painful thumb CMC joint as well as for the patient who is considering joint arthrodesis because the stabilization provided simulates the postoperative condition.

For the thumb whose function is impaired secondary to medial instability at the IP joint, a dorsal gutter splint may be applied. This static functional splint extends dorsally from the tip of the thumb to the base of the proximal phalanx. It provides IP joint support during functional pinch activities (57).

Tendon Repairs

Splinting is essential during recovery and rehabilitation in the treatment of a patient with a tendon repair. The primary goal of rehabilitation after primary repair of a severed tendon is to restore tendon gliding and assist in regaining maximum function. Initially, static splints are used for protection to restrict motion. Later, dynamic splints can be used to increase ROM and to provide stretch to scar tissue.

Flexor Tendon Repairs

Splints are designed to maintain early passive mobilization while at the same time allowing for maximal function for the remainder of the hand. Immediately after surgery, the patient is fitted with a dorsal protective splint for the entire wrist and hand. This splint is designed so that it supports the digit in the position of the tendon repair. Room is allowed between the dorsum of the finger and the splint so as to allow for passive extension exercises with the splint in place. This space should allow for 20° to 30° of passive extension at both the proximal and distal interphalangeal (DIP) joints, which serves as an outer limit for passive extension exercises to prevent excess tension.

The uninjured digits are also blocked from extension and they are gently placed into a position of full MCP flexion (90°) and complete PIP extension (0°). This position maintains the collateral ligments in their lengthened state and decreases the later possibility of joint stiffness in the uninjured fingers due to the period of immobilization and reaction to injury. The wrist is maintained in 20° to 30° of flexion. Once the initial period of immobilization has been completed, the splint is cut so that it resembles a dorsal protective splint. If PIP joint contractures are evident at an early stage, a dynamic PIP extension splint with a static MCP flexion base may be fabricated. This splint puts little stress on the tendon anastamosis and is very effective in increasing extension of the PIP joint early in the course of recovery.

Finger caps or stalls are fabricated from polyform and are shaped around the tip of the finger to the level of the PIP joint. A finger stall is shaped in a tubular fashion along the length of the finger but ends just distal to the volar crease of the DIP joint. With the finger stall in place, the patient is able to work on isolated profundus motion (DIP motion).

Extensor Tendon Injuries

Clinically, there is less difficulty recovering function after an extensor tendon laceration. After immobilization, the primary precaution is avoidance of sudden gripping or heavy lifting, which could cause tendon rupture. If passive ROM is limited, the patient may be fitted with a dynamic PIP flexion splint and a dynamic DIP flexion splint.

Injuries at the DIP joint level will result in a mallet finger deformity. Acute injuries are usually treated with immobilization with a finger stall or splint. Injuries at the PIP joint level are more complex due to the arrangement of the extensor mechanism in the lateral bands. Lacerations at the PIP joint may develop into a boutonniere deformity if not immobilized or left unrepaired. A static finger extension splint is often used to provide the necessary immobilization of the finger itself. As further healing occurs, a dynamic PIP flexion splint may be needed to aid in recovery of joint mobility with use of a static extension splint at night.

Peripheral Nerve Injury

Orthotics in peripheral nerve injuries are used (a) to keep denervated muscles from remaining in an overstretched position, (b) to prevent joint contractures or the development of strong substitution patterns, and (c) to improve functional use of the hand (60). Immediately after injury, tension on the healing nerve tissues should be prevented to allow for adequate healing. Thereafter, gliding of the tendon and joint takes precedence because strict immobilization will often result in long-term restriction of full movement. Specific factors required for a proper orthotic prescription in peripheral nerve injury include an understanding of the direct motor and sensory deficits, as well as losses that may be caused indirectly by the lesion (such as contractures) all coupled with knowledge of the orthotic armamentarium. Compensatory muscle patterns for each lesion may differ; therefore, so will the orthotic approaches to each patient. When prescribing an orthosis for any type of lesion, one should outline the losses from the injury, whether functional substitution is available, and if not, what orthosis can provide for the functional objectives (Table 25-3). Motor deficit defects are the easiest to provide with compensatory orthotics because devices can assist or provide the needed function. Sensory disturbances and pain are more difficult to improve, but may be reduced by external stabilization that protects irritated tissue.

There is certainly no shortage of orthoses available. It is generally advisable to avoid prescribing cumbersome and complex orthoses. All losses do not need compensation—only those functionally important to the patient. In some instances, an orthosis may be prescribed for management of only the most functionally important deficit associated with the condition. For example, in a case of a proximal radial nerve lesion (above the spiral groove), there is weakness of the elbow, wrist, and finger extensors; the orthosis usually prescribed will reduce hand and wrist disability but will not effect elbow extension or forearm supination, which are also weak. If the patient requires these functions, a more complex orthosis can be prescribed. An important issue to consider before prescribing an orthosis is the etiology of and prognosis for the neuropathy. If the injury is neuropraxic and likely to recover quickly, then a prefabricated orthotic may be used rather than prescribing a complex and costly custom-made orthosis.

Radial Nerve Injury

Radial nerve damage above the elbow affects all wrist and finger extensors, compromising all prehension patterns. The primary functional loss is the inability to stabilize the wrist in extension so that one can use the finger flexors to their maximum function. With lesions at the elbow, the extensor carpi radialis longus already may be innervated, allowing some extension to take place with radial deviation, because the extensor carpi ulnaris is innervated distal to the elbow. With unstable MCP joints, the ulnar innervated interossei and the ulnar and median supplied lumbricals expend most of their force flexing the MCP joints, with little power left to extend the distal joints. With the MCP joints supported, however, the intrinsics can straighten the IP joints actively.

Orthotic Management

Patients with radial nerve palsy have the potential for relatively normal use of the hand using a splint that harnesses the wrist to allow the finger flexors to function. The ideal splint allows tenodesis action; finger extension with wrist flexion, and wrist extension with finger flexion. A proper splint protects against overlengthening of paralyzed wrist extensors and shortening of flexors.

High Lesions

Substitution for elbow loss is rarely indicated. A forearm-based volar or dorsal static wrist extension splint with dynamic extension outriggers for the fingers and thumbs should be supplied soon after the injury. The outriggers should be securely attached and placed directly over the proximal phalanges so as to allow a dynamic extension force to be applied perpendicular to the phalanges. Finger extension is achieved by the patient, allowing the wrist to flex as the statically suspended proximal phalangeal area pulls the MCP joint into extension. The thumb is not always included with an outrigger, so as to avoid cumbersomeness. An outrigger for the thumb may be used to avoid a substitute motion for extension through use of the abductor pollicis brevis and adductor pollicis muscles.

Low Injury

In posterior interosseous nerve palsy, wrist extension is usually spared, although with radial deviation. Attempted finger extension will demonstrate MCP flexion and IP extension (intrinsic plus hand), because of loss of the extensor digitorum. The splint used for a low radial nerve injury is similar to that used for a high injury. This is a static wrist support splint (maintains the wrist in approximately 30° of hyperextension) and can be used with the MCP joints supported in extension and the thumb extended and radially abducted (the functional position). Alternatively, a dynamic splint allows the wrist to flex and causes finger extension as the suspended PIP area pulls the MCP joints into extension.

TABLE 25-3. *Orthotics in peripheral nerve injuries*

Nerve injured	Motor deficits	Deformities	Orthotic objectives	Orthotic
• Proximal radial	• Elbow extension • Weak forearm supination • Wrist extension • 2–5 MCP joint ext • Thumb extension	• Wrist drop • MCP and IP ext contr • Thumb web space contracture • Flattening of palmar arch	• Prevent wrist drop • Assist wrist extension • Assist thumb abd/ext • Maintain thumb web space • Maintain transverse palmar arch	• Forearm-based dorsal or volar static wrist extension splint wrist extension splint with dynamic extension outriggers for the fingers • May also need thumb outrigger
• Distal radial	• Wrist extension (may be partial) • 2.5 MCP joint ext • Thumb abd/ext	• Wrist drop • MCP/IP ext contracture • Flattening of palmar arch	• Prevent wrist drop • Maintain thumb web space • Maintain transverse palmar arch • Assist wrist extension • Assist thumb abd/ext	• As above with static wrist extension, only as needed
• Proximal median	• Forearm pronation • Wrist palmar flex • Weak wrist radial deviation • Flexion of 2 and 3 MCP joints • Thumb opposition and IP flexion • Flex 2 and 3 IP joint • Thumb MCP flex and abduction	• Forearm and thenar atrophy • Thumb on finger plane • Thumb web space contracture • Flattening of transverse palm arch	• Maintain thumb web space • Maintain transverse palmar arch • Maintain thumb in abd/opp • Assist MCP and IP flexion • Reduce pain by limiting wrist and thumb motion	• Thumb spica splint • Resting hand splint • Tendon transfer
• Distal median	• Thumb opposition • Weak thumb flex and abduction • First 2 lumbrical weakness	• Thenar atrophy • Thumb on finger plane • Thumb web space contracture	• Maintain thumb web space • Maintain thumb in abduction and opposition • Reduce pain by limiting wrist and thumb motion	• Soft dynamic thumb abduction splint • Thumb spica splint • C-bar • Opponens bar to stabilize the thumb in opposition
• Proximal ulnar	• Weak wrist flexion • Wrist ulnar dev • 4 and 5 DIP flex • 5 and 5 IP ext • 2–5 MCP abd/add • 5th finger opposition • Thumb adduction	• Interossei atrophy • Hypothenar atrophy • 5th MCP abd contr • Flattening of trans palm arch • During pinch, 1st IP hyperflexes and/or 1st MCP hyperextends • Partial "claw hand"	• Stabilize 1st MCP • Limit 4th and 5th MCP ext • Maintain trans palm arch • Improve grasp	• Any splint that blocks the MP joint from fully extending including • Rigid static dorsal splint • Rigid dynamic volar splint • Soft dynamic splint • PIP static or dynamic extension splint
• Distal ulnar	• 4th and 5th MCP flex when IP ext • 4th and 5th IP felx • 2–5 MCP abd and add • 5th finger opposition • Thumb adduction	• Interossei atrophy • Hypothenar atrophy • Partial "claw hand" • During pinch, 1st IP hyperflexes and/or 1st MCP hyperext • 5th MCP abd contr • Flattening of trans palm arch	• Limit 4th and 5th MCP ext • Prevent 4th and 5th PIP flex contracture • Stabilize 1st MCP • Maintain trans palm arch • Improve grasp	• As above in proximal ulnar

DIP, distal interphalangeal; IP, interphalangeal; MCP, metacarpophalangeal; PIP, proximal interphalangeal.

Median Nerve Injury

Severe dysfunction of the median nerve is functionally devastating, more than any other lesion, because it innervates many muscles in the forearm and hand, as well as most of the thumb muscles. Important sensation on the palmar aspect of the hand is also lost. Table 25-3 lists the motor loss, deformities, and orthotic objectives in median nerve injuries.

High Lesions

High median nerve injuries are seen at or near the elbow. In these lesions, there is loss of the flexor digitorum profundus (FDP) muscle of the index and long fingers as well as flexor digitorum superficialis muscle to all fingers, allowing only gross function of the hand. Because the recovery is poor, splinting of this level of deformity to maintain passive ROM is appropriate in preparation for tendon transfers.

Low Lesions

Adduction contractures of the thumb (due to unopposed action for the adductor pollicis muscle) are the most common deformity after a low lesion of the median nerve, and a splint can be provided to hold the first metacarpal abducted from the hand. Splinting not only prevents the opponens pollicus and abductor pollicus brevis from resting in a stretched position but also maintains a soft-tissue length of the first web space and provides a force to balance the pull of the normal adductor pollicis. A C-bar design has been traditionally recommended (61). An opponens bar on the proximal phalanx of the thumb stabilizes it in opposition to the index and middle fingers, therefore allowing full wrist movement and IP flexion of the thumb. Daytime splinting with a leather or thermoplastic material, to stabilize the thumb in an opposed position, can be used along with a more sturdy night splint.

Patients with carpal tunnel syndrome are most frequently prescribed a volar wrist orthosis, keeping the wrist between neutral and 10° of extension. For more proximal lesions, a long opponens splint with wrist control, or a finger- or wrist-driven prehension orthosis with closing achieved by the fourth and fifth digits, can be used. However, the patient may prefer not to use this orthosis because lateral prehension is still possible through muscles innervated by the ulnar nerve.

Ulnar Nerve Injuries

High Lesions

In a high-level ulnar nerve lesion, because of the absence of tension from the FDP and all the intrinsics of the ring and little finger, the clawing in the hand is not as obvious. There is no difference needed for splint designs for the different levels of lesion. In a high lesion, one must instruct the patient to maintain full passive interphalangeal flexion of the ring and little fingers when the profundi are absent.

Low Lesions

In an ulnar nerve injury at the wrist, there is a denervation of the majority of the intrinsic muscles of the hand. The greatest functional loss is the inability to open the hand in a large span to handle objects. At the thumb, the loss of the powerful adductor and the deep head of the flexor pollicis brevis removes some of the supporting forces of MCP joint during pinching. The deformity at the thumb can rarely be assisted by splinting.

The goal in splinting ulnar nerve palsy is to prevent overstretching of the denervated intrinsic muscle of the ring and little fingers. The MCP joints must be prevented from fully extending. Any splint that blocks the MCP joint in slight flexion prevents a claw deformity and allows the intrinsic extensors to transmit force into the dorsal hood mechanism of the finger. Blocking the MCP joints may be incorporated into an immobilization splint. Blocking of the MCP joint extension also may be accomplished by a dynamic splint with cuffs for the fourth and fifth fingers.

A basic requirement is protection of the architectural integrity of the hand before fixed contractures develop. The palmar arch needs to be supported, not only so that the fingers may assume the most functional position, but also so that the fourth and fifth fingers do not get in the way of the first three fingers. Because two thirds of the palmar surface of the hand still has normal sensation, splints for ulnar nerve lesions should cover a minimal surface of the hand. Finger flexion range also should remain unimpeded.

Splints recommended for ulnar nerve lesions include a basic opponens orthosis with fourth and fifth MCP extension stop (lumbrical bar) set at roughly 30° of flexion. A bar on the side of the splint can limit radial deviation for patients with proximal lesions, although this is rarely needed. Similar splinting is used in proximal and distal lesions; however, with absence of the pull from the FDP and all the intrinsics of the ring and little fingers, the clawing in the high ulnar lesions is not as obvious. As the FDP reinnervates, clawing becomes more evident and splinting becomes even more important.

Shoulder Slings

Shoulder slings are used to prevent shoulder subluxation in patients with brachial plexus injuries (62–64), polymyositis (65), hemiplegia (66), and central cord syndrome injuries (63). Some sling supports, such as the universal hemiplegic sling, immobilize the whole arm. These slings restrict active motion of the shoulder by keeping the humerus in adduction and internal rotation and placing the elbow into flexion (67). These slings are designed to remove the weight of the arm from the shoulder but do not approximate the humeral head back into the glenoid fossa. These slings also reinforce synergy patterns and fail to provide motor or sensory feedback (68). Other slings support the shoulder but leave the rest of the arm free for function (65,67,68). Although there are numerous styles of slings, there is no consensus as to which type of sling is best for a particular goal or whether a sling should be used for the subluxed shoulder.

In using any sling, it must not prevent function that the patient has and should not create new problems such as edema in the dependent hand, positioning in patterns of spasticity, or pulling the humerus out of the glenoid fossa. Rigid arm boards are often preferred to the use of the sling for the wheelchair-bound patient because they allow the humeral head to approximate the glenoid fossa at a more natural angle, and they elevate the hand so that edema is less likely to occur (66,69–72). An alternative to an armboard is the use of a wheelchair lapboard, which can be used when a patient has decreased trunk control, visual field deficits, or need for a work surface (73).

Spasticity

Splinting in spasticity employs the principle of prolonged muscle stretch to reduce spasticity. Other treatment principles incorporated into splinting designs for the spastic patient include positioning opposite to patterns of spasticity to inhibit or prevent development of increased tone (66), tactile stimulation to facilitate antagonists and inhibit the spastic muscles, and quick stretch to facilitate hypotonic muscles. The splint must incorporate both the wrist and fingers in order to stretch the long finger flexor muscles. Hand splints for spasticity include dorsal or volar spasticity reduction splints. These splints are molded to provide 30° of wrist extension, 45° of MCP flexion and full interphalangeal extension, finger abduction, and thumb extension and abduction. This position duplicates the spasticity-inhibiting pattern of Bobath. The finger abduction splint for the spastic hand may be constructed of a block of foam with holes punched through the foam to allow insertion of the fingers in an abducted position.

Spinal Cord Injury

C1–C3 Level

Long Opponens

A long opponens splint is a static splint used to prevent contracture, immobilize the wrist, and provide support to the palmar transverse arches, thumb, and web space. It is applied to the volar surface and extends from the forearm to the CMC joint. A support bar can be provided on the volar, dorsal, or radial surface. The wrist is positioned in 20° to 30° of extension and 5° to 10° of ulnar deviation and thumb opposition (74).

Resting Hand Splint

A resting hand splint, which was already discussed in the arthritis section, is also a static splint used to immobilize the wrist, finger, and thumb. The resting hand splint provides more support for the fingers due to the extended support to the finger tips.

Spiral Splints

A spiral splint is a static splint used to support the wrist and palmar arch and to pronate the forearm. The orthosis spirals from the forearm volar and dorsal surface to the distal transverse arch, allowing the fingers and thumb to be free from support. Additional support can be added to maintain the thumb in opposition if needed. The use of clear material that spirals around the extremity and leaves the fingers free is cosmetically appealing. A cuff can be adapted to the palmar surface to assist with functional activities such as feeding, grooming, or using a computer. However, spiral splints are difficult to don and doff and can create skin pressure problems due to firm material that spirals around the upper extremity. Spiral splints are also relatively costly to fabricate.

C4 Level

Mobile Arm Support (Formerly called Balanced Forearm Orthosis)

A mobile arm support (MAS) is a dynamic orthosis that assists and/or substitutes for weak muscles of the shoulder, elbow, and forearm in order to use the hand for functional activity. The main requirement of an MAS is to support the arm weight, counteract and balance the force of gravity, and allow controlled movements (75). A neutral position needs to be established in order to use the MAS effectively. A properly balanced MAS maintains the forearm in a position of 45° from horizontal and the upper arm in approximately 45° of shoulder abduction and flexion without patient effort (74). In order for the MAS to operate appropriately, the client must have the following shoulder movements while positioned in the MAS: depression and elevation, external and internal rotation, and horizontal adduction and abduction of the humerus. The power to operate an MAS comes from the client's musculature; however, an active MAS has an external power unit to substitute for weakness.

An MAS can be attached by brackets to a wheelchair. A proximal swivel arm is then placed into the brackets, which allows the humeral motion. A distal swivel arm is attached to the proximal arm, which allows elbow motion within the horizontal plane. A forearm trough maintains the position of the upper extremity on the distal arm.

Power Tenodesis

A power tenodesis is a dynamic splint using external power in order to provide prehension at the fingertips when there is less than fair grade of wrist extension. It positions the wrist in 15° of extension, the thumb in abduction and partial opposition, MCP and interphalangeals of the thumb in extension, and the second and third digits in a semiflexed position at the MCP and PIP joints. The pads of the second and third digits meet the pad of the thumb in opposition in order to elicited a pinch. Two types of external power can be used:

1. Battery and cable. The battery cable extends to the finger pad switch, which is connected to the battery and accessed to operate the power to open and close the fingers.
2. CO_2 and McKibben muscle. The McKibben artificial muscle operates the fingertips due to its attachment to the cable. CO_2 is pushed into the muscle through the activation of a pneumatic valve, which causes the shortening of the muscles and elicits finger closure. The sec-

ond activation causes the release of CO_2 from the muscle, resulting in relaxation and opening of the fingers.

Economy Wrist Support (ADL Wrist Support)

The economy wrist support is a static splint used to maintain the wrist in neutral position. It is a dorsal splint that starts from the mid-forearm and extends to just below the CMC joint with three points of support: forearm, wrist, and palmar arch. A palmar cuff is built into the palmar arch support to allow eating utensils or self-care equipment to be inserted for assistance with ADL. There are two main problems noted with this splint over time: (a) lack of ulnar wrist support, which will cause ulnar deviation, and (b) lack of support in the area of the palmar arches.

C5 Level

Ratchet Type Flexor Hinge Orthosis

The ratchet flexor hinge orthosis is a dynamic, externally powered orthosis. This splint is appropriate when the client has no active wrist extension. The ratchet splint allows the fingers to open and close once the client passively engages the ratchet mechanism by applying pressure external to the wrist to lock it in extension. It is important for the client to be able to use the other hand or lateral wrist to operate the ratchet button during the grasping motion.

C6 Level

Wrist-Driven Flexor Hinge (or Tenodesis) Splint

A wrist-driven flexor hinge orthosis is a dynamic splint that uses active wrist extension in order to flex the fingers for prehension. This elicited movement is known as tenodesis because it takes advantage of the finger flexor tendons.

RIC Tenodesis Orthosis

The RIC tenodesis orthosis is an inexpensive splint that is easily fabricated and made from high- or low-temperature thermoplastic material. It consists of a three-piece wrist and hand splint: a contoured cuff around the forearm with one Velcro strap to secure the piece, a short opponens splint to provide thumb opposition, and a dorsal cover over the second and third digits in a slightly flexed position at PIP and DIP joints. The lever is a nonrigid material made from either a cord or chain in combination with Velcro. The cord attaches from the volar surface to the finger piece, connects to the center of the palmar arch, and then to the volar forearm sling. The Velcro strap on the forearm sling may be adjusted to shorten or lengthen the cord for specific wrist positions.

Short Opponens Splint

A short opponens splint is a static splint used to maintain an adequate web space with opposition of the thumb for prehension activities. A short opponens splint is used for patients who have active wrist extension against gravity. The thumb is positioned in opposition under the second digit with the pad of the thumb exposed for three-point pinch.

A universal cuff is a 1-inch strap that fits around the dorsal/palmar surface of the hand below the metacarpal joint. A cuff is located on the palmar surface in order to insert utensils, grooming devices, or computer devices to assist with ADL.

C7 Level

MCP flexion and MCP extension orthoses are appropriate when wrist strength is a grade of 4/5; however, flexors and extensors of the fingers are weak. Both splints use a mechanical activator that is located on the radial side of the orthosis and assists with finger flexion and extension. Both splints are similar in positioning to the tenodesis splint, except that there is no wrist support. The thumb is maintained in opposition with the second and third digits in a semiflexed position. When using the MCP flexion splint, muscle strength of 4/5 is needed for finger extension; however, little or no finger flexion is needed. The MCP extension splint conversely requires a grade of 4/5 finger flexion, and little finger extension is needed.

Other Common Wrist and Finger Orthoses

Static volar and dorsal wrist splints are used primarily to support and immobilize the wrist. The gutter splint also can be used to control radial and ulnar deviation.

Splint	Indications
Static	
Volar	Carpal tunnel release, wrist fractures, RSD, tendonitis/ tenosynovitis, ganglion cyst
Dorsal	Ganglion, tendinitis/tenosynovitis, flexor tendon injuries
Ulnar/radial gutter	Distal forearm fractures, tendinitis/ tenosynovitis, wrist fusion, congenital club hand
Dynamic	Volkman's contracture, Colles' fracture, dorsal synovectomy, radial nerve injury

Thumb

The thumb spica splint is used to immobilize and protect the thumb. It can be used for a variety of injuries, including scaphoid fracture, gamekeeper's thumb, Bennett's fracture, deQuervain's tenosynovitis, and for sprains, dislocations, and tendon transfers. A dynamic thumb splint can be created by using an outrigger on a wrist orthosis. It is often used in replantation, crush injury, and nerve and tendon repair.

Finger

Static finger splints have been described elsewhere in this chapter. At the MCP joint, splints can be dorsal or volar, and in trauma they can be used for the following conditions: mallet finger, volar plate injury, ligament tears, digit amputation, and tendon repairs. Dynamic MCP flexion splints are used for fractures, crush injuries, replantation, collateral ligament tightness, swan-neck deformity, and nerve injury. Dynamic MCP extension splints are used for flexion contractures and boutonniere deformities.

REFERENCES

1. *Dorland's medical dictionary.* Philadelphia: WB Saunders, 1985.
2. McCullough NC III. Biomechanical analysis systems for orthotic prescriptions. In: *Atlas of orthotics.* St. Louis: CV Mosby, 1975.
3. Harris EE. A new orthotics terminology: a guide to its use for prescription and fee schedule. *Orthop Prosthet* 1973; 27:6.
4. Lunsford TR, Davidson M, Lunsford BR. The effectiveness of four contemporary cervical orthosis in restricting cervical motion. *J Prosthet Orthop* 1994; 6:93–99.
5. Nash CL. Current concepts review. Scoliosis bracing. *J Bone Joint Surg [Am]* 1981; 62:848–852.
6. O'Brien J. Clinical studies with the halo pelvic apparatus: an experimental and clinical investigation. *Acta Orthop Scand* 1975; 163(suppl): 1–188.
7. O'Brien JP, Yan ACMC, Hodgson AR. Halo-pelvic traction: a technique for severe spinal deformities. *Clin Orthop* 1973; 93:179–190.
8. Garfin SR, Botte MJ, Waters RL, Nickel VL. Complications in the use of halo fixation device. *J Bone Joint Surg [Am]* 1986; 68:320–325.
9. Fisher SV, Bowar JF, Essam AA, Gullikson G. Cervical orthoses effect on cervical spine motion: roentgenographic and goniometric method of study. *Arch Phys Med Rehabil* 1977; 58:109–115.
10. Hartman JT, Palumbo F, Hill BJ. Cineradiography of the braced normal cervical spine: a comparative study of five commonly used cervical orthoses. *Clin Orthop Rel Res* 1975; 109:97–102.
11. Johnson RM, Hart DL, Simmons EF, et al. Cervical orthosis: a study comparing their effectiveness in restricting cervical motion in normal subjects. *J Bone Joint Surg [Am]* 1977; 59:332–339.
12. Koch RA, Nickel VL. The halo vest: an evaluation of motion & forces across the neck. *Spine* 1978; 3:103–107.
13. Lysell E. Motion of the cervical spine [Thesis]. An experimental study on autopsy specimans. *Acta Orthop Scand Suppl* 1969; 123:1.
14. Colachis SC, Strohm BR, Ganter EL. Cervical spine motion in normal women. *Arch Phys Med Rehabil* 1973; 5:161–169.
15. Carter VM, Fasen JM, Roman J, et al. The effect of a soft collar, used normally recommended or reversed, on three planes of cervical range of motion. *J Orthop Sports Phys Ther* 1996; 23:209–215.
16. Graziano AF, Scheidel EA, Clin Jr, Baer LJ. A radiographic comparison of prehospital cervical immobilization methods. *Ann Emerg Med* 1987; 16:1127–1131.
17. Solot JA, Winzelberg GC. Clinical and radiological evaluation of vertebrace extrication collars. *J Emerg Med* 1990; 8:79–83.
18. Perry J, Nickel VL. Total cervical spine fusion for neck paralysis. *J Bone Joint Surg* 1959; 41:37–59.
19. Botte MJ, Byrne TP, Abrams RA, Garfin SR. The halo skeletal fixator: current concepts of application and maintenance. *Orthopedics* 1995; 18:463–471.
20. Wolf JW, Jones HC. Comparison of cervical immobilization in halo-casts and halo-vest jackets. *Orthop Trans* 1981; 5:118.
21. Lind B, Sihlbom H, Nordwell A. Forces and motions across the neck in patients treated with halo-vest. *Spine* 1988; 13:162–167.
22. Wang GJ, Meskal JT, Albert T, et al. The effect of halo-vest length on stability of the cervical spine: a study in normal subjects. *J Bone Joint Surg [Am]* 1988; 70:357–360.
23. Botte MJ, Byrne TP, Garfin SR. Application of the halo devices for immobilization of the cervical spine utilizing an increased torque pressure. *J Bone Joint Surg [Am]* 1987; 69:750–752.
24. Rizzolo SJ, Piazza MR, Cotler JM, et al. The effect of torque pressure on halo pin complication rates: a randomized prospective study. *Spine* 1993; 18:2163–2166.
25. Olson RS. Halo skeletal traction pin site care: toward developing a standard of care. *Rehabil Nurs* 1996; 21:243–246.
26. Celeste S, Folcik M, Dumas K. Identifying a standard for pin site care using the quality assurance approach. *Orthop Nurs* 1984; 3:17–24.
27. Garfin SR, Botte MJ, Waters RL, Nickel VL. Complications in the use of the halo fixation device. *J Bone Joint Surg [Am]* 1986; 68:320–325.
28. Williams FH, Nelms DK, McGaharan KM. Brain abscess: a rare complication of halo usage. *Arch Phys Med Rehabil* 1992; 73:490–492.
29. Rosenblum D, Ehrlich V. Brain abscess and psychosis as a complication of a halo orthosis. *Arch Phys Med Rehabil* 1995; 76:865–867.
30. Wetzel FT, Dunsieth NW, Kuhlengel KR, Paul EM, Lahey DM. The effectiveness of the cervical halo: open versus closed ring: a preliminary report. *Paraplegia* 1995; 33:110–115.
31. Maiman D, Millington P, Novack S, et al. The effect of the thermoplastic minerva body jacket on cervical spine motion. *Neurosurgery* 1989; 25:363–368.
32. Pringle RG. Review article: Halo vs Minerva—which orthosis? *Paraplegia* 1990; 28:281–284.
33. Benzel EC, Haden TA, Saulsberg CM. A comparison of the minerva and halo jackets for stabilization of the cervical spine. *J Neurosurg* 1989; 70:411–414.
34. Sharpe KP, Rao S, Ziogas A. Evaluation of the effectiveness of the Minerva cervicothoracic orthosis. *Spine* 1995; 20:1475–1479.
35. Gaskill SJ, Marlin AE. Custom fitted thermoplastic minerva jackets in the treatment of cervical spine instability in preschool age children. *Pediatr Neurosurg* 1990; 16:35–39.
36. Fidler MW, Plasmans CMT. The effects of four types of supports on the segmental mobility of the lumbosacral spine. *J Bone Joint Surg* 1983; 65:943–947.
37. Lantz SA, Schultz AB. Lumbar spine orthosis wearing. Restriction of gross body motion. *Spine* 1986; 11:834–837.
38. Sypert GW. External spinal orthotics. *Neurosurgery* 1987; 20:642–649.
39. Axelsson P, Johnsson R, Stromqvist B. Lumbar orthosis with unilateral hip immobilization: effect on intervertebral mobility determined by Roentgen stereophotogrammetric analysis. *Spine* 1993; 18:876–879.
40. Bussel M, Merritt J, Fenwick L. Spinal orthoses. In: Redford JB, Basmajian JV, Trautman P, eds. *Orthotics: clinical practice and rehabilitation technology.* New York: Churchill-Livingstone, 1995; 71–102.
41. Fisher SV, Winter RB. Spinal orthoses in rehabilitation. In: Braddom RL, ed. *Physical medicine and rehabilitation.* Philadelphia: WB Saunders, 1996; 359–380.
42. Redford JB, Patel AT. Orthotic devices in the mangement of spinal disorders. *Phys Med Rehabil State Art Rev* 1995; 9:709–724.
43. Meyer PR. Fractures of the thoracic spine: T1–10. In: Meyer PR Jr, ed. *Surgery of spine trauma.* New York: Churchill-Livingstone 1989; 525–571.
44. Nachemson AL. Orthotic treatment for injuries and diseases of the spinal column. *Phys Med Rehabil State Art Rev* 1987; 1:11–24.
45. Hanley EN, Eskay ML. Thoracic spine fractures. *Orthopedics* 1989; 12:684–696.
46. Jones RF, Snowden E, Coan J, et al. Bracing of thoracic and lumbar spine fractures. *Paraplegia* 1987; 25:386–393.
47. McEvoy R, Bradford D. The management of burst fractures of the thoracic and lumbar spine—experience in 53 patients. *Spine* 1985; 10: 631–637.
48. Walsh NE, Schwartz RK. The influence of prophylactic orthoses on abdominal strength and low back injury in the workplace. *Am J Phys Med Rehabil* 1990; 69:245–250.
49. Long C, Schutt AH. Upper limb orthotics. In: Redford JB, ed. *Orthotics etcetera,* 3rd ed. Baltimore: Williams & Wilkins, 1986; 198.
50. Calliet R. *Hand pain & impairment.* Philadelphia: FA Davis, 1982.
51. Shafer AA. *Common problems, useful solutions in hand rehabilitation.* Dedham, MA: Amed, 1986.
52. Dovelle S, Hecter PK, McFaul TV. A dynamic finger flexion loop. *Am J Occup Ther* 1988; 42:535–537.
53. Dovelle S, Hecter PK, Phillips PD. A dynamic traction splint for the management of extrinsic tendon tightness. *Am J Occup Ther* 1987; 11: 123–125.
54. Souter WA. Splintage in the rheumatoid hand. *Hand* 1971; 3:144.
55. Melvin JL. *Rheumatic disease: occupational therapy and rehabilitation.* Philadelphia: FA Davis, 1977; 165.
56. McCann VH, Philips CA, Quigley TR. Preoperative and post-operative

management. The role of the allied health professional. *Orthop Clin North Am* 1975; 6:900.

57. Bennett RL. Orthotic devices to prevent deformities of the hand in rheumatoid arthritis. *Arthritis Rheumatism* 1965; 8:1011.
58. Philips CA. Hand therapy in the early stages of rheumatoid arthritis. In: Hunter A, ed. *Rehabilitation of the hand.* St. Louis: CV Mosby, 1978.
59. Fess EE, Gettle KS, Strickland JW. Hand splinting: principles and methods. St. Louis: CV Mosby, 1981.
60. Colditz JC. Splinting for radial nerve palsy. *J Hand Ther* 1987; 1: 39–42.
61. Bunnell S. *Surgery of the hand.* Philadelphia: JB Lippincott, 1956.
62. DeVore GI. A sling to prevent a subluxed shoulder. *Am J Occup Ther* 1970; 21:580–581.
63. Kohlmeyer K, Weber C, Yarkony G. A new orthoses for central cord syndrome and brachial plexus injuries. *Arch Phys Med Rehabil* 1990; 71:1006–1009.
64. Robinson C. Brachial plexus lesions. Part 2: Functional splintage. *Br J Occup Ther* 1986; 19:331–334.
65. Neal MR, Williamson J. Collar sling for bilateral shoulder subluxation. *Am J Occup Ther* 1980; 34:100–101.
66. Bobath B. *Adult hemiplegia: evaluation and treatment.* London: William Heinemann Medical, 1990.
67. Sullivan B, Rogers S. Modified bobath sling with distal support. *Am J Occup Ther* 1989; 43:47–49.
68. Moodie NB, Brisbin J, Morgan AM. Subluxation of the glenohumeral joint in hemiplegia. Evaluation of supportive devices. *Physiother Can* 1986; 38:151–157.
69. Ferreri J, Tumminella J. A swivel cock-up splint type arm trough. *Am J Occup Ther* 1974; 28:359.
70. Goold NJ. A versatile wheelchair armrest attachment. *Am J Occup Ther* 1976; 30:502–504.
71. Iveson F, Phillips M, Ream WD. A removal arm trough for wheelchair patients. *Am J Occup Ther* 1972; 26:269.
72. Salo RF. A hammock wheelchair armrest. *Am J Occup Ther* 1978; 32: 525.
73. Walsh M. Half-lapboard for hemiplegic patients. *Am J Occup Ther* 1987; 44:533–535.
74. Trombly CA. *Occupational therapy for physical dysfunction,* 3rd ed. Baltimore: Williams & Wilkins, 1989.
75. Malick MJ. *Manual on static hand splinting.* Pittsburgh: Hamarville Rehabilitation Center, 1972.
76. Ducker TB. Restriction of cervical spine motion by cervical collars [Abstract]. *Proceedings of 58th Annual Meeting of the American Association of Neurological Surgery*, Park Ridge, IL, 1990.
77. Johnson RM, Owen JR, Callahan RA. Cervical orthoses: a guide to their selection and use. *Clinical Orthop Rel Res* 1981; 154:34–45.

Rehabilitation Medicine: Principles and Practice, Third Edition,
edited by Joel A. DeLisa and Bruce M. Gans.
Lippincott–Raven Publishers, Philadelphia © 1998.

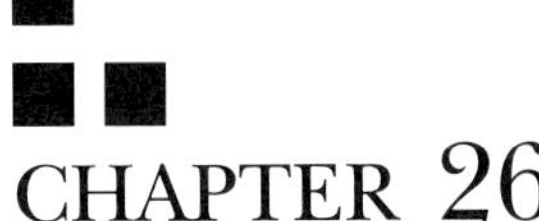

CHAPTER 26

Lower Extremity Orthotics, Shoes, and Gait Aids

Kristjan T. Ragnarsson

Orthotics is the systematic pursuit of straightening and improving function of the body or body parts by the application of an orthosis to the outside of the body. The term "orthosis" may refer to a number of devices with a more restricted or specific meaning, such as braces, splints, calipers, and corsets. Depending on the design, an orthosis may totally immobilize a joint or body segment, restrict movement in a given direction, control mobility, assist with movement, or reduce weight-bearing forces. In the presence of weak or paralyzed muscles, orthotic immobilization of a joint or an entire limb provides support. In the presence of unbalanced muscle forces, an orthosis prevents the generation of a deformity or joint contracture. In the presence of inflamed or injured musculoskeletal segments, an orthosis reduces pain and allows healing. Extension of an orthosis to a healthy body part can transfer or redistribute the weight-bearing forces, thereby reducing the actual load on a long bone or whole limb. This may help to relieve pain and allow healing of injured parts. The primary principle behind the prescription of an orthosis is the improvement of function.

Before an orthosis is prescribed, the precise functions it is meant to improve must be determined. The physician needs to know the indications for prescribing a specific orthosis, the anatomy and neuromuscular function, and the functional and biomechanical deficits present. The physician also must thoroughly understand the mechanical principles of orthotic application, the materials used in fabrication, the various designs that are available, and the training that the patient must receive, both before and after receiving the orthosis. Finally, the physician needs to be aware of the cost of the orthosis and the patient's financial means, carefully judging whether the benefits to be obtained will justify the cost.

K. T. Ragnarsson: Department of Rehabilitation Medicine, The Mount Sinai Medical Center, New York, New York 10029.

Whereas the indications for prescribing and using an orthosis may be obvious, contraindications are more subtle. The use of an orthosis should be discontinued when it causes pain, reduces function, worsens posture or gait, causes emotional distress, or when more effective results may be achieved by physical therapy or relatively minor surgical procedures. Allergy to the orthotic materials, restriction of peripheral circulation, or development of pressure sores requires immediate alteration or adjustment of the orthosis. Although an orthosis may significantly improve mobility and self-sufficiency, it also is a visible reminder of a lasting or permanent disability. Cosmetic appearance and comfort of the orthosis are two factors that will ease the patient's adjustment to the disability and facilitate acceptance of the device.

MATERIALS AND MECHANICS

A wide variety of materials have been used to fabricate orthotic appliances. Some of them have been used for centuries, such as metal, rubber, leather, and canvas, whereas others have been developed more recently, such as plastics and synthetic fabrics. When the appropriate materials are selected for an orthotic device, their strength, durability, flexibility, and weight need to be considered carefully. The orthotic design should be simple, inconspicuous, comfortable, and as cosmetic as possible. It should adhere to the basic principle of distributing forces over a sufficiently large surface area. Parts that are in contact with the body should be accurately contoured and padded.

The choice of orthotic material depends on the clinical purpose and the characteristics of the patient. Traditional orthotic devices use metals to provide strength and durability with straps and padding made of leather (Fig. 26-1). The metals primarily used are steel and aluminum, mostly in alloy forms with various other metals to further increase the strength of the orthosis and to resist corrosion. Although metal orthoses are heavy and are unappealing, they are adjustable, which allows them to accommodate for growth and the changing needs of the patient.

Orthoses that are made of plastic (Fig. 26-2) generally are somewhat lighter and closer fitting because they can be molded directly to the body or over a plaster replica of the body part. The close fit of the plastic orthosis provides wider distribution of the corrective forces than is possible with a metal orthosis. Comfort may be increased by adding foam liners on the inside of the orthosis. Based on the weight of the patient, the use of the orthosis, the specific type of plastic used, and the design of the orthosis, plastic materials generally provide adequate strength and durability. Plastic orthoses generally are not adjustable in length, but some materials allow reshaping when heated to accommodate or provide relief at pressure points. Plastic orthoses usually are fitted with metal joints or flexible spring-loaded plastic bars because plastic joints are not as durable.

Two major types of plastic materials are used in orthotics: thermosetting and thermoplastic materials. Thermosetting plastics—for example, formaldehyde, epoxy, and polyester resins—typically are used as laminates in a laminated form. They require heat to harden but do not soften with subsequent heating. Thermoplastics soften when they are heated, making the material moldable. Subsequent heating will soften the material for further molding, and lowering the temperature hardens the material once again. Low-temperature thermoplastics, such as Orthoplast and Plastazote, become workable at temperatures that are just above the body temperature. This allows quick fabrication and molding directly on the body. Unfortunately, these materials lack strength and durability and therefore are not indicated for long-term use. The high-temperature thermoplastics, such as polyethylene, polypropylene, copolymers, ortholene, and vinyl polymers, require heating to 150°F or more to make them workable. Fabrication of an orthosis made of any of these materials requires an exact plaster replica of the body part. The heated plastic is then applied to the replica for proper molding. These materials generally are strong and durable, and they have a "good memory," returning to their original position after flexible deformation. The orthosis provides support and may also give a spring-action assist force. Most plastic orthoses designed for long-term use are made of high-temperature thermoplastics.

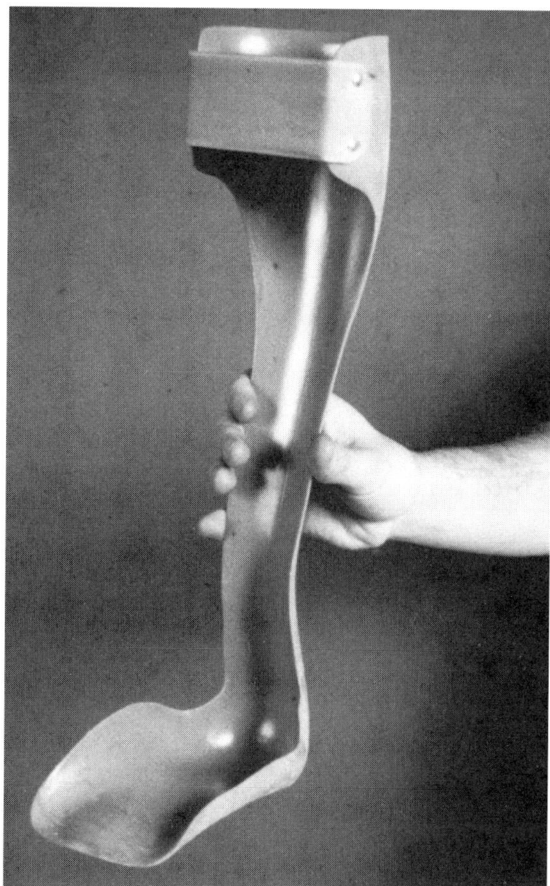

FIG. 26-2. Plastic leaf-spring ankle–foot orthosis.

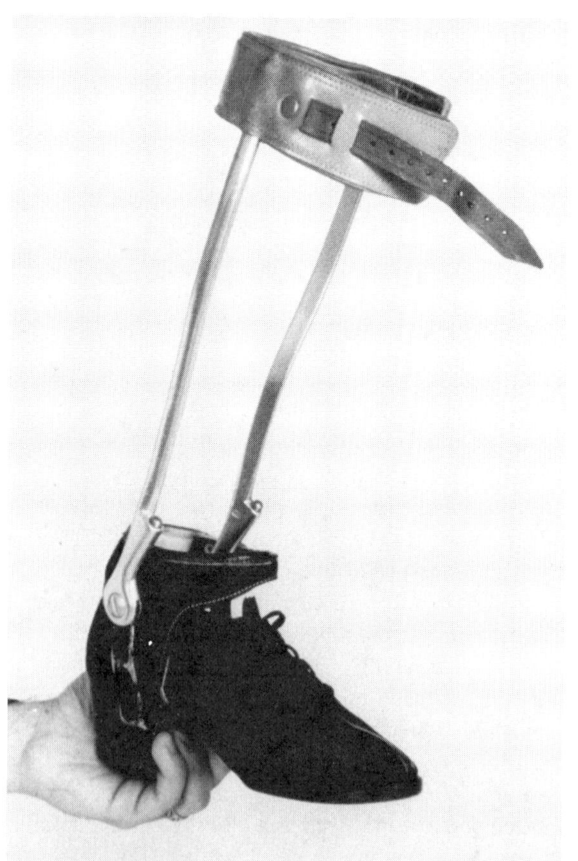

FIG. 26-1. Kienzak ankle–foot orthosis with a medial T-strap to control vagus.

TERMINOLOGY

The lexicon of terms used to describe orthotics was very confusing; often, clinicians used different terms to describe even the most basic device. Devices or parts of orthoses were given names that might describe their purpose, the body part to which they were applied, the inventor of the device, or where they were developed. To facilitate communication and minimize the use of acronyms, a logical, easy-to-use system of standard terminology was developed. This system uses the first letter of each joint that the orthosis crosses in correct sequence, with the letter "O" for orthosis at the end. Thus, the more common orthoses would be named AFO (ankle–foot orthosis), KAFO (knee–ankle–foot orthosis), and KO (knee orthosis). A properly written orthotic prescription does not just state the name of the orthosis; it also is necessary to state the desired function to be obtained, the specific material from which the device is to be made, and the specific design and construction that is to be employed.

SHOES AND FOOTWEAR

The basic function of commercial shoes is to protect the feet from rough walking surfaces, the weather, and the environment as well as to provide support for the feet during standing and walking. To improve comfort and function, special shoes are commercially available for certain unusual or abnormal foot activities, mostly for recreational use and for pathologic foot conditions. The clinician frequently fails to appreciate the importance of comfortable and well-fitting shoes. Foot problems that easily could be corrected by prescription of proper shoes or shoe modifications frequently interfere with optimum functional performance.

Components

The parts of a shoe (Fig. 26-3) consist of the sole, the heel, the upper, the linings, and reinforcements. Each component can be made of a wide variety of materials and designs, depending on the quality and specific use of the shoe.

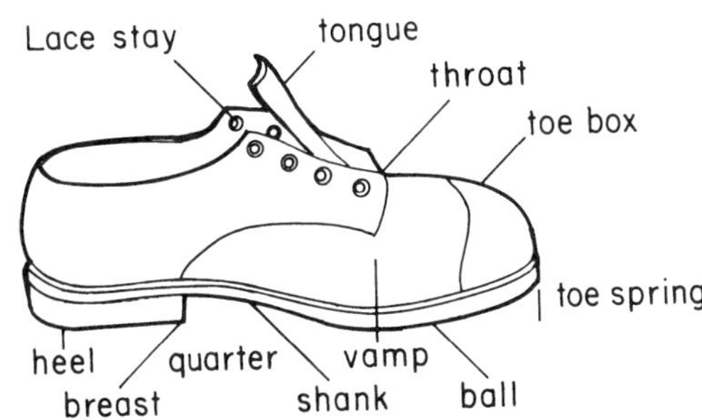

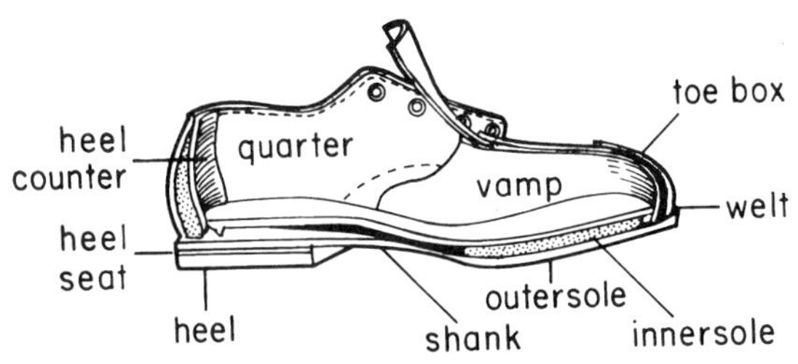

FIG. 26-3. Shoe components.

The sole is the bottom part of the shoe. It is divided into the outer sole, or the surface that touches the ground, and the inner sole, the part closest to the foot and to which the upper and the outer sole are attached. Sometimes a compressible filler made of cork or latex separates the inner from the outer soles. It is preferable that both the inner and the outer soles be made of leather of variable thickness. Leather soles best maintain proper fit and are especially indicated if shoe modifications are required. Rubber soles make modifications more difficult and have the additional drawback of eliminating a large ventilating surface, which may result in excessive sweating and skin problems. The greater friction coefficient of rubber soles may also cause the shoe to stop abruptly on heel strike, thrusting the foot forward into the forepart of the shoe. The widest part of the sole is at the metatarsal heads and is called the ball. The narrowest part of the sole, between the heel and the ball, is called the shank. The shank usually is reinforced by a strip of metal, leather, fiberboard, or other firm material. The external heel seat is the posterior part of the sole to which the heel is secured. The toe spring is attached to the outer surface, between the outer sole and the floor. The purpose of the toe spring in the design of the shoe is to cause a rocker effect during push-off and to reduce wrinkling of the upper.

The heel is attached to the outer sole under the anatomic heel and is made of leather, wood, plastic, rubber, or metal. The heel block, which is fastened to the heel seat, is made of a firm material, but the plantar surface is usually made of hard rubber. The anterior surface of the heel is called the breast. The height of the heel is measured in eighths of an inch at the breast. The height and design of the heel vary greatly. The flat heel has a broad base and measures 0.75 to 1.25 inches in height. A Thomas heel is flat and has a medial extension to support a weak longitudinal foot arch. A military heel has a slightly narrower base and measures 1.25 to 1.375 inches in height. A Cuban heel has a still narrower base but is higher. Heels up to 2 to 3 inches high are available, but they are mainly used for fashionable appearance rather than for extended walking. Shoes with lower heels, no heels, or negative heels also exist. A spring heel, which has a heel height of only $\frac{1}{8}$ to $\frac{3}{16}$ inch, is placed under the outer sole and thus eliminates the heel breast. This type of heel is common on shoes for infants and children up to 3 years of age. Many athletic shoes, including running shoes, have no heels because one can run faster without heels. The negative heel popularized on the earth shoe provided comfort for some people. The clinician needs to be aware that the height of the heel affects foot and ankle positions as well as the general posture of the trunk. Heel height may thus be a factor in certain clinical conditions, such as shortening of gastrocnemius and low back pain. High heels, especially those with a tapered, narrow striking point, make the ankle and foot more unstable and thereby contribute to ankle injuries and falls.

The upper is that part of the shoe that is above the sole. It is most commonly made of leather, although any soft and durable material may be used. Leather is found to be most comfortable because it allows evaporation and absorption of moisture and molds well to the shape of the foot. The upper consists of the vamp, quarters, and lace stay. The vamp is the anterior portion of the upper, which covers the toes and the instep. The tongue, a strip of leather lying under the laces, and the throat, the opening at the base of the tongue, are parts of the vamp. Anteriorly, the vamp has a reinforced toe box or toe cap to maintain appearance and to protect the toes against trauma. The lace stay, or the portion containing the eyelets for laces, is usually part of the vamp, but it may be part of the quarters.

The two quarters make up the posterior part of the shoe. The quarters usually are reinforced by the heel counter, which stabilizes the foot by supporting the calcaneus and gives structural stability to the shoe. The counter usually extends anteriorly to the heel breast, but it may extend further forward or upward on specially made shoes. It, like the toe box, is made of firm leather or synthetic material. Laterally, the quarter is cut lower to avoid infringing on the lateral malleolus. Sometimes a band of leather, referred to as a collar, is stitched to the top of the quarters to reduce pistoning or to prevent the shoe from failing off. The linings are made of leather, cotton, or canvas and should be used in all portions of the shoe that are in contact with the foot to absorb perspiration and smooth the contact area, thus providing added comfort.

Fabrication

Shoes are built around a positive model or replica of the weight-bearing foot, which is called a last (1). The last, which is made of solid rock maple or plastic materials, determines the fit, the walking comfort, the appearance, and the style of the shoe. Usually the last has a slight forefoot inflare. Other common lasts include the broad-toe last with a straight medial border that extends from the heel to the toe; the juvenile symmetric straight last, which can be bisected into nearly equal right and left halves; and the orthopaedic last with special features designed to accommodate various structural and anatomic problems (e.g., varus, valgus).

During fabrication, the insole is nailed to the last, the lining is tucked to the inner sole rim, and the reinforcements (i.e., counter, toe box) are attached. The upper of the shoe is softened by humidity for easier molding and fitted snugly to the last to adapt to its every detail and then nailed or glued to the inner sole. Finally, the outer sole and heel are attached. The Goodyear welt construction of shoes is a method used in production of high-quality shoes in which the upper is sewn to the sole. This method provides a perfectly smooth inner surface, comfort, and a strong shoe that retains its shape and is easy to modify and repair. Unfortunately, these shoes tend to be bulky, heavy, and less flexible.

Types and Styles

There are innumerable shoe types and styles (Fig. 26-4), although basic designs are relatively few. The basic designs are mainly determined by the shape of the upper, especially the design of the toe and the height of the quarters. On low-quarter shoes, or the Oxford, the quarters extend approximately 1 inch below the malleoli and do not restrict ankle or subtalar motions. In high-quarter shoes, the quarters may cover the malleoli, either just barely, as in the chukka shoe, or by 2 inches or more, as in boots. This style prevents piston action during walking and back-and-forth sliding of the foot. In addition, it provides medial–lateral stability at the ankle and subtalar joints and resistance to plantar flexion. The most common throat style is the blucher type, in which the lace stay is not directly fastened to the vamp. This style gives a wide opening for the foot for easy insertion and greater adjustability over the midfoot. The bal-type (Balmoral)

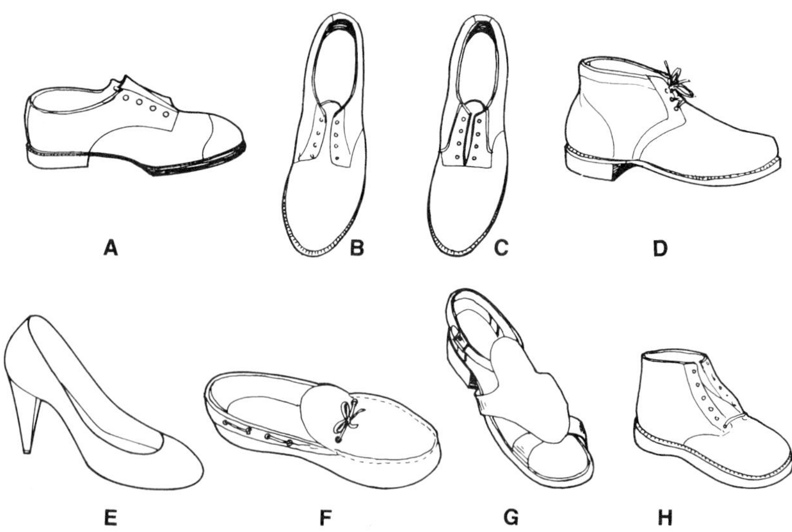

FIG. 26-4. Shoe types and styles. **A:** Oxford or low quarter. **B:** Blucher-type Oxford. **C:** Bal-type Oxford. **D:** Chukka or high quarter. **E:** Pump. **F:** Moccasin. **G:** Sandal. **H:** Child's.

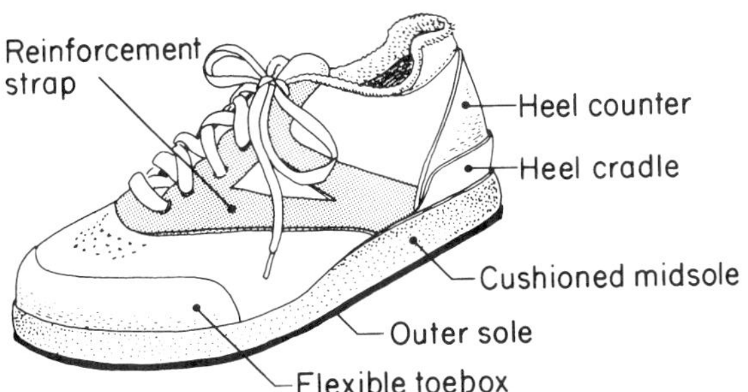

FIG. 26-5. Components of an athletic shoe.

throat, which has the face stay attached directly to the vamp, does not provide such easy foot access. A lace-to-toe shoe, often referred to as a surgical shoe, allows exposure of the entire foot by opening up to the toes. Shoe closure usually is accomplished by cotton laces, which thread through two or more pairs of eyelets, although closure also can be achieved by buckles, zippers, velcro flaps, or elastics.

Athletic shoes (Fig. 26-5) have changed dramatically in design and new materials that have been introduced and used in their fabrication in recent years. Except for their sporty appearance, modern athletic shoes have little in common with old-fashioned sneakers, which were made primarily of a canvas upper and a rubber sole and provided little foot support. Different sports may require different shoe design features for optimal performance and comfort. The sole of a good athletic shoe is stiff at the heel and at the shank but very flexible at the forefoot, where it should bend easily at the ball. The outer sole usually is made of highly durable rubber compounds that provide a good grip on the ground, whereas the inner sole is designed to fit the contours of the foot closely. Between the outer and inner soles, gel- or foamlike materials are placed for cushioning to dampen shocks to the foot. The outer sole often is designed to flare out laterally at the heel and toward the midfoot to improve mediolateral stability at the ankle and to ensure the foot is flat as it strikes the ground in the normal slightly supinated position. Rising up from the rear sole to a height of approximately 0.5 inch is a heel cradle, which further increases mediolateral motion control and hind foot stability. The rigid and noncompressible heel counter provides added stability, but for athletes with a tendency to recurrent ankle sprains, there is the option of using high-top shoes. The upper is reinforced in the midfoot area for maximum stability and to resist excessive side-to-side motion. Such reinforcement is obtained by adding bands, stabilized lacing systems, and motion control straps. In addition to their use in various sports, athletic shoes frequently are used by the elderly and people with gait disorders because they are lightweight and provide excellent foot stability.

Children's shoes (see Fig. 26-4) generally are designed similarly to those for adults. During infancy, shoes are important primarily for foot protection and therefore should be lightweight, flexible, and quadrangularly shaped to conform to the normal foot shape. The soles should be soft and flexible for the crawling child to allow easy bending and to minimize forced inversion or eversion of the foot. Rigid shoes are not necessary for normal development of feet. Children who habitually go barefoot usually have healthy feet that are supple, flexible, and mobile (2). Toddlers up to 3 years of age usually are fitted with shoes that are somewhat more rigid than infants' shoes, although these still must be flexible to permit foot mobility and light in weight to reduce energy cost. The upper should be made of soft leather or permeable fabric to allow evaporation; the toe box should be broad, the medial border relatively straight, and the heel counter firm and snug. The sole should be firm and reinforced at the shank, and its friction should be similar to the bare foot's (i.e., it should be neither slippery nor slide-resistant). The heel should be flat or of the low-spring type. A high-top design may be helpful to keep the shoe from slipping off during running and jumping. For the remainder of the growing years, proper footwear clearly continues to be of great importance. At least a half-inch of space should be allowed between the shoe and the longest toe on weight bearing, whereas the heel of the shoe upper should fit snugly and comfortably without excessive gaping. Excessively worn or ill-fitting children's shoes should be discarded, and other people's shoes (i.e., hand-me-downs) should not be used.

Fitting

The first requirement of a shoe is that it fits and does not cause pain, skin problems, or deformities. Both feet should be measured, and the shoes tried on both feet in case of size discrepancy, and the shoe size should be chosen that is most comfortable for the larger foot. Footwear preferably should be purchased at the end of the day, when the feet often are slightly swollen. When shoes are fitted, each shoe should be judged individually in a fully weight-bearing position. The shoe should fit snugly enough not to fall off but be loose enough to adapt to the size and shape of the foot, which change with climate, ambient temperature, time of day, body position, and weight-bearing whether the person is lying, sitting, or standing. Because the foot expands with weight bearing, shoes initially should be carefully tested for fit, both in length and width, not only by standing but by walking or running several steps and stopping short. The real proof of fit, however, is if the shoe is comfortable after hours of continuous wear or walking. An old piece of advice is to find a comfortable pair of shoes and then take one size larger.

In length, the shoes should extend at least a half-inch beyond the longest toe, usually the hallux or the second toe. The heel-to-ball distance of the foot and the shoe should be equal. Thus, the first metatarsal joint should be located at the inner curve of the shoe, and on toe dorsiflexion, the shoe should bend easily, and the toe break should run directly across the ball. The widest part of the shoe, the ball, should coincide with the broadest part of the foot, leaving enough free space madial and lateral to the heads of the first and fifth metatarsal bones, respectively. The transverse arch of the foot should function normally, weight should be evenly distributed, and no sliding of the forefoot within the shoe should occur. The medial and lateral quarters should not gap, and the heel counter should close around the heel bone without bulges, allowing only a small amount of pistoning. Some pistoning usually is unavoidable in a shoe with a rigid sole and heel counter. The height of the vamp should be adequate to prevent pressure or irritation over the toes and the instep. The height of the quarters should be sufficient to hold the shoe securely on the foot. If the quarters are too high, they can cause irritation of the malleoli.

Different shoe sizes are commercially available and are marked by numbers to indicate length and by letters to indicate width. The numbers used in the United States and Europe are different, as are the numbers used to indicate the sizes of men's, women's, and children's feet. Sizes often vary from one manufacturer to another. In the United States, the smallest shoe is infant size 000, and the largest is a man's size 16. Most shoe stores, however, carry only men's shoe sizes up to 14 or 15 and women's sizes up to 12 or 13. Larger sizes are available in specialty shoe stores, or they may be special ordered. The shoe widths measured at the ball are available in different sizes, ranging from A, which is narrow, to E, which is wide. Each size represents a 0.25-inch increase in width. Few shoe stores stock shoes of extreme width. Shoe depth is not fabricated in different sizes, although extra-depth shoes and shoes with adjustable insoles are available to accommodate foot abnormalities and shoe inserts.

Modifications

Stock shoes may require minor or major modifications by various methods to support the abnormal foot during weight bearing, to reduce pressure on painful areas, and to limit motion of weak, unstable, or painful joints. For these purposes, the clinician may select a special type of shoe, order certain alterations in the construction of the shoe, or apply corrections directly to the foot. The clinician needs to make an accurate diagnosis of the problem, have a clear understanding of why corrections are needed, and write a specific prescription that is best accompanied by a simple drawing to clarify the request. Although certain simple external modifications may be applied easily to many types of commercial shoes, welt shoes are more suitable to work with, especially for major internal modifications, because the shoe structure is not altered by removing and reattaching the sole to the upper. Orthopedic shoes are welt shoes made of good leather, with relatively thick soles, a high and wide toe box, extended medial heel counter, rigid wide steel shank, and a Thomas heel. They are the most frequently prescribed shoes for foot problems requiring shoe modification, and they also are regarded as high-quality footwear for normal feet. Extra-depth orthopedic shoes are made commercially and are widely available. They offer removable insoles, which allow the placement of most foot orthoses (FOs) without compromising fit or comfort. Moldable shoes have uppers that are constructed from thermoplastic materials that can be reshaped when heated to accommodate minor and moderate foot deformities.

A fixed deformity needs accommodation, using the shoe to bring the weight-bearing surface to the foot, whereas a flexible deformity may be actively corrected. Adults usually have relatively fixed deformities requiring passive stabilization, but young children have flexible deformities that may be corrected actively by proper shoe prescription if they are minor or moderate. In more severe cases, serial plaster cast and surgical operations may be required.

Internal

Shoe modifications can be classified as either internal (i.e., those that are inserted into the inner surface of the shoe or sandwiched between shoe components) or external (i.e., those that are attached to the sole or heel). Internal modifications are mechanically more effective. Although they generally are made of soft materials, they are less well tolerated because they reduce the size of the shoe and distort the inner sole. They may be removable or built-in as an integral part of the shoe. Internal shoe corrections include steel shanks, cookies (e.g., scaphoid and metatarsal pads), interior heel lifts and wedges, extended or reinforced heel counters, and protective metal toe boxes. Steel shanks can be used to support a weak longitudinal arch, but if this is insufficient, a cookie made of firm materials such as leather or rubber may be placed along the medial border of the insole at the talonavicular joint. Scaphoid pads also provide additional longitudinal arch support but are made of compressible material. They are prescribed for people who cannot tolerate the firmness of a cookie. The longitudinal arch support of a cookie or scaphoid pad is improved further by insertion of a long medial counter made of rigid leather. Metatarsal pads, which are commercially available in many sizes, may be positioned inside the shoe just proximal to the metatarsal heads to protect and reduce pressure on the second, third, and fourth metatarsal heads by transferring force to their bone shafts. A sesamoid or dancer's pad is thicker and broader, and extends medially to the proximal part of the first metatarsal head. Thus, it provides greater support for more severe cases of metatarsalgia. Heel elevations of more than 0.25 inch should be placed externally. Interior heel wedges of $\frac{1}{16}$ to $\frac{1}{8}$ inch in height may be placed on either the medial or lateral half of the interior heel.

External

External shoe modifications (Fig. 26-6) include sole and heel wedges, flanges and elevations, metatarsal and rocker bars, and different types of heel designs. Wedges are constructed of leather and positioned under the outer sole or heel. Sole and heel wedges usually are placed medially, but

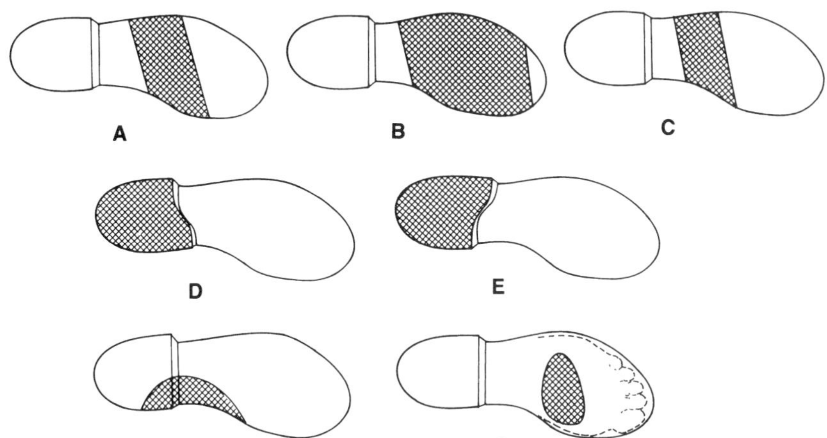

FIG. 26-6. Common shoe modifications (plantar views). **A:** Metatarsal bar. **B:** Rocker bar. **C:** Denver bar. **D:** Thomas heel. **E:** Reverse Thomas heel. **F:** Scaphoid (navicular) pad insert. **G:** Metatarsal pad insert.

occasionally they are placed laterally to shift the body weight from that side of the foot to the other. Flanges or flare-outs are ¼-inch-wide medial or lateral extensions of the sole or heel that provide stability. A lateral flange provides a lever arm, which ensures a foot flat in the presence of excessive inversion or varus deformity. Such small lateral flanges are seen on most commercially available running shoes, where they are intended to prevent inversion sprains.

Elevations (i.e., lifts) of the sole and heel are prescribed for leg length discrepancies. Leg length discrepancies of less than a half-inch generally do not require a shoe modification, but a greater discrepancy should be corrected to make the pelvis level. It may not be necessary or even desirable to provide an elevation for the total leg length to be equal on both sides. If an elevation of more than ¼ inch is required, these should be applied externally. Elevations up to 1 inch in height can be added exclusively to the heel. When elevation of greater than 1 inch is indicated, it has to be applied to both the heel and sole of the shoe. The height of the elevation must be greatest at the heel and taper off from the ball of the shoe to the toe. Elevations greater than 1 inch should be made of lightweight materials, such as layered cork.

A metatarsal bar (i.e., anterior heel) made of leather or rubber may be attached transversely to the outer sole immediately proximal to the metatarsal heads to relieve pressure on them and to reduce pain. A rocker bar is similarly placed but extends distally beyond the metatarsal heads. It also relieves pressure on the metatarsal heads and reduces metatarsal phalangeal flexion on push-off by providing a smooth plantar roll to toe-off. It thus may improve gait when painful or paralytic conditions prevent good push-off. A Denver bar is placed under the metatarsal bones to support the transverse arch extending from the metatarsal heads anteriorly to the tarsal–metatarsal joints posteriorly.

External heel modifications are of several kinds. Already mentioned are heel elevations, wedges, and flanges. The Thomas heel (see Fig. 26-6) or the orthopedic heel is similar in design and material to the regular flat heel but has an anteromedial extension to provide additional longitudinal arch support. This extension may be of variable length, depending on the extent of support required, and its effect may be augmented further by a medial wedge or a Thomas heel wedge. A reverse Thomas heel is an anterolateral extension to support a weak lateral longitudinal arch, but this variety is rarely used. Occasionally, compressible, resilient materials are inserted into the heel (i.e., solid ankle cushion heel), usually in conjunction with a rocker bar for a cushioning effect on heel strike. The result is a simulation of plantar flexion with minimal ankle movement, while the rocker bar provides smooth push-off. Thus, a more natural gait may be obtained in certain clinical conditions despite relative immobilization of the foot and ankle.

LOWER EXTREMITY ORTHOSES

Foot Orthoses

Foot orthoses are removable foot supports made of variable materials placed inside the shoe to manage different foot symptoms and deformities. They have the advantage over shoe modifications in that they can be transferred from shoe to shoe, may be modified without disturbing the shoe, and are more durable than the modified shoe. Although commercially available arch supports exist, such devices are relatively ineffective. Therefore, custom-made FOs are preferred when maintenance of a specific foot alignment over long periods of time is indicated. The usual clinical indications for FOs are to relieve pressure on areas that are painful, ulcerated, scarred, or callused, to support weak or flat longitudinal or transverse foot arches, and to control foot position and thus affect the alignment of other lower limb joints.

Soft or flexible FOs are made from leather, cork, rubber, soft plastics, and plastic foam. Many of these are commercially available and used for simple problems, but they are a poor choice for more severe conditions. The soft FOs usually are fabricated in full length from heel to toe with increased thickness where weight bearing is indicated and relief where no or little pressure should occur. Rubber FOs generally are least acceptable because of poor permeability for evaporating perspiration, lack of molding properties, and excessive compression on weight bearing. Materials that provide best cushioning tend to wear out fast and therefore may require frequent replacement. Numerous kinds of thermoplastic polyethylene foams, such as Plastazote, are available in different densities and thicknesses. They commonly are used for ischemic, insensitive, ulcerated, and arthritic feet. After heating, some of these materials can be molded conveniently directly on the foot, but others with high specific heat require the use of a positive model of the foot. The softer-grade materials tend to bottom out early and may require a latex cork backing to prolong usefulness. Some of these materials have a high friction coefficient and may have to be covered on the foot side with softer material to reduce shear.

The semirigid and rigid FOs come in a variety of materials such as leather, cork, and metals, but most commonly they are made of solid plastics, which allow minimal flexibility. Optimal fabrication requires applying a plaster-of-Paris cast on the patient's feet, removing it, and making a positive replica of the foot on which the orthosis can be accurately molded. These orthoses generally extend from the posterior end of the heel to the metatarsal heads (i.e., three-quarter length) and may have medial and lateral flanges. They are molded to provide support under the longitudinal arch and metatarsal area and to provide relief for painful or irritated areas. The most rigid FOs are made of metal, usually steel or duraluminum, covered with leather, and molded on a positive cast of the patient's foot (e.g., Whitman, Mayer, and Shaffer plates; Boston arch support).

Management of Foot Conditions

Numerous clinical foot problems and deformities are managed best by modification of shoes or fabrication of an FO. The most common of these conditions are listed in Table 26-1 with the suggested shoe modifications. No single remedy or combination of remedies can serve for all cases and instances. Each case has to be judged individually, and other shoe modifications and different interventions considered. Very frequently, a custom-made FO or AFO may negate the necessity for shoe modification, and surgery may be required to obtain optimal correction. Strappings, paddings, and appliances may be applied directly to the foot and toes to correct deformities and protect tender areas such as corns, calluses, ulcers, nails, and bony outgrowths from excessive friction or pressure. Before padding, excess corns, calluses, and nails should be removed.

The clinician prescribing shoes, shoe modifications, and FOs needs to be thoroughly familiar with the normal anatomy, biomechanics, and development of the foot, diagnosis and management of pathologic conditions affecting the foot, as well as the terminology, mechanisms, and manufacture of shoes, their components, and modifications. The clinician needs to educate the patient with foot disorders about foot care and footwear needs. Before and after shoe modifications are applied and periodically thereafter, the shoe and the foot should be examined carefully to ensure proper fit, comfort, and mechanics.

Loss of sensation in the feet often occurs in persons with diabetes mellitus and polyneuropathy. This may result in poor sensory feedback regarding plantar pressures during standing and walking, which in turn may lead to tissue breakdown, ulcer formation, and eventual limb loss (3). Plantar pressures recorded under the posterior and anterior heels and the first metatarsal region of insensate feet have been found to be greater than those in sensate feet (3). Plantar ulcers in diabetic persons have been noted to develop consistently at the site of maximum plantar loading (4–7), and therefore, it is of great importance to provide proper and even redistribution of the plantar pressures through use of therapeutic shoes and custom molded insoles (8,9). Modestly priced athletic shoes have been found to be more effective in reducing plantar pressures in diabetic persons than the more expensive leather-soled oxford shoes (10). Prevention and care of diabetic foot ulcers must emphasize patient education, glycemic control, and careful daily foot hygiene in addition to providing appropriate footwear (11).

The use of FOs and external modifications of athletic or prescription shoes is an important component of the prevention and management of foot and ankle injuries in sports (12) and in the elderly. Athletes not only are at a greater risk of injury than the general population but also have a tendency to treat themselves, look for quick and easy solutions, resume activity before healing is complete, and disregard pain as a symptom of reinjury (12). For the elderly, painful foot problems frequently make walking difficult, and diminished foot proprioception may contribute to the high frequency of falls in this age group (13). Wearing of appropriate footwear and provision of good foot care may do much to keep the elderly population safely ambulatory.

Ankle–Foot Orthoses

Ankle–foot orthoses (AFOs) are most commonly prescribed for muscle weakness affecting the ankle and subtalar joints (14), such as weakness of dorsi and plantar flexors, invertors, and evertors. Such AFOs also can be prescribed for prevention or correction of deformities of the foot and ankle and reduction of weight-bearing forces. In addition to having mechanical effects on the ankle, the AFOs also may affect the stability of the knee by varying the degree of plantar- or dorsiflexion at the ankle. An ankle fixed in dorsiflexion will provide a flexion force at the knee and thus may help to prevent genu recurvatum; a fixed plantarflexion will provide an extension force that may help to support a weak knee during the stance phase of gait.

Although traditional metal orthoses still are prescribed, plastic AFOs have become more common. They may be fabricated from either thermoplastic or thermosetting materials, depending on the function required. Inexpensive, ready-

TABLE 26-1. *Clinical foot condition and suggested modifications of the orthopedic shoe*

Clinical condition	Objectives of modifications	Modifications
Limb shortening	Provide symmetric posture Improve gait	Heel elevation: If <½ in: internal If >½ in: external Heel and sole elevation (if >1 in) Rocker bar High-quarter shoe
Arthritis, fusion, or instability of ankle and subtalar joints	Support and limit joint motion Accommodate deformities Improve gait	High-quarter shoe Reinforced counters Long steel shank Rocker bar SACH heel
Pes plano-valgus	Reduce eversion Support longitudinal arch	For children: High-quarter shoe with broad heel, long medial counter, and medial heel wedge For adults: Thomas heel with medial high wedge Medial longitudinal arch support with cookie or scaphoid pad
Pes equinus (fixed)	Provide heel strike Contain foot in shoe Reduce pressure on MT head Ease putting on of shoe Equalize leg length	High-quarter shoe, expecially for children Heel elevation Heel and sole elevation on other shoe Modified lace stay for wide opening Medial longitudinal arch support Rocker bar, occasionally
Pes varus	Obtain realignment for flexible deformity Accommodate a fixed deformity Increase medial and posterior weight bearing on foot	High-quarter shoe Long lateral counter Reverse Thomas heel Lateral sole and heel wedges for flexible deformity Medial wedges for fixed deformity Lateral sole and heel flanges Medial longitudinal arch support
Pes cavus	Distribute weight over entire foot Restore anteroposterior foot balance Reduce pain and pressure on MT heads	High-quarter shoe High toe box Lateral heel and sole wedges Metatarsal pads or bars Molded inner sole Medial and lateral longitudinal arch support
Calcaneal spurs	Relieve pressure on painful area	Heel cusion Inner relief in heel and fill with soft sponge
Metatarsalgia	Reduce pressure on MT heads Support transverse arch	Metatarsal or sesamoid pad Metatarsal or rocker bar Inner sole relief
Hallux valgus	Reduce pressure on 1st MTP joint and big toe Prevent forward foot slide Immobilize 1st MTP joint Shift weight laterally	Soft vamp with broad ball and toe Relief in vamp with cut-out or balloon patch Low heel Metatarsal or sesamoid pad Medial longitudinal arch support Soft vamp
Hallus rigidus	Reduce pressure and motion of 1st MTP joint Improve push off	Long steel spring in sole Sesamoid pad Metatarsal or rocker bar Medial longitudinal arch support
Hammer toes	Relieve pressure on painful areas Support transverse arch Improve push off	Soft-vamp, extra-depth shoe with high toe box or balloon patch Metatarsal pad
Foot shortening (unilateral)	Fit shoe to foot	Extra inner sole and padded tongue for difference of less than one size Shoes of split sizes or custom-made
Foot fractures	Immobilize fractured part	Long steel shank Longitudinal arch support Metatarsal pad Metatarsal or rocket bar

MT, metatarsal; MTP, metatarsophalangeal; SACH, solid ankle cusion heel.

to-use AFOs are widely available and useful for minor or temporary deficits, but custom-made orthoses molded on a replica of the foot, ankle, and leg are indicated for more severe and permanent deficits. Plastic AFOs are worn inside the shoe and consist of the footplate, an upright component, and a velcro calf strap. The shoe that attaches the orthosis to the foot has to have secure closures. Although these orthoses can be changed from shoe to shoe, it is important that all shoes worn have the same heel height to provide equal biomechanical effects at the ankle and knee. The footplate in a custom-made AFO may be accurately molded to provide all the functions of a molded FO; at the least, it should always support the metatarsal and longitudinal foot arches.

The upright components on plastic AFOs vary in design, depending on the desired function, but usually these extend from the footplate without a joint mechanism to the upper calf approximately 1 to 2 inches below the head of the fibula. A plastic AFO can be fabricated to control plantarflexion, dorsiflexion, or inversion or eversion of the ankle, depending on the design, built-in position of the orthosis, thickness of the material used, and location of the trim lines. A plastic leaf-spring orthosis (PLSO) probably is the most commonly prescribed type of AFO (see Fig. 26-2). It substitutes for weakness of ankle dorsiflexors and provides some mediolateral stability. An associated strong tendency for ankle inversion, as often seen in hemiplegics, may be counteracted by increasing the rigidity of the upright component at the ankle and increasing the lateral support at the calf. Severe spasticity of the ankle may require prescription of a solid-ankle plastic AFO (Fig. 26-7). Most ready-to-wear AFOs are of the PLSO or solid-ankle varieties. A plastic spiral AFO may be prescribed effectively for concomitant weakness of both dorsiflexors and plantarflexors of the ankle when spasticity is absent or insignificant. In recent years, plastic AFOs have been fabricated in the more traditional design of double uprights and a foot, including articulations and stops.

Metal AFOs usually have both medial and lateral uprights with an ankle joint mechanism. The uprights are attached to the shoe by a stirrup and secured to the calf by a padded leather-covered calf band, leather strap, and a buckle. Sturdy shoes, such as orthopedic shoes, are required for metal orthoses. The stirrups usually are attached directly to the shoe between the sole and the heel, although a footplate inside the shoe occasionally is used. The upper end of the stirrup connects with the uprights at the ankle joint. The solid stirrup is used most commonly and provides the most rigid and least bulky shoe attachment. The split stirrup allows transfer of the plate, both made of molded plastic but connected by two hinged metal joints at the ankle. This development has been fabricated by improved ankle joint designs with narrower profiles and interchangeable disks to determine the permitted angles of dorsi- and plantarflexion orthosis to any shoe with a flat caliper insertion.

Different ankle joint mechanisms allow fixed, limited, or full dorsiflexion or plantarflexion. The Klenzak ankle joint orthosis (see Fig. 26-1), permits assistance of ankle motion

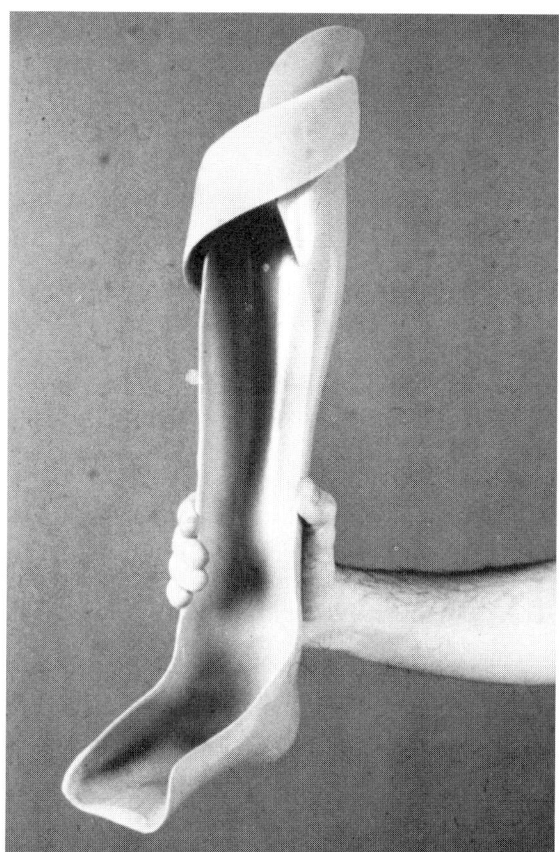

FIG. 26-7. Plastic solid ankle–foot orthosis.

in dorsiflexion by inclusion of a spring. A plantarflexion stop can induce knee flexion, whereas a dorsiflexion stop induces a knee extension force during the stance phase of gait. The round caliper is a design that attaches uprights without ankle joints to the shoe by a metal plate, but the uprights are easily detachable from the shoe. Motion occurs where the uprights are inserted into the sole of the shoe at a considerable distance from the axis of the anatomic ankle joint. The round caliper often is prescribed for children with cerebral palsy who have difficulty putting on an orthosis. T-straps (see Fig. 26-1) may be attached to the shoe medially or laterally to control valgus (i.e., eversion) or varus (i.e., inversion) and are buckled around the contralateral upright to apply a counteracting force.

A variety of prefabricated AFOs are available for prevention of foot and ankle deformities. Such AFOs are frequently prescribed for neurologic conditions when there is a risk of Achilles tendon shortening, but they may also be helpful in the management of plantar fasciitis and heel pain (15). They are usually worn at night only and are not designed for weight bearing.

Standard Knee–Ankle–Foot Orthoses

Below the knee, the components of the standard KAFO are the same as those of metal or plastic AFOs, except that

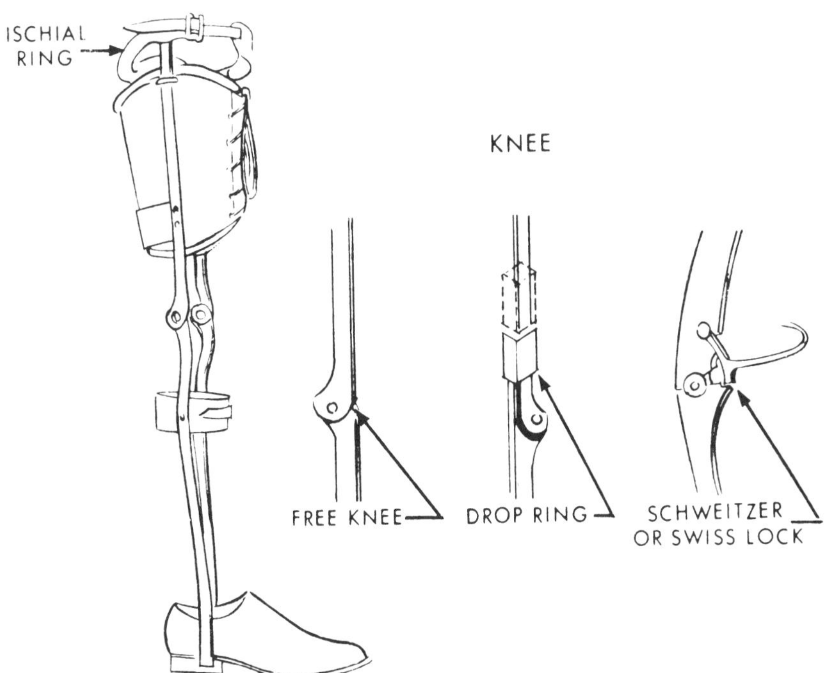

FIG. 26-8. Conventional knee–ankle–foot orthosis with variations of kneelocks. (From American Academy of Orthopedic Surgeons. *Atlas of orthotics.* St Louis: CV Mosby, 1975.)

the uprights extend to the knee joint, where they join the thigh uprights (Fig. 26-8). Although the anatomic knee joint has a changing axis of rotation, polycentric designed knee joints have few clinical applications because during ambulation the orthotic knee joint usually is locked. A free knee joint is indicated when mediolateral instability or genu recurvatum is present but knee extension strength is adequate for weight bearing.

If knee extensors are weak, and buckling occurs, a knee lock or offset joint is indicated. The drop-ring lock is used most commonly. It is placed on the lateral upright bar and drops over the joint when it is fully extended. A spring-loaded pull rod may be added to the ring to ease locking and unlocking, especially when the patient is unable to reach the knee. A cam lock with a spring-loaded cam that fits into a groove in full extension is easier to release but gives good stability and may be used in severe spasticity. A bail lock (i.e., Swiss lock) is a lever bow that snaps into locked position on full extension and unlocks automatically when pressed upward against an object, such as a chair. In the presence of a knee flexion contracture, an adjustable knee joint may be indicated using either a fan or dial lock. In the absence of knee flexion spasticity or contracture, a posteriorly offset knee joint provides a stable knee during stance but allows flexion during the swing phase.

Even when mechanically locked, the knee with weak extensors would bend on weight bearing if not stabilized by straps above and below the patella or by a patellar strap, a soft leather pad covering the kneecap and fastened with four adjustable straps to the uprights. The thigh uprights are connected by a rigid, padded upper thigh band with an anterior soft closure. This band should be 1.5 inches below the ischium, unless ischial rest is prescribed. Usually, a second, rigid lower thigh band also is used with soft anterior straps.

The Scott–Craig orthosis eliminates the lower thigh and calf bands, which makes it easier to put on and remove (Fig. 26-9) (16). It consists of two uprights with four rigid connections: posterior rigid upper thigh band, bail-type knee lock, rigid anterior upper tibial band with soft posterior strap, and at the lower end, a stirrup with a rigid sole plate built into the shoe extending to the metatarsal heads. It is connected to the uprights by double-stop (Becker) ankle joints that are adjusted to place the orthosis in 5° of dorsiflexion for optimum balance (17). The shoe sole is perfectly flat from the heel to the metatarsal bar, where it becomes slightly rounded to the toe. Properly adjusted, the orthosis should stand balanced on its own. It is a stable orthosis that biomechanically functions as the standard KAFO.

Modified Knee–Ankle–Foot Orthoses

Plastic laminated knee–ankle–foot orthoses (KAFOs) may incorporate standard ankle and knee components, but the uprights and bands are made of skin-colored laminated plastic that closely fits the limb and is lightweight (Fig. 26-10). The thigh piece is a quadrilaterally shaped posterior thigh shell with or without an ischial weight-bearing seat closed anteriorly by a plastic band and a velcro strap. A suprapatellar or pretibial shell provides knee extension force, which eliminates the need for patellar strap and provides mediolateral knee stability. At the lower end, the uprights are connected to a molded plastic footplate to be worn inside a shoe.

A plastic laminated supracondylar KAFO is indicated for

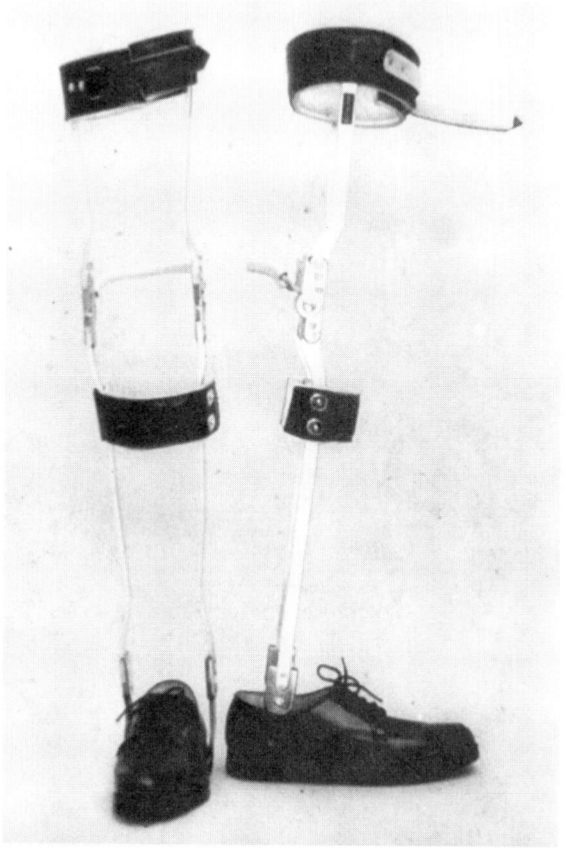

FIG. 26-9. The Scott–Craig knee–ankle–foot orthosis.

patients who lack knee and ankle muscle power but have normal hip extensors, full knee extension, and no spasticity (17). A molded footplate and a solid ankle design immobilize the foot and ankle in equinus, which produces a knee extension force during stance. Genu recurvatum is controlled by a supracondylar anterior shell and a counteracting popliteal shell posteriorly. The absence of a mechanical knee joint allows free knee flexion during swing phase with better gait pattern and reduced energy cost.

Lightweight modular KAFOs have been designed for quick and easy assembly and provided for children with Duchenne Muscular Dystrophy in order to extend their walking ability (18). Such a KAFO consists of a plastic thigh piece and an AFO, both available in several prefabricated sizes. The two components are joined at the knee by a metal joint system with an automatic ring or bail locks.

Knee Orthoses

Knee orthoses are prescribed to prevent genu recurvatum and to provide mediolateral stability. As such they may be used during sports and other physical activities to provide functional support for unstable knees or during the rehabilitation phase following injury or surgery on the knee. The use of KOs for the prevention of knee injury in athletes is controversial (19). Numerous designs of KOs are available, a development enhanced by the growing field of sports medicine. Most KOs consist of two uprights, free or adjustable knee joints, and thigh and calf cuffs. The Swedish knee cage

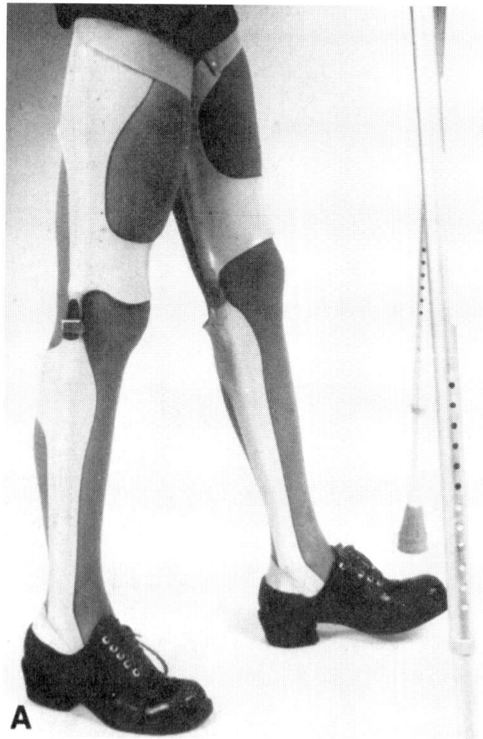

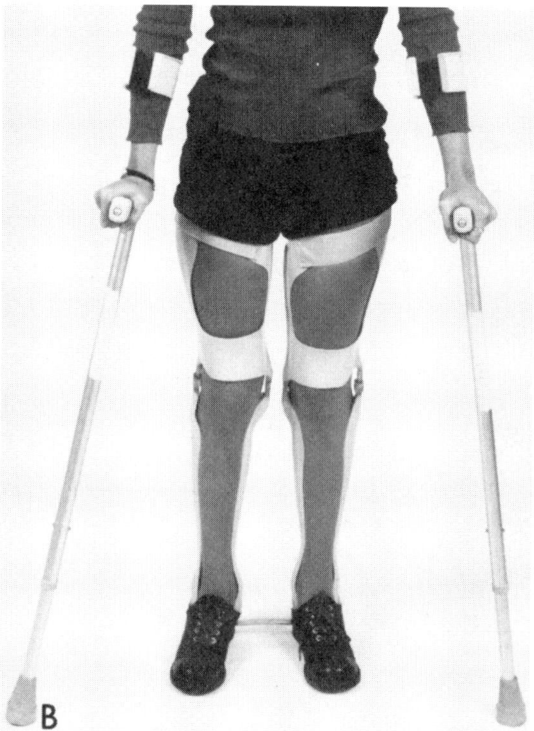

FIG. 26-10. Plastic-laminated knee–ankle–foot orthoses viewed from side **(A)** and front **(B)**.

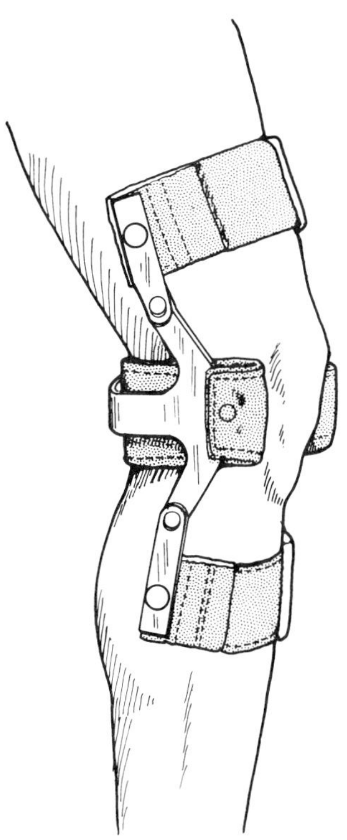

FIG. 26-11. The Swedish knee cage is an example of a knee orthosis.

(Fig. 26-11) prevents recurvatum but permits flexion. The three-way knee stabilizer orthosis looks similar and gives good control of structural knee instability in the lateral, medial, and posterior directions and is indicated for genu valgum, varus, and recurvatum. The standard KOs have short lever arms and may not be effective when strong forces are required for control. They also have a tendency to slip down. Numerous KO designs with longer lever arms and, often, derotational components have been commercially fabricated and prescribed for advanced physical activities and athletics.

Hip–Knee–Ankle–Foot Orthoses

Hip–knee–ankle–foot orthoses consist of the same components as described for the standard AFOs and KAFOs, with the addition of an attached lockable hip joint and a pelvic band to control movements at the anatomic hip joint. The hip joint usually has a ring drop lock. The pelvic band, which may be unilateral or bilateral, encompasses the pelvis between the iliac crest and greater trochanter laterally, curves down over the buttocks, and then passes up again over the sacrum. The indications for prescribing a pelvic band have been controversial because several studies indicate that it increases lumbar excursion and displacement of gravity during ambulation, and thus, energy cost may be greater. For most paraplegics, pelvic bands probably are not necessary, although they may improve standing balance, especially if spasticity is severe.

The Louisiana State University reciprocating gait orthosis (Fig. 26-12) provides bilateral KAFOs with posterior offset knee joints, knee locks, posterior plastic ankle–foot and thigh pieces, a custom-molded pelvic girdle, and special thrust-bearing hip joints, coupled together with a cable and conduit, and a thoracic extension with velcro straps (20,21). The cable coupling mechanism provides hip stability by preventing simultaneous bilateral hip flexion, yet allows free hip flexion coupled with reciprocal extension of the contralateral hip when a step is attempted. Using two crutches, paraplegics are able to ambulate with a four-point gait pattern. This orthosis also has been tested and used in conjunction with a functional electric stimulation system to facilitate paraplegic ambulation.

Fracture Orthoses

Orthoses of different designs have been used in the management of fractures (22). By definition, a plaster-of-Paris cast applied to a fractured limb is an orthosis that provides rigid immobilization while healing occurs. The term "frac-

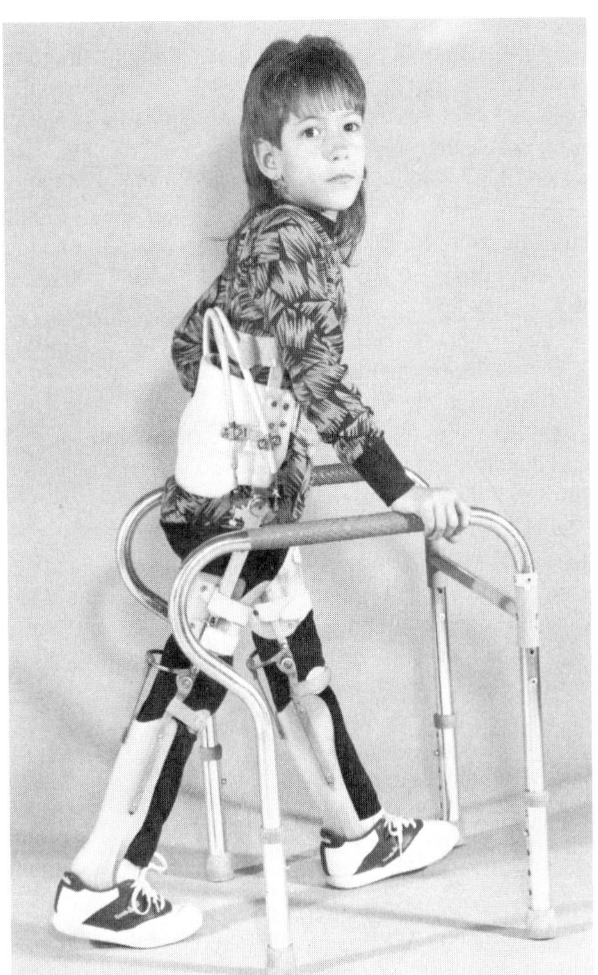

FIG. 26-12. Louisiana State University reciprocating gait orthosis. (Courtesy of Durr-Fillauer Medical, Chattanooga, TN.)

ture orthosis,'' however, refers to a concept of management based on the hypothesis, supported by considerable clinical evidence, that mobilization of adjacent joints does not impede healing of fractures, that functional activity stimulates osteogenesis, and that rigid immobilization of fractures is not a prerequisite for healing. Even when this management concept is applied, all fractures initially are immobilized either by traction or in conventional casts while the acute pain and swelling associated with the injury subsides and early healing takes place. Such immobilization should be maintained for at least 3 weeks, but no more than 6 weeks, before the fracture orthosis is applied. The initial immobilization is done to minimize leg shortening, but the lowest incidence of leg shortening has been found in those patients who have had fracture orthoses applied 2 to 4 weeks postinjury.

Problems associated with fracture orthoses are increased angulation of the bone and refracturing, both of which are rare. Fracture orthoses have been used most often to treat fractures of the shafts of the tibia and femur when internal fixation is unnecessary, contraindicated, or refused by the patient and when healing is significantly delayed or does not occur. Fracture orthoses are contraindicated when satisfactory alignment of the fracture cannot be obtained or maintained.

Initial efforts to use orthotic devices for lower extremity fractures were inspired by prostheses for lower extremity amputees. Three basic components are required for fabrication of a fracture orthosis: a cylinder, footplate, and joint mechanisms. The cylindrical component closely fits the fractured limb to provide a hydraulic mechanism that will promote stability for the bony structures and resist shortening. The vertical load of weight bearing is offset by lateral and oblique forces from an essentially incompressible fluid chamber that is created by the encasing cylindrical orthotic component. Most proximally on the orthosis, a weight-bearing surface may be provided, such as a patellar tendon-bearing socket or ischial seat, to reduce further the pressure on the fracture site. This mechanism is far less important in the distribution of weight-bearing pressures than the hydraulic mechanism mentioned. The cylindrical components usually are made of plaster-of-Paris cast or low-temperature thermoplastics (Orthoplast). The second major component of a fracture orthosis is a footplate, which is to be worn inside a shoe. The footplate usually is prefabricated and made of plastic, although custom-made footplates occasionally are made. The footplate usually is attached to the cylindrical component by simple plastic hinges rather than metallic joints. Similar joint mechanisms may be used for the knee, connecting the above- and below-knee pieces.

Appropriately designed and fitted, fracture orthoses allow functional ambulation with progressively increasing weight bearing. Absence of pain, good callus formation, and lack of gross motion at the fracture site indicate that the fracture is stable. The fracture is considered healed when full weight bearing is tolerated and radiographs show that the fracture is obliterated with evidence of good callus formation and consolidation. Fractures of the tibial shaft generally do not require surgical intervention and heal spontaneously. After 2 to 4 weeks of immobilization in a long leg cast, most patients with closed tibial fractures are ready for active range of motion of the knee and ambulation with increased weight bearing. Fractures of the distal tibia can be treated with a below-knee orthosis with a patellar tendon indentation for weight bearing (Fig. 26-13). Fractures of the proximal tibia, especially those involving the knee joint, generally require a thigh piece that is connected to the leg portion with a polycentric knee joint. Closed transverse fractures of the midfemoral shaft generally are best treated with intramedullary nailing, but for some open, severely comminuted, or oblique femoral fractures, management with fracture orthoses may present a better approach (23). Fractures of the mid- or distal femoral shaft are managed more successfully with fracture orthoses than are fractures of the proximal femoral shaft because of the latter's strong tendency to produce varus angulation and malalignment. The thigh component of the orthosis resembles that of the quadrilateral above-knee prosthesis with an ischial seat and a three-point fixation contour that resists varus angulation (Fig. 26-14). The thigh component is connected to the calf piece by freely moving metal or plastic joints. The calf piece is attached to a footplate by joints, as seen in the tibial fracture orthosis (see Fig. 26-13).

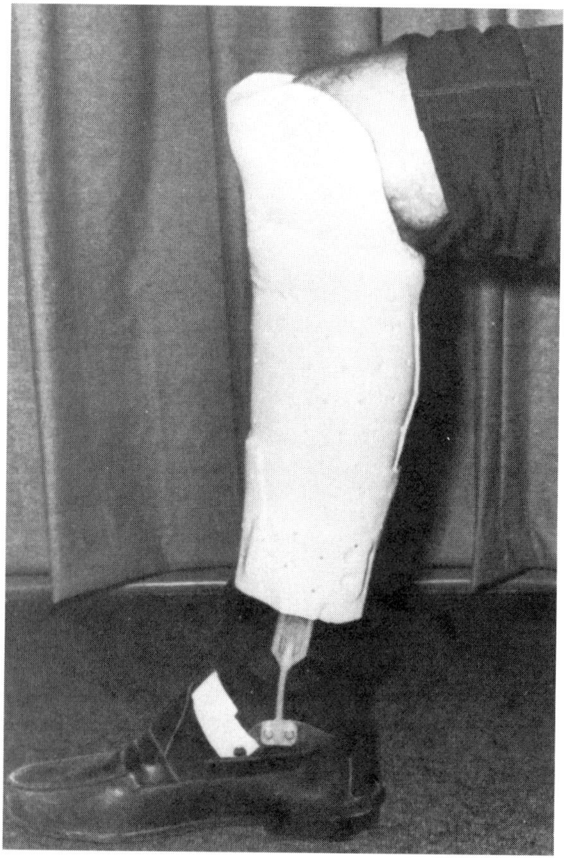

FIG. 26-13. Orthosis for fracture of the tibia. (From American Academy of Orthopedic Surgeons. *Atlas of orthotics.* St Louis: CV Mosby, 1975.)

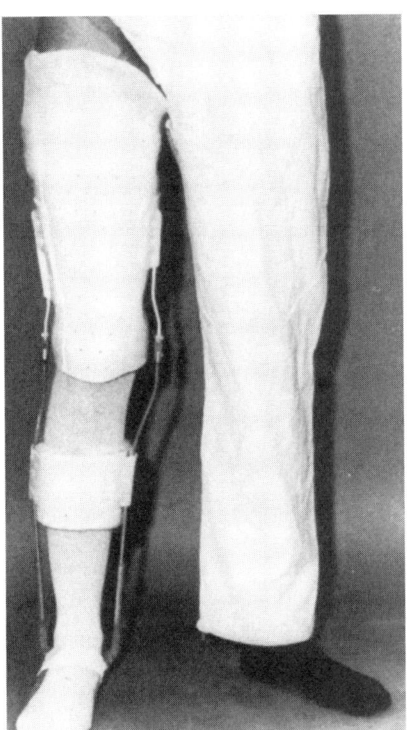
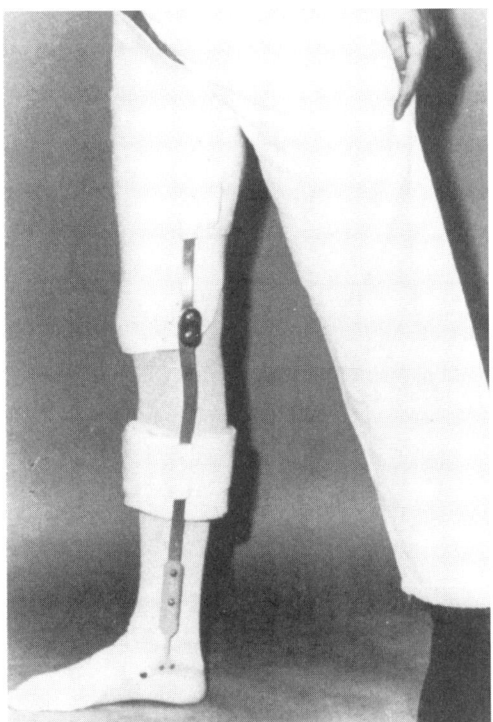
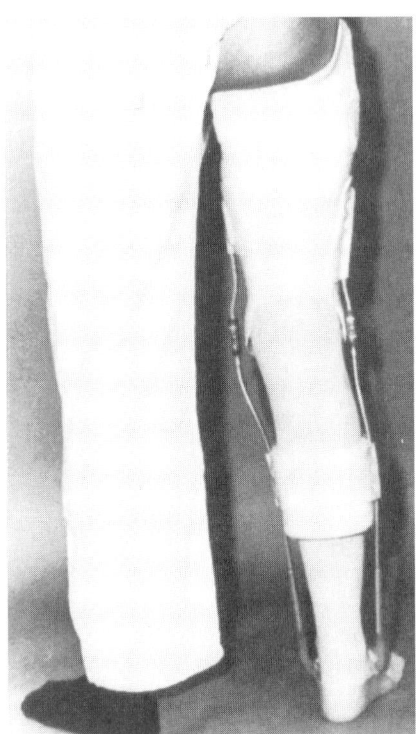

A,B C

FIG. 26-14. Front **(A)**, side **(B)**, and rear **(C)** views of an orthosis for fracture of the distal femur. (From American Academy of Orthopedic Surgeons. *Atlas of orthotics*. St Louis: CV Mosby, 1975.)

Occasionally, fracture orthoses are used in the management of fractures of the forearm and wrist as a therapeutic alternative to other means of external or internal fixation. A cylindrical forearm component is attached by a joint mechanism to a handpiece. Active use of muscles and joints is encouraged, although weight bearing generally is not indicated because it may not be necessary.

GAIT AIDS

Canes

Canes, when properly used, will increase base of support, decrease loading and demand on the lower limb and skeletal structures, provide additional sensory information, and assist with acceleration and deceleration during locomotion. Canes are prescribed for various disabilities to improve balance, to decrease pain, to reduce weight-bearing forces on injured or inflamed structures, to compensate for weak muscles, and to scan the immediate environment. Pathologic conditions affecting the upper limbs may interfere with the use of canes and crutches or warrant prescription of specially designed gait aids.

The total length of a properly measured cane should equal the distance from the upper border of the greater trochanter to the bottom of the heel of the shoe. The patient should be able to stand with the cane with the elbow flexed at 20° to 30° and both shoulders level. The patient should be instructed in the proper use of the cane—to hold the cane in the hand opposite the affected limb and to advance the cane and the affected leg in a three-point gait pattern. When ascending stairs the good leg is advanced first, but when descending, the cane and the affected leg lead.

Canes are most commonly made of hardwood or aluminum but can vary in design (Fig. 26-15). All canes should be fitted with a deeply grooved 1- to 2-inch-wide rubber tip for good traction and safety, and the clinician should check these regularly for wear. The common C handle or crook-top cane is inexpensive, but this type of handle may be uncomfortable and difficult to grasp, especially for those with hand problems. Additionally, the weight-bearing line falls behind the shaft of the cane, thus reducing its supportive value. A functional handle that fits the grip, conforms to the natural angle of the hand, and is more centered over the shaft of the cane is more comfortable and provides better support. Wide-based canes made of metal provide a wider area of support. These designs consist of three or four short legs attached to a single upright shaft with a molded or wooden handle. Several base widths are available, and the length of the shaft is adjustable. Wide-based canes are prescribed for persons with greater degrees of impaired balance, preferably only for temporary use, because these canes often are heavy and awkward in appearance.

Crutches

The indications for prescribing a pair of crutches are similar to those for canes, but the clinical deficits usually are

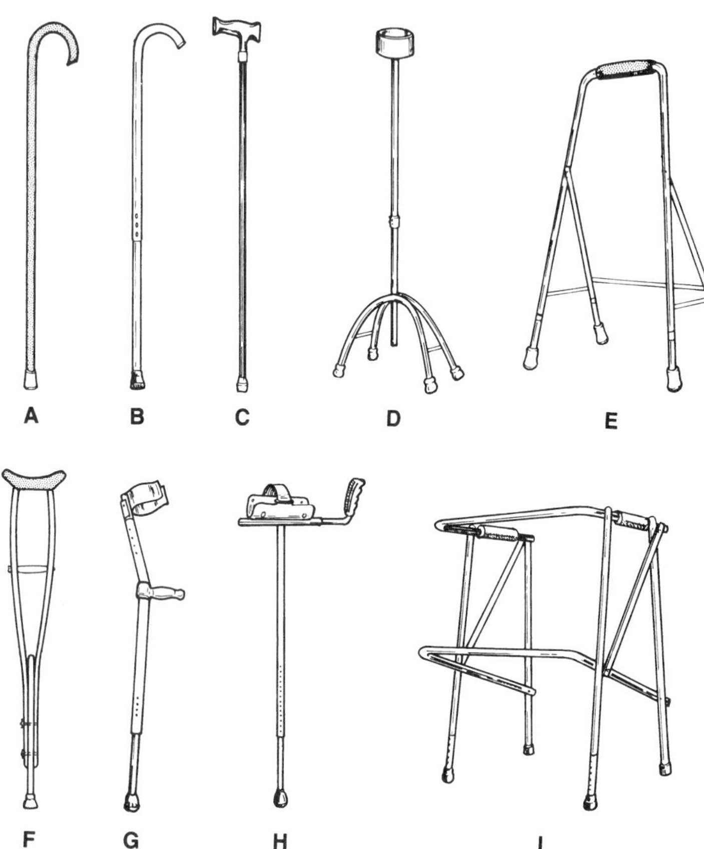

FIG. 26-15. Canes, crutches, and walkers. **A**: C-handle or crook-top cane. **B:** Adjustable aluminum cane. **C:** Functional grip cane. **D:** Adjustable wide-base quad cane. **E:** Hemiwalker. **F:** Adjustable wooden axillary crutch. **G:** Adjustable aluminum Lofstrand crutch. **H:** Forearm support or platform crutch. **I:** Walker or walkerette.

greater. Good strength of the upper limbs usually is required because persons needing crutches tend to require them more for weight bearing and propulsion than for balancing or as sensory aids. For effective crutch walking, the upper limb joints should have good range of motion, and the key muscle groups (i.e., shoulder flexors and depressors, elbow and wrist extensors, finger flexors) should be strong. Axillary crutches (see Fig. 26-15) are the most commonly prescribed crutches in the United States. The wooden axillary crutch is easily adjustable and made of hardwood with two upright shafts connected by a padded axillary piece on top, a handpiece in the middle, and an extension piece below. The extension piece and shafts have numerous holes at regular intervals so the total length of the crutch and the height of the handles may be adjusted. A large, soft rubber suction tip is attached to the extension piece to allow total contact with the floor. Metal axillary crutches consist of a single contoured tubular structure, which can be adjusted by telescoping and push-button positions. A functional handle is adjustable in height.

When a person is measured for axillary crutches, the total length of the crutch and the height of the handle are the two main dimensions to be considered. The handle height is measured in the same manner as with canes, but the total length of the crutch should be equal to the distance from the anterior fold of the axilla to either a point 6 inches anterolaterally from the foot or to the bottom of the heel, plus 1 or 2 inches.

The popular Lofstrand crutch (see Fig. 26-15) consists of a single aluminum tubular shaft, adjustable in length, a molded handpiece, and a forearm piece bent posteriorly just above the handpiece. The forearm piece, also adjustable in length, extends to 2 inches below the elbow, where a forearm cuff with a narrow anterior opening is attached. This crutch is lightweight, easily adjustable, and gives freedom for hand activities because the handpiece can be released without loosing the crutch. It requires, however, greater skills than the axillary crutch, good strength of the upper limbs, and adequate trunk balance for safe ambulation.

The Canadian elbow extensor crutch (i.e., triceps crutch) has a single aluminum upright shaft attached to bilateral uprights, which extend to above the elbow. These are connected by a handle and two half cuffs, one below and one above the elbow. This crutch rarely is prescribed but may benefit those with triceps weakness.

Forearm support (i.e., platform) crutches (see Fig. 26-15) may be prescribed when clinical conditions of the forearm, wrist, or hands prevent safe or comfortable weight bearing, such as in the presence of arthritis of the elbow, wrist, or hand, fractures of forearm or hand, or weakness of triceps or grasp.

Walkers

Walkers provide a wider and more stable base of support than do either canes or crutches (see Fig. 26-15). They may be prescribed for patients requiring maximum assistance with balance, the elderly, the fearful, and the uncoordinated. The patient must have good grasp and arm strength bilaterally, although forearm supports can be used as above. Walkers are conspicuous in appearance and interfere with development of smooth reciprocal gait patterns. Although they are very useful during rehabilitation, care should be taken that the patient does not become emotionally dependent on the balance stability provided by the walker. Walkers are available in various sizes, are adjustable in height, and come in different designs, such as folding, rolling, reciprocal, or stair walkers.

REFERENCES

1. Zamosky I, Licht S, Redford JB. Shoes and their modifications. In: Redford JB, ed. *Orthotics etcetera.* Baltimore: Williams & Wilkins, 1980; 368–431.
2. Staheli LT. Shoes for children: a review. *Pediatrics* 1991; 88:371–375.
3. Zhu H, Wertsch JJ, Harris GF, Alba HM, Price MB. Sensate and insensate in-shoe plantar pressures. *Arch Phys Med Rehabil* 1993; 74: 1362–1368.
4. Stokes IAF, Fairs IB, Hutton WC. The neuropathic ulcer and loads on the foot in diabetic patients. *Acta Orthop Scand* 1975; 46:839–847.
5. Cavanagh PR, Hennig EM, Rodgers MM, Sanderson DJ. The measurement of pressure distribution on the plantar surface of diabetic feet. In: Whittle M, Harris D, eds. *Biomechanical measurements in orthopaedic practice.* Oxford: Clarendon Press, 1985; 159–166.
6. Duckworth T, Boulton AJM, Betts RP, Franks CI, Ward JD. Plantar pressure measurements and the prevention of ulceration in the diabetic foot. *J Bone Joint Surg* 1985; 67B:79–85.
7. Boulton AJM, Betts RP, Franks CI, Ward JD, Duckworth T. The natural history of foot pressure abnormalities in neuropathic diabetic subjects. *Diabetic Res* 1987; 5:73–77.
8. Lord M, Hosein R. Pressure redistribution by molded inserts in diabetic footwear: A pilot study. *J Rehabil Res Dev* 1994; 31:214–221.
9. Chen RCC, Lord M. A comparison of trial shoe and shell shoe fitting techniques. *Prosthet Orthot Int* 1995; 19:181–187.
10. Perry JE, Ulbrecht JS, Derr JA, Cavanagh PR. The use of running shoes to reduce plantar pressures in patients who have diabetes. *J Bone Joint Surg* 1995; 77a:1819–1828.
11. Birrer RB, Dellacorte MP, Grisafi PJ. Prevention and care of diabetic foot ulcers. *Am Fam Physician* 1996; 53:601–611.
12. Janisse DJ. Indications and prescriptions for orthoses in sports. *Orthop Clin North Am* 1994; 25:95–107.
13. Robbins S, Waked E, McClaran J. Proprioception and stability: Foot position awareness as a function of age and footwear. *Age Aging* 1995; 24:67–72.
14. Lehmann JF. Biomechanics of ankle foot orthoses: prescription and design. *Arch Phys Med Rehabil* 1979; 160:200–207.
15. Ryan J. The use of posterior night splints in the treatment of plantar fasciitis. *Am Fam Physician* 1995; 52:891–898.
16. O'Daniel WE, Hahn HR. Follow-up usage of the Scott–Craig orthosis in paraplegia. *Paraplegia* 1981; 19:373–378.
17. Lehneis HR. New developments in lower limb orthotics through bioengineering. *Arch Phys Med Rehabil* 1972; 53:303–310.
18. Taktak DM, Bowker P: Lightweight modular knee–ankle–foot orthosis for Duchenne muscular dystrophy: design, development and evaluation. *Arch Phys Med Rehabil* 1995; 76:1156–1162.
19. Podesta L, Sherman MF. Knee bracing. *Orthop Clin North Am* 1988; 19:737–745.
20. Douglas R, Larson PF, D'Ambrosia R, McCall RE. The LSU reciprocation-gait orthosis. *Orthopedics* 1983; 6:834–839.
21. Durr-Fillauer Medical, Inc. *LSU reciprocating gait orthoses: A pictorial description and application manual.* Chattanooga, TN: Durr-Fillauer Medical, Inc., 1983.
22. Sarmiento A, Sinclair WF. *Atlas of orthotics: biomechanical principles and application.* St Louis: CV Mosby, 1975; 245–254.
23. St Pierre RK, Holmes HE, Flemming LL. Cast bracing of femoral fractures. *Orthopedics* 1982; 5:739–745.

Rehabilitation Medicine: Principles and Practice, Third Edition,
edited by Joel A. DeLisa and Bruce M. Gans.
Lippincott–Raven Publishers, Philadelphia © 1998.

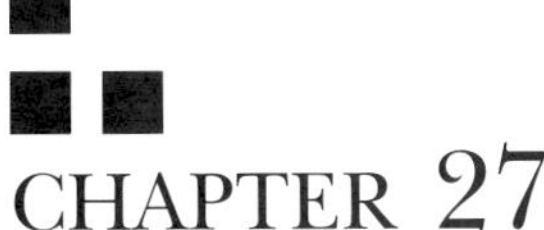

CHAPTER 27

Upper and Lower Extremity Prosthetics

James A. Leonard, Jr. and Robert H. Meier III

The rehabilitation of the person with limb loss requires the skills of many health care professionals: orthopedic surgeon, general or vascular surgeon, physiatrist, prosthetist, physical therapist, occupational therapist, social worker, psychologist, and vocational counselor. Ideally, these health care specialists function together as an integrated team. In particular, teams in regional amputee or prosthetic centers who see a large number of amputees are able to provide the optimum in prosthetic rehabilitation as a result of their combined experience (1).

Advances in the care and prosthetic restoration of the amputee have always come from multiple arenas: development in new surgical techniques, improvements in the preoperative and postoperative management, advances in prosthetic technology, and better understanding of the psychosocial implications of limb loss. In the last several years, it has been the areas of prosthetic designs, material technologies, and fabrication techniques for prosthetic construction and engineering technologies that have seen the greatest number of advances. These new developments have not replaced previous technology and techniques but have been added to the options available to the clinic team in prescribing the most appropriate prosthesis for the individual patient.

If rehabilitation programs for the person with an amputation are to provide a useful service, they must focus on the person who has experienced such a catastrophic loss. A prosthesis can be fabricated for almost every level of amputation, but it may not meet the amputee's perceived needs. It is the art of assisting the individual with an amputation to meet these needs that is the foundation of this specialized area of rehabilitation. Seldom is the prosthesis the desired replacement of the lost body part. Tempering expectation with reality, however, is an essential part of the rehabilitation experience. Assuring that the most comfortable, cosmetic, and functional prosthesis has been made available is only a part of working with the amputee. These rehabilitation programs should be designed to place the focus on the individual's adaptation to the loss of a limb and not just focus on the provision of a prosthetic substitute. Guidance also must be given in the proper use and care of the prosthesis. The true test of the rehabilitation program is the manner in which the amputee incorporates the prosthesis into his or her life style.

J. A. Leonard, Jr.: Department of Physical Medicine and Rehabilitation, University of Michigan Medical Center, Ann Arbor, Michigan 48104-0042.

R. H. Meier III: O'Hara Regional Center for Rehabilitation, Denver, Colorado 80204.

ACQUIRED AMPUTATIONS

Incidence and Etiology

The etiology of limb loss and the associated medical conditions often are important considerations in developing a management program for the amputee. Loss of limb generally is divided into two broad categories: acquired and congenital. Congenital deficiencies are discussed later in this chapter.

The loss of part or all of an extremity as the direct result of trauma or by surgery is known as an acquired amputation. Surgical amputations are performed for disease, benign or malignant tumors, and for traumatic injuries to the extremities without hope of salvage. Review of data collected for 1993 by the National Center for Health Statistics (NCHS) provides estimates of the prevalence of 1,546,000 people with major limb amputations (excluding loss of tip of fingers or toes) in the United States (2). Earlier work by the NCHS in 1977 provides the most detailed breakdown available for the United States in the level of amputation, socioeconomic data, age, geographic distribution, and use of a prosthesis (3,4). In 1993, it is estimated that 127,000 amputations were performed in acute-care nonfederal hospitals, the majority in the lower extremity. Of the 98,000 lower extremity amputations, 42,000 were toe or partial foot amputations, 29,000 were at the transtibial (below-knee) level, and 25,000 were at the transfemoral (above-knee) level (5). The approximately 6:5 ratio of transtibial to transfemoral amputations varies from previous reports by other studies that suggest a ratio of approximately 2:1 (6). The studies noting more transtibial amputations may be biased in that these data were generated from prosthetic centers where patients were being actively fitted with prostheses. The reader is referred to the works by Moore and Malone, Murdoch and Wilson, and Sanders for a detailed discussion of lower extremity amputation statistics (7–9).

Trauma is the leading cause of acquired amputation in the upper extremity (approximately 75%), occurring primarily in men aged 15 to 45 years. Disease and tumors are responsible for about equal numbers of the remaining acquired upper extremity amputations. In the lower extremity, disease states account for approximately 75% of all acquired amputations, with complications of diabetes and peripheral vascular disease far and away accounting for most of these, especially in the 60 years and over population. Trauma is the next most common cause for lower extremity amputation (20%), followed by tumors (5%). Among children aged 10 to 20 years, however, tumor is the most frequent cause of all amputations in both the upper and lower extremities (6,9,10).

Amputation Surgery

Amputations frequently occur after extensive medical and surgical effort has been expended to salvage the involved extremity. In such a setting, amputation surgery may be mistakenly considered by the health care team rendering the acute care to be a course of last resort—in other words, a failure of modern medicine. Amputations may be performed by less experienced members of the surgical team, and the healing and final result of the residual limb may be less than optimum. To provide the best potential for rehabilitation and prosthetic restoration, amputation surgery must be approached as a reconstructive procedure. Careful attention must be given to the management of the various tissues involved, such as beveling the ends of bones. The nerves are sharply transected and allowed to retract into proximal soft tissues so that they do not become adherent in scar or remain in a location where they might be traumatized by a prosthesis. Appropriate myofascial closure of the muscle or myodesis provides for good control of the remaining bone in the residual limb, and appropriate placement of the skin incision line avoids bony prominences and adherence to underlying bone. Such attention to detail will result in a well-shaped residual limb that can be best fitted with a prosthesis and permit maximum prosthetic function (11).

In performing an amputation, one must give careful consideration to the level of amputation. In general, the approach is to save as much length as possible. A level must be chosen that will ensure good healing of the surgical incision with adequate full-thickness skin coverage, although skin grafts in nonvascular amputees have been used successfully to preserve length. In patients with vascular disease, noninvasive vascular studies such as ankle-brachial indices, Doppler waveform analysis, and xenon washout studies are but a few of the techniques available to help predict which levels of lower extremity amputation will heal successfully. Often, however, the final decision in choosing the level of amputation in the vascular patient cannot be made until the time of surgery, when the amount of blood flow in the tissues at the level of proposed amputation actually can be observed (7,8,12,13). Function with a prosthesis after an amputation also must be taken into account when choosing an amputation level. Sometimes a slightly shorter residual limb can be fitted with a more functional and cosmetic prosthesis, making, for example, a long transhumeral amputation preferable to an elbow disarticulation.

In the lower extremity, the following are the preferred levels of amputation:

- Toe amputations
- Ray resections
- Transmetatarsal amputations
- Syme amputation (i.e., disarticulation of the foot)
- Transtibial amputation (i.e., at a level proximal to the junction of the middle and distal thirds of the leg)
- Knee disarticulation
- Transfemoral amputation (i.e., at a level 8 cm or more proximal to the level of the knee joint so that the femoral condyles are excised)
- Hip disarticulation (i.e., short transfemoral amputations at or proximal to the greater trochanter are considered functionally as a hip disarticulation)
- Hemipelvectomy

In the upper extremity, the following are the preferred levels of amputation:

- Finger or thumb amputation
- Ray resection
- Transmetacarpal resection
- Wrist disarticulation
- Transradial amputation
- Elbow disarticulation
- Transhumeral amputation (i.e., 6.5 cm or more proximal to the elbow joint)
- Shoulder disarticulation
- Forequarter amputation (interscapulothoracic disarticulation)

Short residual limbs may be lengthened by using bony techniques such as the Ilizarov or free fibular grafts (14–18). Also, soft tissue coverage of the residual limb has been enhanced with the use of microvascular myocutaneous free flaps and skin expanders (19–22).

PATIENT EVALUATION AND MANAGEMENT

The interaction of the health care team working with the patient to achieve the goal of prosthetic restoration and rehabilitation can be referred to as prosthetic management. The process of prosthetic rehabilitation has been described in nine phases by Meier (23) (Table 27-1). Prosthetic manage-

TABLE 27-1. *Phases of amputee rehabilitation*

Phase	Hallmarks
1. Preoperative	Assess body condition, patient education, discuss surgical level, postoperative prosthetic plans
2. Amputation surgery, reconstruction	Length, myoplatic closure, soft-tissue coverage, nerve handling, rigid dressing
3. Acute postsurgical	Wound healing, pain control, proximal body motion, emotional support
4. Preprosthetic	Shaping and shrinking amputation stump, increasing muscle strength, restoring patient locus of control
5. Prosthetic prescription and fabrication	Team consensus and prosthetic prescription, experienced limb fabrication
6. Prosthetic training	Increase wearing of prosthesis and mobility skills
7. Community integration	Resume roles in family and community activities; regain emotional equilibrium and health coping strategies; pursue recreational activities
8. Vocational rehabilitation	Assess and plan vocational activities for future. May need further education, training or job modification.
9. Follow-up	Provide lifelong prosthetic, functional, medical, and emotional support; provide regular assessment of functional level and prosthetic problem solving

Modified from Esquenazi A, Meier RH. Rehabilitation in limb deficiency. 4. Limb amputation. *Arch Phys Med Rehabil* 1996; 77:S18–28, with permission of WB Saunders.

ment is a process that follows a temporal sequence that, for the sake of convenience, can be divided into distinct segments in this chapter: preprosthetic management, prosthetic fitting and training, and prosthetic follow-up care. This staging and use of the hallmarks permits the rehabilitation physician to assess the amputee and plan the rehabilitation program.

Preprosthetic Management

Preoperative

Preprosthetic management begins when the decision to perform an amputation is made, when a patient initially is evaluated after a traumatic amputation, or when a child is born with a congenital skeletal deficiency. It ends with the fitting of a provisional or definitive prosthesis. If the patient can be evaluated by members of the prosthetic team before amputation, the optimum of care can be provided. Evaluation should assess and document the patient's range of motion and strength in the involved as well as the noninvolved extremities, mobility and ambulation, activities of daily living and self-care skills, social support, and the patient's reaction to the planned surgery. It is also important to inquire about the patient's needs and desires for postoperative vocational and avocational activities. Ideally, the patient should be seen before the amputation to give him or her information about the rehabilitation and prosthetic restoration process following surgery. This often will help allay some of the fears the patient may have about his or her life after surgery. This is the best time to start therapy programs for range of motion, conditioning exercises, correct positioning of the residual limb, ambulation with gait aids, instructing the patient in relaxation techniques, and activities of daily living that will continue after surgery. The patient often is more able to absorb and comply with a therapy program during the preoperative period than during the early postoperative period, when incisional pain, medication, or apprehension may interfere with the ability to participate in the therapy program.

Postoperative

The postoperative goals of preprosthetic management are the following:

- Healing of the incision
- Pain control
- Preparation of the residual limb for prosthetic fitting
- Maintaining range of motion, especially in the remaining proximal joints of the amputated extremity
- Independent mobility
- Independence in self-care and activities of daily living
- Education about prosthetic fitting and care
- Support for the adaptation to the changes resulting from the amputation

In the postoperative therapy program, certain muscle strengthening should be emphasized. In the Syme, transtibial, knee disarticulation, or transfemoral amputee, strengthening of the gluteus medius and gluteus maximus muscles should be accomplished in addition to strengthening of any residual hamstring or quadriceps muscles. In the upper limb amputee, proximal shoulder girdle muscle strengthening should be taught, emphasizing the trapezius, serratus anterior, pectoralis major, as well as any residual deltoid and biceps function.

The response to amputation has been compared to the grieving process in that the amputee experiences identifiable stages of denial, anger, depression, coping, and acceptance. Not every person will progress through these stages or ultimately adapt to the loss. The etiology of the amputation may contribute significantly to the patient's response to the limb loss. The person's ultimate response to the psychosocial impact of limb loss is determined by many factors, including the person's life experience and inner strengths, the quality of the social support systems available to the person, the comprehensive care provided by the prosthetic team, and the functional outcome that is achieved through rehabilitation (24).

Residual Limb Care

In addition to maintaining range of motion and strength, postoperative treatment includes shaping of the residual limb and reduction of soft tissue volume. Sterile soft dressings commonly used after amputation surgery do little to protect, shape, or shrink the residual limb. Soft dressings may prevent optimal healing because they allow the development of postoperative edema. The shrinking and shaping process can be accomplished in one of several ways, all of which can be used in the early postoperative period without compromise to wound healing if carefully done. Postoperative dressings such as elastic bandage wraps, elastic stockinette (Compresso-Grip, Knit Rite, Kansas City, MO), residual limb (i.e., stump) shrinkers, or Unna paste casts can be used quite successfully (25). The use of elastic bandage wraps requires considerable cooperation, skill, and attention on the part of the patient, family, or medical staff because the wraps need to be reapplied frequently and carefully to be successful.

With an experienced team, immediate postoperative rigid dressing may be the preferred method of amputation wound care. It can be either removable or nonremovable (26–28). Ideally, the rigid dressing should be applied immediately after surgery in the operating room, before postoperative edema has a chance to develop. By limiting postoperative swelling, the rigid dressing helps to promote wound healing and limit postoperative pain. Typically, a nonremovable rigid dressing is taken off and changed 5 to 10 days after surgery. A removable rigid dressing may be taken off and replaced whenever the wound needs to be viewed but must be replaced immediately, before edema has a chance to develop. The rigid dressing has the additional advantages of providing some protection for the extremity in case of a fall, and, if properly designed, it can serve as a socket to which temporary components can be attached, thus creating a preparatory prosthesis.

The preprosthetic phase of management, before definitive prosthetic fitting, can typically last 6 to 10 weeks for the dysvascular lower extremity amputee, a considerably shorter period of time for the traumatic lower extremity amputee, and 3 to 6 weeks for the upper extremity amputee (29).

Prosthetic Fitting

The prosthetic-fitting period of care begins when the residual limb is ready for casting and a prescription has been developed for a preparatory or definitive prosthesis. This period continues until the completion of training in the use of the prosthesis. Input from all members of the team, especially the patient, will result in the most appropriate prosthetic prescription. The prosthetic prescription takes into account the needs, objectives, and abilities of the amputee and selects from the available prosthetic designs and components.

Prosthetic fitting presumes that an amputee is a candidate for a prosthesis or wishes to be fitted with a prosthesis. Not all amputees are candidates for prosthetic fitting. There are no hard and fast rules regarding who is or is not a prosthetic candidate, but there are some general guidelines that can be followed. An amputee should have reasonable cardiovascular reserve, adequate healing, skin coverage, range of motion, muscle strength, motor control, and learning ability to achieve useful prosthetic function. A poor candidate for functional prosthetic fitting would be a vascular lower extremity amputee with an open or poorly healed incision, a transfemoral amputee with a 45°-flexion contracture at the hip, or a transradial amputee with a flail elbow and shoulder. Lower extremity amputees who can walk with a walker or crutches without a prosthesis usually possess the necessary balance, strength, and cardiovascular reserve to walk with a prosthesis. Generally, bilateral short transfemoral amputees over the age of 45 years are considered to be unlikely candidates for full-length prosthetic fitting. Additional medical problems such as severe coronary artery disease, pulmonary disease, severe polyneuropathy, or multiple-joint arthritis may result in an amputee who could be fitted with a prosthesis but who may not be a functional prosthetic user. Patients whose prognoses are poor, life expectancies are short, or disease and treatments result in significant fluctuations in body weight are not good candidates. In borderline cases, it may be necessary to proceed with actual prosthetic fitting to determine eventual prosthetic function. The use of a less costly preparatory prosthesis is appropriate before a decision is made about fitting such a person with a more costly definitive prosthesis.

Once it is thought that an amputee is a prosthetic candidate, a decision is made on the purpose of prosthetic fitting. The prosthesis can be functional, cosmetic, or both. Prostheses that are intended to replace function never totally replace the function of the body part that has been amputated. Each prosthetic component provides a different type of functional capability. A prosthesis might be designed to meet specific vocational, recreational, or social needs. It is important that the prosthetic team spend time reviewing the activities of daily living and the vocational and avocational activities for which the prosthesis is to be used. In the case of young children, a prosthesis often is necessary for the progression of normal development.

Patients who are not candidates for functional prosthetic use may choose to have a cosmetic prosthesis. These cosmetic prostheses can be fabricated to have an appearance similar to that of the opposite limb.

The next decision is when to fit the prosthesis. For the acquired upper extremity amputee, there is evidence that early fitting ensures better functional prosthetic use and return to preamputation activity levels and occupation. Malone and colleagues describe the 30 days following upper extremity amputation as the "golden period" during which prosthetic fitting should occur to ensure good prosthetic outcome (30). Prosthetic fitting for the upper extremity amputation after this 30-day period has resulted in a significant reduction in prosthetic acceptance and use and a much lower rate of return to previous occupational activity levels. A preparatory prosthesis—either conventional or myoelectric—can be applied immediately in the operating room but will not achieve a better outcome over early fitting (i.e., 7 to 30 days after surgery). The definitive upper extremity prosthesis should be fit when the residual limb is well healed and shaped and the limb volume has stabilized.

The timing of prosthetic fitting for the lower extremity is more controversial than for the upper extremity. Because the majority of lower extremity amputations in the United States occur as the result of complications of peripheral vascular disease, primary wound healing at the amputation site is of paramount importance. At one time, immediate postoperative fitting of a rigid dressing and pylon prosthesis was advocated to speed rehabilitation for the lower extremity amputee (26). Because of the limited number of people with the necessary experience and skill to fabricate this type of prosthesis properly, immediate fitting with a pylon is no longer recommended for vascular amputees; improperly done, this technique may jeopardize primary wound healing and may contribute to reamputation at more proximal levels secondary to compromised wound healing. If properly fabricated and applied, however, an immediate postoperative prosthesis can be used safely for ambulation with partial weight bearing (31). Immediate fitting in the younger traumatic amputee has been more successful and is a reasonable method of treatment. For the lower extremity amputee, whether vascular or nonvascular, early preparatory prosthetic fitting is currently a more accepted form of prosthetic management. Vascular amputees tend to have fewer complications with provisional prostheses when the socket of the provisional prosthesis is a custom-fabricated thermoplastic or laminated socket rather than plaster socket because of the better fit.

Prosthetic Fabrication

Considerable progress has occurred in prosthetic fabrication during the past decade. Improved materials, new designs, and better fitting techniques have resulted in prostheses that are lighter and stronger and provide improved comfort, function, and cosmesis.

Preparatory Prosthesis

In the past, a temporary, provisional, or preparatory prosthesis used a socket usually made from conventional or synthetic plaster bandages (Fig. 27-1). Today, more provisional sockets are being made from thermoplastics (Fig. 27-2). Although some of these thermoplastic sockets come in various preformed sizes, most thermoplastic sockets are custom-made because they provide a better fit. Because the plastic must be heated in an oven to 300°F or higher to be moldable, the socket must be formed over a positive mold of the residual limb. The prosthetist must make a cast of the residual limb, modify the resulting positive mold, and then vacuum-form the provisional socket, often over a foam liner. In contrast, the plaster provisional socket can be constructed by a physician, prosthesist, or therapist, is less durable than a thermoplastic socket, and will need several changes and modifications to maintain an adequate fit. A new option that combines the convience of plaster with the advantages of a custom thermoplastic provisional socket is the use of preformed sockets made of a carbon fiber and fiberglass-reinforced water-activated polymer. These water-activated polymer sockets permit a lightweight durable socket to be molded directly on the amputee's residual limb (Icex socket, Össur, USA, Carpentaria, CA; and Alps Socket Pro, Alps South Corp., St. Petersburg, FL), providing a custom lightweight relatively durable prosthetic socket within hours and reducing both the time and labor required for a prosthetist to produce a custom laminated or thermoplastic provisional socket. All of these sockets can be attached to modular prosthetic components as necessary to complete the provisional prosthesis.

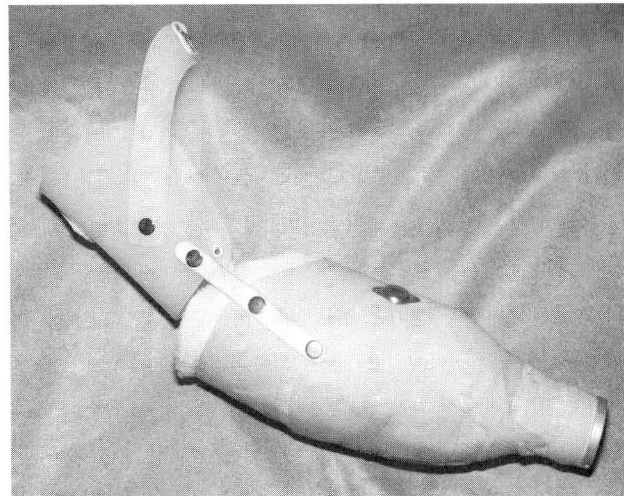

FIG. 27-1. Synthetic plaster transradial postoperative provisional prosthesis.

Definitive Prosthesis

When the shaping and shrinking process has been completed and the residual limb volume has stabilized, a definitive or permanent prosthesis is made. This usually follows these steps:

1. Cast the residual limb.
2. Make a plaster positive mold of the residual limb.
3. Modify the plaster positive, removing plaster from the pressure-tolerant areas and adding plaster to the pressure-sensitive areas of the residual limb.
4. Fabricate a check socket over the modified plaster positive.
5. Trial-fit the check socket with modification of the check socket as necessary to ensure an adequate, comfortable fit.

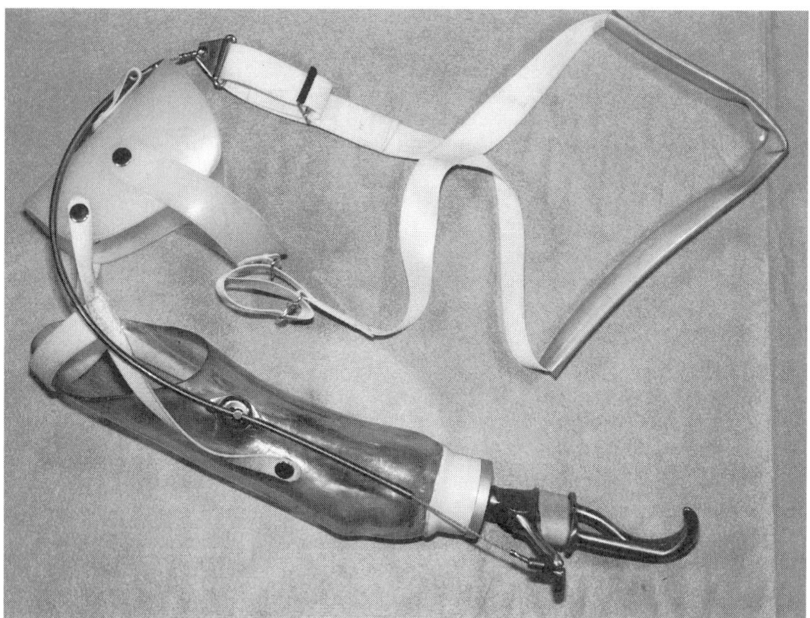

FIG. 27-2. Thermoplastic transradial provisional prosthesis.

6. Make a new plaster positive mold from the check socket.
7. Fabricate the final thermoplastic or laminate socket over the new plaster positive.

Now, computer aided design-computer assisted manufacturing (CAD-CAM) technology can be used as either an adjunct or an alternative to several of the more traditional steps of socket fabrication listed above. Computerized equipment can be used to digitize the residual limb directly or a cast of the residual limb (negative mold) to provide a positive computer model of the residual limb. This digitized image can be modified on the computer much as the plaster positive in step 3 above. A computer-controlled milling machine then creates a positive model that will be used to create the check socket. Additional modifications can be made directly to the computer model to provide additional positive models for revised sockets (32,33).

Although the use of a clear check socket has become the norm for lower extremity prosthetic fabrication, the final prosthetic socket may be fabricated directly over the modified plaster positive mold (i.e., step 3 above) and then fit on the patient with additional modifications being made directly to the final socket. A clear thermoplastic sheet (e.g., Lexan, G.E. Plastics, Pittsfield, MA; Duroplex, Durr-Fillauer, Chattanooga, TN; Surlyn, Bixby Plastics, Newbury Port, MA) or cone (e.g., Orthoglass, Otto Bock, Minneapolis, MN) is vacuum-formed over the modified positive and then the fit is checked on the patient. Because the check socket is clear, areas of excessive pressure or of noncontact between the socket and residual limb will be seen on direct observation. The fit can be modified quickly to achieve the desired optimum fit of the socket; a new positive mold can be made for the fabrication of the definitive socket. Clear thermoplastic check sockets also have become the mainstay in upper extremity prosthetic fittings as well (Fig. 27-3). The thermoplastic check socket can be used with a suspension system and other prosthetic components attached to provide a temporary prosthesis. This temporary prosthesis is useful for further evaluating the fit of the socket, the resulting function, or for ease in adjusting placement of other prescribed prosthetic components, such as electrodes in a myoelectric prosthesis.

The majority of definitive prosthetic sockets and external supporting frames are still fabricated from thermosetting resins, either polyester or acrylic. In the fabrication of these laminated sockets, resins are drawn under vacuum into a fabric stockinette, usually Dacron or nylon, which provides reinforcement to the plastic. Other reinforcing fabric materials such as graphite fibers and Kevlar are available to provide extremely lightweight but strong laminations. More prosthetists are using thermoplastics and vacuum-forming tech-

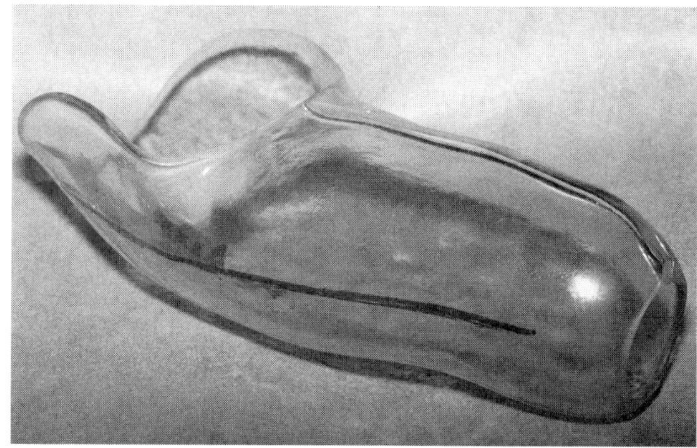

FIG. 27-3. A transradial clear thermoplastic check socket.

TABLE 27-2. *Advantages and disadvantages of various upper limb prostheses*

Type	Pros	Cons
Cosmetic (passive)	Most lightweight Best cosmesis Least harnessing	High cost if custom made Least function Low-cost glove stains easily
Body powered	Moderate cost Moderately lightweight Most durable Highest sensory feedback	Most body movement to operate Most harnessing Least satisfactory appearance
Externally powered (myoelectric and switch control)	Moderate or no harnessing Least body movement to operate Moderate cosmesis More function-proximal levels	Heaviest Most expensive Most maintenance Limited sensory feedback
Hybrid (cable elbow/electric TD)	All-cable excursion to elbow Increased TD pinch	Electric TD weights forearm (harder to lift) Good for elbow disarticulation (or long above elbow)
Hybrid (electric elbow/cable TD)	All-cable excursion to TD Low effort to position TD Low maintenance TD	Least cosmesis Lower pinch force for TD

TD, terminal device.

Modified from Esquenazi A, Leonard JA, Meier RM, et al. 3. Prosthetics. *Arch Phys Med Rehabil.* 1989; 70(Suppl):207.

niques in the fabrication of definitive prosthetic sockets with good success.

Prosthetic Construction Design

Prosthetic construction can be either exoskeletal or endoskeletal. Exoskeletal design is the more traditional construction, comprising a rigid plastic lamination over a filler material of wood or foam, which has been shaped to provide the cosmetic appearance of the prosthesis. It is the outer plastic lamination that provides the strength and durability for the prosthesis.

Endoskeletal design uses internal modular components and tubing to provide the strength for weight-bearing capabilities. The cosmetic appearance is provided by shaped foam covers slipped over the modular components. The modular design of the components of the endoskeletal system allows for relatively easy changing of the components or alignment of the prosthesis after final fabrication has been completed. These changes are more difficult with an exoskeletal prosthesis. An endoskeletal prosthesis is usually lighter, especially if lighter thermoplastic sockets and lightweight titanium or graphite modular components are used.

UPPER EXTREMITY PROSTHESES

A prescription for an upper extremity prosthesis must describe the choice of socket, joint components, terminal device, method of suspension, and control system. As previously mentioned, a detailed history of the person's preferred activities is necessary to make a proper selection of the available options.

An upper extremity prosthesis attempts to replace very complex functions. A significant portion of these functions are accomplished with the hand, which is positioned for functional activities by the coordinated movements of the muscles and joints in the extremity proximal to the hand. Once positioned in space, the hand is able to perform tasks ranging from those requiring fine dexterity with light prehensile forces to gross grasping movements with great prehensile forces, all the while providing multiple levels of sensory feedback to allow modulation of the prehensile activity. The level of dexterity and functional capability is greatest in the dominant upper extremity.

Typical prosthetic replacement for the upper extremity can replace several of the grasping and manipulating functions of the hand and allow movement of proximal prosthetic joints to position the terminal device in space, but it does not provide sensory feedback directly from the terminal device. The functional use of a prosthesis in a unilateral amputee seldom approaches a level of skill and dexterity equal to that of the limb it has replaced. When the dominant upper extremity has been amputated, the amputee usually transfers the role of dominant function to the remaining upper extremity, and the prosthesis serves in the role of assisting in bimanual function. In general, the more distal the amputation, the more functional the person is with the prosthesis because more control is provided by the proximal muscles and joints of the extremity.

Upper extremity prostheses can be divided into three

groups: body-powered or conventional, externally powered or electric, and passive or cosmetic. The advantages and disadvantages for each of the three general types of upper limb prostheses are presented in Table 27-2.

Body-Powered Prostheses: Components

All conventional body-powered upper extremity prostheses have these component parts:

- Terminal device or devices
- Interposing joints as needed by the level of amputation
- Socket
- Suspension
- Control system

Prostheses for amputation levels proximal to the hand/wrist will have a terminal device, wrist unit, suspension harness, and control system. Terminal devices for body-powered prostheses can be hooks, functional hands, cosmetic hands, or special terminal devices for specific function (e.g., bowling ball terminal device, golf club holder). The most commonly used functional terminal devices (i.e., hooks or hands) are voluntary opening, with springs or rubber bands providing prehensile forces. Voluntary-closing terminal devices allow the amputee to provide and control a variable prehensile force transmitted through the control cable to the terminal device. They also provide greater proprioceptive input by means of the force exerted on the control cable. Many different voluntary-opening hook designs are available for various functional applications, the most commonly prescribed being the Dorrance 5X, 5XA, and 7 (Hosmer Dorrance, Campbell, CA). Functional prosthetic hands are heavier than the hooks and frequently do not provide as much function. Passive (cosmetic) hands are lighter than functional hands and can be passively positioned but provide little if any function. Both of these hands are covered by a cosmetic glove that has been tinted to approximate the appropriate skin color.

Wrist units provide a receptacle for connecting the terminal device to the prosthesis and permit prepositioning of the terminal device for functional activities (i.e., supination–pronation for all units or flexion if the appropriate unit is used). Wrist units control terminal device rotation by either friction or a locking mechanism. The appropriate wrist unit design can be chosen as needed for the individual amputee. A quick-disconnect wrist unit permits an easy interchange of different terminal devices, such as a hook for a hand. A wrist flexion unit permits several positions of flexion to allow the terminal device to be placed in an optimal position to provide function. A locking wrist unit enhances the use of the terminal device with heavier objects or where leverage with the terminal device is important for function.

The socket of a conventional upper extremity prosthesis is suspended by a harness system—usually a figure-8 harness—to which the control cables are attached. A shoulder saddle with a chest strap is an alternative suspension that permits carrying heavier loads with the prosthesis. Socket designs such as a suction socket or a self-suspending socket (e.g., Muenster) can provide partial or complete suspension. If the socket provides complete suspension for the prosthesis, then a figure-9 harness can be used for the control cable to provide body power for terminal device operation.

Additional details regarding componentry, sockets, suspension, and control systems are discussed where appropriate in the following sections pertaining to particular levels of amputation.

Prostheses by Level of Amputation

Partial Hand

For partial hand/wrist amputations (e.g., phalanges, ray resections, transmetacarpal, transcarpal), a prosthesis may not be necessary. Surgical reconstruction may be a more appropriate choice of treatment to preserve or enhance function while maintaining sensation in the residual partial hand. Often all that is necessary to restore function for this level of amputation is an opposition post, either fixed or adjustable, that permits prehension of objects while at the same time providing sensory feedback from the skin of the remaining portion of the hand. A cosmetic alternative can be provided for this level of amputation; however, a prosthesis that covers sensate skin is often discarded in favor of greater function and the use of remaining sensation.

Wrist Disarticulation

A wrist disarticulation spares the distal radial–ulnar articulation and thus preserves full forearm supination–pronation. Socket designs for this level are tapered and flattened distally to form an oval that allows the amputee fully to use active supination–pronation, thus avoiding having to preposition the terminal device for functional activities. A special thin wrist unit is used to minimize the overall length of the prosthesis because of the extremely long residual limb. If cosmesis is of importance to the amputee, a long transradial amputation may be a more appropriate amputation level. The socket is attached to a triceps pad by flexible elbow hinges, and the harness attaches to the triceps pad.

Transradial Amputations

Transradial amputations are classified by the length of bony forearm remaining: very short (<35%), short (35% to 55%), and long (55% to 90%). Long transradial residual limbs retain from 60° to 120° of supination–pronation, and short transradial residual limbs retain less than 60°. Flexible elbow hinges are used for these two levels of amputation to attach the socket to the triceps cuff. For very short transradial amputation levels, rigid hinges generally are used. This can be accomplished by using external metal joints attached to the socket and cuff or by directly attaching a modified plastic triceps cuff to the socket itself. With transradial amputations, in which range of motion is limited at the elbow, polycentric elbow joints or a split socket with step-up hinges can be used to provide additional flexion. Additional flexion is gained with the use of these elbow hinges, but there is a resultant loss of elbow flexion power and a decrease in the amputee's ability to actively lift weight with the prosthesis (see Case 27-1).

Elbow Disarticulation

Elbow disarticulation sockets are flat and broad distally to conform to the anatomic configuration of the epicondyles of the distal humerus. This design provides the amputee with active rotation of the prosthesis (internal and external rotation of the humerus). The length of the socket requires the use of external elbow joints, with a cable-operated locking mechanism on the medial joint. The harness is either a figure-8 or a shoulder saddle and chest strap. The control system for this level uses two separate cables; one activates the elbow lock, and the other cable is a fair-lead control system that has one cable with two functions: it provides power for elbow flexion when the elbow is unlocked and provides tension that will open the terminal device when the elbow is locked.

Transhumeral Amputations

Transhumeral amputations also are classified by the length of residual humerus: humeral neck (<30%), short transhumeral (30% to 50%), and standard transhumeral (50% to 90%). In transhumeral amputations with residual limb lengths greater than 35%, usually the proximal trimline of the socket extends to within 1 cm of the acromion, and the socket is suspended by either figure-8 or shoulder saddle and chest strap suspension systems. Sockets for residual limbs shorter than 35% should have the proximal trimline extend 2.5 cm medial to the acromion. This socket design often can be suspended with only a chest strap, but other harness systems can be used if appropriate. A suction socket suspension is another option available for suspension of transhumeral prostheses. This form of suspension, when used with conventional harnessing systems, may provide for better prosthetic control, especially for the shorter transhumeral amputation levels. Suction socket suspension, when combined with externally powered myoelectric components, results in a transhumeral prosthesis that is self-suspending and free of any harness.

The use of an internal elbow joint is preferred in a transhumeral prosthesis because of greater mechanical durability. If the level of amputation is 4 cm or more proximal to the level of the epicondyles, then an internal elbow unit can be used. A transhumeral residual limb with bony or soft tissue length that extends more distally than this will require a prosthesis with external elbow joints to maintain the elbow joint center equal to that on the nonamputated side. Internal elbow units have a turntable that allows passive internal or exteral rotational positioning of the forearm shell and the terminal device. Elbow spring-lift assist units also are available for internal elbow units to help counterbalance the weight of the forearm and make elbow flexion easier for the amputee. The control system is the same dual-control cable system used for the elbow disarticulation level (see Case 27-2).

Shoulder Disarticulation/Forequarter Amputations

For shoulder disarticulation and forequarter amputation, the socket extends onto the thorax to suspend and stabilize the prosthesis. The portion of the thorax covered by the socket is more extensive for the forequarter amputation. In some cases an open-frame socket rather than a plastic laminated socket is chosen for these levels to reduce prosthetic weight and to minimize heat buildup by reducing the amount of skin coverage.

Prosthetic components are similar to those for the transhumeral prosthesis with the addition of a shoulder unit, which allows passive positioning of the shoulder joint in flexion–extension and abduction–adduction. These sockets are suspended by chest straps attached anteriorly and posteriorly to the socket. The control system is a triple-cable system in which three cables each provide a distinct function. One cable, attached to the forearm shell and an axilla loop, provides active elbow flexion when the opposite humerus is flexed. A second cable, attached to the terminal device and the chest strap, provides terminal device opening with chest expansion. A third cable, attached to the elbow lock and a nudge control, locks and unlocks the elbow when the nudge control is depressed by the chin or opposite hand.

The difficulty in providing body-powered control motions of sufficient strength is a reason for considering externally powered prostheses for these proximal levels of amputations.

It is important to consider a passive, cosmetic prosthetic restoration for selected patients. These cosmetic prostheses can be fabricated to have an appearance similar to that of the opposite limb. The most lifelike of the cosmetic prostheses are labor intensive and made of hand-tinted silicone. There are only a few prosthetists or anaplastologists in this country who specialize in this art form of prosthetic fabrication.

Externally Powered Prostheses

In North America, external power for upper extremity prostheses is provided by small electric motors incorporated into the prosthesis to control various functions. Reliable external power units are available for terminal device operation, wrist rotation, and elbow flexion–extension. These electric motors can be controlled by myoelectric signals, switches, or even acoustic signals (23,29,34–38). Externally powered prostheses can provide not only greater prehensile forces than the body-powered prostheses but also proportional prehension. Externally powered prostheses may provide more elbow function, especially in the short transhumeral or more proximal level amputee in whom control motion or strength may be limited.

Switch-Controlled Prostheses

For switch-controlled prostheses, small microswitches are incorporated either inside or outside the prosthetic socket and are operated on contact by the amputee. Pull switches incorporated into conventional harness-and-cable control systems also are available to control prosthetic function.

Myoelectric Prostheses

Myoelectrically controlled prostheses are the most appealing of the externally powered prostheses. In the case of the transradial level amputation, the prosthesis has a self-suspending socket that eliminates the need for a harness (Fig. 27-4).

A myoelectrically controlled prosthesis has a set or sets of electrodes embedded in the prosthetic socket. These electrodes make contact with the skin and detect muscle action potentials from a voluntarily contracting muscle in the residual limb. The detected electrical signal is then amplified and rectified. The final signal is then capable of turning on an electric motor to provide a function (e.g., terminal device operation, wrist rotation, elbow flexion). Several different systems are available to process myoelectric signals. One system uses two sets of electrodes and amplifiers to control motion, one for a motion in one direction and one for the opposite motion (i.e., terminal device opening and terminal device closing). The single-site control system system uses one set of electrodes for both motions (37). In this system it is the strength of voluntary contraction (i.e., amplitude of the myoelectric signal) that will control which motion will occur; a weak contraction will close the terminal device and a strong contraction will open the terminal device. The single-site control system allows an amputee with only one good control site (i.e., site of a strong reproducible voluntary contraction) in the residual limb to operate a myoelectrically controlled prosthesis. A single-site system also will allow an amputee to use two control sites to power two different functions, as in terminal device operation and wrist rotation.

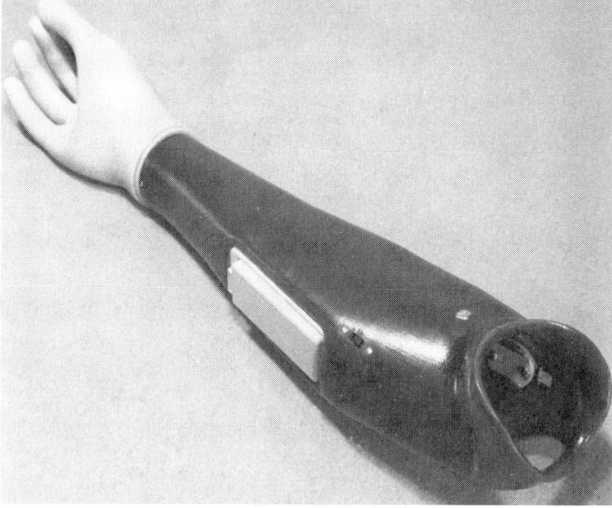

FIG. 27-4. Self-suspending transradial myoelectric prosthesis without cosmetic glove on the prosthesis. The Otto Bock myoelectric hand with outer shell (Minneapolis, MN) is seen in the **top left** of the photograph. The removable rechargeable battery is in the midforearm of the prosthesis. The myoelectric electrode controlling hand opening (i.e., extensor surface) is seen inside the self-suspending socket **(bottom right)**.

In some systems the strength of contraction controls the speed of the function controlled. The Liberty Mutual or Boston elbow (Liberty Mutual, Boston, MA) is a proportional electric elbow that will flex or extend faster in direct proportion to the increasing amplitude of the contraction within the control muscle. The most sophisticated and expensive of the current myoelectric systems is the Utah elbow (Fig. 27-5) developed by Motion Control (Salt Lake City, UT). This system uses microprocessor technology and two sets of electrodes to provide for both elbow function and terminal device operation. This system also allows for a free-swing phase of the elbow joint to provide a normal cosmetic arm swing when walking.

The major obstacles to prescription of myoelectrically controlled prostheses are their cost, reliability, and weight. These systems are expensive because of large research and development costs, limited production, and small consumer market. Thus, no significant reductions in myoelectric cost should be expected. Reliability was a significant issue when these systems were first introduced. Today, the reliability is much improved, and local prosthetists are able to make many of the adjustments or repairs necessary to keep the units functioning rather than having to return them to the manufacturer. The Utah elbow was designed with field serviceability in mind in that it has a limited number of easily and quickly replaced modular components. Myoelectric prostheses generally are heavier than their equivalent conventional prostheses because of the additional motors, batteries, and electrodes. Myoelectric prostheses occasionally are rejected because of the increased weight.

Myoelectric prosthetic components are available that may be fitted to a wide range of people, from infants to adults. The age at which to fit children with a myoelectric prosthesis is a controversial and complex issue beyond the scope of this chapter (see Table 27-9 at the end of this chapter). This subject is reviewed in detail elsewhere (29,39,40). The majority of myoelectric terminal devices and components have been designed and manufactured for adult sizes in view of the significant costs involved with their production.

Most myoelectric terminal devices tend to be hands, but some electric hook designs are available. Myoelectrically controlled prostheses can and have been fit immediately after surgery (41), but it generally is recommended that myoelectric fittings be delayed until the residual limb is completely healed and the limb volume has stabilized sufficiently. Myoelectric prosthetic fitting that has occurred before stabilization of the residual limb volume may lead to frustration of the amputee because of poor socket fit and skin electrode

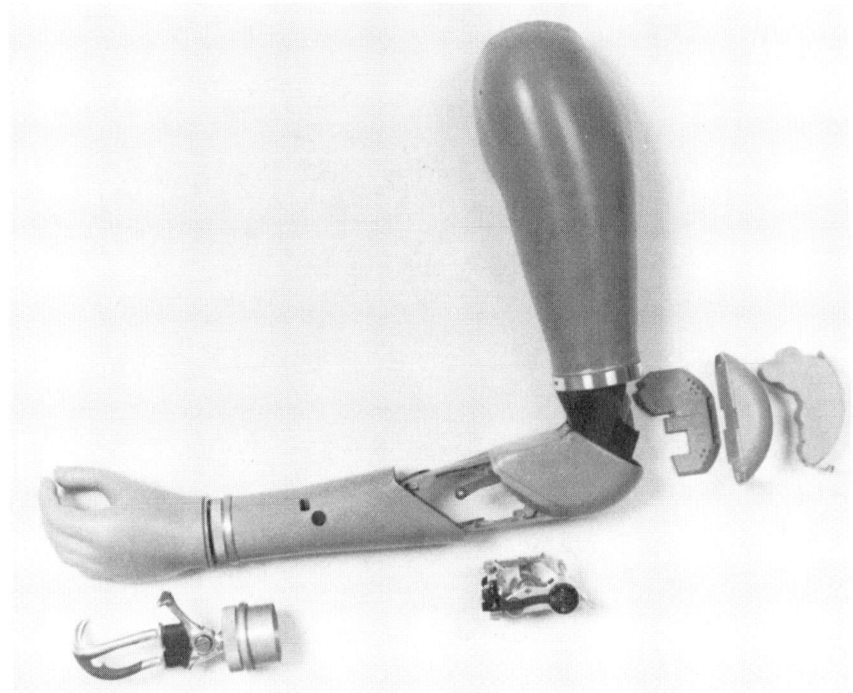

FIG. 27-5. Utah elbow system. Shown are the controller electronics, battery, motor, and terminal device options. A myoelectric hand is attached to the prosthesis. The voluntary opening hook terminal device is available if body power is to be used for terminal device control. (Courtesy of Motion Control, Salt Lake City, UT.)

contact, both of which occur with reducing limb volume, and may necessitate an early replacement of the prosthetic socket. Myoelectric components have been combined with body-powered components to result in a hybrid prosthesis, which may provide better function for some amputees than either myoelectric or body power control used alone.

Final Prosthetic Evaluation and Control Training

After the prosthesis has been fabricated, it should be checked by the members of the prosthetic team to make sure that the fit is comfortable and that the control system is properly adjusted for maximum functional operation. The amputee should then initiate a program of prosthetic training with the therapist, usually in the outpatient setting. This training should include instruction in how to put on and remove the prosthesis, wearing and care of limb socks, opening and closing of the terminal device, grasping and releasing objects, transferring objects, and prepositioning of the terminal device for functional activities. As skills progress for the basic uses of the prosthesis, activities of daily living, homemaking, and occupational and recreational activities should be undertaken and simulated in the training sessions. The amputee should be given a home program with specific goals to be achieved between the outpatient training sessions. Upper extremity amputees must be cautioned to remove their prosthesis frequently to check for signs of excessive pressure or irritation that may occur with poor socket fit or overuse until skin tolerance increases. Initially, the patient should wear the prosthesis for only 15 to 20 minutes before checking the skin. If no problems are apparent, wearing time is gradually increased during the first few days of wear and thereafter more quickly. With good skin tolerance, an upper extremity amputee can wear the prosthesis for an entire day within a week or so of receiving it.

Control training for externally powered prostheses is more complex than for body-powered upper extremity prostheses. The same goals as outlined for conventional prostheses are appropriate for myoelectrically controlled prostheses. In addition, the amputee must learn to separate, modulate, and sustain voluntary muscle contractions in the muscles selected to control the powered functions of the prosthesis. As for conventionally powered prostheses, a home program to practice and enhance prosthetic control skills should be outlined to achieve independent function.

Adults and older children can be expected to practice specific tasks and routines both in therapy and at home as outlined by the therapist to achieve the necessary skills for independent function. The training time in a young child with an upper extremity prosthesis will be significantly longer than that for an adult or older child.

In adults, unilateral upper extremity basic training should provide for a minimum of the following times: 5 hours for transradial, 10 hours for transhumeral, and 15 hours or more for shoulder disarticulation. Basic prosthetic training usually occurs in a short period of time spent under the guidance of a therapist. Prosthetic learning occurs over a lifetime of use, however, as the amputee continues to be challenged with new bimanual experiences. The amputee becomes the problem solver and develops new use patterns that are most efficient for his or her activity needs. Training with an externally powered (electric) prosthesis often requires more time than with a body-powered prosthesis because more exacting individual muscle motions and quantity of muscle contraction are required in the control of the prosthesis.

Bilateral Upper Extremity Amputations

The bilateral upper extremity amputee is immediately faced with the loss of ability to perform almost every activity of daily living. Early restoration of any activity of daily living is important. Providing a utensil cuff, which can be attached to a residual arm, can assist the patient with feeding and toothbrushing.

With the bilateral amputee, early prosthetic fitting should be accomplished even with temporary or preparatory prostheses. In the bilateral amputee, dominance usually is assumed by the longer residual limb. Special component considerations apply in this case. Wrist flexion units, at least on the dominant side or perhaps bilaterally, will permit midline activities such as shirt buttoning, belt buckling, and toileting. Also, wrist rotator units, which provide automatic terminal device positioning, provide for easier bilateral prosthetic use.

Special toileting techniques must be taught for patient independence. In addition, foot skills should be reviewed, and lower extremity mobilizing exercises should be performed.

Upper Extremity Prosthetic Follow-Up

The routine follow-up visits to the clinic for a new amputee should occur initially 4 to 6 weeks after receipt of the prosthesis, then at 3 months, then at 6 months, and then at yearly intervals. Additional clinic visits should occur whenever a problem arises. At these follow-up visits, the amputee's use and function with the prosthesis should be reviewed, any difficulties or problems resolved, the fit and condition of the prosthesis evaluated, and the condition of the residual limb noted. If necessary, additional therapy may be suggested, repairs to the prosthesis made, medical problems with the residual limb attended to, and a new prosthesis prescribed if indicated. With average use, an upper extremity prosthesis can be expected to be worn for 3 to 5 years before total replacement is necessary. The socket itself may need to be replaced more frequently than the other components.

Although our emphasis has been on prosthetic restoration, the focus of rehabilitation should remain on the amputee and his or her desired life-style following limb loss. Many amputees do well without the aid of a prosthesis and should not be viewed as having failed if they choose not to wear a prosthesis.

LOWER EXTREMITY PROSTHESES

The functions provided by a lower extremity prosthesis are weight bearing, locomotion, and cosmesis. These functions are less complex and more uniform from amputee to amputee than those of an upper extremity prosthesis. Because weight bearing is a major concern in a lower extremity prosthesis, distribution of forces at the interface between the skin of the residual limb and the socket of the prosthesis is critical. The residual limb–socket interface is the major site of lower extremity prosthetic fitting problems and the reason for most lower extremity prosthetic modifications. The second major function, locomotion, should allow the amputee to walk with as normal a gait as possible. The cosmetic effect of a lower limb prosthesis should be considered a function of prosthetic use when seated, standing, walking, and running.

Componentry

The prosthetic prescription must balance the amputee's need for stability, safety, mobility, function, durability, and cosmesis as well as available resources/financial sponsorship. The availability of prosthetic services also must be considered because some components require more frequent maintenance than others. A lower extremity prosthetic prescription should describe the construction design, socket type, suspension method, appropriate joint components, and prosthetic foot.

Socket types, suspension systems, and joint components of a prosthesis are specific for the particular level of amputation and are discussed for each of the appropriate amputation levels to follow.

Prosthetic Feet

All prostheses for amputations at or proximal to the ankle require the use of a prosthetic foot. There are many different designs of prosthetic feet available (42,43). Specially modified versions of several of the following prosthetic feet are available for Syme amputation prostheses (see section on Syme amputation prosthesis).

The solid ankle cushion heel (SACH) foot is the most commonly used prosthetic foot because it is durable, lightweight, inexpensive, and easily interchanged to accommodate shoes of different heel heights. The presence of a compressible heel and wooden keel in this foot design allow it to simulate the motions of the ankle in normal walking without actual ankle movement occurring. The compressibility of the heel permits the SACH foot to accommodate partially for uneven terrain, but this foot is best suited for flat, level surfaces.

A single-axis foot permits movement of the foot–ankle complex in one plane. Movement occurs in the plantarflexion–dorsiflexion axis. If the plantarflexion movement occurs easily, an extension moment occurs on the tibia, enhancing knee extension and thereby enhancing knee stability. The movement is controlled by the use of adjustable internal rubber bumpers that provide resistance to dorsiflexion and plantarflexion. This foot is usually heavier than the SACH foot, and the internal components need periodic adjustment or replacement. This foot usually is not used with a transtibial prosthesis but with prostheses for more proximal amputation levels that require additional knee control or stability.

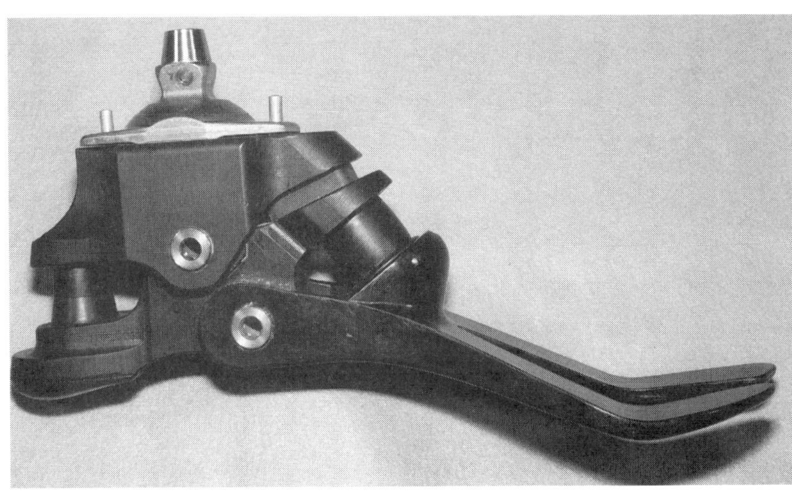

FIG. 27-6. TruStep composite carbon fiber multiaxial foot. Three bumpers can be seen, one plantarflexion bumper and two dorsiflexion bumpers.

Using a movable ankle is especially helpful in the bilateral lower extremity amputee because of the improved knee stability.

Multiaxis prosthetic feet are being prescribed more frequently for the amputee who is involved in athletic activities or who walks on uneven terrain. The advantage of the multiaxis foot is that it offers some controlled movement in the normal anatomic planes of the ankle: dorsiflexion–plantarflexion, inversion–eversion, and rotation. A number of different foot designs are available to provide this multiaxial motion. Some of the prosthetic feet accomplish this movement without the use of mechanically moving parts; they rely instead on the inherent flexibility of the materials and design of the foot. Other multiaxis feet use mechanical systems to provide this mobility such as the relatively lightweight TruStep (Fig. 27-6) composite foot (College Park Industries, Inc., Fraser, MI). The additional mechanical components necessary for the movement in these feet add to their overall weight and may require frequent maintenance, especially in the very active amputee. For the active amputee, however, the improved balance, coordination, and function provided by these feet generally outweigh the disadvantages of increased weight and more frequent maintenance. A suggested schema for the selection of the most appropriate prosthetic foot has been proposed by Esquenazi and Torres (43) (Table 27-3).

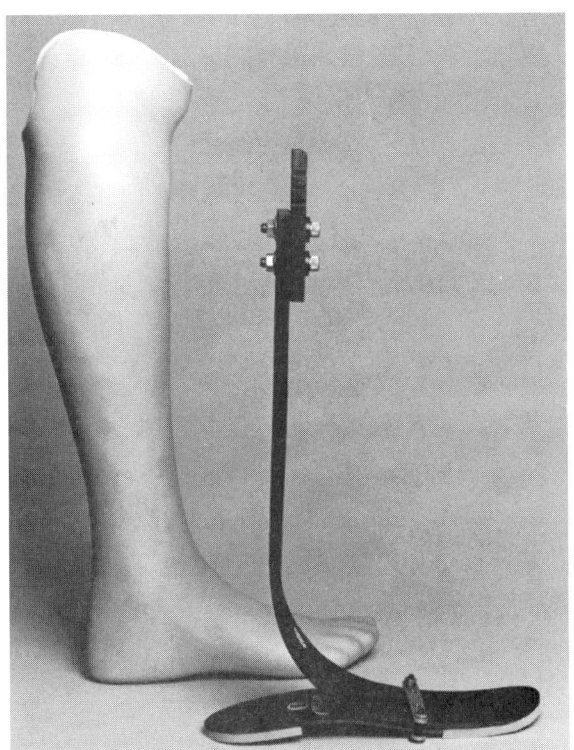

FIG. 27-7. Flex-Foot prosthetic foot and shank component with and without cosmetic foam cover. The flexibility of the carbon fiber epoxy foot and shank gives it the ability to store and return energy. (Courtesy of Flex-Foot, Aliso Viejo, CA.)

Major advances in lower extremity prosthetic component design continue in the development of dynamic response (i.e., energy-storing) prosthetic feet such as the Flex-Foot feet (Figs. 27-7 and 27-8), the Springlite feet (Salt Lake City, UT), Seattle Limb System feet (Fig. 27-9), Endolite foot (Endolite, N.A., Centerville, OH), and the Carbon Copy II and III feet (Fig. 27-10). The design of these feet incorporates the use of resilient, flexible, energy-storing materials. Energy is stored in the foot at the time of heel strike as the weight of the body either compresses or flexes the resilient material within the foot and is returned to the amputee at the time of push-off as the components of the energy-storing foot return to their normal shape or configuration. The resiliency of these feet makes them particularly suitable for amputees involved in activities requiring running and jumping. Many amputees report they believe that they are more functional with a prosthesis with a dynamic response foot. It has been assumed that these prosthetic foot designs make prosthetic ambulation more efficient and require less energy consumption by the amputee. The data on the effect of dynamic response feet on the energy expenditure of prosthetic

TABLE 27-3. *Recommended foot-ankle systems according to level of amputation*

	Weight (g)	Below-knee sedentary	Above-knee sedentary	Symes sedentary	Bilateral sedentary	Below-knee active	Above-knee active	Symes active	Bilateral active
Carbon Copy II	495	2	1	2	1	3	3	2	2
Carbon Copy III	900	2	NA	NA	0	3	NA	NA	3
Dynamic	550	1	1	NA	1	1	2	NA	1
Flex-Foot	900	0	0	NA	1	3	3	NA	2
Flex-Walk	550	1	1	NA	1	3	1	NA	3
Flex Symes	900	NA	NA	1	NA	NA	NA	3	NA
Graph-Lite	600	1	2	NA	1	2	2	NA	2
Greissinger	850	1	1	NA	1	1	2	NA	1
Icelandic	500	?	?	NA	?	?	?	NA	?
Endolite with ankle	800	0	0	NA	1	1	2	NA	1
Multiflex	540	3	3	NA	3	2	2	NA	2
Quantum	540	2	2	2	2	1	1	1	1
RAX	425	2	1	NA	12	1	1	NA	1
Sabolich	500	0	0	NA	0	3	3	NA	2
S.A.F.E. I & II	750	1	1	2	1	2	1	3	2
Seattle Light with ankle	715	1	1	NA	1	2	1	NA	2
Seattle Light	470	3	3	2[a]	2	2	1	1[a]	2
Spring-Lite	900	0	0	NA	0	3	3	NA	2
STEN	685	1	0	NA	0	1	0	NA	1

[a] To be used without ankle.

0, Not recommended; 1, good; 2, very good; 3, excellent, NA, not available.

From Esquenazi A, Torres MM. Prosthetic feet and ankle mechanisms. *Phys Med Rehabil Clin* 1991; 2:299–309, with permission of WB Saunders.

ambulation are still mixed (44–48). The original designs of several of these feet were quite heavy, but newer designs of several of these feet have resulted in significant reduction in weight, making them an option for the geriatric amputee, for whom prosthetic weight often is a consideration. The reduction of weight and the shift of the center of mass of the prosthesis from the foot closer to the socket with the lightweight Flex-Foot and Springlite also aids in reducing energy expenditure.

Prosthesis by Level of Amputation

Partial Foot Amputations

Partial foot amputations involving the forefoot, such as toe amputations, ray resections, and transmetatarsal amputations, generally require only shoe fillers or shoe modifications. The shoe modifications required may include the addition of a spring steel shank extending to the metatarsal heads, a rocker sole, and padding of the tongue of the shoe to help hold the hindfoot firmly in the shoe. Transtarsal amputations (e.g., Chopart, Lisfranc, Boyd) are not the most desirable levels of elective amputation but will have better functional results if there are active dorsiflexion and plantarflexion, balanced musculature, with normal skin and heel pad present. The best prosthetic option for a hindfoot amputation is the use of a custom prosthetic foot with a self-suspending split socket, which allows a regular low-quarter shoe to be worn (49). A posterior leaf-spring ankle–foot orthosis is another alternative.

Syme Amputation

A Syme level amputation is the next proximal site of amputation and is often preferred to one at the transtarsal level. Preservation of the articular cartilage covered by the heel pad allows for direct end-bearing on the residual limb. This advantage is frequently proposed as the primary reason for choosing this level of amputation because the amputee can stand easily and walk on the end of the residual limb without wearing a prosthesis.

The distal bulbous end of the leg, which results from the flaring of the tibia and fibula at the malleoli, has led to socket designs that are self-suspending. The classic socket designs have been either posterior or medially opening Canadian Syme prostheses. Both entail removal of a portion of the distal total contact socket wall to allow the bulbous distal residual limb to pass through the narrower, more proximal portion of the socket. The socket wall is then replaced to provide the necessary suspension. The major disadvantage with this level of amputation is the poor cosmesis of the prosthesis. The distal bulbous end of the residual limb is further accentuated by the prosthesis.

Newer socket designs that incorporate either an expandable air suspension chamber inside the socket or a thin removable expandable inner socket liner provide a more cosmetically acceptable prosthetic design. Because there is no need to remove a section from the socket wall, the structural integrity is maintained with these new designs, resulting in a prosthetic socket that can be thinner, lighter, and stronger. Several prosthetic feet are available for a Syme prosthesis,

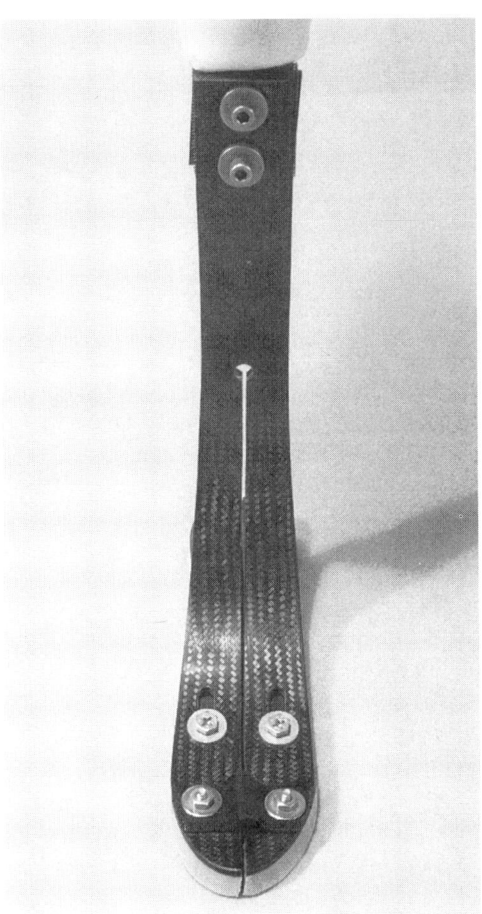

FIG. 27-8. Split-toe Flex-Foot design (Aliso Viejo, CA) permits inversion–eversion motion of the graphite pylon foot not possible with the standard design. The split in the foot continues through the heel as well (not shown).

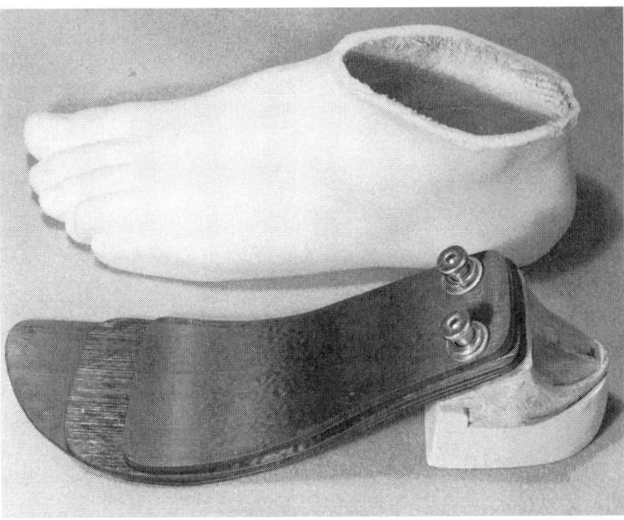

FIG. 27-10. Carbon Copy III foot. The series of interchangeable graphite plates that make up the keel of this foot rest on a compressible heel (*foreground*). In the background is the cosmetic cover for the foot. This system is completed with special adjustable graphite pylon and foam filler for the top of the foot. (Courtesy of Ohio Willow Wood, Mt. Sterling, OH.)

including the Syme SACH foot, Carbon Copy Syme foot (Ohio Willow Wood, Mt. Sterling, OH), Seattle Syme foot (Seattle Limb Systems, Seattle, WA), and the Syme Flex-Foot (Flex-Foot, Aliso Viejo, CA). Prosthetic feet are discussed further in the following section.

Transtibial Amputations

The standard socket used for the average transtibial amputee is the total-contact patellar tendon-bearing (PTB) socket that bears weight over the entire surface of the residual limb, with more weight bearing in the area of the patellar tendon

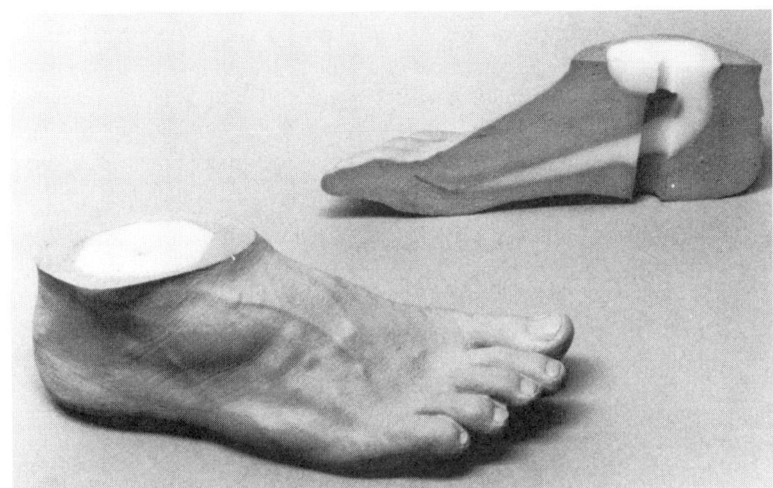

FIG. 27-9. Seattle foot. The sagittal section demonstrates the flexible keel of this foot. (Courtesy of Seattle Limb Systems, formerly Model Instrument Development, Seattle, WA.)

and the tibial flare and reduced weight bearing over the bony prominences such as the tibial crest, distal end of the tibia, and the head of the fibula. The PTB socket may be windowed to decrease pressure over certain areas of the residual limb. This design includes an inner flexible thermoplastic socket wall, and the design is referred to as an Icelandic Scandinavian New York (ISNY) socket (Fig. 27-11). A liner can be added to the socket to protect fragile or insensate skin, to reduce shear forces, provide a more comfortable socket for tender residual limbs, or accommodate for growth. Liners can be made of closed-cell thermoplastic foams, rubber covered with leather, or silicone gels. Originally slicone gel liners needed to be covered with leather to maintain their shape and provide some durability. There are now several types of gel liners that provide for excellent shear absorption at the interface. These liners are readily available as impregnated sheaths that can be worn inside virtually any nonsuction socket. They are also available as stock suspension liners (see below) from several manufactures or can be custom fabricated for individuals with particularly difficult skin–socket interface problems such as can occur with residual limbs covered with a split-thickness skin graft.

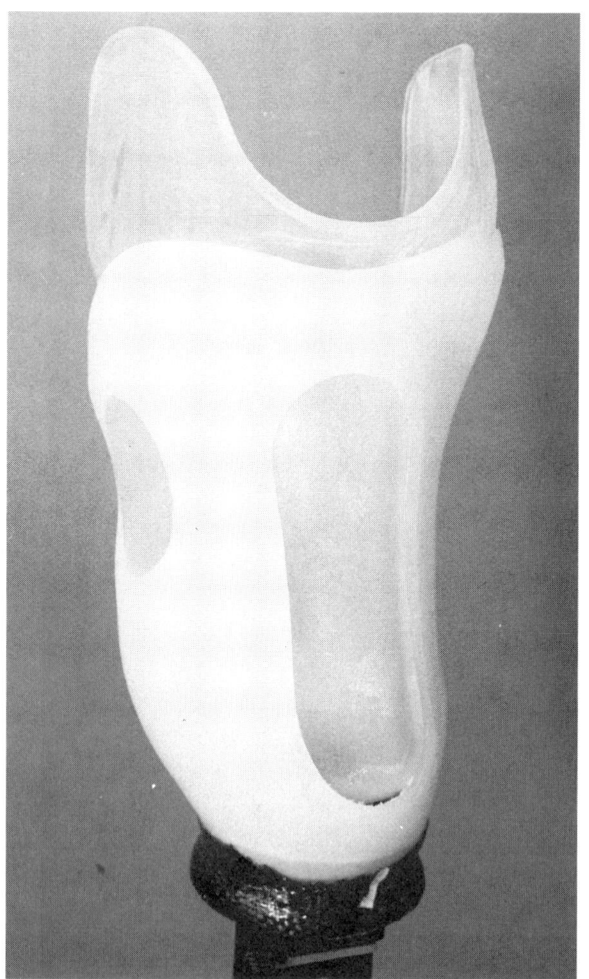

FIG. 27-11. The Icelandic Scandinavian New York (ISNY) below-knee socket. The rigid outer frame is windowed to provide relief for the head of the fibula and crest of the tibia.

A supracondylar cuff is the most common traditional form of suspension for a transtibial prosthesis. Alternative options for suspension include thigh corsets with knee joints, waist belt and forkstrap (i.e., Y-strap), supracondylar medial wedge suspension, and rubber or neoprene sleeve suspension. More and more transtibial prostheses are of a self-suspending design that can be accomplished in various manners. The silicone suction suspension (3-S) and other similar gel suspension liner designs includes a stock or custom-formed silicone or other gel material liner with an attached distal pin that locks into a receptacle in the bottom of the socket/shank (see Figs. 27-12 and 27-13). Several brands of commercially available silicone-like suspension sleeves (Alps, Alps South Corp., St. Petersberg, FL; Alpha-1, Ohio Willow Wood, Mt. Sterling, OH; Iceross, Cascade Orthopedic, Chester, CA) are available. With the developement of the new types of gel liners, there has been renewed interest in development of suction suspension systems utilizing one-way valves to assist in creating a vacuum inside the transtibial socket to reduce pistoning and improve hemodynamics in the residual limb as originally discussed by Koepke et al. when they introduced the concept of the silicone gel liner and latex sleeve suspension system in late 1960s (50). The patellar tendon supracondylar (PTS) socket design is another popular method for self-suspension. Ankle rotator units are available for those amputees who require absorption of axial torque, such as golfers or boaters. The selection of a prosthetic foot completes the transtibial prosthesis prescription (see Case 27-3).

Knee Disarticulation

Knee disarticulation level amputations have some of the same advantages and disadvantages as the Syme level amputation. This level provides a wide, flat surface for end-bearing within a prosthesis and an anatomic configuration ideal for a self-suspending socket. The bulbous distal end of a knee disarticulation residual limb presents some of the same cosmetic concerns that are present with the Syme residual limb. More significantly, however, the knee disarticulation level of amputation presents the problem of trying to maintain equal knee centers between the amputated and nonamputated lower extremities. The development of special knee units, such as the older Orthopedic Hospital Copenhagen disarticulation knee unit and the four-bar linkage knee units, has resulted in a prosthesis with nearly equal thigh lengths, leg lengths, and knee centers, thereby making knee disarticulation level amputations more cosmetically acceptable.

Transfemoral Amputations

Research after World War II led to the development of the total-contact quadrilateral socket. This design replaced the plugfit socket as the standard for the transfemoral prosthesis. For years the quadrilateral socket was the only socket design used for transfemoral prostheses. Now, two newer socket de-

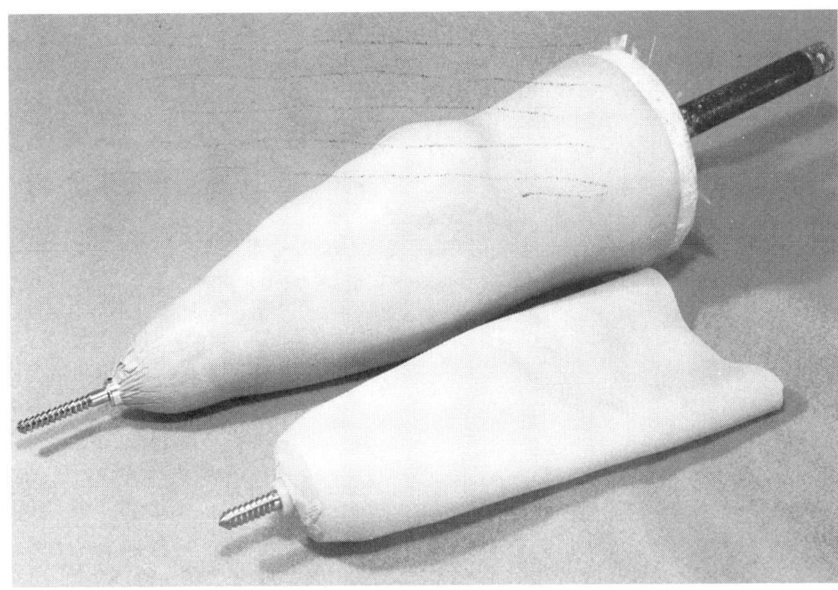

FIG. 27-12. Silicone suspension liners used with the 3-S suspension system. The top liner, on the plaster positive, is a custom liner. The bottom liner is a commercially available Iceross liner (Cascade Orthopedic, Chester, CA). The suspension or shuttlecock pin is to the left at the distal end of each liner.

signs are being used more frequently for transfemoral prostheses: the ischial containment socket with a narrow medial–lateral configuration and the transfemoral frame socket with flexible liner, also known as the ISNY socket (51).

The ischial containment, narrow medial–lateral design, also known as normal shape normal alignment (NSNA) or contoured adducted trochanter-controlled alignment method (CATCAM), was developed to provide for a more normal anatomic alignment of the femur inside the prosthesis (Fig. 27-14) (52–55). The ischial tuberosity is controlled inside the socket to stabilize the relationship between the pelvis and the proximal femur rather than allowing the tuberosity to sit on the top of the posterior brim as in the quadrilateral socket. To control the pelvis, the lateral and posterior trimlines of the socket brim are more proximal than the quadrilateral socket. This higher trimline also results in better control

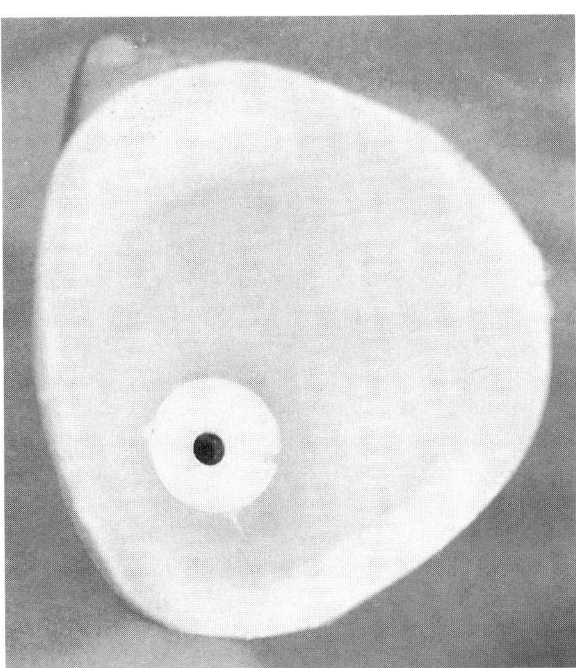

FIG. 27-13. Transtibial prosthetic socket with receptacle for the 3-S suspension pin of a silicone suspension liner seen at the bottom of the socket.

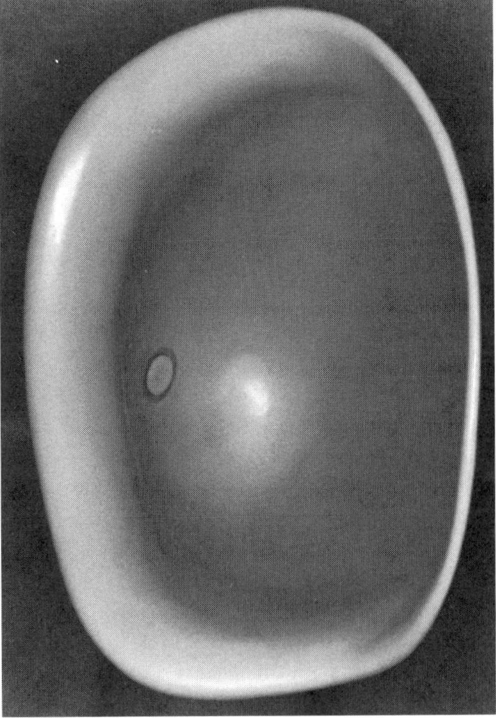

FIG. 27-14. Narrow medial–lateral transfemoral socket (NSNA design) viewed from above. The valve seen distally is on the medial aspect of the socket.

of the residual limb, particularly for short transfemoral amputations.

The original Scandinavian flexible socket was designed to have a total-contact thermoplastic inner socket supported by a graphite-reinforced, laminated open framework. It is more common to find the frame to be intact circumferentially with or without fenestrations to provide greater structural stability (Fig. 27-15). The frame can be constructed of either laminated or thermoplastic material. Either the traditional quadrilateral socket or the ischial containment, narrow medial–lateral socket shapes can be used with this type of socket design. The socket is flexible because of the characteristics of the thermoplastic material used to form the inner socket. As Thermoflex warms to body temperature, it becomes even more flexible (Figs. 27-15). Amputees report that the irritation noted in the groin region from the proximal socket brim is resolved with this more flexible plastic liner. The advantages of the frame–flexible liner type of socket design are threefold: increased comfort because the socket is able to change configurations owing to the flexibility of the material; increased proprioceptive feedback and prosthetic control because the socket wall moves with the contracting muscles in the residual limb; and direct observation of the residual limb–socket interface in both static and dynamic situations, because the socket can be made of transparent material. Better prosthetic socket fit can be achieved because fitting problems are directly observed and corrected.

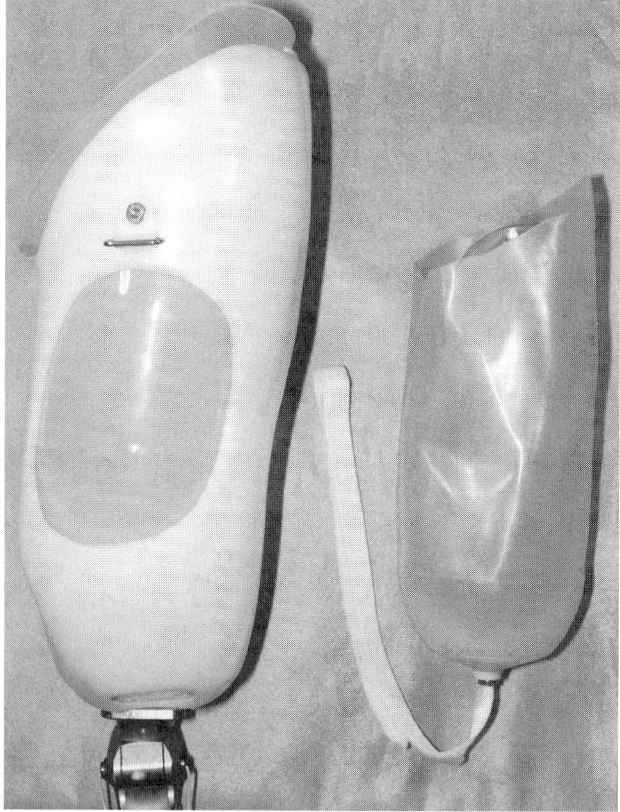

FIG. 27-15. Thermoplastic ischial containment transfemoral frame socket with Thermoflex liner. The flexible liner extends proximally above the brim of the frame. The anterior windowing over the quadriceps muscle is seen. The Alps suspension liner with distal dacron strap (used in place of a pin, see Fig. 27-12) to secure the silicone supension liner in the socket is to the right of the socket. The dacron strap is passed through a hole in the distal end of the socket and secured through the proximal D-ring on the anterior proximal socket.

Several options are available for suspension of transfemoral prostheses, but the use of a suction socket usually is preferred. The use of a suction socket, however, requires a stable residual limb volume. Increase in residual limb volume will prevent the amputee from fitting completely in the socket, and a reduction in residual limb volume will result in a loss of suction and suspension, making it impossible for the amputee to wear the prosthesis. A suction socket is worn without a sock on the residual limb. Two methods may be used to don the suction transfemoral socket. The most common method uses a stockinette pull sock. An alternative method, now used more frequently, is a wet mount (i.e., fit): a cream or gel is applied to the residual limb skin, and the limb is slipped into the socket. The remaining air is released through the suction valve, creating a small vaccuum, which holds the socket on the limb (Fig. 27-14). The use of a silicone/gel suspension liner with strap or pin attachment (3-S suspension system), depending on the length of the residual limb, can also provide a beltless pseudosuction type of suspension (Figs. 27-15). For many amputees, this suspension system provides the security and lack of pistoning achieved with a traditional suction suspension, but with the ease of donning of a belt-suspended prosthesis. Socks can be added over the suspension liner to accommodate for volume change of the residual limb just as for transtibial amputees utilizing the 3-S system. If need be, an auxillary belt suspension can be used with this suspension system just as with other true suction suspensions. The use of a hypobaric sock, a conventional limb sock with an impregnated silicone band near the proximal end of the sock, can provide complete or partial suction suspension in those transfemoral amputees with fluctuating residual limb volume. The silicone band provides a seal to prevent air leak just as the skin does in a conventional suction socket. Varying the number of hypobaric sock plies permits accommodation for changing residual limb volume secondary to limb shrinkage or weight change. Commonly, an auxiliary suspension system will be needed with hypobaric suspension. A Silesian belt can be used either as an auxiliary form of suspension with a suction socket or as the primary form of suspension. A standard Silesian belt attaches to the anterior and lateral portions of the proximal prosthetic socket and passes over the opposite iliac crest. A total elastic suspension (TES) belt functions much like a Silesian belt in that it can be either an auxiliary or primary form of suspension. The TES belt is made of the same neoprene material used for transtibial suspension sleeves. It slips over the outside of the prosthetic socket and surrounds the waist above the iliac crests to provide suspension. Many amputees find the TES belt to be more comfortable than the

Silesian belt. Other amputees find the TES belt, because it is elastic, to be a less secure suspension than the Silesian belt. A pelvic band and belt with hip joint is a third alternative for suspension of a transfemoral prosthesis. Suspending a transfemoral prosthesis is easiest with this method. The pelvic band is closely contoured about the anterior iliac crest on the side of the amputation to discourage rotation of the prosthesis on the residual limb during ambulation. Use of a hypobaric sock with a belt suspension system is another alternative available to help control rotation of the prosthesis on the residual limb that frequently occurs with these suspension systems. Occasionally, an amputee who would be a candidate for a pelvic band and belt suspension will not be able to wear a belt around the waist (i.e., a person who has a subcutaneous axillary femoral bypass graft that cannot be compressed by a waist belt); he or she will require the use of a shoulder belt or suspender suspension for the prosthesis.

The distal end of the transfemoral residual limb should be at least 8 cm proximal to the level of the distal end of the femur and above the condyles of the femur to allow the use of a conventional internal prosthetic knee joint. Several different designs of prosthetic knee joints are available. The prosthetic knee provides several important functions: stability during stance (to prevent knee buckling), either through alignment or mechanical means [i.e., stance phase control, friction brake (safety knee), or a lock], and knee motion during swing to permit easy clearance of the toe and adequate flexion to allow the knee to bend when sitting. The knee unit should control the heel rise of the shank, assisting or resisting the acceleration and deceleration of the shank during swing phase. A single-axis constant-friction unit is used most commonly. Hydraulic or pneumatic knee units are available that can provide either swing phase control or swing and stance phase control for amputees who are very active and change their cadence frequently. For amputees who have difficulty maintaining knee stability during stance, locking knees and safety knees are available. Multiaxial four- and six-bar knee units provide for increased stability during stance while at the same time providing a moving center of knee rotation approaching that of the anatomic knee joint, all with a low profile that helps maintain an equal prosthetic knee center with the nonamputated lower extremity for long transfemoral or knee disarticulation prostheses. The four-bar design is the lighter of the two designs and is illustrated in Figure 27-16 (23).

Thigh rotators are available for people who have a need or desire to cross their legs or to be able to sit on the floor (Fig 27-17). All of the prosthetic feet mentioned in the transtibial amputation section are available for use, as appropriate, with transfemoral prostheses. A single-axis foot that permits quicker plantarflexion of the prosthetic foot at heel strike can improve knee stability in amputees who demonstrate a tendency to buckle the knee in early stance, although with proper choice of knee unit and alignment, this is seldom necessary (see Case 27-4).

Hip Disarticulation/Hemipelvectomy

Amputees with less than 5 cm of residual femur usually are fitted as hip disarticulation level amputees. The standard

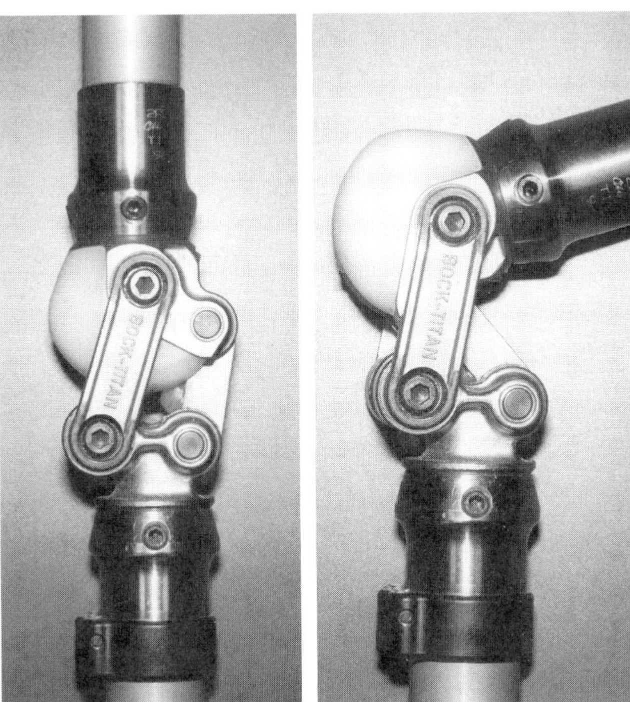

FIG. 27-16. A: Four-bar knee unit fully extended. Note the multiple pivot points (axes) of this joint. **B:** Four-bar knee unit flexed almost 90°. Note change in orientation of the several axes of the joint as well as the low profile of the knee when flexed.

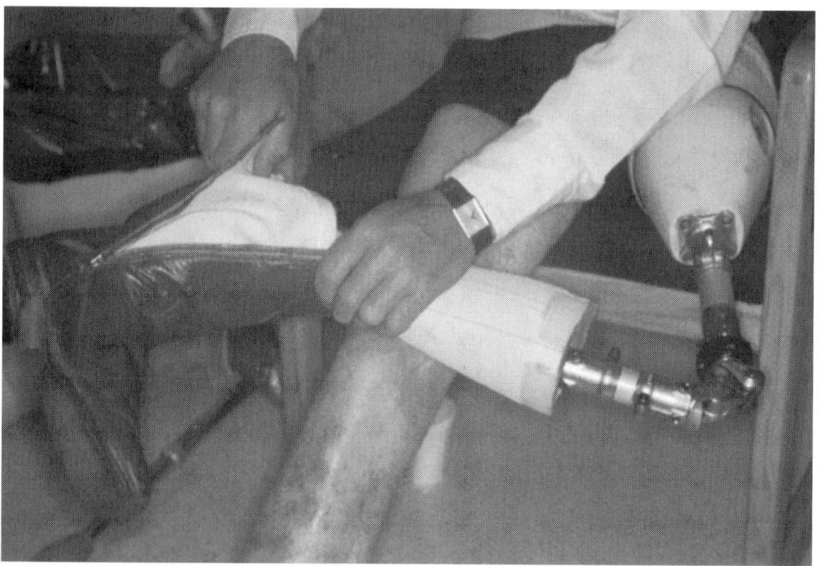

FIG. 27-17. The presence of the thigh rotator on this transfemoral prosthesis allows this man to put on his boot more easily.

prosthesis for a hip disarticulation is the Canadian hip disarticulation prosthesis. The socket of this prosthesis encloses the hemipelvis on the side of the amputation and extends around the hemipelvis of the nonamputated side, leaving an opening for the nonamputated lower extremity. There is a flexible anterior wall with an opening that allows the prosthesis to be donned. Weight is borne on the ischial tuberosity of the amputated side. Endoskeletal prosthetic components are preferred for this level of amputation to reduce the overall weight. The endoskeletal hip joint has an extension assist, as does the knee unit, which usually is a constant-friction knee. Endoskeletal components may be made from aluminum, titanium, or carbon graphite composite materials. Traditionally, a single-axis or SACH foot with a soft heel have been the most common choice for the prosthetic foot. The newer lightweight foot–ankle combination such as the Endolite foot/ankle complex or the Endolite ankle with a Seattle Lite foot may be a better option for this level. A cosmetic cover completes the prosthetic prescription. If necessary, locking hip or knee joints can be used.

The prosthesis for a hemipelvectomy resembles that for the hip disarticulation except in the interior configuration of the socket. In the hemipelvectomy, most of the weight is borne by the soft tissues on the amputated side, with some of the weight being borne by the sacrum, the rib cage, and the opposite ischial tuberosity.

Final Prosthetic Evaluation

After the prosthetist has statically and dynamically aligned the prosthesis and ensured the fit of the socket, the amputee should be seen for final prosthetic evaluation by the entire clinical team. At this time the prosthesis is evaluated for appropriate fit, alignment, and length. Minor adjustments in alignment and length can be made at the time of this evaluation, before the completion of the definitive prosthesis, if the prosthesis is an exoskeletal design and still on the alignment fixture, or if it is an endoskeletal prosthesis.

Gait Training

After completing the final prosthetic evaluation, a new amputee will require a period of gait training to learn how to function using the prosthesis. This training takes place with the supervision of the physical therapist. For the new amputee it may be appropriate to have the initial gait training occur while the prosthesis still is capable of being adjusted, to permit minor adjustments in alignment or length that may become apparent through the gait-training process. The amputee is instructed in how to put on and take off the prosthesis, how to determine the appropriate ply and number of limb socks to be worn, when and how to check the skin for evidence of irritation, and how to clean and care for the prosthesis. Gait training often occurs on an outpatient basis and may last from 1 week to 1 month, or more, with three to five visits per week. The more proximal levels of amputation require more lengthy gait training.

After the amputee has learned to put on the prosthesis, he or she initially is taught to shift weight onto the prosthesis while working in the parallel bars. Balance training also occurs in the early phase of prosthetic training while still in the parallel bars. Developing the most benefit from using a dynamically responsive (i.e., energy-storing) prosthetic foot requires special attention to careful, knowledgeable gait training. More emphasis must be placed on loading the prosthetic toe from the heel-off to toe-off phase of stance. In addition, better functional cosmesis can be achieved if training includes attention to equal step length and even cadence. Once weight shifting and balance activities with the prosthesis have been mastered, a program of progressive ambulation begins in the parallel bars and progresses to the most independent level of ambulation, using a walker, crutches, or cane, or walking unassisted. Early gait training should also focus on gaining knee stability, equal step lengths, and avoiding lateral trunk bending. Following mastery of ambulation on flat, level surfaces, techniques for managing uneven terrain, stairs, ramps, curbs, and falling and getting up off the ground are learned. Moving from a walker to less cumbersome gait aids can be achieved for most leg amputees. Transfer activities also should be reviewed as part of the gait training. Basic gait training is insufficient for achieving maximal prosthetic function. With the appropriate therapy and a well-fitted prosthesis, most transtibial and transfemoral amputees can achieve high levels of prosthetic function. In addition, prosthetic training should include how the prosthesis will function for driving, recreation, and vocational pursuits.

Wearing tolerance for the prosthesis gradually must be increased. Initially, the amputee will wear the prosthesis only for 15 to 20 minutes, removing it to check the condition of the skin. As the skin's ability to tolerate increased pressure with weight bearing increases, the length of wearing time gradually is increased. Several weeks may be required before the amputee is able to wear the prosthesis full time. The amputee may take the prosthesis home when safe and independent ambulation has been demonstrated and residual limb skin checks are assured.

Lower Extremity Prosthetic Follow-Up

The frequency of follow-up visits for lower extremity amputees is similar to that for upper extremity amputees. During the initial 6 to 18 months, most amputees will experience rapid loss of residual limb volume, resulting in a prosthetic socket that will be too large. During this period of time, return visits to the clinic or prosthetist should occur at intervals frequent enough to ensure that this loss of residual limb volume is being compensated for adequately by the use of additional limb socks or by appropriate modifications of the prosthetic socket. It is usual for a new amputee to require replacement of the prosthetic socket during this time period because of the significant loss of soft tissue volume. At the follow-up clinic visits the condition of the residual limb, the prosthesis, the amputee's gait (Table 27-4), and the level of function are reviewed (56). Appropriate medical treatment, prosthetic modifications, or additional therapy are prescribed as needed. When the residual limb volume has stabilized sufficiently and the amputee is doing well with the prosthesis, yearly visits to the amputee clinic are appropriate. Once the residual limb has stabilized, the average life expectancy for a lower extremity prosthesis before replacement should be 3 to 5 years.

SPECIAL PROSTHETIC ISSUES

Phantom Sensation and Phantom Pain

All people with acquired amputations experience some form of phantom sensation, which is the awareness of a nonpainful sensation in the amputated part (57). This sensation is most prominent in the period immediately after amputation and gradually diminishes in intensity over time but can persist throughout the amputee's life. Phantom pain is the awareness of pain in the portion of the extremity that has been amputated. It may be diffuse throughout the entire amputated extremity, or it may be restricted to the distribution of a single peripheral nerve. The occurrence of phantom pain generally is considered to be a significant problem in only 5% or less of the total amputee population, but some authors have noted that phantom pain has been reported by more than three-quarters of all amputees at some time during their life after amputation (23,57). In the early postoperative period, phantom pain may be significantly reduced with the use of amitriptyline or other tricyclic antidepressants in low doses at bedtime. Gabapentin, currently being used to treat several forms of acute and chronic musculoskeletal and neurogenic pain, seems to have a role in the management of phantom limb pain. At present it appears to have benefit as a second-line medication for phantom pain either alone or in combination with low-dose tricyclic antidepressants. Range-of-motion exercises, relaxation exercises, and gentle massage of the residual limb also may help reduce phantom pain. For chronic phantom pain, many therapeutic modalities have been suggested and tried with varying rates of success (23,57,58). Often, the treatment modalities employed, either medical or surgical, do not provide long-lasting relief. The various forms of therapy attempted to treat phantom pain have been reviewed by Sherman (59,60).

Residual limb pain should be differentiated from phantom pain and is usually caused by maldistribution of forces in the prosthetic socket. This pain occurs in the remaining part of the limb and results from excessive pressures applied to the soft tissues. Usually, prosthetic modifications, changing the numbers of stump socks, or the addition of a gel interface can provide pain relief.

Neuroma formation may also account for the onset of residual limb pain. If a neuroma is palpated and reproduces the pain, the neuroma can be injected with a local anesthetic combined with steroids as a diagnostic and therapeutic procedure. If this injection relieves pain for a minimum of several days, the injection can be repeated again. If recurrent injection does not provide prolonged relief, some practitioners have injected phenol for longer pain relief. If the neuroma is quite large or injection does not relieve the pain for any significant period of time, surgery may be indicated. However, following the neuroma resection, the neuroma will reform and, on occasion, again become symptomatic (see Chapter 56, Treatment of the Patient with Chronic Pain, for additional information).

Dermatologic Disorders

Numerous problems with the skin on the residual limb can occur, such as hyperhidrosis, folliculitis, allergic dermatitis, or breakdown of the skin at the site of adherent scars

TABLE 27-4. *Some common gate abnormalites seen with lower extremity amputees/prostheses*

Transfemoral prostheses		
Observed gait abnormality	Possible cause	Suggested modification
Prosthesis abducted	Prosthesis too long Abduction contracture of hip Adductor roll Medial groin irritation from prosthetic brim	Shorten prosthesis appropriately Physical therapy to reduce contracture Contain adductor roll in socket, shrinker Modify socket brim—reduce irritation
Knee buckling at heel strike	Incorrect TKA alignment—knee center forward Excessive foot dorsiflexion Excessive heel height—changed shoe	Realign prosthesis to move knee center posterior to TKA Correct foot alignment Replace with shoe of proper heel height—one used for alignment
Prosthetic foot rotated	Prosthesis donned in internal or external rotation Inadequate suspension Poor socket fit	Redon prosthesis correctly Improve suspension Correct socket fit—provide adequate relief for muscle contours
Vaulting on other leg or circumduction of prosthesis during swing phase	Prosthesis too long Prosthetic knee does not flex freely Fear of knee buckling—knee unit functions ok	Shorten prosthesis Adjust/replace knee unit Consider a more stable knee unit
Whips	Improper position of knee Medial whip—knee too externally rotated Lateral whip—knee too internally rotated Prosthesis donned incorrectly	Adjust knee for proper alignment Redon prosthesis correctly
Excessive drop of pelvis on contralateral side during prosthetic stance	Weak ipsilateral hip abductors Hip abduction contracture Prosthetic socket in too much abducton	Strengthen hip abductors Reduce/eliminate contracture Realign socket
Excessive lumbar lordosis or stands/walks with a flexed posture at the hips	Hip flexion contracture Socket not flexed enough for contracture	Eliminate contracture Preflex prosthetic socket more

Transtibial amputees/prostheses		
Observed gait abnormality	Possible cause	Suggested modification
Medial thrust of knee—stance	Foot too far outset	Realign foot position
Lateral thrust of knee—stance	Foot too far inset	Realign foot position
Excessive heel rise—toe off	Toe lever too long Keel too stiff Dorsiflexion bumper to rigid	Shorten toe lever by adjusting foot position Choose foot with lower weight rating or a different foot design Replace with softer bumper
Excessive heel contact—heel strike	Heel too soft Compresible heel worn out Plantar flexion bumper too soft/worn	Replace with proper foot/weight rating Replace with new foot Replace with proper or new bumper
Excessive knee flexion—heel strike	Too much socket flexion Foot in too much dorsiflexion Short toe lever—long heel lever Soft/worn dorsiflexion bumper	Realign socket Realign foot Correct foot position Replace firmer or new bumper
Pelvis not level	Prosthesis too long/too short Too many/too few limb socks	Adjust prosthesis to proper length Use correct number of limb socks
Excessive pistoning—swing	Inadequate suspension	Correct suspension problems

or split-thickness skin grafts (61,62). Skin problems can be minimized by instructing the amputee carefully to wash and dry the residual limb daily and to wear natural-fiber limb socks that are absorbent to minimize the moisture inside the socket to prevent skin maceration. At times it is appropriate to use nylon, polyamide, or gel sheaths between the skin and the limb sock to reduce shear forces that can cause skin breakdown.

Hyperhidrosis can be controlled successfully by using concentrated antiperspirants, such as Drysol (Person & Covey, Glendale, CA), on the residual limb. Folliculitis may require the use of antibiotics, and sebaceous cysts may require surgical drainage or excision. Allergic dermatitis can result from the detergents used to wash the limb socks and may require only that the detergent be changed. Also, the use of scented lotions to moisturize the skin may result in an allergic dermatitis secondary to the active ingredients in the scent. The use of gel sheaths and liners and suspension liners may result in contact dermatitis and fungal infections. These liners can create a moist warm environment that favors fungal infections, and prevention requires meticulous care of the skin. Some amputees' contact dermatitis seen in conjuction with the use of these liners may be caused by an allergic reaction to the liner material, but in most cases the rash is usually secondary to a residue of a soap or other substance used to clean the liner. In rare cases, the dermatitis may result from the materials used to fabricate the prosthetic socket, in which case a new prosthetic socket must be fabricated from nonallergenic materials. If allergy to a component of the prosthesis is suspected, confirmation with a patch test for 24 to 48 hours with a small piece of the suspected material on the forearm may be most helpful in guiding treatment decisions.

Socket Fit

Socket comfort, which is related to socket fit, is one of the most important aspects of prosthetic acceptance and function. Both upper and lower extremity amputees can have problems with socket fit. The usual reasons for changes in socket fit are weight gain or weight loss and soft tissue atrophy resulting in changes of the limb contour. Frequently, minor problems in socket fit can be handled by modifications to an existing prosthetic socket or with the the use of growth liners. Significant changes in socket fit will require a new prosthetic socket.

One specific problem that can result from poor socket fit for the lower extremity amputee that is not typically encountered with the upper extremity amputee, is a choke syndrome. This situation results when the prosthetic socket is tight circumferentially in the proximal region and there is lack of good distal contact between the residual limb and the socket. The proximal constriction results in obstruction of venous outflow, producing edema of the distal end of the residual limb where socket contact is not present. Usually this area of edema produces a circular, well-circumscribed margin. If the choke syndrome is allowed to progress, the edema will progress to induration, erythema, breakdown, and drainage. The area of choke is quite tender to palpation and is prone to developing cellulitis if there is an open lesion. If a choke syndrome becomes chronic, the tissues involved on the distal residual limb can become brownish-orange in color as the result of pigments (e.g., hemosiderin) from extravasated red blood cells that accumulate in the tissues. This pigmentation usually is permanent, even if the choke syndrome ultimately is resolved. The tissues in a chronic choke syndrome also can take on a verrucous appearance. The appropriate treatment for a choke syndrome is to relieve the proximal constriction and to restore total contact distally between the residual limb and the socket (61,62).

Functional Outcomes with Prostheses

Assessing functional outcomes for prosthetic rehabilitation has not been standardized in prosthetic rehabilitation centers in the United States. Yet, developing these outcomes would be useful in comparing prosthetic designs, the costs of prosthetic rehabilitation care, and the idealized levels of function for the person with an amputation. Using a checklist for prosthetic functional outcomes can be useful, but in addition, it is important to assess the vocational, avocational, and perceived quality of life achieved with prosthetic rehabilitation.

A proposed checklist for prosthetic functional outcome at the major levels of arm and leg loss is presented in Tables 27-5 through 27-8. These are idealized lists of expected function. Some amputees will not be able to achieve all of the desired function because of comorbid factors, prosthetic issues, or insufficient motivation to achieve these things. However, most amputees should be able to achieve these idealized functions. Neither age nor a history of cardiopulmonary disease should be an excuse for the rehabilitation team to end the rehabilitation program before the person has

TABLE 27-5. *Functional outcomes for transradial prosthetic restoration*

1. Independent in donning and doffing prostheses
2. Independent in all activities of daily living
3. Can write legibly with remaining hand
4. Has comfortably switched dominance (if necessary)
5. Drives
6. Has returned to work (same or modified job)
7. Can perform one-handed activities
8. Uses a button hook easily
9. Has prepared a meal
10. Has been evaluated for adaptive equipment for the kitchen and in performing ADL
11. Has performed carpentry and automotive activities (if done prior to amputation)
12. Wears prostheses during all waking hours
13. Utilizes prosthesis for bimanual activities for at least 25% of manual activities

ADL, activities of daily living.

TABLE 27-6. *Functional outcomes for transhumeral prosthetic restoration*

1. Independent in donning and doffing prostheses
2. Independent in all activities of daily living
3. Can write legibly with remaining hand
4. Had comfortably switched dominance (if necessary)
5. Drives
6. Has returned to work (same or modified job)
7. Can perform one-handed activities
8. Uses a button hook easily
9. Has prepared a meal
10. Has been evaluated for adaptive equipment for the kitchen and in performing ADL
11. Has performed carpentry and automotive activities (if done prior to amputation)
12. Wears prostheses during all waking hours
13. Utilizes prosthesis for bimanual activities for at least 25% of manual activities

ADL, activities of daily living.

achieved these levels of function. If an item on the functional outcome list is not achieved, a notation of the reason for not achieving that item of function should be made.

In addition to these checklists of function, a quality-of-life questionnaire should also be employed to determine the amputee's perception of life following prosthetic rehabilitation. The amputee's resumption of previous activities and their postamputation role in the family and the community should be assessed during periods of follow-up.

Pediatric Limb Deficiency or Amputation

The absence of part or all of an extremity at birth is more appropriately referred to as a congenital skeletal deficiency rather than a congenital amputation. The Birth Defects Monitoring Program, a national program monitoring congenital malformations for the United States, reports the incidence of these congenital upper and lower limb reduction deformities at 303 for 1986–1987, or 2.41 per 10,000 births (upper limb, 1.58 per 10,000 births; lower limb, 0.83 per 10,000 births) (63). When a child is born with an absent or malformed limb, the question ''Why?'' is always asked, but often no etiology can ever be identified. A few genetically determined syndromes such as Holt-Oram, Fanconi syndrome, and thrombocytopenia–absent radius have been associated with skeletal deficiencies (29,40,64–66). Congenital amniotic bands occasionally have been implicated, but no clear understanding of how these occur has been reached. Exposure to teratogenic agents during limb development, such as thalidomide and excessive radiation, has been identified as resulting in limb defects at birth (64,65).

Multiple systems for classifying congenital limb deficiencies have been proposed in both Europe and North America, but no one system has been universally accepted. In the United States some form of the Frantz–O'Rahilly system is most commonly used. The ISPO Dundee Classification System was developed by a group of international experts with the hope that it would become the standard for classification of congenital limb deficiencies. The fact that this has not occurred has made data collection for epidemiologic and etiologic purposes difficult. Classification of congenital limb deficiencies often is confused further when congenital deficiencies are described in the same terms used for acquired amputations, such as ''transradial'' or ''transtibial.'' The use of similar terminology occurs either because the congenital deficiency appears similar to an acquired amputation or be-

TABLE 27-7. *Functional outcomes for transtibial prosthetic restoration*

1. Ambulation with prosthesis on level and uneven surfaces, stairs, ramps and curbs
2. Ambulation with minimal or no gait aids
3. Independent with dressing
4. Independent in donning and doffing prosthesis
5. Independent in stump wrapping or applying a shrinker
6. Able to drive
7. Can participate in shopping activities
8. Has returned to previous work, with or without modifications
9. Can stand for up to two continuous hours
10. Can sit for up to two continuous hours
11. Can arise from the kneeling position
12. Comfortable with falling techniques and can arise from the floor
13. Can hunt, fish, run, bicycle (if part of previous lifestyle)
14. Knows how to purchase properly fitting footwear for the remaining foot
15. Knows proper skin and nail care for remaining foot
16. Can safely perform aerobic conditioning program
17. Climbs stairs foot over foot

TABLE 27-8. *Functional outcomes for transfemoral prosthetic restoration*

1. Ambulation with prosthesis on level and uneven surfaces, stairs, ramps and curbs
2. Ambulation with minimal or no gait aids
3. Independent with dressing
4. Independent in donning and doffing prosthesis
5. Independent in stump wrapping or applying a shrinker
6. Able to drive
7. Can participate in shopping activities
8. Has returned to previous work, with or without modifications
9. Can stand for up to two continuous hours
10. Can sit for up to two continuous hours
11. Can arise from the kneeling position
12. Comfortable with falling techniques and can arise from the floor
13. Can hunt, fish, run, bicycle (if part of previous lifestyle)
14. Knows how to purchase properly fitting footwear for the remaining foot
15. Knows proper skin and nail care for remaining foot
16. Can safely perform aerobic conditioning program
17. Stairs are generally climbed one at a time
18. Can run (if amputee desires, has adequate cardiopulmonary reserve and residual limb length)
19. Uses no more than a cane for ambulation

TABLE 27-9. *Pediatric prosthetic fitting*

Level of pediatric amputation	Age for prosthetic fitting	Developmental milestones	Prosthetic prescription
Transradial	6 months	Child can sit and reaches across midline for bimanual manipulation of objects	Body-power—Passive mitt TD, plastic laminate, self-suspending socket
	9 months		External-power—"Cookie crusher," single-site control
	18 months		Go to two state control
Transhumeral	6 months	Same as transradial	Body-power—Passive mitt and elbow; activate elbow at 18 months.
	24 months		External-power—Variety Village elbow with two-state control
Transtibial	9–12 months	Child pulls to stand	PTB, plastic laminate, supracondylar strap, SACH foot. Pediatric dynamic responsive feet now available for use.
Transfemoral	9–12 months	Child pulls to stand	Narrow M-L, ischial containment with no knee unit; suspension with Silesian bandage; add knee unit at 18 months

PTB, patellar tendon-bearing; SACH, solid ankle cushion heal; TD, terminal device.

cause a congenital skeletal deficiency has undergone a surgical conversion to accommodate appropriate prosthetic restoration. Surgical conversion has been estimated to be necessary in the management of 50% of lower extremity congenital deficiencies and only 8% of upper extremity deficiencies (67).

When amputations are performed in children for disease, tumor, or trauma or to surgically convert a congenital skeletal deficiency to a level more appropriate for prosthetic fitting, a disarticulation level amputation is preferred rather than an amputation through a long bone when the resulting level of function with a prosthesis will be similar. Approximately 12% of children with acquired amputations experience a condition known as bony overgrowth. Bony overgrowth is the appositional deposition of bone to the end of the amputated long bone. This bone growth results in a spikelike formation at the end of the bone that has a thin cortex and no medullary canal. The bone frequently grows faster than the overlying skin and soft tissues; a bursa may develop over the sharp end, or the bone actually may protrude through the skin with subsequent development of cellulitis and osteomyelitis. Overgrowth is seen most frequently in the humerus, fibula, tibia, and femur, in that order. It has been reported in the congenital limb deficiencies, but rarely. Several treatment approaches have been advocated for the management of this problem, all with limited success. The technique proposed by Marquardt in which the distal end of the bone is capped with a cartilage epiphysis is the best of the surgical options available to manage this problem (67).

For the child with a congenital skeletal deficiency, the initial prosthesis for the upper extremity usually is fitted when the child has attained independent sitting balance, or at approximately 6 months of age (Table 27-9). For the lower extremity, the initial prosthesis is fitted when the child begins to pull to a stand, which generally is between 9 and 14 months. Young children and infants usually learn to use their prostheses by incorporating them as part of play activities rather than through specific exercises. Prosthetic training periods for children may last only for several minutes at a time because of limited attention span, and they may require much longer periods of free play interspersed between actual training sessions. It is important that parents be instructed in techniques to help their children attain the necessary prosthetic skills because much of the training in the use of the prosthesis will occur in the home rather than in the clinic.

PROSTHETIC PRESCRIPTION EXAMPLE CASES

The prosthetic prescriptions presented for these cases are as examples only. They do not represent the standard or typical prosthetic prescriptions for these levels of amputation. The authors want to be clear that a specific prosthetic prescription must be tailored to meet the specific needs of an individual amputee. The examples presented here serve to highlight the decision process that might be followed to arrive at an appropriate prosthetic prescription.

Case 27-1: Transradial

A 24-year-old right-handed man sustains a work-related crush injury to his right hand, resulting in a long transradial level of amputation. He plans to return to work operating a drill press.

Possible prosthetic prescriptions include:

Body power
Double-wall plastic laminate socket
Quick-change locking wrist unit

No. 7 (heavy duty, "Farmer's hook") terminal device
Flexible elbow hinges
Triceps pad
Figure-8 harness for suspension
Bowden single control cable
External power
Double-wall plastic laminate socket with self-suspending design
Otto Bock Greifer (myoelectric hook) terminal device

In this person, body power will be lightest in weight, most durable, and least expensive. If more than 6 to 7 pounds of pinch force are necessary from the terminal device for functional activities, the Greifer will provide up to 35 pounds of pinch force.

Case 27-2: Transhumeral

A 35-year-old right-handed female homemaker sustains a short transhumeral level of amputation following a motor vehicle accident.

Possible prosthetic prescriptions include:

Body power
Double-wall plastic laminate socket
Constant-friction wrist unit
No. 5XA (lightest weight) terminal device
Internal, alternating locking elbow with turntable
Figure-8 harness
Bowden double control cable
External power
Double-wall plastic laminate socket
Otto Bock myoelectric hand
Utah myoelectric elbow
Figure-8 harness

In this person, because of the short residual limb, external power may be more comfortable and functional but will be heavier and much more expensive than body power.

Case 27-3: Transtibial

A 72-year-old retired man with type II diabetes and peripheral vascular disease has a transtibial amputation for an infected nonhealing ulcer and gangrenous foot.

Possible prosthetic prescriptions include:

Provisional
Total contact patellar tendon-bearing (PTB) thermoplastic socket
Foam liner (soft insert)
Neoprene sleeve suspension
Lightweight alignable shank
SACH foot
Definitive
Exoskeletal design prosthesis
Total-contact laminated PTB socket
Silicone suction suspension (3-S)
Lightweight multiaxial foot

The provisional prosthesis is a lightweight design that provides a stable support base on which to learn to walk with a prosthesis. The soft liner will make modifications for changes in residual limb volume that are expected to occur easier to accomplish. An exoskeletal design with multiaxis foot was chosen for the definitive prosthesis in consideration of the individual's desire to return to his gardening activities, which required a prosthesis that was more durable and stable on uneven ground with a secure suspension system that would not be torn up when kneeling with the prosthesis.

Case 27-4: Transfemoral

A 28-year-old female daycare teacher sustained an open comminuted distal femur fracture while mountain climbing ultimately had a midthigh level transfemoral amputation after developing osteomyelitis.

Possible prosthetic prescriptions include:

Provisional
Total contact thermoplastic ischial containment socket
TES belt suspension
Hydraulic knee unit
Lightweight dynamic-response foot
Cosmetic foam cover
Definitive
Total-contact carbon fiber reinforced ischial containment suction frame socket with Thermoflex liner
Thigh rotator
Swing and stance phase-control hydraulic knee unit
Split-toe Flex-Foot
Cosmetic foam cover

The provisional prosthesis, an endoskeletal design with a nonsuction socket, belt suspension, and hydraulic knee unit, was chosen to allow easy accommodation for anticipated major changes in residual limb volume that were expected to occur quickly with prosthetic use while at the same time recognizing this individual's high level of physical activity. The cosmetic cover was added to the provisional prosthesis, not usually done, recognizing her work with small children and her desire not to scare them with the prosthesis. The changes in the definitive prosthesis reflected the individual's desire to eliminate the belt suspension, achieve a more secure suspension, and accommodate to her recreational and competitive sports activities. The thigh rotator was added so that she could sit on the floor and work with the children in her class.

REFERENCES

1. Malone JM, Moore WS, Goldstone J, Malone SJ. Therapeutic and economic impact of a modern amputation program. *Ann Surg* 1979; 189:798–802.
2. United States Department of Health and Human Services. *Vital and health statistics: current estimates from the National Health Interview*

Survey, 1993. Series 10, 190. Washington, D.C.: US Government Printing Office, 1994; 94.

3. United States Department of Health and Human Services. *Vital and health statistics: prevalence of selected impairments: United States-1977. Series 10, 134.* Washington, D.C.: US Government Printing Office, 1981; 14–17,28–29.
4. United States Department of Health and Human Services. *Vital and health statistics: use of special aids: United States, 1977. Series 10, 135.* Washington, D.C.: US Government Printing Office, 1980; 12–13,15–16,23–25.
5. United States Department of Health and Human Services. *Vital and health statistics: detailed diagnoses and procedures, National Hospital Discharge Survey, 1993. Series 13, 122.* Washington, D.C.: Government Printing Office, 1995; 134.
6. Kay HW, Newman JD. Relative incidences of new amputations: statistical comparisons of 6,000 new amputees. *Orthot Prosthet* 1975; 29: 3–16.
7. Moore WS, Malone JM, eds. *Lower extremity amputation.* Philadelphia: WB Saunders, 1989.
8. Murdoch G, Wilson AB. *Amputation surgical practice and patient management.* Boston: Butterworth Heinemann, 1996.
9. Sanders GT. *Lower limb amputations: a guide to rehabilitation.* Philadelphia: FA Davis, 1986.
10. Glattly HW. A statistical study of 12,000 new amputees. *South Med J* 1964; 57:1373–1378.
11. Friedman LW. *The surgical rehabilitation of the amputee.* Springfield, IL: Charles C Thomas, 1978.
12. Banerjee SN, ed. *Rehabilitation management of amputees.* Baltimore: Williams & Wilkins, 1982.
13. Burgess EM, Matsen FA III. Determining amputation levels in peripheral vascular disease. *J Bone Joint Surg [Am]* 1981; 63A:1493–1497.
14. Kour AK, Seo JS, Pho RW. Combined free flap, Ilizarov lengthening and prosthetic fitting in the reconstruction of a proximal forearm amputation—a case report. *Ann Acad Med* 1995; 24(Suppl):135–137.
15. Vavylov VN, Kalakutsky NV, Agrachyova IG. Reconstruction of very short humeral stumps. *Ann Plast Surg* 1994; 32:145–147.
16. Stricker SJ. Ilizarov lengthening of a posttraumatic below elbow amputation stump. A case report. *Clin Orthop* 1994; 306:124–127.
17. Moss AL, Waterhouse N, Townsend PL, Hannon MA. Lengthening of a short traumatic femoral stump. *Injury* 1985; 16:350–353.
18. Perrson BM, Broome A. Lengthening a short femoral stump. *Acta Orthop Scand* 1994; 65:99–100.
19. Shenaq SM, Krouskop T, Stal S, Spira M. Salvage of amputation stumps by secondary reconstruction utilizing microsurgical free tissue transfer. *Plast Reconstr Surg* 1987; 79:861–870.
20. Rees R, Shack B, Hulsey T, Lynch J. A new technique for reconstruction of an open above-knee amputation. *Plast Reconstr Surg* 1983; 72: 882–886.
21. Kasabian AK, Glat PM, Eidelman Y, Colen S, Longaker MT, Attinger C, Shaw W. Salvage of traumatic below-knee amputation stumps utilizing the filet of foot free flap: critical evaluation of six cases. *Plast Reconstr Surg* 1995; 96:1145–1153.
22. Rees RS, Nanney LB, Fleming P, Cary A. Tissue expansion: its role in traumatic below-knee amputations. *Plast Reconstr Surg* 1986; 77: 133–137.
23. Esquenazi A, Meier RH. Rehabilitation in limb deficiency. 4. Limb amputation. *Arch Phys Med Rehabil* 1996; 77:S18–S28.
24. Friedman LW. *The psychological rehabilitation of the amputee.* Springfield, IL: Charles C Thomas, 1978.
25. MacLean N, Fick GH. The effect of semirigid dressings on below-knee amputations. *Phys Ther* 1994; 74:668–673.
26. Burgess EM, Romano RL, Zetti JH. *The management of lower extremity amputations.* Washington, D.C.: US Government Printing Office, 1969.
27. Leonard JA, Andrews KL. Rigid removable dressings, immediate post-operative prostheses, and rehabilitation of the amputee. In: Ernst CB, Stanley JC, eds. *Current therapy in vascular surgery.* Philadelphia: BC Decker, 1991; 708–712.
28. Wu Y, Krick H. Removable rigid dressing for below-knee amputees. *Clin Prosthet Orthot* 1987; 11:33–44.
29. Atkins DJ, Meier RH, eds. *Comprehensive management of the upper-limb amputee.* New York: Springer-Veriag, 1989.
30. Malone JM, Fleming LL, Robenson J, et al. Immediate, early, and late postsurgical management of upper-limb amputation. *J Rehabil Res Dev* 1984; 21:33–41.
31. Folsom D, King T, Rubin JR. Lower-extremity amputation with immediate postoperative prosthetic placement. *Am J Surg* 1992; 164: 320–322.
32. Oberg T, Lilja M, Johansson T, Karsznia A. Clinical evaluation of transtibial prosthesis sockets: a comparison between CAD CAM and conventionally produced sockets. *Prosthet Orthot Int* 1993; 17: 164–171.
33. Houston VL, Mason CP, Beattie AC, LaBlanc KP, Garbarini M, Lorenze EJ, Thongpop CM. The VA-Cyberware lower limb prosthetics–orthotics optical laser digitizer. *J Rehabil Res Dev* 1995; 32:55–73.
34. Barry DT, Leonard JA, Gitter AJ, Ball RD. Acoustic myography as a control signal for an externally powered prosthesis. *Arch Phys Med Rehabil* 1986; 67:267–269.
35. Sears HH, Shaperman J. Proportional myoelectric hand control: an evaluation. *Am J Phys Med Rehabil* 1991; 70:20–28.
36. Scott RN. Myoelectric control systems research at the Bio-Engineering Institute, University of New Brunswick. *Med Prog Technol* 1990; 16: 5–10.
37. Scott RN, ed. *Progress report no. 17: myoelectric control systems.* Fredrickton, NB: University of New Brunswick, 1980.
38. Michael JW. Upper limb powered components and controls: current concepts. *Clin Prosthet Orthot* 1986; 10:66–77.
39. Scott RN, ed. *4. Myoelectric prostheses for infants.* Fredrickton, NB: University of New Brunswick, 1992.
40. Jain S. Rehabilitation in limb deficiency. 2. The pediatric amputee. *Arch Phys Med Rehabil* 1995; 77:S9–S13.
41. Malone JM, Childers SJ, Underwood J, et al. Immediate postsurgical management of upper extremity amputation: conventional, electric, and myoelectric prostheses. *Orthot Prosthet* 1981; 35:1–9.
42. Edelstein JE. Current choices in prosthetic feet. *Crit Rev Phys Rehabil Med* 1991; 2:213–226.
43. Esquenazi A, Torres MM. Prosthetic feet and ankle mechanisms. *Phys Med Rehabil Clin* 1991; 2:299–309.
44. Michael J. Energy-storing feet: clinical comparison. *Clin Prosthet Orthot* 1987; 11:154–168.
45. Gitter A, Czerniecki JM, DeGroot DM. Biomechanical analysis of the influence of prosthetic feet on below knee amputee walking. *Am J Phys Med Rehabil* 1991; 70:142–148.
46. Colborne GR, Naumann S, Longmuir PE, Berbrayer D. Analysis of mechanical and metabolic factors in the gait of congenital below knee amputees. A comparison of the SACH and Seattle feet. *Am J Phys Med Rehabil* 1992; 71:272–278.
47. Casillas JM, Dulieu V, Cohen M, Marcer I, Didier JP. Bioenergetic comparison of a new energy-storing foot and SACH foot in traumatic below-knee vascular amputations. *Arch Phys Med Rehabil* 1995; 76: 39–44.
48. Lehmann JF, Price R, Boswell-Bessette S, Dralle A, Questad K. Comprehensive analysis of dynamic elastic response feet: Seattle Ankle/Lite foot versus SACH foot. *Arch Phys Med Rehabil* 1993; 74:853–861.
49. Hayhurst DJ. Prosthetic management of a partial-foot amputee. *Inter-Clin Info Bull* 1978; 17:11–15.
50. Koepke GH, Giacinto JP, McUmber RA. Silicone gel below-knee amputation prosthesis. *Inter-Clin Info Bull* 1971; 12:13–15.
51. Jendrzejczyk DJ. Flexible socket systems. *Clin Prosthet Orthot* 1985; 9:27–31.
52. Gottschalk FA, Kourosh S, Stills M, McClellan B, Roberts J. Does socket configuration influence the position of the femur in above knee amputation? *J Prosthet Orthot* 1989; 2:94.
53. Gottschalk FA, Stills M. The biomechanics of transfemoral amputation. *Prosthet Orthot Int* 1994; 18:12–17.
54. Long IA. Normal shape-normal alignment (NSNA) above-knee prosthesis. *Clin Prosthet Orthot* 1985; 9:9–14.
55. Sabolich J. Contoured adducted trochanteric-controlled alignment method (CAT-CAM): introduction and basic principles. *Clin Prosthet Orthot* 1985; 9:15–26.
56. Czerniecki JM. Rehabilitation in limb deficiency. 1. Gait and motion analysis. *Arch Phys Med Rehabil* 1996; 77:S3–S8.
57. Sherman RA, Tippens JK. Suggested guidelines for treatment of phantom limb pain. *Orthopedics* 1982; 5:1595–1600.
58. Lundeberg T. Relief of pain from a phantom limb by peripheral stimulation. *J Neurol* 1985; 232:79–82.

59. Sherman RA. Published treatments of phantom limb pain. *Am J Phys Med* 1980; 59:232–244.
60. Sherman RA, Sherman CJ, Gail NA. Survey of current phantom limb treatment in the United States. *Pain* 1980; 8:85–99.
61. Levy SW. *Skin problems of the amputee.* St Louis: Warren H Green, 1983.
62. Spires MC, Leonard JA. Prosthetic pearls: solutions to thorny problems. *Phys Med Rehabil Clin* 1996;7:509–526.
63. Edmonds LD, James LM. Temporal trends in the prevalence of congenital malformations at birth based on the birth defects monitoring program: United States, 1979–1987. *CDC Surveil Summ Morbid Mortal Weekly Rep* 1990; 39(SS4):19–23.
64. Kalamchi A, ed. *Congenital lower limb deficiencies.* New York: Springer-Verlag, 1989.
65. Setoguchi Y, Roseufelder R. *The limb deficient child,* 2nd ed. Springfield, IL: Charles C Thomas, 1982.
66. Setoguchi Y. The management of the limb deficient child and its family. *Prosthet Orthot Int* 1991; 15:78–81.
67. Bowker JH, Michael JW. *Atlas of limb prosthetics: surgical, prosthetic, and rehabilitation principles. American Academy of Orthopedic Surgeons,* 2nd ed. St. Louis: CV Mosby, 1992.

Rehabilitation Medicine: Principles and Practice, Third Edition,
edited by Joel A. DeLisa and Bruce M. Gans.
Lippincott–Raven Publishers, Philadelphia © 1998.

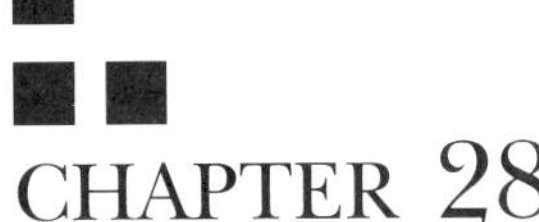

CHAPTER 28

Therapeutic Exercise

Martin D. Hoffman, Lois M. Sheldahl, and William J. Kraemer

The term ''therapeutic'' relates to the treatment of disease or physical disorder, and ''exercise'' refers to bodily exertion for the sake of training or improvement of health. This chapter on ''therapeutic exercise'' therefore addresses the use of activities requiring physical exertion in the treatment and prevention of illness and disabling conditions. The pertinent exercises considered in this chapter include those to develop endurance, strength, range of motion, and proprioception.

The use of therapeutic exercise in the treatment of injuries is not a new concept. Hippocrates (460–370 B.C.) reportedly advocated exercise as an important factor in the healing of injured ligaments, and the Hindus and Chinese used therapeutic exercise in the treatment of athletic injuries as early as 1000 B.C. Today, the various types of exercise probably account for the most commonly used treatments in the field of physical medicine and rehabilitation. Therefore, it is important for clinicians in the field to have a thorough understanding of this area.

The concepts forming the basis for therapeutic exercise come from studies in basic physiological science and applied exercise physiology. In recent years, epidemiologic investigations have provided additional insight into the importance of exercise in prevention of disease. Consequently, much of this chapter is devoted to this basic information that provides the foundation for the clinical use of exercise.

BASIC CONCEPTS AND DEFINITIONS

Force, Tension, and Torque

Several terms are used in discussing the forces generated by muscular contraction. *Force* can be thought of as a push or pull acting on an object. As a vector quantity, force has both direction and magnitude. The force exerted on an object through muscular contraction can be readily measured with strain gauges or load cells. During muscular contractions, *tension* is developed in the muscle that generates forces at the insertion sites of the muscle. Muscle tension cannot be directly measured without invasive instrumentation. *Torque* is a measurement of the effectiveness of a force in producing rotation about an axis. Torque is equal to the product of a force times the perpendicular distance between the site of force application and the axis of rotation (Fig. 28-1). Torque is commonly measured in the clinical setting.

M. D. Hoffman: Department of Physical Medicine and Rehabilitation, Medical College of Wisconsin, Milwaukee, Wisconsin 53295.
L. M. Sheldahl: Department of Medicine, Veterans Administration Medical Center, Medical College of Wisconsin, Milwaukee, Wisconsin 53295.
W. J. Kraemer: Department of Applied Physiology, Center for Sports Medicine, The Pennsylvania State University, University Park, Pennsylvania 16802.

Energy, Work, and Power

Work is the product of a force times the distance through which the force is exerted, and *energy* is the capacity to perform work. In animals, energy is expended in performing work by the degradation of foodstuffs through chemical reactions. Although the terms work and energy are used interchangeably, it should be recognized that it is possible to expend energy but perform no mechanical work. *Power* is the rate of performing work and is calculated by dividing the work by the time required to perform the work.

Strength and Types of Muscle Contractions

Strength of contraction can be measured as either a force or torque. Therefore, maximal strength is the maximal force or torque that can be exerted by a muscle. When defining the strength of a contraction, it is important to specify the type of contraction and velocity of movement.

Muscle contractions can be divided into static and dynamic. *Static* (or *isometric*) contractions are those in which there is no movement of the load on which the muscle is acting. Classically, this type of contraction has been described as resulting in no change in muscle length; however, there may be internal reductions in muscle length associated

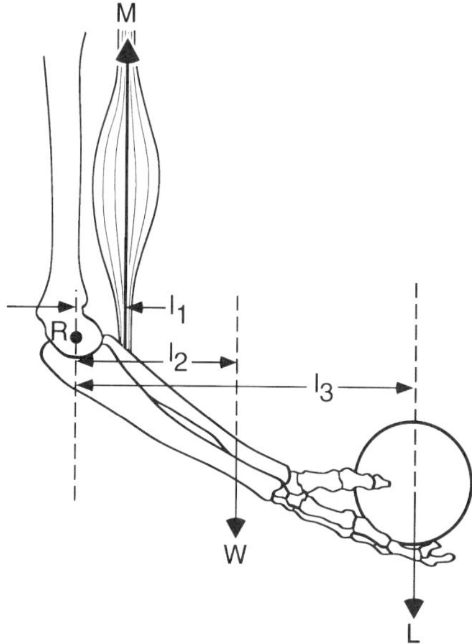

FIG. 28-1. The torque acting at the elbow can be calculated from $W \times l_2 + L \times l_3$, which is also equal to $M \times l_1$, where W is the forearm weight and l_2 identifies the center of mass of the forearm.

with lengthening of elastic elements in series with the muscle.

Dynamic contractions are divided into several subgroups because muscles may contract in lengthening or shortening fashions, and the resistance may be applied in various manners. If a muscle shortens as it contracts, it is referred to as a *concentric* contraction, and if it lengthens, it is called an *eccentric* contraction. The term *isotonic* contraction implies that the tension of the muscle remains constant throughout the movement. However, achieving this condition, or for that matter even that of a constant torque exerted by the muscle, is rare. For practical purposes the term isotonic contraction refers to a dynamic contraction with a constant load, but the more appropriate term for these types of contractions that has been adopted in the literature is *dynamic constant external resistance.* An *isokinetic* contraction is one in which the movement is performed at a constant angular velocity but the load, resistive force, or muscle tension may vary. Both isotonic and isokinetic contractions can be performed concentrically or eccentrically.

Oxygen Uptake

Oxygen uptake ($\dot{V}O_2$) is a measure of the rate of oxygen utilization for the production of energy. This measure is typically reported in units of liters per minute or milliliters per kilogram body mass per minute. Another commonly used measurement unit for oxygen uptake is the *metabolic equivalent* (MET). One MET is equal to 3.5 ml/kg per minute, which is approximately the resting metabolic rate. *Maximal oxygen uptake* ($\dot{V}O_{2max}$) is the maximal rate at which an individual can utilize oxygen. Classically, this is determined as the rate of oxygen uptake at which no further increase occurs despite an increase in dynamic work rate by the individual (Fig. 28-2). The term peak $\dot{V}O_2$ is often referred to when it is recognized that the highest attainable $\dot{V}O_2$ was not reached by the individual because of the mode of exercise being used, the testing protocol, or inadequate motivation.

METABOLIC FUNDAMENTALS

Part of adaptation to regular exercise is the development of the energy systems most involved in the type of training being used. Therefore, to condition an individual optimally for participation in a particular activity or sport, an exercise program should be designed to increase the physiological capacity of the energy systems most important to that activity. For this reason, it is valuable to have an understanding of how energy is derived for muscular contraction.

The immediate usable form of chemical energy for all muscular contraction is ATP. ATP is supplied to the muscle through three systems: (a) the adenosine triphosphate–creatine phosphate (ATP-CP) system, (b) the anaerobic glycolysis system, and (c) the aerobic system. The relative utilization of the three systems depends on the intensity and duration of the exercise (Table 28-1).

Anaerobic Metabolism

Anaerobic metabolism refers to a series of chemical reactions that do not require the presence of oxygen. Two of the systems that supply energy for muscular contraction are anaerobic.

The ATP-CP System

ATP and CP are high-energy phosphagen compounds stored within the muscle and ready for immediate use. The breakdown of ATP produces adenosine diphosphate (ADP), inorganic phosphate, and energy used in muscular contraction. Creatine phosphate is broken down to create energy that is used to reform ATP.

This system provides an immediate source of energy for the muscle and has a large power capacity. In other words, a large amount of energy per unit time can be supplied through this system. However, because of the small stores of ATP and CP, the total capacity for work with the ATP-CP system is limited. In fact, the energy resources from the ATP-CP system will be exhausted in 30 seconds or less during an all-out bout of exercise (3,4).

Anaerobic Glycolysis System

Glycolysis refers to a series of reactions resulting in the breakdown of carbohydrate into pyruvate or lactate. Anaerobic glycolysis means that this breakdown of carbohydrate is performed in the absence of oxygen. Without oxygen, glycolysis produces lactate.

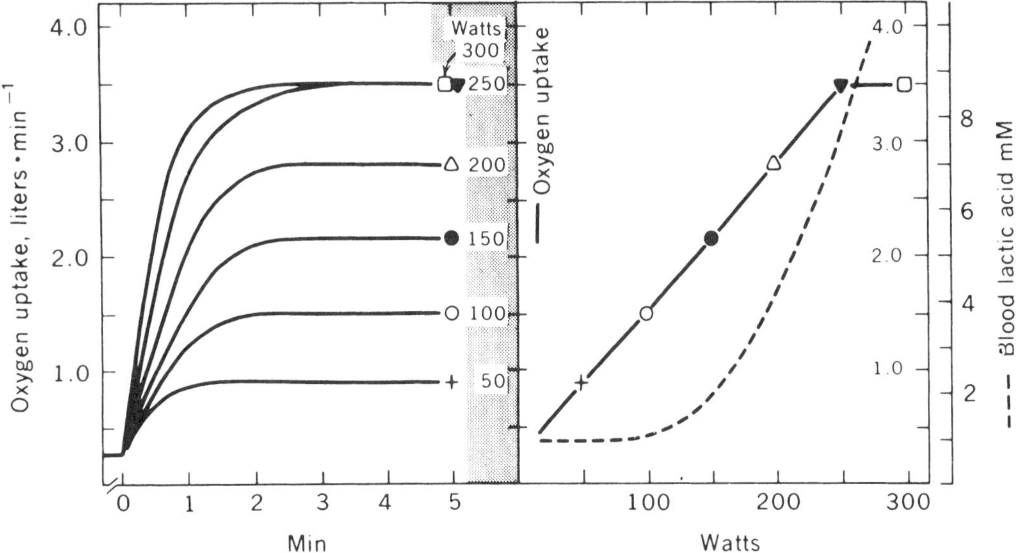

FIG. 28-2. Schematic demonstration of the determination of maximal oxygen uptake. **Left:** Oxygen uptake increases during five minute exercise stages on a bicycle ergometer at different work loads (noted within the **shadowed area**). **Right:** Oxygen uptake at each workload measured after 5 minutes, plotted in relation to workload. Note that there was no additional increase in oxygen uptake between the 250-W and 300-W workloads. Maximal oxygen uptake is 3.5 liters/min. Blood lactic acid concentrations across each workload are also demonstrated. (With permission from Astrand PO, Rodahl K. *Textbook of work physiology: physiological basis of exercise, 3rd ed.* New York: McGraw-Hill, 1986.)

During maximal exercise that lasts 1 to 3 minutes, lactic acid accumulates in the muscles and blood. When the concentration of lactic acid is high enough, nerve endings are stimulated, resulting in the sensation of pain. In addition, the lactic acid within the muscle cell inhibits the production of more ATP (5) and the binding of calcium to troponin (6), which is part of the series of events leading to muscle contraction. Therefore, the amount of energy obtained from the anaerobic glycolysis system is limited by these effects. Nevertheless, the anaerobic glycolysis system is extremely important because it can provide a rapid supply of energy. It can also produce a larger amount of energy than the ATP-CP system even though it cannot supply the muscle with as much energy per unit time as the ATP-CP system.

Aerobic Metabolism

In the presence of oxygen, glycolysis produces pyruvate, which is further metabolized through the tricarboxylic acid (TCA) cycle (also known as the Krebs or citric acid cycle) and electron transport system to yield carbon dioxide, water, and energy. Relative to anaerobic glycolysis, the energy produced from a given amount of carbohydrate is about 13 times greater through aerobic metabolism. Furthermore, there are no fatiguing or painful by-products through aerobic metabolism, and not only carbohydrate but fats and proteins may be metabolized aerobically. Although the ability to metabolize fat means that this system provides a virtually unlimited source of energy, aerobic metabolism provides energy at the slowest rate of the three energy systems.

The Energy Continuum

All three energy systems supply a portion of energy to the body at all times. However, one energy system may predominate during a particular activity. Which energy systems are predominant during a given activity depends on the rate of energy (power) requirement during the activity (Fig. 28-3). In activities performed at maximal intensity for only a few seconds, most of the ATP is supplied by the ATP-CP

TABLE 28-1. *Characteristics of the three metabolic systems*

Metabolic system	Substrate (fuel)	Oxygen required	Speed of ATP mobilization	Total ATP production capacity
Anaerobic metabolism				
ATP-CP system	Stored phosphagens	No	Very fast	Very limited
Glycolysis	Glycogen/glucose	No	Fast	Limited
Aerobic metabolism	Glycogen/glucose, fats	Yes	Slow	Virtually unlimited

ATP adenosine triphosphate; ATP-CP, adenosine triphosphate—creatine phosphate.

Adapted from Fox EL, Mathews DK. *The physiological basis of physical education and athletics.* Philadelphia: WB Saunders, 1981.

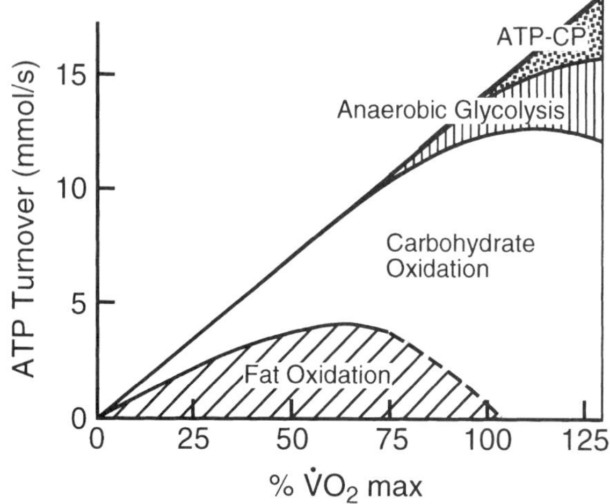

FIG. 28-3. Relative importance of the different metabolic systems as a function of exercise intensity. (Adapted from Sahlin K. Metabolic changes limiting muscle performance. In: Saltin B, ed. *Biochemistry of exercise VI.* Champaign, IL: Human Kinetics, 1986; 323–343.)

system. Activities of lower intensity, such as those at a maximal effort that can be sustained for 1 to 2 minutes, primarily rely on the anaerobic glycolysis system. Longer-duration, lower-intensity activities that may last several minutes or hours are supplied almost entirely through aerobic metabolism.

During a graded exercise test, blood lactate concentration remains relatively constant until a critical work rate is reached, at which time lactate begins to accumulate in the blood (Fig. 28-2). This accumulation does not indicate the onset of anaerobic glycolysis but rather is the result of the rate of lactate production exceeding its rate of removal.

Fuel Utilization

The three fuels that may be used to generate ATP for muscular contraction are carbohydrate, fat, and protein. These fuels differ in the amount of oxygen required for metabolization to the end products of carbon dioxide and water (Table 28-2). Thus, the amount of carbon dioxide produced relative to the amount of oxygen utilized (the respiratory quotient [RQ]) differs among fuels. During exercise, this ratio is referred to as the respiratory exchange ratio (RER) rather than RQ. This distinction is made because the rate of carbon dioxide exhalation increases out of proportion to metabolism whenever metabolic acidosis exists, as occurs at high exercise intensities. Metabolic acidosis is buffered by the bicarbonate system with nonmetabolic carbon dioxide produced as a byproduct. Therefore, at maximal exertion during dynamic exercise, an RER greater than 1.1 is expected. In fact, an RER greater than 1.1 is frequently used as a criterion to assess whether maximal exertion was achieved with graded dynamic exercise testing.

TABLE 28-2. *Characteristics of the different metabolic substrates*

Fuel	Energy content (kcal/g)	Oxygen equivalent (kcal/liter)	Respiratory quotient (RQ)
Carbohydrate	4.1	5.0	1.00
Fat	9.3	4.7	0.70
Protein	4.3	4.4	0.80

Because fat serves as the primary form of stored energy in the body, it is fortunate that it has a caloric density that is much higher than carbohydrate (9.3 compared with 4.1 kcal/g). However, slightly less energy (4.7 compared with 5.0 kcal/liter) is produced from every liter of oxygen when fat is used compared with carbohydrate. Amino acids can also be metabolized to produce energy for muscular contraction, although this contribution is generally negligible.

The fuel used during exercise is influenced by several factors including the exercise intensity and duration, preexercise diet, mode of exercise, and level of fitness. As the intensity of the exercise is increased, the predominant fuel source shifts toward carbohydrate. This is partly because ATP production shifts toward anaerobic metabolism during high-intensity exercise and carbohydrate is the only fuel available for anaerobic glycolysis. Carbohydrates are made available to the contracting muscle through mobilization of muscle and liver glycogen stores as well as through ingested carbohydrates that are circulating in the bloodstream.

Exercise duration also has an effect on the fuel utilization pattern. Fat usage gradually increases during long bouts of exercise. Free fatty acids are made available to the contracting muscle through lipolysis of triglycerides within extramuscular (e.g., adipose) and muscular stores. The type of diet consumed before exercise affects fuel utilization during exercise. During prolonged exercise, carbohydrate is more

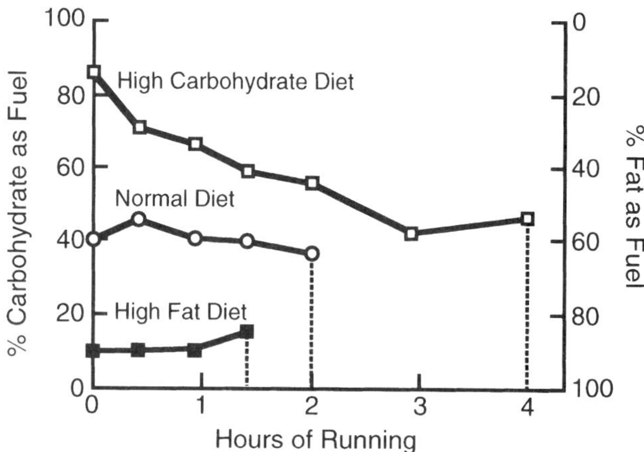

FIG. 28-4. Effect of three different diets on fuel source used during running. *Vertical bars* represent the points at which exhaustion occurred. (Based on data from Christensen EH, Hansen O. Arbeitsfahigkeit und Ermahrung. *Skand Arch Physiol* 1939; 8:160–175.)

likely to be used when one has been eating a diet rich in carbohydrates (Fig. 28-4).

The mode of exercise can also influence the fuel source used during exercise. Exercise that localizes the work to a small muscle mass will tend to use a greater proportion of carbohydrate as fuel.

Finally, training status can affect the composition of the fuel used during exercise. Adaptations to endurance training increase the ability of muscles to use free fatty acids as a fuel and spare glycogen (9,10).

MUSCLE PHYSIOLOGY

Structure and Function of Muscle

Morphology

Skeletal muscle is made up of structural and functional subunits as displayed in Figure 28-5. The largest subunit of a muscle is the fascicle. Within the fascicle is found anywhere from one to hundreds of muscle fibers, the individual muscle cells. At each of these structural levels is a different connective tissue covering.

Myofibrils are found within the muscle cells. The smallest functional subunit of the myofibril is the sarcomere. Sarcomeres are aligned end to end to form a myofibril. Myofibrils contain two basic protein filaments, a thicker one called myosin and a thinner one called actin. These proteins are arranged in such a way as to give skeletal muscle its striated appearance. Sarcomeres run from one Z-line to the next Z-line.

Sliding Filament Theory

The primary function of muscle is to shorten and develop tension. The sliding filament theory (Fig. 28-6) provides an explanation of how muscle fibers shorten and so develop tension.

On stimulation from the motor axon, calcium ions are released from storage in the sarcoplasmic reticulum, exposing active binding sites on the actin and allowing ac-

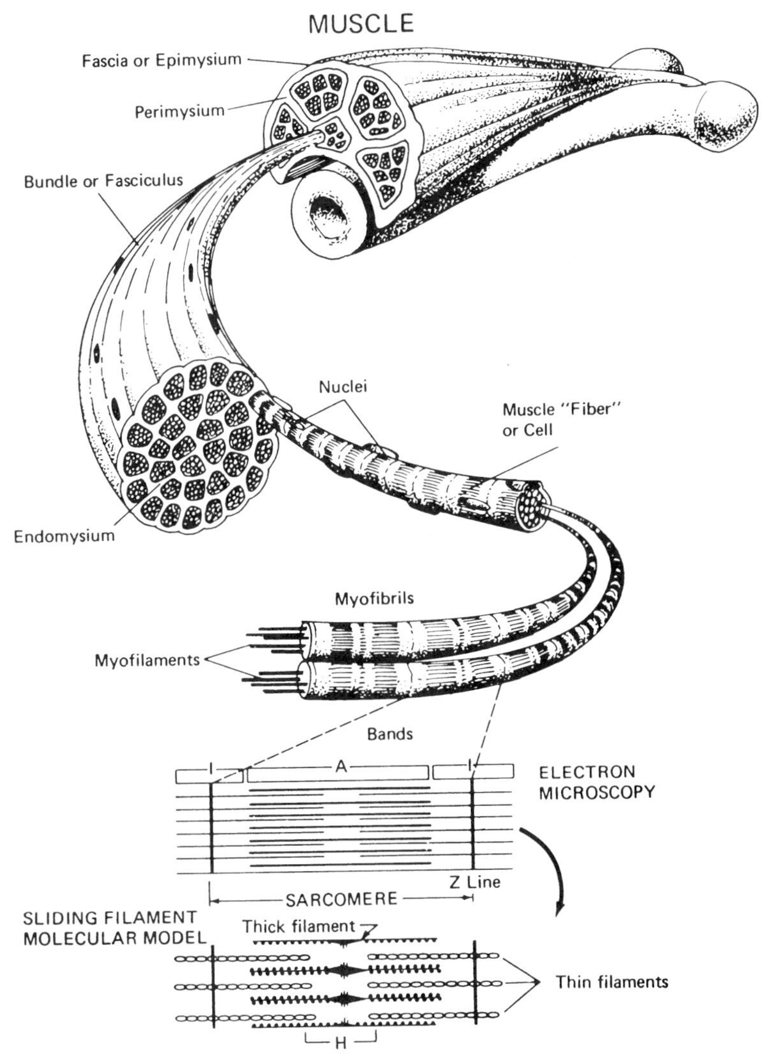

FIG. 28-5. Structural and functional subunits of skeletal muscle. (With permission from Lamb DR. *Physiology of exercise: Responses and adaptations, 2nd ed.* New York: Macmillan, 1984.).

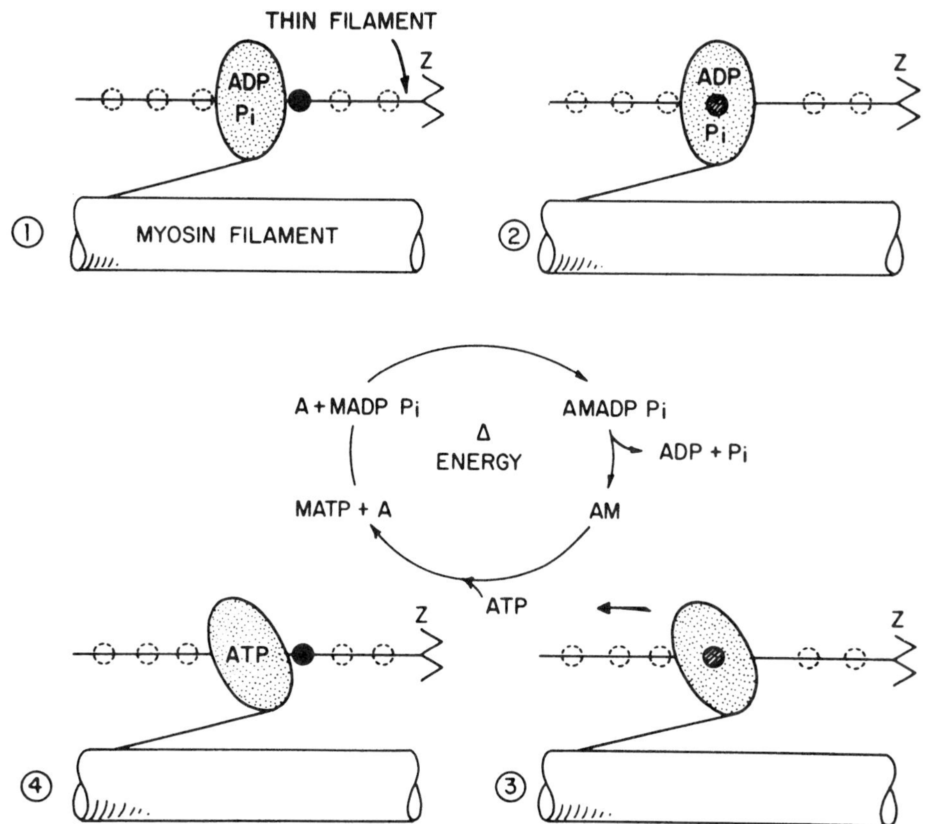

FIG. 28-6. Postulated mechanism of cross-bridge formation and cycling by actin and myosin filaments. The head of the myosin filament is stippled and forms the cross-bridge between the two filaments. Active sites on the actin (thin) filament are outlined by *broken circles*. **1:** No bonds between filaments. **2:** Initial attachment of myosin head to one of the active sites on the actin filament. This attachment takes place only in the presence of Ca^{2+} ions. **3:** Formation of strong actin–myosin bond. This process causes a conformational change in the angle of the myosin head, which produces a relative movement of actin and myosin filaments across one another. ADP and phosphate ions are lost from the myosin; **4:** If ATP is available, the actin–myosin bond can be broken. Subsequent hydrolysis of the ATP by the myosin ATPase returns the cycle to stage **1**. If no ATP is available, the actin–myosin bond remains intact, as in muscular rigor. (From Gordon AM. Muscle. In: Ruch T, Patton H, eds. *Physiology and biophysics, vol IV.* Philadelphia: WB Saunders, 1982; 170–260, reprinted by permission of W.B. Saunders Co.)

tin–myosin cross-bridge formation. Once the actin–myosin bonds are formed, a conformational change in the angle of the myosin head occurs, causing the actin filaments to be pulled over the myosin filaments and shorten the sarcomere.

For more shortening to occur, ATP is required to break the actin–myosin bond and allow binding of myosin to another actin site closer to the Z-line. The conformation change of the myosin head then occurs resulting in further shortening.

Relaxation of the muscle occurs when stimulation ends. This triggers the active pumping of calcium back into the sarcoplasmic reticulum. The result is a loss of active binding sites on the actin so actin–myosin cross-bridges are broken, and the muscle relaxes.

Mechanical Model

A useful model to understand the mechanical properties of muscles is shown in Figure 28-7. This model consists of the contractile element with both series and parallel elastic elements. The contractile element actively generates force and represents the interaction between actin and myosin filaments. The elastic elements are purely passive components acting as mechanical springs. The series elastic element represents the tendinous insertions of muscle, and the parallel

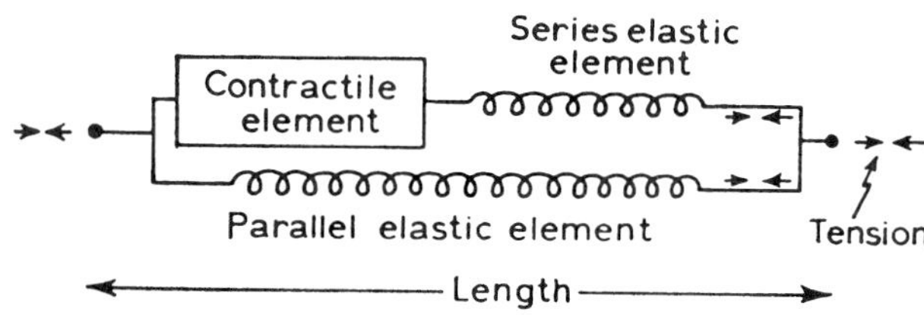

FIG. 28-7. Mechanical model of muscle consisting of a contractile element and two elastic elements. (From Roberts TDM. *Neurophysiology of postural mechanics.* London: Butterworth, 1978.)

TABLE 28-3. *Motor unit type, contractile properties, and metabolic properties of muscle fibers*

	Type I: Slow oxidative (SO)	Type IIA: Fast, oxidative glycolytic (FOG)	Type IIB: Fast glycolytic (FG)
Motor unit type	S	FR	FF
Oxidative capacity	High	Moderately high	Low
Glycolytic capacity	Low	High	Highest
Contractile speed	Slow	Fast	Fast
Fatigue resistance	High	Moderate	Low
Motor unit strength	Low	High	High

FF, fast-fatiguable; FR, fast-fatigue resistant.

elastic element represents the connective tissue surrounding the various subunits of the muscle.

Muscle Fiber Types

Skeletal muscles contain a mixture of muscle fiber types that can be distinguished by their physical and biochemical characteristics. Unfortunately, the nomenclature for classification of muscle fibers has not developed in a uniform manner. Table 28-3 displays the different classification systems and fiber type characteristics.

Recognition that there may be differences in muscles dates back to observations that fowl has meat that is "red" and "white." It has since been learned that the different properties of muscles extend beyond the muscle fiber to the level of the motor unit. Based on contraction speed following a stimulus to the nerve axon, two main categories of motor units can be distinguished—fast units and slow units. Peak tension and relaxation are achieved more rapidly for fast units than slow units (Fig. 28-8). Units with a fast contraction time are composed of muscle fibers with relatively large fiber diameters and are innervated by large, fast-conducting motor neurons. These units also have a larger number of muscle fibers. Compared with the slow units, the fast units produce higher tensions. These fast units are further subdivided into fast fatiguable (FF) units, which fatigue relatively easily, and fast fatigue-resistant (FR) units, which have a high resistance to fatigue similar to the slow units.

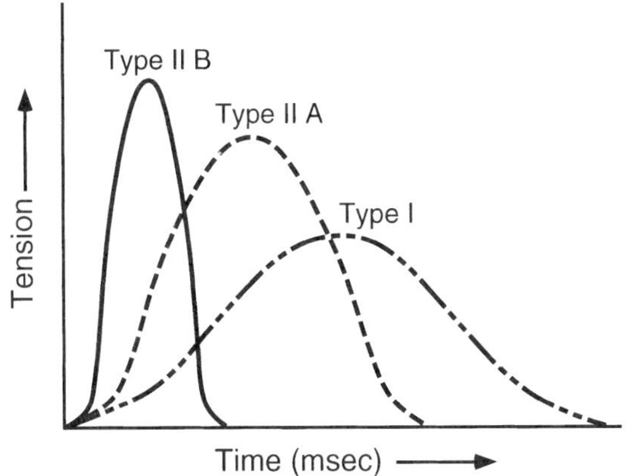

FIG. 28-8. Schematic representation of rate of tension generation and force production with different fiber types. The speed of contraction and force are greatest for type II fibers.

Although the number of fibers per unit and the fiber diameter are larger with fast units, these factors do not fully explain the differences in force production of fast and slow units. It is thought that there are also differences in the mechanism of force production within the fibrils (14).

All fibers from a given motor unit have the same histochemical characteristics. Slow units innervate type I (slow oxidative [SO]) fibers. These fibers are characterized by high activities of succinic dehydrogenase and nicotinamide adenine dinucleotide dehydrogenase, enzymes involved in the major pathways for oxidative metabolism. The type I fibers are also richly supplied by capillaries. As a result, these fibers are suited well for performance of low-intensity, long-duration activities.

Those fibers innervated by fast motor units (fast-twitch or type II fibers) have a high activity of myofibrillar ATPase, the enzyme that breaks down ATP to release energy for contraction. They also have a high capacity for anaerobic metabolism as demonstrated by the high levels of glycogen and phosphorylase. Phosphorylase is an enzyme that is involved in the breakdown of glycogen. As a result, these fibers are suited for performance of high-intensity, short-duration work. Subgroups of fast-twitch fibers include type IIB (fast, glycolytic [FG]) and type IIA (fast, oxidative glycolytic [FOG]) fibers which correspond with FF and FR motor units types, respectively. Compared with the type IIB fibers, the type IIA fibers have a higher activity of oxidative enzymes and a richer capillary supply.

The advantage of having different types of muscle fibers within a muscle is that the characteristics of the muscle are extended beyond that of any single fiber type. It is the proportion of muscle fiber types within a muscle that gives muscles the properties that make them suitable for different functions.

Factors Affecting Muscle Function

Muscle function is affected by a number of factors. It is well recognized that these factors include the state of training and degree of fatigue of the muscle. The specific adaptations of muscle to exercise training, and the relationship of fatigue with muscle function are discussed in later sections. In this section, the interaction of other muscular, neural, and mechanical factors affecting muscle function are discussed.

Muscular Factors

Cross-Sectional Area

Muscle size is one of the most obvious factors affecting strength. In isolated as well as intact muscles, maximal strength is related to the cross-sectional area of the muscle. This relationship probably is related to the greater quantities of actin and myosin and, therefore, greater numbers of cross-bridges that can be activated to produce force when the muscle is larger. Muscles can produce 10 to 20 N/cm^2 of cross-sectional area (15).

Numerous studies have demonstrated changes in muscle cross-sectional area that occur in conjunction with strength changes produced by resistance training or detraining. Nevertheless, strength and muscle cross-sectional area do not change in parallel. It is clear that cross-sectional area of the muscle does not fully account for differences in strength among individuals.

Muscle Fiber Type

As described above, the maximal force and power generation of a muscle is related to the percentage of fast twitch fibers. In other words, muscle that has a high percentage of fast twitch fibers will generate a greater maximal force than the same size muscle with a lower percentage of these fibers.

Neural Factors

Motor Learning and Recruitment

The importance of neural factors in affecting muscular strength has been recognized through the dissociation between changes in strength and muscle size during a strength-training program. The gains in strength during the first few weeks of such training occur without any change in muscle size (16,17). The general consensus is that these early changes reflect neural adaptations that may include improved muscle activation and improved task performance from motor learning and coordination (18). Greater details on the neural adaptations that result from strength training are discussed in the section on strength-training adaptations.

Inhibitory Reflexes

Neural factors may also play a role in inhibition of muscle contraction. A protective reflex mechanism is thought to operate through the Golgi tendon organs that may be of particular importance when large amounts of force are being generated (19,20). Reflex inhibition of muscle contraction can also result through other sensory nerve endings. For instance, it has been demonstrated that quadriceps muscle inhibition is mediated through afferent activity of intracapsular receptors (21). It is also likely that muscle contraction is inhibited through pain reflexes (22–24).

Protective reflex mechanisms are also thought to be involved in what has been called the bilateral deficit. The force developed during bilateral contractions of a given muscle group is less than the sum of the forces developed by each limb independently (25,26). A reduced motor unit stimulation is associated with this bilateral deficit (27).

It may be possible to reduce the influence of protective reflexes through strength training. Hypnosis was shown to increase maximal force produced during forearm flexion by 17% among non-resistance-trained individuals, whereas there was no significant change in a strength-trained individual (28). It was concluded that strength training may induce an inhibition of the protective reflex mechanisms. Furthermore, the bilateral deficit has been shown to be reduced through training with bilateral contractions (29).

The protective reflexes may be reduced in another way. Strength of a muscle group is increased when its activity is immediately preceded by contraction of the antagonist muscle group (30). The precontraction is thought to reduce the neural protective mechanism, allowing a greater force production.

Mechanical Factors

Force–Velocity Relationship

The maximum force a muscle can exert is dependent on the speed at which it is contracting. The maximal isometric force of a muscle is always greater than the force that can be exerted during shortening, and the maximal force exerted during lengthening is always greater than that exerted during isometric contraction. This relationship is displayed in Figure 28-9.

It is thought that the shape of the force–velocity curve is explained on the basis of the sliding filament theory of muscle contraction (14). During a maximal isometric contraction, all cross-bridges are formed. However, during shortening, there is an increase in the rate of detachment of cross-bridges and an increase in the number of attached cross-bridges that exert negative force. The result is a decrease in the total force exerted when the muscle is shortening. During lengthening contractions, the rate of detachment of cross-bridges is slower than during a shortening contraction at the

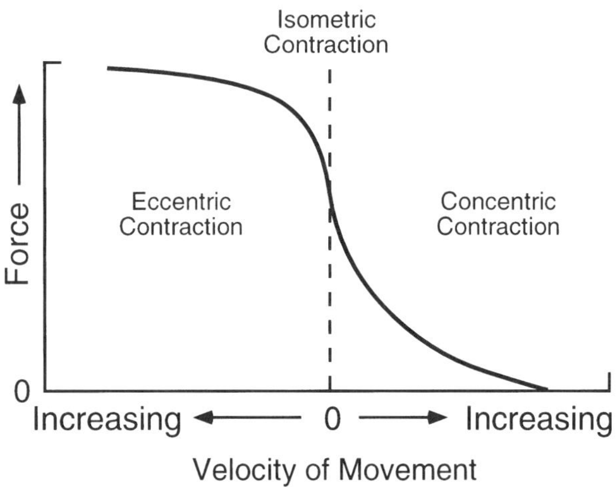

FIG. 28-9. Schematic relationship between maximal muscular force and velocity of movement.

same velocity. The effect is that cross-bridges are forcibly detached, and a greater force is exerted than during shortening contractions.

Positive Versus Negative Work

Besides the difference in maximal force production through concentric and eccentric contractions, there is also a difference in energy cost for performing work through concentric (positive work) and eccentric (negative work) contractions. The energy cost for negative work is dramatically less than that for performing the same amount of positive work (Fig. 28-10). This phenomenon is thought to be linked to the requirement for ATP for the detachment and resetting of the cross-bridges in concentric work but not in eccentric work (Fig. 28-11).

Short-Range Stiffness

When a maximally activated muscle is forcibly lengthened, the force produced by the muscle is greater than that produced isometrically (Fig. 28-9). However, the situation may be different when the muscle is contracting submaximally. Forced lengthening of a partially contracted muscle results in an initial resistance greater than that produced isometrically, but the resistance may then fall below that produced isometrically (34). This phenomenon is referred to as short-range stiffness and is thought to be accounted for as follows. The rapid rise in tension at the beginning of forced lengthening results from stretch of attached actin–myosin cross-bridges. The stiffness of the muscle is very high while the cross-bridges are still attached. However, once the cross-bridges begin to dissociate, it is thought that the formation of new cross-bridges occurs more slowly in a partially activated muscle, and so the number of attached cross-bridges and the force produced are diminished.

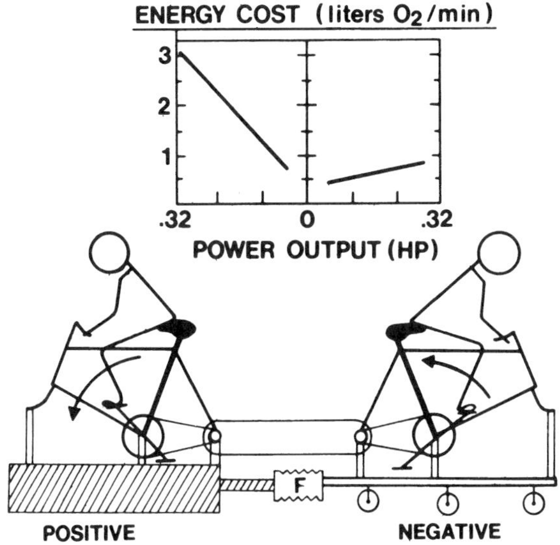

FIG. 28-10. Demonstration of the difference in energy cost between positive and negative work. The two subjects pedaled coupled bicycles with one pedaling forward (performing positive work) and the other providing the resistance as the cranks rotated backwards (performing an equal amount of negative work). **Graph inset** shows the differences in energy costs across the examined power outputs. (From Cavanagh PR, Kram R. Mechanical and muscular factors affecting the efficiency of human movement. *Med Sci Sports Exerc* 1985; 17:326–331, reprinted by permission of Williams & Wilkins. Figure based on data from Abbott BC, Bigland B, Ritchie JM. The physiological cost of negative work. *J Physiol* 1952; 117:380–390.)

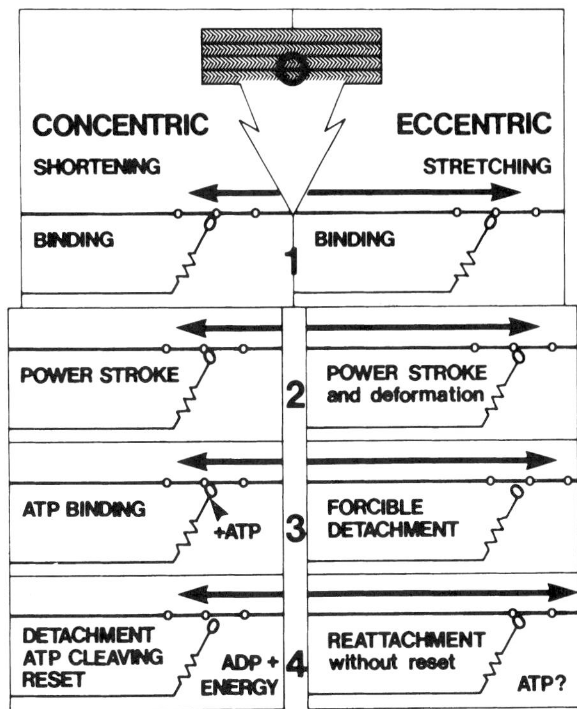

FIG. 28-11. Schematic comparison of the cross-bridge formation and cycling during concentric and eccentric work. ATP is required for the detachment and resetting of the cross-bridges in concentric work but not in eccentric work. (From Cavanagh PR, Kram R. Mechanical and muscular factors affecting the efficiency of human movement. *Med Sci Sports Exerc* 1985; 17:326–331, reprinted by permission of Williams & Wilkins. Figure based on data from White DCS. Muscle mechanics. In: Alexander RMcN, Goldspeak G, eds. *Mechanics and energetics of animal locomotion.* London: Chapman and Hall, 1977; 23–56.)

Short-range stiffness is important in the initial part of the response of a limb to a disturbing force. For instance, partial contraction of agonist and antagonist muscles about a joint increases the mechanical stiffness of the joint and can provide considerable resistance to pertubating forces such as those that might be encountered while walking across a crowded room with a full glass.

Muscle Orientation and Attachment

The distance a tendon is inserted from the axis of rotation affects the torque generated by that muscle. For a given

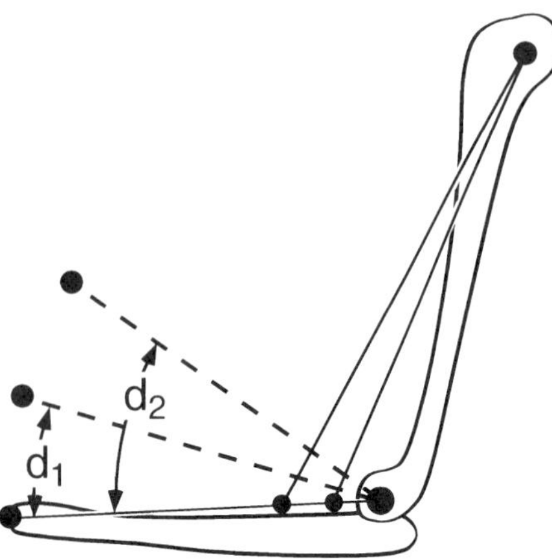

FIG. 28-12. Schematic representation of the effect of tendon insertion site on excursion. The excursion from a more proximally inserted muscle may be double that of a more distally inserted muscle for the same amount of shortening. Whereas a tendon insertion closer to the center of rotation will allow greater excursion, torque production will be reduced for a given tension developed in the muscle.

tension developed by a muscle, a tendon insertion farther from the center of rotation will allow greater torque production, although angular range will be reduced (Fig. 28-12). This anatomic effect allows some muscles to be more suited for production of large forces than others. Small anatomic variations may also account for some of the performance differences among individuals.

Length–Tension Relationship

The tension produced by a muscle is affected not only by the contractile elements but also by passive stretch of the elastic elements (Fig. 28-7). When relaxed muscle is passively stretched beyond its resting length, tension progressively develops (Fig. 28-13). Maximal contraction of the muscle at different lengths yields another length–tension curve. Subtraction of the passive tension from the total tension of the contracting muscle yields a closer representation of the actual tension produced by the contractile elements. The greatest tension generated by the contractile mechanism is at the resting length of the muscle, and the greatest total tension is at a length slightly longer than resting length.

The influence of length on the force produced by the contractile mechanism is related to the way in which the actin and myosin filaments interact at the sarcomere level. Figure 28-14 shows the length–tension relationship for a single muscle fiber and the overlap of the actin and myosin filaments in a single sarcomere. As the overlap between actin and myosin increases, so does the tension production. Maximal tension is developed at lengths yielding maximal contact of actin and myosin filaments. As the sarcomere length decreases further, the actin filaments begin to overlap. It is believed that this interferes with cross-bridge formation and causes a decline in tension development. Variations among sarcomeres and muscle fibers cause the length–tension curve to be more rounded for a whole muscle.

An example of the effect of muscle length on force production is apparent by the position of the wrist during a hand grip. While gripping, the wrist is maintained in extension by contraction of the wrist extensor muscles of the forearm. This allows the finger flexor muscles to be at a more optimal part of the length–tension curve. In this way, a more powerful hand grip is produced.

Leverage Effect

The leverage effect relates to the mechanical advantage offered by the angle of tendon insertion. The torque produced by a muscle is dependent on the sine of the insertion angle. When the insertion angle is 90°, the torque production is greatest for a given tension in the muscle.

Torque production is the net result of the length–tension relationship and the leverage effect. As a result of the force–velocity relationship, the torque production for a given movement is also dependent on the velocity of movement. Figure 28-15 displays an isokinetic torque curve for a movement commonly tested in the clinical setting.

Force Transmission

A manner in which muscle force transmission is thought to vary without changing the tension developed in the muscle fibers is through a change in the elastic elements described in the mechanical model discussed previously (Fig. 28-7). A decrease in the elasticity of these elements would allow

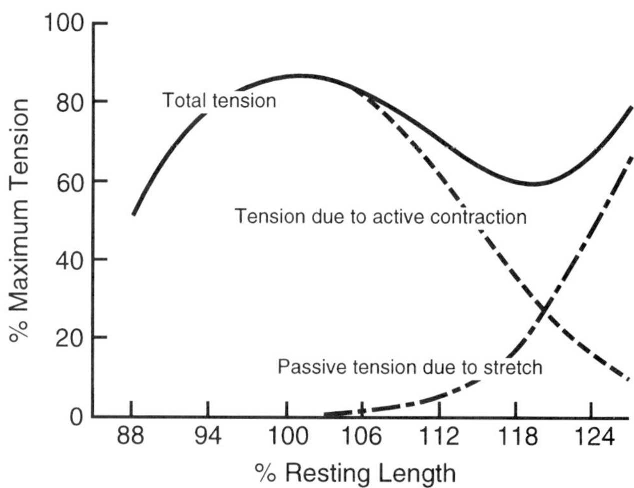

FIG. 28-13. Length–tension diagram for passive stretch of an unstimulated muscle and total tension when the muscle is maximally stimulated. Active tension resulting solely from muscular contraction is obtained by subtracting the passive-stretch curve from the total-tension curve. Normal resting length is 100%. (Redrawn from Schottelius BA, Senay LC. Effect of stimulation-length sequence on shape of length–tension diagram. *Am J Physiol* 1956; 186:127–130.)

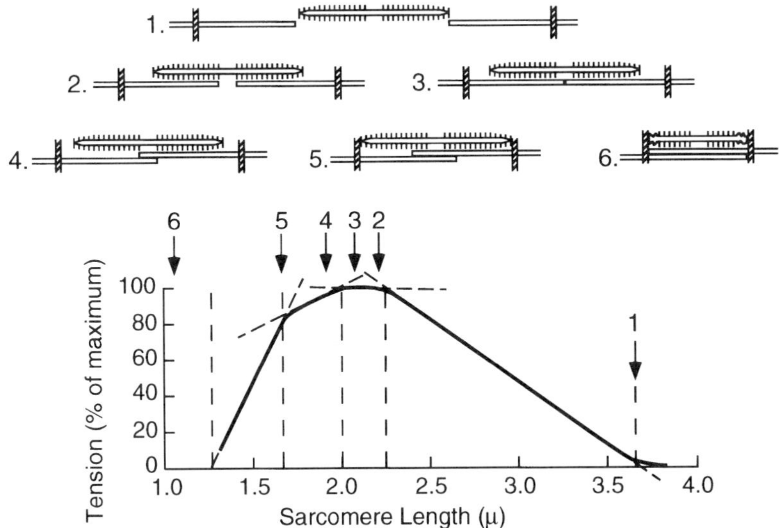

FIG. 28-14. Relationship between sarcomere length and tension generation. The amount of overlap between actin and myosin filaments within each sarcomere is shown; the length of each sarcomere is given above, and the tension for each condition is shown below. Maximal tension is produced when there is the greatest overlap between filaments *(points 2 and 3)*. Tension drops if the overlap is less or if the actin filaments contact each other. (Adapted from Gordon AM, Huxley AF, Julian FJ. The variation in isometric tension with sarcomere length in vertebrate muscle fibres. *J Physiol* 1966; 184:170–192.)

a greater proportion of the force generated by the sarcomere to be transmitted to the skeletal system. With training, tensile strength of connective tissue is known to increase (38). Such changes may improve force transmission of a muscle.

Elastic Storage and Recovery

Storage and recovery of elastic energy in the muscle–tendon unit occurs when an active prestretch immediately precedes a shortening contraction. This combination of eccentric and concentric contractions is a natural type of movement that has been referred to as the ''stretch-shortening cycle'' (39,40) and allows a greater concentric force production or power output than when the prestretch does not occur. In effect, this phenomenon modifies the length–tension curve so that at a given muscle length, the force produced is greater than without the prestretch. The precise location and mechanism of the elastic storage is not clear, but it has been attributed to compliance of the cross-bridges and connective tissue.

The greater force from a concentric contraction when immediately preceded by an eccentric contraction is a common feature of normal movement. An example of the use of elastic storage in this manner is the knee and hip flexion that

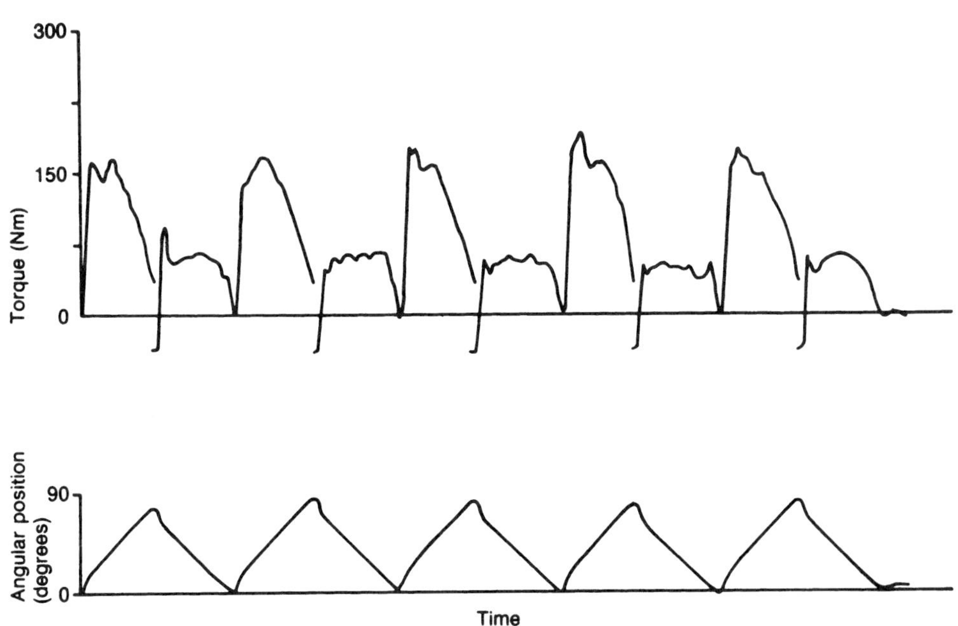

FIG. 28-15. Real-time display of gravity-corrected torque and angular position during a knee extension–flexion isokinetic test. (From Baltzopoulos V, Brodie DA. Isokinetic dynamometry: applications and limitations. *Sports Med* 1989; 8:101–116.)

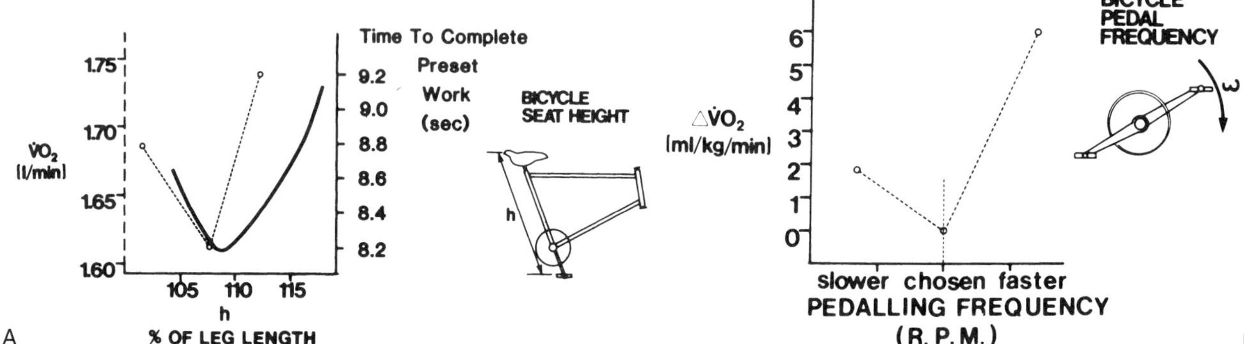

FIG. 28-16. A and B: Optimal phenomenon in bicycling. Both seat height and pedaling frequency show an optimal point at which energy cost for producing a given power output is minimized. Maximal power output is also related to seat height by a parabolic curve. (From Cavanagh PR, Kram R. Mechanical and muscular factors affecting the efficiency of human movement. *Med Sci Sports Exerc* 1985; 17:326–331, reprinted by permission of Williams & Wilkins. Figure based on data from Nordeen-Snyder K. The effect of bicycle seat height variation upon oxygen consumption and lower limb kinematics. *Med Sci Sports* 1977; 9:113–117; Hamley EJ, Thomas V. Physiological and postural factors in the calibration of the bicycle ergometer. *J Physiol* 1967; 191:55P–57P; Hagberg JM, Mullin JP, Giese MD, Spitznagel E. Effect of pedaling rate on submaximal exercise responses of competitive cyclists. *J Appl Physiol* 1981; 51:447–451.)

occurs immediately before jumping. The most dramatic example of the use of elastic storage and recovery to affect the energy cost of movement is seen with the big red kangaroo. This animal actually uses less energy per unit time as its speed increases as a result of greater use of elastic storage and recovery (41).

Optimal Phenomena

The mechanical properties of muscles are important in accounting for what has been referred to as "optimal phenomena" (31). One such phenomenon is how the aerobic demand of riding a bicycle at a given power output is altered by the seat height. A height can be identified that minimizes aerobic demand and maximizes power output (Fig. 28-16). Another example of optimal phenomena in cycling relates to pedaling rate. There is a pedaling frequency at which the aerobic demand to generate a given power output is minimized (Fig. 28-16). Individuals also have a stride length that optimizes the aerobic demands of running (Fig. 28-17) and a walking speed that optimizes the aerobic demands for walking a given distance (Fig. 28-18).

The critical observation to understanding these optimal phenomena has come from the work of Hill (47). He showed that the force–velocity curve could be used to generate a power–velocity curve that shows a point of optimality (Fig. 28-19). Then, by considering the energy cost of developing muscle tension under various conditions, a muscle efficiency–velocity curve was generated that also showed a point of optimality. Thus, the changing of pedaling or stride rate can be considered as moving along the velocity axis of the muscle-efficiency curve. The interaction of the length–tension relationship is also important for some of the optimal phenomena.

Muscular Fatigue and Endurance

Endurance and work intensity are related by hyperbolic functions as demonstrated in Figures 28-20 and 28-21. At high intensities, work can be continued for only short durations, whereas at low intensities, work can be continued much longer. The portion of the curve approaching the time axis is predominantly determined by the capacity for aerobic metabolism, whereas the portion of the curve approaching the intensity axis is predominantly determined by the capacity for anaerobic metabolism. The portion with greatest curvilinearity is determined by a combination of aerobic and anaerobic capabilities.

Most exercise is performed at submaximal levels. At the

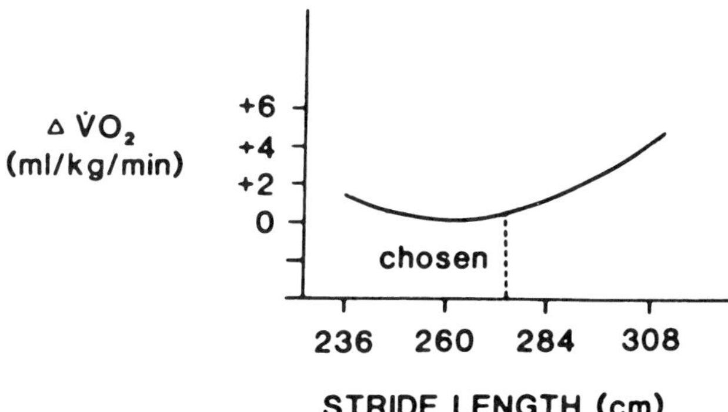

FIG. 28-17. Optimal phenomena in running. For a given running speed, there is a stride length at which energy cost is minimized. The freely chosen stride length is typically close to optimal. (From Cavanagh PR, Williams KR. The effect of stride length variation on oxygen uptake during distance running. *Med Sci Sports Exerc* 1982; 14:30–35, reprinted by permission of Williams & Wilkins.)

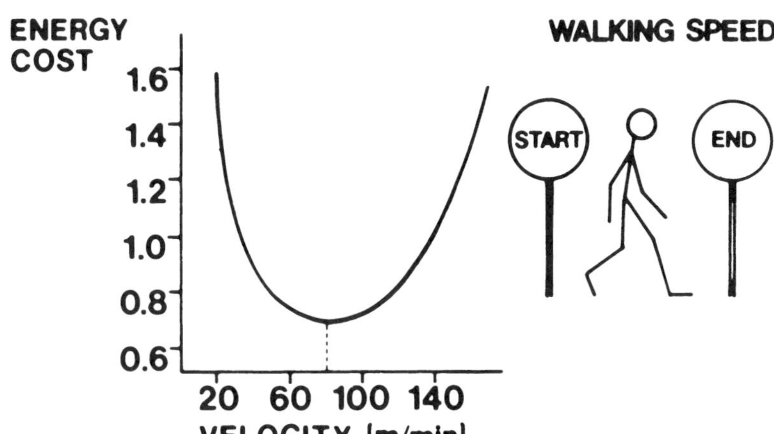

FIG. 28-18. Optimal phenomena during walking. A speed exists at which energy cost per unit distance is minimized. Energy cost is shown here in units of kilocalories per kilogram body mass per meter traveled. (From Cavanagh PR, Kram R. Mechanical and muscular factors affecting the efficiency of human movement. *Med Sci Sports Exerc* 1985; 17:326–331, reprinted by permission of Williams & Wilkins. Figure based on data of Ralston JH. Energy–speed relation and optimal speed during level walking. *Int Z Angew Physiol* 1958; 17:277–283.)

onset of exercise, there is little sense of effort, but as the exercise is continued, performance is eventually reduced. This has led to the concept that fatigue is delayed in onset. However, the maximal force one can generate begins to decline from the onset of even submaximal work with the same muscle group (Fig. 28-22). Therefore, it may be preferable to think of fatigue as ''any reduction in the maximal force-generating capacity'' (52).

Another conceptual issue relates to the common belief that fatigue is a failure of normal physiological function. Perhaps it is more appropriate to consider fatigue as a protective mechanism for survival. Fatigue prevents the onset of irreversible muscle rigor and protects the subsequent recovery process.

The causes of fatigue have received considerable attention but have not been clearly established. It is evident that multiple factors are involved, and the relative importance of each is dependent on the fiber type composition of the contracting muscle, the intensity, type, and duration of the contractile activity, and the individual's fitness and motivation level. For instance, the fatigue experienced from high-intensity short-duration exercise such as weight lifting is dependent on factors different from those causing fatigue during low-intensity long-duration endurance exercise.

In daily life, a reduction in power output is frequently limited by central neural drive. Nevertheless, when motiva-

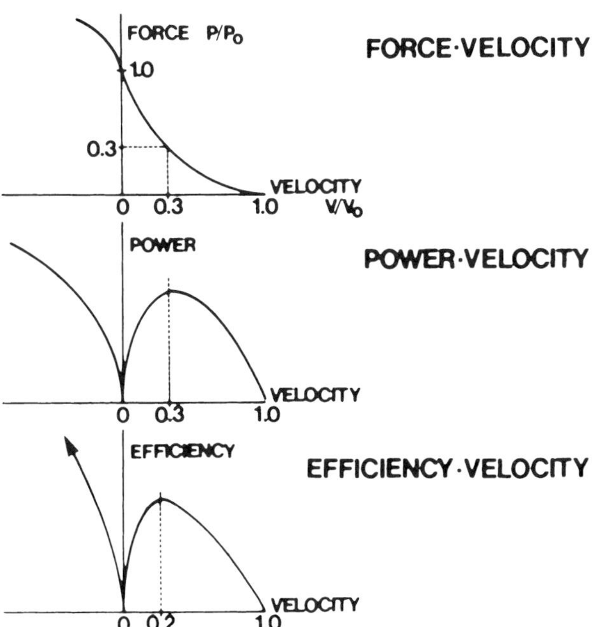

FIG. 28-19. Optimal phenomena can be explained by derivations from the force–velocity relationship. The power–velocity curve is obtained from the product of force and velocity and demonstrates an optimal point. Energetic data allow generation of the efficiency–velocity curve, which also shows an optimal point. (From Cavanagh PR, Kram R. Mechanical and muscular factors affecting the efficiency of human movement. *Med Sci Sports Exerc* 1985; 17:326–331, reprinted by permission of Williams & Wilkins. Figure based on Hill AV. The maximal work and mechanical efficiency of human muscles and their most economical speed. *J Physiol* 1922; 56:19–41.)

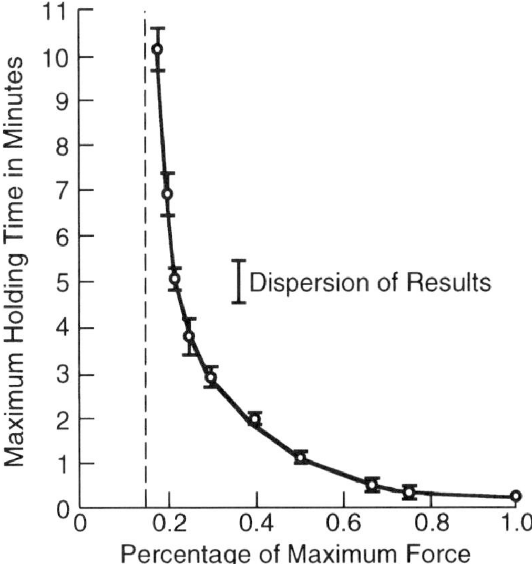

FIG. 28-20. Isometric endurance as a function of percentage of maximal strength. (Adapted from Rohment W. Ermittlung von erholungspausen fur statische arbeit des menschen. *Int Z Angew Physiol* 1960; 18:123–164.)

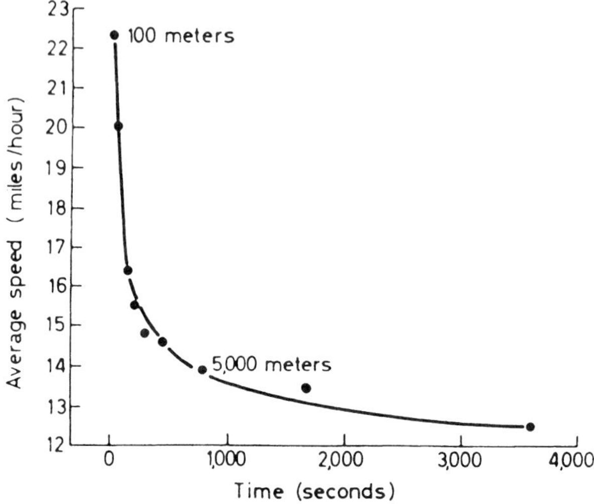

FIG. 28-21. Relationship of running speed to exercise duration for world record runs. (From Simonson E. Recovery and fatigue. In: Simonson E, ed. *Physiology of work capacity and fatigue.* Springfield, IL: Charles C Thomas, 1971; 440—458, reprinted by permission of Charles C. Thomas, Publisher, Ltd., Springfield, Illinois. Figure based on data from Lloyd BB. World running records as maximal performances: oxygen debt and other limiting factors. *Circ Res* 1967; 20–21[Suppl 1]:I218–I226.)

tion is high, the primary sites of muscular fatigue are thought to be within the muscle cell rather than the central nervous system or the neuromuscular junction. Specifically, it is thought that fatigue may result from disturbances in the surface membrane, excitation–contraction coupling, or metabolic events (53).

ACUTE PHYSIOLOGICAL RESPONSES TO EXERCISE

Dynamic Exercise

Acute physiological adjustments occur in most bodily systems with dynamic exercise. Collectively, these adjustments increase the availability of oxygen and nutrients to the active muscle cells, remove exercise-induced metabolic byproducts (e.g., carbon dioxide, lactate, heat), and maintain an appropriate internal milieu (pH, body fluid, etc.) for bodily function.

Dynamic work effort is typically expressed in either absolute units (e.g., $\dot{V}O_2$ in liters per minute) or relative units (e.g., percentage of an individual's $\dot{V}O_{2max}$). Absolute units provide a measure of work performed per unit time, whereas relative units reflect the degree of effort or how strenuous the work feels. Most physiological changes with exercise are primarily proportional to relative work units (54). This includes heart rate, ventilation, sympathetic/parasympathetic

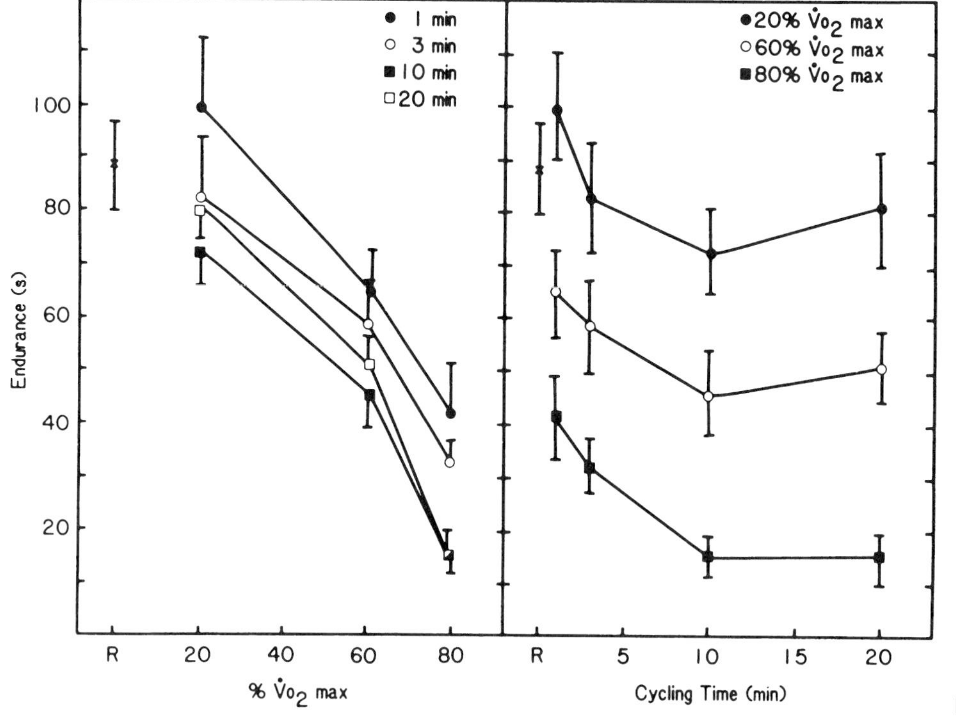

FIG. 28-22. Effect of leg cycling at different intensities and durations on endurance of isometric knee extension at 40% of rested maximal voluntary contraction. **Panel A** shows the data as a function of the workload, and **panel B** shows the data as a function of duration of cycling. Mean isometric endurance in the rested state is displayed at *R*. (With permission from Hoffman MD, Williams CA, Lind AR. Changes in isometric function following rhythmic exercise. *Eur J Appl Physiol* 1985; 54:177–183.)

nerve outflow, circulating hormones, and core temperature. The one parameter that rises more in proportion to absolute work performed than relative intensity is cardiac output, which increases about 5 to 6 liters/min for each 1 liter/min rise in $\dot{V}o_2$ (55).

Many of the cardiovascular adjustments to dynamic exercise are regulated by changes in autonomic nervous activity outflow (56–59). Parasympathetic tone exists at rest, and its withdrawal at the onset of exercise allows heart rate to rise. When work intensity reaches about 50% $\dot{V}o_{2max}$, parasympathic withdrawal appears to be exhausted, and any further rise in heart rate is totally dependent on increased sympathetic nerve activity. In addition to increasing heart rate, sympathetic nerve activity increases myocardial contractility, mobilizes nutrients, influences several circulating hormone levels, and contributes to blood flow redistribution by vasoconstriction in inactive regions. Although muscle sympathetic nerve activity appears to increase in the working muscles, metabolic byproducts override this vasoconstriction effect to produce vasodilation. Control of the autonomic nervous system during exercise originates from both central and peripheral receptors located in the motor cortex, ergoreceptors, and arterial baroreceptors (59–61).

The rise in cardiac output (about four- to sixfold at maximal effort) with upright exercise stems from a rise in heart rate (two- to threefold) and stroke volume (about 50%) (55,62). The rise in stroke volume results from increased myocardial preload and contractility (55,63,64). Preload increases as a result of enhanced venous return, which is brought on by venoconstriction and muscle contraction. An increase in contractility leads to more complete emptying of the heart (i.e., decreased left ventricular end-systolic volume), whereas an increase in preload increases left ventricular end-diastolic volume; the net effect is increased stroke volume.

Up to 80% of cardiac output can be distributed to the active muscles at maximal effort compared to only about 20% of cardiac output being distributed to the muscles at rest. As illustrated in Figure 28-23, this marked blood flow redistribution is accomplished by arterial vasodilation in the active muscles and arterial vasocontriction in other vascular regions (e.g., splanchnic, inactive muscle, renal) (1,55,62,66). Total systemic vascular resistance declines progressively with increasing work intensity. The precise mechanisms leading to vasodilation in the active muscle remain debatable but likely stem from changes in several local factors including potassium, hydrogen ion, endothelium-relaxing factor, adenosine, osmolarity, and others (67,68).

Oxygen extraction rate is high within the active muscle. This, combined with the increased percentage of blood flow directed to the muscles, leads to an approximately threefold increase in arteriovenous oxygen difference at maximal exercise (55).

Systolic blood pressure rises progressively with increased dynamic work load while diastolic blood pressure generally remains relatively unchanged. The net effect is a modest increase in mean arterial blood pressure (usually less than 20 mm Hg).

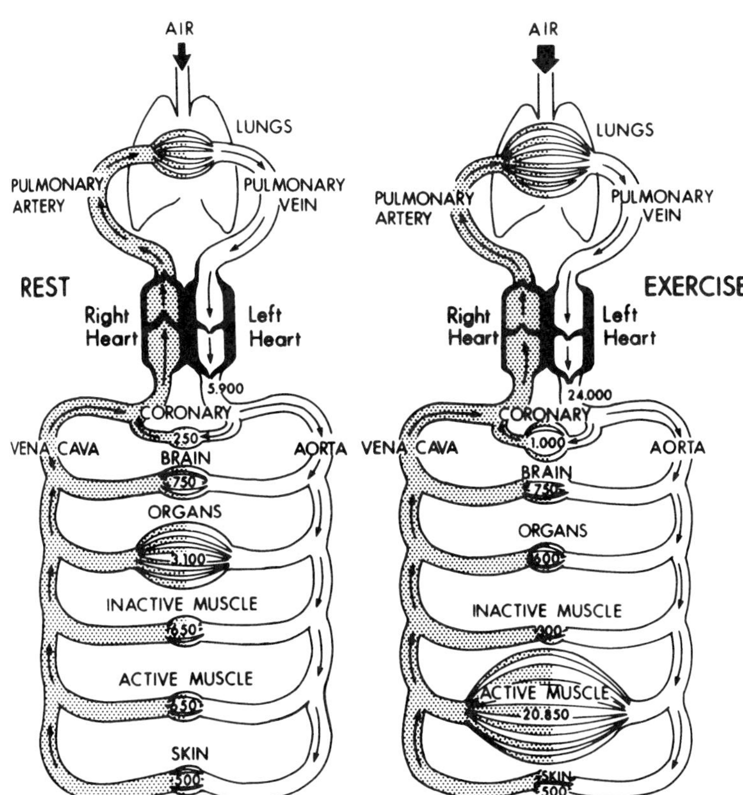

FIG. 28-23. Schematic representation of the blood flow and distribution at rest and during maximal dynamic exercise. Exercise results in increases in blood flow to the exercising muscles and the coronary circulation but in reduced flow to the organs. Blood flow rates are indicated in milliliters per minute. (From Mitchell JH, Bloomqvist G. Maximal oxygen uptake. *N Engl J Med* 1971; 284:1018–1022, reprinted by permission of *The New England Journal of Medicine.*)

Ventilation rises linearly with $\dot{V}O_2$ up to the anaerobic threshold (69,70). At and above the anaerobic threshold, ventilatory volume and carbon dioxide output ($\dot{V}CO_2$) rise out of proportion to metabolism because of the CO_2 produced from the bicarbonate buffering system (69,70). The changes in the relationship among $\dot{V}O_2$, ventilation, and $\dot{V}CO_2$ with graded exercise testing is used to assess the anaerobic threshold noninvasively (69,70). The significance of determining the anaerobic threshold is that it provides an index of tolerance for sustained work and can be used in prescribing exercise intensity for aerobic training.

Considerable amounts of heat can be produced during exercise, as about 75% of the energy with aerobic metabolism is released as heat. Heat is transported to the skin surface via the cardiovascular system and dissipated via convection, radiation, conduction, and evaporation. Body core temperature rises with exercise, which aids in heat dissipation by increasing the heat flow gradient from the core to the skin (71,72). Reflex and locally mediated arterial vasodilation allows greater blood flow to be directed to the cutaneous vascular bed (59,73,74). This increased blood flow is accomplished in part by blood flow redistribution away from splanchnic and renal arterial vascular beds (59,74). Increased cutaneous venous compliance permits increased cutaneous blood volume and surface flow, which enhance heat dissipation at the skin surface (74,75). Increased cutaneous blood volume may lead to reduced venous return, left ventricular end-diastolic volume, and stroke volume. Heart rate can rise to compensate for the lower stroke volume as long as maximal heart rate is not attained. The sequence of events associated with heat stress during exercise is referred to as "cardiovascular drift" (73,75,76). Some cardiovascular drift typically occurs with prolonged (e.g., >60 minutes) exercise in a thermoneutral environment, although the magnitude is much greater in hot and/or humid environments because of the greater cutaneous blood flow and blood volume circulatory demands for heat removal. In a hot environment, the skin-to-environment temperature gradient for dissipating heat via convection, radiation, and conduction is reduced or even reversed if air temperature is greater than skin temperature. Similarly, the ability to dissipate heat via evaporation is proportional to the magnitude of the water pressure gradient existing between the skin and environment.

Sustained levels of high work intensity, especially when performed in combination with heat stress, can lead to high rates of sweat loss reaching 2 to 3 liters/hour. These rates of sweating can lead to dehydration and subsequent sequelae of decreased total blood volume, blunted cardiac output reserve, reduced thermoregulatory capacity, and decreased work tolerance (75,77–80). To help prevent serious dehydration, fluids should be consumed during sustained exercise. This should occur even in the absence of thirst because a person can lose up to 2% of body water before feeling thirsty (73,77). A number of hormones involved in fluid regulation are altered during exercise, including increases in plasma renin activity, aldosterone, arginine vasopressin, and atrial natriuretic peptide (78,80–85).

Static Exercise

The hemodynamic responses to static exercise are related to the percentage of maximal voluntary contraction (MVC) and the amount of muscle mass involved in the contraction (86). Increases in $\dot{V}O_2$, cardiac output, and heart rate are typically modest during static exercise compared with dynamic exercise (Fig. 28-24). Additionally, total peripheral vascular resistance does not decrease, and stroke volume typically fails to rise as occurs with dynamic exercise (62). Blood flow through the active muscle is dependent on a balance between metabolically induced vasodilation and mechanical restriction of flow associated with contraction of the surrounding muscle. At high static efforts, blood flow through the active muscle is restricted and may be completely occluded (88). Reduced muscle blood flow relative to metabolic demands results in greater reliance on anaerobic metabolism and consequently earlier onset of fatigue than occurs with dynamic exercise. Mechanical and metabolic activation of skeletal muscle afferent nerve fibers during static exercise evokes a pressor response that leads to a significant increase in blood pressure, especially mean and diastolic blood pressures (89). For this reason, static exercise is often viewed as placing primarily a pressure load on the left ventricle, whereas dynamic exercise is viewed as placing more of a volume load on the left ventricle (90,91).

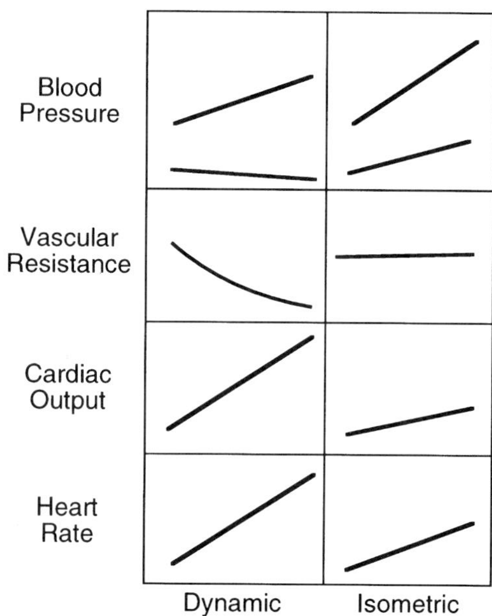

FIG. 28-24. Schematic comparison of hemodynamic responses to dynamic and isometric exercise. (Adapted from Hanson P, Rueckert P. Hypertension. In: Pollock ML, Schmidt DH, eds. *Heart disease and rehabilitation, 3rd ed.* Champaign, IL: Human Kinetics, 1995; 343–356.)

EFFECTS OF INACTIVITY AND IMMOBILIZATION

Inactivity and immobilization are commonly utilized in the management of many medical conditions. Although inactivity and immobilization are frequently necessary and appropriate treatments, there may be adverse consequences to these measures. Accordingly, complete or prolonged inactivity should be avoided when possible.

The adverse effects of restricted activities should be understood so that they may be minimized. Complete rehabilitation requires not only recovery of the injured tissue from the illness but also recovery from the secondary effects that the injury or illness has induced on other parts of the body. Minimization of these secondary effects will allow an individual to optimally return to desired activities.

Aerobic Capacity

It is well recognized that prolonged bed rest results in deconditioning. Saltin and co-workers (92) demonstrated a 27% decrease in $\dot{V}O_{2max}$ of normal, healthy young men after a 3-week period of bed rest (Fig. 28-25). Some of the deleterious effects of bed rest on cardiovascular function can present rather quickly. For instance, a reduction in plasma volume occurs after only one or two days of bed rest and results in a lower maximal stroke volume and cardiac output (93). Furthermore, it is important to recognize that the rate of recovery of cardiorespiratory fitness may be even slower than the rate of loss that occurs during deconditioning (92).

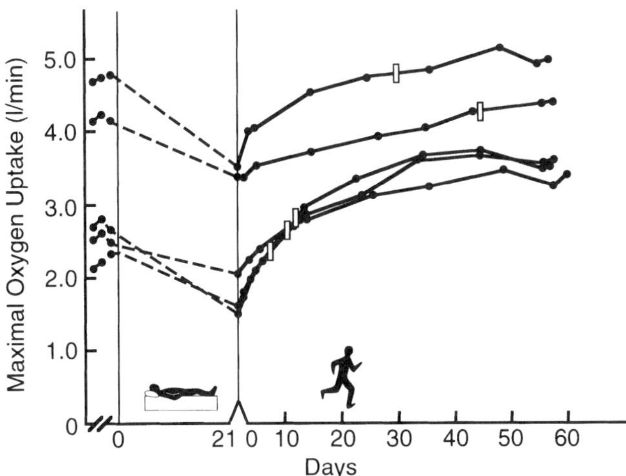

FIG. 28-25. Individual data demonstrating the changes in maximal oxygen uptake with 21 days of bed rest followed by an aerobic training program. The bars mark the time during the training period at which the maximal oxygen uptake had returned to baseline values before bed rest. (Redrawn from Saltin B, Blomqvist G, Mitchell JH, Johnson RL, Wildenthal K, Chapman CB. Response to exercise after bed rest and after training; a longitudinal study of adaptive changes in oxygen transport and body composition. *Circulation* 1968; 38: VII1–VII67.)

Muscular Strength and Endurance

Several studies have demonstrated a significant reduction in muscular strength and endurance following immobilization (94). It has been shown that strength can drop by as much as 20% to 30% during only 7 to 9 days of complete immobilization (95,96). Bed rest has been found to decrease strength by 1.0% to 1.5% per day (96). It appears to be the type I (slow twitch) fibers that are particularly affected in the early stages of immobilization, with a decrease in fiber diameter and percentage of type I fibers and a decrease in oxidative enzymes (94,97). As a result of these changes, muscular endurance is seriously reduced along with strength.

Restricted activities following a local injury may also induce undesirable changes that are rather distant from the site of injury. For instance, the strength and recruitment patterns of the hip musculature have been shown to be altered for several months after an ankle sprain (98,99).

Bone, Joints, and Soft Tissue

Immobilization results in considerable changes to the bone, cartilage, joint, and soft tissue. Inactivity results in atrophy and a reduction in the fracture threshold of bone (100). These changes actually begin to develop within the first few days of inactivity as evidenced by increased urinary and fecal excretion of calcium and phosphorus (93,101).

Fibrous connective tissue undergoes biochemical and mechanical changes from immobilization. Ligaments have been shown to have chemical changes after just 2 weeks of immobilization (102). Bone–ligament–bone preparations of primates have been found to have a decrease in load to failure and an increase in extensibility present after 8 weeks of immobilization (103,104). Furthermore, recovery was still incomplete 12 months after resumption of activity. The return of strength to surgically repaired ligaments is also hampered by immobilization compared with exercise (38).

Joints are also affected by immobilization. Periarticular connective tissue becomes less extensible through inactivity (105–107). Articular cartilage is especially susceptible to the effects of immobility and disuse because cartilage receives its nutrition through joint motion and compression. Rabbit studies have shown changes in the histologic characteristics of cartilage after just 1 to 2 days of immobilization (108) and irreversible degenerative changes to cartilage after 8 weeks of immobilization (106).

Proprioception and Coordination

Coordination of multimuscular activities is a learned, trainable skill required in performing daily activities. The neural patterns used to perform certain skilled activities are thought to be adversely affected by immobilization (109). This is supported by the findings of a decrease in integrated electromyographic activity and reduced synchronization of contraction after immobilization and detraining (110).

Proprioceptive sensation is important in making coordinated movements. Direct damage to proprioceptive receptors arising from muscles, joint capsules, ligaments, and skin as a result of injury or surgical procedures may result in a decrease in proprioceptive ability (111,112). Prolonged inactivity delays recovery of proprioception.

AEROBIC EXERCISE

Benefits Derived from Aerobic Exercise

Many studies have shown that inactive people increase functional work capacity with aerobic exercise training. This can be especially beneficial for those with limited work reserve because of age, disease, or disability (113–115). Aerobic training enables one to be more active in normal daily routines, maintain greater independence in older age or with disabilities, and resume activities including occupational work after a cardiac event (113,116–121). Shephard (113) estimated that remaining physically active into old age can allow one to maintain functional independence for 10 to 20 years longer than if one is inactive (Fig. 28-26).

Several studies have indicated that regular physical activity improves sense of well-being (122,123). Changes that have been postulated to contribute to this include reduced psychological stress, improved tolerance for activities of daily living, and hormonal changes (e.g., rise in endorphins). In addition, regular aerobic exercise may help improve quality of life by protecting people from development of disabling diseases such as heart disease, diabetes, and cancer as well as enabling people with diseases to regain functional work tolerance. Freedom from disease and ability to function independently into old age are important factors in quality of life.

It has been suggested that physical activity may be the most important variable in reducing overall lifetime morbidity (117). It is clear that health can be improved in many ways through regular aerobic exercise training.

Primary and Secondary Prevention of Heart Disease

Physical inactivity is considered a major risk factor for the development of heart disease (115,124,125). Many epidemiologic studies (126–131) have shown that people who are physically inactive have a higher incidence of heart disease than those who are physically active. Based on meta-analysis studies, the estimated risk is approximately two times greater for inactive compared to active people (132,133). In fact, this risk approaches that for hypertension and hypercholesterolemia. Because physical inactivity affects a greater number of people than any other single heart disease risk factor, the significance of physical inactivity is especially noteworthy.

In secondary prevention, meta-analysis of randomized trials of cardiac rehabilitation indicates a 20% to 25% reduction in mortality in those who participated in cardiac rehabilitation versus those who did not (134,135). The independent influence of exercise conditioning on mortality remains uncertain, as several of these programs included education and advice on modifying other risk factors.

Reduced incidence of cardiovascular disease through physical activity certainly could have important societal implications. The estimated cost of cardiovascular disease in the United States was $138 billion in 1995 (136). If the prevalence rates remain the same, future health care costs could escalate with the projected rise in number of Americans older than 65 years. A regular program of exercise, combined with other healthy lifestyle habits, has tremendous potential in curtailing future health care costs. The nation's health care goals for the year 2000, published in the Healthy People 2000 Program, are aimed at encouraging Americans to adopt healthier lifestyle habits including greater participation in a regular program of exercise (137).

The mechanism by which physical activity reduces the risk of heart disease is not entirely clear. Some of the reduced risk stems from its impact on improving other risk factors such as lipids, blood pressure, obesity, diabetes, and psychological stress (115). Physical inactivity remains, however,

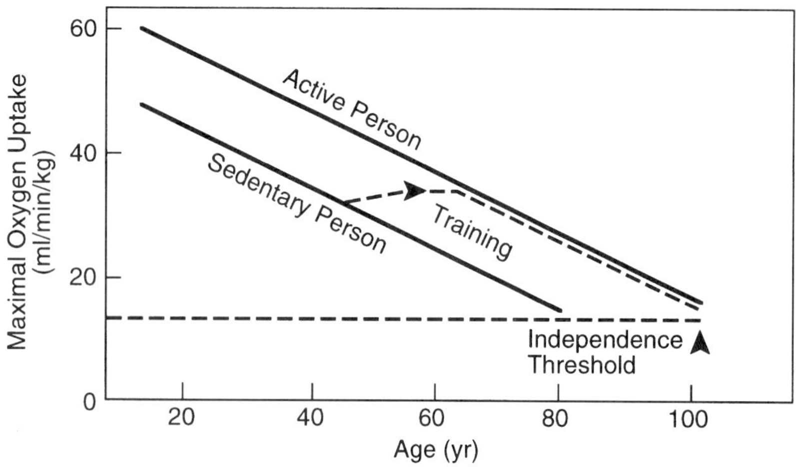

FIG. 28-26. Demonstration of the effect of aerobic training on improving aerobic capacity and delaying its drop to a threshold where independent function can no longer be sustained. (Adapted from Shephard RJ. Exercise and aging: extending independence in older adults. *Geriatrics* 1993; 48:61–64.)

an independent risk factor for coronary artery disease after statistical adjustment for other risk factors.

The exercise threshold required for primary and secondary prevention remains at issue (115,138,139). For many years, the primary recommendation was to participate in an aerobic exercise program. More recently, health organizations have revised their recommendations to acknowledge the benefit of physical activities that may not meet the aerobic criteria (115). Inactive people have been encouraged to accumulate at least 30 minutes of moderate exercise most, and preferably all, days of the week (115). This 30 minutes can be accumulated from activities performed throughout the day such as climbing stairs, gardening, playing with children, etc. This change in recommendations stems from (a) epidemiologic studies showing reduced incidence of heart disease in physically active people including those who were not necessarily participating in an aerobic exercise program, (b) the failure of many people to adopt long-term aerobic exercise programs because of a variety of factors including discomfort with higher intensity effort, and (c) the low levels of physical activity required in our normal daily activities (115). Although the magnitude of benefits in terms of prevention are likely to be dose-related, benefits are first contingent on long-term compliance to a regular program of physical activity. Short-term participation (e.g., 3 or 6 months) has minimal or no benefit in preventing disease (115).

Blood Pressure Regulation

Hypertension is a major risk factor for heart disease. Regular exercise is associated with improved blood pressure control (115,140–143). Decreases of 8 to 10 mm Hg in systolic blood pressure and 5 to 8 mm Hg in diastolic blood pressure have been observed with regular exercise training in those with hypertension. Debate still exists regarding the type of exercise program that produces the best blood-pressure-lowering effect. Some data suggest that higher-intensity exercise or more frequent exercise is less effective than lower levels of exercise (87). Questions also exist as to the relative importance of exercise independent of weight loss on lowering blood pressure (144–146).

Lipid Management

Most studies indicate that aerobic exercise training lowers plasma triglycerides and raises high-density lipoprotein (HDL) cholesterol (115,147–149). Importantly, increased ratios of HDL/LDL cholesterol and HDL/total cholesterol are associated with decreased risk for development of coronary artery disease. Questions remain regarding the threshold of exercise needed to produce changes in HDL-cholesterol (148,150–153). Most data suggest a dose-dependent relationship (148,151–153). Recently, a threshold of about 7 miles/week was reported for detection of an increase in HDL-cholesterol in healthy men (151). This threshold corresponds to a brisk walk or moderate jog of about 30 minutes three to five times weekly. Although lipid changes are associated with long-term participation in an exercise program, a single bout of exercise may also produce some short-term beneficial lipid changes (154,155).

Weight Control

The incidence of obesity is rising within industrialized countries. More than 33% of the U.S. population is considered obese (156,157). Especially disconcerting is the rising number of obese children. Obesity carries many health risks including heart disease, diabetes, hypertension, dyslipidemia, and cancer (158). When the body mass index (body mass in kilograms/height in meters squared) increases above 27, mortality increases sharply (158,159).

Most population studies show an inverse relationship between obesity and physical activity (115). Although many overweight people periodically lose significant amounts of fat through diet alone, most regain this weight (160). In fact, many obese individuals undergo a weight loss/weight regain cycle (yo-yo weight pattern) many times in a lifetime. Rather than trying to lose weight through diet alone or exercise alone, a combination of moderate diet restrictions and increased regular exercise results in the best long-term weight management plan (161). Exercise seems to be especially important in long-term maintenance of weight loss (115,159). The most appropriate combination of intensity, duration, frequency, and mode of exercise to recommend for weight loss remains uncertain but will likely vary depending upon percent body fat, age, and presence/absence of orthopedic or other medical complications (161–163). In addition to fat loss, increased physical activity may help maintain or increase lean body tissue during weight loss.

Diabetes Prevention

Diabetes is a risk factor for cardiovascular disease. Regular exercise is advocated in the primary prevention of non-insulin-dependent diabetes mellitus (NIDDM) (164,165). A major benefit of exercise is that it increases insulin sensitivity (166–168). This effect is seen after a single bout of exercise, suggesting an acute effect (167,169). If exercise is performed regularly, this acute benefit is maintained chronically. Improved insulin sensitivity may decrease insulin requirements and provide better glucose regulation (170). Exercise may also decrease the incidence of NIDDM through weight, lipid, and blood pressure control (171–173). One study has suggested that for each 500 kcal/day increase in energy expenditure, the age-adjusted risk of NIDDM can be reduced by 6% (165).

The intensity, frequency, and duration of exercise needed to provide protection against the development of NIDDM or improve control of NIDDM remains uncertain. Most studies showing benefits have utilized an aerobic exercise program. Moderate to high-intensity exercise (≥5.5 METs) performed ≥40 min/week was recently found to reduce the incidence of NIDDM, whereas lower levels of exercise, regardless of duration, did not provide protection (173). These results suggest that a threshold of exercise must be achieved in terms of intensity and duration.

Maintenance of Bone Density

Osteoporosis is a major health problem, especially among elderly women. Regular physical activity generally is associated with greater bone density (174–181). In addition, exercise habits during peak bone-forming years appear to impact on bone density years later (176,181). The mechanism(s) by which exercise increases bone density are incompletely understood. Weight-bearing appears to be an important stimulus, although muscle contraction without weight-bearing may also promote bone density (174,175,177–179). In women, very high-intensity training can lead to amenorrhea and reduced bone density (182), an effect believed to be related to decreased estrogen levels.

Increased Fibrinolytic Activity

Exercise has several effects on coagulation factors. Regular exercise reportedly lowers the risk of thrombosis by impacting on hematocrit, fibrinogen, platelet function, and fibrinolysis (115,183–186). Although most types of chronic exercise appear beneficial, very large amounts of high-intensity exercise may increase platelet adhesiveness and aggregability in some individuals (186,187).

Improved Sleep

Epidemiologic studies indicate that regular physical activity may be beneficial in improving sleep quality and reducing sleepiness during normal waking hours (188). The mechanism(s) by which exercise impacts on sleep remains uncertain.

Enhanced Immune Function

Exercise training appears to have a beneficial impact on the immune system although excessive training may disrupt normal immune function (189–192).

Reduced Cancer Risk

A growing number of studies are showing that increased physical activity is associated with reduced risk of colon and perhaps breast, prostate, and lung cancer (127,193,194).

Physiological Adaptations to Aerobic Conditioning

Aerobic exercise training produces many physiological adaptations (Table 28-4). An important adaptation is increased work capacity or $\dot{V}O_{2max}$. The majority of studies indicate that sedentary people within diverse populations (age, gender, income, ethnic background, health status) will experience ≥15% improvement in $\dot{V}O_{2max}$ within 3 months of starting aerobic training (55,62,115,195,196). This increase is caused about equally by central cardiovascular adaptations that raise maximal cardiac output and peripheral adaptations that enhance oxygen extraction from the circulating blood (62).

TABLE 28-4. *Physiological adaptations to aerobic exercise training as observed in resting and exercise states*

	Rest	Submaximal exercise	Maximal exercise
Aerobic power	No change	No change	Increase
Heart rate	Decrease	Decrease	Decrease
Stroke volume	Increase	Increase	Increase
Cardiac output	No change	No change	Increase
Myocardial O_2 demand	Decrease	Decrease	No change
Ventilation	No change	Decrease	Increase
Arteriovenous O_2 difference	No change	Increase	Increase
Blood lactate concentration	No change	Decrease	Increase
Muscle blood flow	No change	Decrease	Increase
Splanchnic blood flow	No change	No change	Decrease
Systolic blood pressure	Decrease	Decrease	No change
Diastolic blood pressure	Decrease	Decrease	No change

Increased oxygen extraction with aerobic training stems from changes within the trained muscle including increased capillary density, capillary–fiber ratio, tissue myoglobin, size and number of mitochondria per muscle cell, and respiratory enzyme capacity per mitochondrion (197–199). These muscular adaptations are believed to raise the anaerobic threshold and improve tolerance for sustained work.

The rise in maximal cardiac output with aerobic conditioning resides in increased stroke volume. Maximal heart rate does not rise and may be even lower in well-conditioned endurance athletes. The mechanism(s) by which maximal stroke volume increases with training is not entirely clear but involves increased cardiac preload and probably enhanced myocardial contractility and relaxation (62,200). Aerobic training causes an increase in total blood volume that partially accounts for the increased cardiac preload. The extent of cardiac adaptations appears to be related to such training factors as the length, intensity, duration, and mode of training and the time of life at which training was initiated. A characteristic finding among elite male endurance athletes is an increased heart size (''athlete's heart'') characterized by increased left ventricular end-diastolic volume and a proportional increase in left ventricular mass and normal wall tension (62,201). Importantly, the enlarged heart of the athlete differs from the enlarged heart in hypertension and congestive heart failure (202). In the elite athlete, left ventricular hypertrophy is eccentric rather than concentric, and ventricular dilation is proportional to wall thickness. Indices of left ventricular diastolic function are typically normal or increased in athletes but impaired in pathologic states (203). The increased heart size in the athlete is believed important in permitting high levels of maximal stroke volume and thereby high functional work tolerance. Although highly trained women frequently show cardiac dimensional adaptations, they rarely demonstrate cardiac dimensional changes outside normal limits (204).

Physiological adaptations to aerobic training may be restricted to the trained muscles when the amount of muscle mass used in the exercise is small (205–207). For instance, the physiological benefits of upper body endurance training appear to be primarily limited to the periphery (205,207). This is attributed to the lower blood flow and cardiac output requirements, which lessen the stimulus for central (i.e., heart) adaptations.

Principles of Aerobic Conditioning

Intensity, duration, and frequency criteria have been established to define aerobic exercise training (208). The recommended exercise intensity range is 50% to 85% of $\dot{V}O_{2max}$ or 60% to 90% of maximal heart rate. This typically translates to perceived exertions of "fairly light" to "hard" (209,210). To achieve these recommended intensities, exercise modes that incorporate a large muscle mass such as walking, running, cycling, swimming, and cross-country skiing are optimal (210,211). Exercise duration should be at least 20 minutes, and exercise frequency should be at least three times per week.

The optimal rate of progression to follow in implementing an exercise program depends on several factors including the individual's current activity levels, functional work reserve, health, age, and exercise goals (208). The primary focus should be on adopting a progression that will result in long-term participation. Attempting to do too much too fast can lead to increased dropout rates as a result of perceived excessive discomfort and/or injuries. The American College of Sports Medicine suggests a progression rate subdivided into three phases, as illustrated in Table 28-5. Exercise programs can be tailored according to personal preferences by selecting various combinations of frequency, duration, and intensity.

Assessment of Aerobic Capacity

The $\dot{V}O_{2max}$ provides a reliable, reproducible measure of dynamic work capacity and cardiovascular fitness. It also provides information regarding medical prognosis in patients with heart disease and can aid in evaluating work resumption after recovery from a cardiac event (91,208,212). Many factors influence $\dot{V}O_{2max}$, including age, gender, chronic levels of exercise, genetics, and disease (91,208). With increasing age, $\dot{V}O_{2max}$ declines about 5% to 10% per decade after age 20 (199,213). The age-related loss is attributed to several factors, including a progressive decline in maximal heart rate, body composition changes (e.g., loss of muscle), decreased physical activity, myocardial and vascular stiffening, and disease with increased age (199,213–215). Gender has an impact on $\dot{V}O_{2max}$, with men having higher values than women when compared at a given age and activity level (91,199). The gender difference is largely attributed to the smaller muscle/whole-body weight ratio, lower hemoglobin, and smaller stroke volume in women (91). Regular aerobic exercise is known to increase $\dot{V}O_{2max}$, with the magnitude of increase being dependent on length of training and intensity of effort. The high levels of $\dot{V}O_{2max}$ observed in elite endurance athletes (e.g., 70 to 85 ml/kg per minute) compared to average young men (e.g., 40 to 50 ml/kg per minute) probably stem from prolonged intense training plus genetic factors that enhance responsiveness to training (199,216,217).

The $\dot{V}O_{2max}$ can be mathematically defined as the product of maximal cardiac output and maximal arteriovenous oxy-

TABLE 28-5. *Example of the progression of an aerobic exercise program for a presumably healthy individual*

Program phase	Week	Exercise frequency (sessions/week)	Exercise intensity (% $\dot{V}O_2$ max or HR reserve)	Exercise duration (min)
Initial stage	1	3	40–50	12
	2	3	50	14
	3	3	60	16
	4	3	60–70	18
	5	3	60–70	20
Improvement stage	6–9	3–4	70–80	21
	10–13	3–4	70–80	24
	14–16	3–4	70–80	24
	17–19	4–5	70–80	28
	20–23	4–5	70–80	30
	24–27	4–5	70–85	30
Maintenance stage	28+	3	70–85	30–45

From American College of Sports Medicine. *ACSM'S guidelines for exercise testing and prescriptions, 5th ed.* Baltimore: Williams & Wilkins, 1995.

gen difference. Considerable debate has existed over the years as to what physiological system limits $\dot{V}O_{2max}$. Most current evidence points to the cardiovascular system (58,199,218–220). A cardiovascular limitation could reside in maximal cardiac output, maximal muscle blood flow, or maintenance of an appropriate arterial perfusion pressure.

Aerobic capacity can be assessed through direct measurement of $\dot{V}O_2$ during maximal exercise or through estimates from maximal or submaximal testing. Direct measurement of $\dot{V}O_{2max}$ is achieved with open-circuit spirometry techniques. In the clinical laboratory setting, $\dot{V}O_{2max}$ is more often estimated based on the peak workload attained, rather than directly measured. If $\dot{V}O_{2max}$ is estimated, it is important to discourage significant handrail support with treadmill testing, as this can lead to a marked overestimation (208,221). Reasonably accurate estimates are possible with treadmill and cycle ergometer testing, as work efficiency is relatively constant among people with these testing modes. Conditions in which work efficiency is altered (e.g., walking with a prosthesis) can significantly reduce the accuracy of estimating $\dot{V}O_2$ based on workload (222).

Treadmill or leg cycle ergometer testing is primarily used to evaluate $\dot{V}O_{2max}$, although arm ergometry testing may be used for those unable to perform leg exercise. Among these test modalities, $\dot{V}O_2$ at peak effort is generally highest with the treadmill, intermediate with leg cycle ergometer, and lowest with the arm ergometer (223–225). Differences in peak $\dot{V}O_2$ between ergometers are largely attributed to differences in amount of muscle used.

Some individuals do not achieve $\dot{V}O_{2max}$ with symptom-limited testing, as the test is stopped before fatigue at the appearance of an adverse sign and/or symptom of another limiting factor (e.g., claudication). Lack of motivation is another common reason for not achieving a true $\dot{V}O_{2max}$.

Supervision of exercise tests requires knowledge of when to stop a test for unreasonable risk and of which individuals should not undergo testing because of contraindications for exercise (208,226). Most clinical laboratories have established end points for graded dynamic exercise testing and contraindications for exercise testing (91,208,226).

A less formal method for assessing tolerance for daily activities or for estimating functional work tolerance is to measure distance walked/jogged in a set time period (e.g., 12 min) (208).

STRENGTH

Importance of Resistance Training

Strength development through resistance training is important for the prevention and rehabilitation of injuries and for improving sports performance (227). Strength is also important for maintenance of functional capacity. With the many physiological conditions that promote catabolic breakdown of the muscle and connective tissues (e.g., aging, injury, disease), resistance training presents the only natural method to offset such wasting conditions.

Physiological Adaptations to Resistance Training

Nervous System Adaptations

Maximal force production from a muscle requires the maximal recruitment of all motor units (228). It has been theorized that untrained individuals may not be able to recruit all motor units voluntarily. Thus, part of the adaptation to resistance training is the development of the ability to recruit all motor units (18). Such neural adaptations are thought to be responsible for the increase in strength that precedes any increase in muscle size during the early phase of a resistance training program.

The central nervous system is also capable of limiting force by engaging inhibitory mechanisms that may be protective in nature. Resistance training may result in changes in the order of fiber recruitment or reduced inhibition.

Muscle Enlargement

During heavy resistance training, motor units containing both type I and type II muscle fibers are recruited and presented with a stimulus for adaptation. As a result, resistance training typically induces increases in the cross-sectional area of both type I and type II muscle fibers. This fiber hypertrophy is translated to increases in the cross-sectional size of the intact muscle, which can be observed after several months of training (229,230).

An upper limit of muscle cell growth has not been determined, but it has been suggested that an ''optimal size'' or ceiling of adaptation may exist for individual muscle fibers after a prolonged period of strength training. Alterations in the neural patterns of activation within the muscle to recruit all the available fibers may be of importance for the intact muscle to achieve maximal hypertrophy (231).

The increase in muscle fiber hypertrophy is thought to occur through remodeling of protein within the cell and an increase in the size and number of myofibrils (232). Increases in the number of actin and myosin filaments along with sarcomere addition contribute to the increase in muscle fiber size. It has been suggested that the packing density of actin increases, but not myosin, as the contractile proteins are added to the outside of the myofibril without altering the cross-bridge configurations (232,233).

The mechanisms and biochemical alterations that mediate the net changes observed with heavy resistance training remain an intense topic of study. Hormonal changes induced by resistance exercise appear to stimulate the uptake of amino acids, yet their incorporation into the contractile unit is not guaranteed. It is possible that contractile proteins accumulate in the muscle fiber either by an increased synthesis or decreased rate of breakdown, or some combination of both. It is clear that muscle fibers are disrupted, and certain fibers damaged, with intense resistance exercise (234). The extent of this damage is less in trained individuals than in untrained individuals. The repair process of remodeling the muscle fiber may well involve a host of regulatory mechanisms (e.g., hormonal and metabolic) interacting with the training status of the individual as well as the availablity of protein.

Hyperplasia is considered to be a possible adaptive strategy (233), but the extent and frequency of this adaptive response remain a topic of debate. It may be that hyperplasia exists but the magnitude of its contribution in even exceptional situations may not be great (<5%). In addition, hyperplasia may not occur equally in all individuals (232).

Muscle Fiber Conversion

Transition within the muscle fiber subtypes from type IIB to type IIA appears to be quite typical with resistance training (235–237), and this conversion begins to occur within about 2 weeks of initiation of training (238). However, any transformation from type I to type II muscle fibers seems less probable (235,236).

It is not known to what extent this early conversion of muscle fibers may contribute to the initial changes in muscle strength. Nervous system alterations may have the most dramatic effects mediating strength changes early in a training program, but other changes are taking place in the remodeling of the muscle fibers that may also have an influence on strength.

Other Adaptations Within the Muscle

It has been demonstrated that strength training can increase the activity of enzymes associated with the ATP-CP energy system (239,240), the anaerobic glycolysis system (239), and the aerobic system (239–241). However, increases in enzyme activity have not been a consistent finding among studies. The design of the strength-training program affects the magnitude of enzyme changes in the muscle. Changes in metabolic enzymes are dependent upon the duration of individual sets rather than the total amount of work performed. For practical application, normal heavy resistance programs will have minimal effect on enzyme activities. However, a training program that calls for resistances that are tolerable for at least 30 seconds will most likely induce increases in the activity of muscle enzymes.

Muscular stores of ATP and CP (242) and glycogen (242) may increase with resistance training, although these changes are not always observed (243). Whether or not these changes occur with resistance training appears to be dependent on pretraining status, muscle group examined, and the type of program performed.

Improved capillarization has been observed with resistance training of untrained subjects (236,243-245), but the time required for this adaptation to take place can be greater than 12 weeks (243,246,247). It is thought that low-intensity/high-volume strength training is more likely to increase capillary density than high-intensity/low-volume training.

Myoglobin content in the muscle may be decreased following strength training (246). Thus, it has been postulated that long-term strength training may depress the ability of the muscle fibers to extract oxygen. Again, the initial state of training as well as the specific type of program that is used may influence the effect of resistance training on myoglobin content.

Few studies have examined the effect of resistance training on mitochondrial density, but the observation of decreased mitochondrial density by one study (248) is consistent with the limited demands for oxidative metabolism placed on the musculature during most resistance-training programs.

Body Compositional Changes

Body compositional changes can occur during short-term (6 to 24 weeks) resistance-training programs. Increases in fat-free mass normally mirror increases in muscle tissue weight, but because of concomitant decreases in fat, total body weight generally increases little over short training periods. The largest gains in fat-free mass that can be expected are a little more than 3 kg (6.6 lb) in 10 weeks of training (227). Though some athletes desire rapid gains in body weight, this is not possible to achieve through gains in muscle mass.

Endocrine System Adaptations

It is apparent that the endocrine system plays a major role in the adaptational responses of skeletal muscle to resistance training. Serum testosterone concentrations have been demonstrated to increase in the first 6 weeks of resistance training and then return to pretraining values (238). During the time that serum testosterone concentrations are elevated, significant changes in the quality of muscle protein occurs. Thus, the endocrine system appears to play an important role in the mediation of protein synthesis or reduced degradation that occurs during some phases of training.

Adaptations to Connective Tissue, Bone, and Cartilage

The adaptations from resistance training allowing greater tension development by the muscles make it important for the strength of ligaments and tendons to also increase in order to avoid damage to these structures. It is now acknowledged that the dense fibrous tissues that make up tendons and ligaments are adaptable, but no research has been done specifically to examine the effects of heavy resistance exercise on these structures (249,250).

Physical activity causes increased metabolism, thickness, weight, and strength of ligaments (38,251). Damaged ligaments regain their strength at a faster rate if physical activity is performed after the injury (38,251). Research involving laboratory animals has demonstrated that endurance-type training increases the amount of force necessary to cause separation at the attachment site of a ligament or tendon to a bone and the musculotendinous junction (38). There is reason to believe that resistance training would produce similar results.

The connective tissue sheaths that surround the entire muscle (epimysium), groups of muscle fibers (perimysium), and individual muscle fibers (endomysium) also adapt to resistance training. These sheaths are of major importance in the tensile strength and elastic properties of muscle, as they form the framework that supports an overload on the muscle. It has been found that muscle hypertrophy is accompanied by an increase in the collagen content of these connective tissue sheaths (252,253), but the amount of connective tissue appears to increase at the same rate as the muscle tissue (254).

Bone adapts to resistance training, but much more slowly than muscle, requiring 6 to 12 months for adaptations to be observed (255). Bone is sensitive to compression and strain. Such forces are common in resistance training and are related to the type of exercise utilized, the intensity of the resistance, and the number of sets performed. Training characterized by high-power exercise movements, heavy resistances, and multiple sets appears to be most likely to produce changes in bone metabolism.

Resistance training has been found to increase the thickness of hyaline cartilage on the articular surfaces of bone (256,257). One major function of hyaline cartilage is to act as a shock absorber between the bony surfaces of a joint. Increasing the thickness of cartilage could facilitate the performance of this shock absorber function.

Peak Oxygen Consumption

The $\dot{V}O_{2max}$ is normally not considered to be significantly affected by heavy resistance training (258,259). However, circuit weight training consisting of performing sets of exercises of 12 to 15 repetitions at 40% to 60% of the one-repetition maximum with short rest periods of 15 to 30 seconds between exercises may produce small increases in $\dot{V}O_{2max}$ (260). A resistance training program designed to increase $\dot{V}O_{2max}$ should consist of a high volume of training and relatively short rest periods between sets and exercises. Even then, the maximal increase in $\dot{V}O_{2max}$ brought about by resistance training is substantially less than the 15% to 20% increase associated with traditional aerobic training programs. Therefore, if a major goal of a training program is to increase $\dot{V}O_{2max}$, some form of endurance training should be included in the program.

Principles of the Exercise Prescription for Enhancing Strength

General Guidelines

A number of factors should be considered in any resistance training prescription (227). These include (a) the choice of exercise, (b) the order of the exercises, (c) the number of sets, (d) the amount of rest taken between sets and exercises, (e) the intensity of the exercise, and (f) the rate of progression of the exercise.

Choice of Exercise

A very basic, but important consideration to remember is that the prescribed exercise must be consistent with the desired goals. In other words, the prescribed exercise should strengthen the muscle groups that are desired to be strengthened.

Order of the Exercises

Typically, the large muscle group exercises or more complex exercises are performed in the beginning of a workout. If a circuit program is being used, it is customary to begin with exercises involving the arms and then move to the leg exercises.

Number of Sets

A resistance training program usually begins with one set of each exercise, and then progresses to three or more sets of each exercise. Typically not over six sets are performed for one exercise movement.

Amount of Rest Between Sets and Exercises

Rest periods are commonly 3 minutes or more when very heavy resistances are used, 2 to 3 minutes when moderate resistances are used, and 1 to 2 minutes when lighter resistances are used. In all cases, one should rest until the exercise can be repeated safely. Short rest periods (<2 minutes) are more stressful and should be used only if one can tolerate the metabolic demands.

Intensity of the Exercise

The intensity of a resistance exercise is frequently described as a percentage of the maximal amount of resistance that can be applied and allow completion of one full repetition of the exercise (the one-repetition maximum [1 RM]). To induce strength gains, an intensity of at least 60% to 65% of the 1 RM is required (261). This means that use of a very light resistance, even if a large number of repetitions are performed, will not result in strength gains.

The maximal number of repetitions that can be performed per set is dependent on the percentage of the 1 RM that is used. The number of repetitions that can be performed at a given percentage of the 1 RM varies with the muscle group involved and the individual. For example, the maximal number of repetitions possible at 60% of 1 RM for the leg press may be 34, whereas for a knee curl it may be 11 (262).

The intensity of a resistance exercise is also commonly

described by the maximal number of repetitions that can be performed with the load. Typically, loads corresponding with 6 to 15 RM are recommended. A 6-RM resistance represents a greater intensity than a 15-RM resistance.

Rate of Progression of the Exercise

Progressive resistance exercise or progressive overload refers to the need to continually increase the stress placed on the muscle as it becomes capable of producing greater force or has more endurance. At the start of a training program, the 15 RM for arm curls might be 40 lb and is a sufficient stimulus to produce an increase in strength. As strength increases with training, 15 repetitions with 40 lb may no longer be a sufficient stimulus to increase strength. If the training stimulus is not increased at this point, no further gains in strength will occur.

To assure that progressive overload to the muscle occurs, the load for the desired training RM should be adjusted upwards as strength is increased. Alternatively, the volume of training performed (i.e., the number of sets and repetitions of a particular exercise) can be increased. Due to the possibility of overtraining, care must be exercised when progressively overloading the muscle. This is especially true when the progressive overload is in the form of an increased volume of training (263). Therefore, as a general rule, rapid increases in the resistance or volume of training, especially for individuals with little resistance training experience, should be avoided. A reasonable guideline is not to increase the resistance for a particular number of repetitions or volume of training more than 2.5% to 5% at any one time.

Program Variation and Periodization

Variation in the training program is important for optimal gains in strength (264–267). Slight variations in the position of the foot, hand, or other body parts that do not affect the safety in performing the exercise can be valuable in producing continued gains in strength (268). Variations may also be achieved through alterations in intensity, volume, the choice of exercises, order of exercise, and amount of rest between sets.

A systematic process to varying a strength training program is called ''periodization'' (269). Its purpose is to avoid overtraining, provide time for physical and mental recovery, and allow continued gains with the training program. Over the past 10 years many systems of program periodization have been developed, and it appears that the key to the general concept is based on the need for variation of the workout stimulus. Variation in the program also enhances long-term adherence by reducing boredom with the exercise program.

Specificity

Speed Specificity

Resistance training produces its greatest strength gains at the movement velocity at which the training is performed. An intermediate training velocity is best if the aim of the program is to increase strength across a wide range of velocities of movement (270). However, training at a fast velocity results in gains in strength at a fast velocity to a slightly greater extent than training at a slow velocity, and vice versa (270,271). Thus, use of velocity-specific training to maximize strength and power gains at a specific velocity may be appropriate in some cases.

Contraction Specificity

If an individual trains isometrically, and progress is evaluated with an isometric muscle contraction, a large increase in strength may seem apparent. However, if this same individual's progress is determined using concentric or eccentric muscle contractions, little or no increase in strength may be demonstrated. This is called testing specificity and indicates that gains in strength are specific to the type of muscle contraction used in training. This specificity of strength gain is related to the individual learning to recruit the muscles to perform a particular type of muscle contraction. Therefore, a training program for a specific activity should use the types of muscular contractions employed in that activity.

Joint Angle Specificity

Studies involving isometric training have demonstrated that if the exercise is only performed at a specific joint angle, strength gains will be realized in a narrow range around that specific joint angle and not throughout the full range of motion of the joint (272–274). The carryover in strength gains from isometric training appears to be approximately 20° to either side of the training angle (275).

Methods to Enhance Strength

Machines Versus Free Weights

The controversy about whether resistance machines or free weights produce the greatest gains in strength and power probably started soon after the first resistance machine was invented, and this controversy has continued since. Advocates of free weights point out that machines allow movement only in a predetermined plane and path of movement, so balancing of the resistance in all directions is not possible. The need to balance the resistance requires the use of muscles not involved in the movement as prime movers. The involvement of these muscles used for maintaining balance is greater with free weights than machines. Advocates of free weights also claim that the need to balance the resistance is more like a sporting event or daily life, where balancing of any resistance moved is needed and, therefore, is an important part of resistance training. Conversely, machine advocates claim that the lack of a need to balance the resistance is good, because it allows greater isolation of the muscles involved in the exercise as prime movers. In addition, machine advocates claim, because movement is allowed only in one plane and direction, it is easier to teach proper exercise technique. Both sides in this controversy use the same facts but interpret them to be positive from their particular point of view. This can lead to confusion when trying to make decisions about which equipment to use in resistance training.

In reality, the relative advantages attributed to machines and free weights can be used to enhance a resistance-training program. Machines allowing movement in only one plane and direction providing isolation of a muscle group are very useful when the goal of the program is to increase strength or power or local muscular endurance of a specific muscle group. Because isolation of a muscle group is possible with machines, they are ideal for rehabilitation programs after an injury, for programs aimed at increasing muscular strength and power of a particular muscle group or joint prone to injury, or in a muscle group that is the weak link in performance of a certain activity. Free weight exercises, where it is necessary to balance the resistance in all directions, are a good choice when the goal of the program is to strengthen total body movements and provide coordination among various muscle groups. Thus, both machine and free-weight exercises have a place in a well-designed resistance-training program.

Isometric Resistance Exercise

Isometric resistance training is normally performed against an immovable object such as a wall, a barbell, or a weight machine loaded beyond the maximal concentric strength. Isometrics can also be performed by having a weak muscle group contract against a strong muscle group. For example, trying to bend the left elbow by contracting the left elbow flexors maximally and resisting the movement by pushing down on the left hand with the right hand with just enough force to stop any movement at the left elbow. The cost of using isometrics can range from minimal, by using a wall as an immovable object, to quite expensive when using a loaded weight machine as the immovable object.

Isometrics came to the attention of the American public in the early 1950s, when Steinhaus (276) introduced the work of two Germans, Hettinger and Muller (277). Hettinger and Muller concluded that gains in strength of 5% per week were produced by one daily isometric contraction of 6 seconds' duration at two-thirds of maximal isometric strength. Gains in strength of this magnitude with such little training time and effort seemed unbelievable. Review of subsequent studies demonstrated that isometric training leads to isometric strength gains but that the gains are substantially less than 5% per week (278). As with other forms of strength training, the strength gains are achieved through a combination of muscular hypertrophy (279,280) and neural adaptations.

Increases in strength from isometric training are related to the number of muscle contractions performed, the duration of the contractions, whether the muscle contractions are maximal or submaximal, and the frequency of training. Most studies involving isometric training manipulate several of these variables simultaneously. As a result, it is difficult to evaluate the importance of any one factor. Enough research has been conducted, however, to allow for some recommendations concerning isometric training.

Increases in strength can be achieved with submaximal isometric muscle contractions (277,279,281,282). However, it is generally believed, and supported by the majority of research, that maximal voluntary muscle contractions are superior to submaximal contractions in bringing about increases in strength (283,284).

Many combinations of number and duration of maximal isometric contractions can result in strength gains. Optimal gains in strength can result from either a small number of long duration contractions or a high number of short duration contractions. As an example, seven daily 1-minute contractions at 30% of maximal isometric strength or 42 3-second maximal isometric contractions per training day over a 6-week training period both resulted in about a 30% increase in isometric strength (282).

It has been concluded that isometric training once every 2 weeks does not cause increases in strength, though it does serve to maintain strength (285). It has also been calculated that, compared with daily training sessions, alternate-day isometric training is 80% as effective and once-a-week training is 40% as effective (285). The exact percentages are controversial, but the superiority of daily training with isometrics is well established (286). To increase maximal strength, the optimal isometric program should consist of maximal isometric contractions performed on a daily basis.

A potential limitation of isometric resistance training relates to joint angle specificity. The literature suggests some practical guidelines for using isometric training to increase strength throughout the entire range of motion. First, the training should be performed at joint angle increments of approximately 10° to 20°. Second, if isometric contractions cannot be performed throughout the entire range of motion, it is best to perform them with the muscle in a lengthened position as opposed to a shortened position.

Dynamic Constant-External-Resistance Exercise

Dynamic constant-external-resistance training is commonly referred to as isotonic training. This type of exercise is one in which the external load or resistance does not change through the movement. Dynamic constant external resistance training can be performed with free weights and exercise machines with nonvariable resistance.

Various combinations of sets and repetitions of this type of training have been demonstrated to induce similar gains in strength during an initial short period of training, especially in untrained individuals. Strength gains have been reported with numbers of sets ranging from one to six and numbers of repetitions per set ranging from one to 20

(235,245,287–295). It has been reported that one set per training session results in 80% of the strength gains of a multiple-set program (296). However, it must be realized that this conclusion relates to untrained subjects over a relatively short duration of training where "learning effects" can result in what appear to be large strength gains.

The optimal frequency of dynamic constant external resistance training sessions is not clearly established. However, the majority of research indicates that three training sessions per muscle group per week is the minimum frequency that causes maximum gains in strength in novice subjects over an initial short training period.

Variable Resistance Exercise

Variable resistance devices usually operate through lever arms, cams, or pulley arrangements to alter the resistance through the movement. The goal of these designs is to match the differences in strength over the range of the movement with the resistance. Proponents of variable-resistance machines believe that by altering the resistance to match the strength curve, the muscle is forced to contract maximally throughout the entire range of motion, resulting in maximal gains in strength. As has been demonstrated with dynamic constant external resistance training, various combinations of sets, repetitions, and training sessions per week can cause significant increases in strength with variable resistance equipment (294,297–304).

Elastic tubing or bands provides another form of variable resistance in common use. While offering an inexpensive method for strength training, the variation in resistance provided through elastic tubing does not correspond with strength curves. The resistance provided by elastic tubing increases as a function of the length of the tubing, whereas strength curves typically show a maximum located midrange in the movement.

Isokinetic Exercise

An isokinetic contraction is one in which the movement is performed at a constant angular velocity. Unlike other types of resistance training, there is no set resistance to meet with isokinetic training. Rather, the velocity of movement is controlled, and any force applied against the machine results in an equal reaction force. This makes it theoretically possible for a muscular contraction to be performed at a continual, maximal force through the full range of motion for the movement. Advocates of isokinetic training believe that the ability to exert maximal force throughout the range of motion leads to optimal strength gains. Another advantage is that the exercise can be limited to concentric contractions, which may minimize muscle soreness. In addition, it may be possible to reduce joint forces by using isokinetic training at high speeds where torque production is reduced.

The research indicates that isokinetic strength training can induce gains in strength through various combinations of velocity of movement, number of repetitions and number of sets. Rather than using a specified number of repetitions, a specified period of time for each set ranging from 20 to 60 seconds has been used (305–310). Another approach has been to continue the set until torque production has dropped to a specified percentage of maximal, usually between 50% and 90% (311,312). It appears that training should be at a velocity between 180° and 240° per second if the goal is to increase strength over a wide range of velocities (271).

Eccentric Training

Eccentric training refers to muscular contractions in which the muscle lengthens in a controlled manner. Eccentric force output is greater than concentric force output (313,314). Because of the greater resistance that can be used during eccentric training, advocates of this technique believe that greater strength gains can occur compared with training that is primarily concentric in nature.

Including an eccentric component during either dynamic constant external resistance training (235,315) or isokinetic training (316,317) appears to allow greater strength gains than when only concentric exercise is performed. However, the majority of evidence indicates that eccentric exercise alone results in no greater gains in isometric, eccentric and concentric strength than dynamic constant external resistance training that involves both a concentric and eccentric component (278,286,318).

Comparison of Different Types of Strength Training

Studies comparing the various types of resistance training typically have several problems, making it difficult to identify the most beneficial type of training for strength gains. A major issue relates to specificity of training. When training and testing are performed using the same type of resistive equipment, a large increase in strength is demonstrated. However, if training and testing are performed with different types of equipment, the increase in strength is substantially less or nonexistent. Problems in comparison also arise in equating total training volume (i.e., sets and repetitions), total work (i.e., total repetitions times resistance) and total training time. These discrepancies make it difficult to prove the superiority of one type of resistance training over another. In addition, the demonstration of differences between types of resistance training may require studies of longer duration than the typical 10 to 20 weeks.

Safety Issues

Resistance training, as with all physical activities, has some inherent dangers. However, the risk of injury while performing resistance training has been demonstrated to be very low. In one study of college football players, the weight room injury rate was demonstrated to be 0.13 injuries per 1,000 athlete exposures (319). A properly designed exercise prescription, the use of proper lifting, spotting and breathing techniques, and good maintenance of equipment help to reduce the chance of injury during resistance training.

Spotting

Proper spotting is necessary to ensure the safety of the participants in a resistance-training program using free weights. Spotters serve to assist the trainee with the exercise and to summon help if an accident does occur. Several factors should be considered when spotting, including (a) the spotter must be strong enough to assist the trainee if needed, (b) during the performance of certain exercises (i.e., back squats), more than one spotter may be necessary to ensure the safety of the lifter, (c) spotters should know the proper technique of the lift they are spotting and proper spotting technique, (d) a spotter should know how many repetitions the trainee is going to attempt, (e) spotters must be attentive at all times to the lifter and to his or her performance of the exercise, and (f) spotters should know how to summon help if an injury does occur. Following these simple guidelines will aid in the avoidance of weight room injuries.

Breathing

Blood pressure rises substantially during the performance of resistance training exercises (254,320). Blood pressure during an isometric contraction in which breathing is allowed is substantially lower than when the contraction is performed simultaneously with a Valsalva maneuver, or when a Valsalva maneuver is performed in the absence of an isometric muscle action. Therefore, Valsalva maneuvers are not recommended during the performance of resistance training exercises.

Normally, it is recommended to exhale during the lifting of the resistance and inhale during the lowering of the resistance during each repetition. During the last few repetitions of a heavy resistance set, some breath holding will invariably occur. However, excessive breath holding should be discouraged.

Proper Technique

Proper lifting technique is a necessary injury prevention measure. This is especially true in exercises that place stress on the lower back region.

Altering the movement used can allow utilization of additional muscles to help perform the exercise. This decreases the training stimulus to the muscles normally associated with a particular exercise. This is another reason why proper lifting technique is important.

Full Range of Motion

Resistance exercises should normally be performed through the full range of motion allowed by the body position and the joints involved. Although no definitive studies are available, it is assumed that to optimally develop strength throughout the full range of motion of a joint, training must be performed through the full range.

Equipment Maintenance

Maintaining equipment in proper operating condition is of utmost importance for a safe resistance training program. Pulleys and cables or belts should be regularly checked for wear and replaced as needed. Equipment should be lubricated as indicated by the manufacturer. Cracked or broken free weight plates or plates in the weight stack of a machine should be replaced. Upholstery should be disinfected daily. The sleeves on Olympic bars should revolve freely so that skin is not torn off of a lifter's hands.

Assessment of Strength

Muscular strength is commonly assessed in the clinical setting through manual muscle testing (321). However, owing to the potential interindividual and intraindividual variations with manual muscle-testing techniques, more objective strength measurement methods may be valuable under some situations. Hand-held devices for recording force production have been in use since at least 1941 (321). These devices measure the amount of force exerted by the examiner against the limb of the patient, and may be especially valuable for providing more objective strength measurements than manual muscle testing at the higher end of the strength range.

Strength may also be easily assessed in the clinical setting through various isometric dynamometers. These devices are available to measure either compressive or tensile forces. Such devices are commonly used for testing isometric hand grip and isometric lifting strength.

Resistance training equipment may also be used to assess strength. The 1 RM can be measured either with free weights or resistance machines. Various isokinetic and isometric machines have also been used to measure strength in the clinical as well as the research setting. The disadvantages of these devices are the cost of the equipment and the time required for performing the tests, but the advantage is that a more objective strength measurement may be obtained.

With all forms of strength testing, the positioning of the body, method of body stabilization, movement speed, and positioning of the testing device must be standardized in order to be able to make comparison with subsequent strength measurements.

RANGE OF MOTION

Importance

It is important to maintain a range of motion adequate to perform one's desired activities. Lost range of motion can interfere with such functional activities as ambulation, self-care, or attendant care. Severe restrictions in range of motion may even produce complications like skin breakdown. Even relatively small reductions in range may result in biomechanical accommodations that place abnormal stress on tissues elsewhere in the body that can induce secondary problems.

While it is clear that restoration and maintenance of a functional range of motion is desirable, the benefits from greater flexibility are not clear. Proponents of stretching have claimed numerous positive effects including the prevention of musculoskeletal injuries and improved performance in sports, reduced postexercise muscle soreness, and improved general well-being. Nevertheless, the objective support for these claims is limited. Pre-exercise stretching has been demonstrated to have no effect on the development of delayed onset muscle soreness (322). It has also recently been demonstrated that running economy is even better among those individuals who have some lower extremity tightness (323,324). This has been suggested to be related to the ability to better utilize elastic storage and recovery and minimize the need for muscle-stabilizing activity. In contrast, the performance of a rebound bench press (no pause between the eccentric and concentric work) among power lifters has been demonstrated to be improved through enhanced flexibility (325). This finding was attributed to a reduction in stiffness of the musculotendinous unit that allowed better utilization of elastic storage and recovery.

Factors Affecting Range of Motion

A number of factors can limit joint range of motion, including tightness of soft tissue structures such as muscle, tendon, ligament, and joint capsule. Involuntary muscle contraction in the form of spasm can also restrict range. The bony contour of the joint is important in determining the full range of motion. When there is abnormal bone growth around a joint, range can be restricted. In addition, intra-articular loose bodies (e.g., bone or cartilage) and excessive fluid can restrict joint range of motion.

Range of motion varies widely among individuals. Regular activities using a full range of motion will help maintain range, but the maintenance of range of motion is specific to the joints that are used. For instance, an individual can have normal range in one joint but have severely restricted range in another. When connective tissue is not stretched, the collagen component gradually shortens. As a result, the periarticular collagen and the connective tissue of the muscle shorten. Furthermore, immobilization of a muscle in a shortened position also causes a decrease in the muscle length through a decrease in the number of sarcomeres in the muscle (326).

Age and sex also seem to affect range of motion. Women tend to have greater range of motion than men, and young individuals tend to have greater range than the elderly. Tissue temperature is another factor affecting range of motion, with warm tissue having greater distensibility than cool tissue (327-329).

Techniques to Assess Range of Motion

Range of motion may be assessed in various ways. Angle measurements can be made with a goniometer, electrogoniometer, or flexometer (330). Flexibility for some movements is also commonly assessed through distance measurements between specific reproducible reference points. One example of this technique would be the assessment of temporomandibular joint motion through measurement of the distance between the upper and lower incisors.

Methods to Improve Range of Motion

Techniques

Restoration of joint range of motion and soft tissue extensibility can be achieved through the utilization of several different stretching techniques and modalities. The three general categories of stretching techniques include ballistic, static, and proprioceptive neuromuscular facilitation (PNF) procedures.

Ballistic stretching is characterized by repetitious bouncing movements where the momentum of a moving body segment is used to generate forces producing a rapid stretch. Fast rates of stretching, as is the case with ballistic stretching, are not advisable, particularly during the early phases of rehabilitation. When fast stretch rates are used, greater tensions are developed, and more energy will be absorbed within the muscle–tendon unit for a given length of stretch (331). As a result, there is a greater risk for injury with this type of stretching. Furthermore, ballistic stretching does not appear to be as effective in enhancing range as other methods of stretching (332,333).

Static stretching involves a slowly applied stretch that is held for several seconds. Proponents of this technique believe that the muscle stretch reflex is minimized through a slow progressive stretch (334). Static stretching is generally easy to perform, can be done voluntarily or received passively by the individual, and has little associated risk of injury. While the optimal time to hold a static stretch and number of stretches that should be performed is not known, experimental studies on animals suggest that the majority of stress relaxation takes place during the initial 12 to 18 seconds, and there is little alteration in muscle–tendon unit lengthening after the fourth stretch (331).

Several stretching techniques use the principles of PNF that were developed by Kabat (335) to aid in the rehabilitation of injured World War II veterans. The concept of these stretching techiques is to enhance relaxation of the muscle to be stretched through reciprocal inhibition and the stretch reflex. The two most common PNF stretching techniques are the contract–relax technique and the agonist contract–relax technique. With the former, the muscle is passively stretched, then contracted for 6 to 8 seconds, and then relaxed and passively stretched further to an increased pain-free range. This process is repeated three to six times. Theoretically, the prestretch contraction of the muscle results in inhibition through Golgi tendon organ reflexes. The agonist contract–relax technique is identical to the contract–relax technique except that the stretch is accompanied by a submaximal contraction of the opposing muscle to the one being stretched. This voluntary contraction of the opposing muscle theoretically results in reciprocal inhibition of the stretched muscle.

When able to participate, the patient can provide valuable feedback to assure that appropriate positioning is used so that the desired tissues are being stretched. The patient should also understand that some discomfort may be required for adequate stretching to result, but prolonged poststretching pain is indicative of an overzealous approach. It also seems to be of considerable importance for the patient and therapist to understand that the most rapid gains in range of motion will be achieved through regular stretching. In some cases, the performance of stretching exercises several times each day is desirable, but there is evidence that increases in range of motion can be achieved through three to five sessions per week (332,333).

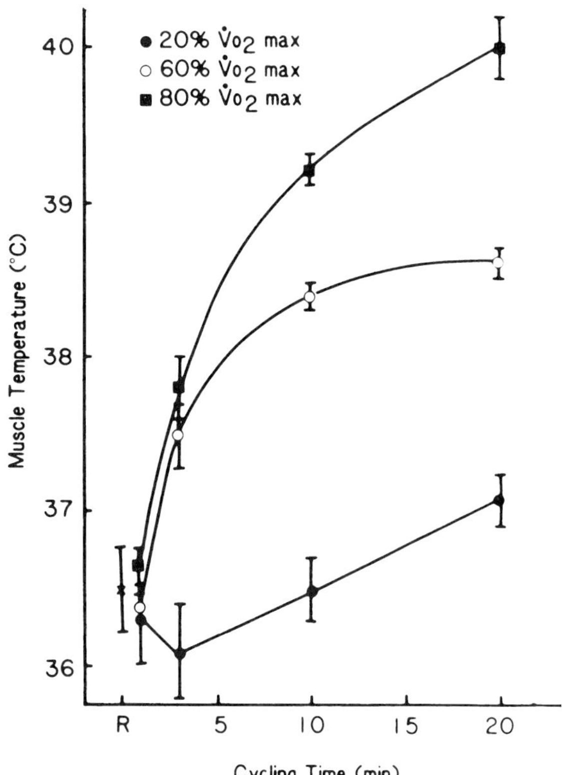

FIG. 28-27. Effect of leg cycling at different intensities and durations on intramuscular temperature of the quadriceps at a depth of 3 cm. The mean resting value is represented at *R*. (With permission from Hoffman MD, Williams CA, Lind AR. Changes in isometric function following rhythmic exercise. *Eur J Appl Physiol* 1985; 54:177–183.)

Modalities

Some modalities may be used to enhance range of motion. Because the distensibility of warm tissue is greater than that of cool tissue (327–329), heat is commonly used before stretching. Ultrasound is the best therapeutic modality for heating deep-lying tissues (336) and can be used effectively as a prestretching treatment when there are no contraindications for its use. One should also take advantage of the elevation in tissue temperature that can be achieved through exercise. For example, the quadriceps intramuscular temperature can be elevated by 2°C after 10 minutes of cycling at a moderate intensity (Fig. 28-27).

Simultaneous stretching and brief application of fluorimethane spray (stretch and spray) or passage of ice along the course of the muscle being stretched has also been advocated as a means to enhance the stretch of muscles (337). When an active trigger point is present, stretching may be enhanced by injection of a small amount of local anesthetic into the trigger point before stretching. The reader is referred elsewhere (337) for a description of the techniques for stretch and spray and trigger point injections.

PROPRIOCEPTION

Importance

Proprioceptive organs provide the central nervous system with information about the position and movement of body parts. Recent work has demonstrated the importance of proprioceptive sensation in the rehabilitation after injuries, and in understanding the etiologies and predisposing factors to injuries and reinjuries.

Decreased joint proprioception has been observed in patients with osteoarthritis, rheumatoid arthritis, and Charcot's disease and is believed to influence the progressive joint deterioration with these disorders (338,339). The risk of falling may also relate to proprioception as measures of postural sway have been demonstrated to relate to the falling risk (340–343).

Much of the work demonstrating the importance of proprioception in rehabilitation comes from the sports medicine literature. The importance of improving proprioception has been demonstrated by the finding of a significantly greater risk of sustaining an ankle injury during soccer among players with abnormal proprioceptive testing compared with those players with normal values (344). The successful return to sport after a ligament injury may be even more dependent on proprioception than on ligament tension (345) .

Factors Affecting Proprioception

Sensation of the position and movement of a joint arise from afferent information originating from muscles, joint capsules, ligaments, and skin. As a result, injuries or disease to these structures may affect proprioception. For instance, reduced proprioception has been shown to be associated with knee (346) and ankle (112,347,348) ligament injuries, rheumatoid arthritis (349), and osteoarthritis (338). The importance of muscle receptors in proprioception has been demonstrated through the finding of impaired reproduction of joint angle after fatiguing contractions of the associated muscles (350).

Disease of the neurologic system may also affect proprioception. Diabetics with cutaneous sensory neuropathy have been shown to have a significant loss of ankle joint proprioception (351).

Decreases in proprioception have also been found with increasing age (338,349,352,353) and may be part of the normal aging process.

Techniques to Assess Proprioception

Methods for accurate and objective assessment of joint movement and position perception have not been adequately developed for widespread clinical use. The most common clinical method of evaluating proprioception is a nonquantitative test of joint position perception consisting of the subject verbally describing the joint position after the examiner passively moves the segment into one of two or more predetermined positions (354). Another nonquantitative testing technique used in the clinical setting involves testing the ability of a person to return a joint to a predetermined joint position.

In the research setting, a number of techniques have been used in the evaluation of proprioception. These research techniques include using an isokinetic dynamometer to quantify angles during reproduction of a predetermined joint position (355,356), matching of joint position with the side contralateral to the one being passively moved or positioned (357–359), and measurement of joint movement perception threshold (111,351,355). Although not exclusively a measure of proprioception, other techniques that may provide related information about balance and coordination include measures of postural sway (360,361) and responses to perturbations that create sway (362).

Techniques to Improve Proprioception

Proprioceptive exercises are performed with the goal of reducing the proprioceptive deficits that may have resulted through injury or disease. There is some evidence for the effectiveness of proprioceptive exercises in that it has been shown that the proprioceptive deficits present after ligament injuries can be reduced (363–365).

Classical lower extremity proprioceptive exercises have used the tilt (teeter or wobble) board. Unidirectional boards may be used initially, followed by multidirectional boards. More functionally specific proprioceptive exercises can also be developed. These activities may include backward and sideways walking and running, or other agility drills.

It should also be noted that elastic bandaging (338) has been shown to improve position sense in those with impaired proprioception. It is thought that this may be achieved through enhancement of the activity of the skin proprioceptors.

THE EXERCISE PRESCRIPTION

General Considerations

The exercise prescription should be a systematic and individualized recommendation about physical activity for development and maintenance of health and fitness and/or treatment of specific conditions. Regardless of the individual's age, functional capacity, or medical conditions, the exercise prescription should include information about the mode, intensity, duration, frequency, and rate of progression of physical activity. Individualization of the exercise prescription is based on considerations of the individual's health history, cardiac risk factors, behavioral characteristics, personal goals, exercise preferences, and specific exercise needs.

The specific purpose of an exercise program will depend on the individual. However, exercise goals generally include (a) to counteract the detrimental physiological effects of previous sedentary living or a transient period of reduced activity associated with disease or injury, and (b) to optimize functional capacity within the physical limitations of medical conditions that may be present. In addition, valuable clinical information for the ongoing treatment of a patient can frequently be elicited through exercise training programs.

Risk Stratification

A concern in advising middle-aged and older people is the risk of sudden cardiac death or other cardiac complications associated with exercise. The incidence of sudden death with exercise is low, but when it occurs in those over 35 years of age, it is usually related to a combination of coronary artery disease and vigorous exercise (366). Importantly, the benefits of exercise conditioning outweigh the small risk of sudden cardiac death or other cardiac complications (115,367,368). Furthermore, regular exercise may help protect against sudden death or myocardial infarction from strenuous physical activities (57,62,115,367).

Risk stratification assists in the decision about how to proceed in developing an exercise program. This is performed through a clinical evaluation that includes identification of the presence of coronary risk factors. The major coronary risk factors are displayed in Table 28-6. Those individuals who have no symptoms suggestive of cardiopulmonary disease (Table 28-7), are apparently healthy, and have no more than one major coronary risk factor are considered at low risk. Those individuals with symptoms sugges-

TABLE 28-6. *Coronary artery disease risk factors*

Positive risk factors	Defining criteria
1. Age	Men >45 years; women >55 or premature menopause without estrogen replacement therapy
2. Family history	Myocardial infarction or sudden death before 55 years of age in father or other male first-degree relative, or before 65 years of age in mother or other female first-degree relative
3. Current cigarette smoking	
4. Hypertension	Blood pressure ≥140/90 mm Hg, confirmed by measurements on at least 2 separate occasions, or on antihypertensive medication
5. Hypercholesterolemia	Total serum cholesterol >200 mg/dL (5.2 mmol/liter) (if lipoprotein profile is unavailable) or HDL <35 mg/dL (0.9 mmol/liter)
6. Diabetes mellitus	Persons with insulin-dependent diabetes (IDDM) who are >30 years of age, or have had IDDM for >15 years, and persons with noninsulin-dependent-diabetes (NIDDM) who are >35 years of age should be classified as patients with disease
7. Sedentary lifestyle/physical inactivity	Persons comprising the least active 25% of the population, as defined by the combination of sedentary jobs involving sitting for a large part of the day and no regular exercise or active recreational pursuits
Negative risk factors	**Defining criteria**
1. High serum HDL cholesterol	>60 mg/dL (1.6 mmol/liter)

It should be noted that (a) it is common to sum risk factors in making clinical judgments. If HDL is high, subtract one risk factor from the sum of positive risk factors, since high HDL decreases coronary artery disease; (b) obesity is not listed as an independent positive risk factor because its effects are exerted through other risk factors (e.g., hypertension, hyperlipidemia, diabetes). Obesity should be considered as an independent target for intervention.

From American College of Sports Medicine. *ACSM'S guidelines for exercise testing and prescriptions, 5th ed.* Baltimore: Williams & Wilkins, 1995.

tive of cardiopulmonary or metabolic disease and/or two or more major coronary risk factors are considered at increased risk. A third category is those with known cardiac, pulmonary or metabolic disease.

Those individuals at low risk can begin moderate exercise (intensities of 40% to 60% of $\dot{V}O_{2max}$) programs without the need for further assessment (Table 28-8). It is also believed that vigorous exercise (intensities over 60% of $\dot{V}O_{2max}$) may be initiated without further assessment among low-risk men 40 years of age or younger and low-risk women 50 years of age or younger. Vigorous exercise in older individuals at low risk should be preceded with a medical examination and exercise test. Those at higher risk but without symptoms may begin a moderate exercise program without a medical examination or exercise test, but should undergo these evaluations if initiating a vigorous exercise program. All others at higher risk or with known disease are advised to undergo a medical examination and exercise test before beginning a moderate or vigorous exercise program.

TABLE 28-7. *Major symptoms and signs suggestive of cardiopulmonary disease*[a]

1. Pain, discomfort (or other anginal equivalent) in the chest, neck, jaw, arms, or other areas that may be ischemic in nature
2. Shortness of breath at rest or with mild exertion
3. Dizziness or syncope
4. Orthopnea or paroxysmal nocturnal dyspnea
5. Ankle edema
6. Palpitations or tachycardia
7. Intermittent claudication
8. Known heart murmur
9. Unusual fatigue or shortness of breath with usual activities

[a] These symptoms must be interpreted in the clinical context in which they appear, because they are not all specific for cardiopulmonary or metabolic disease.

From American College of Sports Medicine. *ACSM'S guidelines for exercise testing and prescriptions, 5th ed.* Baltimore: Williams & Wilkins, 1995.

For individuals who have recently experienced a cardiac event, participation in a supervised exercise program within a cardiac rehabilitation program is an effective and safe way of initiating an exercise program and then progressing to an aerobic intensity threshold (369). Surveys indicate low morbidity and mortality rates associated with supervised exercise programs (370–372). A 1986 report derived from a survey among multiple centers indicated a major complication rate of one per 81,101 patients (371).

In children and young adults, deaths associated with physical activities are uncommon but, when they occur, are generally related to congenital heart disease or acquired myocarditis (115,373). Individuals with known congenital heart disease should generally be encouraged to remain physically active but refrain from vigorous and competitive athletics (115). Screening for detection of cardiac abnormalities in young people prior to participation in sports appears to be of limited value (373).

Injury and Illness Precautions

It is important that exercise programs are designed to avoid inducing or exacerbating health problems. Although any exercise carries some risk of injury, the risk can be

TABLE 28-8. *Indications for medical examination and clinical exercise testing prior to exercise participation*

	Apparently healthy		Increased risk[a]		
Exercise intensity	Younger[b]	Older	No symptoms	Symptoms	Known disease[c]
Moderate[d]	No	No	No	Yes	Yes
Vigorous[e]	No	Yes	Yes	Yes	Yes

[a] Persons with two or more risk factors (see Table 28-6) or one or more signs or symptoms (see Table 28-7).

[b] Persons with known cardiac, pulmonary, or metabolic disease.

[c] Younger implies ≤40 years for men, ≤50 years for women.

[d] Moderate exercise is defined as an intensity of 40–60% maximal oxygen uptake; if intensity is uncertain, moderate exercise may alterantely be defined as an intensity well within the individual's current capacity, one which can be comfortably sustained for a prolonged period of time, that has a gradual initiation and progression, and is generally noncompetitive.

[e] Vigorous exercise is defined as an intensity >60% maximal oxygen uptake; if intensity is uncertain, vigorous exercise may alternately be defined as exercise intense enough to represent a substantial cardiorespiratory challenge or if it results in fatigue within 20 minutes.

Adapted from American College of Sports Medicine. *ACSM's guidelines for exercise testing and prescriptions, 5th ed.* Baltimore: Williams & Wilkins, 1995.

extremely minimal through individualization of the exercise prescription. It is recognized that an increased risk of musculoskeletal injury is associated with weight bearing activities, high exercise intensities and volume, previous history of injury, biomechanical abnormalities, and a rapid increase in exercise participation. Injury risk can be minimized by avoidance of weight bearing activities in those predisposed to musculoskeletal injuries because of obesity, previous injury or biomechanical abnormalities, selection of appropriate footwear, and gradual increases in physical activity.

The effect of exercise on immune function is not completely understood. There is some evidence that regular aerobic exercise enhances immune function, but that strenuous exercise may transiently impair immune status (189–192). Furthermore, the effect of exercise on the progression of existing infectious diseases like viral respiratory infections is not well understood. Myocarditis can develop when individuals continue to exercise in the presence of such illnesses. Therefore, it is generally recommended that strenuous exercise be avoided in the presence of fever or myalgia.

Environmental Factors

Hot and/or humid conditions can increase the health risk associated with exercise. In extreme conditions of exercise and environmental heat stress, competition for blood flow between muscle and cutaneous vascular beds can lead to reduced ability to exercise and/or thermoregulate. Serious heat disorders with exercise are more common in competitive events where the drive to perform well can override normal signals to stop or decrease work levels. Due to the potential health hazards of exercise performed in hot/humid environmental conditions, some organizations or groups cancel events or release warnings regarding activity participation based on environmental conditions. When participating in activities performed in a hot environment, people should monitor their ability to respond physiologically to the combined stressors. Heart rate tracks upward and rating of perceived effort typically rises in relation to the body heat load. Thus, these parameters can provide important feedback information in regulating work level in a hot environment (73,76).

The importance of fluid intake during sustained exercise should be emphasized. Anyone planning to compete in an endurance-type activity combined with heat stress should undergo heat acclimation prior to competition. Daily exercise in the heat for seven to ten days will significantly improve ability to thermoregulate (73). Some of the physiological adjustments with acclimation include improved sweating (earlier onset and increased capacity), decreased loss of electrolytes, and increased blood volume. As a consequence of acclimation, physiological strain during exercise combined with heat is reduced as evidenced by a lower heart rate and core temperature (73). A position statement issued by the American College of Sports Medicine on preventing heat problems with distance running serves as a useful guide for avoiding heat-related problems with exercise (374).

In extremely cold environments, it is important to provide protection against hypothermia and cold injuries to exposed skin. Appropriate clothing and protection of the hands and face can allow comfortable continuation of exercise under quite extreme conditions.

Concerns regarding the safety of exercise at altitude have been raised, especially for patients with ischemic heart disease (375,376). Typically, work capacity is reduced at high altitudes due to lower oxygen availability. This effect is seen starting at about 1,500 m and further reduced about 6 to 10% per additional 1000 m ascent. Most resort areas and major highways are located at <4000 m. Minimal information is available regarding the safety of exercise at altitude for patients with cardiopulmonary diseases, although it appears that exercise is safe for many cardiac patients, at least up to moderate altitudes (375). Since work capacity often is reduced at altitude, the amount of absolute work that can be performed at a prescribed index of myocardial work (i.e., rate-pressure product) will be lower at high altitude compared with sea level. Due to the impact on work capacity, heart rate and perceived effort provide better indices to gauge work level than absolute work units. Due to the improved oxygen carrying capacity brought on during the first few days of exposure to altitude, individuals should be encouraged to delay vigorous physical activities upon immediately arriving at high altitudes.

Safety issues regarding exercise combined with air pollution have been raised. As reviewed elsewhere (73,376), minimal information is available regarding the impact of many air pollutants on work tolerance or cardiovascular responses to exercise. Since air pollutants can impact on oxygen carrying capacity and lung function, communities often issue ozone alerts when the ozone level reaches a critical threshold. These alerts often advise people, especially those with coronary artery and pulmonary diseases, to avoid outdoor exercise. The long-term health effects of repeated exercise combined with air pollution remain unclear.

Other environmental factors may also impact certain types of exercise. For instance, uneven or soft terrain and the presence of wind may substantially increase physiological demands (377,378) and necessitate that absolute work rates be adjusted downward. For some individuals, it is important to also consider the risk of falling presented by the exercise environment.

Equipment

A multitude of devices are on the market for use in strength and aerobic training. Special devices are also available for stretching and proprioceptive exercises. Special exercise equipment items are often used in the clinical setting and may be quite advantageous under some circumstances. Nevertheless, it is generally desirable to develop exercise programs that can be continued by the patient outside the clinical setting. This frequently means developing exercise programs that are not reliant upon special equipment. For strength training this may mean that exercises need to be designed that use body weight, readily available items found at home, or elastic tubing as the resistive force. Maintenance and development of aerobic conditioning can also be achieved through many different modes of exercise. When walking and running are appropriate options for an individual, these modes of exercise can certainly be as beneficial as other forms of exercise (210) and do not require any special equipment. Viable alternatives for some individuals may include the use of community resources, or purchase of exercise equipment for use at home.

Compliance

Exercise requires participation by the individual performing the exercise. This is sometimes a challenging concept to overcome when working with some patients who have grown accustomed to the classical medical model of passively accepting the treatment provided by their clinicians. Instilling an understanding of the concept that the individual needs to be a participant in the exercise program, along with a basic understanding of exercise, is critically important for success of the exercise program.

Often patients do not understand the differences between stretching and strengthening, and between exercises to develop strength and those to develop aerobic capacity. For strength gains to occur, it is important for the patient to understand that the muscles need to be voluntarily contracted against resistance. Whether the exercise is for strengthening, aerobic conditioning or stretching, patients need to realize that some discomfort is required for success, but should also recognize the difference between an appropriate level of discomfort and signals of over zealousness.

When exercise is initiated too aggressively, the transient exacerbation of symptoms or delayed onset muscle soreness may be discouraging to the patient. Post-exercise cryotherapy to local areas of inflammation may control exacerbations of symptoms. Restriction in the use of exercises involving eccentric contractions may also limit the development of delayed onset muscle soreness.

Another important concept for the patient to understand is that the desired changes resulting from an exercise program may not occur in a few days or even a few weeks. The patient must commit to a regular and consistent exercise routine for success. Adherence to a supervised exercise program depends upon the personality characteristics of the patient, various aspects of the rehabilitation setting, and the quality of the relationship developed between the patient and clinicians (379). Motivation of the patient is an essential element to success. Education and goal setting play an important role in developing and maintaining motivation. After completion of a supervised exercise program, compliance may be improved through regular follow-up appointments. During these visits, the exercise program may be modified and advanced as appropriate.

Health benefits associated with physical activity are largely dependent on long-term adherence to regular participation. Unfortunately, many people who initiate an exercise program do not continue long-term. Drop-out rates from supervised programs remain high and are even higher for individuals after leaving a supervised program.

Approximately one in four adults report no leisure-time activity and an additional one-third do not get enough physical activity to obtain health benefits (115). Most teenagers do not participate in vigorous activities and about 50% do not participate in physical education classes at school (115). Sedentary living is more common among Americans who have less education and are economically or socially disadvantaged (115,380). To achieve the exercise objectives established in the Healthy People 2000 Program, considerable change in physical activity participation is needed. Although there are indications of improved public awareness of the benefits associated with regular physical activity, this awareness has not yet translated into substantial improvement in physical activity levels among those who are sedentary (381–384). The recent release of the Surgeon General's report on physical activity emphasizes the importance of increasing physical activity levels among all Americans (385).

In implementing exercise programs for long-term compliance, it is important that individuals find physical activities that they are willing to undertake on a regular basis. The appropriate mode of activity, intensity, frequency, and duration to recommend is best determined by learning the individual's exercise preferences (115).

For many people, encouraging them to build greater physical activity into their normal "routines" and/or to participate in sport activities may be more effective in increasing habitual physical activity than encouraging participation in more traditional aerobic modes such as running or ergometry. Sport activities are more enjoyable for some and may thereby lead to better compliance. Electing to perform home activities in a manner more conducive to health benefits (e.g., using a walk-behind mower rather than a rider mower, use the stairs rather than the elevator) is a convenient and inexpensive way to increase physical activity levels (115,386). When combined with a walk/jog or some other type of exercise program, recreational and home activities can add welcomed variety and thereby enhance compliance to a regular program of exercise.

Attitudinal and behavioral factors within different population subgroups (ethnic background, socioeconomic status, gender, age, disease) can influence motivation for, and ability to sustain, physical activities (115,387–389). If an individual perceives that a recommended physical activity is inappropriate for them due to age, gender or some other factor, the person is likely to be more resistant to accepting advice.

Compliance to a regular program of physical activity is most likely if the individual perceives a benefit, the activity is enjoyable or acceptable, the individual feels safe and competent with the activity, the activity is convenient or fits into the daily schedule, costs are minimal, negative perceptions are minimized, and if the individual recognizes the benefit of performing daily activities in ways that incorporate more physical activity (115). Further work is required to develop better strategies for improving exercise compliance, especially among subpopulations where physical activity participation is low such as those who are socioeconomically deprived (115,382,383).

EXERCISE PRESCRIPTION IN SPECIAL POPULATIONS

Considerations in Chronic Disease States

Exercise is an important component of the management of many medical and disabling conditions. Additionally, many of the individuals treated in the rehabilitation setting with exercise will have concomitant medical conditions or disabilities that will affect the design of an exercise program, and their responses and adaptations to exercise. Special considerations in the design of exercise programs are often required when disease or disability are present.

The interaction between exercise and the given medical condition is important to understand so that the potential adverse effects of exercise may be avoided. In general, the exercise program must not interfere with the standard medical treatment of a disease state, and must be individualized in accordance with the presence and severity of the medical condition. Considerations relative to some of the common medical conditions and disabilities encountered in the rehabilitation setting are discussed below.

Cardiac Disease

Cardiac disease is a common condition among individuals treated in the rehabilitation setting. While exercise can generally be performed by those individuals with cardiovascular disease, it is important to recognize the presence and extent of disease prior to initiating exercise. This knowledge allows the development of a safe exercise program for the individual. Risk stratification (discussed above) assists in the process of developing a safe exercise program.

The general guidelines for aerobic exercise already discussed are applicable for patients with stable cardiac disease. In patients with ischemic changes, angina or arrhythmias during exercise, an exercise intensity 10-15 beats per minute below the ischemic, angina and dysrhythmic thresholds should be prescribed. When an individual is at high risk for cardiac events during exercise (Table 28-9), a more cautious approach is warranted with regard to the exercise intensity and level of supervision, and electrocardiographic and blood

TABLE 28-9. *Characteristics of cardiac patients associated with an increased risk for cardiac events during exercise*

Clinical status
Multiple myocardial infarctions
Poor left ventricular function (ejection fraction <40% at rest)
History of chronic congestive heart failure
Rest or unstable angina pectoris
Complex dysrhythmias
Left main coronary artery or three vessel atherosclerosis on angiography
Exercise test response
Low exercise tolerance (<4 METs)
Low peak heart rate off drugs (<120 beats/min)
Severe ischemia (ST depression >2 mm)
Angina pectoris at low heart rate or workload
Inappropriate systolic blood pressure response (decrease with increasing workloads)
Complex cardiac dysrhythmias, especially in patients with poor left ventricular function
Exercise training participation
Exercises above prescribed limits

MET, metabolic equivalent.

Adapted from American College of Sports Medicine. *ACSM's guidelines for exercise testing and prescriptions, 4th ed.* Philadelphia: Lea & Febiger,1991.

pressure monitoring should be considered. Gradual and prolonged cool-downs are particularly important in the population with known cardiac disease for reducing the risk of arrhythmias and post-exercise hypotension from blood pooling in the lower extremities.

Resistance training can be performed by most patients with stable cardiac disease as long as a significant dynamic work component is involved. Exclusion criteria for resistance training include congestive heart failure, severe valvular disease, poor left ventricular function, uncontrolled dysrhythmias and peak exercise capacity under 5 METs (390). When exercise intensity monitoring is warranted, the rate-pressure product may be a better indicator of ischemic threshold during resistance exercise than heart rate. For an accurate determination of the rate-pressure product, blood pressure needs to be taken while the muscular contractions are performed since blood pressure decreases rapidly upon release of the resistive load.

Diabetes

The diabetic individual can present many challenges in developing an exercise program. Problems associated with diabetes include cardiovascular disease, peripheral neuropathy, peripheral vascular disease, autonomic dysfunction, renal disease and retinopathy. Because of the high risk of cardiovascular disease in diabetics, exercise testing prior to the initiation of an exercise program is advisable (390).

The most common problem experienced by exercising diabetics is hypoglycemia. This can result from the presence of too much insulin, or accelerated absorption of insulin from the injection point. This is most likely to occur when short acting insulin is used and injected near the active muscle mass. It is therefore important that type I (insulin-dependent or juvenile-onset) diabetics be under adequate regulation before initiating an exercise program. Table 28-10 lists recommendations that have been provided to minimize the risk of hypoglycemic events among diabetics. An important component of the exercise prescription for the diabetic involves education on these precautions.

TABLE 28-10. *Recommended precautions for diabetics to avoid hypoglycemic reactions associated with exercise*

1. Frequently monitor blood glucose at the initiation of an exercise program.
2. Decrease the insulin dose (by 1–2 units) or increase carbohydrate intake (10–15 g per half-hour of exercise) prior to an exercise bout.
3. Inject insulin in an area such as the abdomen that is not active during exercise.
4. Avoid exercise during periods of peak insulin activity.
5. Eat carbohydrate snacks before and during prolonged periods of exercise.
6. Be knowledgeable of the signs and symptoms of hypoglycemia.
7. Avoid exercising alone.

Adapted from American College of Sports Medicine. *ACSM's guidelines for exercise testing and prescriptions, 4th ed.* Philadelphia: Lea & Febiger,1991.

It is recommended that the diabetic be attentive to the importance of using proper footwear and the practice of good foot hygiene. It should be recognized that diabetics on beta-blocking agents may be unable to experience hypoglycemic symptoms and/or angina. Additionally, it is important for the diabetic to take precautions to avoid hyperthermia that may result from impaired sweating.

The general exercise guidelines for aerobic exercise discussed above are applicable for the diabetic individual. However, it is important to recognize that the use of heart rate for establishing exercise intensity may be inappropriate for those diabetics with autonomic neuropathy and chronotropic insufficiency. In these cases, the use of perceived exertion to establish intensity may be more appropriate. The recommended mode of exercise also requires some consideration. Avoidance of weight-bearing activities in order to minimize foot irritation is important for obese diabetics. Also, those with advanced retinopathy should not use exercise modes that cause excessive jarring or a marked increase in blood pressure.

Obesity

Weight loss is achieved through a negative caloric balance. This is best accomplished from a combination of reduced caloric intake and increased caloric expenditure (161). Exercise increases overall energy expenditure, and so is recommended as a component of the treatment of obesity.

Individuals who are overweight are generally sedentary and are likely to have negative connotations about exercise. Exploration of the past history with exercise by these individuals is important in developing future exercise compliance. Other problems associated with exercise in obesity include muscle soreness and orthopedic injury. As a result, aerobic exercise programs for obese individuals should utilize activities that minimize joint stress, such as walking, cycling, rowing, stair climbing and exercise in water.

Arthritis

The exercise program for individuals with arthritis must be adjusted depending upon the state of the disease. When the disease activity is high in those with rheumatoid arthritis, activity may need to be minimized to avoid tissue damage. The use of short duration, frequent sessions may be tolerated and allow one to minimize the adverse effects of inactivity and maintain range of motion even during high disease activity. The use of non-weight bearing and low impact activities are recommended to limit joint stress. Swimming and cycling may be the best tolerated exercise modes by those with arthritis. Resistance training and range of motion activities are also particularly important to optimize joint stability and movement patterns.

Peripheral Vascular Disease

Peripheral arteriosclerosis is associated with hypertension and hyperlipidemia, and is frequently observed in patients with coronary artery disease, cerebrovascular disease and diabetes. Because of the common association of peripheral arteriosclerosis with coronary artery disease, these patients are generally advised to undergo exercise testing prior to initiating an exercise program. A discontinuous testing protocol will likely optimize the testing results. Because of the limitations by leg discomfort with treadmill or cycle ergometry testing, arm ergometry may be required to achieve adequate myocardial stress.

Walking is the preferred mode of exercise training for induction of functional changes, but non-weight bearing activities may be better tolerated initially by these patients. Exercise sessions should use interval training at intensities that elicit the most leg discomfort tolerable to the patient. Initially, the sessions should be 20-30 minutes twice a day, and progress to 40-60 minutes in one session each day. As functional capacity improves, the exercise intensity should be increased so that central cardiovascular adaptations are more likely to be induced.

Spinal Cord Injury

Spinal cord injury affects exercise capacity through its alteration of the amount of functioning muscle mass, and through compromise of the autonomic nervous system affecting cardioacceleration, blood flow redistribution and thermoregulation. These issues are important from the standpoint of exercise capacity, potential training adaptations and safety during exercise.

Depending on the extent and level of the lesion, spinal cord injury can limit the functional muscle mass to the upper body. This limitation reduces the aerobic demands that can be induced during training. While it is clear that endurance training with the upper body can enhance peak $\dot{V}O_2$ and work capacity during exercise, it is likely that most or all of the changes are achieved through peripheral rather than central adaptations (205,207). This means that spinal cord injury may prevent or severely limit the ability to achieve central cardiovascular adaptations.

Complete lesions of the spinal cord will also have an effect on the autonomic nervous system. Loss of sympathetic cardiac innervation from lesions above the sixth thoracic level can limit maximal heart rate to 110-130 beats per minute (391). Lesions at the cervical and thoracic levels can impair control over regional blood flow during exercise causing venous blood pooling in the legs and abdomen, and consequently a reduced preloading of the heart. Stroke volume and cardiac output at a given oxygen uptake during exercise tend to be reduced in those with spinal cord injury (392,393). Furthermore, thermoregulatory ability is impaired through loss of sympathetic nervous system control for vasomotor and sudomotor responses in the areas of the insensate skin (394).

Exercise testing prior to the initiation of an exercise program may have a somewhat greater role in the spinal cord injured than the general population. Besides assisting in the recognition of the presence of coronary artery disease, exercise testing in spinal cord injury may also assist in assuring that the individual will not have serious problems with hypotension during exercise. Exercise testing may have additional importance since classical symptoms of angina pectoris may be absent in quadriplegics because most of the visceral afferents from the heart enter the spinal cord at the upper thoracic levels. Exercise testing will generally be performed using arm or wheelchair ergometry.

Despite the physiological limitations, spinal cord injured individuals have demonstrated that they can safely participate in many activities such as long distance wheelchair propulsion, swimming, kayaking and cross-country skiing on sit skis. Wheelchair propulsion and wheelchair or arm crank ergometry are common training modes. Recent research has suggested that lower body compression (395-397), functional electrical stimulation of the paralyzed lower limbs (398,399) or supine body position (400), concomitant with upper body exercise may enhance venous return and cardiac output and provide a greater chance for central training adaptations.

The intensity and duration guidelines for cardiovascular training in the apparently healthy appear to be reasonable for the spinal cord injured (391). Autonomic dysreflexia and hypotension are potentially serious complications that may present with exercise in this population. The potential thermoregulatory problems of the spinal cord injured should also prompt caution in hot conditions. Nevertheless, the overall risk of serious problems from participating in appropriately structured exercise programs appears to be low for the spinal cord injured.

Postpoliomyelitis Syndrome

The fear of increasing muscle weakness from overuse has been a concern about the use of exercise in individuals who have post-polio sequelae. However, it now appears that these individuals can generally exercise without adverse effects. Individuals with post-polio sequelae generally seem to respond to endurance training in a manner similar to healthy adults (401–404). Likewise, it has been demonstrated that resistance training can enhance strength without complications in individuals with post-polio sequelae (405). Nevertheless, it is recommended that careful individual monitoring, including occassional muscle function tests, be performed during the physical training of individuals with post-polio sequelae (403).

Multiple Sclerosis

Concerns about the safety of exercise in those with multiple sclerosis have centered around the potential adverse effects from the autonomic dysfunction that may accompany the disease, and the potential exacerbation of the disease through thermal stress. Unfortunately, very little is known about the effects of multiple sclerosis on the physiological responses to exercise, or the effects of exercise on the disease process (406). There is encouraging evidence that some individuals with multiple sclerosis can perform endurance exercise to levels above the anaerobic threshold without development of significant or persistent neurologic symptoms (407), that aerobic training can induce beneficial cardiovascular adaptations (408), and that strength gains can be achieved through resistance training (409). Nevertheless, until more scientific investigation is completed, a conservative approach to exercise is warranted in the multiple sclerosis patient.

Cancer

Exercise is becoming an accepted component of rehabilitation of patients with cancer. Besides counteracting the effects of inactivity and improving psychological status (410), there is some evidence that immune function may be improved through moderate levels of exercise (189-192).

A number of problems may interfere with the exercise program of individuals with cancer. Cancer treatments may induce cytotoxicity, immunologic suppression, bleeding disorders and anemia. Some chemotherapeutic agents induce direct cardiac or pulmonary damage that affect exercise performance. Difficulties in maintaining nutritional needs, adequate hydration and electrolyte balance may also be problematic. Other side effects such as fatigue and infection may seriously impact exercise programs.

The general guidelines for aerobic exercise training discussed above are appropriate for individuals with cancer, but the intensity should usually be at the lower end of the range. Patients with known or potential malignancies affecting bone, particularly the spine, pelvis, femur and ribs, should use non-weightbearing modalities. When the risk of bruising, fractures and balance problems are increased, resistance exercise should be performed on machines rather than with free weights. It has also been recommended that patients with low platelet counts should avoid resistance training for 36 hours prior to blood draws for enzyme studies since there may be an effect of resistance training on those enzymes that are sometimes used to follow the clinical course of patients (208).

Considerations in Selected Groups Within the Able-Bodied Population

Pregnant women, children, and the elderly possess unique physical, physiological and behavioral characteristics that need to be considered in the design of exercise programs.

Pregnancy

Concerns about exercise during pregnancy have related to the competition between the exercising maternal muscle and the fetus for blood flow, oxygen delivery and glucose availability, and issues related to heat dissipation. Presently though, there is no evidence in humans to indicate that healthy pregnant women need to limit their exercise intensity for fear of adverse effects.

TABLE 28-11. *Contraindications for exercising during pregnancy*

1. Pregnancy induced hypertension
2. Preterm rupture of membrane
3. Preterm labor during the prior or current pregnancy
4. Incompetent cervix
5. Persistent second- to third-trimester bleeding
6. Intrauterine growth retardation

From American College of Obstetricians and Gynecologists. *Exercise during pregnancy and postpartum period* (Techinical Bulletin 28-189). Washington, D.C. Author, 1994

Contraindications for exercise during pregnancy have been established (Table 28-11). For women who do not have risk factors for adverse maternal or perinatal outcomes, the American College of Obstetrics and Gynecology has provided exercise recommendations (Table 28-12). Within these recommendations, and equipped with the understanding of signs and symptoms for discontinuing exercise (Table 28-13), exercise during pregnancy is felt to be safe.

Those women who exercise regularly and become pregnant can continue their training program. Those women beginning a new strenuous exercise program after becoming pregnant are advised to receive physician authorization and begin low intensity and low or non-impact activities.

Children

Children are anatomically, physiologically and psychologically immature, so special precautions should be applied when designing exercise programs for this group. Concern has been raised about the risk of overuse injuries and damage to the epiphyseal growth plates if the amount of exercise is excessive (413). There is also concern about the ability of children to adapt to thermal stress. Children are physiologically less tolerant of heat than adults because of a higher threshold for sweating, a lower output of the heat-activated sweat glands and a slower acclimatization to heat (414).

Aerobic exercise programs for children should increase the quantity of exercise gradually, assure the use of appropriate footwear, and take precautions in high environmental temperatures that include limiting strenuous prolonged exercise, providing good hydration and encouraging the use of light clothing.

It has been concluded that children can induce significant strength gains through resistance training (227). Resistance training by children should be performed under close adult supervision, with maximal resistance being avoided and proper lifting techniques being stressed.

Elderly

When designing an exercise program for older adults, the possibility that a latent or active disease process may be present must be considered. Exercise testing should be performed prior to beginning a vigorous exercise program as outlined in Table 28-8. The exercise prescription must be individualized based upon health status and individual goals.

A conservative approach to exercise is generally warranted in the elderly since many older persons suffer from a variety of medical problems. Aerobic exercise sessions may initially need to be divided into short bouts and the mode of exercise should not impose significant joint stress. Due to the variability in maximal heart rate in persons over 65 years of age, the use of age predicted maximal heart rates for exercise prescriptions is not recommended.

TABLE 28-12. *Recommendations for exercise in pregnancy and postpartum*

1. During pregnancy, women can continue to exercise and derive health benefits from mild to moderate exercise routines. Regular exercise (at least three times per week) is preferable to intermittent activity.
2. Women should avoid exercise in the supine position after the first trimester. Such a position is associated with decreased cardiac output in most pregnant women. Because the remaining cardiac output will be preferentially distributed away from splanchnic beds (including the uterus) during vigorous exercise, such regimens are best avoided during pregnancy. Prolonged periods of motionless standing should also be avoided.
3. Women should be aware of the decreased oxygen available for aerobic exercise during pregnancy. They should be encouraged to modify the intensity of their exercise according to maternal symptoms. Pregnant women should stop exercising when fatigued and not exercise to exhaustion. Weightbearing exercises may under some circumstances be continued at intensities similar to those prior to pregnancy throughout pregnancy. Non-weightbearing exercises, such as cycling or swimming, will minimize the risk of injury and facilitate the continuation of exercise during pregnancy.
4. Morphologic changes in pregnancy should serve as a relative contraindication to types of exercise in which loss of balance could be detrimental to maternal or fetal well-being, especially in the third trimester. Further, any type of exercise involving the potential for even mild abdominal trauma should be avoided.
5. Pregnancy requires an additional 300 kcal/day in order to maintain metabolic homeostasis. Thus, women who exercise during pregnancy should be particularly careful to ensure an adequate diet.
6. Pregnant women who exercise in the first trimester should augment heat dissipation by ensuring adequate hydration, appropriate clothing, and optimal environmental surroundings during exercise.
7. Many of the physiological and morphological changes of pregnancy persist 4 to 6 weeks postpartum. Thus, pre-pregnancy exercise routines should be resumed gradually based upon a woman's physical capability.

From American College of Obstetricians and Gynecologists. *Exercise during pregnancy and postpartum period* (Techinical Bulletin 28-189). Washington, D.C.: Author, 1994.

TABLE 28-13. *Reasons for pregnant women to discontinue exercise and consult a physician*

1. Any signs of bloody discharge from the vagina
2. Any 'gush' of fluid from the vagina (premature rupture of membranes)
3. Persistent contractions (>6 to 8/hour) which may suggest onset of premature labor
4. Unexplained abdominal pain
5. Absence of fetal movement
6. Sudden swelling of the ankles, hands and face
7. Persistent, severe headaches and/or visual disturbance
8. Unexplained spells of faintness or dizziness
9. Swelling, pain, and redness in the calf of one leg (phlebitis)
10. Elevation of pulse rate or blood pressure which persists after exercise
11. Excessive fatigue, palpitations, chest pain
12. Insufficient weight gain (<1.0 kg/month during last 2 trimesters)

From Wolfe LA, Hall P, Webb KA, Goodman L, Monga M, McGrath MJ. Prescription of aerobic exercise during pregnancy. *Sports Med* 1989; 8:273–301.

Resistance training can be of considerable benefit to the elderly (415). Like the aerobic exercise prescription, resistance training programs need to be individualized. Resistance training should be initiated with close supervision and minimal resistance.

Maintenance of a functional range of motion is also particularly important for the elderly. As for younger individuals, stretching exercises should be preceded with a warm-up to increase the soft tissue temperature.

REFERENCES

1. Astrand PO, Rodahl K. *Textbook of work physiology: physiological basis of exercise, 3rd ed.* New York: McGraw-Hill, 1986.
2. Fox EL, Mathews DK. *The physiological basis of physical education and athletics.* Philadelphia: WB Saunders, 1981.
3. Goldspink G, Larson RE, Davies RE. The immediate energy supply and the cost of maintenance of isometric tension for different muscles in the hamster. *Z Vergl Physiol* 1970; 66:389–397.
4. Meyer RA, Terjung RL. Differences in ammonia and adenylate metabolism in contracting fast and slow muscle. *Am J Physiol* 1979; 237: C11–C18.
5. Trivedi B, Danforth WH. Effect of pH on the kinetics of frog muscle phosphofructokinase. *J Biol Chem* 1966; 241:4110–4112.
6. Nakumura Y, Schwartz S. The influence of hydrogen ion concentration on calcium binding and release by skeletal muscle sarcoplasmic reticulum. *J Gen Physiol* 1972; 59:22–32.
7. Sahlin K. Metabolic changes limiting muscle performance. In: Saltin B, ed. *Biochemistry of exercise VI.* Champaign, IL: Human Kinetics, 1986; 323–343.
8. Christensen EH, Hansen O. Arbeitsfahigkeit und Ehrnahrung. *Skand Arch Physiol* 1939; 8:160–175.
9. Martin WH III. Effects of acute and chronic exercise on fat metabolism. *Exerc Sport Sci Rev* 1996; 24:203–231.
10. Henriksson J. Training induced adaptations of skeletal muscle and metabolism during submaximal exercise. *J Physiol* 1977; 270: 661–675.
11. Lamb DR. *Physiology of exercise: responses and adaptations, 2nd ed.* New York: Macmillan, 1984.
12. Gordon AM. Muscle. In: Ruch T, Patton H, eds. *Physiology and biophysics, Vol IV.* Philadelphia: WB Saunders, 1982; 170–260.
13. Roberts TDM. *Neurophysiology of postural mechanics.* London: Butterworth, 1978.

14. Rothwell JC. *Control of human voluntary movement*. Rockville, MD: Aspen Publishers, 1987.
15. Zierler KL. Mechanism of muscle contraction and its energetics. In: Mountcastle VB, ed. *Medical physiology, 13th ed.* St Louis: CV Mosby, 1974; 77–120.
16. Ikai M, Fukanaga T. A study on training effect on strength per cross-sectional area of muscle by means of ultrasonic measurement. *Eur J Appl Physiol* 1970; 28:173–180.
17. Moritani T, deVries HA. Neural factors versus hypertrophy in the time course of muscle strength gain. *Am J Phys Med* 1979; 58:115–130.
18. Enoka RM. Muscle strength and its development: new perspectives. *Sports Med* 1988; 6:146–168.
19. Caiozzo VJ, Perrine JJ, Edgerton VR. Training-induced alterations of the *in vivo* force–velocity relationship of human muscle. *J Appl Physiol Respir Environ Exerc Physiol* 1981; 51:750–754.
20. Wickiewicz TL, Roy RR, Powell PL, Perrine JJ, Edgerton VR. Muscle architecture and force–velocity relationships in humans. *J Appl Physiol Respir Environ Exerc Physiol* 1984; 57:435–443.
21. Spencer JD, Hayes KC, Alexander IJ. Knee joint effusion and quadriceps reflex inhibition in man. *Arch Phys Med Rehabil* 1984; 65: 171–177.
22. Stener B. Reflex inhibition of quadriceps elicited from subperiosteal tumour of femur. *Acta Orthop Scand* 1969; 40:86–91.
23. Stener B, Peterson I. Electromyographic investigation of the reflex effects upon stretching the partially ruptured medial collateral ligament of the knee joint. *Acta Chir Scand* 1962; 124:396–415.
24. Swearingen RL, Dehne E. A study of pathological muscle function following injury to joint. *J Bone Joint Surg* 1964; 46:1364.
25. Ohtsuki T. Decrease in grip strength induced by simultaneous bilateral exertion with reference to finger strength. *Ergonomics* 1981; 24: 37–48.
26. Secher NH, Rorsgaard S, Secher O. Contralateral influence on recruitment of curanized muscle fibers during maximal voluntary extension of the legs. *Acta Physiol Scand* 1978; 130:455–462.
27. Vandervoot AA, Sale DG, Moroz J. Comparison of motor unit activation during unilateral and bilateral leg extension. *J Appl Physiol Respir Environ Exerc Physiol* 1984; 56:46–51.
28. Ikai M, Steinhaus AH. Some factors modifying the expression of human strength. *J Appl Physiol* 1961; 16:157–163.
29. Secher NH. Isometric rowing strength of experienced and inexperienced oarsmen. *Med Sci Sports* 1975; 7:280–283.
30. Caiozzo VJ, Laird T, Chow K, Prietto CA, McMaster WC. The use of precontraction to enhance the *in-vivo* force velocity relationship. *Med Sci Sports Exerc* 1983; 14:162.
31. Cavanagh PR, Kram R. Mechanical and muscular factors affecting the efficiency of human movement. *Med Sci Sports Exerc* 1985; 17: 326–331.
32. Abbott BC, Bigland B, Ritchie JM. The physiological cost of negative work. *J Physiol* 1952; 117:380–390.
33. White DCS. Muscle mechanics. In: Alexander RMcN, Goldspink G, eds. *Mechanics and energetics of animal locomotion*. London: Chapman and Hall, 1977; 23–56.
34. Joyce GC, Rack PMH, Westbury DR. The mechanical properties of cat soleus muscle during controlled lengthening and shortening movements. *J Physiol* 1969; 204:461–474.
35. Schottelius BA, Senay LC. Effect of stimulation-length sequence on shape of length–tension diagram. *Am J Physiol* 1956; 186:127–130.
36. Gordon AM, Huxley AF, Julian FJ. The variation in isometric tension with sarcomere length in vertebrate muscle fibres. *J Physiol* 1966; 184:170–192.
37. Baltzopoulos V, Brodie DA. Isokinetic dynamometry: applications and limitations. *Sports Med* 1989; 8:101–116.
38. Tipton CM, Matthes RD, Maynard JA, Carey RA. The influence of physical activity on ligaments and tendons. *Med Sci Sports* 1975; 7: 165–175.
39. Komi PV. Physiological and biomechanical correlates of muscle function: effects of muscle structure and stretch–shortening cycle on force and speed. *Exerc Sport Sci Rev* 1984; 12:81–121.
40. Norman RW, Komi PV. Electromechanical delay in skeletal muscle under normal movement conditions. *Acta Physiol Scand* 1979; 106: 241–248.
41. Taylor CR, Heglund N, Maloiy GMO. Energetics and mechanics of terrestrial locomotion. *J Exp Biol* 1982; 97:1–21.
42. Nordeen-Snyder K. The effect of bicycle seat height variation upon oxygen consumption and lower limb kinematics. *Med Sci Sports* 1977; 9:113–117.
43. Hamley EJ, Thomas V. Physiological and postural factors in the calibration of the bicycle ergometer. *J Physiol* 1967; 191:55P–57P.
44. Hagberg JM, Mullin JP, Giese MD, Spitznagel E. Effect of pedalling rate on submaximal exercise responses of competitive cyclists. *J Appl Physiol* 1981; 51:447–451.
45. Cavanagh PR, Williams KR. The effect of stride length variation on oxygen uptake during distance running. *Med Sci Sports Exerc* 1982; 14:30–35.
46. Ralston JH. Energy–speed relation and optimal speed during level walking. *Int Z Angew Physiol* 1958; 17:277–283.
47. Hill AV. The maximal work and mechanical efficiency of human muscles and their most economical speed. *J Physiol* 1922; 56:19–41.
48. Rohment W. Ermittlung von erholungspausen fur statische arbeit des menschen. *Int Z Angew Physiol* 1960; 18:123–164.
49. Simonson E. Recovery and fatigue. In: Simonson E, ed. *Physiology of work capacity and fatigue*. Springfield, IL: Charles C Thomas, 1971;440–458.
50. Lloyd BB. World running records as maximal performances: oxygen debt and other limiting factors. *Circ Res* 1967; 20–21(Suppl 1): I218–I226.
51. Hoffman MD, Williams CA, Lind AR. Changes in isometric function following rhythmic exercise. *Eur J Appl Physiol* 1985; 54:177–183.
52. Bigland-Ritchie B, Bellemare F, Woods JJ. Excitation frequencies and sites of fatigue. In: Jones NL, McCartney N, McComas AJ, eds. *Human muscle power*. Champaign, IL: Human Kinetics, 1986; 197–213.
53. Fitts RH. Cellular mechanisms of muscle fatigue. *Physiol Rev* 1994; 74:49–94.
54. Lewis S, Taylor WF, Graham RM, Pettinger WA, Schutte JE, Blomqvist CG. Cardiovascular responses to exercise as a function of absolute and relative workload. *J Appl Physiol* 1983; 54:1314–1323.
55. Blomqvist CG. Clinical exercise physiology. In: Wenger NK, Hellerstein HK, eds. *Rehabilitation of the coronary patient*. New York: John Wiley & Sons, Inc, 1984; 179–196.
56. Hammond HK, Froelicher VF. Normal and abnormal heart rate responses to exercise. *Prog Cardiovasc Dis* 1985; 27:271–296.
57. Paterson DJ. Antiarrhythmic mechanisms during exercise. *J Appl Physiol* 1996; 80:1853–1862.
58. Rowell LB, O'Leary DS. Reflex control of the circulation during exercise: chemoreflexes and mechanoreflexes. *J Appl Physiol* 1990; 69:407–418.
59. Shepherd JT. Circulatory response to exercise in health. *Circulation* 1987; 76(Suppl VI):VI3–VI10.
60. Mitchell JH. Neural control of the circulation during exercise. *Med Sci Sports Exerc* 1990; 22:141–154.
61. Mitchell JH, Kaufman MP, Iwamoto GA. The exercise pressor reflex: its cardiovascular effects, afferent mechanisms, and central pathways. *Annu Rev Phyiol* 1983; 45:229–242.
62. Buttrick PM, Scheuer J. Exercise and the heart: acute hemodynamics, conditioning training, the athlete's heart, and sudden death. In: Schlant RC, Alexander RW, eds. *The heart, 8th ed*. New York: McGraw-Hill, 1994; 2057–2066.
63. Braunwald E, Sonnenblick EH, Ross J Jr, Glick G, Epstein SE. An analysis of the cardiac response to exercise. *Circ Res* 1967; 20–21(suppl I):I44–I58.
64. Higginbotham MB, Morris KG, Williams RS, McHale PA, Coleman RE, Cobb FR. Regulation of stroke volume during submaximal and maximal upright exercise in normal man. *Circ Res* 1986; 58:281–291.
65. Mitchell JH, Blomqvist G. Maximal oxygen uptake. *N Engl J Med* 1971; 284:1018–1022.
66. Rowell LB. *Human cardiovascular control*. New York: Oxford University Press, 1993.
67. Hudlicka O, Khelly F. Metabolic factors involved in regulation of muscle blood flow. *J Cardiovasc Pharmacol* 1985; 7(Suppl 3): S59–S72.
68. Johnson PC. Autoregulation of blood flow. *Circ Res* 1986; 59: 483–495.
69. Wasserman K. Determinants and detection of anaerobic threshold and consequences of exercise above it. *Circulation* 1987; 76(Suppl VI): VI29–VI39.
70. Wasserman K, Beaver WL, Whipp BJ. Gas exchange theory and the

lactic acidosis (anaerobic) threshold. *Circulation* 1990; 81(Suppl II): II14–II30.

71. Nielsen B, Nielsen M. Body temperature during work at different environmental temperatures. *Acta Physiol Scand* 1962; 56:120–129.
72. Saltin B, Hermansen L. Esophageal, rectal, and muscle temperature during exercise. *J Appl Physiol* 1966; 21:1757–1762.
73. Folinsbee LJ. Heat and air pollution. In: Pollock ML, Schmidt DH, eds. *Heart disease and rehabilitation, 3rd ed.* Champaign, IL: Human Kinetics, 1995; 327–342.
74. Rowell LB. Cardiovascular adjustments to thermal stress. In: *Handbook of physiology, sect 2, vol III: The cardiovascular system, Chapter 27: Peripheral circulation and organ blood flow.* Bethesda, MD: American Physiological Society, 1983; 967–1023.
75. Johnson JM. Exercise and the cutaneous circulation. *Exerc Sport Sci Rev* 1992; 20:59–97.
76. Sheldahl LM, Wilke NA, Dougherty S, Tristani FE. Cardiac response to combined moderate heat and exercise in men with coronary heart disease. *Am J Cardiol* 1992; 70:186–191.
77. Costill DL, Miller JM. Nutrition for endurance sport: carbohydrate and fluid balance. *Int J Sports Med* 1980; 1:2–14.
78. Montain SJ, Coyle EF. Influence of graded dehydration on hyperthermia and cardiovascular drift during exercise. *J Appl Physiol* 1992; 73:1340–1350.
79. Nadel ER, Fortney SM, Wenger CB. Effect of hydration state on circulatory and thermal regulations. *J Appl Physiol* 1980; 49:715–721.
80. Noakes TD. Fluid replacement during exercise. *Exerc Sport Sci Rev* 1993; 21:297–330.
81. Altenbirch HU, Gerzer R, Kirsch KA, Weil J, Heyduck B, Schultes I, Rocker L. Effect of prolonged physical exercise on fluid regulating hormones. *Eur J Appl Physiol* 1990; 61:209–213.
82. Galbo H. *Hormonal and metabolic adaptation to exercise.* New York: Thieme, 1983.
83. Kjaer M. Regulation of hormonal and metabolic responses during exercise in humans. *Exerc Sport Sci Rev* 1992; 20;161–184.
84. Sheldahl LM, Tristani FE, Connelly TP, Levandoski SG, Skelton MM, Cowley AW Jr. Fluid-regulating hormones during exercise when central blood volume is increased by water immersion. *Am J Physiol* 1992; 262:R779–R785.
85. Wade CE, Freund BJ. Hormonal control of blood volume during and following exercise. In: Gisolfi CV, Lamb DR, eds. *Perspectives in exercise science and sports medicine. Vol 3. Fluid homeostasis during exercise.* Indianapolis: Benchmark Press, 1990; 207–241.
86. Lewis SF, Snell PG, Taylor WF, Hamra M, Graham RM, Pettinger WA, Blomqvist CG. Role of muscle mass and mode of contraction in circulatory responses to exercise. *J Appl Physiol* 1992; 73:1590–1597.
87. Hanson P, Rueckert P. Hypertension. In: Pollock ML, Schmidt DH, eds. *Heart disease and rehabilitation, 3rd ed.* Champaign, IL: Human Kinetics, 1995; 343–356.
88. Lind AR, Williams CA. The control of blood flow through human forearm muscles following brief isometric contractions. *J Physiol* 1979; 288:529–547.
89. Williamson JW, Olesen HL, Pott F, Mitchell JH, Secher NH. Central command increases cardiac output during static exercise in humans. *Acta Physiol Scand* 1996; 156:429–434.
90. Longhurst JC, Mitchell JH. Does endurance training benefit the cardiovascular system? *J Cardiovasc Med* 1983; 8:227–236.
91. Fletcher GF, Balady G, Froelicher VF, Hartley LH, Haskell WL, Pollock ML. Exercise standards. A statement for health professionals from the American Heart Association. *Circulation* 1995; 91:580–615.
92. Saltin B, Blomqvist G, Mitchell JH, Johnson RL, Wildenthal K, Chapman CB. Response to exercise after bed rest and after training: a longitudinal study of adaptive changes in oxygen transport and body composition. *Circulation* 1968; 38:VII1–VII67.
93. Greenleaf JE, Kozlowski S. Physiological consequences of reduced physical activity during bed rest. *Sport Sci Rev* 1982; 84–119.
94. Appell H-J. Muscular atrophy following immobilization: a review. *Sports Med* 1990; 10:42–58.
95. Miles MP, Clarkson PM, Bean M, Ambach K, Mulroy J, Vincent K. Muscle function at the wrist following 9 d of immobilization and suspension. *Med Sci Sports Exerc* 1994; 26:615–623.
96. Mueller EA. Influence of training and of inactivity on muscle strength. *Arch Phys Med Rehabil* 1970;51:449–462.
97. Booth FW, Gollnick PD. Effects of disuse on the structure and function of skeletal muscle. *Med Sci Sports Exerc* 1983; 15:415–420.
98. Beckman SM, Buchanan TS. Ankle inversion injury and hypermobility: effect on hip and ankle muscle electromyography onset latency. *Arch Phys Med Rehabil* 1995; 76:1138–1143.
99. Nicholas JA, Strizak AM, Veras G. Limb involvement with lower extremity injury. *Am J Sports Med* 1976; 4:241–245.
100. Booth FW, Gould EW. Effects of training and disuse on connective tissue. *Exerc Sport Sci Rev* 1975; 3:83–112.
101. Deitrick JE, Whedon GD, Shorr E. Effects of immobilization upon various metabolic and physiological functions of normal men. *Am J Med* 1948; 4:3–36.
102. Gamble JG, Edwards CC, Max SR. Enzymatic adaptations in ligaments during immobilization. *Am J Sports Med* 1984; 12:221–228.
103. Noyes FR. Functional properties of knee ligaments and alterations induced by immobilization: a correlative biomechanical and histological study in primates. *Clin Orthop Rel Res* 1977; 123:210–242.
104. Noyes FR, Torvik PJ, Hyde WB, DeLucas JL. Biomechanics of ligament failure II. An analysis of immobilization, exercise, and reconditioning effects in primates. *J Bone Joint Surg* 1974; 56A:1406–1418.
105. Enneking WF, Horowitz M. The intra-articular effects of immobilization on the human knee. *J Bone Joint Surg* 1972; 54A:973–985.
106. Finsterbush A, Friedman B. Reversibility of joint changes produced by immobilization in rabbits. *Clin Orthop Rel Res* 1975; 111:290–298.
107. Woo SL-Y, Matthews JV, Akeson WH, Amiel D, Convery FR. Connective tissue response to immobility: correlative study of biomechanical and biochemical measurements of normal and immobilized rabbit knees. *Arthritis Rheum* 1975; 18:257–264.
108. Troyer H. The effect of short-term immobilization on the rabbit knee joint cartilage: a histochemical study. *Clin Orthop Rel Res* 1975; 107: 249–257.
109. Rutherford OM. Muscular coordination and strength training: implications for injury rehabilitation. *Sports Med* 1988; 5:196–202.
110. Sale DG. Neural adaptation in strength and power training. In: Jones NL, McCartney N, McComas AJ, eds. *Human muscle power.* Champaign, IL: Human Kinetics, 1986; 289–307.
111. Barrack RL, Skinner HB, Buckley SL. Proprioception in the anterior cruciate deficient knee. *Am J Sports Med* 1989; 17:1–6.
112. Garn SN, Newton RA. Kinesthetic awareness in subjects with multiple ankle sprains. *Phys Ther* 1988; 68:1667–1671.
113. Shephard RJ. Exercise and aging: extending independence in older adults. *Geriatrics* 1993; 48:61–64.
114. Clausen JP, Trap-Jensen J. Heart rate and arterial blood pressure during exercise in patients with angina pectoris. Effects of training and of nitroglycerin. *Circulation* 1976; 53:436–442.
115. NIH Consensus Development Panel on Physical Activity and Cardiovascular Health. Physical activity and cardiovasclar health. *JAMA* 1996; 276:241–246.
116. Fentem PH. Exercise in prevention of disease. *Br Med Bull* 1992; 48: 630–650.
117. Fries JF. Physical activity, the compression of morbidity, and the health of the elderly. *J R Soc Med* 1996; 89:64–68.
118. Fries JF, Singh G, Morfeld D, Hubert HB, Lane NE, Brown BW Jr. Running and the development of disability with age. *Ann Intern Med* 1994; 121:502–509.
119. Hiatt WR, Wolfel EE, Meier RH, Regensteiner JG. Superiority of treadmill waking exercise versus strength training for patients with peripheral arterial disease. Implications for the mechanism of the training response. *Circulation* 1994; 90:1866–1874.
120. Stawbridge WJ, Cohen RD, Shema SJ, Kaplan GA. Successful aging: predictors and associated activities. *Am J Epidemiol* 1996; 144: 135–141.
121. Young DR, Masaki KH, Curb JD. Associations of physical activity with performance-based and self-reported physical functioning in older men: the Honolulu Heart Program. *J Am Geriatr Soc* 1995; 43: 845–854.
122. Blumenthal JA, Fredrikson M, Kuhn CM, Ulmer RL, Walsh-Riddle M, Appelbaum M. Aerobic exercise reduces levels of cardiovascular and sympathoadrenal responses to mental stress in subjects without prior evidence of myocardial ischemia. *Am J Cardiol* 1990; 65:93–98.
123. Lavie CJ, Milani RV, Littman AB. Benefits of cardiac rehabilitation and exercise training in secondary coronary prevention in the elderly. *J Am Coll Cardiol* 1993; 22:678–683.
124. Bernadet P. Benefits of physical activity in the prevention of cardiovascular diseases. *J Cardiovasc Pharm* 1995; 25(Suppl 1):S3–S8.
125. Pate RR, Pratt M, Blair SN, et al. Physical activity and public health.

A recommendation from the Centers for Disease Control and Prevention and the American College of Sports Medicine. *JAMA* 1995; 273: 402–407.
126. Blair SN, Kampert JB, Kohl HW III, Barlow CE, Macera CA, Paffenbarger RS Jr, Gibbons LW. Influences of cardiorespiratory fitness and other precursors on cardiovscular disease and all-cause mortality in men and women. *JAMA* 1996; 276:205–210.
127. Blair SN, Kohl HW III, Paffenbarger RS Jr, Clark DG, Cooper KH, Gibbons LW. Physical fitness and all-cause mortality. A prospective study of healthy men and women. *JAMA* 1989; 262:2395–2401.
128. Lakka TA, Venalainen JM, Rauramaa R, Salonen R, Tuomilehto J, Salonen J. Relation of lesiure-time physical activity and cardiorespiratory fitness to the risk of acute myocardial infarction in men. *N Engl J Med* 1994; 330:1549–1554.
129. Paffenbarger RS Jr, Hyde RT, Wing AL, Hsieh CC. Physical activity, all-cause mortality, and longevity of college alumni. *N Engl J Med* 1986; 314:605–613.
130. Paffenbarger RS Jr, Hyde RT, Wing AL, Lee IM, Jung DL, Kampert JB. The association of changes in physical-activity level and other lifestyle characteristics with mortality among men. *N Engl J Med* 1993; 328:538–545.
131. Sandvik L, Erikseen J, Thaulow E, Erikssen G, Mundal R, Rodahl K. Physical fitness as a predictor of mortality among healthy, middle-aged Norwegian men. *N Engl J Med* 1993; 328:533–537.
132. Berlin JA, Colditz GA. A meta-analysis of physical activity in the prevention of coronary heart disease. *Am J Epidemiol* 1990; 132: 612–628.
133. Powell KE, Thompson PD, Caspersen CJ, Kenrick JS. Physical activity and the incidence of coronary heart disease. *Annu Rev Public Health* 1987; 8:253–287.
134. O'Connor GT, Buring JE, Yusulf S, Goldhaber SZ, Olmstead EM, Paffenbarger RS Jr, Hennekens CH. An overview of randomized trials of rehabilitation with exercise after myocardial infarction. *Circulation* 1989; 80:234–244.
135. Oldridge NB, Guyatt GH, Fischer ME, Rimm AA. Cardiac rehabilitation after myocardial infarction: combined experience of randomized clinical trials. *JAMA* 1988; 260:945–950.
136. American Heart Association. *Heart and stroke facts: 1995 statistical supplement*. Dallas: American Heart Association, 1994.
137. Public Health Service. *Healthy people 2000: national health promotion and disease prevention objectives*. Washington, D.C.: US Department of Health and Human Services, DHHS publication (PHS) 91-50212, 1991.
138. Kokkinos PF, Narayan P, Colleran JA, Pittaras A, Notargiacomo A, Reda D, Papademetriou V. Effects of regular exercise on blood pressure and left ventricular hypertrophy in African-American men with severe hypertension. *N Engl J Med* 1995; 333:1462–1467.
139. Lemaitre RN, Heckbert SR, Psaty BM, Siscovick DS. Leisure-time physical activity and the risk of nonfatal myocardial infarction in postmenopausal women. *Arch Intern Med* 1995; 155:2302–2308.
140. Fagard RH. Prescription and results of physical activity. *J Cardiovasc Pharm* 1995; 25(Suppl 1):S20–S27.
141. Fagard RH, Tipton CM. Physical activity, fitness, and hypertension. In: Bouchard C, Shephard RJ, Stephens T, eds. *Physical activity, fitness, and health: international proceedings and consensus statement*. Champaign, IL: Human Kinetics, 1994; 633–655.
142. Paffenbarger RS Jr, Wing AL, Hyde RT, Jung DL. Physical activity and incidence of hypertension in college alumni. *Am J Epidemiol* 1983; 117:245–257.
143. Palatini P, Graniero GR, Mormino P, Nicolosi L, Mos L, Visentin P, Pessina AC. Relation between physical training and ambulatory blood pressure in stage I hypertensive subjects. Results of the HARVEST Trial. *Circulation* 1994; 90:2870–2876.
144. Cox KL, Puddey IB, Morton AR, Burke V, Beilin LJ, McAleer M. Exercise and weight control in sedentary overweight men: effects on clinic and ambulatory blood pressure. *J Hypertens* 1996; 14:779–790.
145. Gilders RM, Voner C, Dudley GA. Endurance training and blood pressure in normotensive and hypertensive adults. *Med Sci Sports Exerc* 1989; 21:629–636.
146. Martin JE, Dubbert PM, Cushman WC. Controlled trial of aerobic exercise in hypertension. *Circulation* 1990; 81:1560–1567.
147. Durstine JL, Haskell WL. Effects of exercise training on plasma lipids and lipoproteins. *Exerc Sport Sci Rev* 1994; 22:477–521.
148. Marrugat J, Elosua R, Covas MI, Molina L, Rubies-Prat J. Amount and intensity of physical activity, physical fitness, and serum lipids in men. *Am J Epidemiol* 1996; 143:562–569.
149. Podl TR, Zmuda JM, Yurgalevitch SM, Fahrenbach MC, Bausserman LL, Terry RB, Thompson PD. Lipoprotein lipase activity and plasma triglyceride clearance are elevated in endurance-trained women. *Metabolism* 1994; 43:808–813.
150. King AC, Haskell WL, Young DR, Oka RK, Stefanick ML. Long-term effects of varying intensities and formats of physical activity on participation rates, fitness, and lipoproteins in men and women aged 50 to 65 years. *Circulation* 1995; 91:2596–2604.
151. Kokkinos PF, Holland JC, Narayan P, Colleran JA, Dotson CO, Papademetriou V. Miles run per week and high-density lipoprotein cholesterol levels in healthy, middle-aged men. *Arch Intern Med* 1995; 155: 415–420.
152. Superko RH. Exercise training, serum lipids, and lipoprotein particles: is there a change threshold? *Med Sci Sports Exerc* 1991; 23:667–685.
153. Williams PT, Wood PD, Haskell WL, Vranizan MA. The effects of running milage and duration on plasma lipoprotein levels. *JAMA* 1982; 247:2674–2679.
154. Ginsburg GS, Agil A, O'Toole M, Rimm E, Douglas PS, Rifai N. Effects of a single bout of ultraendurance exercise on lipid levels and susceptibility of lipids to peroxidation in triathletes. *JAMA* 1996; 276: 221–225.
155. Hicks AL, MacDougall JD, Muckle TJ. Acute changes in high-density lipoprotein cholesterol with exercise of different intensities. *J Appl Physiol* 1987; 63:1956–1960.
156. Pi-Sunyer FX. The fattening of America (editorial). *JAMA* 1994; 272: 238–239.
157. Kuczmarski RJ, Flegal KM, Campbell SM, Johnson CL. Increasing prevalence of overweight among US adults: the National Health and Nutrition Examination Surveys, 1960 to 1991. *JAMA* 1994; 272: 205–211.
158. Manson JE, Willett WC, Stampfer MJ, et al. Body weight and mortality among women. *N Engl J Med* 1995; 333:677–685.
159. Byers T. Body weight and mortality (editorial). *N Engl J Med* 1995; 333:723–724.
160. Grodstein F, Levine R, Troy L, Spencer T, Colditz GA, Stampfer MJ. Three-year follow-up of participants in a commerical weight loss program. *Arch Intern Med* 1996; 156:1302–1306.
161. Blix GG, Blix AG. The role of exercise in weight loss. *Behav Med* 1995; 21:31–39.
162. Brownell KD, Marlatt GA, Lichtenstein E, Wilson GT. Understanding and preventing relapse. *Am J Physiol* 1986; 41:765–782.
163. Tremblay A, Simoneau JA, Bouchard C. Impact of exrcise intensity on body fatness and skeletal muscle metabolism. *Metabolism* 1994; 43:814–818.
164. Blake GH. Control of type II diabetes. *Postgrad Med* 1992; 92: 129–137.
165. Helmrich SP, Ragland DR, Leung RW, Paffenberger RS. Physical activity and reduced occurrence of non insulin dependent-diabetes mellitus. *N Engl J Med* 1991; 325:147–152.
166. Donahue RP, Orchard TJ, Becker DJ, Kuller H, Drash AL. Physical activity, insulin sensitivity, and the lipoprotein profile in young adults: the Beaver County Study. *Am J Epidemiol* 1988; 27:95–103.
167. King DS, Baldus PJ, Sharp RL, Kesl LD, Feltmeyer TL, Riddle MS. Time course for exercise-induced alterations in insulin action and glucose tolerance in middle-aged people. *J Appl Physiol* 1995; 78: 17–22.
168. King DS, Dalsky GP, Clutter WE, Young DA, Staten MA, Cryer PE, Holloszy JO. Effects of exercise and lack of exercise on insulin sensitivity and responsiveness. *J Appl Physiol* 1988; 64:1942–1946.
169. Hicks AL, MacDougall JD, Muckle TJ. Acute changes in high-density lipoprotein cholesterol with exercise of different intensities. *J Appl Physiol* 1987; 63:1956–1960.
170. Barnard RJ, Lattimore L, Holly RG, Cherny S, Pritikin N. Response of noninsulin-dependent diabetic patients to an intensive program of diet and exercise. *Diabetes Care* 1982; 5:370–374.
171. Kriska AM, Blair SN, Pereira MA. The potential role of physical activity in the prevention of non-insulin-dependent diabetes mellitus: the epidemiological evidence. *Exerc Sport Sci Rev* 1994; 22:121–143.
172. Lehmann R, Vokac A, Niedermann K, Agosti K, Spinas GA. Loss of abdominal fat and improvement of the cardiovascular risk profile by regular moderate exercise training in patients with NIDDM. *Diabetologia* 1995; 38:1313–1319.

173. Lynch J, Helmrich SP, Lakka TA, Kaplan GA, Cohen RD, Salonen R, Salonen JT. Moderately intense physical activities and high levels of cardiorespiratory fitness reduce the risk of non-insulin-dependent diabetes mellitus in middle-aged men. *Arch Intern Med* 1996; 156: 1307–1314.
174. Gutin B, Kasper MJ. Can vigorous exercise play a role in osteoporosis prevention? A review. *Osteoporos Int* 1992; 2:55–69.
175. Hughes VA, Frontera WR, Dallal GE, Lutz KJ, Fisher EC, Evans WJ. Muscle strength and body composition: assocations with bone density in older subjects. *Med Sci Sports Exerc* 1995; 27:967–974.
176. Kohrt WM, Snead DB, Slatopolsky E, Birge SJ Jr. Additive effects of weight-bearing exercise and estrogen on bone mineral density in older women. *J Bone Miner Res* 1995; 10:1303–1311.
177. Kriska AM, Sandler RB, Cauley JA, LaPorte RE, Hom DL, Pambianco G. The assessment of historical physical activity and its relation to adult bone parameters. *Am J Epidemiol* 1988; 127:1053–1063.
178. Michel BA, Bloch DA, Fries JF. Weight-bearing exercise, overexercise, and lumbar bone density over age 50 years. *Arch Intern Med* 1989; 149:2325–2329.
179. Orwoll ES, Ferar J, Oviatt SK, McClung MR, Huntington K. The relationship of swimming exercise to bone mass in men and women. *Arch Intern Med* 1989; 149:2197–2200.
180. Pocock N, Eisman JA, Yeates MG, Sambrook PN, Ebert S. Physical fitness is a major determinant of femoral neck and lumbar spine bone mineral density. *J Clin Invest* 1986; 78:618–621.
181. Ulrich CM, Georgiou CC, Snow-Harter CM, Gillis DE. Bone mineral density in mother–daughter pairs: relations to lifetime exercise, lifetime milk consumption, and calcuim supplements. *Am J Clin Nutr* 1996; 63:72–79.
182. Rencken ML, Chesnut CH III, Drinkwater BL. Bone density at multiple skeletal sites in amenorrheic athletes. *JAMA* 1996; 276:238–240.
183. Stratton JR, Chandler WL, Schwartz RS, et al. Effects of physical conditioning on fibrinolytic variables and fibrinogen in young and old healthy adults. *Circulation* 1991; 83:1692–1697.
184. Szymanksi LM, Pate RR, Durstine JL. Effects of maximal exercise and venous occlusion on fibrinolytic activity in physically active and inactive men. *J Appl Physiol* 1994; 77:2305–2310.
185. Wang JS, Jen CJ, Chen H. Effects of exercise training and deconditioning on platelet function in men. *Arterioscler Thromb Vasc Biol* 1995; 15:1668–1674.
186. Wang JS, Jen CJ, Kung HC, Lin LJ, Hsiue TR, Chen H. Different effects of strenuous execise and moderate exercise on platelet function in men. *Circulation* 1994; 90:2877–2885.
187. Todd MK, Goldfarb AH, Kauffman RD, Burleson C. Combined effects of age and exercise on thromboxane B_2 and platelet activation. *J Appl Physiol* 1994; 76:1548–1552.
188. O'Connor PJ, Youngstedt SD. Influence of exercise on human sleep. *Exerc Sport Sci Rev* 1995; 23:105–134.
189. Cannon JG. Exercise and resistance to infection. *J Appl Physiol* 1993; 74:973–981.
190. Nieman DC, Buckley KS, Henson DA, et al. Immune function in marathon runners versus sedentary controls. *Med Sci Sports Exerc* 1995; 27:986–992.
191. Sen CK. Oxidants and antioxidants in exercise. *J Appl Physiol* 1995; 79:675–686.
192. Shephard RJ, Rhind S, Shek PN. The impact of exercise on the immune system: NK cells, interleukins 1 and 2, and related responses. *Exerc Sport Sci Rev* 1995; 23:215–241.
193. Lee IM. Physical activity, fitness, and cancer. In: Bouchard C, Shephard RJ, Stephens T, eds. *Physical activity, fitness, and health: international proceedings and consensus statement.* Champaign, IL: Human Kinetics, 1994; 814–831.
194. White E, Jacobs EJ, Daling JR. Physical activity in relation to colon cancer in middle-aged men and women. *J Epidemiol* 1996; 144: 42–50.
195. Lavie CJ, Milani RV. Effects of cardiac rehabiliation program on exercise capacity, coronary risk factors, behavioral characteristics, and quality of life in a large elderly cohort. *Am J Cardiol* 1995; 76: 177–179.
196. Sheldahl LM, Tristani FE, Hastings JE, Wenzler RB, Levandoski SG. Comparison of adaptations and compliance to exercise training between middle-aged and older men. *J Am Geriatr Soc* 1993; 41: 795–801.
197. Holloszy JO, Coyle EF. Adaptations of skeletal muscle to endurance exercise and their metabolic consequences. *J Appl Physiol* 1984; 56: 831–838.
198. Hurley BF, Hagberg JM, Allen WK, Seals DR, Young JC, Cuddihee RW, Holloszy JO. Effect of training on blood lactate levels during submaximal exercise. *J Appl Physiol* 1984; 56:1260–1264.
199. Joyner MJ. Physiological limiting factors and distance running: influence of gender and age on record performances. *Exerc Sports Sci Rev* 1993; 21:103–133.
200. Shulman SP, Fleg JL, Goldberg AP, et al. Continuum of cardiovacular performance across a broad range of fitness levels in healthy older men. *Circulation* 1996; 94:359–367.
201. Maron BJ. Structural features of the athlete's heart as defined by echocardiography. *J Am Coll Cardiol* 1986; 7:190–203.
202. Maron BJ, Pelliccia A, Spirito P. Cardiac disease in young trained athletes: insights into methods for distinguishing athlete's heart from structural heart disease with particular emphasis on hypertrophic cardiomyopathy. *Circulation* 1995; 91:1596–1601.
203. Fouad FM. Left ventricular diastolic function in hypertensive patients. *Circulation* 1987; 75(Suppl I):I48–I55.
204. Pelliccia A, Maron BJ, Culasso F, Spataro A, Caselli G. Athlete's heart in women. Echocardiographic characterization of highly trained elite female athletes. *JAMA* 1996; 276:211–215.
205. Clausen JP, Trap-Jensen J, Lassen NA. The effects of training on the heart rate during arm and leg exercise. *Scand J Clin Lab Invest* 1970; 26:295–301.
206. Davies CT, Sargeant AJ. Effects of training on the physiological responses to one- and two-leg work. *J Appl Physiol* 1975; 38:377–375.
207. Magel JR, McArdle WD, Toner M, Delio DJ. Metabolic and cardiovascular adjustment to arm training. *J Appl Physiol* 1978; 45:75–79.
208. American College of Sports Medicine. *ACSM's guidelines for exercise testing and prescription, 5th ed.* Baltimore: Williams & Wilkins, 1995.
209. Pollock ML, Wilmore JH. *Exercise in health and disease: evaluation and prescription for prevention and rehabilitation, 2nd ed.* Philadelphia: WB Saunders, 1990.
210. Zeni AI, Hoffman MD, Clifford PS. Energy expenditure with indoor exercise machines. *JAMA* 1996; 275:1424–1427.
211. Hoffman MD, Kassay KM, Zeni AI, Clifford PS. Does the amount of exercising muscle alter the aerobic demand of dynamic exercise? *Eur J Appl Physiol* 1996; 74:541–547.
212. Froelicher VF, Umann TM. Exercise testing: clinical applications. In: Pollock ML, Schmidt DH, eds. *Heart disease and rehabilitation, 3rd ed.* Champaign, IL: Human Kinetics, 1995; 57–80.
213. Buskirk ER, Hodgson JL. Age and aerobic power: the rate of change in men and women. *Fed Proc* 1987; 46:1824–1829.
214. Fleg JL, Lakatta EG. Role of muscle loss in the age-associated reduction in $\dot{V}O_{2max}$. *J Appl Physiol* 1988; 65:1147–1151.
215. Hagberg JM. Effect of training on the decline in $\dot{V}O_{2max}$ with aging. *Fed Proc* 1987; 46:1830–1833.
216. Bouchard C, Dionne FT, Simoneau JA, Boulay MR. Genetics of aerobic and anaerobic performances. *Exerc Sport Sci Rev* 1992; 20:27–58.
217. Fagard R, Bielen E, Amery A. Heritability of aerobic power and anaerobic energy generation during exercise. *J Appl Physiol* 1991; 70: 357–362.
218. Ekelund LG, Holmgren A. Central hemodynamics during exercise. *Circ Res* 1967; 20–21(Suppl I):I33–I43.
219. Saltin B, Strange S. Maximal oxygen uptake: "old" and "new" arguments for a cardiovascular limitation. *Med Sci Sports Exerc* 1992; 24: 30–37.
220. Vanoverschelde JLJ, Essamri B, Vanbutsele R, D'Hondt AM, Cosyns JR, Detry JMR, Melin JA. Contribution of left ventricular diastolic function to exercise capacity in normal subjects. *J Appl Physiol* 1993; 74:2225–2233.
221. Manfre MJ, Yu GH, Varma AA, Mallis GI, Kearey K. The effect of limited handrail support on total treadmill time and the prediction of $\dot{V}O_{2max}$. *Clin Cardiol* 1994; 17:445–450.
222. Berry MJ, Brubaker PH, O'Toole ML, et al. Estimation of $\dot{V}O_2$ in older individuals with osteoarthritis of the knee and cardiovascular disease. *Med Sci Sports Exerc* 1996; 28:808–814.
223. Franklin BA, Vander L, Wrisley D, Rubenfire M. Aerobic requirements of arm ergometry: implications for exercise testing and training. *Physician Sportsmed* 1983; 11:81–90.
224. Gleim GW, Coplan NL, Scandura M, Holly T, Nicholas JA. Rate pressure product at equivalent oxygen consumption on four different exercise modalities. *J Cardiopulm Rehabil* 1988; 8:270–275.

225. Levandoski SG, Sheldahl LM, Wilke NA, Tristani FE, Hoffman MD. Cardiorespiratory responses of coronary artery disease patients to arm and leg cycle ergometry. *J Cardiopulm Rehabil* 1990; 10:39–44.
226. Pina IL, Balady GJ, Hanson P, Labovitz AJ, Madoona DW, Myers J. Guidelines for clinical exercise testing laboratories. A statement for healthcare professionals from the Committee on Exercise and Cardiac Rehabilitation, American Heart Assocation. *Circulation* 1995; 91: 912–921.
227. Fleck SJ, Kraemer WJ. *Designing resistance training programs, 2nd ed.* Champaign, IL: Human Kinetics, 1997.
228. Sale DG. Neural adaptation to strength training. In: Komi PV, ed. *Strength and power in sports. The encyclopaedia of sports medicine.* Oxford: Blackwell, 1992; 249–265.
229. Billeter R, Hoppeler H. Muscular basis of strength. In: Komi PV, ed. *Strength and power in sports. The encyclopaedia of sports medicine.* Oxford: Blackwell, 1992; 39–63.
230. Booth FW, Thomason DB. Molecular and cellular adaptation of muscle in response to exercise: perspective of various models. *Physiol Reviews,* 1991; 71:541–585.
231. Hay JG. Mechanical basis of strength expression. In: Komi PV, ed. *Strength and power in sports. The encyclopaedia of sports medicine.* Oxford: Blackwell, 1992; 197–210.
232. MacDougal JD. Hypertrophy or hyperplasia. In: Komi PV, ed. *Strength and power in sports. The encyclopaedia of sports medicine.* Oxford: Blackwell, 1992; 230–238.
233. Antonio J, Gonyea WJ. Muscle fiber splitting in stretch-enlarged avian muscle. *Med Sci Sports Exerc* 1994; 26:973–977.
234. Kraemer WJ, Dziados JE, Marchitelli LJ, et al. Effects of different heavy-resistance exercise protocols on plasma β-endorphin concentrations. *J Appl Physiol* 1993; 74:450–459.
235. Dudley GA, Tesch PA, Miller BJ, Buchanan P. Importance of eccentric actions in performance adaptations to resistance training. *Aviat Space Environ Med* 1991; 62:543–550.
236. Hather BM, Tesch PA, Buchanan P, Dudley GA. Influence of eccentric actions on skeletal muscle adaptations to resistance training. *Acta Physiol Scand* 1991; 143:177–185.
237. Kraemer WJ, Patton J, Gordon SE, et al. Compatibility of high intensity strength and endurance training on hormonal and skeletal muscle adaptations. *J Appl Physiol* 1995; 78:976–989.
238. Staron RS, Karapondo DL, Kraemer WJ, et al. Skeletal muscle adaptations during the early phase of heavy-resistance training in men and women. *J Appl Physiol* 1994; 76:1247–1255.
239. Costill DL, Coyle EF, Fink WF, Lesmes GR, Witzmann FA. Adaptations in skeletal muscle following strength training. *J Appl Physiol* 1979; 46:96–99.
240. Exner GU, Staudte HW, Pette D. Isometric training of rats—effects upon fast and slow muscle and modification by an anabolic hormone in female rats. *Pflugers Arch* 1973; 345:1–4.
241. Grimby G., Bjorntrop P, Fahlen M, et al. Metabolic effects of isometric training. *Scand J Clin Lab Invest* 1973; 31:301–305.
242. MacDougall JD, Ward GR, Sale DG, Sutton JR. Biochemical adaptation of human skeletal muscle to heavy resistance training and immobilization. *J Appl Physiol* 1977; 43:700–703.
243. Tesch PA, Thorsson A, Colliander EB. Effects of eccentric and concentric resistance training on skeletal muscle substrates, enzyme activities and capillary supply. *Acta Physiol Scand* 1990; 140:575–580.
244. Frontera WR, Meredith CM, O'Reilly KP, Knuttgen HG, Evans WJ. Strength conditioning in older men: skeletal muscle hypertrophy and improved function. *J Appl Physiol* 1988; 64:1038–1044.
245. Staron RS, Malicky ES, Leonardi MJ, Fakel JE, Hagerman FC, Dudley GA. Muscle hypertrophy and fast fiber type conversions in heavy resistance-trained women. *Eur J Appl Physiol Occup Physiol* 1989; 60:71–79.
246. Tesch PA. Short- and long-term histochemical and biochemical adaptations in muscle. In: Komi PV, ed. *Strength and power in sports. The encyclopaedia of sports medicine.* Oxford: Blackwell, 1992; 239–248.
247. Tesch PA, Hjort H, Balldin UI. Effects of strength training on G tolerance. *Aviat Space Environ Med* 1983; 54:691–695.
248. MacDougall JD, Sale DG, Moroz JR, Elder GCB, Sutton JR, Howard H. Mitochondrial volume density in human skeletal muscle following heavy resistance training. *Med Sci Sports* 1979; 11:164–166.
249. Stone MH. Connective tissue and bone response to strength training. In: Komi PV, ed. *Strength and power in sports. The encyclopaedia of sports medicine.* Oxford: Blackwell, 1992; 279–290.
250. Zernicke RF, Loitz BJ. Exercise-related adapations in connective tissue. In: Komi PV, ed. *Strength and power in sports. The encyclopaedia of sports medicine.* Oxford: Blackwell, 1992; 77–95.
251. Staff PH. The effect of physical activity on joints, cartilage, tendons and ligaments. *Scand J Soc Med* 1982; 29(Suppl):59–63.
252. Laurent GJ, Sparrow MP, Bates PC, Millward DJ. Collagen content and turnover in cardiac and skeletal muscles of the adult fowl and the changes during stretch-induced growth. *Biochem J* 1978; 176: 419–305.
253. Turto H, Lindy S, Halme J. Protocollagen proline hydroxylase activity in work-induced hypertrophy of rat muscle. *Am J Physiol* 1974; 226: 63–65.
254. MacDougall JD, Tuxen D, Sale DG, Moroz JR, Sutton JR. Arterial blood pressure response to heavy resistance exercise. *J Appl Physiol* 1985; 58:785–790.
255. Conroy BP, Kraemer WJ, Maresh CM, Dalsky GP. Adaptive responses of bone to physical activity. *Med Exerc Nutr Health* 1992; 1(2):64–74.
256. Holmdahl DC, Ingelmark RE. Der bau des gelenknorpels unterverschiedenen funktionellen verhaltnissen. *Acta Anat* 1948; 6:113–116.
257. Ingelmark BE, Elsholm R. A study on variations in the thickness of the articular cartilage in association with rest and periodical load. *Uppsala Lakaretorenings Foxhandlingar* 1948; 53:61–64.
258. Fahey TD, Brown CH. The effects of anabolic steroid on the strength, body composition and endurance of college males when accompanied by a weight training program. *Med Sci Sports* 1973; 5:272–276.
259. Lee A, Craig BW, Lucas J, Pohlman R, Stelling H. The effect of endurance training, weight training and a combination of endurance and weight training upon the blood lipid profile of young male subjects. *J Appl Sport Sci Res* 1990; 4:68–75.
260. Gettman LR, Pollock ML. Circuit weight training: a critical review of its physiological benefits. *Phys Sportsmed* 1981; 9:44–60.
261. McDonagh MJN, Davies CTM. Adaptive response of mammalian skeletal muscle to exercise with high loads. *Eur J Appl Physiol* 1984; 52:139–155.
262. Hoeger WWK, Barette SL, Hale DF, Hopkins DR. Relationship between repetitions and selected percentages of one repetition maximum. *J Appl Sport Sci Res* 1987; 1:11–13.
263. Stone MH, O'Bryant H, Garhammer JG, McMillian J, Rozenek R. A theoretical model for strength training. *Natl Strength Cond Assoc J* 1982; 4:36–39.
264. Matveyev L. *Fundamentals of sports training.* Moscow: Progress, 1981.
265. O'Bryant HS, Byrd R, Stone MH. Cycle ergometry performance and maximum leg and hip strength adaptations to two different methods of weight-training. *J Appl Sport Sci Res* 1988; 2:27–30.
266. Stone MH, O'Bryant H, Garhammer JG. A hypothetical model for strength training. *J Sports Med Phys Fitness* 1981; 21:342–351.
267. Willoughby DS. The effects of mesocycle-length weight training programs involving periodization and partially equated volumes on upper and lower body strength. *J Strength Cond Res* 1993; 7(1):2–8.
268. Garhammer, J. Equipment for the development of athletic strength and power. *Natl Strength Cond Assoc J* 1981; 3:24–26.
269. Fleck SJ, Kraemer WJ. *Periodization breakthrough.* New York: Advance Research Press, 1996.
270. Kanehisa H, Miyashita M. Effect of isometric and isokinetic muscle training on static strength and dynamic power. *Eur J Appl Physiol* 1983; 50:365–371.
271. Kanehisa H, Miyashita M. Specificity of velocity in strength training. *Eur J Appl Physiol* 1983; 52:104–106.
272. Gardner G. Specificity of strength changes of the exercised and nonexercised limb following isometric training. *Res Q* 1963; 34:98–101.
273. Meyers CR. Effect of two isometric routines on strength, size and endurance in exercised and non-exercised arms. *Res Q* 1967; 38: 430–440.
274. Williams M, Stutzman L. Strength variation throughout the range of motion. *Phys Ther Rev* 1959; 39:145–152.
275. Knapik JJ, Mawdsley RH, Ramos MU. Angular specificity and test mode specificity of isometric and isokinetic strength training. *J Orthop Sports Phys Ther* 1983; 5:58–65.
276. Steinhaus AH. *Some selected facts from physiology and the physiology of exercise applicable to physical rehabilitation.* Paper presented to the Study Group on Body Mechanics, Washington, D.C., 1954.

277. Hettinger R, Muller E. Muskelleistung und Muskeltraining. *Arbeits Physiol* 1953; 15:111–126.
278. Fleck SJ, Schutt RC. Types of strength training. *Clin Sports Med* 1985; 4:159–169.
279. Davies J, Parker DF, Rutherford OM, Jones DA. Changes in strength and cross sectional area of the elbow flexors as a result of isometric strength training. *Eur J Appl Physiol* 1988; 57:667–670.
280. Garfinkel S, Cafarelli E. Relative changes in maximal force, EMG, and muscle cross-sectional area after isometric training. *Med Sci Sports Exerc* 1992; 24:1220–1227.
281. Alway SE, Sale DG, MacDougall JD. Twitch contractile adaptations are not dependent on the intensity of isometric exercise in the human triceps surae. *Eur J Appl Physiol* 1990; 60:346–352.
282. Davies CTM, Young K. Effects of training at 30 and 100% maximal isometric force on the contractile properties of the triceps surae of man. *J Physiol* 1983; 36:22–23.
283. Rasch P, Morehouse L. Effect of static and dynamic exercises on muscular strength and hypertrophy. *J Appl Physiol* 1957; 11:29–34.
284. Ward J, Fisk GH. The difference in response of the quadriceps and biceps brachii muscles to isometric and isotonic exercise. *Arch Phys Med Rehabil* 1964; 45:612–620.
285. Hettinger R. *Physiology of strength.* Springfield, IL: Charles C Thomas, 1961.
286. Atha J. Strengthening muscle. *Exerc Sport Sci Rev* 1981; 9:1–73.
287. Berger RA. Effect of varied weight training programs on strength. *Res Q* 1962; 33:168–181.
288. Berger RA. Optimum repetitions for the development of strength. *Res Q* 1962; 33:334–338.
289. Berger RA. Comparative effects of three weight training programs. *Res Q* 1963; 34:396–398.
290. Graves JE, Pollock ML, Leggett SH, Braith RW, Carpenter DM, Bishop LE. Effect of reduced frequency on muscular strength. *Int J Sports Med* 1988; 9:316–319.
291. Häkkinen K, Alén M, Komi PV. Changes in isometric force- and relaxation-time, electromyographic and muscle fibre characteristics of human skeletal muscle during strength training and detraining. *Acta Physiol Scand* 1985; 125:573–585.
292. Henderson JM. The effects of weight loadings and repetitions, frequency of exercise and knowledge of theoretical principles of weight training on changes in muscular strength. *Dissertation Abstr Int* 1970; 31A:3320.
293. O'Shea P. Effects of selected weight training programs on the development of strength and muscle hypertrophy. *Res Q* 1966; 37:95–102.
294. Sale DG, MacDougall JD, Jacobs I, Garner S. Interaction between concurrent strength and endurance training. *J Appl Physiol* 1990; 68: 260–270.
295. Withers RT. Effect of varied weight-training loads on the strength of university freshmen. *Res Q* 1970; 41:110–114.
296. American College of Sports Medicine. The recommended quantity and quality of exercise for developing and maintaining cardiorespiratory and muscular fitness in healthy adults. *Med Sci Sports Exerc* 1990; 22:265–274.
297. Ariel G. Barbell vs dynamic variable resistance. *US Sports Assoc News* 1977; 1:7.
298. Braith RW, Graves JE, Leggett SH, Pollock ML. Effect of training on the relationship between maximal and submaximal strength. *Med Sci Sports Exerc* 1993; 25:132–138.
299. Coleman AE. Nautilus vs universal gym strength training in adult males. *Am Cor Ther J* 1977; 31:103–107.
300. Gettman LR, Culter LA, Strathman T. Physiological changes after 20 weeks of isotonic vs isokinetic circuit training. *J Sports Med Phys Fitness* 1980; 20:265–274.
301. Graves JE, Pollock ML, Jones AE, Colvin AB, Leggett SH. Specificity of limited range of motion variable resistance training. *Med Sci Sports Exerc* 1989; 21:84–89.
302. Hurley BF, Seals DR, Ehsani AA, et al. Effects of high-intensity strength training on cardiovascular function. *Med Sci Sports Exerc* 1984; 16:483–488.
303. Peterson JA. Total conditioning: A case study. *Athletic J* 1975; 56: 40–55.
304. Stone MH, Johnson RC, Carter DR. A short term comparison of two different methods of resistance training on leg strength and power. *Athletic Training* 1979; 14:158–160.
305. Bell GJ, Petersen SR, Maclean I, Reid DC, Quinney HA. Effect of high velocity resistance training on peak torque, cross sectional area and myofibrillar ATPase activity. *J Sports Med Phys Fitness* 1992; 32:10–17.
306. Bell GJ, Petersen SR, Wessel J, Bagnall K, Quinney HA. Adaptations to endurance and low velocity resistance training performed in a sequence. *Can J Sport Sci* 1991; 16:186–192.
307. Bell GJ, Snydmiller GD, Neary JP, Quinney HA. The effect of high and low velocity resistance training on anaerobic power output in cyclists. *J Hum Movement Stud* 1989; 16:173–181.
308. Lesmes GR, Costill DL, Coyle EF, Fink WJ. Muscle strength and power changes during maximal isokinetic training. *Med Sci Sports* 1978; 4:266–269.
309. Petersen SR, Miller GD, Quinney HA, Wenger HA. The effectiveness of a mini-cycle on velocity-specific strength acquisition. *J Orthop Sports Phys Ther* 1987; 9:156–159.
310. Seaborne D, Taylor AW. The effect of speed of isokinetic exercise on training transfer to isometric strength in the quadriceps. *J Sports Med* 1984; 24:183–188.
311. Fleck SJ. Varying frequency and intensity of isokinetic strength training. *Dissertation Abstr Int* 1979; 39:2126A.
312. Smith MJ, Melton P. Isokinetic versus isotonic variable resistance training. *Am J Sports Med* 1981; 9:275–279.
313. Rizzardo M, Bay G, Wessel J. Eccentric and concentric torque and power of the knee extensors of females. *Can J Sport Sci* 1988; 13: 166–169.
314. Tesch PA, Dudley GA, Duvoisin MR, Hather BM, Harris RT. Force and EMG signal patterns during repeated bouts of concentric or eccentric muscle actions. *Acta Physiol Scand* 1990; 138:263–271.
315. Häkkinen K, Komi PV, Tesch PA. Effect of combined concentric and eccentric strength training and detraining on force–time, muscle fiber and metabolic characteristics of leg extensor muscles. *Scand J Sports Sci* 1981; 3:50–58.
316. Colliander EB, Tesch PA. Effects of eccentric and concentric muscle actions in resistance training. *Acta Physiol Scand* 1990; 140:31–39.
317. Lacerte M, deLateur BJ, Alquist AD, Questad KA. Concentric versus combined concentric–eccentric isokinetic training programs: effect on peak torque of human quadriceps femoris muscle. *Arch Phys Med Rehabil* 1992; 73:1059–1062.
318. Clarke DH. Adaptations in strength and muscular endurance resulting from exercise. *Exerc Sport Sci Rev* 1973; 1:73–102.
319. Zemper ED. Four year study of weight room injuries in a national sample of college football teams. *Natl Strength Cond Assoc J* 1990; 12(3):32–34.
320. Fleck SJ, Dean LS. Resistance-training experience and the pressor response during resistance exercise. *J Appl Physiol* 1987; 63:116–120.
321. Kendal FP, McCreary EK, Provance PG. *Muscles: testing and function, 4th ed.* Baltimore: Williams & Wilkins, 1993.
322. High DM, Howley ET, Franks BD. The effects of static stretching and warm-up on prevention of delayed-onset muscle soreness. *Res Q Exerc Sport* 1989; 60:357–361.
323. Craib MW, Mitchell VA, Fields KB, Cooper TR, Hopewell R, Morgan DW. The association between flexibility and running economy in sub-elite male distance runners. *Med Sci Sports Exerc* 1996; 28:737–743.
324. Gleim GW, Stachenfeld NS, Nicholas JA. The influence of flexibility on the economy of walking and jogging. *J Orthop Res* 1990; 8: 814–823.
325. Wilson GJ, Elliot BC, Wood GA. Stretch shorten cycle performance enhancement through flexibility training. *Med Sci Sports Exerc* 1992; 24:116–123.
326. Herring SW, Grimm AF, Grimm BR. Regulation of sarcomere number in skeletal muscle: a comparison of hypotheses. *Muscle Nerve* 1984; 7:161–173.
327. Noonan TJ, Best TM, Seaber AV, Garrett WE. Thermal effects on skeletal muscle tensile behavior. *Am J Sports Med* 1993; 21:517–522.
328. Strickler T, Malone T, Garrett WE. The effects of passive warming on muscle injury. *Am J Sports Med* 1990; 18:141–145.
329. Warren CG, Lehmann JF, Koblanski JN. Elongation of rat tail tendon: effect of load and temperature. *Arch Phys Med Rehabil* 1971; 52: 465–484.
330. Leighton JR. The Leighton flexometer and flexibility test. *J Assoc Phys Ment Rehabil* 1966; 20:86.
331. Taylor DC, Dalton JD, Seaber AV, Garrett WE. Viscoelastic properties of muscle–tendon units: the biomechanical effects of stretching. *Am J Sports Med* 1990; 18:300–309.

332. Sady SP, Wortman M, Blanke D. Flexibility training: ballistic, static or proprioceptive neuromuscular facilitation? *Arch Phys Med Rehabil* 1982; 63:261–263.
333. Wallin D, Ekblom B, Grahn R, Nordenborg T. Improvement of muscle flexibility—a comparison between two techniques. *Am J Sports Med* 1985; 13:263–268.
334. Anderson B, Burke ER. Scientific, medical, and practical aspects of stretching. *Clin Sports Med* 1991; 10(1):63–86.
335. Kabat H. Studies on neuromuscular dysfunction: XV. The role of central facilitation in restoration of motor function in paralysis. *Arch Phys Med Rehabil* 1952; 33:521–533.
336. Lehmann JF, Warren CG, Scham SM. Therapeutic heat and cold. *Clin Orthop Rel Res* 1974; 99:207–245.
337. Travell JG, Simons DG. *Myofascial pain and dysfunction, Vol 1*. Baltimore: Williams & Wilkins, 1983.
338. Barrett DS, Cobb AG, Bentley G. Joint proprioception in normal, osteoarthritic and replaced knees. *J Bone Joint Surg* 1991; 73B:53–56.
339. Barrack RL, Skinner HB, Cook SD, Haddad R. Effect of articular disease and total knee arthroplasty on knee position sense. *J Neurophysiol* 1983; 50:684–687.
340. Lichtenstein MJ, Shields SL, Shiavi RG, Burger MC. Clinical determinats of biomechanics platform measures of balance in aged women. *J Am Geriatr Soc* 1988; 36:996–1002.
341. Lord SR, Sambrook PN, Gilbert C, et al. Postural stability, falls and fractures in the elderly: results from the Dubbo Osteoporosis Epidemiology Study. *Med J Aust* 1994; 160:684–691.
342. Maki BE, Holliday PJ, Fernie GR. Aging and postural control: a comparison of spontaneous- and induced-sway balance tests. *J Am Geriatr Soc* 1990; 38:1–9.
343. Topper AK, Maki BE, Holliday PJ. Are activity based assessments of balance and gait in the elderly predictive of risk of falling and/or type of fall? *J Am Geriatr Soc* 1993; 41:479–487.
344. Tropp H, Ekstrand J, Gillquist J. Stabilometry in functional instability of the ankle and its value in predicting injury. *Med Sci Sports Exerc* 1984; 16:64–66.
345. Barrett DS. Proprioception and function after anterior cruciate reconstruction. *J Bone Joint Surg [Br]* 1991; 73B:833–837.
346. Corrigan JP, Cashman WF, Brady MP. Proprioception in the cruciate deficient knee. *J Bone Joint Surg* 1992; 74B:247–250.
347. Glencross D, Thornton E. Position sense following joint injury. *J Sports Med* 1981; 21:23–27.
348. Tropp H, Odenrick P, Gillquist J. Stabilometry recordings in functional and mechanical instability of the ankle joint. *Int J Sports Med* 1985; 6:180–182.
349. Ferrell WR, Crighton A, Sturrock RD. Position sense at the proximal interphalangeal joint is distorted in patients with rheumatoid arthritis of finger joints. *Exp Physiol* 1992; 77:675–680.
350. Skinner HB, Wyatt MP, Hodgdon JA, Conard DW, Barrack RL. Effect of fatigue on joint position sense of the knee. *J Orthop Res* 1986; 4: 112–118.
351. Simoneau GG, Derr JA, Ulbrecht JS, Becker MB, Cavanagh PR. Diabetic sensory neuropathy effect on ankle joint movement perception. *Arch Phys Med Rehabil* 1996;77:453–460.
352. Skinner HB, Barrack RL, Cook SD. Age-related decline in proprioception. *Clin Orthop Rel Res* 1984; 184:208–211.
353. Skinner HB, Barrack RL, Cook SD, Haddad RJ. Joint position sense in total knee arthroplasty. *J Orthop Res* 1984; 1:276–283.
354. Bates B. *A guide to physical examination and history taking*. Philadelphia: Lippincott, 1987.
355. Barrack RL, Skinner HB, Cook SD. Proprioception of the knee joint: paradoxical effect of training. *Am J Phys Med* 1984; 63:175–181.
356. Steele GJ, Harter RA, Arthur JT. Comparison of functional ability following percutaneous and open surgical repairs of acutely ruptured Achilles tendons. *J Sports Rehabil* 1993; 2:115–127.
357. Barenberg RA, Shefner JM, Sabol JJ Jr. Quantitative assessment of position sense at the ankle: a functional approach. *Neurology* 1987; 37:89–93.
358. Ferrell WR, Smith A. The effect of loading on position sense at the proximal interphalangeal joint of the human index finger. *J Physiol* 1989; 418:145–161.
359. McNair PJ, Marshall RN, Maguire K, Brown C. Knee joint effusion and proprioception. *Arch Phys Med Rehabil* 1995; 76:566–568.
360. Friden T, Zatterstrom R, Lindstrand A, Moritz U. A stabilometric technique for evaluation of lower limb instabilities. *Am J Sports Med* 1989; 17:118–122.
361. Hughes MA, Duncan PW, Rose DK, Chandler JM, Studenski SA. The relationship of postural sway to sensorimotor function, functional performance, and disability in the elderly. *Arch Phys Med Rehabil* 1996; 77:567–572.
362. Brunt D, Andersen JC, Huntsman B, Reinhert LB, Thorell AC, Sterling JC. Postural responses to lateral pertubation in healthy subjects and ankle sprain patients. *Med Sci Sports Exerc* 1992; 24:171–176.
363. Freeman MAR, Dean MRE, Hanham IWF. The etiology and prevention of functional instability of the foot. *J Bone Joint Surg [Br]* 1965; 47:678–685.
364. Gauffin H, Tropp H, Odenrick P. Effect of ankle disk training on postural control in patients with functional instability of the ankle joint. *J Sports Med* 1988; 9:141–144.
365. Tropp H, Ekstrand J, Gillquist J. Factors affecting stabiliometry recordings of single limb stance. *Am J Sports Med* 1984; 12:185–188.
366. Maron BJ, Poliac LC, Roberts WO. Risk of sudden death associated with marathon running. *J Am Coll Cardiol* 1996; 28:428–431.
367. Mittleman MA, Maclure M, Tofler GH, Sherwood JB, Goldberg RJ, Muller JE. Triggering of acute myocardial infarction by heavy physical exertion. Protection against triggering by regular exertion. *N Engl J Med* 1993; 329:1677–1683.
368. Willich SN, Lewis M, Lowel H, Arntz HR, Schubert F, Schroder R. Physical exertion as a trigger of acute myocardial infarction. *N Engl J Med* 1993; 329:1684–1690.
369. Agency for Health Care Policy and Research. *Clinical practice guideline number 17: cardiac rehabilitation.* US Department of Health and Human Services, AHCPR publication number 96-0672, 1995.
370. Haskell WL. Cardiovascular complications during exercise training of cardiac patients. *Circulation* 1978; 57:920–924.
371. Van Camp SP, Peterson RA. Cardiovascular complications of outpatient cardiac rehabilitation programs. *JAMA* 1986; 256:1160–1163.
372. Vongvanich P, Paul-Labrador MJ, Merz CNB. Safety of medically supervised exercise in a cardiac rehabilitation center. *Am J Cardiol* 1996; 77:1383–1385.
373. Maron BJ, Shirani J, Poliac LC, Mathenge R, Roberts WC, Mueller FO. Sudden death in young competitive athletes. Cinical, demographic, and pathological profiles. JAMA 1996; 276:199–204.
374. American College of Sports Medicine. Position statement: prevention of thermal injuries during distance running. *Med Sci Sports Exerc* 1984; 16:ix–xiv.
375. Grover RF, Reeves JT, Rowell LB, Piantadoski CA, Saltzman HA. The influence of environmental factors on the cardiovascular system. In: Schlant RC, Alexander RW, eds. *The heart, 8th ed.* New York: McGraw-Hill, 1994; 2117–2132.
376. Sheldahl LM, Wilke NA, Tristani FE. Evaluation and training for resumption of occupational and leisure-time activities in patients after a major cardiac event. *Med Exerc Nutr Health* 1995; 4:273–289.
377. Pugh LGCE. The influence of wind resistance in running and walking and the mechanical efficiency of work against horizontal or vertical forces. *J Physiol* 1971; 213:255–276.
378. Zamparo P, Perini R, Orizio, Sacher M, Ferretti G. The energy cost of walking or running on sand. *Eur J Appl Physiol* 1992; 65:183–187.
379. Fisher AC. Adherence to sports rehabilitation programmes. *Sports Med* 1990; 9:151–158.
380. Caspersen CJ, Merritt RK. Physical activity trends among 26 states, 1986–1990. *Med Sci Sports Exerc* 1995; 27:713–720.
381. Crespo CJ, Keteyian SJ, Heath GW, Sempos CT. Leisure time physical activity among US adults: results from the third National Health and Nutrition Examination Survery. *Arch Intern Med* 1996; 156: 93–98.
382. McGinnis JM. Healthy People 2000 at mid decade. *JAMA* 1995; 273: 1123–1129.
383. Young DR, Haskell WL, Taylor CB, Fortmann SP. Effect of community health education on physical activity knowledge, attitudes, and behavior. The Stanford Five-City Project. *Am J Epidemiol* 1996; 144: 264–274.
384. Yusuf HR, Croft JB, Giles WH, Anda RF, Casper ML, Caspersen CJ, Jones DA. Leisure-time physical activity among older adults. United States, 1990. *Arch Intern Med* 1996; 156:1321–1326.
385. Surgeon General of the Public Health Service. *Surgeon General's report on physical activity and health* (S/N 017-023-00196-5). Washington, D.C.: US Public Health Service; 1996.

386. Sheldahl LM, Wilke NA, Hanna RD, Dougherty SM, Tristani FE. Responses of people with coronary artery disease to common lawn-care tasks. *Eur J Appl Physiol* 1996; 72:357–364.
387. Dishman RK, Buckworth J. Increasing physical activity: a quantitative synthesis. *Med Sci Sports Exerc* 1996; 28:706–719.
388. Gordon NF, Scott CB. Exercise intensity prescription in cardiovascular disease. *J Cardiopulm Rehabil* 1995; 15:193–196.
389. Sallis JF, Hovell MF, Hofstetter CR. Predictors of adoption and maintenace of vigorous physical activity in men and women. *Prev Med* 1992; 21:237–251.
390. American College of Sports Medicine. *ACSM's guidelines for exercise testing and prescription, 4th ed.* Philadelphia: Lea & Febiger, 1991.
391. Hoffman MD. Cardiorespiratory fitness and training in quadriplegics and paraplegics. *Sports Med* 1986; 3:312–330.
392. Davis GM. Exercise capacity of individuals with paraplegia. *Med Sci Sports Exerc* 1993; 25:423–432.
393. Davis GM, Shephard RJ. Cardiovascular fitness in highly active versus inactive paraplegics. *Med Sci Sports Exerc* 1988; 20:463–468.
394. Hopman MTE, Oeseburg B, Binkhorst RA. Cardiovascular responses in persons with paraplegia to prolonged arm exercise and thermal stress. *Med Sci Sports Exerc* 1993; 25:577–583.
395. Hoffman MD, Sheldahl LS, Wenzler RB. Cardiovascular responses in paraplegics during exercise with lower extremity compression. *Clin Res* 1987; 35:287a.
396. Hopman MTE, Oeseburg B, Binkhorst RA. The effect of an anti-G suit on cardiovascular responses to exercise in persons with paraplegia. *Med Sci Sports Exerc* 1992; 24:984–990.
397. Pitetti KH, Barrett PJ, Campbell KD, Malzahn DE. The effect of lower body positive pressure on the exercise capacity of individuals with spinal cord injury. *Med Sci Sports Exerc* 1994; 26:463–468.
398. Davis GM, Servedio FJ, Glaser RM, Gupta SC, Suryaprasad AG. Cardiovascular responses to arm cranking and FNS-induced leg exercise in paraplegics. *J Appl Physiol* 1990; 69:671–674.
399. Hooker SP, Figoni SF, Rodgers MM, et al. Metabolic and hemodynamic responses to concurrent voluntary arm crank and electrical stimulation leg cycle exercise in quadriplegics. *J Rehabil Res Dev* 1992; 29:1–11.
400. McLean KP, Skinner JS. Effect of body training position on outcomes of an aerobic training study on individuals with quadriplegia. *Arch Phys Med Rehabil* 1995; 76:139–150.
401. Birk TJ. Poliomyelitis and post-polio syndrome: exercise capacities and adaptation—current research, furture directions, and widespread applicability. *Med Sci Sports Exerc* 1993; 25:466–472.
402. Dean E, Ross J. Modified aerobic walking program: effect on patients with postpolio syndrome symptoms. *Arch Phys Med Rehabil* 1988; 69:1033–1038.
403. Ernstoff B, Wetterqvist H, Kvist H, Grimby G. Endurance training effect on individuals with postpoliomyelitis. *Arch Phys Med Rehabil* 1996; 77:843–848.
404. Jones DR, Speier J, Canine K, Owen R, Stull GA. Cardiorespiratory responses to aerobic training by patients with post-poliomyelitis sequelae. *JAMA* 1989; 261:3255–3258.
405. Einarsson G. Muscle conditioning in late poliomyelitis. *Arch Phys Med Rehabil* 1991; 72:11–14.
406. Ponichtera-Mulcare JA. Exercise and multiple sclerosis. *Med Sci Sports Exerc* 1993; 25:451–465.
407. Kosich D, Molk B, Feeney J, Petajan JH. Cardiovascular testing and exercise prescription in multiple sclerosis patients. *J Neurol Rehabil* 1987; 1:167–170.
408. Schapiro RT, Petajan JH, Kosich D, Molk B, Feeney J. Role of cardiovascular fitness in multiple sclerosis. *J Neurol Rehabil* 1988; 2:43–49.
409. Gehlsen GM, Grigsby SA, Winant DM. Effects of an aquatic fitness program on the muscular strength and endurance of patients with multiple sclerosis. *Phys Ther* 1984; 64:653–657.
410. Friedenreich CM, Courneya KS. Exercise as rehabilitation for cancer patients. *Clin J Sports Med* 1996; 6:237–244.
411. American College of Obstetricians and Gynecologists. *Exercise during pregnancy and the postpartum period* (Technical Bulletin 28-189). Washington, D.C.: ACOG, 1994.
412. Wolf LA, Hall P, Webb KA, Goodman L, Monga M, McGrath MJ. Prescription of aerobic exercise during pregnancy. *Sports Med* 1989; 8:273–301.
413. Micheli LJ. Pediatric and adolescent sports injuries. *Exerc Sport Sci Rev* 1986; 14:349–351.
414. Bar-Or O. Climate and the exercising child—a review. *Int J Sports Med* 1980; 1:53–65.
415. Fiatarone MA, O'Neill EF, Ryan ND, et al. Exercise training and nutritional supplementation for physical frailty in very elderly people. *N Engl J Med* 1994; 330:1769–1775.

Rehabilitation Medicine: Principles and Practice, Third Edition, edited by Joel A. DeLisa and Bruce M. Gans. Lippincott–Raven Publishers, Philadelphia © 1998.

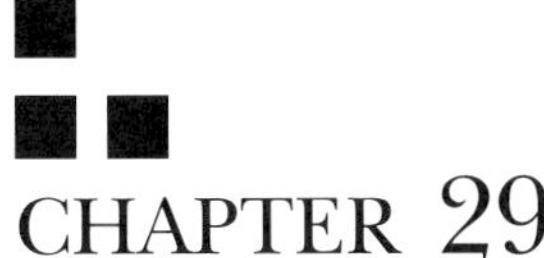

CHAPTER 29

Assistive Technology for Rehabilitation and Reduction of Disability

James R. Swenson, Laura L. Barnett, Bonnie Pond, and Andrew A. Schoenberg

The goals of medical rehabilitation are to return the disabled individual to his or her maximum degree of physical independence, psychosocial adjustment, and vocational productivity. Treatment strategies commonly used include complete reversal of the medical impairment; reduction of the medical impairment by using medical, surgical, or rehabilitation treatment; substitution for lost function by utilization of the person's residual function or, finally, the use of devices that will assist the person to overcome some of the disabilities.

The discipline of using devices to improve function is known as assistive technology. Assistive technology is defined as any item, piece of equipment, or product system, whether acquired commercially off the shelf, modified, or customized, that is used to increase, maintain, or improve functional capabilities of individuals with disabilities (1). Assistive technology (AT) is a broad term that includes a large variety of items such as walkers, mechanical lifts, communication devices, and environmental control units. The careful selection of and training in the use of assistive technology devices can greatly increase the quality of life of many disabled individuals by decreasing or eliminating many of the barriers to independence.

This chapter covers the basic principles of evaluation and funding for AT, information on AT products, computers and computer-based adaptations, augmentive and alternative communication (AAC) devices, environmental control units (ECU), AT for vision and hearing disabilities, automobile adaptations, home environment and vocational AT, and a brief review of robotics and neuroprosthetics.

J. R. Swenson: Department of Physical Medicine and Rehabilitation, University of Utah School of Medicine, Salt Lake City, Utah 84132.

L. L. Barnett and B. Pond: Department of Rehabilitation Services, University of Utah Hospital, Salt Lake City, Utah 84132.

A. A. Schoenberg: Department of Physical Medicine and Rehabilitation, University of Utah Hospital, Salt Lake City, Utah 84132.

INFORMATION SOURCES

Reading the ever-increasing supply of information on AT has become a formidable task. One role of the AT practitioner is to provide information regarding the latest devices to clients and patients. Competent AT providers study and review a variety of government publications, vendor catalogs, scientific journals, and electronic libraries to keep abreast of new developments and devices in assistive technology.

One particularly comprehensive electronic library on assistive technology for the disabled is Co-Net, which is available on CD-ROM from The Trace Research and Development Center at the University of Wisconsin–Madison (2). Co-Net includes four libraries on disability issues: AbleData, Cooperative Service Directory, Publications and Media, and Text Library.

The AbleData library contains information on more than 23,000 devices as well as programs for searching and finding the desired devices by type, name, and manufacturer. The Cooperative Service Directory contains a comprehensive list of private and public organizations serving the disabled community, with contact information and types of services provided. It allows users to sort for agencies close to their home. The Publications and Media library is a bibliography on disability topics such as references on funding, disability statistics, information on referral sources, and specialized AT areas such as functional electrical stimulation. The Text Library contains texts of important government publications such as the ADA, current disability laws, and telecommunications access issues.

SERVICE DELIVERY AND EVALUATION

Assistive technology services may be delivered in a wide variety of settings, including comprehensive medical rehabilitation centers, university-affiliated clinics, state agency-based AT programs, private rehabilitation engineering and technology firms, and nonprofit disability organizations (3). Information, demonstration, and referral services are also available from many AT centers sponsored by the Federal Government. Durable medical equipment suppliers provide information, demonstrations, and support for various assistive technology products. Because AT is a relatively new field, consumers may encounter difficulty locating experienced professionals to deliver AT services.

A multidisciplinary model of service delivery is preferred for complex client needs, as it provides a larger pool of resources and expertise. The client's functional goals are central to the evaluation of his or her needs. The team of professionals may include an occupational therapist, rehabilitation engineer, physical therapist, speech/language pathologist, physiatrist, case manager, and funding specialist. Special educators are often included when dealing with clients whose AT goals include participation in educational programs. The team may also include family members, care providers, and others who are involved with the client.

The AT team initiates a comprehensive evaluation of a client (see Fig. 29-1). The initial step is to gather background information, including a recent medical history and physical examination; cognitive and language testing; visual, hearing, and speech assessments; and information on AT devices currently and previously used. A clear understanding of the client's functional abilities is essential. Information regarding the client's current seating and positioning problem is helpful. Seating problems may need to be resolved before provision of other AT services.

The client should be asked what tasks he or she would like to accomplish using technology and what increase in functional independence is anticipated. Initial information about possible funding sources is also gathered. The client will be asked to bring current assistive devices, including glasses and hearing aids, to the evaluation.

Once the client's goals and expectations are established, an assessment of physical skills, mobility, cognitive and linguistic skills, and sensory function is performed using either formal evaluation tools or functional tasks. The team, with client's input, then develops a list of criteria for selection of the AT device (4). This list of criteria is compared with available devices to determine the best possible match.

The AT professional can arrange a device trial to determine whether the device selected will achieve the expected functional goal. For more complex AT systems, a trial period of several weeks may be needed before the decision to purchase is made. Intervention may be needed during this time for device adaptation and further training.

When the client makes a final decision for purchase of a device, the case manager or funding specialist assists the family in locating sources of funding and dealing with third-party payers. The evaluation report is a key part of the funding process and must be complete and timely. Requests for funding include medical prescription, equipment specifications, costs, functional goals, medical diagnoses, vendor information, and costs of training, follow-up, and maintenance.

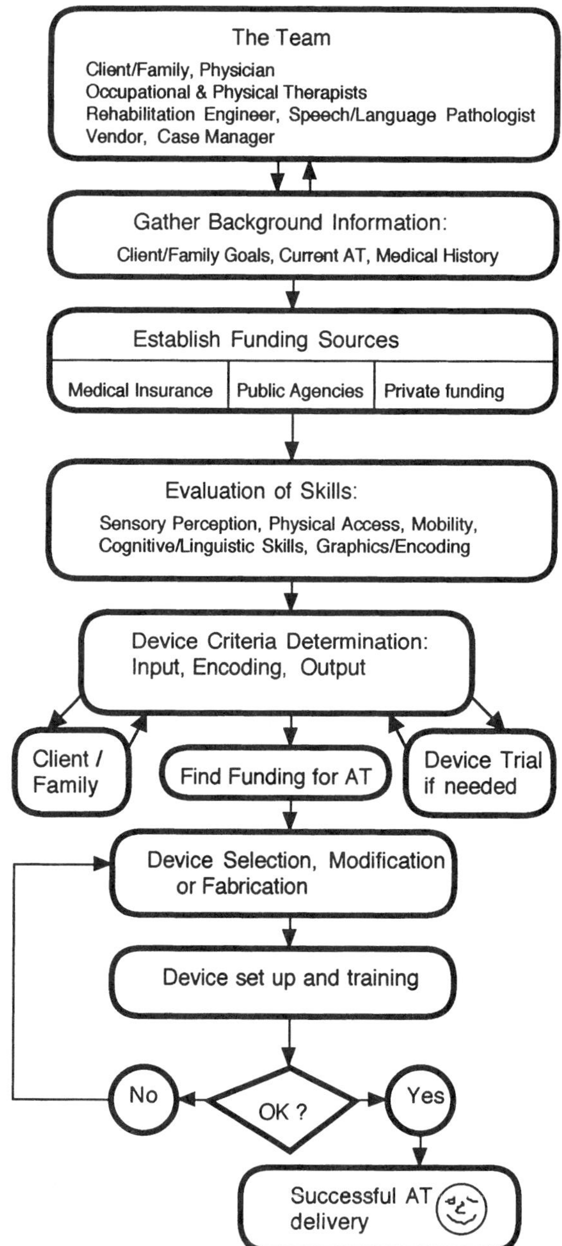

FIG. 29-1. Process diagram showing steps and sequences in assessment and effective delivery of assistive technology.

The funding sources for assistive technology fall into several basic categories (see Table 29-1). One source to be investigated is private or government medical insurance. Medical insurance defines assistive technology as medical equipment necessary for treatment of a specific illness or

TABLE 29-1. *Funding alternatives for assistive technology*

Private funding	Government funding
Private health insurance	Medicare
Casualty insurance	Medicaid
Disability insurance	Vocational rehabilitation
Charitable organizations	Independent living centers
Disability-related nonprofit organizations	Veterans Administration
Churches	CHAMPUS
Service groups	Individuals with Disabilities Education Act
Equipment loan programs	Children with special health care needs
Low-interest loan programs	State or local educational programs

CHAMPUS, Civilian Health and Medical Programs of Uniformed Services.

injury. A physician's prescription is usually required. Assistive technology is usually covered under policy provisions for durable medical equipment, orthotics and prosthetics, or daily living and mobility aids. With private insurance, AT providers request funding under the specific provisions of the individual policy, appealing any denials and offering medical justification for coverage. With government insurance policies, such as Medicaid and Medicare, coverage is based on existing law and regulations. Information on covered services and how to request funding is available from the Medicaid programs in individual states and from the Health Care Financing Administration for Medicare. Assistive technology professionals should continually advocate for adequate coverage of AT in all health care plans.

Funding of assistive technology is also available from other federal and state government entities, such as the Veterans Administration, State Vocational Rehabilitation, Rehabilitation Services Administration, State Independent Living Rehabilitation Centers, and State Education Services. Local school districts may fund assistive technology for children. Each agency or program sets criteria for the funding of assistive technology based on the goals of the agency and the purpose of the technology. For example, vocational rehabilitation agencies generally pay for devices to facilitate gainful employment (including homemakers), and education program funding is directed toward enhancing the client's performance in school. Private funding is available through subsidized loan programs, churches, charitable organizations, and disability-related nonprofit groups. The AT provider must keep abreast of the requirements of various funding sources in order to direct the client to appropriate organizations. Often a combination of funding from several sources is needed to reduce out-of-pocket costs. Because funding for replacement of AT devices is difficult to obtain, careful selection of the initial device is required. Providers can also assist clients by considering funding when making equipment recommendations by including both low- and high-cost alternatives with their advantages. Funding is generally available for assistive technology, but persistence and advocacy by the AT provider are required for success (5,6).

Once the device has been delivered, the vendor or AT professional needs to customize the equipment, if required, and train the client and care providers in the operation of the device. With more complex assistive technology, such as computer access or augmentative communication, an extended period of training and therapy is required. Follow-up by the AT provider on a regular basis is helpful in order to adapt the device for the user's changing needs, facilitate maintenance as needed, and prevent abandonment of the device.

The problem of assistive technology abandonment is serious. One study showed 5.2% of devices were discarded within the first 3 months, 17.8% within the first 5 years, and 29% overall. Some common reasons for abandonment included failure to consider the client's preference, poor device performance, and changing needs of the client (7). Follow-up services decrease abandonment.

COMPUTERS AND COMPUTER-BASED ADAPTATIONS

Computers and devices based on digital information storage and processing are playing an increasing role in the rehabilitation process. Figure 29-2 illustrates the types of computer functions that are typically used in rehabilitation. Rehabilitation professionals use computers in the therapy process to manage patient information and progress (8), assist in cognitive rehabilitation (9), facilitate motor skills training (10), and provide environmental control. Computers are used as substitutes for impaired, absent, or lost sensory, motor, and communication functions. Computers can also improve the lives of people with disabilities by enhancing vocational, educational, and recreational opportunities.

Computer technology is changing very rapidly in the direction of higher performance, expanded storage and memory, faster processing speed, more complex operating systems, and more powerful applications software. The operating systems have changed from keyboard control to graphic user interface (GUI) (11) input by a mouse or other cursor control devices. Conceptually this has simplified many control functions of the computer, eliminating the need to use complex keyboard commands. However, the GUI control systems require intact vision, functional upper extremity

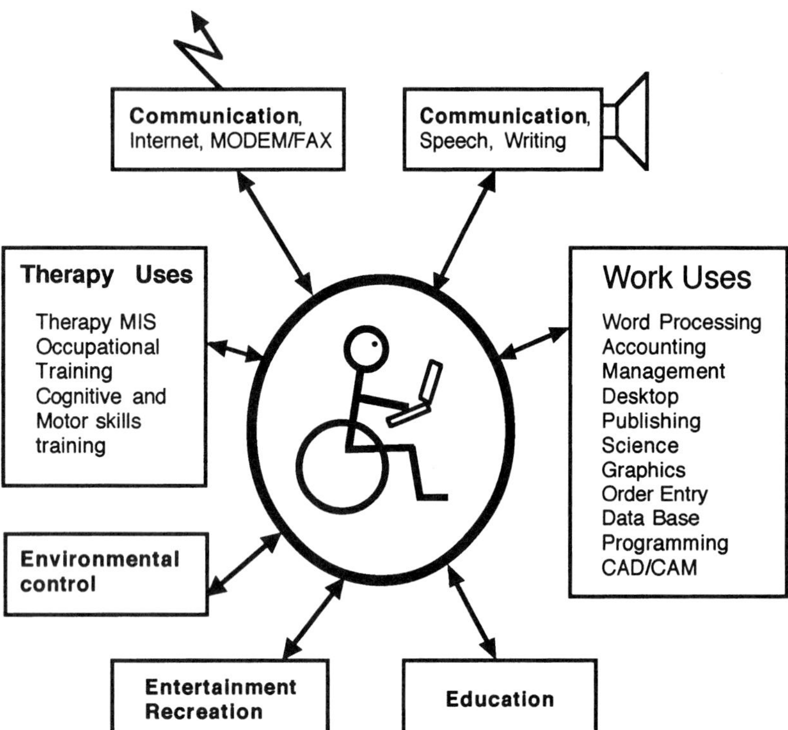

FIG. 29-2. Computer functions and uses in rehabilitation.

control, and good eye–hand coordination for controlling the cursor on the screen.

The major operating system vendors have collaborated with the U.S. government to make computers more accessible to those with disabilities (12). Access DOS (IBM), and Access Pack (Microsoft), are software accessibility packages for the disabled. Current operating systems incorporate a variety of accessibility features such as image enlargement and keyboard commands for menu selection.

Computer Selection

The selection of an appropriate computer and software for any person, including one with a disability, should first focus on the needs or functions that are desired. Word processors, data bases, spreadsheets, and telecommunication packages are the basic software programs for most computer users. Software for these basic programs are frequently combined in an integrated package. When a client desires more complex programs such as multimedia, computer-aided design (CAD), and other graphic programs, a higher performance computer is required. If the client has a need for speech recognition programs, a computer with large memory and high speed is required.

Input and Control Considerations

When choosing an input control method first consider the simple methods of keystroke entry and enhancement with a standard keyboard and then proceed to explore alternative methods of entering alphanumeric information with a standard mouse. If these are not successful, consider alternative input devices designed for persons with disabilities.

When individual finger function is impaired, single-finger or pointer typing aids can be used, such as a typing cuff. When upper extremity function is impaired, mouth sticks or head-mounted pointers are possible choices. These aids are usually combined with word prediction, abbreviation expansion software, and "sticky keys," which is a modification of certain function keys to remain on until another key is depressed. This allows single-digit input of two key commands. Control of the cursor can be provided by a trackball or trackpad, which can be operated with the pointing device. Modifications for single-finger typing are relatively inexpensive.

When limb movement is not functional, electronic head-motion-sensing devices based on infrared, ultrasound, or light beam technology can be used to control the movement of the cursor on the monitor. These devices are usually combined with a software package that includes a virtual keyboard displayed on the monitor. Pointing the beam at the key on the monitor and activating a switch enters a letter or symbol.

For those unable to control a standard keyboard, specialized membrane keyboards are available (Fig. 29-3). The key size and function can be programmed to the user's needs. Some have the capability for customized macro functions in which a single key can represent an entire phrase or activate complex control functions such as printing, faxing, or cursor control. Keyboard and key function modifications are pro-

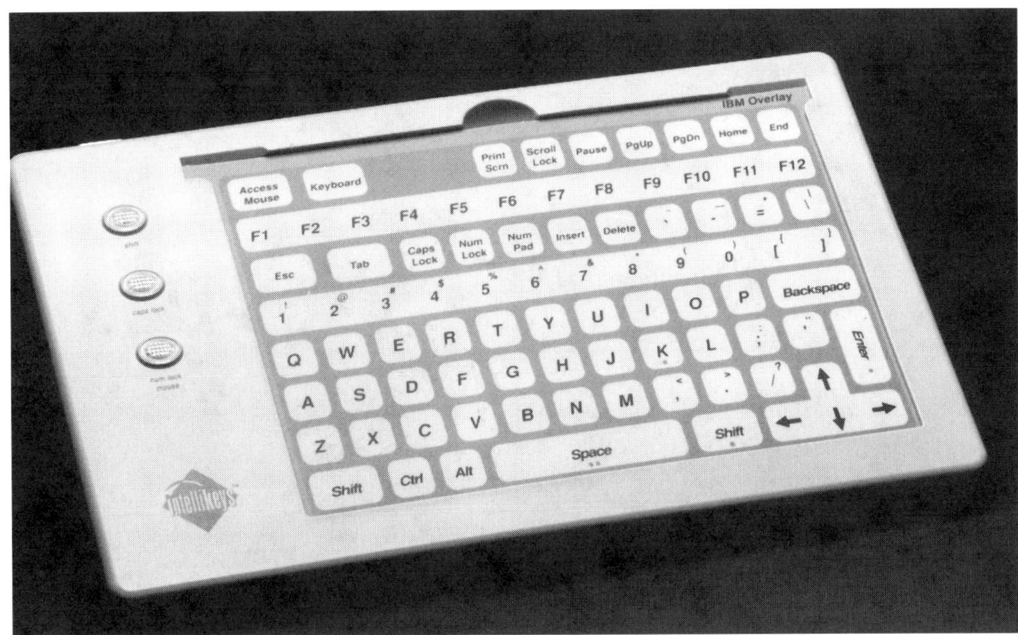

FIG. 29-3. Intellikeys (Intellitools, Novato, CA) is a programmable membrane keyboard.

vided to reduce erroneous activation of keys. Intellikeys (Intellitools, Novato, CA) is an example of a versatile membrane keyboard that is programmable and comes with many standard keyboard overlays. Membrane-type keyboards are more expensive than standard keyboards.

An alternative to programmable membrane keyboards is the touch screen, which mounts on the monitor face of a desktop computer. Touch screens are also incorporated into some laptop computers.

Single-handed keyboards are useful for persons with amputation and hemiplegia. They are also useful for people with visual impairments who have difficulty using braillers or other tactile-oriented keyboards. The keyboard design may incorporate wrist support or a key arrangement that conforms to the neutral position of the wrist. Single-handed keyboards require good client cognitive function and dexterity. Single-handed "chordic" keyboards allow characters to be entered using various combination of seven keys and allow typing speed up to 50 words per minute (13). Adequate training is required for clients using these special keyboards.

When motor function is impaired to the extent that the client cannot select choices on a two-dimensional screen or special keyboard, as in severe CP, ALS, or MS, input using switch control may be the remaining option. Selection of an appropriate switch for a severe motor disability is an important aspect of a successful input adaptation.

Two of the switches commercially available are shown in Figures 29-4 and 29-5. Because of their reliability and low cost, mechanical switches are the preferred choice if the client has enough movement and force for switch activation. Switches may be activated by one's head or any extremity. A pneumatic sip-and-puff switch may be considered in clients without extremity control or when head movement is unreli-

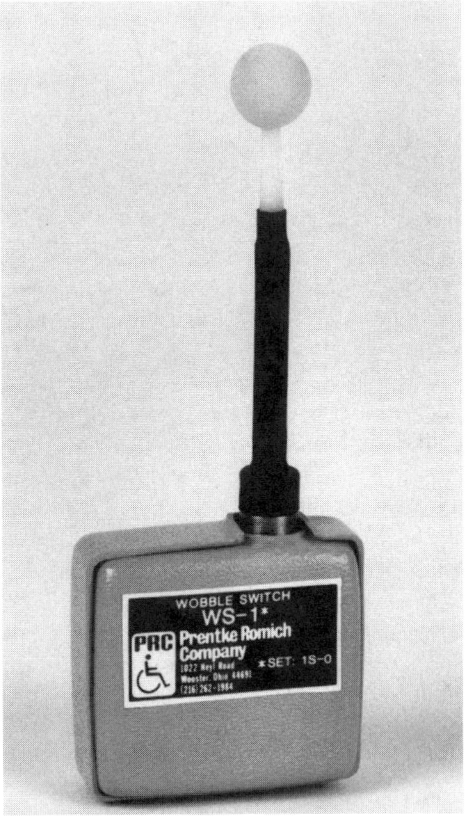

FIG. 29-4. The Wobble Switch (Prentke Romich Co., Wooster, OH) is a simple mechanical switch that can be activated by gross movements in any direction.

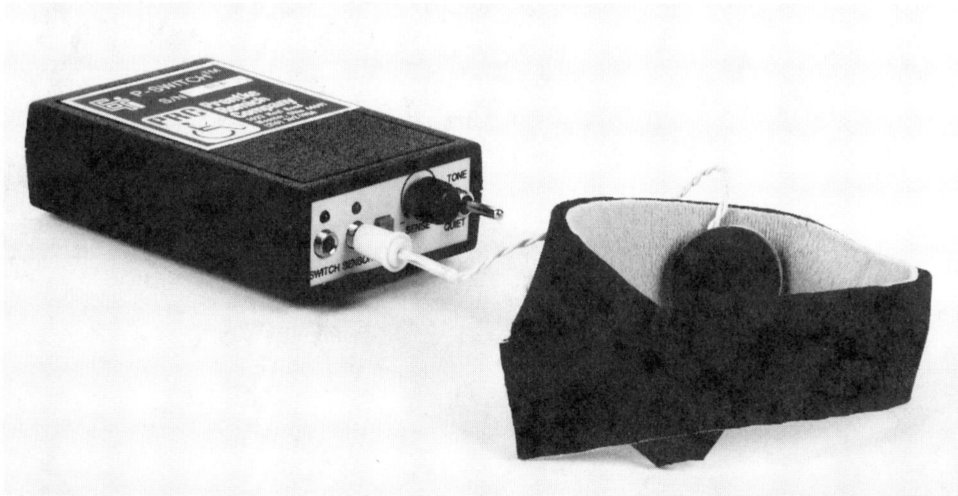

FIG. 29-5. The P-Switch (Prentke Romich Co., Wooster, OH) is a very sensitive switch designed to detect small controlled muscle movements.

able or weak. A sip-and-puff switch is a dual switch activated by changes in air pressure produced by sipping or puffing on a straw. Optical switches that rely on breaking a beam of light by eye blink or lip movement are considered for the most severe cases of motor paralysis. Electromyographic control of switches can be used in rare instances. Switch mounting and placement are essential for successful use of switches.

Morse code is an effective method of input for those with good cognitive function but poor motor control. Morse code, using one switch for dot and another for dash, frequently is successful where direct selection has failed. Morse code requires a special interface to the computer, which converts the dot-dash code to the character codes required by the computer. Specialized software is required to implement the Morse code and usually is included in the purchase of the hardware interface (14).

Single-switch scanning is the slowest of the input methods but provides an alternative for those who cannot use Morse code or other methods of input. Scanning involves some type of virtual keyboard or other graphic communication symbols displayed on the computer monitor. To make a selection, the client must hit the switch when the desired letter or symbol is highlighted. Good timing is required, particularly if scanning is set to a fast rate. Cognitive difficulty must also be considered in scanning if many choices are displayed.

Word Prediction and Abbreviation Expansion

When input rate is slow (such as single-digit typing, Morse code, or scanning), accelerating the input process is desirable. Many software programs have been developed that use word prediction and abbreviation expansion. In word prediction, the computer generates a list to predict the next words to be entered, based on word frequency and grammar. Word prediction requires good client literacy, cognition, and visual function. The client needs to rapidly scan, recognize, and select a word from a displayed list. Word prediction should be considered where input typing rates are slow. When visual scanning is impaired, several software programs have the option of using speech synthesizers to auditorially scan the displayed word list (15,16). Abbreviation expansion and macro capability are included in many of the specialized software programs. These programs allow two or three key strokes to represent a desired message (i.e., "Hi, my name is Jane Doe") or computer command such as print and save a document. Simple Morse code sequences can also be customized to represent desired messages.

Speech Input

Speech recognition as a computer input method is an increasingly effective solution for upper-extremity-impaired clients who have consistent speech, adequate vision, and cognition. Basic computer control commands consisting of dual or triple words are preprogrammed and are user independent. For the larger vocabularies used in word processing, the client must train the computer to his or her own voice. Words must be pronounced consistently with stops between words. Most systems require that the user recognize and immediately correct words that have been misrecognized by the computer. Newer systems circumvent this problem by recording the speech digitally and allow for later correction of dictation by either the original speaker or an alternate person who may have better spelling and typing skills. Individuals with both speech and motor impairment require special adaptations of software and training protocols to benefit from the speech recognition technology (17).

Speech recognition is also an option for visually impaired clients. However, special provision must be made to generate auditory feedback on what has been recognized and/or predicted by the computer. Headphones are recommended to prevent the speech output from entering the microphone that is used for speech input. Dedicated, computer-based sound or speech recognition devices for specialized functions are also available. Speech or sound recognition has also been used to control the environment, activate switches, and dial telephone numbers.

Computer Output Modes

Modern personal computers incorporate "multimedia" capability that can use a combination of video, sound, and graphics to create dynamic displays of information. Many of the adaptations used by persons with disabilities, such as enlarged images and text-to-speech synthesis, are increasingly incorporated into computer software. The newer operating systems, for example, allow the user to program a mouse button to perform specialized functions such as enlarging selected areas of the computer's display. Thus, specialized programs for enlarging text and graphics are often not needed.

Speech output is an essential component of many assistive technology applications, including screen and text readers for the blind, augmentative communication devices for the speech impaired, and adaptive computer software for the learning disabled.

Speech output may be produced electronically by two different methods: digital recording and speech synthesis. Digital recording is a method in which human speech is recorded into the device, the speech sample is digitized for electronic storage, and the sample can then be replayed. Digitized speech is available in a number of communication devices and computer software applications. Advantages of digitized speech for communication applications include increased intelligibility of the speech output, ease of matching for gender and age, and ease of recording. Disadvantages of digitized speech include a large amount of electronic memory required to store the speech sample and the limitation in vocabulary, since only what has been recorded may be retrieved. In order to obtain text-to-speech capability, in which typed text may be transformed into speech, speech synthesis is required. Synthesizers vary greatly in price and intelligibility. Recent studies indicate that DECtalk (Digital Equiptment Co., Maryland, CA) and Macintalk Pro (Apple Computer, Inc., Cupertino, CA) offer the most intelligible speech (18).

AUGMENTATIVE AND ALTERNATE COMMUNICATION

Augmentative and alternative communication (AAC) refers to a variety of approaches designed to support, enhance, or augment the communication of individuals who are not independent, verbal communicators in all situations (19). Congenital conditions most commonly requiring AAC include cerebral palsy, mental retardation, autism, developmental verbal apraxia, and developmental language disorders (20). Acquired conditions for which AAC is often used include traumatic brain injury, stroke, amyotrophic lateral sclerosis, tetraplegia, and multiple sclerosis (21). Augmentative communication has also been successfully used for individuals who are temporarily nonspeaking as a result of ventilator dependence (22).

Augmentative and alternative communication includes a broad range of techniques appropriate for individuals with varied levels of cognitive, linguistic, and physical ability. No strict set of cognitive or physical prerequisites must be achieved in order to be a candidate for augmentative communication. Specific AAC techniques that match the individual's needs and abilities are chosen on the basis of a comprehensive evaluation. An individual need not be totally unable to produce speech in order to benefit from AAC but may use augmentative communication strategies to supplement partially intelligible or slow speech. Research indicates that augmentative communication will not hamper development or return of natural speech production capability. In fact, several studies show improvement in speech production, language skills, and behavior following intervention with AAC (23). Current research and experience support the practice of preschool intervention with children to facilitate communication development (24).

Augmentative communication approaches may be described along a continuum from low-tech strategies to high-tech approaches. Low-tech AAC strategies have been in use for many years, with clinical documentation beginning in the 1950s (25). Low-tech approaches commonly include an array of objects, pictures, letters, or symbols that are accessed by pointing, eye gaze, or partner-assisted scanning. For example, a ventilator-dependent patient may spell out words by pointing to an alphabet board. A student with mental retardation may communicate by pointing to pictures in a notebook. A patient with ALS may indicate basic needs by directing his gaze to a symbol on an eye gaze (etran) board.

Low-tech augmentative communication methods are generally inexpensive. They are easily adapted to a specific user's needs and may be quickly altered as needs change. Low-tech systems generally offer less functional independence because more knowledge and skill are often required of the conversation partner. Individuals who use a high-tech communication system frequently rely on a low-tech method to provide a backup in case of equipment breakdown or to communicate in environments where high-tech equipment cannot be safely and conveniently operated.

Use of high-tech AAC systems dates from the development of the microcomputer in the 1970s (25). Associated developments in electronics and speech synthesis allowed the manufacture of devices with voice output at a reasonable cost. Currently a large number of high-tech AAC systems are available to meet the needs of consumers. Many current AAC systems are based on commercially available laptop computers, while other systems are "dedicated" devices designed solely as communication aids. High-tech AAC systems generally allow faster, more effective communication of a larger range of messages with less assistance from the listener. A comprehensive professional evaluation is needed to select the most appropriate device for a particular individual. The evaluation should include assessment of physical access methods, and vocabulary representation, retrieval, and selection.

Physical Access Methods

The various input methods for access described in the computer access section can be applied to operate a communication device (direct selection, single-switch scanning, optical head pointing, Morse code). Access methods for a specific individual are chosen on the basis of the person's physical and cognitive skills and limitations. Input methods may also be evaluated on the basis of speed and accuracy. Both decreased speed and frequent errors limit communication opportunities for clients using AAC because listeners are often unwilling to wait during message generation and correction.

Vocabulary Representation and Retrieval

The purpose of an AAC system is the expression of meaning from one person to another. This meaning may range from a routine request for assistance to the expression of an emotional or abstract idea. Efficient retrieval and representation of such a wide range of meanings has presented a challenge in the development of augmentative communication systems.

Currently available systems vary greatly in vocabulary storage and retrieval (encoding) strategies, but all systems are based on communication symbols. Symbols vary in their transparency (guessability) and translucency (learnability). In order to select a set of symbols for a communication system, the transparency and translucency of the symbol are matched to the client's cognitive and perceptual abilities. For individuals with severe cognitive impairments, vocabulary may be represented as objects (26). For example, a client might point to a glass to receive a drink of water. Actual photographs of objects or activities may also be used to represent vocabulary. Line drawings, though somewhat less learnable than photographs, may be more easily discriminated by persons with visual impairments.

A number of pictographic symbol sets have been used successfully in AAC intervention, including Picture Communication Symbols (Mayer Johnson Co., Solana Beach, CA), Blissymbols (Blissymbolics Communication International, Toronto, Ontario) and DynaSyms (Sentient Systems Technology, Pittsburg, PA). See Figure 29-6 for sample communication symbols. The reader is directed to an excellent review of these picture systems and related research in Beukelman and Miranda (27). A number of picture systems include single word labels on each symbol to facilitate development of sight reading.

Orthographic (letters and numbers) symbols are a preferred choice for individuals who are literate or have the potential to become literate. Orthographic symbols may be used to spell an unlimited range of messages and communicate complex and novel ideas. Letters and numbers may also be combined as abbreviations to represent frequently used messages. However, because spelling is quite slow in conversation, individuals who use orthographic symbols may also use pictographic symbols to represent a portion of their vocabulary. Nonvisual symbols such as Morse code and Braille may also be used to spell messages with AAC systems.

Communication symbols may be organized in a number of different ways on AAC devices. When strictly orthographic

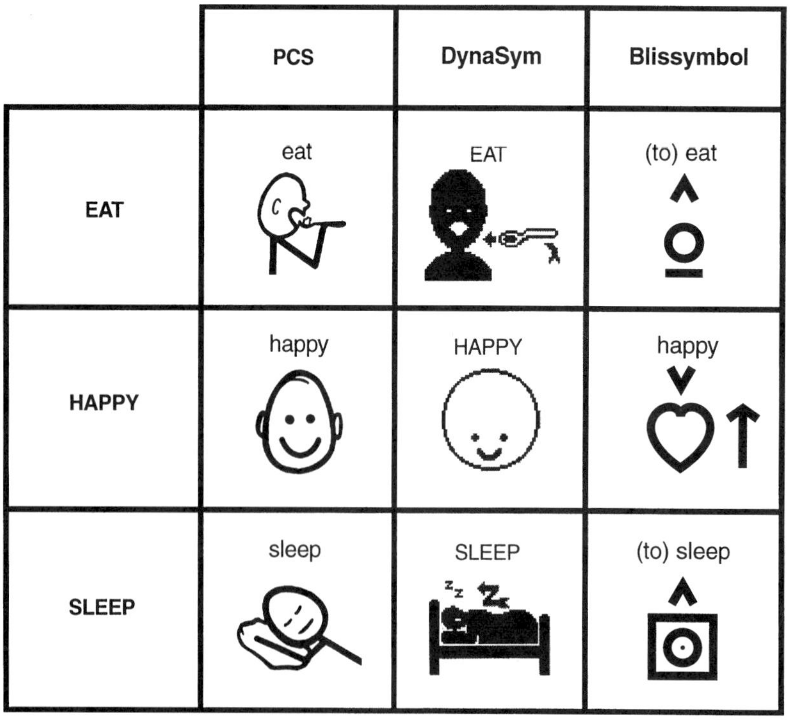

	PCS	DynaSym	Blissymbol
EAT	eat	EAT	(to) eat
HAPPY	happy	HAPPY	happy
SLEEP	sleep	SLEEP	(to) sleep

FIG. 29-6. Communication symbols. Three concepts are represented in various communication symbol systems: Picture Communication Symbols (Mayer Johnson Co., Solana Beach, CA), Dynasyms (Sentient Systems Technology, Pittsburgh, PA), and Blissymbols (Blissymbolics Communication International, Toronto, Ontario, Canada).

symbols are used, they may be organized in alphabetical order or in the standard keyboard arrangement. Special scanning arrays have also been developed to increase speed by organizing letters according to frequency of use. When pictographic symbols are used to represent single words or complete messages, the issue of vocabulary organization becomes more complex. Vocabulary is best organized in a way that facilitates learning, recall, and message construction for that particular client.

Low-tech communication boards and many high-tech AAC devices utilize communication displays in which each symbol occupies a fixed place on the display. The size and number of symbols on the fixed display are determined by the cognitive, physical, and perceptual abilities of the user. The size of the display and the number of symbols are necessarily limited, and thus vocabulary capacity is limited. With low-tech displays, users often develop many pages or overlays for their communication system to expand the vocabulary. With high-tech devices the need for more vocabulary has been addressed in two major ways. In a level/location system, vocabulary items are divided into several groups (or levels). A separate overlay is prepared for each level with symbols placed in the various locations on the overlay. The device is then programmed with vocabulary for each level. Depending on the user and the device, assistance may be needed to change overlays.

The second means of storing a large amount of vocabulary using a limited number of keys is symbol sequencing. With this method a word or message is stored under a combination of keys. Vocabulary may be stored under letter combinations using abbreviation expansion; however, given the high likelihood of conflicting abbreviations and the difficulty in recalling a great number of abbreviations, this method is impractical for very large vocabularies. Sequencing may also be accomplished using pictographic symbols. Semantic compaction or Minspeak is a method developed by Bruce Baker (28) in which multimeaning icons are sequenced to represent word-, phrase-, or sentence-level vocabulary. A meaningful relationship is developed between the icon and the stored vocabulary, facilitating recall. Effective use of semantic compaction requires the ability to associate several meanings with an icon and to recall many icon sequences. However, once learned, the vocabulary is available from a single fixed display, facilitating rapid, linguistically complete communication. Many AAC users, particularly those who are nonspeaking as a result of cerebral palsy, have developed excellent communication skills using Minspeak-based systems (see Fig. 29-7, for example).

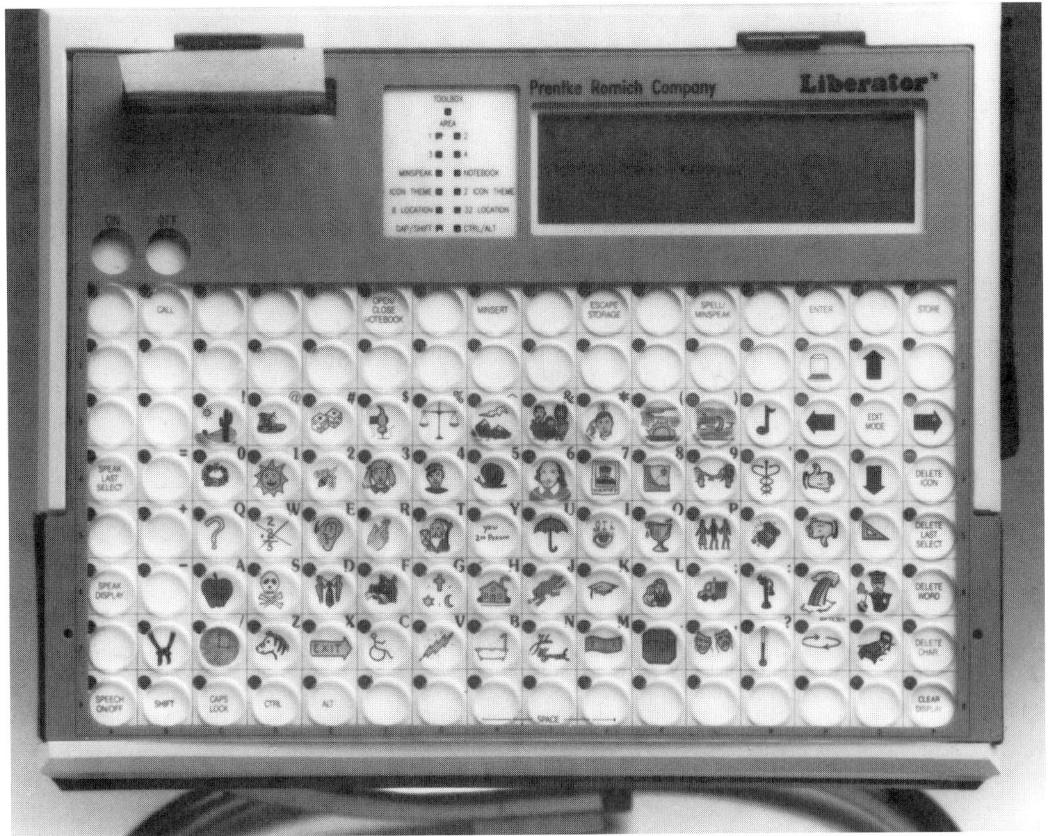

FIG. 29-7. The Liberator (Prentke Romich Co.) is a fixed display device that uses Minspeak to represent and retrieve vocabulary. Words or phrases are retrieved by activating sequences of multimeaning Minspeak icons. Lights on the keyboard display facilitate recall by indicating where vocabulary is stored.

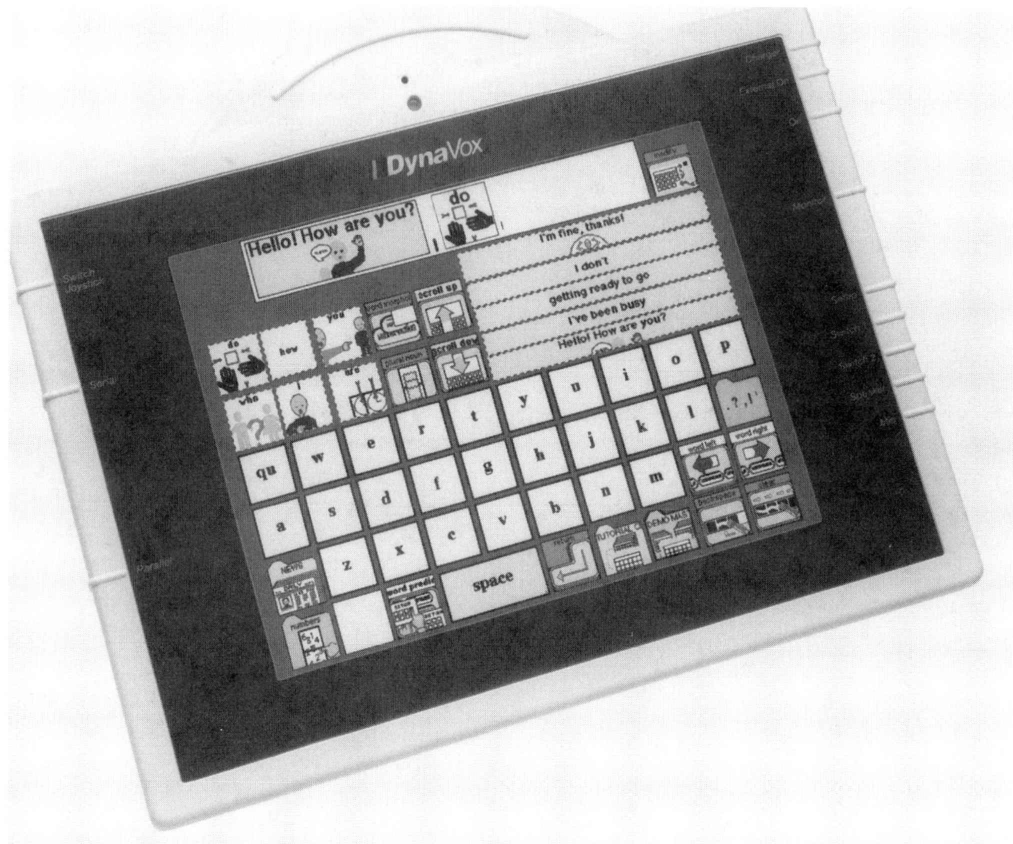

FIG. 29-8. The Dynavox (Sentient Systems Technology, Pittsburgh, PA) is a dynamic screen communication device. Screens of letters or communication symbols are linked together to allow access to a large vocabulary.

A dynamic display is one that can present a changing set of symbols to the user (see Fig. 29-8, for example). Dynamic displays now allow the levels and locations of the earlier systems to be accessed easily from the computer screen, eliminating the need for changing overlays. Each level (or page) in the communication system can be custom designed for the user, with the size, number, and color of symbols selected based on the user's needs. The pages may be linked together to provide faster access during communication. By using the dynamic levels/locations system, the number of choices presented to the user in each screen may be controlled, and vocabulary may be organized to meet the user's specific needs. However, the user must visually scan each screen to make a selection, which may interrupt the speaking task and interfere with the development of more automatic motor movements. Dynamic display software used with dedicated devices or portable computers represents a rapidly growing segment of the AAC market.

Vocabulary Selection

The actual content of the communication system vocabulary is the most critical issue in the eventual success or failure of the AAC intervention. The most elaborate technical device will be of no use unless the user can express what he thinks, feels, and desires. Selection of vocabulary has different implications for literate and nonliterate AAC users. As previously discussed, literate individuals should have access to orthographic symbols on the communication display, allowing them to spell out any message. The additional nontext vocabulary included on such systems can be described as ''acceleration/timing'' vocabulary, designed to increase communication rate and improve timing in conversation, allowing retrieval of messages with fewer keystrokes (29).

For individuals who are preliterate or who are unlikely to develop or regain literacy, vocabulary selection is a defining process. The vocabulary included on the communication device defines how the AAC user will interact with others, determines the content of the interaction, and affects the success of each communication attempt. For example, an adult whose communication display includes only requests for basic needs will be unable to ask simple conversational questions (''What's going on?'') or comment on choices (''I don't like that''). With children, the selection of vocabulary powerfully affects the development of language and literacy skills. Children need access to a wide variety of language concepts and grammatic forms at an appropriate developmental level in order to develop good language skills as a foundation for literacy.

Some currently available AAC systems include preprogrammed vocabularies designed with language development and communication functions in mind. These standard vocabularies must be taught to the user and customized for individual needs. With other systems the responsibility for selecting, organizing, and programming vocabulary rests on the AAC user and various care providers. Because of the complex language, learning, and interaction issues involved, the assistance of a speech language pathologist, special educator, or other professional with expertise in vocabulary selection and training is essential. Close coordination is also needed between the user and support personnel so that vocabulary can be frequently updated. Most augmented communicators also need ongoing training in communication skills using their AAC system. Success in use of an augmentative communication system depends on careful selection of an appropriate device or technique, continuous attention to vocabulary selection, and effective training in system use.

ENVIRONMENTAL CONTROL UNITS

Individuals with physical and cognitive limitations often require alternate means of manipulating or accessing objects in their environment. These objects may include a lamp, television, or hospital bed. Many physical and cognitive limitations provide barriers to independence in one's environment. Environmental control is an area of assistive technology that deals with overcoming these barriers. An ECU is a system, unit, or device that provides a link between a person's motor abilities and the environment. A common example of an ECU is a hand-held remote control for the television. This device eliminates the need to move to the television to access the desired channels or volume and eliminates a potential barrier for some individuals with physical disabilities. A more specialized ECU is one controlled by voice activation. Individuals with impaired or absent motor abilities could utilize their intact speech to become more independent. There are a variety of speech-controlled devices for persons with disabilities that can assist individuals to gain independence.

Five elements make up an environmental control unit; these include, (a) the switch device, (b) control device, (c) connections, (d) target device, and (e) feedback device (30). The switch device (a) is the input device activated by the user to send the command signal to the environmental control unit or control device. The control device (b) transforms and transmits the signal and sends it to the target device to perform a function. This signal transmission is achieved by connections (c), such as wires, radio waves, or infrared signals. The target device (d) can be a household appliance, telephone, radio, or any item using electrical power. The feedback device (e) provides a signal, auditory or visual, to the user about the status of the target device or command given. Referring to the above example of a hand held remote control: The hand held remote is the switch device; the infrared signals are the connections; the television is the control device and the target device; and the channel number display and sound level give the user the needed feedback.

Environmental control systems can be divided into three categories. Centralized systems have a direct connection between the target device and the control device via a cord. Modular systems are wireless and utilize infrared signals, radio waves, or existing household wiring as the connection. Master systems combine the technology of both centralized and modular systems (31). The Control 1 (Prentke Romich Co., Wooster, Ohio) is an example of a master system. In a hospital environment, the control device has direct connection to the nurse call switch, television control, and hospital bed control via cord connectors. A user can also activate a radio, fan, and light via a wireless modular device.

Infrared signals are commonly used as the connector on remote television controllers. Infrared signals are sent in direct line between the control and target device. Some controllers are Universal Controllers, which can be programmed to control different infrared compatible devices by using a provided manufacturer code. A possible disadvantage for some users is that the infrared controller needs to be in direct line of sight with the target device. However, relay devices are available.

Computer based environmental control systems are popular for both individuals with and without disabilities. A user can access a wide variety of devices such as security lights, coffee pots and home stereo systems through their computer. Some radio signal systems have an interface for home computers which may provide as many options as a dedicated environmental control master system designed for people with disabilities. Many users with disabilities may be able to obtain funding for a computer for school or work and add software to create their own environmental control system at less cost.

To choose the most appropriate ECU several questions need to answered. What environment(s) will the client be in, and how much time is spent in each environment? A client who spends the day sitting in a powered wheelchair to increase mobility would need a more portable system with the capability to control many types of target devices. Mobile systems need wireless connectors.

What target devices need to be accessed? A client who wishes to control only a few devices such as a television and VCR could use a smaller and less expensive system or device such as a universal controller. A client who wants to control multiple devices in multiple locations may need a computer-based radio signal system to meet their needs.

Will the client's needs and abilities be changing? Change in client needs may require different input methods and types of target devices. A newly injured client may initially use a pneumatic switch and eventually be able to control a rocker switch.

What are the client's physical, cognitive and sensory abilities? Each part of an environmental control system varies in complexity. The abilities of the user need to be assessed to ensure success in device use. Addressing the above questions initially can assist the therapist to choose the most appropriate system and decrease chances that an ineffective device is selected.

Appropriately prescribed environmental control units can result in a more productive and satisfying life style. In the hospital setting, ECUs allow patients to experience independence and decrease the level of nursing supervision. In the home, an ECU may allow a client to spend more time without caregiver assistance. Occupational therapists and rehabilitation engineers can provide recommendations on positioning and setup of the ECU to maximize client usage.

In addition to dedicated ECUs, many consumer products may provide effective environmental control at a lower cost. A telephone with an enlarged key pad, a speaker phone, and a cordless telephone are examples of inexpensive consumer products which may be used to provide environmental control. The enlarged keypad would benefit users with visual, tactile, or fine motor deficits. Speaker phones may benefit individuals with decreased upper extremity strength or endurance to hold the receiver. Telephone headsets or ear pieces may also assist with this impairment. A cordless phone or phone headset promotes energy conservation for people with low endurance eliminating extra trips across a room to the telephone. The use of luxury, energy-saving devices to reduce medical disability must be carefully explained to funding sources.

Another helpful device that is inexpensive and may be found at a hardware store is a timer switch. Timers can control lights inside and outside the home, creating an occupied home look from the outside and decreasing the need for daily trips around the home to turn lights on and off. For individuals with arthritis or fine motor impairments, touch lights have become an increasingly popular item. Converters are available to convert a lamp with a standard switch into a touch lamp. The user simply touches the lamp base to activate/deactivate the light.

Security and safety issues are important when making recommendations for some clients to live alone in their own home or remain at home alone when caregivers are away. A cordless phone kept with the client can be used to call for help in case of emergency. A variety of personal assistance systems are also available. One example is the X-10 Personal Assistance System (X10 Inc., Closter, NJ), which provides the user with a one-button radio frequency transmitter to be worn around the neck. Depression of the alarm button activates a home-located alarm receiver, which then calls up to four telephone numbers stored within the control device. When the switch alarm receiver is activated, the first number is dialed. If no one answers, it will proceed to the next number and continue until someone answers and presses "0" on the keypad. At that time, a prerecorded message will play. The receiver of the call may also activate a built-in microphone and listen in on the caller to monitor the situation.

Personal assistance services are also available. A client subscribes to a local service center and is provided with a one-button radio frequency transmitter to be worn around the wrist or neck. This can be activated to initiate an emergency call to the local service center. As the service center receives the call they call a prearranged contact person to check on the client. They may also call the appropriate local emergency personnel.

INTEGRATION OF AT SYSTEMS

Clients with AT needs may require the use of more than one type of system. For example, a nonspeaking client with cerebral palsy may require use of an AAC system and an ECU while seated in a power wheelchair. When several types of assistive technology are used together, the client may choose to integrate the systems. Integration of AT systems may achieve better access, improve appearance and promote more independent use of the technology. However, integrated systems are more difficult to design, implement, and maintain. Because integration often requires custom designed components, integrated systems may also be more expensive. Assistive technology systems may be integrated in the areas of input, device mounting and power supply.

Once an optimal method of input is identified for each device, a client may be able to use this method to operate more than one AT device. For example, a client who uses Morse code with bilateral head switches for communication with a laptop computer may use those same input switches to operate a power chair and ECU. This integration is achieved using different control modes in the wheelchair operating system (32). When the power chair is stopped, the client may change to a designated mode to access the ECU. The client then may also access the communication device by changing to its designated mode. Only one mode may be accessed at a given time.

Placement of AT devices within the client's environment is referred to as mounting. When AT devices are mounted for a client, careful planning is needed to allow safe, effective, and independent access to each device. For example, a client using an augmentative communication device with a power wheelchair may need a custom laptray to allow access to both the wheelchair joystick and the communication device keyboard. A client in bed may need overhead mounting of an environmental control system that does not block visual access to a computer monitor.

The AT systems may also be integrated by using a common power source. For example, a client in a power wheelchair may use the wheelchair battery for power to run a laptop computer. Because of the electrical current involved, such adaptations must be made by a vendor or engineer qualified in electrical safety.

ASSISTIVE TECHNOLOGY FOR VISION AND HEARING DISABILITIES

A wide variety of assistive technology has been developed to assist clients with visual and/or hearing impairment. In the case of mild or moderate visual or hearing impairment, assistive technology serves to augment a limited sensory pathway. For clients with severe sensory impairments, the technology provides input through an alternative sensory pathway. For example, a client with low vision might use a magnification system to increase the size of written text, thus augmenting the visual pathway. A blind person might use a computer with speech synthesis to access the screen display, thus substituting the auditory pathway for vision.

In evaluating an individual with a vision or hearing disability for assistive technology, the AT provider must consider the exact nature and extent of the sensory impairment, the age of onset, and the prognosis in order to recommend an appropriate assistive device.

Individuals with some functional residual vision often benefit from devices that adapt and magnify visual stimuli for easier perception (namely, eyeglasses and magnifying lenses). Closed-circuit television systems (CCTV) use a video camera with a video monitor to magnify text from a book or other document for display on a video screen. Computer software is also available to magnify screen text and graphics.

Persons with no functional vision must rely on alternative pathways for receiving information. One such alternative method is Braille, a system of embossed dots displayed in a cell three dots high and two dots across (33). Each cell represents a print character. A variety of note-taking devices and Braille printers are available. Braille keyboards are available for entering information into a computer. Braille cell displays are also available to display text from the computer screen.

Speech output provides an additional alternative for the visually impaired. Speech synthesizers paired with computer software for screen reading and screen navigation provide access to any text appearing on the computer screen, and give spoken feedback regarding the position of the cursor, and contents of menus. Talking books provide an audio tape version of written materials. In order to assist blind persons with community mobility, some communities have implemented talking signs which provide auditory cues for mass transit, public facilities, and traffic lights (34).

Heavy reliance on graphics in computer software has presented an obstacle for persons with visual impairments. Alternative methods under exploration at this time include tactile display of graphical data, allowing blind persons to explore two-dimensional graphs with specialized instruments (35). Tactile display of pictorial information using raised images is also under development (36).

Assistive technology for persons with hearing impairment is focused in the areas of sound amplification, visual telecommunications, alerting systems, and television captioning. Individuals with some residual hearing often benefit from personal amplification devices such as hearing aids, which are customized for the individual based on the results of audiometric testing. In public settings such as conference facilities or concert halls, hard-of-hearing persons may use assistive listening devices that amplify the auditory information from the public address system. Sound is transmitted from the PA system to the listener's receiver via infrared or FM signals and can then be volume adjusted.

Telecommunications for the deaf are based on the Text Telephone (TTD). The TTD is a device used to transmit text from one location to another using the telephone lines. The TTD consists of a teletypewriter (TTY) and a telephone modem. Two individuals with TTDs in their home can converse over the telephone lines independently. When a deaf person with a TTD wishes to speak to a person who does not have a TTD, a relay service is used to interpret the message. Specialized software is also available to facilitate connections between regular computer modems and TTYs.

Individuals with little or no residual hearing may need alerting systems to function safely and independently in a variety of environments. These devices change ordinary environmental auditory signals such as a doorbells, smoke alarm, or alarm clock into tactile or visual signals.

Much of the media presented via television, multimedia software, and the Internet includes auditory signals, which are impossible for severely hearing impaired individuals to interpret. Captioning takes these auditory signals and presents them as text, which is then displayed on the television screen. Captioning is available for broadcast television and for videos. Beginning in July 1993, all televisions sold in the United States are required to include internal decoders for closed captioning.

Deaf-Blind

Persons who have both visual and hearing impairment require a variety of creative assistive technology solutions. In many cases, the devices used by the deaf and the blind may be combined. For example, a refreshable Braille display may be used in conjunction with a TTD for telecommunications. A device called Dexter has also been developed for telecommunications and face-to-face conversation for the deaf-blind. Dexter is a robotic finger spelling hand which transforms text input into the American manual alphabet. The user places his hand over Dexter to read the finger spelled message (37). Alarms that use vibration instead of sound are also available.

NEUROPROSTHETICS

Neuroprosthetics refers to a broad area of substituting for lost neural function by means of devices that electrically stimulate the nervous system. This section briefly reviews progress and expected advances in the area of restoring the lost sensory functions of hearing and vision.

Cochlear Prosthesis

The cochlear prosthesis is a device that can restore hearing in deaf persons to a level where spontaneous speech reception and telephone conversation is possible (38). It is one of the more successful applications of multichannel electrical stimulation of the nervous system (39). In this case, the electrode is implanted into the cochlea near the auditory nerve. For the prosthetic device to be successful, a significant number of nerve fibers of the auditory nerve must be functional (40). An external speech processor with a microphone transforms the speech sounds into patterns of electrical stimulation pulses applied to the implanted electrode. The deaf person perceives a resultant sound pattern, which the brain learns to interpret as speech (see Chapters 12 and 70).

Vision Prosthesis

Restoration of vision in completely blind persons by direct stimulation of the visual cortex has been a subject of research for more than 30 years (41). Experiments are being conducted with implanted electrode arrays in both animals and humans. It is established that humans perceive both white and colored dots when the visual cortex is electrically stimulated (42). It is postulated that an array of electrodes (100 to 1,000) could produce visual precepts not unlike an electronic scoreboard. With proper processing of video information from a miniature video camera worn by the blind person, navigational information such as street names as well as basic outlines of structures in the environment could be successfully transmitted to the brain (43).

Much research remains to be done in the area of technology, surgical implant methods, and psychosensory physiology. Biomaterial compatibility for long-term implantation in the brain is a major problem. The ability of the visual system to adapt to an unfamiliar and nonbiological stimulation pattern is uncertain. Nevertheless, the positive experience gained with the ''artificial ear'' encourages further research and development for an ''artificial eye.''

TRANSPORTATION

Rehabilitation and reintegration of a person with a disability into the larger community requires transportation modifications. Federal guidelines and standards for public transportation mandate wheelchair access for the disabled. This includes wheelchair lifts and wheelchair securement in public transportation vehicles. With the advent of Americans with Disabilities Act, more public transportation is being made accessible.

Vehicle Adaptations

Individuals with physical disabilities may achieve transportation independence through use of adaptations designed for vehicle access and driving control. Vehicles can be modified to accommodate wheelchair storage, lifts, and ramps. Wheelchair tie-downs for securement are also available. Both minivans and full-size vans are able to accommodate an electric wheelchair lift. Powered wheelchair lifts allow the client to position him- or herself on the lift and use a control switch to raise or lower the lift to enter or exit the van. These lifts should also have manual controls in the event of power failure. Portable ramps can also be used for wheelchair access into a van.

Wheelchair storage is an issue for both drivers and passengers. Some vans provide room for up to four wheelchairs. Automobile storage for wheelchairs may be in the trunk or passenger areas. External storage devices include trunk- or roof-mounted racks.

Driving control devices vary from ignition key holders and door openers to alternate steering, brake, and accelerator controls. Some steering modifications include spinner knobs, quad-grip gloves, and other grip-assist devices. Reduced-effort steering systems and/or braking systems can be installed by vehicle manufacturers. For individuals with impaired lower extremity function, hand controls are available for brake and accelerator pedal adaptations. A left-foot accelerator pedal can be used for those with right leg impairments (44). Accessories and modifications for turn signals, light switches, and other console features are also available.

Driver Training and Evaluation Issues

Many patients engaged in the rehabilitation process have a personal desire to drive a car. This need is as important as wheelchair mobility or independence in daily living skills. Medical evaluation for driving readiness should include assessment of physical skills, neurologic, sensory, and cognitive function, seizure status, and any other medical conditions that would impair driving safety and skills. The physician must know the state's medical requirements for driving. Driving involves complex and rapid decision making in response to environmental events while carrying on automatic driving tasks such as steering, braking, and acceleration (45). A clinical driving evaluation assesses visual acuity and perception, reaction times, cognition, motor skills, and driving knowledge. If the client uses a wheelchair, additional data are gathered to determine the position of the vehicle controls. If the assessment indicates that on-the-road driving can be performed, the test vehicle is modified or adjusted for the particular client. The evaluation process involves off-road testing of basic driving functions and familiarization with modified controls. Adequate practice with the modified controls in a low-traffic area may be needed before the client proceeds to driving in busy traffic areas. Comprehensive criteria have been developed to determine readiness for driving and specifications of car and van modifications. The evaluator will write recommendations for necessary car modifications and identify vendors to supply necessary equipment (46).

Disabled drivers must be able to deal with emergency situations such as the need for medical attention and equipment breakdown when on the road. Many clients with adequate upper extremity function carry cellular phones or citizens band radios during travel in remote areas. Adaptations of telecommunications equipment for persons with disabilities, such as specialized mounting and access modifications, need to be considered in specifying vehicle modifications. Auditory detection and localization of sirens must also be assessed for clients with hearing impairments. A number of devices for siren detection are available for hearing-impaired individuals.

ASSISTIVE TECHNOLOGY WITHIN THE HOME ENVIRONMENT

When a disability interferes with basic activities of daily living (ADL), there are many AT options that can substitute for lost functions. Occupational therapists often use adaptive equipment when treating individuals with limited independence in activities of daily living. Adaptive equipment can be categorized by type of physical limitations. There are extremity extenders that enable individuals with limited reach or mobility to pick up items, reach items, or communicate. An example of each would be a reacher to pick up items dropped on the floor, a dressing stick that would enable one to place pants over his or her feet, or a mouth stick to allow someone to type or write without the use of upper extremities.

The second category of adaptive equipment, fine motor devices, include items to accommodate for limited hand use. Handles of utensils, writing instruments, and grooming aids can be built up with foam, plastic, or other materials for those with limited grasping ability. A universal cuff could be used for a client with impaired grasp. This cuff encircles palm of the hand and has a slot to contain a utensil or writing instrument.

A third category would include task-specific devices designed primarily for one use. A button hook allows someone with limited hand function to hook and unhook buttons. A plate guard is an item that attaches to the rim of a plate to prevent food from spilling off. It also assists users in putting food onto the utensil. A wash-mitt fits over the hand to allow individuals with limited grasp to wash their face and body. A pan holder to prevent rotation of the pan while stirring promotes one handed cooking.

Because of the abundance of effective inexpensive consumer products for ADL and homemaking tasks, there is little high-tech ADL equipment on the market. In general, high-tech equipment is more expensive, contains electronic circuits, and is not mass produced. When a low-tech device will not perform the complex task involved, high-tech devices may be used. An example of high-tech equipment is an electronic feeder. It is designed to scoop food onto a utensil, using a mechanical arm and plate guard, and bring the utensil to the user's mouth. This device is used primarily by clients with nonfunctional upper extremities, so the feeder is activated by shoulder or head movements. A cup holder is present to allow the user to drink from a long straw. Once the food and drink are set up by the caregiver, the user can be independent with the self-feeding task, resulting in increased self esteem, independence and enjoyment of the meal.

Another high-tech ADL device is the electronic page turner. An electronic page turner is a bookstand with an automated system to turn the pages. Page turners vary depending on the thickness of the reading material used, power source, and other features. Some devices can turn pages forward and back, whereas others only turn forward. Page turners are typically activated by mechanical switches. Text must lie flat within the stand and may need to be less than 2 inches thick.

ASSISTIVE TECHNOLOGY FOR VOCATIONAL MANAGEMENT

Many persons with disabilities inquire about available technology that would allow them to resume education or work. Literature on the availability and cost of job accommodation is considerable. This section discusses assistive technology for the workplace.

Specialized desks and adjustable-height tables and chairs are available for those working in office settings. The prevention of job-related injuries to the back, neck, and wrist can be accomplished with wrist supports, keyboard adaptations, and adjustable tables and chairs. Various devices for facilitating computer access and reducing fatigue of the motor and visual system are available. Ergonomic keyboards are often prescribed for clients with carpal tunnel syndrome and other repetitive motion injuries. These include split or folded QWERTY keyboards (47) as well as single-handed keyboards (13). Monitor supports, which allow the monitor to be placed at the desired distance, elevation, and angle, and adjustable arm rests and/or wrist supports are other common workplace adaptations. These devices can be purchased from local office supply stores at relatively modest cost. Antiglare screens are useful for many people whose work demands long hours of gazing at the monitor. When low vision is a problem, whole-screen enlarging lenses are available. Adapted office equipment includes talking calculators with large buttons, no-hands speaker phones, electric staplers, and all types of paper and file folder management devices for people with reduced finger and hand function.

For those working in an industrial setting, a wide variety of adapted tools have also been developed. This includes automotive, electronic, manual, power, and measuring tools. Specialized adaptive devices and work stations are available for many occupations. A significant source of custom job accommodation information in the area of product manufacturing can also be found in the transactions of RESNA (Arlington, VA) (48) and Trace (2).

Information about modification of tractors and other agricultural machinery to aid agricultural workers with physical disabilities is available from Purdue University (49). This occupation-specific information is beyond the scope of this chapter.

ROBOTICS

Much research and development has been conducted in applying robotic technology to augment function for those with physical disabilities (50). A good overview of the current state of robotics in rehabilitation research was published in a special issue of the *IEEE Transactions on Rehabilitation Engineering* (51–53). There has been no lack of effort both in North America and in Europe to apply robotics to people with disabilities. Robotics devices for those with physical disabilities range in price from $1,500 to $60,000. The cost increases dramatically with the number of degrees of freedom provided by the robot, ranging from two to six. Degrees of freedom refer to the ability of the robot arm to move a grasped object in a three-dimensional space. Three degrees of freedom are required for arbitrary positioning in space. If the object needs also to be rotated each rotation axis adds another degree of freedom. Repetitive tasks which require the same motion repeatedly and do not have to adapt to changing environmental conditions are the easiest to implement. An example would be a robot arm set up to perform basic feeding functions for someone with quadriplegia (50). A more challenging task is to have the robot perform multiple functions such as required in running an office. This RAID robot arm has a large area of operation for selecting files, opening books and files, and manipulating papers in an office setting (53). The clinical acceptance of robotic aids by persons with disabilities will depend on future improvements in robotic technology. This includes (a) better methods of volitional control of many degrees of freedom, (b) development of force and position feedback in addition to the visual feedback that currently predominates, (c) increased reliability and safety, and (d) justification of the cost based on effectiveness of the robot in increasing productivity and independence.

For more information on this active area of research and development, consult the various centers described in the quoted references or RESNA—Special Interest Group in Robotics and Mechatronics (54).

FEDERAL PROGRAMS

Acceptance and usage of AT have been promoted by several pieces of Federal legislation, beginning with the Rehabilitation Act of 1973, which established vocational rehabilitation on a national and state basis. With vocational rehabilitation came the realization that assistive technology was needed to facilitate return of disabled persons to work. The landmark Americans With Disabilities Act of 1990 extended the Rehabilitation Act to all private and public institutions. It clearly mandated that discrimination against individuals with a disability should be discontinued in both hiring and promoting people in the workplace if the person was otherwise qualified for the job. Among the many features of that act was the requirement that employers needed to provide and fund reasonable accommodations for individuals with disabilities. Reasonable accommodations include job restructuring and modification of equipment. The definition of reasonable accommodations and the cost to be borne by the employer are still being discussed and are in a state of evolution. Key legislative features also included accessibility for transportation and public accommodations in state and local government buildings. The Individuals with Disabilities Education Act of 1990 helped remove many of the barriers in the classroom setting and mandated the accommodations and services to be provided in the classroom for students with disabilities. The Technology-Related Assistance for Individuals with Disability Acts of 1988 placed specific emphasis on the use of assistive technology as part of the continuum of services.

REFERENCES

1. Technology-related Assistance for Individuals with Disabilities Act of 1988, PL100-407, 29 USC 2202 (3).
2. Trace Research & Development Center, University of Wisconsin–Madison, s-151 Waisman Center, Madison, WI 53705-2280. Web site: http://trace.wisc.edu.
3. Hobson DA. RESNA: Yesterday, today, and tomorrow. *Assist Technol* 1996; 8:131–143.
4. Cook AM, Hussey SM. *Assistive technologies: principles and practices.* St Louis: CV Mosby, 1991.
5. Hoffman A. Funding: How you can make it work. In: Coston C, ed. *Planning and implementing augmentative communication service delivery: proceedings of the national planners conference on assistive device service delivery.* Washington, D.C.: RESNA, 1988; 64–74.
6. Wallace J. Creative financing of assistive technology. In: Flippo K, Inge K, Barcus JM, eds. *Assistive technology: a resource for school, work and community.* Baltimore: Paul H. Brookes, 1995; 245–268.
7. Phillips B, Zhao H. Predictors of assistive technology abandonment. *Assist Technol* 1993; 5:36–45.
8. Treviranus J. Mastering alternative computer access: the role of understanding, trust, and automaticity. *Assist Technol* 1994; 6:26–41.
9. Batt RC, Lounsbury PA. Teaching the patient with cognitive deficits to use a computer. *Am J Occup Ther* 1990; 44:364–367.
10. Downing A, Martin B, Stern L. Methods for measuring the characteristics of movements of motor-impaired children. *Assist Technol* 1990; 2:131–141.
11. Shein F, Galvin R, Hammann G, Treviranus J. Scanning the Windows desktop without mouse emulation. *Proc RESNA Conf* 1994; 14: 391–393.
12. Vanderheiden GC. Guidelines for the design of consumer products to increase their accessibility to persons with disabilities. *Proc RESNA Conf* 1991; 11:187–189.
13. Product Preview. BAT personal keyboard permits one-handed typing. *Closing the Gap* 1994; 13(2):1–4.
14. Blavat VT. Keyboard emulation via Morse code entry: a comparison of configuration parameters across four systems. *Closing the Gap* 1996; 15(2):1–28.
15. Hortsmann-Koester H, Levine SP. Modeling the speed of text entry with a word prediction interface. *IEEE Trans Rehabil Eng* 1994; 2: 177–187.
16. Klund J, Novak M. If word prediction can help, which program do you choose? *Closing the Gap* 1996; 15(3):1–16.
17. Bowes DR. Adapting speech input computing for individuals with speech impairments. *Proc RESNA Conf* 1995; 15:400–402.
18. Ruprecht SL, Beukelman DR, Vrtiska H. Comparative intelligibility of five synthesized voices. *Augment Altern Commun* 1995; 11:244–247.
19. Beukelman DR, Yorkston KM, Dowden PA. *Communication augmentation: a casebook of clinical management.* San Diego: College-Hill Press, 1985.
20. Mirenda P, Mathy-Laikko P. Augmentative and alternative communication applications for persons with severe congenital communication disorders: an introduction. *Augment Altern Commun* 1989; 5:3–13.
21. Beukelman DR, Yorkston KM. Augmentative and alternative communication for persons with severe acquired communication disorders: an introduction. *Augment Altern Commun* 1989; 5:42–48.
22. Fried-Oken M, Howard JM, Stewart SR. Feedback on AAC intervention from adults who are temporarily unable to speak. *Augment Altern Commun* 1988; 7:43–50.

23. Silverman FH. *Communication for the speechless.* Englewood Cliffs, NJ: Prentice-Hall, 1995.
24. Kangas K, Lloyd LL. Early cognitive skills and prerequisites to augmentative and alternative communication: what are we waiting for? *Augment Altern Commun* 1988; 4:211–221.
25. Zangari C, Lloyd LL, Vicker B. Augmentative and alternative communication: an historic perspective. *Augment Altern Commun* 1994; 10: 27–59.
26. Rowland C, Schweigert P. Tangible symbols: symbolic communication for individuals with multisensory impairments. *Augment Altern Commun* 1989; 5:226–234.
27. Beukelman DR, Mirenda P. *Augmentative and alternative communication.* Baltimore: Paul H Brookes, 1992.
28. Baker B. Semantic compaction for sub-sentence vocabulary units compared to other encoding and prediction systems. *Proc RESNA Conf* 1987; 10:118–120.
29. Beukelman D, Mcginnis J, Morrow D. Vocabulary selection in augmentative and alternative communication. *Augment Altern Commun* 1991; 7:171–185.
30. Haataja S, Saarnio I. An evaluation procedure for environmental control systems. *Proc RESNA Conf* 1990; 13:25–26.
31. Dickey R, Shealey SH. Using technology to control the environment. *Am J Occup Ther* 1987; 41:717–721.
32. Caves KM, Gross K. Integrated systems. In: Hammel J, ed. *Assistive technology occupational therapy: a link to function.* Bethesda, MD: American Occupational Therapy Association, 1996; 1–24.
33. Rothstein R, Everson JM. Assistive technology for individuals with sensory impairments. In: Flipps K, Inge K, Barcus JM, eds. *Assistive technology: a resource for school work and community.* Baltimore: Paul H Brookes, 1995; 105–132.
34. Therrien DJ, Tippin S, Groff C, Belcher S. Bus stop locator: an application of audible signage technology. *Proc RESNA Conf* 1996; 16: 481–483.
35. Fritz JP, Barner KE. Design of a haptic graphing system. *Proc RESNA Conf* 1996; 16:158–160.
36. Way T, Barnet K. Towards automatic generation of tactile graphics. *Proc RESNA Conf* 1996; 16:161–163.
37. Gilden D. Deaf-blind users grasp the idea with Dexter, a prototype robotic fingerspelling hand. *Proc RESNA Conf* 1996; 16:164–166.
38. Eddington DK, Orth JL. Speech recognition in a deaf subject with a portable, multichannel cochlear implant system. *Adv Audiol* 1984; 2: 61–67.
39. O'Malley Teeter J. A review of the functional electrical stimulation equipment market. *Assist Technol* 1992; 4:40–45.
40. Loeb GE, Byers CL, Rebscher SJ, Casey DE, et al. Design and fabrication of an experimental cochlear prosthesis. *Med Biol Eng Comput* 1983; 21:241–254.
41. Brindley GS, Lewin WS. The sensations produced by electrical stimulation of the visual cortex. *J Physiol* 1968; 196:479–493.
42. Hambrecht TF. Microstimulation of the human visual cortex: experiments towards a functional visual prosthesis. Experiments towards visual prosthesis. In: *Proceedings of the RESNA '96 Conference. Supplement: Research Symposium: Recent developments in neuroprosthetics: progress towards functional artificial vision.* Washington, D.C.: RESNA, 1996; 4–6.
43. Horch K, Cha K, Normann R. Simulation of a phosphene based visual field: psychophysics of pixelized vision. In: *Proceedings of the RESNA '96 Conference. Supplement: Research symposium: Recent developments in neuroprosthetics: progress towards functional artificial vision.* Washington, D.C.: RESNA, 1996; 11–16.
44. Shipp M. *Adaptive driving devices and vehicle modifications.* Ruston, LA: Louisiana Tech University, 1988.
45. Kerr CM III, Irwin E. Driver assessment and training of the disabled client. In: Smith RV, Leslie JH Jr, eds. *Rehabilitation engineering.* Boca Raton, FL: CRC Press, 1990; 317–321.
46. Kerr CM III, Irwin E. Driver assessment and training of the disabled client. In: Smith RV, Leslie JH Jr, eds. *Rehabilitation engineering.* Boca Raton, FL: CRC Press, 1990; 321–434.
47. Kramer H. *Using assistive technology to adapt the computer for individuals with repetitive motion injuries and chronic pain. Handout summary.* Lakewood, CO: Colorado Easter Seal Society Center for Adapted Technology, 1996; 1–14.
48. Vanderheiden GC. Use of multiple parallel interface strategies to create a seamless accessible interface for next-generation information systems. *Proc RESNA Conf* 1994; 14:508–510.
49. Field B, Kirkpatrick E, Newman M, eds. *Breaking new ground.* West Lafayette, IN: Breaking New Ground Resource Center, Purdue University, 1996; 14(2).
50. Harwin WS, Rahman R, Foulds RA. A review of design issues in rehabilitation robotics with reference to North American research. *IEEE Trans Rehabil Eng* 1995; 3:3–13.
51. Kawamura K, Bagchi S, Iskarous M, Bishay M. Intelligent robotic systems in service of the disabled. *IEEE Trans Rehabil Eng* 1995; 3: 14–21.
52. Erlandson RF. Applications of robotic/mechatronic systems in special education, rehabilitation therapy, and vocational training: a paradigm shift. *IEEE Trans Rehabil Eng* 1995; 3:22–34.
53. Dallaway JL, Jackson RD, Timmers HA. Rehabilitation robotics in europe. *IEEE Trans Rehabil Eng* 1995; 3:35–45.
54. Mahoney RM. Report from the chair. In: *Rehabilitation Robotics Newsletter* 1996(winter/spring); 3–4.

Rehabilitation Medicine: Principles and Practice, Third Edition,
edited by Joel A. DeLisa and Bruce M. Gans.
Lippincott–Raven Publishers, Philadelphia © 1998.

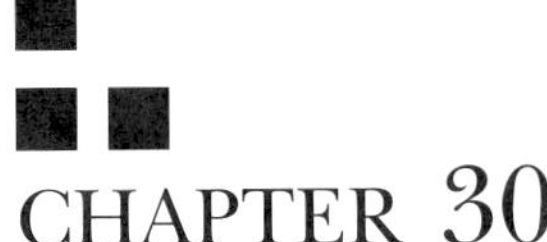

CHAPTER 30

Wheelchair Prescription and Adaptive Seating

Donald M. Currie, Karen Hardwick, and Rebecca A. Marburger

Few areas of medical practice demand more creativity in applying kinesiologic, pathophysiological, and technical knowledge to meet the needs of a patient and family in their unique physical and psychosocial environments than prescribing and solving problems related to wheelchairs and adaptive seating. The purpose of this chapter is to provide a framework for a systematic approach to the patient that will ensure a final result that best meets the patient's needs for mobility, positioning, and function. We present a structured checklist that the entire rehabilitation team, including the patient and family, can use for communication, creative decision making, and problem solving. With this approach the entire process from problem identification and goal setting to delivery of equipment, training, and follow-up can be done as a team effort, with the most effective and efficient results for those rehabilitation patients who must use wheelchairs or special positioning devices for all or part of their time out of bed.

Selection and prescription of a wheelchair and adaptive seating should be a team process, even for simple prescriptions. Each member of the team has a unique perspective and role. Sometimes only two or three team members need to be involved. For complex patients, the team may include any combination of the following members:

- Physiatrist and other physicians
- Occupational therapist (OT)
- Physical therapist (PT)
- Speech-language pathologist
- Nurse
- Orthotist
- Rehabilitation engineer
- Technician
- Schoolteacher and other educational professionals
- Durable medical equipment provider
- Representative from insurance company or other funding agency
- Social worker
- Case manager
- Vocational rehabilitation counselor

As integral team members, the patient and his or her family and personal care attendants should be maximally involved in decision making.

The physiatrist has the broadest perspective on the medical, rehabilitation, and technical aspects of the case and should review all medical problems, goals, and plans that might relate to seating and mobility. He or she will sign and take responsibility for the prescriptions written to meet the patient's needs and must often write letters of medical necessity to explain to payers why the equipment prescribed is needed.

The OT is an expert consultant on functional evaluation, control of tone and reflexes, goal setting, and problem solving. He or she often is the technical expert for seating and positioning technology that will be used. The OT will evaluate and select from the many control systems available if a powered wheelchair is prescribed. He or she helps train the patient in the use of the equipment for functional activities. Many OTs have special training in swallowing and feeding evaluations—important because the adaptive seat often is an important component of the feeding program for severely disabled patients.

The PT assumes some of these roles on some seating teams. As the mobility and transfer expert, he or she selects components for optimal mobility and transfers and trains the patient in these functional activities (see Chapter 13, Fig. 13-4).

The speech-language pathologist determines how seating affects communication. He or she is the expert for evaluating

D. M. Currie: Department of Rehabilitation Medicine, University of Texas Health Science Center at San Antonio, San Antonio, Texas 78284-7798.
K. Hardwick: Department of Habilitation Therapies, Austin State School, Austin, Texas 78767.
R. A. Marburger: Department of Occupational Therapy, Austin State School, Austin Texas 78703.

and selecting augmentive and alternative communication systems or devices that will be used with and must be compatible with the seating/mobility system. The speech-language pathologist may evaluate swallowing problems and advise on the effects of the seating/mobility system and body position on swallowing and nutrition.

The orthotist may be involved in molding for and fabricating custom-contoured seats. In addition to fabricating spinal or other orthoses, the orthotist provides expert consultation on how orthoses must function and interact with the seating/mobility system.

A rehabilitation engineer may be involved in evaluation of human–machine interactions as they apply to seating or function while in the seat. He or she may offer technical advice and assistance in solving problems with a wheelchair or adaptive seat and may be involved in research, development, and design related to customized seating and mobility components. A technician usually does the actual assembly, fabrication, and maintenance.

Schoolteachers and other educators know what functions the patient must be able to perform in the classroom and anticipate functions that will be needed for employment if that is a goal. They have observed the patient for many hours and have insights about positions of optimal function, sitting endurance, daily routine, and the use of other positioning and mobility devices.

The durable medical equipment dealer provides the wheelchair or the base for the special seat. He or she may be able to lend equipment for a trial period before it is ordered, may keep the team abreast of new technology, and may be the expert consultant about such information as the effect on warranties if components are mixed or modified. He or she should assemble the components according to the specifications of the prescription, check out fit and safe operation of components on delivery, and instruct the patient in the basic use and maintenance of the equipment when it is delivered.

The insurance companies or funding agencies are vital to this process. Good communication with their representatives and medical advisors often makes possible the purchase of expensive equipment that would be denied if it were not prescribed according to the restrictions, guidelines, and appeals processes of the company or agency.

The social worker or caseworker communicates with the patient and the rest of the team about important factors related to the use of seating/mobility equipment, such as architectural barriers or the cooperation of landlords. He or she usually is the liaison between the funding provider and the rest of the team and may be able to coordinate multiple funding providers, including volunteer organizations, to pay for needed equipment that the patient could not afford otherwise.

The vocational rehabilitation counselor is the consultant for use of the seating/mobility device in the workplace. Many vocational counselors also control funds that can help pay for equipment that can enable the patient to become employable either competitively or noncompetitively.

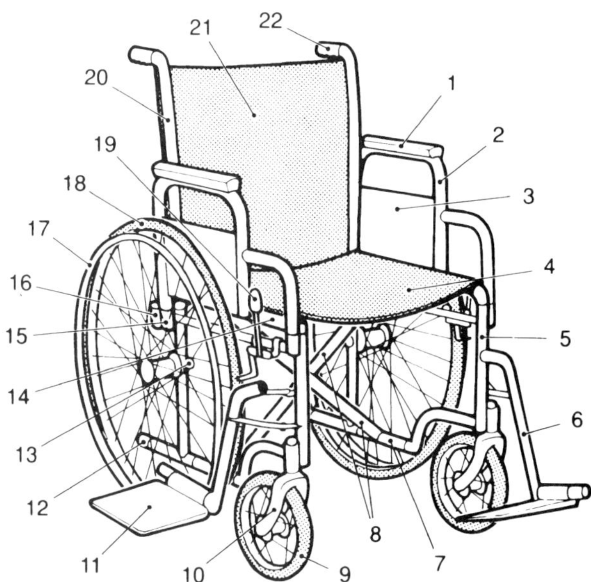

FIG. 30-1. Wheelchair terminology. A drawing such as this one can be used to teach the patient, family, and other team members the terminology they need to know to function as informed members of the seating team. In this case, the various parts of a typical outdoor sling-seat wheelchair are enumerated: *1*, arm pad; *2*, desk-style removable arm rest; *3*, clothes guard; *4*, sling seat; *5*, down tube; *6*, foot rest; *7* bottom rail; *8*, cross brace, X bar, or X frame; *9*, caster; *10*, caster fork; *11*, footplate; *12*, tipping lever; *13*, axle; *14*, seat rail; *15*, arm rest bracket or hole for non-wrap-around arm rest; *16*, arm rest bracket or hole for wrap-around arm rest; *17*, handrim; *18*, wheel; *19*, wheel lock, brake lever; *20*, back post; *21*, sling back; *22*, push handle.

The patient and his or her family and personal care attendants know what they need from a positioning/mobility system for optimal function in their environments. Pictures and drawings, such as Figure 30-1, can be used to explain unfamiliar terminology. The SEAT × 2 checklist (Table 30-1)

TABLE 30-1. *The SEAT × 2 checklist*

Support (*SCALPS*)
  for *S*afety and *C*omfort/*C*osmesis
  of *A*rms, *L*egs, *P*elvis, *S*pine and head
*S*kin
*E*asy propulsion
*E*asy transfers
*A*lteration of tone
*A*ccommodation (*GrOW FAST*)
  of *Gr*owth,
  of *O*ther (i.e., miscellaneous requirements, such as feeding, suctioning, and ventilation equipment),
  of *W*orsening medical condition,
  of *F*unctional *A*ctivities,
  of *S*tructural deformities,
  of *T*echnology
*T*ransportability with safe tie-downs
*T*errain

is used so the team can jointly understand, prioritize, and agree on goals that can be accomplished with wheelchairs and special seating. As the patient and family answer questions related to the checklist, they provide the rest of the team with information necessary to choose the seating/mobility system that will best achieve the high-priority goals for that patient. Thus informed, they can become important decision makers in the selection and use of the equipment.

The seating team should be flexible. Where certain team members are unavailable, other team members may assume their ordinary roles. Only two or three permanent members are necessary. These can invite other members on a case-by-case basis as needed to meet the requirements of the patient and most efficiently use the time and expertise of all members of the team. The permanent members can communicate with flexible members to obtain all the expertise and information needed to provide the optimal seating/mobility device.

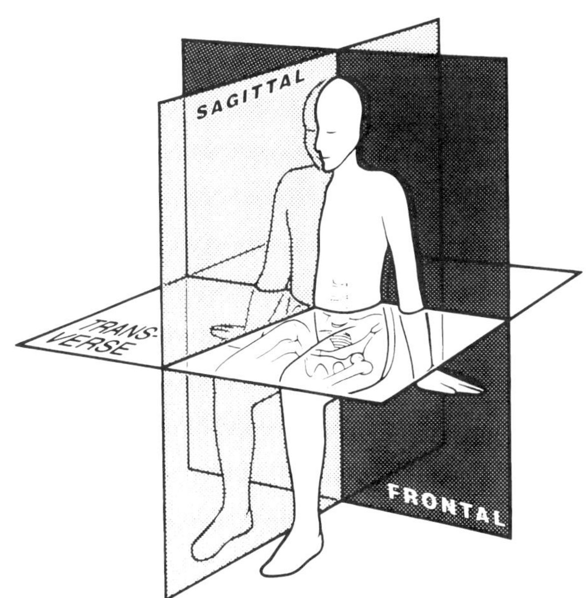

FIG. 30-2. Anatomic planes of the seated body. The symmetric normal sitting posture may not be attainable by many patients, who require special seating.

THE SEAT × 2 CHECKLIST

The SEAT × 2 checklist, with its framework of two *S*s, two *E*s, two *A*s, and two *T*s, can serve as a memory aid for the clinician and, even more important, as a communication tool for the entire team (see Table 30-1).

Table 30-1 includes acrostic memory aids to help ensure that all problems and goals related to the optimal prescription are considered. The knowledge and expertise of all the team members are shared using this communication tool in order to select the components that can best achieve the goals for seating, mobility, and function for the patient. It is especially useful in communicating with and educating patients and their families and caregivers about special seating so that they become informed members of the seating team; the educated user often is in the best position to make appropriate decisions about his or her wheelchair (1).

Support

The first *S* in SEAT is for support. The SCALPS acronym, for *s*afety, *c*omfort and *c*osmesis, *a*rm support, *l*eg support, *p*elvic support, and *s*pinal/head support, reminds the team to consider how to support all body parts in the safest, most comfortable, most cosmetic, and most functional manner possible (see Table 30-1). If deformities are mild, the goal usually is to support the patient with the body aligned in the normal symmetric sitting posture shown in Figure 30-2. This often is not the most functional or comfortable sitting posture for a person with a severe disability.

Safety

Safety is important. A wheelchair can be dangerous, and wheelchair safety has not kept pace with improved wheelchair performance in other areas (2). Falling, either tipping over or falling out of a wheelchair, is the most common cause of injury related to wheelchairs (2,3).

Forward is the most common direction of tipping or falling in standard wheelchairs, but powered scooters and carts are at particular risk of sideways tips and falls (3). Many falls occur in association with going down ramps (3). A patient with abnormal tone or movements and loss of motor control can accidentally injure himself or herself, or even be killed, by slipping out of the proper position and becoming asphyxiated by seat belts or other straps, or can accidentally move the chair to a place of danger if it cannot be locked or controlled (4–6).

A patient who is transported by a motor vehicle while in the wheelchair is at risk for injury if the vehicle is involved in an accident or must stop or maneuver quickly.

Wheelchair safety can be improved by improved injury reporting, improved safety standards, and the placing of a high priority on safety by manufacturers, prescribers, and purchasing groups (3,7).

Wheelchair stability in the sagittal plane is most influenced by the position of the rear axle, the fore-and-aft position and height of the seat, the diameter and position of the casters, and the position of any loads carried in the wheelchair (8–11).

As the rear axle position is moved forward, the position most patients prefer for ease of pushing, static stability is decreased to the rear so that the chair will tip backward more easily when accelerating quickly or going up ramps. Conversely, if the rear axle is moved backward, stability is increased and backward tipping is reduced for the user who is elderly or has poor trunk stability (12).

The addition of antitip devices also can be used to prevent the chair from tipping backward (13).

A rearward wheel placement is required for amputees because loss of the mass of the lower extremities puts the sitting center of mass farther backward. Thus, a wheelchair with a far rearward axle position is called an amputee wheelchair.

The position and diameter of the front caster, the seat position, and the locations of extra loads carried by the patient are the most important factors related to the most common tips or falls—those in the forward direction. Forward tips and falls are less likely with larger casters placed more forward, low and rearward seat position, and carrying loads under or behind the seat rather than setting them on the footrests (14). However, some users prefer the better turning maneuverability achieved by using small casters placed more rearward.

The width of separation of the points where the large wheels contact the ground affects lateral stability. Adjusting the camber, the angle between the plane of the wheels and a line perpendicular to the floor, to approximately 7° will maximize lateral stability without making the chair too wide. On many wheelchairs the camber can be adjusted. The use of camber to increase stability is especially important for some sports uses that require quick turns or long reaches over the side of the chair.

Wheel locks are a necessary safety feature for most users. Wheel lock variations include low positioning for very active users who have a long pushing stroke, extending handles for those who require greater ease of setting and releasing, and changing the direction of setting and releasing so that locking is effected by a pushing or pulling movement (Fig. 30-3). A specialized variation of the wheel lock is a simple spring-loaded accessory called a *grade aid* that allows the chair to move forward only (Fig. 30-4). These devices are engaged only on uphill grades. They can enable weaker pushers to ascend hills they could not otherwise negotiate. They should not be used for strong pushers, however, because they can become accidentally engaged while the user is performing a wheelie, thus causing a backward-tipping fall.

A special case of wheelchair safety and injuries relates to wheelchair sports. Wheelchair racing is a high-risk sport for injuries (15). Some of the injuries seen are unusual in other settings—for example, hyperthermia, bladder infections, and soft tissue injuries to the shoulders (16). Prolonged periods of high strain were found only during sports activities in one study (17). Entrapment neuropathies of the median nerve at the carpal tunnel and ulnar nerve at the elbow and of the deep ulnar branch at the wrist are common in wheelchair athletes (18–20). There is controversy about the efficacy of hand protection in prevention of these problems.

Comfort and Cosmesis

Comfort is important for all patients, especially those with intact sensation. It may be difficult to determine what is comfortable for the patient with cognitive or sensory impairments.

Cosmesis is important for all patients, even those with severe or profound cognitive disabilities. Even if the patient is unaware of appearance, the family or other caretakers will want the best appearance possible. An attractive, nonobtrusive wheelchair can be a major determinant of self-esteem. Good appearance in the seat may even influence caregivers to attend to a patient's needs more diligently. Esthetic considerations are important in prescribing powered mobility

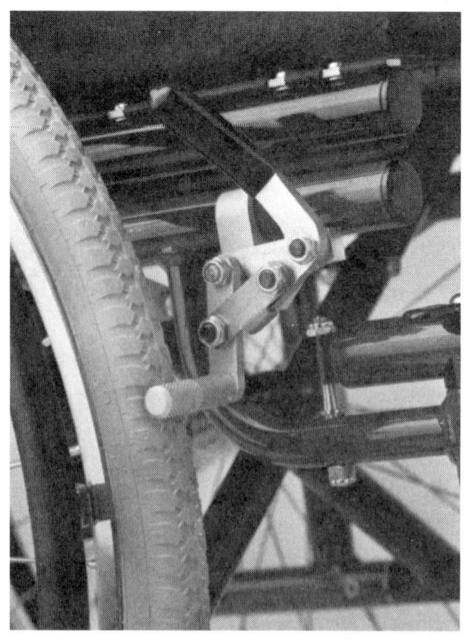
A

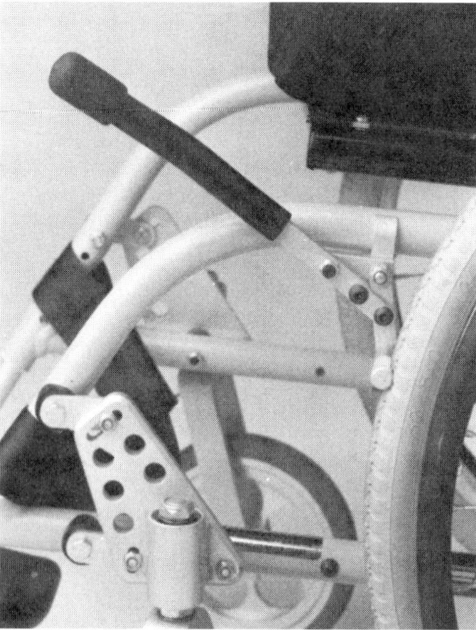
B

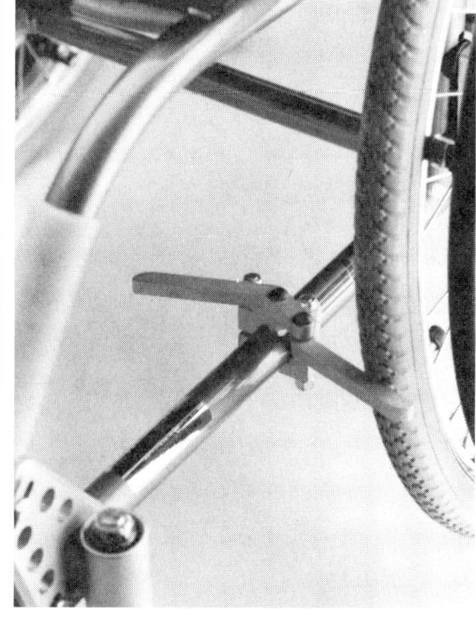
C

FIG. 30-3. Brake options. **A:** Pull-to-lock high brakes. **B:** Push-to-lock high brakes with extension. **C:** Low brakes.

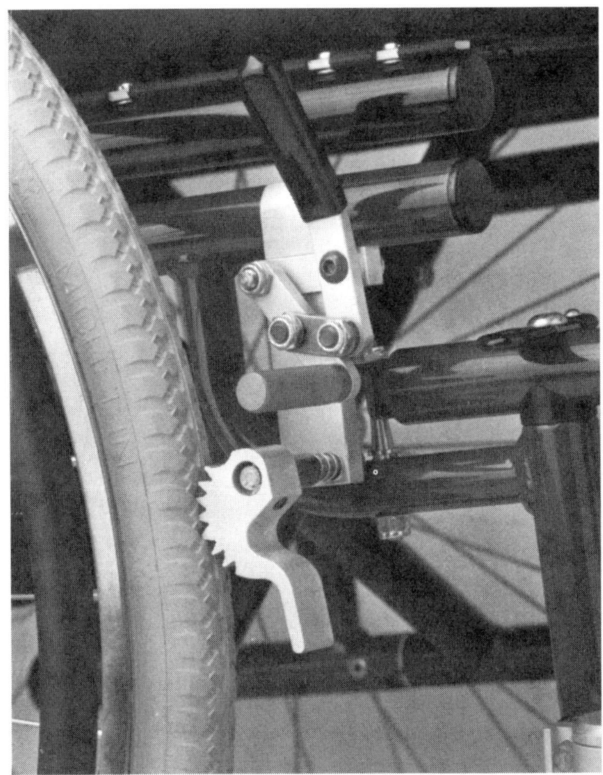

FIG. 30-4. A grade aid has spring-loaded teeth that allow forward movement but prevent the wheelchair from rolling backward while ascending ramps or inclines.

systems. The user who requires this type of chair centers interpersonal communication and relationships around speech and facial expressions; therefore, it is imperative that the head and face not be encumbered or surrounded by machinery. Another important esthetic consideration is the desirability of concealing or enclosing wires, tubes, gears, motors, clamps, and other devices in rounded, smooth, unobtrusive casings so that attention is drawn appropriately to the person in the chair rather than to the machinery that surrounds him or her. Another cosmetic consideration is noise. The quieter the function of the device, the less attention it will draw to itself, and the more effective it will allow the user to be. Another consideration is the use of clothing protectors to keep the clothes from getting dirty or torn while wheeling outside. Clothing protectors can be part of the armrests or lightweight plastic panels or fabric triangles laced to the seat and back upholstery.

Arm Support

Arm support varies greatly from patient to patient. If upper extremity function is normal, the goal may be to eliminate all parts that interfere with arm movement and hand function or with manual propulsion of the wheelchair. Athletic wheelchair users may want to eliminate arm rests and may even choose to eliminate wheel locks because they present a hazard to the thumbs and hands during vigorous pushing. For other users, arm rests can aid significantly in transfers, weight shifts, reducing ischial pressure by bearing some of the body weight on the arms, maintaining balance, and increasing comfort. For those who bear weight on the arms, selecting arm rests that are supportive and adjustable in height facilitates weight-shifting maneuvers. Patients with poor trunk control may need arm rests for stability. Wheelchair arm rests may be removable or fixed. Usually a swing-away or removable arm rest is required if the user cannot stand to transfer. Support of the arm of the seated hemiplegic patient with an arm trough may be an important measure to prevent or treat shoulder problems. The child or adult with severe spasticity, a startle reflex, strong tonic labyrinthine reflex, or movement disorder needs some type of arm restraint to prevent accidental injury to self or others.

Leg Support

Leg support also may vary, from elimination of support, to allow free movement of the lower extremity for propulsion or other function, to restraint, to prevent injury to self or others. The seat surface, be it hammock, firm, or molded, supports the thighs. The lower legs usually do not require direct support if there is proper support of the thighs and feet. The purpose of leg supports and foot rests is to afford protection, proper positioning, and maximal balance. The height of foot rests should enable the foot to be supported sufficiently to maintain circulation to the lower extremities and keep the ankle in a neutral position but not so high as to force more weight backward onto the ischial tuberosities and increase the risk of pressure sores (21).

A wide variety of foot rests and leg rests is available, all with advantages and disadvantages. The term leg rest means *elevating* leg rest to most manufacturers and durable medical equipment suppliers. Elevating leg rests often are used to treat lower extremity edema, injury, or a stiff knee. In the long run, however, these problems should be managed in another way if possible, because elevating the leg rests results in decreased forward static stability, increased rolling resistance, and more difficulty maneuvering in tight places (14).

Abductor wedges or pommels may be needed if there is excessive adductor tone. They should not be used to hold the pelvis back in the seat except in rare instances. They interfere with many functions (e.g., transfers, use of a urinal). If an abductor wedge is removable, it or any other removable part can be secured to the chair with a chain or tether to prevent loss. A barrel-shaped seat shows promise for improved hip stabilization in children with cerebral palsy (22).

Pelvic Support

Pelvic support is considered the key to proper support of the entire body for most patients with brain disorders (23). A firm seat is indicated for many but not all patients. A

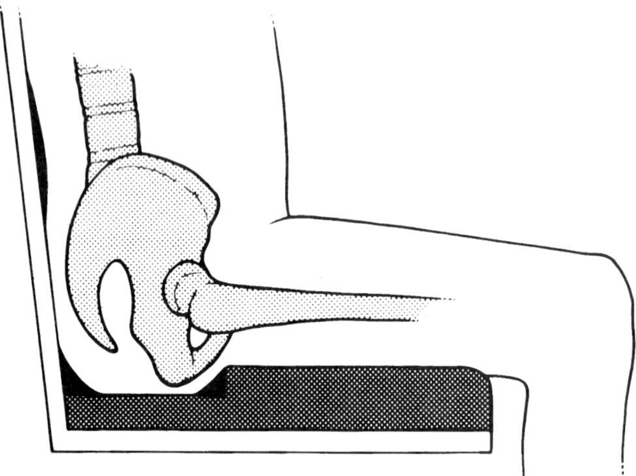

FIG. 30-5. A foam wheelchair cushion with an ischial ledge cutout prevents the pelvis from sliding forward and tilting posteriorly into a sacral-seating position. The edge of the foam is soft and compresses under the body weight, so it does not cause an ischial decubitus ulcer.

fabric sling or hammock seat is lighter and may be more functional for some. An ischial ledge may be built into the seat or cushion to prevent the ischial tuberosities from sliding forward (Fig. 30-5). Cushions affect pelvic support, pressure distribution, and stability. Most patients with a significant pelvic obliquity require a custom-molded seat.

Spinal and Head Support

Support of the spine and head may vary from a very short fabric sling back that provides almost no support at all for the patient with no spinal deformity, normal trunk control, and strong arms, to a custom-molded back with special head supports. Wheelchair back height should be sufficient to support the user in good posture and prevent fatigue over an extended time while affording as much movement as possible. In all cases, the back should provide good support for the lumbar spine. An adjustable back height sometimes is desirable for the user with varying needs throughout the day. It is important that the wheelchair back does not force the user into poor posture. Push handles may be attached to the back or base of a wheelchair. Many users prefer not to have push handles because they connote a certain amount of dependence; however, if the user spends a significant amount of time being pushed, push handles are required. Often the seat can be designed to place the patient in a position where gravity helps stabilize the trunk and head in the contours of the seat. With such a design, multiple restraining straps, halos, and pads can be eliminated. This concept of creatively using gravity as a friend rather than foe is discussed further in the section on the minimalist approach to custom-molded seating for the severely involved patient. If further support is required, thoracic pads and a chest belt or other type of chest support may be used if position cannot be controlled in any other way. Restraining a person in a wheelchair with straps makes effective weight-shifting maneuvers for pressure relief almost impossible and should be used only when absolutely necessary to maintain acceptable posture and stability. However, the use of neoprene belt chest straps for certain patients, especially individuals with low thoracic paraplegia, improves functional reach (24).

Skin

The second *S* in SEAT × 2 refers to skin. The skin over bony prominences is especially susceptible, but other areas may be damaged by any part of the chair that contacts the body, or if the skin has been damaged by the disabling condition, as in patients with burns or scleroderma. Providing total body contact over a wide surface area and using soft materials for those parts of the seat that are in contact with the body are strategies to distribute pressure and reduce shear forces.

Wheelchair cushions are the most commonly used means of protecting the skin. In using wheelchair cushions, the two major functions of distributing weight over the greatest area, thus minimizing skin pressure at bony prominences, and providing a stable seating base often must be balanced against one another (25).

Other wheelchair cushion considerations include weight, durability, ease of cleaning, cost, heat dispersion, ventilation, and appearance. A multichambered villous pneumatic cushion may provide the best pressure relief but provides very little seating stability (26).

A firm, contoured foam cushion provides good stability, but the pressure relief provided by this type of cushion is not adequate for some people. A cushion that uses a gel-filled bladder over a firm, contoured foam base can be used in an attempt to optimize both stability and pressure relief and is adequate for some users. Newer, multidensity carved foam cushions and honeycomb hydrocarbon plastic cushions (StimuLite, Supracor, San Jose, CA) also show promise in combining maximum stability with adequate pressure relief (27).

StimuLite cushions are durable, washable, easily maintained, and provide excellent ventilation. As people with disabilities age, it is important to monitor them carefully because they may lose tissue over bony prominences with a resultant higher risk for decubitus ulcers (28). If this occurs, a cushion with better pressure distribution should be used.

Allergic reactions to materials in direct contact with the skin may occur. Body temperature and sweating often become important considerations, especially for more severely disabled patients in hot climates. Encasing much of the body in a seating system that provides good support interferes with the normal dissipation of body heat.

Intermittent relief of pressure is necessary to prolong sitting time safely and comfortably. If the patient is unable to relieve pressure independently, the seat should be equipped to recline or tilt-in-space (Figs. 30-6 and 30-7). Manual tilt-

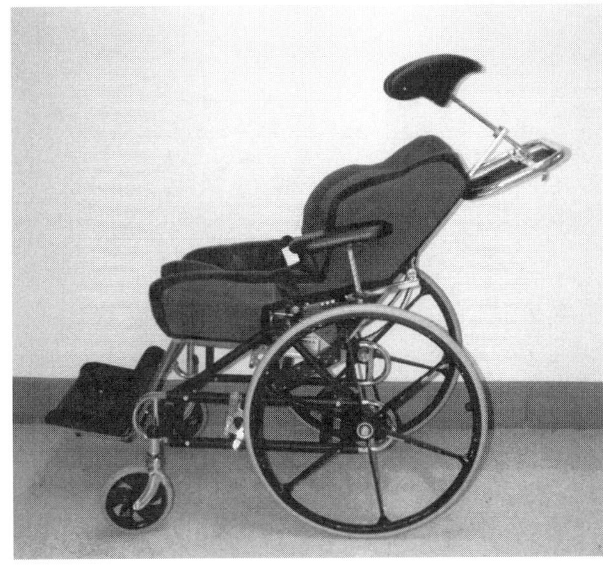
A

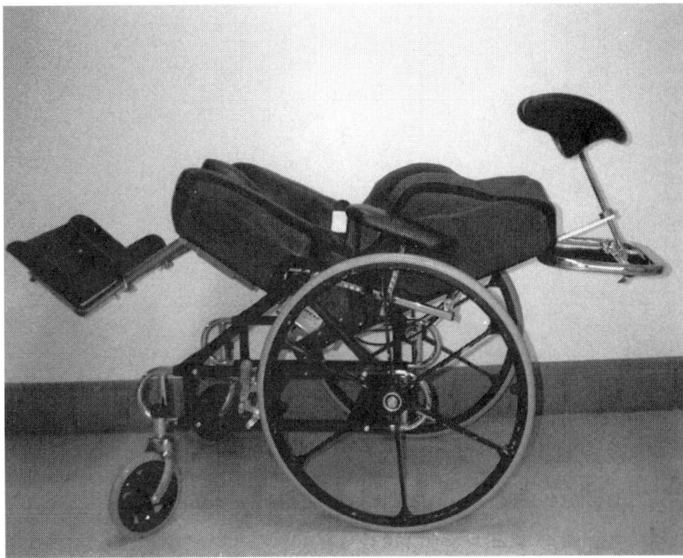
B

FIG. 30-6. A custom-molded seat with a manual tilt-in-space mechanism. **A**: Upright position. **B:** Tilted position.

ing mechanisms are controlled by an attendant caretaker. Power tilt mechanisms can be controlled by the patient. The back only may recline. The recline mechanism may be powered and paired with electric foot rests and supportive arm and head rests (29).

When prescribing a reclining system, the clinician must pay careful attention to shear forces produced by the reclining process (30,31).

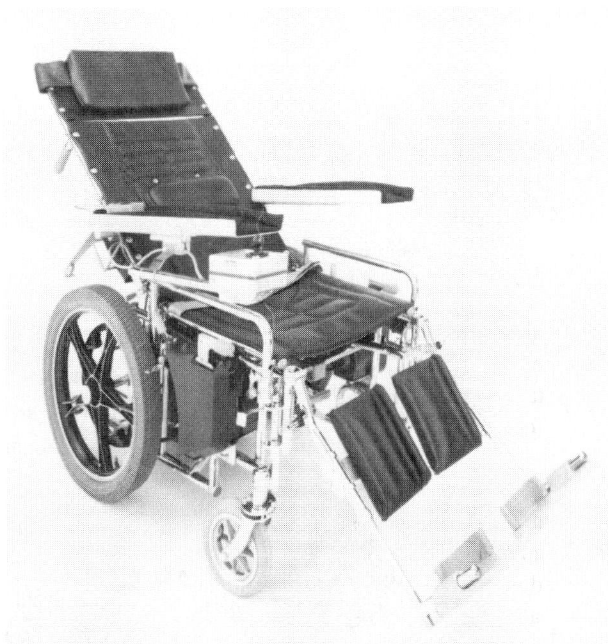

FIG. 30-7. A reclining wheelchair can be useful for a person who cannot adequately shift his or her own weight. Arm rests and leg rests must provide support for the limbs in all positions.

Shear is the sliding force of the skin rubbing against the seat. If shear forces are not minimized, the process of reclining and resuming the upright posture tends to slide the buttocks forward on the seat into a poor sitting position, especially when there is significant spasticity. This can lead to pressure sores or even skeletal deformity. Shear forces are controlled in one of four ways:

1. Maintain the seat-to-back angle by tilting the entire seat rather than reclining the back.
2. Align the axis of movement of the reclining back with the anatomic axis of hip flexion and extension.
3. Slide the back of the chair downward while reclining.
4. Slide the seat of the chair anteriorly while reclining.

Each method has its advantages and drawbacks for various patient problems. An important consideration is that all powered recline and tilt systems add 1 to 2 inches to the height of the seat above the floor. This increase may prevent the user from rolling under tables or going through a van door without being reclined. Tilt-in-space usually provides better repositioning than a reclining back when the upright position is resumed.

The position of the body greatly affects the ability of any cushion to lower tissue interface pressure and shear (31–33). This fact is used in certain weight-shifting maneuvers, such as leaning forward or sideways (33).

Computerized technology is used to measure pressure and shear, to develop and test computer models to predict the effects of various positions and activities on the skin, and to develop a ''smart'' cushion that can sense pressures at various parts of the tissue interface and then adjust its shape to lower the pressure at the desired locations (31,34,35).

Commercial systems, recently made available, can provide lateral tilting in the frontal plane. Lateral tilting mecha-

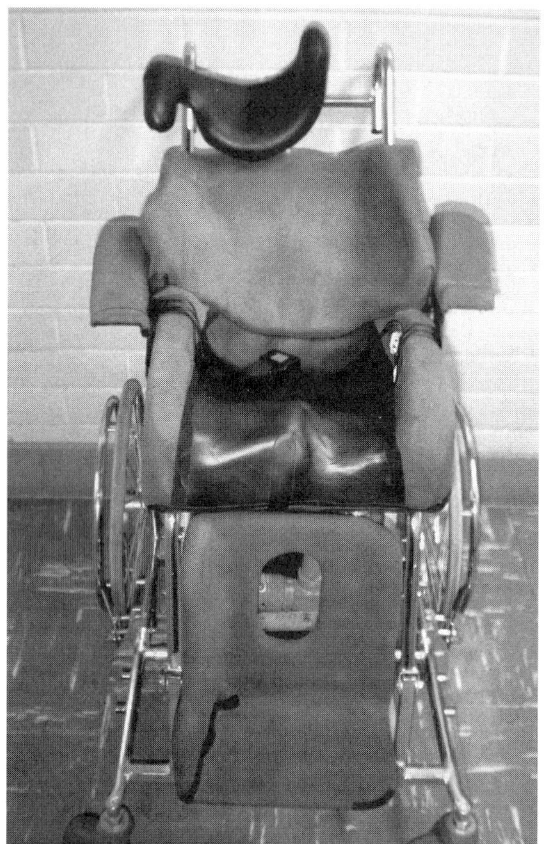
A

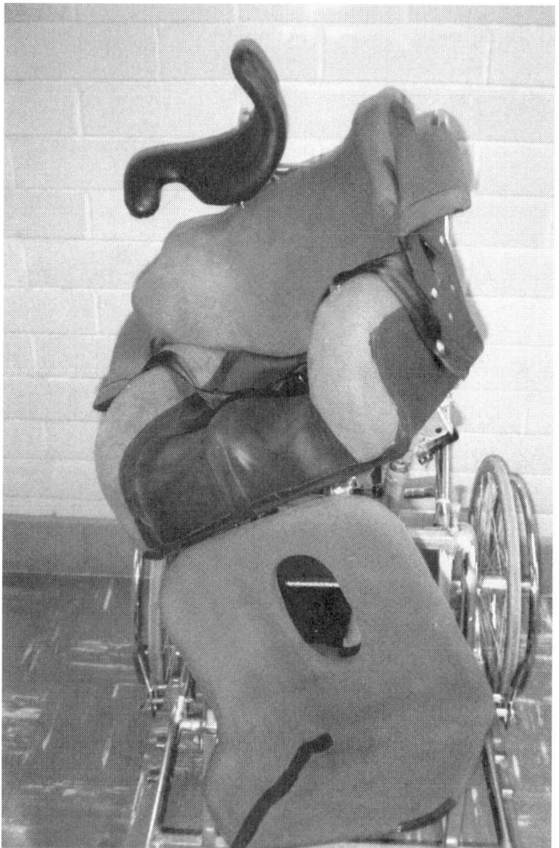
B

FIG. 30-8. A: A custom-molded seat with a manual lateral tilt-in-space mechanism in the upright position. **B:** The laterally tilted position was shown to improve gastric emptying on radiographic studies of the patient who uses this chair. Its use reduced gastroesophageal reflux and eliminated recurrent episodes of aspiration pneumonia.

nisms may improve function or facilitate care of a few selected patients (Fig. 30-8). Regardless of the method used to shift weight, some patients may benefit from the use of a timed visual or audio reminder to perform weight-shifting maneuvers (36). Many inexpensive wrist watches have self-resetting countdown timers with an alarm sound that can provide such a reminder at any desired interval for less than $30.00.

Easy Propulsion

Easy self-propulsion is essential to make the patient as functional as possible. Pushing with any combination of arms and legs is possible for manual mobility, and there are a wide variety of configurations and accessories to facilitate various capabilities and limitations. If manual propulsion is impossible or is too difficult or slow to be functional, power mobility should be used if the patient is otherwise competent. For example, manual propulsion by most persons with complete C6-spared quadriplegia or higher is too slow to be functional, so powered wheelchairs should be prescribed for these persons (37). Various equipment for manual and power mobility is discussed below.

The seat height relative to the rear axle and handrim is important in maximizing the efficiency of wheeling, particularly for users who are tall or have short arms in proportion to their trunk height (38). Raising the seat lessens the overall stability of the chair, however. An adjustable axle plate allows adjustment of the important parameters of seat height and position of the wheels in relation to the patient's arms and hands (Fig. 30-9).

Although all agree that wheelchair weight is important when considering transportability, some research shows that weight has little effect on the overall energy cost of wheeling (39,40). This may be true for wheeling on level surfaces, but wheelchair weight does have an effect on ease of propulsion uphill. If folding frames are used, precise wheel alignment may be difficult to maintain, with a resultant increased rolling resistance and decreased efficiency of pushing (41).

Rigid frames maintain wheel alignment better than folding frames and thus provide the least rolling resistance. The inconvenience of rigid frames, however, makes them unacceptable to some wheelchair users. Placing the rear axle more forward makes a wheelchair easier to push (42,43). It also is easier to keep the chair on a straight line on a side slope, and the casters roll over bumps more easily because

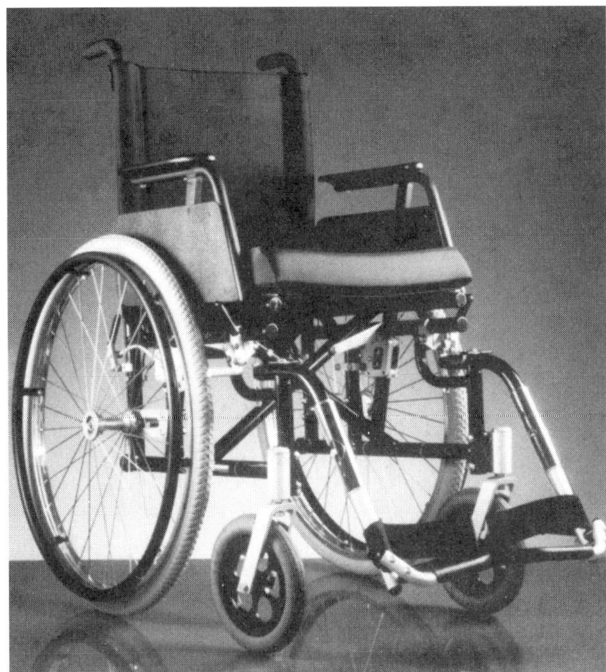

FIG. 30-9. An axle plate allows adjustment of rear wheel location to accommodate various needs, such as raising or lowering the seat height above the floor, changing the camber of the wheels, or moving the wheels forward for easier pushing or backward for more stability. The quick-disconnect axles make this chair easier to transport.

they are bearing less weight. As noted above, however, a more rearward wheel position with its increased rearward stability may be safer for some users. In general, the active person with good trunk stability will use a more forward wheel position, whereas a person with a higher-level disability requires more rearward placement. As a person progresses in rehabilitation, optimal wheel placement may change. A cambered wheel is easier to push than a vertical wheel for most patients.

The type of wheels and tires has an effect on ease of self-propulsion. Solid, smooth tires are best on smooth, hard indoor floors such as those found in hospitals or nursing homes. Pneumatic tires give a smoother ride outdoors on uneven ground, and treaded tires will improve traction (44).

Flat tires are a problem with pneumatic tires, but this problem can be minimized by using thorn-resistant tubes or replacing the tubes with flat-free solid inserts; however, these inserts provide a harder ride and add weight to the chair.

The type of handrim used influences ease of self-propulsion. For high speeds, a small-diameter, smooth rim close to the hub is preferred. For power and maneuverability, a larger-diameter rim is indicated. Rubberized coatings for the handrims improve gripping and appearance but may wear off (45). With time, coatings may discolor the hands or become rough and injure the hands. A pair of sports gloves often is the best way to improve gripping the handrims. Rim projections (knobs) are sometimes useful for a person with quadriplegia and may be varied in spacing and angle. Positioning the handrims close to the wheels may allow the hands to contact the side walls of the tires for increased traction without touching the treads directly. Training using progressive resistive exercises improves self-propulsion using the arms in some patients (46).

Persons with hemiplegia propel using the good hand and foot together, so the height of the seat above the ground must be appropriate for the pushing foot to reach the ground. A simple modification of the cushion allowing better extension of the pushing hip improves propulsion for hemiplegic individuals (47).

Propulsion using levers or cranks instead of the handrims has theoretical advantages in terms of mechanical efficiency, but practical limitations related to maneuverability have thus far limited the usefulness of levers and cranks (48–50).

Propulsion using powered wheelchairs is most functional for many users (37). Users of powered wheelchairs must have sufficient vision, judgment, and motor control to operate the equipment safely. Experimental control systems that also guide the wheelchair may become useful in some settings in the future (51).

Easy propulsion must also be considered for family members or personal care attendants who will push a manual wheelchair when the user is tired or unable to self-propel. Push handles should usually attach to the frame rather than the seat back of tilting or reclining wheelchairs because handles attached to the seat back become too low for comfortable pushing when these chairs are tilted or reclined. Push handles that fold, telescope, or can be easily removed are now available and are useful for many users

Easy Transfers

Easy transfers are essential whether the patient transfers independently or with partial or total assistance. Other equipment may be needed to achieve the goal of easy transfers (e.g., mechanical lifts, a sliding board). Transfer training is essential whichever equipment is used. One should also prescribe a sliding board storage pocket whenever a sliding board is prescribed.

Alteration of Tone and Reflexes

Alteration of abnormal tone and primitive reflexes is an important goal for many patients with brain disorders. Strategies to reduce hypertonicity include providing enough stability for the patient to feel posturally secure, correct position of the head, comfortable correct position of the lower extremities, and correct use of gravity. Hypotonicity requires support and use of gravity.

Accommodation

Accommodation of many factors is necessary. The *GrOW FAST* acronym helps all of the members of the team to remember to consider the most important factors that must be accommodated (see Table 30-1):

*Gr*owth is an important consideration for children. Size changes may also be important for an adult whose weight is unstable.

*O*ther refers to special needs (e.g., feeding tubes, ostomies, a portable ventilator, a suctioning apparatus, an oxygen cylinder).

*W*orsening medical condition refers to diagnoses where progressive deterioration is predictable, most often progressive neuromuscular diseases. Worsening of the patient's condition must also be considered for aging patients, especially those with dementia, and for aging of personal care attendants who must lift and transport a patient's wheelchair.

*F*unctional *a*ctivities include all the usual activities of daily living as well as specialized vocational, recreational, sports, and educational activities. For example, for those involved in sports, no single chair is adequate. Prescription of sports wheelchairs is highly specialized and should be done by practitioners who are well versed in the biomechanics, physical requirements, safety considerations, and competitive principles of the sports for which the chairs are to be used. Most users who are active in wheelchair sports require individualized wheelchairs for different sports. Few standardized measures of function include the instrumental activities of daily living, which may be important for the wheelchair user (see Chapter 7) (52).

For most users, function is optimized by having the narrowest chair possible that will allow adequate seat width. Wrap-around arm rests help to decrease chair width but are more difficult to replace after removal for transfers. Some folding chairs have the capability of using a crank device to partially fold the chair with the user sitting in it, thus temporarily narrowing the chair to go through a doorway. The safety of such devices, however, must be carefully monitored in each individual situation (53).

*S*tructural deformities and contractures of the spine or lower extremities usually require a custom-molded seat.

*T*echnology needs vary greatly from patient to patient and range from such high-technology items as computers or environmental control systems to low-technology items such as a lap tray or rollers on the foot rests to assist in opening doors (Fig. 30-10) (see Chapter 29).

Transportability

Transportability refers to how the wheelchair and seating system are moved and transported when the patient is not seated in them. This is the goal for which weight of the equipment chosen is most important. If the patient is transported in the wheelchair or seat, a safe tie-down system is important. Most wheelchair tie-down systems, however, provide far less safety than seat belts and air bags, and few have had adequate crash testing (54).

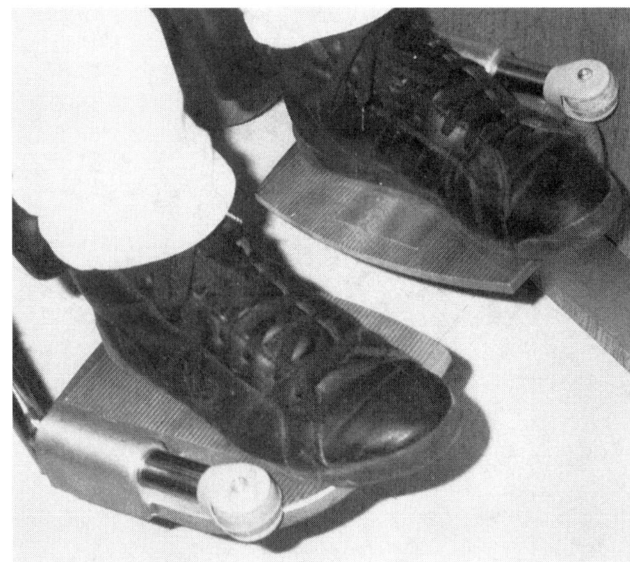

FIG. 30-10. Door-opening foot rest rollers.

Terrain

Terrain over which the wheelchair will be used always must be considered. Information from the patient and caretakers is essential for correct selection of appropriate size and configuration of wheels, tires, tubes, or flat-free inserts for the individual patient. Specialized suspensions and shock-absorbing equipment may be indicated for heavy patients or for those who must negotiate rough terrain. The use of larger or pneumatic casters, or both, often is necessary to negotiate rough terrain.

EVALUATION

The purpose of the evaluation for seating and mobility is to identify all factors that will influence the selection of an appropriate system so that the best decisions can be made about the seating/mobility prescription and training for the individual patient. Evaluation begins with a thorough review of the following:

- Medical, surgical, and seating history
- Diagnosis
- Precautions that are necessary when dealing with certain physical conditions or diseases
- Prognosis for future physical or functional ability
- Prevention of the problems associated with impaired mobility

For example, muscular dystrophy predictably influences the choice of seating system because the course of disease results in impaired respiratory function and declining ability to perform independent weight shifting to protect the skin. Conditions that are characterized by lack of sensation must be accommodated through attention to pressure distribution and shear on weight-bearing surfaces. Conditions that result in abnormalities of muscle tone may require attempts to normalize tone, provide support against gravity, and accommodate fixed deformities.

Medical History

A good starting point is to ask the patient, family, and caregivers their understanding and expectations of the purpose of the seating/mobility evaluation. What would they like to see accomplished as a result of the evaluation and the use of any equipment that will be prescribed? Knowing the patient's and family's expectations will avoid misunderstandings.

The medical diagnosis often, but not always, explains the disability that causes the patient to need a wheelchair or adaptive seat. A knowledge of the natural course of the underlying conditions will direct the clinicians to ask questions about problems known to be associated with the diagnosis, especially those that will influence decisions about seating and mobility. For example, for a spinal-cord-injured patient, specific questions about decubitus ulcers and other skin lesions, spasticity, contractures and other deformities, urinary incontinence, and orthostatic hypotension must be explored. With the child with cerebral palsy, problems related to vision, convulsions, and cognitive status as well as muscle tone, musculoskeletal contractures and deformities, and nutritional status must be explored. Similarly, knowledge of the usual course of progression and potential complications of a neuromuscular disease guides the physician member of the seating team to ask questions that will pinpoint problems that can influence the current choice of seat and possibly prevent predictable complications later. Refer to Table 30-2 for a list of items on the review of systems that commonly influence the seating/mobility decisions.

Surgical History

In addition to an inventory of past operations, questions should be asked about any future surgery that has been discussed or planned. For example, spinal surgery for scoliosis may completely change the type of adaptive seat to be used and the timing of the prescription. A gastrostomy or urinary or intestinal diversion will influence the choice of body positions, restraint straps, or expected growth or weight gain. Questions also should be asked about fractures, serious injuries, and decubitus ulcers.

Seating History

Questions should be asked about all seats and positioning aids used now and in the past. What was good about methods and equipment that were used? What were the major limitations and shortcomings of past seating/mobility equipment? How many hours at a time and per day does the patient sit in various equipment? In what position, and where, does the patient eat? What dangerous situations have occurred related to seating—for example, injuries to extremities, tipping of or falls from a wheelchair, or straps choking the patient or threatening the airway? Reviewing each item of the SEAT × 2 checklist as it relates to seating/mobility equipment used in the past is an easy way to assure taking a complete seating history (see Table 30-1).

TABLE 30-2. *Seating and mobility: review of systems*

Skin
- Sensory status
- Cutaneous allergies
- Decubitus ulcers
- Scars and other lesions (e.g., rashes, infection, diabetic lesions)
- Sweating or excessive skin dryness
- Urinary or fecal soiling

Cardiopulmonary and circulatory
- Pneumonia
- Restrictive lung disease, especially with spinal deformity or weakness
- Chronic obstructive pulmonary disease
- Aspiration
- Exercise tolerance
- Need for resuscitation
- Poor circulation (i.e., cold or discolored feet)
- Edema of feet and legs
- Arterial or venous insufficiency

Gastrointestinal
- Nutrition and weight control
- Swallowing
- Tube feeding
- Use of diapers
- Bowel habits and control
- Gastroesophageal reflux and gastric emptying
- Ostomies

Renal
- Urinary control
- Renal function
- Urinary tract infection
- Urinary tract stones
- Use of catheters or urinals while sitting
- Diversions and ostomies

Endocrine
- Diabetes
- Growth

Neurologic
- Mental status and behavior
- Cognitive function—educational and vocational history and expectations
- Muscle tone
- Special senses
- Somatic sensation
- Movement disorders
- Seizures
- Drooling and swallowing

Musculoskeletal
- Spinal deformity
- Hip dislocation, subluxation, dysplasia
- Deformities and contractures of limbs
- Leg length discrepancies, true or apparent

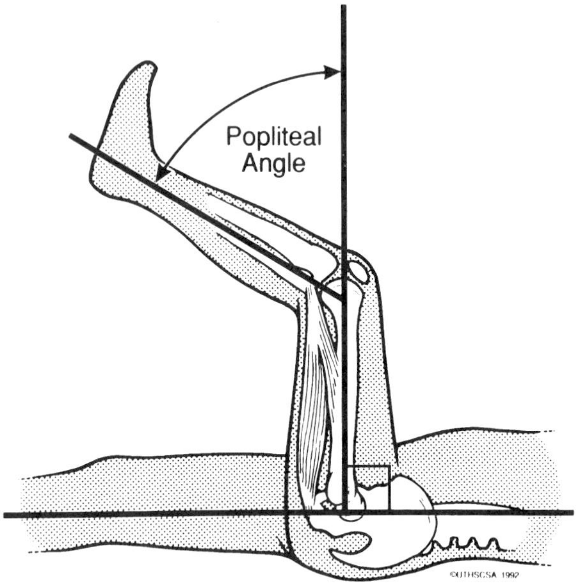

FIG. 30-11. The popliteal angle test for hamstring contracture. The patient is supine with the hip flexed 90° and the pelvis stabilized by the contralateral thigh. The knee is extended to the point of resistance. The angle between the leg and vertical is the popliteal angle.

Bed Examination

The patient should be examined lying on the examination table and sitting, both on a firm, flat surface and in any seat currently being used (55).

It is tempting to defer the examination on the examination table with severely involved patients because they are difficult to transfer. Considerable time often is required to relax spastic tone to be able to assess accurately joint range of motion. The temptation to defer the bed examination must nevertheless be resisted because this part of the examination often discloses problems that must be taken into account in prescribing an appropriate wheelchair or adaptive seat. Particular attention should be paid to measuring hip flexion and hamstring length. The popliteal angles should be measured to assess for hamstring tightness; straight leg raising cannot be used in patients with a knee flexion contracture (Fig. 30-11) (56).

Sitting Examination

Physical and Functional Considerations

Some of the following physical problems may be encountered in seating adults and children with mobility impairment:

- Abnormal muscle tone
- Dominant primitive reflex patterns
- Complex medical conditions
- Skeletal deformities
- Poor muscle strength
- Large or small body size or unusual proportions
- Extremes of age
- Limited ranges of joint motion

Functional considerations in seating may include transfer skills, living and work environments, the person's need for comfort and rest while maintaining optimal positioning for mobility and work, and cosmetic factors that can dramatically affect self-esteem and treatment by others (57,58).

A number of approaches and classifications have been developed to assist in the evaluation process. One method of classification addresses the level of sitting ability (59,60). Others address the degree of skeletal deformity and pathologic muscle activity (61,62).

Regardless of the approach used, similar basic principles for evaluating body structure and function provide a framework for most of the seating evaluation. These areas of evaluation include careful neuromusculoskeletal examination of the extremities, pelvis, spine, and head. Sitting is examined with the person seated on a flat surface and in any wheelchair or seating system currently used. If available, a simulator chair can be used to evaluate the patient sitting in an ideal position (Fig. 30-12). Special evaluations also may be performed, such as skin-interface pressure measurement or assessments for augmentive communication or control systems for powered mobility.

Areas of Evaluation

Pelvis

Attention usually is directed first to the pelvis (62). Abnormalities of the pelvis have profound effects on seating because of the role of the pelvis in weight bearing, weight shifting, and alignment (63). Attention should be paid to anterior and posterior tilt, lateral symmetry, and rotation because restriction in any direction will cause changes throughout the body (64).

In some people with cerebral palsy or other neuromuscular disorders, however, orientation of the head, neck, and body relative to the vertical plane may be the logical starting point because of the influence of head position on muscle tone and posture (65).

Posterior pelvic tilt is a common disorder of pelvic alignment in people with abnormal muscle tone (Fig. 30-13). Exaggerated posterior tilt usually is caused by overactivity in the hip extensors with tight hamstrings and hypotonic low back extensors. This combination of forces makes assumption and maintenance of optimal pelvic positioning difficult (66).

The pull of the spastic hamstrings on the pelvis causes the pelvis to tilt posteriorly and the lumbar spine to flex. Consequently, a normal lordotic lumbar curve does not occur, which affects total spinal alignment and function (66). Pelvic inflexibility can occur even in children with low muscle tone and no obvious limitation in range of motion (67). In such cases, the adaptive seat usually should accommodate

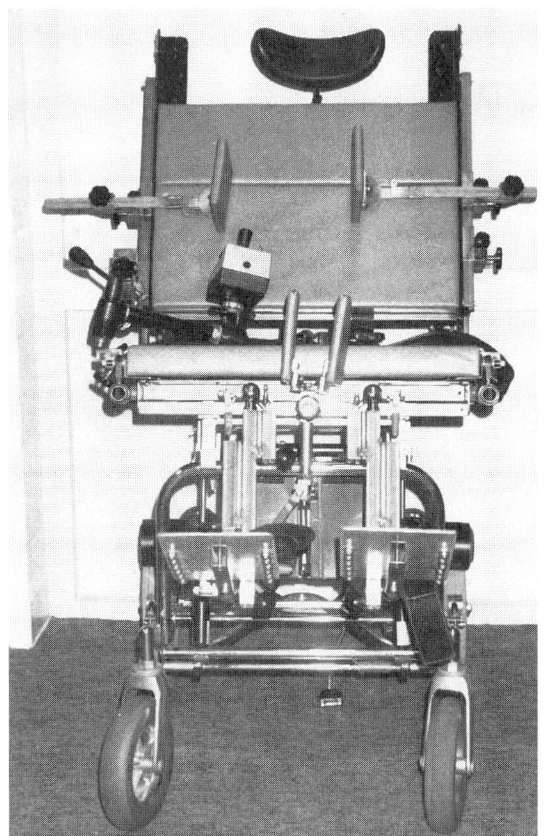

A

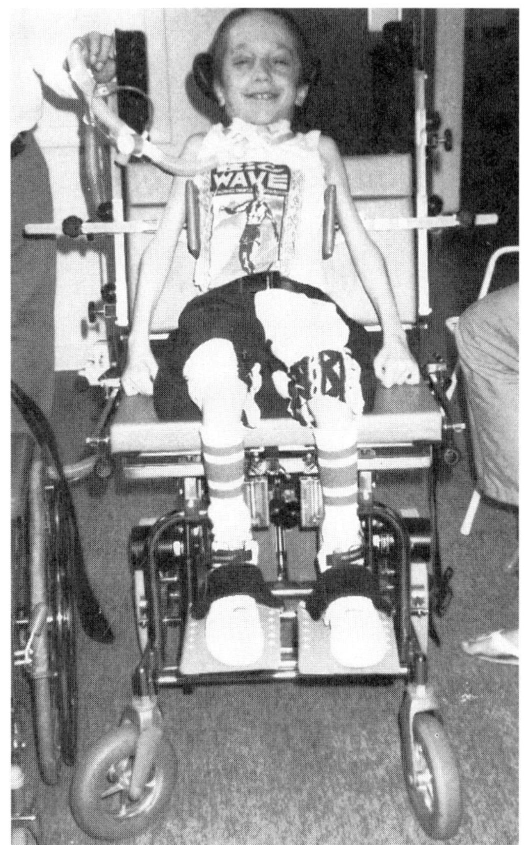

C

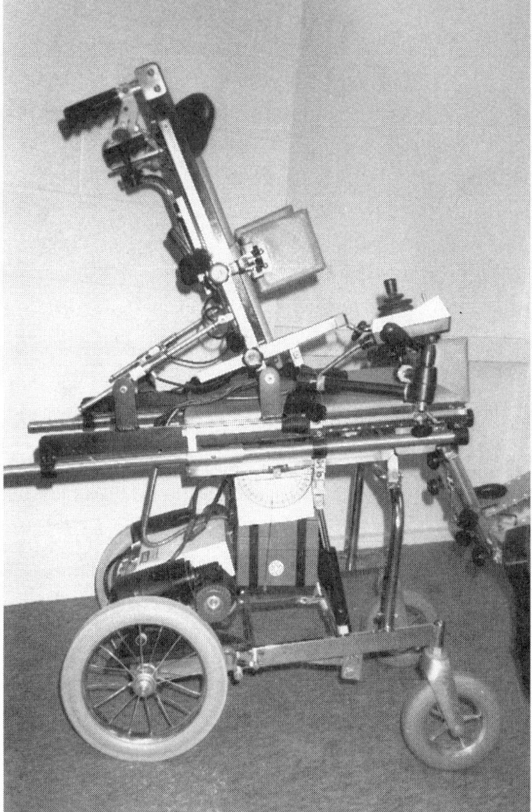

B

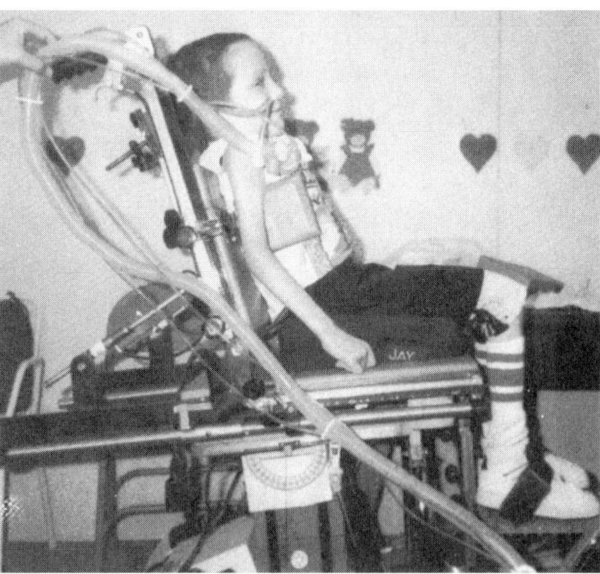

D

FIG. 30-12. A–D: A planar simulator wheelchair is capable of adjustment to accommodate almost any size patient from infant to adult. All angles (i.e., recline, tilt-in-space, knee flexion, foot position) are adjustable. Many accessories can be added to support the body. The chair is powered with multiple control options that can be used to assess a patient's ability to operate switches or train a patient to use the control system before the prescription is written.

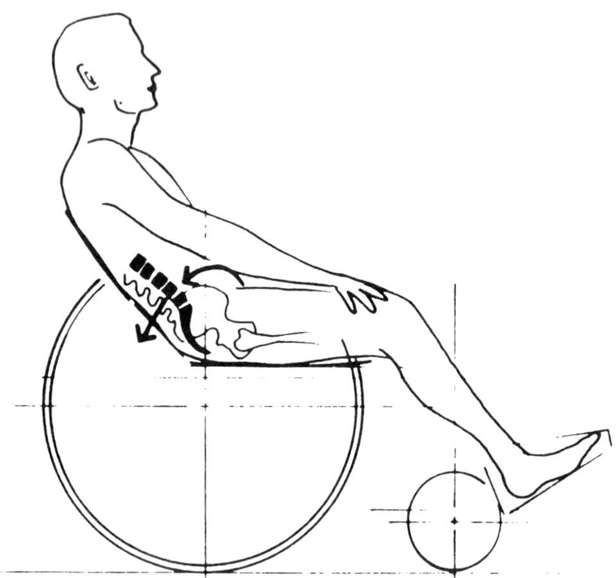

FIG. 30-13. Posterior pelvic tilt.

rather than attempt to correct or prevent spinal deformity (68).

Anterior pelvic tilt describes inclination of the pelvis in the sagittal plane forward of its neutral position (Fig. 30-14) (69). Anterior tilt may be caused by hypotonicity of trunk musculature, shortening of low back extensors, tightening of the iliotibial bands, or tight hip flexors (23,69,70). If this position is maintained, shoulder girdle movement will be restricted, and upper extremity function will be impaired (71).

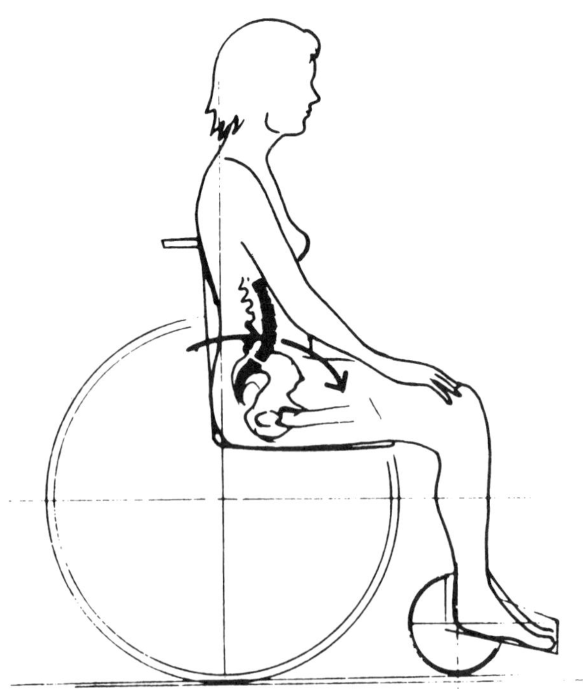

FIG. 30-14. Anterior pelvic tilt.

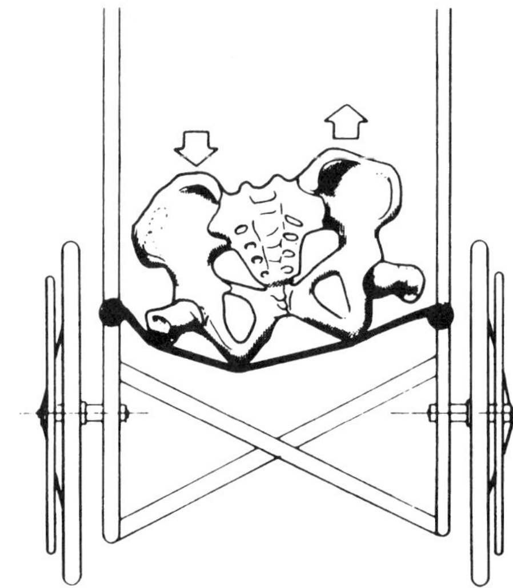

FIG. 30-15. Pelvic obliquity.

Pelvic obliquity is a slanting or inclination of the pelvis in the frontal plane such that it is not horizontal when the person is standing or sitting (Fig. 30-15). It may be caused by imbalanced posture or muscle tone, scoliosis, hip dislocation, or surgery (72). It often is seen in combination with scoliosis. In a long thoracolumbar C-curve, the pelvis may form part of the curve. Other factors that predispose a person to pelvic obliquity include hip adduction contracture, weak hip abductors, or hip dislocation or subluxation (70,73).

Pelvic rotation refers to movement of the pelvis around the longitudinal axis of the body in the transverse plane (Fig. 30-16). In the presence of a dislocated hip, the pelvis usually is rotated posteriorly on the side of dislocation.

The *windswept hip* phenomenon is one of the most difficult pelvic problems to treat (Fig. 30-17) (72–74). This rather characteristic posture often is part of a more complex pattern of deformity that includes hip dislocation, pelvic obliquity, pelvic rotation, and scoliosis. A windswept deformity combines flexion with abduction–external rotation on one hip and adduction–internal rotation of the opposite hip (72). The typical deformity is manifested by a scoliosis convex away from the side on which the hip is dislocated, adduction of the dislocated leg, and abduction of the other leg with an apparent leg length discrepancy (69,75). There is some disagreement among clinicians over the etiologic factors and sequence of events leading to the windswept hip deformity. Letts and colleagues name hip dislocation as the first deformity, followed by pelvic obliquity in which the pelvis is tilted upward on the side of the dislocation with progressive scoliosis (see Fig. 30-17) (73,74). Early, aggressive conservative measures to prevent contractures of the hip joint and keep the hips reduced plus surgical release when indicated may slow or prevent this complex pattern of deformity (69). If there are fixed contractures and the dislocated hip is not painful, however, or if a surgical procedure is too risky or declined by the patient, the most appropri-

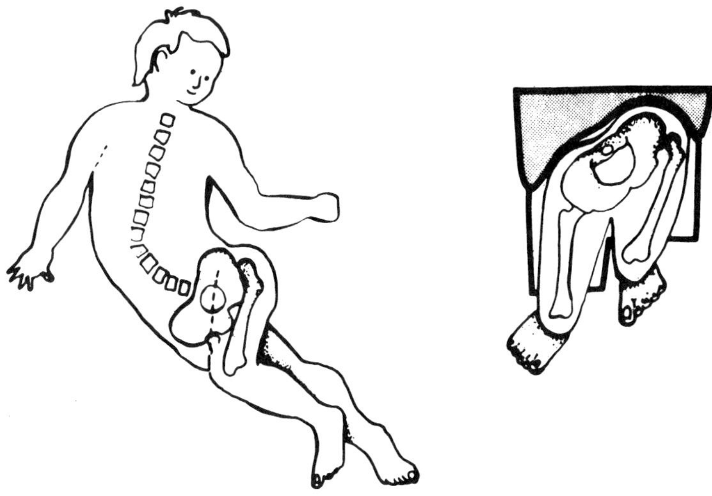

FIG. 30-16. Pelvic obliquity frequently has a rotatory component that compounds the difficulty in obtaining stable seating. (From Letts M, Rang M, Tredwell S. Seating the disabled. In: *American academy of orthopaedic surgeons: atlas of orthotics, 2nd ed.* St Louis: CV Mosby, 1985; 447.)

ate course of management is to accommodate the deformities in a seating system (73).

Spine

The most common skeletal deformity seen in seating is *scoliosis.* Curvature of the spine is described in terms of the direction of the convexity of the curves and the areas of spinal involvement (72). The curves can be structural or functional and can be found in combination. Curves are considered functional when they can be corrected by lateral bending of the spine toward the convexity. Generally, when the curve is functional, very little vertebral rotation will be present (76). Curves are considered to be structural when alterations in the anatomy of the spine limit its flexibility and correction is not possible. The apical vertebra usually is most rotated and is the last to alter its inclination (76). Scoliosis rarely is isolated as a factor in seating but is accompanied by deformities or dysfunction in head and pelvic position. A person with scoliosis may exhibit any or a combination of the following postural components:

- Uneven shoulders
- Prominence of one scapula
- Asymmetry of the pelvis
- Asymmetry of the rib cage
- Kyphosis with forward-flexed head
- Other compensatory head positions

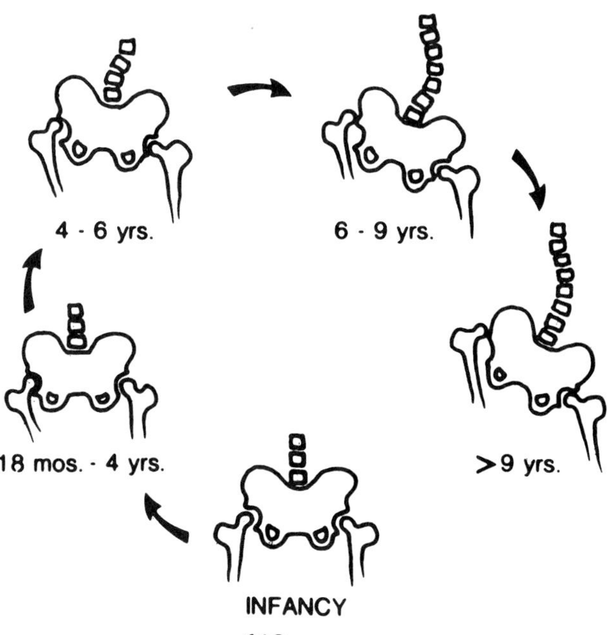

FIG. 30-17. The genesis of the windswept hip phenomenon. (From Letts M, Shapiro, L, Mulder K, Klassen O. The windblown hip syndrome in total body cerebral palsy. *J Pediatr Orthop* 1984; 4:55–62.)

Once a structural curve develops, support is necessary to try to control progression of the curve rather than correct it. Orthotic or surgical management should be used for correction. Assessment should include determining the support needed to provide alignment, comfort, and function, recalling that spinal curvature also can affect gastrointestinal and pulmonary functions (72,77).

Other spinal deformities that require evaluation for seating systems include kyphosis and lordosis. *Kyphosis* is abnormal posterior curvature of the upper chest and thoracic spine (72). Abnormal kyphosis may be an accentuation of the convexity of the thoracic spine beyond the normal 20° to 40° curve or may extend to the normally lordotic lumbar spine (72). In sitting, people with kyphosis often exhibit increased lordosis of the cervical spine with hyperextension of the head and protraction of the scapula. This forward head position places the trachea in a dependent position that may leave the airway vulnerable to aspiration during swallowing. *Lordosis* is characterized by an abnormal anterior curvature of the lower portion of the spine (76). Hyperlordosis is associated with an anterior pelvic tilt and, usually, hip flexion contractures and abdominal muscle weakness. The extensor muscles of the low back also become contracted. In sitting, the person may strive to maintain balance by hyperextending the neck and retracting the shoulder girdle (72). This posture interferes with upper extremity function.

Head

Head position is critical because of the influence of the head on primitive reflexes, muscle tone, upper extremity function, swallowing, and visual orientation (78).

A person's head position often dictates the overall body tone, particularly in the trunk and upper extremities and shoulder girdle (65,79). Reclining a person with the head in the same plane as the trunk may result in increased trunk and shoulder girdle extensor tone because of the effects of the supine tonic labyrinthine reflex (80). Hyperextension can be caused by extensor hypertonicity, severe generalized hypotonicity, or poor flexor control (81). Rotation can be a result of the asymmetric tonic neck reflex or residual rooting reflex initiated by stimulation to the cheek. Forward flexion can be caused by domination of primitive flexor tone or severe or profound retardation with sensory deficits such as cortical blindness. Evaluation should be directed toward uncovering the causative factor of head misalignment to provide an appropriate seating prescription.

Upper and Lower Extremities

The upper and lower extremities must be assessed in the various positions and degrees of support that will be available in the seating/mobility system because of the effects of gravity and support on limb function and tone (82–84).

Areas of evaluation in the upper extremities include the following:

- Range of motion and strength
- Grasp patterns
- Eye–hand coordination
- Joint stability
- Movement patterns
- Functional use of the hands

Upper extremity structure and function may influence propulsion, weight shift, and transfers as well as other necessary activities. Function must be assessed to determine the extent of support, restraint, or other modifications required to promote optimal independence (63,85,86).

Areas of concern in the lower extremities include range of motion, joint stability, movement patterns, and function, especially foot propulsion, weight bearing, and transfers (87).

Range of motion, especially the popliteal angle, is extremely important in the design of the mobility system because of the effects of tight hamstrings on pelvic position, transfers, and propulsion. If the hips flex less than 90°, a larger seat-to-back angle or, in severe cases, a straddle seat is required (88).

Evaluation should address foot, ankle, leg, and hip deformity in terms of the amount of support or accommodation required. An example in which joint stability would be an important consideration is exacerbating a dislocated hip by using knee blocks to prevent the pelvis from sliding forward on the seat. Abnormal or excessive movement or muscle tone should be addressed in terms of support needed to normalize tone and inhibit reflex patterns. Additional factors in lower extremity assessment may include medical concerns such as dependent edema, impaired distal pulses, venous stasis, and foot or leg ulcers.

Complex Medical Conditions

Complex medical problems may affect evaluation of seating and positioning because of the relationship between body position and certain physiological functions. Some patients may require passive positioning to inhibit gastroesophageal reflux and facilitate gastric emptying. Seating for these people might include both reclined and upright positions as well as lateral tilt following meals (see Figs. 30-6 and 30-8). People with restrictive lung disease, aspiration, and other pulmonary conditions may require varied therapeutic positioning for good pulmonary toilet. The seating approach in these patients may include proper trunk support without restriction to the movement of ribs, regular change in position in space, and strategies to relax muscle tone.

Aging and dementia present further challenges to the provision of appropriate seating because of the unique probems brought about by chronic debilitating influences on physical and mental health. Seating for a common problem such as kyphosis might focus on placing the individual in a slightly reclined position to move the trachea out of the dependent position to prevent aspiration. A factor associated with dementia is the loss of depth perception, which creates a strong fear of movement. Seating must address this fear by providing security through more surface contact and comfort through cushioning. Other concerns include loss of alertness, fluctuating skill levels, loss of bone mass, thinning of the skin, and impairments in judgment that influence safety (89).

Functional Considerations

Evaluation of seating, positioning, and mobility systems must address functional considerations as well as medical and physical concerns (90,91). Areas of specific importance include the following:

- transfer skills and methods
- size and arrangement of living and work environments
- need for rest and change of position to maintain comfort
- type of transportation available
- type of propulsion used
- optimal positioning for mobility and work
- cosmetic factors that can affect self-esteem and treatment by others (67)

The patient's functional skills directly influence the type of wheelchair chosen and the components and accessories prescribed (92–96). Factors to consider in evaluation of transfer skills may include the height of seat, type of transfers done, amount of energy or physical assistance required, type of mechanical lift used, balance point of the system, and type and adjustability of the accessories. Evaluation of the work or living environment should address the size and layout of permanent structures, the amount of room needed to move or use a particular system, and the configuration of work surfaces. Postural control and upper extremity function may be improved in the antigravity position when the longitudinal axis of the trunk and head tilts anterior to the fulcrum at the ischial tuberosities (97). Work postures in the antigravity position are tiring for individuals with poor postural mechanisms and must be punctuated with periods of rest. The ability to change positions in order to maintain comfort may be assessed. A patient able to tolerate upright sitting for only a short time can take frequent, brief rests in a tilted position and thus be able to work through the day. Another area of evaluation concerns preferences in color, design, and appearance. Equipment with poor cosmesis may end up not being used by the patient.

Mobility of the wheelchair both in terms of propulsion as well as transportation of the system from one location to another is an essential part of the functional evaluation (98,99). The dimensions, weight, center of gravity, and accessories of the wheelchair must be compatible with or adaptable to the available modes of transportation (94). Assessment of propulsion must include motor coordination, grasp pattern, strength, endurance, and cognitive ability for both manual and powered mobility (100,101).

The person's physical capability and ability to interface with the equipment must be evaluated. Additional factors that must be assessed when powered mobility is being considered include identification of appropriate access and control sites, and level of electronic sophistication (see Chapter 29).

Powered mobility may be appropriate for people who cannot achieve energy-efficient mobility in a manual wheelchair (102–104). In general, powered wheelchairs are less transportable than manual chairs.

There are five general types of configurations available for powered mobility: the traditional belt-driven chair, the modular powered base, the portable folding powered wheelchair, the scooter, and add-on power devices. The traditional belt-driven chair is durable and stable and can support all types of control systems and most seating options. Its advantages include a smaller turning radius than the powered-base chairs and an option to lower the frame and allow the user to fit under many desks and tables.

The powered-base chair generally is more durable and may have advantages for the user who drives frequently outdoors. It also can accommodate most types of seating and control systems. Like the traditional belt-driven chair, it requires a van and wheelchair lift or ramp to attain community mobility, and almost all curbs and stairs must be ramped.

The folding powered chair is lighter in weight and has removable batteries. Transportability is its major advantage. It cannot support a powered recline or tilt system or other specialized seating options and is less powerful and less durable than the belt-driven or powered-base chair. Add-on power devices can be useful in some instances where most wheelchair propulsion is done manually but powered assistance is required for ramps or long distances (105).

There are a number of three-wheel and four-wheel scooters available in several sizes and prices. They generally are most useful for people with normal neuromuscular function who are partially ambulatory but have limited stamina. They generally are durable for indoor and outdoor use and may be disassembled for transport in an automobile trunk. The golf-cart-like appearance often is cosmetically more acceptable to elderly people with little tolerance for their disability. They are seldom adequate for a person with significant neuromuscular dysfunction because transfers into and out of scooters require significant lower extremity control and near-normal upper extremity function to manage the controls.

There are a variety of control systems that permit severely handicapped people to operate powered mobility systems (106). The factors influencing the choice of control systems include spasticity, weakness or paralysis, tremor, impaired coordination, poor vision, visual field neglect, sensory deficits, impaired perceptual function, and cognitive function. Evaluation of the person's abilities should result in appropriate selection of the control site, which may include any extremity, the head, chin, and tongue as well as the eyebrows, the voice, the breath, extraocular motion, and any muscle the person can contract voluntarily (107). An ideal method of evaluation would involve use of a powered simulator wheelchair with a variety of control options (see Fig. 30-12).

Primary wheelchair control (i.e., acceleration, braking, turning) is controlled most often by a joystick that can be positioned to be controlled by either hand, chin, or a lower extremity. For people whose head control is not adequate for joystick movement, a pneumatic switch control system operated by sip and puff may be indicated. Control using a pneumatic switch is less direct, and wheelchair speed usually must be slower to compensate for this type of system. Voice-activated controls have been available for a number of years but have not yet proved as useful as the available electromechanical control systems. Other systems such as eye position control, ultrasound or mechanically mediated head position control, and muscle electrical activity control have shown promise but have yet to prove to be generally advantageous for a significant proportion of users. It often is cost effective to incorporate environmental control and communication functions into wheelchair controls. In these cases, evaluation of compatibility with computers, environmental controls, and communication devices is required.

Electric wheelchairs are powered by lead acid or gel cell batteries. The advantage of gel cell batteries is their relative stability and lower free-hydrogen production, making them safer for airline travel and for use around open flames. Battery life depends on wheelchair use and the number of secondary devices powered by the wheelchair batteries, but generally wheelchair batteries will require recharging nightly (108). Motors vary widely in power and durability. Speed is a function of the motor and power linkage and usually can be adjusted to suit the user's needs.

GOALS OF WHEELCHAIR PRESCRIPTION AND ADAPTIVE SEATING

The purpose of the evaluation of the patient who needs a wheelchair or adaptive seating is to write prescriptions that will best meet that person's needs. Sometimes the seating and mobility goals can be best achieved by modifying or repairing the current wheelchair or seating system rather than by prescribing new equipment.

The first step is to identify all problems that relate to seating. The next steps are to identify and prioritize goals to be achieved by the use of special seating or a wheelchair. Equipment is then selected and a detailed prescription developed to best achieve the goals, with emphasis on the higher-priority goals. If available equipment and technology cannot achieve all the desired goals, only lower-priority goals should be sacrificed so that all high-priority goals are achieved. For example, a spinal-cord-injured paraplegic woman may be able to learn to lift her wheelchair into her automobile to complete a car transfer only if the wheelchair is very light in weight. If her spine is straight and stable and her pelvis is level, a sling seat and back might be adequate for support, even though a firm seat and back would give slightly better support. In this case, transportability is a more important goal for her total function than support, so a lightweight wheelchair with a sling seat and back should be prescribed.

The information in Table 30-3 can be helpful to rank goals according to different priorities for three different diagnostic categories. Cerebral palsy, traumatic brain injury, and stroke have been combined as brain lesion. Spinal cord injury has been subdivided into paraplegia and quadriplegia. Although the priorities will vary for individual patients, these rankings can serve as a starting point for the team. The knowledge and expertise of each team member are then used to select equipment that will best balance the patient's needs for seating, mobility, and function.

From Goals to Prescriptions

In the next step, the seating team, including the patient, family, and caregivers, discusses the equipment options that

TABLE 30-3. *The SEAT × 2 checklist of goals of special seating for specific disabilities*

Goal	SCI paraplegia	SCI quadraplegia	Brain lesion	Muscular dystrophy
*S*upport (SCALPS)				
*S*afety (restraints and stability)	+	+ +	+ +	+ +
*C*omfort and cosmesis	+/−	+ /−	+ +	+ +
*A*rms	−	+	+ +	+ +
*L*egs	+	+	+ +	Often rejects foot rests
*P*elvis	+	+ +	+ +	+
*S*pine and head	Depends on level	+/−	+ +	+
*S*kin				
Pressure distribution	+	+ +	+/−	+ (for comfort)
Pressure relief	+	+ +	+/−	+ + (for comfort)
*E*asy propulsion	+	+ + to − (may need power)	+ to −	+ + (need power)
*E*asy transfers	+	+	+	+ + (for attendant)
*A*lteration of tone	−	−	+ +	−
*A*ccommodation (GrOW FAST)				
of *Gr*owth	+ /−	+/−	+	+
of *O*ther	Individualize	Individualize	Individualize	Individualize
of *W*orsening (i.e., progressive) disease	−	−	−	+
of *F*unctional *A*ctivities (i.e., ADL needs)	+	+	+	+ +
of *S*tructural deformities and contractures	+/−	+/−	+ +	+
of *T*echnology	+/−	+ +	+/− to + +	+
*T*ransportability	For patient	For patient or attendant	For attendant	For attendant or family
*T*errain	+	+	+	+

+ + , usually important; + , often important; +/−, sometimes important; −, usually not important
ADL, activities of daily living; SCI, spinal cord injury.

TABLE 30-4. *Strategies and equipment used to achieve goals*

Support	
Safety and stability	Protect patient from injury to self or others (e.g., with restraints, antitip devices); wide base, cambered wheels, and durable frames that won't break
Comfort and cosmesis	Balance snug fit with free movement (see Skin); allow patient to make cosmetic choices
Arms	Arm rests, wrist straps, trays
Legs	Abductor wedges, adductor pads, straps, contoured seat, foot rests, leg rests, shoe holders, custom foot guards, door guards
Pelvis and trunk	Seat belts (45° or other), ischial ledge, limbar pad, pelvic positioners, knee block, seat-to-back angle, custom contour seat; consider 90° or greater knee flexion, tilt-in-space, scoliosis pads, Danmar chest support, H-strap, curved or sectional back, custom back, lap tray, arm rests, shoulder retractors, trunk orthoses
Spine and head	High-back, curved, or shaped-back Otto Bock head support, three piece head support, collar, head, straps, halos, head harness, custom head support, recline or tilt, Hensinger collar
Skin	Cushions (including pressure evaluations), custom-molded seats, foot rests, arm rests, trunk supports, push-ups, weight shifts, tilt-in-space, or recline
Easy self-propulsion	Lightweight equipment, position of wheels, high-friction-coated handrims, power, proportional control, projections, grade aids, back height and width
Easy transfers	Swing-away and detachable positioners, supports, accessories, and hardware; wheel position, mechanical lifts, van or bus lifts, sliding boards, training or attendants, seat height
Accommodation	
of Growth	Brands that accommodate growth (e.g., X—L), modular and sectional components
of Other	Feeding tubes, special feeding needs, ventilator, medical supplies, schoolbooks, crutch holders
of Worsening disease	Consider prognosis
of Functional Activities	Consider ADLs, architecture of home and workplace, and recreational activities
of Structural deformities	90° foot rests, windswept hips, hip extension contractures, recline, customized seat, back, and foot rests
of Technology	Braces, environmental control units, lifts (van dimensions), ventilators, control systems and mounting hardware, communication devices, positioning hardware, desks and tables, computer work stations, tilt-in-space hardware
Alteration of tone	Head position, hip position, skin support and comfort, stable and click-in-place hardware, short foot rests, inhibitive casts or braces
Transportability	Lightweight, removable and modular parts, folding, dimensions compatible with van and lifts (especially height of van and car doors), mechanical lifts
Terrain	Brakes, grade aids, pneumatic tires, Davis forks, heavy-duty power bases (e.g., Fortress), hard inserts, large casters

ADL, activities of daily living.

can achieve the seating goals of that patient. It is extremely helpful to have a collection of equipment that the patient can try out before definitive prescriptions are written. Even if the fit is not perfect, adaptations can be made with pillows, cushions, and bolsters to give the patient the feel of the equipment being considered. Most clinics cannot keep a large bank of equipment, but all can keep pictures of a wide variety of wheelchairs and adaptive seating and positioning equipment. All seating clinics should cultivate good relationships with durable medical equipment dealers who can lend equipment to a patient on a trial basis, or at least allow a trial of equipment in the store. A simulator wheelchair also can be an invaluable tool at this stage, as discussed in the section on planar seating.

After a patient has tried out equipment, a final decision is made by the whole team. The physician writes a detailed prescription system, including all relevant components and accessories (Table 30-4).

When the equipment is received, final fitting is necessary. The durable medical equipment provider and the OT often work together to assemble the components and ensure that they fit. The OT and PT, and sometimes other team members, train the patient, family, and caregivers in the proper use of the equipment until it is being used properly, and the follow-up period begins.

Planar Seating

The seating needs of many patients can be met by seats with flat surfaces in contact with the body. The most common flat seating surface is tautly stretched fabric, as in the typical folding, sling-seat/sling-back wheelchair (see Fig. 30-1). Padded, solid, flat seats and backs may be fabricated from plywood or plastic and upholstered foam rubber soft enough to conform to the body contours when compressed by the person's body weight.

A planar simulator chair can be used to determine whether a planar seat will work for an individual patient (see Fig. 30-12). In our experience, use of this simulator has enabled prescription of planar seating for people originally referred for custom-molded seating, by using correct adjustment of seat-to-back angle and tilt-in-space and correct use of accessories such as cushions, foot rests, and trunk and head supports.

Some advantages of planar seating are low cost, simplicity and reliability, good accommodation of growth, light weight, easy transportability, flexibility, and a wide array of commercially available systems. Planar seats are relatively easy to prescribe (109,110). The major disadvantage is inadequate support or pressure distribution for people with severe deformities or abnormal tone.

Modular, Noncustomized Component Seating Systems

These systems are not used as often as planar or customized seating in most centers, primarily because they require the seating clinic to maintain a large inventory of relatively expensive components, and because most patients whose needs cannot be met by variations of planar seats require customized seating systems. Examples of modular seating systems include the CP seat and the Winnipeg modular wheelchair insert system (111). Variations of these modular systems more often used with adults include the Jay Modular Seat and Back (Jay Medical, Boulder, CO) and the Design-A-ROHO kit (ROHO, Belleville, IL).

Customized Seats

Providing successful seating and mobility systems for people with severely handicapping conditions often requires customization (112). Whenever a person with physical and functional limitations is unable to be served adequately by use of standard seating approaches because of the complex interplay of factors affecting selection of a seating system, customization often is the answer (113–116).

The custom-seating approach seeks to provide appropriate fit and design to maximize comfort, support, and function and may include the use of multiple positions in space and contouring (71,117–126). The patient's degree of dysfunction should directly influence the extent of intervention (127,128). Other considerations in prescribing a customized system include application of esthetic principles, appropriate selection of wheelchair frames, and cost factors (129,130).

Design and Fit of Customized Seating Systems

Appropriate design and fit of customized seating systems should begin with the person's physical structure and muscle tone. Structural abnormalities that affect seating include scoliosis, kyphosis, lordosis, limb contractures, dislocations, and other bony and soft tissue deformities. It is important that a seating system not be used primarily for correction; rather, it should provide support and comfort. A seating system prescribed for corrective purposes initially may appear to provide a good seating position. Over a period of a few hours, however, the person may attempt to escape discomfort with a resultant poor fit that actually increases deformity. For example, for a seating system to be tolerated over time, an abnormal pelvic position frequently must be accommodated. If the pelvis is supported initially in a position of comfort, often allowing the pelvis to tilt posteriorly, abnormal tone may decrease with an actual improvement in pelvic flexibility. The seat-to-back angle can be readjusted subsequently to a more neutral pelvic position (131).

Other functions of a customized seating system are to achieve and maintain optimal positioning to normalize muscle tone, inhibit the influence of abnormal postural reflexes, decrease effort during functional activities, achieve comfort, and align internal structures (129,132–134).

Positioning for optimal function often deviates from the normal symmetric sitting posture. Severe neurologic impairment and orthopedic deformity frequently result in midline shift, rotation of body parts, and uneven weight-bearing surfaces. Musculoskeletal misalignment affects not only external appearance and movement but can influence the function of internal organs controlling respiratory, cardiac, circulatory, digestive, and eliminative activity (130,135). Appropriate positioning may improve physiological function. For example, appropriate positioning is necessary to achieve optimal respiratory function if the person has severe scoliosis causing restrictive pulmonary disease (136).

Contouring

Contouring is used to distribute body contact evenly over a large surface area for people who have skeletal deformity or who have imbalanced muscle tone that requires external stability (137). Contouring can be accomplished by many methods; these include sculpting blocks of foam, adjustable modular linkage systems (Matrix, Matrix USA, Indianapolis, IN), enclosed bead systems (Bead Seat, Pyramid Rehab, Memphis, TN), direct foam-in-place, indirect foam-in-place, commercially fabricated contouring (Pin Dot, Niles, IL), Carapace, Summit Systems, Otto Bock (Otto Bock, Minneapolis, MN), computer shape sensing (Pin Dot), and others (116,138). The use of contouring can increase function by supporting the person so that attention and available strength can be directed toward activity and away from the need to maintain stability. Contoured seats may require modification for growth, weight gain or loss, and changing body shape.

Sculpting blocks of foam was one of the first methods used to achieve contouring. This method is time consuming, and a high level of artistic ability is required to look at the patient and sculpt a seat or back that exactly fits the patient's contours. Modular linkage systems provide a prefabricated system with a wide range of adjustability (139). These systems require many man-hours to assemble and maintain shape. Their use is limited mainly to seating smaller, lighter people or providing support to individual body parts rather than the whole patient. The enclosed bead system, a viscous, moldable material (i.e., polystyrene beads mixed with epoxy) encased in a flexible latex covering, can be shaped directly around a person. This system is a self-contained unit that allows custom contouring and some simulation in the absence of a molding frame (140).

Drawbacks include the short time available to mold the shape after introduction of the epoxy, limited depth for contouring, and a relatively hard finished surface that is difficult to cushion and modify effectively. Direct foam-in-place, in which foam-producing chemicals are poured into a bag placed under and around a person, forms total contact contouring around the body (141).

This method is fast, relatively inexpensive, and provides a seating surface that is comfortable and reduces interface pressure. The method has some important limitations, however. It is difficult to use direct foam-in-place with people with increased muscle tone, sensitivity to heat, or whose position is difficult to maintain. People who are large or heavy present a challenge when using traditional foam-in-place technique because of the necessity of suspending and holding them in a precise position for a period of time before the foam sets. Movement during the foaming process can disrupt the chemical reactions, causing hard spots in the surface of the foam.

Indirect foam-in-place, commercially contoured seats, and computer-generated shape sensing require use of a custom-molding frame to simulate the optimum seated position and produce a model of the person's body (142).

The amount and type of support needed, the effects of the support on muscle tone, the effects of gravity and position in space, and the ability of the system to provide the desired results over a period of time may be assessed before the final prescription is written.

Indirect foam-in-place overcomes many of the difficulties encountered using direct foam-in-place. A molding frame is used to simulate the optimal seat (Fig. 30-18). The patient is moved, and a plaster cast is made directly on the molding frame. The cast is used as the mold for the foam. This process can be completed on site, or the cast can be sent out for commercial fabrication of the product. Both methods have all the advantages of direct foam-in-place as well as the following advantages:

- Problems with patient size and movement are eliminated.
- The plaster model can be modified.

Indirect foam-in-place performed on site allows use of varied densities of foam to address skin sensitivity or pressure considerations, less waste of foam than with direct foam-in-place, completion on site, and ready modification of the completed system (142).

The disadvantages of this method lie in less durability than commercially fabricated systems and the need for rather extensive fabricating facilities and skill. Commercially fabricated systems require the plaster model to be mailed to the central fabrication facility; delivery may take several weeks. The finished product is durable and attractive but cannot be modified or refitted on site; rather, it must be returned to the company.

Computer shape sensing produces contoured seating components by use of evaluation data that are fed into a machine that produces a facsimile. One method involves use of a mechanical shape sensor in which the person sits on sensors embedded in a foam cushion. A cable is attached to the sensors, which are depressed according to the person's contours. A digital printout is produced that is optically scanned by a machine. The machine produces a finished cushion that corresponds to the contour information recorded on the printout. A different method uses a bead-filled fitting chair. A stylus is passed over the contours left in the bead bag by the person. Digitized data are produced and fed into a machine that produces a contoured cushion. These methods are designed to produce a seat that should conform directly to the person and evenly distribute pressure (106).

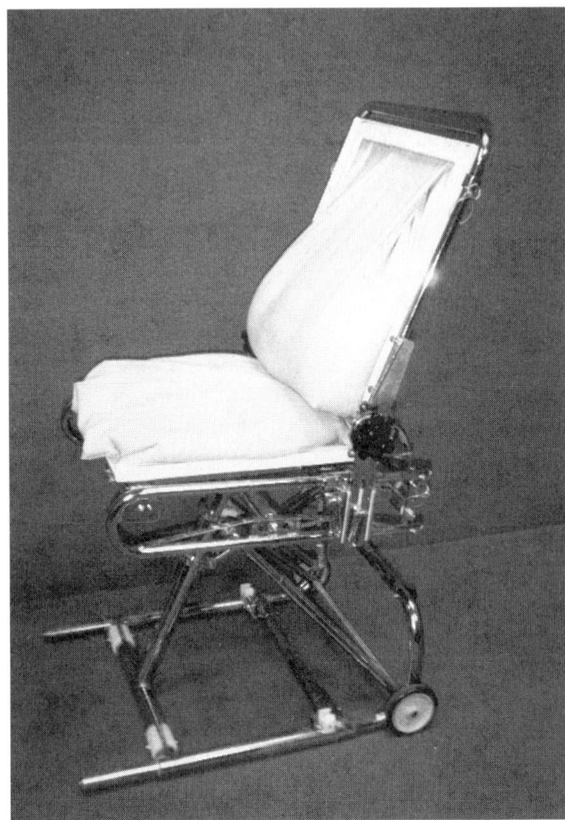

FIG. 30-18. Pin-dot molding frame (Pin Dot Products, Niles, IL) is used to simulate the optimal seat in the indirect foam-in-place method of contouring.

Position in Space

The use of multiple positions in space can enable a person with limited endurance to work and rest in the same seating system. In this discussion, the term recline refers to inclination of the seat back only. Recline is seldom used because of the problem of shear, which is only partially resolved by the use of zero-shear components. Tilt-in-space refers to changing the position in space without changing the seat-to-back angle. By using tilt-in-space, the person may work or eat in an upright or anteriorly tilted position for short periods of time (143,144), return to a neutral position, and, through additional posteriorly tilted positions, rest as needed without having to be removed from the seating system. One benefit of using variable tilt-in-space is that the schedules of people with severe disabilities and low physical endurance can be adapted to meet their medical needs. Meticulous skin care and regular positioning out of the seating system still are mandatory. Other important issues in the use of position in space include the therapeutic use of gravity, both to limit its effects on skeletal deformity and function and to assist in maintaining position and the effect of head position on primitive reflexes. Recently a few durable medical equipment manufacturers have begun to produce laterally tilting wheelchairs. Laterally tilting chairs can be used to mechanically enhance gastric emptying, provide alternate weight bearing surfaces, and use gravity to inhibit skeletal deformity.

Appropriate use of contouring and position in space can reduce the need for multiple straps, lap boards, knee blocks, and other devices used to maintain people in their seating systems. Reducing the number of these restraints can improve comfort, appearance, and function by freeing the person's arms from acting as stabilizers.

Other Considerations

Attention to appearance is very important. The minimalist approach focuses on removal of extraneous, visible parts of the wheelchair. This approach provides strength and durability, minimizes the need for restraints, and ensures a fit that allows the person, rather than the equipment, to be the focus of visual attention. This principle fosters normalization by deemphasizing adaptive devices.

Financial concerns must be considered because many insurance companies and government programs limit coverage of medical equipment. Adaptations can be made, however, to most commercial wheelchair frames to enable existing systems to meet a variety of needs. If funding cannot be procured to purchase a multioption mobility system, adaptations may be made at a reasonable cost to increase the usefulness of the existing system. It is important to address warranty status of any equipment before permanent changes are made.

Alternate Positioning Devices

No matter how well a contoured system fits a person, alternate positioning out of the wheelchair is essential for skin integrity, circulation, movement, and comfort. Alternate positioning can be as simple as moving to a standard dining room chair for meals or an easy chair for leisure activities. Alternate positioning may involve bed rest or use of customized positioning equipment (112). Depending on the severity of the patient's condition, specific night positioning may be indicated for aggressive management of deformity (145,146).

Follow-Up and Maintenance

Follow-up and maintenance are an essential part of the wheelchair evaluation and prescription. Follow-up should occur after the person has had the opportunity to use the seating or mobility system in the daily environment. This process should address both fit and functional use of the equipment. Contact between the team and patient should occur within a month even if changes are unnecessary. The first year a system is used is especially critical. Although customized positioning equipment will not change bony deformities, soft tissue changes may alter body configuration and require modifications. Children may need follow-up as often as every 3 or 4 months because of growth and their developing neuromotor status. Adult seating systems should be evaluated at least annually.

In addition to follow-up, maintenance should occur on a regular basis to ensure continued fit, usefulness, and safety of the equipment. Products constructed of foam must be checked regularly because the pressure-relieving properties of foam change over time depending on the quality of the material and the care and use of the system. Batteries must be charged and maintained according to the manufacturer's schedule to minimize expense and inconvenience. If people are unable to perform their own maintenance, these services usually are available through a local medical equipment dealer.

Special Seating Teams and Clinics

Patients with the need for specialized seating or mobility equipment are complex to evaluate and require the use of technologies that are rapidly changing. For these reasons, speciality seating clinics have developed. The models for speciality seating clinics include the use of an extensive interdisciplinary team that is center based (147), the use of a very small permanent team with flexible team members, mobile seating evaluation units (148–150), and a central clinic with satellite clinics.

Most specialized seating clinics devote 1.5 to 2 hours to the initial evaluation of the patient. The time is used for the following procedures:

- Take a history and perform the physical examination.
- Set up simulations for positioning, manual propulsion, and powered mobility.
- Set seating goals and rank them according to the priorities of the team, particularly of the patient and family.
- Try out equipment or look at pictures of equipment.
- Arrive at a final decision so that prescriptions, reports, and letters of medical necessity can be written.

Refer to a speciality seating clinic if the patient has severe neurologic involvement or orthopedic deformities, is at high risk for decubitus ulcers or has a history of recurrent decubitus ulcers, may require a complicated or specialized seating system (e.g., sports or racing chairs, extra-wide or heavy-duty chairs, tilt-in-space to provide pressure relief), has never had a satisfactory seating system in the past despite multiple attempts, or when simulations need to be set up that require the special equipment found only in the specialty seating clinic. Simulations include the use of planar simulator chairs, custom molding frames, and the use of wheelchairs with various interchangeable control systems that a severely involved client can try out. If 90° knee flexion is required in an adult because of tight hamstring muscles, the specialty team clinic can recommend technology that is available to accommodate this position and best meet other seating goals. If there simply is uncertainty about whether some other seating system or base might be better than what has been used in the past, or if the patient has special mobility or living needs dictated by a small car, small van door, small house or mobile home, or unusual architectural barriers in the home or workplace, the seating clinic can help solve problems related to these factors.

REFERENCES

1. Jebsen RH. Essentials of wheelchair prescription. *Northwest Med* 1968; 67:755–758.
2. Gray B, Hsu JD, Furumasu J. Fractures caused by falling from a wheelchair in patients with neuromuscular disease. *Dev Med Child Neurol* 1992; 34:589–592.
3. Kirby RL, Ackroyd-Stolarz SA. Wheelchair safety—adverse reports to the United States Food and Drug Administration. *Am J Phys Med Rehabil* 1995; 74:308–312.
4. Calder CJ, Kirby RL. Fatal wheelchair-related accidents in the United States. *Am J Phys Med Rehabil* 1990; 69:184–190.
5. Kirby RL, Ackroyd-Stolarz SA, Brown MG, Kirkland SA, MacLeod DA. Wheelchair-related accidents caused by tips and falls among noninstitutionalized users of manually propelled wheelchairs in Nova Scotia. *Am J Phys Med Rehabil* 1994; 73:319–330.
6. Kirby RL. Nonfatal wheelchair-related accidents reported to the National Electronic Injury Surveillance System. *Am J Phys Med Rehabil* 1994; 73:163–167.
7. Kirby RL, Coughlin SG, Christie M. Could changes in the wheelchair delivery system improve safety? *Can Med Assoc J* 1995; 153: 1585–1591.
8. Kirby RL, Ashton BD, Ackroyd-Stolarz SA, MacLeod DA. Adding loads to occupied wheelchairs: effect on static rear and forward stability. *Arch Phys Med Rehabil* 1996; 77:183–186.
9. Cooper RA, Stewart KJ, VanSickle DP. Evaluation of methods for determining rearward static stability of manual wheelchairs. *J Rehabil Res Dev* 1994; 31:144–147.
10. Kirby RL, Ackroyd-Stolarz SA, Charlebois PB. Influence of seat position on the static and dynamic forward and rear stability of occupied wheelchairs. *Arch Phys Med Rehabil* 1993; 74:977–982.
11. Kirby RL, McLean AD, Eastwood BJ. Influence of caster diameter on the static and dynamic forward stability of occupied wheelchairs. *Arch Phys Med Rehabil* 1992; 73:73–77.
12. Hunter J. Energy costs of wheelchair propulsion by elderly and disabled people. *Int J Rehabil Res* 1987; 10:50–54.
13. Kirby RL, Thoren FA, Ashton BD, Ackroyd-Stolarz SA. Wheelchair stability and maneuverability: effect of varying the horizontal and vertical position of a rear-antitip device. *Arch Phys Med Rehabil* 1994; 75:525–534.
14. Kirby RL, Atkinson SM, MacKay EA. Static and dynamic forward stability of occupied wheelchairs: influence of elevated footrests and forward stabilizers. *Arch Phys Med Rehabil* 1989; 70:681–686.
15. Taylor D, Williams T. Sports injuries in athletes with disabilities: wheelchair racing. *Paraplegia* 1995; 36:296–299.
16. Wilson PE, Washington RL. Pediatric wheelchair athletics: sports injuries and prevention. *Paraplegia* 1993; 31:330–337.
17. Janssen TW, van Oers CA, van der Woude LH, Hollander AP. Physical strain in daily life of wheelchair users with spinal cord injuries. *Med Sci Sports Exerc* 1994; 26:661–670.
18. Dozono K, Hachisuka K, Hatada K, Agata H. Peripheral neuropathies in the upper extremities of paraplegic wheelchair marathon racers. *Paraplegia* 1995; 33:208–211.
19. Burnham RS, Steadward RD. Upper extremity peripheral nerve entrapments among wheelchair athletes: prevalence, location, and risk factors. *Arch Phys Med Rehabil* 1994; 75:519–524.
20. Burnham R, Chan M, Hazlett C, Laskin J, Steadward R. Acute median nerve dysfunction from wheelchair propulsion: the development of a model and study of the effect of hand protection. *Arch Phys Med Rehabil* 1994; 75:513–518.
21. Frank TG, Abel EW. Design and evaluation of footrests for hospital wheelchairs. *J Biomed Eng* 1990; 12:333–339.
22. Clark AM, Redden JF. Management of hip posture in cerebral palsy. *J R Soc Med* 1992; 85:150–151.
23. Bergen AP, Colangelo C. *Positioning the client with central nervous system deficits: the wheelchair and other adapted equipment, 2nd ed.* Valhalla, NY: Valhalla Rehabilitation Publication, 1985.
24. Curtis KA, Kindlin CM, Reich KM, White DE. Functional reach in wheelchair users: the effects of trunk and lower extremity stabilization. *Arch Phys Med Rehabil* 1995; 76:360–367.
25. Ferguson-Pell MW, Wiklei JC, Reswich JBV, Barbenel JCP. Pressure sore prevention for the wheelchair-bound spinal cord injured patient. *Paraplegia* 1983; 18:42–51.
26. Fisher SV, Patterson R. Long term pressure recordings under the ischial tuberosities of tetraplegics. *Paraplegia* 1983; 21:99–106.
27. Springle SH, Faisant TE, Chung KC. Clinical evaluation of custom-contoured cushions for the spinal cord injured. *Arch Phys Med Rehabil* 1990; 71:655–658.
28. Garber SL, Krouskop TA. Body build and its relationship to pressure distribution in the seated wheelchair patient. *Arch Phys Med Rehabil* 1982; 63:17–20.
29. Merbitz CT, King RB, Bleiberg J. Continuous direct recording of wheelchair pressure relief behavior. *Arch Phys Med Rehabil* 1983; 64:490–491.
30. Pritham CH, Leiper CI. A method for custom seating of the severely disabled. *Orthot Prosthet* 1981; 35:19–26.
31. Hobson DA. Comparative effects of posture on pressure and shear at the body–seat interface. *J Rehabil Res Dev* 1992; 29:21–31.
32. Koo TK, Mak AF, Lee YL. Posture effect on seating interface biomechanics: comparison between two seating cushions. *Arch Phys Med Rehabil* 1996; 77:40–47.
33. Park CA. Activity positioning and ischial tuberosity pressure: a pilot study. *Am J Occup Ther* 1992; 46:904–909.
34. Todd BA, Thacker JG. Three-dimensional computer model of the human buttocks, *in vivo*. *J Rehabil Res Dev* 1994; 31:111–119.
35. Kwiatkowski RJ, Inigo RM. A closed loop automated seating system. *J Rehabil Res Dev* 1993; 30:393–404.
36. White GW, Mathews RM, Fawcett SB. Reducing risk of pressure sores: effects of watch prompts and alarm avoidance on wheelchair push-ups. *J Appl Behav Anal* 1989; 22:287–295.
37. Newsam CJ, Mulroy SJ, Gronley JK, Bontrager EL, Perry J. Temporal–spatial characteristics of wheelchair propulsion. Effects of level of spinal cord injury, terrain, and propulsion rate. *Am J Phys Med Rehabil* 1996; 75:292–299.
38. Hughes CH, Weimar WH, Sheth PN, Brubaker CE. Biomechanics of wheelchair propulsion as a function of seat position and user-to-chair interface. *Arch Phys Med Rehabil* 1992; 73:263–269.
39. Stoboy H, Rich BW, Lee M. Workload and energy expenditure during wheelchair propelling. *Paraplegia* 1971; 8:223–230.
40. Bednarczyk JH, Sanderson DJ. Limitations of kinematics in the assessent of wheelchair propulsion in adults and children with spinal cord injury. *Phys Ther* 1995; 75:281–289.
41. Ruggles DL, Cahalan T, An KN. Biomechanics of wheelchair propulsion by able-bodied subjects. *Arch Phys Med Rehabil* 1994; 75: 540–544.
42. Brubaker CE. Wheelchair prescription: an analysis of factors that affect mobility and performance. *J Rehabil Res Dev* 1986; 23:19–26.
43. Masse LC, Lamontagne M, O'Riain MD. Biomechanical analysis of wheelchair propulsion for various seating positions. *J Rehabil Res Dev* 1992; 29:12–28.
44. Gordon J, Kauslarich JJ, Thacker JG. Tests of two new polyurethane foam wheelchair tires. *J Rehabil Res Dev* 1989; 26:33–46.
45. Gaines RF, La WH. Users' responses to contoured wheelchair handrims. *J Rehabil Res Dev* 1986; 23:57–62.
46. O'Connell DG, Barnhart R. Improvement in wheelchair propulsion in pediatric wheelchair uers through resistance training: a pilot study. *Arch Phys Med Rehabil* 1995; 76:368–372.

47. Cron L, Sprigle S. Clinical evaluation of the hemi wheelchair cushion. *Am J Occup Ther* 1993; 47:141–144.
48. Van der Woude LH, van Kranen E, Ariens G, Rozendal RH, Veeger HE. Physical strain and mechanical efficiency in hubcrank and handrim wheelchair propulsion. *J Med Eng Tech* 1995; 19:123–131.
49. Van der Woude LH, Veeger HE, de Boer Y, Rozendal RH. Physiological evaluation of a newly designed lever mechanism for wheelchhairs. *J Med Eng Tech* 1993; 17:232–240.
50. Hughes CJ, Weimar WH, Sheth PN, Brubaker CE. Biomechanics of wheelchair propulsion as a function of seat position and user-to-chair interface. *Arch Phys Med Rehabil* 1992; 73:263–269.
51. Wakaumi H, Nakamura K, Matsumura T. Development of an automated wheelchair guided by a magnetic ferrite marker lane. *J Rehabil Res Dev* 1992; 29:27–34.
52. Lawton MP, Mass M, Fulcomer M, Kleban MH. A research and service oriented multi-level assessment instrument. *J Gerontol* 1982; 37: 91–99.
53. Stewart CP, Carus DA, Kerr G. Development of a universal wheelchair narrower. *Prosthet Orthot Int* 1989; 13:39–41.
54. Marks J. Wheelchairs and vans: do they belong together? In: *Proceedings of the annual assembly of the American Academy of Physical Medicine and Rehabilitation*, Orlando, FL, Oct 18–23, 1987. Chicago: American Academy of Physical Medicine and Rehabilitation, 1987; 256–269.
55. Letts RM. *Principles of seating the disabled.* Boca Raton, FL: CRC Press, 1991.
56. Bleck EE. Orthopaedic management in cerebral palsy. *Clin Dev Med* 1987; 99/100:52–53.
57. Farber SD. *Neurorehabilitation: a multisensory approach.* Philadelphia: WB Saunders, 1982; 248–258.
58. Hulme JB, Gallacher K, Walsh J, Niesen S, Waldron D. Behavioral and postural changes observed with use of adaptive seating devices by clients with multiple handicaps. *Phys Ther* 1987; 67:1060–1067.
59. Hoffer M. Basic considerations and classifications of cerebral palsy. In: Stolov WC, Clowers MR, eds. *Handbook of severe deformity.* Washington, D.C.: United States Department of Education, Rehabilitation Services Administration, 1981; 96–102.
60. Mulcahy CM. An approach to the assessment of sitting ability. *Br J Occup Ther* 1986; 49:368.
61. Kendall FP, Kendall-McCreary E. *Muscles testing and function, 3rd ed.* Baltimore: Williams & Wilkins, 1983.
62. Hobson DA, Trefler E. Towards matching needs with technical approaches in specialized seating. In: *Proceedings of the second international conference on rehabilitation engineering.* Ottawa: RESNA, 1984; 486–488.
63. Boehme R. *Improving upper body control.* Tucson, AZ: Communication Skill Builders, 1988.
64. Hundermark LM. Evaluating the adult with cerebral palsy for specialized adaptive seating. *Phys Ther* 1985; 65:209–212.
65. Nwaobi OM. Effects of body orientation in space on tonic muscle activity of patients with cerebral palsy. *Dev Med Child Neurol* 1986; 28(4):41–44.
66. Monahan LC, Taylor SJ, Shaw CG. Pelvic positioning: another option. In: *Proceedings of the fifth international seating symposium: seating the disabled.* Memphis, TN: University of Tennessee, Rehabilitation Engineering Program, 1989; 32–38.
67. Hardwick KD, Feichtinger L. Issues in evaluation and fabrication of seating mobility systems for multiply handicapped individuals. In: *Proceedings of the seventh international seating symposium: seating the disabled.* Memphis, TN: University of Tennessee, Rehabilitation Engineering Program, 1991; 75–78.
68. Eberle CF. Pelvic obliquity and the unstable hip after poliomyelitis. In: *Proceedings of the third international symposium: seating the disabled.* Memphis, TN: University of Tennessee Center for the Health Sciences, Rehabilitation Engineering Program, 1987; 300–304.
69. Henderson B. *Seating in review: current trends for the disabled, 4th ed.* Winnipeg: Otto Bock, 1989.
70. Samilson RL, Bechard R. Scoliosis in cerebral palsy: incidence, distribution of curve patterns, natural history, and thoughts on etiology. *Curr Pract Orthop Surg* 1973; 5:183–205.
71. Ward D. *Positioning the handicapped child for function, 2nd ed. (rev).* St Louis: Phoenix Press, 1984.
72. Fraser BA, Hensinger RN, Phelps JA. *Physical management of multiple handicaps: a professional guide, 2nd ed.* Baltimore: Paul H. Brookes, 1990.
73. Letts M. Seating the disabled. In: *Proceedings of the third international symposium: seating the disabled.* Memphis, TN: University of Tennessee Center for the Health Sciences, Rehabilitation Engineering Program, 1987; 7–23.
74. Letts M, Shapiro L, Mulder K, Klassen O. The windblown hip syndrome in total body cerebral palsy. *J Pediatr Orthop* 1984; 4:55–62.
75. Tredwell SJ. The basic approach to seating. In: *Proceedings of the fourth international seating symposium (syllabus).* Vancouver: Division of Continuing Education in the Health Sciences, University of British Columbia, 1988; 60–69.
76. Benson DR. The back: thoracic and lumbar spine. In: D'Ambrosia RP, ed. *Musculoskeletal disorders: regional examination and differential diagnosis.* New Orleans: Louisiana State University, School of Medicine, Department of Orthopaedic Surgery, 1986; 287–365.
77. Nwaobi OM, Smith P. Effect of adaptive seating on pulmonary function in children with cerebral palsy. In: *Proceedings of the RESNA ninth annual conference.* Minneapolis, MN: RESNA, 1986; 384–385.
78. O'Brien M, Tsurumi K. The effect of two body positions on head righting in severely disabled individuals with cerebral palsy. *Am J Occup Ther* 1983; 37:673–680.
79. Nwaobi OM, Brubaker CE, Cusick B, Sussman MD. Electromyography investigation of extensor activity in cerebral palsied children in different seating programs. *Dev Med Child Neurol* 1983; 25:175–183.
80. Taylor SJ. Evaluating the client with physical disabilities for wheelchair seating. *Am J Occup Ther* 1987; 41:71–76.
81. Trefler E, Taylor S. Decision making guidelines for seating children with cerebral palsy. In: Trefler E, Tooms RE, Hobson DA, eds. *Seating for children with cerebral palsy: a resource manual.* Memphis, TN: University of Tennessee Center for the Health Sciences, Rehabilitation Engineering Program, 1984; 55–76.
82. Nwaobi O, Hobson D, Trefler E. Hip angle and upper extremity movement time for children with cerebral palsy. In: *Proceedings of the RESNA eighth annual conference.* Memphis, TN: RESNA, 1985; 39–41.
83. Nwaobi OM. Seating orientations and upper extremity function in children with cerebral palsy. *Phys Ther* 1987; 67:1209–1212.
84. Nwaobi OM, Cusick B. The effect of hip flexion angle on the electrical activity of the hip adductors in cerebral-palsied children. Unpublished report, cited in Nwaobi OM. Effects of body orientation in space on tonic muscle activity of patients with cerebral palsy. *Dev Med Child Neurol* 1986; 28(4):41–44.
85. Nwaobi OM. Nondominant arm restraint and dominant arm function in a child with athetoid cerebral palsy: electromyographic and functional evaluation. *Arch Phys Med Rehabil* 1987; 68:837–839.
86. Trefler E. Arm restraints during functional activities. *Am J Occup Ther* 1982; 67:599–600.
87. Stokes IAF, Abery JM. Influence of the hamstring muscles on lumbar spine curvature in sitting. *Spine* 1980; 5:525–528.
88. Currie DM, Ysla R. Electric cart modification for boy with hip extension contractures. *Arch Phys Med Rehabil* 1982; 63:588–589.
89. Trefler E, Hobson D, Taylor S, Monahan L, Shaw G. *Seating and mobility for persons with physical disabilities.* Tucson: Therapy Skill Builders, 1993.
90. Allen VR. Basic considerations in adapted equipment design. In: *Proceedings of the second international conference on rehabilitation engineering.* Ottawa: RESNA, 1984; 316–317.
91. Hill JP, Presperin J. Deformity control. In: Intagliata S, ed. *Spinal cord injury: a guide to functional outcomes in occupational therapy. Rehabilitation Institute of Chicago procedure manual.* Rockville, MD: Rehabilitation Institute of Chicago, 1986; 49–85.
92. Hulme JB, Shaver J, Archer S, Mullette L, Eggert C. Effects of adaptive seating devices on the eating and drinking of children with multiple handicaps. *Am J Occup Ther* 1987; 41:81–89.
93. Murphy TE. The positioner chair: a classroom chair for children with a forward tilting seating. In: *Proceedings of the fifth international seating symposium: seating the disabled.* Memphis, TN: University of Tennessee, Rehabilitation Engineering Program, 1989; 23–28.
94. LeVine SP, Borenstein J, Koren Y. The Navchair control system for automatic assistive wheelchair navigation. In: Presperin JJ, ed. *Proceedings of the 13th annual conference on rehabilitation engineering.* Washington, D.C.: RESNA, 1990; 193–194.

95. Caudrey DJ, O'Mara NA. Hand function in cerebral palsy: the effect of hip flexion angle. *Dev Med Child Neurol* 1984; 26:601–606.
96. Wright C, Nomura M. Positioning and motor control. *The Exceptional Parent* 1985; 15:40–42.
97. Myhr U, von Wendt L. Improvement of functional sitting position for children with cerebral palsy. *Dev Med Child Neurol* 1991; 33: 246–256.
98. Stout JP, Bull MJ, Stroup KB. Safe transport for children with disabilities. *Am J Occup Ther* 1989; 43:31–36.
99. Shaw G. Vehicular transport safety for the child with disabilities. *Am J Occup Ther* 1987; 41:35–42.
100. Bossingham DH. Wheelchairs and appliances. *Clin Rheum Dis* 1981; 7:395–415.
101. Bossingham DH, Russell P. The usefulness of powered wheelchairs in advanced inflammatory polyarthritis. *Rheumatol Rehabil* 1980; 19: 131–135.
102. Butler C. Effects of powered mobility on self-initiated behaviors of very young children with locomotor disability. *Dev Med Child Neurol* 1986; 28:325–332.
103. Butler C. Powered mobility for very young disabled children. *Dev Med Child Neurol* 1983; 25:472–474.
104. Chase J, Bailey DM. Evaluating the potential for powered mobility. *Am J Occup Ther* 1990; 44:1125–1129.
105. Cremers GB. Hybrid-powered wheelchair: a combination of arm force and electrical power for propelling a wheelchair. *J Med Eng Technol* 1989; 13:142–148.
106. Marinic J, McAdam W, Pizey G, Slagerman M. Otto Bock shape system for seating. In: *Proceedings of the seventh international seating symposium: seating the disabled.* Memphis, TN: University of Tennessee Center for the Health Sciences, Rehabilitation Engineering Program, 1991; 103–105.
107. Barker MR, Hastings W, Flanagan K. The control evaluator and training kit: an assessment tool for comparative testing of controls. In: *Proceedings of the sixth annual comference on rehabilitation engineering.* Washington, D.C.: RESNA, 1983; 159.
108. Kauzlarich JJ. Wheelchair batteries: II. Capacity, sizing and life. *J Rehabil Res Dev* 1990; 27:163–170.
109. DeLisa JA, Greenberg S. Wheelchair prescription guidelines. *Am Fam Physician* 1982; 25:145–150.
110. Britell CW. Wheelchair prescription. In: Kottke FJ, Lehmann JF, eds. *Krusen's handbook of physical medicine and rehabilitation, 4th ed.* Philadelphia: WB Saunders, 1990; 548–563.
111. Letts RM. *Principles of seating the disabled.* Boca Raton, FL: CRC Press, 1991.
112. Pope PM, Booth E, Gosling G. The development of alternative seating and mobility systems. *Physiother Pract* 1988; 4:78–93.
113. Holte RN. A brief guide to postural seating technology. In: Enders A, ed. *Technology for independent living sourcebook.* Bethesda, MD: RESNA, 1984; 159–162.
114. Jones CK. The use of molded techniques for fitting C5-6 spinal cord injured five or more years post injury. In: *Proceedings of the third international symposium: seating the disabled.* Memphis, TN: University of Tennessee Center for the Health Sciences, Rehabilitation Engineering Program, 1987; 189–192.
115. Montgomery PC, Cashin H. Seating device for multiply handicapped infants. *Phys Ther* 1985; 65:1069–1070.
116. Nwaobi OM. Biomechanics of seating. In: Trefler E, ed. *Seating for children with cerebral palsy: a resource manual.* Memphis, TN: University of Tennessee Center for the Health Sciences, Rehabilitation Engineering Program, 1984; 37–54.
117. Forbes MJ, Holte RN, Paul IT, Vankampen E. A comparison of three custom seating techniques. In: *Proceedings of the international conference in rehabilitation engineering.* Toronto: RESNA, 1980; 147–152.
118. Ford F. Neuromotor function as it relates to therapeutic seating. In: Trefler E, ed. *Seating for children with cerebral palsy: a resource manual.* Memphis, TN: University of Tennessee Center for the Health Sciences, Rehabilitation Engineering Program, 1984; 10–23.
119. Pope PM. A study of instability in relation to posture in the wheelchair. *Physiotherapy* 1985; 71:124–136.
120. Shaw G, Monahan L, Taylor S, Wyatte D. Peak seating pressure for institutionalized elderly wheelchair users. In: *Proceedings of the seventh international seating symposium: seating the disabled.* Memphis, TN: University of Tennessee, Rehabilitation Engineering Program, 1991; 151–156.
121. Shields RK, Cook TM. Effect of seat angle and lumbar support on seated buttock pressure. *Phys Ther* 1988; 68:682–686.
122. Siegel IM, Silverman M. Fully contoured seating for the wheelchair-bound patient with neuromuscular disease. *Phys Ther* 1983; 63: 1625–1626.
123. Trefler E, Hanks S, Huggins P, Chiarizzo S, Hobson D. A modular seating system for cerebral-palsied children. *Dev Med Child Neurol* 1978; 20:199–204.
124. Trefler E, Nickey J, Hobson DA. Technology in the education of multiply handicapped children. *Am J Occup Ther* 1983; 37:381–397.
125. Trefler E, Monahan L, Nwaobi OM. Functional arm restraint for children with athetoid cerebral palsy. In: *Proceedings of the RESNA ninth annual conference.* Minneapolis, MN: RESNA, 1986; 60–61.
126. Jones SL. Issues to consider for postural health. *Physiother Can* 1988; 40:172–174.
127. Krouskop TA, Garber SL, Pugh S. Issues in seating and positioning spinal cord injured persons. In: *Proceedings of the third international symposium: seating the disabled.* Memphis, TN: University of Tennessee, Rehabilitation Engineering Program, 1987; 176–184.
128. Chari VR, Kirby RL. Lower limb influence on sitting balance while reaching forward. *Arch Phys Med Rehabil* 1986; 67:730–733.
129. Hilbers PA, White TP. Effects of wheelchair design on metabolic and heart rate responses during propulsion by persons with paraplegia. *Phys Ther* 1987; 67:1355–1398.
130. Medhat MA. Terminology for positioning, seating and chair systems parameters. In: *Proceedings of the fifth international seating symposium: seating the disabled.* Memphis, TN: University of Tennessee, Rehabilitation Engineering Program, 1989; 120.
131. Bleck EE. Orthopaedic management in cerebral palsy. *Clin Dev Med* 1987; 99/100:186–190.
132. Brunswic M. Ergonomics of seat design. *Physiotherapy* 1984; 70: 40–43.
133. Carlson JM, Lonstein J, Beck KO, Wilkie DC. Seating for children and young adults with cerebral palsy. *Clin Prosthet Orthot* 1987; 11(3):137–158.
134. Mulcahy CM, Pountney TE. The sacral pad. *Physiotherapy* 1986; 72: 473–474.
135. Nwaobi OM, Smith P. Effect of adaptive seating on pulmonary function of children with cerebral palsy. *Dev Med Child Neurol* 1986; 28: 351–354.
136. Cullen CA. Contoured components on adaptive seating devices. *Clin Manage* 1985; 6(5):12–15.
137. Moore S, Bergman JS, Edwards G, Cowsar D, Echols SD, Forbes J. The DESEMO customized seating support: custom-molded seating for severely disabled persons. *Phys Ther* 1982; 62:460–463.
138. Cooper DG, Hawkes E. The MERU shapeable matrix support surface for children and adults. In: *Proceedings of the second international conference on rehabilitation engineering.* Ottawa: RESNA, 1984; 475–476.
139. Hobson DA, Taylor S, Shaw G. The bead matrix insert system: a four year follow up clinical report. In: *Proceedings of the third international symposium: seating the disabled.* Memphis, TN: University of Tennessee Center for the Health Sciences, Rehabilitation Engineering Program, 1987; 70–74.
140. Wengert ME, Margolis SA. Application of a foam-in-place seated positioning system for the non-ambulatory elderly. In: *Proceedings of the fifth international seating symposium: seating the disabled.* Memphis, TN: University of Tennessee, Rehabilitation Engineering Program, 1989; 197–199.
141. Shapcott N, Bar C. Seating simulation as an aid to assessment. In: *Proceedings of the RESNA thirteenth annual conference.* Washington, D.C.: RESNA, 1990; 111–112.
142. Hardwick KD, Feichtinger L. Innovative uses of existing technology. In: *Proceedings of the RESNA thirteenth annual conference.* Washington, D.C.: RESNA, 1990; 407–408.
143. Bendix T, Biering-Sorensen F. Posture of the trunk when sitting on forward inclining seats. *Scand J Rehabil Med* 1983; 15:197–203.
144. Post KM, Murphy TE. The use of forward sloping seats by individuals with disabilities. In: *Proceedings of the fifth international seating symposium: seating the disabled.* Memphis, TN: University of Tennessee, Rehabilitation Engineering Program, 1989; 54–60.

145. Bell EJ. Management and prevention of certain deformities in cerebral palsy. *Physiotherapy* 1987; 73:368–370.
146. Chevez JV. The impact of OBRA '87 guidelines on resident body positioning in long-term-care facilities. *Gerontology (Spec int sect newslett)* 1991; 14:1–4.
147. Shapcott N, Kessel M, Hobson D. Service delivery at the University of Tennessee Rehabilitation Engineering Program. In: *Proceedings of the RESNA ninth annual conference.* Minneapolis, MN: RESNA, 1986; 148–150.
148. Dodds R. Rehabilitation technology services: a mobile rehabilitation engineering department. In: *Proceedings of the RESNA tenth annual conference.* San Jose, CA: RESNA, 1987; 13–14.
149. Anderson MA, Anderson LL. Rehabilitation technology service delivery utilizing a mobile system: the Kansas model. In: *Proceedings of the RESNA twelfth annual conference.* New Orleans, LA: RESNA, 1989; 214–215.
150. Mundy P, Phripp T. A service delivery model for the provision of specialized seating. In: *Proceedings of the RESNA ninth annual conference.* Minneapolis, MN: RESNA, 1986; 137–139.

Rehabilitation Medicine: Principles and Practice, Third Edition,
edited by Joel A. DeLisa and Bruce M. Gans.
Lippincott–Raven Publishers, Philadelphia © 1998.

CHAPTER 31

Pharmacotherapy of Disability

Todd P. Stitik, Robert Klecz, Ross O. Zafonte, and David S. Klein

A variety of medications from diverse classes are used by the practicing physiatrist. Although this chapter does not purport to be an all-inclusive detailed source of information on each and every medication used by physiatrists, it has been written in enough detail that the practitioner can conveniently locate useful information on common physiatric applications, the mechanism of action, basic pharmacokinetics, relevant dosing, side effects, and drug interactions for many of them. Although most of the medications are widely used in other areas of medicine and therefore are not exclusive to physical medicine and rehabilitation, they are discussed as much as possible as they uniquely pertain to this field. Much of the information has been put into tabular form so that it is user friendly and provides the rehabilitation specialist with one focused source to refer to rather than one that provides very general information in which the relevant details must be sorted out. Although the tables list most of the medications from the various categories, all of them could not be included because of space constraints.

Even though many medications are at times mentioned by their specific trade names, and certain biases based on the authors experiences are presented, this does not necessarily endorse the use of one product over another.

ANALGESICS

Perhaps the major theme in many outpatient physiatric practices is the treatment of pain from various musculoskeletal injuries and conditions, and pain caused by neurogenic disorders. Thus, the physiatrist should be very familiar with analgesics. Although analgesics have been grouped into specific categories according to use (Table 31-1), there is a large degree of overlap.

Analgesic Agents Typically Used for Musculoskeletal Pain

Analgesic medications that are generally used for pain of musculoskeletal etiology include acetaminophen, narcotic analgesics, nonsteroidal anti-inflammatory drugs (NSAIDs), and tramadol (Ultram). Of these, NSAIDs are the most commonly used medications worldwide (1), and their use will probably become even more widespread now that some of the more popular anti-inflammatories have become available over the counter. In attempting to self-medicate, however, patients are often confused as to the exact class of medication they are taking. A common misconception among patients is that they are taking a muscle relaxant when, in reality, they are taking an over-the-counter NSAID. Tylenol, the most popular form of acetaminophen, has gained acceptance as an analgesic especially for patients with arthritis with the publication of an article that compared it with NSAIDs for the treatment of pain of osteoarthritis (2). There has been a recent surge in the use of narcotics for the treatment of chronic pain conditions. Tramadol is still finding its place into everyday practice and may very well become one of the most commonly prescribed analgesics in the United States as it has in parts of Europe.

Acetaminophen (Tylenol)

Relevance to Physiatry

Although acetaminophen is unsatisfactory as a single agent in patients requiring a powerful analgesic, it can be an excellent yet often forgotten adjuvant medication or primary medication for mild to moderate painful conditions. It ap-

T. P. Stitik: Department of Physical Medicine and Rehabilitation, University of Medicine and Dentistry of New Jersey, New Jersey Medical School; and Doctors Office Center, Newark, New Jersey 07103.
R. Klecz: River Edge, New Jersey 07661.
R. O. Zafonte: Traumatic Brain Injury Unit, Department of Physical Medicine and Rehabilitation, Wayne State University, Rehabilitation Institute of Michigan, Detroit, Michigan 48201.
D. S. Klein: Shenandoah Valley Pain Clinic, Staunton, Virginia 24461.

TABLE 31-1. *Analgesics and other agents used to manage pain*

Agents generally used for musculoskeletal pain	Agents generally used for neurogenic pain
Acetaminophen	Capsaicin (Zostrix)
Muscle relaxants	Carbamazepine (Tegretol)
Narcotic analgesics	Gabapentin (Neurontin)
Nonsteroidal anti-inflammatory drugs (NSAIDs)	Mexitil (Mexilitene)
Tramadol (Ultram)	Phenytoin (Dilantin)
	Tricyclic antidepressants

pears to have a good role in patients with osteoarthritis who require long-term analgesic use (2). This is particularly true in the later stages of osteoarthritis, where underlying inflammation is probably not playing a major role. It can be extremely valuable for patients who can not tolerate the gastrointestinal (GI) side effects of NSAIDs and in whom the dizziness associated with tramadol or the various side effects with narcotics are interfering with rehabilitation. It is often used in the pediatric rehabilitation setting because it is not associated with Reye syndrome.

Acetaminophen is also combined with various narcotic analgesics as well as with butalbital and caffeine (Fioricet or Esgic). These later two agents are used for the treatment of headaches.

Mechanism of Action and Pharmacokinetics

Although acetaminophen, like the NSAIDs, inhibits the cyclooxygenase enzyme and thereby diminishes prostaglandin synthesis, it is unclear why acetaminophen fails to exert antiinflammatory effects. Because it has comparable analgesic and antipyretic effects, however, it has been proposed that acetaminophen preferentially inhibits central nervous system (CNS) prostaglandins without affecting prostaglandin levels at peripheral sites of inflammation (3).

Rapid and almost complete absorption occurs from the upper gastrointestinal tract. Part of the drug is bound by plasma proteins, but the unbound portion exerts the therapeutic effects. Metabolism then occurs in the liver, and excretion is via the kidney.

Preparations and Dosing

Tylenol is by far the most popular brand of acetaminophen; thus, the trade name Tylenol is very often used interchangeably with the generic term acetaminophen. Tylenol is dosed at 325 mg to 650 mg q4h prn, whereas extra-strength Tylenol (ES-Tylenol) contains 500 mg of acetaminophen and is dosed at 500 mg q3h or 1,000 mg q6h. The maximum allowable daily dose in a patient with normal hepatic function is 4 g (12 regular-strength or 8 extra-strength Tylenol tablets). It is also available as a capsule, gel cap, liquid, and suppository.

Relevant Side Effects and Drug Interactions

Unlike aspirin, there seems to be no association between usual therapeutic doses of acetaminophen and GI irritation. When it is taken in excess (15 g or more), an intermediary substance of metabolism (N-acetylbenzoquinoneimine) can induce fatal hepatic necrosis via its action on particular hepatic proteins. In addition, renal toxicity, hepatic toxicity, and thrombocytopenia can occur in patients who can not clear the drug normally because of renal and/or hepatic impairment. Acetaminophen has never been associated with Reye syndrome, and, in contrast to adults, overdosage in children less than 6 years of age is rarely associated with hepatotoxicity.

Unlike aspirin, it does not antagonize the effects of uricosuric agents, but large doses can potentiate the effect of oral anticoagulants.

Narcotic Analgesics

Relevance to Physiatry

Narcotic analgesics are also known as opiate or opioid analgesics because some are derived from opium. They comprise the most potent and the most potentially dangerous class of analgesics. They are generally indicated for moderate to severe pain, especially that which is dull and constant rather than sharp and intermittent. Although these agents are particularly effective when given at constant intervals rather than on a prn basis, they have been utilized quite successfully in patient-controlled analgesia systems. Other pertinent physiatric uses include the control of diarrhea and cough, particularly in patients with a nonproductive cough that is interfering with sleep and thus with rehabilitation efforts. Potential side effects, which are discussed in more detail below, can impact on a patient's ability to participate in a rehabilitation program.

Mechanism of Action and Pharmacokinetics

There are three separate families of endogenous opioids: endorphins, enkephalins, and dynorphins; and three primary opioid receptor types: mu, kappa, and delta. Each of the receptors has a different distribution within the CNS and can cause slightly different physiological responses when it is activated. Although the exact biochemical alterations that follow the drug–receptor binding are not completely clear, the basic mechanism of analgesia is inhibition of pain impulse transmission to higher centers and alteration of the patient's perception of pain. Narcotic analgesics can be classified on the basis of their interaction with the receptor, i.e., agonist, antagonist, and mixed agonist/antagonist.

Several different routes of administration can be employed and include the oral (PO), intramuscular (IM), intravenous (IV), subcutaneous (SC), intranasal, and transdermal routes. Most drug metabolism then occurs in the liver, but some also occurs in the kidney, lung, and central nervous system. Metabolites are ultimately excreted into the urine. Short-acting agents generally peak in 30 to 60 minutes and last 4 hours, whereas sustained-release agents peak by 2 to 3 hours and last 12 hours.

Preparations and Dosing

A generally accepted strategy when administering narcotic analgesics is to use a short-acting preparation in order to titrate the dose before starting a long-acting agent. Long-acting agents will obviously be more convenient for patients, and their sustained effect should help to prevent the peaks and troughs in serum medication concentrations that are inherent with short-acting medications. By maintaining analgesic efficacy through the night, long-acting medications could also help prevent awakening by pain, thus allowing patients to get an otherwise uninterrupted night of sleep, which should help with a rehabilitation program. Some of the narcotic preparations of particular importance to the physiatrist, along with their usual dosage ranges and relative potencies (where known and where applicable), are shown in Table 31-2 and are discussed below. Because of significant first-pass metabolism with oral dosing, required oral doses are larger than parenteral ones.

Codeine Preparations

In addition to its use as a mild to moderately strong analgesic, codeine is a powerful antitussive. After oral, IM, or SC administration, it is partly demethylated to morphine and partly converted to norcodeine. These compounds are then conjugated in the liver, and most are excreted into the urine. Adverse effects are typical of other narcotics with perhaps a somewhat increased frequency of CNS side effects. In addition, some codeine-containing preparations such as the various forms of Tylenol with codeine contain sodium metabisulfite, a preservative notorious for its propensity to cause allergic reactions including anaphylaxis in susceptible patients. Thus, codeine *per se* is not infrequently mistakenly identified as the allergen by the patient or physician.

Fentanyl Transdermal (Duragesic)

Fentanyl is a powerful opioid agonist that can be delivered transdermally using a patch that lasts for 72 hours or transmucosally by a lollipop formulation (Fentanyl Oralet) that has recently been developed. The fentanyl patch is generally used in patients with chronic pain syndromes who can not be managed with nonopioids or prn dosing of short-acting

TABLE 31-2. *Narcotic analgesics*

Narcotic class/subclass/generic (trade) name	Usual dosage range (time in hours)	Relative potency PO (IM)
Agonists		
Codeine	15–60 mg PO q4–6; 15–60 mg IM q4–6	200 (120)
Fentanyl transdermal (Duragesic patch)	1 patch q72	
Hydromorphone (Dilaudid)	2 mg PO q4–6; 3 mg PR q6–8	1.5
Meperidine (Demerol)	1–1.8 mg/kg PO or IM q3–4 up to 150 mg	300 (75)
Morphine sulfate elixir (Roxanol)	10–30 mg PO q4	60
Morphine sulfate, sustained release (MS Contin)	30 mg PO q8–12	60
Oxycodone, immediate release (OxyIR; Roxicodone)	5 mg PO q6	30
Oxycodone, sustained release (Oxycontin)	10–40 mg PO q12	30
Propoxyphene (Darvon, Dolene)	65 mg PO q4	130
Partial agonists		
Butorphanol nasal spray (Stadol NS)	1 mg (1 spray per nostril) q3–4	
Pentazocine (Talwin NX) (Pentazocine 50 mg and Naloxone 0.5 mg)	1 tab PO q3–4	N/A
Analgesic combinations		
Narcotic/acetaminophen		
Darvocet (propoxyphene/acetaminophen) (N-50, 50/325 mg; N-100, 100/650 mg)	1–2 tabs PO q4	N/A
Lortab (hydrocodone/acetaminophen) (2.5/500 mg, 5/500 mg, 7.5/500 mg)	1–2 tabs PO q4–6	N/A
Lorcet (hydrocodone/acetaminophen) (5/500 mg)	1 tab PO q6	N/A
Percocet (oxycodone/acetaminophen) (5/325 mg)	1 tab PO q6	N/A
Tylenol with codeine tabs (Tylenol/codeine) (Tylenol #2, 300/15 mg; #3, 300/30 mg; #4, 300/60 mg)	1–2 tabs PO q4–6	N/A
Vicodin (hydrocodone/acetaminophen) (5/500 mg), Vicodin-ES (7.5/750 mg)	1–2 tabs PO q4–6, or 1 tab PO q4–6 (ES)	N/A
Narcotic/aspirin		
Darvon (propoxyphene/ASA/caffeine) (65/389/32.4 mg)	1 tab PO q4	N/A
Percodan (oxycodone/aspirin) (5/325 mg)	1 tab PO q6	N/A

IM, intramuscular; PO, oral.

Modified from Green SM, ed. *The 1997 Tarascon pocket pharmacopoeia.* Loma Linda, CA: Tarascon Publishing, 1997; and Levy MH. *Pharmacologic management of cancer pain.* Philadelphia: WB Saunders, 1994.

opioids. Because of its potential for significant respiratory depression, its rather slow onset of action, and the fact that its side effects may not be as easily reversible as those of oral narcotics, it should not be used for acute pain syndromes. In addition, when opioid therapy is initiated, the lowest dose (25 μg/hr) should be selected. Other available doses are as follows: 50 μg/hr (5.0 mg); 75 μg/hr (7.5 mg); 100 μg/hr (10 mg). For patients who are already on opioids, the opioid dose should be expressed in terms of the equianalgesic morphine dose (Table 31-2), and this should then be converted to the equivalent Duragesic dose as can be determined by looking this up in a standard table. In addition, the physiatrist should become familiar with other details of Duragesic use including dosage titrations, the concomitant use of other analgesics, and weaning patients from the patch. It can be subject to abuse because, although the patch is inactivated when it is removed from the skin and is therefore not transferrable between patients, it can serve as a drug reservoir, as the liquid medication can be withdrawn from the patch by using a tuberculin syringe.

Meperidine (Demerol)

There are at least two reasons why neither oral nor parenteral meperidine is a preferred narcotic. First, it has a short duration of action and thus necessitates frequent dosing with the inherent peaks and troughs in serum concentrations. Secondly, normeperidine, a toxic metabolite that can provoke seizures and other forms of central nervous system excitation such as anxiety, tremors, and myoclonus, accumulates with prolonged use (more than several days), particularly in patients with compromised renal function. In fact, normeperidine accumulates just as much with oral doses as with IV doses, even though oral doses have only about 25% of the analgesic effect. Unfortunately, naloxone (Narcan) not only fails to reverse these effects but may actually worsen them.

Oxycodone Preparations

Oxycodone is a morphine derivative that is found in several combination analgesic products and is now also available in a short-acting immediate-release form and in a longacting form. OxyIr is the immediate-release form of oxycodone HCl (5-mg doses), whereas Oxycontin is the long-acting oxycodone preparation. In patients undergoing rehabilitation programs, OxyIr, like MsIR, can be used to premedicate patients 1 hour before their therapy session. It can also be used to treat breakthrough pain at one-fourth to one-third the 12-hour dose of Oxycontin. When it is used in this fashion, if more than two rescue doses are needed in any 24-hour period, one should strongly consider increasing the dose of Oxycontin. Unlike fixed-combination opioid analgesics that are combined with acetaminophen or aspirin, Oxycontin is not limited by the potential for toxicity associated with increasing doses of aspirin or acetaminophen. Besides the obvious advantages of having a long half-life, it should be better tolerated because more constant blood levels are maintained, whereas narcotic side effects in general are most often associated with high peak serum drug levels.

Partial Agonists (Mixed Agonists–Antagonists)

Partial narcotic agonists act at opioid receptors in both an agonistic and antagonistic fashion. This class of medications does not seem to offer any advantage over opioid agonists other than a diminished risk of respiratory depression. And even this is of diminishing benefit as tolerance to this side effect occurs with time for narcotic agonists. Partial narcotic agonists are occasionally useful in patients unable to tolerate other opioids. There is no obvious specific advantage of this medication class in rehabilitation patients. Although pentazocine (Talwin) is the prototypic partial agonist, another partial agonist, Stadol, offers the flexibility of intranasal administration.

Relevant Side Effects and Drug Interactions

Addiction, tolerance, and physical dependence are three terms that are often confused with one another. *Addiction* can be defined as the habitual use of a substance in order to achieve a certain effect that the patient perceives as pleasurable. Fear of addiction is perhaps the major reason physicians tend to underprescribe narcotics.

Tolerance refers to the phenomenon of more drug being needed to produce a given effect. One may need to explain this to patients and families in order to quell the anxiety that often develops when a patient's narcotic dosage requirement increases after he or she has been on the medication for approximately a month. Specifically, although tolerance probably begins to occur after the first dose, it does not become apparent until 2 to 3 weeks after the medication is begun, and it generally lasts 1 to 2 weeks after the medication is removed. In contrast, some feel that if the medication doses are matched closely with the patient's needs, then addiction never develops because no excess medication is present to cause euphoria. An advantage of tolerance is that it also occurs with essentially all narcotic side effects (except constipation). Because there is incomplete cross-tolerance among the different narcotics, better analgesia can often be obtained by simply switching to another agent.

Physical dependence refers to the fact that withdrawal occurs if the drug is suddenly stopped. The onset and duration of withdrawal symptoms correlate with the half-life of the drug. As with addiction, some feel that if the medication doses are matched closely with the patient's needs, then physical dependence never develops. However, most patients who take opioids for more than 1 month develop at least some degree of physical dependence. In order to avert withdrawal symptoms in physically dependent patients, guidelines have been developed for weaning patients from an opioid (6). If withdrawal should still develop, autonomic symptoms can be blunted with the use of transdermal clonidine (Catapres-TTS) at a dose of 0.1 to 0.2 mg/day. Because a patient going through withdrawal might complain of only relatively mild nonspecific muscle aches and pains, withdrawal should always be kept in mind as a possibility when patients are taken off of narcotics.

Although narcotic analgesics have achieved notoriety for their addictive potential and sometimes fatal side effect profile, constipation is the most common narcotic side effect. Unlike most other narcotic side effects, tolerance does not develop to constipation. Because constipation can have such a profound unfavorable effect, some propose that all patients who are begun on narcotics should be begun on laxatives prophylactically, and if constipation still develops, it should be treated aggressively. Other gastrointestinal side effects include nausea and vomiting. In contrast to prophylaxis against constipation, nausea prophylaxis is not routinely given because tolerance to nausea usually develops. If nausea should develop, treatment of this depends on its underlying etiology. For example, if the nausea is actually secondary to constipation associated with the narcotic, then the constipation should be treated. In contrast, if nausea is a primary effect of the medication, i.e., stimulation of the chemotrigger zone, then prochlorperazine (Compazine) is generally regarded as the first-line agent. If the patient is still nauseous, then haloperidol (Haldol) would be a good second choice. If the patient is nauseous and agitated, then chlorpromazine (Thorazine) might be the agent of choice because of its strong sedative effects.

Nausea can also be caused by gastric outlet obstruction from the antimotility effect of opioids. In this setting, metoclopramide (Reglan) or cisapride (Propulsid) could be tried. In terms of adjuvant pain medications in a patient who is nauseous because of narcotics, an agent with a nonoral route of administration would be appropriate.

Common CNS side effects include both sedation and euphoria. Sedation can be counteracted by the use of CNS stimulants such as caffeine, dextroamphetamine, and ritalin, but euphoria is more difficult to control and largely accounts for the strong addictive potential of narcotics. Cardiopulmonary untoward effects include orthostatic hypotension to a degree that can create considerable difficulty in rehabilitating patients who are undergoing transfer and ambulation training. Another CNS side effect is respiratory depression, which can be severe enough to cause respiratory arrest. Tolerance develops to this, however, and explains the well-known phenomenom of why a large narcotic dose that would be fatal to a narcotic-naive patient is well tolerated by a habitual user.

Nonsteroidal Anti-inflammatory Drugs

Relevance to Physiatry

The NSAIDs are an effective alternative to narcotics for pain of mild to moderate severity and are an alternative to steroids for the control of inflammation. NSAIDs can also be used concomitantly with narcotics so that lower doses of narcotics are needed to achieve the same degree of pain relief with fewer side effects. Analgesia with NSAIDs is achieved at relatively low doses, whereas an anti-inflammatory effect requires somewhat higher doses. Perhaps the major advantage of this medication class over narcotics is that pain relief is attained without significant sedation; thus, there is generally little to no interference with rehabilitation efforts. In fact, these medications can be particularly useful for premedicating patients before therapy if pain has been adversely affecting performance. Compared to corticosteroids for the treatment of inflammatory conditions, NSAIDs can be used for relatively long time periods, usually without well-publicized steroid side effects such as osteoporosis and weight gain. They have largely replaced aspirin (ASA) for musculoskeletal pain.

Although numerous NSAIDs are now available, they all share a basic common mechanism of action as well as a basic side effect profile. Most agents, however, have at least one characteristic that makes them somewhat unique. Clinical superiority is difficult to demonstrate in many cases, however. Physiatrists should become familiar with at least one agent from each of the NSAID classes so that one can readily change to another class in case of medication side effects or lack of efficacy.

Future developments in this area of pharmacotherapy might involve the widespread clinical use of leukotriene inhibitors. These agents inhibit leukotriene synthesis by blocking the lipoxygenase enzyme. Leukotrienes are derived from arachadonic acid and contribute to the inflammatory response by increasing vascular permeability and by exerting a chemotactic effect on PMNs. Thus, blocking leukotriene synthesis provides a mechanism for controlling inflammation. Although leokotriene inhibitors are currently indicated only for the prophylaxis and chronic treatment of asthma (7), they might eventually be used either in combination with or instead of NSAIDs.

Mechanism of Action and Pharmacokinetics

Like ASA, the prototypic medication in this category, NSAIDs exert most, if not all, of their effects by inhibiting cyclooxygenase, a key enzyme involved in the synthesis of prostaglandins and other related compounds such as thromboxanes and leukotrienes. Prostaglandins help to regulate cellular function and are produced from the arachidonic acid found in the cell walls of all cells in the body except RBCs. The four primary properties of these medications include analgesia (for mild to moderate pain), anti-inflammatory effects, antipyresis, and anticoagulant effects.

Depending on the route of administration, NSAIDs are generally absorbed in the upper GI tract; a large percentage is then bound to plasma protein, and the unbound drug exerts its effects. Metabolism takes place in the liver, and excretion occurs via the kidney. Both short-acting and long-acting

NSAIDs (half-lives of 30 to 50 hours at steady state) exist. Although the clinical significance of drug accumulation of long-acting agents in terms of toxicity is unclear, the potential for this has been examined in detail for two long-acting agents, oxaprozin and piroxicam (8).

Preparations and Dosing

Table 31-3 shows a classification scheme according to chemical structure, provides key information about the individual NSAIDs, and lists over-the-counter (OTC) preparations as well as those available in transdermal (TD) form through compounding pharmacies. Additional information about each of the NSAID classes is as follows:

Salicylates. These include ASA and the three NSAIDs that comprise the group of nonacetylated salicylates. Compared to other classes of NSAIDs, nonacetylated salicylates are relatively weak in potency. What is lost in therapeutic potency is gained, however, in a favorable side effect profile.

TABLE 31-3. *NSAIDs*

Class, generic (trade) name	Dose (oral, mg)	Other (properties and side effects)
Salicylates, acetylated		
Aspirin (Ecotrin, Empirin, Bayer)	650 q4–6h	Especially used for antipyresis and anticoagulation; nonprescription; combined with narcotics and muscle relaxants; allergy, especially if nasal polyps, hay fever, asthma; GI toxicity, but enteric-coated and buffered forms exist; Reye syndrome
Salicylates, nonacetylated		
Diflunisal (Dolobid)	1,000 load, then 500 bid	Weak anti-inflammatory effect; lacks antipyretic activity
Salsalate (Disalcid, Salflex)	3,000/day in divided doses	Weak anti-inflammatory effect; no platelet inhibition
Salicylate combination (Trilisate)	500–1,000 q4–8h	Weak antiinflammatory effect; ? no ASA-allergic reactions
Propionic acids		
Fenoprofen (Nalfon)	200–600 tid–qid	Short $T_{1/2}$ and frequent dosing; frequent but mild GI side effects
Flurbiprofen (Ansaid)	50–100 bid–qid	Available in ophthalmic solution (Ocufen); TD form available
Ibuprofen (Motrin)	600–800 tid–qid	Inexpensive and widely used; short $T_{1/2}$ and frequent dosing; OTC forms include Advil, Nuprin, Rufen; transdermal form available
Ketoprofen (Orudis, Oruvail)	50–75 tid; 200 qd	Accumulates if poor renal function; OTC form is Orudis-KT; TD form available
Naproxen (Naprosyn, EC-Naprosyn)	250–500 bid; 375–500 bid	High incidence GI side effects; ? advantage of enteric-coated form, although expensive; OTC form is Aleve
Naproxen-Na (Naprelan, Anaprox)	750–1,000 qd; 275–550 bid	Naprelan utilizes Intestinal Protective Drug Absorption System (IPDAS): immediate and sustained-release components
Oxaprozin (Daypro)	600 bid; 1,200 qd	Long $T_{1/2}$ allows qd or bid dosing
Acetic acids		
Diclofenac (Cataflam, Voltaren, Voltaren-XR)	50 bid–tid, 100 qd	LFT monitoring suggested if use is prolonged; side effects in up to 20%
Etodolac (Lodine, Lodine-XL)	200–400 tid–qid; 400–600 qd	Short $T_{1/2}$ necessitates frequent dosing; ? gastric-sparing properties
Indomethacin (Indocin, Indocin-SR)	25–50 tid; 75 qd	Most potent and toxic NSAID; PR preparation; drug of choice in ankylosing spondylitis; dose-related side effects in up to 25–50%; CNS/hematologic toxicity
Ketorolac (Toradol)	10 qid (PO); 15–60 (IM)	FDA-approved for only five consecutive days; GI bleeding at higher doses; rapid analgesia with IM form
Nabumetone (Relafen)	500–750 bid	Long $T_{1/2}$ allows qd or bid dosing; nonacidic prodrug
Sulindac (Clinoril)	150–200 bid	Prodrug; ? renal-sparing but may be more GI toxic
Tolmetin (Tolectin)	200–600 tid–qid	Short $T_{1/2}$ requires frequent dosing; frequent GI toxicity
Fenemates		
Meclofenamate (Meclomen)	50 tid–qid	Short $T_{1/2}$ requires frequent dosing; diarrhea common
Mefenamic acid (Ponstel)	250 qid	Short $T_{1/2}$ requires frequent dosing; used for dysmenorrheic pain
Oxicams		
Piroxicam (Feldene)	20 qd	Long $T_{1/2}$ permits qd dosing; accumulation in elderly may result from enterohepatic recirculation; dermatologic side effects

bid, twice a day; CNS, central nervous system; FDA, Food and Drug Administration; GI, gastrointestinal; IM, intramuscular; NSAID, nonsteroidal anti-inflammatory drug; OTC, over-the-counter; PO, oral; qid, four times a day; $T_{1/2}$, half-life; tid, three times a day; TD, transdermal.

This has been especially shown in terms of GI irritation, platelet inhibition, and allergic reactions. Within this medication category, however, it is not clear that any one particular agent offers any particular advantage over the other two.

Propionic Acids. This is perhaps the most popular class of NSAIDs, largely because of the widespread use of ibuprofen for the last 20-plus years and the fact that ibuprofen has been available OTC.

Acetic Acids. This class includes the most potent and therefore also the most potentially toxic group of NSAIDs. It also includes the two NSAIDs that can be administered via IM and PR routes and includes the two NSAIDs that are actually prodrugs and therefore are converted into the active form after absorption.

Fenamates. Significant GI toxicity is associated with meclofenamate, whereas mefanamic acid has been marketed for the treatment of dysmenorrheic pain.

Oxicams. The representative agent from this group has a very long half-life and therefore allows true once-daily dosing but has also been associated with severe dermatologic reactions such as exfoliative dermatitis and pemphigus vulgaris.

Relevant Side Effects and Drug Interactions

Gastrointestinal side effects are the most frequently observed form of NSAID-related toxicity and especially occur in older patients and in those with a prior history of peptic ulcer disease. Because of the widespread use of these medications and the relatively high incidence of GI side effects, NSAID-induced GI pathology is the most prevalent adverse drug reaction in the United States (9). The following statistics are based on an estimated 17 million NSAID users in the United States (1):

- Twenty-five percent of patients experience upper GI symptoms including heartburn, bloating, or cramping, and 10% to 15% experience diarrhea.
- Endoscopic studies performed after 12 weeks of NSAID therapy have shown the following, generally asymptomatic, findings:
  –Gastric: 40% prevalence of erosions and 15% prevalence of ulcers.
  –Duodenal: 15% prevalence of erosions and 5% prevalence of ulcers.
- Relative risks while on NSAID therapy are as follows:
  –Three to four times increased risk of ulcer bleeding or perforation.
  –Five times increased rate of hospitalization or death from a GI complication.

Despite these alarming numbers, it should be kept in mind that the above data pertain to long-term use of NSAIDs rather than the few weeks of therapy that most patients with acute musculoskeletal problems receive, and there appears to be considerable variation among the NSAIDs in causing GI side effects (10).

Gastrointestinal side effects occur both as direct mucosal irritant effects and via the systemic effect of prostaglandin inhibition because prostaglandins normally protect the lining of the GI tract by stimulating the production of a gastric mucosal barrier. The direct irritant effect varies widely among NSAID preparations and obviously depends on the route of administration, whereas the systemic effect will occur whether the drug is given PO, PR, or IM and whether the drug is a prodrug or if it is enteric coated. There is laboratory evidence, however, that differences in the systemic effects of NSAIDs on prostaglandin metabolism do exist (1). The metabolic breakdown of the different NSAIDs might also in part dictate the medication's GI side effect profile. In particular, those NSAIDs, such as indomethacin, diclofenac, naproxen, piroxicam, and sulindac, that undergo extensive biliary excretion of active metabolites might predispose to increased GI toxicity (1). The proposed mechanism is that biliary excretion provides longer contact with gastric mucosa. In addition to their direct mucosal irritation and impaired platelet aggregation from prostaglandin inhibition, NSAIDs can cause preexisting ulcers to bleed. In response to this high frequency of adverse effects, several strategies can be used to prevent GI toxicity:

1. It is generally recommended that these medications be taken with meals so that absorption is delayed and food is present to directly protect the mucosa from the stomach's acid environment.
2. Some of the preparations are now enteric-coated so that absorption occurs in the duodenum rather than in the stomach.
3. In cases of prior significant gastrointestinal toxicity from NSAIDs, or in patients with a prior history of peptic ulcer disease, it is not uncommon to give other medications including antacids, H_2 blockers, misoprostyl, omeprazole, and sucralfate concomitantly (Table 31-4).

Although this is a hotly debated topic that is far from settled, some generalizations can be made. For example, it is typically felt that the treatment of NSAID-induced gastric ulcers is more difficult than that of NSAID-induced duodenal ulcers. Thus, more intensive or prolonged acid-reduction therapy has been suggested in the setting of gastric ulcers caused by NSAIDs.

It would be quite useful to identify those patients who are at particular risk for NSAID-induced GI side effects, especially because the majority of NSAID-induced ulcers are asymptomatic, and bleeding is often the initial symptom. Unfortunately, periodic fecal occult blood testing is not felt to be helpful in screening for NSAID-induced ulcers because of the high frequency of positive tests (1). As of now, there is epidemiologic support for only a few risk factors, including a history of previous NSAID-induced ulcer complication, prior ulcer disease, advanced age (>75), and concomitant corticosteroid or anticoagulant use. Of note, smoking in the absence of other risk factors does not appear to increase the risk of NSAID-induced ulceration or bleeding (1).

TABLE 31-4. *Agents for prophylaxis and treatment of upper GI toxicity caused by NSAIDs*

Medication	Dose range	Gastric ulcers (NSAID-induced)	Duodenal ulcers (NSAID-induced)
Antacids	Standard	Not preventative	Not preventative
H_2 blockers	Standard	Not preventative	Preventative
	High dose	? Preventative	Preventative
Misoprostol (Cytotec)	Standard (200 μg qid)	Preventative (FDA-approved)	Preventative
	Low dose (200 μg bid–tid)	? Preventative	? Preventative
Omeprazole (Prilosec)	Standard	Not preventative	? Preventative
Sucralfate (Carafate)	Standard	Not preventative	Healing (if NSAIDs stopped)

FDA, Food and Drug Administration; GI, gastrointestinal; NSAIDs, nonsteroidal anti-inflammatory drugs.

Less common GI side effects involve the esophagus, the nonduodenal portion of the small bowel, the colon, and the liver. Esophageal side effects include esophagitis and benign esophageal strictures. As in the duodenum, the remainder of the small bowel can undergo ulcerations and erosions in response to NSAIDs. In addition, it can develop characteristic weblike strictures. As in the small bowel, the colon can develop ulcerations and erosions, and there can be unmasking of irritable bowel disease. Hepatic toxicity is quite rare except in patients with preexisting liver disease. Clinically significant hepatic enzyme elevations have been shown with some agents, particularly diclofenac, and it is therefore suggested that hepatic enzyme levels be monitored when this NSAID is being taken. The optimal timing for measuring these levels has yet to be determined.

Renal side effects comprise the next major category of toxicity and can especially occur in patients with preexisting kidney disease or in those situations such as congestive heart failure and hypovolemia where renal blood flow may already be compromised. Examples of NSAID-induced renal toxicity include acute renal failure, nephrotic syndrome, and interstitial nephritis. It has been suggested but not proven that sulindac is somewhat renal-sparing compared to other NSAIDs (11).

True allergic reactions to NSAIDs occur in 1% of the population and cover the entire spectrum from simple skin rashes and rhinitis to anaphylaxis. The NSAIDs, other than perhaps trilisate, should not be used in aspirin-allergic patients because of the potential for cross-reactions, which are believed to range from an incidence of 5% for ibuprofen and mefanamic acid to 100% for indomethacin (12). Cross-sensitivity also occurs between ASA and high doses of acetaminophen.

Because of a theoretical possibility of impaired fracture healing from prostaglandin inhibition, there has been some controversy in the literature regarding the use of NSAIDs in this patient population (13,14). Practitioners generally believe that it is unnecessary to withhold anti-inflammatories from patients who have suffered a fracture or have undergone an ORIF and are experiencing mild to moderate pain because impaired fracture healing with NSAIDs probably does not occur to any clinically significant degree.

Tramadol HCl (Ultram)

Relevance to Physiatry

Tramadol is a synthetic analgesic that was originally marketed in 1977 in Germany, where it is currently the largest-selling prescription analgesic for acute and chronic pain (15). It was approved in the United States by the Food and Drug Administration (FDA) in 1993 for the treatment of moderate to moderately severe pain.

Tramadol's exact role in physiatry, as in other areas of medicine, is still being determined. Its favorable pharmacokinetics, i.e., relatively rapid onset of action followed by a slow, steady decline in efficacy, and its low side effect profile make it potentially very useful in the treatment of both acute and chronic pain. In particular, its good efficacy in cancer patients with pain from bone metastases (16,17) suggests that it can be tried in appropriate patients enrolled in cancer rehabilitation programs. In acute pain situations, its onset of analgesic action within 1 hour is also of benefit. It offers the advantages of not being classified as a controlled substance, and it acts synergistically with NSAIDs without worsening their side effect profile.

It has been shown that tramadol at the 50-mg dose is comparable in pain relief to Tylenol #3. In chronic malignant pain, two studies have found it to offer some benefits (16,17). Trials have also been conducted in patients with acute pain; however, these have largely been done in the settings of postcesarean section, gynecologic surgery, and oral surgery rather than for musculoskeletal or peripheral neurogenic pain scenarios.

Because tramadol (75-mg dose) was not found to affect one's physical working capacity as measured by a cycle ergometer in healthy volunteers, nor was it found to affect psychomotor performance as measured by an "eye-to-hand coordination" test, it may be particularly advantageous over opioids for injured workers who are being returned to their jobs (18).

In traumatic brain injury patients, however, it may increase a patient's risk of convulsions, especially for those who are taking medications that otherwise lower seizure threshold or who have or are recovering from a central nervous system infection.

Mechanism of Action and Pharmacokinetics

Tramadol has a synergistic dual mechanism of action of both an opioid and a monoamine reuptake inhibitor (15): (a) It acts as a synthetic analog of codeine that occupies opiate receptors but with an affinity ten times less than codeine, and it is only partially antagonized by naloxone; (b) It also acts as a tricyclic antidepressant in modifying the transmission of pain impulses by blocking the reuptake of the monoamines norepinephrine and serotonin, and by enhancing neuronal serotonin release.

Tramadol is absorbed through the GI tract, and a mean peak plasma concentration occurs after 1.5 to 2 hours. (Intravenous, IM, SC, and PR preparations are available for clinical use in Europe but not in the United States at the time of this writing.) There is low serum protein binding, and extensive first-pass metabolism occurs in the liver, where it is converted to several metabolites (19). Eventually, 30% of the unchanged drug is excreted in the urine, and 60% is excreted as metabolites (16). The analgesic effect appears at 30 minutes, peaks at approximately 2 hours, and then slowly declines to the point where it is ineffective at approximately 6 hours after the dose (19). Combination analgesic products, in contrast, often exhibit a rapid onset of action followed by a steep decline in analgesic effect. It has a half-life ($T_{1/2}$) of 6.3 hours; thus, steady state occurs within 2 days if it is taken qid.

Preparations and Dosing

The dose of tramadol in the form of capsules or oral drops is 50 to 100 mg every 4 to 6 hours, with a maximum total daily dose of 400 mg. Dosing adjustments are needed in patients older than 75 (no more than 300 mg per day), those with a creatinine clearance of less than 30 ml/min (q12h dosing and maximum daily dose of 200 mg) and those with hepatic cirrhosis. Although the usual starting dose is 50 to 100 mg, it can be useful to have the patient take half this amount in order to avoid first-dose nausea. If there is inadequate analgesia within the first 60 minutes, another 25 to 50 mg can be taken. An alternative strategy is to begin with an initial 100-mg dose for more severe acute pain. If side effects such as dizziness or nausea do eventually occur, the patient should halve the maintenance dose in order to determine whether there is adequate analgesia with acceptable side effects. Abrupt discontinuation is not recommended because of the possibility of withdrawal.

Relevant Side Effects and Drug Interactions

In contrast to the synergistic analgesic effects of stimulation of opioid and nonopioid receptors, side effects (19–21) occur in an additive or less-than-additive manner. Nausea and dizziness are the most common ones, followed by sedation, dry mouth, and sweating. Traditional opioid side effects such as respiratory depression (especially with the IV form), cardiac depression, and constipation are rarely seen. Because euphoria does not seem to be a common effect, there is a low psychological dependency and abuse potential. In addition, there is a low probability of tolerance to the analgesic effect. Withdrawal can be seen but is not as severe as that seen with opioids. There have been, to date, two long-term safety studies in patients with chronic, nonmalignant pain; these found that tolerance was insignificant, as there was a slight but insignificant dose escalation (16,17).

Drug interactions include seizures when tramadol is used concurrently with medications capable of lowering the seizure threshold. Drugs that exert a clinically significant effect on its metabolism include carbamazepine and rifampin. Carbamazepine so markedly induces the metabolism of tramadol that up to twice the usual dose of tramadol might be required for those patients who are taking both medications. Because of low protein binding, it does not appear to interact with anticoagulants or oral hypoglycemics.

DRUGS OTHER THAN ANALGESICS

Agents Used to Treat Musculoskeletal Pain

Muscle Relaxants

Relevance to Physiatry

Muscle relaxants are generally reserved for short-term use in painful musculoskeletal conditions. Unlike antispasticity agents, muscle relaxants are not indicated for true skeletal muscle spasticity. The various drugs that comprise the category known as muscle relaxants act to diminish muscle excitability and thus decrease the pain associated with increased muscle tension but are not felt to directly relax tense skeletal muscle. The sedation that generally accompanies their use needs to be taken into consideration when these agents are prescribed. One may want to prescribe these for nighttime use only and preferentially use the shorter-acting agents. Unlike true antispasticity agents, these agents generally do not decrease muscle strength to a significant degree.

Mechanism of Action

Muscle relaxants are part of several different medication groups (Table 31-5); thus, no one mechanism of action or set of pharmacokinetic rules exists. A common theme, however, is that they somehow interfere with the following sequence of events (22):

1. Nociceptive input from skeletal muscles after injuries and during inflammatory states travels afferently along IA nerve fibers to the spinal cord.
2. This results in the stimulation of alpha motor neurons, which in turn causes skeletal muscle contraction and leads to the accumulation of metabolites such as lactate.
3. Lactate in particular then further stimulates the alpha motor neuron.

TABLE 31-5. *Muscle relaxants*

Generic (trade) name	Structural analog	Dose (mg)	Other properties and side effects
Single agents			Sedation is generally the most common side effect
Carisoprodol (Soma, Rela)	Meprobamate (Equanil, Miltown)	350 PO tid and h/s	? Mechanism; sedation; first-dose idiosyncratic reactions; contraindicated in acute intermittent porphyria
Chlorzoxazone (Paraflex, Parafon Forte)	None	250–500 PO tid–qid	Inhibits multisynaptic reflex arcs at spinal cord and subcortical areas; rare GI side effects including bleeding and unpredictable fatal hepatotoxicity
Cyclobenzaprine (Flexeril)	Tricyclic antidepressants	10-20 PO tid	Widely used; plasma levels vary widely; sedation and anticholinergic side effects
Diazepam (Valium)	Benzodiazepines	2–10 PO tid–qid	Also used as an antispasticity agent
Metaxalone (Skelaxin)	None	800 PO tid–qid	Paradoxic CNS excitation; hematologic toxicity, especially hemolytic anemia; avoid if hepatic dysfunction
Methocarbamol (Robaxin)	Mephenesin (first muscle relaxant)	1,000 PO/IM/IV qid	First use loading dose 1,500 mg qid for 48–72 hr; IM form inconvenient because half must be injected into each buttock
Orphenadrine (Norflex)	Antihistamines	100 PO bid; 60 IV/IM bid	Anaphylaxis reported in some asthmatics given IM/IV preparations
Muscle relaxant/analgesic			Addition of ASA and caffeine is based on a presumed synergistic effect with the muscle relaxant
(Norgesic, Norgesic Forte)		1–2 tabs PO tid–qid	Norgesic (Norgesic Forte) contains (mg) orphenadrine 50 (100)/ASA 385/caffeine 30
(Soma Compound)		1–2 tabs PO qid	Contains (mg) carisoprodol 200/ASA 325
(Soma Compound with Codeine)		1–2 tabs PO qid	Contains (mg) carisoprodol 200/ASA 325/codeine 16; potentially quite sedative
(Robaxisal)		2 tabs PO qid	Contains (mg) methocarbimal 400/ASA 325

ASA, aspirin; bid, twice a day; CNS, central nervous system; GI, gastrointestinal; h/s, bedtime; IM, intramuscular; IV intravenous; PO, oral; qid, four times a day; tid, three times a day.

Medications

Medications of this class are listed in Table 31-5.

Agents Used to Treat Neurogenic Pain

Antidepressants: Tricyclic Antidepressants and Trazodone (Desyrel)

Relevance to Physiatry

Besides being used for the treatment of depression that is not infrequently associated with disabling conditions (e.g., poststroke depression) and injuries, the major physiatric application of these agents is the treatment of neurogenic pain and chronic pain syndromes. Of the tricyclic antidepressants (TCAs), amitriptyline and nortriptyline are probably the two most popular agents. Trazodone is an antidepressant agent that is chemically unrelated to other known antidepressants and is sometimes substituted in those patients who are intolerant to the anticholinergic side effects of TCAs.

When TCAs have been used for neurogenic pain, an analgesic effect has been reported in 50% to 60% of patients (3). In the treatment of chronic pain, some have contended that these medications act via their effect on the depression that is often present in these patients (23). Intuitively, one would expect that this is accurate because a depressed patient is much less motivated to engage in a rehabilitation program compared with a nondepressed patient. However, there is evidence that antidepressants can be of use even if the patient does not have any symptoms of depression (24). An alternate theory is that these agents work in chronic pain patients by improving their sleep patterns (24). However, they have also been shown to be effective even in the absence of an effect on sleep (24). Elderly and otherwise medically fragile patients should probably be begun on nortriptyline rather than amitriptyline, given nortriptyline's superior side effect profile. Orthostatic hypotension is a relatively common initial side effect of TCAs that can interfere greatly with rehabilitation.

Mechanism of Action and Pharmacokinetics

The TCAs increase aminergic transmission by inhibiting the reuptake of norepinephrine and serotonin at the presynaptic terminals of nerve endings. In doing this, they cause an elevation of the pain threshold in both depressed and nondepressed patients. The dose required to raise the pain threshold is usually lower than that required to treat primary depression. These agents are rapidly absorbed and metabolized and then excreted into the urine. Nortriptyline is a demethylated active metabolite of amitriptyline that is also available as an individual agent.

Trazadone's exact mechanism of action in humans is not yet fully understood, but in animals it selectively inhibits serotonin uptake. It is well absorbed after oral ingestion and has a variable clearance that may lead to accumulation in some patients.

Preparations and Dosing

Available dosage preparations are listed in Table 31-6.

Relevant Side Effects and Drug Interactions

Side effects of TCAs are mainly related to their anticholinergic and antihistaminergic properties as well as their potentiation of adrenergic drugs. Common anticholinergic side effects include dryness of mouth, blurred vision, tachycardia, constipation, and urinary retention; less common anticholinergic side effects are disorientation and confusion. The main antihistaminergic side effect is sedation, thus explaining why these agents are often prescribed as a single bedtime dose. They also exert some quinidine-like effects on the heart, including prolongation of atrioventricular conduction time. Other less common side effects include leukopenia and an increased appetite for carbohydrates with resultant weight gain. In general, nortriptyline tends to be better tolerated.

Trazodone also possesses some anticholinergic effects, but these are less than those of the tricyclic antidepressants. Trazodone has been associated with priapism that in many cases required surgical intervention and in some cases resulted in permanent impairment of erectile function. Occasional and clinically insignificant low WBC and neutrophil counts have been found.

The TCAs should not be used in patients taking monoamine oxidase inhibitors (MAOIs) and should only be instituted cautiously in patients who have been off of MAOIs for at least 2 weeks. The concomitant use of TCAs and MAOIs can cause hyperpyretic crises, seizures, and death. The TCAs should also be used cautiously in patients taking other anticholinergic medications, neuroleptics, or CNS depressants. Cimetidine can cause significant increases in the concentrations of TCAs by reducing their hepatic metabolism. Perhaps not well known is the recommendation that in local anesthetic solutions that contain epinephrine be used with caution in patients taking TCAs (11).

It is not known whether interactions occur between trazodone and monoamine oxidase inhibitors. Trazodone can increase serum digoxin and phenytoin levels and can cause either an increase or a decrease in prothrombin times in patients on warfarin.

Capsaicin (Zostrix; Zostrix-HP)

Relevance to Physiatry

Capsaicin has been used most often for the temporary relief of pain in patients with rheumatoid arthritis, osteoarthritis, postherpetic neuralgia, and diabetic neuropathy. It offers the physiatrist a readily available analgesic medication with an alternative route of administration. In order to maximize the probability that the patient will not prematurely discontinue it because of the frequent initial occurrence of stinging at the application site, it might be best to begin with the 0.025% concentration and then change to the HP formulation (0.075%) as needed. Capsaicin is becoming more frequently used by the general public since it became available over the counter and is even being advertised as a sports cream for muscle soreness as well as for arthritic pain.

Mechanism of Action and Pharmacokinetics

Capsaicin is a naturally occurring compound that has been extracted from plants of the Solanaceae family and is believed to exert its analgesic effect by locally depleting and preventing the reaccumulation of substance P, an endogenous neuropeptide that is involved in pain impulse transmission from the skin and joints. Capsaicin has been formulated into a cream that is applied directly to the skin, through which it is absorbed.

Preparations and Dosing

Capsaicin is available in a concentration of 0.025% (Zostrix) and 0.075% (Zostrix-HP) and should be applied to affected sites three to four times per day.

TABLE 31-6. *Antidepressants used in the treatment of neurogenic pain*

Generic (trade) name	Dose for neurogenic pain (mg)	Other properties and side effects
Amitriptyline (Elavil, Endep)	10–100 h/s (150–300/day)	Injectable form available
Nortriptyline (Aventyl, Pamelor)	10–30 h/s (50–150/day)	First metabolite of amitriptyline; fewer side effects
Trazodone (Desyrel)	50–150 h/s (400–600/day divided bid)	Priapism that can be severe; fewer anticholinergic side effects than for TCAs

TCAs, tricyclic antidepressants.

Relevant Side Effects and Drug Interactions

Transient warm stinging or burning at the application site is quite common, particularly with the HP formulation. This generally disappears after the first few days of use but can be so intense that it causes patients to self-discontinue it. No specific drug interactions have been reported.

Membrane-Stabilizing Agents

Carbamazepine (Tegretol)

Relevance to Physiatry

Neurogenic pain of a shooting or stabbing quality is most likely to respond to carbamazepine. A classic example of this type of pain is that from neuromas in amputee patients. Carbamazepine's relative lack of CNS side effects compared to other membrane-stabilizing agents offers an obvious advantage to patients attempting to perform functional activities. However, the need for laboratory monitoring of potential toxicity is a drawback.

Mechanism of Action and Pharmacokinetics

Its mechanism of action for relief of neurogenic pain is not completely known. It is well absorbed, highly plasma protein bound, and has a variable $T_{1/2}$ because it induces its own metabolism.

Preparations and Dosing

Carbamazepine is available in chewable tablets, tablets, and suspension formulations. As a neurogenic pain medication, it is dosed starting at 100 mg bid and increased gradually if needed up to 400 mg tid. If it is to be used for prolonged periods of time, its dose should be reduced to the minimum effective one. An extended-release form, Tegretol-XR, can be given bid using the same total daily milligram dose as the non-extended-release form. It is important that the patient swallows the intact extended-release tablet without chewing it or the sustained-release effect will be lost.

Relevant Side Effects and Drug Interactions

Bone marrow suppression, hepatotoxicity, and, to a lesser degree, renal dysfunction have been associated with carbamazepine. Pretreatment complete blood cell count (CBC), LFTs, blood urea nitrogen (BUN), and urinalysis as well as possibly a pretreatment reticulocyte count and serum iron level are recommended. Although exact guidelines have not been developed, periodic monitoring of at least the CBC and LFTs should also be performed, and if toxicity is detected, serious consideration should be given to discontinuing the medication. The value of monitoring serum carbamazepine levels is less clear when it is being used to treat neurogenic pain, compared to when it is being used for seizures.

Because of the significant degree of hepatic enzyme induction caused by carbamazepine, it has both the potential of affecting the serum levels of a wide variety of medications and having its serum levels affected by other medications, as shown in Table 31-7. Given this tremendous potential for drug interactions, it is best to consult an appropriate reference book before starting the patient on it.

Gabapentin (Neurontin)

Relevance to Physiatry

Neurontin has been most often employed as an adjuvant antiepileptic agent for partial seizures with or without secondary generalization. Its main physiatric use is in the treatment of chronic neurogenic pain such as radiculopathy. Although it is not yet FDA-approved for this indication, it offers a reasonable alternative to patients who continue to have radicular symptoms despite treatment with other medications such as NSAIDs, oral corticosteroids, epidural ste-

TABLE 31-7. *Potential drug interactions with carbamazepine*

Interaction	Decreased serum level	Increased serum level
Medications whose serum levels are affected by carbamazepine	Acetaminophen, alprazolam, clonazepam,clozapine, dicumarol, ethosuximide, doxycycline, haloperidol, methsuximide, oral contraceptives, phensuximide, phenytoin, theophylline, tramadol, valproate, warfarin	Clomipramine, phenytoin, primidone
Medications that affect serum carbamazepine levels	Cisplatin, doxorubicin, felbamate, phenobarbital, phenytoin, primidone, rifampin, theophylline	Calcium channel blockers, cimetidine, clarithromycin, erythromycin, danazol, fluoxetine, isoniazid, itraconazole, ketaconazole, loratadine, macrolides, niacinamide, nicatinamide, propoxyphene, terfenadine, troleandomycin, valproate

roid injections, narcotic analgesics, TCAs, and tramadol. In particular, it tends to be much less sedating than TCAs; thus, it may ultimately play a major role in the treatment of other types of neurogenic pain such as those related to peripheral neuropathies. There have been case reports that have described pain relief for patients with neuropathic pain, but published controlled studies are lacking (25). It is also being investigated for spasticity reduction in patients with spinal cord injury (26). Its apparent lack of drug interaction may prove to be a major advantage.

Mechanism of Action and Pharmacokinetics

This medication is classified as an anticonvulsant whose exact mechanism of action is not completely understood. Because γ-aminobutyric acid (GABA) is the major excitatory neurotransmitter in the central nervous system, Neurontin was originally developed as an antiseizure medication that was to inhibit GABA receptors. Although it is structurally related to GABA, it does not interact with GABA receptors, it is not metabolically converted into GABA or a GABA agonist, and it does not inhibit GABA uptake or GABA degradation. It apparently does not bind to other common receptors including benzodiazepine, glutamate, N-methyl-D-aspartate (NMDA), glycine, beta-adrenergic, cholinergic, muscarinic, nicotinic, histaminic, serotinergic, dopaminergic, calcium channels, or sodium channels (11). One hypothesis is that it acts by altering the concentration or metabolism of cerebral amino acids (27). There is some evidence that it particularly affects polysynaptic reflexes; thus, it may act by raising the interneuron pool threshold (26). This highly water-soluble drug is rapidly absorbed from the GI tract, after which it is not protein bound, is not metabolized by the liver, and is excreted unchanged in the urine. Because its elimination $T\frac{1}{2}$ is from 5 to 9 hours, it should be taken in three divided doses.

Preparations and Dosing

The usual dosage range varies from 900 to 1,800 mg in divided doses tid with a maximum of 3,600 mg/day. When a patient is started on gabapentin, it is recommended that a 300-mg dose be given h/s on day 1, followed by bid dosing on day 2, and then to tid dosing on day 3. It is felt that this regimen will help the patient to accommodate to the CNS side effects described below.

Relevant Side Effects and Drug Interactions

Its main side effects relate to CNS depression, including its potential for somnolence (24.4%), dizziness (20.3%), and ataxia (17.4%) (11). These side effects are generally transient in nature and usually resolve within 2 weeks of onset. There have been only rare reports of adverse events that required discontinuation of gabapentin. These have included rash, leukopenia to less than 3,000/mm^3, increased BUN, thrombocytopenia, and ECG changes. Given the rarity of these events, routine laboratory monitoring and monitoring of gabapentin levels are not indicated.

There are no known drug interactions between gabapentin and other medications, including antiepileptic medications and oral contraceptives. The two exceptions are cimetidine, which slightly decreases renal gabapentin excretion to a degree that is not felt to be clinically significant, and Maalox, which reduces gabapentin's bioavailability by about 20%. The lack of drug–drug interactions is not suprising because gabapentin is not appreciably metabolized, does not induce hepatic enzymes, and does not undergo tubular secretion by the pathway that is blocked by probenecid.

Clonazepam (Klonopin)

Relevance to Physiatry

Perhaps the two main physiatric applications of this medication are for the treatment of neurogenic pain syndromes, particularly trigeminal neuralgia, and for the treatment of selected movement disorders. For trigeminal neuralgia, it has been used in those patients who are either intolerant to or who have failed carbamazepine, baclofen, and phenytoin. In terms of movement disorders, it has been used for the treatment of sleep-related nocturnal myoclonus, and there are studies to support its use in the treatment of restless legs syndrome (uncontrollable movements of the legs without myoclonic jerks) (28). It is also used as an alternative for the treatment of absence and myoclonic seizures, and there have been anecdotal reports of its use in tardive dyskinesia (28).

Mechanism of Action and Pharmacokinetics

Like other benzodiazepines, clonazepam potentiates the inhibitory effects of GABA. It is well absorbed orally, is highly bound to plasma proteins, and is metabolized in the liver.

Preparations and Dosing

This medication is available in tablets containing 0.5, 1, or 2 mg. For the above uses, clonazepam is begun at 0.5 mg h/s or tid and increased to 2 mg tid as needed.

Relevant Side Effects and Drug Interactions

As is true for other benzodiazepines, long-term use of clonazepam can cause psychological as well as physical addiction. Withdrawal symptoms include a flu-like syndrome, and abrupt discontinuation of high doses used chronically can lead to convulsions. In contrast, ataxia and personality changes tend to occur early in the treatment course and may partially subside with long-term administration. Caution should be exercised when it is given with other CNS depressants.

Mexiletine HCl (Mexitil)

Relevance to Physiatry

Mexiletine was originally used for the treatment of life-threatening ventricular arrhythmias. More recently, non-FDA-approved uses for this medication have also been uncovered. For example, it has been found to be effective in treating pain caused by alcoholic peripheral neuropathy and for pain of diabetic neuropathy (29,30), particularly in those patients complaining of stabbing or burning pain, heat sensations, or formication (31). Small studies have shown some benefit in various other conditions including phantom pain in amputee patients (32), pain of central origin such as the thalamic pain syndrome (33), multiple sclerosis complicated by painful dysesthesias (34), and in the treatment of paramyotonia congenita and Thomsen–Becker myotonia (35). In addition, there is a case report of its beneficial effect on fecal incontinence in patients with myotonic muscular dystrophy (36). In contrast, it has been tried in spinal cord injury patients with spinal dysesthetic pain and trigeminal neuralgia but has not been found to be helpful in these conditions (37,38).

Mechanism of Action and Pharmacokinetics

Mexiletine is a structural analog of lidocaine in that it is a class I subclass B antiarrhythmic agent that acts by blocking sodium channels in nerve and muscle cell membranes. It is rapidly and well absorbed (80% to 90% bioavailability) from the GI tract and then is highly bound to plasma proteins before being extensively metabolized by the liver. About 10% is excreted unchanged into the urine.

Preparations and Dosing

For the control of cardiac arrhythmias, doses ranging from 200 mg to 400 mg every 8 hours are used. For painful alcoholic peripheral neuropathy, the minimum effective dose is 300 mg/day, and the usual effective dose is 450 mg/day divided tid.

Relevant Side Effects and Drug Interactions

The three main categories of side effects include gastrointestinal, neurologic, and cardiovascular. Gastrointestinal side effects include nausea, anorexia, and gastric irritation and can be found in up to 40% of patients. Like other class I drugs, it is also associated with dizziness, visual disturbances, and nausea in up to 10% of patients. In addition, tremor and coordination difficulties have been described. In patients with a normal cardiac conduction system, it has a minimal effect on cardiac impulse generation and propagation despite its use as an antiarrhythmic drug. In patients with abnormal cardiac conduction, the most common side effect is aggravation of cardiac rhythm disturbances. In fact, it is contraindicated in the presence of second- or third-degree heart block in patients without a pacemaker. Phenytoin and rifampin induce the hepatic metabolism of mexiletine, whereas mexiletine may increase the plasma levels of theophylline. Because caffeine clearance is reduced 50% by mexiletine, it can potentially interact with caffeine-containing medication compounds.

Phenytoin (Dilantin)

Relevance to Physiatry

Besides its well-known use as an antiepileptic agent, this agent is also used for patients with painful neuropathies in whom there is intolerance to carbamazepine or amitriptyline or in whom these medications have been unsuccessful. Ataxia caused by phenytoin toxicity can cause great difficulties with transfer, ambulation, and elevation training.

Mechanism of Action and Pharmacokinetics

Phenytoin is believed to exert its membrane-stabilizing effects by inhibiting sodium entry into neurons both at rest and during excitation. After entering the plasma, it is highly protein bound, metabolized via hydroxylation in the liver, and most is excreted into the bile as inactive metabolites that are then reabsorbed and excreted into the urine by glomerular filtration and tubular secretion.

Preparations and Dosing

Phenytoin is available as extended-release capsules, tablets, an injectable form, and as an oral suspension. When used for neurogenic pain syndromes, the required doses are significantly less than those used in the treatment of seizure disorders (100 mg tid or qid or 300 mg qd for the extended-release capsules). At these higher doses, it can be important to monitor serum levels of the medication because there is saturation of the metabolic pathways; thus, the half-life of the drug increases as the plasma concentrations rise. Stated another way, further increases in dose cause greater than expected plasma drug levels.

Relevant Side Effects and Drug Interactions

Unwanted effects of phenytoin can be classified into three different categories, including toxic effects, true side effects, and idiosyncratic reactions. Toxic effects generally occur at plasma levels between 20 and 40 μg/ml and include sedation, ataxia, and nystagmus. A peripheral neuropathy that primarily affects sensory nerve fibers can occur if serum levels are allowed to climb. However, because the dose used for neurogenic pain is generally low, toxic side effects are usually not encountered. True side effects usually require

TABLE 31-8. *Potential drug interactions with phenytoin*

Drugs that can interfere with phenytoin absorption	Antacids (calcium-containing), Moban brand chloride
Drugs that can raise phenytoin levels	Alcohol (acute intake), amiodarone, chloram poxide, diazepam, dicumarol, disulfirar suximide, fluoxetine, halothane, H_2 anta Iphenidate, phenothiazines, phenylbutaz cinimides, sulfonamides, tolbutamide, ticlid (?), trazodone
Drugs that can decrease phenytoin levels	Alcohol (chronic abuse), carbamazepine, reserpine, sucralfate
Drugs that can raise or decrease phenytoin levels	Phenobarbital, sodium valproate, valproic acid
Drugs whose serum levels can be raised or decreased by phenytoin	Phenobarbital, sodium valproate, valproic acid
Drugs whose efficacy is impaired by phenytoin	Corticosteroids, coumarin anticoagulants, digitoxin, doxycycline, estrogens, furosemide, oral contraceptives, quinidine, rifampin, theophylline, vitamin D

long-term use of the medication and include osteomalacia and hypocalcemia secondary to interference with vitamin D metabolism, megaloblastic anemia from lowered serum folate levels, hirsutism, and gingival hyperplasia as a result of interference with fibroblastic activity. Idiosyncratic reactions include blood dyscrasias and a rare clinical picture that resembles malignant lymphoma. See Table 31-8 for potential drug interactions.

Agents Used to Treat Skeletal Pain

Anti-Bone-Resorption Agents

Relevance to Physiatry

As the general public and physicians themselves become more aware of the necessity to prevent, diagnose, and treat osteoporosis, physiatrists are becoming more actively involved in the care of patients with this disorder. Although some physiatrists limit their involvement to the prescription of therapeutic exercise, others prescribe medications to prevent and treat this condition. In addition to calcium and vitamin D dietary supplementation, there are three major classes of anti-bone-resorption medications, including biphosphonates, calcitonin preparations, and estrogens as shown in Table 31-9. As an alternative to prescribing these agents individually, there are data that the combined use of estrogen and etidronate is more effective than either therapy alone, and a study on the combined use of estrogen and alendronate is under way (39). Bone-forming agents such as sodium fluoride are not approved for use at the time of this writing because of lack of data proving efficacy and the concern that long-term therapy might actually increase the risk of hip and vertebral fractures because the new bone that is formed is brittle (39,40).

Anticoagulants and Antithrombotics

Anticoagulants

Relevance to Physiatry

These medications are primarily used for prophylaxis against abnormal, excessive clot formation within the vascular system. In general, they affect the function and synthesis of various clotting factors, thus reducing the tendency toward clot propagation and the risk of developing a deep vein thrombus (DVT) or pulmonary or cerebral embolus. The incidence of thromboembolic phenomena has been reported widely, and patients at risk for developing thromboembolic phenomena are frequently encountered in the rehabilitative setting (41,42). Included are those following spinal cord injuries, strokes, multiple trauma, as well as hip and knee arthroplasties. Thus, measures to reduce this risk, including anticoagulation and conservative means to stimulate blood flow in the legs, such as with external compression devices, are warranted in appropriate patients. It has been suggested that patients with proximal DVT or pulmonary embolus be treated similarly (43).

Whenever a patient is on anticoagulants, it is important to include this information in the therapy prescription so that the therapist can take appropriate precautions to prevent patient falls. This also alerts the therapist to monitor closely and report potential signs of bleeding, such as a newly swollen joint, because this may represent a hemarthrosis.

Anticoagulants can be administered either parenterally or orally. Heparin and, more recently, low-molecular-weight heparin (LMWH) are the major parenteral anticoagulants. The intravenous use of anticoagulants is usually associated with the treatment of acute thromboembolic phenomena, whereas subcutaneous administration is more common for prophylaxis. However, there is evidence that supports the use of subcutaneously administered LMWH in cases of acute proximal DVT, and in selected patients, it may be as effective and safe as treatment with intravenous heparin (44,45).

Fixed low-dose heparin therapy has been extensively studied in various patient groups and has been shown to be an inexpensive and feasible form of treatment that is not associated with an increased risk of major hemorrhage (46,47). More recently, LMWH has been shown to be more effective than fixed low-dose heparin in DVT prophylaxis in various clinical situations and is associated with only a low risk of bleeding (46,48,49).

With respect to oral anticoagulation, warfarin is by far the

TABLE 31-9. *Anti-bone-resorption medications*

Medication class: mechanism of action	Effectiveness	Preparation and dosing	Other properties and side effects
Biphosphonates (diphosphonates) bind to the surface of bone and inhibit osteoclastic bone resorption	Bone loss resumes if alendronate is stopped; adequate calcium and vitamin D are important	First generation, etidronate (Didronel), 400 mg PO qd for 14 days, then repeat every third month; second generation, alendronate (Fosamax) 10 mg PO qd	Upper GI side effects, especially if not taken on an empty stomach; long-term effects of drug accumulation in bone being studied; etidronate impairs bone mineralization if not used cyclically
Calcitonins directly inhibit osteoclast activity (greater efficacy with salmon preparation than human calcitonin)	Reduce bone loss in both early and established osteoporosis; reduce fractures in established osteoporosis; effect possibly wanes after 18–24 months of therapy; unknown long-term usefulness	Calcimar, 100 U SC qd; miacalcin, 100 U SC qd; miacalcin nasal spray, 200 U qd	Nausea, flushing, and injection site inflammation with the SC preparations; infrequent nasal symptoms such as stuffiness, rhinorrhea, and rhinitis with intranasal form
Estrogens suppress bone resorption	Prevent bone loss in early menopause; possibly effective in established osteoporosis; no significant difference between oral and transdermal preparations; bone loss resumes quickly if discontinued	Conjugated estrogens (Premarin), 0.625 mg PO qd; estropipate (Ogen), 0.625 mg PO qd; estradiol (Estrace), 0.5, 1.0 mg PO qd; estradiol (Estraderm), 0.05, 0.1 mg TDS biw	Breast swelling and tenderness in older women at the onset of treatment; should not be given to women with unexplained uterine bleeding, breast masses of ? significance, and/or history of previous breast or endometrial cancer

biw, biweekly; GI, gastrointestinal; PO, oral; SC, subcutaneous; TDS, transdermal system.

most commonly used medication. Thus, the primary focus of further discussion of oral anticoagulants is limited to this drug. The use of oral anticoagulants in DVT prophylaxis following hip or knee arthroplasty has been well established (46,50). Although its efficacy in preventing DVT in orthopedic patients may be somewhat less than that of LMWH, it is the mainstay of treating documented thromboembolism following initial heparin treatment (50). Another important indication for oral anticoagulation is stroke prophylaxis, especially in the presence of atrial fibrillation (51,52). Specifically, it has been demonstrated that oral anticoagulation is associated with a significant risk reduction of stroke and that it is more efficacious than ASA in preventing stroke in the presence of atrial fibrillation (52).

Mechanism of Action and Pharmacokinetics

Heparin affects the clotting mechanism by increasing the activity of antithrombin III, thus inactivating several clotting factors, primarily thrombin and factor Xa. This ultimately causes inhibition of fibrin formation and hence prevents a stable clot from developing. With low-dose heparin therapy, the primary anticoagulant mechanism is through prevention of the conversion of prothrombin to thrombin via inactivation of factor Xa. After subcutaneous injection, the onset of activity is between 20 and 60 minutes, with peak plasma levels occurring between 2 and 4 hours. Heparin is ultimately metabolized by the liver and the reticuloendothelial system.

Of the LMWH preparations, enoxaparin (Lovenox) has recently been approved in the United States for DVT prophylaxis following hip and knee arthroplasties, and dalteparin (Fragmin) has been approved for DVT prophylaxis in patients undergoing abdominal surgery who are also at particular risk of thromboembolic complications. After subcutaneous injection, the maximal effectiveness occurs between 3 and 5 hours, and the activity persists for about 12 hours.

Warfarin interferes with the action of vitamin K by inhibiting the hepatic synthesis of coagulation factors II, VII, IX, and X. Its effect is detectable once the baseline level of these factors already in circulation starts to be depleted by metabolic degradation. After oral administration, the maximal concentration in the plasma is achieved between 1 and 9 hours. Almost all of the medication (97%) is bound to the plasma albumin. The initial effect is apparent in 24 hours, but the peak effect occurs between 3 and 4 days and lasts for about 4 to 5 days. It is metabolized in the liver and has a half-life of around $2\frac{1}{2}$ days.

Preparations and Dosing

Although heparin is a mucopolysaccharide that is naturally synthesized in the body, the form of heparin used for therapeutic purposes is derived from porcine intestinal mucosa or bovine lung. Because of its molecular size, heparin administered orally would not be absorbed readily from the gastrointestinal tract. It is thus administered either by deep subcutaneous injection or intravenously. The dosage of heparin sodium, when used in fixed low-dose therapy for the prevention of deep venous thrombosis, is typically 5,000 units SC every 8 to 12 hours. During fixed low-dose heparin therapy, it is not necessary to monitor the activated partial thromboplastin time (aPTT), because this index is essentially unaffected. However, this monitoring is required during full-dose therapy, which is most commonly utilized during the initial treatment of acute proximal DVT or PE. In this instance, unfractionated heparin is given intravenously, initially as a bolus followed by continuous infusion. Subsequently, the aPTT is monitored at frequent intervals, and the infusion rate of the heparin is adjusted to maintain the value between 1.5 and 2.5 times the control value (53). Several other specific approaches used for dosing heparin intravenously have also been described (53–56).

The LMWH is derived from unfractionated heparin through depolymerization and has a higher ratio of anti–factor Xa to anti–factor IIa activity than pure unfractionated heparin. The LMWH is associated with lower incidences of bleeding complications as reported by the manufacturers. The recommended dosage for enoxaparin (Lovenox) is 30 mg SC every 12 hours, with treatment initiated within 24 hours and usually lasting for up to 14 days postoperatively. Dalteparin (Fragmin) is given subcutaneously, 2,500 IU, 1 to 2 hours before abdominal surgery and is continued daily for 5 to 10 days postoperatively.

As stated above, the most commonly utilized oral anticoagulant is warfarin sodium (Coumadin, Panwarfin). The dosage of warfarin is individualized and is based on monitoring the therapeutic efficacy by regular prothrombin time (PT) assessments. Because of significant variability in thromboplastin reagents used in making these assessments among laboratories, a common standardized scale, known as the International Normalized Ratio (INR), was developed to factor in this variability and allow for more accurate monitoring of therapeutic efficacy regardless of the reagents used. Typically, for prophylaxis and also for the treatment of thromboembolism, the manufacturer recommends maintaining an INR of 2.0 to 3.0. This includes prophylaxis against embolism associated with atrial fibrillation and biological heart valve replacements. The effectiveness of anticoagulation within this range is essentially equivalent to that of higher dosages, yet with fewer hemorrhagic events (57). A higher INR (2.5 to 3.5) is suggested with mechanical heart valves (58).

The usual starting dose of warfarin is from 5 to 10 mg orally per day (for those rare patients in whom oral administration is not feasible, warfarin may be given by intramuscular or intravenous injection). Larger loading doses should be avoided, when possible, given the increased risk for hemorrhage. It is also prudent to start with lower loading doses in the elderly or debilitated or in those who are known to be sensitive to warfarin. Oral anticoagulation is usually initiated at the time of heparin treatment, is overlapped with it for about 4 to 5 days in order for the INR to increase to 2.0 to 3.0, and is then continued alone for a variable time period that depends on the underlying condition. For instance, the common practice in treating orthopedic patients is to discontinue the anticoagulant before discharge home or when the patient is fully ambulatory. However, there is evidence to support treatment for a longer period of time in order to further reduce DVT risk (42,59).

If oral anticoagulants are used concomitantly with heparin, the PT should be checked at least 5 hours following the last intravenous dose and 24 hours following the last subcutaneous dose of heparin. These time periods are recommended because heparin itself can prolong the one-stage PT.

Relevant Side Effects and Drug Interactions

The adverse effects of greatest concern with heparin are those related to hemorrhagic phenomena, most commonly presenting as bruising, petechiae, epistaxis, and gastrointestinal as well as urinary tract bleeding. The administration of heparin should obviously be done with extreme caution in patients at increased risk for bleeding, including those that are already taking drugs that affect platelet function such as salicylates, NSAIDs, and dipyridamole. Another potential problem is heparin-induced thrombocytopenia from either a direct effect on platelets or by an immunologic response. Thus, it is important to monitor complete blood counts, especially at the start but also at regular intervals during treatment. Other adverse effects that may occur include local irritation (especially with deeper injections; thus, the need to avoid intramuscular injection) and hypersensitivity reactions.

Hemorrhage is also the most common adverse effect of oral anitcoagulants. As for parenteral anticoagulants, it presents most commonly as gastrointestinal or genitourinary bleeding. The risk of hemorrhagic complications is reduced by close monitoring of therapeutic efficacy (PT and INR). Skin necrosis, a relatively rare but potentially hazardous reaction, may develop in susceptible individuals such as those patients with protein C deficiency because there is normally local thrombosis that occurs within the first few days of initiating coumadin. The concurrent administration of heparin for the first 5 to 7 days of anticoagulation reduces the risk of this reaction.

Many drugs can alter the therapeutic efficacy of warfarin. Those that may increase the PT include acetaminophen, ASA, NSAIDs, phenytoin, sulfonamides, and thyroid supplements. Those that can decrease the PT include adrenocorticosteroids, antacids, antihistamines, carbamazepine, haloperidol, and vitamin C. Others, including diuretics and H_2 blockers, may cause either an increase or decrease in the PT.

Antithrombotics

Relevance to Physiatry

These medications are also referred to as antiplatelet drugs, given their primary effect of inhibiting platelet aggregation. The typical agents in this group include ASA, dipyridamole, and ticlopidine. The use of ASA in appropriate patients has been associated with significant reductions in the risk of thrombotic vascular events, namely stroke and myocardial infarction (60). Aspirin is in fact an important medication for the secondary prevention of ischemic stroke. Some studies even indicate that low-dose ASA therapy is of equal benefit but with fewer side effects (61,62). Ticlopidine is also useful in ischemic stroke prevention, but its use has been limited to certain circumstances. Specifically, evidence supports its use in women with recent TIAs, patients in whom prior ASA use failed to prevent stroke, in those intolerant to ASA, and in patients with vertebrobasilar disease or with hypertensive cardiovascular disease without significant carotid disease (63). In terms of antithrombotic therapy, dipyridamole has not been proven to provide any benefit over ASA (60).

Medications

Medications in this class are described in Table 31-10.

Cardiovascular Medications

Medications that affect the cardiovascular system are very frequently encountered in the rehabilitative setting, especially in the elderly population. It is not uncommon for the physiatrist to make adjustments in these medications, especially while the patient is being cared for on an inpatient rehabilitation unit. Because these medications can have a such a profound impact on the patient's medical status and general well-being, it is important for the physiatrist to have a basic knowledge of the types of medications used, their indications, and their effects.

Alpha Blockers

Relevance to Physiatry

Although the primary general medical uses of alpha blockers are for the treatment of hypertension and prostate-related bladder outlet obstruction, in physiatry they are also utilized for the control and prevention of vascular manifestations of autonomic dysreflexia (64). In addition, phenoxybenzamine can also be utilized in reflex sympathetic dystrophy (RSD) because it affects both types of alpha receptors, thus leading to a chemical sympathectomy. The frequent occurrences of orthostatic hypotension and reflex tachycardia during the first few days of initiating treatment (especially the first-dose phenomenon) should be taken into account, as should the fact that postural hypotension can also occur following rapid increases in the dosage, during the established use of these medications, or following the addition of a second antihypertensive medication. The clinical use of alpha-2 blockers is limited and is still being determined. For example, yohimbine (Yocon) is thought to be of benefit in treating psychogenic impotence, diabetic neuropathy, and postural hypotension (65).

TABLE 31-10. *Antiplatelet agents*

Generic (trade) name	Mechanism of action	Dose (mg)	Other properties and side effects
Aspirin	Inhibits thromboxane A_2 synthesis and thus ability of platelet aggregation	81–325 PO qd	Regular, buffered, and enteric-coated; avoid using with ticlopidine
Ticlopidine (Ticlid)	Time- and dose-dependent inhibition of platelet aggregation and release of granules, which impedes ADP-induced platelet–fibrinogen binding. Maximal effect occurs by the eighth to 11th days of use; need 2-week discontinution for return of normal platelet function	250 PO bid (as with ASA, higher doses associated with greater likelihood of adverse effects, but antithrombotic effect is the same) (19)	Contraindicated for hypersensitivity, neutropenia, thrombocytopenia, hemostatic disorder, or severe liver impairment; rash and diarrhea are relatively common; reversible neutropenia (2.4%); thus, monitor CBC biweekly for 3 months; phenytoin and propranolol levels might be increased by ticlopidine
Dipyridamole (Persantine)	Increases platelet cAMP, thus, less adherence, aggregation, and enzymatic activity	75–100 PO qid	Vasodilation, thus use caution in those with hypotension; diarrhea, vomiting, flushing, or pruritus

ADP, adenosine 5' disphospate; ASA, aspirin; cAMP, 3',5'cyclic adenosine monophosphate; CBC, complete blood cell count; PO, oral.

TABLE 31-11. *Cardiac medications acting on the sympathetic nervous system*

Generic (trade) name	Dose (mg)	Other properties and side effects
Alpha agonists		
Clonidine hydrochloride (Catapres, Catapres-TTS)	Oral, 0.1 bid up to 2.4 mg/day; patch, 0.1–0.3/day; change qwk	Renally metabolized; also used to blunt autonomic symptoms from narcotic withdrawal
Guanfacine hydrochloride (Tenex)	0.5–1.0 PO/day up to 3.0/ day	Taken h/s to avoid daytime somnolence; renal metabolism
Guanabenz acetate (Wytensin)	4 PO bid and increased prn by 4/day up to 32/day	Hepatically metabolized
Methyldopa (Aldomet)	250 PO bid up to 2,000/day	First metabolized in the brain to methylnorepinephrine, which activates alpha-2 receptors; parenteral form also available
Alpha-1 antagonists		Orthostatic hypotension, especially first dose
Doxazosin (Cardura)	Start 1 PO qd; maximum 16 PO qd	Newest agent of this class
Prazosin (Minipress)	Start 1 PO bid–tid; maximum 40 PO qd	If peripheral edema, can switch to Minizide (prazosin/polythiazide), 1 tab PO bid
Terazosin (Hytrin)	Start 1 PO qh/s; maximum 20 PO qd	Not available in combination with a diuretic

bid, twice a day; PO, oral; qd, every day; qh/s, at bedtime; tid, three times a day.

Medications

These agents are listed in Table 31-11.

Alpha-2 Agonists

Relevance to Physiatry

The common indication for these medications is the treatment of hypertension, either alone or in combination with other antihypertensive medications. They may be used in acute autonomic dysreflexia refractory to other measures and medications and also in the prevention of its recurrence (64). Because of their centrally acting mechanism, they may cause drowsiness, a definitely untoward effect when attempting to objectively monitor the progress of a patient with altered mental status (e.g., early traumatic brain injury or stroke). In addition to its antihypertensive properties, one of the alpha agonists, clonidine, is useful in the treatment of pain from RSD and in the treatment of spasticity, especially when delivered by patch (66). The exact mechanism of this latter effect is not fully understood. The CNS side effects can interfere with rehabilitation efforts. The FDA has recently released tizanidine hydrochloride (Zanaflex), a new alpha-2 agonist developed primarily for the management of spasticity. Its advantage over clonidine primarily is its much lower incidence of hypotensive side effects.

Medications

Table 31-11 lists drugs in this category.

Angiotensin-Converting Enzyme Inhibitors

Relevance to Physiatry

Although there are no unique physiatric uses for these agents, angiotensin-converting enzyme inhibitors (ACEIs) will probably become even more commonly used now that it has been shown that they exert a renal-protective effect in diabetics (67). A related and recently available class of medications whose role has yet to be established are the angiotensin II receptor antagonists. An advantage of these in patients enrolled on rehabilitation programs is their relative lack of cardiovascular side effects compared to other agents.

Medications

Losartan (Cozaar) is the only angiotensin II receptor antagonist that is FDA-approved at the time of this writing for the treatment of hypertension. The typical dosage of losartan is 50 mg daily by mouth, initially, with a maximum dosage of 100 mg daily. Table 31-12 lists ACEIs presently available.

TABLE 31-12. *Angiotensin-converting enzyme inhibitors*

Generic (trade) name	Oral dose (mg)
Benazepril (Lotensin)	HTN: 10 qd, up to 80 daily
Captopril (Capoten)	HTN: 25 bid–tid, up to 450 daily; CHF: 6.25–12.5 tid
Enalapril (Vasotec)	HTN: 5 qd–bid, up to 40 daily; CHF: 2.5 qd–bid, up to 40 daily
Fosinopril (Monopril)	HTN: 10 qd, up to 80 daily
Lisinopril (Prinivil, Zestril)	HTN: 10 qd, up to 40 daily; CHF: 5 qd, up to 20 daily
Moexipril (Univasc)	HTN: 7.5 qd, up to 30 daily
Quinapril (Accupril)	HTN: 10 qd, up to 80 daily; CHF: 5 bid, up to 20–40 daily
Ramipril (Altace)	HTN: 2.5 qd, up to 20 daily

bid, twice a day; CHF, congestive heart failure; HTN, hypertension; qd, everyday; tid, three times a day.

Antiarrhythmic Medications

Relevance to Physiatry

The physiatrist is likely to encounter patients who are regularly taking antiarrhythmics. This is particularly true of

TABLE 31-13. *Antiarrhythmic medications*

Class	Electrophysiological effect	Arrhythmia indications	Examples
I	Block sodium channels		
A			Quinidine, procainamide, disopyramide
B		Ventricular dysrhythmias	Lidocaine, tocainide, mexiletene, phenytoin
C		Ventricular dysrhythmias	flecainide and encainide
II	Block beta-adrenergic receptors	SVT, PVCs	Beta blockers
III	Prolong membrane repolarization	Ventricular dysrhythmias, recurrent ventricular fibrillation, or unstable V-tach	Bretylium, sotalol, amiodarone
IV	Block calcium channels	SVT especially PSVT; rapid ventricular rate in A-fib	Calcium channel blockers

PVC, premature ventricular contraction; PSVT, paroxysmol supraventricular tachycardia; SVT, supraventricular tachycardia.

patients undergoing cardiac rehabilitation. Thus, a basic understanding of these medications along with their classification scheme is important.

Medications

Drugs in this group are listed in Table 31-13.

Beta Blockers

Relevance to Physiatry

The physiatrist should understand the reason(s) for which a referred patient may be on a given beta blocker. This is especially important in treating patients following myocardial infarction or with cardiac arrhythmias. In the former, during the second phase of a three-phase cardiac rehabilitation program, a therapeutic exercise program of appropriate intensity for a patient on beta blockers would be based on a percentage of the symptom-limited heart rate or of the maximum workload performed on exercise stress test rather than being based on absolute heart rate (68). In general, beta blockers tend to impair a patient's tolerance to exercise.

Most commonly, these medications are used in the treatment of hypertension, angina pectoris, and cardiac arrhythmias. In addition to these uses, beta blockers have also been employed in the treatment of migraine headaches, heightened metabolic turnover states such as thyrotoxicosis, and may be of benefit in treating chronic or recurrent aggression associated with traumatic brain injury (69).

Medications

Table 31-14 lists drugs in this class.

Calcium Channel Blockers

Relevance to Physiatry

These medications are commonly encountered in the physiatric setting, given their efficacy and convenient dosing preparations for the treatment of hypertension. The frequency of use may be diminishing with the expanded role of ACEIs, particularly in diabetic patients, and the recent controversy involving the use of regular, short-acting, nifedipine (70). One physiatric-specific use has been sublingual Procardia for rapid lowering of blood pressure in patients with autonomic dysreflexia. Side effects such as orthostatic hypotension, peripheral edema, and headache can be annoying. The physiatrist should be careful in ordering physical therapy modalities such as the whirlpool or Hubbard tank that can worsen vasodilation in any patient who is already taking a calcium channel blocker or other vasodilator.

Medications

Medications in this group are listed in Table 31-15.

Cardiac Glycosides

The cardiac glycosides consist of digitalis, digoxin, digitoxin, and deslanoside. Because digitalis is the prototype agent, discussion focuses on it. Although digitalis may be useful in improving cardiac functioning in some patients, which sometimes allows them to tolerate activity better, there may be potentially devastating effects that can result from their use. The physiatrist should have a high index of suspicion for early signs (particularly nausea) of digitalis toxicity in addition to periodically monitoring the efficacy of treatment and serum levels of the medication as well as serum electrolytes. The primary uses for cardiac glycosides include the treatment of congestive heart failure and control of ventricular rate in atrial fibrillation. Maintenance doses of digoxin (Lanoxin, Lanoxicaps) are generally in the range of 0.125 to 0.25 mg per day but can vary depending on toxicity and the underlying condition.

Diuretics

Relevance to Physiatry

In addition to the primary indications for diuretic use including hypertension and certain forms of edema, there are

TABLE 31-14. *Beta blockers*

Generic (trade) name	Oral dose (mg)	Indications and unique properties
Beta-1 selective		
Acebutolol (Sectral)	200 bid to 400 qd up to 1,200 qd	Arrhythmias, hypertension
Atenolol (Tenormin)	50 qd up to 100 qd	Angina, hypertension
Betaxolol (Kerlone)	10 qd up to 20 qd	Hypertension
Bisoprolol (Zebeta)	5 qd up to 20 qd	Hypertension
Metoprolol (Lopressor, Toprol XL)	50 bid up to 450 daily or 50–100 qd up to 400 daily	Angina
Beta (nonselective)		
Carteolol (Cartrol)	2.5 qd up to 10 daily	Hypertension
Labetalol (Trandate, Normodyne)	100 bid up to 2,400 daily	Hypertension; posesses alpha-1 antagonistic effects
Nadolol (Corgard)	40 qd up to 320 daily	Hypertension, angina
Penbutolol (Levatol)	20 qd up to 80 daily	Hypertension
Pindolol (Visken)	5 bid up to 60 daily	Hypertension; mild intrinsic beta-mimetic properties
Propranolol (Inderal, Inderal-LA)	40 bid up to 640 daily	Hypertension, angina, post-MI arrhythmias
Sotalol (Betapace)	80 bid up to 640 daily	Atrial fibrillation, life-threatening ventricular arrhythmias
Timolol (Blocadren)	10 bid up to 60 daily	Hypertension, post-MI arrhythmias

bid, twice a day; MI, myocardial infarction; qd, every day;

also other conditions that the physiatrist may encounter that warrant the use of diuretics. For instance, in the acute treatment of hypercalcemia secondary to immobilization (e.g., spinal cord injury), furosemide, in addition to hydration, may be of benefit (71). Diuretics may also facilitate the mobilization of fluid in early lymphedema but should not be used regularly for chronic treatment of this condition (72). In contrast, diuretic-associated orthostatic hypotension is a troublesome potential problem, particularly in those patients who are undergoing transfer, gait, and elevation training.

Medications

These drugs are described in Table 31-16.

Nitrates

Relevance to Physiatry

Organic nitrate use is commonly encountered in inpatient rehabilitative settings, where there are many patients with coronary artery disease. In addition to their use in angina,

TABLE 31-15. *Calcium channel blockers*

Generic (trade) name	Oral dose (mg)	Other properties and side effects
Amlodipine (Norvasc)	2.5–5 qd, up to 10 daily	Indicated for hypertension, stable and variant angina
Bepridil (Vascor)	200 qd, up to 400 daily	Indicated for stable angina
Diltiazem (Cardizem, Cardizem SR, Cardizem CD, Dilacor XR)	30 qid, up to 360 daily; 60–120 bid, up to 360 daily; 180–240 qd, up to 540 daily	Indicated for hypertension (extended preparations), stable and variant angina (can also be use IV for rapid atrial fibrillation)
Felodipine (Plendil)	5 qd, up to 10 daily	Indicated for hypertension
Isradipine (DynaCirc)	2.5 bid, up to 20 daily	Indicated for hypertension
Nicardipine (Cardene, Cardene SR)	20 tid, up to 120 daily; 30 bid, up to 120 daily	Indicated for hypertension (SR form) and stable angina
Nifedipine (Procardia, Adalat, Procardia XL, Adalat CC)	10 tid, up to 120 daily; 30–60 qd, up to 120 daily	Indicated for stable and variant angina; hypertension
Nimodipine (Nimotop)	60 q4h for 21 days	Indicated only for reduction of cerebral vasospasm following subarachnoid hemorrhage; must start within 96 hr of the bleed
Nisoldipine (Sular)	20–60 qd	Indicated for hypertension
Verapamil (Isoptin, Calan, Isoptin SR, Calan SR, Verelan)	80 tid, up to 360 daily; 240 qd, up to 480 daily	Indicated for hypertension; can also be used IV for treatment of SVT, although it has been replaced by adenosine for this indication

bid, twice a day; hr, hour; IV, intravenous; qd, everyday; tid, three times a day

TABLE 31-16. *Diuretics*

Generic (trade) name	Dose (mg)	Other properties and side effects
Thiazide		Sulfur-containing; thus, allergy potential
Chlorthiazide (Diuril)	250–500 PO qd to bid	Available in suspension for pediatric dosing
Chlorthalidone (Hygroton)	25–100 PO qd	Rarely used
Hydrochlorothiazide (HCTZ, Esidrix, Oretic, Hydrodiuril)	25–200 PO qd	Main use is for hypertension, alone or combined with other antihypertensives
Indapamide (Lozol)	1.25–5.0 PO qd	Technically an indoline; main use is for HTN
Metolazone (Zaroxolyn)	5–20 PO qd	Used with loop diuretics in edema states refractory to maximum doses of loop diuretics
Loop		Used when rigorous diuresis is needed
Bumetanide (Bumex)	0.5–2.0 PO qd; 0.5–1 IV/IM	1 mg is equivalent to 40 mg furosemide
Ethacrynic acid (Edecrin)	25–100 PO qd to bid; 0.5–1 mg/kg IV up to 50	
Furosemide (Lasix)	20–80 PO qd to bid; 1 mg/kg IV up to 20–40	Most commonly used loop diuretic
Torsemide (Demadex)	5–20 PO/IV qd	Equal efficacy with oral and IV doses
Potassium-sparing		Possible hyperkalemia, especially if used with ACEIs
Amiloride (Midamor)	5–10 PO qd	Rarely used; lack mineralocorticoid side effects
Spironolactone (Aldactone)	25–50 PO qd to bid	Aldosterone antagonist
Triamterene (Dyrenium)	100 PO bid	Rarely used; lack mineralocorticoid side effects

ACEIs, angiotensin-converting enzyme inhibitors; bid, twice a day; IM, intramuscular; IV, intravenous; PO, oral; qd, every day.

oral or transdermal nitrates may help to reduce acute blood pressure elevations such as in autonomic dysreflexia. The physiatrist should also be well acquainted with possible deleterious effects that nitrates may have in a patient undergoing an intensive rehabilitative program. In particular, it is important to prevent orthostatic hypotension and tachycardia through measures such as gradual position changes, especially in the mornings, and having the patient avoid prolonged standing if lower extremity strength is diminished.

Medications

Organic nitrates are listed in Table 31-17.

Corticosteroids

Relevance to Physiatry

The corticosteroid property of most use in physiatry is the powerful anti-inflammatory effect rather than the mineralocorticoid or androgenic/estrogenic effects. In particular, they are used in the injectable form for office-based procedures, in short tapering courses for radiculopathy and other localized musculoskeletal conditions, and are used chronically for systemic inflammatory conditions. Although controversial because their efficacy has never be proven, corticosteroids are sometimes administered by therapists transdermally via iontophoresis or phonophoresis. Besides their therapeutic uses, physiatrists also ultimately care for many patients who have developed corticosteroid-related side effects (especially osteoporosis and avascular necrosis leading to joint replacement) from chronic use.

Mechanism of Action and Pharmacokinetics

Corticosteroids bind to receptors within a target cell's nucleus and cause the cell to alter its usual protein synthesis. These altered proteins then exert various effects in the body, some of which can be used to therapeutic advantage and others of which can lead to troublesome side effects. Corticosteroids can be classified as mineralocorticoid, androgenic/estrogenic, and glucocorticoid depending on their predominant effect in the body.

At physiological as opposed to pharmacologic doses, the glucocorticoid class of corticosteroids exert antiinflammatory and immunosuppressive effects via the following mechanisms:

1. Inhibition of prostaglandin and leukotriene synthesis, probably by preventing the release of arachadonic acid from phospholipids rather than by inhibiting cyclooxygenase as NSAIDs do.
2. Inhibition of chemotactic factor release, leading to a diminished attraction of WBCs to the sites of inflammation.
3. Decrease in circulating lymphocytes and monocytes.
4. Reduction of vascular permeability by acting as direct vasoconstrictors or by inhibiting the release of vasodilators such as histamines and kinins.
5. Stabilization of lysosomal membranes (occurs only at higher steroid doses).

Oral glucocorticoids are absorbed through the GI tract, metabolized by the liver, and excreted by the kidneys at a rate that is proportional to the particular agent's water solubility.

TABLE 31-17. *Nitrates*

Generic (trade) name	Dose
Isosorbide dinitrate	
tablets (Isordil, Sorbitrate)	10–40 mg PO tid at least 6 hr apart
sublingual tablets (Isordil, Sorbitrate)	1 tab (2.5–10 mg) SL prn
sustained release (Isordil Tembids, Dilatrate SR)	40–80 mg PO bid to tid
Isosorbide mononitrate	
tablets (ISMO, Monoket)	20 mg PO bid at least 7 hr apart
extended release (Imdur)	30–240 mg PO qd (start with 30–60 PO qd)
Nitroglycerin	
ointment 2% (Nitro-Bid, Nitrol)	Start 0.5 inch q8; maintenance 1–2 inches q8h; maximum 4–5 inches q 4 hrs. (15 mg/inch)
spray (Nitrolingual)	1–2 oral sprays prn
sublingual (Nitrostat)	0.4 mg SL
sustained release (Nitro-Bid)	Start 2.5 mg PO bid to tid and titrate up
transdermal (Deponit, Minitran, Nitro-Dur, Nitrodisc, Transderm-Nitro)	1 patch 12–16 hr/day

bid, twice a day; PO, oral; qd, every day; SL, sublingual; tid, three times a day.

Preparations and Dosing

Perhaps the two most commonly used oral steroid preparations in many physiatric practices are prednisone and the Medrol dose pack. One dose pack starts the patient at 24 mg of Medrol (equivalent to 30 mg of prednisone) and tapers off over 7 days. A dose pack is a convenient form in which to prescribe a short tapering course of oral steroids because the instructions are both easy for the physician to explain to the patient and for the patient to follow. That is, the patient simply takes the daily packet of medication into which the tapering dose has already been set up. This eliminates the need for the patient to have to count out a certain number of pills each day and will probably increase compliance because it eliminates the feeling by many patients that taking seven pills at once, for example, is "just too much, no matter what the doctor says." Two potential drawbacks, however, are the expense of a Medrol dose pack compared to generic prednisone and the fact that a Medrol dose pack provides a peak equivalent prednisone dose of only 30 mg. A higher-strength dose pack, the Sterapred DS 12 day Unipak, delivers peak prednisone doses of 60 mg but involves qid dosing.

The most commonly used injectable agents are betamethasone (Celestone), dexamethasone (Decadron), and methylprednisolone (Medrol). When selecting a given agent, equivalent doses relative to cortisone, relative antiinflammatory potency, relative mineralocorticoid potency, and duration of action need to be considered (Table 31-18) (4,73). For comparison, physiological steroid doses are equivalent to 30 mg/day of hydrocortisone (7.5 mg day of prednisone), whereas stress doses are equivalent to 300 mg/day of hydrocortisone (75 mg/day of prednisone).

The following guidelines should be considered when prescribing corticosteroids (28,73):

1. Use these only after less toxic therapy has proven to be ineffective.
2. Use the smallest amount of corticosteroid that is able to control symptoms because the severity of side effects is proportional to the dose.
3. Administer the corticosteroid locally rather than systemically whenever possible.
4. For those patients receiving short-term corticosteroids, it is best to use daily corticosteroid treatment with once-per-day dosing (preferably in the morning). In contrast, using qid dosing of one-fourth the daily dose is not only inconvenient, it also causes considerably more adrenal suppression.
5. It can be helpful not to refer to these medications as steroids because of the negative connotations that this word has. Instead, refer to the medication as cortisone or prednisone. These words, however, may already have enough negative connotations of their own. If the patient is offering some resistance to taking the medication, the physician can emphasize that possible side effects with prednisone, including osteoporosis and truncal obesity, are seen with chronic use and not with a short course.
6. Because oral steroids typically cause a metallic taste, forewarning the patient of this can certainly avoid unnecessary patient distress as well as unnecessary phone calls to the physician.
7. For those patients receiving long-term steroids, alternate-day therapy is desirable because the hypothalamic–pituitary–adrenal axis has a chance to recover on the alternate morning while the anti-inflammatory effects persist longer than the physical presence of steroids and their metabolic effects. The likelihood of developing secondary adrenal insufficiency is determined by the dose, potency, and duration of exogenous glucocorticoids. Although it is impossible to predict the exact glucocorticoid dose that will cause adrenal suppression, some guidelines for doses capable of causing this are as follows: (a) doses equivalent to 100 mg hydrocortisone (25 mg prednisone) daily for 3 days; (b) doses equivalent to 30 mg hydrocortisone (7.5 mg prednisone) daily for 30 days.

TABLE 31-18. *Corticosteroid preparations*

Corticosteroid generic (trade) name	Route	Equivalent oral dose (mg)	Relative potencies: anti-inflammatory (mineralocorticoid)	Relative duration[a]
Betamethasone (Celestone)	PO/IM	0.6–0.75	20–30 (0)	L
Cortisone (Cortone)	PO	25	0.8 (2)	S
Dexamathasone (Decadron)	PO/IM/IV	0.75	20–30 (0)	L
Hydrocortisone (Cortef, Cortisol, Solu-Cortef)	PO/IM/IV	20	1[b] (2)	S
Methylprednisolone (Medrol, Medrol Dosepack, SoluMedrol)	PO/IM/IV	4	5 (0)	I
Prednisolone (Hydeltra)	PO/IM/IV	5	4 (1)	I
Prednisone (Deltasone, Orasone, Sterapred Unipak, Sterepred DS Unipak)	PO	5	4 (1)	I
Triamcinolone (Aristocort, Kenacort, Kenalog)	PO/IM	4	5 (0)	I

IM, intramuscular; IV, intravenous; PO, oral.
[a]I, intermediate; L, long; S, short.
[b]Cortisol is used as the reference because it is the major glucocorticoid produced in the body.

8. Rather than simply discontinuing steroids, wean patients off them over a course of weeks to months if they have been receiving them for more than several weeks. One can refer the patient to an endocrinologist for testing of their adrenal responsiveness to ACTH or for metyrapone or insulin tolerance testing if it is unclear whether they are adrenally suppressed. Recovery of adrenal function is variable, and even after appropriate treatment, relative adrenal suppression can last up to 1 year.
9. When corticosteroid injections are administered, general principles have been suggested in order to diminish the chance of arthropathy from the possible catabolic effect of repeated intra-articular use of corticosteroids or steroid-induced crystal arthropathy and to avoid the possibility of tendon rupture: (a) limit the number of intra-articular corticosteroid injections to no more than four per year and 20 in a lifetime for a given joint (74); (b) never inject directly into a tendon and avoid peritendinous injection of the Achilles and patellar tendons, as tendon rupture can occur from the catabolic effect of corticosteroids on proteins and the inhibition of collagen synthesis.
10. The choice of injectable corticosteroid agent depends in part on the underlying condition being treated. For example, for acute or subacute conditions in which a relatively fast effect is desired, a short-acting and therefore rapid-onset agent is preferable. In contrast, long-acting agents are preferable for chronic inflammatory conditions in which long-term suppression of inflammation is the goal.
11. Dosing guidelines for injectable steroids have been suggested as follows (73): (a) large joints (e.g., glenohumeral, knee, hip), 40 mg of methylprednisolone or equivalent; (b) intermediate joints (e.g., elbow, ankle), 20 to 30 mg of methylprednisolone or equivalent; (c) small joints (e.g., phalangeal joints), 10 to 20 mg of methylprednisolone or equivalent.
12. Epidural steroid injections should probably be performed only with preservative-free corticosteroid preparations such as betamethasone (Celestone) because accidental subarachnoid injection can theoretically lead to arachnoiditis. One must also be careful not to use a local anesthetic preparation that contains a preservative because it can cause flocculation of the betamethasone.

Relevant Side Effects and Drug Interactions

Although not a true side effect, yet a major potential problem with the use of corticosteroids, is the fact that these medications often just mask the inflammation associated with a given disease rather than effecting a cure. Thus, there is a tendency for patients to ignore the underlying disorder when they are feeling better from the anti-inflammatory effects of corticosteroids. A classic example is the patient who has received a subacromial steroid injection and then immediately resumes the repetitive overhead activity that led to shoulder impingement in the first place.

Most of the true side effects occur after prolonged administration, and many of these are basically manifestations of Cushing syndrome as shown in Table 31-19. Simple routine

TABLE 31-19. *Corticosteroid side effects*

Organ system	Side effect
Central nervous system	Behavior and mood alteration
Cardiovascular	Fluid retention; hypertension
Endocrine/metabolism	Adrenal atrophy; amenorrhea; appetite increase; glucose tolerance impairment; hypernatremia and hypokalemia
Gastrointestinal	Aggravation of peptic ulcer disease
Musculoskeletal	Avascular necrosis; bone demineralization; steroid myopathy
Skin/cosmetic	Acne, buffalo hump, moon face, hirsuitism, skin thinning

glucose monitoring along with adjustments in the dose of insulin or oral hypoglycemic agent should be recommended when a corticosteroid injection is administered to a diabetic patient. Two of the more interesting and pertinent catabolic side effects listed in the table are steroid myopathy and avascular necrosis. In fact, those practitioners who routinely perform electromyography (EMG) are probably familiar with the request from referring physicians to rule out steroid myopathy. Avascular necrosis of the femoral or humeral heads is an idiosyncratic event that can occur after a short course of prednisone but is fortunately quite rare.

Skin depigmentation and subcutaneous atrophy are possible dermatologic complications that can occur whenever corticosteroids are injected but can be minimized by using an injection needle other than the one used to draw up the medication and/or mixing a vehicle into the solution such as a local anesthetic or normal saline. Skin thinning can occur with chronic oral corticosteroid use.

Allergic reactions including anaphylactoid and true anaphylaxis have been reported in patients receiving a corticosteroid injection (73). Some allergic reactions have even been reported up to a week after an injection, presumably caused by gradual systemic absorption of the medication.

Acceleration of corticosteroid metabolism with subsequent diminution in effect occurs from medications that induce hepatic microsomal enzymes, such as phenobarbital, phenytoin, carbamazepine, and rifampin. In contrast, the potency of corticosteroids is increased by those medications such as NSAIDs, oral contraceptives, and exogenous estrogens, which exert similar effects. Some practitioners discontinue NSAIDs while a patient is receiving a course of corticosteroids because of the presumed increased potential for GI toxicity.

Gastrointestinal Medications

Antiemetics

Relevance to Physiatry

When patients are nauseated, it is very difficult for them to participate in a rehabilitation program in a meaningful way. Nausea can be particularly prevalent in patients enrolled in cancer rehabilitation programs who are receiving chemotherapy. Nausea should always evoke suspicion of early digoxin toxicity in patients taking cardiac glycosides.

Medications

Antiemetic drugs are listed in Table 31-20.

Medications That Act by Affecting Gastrointestinal Motility

Relevance to Physiatry

Abnormally slow gastrointestinal transit (e.g., diabetic gastroparesis) can especially occur in patients with diabetes mellitus. Because the average physiatrist not infrequently treats diabetics, one may find it necessary to begin a patient on a promotility agent. The two most commonly used agents that affect GI motility are cisapride and metaclopramide.

Medications

Medications in this group are listed in Table 31-21.

Antidiarrheal Drugs

Relevance to Physiatry

Diarrhea is not an uncommon complaint among hospitalized patients. This condition obviously can interfere with a

TABLE 31-20. *Antiemetics*

Medication and mechanism of action	Generic (trade) name	Dose (mg)	Other properties and side effects
Phenothiazines: act at the chemoreceptor trigger zone and the vomiting center	Prochlorperazine (Compazine)	5–10 PO/IM tid–qid	Antidopaminergic: extrapyramidal reactions and neuroleptic malignant syndrome possible
	Promethazine (Phenergan)	1/kg up to max 25–50 PO/IM/PR q4–6h	IV form also available, lacks effect on dopamine, antihistaminergic
	Thiethylperazine (Torecan)	10 PO/IM q8h	Same as for prochlorperazine
Antihistamines: act at the chemoreceptor trigger zone and the vomiting center	Dimenhydrinate (Dramamine)	50 PO/IM/IV q4h	Sedating; transdermal preparation no longer commercially available
Other: act at the chemoreceptor trigger zone and the vomiting center	Trimethobenzamide (Tigan)	250 PO tid–qid; 200 IM/PR q6–8h	Hypersensitivity and Parkinson-like symptoms have been reported
Cannabinoids	Dronabinol (Marinol)	Dosage varies	Chemotherapy-related nausea
Selective serotonin reuptake inhibitors: block the 5-HT_3 serotonin receptor	Granisetron (Kytril)	1 PO bid × 1 day	Chemotherapy-related nausea
	Ondansetron (Zofran)	8 PO bid × 2 days	Chemotherapy-related nausea

bid, twice a day; IM, intramuscular; PO, oral; PR, rectally; qid, four times a day; tid, three times a day.

TABLE 31-21. *Medications affecting gastrointestinal motility*

Mechanism of action, generic (trade) name	Dose (mg)	Other properties and side effects
Antidiarrheal: Opioid		
Diphenoxylate/atropine (Lomotil)	2.5–5 PO tid–qid	Atropine limits abuse potential (schedule 5) but adds to possible side effects; liquid also available
Loperamide (Imodium)	4 PO initially, then 2 prn (max 16 mg/day)	Haloperidol derivative, resembles meperidine structurally; no known abuse potential; elixir available
Promotility: Cholinergic		
Cisapride (Propulsid)	10–20 PO qid	Fatal dysrhythmias can occur if used with ketoconazole, itraconazole, erythromycin, fluconazole, clarithromycin
Metaclopramide (Reglan)	10–30 PO qid 30 min before meals and h/s	Dopamine receptor antagonist; thus, CNS side effects and extrapyramidal reactions; IV/IM/elixir also available

CNS, central nervous system; h/s, at bedtime; IM, intramuscular; IV, intravenous; PO, oral; prn, as required; qid, four times a day; tid, three times a day.

course of rehabilitation. Therefore, medications are commonly used for the short-term management of acute, nonspecific diarrhea and may also be used for chronic diarrhea associated with inflammatory bowel disease. They should be avoided, however, when diarrhea is suspected to be the result of obstructive jaundice, fecal impaction, or an infectious processes with toxin production. The two most commonly used antidiarrheal agents for hospitalized patients are diphenoxylate with atropine (Lomotil) and loperamide (Imodium).

Medications

Drugs in this group are named in Table 31-21.

Medications That Reduce Gastric Acid Secretion

Relevance to Physiatry

Besides their use in the prevention and treatment of NSAID-induced gastrointestinal pathology, which was discussed earlier, these medications are also used for idiopathic gastric and duodenal ulcers as well as for gastroesophageal reflux disease. Other than cimetidine, which can cause CNS changes in the elderly, these medications are usually well tolerated and do not seem to interfere with patients undergoing rehabilitation.

Medications

Drugs that inhibit gastric acid secretion are listed in Table 31-22.

Laxatives

As is true for diarrhea, constipation can also have a significant negative impact on a patient's rehabilitation progress. Laxatives can be used to facilitate or restore regular bowel movements in patients suffering from constipation. There is a large choice of available preparations, as shown in Table 31-23, and their effects range from mild, as with the use of bulking agents, to more aggressive, such as can be achieved with hyperosmolar preparations. They should be used with caution in the presence of nausea, vomiting, or unexplained abdominal pain.

Hypnotics

Insomnia is frequently associated with life stressors such as injury or illness and can significantly interfere with a patient's rehabilitation by producing daytime lethargy, irritability, difficulties with concentration, etc. Hence, treatment of insomnia can play an important role in the overall management of a patient. Although conditions such as fibromyalgia and chronic fatigue syndrome are strongly associated with a sleep disturbance, hypnotics should not be used routinely in patients with these conditions (75). Their use, however, in acute care and rehabilitation settings is quite common.

Benzodiazepines

Mechanism of Action and Pharmacokinetics

These agents exert hypnotic and anxiolytic effects by binding nonselectively to the GABA-BZ receptor complex, particularly in the limbic system, the thalamus, and the hypothalamus. In doing so they reduce delta sleep. Those benzodiazepines that are used for insomnia are generally well absorbed, undergo very little first-pass metabolism, are highly metabolized by the liver, are excreted with short elimination half-lives, and their metabolites do not accumulate.

Preparations and Dosing

Temazepam (Restoril) is perhaps the most widely used agent for the treatment of insomnia in this class. A dosing range of 7.5 to 30 mg at bedtime is recommended for this schedule IV drug.

TABLE 31-22. *Medications that act by reducing gastric secretion*

Mechanism of action	Generic (trade) name	Oral dose (mg)	Other properties and side effects
H_2 blockers: Block histamine H_2 receptors of gastric acid-producing parietal cells	Cimetidine (Tagamet)	800 h/s or 400 bid	Because of the change in gastric fluid acidity as a result of H_2 blockers, GI absorption of various drugs can be altered; IV form also available; cimetidine has somewhat greater incidence of side effects, especially headache, dizziness, nausea, and myalgias; in the elderly and those with impaired renal function, CNS disturbances can occur; only cimetidine interferes with cytochrome P-450 activity and thus increases half-lives of many meds
	Famotidine (Pepcid)	40 h/s or 20 bid	IV form also available
	Nizatidine (Axid)	300 h/s or 150 bid	
	Ranitidine (Zantac)	300 h/s or 150 bid	IV form also available
Proton pump inhibitors: Decrease gastric acid secretion by inhibiting the parietal cell membrane enzyme that actively transports hydrogen ions out of the cell	Lansoprazole (Prevacid)	15 to 30 qd	Used primarily for prevention of gastric ulcers secondary to ASA or NSAIDs in high-risk patients; well tolerated but sometimes associated with nausea, diarrhea, headache, dizziness, and possible bacterial colonization in the stomach as a result of the elevation in gastric fluid volume; inhibition of the metabolism of medications transformed by cytochrome P-450
	Omeprazole (Prilosec)	20 to 40 qd	Same as for Prevacid
Prostaglandin analogs: Reduces gastric acid secretion and has mucosal protective properties	Misoprostol (Cytotec)	100–200 μg qid	Diarrhea very common; not to be used in women of child-bearing age because of abortifactant properties; no known drug interactions

ASA, aspirin; bid, twice a day; CNS, central nervous system; GI, gastrointestinal; h/s, at bedtime; IV, intravenous; NSAID, nonsteroidal anit-inflammatory drug; qd, everyday; qid, four times a day;

Relevant Side Effects and Drug Interactions

Daytime drowsiness, headache, and fatigue were the three most frequently reported side effects in controlled clinical studies of patients who received temazepam at bedtime (11). As with all benzodiazepines, dependence and rebound insomnia can develop, particularly if it is used regularly for more than a few weeks, and patients should be cautious if they are taking other CNS depressants.

Zolpidem Tartrate (Ambien)

Mechanism of Action and Pharmacokinetics

Zolpidem is unique in that its chemical structure is unrelated to those of benzodiazepines, barbiturates, and other hypnotic agents. It preferentially binds to the omega-1 subunit of the GABA-BZ receptor complex, whereas benzodiazepines nonselectively bind to all three of the omega subunits. Zolpidem's binding is believed to be responsible for its selective hypnotic effect yet lack of anticonvulsant, anxiolytic, and muscle relaxant properties that are seen with benzodiazepines. In terms of the hypnotic effect of zolpidem, there is relative preservation of sleep architecture both in otherwise healthy patients and in patients with acute or chronic insomnia.

Zolpidem is rapidly absorbed from the GI tract and achieves a mean peak serum level in approximately 1½ hours. It is then converted to inactive metabolites, which are eliminated by the kidneys with a mean elimination half-life of approximately 2½ hours. It has not been found to accumulate when it was studied in young subjects who used the medication (20 mg) on a nightly basis for 2 weeks, nor was it found to accumulate in the elderly who used it (10 mg) nightly for 1 week (11). This is a desirable characteristic of a hypnotic agent, as accumulation can lead to daytime sedation.

Preparations and Dosing

Zolpidem is classified as a schedule IV controlled substance. The usual nighttime dose is 10 mg immediately before bedtime in nonelderly patients and 5 mg immediately before bedtime in the elderly and in patients with hepatic insufficiency. Doses greater than 10 mg are not recommended.

Relevant Side Effects and Drug Interactions

In controlled clinical trials, the most commonly observed adverse effects seen at statistically significant differences from placebo-treated patients associated with the short-term use (up to ten nights) of zolpidem were daytime drowsiness

TABLE 31-23. *Laxatives*

Mechanism of action	Generic (trade) name	Dose	Other properties and side effects
Bulking agents: contain natural fiber, which increases fecal H_2O capacity and enhances bacterial floral growth	Psyllium (Metamucil, Fiberall); methylcellulose (Citrucel)	1 tsp PO qd–tid; 1 tbsp PO qd–tid	Gritty texture prohibits use in some patients
Colonic stimulants ("irritant cathartics") act on colonic and rectal sensory nerve endings on mucosal contact; peristalsis and subsequent purging then occur by parasympathetic reflexes	Bisacodyl (Dulcolax); cascara sagrada (Cascara); castor oil (Purge); senna (Senokot) tablets (8.6 mg/tab) or syrup (8.8 mg/tsp)	10 mg PO/PR prn; 325 mg PO qh/s; 15–30 ml PO qh/s; 2–4 tabs PO qd–bid/ or 10–15 ml PO qh/s	Dulcolax affects fluid and electrolyte absorption throughout the intestine; Cascara and Senokot act on the large intestine, so there is a delayed effect of approximately 8 hr and may cause urinary discoloration; Castor oil intestinally hydrolyzed to a cathartic (ricinoleic acid)
Combination products	Docusate/casanthranol (Peri-Colace); senna/docusate (Senokot-S tabs); milk of magnesia/cascara	1–2 caps qh/s; 15–30 ml qh/s; 2 PO qd or 4 PO bid	Pericolace capsule, 100 mg docusate/30 mg casanthranol; Pericolace liquid, 60 mg docusate/30 mg casanthranol per 15 ml
Hyperosmolar agents ("bulk cathartics") cause H_2O secretion into the colon and rectum, leading to loosening and facilitated expulsion of feces	Sodium biphosphanate (Fleet enema, Fleet Phospho-soda, Fleet Bisacodyl supp., Fleet Bisacodyl tabs); magnesium citrate soda; magnesium hydroxide (milk of magnesia)	1 PR; 45 ml; 1 PR; 4 tabs; 200–300 ml PO; 5–15 ml PO q6 prn	Because of their osmotic concentration, hyperosmolar agents should be avoided in acute congestive heart failure and used with caution with impaired renal function, heart disease, and electrolyte imbalances; Fleet products usually used as bowel preps 3 hr before a procedure
Miscellaneous agents	Glycerin suppositories; lactulose (Chronulac)	1 PR; 30 ml qh/s	Glycerin stimulates rectal contraction within 15–30 min via hyperosmotic and irritant actions; lactulose is a synthetic disaccharide that is converted by colonic bacteria to short-chain organic acids that cause colonic fluid accumulation
Stool softeners: surfactant increases stool H_2O absorption as it descends the lower GI tract	Docusate sodium (Colace): capsules (100 mg); syrup/liquid (20 mg/5 ml); microenema (200 mg/5 ml)	100 mg PO qd–tid	May not see the effect until 1 to 3 days; begin with the highest dose and then reduce when the first bowel movement occurs

GI, gastrointestinal; PO, oral; PR, rectally; prn, as required; qh/s, every bedtime; qd, everyday; tid, three times a day.

(2%), dizziness (1%), and diarrhea (1%), whereas those associated with long-term use (28 to 35 nights) were dizziness (5%) and drugged feelings (3%) (11). Increased wakefulness during the last third of sleep after several weeks of use was not felt to occur with zolpidem as with other hypnotics that have a short elimination half-life. Zolpidem has the potential for causing excessive CNS depression when used along with other CNS depressants.

Hypoglycemics

Insulin preparations are listed in Table 31-24; oral hypoglycemics, which include sulfonylureas and biguanides, are listed in Table 31-25.

Diabetes mellitus is often present in patients under the care of a physiatrist. Proper glucose control is important both acutely, in order to avoid uncontrolled blood sugar elevations or hypoglycemic reactions, and chronically, in order

TABLE 31-24. *Insulin preparations*

Insulin class	Generic (trade) name	Pharmacokinetic properties		
		Initial effect	Peak action	Duration
Short-acting	Regular (Semilente)	30–60 min 2–4 hr	8 hr	
Intermediate-acting	NPH (Lente)	1–2 hr	6–12 hr	18–24 hr
Long-acting	Protamine zinc insulin suspension (Ultralente)	4–6 hr	16–20 hr	Up to 36 hr

to avoid long-term complications (76,77). The effects of exercise on blood glucose levels must be taken into account as patients who have not regularly exercised are enrolled into therapy programs. In addition to insulin and traditional oral hypoglycemics, a newer agent known as metformen is now available and is generally used in patients in whom dietary control alone is inadequate or there has been a partial or failed response to sulfonylureas.

Local Anesthetics

Relevance to Physiatry

Local anesthetics are frequently administered in the outpatient physiatric setting before performing a variety of procedures and are also used in diagnostic nerve blocks. Both short-acting and long-acting forms are available. Although lidocaine is the most commonly used agent for percutaneous infiltration anesthesia as well as for diagnostic blocks and injections, long-acting local anesthetics such as bupivacaine are also used for procedures in which at least several hours of analgesia are desired. A classic example is the shoulder impingement test in which the physiatrist may inject a long-acting local anesthetic along with a corticosteroid preparation into the subacromial bursa of a patient who has had a good response to lidocaine. The long-acting anesthetic is used so that the patient can receive additional hours of analgesia and bridge the time gap between the pain relief from the lidocaine and that of the corticosteroid. Local anesthetics are also generally added to corticosteroids for intra-articular injection so that the joint can be more fully bathed and so that the patient can achieve some immediate pain relief for the purpose of providing treatment feedback to the physician (73). Lidocaine in concentrations of either 0.5% or 2% is often a component of proliferant solutions used in prolotherapy (73).

Mechanism of Action and Pharmacokinetics

Although local anesthetics can be classified as either esters (e.g., procaine) or amides (e.g., bupivacaine and lidocaine), both classes interfere with nerve conduction by a mechanism of action that is not completely understood (73). At the cellular level, they appear to compete with calcium for binding to a receptor that controls sodium flux across the cell membrane (78). When this occurs, the rate of depolarization of the action potential slows, as does propagation of the nerve impulse (11). Overall, they affect small, unmyelinated fibers before affecting larger, myelinated fibers. Thus, the order of function loss following blockade is (a) pain, (b) temperature, (c) touch, (d) proprioception, (e) skeletal muscle tone.

Those of the ester class are quickly hydrolyzed in the plasma by the pseudocholinesterase enzyme, whereas amides are metabolized in the liver. Serum levels peak at approximately 5 to 25 minutes, depending on the administration route (73). Metabolites and unchanged drug are then excreted into

TABLE 31-25. *Oral hypoglycemic agents*

Class	Generic (trade) name	Dose (mg)	Other properties and side effects
Sulfonylureas (short-acting)	Tolbutamide (Oramide, Orinase); tolazamide (Tolamide, Tolinase)	Tolbutamide, start 250–500/day; max 3,000/day (daily or divided into two doses); tolazamide, start at 100–250/day, max 750–1,000	Duration up to 10 hr
Sulfonylureas (long-acting)	Acetohexamide (Dymelos); Chlorpropamide (Diabenese); glipizide (Glucotrol); glyburide (DiaBeta, Micronase)	Acetohexamide, start at 250 daily up to 1,500 per day, in two divided doses; chlorpropamide, start at 100 to 250 qd, up to 750 to 1,000; glipizide, start at 5 qd, up to max 40/day (divided into two daily doses once more than 15 per day is required); glyburide, start 2.5 to 5 up to max 20 qd	Chlorpropamide has a very long duration, up to 24 hr, making it relatively dangerous, especially in the elderly; duration up to 10 hr
Biguanide	Metformin (Glucophage)	Start at 500 qd to bid with meals and may gradually increase to maximum of 2,550/day	Avoid in renal insufficiency; may cause lactic acidosis

bid, twice a day; qd, every day.

the urine. The duration of action of agents from either class is greatly prolonged if the solution contains epinephrine because of epinephrine's potent vasoconstrictor effect.

Preparations and Dosing

Two of the most commonly used local anesthetics in physiatric practice are reviewed in Table 31-26. Although additional concentrations are also available, those that are most relevant to percutaneous infiltration anesthesia are listed. The maximum doses for percutaneous infiltration shown in the table are guidelines, and the doses should ideally be individualized for each patient on the basis of several factors including the size and physical status of the patient as well as the usual rate of systemic absorption from a particular injection site. In general, the lowest concentration and smallest dose that will achieve a given effect should be used. When doses larger than those shown in the table are given, preparations containing epinephrine are preferred. The reader is referred to other sources for dosing guidelines for other specific procedures such as nerve blocks, tendon sheath injections, bursal injections, and epidural steroid injections. Of note, preservative-free local anesthetic solutions must be used for epidural injections because the safety of preservatives in the epidural and subarachnoid spaces is not completely known (73).

Bupivacaine (Marcaine, Sensorcaine). For reasons discussed above, bupivacaine is especially used with corticosteroids in the injection solution for procedures in which a prior lidocaine test injection has given good pain relief. When bupivacaine is used for intra-articular injections, some recommend that it be restricted to non–weight-bearing joints so that the patient does not inadvertently traumatize the joint while it is under the effects of this long-acting anesthetic.

Lidocaine (Xylocaine). Because of its more favorable side effect profile, lidocaine has replaced procaine (Novocain) in both medicine and dentistry as the short-acting local anesthetic of choice. In addition to the above-listed 0.5% and 1% solutions, a 2% concentration is also available and is especially useful for procedures in which total injection volumes should be minimal, such as a digital nerve block or AC joint injection.

In addition to the injectable local anesthetics, topical preparations are also available. For example, EMLA Cream is composed of prilocaine (an amide local anesthetic that goes under the trade name Citanest) and lidocaine at concentrations of 2.5%. It can be used to anesthetize the skin before a needle-stick procedure. At least four European studies to date have compared EMLA Cream applied for at least 1 hour with placebo cream, ethyl chloride, subcutaneous lidocaine, and intradermal lidocaine before IV cannulation. In these studies, it was found to be more efficacious than placebo cream and ethyl chloride, comparable to subcutaneous lidocaine, and less effective than intradermal lidocaine, yet still preferable to lidocaine infiltration (11).

Relevant Side Effects and Drug Interactions

Although local anesthetics predominantly affect the circumscribed area into which they have been administered, they nonetheless are absorbed from this site and can therefore also exert systemic effects on both the cardiovascular and central nervous systems. Any CNS toxicity tends to occur earlier than cardiovascular toxicity and may manifest either as excitation in the form of seizures or at even higher levels as central respiratory depression. At nontoxic concentrations, local anesthetics act as antiarrhythmics, whereas at toxic levels, they are pronation-arrhythmic and exert a negative inotropic effect. The full-blown picture of local anesthetic toxicity consists of salivation and tremor, convulsions, and coma associated with hypertension and tachycardia followed by hypotension.

True allergic reactions to amide local anesthetics such as lidocaine and bupivacaine are quite rare. In contrast, allergic reactions are more common with ester local anesthetics such as procaine. There does not appear to be a cross sensitivity among these two classes of local anesthetics.

Certain technique-related precautions should be observed in injecting local anesthetics in order to avoid inadvertent toxic serum levels. In addition, doses should be adjusted depending the type of procedure being performed because this in part dictates the potential serum level of lidocaine. For example, high serum concentrations occur after intercostal nerve blocks because the intercostal regions are highly vascu-

TABLE 31-26. *Commonly used local anesthetics*

Generic (trade) name	Applicable preparations and concentrations	Onset (duration) of action	Usual dosage (ml), bursal injection[a]	Usual dosage (ml), joint injection, small (large) joint	Maximum dosage, percutaneous infiltration
Bupivacaine (Marcaine, Sensorcaine)	0.25% or 0.5%, with epinephrine	5 min (2–4 hr)	(A) 2½–4½; (IP) 4–4½; (Ish) 2½–4; (SA) 4–6; (T)4½–9	1–2 ml (2–4 ml)	Up to 70 ml (up to 90 ml with epinephrine)
Lidocaine (Xylocaine)	0.5% or 1%, with epinephrine	½–1 min (1½ hr)	(A) 2½–4½; (IP) 4–4½; (Ish) 2½–4; (SA) 4–6; (T) 4½–9	1–2 ml (2–4 ml)	Up to 60 ml (up to 100 ml with epinephrine)

[a] (A), anserine bursa; (IP), iliopectineal bursa; (Ish), ischial bursa; (SA), subacromial bursa; (T), trochanteric bursa.

larized, whereas the lowest occur after subcutaneous administration (11). The epidural region is another highly vascular region from which dangerously high serum concentrations can occur. In general, the smallest dose that can produce effective anesthesia should be used in injecting local anesthetics into these regions. Lumbar and caudal epidural steroid injections are procedures that in particular have the potential to produce significant toxicity from inadvertent intrathecal administration. Other factors involved in the potential for local anesthetic toxicity are extremes of age and acute illness. In addition, because the amide group of local anesthetics are metabolized in the liver, they should be used cautiously in patients with hepatic dysfunction or with reduced hepatic blood flow (e.g., congestive heart failure [CHF]) (73).

In an effort to prolong the effect of the local anesthetic and to help prevent potential systemic side effects, epinephrine is sometimes added at a concentration that varies from 2 to 10 μg/ml (i.e., 1:500,000 to 1:100,000). However, when epinephrine is also present, additional side effects such as anxiety, tachycardia, and hypertension may occur. At times, the presence of these side effects can be of use in monitoring for inadvertent placement of an injection. For example, when performing an epidural injection, their presence during the test dose suggests that the solution has reached the intrathecal space. Epinephrine solutions also contain the potential allergen sodium metabisulfite. Although the incidence of sulfite sensitivity in the general population is unknown, it is probably relatively low. Tissue ischemia from epinephrine can occur when it is injected into areas that are supplied by end arteries (e.g., digits) or have a compromised blood supply. An increased incidence of injection pain and wound infection can occur when epinephrine is present (73).

The CNS side effects of local anesthetics are additive when these drugs are given along with CNS depressants (73). Local anesthetics can potentially enhance the action of neuromuscular blocking agents. Local anesthetic solutions containing epinephrine should not be administered to patients taking MAOIs or TCAs because of the potential for severe hypertension.

Respiratory Medications: Decongestants, Expectorants, and Mucolytics

Respiratory tract disorders and infections are not uncommon to both inpatients an outpatients involved in rehabilitation programs. A variety of medications are used in managing these conditions (see Table 31-27). Decongestants are used to treat upper respiratory congestion and increased mucosal secretion that occurs in colds, seasonal allergies, or infections. Particularly when combined with postural drainage and percussion, expectorants and mucolytics are useful in facilitating pulmonary toilet through improving the quality and expulsion of mucus in order to prevent airway occlusion and subsequent complications resulting from it. Selective beta-2 adrenergic agonists are useful in the treatment of reversible airway obstruction in patients with bronchial asthma or chronic obstructive pulmonary disease (COPD). Their use in exercise-induced asthma has direct physiatric application. Anticholinergic medications can be of benefit in relieving bronchoconstriction, particularly in COPD.

Medications Used to Treat Agitation

Patients suffering from traumatic brain injury (TBI) often experience agitation during their recovery. It is imperative that the preliminary steps of neuromedical assessment and behavioral management be performed before attempting to treat agitation with medication. It is also important to subsequently use an adequate and objective measure of agitation such as the Agitated Behavior Scale in order to evaluate the medication's effectiveness (79). Medications that can impair cognition are listed in Table 31-28.

A key step in the assessment and treatment of agitated behaviors is the consideration of underlying sleep disorders. Although sedating serotonergic agents such as trazodone may be most helpful in sleep initiation disorders (80), Boyeson has reported a potential concern with the use of serotonergic agents in animals. However, there is no convincing evidence of adverse impact on human neurologic recovery (81).

Anticonvulsants such as carbamazepine and valproic acid have been recommended for the treatment of agitated behaviors (82). Although they have a relatively equal efficacy, there is some suggestion that carbamazepine has a lower side effect profile.

The TCAs, specifically the more sedating TCA amitriptyline, has been advocated by Jackson (83). Other TCAs (doxepin, nortriptyline, desipramine, and protriptyline) have also been considered successful in the treatment of agitation.

Lithium, a monovalent cation that is administered as either lithium citrate or lithium carbonate, has efficacy in the treatment of impulse control and explosive disorder. Hass also reported the use of lithium in a traumatic brain injury patient with behavioral disturbance (84). One must be well aware of its potentially serious side effect profile (85).

Buspirone, an anxiolytic agent whose mechanism of action is not clearly understood, has been reported to be helpful in the treatment of posttraumatic agitation (86). Its slow onset limits its utility in the acutely agitated patient.

Other medications that have been tried include two groups that are generally not thought of as having psychoactive properties *per se*. Gualtieri and Evans have reported a significant success in the treatment of agitation with amantadine (87), and lipophilic beta blockers that cross the blood-brain barrier have been useful in the treatment of aggressive behaviors (88). Table 31-29 lists drugs used to treat agitation.

Medications Used for Disorders of Arousal and Attention

Relevance to Physiatry

Conditions that are likely to be encountered by the physiatrist and that can cause problems with attention and arousal

TABLE 31-27. *Respiratory medications*

Medication class and mechanism	Generic (trade) names	Dose	Other properties and side effects
Anticholinergics: relieve bronchoconstriction via antagonism of muscarinic cholinergic receptors	Ipratropium bromide (Atrovent)	2 puffs (by metered-dose inhaler) qid, up to 12 puffs per 24 hr; maximal clinical effects in 30–90 min and last for 4 hr	Most cause significant systemic side effects because of easy absorption; fewer side effects with ipratropium because very little respiratory or GI absorption
Decongestants (alpha-1 adrenergic agonists): nasal mucosa blood vessel vasoconstriction, thus decreased secretion and congestion	Ephedrine, epinephrine, naphazoline, oxymetazoline, phenylephrine, phenylpropanolamine, pseudoephedrine (Sudafed), tetrahydrozoline, and xylometazoline	Depends on the particular preparation	Uses, decrease in secretions and congestion, also used in combination with agents such as expectorants, antitussives, or antihistamines; side effects, H/A, dizziness, increased BP, and palpitations
Expectorants: not clearly understood how they enhance respiratory tract secretion production, making it easier to advance sputum upwards	Guaifenesin (Robitussin), terpin hydrate	5–20 cc PO q4h; 5–10 cc PO tid–qid	Usually given orally, either alone or in combination with other respiratory agents; GI distress, especially in high doses; in extended usage, hose containing iodide may cause iodism, hypothyroidism or hypersensitivity
Mucolytics: decrease mucus viscosity by splitting mucoprotein disulfide bonds	Acetylcysteine (Mucomyst, Mucosol)	6–10 cc 10% or 3–5 cc 20% solution; nebulized form q6–8h	Possible nausea and vomiting, stomatitis, or rhinorrhea
Selective beta-2 adrenergic agonists: affinity for beta-2 adrenergic receptors in bronchiolar smooth muscles	Albuterol (Proventil, Ventolin), bitolterol (Tornalate), isoetharine (Bronkosol, nebulized; Brokometer, inhaled), metaproterenol (Alupent, Metaprel), pirbuterol (Maxair)	Response rate varies with administration mode: rapid response to aerosol inhalation or subcutaneous injection; delayed but longer if given orally	Tachycardia, arrhythmias, and myocardial ischemia, especially with underlying cardiac disease

BP, blood pressure; GI, gastrointestinal; H/A, headache; qid, four times a day; tid, three times a day.

TABLE 31-28. *Medication classes that can impair cognition*

Anticholinergic agents
Anticonvulsants
Antiemetics
Antipsychotics
Beta-adrenergic blockers
Benzodiazepines
Barbiturates
Central-acting antihypertensive agents
Gastric motility agents (e.g., metaclopramide)
Cardiac glycosides
H_2 blockers
Hypnotics
Opiates
Xanthine derivatives (e.g., aminophylline)

include but are not limited to TBI, certain types of cerebrovascular accidents, and Alzheimer disease. Because successful rehabilitation can be quite difficult in these patients, attempts have been made to used medications that can counteract poor arousability and improve an inadequate attention span. Before attempting to use stimulant medication, an important first step in patient management is the discontinuation of any potentially sedating medications.

Although some agents have been described as beneficial in hemineglect syndromes (89), aphasia (90), and slow to recover or minimally responsive states (91), treatment is often simply based on case reports and limited research.

Medications

Table 31-20 lists drugs used for these indications. Direct-acting stimulants such as amphetamine, methyl-

TABLE 31-29. *Medications used to treat agitation*

Generic (trade) name	Oral dose guidelines (mg)[a]	Mechanism of action	Other properties and side effects
Amantadine (Symmetrel)	100–400 divided qd or bid	Pre- and postsynaptic dopaminergic facilitation	Hallucinations, insomnia, seizures; other uses: influenza A treatment and prophylaxis, Parkinson disease, and drug-induced extrapyramidal reactions
Amitriptyline (Elavil, Endep)	25–100 qh/s or divided tid	Noradrenergic potentiation	Anticholinergic side effects
Buspirone (BuSpar)	15–60 divided bid	Unclear; may affect serotonin and/or dopamine	Dizziness, nausea, headache, paradoxical nervousness/excitation
Carbamazepine (Tegretol)	400–1,600 divided bid or tid	Stabilizes neuronal membranes	Bone marrow suppression; hepatic toxicity; see Table 31-7 for interactions
Lithium carbonate (Eskalith, Lithane, Lithobid, Lithonate)	600–900 divided tid to qid (or bid with controlled-release tabs)	Stabilizes neuronal membranes; effect on adenylate cyclase	Multiple potential side effects and drug interactions including paradoxic agitation and restlessness
Propranolol (Inderal)	60–420 divided bid	Beta-adrenergic blockade, presynaptic noradrenergic effect	Usual beta-blocker side effects
Trazodone (Desyrel)	50-600 qh/s or divided bid	competitive inhibitor of serotonin reuptake	Dizziness, drowsiness, dry mouth, hypotension, nervousness, priapism (1/10,000); increased digoxin and phenytoin levels; altered PT level in coumadinized patients
Valproic acid (Depakene)	15 to 60 mg/kg per day divided tid	Unknown; possibly increases GABA levels in the brain	GI; various CNS including hallucinations, tremor, and ataxia; hepatic, others

bid, twice a day; CNS, central nervous system; GI, gastrointestinal; PT, prothrombin time; qh/s, every bedtime; qid, four times a day; tid, three times a day.

[a]Doses listed in the table are guidelines and should be individualized according to side effects and response.

phenidate, and pemoline increase presynaptic noradrenergic release. In contrast, amantadine has both pre- and postsynaptic effects, levodopa and levodopa/carbidopa are converted to dopamine, (92) and bromocriptine and pergolide are direct postsynaptic dopamine agonists. In some conditions, it can be advantageous to combine medications with different modes of action.

Medications That Affect Cognition and Memory

Relevance to Physiatry

As is true for disorders of attention and arousal, conditions that can impair cognition and memory can also significantly diminish a patient's rehabilitation potential. In addition, medications that can potentially impair neurological recovery always need to be avoided if possible in this patient population. In fact, many medications may induce sedation or memory dysfunction or decrease overall arousal. A partial list of potentially impairing medications is noted in Table 31-28, and some of these are discussed in more detail below.

Commonly encountered anticonvulsant agents include phenytoin, carbamazepine, phenobarbital, and valproic acid. The main concern regarding side effects in the traumatic brain injury setting pertains to deleterious effects on cognition. In particular, long-term use of phenytoin has been reported to have negative cognitive effects (93). The negative impact of phenobarbital on cognition is well documented, and this medication should not be a first choice as anticonvulsant therapy in the brain injury survivor. Glenn and Wroblewski have advocated the use of carbamazepine or valproic acid as preferable agents in the treatment of posttraumatic seizures because of the suggestion that they have fewer cognitive side effects (94). However, controversy remains as to the relative cognitive disturbance each one of these agents may cause (95). Second-generation anticonvulsants such as gabapentin (see above) and lamotrigine are now available but to date have been approved only as adjuvant agents rather than as monotherapy (96). Vigabatrin carries unique NMDA antagonist qualities but is not yet available in the United States. The effects of this agent on cognition in brain injury is not well described (97). Recent recommendations have advocated that anticonvulsant prophylaxis may be warranted only for the first week after injury (98–100). Although anticonvulsant prophylaxis remains a point of discussion, no

TABLE 31-30. *Medications used for disorders of attention and arousal*

Generic (trade) name	Oral dose (mg)	Mechanism of action	Other properties and side effects
Amantadine (Symmetrel)	100–400 divided qd or bid	Pre- and postsynaptic dopaminergic facilitation	See Table 31-26
Bromocriptine (Parlodel)	5–60 qd	Direct dopamine agonist	Nausea, hypotension, hallucinations; other uses: hyperprolactinemia, acromegaly, and Parkinsonism
Dextroamphetamine (Dexedrine)	5–60 qd divided q4–6h (avoid h/s)	Presynaptic noradrenergic and dopamine release	Hypertension, tachycardia, behavioral disturbance; other uses: ADD and narcolepsy
Carbidopa/levodopa (Sinemet)	25/100 tid; 25/250 up to 8 tabs per day	Presynaptic agonist	Nausea, vomiting, hypotension, seizures, hallucinations; other uses: Parkinson disease/Parkinsonism
Methylphenidate (Ritalin)	5–80 divided bid or tid	Presynaptic noradrenergic and dopamine release	Arrhythmias, hypertension; other uses: ADD and narcolepsy
Pemoline (Cylert)	18.75–112.5 qAM	Noradrenergic and dopamine release	Liver dysfunction; behavioral disturbance; other use: ADD
Pergolide (Permax)	1–4 divided tid	Direct dopamine agonist	Nausea, hypotension; other use: Parkinson dieases
Selegiline (Eldepryl)	5–10 divided bid	MAO-B inhibitor	Various food and drug interactions; other use: Parkinson disease

ADD, attention deficit disorder; bid, twice a day; h/s, at bedtime; qAM, every morning; qd, everyday; tid, three times a day.

clear evidence exists to support long-term prophylaxis. The role of anticonvulsant prophylaxis in patients with penetrating head trauma remains controversial.

Centrally acting antihypertensives such as methyldopa may have a significantly sedating effect. In addition, although clonidine has been advocated for treatment of spasticity and agitation, it may produce impaired cognition (101). Beta blockers that cross the blood–brain barrier have been useful in the treatment of agitation (102); however, they may also produce significant sedation (103). Calcium channel antagonists have been implicated as agents that may decrease dopaminergic neurotransmission and have an effect on motor recovery (104).

Benzodiazepines readily cross the blood–brain barrier and produce antegrade amnesia and anxiolysis. They are noted to decrease new learning and memory and have been reported to produce increased confusion and agitation (105). Thus, their routine use in the traumatic brain injury survivor is generally not recommended.

Neuroleptics block dopamine in addition to serving as cholinergic and adrenergic antagonists. Because monoamines such as dopamine appear to be decreased after brain injury (106), the use of agents that also decrease monoamines is somewhat counterintuitive. Feeney first raised concerns that neuroleptics may impair recovery after brain injury (107). Gualteri has since stated that neuroleptics are relatively contraindicated in brain injury patients (108). Potential neuroleptic side effects include extrapyramidal movement disorders, the neuroleptic malignant syndrome, a lowered seizure threshold, and an impairment of new learning and memory. In a small study, Rao noted little impact on recovery by the neuroleptic haloperidol (109). Glenn nonetheless recommends reserving antipsychotic agents for short-term situations where patients remain a danger to self or others (110). Perhaps a reasonable recommendation is that neuroleptic medications not be considered agents of first choice in the treatment of traumatic brain injury patients with behavioral disturbance.

Atypical antipsychotics (risperidone and clozapine) are newer agents with both dopaminergic and serotonergic blocking properties (111). They appear to have a lower potential for extrapyramidal side effects, but their effect on cognitive outcome in the brain injury survivor is unclear.

Gastrointestinal agents such as histamine H_2 blockers (cimetidine, rantidine, famotidine, and naziditine) have been implicated as having sedative potential in the elderly as well as in the patient with central neurologic injury (112). The mechanism for this may be central cholinomimetic effects of these medications. Metaclopramide has significant dopamine D_2 antagonist effects and can thus potentially produce impaired cognitive responses (113). In addition, metaclopramide has been associated with extrapyramidal side effects.

In contrast to avoiding those medications that can cause negative effects, physiatrists have been quite interested in agents that can potentially improve a patient's intellectual abilities. Although no clearly efficacious treatment is available yet, the following agents have been investigated.

Medications

Because acetylcholine is the neurotransmitter most purely associated with memory, attempts to enhance acetylcholine by acetylcholinesterase inhibition has been the most promising venue (114). Tacrine (Cognex), which works as an acetylcholinesterase inhibitor, is now approved for use in the Alzheimer population (115). No clinical trial with tacrine has yet been done in brain injury patients, however. In a case-control trial, McLean reported the effectiveness of oral physostigmine, another anticholinesterase medication.

Other medications include piracetam, a nootrope (toward the mind) agent that has shown promise in the treatment of memory disorders (116,117), vasopressin, an antidiuretic hormone analog that has been proposed as a medication to enhance general cognition (118,119), and amphetamines. The latter have an inferred beneficial effect in TBI in animals and humans, perhaps improving both cognitive and motor recovery (120,121).

Medications Used in the Management of Heterotopic Ossification

Relevance to Physiatry

Heterotopic ossification (HO) has been referred to as paraosteoarthropathy, ectopic ossification, and myositis ossificans. It occurs in several groups of patients cared for by physiatrists. For example, HO resulting from traumatic brain injury usually is para-articular and occurs in one plane around a joint (122). Reports regarding the prevalence of HO have been hampered by the various assessment measurements that were employed. The prevalence of clinically significant HO is believed to be between 10% and 20%, with fewer than 10% experiencing true joint ankylosis. In a retrospective review, the most common sites identified with HO involvement in TBI patients were the hip, elbow, and shoulder (123).

Diphosphonates

Diphosphonates, specifically etidronate disodium, have been proposed as agents that may be helpful in the prevention of neurogenic HO, but clear proof regarding the long-term effectiveness of etidronate disodium is lacking. Spielman, however, has suggested that patients with long-term immobilization and spasticity are most likely to benefit from etidronate disodium treatment (124). In contrast, diphosphonates have not been found to reduce HO after total hip arthroplasty (125,126), and they may not be effective in patients in whom significant bone formation has already begun. Standard dosage has been 10 mg/kg for 2 weeks followed by 20 mg/kg for 10 weeks. Heterotopic ossification tends to form over a 6-month time period; therefore, doses of 20 mg/kg over 6 months have been advocated (127). Use of these for longer duration has produced spontaneous fractures in dogs (128). It has been noted to cause GI symptoms (nausea, vomiting, diarrhea) as its most prominent side effect (129).

NSAIDs and Coumadin

The NSAIDs, particularly indomethacin, have been advocated as prophylactic agents to prevent HO formation after hip replacement and after acetabular fracture surgery (130), although proof of their effectiveness in patients with neurogenic HO is lacking. There are reports of coumadin as a medication that may have efficacy in the prevention and management of HO (131).

TRANSDERMAL MEDICATIONS

Transdermal drug delivery is hardly a novel concept, as it has long been appreciated that the skin is not a tight barrier to chemical entry. When applied directly to or over a targeted tissue or area, medications can be delivered to the desired structure at high concentrations, yet with minimal potential for systemic side effects. In contrast, when the bloodstream is relied on to deliver a medication to a target tissue, only a small percentage of the administered dosage reaches that

TABLE 31-31. *Topical NSAIDs*

Agent (concentrations)	Dosing (hr)	Suggested uses	Reported side effects
Flurbiprofen (5%)	q6	Disorders involving deep tissues such as the shoulder capsule and knees	Skin irritation, photosensitivity
Ibuprofen/urea gel (10%)	q4–6	Sprains, enthesopathies such as tendinitis and periostitis, pain caused by fractured finger, toe, rib	Dizziness, vertigo, skin dryness
Ketoprofen (1–10%)	q6–8	Arthralgias caused by osteoarthritis, rheumatoid arthritis, costochondritis, TMJ dysfunction, trochanteric bursitis	Same as for flurbiprofen (137,138)
Piroxicam (0.5%) with ibuprofen/urea gel	qd–q12	Not specified	Not specified
Piroxicam (0.5%) with flurbiprofen (0.5%)	qd–q12	DJD of the knee and elbow; trochanteric bursitis	Contact dermatitis, photosensitivity

DJD, degenerative joint disease; NSAIDs nonsteroidal anti-inflammatory drugs; TMJ, temporomandibular joint.

TABLE 31-32. *Transdermal membrane-stabilizing agents*

Agent (concentration)	Dosing (hr)	Suggested uses	Miscellaneous
PTH suspended solutions (5%,10%)	q6	Trigeminal neuralgia (5%) (139); RSD, carpal tunnel syndrome, tarsal tunnel syndrome, facial neuralgia, Morton metatarsalgia, postherpetic neuralgia	Use in modest amounts and rub in for at least 2 min to ensure proper penetration
PTH with carbamazepine or PTH with amitriptyline	q6	Trigeminal neuralgia; TMJ syndromes	Can use extraorally or intraorally
Baclofen suspended solution (2%,4%)	q6	Pain caused by fibromyalgia, especially in the neck, shoulders, arms, and lower legs	Expensive; does not penetrate deeply enough to be effective for pain in the low back, hips, and deep structures of the shoulders
Quinine (2–4%)	q6	Pain caused by fibromyalgia	Allergenic, not widely used

PTH, phenytoin; RSD, reflex sympathetic dystrophy; TMJ, temporomandibular joint.

tissue. Even when a medication is delivered intravenously and the variable of absorption is largely eliminated, distribution to the entire body is still at issue. When a medication is delivered directly to a target tissue, issues of digestion are eliminated, volumes of distribution are decreased, and local concentrations are increased, while the remainder of the body is spared from medication-induced side effects.

Minimization of the need for oral medications, injections, and hospital procedures results in cost savings. The topical use of properly formulated medications can result in extremely rapid and effective responses, and when viewed with regard to the elimination of medications that are administered to treat side effect problems, cost effectiveness is even more apparent.

Transdermal formulations consist of transdermal vehicles and enhancers, which pull the drug through the skin, combined with an appropriate pharmaceutical, chosen for suitability in the transdermal vehicle and appropriate for the target tissue. The formulation of these requires consideration of chemical reactivity, physician characteristics, partition coefficient, and stability.

Transdermal agents are useful adjuncts to oral medications, injections, and physical modalities in the treatment of pain disorders. Discussed earlier in this chapter were several analgesic medications that are already commercially available by the transdermal route, including capsaicin, EMLA, and fentanyl. Analgesic medications that are currently available in transdermal form only through compounding pharmacies and are potentially most relevant to physiatry include anti-inflammatories and membrane-stabilizing agents (Tables 31-31 and 31-32). Topical anti-inflammatories have been available in Europe for many years (132,133). The vasodilatory agent guanethidine, in 2% and 4% preparations, has been used with 4% lidocaine to treat RSD of the upper extremity and lower extremity, respectively (134–136). Other commercially available transdermal medications include catapress, nitroglycerin, scopolamine, and hormones. In addition, if one were to include transmucosal medications, such as ophthalmologic topicals, suppositories, and nasal sprays, the list of transdermal agents would also include anticholinergics, antiemetics, antibiotics, and more.

REFERENCES

1. Bjorkman DJ. Nonsteroidal anti-inflammatory drug-induced gastrointestinal injury. *Am J Med* 1996; 101(1A):25S–32S.
2. Bradley JD, Brandt KD, Katz BP, Kalasinski LA, Ryan SI. Comparison of an antiinflammatory dose of ibuprofen, an analgesic dose of ibuprofen, and acetaminophen in the treatment of patients with osteoarthritis of the knee. *N Engl J Med* 1991; 325(2):87–91.
3. Flower RJ, Vane JR. Inhibition of prostaglandin synthetase in brain explains the anti-pyretic action of paracetamol (4-acetamidophenol). *Nature* 1972; 240:410.
4. Green SM, ed. *The 1997 Tarascon pocket pharmacopoeia.* Loma Linda, CA: Tarascon Publishing, 1997.
5. Levy MH. *Pharmacologic management of cancer pain.* Philadelphia: WB Saunders, 1994.
6. Max MB, Payne R, Edwards WT, et al. *Principles of analgesic use in the treatment of acute pain and cancer pain, 3d ed.* Chicago: American Pain Society, 1993.
7. Accolate (zafirlukast) full prescribing information, Zeneca Pharmaceuticals, Wilmington, DE, 1996.
8. Tolbert D. Predicted versus actual steady-state plasma levels for oxaprozin, a new nonsteroidal anti-inflammatory drug. *Drug Ther* 1993; March(Suppl):47–51.
9. Singh G, Ramey DR, Morfeld D, et al. Gastrointestinal tract complications of nonsteroidal anti-inflammatory drug treatment in rheumatoid arthritis. *Arch Intern Med* 1996; 156:1530–1536.
10. Griffin MR, Piper JM, Daugherty JR, Snowden MRI, Ray W. Nonsteroidal antiinflammatory drug use and increased risk for peptic ulcer disease in elderly persons. *Ann Intern Med* 1991; 114:257–263.
11. Product information. In: Sifton DW, ed. *Physician's desk reference.* Montvale, NJ: Medical Economics Company, 1997.
12. Settipane GA. Aspirin and allergic diseases: a review. *Am J Med* 1983; 74(6A):102–109.
13. Allen HL, Wase A, Bear WT. Indomethacin and aspirin: effect of non-steroidal antiinflammatory agents on the rate of fracture repair in the rat. *Acta Orthop Scand* 1980; 51:595–600.
14. Altman RD, Latta LL, Keer R, Renfree K, Hornicek FJ, Banovac K. Effects of nonsteroidal antiinflammatory drugs on fracture healing: a laboratory study in rats. *J Orthop Trauma* 1995; 9(5):392–400.
15. Gibson TP. Pharmacokinetics, efficacy, and safety of analgesia with a focus on tramadol HCl. *Am J Med* 1996; 101(1A):47S–53S.
16. Osipova NA, Novikov GA, Beresnev VA, Loseva NA. Analgesic effect of tramadol in patients with chronic pain: a comparison with prolonged-action morphine sulfate. *Curr Ther Res* 1991; 50:812–821.
17. Rodrigues N, Rodrigues PE. Tramadol in cancer pain. *Curr Ther Res* 1989; 46:1142–1148.
18. Muller-Limmroth W, Krueger H. The effect of tramadol on psychic

and psychomotor performance in man [Ger]. *Arzneim-Forsch (Drug Res)* 1978; 28:179–180.

19. Raffa RB. A novel approach to the pharmacology of analgesics. *Am J Med* 1996; 101(1A):40S–46S.
20. Houmes RJM, Voets MA, Verkaaik A, et al. Efficacy and safety of tramadol versus morphine for moderate and severe postoperative pain with special regard to respiratory depression. *Anesth Analg* 1992; 74: 520–514.
21. Lee CR, McTavish D, Sorkin EM. Tramadol: a preliminary review of its pharmacodynamic and pharmacokinetic properties, and therapeutic potential in acute and chronic pain states. *Drugs* 1993; 46(2): 313–340.
22. Ciccone CD. Skeletal muscle relaxants. In: Wolf SL, ed. *Pharmacology in rehabilitation, 2nd ed.* Philadelpha: FA Davis, 1996; 62.
23. Sullivan MJ, Reesor K, Mikail S, Fisher R. The treatment of depression in chronic low back pain: Review and recommendations. *Pain* 1992; 50:5–13.
24. McQuay HJ, Carroll D, Glynn CJ. Low dose amitriptyline in the treatment of chronic pain. *Anaesthesia* 1992; 47(2):646.
25. Galer BS. Neuropathic pain of peripheral origin: advances in pharmacologic treatment. *Neurology* 1995; 45(Suppl 9):S17–S25.
26. Priebe MM, Sherwood AM. A quantitative study of the effects of gabapentin on spasticity. In: *Proceedings of the American Paraplegia Society 42nd Annual Conference*, Las Vegas, 1996; 26.
27. Taylor CP. Emerging perspectives on the mechanism of action of gabapentin. *Neurology* 1994; 44(6 Suppl 5):S10–S16.
28. American Medical Association Department of Drugs, Division of Drugs and Technology. *Drug evaluations, 6th ed.* Chicago: American Medical Association, 1986.
29. Stracke H, Meyer UE, Schumacher HE, et al. Mexiletine in the treatment of diabetic neuropathy. *Diabetes Care* 1992; 15(11): 1550–1555.
30. Dejgard A, Petersen P, Kastrup J. Mexiletine for treatment of chronic painful diabetic neuropathy. *Lancet* 1988; 1:9–11.
31. Nishiyama K, Sakuta M. Mexiletine for painful alcoholic neuropathy. *Intern Med* 1995; 34(6):577–579.
32. Davis RW. Successful treatment for phantom pain. *Orthopedics* 1993; 16(6):691–695.
33. Awerbuch GI, Sandyk R. Mexiletine for thalamic pain syndrome. *Int J Neurosci* 1990; 5(2–4):129–133.
34. Okada S, Kinoshita M, Fujioka T, Yoshimura M. Two cases of multiple sclerosis with painful tonic seizures and dysesthesia ameliorated by the administration of mexiletine. *Jpn J Med Sci Biol* 1991; 30(4): 373–375.
35. Jackson CE, Barohn RJ, Ptacek LJ. Paramyotonia congenita: abnormal short exercise test, and improvement after mexiletine therapy. *Muscle Nerve* 1994; 17(7):763–768.
36. Hayashi T, Ichiyama T, Tanaka H, et al. Succesful treatment of incontinence of feces in myotonic muscular dystrophy by mexiletine. *No to Hattatsu [Brain Dev]* 1991; 23(3):310–312.
37. Chio-Tan FY, Tuel SM, Johnson JC, et al. Effect of mexiletine on spinal cord injury dysesthetic pain. *Am J Phys Med Rehabil* 1996; 75(2):84–87.
38. Pascual J, Berciano J. Failure of mexiletine to control trigeminal neuralgia. *Headache* 1989; 29(8):517–518.
39. Rakel RA. *Conn's current therapy 1997.* Philadelphia: WB Saunders, 1997.
40. Riggs BL, Hodgson SF, O Fallon WM. Effect of fluoride treatment on fracture rate in postmenopausal osteoporosis. *N Engl J Med* 1990; 322:802–810.
41. Green D,Hull RD, Mammen EF, Merli GJ, Weingarden SI, Yao JS. Deep vein thrombosis in spinal cord injury; summary and recommendations. *Chest* 1992; 102(Suppl):633S–635S.
42. Trowbridge A, Boese CK, Woodruff B, et al. Incidence of posthospitalization proximal deep vein thrombosis after total hip arthroplasty: a pilot study. *Clin Orthop* 1994; 299:203–208.
43. Huisman MV, Buller HR, ten Cate JW, et al. Unexpected high prevalence of silent pulmonary embolism in patients with deep venous thrombosis. *Chest* 1989; 95:498–502.
44. Levine M, Gent M, Hirsh J, et al. A comparison of low-molecular-weight heparin administered primarily at home with unfractionated heparin administered in the hospital for proximal deep- vein thrombosis. *N Engl J Med* 1996; 334:677–681.
45. Koopman MMW, Prandoni P, Piovella F, et al. Treatment of venous thrombosis with intravenous unfractionated heparin administered in the hospital as compared with subcutaneous low-molecular-weight heparin administered at home. *N Engl J Med* 1996; 334:682–687.
46. Clagett GP, Anderson FA Jr, Heit J, et al. Prevention of venous thromboembolism. *Chest* 1995; 108(Suppl):312S–334S.
47. Collins R, Scrimgeour A, Yusuf S, et al. Reduction in fatal pulmonary embolism and venous thrombosis by perioperative administration of subcutaneous heparin: an overview of results of randomized trials in general, orthopedic, and urologic surgery. *N Engl J Med* 1988; 318: 1162–1173.
48. Green D, Chen D, Chmiel JS, et al. Prevention of thromboembolism in spinal cord injury: the role of low molecular weight heparin. *Arch Phys Med Rehabil* 1994; 75:290–292.
49. Green D, Hirsh J, Heit J, et al. Low molecular weight heparin: a critical analysis of clinical trials. *Pharmacol Rev* 1994; 46:89–109.
50. Imperiale TF, Speroff T. A meta-analysis of methods to prevent venous thromboembolism following total hip replacement. *JAMA* 1994; 271:1780–1785 [Erratum, *JAMA* 1995; 273:288].
51. Chimowitz MI, Kokkinos J, Strong J, et al. The warfarin–aspirin asymptomatic intracranial disease study. *Neurology* 1995; 45: 1488–1493.
52. Stroke Prevention in Atrial Fibrillation Investigators. Warfarin compared to aspirin for prevention of thromboembolism in atrial fibrillation. *Lancet* 1994; 343:687–691.
53. Ginsberg JS. Management of venous thromboembolism. *N Engl J Med* 1996; 335:1816–1828.
54. Raschke RA, Reilly BM, Guidry JR, et al. The weight-based heparin dosing nomogram compared with a standard care nomogram: a randomized controlled trial. *Ann Intern Med* 1993; 119:874–881.
55. Cruickshank MK, Levine MN, Hirsh J, et al. A standard heparin nomogram for the management of heparin therapy. *Arch Intern Med* 1991; 151:333–7.
56. Hull RD, Raskob GE, Rosenbloom D, et al. Optimal therapeutic level of heparin therapy in patients with venous thrombosis. *Arch Intern Med* 1992; 152:1589–1595.
57. Hirsh J, Dalen JE, Deykin D, et al. Oral anticoagulants: mechanism of action, clinical effectiveness, and optimal therapeutic range. *Chest* 1992; 102(Suppl): 312S–325S.
58. Stein PD, Alpert JS, Copeland J, et al. Antithrombotic therapy in patients with mechanical and biological prosthetic heart valves. *Chest* 1992; 102(s):445s–455s.
59. Bergqvist D, Benoni G, Bjorgell, O, et al. Low-molecular-weight heparin (Enoxaparin) as prophylaxis against venous thromboembolism after total hip replacement. *N Engl J Med* 1996; 335:696–700.
60. Antiplatelet Trialists Collaboration. Collaborative overview of randomised trials of antiplatelet therapy. I: Prevention of death, myocardial infarction, and stroke by prolonged antiplatelet therapy in various categories of patients. *Br Med J* 1994; 308:81–106.
61. The SALT Collaborative Group. Swedish low-dose trial (SALT) of 75 mg aspirin as secondary prophylaxis after cerebrovascular ischaemic events. *Lancet* 1991; 338:1345–1349.
62. Dutch TIA Trial Study Group. A comparison of two doses of aspirin in patients after a transient ischemic attack or minor ischemic stroke. *N Engl J Med* 1991; 325:1261–1266.
63. Grotta JC, Norris JW, Kamm B. Prevention of stroke with ticlopidine: who benefits most? *Neurology* 1992; 42:111–115.
64. Braddom RL, Rocco JF. Autonomic dysreflexia. *Am J Phys Med Rehabil* 1991; 70:234–241.
65. Reid D, Morales A, Harris C, et. al. Double-blind trial of yohimbine in treatment of psychogenic impotence. *Lancet* 1987; 2:421–423.
66. Yablon SA, Sipski ML. Effect of transdermal clonidine on spinal spasticity: A case series. *Am J Phys Med Rehabil* 1993; 72: 154–157.
67. Lewis E, Hunsicker L, Bain R, Rohde R. The effect of angiotensin-converting-enzyme inhibition on diabetic nephropathy. *N Engl J Med* 1993; 329:1456–1462.
68. Flores AM. Hospital-based cardiac rehabilitation. In: Halar E, ed. *Cardiac rehabilitation part II. PM&R clinics of North America.* Philadelphia: WB Saunders, 1995; 243–261.
69. Bell KR, Cardenas DD. New frontiers of neuropharmacologic treatment of brain injury agitation. *Neurorehabilitation* 1995; 5:223–244.
70. Grossman E, Messerli FH, Grodzicki T, et al. Should a moratorium

be placed on sublingual nifedipine capsules given for hypertensive emergencies and pseudoemergencies? *JAMA* 1996; 276:1328–1331.
71. Maynard FM. Immobilization hypercalcemia following spinal cord injury. *Arch Phys Med Rehabil* 1986; 67:41–44.
72. Ernst CB, Stanley JC, ed. *Therapy in vascular surgery,* 2nd ed. Philadelphia: BC Decker, 1991.
73. Lennard TA. *Physiatric procedures in clinical practice*. Philadelphia: Hanley and Belfus, 1995.
74. Porter DR, Sturrock RD. Fortnightly review: medical management of rheumatoid arthritis. *Br Med J* 1993; 307:425.
75. Moldofsky H, Lue FA, Mously C, et al. The effect of zolpidem in patients with fibromyalgia: a dose ranging, double blind, placebo controlled, modified crossover study. *J Rheumatol* 1996; 23(3):529–533.
76. Reichard P, Nilsson B-Y, Rosenquist U. The effect of long-term intensified insulin treatment on the development of microvascular complications of diabetes mellitus. *N Engl J Med* 1993; 329:304.
77. The Diabetes Control and Complications Trial Research Group. The effect of intensive treatment of diabetes on the development and progression of long-term complications in insulin-dependent diabetes mellitus. *N Engl J Med* 1993; 329:977.
78. Goth A. *Medical pharmacology, 10th ed.* St Louis: CV Mosby, 1981.
79. Corrigan J. Development of a scale for assessment of agitation following traumatic brain injury. *J Clin Exp Neuropsychol* 1989; 11: 261–277.
80. Zafonte R, Mann N., Fichtenberg N. Sleep disturbance in traumatic brain injury: pharmacologic options. *Neurorehabilitation* 1996; 7: 189–195.
81. Boyeson M, Harmon R. Effects of trazodone and desipramine on motor recovery in brain injured rats. *Am J Phys Med Rehabil* 1993; 72:286–294.
82. Barrat E. The use of anticonvulsants in aggression and violence. *Psychopharmacol Bull* 1993; 29:75–81.
83. Jackson R, Corrigan J, Gribble M. Amitriptyline for agitation in head injury. *Arch Phys Med Rehabil* 1985; 66:180–181.
84. Hass J, Cope N. Neuropharmacologic management of behavioral sequelae in head injury: a case report. *Arch Phys Med Rehabil* 1985; 66:472–474.
85. Glenn M, Joseph A. The use of lithium for behavioral and affective disorders after traumatic brain injury. *J Head Trauma Rehabil* 1987; 2:68–76.
86. Gultieri C. Buspirone: Neuropsychiatric effects. *J Head Trauma Rehabil* 1991; 6:90–92.
87. Gualtieri C, Evans R. Stimulant therapy for the neurobehavioral sequelae of traumatic brain injury. *Brain Inj* 1988; 2:273–290.
88. Elliot F. Propranolol for the control of belligerent behavior following acute brain damage. *Ann Neurol* 1977; 1:489–491.
89. McNeny R, Zasler N. Neuropharmacologic management of hemi-inattention after brain injury. *Neurorehabilitation* 1991; 1:72–78.
90. Crimson M. Childs A, Wilcox R. The effect of bromocriptine on speech dysfunction in patients with diffuse brain injury. *Clin Neuropharmacol* 1988; 11:462–488.
91. Haig A, Ruess J. Recovery from vegetative state of six months duration associated with sinemet. *Arch Phys Med Rehabil* 1990; 71: 1081–1083.
92. Schamanke T, Avery R, Barth T. The effects of amphetamine on recovery of function after cortical damage in the rat depend on behavioral requirements of task. *J Neurotrauma* 1996; 13:293–307.
93. Dimken S, Temkin N, Miller B. Neurobehavioral effects of phenytoin prophylaxis for posttraumatic seizures. *JAMA* 1991; 265:1271–1277.
94. Glenn M, Wrobleski B. Anticonvulsants for prophylaxis of post-traumatic seizures. *J Head Trauma Rehabil* 1986; 1:73–74.
95. Masagli T. Neurobehavioral effects of phenytoin, carbamazepine, and valproic acid: implications for use in traumatic brain injury. *Arch Phys Med Rehabil* 1991; 71:219–226.
96. Britton J, So E. Selection of antiepileptic drugs: A practical approach. *Mayo Clin Proc* 1996; 71:778–786.
97. Rogawski M, Porter R. Antiepileptic drugs: pharmacologic mechanisms and clinical efficacy with consideration of promising developmental compounds. *Pharmacol Rev* 1990; 42:223–227.
98. Yablon S. Post-traumatic seizures. *Arch Phys Med Rehabil* 1993; 74: 983–1001.
99. Temkin NA. Randomized double-blind trial following severe head injury; implications for clinical trials and prophylaxis. *N Engl J Med* 1990; 323(8):497–502.
100. Bullock R, Chestnut R. Clifton R, et al. Brain Injury Foundation. *Guidelines in the management of severe head injury*. New York: Author, 1995.
101. Donovan W, Carter E, Ross C, Wilkerson M. Clonidine effect on spasticity: A clinical trial. *Arch Phys Med Rehabil* 1988; 69:193–194.
102. Yudofsky S, Siver J. Propranolol in the treatment of rage and violent behavior in patients with chronic brain syndromes. *Am J Psychiatry* 1981; 138:218–220.
103. Horn L. Atypical medications for the treatment of disruptive aggressive behavior in the brain-injured patient. *J Head Trauma Rehabil* 1987; 2(4):18–28.
104. Mena M, Garcia de Yebenes M, Tabernero C, et al. Effects of calcium antagonists on the dopamine system. *Clin Neuropharmacol* 1995; 18(5):410–426.
105. Gualtieri C. The psychopharmacology of traumatic brain injury. In: Gualtieri C, ed. *Neuropsychiatry and behavioral pharmacology*. New York: Springer Verlag, 1991.
106. Feeney D, Gonzalez A, Law W. Amphetamine, haloperidol, and experience interact to affect rate of recovery from motor cortex injury. *Science* 1982; 217:855–857.
107. Van Worekum T, Mildehound J, Gottschal T, Nicolai G. Neurotransmitters in the treatment of head injuries. *Eur Neurol* 1982; 21: 227–234.
108. Silver J, Yudofsky S. Psychopharmacological management of destructive behavior after traumatic brain injury. *J Head Trauma Rehabil* 1994; 9(3):43–60.
109. Rao N, Jellinek M, Woolston D. Agitation in closed head injury: haloperidol effects on rehabilitation outcome. *Arch Phys Med Rehabil* 1985; 66:30–34.
110. Wrobleski B, Glenn M. Pharmacologic treatment for survivors of severe brain injury. In: Levin H, Benton A, Muizelaar J, Eisenberg H, eds. *Catastrophic brain injury*. New York: Oxford University Press, 1996, 93–120.
111. Elovic E. Atypical antipsychotics: risperidone and clozapine. *J Head Trauma Rehabil* 1996; 11:89–92.
112. Sedman A. Cimetidine–drug interactions. *Am J Med* 1984; 76: 109–112.
113. Myers Mary Ann. Gastrointestinal complications of traumatic brain injury. In: Horn L, Zasler N, eds. *Medical rehabilitation of traumatic brain injury*. Philadelphia: Haley and Belfus, 1996, 515–538.
114. McLean A, Cardenas D, Haselkorn J. Cognitive psychopharmacology. *Neurorehabilitation* 1993; 3:1–14.
115. Farlow M, Gracon S, Hershey L. A controlled trial of tacrine in Alzheimer's disease. *JAMA* 1992; 268:2523–2529.
116. McLean A, Cardenas D, Bergres D. Placebo controlled study of pramiracetam in young males with memory and cognitive problems resulting from head injury and anoxia. *Brain Inj* 1991; 5:375–380.
117. Moline K. Cognitive enhancing drugs. *Headlines* 1992; May/June: 22–23.
118. Koch-Hendrickson N, Nielsen H. Vasopressin in postraumatic amnesia. *Lancet* 1981; 3:38–39.
119. Jenkins J, Mather H, Couglan A. Desmopressin and desglycinamide vasopressin in post-traumatic amnesia. *Lancet* 1981; 3:39.
120. Feeney D, Hovda D. Amphetamine and apomorphine restore tactile placing after motor cortex injury in the cat. *J Psychopharmacol* 1983; 79:67–71.
121. Kaelin D, Cifu D, Matthies B. Methylphenidate for hypoarousal in the brain injured adult. *Arch Phys Med Rehabil* 1994; 75(9):1030.
122. Garland D. Heterotopic ossification. *Phys Med Rehabil State Art Rev* 1993; 7:611–622.
123. Garland D, Blum C, Waters R. Periarticular heterotopic ossification in head injured adults: incidence and location. *J Bone Joint Surg Am* 1980; 62A:1143–1146.
124. Speilman G, Gennarelli T, Rodgers C. Disodium etidronate: Its role in preventing heterotopic ossification in severe head injury. *Arch Phys Med Rehabil* 1983; 64:539–543.
125. Thomas BJ, Amstutz HC. Results of the administration of diphosphonate for the prevention of heterotopic ossification after total hip arthroplasty. *J Bone Joint Surg Am* 1985; 67A:400.
126. Thomas BJ, Amstutz HC. Prevention of heterotopic bone

formation: clinical exposure with diphosphonate. *Orthop Trans* 1986; 10:545.
127. Garland D. A clinical perspective of common forms of acquired heterotopic ossification. *Clin Orthop* 1991; 263:13–29.
128. Flora L, Hassing G, Cloyd C. The long-term skeletal effects of EHDP in dogs. *Bone* 1981; 3:289–300.
129. Hammond F, Francisco G. Heterotopic ossification prophylaxis. *J Head Trauma Rehabil* 1996; 11:80–88.
130. Schmidt S, Kjaersgaard-Anderson P, Pederson N. The use of indomethacin to prevent the formation of heterotopic ossification after total hip replacement. *J Bone Joint Surg* 1988; 70A:834–838.
131. Buschbaker R. Heterotopic ossification: a review. *Crit Rev Phys Rehabil Med* 1992; 4:199–213.
132. Baixauli F, Ingles F, Alcantara P, Navarrete R, Puchol E, Vidal F. Percutaneous treatment of acute soft tissue lesions with naproxen gel and ketoprofen gel. *J Intern Med Res* 1990; 18:372–378.
133. Gevi M, Merlo M. Ketoprofen lysine by topical route in sports traumatology. *Curr Ther* 1983; 34:844–850.
134. Klein DS. Treatment of pain due to malignancy. *Prog Anesthesiol* 1991; 5:186–200.
135. Klein DS. Transdermal use of guanethidine for reflex sympathetic dystrophy. *Neuropractice* 1995; 6:4.
136. Ramamurthy S, Hoffman J. Intravenous regional guanethidine in the treatment of reflex sympathetic dystrophy/causalgia: a randomized, double-blind study. Guanethidine Study Group. *Anesth Analg* 1995; 81:718–723.
137. Mozzanica N, Pigatto PD. Contact and photocontact allergy to ketoprofen: clinical and experimental study. *Contact Dermat* 1990; 23: 336–340.
138. Valsecchi R, Falgheieri G, Cainelli T. Contact dermatitis from ketoprofen. *Contact Dermat* 1983; 9:163–164.
139. Zajrzewsja JM, Patsalos PN. Drugs used in the management of trigeminal neuralgia. *Oral Surg Oral Med Oral Pathol* 1992; 74:439–450.

Rehabilitation Medicine: Principles and Practice, Third Edition, edited by Joel A. DeLisa and Bruce M. Gans. Lippincott–Raven Publishers, Philadelphia © 1998.

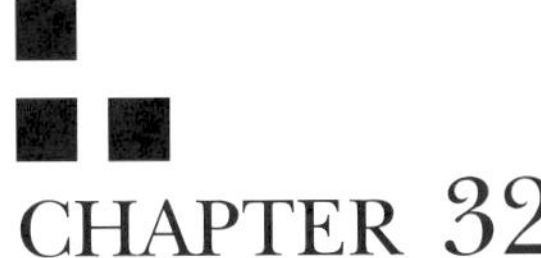

CHAPTER 32

Nutrition in Physical Medicine and Rehabilitation[1]

Faren H. Williams, Barbara Hopkins, Ingeborg Swanson, and Jeanne L. Beer

Good nutrition can optimize rehabilitation efforts in both the acute care and the long-term care settings. A wide variety of nutritional problems are seen because of the diverse diseases and injuries that result in disabilities. Some patients have congenital problems, and others acquire disabilities after accidents or associated with aging. This chapter discusses some of the special nutritional needs of disabled persons. Basic nutritional principles are discussed, and special needs for different groups of disabled people are identified.

BASIC PRINCIPLES OF NUTRITION MANAGEMENT

Nutritional science involves the study of food, the nutrients that food contains, and the way in which food supports health and life. The goal of nutrition management is to ensure that an individual has a diet containing all the necessary substances in the amounts appropriate for that person and is accessible and acceptable to the person.

Malnutrition exists when a person has a poor nutritional status. Historically, malnutrition has been considered primarily to be the result of a lack of one or more nutrients in the diet. The problems of excessive and unbalanced nutrient intake, however, have become evident as life expectancy increases, food supplies in the developed nations of the world have stabilized at abundant levels, and the metabolic bases of chronic disease states have been identified. Thus, any one of three conditions can result in suboptimal function secondary to malnutrition:

1. Nutrient deficiency (undernutrition). This condition develops when insufficient amounts of one or more nutrients are taken in to meet metabolic needs.
2. Nutrient excess (overnutrition). This condition is the result of an excessive intake of one or more nutrients.
3. Nutrient imbalance. This condition develops when a person consumes a diet that is not balanced in nutrients. Therefore, some nutrients might be consumed in excessive amounts and others in insufficient amounts.

The development of malnutrition follows a continuum that initially develops as body stores of a nutrient are changed from a condition of balance to one of imbalance, involving depletion or excess of one or more nutrients. Further imbalance of nutrient intake then leads to alterations of metabolism at the biochemical level. If the imbalance continues, overt disease will result.

FOOD COMPOSITION

Food is made up of chemical substances. Those that must be consumed by living organisms to sustain life are known as nutrients. Other substances that may affect health and function are present in some food. An adequate diet is achieved by balancing the substances in food in amounts appropriate for a given person.

Nutrients

Nutrients include six major categories of chemical compounds:

1. Water
2. Proteins

[1]Sections of this chapter are from "Nutrition" by Donna Frankel, which appeared in DeLisa JA, Gans BM, et al., eds. *Rehabilitation medicine: principles and practice, 2nd ed.* Philadelphia: JB Lippincott, 1993.

F. H. Williams: Department of Rehabilitation Medicine, University of Washington, Seattle, Washington 98195; and Virginia Mason Medical Center, Seattle, Washington 98111.

B. Hopkins: Department of Nutrition, Georgia State University, College of Health and Human Sciences, Atlanta, Georgia 30303.

I. Swanson and J. L. Beer: Department of Nutrition Services, Virginia Mason Medical Center, Seattle, Washington 98111.

3. Carbohydrates
4. Fats
5. Vitamins
6. Minerals

The specific categories of nutrients are based on their chemical composition. Water is the most basic compound essential for life, comprising more than 50% of total body mass, and is an integral part of cell structures and the basic medium for body fluid. Protein, carbohydrates, and fats share the function of supplying energy. In addition, each has a unique chemical composition and, thus, they serve different functions in areas of body composition, cell structure, and metabolic activity. Vitamins are divided into two categories, based on their solubility in fat or water. Many of the vitamins function primarily as cofactors for enzymatic reactions to support metabolic needs of the body. The fat-soluble and some of the water-soluble vitamins are stored in the body to some extent, so that not all vitamins must be obtained daily to maintain balanced nutrition. Minerals include inorganic elements, classified according to the relative quantities required for health (Table 32-1).

Although all nutrients are considered essential to life, the amounts of some nutrients necessary for health are variable because functions overlap. An example of this variability is the proportion of protein, fats, and carbohydrates needed for health. Because all share the function of providing energy to the body, the proportions of these three nutrients in the diet can vary. However, protein and fats have unique roles. There is a basic essential requirement for these substances in the diet not reflected in energy requirements because the body is unable to make the basic components of protein (specific essential amino acids) and of fats (specific essential fatty acids) (1,2). But when amino acids are used for energy, they must be modified chemically in the liver to remove the nitrogen. This process requires more calories, and the ability to remove nitrogen and excrete it has finite limits, which if exceeded may lead to increased ammonia in the body. Therefore, protein can be harmful if it is the only source of

TABLE 32-1. *Vitamins and minerals*

Nutrient	Major Function(s)
Water-soluble vitamins	
Thiamin (B_1)	Coenzyme in carbohydrate metabolism; nerve function
Riboflavin (B_2)	Coenzyme in citric acid cycle, fat metabolism, and electron transport chain
Niacin (B_3)	Coenzyme in citric acid cycle, fat metabolism, and electron transport chain
Biotin	Coenzyme in glucose production and fat synthesis
Pyridoxine	Coenzyme in protein metabolism, neurotransmitter and hemoglobin synthesis
Pantothenic acid	Coenzyme in citric acid cycle and fat metabolism (synthesis and beta-oxidation)
Folate	Coenzyme in RNA and DNA synthesis
Vitamin B_{12}	Coenzyme in folate metabolism, nerve function
Vitamin C	Collagen synthesis; hormone and neurotransmitter synthesis; antioxidant
Fat-soluble vitamins	
Vitamin A (retinoids and provitamin A carotenoids)	Vision; growth; cell differentiation; immunity; antioxidant
Vitamin D	Absorption of calcium and phosphorus; bone maintenance
Vitamin E	Antioxidant
Vitamin K	Blood clotting
Major minerals (>100 mg/day)	
Calcium	Bone and tooth structure; blood clotting; muscle contractions; nerve transmission
Phosphorus	Bone and tooth structure; intermediary metabolism; membrane structure; ATP
Sodium	Major extracellular cation; nerve transmission; regulate fluid balance
Potassium	Major intracellular cation; nerve transmission
Magnesium	Bone structure; enzyme function; nerve and muscle function; ATP
Chloride	Major extracellular anion; nerve transmission
Sulfur	Part of vitamins and amino acids; acid–base balance
Minor minerals (<20 mg/day)	
Iron	Part of hemoglobin and myoglobin; immunity
Cobalt	Part of vitamin B_{12}
Manganese	Functions in carbohydrate and fat metabolism; superoxide dismutase
Molybdenum	Cofactor for several enzymes
Fluoride	Strengthens tooth enamel
Copper	Iron metabolism; superoxide dismutase; nerve and immune function; lipid metabolism; collagen
Zinc	Cofactor in hundreds of enzyme systems; protein synthesis; growth; immunity; superoxide dismutase; alcohol metabolism
Iodine	Synthesis of thyroid hormone
Selenium	Antioxidant function as component of glutathione peroxidase
Chromium	Glucose tolerance

ATP, adenosine triphosphate; DNA, deoxyribonucleic acid; RNA, ribonucleic acid.

energy. Optimal ratios of these three substances should be achieved with a balanced diet.

Another major factor affecting the requirements of various nutrients is the body's ability to store them. Fats and any other excess energy from carbohydrates or proteins are stored as adipose tissue except for minimal quantities of carbohydrate stored as glycogen. The glycogen must be produced from absorbed food substances or from the glycerol component of fat stores. Excess protein results in the conversion of carbon skeletons to fat, and when protein in the diet is limited, the protein of skeletal muscle wil be broken down to meet the metabolic requirements of life-sustaining functions.

Other Components of the Diet

Fiber

Fiber refers to carbohydrates and related substances in the diet that are not digestible; therefore, it is not classified as a nutrient. However, fiber does perform several physiological functions in the gastrointestinal system (3). The primary properties of fiber in the gut seem to be its hydrophilic capacity, which increases stool bulk and decreases transit time, and its ability to bind other dietary substances, so that changes in the fiber content of the diet will alter absorption and bioavailability of both nutrients and toxins. These functions may sound simple, but the overall impact of fiber in the diet is diverse and varies with the type of fiber consumed. The physiological consequences have been shown to affect the control of diabetes mellitus, disorders of lipid metabolism, and obesity. Fiber content of the diet may also affect the incidence of some cancers.

Another positive aspect of fiber ingestion is fiber fermentation. All fibers, except lignin, can be fermented by the gut bacteria and produce components known as short-chain fatty acids (SCFAs). The three most common fatty acids produced are propionate, acetate, and butyrate. Each of them provides energy to the colonocytes, but only butyrate has trophic effects on the colonocytes. The more soluble the fiber (pectins, gums, mucilages), the greater the SCFA production.

Cholesterol

Cholesterol is a member of the sterol group of organic compounds. It is derived from fats and can be synthesized endogenously in quantities sufficient to meet metabolic demand. It is an integral part of cell structures and a precursor of some hormones and vitamin D. Cholesterol is present in some foods and is absorbed during the process of digestion. Dietary sources of cholesterol may be associated with the development of atherosclerosis, but it is not known whether disabled people are affected to the same extent.

DIETARY STANDARDS

Dietary standards serve as guidelines for the amounts of essential nutrients that should be consumed to ensure good health. They are not minimum requirements. The dietary standards used in the United States are the Recommended Dietary Allowances (RDAs) (Table 32-2). The RDAs are designed to meet the needs of most healthy people. They are updated as needed by the Food and Nutrition Board of the National Academy of Sciences, with the most recent publication in 1989. The RDAs are grouped according to age and gender.

DIETARY RECOMMENDATIONS

The purpose of dietary recommendations is to translate the information about nutrients required for health and the nutrient composition of food into the amount and type of food that should be consumed to meet nutritional needs. Two commonly used methods are the Dietary Guidelines for Americans and the Food Guide Pyramid (Figs. 32-1 and

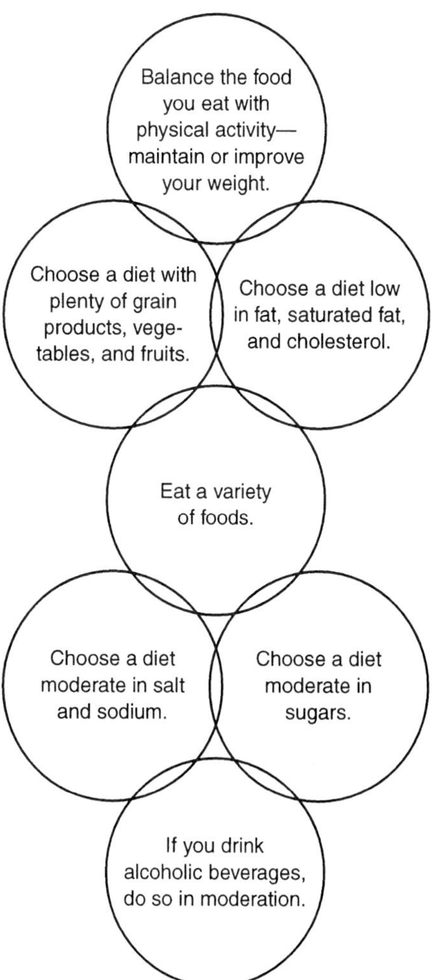

FIG. 32-1. Dietary guidelines for Americans. (From U.S. Department of Agriculture, U.S. Department of Health and Human Services, 1995.)

TABLE 32-2. *Recommended dietary allowances*[a]

			Fat-soluble vitamins				Water-soluble vitamins							Minerals						
	Age	Protein (g)	A (μg RE[b])	D (μg)	E (mg)	K (μg)	C (mg)	Thiamin (mg)	Riboflavin (mg)	Niacin (mg)	B_6 (mg)	Folate (μg)	B_{12} (μg)	Calcium (mg)	Phosphorus (mg)	Magnesium (mg)	Iron (mg)	Zinc (mg)	Iodine (μg)	Selenium (μg)
Infants	0–6 mos	13	375	7.5	3	5	30	0.3	0.4	5	0.3	25	0.3	400	300	40	6	5	40	10
	6–12 mos	14	375	10	4	10	35	0.4	0.5	6	0.6	35	0.5	600	500	60	10	5	50	15
Children	1–3 yrs	16	400	10	6	15	40	0.7	0.8	9	1.0	50	0.7	800	800	80	10	10	70	20
	4–6	24	500	10	7	20	45	0.9	1.1	12	1.1	75	1.0	800	800	120	10	10	90	20
	7–10	28	700	10	7	30	45	1.0	1.2	13	1.4	100	1.4	800	800	170	10	10	120	30
Boys/men	11–14 yrs	45	1,000	10	10	45	50	1.3	1.5	17	1.7	150	2.0	1,200	1,200	270	12	15	150	40
	15–18	59	1,000	10	10	65	60	1.5	1.8	20	2.0	200	2.0	1,200	1,200	400	12	15	150	50
	19–24	58	1,000	10	10	70	60	1.5	1.7	19	2.0	200	2.0	1,200	1,200	350	10	15	150	70
	25–50	63	1,000	5	10	80	60	1.5	1.7	19	2.0	200	2.0	800	800	350	10	15	150	70
	51 +	63	1,000	5	10	80	60	1.2	1.4	15	2	200	2.0	800	800	350	10	15	150	70
Girls/ women	11–14 yrs	46	800	10	8	45	50	1.1	1.3	15	1.4	150	2.0	1,200	1,200	280	15	12	150	45
	15–18	44	800	10	8	55	60	1.1	1.3	15	1.5	180	2.0	1,200	1,200	300	15	12	150	50
	19–24	46	800	10	8	60	60	1.1	1.3	15	1.6	180	2.0	1,200	1,200	280	15	12	150	55
	25–50	50	800	5	8	65	60	1.1	1.3	15	1.6	180	2.0	800	800	280	15	12	150	55
	51 +	50	800	5	8	65	60	1.0	1.2	13	1.6	180	2.0	800	800	280	10	12	150	55
Pregnant/ lactating																				
		60	800	10	10	65	70	1.5	1.6	17	2.2	400	2.2	1,200	1,200	320	30	15	175	65
First 6 mos	65	1,300	10	12	65	95	1.6	1.8	20	2.1	280	2.6	1,200	1,200	355	15	19	200	75	
Second 6 mos	62	1,200	10	11	65	90	1.6	1.7	20	2.1	260	2.6	1,200	1,200	340	15	16	200	75	

μg, micrograms; mg, milligrams; g, grams.

[a]The Recommended Dietary Allowances, expressed as average daily intakes over time, were established by the Food and Nutrition Board, National Academy of Sciences. The recommendations are intended to provide for individual variations among most normal persons as they live in the United States under usual environmental stresses. As always, the best eating style is based on a balanced diet of a variety of foods. That way, you'll be sure to get the required nutrients, even those for which requirements have been less well defined.

[b]μg RE, micrograms retinol equivalents.

Adapted with permission from *Recommended Dietary Allowances, 10th ed.* © 1989 by the National Academy of Sciences, published by National Academy Press, Washington, DC.

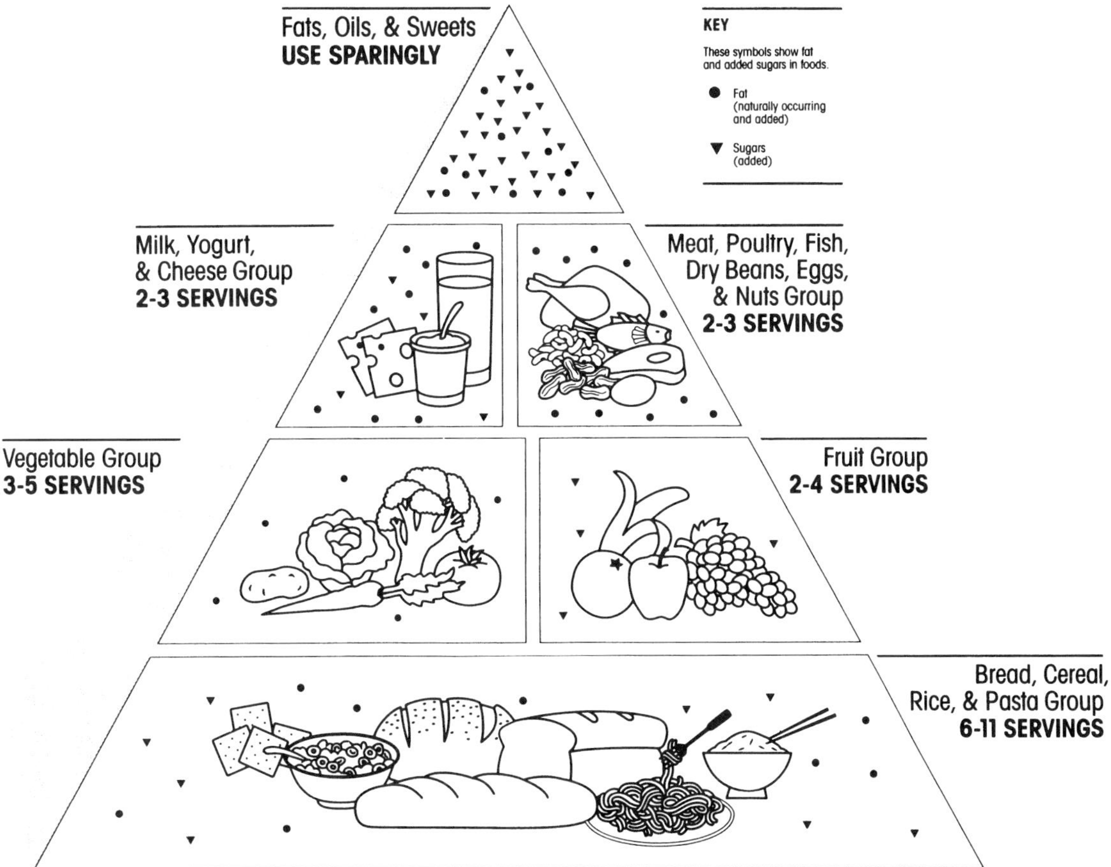

FIG. 32-2. The food guide pyramid is a general guideline to what a person should eat each day in order to get needed nutrients as well as the right amount of calories to maintain a healthy weight. It emphasizes foods from the five food groups shown in the three lower sections of the pyramid. (From U.S. Department of Agriculture and the U.S. Department of Health and Human Services.)

32-2). Both of these methods are designed to promote good health and disease prevention. The Dietary Guidelines offer suggestions for food choices and emphasize the importance of variety and moderation. The Food Guide Pyramid recommends a diet plan based on servings from five food groups.

ASSESSMENT OF NUTRITIONAL STATUS

The assessment of nutritional status helps determine the presence of malnutrition or risk for malnutrition. It involves the gathering and interpretation of data from which the effect of disease, injury, other stressors, and nutritional intervention can be monitored over time. Screening is used to identify individuals who need full nutrition assessment. For comprehensive nutrition assessment, there needs to be direct measurement or estimation of food and nutrient intake and the use of subjective and objective measures of the clinical, anthropometric, biochemical, and physiological status of the person. Appropriate assessment techniques may vary depending on the goals of the assessment.

Screening for Nutritional Risk

In daily clinical practice it is necesary to be able to identify subjects at risk for malnutrition. There is a tendency to focus on the specifics of food intake alone, but the development of malnutrition is multifactorial, and one needs to identify all the potential factors to successfully treat it (Fig. 32-3). People are at risk of going from well nourished to malnourished when any one of these factors is altered. Screening is important to determine which people need more intensive nutritional assessment and intervention.

For routine screening, a simple checklist can rapidly identify those with new risk factors and serve as a guide for referral to a registered dietitian, who can do a more detailed assessment and make recommendations to prevent further nutritional problems (Fig. 32-4).

Evaluation of Food/Nutrient Intake

A record of food intake is necessary to determine the nutrient content of the food actually consumed. The nutrient

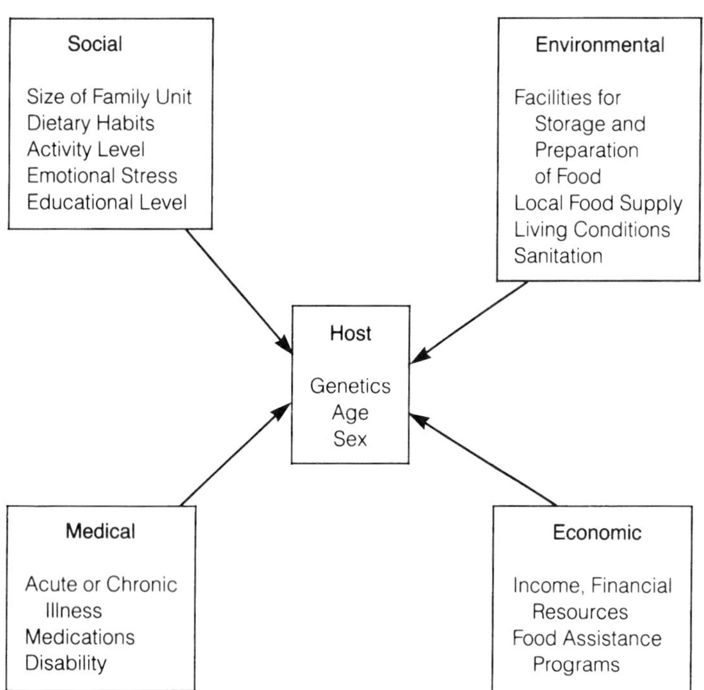

FIG. 32-3. Multifactorial etiology of malnutrition. (From Frankel DL. Nutrition. In: DeLisa JA, Gans BM, et al., eds. *Rehabilitation medicine: principles and practice, 2nd ed.* Philadelphia: JB Lippincott, 1993; 599.)

intake is compared with standards so that adequacy of the diet can be determined. Various methods exist for obtaining this information, all of which have advantages and limitations (4–6).

Collection Methods

Several of the more common collection methods are reviewed here, with the intention of concentrating on both their strengths and weaknesses. Information of this type is crucial to selecting the type of data collection needed to meet the needs of any given patient care situation (31).

Has there been a change in any of the following?

1. Income ______
2. Living Situation ______
3. Source of Food ______
4. Medical Condition ______
5. Physical Activity ______
6. Transportation ______
7. Employment Status ______
8. Eating Habits ______

FIG. 32-4. Screening for risk of malnutrition. If there is a change in any of these factors since the patient was last evaluated, there is a new risk of malnutrition, and further screening of nutritional status should be undertaken. (From Frankel DL. Nutrition. In: DeLisa JA, Gans BM, et al., eds. *Rehabilitation medicine: principles and practice, 2nd ed.* Philadelphia, JB Lippincott, 1993; 599.)

Twenty-Four Hour Food Recall

The registered dietitian, trained dietetic technician, or family member interviews the patient to determine what foods and fluids have been consumed in the previous 24 hours. This is an extremely easy method, but the assumption is that one's intake is "typical" of every day. Possible errors include lack of memory, inability to estimate portions, and inaccurate reporting.

Food Record Diary

The food and fluid consumed over several (usually 3 to 7) days can be recorded. Because food habits vary, especially between weekdays and weekends, it is important to know what specific days have been included. Records are kept by each patient or by the patient's caregiver. Accuracy is increased if portions are measured or weighed as prepared and waste is subtracted.

Food Frequency Record

The frequency with which major groups of foods are consumed (i.e., daily, weekly, monthly, sporadic, or never) can be surveyed. A standard portion size provides the base against which the number of portions for a given time interval are determined. Information is obtained through a questionnaire or interview. It is often used with a 24-hour recall.

Observation of Food Intake

This method may be most pracical for hospitalized patients or those in residential facilities. In this case, the caregiver actually observes the food intake.

Alcohol and Other Food Supplements

It is important to obtain information on ethanol consumption and use of nutritional supplements as part of the survey. It may be helpful to have information about minerals in the water supply. Sodium content of the diet may be highly variable, even within communities, because of variations in the water supply or use of water softeners. If supplements are consumed, it is important to get information on their nutrient content directly from packaging material or the manufacturer because combinations and amounts of ingredients vary among brands.

The reliability of any of the methods will increase with repetition. Through the use of a combination of food intake survey methods, increased reliability can be achieved (7). By combining a food intake survey with the measurement of related biochemical parameters, it is possible to validate the accuracy of the dietary intake information. This approach has been applied successfully to the study of dietary protein intake (8).

Adequacy of Food/Nutrient Intake

The dietary information collected by methods such as those reviewed previously must be translated into information about nutrient composition to determine the adequacy of intake. Methods that assess frequency of food or food group intakes usually are evaluated for nutrient content by comparing the patient's diet pattern with standard intake patterns, as mentioned earlier. If a significant imbalance is evident, there is indication of possible malnutrition, which may be related to poor dietary habits.

When actual food intake is recorded or recalled, it may be compared against patterns of food intake with food surveys, or specific nutrient/energy content may be calculated by information available from food composition tables (9–11). Historically, this was a tedious task, but computer software now transforms food intake data into nutrient intake. There are some potential sources of error. These include nutrient content differences depending on where the food was produced and how it was stored and prepared. Information in food composition tables is based on average data from small samples; therefore, one must use some caution in interpreting the data. If one conducts metabolic balance studies, then nutrient analysis is done on the actual food being consumed.

Balance Studies

Another method for determining the adequacy of food/nutrient intake is that of energy/nutrient balance studies. The assumption is that the optimally nourished person is in a state of equilibrium, with the amount of energy/nutrients used or lost in daily metabolic activity being replaced by energy/nutrients in the diet. When a person is in a physiological stage of growth or tissue repair, it is necessary for the balance to become positive, taking in a greater amount of energy/nutrients. For healthy weight loss, it is necessary for energy balance to become negative, but without loss of lean body mass. Balance for energy and nutrients fluctuates with time, but over a given period, a day or week, the dietitian can assess the overall direction of balance. The measures of energy, nitrogen, and fluid balance have multiple direct clinical applications in the day-to-day nutrition management of a patient.

Energy Balance

Energy is necessary for all activities of life, including the internal work of metabolic processes for maintenance and repair of bodily tissues and the external work done by a person on the environment. The optimal state of nutrition with regard to energy is one of equilibrium. In the person who is growing, either naturally or recovering from an injury to body tissue, energy balance must be positive. If the energy (caloric) intake is inadequate, then body tissues will be metabolized for transformation into energy. Conversely, consumption of excessive amounts of energy (calories) will lead to excess adipose tissue.

The major sources of energy in the diet are carbohydrates, protein, and fat (Table 32-3). Ethanol, too, is a source of energy and may provide significant calories for some individuals. The traditional unit for expression of energy content of foods and energy requirements is the kilocalorie, commonly referred to as a calorie. It is the amount of heat necessary to raise the temperature of 1 kg of water from 15°C to 16°C. The energy content of foods and nutrients has been determined through calorimetric techniques and is used to calculate the energy value of food consumed (9–11). A reasonable estimate of energy sources in the diet is necessary to prevent insufficient or excessive energy intake. The estimate needs to be made in the context of the clinical situation to avoid under- or overfeeding.

In a steady state, energy requirements can be determined by weighing someone over time and using predictive equations. If the weight remains stable, then one's energy needs can be calculated. If the person is gaining or losing weight, then the energy intake is either excessive or deficient, respectively. Routine weights are helpful for management of long-term dietary goals and for educational purposes. Body

TABLE 32-3. *Sources of energy in the diet*

	kcal/g (average)
Carbohydrates	4.0
Protein	4.0
Fat	9.0
Ethanol	7.1

Adapted from Silberman H, Eisenberg D. Evaluation of nutritional status. In: Silberman H, Eisenberg D, eds. *Parental and enteral nutrition for the hospitalized patient.* Norwalk, CT: Appelton-Century-Crofts, 1982; 37.

weight also reflects hydration status, with 1 liter being equivalent to approximately 2 pounds. When weight gain is too fast or too excessive, then fluid shifts should be suspected and appropriate labs checked. Adjustments should be made by closely monitoring the clinical situation and nutrition management, i.e., amount of calories and nutrients being provided to the patient.

It is ideal to have a direct measurement tool. For basic research, direct calorimetry is the most accurate method for the determination of energy expenditure. It requires that the patient be in an insulated chamber. The amount of heat given off directly is determined by temperature measures. The heat removed by vaporization of water from the body surface is calculated from information obtained by measuring the amount of moisture added to the air in the chamber (12). This is too cumbersome, expensive, and demanding for clinical applications.

The technique of indirect calorimetry allows the calculation of energy expenditure through the estimation of heat production from measures of gaseous exchange (i.e., oxygen consumed or carbon dioxide produced) during normal respiration (13,14). With the development of portable equipment for gaseous sampling and analysis, it is possible to apply this technique clinically, as an aid to direct determination of energy expenditure in both the acutely ill patient and the patient with chronic disability, during rest and activity (15–26). Indirect calorimetry is applied mostly in the determination of resting energy expenditure (REE), with additional calories added to cover the demands of both metabolic and physical activity by estimation and clinical monitoring.

Nitrogen Balance

Nitrogen balance reflects the protein status equilibrium of the body; and therefore, provides useful information for monitoring the adequacy of nutrition support. It is most important in patients with high rates of metabolic activity, such as those with head trauma, and patients requiring supplemental feedings.

To assess nitrogen balance, the clinician measures the nitrogen content of the diet plus supplements and the nitrogen content of material lost from the body (through urine and feces) and determines the difference between intake and output. Measures of nitrogen intake can be determined accurately in the hospital setting for patients on total enteral or parenteral feedings because the amount of substrate administered and its protein or nitrogen content are known. However, it is more difficult to accurately determine the amount of nitrogen for patients eating regular meals, and extremely difficult to calculate nitrogen losses. Twenty-four-hour urine collections are needed to do nitrogen balance studies. The urinary urea nitrogen content can be measured, and a correction factor applied for nonurea nitrogen. Additional estimates are used for approximation of the nonurea nitrogen losses in feces and skin. These formulas will be inaccurate in patients with protein-losing enteropathy and those with burns, decubitus ulcers, or abscesses. Those patients lose protein and nitrogen secondary to fluid exudate or necrotic tissue sloughs, and those losses are hard to calculate. There are some nitrogen balance equations that can be helpful.

Fluid Balance

Fluid balance is monitored in the acute hospital by measuring fluid intake, urine output, and body weight. A clinical assessment for edema and dehydration is also helpful. With diarrhea, vomiting, or fever, fluids in excess of output may be required. Fluid balance is affected by hepatic and renal function through the role of plasma proteins and electrolytes in the distribution of body fluid between body compartments. When patients have a neurogenic bladder, fluid intake needs to be spread out during the day so fluid shifts are minimized.

CLINICAL EVALUATION

The clinical history and examination are extremely valuable in identifying people with nutritional problems. Baker (27) studied general surgical patients and found a high correlation between clinical assessment and nutritional status (28).

Historical Information

Much information regarding nutritional status can be obtained from questions asked as part of the general medical history. Of particular concern is information about the following:

- Change in body weight, especially if this was not the result of specific dietary intervention
- Change in appetite or eating habits
- Change in activity level
- Change in gastrointestinal function
- Presence of acute or chronic medical-surgical problems
- Specific feeding or swallowing problems
- Regular medication or supplement use

A sample of questions is presented in Figure 32-4. There are several examples of historical surveys in the literature that either stand by themselves or are used in conjunction with objective data (7, 29–31).

Physical Examination

Specific physical changes associated with nutrient deficiencies are rarely seen in developed countries, but there are abnormalities on physical examination that should alert the clinician to the potential for malnutrition. The physical consequences of specific nutrient deficiency may be seen most frequently in patients on long-term nutritional support with manufactured nutritional supplements or elemental formulations (32). The physiological manifestations of specific nutrient excesses have been identified in people who take large amounts of nutritional supplements. An awareness of specific findings is important. Some of these specific findings are given in Table 32-4.

TABLE 32-4. *Nutrition assessment: physical findings*

Clinical findings	Possible nutritional causes
Hair	
Dyspigmentation (flag sign)	Protein deficiency
Easily plucked	Protein deficiency
Sparse	Protein, biotin, zinc deficiency
Corkscrew hairs	Vitamin C deficiency
Nails	
Spoon nails (koilonychia)	Iron deficiency
Brittle nails	Iron deficiency; excess vitamin A
Traverse ridging	Protein deficiency
Skin	
Scaling	Vitamin A, essential fatty acid, zinc deficiency
Follicular hyperkeratosis	Vitamin A deficiency
Petechiae	Vitamin A, C deficiency
Purpura	Vitamin C, K deficiency
Yellow coloration	Excess carotene
Pellagrous dermatitis	Niacin deficiency
Cellophane appearance	Protein deficiency
Eyes	
Night blindness	Vitamin A deficiency
Bitot spots	Vitamin A deficiency
Papilledema	Vitamin A excess
Pale conjunctivae	Iron deficiency
Mouth	
Angular stomatitis	Riboflavin, niacin, pyridoxine deficiency
Cheilosis	Riboflavin, niacin, pyridoxine deficiency
Tongue	
Pale, atrophic	Iron deficiency
Atrophic lingual papillae	Riboflavin, niacin, folate, vitamin B_{12}, protein, iron deficiency
Glossitis (scarlet)	Riboflavin, niacin, folate, vitamin B_{12} deficiency, pyridoxine
Hypogeusia	Zinc deficiency
Gums	
Spongy, bleeding	Vitamin C deficiency
Musculoskeletal	
Beading of ribs	Vitamin D deficiency
Muscle wasting	Protein-calorie malnutrition
Tenderness	Vitamin C deficiency
Neurologic	
Confusion	Thiamin, niacin, vitamin B_{12} deficiency
Ophthalmoplegia	Thiamin, phosphorus deficiency
Peripheral neuropathy	Thiamin, pyridoxine, vitamin B_{12} deficiency
Tetany	Calcium deficiency
Other	
Cardiomegaly	Thiamine deficiency
Cardiomyopathy	Selenium deficiency
Hepatomegaly	Protein malnutrition
Edema	Protein, thiamin deficiency
Thyroid enlargement	Iodide deficiency

Adapted from Lee RD, Nieman DC. *Nutritional assessment, 2nd ed.* St Louis: CV Mosby, 1996; and Whitney EN, Cataldo CB, Rolfes SR. *Understanding normal and clinical nutrition.* New York: West Publishing, 1994.

Physical findings can reflect three different stages in the development of malnutrition. First, the integrity of body tissues with a rapid turnover, such as skin and mucous membranes, reflects the adequacy of recent nutrition support. Second, the condition of body tissues that have developed over time, such as hair and nails, may reflect changes in nutritional status during variable growth periods. Third, the proportions of body tissues that serve as reservoirs of nutrients, such as skeletal muscle and adipose tissue, reflect chronic nutritional status. With severe malnutrition, the physician may find changes in the size or function of specific organ systems that can be observed on clinical examination.

Evaluation of Body Composition

Knowledge of body composition is important both as a measure of nutritional status (i.e., is it optimal or not?) and as a basis on which to estimate nutrient and caloric needs, because energy and nutrient requirements to maintain lean body mass are greater per kilogram of tissue than are the requirements to maintain adipose tissue mass. Major compartments of the body include lean body mass, intracellular fluid, extracellular fluid, and body fat. The methods used to determine body composition vary depending on the number of body compartments considered and other variables that must be understood to use body composition studies for nutritional assessment (33–35).

Anthropometric Measures

Measures of body size, weight, and proportions all are anthropometric techniques useful in assessing and following nutritional status. The most widely recognized measures are those of height and weight. These measurements should be routinely obtained and recorded. Other anthropometric techniques include skinfold thickness measures, from which one can calculate estimates of total body fat stores; bony measures, such as elbow breadth, arm span, and leg length to estimate frame size, stature, or skeletal mass; and limb circumference, which can be combined in a formula with skinfold thickness to yield an estimate of muscle mass. These techniques allow the health care provider to obtain objective measures with relatively simple, low-risk, noninvasive, low-cost techniques. These techniques may appear deceptively simple, but there is significant potential for erroneous data collection if meticulous attention is not paid to anatomic detail and if the average of repeated measurements is not used (36–40).

The information gained from anthropometric measures can be used in the nutritional management of patients in several ways:

1. It can provide the basis for comparing a person with a group normal standard, classifying a person as to his or her relative position within a group (i.e., patient A weighs less than the average person of the same gender and height).

2. It is theoretically possible to estimate the size of specific body compartments, such as skeletal muscle mass and subcutaneous fat tissue. However, the formulas for extrapolation are less than perfect and have been derived primarily from information gained from studies of physiologically normal people (34–39).
3. It can provide baseline information from which to monitor change over time and, thus, the effectiveness of nutritional intervention and long-term nutrition management (i.e., patient A has gained 2 lb in the past month).

The clinician must recognize potential sources of error when using anthropometric data. It is important to understand factors that affect anthropometric measures. Changes in body weight with time will reflect hydration status, total body tissue mass, or both. Edema secondary to venous stasis, hypoalbuminemia, or both can result in falsely increased skinfold thickness and limb girth measures. Conversely, relative dehydration may falsely decrease these values. In the presence of abnormal tissue, such as heterotopic ossification, the basic assumptions regarding the meaning of the data no longer apply, so results can be misleading. With control of these variables, repetitive measures can be of value in assessing changes over time. It is necessary to understand the basic assumptions made in establishing the standards against which results are compared (39–42).

Other Methods

Standard laboratory techniques for estimating body composition include measures of body density by underwater weighing, air displacement, estimates of specific body compartment sizes by multiple isotope dilution techniques, radiographic estimates of fatty tissue layers and bony sizes, creatinine–height index, whole-body liquid scintillation counting to determine total body potassium content, and bioelectric impedance (43–47). Body composition can be studied with ultrasound and computerized tomographic scanners to determine sizes of specific body tissue layers and organs (48). Other techniques under assessment include infrared interactance (49), dual-photon absorptiometry (50), dual-energy x-ray absorptiometry (47), and neutron inelastic scattering (51).

Biochemical Data

The assessment of nutrition status includes the use of several protein markers (Table 32-5A). Although they have limitations, they provide some objective data on protein status and clinical outcome. Heme protein is useful in determining the presence of anemia. Additional tests confirm the presence of a nutritional anemia (Table 32-5B).

One type of physiological functional assessment technique that seems of particular interest is applying measures of skeletal muscle function to the assessment of nutritional status. Both the force of contraction with rapid repetitive stimuli and the maximal relaxation rate of the abductor pollicis brevis have been studied for this purpose. Suboptimal performance was found in malnourished patients with chronic renal failure (52). In a small group of obese patients, skeletal muscle function became abnormal during a 2-week period of a very low-calorie diet (400 kcal/day) and persisted during an additional 2 weeks of fasting. Function returned to normal after a 2-week period of refeeding. Standard parameters of nutritional status, including serum albu-

TABLE 32-5A. *Objective biochemical measurement of nutrition status: assessment of protein status*

Protein marker	Reference range	Half-life	Remarks
Albumin	3.5–5.0 g/dl Clinical significance: Mild depletion: 2.8–3.49 g/dl Moderate depletion: 2.1–2.79 g/dl Severe depletion: <2.1 g/dl days	20	Decreased in protein malnutrition, metabolic stress, liver disease, overhydration, nephrotic syndrome, protein-losing enteropathies; increased in dehydration
Transferrin	200–300 mg/dl Clinical significance Mild depletion: 150–200 mg/dl Moderate depletion: 100–150 mg/dl Severe depletion: <100 mg/dl	8 days	Decreased in protein malnutrition, chronic infections, acute catabolic states protein-losing enteropathies, nephropathy; increased in iron-deficiency anemia, pregnancy, acute hepatitis
Transthyretin (prealbumin)	16–35 mg/dl Clinical significance Mild depletion: 10–15 mg/dl Moderate depletion: 5–10 mg/dl Severe depletion: <5 mg/dl	48 hr	Decreased in acute catabolic states, protein-losing enteropathies; increased in chronic renal failure
Retinol-binding protein	3.0–6.0 mg/dl	5–7 hr	Decreased in vitamin A deficiency, acute catabolic states, postsurgery; increased in chronic renal failure
Insulin-like growth factor (IGF-1)	0.01–0.04 mg/dl	2 hr	Decrease with starvation and quickly respond to refeeding
Fibronectin	22–40 mg/dl	15 hr	Possible role during nutrition repletion

Adapted from Lee RD, Nieman DC. *Nutritional assessment, 2nd ed.* St Louis: CV Mosby, 1996; and Heymsfield SB, Tighe A, Wang ZM. Nutrition assessment by anthropometric and biochemical methods. In: Shils ME, Olson JA, Shike M, eds. *Modern nutrition in health and disease, 8th ed.* Philadelphia: Lea & Febiger, 1994.

TABLE 32-5B. *Objective biochemical measurement of nutrition status: Nutrition-related anemias*

Nutritional anemia	Parameters
Iron deficiency	↓RBC, ↓Hgb, ↓MCV, ↓MCH, ↓MCHC, ↑Transferrin, ↑TIBC, ↓Ferritin
Macrocytic	
Folate deficiency	↓RBC, ↓Hgb, ↑MCV, ↑MCH, nl MCHC, ↓Serum folate, ↓Red cell folate
Vitamin B_{12}	↓RBC, ↓Hgb, ↑MCV, ↑MCH, nl MCHC, ↓Serum B_{12}

Hgb, hemoglobin; MCH, mean corpuscular hemoglobin; MCHC, mean corpuscular hemoglobin concentration; MCV, mean corpuscular volume; nl, normal; RBC, red blood cell; TIBC, total iron-binding capacity.

min and transferrin values, creatinine–height index, anthropometric measures, and total body nitrogen and potassium levels, did not change during this study (53). One study has shown grip strength to be a more sensitive indicator of general nutritional status in surgical patients than standard anthropometric measures or serum albumin (54). These studies describe innovative methods for assessing nutritional status.

APPLICATION OF PRINCIPLES OF NUTRITION MANAGEMENT IN THE PRACTICE OF REHABILITATION MEDICINE

Risk of Nutrition Problems

Disability results from physiological alterations of the physical and/or mental capacity or function of the patient. Thus, by definition, people with new onset of disability, through illness or injury, are at risk for the development of malnutrition (Fig. 32-5). The need for specific attention to nutritional status and nutritional support in patients admitted to rehabilitation units has been studied. Those patients with abnormal nutrition assessments have increased morbidity and mortality (55). As the patients with disabilities become more chronic, it cannot be assumed that nutrition status and requirements for nutrients stabilize. The homeostatic balance in people living with chronic disability is more precarious than that in able-bodied individuals. With musculoskeletal and neurologic abnormalities, there are changes in body composition. Other factors affecting the person's nutrition are acute or chronic illness and use of medication.

Check if answer to question is yes. Nutrition risk increases as the number of checks increases.

1. Are you on a special diet? ______
2. Have you had a change in your eating habits? ______
3. Has your weight changed? ______
4. Do you have any cravings or desires for specific foods, liquids, or other substances to eat or drink? ______
5. Has your appetite changed? ______
6. Do you eat most of your food away from home? ______
7. Are you experiencing any of the following? ______
   a. Difficulty seeing at night? ______
   b. Dry skin or rashes? ______
   c. Nausea or vomiting? ______
   d. Constipation or diarrhea? ______
   e. Swelling of legs? ______
   f. Change in hair color, texture, or thickness (other than chemically or mechanically induced by hair care)? ______
   g. Yellow skin or eyes? ______
   h. Easy bruising? ______
   i. Swollen, tender joints? ______
   j. Poor healing of minor cuts or scratches? ______
8. Have you been ill or had surgery? ______
9. Are you taking any medicines or supplements? ______
10. Do you avoid any foods, liquids, or additives because of allergies or bad reactions? ______

FIG. 32-5. Historical information suggesting nutritional risk. (From Frankel DL. Nutrition. In: DeLisa JD, Gans BM, et al., eds. *Rehabilitation medicine: principles and practice, 2nd ed.* Philadelphia: JB Lippincott, 1993; 602.)

TABLE 32-6. *Effects of infection on nutrient requirements*

1. Nutrient losses: most nutrients, especially intracellular minerals and nitrogen. Exception is retention of water and salt after initial losses.
2. Increased metabolic rate from fever.
3. Decreased food intake secondary to anorexia.
4. Functional nutrient loss secondary to overuse, diversion, and sequestration of nutrients.
5. Hypermetabolism and accelerated use of cellular energy with phagocytosis

From Biesel WR. Infectious diseases. In: Schneider HA, Anderson CE, Coursi DB, eds. *Nutritional support of medical practice, 2nd ed.* Philadelphia: JB Lippincott, 1983; 443–457.

Acute or Chronic Illness

Acute or chronic illnesses may affect nutritional status by altering the body's metabolic activity, changing the bioavailability of nutrients, changing body composition, or changing the activity level (56–59).

Some conditions are seen more frequently in disabled people. One is decubitus ulcers. With ulcers, there is an increased loss of nutrients through dead tissue and seepage of body fluids. It is not possible to measure these losses clinically, but the needs for increased nutrition for healing are well documented. Respiratory tract and urinary tract infections are commonly seen in the disabled. Energy requirements are greater as body temperature rises. Please refer to Table 32-6 for effects of infection on nutrient requirements.

Gastrointestinal tract symptoms or anorexia, early satiety, bloating, and constipation are reported in more than 50% of people with chronic obstructive pulmonary disease (COPD) (58). One survey of people with spinal cord injury demonstrated that 23% had at least one hospital admission for gastrointestinal complaints after recovery from the acute injury, and 27% had recurrent symptoms sufficient enough to require chronic treatment or alter life-style (60). Gastroesophageal reflux is encountered frequently in children with developmental disability (20,61,62).

Use of Medication

Patients with disabilities are often on medications. Food intake, nutritional status, and efficacy of pharmaceutical agents are interrelated. Food and nutrients can interact with drugs to alter absorption, metabolism, or drug excretion. Drugs can affect nutritional status by their effect on appetite, gastrointestinal function, emotions, renal metabolism, and hepatic metabolism.

Information about drug–nutrient interactions can be obtained from a pharmacist or registered dietitian (63). Other good sources of information are the *Physicians' Desk Reference* or drug information sheets. There are an increasing number of references pertaining to this topic (64–69). One may need to change the medication if there is a potential interaction. Other changes may include administering the drug at a different time, altering the diet, adding nutrition supplements, or a combination of these things.

Other Nutrition Problems

With chronic disease or disability, there may be reduced reserves in the body to tolerate other stresses. Functional disability from chronic disease may be aggravated by other factors, some of which may be partially controlled through dietary means. People with mobility impairment may expend less calories and be more prone to excessive weight gain. The resulting obesity may add to the mobility impairment.

The multidisciplinary rehabilitation team can assist with nutritional support by identifying each patient's individual needs. It is helpful to have a dietitian who attends weekly rehabilitation conferences as an integral member of the team.

Because of the decreased length of acute hospital stays, there may be more nutritional problems identified among rehabilitation patients. It is important to identify these problems early, so nutrition intervention can occur as soon as possible, thereby decreasing mortality and morbidity (57,59,70–82).

People with chronic disease and disability may turn to alternative treatment regimens, which fosters charlatans and quacks. The focus is often on nutrition "supplementation" or "diet" therapy. Although supplementation may be beneficial, excessive supplements may cost patients precious dollars and provide little benefit. In some cases, nutritional imbalances may be caused by some of these additional therapies (83). The health care provider should ask patients about other alternative therapies and demonstrate a willingness to work with patients who choose to explore other options. This allows the medical practitioner to maintain his or her rapport with the patient and may result in the patient receiving the most optimal nutrition therapy.

Food Accessibilty

Many factors are involved in optimizing nutritional status (Fig. 32-3). Changes in any of these factors can change one's access to food, which can affect one's nutritional status significantly. Rehabilitation involves maximizing one's level of independence physically, emotionally, and economically. With transportation, access to shopping, kitchen modifications, adaptive utensils, and more prepared foods available, the disabled person can achieve more independence. Some people will continue to need help with shopping or food preparation, but with that assistance they can live independently.

Nonphysiological Factors

Nonphysiological factors are influenced by disability and can be instrumental in the development of malnutrition. Although the primary physiological reason for eating is to meet the metabolic requirements of the body, actual food consumed is affected by the factors discussed below.

Economic Status

People in developed countries purchase most of their food. With disability, there is often a loss of income and an increase in medical expenses. Because quality of diet may be directly related to income, there may be a change in the variety of nutritious food available for consumption. Limited finances could also limit transportation, resulting in reduced opportunity for shopping. When there are competing financial obligations, one may compromise the variety and quality of food purchased.

Environment

Temperature and humidity extremes have an impact on nutrition requirements. In very hot or cold climates, one's nutritional requirements change. The same is true when one is using an air–fluidized mattress sytem for prevention or healing of skin decubiti. With the increased temperature and constant flow of air, one's fluid requirements are increased. Patients using these mattresses are often debilitated and malnourished, so it is even more imperative that they have all of the nutrients required for promotion of health and healing.

Place of Residence

When a person lives in a private residence, his or her proximity and access to stores, as well as facilities for food storage and preparation, influence the food intake. If an attendant is required to care for someone at home, it is important that the attendant be included in discharge education. Nutrition status of dependent persons correlates with the nutrition knowledge and resources of the family (84,85). Education and social interventions may be needed to achieve optimal nutrition.

If a person lives in an institution, the food presentation and taste as well as the dining facilities and congeniality of others there may influence how well one eats. Regulations include attention to providing balanced meals and evaluation of one's functional status and health maintenance. Despite these regulations, there are variabilities in nutrition management in these settings (86). The support staff responsible for feeding patients in institutions need to understand basic nutrition principles to maintain optimal nutrient intake for disabled patients. Nutrition education for institutional staff has been shown to have a positive effect on the resident's nutritional status (87,88).

Social Factors

Food and beverages, including alcohol, are present at most social gatherings. Choices are based on taste, convenience, and cost, resulting in a relative abundance of foods high in fat, salt, and sugar. Thus, a more active social life may promote poor nutrition habits, with consumption of foods high in calories but with low nutrient density. Conversely, people who are alone and associate eating with socialization may not eat adequately.

Massive advertising campaigns for food products influence food intake, encouraging the consumption of more manufactured foods with variable nutrition content. Food is sometimes used as a reward for good behavior, or it may be seen as a punishment for people with significant feeding disorders. Values are then attributed to food and may have a significant impact on food consumption.

When patients become more dependent because of acute or chronic illness or a severe handicap, they may have decreased appetite and reduced food choices. Food may become the object of a power struggle rather than a basic need for health. Some problems related to food and nutritional status can be prevented by allowing the disabled person to have a choice in food selection or preparation. In some cases, a more comprehensive behavioral management approach to nutrition management is required (89,90).

Physiological Factors

The major physiological factors contributing to food accessibility include mobility, upper extremity function, communication skills, cognitive function, and oral-motor/swallowing skills. Losing the ability to feed oneself has major implications for living independently. The rehabilitation team helps to evaluate all of the physiological factors and tries to address them to the extent possible.

Upper extremity function is necessary for self-feeding (refer to Table 32-7). When one loses some function, there are multiple ways to compensate (91,92). Loss of fine motor coordination and ataxia may compromise independence in self-feeding. Environmental control systems and robotic technology may help resolve some feeding problems related to upper extremity impairment. These devices may have limited application in the patient with tremors or ataxia. Devices also must be as discrete and cosmetic as possible (93).

Oral-motor/swallowing function must be intact for eating and requires integrity of anatomic structures, appropriate control of oral musculature, and coordinated peristaltic action in the esophagus. A comprehensive evaluation includes observation of the oral/pharyngeal phase of swallowing, evaluation of body position, assessment of primitive reflexes, and a feeding trial with foods of different consistencies. The latter should help determine the patient's aspiration risk. It is important to record length of time required to eat a meal, as a patient may be able to swallow adequately but tire too quickly to consume adequate nutrients and calories within a reasonable time (94–97). The major complications of oral-motor/swallowing dysfunction include undernutrition and aspiration pneumonia, both of which can compromise the outcome of rehabilitation efforts.

Patients may perceive feeding problems or deny having

TABLE 32-7. *Motions of the upper extremity necessary for self-feeding*

Body part	Motion	Purpose	Substitution	Loss	Device used to compensate
Hand	Palmar prehension	Pick up and hold utensil	1. Lacing spoon between fingers 2. Adduction of fingers	Minimal	1. Utensil interlaced in fingers (some shaping may be necessary) 2. Moleskin or tape over handle to prevent slipping
	Lateral prehension to middle finger (modified lateral pinch)		3. Hook grasp	Moderate	3. Build-up handle (wood, sponge, or other material) 4. Grip-shaped handles 5. Handle with horizontal and vertical dowels (pegged handle) 6. Handle with finger rings
				Severe	7. Warm Spring–type short opponents with C-bar and utensil attachment 8. Plastic and metal holder
				Complete	9. ADL (universal) cuff 10. Prehension orthosis • Manually operated • Power operated
Wrist	Stabilization (slight flexion and extension of radial and ulnar deviation normally used depending on whether grasp is hook or pinch)	Positioning of hand for optimal function (to prevent wrist flexion)	1. Use of finger or thumb extensors	Partial stability Complete	1. ADL wrist support dorsal (leather with spring steel insert) 2. Flexible, adjustable nylon wrist support or Klenzac joints 3. Tubular spring-clip (ADL) orthosis 4. Cock-up splint, rigid palmar 5. Warm Springs–type long opponents
Forearm	Pronation	Place food on utensil	1. Shoulder abduction and internal rotation 2. Raise forearm to vertical position and then rotate	Partial or complete	1. Swivel spoon 2. Bent fork or spoon
	Supination	Keep utensil level while putting food in mouth to avoid spill	3. Shoulder adduction and external rotation		1. Swivel spoon 2. Placing fork or spoon over thumb, use thumb extensors
Elbow	Flexion of forearm	Raising hand to mouth	1. Use of knee 2. Shoulder abduction 3. Trunk flexion	Partial or complete	1. Balanced forearm orthosis (ball-bearing feeder) 2. Overhead sling with feeder attachment
	Extension	Lowering hand to plate	4. Rock forearm to edge of table		3. Overhead sling with built-up lapboard 4. Long-handled utensil 5. Functional arm orthosis
Shoulder	Stabilization against hyperextension and internal rotation in position of • Slight flexion • Slight abduction	Provides positioning and assists in raising hand to level of mouth	1. Trunk flexion 2. Prop elbow on table	Partial or complete	1. Pillow behind upper arm 2. Overhead sling 3. Balanced forearm orthosis 4. Functional arm orthosis 5. Hyperextension stop

ADL, activities of daily living.

From Zimmerman ME. Activities of daily living. In: Willard HS, Spackman GS, eds. *Occupational therapy, 4th ed.* Philadelphia: JB Lippincott, 1971; 228.

any problems. Either situation may affect nutritional status (97). Signs and symptoms of dysphagia include difficulty articulating words, decreased tongue mobility, facial weakness, weak or hoarse cough, decreased gag reflex, impaired sensitivity in the mouth or face, coughing and choking during or after meals, a wet or gurgled voice quality, pockets of food in the mouth, unexplained weight loss or lack of interest in eating, and chart notes that indicate the need for total assistance with feeding.

Feeding management systems are only as successful as their acceptance by those using them (the disabled person and others involved with his or her care). Try to feed patients foods they like but that are modified appropriately in consistency. Let patients experience all the flavors of foods served by feeding each item separately, not all mixed together.

The economic, social, and psychological status of the disabled person must be given equal consideration and related to the physical or cognitive disabilities present. A high-tech feeding device must be accepted and affordable. For some individuals, especially ones who live alone, having a personal assistant for feeding may be more optimal as he or she will provide needed socialization.

Alternate Feeding Routes

People who cannot take in sufficient nutrients orally may need to be fed by an alternate route, either enteral or parenteral, or a combination. Both physiological and psychological factors contribute to decisions regarding alternate feeding routes. Some patients may have a decreased appetite or feeding disturbances related to psychological factors. These routes allow for adequate nutrients and calories and may be a partial or complete means of nutritional support. Alternate feeding routes may be used to provide excess nutrients needed for additional demands or to prevent malnutrition in a person with severe feeding or gastrointestinal function disturbances.

The importance of alternate feeding routes in patients with major trauma or burns is well established (15,19,22,24, 26,82,98–105). The effectiveness of alternate feedings routes in patients who have started to recover or have more chronic problems is not as well studied (106–109).

Enteral feeding is an integral part of the nutrition management of children with severe neurologic impairments (94,110–112). In children and teenagers with cystic fibrosis, enteral feeding supplements improve total body nitrogen (113).

There are some risks associated with alternate feeding routes. These routes bypass the homeostatic control mechanisms of the body that regulate food and fluid intake. Objective monitors must be used routinely to assess the adequacy of nutritional support to avoid over- or underfeeding (71).

Monitoring should include daily records of intake and output, frequent weight checks, and monitoring of vital signs. Nitrogen balance, fluid balance, serum electrolytes, glucose, blood urea nitrogen, creatinine, and hepatic enzyme levels may need to be evaluated regularly. Indirect calorimetry has improved the ability to provide appropriate calories for people dependent on alternative feeding routes.

Any decisions regarding alternate feeding routes are multifactorial and include the needs and wants of the patient and family and the capacity of the health care delivery system. An in-house nutrition support team is very helpful to implement specific guidelines and protocols for providing nutrition through alternative feeding methods. Some nutrition support teams are available for consultation after discharge from the hospital. The team greatly enhances the success of this technology while decreasing the complications (32,71,82,101,114–120).

Enteral Feeding

Enteral feeding uses the gastrointestinal tract as the site of food intake but bypasses any proximal obstacles to feeding that might exist. Blenderized food, liquid nutritional supplements, or elemental nutrient solutions are delivered directly to either the stomach or the small intestine. Enteral routes include nasogastric, nasoenteric, esophagogastric, gastrostomy, and jejunostomy. When oral feeding is impossible or limited, or one cannot move food through proximal structures of the gastrointestinal tract despite normal oral function, enteral feeding should be considered. It allows safe administration and absorption of dietary substances, provided there is sufficient gastrointestinal function. Enteral feeding is the least expensive alternate feeding route, has lower risks of complications from access or induced metabolic abnormalities, and provides the most physiological approach to alternative feeding.

Products for enteral feeding are numerous, and appropriate formula selection requires knowledge about the specific nutritional needs of the patient, awareness of digestive and absorptive capabilities, and knowledge about the potential effects of formulas on GI, metabolic, and immunologic functions. Formulas can be classified according to specific characteristics. Because protein is the most significant formula component, it seems reasonable to classify formulas according to the type of protein present, with subcategories describing formula characteristics. Types of protein include intact, hydrolyzed, and amino acids.

The primary risk for tube feedings is aspiration. With a depressed gag reflex or impaired swallow, there is no natural protective mechanism to prevent aspiration pneumonia, especially with gastroesophageal reflux or proximal placement of the tube.

The direct gastrostomy or jejunostomy routes are considered most desirable when tube feedings will be needed for a prolonged time. These routes may decrease some of the problems associated with gastroesophageal reflux and are more cosmetic. Other techniques for placement or small tubes are percutaneous (100,116,121). The advantages of percutaneous insertion are the ability to start tube feedings less than 24 hours after surgery and avoidance of general anesthesia with its risks. Large-bore tubes placed surgically (e.g., Janeway gastrostomy, esophagogastrostomy procedures), with the creation of a permanent stoma, have the advantage of being easily inserted and removed so the tube needs to be in place only during mealtimes (116,122). Placement of the tube through a jejunostomy minimizes the risk of aspiration. The disadvantages of more distal placement of the feeding tubes are related to the decreased absorptive capacity of the remaining gut, including less tolerance of high-osmolar loads and altered absorption of some pharmaceutical agents and nutrients.

The rate of administration may be intermittent bolus or continuous drip and depends on the needs and tolerance of the patient, the staff, and the equipment available. Continuous drip requires a mechanical pump to control flow rate, which may limit activity to some extent. Activity tolerance may be limited by the physiological response to a full stomach. Bolus feedings can be problematic because of limited gastric capacity and delayed gastric emptying. When possible, continuous drip feedings, limited to the late evening and night, provide a means of minimizing complications while maximizing patient freedom. Patients receiving gastric feedings while in bed should have the head elevated. One complication is the potential for shear forces, which may compromise skin care.

Parenteral Feeding

Parenteral feeding uses the venous system for direct delivery of elemental forms of nutrients to the body. It is generally done through a central venous access line, which allows for the administration of the entire day's nutrient requirements, but peripheral venous access may be used in limited circumstances. Total parenteral nutrition (TPN) is indicated when the gut is nonfunctional or must be free of food for extended periods of time. Parenteral supplementation is indicated when gastrointestinal function is temporarily interrupted or in the presence of hypermetabolic states that require nutrients in excess of the absorptive capacity of the gut.

Nutrients are delivered in elemental forms. Initial estimates of nutrient requirements were extrapolated from the RDAs, which were established based on administration of food through the gut. Bypassing the gut means the loss of nutrients made by gastrointestinal bacteria and absence of first-pass hepatic metabolism of nutrients, which normally are absorbed from the gut into the portal vein and delivered directly to the liver with oral and enteral feedings. Therefore, patients dependent on parenteral feeding require close observation and frequent monitoring of nutritional status. Complications from nutrient deficiency and nutrient excess have been identified in patients receiving parenteral feeding. The optimal elemental composition of parenteral solutions varies widely, and recommendations are modified on a regular basis as research and experience with parenteral nutrition continue (22,32,115,119,120,123).

There are risks associated with the delivery of parenteral alimentation through a central venous line. With catheter insertion, there is the risk of pneumothorax. Routine use of the catheter may result in infection or contaminated substrate. Fluid and electrolyte balance must be closely monitored. The optimal ratio of carbohydrate and protein must be achieved so that nitrogen retention is optimized without placing excessive metabolic demands on the liver and kidneys for amino acid metabolism and elimination of nitrogenous waste products. The requirement of sufficient lipid to supply essential fatty acids has been recognized for several years, but the value of lipids in relatively significant quantities is still a subject of research (123,124). The ratio of the basic nutrients that provide energy affects the amount of substrate and fluid required because lipids are a more concentrated source of calories than carbohydrates or protein. Carbohydrate metabolism is associated with greater carbon dioxide production than lipid metabolism, a factor recognized to contribute significantly to carbon dioxide levels, and may affect respiratory drive in some patients with respiratory compromise (74,78,125). Severely burned patients have an increased incidence of sepsis when receiving nutrition solely through parenteral access. This problem may be the result of loss of gut integrity from disuse, with subsequent movement of intestinal bacteria into the circulation (126,127).

Complications

Often it is impossible to deliver a full day's nutrient requirements through a peripheral line. Peripheral venous supplementation is indicated in specific situations, such as a temporary interruption of oral feeding (119).

The psychological impact of the long-term use of alternate feeding routes in cancer patients has been reviewed (128). Enteral routes are less problematic than parenteral ones. Psychological problems associated with enteral feeding include gustatory deprivation, dry mouth, and tube-related discomforts. With parenteral feeding, problems have been identified in regard to the loss of normal eating ability and associated body image changes as well as depression and decreased sexual activity. For some there is stress associated with fear of the apparatus, its maintenance, and its function.

Transitional Feeding

At some point it may be desirable to reintroduce oral feedings. Several factors (129) have been identified when this step is considered. One is resolution of the medical problem for which the tube feeding was introduced; others are adequate oral-motor/swallowing skills to support oral food intake and the patient and caregiver readiness.

Children who have been enterally fed from birth have had feeding problems associated with the change from enteral to oral feeding (130). These children may not have developed chewing skills. To prevent these problems, children should receive oral-motor/swallowing stimulation even while receiving all their nutrition enterally.

A gradual transition period from enteral to oral food intake ensures more success.

1. Normalize tube feedings to approximate meals/snacks.
2. Alter feeding schedule to promote hunger.
3. Reduce tube feeding by 25% of calories.
4. Provide adequate fluids.
5. Decrease tube feedings as oral intake increases.

When moving patients from TPN to enteral feedings, Winkler et al. found that patients were able to maintain body weight and continue to improve plasma proteins with TPN after tolerating 60% of caloric requirements by the oral/enteral route (131).

Assessment and Nutritional Status in the Rehabilitation Population

Food/Nutrient Intake

Because there are changes in metabolic demand and activity with disability, current reference standards for food

(RDAs) are not entirely appropriate for the diverse problems seen in this population group.

The food/nutrient intake of children with disabilities has been extensively studied. There are similarities in various studies, indicating that food/nutrient intake varies widely. Poor diets may be related to the disability itself or to associated feeding difficulties (84,85,94). Other factors such as family income (84), educational level of the parents (85), and quality of the food offered to children living in institutions (132) are significant in determining the adequacy of food/nutrient intake. Level of dietary supplements (85,133) and amount of salty, high-fat, and sweet foods consumed affect diet quality (133). These same factors affect the diets of healthy children; thus, a physical or mental disability alone does not result in poor dietary habits.

There are wide individual variations in caloric and nutrient intake of disabled adults, as identified by dietary surveys (134–137). People with physically disabling chronic illness (138,139) consume relatively fewer calories, whereas adults with mental retardation take in more calories (140). Litchford and Wakefield (88) identified a strong correlation between the knowledge of caregivers and the adequacy of diets of mentally retarded adults. Dysgeusia and xerostomia are significant factors in the adequacy of diets (141,142).

Bowman and Rosenberg summarize multiple dietary surveys of the elderly (143). Average energy intakes are below two-thirds of the RDAs, but fewer than 10% have intakes of calcium, iron, vitamin A, and water-soluble vitamins below two-thirds of the RDAs. In elderly veterans, dietary adequacy was correlated to a greater extent with the self-perception of chewing problems than with clinically determined dental status or the degree of social isolation (108).

Food/Nutrient Requirements

Food/nutrient requirements vary with the effects of multiple factors, including body size, body composition, activity level, environmental conditions, presence of illness or injury, medication usage, metabolic activity, body temperature regulation, and amount of specific types of body tissues (14,56). The effect of disability on energy balance has been studied more than its effect on any specific nutrient requirement.

With sudden traumatic changes, such as amputation, there may be a dramatic change in body size or metabolism. Slower changes in body composition may occur after problems, such as spinal cord injury, related to the amount of muscle atrophy. To estimate the effect of altered body size on energy requirements one must consider:

1. The time period during which the body is undergoing physiological adaptation to the disabling condition.
2. The time period after physiological adaptation required for body size to stabilize at a new level.

The onset of disability often affects the metabolic activity of the body. After acute trauma, there is an increase in metabolic requirements associated with the body's stress reaction. There is a catabolic phase with negative nitrogen balance, which may not be entirely reversible even with optimal nutritional support (19,26,73,82,101,121,139). In the hypermetabolic patient, it is important to avoid iatrogenic stress from exogenous protein loads that exceed the metabolic capacity of the body for anabolic purposes. The optimal level of protein support in the initial stages after severe trauma or acute illness has yet to be determined (17,22,99,104,105). Barbiturate therapy in acute head injury has been shown, in one study, to decrease nitrogen excretion (21). Clifton and colleagues have demonstrated that use of a standard correction factor may underestimate total urinary nitrogen excretion when a major catabolic insult has occurred (19); therefore, accuracy in determining nitrogen balance in such cases requires the direct measurement of nonurea nitrogen in the urine. Acutely, it may not be possible to achieve positive energy and nitrogen balance.

After the acute injury, there is an adaptive period during which further adjustments of energy consumption and metabolism occur. This adaptation is followed by a period of relative stability when the steady state of body composition and activity has been achieved (39,132,144,145).

Disabled and healthy people have variable levels of physical activity. Spinal cord patients too have variable activity levels, but they may be further affected by the presence or absence of spasticity. A paraplegic who walks expends more energy than one who is wheelchair dependent. Energy expenditure may vary with different types of prosthetic devices or orthoses (23).

Children with cerebral palsy may have spasticity, which inhibits purposeful movement and results in lower activity levels, whereas those with athetoid forms may have higher activity levels (146–148). To assess energy needs in stable disabled children, it is important to consider requirements for normal growth. These energy requirements are related to both height and physical mobility status (148).

Formulae have been used to estimate the energy needs of disabled people, both acutely after injury (20,144) and at later stages in recovery (106,134–136). Critical assessments of these formulas demonstrate a significant variation from actual energy expenditure, as determined by direct and indirect measures (13,149). Errors are significant with traumatic injuries, such as spinal cord injury (150), head injury (19,142), and burns (37,152).

Indirect calorimetry measures are being used more frequently. It is practical and provides better accuracy than formulas, especially acutely (15–26). For more chronic patients, it is more feasible to rely on formulas to estimate caloric and nutrient requirements. Because of the inaccuracies, close clinical monitoring is indicated.

Nutrition Status Parameters

One's nutritional status needs to be assessed to determine the appropriate nutrition intervention. The traditional parameters of nutritional status may not be applicable to persons with disability. It is not clear whether physiological adaptations to disability result in changes of body composition or biochemical function because of the specific disability/illness or as a result of malnutrition. Finally, one needs to investigate whether altered measures of nutritional status in the disabled reflect an imbalance of diet or a change in absorption, metabolism, or excretion related to the disability.

Presently information obtained regarding nutritional status measures only where the disabled person stands in relation to standards for able-bodied persons. These standards are not applicable to a spinal-cord-injured patient who loses muscle mass in the paretic muscles or to an amputee who loses part of his or her body mass. Thus, serum creatinine is lowered but may not reflect impairment of renal function. To accurately assess renal function, one needs a creatinine clearance measurement. The implications for determining appropriate dosages of medications with renal elimination and potential for renal impairment are significant.

Changes in body composition alter the physiological activity of some pharmaceutical agents. Water-soluble medications are distributed throughout the total-body water compartment; fat-soluble medications are stored in fat. As a result of altered body composition, there may be changes in both the half-life and the effective serum levels of a medication. The futher body composition moves from "normal," the more important it is to monitor dosages of medications, with serum levels or astute clinical observations to monitor for potential toxicity.

Measurements of serum albumin reflect plasma oncotic pressure, which affects the distribution of body fluids and the active levels of drugs that bind to albumin.

Measures of Body Composition

The "ideal" body composition for persons with disability has not been defined, and such a definition may be difficult because of the multitude of problems that result in disability. The main clinical use for body composition in nutrition management of the disabled is to define baseline and monitor overall clinical condition and function. Studies of body composition in spinal-cord-injured persons (145,152–154) have shown the following:

- There is generally a depletion of lean body mass.
- There is a tendency toward an increased proportion of body fat.
- There is an increase in total body fluid.
- There is a high degree of intersubject variability.

Initially, spinal-cord-injured patients lose weight, but there is significant variability of the weight at which patients stabilize (134,136,144,145,155). Some have recommended that these patients weigh less than their ideal weight by 10 to 20 lb to facilitate improved mobility (156). Others have suggested that spinal cord patients who weigh less than 10% below the mean for ideal body weight are at risk for malnutrition (136,155). There are no studies to support these conclusions, and the optimal weight-for-height standard after spinal cord injury has not yet been determined. It will probably vary depending on the degree of paralysis and extent of spasticity, which helps to maintain some muscle tone and mass. In paraplegics, there will be a disproportionate increase in muscle mass in the more exercised upper extremities.

Some have concluded that patients with ALS who have lost more than 10% of their body weight are underweight and at nutritional risk (139). But it is natural that with loss of functioning muscle, as in ALS or spinal cord injury, there will be loss of weight unless there is an increase in body fat or water. The latter would result in an imbalance of lean body mass relative to other body compartments, which is consistent with a poorer nutritional status.

Determining height requires alternative measures in people with contractures or other physical deformities (157).

Combining serial weights with arm circumference and skinfold thickness allows the clinician to follow changes in the proportion of lean body mass compared with fat. Body weight is easily measured, but there is potential for error with patients being weighed at different times of the day, by different individuals using slightly different techniques, or with different scales. All scales need to be calibrated routinely.

Some innovative techniques to determine body composition have helped to evaluate the effects of chronic illness on body composition. Dual-photon absorptiometry has been used to measure the distribution and time course of changes in bone mineral content after paraplegic spinal cord injury. Bone mass was lost, initially, in the proximal tibia and femoral neck, stabilizing at a lower level 2 years postinjury. No change was seen in the spine or distal forearm bones (158). Bioelectric impedance has been shown to be more effective in estimating fat-free mass than skinfold thickness in people with COPD (159). Other work with cancer and renal patients is ongoing (47,160,161).

Children with myelomeningocele have been studied. They have normal body composition until age 2 to 3; but after age 4, there is a significant depletion of body cell mass and total body water and an increased percentage of body fat. The total body water is present disproportionately in the extracellular compartment.

Biochemical and Physiological Measures

Of the static biochemical measures, albumin has consistently been a predictor of outcome for acute medical management and rehabilitation (162–164). Other functional measures need to be evaluated for this population.

Clinical Application of Nutrition Management in Selected Disabilities

Chronic Obstructive Pulmonary Disease

Donahoe and Rogers have summarized the research investigating the role of nutrition in health and longevity of people with COPD (58). The most consistent nutritional predictor of mortality is a body weight less than 90% of the ideal. By indirect calorimetry, it has been shown that the REE as a percentage of predicted metabolic requirements in the underweight group is greater than that in the normal-weight group (25,165). The reason for inadequate dietary intake remains obscure. It is possible that many of the symptoms associated with COPD (e.g., anorexia, early satiety, dyspnea, fatigue, bloating, constipation, dental problems) contribute to dietary inadequacy. Demonstrations of successful refeeding rule against impaired nutrient utilization (109,166). Weight gain can be achieved with close attention to nutritional intake. With adequate calories for energy expenditure, there does not seem to be a problem with variations in carbon dioxide production as a consequence of the ratio among dietary fat, protein, and carbohydrates (58). It is difficult to maintain that weight gain, as losses can occur rapidly during exacerbations of the disease. There is a decrease in respiratory muscle strength with undernutrition (109,167), which reverses with short-term refeeding and weight gain (109). Improved immune function with refeeding after recent weight loss has been reported in nine patients with COPD (166). Peak exercise performance and ventilatory muscle strength are reduced in COPD patients who weigh less than 90% ideal body weight (167). Walking distance was found to be proportional to serum albumin and creatinine–height index (168). Because these studies involved a small number of subjects, other more definitive studies on larger populations need to be done before generalizations can be made.

Cerebral Palsy

Growth failure, decreased height and weight for age, is seen in most chidlren with cerebral palsy (61,112). Multiple factors contribute to poor food intake in these children. These include poor dentition, refusing food, oral motor dysfunction, including involuntary tongue thrust and delayed or absent initiation of the swallowing reflex, vomiting, rumination, and gastrointestinal reflux because of abnormal peristalisis and lower esophageal sphincter dysfunction. Mechanical oral-motor problems cannot always be overcome, especially if the feeding time needed to consume adequate calories becomes too excessive (94). With enteral feedings as supplementation, these children can achieve more normal growth (112), although optimal growth parameters for these children have not been established. Nutrition supplements should be started within 1 year of central nervous sytem (CNS) insult. When children are within 8 years of the CNS insult and significantly small for age, both height and weight, they can achieve within 90% of ideal height with the additional of enteral feedings. After 8 years, weight may increase, but height will not change as significantly (111). Thus, the need for early aggressive nutritional support. Some caregivers, however, may prefer that the children remain smaller because of the mobility dependence and physical care issues.

Nutritional Implications of Specific Clinical Problems

Urinary Tract Stones

Patients with a neurogenic bladder have an increased incidence of urinary tract stones. The causes of these stones are multifactorial (169–171). The increased rate of calcium loss from bone after spinal cord injury and immobilization is well known and difficult to control (172–175). Diet may be critical in some instances. Recommendations for dietary modification include a low-calcium diet (400 to 500 mg/day), a low-sodium diet, and the combination of thiazides and a low-calcium diet (169,176). Some postulate that a high-protein diet, which helps control the adverse effects of nitrogen depletion, may increase calcium excretion in the urine (177). There is no conclusive evidence that control of hypercalciuria will decrease the incidence of stone formation.

There has been concern about the potential for oxalate stone formation in the urinary tract of patients taking in large amounts of vitamin C (i.e., several grams). The increase in urinary oxalate excretion associated with high vitamin C intake may be an artifact induced by the laboratory assay (178,179). Patients with neurogenic bladders continue to use vitamin C supplementation, but without conclusive evidence regarding its benefit.

Sufficient fluid intake to support adequate urine volume (2 to 2.5 liters/day) will keep the urine dilute and decrease the tendency of substances to crystallize out because of high concentration (180). This fluid output is difficult to maintain in patients managed with intermittent catheterization. Thus, the tendency to form stones is only one factor in deciding optimal fluid intake for patients with neurogenic bladders.

The pH of the urine can be manipulated to reduce the tendency to form stones. It is best controlled with medication, as it is difficult to change the urine pH with dietary methods (65).

Decubitus Ulcers

Skin breakdown continues to be a significant cause of morbidity and is an expensive complication of disability. There are multiple studies pertaining to this problem, but prevention is difficult to achieve. The immediate cause of decubitus ulcers is excess pressure on the skin surface, but cells break down because of inability to sustain metabolism. The latter occurs because of poor delivery of nutrients and poor removal of waste products. Thus, local cellular nutrition imbalance is a significant factor that contributes to this problem.

Nutritional needs are increased for healing of a decubitus ulcer, and fluid containing proteins, vitamins, and minerals is continuously lost through the open wound surface. It is important that these patient's nutritional status be monitored closely, with adjustments made in the diet as indicated.

Edema

When there is decreased muscle activity, edema from venous pooling occurs in dependent limbs. It is important to determine whether the edema is related to venous pooling versus decreased plasma oncotic pressure. In the latter case, one's serum albumin will be low.

Nonpharmacologic treatment of edema involves elevation of the dependent extremities or compression with elastic stockings. Some clinicians give diuretics or decrease sodium intake to help control edema. There are two problems with these methods:

1. Patients with flaccid paralysis and decreased lean body mass have a decreased total body potassium. With use of potassium-wasting diuretics, the levels of potassium depletion may be dangerous. Serum potassium levels need to be monitored closely when diuretics are used.
2. Decreased plasma volume may also aggravate the tendency toward orthostatic hypotension, especially in patients with poor cardiovascular response to postural changes.

Constipation

Standard bowel programs used on rehabilitation units are excellent in controlling neurogenic bowel syndromes. One important aspect is having a regular source of fiber in the diet or as a supplement (e.g., psyllium). Up to 30 g/day of fiber may be needed to control constipation in disabled people, especially if there is a combination of immobility and previous laxative abuse (181). Successful alteration of fiber intake in the diet generally requires individual dietary instruction.

Some patients fail a bowel program. In these cases, the failure may be related to inadequate fluid intake. Increasing fluid intake to 1.5 to 2 liters/day will usually help the bowel problems but may make management of a neurogenic bladder more difficult.

Obesity

Obesity is often a problem among the disabled with a significant decrease in activity level or if there is a brain insult with associated cognitive impairment, such as decreased initiation for eating or altered satiety levels. Successful nutritional intervention may require application of behavioral techniques to control food intake as well as a general understanding of the caloric content of foods and how to modify them in one's diet.

Obesity is a common form of malnutrition among the elderly, and malnutrition may occur in association with obesity. The risk of myocardial infarction, stroke, hypertension, non-insulin-dependent diabetes mellitus, osteoarthritis, and some types of cancer is increased with obesity.

Adults with burns have increased respiratory and cardiac morbidity and mortality, disproportionate to burn size, burn location, and age. Those factors may contribute to obesity.

Elderly

The elderly may have impairments in their functional activities of daily living, which may limit their access to different types of food. Limited finances and social isolation may lead to decreased nutrient intake. Many elderly may be overweight but have dietary lipid intakes above recommended levels and have decreased calcium and folic acid intakes. Accurate information regarding food intake is essential in evaluating the nutritional status of this group. Special services such as meals on wheels may help to optimize nutrition intake.

REFERENCES

1. Jackson AA. Aminoacids: essential and non-essential? *Lancet* 1985; 1:1034–1037.
2. Lands WEM. Renewed questions about polysaturated fatty acids. *Nutr Rev* 1986; 44:189–195.
3. Vahouny GV. Conclusions and recommendations of the Symposium on Dietary Fibers in Health and Disease, Washington, D.C., 1981. *Am J Clin Nutr* 1982; 35:152–156.
4. Smicklas-Wright H, Guthrie HA. Dietary methodologies: their uses, analyses, interpretations, and implications. In: Simko MD, Cowel C, Gilbride JA, eds. *Nutrition assessment: a comprehensive guide for planning intervention.* Rockville, MD: Aspen Systems, 1984; 119–138.
5. Wotecki CE. Improving estimates of food and nutrient intake: applications to individuals and groups. *J Am Diet Assoc* 1985; 85:295–296.
6. Wotecki CE. Dietary survey data: sources and limits to interpretation. *Nutr Rev* 1986; 44(Suppl):204–213.
7. Kalisz K, Kevall S. A nutritional interview for clients with development disorders. *Ment Retard* 1984; 22:279–288.
8. Bingham SA, Cummings JH. Urine nitrogen as an independent validatory measure of dietary intake: a study of nitrogen balance in individuals consuming their normal diet. *Am J Clin Nutr* 1985; 42:1276–1289.
9. Adams CF. *Nutritive value of American foods in common units. Agriculture Handbook No. 456, United States Dewpartment of Agriculture.* Washngton, D.C.: US Government Printing Office, 1975.
10. Pennington JAT, Church HN. *Bowes and Church's food values of portions commonly used, 15th ed.* Philadelphia: JB Lippincott, 1989.
11. Watt BK, Merrill AL. *Composition of foods: raw, processed, prepared. Agriculture Handbook No. 8, United States Department of Agriculture.* Washngton, D.C.: Government Printing Office, 1963.
12. Goodhart RS, Shils ME, eds. *Modern nutrition in health and disease, 6th ed.* Philadelphia: Lea & Febiger, 1980.
13. Silberman H. *Parenteral and enteral nutrition. 2nd ed.* Norwalk. CT: Appleton-Century-Crofts, 1982.
14. Shils ME. Food and nutrition related to work, exercise and environmental stress. In: Goodhart RS, Shils ME, eds. *Modern nutrition in health and disease, 6th ed.* Philadelphia: Lea & Febiger, 1980; 814–851.
15. Cunningham JJ, Lydon MK, Russell WE. Calorie and protein provision for recovery from severe burns in infants and young children. *Am J Clin Nutr* 1990; 51:553–557.
16. Moore R, Najarian MP, Konvolinka CW. Measured energy expenditure in severe head trauma. *J Trauma* 1989; 29:1633–1636.
17. Saffle JR, Larson CM, Sillivan J. A randomized trial of indirect calorimetry-based feeding in thermal injury. *J Trauma* 1990; 30:776–783.
18. Allard JP, Pichard C, Hoshino E, et al. Validation of a new formula for calculation of the energy requirements of burn patients. *J Parent Ent Nutr* 1990; 14:115–118.
19. Clifton GL, Robertson CS, Contant CF. Enteral hyperalimentation in head injury. *J Neurosurg* 1985; 62:186–193.
20. Dickerson RN, Guenter PA, Gennearelli TA, Dempsey DT, Mullen

JL. Brief communication: increased contribution of protein oxidation to energy expenditure in head-injured patients. *J Am Coll Nutr* 1990; 9:86–88.

21. Fried RC, Dickerson RN, Guenter PA, et al. Barbiturate therapy reduced nitrogen excretion in acute head injury. *J Trauma* 1989; 29: 1558–1564.
22. Kelly K. Advances in perioperative nutritional support. *Med Clin North Am* 1993; 77(2):465–475.
23. Merkel KD, Miller NE, Merritt JL. Energy expenditure in patients with low-, mid-, high-thoracic paraplegia using Scott-Craig knee–ankle–foot orthoses. *Mayo Clin Proc* 1985; 60:165–168.
24. Saffle JR, Medina E, Raymond J, et al. Use of indirect calorimetry in the nutritional management of burned patients. *J Trauma* 1985; 25: 32–39.
25. Schols AMWJ, Soeters PB, Mostert R, Saris WHM, Wouters EFM. Energy balance in chronic obstructive pulmonary disease. *Am Rev Respir Dis* 1991; 243:1248–1252.
26. Turner WW. Nutritional considerations in the patient with disabling brain disease. *Neurosurgery* 1985; 16:707–713.
27. Baker JP, Detsky AS, Wesson ED, et al. Nutritional assessment: a comparison of clinical judgment and objective measurements. *N Engl J Med* 1982; 306:969–972.
28. Shils ME. Nutrition assessment in support of the malnourished patient. In: Simko MD, Cowell C, Gilbride JA, eds. *Nutrition assessment: a comprehensive guide for planning intervention.* Rockville, MD: Aspen, 1984.
29. Christensen KS, Gstundtner KM. Hospital-wide screening improves basis for nutrition intervention. *J Am Diet Assoc* 1985; 85:704–706.
30. Hunt DR, Maslovitz A, Rowlands BJ, Brooks B. A simple nutrition screening procedure for hospital patients. *J Am Diet Assoc* 1985; 85: 332–335.
31. Webb P, Sangal S. Sedentary daily expenditure: a base for estimating individual energy requirements. *Am J Clin Nutr* 1991; 53:606–611.
32. Evans MJ. The role of total parenteral nutrition in critical illness: guidelines and recommendations. *AACN Clin Issues Crit Care Nurs* 1994; 5(4):476–484.
33. Heymsfield SB, Wang J, Lichtman S, Kamen Y, Kehyias J, Pierson RN Jr. Body composition in elderly subjects: a critical appraisal of clinical methodology. *Am J Clin Nutr* 1989; 50:1167–1175.
34. Johnston FE. Relationships between body composition and anthropometry. *Hum Biol* 1982; 54:221–245.
35. Mackie A, Hannan WJ, Tothill P. An introduction to body composition models used in nutritional studies. *Clin Phys Physiol Meas* 1989; 10:297–310.
36. Williams SR. *Nutrition and diet therapy, 5th ed.* St. Louis: CV Mosby, 1985.
37. Barlett HL, Puhl SM, Hodgson JL, Buskirk ER. Fat-free mass in relation to stature: ratios of fat-free mass to height in children, adults, and elderly subjects. *Am J Clin Nutr* 1991; 53:1112–1116.
38. Dixon JK. Validity and utility of anthropometric measurements: A survey of cancer outpatients. *J Am Diet Assoc* 1985; 85:439–444.
39. Himes JH, ed. *Anthropometric assessment of nutritional status.* New York: Wiley-Liss, 1991.
40. Abernathy RP. Body mass index: determination and use. *J Am Diet Assoc* 1991; 91:843.
41. Frisancho AR. New standards of weight and body composition by frame size and height for assessment of nutritional status of adults and the elderly. *Am J Clin Nutr* 1984; 40:808–819.
42. Willet WC, Stampfer M, Manson JA, VanItallie T. New weight guidelines for Americans: justified or injudicious? *Am J Clin Nutr* 1991; 53:1102–1103.
43. Bistrian BR, Blackbrn CL, Sherman M, Scrimshaw NS. Therapeutic index of nutritional depletion in hospitalized patients. *Surg Gynecol Obstet* 1975; 141:512–516.
44. Forbes GB, Bruining GJ. Urinary creatininbg excretion and lean body mass. *Am J Clin Nutr* 1976; 29:1359–1366.
45. Grande F, Keys A. Body weight, body composition and calorie status. In: Goodhart RS, Shils MD, eds. *Modern nutrition in health and disease, 6th ed.* Philadelphia: Lea & Febiger, 1980; 3–34.
46. Szeluga DJ, Stuart RK, Utermohlen V, Santos GW. Nutritional assessment by isotope dilution analysis of body composition. *Am J Clin Nutr* 1980; 40:847–854.
47. Svendsen OL, Haarbo J, Heitmann BL, Gotfredsen A, Christiansen C. Measurement of body fat in elderly subjects by dual-energy S-ray absorptiometry, bioelectrical impedance, and anthropometry. *Am J Clin Nutr* 1991; 53:1117–1123.
48. Heymsfield SB, McManus CB. Tissue components of weight loss in cancer patients: a new method of study and preliminary observations. *Cancer* 1985; 55:238–249.
49. Conway JM, Norris KH, Bodwell CE. A new appraoch for the estimation of body composition: infrared interactance. *Am J Clin Nutr* 1984; 40:1123–1130.
50. Mazess RB, Peppler WW, Gibbons M. Total body composition by dual-photon (^{153}Gd) absorptiometry. *Am J Clin Nutr* 1984; 40: 834–839.
51. Kehayias JJ, Heymsfeld SB, LoMonte AF, Wang J, Pierson RN Jr. *In vivo* determination of body fat by measuring total body carbon. *Am J Clin Nutr* 1991; 53:1339–1344.
52. Berkelhammer CH, Leiter LA, Jeejeebhoy KN, et al. Skeletal muscle function in chronic renal failure: an index of nutritional status. *Am J Clin Nutr* 1985; 42:845–854.
53. Russell DMcR, Leiter LA, Whitwell J, et al. Skeletal muscle function during hypocaloric diets and fasting: a comparison with standard nutritional assessment parameters. *Am J Clin Nutr* 1983; 37:133–138.
54. Hunt DR, Rowlands BJ, Johnston D. Hand grip strength: a simple prognostic indicator in surgical patients. *J Parent Ent Nutr* 1985; 9: 701–704.
55. Baugh E. Actions to improve nutrition care on a general rehabilitation unit. *J Am Diet Assoc* 1985; 85:1632–1634.
56. Food and Nutrition Board. *Recommended dietary allowances, 10th ed.* Washington. D.C.: National Academy Press. 1989.
57. Dickerson JWT. Vitamin requirements in different clinical conditions. Bibl Nutr Dieta 1985; 35:44–52.
58. Donahoe M, Rogers RM. Nutritional assessment and support in chronic obstructive pulmonary disease. *Clin Chest Med* 1990; 11: 487–504.
59. Wretlind A. Nutrient requirements in various clinical conditions. *Bibl Nutr Dieta* 1985; 35:31–43.
60. Stone JM, Nino-Murcia M, Wolfe AV, Perkash I. Chronic gastrointestinal problems in spinal cord injury patients: a prospective analysis. *Am J Gastroenterol* 1990; 85:1114–1119.
61. Fee MA, Charney EB, Robertson WW. Nutritional assessment of the young child with cerebral palsy. *Infants Young Child* 1988; 1:33–40.
62. Morris MJ, Ingram DH, Howison M, Kaltreider C, Nichter CA. The disabled child. In: Gines DJ, ed. *Nutrition management in rehabilitation.* Rockville, MD: Aspen Publications, 1990; 109–137.
63. Murray JJ, Healy MD. Drug-nutrient interactions: a new responsibility for the hospital dietitian. *J Am Diet Assoc* 1991; 91:66–73.
64. Awad AG. Diet and drug interactions in the treatment of mental illness: a review. *Can J Psychiatry* 1984; 29:609–613.
65. Hansten PD. *Drug interactions, 5th ed.* Philadelphia: Lea & Febiger, 1985.
66. O'Brien RY. Spinal cord injury. In: Gines DJ, ed. *Nutrition management in rehabilitation.* Rockville, MD: Aspen Publications. 1990; 159–174.
67. Roe DA. *Drug-induced nutritional deficiencies, 2nd ed.* Westport, CT: Avi Publishing, 1985.
68. Roe DA. *Diet and drug interactions.* New York: Van Nostrand Reinhold, 1989.
69. Wolman PG. Arthritis. In: Gines DJ, ed. *Nutrition management in rehabilitation.* Rockville, MD: Aspen Publications, 1990; 245–270.
70. Grant JP, Custer PB, Thurlow J. Current techniques of nutritional assessment. *Surg Clin North Am* 1981; 64:437–463.
71. MacBurney M, Wilmore DW. Rational decision making in nutritional care. *Surg Clin North Am* 1981; 61:571–582.
72. Solomons NW, Allen LH. The functional assessment of nutritional status: principles, practice and potential. *Nutr Rev* 1983; 41:33–50.
73. Caldwell MD, Kennedy-Caldwell C. Normal nutritional requirements. *Surg Clin North Am* 1981; 61:489–507.
74. Barton RG. Nutrition support in crtiical illness. *Nutr Clini Pract* 1994; 9(4):127–139.
75. Haider M, Haider SQ. Assessment of protein-calorie malnutrition. *Clin Chem* 1984; 30:1286–1299.
76. Hannaman KN, Penner SF. A nutrition assessment tool that includes diagnosis. *J Am Diet Assoc* 1985; 85:607–609.
77. Jensen TG, Long JM III, Dudrick SJ, Johnston DA. Nutritional assessment indications of postburn complications. *J Am Diet Assoc* 1985; 85:68–72.

78. Kaminski MV Jr, Blumeyer TH. Metabolic and nutritional support of the intensive care patient. Ascending the learning curve. *Crit Care Clin* 1993; 9(2):363–376.
79. Blackburn GL, Thornton PA. Nutritional assessment of the hospitalized patient. *Med Clin North Am* 1979; 63:1103–1115.
80. Burton BT, Foster WR. Health implications of obesity: an NIH consensus development conference. *J Am Diet Assoc* 1985; 85: 1117–1121.
81. Dickhaut SC, DeLee JC, Page CP. Nutritional status: importance in predicting wound healing after amputation. *J Bone Joint Surg* 1984; 66:71–75.
82. Kudsk KA, Stone JM, Sheldon GF. Nutrition in trauma and burns. *Surg Clin North Am* 1982; 62:183–192.
83. Sibley WA. *Therapeutic claims in multiple sclerosis, 2nd ed.* New York: Demos Publications, 1988.
84. Bryan AH, Anderson EL. Dietary and nutritional problems of crippled children in five rural counties of North Carolina. *Am J Public Health* 1965; 55:1545–1554.
85. Gouge AL, Ekwall SW. Diets of handicapped children: physical, psychological, and socioeconomic correlations. *Am J Ment Defic* 1975; 80:149–157.
86. Cunningham K, Gibney MJ, Kelly A, Kevany J, Mulcahy M. Nutrient intakes in long-stay mentally handicapped persons. *Br J Nutr* 1990; 64:3–11.
87. Magnus MH, Roe DA. Computer instruction in drug-nutrient interactions in long term care. *J Nutr Educ* 1991; 23:10–17.
88. Hull MA, Kidwell J. Feeding skills and weight gain in institutionalized adults with severe handicaps. *Dietet Dev Psychiatr Dis* 1988;7(2).
89. White W, Kamples G. Dietary noncompliance in pediatric patients in the burn unit. *J Burn Care Rehabil* 1990; 11:167–174.
90. McCarran MS, Andrasik F. Behavioral weight-loss for multiple-handicapped adults: assessing caretaker involvement and measures of behavior change. *Addict Behav* 1990; 15:13–20.
91. Loosen BM. Self-help aids. In: Redford JB, ed. *Orthotic etcetera, 2nd ed.* Baltimore: Williams & Wilkins, 1980; 650–681.
92. Zimmerman ME. Activities of daily living. In: Willard HS, Spackman GS, eds. *Occupational therapy, 4th ed.* Philadelphia: JB Lippincott, 1971; 228.
93. Broadhurst MJ, Stammers CW. Mechanical feeding aids for patients with ataxia: design considerations. *J Biomed Eng* 1990; 12:209–214.
94. Gisel EG, Patrick J. Identification of children with cerebral palsy unable to maintain a normal nutritional state. *Lancet* 1988; 1:283–285.
95. Stratton M. Behavioral assessment scale of oral functions in feeding. *Am J Occup Ther* 1981; 35:719–721.
96. Kenny DJ, Koheil RM, Greenberg J, et al. Development of a multidisciplinary feeding profile for children who are dependent feeders. *Dysphagia* 1989; 4:16–28.
97. Gordon SR, Kelley SI, Sybyl JR, et al. Relationship in very elderly veterans of nutritional status, self-perceived chewing ability, dental status, and social isolation. *J Am Geriatr Soc* 1985; 33:334–339.
98. Pfisterer M, Lessire H, Kleine R, Nolte G, Puchstein C. Caloric requirements in burned patients. *Acta Anaesthesiol Belg* 1989; 40: 187–194.
99. Dominioni L, Trocki O, Fang CH, et al. Enteral feeding in burn hypermetabolism: nutritional and metabolic effects of different levels of calorie and protein intake. *J Parent Ent Nutr* 1985; 9:269–279.
100. Gay F, et Nawar A, Van-Gossum A. Percutaneous endoscopic gastrostomy. *Acta Gastroenterol Belg* 1992; 55(3):285–294.
101. Kudsk KA, Stone JM, Sheldon GF. Nutrition in trauma. *Surg Clin North Am* 1981; 61:671–679.
102. Rapp RP, Young B, Twyman D, et al. The favorable effect of early parenteral feeding on survival in head-injured patients. *J Neurosurg* 1983; 58:906–912.
103. Twyman D, Young AB, Ott L, et al. High protein enteral feedings: a means of achieving positive nitrogen balance in head injured patients. *J Parent Ent Nutr* 1985; 9:679–684.
104. Enzi G, Casadei A, Sergi G, Chiarella A, Zurlo F, Mazzoleni F. Metabolic and hormonal effects of early nutritional supplementation after surgery in burn patients. *Crit Care Med* 1990; 18:719–721.
105. Chiarelli A, Enzi G, Casadei A, Baggio B, Valerio A, Mazzoleni F. Very early nutrition supplementation in burned patients. *Am J Clin Nutr* 1990; 51:1035–1039.
106. Bildsten C, Lamid S. Nutritional management of a patient with brain damage and spinal cord injury. *Arch Phys Med Rehabil* 1983; 64: 382–383.
107. Newmark SR, Simpson S, Daniel P, et al. Nutritional support in an inpatient rehabilitation unit. *Arch Phys Med Rehabil* 1981; 62: 634–637.
108. O'Gara JA. Dietary adjustments and nutritional therapy during treatment of oral-pharyngeal dysphagia. *Dysphagia* 1990; 4:109–112.
109. Whittaker JS, Ryan CF, Buckley PA, Road JD. The effects of refeeding on peripheral and respiratory muscle function in malnourished chronic obstructive pulmonary disease patients. *Am Rev Respir Dis* 1990; 142:283–288.
110. Isaacs JS. Neurologically impaired children fed by gastrostomy. *Diet Dev Psychiatr Dis* 1991; 9:1–3.
111. Sanders KD, Cox K, Cannon R, et al. Growth response to enteral feeding by children with cerebral palsy. *J Parenter Enteral Nutr* 1990; 14:23–26.
112. Shapiro BK, Green P, Krick J, Allen D, Capute AJ. Growth of severely impaired children: neurological versus nutritional factors. *Dev Med Child Neurol* 1986; 28:720–733.
113. Gaskin KJ, Waters DL, Baur LA, Soutter VL, Gruca MA. Nutritional status, growth and development in children undergoing intensive treatment for cystic fibrosis. *Acta Paediatr Scand [Suppl]* 1990; 366: 106–110.
114. Taylor KB, Anthony LE. *Clinical nutrition.* New York: McGraw-Hill, 1983.
115. Mattox TW, Bertch KE, Mirtallo JM, Straugsberg KM, Cuddy PG. Recent advances: parenteral nutrition support. *Ann Pharmacother* 1995; 29(2):174–180.
116. Boyes RJ, Kruse JA. Nasogastric and nasoenteric intubation. *Crit Care Clin* 1992; 8(4):865–878.
117. Moore MC, Greene HL. Tube feeding of infants and children. *Pediatr Clin North Am* 1985; 32:401–417.
118. Rombeau HL, Caaldwell MD. *Clinical nutrition: enteral and tube feeding, 2nd ed.* Philadelphia: WB Saunders, 1990.
119. Driscoll DF, Bistrian BR. Special considerations required for the formulation and administration of total parenteral nutrition therapy in the elderly patient. *Drugs Aging* 1992; 2(5):395–405.
120. Wesley JR, Coran AG. Intravenous nutrition for the pediatric patient. *Semin Pediatr Surg* 1992; 1(3):212–230.
121. DiLorenzo J, Dalton B, Miskovitz P. Percutaneous endoscopic gastrostomy. *Postgrad Med* 1992; 91(1):277–281.
122. Tealey AR. Percutaneous endoscopic gastrostomy in the elderly. *Gastroenterol Nurs* 1994; 16(4):151–157.
123. Fleming CR. Hepatobiliary complications in adults receiving nutrition support. *Dig Dis* 1994; 12(4):191–198.
124. Bell SJ, Mascioli EA, Bistrian BR, Babayan VI, Blackburn GL. Alternative lipid sources for enteral and parenteral nutrition: long- and medium-chain triglycerides, structured triglycerides, and fish oils. *J Am Diet Assoc* 1991; 91:74–78.
125. Irwin MM, Openbrier DR. A delicate balance: strategies for feeding ventilated COPD patients. *Am J Nurs* 1985; 85:274–280.
126. Alexander JW, Gottschlich MM. Nutritional immunomodulation in burn patients. *Crit Care Med* 1990; 18(Suppl):149–153.
127. Lipman TO. Bacterial translocation and enteral nutrition in humans: an outsider looks in. *J Parent Ent Nutr* 1995; 19(2):156–165.
128. Padilla GV, Grant MM. Psychological aspects of artifical feeding. *Cancer* 1985; 55:301–304.
129. Glass RP, Lucas B. Making the transition from tube feeding to oral feeding. *Nutr Focus* 1990; 5:1–6.
130. Illingworth RS, Lister J. The critical or sensitive period, with special reference to certain feeding problems in infants and children. *J Pediatr* 1964; 65:839–847.
131. Winkler MF, Pomp A, Caldwell MD, Albina JE. Transitional feeding: the relationshp between nutritional intake and plasma protein concentrations. *J Am Diet Assoc* 1989; 89:969–970.
132. Berg K. Somatic adaptation in cerbral palsy: summary and general discussion. *Acta Paediatr Scand [Suppl]* 1971; 204:81–93.
133. Brown JE, Davis E, Flemming PL. Nutritional assessment of children with handicapping conditions. *Ment Retard* 1979; 17:129–132.
134. Barboriak JJ, Rooney CB, El Ghatit AZ, et al. Nutrition in spinal cord injury patients. *J Am Paraplegia Soc* 1983; 6:32–36.
135. Newmark SR, Sublett D, Black J, Geller R. Nutritional assessment in a rehabilitation unit. *Arch Phys Med Rehabil* 1981; 62:279–282.

136. Peiffer SC, Bluse P, Leyson JFJ. Nutritional assessment of the spinal cord injured patient. *J Am Diet Assoc* 1981; 78:501–505.
137. Hodges P, Sauriol D, Man SFP, et al. Nutrient intake of patient with cystic fibrosis. *J Am Diet Assoc* 1984; 84:664–669.
138. Hewson DC, Pyhillips MA, Simpson KE, et al. Food intake in multiple sclerosis. *Hum Nutr Appl Nutr* 1984; 38A:355–367.
139. Slowie LA, Paige MS, Antel JP. Nutritional considerations in the management of patients with amyotrophic lateral sclerosis (ALS). *J Am Diet Assoc* 1983; 83:44–47.
140. Green EM, McIntosh EN. Food and nutrition skills of mentally retarded adults: assessment and needs. *J Am Diet Assoc* 1985; 85: 611–613.
141. Mattes-Kulig DA, Henkin RI. Energy and nutrient consumption of patients with dysgeusia. *J Am Diet Assoc* 1985; 85:822–826.
142. Rhodus NL, Brown J. The association of xerostomia and inadequate intake in older adults. *J Am Diet Assoc* 1990; 90:1688–1692.
143. Bowman BB, Rosenberg IH. Assessment of the nutritional status of the elderly. *Am J Clin Nutr* 1982; 35:1142–1141.
144. Cos SAR, Weiss SM, Posuniak EA, et al. Energy expenditure after spinal cord injury: an evaluation of stable rehabilitating patients. *J Trauma* 1985; 25:419–423.
145. Greenway RM, Houser HB, Lindan O, Weir DR. Long-term changes in gross body composition of paraplegic and quadriplegic patietns. *Paraplegia* 1969; 7:301–318.
146. Berg K, Olsson T. Energy requirements of school children with cerebral palsy as determined from indirect calorimetry. *Acta Paediatr Scand [Suppl]* 1971; 240:71–80.
147. Culley WJ, Middleton TO. Caloric rquirements of mentally retarded children with and without motor dysfunction. *J Pediatr* 1969; 75: 380–384.
148. Eddy TP, Nicholson AH, Wheeler DF. Energy expenditures and dietary intake in cerebral palsy. *Dev Med Neurol* 1965; 7:377–386.
149. Daly JM, Meymsfield SB, Head CA, et al. Human energy requirements: overestimation by widely used prediction equation. *Am J Clin Nutr* 1985; 42:1170–1174.
150. Kearns PJ, Pipp TL, Quick M, Campolo M. Nutritional requirements in quadriplegics (abstract). *J Parent Ent Nutr* 1982; 6:577.
151. Turner WW, Ireton CS, Hunt JL, Baxter CR. Predicting energy expenditures in burned patients. *J Trauma* 1985; 25:11–16.
152. Chantraine A, Delwaide PA. Hydroelectrolytic determination in paraplegics. *Paraplegia* 1976; 14:138–145.
153. Claus-Walker J, Halstead LS. Metabolic and endocrine changes in spinal cord injury: I. The nervous system before and after transection of the spinal cord. *Arch Phys Med Rehabil* 1981; 62:595–601.
154. Kuhlemeier KV, Milelr JM III, Nepomuceno CS. Insensible weight loss in patients with spinal cord transection. *Paraplegia* 1976; 14: 195–201.
155. Mirahmadi MK, Barton CH, Vaziri ND, et al. Nutritional evaluation of hemodialysis patients with and without spinal cord injury. *Am J Paraplegia* 1983; 6:36–40.
156. Pierce DS, Nickel VH. *The total care of spinal cord injuries.* Boston: Little, Brown & Co., 1977.
157. Feucht S. Assessment of growth. *Nutr Focus* 1989; 4:1–8.
158. Biering-Sorensen F, Bohr JJ, Schaadt OP. Longitudinal study of bone mineral content in the lumbar spine, the forearm and the lower extremities after spinal cord injury. *Eur J Clin Invest* 1990; 20:330–235.
159. Schols AMWJ, Wouters EFM, Soeters PB, Westerterp KR. Body composition by bioelectrical-impedance analysis compared with deuterium dilution and skinfold anthropometry inpatients with chronic obstructive pulmonary disease. *Am J Clin Nutr* 1991; 53:421–424.
160. Panzetta F, Guerra U, d'Angelo A, et al. Body composition and nutritional status in patients on continuous ambulatory peritoneal dialysis (CAPD). *Clin Nephrol* 1985; 23:18–25.
161. Shizgal HM. Body composition of patients with malnutrition and cancer: summary of methods of assessment. *Cancer* 1985; 55:250–253.
162. Foster MR, Heppenstall RB, Friedenberg ZB, Hozack WJ. A prospective assessment of nutritional status and complications in patients with fractures of the hip. *J Orthop Trauma* 1990; 4:49–57.
163. Sullivan DH, Patch GA, Walls RC, Lipschitz DA. Impact of nutrition status on morbidity and mortality in a select population of geriatric rehabilitation patients. *Am J Clin Nutr* 1990; 51:749–958.
164. Sullivan DH, Walls RC, Lipschitz DA. Protein-energy undernutrition and the risk of mortality within 1 y of hospital discharge in a select population of geriatric rehabilitation patients. *Am J Clin Nutr* 1991; 53:599–605.
165. Wilson DO, Donahoe M, Rogers RM, Pennock BE. Metabolic rate and weight loss in chronic obstructive lung disease. *J Parent Ent Nutr* 1990; 14:7–11.
166. Fuensalida CE, Petty TL, Jones ML, et al. The immune response to short-term nutritional intervention in advanced chronic obstructive pulmonary disease. *Am Rev Respir Dis* 1990; 142:49–56.
167. Gray-Donald K, Gibbons L, Shapiro SH, Martin JG. Effect of nutritional status on exercise performance in patients with chronic obstructive pulmonary disease. *Am Rev Respir Dis* 1989; 140:1544–1548.
168. Rutan RL, Herndon DN. Growth delay in postburn pediatric patients. *Arch Surg* 1990; 125:392–395.
169. Abraham PA, Smith CL. Medical evaluation and management of calcium nephrolithiasis. *Med Clin North Am* 1984; 68:281–299.
170. DeVivo MJ, Fine PR, Cutter GR, Maetz HM. The risk of renal calculi in spinal cord injury patients. *J Urol* 1984; 131:857–860.
171. Robertson WG, Peacock M. Metabolic and biochemical risk factors in renal stone disease. *Contrib Nephrol* 1984; 37:1–4.
172. Claus-Walker J, Spencer WA, Careter RE, et al. Bone metabolism in quadriplegia: dissociation between calciuria and hydroxyprolinuria. *Arch Phys Med Rehabil* 1975; 56:327–332.
173. Kaplan PE, Gandhavadi B, Richards L, Goldschmidt J. Calcium balance in paraplegic patients: influence of injury duration and ambulation. *Arch Phys Med Rehabil* 1978; 59:447–450.
174. Maynard FM, Imai K. Immobilization hypercalcemia in spinal cord injury. *Arch Phys Med Rehabil* 1977; 58:16–24.
175. Naftchi NE, Viau AT, Sell GH, Lowman EW. Mineral metabolism in spinal cord injury. *Arch Phys Med Rehabil* 1980; 61:139–142.
176. Lamid S, El Ghatit AZ, Melvin JL. Relationship of hypercalcuria to diet and bladder stone formation in spinal cord injury patients. *Am J Phys Med* 1984; 63:182–187.
177. Fellstrom B, Danielson BG, Karlstrom B, et al. Urinary composition and supersaturation on a high protein diet. *Contrib Nephrol* 1984; 37: 27–30.
178. Fituri N, Allawi N, Bentley M, Costello J. Urinary and plasma oxalate during ingestion of pure ascorbic acid: a reevaluation. *Eur Urol* 1983; 9:312–315.
179. Hoffer A. Letter: ascorbic acid and kidney stones. *Can Med Assoc J* 1985; 132:320.
180. Power C, Barker DJP, Nelson M, Winter PD. Diet and renal stones: a case-control study. *Br J Urol* 1984; 56:456–459.
181. Burr M, Alton M. Constipation in immobile patients. *Med J Aust* 1984; 1:446–447.

ADDITIONAL READINGS

Brose L. Prealbumin as a marker of nutritional status. *J Burn Care Rehabil* 1990; 11:372–375.

Center for Science in the Public Interest. *New American eating guide.* Washington, D.C.: Center for Science in the Public Interest, 1988.

Clark HD, Hoffer LJ. Reappraisal of the resting metabolic rate of normal young men. *Am J Clin Nutr* 1991; 53:21–26.

Curtin HC, Harvey RF, Jellinek HM. Role of the clinical nutritionist as a member of a rehabilitation team. *Nutr Supp Serv* 1982; 2:25–31.

Dietz WH, Bandini L. Nutritional assessment of the handicapped child. *Pediatr Rev* 1989; 11:109–115.

Duyff RL. The adequate diet—the prudent diet. In: Howard RB, Herbold NH, eds. *Nutrition in clinical care, 2nd ed.* New York: McGraw-Hill, 1982; 13–39.

Dwyer JT. Concept of nutritional status and its measurement. In: Himes JH, ed. *Anthropometric assessment of nutritional status.* New York: Wiley-Liss, 1991; 5–28.

Dwyer J, Foulkes E, Evans M, Ausman L. Acid–alkaline diets: time for assessment and change. *J Am Diet Assoc* 1985; 85:841–845.

Ernst ND. NIH consensus development conference on lowering blood cholesterol to prevent heart disease: implications for dietititans. *J Am Diet Assoc* 1985; 85:586–588.

Hecht JS, Grabois M, Kunioki S, Hart WD. Nutritional assessment of newly spinal cord injure patients (abstract). *Arch Phys Med Rehabil* 1981; 62: 527.

Henley M. Feed that burn. *Burns* 1989; 15:351–361.

Hildreth MA, Herndon DN, Desai MH, Duke MA. Caloric needs of adolescent patients with burns. *J Burn Care Rehabil* 1989; 10:523–526.

Isaacs JS, Davis BD, La Montagne MJ. Transitioning the child fed by gastrostomy into school. *J Am Diet Assoc* 1990; 90:982–985.

Joint FAO/WHO/UNU Expert Consultation. *Energy and protein requirements. WHO Technical Reports Series 724.* Geneva: WHO, 1985.

Lamden MP, Chrystowski GA. Urinary oxolate excretion in man following ascorbic acid ingestion. *Proc Soc Exp Biol Am* 1954; 85:190–192.

Margen S. Evaluation of nutritional status in the outpatient setting. *Med Clin North Am* 1979; 63:1095–1101.

McClain L, Todd C. Food store accessibility. *Am J Occup Ther* 1990; 44: 487–491.

Moolton SE. Bedsore in the chronically ill patients. *Arch Phys Med Rehabil* 1972; 53:430–438.

NIH Consensus Development Conference Statement. Lowering blood cholesterol to prevent heart disease. *Arteriosclerosis* 1985; 5:404–412.

O'Keefe KP. Complications of percutaneous feeding tubes. *Emerg Med Clin North Am* 1994; 12(3):815–826.

Oser BL. Chemical additives in foods. In: Goodhart RS, Shils ME, eds. *Modern nutrition in health and disease, 6th ed.* Philadelphia: Lea & Febiger, 1980; 506–519.

Payne-James JJ, Khawaja HT. First choice for total parenteral nutrition: the peripheral route. *J Parent Ent Nutr* 1993; 17(5):468–478.

Pennington JAT. Considerations for a new food guide. *J Nutr Educ* 1981; 13:53–55.

Pike RL, Brown ML. *Nutrition: an integrated approach, 2nd ed.* New York: John Wiley & Sons. 1975.

Pi-Sunyer FX, Woo R. Laboratory assessment of nutritional status. In: Simko MD, Cowel C, Gilbride JA, eds. Nutrition assessment: a comprehensive guide for planning intervention. Rockville, MD: Aspen Systems, 1984; 139–174.

Purdue GF, Hunt J, Lang ED. Obesity: a risk factor in the burn patient. *J Burn Care Rehabil* 1990;11:32–34.

Rayan GM, McCormack ST, Hoelzer DJ, Schultz RT. Nutrition and the rheumatoid hand patient. *J Okla State Med Assoc* 1989; 82:505–509.

Rosa AM, Shizgal HM. The Harris Benedict equation reevaluated: resting energy requirements and body cell mass. *Am J Clin Nutr* 1984; 40: 168–182.

Sauberlich HE, Skala JH, Dowdy RP. *Laboratory tests for the assessment of nutritional status.* Cleveland: CRC Press, 1974.

Schaumberg H, Kaplan J, Windebank A, et al. Sensory neuropathy from pyridoxine abuse: a new megavitamin syndrome. *N Engl J Med* 1983; 309:445–448.

Schols AMWJ, Mostert R, Soeters PB, Greve LH, Wouters EFM. Nutritional state and exercise performance in patients with chronic obstructive lung disease. *Thorax* 1989; 44:937–941.

Shepherd K, Roberts D, Golding S, Thomas BJ, Shepherd RS. Body composition in myelomeningocele. *Am J Clin Nutr* 1991; 53:1–6.

Shuran M. Nelson RA. Quantitation of energy expenditure by infrared thermography. *Am J Clin Nutr* 1991; 53:1361–1367.

Siddell EP, Broman RD. A national survey of neonatal intensive-care units: criteria used to determine readiness for oral feedings. *J Obstet Gynecol Neonat Nurs* 1994; 23(9):783–789.

Simko MD, Cowell C, Gilbride JA. *Nutrition assessment: a comprehensive guide for planning intervention.* Rockville, MD: Aspen Systems, 1984.

Solomons NW. Assessment of nutritional status: functional indicators of pediatric nutriture. *Pediatr Clin North Am* 1985; 32:319–334.

Strohmeyer SL, Massey LK, Davison MA. A rapid dietary screening device for clinics. *J Am Diet Assoc* 1984; 84:428–432.

Tuckerman MM, Turco SJ. *Human nutrition.* Philadelphia: Lea & Febiger, 1983.

Tweng RYL, Sullivan MA, Downes NJ. A proposed method for the nutritional rating of foods. *J Nutr Educ* 1986; 18:67–74.

Underwood BA. Evaluating the nutritional status of individuals: A critique of approaches. *Nutr Rev* 1986; 44(Suppl):213–224.

Uretsky SD. It beats the truth. *Am J Hosp Pharm* 1987; 44:2373–2374.

VanLandingham SB, Key JC, Symmonds RE. Nutritional support of the surgical patient. *Surg Clin North Am* 1982; 62:321–331.

Rehabilitation Medicine: Principles and Practice, Third Edition, edited by Joel A. DeLisa and Bruce M. Gans.
Lippincott–Raven Publishers, Philadelphia © 1998.

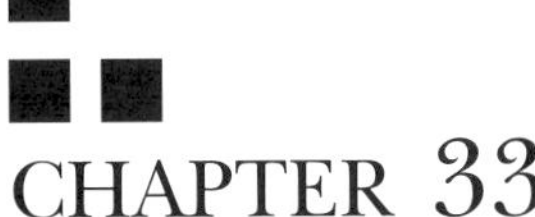

CHAPTER 33

Recreation and Sport for People with Disabilities

Kenneth J. Richter, Claudine Sherrill, B. Cairbre McCann, Carol Adams Mushett, and Susan M. Kaschalk

As rehabilitationists we have a much larger mandate than just diagnosing and treating diseases and their consequences. We truly need to care for patients (1). We have all at one time or another heard during rehabilitation conferences that the person we are caring for ''just is not motivated,'' but there is an old maxim in rehabilitation that ''everyone is motivated, just to different things.'' We need to keep this in mind and have a person orientation, not just a disease orientation. Especially in this time of physician-assisted suicide (2), we need to keep sight of the human issues involved. As rehabilitationists we hopefully expand the life options available to people with disabilities. In doing so we need to help a person discover what is important to him or her. In a very real sense it is not just medical issues we are addressing, but human issues (3). Why would people want to learn to walk if they have no place to walk to? Why would people want to get dressed if they have nothing to get dressed up for? Although some individuals find meaning in religion, others find meaning in art, poetry, gardening, or sports. By understanding the options available, individuals with disabilities are hopefully able to find that which will give meaning to their lives. As Nietzsche said, ''One who has a why will find a how'' (4). Life needs to have ''want to's'' not just ''have to's'' (5).

K. J. Richter: Department of Recreation Medicine, St. Joseph Mercy at Oakland, Michigan State University, Pontiac, Michigan 48341.

C. Sherrill: Department of Kinesiology, Texas Woman's University at Denton, Denton, Texas 76204.

B. C. McCann: Department of Rehabilitation Medicine, Maine Medical Center, Portland, Maine 04102-3175.

C. Adams Mushett: Department of Kinesiology and Health, Georgia State University, College of Education, Atlanta, Georgia 30303.

S. M. Kaschalk: St. Joseph Mercy Hospital, Pontiac, Michigan 48320.

Although there are significant benefits to recreation and sport, such as the avoidance of the negative consequences of a sedentary life (6), we feel that the existential issue mentioned above is the most important value of recreation and sport. The maximization of life is much more than just the minimization of disease. It is more than just the prevention of secondary, unnecessary disability, it is the reaching of life's potential, the effect of which reaches far beyond the individual to all of society (7). It is the responsibility of the rehabilitation specialist to assist persons with disabilities to achieve their maximum potential in every sphere of their lives. Promotion of recreation and sport are necessary to accomplish this. We must move beyond just disease and trauma.

HISTORY OF SPORTS FOR PEOPLE WITH DISABILITIES

The history of sports for people with disabilities can be reviewed from two perspectives: the medical and the sports model. Sports activities today exhibit influences from both these origins (8).

Viewed from the medical standpoint, sports had its origins in the related activities of gymnastics, and in the concept of exercise being therapeutic and contributing to fitness and health. These beginnings are well described by Guttman in his *Textbook of Sport for the Disabled* (9). Later, therapeutic exercises, including group activities, became recognized as a fundamental part of the orthopedic management of fractures (10). The use of sports as a further motivation to enhance the physiologic and anatomic aspects of musculoskeletal healing and strengthening was a further natural development. The step from group gymnastics, sports, and exercises took place when Guttman incorporated sports activities into the total program of rehabilitation for patients with spinal cord injury (11).

Organized Sports

Guttman's efforts led directly to the creation of an international sports movement for spinal cord injured, which sponsored the first international games for people with disabilities in 1952. This movement was identified for many years as the International Stoke Mandeville Games Federation (ISMGF). Its name changed more recently to International Stoke Mandeville Wheelchair Sports Federation (ISMWSF) (Fig. 33-1).

Other organizations developed their identity with specific disability groups, such as blind, deaf, cerebral palsy, and amputee. Within these organizations, control of the direction, staffing, and goal setting were made by persons who, for the most part, came from the medical or educational systems.

The U.S. disabled sports movement was sparked by Ben Lipton, director of the Bulova School of Watch Making, in New York. He established the U.S. National Wheelchair association (NWAA) in 1957, which sponsored the annual national wheelchair games, which for many years was held on the grounds of the Bulova school. In recent years the NWAA has been renamed Wheelchair Sports USA. There was another quite separate and distinct influence that led to a change in the character and direction of sports for people with disabilities. This was based on the concepts of the value of sports in its own right, and the perceived need to identify the participants as true sportsmen and -women, rather than part of a rehabilitation process. This effort has led to the development of an international governing body, the International Paralympic Committee (IPC), which is associated with the Olympic movement. Through this development, the Paralympic Games have gained stature and have served as the showcase for the elite performers in disabled sports. In the 1996 Paralympic Games in Atlanta, 3,500 competitors from almost 120 countries participated. This development has led to a close link between national governing bodies for Paralympic sports and the Olympic sports movement. There is a concern that an emphasis on elite level sports (Paralympics) will dilute the financial resources available for developmental or entry-level sports, although on the other hand, there could be a beneficial trickle-down effect (Table 33-1).

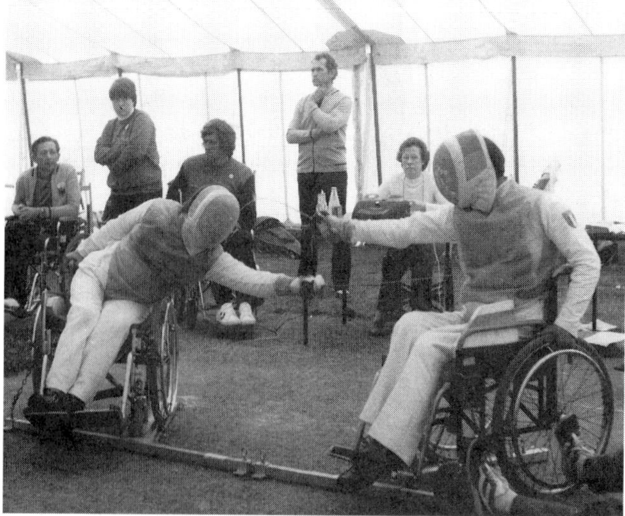

FIG. 33-1. Fencing at the International Stoke Mandeville Games.

TABLE 33-1. *Sports in which individuals with disabilities frequently engage*

All-terrain vehicles	Football	Showdown
Aquatics	Goal ball	Snow skiing
Archery	Golf	Skydiving
Basketball	Gymnastics	Slalom
Beep baseball	Hunting	Sledge hockey
Blowdarts	Ice skating	Snowmobiling
Boating	Ice sledding	Soccer
Boccia	Lawn bowling	Softball
Bowling	Martial arts	Table tennis
Cross country	Powerlifting	Team handball
Cycling	Power soccer	Tennis
Equestrian	Quad rugby	Track
Fencing	Racquetball	Volleyball
Field events	Road racing	Waterskiing
Fishing	Roller skating	Weight training
Fitness programs	Rugball	Wilderness experiences
Floor hockey	Scuba diving	
Flying	Shooting	Wrestling

Reprinted with permission from Sherrill C. *Adapted education, recreation, sport,* 5th ed. Dubuque, IA: WCB/McGraw-Hill, 1998.

Disability Group Sports Versus Integrated Disability Sports

Sports development at all levels, until recently, has been mostly identified with specific disability groups. Wheelchair sports, which is primarily for people with spinal cord injuries and bilateral lower extremity amputations, developed through an organizational structure at international, national and local levels, that is, from the Stoke Mandeville organization down to the local community group.

Cerebral palsy sports achieved its own American identity in 1978, when a U.S. National Sports organization, the National Association of Sport for Cerebral Palsy, was formed, facilitating regional and national competitions. This in turn led to the creation of a national team, which competed internationally for the first time in 1978. In 1987, cerebral palsy sports was reorganized as the U.S. Cerebral Palsy Athletic Association (USCPAA).

Amputee sports developed through several separate pathways. Winter sports offered the opportunity for unilateral amputees to ski, using some simple pole modifications, usually not using the prosthesis. In more recent years technical developments led to the participation of bilateral lower limb amputees in sled, and mono-skiing downhill events. Summer sports for amputees developed differently in Europe than in the United States. In Europe the emphasis was on the use of prostheses in sports as much as possible in field and track events, whereas in the United States, initially, amputees participating in sports favored the wheelchair route to competition. The development of technically more sophisticated prostheses, such as energy storage foot and ankle systems, has resulted in significantly more amputees participating in sports with their prostheses (e.g., in track events). Bilateral above-knee amputees, who represent a higher degree of impairment, continue to usually compete in wheelchair sports such as track and field and basketball. National Handicap Sports (NHS), which recently became Disabled Sports/USA, is the U.S. organization that represents amputees in competitive sports activities.

The most recent trend in organizing sports at the international level involves an attempt to integrate all types of locomotor disability into one system. This effort is being driven by the IPC in an attempt to reduce the multiplicity of athlete classes and events and ease the problem for sports organizers. Initial enthusiasm for the idea has subsequently been tempered by the realization that both the quality of performance and the actual level of performance are so variable that it may be meaningless to attempt to compare athletes with such diverse types of impairment in one competition. It has been likened to comparing apples with oranges and ending up with grapefruit.

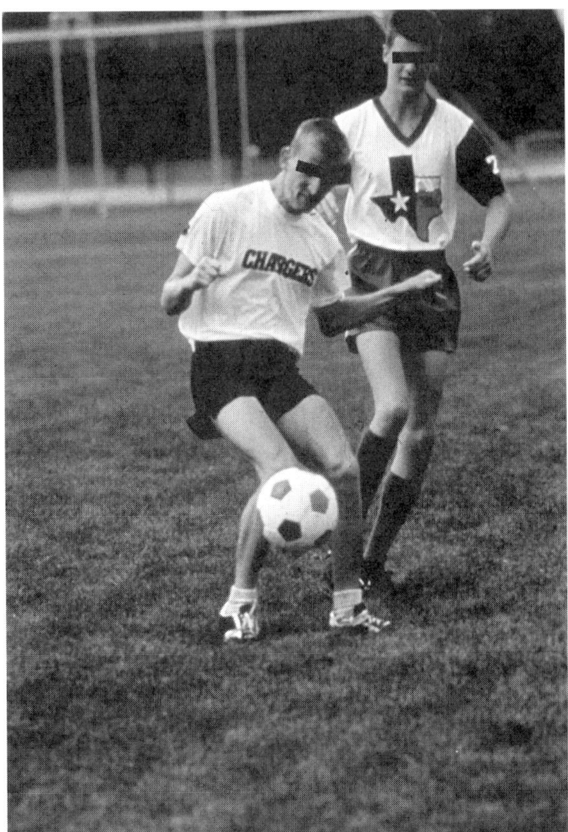

FIG. 33-2. Elite soccer players with cerebral palsy in action.

Involvement of People with Disabilities in Able-Bodied Sports

Some disabled athletes have been able to compete in able-bodied sports despite significant impairment. They have achieved this integration by succeeding in overcoming the effects of the impairment. Such success in this very special group reflects the individual's drive and motivation, which enables him or her to break this particular barrier and has also demonstrated the resiliency and adaptability of human neuromuscular and musculoskeletal systems. Interestingly, in 1960, the year of the first Paralympics, a boxer with a below-knee amputation was denied entrance into the Olympic trials because it was felt his lightweight prosthesis would give him an unfair advantage over able-bodied boxers by dropping him into a lighter weight class.

IMPACT OF EXERCISE IN SPORTS FOR PEOPLE WITH DISABILITIES

The impact of vigorous physical activity on people with disabilities and their families is the same as for able-bodied people, except perhaps more significant because the need is greater. The impact can be positive or negative, depending on the goals of the individual, the respect accorded the body, and the personal meaning of activity outcomes. Several professions exist to maximize positive outcomes and minimize negative outcomes. This is typically achieved by teaching individuals with disabilities the importance of physical exercise and sport involvement, helping them develop the skills and fitness for success, supporting them in finding and/or initiating sport activity that meets personal needs and interests, and helping them to achieve goals and stay involved during all seasons of the year at a level equal to or exceeding the recommendations of the Surgeon General (6). Two of the key professions in this endeavor are adapted physical education and therapeutic recreation. As rehabilitationists, it is important that we become familiar with these professionals and what they have to offer (Fig. 33-2).

EDUCATION

Schools increasingly are working with parents and hospital and community personnel to assure that children with disabilities are socialized into healthy, active life-styles that maximize opportunities for development of self-worth and generalized well-being. Of particular importance is socialization into sports (i.e., acquiring the attitudes, fitness, and skills that the majority of children and youth in American society possess and value). Adapted physical activity is the school-based profession that assumes responsibility for socializing children into healthy, active life-styles with strong sports interests and involvement. Rehabilitationists and others concerned with recreation and sports opportunities for persons with disabilities need to understand the adapted physical activity profession and to work closely with adapted physical educators to assure that students are provided appropriate physical education and sport experience.

Appropriate physical education and sports may be in regular physical education classes with support services provided by adapted physical education specialists or in separate settings where adapted physical educators teach specific skills in wheelchair, blind, amputee, or cerebral palsy sports. Most students benefit from opportunities to learn in both mainstream and separate settings. In the latter, they should be exposed to adult athletes with disabilities who can serve as role models and help them make the transition from school to community recreation and sports.

Many students with disabilities are still denied opportunities to learn and practice appropriate sports activities in school. School districts that do not employ adapted physical education specialists seldom have anyone on staff who is knowledgeable about appropriate disability sports programming and who can advocate for sports opportunities for students with disabilities. Physicians and rehabilitationists are needed to advocate for appropriate school physical education and sports for students with disabilities. The following section aims to present information needed to understand adapted physical education and to develop cooperative, collaborative services between school, health care, and agency personnel.

The adapted physical education professional in the school's physical education program is the individual responsible for ascertaining that fitness, sports, dance, aquatics, and other physical activities conducted by schools meet the individual needs of students with health impairments, disabilities, or developmental coordination disorder. With the increase of managed care, many of the rehabilitation functions that were performed in the medical setting may shift to the educational arena. The legal basis of adapted physical education service delivery is addressed in Public Law 101-476 (12), the Individuals with Disabilities Education Act of 1990, which is a reauthorization of the Education of the Handicapped Act of 1970.

The specific clause within the law that has promoted the growth of adapted physical education as a public school service delivery area is the definition of special education [Section 1401, (12)]. This definition states that special education is specially designed instruction, at no cost to parents or guardians, to meet the unique needs of a child with a disability, including (a) instruction conducted in the classroom, in the home, in hospitals and institutions, and in other settings; and (b) instruction in physical education (12).

The law thus makes physical education for individuals with disabilities a direct service that is an integral part of the individualized education program (IEP) process for students 3 to 21 years of age. This instructional service is required, whereas other services that also pertain to motor development (e.g., occupational and physical therapy, recreation and leisure services) in the schools are related and optional, depending on the discretion of members of the IEP team.

The rules and regulations for implementing PL 101-476 state that students with disabilities must be afforded the opportunity to participate in the regular physical education program available to nondisabled students unless (a) the student is enrolled full time in a separate facility or (b) the student needs specially designed physical education instruction as prescribed in his or her annual IEP by a multidisciplinary assessment team.

Specially designed physical education, according to the law, may be called adapted physical education, special physical education, movement education, or motor development (12).

The rules and regulations for implementing PL 101-476 also define "physical education." The term, according to the law, means the development of physical and motor fitness, fundamental motor skills and patterns, and skills in aquatics, dance, and individual and group games and sports (including intramural and lifetime sports) (12). The latter not only includes motor skills but also encompasses knowledge of rules, strategies, sportsmanship, and support resources, as well as development of adapted behavior skills for lifespan use of community facilities and maintenance of health, fitness, and leisure practices that enrich and improve quality of life.

Adapted physical education services may be delivered in regular physical education classes, in separate classes, or in one-to-one tutorial settings. The best arrangement for many students is instructional time divided between a regular class of reasonable size (i.e., no more than 20 students in a class) and an adapted class or resource room. The adapted class should provide individual or small group instruction in skills needed for motor success and peer group acceptance in regular instructional and after school programs, as well as training in wheelchair, blind, amputee, or cerebral palsy sports required for participation with local disability sport groups and for involvement in the worldwide Paralympic movement.

The competencies needed to deliver school adapted physical education services have been specified by the National Consortium for Physical Education and Recreation for Individuals with Disabilities (NCPERID), which is establishing a national certification examination, and by numerous other organizations and leaders (13–16). Worldwide, the International Federation of Adapted Physical Activity (IFAPA) and regional affiliates promote preservice, inservice, and continuing education of high-quality adapted physical education specialists, regular physical educators, and related services personnel. The official journal of IFAPA is the *Adapted Physical Activity Quarterly*, which has been published by Human Kinetics since 1984.

Several other organizations offer resources for help in adapted physical education service delivery. The American Alliance for Health, Physical Education, Recreation, and Dance (AAHPERD), the organization in which most physi-

TABLE 33-2. *International sport organizations and U.S. equivalents with dates of founding*

International	United States	Population served
Comite International des Sports des Sourds (CISS), 1924	American Athletic Association for the Deaf (AAAD), 1945	Sports for deaf athletes (i.e., hearing loss of 55 decibels or greater in the better ear)
International Stoke Mandeville Wheelchair Sports Federation (ISMWSF), 1957	Wheelchair Sports, USA (WS, USA)	Wheelchair sports for spinally impaired
International Sports Organization for the Disabled (ISOD), 1963	No equivalent. The United States has three separate organizations: Disabled Sports/USA (DS/USA) has governed amputee sports since 1989 U.S. Les Autres Sports Association (USLASA), 1986 Dwarf Athletic Association of America (DAAA), 1986	Wheelchair and ambulatory sports for amputees (nine classes) and others (six classes)
Cerebral Palsy International Sports and Recreation Association (CP-ISRA), 1978	U.S. Cerebral Palsy Athletic Association (USCPAA), 1978	Wheelchair and ambulatory sports for eight cerebral palsy classes
International Blind Sports Association (IBSA), 1981	U.S. Association for Blind Athletes (USABA), 1976	Sports for three classes of visual impairment
Special Olympics International (SOI), 1968	SOI, 1968	Sports for athletes with mental retardation
International Sports Federation for Persons with Mental Handicap (INASFMH), 1986	No U.S. equivalent	Sports for athletes with mental handicaps, also called learning difficulties

Disabled Sports/USA, called National Handicapped Sports (NHS) until 1995, is a powerful U.S. sport organization that governs winter sports and other events for several disability groups. Wheelchair Sports, USA was called the National Wheelchair Athletic Association (NWAA) until 1994. CISS (French) translates into International Committee of Sports of Silence.

Reprinted with permission from Sherrill C. *Adapted education, recreation, sport,* 5th ed. Dubuque, IA: WCB/McGraw-Hill, 1998.

cal educators maintain membership, has a structure called the Adapted Physical Activity Council (APAC) that develops policy and conducts annual meetings specifically on adapted physical education service, professional preparation, issues, and trends at annual conferences. Adapted physical activity specialists are taught to work closely with staff and athletes of disability sports organizations (e.g., Disabled Sports/USA, United States Cerebral Palsy Athletic Association). Lists of these and other organizations appear in the appendices of most adapted physical education textbooks (Table 33-2).

University-based teacher training programs have offered opportunities for learning adapted physical education competencies since the early 1900s (17). The knowledge base for this field originally came from Swedish medical and educational gymnastics (18,19). From the 1920s through the 1950s, courses, textbooks, and service delivery were called corrective or individualized physical education (20–22). In 1952, the AAHPERD officially adopted the term "adapted physical education" and encouraged the development of this curricular area in public schools. Today over 20 textbooks exist to guide basic teacher training in adapted physical education. The best known of these are by Sherrill (16), Winnick (23), and Block (24).

Most universities require courses and practicum work in adapted physical education of all individuals preparing for physical education teacher certification. This enables regular physical educators in mainstream classes to adapt activities to meet the individual needs of students. Several universities also offer master's and doctoral degrees in adapted physical education, which prepare specialists for public schools and universities. Adapted physical education specialists in public schools assist regular educators, provide motor development assessment and consultant services, teach students with severe disabilities in resource rooms or separate settings, conduct after-school disability sports programs, and work with families in facilitating home-school-community cooperative programming to assure healthy, active life-styles for all students (Fig. 33-3).

RECREATION

Sports is only a subset of the much larger field of recreation. As Mark Twain said about recreation, "Play consists of whatever a body is not obliged to do" (25). But recreation's value to life in general and rehabilitation in specific is exemplified by its root word "creation."

"To rehabilitate is to restore the power or capacity for living . . . living does not signify merely biological life and function but it takes on a qualitative dimension. It is the

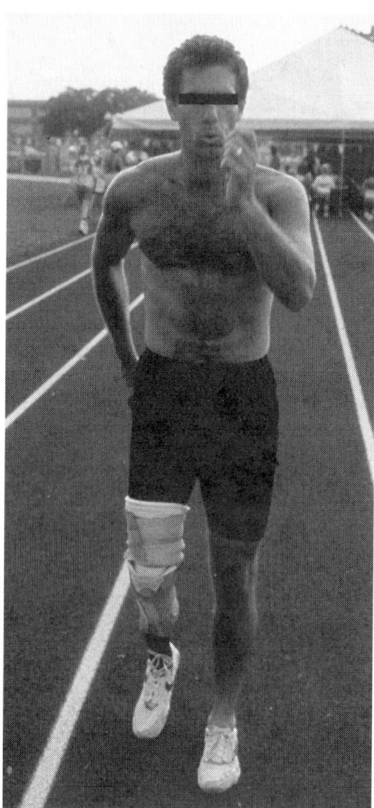

FIG. 33-3. A world record breaking sprinter and long jumper.

restoration of the power of living well, living meaningfully that rehabilitation essentially seeks'' (26). According to Datillo and Kleiber, '' . . . A purpose not only of TR (therapeutic recreation), but of leisure services in general, is to engender enjoyment. For whatever additional benefits enjoyment may bring, it is, in and of itself, a major rationale for the provision of leisure services. Leisure professionals seek to identify the factors that interfere with and prohibit enjoyment, those that facilitate enjoyment, and other benefits that accrue to people who enjoy themselves'' (27).

Datillo and Kleiber further linked enjoyment to higher levels of self-determination and quality of life (27). This theme is further reflected in the definition statement of the American Therapeutic Recreation Association: ''The primary purposes of treatment services, which are often referred to as recreational therapy, are to restore, remediate, or rehabilitate in order to improve functioning and independence as well as reduce or eliminate the effects of illness or disability'' (28).

Therapeutic recreation is holistic and eclectic in its approach. The therapeutic recreation professional is concerned with the total person, not just an isolated problem or limitation (29). Therapeutic recreation services are action oriented and focus on the patient/client's experience, not on the activity. It is purposeful intervention, not merely diversionary. The process includes assessment, treatment planning, implementation, and evaluation. According to Austin and Crawford, ''Therapeutic Recreation is a means, first to restore oneself or regain stability (health protection), and second, to develop oneself through leisure as a means to self-actualization (health promotion)'' (30).

Therapeutic recreation uses leisure experiences to provide and facilitate opportunities for self-determination and empowerment. Austin and Crawford asserted that ''Typical outcomes of Therapeutic Recreation interventions include increasing personal awareness, increasing interpersonal or social skills, developing leisure skills, decreasing stress, improving physical fitness and functioning, developing feelings of positive self-regard, self-efficacy perceived control, pleasure, and enjoyment'' (30).

Therapeutic recreation services are delivered in a variety of environments, including inpatient and outpatient rehabilitation, psychiatry, substance abuse treatment, pediatric hospitals, residential and independent living centers, prisons, public schools, public recreation departments, and numerous other public and private agencies. Services are delivered across the life span. Children, adolescents, adults, and senior citizens receive the benefits of therapeutic recreation.

Perhaps the most critical intervention typically provided by therapeutic recreation in the rehabilitation environment is community reintegration training. Just as hospitals are expanding beyond traditional boundaries, so is therapeutic recreation. Community reintegration is defined as the frequency, variety, and intensity to which one resumes and maintains involvement and activity outside the home after the onset of a disability or chronic illness. Reintegration is neither automatic nor spontaneous. Barriers to successful reintegration of an individual into his or her community include self-image and self-esteem, family attitudes and support, self-care limitations, financial resources, equipment limitations, transportation, and physical barriers.

It is important to note that the degree or severity of disability only minimally affects one's ability to resume normalized community activity. The most critical factors in successful reintegration are attitude and self-concept and the ability to effectively apply and utilize adaptive techniques and equipment in the real world environment. Individualized, goal-oriented community therapy provides patients with the opportunity to risk and to achieve a level of success that is reflective of a heightened self concept. Community reintegration education for inpatients undergoing rehabilitation accomplishes the following goals:

1. It breaks down the psychological fears that block the patient's openness to traditional treatment.
2. It increases the patient's motivation for developing skills for independence by providing the patients with the opportunity to see what is attainable.
3. It gives a sense of relevance to therapy by clearly demonstrating why rehabilitation techniques are valid and significant.
4. It assists the newly disabled person in redefining and re-evaluating himself or herself and his or her disability

in a positive sense, and how that disability will impact on quality of life.

5. It places the rehabilitation patient in a proactive position to identify and overcome potential problems that may occur after discharge.

When limited to the rehabilitation hospital environment, traditional therapies simply cannot address the scope and complexity of skills necessary to resume normal community activity. A rehabilitation patient's ability to resume normalized activities within his or her community is further limited by the presence of inaccurate, outdated, and negative stereotypes of people with disabilities. This lack of understanding has perpetuated the belief that disabled means unable, and that people with disabilities should be protected or isolated from potential risks of failure. Unfortunately, when individuals are sheltered from potential failure, they are also robbed of the opportunities for success and a normalized life-style. Early intervention will help to prevent the development of unhealthy patterns of inactivity and isolation often seen after discharge.

Community training is equally important for individuals with congenital disabilities who may not present in the traditional acute inpatient environment. People define themselves in a variety of dimensions or categories such as physical appearance, athletic ability, romantic appeal, academic competence, and so on (31). The complexity is further shown in the realization that self-concept is the product of the continuous interaction of the individual and his or her environment. These separate dimensions are inter-related in that our self-concept in one category can influence our self-concept in another area. Hamachek suggested that the interconnectedness of our emotional circuitry and the absence of watertight compartments for the self-concept allows what is felt in one dimension to overflow into other dimensions of the self (32). Based on the individual's life experiences, interactions with others, and his or her own personal values, the individual develops a positive or negative orientation to each dimension that is weighted in its importance to the individual's global self-worth (31). Therefore, it is imperative that individuals with congenital disabilities receive normalized social, recreational, educational, and athletic opportunities.

Perhaps Stephen W. Hawkings said it best in his message to the athletes at the opening ceremonies of the 1992 Paralympic Games in Barcelona, Spain: "Each one of us has within us a spark of fire, a creative force. Some of us have lost the use of parts of our bodies, through accident or illness, but that is really of minor significance. It is just a mechanical problem. The important thing is that we have the human spirit, the ability to create. This creativity can take on many forms, from theoretical physics to physical achievement. The important thing is that one should be stretched to be outstanding in some field" (Fig. 33-4).

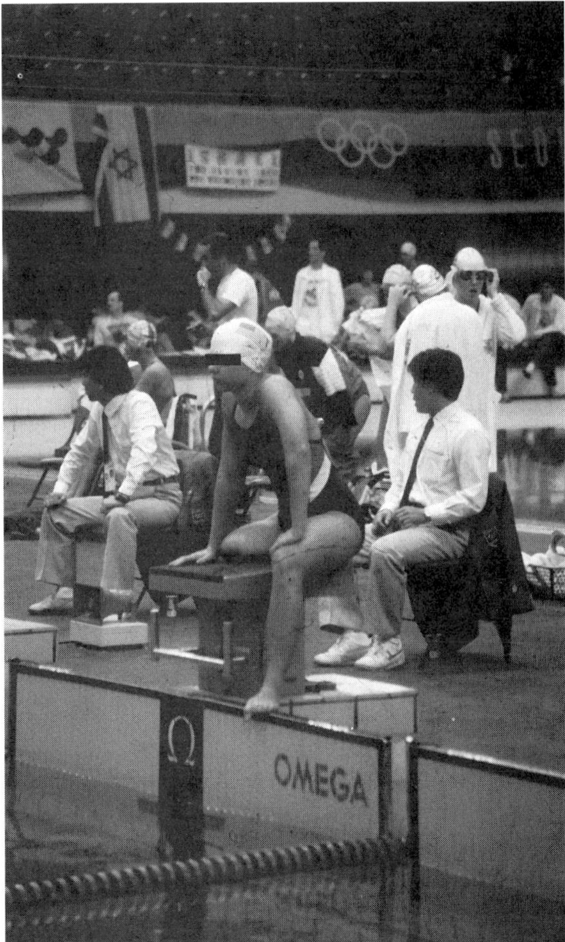

FIG. 33-4. A paralympic swimmer in Seoul, Korea.

SPORTS MEDICINE AND SCIENCE IN SPORTS FOR ATHLETES WITH DISABILITIES

The development of a sports science and medicine dimension has been an important part of the history of sports for people with disabilities. In the early development, the first scientific publications were in the context of the therapeutic value of sports for people with disabilities (33). The work capacity of persons with a spinal injury was reported by Kottke in some of the earliest studies on this subject (34), but it was not until much later, beginning in the 1970s, that the actual work capacity of wheelchair athletes was first studied (35). Since then, there have been numerous studies reported, both in the spinal literature and in the sports scientific literature. Such studies have continued to shed light on the physical performance potentials of wheelchair athletes with spinal injury. There was early mention of sports-related injuries in a report from the 1976 Olympiad (36). A more extensive recent study was reported in 1992 (37). There is ongoing interest and study of chronic musculoskeletal injuries related to participation in sports for disabled individuals (38). From these diverse beginnings, sports for people with disabilities has developed to several levels (Fig. 33-5):

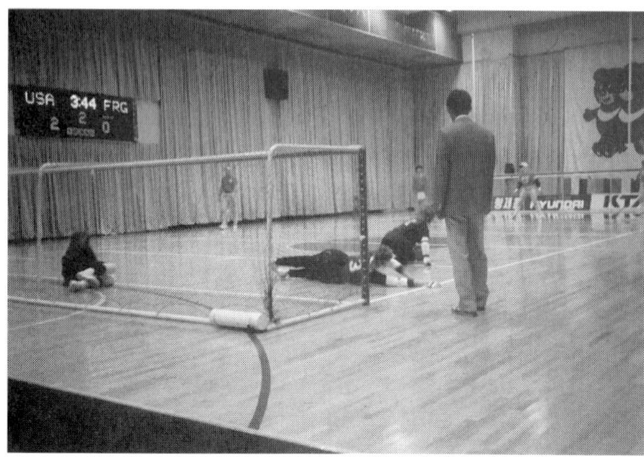

FIG. 33-5. Athletes with visual impairment playing goalball.

1. As a rehabilitation tool to assist in achieving maximum physical function as well as psychological and social benefits.
2. Recreational sports affording people with disabilities an opportunity to enjoy sport for sport's sake, often in an integrated fashion with nondisabled individuals.
3. Sports for fitness and health, involving pleasurable exercise in a sports environment.
4. Competitive sports at several levels of involvement, such as road racing in marathons, competing in club competitions, or participating in wheelchair sports team activities at the local and regional level, while offering an opportunity to gain access to international competition.

PHYSIOLOGIC BENEFITS

The physiologic benefits of regular physical activity for people with disabilities are believed to be similar to those published by the American College of Sports Medicine for the general population (39). These include improvement in cardiovascular function, reduction in coronary artery disease risk factors, and decreased mortality and morbidity (40). The sparse research on disability, sports, and health benefits has been summarized by Shephard (41,42), Rimmer (43), Nelson and Harris (44), McCubbin (45), and Durstine and colleagues (46).

When surveyed, athletes with disabilities state that fitness and health rank first among the many contributions that sports make to their lives (47,48). Illustrative of research that documents the very high levels of physiologic function that wheelchair athletes can reach is work by Veeger and colleagues (49). Research also indicates that athletically active persons in wheelchairs have fewer kidney infections, skin breakdowns, and other medical complications than their sedentary peers (50). Observation of athletes with disabilities at World Games and Paralympics substantiates what research does not yet make available. Athletes, regardless of type of disability, appear to have optimum fitness and health.

There is much research to document that habitual physical activity is missing in the lives of most persons with disabilities (51–53). LaPlante, for instance, at a National Institutes of Health symposium conducted in conjunction with the 1996 Paralympics, noted that only 28% of adults with limitations engage in regular intense exercise (i.e., sustained large muscle activity for 20 minutes or more each bout, a minimum of 5 days a week).

Research has noted the psychosocial benefits of sports for individuals with disabilities (47,54–56). Chief among these is self-esteem or enhancement of the sense of self. Hutzler and Bar-Eli (54) summarized early research as follows:

> In general, the studies reviewed reveal significant positive changes varying in intensity and duration in the self-concept of disabled populations after sports participation sessions. In addition, significantly higher values of self-concept were observed among disabled people regularly participating in sports compared with sedentary, inactive disabled individual.

Sherrill (47), after interviewing over 300 adult athletes with cerebral palsy or visual impairments, concluded that almost all athletes believe that sports are a means of affirming their competence and helping others to focus on their abilities rather than their disabilities. Adult athletes, with the exception of females with cerebral palsy and males with visual impairments, also score higher on self-regard scales than the normal values for able-bodied people (55). Most exciting perhaps, are findings showing that young athletes with disabilities, 9 to 18 (mean 13.94) years of age, have mean scores on eight different self-concept scales that are close to those of able-bodied youth (57). In contrast, most individuals with disabilities who are not involved in sports have low self-concepts (58).

Internal locus of control, inner-directedness, self-direction, self-efficacy, and well-being are associated with sports involvement. Highly active men with paraplegia (42) and male quadriplegic rugby players (59) score high on internal locus of control. Elite male wheelchair athletes score higher on measures of inner directedness than do able-bodied athlete normative groups (60) and sedentary individuals with spinal cord injury (61). Elite women wheelchair racers describe the positive contribution of sports to self-direction, self-efficacy, and self-esteem (62). Wheelchair tennis players score high on self-efficacy and well-being (63). Self-efficacy, for athletes with disabilities, is strongly associated with social support of family and friends (64). Indeed, a major outcome of competitive sports involvement is emotional strength built on experiencing the social support of significant others (65).

Athletes with a disability also perceive their varying mood states (vigor, tension, depression, anger, fatigue, and confusion) as mentally healthy (55,66). Several studies indicate that scores of athletes on scales of perceived well-being are superior to able bodied norms and to scores of sedentary people with disabilities (55). This supports research that links regular, vigorous physical activity and related social interactions with good mental health.

SOCIALIZATION INTO SPORTS

Sports socialization is the process of becoming involved in sports, learning sports roles and values, and acquiring a sporting identity. The process, of course, is different for people with and without disabilities and for people with congenital and acquired disabilities (67,68). Able-bodied children are typically socialized into sports primarily by their parents who enroll them in organized sports programs between 4 and 8 years of age and strongly encourage their sports interests and abilities. In contrast, the sports socialization of children with congenital disabilities is constrained by parents' and teachers' lack of knowledge about sports in relation to disability and by a tendency toward overprotection (16). Athletes with cerebral palsy and blindness report that friends and agency personnel have influenced their sports socialization more than family members (68); also, many athletes report personal responsibility for involving themselves in sports, noting many barriers to socialization.

Athletes with acquired disabilities report discontinuous sports socialization with disease or injury interrupting and/or changing the nature of their sports involvement (67). Time of onset is very important in that the older the child, the more likely his or her sports socialization will continue along its original path. Athletes also emphasize the importance of strong sports programs in rehabilitation hospitals and centers. Programs that employ sports directors with disabilities are especially valuable in that they provide role models.

EXERCISE TECHNIQUES AND TRAINING

There are different types of training techniques, each offering a specific benefit to the exerciser. The rehabilitation specialist can help the exerciser increase his or her performance by using the most appropriate technique. Specificity training incorporates training techniques and uses physiologic systems that are similar to the sporting activity of the performance. The body's adaptation is specific to the type of training performed. Because training specificity incorporates mechanical and metabolic systems (69), training programs should be specific to the energy system (i.e., adenosine triphosphate–creatine phosphate [ATP-CP], anaerobic glycolysis, aerobic) (70) used in the sporting activity system, moving from general to more specific as the sporting event approaches. Training also should be specific to the muscular force and movements of the sport at hand (70). For example, an athlete who competes in the wheelchair 100-meter race should train by using an arm ergometer or wheelchair to perform short-duration, high-intensity activities. The more similar the training program is to the specific sport, the better prepared the athletes will be for the sport leading to an increased performance (71).

The concept of the overload principle is to increase the body's stress or exercise load higher than it is normally used to handling in order to increase the body's ability (69,71). This results in the body increasing its ability to handle the stress. This is obvious in strength-gaining activities. If the body is used to lifting 50 kg at 10 repetitions, the overload principle would increase the weight to 75 kg at 10 repetitions or keep the weight at 50 kg and increase the repetitions to 15. Progressive increases in overload should be monitored for each individual athlete. Overload may not always be appropriate and or it may need to be carefully monitored with certain medical conditions such as progressive neurologic disorders (69).

During periods of training, especially intensive training, the body requires appropriate rest periods. Rest and recovery periods should be built into the training program as well as the competition season (69,70). This rest period may mean that the athlete discontinues sports altogether or the athlete may become involved in other types of activities at a decreased intensity (70). It is important to determine rest periods on an individual basis and incorporate overload/recovery schedules as needed via utilization of periodization.

Periodization is a graduated training technique incorporating a cycling of specificity, intensity, and volume of training to achieve peak levels of fitness for the most important competitions (71,72). Improving in an exercise requires a balance between overload (exercise) and recovery (rest) periods. The concept of periodization, a training plan of divide and conquer, allows the body to build up to predetermined exercise goals while preventing overtraining (71). To do this, the training is broken down into cycles with each cycle containing different amounts of general fitness and sports specific conditioning objectives. Each cycle is broken down into phases that include preseason, in-season, and off-season training (70,71). The training cycle may begin with a high volume and low intensity of general conditioning to develop an apparent base, gradually moving to low-volume, high-intensity sport-specific and skill training. Additionally, each cycle includes appropriate rest periods to allow recovery.

The principles of training and periodization, we feel, are the same for all athletes whether they have a disability or not. It is the application of these principles that must be individualized. If an athlete is at a performance plateau, it often means that the intensity/recovery training equation is wrong for that athlete. Because the optimal equation for each athlete is unique, training must be carefully monitored to ensure that progress is continuing or the training regiment of overload and recovery may need changing.

When planning exercise for individuals with a disability, training techniques should take into consideration the individual's abilities and safety precautions specific to the individual's disability. Training programs may need to be modified, especially for individuals with progressive disorders or individuals who fatigue after exercise (69). Although the proper amounts of exercise for individuals with many of the progressive disorders may help maintain the individual's functional abilities, during an exacerbation exercise should be discontinued or significantly modified (69). An individual with postpolio syndrome or muscular dystrophy may encounter an overuse weakness if training is too intensive (73).

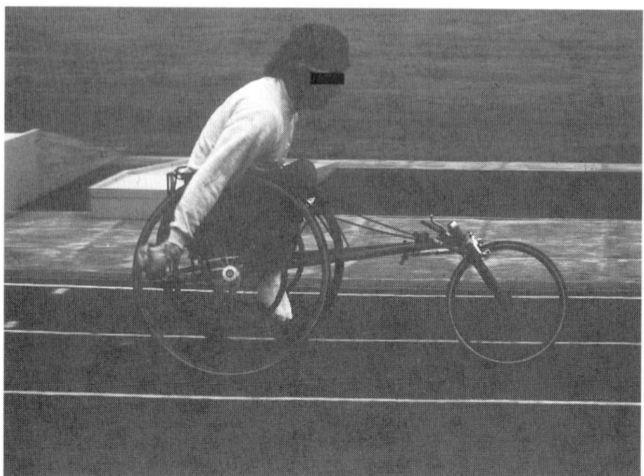

FIG. 33-6. Athlete in a racing chair.

Additionally, the symptoms of an individual with multiple sclerosis may be exacerbated with an increase in core body temperature. Exercisers with disabilities such as spinal cord injuries, Down syndrome, and cerebral palsy may not be able to tolerate conditions of heat or cold during outdoor training or competitions (74). During strength training, individuals with an amputation who have a prosthesis should apply force though the long axis of the limb only in order to decrease the chance of stress to the limb (69).

Exercise is like medicine: with the proper dose it can be a beneficial and enjoyable part of an individual s life (Fig. 33-6).

CONTROVERSIES IN SPORTS FOR ATHLETES WITH DISABILITIES

Performance Potentials and Classification

The Concept

Classification is a critical and very controversial component of competitive sports among disabled athletes. It enables the athlete to be grouped with others whose performance lies in a somewhat similar range. This is meant to ensure fair competition among athletes with similar potential, so that there is a realistic opportunity to succeed in competition. The concept of classification is not unique to sports for people with disabilities. In the able-bodied arena, competitors are classified by gender, age, and weight in certain sports, and the use of handicap enables persons with differing abilities to compete against one another. In sports for people with disabilities, classification is necessary because of the wide range of impairment and the resultant wide range of sports performance (Fig. 33-7).

The Process

Early examples of classification were in wheelchair sports, where the initial number of classes was two, identified as "high" and "low" paraplegics. In amputee sports, various levels of amputation led to different classes, such as above knee or below knee. In cerebral palsy sports, the qualitative difference in motor performance between an athetoid, spastic hemiplegic, or diplegic competitor necessitated separate competitive events.

Over time, with increasing numbers, and wider range of competitors, increasing levels of performance and competition, the classification system became more complex. Additional classes were added where it was determined that performance potential significantly exceeded the range of existing classes. In recent years there has been an attempt to combine in one system competitors with quite different disability profiles. For example, a competitor with cerebral palsy might be classified to compete against a competitor with a spinal cord injury or an amputation.

The process of classification is necessary in competition, whereas it is not particularly relevant in recreational sports or in health or fitness sports. At the elite level of competition, now defined as Paralympic sports, classification is most critical because the classification process is a key determinant of competition results. In some sports, classification is not so critical. In archery and shooting, where dynamic trunk or leg control is not so critical, it has been determined that two classes—tetraplegic and paraplegic—are sufficient to allow fair and meaningful competition.

Classification by Disability Group

Classification was originally applied within specific disability groups (e.g., spinal injured, amputee, cerebral palsy) because most competition took place separately within these disability groups. Classification for spinal cord–injured athletes has the longest history since the first wheelchair competitions in the Stoke Mandeville spinal cord hospital in 1942.

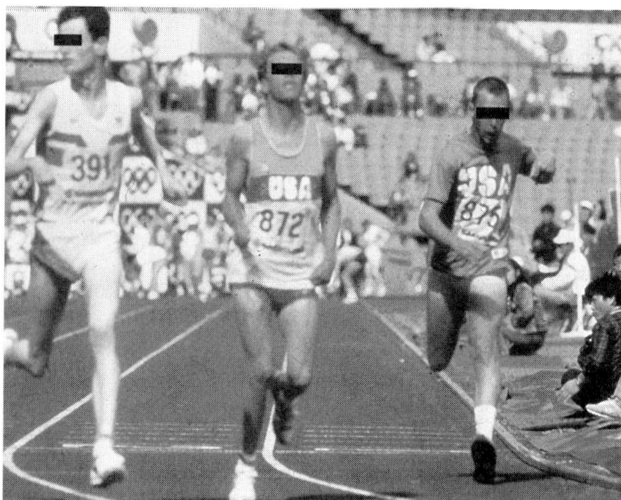

FIG. 33-7. Sprinters at the finish line in Assen, Holland at the 1990 World Championships. They are CP-ISRA class 6 (athetoid characteristics).

The process was fundamentally a medically based determination of impairment and level of injury, and at one time included eight levels that were considered significant. Amputee classification continues to be based on the anatomic determinants of limb loss. Cerebral palsy classification has been more difficult. The consideration of movement disorder, spasticity, and severity of involvement has made it more difficult to define or create a continuum of impairment, such as is possible in spinal cord injury. In cerebral palsy sports, at the moment, there are four wheelchair classes and four standing classes.

Classification for Individual Sports

In 1992 there began a shift away from the classification focus on the individual athlete profile to a greater emphasis on the analysis of individual sports performance. This shift coincided with a sports philosophy that has attempted to distance itself from what may be perceived as medical influence or identification. It represented a desire to characterize sports for people with disabilities as a pure sports movement without relationships to rehabilitation or therapy. Unfortunately this tends to separate the elite from the developmental sports movement because for many people with disabilities the first opportunity to engage in adapted physical activities such as sports occurs within the medical system as part of rehabilitation. There has also been a desire to become integrated with able-bodied sports and with sports specialists, such as trainers and coaches of the able bodied. This has been termed ''vertical integration.'' Many high-performance athletes hope to become totally identified with the ''legitimate'' sports movement, with a desire to shed the identity of medical need or support. As many sportsmen and -women with disabilities have said, they wish to gain recognition on the sports pages of the newspapers rather than in the human interest section (Fig. 33-8).

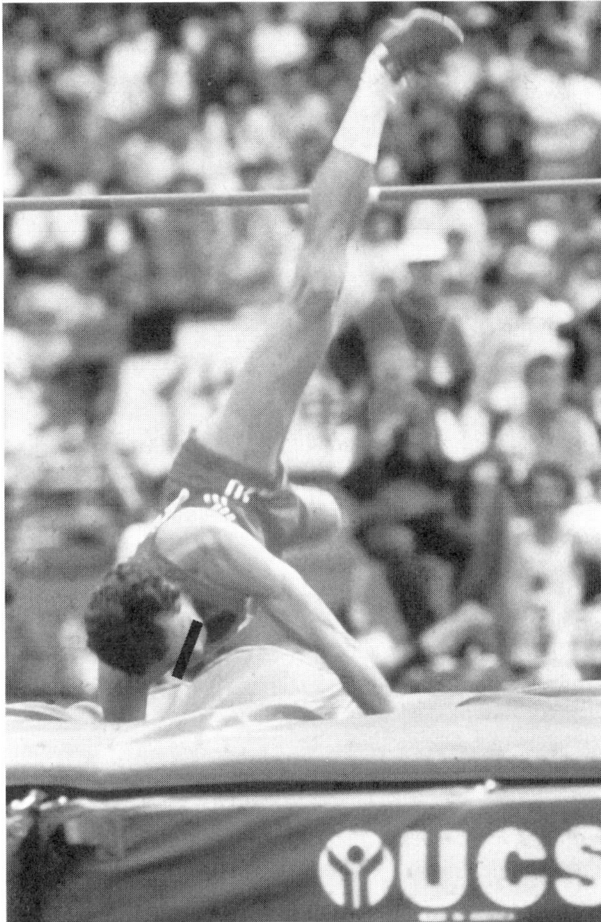

FIG. 33-8. A Canadian athlete with an above-the-knee amputation, cleared over 6 feet 8 inches on the high jump.

The Physician's Role in the Process

There has been a recent challenge to the fundamental concept that identification of impairment best determines the classification of the athlete. Rather, it is believed that observation of the athlete during competition allows the experienced and skilled observer to determine the class relevant to the sport.

This questions the need for physician involvement in a sports-centered task. The task of grouping athletes in competition is seen to be better suited to a team of fellow athletes, coachs, and sports technical experts, who are knowledgeable in the specific sport. It is claimed that athletes can be fairly classified for competition in any sport by observation of the individual's posture, movement pattern, and skill portrayal while engaging in the sport, without the need for assessment of such factors as muscle strength, tone, or joint range.

The desire to consolidate athlete competition across disability lines is quite contentious when it seems evident to some that a competitor with cerebral palsy with either spasticity or athetosis exhibits fundamental motor characteristics and performance parameters of a totally different character compared with an amputee or a person with spinal cord trauma (75). In sports scientific terms, the actual athlete performance has little comparative meaning to another athlete's performance, in the absence of an impairment analysis, which reveals what physical resources the athlete has (76) (Fig. 33-9).

There is a sense that the attempt to group all disabilities together in one competition system is driven by an administrative desire for convenience in competition and a further desire to integrate sports for disabled into the Olympic movement in as simple a fashion as possible. As sports for people with disabilities have grown and prospered, the opportunity for physiatrist involvement seems obvious at a number of levels. The relationship of impairment to performance as applied to sports/athlete classification is a field in which interested physiatrists have a great role to play.

Boosting

The term ''boosting'' was originated by tetraplegic wheelchair athletes to describe a process that they discovered aug-

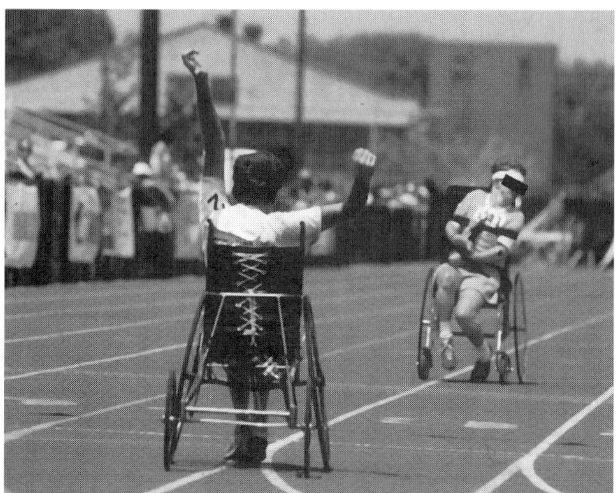

FIG. 33-9. Examples of different propulsion styles in athletes. USCPAA class II lower.

mented performance in certain competitions. It involves the triggering of autonomic dysreflexia, long recognized as a serious complication or emergency in spinal cord injury management (77). Individuals with high thoracic or cervical level spinal cord injury are at risk of this occurrence because of the disruption of autonomic sympathetic pathways. As a result, the control and modulation of autonomic responses to peripheral stimuli is lost, and the well-recognized clinical syndrome of hypertension, tachycardia, flushing, and goose pimples result.

In 1993 it first became known that tetraplegic athletes were using this response to improve performance in competition, most notably in wheelchair track events. Burnham and colleagues first confirmed this in an experimental laboratory study. The results of their study were subsequently presented and discussed in depth in an international meeting in Edmonton, Alberta, devoted to sports for people with disabilities (78). A presentation by a world class tetraplegic athlete was of particular interest as he described his personal experience in using this response to enhance performance, while informing the audience that it was currently a technique almost universally used by tetraplegic athletes. The mechanisms used to induce dysreflexia primarily include bladder distention, induced by catheter clamping and ingestion of large volumes of fluid before an event, or by nociceptive stimulation, such as sitting on the arm of a wheelchair (79). Burnham's studies demonstrated that race time was reduced by 9.7%, whereas oxygen consumption (VO_2) was significantly increased, in association with the increased blood pressure. A study of the improvement in race times in tetraplegic classes between the Paralympics in Seoul (1988) and Barcelona (1992) (Table 33-3) might suggest that some of this marked improvement was the result of boosting.

As a result of these disclosures, a dilemma has been created for the disabled sports movement. The practice falls outside doping as currently defined. There are two concerns. The fact of unfair advantage or cheating by those willing to take the risk is obvious. Nevertheless, there is some argument as to whether it should be ranked with drug doping as an offense. Proponents of the practice appeal to the notion of regaining some element of "normalcy" in that the ultimate performance gained does not go beyond the physiologic norms of autonomic function of the paraplegic competitor.

The more acute concern is about serious consequences, including death, which may occur if this practice continues unchecked. Other than checking competitors at the starting line for clinical evidence of dysreflexia, it is difficult to know how one can deal with the process. Competitors have developed a great capability of "turning on" this syndrome, such as by clamping a catheter or timing an ingestion of fluid at a measured time before the start of an event. This issue is currently being studied by the sports medicine and science committee of the involved international sports federation for wheelchair sports.

Heat Problems

In 1996 the Paralympics were held in Atlanta, Georgia, during the heat of a typical Georgia summer. There were no major difficulties with heat intolerance, but there could have been if athletes and staff were not aware of the issue (80,81). The susceptibility to heat intolerance is due to multiple factors, including decrease in sensory awareness, sympathetic nervous system dysfunction, and a deficient body mechanism for warming and cooling (82). This susceptibility primarily affects the athlete with a spinal cord injury but also may be found in athletes with other disabilities such as cerebral palsy, obesity, and Down syndrome (74). The most vulnerable athletes are those with a spinal injury above the eighth thoracic level (83,84). In addition, these athletes may be on medications such as anticholinergics, which increase their vulnerability (85). In Atlanta this was addressed by attentive focus to hydration, encouraging the consumption of 1 to 2 cups of fluids every 10 to 15 minutes during competition and training (86). Practical aspects such as providing shade, using light clothing and hats, and attaching water bottles to training wheelchairs were found to be helpful.

It is particularly important to be aware of dehydration in athletes with a swallowing disorder. This may be manifested by drooling in a condition such as cerebral palsy. These athletes not only have a difficult time taking the fluids but may have a significant fluid loss from the lost saliva. Like every athlete, they need to monitor the volume and color of

TABLE 33-3. *Improvement in tetraplegic race times: boosting paralympic performance—100-meter tetraplegic classes*

	Seoul, 1988	Barcelona, 1992
Cervical 6	24.22 seconds	23.16 seconds
Cervical 7	20.39 seconds	18.24 seconds

their urine output and additionally need to attend to swallowing strategies.

Seizures

Seizures are sometimes a concern in athletes with disabilities (87). This has long been an area of controversy, and we feel undue restrictions. As recently as 1996, an official committee of the American Medical Association recommended keeping individuals with seizures from participating in a variety of sports ranging from football to tennis and track and field (88). The concern has been that sporting activities would increase the risk of seizures. Indeed, stress with its concomitant release of epinephrine as well as hypoglycemia, hypoxia, dehydration, electrolyte imbalance, and hyperventilation, are factors that could occur during athletic competition and are known to increase seizure activity (89). However, as Lennox said in 1941, Physical and mental activities seem to be an antagonist of seizures (90). Problems such as hypoglycemia, dehydration, and electrolyte disorder can be avoided with appropriate nutritional and fluid intake. Hyperventilation, which occurs in the laboratory and stimulates seizures, is an artificial phenomenon and not the physiologic response of hyperventilation on the athletic field. In the laboratory setting the hyperventilation results in a decrease in the pCO_2, causing the pH to increase, which results in a vasoconstriction in the cerebral vessels and local hypoxia. This results in lowered seizure threshold. However, on the athletic field the hyperventilation is in direct response to the metabolic demands of exercise, including the lactic acidosis. There is no alkalosis that occurs. If one suspects that this is a rare instance of sports precipitating a seizure, one should consider obtaining an exercise electroencephalogram (91).

In fact, athletes usually experience fewer epileptic activities during exercise (92–94). The antiseizure medications may have negative effects on attention in athletes (87). Although these problems usually can be addressed and have not been found to have significant negative impact on athletic performance when seizures do occur in the sporting arena, the usual techniques of treatment should be used (95,96). However, in the athletic arena, with a potentially dehydrated athlete, it is sometimes difficult to get intravenous access. Use of intrarectal administration of diazepam may be an option in this case (97–99).

Drugs

It is common for athletes with disabilities to use prescribed medications for asthma, seizures, hyperactivity, spasticity, and other conditions. One needs to be aware of the indications, contraindications, side effects, and possible synergistic effects of using multiple medications in the sports and recreation setting.

There are very significant social and legislative problems regarding drug use. For example, athletic organizations, such as the U.S. Olympic Committee (USOC) and the International Olympic Committee (IOC), have their own drug regulations. The use of anticonvulsants is banned in athletes in shooting events, although this has never been proven to be a performance enhancer (100). As rehabilitationists we need to be aware of these issues, not only to legislate for rational restrictions but also to counsel athletes. An up-to-date list of banned medications can be obtained from the USOC Drug Control Hotline at (800) 233-0393.

In 1992 at the Barcelona Paralympics, the U.S. Wheelchair Basketball team lost a gold medal because one of the participants was found to be using propoxaphene, a banned substance, which does have a possible legitimate use in individuals with spinal cord injury in the treatment of hyperhidrosis (87,101). Inexplicably, codeine is permitted by both the USOC and IOC. As rehabilitationists with interest in sports medicine, we need to be aware of the political affairs and hopefully give input to make things even more rational.

Spasticity

There has long been a concern among those with a neurodevelopmental background (102) and other professionals (103) that athletes with spasticity of cerebral origin should not become involved in competitive sports. However, although it is clear that stress, such as may occur in sports, causes a transient increase in spasticity, the more important question is what happens during the long term (104). For almost 20 years there have been international competitions under the auspices of the Cerebral Palsy International Sports and Recreation Association for athletes with cerebral palsy and related conditions such as stroke and head injury. The anecdotal evidence has been that there has been a very positive, not negative, effect on the participants. The scientific literature also has reports and studies that have shown the benefits of sports and vigorous exercise, including resistance training in athletes with spasticity of cerebral origin (105–111). In fact, these works have shown that individuals with spasticity of cerebral origin not only have the durability to participate in sports and resistive exercise, but they show benefit. The spasticity appears to habituate to the stress stimulus and that improvement can certainly be made (112). There are still many areas that need to be addressed. There is not just a question of doing away with old superstitions, but we need to develop new knowledge through research to answer many questions. What is the most effective way to train a spastic muscle for functional strength and endurance? Are there unique issues of periodization of exercise in athletes with cerebral palsy? What are the long-term consequence of exercise and sports for individuals with spasticity of cerebral origin? However, although research needs to be performed we strongly feel that it has been shown that sports and exercise is a positive activity for individuals with spasticity of cerebral origin, and we strongly encourage medical and educational communities to promote sports and exercise as options for these people.

INJURIES AND MEDICAL ISSUES

Unfortunately, perceptions on the risk of sports participation by individuals with disabilities has been based more on intuition and beliefs than on facts. We have observed that physicians often make one of two diametrically opposed errors when evaluating the potential sports risk for an individual with a disability. One error is assuming that sports for athletes with disabilities cannot be too rigorous or risky; therefore, anybody should be allowed to compete. Another error is assuming that an individual with a disability is so fragile that any type of competition is prohibitively risky. Obviously, as rehabilitation physicians with a sporting interest, we must attempt to determine what the real risks are. Athletes must be evaluated objectively and fairly to appraise them of any potential risks while not needlessly preventing them from participating. To be effective in doing this requires a knowledge of both disability issues as well as sports and sports medicine. Health-care providers must realize that sports are activities in which injuries are indeed expected and need to be addressed promptly and appropriately. Researchers have demonstrated that the injury risk in an athlete with a disability is essentially the same as the injury risk for the so called able bodied athlete (37,105,113–115). In fact as shown by epidemiologic investigation of the Athletes with Disabilities Injury Registry (ADIR), the risk of injury per athletic exposure for an athlete with disability is similar to that of an athlete without a disability (114). However, the ADIR study also showed that the risk of a more serious injury was greater for an athlete with a disability. Some of the reason for the more serious injuries, which are defined as a longer period away from sports, may be secondary to inadequate coaching and poor medical access (116) (Fig. 33-10).

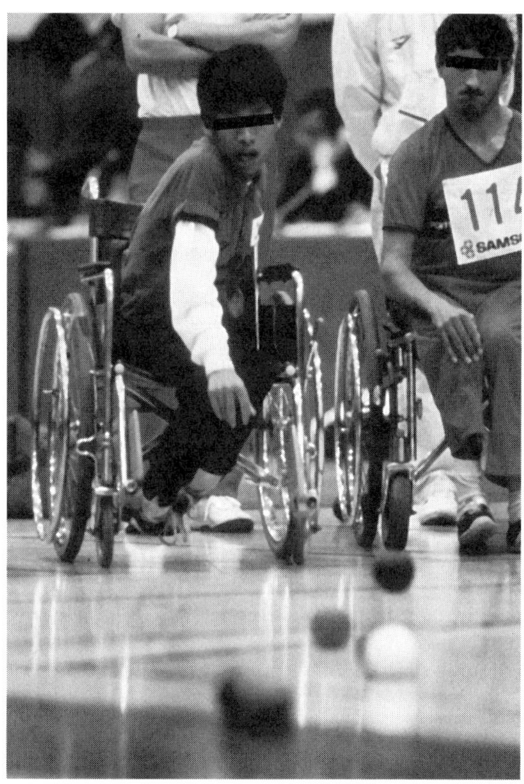

FIG. 33-10. Paralympic boccia players. Boccia is one of the most rapidly developing sports.

Wheelchair Athletes

Athletes with disabilities experience athletic-related injuries that are specific to the demands and risks of their sport. The most common injuries were strains and muscular injuries of the upper extremity (117,118). Many of these injuries are understandable. Because hands are used continuously for propulsion, blisters of the fingers and thumbs may develop. Overuse entrapment syndromes may occur (119), although their risk does not seem to be high when compared with their occurrence in nonathletes with disabilities (120). A major concern is overuse injury cumulative trauma disorders, particularly of the shoulder. Wheelchair propulsion is increased by increasing the speed and force of the impulse supplied to the hand rim. Wheelchair design changes (lowering the seat height to allow for a low center of gravity) may contribute to more injuries because the decreased seat height may place the elbow and upper arm in contact with the wheel, where a friction burn can occur. Fractures of the metacarpals and phalanges are possible from falls and collisions with other wheelchairs that may occur in sports such as wheelchair basketball. Researchers have estimated that although stroke technique may vary, the hands of some athletes are in contact with the hand rim for 270°(121). The rotator cuff is vulnerable from overuse injuries, which result in tendinitis or impingement syndrome. Many of these injuries may be prevented through the use of not only reasonable training programs with appropriate progression and periodization, but also special attention to the balance of the shoulder girdle musculature. In wheelchair athletes the anterior musculature often needs to be stretched, and the posterior musculature, especially the external rotators and the scapular adductors, need to be strengthened (122). By the nature of wheelchair propulsions, the wheelchair athlete tends to overdevelop the anterior musculature with a relatively weak posterior musculature. Therefore, exercises that strengthen posterior musculature, such as a rowing machine, may be beneficial in preventing this injury from occurring (Fig. 33-11).

Athletes with an Amputation

Although there is still some unfounded concern that an athlete with an amputation should not be having stress resistance developed through the prosthesis (123,124), experience clearly shows that this is not a valid concern. The amputee is at risk of developing various skin irritations or breakdowns from sports. However, with the use of appropriate padding within the prosthesis and friction eliminating

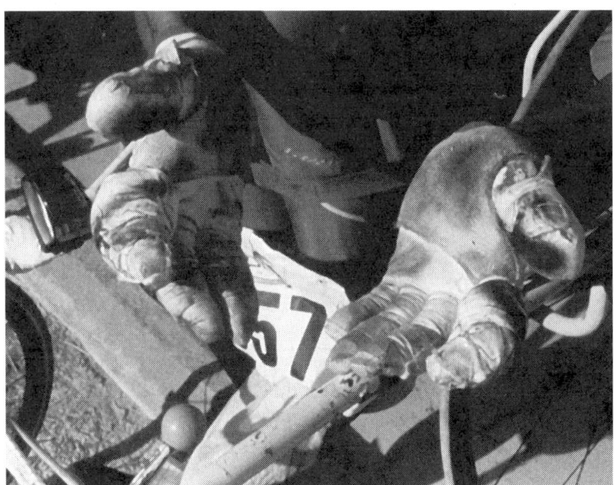

FIG. 33-11. Gloves reflecting the intensity of action of a wheelchair racer.

material, such as silicone liners, over these irritated areas, sports can be performed safely.

Athletes with Cerebral Palsy

Seizures are relatively frequent in individuals with cerebral palsy. Fifteen percent of the athletes on the Paralympic team had seizure conditions (87), although in actuality seizures have not turned out to be a problem. As outlined in a previous section, participation in sports tends to cause an increase in lactic acid (particularly if it is an aerobic sport), which lowers pH and leads to more stable membranes and less risk of seizure (87).

Athletes with cerebral palsy who use wheelchairs have shoulder and upper extremity injuries that are similar to those of spinal cord–injured athletes (114), whereas ambulatory athletes tend to have more knee injuries, as is common in all ambulatory athletes (114).

Athletes with Visual Impairment

Athletes with visual impairment do not have the visual cues in relation to road surfaces and conditions that could lead to injuries, such as walls, curbs, etc. Many events use a guide runner to assist the athlete with a visual impairment. However, the athletes may have different biomechanics because of changes in stepping frequency, stride length, and a prolonged stance phase, and excessive break in acceleration forces have been noted (37). Athletes with a visual impairment may expend more energy performing a task because of a lack of visual cues. This can lead to earlier fatigue and the potential of overuse injuries (Fig. 33-12).

Athletes with Mental Impairment

Although few athletes with Down syndrome compete in the Paralympics, there is an increased awareness of sports concerns for individuals with this condition (125). Due to the physical appearance of the athletes, it is the most recognized form of mental retardation. However, many orthopedic problems, often unrecognized, must be addressed. These include pes planus, patella instability, and atlantoaxial instability (126). Cervical instability has generated the most discussion and concern. In 1983, Special Olympics International (SOI) issued directives to all medical personnel, coaches, parents, and athletes restricting participation of athletes with Down syndrome until they had received medical examinations for atlantoaxial instability. This concern arose after detecting collagen and subsequently ligamentous laxity in a number of athletes. Researchers noted a prevalence of 10% to 20% of cervical spine instability (127–130). It either can be completely asymptomatic or can result in myelopathic changes including pain and motor deterioration. The Special Olympics in general now restricts these athletes from participating in activities that could produce hyperextension, hyperflexion, or direct pressure on the upper spine (130). Radiographic evidence must be presented to demonstrate normal atlantoaxial stability and no bony abnormalities for athletes to participate without any sports restrictions. Permanent

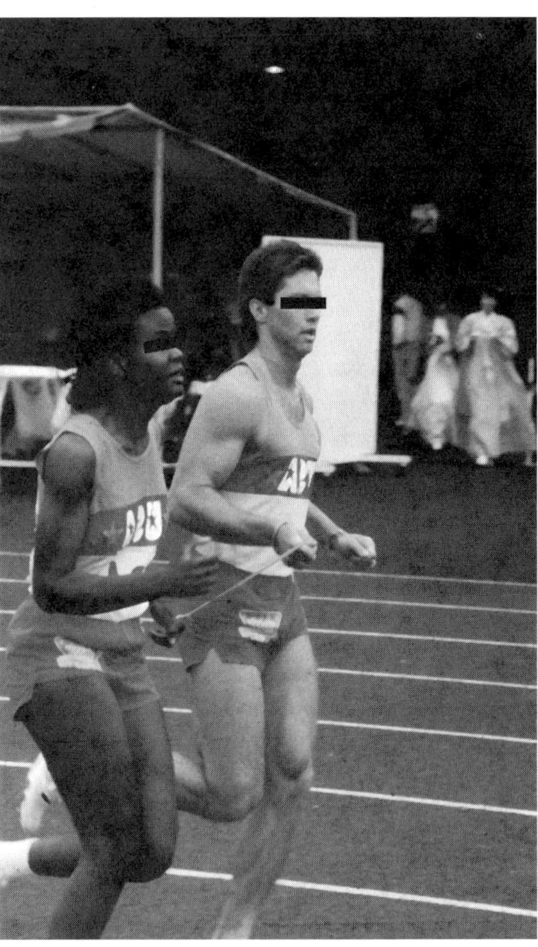

FIG. 33-12. Distance runner from IBSA with her guide runner. Note the cord attaching the two, but there must be very synchronized running styles.

sports restrictions are placed on athletes who illustrate positive radiographic evidence for cervical instability.

Multiple Sclerosis

The key sports restriction in athletes with multiple sclerosis is not to induce overfatigue and especially not to allow undue increases in the body core temperature because these may lead to an exacerbation of the condition (131). In this light it is advisable to counsel athletes with multiple sclerosis not to participate under conditions where core temperature will increase. Swimming is a particularly good sport for the individual with multiple sclerosis because the relative cool water temperature with a high specific heat actually tends to cool the athlete and therefore prevents increase in body core temperature.

Asthma

Asthma is a common disorder. Over 15% of the U.S. Olympic team competing in Los Angeles had asthma or exercise-induced asthma (132,133). Athletes who have this condition can minimize it by avoiding exercise during times of high pollution, such as during the heat of the day when the ozone level is higher. They often do better with a gradual, slow warm-up period. Dry air tends to aggravate broncospasms, and humid air tends to reduce them. Swimming is often an excellent exercise and sport option for asthmatics. The use of long-acting inhaled broncodilators such as albuterol is very affective in acute situations, whereas in a chronic situation use of anti-inflammatories such as nedocromil sodium or inhaled steroids are often very effective. Elite athletes on inhaled steroids must notify the USOC of their use of these medications.

Diabetes

Exercise is a key component in the treatment of insulin-dependent diabetes mellitus and non–insulin-dependent diabetes mellitus. Although there are potential problems such as the loss of glycemic control, with regular activity insulin requirements may change. Insulin may need to be decreased 1 to 2 units and or carbohydrate intake may be increased by 10 to 15 g of additional carbohydrates for every half hour of exercise. (134). It is recommended for diabetic athletes that 60% of calories consumed come from carbohydrates (135). For prolonged activities, 5 to 20 g of carbohydrates should be consumed for every 20 minutes of exercise. Individuals should be encouraged to eat 30 to 60 minutes before initiating activity. Because exercise may lower blood sugar levels for 24 to 48 hours after completion, additional carbohydrate should be consumed after completion of the activity. For prolonged and or exhaustive exercise, individuals should consume 1.5 g of carbohydrate per kilogram of body weight within 30 minutes postexercise and follow up with 1.5 g of carbohydrate per kilogram body weight 1 to 2 hours later (136). Blood glucose levels should be monitored before, during, and after exercise. Consideration should be given not only to the level but also to the rate at which blood glucose levels may change. An increase or decrease of blood glucose level in a short period of time may represent an unstable condition for exercising (137,138). If hypoglycemia occurs during exercise, the athlete should ingest a high-glucose drink or food and, if necessary, discontinue the activity (139). Frequently hypoglycemia may occur due to escalated absorption of insulin that has been injected into an active muscle. This is especially true when using short-acting insulin. The best injection sites are the buttocks and abdomen, where there is more adipose tissue and less active muscle being used (139).

Hyperglycemia is another complication that may occur during exercise. If blood glucose levels are over 250 mg/dl, the individual should monitor urine output for the presence of ketones (140). If ketones are present, exercise should be postponed. Individuals participating in prolonged cardiovascular activity may find that if glucose levels are over 200 mg/dl and no ketones are present, blood glucose levels may increase due to inadequate insulin absorption. These individuals may find it necessary to inject additional short-acting insulin before exercise at a rate of 2 units per 50 mg/dl over 200 mg/dl.

Diabetic athletes are more vulnerable during exercise in excessive heat. This may lead to dehydration, which should be avoided by drinking plenty of water. Because the body's thirst mechanism is lessened with exercise (137), cool, plain water should be consumed before, during, and after exercise. For activities lasting longer that 60 to 90 minutes, a fluid-replenishing drink such as Gatorade or diluted fruit juice may be necessary (137).

Individuals with diabetes should be encouraged to wear proper footwear and practice good foot hygiene. It may be helpful to obtain several pairs of exercise footwear and alternate shoes periodically to redistribute pressure points (141). Injuries to the foot, such as blisters or infections should be treated immediately. The diabetic athlete should always carry easily accessible glucose as well as medical alert information identification when exercising. If glucose levels are unstable, the individual should be encouraged to exercise with a partner who can provide or call for assistance (142).

An individual with diabetes should avoid prolonged isometrics or heavy resistance exercises, which increase blood pressure if retinopathy is present (139). Physicians should be aware that an individual on beta-blockers may be unable to experience symptoms of hypoglycemia and/or angina.

Obesity

Obesity is a common condition in American society. Unfortunately, it is a common cause of primary and secondary disabilities. As rehabilitationists, we must confront this epidemic. A high level of success is noted with an exercise program that increases caloric expenditure when joined with a decrease in caloric intake (143,144). It has been shown that one should not only decrease total calories consumed but also concentrate on reducing dietary fat to 20% to 30% of total calories for the most success (137). Exercise for the obese population should concentrate on the frequency of sessions. Initially, low-intensity, high-duration exercise should be performed five times a week to yield the best results. Low-intensity exercise may be more effective in decreasing fat stores than more intense exercise because at lower intensity, lipid mobilizing systems provide energy whereas the carbohydrate system is used during intense exercise. Intensity should be 50% of maximum for 45 to 60 minutes (137). Appropriate types of exercise include walking, recumbent cycling, and water exercise, as well as using a stair climber and rowing machine. The goal of exercise for this population is to increase caloric expenditure while decreasing problems such as joint and orthopedic trauma. Although water activities and cycling may be easier on the joints, water activities are often a good choice for conditioning but not for weight loss compared with land exercise because of the relatively low increase in core temperature; therefore, the metabolic rate increases little (145). Research suggests that adherence to an exercise program and compliance with exercise are more likely when individuals are involved in a supervised exercise program (137). Although more intense exercise may have more health benefits (146), the greatest health benefits may be observed in previously sedentary individuals who begin to practice any kind of exercise.

CONCLUSION

As discussed in this chapter, sports and recreation are valuable options for people with disabilities. The risks are real, but reasonable. In most cases, the risks are outweighed by tremendous benefits that are not only physiologic in nature, but also existential, psychological, and social.

ACKNOWLEDGMENT

We thank Marie Laidler for her clerical assistance.

REFERENCES

1. Barbour A. *A critique of the medical model*. Stanford, CA: Stanford University Press, 1995.
2. Orentlicher D. The legalization of physician-assisted suicide. *N Engl J Med* 1996; 335:663–667.
3. Cassell EJ. *The nature of suffering and the goals of medicine*. New York: Oxford University Press, 1991.
4. Frankl V. *The doctor and the soul from psychotherapy to logotherapy*, 2nd ed. New York: Vintage Books, 1986.
5. Richter KJ, Kaschalk SM. The future of therapeutic recreation: an existential outcome. In: Sylvester C, ed. *Philosophy of therapeutic recreation: ideas and issues*. Vol. 2. Arlington, VA: National Recreation and Park Association, 1996; 86–91.
6. *US Department of Health and Human Services Physical Activity and Health: A report of the Surgeon General*. Atlanta, GA: US Department of Health and Human Services, Center for Disease Control and Prevention, National Center for Chronic Disease Prevention and Health Promotion, 1996.
7. Wyeth DO. Breaking barriers and changing attitudes. *JOSM* November 1989; 5–10.
8. McCann C. Sports for the disabled: the evolution from rehabilitation to competitive sport. *Br J Sports Med* 1996; 30:279–280.
9. Guttman L. *Textbook of sport for the disabled*. Aylesbury, England: HM & M, 1976.
10. Watson-Jones R. Principles of rehabilitation after fractures and joint injuries. In: *Fractures and joint injuries*. Edinburgh, Scotland: ES Livingstone, 1955; 1019–1038.
11. Guttman L. Sport. In: *Spinal Cord Injuries: Comprehensive Management and Research*, 2nd ed. Oxford, England: Blackwell Scientific, 1976; 617–628.
12. Congressional Record. Public Law 101-476.
13. National Consortium for Physical Education and Recreation for Individuals with Disabilities. *Adapted physical education national standards*. Champaign, IL: Human Kinetics, 1995.
14. American Alliance for Health, Physical Education, Recreation, and Dance. *Guidelines for professional preparation programs for handicapped*. Washington, DC: Author, 1973.
15. Sherrill C. *Leadership training in adapted physical education*. Champaign, IL: Human Kinetics, 1988.
16. Sherrill C. *Adapted physical activity, recreation, and sport: Crossdisciplinary and lifespan*, 5th ed. Dubuque, IA: McGraw-Hill, 1998.
17. Sherrill C, DePauw K. Adapted physical activity and education. In: Massengale JD, Swanson RA, eds. *History of exercise and sport science*. Champaign, IL: Human Kinetics, 1997; 39–108.
18. Posse N. *The Swedish system of educational gymnastics*. Boston, Lee & Shepard, 1890.
19. Nissen H. *ABC of Swedish educational gymnastics*. New York: Educational Publishing, 1892.
20. Lowman C, Colestock E, Cooper H. *Corrective physical education for groups*. New York: Barnes, 1928.
21. Stafford G. *Preventive and corrective physical education*. New York: Barnes, 1928.
22. Rathbone J. *Corrective physical education*. Philadelphia: WB Saunders, 1934.
23. Winnick J. *Adapted physical education and sport*, 2nd ed. Champaign, IL: Human Kinetics, 1995.
24. Block ME. *A teacher's guide to including students with disabilities in regular physical education*. Baltimore: Paul H Brookes, 1994.
25. Twain M, ed. *The wit and wisdom of Mark Twain*. Philadelphia: Running Press, 1991.
26. Jennings B. Healing the self: The moral meaning of relationships in rehabilitation. *Am J Phys Med Rehabil* 1993; 72:401–404.
27. Datillo J, Kleiber DA. Psychological perspectives for therapeutic recreation research: the psychology of enjoyment. In: Malkin MJ, Howe CZ, eds. *Research in therapeutic recreation: concepts and methods*. State College, PA: Venture, 1993; 57–76.
28. American Therapeutic Recreation Association. Definition Statement. 1993.
29. Austin DR. *Therapeutic recreation: process and techniques*, 2nd ed. Champaign, IL: Sagamore, 1991.
30. Austin DR, Crawford ME, eds. *Therapeutic recreation: an introduction*. Englewood Cliffs, NJ: Prentice Hall, 1995.
31. Phillips DA, Zigler E. Self-concept theory and its practical implications. In: Yawkey TD, ed. *Self-concept of the young child: an anthology*. Provo, UT: Frnds of the Libry, 1980; 111–122.
32. Hamachek DE. *Encounters with the self*, 3rd ed. Fort Worth, TX: Holt, Rinehart & Winston, 1987.
33. Guttman L. Experimental studies on the value of archery in paraplegia. *Paraplegia* 1973; 11:105–110.
34. Kottke FJ, Kubicek WG, Olson ME, Hastings RH. Studies on the parameters of cardiovascular performance of quadriplegic patients. *Arch Phys Med Rehabil* 1963; 44:635–644.
35. Hullman K-D, List M, Matthes D, Wiese G, Zika D. Spiroergometric and telemetric investigations during the International Stoke Mandeville Games 1972 in Heidenberg. *Paraplegia* 1975; 13:109–123.
36. Jackson RW, Erickson FA. Sports for the physically disabled. The 1976 Olympiad. *Am J Sports Med* 1979; 7:293–296.
37. Ferrara MS, Buckley WE, McCann BC, Limbird TJ, Powell J, Robl R. The injury experience of the competitive athlete with a disability: prevention implications. *Med Sci Sports Exerc* 1992; 24:184–188.

38. Jokl E. *The clinical physiology of physical fitness and rehabilitation*. Springfield, IL: Charles C Thomas, 1958.
39. American College of Sports Medicine. *Guidelines for exercise testing and prescription*. Baltimore: Williams & Wilkins, 1995.
40. Rimmer JH, Braddock D, Pitetti KH. Research on physical activity and disability: an emerging national priority. *Med Sci Sports Exerc* 1996; 28:1366–1372.
41. Shephard RD. Exercise physiology and fitness in athletes with disabilities: an overview. In: Steadward RD, Nelson ER, Wheeler GD, eds. *Vista '93—the outlook*. Edmonton, Canada: University of Alberta, 1994; 19–45.
42. Shephard RD. *Fitness in special populations*. Champaign, IL: Human Kinetics, 1990.
43. Rimmer JH. *Fitness and rehabilitation programs for special populations*. Dubuque, IA: Brown & Benchmark, 1994.
44. Nelson MA, Harris SS. The benefits and risks of sports and exercise for children with chronic health conditions. In: Goldberg, ed. *Sports and exercise for children with chronic health conditions*. Champaign, IL: Human Kinetics, 1995.
45. McCubbin J. Physical fitness assessment and program considerations for persons with cerebral palsy or amputations: a review of research. In: Steadward RD, Nelson ER, Wheeler GD, eds. *Vista '93—the outlook*. Edmonton, Canada: University of Alberta, 1994; 58–70.
46. Durstine LP, Painter P, Bloomquist LE. *Exercise management for persons with chronic diseases and disabilities*. Indianapolis: American College of Sports Medicine (in press).
47. Sherrill C Social and psychological dimensions of sports for disabled athletes. In: Sherrill C, ed. *Sport and disabled athletes*. Champaign, IL: Human Kinetics, 1986; 21–33.
48. Brasile FM, Hedrick BN. A comparison of participation incentives between adult and youth wheelchair basketball players. *Palaestra* 1991; 7:40–46.
49. Veeger HEJ, Yahmed MH, van der Woude LHV, Charpentier P. Peak oxygen uptake and maximum aerobic power output of Olympic wheelchair-dependent athletes. *Medic Sci Sports* 1991; 23:1201–1209.
50. Stotts KM. Health maintenance: paraplegic athletics and nonathletes. *Arch Phys Med Rehabil* 1986; 67:109–114.
51. Santiago MC, Coyle CP, Kinney WB. Aerobic exercise effect on individuals with physical disabilities. *Arch Phys Med Rehabil* 1993; 74:1192–1198.
52. Glasser RW, Davis GM, Wheelchair-dependent individuals. In: Franklin BA, Gordon S, Timmis GC, eds. *Exercise in modern medicine*. Baltimore: Williams & Wilkins, 1989; 237–267.
53. Rimmer JH, Braddock D, Pitetti KH. Research on physical activity and disability: an emerging national priority. *Med Sci Sports Exerc* 1996; 28:1366–1372.
54. Hutzler Y, Bar-Eli M. Psychological benefits of sports for disabled people: a review. *Scand J Med Sci Sports* 1993; 3:217–228.
55. Sherrill C, Williams T. Disability and sport: psychosocial perspectives on inclusion, integration, and participation. *Sport Sci Rev* 1996; 5: 42–64.
56. Wheeler GD, Malone LA, VanVlack S, Nelson ER, Steadward RD. Retirement from disability sport: A pilot study. *Adapt Phys Activity Q* 1996; 13:382–399.
57. Sherrill C, Hinson M, Gench B, Kennedy SO, Low L. Self-concepts of disabled youth athletes. *Percept Motor Skills* 1990; 70:1093–1098.
58. Sherrill C. Disability identity and involvement in sport and exercise. In: Fox K, ed. *The physical self: from motivation to well-being*. Champaign, IL: Human Kinetics, 1997; 257–286.
59. Fagan W, Sherrill C, French R. Locus of control of quad rugby players and able-bodied men. *Clin Kinesiol* 1994; 49:53–57.
60. Sherrill C, Silliman L, Gench B, Hinson M. Self-actualization of elite wheelchair athletes. *Paraplegia* 1990; 28:252–260.
61. Ridgway ME, Boyd RL. Self-actualization of able-bodied and wheelchair male college students. *Braz Int J Adapt Phys Educ Res* 1994; 1:1–17.
62. Wuerch G, Sherrill C. Sport as empowerment: perspectives of women wheelchair road racers. (Submitted for publication).
63. Greenwood CM, Dzewaltowski DA, French R. Self-efficacy and psychological well-being of wheelchair tennis participants and wheelchair nontennis participants. *Adapt Phys Activity Q* 1990; 7:12–21.
64. Martin JJ, Adams-Mushett CA, Smith KL. Athletic identity and sport orientation of adolescent swimmers with disabilities. *Adapt Phys Activity Q* 1995; 12:113–123.
65. Martin JJ, Mushett CA. Social support mechanisms among athletes with disabilities. *Adapt Phys Activity Q* 1996; 13:74–83.
66. Campbell E, Jones G. Psychological well-being in sport participants and nonparticipants. *Adapt Phys Activity Q* 1994; 11:404–415.
67. Williams T. Disability sport socialization and identity construction. *Adapt Phys Activity Q* 1994; 11:14–31.
68. Sherrill C, Rainbolt W, Montelione T, Pope C. Sport socialization of blind and cerebral palsied elite athletes. In: Sherrill C, ed. *Sport and disabled athletes*. Champaign, IL: Human Kinetics, 1986; 189–195.
69. Disabled sports training book. In: Miller PD, ed. *Fitness programming and physical disability*. Champaign, IL: Human Kinetics, 1995; 73.
70. Kibler WB, Chandler TJ. Sports specific conditioning. *Am J Sports Med* 1994; 22:424–432.
71. Baechle TR, ed. *Essentials of strength training and conditioning*. National Strength and Conditioning Association. Champaign, IL: Human Kinetics, 1994.
72. Liow DK, Hopkins WG. Training practices of athletes with disabilities. *Adapt Phys Activity Q* 1996; 13:372–381.
73. Peach PE. Overwork weakness with evidence of muscle damage in a patient with residual paralysis from polio. *Arch Phys Med Rehabil* 1990; 71:248–50.
74. Pickering GW. The vasomotor regulation of heat loss from the skin in relation to external temperature. *Heart* 1932; 115–135.
75. Richter KJ, Ferrara MS, Adams-Mushett C, McCann BC. Integrated swimming classification: a faulted system. *Adapt Phys Activity Q* 1992; 9:5–13.
76. McCann BC. The medical disability-specific classification system in sports. In: Steadward RD, Nelson ER, Wheeler GD, eds. *Vista '93—the outlook*. Edmonton, Canada: Rick Hansen Centre, 1994; 275–288.
77. Bloch RF. Autonomic dysfunction. In: Bloch RF, Basbaum M, eds. *Management of spinal injuries*. Baltimore: Williams & Wilkins, 1986; 149–163.
78. Burnham R, Wheeler G, Bhambhani Y, Belanger M, Erickson P, Steadward R. Intentional induction of autonomic dysreflexia among quadriplegic athletes for performance enhancement: efficacy, safety, and mechanisms of action. In: Steadward RD, Nelson ER, Wheeler G, eds. *Vista '93—the outlook,* Edmonton, Canada: Rick Hansen Centre, 1994; 224–249.
79. Raymond S. Boosting. In: Steadward RD, Nelson ER, Wheeler GD, eds. *Vista '93—the outlook*. Edmonton, Canada: Rick Hansen Centre 1994; 242–249.
80. Benzinger TH. Heat regulation coma: homeostasis of central temperature in man. *Physiol Rev* 1969; 49:671–759.
81. Randall WC, Rawson RO, McCook RD, et al. Central peripheral factors in dynamic thermoregulation. *J Appl Physiol* 1963; 26:61–64.
82. Letha Y, Hunter-Griffin LC. *Athletic training in sports medicine,* 2nd ed. The American Academy of Orthopedic Surgeons, Rosemont, IL; 1991.
83. Colachis SC III, Otis SM. Thermal regulation and fever in SCI. *Am J Phys Med Rehabil* 1995; 74:114–119.
84. Simon E. Temperature regulation: the spinal cord is the sight of extra hypothalamic thermoregulator functions. *Rev Physiol Biochem Pharmacol* 1974; 71:1–76.
85. Downey RJ, Downey JA, Newhouse E, et al. Hypothermia in a quadriplegic: evidence for a peripheral action of haloperidol in malignant neuroleptic syndrome. *Chest* 1992; 101:1728–1730.
86. Downey JA, Chiodi HP, Darling RC. Central temperature regulation in the spinal man. *J Appl Physiol* 1967; 22:91–94.
87. Richter KJ. Seizures in athletes. *J Osteo Sports Med* 1989; 3:19–23.
88. *Medical evaluation of the athlete: a guide*. AMA Committee on the Medical Aspects of Sports, 1976.
89. Temkin NR, Davis GR. Stress risk factors for seizures among adults with epilepsy. *Epilepsia* 1984; 25:450–456.
90. Lennox, WG. *Science and seizures*. New York: Harper & Rowe, 1941; 134.
91. Ogunyemi AO, Gomez MR, Klass DW. Seizures induced by exercise. *Neurology* 1988; 38:633–634.
92. Livingston S, Thurmon W. Participation of epileptic patients in sports. *JAMA* 1973; 224:236–238.
93. Cowart US. Should epileptics exercise? *Phys Sports Med* 1986; 14: 183–191.
94. Gotze W, Kubicki S, Munter M, Teichmann J. Effect of physical

exercise on seizure threshold: investigation by electroencephalographic telemetry. *Dis Nervous Syst* 1967; 28:664–667.

95. Mitchell WG. Status epilepticus and acute repetitive seizures in children, adolescents, and young adults: etiology, outcome, and treatment. *Epilepsia* 1996; 37(suppl 1):S74–S80.
96. Mattson RH. Parental antiepileptic/anticonvulsant drugs. *Neurology* 1996; 46(suppl 1):8–13.
97. Knudsen FU. Plasma, diazepam and intra-rectal administration solution and by suppository. *Acta Paediatr Scand* 1977; 66:563–567.
98. Krag, et al. Blood level of diazepam, apozepam, in adults after rectal administration, In: Dam M, Gram L, Penry JK, eds. *Advances in epileptology: XII. Epilepsy in a national symposium*. New York: Raven, 1981; 569–573.
99. Minagawa K, Miura H, Mizuno S, et al. Pharamacokinetics of rectal diazepam in the prevention of recurrent febrile convulsions. *Brain Dev* 1986; 8:53–59.
100. Richter KJ. The drug dilemma: IOC, IPC, or perplexity? International Paralympic Congress Lecture. Atlanta Paralympics, Atlanta, Georgia, August 15, 1996.
101. Anderson LS, Biering-Sorensen F, Muller PG, Jensen IL, Aggerbeck B. The prevalence of hyperhidrosis in patients with spinal cord injuries and an evaluation of the effect of dextropropoxyphene hydrochloride in therapy. *Paraplegia* 1992; 30:184–191.
102. Bobath B. Motor development: its effect on the general development and application of treatment for cerebral palsy. *Physiotherapy* 1971; 57:526–532.
103. Huberman G. Organized sports activities with cerebral palsy. *Adolesc Rehabil Lit* 1976; 37:103–106.
104. Richter KJ, Gaebler-Spira D, Mushett CA. Annotation: sport and the person with spasticity of cerebral origin. *Dev Med Child Neurol* 1996; 38:867–870.
105. Richter KJ, Hyman DC, Mushett, CA, Ellenberg MD, Ferrara MJ. Injuries in world class cerebral palsy athletes of the 1988 Seoul Korea Paralympics. *J Osteo Sports Med* 1991; 5:15–18.
106. McCubbin J, Shasby G. Effects of isokinetic exercises in adolescents with cerebral palsy. *Adapt Phys Activity Q* 1985; 2:56–64.
107. Horvat M. Effects of a progressive resistance training program on an individual with spastic cerebral palsy. *Am Correct Ther J* 1987; 41: 7–11.
108. Damiano DL, Vaughan CL, Abel MF. Muscle response to heavy resistive exercise in children with spastic cerebral palsy. *Dev Med Child Neurol* 1995; 37:731–739.
109. Inaba M, Edberg E, Montgomery JN, Gillis MK. Effectiveness of functional training of active exercise and resistive exercises for patients with hemiplegia. *Phys Ther* 1973; 53:28–35.
110. Holland LJ, Steadward RD. Effects of resistance training in flexibility and strength, spasticity/muscle tone and range of motion in elite athletes with cerebral palsy. *Palestra* 1990; summer:27–31.
111. Mushett CA, Wyeth DO, Richter KJ. Cerebral palsy, traumatic brain injury, and stroke. In: Goldberg B, ed. *Sports and exercise for children with chronic health conditions*. Champaign, IL: Human Kinetics, 1995; 123–134.
112. Jankowski LW, Solomon J. Aerobic and neuromuscular training: the effect of the capacity, efficacy, and fatiguability of patients with traumatic brain injuries. *Arch Phys Med Rehabil* 1990; 71:500–504.
113. Birrer RB. The Special Olympics: an injury overview. *Phys Sports Med* 1985; October:15–18.
114. Ferrara MS, Buckley WE. Athletes with disabilities injury registry. *Adapt Phys Activity Quarterly* 1996; 13:50–60.
115. McCormick DP. Injuries in handicapped alpine ski racers. *Phys Sports Med* 1985; 13:93–97.
116. Taylor D, Williams T. Sports injuries in athletes with disabilities wheelchair racing. *Paraplegia* 1995; 33:296–299.
117. Curtis KA, Dillon DA. Survey of wheelchair athletic injuries: common patterns and prevention. *Paraplegia* 1985; 23:170–175.
118. Ferrara MS, Davis R. Injuries to elite wheelchair athletes. *Paraplegia* 1990; 28:335–341.
119. Jackson DL, Hynninen BC, Caborn DNM, McLean J. Electrodiagnostic study of carpal tunnel syndrome in wheelchair basketball players. *Clin J Sports Med* 1996; 6:27–31.
120. Boninger ML, Robertson RN, Wolff M, Cooper RA. Upper limb nerve entrapments in elite wheelchair racers. *Am J Phys Med Rehabil* 1996; 75:170–176.
121. Gehlsen GM, Davis RW, Bahmond R. Intermittent velocity and wheelchair performance characteristics. *Adapt Phys Activity Q* 1990; 7:219–230.
122. Burnham RS, May L, Nelson E, Steadward RD, Reid DC. Shoulder pain in wheelchair athletes—the role of muscle imbalance. *Am J of Sport Med* 1993; 21:238–242.
123. Disabled sports training book. In: Miller PD, ed. *Fitness programming and physical disability*. Champaign, IL: Human Kinetics, 1995.
124. Richter KJ. Book review of *Fitness programming and physical disability*. *Ther Rec J* 1996; 30:150–151.
125. Fernhall B, Pitetti KH, Rimmer J, et al. Cardiorespirator capacity of individuals with mental retardation including Down syndrome. *Med Sci Sports Exerc* 1997; 29:366–371.
126. Hudson PB. Preparticipation screening of Special Olympic athletes. *Phys Sports Med* 1988; 16:97–104.
127. Atlantoaxial instability in Down's syndrome orthopedic clinics in North America. *Phys Sports Med* 1984; 74:152–154.
128. Diamond LS, Lynne KD, Sigman B. Orthopedic disorders in patients with Down's syndrome. *Orthop Clin North Am* 1981; 12:57–71.
129. Hreidarsson S, Magren G, Singer H. Symptomatic atlantoaxial dislocation in Down's syndrome. *Pediatrics* 1982; 69:568–571.
130. Special Olympic summer sports rules: #6. Participation by individuals with Down's syndrome who suffer from the atlantoaxial dislocation condition. Washington, D.C., 1992, revised 1995.
131. Olgiati R, Jacquet J, DiPrampero PE. Energy cost of walking and exertional dyspnea in multiple sclerosis. *Am Rev Respir Dis* 1986; 134:1005–1010.
132. Pierson WE, Voy RO. Exercise induced broncho-spasm in the XXIII Summer Olympic Games. *NE Reg Allergy Pro* 1988; 9:209–213.
133. Voy RO. US Olympic Committee experience with exercise induced bronchospasm. *Med Sci Sports Exerc* 1986; 18:328–330.
134. Nathan DM, Madnek SF, Delahanty L. Programming pre-exercise snacks to prevent post-exercise hypoglycemia in intensively treated insulin-dependent diabetics. *Ann Intern Med* 1985; 102:483–486.
135. Position of the American Dietetic Association and the Canadien Dietetic Association: nutrition for physical fitness and athletic performance for adults. *J Am Diet Assoc* 1993; 93:691–696.
136. Ivy JL, Katz AL, Cutler CL, Sherman WM, Coyle EF. Muscle glycogen synthesis after exercise; effect of time of carbohydrate ingestion. *J Appl Physiol* 1988; 64:1480–1484.
137. Ruderman N, Devlin J, eds. *The health professional's guide to diabetes and exercise*. Denver, CO: American Diabetes Association, 1995; 42–130.
138. Hall M. Sport and diabetes. *Br J Sports Med* 1997; 31:3.
139. Horton ES. Role and management of exercise in diabetes mellitus. *Diabetes Care* 1988; 11:201–211.
140. Wilberg-Henriksson H. Exercise and diabetes mellitus. *Exerc Sport Sci Rev* 1992; 20:330–368.
141. Ferrara MS, Richter KJ, Kaschalk SM. Sport for the athlete with a physical disability. In: Scuderi G, McCann P, Bruno P, eds. *Sports medicine: principles of primary care*. Philadelphia: Mosby-Year Book, 1997; 598–608.
142. American College of Sports Medicine and American Diabetes Association (Joint Position Statement). Diabetes mellitus and exercise. *Medicine and Science in Sports and Exercise* 1997; 12:i–vi.
143. Bennett WI. Beyond overeating. *N Engl J Med* 1995; 332:673–674.
144. Leibel RL, Rosenbaum M, Hirsch J. Changes in energy expenditure resulting from altered body weight. *N Engl J Med* 1995; 332:621–28.
145. Pate RR, Blair SN, Durstine JL, et al. *Guidelines for exercise testing and prescription: ACSM*, 4th ed. Philadelphia-London: Lea & Febiger, 1991.
146. Lee I, Hsieh C, Paffenbarger RS Jr. Exercise intensity and longevity in men. *JAMA* 1995; 273:1179–1184.

Rehabilitation Medicine: Principles and Practice, Third Edition,
edited by Joel A. DeLisa and Bruce M. Gans.
Lippincott–Raven Publishers, Philadelphia © 1998.

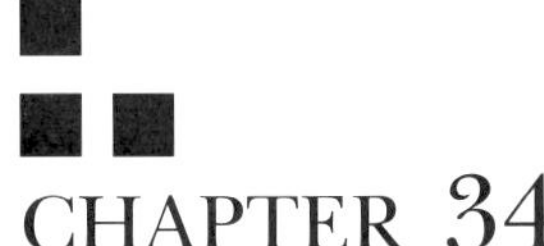

CHAPTER 34

Complementary and Alternative Medicine

Samuel C. Shiflett, Nancy E. Schoenberger, Bruce J. Diamond, Sangeetha Nayak, and Ann C. Cotter

The term ''alternative medicine'' refers to a broad range of treatments and practices that are generally not used or recommended within the context of the mainstream biomedical community. In this sense, a technique is defined as alternative through a social normative process (1). If the prevailing biomedical community within a particular country or culture accepts it, it is conventional; if it does not accept it, it is alternative. For example, some therapies, such as herbal therapies, that are considered alternative in the United States are a part of mainstream medical practice in many European countries. Using the same normative approach, some therapies that are routinely used in physical medicine and rehabilitation (PM&R), such as biofeedback, would still be considered alternative in the context of the broader biomedical community.

S. C. Shiflett: Departments of Psychiatry and Physical Medicine and Rehabilitation, University of Medicine and Dentistry of New Jersey, New Jersey Medical School, Newark, New Jersey 07103; and Center for Research in Complementary and Alternative Medicine, Kessler Medical Rehabilitation and Education Corporation, West Orange, New Jersey 07052.

N. E. Schoenberger: Departments of Psychiatry and Physical Medicine and Rehabilitation, University of Medicine and Dentistry of New Jersey, New Jersey Medical School, Newark, New Jersey 07103; and Kessler Medical Rehabilitation and Education Corporation, West Orange, New Jersey 07052.

B. J. Diamond: Departments of Physical Medicine and Rehabilitation and Research, University of Medicine and Dentistry of New Jersey, New Jersey Medical School, Newark, New Jersey 07103; and Kessler Medical Rehabilitation and Education Corporation, West Orange, New Jersey 07052.

S. Nayak: Research Department, Kessler Medical Rehabilitation and Education Corporation, West Orange, New Jersey 07052.

A. C. Cotter: Department of Physical Medicine and Rehabilitation, University of Medicine and Dentistry of New Jersey, New Jersey Medical School, Newark, New Jersey 07103; and Physical Medicine and Rehabilitation Service, Veterans Administration Medical Center, East Orange, New Jersey; and Center for Complementary and Alternative Medicine, Kessler Medical Rehabilitation and Education Corporation, West Orange, New Jersey 07052.

There are at least two other meanings of the term ''alternative.'' First, many, but by no means all, alternative therapies postulate an underlying model of action or of the nature of the body and of the physical world that is completely different from the standard Western scientific understanding of the physiology and anatomy of the human body, and of the nature of matter and energy. Consequently, those techniques that do not have an underlying model or obvious mechanism of action that is consistent with Western scientific thought are often rejected as mere superstition. Second, the term ''alternative'' is frequently used to refer to a technique that is used instead of conventional medical treatment. For this reason, the term ''complementary medicine'' has become popular because it connotes the idea that several therapies, both conventional and unconventional, may be used together to complement each other in the treatment of a medical problem. The phrases complementary and alternative medicine (CAM) and unconventional therapies will be used interchangeably to refer to practices and therapies that are not commonly used in mainstream medicine within the United States.

After World War II, the distinctive field of PM&R evolved in response to the fact that mainstream medicine was not providing adequate care and treatment for patients who had sustained injuries to the musculoskeletal and central nervous systems. In his pioneering book, *The Knife Is Not Enough,* Dr. Henry H. Kessler clearly espoused the need for what are today called complementary and alternative therapies (2). He included not only physical and dietary interventions in his multidisciplinary approach, but he also recognized the important role that spirituality plays in healing. This approach has marked PM&R with more openness to alternative therapies than other specialties.

Because of limited space, this chapter will focus primarily on CAM therapies applied to injury to the central nervous system: stroke, traumatic brain injury, and spinal cord injury. The goals of this chapter are (a) to provide a brief introduc-

TABLE 34-1. *Complementary and alternative techniques*

Categories of complementary and alternative medicine	Examples
Alternative medical systems	
Traditional indigenous systems	Ayurvedic medicine, Native American medicine, traditional Chinese medicine
Unconventional western systems	Homeopathy, environmental medicine, naturopathy
Bodywork	
Acupoint therapies	Acupuncture, acupressure, reflexology
Manual manipulation methods	Massage, craniosacral therapy, polarity therapy, applied kinesiology, structural integration (Rolfing)
Mind–body intervention	
Mind methods	Meditation, hypnosis, biofeedback, imagery, support groups, music therapy, art therapy, animal-assisted therapy
Body/movement methods	Yoga, tai chi, Feldenkrais method, Alexander technique, Pilates method, dance therapy
Religion and spirituality	Prayer, spiritual healing
Biofield energy techniques	Therapeutic touch, Reiki, Qigong, laying-on of hands
Electromagnetic applications	Unconventional uses of electrical and magnetic stimulation
Diet/nutritional supplements	
Special diet therapies	Ornish, fasting, folk and cultural foods
Nutritional supplements	High-dose vitamin/mineral supplements, choline, DHEA
Phytotherapy (herbals)	Plant-derived preparations such as ginkgo biloba extract, Oriental herbs
Pharmacologic approaches	EDTA chelation therapy, hyperbaric oxygen therapy, DMSO

DHEA, dehydroepiandrosterone; DMSO, dimethyl sulfoxide; EDTA, ethylenediamine-tetraacetic acid.

tion to the major alternative therapies that may be used by rehabilitation patients, so that the rehabilitation professional can discuss them with patients in an informed manner when the subject arises; and (b) to provide summaries of the research status regarding efficacy and safety of some of the more commonly encountered unconventional therapies for those techniques that have been subjected to such study. The mention of the technique does not constitute a recommendation or any acknowledgment of research evidence of effectiveness and safety.

Table 34-1 presents a category system useful for organizing the various complementary and alternative techniques applicable to the rehabilitation process. Under each modality are listed the specific techniques that we have encountered being used or recommended for outcomes associated with central nervous system injury. These techniques represent a subset of all CAM therapies.

TRADITIONAL (ETHNIC) MEDICINE AND ALTERNATIVE SYSTEMS OF MEDICAL PRACTICE

Alternative healing systems usually involve a set of practices and remedies that include a number of different modalities and are based on an underlying model of the healing process, which may or may not correspond to conventional medical models. Alternative systems of medicine include such practices as naturopathic medicine and homeopathy, as well as traditional and ethnic medical approaches. Naturopathy is a system that stresses health maintenance and disease prevention through patient education and acceptance of responsibility for one's own health. Underlying the various treatments in naturopathic medicine is the belief in the healing power of nature and the innate intelligence of the body that strives for health. Homeopathy is a method of innate self-healing that relies on small doses of highly diluted medicinal substances. An underlying assumption in the system is the principle of similars, which postulates that substances causing symptoms similar to those of the presenting disease have the capacity to cure that disease. Indigenous systems, such as Ayurveda (the medical tradition from India), traditional Chinese medicine (TCM), and Native American health care, etc., may be included in this category and involve systems of medicine that have been in use for centuries and have emerged over time in the context of a specific ethnic or cultural group. Little research has been conducted on any of these systems of care as a whole. Rather, each modality used within that system tends to be studied in isolation. For example, TCM includes in its medical practices the arts of acupuncture, herbal medicine, massage, bioenergy healing, meditation, and movement therapy. To simplify presentation of the material here and to reflect the manner in which these treatment modalities are typically studied in scientific research projects, we will focus on specific treatment techniques, rather than on their underlying medical system. In doing so, we acknowledge the fact that we may be doing a disservice to understanding the holistic approach that is the basis of most of these systems.

BODYWORK

Bodywork refers to therapies that are used to improve the structure and function of the human body by directly contacting the skin and generally involve manipulation of the musculoskeletal structure. Although often considered to be unconventional in mainstream medicine, many forms of physical manipulation have been used for years in the field of PM&R, including massage and physical therapy. There are numerous variations of this basic modality, and a detailed discussion of this general approach is presented in Chapter 22. Less conventional bodywork concepts and techniques are discussed in this chapter. An excellent introduction to a number of bodywork, mind-body, and energy techniques applied to the rehabilitation process can be found elsewhere (3).

Acupuncture

Acupuncture has been used in TCM for over 3,000 years, generally in conjunction with other techniques, including herbal medicine and massage. A concept that is central to its use is the idea that the basis for life is qi (pronounced chee), the vital life energy that runs through the body in 12 major pathways or channels called meridians. These channels correspond to the major organ functions of the body. Illness is believed to result from an improper amount of or imbalance in this energy. By inserting thin, noncutting needles into specific points along these meridians, it is believed that the energy flowing in these meridians can be corrected and balanced in the sickly person (4,5). From the perspective of Western medicine, these meridians have not been shown to correspond to any known anatomic or physiologic systems.

In recent years, a number of new forms of acupuncture have emerged that have varying degrees of similarity to TCM acupuncture. Attempts to understand the effects of acupuncture from a conventional physical model have resulted in the emergence of Western acupuncture, which postulates that biochemical substances, such as endorphins, or electrophysiologic changes induced by the insertion of the needles mediate any observed change in function (rather than affecting the life force). Choice of acupuncture points is based more on conventional Western diagnoses rather than on traditional Chinese methods of diagnosis; consequently, some purists feel that Western acupuncture is a treatment modality distinct from TCM acupuncture. In addition, some forms of acupuncture involve sending a low-voltage electric current across the needles to strengthen the effects of the needles (electroacupuncture or transcutaneous electrical nerve stimulation [TENS] acupuncture). Other forms of acupuncture include auricular acupuncture, scalp acupuncture, Korean hand acupuncture, and laser acupuncture, which uses a high-wavelength and low-energy laser (6).

Acupuncture has been used to treat various neurologic diseases and conditions, including paralysis, acute partial ischemic stroke, stroke during the subacute phase, cerebrovascular disease, aphasia, parkinsonism, and multiple sclerosis. Research on the effectiveness of acupuncture is abundant, although many of the reports involve case studies rather than controlled research protocols. Several studies have reported that acupuncture has shown efficacy in the treatment of stroke. For example, it has been hypothesized that the sensory stimulation of traditional acupuncture points with needles and electrostimulation may promote the restructuring and consolidation of coordinated motor function of affected limbs in the stroke patient, thus serving to enhance the recovery of postural control (7). Severe hemiparetic patients who were receiving acupuncture were reported to have recovered faster and to have displayed significant improvements in balance, mobility, and quality of life scores versus a nontreatment control group (8).

Acupuncture has been reported to work best when used as early as possible on stroke patients, and it appears to be more effective with stroke patients if their lesions are singular, shallow, and with a small focus, instead of large, bilateral lesions with deep multiple foci (9). In a study of paralysis in chronic and acute stroke patients, acupuncture appeared to induce improvement in most patients, but the best outcome was found in the acupuncture group given treatment less than 3 months after stroke onset, with greater efficacy reported when treatment was administered less than 36 hours after the stroke (10). This same study also reported that patients exhibiting a beneficial response to treatment had damage to less than half of the motor pathway areas, as seen on computed tomography scans, and that this damage did not involve the periventricular white matter areas (which contain many descending pyramidal tract pathways) (10).

Research using animal models has reported that rats treated with electro-acupuncture exhibit spontaneous sprouting of severed sciatic nerve tissue, with a 14% to 30% increase in regeneration rate compared with the no-treatment group (11). Thus, acupuncture appeared to induce regeneration in nerve tissue. Furthermore, results from rat models, in which spinal cord contusion was induced, suggest that electro-acupuncture applied 1 hour after spinal cord injury decreased posttraumatic sequelae (12).

Acupuncture generally has been found to be safe, and the rare complications can be minimized by using licensed practitioners (13). Overall, acupuncture shows promise as an alternative treatment modality, but its efficacy must be substantiated in rigorously designed clinical studies.

Acupressure

Acupressure is a technique based on the concept of meridians and acupoints, but instead of needle insertion, pressure is applied to the acupoint. There is some evidence that acupressure may help alleviate pain, nausea, and motion sickness, but the evidence is not strong (14–16). Its usefulness in treating neurologic injury is undocumented. Furthermore, the assumption that acupressure works in the same manner as acupuncture may be unwarranted because the mechanics of inserting a needle may be quite different from pressure on the same point. Nevertheless, its similarity to trigger point therapy and related treatment modalities involving pressure suggests that it may have some utility, especially in patients reluctant to have needles inserted. The Japanese version of acupressure is called shiatsu and is often used in conjunction with other massage techniques.

Reflexology

Reflexology is a point-pressure modality. This technique is based on the concept that the body is represented in zones on the hands and the feet and that pressure on specific points ''reflexively'' adjusts problems in the areas of the body represented by the point being manipulated. These zones may correspond to the meridians in TCM (17). Although reflexology has shown some efficacy in improving general health and feelings of well-being, its ability to treat neurologic injury is unknown. It is sometimes used as a part of a more general approach referred to as sensorimotor development, which uses a number of different techniques that attempt to re-establish the neurologic connections between the brain and motor system (18) and has been applied to stroke, brain injury, and childhood developmental disorders, including cerebral palsy and Down syndrome.

Craniosacral Therapy

Craniosacral therapy is a gentle, noninvasive manipulative technique applied to the spinal cord and cranium to correct disruptions in the craniosacral rhythmic activity. This activity is believed to be disrupted in spinal cord and traumatic brain injury, and so one of the major focuses of this technique has been this type of injury (19,20). The technique has been in use for over 20 years, and Upledger (19,20) has reported success in treating chronic pain, chronic brain dysfunction, spasticity and other conditions associated with spinal cord injury. A number of other conditions also have been treated with this technique, but there is little formal research supporting its efficacy.

Polarity Therapy

This is a method of energy manipulation that is based on the principle that every cell has both negative and positive poles. Subtle touch or pressure is applied on specific points to harmonize the flow of energy through the body and to enhance the body's structural balance (21).

Applied Kinesiology

Applied kinesiology is a method of diagnosis and treatment that assumes that muscles are related to specific organs, and the state of the muscle reflects the general state of its associated organ or system. Testing for weak or strong muscles permits a diagnosis and specific treatment involving one or more of several techniques, including pressure on acupoints, spinal manipulation, and nutritional adjustment (22,23). The technique is used extensively by chiropractors and osteopaths as well as other bodywork specialists and can be used to correct structural imbalances, joint problems, and musculoskeletal problems. A similar technique, called Touch for Health, is oriented more to non–health-care professionals (24).

MIND–BODY INTERVENTIONS

The basic premise of mind–body interventions is that the mind is not dualistically distinct from the body. The mind and body are assumed to be integrally related such that the mind influences the body and, in turn, is influenced by it. Mind or mental techniques include visual imagery, art and music therapy, biofeedback, hypnosis, meditation, and prayer, all of which act directly on the mind to alter its state and indirectly on physical conditions affected or controlled by the mind, such as hypertension and pain. A discussion of biofeedback is presented in Chapter 21. In this context, body techniques (in contrast to bodywork techniques), are basically movement therapies, and include such techniques as yoga, tai chi, and dance therapy. They can affect the body directly and also are used to alter the state of the mind, most often to treat mental conditions such as depression, anxiety, and stress. The use of yoga and tai chi in the treatment of pain and musculoskeletal conditions is becoming increasingly commonplace. Techniques described in greater detail in this section have shown some indication that they may have a rehabilitation-related benefit above and beyond their beneficial impact on mood.

Hypnosis

Hypnosis is effective as a treatment for psychological issues and symptoms (25). When psychological factors interfere with patients' progress in rehabilitation, hypnotherapy can improve mood and attitudes, increase motivation and feelings of self-efficacy, and decrease negative behaviors so that physical rehabilitation can produce greater functional improvement. In light of substantial evidence that hypnosis can affect physiologic functioning, some advocates have suggested that there may be physical changes after hypnotic treatment of stroke and neurologic disorders that are not mediated by psychological variables (26).

There are some limited examples in the research literature of hypnotherapy in the treatment of stroke, spinal cord injury, and traumatic brain injury. Most published reports are case studies, and many of them focus on the psychological aspects of rehabilitation, including motivation, compliance, self-efficacy, self-control, and anxiety (27,28). A few reports target physical symptoms, including hemiplegia, spasticity, and speech impairment. In case reports of patients treated with hypnosis after a stroke, increased movement in hemiplegic limbs and improved ambulation were observed (26,29,30), as well as the return of normal speech (26,30). One young man who was treated with hypnosis and self-hypnosis after spinal cord injury reported showing decreased phantom pain in his paralyzed arm, allowing a return to work (31), and another showed improved strength, decreased pain, and increased functional use of his arms (32). Attempts to treat spasticity have apparently been less successful (33).

Hypnosis was used in the treatment of headache or vertigo after brain injury in a sample of 155 patients. Almost half of the patients reported resolution of symptoms, and another 20% experienced significant symptom reduction (34). Outcome was best for those who had been injured less than 6 months before treatment. In two cases, reports of young people with traumatic brain injuries, hypnotic treatment was followed by increased interaction with others, improved mood, increased participation in treatment, and substantial gains in physical therapy (26).

Although these studies are encouraging, the lack of control conditions makes the results inconclusive. In the stroke and brain injury case studies, for example, results are confounded because they occurred during the first year after the accident, a period during which spontaneous recovery is still probable.

Meditation

In some form, meditation has long been used in many cultures, both Eastern and Western. Originally, it was tied to religious practices and was performed with spiritual goals of enlightenment and closeness with a deity. Modern forms of meditation have separated the techniques from their religious contexts, and the goals for which meditation is used have become more concrete, for example, decreased anxiety and improved health. Although there are many forms of meditation, most are intended to create a state of physical and mental relaxation, and people sit or lie quietly while focusing on one or two stimuli, such as their breathing patterns, a word, or an image.

There has been extensive research on the impact of meditation on physical and psychological problems. The most robust finding is the success of meditation for reducing hypertension (35–38), and there is also evidence of reduction in cholesterol level (39). Research evidence for the effectiveness of meditation in the rehabilitation process is extremely limited. Yoffe (40) wrote an anecdotal report about her experiences after a stroke at 30 years of age that resulted in hemiplegia. She feels that the meditation process was directly responsible for her ability to walk without a cane or leg brace 9 months after her stroke and, based on her experience, has developed a treatment program for stroke patients that includes meditation as a core component. Her progress cannot be conclusively attributed to meditation, however, because spontaneous recovery can occur for at least a year after stroke.

Given the success of meditation for reducing hypertension and the fact that hypertension is a predisposing factor for stroke and recurrence of stroke, it seems reasonable to conclude that meditation may be effective in reduction of risk for stroke. Although no studies were located that address the issue of stroke prevention specifically, regular practice of transcendental meditation in a group of elderly nursing home residents (a) significantly reduced systolic blood pressure and (b) significantly increased 3-year survival rates when compared with simple relaxation and no treatment. One hundred percent of the transcendental meditation group were alive after 3 years versus 68% of the no-treatment group (41). Meditation has been shown to improve cognitive functioning in college students and elderly adults who have no history of head injury (41,42). However, its applicability to head-injured patients is unknown.

Music Therapy

Music therapy is a rapidly evolving field with many clinical applications, especially in the rehabilitation of stroke and brain-injured patients having difficulty in communication and emotional expression (43). One of the advantages of music therapy lies in the diversity of techniques it has to offer and its applicability to a range of clinical symptoms and etiologies. It is helpful in minimizing stress and anxiety, improving mood and level of comfort, reducing feelings of isolation, encouraging verbal and nonverbal communication, and improving immune functioning (44,45). Research with traumatic brain injury patients suggests that music therapy can aid in muscular coordination (46,47); a variety of motor symptoms, including rigidity, spasticity, tremor, and ataxia (47); and emotional empathy (48). Music therapy has been used in conjunction with physical rehabilitation in spinal cord injury as well as brain injury and stroke (49). Although there is a large literature on the usefulness of music therapy as a general therapeutic modality, data substantiating its beneficial effects in rehabilitation of stroke and brain injury are limited.

Prayer and Spiritual Healing

Prayer is discussed here as a mental process outside the context of any particular religious system. There are a number of studies that demonstrate the efficacy of prayer for nonhuman subjects, including mice, yeast, bacteria, fungi, flagellates, plants, and seeds, as well as for in vitro samples of human tissue, such as red blood cells and cancer cells (50). Comparatively, there are fewer studies involving human subjects, and the research methodology is generally weaker (51–53). Nevertheless, approximately one half of the stronger studies showed some positive effect due to prayer. One of the best controlled studies (a randomized, double-blind study in which neither the patients, nurses, nor doctors knew the group assignment of patients) demonstrated a strong, beneficial effect of prayer on coronary care unit patients. The prayed-for group was less likely to require antibiotics or endotracheal entubation, were less likely to develop pulmonary edema, and were less likely to die (54).

Animal Assisted Therapy

Pet therapy, also referred to as animal-assisted therapy (AAT), has its origins during World War I when pets were brought into an Air Force convalescence center to offer companionship to servicemen. The research literature indicates that patients benefit socially (e.g., interact more with other people), physically (e.g., decreased cardiovascular risk and blood pressure), and psychologically (e.g., improved sense of well-being and self-esteem) from interacting with animals (55–58). It is argued that contact with animals provides patients with a unique aspect of healing that is separate from that provided by medications and other forms of treatment and human contact.

Another area that involves the use of animal-assisted therapy is therapeutic riding for the physically handicapped, including individuals with cerebral palsy, multiple sclerosis, spinal deformities, paraplegia, muscular dystrophy, and lumbago. Therapeutic riding, as applied to rehabilitation, involves three major areas of concentration (59):

1. Hippotherapy is a passive form of horse riding where the patient allows the horse to move the rider. The movement of the horse exercises both sides of the patient's body, approximating a human gait.
2. Riding therapy is a more active form of hippotherapy and involves the practice of physiotherapeutic exercise on horseback.
3. Riding for rehabilitation is the next step for the patient after he or she has been involved with hippotherapy or riding therapy. Here the patient makes the transition to taking more control of the horse and improving coordination.

A study of 67 paraplegic and quadriplegic patients who participated in an 18-month hippotherapy program reported that the program had lasting effects in many areas, including decreased spasticity, easier catheterization, improved bowel functioning, more balanced mood, and improved sleep (60).

One of the chief concerns about bringing animals into a hospital/health-care setting has been the transmission of zoonoses (61,62). However, this is a concern that can easily be remedied by careful screening and appropriate immunization of the animals before therapy. In addition, the animals need to be screened for biting and scratching and must be constantly accompanied by a program host or supervisor (61,62). Allergy to horses has occasionally been observed in disabled children participating in therapeutic riding sessions (63). Nevertheless, successful programs have been instituted in a number of acute rehabilitation settings.

MOVEMENT THERAPIES

Described here are five of the more popular movement techniques in use today: yoga, tai chi, the Alexander Technique, the Feldenkrais method, and the Pilates (pi-*la*-tes) technique. These techniques are similar in that they aim to improve a patient's kinesthetic awareness, awareness and control of breathing, and ease, control, and joy in everyday movement. All may be useful for a wide spectrum of patients from severely physically challenged to high-performance athletes.

Yoga and tai chi, the oldest techniques described, are frequently referred to as mind–body techniques because they actively seek to balance both physical and nonphysical aspects of the person. Both encourage a relaxed focus, are meditative in nature, and are part of a larger philosophy or way of life. Both derive from a broader system of health with an underlying model that is not easily integrated into Western biomedical models. The other three techniques described take a more functional approach, were developed in the early and middle parts of the 20th century, and to some extent were influenced by the older, Eastern approaches. All of the techniques take a less focal and more global approach to rehabilitation of specific conditions based on the rationale that the whole body is involved in all movement. For a discussion of other therapeutic exercise techniques, see Chapter 28.

Yoga

Yoga is an ancient Indian art first brought to this country in the mid-1800s. In Sanskrit, the word "yoga" means union (with God), is a way of life involving a number of different spiritual practices or yogas, and encompasses ethical conduct, social responsibility, nutrition, and physical health practices. The branch of yoga that is best known in the West is hatha yoga, and is often simply referred to as yoga. It is practiced for the achievement of physical strength, flexibility, and relaxation through postures known as asanas (*a*-sana), which are maintained for a specific period of time, from several seconds to several minutes. Pranayama (pra-na-*ya*-ma), or breathing techniques, and meditation are also often practiced along with hatha yoga.

Yoga has been extensively studied both in India and the West, with thousands of studies reporting positive health effects, including lowering of blood pressure (64) and decreased cholesterol levels (65). Yoga has been applied to programs for rheumatoid arthritis (66), osteoarthritis (67), chronic back pain (68), cardiac rehabilitation (69), carpal tunnel syndrome (67), and improved athletic performance (70). Yoga may easily be integrated into the office setting with an instructor who is experienced in teaching students with neurologic and orthopedic conditions. Yoga classes are a convenient way to transition from the physical therapy supervision to a home-based program.

Tai Chi

Tai chi is a form of postures and movements that dates back to the 17th century in China. Tai chi is made up of a series of linked contrasting movements, with constant weight shifting from one leg to another, changing of direction, and moving the arms in space. Specific postures are moved through with the focus on achieving balanced, graceful movement. Because it is a slow, rhythmic, weight-bearing exercise, participants are able to improve balance, coordination, concentration, and relieve stress in a safe manner. Reports on the benefits of tai chi include improved cardiorespiratory function, improved strength and balance, decreased falls in the elderly (71–73), and improved psychological parameters (74). Improved strength and energy have occurred in patients with chronic fatigue syndrome (75).

Movement Awareness Techniques

The Alexander technique attempts to improve cervical posturing by focusing on developing a balance between the head and neck in static and dynamic situations, as well as proper breathing (76). Most sessions are one on one, with the practitioner directing the student verbally and with light touch into postures that will help him or her to experience the state of being in proper alignment. Alexander practitioners are consulted for any patient with postural difficulties, chronic and occupational back and neck pain, or for improved performance in athletics and the performing arts.

The Feldenkrais method represents a specific integration of physics, Judo, yoga, and various movement philosophies designed to help overcome physical impairments (77). It is based on the capacity of humans to learn movement. The technique helps patients realize they have choices in movement, so they can learn to use efficient and pain-free movement. There are two variations of the technique. Awareness Through Movement is a verbally directed lesson taught in a group format in which movements are gentle and slow, within comfort range. Lessons are based on a function (getting up from a chair, rolling from supine to prone). The second variation, Functional Integration, is a one-on-one, hands-on technique in which the practitioner gently guides the student through various movement sequences. Feldenkrais has been used successfully with various neurologic conditions, including cerebral palsy, hemiplegia, and multiple sclerosis.

The Pilates method was developed by Joseph Pilates during and after World War I as a result of his contact with disabled soldiers. The technique is now used by both high-level athletes and those undergoing rehabilitation with such diverse diagnoses as spinal cord injury, multiple sclerosis, and arthritis. The technique is characterized by education in the use of proper body mechanics in all movements, truncal and pelvic stabilization, coordinated breathing, and eccentric muscle contractions to promote strengthening with minimal increase in bulk. A typical rehabilitation program using a Pilates-based approach may not begin by focusing on the area that is injured but by teaching exercises to enhance awareness that the body works as a whole and that the injured part is the weak link in the whole kinetic chain (78). Attention is directed to conditioning the entire musculoskeletal system while the patient is rehabilitating from injury. Exercises are performed with little or no resistance until strength and awareness are developed and successively more challenging tasks are added.

ENERGY HEALING TECHNIQUES

Biofield energy healing is one of the more controversial of the unconventional modalities because it postulates the existence of a subtle energy field within and around the body that cannot be measured by standard biomedical instrumentation and does not correspond to any form of physical energy currently known to science. Although unknown in modern biomedical science, the existence of this subtle energy is an integral part of almost every traditional ethnic medical system, and the concept dates back thousands of years. The energy field is also known as the vital life force in Western metaphysical traditions, and as qi or chi (Chinese), ki (Japanese), and prana (Sanskrit) in Eastern traditions. All of the techniques have as a basic underlying concept the idea that illness is a result of, or at least associated with, imbalances and blockages in this energy field.

The various techniques included in this group of therapies involve a practitioner placing his or her hands on or near the physical body and either actively or passively altering the energy in the person being treated by means of the energy flowing through the practitioner. Although physical touch is involved, its purpose is to transmit the energy, not to manipulate the skin, muscle, or other organ, and the mechanism of action is quite different from that usually proposed in manual manipulation techniques. However, it should be noted that a number of techniques have been developed during the past few decades that combine physical manipulation with subtle energy healing, and in traditional systems of medicine such as TCM, massage and energy healing, although seen as separate techniques, are most often used together. Although generally used to promote the overall health of the individual, these techniques often have been used to treat specific diseases and medical conditions, including stroke and brain injury.

Therapeutic Touch

Therapeutic touch is a technique first described in 1979 and developed by a nurse academician, Dolores Krieger, at New York University, and Dora Kunz, a natural healer. Based on the idea that the human energy field extends beyond the skin, the practitioner uses the hands as sensors to locate problems, and then serves as a conduit for universal energy, consciously transferring energy into the client's energy field in rhythmic, sweeping motions (79). This technique can be used with or without touching the body. It is taught in over 80 universities in over 30 countries (21).

Qigong

Qigong (pronounced chee-*kung*) is an ancient philosophical system of harmonious integration of the human body with the universe (80). The word "qigong" is derived from the word "qi," which refers to the vital breath, or life force, and "gong" which means discipline, work, or skill. When qigong is practiced, the goal is to balance the qi or vital energy within the body, thus preventing or curing illness. In self-administered qigong (internal qigong), the individual uses a variety of means, including breathing, visualization, and physical movements to bring the qi into balance. Qi also can be directed into a person by a trained master, who consciously emits the qi from his or her body into another person (external qigong).

The general healing nature of the qi is such as to suggest that it can be applied with some success to almost any medical or health problem. McGee and Chow relate a number of case studies for many different conditions, including stroke, paralysis, and cerebral palsy (81). However, rigorous research is sparse. Two studies from China pertain to paralysis and spinal cord injury. In one study, 43 paralysis patients (19 hemiplegia; 24 paraplegia) were treated with emitted qi from several qigong masters (82). Treatment also included massage of certain acupoints and performance of qigong exercises that had been adjusted for physical limitations due to the paralysis. Results indicated that there were improvements in various functional indicators, including range of motion, walking, activities of daily living, and in various psychosomatic symptoms. In an animal study, young pigs with surgically induced spinal cord injury received either Ba Gua induction qigong or no treatment (83). After 89 days, 91% of the pigs receiving qigong could walk, whereas 0% of pigs in the control group could walk. The quality of these two studies is not known because the information is based only on brief abstracts of conference presentations; however, the use of control groups suggests that they may be reasonably well-controlled studies.

In addition to research evidence, there are a number of practitioners and at least one hospital in the Far East that specialize in the use of qigong to treat paralysis and other neurologic disorders. For example, the Army General Qigong Hospital in Beijing, China, focuses on the treatment of paralysis using qigong. Walker claims that thousands of paralysis patients have been treated at this hospital, with 90% showing some improvement and 46% experiencing complete recovery from their paralysis (84).

Reiki

Reiki (pronounced *ray*-key) is a form of energy healing that usually involves a practitioner laying his or her hands lightly on specific locations on the body of the person being treated, allowing the ki or vital life force, to flow through the Reiki practitioner into the body of the patient being treated (85). Having originated in Japan in the 1800s, Reiki has become an increasingly popular and accessible healing technique throughout the Western world. It also can be administered from a distance (absent healing) or self-administered. Despite many anecdotal reports of its effectiveness in a variety of health problems, there has been little research.

ELECTROMAGNETIC APPLICATIONS

In recent years, a number of different electromagnetic techniques have been applied to the treatment of wounds, ulcers, swelling, bone fractures, pain, and mood disorder, among other medical conditions. Although still thought of as alternative by many health-care providers, the status of this modality as an alternative therapy is debatable, with these treatments available in a limited but growing number of conventional health-care settings. Within the rehabilitation community, these techniques are now so well integrated into multidisciplinary treatment protocols that they are, for all practical purposes, conventional. The use of magnets in the treatment of musculoskeletal pain has become very popular in the past few years, but there is currently no research-based evidence for its effectiveness. Chapter 24 presents a discussion of functional electrical stimulation and related techniques.

DIET/NUTRITIONAL SUPPLEMENTS

Dietary and nutritional therapy involves the regulation of diet and direct nutritional intervention to optimize metabolic, cardiovascular, neurologic, or immune system functioning and is often recommended as a preventative therapy for specific conditions. In terms of central nervous system injury, supplementation involving so-called smart vitamins and minerals, such as choline (lecithin) has been recommended for brain injury and stroke patients. Other substances, such as bromelain (pineapple extract), vitamin E, coenzyme Q-10, ginger, fish oil, garlic, and soy protein, have been suggested as ways to improve cardiovascular functioning, thus reducing risk of cardiovascular and cerebrovascular accidents. In rehabilitation, they have been suggested as ways to reduce the risk of a subsequent occurrence of cerebrovascular accident. The importance of dietary regulation is discussed in Chapter 32.

PHYTOTHERAPIES: THERAPIES USING HERBS AND PLANT MATERIALS

Herbal medicine involves the use of whole plant material, such as the root, stem, flower, extract, etc. Plant materials are by far the oldest form of medication and are part of virtually all indigenous medical traditions. Plant materials can be directly ingested, inhaled, or applied topically. Herbal medicine, like conventional pharmaceutical drugs, is believed to work either due to the action of a specific chemical in the herb or the synergistic interaction between various components of the plants. Indeed, numerous medications and pharmaceutical compounds have their origin in substances originally isolated from plants. Some herbs and plant materials appear to have useful medicinal effects of relevance to rehabilitation, with reported effects on vascular elasticity, platelet activating factor, and cognitive functioning. Despite being natural, not all plants and herbs are safe for human consumption and should be used only with full knowledge of the nature and effects of the plant component in question and their possible interactions with a patient's medications.

Chinese Herbal Medicine

Chinese herbs and other plants have been used in medical treatments for thousands of years. There are currently hundreds of natural substances available for use, and most herbal prescriptions contain upwards of 15 ingredients, which makes it difficult to identify the effects of specific components.

A number of botanical extracts have been identified as beneficial in the treatment of cerebral ischemia, cerebral thrombosis, and stroke. These substances are generally used as elements of complex decoctions. No controlled clinical trials of their efficacy have been located, but some may exist in the Chinese or Japanese language literatures. One study compared the effectiveness of Chinese herbal medicines with conventional Western medicine in the treatment of hemorrhagic stroke (86). Results indicated significantly greater survival rate and improvement in symptoms in the group treated with herbal medicine compared with Western medicine.

Ligusticum Chuanxiong (LC) was recommended for the treatment of stroke as early as the Tang Dynasty (A.D. 581 to 682) (87). Herbal prescriptions containing it or its active ingredient *Ligusticum wallichii* (tetramethylpyrazine) have been successful in reducing the harmful effects to patients with cerebral ischemia or stroke, according to clinical reports (87–90). LC appears to act by decreasing platelet aggregation and thrombus formation, thereby increasing cerebral blood flow (91). In addition, there is a small amount of research into many other medicines that have been used to treat stroke-related problems, including Ginseng ZaiZao Wan and Huo Luo Dan compounds for aphasia and hemiplegia (91), motherwort (92), jia-wei-gui-pi-tang (Kamikihi-To in Japanese) (93), oren-gedoku-to (94), and Tsumura-Zokumeito (95,96). Ding and He (91) provide general guidelines for treatment of brain injury, including the use of An Gong Niu Huang Wan and Su He Xiang Wan prescriptions to reverse coma resulting from brain stem injury. Several animal studies show that animals treated with *Radix salviae miltiorrhizae* before ligation-induced ischemia had decreased mortality, decreased neuronal damage, and decreased edema when compared with untreated animals (97–102).

The main safety issue involved in herbal medicine is the potential toxicity of one or more ingredients in a decoction. Because many of these substances have been used for centuries without reports of serious negative consequences, the risk is estimated to be low. However, contamination of herbs produced in the Far East has occasionally occurred, and purity of these herbal preparations must be ascertained before use. Use of these herbs should always be supervised by an expert in Chinese herbal medicine.

Ginkgo Biloba

The leaf of the Ginkgo tree has been part of the traditional Chinese pharmacopoeia for 5,000 years. A standardized extract of the Ginkgo leaf is widely used in Asia and in Germany and France, and is increasingly being used in the United States. It is one of the most commonly prescribed medications in Germany (103). Ginkgo biloba extract (GBE) has been evaluated in both animal and human models. It shows promise in treatment of some of the most salient and debilitating symptoms associated with stroke, traumatic brain injury, cerebral vascular insufficiency, senile dementia, and the effects of normal aging. Ginkgo biloba has been used in the treatment of ischemia (i.e., inadequate oxygenation/reperfusion) (104) and memory/information processing impairments that may be observed in older people and in patients with Alzheimer's disease (105,106). Research into the mechanisms of action of Ginkgo biloba suggests that it may improve arterial and vascular elasticity (107). In addition, evidence derived from animal models and clinical studies supports the idea that Ginkgo biloba acts as an anti–platelet-activating factor (104). Taken together, these findings suggest that Ginkgo biloba can play a role in treating the symptoms of cerebrovascular disease during both acute and chronic stages.

Although the duration of treatment and the window of time required to demonstrate efficacy has varied across studies, improvement generally has been observed within 4 to 12 weeks (108,109). No serious side effects have been observed in clinical trials, but in rare cases patients have shown allergic skin reactions, headache, and mild gastrointestinal upset (110). Despite the fact that patients taking GBE are often receiving a variety of medications, there are no known drug interactions (110).

PHARMACOLOGIC APPROACHES AND ALTERNATIVE USES OF CONVENTIONAL THERAPIES

This category refers to a broad group of drugs and conventional treatments approved for one type of medical condition, but which are believed to have beneficial effects on other conditions that have not been approved by the U.S. Food and Drug Administration (FDA) (e.g., the use of anticonvulsants for the treatment of pain). Although physicians are theoretically permitted to prescribe medications for nonapproved conditions, many are reluctant to do so, even if they are aware of the potential beneficial effects, because of fear of malpractice lawsuits, possible investigation by the FDA, or punishment by their local licensing agency, including license revocation. Consequently, even though these alternative uses of conventional prescription medical treatments are available under a doctor's supervision, they are sometimes difficult to obtain because so few physicians know about them or are willing to prescribe them. Two techniques that seem to show promise are presented here.

Dimethyl Sulfoxide

Dimethyl sulfoxide (DMSO) has been used for years as an anti-inflammatory by veterinarians, sports trainers, and

Olympic athletes (111). It is most widely used as a topical analgesic, in a 70% DMSO, 30% water solution. Burns, cuts, and sprains have been treated with DMSO, and relief is reported to be almost immediate, lasting up to 6 hours (111). DMSO is approved by the FDA for the treatment of only one medical condition: interstitial cystitis. However, results from a series of studies suggest that DMSO may lower intracranial pressure, stabilize blood pressure, and increase blood flow to areas of injury (111–114). DMSO has been used with human patients suffering severe head trauma, with encouraging results (114). Its possible effectiveness in dissolving clots in stroke also has been suggested by de la Torre (quoted in Muir [111]). Despite early concerns, it appears to be safe when used with standard cautions. Its main drawback seems to be that it usually leaves an odd taste in the mouth (even when applied topically) and may cause an unpleasant breath odor, somewhat akin to garlic. More research is clearly needed.

Hyperbaric Oxygen Therapy

Hyperbaric oxygen (HBO) therapy is defined as the treatment of a patient entirely enclosed within some type of chamber that forces the patient to breathe oxygen at a pressure greater than sea level in order to achieve high arterial and tissue oxygen tensions (115). In the past, hyperbaric oxygen has been used to treat bubble-related diseases, decompression sickness, and air embolism.

A problem for stroke patients is the deprivation of oxygen in key brain areas due to an interruption of blood flow. HBO therapy has been advocated in these circumstances because it may enhance neuronal viability by its ability to increase the amount of dissolved oxygen in the blood without changing blood viscosity (116). HBO therapy also may have other beneficial effects, such as reducing brain edema after injury without impairing tissue oxygen delivery (117).

In a large study by Neubauer and End (118), 122 patients with stroke due to thrombosis were treated with HBO in addition to standard treatment. In the bedridden group, 64% of the patients showed improvement in ability to use a wheelchair or to walk with or without aids. In the wheelchair group, 71% of the patients showed improved ambulation. In the group categorized as walking with aids, 56% of the patients improved enough to walk independently. However, in a study of HBO therapy for the treatment of acute ischemic stroke in patients who had experienced middle cerebral artery occlusion, the results were mixed (119). In addition, there have been a number of animal studies and isolated small clinical/case-based studies, but no major study showing the benefit of this treatment for wide scale application. In general, existing research suggests that HBO therapy in patients with stroke may be beneficial, but additional research is clearly needed.

Research on the use of hyperbaric oxygen in brain injury and spinal cord injury is less encouraging than in stroke. In general, the limited research suggests that HBO therapy may speed up the healing process and lower the mortality rate, but may not substantially improve functioning (120–124).

Use of CAM Techniques in the Physiatric Setting

The judicious use of complementary therapies to supplement standard medical interventions has been a hallmark of physiatric rehabilitation, often under the supervision of a multispecialty team of caregivers. This holistic approach has flourished because it is effective and provides for interventions not otherwise available in standard medical settings. The message of this chapter is that there may be a number of other promising therapies that can be integrated into this approach. Some techniques, such as acupuncture, phytotherapies, and nutritional supplementation, already have bodies of research that suggest their usefulness in this setting. Other techniques appear promising based on anecdotal reports and case studies but have not yet been adequately documented.

By becoming familiar with these alternative approaches, the rehabilitation caregiver can have informed conversations with patients and begin to consider the possibility of using one or more techniques as adjuncts to existing treatment protocols, when evidence suggests the potential utility and safety of the technique. This process begins with becoming acquainted with possible methods for treating a focal condition. The techniques discussed in this chapter represent only a sampling of the many potentially useful complementary therapies available for use in a rehabilitation setting. In the past, locating information on the various therapies would have been a difficult task, but today there is a rapidly growing body of information easily available to a rehabilitation specialist that help facilitate this process (e.g., Vickers [125] and Davis [3]). Davis, in particular, gives useful suggestions for integrating a number of complementary therapies into the rehabilitation process.

Once an approach has been tentatively identified, it is necessary to identify a reputable practitioner. There are often professional associations of alternative practitioners (e.g., the American Academy of Medical Acupuncture and the American Holistic Medical Association) that can provide referrals to local practitioners and also can attest to the training and certifications received by its membership. For some of these treatments (e.g., acupuncture), many states have licensing laws regulating their practice. Local and national alternative life-style resource directories have become commonplace and are good sources of potential practitioners, but the issue of credentials and competence should be addressed. Pragmatic issues must be considered. Many therapies may not be reimbursable through insurance. Cost of treatment, including length and number of treatments, will affect decisions, especially if not covered by insurance. The ability to directly monitor treatment or to provide it on the premises of the rehabilitation facility will probably be a factor in many medical problems. Some therapies can be given in group settings, and others require one-on-one treatment.

Next, communication with the practitioner is essential,

including an assessment of their knowledge of the medical condition they might be asked to treat, as well as their awareness of standard practices in medical and rehabilitation settings. Involvement of the patient is also an important part of the process of deciding whether to try an alternative technique, and if so, which one. Careful monitoring and documentation of progress, safety issues, side effects, and related matters is essential, not only for the protection of the patient, but also because, from time to time, case study reports to the scientific literature may be warranted, either to encourage further exploratory use of the technique or to discourage its use if undesired results occur. In this way, the field of PM&R can move forward in innovative treatment of patients while continuing to provide the highest levels of care and safety.

ACKNOWLEDGMENT

We thank Dr. John Moldover and Diane Zeitlin for their valuable comments during preparation of this chapter.

REFERENCES

1. Jonas W. Office of Alternative Medicine. Advisory Council address. *Complementary Alternative Med NIH* 1996; 3:1.
2. Kessler HH. *The knife is not enough.* New York: WW Norton, 1968.
3. Davis CM, ed. *Complementary therapies in rehabilitation.* Thorofare, NJ: SLACK, 1997.
4. Vincent CA, Richardson PH. Evaluation of therapeutic acupuncture: concepts and methods. *Pain* 1986; 24:1–13.
5. O'Connor BB. Vernacular health care responses to HIV and AIDS. *Alternative Ther* 1995; 88:119–202.
6. Naeser MA, Alexander MP, Stiassny-Eder D, et al. Laser acupuncture in the treatment of paralysis in stroke patients. *Am J Acupunct* 1995; 23:13–28.
7. Magnusson M, Johansson K, Johansson BB. Sensory stimulation promotes normalization of postural control after stroke. *Stroke* 1994; 25: 1176–1180.
8. Johansson K, Lindgren I, Widner H, Wiklund I, Johansson BB. Can sensory stimulation improve the functional outcome in stroke patients? *Neurology* 1993; 43:2189–2192.
9. Chen YM, Fang YA. 108 cases of hemiplegia caused by stroke. *Acupunct Electrother Res* 1990; 15:9–17.
10. Naeser MA, Alexander MP, Stiassney-Eder D, Galler V, Hobbs J, Bachman D. Acupuncture in the treatment of paralysis in chronic and acute stroke patients—improvement correlated with specific CT scan lesion sites. *Acupunct Electrother Res* 1994; 19:227–249.
11. Bensoussan A. Does acupuncture therapy resemble a process of physiological relearning? *Am J Acupunct* 1994; 22:137–144.
12. Politis MJ, Korchinski MA. Beneficial effects of acupuncture treatment following experimental spinal cord injury. *Acupunct Electrother Res* 1990; 15:37–49.
13. Shiraishi S, Gotu I, Koroiwa Y, Nishio S, Kinoshita K. Spinal cord injury as a complication of an acupuncture. *Neurology* 1979; 29: 1180–1182.
14. O'Brien B, Relyea MJ, Taerum T. Efficacy of P6 acupressure in the treatment of nausea and vomiting during pregnancy. *Am J Obstet Gynecol* 1996; 174:708–715.
15. Ho CM, Hseu SS, Tsai SK, Lee TY. Effect of P6 acupressure on prevention of nausea and vomiting after epidural morphine for post-cesarean section pain relief. *Acta Anaesthesiol Scand* 1996; 40: 372–275.
16. Belluomini J, Litt RC, Lee KA, Katz M. Acupressure for nausea and vomiting of pregnancy: a randomized, blinded study. *Obstet Gynecol* 1994; 84:245–248.
17. Dougans I, Ellis, S. *The art of reflexology.* Rockport, MA: Element Books, 1992.
18. American Academy for Human Development. *The developmentalist.* Piqua, OH: American Academy for Human Development, 1995.
19. Upledger JE, Vredevoogd JD. *Craniosacral therapy.* Seattle, WA: Eastland, 1983.
20. Upledger JE. Craniosacral therapy. *Phys Ther* 1995; 75:328–330.
21. Collinge W. *The American Holistic Health Association guide to alternative medicine.* New York: Warner, 1996.
22. Goodheart G. *You'll be better: the story of applied kinesiology.* Geneva, OH: AK Printing, 1964.
23. Valentine T, Valentine C. *Applied kinesiology.* Rochester, VT: Inner Traditions, 1989.
24. Thie JF. *Touch for health.* Van Nuys, CA: TH Enterprises, 1987.
25. Rhue JW, Lynn SJ, Kirsch I, eds. *Handbook of clinical hypnosis.* Washington, D.C.: American Psychological Association, 1993.
26. Crasilneck HB, Hall JA. The use of hypnosis in the rehabilitation of complicated vascular and post-traumatic neurological patients. *Int J Clin Exp Hypn* 1970; 18:145–159.
27. Appel PR. Clinical applications of hypnosis in the physical medicine and rehabilitation setting: three case reports. *Am J Clin Hypn* 1990; 33:85–93.
28. Sullivan DS, Johnson A, Bratkovitch J. Reduction of behavioral deficit in organic brain damage by use of hypnosis. *J Clin Psychol* 1974; 30:96–98.
29. Holroyd J, Hill A. Pushing the limits of recovery: hypnotherapy with a stroke patient. *Int J Clin Exp Hypn* 1989; 37:120–128.
30. Manganiello AJ. Hypnotherapy in the rehabilitation of a stroke victim: a case study. *Am J Clin Hypn* 1986; 29:64–68.
31. Sthalekar HA. Hypnosis for relief of chronic phantom pain in a paralysed limb: a case study. *Aust J Clin Hypnother Hypn* 1993; 14:75–80.
32. Lucas D, Stratis DJ, Deniz S. Hypnosis in conjunction with corrective therapy in a quadriplegic patient: a case report. *Am Correct Ther J* 1981; 35:16–20.
33. Chappell DT. Hypnosis and spasticity in paraplegia. *Am J Clin Hypn* 1964; 7:33–36.
34. Cedercreutz C, Lahteenmaki R, Tulikoura J. Hypnotic treatment of headache and vertigo in skull injured patients. *Int J Clin Exp Hypn* 1976; 24:195–201.
35. Benson H. Systemic hypertension and the relaxation response. *N Engl J Med* 1977; 296:1152–1156.
36. Hafner RJ. Psychological treatment of essential hypertension: a controlled comparison of meditation and meditation plus biofeedback. *Biofeedback Self Regul* 1982; 7:305–316.
37. Schneider RH, Alexander CN, Wallace RK. In search of an optimal behavioral treatment for hypertension: a review and focus on transcendental meditation. In: Johnson EH, Gentry WD, Julius S, eds. *Personality, elevated blood pressure, and essential hypertension.* Washington, D.C.: Hemisphere, 1992.
38. Wallace RK, Silver J, Mills P, Dillbeck MC, Wagoner DE. Systolic blood pressure and long-term practice of the Transcendental Meditation and TM-Sidhi program: effects of TM on systolic blood pressure. *Psychosom Med* 1983; 45:41–46.
39. Cooper MJ, Aygen MM. A relaxation technique in the management of hypercholesterolemia. *J Hum Stress* 1979; 5:24–27.
40. Yoffe E. Meditate away paralysis. *Nat Health* 1995:50–52.
41. Alexander C, Langer,EJ, Newman RI, Chandler HM, Davis JL. Transcendental meditation, mindfulness, and longevity: an experimental study with the elderly. *J Pers Soc Psychol* 1989; 57:950–964.
42. Dillbeck MC, Assimakis PD, Raimondi D, Orme-Johnson DW, Row R. Longitudinal effects of the transcendental meditation and TM-Sidhi program on cognitive ability and cognitive style. *Percept Mot Skills* 1986; 62:731–738.
43. Purdie H, Baldwin S. Models of music therapy intervention in stroke rehabilitation. *Int J Rehabil Res* 1995; 18:341–350.
44. Lane D. Music therapy: gaining an edge in oncology management. *J Oncol Management* 1993: 2;42–46.
45. Lane DL. The effect of a single music therapy session on hospitalized children as measured by salivary immunoglobulin A, speech pause time, and a patient opinion likert scale. Unpublished doctoral dissertation, Case Western Reserve University, Cleveland, Ohio, 1991.
46. Aldridge D, Gustorff D, Hannich HJ. Where am I? Music therapy applied to coma patients. *J R Soc Med* 1990; 83:345–346.
47. Kearney S, Fussey I. The use of adapted leisure materials to reinforce correct head positioning in a brain-injured adult. *Brain Inj* 1991; 5: 295–302.

48. Eslinger P. Music therapy and brain injury. Unpublished report to the Office of Alternative Medicine at the NIH, Bethesda, Maryland, 1993.
49. Staum MJ. Music for physical rehabilitation: an analysis of the literature from 1950–1986 and applications for rehabilitation settings. In: Furman CE, ed. *Effectiveness of music therapy procedures: documentation of research and clinical practice.* Washington, D.C.: National Association for Music Therapy, 1988; 65–104.
50. Benor DJ. Survey of spiritual healing research. *Complement Med Res* 1990; 4:9–33.
51. Collipp PJ. The efficacy of prayer: a triple-blind study. *Med Times* 1969; 97:201–204.
52. Dossey L. *Healing words: the power of prayer and the practice of medicine.* San Francisco: Harper Collins, 1993.
53. Joyce CRB, Welldon RMC. The objective efficacy of prayer. A double-blind clinical trial. *J Chronic Dis* 1965; 18:367–377.
54. Byrd RC. Positive therapeutic effects of intercessory prayer in a coronary care unit population. *South Med J* 1988; 81:826–829.
55. Friedmann E, Katcher AH, Thomas SA, Lynch JJ, Messent PR. Social interaction and blood pressure. Influence of animal companions. *J Nerv Ment Dis* 1983; 171:461–465.
56. Beck AM. The therapeutic use of animals. *Vet Clin North Am Small Anim Pract* 1985; 15:365–375.
57. Fick KM. The influence of an animal on social interactions of nursing home residents in a group setting. *Am J Occup Ther* 1992; 47: 529–534.
58. Cole KM, Gawlinski A. Animal-assisted therapy in the intensive care unit: a staff nurse's dream come true. *Nurs Clin North Am* 1995; 30: 529–537.
59. Biery MJ. Riding and the handicapped. *Vet Clin North Am Small Anim Pract* 1985; 15:345–354.
60. Exner G, Engelmann A, Lange K, Wenck B. Basic principles and effects of hippotherapy within the comprehensive treatment of paraplegic patients. *Rehabilitation (Stuttg)* 1994; 33:39–43.
61. Hudson T. Screening builds in safety for pet visits. *Hospitals* 1990; 64:81–82.
62. Strickland DA. Furry therapists boost staff, too. *Med World News* 1991; January:47.
63. Lelong M, Castelain MC, Bras C, et al. An outbreak of allergy to horses in children: a review of 56 recent cases. *Pediatrie* 1992; 47: 55–58.
64. Sundar S, Agarwal SK. Role of yoga in the management of essential hypertension. *Acta Cardiol* 1984; 39:203–208.
65. Ornish D. Can lifestyle changes reverse coronary heart disease? *Lancet* 1990; 336:129–132.
66. Haslock I, Monro R, Nagarathna R, Nagendra HR, Raghuram NV. Measuring the effects of yoga in rheumatoid arthritis. *Br J Rhematol* 1994; 22:787–788.
67. Garfinkel MS, Schumacher HR, Husain A, Levy M, Reshetar RA. Evaluation of a yoga based regimen for treatment of osteoarthritis of the hands. *J Rheumatol* 1994; 21:2341–2343.
68. Schatz M. *Back care basics.* Berkeley: Rodmell Press, 1992.
69. Levy JK. Standard and alternative adjunctive treatments in cardiac rehabilitation. *Tex Heart Inst J* 1993; 20:198–212.
70. Raju PS, Madhavi S, Prasad KV, et al. Comparison of the effects of yoga and physical exercise in athletes. *Ind J Med Res* 1994; 100: 81–86.
71. Province MA, Hadley EC, Hornbrook MC, et al. The effects of exercise on falls in elderly patients: a preplanned meta-analysis of the FICSIT trials. *JAMA* 1995; 273:1341–1347.
72. Wolf S, Barhnart HX, Kutner NG, et al. Reducing frailty and falls in older persons: an investigation of t'ai chi and computerized balance training. *J Am Geriatr Soc* 1996; 44:489–497.
73. Wolfson LW, Whipple R, Derby C. Balance and strength training in older adults: intervention gains and t'ai chi maintenance. *J Am Geriatr Soc* 1996; 44:498–506.
74. Plummer JP. Acupuncture and homeostasis: physiological, physical, and psychological. *Am J Chin Med* 1981; 9:1–14.
75. Cheu J, DeMasi I. Personal communication, 1997.
76. McGowan D, Alexander FM, eds. *Alexander technique: original writings of F.M. Alexander—constructive conscious control.* Burdett, NY: Larson, 1996.
77. Feldenkrais M. *Awareness through movement: health exercises for personal growth.* New York: Harper, 1972.
78. Loosli AR. Knee rehabilitation for dancers using a Pilates based technique. *Kinesiol Med Dance* 1992; 14:1–12.
79. Krieger D. *The therapeutic touch. How to use your hands to help or to heal.* Englewood Cliffs, NJ: Prentice-Hall, 1979.
80. Eisenberg D, Wright TL. *Encounters with Qi.* New York: Viking Penguin, 1987.
81. McGee CT, Chow EPY. *Miracle healing from China: qigong.* Coeur d'Alene, ID: MediPress, 1994.
82. Huang M. Effect of emitted qi combined with self-practice of qigong in treating paralysis [Abstract]. First World Conference for Academic Exchange of Medical Qigong, Beijing, China, 1988.
83. Wan S, et al. Repeated experiments by using the emitted qi in treatment of spinal cord injury. (Abstract) Second World Conference for Academic Exchange of Medical Qigong, Beijing, China, 1994.
84. Walker M. The healing powers of qigong (chi kung). *Townsend Letter for Doctors* April, 1994.
85. Rand WL. *Reiki: the healing touch.* Southfield, MI: Vision Publications, 1991.
86. Lin Y, Ren J. Study on application of the principle of eliminating stasis and refreshing spirit for acute stage of hemorrhagic apoplexy. *J Tradit Chin Med* 1994; 14:92–97.
87. Chen K, Chen K. Ischemic stroke treated with Ligusticum chuanxiong. *Chin Med J* 1992; 105:870–873.
88. Anonymous. Danshen in ischemic stroke. *Chin Med J* 1977; 3: 224–226.
89. Chen K, Song J. Progress of research on ischemic stroke treated with Chinese medicine. *J Tradit Chin Med* 1992; 12:204–210.
90. Guo SK, Chen KJ, Qian ZH, Weng WL, Qian MY. Tetramethylpyrazine in the treatment of cardiovascular and cerebrovascular diseases. *Planta Med* 1983; 47:89.
91. Ding Y, He X. Traditional Chinese herbs in treatment of neurological and neurosurgical disorders. *Can J Neurol Sci* 1986; 13:210–213.
92. Kuang P, Zhou X, Zhang F, Lang S. Motherwort and cerebral ischemia. *J Tradit Chin Med* 1988; 8:37–40.
93. Nishizawa K, Inoue O, Saito Y, Suzuki A. Protective effects of kami-kihi-to, a traditional Chinese medicine, against cerebral ischemia, hypoxia and anoxia in mice and gerbils. *Jpn J Pharmacol* 1994; 64: 171–177.
94. Mori M, Hojo E, Takano K. Action of oren-gedoku-to on platelet aggregation in vitro. *Am J Chin Med* 1991; 19:131–133.
95. Goto K, Suekawa M, Aburada M, Hosoya E. Pharmacological study of TJ-8007 (Tsumura-Zokumeito) (I): protective effects of TJ-8007 against anoxic brain damage. *Nippon Yakurigaku Zasshi* 1987; 89: 355–363.
96. Goto K, Suekawa M, Hosoya E. Pharmacological study of TJ-8007 (tsumara-zokumeito) (II): protective effect of TJ-8007 against cerebral ischemia. *Nippon Yakurigaku Zasshi* 1989; 93:255–260.
97. Kuang P, Pu C, Liu Z, Yin W, Zhang F, Liu Y. Cerebral infarction in a bilateral common carotid artery ligation model protected by radix salviae miltiorrhizae. *J Tradit Chin Med* 1986; 6:121–124.
98. Kuang P, Wu W, Zhang F, Liu J, Pu C. The effect of radix salviae miltiorrhizae on vasoactive intestinal peptide in cerebral ischemia: an animal experiment. *J Tradit Chin Med* 1989; 9:203–206.
99. Kuang P, Wu W, Liu J, Zhang F, Pu C. The effect of radix salviae miltiorrhizae (RSM) on substance P in cerebral ischemia-animal experiment. *J Tradit Chin Med* 1991; 11:123–127.
100. Kuang P, Wu W, Zhu K. Evidence for amelioration of cellular damage in ischemic rat brain by radix salviae miltiorrhizae treatment-immunocytochemistry and histopathology studies. *J Tradit Chin Med* 1993; 13:38–41.
101. Kuang P, Li Z, Zhang F, Tao Y, Liu J, Wu W. Protective effect of radix salviae miltiorrhizae composita on cerebral ischemia. *J Tradit Chin Med* 1995; 15:135–140.
102. Wu W, Kuang P, Zhu K. The effect of radix salviae miltiorrhizae on the changes of ultrastructure in rat brain after cerebral ischemia. *J Tradit Chin Med* 1992; 11:183–186.
103. Anonymous. Ginkgo biloba extract: over 5 million prescriptions a year. *Lancet* 1989; 334:1513–1514.
104. Braquet P, Paubert-Braquet M, Koltai M, Bourgain R, Bussolino F, Hosford D. Is there a case for PAF antagonists in the treatment of ischemic disease? *TIPS* 1989; 10:23–30.
105. Vorberg G. Ginkgo biloba extract (GBE): a long-term study of chronic cerebral insufficiency in geriatric patients. *Clin Trials J* 1985; 22: 149–157.

106. Kleijnen J, Knipschild P. Ginkgo biloba for cerebral insufficiency. *Br J Clin Pharmacol* 1992; 34:352–358.
107. Christen Y, Costentin J, Lacour M, eds. Effects of ginkgo biloba extract (Egb 761) on the central nervous system. IPSEN Institute International Symposium, Montreaux, Switzerland, 1991.
108. Mouren X, Caillard P, Schwartz F. Study of the antiischemic action of Egb 761 in the treatment of peripheral arterial occlusive disease by TcPo2 determination. *Angiology* 1994; 45:13–17.
109. Witte S, Anadere I, Walitza E. Improvement of hemorheology with ginkgo biloba extract. Decreasing a cardiovascular risk factor. [German]. *Fortschr Med* 1992; 110:247–250.
110. Kleijnen J, Knipschild P. Ginkgo biloba. *Lancet* 1992; 340: 1136–1139.
111. Muir M. DMSO: Many uses, much controversy. *Alternat Complement Ther* 1996; 3:231–236.
112. de la Torre JC, Rowed DW, Kawanage HM, Mullan S. Dimethyl sulfoxide in the treatment of experimental brain compression. *J Neurosurg* 1972; 38:345–354.
113. de la Torre JC, Kawanaga HM, Johnson CM, Goode DJ, Kajihara K, Mullan S. Dimethyl sulfoxide in central nervous system trauma. *Ann N Y Acad Sci* 1975; 243:362–389.
114. Karaca M, Bilgen UY, Akar M, de la Torre JC. Dimethyl sulphoxide lowers ICP after closed head trauma. *Eur J Clin Pharmacol* 1991; 40:113–114.
115. Davis JC. Hyperbaric oxygen therapy. *J Intensive Care Med* 1989; 4:55–57.
116. Mink RB, Dutka AJ. Hyperbaric oxygen after global cerebral ischemia in rabbits reduces brain vascular permeability and blood flow. *Stroke* 1995; 26:2307–2312.
117. Sukoff MH, Ragatz RE. Hyperbaric oxygenation for the treatment of acute cerebral edema. *Neurosurgery* 1982; 10:29–38.
118. Neubauer RA, End E. Hyperbaric oxygenation as an adjunct therapy in strokes due to thrombosis. A review of 122 patients. *Stroke* 1980; 11:297–300.
119. Nighoghossian N, Trouillas P, Adeleine P, Salord F. Hyperbaric oxygen in the treatment of acute ischemic stroke. *Stroke* 1995; 26: 1369–1372.
120. Neubauer RA, Gottlieb SF, Pevsner H. Hyperbaric oxygen for treatment of closed head injury. *South Med J* 1994; 87:933–936.
121. Rockswold GL, Ford SE. Preliminary results of a prospective randomized trial for treatment of severely brain-injured patients with hyperbaric oxygen. *Minn Med* 1985; 68:533–535.
122. Rockswold GL, Ford SE, Anderson DC, Bergman TA, Sherman RE. Results of a prospective randomized trial for treatment of severely brain-injured patients with hyperbaric oxygen. *J Neurosurg* 1992; 76: 929–934.
123. Clifton GL. Hypothermia and hyperbaric oxygen as treatment modalities for severe head injury. *New Horizons* 1995; 3:474–478.
124. Gamache FW, Myers RAM, Ducker TB, Cowley RA. The clinical application of hyperbaric oxygen therapy in spinal cord injury: a preliminary report. *Surg Neurol* 1980; 15:85–87.
125. Vickers AJ. *Complementary medicine and disability.* London: Chapman & Hall, 1993.

Rehabilitation Medicine: Principles and Practice, Third Edition,
edited by Joel A. DeLisa and Bruce M. Gans.
Lippincott–Raven Publishers, Philadelphia © 1998.

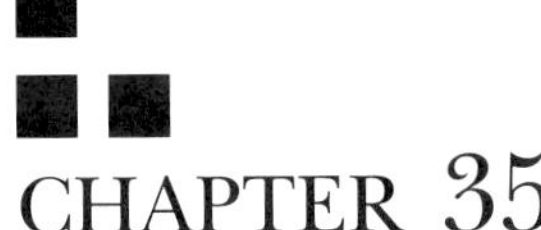

CHAPTER 35

Aquatic Rehabilitation

Bruce E. Becker and Andrew J. Cole

INTRODUCTION AND BRIEF HISTORY

Historical Applications

Throughout all recorded history, the sick and suffering have resorted to springs, baths, and pools for their soothing, healing, and powerful effects. "Taking the waters," soaking in baths and pools, and resting at places called spas played an important social and spiritual role in the river valley civilizations of Mesopotamia, Egypt, India, and China. Ritual bathing pools were widely used for individual and social renewal and healing. Healing water rituals also appeared in ancient Greek, Hebrew, Roman, Christian, and Islamic cultures (1). During the Middle Ages in Europe, the beginnings of formal resorts formed for the purposes of healing began to emerge. These became the progenitors of the current group of European spas. Dr. Sidney Licht, a physiatrist and founding member of the American Society of Medical Hydrology and Climatology, has defined a spa as a "place where mineral containing waters flow from the ground naturally, or to which it is pumped or conducted, and is there used for therapeutic purposes" (2).

In the decades before the American Civil War, major health reforms swept the nation, and numerous hydropathic establishments, institutes, and medical colleges were built for the practice of Water Cure—cold water bathing. The American Medical Association Committee on Sanitaria and Springs published its first national report on sanitaria in 1880. At the turn of the century, medical men such as Simon Baruch, John Harvey Kellogg, and Guy Hinsdale regularly conducted clinical hydrotherapeutic experiments and prescribed aquatic therapeutics. Baruch established the American medical standards for hydrotherapy in *The Principles and Practice of Hydrotherapy,* and in 1921, shortly before he died, Baruch published his last book, *An Epitome of Hydrotherapy.*

Although most writings concerned the internal and external curative benefits of the waters, baths, and pools, limited emphasis was placed on water exercise. In 1911, Charles LeRoy Lowman began using therapeutic tubs to treat spastic patients and those with cerebral palsy. Lowman had founded the Orthopaedic Hospital in Los Angeles in 1913, later to become Rancho Los Amigos. He visited the Spaulding School for Crippled Children in Chicago, where he observed paralyzed patients exercising in a wooden tank. Upon his return to California, he transformed the hospital's lily pond into two therapeutic pools (3,4). He also made a motion picture showing the various types of cases treated with pool therapy. At Warm Springs, Georgia, LeRoy Hubbard developed his famous tank, and in 1924 Warm Springs received its most famous aquatic patient, Franklin D. Roosevelt.

At Saratoga Springs, New York, financier Bernard M. Baruch, Roosevelt's friend and the son of Dr. Simon Baruch, headed a special commission to plan a scientific American spa (5). The commission studied spa design, natural treatments, and efficient operations based on what was then felt to be the sound medical and scientific care for chronically ill patients, especially those suffering from cardiac, vascular, and circulatory ailments, and selected Dr. Walter S. McClellan to be the Medical Spa Director (6). The same year (1931), Dr. W.E. Fitch, McClellan, and several other spa doctors, scientific directors, and spa general managers met at French Lick Spa to organize "an association which would be of mutual benefit to everyone interested in the advancement of (Medical) Hydrology in this country" (7). A wealth of information, research, and articles on health resort medicine, spa therapy, and pool treatments appeared in professional journals during the 1930s. At Northwestern University Medical School in Chicago, Dr. John S. Coulter presented lectures on physical therapy that he placed within the history of spa medicine (8). In 1933 the Simon Baruch Research

B. E. Becker: Department of Physical Medicine and Rehabilitation, Wayne State University, Rehabilitation Institute of Michigan, Detroit, Michigan 48201.

A. J. Cole: Puget Sound Sports and Spine Physicians, Seattle, Washington 98122.

Institute of Balneology at Saratoga Springs Spa was established, and the facility began the printing of their scientific bulletin: *The Publications of Saratoga Spa.* At Hot Springs, Arkansas, a warm swimming pool was installed for special underwater physical therapy exercises and pool therapy treatments with chronic arthritic patients (9–11). By 1937, Dr. Charles LeRoy Lowman published his *Technique of Underwater Gymnastics: A Study in Practical Application,* in which he detailed pool therapy methods of specific underwater exercises that "carefully regulated dosage, character, frequency, and duration for remedying bodily deformities and restoring muscle function" (12). During the 1950s the National Foundation for Infantile Paralysis supported the corrective swimming pools and hydrogymnastics of Charles L. Lowman and the therapeutic use of pools and tanks for the treatment of poliomyelitis. In 1962, Drs. Sidney Licht, Herman Flax, Sigmund Foster, William Erdman, Lucille Eising, J. Wayne McFarland, Jens Henriksen, and Richard Gubner organized the American Society of Medical Hydrology and Climatology (ASMH), which traditionally continues to meet at the annual meeting of the American Academy of Physical Medicine and Rehabilitation.

Current Trends and Uses

With the end of the polio epidemic and the rise of newer and more exciting technology in rehabilitative therapeutics, the use of the aquatic environment in rehabilitation waned. Medical hydrology became a smaller and smaller component of physiatric and physical therapy training. Principles of medical hydrology and aquatic rehabilitation that were formerly an important part of a therapist's training program were de-emphasized. Since the mid-1980s, the increase in health-care costs, constraints on physical therapy utilization under managed care, coupled with an emerging public understanding of the value of aquatic rehabilitation and better training within the rehabilitative professions have begun to drive a broader utilization of aquatic therapies. Fortunately, basic science research in the biologic effects of immersion accelerated during the late 1960s for two fortuitous reasons. Water was recognized as a wonderful surrogate for the weightlessness of space, and as we prepared to place humans outside gravity, it became essential to forecast the effects of space flight. At the same time, Murray Epstein and other endocrinologists realized that aquatic immersion was a benign means of simulating central volume expansion to better understand volume homeostasis. The end result of these research efforts has been that aquatic therapy has a considerable foundation of high-quality basic science research.

THE PHYSICS OF WATER AND ITS RELATIONSHIP TO AQUATIC REHABILITATION

Density and Specific Gravity

Density is defined as mass per unit volume, and is given the Greek letter rho (ρ). The relationship of ρ to mass and volume is characterized by the following formula:

$$\rho = m/V$$

where m is the mass of a substance whose volume is V. Density is measured in the international system by kilogram/m^3 and occasionally as g/cm^3. Density is a temperature-dependent variable, although much less so for solids and liquids than for gases. In addition to density, substances are defined by their specific gravity, the ratio of the density of that substance to the density of water. Water has a specific gravity equal to 1.00 at 4°C by definition. Although the human body is mostly water, the body's density is slightly less than water and averages a specific gravity of 0.974, with males averaging higher density than females. Lean body mass, which includes bone, muscle, connective tissue, and organs, has a typical density near 1.10, whereas fat mass, which includes both essential body fat plus fat in excess of essential needs, has a density of about 0.90 (13). Consequently, the human body displaces a volume of water weighing slightly more than the body, forcing the body upward by a force equal to the volume of the water displaced.

Hydrostatic Pressure

Pressure is defined as force per unit area, where the force F by convention is understood to act perpendicularly to the surface area A. This relationship is:

$$P = F/A$$

The standard international unit of pressure is called a pascal (Pa), after the French scientist Blaise Pascal, and is measured in Newtons/m^2, dynes/cm^2, kg/m^2, and pounds per square inch. Fluids have been experimentally found to exert pressure in all directions. At a theoretical point position immersed in a vessel of water, the pressure exerted upon that point is equal from all directions. Obviously, if unequal pressure were being exerted, the point would move until the pressures were equalized upon it. Pressure is directly proportional to both the liquid density and to the immersion depth, when the fluid is incompressible, as water is at the depths used in therapeutic environments. Because pressure responds not only to the fluid depth but also to any force exerted on its surface, the pressure of the Earth's atmosphere is an important contributor to the total force from immersion. Water exerts a pressure of 22.4 mm Hg for every foot of water depth, which translates to 0.73 mm Hg/cm or slightly under 2 mm Hg per inch of H_2O depth. Thus, a body immersed to a depth of 48 inches is subjected to a distal pressure equal to 88.9 mm Hg, far greater than venous or lymphatic pressures. This external compressive force significantly aids the resolution of edema in an injured body part.

Buoyancy

Buoyancy causes immersed objects to have less apparent weight than the same object on land. Buoyancy, a force opposite to gravity, acts on the object with a force generated by the volume of H_2O displaced. This principle was discovered by Archimedes (287 to 212 B.C.) and is the reason why water can be used to advantage in the management of medical problems requiring weight off-loading. A human with a specific gravity of 0.97 will reach floating equilibrium when 97% of his or her volume is submerged.

Because the force of buoyancy is an upward force, there are important consequences in the therapeutic aquatic environment. The center of gravity is a point at which all force moments are in equilibrium. For a human being standing in the "anatomical" position, this point is located slightly posterior to the mid-sagittal plane and at the level of the second sacral vertebra, because the human body is nonuniform with respect to density. The lungs obviously are less dense than the lower limbs, for example. The center of buoyancy is defined as the center of all buoyancy force moments summating each body segment. Typically, the human center of buoyancy is in the mid-chest. The difference between the center of gravity (a downward force) and the center of buoyancy (an upward force) may generate rotational torque.

Water in Motion

Flow Characteristics

When water moves smoothly, in layers moving at the same speed, the water is defined as in laminar or streamline flow. When water moves more rapidly, even minor oscillations create uneven flow, and parallel paths are knocked out of alignment, resulting in turbulent flow. Within the mass of water, flow patterns arise that run dramatically out of parallel. These paths are called eddy currents. An example of the latter are the eddy currents that form in the blood stream behind artery walls encrusted with cholesterol plaque. Turbulent flow absorbs energy at a much greater rate than streamline flow, and the rate of energy absorption is determined by the internal friction within the fluid. This internal friction is called viscosity. The major determinants of water motion are viscosity, turbulence, and speed. Flow rates decrease when turbulence occurs, largely due to the significant nonlinear increase in internal friction in the fluid. The onset of turbulent flow obviously is a function of fluid velocity, but it is also related to fluid density, viscosity, and enclosure radius. The transition from laminar flow to turbulent flow often occurs abruptly with increasing velocity.

Viscosity and Drag

Viscosity refers to the magnitude of internal friction specific to the fluid. As layers of fluid molecules are set into motion, molecular attraction creates resistance to movement and is detected as friction. Energy must be exerted to create movement, and as in the first law of thermodynamics, energy is never lost but rather transformed and stored as potential or kinetic energy. Some energy is transformed into heat,

TABLE 35-1. *Coefficients of viscosities for a variety of fluids*

Fluid	Temperature (°C)	Coefficient of viscosity η (Pa · s)
Water	0	1.8×10^{-3}
Whole blood	37	4×10^{-3}
Blood plasma	37	1.5×10^{-3}
Engine oil (SAE 10)	30	200×10^{-3}
Glycerin	20	$1{,}500 \times 10^{-3}$
Water vapor	100	0.013×10^{-3}

some into kinetic energy, and some may be stored as potential energy by increasing surface tension. Fluids are in part defined by individual viscosity, expressed quantitatively as the coefficient of viscosity (η) (Table 35-1). The greater the coefficient, the more viscous the fluid and the more the force that is required to create movement within the fluid. This force is proportionate to the number of molecules of fluid set into motion and the velocity of movement. Because velocity is described by distance/time, viscosity is the first time-dependent property. An equation that expresses this relationship must define the volume of the fluid in motion, measured as the area (A), depth (l), and velocity (v) of the motion. The SI unit of measurement of viscosity is called a poise, after the French scientist J.L. Poiselle (1799 to 1869), who studied the physics of blood circulation.

Water is intermediate in viscosity as liquids go, but still presents much resistance to movement. Under turbulent flow conditions, this resistance increases as a log function of velocity. The greatest surface area drag on a swimming man is his head, although the negative pressure following the swimmer causes the greatest force resisting forward movement. There is turbulence produced by fast-moving body surface areas and a drag force produced by the turbulence behind. Viscosity, with all its attendant physical properties, is a quality that makes water a useful strengthening medium. Viscous resistance increases as more force is exerted against it, but resistance drops to zero almost immediately upon cessation of force because there is only a small amount of inertia (viscosity effectively counteracts inertial momentum). Thus, when a rehabilitating person feels pain and stops movement, the force decreases precipitously, and water viscosity damps movement almost instantaneously. This allows great control of strengthening activities within the envelope of patient movement comfort.

Specific Heat

Water is used therapeutically in all three of its thermal states: solid, liquid, and gas. A major reason for its usefulness lies in the physics of aquatic thermodynamics. All substances on earth possess energy stored as heat. This energy is measured in a quantity called a calorie (cal). A calorie is defined as the heat required to raise the temperature of 1 g of water by 1°C (e.g., from 14.5 to 15.5°C). The energy required to raise temperature is defined in kilocalories, the amount of energy required to raise one kilogram of water 1°C, and this unit by convention is termed a Calorie (with a capital C) (Cal). This is the unit in which food energy content is measured. The British system measures heat energy in British Thermal Units (BTU), the amount of energy required to raise 1 pound of water 1°F (1 BTU = 0.252 Cal). A mass of water possesses a measurable amount of stored energy in the form of heat. Energy stored may be released through a change to a lower temperature, or additional energy may raise the water temperature. The formula defining the quantity of energy required or released is:

$$Q = mc\Delta T^\circ$$

where m equals the mass of water, c equals the specific heat capacity of the fluid, and ΔT° equals the change in temperature. The work required to produce this energy is called the mechanical equivalent of heat and is measured in joules (J). One Calorie is equivalent to 4.18×10^3 J. A body immersed in a mass of water becomes a dynamic system. If the temperature of the water exceeds the temperature of the submersed body, the system equilibrates to a different level, with the submersed body warming through transference of heat energy from the water, and the water cooling through loss of heat energy to the body. By the first law of thermodynamics, the total heat (and thus energy) content of the system remains the same. Energy applied to this system increases the kinetic energy of some of the molecules, and when high kinetic energy molecules collide with lower kinetic energy molecules, they transfer some of their energy, increasing and equilibrating the total energy of the system. Water is defined as having a specific heat capacity equal to 1.00. Air, in contrast, has a far lower specific heat capacity = 0.001. Thus, water retains heat 1,000 times more than an equal volume of air.

Thermal Energy Transfer

The therapeutic utility of water is greatly dependent on both its ability to retain heat and its ability to transfer heat energy. Exchange of energy in the form of heat occurs in three ways: conduction, convection, and radiation. Conduction may be thought of as occurring through molecular collisions occurring over a small distance. Substances vary widely in their ability to conduct heat. Convection requires the mass movement of large numbers of molecules over a large distance (i.e., fluid flow). Heat transfer across a gradient is measured by the amount of heat in calories transferred per second across an imaginary membrane. Liquids and gases are generally poor conductors but good convectors. Water is an efficient conductor of heat and transfers heat 25 times faster than air. Radiation transfers heat through the transmission of electromagnetic waves. The rate of radiant energy transfer from a body is proportional to the fourth power of its temperature in degrees Kelvin. It is also proportional to surface area, to the emissivity of the material, and to the second power of the distance between the energy-radiating and energy-absorbing bodies. The thermal conductive property of water, in combination with water's high specific heat, makes its use in rehabilitation versatile as it retains heat or cold while transferring it easily to the immersed body part.

BIOLOGIC ASPECTS OF AQUATIC REHABILITATION

Circulatory System Effects

Water begins to exert pressure on the body immediately upon immersion. Pressure in the venous and lymphatic side of the circulation is much lower than pressure on the arterial side of the system. Venous and lymphatic pressures vary, depending on the part of the body and its vertical relationship to the heart but are in part controlled by the system of valves within both systems, which prevents backflow. These one-way valves act to divide the large vertical column fluid into many short columns with little vertical height. This allows much lower hydrostatic pressure gradients inside the vessel wall, so that the maximum venous pressure is 30 mm Hg peripherally, decreasing steadily as blood travels toward the right atrium, which has a negative pressure of −2 to −4 mm Hg. The role of these valves in maintaining a low pressure system is critical, as can be observed when they fail, creating venous varicosities due to the lack of sufficient vessel wall strength to support the increased height of the fluid column. Consequently, venous and lymphatic return is sensitive to external pressure changes, including compression from surrounding muscles and from external water pressure. During water immersion, hydrostatic pressure displaces blood upward through this one-way system, first into the thighs, then into the abdominal cavity vessels, and finally into the great vessels of the chest cavity and into the heart. Central venous pressure begins to increase with immersion to the xiphoid and increases until the body is completely immersed. Right atrial distension occurs while pressure increases by 14 to 18 mm Hg during immersion to the neck, going from about −2 to −4 mm Hg to −14 to −17 mm Hg (14,15). The transmural pressure gradient of the right atrium increases significantly, measured by Arborelius and others at 13 mm Hg, going from 2 mm Hg to 15 mm Hg. Extra systoles may result, especially early into immersion (15).

Pulmonary blood flow increases with increased central blood volume and pressure. Mean pulmonary artery wedge pressure increases from 5 mm Hg on land to 22 mm Hg during immersion to the neck (15). Most of the increased pulmonary blood volume is distributed in the larger vessels of the pulmonary vascular bed, and only a small percentage (5% or less) at the capillary level. This is validated by the fact that the diffusion capacity of the lungs changes very little.

Central blood volume increased by 0.7 L in Arborelius' classic study (15). This represents a 60% increase in central volume, with one third of this volume taken up by the heart and the remainder by the great vessels of the lungs. Cardiac volume increases 27% to 30% with immersion to the neck (16), but the heart is not a static receptacle. The healthy cardiac response to increased volume (stretch) is to increase the force of contraction. As the myocardium stretches, an improved actin/myosin filament relationship is produced, enhancing the myocardial efficiency (Starling's Law) (17). Mean stroke volume increases 35% on average with immersion to the neck from a resting baseline of about 71 ml/beat, to about 100 ml/beat, which is close to the exercise maximum for a sedentary deconditioned individual on land (14,18). There is both an increase in end-diastolic volume and a decrease in end-systolic volume (14). Stroke volume is one of the major determinants of the increase in cardiac output seen with training because heart rate response ranges remain relatively fixed (18).

Most of the changes are temperature dependent, with cardiac output increasing progressively with increasing water temperatures. Weston found cardiac output to increase by 30% at 33°C rising to 121% at 39°C (16). There is considerable individual variance in the many studies assessing this phenomenon.

As cardiac filling and stroke volume increase with deeper immersion from symphysis to xiphoid, the heart rate typically decreases (19). This decrease is variable, with the amount of decrease dependent on water temperature. Typically, at average pool temperatures the rate decreases by 12% to 15% (19). There is a significant relationship between water temperature and heart rate. At 25°C, the heart rate decreases by approximately 12 to 15 beats/min (17), whereas at thermoneutral temperatures the rate decrease is less than 15%, and in warm water the rate generally increases significantly, contributing to the major increase in cardiac output at high temperatures (8,18). The reduction variability is believed to be related to decreased peripheral resistance at higher temperatures and increased vagal effects.

The most efficient way for the heart to deliver more blood during exercise is to increase stroke volume. Maximal myocardial oxygen consumption efficiency (peak heart muscle efficiency) occurs when stroke volume increases because the heart rate increase is a less efficient means of increasing output (17,19). Thus, as cardiovascular conditioning occurs, cardiac output increases are achieved with smaller increases in heart rate but greater stroke volumes. This is the reason that conditioned athletes are able to maintain lower pulse rates for a given cardiac output, when compared with matched deconditioned individuals (17).

Several studies have validated the use of aquatic environments in cardiovascular rehabilitation after infarct and ischemic cardiomyopathy by actively rehabilitating heart patients in an aquatic environment (20,21). Tanaka found that a single immersion in a very hot water (41°C) bath decreased both pulmonary wedge pressure and right atrial pressure by nearly 30%, and over a period of 1 month of daily therapy patients showed nearly a 30% increase in ejection fraction, significantly improving by one and sometimes two New York Heart Association classifications.

Because the ultimate purpose of the heart as an organ is to pump blood, its ultimate measure of performance is the amount of blood pumped per unit time. Cardiac output is the product of stroke volume times pulse rate per unit time. Submersion to the neck increases cardiac output by more than 30% (14). Output increases by about 1,500 ml/min, of which 50% is directed to increased muscle blood flow (14). Normal resting cardiac output is approximately 5 L/min. Maximum output in a conditioned athlete is about 40 L/min, which is equivalent to 205 ml/beat times 195 beats/min. Maximum output at exercise for a sedentary individual on land is approximately 20 L/min, equivalent to 105 ml/beat times 195 beats/min (18). Because immersion to the neck produces a cardiac stroke volume of about 100 ml/beat, a resting pulse of 86 beats/min produces a cardiac output of 8.6 L/min and is already producing increased cardiac work. The increase in cardiac output appears to be somewhat age dependent, with younger subjects demonstrating greater increases (59%) than older subjects (22%) (22). The increase is also highly temperature dependent, varying directly with temperature increase from 30% at 33°C to 121% at 39°C (23). Recent research has shown that conditioned athletes demonstrate an even greater increase in cardiac output than untrained control subjects during immersed exercise and that this increase was sustained for longer periods than in the control group (24). Therefore, the myth that water exercise is not aerobically efficient is faulty; it may be an ideal cardiovascular conditioning medium. There is an emerging body of research on water exercise–induced cardiac output, but significant work needs to be done to delineate the effects of age, gender, temperature, and conditioning, as well as to explain the significant individual response variations. The cascade of cardiovascular responses to immersion are shown in Figure 35-1.

During immersion to the neck, systemic vascular resistance decreases by 30% (14). Diminished sympathetic vasoconstriction produces this decrease, with peripheral venous tone decreasing by 30% from 17 mm Hg to 12 mm Hg at thermoneutral temperatures (25). Total peripheral resistance decreases during the first hour of immersion and remains low for several hours thereafter. This decrease is related to temperature, with higher temperatures producing greater reductions. This resistance drop decreases end-diastolic pressures. Immersed systolic pressures increase with increasing workload as they do on land, but these increases appear to be reduced in magnitude when compared with equivalent land-based work (26). Venous pressures also decrease during immersion because less vascular tone is required to support the system.

The effect of immersion on blood pressure has been quite extensively studied. A consistent finding has been the rather striking individual variation, but trends have emerged that

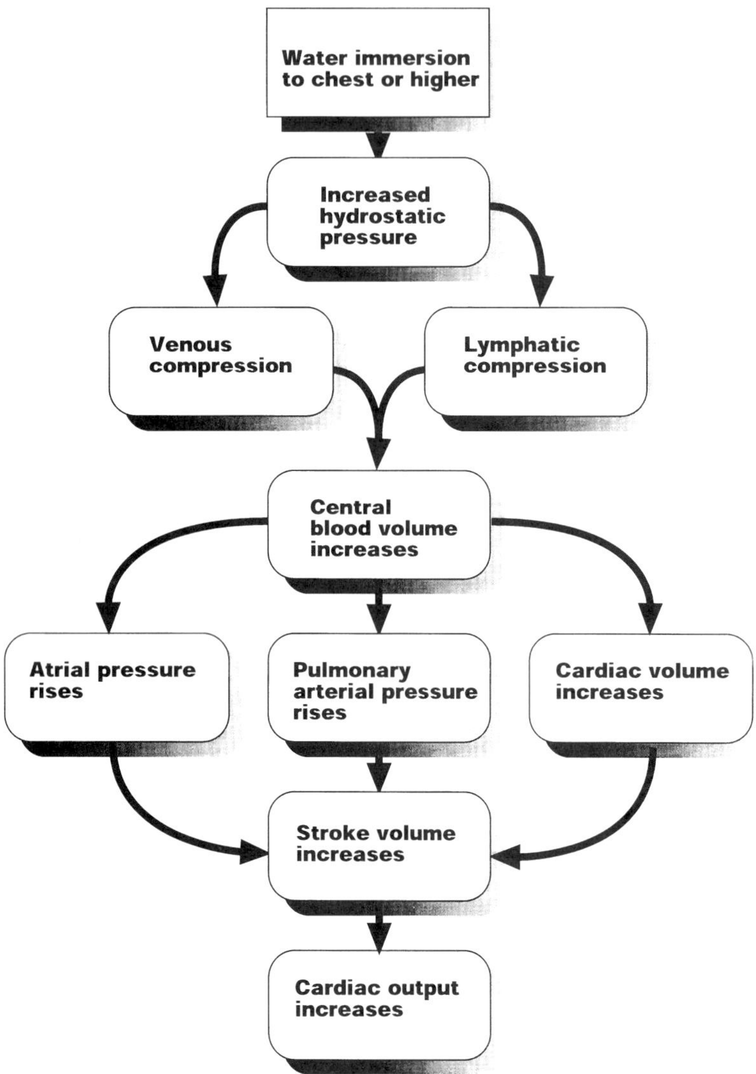

FIG. 35-1. Cardiovascular schematic.

are useful. Very short-term immersion (10 minutes) in thermoneutral temperatures has been found to slightly increase both systolic and diastolic pressures, perhaps as part of the thermal accommodation process (26). Other studies conducted in carefully controlled environments have found no effects or actual decreases in pressures during longer immersion periods more typical of therapeutic sessions (27). In an important study for aquatic rehabilitation, Corruzi et al. found that longer immersion produced significant decreases in mean arterial pressure, with sodium-sensitive hypertensive patients showing even greater decreases (18 to 20 mm Hg) than normotensive patients, and sodium-insensitive patients showing smaller decreases (5 to 14 mm Hg) (28). No studies have demonstrated consistent sustained increases in systolic pressure with prolonged immersion, although several have found no significant decrease. Based on a substantial body of research, the therapeutic pool appears to be both a safe and potentially therapeutic environment for both normotensive and hypertensive patients, with both sodium-sensitive and insensitive hypertensives demonstrating decreases in pressure during therapeutically customary periods of immersion (29).

In 1989, Gleim and Nicholas found that oxygen consumption (VO_2) was three times greater at a given running speed (53 m/min) in water than on land (26). Thus, looking at the reverse effect of this fact, during water walking and running, only one half to one third the speed was required to achieve the same metabolic intensity as on land (30). It is important to note that the relationship of heart rate to VO_2 parallels the relationship extant during land-based exercise, even with accounting for the heart rate decrease in water. Consequently, metabolic intensity in water may be predicted as on land from monitoring heart rate.

Pulmonary System Effects

The pulmonary system is profoundly affected by immersion of the body to the level of the thorax. Part of the effect is due to the shift of blood into the chest cavity, and part is due to compression of the chest wall itself by water. The combined effect is to alter pulmonary function, increase the work of breathing, and change respiratory dynamics.

Functional residual capacity reduces to about 54% of the normal value with immersion to the xiphoid (31). Most of this loss is due to reduction in expiratory reserve volume (ERV), which decreases by 75% at this level of immersion (32). The change in this volume may be readily experienced at poolside: while sitting on the edge of the pool exhale normally, and then expel the rest of the reserve volume forcibly. Enter the water to neck level, and perform the same experiment—the difference is very perceptible. Little air remains to exhale at the endpoint of relaxed exhalation. ERV is reduced to 11% of vital capacity, equal to breathing at a negative pressure of −20.5 cm H_2O (30). There is some loss of residual volume, which decreases by 15% (30). Vital capacity decreases by about 6% to 9% when comparing neck submersion to controls submerged to the xiphoid (30,33). About 50% to 60% of this vital capacity reduction is due to increased thoracic blood volume, and 40% to 50% is due to hydrostatic forces counteracting the inspiratory musculature (30,33). Pressure on the rib cage shrinks the rib cage circumference by approximately 10% during submersion (33). The reduction in vital capacity does appear to fluctuate somewhat with temperature, with cooler water immersion (25°C) producing a greater decrease and warm water immersion (40°C) a *smaller decrease* (34). Figure 35-2 depicts the changes in pulmonary function during immersion.

The ability of the alveolar membrane to exchange gases is called diffusion capacity. Diffusion capacity of the lungs is reduced slightly, as is partial pressure of oxygen (PO_2) as the lung beds become distended with blood shifted from the extremities and abdomen. Total intrapulmonary pressure shifts to the right by 16 cm H_2O (33). This causes airway resistance to the movement of air to increase by 58% or more resulting from reduced lung volume (33). Expiratory flow rates are reduced, increasing the time to move air into and out of the lungs. Chest wall compliance is reduced due to the pressure of water on the chest wall, increasing pleural pressure from −1 to +1 mm Hg (14).

The combined effect of all these changes is to increase the total work of breathing. The total work of breathing for a tidal volume of 1 L increases by 60% during submersion to neck. Three quarters of this effort is attributable to an increase in elastic work (redistribution of blood from the thorax) and the rest to dynamic work (hydrostatic force upon the thorax) (33). Thus, for an athlete accustomed to land-based conditioning exercises, a program of water-based exercise results in a significant workload challenge to the respiratory apparatus. In the authors' experience, this challenge can raise the efficiency of the respiratory

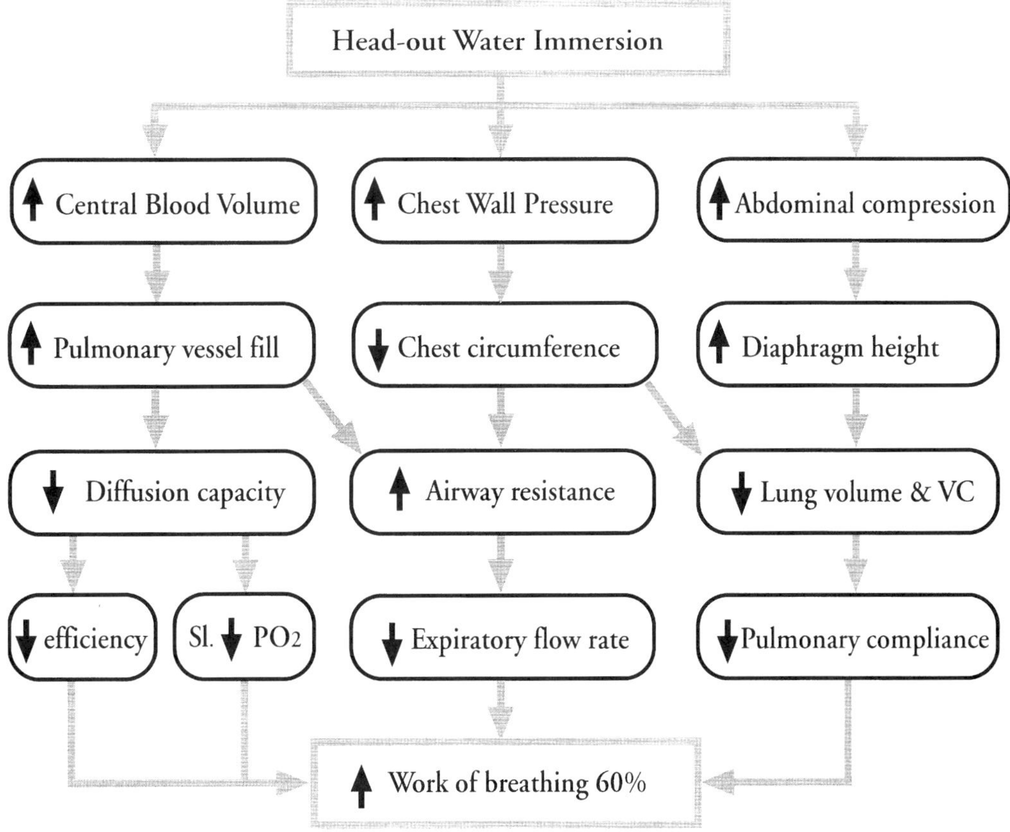

FIG. 35-2. Effects of immersion on respiration.

system if the time spent in water conditioning is sufficient to achieve respiratory apparatus strength gains.

Musculoskeletal Effects

Joint Effects

As the body gradually immerses, water is displaced, creating a progressive off-loading of the immersed joints. With neck immersion, only about 15 pounds of compressive force (the approximate weight of the head) is exerted on the spine, hips, and knees. A person immersed to the symphysis pubis has effectively off-loaded 40% body weight, and when further immersed to the umbilicus, approximately 50%. Xiphoid immersion produces 60% or more off-loading, depending on whether the arms are overhead or beside the trunk. A body suspended or floating in water essentially counterbalances the downward effects of gravity by the upward force of buoyancy. This effect may be of great therapeutic utility. For example, a fractured pelvis may not become mechanically stable under full body loading for a period of many weeks, but with water immersion, gravitational forces may be partially or completely offset so that only muscle torque forces are present on the fracture site(s), allowing "active-assisted" range of motion activities, gentle strength building, and even gait training.

The effects of buoyancy and water resistance make possible high levels of energy expenditure with relatively little movement and strain on lower extremity joints (35,36). Off-loading occurs as a function of immersion, as was extensively discussed earlier, but the water depth chosen may be adjusted for the amount of loading desired. The spine especially is well protected during aquatic exercise programs, facilitating early rehabilitation.

Shallow water vertical exercises generally approximate closed-chain exercise, but with reduced joint loading because of the partial buoyancy counterforce. Deep water exercises more generally approximate an open chain system, as do horizontal exercises such as swimming. Paddles and other resistive equipment tend to close the kinetic chain. However, aquatic programs offer the ability to damp the force of movement instantaneously because of the viscous properties of water.

The force exerted against the floor by the walking body is counteracted by the ground. This force is termed ground reaction force and may easily be measured through a force plate. It has been found to differ substantially during walking in chest-deep water. Force plate tracings of the pressure generated during a gait cycle on dry land compared with chest deep water walking are substantially reduced in magnitude by more than 50%, are generated more slowly, and the forces are transmitted over a longer time interval during water walking (30). Clinically, this means that less joint compression is produced, and impact strain is diminished.

Water immersion causes significant effects on blood circulation through muscle tissue. These effects are caused by the compressive effects of immersion as well as by the reflex regulation of blood vessel tone. To resist blood pooling during dry conditions, sympathetic vasoconstriction tightens the resistance vessels of skeletal muscle. Immersion pressure removes the biologic need for vasoconstriction, thus increasing muscle blood flow. During immersion, it is likely that most if not all of the increased cardiac output is redistributed to skin and muscle rather than to the splanchnic beds (33). Resting muscle blood flow has been found to more than double during immersion to the neck, and with this increased perfusion, muscle tissue washout was found to increase 130% above dry land clearance (37). Thus, oxygen delivery is significantly increased during immersion, as is the removal of muscle metabolic waste products. Hydrostatic forces add an additional circulatory drive to drive out edema, muscle lactate, and other metabolic end products.

Renal and Endocrine Effects

Because aquatic immersion produces central volume expansion in a pharmacologically and physiologically noninvasive manner, aquatic immersion serves as an excellent model for volume homeostasis. Aquatic immersion creates many effects on renal blood flow, on the renal regulatory systems, and on the endocrine systems. These effects have been studied extensively in both the American and international literatures. Murray Epstein, one of the most skilled and prolific researchers in studying immersion effects on the human, published an exhaustive summary of these effects in 1992 (36). The flow of blood to the kidneys increases immediately upon immersion. This causes an increase in creatinine clearance, a measure of renal efficiency, initially upon immersion (36). Renal sympathetic nerve activity decreases due to the vagal response caused by left atrial distension, as discussed earlier in this chapter, and this decrease in sympathetic nerve activity increases renal tubular sodium transport (38). Calculated renal vascular resistance decreases by about one third (36). Renal venous pressure increases almost twofold (36). Sodium excretion increases 10-fold in individuals with normal total-body sodium, and this sodium excretion is accompanied by free water, creating a major part of the diuretic effect of immersion. This increase in sodium excretion is a time-dependent phenomenon. Sodium excretion also increases as a function of depth, due to the shifting of circulating central blood volume (36). Potassium excretion also increases with immersion (27). The renal effects of immersion are shown in Figure 35-3.

Renal function is largely regulated by the hormones renin, aldosterone, and antidiuretic hormone (ADH), by the dopa-dopamine system, and by the atrial naturetic peptide (ANP) system. All these hormones are greatly affected by immersion (Fig. 35-4). Aldosterone controls Na^+ reabsorption in the distal renal tubule, and accounts

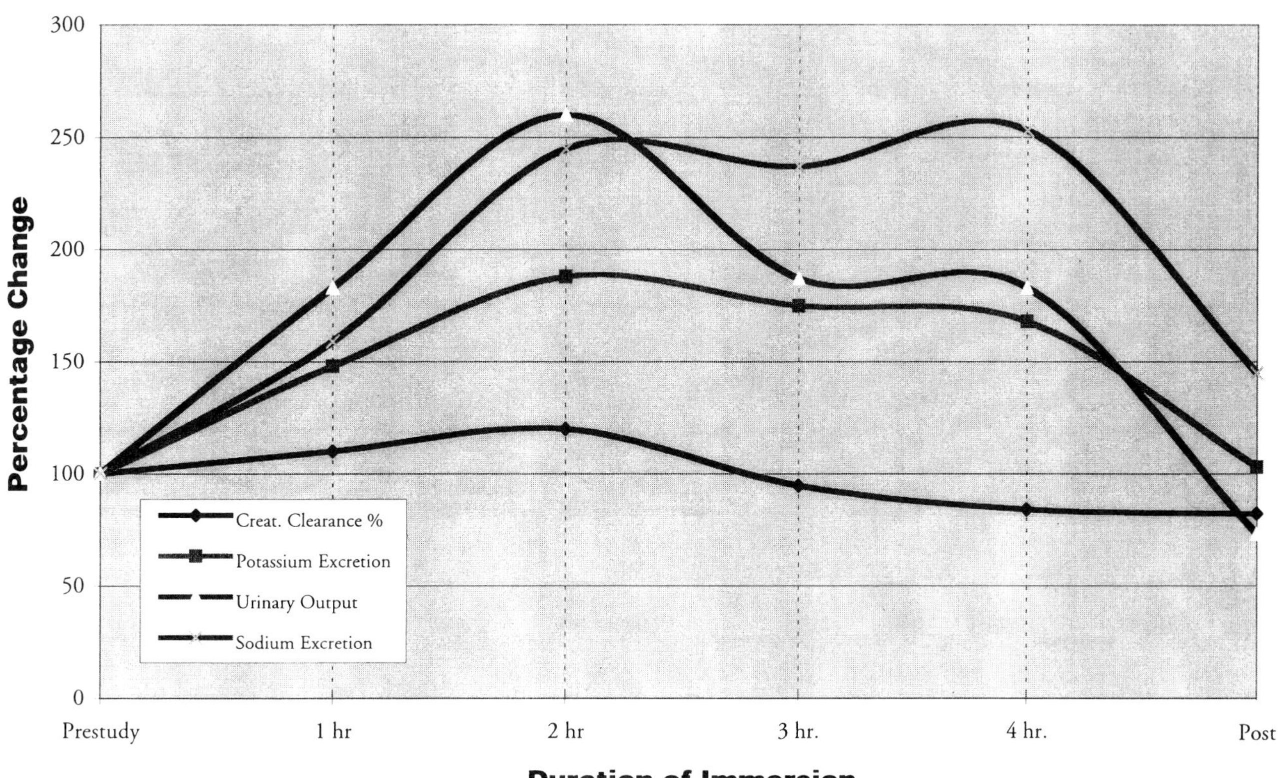

FIG. 35-3. Renal function changes during immersion.

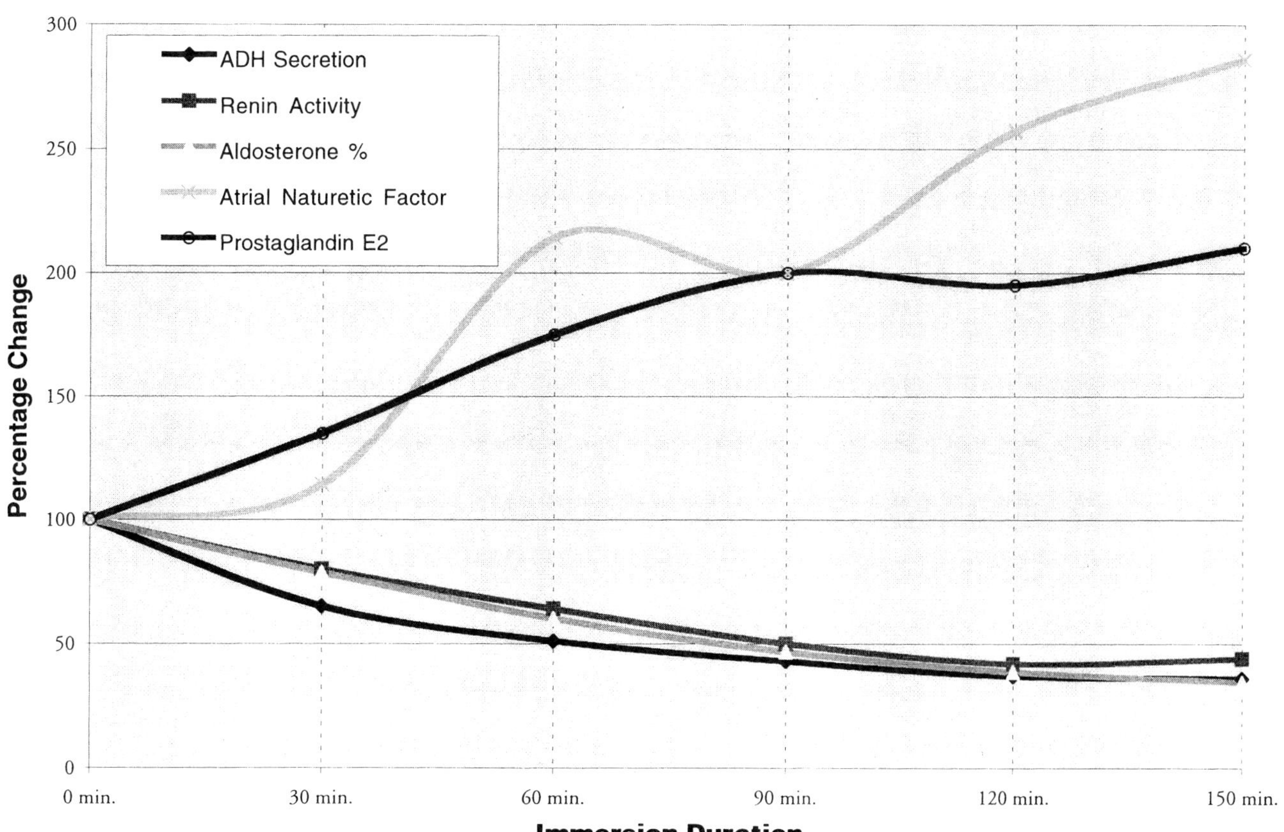

FIG. 35-4. Renal hormone responses to immersion.

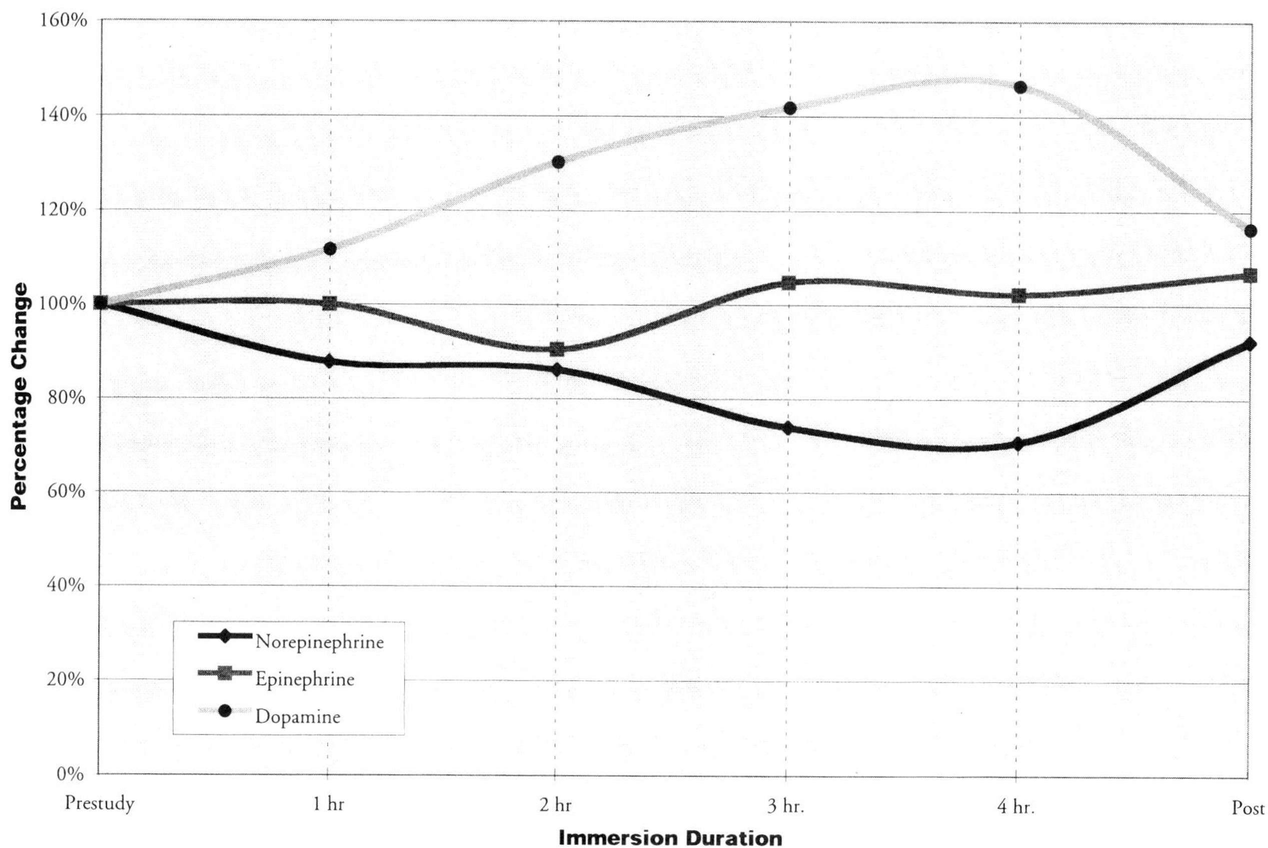

FIG. 35-5. Catecholamine responses to immersion.

for most of the Na^+ loss with immersion (16,36). ADH release is significantly suppressed with immersion by 50% or more and is the other major contributor to diuresis. Another factor important in sodium regulation is atrial naturietic peptide (ANP) which has both sodium excretion–facilitating and diuretic activity. ANP relaxes vascular smooth muscle and inhibits production of aldosterone. Immersion produces a prompt and continuing increase in ANP (27). Renal prostaglandin E secretion increases steadily through the first 2 hours of immersion, and then decreases gently over the next 3 hours. Plasma renin activity is reduced by 33% to 50% at 2 hours of immersion to the neck (36). Overall, immersion-induced central volume expansion causes an increase in urinary output accompanied by significant sodium and potassium excretion, beginning almost immediately upon immersion, steadily increasing over several hours of immersion. This may cause a decrease in blood pressure, and the resultant decrease may be sustained over a period of several to many hours. Immersion was historically one of the few effective ways of treating congestive heart failure noninvasively before the discovery of digitalis.

Accompanying the renal hormone effects are changes in the autonomic nervous system neurotransmitters, collectively called catacholamines, which act to regulate vascular resistance, cardiac rate, and force. The most important of these are epinephrine, norepinephrine, and dopamine. Catecholamine levels begin changing immediately upon immersion (Fig. 35-5) (39,40).

REHABILITATIVE APPLICATIONS

Arthritis and Related Disorders

The value of the aquatic environment has a longer history in the management of the arthritic diseases than in almost any other disease group. The losses that accompany chronic joint disease are many: loss of strength, loss of joint mobility and stability, and ultimately loss of functional capacity. It has been noted that rheumatoid patients as a group have lower than expected aerobic capacity and physical performance, with overall muscle strength 60% below that of age-matched control subjects. These deficits respond promptly to active rehabilitation, with well-tailored strengthening and endurance programs achieving gains in physical performance levels in as brief a time as 6 weeks (36). Long-term exercise regimens in rheumatoid patients over many years have been proven to be well tolerated, with resultant improvement in functional and other outcome measures (41).

Because patients with arthritis have been shown to have decreased endurance, these individuals should participate in some form of aerobic exercise to enhance their overall fitness. Studies have demonstrated the benefits of aerobic exercise for many conditions, including fibromyalgia pain (42), rheumatoid arthritis (38,43), lupus (44), and osteoarthritis (45). Low-impact exercise has been shown to be more efficacious than medications in the self-management of osteoarthritis (46). Because the safest medium to reduce impact is the pool, the incorporation of aquatic exercise and/or swimming provides an advantageous alternative to manage arthritic symptoms. This argument has been substantiated in two studies of patient groups, with nonacute rheumatoid and osteoarthritis participating in water exercise regimens. In a study of rheumatoid patients, Danneskiold-Samsoe et al. found markedly increased isometric and isokinetic muscle strength of the quadriceps after only moderate training in the pool. Other gains included an increase in aerobic capacity, freedom of movement, and a higher degree of independence in activities of daily living (47). Bunning et al. concluded that pool therapy was both efficacious and achieved high compliance for those with osteoarthritis and that aquatic exercise should be the cornerstone of active rehabilitation for severe arthritis. Patients who participated in the study exhibited significant improvements in aerobic capacity and walk time and physical activity level, and were less depressed than controls (48).

The Arthritis Foundation, in conjunction with the YMCA, has developed a series of aquatic exercise regimens and classes for groups and individuals and certifies instructors. Training materials are available through the Arthritis Foundation (49). The original program was developed in 1983, revised in 1989 and 1996, and includes range of motion, strengthening, and endurance-building exercises. Swimming skills are unnecessary. The certification process is sufficient so that the medical practitioner may feel comfortable referring a patient to the program, and the authors' experience has been that patient adherence has been high, therapeutic value significant, and cost to the patient low. The Arthritis Foundation has developed two other programs: PACE (People with Arthritis Can Exercise), a community-based group program, and Joint Efforts, a gentle exercise program for sedentary older adults.

Spine Rehabilitation

Accurate diagnosis of patients spinal injuries and observation of their initial responses to land-based or aquatic stabilization programs helps determine further therapeutic exercise treatment. A transition from dry to wet exercise conditions eliminates dry land risks, establishes a supportive training environment, provides a new therapeutic activity, decreases the risk of peripheral joint injury, and allows a return to prior activity. Moving from dry to wet environments also should be considered if patients cannot tolerate axial or gravitational loads; they require increased support in the presence of a strength or proprioceptive deficit (50); or they are at risk of a compression fracture due to decreased bone density (48). Remaining in a water-supported environment is appropriate if a dry environment exacerbates symptoms or if patients prefer water. Transition from a wet to a dry environment should occur if patients are doing well in the water but must return to land to meet functional training needs efficiently and attain their ultimate competitive goals (51,52).

The aquatic rehabilitation programs that will be reviewed are based on dynamic lumbar, thoracic, and cervical stabilization techniques that have been previously described for land programs (53,54). Dynamic land-based stabilization training is a therapeutic exercise program that helps patients gain dynamic control of segmental spine forces; eliminates repetitive injury to motion segments (i.e., discs, zygapophyseal joints, and related structures); encourages healing of injured motion segments; and possibly alters the degenerative process. The underlying premise is that motion segments and supporting soft tissues react to minimize applied stresses and reduce risk of injury (53,54). The goals of aquatic stabilization exercise and swimming programs incorporate these elements but take into account the unique properties of water so that risk of spine injury is reduced. Aquatic stabilization programs help develop patients' flexibility, strength, and body mechanics so that a smooth transition to aquatic stabilization swimming programs or other spine-stabilized activities may occur. Such programs can help first-time swimmers or patients who previously swam (55,56).

Graded elimination of gravitational forces through buoyancy allows patients to train with decreased yet variable axial loads and shear forces. In essence, water increases the safety margin of patient postural error by decreasing the compressive and shear forces on the spine. Velocity can be controlled better by water resistance, viscosity, buoyancy, and training devices. Buoyancy increases the range of training positions. The psychological outlook of athletes may be enhanced because rehabilitation occurs in their competitive environment. Many believe that pain attenuation takes place in the water because of the sensory overload generated by hydrostatic pressure, temperature, and turbulence (57).

Aquatic Spine Stabilization Techniques

The spine stabilization principles discussed for land programs also apply to aquatic programs. Certain exercises that can be performed on land cannot be reproduced in water and vice versa. Aquatic programs can be designed for patients who cannot train on land or for those whose land training has reached a plateau. Richard Eagleston first described aquatic stabilization in 1989 (58).

Eight core aquatic stabilization exercises with four levels of difficulty have been developed to provide graded training of stabilization skills (55,59). Programs must be customized to meet the needs of each patient's unique spine pathology, related musculoskeletal dysfunctions, and comfort with the aquatic environment. Also, patients who have had joint replacements require particular care during positioning in the water because the replacements can change the center of buoyancy and may cause patients to sink due to high specific gravity (60). When a program is mastered, a more advanced program is provided. Eventually, if a patient wants to incorporate a swimming program, a series of transitional aquatic stabilization exercises are initiated. These help to establish a spine-stabilized swimming style that minimizes the risk of further spine injury and helps maximize swimming performance (61,62).

Spine-Stabilized Swimming Programs

Once a patient's stabilization skills have progressed to the point when swimming is possible, a thorough analysis of stroke technique and its effect on spine motion is critical (46). The following overview focuses on lumbar spine injury and indicates the role that the cervical spine plays in the mechanics of lumbar aquatic motion.

Analysis of stroke mechanics, like gait analysis, should be performed in an ordered, sequential manner so that all deficits and their relationships are carefully and fully scrutinized. Typically, the analysis begins at the head and progresses distally.

Prone Swimming

During prone swimming the patient's head should be midline. Breathing should occur by turning the head, i.e., rotating the head along the axial plane. There should be no craning (i.e., suboccipital cervical extension and rotation) or cervical extension and rotation (C2–C7). Body roll also contributes to proper breathing mechanics and is essential to minimize dysfunctional cervical positioning and subsequent pain. The cervical spine should be kept in the neutral position along the sagittal plane because excessive extension causes the legs and torso to drop in the water, and excessive flexion can cause a struggle for air (63,64).

The upper body arm position is evaluated by stroke phase. Freestyle is made up of three phases. The entry phase includes hand entry and hand submersion (ride). The pull phase incorporates insweep, outsweep, and finish components. The recovery phase includes the exit and arm swing. Several stroke defects can cause poor lumbar mechanics. If the arm abducts beyond 180°, lateral lumbar flexion and rotation are produced. During the pull phase, decreased body rotation can cause lateral lumbar flexion and rotation that stress the lumbar motion segments, particularly the annular fibers surrounding the nucleus pulposus. Inadequate strength in the triceps during the finish phase results in low arm recovery, which in turn generates secondary lateral flexion and rotation through the lumbar spine. During recovery, inadequate body roll causes the neck to crane, which results in a struggle for air and accompanying lateral flexion and rotation through the lumbar spine (Table 35-2).

The aquatic environment provides numerous advantages to assist rehabilitation of patients with spine pain. A series of aquatic stabilization exercises have been designed that incorporate the intrinsic properties of water and enhance rehabilitative efforts. When these exercises are mastered, injured patients can soon advance to spine-safe swimming or

TABLE 35-2. *Freestyle stroke defects*

Primary peripheral joint stroke defect	Secondary effect	Spine reaction
Head high	Lower body sinks	Increased cervical extension Increased lumbar extension
Head low	Upper body sinks	Increased lumbar flexion
Crane breathing	Lower body sinks Contralateral shoulder sinks	Increased cervical and suboccipital extension Increased cervical rotation Increased lumbar lateral flexion and rotation
Crossover hand entry	Lateral body movement	Increased lumbar lateral flexion and rotation
Wide hand entry	Contralateral shoulder roll	Increased cervical rotation Increased lumbar lateral flexion and rotation
Inefficient pull power	Upper body sinks Difficulty breathing	Increased cervical rotation Increased cervical extension Increased lumbar extension Increased lumbar lateral flexion and rotation
Increased hip flexion	Decreased kick propulsion Lower body sinks	Increased cervical extension Increased lumbar extension Increased lumbar lateral flexion and rotation
Crossover kick	Decreased kick propulsion Increased hip roll Lower body sinks	Increased cervical extension Increased lumbar extension Increased compensatory lumbar lateral flexion and rotation
Increased knee flexion	Decreased kick propulsion Lower body sinks	Increased cervical extension Increased lumbar extension
Increased ankle dorsiflexion	Decreased kick propulsion Increased hip roll Lower body sinks	Increased cervical extension Increased lumbar extension Increased compensatory lumbar lateral flexion and rotation

Data from Aquatechnics Consulting Group, Inc., Aptos, CA.

other high-level aquatic training activities (65). Swimming programs, in particular, require that close attention be directed to proper swim-stroke biomechanics and to the effect that abnormal mechanics may have on the spine. This attention ensures the most rapid rehabilitation of painful spinal disorders.

Neurologic Disorders

The advantages of the aquatic environment in the rehabilitation of neurologic disease have been noted for many centuries. Roosevelt's rehabilitation at Warm Springs, Georgia, is common knowledge. The use of pool exercises for spinal injury rehabilitation is a mainstay at many rehabilitation centers, and Sir Ludwig Guttman built a central focus for aquatics in the Spinal Injury Unit at Stoke-Mandeville. Throughout the United States, the Easter Seals organization has focused the rehabilitation of children with cerebral palsy through pool-based programs.

From a technical standpoint, there is little difference in the aquatic techniques used in neurologic rehabilitation, with some disease-specific exceptions. Patients with multiple sclerosis may benefit greatly from aquatic programs, because of the ability of water to prevent core temperature increase during exercise, but the pool temperature should be cool to start, below thermoneutral, and the authors have found ideal pool temperatures for patients with multiple sclerosis to be in the range of 25°C to 28°C (77°F to 82°F). In contrast, spinal-injured patients lacking thermoregulatory capacity require much higher temperatures, in the range of 35°C to 37°C (95°F to 98°F). All neurologically impaired individuals obviously require close monitoring for poolside or in-water personnel. Patients with normal thermoregulatory ability and tolerance may be safely treated between 28°C and 35°C.

The techniques developed at Bad Ragaz and the methods developed by James McMillan, which have been called the Halliwick Method because of their initial development and use at the Halliwick School for Crippled Girls in England, have extensive history in the management of cerebral palsy rehabilitation. Their description is beyond the limitations of this chapter but are thoroughly described elsewhere (66,67). Essentially, the techniques use the properties of buoyancy, warmth, and careful body positioning to achieve reduction in muscle tone. The patient is floated through the use of buoyant rings to support arms, legs, and head as clinically warranted. These techniques are valuable in spinal injury rehabilitation as well and have been used in hemiplegia following stroke.

TECHNICAL ISSUES

Facility Options

Health Facility Pools

Aquatic facilities located within health-care facilities are generally warm water pools rarely offering temperature adjustability and are shallow in depth, rarely exceeding 4.5 feet deep, and are usually in-ground construction. They often offer ramp access or may use slings to gain access for disabled individuals. The pools are usually small, due to constrains imposed by expensive space and construction. Although warm water is more comfortable for low-level activities and acute rehabilitation, it is not ideal for patients with multiple sclerosis, and it makes high-level activities exhausting. Pool size limits high-level activities as well, and often group therapy must be done in small groups only. Staff is medically knowledgable, but often varies in aquatic skill sophistication. Facility-based pools are suitable for the acute rehabilitation of orthopedic populations, neurologic rehabilitation (with the exception of patients with multiple sclerosis due to water temperature), and arthritis rehabilitation. Common appropriate techniques include Bad Ragaz, Halliwick, aquatic spine stabilization, Red Cross arthritis, and low-level conditioning programs.

Community Pools

Community pools nearly always use cool water, vary in depth often to 9 feet, usually offer stair or ladder access, and are in-ground designs. Varied depths make a wide range of programs possible, both horizontal and vertical, although the cool water precludes sedentary activities. Staff size is usually limited, and without medical sophistication. These facilities are ideal for transitioning patients from the acute health facility pool, especially to group activities such as aquaerobics, low back classes, arthritis classes, or general conditioning. Because of access difficulty and cool water, they are often difficult for populations with severe physical limitations.

Hot Tubs, Spas, and Therapeutic Tanks

These facilities usually feature hot water, are small in size, very shallow, rarely exceeding 3 in depth, and are often above-ground designs. Most offer added turbulence through jets and temperature adjustability through a narrow range. Although the high temperature is useful for acute treatments, patients quickly elevate their core temperatures even when not exercising. Hot tubs and spas are suitable for acute joint rehabilitation, relaxation, and limited arc movements. Staff is varied in skill level, but often does not come from a therapy background.

Deep Water Environments

Deep water environments, including therapeutic tanks, may be deeper, cooler, and facilitate suspended activities for avoidance of weight bearing. These environments are very adaptable, permitting even high-level conditioning, including aqua-running, cross-country skiing, and ballet movements, if the temperature can be brought to an appropriate level. Tethering may be used to stabilize the immersed individual during exercise. Swimming skill is not required, although tank use usually requires flotation and always requires immediate supervision. Deep water facilities are ideal for athletic rehabilitation, rehabilitation of early fractures when weight bearing is precluded, and high-level conditioning activities. Staff tends to come from an athletic training background.

Techniques in Current Use

Treatment Schools of Thought

These include Bad Ragaz (66), Halliwick (67), and Watsu. All of these methods of aquatic therapy are techniques consisting of a developmental and progressive set of structured exercises. The first two are primarily intended for neurologic impairment, and the latter is an offshoot of shiatsu massage technique and was not originally developed for medical therapy, although more recently it has been found useful in the management of cerebral palsy.

Specialized Equipment

Flotation Devices

A broad range of flotation devices have been developed for aquatic rehabilitation. For central trunk flotation, Neoprene vests and foam waist-belts are the most commonly used. Bad Ragaz techniques use foam rings that are placed around arms and legs or under the head. Kick boards, leg floats, vinyl foam flexible buoys, and combinations of the above are all important pieces of the aquatic rehabilitation armamentarium if a broad base of patients is to be treated.

Resistive Devices

As strengthening proceeds, the natural resistance of the water may be augmented through devices to increase the surface area of the moving part. Finned dumbells, finned boots, kick boards, and flotation devices all may be used to add resistance to movement.

Performance Measurement Tools

Water is a more challenging environment for the therapist wishing to quantify performance. Waterproof heart rate monitors are useful, and as in the spine section, quantifying time, resistance, and movement freedom can add quantification (65). The authors have found standardized exercise log sheets to be useful. These sheets are completed during the treatment session and monitored during subsequent visits as well as in outpatient medical visits. If properly created, they may be used as a clinic progress note, providing support for reimbursement processes.

SUMMARY

The decline in utilization of the aquatic environment has been to the disadvantage of patients. This environment offers significant benefit, a wide margin of therapeutic safety, and cost effectiveness to a great variety of clinical situations. In a time of scrutiny of health-care expenditures, it becomes critical to find safe, inexpensive treatment modalities for common problems. We must find methods that are suitable for self-management regimens, ideally across a large variety of clinical concerns, and which may be easily learned by the patient. These methods should have the added advantages of high patient compliance and consistency. The aquatic environment offers a significant step toward these goals. Aquatic therapy is a scientifically grounded, useful approach to a broad range of rehabilitative problems from acute to chronic, and patients find it helpful and pleasurable. Although specific aquatherapeutic approaches are plentiful, many problems lend themselves to creative aquatic-based solutions as well. Successful rehabilitation may occur with a high safety margin and at low cost, especially when community pools are used, and professional extender personnel may be used for group programs, further decreasing cost while increasing regimen adherence (68).

REFERENCES

1. deVierville JP. A history of aquatic rehabilitation. In: Becker BE, Cole AJ, eds. *Comprehensive aquatic therapy*. Newton, MA: Butterworth-Heinemann, 1997.
2. Licht S, ed. *Medical hydrology*. Vol. 7. The Physical Medicine Library. Baltimore, MD: Waverly, 1963.
3. Lowman CL. *Technique of underwater gymnastics: a study in practical application*. Los Angeles: American Publications, 1937; 4.
4. Lowman CL. *Therapeutic use of pools and tanks*. Philadelphia: WB Saunders, 1952.
5. Groedel FM. *The mineral springs and baths at Saratoga Springs*. Saratoga Springs, NY: Saratoga Springs Commission, 1932; 5.
6. McClellan WS. What is being done at New York State's great enterprise: Saratoga Springs. *J Am Med Hydrol* 1932; 1:27–30.
7. The American Society of Medical Hydrology. Minutes of Working Committee. French Lick Springs Hotel, December 4, 1931.
8. Coulter JS. *Physical therapy, clio medica; a series of primers on the history of medicine*, Vol. 7. New York: P. B. Hoebner, 1932. (Reprinted by AMS Press: New York, 1978.)
9. Smith EM. Underwater therapy in chronic arthritis. *Archives Phys Ther X-Ray Radium* 1935; 16:534–536.
10. Martin LG. Underwater physiotherapy and pool therapy. Presented to the 58th Annual Session of the Arkansas Medical Society, Hot Springs National Park, AR, May 2–4, 1933.
11. Smith EM. Hydrotherapy in arthritis—underwater therapy applied to chronic atrophic arthritis. Presented to the 14th Annual Session of the American Congress of Physical Therapy, Kansas, MO, September 11, 1935.
12. Lowman CL. Preface. In: *Technique of underwater gymnastics: a study in practical application*. Los Angeles: American Publications, 1937; 4.
13. Bloomfield J, Fricker P, Fitch K. *Textbook of science and medicine in sport*. Champaign, IL: Human Kinetics Books, 1992; 5.
14. Arborelius M, Balldin UI, Lilja B, Lundgren CE. Hemodynamic changes in man during immersion with the head above water. *Aerospace Med* 1972; 43:593–599.
15. Risch WD, Koubenec HJ, Beckmann U, et al. The effect of graded immersion on heart volume, central venous pressure, pulmonary blood distribution and heart rate in man. *Pflugers Arch* 1978; 374:117.
16. Weston CFM, O'Hare JP, Evans JM, Corrall RJM. Haemodynamic changes in man during immersion in water at different temperatures. *Clin Sci Lond* 1987; 73:613–616.
17. Evans BW, Cureton KJ, Purvis JW. Metabolic and circulatory responses to walking and jogging in water. *Res Q* 1978; 49:442–449.
18. Dressendorfer RH, Morlock JF, Baker DG, Hong SK. Effects of head-

out water immersion on cardiorespiratory responses to maximal cycling exercise. *Undersea Biomed Res* 1976; 3:183.

19. Haffor AA, Mohler JG, Harrison AC. Effects of water immersion on cardiac output of lean and fat male subjects at rest and during exercise. *Aviat Space Environ Med* 1991; 62:125.
20. McMurray RG, Fieselman CC, Avery KE, Sheps DS. Exercise hemodynamics in water and on land in patients with coronary artery disease. *Cardiopulmonary Rehabil* 1988; 8:69–75.
21. Tei C, Horikir Y, Park JC, et al. Acute hemodynamic improvement by thermal vasodilation incongestive heart failure. *Circulation* 1995; 91: 2582–2590.
22. Tajima F, Sagawa S, Iwamoto J, et al. Renal and endocrine responses in the elderly during head-out immersion. *Am J Physiol* 1988; 254: R977–R983.
23. Weston CFM, O Hare JP, Evans JM, Corrall RJM, Haemodynamic changes in man during immersion in water at different temperatures. *Clin Sci Lond* 1987; 73:613–616.
24. Claybaugh JR, Pendergast DR, Davis JE, Akiba C, Pazik M, Hong SK. Fluid conservation in athletic responses to water intake, supine posture, and immersion. *J Appl Physiol* 1986; 61:7–15
25. Epstein M. Cardiovascular and renal effects of head-out water immersion in man. *Circ Res* 1976; 39:620–628.
26. Gleim GW, Nicholas JA. Metabolic costs and heart rate responses to treadmill walking in water at different depths and temperatures. *Am J Sports Med* 1989; 17:248–252.
27. Epstein M, Lifschitz D, Hoffman D, Stein J. Relationship between renal prostaglandin E and renal sodium handling during water immersion in normal man. *Circ Res* 1979; 45:71–80.
28. Coruzzi PAA, Novarini A, Biggi A, Lazzeroni E, et al. Low pressure receptor activity and exaggerated naturiesis in essential hypertension. *Nephron* 1985; 40:309–315.
29. Corruzi P, Musiari L, Mossini GL, Ceriati R, Novarini A. Water immersion and salt-sensitivity in essential hypertension. *Scand J Clin Lab Invest* 1993; 53:593–599.
30. Nakazawa K, Yano H, Miyashita M. Ground reaction forces during walking in water. In: Miyashita M, Mutoh Y, Richardson AB, eds. *Medicine and science in aquatic sports. 10th FINA World Sport Medicine Congress.* Basel, Switzerland: S Karger AG, 1994; 28–35.
31. Agostoni E, Gurtner G, Torri G, Rahn H. Respiratory mechanics during submersion and negative pressure breathing. *J Appl Physiol* 1966; 21: 253.
32. Hong SK, Cerretelli P, Cruz JC, Rahn H. Mechanics of respiration during submersion in water. *J Appl Physiol* 1969; 27:535–536.
33. Epstein M. Renal effects of head out immersion in humans: a 15-year update. *Physiol Rev* 1992; 72:563–621.
34. Choukroun ML, Varene P. Adjustments in oxygen transport during head-out immersion in water at various temperatures. *J Appl Physiol* 1990; 68:1475–1480.
35. Harrison RA, Hillman M, Bulstrode S. Loading of the lower limb when walking partially immersed. *Physiotherapy* 1992; 78:165–166.
36. Beals C. A case for aerobic conditioning exercise in rheumatoid arthritis [Abstract]. *Clin Res* 1981; 29:780.
37. Balldin UI, Lundgren CEG, Lundvall J, Mellander S. Changes in the elimination of ^{133}xenon from the anterior tibial muscle in man induced by immersion in water and by shifts in body position. *Aerospace Med* 1971; 42:489.
38. Ekdahl C, Anderson SI, Mortotz V, et al. Dynamic versus static training in patients with rheumatoid arthritis. *Scand J Rheumatol* 1990; 19: 17–26.
39. Grossman E, Goldstein DS, Hoffman A, Wacks IR, Epstein M. Effects of water immersion on sympathoadrenal and dopa-dopamine systems in humans. *Am J Physiol* 1992; 262:R993–R999.
40. Krishna GG, Danovitch GM, Sowers JR. Catecholamine responses to central volume expansion produced by head-out water immersion and saline infusion. *J Clin Endocrinol Metab* 1983; 56:998–1002.
41. Nordemar R. Physical training in rheumatoid arthritis: a controlled long-term study. II. Functional capacity and general attitudes. *Scand J Rheumatol* 1981; 10:25–30.
42. McCain G. Non-medical treatment in primary myalgia. *Rheum Dis Clin North Am* 1989; 15:73–90.
43. Perlman SG, Connell K, Alberti J, et al. Synergistic effects of exercise and problem solving education for rheumatoid arthritis patients. *Arthritis Rheum* 1987; 30(suppl):13.
44. Robb-Nicholson C, Daltroy E, Eaton H, et al. Effects of aerobic conditioning in lupus fatigue: a pilot study. *Br J Rheumatol* 1989; 28: 500–505.
45. Bunning RD, Materson RS. A rational program of exercise for patients with osteoarthritis. *Semin Arthritis Rheumatism* 1991; 21(suppl 2): 33–43.
46. Hampson SE, Glosgow RE, Zeiss AM. Birskovich SF, Foster L, Lines A. Self management of osteoarthritis. *Arthritis Care Res* 1993; 6: 17–22.
47. Danneskiold-Samsoe B, Lyngberg K, Risum T, Telling M. The effects of water exercise therapy given to patients with rheumatoid arthritis, *Scand J Rehabil Med* 1987; 19:31–35.
48. Goldstein E, Simkin A, Epstein L, Peritz E. The influence of weight-bearing water exercises on bone density of post-menopausal women. Unpublished results, Zimmer College of Physical Education, Jerusalem, 1995.
49. The National Arthritis Foundation, 1330 W. Peachtree, Atlanta GA 30309. Information regarding the nearest Arthritis Aquatic program may be located through the Arthritis Info-line at 1-800-283-7800.
50. Minor MA, Hewett JE, Webel RR, et al. Efficacy of physical conditioning exercise in patients with rheumatoid arthritis and osteoarthritis. *Arthritis Rheum* 1989; 32:1396–1405.
51. Cole AJ, Campbell DR, Berson D, et al. Swimming. In: Watkins RG, ed. *The spine in sports.* St. Louis: CV Mosby, 1996; 362–385.
52. LeFort SM, Hannah TE. Return to work following an aquafitness and muscle strengthening program for the low back injured. *Arch Phys Med Rehabil* 1994; 75:1247–1255.
53. Saal JA, Saal JS. Later stage management of lumbar spine problems. *Phys Med Rehabil Clin North Am* 1991; 2:205–221.
54. Saal JA. Dynamic muscular stabilization in the nonoperative treatment of lumbar pain syndromes. *Orthop Rev* 1990; 19:691–700.
55. Cole AJ, Moschetti ML, Eagleston RE. Getting backs in the swim. *Rehabil Mgmt* 1992; 5:62–71.
56. Cole AJ, Herring SA. The role of the physiatrist in the management of lumbar spine pain. In: Tollison DC, ed. *The handbook of pain management,* 2nd ed. Baltimore: Williams & Wilkins, 1994; 85–95.
57. Constant F, Collin JF, Guillemin F, Boulangé M. Effectiveness of spa therapy in chronic low back pain: a randomized clinical trial. *J Rheumatol* 1995; 22:1315–1320.
58. Eagleston R. Aquatic stabilization programs. Presented at the Conference on Aggressive Nonsurgical Rehabilitation and Lumbar Spine and Sports Injuries. San Francisco Spine Institute, March 23, 1989, San Francisco, California.
59. Cole A, Eagleston R, Moschetti M. Spine pain: rehabilitation strategies. In: Becker B, Cole A, eds. *Comprehensive aquatic therapy.* New York: Butterworth-Heinemann, 1997; 73–102.
60. Brewster NT, Howie CR. That sinking feeling. *Br Med J* 1992; 305: 1579–1580.
61. Cole AJ, Moschetti ML, Eagleston RA. Swimming. In: White AH, ed. *Spine care.* St. Louis: CV Mosby, 1995; 727–745.
62. Cole AJ, Campbell DR, Berson D, et al. Swimming. In: Watkins RG, ed. *The spine in sports.* St. Louis: CV Mosby, 1996; 362–385.
63. Maglisco E. *Swimming even faster.* Sunnyvale, CA: Mayfield, 1993.
64. Cole AJ, Moschetti ML, Eagleston RE. Getting backs in the swim. *Rehabil Mgmt* 1992; 5:62–71.
65. Wilder RP, Brennan D, Schotte DE. A standard measure for exercise prescription for aqua running. *Am J Sports Med* 1993; 21:45–48.
66. Garrett G, Bad Ragaz ring method. In: Ruoti RG, Morris DM, Cole AJ, eds. *Aquatic rehabilitation.* Philadelphia: Lippincott–Raven, 1996; 289–304.
67. Cunningham J. Halliwick method. In: Ruoti RG, Morris DM, Cole AJ, eds. *Aquatic rehabilitation.* Philadelphia: Lippincott–Raven, 1996; 305–331.
68. Becker BE. Motivating adherence in the rehabilitation setting. *J Back Musculoskeletal Med* 1991; 1:37–48.

PART III

Major Rehabilitation Problems

Rehabilitation Medicine: Principles and Practice, Third Edition,
edited by Joel A. DeLisa and Bruce M. Gans.
Lippincott–Raven Publishers, Philadelphia © 1998.

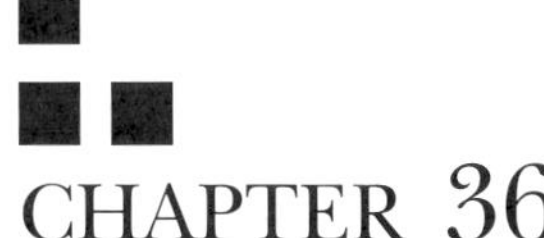

CHAPTER 36

Primary Care for Persons with Disability

William L. Bockenek, Nancy Mann, Indira S. Lanig, Gerben DeJong, and Lee A. Beatty

The issue of providing quality of medical care to all persons has been brought to the forefront with the current changes in medicine and health-care reform. In addition, terms such as "cost containment," "appropriate utilization of resources," and "quality management" are heard by practicing physicians on a daily basis concerning their patient care interactions. The impetus to make changes in our current health-care system also has been affected by economic issues (1). Health costs have increased exponentially in recent years. The proportion of the gross national product spent on health care was 4.7% in 1947, 12.2 % in 1990, and is predicted to be 15% in the year 2000 (1). Even though health-care costs have risen significantly, patients' health outcome and satisfaction have not risen proportionately. When the United States was compared with numerous other countries with respect to health outcomes and satisfaction in relation to cost, the United States ranked lowest of the nations studied, compared with countries such as The Netherlands that are among the best (1). When the same countries were compared with respect to their percentage of primary care physicians, the results were similar, with the United States having the smallest percentage of primary care physicians, and the countries with greatest satisfaction having the greatest percentage of primary care physicians.

W. L. Bockenek: Spinal Cord Injury Program and Department of Physical Medicine and Rehabilitation, Charlotte Institute of Rehabilitation, Carolinas Medical Center, Charlotte, North Carolina 28203.

N. Mann: Department of Physical Medicine and Rehabilitation, Wayne State University School of Medicine, Rehabilitation Institute of Michigan, Detroit, Michigan 48201.

I. S. Lanig: Department of Physical Medicine and Rehabilitation, University of Colorado Health Science Center, Craig Hospital, Englewood, Colorado 80110.

G. DeJong: Department of Family Medicine, National Rehabilitation Hospital Research Center, Georgetown University, Washington, D.C. 20010.

L. A. Beatty: Department of Family Medicine, University of North Carolina at Chapel Hill, School of Medicine, Mount Holly, North Carolina 28120.

Although there is great consensus in the United States and abroad that primary care is a critical component of any health-care system, there is considerable imbalance between primary and specialty care in the United States (2). The proportion of specialists in the United States is over 70% of all patient care physicians, whereas in other industrialized countries 25% to 50% of physicians are specialists (2).

Further work has shown that based on staffing patterns in classic health maintenance organizations (HMOs), there are about 3.1 times more pathologists, 2.5 times more neurosurgeons, 2.4 times more general surgeons, 2.0 times more cardiologists and neurologists, 1.9 times more gastroenterologists, 1.8 times more ophthalmologists, and 1.5 times more radiologists in the nation than would be needed (2). Furthermore, the interest of medical students in primary care careers decreased from 36% in 1982 to 14% in 1992 (2). Although it is clear that there is a plethora of specialists and a need for greater primary care services, considerable room for debate remains on its true impact on health-care costs and quality of patient care.

Beginning in the late 1980s and continuing to the present, recognition of the difficulties that persons with disabilities face in accessing quality health care has become apparent. Although the medical literature is relatively sparse on this issue, multiple conferences and publications have addressed this topic. Although the Association of Academic Physiatrists (AAP) and the American Academy of Physical Medicine and Rehabilitation (AAPM&R) have both developed position statements on the provision of primary care services to persons with disabilities lending their support to physiatrists who choose to provide these services, there is a variety of opinions among practitioners as to how these services are best provided (3,4).

This chapter provides an overview of the primary care issue, with special emphasis on persons with disabilities, as well as a discussion on issues in health promotion in persons with disabilities. A practical approach to primary medical care in a general population that can easily be adapted to persons with disabilities follows. The chapter concludes with a review of several models of primary care currently in place and describes management issues more specific to those with disabilities.

Definitions of Primary Care

The Health Resources and Services Administration has defined primary care based on the following three anchoring principles: (a) the routine medical care and services people receive on first contact with the health-care system for a particular health incident, i.e., prevention, maintenance, diagnosis, limited treatment, management of chronic problems, and referral; (b) assumption of longitudinal responsibility for the patient regardless of the presence or absence of disease (i.e., all of a person's health-care needs—physical, psychological, and social—are met); and (c) integration of other health resources when necessary (gatekeeper function) (5).

The Institute of Medicine (6) has provided a definition as well, which states that primary care is the provision of integrated, accessible health-care services by clinicians who are accountable for addressing a large majority of personal health-care needs, developing a sustained partnership with patients, and practicing in the context of family and community. ''Integration'' includes comprehensive, coordinated and continuous services. ''Accessibility'' refers to eliminating geographical, financial, and cultural barriers to seeing the caregiver. ''Health-care services'' includes hospitals, nursing homes, office, school, home, and intermediate care facilities. ''Clinicians'' can be physicians, nurse practitioners, physician assistants, or similar health-care practitioners. ''Accountable'' refers to the clinician being responsible for quality of care, patient satisfaction, efficient use of resources, and ethical behavior. ''Majority of personal health-care needs'' describes the full spectrum of physical, mental, emotional, and social concerns. ''Sustained partnership'' is a long-term relationship that includes health promotion, disease prevention, and the management of disease itself. ''Context of family and community'' includes an understanding of the patient's social background and support systems.

Primary care may be distinguished from specialty care by the time, focus, and scope of services provided to the patients (2). Primary care as noted above is first-contact care on entry into the health-care system. Specialty care generally follows primary care upon referral from the primary care provider. Whereas primary care addresses the person as a whole, specialty care usually focuses on specific diseases or organ systems. Because primary care providers see patients at their initial interface with the health-care system, they are presented with a variety of symptoms and concerns that may represent early stages of disease that are not yet easily classified into specific diseases or organ systems. Through the various roles of the primary care provider, but especially the gatekeeper function, referral to specialty care occurs when organ or diagnostic specific disease is identified that is beyond the scope of services provided by the primary care provider. Although primary care is comprehensive in scope and is present throughout the continuum of care, specialty care tends to be limited to specific illness episodes, the organ system involved, or the disease process identified.

Primary Care Issues in Graduate Medical Education

Three specialties typically are thought of as primary care fields. The largest is general internal medicine, followed by general pediatrics and family practice. In 1990 there were 240,000 primary care physicians or 39% of the total U.S. physician population. However, of these 240,000 physicians, only 76% considered themselves in ''general practice'' (29.8% of all U.S. physicians). Obstetrics and gynecology, although regarded by the American College of Obstetrics and Gynecology and the American Medical Association as a primary care provider for women, does not traditionally fulfill this role because it does not meet the ''whole body'' medicine criterion often cited as the standard for judging whether a specialty offers primary care (7).

In its third report (8), the Council on Graduate Medical Education (COGME) stated that generalist physicians are trained, practice, and receive continuing education in a broad set of competencies to care for the entire population in office, hospital, and residential settings; provide comprehensive age- and gender-specific preventive care; evaluate and diagnose common complaints; treat common acute conditions; provide ongoing care for chronic illnesses and behavior problems; and seek appropriate consultation for other needed specialized services. Given these required competencies, COGME concluded that family physicians, general internists, and general pediatricians are properly trained to function as generalist physicians. Although other physicians provide elements of primary care, COGME also noted that physicians who are broadly educated as generalist physicians provide more comprehensive and cost-effective care than do other specialists and subspecialists (9).

The recent emphasis on health-care system reform has sparked the decades-old debate as to who is a generalist physician and has re-emerged with important implications for physician work-force policy and medical education (9). In its third report (8), COGME recommended that the nation set a goal that at least 50% of all physicians be practicing generalist physicians. The Association of American Medical Colleges (AAMC) recommended that a majority of graduating medical students be committed to generalist careers (10). Both COGME and the AAMC define generalist physicians as residents who complete a 3-year training program in either family medicine, internal medicine, or pediatrics, and who do not subspecialize. Given the enhanced role and growing prestige of the generalist physician and the increased emphasis on primary care, other physician groups including PM&R have suggested that they be included in this category (3,9).

In its recently completed fourth report (11), COGME stated that the designation of a specialty being included as primary care should be based on an objective analysis of training requirements in disciplines that provide graduates with broad capabilities for primary care practice. A recent report (9) analyzed the training requirements of numerous specialties, including those typically thought of as primary care specialties (family practice, internal medicine, pediatrics) and several that have recently proposed inclusion as a primary care specialty (emergency medicine and obstetrics and gynecology). Only the previously established primary care fields actually prepared their residents in the broad competencies required for primary care practice. Althgough PM&R was not included in the analysis, based on the current training requirements and a similar analysis, it would not fulfill the necessary training needs.

Generalist Versus Specialist

Although it is well accepted that there is an imbalance between primary and specialty care, numerous arguments have been advanced by advocates of both the generalist and specialist perspectives (2,8,12). The generalist perspective points to the research that supports the efficacy of primary care and indicates that generalists have broader medical knowledge and skills; are better trained in psychosocial, preventive, and community aspects of care; and provide less costly care and are more accessible, factors that make them preferable to specialists as primary care providers (12). In addition, the generalists' cross-disciplinary skills provide for more efficient referral patterns when using their gatekeeper function.

Specialists, on the other hand, assert that their training before subspecialization is equivalent to generalists, allowing them to deal with primary care issues (similar to generalists) as well as manage problems within their specialty (that generalists might have to refer elsewhere) (12). Numerous studies support the specialist viewpoint that primary care can be provided in an efficient and cost-effective manner by the same practitioner who provides more sophisticated, specialized, and up-to-date medical services (12).

Meeting the Post-Rehabilitation Health-Care Needs of People with Disabilities

The traditional distinctions between primary care and specialty care become much less clear when we consider the ongoing post-rehabilitative health-care needs of people with disabilities (7). Here the boundaries between primary and specialty care overlap considerably. It is not clear where one ends and the other begins. The handoff from rehabilitative care in the rehabilitation center to primary care in the community is not straightforward. This is best understood when we consider the nature of the ongoing health-care needs of people with disabilities and why many primary care issues have significant rehabilitative or functional content.

It is difficult to generalize about the ongoing health-care needs of people with disabilities, in part because different disabling conditions have widely varying pathophysiologies, comorbidities, and functional consequences. These differences often obscure the fact that people with disabilities experience most of the same health conditions experienced by people without disabilities. However, people with disabilities are at greater risk for certain common health conditions than are those in the general population, often experience these conditions differently, and may require a somewhat different and extended therapeutic regimen that takes into account both their underlying impairment and their functional limitations. However, people with disabilities observe that many health-care providers are often unable to look beyond the disabling condition to address the health problem that precipitated the provider–patient encounter in the first place.

Six Characterizations

There are many ways one can characterize the ongoing health-care needs of people with disabilities relative to those without disabilities. At the risk of overgeneralization, we note six ways in which the ongoing health-care needs of people with disabilities are different from those in the general population. These characterizations are limited mainly to people with the types of conditions commonly seen in inpatient rehabilitation settings (13,14).

First, people with disabilities generally have a thinner margin of health that must be carefully guarded if medical problems are to be averted (15). This observation applies to health conditions that people with disabilities share with the nondisabled population (e.g., upper respiratory infection, pneumonia) as well as conditions more likely to appear among people with disabling conditions (e.g., urinary tract infections, renal failure, pressure sores). It should be emphasized that people with disabilities are not "sick" and that most are generally very healthy. However, their impairments and functional limitations often render them more vulnerable to certain health problems.

Second, people with disabilities often do not have the same opportunities for health maintenance and preventive health as those without disabilities. For example, people with mobility limitations usually have fewer opportunities to participate in aerobic activity needed for good cardiovascular health, and people with paralysis may not be able to detect certain health conditions early because they cannot experience pain in certain body regions (15).

Third, people with disabilities who acquired their impairment early in life may experience onset of chronic health conditions earlier than people in the general population. For example, it is believed that people with long-standing mobility limitations are likely to have an earlier onset of coronary artery disease than the general population. Likewise, people with mobility limitations may experience an earlier onset of adult diabetes because of obesity and may experience an earlier onset of renal disease (e.g., pyelonephritis) because of a neurogenic bladder (16).

Fourth, people with disabilities who acquire a new health condition, apart from their original impairment, are likely to experience secondary functional losses. Thus the functional consequences of a new chronic health condition are usually more significant for a person who already has a disabling impairment. The onset of exertional angina, for example, may require that the person upgrade from a manual to an electric wheelchair and from a conventional automobile to an adapted van.

Fifth, people with disabilities may require more complicated and prolonged treatment for a given health problem than do people without disabilities. For example, using a plaster cast for a broken leg may be complicated by the individual's vulnerability to a pressure sore when the individual has no sensation in the lower limbs. Likewise, a person with a disability may require a longer recovery period after an acute episode of illness or injury because of preexisting functional limitations that limit a person's participation in various therapies (e.g., using a treadmill or exercise bicycle after an acute myocardial infarct).

And sixth, people with disabilities may need durable medical equipment and other assistive technologies that require some level of functional assessment. Today these devices are often prescribed by physicians who have only a rudimentary understanding about the fit between various types of equipment and the needs of the individual consumer. A poor fit between the individual and an assistive device can reduce functional capacity and may induce the individual to abandon the device, the combination of which is wasteful for both the individual and for society.

These six characterizations are not exhaustive. A more complete characterization will be important in sorting out the respective roles of traditional primary care disciplines and the various specialty disciplines in managing the health-care needs of people with disabilities. The six characterizations point out that traditional distinctions lose their meaning when managing the health-care needs of a person with a disabling or chronic health condition.

Impact on Health-Care Utilization and Expenditures

These six characterizations are borne out in the higher-than-average rates of health-care utilization and expenditures among people with disabilities. A subset of the disabled population, namely those with limitations in activities of daily living (ADLs), i.e., the kinds of people with disabilities commonly seen in inpatient rehabilitation centers, use far more health services than do those without ADL limitations. Results from the 1987 National Medical Expenditure Survey, the most exhaustive population-based health-care utilization survey to date, found that working-age people with ADL limitations, compared with people without ADL limitations, spend, on average, in any one year, 12 times more days in a hospital and incur 7.4 times more overall health-care expenditures (17) (Figs. 36-1 and 36-2).

It should be emphasized that these ratios are averages that

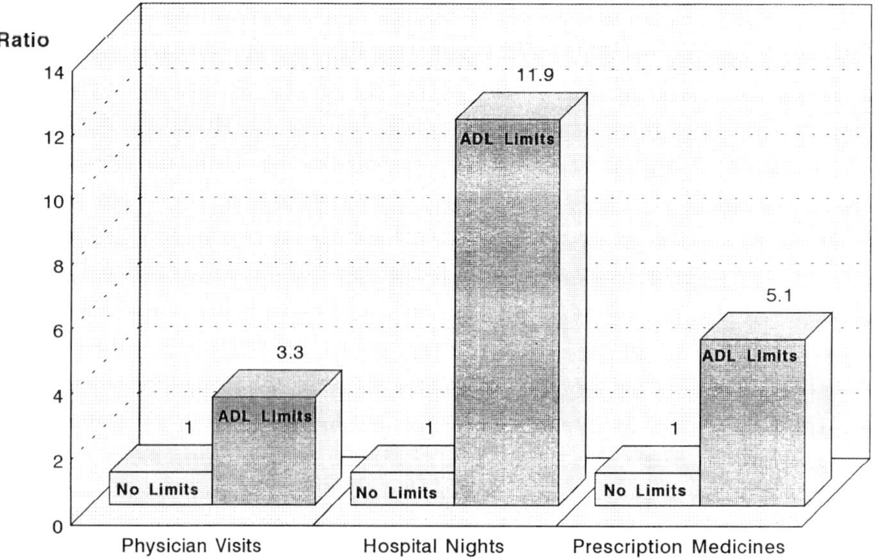

FIG. 36-1. Relative per capita health-care utilization in working-age population by ADL limitation. (From NRH Research Center. Computed from National Medical Expenditures Survey, 1987.)

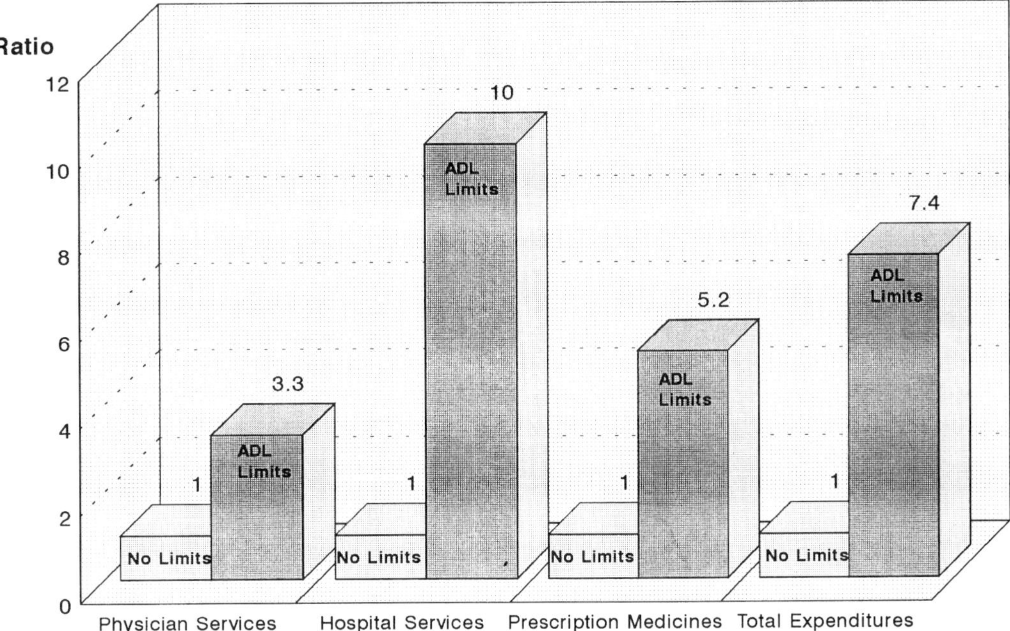

FIG. 36-2. Relative per capita health-care expenditures in working-age population by ADL limitation. (From NRH Research Center. Computed from National Medical Expenditures Survey, 1987.)

mask wide variations in relative health-care expenditures. Among people with ADL limitations, 30% account for 87% of total health-care expenditures within this subpopulation. This distribution is remarkably consistent across subpopulations and within the total population, where 30% of the total population account for 90% of total health-care expenditures (17). The point to be underscored is that people with disabilities, particularly those with ADL limitations, use disproportionately more health-care expenditures.

Access to Primary Care

Many of the secondary health conditions experienced by people with disabilities are entirely preventable through scrupulous health maintenance strategies and timely interventions by knowledgeable practitioners before new health conditions become emergent or even life-threatening (18,19). People with disabilities often express frustration about their access to primary care providers who are knowledgeable about the management of secondary health conditions and the impact of these new health conditions on their functional capacities (15,20,21). People with disabilities often remark that they must spend considerable effort educating their primary care providers about their disability and how it needs to be taken into consideration when new health condition are addressed (22,23).

In a survey of 607 respondents with disabilities (e.g., spinal cord injury, multiple sclerosis, cerebral palsy, postpolio) in the Washington, D.C. area, it was found that many people had difficulty finding a physician who was knowledgeable about their health-care needs (22). Respondents who had a previous rehabilitation experience often indicated that they consulted with their original physiatrist when they were not confident about a therapy recommended by their primary care physician. Respondents also reported that many physician offices were not fully accessible, as in the case of examining tables that failed to accommodate the transfer requirements of wheelchair users.

In subsequent interviews with primary care providers in the Washington, D.C. area, it was also found that many preferred to serve only a very limited number of people with disabilities because people with disabilities often took longer to process in the course of an ordinary office visit and slowed down a busy office practice (24). With rapid growth of capitation-based managed care since then, primary care physicians have even less incentive to serve high-use populations such as people with disabilities.

Multidimensional Character of the Issues

This brief review illustrates how the boundary issues between primary and specialty care in the case of people with disabilities need to be addressed at several different levels. First there is the issue of the functional and rehabilitative implications inherent in many primary care encounters. Second, there is the issue of knowledge base and whether traditional primary care providers are adequately equipped to address the needs of people with disabilities. Third, there is the issue of whether primary care providers have the facilities to accommodate people with disabilities. And fourth, there is the issue of whether our systems of health-care financing discourage providers, primary care or otherwise, from addressing the primary health-care needs of people with disabilities.

PHYSICAL MEDICINE AND REHABILITATION AS A PRIMARY CARE SPECIALTY

With these issues in mind, the issue of PM&R as a primary care specialty can now be brought into focus. PM&R is the medical specialty that deals with the needs of severely disabled persons. Primary care physicians often refer these patients after a catastrophic illness. When these patients require comprehensive inpatient rehabilitation, the physiatrist usually serves as their primary caregiver during their relatively short hospital stay but subsequently refers the patient back to the referring physician for follow-up general medical care. Follow-up visits at the physiatrist's office typically deal with rehabilitation issues (7).

On the other hand, patients with spinal cord and brain injuries often present from referring specialists, i.e., neurosurgeons and orthopedic surgeons, with no regular primary care physician. After hospitalization, their follow-up care and health maintenance to prevent rehospitalization become major issues. Physicians in spinal cord and brain injury centers often choose to become the primary care physicians for these patients. Due to the specialized and often complex medical needs of the person with severe disability, primary care physicians in the community often welcome the physiatrist's involvement and encourage their assistance in providing for the primary care needs of their shared patients (7).

Primary care services are often requested by those persons with severe disability to be performed at the rehabilitation facility. In a recent survey (25) of 144 outpatients with spinal cord injury, it was found that 48% considered their rehabilitation physician as their primary care physician. Fifty-one percent of persons also requested that all of their general medical care be provided by the physicians at the rehabilitation facility. The primary reasons for these requests included maintaining continuity of care with the physician that the patients felt most understood their specialized needs as well as easier integration with the rehabilitation hospital for other ancillary health needs (e.g., seating clinic, physical and occupational therapy).

Although it appears that many patients would like their primary care needs met by the physiatrists, there is not a clear consensus of whether this is a practical approach to the issue of providing this care. The problems described in developing PM&R as a primary care specialty were outlined partially earlier in this chapter. Additional considerations include manpower or work-force issues, the preferences professed by current practitioners in the field as well as those in training, and concerns dealing with PM&R residency curricula and the ability to provide adequate training in primary care issues based on our present residency requirements.

As previously noted, it is widely believed that there is a shortage of generalists. If 20% of medical graduates each year train to be generalists, then 50% of all physicians will be considered primary care practitioners by the year 2040 (26). There are several ways to reach the goals previously set forth by COGME (8) and the AAMC (10). They include having more medical school graduates enter primary care fields, reducing the number of specialty residency positions, and encouraging current practitioners in subspecialties to broaden the scope of their practice to include a more primary care role (27). An additional option is to change the current curriculum of some of our residency programs to include more adequate training in primary care issues.

A recent work-force study was performed to determine the current and future manpower needs for the PM&R practitioner (28). The model was based on the assumption that current residency capacity as well as utilization of physiatry skills remains constant at its 1994–1995 level. The results were that the demand for physiatrists will continue to exceed supply, on average, through the year 2000. Excess supply has emerged and will continue to emerge in selected geographic areas early in the 21st century. In order to maintain a level of demand, it was recommended in this report that the field should emphasize the role of physiatrists in providing efficacious and cost-effective health care. An additional option would be to further broaden the scope of practice to include primary care services.

Unfortunately, there are several issues that will likely dampen the success of this effort. The above work force projection is based on the premise that managed care will continue to grow at a moderate level. Estimates of HMO growth show that in 1994 it was at a level of 20% and is expected to increase to 36% by the year 2000 and to 53% by 2015 (28). PM&R is not typically designated as a primary care provider in our current HMO and managed care systems. In addition, even if PM&R were designated as a primary care provider for persons with severe disability, it is unlikely that this would have a significant impact on the shortage of generalists. The total percentage of currently practicing physiatrists as compared with the total number of U.S. physicians is less than 1% (7). Based on our current training capacity, it is doubtful that there will ever be the number of physiatrists necessary to provide direct primary care for the large majority of persons with disability (7).

Some of the above assumptions are based on the premise that current practitioners and those in training in PM&R are willing to provide primary care services. A recent survey (27) of 106 PM&R physicians (55 physiatrists and 51 PM&R residents) showed that only 39% agreed that PM&R

should be designated as a primary care specialty. The majority also felt that these services should be restricted to those with severe disability (e.g., spinal cord and brain injury). Overall, 53% felt that physiatrists are competent in providing general medical care, but only 38% were convinced that the current 4-year PM&R residency sufficiently prepares physiatrists to assume the role of a primary care provider.

Current PM&R training and residency curricula do not place a great focus on several areas that are essential to providing primary care services. These include health promotion and education, as well as preventive services (7). Significant changes would need to occur in our current residency requirements to provide the above training. This would likely require extension of our current 4-year training requirement as well as substantial adjustments to our current residency experiences. A series of recommendations (29) for changes in the current PM&R residency curriculum have been proposed to assist PM&R residency programs in providing for education in the provision of primary care. These include applying general preventive care principles and interventions to those with disabilities, expanding the role of "continuity clinics," publishing a "study guide" on the topic of primary care for the disabled similar to the study guides currently published by the AAPM&R, and providing continuing education on common medical problems seen in the disabled and nondisabled population. Additional consideration was given to developing special or added qualifications in primary care for the disabled or expanding the availability of double board certification (current combined programs involve internal medicine and pediatrics) to include family practice. Proposals such as these would require significant changes in our current training programs that may ultimately result in a negative impact on the continued growth and attractiveness of our field (7). Changes such as increasing the length of residency training and altering "quality of life issues" for residents and practicing physiatrists (the three "L's" of primary care: low pay, long hours, low prestige) may be viewed as adverse by prospective PM&R residents (7). In fact, this may ultimately lead to further limitation of the accessibility of care to those persons with severe disabilities.

Other potential options to ensure provision of primary care services to those with severe disabilities include collaboration with other medical specialties as well as allied health providers. Several "models" have been developed that include close working relationships of physiatrists with internal medicine specialists as well as physician extenders such as nurse practitioners (21). The nature of this collaboration can be achieved in numerous ways; however, at a minimum it should include physiatric education of the other primary care providers and team ventures with them to provide primary care for this population (7). A more detailed description of these types of collaborations is provided later in this chapter.

HEALTH PROMOTION IN PERSONS WITH DISABILITIES

The overall life course health profile of an individual with a disabling condition is the result of interaction among our disability management strategies, general health-care practices, biologic and socioenvironmental factors, and life-style behaviors. Therefore, when physiatrists address the longitudinal health-care needs of those with chronic disabilities, they must view disability-related health management and general health-promoting strategies as equally important components of care. In order to do this, they must enhance their frames of reference and incorporate the concepts of health promotion and secondary condition risk reduction.

Health Promotion and Related Models

Health promotion has several features that overlap with both primary care and medical rehabilitation. Most notable, all three emphasize education and encouragement of self-responsibility, and all address the potential or actual impact of a given physical or cognitive/emotional condition across several dimensions of health. Finally, all address both health maintenance and disease prevention so as to enhance and protect functional capacity over the life span.

As a general concept, health promotion describes all efforts directed toward helping individuals modify their life-styles and behavior so as to promote a state of optimal health. Health promotion *per se* is not disease or health problem specific. However, the most important health-promoting behaviors recommended are proper nutrition, weight control, smoking cessation, stress management, physical fitness, elimination of any drug or alcohol misuse, disease and injury prevention, development of social support, and maintenance of a regularly scheduled health surveillance plan to monitor health status (30–33). These behaviors emphasize enhancement of health status in the absence of a specific health threat (31).

Early twentieth century definitions of optimal health emphasized freedom from disease and issues related to hygiene. However, contemporary definitions of health typically reflect its complex multidimensional nature, incorporating themes related to disease, environment, capacity or potential, and effective coping (34). Indeed, the Department of Health and Human Services defined optimal health as having a "full range of functional capacity at each life stage, allowing one the ability to enter into satisfying relationships with others, to work, and to play" (35).

These multidimensional definitions of health find parallels in the International Classification of Impairments, Disabilities, and Handicap model of disablement (36) and its variations (37–39). These models of the disablement process attempt to describe the "health impact" of disease or injury in three principle domains of the human experience. Specifically, attention is directed to the impact on the organ level (impairment), the impact on the performance of routine tasks, skills, and human behaviors (disability), and the impact on social role performance, community integration, and opportunity (handicap). Several models (37,39) have attempted to incorporate biologic, environmental, life-style, and behavioral influences on the disabling process and the interaction with quality of life/perceptions of personal well-being. In addition, various investigators (40–43) have proposed that a more complete accounting of the health impact of a given injury or disease also requires inclusion of a fourth domain: subjective well-being—reflecting an individual's own assessment of health, life satisfaction, and other life experiences rather than the objective nature of these experiences. The merging of contemporary definitions of health, the physiatry-oriented models of disablement, and the disabled individual's own perceptions of well-being can provide a conceptual framework upon which specific health-promoting and secondary condition risk reduction strategies can be formulated within the context of chronic disability.

Health Protection and Secondary Risk Reduction

Intimately related to health promotion is health protection. Health-protecting behaviors, although overlapping to some degree with health-promoting behaviors, emphasize preventive measures that guard or defend an individual against specific injuries or illnesses (44,45). Public health interventions designed to protect health have traditionally been conceptualized as primary, secondary, and tertiary preventive measures. Primary prevention refers to those activities undertaken to reduce the circumstances that would result in the subsequent development of a disease process or illness. It addresses risks. Attention can be directed to the host (e.g., immunization, counseling on life-style behaviors), to the environment (e.g., elimination of physical hazards), or to a specific agent, if one is identified (e.g., contaminated water). Secondary prevention emphasizes the early detection and prompt intervention against asymptomatic disease processes in evolution. Screening efforts characterize this level of prevention. Tertiary prevention attempts to minimize disability from existing disease through medical treatment, education, and rehabilitation. Efforts to prevent the development of secondary conditions (i.e., secondary impairments, disabilities, or handicaps) known to occur in those with specific disabilities incorporate principles from all three of these traditional models of prevention/health protection (37,46). Expansion of these public health concepts for application among those with disabilities can provide additional conceptual grounding for the development of disability-specific prevention protocols. Specifically, primary prevention for those with an existing disability should include appropriately tailored measures to eliminate risk factors for chronic conditions not necessarily directly related to their primary disability. Interventions may include protocols for health-promoting activities such as smoking cessation, weight control, reduction of substance abuse, increasing physical exercise if feasible, and screening for age- and gender-specific carcinoma (39). Tailoring of these measures includes deliberate attention to the economic, logistic, architectural, and attitudinal obstacles to primary health care often encountered by persons with disabilities.

Secondary prevention measures in those with chronic disability should focus on ongoing anticipatory strategies to minimize the adverse health impact over time of the primary disability, superimposed aging issues, or new injuries. Emphasis is placed on early detection of secondary conditions that, if left unaddressed, can have deleterious effects on organ systems, performance of ADLs, and/or community reintegration over time (37,39). Tertiary prevention measures are then activated when appropriate.

Tertiary prevention incorporates ongoing interval efforts to maximize and maintain functional capacity over the life course. Education in new skills and equipment is pursued as functional abilities change. Strategies to combat secondary handicaps are pursued with attention directed to stabilizing or improving access to comprehensive specialized care, and stabilizing access to personal care assistance/support services. Additional attention may be given to ongoing vocational rehabilitation and problem solving the socioeconomic disincentives and obstacles often experienced by disabled individuals seeking a place in the work force.

Building a Knowledge Base

Thoughtful advice and counsel (i.e., patient education) about behaviors, life-style, and self-care practices that influence overall health can have far greater impact on health and longevity than specific screening tests or procedures (47). It is for this reason that emphasis on awareness and education is at the crux of health promotion activities. However, the success of health promotion educational efforts depends on a variety of issues that can be grouped into three categories: (a) issues related to health-care professionals themselves, (b) issues related to the patient, and (c) issues related to clinical/environmental circumstances (48). Comments here are limited to the first category. Specifically, addressing the former, rehabilitation professionals may lack self-efficacy regarding their knowledge base and skills necessary for education and motivating individuals in health-promoting behaviors. Additionally, their own personal health enhancement beliefs and practices, their underestimating of patient interest or motivation, or their overestimating of patient knowledge will also influence the nature of clinical encounters and related patterns of education or referral (48–50). Continuing education activities, collaboration with primary care providers in the community, hands-on skills training, small group discussion, and case studies can be useful to physiatrists interested in building their knowledge base over time (51).

In order to facilitate effective patient education and behavioral change, the rehabilitation professional must have a clear understanding of available epidemiology assessment and intervention information related to commonly encountered disability-related and general health-related issues. Upon establishing this knowledge base, the physiatrist who so chooses can then routinely pose and answer the following questions during routine medical encounters:

1. What are potential disability-related or general health-related problems of which the patient should be aware?
2. What steps are necessary to clarify if the patient is at risk for specific conditions?
3. Is the problem present?
4. If present, what should be done?

Questions 1 and 2 require knowledge of (a) available epidemiologic data and risk factor information and (b) specialty-specific technical assessment skills. Question 3 requires skills in interpretation of the data secured, and Question 4 requires knowledge in appropriate education and therapeutic intervention options (35,48,52).

The Interdisciplinary Assessment of Health

A systematic health assessment is necessary to establish and document an individual's current health status, life-style practices, and psychosocial variables that can influence health. Thereafter, goals can be established and pursued in a manner appropriate to the individual's unique circumstances, resources, and personal desires (46). Particular attention must be directed to the social and environmental aspects of disability that are typically of a magnitude sufficiently significant to greatly influence health-promoting activities (15,51,53,54).

Health risk appraisal or health status assessment instruments are often used in the general population in risk factors assessment, education, and behavioral change programs. However, there are no such validated instruments for use in the disabled populations. Additionally, concerns have been raised regarding the validity and reliability of the data yielded by some of these instruments, even in the nondisabled population (55). Nonetheless, simple icebreaker type health status assessments designed for use in the general population can be used to stimulate interest and initiate health promotion discussions between disabled individuals and rehabilitation professionals. Additionally, despite the current lack of valid and reliable health risk appraisal instruments for those with disabilities, the adoption of certain general health risk assessment principles related to smoking, weight control, nutrition, physical activity, cancer screening, and family history risk factors for disease seems appropriate for those with chronic disabilities (46). In addition, there is a fair degree of consensus in the medical rehabilitation literature on the core concepts that should be incorporated into disability-specific health status assessments (51,53,55). Table 36-1 provides a partial list of health assessment questions appropriate for individuals with physical disabilities. The following section reviews specific general health-promoting activities that should be addressed and encouraged during physiatric encounters wherein the physiatrist is the functional primary provider.

SPECIFIC GENERAL HEALTH PROMOTING ACTIVITIES

Smoking Cessation

Smoking only further compromises a disabled person's already impaired physiologic reserves for good health. Therefore, it is vitally important for physiatrists to encourage and help every patient they encounter who smokes, to quit. Cigarette smoking is the single most preventable cause of death and disability in the United States (56). It is known to cause heart disease, stroke, and chronic obstructive pulmonary disease (57). Approximately 25% of adult Americans smoke cigarettes (58). Over 400,000 Americans die from tobacco use each year—more than the number of individuals who die from acquired immunodeficiency syndrome, cocaine, heroin, gang violence, alcohol, fires, automobile accidents, driving under the influence, suicide, and homicide combined (57). Numerous studies have demonstrated that physicians' advice is a strong motivator and that their efforts to encourage patients to quit do make a difference (59–61). Unfortunately, only half of smokers report that their primary care physicians in the previous year have even asked about their smoking status during the past year (62).

This lack of physician attention to smoking status and smoking cessation recommendations is particularly disturbing in light of the fact that options for office practice–based smoking cessation strategies are readily available from a variety of sources (63,64). Most notably, in 1996 the Centers for Disease Control (CDC) and the Agency for Health Care Policy and Research (AHCPR) produced clinical practice guidelines on smoking cessation (65). Emphasis was placed on assessment and intervention strategies designed to be brief, requiring 3 minutes or less of direct clinician time. Physicians were encouraged to include smoking status (current, former, never) on the vital signs stamp at every clinic/office visit. Nicotine replacement therapy (patch or gum) was recommended for smoking cessation unless special circumstances were present, such as pregnancy, the early post–myocardial infarction period, serious arrhythmias, or severe angina pectoris. The practice guidelines recommend that clinicians acknowledge that the majority of smokers who quit smoking will gain weight. Patients should be told that most individuals will gain less than 10 pounds, although a small minority may gain substantially more (66,67). Follow-up for positive reinforcement or prebehavioral change encouragement over time is encouraged. The physiatrist and interdisciplinary team, in particular, are often in a relationship with patients wherein cross-discipline reinforcement and follow-through can be instituted during routinely scheduled inpatient or outpatient clinical encounters.

TABLE 36-1. *Health promotion assessment and health maintenance activities in those with chronic disabilities: secondary impairment and secondary disability screening and early detection activities*

Physical health functions	
Respiratory	Smoking/exposure to second-hand smoke Influenza and pneumococcal vaccine status, particularly in those with advanced age higher levels of paraplegia/tetraplegia, or neuromuscular compromise that influences muscles of respiration Fund of knowledge regarding management of early signs of chest congestion Access to assistance with secretion mobilization Posture/kyphosis/truncal spasticity/abdominal distention/obesity problems that can have potential impact on chest expansion/respiratory function Aspiration risk/gastroesophageal reflux Forced vital capacity and forced expiratory volume in one second Aging-related phenomena
Cardiovascular	Risk factors: family history, physical inactivity/decreased exercise capacity, dyslipidemia, abnormal carbohydrate metabolism, obesity, smoking, impaired peripheral circulation, hypertension Exercise practices in individuals capable of exercise/adapted exercise Fund of knowledge regarding diet, weight control, physical activity options, and smoking cessation resource options
Skin	Fund of knowledge on risk factors for skin breakdown and how to resolve early problems
Frequency of pressure reliefs	Frequency of visual skin inspections
	Moisture issues/fecal or urinary incontinence/friction Age and condition of wheelchair cushion/seating system Posture/pelvic obliquity/spasticity-induced shearing and pressure issues Weight/nutritional status and impact on skin vulnerability Transfer skills Pedal edema/shoe or orthotic trimlines and fit Palmar skin protection Cigarette smoking Sunscreen utilization Aging-related changes
Neuromusculoskeletal	Upper extremity neuromusculoskeletal pain issues with or without current functional impact (rotator cuff) pathology; shoulder, elbow, wrist or phalangeal joint contractures; ulnar and median nerve entrapment syndromes Lower extremity/axial skeleton degenerative changes with impact on ambulation skills Osteoporosis Spasticity/tone related impact on transfer safety, posture, or shearing phenomenon on skin Stability of sensory/motor profile Charcot joint arthropathy with impact on trunk stability/dysreflexia patterns/pain issues Neuropathic pain phenomena (new onset versus stable pattern; functional impact) Motor coordination Activities to enhance strength, endurance and flexibility
Genitourinary	Bladder hygiene/bladder management technique and equipment/ supplies/adjunct therapies Infection/incontinence rates Urinary tract stone formation (upper and lower tracts) Genitourinary system surveillance history to date Gynecologic history, including Papanicolaou smear/bimanual examination/amenorrhea/ breast self-examination habits/postmenopausal hormone replacement Prostate health assessment Fertility and sexuality concerns
Gastrointestinal	Bowel evacuation technique/duration/predictability Early identification of hypomobility patterns Latex allergy response Nutrition and hydration Anticholinergic use for detrusor hyperreflexia Gallstone disease Colon cancer (age specific) Symptomatic hemorroids (bleeding; dysreflexia inducing)

(continued)

TABLE 36-1. *Continued.*

Functional status	Interval changes in function secondary to changes in strength, endurance, balance, vision, hearing, hypotension, fatigue levels, pain status, cognition, polypharmacy, access to personal care assistance/transportation/health-care resources in community, or life stressors Mobility Cognitive intellectual Communication Social attitudinal Depression Knowledge base regarding physical activity/exercise options appropriate for the nature of their disability Family and social support systems Support systems for primary care providers/family
Nutritional assessment	History and physical examination Body weight HDL-C/LDL-C, fasting serum glucose Swallowing difficulties Functional, economic, or environmental influences on dietary habits/adequacy of nutrient intake Medication effect on appetite/bowels Nutrition intake/diet composition
Tobacco, alcohol and substance use evaluation	Smoking/second-hand smoke exposure CAGE screening questionnaire/brief MAST screening tool Adult immunizations Dental health Ocular health

Adapted with permission from Lanig IS. *A practical guide to health promotions after spinal cord injury.* Gaithersburg, MD: Aspen, 1996; 55.

Nutrition and Weight Control

For many individuals with chronic disability, the promotion and protection of their nutritional health can be compromised by a variety of physical and socioeconomic difficulties. Bulbar signs/swallowing difficulties, limitations in upper extremity function, income restrictions, and food procurement and preparation difficulties are several confounding variables that can adversely impact food selection and consumption.

Mounting scientific evidence, however, has underscored the direct relationship between diet and health (68). Poor diet has been implicated or identified as risk factors in several chronic diseases that have become the leading causes of death in the United States: heart disease, diabetes, stroke, and some forms of cancer. In response to these, numerous health agencies—most notably the U.S. Department of Health and Human Services, American Heart Association, and National Cancer Institute—have proposed dietary guidelines for the American population (69–71).

For those with disabilities, nutritional health-related secondary conditions can manifest themselves in the form of compromised skin integrity, increased skin vulnerability from cachexia, suboptimal wound healing capacity, adult-onset glucose intolerance and dyslipidemias (72), bowel evacuation problems, fluid intake–related genitourinary tract difficulties, and functional compromise associated with weight gain. Identifying and reducing environmental, socioeconomic, and disability-related physiologic or functional skills risk factors for poor nutritional health often require a team approach (73).

Physiologic and body composition differences in many individuals with chronic disability influence the reliability and utility of standard nutritional assessment tools. Basic biochemical and clinical assessment can be pursued based on principles described elsewhere in this text. Data relating to dietary history, social situation history, and functional status components of the nutritional health assessment can be obtained through the interdisciplinary treating team's collaborative efforts. Action plans can be proposed based on the assembled data.

Physical Fitness

The cycle of disability has been characterized as a vicious cycle wherein physical disability and dysfunction → functional motor impairment → inability to exercise → physical inactivity → deconditioning → medical complications → additional/perpetuated physical disability/dysfunction (74). Health promotion and related educational efforts for those with disabilities would therefore be incomplete without the provision of a physical fitness component. Exercise regimens adapted to the characteristic limitations or physiologic vulnerabilities created by their specific impairments/disabilities are a must.

Physical fitness encompasses the physiologic attributes of (a) cardiopulmonary fitness, (b) muscular strength, (c) muscular endurance, (d) flexibility, and (e) body composition. Training principles and programs for those with disabilities have steadily been investigated and/or developed in recent years (30,75–82).

In 1996 the Surgeon General's Report on Physical Activity and Health included an unprecedented section specifically directed to persons with disabilities (83). Benefits of physical activity, including improvements in stamina, muscle strength, promotion of general feelings of well-being, and modulation of joint swelling and pain associated with arthritis, were cited. The importance and positive correlation of social support and the regular physical activity in those with disabilities was noted.

However, for many with disabilities, physical fitness cannot be defined in terms of the traditional conceptions of fitness in the general population. Rather, it must be defined in a broader sense that encompasses not only appropriately modified descriptions of endurance, strength, and flexibility, but also (a) conscientious nutritional health practices to nourish the body, (b) health practices and medical follow-up to minimize the risk of secondary impairments and disabilities, and (c) a balanced commitment to maximizing functional capabilities in both necessary and discretionary activities of daily living (84).

Well-planned, clinically sound physical exercise can improve cardiovascular and/or peripheral muscle endurance, enhance strength and coordination, and improve flexibility in many individuals with chronic disabilities. Therefore, despite a variety of practical challenges often articulated, the interdisciplinary team should systematically evaluate and recommend physical exercise activities for most individuals with chronic disability. In those with neuromuscular disease, there is a common concern that strength and endurance exercises have the potential to create exercise-induced weakness (85,86). This concern can be tempered through specific recommendations for nonfatiguing intensity and duration of exercise activities and with monitoring of functional capacity after introduction of regular exercise activities (87,88). For those with arthritis, isometric exercise programs can often maintain strength if pain and inflammation with movement is particularly problematic. However, attention must be directed to maintaining functional range of motion. Overall, strength and endurance programs for individuals with arthritis have been shown to result in better disease outcomes (89,90). Exercise programs to reverse deconditioning associated with multiple sclerosis can be beneficial to those with stable or mild to moderately impaired neurologic profiles. Attention should be directed to balancing frequency, duration, and time of day so that the exercise activity does not compromise the individual's ability to perform activities of daily living (91). For those with spinal cord injury, the level of injury will influence the cardiovascular response to exercise. Generally speaking, the higher the level of injury, the more likely a significant reduction in cardiopulmonary capacity and fitness as compared with those of the nondisabled population (92,93). However, the gains in peripheral muscle strength and endurance often enhance functional capacity and should therefore be encouraged. Recommendations for adaptation of exercise equipment and regimen to accommodate weakness, sensory deficits or orthopedic limitations created by various disabilities is increasingly more available through a variety of resources.

Screening for Substance Abuse

The importance of screening for drug and alcohol abuse in the disabled population is necessitated by both the impact of these substances on bodily functions and by the behavioral aberrations associated with excessive use (94). A large percentage of individuals admitted to rehabilitation services with neurotrauma were intoxicated at the time of injury and often had preinjury histories of hazardous ethanol consumption patterns (95–99). Additionally, for some individuals with chronic disabilities, maladaptive coping may include intemperate or frankly abusive alcohol consumption. For others, excessive alcohol consumption may be a form of maladaptive self-medication for chronic pain phenomena. Finally, given the high prevalence of alcoholism found in the community-based general population studies and the morbidity and mortality associated with alcohol abuse and dependency, public health agencies recommend that screening for alcoholism should be a routine part of every medical evaluation (47). One first seeks to help the problem drinker acknowledge the problem, understand its consequences, and recognize the need for treatment. Thereafter, attention shifts to negotiating and carrying out an acceptable, customized treatment plan (100).

The CAGE questionnaire was designed as an easy, expedient instrument to evaluate a patient's alcohol usage and to determine if further assessment is necessary (101). Although a limitation of this instrument is that it relies on self-report, it appears that those who drink intemperately are more inclined to give accurate responses to CAGE questions when they are part of a series of life-style questions that include diet, exercise habits, smoking, and safe sex practices (102–104). The CAGE interview questions are shown in Table 36-2. The *italicized* words in the CAGE interview questions reflect adaptations made to include drug use screening questions. The CAGE adapted to include drugs is called the CAGE-AID. Other screening tools that have been shown to be useful in health screening activities include the 25-question Michigan Alcoholism Screening Test (MAST) (105), the 10-question brief MAST (106), and the World Health Organization Alcohol Use Disorders Identification Test (AUDIT) (107,108). The AUDIT attempts to identify drinkers whose consumption patterns place them at risk for direct or indirect medical problems and alcohol dependency before frank dependency has developed.

Formal diagnosis of alcohol dependence or abuse involves tracking the quantity and duration of consumption, identifying physiologic manifestation of ethanol addiction, loss of control over drinking, and damage to physical health and social functioning (100). Routine screening may facilitate early detection of hazardous consumption patterns before frank dependency or abuse develops. Hazardous consumption has been defined as four or more drinks per day in

TABLE 36-2. *The CAGE/CAGE-AID questions*

The original CAGE questions appear in plain type. The adaptations to include drugs (CAGE-AID) are indicated in *italics.* The CAGE or CAGE-AID should be preceded by these two questions:
1. Do you drink alcohol? If yes, how much? How often?
2. Have you ever experimented with drugs? Which ones?

If the person has experimented with drugs, ask the CAGE-AID questions. If the patient only drinks alcohol, ask the CAGE questions.

CAGE and CAGE-AID questions
1. In the last three months, have you felt you should cut down or stop drinking or *using drugs?*
   Yes No
2. In the last three months, has anyone annoyed you or gotten on your nerves by telling you to cut down or stop drinking or using *drugs?*
   Yes No
3. In the last three months, have you felt guilty or bad about how much you drink or *use drugs?*
   Yes No
4. In the last three months, have you been waking up wanting to have an alcoholic drink or *use drugs* (eye-opener)?
   Yes No

Each affirmative response earns one point. One point indicates a possible problem.
Two points indicate a probable problem.

men and two or more drinks per day in nonpregnant women (109–111). A "drink" is defined as approximately 12 ounces of beer, 5 ounces of wine, or 1.5 ounces of distilled liquor—the equivalent of 0.6 ounces of ethanol.

Once a problem is identified, a multifaceted, personalized, long-term management plan operationalized in collaboration with available community resources and family should be pursued. Transportation issues, architectural and attitudinal barriers within community-based resource facilities, and sometimes united social support are specific challenges to systematic management in those individuals with both chronic disability and substance abuse problems.

PRIMARY MEDICAL CARE IN THE GENERAL POPULATION

Within the past two decades in the United States there has been a resurgence of interest in primary medical care. Poor or rural patients confront a monolithic health-care system that has become too centralized, too costly, and inaccessible. Even patients with adequate financial and social resources have found it increasingly difficult to navigate by self-referral through the complex, technologically intimidating medical system that characterizes subspecialty care. Managed care organizations use generalist physicians and physician extenders to deliver services that, they argue, provide health care that is more accessible and less costly than specialist care and which is equally effective as specialty care in health outcomes (112).

As discussed earlier in the chapter, the term "primary care" has received many definitions by various medical organizations (5,6). However, most would agree that primary medical care has the following interdependent key components: first contact, continuity, comprehensiveness, and coordination of patient care, as well as care provided within a family and community context. This definition, paraphrased from a defining statement developed by the American Academy of Family Physicians, also serves well for other primary care providers such as general internists and general pediatricians. Within this framework of comprehensive and coordinated service, general providers must continually address these patient care issues:

- Disease prevention and health promotion
- Prospective care and disease/injury risk reduction
- Organization of the medical care team
- Recognition and management of family and community issues that affect the patient's health

An exhaustive report of these primary care topics is beyond the scope of this chapter. We intend to present an overview of those health-care issues that a modern generalist faces every day in his or her office and community with the knowledge that these same issues also will apply to those with disability and that the information provided may overlap with that previously presented.

Disease Prevention and Health Promotion

Over the past half century, specialty care has developed and championed an imposing array of technology and procedures for the diagnosis and treatment of existing disease. Paradoxically, many of the most serious maladies seen in clinical practice can be either averted, postponed, or reduced by prevention programs. Thus, a fundamental principle of primary care is the integration of preventive care and health promotion into clinical practice.

Primary care physicians have a number of helpful resources to assist them in developing preventive programs for their community and patient population.

In 1984, the U.S. Department of Health and Human Services commissioned the U.S. Preventive Services Task Force, an expert panel of preventive care researchers and clinicians, to publish its *Guide to Clinical Preventive Services* in 1989 and issued an update in 1995 (113). The *Guide* reports on the scientific assessment of the effectiveness of various interventions such as screening tests, counseling, and immunization/chemoprophylaxis. The panel reached several important conclusions regarding preventive services:

1. The most effective interventions are those that address the life-style choices and health practices of patients.
2. Proper selection of screening tests must include the patient's individual risk profile to assure cost effectiveness and reduction of potential adverse effects from the screening intervention.
3. Traditional clinical activities such as diagnostic testing

(i.e., routine blood panels) may be of less patient value than life-style counseling and patient education. This ''paradigm shift'' in clinical practice has tremendous implications for the training and role of primary care providers.

4. The importance of life-style choice in preventing disease implies a vastly changing role for patients as well. Patients will need to become the principal ''effector'' in primary disease prevention rather than a ''consumer'' of health-care services. Providers will thus need to develop skills in empowering patients to change adverse behaviors. Providers also will need to recognize and explore individual patients' health beliefs, which, if unidentified, will place major communication barriers between patient and provider.
5. Preventive services must be addressed or offered each time there is any provider/patient interaction—during sick visits as well as well visits. This longitudinal model will require good medical record-keeping and effective prompts and reminders for both physician and patient.
6. Much more outcomes- and evidence-based research is needed to establish proven effective interventions for many prevention systems. As can be seen in the accompanying preventive care schedules, there is limited consensus on many important recommendations.
7. Techniques and methodology for evaluating the effectiveness of prevention strategies need to be refined and standardized so that practicing clinicians can easily conclude if a preventive service is applicable to his own clinical setting.

The Clinician's Handbook of Preventive Services was created in 1994 for the U.S. Public Health Service. This concise and practical reference includes preventive services developed by the above task force, plus recommendations from other major U.S. health authorities, including CDC, National Institutes of Health, American Cancer Society, and American Heart Association, as well as professional organizations such as the American Academy of Family Physicians and the American Academy of Pediatrics (114) (Figs. 36-3 and 36-4).

Prospective Care and Risk Reduction

The care of patients with chronic illness is becoming more aggressive as prospective investigations demonstrate reduc-

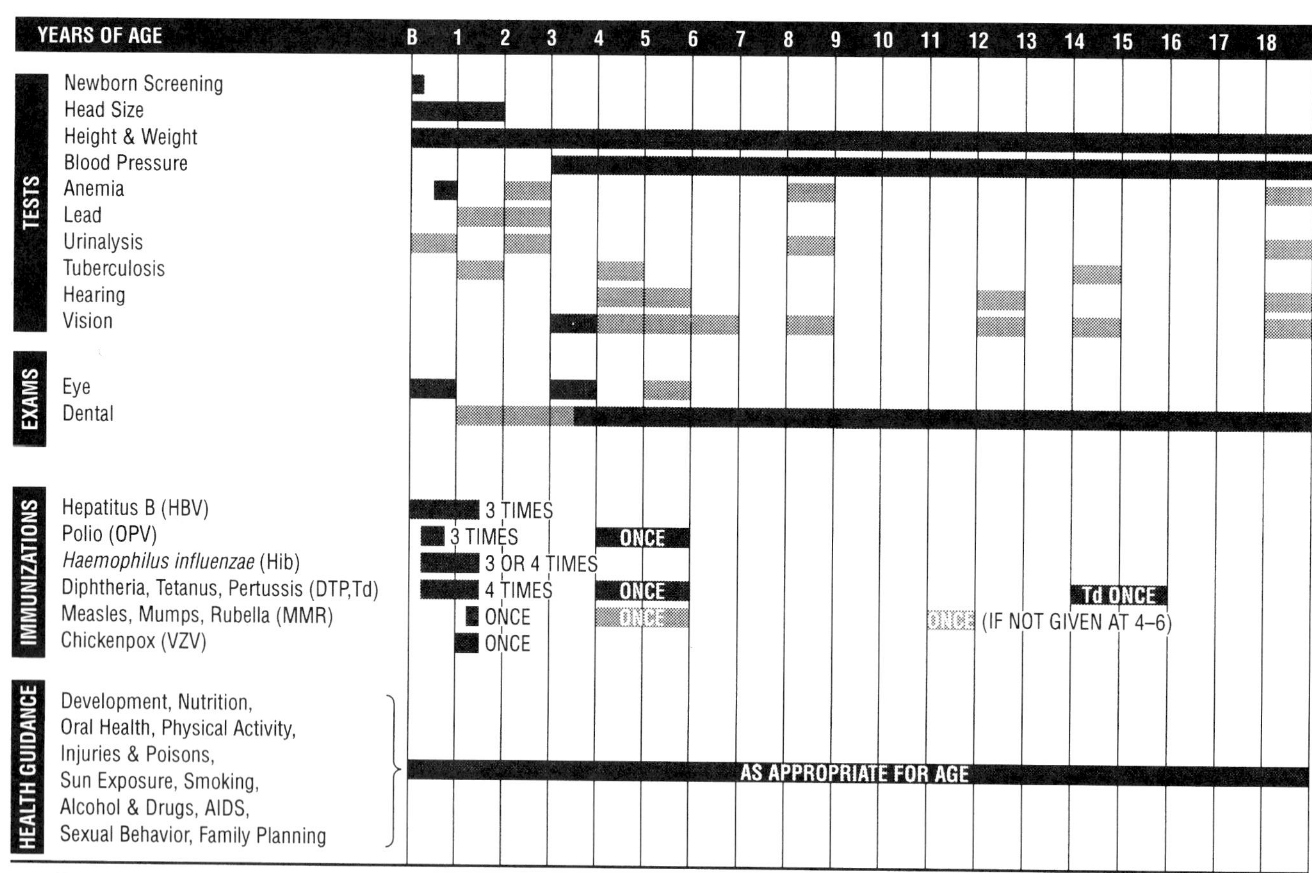

FIG. 36-3. Child preventive care time lines: Recommendations of major authorities (e.g., U.S. Public Health Service, Centers for Disease Control, National Institutes of Health, American Cancer Society, and American Heart Association).

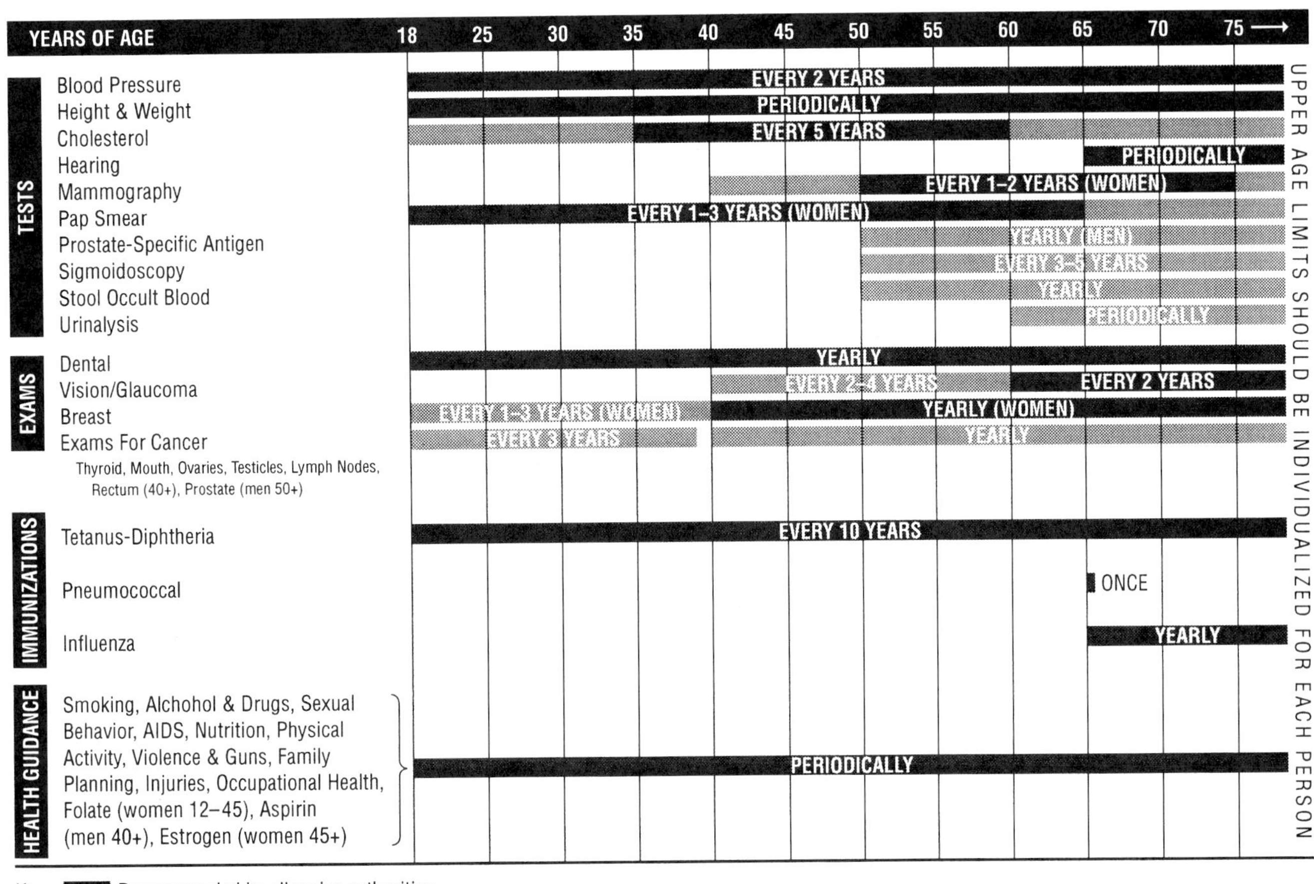

FIG. 36-4. Adult preventive care time lines: Recommendations of major authorities (see Fig. 36-3).

tion of target organ disease by careful adherence to clinical guidelines. The Agency for Health Care Policy and Research, national treatment consensus groups such as the Joint National Committee on Detection, Evaluation, and Treatment of High Blood Pressure, and regional managed care organizations publish clinical policy for the evaluation and management of chronic diseases (115).

Due to a growing national interest with sports medicine and a concern for workplace injuries, primary care medicine also has turned its attention to recurrent injuries. These ailments, although not usually life shortening like chronic diseases, have a major impact on quality of life and business productivity.

The following are selected primary care issues that are undergoing a major shift away from their past preoccupation with the treatment of irreversible sequelae toward the present development of disease deterrence through risk modification:

Hypertension

Adequate treatment reduces a patient's risk for stroke, coronary artery disease, abdominal aortic aneurysm, peripheral vascular disease, hypertensive retinopathy, congestive heart failure, and renal failure. Hypertension is defined as persistent elevation of diastolic pressure at or above 90 mm Hg and/or persistent elevation of systolic pressure above 140 mm Hg (115). Mounting evidence strongly supports treatment of isolated systolic hypertension in the elderly for the prevention of stroke (116). First-line agents include diuretics, acetylcholinesterase (ACE) inhibitors, and long-acting calcium channel blockers. Studies from the early 1990s concluded that short-acting calcium channel blockers increase morbidity and mortality and thus should be avoided.

Diabetes Mellitus

Prospective trials conclude that intensive insulin therapy in insulin-dependent diabetic patients may prevent chronic complications of diabetes, including retinopathy, neuropathy, and nephropathy (117). The goal of this intensified insulin therapy is to achieve a near-euglycemic state. This meticulous blood glucose control thus dictates a motivated, well-informed patient and a close doctor–patient relationship. For non–insulin-dependent diabetes, a chronic disorder characterized by relative insulin resistance in the peripheral tissues and reduction of body fat through diet and exercise is by far the most important treatment (118,119). Although prospective trials have not yet been published, most authorities believe that close control of blood glucose levels in diabetic patients will significantly reduce the burden of nephropathy, renal failure, coronary artery disease, and neuropathy-associated limb amputation.

Atherosclerotic Cardiovascular Disease

Mortality from stroke and heart attack is decreasing in many western hemisphere nations, including the United States. Authorities theorize that this decline is primarily due to a reduction in cigarette smoking and better treatment of hypertension. However, cardiovascular disease is still the number one cause of premature death and disability in the United States. Although progress has been made, prospective care should expand risk reduction efforts to include aggressive treatment of hypercholesterolemia, obesity, and inactivity, which are the other major independent, controllable risk factors for atherosclerosis. For those patients who have survived myocardial infarction, there are therapies that reduce the chance of further morbidity and mortality. Aspirin in a recommended dose of 80 to 325 mg a day reduces the risk of a second heart attack. Beta-blockers also have been shown to reduce the risk of subsequent myocardial infarction. For heart attack patients who have ejection fractions of 30% or less, ACE inhibitor treatment, even in the absence of hypertension, results in less left ventricular failure and fewer episodes of future ischemia (120).

Cancer

For patients with adequate access to care, many cancers are curable and some malignancies are becoming treatable chronic diseases. Prospective epidemiologic studies suggest that reduction of dietary fat will decrease the incidence of some cancers, including breast and colon cancer. Early detection of breast cancer through mammography and self-detection has led to a reduction in morbidity and mortality. Hormone receptor antagonists such as tamoxifen reduce breast cancer recurrence in women over 50 years of age who have positive axillary lymph nodes (121). Treatment for lung cancer, now the leading cause of cancer death for both men and women, is still discouraging, which underscores the need for smoking prevention and cessation.

Infectious Diseases

Human immunodeficiency virus (HIV) infection has had an overwhelming impact on the lives, anxieties, and behaviors of Americans. It has also significantly affected how clinicians practice medicine. Primary care providers have incorporated HIV risk assessment, including high-risk behavior assessment, into their review of systems and patient education programs (122). Strategies for reduction of blood-borne pathogen risk is now commonplace in medical facilities and many businesses. The resurgence of tuberculosis invokes thoughtful pause from the clinician who is evaluating a cough and fever presentation previously regarded as mundane.

Women's Health

Morbidity and mortality, both for the expectant mother and fetus, are still unacceptably high in this country. Most authorities conclude that obstetric complications could be significantly reduced by improving access to prenatal care. Studies published in the past decade have shown that adequate dietary folate and avoidance of alcohol during pregnancy will reduce the incidence of fetal anomalies.

The major advance in prospective care for women during the last two decades is hormone replacement therapy (HRT). In postmenopausal women, HRT increases HDL cholesterol, lowers LDL cholesterol, and reduces premature mortality from ischemic heart disease. HRT significantly delays bone resorption, thus reducing osteoporosis, a leading cause of morbidity and suffering in older women. In addition, HRT decreases perimenopausal vasomotor symptoms such as hot flushes and may ameliorate mood disorders associated with the climacteric. New treatment regimens, such as the continuous/combined estrogen–progestin protocol, are convenient and avoid the risk of endometrial hyperplasia/cancer in women with an intact uterus (123). Conflicting evidence exists regarding the association of HRT with an increased risk of breast cancer. As of this writing, some longitudinal studies show at most a 40% increase in breast cancer associated with HRT, and other studies conclude no association (124). This possible HRT complication contrasts with the documented severalfold reduction in cardiovascular mortality and osteoporosis achieved through hormone replacement treatment.

Osteoporosis

Prevention or reduction of osteoporosis has become a public health priority as the United States prepares for a burgeoning elderly population due to the aging of the large post–World War II generation. Osteoporotic hip fractures cause a serious burden of complications, including a 30% incidence of nursing home placement (125). Approximately 50% of women over 80 years of age who become nonambulatory have an ensuing mean survival of about 6 months. Multiple vertebral compression fractures compromise a woman's respiratory reserve and adversely affect balance, thus increasing risk for falls. HRT, especially if initiated within the first 3 years after menopause and if coupled with at least 1,200 to 1,500 mg of elemental calcium daily, is the most effective deterrent of osteoporosis. Other important risk reduction interventions are weight-bearing exercise, maintenance of ideal body weight and good general nutrition, avoidance of cigarettes and excessive alcohol, avoidance of high-dose diuretics, and avoidance of excessive thyroid replacement. New treatment regimens, including nasal calcitonin and biphosphonates, may retard progression of existing osteoporosis and may be useful HRT substitutes for women who cannot or will not take estrogen (126).

Low Back Injuries

A leading cause of missed days in the workplace, acute low back pain has not yet received the scientific inquiry and educational priority that it deserves. A recent report revealed that treatment from family physicians, orthopedists, and chiropractors had equal success in resolving uncomplicated acute low back pain (127). However, ambulatory patients surveyed in the study were significantly more satisfied with the care they received from chiropractors, probably due to the chiropractors' more thorough physical examination and patient education efforts. This study's conclusions should not be surprising because undergraduate and resident medical education programs have not adequately stressed orthopedic examination and patient education techniques. The Agency for Health Care Policy and Research recently published clinical guidelines for the evaluation and management of acute low back pain (128). Authorities propose that prevention programs emphasizing weight reduction, proper lifting techniques, ergonomic design of the home and workplace, and strengthening and flexibility enhancement will reduce the incidence of this common illness.

Overuse Injuries

Sports-related and work-related overuse injuries present principally in ambulatory medical settings. Therefore, primary medical care providers should be familiar with their evaluation and management.

Sports

Exercise is an important risk reducer for the chronic diseases mentioned above. Providers should know how to manage the adverse reactions (overuse injuries) of an exercise prescription, just as they should know how to manage the adverse reactions of medication. Common running and walking overuse injuries include metatarsal and tibial stress fractures, metatarsalgia and Morton's neuroma, shin splints, patellofemoral pain syndrome, infrapatellar tendinitis, Achilles tendinitis, pes anserine bursitis, and iliotibial band friction syndrome. Although overuse injuries of the lower extremities are usually precipitated by improper training techniques and excessive exercise duration or intensity, sports medicine practitioners now know that the root cause is often biomechanical imbalances such as overpronation and inflexibility (129). Thus, a working knowledge of strength and flexibility assessment, biomechanical foot disorders, and proper athletic shoe prescription is an essential requirement of the modern primary care provider.

Repetitive Injuries in the Workplace

Because primary care providers aim to view patients in the full context of their home and work, occupational medicine issues are an integral component of comprehensive health care. For example, our "keyboard society" has hastened a dramatic increase in the reporting of carpal tunnel syndrome cases. Primary care providers must become well versed in the assessment, conservative treatment, and knowledgeable referral of patients with carpal tunnel syndrome and other work-related repetitive injuries.

Trauma-Related Injuries

Motor Vehicle Injuries

In 1993, motor vehicle crash–related injuries were the eighth leading cause of death in the United States (130). Motor vehicle fatality rates are highest for young and elderly adults, whereas injury rates peak in young adulthood (130,131). Although alcohol-related traffic fatality rates have declined by more than one third since 1979 (132), alcohol use remains an important risk factor for motor vehicle injuries. Evidence also indicates that impairment with drugs other than alcohol also may play an important role in traffic injuries and deaths, although the relationship is not as well defined as for alcohol. In addition to driving while impaired by alcohol or drugs, failing to use occupant protection (e.g., safety belts, child safety seats, motorcycle helmets) is also an important risk factor for motor vehicle injury (133). Substance abuse screening and intervention are likely to be efficacious in reducing motor vehicle injuries and fatalities, whereas the use of occupant restraints has been shown to reduce the risk of motor vehicle injury and death (133).

Recommendations (133) from the U.S. Preventive Services Task Force for the prevention of motor vehicle related injuries are listed as follows:

1. Clinicians should regularly urge their patients to use lap and shoulder belts for themselves and their passengers while riding in automobiles, including automobiles equipped with air bags.
2. Operators of vehicles carrying infants and toddlers should be urged to install and regularly use federally approved child safety seats in accordance with the manufacturer's instructions and the child's size.
3. Those who operate or ride on motorcycles should be counseled to wear approved safety helmets.
4. All patients should be counseled regarding the dangers of operating a motor vehicle while under the influence of alcohol or other drugs, as well as the risks of riding in a vehicle operated by someone who is under the influence of these substances.

Household and Recreational Injuries

Unintentional injuries accounted for nearly 89,000 deaths in the United States in 1993, half of these being related to household, recreational, and other etiologies unrelated to motor vehicles (130). Falls, poisoning, fires and burns, drowning, suffocation and aspiration, firearms, and bicycling cause nearly two thirds of these deaths (134). Almost 90% of deaths relating to sports and recreation occur during swimming, boating, bicycling, riding off-road vehicles such as all-terrain vehicles, or using firearms (134). All of the above are also common causes of nonfatal injuries, with falls being the most common (133).

Recommendations (133) from the U.S. Preventive Services Task Force for the prevention of household and recreation related injuries are listed as follows:

1. Parents should be counseled on measures to reduce the risk of unintentional injuries to their children from residential fires and hot tap water, drowning, poisoning, bicycling, firearms, and falls.
2. Homeowners should install smoke detectors in appropriate locations and test the devices periodically to ensure proper operations. Encourage the use of flame-resistant nightwear during sleep, and reduce or cease smoking in the home.
3. Households are advised to keep a 1-ounce bottle of ipecac, display the telephone number of the local poison control center, and place all medications, toxic substances, and matches in child-resistant containers.
4. Bicyclists and parents of children who ride bicycles should be counseled about the importance of wearing approved safety helmets and avoiding riding bicycles in motor vehicle traffic.
5. Families should be encouraged to install fences with gates around swimming pools.
6. All windows that pose high risk for falls should have window guards.
7. All residents of homes with swimming pools, young children, or elderly persons should be encouraged to learn cardiopulmonary resuscitation and maneuvers to manage choking incidents.
8. Remove firearms from the home or at a minimum keep them unloaded in a locked compartment separated from the ammunition.
9. Elderly patients should be counseled on measures to reduce the risk of falling, including exercise (particularly training to improve balance), safety-related skills and behaviors, and environmental hazard reduction, along with monitoring and adjusting medications.

Organization of the Medical Care Team

Managed care has dramatically and irrevocably changed the delivery of health care in the United States. Managed care organizations now carefully define the roles of their primary care providers and specialty providers. Powerful practice management computer data bases are being developed that track patient populations, case mix and levels of service acuity, resource utilization, prescribing patterns, referral patterns, individual practice profiles, and treatment outcomes. Individual practices, regional health-care systems, and Fortune 500 health-care conglomerates are implementing continuous quality improvement programs.

A new concept in managed care delivery that depends on continuous quality improvement for its success is called disease state management (135). This health-care organization model targets high-cost and high-volume diagnoses and those conditions that tend to have wide variations in provider practices and resource utilization. The intention of disease state management is to improve outcomes while maintaining or lowering overall costs. The process of disease state management must include evidence-based clinical policies, an accurate and complete data base that can measure the well-defined outcomes, and a team-oriented, multidisciplinary approach. The multidisciplinary approach will require careful and extensive communication between generalist and specialist members of the team (136). Advocates of this organizational system recognize that its success critically depends on a sophisticated information system and the rapid development of evidence-based clinical policies that focus on patient outcomes. Unfortunately, outcome studies in primary care need further development. Thus, outcome-based research will be an important research objective for primary care scholarship.

Family and Community Issues

Primary care providers assess and treat patients within the context of their family and community. Indeed, comprehensive longitudinal care is incomplete and ineffective without addressing the meshwork of stresses and supports that surround individual patients (137). Quality primary care addresses and explores the following family/community issues:

The family circle
Patient birth order
Family genogram
Childhood traumas, expressed and suppressed
Family violence
Marital history and marital stresses
Chronic illness in other family members
Family organization and identity (chaotic?, crisis-oriented?, nurturing?, etc.)
Educational level of the patient
Educational resources available for the patient and family
Child day-care services
Health belief models expressed by the patient and family members
Timing of illnesses in a patient's life cycle stage
Patient's work/employment history
Co-worker stress/support
Patient hobbies and stress relievers
Patient's pets
Home safety

Neighborhood safety
Family and nonfamily members living in the same household
Transportation availability
Services and support for persons with disabilities
Financial resources
Legal difficulties and legal aid services
Spiritual support (and stress)
Recreation resources
Available community health and counseling agencies
Self-help and support groups
Respite care for families of the elderly
Elderly day-care programs
Extended care facilities
Rehabilitative services
Hospice

Patient Management Protocols and Clinical Policies

Comprehensive descriptions of common disease management protocols are beyond the scope of this chapter. Detailed clinical guidelines for a number of primary care conditions have been published by the Agency for Health Care Policy and Research. Here are some examples of available monographs[1]

Pressure ulcers in adults
Managing early HIV infection
Managing urinary incontinence
Heart failure: evaluation and care of patients with left ventricular systolic dysfunction
Middle ear fluid in young children
Depression in primary care

MODEL PROGRAMS FOR PROVIDING PRIMARY CARE FOR PERSONS WITH DISABILITIES

Few models are currently in place in the United States that provide comprehensive primary care for adults with physical disabilities. Many multidisciplinary pediatric programs provide care for children with disabilities, but few of these programs incorporate long-term primary care management. Many rehabilitation providers are currently exploring the development of primary care programs as a response to unmet needs in their patient populations.

Barriers

There are multiple barriers to access of appropriate health-care services for adults with disability (19). Individuals with physical or cognitive challenges often have complex medical management needs (23). Few clinicians have had experience managing the long-term care needs of this population (15). Little exposure to the specific needs of the person with disability occurs in most primary care residency programs. This lack of experience may result in attitudinal barriers that can impact the health-care choices primary care practitioners make for their patients. In addition, there are major financial disincentives for physicians caring for this complex population. Rarely, do the care needs of these adults fit the typical time framework allotted for outpatient visits (20,138).

Physical access to health care remains a barrier for the person with a disability. Outpatient offices may not be wheelchair accessible. Examination rooms are frequently too small to accommodate patients, their mobility devices, and their families and/or caretakers. Many of the staff in community-based outpatient settings are not familiar with transfer techniques, and examination tables often do not adjust to heights that facilitate transfers. This may lead to inadequate physical examinations with patients being examined in their wheelchairs.

Lack of reliable transportation also can inhibit access to timely primary care (139). Patients without access to transportation often use the emergency room for all outpatient care, which leads to inappropriate and fragmented care as well as increasing the cost of care. This leads to a lack of adequate coordination of care, which as noted previously is an essential factor in promoting wellness and providing for optimal utilization of resources.

Physiatric Model

Many physiatrists provide primary care to a proportion of their patients with severe disability (27). This is especially common among physiatrists who follow large numbers of patients with spinal cord injuries and traumatic brain injuries. Many of these patients are young and did not have consistent primary care providers before injury. Multiple barriers can limit the ability to establish new primary care access after injury. Most of the PM&R primary care providers do not have structured primary care programs that can provide a full range of primary care services. They tend to provide medical management on an as-needed basis with coverage provided by emergency departments when they are not available. Few current PM&R providers have an adequate support system established to facilitate the provision of efficient comprehensive primary care management. No physiatric-based primary care programs currently provide services on a capitated, risk-sharing basis.

Home Care Model

Boston's Community Medical Group (BCMG) was established in 1983 as an outgrowth of the Urban Medical Group (UMG). UMG was established in Boston in 1978 by a group of Boston area physicians, nurse practitioners, and physician assistants to provide continuous primary care to inner-city nursing home residents and frail home-bound older adults (140). In cooperation with a center for independent living, BCMG set forth to provide these same benefits to younger

[1] To obtain a list of monographs or to order guideline products, write: AHCPR Publications Clearinghouse, P.O. Box 8547, Silver Spring, MD, 20907. Ordering is also available through the Internet.

adults living independently with major disabilities, including spinal cord injury, cerebral palsy, traumatic brain injury, and other neurologic diseases. Primary care services are provided in the patients' homes, ambulatory care sites, hospitals, and long-term care facilities. A team approach is used but with heavy reliance on nurse practitioners as the providers of first-contact care and gatekeeper functions. Initially this program functioned on a fee-for-service basis via a unique contract with their state Medicaid program; however, beginning in April 1992, BCMG converted to a prepaid capitated method of payment (141).

In 1996, the program was providing comprehensive care for 171 people with major disabling conditions as noted above (141). A primary care physician and nurse practitioner perform an initial comprehensive evaluation of each new patient and develop a plan of medical, nursing, rehabilitation, and social care which the nurse practitioner then implements. The nurse practitioner evaluates all new medical problems and provides home visits. The primary physician maintains direct responsibility for supervising the nurse practitioner via regular meetings and emergency consultation. Emergency access is available 24 hours per day (142).

Physiatrist–Internist Collaborative Practice Model

Several programs are being developed using a physiatrist–internist collaborative practice model (21). In 1990, Schwab Rehabilitation Hospital developed a unique relationship with a not-for-profit, community-based agency (Anixter Center) that serves over 1,500 disabled children and adults each year. In order to provide health-care services in a coordinated and accessible way to individuals with physical, cognitive, and developmental disabilities, Schwab developed an outpatient health-care center located on-site at Anixter Center. This program uses the services of an internal medicine specialist to provide primary medical services and a physiatrist to provide physical medicine services and rehabilitation prescription and referral. Health maintenance and preventive services are provided on a regular basis, obviating costly hospitalizations that may occur after long delays for identification and treatment of medical problems.

In addition to primary care and physiatric services, the program provides on-site specialty consultations including obstetrics and gynecology, neurology, psychiatric and psychological services, podiatry care, wheelchair assessments, health promotion and screening, audiology evaluations, nutritional counseling, and orthotic/prosthetic evaluations. If inpatient hospitalization is required for their clients, care is coordinated by one physician familiar with their medical and rehabilitative needs. Additional services provided at Anixter Center, to add to its holistic approach to treatment, include vocational evaluation and training, addiction recovery, independent living training, job placement, and residential and in-home support services via numerous satellite facilities throughout the Chicago area. This is a fee-for-service program that provides care for over 500 client visits per month.

Another program using a physiatrist–internist collaborative practice model was developed at the Rehabilitation Institute of Michigan (RIM) to provide coordinated primary care for individuals with physical disabilities. The program focused on addressing key concerns of patient access and care coordination (143).

The population is predominantly of a younger age group with 77% of the patients less than 50 years of age. Eighty percent of the patients belong to the traumatic brain injury, spinal cord injury, and young stroke diagnostic groups. Adults with childhood-onset disabilities, including cerebral palsy and myelomeningocele, are a growing segment of the population because the program makes a good transition from comprehensive multidisciplinary pediatric programs.

There is a high frequency of patients with physical impairments including hemiplegia/paresis, paraplegia/paresis, and tetraplegia/paresis. A large percentage of the population has coexisting cognitive deficits. This has clearly impacted on the educational needs of patients and families. Cognitively impaired patients may need a great deal of family support to follow medical recommendations. This may include educating multiple family members who assist a patient in his or her home environment. Unfortunately, persons with cognitive disabilities are often labeled as noncompliant when in fact they may not be able to problem solve in unusual situations such as a missed doses or lost medications. Twenty-four hour access to a health-care provider who understands the patient's deficits can improve patient follow-through on treatment recommendations in these situations.

Educational status and family support are sentinel factors in the health maintenance of the person with a disability. Approximately 57% of these primary care patients live with other family members. The vast majority (94%) do not have a spouse. A significant percentage (22%) live alone, and 48% have not received their high school diploma.

The first goal of the program was to improve access to primary care for Medicaid recipients with major physical impairments, enhancing health status and reducing overall cost. The availability of transportation has a major impact on access to health-care services. The "do not show" (DNS) rate for patients where transportation was provided and arranged for by the primary care program coordinator was 0.8%. Patient DNS rate was 12% for patients who did not qualify for transportation services. After discontinuation of the transportation program (for budgetary reasons), the DNS rate for patients previously receiving transportation increased to 44%. Others have reported that many persons with disability use the emergency department as their primary care provider because of the availability of ambulance transportation (139).

The second goal of the program was to coordinate the delivery of rehabilitation services with the delivery of general medical and preventive care for Medicaid recipients with major physical impairments to improve the quality of care they receive. The clinical care delivery model is based on a physiatrist–internist collaborative practice (7). On the initial visit to the program, comprehensive evaluations are performed by both the internist and physiatrist, focusing on general health status, risk factors, preventive care needs, functional status, psychosocial status, and functional goals. The physician extender (a physician assistant or advanced practice nurse) assists with initial record review, history taking, physical examination, and patient education. A collaborative management plan is established, and follow-up visits are planned.

The initial concept for the RIM program was a multispecialty interdisciplinary model with specialty physicians on site in the clinic on a regularly scheduled basis (21). As the model evolved with protocol development, it moved toward a collaborative practice model with specialty consultation as needed. Urology evaluations are available on site because of a large population with spinal cord injury. The collaborative development of protocols with specialty physicians and surgeons has included pathways to facilitate the efficiency of the consultation process, including preconsultation information gathering and testing when appropriate.

The program provides patients with 24-hour, 7-days-per-week physician access via an answering service, with the internist and physician extender rotating coverage. Patients can be seen on an urgent basis during the week. Special arrangements with the emergency department have been established to manage urgent needs at night and on weekends.

It was initially expected that patients would enter the program after all inpatient and outpatient rehabilitation programs had been completed, with a focus on primary care issues. However, it was found that the program has been serving a significant number of patients with acute rehabilitation needs who were discharged from acute inpatient rehabilitation after onset of a new disability. This trend is likely to continue because patients discharged from acute rehabilitation settings often have difficulty returning to their previous primary care providers (18). Also, many patients did not have consistent primary health-care providers before their injury. This trend resulted in a high utilization of therapy services during the first year of the program. Therapy utilization has been needed for both postacute intervention for new-onset disabilities, unrecognized problems, and treatment of the observed potential for further functional improvement.

One potential area for cost saving and improving continuity of care has been a focus on decreasing use of emergency department services. Patients are required to contact the program before going to the emergency department. This has been a difficult behavior to establish in many of the patients who have used the emergency department as their primary care provider in the past. In the initial 18 months of the program, 76% of patients did not contact the program before an emergency department visit. The emergency department is required to contact the program before providing any medical care. This has improved management of acute medical problems and markedly decreased use of the emergency department.

The major lessons learned from the initial implementation of the program relate to time. The time necessary for initial office visits was even greater than initially expected. Initial evaluations averaged 2.5 hours. Half of the follow-up visits lasted 15 to 45 minutes, not including documentation time. The team clearly felt that time spent on the initial visit obtaining as complete a data base as possible was the major factor in improving management of long-term primary care needs.

The initial outcomes of the program have included a focus on prevention and health maintenance, not just crisis intervention. It has helped to shift patient management out of the high-cost settings of the emergency department and inpatient care, and into that of outpatient care. Careful evaluation and optimization of the number of medications and frequency of administration have improved compliance, especially for patients with cognitive impairments. The collaborative practice model in a rehabilitation setting has allowed for the integration of functional goals into the health maintenance paradigm. The program has facilitated longer term follow-up related to achievement of vocational goals, driving, community reintegration, and recreation and leisure skills.

There is a need to develop similar programs to provide coordinated, comprehensive primary care services for adults with a wide range of disabilities. There are several options for program design, but it is clear that a structured support network of coordinated services is essential. This population uses a proportionally greater degree of resources than the general population, but long-term cost savings can be achieved by shifting care from high-cost inpatient and emergency department settings to outpatient and community settings. Initially, however, there is an increase in service utilization as unmet needs are identified.

Primary care programs for persons with disabilities need to anticipate greater time allocation per patient visit than traditional primary care models. Inclusion of the patient's support system in the primary care process is essential to facilitate follow-through in the home and community. Cognitive deficits are a frequent impairment requiring a strong focus on patient and caregiver education.

CONCLUSION

All of us, including persons with disabilities, want the same things for ourselves and our families: a compassionate, knowledgeable, available physician to help us maintain our health when we are well and to manage our minor illnesses when we are sick, and the best specialists available when we have a major acute or chronic medical problem (7). In this chapter we have reviewed some of the obstacles that those with disabilities endure to achieve the above ideal. It is not expected that the field of physical medicine and rehabilitation will be declared a primary care specialty, nor would this be a viable solution to providing primary care services for all of those with disabilities. However, one of the goals of writing this chapter was to provide to those physiatrists who currently perform continuity of care and gatekeeper functions some guidelines as well as resources to continue to provide state-of-the-art primary care. The majority of practicing physiatrists, however, do not fulfill this role.

Our health-care system is changing rapidly, and in order to assist our patients with disabilities to achieve optimal health, we need to frequently re-evaluate and modify our methods of health-care delivery. The last section of this chapter provided alternatives and models for the provision of primary care services in this population. These programs have become very successful within their own health-care systems but may not directly apply to all practitioners interested in providing these services. At a minimum, rehabilitation care providers should collaborate with existing primary care providers, including generalist physicians and physician extenders, to achieve the goal of providing adequate, high-quality primary care for persons with disabilities. This collaboration could include educating primary care providers on physiatric issues and team ventures with them to provide primary care for this population.

REFERENCES

1. Williamson JW, Walters KW, Cordes DL. Primary care, quality improvement, and health systems change. *Am J Med Qual* 1993; 8: 37–44.
2. Shi L. Balancing primary versus specialty care. *J R Soc Med* 1995; 88:428–432.
3. American Academy of Physical Medicine and Rehabilitation. AAPM&R position on physiatrists as primary care providers. *AAPM& R handbook.* Chicago: American Academy of Physical Medicine and Rehabilitation, 1993; 1–4.
4. Bockenek WL, Currie DM. Physical medicine and rehabilitation as a primary care specialty? A report from the Association of Academic Physiatrists Academic Affairs committee. *AAP Newsletter* 1993:5–7.
5. Status and future. Health Research and Services Administration National Research Service Awards Program, April 17, 1991.
6. *Defining primary care: an interim report.* Washington, D.C.: National Academy Press, 1994.
7. Bockenek WL, Currie DM. Physical medicine and rehabilitation as a primary care specialty: commentary. *Am J Phys Med Rehabil* 1994; 73:58–60.
8. Rivo ML, Satcher D. Improving access to health care through physician work force reform: direction for the 21st century. Third report of the Council on graduate medical education. *JAMA* 1993; 270: 1074–1078.
9. Rivo ML, Saultz JW, Wartman SA, Dewitt TG. Defining the generalist physician training. *JAMA* 1994; 271:1499–1504.
10. Association of American Medical Colleges. AAMC policy on the generalist physician. *Acad Med* 1993; 68:1–6.
11. Council on Graduate Medical Education. *Fourth report: recommendations to improve access to health care through physician work force reform.* Rockville, MD: U.S. Public Health Service, Health Resources and Services Administration, Bureau of Health Professions, 1993.
12. Gabriel SE. Primary care: specialists or generalists. *Mayo Clin Proc* 1996; 71:415–419.
13. DeJong G, Brannon RW, Batavia AI. Financing health and personal care. In: Whiteneck GG, Charlifue SW, Gerhart KA, et al., eds. *Aging with spinal cord injury.* New York: Demos Publishers, 1993; 275–294.
14. DeJong G. Primary care for persons with disabilities: an overview of the problem. *Am J Phys Med Rehabil* 1997; 76(suppl):2–8.
15. Institute of Medicine, Committee on a National Agenda for Prevention of Disabilities Disability in America. In: Pope AM, Tarlov AR, eds. *Toward a National Agenda for Prevention.* Washington, D.C.: National Academy Press, 1991.
16. Bauman WA. The endocrine system. In: Whiteneck GG, Charlifue MA, Gerhart KA, et al., eds. *Aging with spinal cord injury.* New York: Demos Publications, 1993; 275–294.
17. National Rehabilitation Hospital Research Center. Health care utilization project team revisits expenditure data. Research Update, fall 1996.
18. American Congress of Rehabilitation Medicine. Addressing the post-rehabilitation health care needs of persons with disabilities. *Arch Phys Med Rehabil* 1993; 74(suppl):8–14.
19. DeJong G, Batavia A, Griss R. America's neglected health minority: working age persons with disabilities. *Milbank Q* 1989; 67(suppl 2): 311–351.
20. Burns TJ, Batavia AI, Smith QW, DeJong G. The primary health care needs of persons with physical disabilities: what are the research and service priorities? *Arch Phys Med Rehabil* 1990; 71:138–143.
21. Gans BM, Mann NR, Becker BE. Delivery of primary care to the physically challenged. *Arch Phys Med Rehabil* 1993; 74(suppl): 15–19.
22. Batavia AI, DeJong G, Burns TJ, Burns QW, Smith SM, Butler D. *A managed care program for working-age persons with physical disabilities: a feasibility study.* NRH Research Center. Washington, D.C.: Robert Wood Johnson Foundation, 1989.
23. Batavia A, DeJong G, Halstead L. Primary medical services for people with disabilities. *Am Rehabil* 1989; 14:4,9–12,26–27.
24. Brannon R, Naierman N, DeJong G. Unpublished report to the Robert Wood Johnson Foundation. Washington, D.C.: National Rehabilitation Hospital Research Center, 1990.
25. Bockenek WL, Blom JM. Health care needs assessment in a population with severe disability. *Am J Phys M Rehabil* 1994; 73:144.
26. Kindig DA, Cultice JM, Mullan F. The elusive generalist physician: Can we reach a 50% goal? *JAMA* 1993; 270:1069–1073.
27. Francisco GE, Chae JC, DeLisa JA. Physiatry as a primary care specialty. *Am J Phys Med Rehabil* 1995; 74:186–192.
28. Hogan PF, Dobson A, Haynie B, et al. Physical medicine and rehabilitation work force study: the supply of and demand for physiatrists. *Arch Phys Med Rehabil* 1996; 77:95–99.
29. Buschbacher RM, DeLisa JA, Kevorkian CG. Commentary: the physiatrist as primary care provider for the disabled. *Am J Phys Med Rehabil* 1997; 76:149–153.
30. Marge M. Health promotion for persons with disabilities: moving beyond rehabilitation. *Am J Health Promotion* 1988; 2:29–35.
31. Pender NJ. *Health promotion in nursing practice, 1982.* Norwalk, CT: Appleton & Lange, 1982.
32. Spellbring AM. Nursing's role in health promotion—an overview. *Nurs Clin North Am* 1991; 26:804–805.
33. USDHHS. *Healthy people 2000 (PHS 91, 50212–50213).* Washington, D.C.: Government Publishing Office, 1991.
34. Noack H. Concepts of health and health promotion. In: Abelin T, Brzezinski ZJ, Carstairs VDL, eds. *Measurement in health promotion and protection.* Copenhagen: World Health Organization Regional Publications European Series 1987; 5–28.
35. Department of Health and Human Services. *Healthy people 2000 (PHS 91, 50212–50213).* Washington D.C.: Government Printing Office, 1991.
36. World Health Organization. *World Health Organization international classification of impairments, disabilities and handicaps: a manual of classification relating to the consequences of disease.* Geneva: World Health Organization, 1980.
37. Pope AM, Tarlov AR, eds. *Disability in America.* Washington, D.C.: National Academy Press, 1991.
38. Nagi SZ. An epidemiology of disability among adults in the United States. Melbank Memorial Fund. *Q Health Society* 1976; 54:439–467.
39. Patrick DL, Richardson M, Starks HE, Rose MA. A framework for promoting the health of people with disabilities. In: Lollar DJ, ed. *Preventing secondary conditions associated with spina bifida or cerebral palsy. Proceedings and recommendations of a symposium, February 17–19, 1994, Crystal City, VA.* Washington: Spina Bifida Association of America, 1994.
40. Fuhrer MJ. Setting the conceptual landscape. In: Graitcer PL, Maynard FM, eds. *Proceedings from the first colloquium on preventing secondary conditions among people with spinal cord injuries.* February 27–28, 1990. Atlanta, GA: U.S. Department of Health and Human Services, Centers for Disease Control and Prevention, 1990; 37–40.
41. Fuhrer MJ. Subjective well-being. Implications for medical rehabilita-

tion outcomes and models of disablement. *Am J Phys Med Rehabil* 1994; 73:358–364.
42. Fuhrer MJ. The subjective well-being of people with spinal cord injury: relationships to impairment, disability, and handicap. *Top Spinal Cord Inj Rehabil* 1996; 1:56–71.
43. Whiteneck GG. Outcome evaluation and spinal cord injury. *Neuro Rehabil* 1992; 2:30–40.
44. Bigbee JL, Jansa N. Strategies for promoting health protection. *Nurs Clin North Am* 1991; 26:895–913.
45. Pender NJ. *Health promotion in nursing practice,* 2nd ed. East Norwalk, CT: Appleton & Lange, 1987.
46. Lanig IS. The interdisciplinary assessment of health. In: Lanig IS, Chase TM, Butt LM, et al. *A practical guide to health promotion after spinal cord injury.* Gaithersburg, MD: Aspen, 1996; 50–77.
47. Mulley AG Jr. Health maintenance and the role of screening. In: Goroll AH, May LA, Mulley AG Jr, eds. *Primary care medicine: office evaluation of the adult patient,* 3rd ed. Philadelphia: JB Lippincott, 1995; 13–16.
48. Lanig IS. Principles of effective patient education. In: Lanig IS, Chase TM, Butt LM, et al. *A practical guide to health promotion after spinal cord injury.* Gaithersburg, MD: Aspen, 1996: 34–39.
49. Green LW, Cargo, M, Ottoson JM. The role of physicians in supporting life style changes. *Med Exerc Nutrition Health* 1994; 3:119–130.
50. Lipetz M, Bussigel M, Bannderman J, Risley B. What is wrong with patient education programs. *Nurs Outlook* 1990; 38:184–189.
51. Gans KM, Jack B, Lasater TM. Changing physicians' attitudes, knowledge, and self efficacy regarding cholesterol screening and management. *Am J Prev Med* 1993; 9:101–106.
52. Pololi LH, Coletta EM, Kern DG, et al. Developing a competency based preventive medicine curriculum for medical schools. *Am J Prev Med* 1994; 10:240–244.
53. Graitcer PL, Maynard FM. *Proceedings from the first colloquium on preventing secondary disabilities among people with spinal cord injuries, February 27–28, 1990.* Atlanta, GA: U.S. Department of Health and Human Services, Centers for Disease Control, 1990.
54. Lollar DJ. *Preventing secondary conditions associated with spina bifida or cerebral palsy. Proceedings and recommendations of a symposium, February 17–19, 1994.* Crystal City, VA: Washington, D.C.: Spina Bifida Association, 1994.
55. Heim C. Health assessment. In: O'Donnell MP, Harris J, eds. *Health promotion in the workplace,* 2nd ed. Albany, NY: Delmar, 1994; 219–239.
56. U.S. Department of Health and Human Services. *Reducing the health consequences of smoking: 25 years of progress. A report of the Surgeon General.* Atlanta, GA: USDHHS, Public Health Service, Centers for Disease Control, Center for Chronic Disease Prevention and Health Promotion, Office on Smoking and Health. DHHS Publication No (PHS) (CDC) 89-8411, 1989.
57. Centers for Disease Control. Cigarette smoking-attributable mortality and years of potential life lost: United States, 1990. *MMWR* 1993; 42:645–649.
58. Centers for Disease Control. Cigarette smoking among adults: United States, 1993. *MMWR* 1994; 43:925–930.
59. National Cancer Institute. Tobacco and the clinician: interventions for medical and dental practice. NIH Publication No. 94-3693. *Monogr Natl Cancer Inst* 1994; 5:1–22.
60. Ockene JK. Smoking intervention: the expanding role of the physician. *Am J Public Health* 1987; 77:782–783.
61. Pederson LL. Compliance with physician advice to quit smoking: a review of the literature. *Prev Med* 1982; 11:71–84.
62. Roberson MD, Laurent SL, Little JM Jr. Including smoking status as a new vital sign: it works. *J Fam Pract* 1995; 40:556–563.
63. Rigotti NA. Smoking cessation. In: Gorroll AH, May LA, Mulley AG, eds. *Primary care medicine: office evaluation and management of the adult patient,* 3rd ed. Philadelphia: JB Lippincott, 1995; 300–308.
64. Glynn TJ, Manley MW. *How to help your patients stop smoking: a National Cancer Institute manual for physicians.* Bethesda, MD: U.S. Department of Health and Human Services, Public Health Service, National Institutes of Health, National Cancer Institute. NIH Publication No. 90-3064, 1990.
65. Fiore MC, Bailey WC, Cohen SJ, et al. *Smoking cessation. Clinical practice guideline No. 18.* Rockville, MD: U.S. Department of Health and Human Services, Public Health Service, Agency for Health Care Policy and Research. AHCPR Publication No. 96-0692. April 1996.
66. Williamson DF, Madans J, Anda RF, Kleinman JC, Giovino GA, Beyers T. Smoking cessation and the severity of weight gain in a national cohort. *N Engl J Med* 1991; 324:739–745.
67. Emont SC, Cummings KM. Weight gain following smoking cessation: a possible role for nicotine replacement in weight management. *Addict Behav* 1987; 12:151–155.
68. Weinsier RL, Morgan SL, Perrin VG. *Fundamentals of clinical nutrition.* St. Louis, MO: Mosby Year Book, 1993.
69. U.S. Department of Health and Human Services, Public Health Service & National Institute of Health. *Cancer prevention research summary: nutrition.* Bethesda, MD: National Cancer Institute, 1985.
70. American Heart Association. Dietary guidelines for healthy American adults: A statement for physicians and health professionals by the Nutrition Committee. Dallas, TX, 1988.
71. Butrum RR, Clifford CK, Lanza E. NCI dietary guidelines: rationale. *Am J Clin Nutr* 1988; 48:888–895.
72. Bauman WA, Spungen AM, Raza M, et al. Coronary artery disease: Metabolic risk factors and latent disease in individuals with paraplegia. *Mt Sinai J Med* 1992; 59:163–168.
73. Lanig IS. Promoting nutritional health. In: Lanig IS, Chase TM, Butt LM, et al. *A practical guide to health promotion after spinal cord injury.* Gaithersburg, MD: Aspen, 1996; 205–229.
74. Figoni SF. *Cycle of disability. National handicapped sports—adapted fitness instructor handbook.* Rockville, MD, 1991;2.
75. Abood DA, Burkhead BJ. Wellness: a valuable resource for persons with disability. *Health Educ* 1988; 19:21–25.
76. Curtis KA, Steadward RD, Weiss MS. Impairment: no barrier to fitness. *Patient Care* 1990; January:130–162.
77. Hjeltnes N, Jensen T. Physical endurance capacity, functional status and medical complications in spinal cord injured subjects with long-standing lesions. *Paraplegia* 1990; 28:428–432.
78. Lockette KF, Keyes AM. *Conditioning with physical disabilities.* Champaign, IL: Human Kinetics, 1994.
79. Micheo WF, Fontera W. Fitness and the disabled. *Bol Assoc Med P R* 1989; 10:447–450.
80. Miller PD, ed. *Fitness programming and physical disability.* Champaign, IL: Human Kinetics, 1991.
81. Reynolds JP. Stepping out of the medical model: fitness and physical therapy. *PT Magazine* 1993; May:24–41.
82. Rimmer JH. *Fitness and rehabilitation programs for special populations.* Champaign, IL: Human Kinetics, 1994.
83. U.S. Department of Health and Human Services. *A report of the Surgeon General: physical activity and health—persons with disabilities.* Atlanta, GA: Centers of Disease Control and Prevention, National Center for Chronic Disease Prevention and Health Promotion, The President's Council on Physical Fitness and Sports, 1996.
84. Chase TM. Physical fitness strategies. In: Lanig IS, Chase TM, Butt LM, et al. *A practical guide to health promotion after spinal cord injury.* Gaithersburg, MD: Aspen, 1996; 243–306.
85. Dangain J, Vrobova G. Response of normal and dystrophic muscles to increased functional demand. *Exp Neurol* 1986; 94:796–801.
86. McCarthy DA, Dale MM. The leucocytosis of exercise: a review and model. *Sports Med* 1988; 6:333–363.
87. Feldman RM. The use of strengthening exercise in post-polio sequelae, methods and results. *Orthopedics* 1985; 8:889–890.
88. Ernstoff B, Wetterquist H, Krist H, Grimby G. Endurance training effect on individuals with post poliomyelitis. *Arch Phys Med Rehabil* 1996; 77:843–848.
89. Fisher NM, Pendergast DR, Gresham GE, et al. Muscle rehabilitation: its effect on muscular and functional performance of patients with knee osteoarthritis. *Arch Phys Med Rehabil* 1991; 72:367–374.
90. Nordemar R, Ekblom B, Zachrisson L, et al. Physical training in rheumatoid arthritis. *Scand J Rheumatol* 1981; 10:17–23.
91. Cobb ND, Dietz MA, Grigsby J, Kennedy DM. Rehabilition of the patient with multiple sclerosis. In: DeLisa JA, Gans BM, Currie DM, et al., eds. *Rehabilitation medicine: principles and practice,* 2nd ed. Philadelphia: JB Lippincott, 1993; 861–885.
92. Davis GM, Jackson RW, Shephard RJ. Sports and recreation for the disabled. In: Strauss RH, ed. *Sports medicine.* Philadelphia: WB Saunders, 1984; 286–304.
93. Drory Y, Ohry A, Brooks ME, Dolphin D, Kellerman JJ. Arm crank

ergometry in chronic spinal cord injured patients. *Arch Phys Med Rehabil* 1990; 71:389–392.

94. Rohe DE. Psychological aspects of rehabilitation. In: DeLisa JA, Gans BM, Currie DM, et al., eds. *Rehabilitation medicine: principles and practice,* 2nd ed. Philadelphia: JB Lippincott, 1993; 131–150.
95. Rohe DE, DePompolo RW. Substance abuse policies in rehabilitation medicine departments. *Arch Phys Med Rehabil* 1985; 66:701–703.
96. Fullerton DT, Harvey RF, Klein MH, Howell T. Psychiatric disorders in patients with spinal cord injuries. *Arch Gen Psychiatry* 1981; 38: 1369–1371.
97. Heinemann AW, Manott BD, Schnoll S. Substance use by persons with recent spinal cord injuries. *Rehabil Psychology* 1990; 35: 217–228.
98. Rimel RW. A prospective study of patients with central nervous system trauma. *J Neurosurg Nurs* 1981; 13:132–141.
99. Heinemann AW, Doll MD, Armstrong KJ, Schnoll S, Yarkony GM. Substance use and receipt of treatment by persons with long-term spinal cord injuries. *Arch Phys Med Rehabil* 1991; 72:482–487.
100. Hanna EZ. Approach to the patient with alcohol abuse. In: Goroll AH, May LA, Mulley AG Jr., eds. *Primary care medicine: office evaluation of the adult patient,* 3rd ed. Philadelphia: JB Lippincott, 1995; 1044–1053.
101. Ewing JA. Detecting alcoholism: the CAGE questionnaire. *JAMA* 1984; 252:1905–1907.
102. Bush B, Shaw S, O'Leary P, Delbanco T, Aronson MD. Screening for alcohol abuse using the CAGE questionnaire. *Am J Med* 1987; 82:231–235.
103. Kitchens JM. Does this patient have an alcohol problem? *JAMA* 1994; 272:1782–1787.
104. Mayfield D, McLeod G, Hall P. The CAGE questionnaire: validation of a new alcohol screening instrument. *Am J Psychiatry* 1974; 131: 1121–1123.
105. Selzer ML. The Michigan Alcoholism Screening Test: the quest for a new diagnostic instrument. *Am J Psychiatry* 1971; 127:1653–1658.
106. Porkony AD, Miller BA, Kaplan HB. The brief MAST: a shortened version of the Michigan Alcoholism Screening Test. *Am J Psychiatry* 1972; 192:3.
107. Saunders JB, Aasland OG, Amundsen A, Grant M. Alcohol consumption and related problems among primary health care patients: W.H.O. collaborative project on early detection of persons with harmful alcohol consumption, I. *Addiction* 1993; 88:349–362.
108. Saunders JB, Aasland OG, Amundsen A, Grant M. Alcohol consumption and related problems among primary health care patients: W.H.O. collaborative project on early detection of persons with harmful alcohol consumption, II. *Addiction* 1993; 88:791–804.
109. Pequingnot G, Tuyns AJ, Berta JL. Ascitic cirrhosis in relation to alcohol consumption. *Int J Psychiatry* 1978; 7:113–120.
110. Rankin JG, Ashley MH. Alcohol-related problems. In: Last JM, Wallace RB, eds. *Public health and preventive medicine,* 12th ed. East Norwalk, CT: Appleton & Lange, 1992; 1039–1975.
111. Skinner HA, Schuller R, Roy J, Israel Y. Identification of alcohol abuse using laboratory tests and a history of trauma. *Ann Intern Med* 1984; 101:847–851.
112. Greenfield S, Nelson EC, Zubkoff M, et al. Variations in resource utilization among medical specialties and systems of care: results from the medical outcomes study. *JAMA* 1992; 267:1624–1630.
113. U.S. Preventive Services Task Force. *Guide to clinical preventive services: an assessment of the effectiveness of 169 interventions. Report of the U.S. Preventitive Services Task Force.* Baltimore: Williams & Wilkins, 1995.
114. *The clinician's handbook of preventive services. Put prevention into practice.* Washington, D.C.: U.S. Public Health Service, U.S. Department of Health and Human Services, 1994.
115. National Institutes of Health: National Heart, Lung and Blood Institute. *The fifth report of the Joint National Committee on Detection, Evaluation, and Treatment of High Blood Pressure.* Bethesda, MD: National Institutes of Health. NIH Publication No. 93-1088, 1993.
116. SHEP Cooperative Research Group. Prevention of stroke by antihypertensive drug treatment in older persons with isolated systolic hypertension. *JAMA* 1991; 265:3255–3264.
117. The Diabetes Control and Complications Trial Research Group. The effect of intensive treatment of diabetes on the development and progression of long-term complications in insulin-dependent diabetes mellitus. *N Engl J Med* 1993; 329:977–986.
118. American Diabetes Association. Standards of medical care for patients with diabetes mellitus. *Diabetes Care* 1994; 17:661–623.
119. Lebovitz HE, Lipsky MS. Management of type II diabetes mellitus. *Am Fam Physician* 1995, monograph 1.
120. Smith SC Jr, Blair SN, Criqui MH, et al. Preventing heart attack and death in patients with coronary disease. *Circulation* 1995; 92:2–4.
121. Harris JR, Lippman ME, Veronesi U, Willett W. Breast cancer, parts I,II,III. *N Engl J Med* 1992; 327:319–328,390–398,473–480.
122. Cohen PT, Snade MA, Volberding PA. *The AIDS knowledge base,* 2nd ed. Boston: Little, Brown, 1994.
123. Mayeaux EJ, Johnson C. Current concepts in post-menopausal hormone replacement therapy. *J Fam Prac* 1996; 43:69–75.
124. Colditz GA, Hankinson SE, Hunter DJ, et al. The use of estrogens and progestins and the risk of breast cancer in postmenopausal women. *N Engl J Med* 1995; 332:1589–1593.
125. Oncken CA. Osteoporosis. In: Rakel RE, ed. *Saunders manual of medical practice.* Philadelphia: WB Saunders, 1996; 707–709.
126. Lufkin EG, Zilkoksi M. Diagnosis and management of Osteoporosis. *Am Fam Physician* 1996, monograph No.1.
127. Carey TS, Garrett J, Jackman A, McLaughlin C, Fryer J, Smucker DR. The outcomes and costs of care for acute low back pain among patients seen by primary care practioners, chiropractors, and orthopedic surgeons. *N Engl J Med* 1995; 333:913–917.
128. Agency for Health Care Policy and Research. *Low back pain problems in adults: assessment and treatment.* Rockville, MD: Agency for Health Care Policy and Research. AHCPR Publication No. 95-0643, 1994.
129. Beatty LA. Plantar fasciitis. In: Rakel RE, ed. *Saunders manual of medical practice.* Philadelphia: WB Saunders, 1996; 814–816.
130. National Center for Health Statistics. *Annual summary of births, marriages, divorces, and deaths: United States, 1993.* Monthly vital statistics report. Vol. 42, no. 13 (suppl). Hyattsville, MD: Public Health Service, 1994.
131. National Highway Traffic Safety Administration. *Traffic safety facts 1992: a compilation of motor vehicle crash data from the Fatal Accident Reporting System and the General Estimates System.* Washington, D.C.: Department of Transportation, 1994.
132. Zobeck TS, Grant BF, Stinson FS, et al. Alcohol involvement in fatal traffic crashes in the United States: 1979–90. *Addiction* 1994; 89: 227–231.
133. Report of the U.S. Preventive Services Task Force. *Guide to clinical preventive services,* 2nd ed. Alexandria, VA: International Medical Publishing, 1996; 643–678.
134. Baker SP, O'Neill B, Ginsburg MJ, et al., eds. *The injury fact book,* 2nd ed. New York: Oxford University Press, 1992.
135. American Academy of Family Physicians. A position paper on disease state management. Compendium of AAFP positions on selected health issues. AAFP, 1996.
136. Lanier DC, Clancy CM. The changing interface of primary and specialty care. *J Fam Prac* 1996; 42:303–305.
137. Benedict S. Role of the community. In: Sloan PD, Slatt LM, Curtis P, ed. *Essentials of family medicine.* Baltimore: Williams & Wilkins, 1993; 31–38.
138. DeJong G. Post-rehabilitation health care for people with disabilities: an update on the 1988 white paper of the American Congress of Rehabilitation Medicine. *Arch Phys Med Rehabil* 1993; 74(suppl): 2–7.
139. Batavia AI, DeJong G, Burns TJ, Smith QW, Melus S, Butler D. *Physical disabilities: a feasibility study.* Washington, D.C.: National Rehabilitation Hospital Office of Research, 1989.
140. Meyers AR, Master RJ. Managed care for high-risk populations. *J Aging Social Policy* 1989; 1:197–215.
141. Meyers AR, Glover M, Master RJ. Primary care for persons with disabilities: the Boston, Massachusetts program. *Am J Phys Med Rehabil* 1997; 76(suppl):37–42.
142. Meyers AR, Cupples A, Lederman RI, et al. A prospective evaluation of the effect of managed care on medical care utilization among severely disabled independently living adults. *Med Care* 1987; 25: 1057–1068.
143. Mann NR. Primary care for persons with disabilities: rehabilitation of Michigans' model program. *Am J Phys Med Rehabil* 1997; 76(suppl): 47–49.

Rehabilitation Medicine: Principles and Practice, Third Edition,
edited by Joel A. DeLisa and Bruce M. Gans.
Lippincott–Raven Publishers, Philadelphia © 1998.

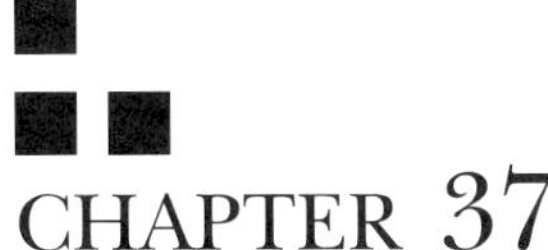

CHAPTER 37

Rehabilitation of the Pediatric Patient

Robert P. Christopher and Bruce M. Gans

The rehabilitation of children with physical impairments both resembles and differs from that established for adults. It is a challenging combination of normal child care and the best of rehabilitation intervention strategies. With the understanding that a child is not merely a miniature adult, and that specific physiologic parameters exist that either complicate or allow unique intervention opportunities, successful aid may be offered. It is only through an understanding of the long-term outcome and consequences of disability in adult life, however, that proper management strategies for the young child may be chosen.

This chapter reviews the scope of disabling disorders that occur in childhood, the specific differences between children and adults that relate to their special needs, and the basic principles of management of disabled children. The specific management of various childhood disorders will be found both within this chapter and within relevant sections of other chapters.

Frequently, a semantic issue comes to the fore in the care of children with physical disabilities: do they require rehabilitation or habilitation? Although it is true that the developing child who has not acquired an ability and then lost it may more accurately be described as needing habilitation, the convention used in this text generalizes all needs, strategies, and services under the term "rehabilitation."

The various disabling disorders that occur in childhood may be characterized according to several parameters of interest, including time of onset and pattern of the natural history of the disease. Disorders that are present from the time of birth are described as congenital if they are not due to known external environmental factors during the birth or postbirth period. Those that occur later are generally considered to be acquired.

Congenital problems may be further specified by cause as either genetic or influenced by some extrinsic factor, even though the effect was expressed in the prenatal period (e.g., fetal alcohol syndrome).

Acquired disabilities usually are the result of trauma (1–3), infection, or other causes. Acquired disorders should not be confused with congenital (i.e., genetic) disorders that are discovered only after birth (e.g., Duchenne muscular dystrophy is usually diagnosed only after 3 years of age but is a genetic disorder detectable at birth).

The temporal pattern of disabling disorders in children may be static, transient, or progressive. The progressive or degenerative disorders of childhood represent a relatively unique class of rehabilitation problems because of the simultaneous occurrence of growth, development, disease progression, and deterioration.

The three most common disabling disorders of childhood seen in a comprehensive rehabilitation setting are cerebral palsy, myelodysplasia, and muscular dystrophy. These and other diseases are categorized by their onset and temporal patterns in Table 37-1. What is known about etiology and epidemiology is shown is Table 37-2. Information about the prevalence of children with disabilities being served by the public school system is shown in Table 37-3. The incidence of most disabling disorders has not changed appreciably in this country in the past 10 years. The exceptions are a known decline in the incidence of children being born with spina bifida--due in part to prenatal detection and therapeutic abortion—and a change in the characteristics, but not numbers, of children developing cerebral palsy. Perinatal brain damage has become more commonly characterized by severe quadriparesis rather than diplegia or total body–involved athetoid patterns (4).

Developmental disabilities in children exert a major impact not only on the child's ability to function in the family and in society, but they also result in 1.5 more doctor visits

R.P. Christopher: Division of Rehabilitation Medicine, University of Tennessee College of Medicine, Memphis, Tennessee 38163.

B.M. Gans: Department of Physical Medicine and Rehabilitation, Wayne State University School of Medicine, Rehabilitation Institute of Michigan, The Detroit Medical Center, Detroit, Michigan 48201-4217.

TABLE 37-1. *Common disabling conditions of childhood: temporal patterns*

Transient	Static	Progressive
Congenital		
Brachial plexus injury	Cerebral palsy	Muscular dystrophy
	Spina bifida	Spinal muscular atrophy
	Retardation	Cystic fibrosis
Acquired		
Guillain-Barré syndrome	Spinal cord injury	Juvenile rheumatoid arthritis
	Traumatic brain injury	Collagen vascular disease
	Traumatic limb amputation	
	Polio	

TABLE 37-2. *Epidemiology of common childhood disabling disorders (per 100,000)*

Diagnosis	Incidence	Prevalence
Cerebral palsy	43	250
Spina bifida	43	40
Muscular dystrophy	1.4	60
Spinal cord injury	5.8	2.7
Traumatic brain injury	600	210
Limb deficiency	38	38
Down syndrome	65	110
Arthritis	220	220

Adapted with permission from Gortmaker SL, Sappenfield W. Chronic childhood disorders: prevalence and impact. *Pediatr Clin North Am* 1984; 31:3–18; Human Services Research Institute. *Summary of data on handicapped children and youth.* Washington, D.C.: US Government Printing Office, 1985; Anderson DW, McLaurin RI. Report on the national head and spinal cord injury survey. *J Neurosurg* 1980; 53(suppl):1–43.

and 3.5 more hospital days per year than for the nondisabled child. In addition, these children typically lose twice the number of school days annually, and there is a 2.5-fold increase in the likelihood of repeating a grade in school when compared with the general population of children. The extent of this impact is much greater in children with multiple disabilities or with either cerebral palsy, seizures, delays in growth and development, or emotional or behavioral problems (5).

THE PEDIATRIC PATIENT: DIFFERENCES TO CONSIDER

Although children may be thought of as small adults, the reality is that adults are merely large children. Maintaining this perspective is perhaps the most fundamental philosophical difference to be emphasized for health professionals who are going to work with disabled children.

Size, Shape, and Weight

The most striking difference between adults and children is size. Knowledge of the patterns of growth and development is key to understanding, anticipating, and managing the difficulties that disabled children experience. In the early years, head circumference, weight, and height are important parameters to monitor. Standard tables of growth and development may be used to record and compare disabled children with the normal population (Tables 37-1 to 37-3).

The pattern of growth shows anticipated bursts and plateaus that are related to gender, age, and even season. Figure

TABLE 37-3. *Number and percentage of students 6–21 years of age served under IDEA Part B and Chapter 1 of ESEA (SOP) by disability: school year 1991–1992*

	IDEA Part B		Chapter 1 (SOP)		Total	
Disability	Number	Percent[a]	Number	Percent[a]	Number	Percent[a]
Specific learning disabilities	2,218,948	98.7	30,047	1.3	2,248,995	100.0
Speech or language impairments	990,016	98.9	10,655	1.1	1,000,671	100.0
Mental retardation	500,986	90.4	53,261	9.6	554,247	100.0
Serious emotional disturbance	363,877	90.8	36,793	9.4	400,670	100.0
Multiple disabilities	80,655	82.0	17,747	18.0	98,402	100.0
Hearing impairments	43,690	71.0	17,073	28.1	60,763	100.0
Orthopedic impairments	46,222	89.4	5,468	10.6	51,690	100.0
Other health impairments	56,401	95.8	2,479	4.2	58,880	100.0
Visual impairments	18,296	75.7	5,873	24.3	24,169	100.0
Deaf-blindness	773	54.3	650	45.1	1,423	100.0
Autism	3,555	68.3	1,653	31.7	5,208	100.0
Traumatic brain injury	285	85.4	45	13.6	330	100.0
All disabilities	4,323,704	96.0	181,744	4.0	4,505,448	100.0

[a] Percentages sum across rows.

Reprinted with permission from Ing CD. *Summary of data on children and youth with disabilities.* Washington, D.C.: US Department of Education, National Institute on Disability and Rehabilitation Research. Office of Special Education Programs, 1993.

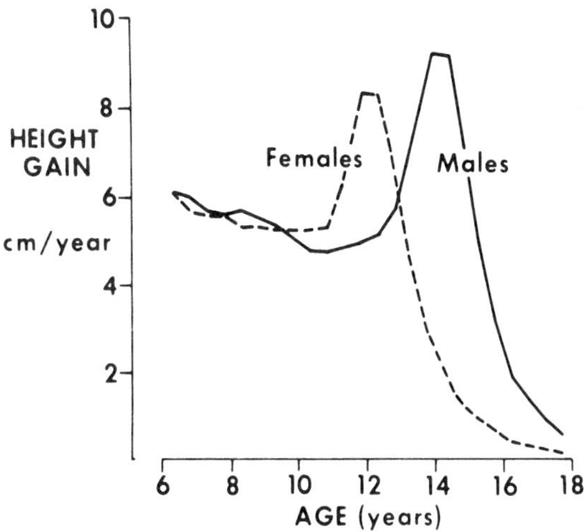

FIG. 37-1. Growth velocity for normal children around the time of puberty. (Reprinted with permission from Tanner JM. *Growth at adolescence.* Oxford, England: Blackwell Scientific, 1962.)

37-1 shows the pattern of height change as a function of age for boys and girls.

The seasonality of growth is shown in Figure 37-2. In summer, growth is faster than in winter, implying that it is wiser to fit new customized orthotic and prosthetic appliances to growing children in the fall, rather than the spring (6).

Patterns of tissue growth vary widely. Knowledge of the growth patterns associated with puberty is important for management and even diagnosis. The specific tissue growth curves shown in Figure 37-3 are useful to remember. This growth may represent a change in contour that, for example, would influence a body jacket design for a pubescent girl.

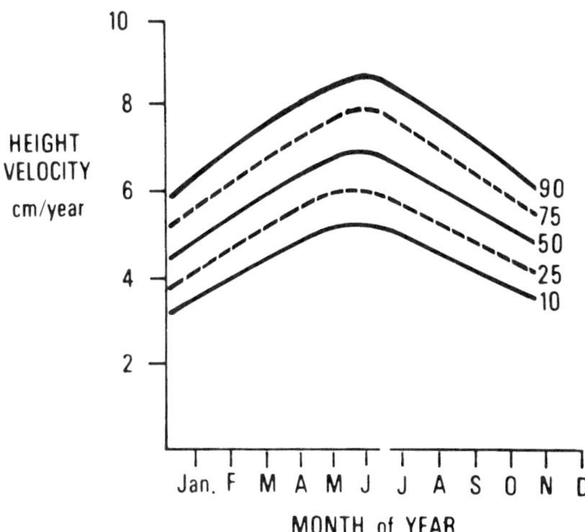

FIG. 37-2. Growth velocity as a function of the time of year in prepubertal boys. (Adapted with permission from Marshall WA. Evaluation of growth rates and height over periods of less than one year. *Arch Dis Child* 1971; 46:414–420.)

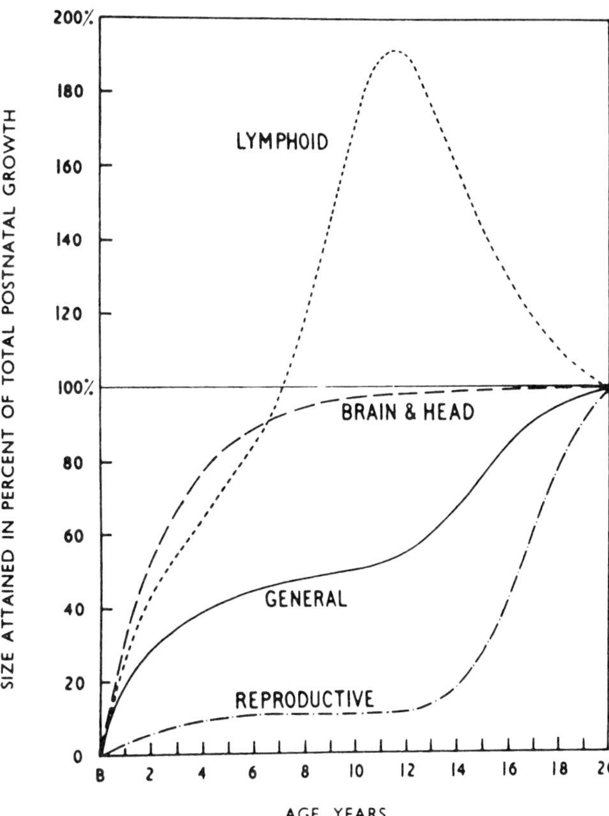

FIG. 37-3. Postnatal growth curves of four major organ systems relative to size attained at 20 years of age. (Reprinted with permission from Tanner JM. *Growth at adolescence.* Oxford, England: Blackwell Scientific, 1962.)

Physiologic Performance

Children vary in accordance with age and size in a number of physiologic parameters. Normal heart rate, respiratory rate, heat transfer behavior, and various chemical assessments all change as a function of age. For example, the serum alkaline phosphatase level may be elevated in an adolescent not because of the presence of an occult heterotopic ossification but rather because of normal bone growth.

The question of enhanced neural plasticity in youth remains open (7,8). Conflicting data appear in the literature to support or reject this concept, but the clinical management implications are generally well accepted: the more treatment that is administered earlier and younger, the better the outcome seems to be.

A number of neurologically mediated reflex behaviors are age and development dependent. For example, the asymmetric tonic neck reflex (ATNR) is a normal behavior when elicited at 2 to 6 months of age, but may be distinctly abnormal when it is persistent and dominant many months later.

Primitive Reflex Patterns

Because they are commonly observed in children with physical disabilities, the major primitive reflex patterns that

TABLE 37-4. *Normal acquisition and regression of primitive reflex behaviors*

Reflex	Age of onset	Age reflex disappears
Moro	Birth	6 months
Palmar grasp	Birth	6 months
Plantar grasp	Birth	9–10 months
Adductor spread of patellar reflex	Birth	7 months
Tonic neck	2 months	5 months
Landau	3 months	24 months
Parachute response	8–9 months	Persists

Reprinted with permission from Swaiman KF, Jacobson RI. Developmental abnormalities of the central nervous system. In: Baker AB, Joynt RJ, eds. *Clinical neurology*. Philadelphia: Harper & Row, 1984.

may either interfere with or facilitate skilled motor actions should be well understood. These motor patterns may be thought of as hard-wired or firm ware in that they represent fundamental, neurally mediated, preferential relationships between body sensors of the internal and external environment and motor patterns. Many of these patterns appear to have offered evolutionary advantages to the organism. Whether this advantage is clear or not, it is sufficient for the treating clinician simply to know of the existence of these patterns.

The primitive reflexes should probably be renamed primitive motor behaviors because they really are stereotypical motor responses and spontaneous patterns of movement. Most of the commonly observed patterns appear to be associated with specific stimuli. The stimuli may be categorized according to proprioceptive, vestibular, or cutaneous senses (9). The times of appearance and disappearance for these reflexes in the developmental sequence are summarized in Table 37-4.

Proprioceptive Patterns

The proprioceptive patterns may depend on trunk, head and neck, and limb positions. The most basic patterns are the flexion and extension synergies of the arms and legs. In the upper extremity, the full flexor pattern shows shoulder adduction, flexion, and internal rotation with elbow flexion, wrist pronation and flexion, and finger and thumb flexion (Fig. 37-4). The thumb is frequently tightly adducted and flexed into the palm. The extensor pattern of the upper extremity shows shoulder extension, relative abduction and external rotation, elbow extension, wrist supination, and finger extension (Fig. 37-5).

Lower extremity patterns are similar. The extension posture of the leg includes hip adduction, extension, and internal rotation, along with knee extension, internal tibial rotation, and equinovarus foot posturing (Fig. 37-6). The flexor pattern consists of hip flexion, abduction and external rotation, knee flexion, external tibial rotation, and calcaneovalgus posturing of the foot (Fig. 37-7).

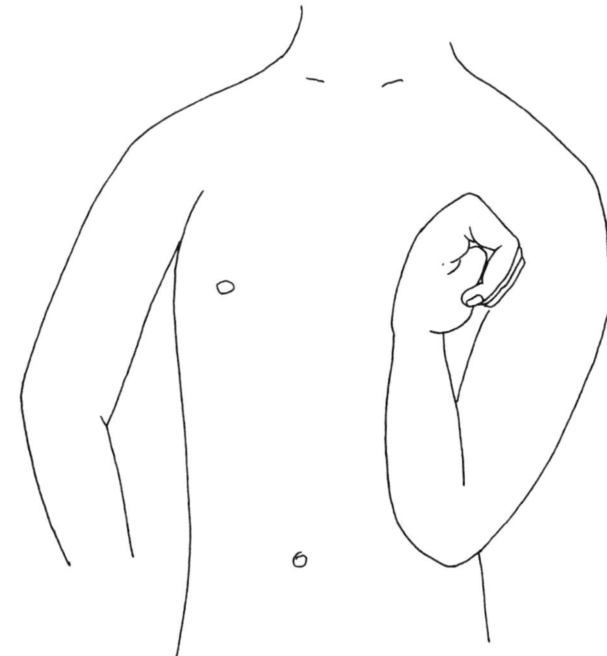

FIG. 37-4. The flexor synergy in the upper extremity.

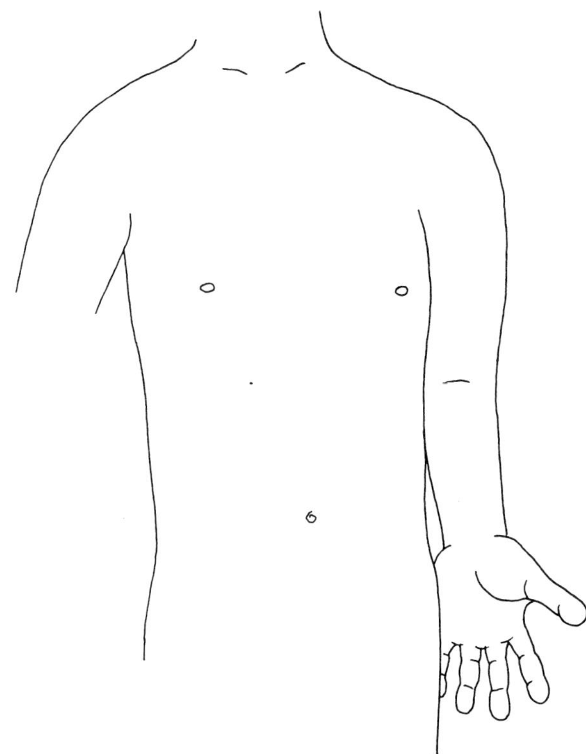

FIG. 37-5. The extensor synergy in the upper extremity.

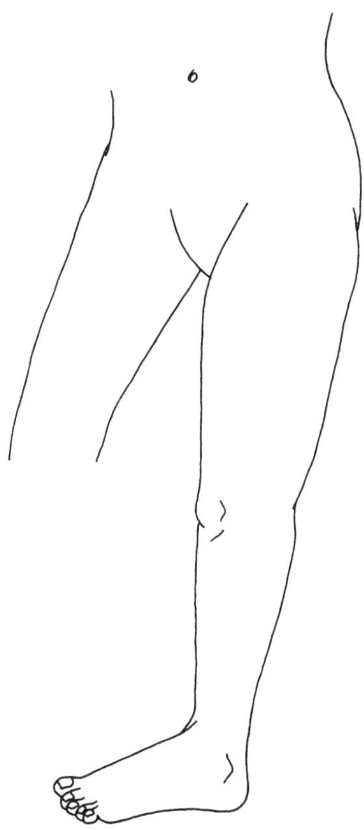

FIG. 37-6. The extensor synergy in the lower extremity.

In both of these postures, the fingers and toes appear to be influential in establishing the dominance of one or the other posture. It is frequently noted that forcing the toes into extension will facilitate a full flexor synergy of the leg. Similarly, placing the flexed thumb in an abducted and extended position will frequently facilitate a full extensor response in the arm.

Lateral rotation of the head on the trunk produces the ATNR (Fig. 37-8). This is the classical fencer's posture of extension in the upper and lower extremities on the nasal side, and flexion of both limbs on the occipital side. The symmetric tonic neck reflex (Fig. 37-9) describes midline effects of flexing and extending the head on the body. Flexion of the head facilitates flexion in the upper extremities and extension of the lower extremities. Extension produces the opposite pattern.

The long spinal reflex posture (Fig. 37-10) relates the reciprocal influence of the upper extremity to the ipsilateral lower extremity. The typical hemiplegic posture of flexion in the arm and extension in the leg is an example of this reflex. On occasion, facilitation of the opposite posture in one limb may be achieved by reversing the pattern in the other limb. For example, a better flexor pattern of the leg during gait may be facilitated in a child by superimposing extension positions of the ipsilateral arm.

The crossed extension reflex describes the influence of the body position across the midline. This pattern promotes symmetry of left and right limbs. Thus, flexion of the left arm will facilitate flexion of the right. One commonly observed result of this reflex is the typical diplegic posture seen in children with cerebral palsy (Fig. 37-11).

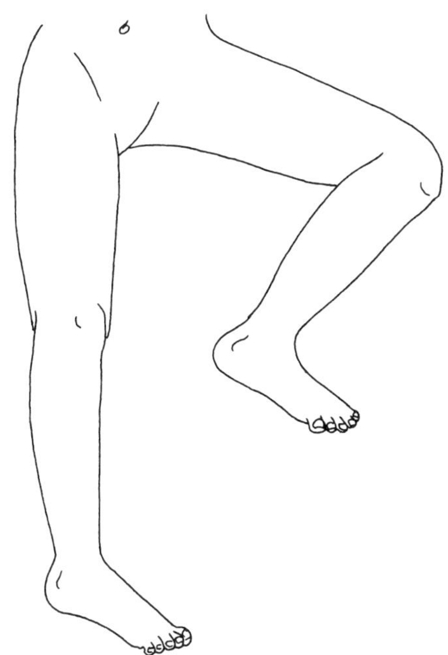

FIG. 37-7. The flexor synergy in the lower extremity.

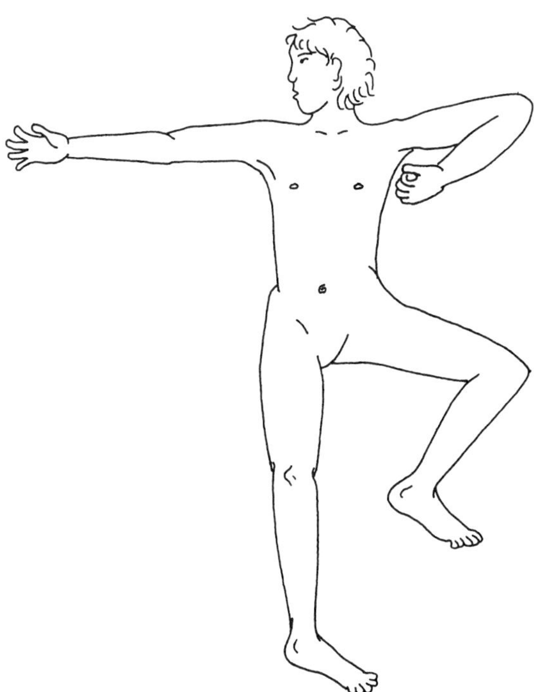

FIG. 37-8. The asymmetric tonic neck reflex.

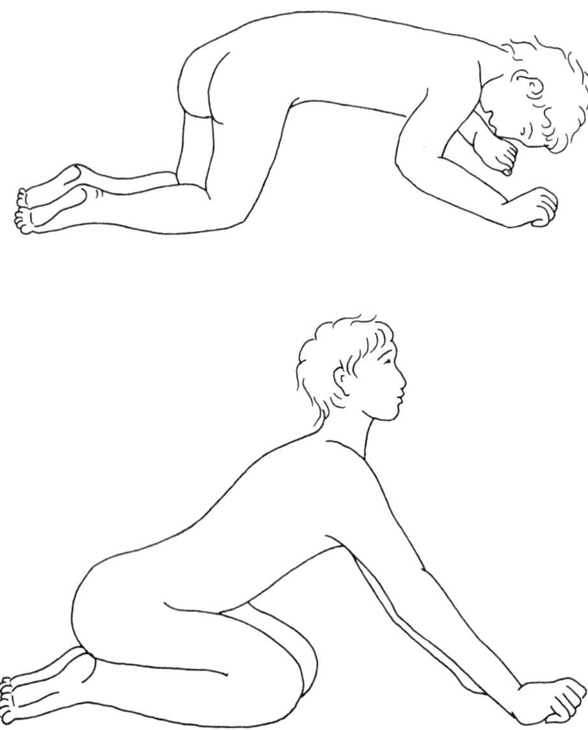

FIG. 37-9. The symmetric tonic neck reflex.

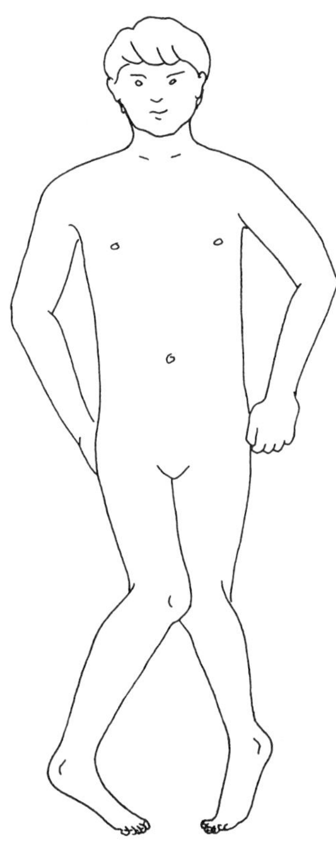

FIG. 37-11. Posture in spastic diplegia due in part to the dominance of the crossed extension reflex.

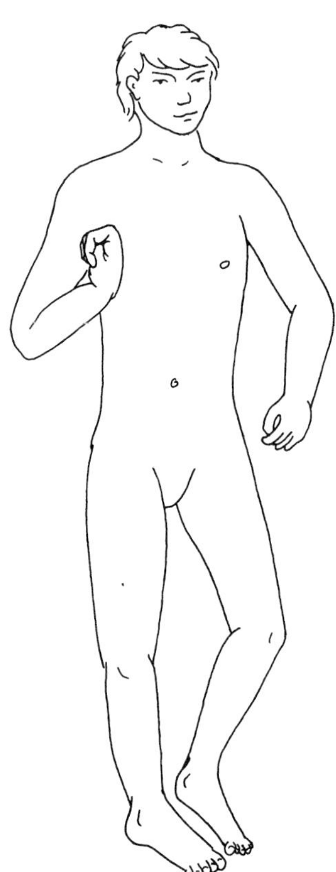

FIG. 37-10. The long spinal reflex posture.

Vestibular Patterns

The vestibular system mediates static postures and dynamic postural reactions. These are important movement patterns that facilitate the development of mobility skills (10).

The most commonly seen static vestibular pattern is the tonic labyrinthine reflex (Fig. 37-12). This pattern, facilitated by the supine position of the head, demonstrates lower extremity symmetrical extension with upper extremity shoulder abduction and external rotation. In the prone posi-

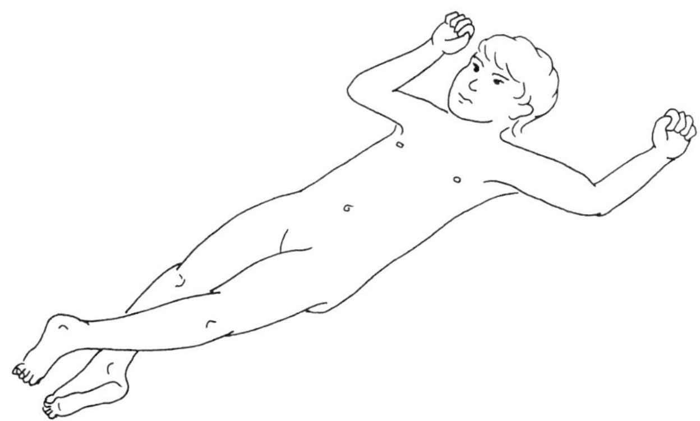

FIG. 37-12. The tonic labyrinthine reflex in the supine position.

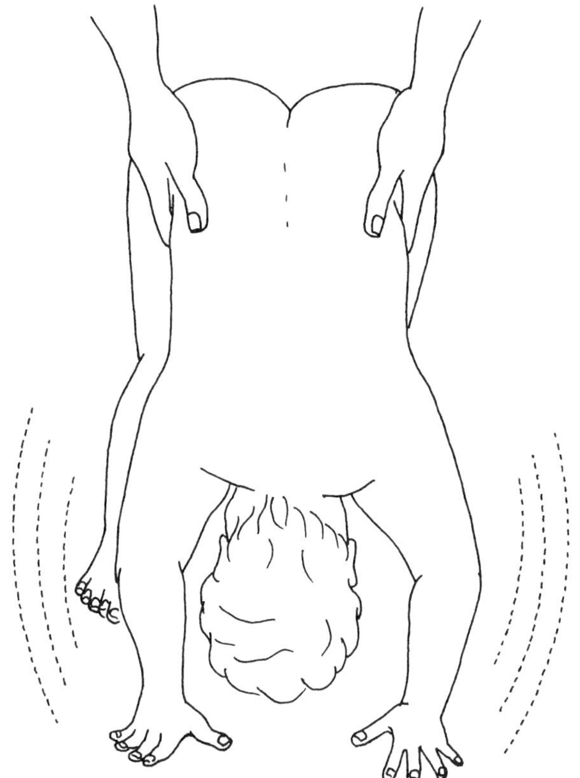

FIG. 37-13. The parachute response is a protective response made to downward motion of the head.

tion, shoulder adduction and internal rotation are accompanied by lower extremity flexor posturing.

The dynamic vestibular reflexes are all variations on the body's tendency to weight-shift to a point of postural stability and to extend the upper limbs to oppose the direction of travel in higher velocity movements or more extreme postural deviations (11). Thus, the protective extension reflexes are seen in all planes. In the inverted position, this postural reaction is called the parachute response (Fig. 37-13) and consists of extension of the upper extremities with downward movement of the head and body.

Cutaneously Mediated Patterns

Cutaneously mediated reflex patterns demonstrate the facilitative relationship between skin tactile receptors and underlying muscle excitation. In general, cutaneous stimulus evokes activation of the muscle groups served by the same sclerotome. In the hand, stroking the palm results in the palmar grasp response. Similarly, in the foot the plantar grasp response occurs with plantar stimulation. Light tactile input to the shin area may evoke a vigorous full flexor response in children with hyperactive cutaneously mediated reflex patterns.

Kinesthetic Patterns

The application of vertical load demand to the legs results in several characteristic primitive reflex postures. In young infants, the stepping response will be seen as a result of both loading one limb (e.g., by vertical suspension) and stimulating the dorsum of the opposite foot, which is presumably a cutaneous influence as well. The positive supporting reaction occurs pathologically in older children when a loading of the suspended child's plantar surface results in a symmetric extension pattern of the lower extremities.

Child Development

Physical growth is accompanied by emotional, functional, cognitive, linguistic, and psychosocial development. Many specific methods of quantifying the state of a child's development have been proposed and are used in various settings (12–19). What is most important is the recognition of the relative separateness of development along a number of dimensions. For example, there may be next to no correlation between motor development and cognitive skill acquisition. Similarly, language and cognitive functions may be largely independent (e.g., the extremely bright but nonspeaking child with athetoid cerebral palsy) (20–22).

Psychosocial Development

Emotional maturation occurs as a function of experience as well as age (23,24). It is quite easy to misinterpret and misjudge the emotional maturity of children with disabilities. Frequently, they may be infantilized by family and caretakers (e.g., a 42-year-old man with severe impairment from cerebral palsy may still be called "Jimmie" instead of "James"). They also may be assumed to be more mature than is really the case, particularly if much of their time has been spent in the company of adults in hospitals and other health-care settings.

Academic achievement must be distinguished from cognitive abilities (25,26). Many children with disabilities experience less than full educational experiences because of a variety of interfering problems, including medical interventions. Formal standardized testing should be used periodically for these children to assess their academic progress.

In many cases, adaptation to a child's disability may really be the parent's adaptation to that disability (27). Children who grow up with a physical limitation usually do not have a sense of loss of ability. It is usually only later, around adolescence, when social sensitivity and maturity cause adaptation problems to surface. In the early years, it is important not to allow an adult's feelings to be projected onto a child. The most effective strategy appears to be to help the child and family identify strengths and abilities the child has, despite the disabilities, to build a sense of confidence and self-worth (28). In many respects, this may be similar to the old adage of encouraging that the glass be seen as half-full rather than half-empty.

Socially, children are substantially different from adults. They commonly have caretakers available (i.e., parents, guardians), and these caretakers are comfortable in that role;

indeed, they have emotionally contracted for it. This is in distinction to the spouse who finds himself or herself responsible for the care of a newly disabled partner. The emotional commitment in this situation is usually an equal, rather than an independent–dependent, relationship. Thus, for more seriously disabled children, returning home is generally feasible because of the availability of loving caretakers (29,30).

COMMON CONCERNS IN TREATING DISABLED CHILDREN

Medical Problems

Although the disabling disorders of childhood are widely varied, they share a number of common issues and potential as well as active problems. This section will review the common problem areas and appropriate management and treatment strategies for them.

Well Child Care

The most important medical perspective is that of well child care, which concerns itself principally with growth, development, nutrition, and prevention of contagious diseases. These areas of concern are translated into traditional pediatric monitoring strategies, including routine periodic assessment of weight, height, head circumference, and certain specific observations. These may include limb length for a child with an amputation; periodic assessment of developmental status, using either a routine screening instrument such as the Denver Development Screening Test or other more sophisticated instruments, depending on the child's specific problems and developmental level; review of food and liquid intake patterns, bowel and bladder function, and nutritional status as determined by growth and chemical evaluations; and review and maintenance of preventive immunization programs.

Immunization deserves special attention in the child with a disability. Surprisingly, the more seriously ill child may slip through the cracks of the well child system and be found to be behind in immunizations. The obvious solution is to ensure by routine practice that immunization histories are reviewed regularly. Many children with serious disabilities are at risk for pulmonary infections. Some of these children should also be offered immunization against pneumococcal infections.

Incontinence

The child with a disability frequently may be observed to be wearing diapers long after it is appropriate from a social development perspective. Many times these children may become continent with the use of classical bowel programs and alternative bladder management strategies. The child should be periodically assessed to be certain that appropriate medical interventions have been offered for both of these functions. Investment in these objectives by the parents and consistency of program implementation between home and school personnel are essential for successful control of incontinence.

Gastroesophageal Reflux

One of the most common intestinal problems encountered in children with neuromuscular impairment is gastroesophageal (GE) reflux (31–35). This may lead to a variety of subtle or dramatic, and occasionally life-threatening, symptoms. In the extreme case, it leads to recurrent aspiration pneumonia, chronic pulmonary disease, and even sudden death. In less severe situations, failure to thrive, difficulty with sleep patterns, and epigastric distress are common. A high index of suspicion should be maintained as to the risk of GE reflux being present, and diagnosis and medical or surgical management should be pursued when appropriate.

Skin Protection

Small children rarely develop decubitus ulcers. This should not be surprising when one remembers that the principal cause of these lesions is excessive external force loads that exceed internal tissue capillary filling pressure. Because children are smaller and lighter, they rarely experience excessive pressure levels for prolonged periods of time. The distribution of subcutaneous fat in children may be a further protective factor in that it more evenly distributes forces in a more tolerable manner. A third factor that may contribute is the general activeness of children as a normal aspect of their play and school behaviors.

There are several specific kinds of skin difficulties. The first is pressure irritation from orthoses, splints, and casts. Children often do not spontaneously report pain from these appliances, even if they are sensate in the area. Careful inspection and diligence on the part of the parents are essential for the prevention of these problems.

One common site of pressure damage in children is the occipital protuberance, from the relatively large mass of the head concentrating pressure over a small bony prominence when the infant or child is supine. Many nondisabled infants may show a loss of hair over the occipital protuberance from prolonged supine lying and side to side movements of their heads. If this is seen in a child with delayed development of head control, the area should be watched closely to prevent skin breakdown.

Skin lesions from a variety of other problems that are not specifically related to the disabling disorder also routinely occur in children. Care should be taken to distinguish between skin lesions that are associated with infectious disease, allergy, and other specific diseases (e.g., dermatomyositis) and those problems relating to urine contamination, pressure, drooling, and shear forces.

Spasticity

Several specific issues regarding spasticity in children deserve mention (see Chapter 40) (36). The drugs used for spasticity management in adults may be used with children, but greater vigilance and monitoring must be maintained by the physician. All of these drugs show more prominent central nervous system (CNS) side effects in children, particularly somnolence. In addition, consistent compliance by children and the parents may be difficult to achieve. Although this may not generally be a problem, it can be problematic in several circumstances.

The child with a seizure disorder may be adversely affected by the sudden withdrawal of diazepam, which was being used for spasticity management and was not recognized for its contribution to epilepsy control. In addition, because children may become physiologically addicted to diazepam, slow withdrawal may be necessary.

Baclofen is also a useful drug in certain situations. However, we have observed several incidences of hallucinations in children both on therapeutic levels and with sudden withdrawal. For these reasons, careful consideration should be made of the ultimate wisdom of drug management for these problems. Continuous intrathecal baclofen provided by an implanted pump has been used for a number of years to control spasticity in adults with spinal cord disorders. Recently, a smaller pump suitable for use in children has become available and is being used with some success in several centers in the United States and Canada (37).

Children tend to be responsive to physical modalities for spasticity management. The use of positioning, exercise, casting and bracing, and a variety of other modalities has been encouraged. However, care should be taken to integrate these management strategies into a child's total daily routine so that normal family, play, and educational experiences continue. There has been a resurgence of interest in the use of therapeutic electrical stimulation in children with spastic hemiplegia. This modality may produce a significant increase in passive ranges of movement with concomitant improvement in upper and lower extremity function when combined with a neurodevelopmental therapeutic exercise program (38).

Surgical intervention for spasticity management has been periodically tried. One approach showing promise is the selective dorsal rhizotomy (see Chapter 40).

Botulinium toxin in very small doses has been injected subcutaneously for treatment of blepharospasm and other types of facial muscle spasm and fasiculations. This drug also has been found to be useful in providing temporary amelioration of spasticity when injected directly into muscle. Much of the initial work was performed in adults, but the results of several recent studies in children with cerebral palsy look very promising (see Chapter 40) (39).

Contractures

Children will develop soft-tissue and joint contractures from immobility, inadequate stretching, constant muscular contractions, and inflammatory disorders of the joints, soft tissue, or skin. Prevention is the best strategy for management. Whenever possible, protective actions such as tone control, spasticity management, proper positioning, appropriate exercise programs, proper handling techniques, and control of the inflammatory disease should be undertaken.

Treatment will depend on the cause of the contracture. For contractures associated with tonic muscular contraction, serial or inhibitive casting is frequently effective (e.g., in the head-injured child). Surgical intervention may be helpful but must be carefully considered in terms of the specific indications for the procedure as well as the potential deleterious effects. Several examples will illustrate this point. The child with athetoid cerebral palsy may present with a dominant extensor synergy of the lower extremities with concomitant hip adduction posturing. In many cases, if the adductors are surgically released, overwhelmingly dominant flexor tone may result, leading to the rapid development of abduction contractures that may be more disabling than the original adduction posturing.

Children with muscular dystrophy frequently show the early development of contractures of the heel cords and an associated toe-toe gait. The unknowing surgeon who releases these contractures will likely eliminate the child's ability to walk. The pathokinesiology of this particular problem shows that the toe gait and equinus posture are necessary to maintain knee extension stability. After this type of surgery, bracing with at least an ankle-foot orthosis is mandatory to re-establish a less functional gait (40).

Scoliosis

The child with a physical disability is at significant risk for the development of a paralytic scoliosis, due to either weakness or trunk tone asymmetry. In either case, preventive maintenance and routine monitoring are the management strategies of choice. The child with a congenital spinal defect or deformity (e.g., spina bifida, congenital hemivertebrae) represents a special case for which aggressive treatment with orthotics and surgery must be considered first.

Physical examination of the back for resting posture, dynamic posture, and flexibility should be performed routinely. For children at particularly high risk, routine x-ray evaluation of the spine is appropriate. The ideal x-ray protocol to detect subtle evidence of spinal inflexibility and early curve includes multiple views. In the supine position, anteroposterior (AP), neutral, and maximal left and right bending views are extremely helpful. Sitting AP and lateral views and, if possible, standing AP films will demonstrate the effects of gravity or tight musculature. Views in and out of spinal orthotics are helpful to determine their efficacy. Occasionally it is useful to take AP sitting views of the patient in a seating device or wheelchair. Assessments made at intervals of 1 to 1.5 years during slow growth periods are sufficient. During rapid growth, closer assessment is required.

Management of a spinal curve depends on the etiologic

factors. For flaccid curves, proper positioning and seating, flexibility exercises, and aggressive orthotic management are appropriate. Curves secondary to asymmetric tone and spasticity are dealt with similarly, although tolerance to each of these may be more limited, making tone control more essential. Early surgical management of spinal curvatures is becoming increasingly more common (41), for example, the boy with muscular dystrophy who can be treated by spinal fusion with intersegmental instrumentation early in the course of the disease, while he is in good condition from a pulmonary perspective, so that he can tolerate the surgery well and return to active functioning in a short period of time.

In any case, care should be taken so that management of the scoliosis does not interfere greatly with the child's capacity to function. The muscular dystrophy patient is a specific example. It has been commonly observed that the optimal management of a spinal deformity may place the child at a mechanical disadvantage to use his weakened upper extremities. In the extreme, the child may have a straight back at the price of useless upper extremities, a questionable trade-off at best.

Hip Development

The hips and pelvis are a common area for musculoskeletal problems. Children are normally born with a degree of hip flexion, anteversion, and coxa valga (42). With normal growth and development, these postures revert to adult norms. Children with any gross motor disorder may show abnormal development in these areas, with either retention or exaggeration of the postures. These may lead to soft-tissue and bony deformities that ultimately will require surgical intervention. Normal developmental aspects of the hip joint range of motion are shown in Figure 37-14 and Table 37-5.

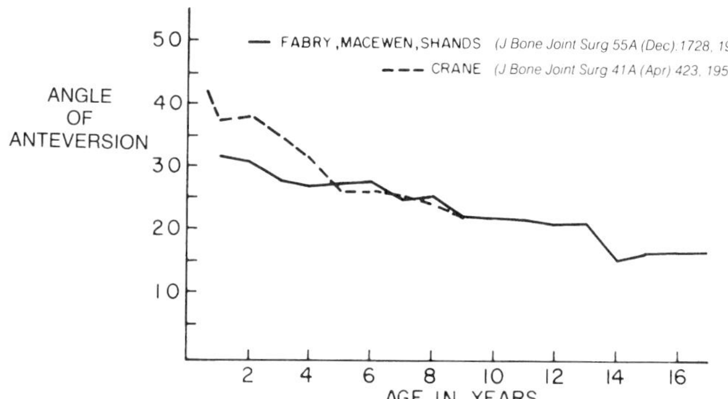

FIG. 37-14. Normal femoral anteversion as a function of age. (Reprinted with permission from Chung SMK. *Hip disorders in infants and children.* Philadelphia: Lea & Febiger, 1981.)

Conservative management of these problems includes facilitation of normal positioning, weight-bearing experience, and range of motion experiences. Many children's centers have found prone and/or supine standers to be helpful in providing the weight bearing necessary for hip joint development, especially in children with poor or absent trunk control. The role of hip orthotics is variable, depending on the specific clinical situation. Objective data confirming or rejecting the benefits of night casts and orthoses of a variety of configurations are limited in the population of children with serious disabilities. Treatment regimens tend to vary more with the regional philosophy than by analysis of objective data.

Asymmetries and obliquities of the pelvis may present profound challenges to the child and caregivers for positioning, seating, and ambulation. Fixed contractures and limitations of pelvic and lower spinal flexibility result in an uneven

TABLE 37-5. *Normal passive range of hip motion in children and adults*

Age	Flexion	Flexion contracture	Abduction in extension	Frog-leg abduction	Internal rotation	External rotation
Newborn	120°–140°	10°–75°, mean 28°		50°–90°, mean 76°	35°–100°[a], mean 62°	45°–110°, mean 89°
6 weeks	120°–140°	6°–32°, mean 19°			16°–36°[b], mean 24°	26°–73°, mean 48°
3 months	120°–140°	1°–18°, mean 7°			15°–35°[b], mean 26°	37°–60°, mean 45°
6 months	120°–140°	−1° to +16°, mean 7°			15°–42°[b], mean 21°	34°–61°, mean 46°
3 years	120°–140°	~ 0°	80°		~ 30°–45°	~ 35°–45°
4 to 10 years	120°–140°	~ 0°	60°–70°		~ 30°–45°[a]	~ 35°–45°
Adults	135°	0°	45°	65°	45°[a] 35°[b]	45° 45°

[a] Measured with hips and knees flexed to 90°
[b] Measured with hips extended and knees flexed to 90°

Reprinted with permission from Chung SMK. *Hip disorders in infants and children.* Philadelphia: Lea & Febinger, 1981; 67.

base for seating and standing. Management is oriented toward identifying the problem, and therapy is aimed at achieving flexibility and accommodating positioning and seating systems to the deformity.

Lower Extremity Development

Major problems seen in the lower extremities are unequal leg length and rotational deformities, such as internal tibial torsion. A variety of factors may lead to these deformities. These problems must first be recognized; then they can be treated by adapting shoes, orthotics, prosthetics, or seating systems as appropriate. Therefore, the routine examination of any child with a physical disability for these alignment and structural conditions is necessary (43).

Common Rehabilitation Problems

Just as there are generic medical problems common to many different diagnoses, so too are there common functional issues. Specific management strategies vary with the particular disease, but the determination of goals and objectives is largely independent of the specific disease.

Communication

The desire and ability to communicate is the highest priority in managing a child with a disability. Although it is not the first developmental milestone achieved by an infant (at least, not as perceived by the parents), communication is essential as a window to the mind. Frequently, the child with serious physical disability is dependent not so much on his or her abilities to physically manipulate the environment as on the ability to control it through communication.

Early on, it is important to keep in mind the fact that language development does not need to follow motor development. Simply put, a child's inability to move well independently does not preclude an ability to think and to communicate. In fact, in some extremes, there may be a complete disparity between motor and communicative development. For example, in severe athetoid cerebral palsy, the child may be totally unintelligible because of the motor deficit, yet if careful testing and assessment through nonvocal communication techniques are performed, normal to superior receptive language and cognitive function are frequently demonstrated.

For children with physical limitations, the use of an augmentative or alternative system or device for communication enhancement may be necessary. These strategies basically convert the available reliable motor abilities of the child into message-sending actions that are understandable by the listener. Specifically, this may mean something as sophisticated as a device that responds to eye position by generating computer-synthesized speech. What is important is not the technology but the identification of the potential for communication and the development of a system that allows a child to live up to his or her communicative potential.

Mobility

Second to communication in priority is the child's ability to control his or her motion in three-dimensional space. Frequently, children are provided with passive transportation instead of the technical ability to achieve independent mobility. From a developmental perspective, newborns start experiencing self-directed movement in space in their cribs, and a child who is crawling and creeping is acquiring substantial knowledge about the world by navigating within it. It is important not only to provide convenient transportation for parents but also to give the child control over his or her own mobility.

A variety of methods provide mobility control. For the child with ambulation potential, various adaptive orthoses and upper extremity aids may be needed. Care should be taken, however, to be critical in assessing both the short-term energy expense of ambulation and also the safety and convenience of this form of mobility. In many cases, although movement of arms and legs may be achieved, it may not be a reasonable or practical means of transportation. Furthermore, many children will literally outgrow their ability to ambulate. Spastic diplegic children frequently lose mechanical advantage and coordination with growth, so that marginal childhood ambulation becomes impractical as the child reaches adolescence or adulthood. Similarly, many children with high lumbar or thoracic paraplegia, as in spina bifida, will lose their ability to ambulate after growth to full adult stature.

Wheeled mobility is possible through the use of many devices. Floor-level devices include the crawling mobile board and caster carts, which provide seated, floor level mobility with large drive wheels. Wheelchairs that are appropriately sized for children are widely available. Some have frames that accommodate growth. The ultralight designs offer mechanical advantages for weaker children who may not be able to propel a regular chair on their own (44).

For the child who is unable to propel a manual wheelchair, there are powered vehicles. Some commercially available battery-powered toy motorcycles and cars may offer socially acceptable and inexpensive options for the occasional user. For primary mobility means, however, true pediatric, powered wheelchairs should be considered (45).

Limited research has been performed that agrees with clinical observations about the age at which a child can control the powered wheelchair (46,47). By 18 months, the child may be able to acquire the eye–hand coordination necessary to control a wheelchair with a joystick. The environment for a young child's driving needs, of course, must be carefully controlled to maintain safety. Furthermore, the chair itself may need to be modified so that excessive velocities cannot be achieved.

Seating and Positioning

Positioning and seating a child with a physical disability are early essential issues that need to be addressed. Although passive seating is the normal first step for infants, as well as for children with tone problems, deformities, or other structural difficulties, these children frequently need adapted seating and positioning systems to allow them to achieve a number of developmental goals (48).

General goals for these devices include the achievement of normalization of tone, symmetric posturing, and proper trunk alignment facilitation. Positioning and seating are often offered as a means to other ends, such as the use of the head or upper extremities for communication, self-care and educational activities, as well as to allow mobility and preservation of good joint alignment (49).

Side-lying devices may facilitate function and maintain trunk flexibility for floor and bed-level activities. Adapted seats are useful for spasticity management and the facilitation of upright activities. Standing devices allow vertical alignment, weight bearing, and experiences in the upright posture. Car seating that is safe from both a postural and a crash safety perspective gives secure travel capacity to the child and family.

The particular positioning or seating device chosen will depend on features, cost, and market availability. For individuals actively involved in the care of children with disabilities, the best arrangement is to have a close working relationship with a dealer in durable medical equipment so that tryouts and assessments of new products are possible.

Self-Care Activities

The acquisition of independent self-care skills is a major component of normal development. Frequently, these skills are delayed in the child with a physical disability. Although physical limitations are often the primary cause, secondary reasons are also common. They include a lack of encouragement from the family to achieve independence and unawareness of the potential for independence through the use of alternative techniques and adaptive aids and devices.

On occasion, expectations for independence may be too demanding. Specifically, the child with an upper extremity deficiency who uses a prosthesis may have unrealistic expectations of function. In many amputee clinics, counseling is necessary to prevent the parents of 3-year-olds from concluding that an upper extremity prosthetic deficiency must exist because their child cannot tie shoelaces yet. Reminding families of appropriate age-related developmental milestones is frequently necessary.

Seriously delayed acquisition of independence may be seen in the myelodysplasia population (50). Studies of this group provide a useful perspective for the analysis of function in children with disabilities. Few methods for the quantified assessment of functional abilities in children exist (51,52).

Education

Whereas vocational rehabilitation is an important consideration for the adult with a disability, special education is important to the child with a disability. The laws and services for children with disabilities vary with state and local school systems, but some common features are present. According to federal law (PL94-142 and PL99-457), the goals of special education are to provide "free and appropriate public education" in the "least restrictive environment" for a child. Part H of PL 99-457 mandates that participating states also provide early intervention services for children with developmental disabilities from birth to 2 years of age. Services that may variably be included in this type of educational program include special education, physical therapy, occupational therapy, speech and language therapy, adaptive physical education, psychological and social work services, and nursing services. In each case, these services become school system responsibilities in that they are necessary for the child to participate in an individualized education program, a specific educational plan with goals, objectives, definition of services, and time frames.

The role of health professionals in the special education system is an advisory and participatory one. Programs developed within a school setting should be consistent with those established out of school, in both the home and other therapy settings. School programs should not let therapeutic goals obscure their educational objectives. Programs that effectively integrate medical rehabilitation needs with those of education are the most effective (53).

Play

Children with disabilities frequently need special assistance in achieving the ability to play successfully. Recreational therapy, music therapy, art therapy, play therapy, and other interventions may be helpful in allowing a child to find mechanisms to express himself or herself and to experiment with future skills and roles (54).

Adapted toys and games are useful. Battery adapters that allow external switch control of any electric or electronic device may give the child with a severe disability the option to play with age-appropriate toys while possessing only limited physical skill.

Children also may need special assistance in experiencing group play. Participation in nursery school programs, play groups, and other endeavors will allow the child to experience play with other children with and without disabilities. Parental counseling and resource identification may be necessary to facilitate these activities.

Social Skills

Children with disabilities are often found to be deficient in adaptive social skills because of a variety of factors, including limited normal childhood experiences and intensive involvement with the health-care community. Efforts may need to be taken to assist a child and family to identify specific behavioral issues and find methods to overcome them. The concept of a child having acquired learned helplessness is useful as a perspective in dealing with these issues.

As these children reach adulthood, they frequently remain in the home setting with their parents long after most young adults have elected to live independently. They also demonstrate a much higher rate of unemployment than their nondisabled counterparts (55).

Parenting Skills

Just as normal child parenting is a challenging experience, so too is parenting a child with a disability. It is further complicated by the challenges of health and social functions experienced by the child and family. Many parents need assistance and guidance in coping with what are really normal parenting issues in their care for the child with a disability.

Common problems include discipline maintenance and difficulty in setting appropriate levels of expectation of responsible behavior. Counseling for the parents on how to distinguish the special limits and expectations that are appropriate for the disability from normal parenting issues, such as control and authority challenging, may be very helpful. Introducing families to parents of other children with disabilities is also a very positive strategy.

Sexuality

Managing the emerging sexuality of a child with a disability requires knowledge, an openness and willingness to discuss, and anticipatory strategies. Many of the early needs of these children are simply for accurate and age-appropriate information about sex and reproduction in general, as well as the child's specific abilities or limitations based on the disability. Frequently, knowledge about the child's sexual and reproductive potential is also needed by the parents.

Education and counseling for the adolescent child are often necessary. Children may express their underlying sexual concerns through other behaviors, including social withdrawal and depression. A high index of suspicion of the need for sexual education and counseling should be maintained by the involved health professional.

Independent Living

A long-term perspective on the child's potential to live independently should be adopted from an early age. Realistic goal setting is the essential first step for any long-term rehabilitation program and for attaining independence. It is frequently possible to distinguish at an early age the child who will need some type of supported living situation in the long term. Helping the family and school system to identify these expectations early on will facilitate appropriate school programming and long-term planning.

It is unfortunately all too frequent that we encounter a seriously developmentally disabled adult 30 to 40 years of age who lives with his or her parents until the parents become infirm or die. Many times there has been inadequate planning for legal, estate, and practical matters that suddenly become crises. The solution to these types of problems is prevention by ensuring that they are anticipated long before they become a reality.

EVALUATION OF THE CHILD WITH A DISABILITY

There are several objectives to be achieved in the evaluation of a child with a disability. Assembling a data base in each of these areas is essential in the development and conduct of a comprehensive habilitation/rehabilitation plan for the child.

1. Determine the type and etiology of the disability.
2. Determine the child's potential to benefit from habilitation/ rehabilitation services.
3. Assess development from birth to the present.
   A. Gross motor
   B. Fine motor
   C. Cognitive
   D. Personal/social
   E. Language
4. Assess the family in terms of their adjustment to the child's disability and their ability to support the habilitation/rehabilitation program.

The first two objectives can be met by means of a careful evaluation by the pediatric rehabilitation physician, including a review of previous medical records and evaluation by other members of the habilitation/rehabilitation team. The data that are developed should be correlated at the team staffing conference chaired by the physician.

The third objective can be achieved by using one or more of a number of development assessment tests to be described in the sections following this discussion. The final objective can be accomplished with an assessment of the family by the team social worker and psychologist along with input from other team members and the physician.

Initial rehabilitation goals and a comprehensive management program to achieve the goals can be developed at the team staffing conference using the assembled data. Involvement of the family is essential in this process. This may be accomplished either by their attendance and participation in staffing conferences or by conducting informing sessions after the conferences. In either case, concurrence of the family with the rehabilitation plan should be obtained and they should be allowed to make suggestions for modifications to the plan based on their personal goals for the child. Preferably, their concurrence should be obtained in writing.

INITIAL EVALUATION BY THE PHYSICIAN

It is essential that the physician establish rapport with the child and family members present. Children are, of course, typically frightened by any encounter with health-care personnel. The environment in which the examination is conducted must be as nonthreatening as the demeanor of the physician. Toys and children's art work are useful tools in creating such an atmosphere. The physician should present as much of a friendly image to the child as possible. Attention to seemingly unimportant factors such as not wearing a white coat in the child's presence and sitting while examining or interviewing the child can have a major impact on the development of a cordial relationship. Other helpful measures include smiling frequently and assuring the child that he or she is not in your office to receive any shots from you. Except in the case of older children, the medical history will be obtained from one or more of the family members. In cases of children with suspected developmental disabilities, a careful review of the pregnancy and birth history as well as the family history is essential. In children with acquired disabilities, detailed information about the illness or injury that produced the disability should be obtained.

Regardless of the cause of the disability, a detailed developmental history should be elicited. This should include not only the ages at which developmental milestones were achieved but also a description, in the family member's own words, as to the effects of developmental deficiencies on the attainment of functional independence skills. Comparing the development of the child with a disability to other children in the family who have shown a normal pattern of development will often facilitate this process. The administration of standard developmental assessment tests will add valuable information in identifying the specific areas of developmental delay in all functional areas.

The initial physical examination by the physician should be as brief as possible. Children are normally rather distractible and have short attention spans. They will usually only be able to cooperate with the examiner for short periods; therefore, it may be necessary to interrupt the examination for short play periods. As much of the examination as possible should be conducted by observation of the child, with actual physical contact between physician and subject kept to a minimum. Much of this can be accomplished while taking the history. Considerable data regarding basic motor skills such as head and trunk control, reciprocal creeping, standing balance, and gait patterns can be obtained in this manner. Play periods are especially useful in collecting this information.

The examining physician must be familiar with techniques of eliciting developmental reflexes and whether they can be considered normal or abnormal at a given age. As brain development continues during the first year of life, these reflexes disappear (Table 37-4). Persistence of them in children provides evidence of abnormal or delayed neurologic development. It is also important for the physician to have an understanding of those developmental reflexes that are normally not present at birth but must develop for the child to attain normal motor function. Protective extension is an example of such a reflex.

Manual muscle testing in a young child is usually not possible. Children less than 5 years of age seldom will consistently cooperate on such testing. Observation of the child during play activities will provide the examiner with information regarding muscle strength. In infants, assessment of muscle function can be obtained by placing the child alternately in positions where the child's extremities can move through range of motion against gravity and with gravity eliminated while encouraging the child to reach for toys placed in their field of vision. Toys that jingle or make other kinds of noise are most useful for this purpose. In the lower extremities, the use of devices that may produce a withdrawal response such as a pin or vibrator can provide data regarding muscle function.

Muscle tone should be assessed not only for the degree of tone (i.e., low, normal or high), but also for the pattern of tone and what activities may trigger abnormal tone. Significant fluctuations in muscle tone should be noted along with a description of factors that seem to cause the fluctuation. For example, in children with spasticity, a marked increase in tone of a given muscle may be produced by a sudden stretch of that muscle or its tendon. In children with athetoid cerebral palsy, tone fluctuations may be produced by startling the child with an unexpected touch or loud noise.

Deviations from normal range of motion in any of the body parts should be recorded. In cases where limitation of range of motion exists, the family should be questioned regarding their observations as to whether such tightness is static or progressive and approximately how long it has been present.

In children of school age and above, the sensory examination including vision and hearing can usually be completed successfully. In younger children and particularly in infants, the sensory examination will primarily consist of the child's response to noxious stimuli such as a pinprick. The response is usually crying and/or withdrawal.

Sensorineural testing in children under 4 years of age will usually be limited to simple screening examinations due to the inability of the child to provide consistent responses to testing. The child's ability to follow objects with his or her eyes combined with observation of spontaneous eye movements or their absence will assist the physician in determining whether more definitive testing is needed. The child's ability to respond or localize sounds will help to make similar determinations with regard to hearing. Vision and hearing testing in infants and younger children suspected of abnormality in these functions will require the use of sophisticated measurement devices by physicians specializing in those areas. Auditory and visual brain stem response testing has proven to be very useful in assessing these functions in children too young to respond to standard screening tests. Older children can be screened for visual and auditory function using the same testing techniques used for adults.

Instruments used in the neurologic examination such as reflex hammers and tuning forks should be shown to the child before they are used. It is often helpful to allow the child to play with them before the testing.

The most critical factor in obtaining useful data from the initial history and physical examination of a child is the development of a cordial relationship with the child and family as early and rapidly as possible during the interview process.

MANAGEMENT OF CHILDHOOD DISABILITY

The strategies of management of the child with a disability are derived from two fundamental knowledge bases. First is the nature of the child's specific physical and functional impairment. Second is a knowledge of normal development and a belief that appropriate management of children with disabilities is to facilitate his or her passage throughout the stages of normal development as much as possible.

Assessment

Development is studied in a number of specific manners, but a simple overview will be sufficient for the purposes of the following discussion. The most powerful concept is that different skill categories may be identified and assessed on a relatively autonomous basis. The major categories of development commonly considered include the following:

- Gross motor
- Fine motor
- Cognitive
- Personal/social
- Language

Each of these aspects of development may be measured according to a number of formal tests and evaluation tools. Four different types of developmental assessment tools exist:

1. Chronologically normalized attainment scales
2. Criterion referenced descriptive tests
3. Physical performance assessments with quantitative assessments of performance levels
4. Functional assessment instruments to describe performance of activities (56)

Developmental Attainment Scales

The most commonly used screening test for developmental attainment assessment is the Denver Developmental Screening Test. This is a survey test instrument that is easy to learn and use and that allows a quick screening for deviations from normal development. It is intended for analysis of normal and near-normal children and is insensitive to increments of developmental progress that may occur in children with severe disabilities.

A second commonly used test is the Bayley Scales of Infant Development, designed for children from birth to 30 months. This tool is also relatively insensitive to increments of change in children with severe disabilities.

Descriptive Tests

Examples of descriptive tests include the Koontz Child Development Program and the Brigance assessments. These tests were developed in response to the need for a tool that would define individual components of an individualized education program.

Performance Analysis

Quantitative analysis of motor performance of children is accomplished by several strategies (57). First is the measurement of physical parameters, such as range of motion and strength, and physiologic parameters, such as heart rate and respiratory rate.

Timed trials of specific activities, such as the Jebson Taylor Hand Function test (58,59), may be useful as norm-referenced comparisons or sequential performance reassessments.

Functional Assessment

Quantitative descriptions of the functional activities of children with disabilities are essential for monitoring and planning rehabilitation programs (60). The Barthel Index (61) has been supplanted by the Functional Independence Measure (FIM) (62) as an example of an adult-oriented instrument. The few pediatric tools currently available include the WeeFIM (63) and the Pediatric Evaluation of Disability Inventory (64). Two notable exceptions are the analytic tool for children with spina bifida described by Sousa and colleagues (50) and the generally useful Tufts Assessment of Motor Performance (TAMP) (65,66). The TAMP provides a method for structured quantitative description of developmentally oriented activities that are commonly performed by children with serious disabilities. This and other similar tools should be routinely incorporated into the diagnostic and analytic reviews of the rehabilitation progress of a child with a disability.

Impact on Growth and Development

Serious disabling impairments will affect a child's growth and development. Only by knowing the likely impact will the health professional be able to anticipate problems and optimize the child's health and function. Upper motor neuron lesions, especially those of the parietal cortex occurring before 4 years of age will result in mild diminishment of corresponding contralateral body growth. The child with hemiplegic cerebral palsy, for example, will show signs of hemihypotrophy of the involved body side. This may include limb, trunk, and even facial asymmetries. Growth is usually not seriously disturbed, but the asymmetry may be notice-

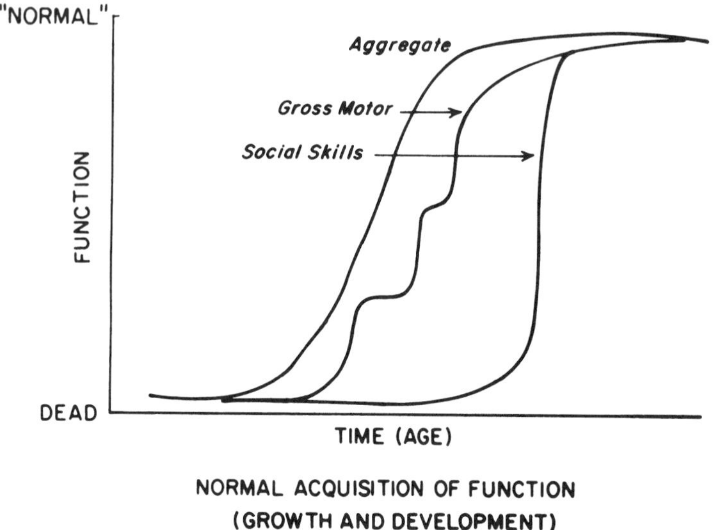

FIG. 37-15. Functional development in normal children as a function of age. In the aggregate, development is thought of as a continuous process, but specific individual skills are acquired in a stepwise fashion.

able. Trunk asymmetries may be mistaken for scoliosis and need careful assessment.

Monitoring of height (67), weight, and head circumference is an important routine management strategy. Use of the normative charts for comparison purposes is appropriate. Significant deviations in the pattern of growth should be noted and explained. Difficulties in growth may be the result of chronic illness, nutritional deficiency, or chronic GE reflux, along with a host of other specific problems.

The presence of a disabling disorder has an obvious impact on the developmental process. In general, the patterns of development may be thought of as mimicking the patterns of adaptation to a disability. Figure 37-15 shows normal development of function along an arbitrary scale of function; Figure 37-16 shows the impact of a congenital disability on that development. Similarly, Figure 37-17 shows the consequences of an acquired disability. In Figure 37-18, the impact of a progressive degenerative disorder is demonstrated. These time patterns of development and progress incorporate recovery, rehabilitation therapy effects, and normal growth and development.

Prediction of Outcome

One of the major responsibilities of the health professional is the establishment of medical and functional prognoses for a child with a disability. From these estimates of outcome, the specific objectives and plans of management can be drawn that will guide the daily activities of the child and family. It is therefore most important to both accurately pre-

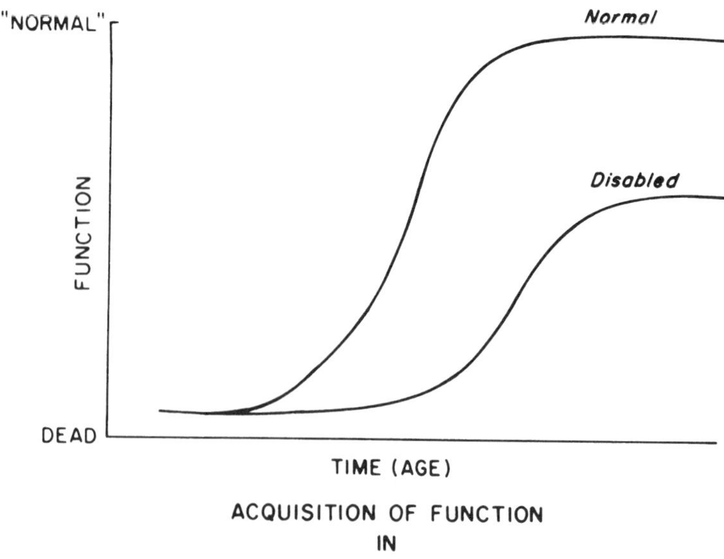

FIG. 37-16. A child with a congenital or early acquired disability shows a slower rate of function acquisition and a lower level of degree of function achieved.

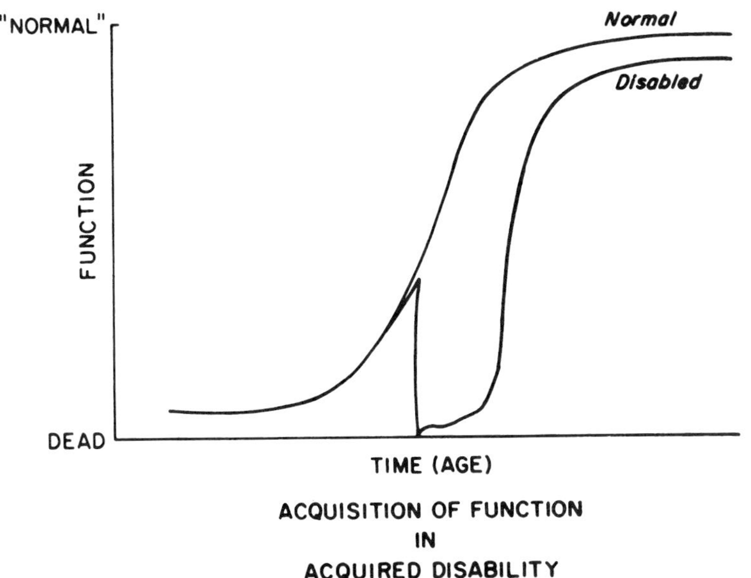

FIG. 37-17. Functional development of a child with a late acquired disability. The normal pattern is interrupted by the onset of the new impairment. Relatively rapid early recovery is followed by continuing improvement due to growth and development, as well as possible continuing recovery.

dict and be cognizant of the limits of predictability for any individual child.

Certain common milestones that are considered major objectives in life should be considered early on. The first of these is the question, Will my child be able to walk? It should be recognized that walking means different things to a medical professional than to a parent. The parent means, Will my child go everywhere he or she wants to, with no assistive devices, no wheelchair, and no help from anyone else? The professional will be more comfortable in distinguishing between a variety of types of walking (e.g., in the house, in the community) and degrees of dependency on devices and other individuals. Initial clarity of predictions should be sought.

The second major question that may or may not be verbalized is, Will my child be able to live independently and earn his or her own living? This is usually closely related to the third question, Will my child be able to marry and have children? Both are major questions that are not easy to answer. It may be useful to guide parents to define what the specific issues related to their child are, and which of them are predictable. By allowing the family to participate in the analysis that may lead to answering the questions, greater comfort with the answers may be derived.

In the case of the child with a degenerative disorder, much more serious questions, such as, How long will my child live? and What will be his or her quality of life? become prominent. The predictions may be obvious, but in our experience they are frequently difficult and evasive. The greatest harm may be done by providing unnecessarily dogmatic projections in either extreme. For the most pessimistic projection, such as when the child is given only a short time to

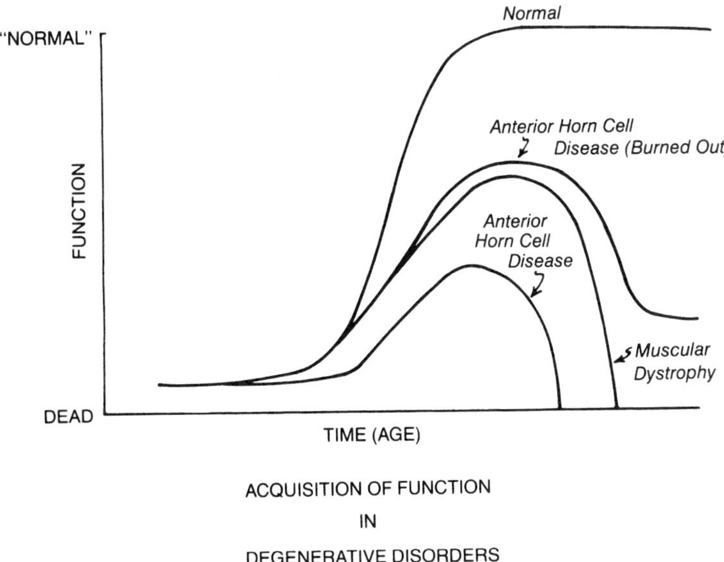

FIG. 37-18. Functional development of a child with a progressive degenerative disorder. In some cases, developmental progress may continue at a less than normal rate while the rate of growth and development exceeds the rate of deterioration from the underlying disease.

live, major difficulties come about when the child survives beyond the expected period. The child and family spend the additional life-time constantly waiting for the end, and, more important, frequently nothing is done to allow the child to grow, achieve goals, or face new challenges, because the family adopts a fatalistic, do-nothing attitude.

At the other extreme, inappropriately optimistic projections will contribute to unrealistic goal setting and will encourage the child and family to set themselves up for failure to achieve objectives, bringing further frustration and emotional pain.

The right approach is to admit uncertainty when it exists, make cautiously optimistic predictions, and move forward with goals that at least provide for comfort and care for both the child and family, and also give some specific positive objectives.

COMMON CHILDHOOD DISABLING DISORDERS

Cerebral Palsy

Cerebral palsy is the most common physical disability of childhood seen in practice by rehabilitation professionals. As such, it serves as a useful teaching model for all brain disorders in childhood, including stroke, head injury, tumor, and infections. Cerebral palsy is defined as a motor disorder occurring because of a lesion that is nonprogressive and occurs in the developing brain (68). This does not preclude other associated problems such as sensory loss, cognitive deficits, language disorders, and so on. Clearly, cerebral palsy is not a specific disease but rather a collection of disorders with some common features.

The various specific forms of cerebral palsy are generally described along four different parameters that usually are specifically correlated. The four parameters are neuroanatomic lesion, etiology, neurologic pattern, and topography of body dysfunction.

The neuroanatomic lesions will be localized to either a physical zone, a blood supply distribution, or a distribution that correlates with cellular metabolic sensitivities. Thus, a vascular lesion will lead to a typical stroke pattern, a depressed skull fracture will lead to local cortical findings, and an ischemic or toxic lesion will show more diffuse deficits according to the cells most affected.

The most common etiologies noted for cerebral palsy include prematurity, ischemia, hypoxemia, hyperbilirubinemia, and external or internal trauma (69,70). The increasing success of newborn intensive care programs in greatly improving the survival rate of low birth weight and very low birth weight infants has resulted in an increase in the prevalence of cerebral palsy. It is estimated that the childhood prevalence of cerebral palsy increased by about 20% between 1960 and 1986 in the United States (71).

The neurologic pattern of loss shows five major types: spasticity, hypotonia, athetosis, ataxia, and mixed patterns. The distinction between these patterns is often difficult, and children frequently appear to evolve from one pattern to another. It is typical, for example, for a hypotonic or floppy infant to evolve toward spasticity, and then perhaps athetoid patterns and finally a mixture of spasticity with athetoid features.

Spasticity in children shows the typical combination of increased resting muscle tone, hyperactive stretch reflexes, clonus, and the spread of reflex responses.

Hypotonia is usually described in children as low tone or floppiness and is demonstrated by low resting muscle tone, diminished stretch reflexes, and, frequently, diminishment of the primitive reflex patterns. It is important to understand that the diagnosis of hypotonia from brain damage is a diagnosis of exclusion. The physician, when confronted with a hypotonic child, must rule out other neuromuscular causes of hypotonia before the diagnosis of cerebral palsy–hypotonia can be established. These would include progressive motor neurone disease, demyelinating neuropathy, motor end plate disorders, and primary muscle disease. Electrodiagnostic studies, muscle enzyme determinations and, if necessary, muscle or peripheral nerve biopsy will assist the physician in identifying the true cause of the low or absent muscle tone.

Athetosis is demonstrated in children by several phenomena that are different from those typically thought of as representative of athetosis in the adult. First is the observation of markedly variable tone. These children may show striking fluctuations in resting tone ranging from flaccidity to opisthotonic rigidity. These changes may or may not be associated with external environmental factors. Associated with the variability of tone is the observation of a strong dominance of primitive reflex patterns throughout the child's motor repertoire. Almost all primitive reflexes are normal findings at certain developmental stages, but their obligatory dominance and preservation over time should never be considered as within normal limits.

Finally, and usually later in development, comes the athetoid movement pattern of writhing and flailing motion. Although these motions are described by some as random actions, they typically are not. Rather, they are poorly learned and even more poorly refined efforts at achieving skilled motor control of the limbs. Careful observation of the child with athetosis will show rather consistent and stereotypical patterns of these so-called adventitious movements.

Ataxia is a less common pattern with both trunk and limb involvement. It is commonly associated with cerebellar damage and is seen frequently as a consequence of traumatic brain injury.

The *mixed pattern* may, in fact, be the most common description for cerebral palsy, even though most investigators have attempted to minimize this category. The typical child shows features of several patterns. For example, the child with athetoid features, such as poor limb control, variable tone, and dominant primitive reflexes, also may show persistently high tone, even though it varies, and soft-tissue contracture. In our experience, the child with pure athetoid patterns will not develop soft-tissue contracture; hence, this child shows a mixed spastic–athetoid pattern.

The distribution of the motor deficit over the body is described by the definition of limbs involved. Thus, *monoplegia* indicates that a single limb is involved; *hemiplegia* indicates that the arm and leg on the same side are affected; and *quadriplegia* means that all four limbs are affected. The term *diplegia* is used when the legs are the major symmetrically involved limbs, and the arms are only subtly affected. The term *paraplegia* is to be avoided, because it implies complete normalcy of the upper limbs. If, in fact, only the lower limbs are involved, the diagnosis of cerebral palsy is most likely incorrect and should be challenged. Quadriplegia also usually implies that trunk, head, and neck control are also deficient. To emphasize the point, the term *total body involved* is sometimes used.

Etiology

The most common neuroanatomic lesion is damage to the germinal matrix zone in the periventricular region of the premature fetus, usually occurring around 24 to 28 weeks of gestational age (72,73). This injury is usually caused by ischemic damage associated with hypoperfusion of the area. That area is susceptible to this type of damage because it is a watershed zone with only marginal blood supply. The lesions tend to be somewhat symmetric, leading to bilateral signs. Furthermore, they occur in the area of those internal capsular tracts that are more heavily involved in the lower extremity's function. As a consequence, the lesions present as spastic diplegia.

Major hypoxic injuries cause diffuse damage to cortical and cerebellar systems, resulting in spastic quadriparesis. There is generally a correlation among the severity of the spasticity, the amount of cognitive dysfunction, and the likelihood for an associated seizure disorder as well.

More selective damage results from hyperbilirubinemia. This previously common form of damage resulted from Rh incompatibility and the resultant erythroblastosis fetalis. As a result of the introduction of RhoGAM and fetal transfusions, the incidence of damage from kenicterus has been drastically diminished. The pattern of these lesions showed a classical triad of athetosis, sensorineural hearing loss, and paralysis of upward gaze (i.e., Parinaud syndrome). Perhaps more important is the frequently noted discrepancy between motor dysfunction, speech dysfunction due to motor difficulties, and the preservation of good cognitive and language function.

More discrete lesions such as cerebral vascular occlusions from emboli or vasculitis result in typical stroke patterns such as hemiplegia. When these occur in infancy and early childhood, their impact on language function is surprisingly minimal. Presumably, shifts of cortical dominance occur as compensatory mechanisms to allow relatively good language function to develop.

The typical relationships between these various parameters and the related clinical syndromes are shown in Table 37-6.

Management

Management of the motor deficit of cerebral palsy requires an understanding of the natural history of the disease and the pattern of motor activity available to the child, as well as a coordinated long-range set of goals.

There are many specific schools of thought about particular therapy programs that may be offered to children. In general, the most effective of these combine knowledge of the reflex behaviors of children with cerebral palsy with knowledge of motor learning.

A variety of specialized therapeutic protocols have been popularized. Little evidence exists, however, to demonstrate the clinical superiority of one over another (74). Leading systems of care include the traditional orthopedic approach of range of motion, stretch, and strengthening; neurodevelopmental treatment (NDT) for motor learning and tone normalization (75); sensory integration (76) for a variety of motor and arousal features; and a variety of other approaches (77). The most commonly used school of therapy in the United States is NDT, as was taught by Berta and Karel Bobath.

Modern therapeutic programs do not rely exclusively on one school of therapy; rather, they draw eclectically upon a variety of techniques and strategies that will optimize the child's ability to function. Above all, providers of therapeutic services need to be aware of the values and limits, as well as the costs and demands, of their interventions, in both financial and human terms. It is important also that they avoid overly burdening the child and family with unlikely or unreasonable therapeutic demands and expectations.

Spinal Dysraphism

One of the most common congenital defects leading to major physical impairment is spinal dysraphism, variously referred to as myelomeningocele, meningomyelocele, myelodysplasia, and spina bifida (78). In general, these disorders represent developmental abnormalities of the spinal axis resulting in spinal cord dysfunction and all the consequences that neurologic disruption typically encompasses, as in spinal cord–injured patients. Representative patterns of the dysraphic state are shown in Figure 37-19.

Etiology

Spinal dysraphism is believed to be of genetic etiology, with both chromosomal and environmental contributing factors. Major risk factors for the development of a dysraphic disorder include a family history of dysraphism and increased maternal or paternal age.

Prenatal diagnosis for mothers at risk includes maternal serum alpha-fetoprotein (AFP) assessment, amniotic fluid

TABLE 37-6. *Classification and patterns of cerebral palsy*

Neurologic	Extent	Severity	Other
Hemiplegia			
Flaccid	Right	Mild	Congenital/acquired
Spastic	Left	Moderately severe	Unknown etiology
		Severe	Epilepsy/no epilepsy
Bilateral hemiplagia	—	Mild	Congenital/acquired
		Moderately severe	
		Severe	Epilepsy/no epilepsy
Diplegia			
Hypotonic	Paraplegic	Mild	Congenital:
Dystonic	Triplegic	Moderately severe	Associated with low birthweight
Rigid/spastic	Paraplegic	Severe	Not low birthweight
			Acquired (rare)
			Epilepsy/no epilepsy
Ataxic diplegia	Paraplegic	Mild	Congenital/acquired:
	Triplegic	Moderately severe	With hydrocephalus and/or spina bifida
	Tetraplegic	Severe	No hydrocephalus/spina bifida
			Epilepsy/no epilepsy
Ataxia	Predominantly	Mild	Congenital/acquired:
	Unilateral (rare)	Moderately severe	With hydrocephalus/spina bifida
	Bilateral symmetrical	Severe	No hydrocephalus/spina bifida
			Hearing loss/no hearing loss
			Epilepsy/no epilepsy
			Disequilibrium syndrome/no disequilibrium syndrome
Dyskinesia	Monoplegic (rare)	Mild	Congenital:
			Kernicterus/no kernicterus
	Hemiplegic (rare)	Moderately severe	Acquired (rare)
	Triplegic	Severe	
	Tetraplegic		

Reprinted with permission from Ingram TTS. Historical review of the definition and classification of the cerebral palsies. In: Stanley F, Alberman E, eds. *Epidemiology of the cerebral palsies.* Philadelphia: JB Lippincott, 1984; 8.

AFP elevations, and ultrasound imaging of the fetus for evidence of anomalous development of the spinal axis. Prenatal diagnosis is, of course, indicated if consideration is being given to termination of the pregnancy if a defect is identified (79).

The risk for spina bifida and other neural tube defects can be reduced if women consume 0.4 mg of folic acid before and during the first trimester of pregnancy (80).

Management

The initial management of a newborn with spinal dysraphism includes decision making with regard to surgical closure of the lesion and assessment for other associated disorders, especially hydrocephalus. The spinal surgery may range from a simple excision of the empty sack with primary closure, to extensive and meticulous neurosurgical untangling of nerve roots and cord, bony reconstruction, and complex plastic surgical flap rotations (81).

The management of hydrocephalus (occurring in 90% of the cases) includes ventricular monitoring by ultrasound while the fontanelle is open and by computed tomography or magnetic resonance imaging thereafter; installation of a ventricular shunt, most commonly to the peritoneum; and monitoring of shunt function through physical examination of the reservoir under the scalp or nuclear scanning of cerebrospinal fluid clearance by the shunt (82,83).

It is important for the physician and his or her management team to recognize that many of these children have neurologic dysfunction above the level of their myelomeningocele even if hydrocephalus is not present. In a Swedish study of 22 neonates investigated prospectively to a median age of 3 years, 19 had a Chiari malformation and 18 developed neurologic dysfunction above the spinal level. Six children developed severe functional impairment of respiration, feeding, and motor performance within the first 3 months of life. Careful monitoring by the rehabilitation team and the medical management team is essential to identify these problems as early as possible and to initiate treatment to correct or control them (84).

The decision to treat or not treat the newborn infant with spinal dysraphism continues to be a complex ethical issue. Objective criteria for determination of indications for not treating (i.e., allowing the infant to die from CNS infection) have been proposed but are still under debate. Increasingly, the clinical tendency is to attempt aggressive surgical intervention in almost all cases (85–87).

Early rehabilitation management concerns include bladder and bowel care, prevention of contractures, hip subluxation or dislocation, prevention of spinal deformity, and encouragement of normal mobility with orthoses and wheelchair use (88).

Infants with significant bladder detrusor sphincter dyssynergia will benefit from an intermittent catheterization program and appropriate monitoring for urologic function (e.g., urodynamic studies, renal scan or intravenous pyelogram, recording of postvoid residuals, periodic urine cultures). Children developmentally around 5 years of age may be taught self-catheterization if no perceptual-motor problems interfere, although they will continue to require supervision for reliability (89).

Bowel flow may be managed with traditional bowel program methods. Occasionally, a flaccid anal sphincter without sufficient tone to retain feces is encountered. When it is developmentally appropriate to establish bowel continence (i.e., to eliminate the use of diapers), efforts at dietary manipulation to enhance stool consistency may be helpful. Outcome studies have demonstrated that when there is compliance by the parents and the child with a toileting intervention that emphasizes patient/family education and a regular, consistently timed, reflex-triggered bowel evacuation, a high rate of success in achieving bowel continence can be obtained. Best results occur when bowel training is instituted before 7 years of age. Presence of the bulbocavernousus and anocutaneous reflexes correlates significantly with achieving continence (90).

Parents should be taught in the newborn nursery to perform effective range-of-motion exercises for all involved limbs and the trunk. In the early years, range of motion that is performed with each diaper change may result in a compliant institution of this home therapy. Bed positioning also should be reviewed to allow passive stretch of tight hip flexors and spinal restrictions.

Early attention to sitting posture is important. The use of adapted infant and child seats may help to minimize kyphoscoliosis. Frequently, a body jacket is effective in controlling spinal alignment against the effects of gravity. Increasingly, early aggressive surgical management (e.g., spinal fusion with intersegmental rod instrumentation) is being selected as the management approach of choice to avoid prolonged external bracing (91). Occasionally, thoracic suspension orthoses for wheelchair positioning are useful.

Early standing with use of a variety of devices is encouraged. A parapodium, standing frame, or knee-ankle-foot orthosis is used. Although few objective studies exist, early standing is believed to enhance hip alignment, bone mineral-

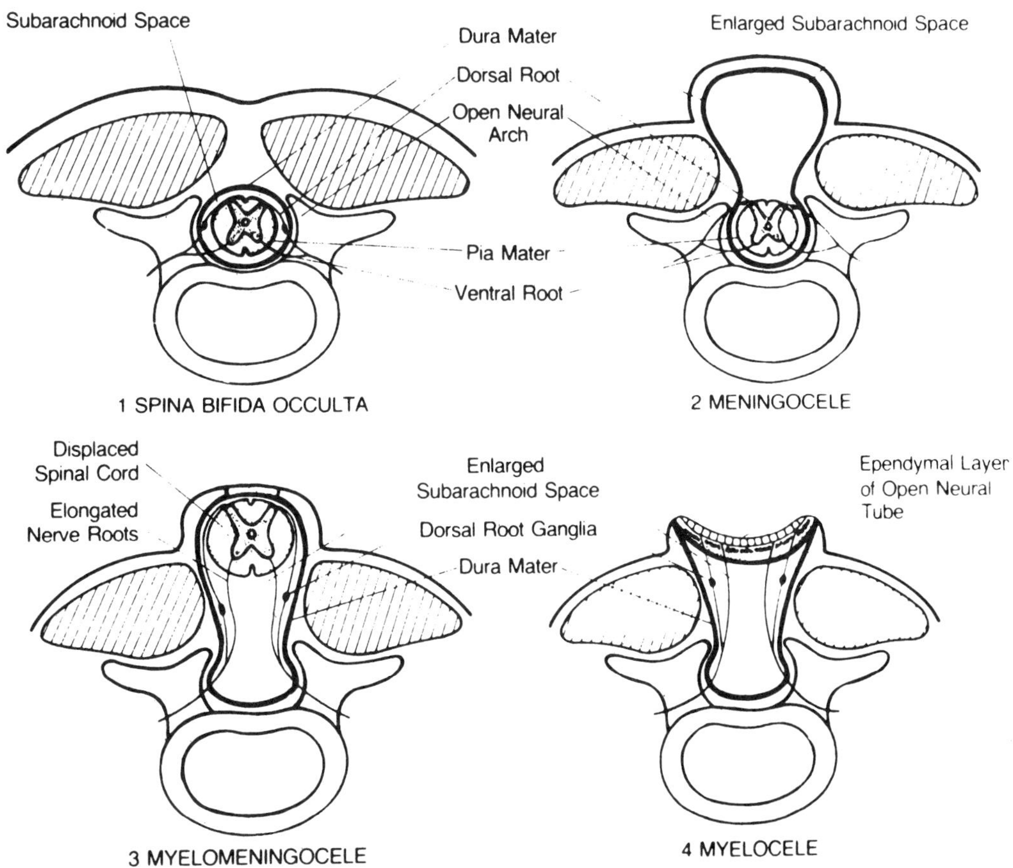

FIG. 37-19. Major patterns of spinal dysraphism. The name of the lesion depends on the contents of the abnormal sac. (Reprinted with permission from Menelaus MD. *Orthopedic management of spina bifida cystica,* 2nd ed. New York: Churchill-Livingstone, 1980.)

ization, urinary function, and psychosocial functioning. The parapodium, swivel walker, reciprocal orthosis, and traditional orthoses for ambulation training are all advocated by various investigators. Moreover, the early institution of good wheelchair skills in parallel with ambulation training offers the needed balance of mobility with ambulation for exercise and function.

Children should be examined for the presence of perceptual motor disorders. These are commonly observed, and their presence, along with a low IQ score, is more likely in a child with a history of shunt malfunctions and repeated infections (92). Frequently, verbal skills may far exceed performance abilities, leading to cocktail party personality behavior. Care should be taken to objectively validate the child's skills and performance of activities, rather than relying on reports by the child.

Later (i.e., adolescent) management focuses on ensuring autonomous self-care skills, including personal hygiene and bladder/bowel care, sexual adaptation, and vocational planning. The specific management techniques differ little from those used for the care of spinal cord-injured patients. The complicating factors are the long-standing behavior patterns that have become entrenched and the frequent presence of mild to moderate cognitive and perceptual deficits. Formerly, chronic renal disease was a source of high fatality for long-term survivors. Given that, for most children, the current long-term prognosis for survival is excellent, the need for long-range planning and vocational rehabilitation is evident (93). It is essential that planning for the transition to adulthood be initiated while the child is still an infant. The model of intervention must be based on developmental concerns and timely issues from infancy through all stages of development to young-adult life. It is only through the careful preparation and utilization of such a developmental and conceptual framework for transition to adulthood that the rehabilitation team, the family, and the individual with spinal dysraphism can feel assured that all of the person's needs are being met (94).

REFERENCES

1. Gans BM, DiScala C. Rehabilitaton of severely injured children. *West J Med* 1991; 154:566–568.
2. Osberg JS, DiScala C, Gans BM. Utilization of inpatient rehabilitation services among traumatically injured children discharged from pediatric trauma centers. *Am J Phys Med Rehabil* 1990; 69:67–72.
3. DiScala C. Osberg JS, Gans BM, et al. Children with traumatic head injury: morbidity and postacute treatment. *Arch Phys Med Rehabil* 1991; 72:662–666.
4. Kiely J, Paneth N. Stanley F. Monitoring the morbidity outcomes of perinatal health services. In: Stanley F, Alberman E. eds. *Epidemiology of the cerebral palsies.* Philadelphia: JB Lippincott, 1984.
5. Boyle CA, Decoufle P, Yeargin-Allsopp M. Prevalence and Health Impact of Developmental Disabilities in US children. *Pediatrics* 1994; 93:399–403.
6. Kaplan SL. Growth: normal and abnormal. In: Rudolph AM, Hoffman JIE, Axelrod S, eds. *Pediatrics,* 17th ed. New York: Appleton-Century-Crofts, 1982.
7. Cotman CW, Nieto-Sampedro M. Gibbs RB. Enhancing the self-repairing potential of the CNS after injury. *Central Nervous System Trauma* 1984; 1:3–14.
8. Young W. A critical overview of spinal injury research. Presented at the First International Symposium on CNS Trauma. *Central Nervous System Trauma* 1984; 1:75–79.
9. Bobath B. *Abnormal postural reflex activity caused by brain lesions,* 3rd ed. Rockville, MD: Aspen, 1985.
10. Bobath B, Bobath K. *Motor development in the different types of cerebral palsies.* London: Heinemann, 1975.
11. Kottke FJ. Neurophysiologic therapy for stroke. In: Licht S, ed. *Stroke and its rehabilitation.* Baltimore: Waverly, 1975.
12. Bayley N. *The Bayley Scales of Infant Development manual.* New York: Psychological Corporation, 1969.
13. Brigance AH. *Brigance diagnostic inventory of early development.* Woburn, MA: Curriculum Associates, 1991.
14. Frankenburg WK, Dodds JB. *The Denver Developmental Screening Test.* Denver: University of Colorado Medical Center, 1969.
15. Gesell A, Amatruda CS. *Developmental diagnosis,* 2nd ed. London: Harper & Row, 1947.
16. Herst J, Wolfe S, Jorgensen G, Pallan S. *Sewall early education developmental profiles,* 2nd ed. Denver: Sewall Rehabilitation Center, 1976.
17. Hoskins TA, Squires JE. Developmental assessment: a test for gross motor and reflex development. *Phys Ther* 1973; 53:117–125.
18. Illingworth RS. *Development of the infant and young child: normal and abnormal,* 8th ed. New York: Churchill-Livingstone, 1987.
19. Koontz CW. *Koontz child development program: training activities for the first 48 months.* Los Angeles: Western Psychological Services, 1974.
20. Berninger VW, Gans BM. Language profiles in nonspeaking individuals of normal intelligence with severe cerebral palsy. *Augmentative Alternative Communication* 1986; 2:56–63.
21. Berninger VW, Gans BM. Assessing word processing capability of the nonvocal, nonwriting. *Augmentative Alternative Communication* 1986; 2:56–63.
22. McCarty SM, St. James P, Berninger VW, Gans BM. Assessment of intellectual functioning across the life span in severe cerebral palsy. *Dev Med Child Neurol* 1986; 28:364–372.
23. Edin JC, Mitchell JR. Normal adolescent growth and development. In: Smith MS, ed. *Chronic disorders in adolescence.* Boston: John Wright, 1983.
24. Gode RO, Smith MS. Effects of chronic disorders on adolescent development: self, family, friends, and school. In: Smith MS, ed. *Chronic disorders in adolescence.* Boston: John Wright, 1983.
25. Bennett FC. Developmental dysfunction and school failure in the adolescent. In: Smith MS, ed. *Chronic disorders in adolescence.* Boston: John Wright, 1983.
26. Lichter P. Educatonal and vocational aspects of chronic disorders in adolescence. In: Smith MS, ed. *Chronic disorders in adolescence.* Boston: John Wright, 1983.
27. Buscaglia L. *The disabled and their parents: a counseling challenge.* Thorofare, NJ: Slack, 1983.
28. Arnold P. Chapman M. Self-esteem, aspirations and expectations of adolescents with physical disability. *Dev Med Child Neurol* 1992; 34: 97–102.
29. Apley J. *Care of the handicapped child.* Philadelphia: JB Lippincott, 1978.
30. Featherstone H. *A difference in the family: life with a disabled child.* New York: Basic Books, 1980.
31. Euler AR, Byrne WJ, Arment ME, et al. Recurrent pulmonary disease in children: a complication of gastroesophageal reflux. *Pediatrics* 1979; 63:47–51.
32. Herbst JJ, Book LS. Bray PF. Gastroesophageal reflux in the near miss sudden infant death syndrome. *J Pediatr* 1978; 92:73–75.
33. Johnson DG, Herbst JJ, Oliveros MA, Stewart DR. Evaluation of gastroesophageal reflux surgery in children. *Pediatrics* 1977; 59:62–68.
34. Meyers WF, Herbst JJ. Effectiveness of positioning therapy for gastroesophageal reflux. *Pediatrics* 1982; 69:768–772.
35. Orenstein SR, Whitington PF, Orenstein DM. The infant seat as treatment fro gastroesophageal reflux. *N Engl J Med* 1983; 309:760–763.
36. Glenn MB, Whyte J. *The practical management of spasticity in children and adults.* Philadelphia: Lea & Febiger, 1990.
37. Albright AL, Neurosurgical treatment of spasticity; selective posterior rhizotomy and intrathecal baclofen. *Stereotactic Funct Neurosurg* 1992; 58:3–13.
38. Hazlewood ME, Brown JK, Rowe PJ, Salter PM. The use of therapeutic

electrical stimulation in the treatment of hemiplegic cerebral palsy. *Dev Med Child Neurol* 1994; 36:661–673.

39. Koman LA, Mooney JF III, Smith B, Goodman A, Mulvaney T. Management of cerebral palsy with botulinum-A toxin: preliminary investigation. *J Pediatr Orthop* 1993; 13:489–495.
40. Johnson EW. Pathokinesiology of Duchenne muscular dystrophy: implications for management. *Arch Phys Med Rehabil* 1977; 58:4–7.
41. Lehman M, Hsu AM, Hsu JD. Spinal curvature, hand dominance and prolonged upper extremity use of wheelchair-dependent DMD patients. *Dev Med Child Neurol* 1986; 28:628–632.
42. Chung SMKL. *Hip disorders in infants and children.* Philadelphia: Lea & Febiger, 1981.
43. Tachdjian MO. *Pediatric orthopedics,* 2nd ed. Philadelphia: WB Saunders, 1990.
44. Gans BM, Hallenborg SC. Advances in wheelchair design. *Phys Med Rehabil State Art Rev* 1987; 1:95–109.
45. Gans BM, Hallenborg SC. Power wheelchairs: making the right choices. *Rx Homecare* 1984; July:32–41.
46. Butler C. Effects of powered mobility on self-initiated behaviors of very young children with locomotor disability. *Dev Med Child Neurol* 1986; 325–332.
47. Butler C, Okamoto GA, McKay T. Motorized wheelchair driving by disabled children. *Arch Phys Med Rehabil* 1984; 65:95–97.
48. Medhat MA, Redford JB. Prescribed seating systems. *Phys Med Rehabil State Art Rev* 1987; 1:111–136.
49. McClenaghan BA, Thombs L, Milner M. Effects of seat-surface inclination on postural stability and function of the upper extremities of children with cerebral palsy. *Dev Med Child Neurol* 1992; 34:40–48.
50. Sousa JC, Gordon LH, Shurtleff DB. Assessing the development of daily living skills in patients with spina bifida. *Dev Med Child Neurol* 1976; 18(suppl 37):43.
51. Gans BM, Mann NR, Hallenborg SC, Haley SC. Tufts assessment of motor performance (TAMP) [Abstract]. *Dev Med Child Neurol* 1986; 28(suppl 53):43.
52. Haley SM, Hallenborg SC, Gans BM. Functional assessment in young children with neurological impairments. *Top Early Childhood Special Educ* 1989; 9:106–126.
53. Chess S, Fernandez P. *The handicapped child in school: behavior and management.* New York: Brunner/Mazel, 1981.
54. Tizard B, Harvey D. *Biology of play.* Philadelphia: JB Lippincott, 1977.
55. Kokkonen J, Saukkonen AL, Timonen E, Serlo W, Kinnunen P. Social outcome of handicapped children as adults. *Dev Med Child Neurol* 1991; 33:1095–1100.
56. Connolly B, Harris S. Survey of assessment tools. *Totline* 1983; 9: 8–11.
57. Lord J, Taggart PJ, Molnar GE. Assessment instruments for evaluation of motor skills in children. In: Redford JB, ed. *Phys Med Rehabil State Art Rev* 1991; 5:389–402.
58. Jebson RH, Taylor N, Trieschmann RB, Trotter MJ, Howard LA. An objective and standardized test of hand function. *Arch Phys Med Rehabil* 1969; 50:311–319.
59. Taylor N, Sand PL, Jebson RH. Evaluation of hand function in children. *Arch Phys Med Rehabil* 1973; 54:129–135.
60. Stengel TJ. Assessing motor development in children. In: Campbell SK, ed. *Pediatric neurologic physical therapy,* 2nd ed. New York: Churchill-Livingstone, 1991; 33–65.
61. Mahoney RI, Barthel DW. Functional evaluation: the Barthel index. *Maryland State Med J* 1965; 14:61–65.
62. Granger CV, Hamilton BB, Sherwin FS. *Guide for the use of the uniform data set for medical rehabilitation.* Buffalo, NY: Research Foundation, State University of New York, 1986.
63. Granger CV, Hamilton BB, Kayton R. *Guide for the use of the functional independence measure (WeeFIM) of the uniform data set for the medical rehabilitation.* Buffalo, NY: Research Foundation, State University of New York, 1988.
64. Feldman AB, Haley SM, Coryell J. Concurrent and construct validity of the Pediatric Evaluation of Disability Inventory. *Phys Ther* 1990; 70:602–610.
65. Haley SM, Ludlow LH, Gans BM, et al. Tufts Assessment of Motor Performance: an empirical approach to identifying motor performance categories. *Arch Phys Med Rehabil* 1991; 72:359–366.
66. Gans BM, Haley SM, Hallenborg SC, et al. Description and inter-observer reliability of the Tufts Assessment of Motor Performance. *Am J Phys Med Rehabil* 1988; 67:202–210.
67. Miller F, Koreska J. Height measurement of patients with neuro-muscular disease and contractures. *Dev Med Child Neurol* 1992; 34:55–60.
68. Ingram TTS. Historical review of the definition and classification of the cerebral palsies. In: Stanley F, Alberman E, eds. *The epidemiology of the cerebral palsies.* Philadelphia: JB Lippincott, 1984.
69. Nelson KB, Ellenberg JH. Antecedents of cerebral palsy. Multi-variate analysis of risk. *N Engl J Med* 1986; 315:81–86.
70. Stanley F, Alberman E, eds. *The epidemiology of the cerebral palsies.* Philadelphia: JB Lippincott, 1984.
71. Bhushan V, Paneth N, Kiely JL. Impact of improved survival of very low birth infants on recent secular trends in the prevalence of cerebral palsy. *Pediatrics* 1993; 91:1094–1100.
72. Wigglesworth J. Brain development and its modification by adverse influences. In: Stanley F, Alberman E, eds. *The epidemiology of the cerebral palsies.* Philadelphia: JB Lippincott, 1984.
73. Cummins SK. Prenatal and perinatal factors and the epidemiology of cerebral palsy: a review. *Physical Med Rehabil State Art Rev* 1991; 5: 403–416.
74. Bower E, McLellan DL. Effect of increased exposure to physiotherapy on skill acquisition of children with cerebral palsy. *Dev Med Child Neurol* 1992; 34:25–39.
75. Bobath K. *A neurophysiological basis for the treatment of cerebral palsy.* Philadelphia: JB Lippincott, 1980.
76. Ayres AJ. *Sensory integration and learning disorders.* Los Angeles: Western Psychological Services, 1972.
77. Scrutton D, ed. *Management of the motor disorders of children with cerebral palsy.* Philadelphia: JB Lippincott, 1984.
78. Molnar GE. Spina bifida: clinical correlations of associated central nervous system malformations. *Phys Med Rehabil State Art Rev* 1991; 5:285–312.
79. Milunsky A, Alpert E. The value of alpha-fetoprotein in the prenatal diagnosis of neural tube defects. *J Pediatr* 1974; 84:889–893.
80. Lary JM, Edmonds LD. Prevalence of spina bifida at birth (United States, 1983–1990: a comparison of two surveillance systems. *MMWR* 1996; 45:15–26.
81. Guthkelch AN. Aspects of the surgical management of myelomeningocele: a review. *Dev Med Child Neurol* 1986; 28:525–532.
82. Schmidt K, Gjerris F, Osgaard O, et al. Antibiotic prophylaxis in cerebrospinal fluid shunting: a prospective randomized trial in 152 hydrocephalic patients. *Neurosurgery* 1985; 17:1–5.
83. Tew B, Evans R, Thomas M, Ford J. The results of a selective surgical policy on the cognitive abilities of children with spina bifida. *Dev Med Child Neurol* 1985; 27:606–614.
84. Dahl M, Ahlsten G, Carlson H, et al. Neurological dysfunction above the cell level in children with spina bifida cystica: a prospective study to three years. *Dev Med Child Neurol* 1995; 37:30–40.
85. Lorber J. Results of treatment of myelomeningocele. An analysis of 524 unselected cases with special reference to possible selection for treatment. *Dev Med Child Neurol* 1971; 13:279–303.
86. McLone DG. Results of treatment of children born with a myelomeningocele. *Clin Neurosurg* 1983; 30:407–412.
87. Shurtleff DB, Hayden PW, Loeser JD, Kronmal RA. Myelodyplasia: decision for death or disability. *N Engl J Med* 1974; 291:1005–1011.
88. McDonald CM. Rehabilitation of children with spinal dysraphism. *Neurosurg Clin North Am* 1995; 6:393–412.
89. Selzman AA, Elder JS, Mapstone TB. Urologic consequences of myelodysplasia and other congenital abnormalities of the spinal cord. *Urol Clin North Am* 1993; 20:485–504.
90. King JC, Currie DM, Wright E, Bowel training in spina bifida: importance of education, patient compliance, age and anal reflexes. *Arch Phys Med Rehabil* 1994; 75:243–247.
91. Menelaus MB. *Orthopedic management of spina bifida cystica,* 2nd ed. New York: Churchill-Livingstone, 1980.
92. McLone DG, Czyzewski D, Raimondi AJ, Sommers RC. Central nervous system infections as a limiting factor in the intelligence of children with myelomeningocele. *Pediatrics* 1982; 70:338–342.
93. Harrington TF, ed. *Handbook of career planning for special needs students.* Rockville, MD: Aspen, 1982.
94. Peterson PM, Rauen KK, Brown J, Cole J. Spina bifida: the transition into adulthood begins in infancy. *Rehabil Nurs* 1994; 19:229–238.

Rehabilitation Medicine: Principles and Practice, Third Edition,
edited by Joel A. DeLisa and Bruce M. Gans.
Lippincott–Raven Publishers, Philadelphia © 1998.

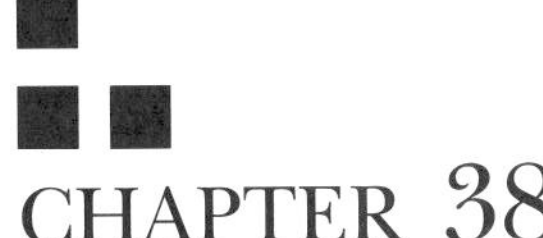

CHAPTER 38

Adults with Congenital and Childhood Onset Disability Disorders

Margaret A. Turk and Robert J. Weber

The issues of secondary conditions and aging in persons with disabilities have become of considerable interest to researchers and clinicians in recent years. Nevertheless, persons with disabilities have been concerned about these issues throughout their lifetimes, and have been questioning health-care professionals about the expectations for lifelong function. For years, children with disabilities and their families have been told that health and functional status, mobility, and musculoskeletal problems essentially stabilize by early adulthood. However, as more people with lifelong mobility impairments live through their adult years, it is apparent that mobility, functional status, and musculoskeletal changes commonly continue in adulthood. In fact, questions and concerns about mobility, function change, and pain are common among the majority of adults with mobility impairments caused by any etiology (1). These ongoing changes occurring in adulthood may be a part of the dynamic aging process, may be related to personal life-style choices, or may be in and of themselves secondary conditions.

There is little published information about aging issues and secondary conditions among persons with congenital and childhood onset mobility impairments. Systematic studies of secondary conditions have only recently been initiated. Most scientific information has only recently been published, and much of the conventional wisdom in this area has been communicated through the network of persons with disabilities. There is minimal information regarding the impact of commonly practiced interventions over a lifetime. Therefore, health-care providers and consumers have limited knowledge from which to base decisions regarding adult health issues and anticipated changes in function in these individuals with disabilities.

This chapter will define secondary conditions and aging as it relates to congenital and childhood onset disabilities; identify common lifelong functional status and health issues of adults with congenital and childhood onset motor impairments; and discuss health promotion strategies in a disability population.

DEFINITIONS

Aging is the conception-to-death series of developmental changes that impact a person's ability to respond to the demands of the environment (2). It encompasses a person's entire lifetime, not just the later stages of life. Aging is not simply a process of becoming older, less functional, and dying. Growth, development, acquisition of skills, maintenance of skills and functional capabilities, repair and replacement, and decline are all parts of aging. During the early stages of aging (infancy, childhood, adolescence), attainment of skills and capabilities is on the rise; in the middle stages (adulthood), maintaining and retaining function is the focus. It is only in the later stages of life that function declines, if disease is not a factor at any of the preceding stages. Aging is also genetically moderated.

The underlying assumption has been that the pattern of aging is the same in persons with lifelong disabilities as it is in the general population. Data to substantiate this assumption are not available. To understand the aging process, one must encompass all the changes that occur in a person from conception until death. Persons with disabilities follow a course of aging, although likely with a slower and lower attainment of skills, and a smaller capacity to adjust to acute

M.A. Turk: Departments of Physical Medicine and Rehabilitation and Pediatrics, State University of New York Health Science Center at Syracuse, Syracuse, New York 13210.

R.J. Weber: Department of Physical Medicine and Rehabilitation, State University of New York Health Science Center at Syracuse, Syracuse, New York 13210.

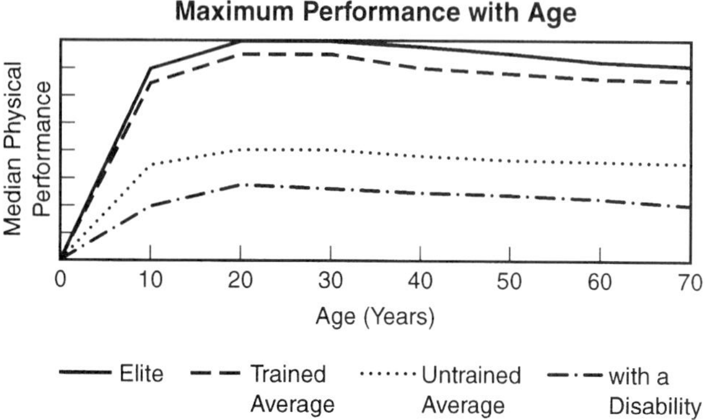

FIG. 38-1. Explanation of aging and performance. Maximum performance (an arbitrary quotient) is achieved after a period of skill attainment, followed by maintenance of skills, and linear decline. As noted, elite and trained individuals achieve significantly higher performance than an untrained average individual. Persons with childhood onset motor impairments have a slower achievement of optimal performace, lower optimal performance level, and quicker and lower performance with age, showing a smaller reserve for acute, recurrent, or chronic limitations to performance. There is still the capability for improved performance with training, as in the nondisabled individual. (Adapted with permission from Fries JF. The compression of morbidity. *Milbank Q* 1983; 61:397–419.)

or intercurrent health or medical and surgical intercedents (Fig. 38-1).

Secondary conditions are impairments, functional limitations, disabilities, diseases, injuries, or other conditions that occur during the life of a person with a disability, where the primary disabling condition is a risk factor for that secondary condition or may alter the standard intervention for prevention or treatment of any health condition (Syracuse Conference, 1994). This is based on the new paradigm that people with disabilities are healthy; that is, a disabling condition does not imply illness and disease. Secondary conditions may be insidiously progressive or have onset in late adolescence or adulthood. They may include progression of pathology or impairment either through complications or through the aging process. There may be variable expression, and some may not be preventable. With better supporting information, some of the reported early aging changes experienced by persons with childhood or congenital-onset disabilities may be considered secondary conditions. They may be modified by environmental or adaptive equipment measures. Secondary conditions may be difficult to identify if there is no index of suspicion by the clinician, or there is an expectation of declining health and function of persons with disabilities as they mature. Commonly reported secondary conditions include pain, contractures, recurrent urinary tract infections, pressure sores, and osteoporosis.

Secondary conditions should not be confused with *associated conditions* or residual deficits. These are terms commonly used to describe conditions that result from the defect, injury, or disease, and often may be considered primary impairments depending on their severity. For cerebral palsy or other brain injuries, the list of associated conditions includes seizures, learning disabilities, mental retardation, sensory problems, and oral motor and communication problems. Some conditions associated with the diagnosis of spina bifida include neurogenic bladder, neurogenic bowel, learning disabilities, mental retardation, and seizures. Persons with a primary disabling condition may have any combination of associated conditions, all of which will impact on their ultimate functional capabilities.

Secondary conditions also do not include other *comorbidities*, that is, other medical conditions unrelated to the primary disabling condition. As an example, persons with cerebral palsy also may develop hypertension or diabetes mellitus should they have the risk factors or genetic predisposition for these conditions.

Health, then, is the absence of disease or illness, beyond the disabling condition. Persons with disabilities should be considered healthy, with a shift of the health-care model from an illness and infirmed paradigm to one of prevention or early identification of secondary conditions, aging issues, and/or comorbidities (Fig. 38-2).

In recent years, a body of literature has accumulated regarding aging and secondary conditions. Spinal cord injury and aging is the best developed with information in the areas of quality of life (3), functional changes over time (4,5), premature and interactive effects of disability and aging (6–8), aging and secondary conditions (9), and psychological adjustment (10), among other issues. Other disability groups that have been studied are cerebral palsy (11), spina bifida (12,13), and polio (14).

Identification of age-related changes and secondary conditions with their risk factors has been better explored (1,15–19) than have prevention or intervention strategies. Recent research has been directed toward maintaining function with age and preventing secondary conditions. The per-

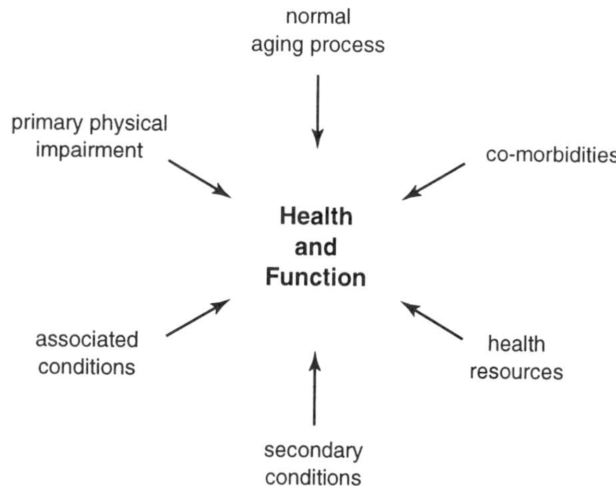

FIG. 38-2. The medical paradigm is changing from illness and disease to health and wellness for persons with disabilities. Multiple factors affect function and health and should be recognized by clinicians who serve persons with disabilities.

son with a disability may have less resilience or reserve against the onset of functional limitations compared with a nondisabled person.

Each factor in the interaction of disability and aging or secondary conditions has the capability to become a negative feedback loop (20), which may lead to further disability or a new medical condition. In effect, as a person with a disability ages, a series of new pathologies, impairments, and functional limitations may become superimposed on the previous ones.

HEALTH AND FUNCTIONAL STATUS: SECONDARY CONDITIONS AND AGE-RELATED CHANGES

The majority of information available regarding adults with congenital and childhood onset motor impairments involves persons with cerebral palsy and spina bifida. This is because of their higher prevalence rates and the many organized pediatric clinics. The accumulated information is a combination of scientifically observed and anecdotal information. Most reported research information is from cross-sectional or convenience samples and represents patient reports and clinical observations, not longitudinal studies using standardized measures. Although there is also supporting information from studies on cross-disability groups, persons with spinal cord injury, and polio survivors, generalization to other disability groups should be considered with caution.

Most problems of adults with congenital or childhood onset motor impairments center around musculoskeletal and physical performance complaints and changes. This is not surprising for a group of people defined by impaired motor function. Although these groups are not homogeneous (i.e., they vary widely in severity and functional capacity), the prevalence of these complaints indicates that musculoskeletal issues have a significant impact on the individual. The clinician therefore should anticipate these complaints and be prepared to identify their cause and manage the problems appropriately.

The personal and social impact of functional changes in performance for adults with congenital and childhood onset mobility impairments will not be addressed. The transition from childhood to adult management and life-styles, goals, and issues also will not be highlighted. However, these aspects should not be ignored, nor can they be easily separated from discussions regarding implications for independence and recognition of changes. People with mobility impairments work hard to meet expectations for achieving independence both for themselves and for parents, professionals, and peers. Changes that compromise these hard-earned achievements can cause a significant emotional injury that should be addressed.

The following listing is designed to provide a core of knowledge to increase awareness of clinically important issues and to encourage further investigation. Table 38-1 provides a guide to commonly occurring secondary conditions and age-related changes for persons with disabilities and prevention strategies.

Health Status

Adults with cerebral palsy report that they enjoy generally good health (16,21). In fact, this self-rated health is comparable with that of the community at large (22). Adults with spina bifida report more health-related problems (e.g., pressure sores, burns, urinary tract infections, obesity) than do individuals with cerebral palsy, but general and comparative health data are not available (12,23). It should be noted that studies of polio survivors or persons with spinal cord injury report elevated cardiovascular system risk factors of hypercholesterolemia, inactivity, smoking, and ischemic heart disease as a leading cause of death in spinal cord injury (14,24,25); these factors and an adverse outcome have not yet been found to be prevalent in aduts with cerebral palsy or spina bifida.

Mortality statistics are limited. In a retrospective review of a British cerebral palsy registry (26), the most common reported cause of death in children and young adults with cerebral palsy was respiratory. In a retrospective time-limited population-based study (27), children with severe or profound mental retardation had an increased risk of dying at a younger age. In a population-based study of adults with cerebral palsy in a mid-sized metropolitan area, persons with cerebral palsy were generally healthy (based on clinical information and self-report), but noted worries and concerns about their health status (16). Spina bifida studies reported in the early 1970s noted survival to adulthood to be 60% to 70% for infants referred to regional centers (28). A more recent study reported a survival rate of 60% for consecutive cases, treated unselectively, within a 16- to 20-year period (29). Shortened life expectancy was reported for persons with developmental disabilities, including mental retardation, severe motor impairments, and in particular a feeding disability, in a state service registry (30).

Age-Related Changes

Information about age-related changes in a nondisabled population is available in the literature. Wide differences exist between individuals in the rate of aging and its effect on their physical function. Different organ systems age at different rates. There is no reason to believe that similar age-related changes will not occur in persons with disabilities. The changes related to the musculoskeletal system and performance should be considered more closely because they may have a more profound expression in persons with long-term motor impairments. Complex performance activities can show greater change with aging because they require coordination and integration of multiple functions (e.g., endurance, sequence of muscle activity, balance, vision). Phys-

TABLE 38-1. *Lifelong motor disabilities, aging, and secondary conditions*[a]

Body system	Pathology, impairment, or other conditions leading to potential secondary conditions	Potential prevention strategies
Skin and subcutaneous tissues	Insensate skin; increased areas of pressure due to poor positioning, obesity, or limited weight shifts because of cognitive, behavioral, or personal care issues; decreased elasticity or turgor in aging with top layer thinning resulting in increased susceptibility to shearing and tearing; urinary or bowel incontinence.	Regular weight shift routine; appropriate seating systems and surfaces; good nutrition and hygiene habits; social or cognitive support to follow through with prevention.
Musculoskeletal system	Decreased strength and endurance; decreased range of motion; pain; osteoporosis (must recognize hereditary and all acquired forms); asymmetric motor performance; overuse or repetitive activities on unprepared system; aging issues of decreased flexibility, strength, endurance, and balance; risk of falls; obesity.	Maintenance of exercise programs (endurance, strength, flexibility); fall avoidance practices; osteoporosis prevention or management—must determine type of osteoporosis and state of clinical/scientific information; use of proper body mechanics and posture; appropriate assistive devices utilization; environmental accessibility; consideration of ergonomically correct work and activity surroundings; use of energy conservation and joint protection techniques.
Cardiovascular system	Hypertension; atherosclerosis (similar risk factors as in nondisabled individuals); limited activity and exercise; deep venous thrombosis and resulting pulmonary emboli—more often an early complication; obesity; age-related changes of slower responsiveness to position or heart rate change.	Health practices to identify risk factors for atherosclerosis (hypertension, smoking, hypercholesterolemia or hyperlipidemia, diabetes, menopause, etc.) and initiation of prevention or management strategies; good nutrition; maintenance of exercise or activity programs.
Genitourinary system	Urinary retention or incontinence; change in urinary function from existing underlying condition (expected or unexpected progressive changes); progressive and chronic kidney filtration changes from poor or unchanged bladder management techniques; chronic urinary tract infections; kidney stones; prostate enlargement; urinary continence changes with menstrual cycle; urinary function changes from aging (e.g., reduced bladder capacity, decreased tissue compliance, reduced flow rate).	Monitoring of fluid intake and output; maintaining regular voiding schedule (e.g., intermittent catheter program, use of medication, timed voiding program); achieving acceptable hygiene program; participation in regular evaluation of urinary management (e.g., urodynamics, renal scans, postvoid residual checks); reporting of urinary habit changes; consideration surgical opinions when appropriate; education in the consequences of urinary management, pros and cons of suggested interventions
Respiratory system	Compromised breathing or cough due to underlying weakness; aspiration; existing obstructive or restrictive pulmonary disease or progression; breathing changes associated with aging (e.g., loss of reserve capacity, decreased tissue compliance); obesity; progressive weakness due to underlying condition; recurrent pneumonia.	Monitoring pulmonary function as appropriate and reporting changes; cessation of smoking or contact with secondary smoke; use of assistive coughing; maintaining exercise or activity program and healthy diet; education of management strategies in progressive conditions; use of vaccinations when appropriate.
Gastrointestinal system	Decreased bowel motility with increased transit time; esophageal reflux; peptic ulcer disease; constipation or obstipation; megacolon; abnormal swallow function; hemorrhoids or risk for hemorrhoids with bowel program; malabsorption.	Good nutrition with diet modification (e.g., consistencies, textures, tastes); maintaining and monitoring routine bowel evacuation with consideration of fiber, fluid, and medication; review of routine medications which could contribute to decreased bowel motility; avoiding overuse of bowel medications; monitoring diet history and weights; reporting changes in bowel evacuation.

[a] This is not an inclusive table and serves as a practical guide only.

Reprinted with permission from Brandt EN Jr, Pope AM, eds. *Enabling America. Assessing the role of rehabilitation science and engineering.* Washington, D.C.: National Academy Press, 1997.

ical work capacity decreases with age, although muscle strength generally is maintained during the adult years. The issues of arthritic changes are complex, but degenerative joint changes in weight-bearing joints are universally noted by 60 years of age in both genders and are hypothesized to be due to "wear and tear." Any predisposing factors (e.g., occupational activities, congenital joint malalignment, hereditary trends) may modify their onset or progression. Postmenopausal osteoporosis and aging-associated osteoporosis (senile osteoporosis) are age-related changes and can clinically present as the basis for fractures.

The impact of these known aging principles on a person with a mobility impairment is not well understood. However, it is known that persons with mobility impairments use more energy to perform mobility activities than their nondisabled peers (31). It has only recently been suggested through cross-sectional and convenience samples that adults with congenital or childhood onset disabilities may show musculoskeletal changes typical of advanced aging earlier than their nondisabled peers (21–23,32). These observations require confirmation through longitudinal controlled studies. Although risk factors may predispose a person to these changes, they are as yet unproven. If these earlier than expected aging changes are confirmed, they should be considered secondary conditions.

Therefore, we should anticipate that persons with congenital or childhood onset disabilities will progress over a disability continuum that includes age-related changes. The traditionally held belief that function is static is no more true for persons with disabilities than it is for persons without disabilities. As adolescents and young adults with disabilities transition to more independence, they and their families must be educated about potential age-related changes. Although speculative, the use of appropriate adaptive equipment (e.g., power and manual wheelchairs, ergonomically correct work stations) as a potential moderator of chronic wear should be discussed. Prevention strategies (e.g., energy conservation, joint protection, exercise) must be considered, and reports of change in function must be evaluated and treated appropriately. However, it must also be recognized that aging alone does not cause dramatic decline in function and that when dramatic decline occurs, specific causes must be sought.

Musculoskeletal Issues

Decreased independence (increased need for assistance) in mobility and self-care is a common complaint of adults with mobility impairments. The reasons for change are varied and may include those related to age changes (e.g., decreased endurance, flexibility, strength, or balance), progressive pathology or secondary conditions (e.g., pain, contractures, spasticity, osteoporosis and fractures, tethering, stenosis), or personal choices (e.g., use of powered mobility to conserve energy). The change in mobility is often a response to a secondary condition or age-related change. Falls also may be such a response. Significant change in mobility or falls should not automatically be accepted as a part of a congenital or childhood onset disabling condition in adult years; treatable etiologies should be sought.

Pain is a typical complaint of adults with mobility impairments, and therefore of adults with spina bifida (23) and cerebral palsy (17,21). Pain may be present for a variety of reasons, and it may be acute, recurrent, or chronic. Increased spasticity, weakness, falls, or progression of contractures or deformities can result from pain, particularly when pain is not reported because of communication difficulties or severe mental retardation. Complaints or indications of pain should be noted by the adult with the mobility impairment or their health-care provider, and evaluation, diagnosis, and intervention should ensue. Pain is often the reason for a change in function, living arrangement, or social interaction.

Pain is usually identified with a specific location, most frequently a joint. Most people report "arthritis" as the etiology, but these pains may originate from either joints or muscles. A good history and clinical examination will help sort out the issues and direct appropriate treatment. Back and leg pain complaints are common in persons with cerebral palsy (17,21,22) and spina bifida (23). Various forms of neck pain are frequently reported in both of these conditions. Although shoulder pain is a prominent problem in persons with spinal cord injury (33,34), it is reported less frequently in persons with cerebral palsy and spina bifida. Joint pain is likely to be related to recurring stresses during walking or other joint-loading activities (e.g., propelling a wheelchair) on normally or abnormally aligned joints that also may have arthritic changes. Degenerative changes have been noted radiographically in dislocated and subluxed hips, not always related to weight-bearing activities, in persons with cerebral palsy (35). Femoral head resection as a treatment strategy for control of pain in hip disease for persons with cerebral palsy is under review (36). Joint fusion has been an accepted intervention, but it may have a negative impact on positioning or on function. Muscle pain or tendinitis may result from functional activities and repetitive motions. Muscular pain is often noted by adults with spasticity as they age, and the spasticity often increases in response to pain. Appropriate management includes initial identification of the problem and its source, traditional interventions (e.g., analgesics, anti-inflammatories, therapy modalities), and re-evaluation of functional activities that may predispose to the pain complaints. There is recent interest in total hip replacements as a treatment option for hip pain from severe arthritis in adults with cerebral palsy, but its lifelong efficacy remains unknown (37). It is most important that treatment strategies are based on the person's history of function, that there is effective input from that person or their care provider, and that practical outcome goals are identified.

Although not common, nerve entrapment is also a cause of pain. The most common nerves and areas of entrapment as reported by adults with developmental disabilities are those susceptible to compression in the nondisabled population: the median nerve at the carpal tunnel and the ulnar nerve in the hand distally and at the elbow. Compression points are often related to use of crutches, transfer techniques, and propelling wheelchairs. Work-related or positional activities also may cause entrapments, just as in the nondisabled population. All hand pain or sensation change does not represent nerve entrapment. Often these complaints are actually problems of repetitive motion or are position related. Although they may be ascribed to carpal tunnel syndrome, they respond poorly to surgery (21). Appropriate testing (including electrodiagnostic testing) is necessary to determine their etiology. Where treatment options are similar for disabled and nondisabled adults, some modification of management will be required if functional independence is changed by or during treatment.

Contractures are a common secondary condition. Their impact on functional status or general health-care needs is variable. Increasing contractures, particularly when associated with pain or increased spasticity, may be an indication of progressing pathology. Aging changes include decreased flexibility, and the clinician must distinguish pathologic causes of increasing contracture through appropriate diagnosis. Charcot joints occur in spina bifida as a result of deformity and impaired sensation. In cerebral palsy, severe motor impairment is associated with scoliosis and other deformities (15). It has been reported in spina bifida that contractures are associated with partial or total dependence (23). Scoliosis seldom progresses during adulthood, but it can cause seating and pressure problems, impaired respiratory function, and pain.

In persons with cerebral palsy, spinal stenosis must be ruled out whenever significant functional change is noted, particularly for change in or loss of walking skills, increased leg spasticity, change in bladder habits, neck pain, vague sensory changes, and (late) change in arm and hand function (38,39). A tethering effect on the spinal cord also occurs, resulting in cranial nerve changes. Some early reports noted a higher risk in those with an athetoid component (40,41); however, more recent reports show these problems are present in spastic forms of cerebral palsy as well. Although it is generally held that stenosis is due to early spondylosis and compression, there also may be a predisposition to it in those with a congenitally narrow canal. Diagnosis is made through imaging studies, whereas comparative evoked potentials also may be helpful in determining neurologic function. Surgical decompression can prevent further, often catastrophic, loss of function but does not assure return of lost function, particularly in cases of long-standing compression with spinal cord atrophy. Postoperative management planning should accommodate change in functional capabilities and care needs. The presence of an athetoid movement component will affect postoperative spine stabilization and possibly head positioning and neck mobility. When no surgical intervention is undertaken, a frank discussion of possible respiratory compromise and the future need for ventilator assistance should be provided.

In persons with spina bifida, the presence of a tethered cord or syringohydromyelia must be ruled out when they experience changes in bladder or bowel habits, strength, sensory level, spasticity, pain (usually backache), progressive scoliosis, or foot deformities. In adults, an antecedent event such as in direct trauma to the back or buttocks often initiates symptoms. Prominent are diffuse leg pain with referral to the anorectal area and changes in bladder or bowel habits; there is usually not progressive deformity noted as is reported in children (42). Diagnostic suspicion should be high for tethered cord in all persons who had immediate closure of the defect (43). The diagnosis is confirmed through evoked potentials, urodynamic studies, and ultrasound or other imaging modalities. However, recent studies report that tethering, cord thinning, lipomas, cavities within the cord, and diastematomyelia are present in some asymptomatic persons with spina bifida so that comparative studies that show internal change are more definitive diagnostically (44). Treatment consists of neurosurgical intervention.

Osteoporosis is a secondary condition associated with mobility impairments, often referred to as secondary osteoporosis of immobilization. This is not the osteoporosis associated with aging (postmenopausal or senile), but a condition noted much earlier in the lives of persons with mobility impairments. Reductions both in weight bearing and in physical activity with associated changes in muscular contraction forces are believed to play an etiologic role. Other contributing factors for osteoporosis in this population include poor nutrition, medications (e.g., phenytoin, barbiturates), and endocrine-related problems. Secondary osteoporosis is a known problem in persons with spina bifida and in persons with cerebral palsy who are categorized as severe and have no effective independent weight bearing, although it is underreported (15). It has been shown that muscle activity is a more important determinant than weight bearing in persons with spina bifida (45). It has never been proven that passive, supported standing has any positive effect on secondary osteoporosis. Fractures of the extremities (not of the vertebrae as is seen in postmenopausal or senile osteoporosis) often are the first signs of significant secondary osteoporosis. Fractures are reported in adults with cerebral palsy and spina bifida (21,23). Unfortunately, treatment options for fractures are often limited because of the poor healing of severely osteoporotic bones with casting or surgical plating. Adequate pain management is of utmost importance. The impact on the individual of functional changes associated with the fracture needs to be addressed. Early recognition of osteoporosis and heightened efforts to protect against fractures in mobility-impaired individuals (e.g., appropriate transfer techniques, protection of distal limbs, fall prevention) are the best management approaches because at present there is no satisfactory prevention or intervention for this type of osteoporosis. The interrelationship of age-related osteoporosis with secondary osteoporosis is unknown.

In order to accomplish their daily routines, adults with mobility impairments often find they must conserve energy. The most practical way to do this is usually by making adjustments in the amount of walking or through use of power mobility aides. Although these adaptations are functional changes, they may not represent pathology, but rather normal aging effects. Normal aging and limited activity reduce physical performance reserve. Because mobility in the face of physical impairment requires vigorous effort, it is sometimes assumed that this alone provides conditioning. However, simply maintaining a daily activity will not enhance endurance or strength beyond that required of the activity. For instance, independent transferring maintains shoulder strength at the minimum level for that activity; it does not create endurance capacity in the arm or prepare one to perform weighted activities above the head. Participation in a fitness or exercise program should be considered, particularly where capability is marginal or waning.

Other Body Systems Issues

Pressure sores are a commonly occurring secondary condition in persons with disabilities. Although not common in cerebral palsy, they are frequent in persons with spina bifida related to their impaired protective sensation. The incidence and location of the sores is directly related to the functional motor level (23,46). Pressure sores are a persistent problem at all ages and do not necessarily decrease with age (12,23). Interestingly, obesity and burns are commonly associated with recurrent and chronic pressure sores (47), and then are themselves acknowledged secondary conditions in spina bifida (12). A study conducted of a self-selected population of adults with spina bifida noted that preventive measures were generally not practiced or were ineffectively practiced in this group (23). Osteomyelitis is a complication of recurrent or chronic pressure sores and ultimately may require amputation for management (12,47).

Urologic problems are reported in both cerebral palsy and spina bifida. In spina bifida, lifelong issues are similar to those for persons with spinal cord injury: routine follow-up, recurrent urinary tract infections, renal calcifications, and renal failure or impairment (12,23,47). Renal failure is a serious secondary condition, and dialysis is an effective treatment in this group. Urinary diversion is associated with adverse affects on both health and renal function (48). Clean intermittent catheterization is an effective long-term management strategy for properly selected persons with neurogenic bladders from spina bifida (48). Urinary incontinence persists into adulthood, can be a socially limiting condition, and is shown in at least one study to be associated with underemployment or unemployment (23). A survey of persons identified in a state registry as having spina bifida reported only a slight majority of the adults had achieved independence in urinary management (12). Neurogenic bladders in adults with cerebral palsy are only infrequently associated with upper tract pathology (49). Some women report that incontinence consistently occurs at a particular point of their menstrual cycle (50). Urinary incontinence can be effectively addressed through well-established diagnostic and intervention approaches. There are no available data that assess the adverse impact of urinary incontinence on social integration in cerebral palsy, but anecdotal support for this association is abundant. In both cerebral palsy and spina bifida, urinary habit changes may indicate other central or spinal pathology. Cognitive function also can affect urinary continence and should be taken into account. Self-imposed prevention strategies to manage incontinence (e.g., extreme fluid restriction, infrequent voiding) can cause other medical conditions. In older men, a high index of suspicion of prostate enlargement as the cause of urinary symptoms should be maintained. In both men and women, urinary incontinence should be identified and addressed regardless of age or other conditions.

Gastrointestinal conditions occur in association with both cerebral palsy and spina bifida. Usually they are chronic rather than new or late-onset problems. Changes in oral motor function affecting eating and swallowing may indicate spinal cord or brain stem pathology. Symptomatic Arnold-Chiari malformation should be considered in spina bifida, and cervical cord stenosis should be ruled out in cerebral palsy. Dental hygiene and health have been reported as problems for adults with cerebral palsy (11,51). Appropriate nutrition is a lifelong goal in persons with disabilities. Growth retardation seen in children with cerebral palsy persists with age (52). Obesity is a problem in spina bifida in adolescence through adulthood. There are higher levels of body fat in women and those not walking (53), and there is a correlation of increased body fat with previous hydrocephalus (54). Although children with cerebral palsy are reported to have multiple gastrointestinal problems (55), studies of adults indicate that these conditions are not common (16,21) despite anecdotally reported concerns (11). Constipation and diarrhea may continue through adulthood; megacolon can develop if management is inadequate. In spina bifida, it has been noted that assistance is commonly required for bowel management, even in adulthood (12,56).

The issues of women's health apply for this population as well, with perhaps even greater questions of access and preventive maintenance programs in addition to reproductive health. Generally, women with disabilities have limited participation in typical health maintenance activities such as routine pelvic examinations, Papanicolaou smears, and breast examinations (57). This is documented for women with cerebral palsy (50), and very likely to be true for women with spina bifida. Although architectural barriers (e.g., inaccessible offices, inaccessible examination tables) may be a part of the problem, attitudinal barriers also contribute. Women with spasticity or contractures may find a pelvic examination to be difficult, painful, and too hurried to allow their effective participation. Health-care providers often consider women with disabilities to be asexual and therefore, not in need of routine obstetric or gynecologic care. However, these women are typically able to conceive and carry pregnancies to term without the expectation of major complications. Although sample sizes are small, studies do indicate there could be associated problems with pregnancies in this group, emphasizing the importance of prenatal care (23,50). In spina bifida, back pain and deterioration in urologic status has been reported to be associated with pregnancy (58).

Latex sensitivity occurs in persons with spina bifida with the incidence of latex antibodies in this group approaching 40% (59). This sensitivity has been noted across disabilities. In children, risk factors for the development of latex sensitization are atopy and atopic dermatitis; risk factors for allergic response are elevated immunoglobulin E to latex, positive history of allergic response to latex contact, and frequent operations (60). This remarkably high level of sensitivity must be considered across a wide range of management (e.g., catheters, condoms, gloves).

Access to Health Care

Access to health care for persons with disabilities has become a more public issue. Access involves environment, attitudes, and systems. Architectural barriers have been addressed through the Americans with Disabilities Act, although accessible health-care provider offices and accessible examination and procedure tables continue to be available on only a limited basis. Attitudinal barriers involve both consumers and providers. Providers may have a limited knowledge regarding persons with lifelong disabilities. This lack of knowledge or understanding is perceived as a lack of caring and interest and as condescension. Through lack of knowledge, providers may in fact make erroneous assumptions of a consumer's cognitive status or ability to understand and make decisions. A consumer with a communication impairment (e.g., hearing impairment, speech production impairment) may need more time to communicate, require an interpreter, or require personal preparation time for the appointment, in order to have his or her needs conveyed. A consumer may avoid routine medical appointments because of bad experiences. Consequently, the consumer may seek help only late in the course of an acute medical condition or change and limit the options of care, increasing the risk for serious complications. In particular, consumers report that their routine health-care providers know little about their disability and its impact on health and function (32).

The present managed care environment may not authorize the increased follow-up care appropriate for persons with disabilities, or may limit access to specialists well versed in issues of lifelong disabilities. This is not to suggest that persons with disabilities are ill and require excess medical care. Rather it is to recognize the need for knowledgeable monitoring and timely intervention to prevent loss of function; to identify secondary conditions, age-related changes, or anticipated health issues; and to implement appropriate intervention and prevention strategies to maintain health and function.

HEALTH AND WELLNESS AGENDA

As a result of the steady improvement in medical care and social support systems during the past 50 years, persons with disabilities are healthy, conducting active and productive lives, and generally living longer. The medical paradigm must now shift from that of illness and disease to one of health and wellness. The health-care delivery system must view persons with disabilities through a typical health maintenance and preventive medicine approach. This requires a change in attitudes and care models. Both prevention and promotion strategies should be used: prevention of activities that lead to illness and disease (e.g., smoking cessation, dietary discretion, routine laboratory and examinations, protected sexual activity) and promotion of activities that improve general well-being (e.g., stress management, exercise) adapted to meet individual requirements and performance. However, positive health behaviors require social, health, and community resources. The more resources a person has, the more likely that individual will engage in health promotion and protective behaviors (61) (Fig. 38-3). Again, access

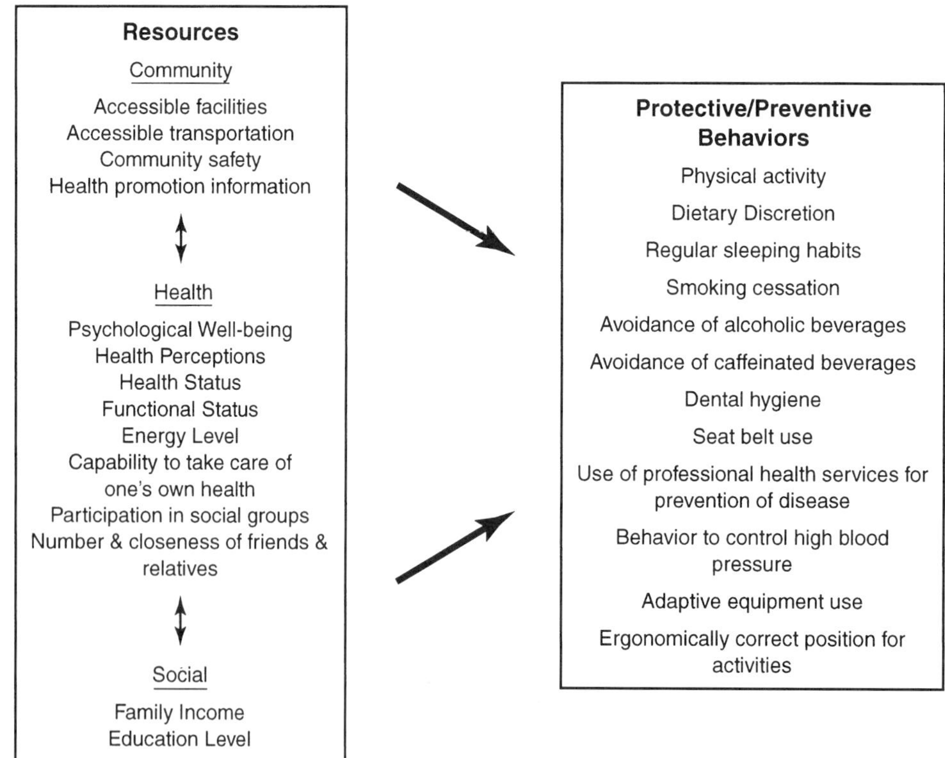

FIG. 38-3. The resource model for persons with disabilities.

is an important issue. Availability of information and the education of consumers are important, but not the most effective public health strategy. To participate in positive health behaviors, one must be interested, ready to make changes, have the needed resources, and a supportive environment. Early involvement of adolescents with mobility impairments in health promotion activities may pave the way for maintaining these behaviors into adulthood.

Because musculoskeletal conditions are the most common age-related changes and secondary conditions that affect performance, it would seem most reasonable to view typical physiatric strategies and interventions as preventive management techniques. Use of adaptive equipment, energy conservation techniques, joint protection, and ergonomic positioning may enhance function, decrease musculoskeletal complaints, and possibly prevent or delay some functional changes. Personal attitudes (of the person with a mobility impairment or their personal support system) may have to change before a person with impaired mobility will consider such assistance or be supported in considering the value of using more supported (less independent) techniques.

Exercise is a well-known health-promoting behavior, and its effects are also positively demonstrated in persons with disabilities (62). Benefits of a regular exercise program include improved fitness, weight reduction, improved mood, and improved sleep. It is also known that persons must be judicious in participating in exercise programs. Of course, care must be taken in prescribing exercise for persons with impaired mobility; they should participate in an appropriate program of exercise or activity, especially keeping in mind their risk factors for musculoskeletal injury. Regular exercise involving repetitive joint-loaded activities (jogging, running) started by young adults without disabilities more often resulted in discontinuation of exercise because of joint pain than for persons who started an exercise program in their middle years. Adults with cerebral palsy tend to report perceived changes in balance and then fear of falling (32), which usually improves with a general fitness program. Exercises, including strengthening exercises, are not contraindicated for persons with spasticity. Generally, adults and young adults with mobility impairments do not participate in routine fitness or exercise programs. This is as much from limited knowledge in this area as well as attitudes of care providers and persons with disabilities relative to exercise as a self-directed nonmedical activity. And, just as in the nondisabled population, priorities for persons with a mobility impairment may not include exercise and fitness.

SUMMARY

Adults with congenital and childhood onset mobility impairments are generally healthy. Not all adults have serious health problems, and many now recognize the aging process as a natural course of events. The most common age-related changes and secondary conditions involve physical performance and the musculoskeletal system. Prevention strategies require knowledge of expected changes and possible risk for changes, recognition of changes that alter function and require intervention, and an understanding of interventions that impact on function. This requires that a person with a mobility impairment have access to knowledgeable health care; environmental, communication, attitudinal, and systems barriers must be overcome.

It is time to reconsider the model of illness and disease for persons with lifelong disabilities. Particularly in the realm of mobility, a health and wellness model should be developed. Use of prevention strategies must be considered in childhood and adolescence to address the more frequent secondary conditions. Programs of fitness and exercise have been proven beneficial in nondisabled groups and disability groups alike. Health promotion strategies should be used for persons with congenital and childhood onset mobility impairments.

REFERENCES

1. Seekins T, Clay J. *Secondary disabilities in a population of adults with physical disabilities served by three independent living centers in a rural state.* Missoula, MT: Research and Training Center on Rural Rehabilitation Services, University of Montana, 1991.
2. Machemer RH. Biology of human aging. In: Machemer RH, Overeynder JC, eds. *Aging and developmental disabilities: an in-service curriculum.* Rochester, NY: University of Rochester, 1993; 1–23.
3. Evans RL, Hendricks RD, Connis RT, et al. Quality of life after spinal cord injury: a literature critique and meta-analysis (1983–1992). *J Am Paraplegia Soc* 1994; 17:60–66.
4. Gerhart KA, Bergstrom E, Charlifue SW, et al. Long-term spinal cord injury: functional changes over time. *Arch Phys Med Rehabil* 1993; 74; 1030–1034.
5. Pentland WE, Twomey LT. The weight-bearing upper extremity in women with long term paraplegia. *Paraplegia* 1991; 29:521–530.
6. Bauman WA, Spungen AM. Disorders of carbohydrate and lipid metabolism in veterans with paraplegia or quadriplegia: a model of premature aging. *Metabolism* 1994; 43:749–756.
7. Lammertse DP, Yarkony GM. Rehabilitation in spinal cord disorders. Outcomes and issues of aging after spinal cord injury. *Arch Phys Med Rehabil* 1991; 72(suppl):309–311.
8. Ohry A, Shemesh Y, Rozin R. Are chronic spinal cord injured patients (SCIP) prone to premature aging? *Med Hypoth* 1983; 11:467–469.
9. Whiteneck GG, Charlifue SW, Gerhart KA, et al. *Aging with spinal cord injury.* New York: Demos, 1993.
10. Krause JS, Crewe NM. Chronologic age, time since injury, and time of measurement: effect on adjustment after spinal cord injury. *Arch Phys Med Rehabil* 1991; 72:91–100.
11. Turk MA, Overeynder JC, Janicki MP, eds. *Uncertain future-aging and cerebral palsy: clinical concerns.* Albany, NY: New York State Developmental Disabilities Planning Council, 1995.
12. Farley T, Vines C, McCluer S, Stefans V, et al. Secondary disabilities in Arkansas with spina bifida [Abstract]. *Eur J Pediatr Surg* 1994; 4(suppl I):39–40.
13. Lollar DL. *Preventing secondary conditions associated with spina bifida or cerebral palsy: proceedings and recommendations of a symposium.* Washington, DC: Spina Bifida Association of America, 1994.
14. Maynard FM, Julius M, Kirsch N, et al. *The late effects of polio: a model for identification and assessment of preventable secondary disabilities: final report.* Bethesda, MD: Centers for Disease Control, 1991.
15. Turk MA, Weber RJ, Pavin M, et al. Musculoskeletal problems among adults with cerebral palsy: findings among persons who reside at a developmental center [Abstract]. *Arch Phys Med Rehabil* 1995; 76: 1055.
16. Turk MA, Weber RJ, Pavin M, Geremski C, et al. Medical secondary conditions among adults with cerebral palsy. *Arch Phys Med Rehabil* 1995; 76:1055.
17. Turk MA, Weber RJ, Geremski CA, et al. Pain complaints in adults with cerebral palsy. *Arch Phys Med Rehabil* 1996; 77:940.

18. Turk MA, Weber RJ, Geremski CA, et al. The reproductive functioning of women with cerebral palsy. *Arch Phys Med Rehabil* 1996; 77:979.
19. Whiteneck GG, Charlifue SW, Frankel HL, et al. Mortality, morbidity and psychosocial outcomes of persons spinal cord injured more than 20 years ago. *Paraplegia* 1992; 30:617–630.
20. Guralnik JM. Understanding the relationship between disease and disability. *J Am Geriatr Soc* 1994; 42:1128–1129.
21. Murphy KP, Molnar GE, Lankasky K. Medical and functional status of adults with cerebral palsy [Abstract]. *Dev Med Child Neurol* 1995; 37:1075–1084.
22. Turk MA, Geremski CA, Rosenbaum PF. *Secondary conditions of adults with cerebral palsy [final report]*. Health Science Center at Syracuse, NY, Centers for Disease Control & Prevention, R04/CCR208516, 1997.
23. Dunne KB, Gingher N, Olsen LM, Shurtleff DB. A survey of the medical and functional status of members of the adult network of the Spina Bifida Association of America. Unpublished, 1984.
24. Ragnarsson KT. The cardiovascular system, aging with spinal cord injury. In: Whiteneck GG, Charlifue SW, Gerhart KA, et al., eds. *Aging with spinal cord injury*. New York: Demos, 1993.
25. Stover SL, Fine PR. Spinal cord injury: the facts and figures. Birmingham, AL: University of Alabama, 1986.
26. Evans PM, Alberman E. *Certified cause of death in children and young adults with cerebral palsy*. London: The London Hospital Medical College, Department of Clinical Epidemiology, 1990.
27. Kudrjavcev T, Schoenberg BS, Kurland, LT, et al. Cerebral palsy: survival rates, associated handicaps, and distribution by clinical subtype (Rochester, MN, 1950–1976). *Neurology* 1985; 35:900–903.
28. Shurtleff DB, Hayden PW, Chapman WH, et al. Myelodysplasia: problems of long-term survival and social function. *West J Med* 1975; 122: 199–205.
29. Hunt GM. Open spina bifida: outcome for a complete cohort treated unselectively and followed into adulthood. *Dev Med Child Neurol* 1990; 32:108–118.
30. Eyman RK, Grossman HJ, Chaney RH, et al. The life expectancy of profoundly handicapped people with mental retardation. *N Engl J Med* 1990; 323:584–589.
31. Williams LO, Anderson AD, Campbell J, et al. Energy cost of walking and of wheelchair propulsion by children with myelodysplasia: Comparison with normal children. *Dev Med Child Neurol* 1983; 25: 617–624.
32. Overeynder JC, Turk MA, Dalton AJ, et al. *I'm worried about the future . . . The aging of adults with cerebral palsy*. Albany, NY: New York State Developmental Disabilities Planning Council, 1992.
33. Sie IH, Waters RL, Adkins RH, et al. Upper extremity pain in the postrehabilitation spinal cord injured patient. *Arch Phys Med Rehabil* 1992; 73:44–48.
34. Subbarao JV, Klopfstein J, Turpin R. Prevalence and impact of wrist and shoulder pain in patients with spinal cord injury. *J Spinal Cord Med* 1994; 18:9–13.
35. Bagg MR, Farber J, Miller F: Long-term follow-up of hip subluxation in cerebral palsy patients. *J Pediatr Orthop* 1993; 13:32–36.
36. Perlmutter MN, Synder M, Miller F, Bisbal R. Proximal femoral resection for older children with spastic hip disease. *Dev Med Child Neurol* 1993; 35:525–531.
37. Buly RL, Huoo M, Root L, et al. Total hip arthroplasty in cerebral palsy: long-term follow-up results. *Clin Orthop Rel Res* 1993; 296: 148–153.
38. Reese ME, Msall M, Owen S, et al. Case reports: acquired cervical spine impairment in young adults with cerebral palsy. *Dev Med Child Neurol* 1991; 33:153–166.
39. Turk MA, Machener RH. Cerebral palsy in adults who are older. In: Machemer RH, Overeynder JC, eds. *Aging and developmental disabilities: an in-service curriculum*. Rochester, NY: University of Rochester, 1993; 111–130.
40. Fuji T, Yonenobu K, Fujiwara K, et al. Cervical radiculopathy or myelopathy secondary to athetoid cerebral palsy. *J Bone Joint Surg [Am]* 1987; 69:815–821.
41. Kidron D, Steiner I, Melamed E. Late onset progressive radiculomyelopathy in patients with cervical athetoid-dystonic cerebral palsy. *Eur Neurol* 1987; 27:164–166.
42. Pang D, Wilberger J. Tethered cord syndrome in adults. *J Neurosurg* 1982; 57:32– 46.
43. Venes JL. Surgical considerations in the initial repair of meningomyelocele and the introduction of a technical modification. *Neurosurgery* 1985; 17:111–113.
44. McEnery G, Borzyskowski M, Cox TCS, Nelville BGR. The spinal cord in neurologically stable spina bifida: a clinical and MRI study. *Dev Med Child Neurol* 1992; 34:342–347.
45. Rosenstein BD, Green WB, Herrington RT, Blum AS. Bone density in myelomeningocele: the effects of ambulatory status and other factors. *Dev Med Child Neurol* 1987; 29:486–494.
46. Harris MB, Banta JV. Cost of skin care in the myelomeningocele population. *J Pediatr Orthop* 1990; 10:355–361.
47. Dorval J. Achieving and maintaining body systems integrity and function: clinical issues. In: Lollar DJ, ed. *Preventing secondary conditions associated with spina bifida or cerebral palsy*. Washington, DC: Spina Bifida Association of America, 1994; 65–77.
48. Koch MO, McDougal WS, Hall MC, et al. Long-term metabolic effects of urinary diversion: a comparison of myelomeningocele patients managed by clean intermittent catheterization and urinary diversion. *J Urol* 1992; 147:1343–1347.
49. Murphy K, Kliever E, Steele BM. Cerebral palsy: neurogenic bladder, treatment and outcomes [Abstract]. *Dev Med Child Neurol Suppl* 1996; 38:7.
50. Turk MA, Weber RJ, Geremski CA, et al. Health and functional characteristics of women with cerebral palsy. *Dev Med Child Neurol Suppl* 1996; 38:19.
51. Swedan NG, Gaebler-Spira DJ. Adults with developmental disabilities: cerebral palsy in adults over 40: lifestyle issues related to aging [Abstract]. *Arch Phys Med Rehabil* 1996; 77:979.
52. Ferrang TM, Johnson RK, Ferrara MS. Dietary and anthropometric assessment of adults with cerebral palsy. *J Am Diet Assoc* 1992; 92: 1083–1086.
53. Shepherd K, Roberts D, Thomas S, Shepherd BJ. Body composition in myelomeningocele. *Am J Clin Nutr* 1991; 53:1–6.
54. Mita K, Akataki K, Itoh K, et al. Assessment of obesity of children with spina bifida. *Dev Med Child Neurol* 1993; 35:305–311.
55. Pugliese JM, Edwards G. *Secondary and associated conditions of children with cerebral palsy or spina bifida [final report]*. United Cerebral Palsy of Greater Birmingham, AL, 1996.
56. Lie HR, Lagergren J, Rasmussen F. Bowel and bladder control of children with myelomeningocele: a Nordic study. *Dev Med Child Neurol* 1991; 33:1053–1061.
57. Nosek MA, Rintala DH, Young M, et al. National study of women with physical disabilities [draft report]. Baylor College of Medicine, Austin, TX, 1996.
58. Dunne KB, Arata M, Grover S, Bryan AD. Pregnancy in women with spina bifida-antenatal complications. *Dev Med Neurol Suppl* 1996; 74:7.
59. Tosi LL, Slater JE, Shaer C. Latex allergy in pediatric spina bifida patients: incidence and implications. *Dev Med Child Neurol* 1993; 69:17.
60. Liebke C, Niggemann C, Wahn U. Sensitivity and allergy to latex in atopic and non-atopic children. *Pediatr Allergy Immunol* 1996; 7: 103–107.
61. Kulbok PP. Social resource, health resources, and preventive behaviors: patterns and predictions. *Public Health Nursing* 1985; 2:67–81.
62. Turk MA. The impact of disability on fitness in women: musculoskeletal issues. In: Krotoski MA, Nosek M, Turk MA, eds. *Women with physical disabilities: achieving and maintaining health and well-being*. Baltimore: Brookes, 1996; 387–405.

Rehabilitation Medicine: Principles and Practice, Third Edition,
edited by Joel A. DeLisa and Bruce M. Gans.
Lippincott–Raven Publishers, Philadelphia © 1998.

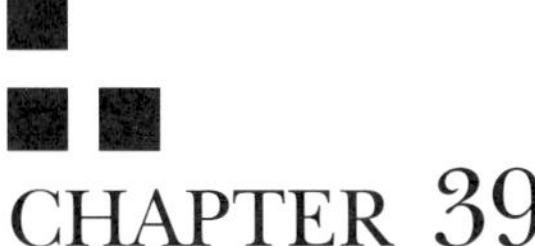

CHAPTER 39

Geriatric Rehabilitation

Gary S. Clark and Hilary C. Siebens

Aging, an integral part of living, typically is accompanied by gradual but progressive physiologic changes and an increased prevalence of acute and chronic illness. Although neither a disease nor disability *per se*, aging nonetheless is associated with a higher incidence of physical impairment and functional disability. Many of these functional difficulties occur from the interactions of decreased physiologic reserve with chronic illness. Recent research suggests effective interventions to prevent, delay, minimize, or reverse such physiologic declines. Appropriate roles for geriatric rehabilitation accordingly include not only intervening to reverse disability caused by specific disease or injury (e.g., stroke, hip fracture), but also contributing to preventive gerontology by virtue of promoting structured physical fitness (i.e., wellness) programs and early rehabilitation for common musculoskeletal disorders to avoid progression to disability (1,2). Unique contributions of rehabilitation to geriatric patients include functional assessment (including evaluation of underlying impairments contributing to disability) with realistic goal setting, interdisciplinary team care, and efficacious adjustment of therapy interventions (e.g., timing, setting, intensity) to prevent, reverse, or minimize disability (3). Given the burgeoning number of older persons living longer, described below, Rusk's observation, as modified by Kottke, becomes ever more relevant: "As modern medicine adds years to life, rehabilitation becomes increasingly necessary to add life to these years" (4).

DEMOGRAPHY AND EPIDEMIOLOGY OF AGING

Demographic Imperative

The context for the increasing interest and concern about health care needs of older adults is found in demographic projections of an expanding elderly population in the United States and other developed countries. At the turn of the century, one of every 25 Americans (4%) was "elderly," which was arbitrarily defined as 65 years of age or older (5). By 1994, there were 33 million people 65 years of age and older, representing 12.6% (one of every eight Americans) of the population (5). Current projections indicate that 68 million, or one of every five Americans (21%), will be 65 years of age or older by the year 2040 (6,7). The peak growth of older persons will occur from 2010 to 2030, when the majority of baby boomers will turn 65, and create the "elder boom" (6).

There is increasing recognition of differences in health-care needs and issues among subgroups of older people. Of particular significance from a health-care standpoint is the rapidly expanding relative proportions of the population age 65 years and older who are 75 to 85 years of age (old-old) and 85 years of age or older (oldest-old). These groups include many of the so-called "frail elderly," with a disproportionately high prevalence of disabilities and consumption of health services (8). In the United States as well as many other countries, the 85-or-older group is the fastest growing segment of the population, both proportionately and in actual numbers (7). Currently comprising approximately 1% of the population (3.2 million), the number of oldest-old is predicted to increase dramatically by the year 2040; projections range from 5.5% of the total population (12.2 million) (6) to 8.0% (17.8 million) (8). Among the 65-or-older population, the oldest-old segment will increase from the current 10% to 18% or more by the year 2040, with perhaps 1 million centenarians (8).

This demographic trend, whereby the percentage of the younger population decreases while that of the older population increases, is referred to as "squaring" of the population pyramid, and results from a combination of decreased fertility and increased longevity (9). Mortality rates in the United States have declined progressively, such that projected life expectancy at birth in 2040 is estimated at 75.0 years for

G.S. Clark: Department of Rehabilitation Medicine, Buffalo General Hospital, Buffalo, New York 14203-1154.

H.C. Siebens: Department of Physical Medicine and Rehabilitation, Harvard Medical School; and Massachusetts General Hospital, Boston, Massachusetts 02114-2696.

men and 83.1 years for women, up from 1990 values of 71.6 and 79.2 years, respectively (6). Elderly people themselves also are living longer: 1990 statistics estimate a longevity at 65 years of age of 15.0 years for men and 19.5 years for women; this is projected to increase further to 17.1 and 22.6 years, respectively, by the year 2040 (7).

The increasingly delayed occurrence of death at all ages appears in large part to be due to delays in onset and lethality of such diseases as stroke, cancer, and myocardial infarction, resulting from improved health-care interventions as well as risk factor reduction (7,10). Increasingly, people are surviving their initial encounter with these previously fatal diseases, resulting instead in chronic illnesses. This latest trend has been deemed the fourth stage of epidemiologic transition (i.e., the postponement of death from degenerative diseases) (11). These significant reductions in mortality are associated with an increasing risk for development of various chronic diseases commonly associated with aging. Certainly the incidence and prevalence of many disabling chronic illnesses increases substantially among older adults, including arthritis, osteoporosis with associated fractures, stroke, amputation, and various neurodegenerative disorders (e.g., Alzheimer's disease, Parkinson's disease) (7,8).

This demographic imperative has far-reaching implications for increasingly limited United States health-care resources and dollars: current national direct costs of medical services for older individuals with chronic conditions is in excess of $470 billion (in 1990 dollars), with a projected near doubling by the year 2050 (7). The old-old and oldest-old groups consume the greatest proportion of resources (8). A disproportionate amount of these health-care costs represent nursing home and other institutional care. In the 65-or-older population as a whole, 3% of men and 6% of women reside in nursing homes. These proportions increase dramatically with age, however, from 1% for 65- to 74-year-old men and women, to 15% of men and 25% of women 85 years of age or older (12). The 85-or-older group comprises 45% of all elderly nursing home residents. Not surprising in view of the preceding, the number of nursing home beds needed by 2040 is projected to increase from the current 1.3 million to over 4 million, with more than half occupied by people 85 years of age or older (8). From another perspective, however, 80% of the 85-or-older population is not in nursing homes, and half of those in nursing homes do not necessarily need to be there because they have chronic disabling disorders that are potentially preventable (13).

Compression of Morbidity

Fries has advanced the concept of rectangularization of both the mortality and morbidity curves, with the prediction of a mean age at death under "ideal societal conditions" of approximately 85 years (14). Fries notes that modern medicine has succeeded in largely eliminating early death from acute diseases, but at the cost of significantly greater medical services needed to care for people developing multiple disabling chronic diseases by virtue of living longer. By postulating that these chronic disabling disorders largely can be prevented or postponed (e.g., with regular exercise, healthier diets, elimination of smoking) in the context of a "fixed" life span, he postulates a concomitant "compression of morbidity" (14). He argues that death and disability will become increasingly unavoidable, with decreasing benefit of medical intervention. The implication is that health-care needs for older people will decrease because they will be healthy until shortly before their demise, and the predicted short duration of predeath morbidity will be expected and accepted with acknowledged futility of medical intervention.

These predictions have sparked a number of controversies. A number of researchers maintain that current mortality data support an expansion rather than a compression of mortality, with a continuing trend toward increased life expectancy at all ages and increasing variability of age at death among older age groups (15,16). Others argue that with this increasing longevity there will be a corresponding increased need for health-care intervention to try to minimize morbidity and resultant disability (17,18). Although a number of reports have documented dramatically increasing health-care costs near the end of life, it should be noted that these are costs of dying, not of aging *per se* (19,20). In fact, there is some evidence suggesting the incremental costs associated with extending life may actually plateau or even decrease (21). This debate comes at a time of focus on cost containment and intense discussion over the feasibility and appropriateness of rationing of health care (22).

There appears to be increasing consensus that the predicted exponential increase in health-care costs can be contained only by preventing or minimizing disability and health complications from those age-dependent disorders that produce the greatest needs for long-term care, including Alzheimer's disease, Parkinson's disease, osteoarthritis, hip fractures, osteoporosis, and peripheral vascular disease (8,20,23). This can be accomplished only by greater research support and efforts to delineate the epidemiology of disability, to determine the fundamental basis of age-associated chronic conditions, and to identify interventions for preventing or delaying resulting disability (13).

Active Life Expectancy

A derivative of research into longevity and epidemiology of aging relates to issues of quality of life, given the well-described increased incidence of frequently disabling chronic disorders such as degenerative neurologic diseases (e.g., Alzheimer's disease, Parkinson's disease), degenerative musculoskeletal conditions (e.g., osteoporosis, osteoarthritis), and multisensory losses (e.g., vision and hearing) (9). One concept that attempts to delineate quality of life for older people has been termed "active life expectancy," referring to the proportion of remaining life span characterized by functional independence (24). Initial estimates suggested that for each additional year of life in old age, approximately 40% of remaining life would be relatively autonomous and functional, with the remaining 60% spent in a disabled or dependent condition (24). More recent studies have expanded on the concept of active life expectancy to evaluate both physical and cognitive impairments, as well as their interrelationships (18,25). A significant gender difference in active life expectancy with aging has been identified (18). At age 65 years, men can expect 82% of their remaining life span (11.9 of 14.4 years) to be disability free, whereas women may experience 13.6 years of active, nonimpaired functioning (73% of their 18.6 years of life expectancy). By 85 years of age, these proportions change to 50% for men (2.6 of 5.2 years) and 35% for women (2.3 of 6.4 years). A further decline is noted by age 95 years, when only 20% of male life expectancy (0.6 of 3.2 years) and 10% of female life expectancy (0.4 of 3.7 years) is lived in an active state (18).

Although the increasing incidence and prevalence of chronic and multiple diseases with aging is well documented, there is no one-to-one correlation between either disease and illness (26) or disease and disability (27). A significant proportion of the elderly are limited in the amount or kind of their usual activity or mobility secondary to chronic impairments: over 60% of adults with functional impairments due to chronic health problems are 65 years of age or older (7). Furthermore, there are often fluctuations in levels of disability in older individuals. In a 2-year follow-up study, a number of older persons who were initially disabled had recovered their functional independence and vice versa (25). Also, the overall health of progressive cohorts of older persons has been changing. Future generations may well be healthier than current generations, partly due to higher levels of education and health awareness (25). However, Kane raises disturbing questions regarding potentially adverse economic, cultural and individual consequences of successfully overcoming the aging (and dying) process and urges ongoing dialogue to further explore these ethical questions (28).

In summary, an increasingly large number of elderly people are living longer and increasingly will develop varying (and changing) degrees of functional disability. The challenge to health-care providers, accordingly, is to try to prevent, reverse, or at least minimize functional impairments resulting from the various chronic and multiple illnesses to which the elderly are prone.

PSYCHOLOGIC AND SOCIAL ISSUES IN AGING

Ageism and Myths of Aging

Butler coined the term "ageism" to describe biased perceptions of older people by the younger population in today's youth-oriented culture, as well as perceptions of old age by the elderly themselves (29). There are a number of prevalent and misleading ageism myths (30). The myth that most elderly live in institutions contrasts with the reality that only about 5% do (12). The common notion that the elderly are not interested in sexual activity is certainly not universally true. Although there is a general change in sexual function with aging, with decreased sexual activity, this is related to multiple variable organic and social changes (31). The majority of elderly maintain some level of sexual interest and activity (32). Another myth that is untrue is that older people want to live with their adult children (33).

A popular misconception is that people experience a progressive decline in intelligence as they age. Although there is a decline in some aspects of fluid intelligence with aging (i.e., intellectual performance as measured by timed cognitive performance tasks, associative memory, logical reasoning, abstract thinking), crystal intelligence (i.e., intellectual performance as measured by tests of verbal abilities in vocabulary, information, and comprehension) is preserved (34). The ability to learn is preserved, albeit at a slower rate.

Ageism also perpetuates the myth that all older people become sick and dependent. As discussed previously, although there is a high incidence and prevalence of disease and often multiple diseases with aging, only a relative minority of older people actually become dependent (Fig. 39-1) (7). Of adults 85 years of age or older, only about 40% require assistance in activities of daily living (ADL) or homemaking. The majority of elderly are cognitively intact, live independently in the community, and are fully independent in ADL (35).

Cumulative Changes

There is increasing awareness of the critical interrelationships, particularly for older people, of physical health, men-

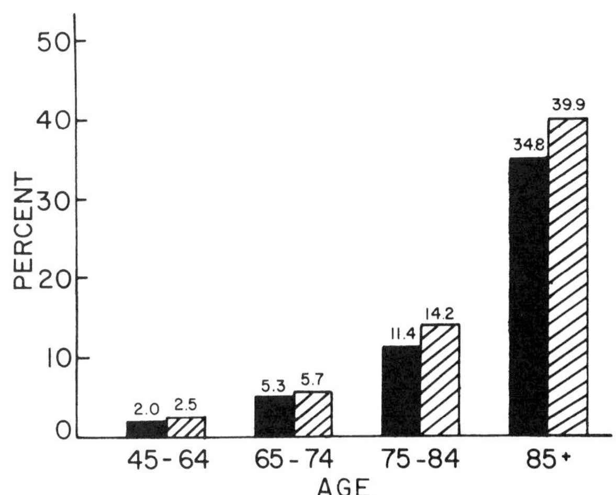

FIG. 39-1. Percentages of adults by age group who require assistance in performing basic activities because of chronic disease (*solid bar:* walking, bathing, dressing, using the toilet, transferring from bed to chair, eating, and going outside) and in home-management activities (*striped bar:* shopping, chores, meals, and handling money). (Reprinted with permission from Rowe JW. Health care of the elderly. *N Engl J Med* 1985; 312:827–835.)

tal health, and life circumstances. The emotional and life stress associated with major losses is well documented (36), and older people may be exposed progressively to multiple significant losses: job, income, health, functional ability and independence, parents, spouse, siblings, children, friends, social roles and status, and self-esteem. There are in fact few norms or defined role expectations regarding appropriate behavior or activities in old age (37). Bereavement, isolation, poverty, illness, and physical disability all are associated with a higher incidence of depression in older adults (38), which in turn is associated with decreased physical and cognitive functioning and increased mortality (39,40).

Social Support Networks

Social support networks include a wide variety of sources that can be categorized as informal (family), semiformal (church, clubs, family doctor, local pharmacist), and formal (health-care system, social service agencies, insurance companies, etc.) (41). Older persons may use supports from a combination of these networks.

Elderly people with children usually live near them and visit frequently; those who do not live close maintain telephone contact (42). Older people without children tend to maintain closer ties with young relatives or with siblings. It is important to consider the extended family, including cousins, in-laws, and others, with regard to support networks, rather than just immediate household members (37). Alienation of old people from their families accordingly also appears to be a myth (42).

Institutionalization of an impaired older person usually is the last resort for families, used only when all other efforts fail (33). Families, rather than the formal system of government and agencies, provide the bulk (up to 90%) of personalized long-term care for their disabled older relatives (43). This includes home health and nursing care, personal care, household maintenance, transportation, cooking, and shopping.

With advancing age, however, older adults tend to have increasingly limited and relatively fragile support systems. Dependency in aging parents results in significant physical, emotional, and financial stresses on their family network (36,43). An alternative support system may evolve gradually over a period of time as the older person loses family support (e.g., death of spouse and siblings, children moving away and unable to actively assist). Such a system might include friends and neighbors in an informal network to assist with shopping, cooking, cleaning, and self-care.

With whatever combination of support systems, a significant additional insult (e.g., onset of a new disease or complication) may overtax an already marginal arrangement. It is commonly observed that as the patient's dependence on the formal network of the health-care system increases, the informal or family network support decreases (41). Furthermore, if the elderly person is hospitalized for a prolonged period, the network(s) may dissipate and may be difficult or impossible to reassemble (43). The critical importance of maintaining the integrity of support networks is illustrated by the observation that for every aged impaired person in a nursing home there are two equally impaired older people living in the community (35,44). The difference is the role played by the latters' informal support systems, providing some 80% of their long-term care.

Increasingly, issues concerning family functioning are being studied. Even when family members are seemingly available to assist older persons, their support cannot always be counted on unless they too receive help. Fortunately, there are an increasing number of studies showing that patients' families can benefit from educational interventions to help prevent weakening in this crucial source of patient support. Caregivers of older patients with cancer and chronic pain are often frustrated, fearful, and anxious. Patient care improved when caregivers were provided with guidelines on what they could do within the home to help the patient (41). Similarly, caregivers of stroke survivors have benefited from more formal teaching (45). Nursing home placement has been delayed by a specific family intervention for patients with Alzheimer's disease (46).

Caregiver burden is another dynamic receiving increasing attention (47). Adding to the physical stress of providing personal care aid may be the unpleasantness of incontinence, or exhaustion due to a relative's sleep disorder. Behavioral problems, such as agitation or impulsivity with poor safety awareness, create proportionately greater caregiver burden than the demands of providing physical assistance (47). Physical and emotional health problems among caregivers have been documented, including depression and immunosuppression. Physical aggression on a caregiver by a patient is not uncommon and may lead to reciprocal abuse (48). Potential intervention strategies include encouraging use of other support systems to augment care provided by family members, as well as the use of respite programs.

Functional Impact

Physically impaired older people tend to become socially isolated, which can result in exacerbation of medical problems, functional deficits, and mental health problems, particularly depression (49). Other factors contributing to a vicious cycle of depression, withdrawal, and functional decline may include the stress of multiple losses, malnutrition, chronic ill health, pain, and adverse drug effects that aggravate depression (36). Unfortunately, dependency too often is fostered by the environment. A classic illustration is the acute hospital setting, where the focus is on routinely providing care and assistance, rather than encouraging self-care (50).

Additional psychosocial barriers can interfere with maintaining or improving functional ability in the elderly. Handicapping sequelae of ageism include devaluation of elderly disabled, by themselves as well as others, lack of interest among health-care professionals in their problems, and limited opportunity for access to appropriate rehabilitation services (49). Further attitudinal obstacles encountered among disabled elderly include the "right of dependency," perceived as earned by virtue of longevity, and the "apathy of fatigue," both physical and emotional, associated with multiple illnesses and hospitalizations (50).

The obvious conclusion, and why rehabilitation plays a key role in restoring function in disabled older people, is the importance of awareness and intervention regarding significant psychoemotional and social factors affecting their health. Many of these can be anticipated and prevented, or at least minimized in terms of their adverse effects. As with any complication, prevention is the best treatment.

BIOLOGY OF AGING

According to Shock, aging "represents the irreversible progressive changes that take place in the performance of a cell, tissue, organ, or total individual animal with the passage of time. As the probability of an individual's death increases with age, most of the changes associated with aging are apt to represent decrements in performance" (51). Strehler categorizes primary aging changes as universal within the species, intrinsic to the organism (i.e., not due to environmental factors), and gradually progressive, excluding stroke and myocardial infarct as normal aging processes (52).

From a clinical and physiological standpoint, normal aging involves a steady decrease in organ system reserves and homeostatic controls, in conjunction with an increase in prevalence of disease (26). Of increasing interest and focus in aging research is the degree to which these processes influence each other, and whether they are indeed interdependent (53).

Successful Aging

Distinctions have been made between aging processes representing "primary aging" (i.e., apparently universal changes that occur with aging, independent of disease and environmental effects), and "secondary aging," which includes lifestyle and environmental consequences and disease as part of the aging syndrome (54). A number of tenets associated with aging research are being reexamined, particularly with the observation that a pathologic process may exaggerate an aging process believed to be normal, even before the disease is detected clinically (54). There is increasing speculation that the nonpathologic processes of aging are distinct but not necessarily independent of the pathologic processes of disease (55).

Most studies of normal aging have focused on the physiological and biochemical changes occurring with aging, with explicit exclusion of disease. However, it is increasingly apparent that such factors as personal habits, diet, exercise, nutrition, environmental exposures, and body composition may have significant impact on observed aging changes (56). Rowe has proposed a conceptual distinction between "successful aging" and "usual aging" (57). He suggests that successful aging could be characterized by minimal or no physiologic losses in a particular organ system and would comprise a relatively small subset of the total normal (i.e., nonpathologic) aging population. The remaining majority of normal older adults demonstrate usual aging, with significant declines in various physiologic functions (56).

The significance of this concept lies in the implications for modifiability of usual aging by virtue of addressing such variables as level of physical activity, frequency of exercise, diet and nutrition, and environmental exposures (55). This principle is demonstrated in studies documenting the effects of exercise, diet, and drugs on the usual aging observations of carbohydrate intolerance (56). Rowe proposes that geriatric research into health promotion initiatives concentrate on increasing the proportion of older adults who "successfully age" by identifying and modifying extrinsic risk factors contributing to usual aging and decreasing the manifestations of "pathologic aging" by preventing or minimizing adverse effects of acquired disease processes (57). This would reinforce the previously described "compression of morbidity," with greater active life expectancy (14,16,18,24,25). Indeed, studies are now beginning to determine which factors distinguish high-functioning older adults from other populations of older adults (58).

Theories of Aging

With continuing research, it appears that there is probably no single cause of aging (55). The concept that comes closest to a unifying theory might integrate hypotheses based on passive (i.e., random) or active processes of genetic programming, perhaps with superimposed nongenetic mechanisms (e.g., environment, lifestyle) that could result in varying individual vulnerability (54,55,57). Certainly this would help explain the well-documented phenomenon of differential aging, whereby different people appear to age at different rates (55,58). Multiple levels of research suggest that rates of aging are affected to varying extents by heredity, lifestyle, environment, occurrence of disease, and psychological coping abilities (13,54,58). Active investigation continues in the areas of neuroendocrine pacemakers, as well as stochastic theories relating to free radicals and DNA damage (59,60).

In view of the apparent multiple mechanisms and levels of aging, it appears unlikely that there will be a single global intervention for life extension. Recent research trends are focusing on potential segmental interventions that may have significant impact on specific components of the aging process (61). One example is the attempt to arrest or reverse the decline in immunocompetence that occurs with aging, thereby delaying the increased susceptibility to infections, with resulting improved quality and quantity of life. The continuing application of new knowledge and techniques in molecular biology, nutrition, endocrinology, exercise physiology, and the neurosciences holds promise for future effective segmental interventions (13,61). A recently advanced hypothesis, based on chaos theory and derived from the field of nonlinear dynamics, applies the concept of measuring decline of complexity of physiologic processes observed with aging, with potential to monitor senescence and test efficacy of interventions (59). A number of studies also have focused on the phenomenon of apoptosis, which refers to the gradual and orderly form of cell death, with evidence suggesting that pathologic stimulation of apoptosis may result in a number of degenerative disorders commonly associated with aging, whereas inhibition appears to be associated with a variety of forms of cancer (62).

PHYSIOLOGY OF NORMAL AGING

The normal aging process involves gradual decreases in organ system capabilities and homeostatic controls that are relatively benign in the absence of disease (26). Although the older person progressively adapts to these changes without need or desire for outside intervention, the steady decreases of physiologic reserves make older adults potentially vulnerable to functional decline from acute and chronic illness (16,54). Characteristics of aging include the following:

Decreased reserve capacity of organ systems, which is apparent only during periods of maximal exertion or stress

Decreased internal homeostatic control (e.g., blunting of the thermoregulatory system, decline in baroreceptor sensitivity)

Decreased ability to adapt in response to different environments (e.g., vulnerability to hypothermia and hyperthermia with changing temperatures, orthostatic hypotension with change in position)

Decreased capacity to respond to stress (e.g., exertion, fever, anemia) (26)

The end result of these age-related declines is an increased vulnerability to disease and injury.

Problems in Study Design

Definition of Normal

A significant concern, in view of the heterogeneity of the aging population, is what is truly normal. There is much variability in rates of aging among healthy elderly and wide variations in individual performance. Further complicating any analysis is a distorted and dispersed normal distribution of skills due to frequency of significantly impaired function from disease (63) or environment and lifestyle (56). More than 80% of the 65-or-older population has at least one chronic disease, and half have two or more disorders (18). Should the relative minority of older people who have escaped serious illness be considered normal aging, as opposed to successful aging? This issue has led to criticisms of some studies as characterizing a supernormal elderly population (64). Katzman suggests that it is more appropriate to define populations of older adults to be studied in terms of either functional abilities or states (e.g., working versus retired, athletic versus sedentary), or by exclusion of specific impairments or disabilities, rather than considering global normality (63).

On the other hand, it is important clinically to be able to differentiate the physiologic consequences of aging (i.e., normal aging) from those of accompanying disease (i.e., pathologic aging) (44). Because detection of disease depends on determination that a patient is other than normal, it is critical to define appropriate age-adjusted criteria for clinically relevant variables in the elderly (64,65). Although many laboratory values do change gradually with aging (65), abnormalities should not be inappropriately attributed to old age (35). A number of age-related changes may resemble the changes associated with a specific disease (55). For example, an age-related decline in glucose tolerance is well documented (53). So dramatic is this change that most people over 60 years of age would be diagnosed as diabetic if traditional criteria, based on studies of primarily younger patients, were applied (64).

Methodology Limitations

A number of methodologic problems are associated with the study of aging. Well recognized are frequent discrepancies in age reporting, with a tendency to distort upwardly (63). This is coupled with difficulties in verifying reported ages, due in part to lost or nonexistent birth records.

A major problem in the design and evaluation of aging studies is the relative validity of both cross-sectional and longitudinal studies (63,64). Cross-sectional studies, although easier and less costly in time and money to perform, tend to overemphasize age changes. This is due in large part to significant differences in educational, nutritional, health, and social experiences of people born in different decades. Contributing further to this distortion is the high proportion of elderly in the United States who were foreign born, with relatively less schooling. This has major implications for studies of psychologic and cognitive changes with aging (63).

A further flaw of cross-sectional studies involves variables related to survival. A selective mortality error is encountered for study populations over 75 years of age, because they represent a sample of biologically superior survivors from a cohort that has experienced at least a 75% mortality rate (64). Another variable is the potential survival benefit of the relatively recent fitness movement, as compared with previous less fitness-conscious cultures (63).

Longitudinal studies tend to underestimate changes due to aging, primarily due to high drop-out rates from death, illness, or relocation. Some studies have experienced as much as a 50% drop-out rate over just a 10-year period (63). On examination, initial scores of survivors usually are found to be higher than initial scores of those who dropped out. This leads to questions of self-selection for relative preservation of function, and again, the issue of supernormals. Subtle changes in methodology over several years may introduce laboratory drifts that are difficult to differentiate from true age-related changes (64). Another problem whenever serial measurements are made is potential distortion due to learning or stress effects.

Mean Versus Maximal Performance

Another concern in the characterization of aging is that a focus on averaged or mean changes in various parameters can hide remarkable individual variation, particularly of peak performance (14). Consider marathon running, which although involving a very select population, does measure maximal performance. A middle-aged male runner with a time of 3.5 hours is in the 99th percentile for his age group, yet not until 73 years of age would that time set an age group record. Although there also is a slow linear decline in maximal performance with aging based on world age-group records, this is only on the order of about 1% per year between the ages of 30 and 70 years (14).

Effects of Age on Organ System Performance

There are several general principles regarding aging effects on performance of various organ systems (51).

Wide Individual Differences in Rate of Aging

Variation between healthy people of the same age is far greater than the variation due to age, and the range of variability increases with aging (14). Linear regressions show average changes with aging, but variation between subjects is so great that it is not possible to determine accurately if age decrements are linear over the entire age span, or whether the rate of decline accelerates in later years (51).

Different Organ Systems Age at Different Rates

There is great variation in the rate of decline for various organ system functions (26). As depicted in Figure 39-2, there is a 60% decline in maximal breathing capacity with aging, but only a 15% decline in nerve conduction velocity and basal metabolic rate. Another demonstration of this principle is the fact that localized cellular growth, aging, and death occur continually in some tissues and organs (e.g., hematopoietic system, skin, mucosa). Furthermore, longitudinal studies have documented that significant decline in function of one organ system (e.g., kidney) does not entail a similar decline in other organ systems (51).

Age Changes with Complex Performances

Complex performances (e.g., running) will show greater changes with aging because of the need to coordinate and integrate multiple organ system functions (e.g., rate, degree and sequence of muscle contraction, balance, proprioception, vision, cardiovascular response), as opposed to simple

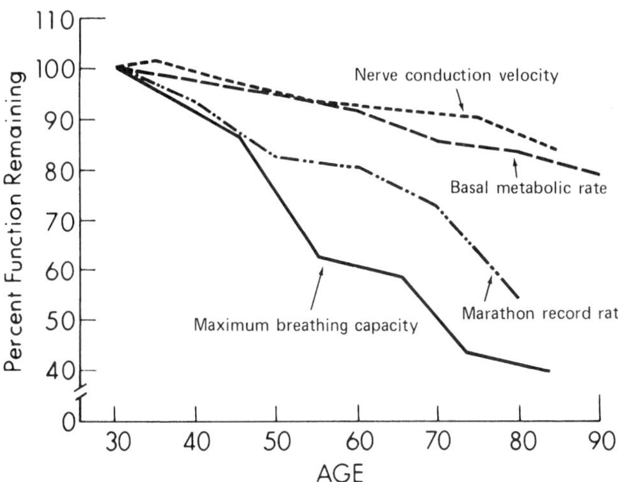

FIG. 39-2. Physiological decrements measured in cross-sectional studies approximate a linear decline with age. (Reprinted with permission from Katzman R. Demography, definitions, and problems. In: Katzman R, Terry R, eds. *The neurology of aging.* Philadelphia: FA Davis, 1983; 1–14.)

performances involving a single system (e.g., renal glomerular filtration) (34,51).

Age Changes in Adaptive Responses

Adaptive responses (e.g., to temperature change) are most affected by aging owing to a decline in effectiveness of physiologic control mechanisms (e.g., sensory-feedback), which is magnified with stress situations (e.g., sudden changes in environment, disease) (26,51,64).

Prevention and Reversibility of Physiologic Decline

There is little question that biologic systems, regardless of direct effects of aging, can be profoundly influenced by environment and lifestyle (26,51). Obvious examples include effects of smoking and sedentary versus active lifestyles. Figure 39-3 illustrates this concept, with the implication that the potential for significant decline increases with aging (26). In further support of this principle, mean hand movement speeds were found to be significantly faster in active 60- to 70-year-olds compared with inactive 20- to 30-year-olds (66).

The modifiability or plasticity of aging is demonstrated by studies in which performance can be bettered despite age, within relatively broad ranges (14). Physical training in the elderly can lower blood pressure and increase cardiac output (67,68). Muscle strength can increase 150% in nursing home residents under systematic resistance training (69). Evidence also suggests that exercise may reverse or retard age-related changes in synaptic function and nerve conduction velocity (70).

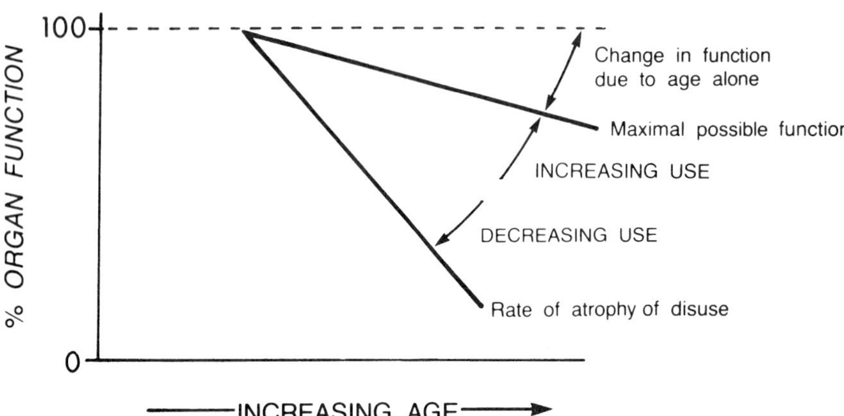

FIG. 39-3. The effect of conditioning and increasing age on organ function. The upper curve represents the maximal possible performance of a given organ system, whereas the lower curve represents the rate of atrophy when the system is never stressed. Organ function always occurs at some point between the two curves. The slope of the upper curve defines the change in function resulting from aging. (Reprinted with permission from Williams ME. Clinical implications of aging physiology. *Am J Med* 1984; 76:1049–1054.)

Functional Implications of Organ System Aging

The clinician must be aware of specific age-related physiologic changes to properly understand disease in the elderly because they significantly influence not only the presentation of disease, but response to treatment and potential complications that often ensue (64). Such knowledge similarly is essential to understand underlying mechanisms of functional deterioration secondary to disease and to formulate effective rehabilitation approaches (44). The following is a summary of clinically significant physiologic changes that occur with aging.

Hematologic System

Although anemia occurs with increasing prevalence with aging, there is increasing evidence that it is not a normal consequence of aging and should be investigated (35,71). Rather, anemia in older people is thought to be due most commonly to malnutrition, blood loss (e.g., bowel polyps, peptic ulcer disease), or malignancy. Another contributing factor may be the high prevalence of chronic diseases with older age, such as chronic infections and chronic inflammatory diseases (e.g., rheumatologic diseases, hepatitis) (44). Although the anemias associated with these conditions commonly are described as "anemia of chronic disease," researchers have demonstrated identical hematologic profiles with acute inflammatory disorders and protein-energy malnutrition (72). It is important to differentiate anemia related to chronic disease, which is characterized by normal or increased iron stores, from iron deficiency states, where iron stores are depleted, because the former does not respond to iron therapy. Recent research, however, suggests that hematopoietic growth factors may offer the potential for a new treatment approach (73).

There appears to be no significant difference between healthy elderly and their younger counterparts in hemoglobin, mean corpuscular volume, serum iron, total iron-binding capacity, vitamin B12, or folate levels; however, elderly have significantly higher ferritin values (74). There is no change in total blood volume or plasma volume with aging (75). Increases in the erythrocyte sedimentation rate and C-reactive protein levels also have been noted with aging.

The functional consequences of anemia can be significant because there is further reduction of reserve capacity. Symptoms of various disease states may appear earlier than otherwise (e.g., orthostatic blood pressure changes, change in anginal pattern with lower exercise tolerance) (75). A very anemic patient may present with a confusional state with the potential for misdiagnosis and mistreatment (76).

There are several physiologic changes with aging that can affect pharmacokinetics, particularly drug distribution. Decreased drug binding for highly protein-bound drugs (e.g., warfarin, meperidine, tolbutamide) may result in a higher unbound, or free, drug concentration with correspondingly magnified actions (77). This effect is even more significant for patients taking multiple drugs because of competition for fewer binding sites.

There also commonly is an altered volume of distribution, due to reduction in total body water and lean body mass, with a relative increase in body fat (77). As a result, water-soluble drugs (e.g., digoxin, cimetidine) tend to have a smaller volume of distribution, with higher plasma concentrations and greater pharmacologic effect (78). Conversely, fat-soluble drugs (e.g., diazepam, phenobarbital) usually have a larger volume of distribution because of relatively greater storage in fatty tissue. This may result in delayed therapeutic effects, with the potential for unexpected delayed toxicity. By the same token, prolonged drug effects are seen after dosage change or discontinuation because of the amount of drug stored in adipose tissue (77).

Gastrointestinal System

The term "presbyesophagus" has been used to describe multiple changes in esophageal function commonly observed with aging, such as delayed esophageal emptying, incomplete sphincter relaxation, and decreased amplitude of peristaltic contractions. Only the latter appears to be a direct result of aging, but it is without clinical significance; the other changes, with potentially significant clinical ramifications, are related to associated disease processes (79). Although decreases in gastric motility and emptying, possibly related to diminished gastric acid secretion, also are observed with aging, it again is not clear whether they represent true aging changes.

Specific age-induced changes in colon function include slightly decreased force and coordination of smooth muscle contraction, as well as impaired rectal perception of feces (80). The high incidence of constipation in older people accordingly is thought to be related to multiple additional factors, such as low dietary fiber and fluid intake, sedentary habits, and various associated diseases interfering with intrinsic bowel function (e.g., parkinsonism, stroke) (80). A variety of medications are constipating, including minerals (e.g., aluminum antacids, iron, calcium), opiates, nonsteroidal anti-inflammatory drugs (NSAIDs), antihypertensives (e.g., calcium channel blockers, clonidine), anticholinergics (e.g., tricyclic antidepressants, neuroleptics, antispasmodics), and sympathomimetics (e.g., pseudoephedrine, isoproterenol, terbutaline) (81).

Fecal incontinence in older people is due most commonly to overflow incontinence secondary to fecal impaction, although other common causes include decreased sphincter tone, cognitive impairments (e.g., from drugs, dementia), or diarrhea (81). Diarrhea among elderly patients results most commonly from fecal impaction, intestinal infection, or drugs (e.g., broad-spectrum antibiotics, digoxin toxicity), but also can be due to chronic laxative abuse (82). More appropriate interventions for bowel regulation include increasing diet fiber, using bulk agents or stool softeners, and avoiding frequent use of enemas or laxatives.

Despite these physiologic changes with aging, little effect is seen on absorption of most orally administered drugs (78). Although there is evidence of altered absorption of dietary thiamine and calcium, drug absorption in general is more significantly affected by concomitant administration of multiple drugs; in particular, antacids and laxatives bind to or reduce dissolution of other medications (77).

Hepatic System

The primary changes in the hepatic system with aging involve progressive decreases in liver size and hepatic blood flow, as well as slowing of hepatic biotransformation, specifically and most consistently microsomal oxidation and hydrolysis (78,80). This can have major implications for circulating concentrations of certain drugs and their metabolites, depending on mode of metabolism and clearance. Drugs with high first-pass clearance (e.g., propranolol, propoxyphene, major tranquilizers, tricyclic antidepressants, antiarrhythmic drugs) are cleared less effectively owing to reduced hepatic blood flow, resulting in greater bioavailability (77,78). These effects can be exacerbated by comorbid processes such as congestive heart failure.

Drugs metabolized by means of phase I biotransformation (i.e., oxidation, reduction, hydrolysis) tend to have prolonged elimination in older people (e.g., diazepam, chlordiazepoxide, prazepam), whereas those undergoing phase II metabolism (i.e., glucuronidation, acetylation, sulfation) generally are not affected by aging changes (e.g., oxazepam, lorazepam, triazolam) (78,83).

It is important to note that studies of drug elimination with aging demonstrate significant differences between people, contributed to by wide interindividual variability, and effects of such factors as smoking, alcohol, caffeine intake, diet, and concurrent use of other medications (78). These changes in hepatic functioning are not reflected in typical liver function tests (84).

Renal System

There are a number of age-related anatomic and physiologic changes in the kidney, including decreases in renal mass, number and functioning of glomeruli and tubules, renal blood flow, and glomerular filtration rate (85). These reductions in renal function have major implications for drug excretion, with prolonged half-lives for those drugs cleared primarily by glomerular filtration (e.g., cimetidine, aminoglycosides, digoxin, lithium, procainamide, penicillin, chlorpropamide) (77,78).

Although there is typically a progressive age-related decrease in creatinine clearance, a corresponding decline in daily urinary creatinine excretion, reflecting decreases in muscle mass, results in no net significant change in serum creatinine level with age (53). As a result, neither serum blood urea nitrogen (BUN), which is dependent on dietary intake and metabolic function, or creatinine is reliable for accurately gauging renal function in older people (86). It should be noted that these changes are mean findings for groups; there is considerable individual variation in the presence and degree of deterioration of renal function with aging (87).

Other common physiologic changes with aging include impaired ability to concentrate or dilute urine, impaired sodium conservation, and decreased ability to excrete an acid load (85). This erosion of reserve capacity allows maintenance of fluid and electrolyte homeostasis under normal conditions, but not with sudden changes in volume, acid load, or electrolyte balance. As a result, older people are more vulnerable to hyponatremia, hyperkalemia, dehydration, and perhaps most seriously, water intoxication (53,88).

Because of difficulty in concentrating urine in conjunction with a blunted thirst mechanism, a hypernatremic state with attendant mental confusion can result if an elderly person is stressed by higher than usual insensible losses (e.g., high or prolonged fever) with poor fluid intake (88). This is pertinent in a rehabilitation setting because patients often are engaged in vigorous activities and may become overheated or dehydrated relatively easily.

Just as older patients are prone to volume depletion when salt deprived, acute volume expansion from an elevated sodium load caused by inappropriate intravenous fluids, dietary indiscretion, or intravenous radiographic contrast dye can result in congestive heart failure, even in elderly patients without pre-existing myocardial disease (89). A further potential complication of the use of radiocontrast materials in the elderly is the risk of acute renal failure, which is exacerbated by the presence of preprocedure dehydration (85). Because renin and aldosterone plasma concentrations are decreased by 30% to 50% in the elderly, with increased susceptibility to hyperkalemia, potassium-sparing diuretics (e.g., spironolactone, triamterene) should be used with great caution (89).

Hyponatremia due to water intoxication may be the most serious electrolyte disorder of geriatric patients (53). Most frequently complicating an acute illness, the clinical picture includes nonspecific signs of depression, confusion, lethargy, anorexia, and weakness. Serum sodium concentrations below 110 mEq/L may result in seizures and stupor. The syndrome of inappropriate antidiuretic hormone secretion, with water retention and hyponatremia, can occur with infections (e.g., pneumonia, meningitis), strokes, various drugs including diuretics, or the stress of anesthesia and surgery (89).

Pulmonary System

Although progressive declines in pulmonary function are observed with aging, in the absence of disease of the pulmonary, cardiovascular, or neuromuscular systems, these declines are reflected primarily as a loss of reserve capacity without major functional limitations (90). However, impaired pulmonary function on spirometric testing identifies increased risk for several common causes of death in older people, including cardiovascular disease, chronic obstructive pulmonary disease (COPD), and lung cancer (91). Changes in pulmonary function observed with aging reflect both effects of aging *per se* on the pulmonary as well as cardiovascular and neuromuscular systems, with the cumulative effects of inhaled noxious agents, especially cigarette smoke and air pollutants, and infectious processes (92).

Progressive decline in a number of pulmonary function tests has been documented with aging, including vital capacity, maximum voluntary ventilation, expiratory flow rate, and forced expiratory ventilation (92). Rather than representing primary pulmonary changes, these declines reflect aging changes in related organ systems, which are stressed by the maximum volitional inspiration and expiration required to complete the tests. Examples include degenerative stiffening of the rib cage (i.e., decreased compliance) in conjunction with weakening of intercostal and abdominal muscles and increased airflow resistance from small airway narrowing due to decreased elasticity (90,91). Residual volume and functional residual capacity increase, related to the loss of elastic recoil, although total lung capacity remains unchanged (91).

Normal gas exchange requires both uniform ventilation of alveoli and adequate blood flow through the pulmonary capillary bed. With increasing age there is a progressive ventilation–perfusion imbalance due to collapse of small peripheral airways with decreased ventilation of alveoli aggravated by obesity and a supine position. Added to this is a mild degree of impaired gas exchange, resulting in a linear decline in pO_2 with aging (91). No changes occur in pCO_2 or pH, and oxygen saturation is normal or only slightly reduced (90).

The reduction in arterial oxygen tension is clinically relevant because it represents a further loss of reserve. Elderly patients are more vulnerable to significant hypoxia from a relatively minor insult (e.g., anemia, congestive heart failure, respiratory infection) because they are closer to the steep slope of the oxygen–hemoglobin dissociation curve (90). This vulnerability is exacerbated further by blunting of central or peripheral chemoreceptor responsiveness: both hypercapneic and hypoxic ventilatory responses markedly diminish with aging, independent of lung mechanics (75). Apparently related to this is the significant increase in sleep-related breathing disorders noted with aging (53).

Maximal oxygen consumption (VO_2max), an overall measure of physical work capacity or fitness, depends on pulmonary ventilation, cardiac output, peripheral circulatory control (i.e., ability to shunt blood to exercising muscles), and muscle mass. Although a progressive decline in VO_2max is observed with aging, this does not appear to be on a pulmonary basis (91,93). In fact, decreases in VO_2max in older adults with mild to moderate chronic obstructive pulmonary disease are due primarily to cardiac deconditioning resulting from limited activity levels (91). Regular exercise to maintain or improve fitness is critical with aging because it is possible to improve fitness with training at any age, and this is associated with reduced vulnerability to stress or disease (67,68,94). The tendency of physicians and society to emphasize decreased activity among older people, in conjunction with obesity and increased recumbency, probably contributes more to poor pulmonary function than aging alone (91).

Although most attention on the high incidence of pneumonia in the elderly is focused on immunologic declines, there appear to be contributing factors relating to the pulmonary system directly or indirectly. Because many pneumonias result from aspiration of the infecting organism, impaired mucociliary function and decreased chest wall compliance with impaired ability to clear aspirated material or secretions probably play a role (91,95). Other nonimmunologic contributing factors may include dysphagia, disruption of the lower esophageal sphincter, various esophageal disorders, and reduced levels of consciousness (92).

Cardiovascular System

A number of established tenets about the aging cardiovascular system have been revised, based on continuing research using more rigorous methodologies to exclude occult disease and control for degree of physical activity. As a result, it now appears that cardiac output at rest and during graded exercise is unaffected by age (53,93). Although resting heart rate does not change with aging, maximal heart rate with exercise does decrease progressively, possibly related to decreased chronotropic responsiveness to adrenergic stimuli (75). The common clinical formula reflecting this decline in maximal heart rate involves subtracting the age from 220 for men, and subtracting (0.6 × age) from 220 for women (96). Increased left ventricular end-systolic volume and decreased ejection fraction with exercise, in conjunction with the diminished heart rate response, suggest that cardiac output during exercise in older people is maintained through increased stroke volume by means of higher left ventricular end-diastolic volumes, using the Frank-Starling mechanism (53).

Another age-associated change is a decrease in the rate of early diastolic filling, with a much greater dependency on late filling through atrial contraction (40). As a result, older people are more vulnerable to deleterious effects of atrial tachycardia or fibrillation and are more susceptible to congestive heart failure (93).

Both cross-sectional and longitudinal studies demonstrate decreases in maximal oxygen consumption with aging, regardless of habitual activity level (97). However, physically active people show significantly smaller decreases in maximal aerobic capacity with aging than do their sedentary counterparts (67). In fact, trained elderly subjects may have greater maximal oxygen consumption than sedentary subjects who are much younger. Furthermore, endurance training, even when begun in old age, can significantly improve exercise capacity (68,94,97). Of clinical relevance is that the energy of walking represents a greater percentage of the total aerobic capacity with advancing age, such that walking becomes a very effective physical conditioning activity (67). Speed of self-selected walking pace was associated with maximal aerobic power independent of age in a cross-sectional study of 84 men who were 19 to 66 years of age (98). Therefore, greater fitness, even in older people, also may be associated with faster walking speeds (94).

Aging is associated with progressive, gradual increases in both systolic and diastolic arterial blood pressure, apparently owing more to loss of arterial elasticity than to neurogenic factors (e.g., increases in circulating norepinephrine) (75). This progressive increase in blood pressure with aging was long regarded as a normal consequence of aging (i.e., without clinical significance) (95). Findings of the Framingham Study, the Hypertension Detection and Follow-Up Program (HDFP), and the Systolic Hypertension in the Elderly Program (SHEP), however, have demonstrated that elevated blood pressure is a significant risk factor for cerebrovascular and cardiovascular diseases, regardless of age (99,100). Prevalence of hypertension in the 60- to 69-year-old group in the HDFP was more than 25% for isolated systolic hypertension (i.e., systolic blood pressure 140 mm Hg or above with diastolic less than 90 mm Hg) and 40% for diastolic hypertension (i.e., diastolic blood pressure 90 mm Hg or above) (99). Stepped-care treatment to maintain blood pressure under 160 mm Hg systolic reduced the incidence of stroke in these people by more than 50% in the HDFP and by 36% in the SHEP, with minimal side effects (100). Based on these findings, hypertension in older adults cannot be considered either normal or acceptable and should be treated with appropriate precautions against potential complications or undesirable side effects (101).

A final age-related physiologic change in the cardiovascular system with important clinical applications is decreased baroreceptor sensitivity (75). This results in a diminished reflex tachycardia on rising from a recumbent position and accounts in part—possibly along with blunted plasma renin activity and reduced angiotensin II and vasopressin levels—for the increased incidence of symptomatic orthostatic hypotension in the elderly, as well as cough and micturition syncope syndromes (102).

Immunologic System

Significant alterations in immunocompetence occur with aging, involving both cellular and humoral immune functions (103). Although the total number of lymphocytes decreases by about 15% in older adults, this does not appear to contribute significantly to the marked decline in immunocompetence (104). There is a decline in lymphocyte proliferation in response to antigen stimulation in older adults, as well as a higher incidence of anergy (103). Age-related shifts have been observed in the regulatory activities of T cells (i.e., fewer T cells with suppressor or helper activity) and monocytes or macrophages (105).

Changes in humoral immunity with aging include increases in circulating autoantibodies and immune complexes, with decreased antibody production (103). The latter is characterized by an attenuated response to immunization, with inability to maintain specific serum antibody levels.

The increased susceptibility of the elderly to infection is a function of both these age-related changes in immune function and the frequency of concomitant factors that further impair host defenses. The latter include diabetes, malignancy, vascular disease, malnutrition, and stress (103,105). Resistance to infection often is compromised further by altered local barriers to infection, such as skin breakdown or an indwelling urinary catheter. Common infectious processes in the elderly include influenza, pneumonia, urinary tract infection, sepsis, herpes zoster, and postoperative wound infections (103).

Of particular clinical relevance is the fact that older people react differently to infections than do their younger counterparts. There is a less active leukocytosis in response to inflammation; the total white blood cell count often is not increased, although usually there is still a shift of the differential count to the left (95,105). The older patient may have less pain or other symptomatology and frequently only a low-grade or absent fever (76).

Endocrine System

The endocrine system also undergoes major changes with aging. There is a gradual decrease in glucose tolerance with aging, although the fasting blood sugar level remains relatively unchanged (53). Accordingly, age-adjusted criteria have been developed (106). This age-related decline in glucose tolerance is due to reduced sensitivity of tissues to the metabolic effects of insulin, or insulin resistance (107). Compounding these physiologic changes with aging are secondary conditions that further reduce tissue sensitivity to insulin, including lifestyle changes (e.g., increased body fat, diet changes, stress), other diseases (e.g., chronic infections, prolonged immobilization), and medications (56).

Of clinical importance is the risk for untreated hyperglycemia, osmotic diuresis, and dehydration, potentially leading to hyperosmolar nonketotic coma or ketoacidosis (95). Certain drugs can cause or potentiate hyperglycemia (e.g., thiazide diuretics, glucocorticoids, tricyclic antidepressants, phenothiazines, phenytoin) (107). Control of serum glucose in older diabetics with oral sulfonylureas or insulin can be fragile, with significant risk for hypoglycemia. Even borderline hyperglycemia appears to result in accelerated atherosclerosis and multiple end-organ involvement, however (53). Of interest is the contribution of obesity and physical inactivity to increased incidence of diabetes in older adults, and the benefits of weight loss and regular exercise in improving control (57,107).

There are multiple other endocrine changes associated with aging. Both production rate and metabolic clearance rate of thyroid hormone decrease with age, such that serum thyroxine (T4) remains constant (53,108). Exogenous doses of T4 as replacement therapy must be adjusted downward, however, to account for the slower clearance. The primary clinical impact of altered thyroid physiology with aging is the need to maintain a high index of suspicion for the unusual presentation of thyroid disease. Presenting signs and symptoms of the older thyrotoxic patient may include palpitations, congestive heart failure, angina, atrial fibrillation, major weight loss associated with anorexia, and diarrhea or constipation (109). Goiter and serious ophthalmopathy frequently are absent (108). Apathetic hyperthyroidism may not be recognized until late in the course of illness: patients appear depressed and withdrawn, with clinical clues of muscle weakness, dramatic weight loss, and cardiac dysfunction (109). Signs and symptoms of hypothyroidism essentially are unchanged with aging, but the diagnosis still may be delayed because of the many similarities between the stereotype of senescence and the hypothyroid state (e.g., psychomotor retardation, depression, constipation, cold intolerance) (108). In view of the higher incidence of hypothyroidism in older adults, routine periodic screening of thyroid function is warranted (109).

The relationships between the hypothalamus, pituitary, and adrenal cortex remain unchanged with age, with preserved diurnal rhythm and stress response (108). Although cortisol production decreases progressively, basal and adrenocorticotrophic hormone–stimulated serum cortisol levels are unchanged with aging. Primary adrenocortical disease is uncommon in the elderly. Significant hyponatremia or hyperkalemia, suggestive of adrenocortical insufficiency, is not uncommon in the elderly but often is secondary to drugs (e.g., thiazide diuretics, chlorpropamide, carbamazepine) (75).

Age-related changes in gonadal function are well documented. There are variable and gradual declines in serum testosterone levels in healthy men with aging, likely due to partial testicular failure, but no indication for routine androgen replacement (53). The postmenopausal declines in estrogen levels are well documented, with clinical expression variably including vasomotor instability syndrome (i.e., hot flashes), atrophic vaginitis, and osteoporosis (35,95). Controversy continues over prophylaxis and treatment of the latter, particularly with regard to potential benefits of dietary supplements and exercise (35). The reader is referred to Chapter 58 for further details.

Thermoregulatory System

Older people have impaired temperature regulation, due to a combination of diminished sensitivity to temperature change and abnormal autonomic vasomotor control. As a result, they have a reduced ability to maintain body temperature with changes in environmental temperature and are vulnerable to both hypothermia and hyperthermia (88,110). The risk of hypothermia is compounded further by impaired thermogenesis (i.e., inefficient sweating), with potential aggravation by a variety of conditions (e.g., hypothyroidism, hypoglycemia, malnutrition) or medications (e.g., ethanol, barbiturates, phenothiazines, benzodiazepines, narcotics) (111). Conversely, diminished sweating is a major contributing factor in heat exhaustion and heat stroke in hot conditions. Hypohidrosis is aggravated by anticholinergics, phenothiazines, and antidepressants (88). Two-thirds of deaths from heat stroke occur in people over 60 years of age, reflecting this impairment in regulatory systems (111). This has major implications for rehabilitation exercise programs, particularly when combined with a tendency for dehydration (67,94).

Sensory System

With aging there is a gradual deterioration of most sensory modalities, including vibratory perception (primarily in the lower extremities), touch sensitivity (as measured by Von Frey hair perception and index finger touch–pressure threshold), and deep pain perception (112).

Deterioration of vision is one of the most recognized changes occurring with aging. The most common visual change with increasing age is a gradual loss of the ability to increase thickness and curvature of the lens to focus on near objects (i.e., presbyopia) and physiologic miosis (113).

Cataract formation, with opacification of the lens, occurs to some degree in 95% of the 65-or-older population. The elderly also are at significantly higher risk for further disease-related visual decrements (e.g., glaucoma, macular degeneration, diabetic retinopathy) (95). The result of these various changes is a loss of visual acuity, decrease in lateral fields of vision, decline in dark adaptation ability and speed of adaptation, and higher minimal threshold of light perception (114). These changes have obvious implications in relation to the higher incidence of falls in the elderly, particularly at night (115,116).

Gradual decline in hearing acuity (i.e., presbycusis) also is characteristic of aging, although again a number of treatable disorders can cause superimposed damage (e.g., wax occluding the outer canal, cholesteatomas, acoustic neuromas) (117). Older people most commonly manifest a conductive hearing loss, possibly due to increased stiffness of the basilar membrane, or distortion of perceived sound with increase in threshold sensitivity, narrow range of audibility, abnormal loudness, and difficulty discriminating complex sounds (95). Continuing advances in hearing aid technology make remediation of such hearing deficits increasingly feasible. Early recognition and treatment of hearing impairments is particularly critical in the presence of cognitive deficits to avoid adverse sequelae of social isolation and development of paranoid ideations or frank psychiatric reactions (117).

Neurologic System

Numerous changes have been noted in the functioning of the neurologic system with aging. The three most important areas of dysfunction accompanying normal aging include decreases in short-term memory, loss of speed of motor activities with slowing in the rate of central information processing, and impairments in stature, proprioception, and gait (34).

The major controversy over neurologic changes with aging concerns cognitive functioning. A significant proportion of the observed decline in fluid intelligence with aging may be related to a decrease in the rate of central information processing (34). Performance on timed motor or cognitive tasks, including abstraction tests (e.g., digit symbol substitution test), reaction time tasks, and other tests requiring speed in processing of new information, deteriorates progressively after 20 years of age. Although there are declines with aging in motor and sensory nerve conduction velocities and rate of muscle contraction, they account for only a fraction of these slowed responses (34).

The primary factor leading to an increased simple reaction time is slowed central processing (118). Choice reaction time, involving additional time for central decision making, is increased to a greater degree in the elderly than simple reaction time. In general, it appears that the more complex the mental task, the greater will be the age effect. Further evidence confirming age-related increases in central processing time includes increased latency of late components of visual, auditory, and somatosensory evoked potentials in older people (34).

Many aspects of learning and memory remain relatively intact during normal aging, including immediate or primary memory as measured by digit span recall, retrieval from long-term storage, storage and retrieval of overlearned material, and semantic memory (119). However, age-related impairments have been documented consistently in tasks involving episodic short-term memory and incidental learning (34). Examples include difficulties with free recall of long (i.e., supraspan) lists of digits or words, and paired associate and serial rate learning, for both visually and verbally presented material. There is evidence that these latter difficulties with short-term memory and learning experienced by the older people are related to slowed central processing. What these investigations indicate (Fig. 39-4) is that older adults are capable of new learning, but at a slower rate (119).

Because much of rehabilitation involves learning, these findings may have major implications for rehabilitation programming for the disabled elderly. This is particularly true in the context of superimposed cognitive deficits, given that intellectual impairment is an important determinant of the effectiveness of a standard geriatric rehabilitation program (120).

A final area of age-related physiologic changes involves posture, proprioception, and gait. In the peripheral nervous

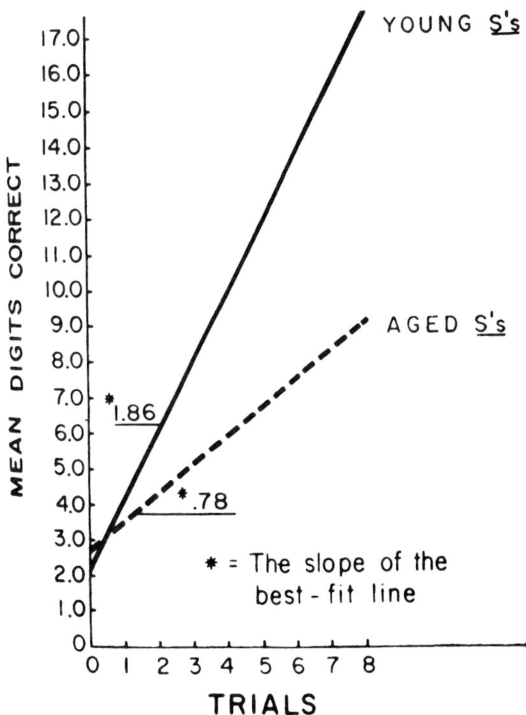

FIG. 39-4. Mean learning curves of young and aged subject *(S's)* asked to recall supraspan digits; the curves are plotted by mean slope and y intercept. (Reprinted with permission from Drachman DA, Leavitt J. Memory impairment in the aged: storage versus retrieval deficit. *J Exp Psychol* 1973; 93:302–308.)

system, declines in nerve conduction velocities already have been discussed. This may relate to the decline in speed of motor activities that occurs with aging, although as previously noted, this is influenced to a great extent by relative level of activity (66). Older people in general also are noted to demonstrate progressive declines in coordination and balance, perhaps related in part to impaired proprioception (34). Another factor that may contribute to these changes is the progressive loss of nigrostriatal neurons with advancing age. The basal ganglia play a major role in control of movement and regulation of muscle tone; in fact, the clinical picture of the aging process resembles Parkinson's disease in some respects, because older people frequently have a flexed posture, muscle rigidity, akinesia, tremor, weak voice, and shuffling gait (70).

This has significant implications for degree of mobility and stability, although there are a number of common, potentially concomitant, pathologic changes that may contribute further to gait problems in the elderly (e.g., vertebral compression fractures with kyphosis, arthritis, degenerative cerebral changes, cerebral infarcts) (34). Table 39-1 summarizes the major physiologic changes that occur normally in the aging neurologic system between the ages of 25 and 75 years.

Musculoskeletal System

The number of motor units decreases with age, as does overall muscle mass, muscle fiber size, number of myofibrils, and concentration of mitochondrial enzymes; these changes occur regardless of level of activity (70,112). Muscle strength is relatively preserved through middle age, with a 20% to 30% loss between the ages of 60 and 90 years. Earlier and greater decrements in maximum power output (i.e., work rate) have been observed, with a 45% decline between the ages of 50 and 80 years (70). Muscle endurance appears to increase or remain stable during aging; this may reflect fiber type regrouping, with increasing type II fiber preponderance with age (112). Significant gains in muscle strength and functional mobility have been demonstrated with a structured, high-intensity resistance exercise program, even in frail nursing home residents up to 96 years of age (69,94).

TABLE 39-1. *Major physiological changes in the neurologic system between 25 and 75 years of age*

Functions	% Decline
Vocabulary, information	None
Comprehension, digit span recall	
Touch sensation, two-point discrimination	
Simple reaction time	<20%
Hand or foot tapping, finger dexterity	
Rising from chair with support 20–40%	
Putting on shirt, cutting with knife	
Speed of handwriting	
Digit symbol substitution	
One-leg standing, eyes open	
Vibration sense, upper extremities	40–60%
Leg flexion	
Vibration sense, lower extremities	>60%
One-leg standing, eyes closed	

Reprinted with permission from Katzman R, Terry R. Normal aging of the nervous system. In: Katzman R, Terry R, eds. *The neurology of aging.* Philadelphia: FA Davis, 1983; 15–50.

The high prevalence of osteoporosis and degenerative joint disease (i.e., osteoarthritis) in the elderly again raises the question about normal physiologic changes versus ubiquitous pathologic processes (35,121). The physiologic changes and sequelae associated with osteoporosis are discussed further in Chapter 58.

Distinction of the disease osteoarthritis from the normal or usual aging changes that occur in weight-bearing joints can be made on a biochemical basis: with osteoarthritis, there are increases in the water content of cartilage and the ratio of chondroitin-4-sulfate to chondroitin-6-sulfate, with decreases in keratin sulfate and hyaluronic acid content—the opposite of what occurs in aging (121). There is a strong relationship between aging and osteoarthritis; however, degenerative joint changes in weight-bearing joints essentially are a universal occurrence in both genders by 60 years of age (35,76). These changes include biochemical alteration of cartilage, especially the proteoglycan component, with reduced ability to bear weight without fissuring, focal fibrillation and ulceration of cartilage, and eventual exposure of subchondral bone (122). The wear and tear hypothesis of osteoarthritis suggests that this process is the result of the cumulative stresses of a lifetime of joint use. Accordingly, primary osteoarthritis results from the stress of repetitive weight loading (e.g., spine, knees) or strain (e.g., distal interphalangeals), whereas secondary osteoarthritis may be related to occupational factors or congenital factors with unusual patterns of stress (e.g., congenital hip dysplasia) (121,122). There appear to be other factors operating, however, because there are specific hereditary trends. Differences in distribution and prevalence occur between genders and races (121). Obesity appears to be a risk factor for knee osteoarthritis in particular, although it is not clear whether this is due to a mechanical or a metabolic etiology.

Genitourinary System

Benign prostatic hyperplasia is an almost universal occurrence in men older than 40 years of age and develops under hormonal rather than neoplastic influence (95). Of note is that the median lobe of the prostate, which is not palpable rectally, can cause a ball-valve obstruction during micturition. Accordingly, after ruling out other etiologies, such as anticholinergic medication side effects, cystoscopy should be considered in patients with persisting obstructive symptomatology but minimal prostatic tissue on rectal examination to detect median lobe hypertrophy (123). Despite an increasing array of evaluative techniques, it remains difficult to predict which patients will progress to urinary retention or obstructive uropathy (124). Usual indications for surgical intervention (e.g., prostatectomy) include increasing obstructive symptoms, recurrent hematuria, bladder calculi, recurrent infections, and postvoid residual volumes greater than 100 ml (123).

Incontinence in the elderly, although increasingly prevalent with advancing age, should be regarded as a symptom of underlying disease; it does not result from the natural aging process (95,124,125). Normal aging probably results in reductions in bladder capacity, ability to postpone voiding, urethral and bladder compliance, maximal urethral closure pressure, and urinary flow rate (125). Postvoid residual volumes are higher, and uninhibited detrusor contractions occur more commonly. Each of these changes predispose older adults to incontinence, but none alone precipitates it. A further causative factor for incontinence in women is loss of the normal posterior urethrovesical angle, which can result from reduced pelvic floor muscle tone from normal aging, multiparity, or surgical manipulation (124). Other common causes of incontinence are listed as follows:

Confusional states
Urinary tract infection
Atrophic urethritis
A wide variety of drugs (e.g., sedatives, anticholinergics, calcium channel blockers)
Limited mobility
Constipation (35)

The primary clinical significance of these predisposing factors is that the new onset or exacerbation of incontinence in an older person is likely due to a precipitating factor outside the urinary tract (125). Usually, remedial intervention can restore continence without necessarily correcting the underlying urologic abnormalities.

Contrary to popular belief, although there is a decrease in sexual function with aging, most older people retain sexual interest and desire, and to a variable extent, capability (31,32). Older men experience a decrease in ability to have psychogenic erections and require more intense physical stimulation for erection; erections may be partial, and orgasm with ejaculation may occur without full engorgement (31). The force of ejaculation is less, along with a less intense sensation of orgasm. Impotence may be caused by a variety of diseases (e.g., diabetes, hypothyroidism) and medications (e.g., antihypertensives, phenytoin, cimetidine) (32). Treatment of impotence in older men has been revolutionized with development of the vacuum tumescent device and advances in penile prostheses (31).

Older women experience postmenopausal changes, including increased fragility of the vaginal wall and attenuation of the excitement phase (e.g., decreased vaginal lubrication) (31). Common sexual difficulties identified included partner's impotence, anorgasmia, decreased libido, and insufficient opportunities for sexual encounters. Despite these changes, most women continue to enjoy sexual intercourse throughout the life cycle (32).

VULNERABILITY OF THE ELDERLY TO FUNCTIONAL DECLINE

Cumulative Functional Sequelae of Disease

The effects of frequently multiple and chronic illnesses usually are gradual over time with cumulative erosion of organ reserves, leaving the elderly person reasonably functional with various adaptations, such as walking more slowly or taking more frequent rests (126). In reality, however, an elderly individual may well be only marginally functional with little or no reserve capacity, so that even a relatively minor superimposed acute complication or disease process (e.g., influenza) may result in functional decompensation (44). Of even greater concern is that this significant functional decompensation may be difficult to reverse even though the intercurrent acute illness is appropriately treated and resolves (127,128).

Older people as a group are more vulnerable to functional sequelae of diseases, for a variety of reasons. They commonly suffer from underreporting of symptomatology related to illness (26,35). Health-care providers may not be trained adequately to evaluate and treat symptoms and signs of functional disability in older patients, and may as a result not recognize the significance of vague and inconsistent symptoms. Older people themselves often exhibit ageism, thinking that such vague symptoms are a natural result of aging (35,129). As a result, the disease process may become quite advanced before care is sought, making treatment much more difficult.

From the older person's viewpoint, the available system of care may seem unresponsive (26). Physician offices frequently are inconveniently located, with inadequate parking and poor access for the physically impaired. A brief encounter with a physician may not allow for development of rapport and full elaboration of symptoms. Busy office staff may be perceived as uninterested or discourteous.

Other issues may contribute further to underreporting of illness. There may be denial of disease coupled with fear of consequences, especially financial (35). Depression is common among older people and may result in the attitude, "What have I got to gain?" (26,40). Increasing isolation, with decreasing opportunities for others to observe and react to changes in appearance or behavior, are additional barriers. Finally, older people may not recognize significant symptoms or seek medical attention because of cognitive impairments, which not infrequently may be secondary to or aggravated by an underlying and potentially reversible disease process (35).

There is often an altered response to illness in the elderly, which contributes to delayed or incorrect diagnosis (76). Many specific diseases present with atypical and nonclassic signs and symptoms. For example, the presentation of a myocardial infarction in an elderly person is less likely to include classic retrosternal chest pain; more often it will involve nausea, dizziness, syncope, or congestive heart failure with decreased activity tolerance (76). Furthermore, a wide variety of diseases may present with similar nonspecific symptoms, including confusion, weakness, weight loss, and general "failure to thrive" (35,130). Accordingly, the differential diagnosis of possible disease processes is much wider in the elderly.

Further confounding accurate elucidation of the underlying illness are the frequent changes in disease patterns and distribution (26). Abnormalities in one organ system often are accompanied by resultant abnormalities in other organ systems. Traditional medical training focuses on disease recognition and treatment in a relatively young population, with emphasis on synthesizing multiple signs and symptoms into a single unifying diagnosis (26,131). The elderly more typically have concurrent symptomatology relating to multiple diseases. Although accurate diagnosis is important, the functional impact of each disease, particularly the cumulative and additive impact of multiple diseases, must be determined (35,44).

There is an increased frequency of many chronic diseases in this population, including anemia, osteoarthritis, osteoporosis, cardiovascular disease, malignancy, and malnutrition. Table 39-2 lists types and patterns of disability associated with various chronic conditions. Palliation and prevention of secondary complications frequently is a more appropriate and realistic goal than is cure of the primary condition (26). There often are atypical and potentially confusing behaviors and responses to treatment, however, secondary to coexisting diseases and decreased functional reserves of multiple organ systems (e.g., affecting drug metabolism and distribution) (77).

Older people also are more prone to a wide variety of concomitant and complicating diseases, which may further cloud diagnosis and treatment decisions. Examples include thrombophlebitis, dehydration, fluid and electrolyte disturbances, adverse drug interactions or toxicity, decubitus ulcers, pneumonia, and general deleterious effects of deconditioning due to inactivity, which occurs earlier and with greater severity in older adults (132–134).

Given these multiple factors, it may prove increasingly important to use different models of disease presentation in older persons (131). In one series of proposed models, the Medical Model, in which the patient's symptoms and signs are fully explained by one disease, is the most basic. The Synergistic Morbidity Model portrays the functional loss that may have suddenly occurred as the result of additive effects of several diseases. In the Attribution Model, a patient might attribute a deterioration in health to an already diagnosed chronic illness when in fact another undiagnosed problem is present (e.g., hypothyroidism superimposed on stroke). In the more complex Causal Chain Model, a medical–psychiatric interaction occurs in which one illness causes another as well as causing functional decrements, with the presenting complaint representing the proverbial last straw of decompensation. Finally, in the Unmasking

TABLE 39-2. *Chronic conditions associated with disability in older adults*

	Association with disability in:			
Characteristics entered into each model	Mobility/exercise tolerance demanding tasks	Upper extremity tasks	Complex household management tasks	Self-care tasks
Age	●		●	
Gender (male)		●		
Angina (nitroglycerine usc)	●	●	●	
Myocardial infarction				●
Congestive heart failure	●			
Stroke	●	●	●	●
Claudication	●		●	
Arthritis	●	●	●	●
Lung disease	●		●	
Depressive symptomology	●	●	●	●
Hearing impairment			●	●
Cognitive impairment: digit symbol substitution	●		●	●
Cancer	●			
Weakness	●	●	●	●
Balance problems, last year	●	●		●
Dizziness, last two weeks				●
BMI (body mass index)[a]		●		●
Weight[a]	●			

● Indicates significant association ($p < 0.01$), adjusting for clinical sites, Minimental State Exam Score, hypertension, visual impairment, diabetes, left ventricular systolic dysfunction by echocardiography, carotid stenosis, grip strength as well as variables in the table.

[a] Increase of 10 lbs.

Reprinted with permission from Fried LP, Guralnik JM. Disability in older adults: evidence regarding significance, etiology, and risk. *J Am Geriatr Soc* 1997; 45:92–100.

Event Model, a stressful external event unmasks an underlying, stable, or slowly progressive chronic condition that had previously been well compensated and unrecognized (131). Models such as these illustrate well the significant and varying complexity of determining exactly what is occurring (and why) in the health of an older person and may be clinically useful in more rapidly and accurately diagnosing and treating older persons with multiple interacting problems.

Effects of Acute Hospitalization

There is increasing recognition of the multiple deleterious effects of acute hospitalization on older people, separate and distinct from sequelae due primarily to their presenting illness (127,135,136). Disorientation due to the foreign hospital environment and relatively infrequent and brief interactions with unfamiliar health-care personnel may contribute to bizarre and inappropriate behavior, including agitation (136). Contributing to this may be relative sensory and social isolation with few familiar environmental cues or social interactions, especially if the patient is confined to a private room or intensive care setting (126). Moreover, there are atypical routines and schedules (e.g., bowel and bladder procedures, blood drawing, vital sign checks at odd hours), which, coupled with unusual noises (e.g., paging, other patients, machines), may contribute to insomnia. A patient with insomnia typically is treated with a sedative medication, which may begin a cycle or cascade of drug side effects and interactions that may adversely affect the patient's health (128,135).

Increased incidence of medical and iatrogenic complications in the older adult is well documented (26,77,131). Drug side effects, complications, and toxicity, together with adverse interactions related to polypharmacy, make up a large proportion of such morbidity (26). There also is a greater frequency of diagnostic and therapeutic misadventures in this age group, related in part to decreased organ reserve with resultant increased vulnerability (135).

There also are a variety of emotional sequelae of hospitalization that may affect health and functional status. Anxiety and confusion relating to the underlying illness and prognosis or just to hospitalization itself may interfere with cooperation with medical treatment or therapy programs (36,49). Depression from similar origins may result in dependency and poor motivation to cooperate or improve function (39). Functional dependency frequently is reinforced during acute hospitalizations, both by the older people who expect hospital staff to assist and by hospital staff who tend routinely to perform self-care tasks without taking the extra time to supervise the patient in performing his or her own self-care (50,127). Documented functional decline after hospitalization for acute medical illnesses also may result from other, as yet unknown, factors (135). On the other hand, brief hospitalization actually may serve as a form of respite for the elderly patient, providing greater social interaction and attention (126).

In addition to significant implications for health care in the hospital setting, these sequelae related to acute hospitalization often affect social support systems and discharge disposition (43,127). The elderly patient may experience loss of confidence or motivation as a result of multiple insults and complications, coupled with erosion of functional abilities from deconditioning (133,134). This in and of itself will put greater stress on often relatively fragile social support systems, making it more difficult for elderly patients to return home to their prior living situation (43).

To try to address these problems, several randomized trials have investigated alternative models attempting to change the organization of care (and outcomes) for older persons during hospitalization. Use of a geriatric consultation team approach did not yield improved outcomes (137). In another randomized clinical trial of 651 patients 70 years of age and older, the experimental patients received care on a special unit, which had the additional components of daily team conferences, active discharge planning, and use of therapy staff for functional training—the core components on typical acute rehabilitation units. Patients in the experimental group were discharged at higher functional levels, and fewer were discharged to skilled nursing facilities (14% versus 22%). Neither cost of hospitalization nor length of stay was increased (138). These studies suggest potential strategies to improve acute hospital care for older persons.

Effects of Deconditioning

Deconditioning can be defined as the multiple changes in physiology induced by physical inactivity and reversed through physical activity (134). Basic exercise physiology is covered well in the literature (139) and is reviewed in Chapter 28. In brief, changes commonly associated with deconditioning are listed as follows:

Decreased maximum oxygen uptake
Shortened time to fatigue during submaximal work
Decreased muscle strength
Decrements in reaction time, balance, and flexibility (134)

That these changes are reversible in older adults has been amply demonstrated through effective muscle-strengthening resistance training programs and comprehensive exercise programs in both nursing homes and the community (69,96,140,141). These programs include exercises for flexibility, muscle strength, and aerobic endurance.

The functional consequences of these changes in older people may be of major clinical significance (132) and may be confused with changes intrinsic to aging or changes from diseases (134). Deconditioning *per se* may account for functional losses when certain threshold values for physical performance are crossed (142). Quadriceps weakness may progress to the point of dependency in getting in and out of a car solely from progressive deconditioning, not related to intrinsic aging or new onset of disease (133). Multiple factors associated with falls may originate from deconditioning or may be exacerbated by deconditioning (143,144). For people living in the community, factors associated with falls include impairments in static balance, leg strength, and hip and ankle flexibility (145,146). In nursing home patients, falls are associated with decreased muscle strength at the knees and ankles (147,148). Weakened muscles also may contribute to other injuries and pain syndromes by allowing abnormal forces to act on bone, joints, ligaments, and tendons. In addition, lack of exercise is being viewed increasingly as a risk factor not only for functional loss but for onset of various disease processes, including cardiovascular disease and diabetes, among others (149).

Deconditioning affecting older people can be differentiated into acute inactivity secondary to bed rest (such as during acute illness) and chronic inactivity from sedentary lifestyles (134). A variety of types and combinations of exercises are available to treat deconditioning; a precise prescription of a therapeutic exercise and activity program, including appropriate precautions and instruction, is essential (94,96). As observed by DeVries, a pioneer in exercise training in older adults, telling patients to get some exercise is like telling them to go take drugs (139). For details on appropriate programming, the reader is referred to texts such as Prime Moves (150), which are dedicated specifically to this topic. Specific strengthening programs have been successfully tested in very elderly patients with associated increased levels of spontaneous physical activity (151). For acutely ill patients it is important to mobilize them as soon as feasible and maintain activity at (almost) all costs.

Psychological issues in maintaining exercise habits are being studied increasingly (96). Currently health professionals can help persons increase their physical activity levels by discussing the issue openly and then helping the patient decide what approach may be most appropriate. One option may be group classes, which offer the benefits of social interaction and support, and perhaps even friendly competition. Exercising on their own at home may be preferable for some, especially if they are self-conscious about their own abilities (152).

MEDICAL MANAGEMENT CONCERNS IN THE DISABLED ELDERLY

Reassessment of Medical Status

Transfer of a patient from an acute medical or surgical service to a rehabilitation unit has been identified as an opportunity for a fresh and objective reassessment of medical status (153). Such an appraisal is even more critical in geriatric rehabilitation and should include confirming the accuracy of referral diagnoses, evaluating for previously unrecognized conditions, and reviewing medications for continuing appropriateness (131). Often a patient's physiologic status has markedly improved or stabilized by the time of transfer, warranting consideration of altering dosage or discontinuing certain medications.

Avoiding Adverse Drug Effects

The incidence of adverse drug reactions approaches 25% in people older than 80 years of age (26). Adverse drug reactions account for 11% to 20% of hospitalizations in people older than 65 years of age and are a frequent cause of mental deterioration (86,154,155). The reasons for drug problems in older adults revolve around five key interrelated areas:

1. Polypharmacy
2. Medications not used as prescribed
3. Increased susceptibility to adverse reactions
4. Altered pharmacokinetics
5. Altered receptor sensitivity

Polypharmacy

Polypharmacy is frequent in older people and often compounded by the frequent use of nonprescription drugs, resulting in preventable adverse drug reactions and unnecessary financial costs (156,157). The average hospitalized Medicare patient receives 10 prescription drugs (84), whereas reviews of institutionalized patients document that up to half of all medication profiles show the potential for clinically important drug interactions (86). Medication histories obtained by physicians often are inaccurate in both inpatient and outpatient settings (158,159), related in part to lack of questioning and underreporting of over-the-counter (OTC) medications, which are used almost as much as prescription medications by older adults (160,161). Over 50% of OTC medications are oral analgesics, with the remainder consisting of cough-and-cold preparations, vitamins, antacids, and laxatives (159,161).

The hospital setting is an excellent one in which to discontinue drugs of questionable value because careful monitoring is possible. Accordingly, all medications should be reviewed carefully on admission, and regularly thereafter. In addition to OTC medications, special attention should be directed to digitalis preparations, NSAIDs, and psychotropic medications (77).

In addition to unawareness of concurrent medications, other factors have been identified as potentially influencing prescribing habits and contributing to polypharmacy in older people. These include pharmaceutical advertising, particularly involving new drugs inadequately tested in older people, and patient and family expectations or even demands for treatment, usually in the form of a prescription (83,157). In one nursing home study, treatments (i.e., medication prescriptions) occurred more often if a patient's problem produced ongoing discomfort for the staff (e.g., agitation); undertreated were conditions in which symptoms were intermittent or had less impact on staff (e.g., arthritis) (162).

Medications Not Taken as Prescribed

Patients do not take medications as prescribed in one third to one half of all cases (163). Patients over 75 years of age who live alone are especially likely to not take medications as prescribed (84). Reasons given by patients in one study for not taking medications included feeling the prescribed dosage was too high and experiencing problematic side effects (164). These patient choices can cause postdischarge deterioration, and patient education before discharge is critical to avoid such problems. Allowing patients to self-medicate in the hospital with flexible administration times may be a useful way to monitor at the very least their understanding and reinforce the need for medications (165). This strategy also may help to decrease the frequency of incorrect drug frequency or dosage, omitted medications, and use of expired medications (166).

Drug toxicity can result when a patient is admitted to the hospital and given all the drugs that have been previously prescribed but were not being taken at home. Such a problem should be suspected when a patient shows a decline in cognitive or functional status 5 to 10 days after admission and other medical workup is unrevealing (167).

Adverse Drug Reactions

Adverse drug reactions appear to be more common in older patients, even when medications are given in the proper dosages (168). This may be related to a relative lack of resiliency in their homeostatic mechanisms (26,77). Although not all adverse drug reactions are avoidable, some investigators suggest that 70% to 90% could be anticipated and prevented (157,162,163). That some patients choose not to adhere to prescriptions given by physicians may in fact help decrease the frequency of adverse drug reactions (164). Serious side effects can occur secondary to OTC medications, especially from antihistamines with anticholinergic side effects, leading to fatigue and confusion even in middle-aged adults (160).

Altered Pharmacokinetics

There are a number of age-related changes in pharmacokinetics, previously reviewed, with significant implications for drug dosing, timing of dosage changes, and potential for unexpected toxicity or interactions. The reader is referred to the previous discussion of organ system aging for hematologic, gastrointestinal, hepatic, and renal systems.

Altered Receptor Sensitivity

Age-related changes in receptor sensitivity to drug effects are a further reason for untoward drug effects in older people. There is evidence that benzodiazepines and warfarin have a greater effect at similar concentrations in the young compared with the elderly (84). Such changes are difficult to evaluate separately from the pharmacokinetic changes related to aging.

The common statement ''go low, go slow'' is sound advice when prescribing drugs for older people. Evaluation of response to drug therapy is critical, and elimination of any unnecessary medicines is essential for improving function in older people. Patient and family education in the use of drugs is particularly important in this population to improve adherence and avoid adverse reactions to medication regimens (165,166).

Managing Common Complications

Incontinence

An all too common complication, devastating to patient self-esteem and family commitment to patient care, is urinary incontinence. For diagnostic classification and evaluation procedures, the reader is referred to Chapter 44. Several recent reviews cover this topic thoroughly (169,170). Treatment for incontinence in the older patient hinges on proper diagnosis, which usually is possible with a complete history of the problem together with careful neurologic, pelvic, rectal, and mental status examinations. Laboratory studies should include urinalysis and culture, serum creatinine or BUN, and a postvoid residual urine volume (169,171). A voiding diary often is helpful in determining the nature of the problem, and cystometrics also may be indicated (125).

Treatment is directed at the cause of the incontinence. Unfortunately, many of the etiologies have no uniformly successful therapy, and there may even be multiple causes. A timed voiding program is useful in many patients, offering toileting opportunities at regular intervals to try to maintain continence (169). Initially, the intervals are very short (e.g., every 15 to 20 minutes), with progressive increase as indicated. Modifications of this technique include Patterned Urge-Response Toileting (PURT) (172) and Functional Incidental Training (FIT) (173), with reports of excellent success in nursing home settings.

Surgical procedures may be useful in the treatment of prostatic hypertrophy and sphincteric incompetence (125,170). Anticholinergics (e.g., propantheline) frequently are useful in the management of detrusor instability, but with the potential risk of retention (171). Other pharmacologic approaches include direct smooth muscle relaxants (e.g., oxybutynin), calcium channel blockers, and imipramine (169,170). Overflow incontinence due to detrusor decompensation may require long-term indwelling catheterization, although intermittent catheterization and cholinergic drugs to stimulate detrusor contraction may be helpful (124). Excellent patient and health-care professional educational materials are available (174,175).

Bowel incontinence may imply severe bilateral brain disease or loss of sensory input from the rectal ampulla (176). Biofeedback has been shown to be helpful in managing sensory bowel incontinence (177,178), but the management of incontinence secondary to diffuse brain disease usually requires a behavioral approach with bowel movements induced by suppositories at regular intervals (176).

Sleep Disorders

Sleep disorders and daytime fatigue are related problems common in the hospitalized elderly person as well as those living in the community (133,135,179). The hospital environment alone can disrupt the sleep cycle, an effect further compounded by the routines of vital signs and medication administration, noises from the ward and neighboring patients, and the depression often associated with the onset of new major chronic illness (135). Sleep deprivation at night leads to fatigue during the day. Napping during the day further disrupts nocturnal sleep patterns, and a vicious cycle can ensue (179).

It is important to document whether insufficient sleep actually is occurring because patients can complain of sleep difficulties when no problem is documented, and they remain alert throughout the day. Simple reassurance in such cases is warranted. In cases of documented sleep disorder, contributing factors such as delirium, medication toxicities, depression, anxiety, restless leg syndrome, chronic pain syndrome, or nighttime medical problems (e.g., congestive heart failure, angina) should be considered (131,135). It is also important to differentiate acute insomnia from chronic insomnia. Acute insomnia (present for less than 1 month) is often related to a stressor (e.g., bereavement) and is treated with support and short-term, intermittent medication. Chronic insomnia (persisting for more than 1 month) should be viewed more as a symptom of another illness (179). Hypnotics should be used judiciously and only if other interventions, such as improved sleep hygiene and treatment of the underlying illness, are unsuccessful.

After addressing these issues, good sleep hygiene practices should be implemented. These include a regular sleep schedule, keeping the patient out of the bed and bedroom until bedtime, a snack before bedtime, daily exercise, relaxing activities in the evening before bedtime, and instruction in mental imagery or deep breathing relaxation techniques to be used as needed in bed at night (180). In addition, patients should not watch clocks during the night. Naps during the day should be avoided unless absolutely needed, briefly after lunch. Only if these interventions fail should a sleep medication be considered. Tricyclic antidepressants can be used in low doses at night to take advantage of sedative side effects, while minimizing anticholinergic activity (e.g., nortriptyline, doxepin) (84). Trazodone, with fewer side effects compared with the tricyclics, may be useful. If a benzodiazepine is used, the choice should be one with a very short half-life (e.g., triazolam, oxazepam) to avoid accumulation with hangover effects. In general, diphenhydramine should be avoided because of anticholinergic effects (77,83). In the patient who remains persistently fatigued without clear organic cause, occult depression should be suspected (76,130). Additional nonmedication treatments that appear promising in older adults include behavioral treatments (like stimulus control to induce good sleep hygiene behaviors), and increased exposure to light (181,182). Recent research suggests potential for use of melatonin as an adjunct in the management of sleep disorders in the elderly (183).

Depression

Depressed mood is a significant problem in older persons and is often missed. Given the importance of improving recognition of depression, several recent reviews have covered the topic in detail (184–186). Rates of major depression vary from 16% to 30% for elderly clinical populations, and prevalence rates in community-dwelling older persons ranges from 2% to 5%. The risk of depression has been estimated to be threefold greater for older persons with disability (39,187). Essential is the distinction, sometimes hard to make, between depressed mood that will respond to supportive counseling and more severe depression requiring more aggressive intervention (e.g., psychotherapy, medication, electroconvulsive therapy) (188). The rehabilitation team should maintain a high index of suspicion for the presence of depression that may require aggressive treatment. Presenting vegetative signs of more severe depression may include the following:

Sleep disturbance
Loss of appetite
Constipation
Impaired concentration
Poor memory
Psychomotor retardation (40)

Symptoms can include depressed mood, poor motivation, fatigue, and suicidal ideation. Other less specific complaints include other somatic symptoms such as pain and ill-characterized dyspnea (38). Depressed patients may appear as if they have a dementia syndrome (184,185).

In many patients with mild reactive depression, the activity and milieu of the rehabilitation unit will alleviate the depression. Progress in therapy and the support of peers and staff often are therapeutic. When the depression is more profound, antidepressants may prove helpful; however, medical contraindications may limit or preclude their use (184). Newer medications such as trazodone and the selective serotonin reuptake inhibitors have low anticholinergic activity and should be considered in addition to those tricyclic antidepressants with the fewest anticholinergic side effects (e.g., doxepin, nortriptyline, desipramine) (185). Doses should be started low, usually at night initially, and increased gradually.

Few studies have investigated the role of psychological and social interventions for older persons (184,186). Depressed outpatient volunteers in generally good health have shown benefits with cognitive behavior, interpersonal and short-term psychodynamic therapies. Clinically, interventions like these are potentially beneficial and require more evaluation, especially because medication alone cannot address the multiple associated issues such as altered life role (especially with disabilities), chronic medical illness, and losses of spouses and close friends (40,186).

Anxiety

Anxiety syndromes are another frequent problem during rehabilitation (189). Symptoms can manifest in multiple systems, as in depression. Careful differential diagnosis is required to distinguish between primary anxiety disorders and those secondary to medical illness or medication. A detailed interview and chronology of onset is needed, and assistance from psychiatry often is needed. Diagnostic categories include adjustment disorder with anxious mood, generalized anxiety disorder, posttraumatic stress disorder, and panic attacks (190). When feasible, nonpharmacologic interventions should first be used, such as behavioral management techniques, physical therapy for muscle relaxation, or psychotherapy (191). Nonetheless, judicious and appropriate medication use is frequently necessary to control anxiety symptoms and facilitate participation in the rehabilitation process. Commonly used options include lorazepam, buspirone, imipramine, and serotonin selective reuptake inhibitors (191).

A baseline anxiety disorder may be exacerbated by hospitalization, leading to agitation with nonpurposeful excessive motor activity. Depression, as well as pre-existing psychoses, can present with agitation (189). The former usually responds to the more sedating tricyclic antidepressants (e.g., doxepin). Paraphrenia is an example of a psychosis occurring in the elderly that often presents with agitation (191). A paranoid psychosis with onset typically late in life, it is characterized by bizarre paranoid delusions in a socially isolated person. Antipsychotics are critical to the management of this problem, coupled with therapeutic alliance with a physician and an attempt to redevelop social contacts for the patient. A history of pre-existing psychiatric disorders always should be sought in the agitated patient. Schizophrenia can continue into old age, although exacerbations respond well to antipsychotics (189).

Delirium

Delirium, a syndrome characterized by the acute onset of fluctuating cognitive deficits in conjunction with attention disorder and disorganized thought, can cause sleep disturbances, hallucinations, and agitation (192). It occurs more often in patients with prior cognitive impairments and can coexist with a dementia, making accurate diagnosis very difficult (193). Any acute medical illness can present in the older person with delirium without the classic signs of the underlying acute illness (131). Infections, dehydration, stroke, hypothermia, uremia, heart or liver failure, and pulmonary emboli are the most common examples of this phenomenon (194). Drug toxicity is another frequent cause of delirium in the elderly, with common offenders including neuroleptics and narcotics (193,194). There is evolving data on factors associated with postoperative delirium states (195). Delirium represents a medical emergency, with significant independent morbidity (196); identifying the cause is critical to its resolution (131).

Pain

Pain is very common in older people, and studies are increasingly focused on the subject (197,198). Prevalence estimates range from 25% to 50% of community-dwelling elderly people and 45% to 80% of nursing home residents (198,199). The consequences of pain are significant and include depression, decreased socialization, sleep disturbance, impaired ambulation, and increased health-care use and costs (197). The pain experienced and reported by older people is no less threatening than that experienced by younger people and must be addressed promptly (198).

Special considerations in managing pain in older persons include difficulty in assessment secondary to patient fears, the higher incidence of comorbid illnesses compared with younger persons, complications in reporting pain in patients with memory and other cognitive impairments, validity difficulties with proxy reporting, and the importance of assessing functional implications of the pain (198,200). Furthermore, physicians understandably tend to attribute new pain to prior conditions. Cognitive impairment does not mask pain at the time of patient questioning, but accurate reporting of past pain is not necessarily reliable (201). Patients may be able to respond appropriately to pain intensity scales concerning current pain, with visual cueing as needed and taking short attention spans into account (202). Special functional considerations include the recognition that advanced and elective activities of daily living may be more sensitive to changes in pain.

Common etiologies of pain in older people include osteoarthritis, cancer, herpes zoster, temporal arteritis, polymyalgia rheumatica, and atherosclerotic peripheral vascular disease (199). Approaches to pain management are similar across age groups and include use of physical modalities (e.g., heat, cold, massage), transcutaneous electrical nerve stimulation (TENS), biofeedback, hypnosis, and distractive techniques (197). Concurrence of depression and pain may occur as in younger persons, requiring direct assessment for depression and intervention if required (185). Of note, older patients with depression are more likely to report pain as a somatic expression of their mood disturbance (201). Medications for pain should be prescribed judiciously and in conjunction with nonpharmacologic approaches (197). Nonsteroidal anti-inflammatory medications are problematic in this population, given the limited study of patients over age 65 (203) and the known fourfold higher risk of peptic ulcer disease (204). Long-term use of opiate analgesics is appropriate for malignant pain and probably in some cases of nonmalignant chronic disabling pain unresponsive to other medications. Tricyclic antidepressants or anticonvulsants may be useful in treating neuropathic pain (197). Physical mobility and activities should be encouraged as much as possible. All these treatments are best administered as part of a multidisciplinary team approach, regardless of the setting (e.g., home, skilled nursing facility, or outpatient department) (198).

A particularly challenging clinical population includes older adults who experience chronic pain, often with repeated failures to respond to traditional medical or surgical treatments. The cognitive–behavioral model of therapy, developed with younger persons, may prove useful in these patients (198). This therapy is safer, more effective, and probably lower in cost than a long-term analgesic regimen, especially if applied early in the course of an evolving pain syndrome. The model divides contributory factors to the pain experience into biomedical variables, psychological variables (e.g., pain coping strategies, depression, personality), and socioenvironmental variables (e.g., social support, spousal criticism). Behavior therapy encourages wellness behaviors, and cognitive therapy helps patients reassess how they view themselves and their pain experience. This model also highlights the importance of assessing family behaviors in the presence of pain. Specific interventions for family coping can be beneficial (45,205). Family and caregiver training, as well as semiformal social supports in the community, may be especially important in the setting of chronic pain in older persons (198). For example, chronic back pain sufferers (typically with associated depression) tend to exhaust their social support (206). Preventing the resulting social isolation would likely improve efficacy of treatment intervention and avoid a cascade of complications (128).

Hypotension

Symptomatic orthostatic hypotension can occur in many older patients after even relatively short periods of bed rest (4,134). It is accordingly a frequent problem during early remobilization of elderly patients in rehabilitation settings. Symptoms can persist if there are underlying problems with blood pressure maintenance related to drug therapy, salt restriction, or autonomic dysfunction (75). Orthostatic hypotension is defined as a decline of 20 mm Hg or more in systolic blood pressure when rising from supine to standing, usually accompanied by symptoms of dizziness or lightheadedness (102).

Evaluation of the patient should include a review of medications (particularly nitrates, antihypertensives, levodopa, diuretics, phenothiazines, and tricyclic antidepressants); examination for autonomic dysfunction (e.g., pupillary response, abnormal sweating, central nervous system disease, response to Valsalva maneuver) or recent fluid loss; and laboratory tests to rule out abnormalities in aldosterone and cortisol levels (76,102,131). Metanephrines should be evaluated when hypotension occurs with episodic hypertension, a hallmark of pheochromocytoma (76).

Treatment for symptomatic orthostasis includes discontinuing any prescribed or OTC medication that could be contributing to the hypotension. The patient should be instructed to exercise (i.e., ankle dorsiflexion) before arising and to stand up slowly while holding onto a support. Thigh-high elastic stockings or an abdominal binder may help minimize lower extremity blood pooling (102). High-sodium diet and fludrocortisone acetate, a synthetic mineralocorticoid, are useful for plasma expansion in the absence of congestive heart failure. Other medications to consider include NSAIDs (which inhibit prostaglandin synthesis), clonidine or midodrine (which are α-2-adrenergic agonists), propranolol (which blocks β-2 vasodilatory receptors), pindolol (which is a β-adrenergic antagonist with intrinsic sympathomimetic activity), or phenylpropanolamine (which is a sympathomimetic) (77,84,102).

Prescription of Rehabilitation Programs

An appropriate therapeutic prescription is critical to the success of rehabilitation program. It must be based on a careful analysis of the patient's current functional limitations, with realistic goal setting in the context of premorbid functioning and anticipated improvement in medical status (207). Specific therapy techniques will be used based on physical status (e.g., neurologic, musculoskeletal, cardiovascular systems) and medical stability, particularly in terms of aerobic capacity. Social and cultural barriers to certain exercises or activities also must be taken into account. The patient should participate in goal setting and understand the relevance of the rehabilitation plan to his or her own goals. Without a strong therapeutic alliance between all health professional team members and the patient (and family), progress will be slow and/or limited.

Functional training approaches usually are well accepted by most older patients because of their obvious relevance and importance. Many therapeutic goals can be achieved by incorporating formal therapy techniques into the context of functional tasks. Examples of this approach include the following techniques:

Remediate perceptual problems during eating or meal preparation
Increase range of motion with dressing training
Strengthen through inclined sanding or woodworking projects
Aerobically condition through adapted competitive sports

Prescription of the rehabilitation program must be tailored to the person to accommodate limitations imposed by comorbid medical problems (208). Cardiovascular (e.g., blood pressure/pulse response, cardiac symptomatology) and pulmonary (e.g., use of oxygen) restrictions should be established if and as appropriate. Weight-bearing limits can be accommodated by means of assistive devices or aquatic therapy. Some patients may have limited exercise tolerance, necessitating flexible therapy scheduling with rest periods. Hunt has delineated a series of practical rehabilitation guidelines (209).

Realistic goal setting is complex in any rehabilitation setting but may be complicated further in older people in two unique respects. First, older adults frequently have potential caregivers (e.g., spouse, siblings, children) who also are approaching retirement and have medical problems of their own; fitness and capability of the proposed caregiver after discharge must be considered in the discharge planning process (43). The second problem relates to the limited remaining life expectancy of the older disabled patient. For example, diabetic amputees over 65 years of age have average survivals of approximately a year (210). In view of the potentially limited longevity, an expedited rehabilitation program to facilitate return home with family would be most appropriate.

A number of potentially negative or counterproductive team dynamics can develop in rehabilitation settings that may interfere with or limit a patient's progress (211). Patients and families tend to trust their health-care providers as the experts who will know and do what is best for them. It is critical that the rehabilitation team maintain vigilance for and strive to counter such negative attitudes as paternalism (e.g., overriding patient goals judged by the team to be unrealistic or inappropriate), arrogance (e.g., presumptive familiarity by addressing patients by their first name without requesting permission or preference), and self-fulfilling prophecies (e.g., patients judged not to have potential for improvement not receiving as much attention or effort as patients felt to have a good prognosis) (211). Other team issues which can impact effectiveness include relative team member roles (either lack of clarity or excess rigidity), communication barriers, or decision-making conflicts. The ongoing challenge for rehabilitation teams is to foster an individual and collective philosophy of respect for and empowerment of the individuals they treat, facilitating functional independence. The latter includes (appropriate) risk-taking (referred to as dignity of risk).

SPECIAL REHABILITATION CONSIDERATIONS FOR DISABLING CONDITIONS IN THE ELDERLY

Dementia

Severe dementia occurs in about 5% of individuals over 65 years of age (with mild to moderate forms in another 10%) and in about 20% of those over 80 years of age (35,110). It is found in more than half of nursing home residents and is the most common precipitating cause of admission (35). Women appear to be affected more frequently than men. Insidious onset of memory loss, loss of abstract reasoning and problem-solving ability, impairment of judgment and orientation, and personality changes with relatively intact alertness and awareness are hallmarks of the disease (212). A patient with early dementia, premorbidly not interfering with daily activities, can become severely disoriented during an acute hospitalization (131,136). This agitated confusion may resolve without any specific therapy in 1 to 2 weeks. Appreciation of this possibility is important with regard to evaluating and working with this population in rehabilitation settings.

Fifty percent to 60% of dementias represent dementia of the Alzheimer type, and another 20% are multi-infarct in origin (110). The remaining large number of potentially reversible causes of dementia include the following conditions:

Subdural hematoma
Brain tumor
Occult hydrocephalus
Syphilis
Hypothyroidism or hyperthyroidism
Hypercalcemia
Vitamin B12 deficiency
Niacin deficiency
Drug toxicity
Depression
Cardiac, renal, or hepatic failure (212)

Diagnostic evaluation always should be performed to rule out these possible causes. Even if one of these potentially treatable etiologies is established, however, reversibility of the dementia may be limited because of permanent damage from the condition (213). Although there are differing guidelines for recommended laboratory tests for evaluating dementia (212), a standard dementia workup, in addition to detailed history and physical examination with cognitive screening, should include at least a complete blood count (CBC), blood chemistry profiles (including electrolytes, creatinine, blood urea nitrogen), erythrocyte sedimentation rate, and thyroid function studies.

Other investigative studies, such as serologic test for syphilis, serum folate, serum cobalamin, drug screening, collagen vascular profile, urinalysis for heavy metals, or computed tomography of the brain, can be undertaken if there is concern that they will clarify the etiology, such as multi-infarct dementia versus Alzheimer's disease (212,214). A trial off all medications probably is warranted in all patients with new onset of dementia. Many clinicians also routinely give a trial of antidepressants to newly identified dementia patients because an occult depression frequently coexists with mild dementia (130,215). Amelioration of the depression may improve overall functioning in this situation.

Patients with moderate or severe dementia can be limited in their new learning in rehabilitation settings because their ability to form new memory is poor. Day-to-day carryover may be limited and makes certain types of therapeutic gains difficult to achieve (120). A rehabilitation trial may still be justified in such situations to clarify learning abilities and to train the family in appropriate care of a patient with a new disability. For instance, the patient may show the ability for procedural learning (learning by performing the activity) even if declarative learning (learning from verbal instruction) is impaired (46,49).

When evaluating the elderly patient for admission to a

rehabilitation program, it is critical to determine the mental status before onset of the new disability by talking to family or others who have observed the patient. Too often the mental status as seen in the acute hospital setting underestimates the patient's cognitive function when healthier and in a more supportive and stimulating environment (such as a rehabilitation unit) (216).

Discharge planning for patients with dementia needs to include family education as to the nature of the patient's cognitive strengths and weaknesses and how to handle potential behavioral problems (46). Community resources for adult day care and respite care programs may be very helpful for families, as well as educational materials like the Agency for Health Care Policy and Research's booklet on early Alzheimer's Disease (217).

Falls

Many of the age-related physiologic declines in multiple organ systems combine to increase dramatically the incidence of falls in the elderly, including visuoperceptual difficulty, postural instability, impaired mobility, orthostatic hypotension, lower extremity weakness, and vertigo due to degenerative or vascular changes in the vestibular apparatus (143,144). Other factors contribute to increase the risk of falling, including environmental hazards, adverse effects of medications, concomitant acute or chronic disease states, depression, apathy, or confusion (110,116,218,219). A model attempting to identify the degree of risk for recurrent falls stratified patients into high and low risk depending on sitting and standing balance, walking ability, and stair climbing (220). In addition, attitudes toward risk were measured, as were social supports and environmental status. Recurrent falls were associated with impaired mobility, attitude toward risk and environmental score.

Prevention of these injurious falls is more problematic. A recent prospective study of 9,516 community-residing white women (average follow-up 4.1 years) found that the likelihood of hip fracture increased in the presence of multiple risk factors and low bone density (221). Suggested possible interventions to decrease risk include maintaining body weight, walking for exercise, avoiding long-acting benzodiazepines, minimizing caffeine intake, and treating impaired visual function. Tai chi reduced risk of multiple falls by 48% in a randomized control trial in community-residing persons 70 years of age and older without chronic illness, many of whom had fallen in the prior year (222). Whether this intervention would work for older persons with chronic illnesses needs to be assessed. In another study of community-dwelling elderly with at least one risk factor for falls, a multifactorial intervention (medication adjustments, behavioral instruction, and exercise) reduced falls from 47% in the control group to 35% in the intervention group (223).

Hip Fracture

Although the majority of falls in older persons fortunately do not result in injury, hip fractures continue to be one of the most serious sequela. Strategies considered for intervention to prevent hip fracture have included both public health initiatives (e.g., emphasizing weight-bearing exercise) and individualized approaches focused on high risk patients (224). The most effective approaches have yet to be worked out. In situations involving rehabilitation of an elderly patient after repair of hip fracture secondary to fall, it is critical to evaluate, and treat, the cause of the incident fall to prevent future recurrence.

A number of controversies involve proper care of the elderly patient after hip fracture. The literature is increasingly evaluating factors affecting outcomes from hip fractures and potential cost-effective changes in practice (225–229).

Issues relating to preoperative decisions include how long to wait for medical stabilization. One guideline suggests that hip fracture patients who have two or fewer comorbidities should have the operation within 2 days of admission, but that a longer delay is beneficial for patients with three or more comorbidities (230).

Several factors affect the decision to operate and what type of surgery. A tendency to treat hip fractures conservatively (i.e., nonsurgically) in demented elderly patients is countered by findings of better function with less morbidity and mortality with surgical management (231). For patients with severe cardiovascular disease that contraindicates general anesthesia, percutaneous pinning with Ender rods under local anesthesia can be performed. Femoral neck fractures can be treated either by resection of the femoral head with endoprosthesis with immediate postoperative weight bearing or by internal fixation with multiple pins with delayed weight bearing. Although intertrochanteric fractures traditionally are managed by internal fixation with nail or compression screw with delayed weight bearing, some studies suggest patients can be mobilized much earlier without complication and with improved morbidity and function (225,228,231).

The postoperative period can be divided into the acute hospital period and posthospital care. The urgency of early mobilization after repair of hip fracture is twofold: the vulnerability to many postoperative complications (e.g., pulmonary problems, thromboembolism, genitourinary sequelae) and the risk of secondary complications from bed rest or relative inactivity (225,226). In one recent study of the acute hospital period after surgical repair of hip fracture, factors associated with discharge to home (which occurred in only 17% of 162 hip fracture survivors) included prior community residing status, age under 85 years, absence of postoperative complications, achieving independence in bed mobility and ambulation with a walker, and a greater number of physical therapy sessions during hospitalization (228).

By far the majority of hip fracture patients in the United States receive post–acute hospital care in other facilities—either acute rehabilitation hospitals/units or skilled nursing facilities. These settings are increasingly necessary as lengths of hospital stay continue to dramatically decline. Which setting is best for which patients is still not clear.

What is necessary during the recuperative phase from hip fracture, in any setting, is close attention to multiple medical problems that can arise (226,227). Optimal length of stay in these settings likewise is not yet clear, and also continues to decline.

Arthritis and Joint Replacements

Management of arthritic conditions in older people, just as in a younger population, must be individualized with close monitoring of benefits (231,232). Treatment principles are comparable, although the balance between rest and activity is much more delicate because of the adverse sequelae of inactivity in the elderly (233). There is evidence that older people with arthritis may respond better to therapeutic programs, and often are more patient and compliant with long-term exercise and activity programs (234). Treatment goals include relief of fear, fatigue, stiffness, and pain, suppressing the inflammatory process, prevention or correction of deformity, and maintaining function (233,234). This is accomplished via a combination of psychological, pharmacologic, physical, and surgical measures.

Important psychological approaches have been developed through the Arthritis Self-Help Course. The multifaceted interventions include education and exercise (235). Part of the benefit may be through improving the patient's ability in relation to managing his or her chronic condition. Successful exercise interventions include programs of focused muscle strengthening (e.g., quadriceps strengthening for osteoarthritis of the knee), general conditioning, and aerobic activities (236–238).

Patients can be educated about the beneficial results of using various assistive devices, such as a firm chair of appropriate height with armrests, built-up handle devices, elevated toilet seat with grab bars, or ambulation aids (e.g., cane, walker), in helping to maintain independent community living. As with any assistive device, having patients try to use various pieces of equipment before purchase will help ensure actual functional use.

Pharmacologic interventions for pain control should start with acetaminophen up to 2 to 4 g/day (239). Codeine or hydrocodone can provide additional analgesia for breakthrough pain. Topical capsaicin cream may be helpful for persistent knee or finger pain. A limited number of intra-articular steroid injections can be considered, but with anticipation of only short-term benefit. NSAIDs may have to be used for control of pain and inflammation, but with great care and close monitoring given the increased risk of acute renal impairments and gastrointestinal bleeding (239). In older patients with a history of gastritis or ulcers who require use of NSAIDs, concurrent administration of misoprostol should be considered (239).

Age should not be a primary factor in considering potential benefits of surgical intervention in the elderly arthritic patient (239). Significant functional gains may be realized with an appropriately timed procedure (e.g., ligament or tendon repair, osteotomy, arthroplasty, prosthetic joint replacement) to improve stability and range or to decrease pain (234). Attention to preoperative and postoperative therapy programs and early mobilization is critical to maximize functional gains and minimize secondary complications from inactivity (233,239). Further details of rehabilitation management, including principles for prescription of medication and therapeutic modalities, can be found in Chapters 59 and 66.

Stroke

Appropriateness of intensive rehabilitation for older stroke patients sometimes is questioned, given limited and sometimes conflicting research data. Studies have variably concluded that age has little or no effect on functional outcomes, that elderly stroke patients may require longer lengths of stay to achieve the same functional gains as younger patients, and that functional outcomes may be similar in differing rehabilitation settings (240–249). The most significant aspects of rehabilitating elderly stroke patients relates to management of their frequent multiple comorbid conditions, as well as to the impact on designing an appropriate therapy program (209,250). Further research is needed to clarify the role, timing, setting and intensity of rehabilitation services for older people after stroke. Chapter 48 reviews concepts of stroke rehabilitation in detail, with reference to older patients.

Amputation

Although a detailed review of rehabilitation of the amputee can be found in Chapters 27 and 60, several aspects require emphasis here. A potential ageist bias leads to the belief that a patient's age should help determine whether or not to prescribe a prosthesis. Other comorbidities rather than age *per se* are the relevant determinants for prosthetic fitting (27,251). A number of studies have documented the successful outcomes of rehabilitation programs for older amputees, including bilateral amputees and amputees with concurrent hemiplegia (251–254). Even in the face of severe medical comorbidity (e.g., cardiovascular disease), a prosthesis still may be both therapeutic and functional, even if only from the standpoint of standing, transfers, or cosmesis (27). For bilateral amputees, although energy costs are significantly higher and ambulation training more difficult, prosthetic fitting still may be useful to allow periodic standing during the day and for walking short distances in the home, which are therapeutic from both an aerobic exercise and psychological standpoint (252). Wheelchair locomotion may be a preferable alternative for longer distance travel at lower energy costs, however. The former rehabilitation criterion of successful crutch ambulation to justify prosthetic prescription is no longer justified (27,251).

Spinal Cord Injury

Although spinal cord injury (SCI) usually is considered a disability occurring primarily in the younger population, there is increasing recognition of its significance for older people. Not only is there a significant incidence of SCI in a growing older population (5.4% in the 61- to 90-year-old age group) (255), but increased survival in an aging population injured earlier in their lives (256). The result is a much higher prevalence of older SCI patients, subject to the usual age-related morbidity and mortality. Similarities have been observed between aging morbidity and that of chronic SCI patients who are not old (257).

Epidemiology of SCI with older age at onset differs from that of younger populations. The etiology of injury is much more likely to be falls (60% in the 75-and-older age group), followed by motor vehicle accidents (32% in the 75-and-older group) (255). Spinal cord injury from metastatic disease and cervical myelopathy occurs primarily in older adults. There is a marked increase in proportionate incidence of quadriplegia (QC) and quadriparesis (QI) in the elderly (67% in the 61- to 75-year-old age group, 88% in the 75-and-older group), as opposed to the more nearly equal distribution between paraplegia (PC) and paraparesis (PI) and QC and QI in younger age groups (255). Elderly SCI patients are three times more likely to be QI as opposed to QC.

There is a progressive disparity in 10-year survival rates between SCI and non-SCI populations with advancing age at injury (255). For those 70 to 98 years of age, the grouped SCI 10-year survival rate is 32%, compared with 48% for their non-SCI counterparts. Life expectancies reported for SCI patients differ depending on whether patients who die before discharge from rehabilitation programs—usually within the first year postinjury—are included in the analysis. If such first-year fatalities are included, life expectancy for SCI patients injured at 60 years of age is 6.5 years for PI, 5.9 years for PC, 4.2 years for QI, and 1.9 years for QC, compared with 20.0 years for the non-SCI population (255). Life expectancies are significantly higher for SCI patients discharged alive from rehabilitation programs (256,258). Older patients with SCI were more likely than their younger counterparts to develop various medical complications, such as pneumonia, gastrointestinal hemorrhage, pulmonary emboli, or renal stones (259). Although overall survival post-SCI is reduced for older adults, with increased morbidity, there does not appear to be a direct relationship between age and functional outcome (260).

These significant life expectancies, and potential for functional gains, make rehabilitation efforts appropriate for all patients following SCI, regardless of age (260). Rehabilitation goals should be comparable with those for a younger SCI population (see Chapter 51), with emphasis on safe care, homemaking and mobility, training a caregiver as needed, and resumption of leisure activities as appropriate.

Disability Prevention in Older Adults

The potential future impact of increased disability as populations age is of major concern to clinicians, health-care administrators, and policy makers. Increasingly, prevention strategies are being proposed both to improve the number of disability-free years of life as well as to contain health-care costs (18,24,25). Some of the themes around prevention can be organized according to the concepts of primary, secondary, and tertiary prevention. Primary prevention involves preventing the onset of a disease (e.g., annual influenza vaccine), whereas secondary prevention involves the diagnosis and treatment of asymptomatic diseases to prevent the development of symptoms (e.g., treatment of hypertension to prevent stroke or myocardial infarction). Tertiary prevention involves treatment once a disease becomes symptomatic to avoid complications (e.g., deep venous thrombosis prophylaxis and appropriate mobilization to prevent skin breakdown in poststroke patients). However, what becomes important in older persons with chronic disease is more prevention of disability or frailty. Frailty as a concept refers to more than older individuals who are dependent in function; it represents a vulnerable state resulting from the balance and interplay of medical and social factors (261). Characteristics of frail older institutionalized persons included female gender, being unmarried, absence of a caregiver, presence of cognitive deficit, functional impairment, and medical condition (diabetes mellitus, stroke, Parkinson's disease) (262). A model for risk factors in the development of frailty has been proposed by Buchner and Wagner (Fig. 39-5) (263). In this model, strategies required to prevent disability in older age involve multiple interventions on living environment and lifestyle (264). These interventions do not easily fall into the traditional categories of primary, secondary, and tertiary prevention.

Another important theoretical model that may help in the development of prevention strategies has been proposed by Lawrence and Jette (265). They have studied the application of a model for the disablement process in 1,048 community residing adults (mean age 74 years) without functional limitations or disabilities. Data were collected over a 6-year period. The model hypothesized a process in which risk factors (age, gender, education, body mass, and physical activity measured as frequency of walking 1 mile) would lead to functional limitations with or without the presence of pathology or impairments. Over time the functional limitations (e.g., inability to walk well) lead to subsequent disability such as inability to go shopping. Guralnik and colleagues likewise found that among nondisabled persons living in the community, impairments in the lower extremity were highly predictive of later disability (266). Studies like these support the role of such interventions as increased physical activity and exercise as types of primary prevention of disability for older persons.

There may in fact be significant overlap of risk factors for multiple problems in older persons. For instance, the risk factors associated with falls, incontinence, and functional dependence are similar—slowed chair stand, decreased arm strength, decreased vision and hearing, and either a high anxiety or depression score (267).

From these types of models successful prevention strate-

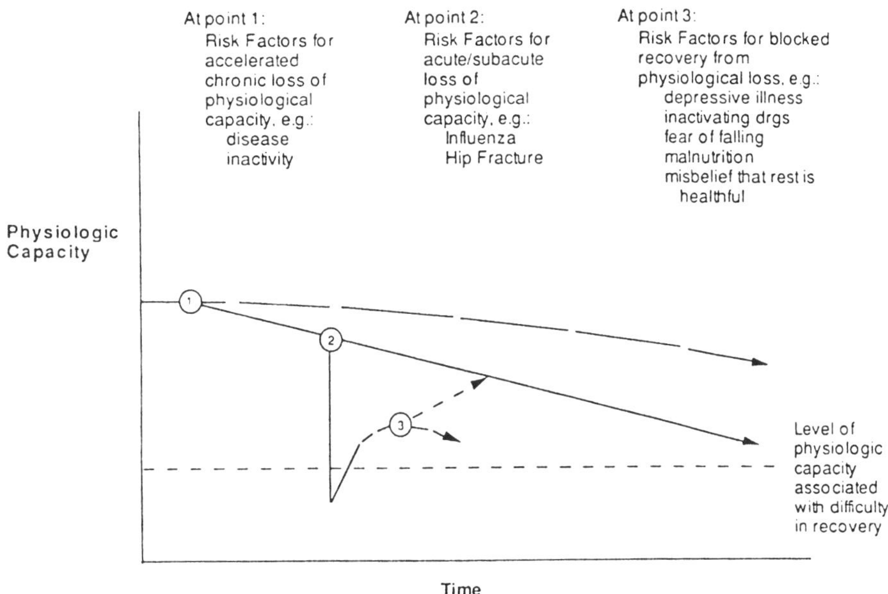

FIG. 39-5. Conceptual model of risk factors for frailty. (From Buchner DM, Wagner EH. Preventing frail health. *Clin Geriatr Med* 1992; 8:1–17.)

gies are being tested, often entailing interventions covering multiple domains. For instance, in fall prevention as previously discussed, studies have shown that incidence of falls can be reduced by appropriate interventions, such as medication adjustments, exercise, safety training, and environmental modifications—all in a single patient if necessary. A comprehensive nurse-practitioner evaluation program for community-residing seniors resulted in a delay in onset of disability and decreased nursing home admission (268). Another study demonstrated that higher self-efficacy was associated with lesser functional decline in persons with diminished physical capacity (269). Research also suggests that self-efficacy—a person's confidence or belief that he or she can achieve a specific behavior or cognitive state—may be modifiable and therefore help guide preventive strategies (270). Identifying which targeted intervention for which specific risk factor in which specific patient will require more research in the years ahead.

Significance of Functional Status in Placement Issues

Reference already has been made to the critical nature of functional status with regard to ability to live independently in the community. Older people often live alone and must perform their own self-care and other daily activities, including homemaking. Issues of safety in this home environment frequently are raised, particularly after an acute adverse event or illness (e.g., a fall with hip fracture). A patient who achieves a level of mobility (i.e., ambulation or transfers) requiring only close supervision or contact guarding because of occasional loss of balance may not be able to safely return home alone. Home-based supervision by an aide, unless paid privately, typically is available only a few hours a day, 5 days a week, for relatively brief intervals. Return to a community setting may be possible if a relative is available to live with this patient. If not, he or she may not even qualify for a boarding home or intermediate care facility; most intermediate care facility admission criteria include independent safe locomotion. This patient accordingly may require a skilled nursing facility (SNF) admission as the only source of 24-hour-per-day supervision available. Unfortunately, alternatives are limited for more homelike settings with other residents of similar functional level.

Role of the Physiatrist in Geriatrics

Physicians from various specialties maintain differing perspectives on their respective roles in geriatrics (271). Physiatrists actually may serve a variety of roles relating to geriatrics, depending on the practice setting. These contributions range from providing primary care in a rehabilitation inpatient hospital setting or subacute (SNF-based) setting (120,272) to consulting in various health-care settings, such as acute care hospital, SNF, day hospital, or home health care (120,229,273). In the latter settings, the physiatrist assesses functional status, formulates realistic goals, coordinates interdisciplinary team care, and monitors efficacy of therapy interventions in reversing disability.

Older people with disabling medical conditions may have difficulty tolerating and participating in an intensive comprehensive medical rehabilitation (CMR) hospital-based program, owing to such factors as severity of deficits, medical comorbidity, and deconditioning. Combined with the quest for least costly health-care alternatives, the ideal system of rehabilitative care would provide for varying levels of intensity and settings (207). Indeed, there is evolving interest in the role and effectiveness of subacute rehabilitation, which provides rehabilitation programs of varying intensity in hospital or SNF settings (248,249).

Another nontraditional setting for rehabilitation is the day hospital, which provides comprehensive, relatively intensive and structured rehabilitation therapies designed to reverse disability and train family members to facilitate maintenance of the patient at home (273,274). This provides a greater intensity of therapy, with a wider array of equipment, under closer medical supervision, than usually is feasible in a home-based treatment program. Day hospitals often allow earlier transition from hospital-based CMR centers to the more familiar and comfortable home setting, with lower health-care costs (273).

There also is increasing interest and program development in augmented home care services, including rehabilitative care (275,276). New and innovative programs to provide intensive, CMR-level rehabilitation services in the home are being developed and tested (277). Such community-based programs may prove cost effective and feasible and help resolve accessibility problems in both urban and rural settings.

These alternative levels and settings of rehabilitation services for older adults provide the potential for a continuum of care, facilitating individually tailored rehabilitative care that can be modified to meet an individual patient's changing needs over time. Further research is required to document the cost effectiveness and benefits of these varied rehabilitation programs, particularly among types of disability and age groups.

REFERENCES

1. Hazzard WR. Preventive gerontology: strategies for healthy aging. *Postgrad Med* 1983; 74:279–287.
2. Steinberg FU. Commentary: principles of geriatric rehabilitation. *Arch Phys Med Rehabil* 1989; 70:67–68.
3. Hoenig H, Mayer-Oakes SA, Siebens H, et al. Geriatric rehabilitation. What do physicians know about it and how should they use it? *J Am Geriatr Soc* 1994; 42:341–345.
4. Kottke FJ. Deterioration of the bedfast patient: causes and effects. *Public Health Rep* 1965; 80:437–450.
5. National Center for Health Statistics, Centers for Disease Control and Prevention. *Health United States, 1993*. Hyattsville, MD: US Public Health Service, 1994. DHHS Publication No. 94-1232.
6. Spencer G. *Projections of the population by age, sex, and race: 1988 to 2080. Current population reports, series P-25, no. 1018*. Washington, DC: United States Bureau of the Census, Government Printing Office, 1989.
7. *Chronic Care in America: A 21st Century Challenge*. Princeton, NJ: Robert Wood Johnson Foundation Publications, 1996.
8. Schneider EL, Guralnik JM. The aging of America: impact of health care costs. *JAMA* 1990; 263:2335–2340.
9. Cassel CK, Brody JA. Demography, epidemiology and aging. In: Cassel CK, Reisenberg DE, Sorenson LB, Walsh JR, eds. *Geriatric medicine*, 2nd ed. New York: Springer-Verlag, 1990; 16–27.
10. Olshansky SJ. Pursuing longevity: delay vs. elimination of degenerative diseases. *Am J Public Health* 1985; 75:754–757.
11. Olshansky SJ, Ault AB. The fourth stage of the epidemiologic transition: the age of delayed degenerative diseases. *Milbank Q* 1986; 64: 355–391.
12. Hing E. *Use of nursing homes by the elderly: preliminary data from the 1985 National Nursing Home Survey. United States Department of Health and Human Services publication (PHS) 87-1250. Advance data from Vital and Health Statistics, no. 135*. Hyattsville, MD: United States Public Health Service, 1987.
13. Fries JF. The sunny side of aging. *JAMA* 1990; 263:2354–2355.
14. Fries JF. Aging, natural death, and the compression of morbidity. *N Engl J Med* 1980; 303:130–135.
15. Rothenberg R, Lentzner HR, Parker RA. Population aging patterns: the expansion of mortality. *J Gerontol* 1991; 46(suppl 2):66–70.
16. Manton KG, Vaupel JW. Survival after the age of 80 in the United States, Sweden, France, England, and Japan. *N Engl J Med* 1995; 333:1232–1235.
17. Schneider E, Brody J. Aging, natural death and the compression of morbidity: another view. *N Engl J Med* 1983; 309:854.
18. Manton KG, Stallard E. Cross-sectional estimates of active life expectancy for the U.S. elderly and oldest-old populations. *J Gerontol* 1991; 46(suppl):170–182.
19. Riley GF, Lubitz JD. Longitudinal patterns of Medicare use by cause of death. *Health Care Finance Rev* 1989; 11:1–12.
20. Experton B, Ozminkowski RJ, Branch LG, Li Z. A comparison by payor/provider type of the cost of dying among frail older adults. *J Am Geriatr Soc* 1996; 44:1098–1107.
21. Lubitz J, Beebe J, Baker C. Longevity and Medicare expenditures. *N Engl J Med* 1995; 332:999–1003.
22. Fisher ES, Welch HG, Wennberg JE. Prioritizing Oregon's hospital resources: an example based on variations in discretionary medical utilization. *JAMA* 1992; 267:1925–1931.
23. Fries JF. The compression of morbidity: near or far? *Milbank Q* 1990; 67:208–232.
24. Katz S, Branch LG, Branson MH, Papsidero JA, Beck JC, Greer DS. Active life expectancy. *N Engl J Med* 1983; 309:1218–1224.
25. Manton KG, Stallard E, Liu K. Forecasts of active life expectancy: policy and fiscal implications. *J Gerontol* 1993; 48(special issue): 11–26.
26. Williams ME, Hadler NM. The illness as the focus of geriatric medicine. *N Engl J Med* 1983; 308:1357–1360.
27. Clark GS, Blue B, Bearer JB. Rehabilitation of the elderly amputee. *J Am Geriatr Soc* 1983; 31:439–448.
28. Kane RS. The defeat of aging versus the importance of death. *J Am Geriatr Soc* 1996; 44:321–325.
29. Butler RN. Age-ism: another form of bigotry. *Gerontologist* 1969; 9: 243–246.
30. Hess BB. Stereotypes of the aged. *J Communication* 1974; 14:76–85.
31. Morley JE, Kaiser FE. Sexual function with advancing age. *Med Clin North Am* 1989; 73:1483–1495.
32. George LK, Weiler SJ. Sexuality in middle and late life. *Arch Gen Psychiatry* 1981; 38:919–923.
33. Stuart MR, Snope FC. Family structure, family dynamics, and the elderly. In: Somers AR, Fabian DR, eds. *The geriatric imperative: an introduction to gerontology and clinical geriatrics*. New York: Appleton-Century-Crofts, 1981; 137–152.
34. Katzman R, Terry R. Normal aging of the nervous system. In: Katzman R, Terry R, eds. *The neurology of aging*. Philadelphia: FA Davis, 1983; 15–50.
35. Rowe JW. Health care of the elderly. *N Engl J Med* 1985; 312: 827–835.
36. Filner B, Williams TF. Health promotion for the elderly: reducing functional dependency. In: Somers AR, Fabian DR, eds. *The geriatric imperative: an introduction to gerontology and clinical geriatrics*. New York: Appleton-Century-Crofts, 1983; 187–204.
37. Medalie JH. The elderly and their families. In: Reichel WR, ed. *Clinical aspects of aging*, 3rd ed. Baltimore: Williams & Wilkins, 1989; 477–486.
38. Kennedy GJ, Kelman HR, Thomas C, Wisniewski W, Metz H, Bijur PE. Hierarchy of characteristics associated with depressive symptoms in an urban elderly sample. *Am J Psychiatry* 1989; 146:220–225.
39. Harris RE, Mion LC, Patterson MB, Frengley JD. Severe illness in older patients: the association between depressive disorders and functional dependency during the recovery. *J Am Geriatr Soc* 1988; 36: 890–896.
40. Covinsky KE, Fortinsky RH, Palmer RM, Kresevic DM, Landefield CS. Relation between symptoms of depression and health status outcomes in acutely ill hospitalized older people. *Ann Intern Med* 1997; 126:417–425.
41. Roy R, Thomas M, Cook A. Social context of elderly chronic pain

patients. In: Ferrell BR, Ferrell BA, eds. *Pain in the elderly*. Seattle: IASP Press, 1996; 111–117.

42. Shanas E. Social myth as hypothesis: the case of family relations of old people. *Gerontologist* 1979; 19:3–9.
43. Brody EM. Informal support systems in the rehabilitation of the disabled elderly. In: Brody SJ, Ruff GE, eds. *Aging and rehabilitation: advances in the state of the art*. New York: Springer-Verlag, 1986; 87–103.
44. Fried LP, Guralnik JM. Disability in older adults: evidence regarding significance, etiology, and risk. *J Am Geriatr Soc* 1997; 45:92–100.
45. Evans RL, Matlock AL, Biship DS, Stranahan S, Pederson C. Family intervention after stroke: does counseling or education help? *Stroke* 1988; 19:1234–1239.
46. Mittelman MS, Ferris SH, Shulman E, Steinberg G, Levin B. A family intervention to delay nursing home placement of patients with Alzheimer disease. *JAMA* 1996; 276:1725–1731.
47. Tsuji I, Whalen S, Finucane TE. Predictors of nursing home placement in community-based long-term care. *J Am Geriatr Soc* 1995; 43: 761–766.
48. Lachs MS, Berkman L, Fulmer T, et al. A prospective community-based pilot study of risk factors for the investigation of elder mistreatment. *J Am Geriatr Soc* 1994; 42:169–173.
49. Kemp B. Psychosocial and mental health issues in rehabilitation of older persons. In: Brody SJ, Ruff GE, eds. *Aging and rehabilitation: advances in the state of the art*. New York: Springer-Verlag, 1986; 122–158.
50. Hesse KA, Campion EW, Karamouz N. Attitudinal stumbling blocks to geriatric rehabilitation. *J Am Geriatr Soc* 1984; 32:747–750.
51. Shock NW. Aging of regulatory systems. In: Cape RDT, Coe RM, Rossman I, eds. *Fundamentals of geriatric medicine*. New York: Raven, 1983; 51–62.
52. Strehler BL. *Time, cells, and aging*, 2nd ed. New York: Academic, 1977.
53. Abrass IB. The biology and physiology of aging. *West J Med* 1990; 153:641–645.
54. Fozzard JL, Metter EJ, Brant LJ. Next steps in describing aging and disease in longitudinal studies. *J Gerontol* 1990; 45:P116–P127.
55. Vijg J, Wei JY. Understanding the biology of aging: the key to prevention and therapy. *J Am Geriatr Soc* 1995; 43:426–434.
56. Rowe JW. Aging reconsidered: strategies to promote health and prevent disease in old age. *Q J Med* 1988; 66:1–4.
57. Rowe JW. Toward successful aging: limitation of the morbidity associated with "normal aging." In: Hazzard WR, Andres R, Bierman EL, Blass JP, eds. *Principles of geriatric medicine and gerontology*. 2nd ed. New York: McGraw-Hill, 1990; 138–141.
58. Seeman TE, Charpentier PA, Berkman LF, et al. Predicting changes in physical performance in a high-functioning elderly cohort: MacArthur studies of successful aging. *J Gerontol* 1994; 49:M97–M108.
59. Lipsitz LA, Goldberger AL. Loss of complexity and aging. Potential applications of fractals and chaos theory to senescence. *JAMA* 1992; 267:1806–1809.
60. Martin GR, Danner DB, Holbrook NJ. Aging—causes and defenses. *Annu Rev Med* 1993; 44:419–429.
61. Schneider EL, Reed JD Jr. Life extension. *N Engl J Med* 1985; 312: 1159–1168.
62. Thompson CB. Apoptosis in the pathogenesis and treatment of disease. *Science* 1995; 267:1456–1462.
63. Katzman R. Demography, definitions and problems. In: Katzman R, Terry R, eds. *The neurology of aging*. Philadelphia: FA Davis, 1983; 1–14.
64. Rowe JW. Clinical research on aging: strategies and directions. *N Engl J Med* 1977; 297:1332–1336.
65. Robbins J, Wahl P, Savage P, Enright P, Powe N, Lyles M. Hematological and biochemical laboratory values in older cardiovascular health study participants. *J Am Geriatr Soc* 1995; 43:855–859.
66. Spirduso WW, Clifford P. Replication of age and physical activity effects on reaction and movement time. *J Gerontol* 1978; 33:26–30.
67. Larson EB, Bruce RA. Health benefits of exercise in an aging society. *Arch Intern Med* 1987; 147:353–356.
68. Naughton J. Physical activity and aging. *Primary Care* 1982; 9: 231–238.
69. Fiatarone MA, Marks EC, Ryan ND, Meredith CN, Lipsitz LA, Evans WJ. High-intensity strength training in nonagenarians: effects on skeletal muscle. *JAMA* 1990; 263:3029–3034.
70. Teravainen H, Calne DB. Motor system in normal aging and Parkinson's disease. In: Katzman R, Terry R, eds. *The neurology of aging*. Philadelphia: FA Davis, 1983; 85–109.
71. Baldwin JG. True anemia: incidence and significance in the elderly. *Geriatrics* 1989; 44:33–37.
72. Lipschitz DA. The anemia of chronic disease. *J Am Geriatr Soc* 1990; 38:1258–1264.
73. Shank WA, Balducci L. Recombinant hemopoietic growth factors: comparative hemopoietic response in younger and older subjects. *J Am Geriatr Soc* 1992; 40:151–154.
74. Lipschitz DA, Udupa KB, Milton KY, Thompson CO. Effect of age on hematopoiesis in man. *Blood* 1984; 63:502–509.
75. Stern N, Tuck ML. Geriatric cardiology: homeostatic fragility in the elderly. *Cardiol Clin* 1986; 4:201–211.
76. Samily AH. Clinical manifestations of disease in the elderly. *Med Clin North Am* 1983; 67:333–344.
77. Goldberg PB, Roberts J. Pharmacologic basis for developing rational drug regimens for elderly patients. *Med Clin North Am* 1983; 67: 315–331.
78. Montemat SC, Cusack BJ, Vestal RE. Management of drug therapy in the elderly. *N Engl J Med* 1989; 321:303–309.
79. Altman DF. Changes in gastrointestinal, pancreatic, biliary, and hepatic function with aging. *Gastroenterol Clin North Am* 1990; 19: 227–234.
80. Shamburek RD, Farrar JT. Disorders of the digestive system in the elderly. *N Engl J Med* 1990; 322:438–443.
81. Castle SC. Constipation: endemic in the elderly? gerontopathophysiology, evaluation, and management. *Med Clin North Am* 1989; 73: 1497–1509.
82. Holt PR. Diarrhea and malabsorption in the elderly. *Gastroenterol Clin North Am* 1990; 19:345–359.
83. Beers MH, Ouslander JG. Risk factors in geriatric drug prescribing: a practical guide to avoiding problems. *Drugs* 1989; 37:105–112.
84. Ouslander JG. Drug therapy in the elderly. *Ann Intern Med* 1981; 95: 711–722.
85. Roy AT, Johnson LE, Lee DB, Brautbar N, Morley JE. Renal failure in older people. *J Am Geriatr Soc* 1990; 38:239–253.
86. Beers MH, Dang J, Hashegawa J, Tamai IY. Influence of hospitalization on drug therapy in the elderly. *J Am Geriatr Soc* 1989; 39: 679–683.
87. Lindeman RD, Tobin J, Shock NW. Longitudinal studies on the rate of decline in renal function with age. *J Am Geriatr Soc* 1985; 33: 278–285.
88. Wongsurawat N. Temperature regulation in the aged. In: Felsenthal G, Garrison SJ, Steinberg FU, eds. *Rehabilitation of the aging and elderly patient*. Baltimore: Williams & Wilkins, 1994; 73–78.
89. Frocht A, Fillit H. Renal disease in the geriatric patient. *J Am Geriatr Soc* 1984; 32:28–43.
90. Keltz H. Pulmonary function and disease in the aging. In: Williams TF, ed. *Rehabilitation in the aging*. New York: Raven; 1984:13–22.
91. Tockman MS. Aging of the respiratory system. In: Hazzard WR, Andres R, Bierman EL, Blass JP, eds. *Principles of geriatric medicine and gerontology*, 2nd ed. New York: McGraw-Hill, 1990; 499–508.
92. Brandstetter RD, Kazemi H. Aging and the respiratory system. *Med Clin North Am* 1983; 67:419–431.
93. Lakatta EG. The aging heart. *Ann Intern Med* 1990; 113:455–466.
94. Frontera WR, Meredith CN. Exercise in the rehabilitation of the elderly. In: Felsenthal G, Garrison SJ, Steinberg FU, eds. *Rehabilitation of the aging and elderly patient*. Baltimore: Williams & Wilkins, 1994; 35–46.
95. Boss GR, Seegmiller JE. Age-related physiologic changes and their clinical significance. *West J Med* 1981; 135:434–440.
96. American College of Sports Medicine. *ACSM's resource manual for guidelines for exercise testing and prescription*. Philadelphia: Lea & Febiger, 1993.
97. Posner JD, Gorman KM, Klein HS, Woldow A. Exercise capacity in the elderly. *Am J Cardiol* 1986; 57:52C–58C.
98. Cunningham DA, Rechnitzer PA, Pearce ME, Donner AP. Determinants of self-selected walking pace across ages 19 to 66. *J Gerontol* 1982; 37:560–564.
99. Borhani NO. Prevalence and prognostic significance of hypertension in the elderly. *J Am Geriatr Soc* 1986; 34:112–114.
100. SHEP Cooperative Research Group. Prevention of stroke by antihypertensive drug treatment in older persons with isolated systolic hyper-

tension: final results of the systolic hypertension in the elderly program (SHEP). *JAMA* 1991; 265:3255–3264.
101. Tjoa HI, Kaplan NM. Treatment of hypertension in the elderly. *JAMA* 1990; 264:1015–1018.
102. Lipsitz LA. Orthostatic hypotension in the elderly. *N Engl J Med* 1989; 321:952–957.
103. Burns EA, Goodwin JS. Immunology and infectious disease. In: Cassel CK, Reisenberg DE, Sorenson LB, Walsh JR, eds. *Geriatric medicine*, 2nd ed. New York: Springer-Verlag, 1990; 312–329.
104. Makinodan T. Immunologic aspects of aging. *Ann Intern Med* 1990; 113:455–466.
105. Felser JM, Raff MJ. Infectious disease and aging: immunologic perspectives. *J Am Geriatr Soc* 1983; 31:802–807.
106. Andres R, Elahi D, Tobin JD, Muller DC, Brant L. Impact of age on weight goals. *Ann Intern Med* 1985; 103:1030–1033.
107. Goldberg AP, Coon PJ. Non–insulin-dependent diabetes mellitus in the elderly: influence of obesity and physical inactivity. *Endocrinol Metab Clin North Am* 1987; 16:843–865.
108. Barzel US. Endocrinology and aging. In: Reichel W, ed. *Clinical aspects of aging*, 3rd ed. Baltimore: Williams & Wilkins, 1989; 373–381.
109. Gambert SR, Tsitouras PD. Effect of age on thyroid hormone physiology and function. *J Am Geriatr Soc* 1985; 33:360–365.
110. Wolfson LI, Katzman R. The neurologic consultation at age 80. In: Katzman R, Terry RD, eds. *The neurology of aging*. Philadelphia: FA Davis, 1983; 221–244.
111. Abrass IB. Disorders of temperature regulation. In: Hazzard WR, Andres R, Bierman EL, Blass JP, eds. *Principles of geriatric medicine and gerontology*, 2nd ed. New York: McGraw-Hill, 1990; 1085–1088.
112. Schaumburg HH, Spencer PS, Ochoa J. The aging human peripheral nervous system. In: Katzman R, Terry R, eds. *The neurology of aging*. Philadelphia: FA Davis, 1983; 111–122.
113. Kasper RL. Eye problems of the aged. In: Reichel W, ed. *Clinical aspects of aging*, 3rd ed. Baltimore: Williams & Wilkins, 1989; 445–453.
114. Wainapel SF. Visual impairments. In: Felsenthal G, Garrison SJ, Steinberg FU, eds. *Rehabilitation of the aging and elderly patient*. Baltimore: Williams & Wilkins, 1994; 327–338.
115. Felson DT, Anderson JJ, Hannan MT, Milton RC, Wilson PW, Kiel DP. Impaired vision and hip fracture: the Framingham study. *J Am Geriatr Soc* 1989; 37:495–500.
116. Tinetti ME. Performance-oriented assessment of mobility problems in elderly patients. *J Am Geriatr Soc* 1986; 34:119–126.
117. Ruben RJ, Kruger B. Hearing loss in the elderly. In: Katzman R, Terry R, eds. *The neurology of aging*. Philadelphia: FA Davis, 1983; 123–147.
118. Walsh DA. Age differences in central perceptual processing: a dichoptic backward masking investigation. *J Gerontol* 1976; 31:178–185.
119. Corey-Bloom J, Wiederholt WC, Edelstein S, Salmon DP, Cahn D, Barrett-Connor E. Cognitive and functional status of the oldest-old. *J Am Geriatr Soc* 1996; 44:671–674.
120. Schuman JE, Beattie EJ, Steed DA, Merry GM, Kraus AS. Geriatric patients with and without intellectual dysfunction: effectiveness of a standard rehabilitation program. *Arch Phys Med Rehabil* 1981; 62: 612–618.
121. Ettinger WH, Davis MA. Osteoarthritis. In: Hazzard WR, Andres R, Bierman EL, Blass JP, eds. *Principles of geriatric medicine and gerontology*, 2nd ed. New York: McGraw-Hill, 1990; 880–888.
122. Scileppi KP. Bone and joint disease in the elderly. *Med Clin North Am* 1983; 67:517–530.
123. Krahn MD, Mahoney JE, Eckman MH, et al. Screening for prostate cancer: a decision analytic view. *JAMA* 1994; 272:773–780.
124. Williams ME, Pannill FC III. Urinary incontinence in the elderly: physiology, pathophysiology, diagnosis, and treatment. *Ann Intern Med* 1982; 97:895–907.
125. Resnick NM, Yalla SV. Management of urinary incontinence in the elderly. *N Engl J Med* 1985; 313:800–805.
126. Cape RDT. The geriatric patient. In: Cape RDT, Coe RM, Rossman I, eds. *Fundamentals of geriatric medicine*. New York: Raven, 1983; 9–15.
127. Hirsch CH, Sommers L, Olsen A, Mullen L, Winograd CH. The natural history of functional morbidity in hospitalized older patients. *J Am Geriatr Soc* 1990; 38:1296–1303.
128. Mold JW, Stein HF. The cascade effect in the clinical care of patients. *N Engl J Med* 1986; 314:512–514.
129. Williamson JD, Fried LP. Characterization of older adults who attribute functional decrements to old age. *J Am Geriatr Soc* 1996; 44: 1429–1434.
130. Sarkisian CA, Lachs MS. Failure to thrive in older adults. *Ann Intern Med* 1996; 124:1072–1078.
131. Fried LP, Storer DJ, King DE, Lodder F. Diagnosis of illness presentation in the elderly. *J Am Geriatr Soc* 1991; 39:117–123.
132. Bortz WMII. Disuse and aging. *JAMA* 1982; 248:1203–1208.
133. Hoenig HM, Rubenstein LZ. Hospital–associated deconditioning and dysfunction. *J Am Geriatr Soc* 1991; 39:220–222.
134. Siebens H. Deconditioning. In: Kemp B, Brummel-Smith K, Ramsdell JW, eds. *Geriatric rehabilitation*. Boston: Little, Brown, 1990; 177–192.
135. Sager JA, Franke TF, Inouye SK, et al. Functional outcomes of acute medical illness and hospitalization in older persons. *Arch Intern Med* 1996; 156:645–652.
136. Warshaw GA, Moore JT, Friedman SW, et al. Functional disability in the hospitalized elderly. *JAMA* 1982; 248:847–850.
137. Reuben DB, Borok GM, Wolde-Tsakid G, et al. A randomized trial of comprehensive geriatric assessment in the care of hospitalized patients. *N Engl J Med* 1995; 332:1345–1350.
138. Landefeld CS, Palmer RM, Kresevic DM, et al. A randomized trial of care in a hospital medical unit especially designed to improve the functional outcomes of acutely ill older patients. *N Engl J Med* 1995; 332:1338–1344.
139. DeVries HA. *Physiology of exercise*. Dubuque, IA: WC Brown, 1980.
140. Frontera WR, Meredith CN, O'Reilly KP, Knuttgen HG, Evans WJ. Strength conditioning in older men: skeletal muscle hypertrophy and improved function. *J Appl Physiol* 1990; 68:329–333.
141. Morey MC, Pieper CF, Sullivan RJ Jr, Crowley GM, Cowper PA, Robbins MS. Five-year performance trends for older exercisers: a hierarchical model of endurance, strength, and flexibility. *J Am Geriatr Soc* 1996; 44:1226–1231.
142. Young A. Exercise physiology in geriatric practice. *Acta Med Scand (Suppl)* 1986; 711:227–232.
143. Lach HW, Reed AT, Arfken CL, et al. Falls in the elderly: reliability of a classification system. *J Am Geriatr Soc* 1991; 39:197–202.
144. Robbins AS, Rubenstein LZ, Josephson KR, Schulman BL, Osterweil D, Fine G. Predictors of falls among elderly people: results of two population-based studies. *Arch Intern Med* 1989; 149:1628–1633.
145. Gehlsen GM, Whaley MH. Falls in the elderly: Part I. gait. *Arch Phys Med Rehabil* 1990; 71:735–738.
146. Gehlsen GM, Whaley MH. Falls in the elderly: Part II. balance, strength and flexibility. *Arch Phys Med Rehabil* 1990; 71:739–742.
147. Tinetti ME. Factors associated with serious injury during falls by ambulatory nursing home residents. *J Am Geriatr Soc* 1987; 35: 644–648.
148. Whipple RH, Wolfson LI, Amerman PM. The relationship of knee and ankle weakness to falls in nursing home residents: an isokinetic study. *J Am Geriatr Soc* 1987; 35:13–16.
149. Fentem PH. Exercise in prevention of disease. *Br Med Bull* 1992; 48: 630–650.
150. Edwards D. *Prime moves: an exercise program for mature adults*. New York: Avery, 1990.
151. Fiatarone MA, O'Neill EF, Ryan DN, et al. Exercise training and nutritional supplementation for physical frailty in very elderly people. *N Engl J Med* 1994; 330:1769–1775.
152. Mills KM, Stewart AL, Sepsis PG, King AC. Consideration of older adults preferences for format of physical activity. *J Aging Phys Activity* 1997; 5:50–58.
153. Steinberg FU. Diagnostic responsibilities of rehabilitation departments: second look. *Arch Phys Med Rehabil* 1981; 62:509.
154. Colt HG, Shapiro AP. Drug-induced illness as a cause for admission to a community hospital. *J Am Geriatr Soc* 1989; 37:323–326.
155. Sinoff GD, Kohn D. Prevalence of adverse drug reactions. *J Am Geriatr Soc* 1990; 38:722–729.
156. Brook RH, Kamberg CJ, Mayer-Oakes A, Beers MH, Raube K, Steiner A. Appropriateness of acute medical care for the elderly: an analysis of the literature. *Health Policy* 1990; 14:225–242.
157. Willcox SM, Himmelstein DU, Woolhandler S. Inappropriate drug prescribing for the community-dwelling elderly. *JAMA* 1994; 272: 292–296.

158. Beers MH, Munekata M, Storrie M. The accuracy of medication histories in the hospital medical records of elderly persons. *J Am Geriatr Soc* 1990; 38:1183–1187.
159. Spagnoli A, Ostino G, Borga AD, D'Ambrosio. Drug compliance and unreported drugs in the elderly. *J Am Geriatr Soc* 1989; 37:619–624.
160. Abrams RC, Alexopoulos GS. Substance abuse in the elderly: over-the-counter and illegal drugs. *Hosp Community Psychiatry* 1988; 39: 822–823.
161. Stoehr GP, Ganguli M, Seaberg EC, Echement DA, Belle S. Over-the-counter medication use in an older rural community: the MoVIES project. *J Am Geriatr Soc* 1997; 45:158–165.
162. Rozzini R, Bianchetti A, Zanett O, Trabucchi M. Are too many drugs prescribed for the elderly after all? *J Am Geriatr Soc* 1989; 37:89–90.
163. Morrow D, Leirer V, Sheikh J. Adherence and medication instructions. *J Am Geriatr Soc* 1988; 36:1147–1160.
164. Cooper JK, Love DW, Raffoul PR. Intentional prescription non-adherence (non-compliance) by the elderly. *J Am Geriatr Soc* 1982; 30: 329–332.
165. Pereles L, Romonko L, Murzyn T, et al. Evaluation of a self-medication program. *J Am Geriatr Soc* 1996; 44:161–165.
166. Hsia Der E, Rubenstein LZ, Choy GS. The benefits of in-home pharmacy evaluation for older persons. *J Am Geriatr Soc* 1997; 45: 211–214.
167. Larson EB, Kukull WA, Buchner D, Reifler BV. Adverse drug reaction associated with global cognitive impairment in elderly persons. *Ann Intern Med* 1987; 107:169–173.
168. Nolan L, O'Malley K. Prescribing for the elderly: Part II. prescribing patterns: differences due to age. *J Am Geriatr Soc* 1988; 36:245–254.
169. Resnick NM. An 89-year-old woman with urinary incontinence. *JAMA* 1996; 276:1832–1840.
170. Ham RJ, Lekan-Rutledge DA. Incontinence. In: Ham RJ, Sloane PD, eds. *Primary care geriatrics*. St. Louis: CV Mosby, 1997; 321–349.
171. National Institutes of Health Consensus Development Conference. Urinary incontinence in adults. *J Am Geriatr Soc* 1990; 38:265–272.
172. Colling J, Ouslander J, Hadley BJ, Eisch J, Campbell E. The effects of patterned urge-response toileting (PURT) on urinary incontinence among nursing home residents. *J Am Geriatr Soc* 1992; 40:135–141.
173. Schnelle JF, MacRae PG, Ouslander JG, Simmons SF, Nitta M. Functional incidental training, mobility performance, and incontinence care with nursing home residents. *J Am Geriatr Soc* 1995; 43:1356–1362.
174. Burgio KC, Pearce KL, Lucco AJ. *Staying dry: a practical guide to bladder control*. Baltimore: Johns Hopkins University Press, 1989.
175. Urinary Incontinence Guideline Panel. *Urinary incontinence in adults: clinical practice guideline. AHCPR publication no. 92-0038.* Rockville, MD: Agency for Health Care Policy and Research, Public Health Service, United States Department of Health and Human Services, 1992.
176. Ouslander JG, Schnelle JF. Incontinence in the nursing home. *Ann Intern Med* 1995; 122:438–449.
177. Marzuk PM. Biofeedback in gastrointestinal disorders: a review of the literature. *Ann Intern Med* 1985; 103:240–244.
178. Wald A. Biofeedback therapy for fecal incontinence. *Ann Intern Med* 1981; 95:146–149.
179. Gottlieb GL. Sleep disorders and their management. *Am J Med* 1990; 88:29S–33S.
180. King AC, Oman RF, Brassington GS, Bliwise DL, Haskell WL. Moderate-intensity exercise and self-rated quality of sleep in older adults—a randomized controlled trial. *JAMA* 1997; 277:32–37.
181. Morin CM, Azrin NH. Behavioral and cognitive treatments of geriatric insomnia. *J Consult Clin Psychol* 1988; 56:748–753.
182. Campbell SS, Dawson D, Anderson MW. Alleviation of sleep maintenance insomnia with timed exposure to bright light. *J Am Geriatr Soc* 1993; 41:829–836.
183. Garfinkel D, Laudon M, Nof D, et al. Improvement of sleep quality in elderly people by controlled-release melatonin. *Lancet* 1995; 346: 541–544.
184. NIH Consensus Development Panel on Depression in Late Life. Diagnosis and treatment of depression in late life. *JAMA* 1992; 268: 1018–1024.
185. Rothschild AJ. The diagnosis and treatment of late-life depression. *J Clin Psychiatry* 1996; 57(suppl 5):5–11.
186. Hirschfeld RM, Keller MB, Panico S, et al. The National Depressive and Manic-Depressive Association consensus statement on the undertreatment of depression. *JAMA* 1977; 277:333–340.
187. Gurland BJ, Wilder DE, Berkman C. Depression and disability in the elderly: reciprocal relations and changes with age. *Int J Geriatr Psychiatry* 1988; 3:163–179.
188. Rapp SR, Davis KM. Geriatric depression: physicians' knowledge, perceptions, and diagnostic practices. *Gerontologist* 1989; 29: 252–257.
189. Flint AJ. Epidemiology and comorbidity of anxiety disorders in the elderly. *Am J Psychiatry* 1994; 151:640–649.
190. Brown CS, Rakel RE, Wells BG. A practical update on anxiety disorders and their pharmacologic treatment. *Arch Intern Med* 1991; 151: 873–884.
191. Martin LM, Fleming KC, Evans JM. Recognition and management of anxiety and depression in elderly patients. *Mayo Clin Proc* 1995; 70:999–1006.
192. Francis J, Martin D, Kapoor WN. A prospective study of delirium in hospitalized elderly. *JAMA* 1990; 263:1097–1101.
193. Schor JD, Levkoff SE, Lipsitz LA, et al. Risk factors for delirium in hospitalized elderly. *JAMA* 1992; 267:827–831.
194. Inouye SK, Charpentier PA. Precipitating factors for delirium in hospitalized elderly persons. Predictive model and interrelationship with baseline vulnerability. *JAMA* 1996; 275:852–857.
195. Marcantonio ER, Goldman L, Mangione CM, et al. A clinical prediction rule for delirium after elective noncardiac surgery. *JAMA* 1994; 271:134–139.
196. O'Keeffe S, Lavan J. The prognostic significance of delirium in older hospital patients. *J Am Geriatr Soc* 1997; 45:174–178.
197. Ferrell BA. Pain management in elderly people. *J Am Geriatr Soc* 1991; 39:64–73.
198. Ferrell BR, Ferrell BA, eds. *Pain in the elderly. A report of the task force on pain in the elderly of the International Association for the Study of Pain.* Seattle: IASP Press, 1996.
199. Ferrell BA, Ferrell BR, Osterweil D. Pain in the nursing home. *J Am Geriatr Soc* 1990; 38:409–414.
200. Nishikawa ST, Ferrell BA. Pain assessment in the elderly. *Clin Geriatr Long Term Care* 1993; 1:15–28.
201. Parmelee PA, Smith B, Katz IR. Pain complaints and cognitive status among elderly institution residents. *J Am Geriatr Soc* 1993; 41: 517–522.
202. Ferrell BA, Ferrell BR, Rivera L. Pain in cognitively impaired nursing home patients. *J Pain Symptom Manage* 1995; 10:591–595.
203. Rochon PA, Fortin PR, Dear KB, Minaker KL, Chalmers TC. Reporting of age in data in clinical trials of arthritis. *Arch Intern Med* 1993; 153:243–248.
204. Griffin MR, Piper JM, Doughtery JR, Snowden M, Ray WA. Nonsteroidal antiinflammatory drug use and increased risk for peptic ulcer disease in elderly persons. *Ann Intern Med* 1991; 114:257–263.
205. Ferrell B, Rivera L. Cancer pain: impact on elderly patients and their family caregivers. In: Roy R, ed. *Chronic pain in old age: an integrated biopsychosocial perspective*. Toronto: University of Toronto Press, 1995.
206. Billings AG, Moos R. The role of coping responses and social resources in attenuating the stress of life events. *J Behav Med* 1981; 4: 139–157.
207. Clark GS, Bray GP. Development of a rehabilitation plan. In: Williams TF, ed. *Rehabilitation in the aging*. New York: Raven, 1984; 125–143.
208. Steinberg FU. Medical evaluation, assessment of function and potential, and rehabilitation plan. In: Felsenthal G, Garrison SJ, Steinberg FU, eds. *Rehabilitation of the aging and elderly patient*. Baltimore: Williams & Wilkins, 1994; 81–96.
209. Hunt TE. Homeostatic malfunctions in the aged. *Br Columbia Med J* 1980; 22:379–381.
210. Bodily KC, Burgess EM. Contralateral limb and patient survival after leg amputation. *Am J Surg* 1983; 146:280–282.
211. Clark GS. Rehabilitation team: process and roles. In: Felsenthal G, Garrison SJ, Steinberg FU, eds. *Rehabilitation of the aging and elderly patient*. Baltimore: Williams & Wilkins, 1994; 439–448.
212. Fleming KC, Adams AC, Petersen RC. Dementia: diagnosis and evaluation. *Mayo Clin Proc* 1995; 70:1093–1107.
213. Clarfield AM. The reversible dementias: do they reverse? *Ann Intern Med* 1988; 109:476–486.
214. Siu AL. Screening for dementia and investigating its causes. *Ann Intern Med* 1991; 115:122–132.

215. McKhann G, Drachman D, Folstein M, Katzman R, Price D. Clinical diagnosis of Alzheimer's disease. *Neurology* 1984; 34:939–944.
216. Beck JC, Benson DF, Scheibel AB, Spar JE, Rubenstein LZ. Dementia in the elderly: the silent epidemic. *Ann Intern Med* 1982; 97:231–241.
217. *Early Alzheimer's disease: recognition and assessment. Consumer Version, Clinical Practice Guideline No. 19.* Rockville, MD: U.S. Department of Health and Human Services, Public Health Service, Agency for Health Care Policy and Research, 1996. AHCPR Publication No. 96-0704.
218. King MB, Tinetti ME. Falls in community-dwelling older persons. *J Am Geriatr Soc* 1995; 43:1146–1154.
219. Lipsitz L. An 85-year old woman with a history of falls. *JAMA* 1996; 276:59–66.
220. Studenski S, Duncan PW, Chandler J, Samsa G, Prescott B, Hogue C, Pearon LB. Predicting falls: the role of mobility and nonphysical factors. *J Am Geriatr Soc* 1994; 42:297–302.
221. Cummings SR, Nevitt MC, Browner WS, et al. Risk factors for hip fracture in white women. *N Engl J Med* 1995; 332:767–773.
222. Wolf SL, Barnhart HX, Kutner NG, et al. Reducing frailty and falls in older persons: an investigation of Tai Chi and computerized balance training. *J Am Geriatr Soc* 1996; 44:489–497.
223. Tinetti ME, Baker DI, McAvay G, et al. A multifactorial intervention to reduce the risk of falling among elderly people living in the community. *N Engl J Med* 1994; 331:821–827.
224. Johnell O, Cooper C, Melton LJ III. Preventive medicine—how do we prevent hip fractures? *Lancet* 1993; Jan 9:89.
225. Koval KJ, Zuckerman JD. Functional recovery after fracture of the hip. *J Bone Joint Dis [Am]* 1994; 76:751–758.
226. Bernardini B, Neinecke C, Pagani M, Grillo A, et al. Comorbidity and adverse clinical events in the rehabilitation of older adults after hip fracture. *J Am Geriatr Soc* 1995; 43:894–898.
227. Kiel DP, Eichorn A, Intrator O, Silliman RA, Mor V. The outcomes of patients newly admitted to nursing homes after hip fracture. *Am J Pub Health* 1994; 84:1281–1286.
228. Guccione AA, Fagerson RL, Anderson JJ. Regaining functional independence in the acute care setting following hip fracture. *Phys Ther* 1996; 76:818–826.
229. Cameron ID, Lyle DM, Quine S. Cost effectiveness of accelerated rehabilitation after proximal femoral fracture. *J Clin Epidemiol* 1994; 47:1307–1313.
230. Zuckerman JD, Skovron ML, Fessel K, Cohen H, Frankel VH. The role of surgical delay in the long-term outcomes of hip fractures in geriatric patients. *Orthop Trans* 1993; 16:750.
231. Hochberg MC, Altman RD, Brandt KD, et al. Guidelines for the medical management of osteoarthritis. Part I. Osteoarthritis of the hip. *Arthritis Rheum* 1995; 38:1535–1540.
232. Hochberg MC, Altman RD, Brandt KD, et al. Guidelines for the medical management of osteoarthritis. Part II. Osteoarthritis of the knee. *Arthritis Rheum* 1995; 38:1541–1546.
233. Ditunno J, Ehrlich GE. Care and training of elderly patients with rheumatoid arthritis. *Geriatrics* 1970; 25:164–172.
234. Nesher G, Moore TL, Zuckner J. Rheumatoid arthritis in the elderly. *J Am Geriatr Soc* 1991; 39:284–294.
235. Lorig K, Mazonson PD, Holman HR. Evidence suggesting that health education for self-managment in patients with chronic arthritis has sustained health benefits while reducing health care costs. *Arthritis Rheum* 1993; 36:439–446.
236. Minor MA. Exercise in the management of osteoarthritis of the knee and hip. *Arthritis Care Res* 1994; 7:198–204.
237. Puett DW, Griffin MR. Published trials of nonmedicinal and noninvasive therapies for hip and knee osteoarthritis. *Ann Intern Med* 1994; 121:133–140.
238. Ettinger WH, Burns R, Messier SP, et al. A randomized trial comparing aerobic exercise and resistance exercise with a health education program in older adults with knee osteoarthritis. *JAMA* 1997; 277: 25–31.
239. Michet CJ, Evans JM, Fleming KC, O'Duffy JD, Jurisson ML, Hunder GG. Common rheumatologic diseases in elderly patients. *Mayo Clin Proc* 1995; 70:1205–1214.
240. Shah S, Vanclay F, Cooper B. Efficiency, effectiveness and duration of stroke rehabilitation. *Stroke* 1990; 21:241–246.
241. Schmidt EV, Smirnov VE, Ryabova VS. Results of the seven-year prospective study of stroke patients. *Stroke* 1988; 19:942–949.
242. Lindmark B. Evaluation of functional capacity after stroke with special emphasis on motor function and activities of daily living. *Scand J Rehabil Med* 1988; 21(suppl):1–40.
243. Granger CV, Clark GS. Functional status and outcomes of stroke rehabilitation. *Top Geriatr Rehabil* 1994; 9:72–84.
244. Wade DT, Langton-Hewer R, Wood VA. Stroke: the influence of age upon outcome. *Age Ageing* 1984; 13:357–362.
245. Granger CV, Hamilton BB, Gresham GE. Stroke rehabilitation outcome study: Part I. general description. *Arch Phys Med Rehabil* 1988; 69:506–509.
246. Granger CV, Hamilton BB, Gresham GE, Kramer AA. The stroke rehabilitation outcome study: Part II. Relative merits of the total Barthel Index score and a four-item subscore in predicting patient outcomes. *Arch Phys Med Rehabil* 1989; 70:100–103.
247. Osberg JS, DeJong G, Haley SM. Predicting long-term outcome among post-rehabilitation stroke patients. *Am J Phys Med Rehabil* 1988; 68:94–103.
248. Keith RA, Wilson DB, Gutierez P. Acute and subacute rehabilitation for stroke: a comparison. *Arch Phys Med Rehabil* 1995; 76:495–500.
249. Kramer AM, Steiner JF, Schlenker RE, et al. Outcomes and costs after hip fracture and stroke: a comparison of rehabilitation settings. *JAMA* 1997; 277:396–404.
250. Garrison SJ. Geriatric stroke rehabilitation. In: Felsenthal G, Garrison SJ, Steinberg FU, eds. *Rehabilitation of the aging and elderly patient.* Baltimore: Williams & Wilkins, 1994; 175–186.
251. Cutson TM, Bongiorni DR. Rehabilitation of the older lower limb amputee: a brief review. *J Am Geriatr Soc* 1996; 44:1388–1393.
252. DuBow LL, Witt PL, Kadaba MP, Reyes R, Cochran V. Oxygen consumption of elderly persons with bilateral below knee amputations: ambulation vs. wheelchair propulsion. *Arch Phys Med Rehabil* 1983; 64:255–259.
253. Wolf E, Lilling M, Ferber I, Marcus J. Prosthetic rehabilitation of elderly bilateral amputees. *Int J Rehabil Res* 1989; 12:271–278.
254. O'Connell PG, Gnatz S. Hemiplegia and amputation: rehabilitation in the dual disability. *Arch Phys Med Rehabil* 1989; 70:451–454.
255. Stover SL, Fine PR, eds. *Spinal cord injury: the facts and figures.* Birmingham, AL: University of Alabama, 1986.
256. DeVivo MJ, Fine PR, Maetz HM, Stover SL. Prevalence of spinal cord injury: a reestimation employing life table techniques. *Arch Neurol* 1980; 37:707–708.
257. Ohry A, Shemesh Y, Rozin R. Are chronic spinal cord injured patients (SCIP) prone to premature aging? *Med Hypotheses* 1983; 11:467–469.
258. DeVivo MJ, Stover SL, Black KJ. Prognostic factors for 12-year survival after spinal cord injury. *Arch Phys Med Rehabil* 1992; 73: 156–162.
259. DeVivo MJ, Kartus PL, Rutt RD, Stover SL, Fine PR. The influence of age at time of spinal cord injury on rehabilitation outcome. *Arch Neurol* 1990; 47:687–691.
260. Yarkony GM, Roth EJ, Heinemann AW, Lovell LL. Spinal cord injury rehabilitation outcome: impact of age. *J Clin Epidemiol* 1988; 41: 173–177.
261. Rockwood K, Fox RA, Stolee P, et al. Frailty in elderly people: an evolving concept. *Can Med Assoc J* 1994; 150:495–498.
262. Rockwood K, Stolee P, McDowell I. Factors associated with institutionalization of older people in Canada: tesing a multifactorial definition of frailty. *J Am Geriatr Soc* 1996; 44:578–582.
263. Buchner DM, Wagner EH. Preventing frail health. *Clin Geriatr Med* 1992; 8:1–17.
264. Lavizzo-Mourey R. Promoting health and function among older adults. In: Hassard WR, Bierman EL, Blass JP, Ettinger WH, Halter JB, eds. *Principles of geriatric medicine and gerontology*. New York: McGraw-Hill, 1994; 213–220.
265. Lawrence RH, Jette AM. Disentangling the disablement process. *J Gerontol* 1996:51B(suppl):173–182.
266. Guralnik JM, Perrucci L, Simonsick EM, Salve ME, Wallace BR. Lower-extremity function in persons over the age of 70 years as a predictor of subsequent disability. *N Engl J Med* 1995; 332:556–561.
267. Tinetti ME, Inouye SK, Gill T, Doucette JT. Shared risk factors for falls, incontinence, and functional dependence. *JAMA* 1995; 273: 1348–1353.
268. Evans LK, Yurkow J, Siegler EL. The CARE program: a nurse-managed collaborative outpatient program to improve function of frail older people. *J Am Geriatr Soc* 1995; 43:1155–1160.
269. Mendes de Leon CF Seeman TE, Baker DI, Riachardson ED, Tinetti ME. Self-efficacy, physical decline, and change in functioning in com-

munity-living elders: a prospective study. *J Gerontol* 1996; 51B(suppl):183–190.

270. Tinetti ME, Powell L. Fear of falling and low self-efficacy: a cause of dependence in elderly persons. *J Gerontol* 1993; 48(Special Issue): 35–38.
271. Kaufman SR, Becker G. Content and boundaries of medicine in long-term care: physicians talk about stroke. *Gerontology* 1991; 31: 238–245.
272. Felsenthal G, Cohen BS, Hilton EB, Panagos AV, Aiken BM. The physiatrist as primary physician for patients on an inpatient rehabilitation unit. *Arch Phys Med Rehabil* 1984; 65:375–378.
273. Cummings V, Kerner JF, Arones S, Steinbock C. Day hospital service in rehabilitation medicine: an evaluation. *Arch Phys Med Rehabil* 1985; 66:86–91.
274. Fisk AA. Comprehensive health care for the elderly. *JAMA* 1983; 249:230–236.
275. Council on Scientific Affairs. Home care in the 1990's. *JAMA* 1990; 263:1241–1244.
276. Grieco AJ. Physician's guide to managing home care of older patients. *Geriatrics* 1991; 46:49–60.
277. Frank JC, Miller LS. Comunity-based rehabilitation for the elderly. In: Felsenthal G, Garrison SJ, Steinberg FU, eds. *Rehabilitation of the aging and elderly patient*. Baltimore: Williams & Wilkins, 1994; 477–485.

Rehabilitation Medicine: Principles and Practice, Third Edition,
edited by Joel A. DeLisa and Bruce M. Gans.
Lippincott–Raven Publishers, Philadelphia © 1998.

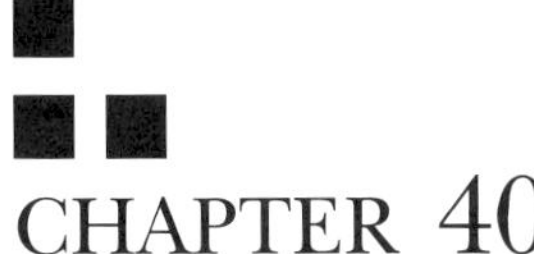

CHAPTER 40

Spasticity and Associated Abnormalities of Muscle Tone

James W. Little and Teresa L. Massagli

To understand spasticity, we must first define muscle tone. Tone is resistance felt by clinicians as they passively move a limb. Spasticity is one type of exaggerated tone, which increases with the velocity of muscle stretch (i.e., velocity-dependent hypertonus); it is due to a hyperactive stretch reflex and is one type of hypertonus that develops after upper motoneuron (UMN) injury (1). Other spinal or brain stem reflexes may become hyperactive, leading to other hypertonus, such as flexor withdrawal spasms or exaggerated tonic neck reflexes. These various types of hypertonus are part of the UMN syndrome and are often accompanied by weakness and impaired motor control. Clinicians try to lessen hypertonus to improve motor control and to reduce spasm effects on sleep, skin breakdown, and pain.

Spasticity and flexor spasms of the UMN syndrome are due to hyperactive spinal reflexes. Some hypertonus of the UMN syndrome is due to imbalance in descending motor control, such as the hemiplegic posture with flexed upper limb and extended lower limb. Other hypertonus or other factors limiting joint motion must be differentiated from spasticity, such as that due to muscle or joint pathology (e.g., myotonia, muscle contracture, myotendinous contracture, or joint capsule tightness), peripheral nerve or spinal cord pathology (e.g., cramp, tetanus, tetany), or other central nervous system (CNS) lesions (e.g., Parkinson's rigidity, tardive dyskinesia).

SIGNS OF SPASTICITY AND HYPERTONUS

The signs of spasticity and hypertonus depend on time postinjury. Spasticity and hypertonus evolve over 3 to 6 months after CNS injury. Spinal reflexes are depressed acutely (i.e., the period of spinal or cerebral shock); they gradually become hyperactive over weeks to months. Later, shortening of muscle fibers (i.e., myotendinous contracture) or joint capsule tightness may add to the hypertonus.

The site and extent of the CNS lesion also affects the spasticity and hypertonus (2,3). Spinal lesions yield only hyperactive spinal reflexes, whereas cerebral lesions yield both hyperactive brain stem and spinal reflexes. The size of the CNS lesion also affects the hypertonus; larger lesions with less recovery of voluntary control lead to more hypertonus. Spasticity and weakness are only mild after pyramidal lesions of the corticospinal tract. Disruption of extrapyramidal cortical–brain stem–spinal pathways is of greater significance in producing spasticity.

The onset of the CNS lesion affects the spasticity and hypertonus (1). With slow-onset lesions (e.g., tumors, spinal stenosis), there is no spinal or cerebral shock. In contrast to acute-onset UMN syndrome, hyperactive reflexes are often the earliest sign of a slowly progressive cerebral or spinal pathology. Paresis appears late in slow-onset UMN syndrome.

Other factors also affect the hypertonus. Limb positioning and use during the appearance of spasticity affect its final manifestations (4). Nociceptive input during the development of hyperactive reflexes increases flexor hypertonus. In infancy, CNS developmental changes alter the pattern of hypertonus.

Spinal Cord Injury

After complete spinal cord injury (SCI), spinal reflexes below the lesion are depressed. This reflex depression is called spinal shock and is due to loss of normal tonic descending facilitation. Over days to months, various neuronal

J. W. Little: Department of Rehabilitation Medicine, University of Washington School of Medicine, Seattle, Washington 98195.
T. L. Massagli: Departments of Rehabilitation Medicine and Pediatrics, University of Washington School of Medicine, Seattle, Washington 98195.

mechanisms increase reflex excitability. Spinal reflexes require 6 months or more to become fully hyperactive (5–7).

After incomplete SCI, spinal reflexes return sooner than after complete SCI. Early hyperreflexia accompanies the return of voluntary movement. Chronically, hypertonus is more disabling in those with minimal sparing of voluntary movement; it is often less severe in those with either complete SCI or with functional voluntary movements (8,9).

Muscle stretch, whether by passive or active limb motion or by tendon tap, elicits reflex contractions. These stretch reflexes are of two varieties: phasic or tonic. Phasic stretch reflexes are elicited by fast but not slow limb motion because the stretch receptor of the IA afferent is velocity sensitive; the reflex muscle contraction fades in seconds because limb velocity slows and the afferent discharge rate decreases (Fig. 40-1). Tonic stretch reflexes are length dependent and likely come from the length-sensitive discharge of group II muscle spindle afferents; the reflex muscle contraction lasts as long as stretch is maintained. Distinguishing phasic and tonic stretch reflexes is important clinically because they respond differently to treatment.

Hyperactive phasic stretch reflexes are seen as:

1. Low-threshold, large-amplitude tendon jerks that often spread to other joints and to the opposite limb
2. Clonus (i.e., repetitive muscle contractions to rapid, maintained stretch), typically observed in ankle plantarflexors, knee extensors, and finger flexors
3. Velocity-dependent hypertonus that often manifests a clasp-knife quality such that passive joint movement results in a sudden giving way of the resistance
4. Extensor spasms, where rapid hip extension (as in going from sitting to supine) elicits a reflex contraction of knee extensors, hip adductors, ankle plantarflexors, and hip extensors and may spread to trunk and upper limb muscles (10)

Hypertonus due to tonic stretch reflexes is less common (Fig. 40-2). Such hyperactive tonic stretch reflexes appear most commonly in flexor muscles and lead to contracture (11).

Another hyperactive spinal reflex after SCI is the flexor withdrawal (i.e., exteroceptive or cutaneomuscular) reflex (Fig. 40-1) (1,8). Noxious input elicits limb flexion. Some flexor spasms are spontaneous, without external stimulus. Uninhibited bladder contractions may elicit some of these

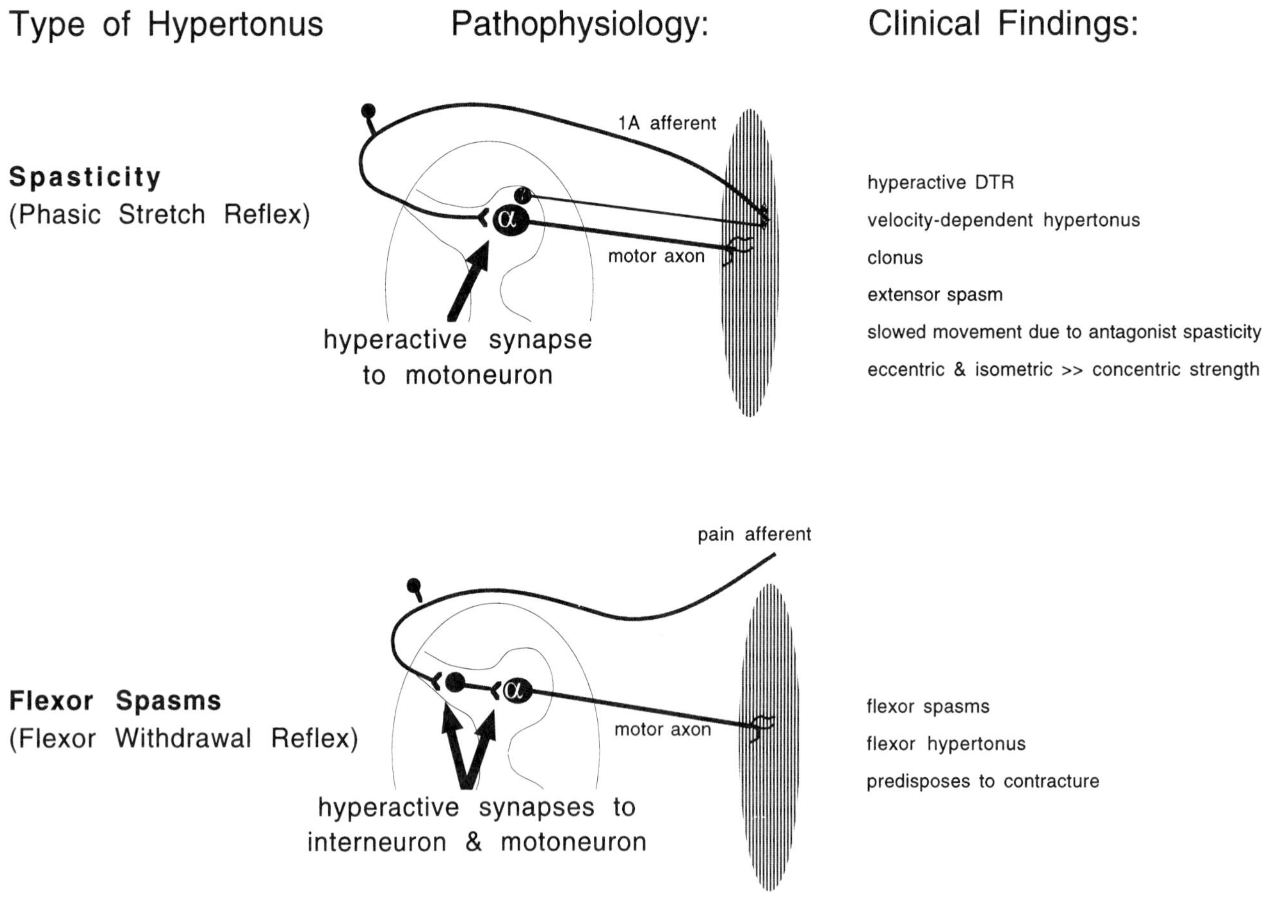

FIG. 40-1. Common types of hypertonus. Two of the most common types of hypertonus after upper motor neuron (UMN) syndrome are the hyperactive phasic stretch reflex (spasticity) and the hyperactive flexor withdrawal reflex (flexor spasms).

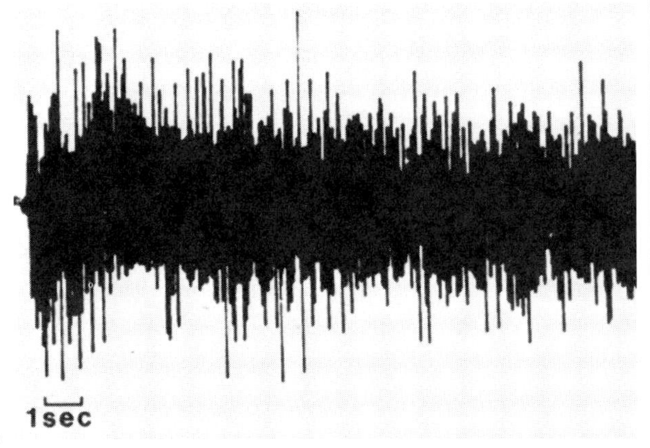

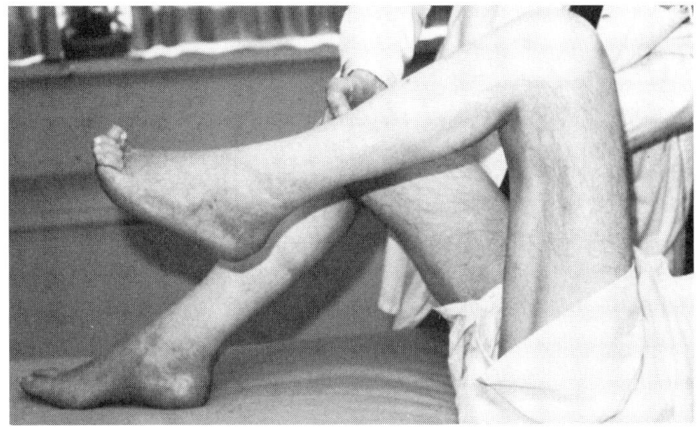

FIG. 40-2. Tonic stretch reflex. Tonic electrical activity from the medial hamstrings elicited by static stretch **(A)** and associated with knee flexion contracture **(B)** in a patient with incomplete spinal cord injury. Electromyographic activity was recorded with surface electrodes overlying the muscle.

spontaneous flexor spasms. Occasionally a limb is in tonic flexor spasm; this is often due to pressure sores, hemorrhoids, paronychia, or other continuous noxious input. A vicious cycle of flexor spasms caused by a pressure sore leads to more noxious stimulation, with more flexor spasms and more skin breakdown (12).

Functionally, the hypertonus of SCI can interfere with self-care, transfers, driving, and sleep and can lead to skin breakdown. After incomplete SCI, hip adductor scissoring and clonus can interfere with gait, but extensor spasms also can aid in standing (Fig. 40-3).

Demyelinating Disease

Spasticity is common and often severe in multiple sclerosis (MS), but its signs are varied (13). Hypertonus, clonus, flexor or extensor spasms, and decerebrate or decorticate rigidity may occur. The hypertonus often is accompanied by contractures, ataxia, weakness, and fatigue (13,14). Lower extremity spasms increase the energy cost of walking (15).

White matter disease in children is usually due to one of the leukodystrophies. Hypertonus, hyperreflexia, and clonus are seen first, then rigidity and exaggerated supraspinal reflexes become prominent, accompanied by contractures (16).

Stroke

After stroke, reflexes and voluntary movement are depressed initially and muscles are flaccid (i.e., cerebral shock). Reflexes begin to return within days to weeks, then become hyperactive over a period of weeks to months (17). They become less hyperactive as voluntary movements recover. This recovery may halt at any point, leaving residual weakness and hyperreflexia.

Spasticity after stroke typically includes velocity-dependent hypertonus, tendon hyperreflexia, and clonus. In contrast to SCI, flexor spasms and other cutaneomuscular hyperreflexia are not as prominent after stroke. Hyperactive tonic neck reflexes or tonic vestibular reflexes may be present.

Synergy, or the cocontraction of flexors or extensors, is common with partial recovery of volitional movements. Associated or synkinetic movements also are common in hemiplegia; movements are accompanied by muscle contraction

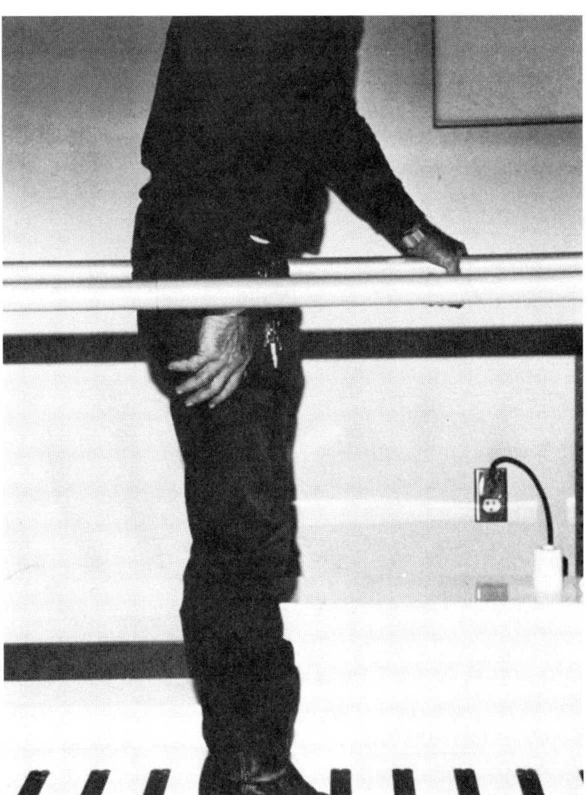

FIG. 40-3. Reflex standing. This patient with T3 traumatic spinal cord injury is motor complete in his lower limbs except for slight voluntary toe movements bilaterally. He can elicit functional lower limb extensor spasms, which he uses to stand beside his pickup truck while he loads and unloads his wheelchair.

on the opposite side or in the other limb on the same side. These synergistic and synkinetic reactions of hemiplegia are exaggerated normal reactions.

Most hemiplegic patients recover some ambulation. Ankle or knee clonus, hip adductor scissoring, deficient hip, knee, and ankle flexion during the swing phase of gait, and exaggerated knee and ankle extension during the stance phase are characteristic of hemiplegic stroke (1,18,19). In the hemiplegic upper limb, flexor tone and movements predominate over extensor.

Traumatic Brain Injury

Various types of hypertonus follow traumatic brain injury (TBI) (20). Decorticate and decerebrate rigidity are common acutely and are prominent when hyperadrenergic ''storming'' is present (i.e., tachypnea, tachycardia, hypertension, and sweating). Rigidity decreases over days to weeks if recovery ensues, but may persist indefinitely after severe trauma. Spasticity emerges after initial cerebral shock as velocity-dependent hypertonus, hyperactive tendon reflexes, and clonus. It may accompany ataxia or rigidity of cerebellar or basal ganglia involvement. Exaggerated tonic neck and vestibular reflexes may be present. As in stroke, hypertonus diminishes with recovery of voluntary movements. Common upper limb impairments include shoulder adduction/internal rotation, elbow flexion/pronation, wrist flexion or extension, clenched fist, and thumb in palm deformity. Common lower limb impairments include hip flexion/adduction, knee extension or flexion, foot equinovarus, and great toe extension.

Decorticate and Decerebrate Rigidity

Mid-brain or bilateral forebrain lesions, whether due to head injury, cerebrovascular accident (CVA), tumor, anoxia, or severe metabolic disorder, result in two stereotyped motor responses: decorticate and decerebrate rigidity. Decorticate rigidity is associated with bilateral forebrain lesions and presents as upper limb flexion and lower limb extension. In decerebrate rigidity, the lesion involves either the diencephalon or mid-brain bilaterally and presents as rigid extension of all limbs, often with neck hyperextension (i.e., opisthotonus). These postures appear immediately after injury, in contrast to spasticity. Decorticate or decerebrate rigidity may be present continuously or wax and wane in appearance. A noxious stimulus often exaggerates the abnormal posture, and tonic neck reflexes may appear superimposed on the underlying hypertonus. These rigid postures are associated with varying degrees of impaired consciousness and tend to resolve if coma lessens.

Cerebral Palsy

Altered muscle tone is an early sign of cerebral palsy (CP) (21). An early hypotonia lasting a few weeks to as long as 1 year after birth evolves to hyperreflexia, clonus, hypertonicity, and abnormal postures, such as scissoring and extension of the lower limbs or persistent flexion and a fisted hand in the upper limbs. Primitive infantile reflexes persist abnormally and become hyperactive. The nature of the movement disorder in spastic CP is a combination of hypertonus, impaired posture, persistent primitive reflexes, upper limb flexor synergies, lower limb extensor synergies, weakness, and abnormal motor control (22–24). Spasticity may coexist with other movement disorders such as athetosis (i.e., involuntary slow writhing), chorea (i.e., involuntary rapid movements), or dystonia (i.e., sustained abnormal postures). Hemiplegia or hemiparesis do not always imply spasticity; in some cases, abnormal motor control and intrinsic muscle changes cause the hemi-syndrome in the absence of velocity-dependent hypertonus (25).

The neurologic abnormalities may lead to muscle shortening, joint capsule tightness, and osseous deformities (26). Common musculoskeletal complications of spastic CP include elbow flexion and pronation contractures, wrist and finger flexion deformities, heel cord tightness with equinovarus or calcaneovalgus, hip flexion and adduction contractures with femoral anteversion, coxa valga, and hip subluxation or dislocation.

PATHOPHYSIOLOGY OF SPASTICITY AND HYPERTONUS

The pathophysiology of spasticity and hypertonus is complex (1,27,28). Different spinal and supraspinal pathways contribute, and multiple neuronal mechanisms lead to the increased reflex excitability.

The Final Common Pathway

The alpha-motoneuron in the spinal cord is the final common path through which all motor output is conveyed. Each motoneuron summates excitation and inhibition from thousands of spinal and supraspinal inputs, and this determines when it will fire. Each discharge of the motoneuron results in a contraction of all its muscle fibers (i.e., the motor unit). Voluntary supraspinal input or reflex spinal input can discharge motoneurons and cause muscle contractions. Spasticity is the appearance of hyperactive spinal stretch reflexes after loss of supraspinal input.

Initially after a CNS lesion, the reflexes are depressed (i.e., cerebral or spinal shock) (Fig. 40-4). This is due to loss of normal descending facilitation. Spinal reflexes have insufficient excitatory input to depolarize the alpha-motoneurons, owing to this spinal or cerebral shock (29). Within days, neuronal mechanisms increase reflex excitability (30). One early mechanism is denervation supersensitivity, which results from increased neurotransmitter receptors or from decreased neurotransmitter inactivation (31,32). Synapse growth by reflex inputs may explain later increases in reflex excitability; the slow growth of new synapses leads to late reflex changes extending over weeks-to-months (30).

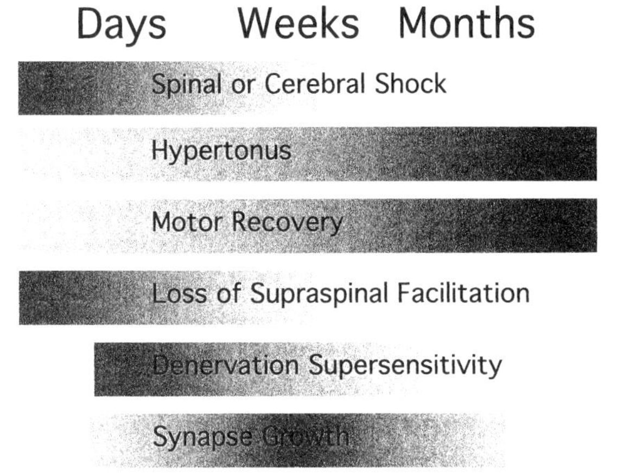

FIG. 40-4. Neuronal mechanisms contributing to hyperreflexia and recovery after upper motor neuron (UMN) injury. The gradual appearance of hyperreflexia and motor recovery over weeks to months after UMN syndrome is likely due to multiple mechanisms that act sequentially, including disinhibition, denervation supersensitivity, and synapse growth.

Some have postulated that spasticity results from loss of normal inhibition in reflex pathways (1,27,28). Such disinhibition fits with decerebrate rigidity, with its immediate-onset extensor hypertonus. The delayed onset of spasticity suggests that neuronal mechanisms other than disinhibition play a greater role in spasticity.

Exaggerated Segmental Reflexes

The muscle spindle has two afferents (IA and II) that respond to muscle stretch. IA afferents respond to velocity of stretch. Group II afferents respond to muscle length. IA afferents are monosynaptic excitatory to alpha-motoneurons of the same muscle and its synergists. Group II fibers are polysynaptic excitatory to flexor motoneurons and inhibitory to extensor motoneurons. Efferent gamma-motoneurons innervate the intrafusal muscle fibers of muscle spindles and maintain tension in the spindle during voluntary contractions; thus, IA and II afferents can respond to muscle stretch even in a shortened muscle. These afferent inputs are altered by inhibition. There is presynaptic inhibition due to inhibitory synapses on the IA afferent endings. There is recurrent inhibition, where alpha-motoneurons send collaterals back to inhibit their own firing through inhibitory interneurons called Renshaw cells. Reciprocal inhibition involves inhibitory interneurons that receive agonist IA afferent input and inhibit alpha-motoneurons to antagonists.

Hyperactive stretch reflexes are due to increased reflex gain and/or lowered reflex threshold (33,34). Reflex gain increases due to (a) denervation supersensitivity in alpha-motoneurons, (b) synapse growth by IA afferents, (c) less presynaptic inhibition on IA terminals (35), or (d) less postsynaptic inhibition (36,37). The long-held view that gamma-motoneuron activity increases after UMN lesions, resulting in increased muscle spindle sensitivity, is no longer accepted (38). Two types of postsynaptic inhibition are more, not less, after SCI: reciprocal inhibition (39) and recurrent inhibition (40). However, reciprocal inhibition is less during voluntary activity, associated with impaired rapid alternating movements (41).

Clonus is attributed to self-sustaining oscillation of phasic stretch reflexes with recurrent bursts of IA afferent discharge and hyperexcitable IA-motoneuronal synaptic transmission (42). Irradiation of tendon reflexes is due to either mechanical spread of the vibration or to increased central excitability of IA afferent connections to synergistic muscles (43). The clasp-knife sign, characteristic of knee extensors, is ascribed to group II muscle spindle afferents from quadriceps femoris muscle, centrally inhibitory to extensor motoneurons (1). Golgi tendon organs (IB afferents) or free nerve endings in muscle may also contribute to clasp-knife inhibition of the stretch reflex (44). Muscle contraction due to muscle shortening, as is often seen in the hamstring muscles after SCI, may be due to group II muscle spindle discharges from the quadriceps femoris muscle as it is stretched; these inputs are excitatory to flexors but inhibitory to extensors (45).

Tonic stretch reflexes imply that tonic stretch of muscle will cause tonic muscle activity. This has been noted in some incomplete SCI and MS patients in hip flexors and knee flexors (11). Group II muscle spindle afferents from flexor muscles may mediate this tonic activity; group II afferents fire tonically in a length-dependent manner, and they facilitate flexor and inhibit extensor motoneurons (46).

Cutaneomuscular (i.e., flexor withdrawal or exteroceptive) reflexes are polysynaptic, polysegmental reflexes to noxious stimuli, mediated by myelinated (A-δ) and unmyelinated (C) fibers, which spread mostly to flexor and less to extensor muscles (1,47). Hyperactive flexor withdrawal reflexes and flexor spasms result from increases in central excitability (48). Joint, muscle, and autonomic afferents also contribute to flexor spasms (49). Denervation supersensitivity, new synapse growth, or disinhibition yield this hyperreflexia. A descending inhibitory pathway, called the dorsal reticulospinal pathway, is known in cats (50). Section of this pathway results in hyperactive flexor reflexes. This dorsal reticulospinal inhibition is abolished after spinal cord but not after cerebral lesions; this may explain more cutaneomuscular and tonic stretch hyperreflexia after spinal cord lesions.

Exaggerated Suprasegmental Reflexes

If the UMN lesion is rostral to the brain stem, then suprasegmental reflexes through the upper spinal cord and brain stem may become hyperactive (e.g., tonic neck and vestibular reflexes). They are particularly prominent after early CNS injury, such as in CP, but they also may develop in adult-onset cerebral injury.

Weakness and Abnormal Voluntary Control

UMN weakness rather than hypertonus can limit voluntary movements (1,51). When spasticity and hypertonus interfere, it is as antagonist cocontraction due to central coactivation (52,53) or as hyperactive segmental reflexes (54). This antagonist cocontraction either mechanically limits agonist motion or results in reciprocal inhibition of agonists (55). Abolishing these antagonist cocontractions via nerve blocks or antispasticity medications can enhance voluntary movements (36,55).

Decorticate and Decerebrate Rigidity

The immediate onset of decerebrate and decorticate rigidity suggests that a disinhibition mechanism is involved. The lesion is in the pons, mid-brain, or diencephalon to cause decerebrate rigidity and involves disinhibition of the reticular formation and lateral vestibular nuclei, which are excitatory to extensor motoneurons. In contrast to the apparent absence of increased gamma-motoneuron activity in spasticity, increased gamma-motoneuron activity does contribute to hyperactive stretch reflexes of decerebrate rigidity (56).

EVALUATING SPASTICITY AND HYPERTONUS

Evaluating the spasticity and hypertonus of UMN syndrome calls for a clinical history, a reflex examination, passive and active limb movements, and a functional examination (Table 40-1).

TABLE 40-1. *Clinical evaluation of spasticity and hypertonus*

Clinical history
Spasm or stiffness interfere?
Spasms useful?
Reflex examination
Hyperactive tendon reflexes?
Flexor spasms or other cutaneomuscular hyperreflexia?
Passive motion examination
Hypertonus? (Ashworth score)
Velocity-dependent hypertonus?
Hypertonus vs. contracture? (+ antagonist EMG if hypertonus)
Clonus?
Active motion examination
Slow with antagonist contraction? = Antagonist spasticity or coactivation
Slow without antagonist contraction? = Weak agonist
Isometric and eccentric contractions stronger than concentric? = Tone-assisted strength
Functional examination
Hypertonus interfere with self-care?
Hypertonus interfere with sitting or standing balance?
Hypertonus interfere with mobility?

EMG, electromyography.

Clinical evaluation of hypertonus after upper motor neuron (UMN) syndrome. The evaluation includes a clinical history, reflex examination, passive and active movement examintion, and a functional examination.

Clinical Evaluation

The clinical history shows the impact of hypertonus. Questions may include:

How often do you have spasms?
Which muscles are involved?
Are the spasms beneficial or detrimental?
What elicits the spasms?
Are the spasms more frequent or more severe than usual?

An increase in spasm frequency or intensity may be an early sign of bladder infection, ureteral stone, acute abdomen, or other noxious input.

The examiner grades the severity and anatomic distribution of hypertonus. The clinician assesses tone, tendon reflexes, cutaneomuscular reflexes, and voluntary movements (57). The Ashworth scale grades severity of hypertonus to passive limb motion, with reasonable interrater reliability (58–60). It is a 5-point rating scale:

0 = normal tone
1 = slight hypertonus, a ''catch'' when limb is moved
2 = mild hypertonus, limb moves easily
3 = moderate hypertonus, passive limb movement difficult
4 = severe hypertonus, limb rigid

Tendon reflex threshold, amplitude, and spread to other muscles are noted. Tendon tap or rapid stretch often elicit clonus; the number of beats is recorded. The examiner notes spontaneous flexor spasms and looks for Babinski and triple flexion (hip, knee, and ankle) responses to the plantar stimulus. Cutaneomuscular reflexes are often lower threshold, larger amplitude, longer duration, and more widespread after UMN lesions.

Voluntary strength is graded on the usual 5-point scale. Isometric strength is often better than concentric strength. Patients may use hyperactive stretch reflexes to facilitate isometric or eccentric strength, ''tone-assisted'' strength (e.g., use lower extremity extensor spasms to stand; Fig. 40-3); concentric contractions are relatively weak because the stretch reflex cannot facilitate these shortening contractions. To assess motor control, the patient rapidly alternates agonist and antagonist contractions. The clinician describes spasticity effects on active movements and deficits of voluntary activation. Simultaneous contraction of other flexors or extensors in the same leg (i.e., synergy) or in the opposite leg (i.e., synkinesis) is described.

Limited speed or range of active motion (ROM) is noted. Antagonist co-contraction limiting voluntary movement may be due to hyperactive antagonist stretch reflexes or antagonist central coactivation; if antagonist spasticity is limiting, then there is mid-range slowing caused by the antagonist spasticity activation. If both passive and active ROM are significantly limited, then surface electromyography (EMG) recording of the antagonist or anesthetic block of the antagonist can be used to distinguish contracture from antagonist muscle cocontraction (61). Tonic neck and vestibular reflexes are assessed by observing effects of head and body position on tone and voluntary movements (62).

Functions compromised by hypertonus are examined, including bed mobility, transfers, walking, and self-care skills

(63). Disability may be due to spasticity and hypertonus, but it also may be due to weakness and contracture. The clinician must correlate the clinical history with the neuromuscular and functional examinations to determine the contribution of hypertonus versus weakness versus contracture to the disability.

Beneficial or Detrimental Hypertonus?

Spasticity and hypertonus can be beneficial or detrimental. Benefits may include:

1. An aid to standing and walking via extensor spasms
2. More strength in isometric and eccentric voluntary contractions, facilitated by hyperactive stretch reflexes, even though concentric contractions are weak
3. Maintained muscle mass due to spasms
4. Maintained bone mineralization due to spasms, despite non–weight bearing and disuse
5. Reduced dependent edema in paralyzed limbs due to spasms
6. Reduced deep vein thrombosis (DVT) risk due to spasms that act as a muscle pump to the veins

Detrimental effects of spasticity and hypertonus include:

1. Impaired standing balance due to clonus, hip adductor scissoring, and flexor spasms
2. Impaired swing phase of gait due to extensor spasms and clonus
3. Slow voluntary movements due to spasticity (i.e., velocity-dependent hypertonus)
4. Skin shear due to flexor and extensor spasms, compromising bed or wheelchair positioning
5. Risk of contracture due to tonic stretch hyperreflexia or flexor spasms
6. Impaired sleep due to spontaneous spasms
7. Impaired perineal hygiene and sexual function due to hip flexor and adductor spasms
8. Interference with driving due to spasms or clonus
9. Pain due to continuous flexor spasms, although most hypertonus is not painful

Other Evaluation Methods

Electrophysiologic and mechanical methods are also available for evaluating spasticity and hypertonus. These quantitative methods can supplement the clinical examination or aid research. The most available method is multichannel EMG. Surface electrodes are taped over selected muscles, and the EMG activity is recorded during passive or active movements or in response to cutaneous stimuli (64,65). This is useful to distinguish contracture from antagonist spasticity and to follow the response to therapy (66,67). Dynamic EMG can distinguish biceps versus brachialis versus brachioradialis hypertonus in TBI patients and plan blocks or surgical releases (68).

Gait analysis involves dynamic EMG recording from lower limb muscles plus joint angle (kinematic) data and ground reaction forces from force plates. The clinical value of gait parameters such as cadence, walking velocity, stride length, joint angular velocity, and the spasticity index in assessing hypertonus is not fully known (69–74). A muscle's spasticity index, defined as EMG activity during its normal off-period of gait divided by its normal on-period, distinguishes normal and spastic subjects (71). Gait analysis can distinguish impairment due to spasticity from that due to weakness, both after stroke and incomplete SCI (74–76). It can aid planning of rehabilitation interventions and orthopedic procedures (69,70,75).

Tibial H reflexes are used to measure reflex excitability. Maximum H reflex amplitude divided by maximum M response (compound muscle action potential) amplitude estimates the proportion of motor units that can be excited reflexively (77). The H/M ratio is higher in spastic patients, implying that a greater percentage of motoneurons are activated via the reflex (6). H reflexes are inhibited during the swing phase of ambulation, but this inhibition is lost in spastic paresis (78). H reflex methods examine only the monosynaptic stretch reflex arc, they are time-consuming and they do not have demonstrated clinical utility.

Electrophysiologic methods are also used to record cutaneomuscular reflexes (79). In spastic patients, cutaneomuscular reflexes show delayed reflexes, disrupted cutaneomuscular organization, and dishabituated reflexes (80–82). Flexor spasms increase in frequency at night, confirming the sleep disruption reported by spastic patients (83).

The pendulum test, recording knee oscillation after dropping the leg from full knee extension, is used to quantify hypertonus. It is reliable on repeated testing, it correlates well with Ashworth scores, and it can be performed with commercially available exercise equipment (84,85). The pendulum test does distinguish hemiplegic spasticity from parkinsonian rigidity (86).

Mechanical recording of muscle torque and angular stiffness correlate with clinical assessments of tone (87,88). The need for complex, expensive equipment has limited such techniques to research facilities. Promising results using a commercially available isokinetic dynamometer and handheld myometer have recently been reported (89,90).

Temporary anesthetic nerve blocks are useful for distinguishing hypertonus from joint capsule tightness and myotendinous contracture. Anesthetic blocks help assess the functional impact of contemplated phenol or alcohol motor-point blocks. Anesthetic nerve blocks only approximate the neurolytic block because they yield sensory loss and more tone reduction than motor point blocks.

Functional effects of spasticity need better assessment (63). Quantitative, reliable measures of mobility and self-care, which are sensitive to changes in spasticity and other hypertonus, are needed to assess the functional benefit of spasticity treatments. Such functional measures may not readily distinguish less spasticity from better strength; functional measures can be combined with more direct measures of spasticity and strength to identify the exact cause for the improved function.

TREATMENT

Stepped Care

Stepped care begins with simple, reversible treatments that have few side effects and proceeds to irreversible treatments that have more side effects (Fig. 40-5). The goal is to minimize adverse effects of hypertonus without compromising function. Attempts to eliminate all hypertonus can lead to worse function by abolishing useful hypertonus and by weakening voluntary movement. Stepped care optimizes function by titrating and individualizing the hypertonus treatments. Stepped care is performed as follows.

First, eliminate nociception. Urinary tract infection, bowel impaction, pressure sore, fracture, paronychia, and acute abdomen are all nociceptive sources that may increase spasticity and hypertonus (12).

Second, provide patient education and adaptive equipment. Explain the beneficial and adverse effects of hypertonus. Teach daily stretch and to move slowly to lessen spasticity. Teach how to use extensor or flexor spasms during transfers or bed mobility. Teach foot protection to prevent skin breakdown due to spasms. Waist or chest straps or contact guarding may be needed if spasms are severe. Tilt-in-space recline mechanisms can lessen the stimulus for spasms, as compared with conventional tilt-back recline mechanisms. Patient education and adaptive equipment can reduce adverse hypertonus and promote function.

Physical Modalities

Daily ROM and static muscle stretch prevent contracture and capsule tightness and reduce stretch reflex hyperactivity (91). Standing is another form of static stretch (92,93). It can reverse early contracture and may reduce stretch reflex excitability; however, it is less effective in normalizing gait (91).

Prolonged muscle stretch with serial casting or orthotics is useful (94–97). Joint ROM can improve, but spasticity and clonus may not diminish. Ankle–foot orthoses can control spastic equinus deformity at the ankle. Medial or lateral T straps or anterior flare of a plastic brace can control varus or valgus. In cerebral palsy, ankle–foot orthoses with tone-reducing features are used to inhibit tonic postures (98–102); such orthoses may improve gait, but hypertonus may not lessen (103,104).

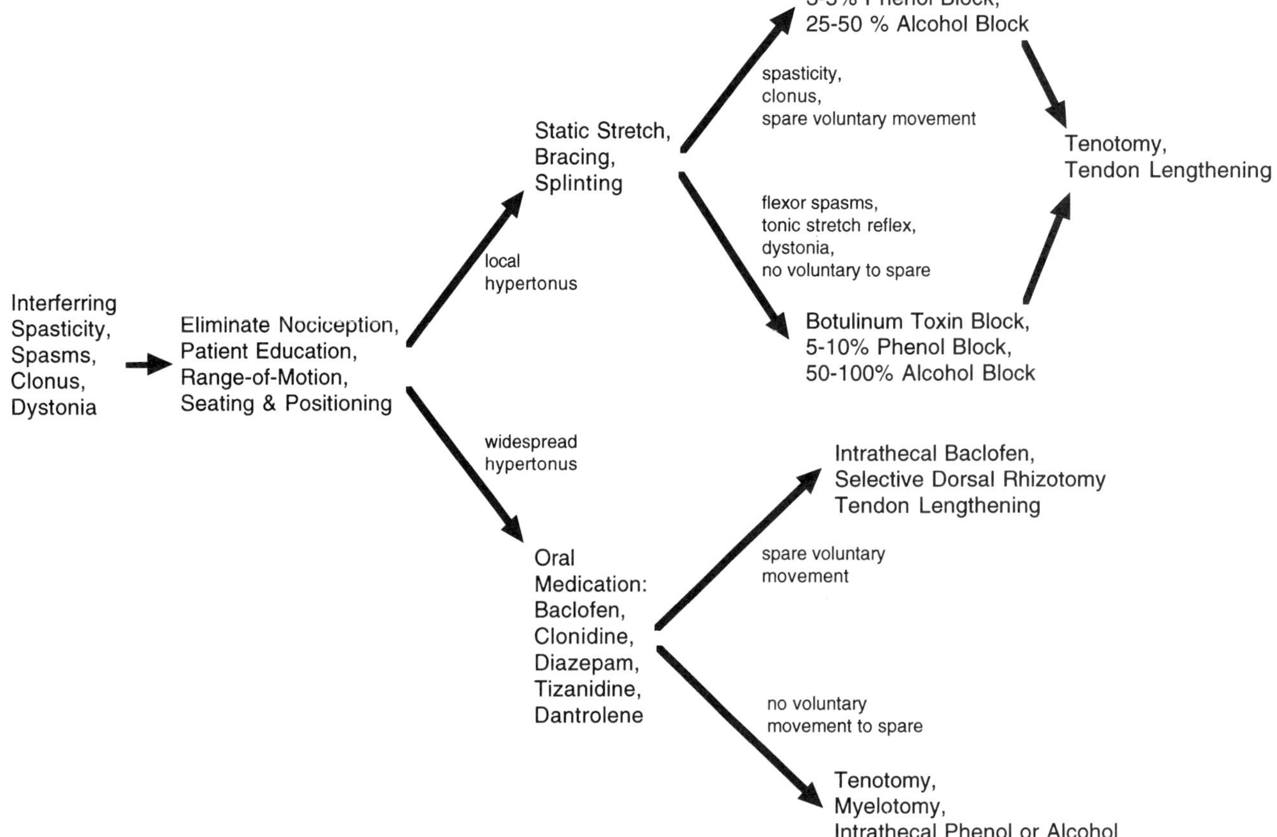

FIG. 40-5. Stepped care for hypertonus of UMN syndrome. Stepped care is individualized and proceeds from reversible treatments with few side effects to irreversible treatments with more side effects.

Biofeedback, using either EMG or joint position sensors, and providing auditory or visual feedback, has reduced spasticity in patients with preserved voluntary motor control, but prolonged use in cerebral palsy did not improve joint ROM (105–107).

Muscle cooling reduces stretch reflex activity and clonus (108). Spasmolytic muscle cooling requires prolonged application for 15 minutes or more. The early effect of skin cooling is to increase hypertonus. Because reduction of spasticity by cooling is only transient, lasting hours, it is not practical for long-term outpatient use. It can aid functional training (94,108).

Electrical stimulation at nearly all levels of the nervous system relieves spasticity. Peripheral stimulation of muscle or nerve for 15 minutes reduces spasticity and clonus for hours, but functional benefits are less clear (109,110). Transcutaneous electrical nerve stimulation decreases spasticity in some SCI patients (111). Spasticity is less for 8 to 72 hours after neuromuscular re-education using agonist–antagonist reciprocating electrical stimulation (112). Rectal electrical stimulation, as used for electroejaculation, relieves spasms for about 8 hours (113). Less hypertonus and more voluntary strength were noted in ankle plantarflexors after peroneal nerve stimulation for 1 year (114).

Medications

There are five widely used oral medicines for spasticity and hypertonus of the UMN syndrome (Table 40-2): baclofen, diazepam, clonidine, tizanidine, and dantrolene. Baclofen acts on inhibitory synapses in the brain and spinal cord that use the neurotransmitter gamma-aminobutyric acid (GABA), binding to GABA-B receptors (115). Baclofen lessens flexor spasms and hyperactive stretch reflexes in hypertonus of spinal origin. It also benefits those with hypertonus from cerebral lesions. Patients whose spasticity is reduced by muscle cooling may benefit most from baclofen (116). The L-baclofen stereoisomer may be more effective than racemic DL-baclofen, but only the latter is clinically available (117). Side effects are generally mild and include drowsiness, nausea, and paresthesias. Patients may report subjective weakness when using baclofen, but isokinetic strengths are unchanged (118). Serum levels may accumulate in patients with renal insufficiency and produce toxicity (119). Rebound spasticity, hallucinations, and withdrawal seizures may occur if the drug is stopped abruptly (120,121). Baclofen is preferred over diazepam in some comparative studies (122,123).

Continuous intrathecal baclofen at doses of 300 to 500 μg/day can eliminate hypertonus in patients with MS, SCI, TBI, and CP, even when oral therapy with baclofen failed (59,124–130). It also eliminates opisthotonus in children with anoxic encephalopathy, but is ineffective against other motor disturbances such as athetosis, ataxia, and dyskinesia. Functional improvements in dressing, transfers, and toileting have been reported in some patients with SCI and MS (125,129). Careful dose titration is required in those who use their hypertonus for standing and walking. Long-term use for years has been successful, but baclofen tolerance develops, necessitating increased dosage or a drug holiday. In some patients receiving prolonged intrathecal baclofen, the dose can be reduced or discontinued with no recurrence of spasticity (131). Side effects may include light-headedness, drowsiness, nausea, hypotension, and weakness. Overdose causes respiratory depression, hypotension, and reversible coma and is best treated by cerebrospinal fluid withdrawal via lumbar puncture and intensive care unit monitoring (132). Pump and catheter malfunction, battery failure every 3 to 5 years, and need for costly continuing refills are limitations of intrathecal baclofen.

Diazepam acts centrally on GABA-A receptors, facilitating GABA-mediated inhibition in the brain and spinal cord (133). Orally, it reduces hypertonus, clonus, and flexor spasms. CNS side effects such as sedation and memory impairment are greater with diazepam than baclofen (120); these limiting CNS effects are most troublesome in head injury or MS patients with impaired mentation. Addiction and respiratory depression are also side effects. The benzodiazepine ketazolam is spasmolytic in MS patients (134).

Dantrolene sodium acts peripherally on excitation–contraction coupling of muscle fibers (135). It blocks calcium ion release from the sarcoplasmic reticulum and thus inhibits muscle contraction. It may selectively reduce stretch reflex hyperactivity and clonus at low doses by preferentially acting on intrafusal over extrafusal muscle fibers. Weakness results at higher doses. Because of its peripheral mode of action, dantrolene often is recommended for CP and other cerebral causes of spasticity. A recent study failed to demonstrate reduced tone or improved function for stroke patients; at 200 mg per day, reduced strength was noted (136). Hepatotoxicity is an uncommon but potentially fatal side effect; this was most common in women over 30 years of age on high daily doses of more than 300 mg for more than 2 months (137). Liver function tests should be monitored.

Clonidine, an alpha-2 agonist, reduces hypertonus and flexor spasms in SCI patients (138–140). It can improve gait in those with spastic paresis (141). Both oral and transdermal forms are effective (142). It can reduce spasm and neuropathic pain when given intrathecally with intrathecal baclofen (143). In one clinical trial, baclofen yielded greater spasticity reduction than clonidine in SCI patients (144). Limited experience suggests some spasmolytic benefit in CVA and CP patients (145). Side effects include postural hypotension, sedation, and depression.

Tizanidine is an alpha-2 agonist that reduces spasticity, clonus, and spasms and may improve voluntary strength (146–150). Tizanidine reduces hypertonus by facilitating presynaptic inhibition through alpha-adrenergic receptors. Tizanidine reduces hypertonus, clonus, and flexor spasms with an efficacy comparable with baclofen; side effects include drowsiness, dry mouth, and hypotension.

Other spasmolytic medications include threonine (151),

TABLE 40-2. *Oral spasmolytic medications*

Medication	Half-life/daily-dose/ route	Metabolism	Site of action	Spasticity effects/ diagnoses benefiting	Common side effects
Baclofen	3.5 hr oral/ 10–80 mg + oral/ oral, intrathecal	Kidney, liver	CNS, GABA-B inhibition	Flexor spasms, spasticity, clonus i.t. effectiveness >> oral/SCI, MS, CVA, TBI, CP	Sedation, confusion, hallucinations, ataxia, weakness, depressed mood, nausea, fatigue withdrawal hallucinations, and seizures
Diazepam	>30 hr oral/ 2–40 mg oral/ oral, intravenous	Liver	CNS, facilitates GABA inhibition	Flexor spasms, spasticity, clonus/SCI, MS, CVA, TBI, CP	Drowsiness, fatigue, ataxia, depression, dizziness, impaired attention, impaired memory
Clonidine	12–16 hr oral/ 0.1–0.4 mg oral/ oral, transdermal	Kidney, liver	CNS, alpha2 adrenergic agonist	Spasticity, clonus, flexor spasms/SCI, CVA, CP	Drowsiness, hypotension, weakness, nausea, constipation, dry mouth, bradycardia withdrawal hypertension
Tizandine	4 hr oral/ 4–36 mg oral/ oral	Liver, kidney	CNS, alpha2 adrenergic agonist	Spasticity, clonus, flexor spasms/SCI, MS, CVA, TBI	Drowsiness, weakness, dizziness, fatigue, hypotension, abnormal liver function tests, dry mouth, visual hallucinations
Dantrolene	9 hr oral/ 25–400 mg oral/ oral	Liver	PNS, blocks Ca^{2+} release in muscle	Spasticity, clonus, flexor spasms/TBI, CVA, MS, SCI	Hepatotoxicity (fatal, nonfatal), weakness, fatigue, drowsiness, diarrhea, nausea, rash

CNS, central nervous system; CP, cerebral palsy; CVA, cerebrovascular accident; GABA, gamma-aminobutyric acid; i.t., intrathecal; MS, multiple sclerosis; PNS, peripheral nervous system; SCI, spinal cord injury; TBI, traumatic brain injury.

The first-line oral medication is usually baclofen. Second-line oral medications are clonidine and diazepam. Third-line medications are tizanidine and dantrolene sodium.

cannabinoids (152,153), chlorpromazine with phenytoin (154), progabide (155), mexiletine (156), cyproheptadine (144,157), orphenadrine (158), gabapentin (159), morphine, and fentanyl. Intrathecal or epidural morphine suppresses lower limb and abdominal spasms, but drug tolerance may develop; intrathecal morphine is used as a drug holiday for intrathecal baclofen (160,161).

Chemical Nerve Blocks

Chemical agents applied to nerves can reduce spasms. Anesthetics (e.g., bupivicaine) block spasms for hours. Phenol (2% to 10% in water, saline, or glycerol) or ethyl alcohol (25% to 100%) block spasms for months to years (162–166). These neurolytic agents are applied to mixed nerves, motor nerve branches, or motor points to relieve spasms. They can be applied to cutaneous nerves to relieve flexor spasms (12). If major mixed nerves with many sensory axons are injected, there is a 10% to 30% risk of painful paresthesias (164,165). Nerves or motor points are located by electrical stimulation through a hypodermic needle, insulated except at the tip; by repositioning the needle and gradually reducing the current until a minimum current is required to elicit a muscle contraction, the clinician can locate the needle tip within 1 to 2 mm of the motor nerve or motor point; alcohol or phenol is then injected. An open procedure allows phenol injection intraneurally. Percutaneous radiofrequency thermocoagulation also abolishes hypertonus (167).

Clonus and velocity-dependent tone respond to blocks with low-concentration phenol (2% to 5%) and alcohol (25% to 50%), which cause more demyelination and less axon degeneration (Table 40-3) (164,166). These low concentration blocks can abolish spasticity, yet partially spare voluntary movement. This may result from slowing of axonal conduction, dispersing the afferent volley and depressing reflexes more than voluntary movements. Such blocks can increase voluntary strength in antagonists by eliminating excess reciprocal inhibition (36). High concentration blocks with phenol (5% to 10%) and alcohol (50% to 100%) that cause more axon degeneration may be more effective for non–velocity-dependent tone, flexor spasms, and dystonia. The site of injection (i.e., mixed nerve, motor branch, or motor point) and volume of injection (i.e., 0.5 to 10 ml per injection site) interact with concentration to yield the final block effect, whether mostly demyelination or mostly axon degeneration (Table 40-3). Transient effects obscure the early results of alcohol and phenol blocks: (a) there is a transient anesthetic effect that wears off in hours, and (b) nociception from the injection can aggravate flexor spasms for several days. Thus, the best assessment of the block effect is obtained at 2 to 3 days postinjection.

Commonly performed motor point blocks are to triceps surae, tibialis posterior, hamstring, and finger and wrist flexor muscles (164,168,169). Subscapularis and pectoralis major motor point blocks can benefit the painful hemiplegic shoulder (170,171). Various nerve blocks, including of the obturator, tibial, musculocutaneous, and paravertebral lumbar spinal nerves, are described (164,172–175). Benefits of nerve blocks include improved strength and speed of movement, more ROM, improved sitting and standing balance, improved perineal hygiene, and better ambulation (164). Tibial nerve blocks for the hemiplegic gait were questioned in a placebo-controlled trial, although the degree of myotendinous contracture and the adequacy of the blocks was not assessed (169). General anesthesia often is necessary in young or uncooperative patients or when severe hypertonus complicates positioning. Repeat nerve and motor point blocks can be performed, but localization may be more difficult (168).

Intramuscular nonselective infiltration (alcohol wash) with 25% to 50% ethanol may benefit (176,177). Muscle is infiltrated at multiple sites without attempts to identify the intramuscular motor points or motor nerves. Triceps surae spasticity is reduced for 2 to 6 weeks. It may be less useful for dystonia and non–velocity-dependent hypertonus. Phenol or alcohol injected intrathecally at the T12/L1 spine can lessen severe lower limb spasms, but voluntary movement, bladder control, and sexual function may be lost (178–181).

Botulinum type A toxin injected into muscle reduces spasticity and other hypertonus (182–184). Toxin is taken up at presynaptic endings of motor axons via endocytosis and prevents release of acetylcholine. The spasmolytic effect develops in 1 to 4 days (183). The block is reversed when motor axons regenerate new neuromuscular junctions, so the effect lasts 2 to 6 months. The maximum recommended dose at one treatment is 400 units (Botox, Allergan, Inc. in U.S.; note that Dysport in U.K. manufactures another botulinum type A toxin with nonequivalent units); the estimated median lethal dose (LD_{50}) in humans is 3,000 to 5,000 units (184). Botulinum toxin is approved by the U.S. Food and Drug Administration for strabismus, blepharospasm, and hemifacial spasm but has been used for spasticity, dystonia, torticollis, and writer's cramp. Direct effect on terminals of alpha motoneurons with weakness and less hypertonus may combine with indirect effects on stretch reflexes via action on gamma motoneuron terminals and on reciprocal inhibition (185,186). Improved ambulation and improved upper limb function may follow botulinum toxin blocks (187,188). Clinical resistance to the toxin can occur with repeat injections; this may be due to antibody formation. Other side effects include weakness, involvement of adjacent muscles, short duration of effect, and cost. Distant clinical effects have not been observed, but single-fiber EMG shows increased jitter in remote muscles (189).

Surgery

Various orthopedic surgeries are used for spasticity and hypertonus, but only after motor recovery is complete

TABLE 40-3. *Chemical nerve blocks: proposed protocols*[a]

Clinical goal (pathophysiologic mechanism)	Neurolytic agent	Concentration	Volume (per site)	Injection site
Abolish spasticity and clonus; spare voluntary movement (demyelinate axons, slow axon conduction, disperse afferent volley)				
Transient effect	Phenol	2–3%	0.5–2 ml	Motor-points
(weeks-months)	Ethyl alcohol	25–50%	2.5–10 ml	i.m. alcohol wash, each quadrant
Semipermanent effect	Phenol	3–5%	2–5 ml	Mixed nerve or motor branches
(months-years)	Ethyl alcohol	25–50%	2–5 ml	Mixed nerve or motor branches
Abolish spasms, dystonia, clonus, and voluntary movement (botulinum toxin irreversibly damages motor terminals; phenol and alcohol degenerate motor axons)				
Transient effect (weeks-months)	Botulinum toxin[b]	40–300 U	10–75 U	Motor-points or blind i.m. injection
Semipermanent effect	Phenol[c]	5–10%	2–5 ml	Mixed nerve or motor branches
(months-years)	Ethyl alcohol[d]	50–100%	2–5 ml	Mixed nerve or motor branches

[a] The optimal neurolytic agent, concentration, volume, and site of injection are yet to be fully established, to achieve these clinical goals.

[b] Do not exceed 400 U of botulinum toxin per day.

[c] Do not exceed 1 g phenol, i.e., 20 ml of 5% phenol; LD_{50} estimated at 8.5 g in adults.

[d] Do not exceed about 50 g ethyl alcohol, i.e., 100 ml of 50% alcohol, to avoid inebriation.

A selective neurolytic block, which abolishes spasticity and clonus but spares voluntary movement, can be achieved with low-concentration alcohol or phenol. Botulinum toxin and higher concentration alcohol or phenol are more effective for tonic stretch hyperreflexia, flexor spasms, and dystonia, but they do not spare voluntary movement in the blocked muscle.

(190,191). These surgeries can improve function, correct deformity, and improve cosmesis. They include tenotomy, tendon lengthening, and tendon transfer. Tendon lengthening and transfers are most useful if voluntary movement is preserved. Lower limb procedures are used in CP, CVA, and TBI to improve borderline ambulation (26,190). Hamstring tenotomy or tendon transfer are used for knee flexion contractures (26,192); improved knee extension range and improved ambulation are reported. Achilles tenotomy or tendon lengthening for equinus deformities (193) and tibialis posterior tenotomy or tendon transfer for varus deformities of the foot are common procedures in CP or CVA hemiplegia; good or excellent results were achieved in 72% of spastic CP subjects after posterior tibialis tendon transfer (194). The SPLATT procedure (split anterior tibialis transfer) involves splitting the tibialis anterior tendon and tunneling the lateral part to the third cuneiform and cuboid bones; this yields some eversion to counteract the inversion of the equinovarus posture. The SPLATT procedure is often combined with Achilles tendon lengthening (195). Adductor tendon section, with or without obturator neurectomy, relieves hip adductor spasms. Iliopsoas tendon or muscle section is used for flexor spasms; more extensive surgery, including pelvic and femoral osteotomies, may be useful in treating painful hip dislocations (196). Subtalar fusion or triple arthrodesis can overcome clonus and extensor hypertonus to improve standing balance and gait (26). When ambulation is borderline, careful preoperative gait analysis is necessary (69,70). Tenotomies or tendon-lengthening procedures may be followed by a recurrence of the original deformity (e.g., equinus), or the alternate deformity (e.g., calcaneus) may develop from overcorrection.

Tendon lengthening, tendon transfers, and selected joint fusions are also useful for upper limb hypertonus (26). Spastic elbow flexors, "clenched fist," and "thumb-in-palm" are managed successfully by surgical release (191,197–199). Anesthetic nerve blocks are useful in assessing the potential benefit of tendon transfer procedures.

Surgery for hypertonus includes peripheral nerve procedures. Peripheral neurectomy abolishes all muscle tone but does not spare voluntary movement. It leads to profound muscular atrophy and sensory loss. Obturator neurectomy to relieve hip adductor spasms is the most common use of this procedure. Selective peripheral neurectomies are performed using microsurgical techniques and intraoperative electrical stimulation (200). This allows selective section of most but not all nerve fibers to a muscle, thus preserving some voluntary muscle activity and lessening atrophy; cutaneous sensory branches are preserved.

Surgery of the CNS is also used to relieve spasticity and hypertonus. Myelotomy involves direct section of the spinal cord in a longitudinal plane using a dorsal approach and dividing it into anterior and posterior halves from T12 to S1. Such a myelotomy divides reflex arcs of the lumbosacral enlargement with reduced hypertonus and yet can spare reflex bladder, reflex bowel, and reflex sexual function by sparing the S2–S3 reflex arcs (201–203). Some spasticity can recur in spared segments.

Another common neurosurgical procedure for spasticity is rhizotomy (204). Section of the posterior roots is easier to perform than section of the anterior roots and does not yield severe muscle atrophy. Posterior rhizotomy disrupts spinal reflex arcs but does not abolish suprasegmental hypertonus. Disadvantages of posterior rhizotomy are sensory loss, associated ataxia, and recurrence of hypertonus. To minimize sensory loss, only portions of each dorsal root are sectioned in selective posterior rhizotomy (205–211). Only those dorsal rootlets are sectioned that show hyperreflexia by intraoperative stimulation and recording. Selective posterior rhizotomy is used primarily in CP and is advocated for two groups of children:

1. Nonambulatory, severely hypertonic children in whom relief of spasticity may aid positioning and daily care
2. Young children with purely spastic CP who have reasonable voluntary motor control and trunk balance, no significant contractures, and who can participate in intensive physical therapy after surgery

A lumbar laminectomy is performed, exposing the cauda equina. Dorsal rootlets are stimulated electrically and sectioned if reflex muscle contraction is observed. Decreased tone occurs in the immediate postoperative period; physical therapy for up to a year is required to see functional change. Improvements in hip, knee, and ankle ROM, as well as in motor function, including sitting, kneeling, crawling, and ambulation, are reported (210,211). Bowel and bladder dysfunction are avoided by sparing the S2–S4 dorsal roots. Rhizotomy requires a multilevel laminectomy, which may lead to progressive spine deformity (212,213). Percutaneous radiofrequency rhizotomies can be performed, thus avoiding laminectomy, but the long-term results have yet to be determined (214,215).

Cordotomy, cordectomy, and cauda equina transection can be performed in extreme cases of spasticity but may be supplanted by intrathecal spasmolytic medications (13,216). Such procedures are not appropriate when useful voluntary motor control is present or when motor recovery is possible. When alpha-motoneurons or the motor axons are destroyed, profound muscle atrophy will result with increased risk of pressure sores.

Epidural electrical stimulation over the dorsal columns reportedly decreases hypertonus in patients with SCI, MS, and spastic hemiplegia, with a carryover effect for a period of hours or days (217–223). More effective control is reported in patients with incomplete than complete SCI, and in those with moderate, not severe, spasms (222,223). Cerebellar stimulation also has been attempted to decrease hypertonus in patients with CP (224–226). Under blinded conditions, no objective evidence for reduced spasticity or functional gains was found for either epidural or cerebellar stimulation (218,225).

In summary, spasticity, flexor spasms, and other hypertonus are part of the UMN syndrome, along with weakness. Spasticity and hypertonus often impair function and compromise quality of life. Physical modalities, medications, chemical nerve blocks, and surgeries can reduce hypertonus and spasticity. The clinician must weigh the beneficial and adverse effects of hypertonus and then select treatments that lessen adverse hypertonus but spare voluntary movement and function.

REFERENCES

1. Burke D. Spasticity as an adaptation to pyramidal tract injury. *Adv Neurol* 1988; 47:401–423.
2. Herman R, Freeman W, Meeks SM. Physiological aspects of hemiplegic and paraplegic spasticity. In: Desmedt JE, ed. *New developments in electromyography and clinical neurophysiology.* Vol. 3. Basel: S Karger AG, 1973; 579–588.
3. Sahrmann SA, Norton BJ, Bomze HA, Eliasson SG. Influence of the site of the lesion and muscle length on spasticity in man. *Phys Ther* 1974; 54:1290–1296.
4. Guttmann L. *Spinal cord injuries.* Oxford, England: Blackwell Scientific, 1976.
5. Michaelis LS. Spasticity in spinal cord injuries. In: Vinken PJ, Bruyn GW, eds. *Handbook of clinical neurology.* Vol. 26. Part II. *Injuries of the spine and cord.* New York: Elsevier, 1976; 477–487.
6. Little JW, Halar EM. H-reflex changes following spinal cord injury. *Arch Phys Med Rehabil* 1985; 66:19–22.
7. Barolat G, Maiman DJ. Spasms in spinal cord injury: a study of 72 subjects. *J Am Paraplegia Soc* 1987; 10:35–39.
8. Little JW, Micklesen P, Umlauf R, Britell C. Lower extremity manifestations of spasticity in chronic spinal cord injury. *Am J Phys Med Rehabil* 1989; 68:32–36.
9. Maynard FM, Karunas RS, Waring WP. Epidemiology of spasticity following traumatic spinal cord injury. *Arch Phys Med Rehabil* 1990; 71:566–569.
10. Kuhn R. Functional capacity of the isolated human spinal cord. *Brain* 1950; 73:1–51
11. Burke D, Gillies JD, Lance JW. Hamstrings stretch reflex in human spasticity. *J Neurol Neurosurg Psychiatry* 1971; 34:231–235.
12. Davis R. Spasticity following spinal cord injury. *Clin Orthop* 1975; 112:66–75.
13. Kraft GH, Freal JE, Coryell JK. Disability, disease duration and rehabilitation service needs in multiple sclerosis: patient perspectives. *Arch Phys Med Rehabil* 1986; 67:164–168.
14. Chen WY, Pierson FM, Burnett CN. Force-time measurements of knee muscle functions of subjects with multiple sclerosis. *Phys Ther* 1987; 67:934–940.
15. Olgiati R, Burgunder JM, Mumenthaler M. Increased energy cost of walking in multiple sclerosis: effect of spasticity, ataxia, and weakness. *Arch Phys Med Rehabil* 1988; 69:846–849.
16. MacFaul R, Cavanagh N, Lake BD, Stephens R, Whitfield AE. Metachromatic leucodystrophy: review of 38 cases. *Arch Dis Child* 1982; 57:168–175.
17. Twitchell T. The restoration of motor function following hemiplegia in man. *Brain* 1951; 74:443–480.
18. Perry J, Giovan P, Harris LJ, et al. The determinants of muscle action in the hemiparetic lower extremity (and their effect on the examination procedure). *Clin Orthop* 1978; 131:71–89.
19. Knutsson E, Richards C. Different types of disturbed motor control in gait of hemiparetic patients. *Brain* 1979; 102:405–430.
20. Mayer NH, Esquenazi A, Wannstedt G. Surgical planning for upper motoneuron dysfunction: the role of motor control evaluation. *J Head Trauma Rehabil* 1996; 11:37–56.
21. Binder H, Eng GD. Rehabilitation management of children with spastic diplegic cerebral palsy. *Arch Phys Med Rehabil* 1989; 70:481–489.
22. Halpern D. Rehabilitation of children with brain damage. In: Kottke FJ, Stillwell GK, Lehmann JF, eds. *Krusen's handbook of physical medicine and rehabilitation,* 4th ed. Philadelphia: WB Saunders, 1990; 746–770.
23. Winters TF Jr, Gage JR, Hicks R. Gait patterns in spastic hemiplegia in children and young adults. *J Bone Joint Surg [Am]* 1987; 69:437–441.
24. Norlin R, Odinrick P. Development of gait in spastic children with cerebral palsy. *J Pediatr Orthop* 1986; 6:674–680.
25. Lin JP, Brown JF, Brotherstone R. Assessment of spasticity in hemiplegic cerebral palsy. II. Distal lower limb reflex excitability and function. *Dev Med Child Neurol* 1994; 36:290–303.
26. Bleck E. *Orthopedic management in cerebral palsy.* London: MacKeith Press, 1987.
27. Young RR, Wiegner AW. Spasticity. *Clin Orthop* 1987; 219:51–62.
28. Katz R, Rymer WZ. Spastic hypertonia: mechanisms and measurement. *Arch Phys Med Rehabil* 1989; 70:144–155.
29. Barnes CD, Joynt RJ, Schottelius BA. Motoneuron resting potentials in spinal shock. *Am J Physiol* 1961; 203:1113–1116.
30. Little JW. Serial recording of reflexes after feline spinal cord transection. *Exp Neurol* 1986; 93:510–521.
31. Sharpless SK. Supersensitivity-like phenomena in the central nervous system. *Fed Proc* 1975; 34:1990–1997.
32. Bach-y-Rita P, Illis LS: Spinal shock: possible role of receptor plasticity and non-synaptic transmission. *Paraplegia* 1993; 31:82–87.
33. Thilmann AF, Fellows SJ, Garma E. The mechanism of spastic muscle hypertonus: variation in reflex gain over the time course of spasticity. *Brain* 1991; 114:233–244.
34. Rymer WZ, Powers RK. Pathophysiology of muscular hypertonia in spasticity. *Neurosurg State Art Rev* 1989; 4:291–301.
35. Nielsen J, Petersen N, Crone C. Changes in transmission across synapses of Ia afferents in spastic patients. *Brain* 1995; 118:995–1004
36. Yanagisawa N, Tanaka R, Ito Z. Reciprocal Ia inhibition in spastic hemiplegia of man. *Brain* 1976; 99:555–574.
37. Leonard CT, Moritani T, Hirschfeld H, Forssberg H. Deficits in reciprocal inhibition of children with cerebral palsy as revealed by H reflex testing. *Dev Med Child Neurol* 1990; 32:974–984.
38. Burke D. Critical examination of the case for or against fusimotor involvement in disorders of muscle tone. In: Desmedt JE, ed. *Motor control mechanisms in health and disease.* New York: Raven, 1983.
39. Ashby P, Wiens M. Reciprocal inhibition following lesions of the spinal cord in man. *J Physiol (Lond)* 1989; 414:145–157.
40. Schefner JM. Neurophysiology of spinal cord injury. In: Young RR, Woolsey RM, eds. *Diagnosis and management of disorders of the spinal cord.* Philadelphia: WB Saunders, 1995:145–152.
41. Boorman GI, Lee RG, Becker WJ, Windhorst UR. Impaired "natural reciprocal inhibition" in patients with spasticity due to incomplete spinal cord injury. *EEG Clin Neurophysiol* 1996; 101:84–92.
42. Rack PMH, Ross HF, Thilmann AF. The ankle stretch reflexes in normal and spastic subjects: the response to sinusoidal movement. *Brain* 1984; 107:637–654.
43. Teasdall RD, Van Den Ende H. The crossed adductor reflex in humans: an EMG study. *Can J Neurol Sci* 1981; 8:81–85.
44. Rymer WZ, Houk JC, Crago PE. Mechanisms of the clasp-knife reflex studied in an animal model. *Exp Brain Res* 1979; 37:93–113.
45. Berardelli A, Hallett M. Shortening reaction of human tibialis anterior. *Neurology* 1984; 34:242–245.
46. Hunt CC, Perl ER. Spinal reflex mechanisms concerned with skeletal muscle. *Physiol Rev* 1960; 40:538–579.
47. Hagbarth KE. Spinal withdrawal reflexes in the human lower limbs. *J Neurol Neurosurg Psychiatry* 1960; 23:222–227.
48. Barolat-Romana G, Davis R. Neurophysiological mechanisms in abnormal reflex activities in cerebral palsy and spinal spasticity. *J Neurol Neurosurg Psychiatry* 1980; 43:333–342.
49. Pederson E, Petersen T, Schroder HD. Relation between flexor spasms, uninhibited detrusor contractions, and anal sphincter activity. *J Neurol Neurosurg Psychiatry* 1986; 49:273–277.
50. Lundberg A. Control of spinal mechanisms from the brain. In: Tower DB, ed. *The nervous system.* Vol. 1. New York: Raven, 1975.
51. Knutsson E. Assessment of motor function in spasticity. *Triangle* 1982; 21:13–20.
52. Ibrahim IK, Berger W, Trippel M, Dietz V. Stretch-induced electromyographic activity and torque in spastic elbow muscles. *Brain* 1993; 116:971–989
53. Corcos DM, Gottlieb GL, Penn RD, et al. Movement deficits caused by hyperexcitable stretch reflexes in spastic humans. *Brain* 1986; 109: 1043–1058.
54. Knutsson E, Martensson A. Dynamic motor capacity in spastic paraparesis and its relation to prime mover dysfunction, spastic reflexes and antagonist co-activation. *Scand J Rehabil Med* 1980; 12:93–106.
55. Knutsson E. Analysis of gait and isokinetic movements for evaluation

of antispastic drugs or physical therapies. In: Desmedt JS, ed. *Motor control mechanisms in health and disease.* New York: Raven, 1983.
56. Brooks VB. *The neural basis of motor control.* New York: Oxford University Press, 1986; 151–159.
57. Priebe MM, Sherwood AM, Thornby JI, Kharas NF, Markowski J. Clinical assessment of spasticity in spinal cord injury: a multi-dimensional problem. *Arch Phys Med Rehabil* 1996; 77:713–716.
58. Ashworth B. Carisoprodol in multiple sclerosis. *Practitioner* 1964; 192:540–542.
59. Penn RD, Savoy SM, Corcos D, et al. Intrathecal baclofen for severe spinal spasticity. *N Engl J Med* 1989; 320:1517–1521.
60. Bohannon RW, Smith MB. Interrater reliability of a modified Ashworth scale of muscle spasticity. *Phys Ther* 1987; 67:206–207.
61. Mizrahi EM, Angel RW. Impairment of voluntary movement by spasticity. *Ann Neurol* 1979; 5:594–595.
62. Stichbury JC. Assessment of disability following severe head injury. *Physiotherapy* 1975; 61:268–272.
63. Hinderer SR, Gupta S. Functional outcome measures to assess interventions for spasticity. *Arch Phys Med Rehabil* 1996; 77:1083–1089.
64. Dimitrijevic M, Sherwood A. Spasticity: medical and surgical treatment. *Neurology* 1980; 30:19–27.
65. Boorman G, Becker WJ, Morrice BL, Lee RG. Modulation of the soleus H-reflex during pedalling in normal humans and in patients with spinal spasticity. *J Neurol Neurosurg Psychiatry* 1992; 55: 1150–1156.
66. McLellan DL, Selwyn M, Cooper IS. Time course of clinical and physiological effects of stimulation of the cerebellar surface in patients with spasticity. *J Neurol Neurosurg Psychiatry* 1978; 41:150–160.
67. Keenan MA, Haider TT, Stone LR. Dynamic electromyography to assess elbow spasticity. *J Hand Surg [Am]* 1990; 15:607–614.
68. Keenan MA, Ahearn R, Lazarus M, Perry J. Selective release of spastic elbow flexors in the patient with brain injury. *J Head Trauma Rehabil* 1996; 11:57–68.
69. Shapiro A, Susak Z, Malkin C, Mizrahi J. Preoperative and postoperative gait evaluation in cerebral palsy. *Arch Phys Med Rehabil* 1990; 71:236–240.
70. Gage JR. The clinical use of kinetics for evaluation of pathological gait in cerebral palsy. *J Bone Joint Surg [Am]* 1994; 76:622–631.
71. Fung J, Barbeau H. A dynamic EMG profile index to quantify muscular activation disorder in spastic paretic gait. *Electroencephalogr Clin Neurophysiol* 1989; 73:233–244.
72. Kadaba MP, Ramakrishnan HK, Wootten ME, Gainey J, Gorton G, Cochran GV. Repeatability of kinematic, kinetic, and electromyographic data in normal adult gait. *J Orthop Res* 1989; 7:849–860.
73. Kirkpatrick M, Wytch R, Cole G, Helms P. Is the objective assessment of cerebral palsy gait reproducible? *J Pediatr Orthop* 1994; 14: 705–708.
74. Knutsson E. Can gait analysis improve gait training in stroke patients. *Scand J Rehabil Med Suppl* 1994; 30:73–80.
75. Kerrigan DC, Glenn MB. An illustration of clinical gait laboratory use to improve rehabilitation management. *Am J Phys Med Rehabil* 1994; 73:421–427.
76. Krawetz P, Nance P. Gait analysis of spinal cord injured subjects: effects of injury level and spasticity. *Arch Phys Med Rehabil* 1996; 77:635–638.
77. Matthews WB. Ratio of maximum H reflex to maximum M response as a measure of spasticity. *J Neurol Neurosurg Psychiatry* 1966; 29: 201–204.
78. Yang JF, Fung J, Edamura M, Blunt R, Stein RB, Barbeau H. H-reflex modulation during walking in spastic paretic subjects. *Can J Neurol Sci* 1991; 18:443–452.
79. Torring J, Pedersen E, Klemar B. Standardisation of the electrical elicitation of the human flexor reflex. *J Neurol Neurosurg Psychiatry* 1981; 44:129–132.
80. Fisher MA, Shahani BT, Young RR. Electrophysiologic analysis of the motor system after stroke: the flexor reflex. *Arch Phys Med Rehabil* 1979; 60:7–11.
81. Dimitrijevic M, Nathan P. Studies of spasticity in man: V. Dishabituation of the flexion reflex in spinal man. *Brain* 1968; 94:349–368.
82. Bathien N, Bourdarias H. Lower limb cutaneous reflexes in hemiplegia. *Brain* 1972; 95:447–456.
83. Pederson E, Klemar B, Torring J. Counting of flexor spasms. *Acta Neurol Scand* 1979; 60:164–169.
84. Price R. Mechanical spasticity evaluation techniques. *Crit Rev Phys Med Rehabil* 1990; 2:65–73.
85. Katz RT, Rovai GP, Brait C, Rymer Z. Objective quantification of spastic hypertonia: correlation with clinical findings. *Arch Phys Med Rehabil* 1992; 73:339–342
86. Brown RA, Lawson DA, Leslie GC, et al. Does the Wartenberg pendulum test differentiate quantitatively between spasticity and rigidity: a study in elderly stroke and Parkinsonian patients. *J Neurol Neurosurg Psychiatry* 1988; 51:1178–1186.
87. Lehmann JF, Price R, de Lateur BJ, Hinderer S, Traynor C. Spasticity: quantitative measurements as a basis for assessing effectiveness of therapeutic intervention. *Arch Phys Med Rehabil* 1989; 70:6–15.
88. Price R, Lehmann JF. Influence of muscle cooling on the viscoelastic response of the human ankle to sinusoidal displacements. *Arch Phys Med Rehabil* 1990; 71:745–748.
89. Engsberg JR, Olree KS, Ross SA, Park TS. Quantitative clinical measure of spasticity in children with cerebral palsy. *Arch Phys Med Rehabil* 1996; 77:594–599.
90. Boiteau M, Malouin F, Richards CL. Use of a hand-held dynamometer and a Kin-Com dynamometer for evaluating spastic hypertonia in children: a reliability study. *Phys Ther* 1995; 75:796–802.
91. Richards CL, Malouin F, Dumas F. Effects of a single session of prolonged plantarflexor stretch on muscle activations during gait in spastic cerebral palsy. *Scand J Rehabil Med* 1991; 23:103–111.
92. Kunkel CF, Scremin AME, Eisenberg B, Garcia JF, Roberts S, Martinez S. Effect of "standing" on spasticity, contracture, and osteoporosis in paralyzed muscles. *Arch Phys Med Rehabil* 1993; 74:73–78.
93. Bohannon RW. Tilt table standing for 30 minutes can reduce spasticity for hours in persons with SCI. *Arch Phys Med Rehabil* 1993; 74: 1121–1122.
94. Giebler KB. Physical Modalities. In: Glenn MB, Whyte J, eds. *The practical management of spasticity in children and adults.* Philadelphia: Lea & Febiger, 1990.
95. Law M, Cadman D, Rosenbaum P, Walter S, Russell D, DeMattaeo C. Neurodevelopmental therapy and upper-extremity inhibitive casting for children with cerebral palsy. *Dev Med Child Neurol* 1991; 33: 379–387.
96. Feldman PA. Upper extremity casting and splinting. In: Glenn MB, Whyte J, eds. *The practical management of spasticity in children and adults.* Philadelphia: Lea & Febiger, 1990.
97. Conine TA, Sullivan T, Mackie T, Goodman M. Effect of serial casting for the prevention of equinus in patients with acute head injury. *Arch Phys Med Rehabil* 1990; 71:310–312.
98. Mills VM. Electromyographic results of inhibitory splinting. *Phys Ther* 1984; 64:190–193.
99. Otis JC, Root L, Kroll MA. Measurement of plantar flexor spasticity during treatment with tone-reducing casts. *J Pediatr Orthop* 1985; 5: 682–686.
100. Watt J, Sims D, Harckham F, Schmidt L, McMillan A, Hamilton J. A prospective study of inhibitive casting as an adjunct to physiotherapy for cerebral-palsied children. *Dev Med Child Neurol* 1986; 28: 480–488.
101. Snook JH. Spasticity reduction splint. *Am J Occup Ther* 1979; 33: 648–651.
102. Hylton N. Dynamic casting and orthotics. In: Glenn MB, Whyte J, eds. *The practical management of spasticity in children and adults.* Philadelphia: Lea & Febiger, 1990.
103. Hinderer K, Harris S, Purdy A, et al. Effects of tone reducing vs. standard plaster casts on gait improvement of children with cerebral palsy. *Dev Med Child Neurol* 1988; 30:370–377.
104. Mossberg KA, Linton KA, Friske K. Ankle-foot orthoses: effect on energy expenditure of gait in spastic diplegic children. *Arch Phys Med Rehabil* 1990; 71:490–494.
105. O'Dwyer N, Neilson P, Nash J. Reduction of spasticity in cerebral palsy using feedback of the tonic stretch reflex: a controlled study. *Dev Med Child Neurol* 1994; 36:770–786.
106. Basmajian JV, Kukulka CG, Narayan MG, et al. Biofeedback treatment of footdrop after stroke compared with standard rehabilitation technique: effects on voluntary control and strength. *Arch Phys Med Rehabil* 1975; 56:231–236.
107. Brown DM, DeBacher GA, Basmajian JV. Feedback goniometers for hand rehabilitation. *Am J Occup Ther* 1979; 339:458–463.
108. Hartviksen K. Ice therapy in spasticity. *Acta Neurol Scand* 1962; 38(suppl 3):79–84.

109. Hazelwood ME, Brown JK, Rowe PJ, Salter PM. The use of therapeutic electrical stimulation in the treatment of hemiplegic cerebral palsy. *Dev Med Child Neurol* 1994; 36:661–673.
110. Seib TP, Price R, Reyes MR, Lehmann JF. The quantitative measurement of spasticity: effect of cutaneous electrical stimulation. *Arch Phys Med Rehabil* 1994; 75:746–750.
111. Bajd T, Gregoric M, Vodovnik L, Benko H. Electrical stimulation in treating spasticity resulting from spinal cord injury. *Arch Phys Med Rehabil* 1985; 66:515–517.
112. Shindo N, Jones R. Reciprocal patterned electrical stimulation of the lower limbs in severe spasticity. *Physiotherapy* 1987; 73:579–582.
113. Halstead LS, Seager SWJ, Houston JM, Whitesell K, Dennis M, Nance PW. Relief of spasticity in SCI men and women using rectal probe electrostimulation. *Paraplegia* 1993; 3:715–721.
114. Stefanovska A, Gros N, Vodovnik L, Rebersek S, Acimovic-Janezic R. Chronic electrical stimulation for the modification of spasticity in hemiplegic patients. *Scand J Rehabil Med Suppl* 1988; 17:115–121.
115. Koella WP. Baclofen: its general pharmacology and neuropharmacology. In: Feldman RG, Young RR, Koella WP, eds. *Spasticity: disordered motor control.* Chicago: Year Book Medical, 1980; 383–396.
116. Knutsson E, Lindblom U, Martensson A. Differences in effects in gamma and alpha spasticity induced by the GABA derivative baclofen (Lioresal). *Brain* 1973; 96:29–46.
117. Albright AL, Barry MJ, Hoffmann P. Intrathecal L-baclofen for cerebral spasticity: a case report. *Neurology* 1995; 45:2110–2111.
118. Smith MB, Surinder PB, Nelson LM, Franklin GM, Cobble ND. Baclofen effect on quadriceps strength in multiple sclerosis. *Arch Phys Med Rehabil* 1992; 73:237–240.
119. Aisen ML, Dietz M, McDowell F, Kutt H. Baclofen toxicity in a patient with subclinical renal insufficiency. *Arch Phys Med Rehabil* 1994; 75:109–111.
120. Roussan M, Terrence C, Fromm G. Baclofen versus diazepam for the treatment of spasticity and long-term follow-up of baclofen therapy. *Pharmatherapeutica* 1985; 4:278–284.
121. Terrence CF, Fromm H. Complications of baclofen withdrawal. *Arch Neurol* 1981; 38:588–589.
122. Cartlidge NEF, Hudgson P, Weightman D. A comparison of baclofen and diazepam in the treatment of spasticity. *J Neurol Sci* 1974; 23: 17–24.
123. From A, Heltberg A. A double-blind trial with baclofen and diazepam in spasticity due to multiple sclerosis. *Acta Neurol Scand* 1975; 51: 158–166.
124. Mueller H, Zierski J, Dralle D, Boerner U, Hoffmann O. The effect of intrathecal baclofen on electrical muscle activity in spasticity. *J Neurol* 1987; 234:348–352.
125 Parke B, Penn RD, Savoy SM, Corcos D. Functional outcome after delivery of intrathecal baclofen. *Arch Phys Med Rehabil* 1989; 70: 30–32.
126. Lazorthes Y, Sallerin-Caute B, Verdie JC, Bastide R, Carillo JP. Chronic intrathecal baclofen administration for control of severe spasticity. *J Neurosurg* 1990; 72:393–402.
127. Meythaler JM, DeVivo MJ, Hadley M. Prospective study on the use of bolus intrathecal baclofen for spastic hypertonia due to acquired brain injury. *Arch Phys Med Rehabil* 1996; 77:461–466.
128. Abel NA, Smith RA. Intrathecal baclofen for treatment of intractable spinal spasticity. *Arch Phys Med Rehabil* 1994; 75:54–58.
129. Azouni P, Mane M, Thiebault JB, Denys P, Remy-Neris O, Bussel B. Intra-thecal baclofen administration for the control of severe spinal spasticity: functional improvement and long-term follow-up. *Arch Phys Med Rehabil* 1996; 77:35–39.
130. Gardner G, Jamous A, Teddy P, et al. Intrathecal baclofen—a multicentre clinical comparison of the Medtronics Programmable, Cordis Secor and Constant Infusion Infusaid drug delivery systems. *Paraplegia* 1995; 33:551–554.
131. Dressnandt J, Conrad B. Lasting reduction of severe spasticity after ending chronic treatment with intrathecal baclofen. *J Neurol Neurosurg Psychiatry* 1996; 60:168–173.
132. Delhaas EM, Brouwers JRBJ. Intrathecal baclofen overdose: report of 7 events in 5 patients and review of the literature. *Intern J Clin Pharm Ther Toxicol* 1991; 29:274–280.
133. Davidoff RA. Mode of action of antispasticity drugs. *Neurosurg State Art Rev* 1989; 4:315–324.
134. Basmajian JV, Shankardass K, Diane Russell. Ketazolam treatment for spasticity: double-blind study of a new drug. *Arch Phys Med Rehabil* 1984; 65:698–701.
135. Ward A, Chaffman MO, Sorkin EM. Dantrolene: a review of its pharmacodynamic and pharmacokinetic properties and therapeutic use in malignant hyperthermia, the neuroleptic malignant syndrome and an update of its use in muscle spasticity. Drugs 1986; 32:130–168.
136. Katrak PH, Cole AM, Poulos CJ, McCauley JC. Objective assessment of spasticity, strength, and function with early exhibition of dantrolene sodium after cerebrovascular accident: a randomized double-blind study. *Arch Phys Med Rehabil* 1992; 73:4–9.
137. Utili R, Boitnott JK, Zimmerman HJ. Dantrolene-associated hepatic injury. *Gastroenterology* 1977; 72:610–616.
138. Nance PW, Shears AH, Nance DM. Clonidine in spinal cord injury. *Can Med Assoc J* 1985; 133:41–42.
139. Maynard FM. Early clinical experience with clonidine in spinal spasticity. *Paraplegia* 1986; 24:175–182.
140. Donovan WH, Carter RE, Rossi CD, Wilkerson MA. Clonidine effect on spasticity: a clinical trial. *Arch Phys Med Rehabil* 1988; 69: 193–194.
141. Stewart JE, Barbeau H, Gauthier S. Modulation of locomotor patterns and spasticity with clonidine in spinal cord injured patients. *Can J Neurol Sci* 1991; 18:321–332.
142. Weingarden SI, Belen JG. Clonidine transdermal system for treatment of spasticity in spinal cord injury. *Arch Phys Med Rehabil* 1992; 73: 876–877.
143. Middleton JW, Siddall PJ, Walker S, Molloy AR, Rutkowski SB. Intrathecal clonidine and baclofen in the management of spasticity and neuropathic pain following spinal cord injury: a case study. *Arch Phys Med Rehabil* 1996; 77:824–826.
144. Nance PW. A comparison of clonidine, cyproheptadine, and baclofen in spastic spinal cord injured patients. *J Am Paraplegia Soc* 1994; 17:150–156.
145. Dall JT, Harmon RL, Quinn CM. Use of clonidine for treatment of spasticity arising from various forms of brain injury: a case series. *Brain Injury* 1996; 10:453–458.
146. Knutsson E, Martensson A, Gransberg L. Antiparetic and antispastic effects induced by tizanidine in patients with spastic paresis. *J Neurol Sci* 1982; 53:187–204.
147. Newman PM, Nogues M, Newman PK, Weightman D, Hudgson P. Tizanidine in the treatment of spasticity. *Eur J Clin Pharmacol* 1982; 23:31–35.
148. Bass B, Weinshenker B, Rice GP, et al. Tizanidine versus baclofen in the treatment of spasticity in patients with multiple sclerosis. *Can J Neurol Sci* 1988; 15:15–19.
149. Hoogstraten MC, van der Ploeg RJ, vd Burg W, Vreeling A, van Marle S, Minderhoud JM. Tizanidine versus baclofen in the treatment of spasticity in multiple sclerosis patients. *Acta Neurol Scand* 1988; 77:224–230.
150. Mathias CJ, Luckitt J, Desai P, Baker H, El Masri W, Frankel HL. Pharmacodynamics and pharmacokinetics of the oral antispastic agent tizanidine in patients with spinal cord injury. *J Rehabil Res Dev* 1989; 26:9–16.
151. Hauser SL, Doolittle TH, Lopez-Bresnahan M, et al. An anti-spasticity effect of threonine in multiple sclerosis. *Arch Neurol* 1992; 49: 923–926.
152. Ungerleider JT, Andyrsiak T, Fairbanks L, Ellison GW, Myers LW. Delta-9-THC in the treatment of spasticity associated with multiple sclerosis. *Adv Alcohol Substance Abuse* 1987; 7:39–50.
153. Meinck HM, Schoenle PW, Conrad B. Effect of cannabinoids on spasticity and ataxia in multiple sclerosis. *J Neurol* 1989; 236: 120–122.
154. Cohan SL, Raines A, Panagakos J, Armitage P. Phenytoin and chlorpromazine in the treatment of spasticity. *Arch Neurol* 1980; 37: 360–364.
155. Rudick RA, Breton D, Krall RL. The GABA-agonist progabide for spasticity in multiple sclerosis. *Arch Neurol* 1987; 44:1033–1036.
156. Jimi T, Wakayama Y. Mexiletine for treatment of spasticity due to neurologic disorders. *Muscle Nerve* 1993; 16:885.
157. Fung J, Stewart JE, Barbeau H. The combined effects of clonidine and cyproheptadine with interactive training on the modulation of locomotion in spinal cord injured subjects. *J Neurol Sci* 1990; 100: 85–93.
158. Casale R, Glynn CJ, Buonocore M. Reduction of spastic hypertonia in patients with spinal cord injury: a double-blind comparison of intra-

venous orphenadrine citrate and placebo. *Arch Phys Med Rehabil* 1995; 76:660–665.
159. Priebe MM, Sherwood AM. A quantitative study of the effects of gabapentin on spasticity. American Paraplegia Society annual meeting, Las Vegas, 1996.
160. Struppler A, Ochs G, Burgmayer B, Pfeiffer HG. The therapeutic use of epidural opioids in flexor reflex spasm. *Electroencephalogr Clin Neurophysiol* 1983; 56(suppl):178.
161. Erickson DL, Lo J, Michaelson M. Control of intractable spasticity with intrathecal morphine sulfate. *Neurosurgery* 1989; 24:236–238.
162. Felsenthal G. Pharmacology of phenol in peripheral nerve blocks: a review. *Arch Phys Med Rehabil* 1974; 55:13–16.
163. Wood KM. The use of phenol as a neurolytic agent: a review. *Pain* 1978; 5:205–229.
164. Glenn MB. Nerve blocks. In: Glenn MB, Whyte J, eds. *The practical management of spasticity in children and adults.* Philadelphia: Lea & Febiger, 1990.
165. Khalili AA, Betts HB. Peripheral nerve block with phenol in the management of spasticity: indications and complications. *JAMA* 1967; 200:1155–1157.
166. Tardieu G, Tardieu C, Hariga J, Gagnard L. Treatment of spasticity by injection of dilute alcohol at the motor point or by epidural route. *Dev Med Child Neurol* 1968; 10:555–568.
167. Beckerman H, Becher J, Lankhorst GF, Verbeek ALM. Walking ability of stroke patients: efficacy of tibial nerve blocking and a polypropylene ankle-foot orthosis. *Arch Phys Med Rehabil* 1996; 77: 1144–1151.
168. Halpern D, Meelhuysen FE. Phenol motor point block in the management of muscular hypertonia. *Arch Phys Med Rehabil* 1966; 47: 659–664.
169. Skeil DA. The local treatment of spasticity. *Clin Rehabil* 1994; 8: 240–246.
170. Chironna RL, Hecht JS. Subscapularis motor point block for the painful hemiplegic shoulder. *Arch Phys Med Rehabil* 1990; 71:428–429.
171. Botte MJ, Keenan MAE. Percutaneous phenol blocks of the pectoralis major muscle to treat spastic deformities. *J Hand Surg [Am]* 1988; 13:147–149.
172. Meelhuysen FE, Halpern D, Quast J. Treatment of flexor spasticity of hip by paravertebral lumbar spinal nerve block. *Arch Phys Med Rehabil* 1968; 49:717–722.
173. Awad EA. Phenol block for control of hip flexor and adductor spasticity. *Arch Phys Med Rehabil* 1972; 53:554–557.
174. Moritz U. Phenol block of peripheral nerves. *Scand J Rehabil Med* 1973; 5:160–163.
175. Keenan MA, Tomas ES, Stone L, Gersten LM. Percutaneous phenol block of the musculocutaneous nerve to control elbow flexor spasticity. *J Hand Surg [Am]* 1990; 15:340–346.
176. Tardieu G, Tardieu C, Hariga J. Selective partial denervation by alcohol injections and their results in spasticity. *Reconstr Surg Traumatol* 1972; 13:18–36.
177. Carpenter EB, Seitz DG. Intramuscular alcohol as an aid in management of spastic cerebral palsy. *Dev Med Child Neurol* 1980; 22: 497–501.
178. Nathan PW. Intrathecal phenol to relieve spasticity in paraplegia. *Lancet* 1959; 2:1099–1102.
179. Cain HD. Subarachnoid phenol block in the treatment of pain and spasticity. *Paraplegia* 1965; 3:75–76,152–160.
180. Swerdlow M. Intrathecal neurolysis. *Anaesthesia* 1978; 33:733–740.
181. Iwatsubo E, Okada E, Takehara T, Tamada K, Akatsu T. Selective intrathecal phenol block to improve activities of daily living in patients wih spastic quadriplegia. *Paraplegia* 1994; 32:489–449.
182. Snow BJ, Tsui JK, Bhatt MH, Varelas M, Hashimoto SA, Caine DB. Treatment for spasticity with botulinum toxin: a double-blind study. *Ann Neurol* 1990; 28:512–515.
183. Cosgrove AP, Corry IS, Graham HK. Botulinum toxin in the management of the lower limb in cerebral palsy. *Dev Med Child Neurol* 1994; 36:386–396.
184. Robinson LR, Wang L. Botulinum toxin injections. *Phys Med Rehabil Clin North Am* 1995; 6:897–900.
185. Priori A, Berardelli A, Mercuri B, Manfredi M. Physiological effects produced by botulinum toxin treatment of upper limb dystonia. *Brain* 1995; 118:801–807.
186. Rosales RL, Arimura K, Takenaga S, Osame M. Extrafusal and intrafusal muscle effects in experimental botulinum toxin-A injection. *Muscle Nerve* 1996; 19:488–496.
187. Dunne JW, Heye N, Dunne SL. Treatment of chronic limb spasticity with botulinum toxin A. *J Neurol Neurosurg Psychiatry* 1995; 58: 232–235.
188. Hesse S, Lucke D, Malezic M, et al. Botulinum toxin treatment for lower limb extensor spasticity in chronic hemiparetic patients. *J Neurol Neurosurg Psychiatry* 1994; 57:1321–1324.
189. Lange DJ, Rubin M, Greene PE, et al. Distant effects of locally injected botulinum toxin: a double-blind study of single fiber EMG changes. *Muscle Nerve* 1991; 14:672–675.
190. Pinzur MS. Surgical correction of lower extremity problems in patients with brain injury. *J Head Trauma Rehabil* 1996; 11:69–77.
191. Botte MJ, Keenan MA. Reconstructive surgery of the upper extremity in the patient with head trauma. *J Head Trauma Rehabil* 1987; 2: 34–45.
192. Keenan MA, Ure K, Smith CW, Jordan C. Hamstring release for knee flexion contracture in spastic adults. *Clin Orthop* 1988; 236:221–226.
193. Graham HK, Fixsen JA. Lengthening of the calcaneal tendon in spastic hemiplegia by the White slide technique: a long-term review. *J Bone Joint Surg [Br]* 1988; 70:472–475.
194. Root L, Miller SR, Kirz P. Posterior tibial-tendon transfer in patients with cerebral palsy. *J Bone Joint Surg [Am]* 1987; 69:1133–1139.
195. Waters RL, Frazier J, Garland DE, Jordan C, Perry J. Electromyographic gait analysis before and after operative treatment for hemiplegic equinus and equinovarus deformity. *J Bone Joint Surg [Am]* 1982; 64:284–288.
196. Brunner R, Baumann JU. Clinical benefit of reconstruction of dislocated or subluxated hip joints in patients with spastic cerebral palsy. *J Pediatr Orthop* 1994; 14:290–294.
197. Keenan MA, Korchek JI, Botte MJ, Smith CW, Garland DE. Results of transfer of the flexor digitorum superficialis tendons to the flexor digitorum profundus tendons in adults with acquired spasticity of the hand. *J Bone Joint Surg [Br]* 1987; 69:1127–1132.
198. Botte MJ, Keenan MA, Gellman H, Garland DE, Waters RL. Surgical management of spastic thumb-in-palm deformity in adults with brain injury. *J Hand Surg [Am]* 1989; 14:174–182.
199. Keenan MA, Ahearn R, Lazarus M, Perry J. Selective release of spastic elbow flexors in patients with brain injury. *J Head Trauma Rehabil* 1996; 11:57–68.
200. Sindou M, Abdennebi B, Sharkey P. Microsurgical selective procedures in peripheral nerves and the posterior root-spinal cord junction for spasticity. *Appl Neurophysiol* 1985; 48:97–104.
201. Laitinen L, Singounas E. Longitudinal myelotomy in the treatment of spasticity of the legs. *J Neurosurg* 1971; 35:536–540.
202. Yamada S, Dayes L, Knierim D, Clark L. Control of mass spasms by longitudinal myelotomy. *Neurosurg State Art Rev* 1989; 4:345–354.
203. Putty TK, Shapiro SA. Efficacy of dorsal longitudinal myelotomy in treating spinal spasticity: a review of 20 cases. *J Neurosurg* 1991; 75:397–401.
204. Nathan PW, Sears TA. Effects of posterior root section on the activity of some muscles in man. *J Neurol Neurosurg Psychiatry* 1960; 23: 10–22.
205. Fraioli B, Guidetti B. Posterior partial rootlet section in the treatment of spasticity. *J Neurosurg* 1977; 46:618–626.
206. Peacock WJ, Arens LJ. Selective posterior rhizotomy for the relief of spasticity in cerebral palsy. *South Afr Med J* 1982; 62:119–124.
207. Sindou M, Mifsud D, Boisson D, Goutelle A. Selective posterior rhizotomy in the dorsal root entry zone for treatment of hyperspasticity and pain in the hemiplegic upper limb. *Neurosurgery* 1986; 18: 587–595.
208. McDonald CM. Selective dorsal rhizotomy: a critical review. *Phys Med Rehabil Clin North Am* 1991; 2:891–915.
209. Abbott R, Forem SL, Johann M. Selective posterior rhizotomy for the treatment of spasticity: a review. *Childs Nerv Syst* 1989; 5:337–346.
210. Vaughan CL, Berman B, Staudt LA, Peacock WJ. Gait analysis of cerebral palsy children before and after rhizotomy. *Pediatr Neurosci* 1988; 14:297–300.
211. McLaughlin JF, Bjornson KF, Astley SJ, et al. The role of selective dorsal rhizotomy in cerebral palsy: critical evaluation of a prospective clinical series. *Dev Med Child Neurol* 1994; 36:755–769.
212. Peter JC, Hoffman EB, Arens LJ, Peacock WJ. Incidence of spinal deformity in children after multiple level laminectomy for selective posterior rhizotomy. *Childs Nerv Syst* 1990; 6:30–32.

213. Crawford K, Karol LA, Herring JA. Severe lumbar lordosis after dorsal rhizotomy. *J Pediatr Orthop* 1996; 16:336–339.
214. Herz DA, Parsons K, Pearl L. Percutaneous radiofrequency foramenal rhizotomies. *Spine* 1983; 8:729–732.
215. Kasdon DL, Lathi ES. A prospective study of radiofrequency rhizotomy in the treatment of posttraumatic spasticity. *Neurosurgery* 1984; 15:526–529.
216. Smolik EA, Nash FP, Machek O. Spinal cordectomy in the management of spastic paraplegia. *Am Surg* 1960; 26:639–645.
217. Illis LS, Sedgwick EM, Tallis RC. Spinal cord stimulation in multiple sclerosis. *J Neurol Neurosurg Psychiatry* 1980; 43:1–14.
218. Gottlieb GL, Myklebust BM, Stefoski D, et al. Evaluation of cervical stimulation for chronic treatment of spasticity. *Neurology* 1985; 35: 699–704.
219. Nakamura S, Tsubokawa T. Evaluation of spinal cord stimulation for postapoplectic spastic hemiplegia. *Neurosurgery* 1985;17: 253–259.
220. Barolat G. Epidural spinal cord stimulation in the management of spasms and spasticity in spinal cord injury. *Neurosurg State Art Rev* 1989; 4:365–370.
221. Cioni B, Meglio M, Prezioso A, Talamonti G, Tirendi M. Spinal cord stimulation (SCS) in spastic hemiparesis. *PACE* 1989; 12:739–742.
222. Dimitrijevic MM, Dimitrijevic MR, Illis LS, et al. Spinal cord stimulation for the control of spasticity in patients with chronic spinal cord injury: 1. clinical observations. *Central Nerv System Trauma* 1986; 3:129–144.
223. Barolat G, Singh-Sahni K, Staas WE, Shatin D, Ketcik B, Allen K. Epidural spinal cord stimulation in the management of spasms in spinal cord injury: a prospective study. *Stereotact Funct Neurosurg* 1995; 64:153–164.
224. Cooper IS, Riklan M, Amin I, et al. Chronic cerebellar stimulation in cerebral palsy. *Neurology* 1976; 26:744–753.
225. Penn RD. Chronic cerebellar stimulation for cerebral palsy: a review. *Neurosurgery* 1982; 10:116–121.
226. Davis R, Gray E, Ryan T, Schulman J. Bioengineering changes in spastic cerebral palsy groups following cerebellar stimulation. *Appl Neurophysiol* 1985; 48:111–116.

Rehabilitation Medicine: Principles and Practice, Third Edition,
edited by Joel A. DeLisa and Bruce M. Gans.
Lippincott–Raven Publishers, Philadelphia © 1998.

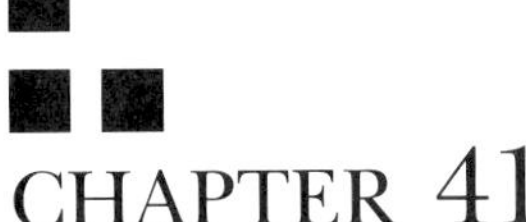

CHAPTER 41

Immobility

Physiological and Functional Changes and Effects of Inactivity on Body Functions

Eugen M. Halar and Kathleen R. Bell

The adverse effects of prolonged bed rest and immobility have become well recognized over the past five decades. Bed rest and immobilization were widely used before 1950 in the management of trauma and acute illness, before their physiologic effects were well understood. It was generally assumed that rest fostered healing of the affected part of the body. What was not appreciated was that physical inactivity can be harmful to the unaffected parts of the body. For example, the immobilization of long bones with a rigid cast has a beneficial effect on bone healing after fractures. However, it may also result in undesirable effects, such as joint contracture and atrophy of the healthy muscles and bones.

Clinical studies on enforced bed rest in normal subjects and on astronauts in zero-gravity conditions (in which their bodies rest from the effects of gravity) have shown significant undesirable effects that may override the therapeutic effects of bed rest in subacute and chronic conditions, impacting complexity and cost of medical treatment as well as functional outcome. Fortunately, many of these complications are easily prevented and, if they occur, easily treated once they are recognized.

Persons who are chronically sick, aged, or disabled are particularly susceptible to the adverse effects of immobility. For example, a healthy subject placed on prolonged bed rest will develop shortening in the musculature of the back and legs, especially those muscles that cross hip and knee joints. In similar circumstances, a patient with motor neuron disease and its accompanying limb weakness or spasticity can be expected to develop the same musculoskeletal complications but at a much accelerated rate. The degree to which each of these hypothetical patients is affected is quite different. The healthy subject may have some degree of stiffness and discomfort, whereas the neurologically impaired subject will likely lose a significant amount of independent functioning. Therefore, the prevention of such complications should be one of the basic principles of any rehabilitation management plan (1).

The effects of immobility are rarely confined to only one body system (Table 41-1). Immobility reduces the functional reserve of the musculoskeletal system, resulting in weakness, atrophy, and poor endurance. Metabolic activity and oxygen extraction in the muscle are reduced, which negatively influences the functional capacity of the cardiovascular system (i.e., cardiac output and work capacity). Immobilization osteoporosis is another complication that has been well documented in studies of astronauts and individuals exposed to prolonged bed rest, and postural hypotension and deep venous thrombosis (DVT) are commonly encountered in bedridden patients. Over time, clinical experience has dictated a move toward earlier mobilization, with a resulting decrease in length of hospitalization and in the incidence of major morbidity associated with the prolonged immobility (2–4).

Deleterious effects of immobility may be grouped together under the general term "deconditioning," which is defined as a reduced functional capacity of the musculoskeletal and other body systems. It should be considered a separate diagnosis from the original condition that led to a curtailment of normal physical activity (Fig. 41-1) (5,6).

This chapter will describe the widespread effects of immobility and review therapeutic and prophylactic approaches to counteract these complications.

E. M. Halar and K. R. Bell: Department of Rehabilitation Medicine, University of Washington Medical Center, Seattle, Washington 98195.

TABLE 41-1. *Adverse effects of immobility*

System(s)	Effect(s)
Musculoskeletal	Contractures Muscle weakness and atrophy Immobilization osteoporosis Immobilization hypercalcemia
Cardiovascular and pulmonary	Redistribution of body fluids Orthostatic hypotension Reduction of cardiopulmonary functional capacity Thromboembolism Mechanical resistance to breathing Hypostatic pneumonia
Genitourinary and gastrointestinal	Urinary stasis, stones, and urinary infections Loss of appetite Constipation
Metabolic and endocrine	Electrolyte alterations Glucose intolerance Increased parathyroid hormone production Other hormone alterations
Cognitive and behavioral	Sensory deprivation Confusion and disorientation Anxiety and depression Decrease in intellectual capacity Impaired balance and coordination

MUSCULOSKELETAL EFFECTS OF IMMOBILITY

Freedom to move our bodies and limbs in the environment around us is an important physical function requiring that the muscles, nerves, bones, and joints be in an optimal physiologic state. Reduction of free joint motion can affect the ability to walk or use the upper extremities, causing impaired mobility and ability to perform activities of daily living. At first, these effects cause minimal functional limitations, and they can easily be overlooked or neglected. Advanced contractures can cause a complete loss of mobility and confinement to bed (7).

For the neurologically impaired or multiple trauma victim, considerations such as preserving functional range of motion (ROM) may seem trivial; however, neglect of these simple factors can be responsible for prolonging hospital stays, increasing the use of health-care resources, and prolonging dependency in mobility and the activities of daily living. Three main types of effects from immobilization are found in the musculoskeletal system: muscle atrophy and weakness, joint contracture, and immobilization osteoporosis (Table 41-1).

Muscle Atrophy and Weakness Due to Disuse

In the recumbent position, muscle activity is minimal because of reduced force of gravity and hypokinesia. Immobility progressively causes a reduction in muscle strength, size, and endurance in addition to producing the perceived weakness associated with cardiovascular deconditioning. Although in most patients these effects are easily reversible, the results may be functionally devastating for those with pre-existing neurologic or musculoskeletal disease (8,9).

With complete rest, a muscle loses 10% to 15% of its strength per week, or about 1% to 3% per day. A patient who maintains total bed rest for 3 to 5 weeks can lose half of his or her muscle strength. This type of muscle weakness is also associated with a reduction in muscle size and with definitive histologic changes (Fig. 41-2) (10–12). At 4 weeks of immobilization, Haggmark et al. found that muscle net weight decreased by 69%. The mean cross-sectional areas of the dark adenosine triphosphatase (ATPase; type II) and light ATPase fibers (type I) were reduced by 46% and 69%, respectively (13,14). Succinate dehydrogenase activity per muscle fiber was increased at the beginning of immobilization, but overall content of this muscle enzyme was reduced significantly at the end of immobilization (15,16). In general, oxidative enzyme activity and content are reduced, as are the number and size of mitochondria (Table 41-2) (17–19).

Metabolic changes in muscle also occur in response to vascular and enzymatic alterations. Although resting energy sourccs arc primarily derived from carbohydrates and fat, nitrogen loss is increased during immobility (Fig. 41-2) (20,21). Restriction of muscular activity reduces protein synthesis and eventually may lead to hypoproteinemia. This protein deficit is aggravated by gastrointestinal mechanisms

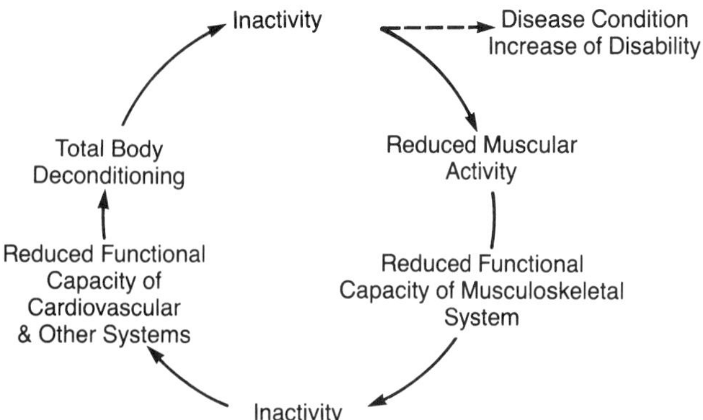

FIG. 41-1. Inactivity, immobility, and prolonged bed rest influence total body functioning.

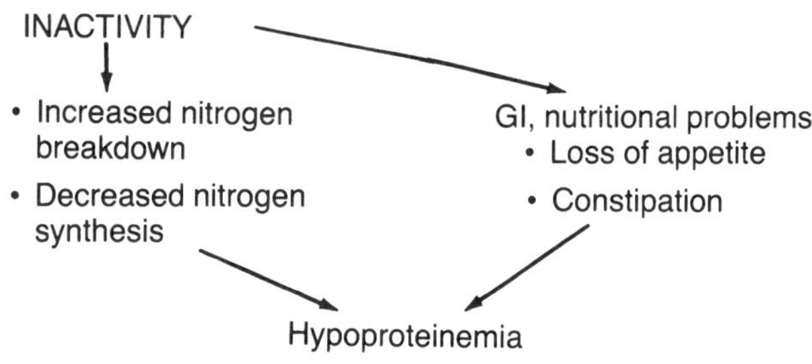

FIG. 41-2. Negative nitrogen balance during prolonged bed rest is caused by a decrease in nitrogen synthesis and increase in nitrogen breakdown and leads to hypoproteinemia. *GI*, gastrointestinal.

TABLE 41-2. *Effect of immobility on skeletal muscle*

Component	Characteristic effect[a]
SDH (succinyl dehydrogenase and other oxidative enzymes)	Decreased aerobic function
Glycogen	Depleted storage levels
CK (creatine kinase)	Depleted storage levels
Sarcomeres	Decreased number in series
Type I and II fiber atrophy	Decreased strength and endurance
Myofibrils	Decreased number Slowed twitch contraction time Reduced maximum twitch and tetanic force
Na-ATPase, K-ATPase	Decreased concentrations of Na and K pumps
VO_2max	Progressive reduction of VO_2max and fitness

[a] The significance of some of these changes remains unclear.

such as loss of appetite, reduced intestinal absorption of protein, and constipation (22). Although daily loss of nitrogen for an immobilized healthy person may reach 2 g, nutritionally depleted persons may lose 12 g/day, and those with long bone fractures may initially lose 8 g/day. Increased nitrogen loss usually begins on the fifth or sixth day of recumbency, with a peak loss in the second week (23,20).

The synthesis of proteins is markedly diminished by inactivity, with the exception of myoglobin, which is increased (17). The number of myofibrils per fiber volume is decreased (20–23). Reduction of muscle activity compromises the blood supply, affecting metabolic activity and muscle endurance. The oxygen supply to the muscle is attenuated, which is associated with increased blood vessel permeability.

A decrease in oxidative enzyme capacity results in a reduction of oxygen extraction from the blood and a lowered tolerance to lactic acid. The above changes and alteration in the shape and size of the end plates and function of the acetylcholine receptors are partly responsible for poor endurance (24,25). Muscle weight loss is usually minimal during the first 2 days of immobility but increases rapidly over the next 10 days. Maximal loss occurs at 8 to 10 days and gradually declines thereafter. This muscle wasting is a result of reduced protein synthesis rather than protein breakdown (26). Collagen synthesis is also reduced, but at a slower rate, producing an increase in the proportion of collagen tissue to muscle (27,28).

Urinary excretion of creatine is minimal under normal conditions (except during pregnancy or in infancy). The excretion of creatine is greater in certain pathologic conditions (e.g., starvation, diabetes, muscular dystrophy, hyperthyroidism, fever, rheumatoid arthritis) as well as during immobility. Prolonged bed rest or weightlessness causes a significant increase in the excretion of both creatine and creatinine, the mechanism of which is not well understood (29,30).

Functional Changes

The reduction of peak muscle tension and the diminution of muscle fiber twitch, as well as tetanic tension, also have been reported to result from immobility. Decreased levels of ATP and glycogen stores, as well as a reduced ability of muscle to use fatty acids after prolonged immobility, leads to reduced endurance (31–33). Generalized muscle weakness may result in poor coordination and quality of movement when the patient is remobilized (4,9).

Along with muscle fiber changes, there is a relative increase in collagen content and cross-linkage, which can lead to muscle rigidity and myogenic contracture (34,35). In the lower limbs, type I muscle fibers, which are active during ambulation, are especially affected. If the quadriceps muscle is immobilized in a shortened position, the deep layer of the vastus intermedius, which is predominantly type I, will show the greatest histochemical change (36). Furthermore, if any extensor muscle is kept in full joint extension, or if flexors are kept shortened in full flexion during immobilization, the number of sarcomeres in series will be reduced (37). This, in turn, reduces the resting length and decreases or increases the force exerted on the muscle during daily activities. Spector and colleagues have shown that the position in which a joint is immobilized has a significant influence on the number of sarcomeres present in the muscle (38). Immobilization in a shortened position can cause muscle fibers to lose 40% of their sarcomeres. Daily stretching of a muscle for half an hour can prevent this loss of sarcomeres in series. For adequate muscle function, stretching to maintain optimal resting length of the muscle is an important factor in the maintenance of normal function (39–41). The rate of atrophy for each muscle is different. The quadriceps, hip, and back extensor muscles atrophy more quickly, decreasing endurance for walking and causing backaches (4,42).

Prevention and Treatment

Fortunately, disuse weakness is relatively simple to prevent. Resumption of normal activities should be encouraged. In addition muscle strength can be maintained with a program of daily muscle contractions of 30% to 50% of maximal tension for several seconds each day (43). Muscle weakness and atrophy also may be prevented by the use of electrical stimulation (44–46). For example, applying local stimulation to the quadriceps while a long leg cast is in place may help preserve muscle bulk and strength and also may shorten rehabilitation time, a factor that may be particularly important in an athlete. A typical program consists of three sessions per day for 30 minutes using direct rectangular biphasic pulse stimulation. In cases in which extensive immobilization results in fixed contracture, prolonged stretching and strengthening is required for several months, and the return of strength may not be complete (42,47).

Immobility and Joint Contractures

A general definition of a contracture is the lack of full active or passive ROM due to joint, muscle, or soft-tissue limitations. A variety of conditions may limit joint movement, including joint pain, paralysis, capsular or periarticular tissue fibrosis, or primary muscle damage. The single factor that contributes most frequently to the occurrence of fixed contractures, however, is the lack of joint mobilization throughout the full allowable range. Prolonged joint immobilization in any position, for any reason, will result in the reduction of resting muscle length, and the shortening of collagen in the joint capsule and other soft tissue (48–50).

Many factors, such as limb position, duration of immobilization, and pre-existing pathology and joint restrictions, affect the rate of contracture development. Edema, ischemia, bleeding, and other alterations to the microenvironment of muscle and periarticular tissue can precipitate the development of fibrosis. Advanced age also must be considered: both muscle fiber loss and a relative increase in the proportion of connective tissue in the body occur in the elderly (6,7,51). In addition, the microvascular changes and relative ischemia found in diabetes mellitus predispose contractures, especially of the hand (52). Contractures that are precipitated by pathologic changes in the joints or muscles may be classified into three groups (Table 41-3): arthrogenic, myogenic, and soft tissue. It is important to remember that all tissues surrounding a joint may become secondarily involved in joint contracture regardless of the initiating disease process.

TABLE 41-3. *Anatomical classification of contractures*

Type of contracture	Causes
Arthrogenic	Cartilage damage, joint incongruency (e.g., congenital deformities), inflammation, trauma, degenerative joint disease, infection, immobilization
	Synovial and fibrofatty tissue proliferation (e.g., inflammation) pain, effusion
	Capsular fibrosis (e g., trauma, inflammation, immobilization)
Soft and dense tissue	Periarticular soft tissue (e. g., trauma, inflammation, immobilization)
	Skin, subcutaneous tissue (e.g., trauma, burns, infection, systemic sclerosis)
	Tendon and ligaments (e.g., tendinitis, bursitis, ligamentous tear and fibrosis)
Myogenic	
Intrinsic, structural	Trauma (e.g., bleeding, edema, immobilization)
	Inflammation (e.g., myositis, polymyositis)
	Degenerative changes (e g., muscular dystrophy)
	Ischemic (e.g., diabetes, peripheral vascular disease, compartment syndrome)
Extrinsic	Spasticity (e.g., strokes, multiple sclerosis, spinal cord injuries and other upper motor neuron diseases)
	Flaccid paralysis (e.g., faulty position, muscle imbalance)
	Mechanical (e.g., faulty position in bed or chair, immobilization and lack of stretch)
Mixed	Combined arthrogenic, soft tissue and muscle contractures noted in a single joint

Mechanical Properties of Connective Tissues

Connective tissue is subdivided into five major groups: (a) loose connective tissue, (b) dense connective tissue (i.e., ligaments), (c) cartilage, (d) bone, and (e) blood vessels. Loose and dense connective tissues are complex, dynamic structures that are important for structural support, stabilization, and movement. It is not well appreciated that these are living, changeable tissues that can adapt both structure and composition in response to a change in environment, particularly to changes in the applied mechanical stresses. An appreciation of the anatomic design is important to fully understand the mechanical properties of both loose and dense connective tissues.

As with all of the connective tissues, dense connective tissues are composed of cells (fibroblasts) and intercellular macromolecules surrounded by polysaccharide gel (extracellular matrix). The intercellular substances, or collagen, impart the mechanical properties of the tissue, whereas the cells are important for homeostasis, adaptation, and repair functions (53).

Collagen

There are two types of intercellular substances in dense connective tissues: collagen fibers and proteoglycans. Fibers in tendons, ligaments, and joint capsules are predominantly of the collagen type, although there is a significant population of elastic fibers in tendons. This is consistent with their function in that tendons have great tensile strength and some elasticity to allow a joint complex to move through both muscle contraction and relaxation. Ligaments, on the other hand, are relatively inelastic and are composed primarily of collagen fibers. Collagen is the most abundant protein in the body and accounts for more than 20% of total body mass. At least 12 different collagens (I–XII) have been identified so far. Each type represents different aggregations of specific polypeptide products of more than 20 different collagen genes (54).

The terminology used in describing the organization and aggregation of collagen molecules is inconsistent and confusing. All collagen molecules have a unique protein conformation known as the triple helix, a result of three constituent polypeptide chains of the collagen molecule coiled together. The synthesis of these chains from amino acids, known as pro alpha-chains, occurs in the rough endoplasmic reticulum of the fibroblast. The precise sequence of amino acids differs between the different types of collagens and accounts for the tissue-specific properties. When the collagen molecules (monomers) are subsequently secreted from the cell, enzymatic cleavage of part of the molecule occurs, and the molecules aggregate in a systematic manner to form fibrils in the extracellular space (54). Collagen fibrils, visible with the electron microscope, are grouped into fibers that are visible with the light microscope. Cross-linking between collagen fibrils is another important structural feature that varies with location and function. The type and strength of collagen cross-linking is the key to tensile strength and is probably altered, depending on the applied mechanical loads. The fibers aggregate into fiber bundles that are grouped together into fascicles. A large number of fascicles form the whole tendon or ligament (55). Like peripheral nerves and striated muscle, there are thin films of loose and dense connective tissues surrounding collagen fiber bundles (endotenon or endoligament), fascicles (peritenon or periligament), and the whole tendon or ligament (epitenon or epiligament). The epitenon or epiligament are thought to be critically important in responding to mechanical loads and injury (56).

In tendons and ligaments, type I collagen predominates, although types III, IV, and VI also have been found. Important variations in collagen diameter have been found in association with site, age, activity level, and repair. Investigations in several animal models and humans alike have demonstrated that changes in collagen diameter, density, and orientation follow Wolff's law: connective tissues orient themselves in form and mass to best resist extrinsic forces. This has been established in response to physiologic conditions (e.g., immobilization or exercise) as well as in response to injury. Changes in collagen are mediated by fibroblasts that are sensitive to mechanical stimuli, enzymes (collagenase and tissue inhibitor of metalloproteinases), and growth factors. These factors shift the dynamic equilibrium toward synthesis or degradation, depending on environmental factors (57).

Proteoglycans

Although proteoglycans make up only about 1% of the dry weight of ligaments and tendons, their functions of lubrication, spacing, and gliding are essential (58). Proteoglycans also impact viscoelastic properties of dense connective tissues. There are several different types of proteoglycans (e.g., hyaluronic acid, chondroitin sulfate, decorin, aggrecan, biglycan) that are specific to site and function. An examination of different regions of a tendon as it traverses around a bony pulley is an excellent example of adaptation of proteoglycans by dense connective tissues. The proximal region of the tendon (at a distance from the bony pulley) is only exposed to tensional forces and contains a scant amount of decorin providing some lubrication to the surrounding collagen fibers. In contrast, the region of tendon that is in contact with bone (and subjected to both compression and tension) contains approximately 10-fold more proteoglycan, most of which is chondroitin sulfate. In other words, the tissue is more like fibrocartilage in the area of compression to best withstand the mechanical forces in that region. Work in animal models has demonstrated that these proteoglycan levels may adjust to environmental cues (53).

Morphological Changes

After trauma, or inflammation of connective tissue, undifferentiated mesenchymal cells start to migrate to the site of injury and gradually change into mature fibroblasts. The fibroblasts travel along fibrin layers, multiply, and develop collagen-producing organelles (54).

These new collagen fibers are usually arranged randomly in loose connective tissue, whereas the collagen fibers in ligaments and tendons are packed and oriented in the direction of force and stretch. The metabolism of collagen is characterized by continuous synthesis and breakdown. If localized synthesis in the muscle or capsule exceeds breakdown, for example, excessive fibrosis will result. Thus, the mechanical properties of the newly formed connective tissue are the result of the amount and quality of collagen produced, the bonding between fibers, and the orientation of the collagen fibers in the tissue (48,49,55).

The balance between synthesis and degradation is disturbed by physical factors such as the lack of stretch that is seen in prolonged immobilization and inactivity. Trauma with bleeding into the soft tissue and muscle, inflammation, degeneration, or ischemia could all trigger an increased synthesis of collagen. In these conditions, additional lack of stretch and mobility may cause the collagen fibers to become more tightly packed (55). In some genetically determined diseases of the collagen metabolism (e.g., Ehlers-Danlos syndrome), the actual production of collagen and the formation of cross-links among the fibers are diminished. On the other hand, collagen degradation is increased in some conditions. In rheumatoid arthritis, for example, the enzyme collagenase is released from polymorphonuclear leukocytes, causing the direct cleavage and destruction of the collagen in joint cartilage. This may explain why patients with rheumatoid arthritis may preserve full ROM in affected joints (59,60).

The collagen in muscle connective tissue provides important functions, such as linking muscle cells and tendons, and is a supportive structure that holds muscle fibers and fascicles together. The synthesis of muscular collagen is influenced by the level of muscular activity and stretching during daily activities. Hence, collagen synthesis in the muscle is greater during activity and reduced during immobility. Immobilization for 1 week causes 21% and 65% decreases in activity of the enzymes prolyl 4-hydroxylase and galactosylhydroxylase glucosyltransferase in nontrained and trained experimental animals, respectively (55–57). The muscle fiber itself contributes little to the development of capsular contracture. However, in myogenic contractures, the muscle membrane (containing type IV collagen), myofibrils, and muscle fibers become shortened, contributing significantly to the limitation of joint ROM (49,50,58).

Muscular Contracture and Lack of Stretch

Myogenic contracture is a shortening of resting muscle length due to intrinsic or extrinsic causes. Intrinsic changes are structural and may be associated with inflammatory, degenerative, or traumatic processes. Extrinsic muscle contracture is secondary, resulting from neurologic abnormalities or mechanical factors. The diagnosis of muscle contracture should be made only after careful physical examination, which should include an evaluation of active and passive ROM. Observing limitation of active ROM alone can lead to an erroneous conclusion of fixed contracture; such limitation also could be due to muscle weakness (38).

Animal studies have indicated that, in the neurologically normal rat, 2 weeks of hind limb immobilization did not result in fixed contractions. However, immobilization for 6 weeks resulted in a 70% reduction of ROM. Five times greater than normal tension was required to achieve end range motion (61).

Muscular dystrophy (MD) is an example of a degenerative process. The most significant histologic changes in this condition are muscle fiber loss, abnormal residual muscle fibers, segmental necrosis of muscle fibers, and increased amounts of lipocytes and fibrosis. The replacement of functional muscle fibers with collagen and fatty tissue in concert with chronically shortened resting muscle length results in contracture (62). In the inflammatory myopathies, muscle fibers are replaced by increasing amounts of collagen and connective tissue in association with lymphocytic infiltration (37,63). Direct muscle trauma also can result in fibrosis. After hemorrhage into a muscle, fibrin deposition occurs. Within 2 to 3 days, the fibrin fibers are replaced by reticular fibers, which then assemble into a loose connective tissue network. If the muscle is kept immobilized, this network rapidly progresses in density and resists stretching. After trauma, external factors such as immobilization result in increases in serum creatine kinase activity, local vascular permeability, swelling, and, eventually, soft-tissue contracture (12).

Among the processes that may cause intrinsic muscle shortening, heterotopic ossification is the only one that involves deposition of bone rather than of collagen. This ossification is most commonly noted after trauma; joint surgery, especially of the hip; spinal cord injury; or other central nervous system injury. The actual initiating factor is unknown. An alteration in local metabolism or blood flow, in connection with the systemic alteration in calcium metabolism that occurs with immobility, may be responsible for initiating this process. Although no truly effective treatment exists, ROM should be aggressively maintained. Surgical resection of the bone may be considered after the bone matures. Surgery for immature heterotopic ossification is often associated with a rebound phenomenon that worsens the extent of previous bone deposition. Prophylaxis can be accomplished through the use of disodium etidronate, a diphosphonate compound that prevents the calcification of ground substance, along with nonsteroidal anti-inflammatory drugs and early mobilization (64).

Extrinsic myogenic contracture is the most common type occurring after multiple injuries and chronic illness, as well as in individuals with disabilities. In planning a therapeutic approach, it is useful to identify the cause of an extrinsic contracture as paralytic, spastic, or biomechanical. If a paralyzed muscle cannot provide adequate resistance to its antagonist muscle across a joint, then the stronger muscle will eventually become shortened. A common example of this is the shortened triceps surae seen in persons with chronic peroneal nerve palsy. Stretch applied to the muscle is essential to prevent contracture in this situation; strengthening of the weak muscle and proper positioning are also vital (30,39).

Similarly, in the presence of spasticity, a dynamic imbalance of muscle control exists across one or more joints. The resting length of spastic muscle is reduced because of increased muscle tone, which encourages faulty joint positioning (Fig. 41-3). It is often clinically difficult to identify the actual onset of structural (intrinsic) changes. If full ROM is unobtainable even after prolonged stretch and tension, then an intrinsic shortening also must be present. Treatment is directed at stretching the abnormal muscle; other antispasticity measures also may be of use, including pharmacologic agents and local nerve or motor point blocks (see Chapter 40).

Mechanical factors also can cause extrinsic muscle contracture. Some degree of muscle shortening is present even in healthy persons who are sedentary, especially in those muscles that cross multiple joints. Two joint muscles in the lower extremities are naturally stretched during ambulation; during bed rest, this does not occur. The back and hamstring muscles are the most commonly shortened; the iliopsoas, rectus femoris, tensor fascia lata, and gastrocnemius are next most likely to shorten. In the upper limbs, the internal rotators of the shoulder are the most frequently contracted. The below-knee amputee with prolonged knee flexion while sitting will develop decreased knee extension due to tight hamstrings and soft tissue behind the knee. On the other hand, the below-knee amputee treated with a rigid postoperative dressing in full knee extension may develop quadriceps muscle tightness that prevents full flexion of the knee.

Patients with muscular dystrophy provide yet another example of contracture aggravated by biomechanical factors (62). In muscular dystrophy, hip extensors often are very weak, forcing the patient into excessive lumbar lordosis: to thrust the center of gravity behind the hip and in front of the knee joints, the patient tends to walk on his toes. Walking on the toes in full ankle plantarflexion prevents natural stretching of the triceps surae from occurring during the stance phase of the gait, encouraging muscle shortening. If

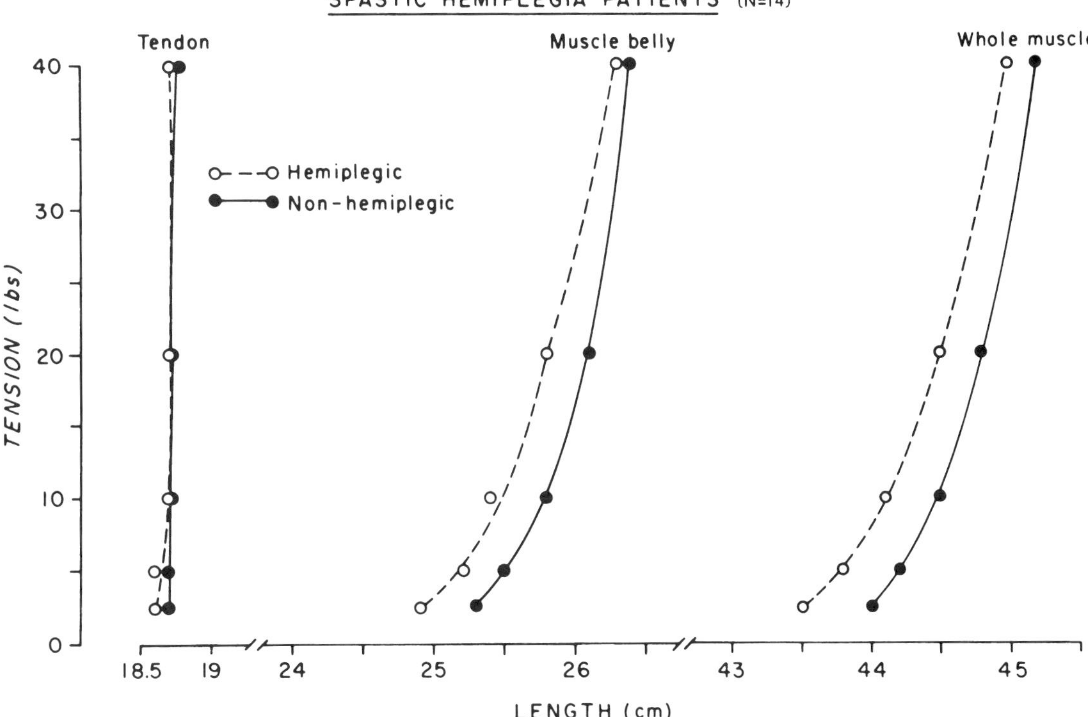

FIG. 41-3. Tension–length diagram of 14 hemiplegic patients with spasticity of the gastrocnemius–soleus muscles. The curve for spastic muscle is shifted to the left; the resting length of muscle belly, but not tendon, is reduced. At 2.5, 5, 10, 20, and 40 pounds of tension, the amount of elongation of spastic and unaffected muscles is not different. This indicated that elongation characteristics are essentially unchanged for spastic muscle, although the resting length of muscle is reduced. the gastrocnemius–soleus muscle belly elongates about 1.5 cm during full dorsiflexion. (With permission from Halar EM, Stolov WC, Venkatesh B, Brozovich FV, Harley JD. Gastrocnemius muscle belly and tendon length in stroke patients and able-bodied persons. *Arch Phys Med Rehabil* 1978; 59:476–484.)

a clinician does not recognize this sequence of events, he or she might assume that weakness and fibrosis are the only reasons for a plantarflexion contracture. A surgical lengthening of the Achilles tendon in such a case will not give the expected improvement. The lengthening of the tendon will actually shorten the muscle belly, decreasing plantarflexor strength and diminishing the ability of these patients to walk on their toes. Because walking on the toes is the only feasible method of ambulation, the result of an ill-advised tendon lengthening may be a wheelchair-dependent patient.

Arthrogenic Contracture

Pathologic processes involving joint components, such as degeneration of cartilage, congenital incongruency of joint surfaces, or synovial inflammation, can lead to capsular tightness and fibrosis. Synovial inflammation and effusion are accompanied by pain that results in limited joint motion and, eventually, in capsular contracture. In experimentally induced acute crystalline arthritis, exercises aggravate synovitis, whereas a short period of immobilization helps to reduce inflammation (65,66). In chronically induced experimental arthritis, however, joints immobilized for several weeks showed much greater destruction of joint cartilage than freely mobilized joints (66). However, short-term immobilization is indicated because of the presence of interleukin-1 in inflammatory synovial fluid. Studies indicate that passive ROM during acute arthritis may increase the release of interleukin-1, promoting interleukin-1 penetration into cartilage and binding to the receptors on the chondrocyte membranes, and inhibiting the production of proteoglycans necessary for protection of cartilage (65–67).

The cartilage loss and pain associated with muscle splinting leads to decrease movement of the joint and a loss in ROM. That pain, not the loss of cartilage, is responsible for the development of contracture and can be illustrated by patients with Charcot joint. These patients lack both pain sensation and proprioception but maintain relatively well-preserved ROM or even hypermobility of the involved joints in the presence of severe destruction of cartilage and joint surfaces (68).

The joint capsule also can lose extensibility as a consequence of collagen fiber shortening due to inadequate joint stretching and positioning in flexion (68,69). In capsular contractures, ROM is compromised in all directions of movement. In arthrogenic contracture and in the later stages of other types of contractures, the periarticular tissue also may undergo histochemical changes (70,71). If repeated trauma or inflammation is present, the collagen metabolism

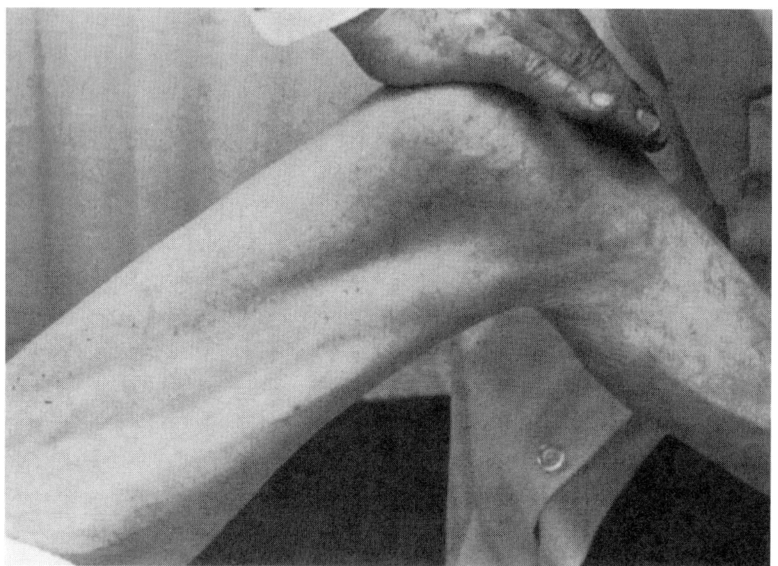

FIG. 41-4. A sequence of contracture development occurred from hip to knee in a patient with traumatic hip fracture treated operatively with pins. Owing to hip flexion contracture and immobility, the hamstrings became tight, causing knee flexion contracture with tightness of posterior capsule and soft tissue. Such a patient must walk on his for her toes, which produces increased energy expenditure.

of the periarticular tissue is altered and is associated with increased production of collagen fibrils in a random pattern of cross-linkage. Proteoglycan content is decreased, leading to joint stiffness and fixed contractures (58,72).

The shoulder and hip joint capsules are more prone than others to contracture. Initiating factors may include bicipital tendinitis, subdeltoid bursitis, rotator cuff damage, spasticity, or poor positioning coupled with immobility. The posterior knee capsule is another common site for capsular shortening, as a consequence of the prolonged flexion seen in patients who use wheelchairs (61,73) (Fig. 41-4).

Soft- and Dense-Tissue Contracture

Cutaneous, subcutaneous, and loose connective tissue around the joint also may become contracted. Trauma to soft tissue with bleeding, for example, can initiate fibrosis, which may progress to contracture if stretching is not provided. In this situation, collagen fibers usually proliferate and are laid down in random arrangements. In contrast to capsular tightness, soft-tissue shortening usually will limit movement in only one plane or axis. Burned skin is particularly susceptible to contracture. During recovery, burns across any joint must be ranged diligently and positioned to oppose the shortening forces of scarred tissue (48,49,59).

Topical steroid and vitamin E applications have failed to reduce soft-tissue contracture or postoperative scar formation after reconstructive joint surgeries. Vigorous active and passive ROM exercises, placement of the joint in a functional resting position, and use of compressive garments should be considered to prevent contractures in burn patients. Here again, adequate stretch and mobilization are important factors in the prevention of fixed contractures (5,30,39).

Ligaments also show biomechanical and biochemical changes during immobility (74). In experimental animals, the rate of growth, length of ligament, and elongational characteristics are influenced by tension applied to the ligament, growth hormones, size of underlying bones, and possibly other unknown factors. A study by Dahners et al. showed that in young, skeletally immature rabbits, the lateral collateral ligament of the knee elongated significantly (140%) when tension was applied for 6 weeks (75). This and other studies indicate that physiologic stretch and tension are important factors in helping both growing and mature ligaments to elongate and to withstand the stresses of weight bearing and mobility. Newton et al. found that ligaments become significantly weaker after prolonged immobilization because of decreased collagen synthesis. In addition, the ligament insertion sites on bone show an increase in osteoclastic activity. During immobility, the fibroblasts of the cruciate ligament may assume a spindle shape with multiple cytoplasmic extensions and demonstrate reduced production of collagen fibrils; resistance to ligament breakage is reduced (76). In a study by Klein, the atrophy of collateral and cruciate ligaments was prevented completely with active ROM exercise in non–weight-bearing limbs. However, this exercise could not prevent a significant bone loss in the femur and tibia of the same experimental animal. This study indicates that active joint motion could prevent ligamentous atrophy but that for full prevention of osteoporosis, weight bearing and exercise of appropriate duration and intensity are important factors of consideration (77,78).

Effects of Contractures on Physical Function

Contractures have major impact in three areas: they interfere with mobility, with the basic activities of daily living, and with nursing care of skin. Lower extremity contractures alter the gait pattern and, in extreme cases, can eliminate ambulation (Fig. 41-4). A hip flexion contracture, for example, reduces hip extension, shortens stride length, and requires the patient to walk on the ball of the foot with increased lumbar lordosis and increased energy consumption. For biomechanical reasons, hip flexion contractures cause the hamstring muscles to shorten, which in turn flexes the knee. It is not uncommon to see a patient with hip contracture develop progressive knee and ankle joint contractures, especially if the joints are not aggressively mobilized. Plantarflexion contractures will cause an absence of heel strike and abnormal push-off, resulting in decreased momentum of forward progression. Hip extension contractures are not frequently encountered. Wheelchair ambulation is impaired by advanced hip and knee extension contractures. Car transfers also may be difficult with the knee fixed in extension. Limitations in upper extremity ROM may lead to impaired reaching, dressing, grooming, eating, and performance of fine motor tasks (5–7). Multiple joint contractures can severely interfere with bed positioning, standing upright, and mobility, making perineal hygiene and skin care difficult. In addition, joint contractures tend to accentuate areas of increased pressure on skin, which may be impossible to prevent without first correcting the contracture. Hip flexion contracture may increase the energy consumption 60% or more during ambulation.

Bed Rest and Low Back Pain

Clinical observations have provided ample support for the theory that prolonged bed rest may cause low back pain, especially after resumption of mobility. This pain is related to several factors, including tightness of the back and hamstring muscles or weakness of the back and abdominal muscles. Any shortening of these muscles will alter spinal alignment and posture. Abdominal and spinal muscle weakness increases spinal curvature and weight bearing on the small apophyseal lumbar joints. Immobilization osteoporosis of the spine also is a possible contributor to the development of back pain (79). Abdominal muscle strengthening exercises as well as strengthening and sensible stretching of paraspinal and hamstring muscles, along with general conditioning, may prevent these complications of bed rest (80,81).

Acute low back pain has been treated with bed rest; however, the therapeutic value of prolonged bed rest has been disproven. In a well-controlled and randomized study, Deyo and colleagues have clearly shown that patients with acute and chronic low back pain who were prescribed 2 days of bed rest subsequently lost less time from work than did patients who received 1 week of bed rest (82,83). There was no difference between the two groups in functional outcome. This study reinforces the principle that prolonged bed rest should not be considered a therapeutic tool in the treatment of low back pain syndrome.

Therapeutic Approach and Management of Contractures

Analysis

The basis for initiating treatment for contractures is a careful determination of the predisposing factors and a knowledge of what joint components or tissues are actually involved. A careful neuromuscular examination emphasizing active and passive ROM is essential. Particular attention should be directed at those muscles crossing two joints. In patients with severe uncontrolled spasticity, it may be necessary to obtain accurate ROM measurements with the use of general anesthesia or local nerve blocks; this is particularly helpful when surgery to repair a decubitus ulcer is contemplated. Of course, the best treatment is prevention, so a careful analysis of positioning and ROM should be undertaken with any patient who is immobilized by disease or by the treatment of disease (39).

Stretch and Restoration of Range of Motion

Once a contracture has developed, the sine qua non for treatment is active and passive ROM exercise combined with a sustained terminal stretch at least twice a day (Table 41-4) (26,37,57,77). For mild contracture, a shorter sustained stretch lasting 20 to 30 minutes may be effective. Prolonged stretches of 30 minutes or more combined with appropriate positioning are necessary for more severe contractures. This generally is more successful when used in combination with the application of heat to the musculotendinous junction or joint capsule. Ultrasound is the most popular heat source for large joints; its properties allow local heating in the presence of metallic implants and rapid increase of tissue temperature to the therapeutic level. Heating of the tissue to 40°C to 43°C will increase the viscous properties of connective tissue and maximize the effect of stretching.

When applying terminal stretch to a joint, the proximal body part should be well stabilized. In many cases, slight distraction of the joint during stretch will prevent joint compression and possible soft-tissue impingement, particularly in the small joints of the hand. The shoulder is commonly a site of contracture, particularly in the adducted and internally rotated position. In this position, the normal downward sliding and rotation of the humeral head on the glenoid fossa does not occur; forced abduction will therefore simply cause painful impingement of the rotator cuff tendon against the acromion. Stretch applied in forward flexion and external rotation will restore some of this motion and should be attempted before abduction.

TABLE 41-4. *Basic principles in the prevention and treatment of contractures*

Prevention
Proper positioning in bed, resting splints
Range-of-motion exercises (active or passive)
Early mobilization and ambulation
CPM (continuous passive motion)
Treatment
Passive range-of-motion exercises with terminal stretch
Prolonged stretch using low passive tension and heat
Progressive (e.g., dynamic) splinting, casting
Treatment of spasticity; pharmacologic, motor point or nerve blocks using phenol, injection of botulinum toxin A
Surgical interventions (e.g. tendon lengthening, osteotomies, joint replacement) (see Table 44-5)
Pain management

Sustained stretch lasting 2 hours or more can be obtained by the use of splinting. Serial casting is the application of plaster or polymer bandages with careful padding over bony prominences. The cast is applied immediately after the use of heat and manual stretch to obtain maximal ROM. After the initial cast has dried and has been worn for 2 to 3 days, it should be removed and the skin checked for pressure areas. The cast can be reapplied every 2 to 5 days. Serial casting is particularly useful for plantarflexion, knee flexion, and elbow contractures. In patients with spasticity, chemical denervation before casting may improve tolerance and decrease the occurrence of skin breakdown. Cutting a cast and placing a wedge to increase tension on the contracted structure is a low-cost alternative to serial casting (84).

Another method of obtaining repeated stretch is dynamic splinting. Movement is allowed, and a spring or elastic band provides tension in the desired direction. This type of splinting is often used in the hand and arm because it allows a measure of function while providing stretch. Another way to provide a form of sustained stretch is to use a continuous passive mobilization (CPM) device (85). The use of these devices has become relatively routine for providing postoperative ROM stretching of the knee, and they also have been adopted for use on other joints. CPM is recommended for the early mobilization of infected joints, synovectomized knees and hips, knee fractures, ligamentous repairs, total knee joint replacement, or any incipient arthrogenic contractures. A study of periosteal joint autografts with postoperative CPM demonstrated a 63% increase in hyaline cartilage formation compared with autograft joints that were immobilized without use of CPM. Early passive mobilization with CPM has been shown to promote the exchange of joint fluid, reduce the need for pain medication after surgery, and prevent contractures in high-risk patients. During CPM therapy, muscles around the joint remain relaxed, and pain is usually minimal. CPM is typically prescribed for 8 to 12 hours a day for a total of 3 to 5 days after surgery. When used alone, CPM is not effective in the treatment of fixed contractures.

To achieve optimal joint position, it sometimes is necessary to lengthen tendons by surgical means (Table 41-5). The benefits and risks of tendon lengthening should be con-

TABLE 41-5. *Surgical treatment of contractures*

Joint	Contracture	Procedure	Comments
Shoulder	Adduction, internal rotation	Subscapularis, pectoralis major tenotomy or lengthening	Postoperative stretching is necessary
Elbow	"Simple" flexion	Open or arthroscopic capsulectomy, biceps tendon lengthening, brachialis myotomy	Compound joint surgery generally not recommended for contractures <30% loss ROM
	Flexion/pronation	Myotomy of brachioradialis combined with z lengthening of biceps tendon	
Wrist and hand	Flexion (may include thumb-in-pain deformity)	Tenotomy of deep and superficial tendons at wrists (transfer of flexor carpi ulnaris to the extensor carpi radialis brevis or extensor carpi radialis longus with pronator releases)	
	"Windblown hand" (flexion contracture and sublaxation of MCP joints)		
	Pronation/wrist flexion		
Hip	Flexion	Psoas tenotomy or z lengthening	
	Adduction	Adductor myotomy	
	Pediatric hip dislocation (hip flexors and adductors)		
Knee	Flexion	Distal hamstring lengthening	May combine with distal rectus femoris transfer
		Posterior capsulotomy, proximal hamstring tenotomy	
		Total knee arthroplasty	
Ankle and foot	Plantar flexion	Lengthening Achilles tendon	Separation of lengthening of gastrocnemius and soleus may preserve strength
	Equinovarus calcaneus deformity	Soft-tissue release, triple arthrodesis	Resection or temotomy of anterior tibial tendon, posterior transfer of anterior tibialis muscle
	Toe flexion	Release of long toe flexors, IP joint arthrodeses	

IP, interphalangeal; MCP, metacarpophalangeal; ROM, range of motion.

sidered carefully. It must be remembered that the muscle belly will remain shortened even though the tendon is longer; therefore, full active ROM may not be restored. Tendon lengthening combined with muscle transfer procedures in spastic or paralytic contractures may give better results because the process attempts to restore equilibrium around the joint; this method is particularly effective at the ankle, using the tibialis posterior muscle. Electromyographic analysis of muscle function before tendon transfer will optimize results. In other situations, such as hip adductor contractures secondary to spasticity, tenotomy may be combined with obturator nerve neurolysis to obtain optimal results (57,66,75). In a chronic fixed joint contracture that interferes with the patient's basic physical functions, the selection of the appropriate surgical procedure is of great importance. Table 41-5 provides the surgical options for different joint contracture management and their surgical treatment (86–88).

Prevention of Contractures

Prevention of contracture in a bed-bound patient starts with the selection of an adequate bed and mattress, proper bed positioning, and a mobility training program. The patient should be moved out of bed as soon as his or her medical condition allows. If bed rest is unavoidable, then bed positioning and bed mobility are incorporated into the patient's nursing management program. A firm mattress is necessary to prevent sagging and avoids excessive hip flexion in a supine position. Moving a footboard 4 inches away from the end of the mattress allows the heel or forefoot to be placed in between, providing pressure relief for the heels or feet. To assist a patient in turning side-to-side or in sitting up, partial side rails for grasp should be a standard part of bed equipment. An overhead trapeze is useful for patients with impaired bed mobility, allowing them to use their upper extremities to help them roll from side to side, scoot up and down, attain a sitting position, and transfer into and out of bed (89).

If a patient with paresis or with otherwise compromised extremities must have prolonged bed rest, a variety of assistive devices are used to keep the joints in functional positions. Because of the recumbent position and weight of the arm, the shoulder tends to assume an adducted and internally rotated position during bed rest. If this position is maintained through the day, and ROM movement is provided for only 15 to 20 minutes daily, the internal rotators and adductors may shorten. With the use of pillows, the shoulder can be maintained effectively in abduction and neutral rotation. A palmar roll or hand splint is used to maintain hand, thumb, and finger joints at optimal position. If flexors of the hand and fingers tighten, a resting splint providing more extension can stretch the contracted muscles (see Chapter 48). For lower extremity positioning, a trochanter roll or derotation bar are used to counteract excessive external rotation. Plantarflexion contractures are best prevented by the use of a splint encompassing the foot, ankle, in neutral position. Provision of daily active or passive ROM and flexibility exercises are essential for prevention of contractures.

Functional Training

The last major area to be considered in the prevention and treatment of contractures is the maintenance and restoration of function. Encouraging the use of the limb for ambulation or other activities will help maintain the function of uninvolved joints as well as focus attention on the normal use of the affected joint. Muscle strengthening should be a primary concern in order to obtain a balance of forces across joints. Electrical stimulation applied to paretic muscles to obtain full muscle contraction can be used to initiate the strengthening process (44–46). Use of electromyographic feedback also may aid the patient in incorporating the weakened muscle appropriately into normal activities. The elimination of poor habits in ambulation and posture, and the use of a strength and endurance program are necessary to prevent recurrent joint contractures (6,32,89).

IMMOBILIZATION OSTEOPOROSIS

Maintenance of skeletal mass depends largely on mechanical loading applied to bone by tendon pull and the force of gravity. Bone mass will increase with repeated loading stresses and will decrease with the absence of muscle activity or with the elimination of gravity (90–93). Certain populations are more susceptible to the effects of muscle inactivity, such as the aging adult or the person with a spinal cord injury. Even in the healthy aging adult, the rate of bone loss exceeds the rate of new bone formation, leading to some degree of osteopenia (93,94). Bone mass begins to decline in the fourth and fifth decades of life, occurring most rapidly in women in the first 5 to 7 years after menopause (95,96). After spinal cord injury, a mismatch also occurs between bone growth and bone loss. Soon after initial injury, for reasons still unclear, osteoblastic activity diminishes and a rapid loss of bone mineral occurs, resulting in severe osteopenia in the paralyzed region of the body (97). Even relatively minor muscle dysfunction can result in bone loss regionally. Persons with rotator cuff ruptures have been shown to have significantly decreased bone mineral density as compared with control arms with bone density proportional to the remaining shoulder function (98).

Immobilization results in a prolonged loss of bone density. Osteopenia due to immobilization is characterized by loss of calcium and hydroxyproline from the cancellous bone of long bone epiphyses and metaphyses. Increased resorption of bone is the primary process responsible for disuse osteoporosis, although the precise nature of this resorption is unknown (93,95). In animal experiments, full body recumbency resulted in loss of both trabecular and compact bone, which remained below baseline 2 months after free activity was allowed (79). These results appear to be true for humans as well. Immobilization of forearms and wrists for a period of almost 5 weeks resulted in significant loss of bone mineral density in both men and women, which was not ameliorated after almost 5 weeks of remobilization and hand therapy

(99). In addition to increased bone resorption, it also appears that weightlessness interferes with bone mineralization. Immobilization osteopenia is a risk factor for hip fracture, especially in elderly patients (96).

The importance of exercise in overcoming inactivity-induced osteopenia should not be overlooked. Disuse osteoporosis can be minimized by the regular use of isometric or isotonic exercises. Ambulation, or at least standing on a tilt table, may retard the loss of calcium. Bourrin and associates studied the effect of controlled exercise on rats immobilized by tail suspension. In all the rats thus treated, there were significant decreases in bone density and bone formation. Abnormalities were especially seen in trabecular bone. Animals who received specific limb exercise in addition to normal remobilization not only recovered bone mass parameters but had improvement in the trabecular patterns; nonexercised animals had persisting trabecular alterations (100). In patient groups at highest risk for significant osteopenia, those either with paralysis or with hormonally based osteoporosis, care should be taken when exercising to prevent fracture. Despite this risk of pathologic fracture, weight-bearing exercise is particularly important to these groups to prevent progression of bone loss. Additionally, in the elderly, exercise targeted at strengthening limb-girdle muscles and lessening the chance of falls is an important adjunct (80,83,92).

Despite a normal serum calcium level, immobilized patients are markedly hypercalciuric. However, adolescent boys after acute spinal cord injury may show a significant hypercalcemia as well. Symptoms of hypercalcemia include anorexia, abdominal pain, nausea, vomiting, constipation, confusion, and, ultimately, coma (101,102). Treatment of immobilization hypercalcemia relies on achieving adequate calcium excretion through hydration with normal and one-half normal saline and diuresis with furosemide. For all immobilized persons, urinary calcium excretion increases above normal levels on the second and third days of recumbency. Maximum loss occurs during the fourth or fifth week when the urinary calcium excretion is double the level of the first week; on the average, calcium loss is 1.5 g/week (93,103). This decrease in total calcium continues even after resumption of physical activity. Three weeks after physical activity is resumed, calcium losses of up to 4.0 g have been measured. This negative calcium balance can last for months and even years (94).

Negative calcium balance can be induced by decreasing physical activity without actual confinement to bed. The sedentary person tends to progressively lose calcium from bone. Several well-controlled studies have shown that normal subjects on a year-long program of exercises will increase their bone mass compared with those who are inactive. Protracted negative balance can lead to secondary complications, such as hip and vertebral bone fractures after minimal trauma or ectopic calcification around the large joints (93,99,104).

Some newer developments in treating or preventing bone loss may have some application for rehabilitating patients. The bisphosphonates are analogues of a naturally occurring bone chemical that inhibit bone resorption, in addition to inhibiting calcium phosphate crystal formation and dissolution (103,105). Pamidronate and clodronate are now used to treat Paget's disease, immobilization-induced hypercalcemia, metastatic bone disease, and other malignancies affecting bone (102,106). One bisphosphonate compound, tiludronate, has been use in paraplegic patients with some efficacy in maintaining bone volume without impairing bone formation. Salmon calcitonin is another compound that has demonstrated some success in maintaining bone density and may be particularly helpful in patient populations who cannot be adequately mobilized (107).

CARDIOVASCULAR AND PULMONARY SYSTEM EFFECT OF IMMOBILITY

Cardiovascular Alteration

During periods of recumbency, the resting heart rate increases by one beat per minute every 2 days, leading to immobilization tachycardia, characterized by an abnormal increase in heart rate on submaximal workloads. Assuming an upright position provokes a significant increase in pulse rate, and the severity of this response is related to the duration of bed rest. A healthy, active person's heart rate increases 13% on getting up from a supine position. But after 3 days, 1 week, and 6 weeks of bed rest, heart rate response increases 32%, 62%, and 89%, respectively (108,109). The heart rate in response to submaximal exercise is also increased after bed rest. Saltin and coworkers found a pulse rate response on submaximal exercise of 129 beats per minutes for active healthy persons, compared with 165 beats per minute after bed rest (89).

Other cardiovascular functions also have been found to change with prolonged bed rest. The stroke volume may decrease 15% after 2 weeks of bed rest, a response that may be related to blood volume reduction. Although heart rate response to submaximal exercises increases progressively, cardiac output on submaximal exercise is reduced (108–110). The alterations of cardiovascular function induced by immobility are frequently referred to as cardiovascular adaptation syndrome (CAS). Diminished cardiac output coupled with peripheral oxygen utilization deficiency causes a decline in maximal oxygen consumption (VO_2max). After 20 days of bed rest, VO_2max may decline by 27%. If a patient with coronary artery disease (CAD) develops CAS, the cardiac ischemia may be aggravated. For example, orthostatic hypotension may precipitate the onset of angina in patients with CAD. One way of preventing CAS is to encourage early ambulation and graded activity. In the 1950s, patients with myocardial infarction were kept in bed for 2 to 3 weeks; today they are encouraged to start walking on the second day (111).

Impaired Cardiovascular Performance

The efficiency of the cardiopulmonary response to muscle demand depends on the frequency with which the maximal work capacity of muscle is approached. Because of interaction between these two systems, the maximal cardiovascular capacity gradually declines with reduced physical activity (108). This decline of cardiovascular function is enhanced in chronically ill and disabled individuals who are immobile.

After 3 weeks of bed rest, the resting pulse increases 10 to 12 beats per minute and the pulse rate increases an average of 35 to 45 beats above normal response after 30 minutes of walking at 3.5 miles per hour up a 10% grade. This represents a 25% decrease in cardiovascular performance (112). There is a gradual elevation of the systolic blood pressure in response to increased peripheral vascular resistance. In addition, the absolute systolic ejection time is shortened, and the diastole filling time reduced, resulting in stroke volume reduction. Work capacity, which is derived from left ventricular pressure and force of ventricular contraction, is also reduced. Overall declines in cardiac output and left ventricular function with prolonged immobility have been reported in several studies (91,109,112).

Pulmonary Alterations

The respiratory complications of immobility are known to be life threatening. Initial pulmonary alterations result from restricted movement of the chest in the supine position and gravity-induced changes in the perfusion of blood through different parts of the lung. When venous pressures and hydrostatic pressure due to gravity are increased in different parts of the lung, then perfusion is also increased. The balance between perfusion and ventilation is altered during recumbency (113). A change of position from upright to supine results in a 2% reduction of the vital capacity, a 7% reduction of total lung capacity, a 19% reduction in residual volume, and a 30% reduction in functional residual capacity (114). Vital capacity and functional reserve capacity may be reduced by 25% to 50% after prolonged bed rest. Mechanisms responsible for this may include diminished diaphragmatic movement in the supine position, decreased chest excursion, progressive decrease in ROM of costovertebral and costochondral joints, and shallower breathing with subsequent increase in respiratory rate (115).

Clearance of secretions is more difficult in a recumbent position. The dependent (i.e., usually posterior) walls accumulate more secretions, whereas the upper parts (i.e., anterior) become dry, rendering the ciliary lining ineffective for clearing secretions and allowing secretions to pool in the lower bronchial tree. The effectiveness of coughing is impaired because of ciliary malfunction and abdominal muscle weakness. Regional changes in the ventilation–perfusion ratio in dependent areas occur when ventilation is reduced and perfusion is increased. This may lead to significant arteriovenous shunting with lowered arterial oxygenation. Atelectasis and hypostatic pneumonia may be the ultimate result of these alterations.

The intercostal and axillary respiratory muscles for deep breathing gradually lose their strength and overall endurance. Treatment or prevention involve early mobilization, frequent respiratory toileting, and frequent position changes. A patient in a recumbent position should be persuaded to perform regular pulmonary toileting and deep breathing and coughing exercises, and to maintain adequate hydration. An incentive spirometer, chest percussion, and postural drainage with oropharyngeal suctioning can prevent aspiration and atelectasis. The presence of pre-existing pulmonary disease requires the use of bronchodilators (see Chapter 55).

Redistribution of Body Fluids

Normally, 20% of total blood volume is contained within the arterial system, 5% in the capillaries, and 75% in the venous system. Immediately upon lying down, 500 ml of blood shifts to the thorax, heart rate decreases, and cardiac output increases by 24%. Estimated cardiac work is increased by approximately 30%. During lengthy periods of bed rest, there is a progressive decline in blood volume, with the maximum reduction on day 14. This reduction in blood volume is due to a reduced hydrostatic blood pressure and decreased secretion of antidiuretic hormone. Plasma volume decreases more than red cell mass, leading to increased blood viscosity and, possibly, to thromboembolic phenomena. The loss of plasma volume after 24 hours is 5%, whereas after 6 and 14 days, the loss is 10% and 20%, respectively, of the pre–bed-rest level (116). The extracellular fluid volume remains unchanged, although longer periods of bed rest will produce a decrease (111,117,118). For normal subjects on bed rest, the reduction of plasma volume can be diminished by exercise. Therapeutic isotonic exercises are almost twice as effective as isometric exercises in preventing plasma volume reduction (119,120).

In addition, a reduction of plasma proteins is noted after prolonged bed rest. Although short periods of intensive exercise produce a small loss of plasma proteins, sustained submaximal exercise actually induces a net gain in plasma protein, which contributes to the stabilization of the plasma volume depletion (121). Hypovolemia, along with circulatory stasis due to bed rest, are important precipitating factors in thrombogenesis.

Postural Hypotension

One of the most dramatic effects of prolonged bed rest is the impaired ability of the cardiovascular system to adjust to the upright position. When a healthy person stands up from a supine position after being confined to bed for several days, 500 ml of blood shifts from the thorax into the legs. As a consequence, the ankle venous pressure increases from 15 cm H_2O in the supine position to 120 cm H_2O in the upright position. Reduced venous return to the heart results from intravascular volume depletion, change in venous compliance, and venous pooling. The end result is decreased stroke volume and cardiac output, and a significant decrease in the systolic blood pressure upon rising. In normal situations, blood pressure decrease is prevented by immediate activation of the adrenergic sympathetic system. Baroreceptors in the right atrium, great thoracic veins, carotid arteries, and aorta trigger adrenergic reflexes, releasing norepinephrine. The increase in plasma norepinephrine levels influences the release of renin and angiotensin II, which in return potentiate the sympathetic response, resulting in an immediate increase in pulse rate and restoration of blood pressure along with prolonged constriction of lower limb and mesenteric blood vessels (122,123).

During prolonged recumbency, the circulatory system is also unable to maintain a stable blood pressure and, for unknown reasons, is unable to mount an adequate sympathetic vasopressive response. Although plasma renin and aldosterone levels remain normal, vasoconstriction is inadequate (124). Several studies indicate that increased beta-adrenergic activity caused by bed rest is to blame for this intolerance (125). This decrease in venous return along with the rapid heart rate, prevents optimal ventricular filling during end diastole. Stroke volume, which depends on diastolic filling, may be insufficient to maintain adequate cerebral perfusion (126–128). The clinical signs and symptoms of postural hypotension are tingling, burning in the lower extremities, dizziness, lightheadedness, fainting, vertigo, increased pulse rate (more than 20 beats per minute), decreased systolic pressure (more than 20 mm Hg), and decreased pulse pressure. In patients with CAD, anginal symptoms may be caused by the decreased coronary blood flow that accompanies inadequate diastolic filling (129).

In healthy people, adaptation to the upright position may be completely lost after 3 weeks of bed rest. A significant increase in heart rate and decrease in systolic pressure may even occur after several days of recumbency in those with sepsis, major trauma, major medical illness, or advanced age (127). The process of restoring the normal postural cardiovascular responses can take 20 to 72 days. Older people take much longer to restore normal blood pressure and heart rate during remobilization.

As a group, patients with tetraplegia are quite susceptible to orthostatic hypotension. When tilted up, they show a significant decrease in mean arterial pressure and an increase in heart rate. Both sympathetic and plasma renin activities, as measured by serum dopamine-beta-hydroxylase and plasma renin radioimmunoassay, are normal or slightly increased. Two possible mechanisms may account for orthostatic hypotension in patients with spinal cord injury. First, the normal increase in plasma norepinephrine that occurs on tilting is delayed in patients with tetraplegia. Second, the successful use of compressive antigravity suits in treating patients with quadriplegia and postural hypotension indicates that venous pooling may play an important role in the occurrence of orthostatic hypotension (130,131).

Early mobilization is the most effective way to counter orthostatic hypotension and should include ROM exercises, strengthening exercises in supine and upright positions, and progressive ambulation. Abdominal strengthening and isotonic–isometric exercises involving the legs are optimal for reversing venous stasis and pooling. Elevating leg rests and reclining backs on wheelchairs are used to assist patients during the reconditioning process. Occasionally a tilt table may be necessary, with the goal of tolerating 20 minutes at 75° of tilt. Supportive garments such as elastic bandage wraps, full-length elastic stockings, and a variety of abdominal binders are used regularly. Beta-blockers such as propranolol may reduce the time needed to restore pulse rate and blood pressure to normal levels after bed rest and reduce the severity of orthostatic intolerance (132,123). Ephedrine and phenylephrine are sympathomimetic agents that help to maintain blood pressure; fludrocortisone (Florinef, Apothcon, Princeton, NJ), a mineralocorticoid, is the next choice of drug to use. Maintaining an adequate salt and fluid intake will prevent any worsening of hypotension secondary to blood volume contraction (89,122,131).

Immobility and Deep Venous Thrombosis

Immobility exposes the patient to two factors that are contained in Virchow's triad and contribute to clot formation: venous stasis and increased blood coagulability. The third factor, injury to the vessel wall, is all that is required to increase the patient's risk for thromboembolism (133). Paralysis and trauma to the lower limbs or pelvis may add to the risk for development of DVT. A direct relationship between the frequency of DVT and the length of bed rest has been observed (134).

In stroke patients, DVT is 10 times more common in the involved extremities than in the uninvolved extremities. In nonambulatory stroke patients, DVT is five times more frequent than in patients who can walk more than 50 feet (135,136). Although the first week of immobilization is the most frequent time for development of DVT, it may occur later during remobilization. When stasis is present, thrombus formation usually starts behind the valve cusp of the deep veins. Stasis may contribute to anoxia and damage of the endothelial cells in the valve pocket, thus adding the third factor for initiating the onset of DVT. Whether stasis alone can result in DVT is not fully confirmed. However, several studies suggest that stasis may lead to increased formation of thrombin, which then leads to platelet aggregation and thrombosis (137). The most common site of DVT formation is the veins in the calf. Usually, such thrombi will attach to the wall of the vein within 1 week; however, 20% of calf thrombi extend to popliteal and thigh veins, and half of these will embolize to the lungs, posing a serious threat to the patient's life (138).

Venous stasis in the lower extremities is mainly due to decreased pumping activity of the calf muscles and increased orthostatic pressure. Other factors that can contribute to stasis are surgery, age, obesity, and congestive heart failure, all of which can lead to abnormal blood flow mechanics. The incidence of DVT in postoperative patients published in 1979 was 29% for those who had general surgery and 44% for those who had hip surgery (134). Also contributing to the likelihood of DVT occurrence in the patient confined to bed is a hypercoagulable state, produced by decreased blood volume and increased blood viscosity and associated with many conditions such as malignancy.

Clinical detection of DVT begins with the observation of signs and symptoms, including edema, tenderness, hyperemia, venous distention, and Homans' sign. When DVT is suspected on clinical grounds, these additional diagnostic studies should be performed:

Doppler ultrasound study may be 95% accurate, depending on the skill of the examiner, but cannot be used to detect thrombi reliably above the level of the femoral vein.

Radionuclide venography is both sensitive and specific for thrombi above the knee, but cannot detect calf thrombi or distinguish between old and new disease unless the patient has a previous study available for comparison.

Contrast venography remains the standard for diagnosis. However, it is invasive, time consuming, painful, and irritating to the venous lining.

Pulmonary emboli are manifested by a sudden onset of dyspnea, tachypnea, tachycardia, or chest pain and often are associated with a pre-existing DVT. Diagnosis rests on arterial blood gases, ventilation–perfusion scans, and pulmonary angiography.

The most common means of preventing thromboembolic complications is to use low-dose subcutaneous injections of heparin (5,000 units twice a day) (139). Other preventive measures include external intermittent leg compression, elastic leg wrappings, active exercise, and early mobilization.

After the diagnosis of DVT is made and treatment with heparin and warfarin is initiated, ambulation can be permitted on the second or third day if the partial thromboplastin time is within the therapeutic range. Recent literature supports the conclusion that 5 to 7 days of bed rest is not necessary for DVT if a therapeutic level of anticoagulation is achieved (140,141).

GASTROINTESTINAL AND GENITOURINARY EFFECTS OF IMMOBILITY

Genitourinary Alteration

Many compromises occur in the physical and metabolic functions of the urinary tract system. Prolonged bed rest contributes to increased incidence of bladder or renal stones and urinary tract infections. Hypercalciuria is a frequent finding in persons who are immobilized. Other important factors include an altered ratio of citric acid to calcium and an increased urinary excretion of phosphorus. In the supine position, urine must flow uphill from the renal collecting systems to be drained through the ureters. Patients often find it difficult to initiate voiding while supine, a situation that is not ameliorated by reduced intra-abdominal pressure secondary to abdominal muscle weakness and deconditioning. Studies have demonstrated less complete voiding in immobilized animals in association with urinary stagnation (142).

Incomplete bladder emptying (e.g., in patients with spinal cord injury or diabetes mellitus) puts the patient at great risk for stone formation (143). The most common types of stones are struvate and carbonate apatite, found in 15% to 30% of immobilized patients. Bladder stones allow bacterial growth and decrease the efficacy of standard antimicrobial treatment. Irritation and trauma to the bladder mucosa by stones can encourage bacterial overgrowth and infection. Urea-splitting bacteria then increase the urine pH, leading to further precipitation of calcium and magnesium (142).

Treatment of these problems lies first in prevention, which includes adequate fluid intake to reduce bacterial colonization, use of the upright position for voiding, and scrupulous avoidance of bladder contamination during instrumentation. Other therapeutic approaches might include acidification of the urine through the use of vitamin C, urinary antiseptics, and, in those populations at highest risk for stone formation, a urease inhibitor. Treatment of stones after they have formed may require surgical removal or the use of ultrasonic lithotripsy. Appropriate antibiotic selection based on urine cultures and sensitivity trials is required to eliminate urinary tract infection. If retention is suspected, postvoiding residual volumes should be measured several times a day with ultrasound scanning devices. After stroke or spinal cord injury, removal of the Foley catheter and initiation of voiding trails should coincide with sitting and ambulation training. A dysfunctional urinary bladder with poor contractility of the detrusor muscle and deficient sphincter coordination will aggravate the adverse effects of immobility.

Gastrointestinal Alterations

Gastrointestinal alterations due to immobility are easily overlooked. Loss of appetite, slower rate of absorption, and distaste for protein-rich foods all lead to nutritional hypoproteinemia. Passage of food through the esophagus, stomach, and small bowel is slowed in the supine position. An upright position increases the velocity of the esophageal waves and shortens the relaxation time of the lower esophagus (144). Thus, sleeping on two or three pillows with upper trunk elevated in bed has therapeutic implications in preventing and treating reflux esophagitis. The transit of food through the stomach is 60% slower in the supine position than when the person is upright (145). Constipation is a common complication that results from the interaction of multiple factors. Immobility causes increased adrenergic activity, which inhibits peristalsis and causes sphincter contraction (146). The loss of plasma volume and dehydration aggravate constipation. In addition, the use of a bedpan for fecal elimination places the patient in a nonphysiologic position, and the desire to defecate is reduced by social embarrassment. The end result is fecal impaction, which requires enemas, manual removal, or, in extreme cases, surgical intervention (147).

Prevention of constipation requires an adequate intake of an appealing, fiber-rich diet, including raw fruits and vegetables, and of liberal amounts of fluids. Stool softeners and bulk-forming agents are helpful in maintaining bowel function. The use of narcotic agents should be limited because they slow peristalsis. Limited use of glycerin or peristalsis-stimulating suppositories, in combination with a regularly timed bowel program, will further assist in the prevention of impaction.

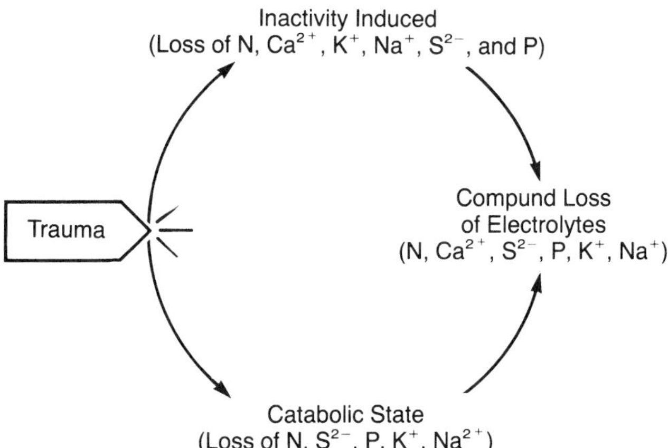

FIG. 41-5. Negative metabolic balance induced by trauma can be aggravated by negative metabolic balance produced by prolonged bed rest and immobility.

METABOLISM AND ENDOCRINE SYSTEM ALTERATIONS RESULTING FROM IMMOBILITY

Daily human energy needs include basal metabolic activity, thermogenesis of food, and the activities of daily living. It is unclear whether the basal metabolism changes during bed rest; this uncertainty stems from inadequate scientific studies on control of factors that could influence the basal metabolic rate during prolonged bed rest (4). Lean body mass decreases during bed rest, and an equal gain in body fat maintains constant total body weight (148). The reduced lean body mass is associated with decreased metabolic activity and maximal oxygen consumption, which further reduces the functional capacity of the musculoskeletal system (28,29).

Electrolyte Balance

Prolonged immobility, especially if associated with the posttraumatic electrolyte changes, will cause an alteration in the metabolic balance of sodium, sulfur, phosphorus, and potassium. A decrease in total body sodium occurs in tandem with the diuresis seen early during bed rest. However, serum sodium levels do not correlate well with the severity of orthostatic hypotension. Hyponatremia is manifested especially in the elderly by lethargy, confusion and disorientation, anorexia, and seizures. Potassium levels progressively decrease during the early weeks of bed rest as well. Immobility alone rarely causes serious electrolyte disturbances, aside from the high calcium levels seen in immobilization hypercalcemia (102). Nevertheless, patients with multiple medical illnesses may be seriously affected by even slight electrolyte abnormalities (Fig. 41-5).

Hormonal Disorders

A lack of physical activity can cause altered responsiveness of hormones and enzymes. Although they may be clinically undetected during early immobility, numerous changes have been demonstrated to occur in the endocrine system. Significant carbohydrate intolerance has been noted as early as the third day of immobility, and peripheral glucose uptake may decline 50% after 14 days (149,150). The duration of immobility correlates proportionally with the degree of carbohydrate intolerance. The glucose intolerance induced by bed rest can be improved by isotonic, but not isometric, exercises of the large muscle groups (151,152). The reason for this intolerance of immobility is not lack of insulin, but rather increased resistance to the action of insulin, resulting in hyperglycemia and hyperinsulinemia. Possible explanations include a reduction in number or affinity of insulin receptors or postreceptor changes in the target cells. Inactivity appears to cause a reduction in insulin-binding sites, predominantly on the muscle membrane (153,154).

A second major hormonal effect is an increase in the serum parathyroid hormone, which is related to hypercalcemia from immobility, although its precise mechanism is unknown (155). Tri-iodothyronine (T3) blood levels are also elevated during immobility (156). In addition, alterations have been reported in androgen levels and spermatogenesis, in growth hormone response to hypoglycemia, in levels of adrenocorticotropic hormone, and in catecholamine secretion from the sympathomedullary system (157,158). Measurements of serum corticosteroid levels during bed rest have been inconclusive. Although the excretion of urinary cortisol is increased, the adrenal gland response to the stimulus of the adrenocorticotropic hormone is reduced after prolonged bed rest. Studies of bed rest for periods of 1 month or more have found that adrenocorticotropic hormone levels were three times higher than baseline and required about 20 days of physical activity to return to normal (158). In contrast, prolonged exercise has been shown to increase plasma hydrocortisone levels and decrease plasma norepinephrine levels. Total cholesterol levels are also increased during immobility (159).

THE NERVOUS SYSTEM AND IMMOBILITY

Sensory deprivation is a silent hazard of prolonged bed rest. Healthy subjects placed on strict bed confinement for 3 hours and required to wear gloves, goggles, and earplugs to reduce sensory input experienced hallucinations and disorientation. During prolonged bed rest, the exposure to social and chronological cues, such as time of day and movement through space, is reduced (160,161). Social isolation alone with preserved mobility can cause emotional lability and anxiety but usually does not cause any intellectual alterations. However, prolonged bed rest and social isolation together produce much greater alterations in mental concentration, orientation to space and time, and other intellectual functions. Restlessness, anxiety, decreased pain tolerance, irritability, hostility, insomnia, and depression may occur during 2 weeks of recumbency and social isolation. Furthermore, judgment, problem solving and learning ability, psychomotor skills, and memory all may be impaired. Perceptual impairment can be altered even after only 7 days of immobility (162,163).

Lack of concentration and motivation, depression, and reduced psychomotor skills may drastically affect the patient's ability to achieve the highest possible level of functioning and independence. These behavioral effects of immobility may result in a lack of motivation and diminish the patient's ability to attain optimal healing and restoration of function. Balance and coordination also are impaired after prolonged immobility, and this effect appears to be due to altered neural control rather than muscle weakness (164,165).

An important strategy in the prevention and treatment of these complications is to apply appropriate physical and psychosocial stimulation early in the course of illness. Options for the treatment of these effects include group therapy sessions, attention to socialization and avocational pursuits during evenings and weekends, and encouragement of family interaction.

CONCLUSIONS

In 1862, the English surgeon John Hilton advocated bed rest as a basic physiologic approach in the treatment of human illnesses. Since that time, bed rest has often been used indiscriminately in the treatment of acute and chronic illnesses. The complications of prolonged bed rest have been increasingly recognized and reported since the mid-1940s. After World War II, clinical investigators, particularly Deitrick and colleagues in 1948 (4), have shown that prolonged bed rest may cause multiple adverse effects in a number of organs and systems. During the 1960s, studies on astronauts greatly advanced our knowledge of the deleterious effects of bed rest and weightlessness, and clinicians are now much more aware of a wide range of adverse effects associated with prolonged bed rest and immobility.

A new era of advocating exercise and cardiovascular conditioning has begun. Studies have indicated that prolonged bed rest and sedentary life-styles have negative effects on human body functioning. These effects are magnified in persons with neurologic disease or in the elderly. The principles advocated by rehabilitation medicine have contributed significantly to the current philosophy on the use and misuse of immobility.

REFERENCES

1. Harper CM, Lyles YM. Physiology and complications of bed rest. *J Am Geriatr Soc* 1988; 36:1047–1054.
2. Downey RJ, Weissman. Physiological changes associated with bed rest and major body injury. In: *Physiological basis of rehabilitation medicine,* 2nd ed. Cambridge, MA: Butterworth-Heinemann, 1994; 448–479.
3. Spencer WA, Vallbona C, Carter RE. Physiologic concepts of immobilization. *Arch Phys Med Rehabil* 1965; 46:89–100.
4. Deitrick JE, Whedon GD, Shorr E. Effects of immobilization upon various metabolic and physiologic functions of normal men. *Am J Med* 1948; 4:3–32.
5. Kottke FJ. The effects of limitation of activity upon the human body. *JAMA* 1966; 196:117–122
6. Hoenig HM, Rubenstein LZ. Hospital-associated deconditioning and dysfunction. *J Am Geriatr Soc* 1991; 39:220–222.
7. Clark LP, Dion DM, Barker WH. Taking to bed: rapid functional decline in an independently mobile older population living in an intermediate-care facility. *J Am Geriatr Soc* 1990; 38:967–972.
8. Booth FW. Effects of limb immobilization in skeletal muscle. *J Appl Physiol* 1982; 52:1113–1118.
9. Booth FW, Gollnick PD. Effects of disuse on the structure and function of skeletal muscle. *Med Sci Sports Exerc* 1983; 15:415–420.
10. Nicks DK, Beneke WM, Key RM, et al. Muscle fibre size and number following immobilization atrophy. *J Anat* 1989; 163:1–5.
11. Eichelberger L, Roma M, Moulder PV. Effects of immobilization on the histochemical characterization of skeletal muscle. *J Appl Physiol* 1958; 12:42.
12. Spector SA. Effects of elimination of activity on contractile and histochemical properties of rat soleus muscle. *J Neurosci* 1985; 5: 2177–2188.
13. Haggmark T, Eriksson E, Lansson E. Muscle fiber type changes in human skeletal muscle after injuries and immobilization. *J Orthop* 1986; 9:181–185.
14. Haggmark T. A study of morphologic and enzymatic properties of skeletal muscles after injuries and immobilization in man [Thesis]. Stockholm, Sweden: Karolinska Institute, 1978.
15. Henriksson R, Reitman JS. Time course of changes in human skeletal muscle succinate dehydrogenase and cytochrome oxidase activities and maximal uptake with physical activity and inactivity. *Acta Physiol Scand* 1977; 99:91–97.
16. Ward GR, MacDougall ID, Sutton IR, et al. Activation of human pyruvate dehydrogenase with activity and immobilization. *Clin Sci* 1986; 70:207–210.
17. Jansson E, Sylven C, Arvidsson I, et al. Increase in myoglobin content and decrease in oxidative enzyme activities by leg muscle immobilization in man. *Acta Physiol Scand* 1988; 132:515–517.
18. Herbison GJ, Jaweed MM, Ditunno JF. Muscle fiber atrophy after cast immobilization in the rat. *Arch Phys Med Rehabil* 1978; 59: 301–305.
19. Appell HJ. Muscular atrophy following immobilization: a review. *Sports Med* 1990; 10:42–58.
20. Mack PB, Montgomery KB. Study of nitrogen balance and creatine and creatinine excretion during recumbency and ambulation of five young adult human males. *Aerospace Med* 1973; 44:739–746.
21. Graham SC, Roland BS, Roy R, et al. Exercise effects on the size and metabolic properties of soleus fibers in hindlimb-suspended rats. *Aviat Space Environ Med* 1989; 60:226–234.
22. Sandler H, Vernikas J, et al. Effects of inactivity on muscle. In: Sandler H, Vernikas J, eds. *Inactivity, physiological effects.* San Diego, CA: Academic, 1986; 77–97.
23. Berg HE, Dudley GA, Haggmark T, et al. Effects: effects of lower limb unloading on skeletal muscle mass and functions in humans. *J Appl Physiol* 1991; 70:1882–1885.

24. Pestronk A, Drachmann B, Griffin IW. Effect of muscle disuse on acetylcholine receptors. *Nature* 1976; 260:352–353.
25. Booth FW, Gollnick PD. Effects of disuse on the structure and function of skeletal muscle. *Med Sci Sports Exerc* 1983; 15:415–420.
26. Ashmore CR, Summers PJ. Stretch-induced growth of chicken muscles: myofibrillar proliferation. *Am J Physiol* 1981:241:C93–97.
27. Wills CA, Caiozzo VL, Yasukawa DI, et al. Effects of immobilization on human skeletal muscle. *Orthop Rev* 1982; 11:57–64.
28. Stuart CA, Shangraw RE, Peters EJ, et al. Effect of dietary protein on bed-rest-related changes in whole-body-protein synthesis. *Am J Clin Nutr* 1990; 52:509–514.
29. Zorbas YG, Andreyev VG, Popescu LB. Fluid-electrolyte metabolism and renal function in men under hypokinesia and physical exercise. *Int Urol Nephrol* 1988; 20:215–223.
30. Goldspink DF. The influence of immobilization and stretch on protein turnover in rat skeletal muscle. *J Physiol* 1977; 264:267–282.
31. Serra G, Tugnoli V, Eleopra R, et al. Neurophysiological evaluation of the muscular hypotrophy after immobilization. *Electromyogr Clin Neurophysiol* 1989; 29:29–31.
32. Duchateau J, Hainaut K. Electrical and mechanical changes in immobilized human muscle. *J Appl Physiol* 1987; 62:2168–2173.
33. Duchateau J, Hainaut K. Effects of immobilization on contractile properties, recruitment and firing rates of human motor units. *J Physiol* 1990; 422:55–65.
34. Baker JH, Matsumoto DE. Adaptation of skeletal muscle to immobilization in a shortened position. *Muscle Nerve* 1988; 11:231–244.
35. Jozsa L, Kannus P, Thoring I, et al. The effect of tenotomy and immobilization on intramuscular connective tissue. *J Bone Joint Surg [Br]* 1990; 72:293–297.
36. Michelsson JE, Aho HJ, Kalimo H, et al. Severe degeneration of rabbit vastus intermedius muscle immobilized in shortened position. *APMIS* 1990; 98:336–344.
37. Williams PE. Use of intermittent stretch in the prevention of serial sarcomere loss in immobilized muscle. *Ann Rheum Dis* 1990; 49: 316–317.
38. Spector SA, Simard CP, Fournier SM, et al. Architectural alterations of rat hind limb skeletal muscle immobilized at different lengths. *Exp Neurol* 1982; 76:94–110.
39. Kottke FJ, Pauley DL, Potka RA. The rationale for prolonged stretching for correction for shortening of connective tissue. *Arch Phys Med* Rehabil 1966; 47:345–352.
40. Holly RG. Barnett CR, Ashmore CR, et al. Stretch-induced growth in chicken wing muscles: a new model of stretch hypertrophy. *Am J Physiol* 1980; 238:C62–71.
41. Robinson GA, Enoka RM, Stuart DG. Immobilization-induced changes in motor unit force and fatigability in the cat. *Muscle Nerve* 1991; 14:563–573.
42. Rutherford OM, Jones DA, Round JM. Long-lasting unilateral muscle wasting and weakness following injury and immobilization. *Scand J Rehabil Med* 1990; 22:33–37.
43. Muller EA. Influence of training and of inactivity on muscle strength. *Arch Phys Med Rehabil* 1970; 51:449–462.
44. Gould N, Donnermeyer D, Pope M, Ashikaga T. Transcutaneous muscle stimulation as a method to retard disuse atrophy. *Clin Orthop* 1982; 164:215–220.
45. Davies CTM, Rutherford IC, Thomas DO. Electrically evoked contractions of the triceps surae during and following 21 days of voluntary leg immobilization. *Eur J Appl Physiol* 1987; 56:306–312.
46. Buckley DC, Kudsk KA, Rose B, et al. Transcutaneous muscle stimulation promotes muscle growth in immobilized patients. *J Parenter Enter Nutr* 1987; 11:547–551.
47. Saltin B, Blomquist G, Mitchell JA, et al. Response to exercise after bed rest and after training: a longitudinal study of adaptive changes in oxygen transport and body composition. *Circulation* 1968; 38(suppl 7):1–55.
48. Amiel D, Woo SL-Y, Harwood FL, et al. The effect of immobilization of collagen turnover in connective tissue: a biochemical-biomechanical correlation. *Acta Orthop Scand* 1982; 53:325–332.
49. Garcia-Bunuel L, Garcia-Bunuel VM. Connective tissue metabolism in normal and atrophic skeletal muscle. *J Neurol Sci* 1980; 47:69–77.
50. Stolov WC, Fry LR, Riddel WM, Weilepp TG Jr. Adhesive forces between muscle fibers and connective tissue in normal and denervated rat skeletal muscle. *Arch Phys Med Rehabil* 1974; 154:208–213.
51. Selikson S, Damus K, Hamerman D. Risk factors associated with immobility. *J Am Geriatr Soc* 1988; 36:707–712.
52. Campbell RR, Hawkins SJ, Maddison PJ, et al. Limited joint mobility in diabetes mellitus. *Ann Rheum Dis* 1985; 44:93–97.
53. Alberts B, Bray D, Lewis J, Raff M, Roberts K, Watson JD. *Molecular biology of the cell.* New York: Garland, 1983; 673–715.
54. Bornstein P, Byers PH. Collagen metabolism. Current concepts (pamphlet). Kalamazoo, MI: Upjohn, 1980.
55. Karpakka J, Vaananen K, Orava S, et al. The effects of preimmobilization training and immobilization on collagen synthesis in rat skeletal muscle. *Int J Sports Med* 1990; 11:484–488.
56. Harper J, Amiel D, Harper E. Collagenases from periarticular ligaments and tendon: enzyme levels during the development of joint contracture. *Matrix* 1989; 9:200–205.
57. Karpakka J, Vaananen K, Vinanen P, et al. The effects of remobilization and exercise on collagen biosynthesis in rat tendon. *Acta Physiol Scand* 1990; 139:139–145.
58. Saamanen AM, Tammi M, Jurvelin J, et al. Proteoglycan alterations following immobilization and remobilization in the articular cartilage of young canine knee (stifle) joint. *J Orthop Res* 1990; 8:863–873.
59. Akeson WH, Garfin S, Amiel D, et al. Para-articular connective tissue in osteoarthritis. *Semin Arthritis Rheum* 1989; 18(suppl 2):41–50.
60. Partridge REH, Duthie TTR. Controlled trial of the effect of complete immobilization of the joints in RA. *Ann Rheum Dis* 1963; 22:91–99.
61. Reynolds CA, Cummings GS, Andrews PD. Effect of non-traumatic immobilization on ankle dorsiflexion stiffness in rats. *J Orthop Sports Phys Ther* 1996; 23:27–33.
62. Johnson EW. Pathokinesiology of Duchenne muscular dystrophy: implications for management. *Arch Phys Med Rehabil* 1977; 54:4–7.
63. Stuart CA, Shangraw RE, Prince MJ, et al. Bed-rest-induced resistance occurs primarily in muscle. *Metabolism* 1988; 37:802–806.
64. Chappard D, Alexandre C, Palle S, et al. Effects of a bisphosphonate (1-hydroxy ethylidene-1, 1 bisphosphonic acid) on osteoclast number during prolonged bed rest in healthy humans. *Metabolism* 1989; 38: 822–825.
65. Van Lent PLEM, Wilms FHA, Van Den Berg WB. Interaction of polymorphonuclear leucocytes with patellar cartilage of immobilized arthritic joints: a scanning electron microscopic study. *Ann Rheum Dis* 1989; 48:832–837.
66. Van Lent PLEM, van den Bersselaar L, van de Putte LBA, et al. Immobilization aggravates cartilage damage during antigen-induced arthritis in mice. *Am J Pathol* 1990; 136:1407–1416.
67. Fam AG, Schumacher HR Jr, Clayburne G. et al. Effect of joint motion on experimental calcium pyrophosphate dihydrate crystal induced arthritis. *J Rheumatol* 1990; 17:644–655.
68. Akeson WH, Amiel D, Ing D, et al. Effects of immobilization on joints. *Clin Orthop* 1987; 219:28–37.
69. Evans EB, Eggers GWN, Butler JK, Blumel J. Experimental immobilization and remobilization of rat knee joints. *J Bone Joint Surg [Am]* 1960; 42:737–758.
70. Behrens F, Krah EL, Oegema TR Jr. Biochemical changes in articular cartilage after joint immobilization by casting or external fixation. *J Orthop Res* 1989; 7:335–343.
71. Finsterbush A, Friedman B. Early changes in immobilized rabbit's knee joint. *Clin Orthop Rel Res* 1973; 92:305–319.
72. Akeson WH, Amiel D, Woo SL-Y. Immobility effects on synovial joints: the pathomechanics of joint contracture. *Biorheology* 1980; 17: 95–110.
73. Amiel D, Frey C, Woo SL-Y, et al. Value of hyaluronic acid in the prevention of contracture formation. *Clin Orthop* 1985; 196:306–311.
74. Noyes FR. Functional properties of knee ligaments and alterations induced by immobilization: a correlative biomechanical and histological study in primates. *Clin Orthop* 1977; 123:210–242.
75. Dahner DE, Sky KE, Muller PR. A study of the mechanisms influencing ligament growth. *J Orthop Res* 1989; 12:1569–1572.
76. Newton PO, Woo SL-Y, Kitabayashi LR, et al. Ultrastructural changes in knee ligaments following immobilization. *Matrix* 1990; 10: 314–319.
77. Klein L, Heiple KG, Torzilli PA, et al. Prevention of ligament and meniscus atrophy by active joint motion in a non-weightbearing model. *J Orthop Res* 1989; 7:80–85.
78. Inoue M, Woo SL-Y, Gomez MA, et al. Effects of surgical treatment and immobilization on the healing of the medial collateral ligament: a

long-term multidisciplinary study. *Connect Tissue Res* 1990; 25: 13–26.
79. Cann CE, Genant HK, Young DR. Comparison of vertebral and peripheral mineral losses in disuse osteoporosis in monkey. *Radiology* 1980; 134:525–559.
80. Lips P, van Ginkel FC, Netelenbos JC, et al. Lower mobility and markers of bone resorption in the elderly. *Bone Mineral* 1990; 9: 49–57.
81. Schneider VS, McDonald J. Skeletal calcium homeostasis and counter measures to prevent disuse osteoporosis. *Calcif Tissue Int* 1984; 36: 151–154.
82. Deyo RA, Diehl AK, Rosenthal M. How many days of bed rest for acute low back pain? *N Engl J Med* 1986; 315:1064–1092.
83. Sinaki M, Offord KP. Physical activity in post-menopausal women: effect on back muscle strength and bone mineral density of the spine. *Arch Phys Med Rehabil* 1988; 69:277–280.
84. Booth BJ, Doyle M, Montgomery J. Serial casting for the management of spasticity in the head-injured adult. *Phys Ther* 1983; 63:1960–1966.
85. Salter RB, Bell RS, Keeley FW. The protective effect of continuous passive motion on living articular cartilage in acute septic arthritis: an experimental investigation in the rabbit. *Clin Orthop* 1981; 159: 223–247.
86. Nene AV, Evans GA, Patrick JH. Simultaneous multiple operations for spastic diplegia. Outcome and functional assessment of walking in 18 patients. *J Bone Joint Surg* 1993; 75:488–494.
87. Delp SL, Statler K, Carroll NC. Preserving planter flexion strength after surgical treatment for contracture of the triceps surae: a computer simulation study. *J Orthop Res* 1995; 13:96–104.
88. Moreno-Alvarez MJ, Espad G, Maldonado-Cocco JA, Gagliardi SA. Longterm followup of hip and knee soft tissue release in juvenile chronic arthritis. *J Rheumatol* 1992; 19:1608–1610.
89. Saltin B, Blomqvist G, Mitchell JH, et al. Response to exercise after bed rest and after training. *Circulation* 1968; 38(suppl VII):1–78.
90. Van-Loon JJ, Bervoets DJ, Burger EH, et al. Decreased mineralization and increased calcium release in isolated fetal mouse long bones under near weightlessness. *J Bone Miner Res* 1995; 10:550–557.
91. Nilsson BE, Westlin NE. Bone density in athletes. *Clin Orthop* 1971; 77:179–182.
92. Marcus R. Relationship of age-related decreases in muscle mass and strength to skeletal status [Review]. *J Gerontol* 1995; 50:86–87.
93. Gross TS, Rubin CT. Uniformity of resorptive bone loss induced by disease. *J Orthop Res* 1995; 13:708–714.
94. Leblanc AD, Schneider VS, Evans HJ. Bone mineral loss and recovery after 17 weeks of bed rest. *J Bone Miner Res* 1990; 5:843–850.
95. Avioli LV. Hormonal alterations and osteoporotic syndromes. *J Bone Miner Res* 1993; 2(suppl):511–514.
96. Perloff JJ, McDermott MT, Perloff KG, et al. Reduced bone mineral content is a risk factor for hip fractures. *Orthop Rev* 1991; 20: 690–698.
97. Uebelhart D, Demiaux-Domenech G, Roth M, Chantraine A. Bone metabolism in spinal cord injured individuals and in others who have prolonged immobilization. A review. *Paraplegia* 1995; 33:669–673.
98. Kannus P, Leppala J, Lehto M, Sievanen H, Heinonen A, Jarvinen M. A rotator cuff rupture produces permanent osteoporosis in the affected extremity, but not in those with whom shoulder function has returned to normal. *J Bone Miner Res* 1995; 10:1263–1271.
99. Houde JP, Schulz LA, Morgan WJ, et al. Bone mineral density changes in the forearm after immobilization. *Clin Orthop* 1995; 317: 199–205.
100. Bourrin S, Palle S, Gentry C, Alexandre C. Physical exercise during remobilization restores a normal bone trabecular network after tail suspension-induced osteopenia in young rats. *J Bone Miner Res* 1995; 10:820–828.
101. Andrews PL, Rosenberg AR. Renal consequences of immobilization in children with fractured femurs. *Acta Paediatr Scand* 1990; 79: 311–315.
102. Gallacher SJ, Ralston SH, Dryburgh FJ, et al. Immobilization related hypercalcemia: a possible novel mechanism and response to pamidronate. *Postgrad Med J* 1990; 66:918–922.
103. Fleisch H. Bisphosphonates in osteoporosis: an introduction. *Osteoporosis Int* 1993; 3(suppl):3–5.
104. Minaire P. Immobilization osteoporosis: a review. *Clin Rheumatol* 1989; 8(suppl 2):95–103.
105. Singer FR, Minoofar PN. Bisphosphonates in the treatment of disorders of mineral metabolism. *Adv Endocrinol Metal* 1995; 6:259–288.
106. Chappard D, Minaire P, Privat C, et al. Effects of tiludronate on bone loss in paraplegic patients. *J Bone Miner Res* 1995; 10:112–118.
107. Tsakalakos N, Magiasis B, Tsekoura M, Lyritis G. The effect of short-term calcitonin administration on biochemical bone markers in patients with acute immobilization following hip fracture. *Osteoporosis Int* 1993; 3:337–340.
108. Taylor HL, Henschel A, Brozek J, et al. Effects of bedrest on cardiovascular function and work performance. *J Appl Physiol* 1949; 2: 223–235.
109. Taylor HL. The effects of rest in bed and of exercise on cardiovascular function. *Circulation* 1968; 38:1016–1017.
110. Convertino VA, Doerr DF, Eckberg DL, et al. Carotid baroreflex response following 30 days exposure to simulated microgravity. *Physiologist* 1989; 32(suppl):67–68.
111. Chobanian AV, Lillie RD, Tercyak A, Blevins P. The metabolic and hemodynamic effects of prolonged bed rest in normal subjects. *Circulation* 1974; 49:551–559.
112. Demida BF, Machinski I. Use of rehabilitation measures for restoration of human physical work capacity after the prolonged limitation of motor activity. *Kosm Biol Aviakosm Med* 1979; 13:74–75.
113. Svanberg L. Influence of posture on the lung volumes ventilation and circulation in normals. *Scand J Clin Lab Invest* 1957; (suppl 25): 1–195.
114. West JB. *Ventilation–blood flow and gas exchange,* 3rd ed. Philadelphia: JB Lippincott, 1977.
115. Craig DB, Wahba WM, Don HF. Airway closure and lung volume in surgical positions. *Can Anaesth Soc J* 1971; 18:92–99.
116. Van Beaumont W, Greenleaf JE, Juhos L. Disproportional changes in hematocrit, plasma volume, and proteins during exercise and bed rest. *J Appl Physiol* 1972; 33:55–61.
117. Greenleaf JE, Van Beaumont W, Brock PJ, Morse JT, Manqseth GR. Plasma volume and electrolyte shifts with heavy exercise in sitting and supine positions. *Am J Physiol* 1979; 236:206–214.
118. Holmgren A, Mossfeldt F, Sjostrand T, Strom G. Effect of training on work capacity, total hemoglobin, blood volume, heart volume and pulse rate in recumbent and upright positions. *Acta Physiol Scand* 1960; 50:73–83.
119. Greenleaf JE, Young HL, Bernauer EM, et al. *Effects of isometric and isotonic exercise on body water compartments during 14 days' bed rest.* Aerospace Medical Association Preprints. Washington, D.C.: Aerospace Medical Association, 1973.
120. Greenleaf JE, Bernauer EM, Young HL, et al. Fluid and electrolyte shifts during bed rest with isometric and isotonic exercise. *J Appl Physiol* 1977; 42:59–66.
121. Zorbas YG, Merkov AB, Nobahar AN. Nutritional status of men under hypokinesia. *J Environ Pathol Toxicol Oncol* 1989; 9:333–342.
122. Greenleaf JE, Wade CE, Leftheriotis G. Orthostatic responses following 30-day bed rest deconditioning with isotonic and isokinetic exercise training. *Aviat Space Environ Med* 1989; 60:537–542.
123. Melada GA, Goldman RH, Luetscher JA, et al. Hemodynamics, renal function, plasma renin and aldosterone in man after 5 to 14 days of bed rest. *Aviat Space Environ Med* 1975; 46:1049–1055.
124. Hyatt KH, Kamenetsky LG, Smith WM. Extravascular dehydration as an etiologic factor in post-recumbency orthostatism. *Aerospace Med* 1969; 40:644–650.
125. Pequinot JM, Guel A, Gauguelin G, et al. Epinephrine, norepinephrine and dopamine during a 4-day head-down bed rest. *J Appl Physiol* 1985; 58:157–163.
126. Stremel RW, Convetino VA, Bernauer EM, Greenleaf JE. Cardiorespiratory deconditioning with static and dynamic leg exercise during bed rest. *J Appl Physiol* 1976; 41:905–909.
127. Lamb LE, Stevens PM, Johnson RL. Hypokinesia secondary to chair rest from 4 to 10 days. *Aerospace Med* 1965; 36:755–763.
128. Robinson BF, Ebstein SE, Beiser GD, at al. Control of heart rate by automatic system. Studies in man on the interrelation between baroreceptor mechanism and exercises. *Circ Res* 1966; 19:400–411.
129. Fareeduddin K, Abelmann WH. Impaired orthostatic tolerance after bed rest in patients with myocardial infarction. *N Engl J Med* 1969; 280:345–350.
130. Vallbona C, Spencer WA, Cardus D, Dale JW. Control of orthostatic hypotension in quadriplegic patients with the use of a pressure suit. *Arch Phys Med Rehabil* 1963; 44:7–18.

131. Vogt FB. Effect of intermittent leg cuff inflation and intermittent exercise on the tilt table response after ten days' bed recumbency. *Aerospace Med* 1966; 37:943–947
132. Robinson BF, Epstein SE, Beiser GD, et al. Control of heart rate by the autonomic system. Studies in man on the interrelation between baroreceptor mechanism and exercises. *Circ Res* 1966; 19:400–411.
133. Gibbs NM. Venous thrombosis of the lower limbs with particular reference to bed rest. *Br J Surg* 1957; 191:209–235.
134. Kudsk KA, Fabian TC, Baum S, et al. Silent deep vein thrombosis in immobilized multiple trauma patients. *Am J Surg* 1989; 158:515–519.
135. Warlow C, Ogston D, Douglas AS. Deep venous thrombosis of the legs after strokes: Part I. incidence and predisposing factors. Part II. Natural history. *Br Med J* 1976; 1:1178–1183.
136. Miyamoto AT, Miller LS. Pulmonary embolism in stroke: prevention by early heparinization of venous thrombosis detected by iodine-125 fibrinogen leg scans. *Arch Phys Med Rehabil* 1980; 61:584–587.
137. Malone PC, Hamer JD, Silver IA. Oxygen tension in venous valve pockets. *Thromb Haemost* 1979; 42:230.
138. Hume M, Sevitt S, Thomas LP. *Venous thrombosis and pulmonary embolism.* Cambridge, MA: Harvard University Press, 1977.
139. Pini M, Pattacini C, Quintaralla R, et al. Subcutaneous vs. intravenous heparin in the treatment of deep venous thrombosis: a randomized clinical trial. *Thromb Haemost* 1990; 64:222–226.
140. Hirsh I. Heparin. *N Engl J Med* 1991.324:1565–1574.
141. Hull RD, Raskob GE, Rosenbloom D, et al. Heparin for 5 days as compared with 10 days in the initial treatment of proximal venous thrombosis. *N Engl J Med* 1990; 322:1260–1264.
142. Anderson RL, Lefever FR, Francis WR, et al. Urinary and bladder responses to immobilization in male rats. *Food Chem Toxicol* 1990; 28:543–545.
143. Leadbetter WF, Engster HE. Problems of renal lithiasis in convalescent patients. *J Urol* 1957; 53:269.
144. Dooley CP, Schlossmacher B, Valenzuela JE. Modulation of esophageal peristalsis by alterations of body position: effect of bolus viscosity. *Dig Dis Sci* 1989; 34:1662–1667.
145. Moore JG, Datz FL, Christin PE, et al. Effect of body posture on radionuclide measurements of gastric emptying. *Dig Dis Sci* 1988; 33:1592–1595.
146. Evans DF, Foster GE, Harcastle JD. Does exercise affect small bowel motility in man. *Gut* 1989; 10–12.
147. Moses FM. The effect of exercise on gastrointestinal tract. *Sports Med* 1990; 9:159–172.
148. Krebs JM, Schneider VS, Evans H, et al. Energy absorption, lean body mass, and total body fat changes during 5 weeks of continuous bed rest. *Aviat Space Environ Med* 1990; 61:314–318.
149. Stuart CA, Shangraw RE, Prince MJ, Peters EJ, Wolfe RR. Bed rest-induced insulin resistance occurs primarily in muscle. *Metabolism* 1988; 37:802–806.
150. Altman DF, Baker SD, McCally M, et al. Carbohydrate and lipid metabolism in man during prolonged bed rest. *Clin Res* 1969; 17:543.
151. Lipman RL, Schnure Jl, Bradley EM, Lecocq FR. Impairment of peripheral glucose utilization in normal subjects by prolonged bed rest. *J Lab Clin Med* 1970; 76:221–230.
152. Dolkas CB, Greenleaf JE. Insulin and glucose responses during bed rest with isotonic and isometric exercise. *J Appl Physiol* 1977; 43: 1033–1038.
153. Mikines KJ, Dela F, Tronier B, Galbo H. Effect of 7 days of bed rest on dose-response relation between plasma glucose and insulin secretion. *Am J Physiol* 1989; 257:43–48.
154. Seider MJ, Nicholson WF, Booth FW. Insulin resistance for glucose metabolism in disused skeletal muscle of mice. *Am J Physiol* 1982; 242:E12–18.
155. Lerman S, Canterbury JM, Reiss E. Parathyroid hormone and the hypercalcemia of immobilization. *J Clin Endocrinol Metab* 1977; 45: 425–488.
156. Balsam A, Leppo LE. Assessment of the degradation of thyroid hormones in man during bed rest. *J Appl Physiol* 1975; 38:216–219.
157. Cockett AT, Elbadawi A, Zemjanis R. The effects of immobilization on spermatogenesis in subhuman primates. *Fertil Steril* 1970; 21: 610–614.
158. Varnikos-Danellis J, Winget CM, Leach CS. *Circadian endocrine and metabolic effects of prolonged bed rest: two 56-day bed rest studies.* NASA Technical Bulletin, No. Tm V-3051. Washington, D.C.: United States National Aeronautic and Space Administration, 1974.
159. Takayama H, Tomiyama M, Managawa A, et al. The effect of physical exercise and prolonged bed rest on carbohydrate, lipid and amino acid metabolism. *Jpn J Clin Pathol* 1974; 22(suppl):126–136.
160. Banks R, Cappon D. Effects of reduced sensory input on time perception. *Percept Motor Skills* 1962; 14:74.
161. Ryback RS, Lewis OF, Lessard CS. Psychobiologic effects of prolonged bed rest (weightlessness) in young healthy volunteers (study 11). *Aerospace Med* 1971; 42:529–535.
162. Downs FS. Bed rest and sensory disturbances. *Am J Nurs* 1974; 74: 434–438.
163. Smith MJ. Changes in judgment of duration with different patterns of auditory information for individuals confined to bed. *Nurs Res* 1975; 24:93–98.
164. Haines RF. Effect of bed rest and exercise on body balance. *J Appl Physiol* 1974; 36:323–327.
165. Trimble RW, Lessard CS. *Performance decrement as a function of seven days of bed rest.* USAF School of Aerospace Medicine Technical Report 70-56. Alexandria, VA: Aerospace Medical Association, 1970.

Rehabilitation Medicine: Principles and Practice, Third Edition,
edited by Joel A. DeLisa and Bruce M. Gans.
Lippincott–Raven Publishers, Philadelphia © 1998.

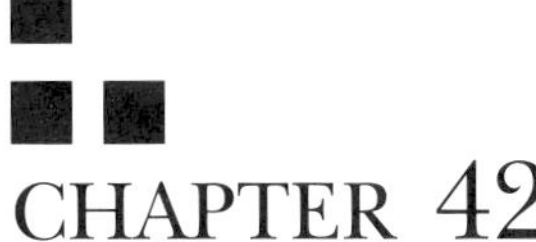

CHAPTER 42

Parkinson's Disease and Other Movement Disorders

Sudesh S. Jain and Gerard E. Francisco

Movement disorders are a group of diseases that are usually classified as extrapyramidal and are associated with involuntary movements or abnormalities of skeletal muscle tone, posture, or both. They are thought to be predominantly caused by lesions within the basal ganglia, are recognized by clinical observation without the need for laboratory testing, are often progressive, and are difficult to treat. Although movement disorders are not frequently encountered in the regular physical medicine and rehabilitation practice, physiatrists should be able to recognize them and appreciate their impact on a patient's health and functional status.

ANATOMY, PHYSIOLOGY, AND NEUROPHARMACOLOGY

Normal voluntary motor control depends on an intricately balanced relationship between cortical, subcortical (including the extrapyramidal system and cerebellum), spinal, and peripheral mechanisms. A basic understanding of the extrapyramidal system provides the basis for the management of patients with movement disorders.

The extrapyramidal system comprises those motor centers that are not part of the pyramidal cortex and tract. These centers include the following: basal ganglia, including the caudate, putamen, and globus pallidus (the amygdala and claustrum are functionally part of the limbic system); subthalamic nucleus; substantia nigra; red nucleus; and the reticular formation of the upper brain stem. The caudate and putamen are referred to as the corpus striatum or neostriatum, and the putamen and globus pallidus are referred to as the lenticular nucleus. The cerebellum is not considered part of the extrapyramidal system.

The anatomic features and connections within the basal ganglia and the cortex are extremely complex and are not completely understood. The reader is referred to neuroanatomy texts for more detail (1). A simplified version of the basal ganglia will be discussed and illustrated here (2) (Fig. 42-1).

Functionally, the basal ganglia can be divided into an afferent and an efferent portion. The corpus striatum (afferent limb of the basal ganglia) receives excitatory input from the cortex and thalamus and dopaminergic input from the substantia nigra. The internal region of the globus pallidus and pars reticularis of the substantia nigra make up the efferent limb of the basal ganglia. Neurons from the various basal ganglia nuclei contribute excitatory and inhibitory impulses. The sum of these impulses is sent to the thalamus via the efferent limb to influence the cortex. A decrease in the pallidothalamic and nigrothalamic discharge will disinhibit the thalamus, causing augmentation of motor movements (3). With modification by the cerebellum, smooth motor control is then coordinated. A direct pathway from the basal ganglia to the alpha or gamma neurons does not exist (4). Dopamine (DA) is believed to be the major neurotransmitter within the nigrostriatal pathway (5).

The function of the basal ganglia in movement has recently become better understood. The cerebral cortex plans the movement, and the basal ganglia, via their connections with the thalamus and cortex, are involved in influencing the direction, course, and amplitude of these movements. Thus, this system provides the postural support necessary

S. S. Jain: Department of Physical Medicine and Rehabilitation, University of Medicine and Dentistry of New Jersey, New Jersey Medical School; Newark, New Jersey 07103; and Department of Clinical Physical Medicine and Rehabilitation, St. Barnabas Medical Center, Livingston, New Jersey 07039.

G. E. Francisco: Brain Injury Program, The Institute for Rehabilitation and Research, Houston, Texas 77030.

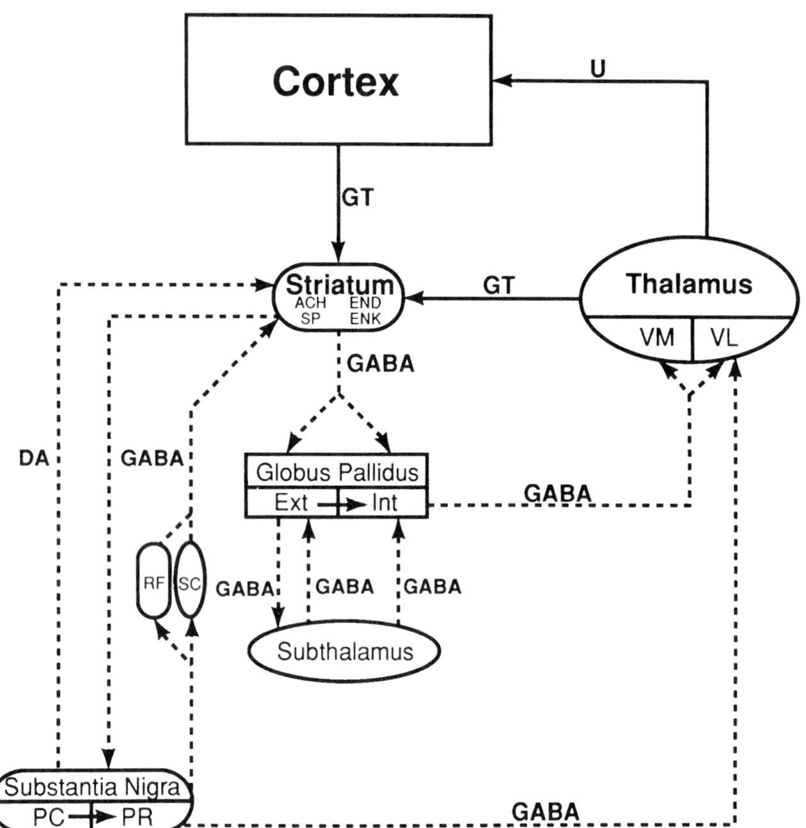

FIG. 42-1. Simplified schematic diagram of the major neuronal connections of the basal ganglia. (—, excitation; --, inhibitory; *ACH*, acetylcholine; *END*, endorphin; *ENK*, enkephalin; *Ext*, external; *GABA*, gamma-aminobutyric acid; *GT*, glutamate; *Int*, internal; *PC*, pars compacta; *PR*, pars reticularis; *RF*, reticular formation; *SC*, superior colliculus; *SP*, substance P; Striatum, caudate and putamen; *U*, unknown; *VL*, ventrolateral; *VM*, ventromedian.)

for execution of voluntary movements and may be involved in the initiation of such movements (6–8).

Basal ganglia function is not solely for control of movement and posture. There is evidence that it may be involved in perceptual and cognitive functions as well (9). It has been suggested that the putamen is involved principally in motor activities and the caudate in more complex functions, including cognition (10,11). Therefore, the motor impairment in Parkinson's disease (PD) may be due to selective DA loss in the putamen, and the cognitive impairment may indicate loss of dopaminergic input to the caudate nucleus.

CLASSIFICATION OF MOVEMENT DISORDERS

Movement disorders can be divided into two clinical categories: those demonstrating a poverty of movement (i.e., hypokinesia) and those displaying excessive abnormal involuntary movements (i.e., hyperkinesia). Tremors may occur in association with either type.

PARKINSONISM

Parkinsonism is an example of hypokinetic disorder. It is one of the most commonly encountered movement disorders in physiatric practice and will be discussed in detail.

Parkinsonism can be divided into three categories (Table 42-1): primary or idiopathic, secondary or symptomatic, and Parkinson's plus.

Primary or Idiopathic Parkinson's Disease

Idiopathic Parkinson's disease (IPD) is a chronic, slowly progressive degenerative disorder of the central nervous system that was first described by James Parkinson in 1817 as paralysis agitans (12). It is characterized by the presence of a resting tremor, rigidity, akinesia, and postural instability (3). However, many other signs and symptoms may be present.

IPD is the most common form of the disease. It affects 1% of the population over 50 years of age in the United States (roughly 0.5 million patients), with an estimated incidence of 40,000 new cases per year (13). Men and women appear to be affected equally (12). Parkinsonism ranks behind cerebrovascular diseases and arthritis as the third most common chronic disease of late adulthood (13). Incidence and prevalence increase with age, with the peak onset between the sixth and eighth decades of life (14). Life expectancy is now near normal (14), but there is a twofold increase in the risk of death that is strongly related to falls due to gait disturbance (15). Common clinical signs and symptoms are noted in Table 42-2.

Tremor is the most common symptom, affecting approximately two thirds of patients with PD. DA depletion may

TABLE 42-1. *Classification of parkinsonism*

Primary or idiopathic Parkinson's disease
Secondary or symptomatic parkinsonism may be due to the following:
- DA antagonists and depletors
- Hemiatrophy–hemiparkinsonism
- Hydrocephalus–normal pressure hydrocephalus
- Hypoxia
- Postencephalitic infections
- Parathyroid dysfunction, metabolic
- Toxic: MPTP, cyanide, CO, Mn
- Trauma
- Tumor
- Vascular: multi-infarct state

Parkinson's plus syndrome: signs of parkinsonism along with other neurologic deficits
- Progressive supranuclear palsy
- Shy Drager syndrome (now called multi-system atrophy/syndrome)
- Cortical basal ganglionic degeneration
- Diffuse Lewy body disease
- Heredodegenerative disease
  - Huntington's disease
  - Wilson's disease
  - Hallervorden Spatz disease
  - Neuroacanthocytosis

CO, carbon monoxide; Mn, menganese; MPTP, 1-methyl-4-phenyl-1,2,3,6-tetrahydropyridine.

cause a loss of inhibitory input to the striatal cholinergic system, allowing excessive excitatory output and facilitating oscillatory loops in the thalamocortical system. Electromyogram (EMG) tracings show rhythmic alternating bursts in agonist and antagonist muscles (16).

Rigidity is an increase in muscle tone that is elicited during passive movement of limbs, neck, or trunk through the entire range of motion. The increased resistance to passive movement is equal in all directions and is usually manifested by a ratchety give during the movement. This cogwheel rigidity is due to underlying tremor even if there is no visible tremor (17).

Flexed posture is seen in patients with PD due to the dominance of the progravity flexor muscles with head bowed, chin toward the chest, kyphotic thorax, protracted shoulders, internally rotated arms with hands in front, and flexion of elbows, knees, and hips.

Bradykinesia refers to slowness of movement, whereas akinesia is the inability to move. Deformities of the hands include ulnar deviations, flexion of the metacarpophalangeal joints and extension of the interphalangeal joints (striatal hands). Inversion of the feet is apparent, and the big toe may be dorsiflexed (striatal toe). There may be lateral tilting of the trunk.

In PD, all aspects of movement are affected, including initiation, execution, and the ability to halt a movement once it has begun. In contrast to the almost unconscious way that

TABLE 42-2. *Clinical signs and symptoms of parkinsonism*

Symptoms	Clinical features
Positive phenomena	
Tremor	Most common symptom. Distal involvement frequency: 3.5 Hz. Suppressed by sleep and activity, increased by fatigue or stress. EMG: rhythmic alternating bursts in agonist and antagonist muscles.
Rigidity	Increase in muscle tone during passive limb movement equal through entire range of motion; increases if contralateral limb is engaged in volition.
Flexed posture	Dominance of progravity flexor muscles (bowed head, chin toward chest, kyphotic thorax, protracted shoulders, internally rotated arms, flexed elbows, knees, and hips).
Negative phenomena	
Bradykinesia	Slowness of movement, masked facies, decreased eye blinking, inability to move. Fatigue. EMG: delayed motor unit recruitment, pauses once recruited, inability to increase firing rate.
Loss of postural reflexes	Tendency to fall to the side (lateral pulsion) or backward (retropulsion); sitting en bloc (collapses in the chair when attempting to sit down)
Postural instability freezing phenomenon	Transient inability to perform a task
Other clinical features	
Fatigue, unexpected weight loss	
Striatal hand (ulnar hand deviation, metacarpophalangeal flexion, interphalangeal extension)	
Striatal toe (foot inversion, big toe dorsiflexion)	
Autonomic dysfunction: orthostatic hypotension, bladder and bowel dysfunction	
Dysfunction of cranial nerves III, VII, and IX; dysphagia; infrequent blinking; difficulty chewing	
Psychosis	
Depression	

EMG, electromyography; IP, interphalangeal; MCP, metacarpophalangeal.

normal persons use their limbs, the patient with PD must consciously force the limb to move.

Movements that do occur are usually slow. EMG studies in patients with PD have shown delays in motor unit recruitment, pauses once recruited, and an inability to increase the firing rate (18). This may necessitate a greater amount of excitatory input from the cortex before movement patterns can be activated. Bradykinesia accounts for many of the disabling characteristics of PD, including the expressionless face and loss of blinking, resulting in a staring expression. Other ocular problems besides reduced eye blinking include restriction of upward gaze, loss of convergence, blepharospasm (involuntary closure of eyelids), and blepharoclonus (fluttering of closed eyelids).

The patient seldom crosses his legs or adjusts body posture when seated in a chair and usually rises slowly to walk. Ambulation is characterized by a small-stepped, shuffling gait pattern with an absence of arm swing, with the patient leaning forward and taking increasingly faster steps to catch up (i.e., festinating gait) with his or her center of gravity.

Pronounced bradykinesia prevents a patient with PD from driving an automobile; foot movement from the accelerator to the brake pedal is too slow. Fatigue in PD may be due to bradykinesia and rigidity. Subtle signs of bradykinesia can be detected even in early parkinsonism if the examiner looks for slowness in shoulder shrugging, lack of gesturing, and decreased armswing. Advanced bradykinesia may interfere with activities of daily living (ADL). Bradykinetic or akinetic states may last seconds, minutes, or hours and are most evident at the onset of activities. Patients may show the ability to make rapid movements (e.g., catch a ball) when experiencing a surge of emotional energy, termed "kinesia paradoxica."

Loss of postural reflexes leads to a tendency to fall to the side (i.e., lateral pulsion) or backward (i.e., retropulsion), because the patient is unable to correct his imbalance through appropriate arm or leg movements. As postural reflexes fail, the patient collapses in the chair when attempting to sit down (sitting en bloc).

Postural instability is probably the least specific and most disabling of all symptoms (13). The gait and postural problems are a result of a combination of bradykinesia, rigidity, loss of anticipatory proprioceptive reflexes and protective reactions to a fall, gait and axial apraxia, ataxia, vestibular dysfunction, and orthostatic hypotension.

Freezing phenomenon (motor block) is the transient inability to perform a task. It most often involves legs when walking but may involve eyelid opening, speaking, or writing. Freezing occurs suddenly and may last only a few seconds with each occurrence. Freezing usually occurs when the patient starts to walk (start hesitation) or attempts to turn while walking, with a fear of inability to deal with barriers such as revolving doors, narrow corridors, or heavily trafficked streets. Stair climbing is usually not as difficult. The combination of freezing and loss of postural reflexes may result in falls, which are responsible for a high incidence of hip fracture in patients with PD.

Patients frequently exhibit additional signs and symptoms. Many of these are due to the illness itself, but some may be secondary to the side effects of drug therapy. Although intellect is often preserved in the early stages, deterioration is seen as the disease progresses, including slowness of thought processes (i.e., bradyphrenia), diminished memory, and personality changes (e.g., passivity, dependency, indecisiveness). Dementia and depression occur, affecting up to two thirds of patients (19). Perceptual motor and visuospatial deficits also have been found during neuropsychological studies (20,21). Dull pain in one shoulder may be an early symptom. Akathisia and restless leg syndrome may be present. Sensory symptoms without objective signs of sensory impairment, e.g., burning and tingling in the region of motor involvement, may be seen. Signs of autonomic dysfunction include orthostasis, increased salivation with drooling, increased perspiration and seborrhea with oily skin, bladder incontinence mostly of the hyperreflexic nature, difficulty in achieving an erection, and decreased gastrointestinal peristalsis. Constipation may represent inactivity or may be a side effect of anticholinergic medication.

Cranial nerve dysfunction may result in difficulty chewing, swallowing (i.e., dysphagia), and blinking secondary to bradykinesia of muscles innervated by cranial nerves III, VII, and IX. Speech is low volume, slow with monotonous tone, and poorly enunciated. Handwriting may be small and cramped (micrographia). Patients may complain of coughing when eating, food sticking in their throat, and difficulty swallowing pills. Reduced pharyngeal peristalsis, delayed swallowing reflex, abnormal lingual control of swallowing, and involuntary reflux from the vallecula and piriform sinuses into the oral cavity may occur (22,23). Silent aspiration may occur without any other swallowing symptomatology. Patients may be unable to cough effectively, which can cause serious problems if respiratory infection develops.

Etiology

The cause of PD is unknown. Research has concentrated on genetics, environmental toxins, and exogenous toxins from cellular oxidative reactions (24). Although monozygotic twins show a low concordance rate for IPD, studies have confirmed that a family history of IPD is strongly associated with the disease, and its increased frequency among the relatives of patients with IPD could be due to genetic or environmental factors. No specific gene has yet been identified. No single environmental factor has emerged as essential, but well-water drinking in rural areas is associated with a double risk of developing IPD. There may be exposure to agricultural insecticides, pesticides, wood pulp, or vegetable farming (25).

A role for environmental toxins is supported by the discovery that 1-methyl-4-phenyl-1,2,3,6-tetrahydropyridine (MPTP), which is a synthetic meperidine derivative causing symptoms similar to those of IPD. However, no specific environmental factor has been identified, and no therapeutic opportunity has been found (26).

Smoking and IPD have been shown to have a negative association, and it has been suggested that tobacco aversion may be part of the premorbid parkinsonian personality (27).

Dietary intake of antioxidants and other oxidative compounds was studied in a population-based case control study by Logroscino et al. (28). It showed increased consumption of animal fats among patients with IPD, which is consistent with the hypothesis that oxidative stress and lipid peroxidation are important in the pathogenesis of the disease. No effect of vitamins with antioxidant activity, either as food or supplements, was observed.

It is hypothesized that neurogenetic disease such as IPD has multifactorial etiologies and occurs predominantly in genetically predisposed subgroups of the general population who have been exposed to cell-specific toxins or protoxins (29).

Pathogenesis

IPD is a disorder of the extrapyramidal system, with a loss of pigmented cells within the substantia nigra (i.e., zona compacta) that produce DA, and degeneration of the nigrostriatal pathway. Microscopically, neuronal dropout and gliosis are seen, as are intracytoplasmic inclusions called Lewy bodies (30).

The core biochemical pathology in parkinsonism is decreased dopaminergic neurotransmission in the basal ganglia. Degeneration of the nigrostriatal DA system results in a marked loss of striatal DA content physiologically, decreased dopaminergic activity in the striatum causes disinhibitation of the subthalamic nucleus and medial globus pallidus, which is the predominant efferent nucleus in the basal ganglia. In drug-induced PD, there is a blockage of DA receptors or depletion of DA storage.

The understanding of the biochemical pathology in IPD has resulted in its pharmacologic treatment using DA replacement therapy. Similarly, the understanding of physiologic changes in basal ganglia has led to surgical intervention such as pallidotomy and thalamotomy.

Diagnosis

Diagnosis of IPD is based on clinical observation but may be difficult in its early stages due to other conditions, e.g. essential tremor, multisystem atrophy, and supranuclear palsy, which may masquerade as IPD.

The clinical factors that most accurately predict IPD are resting tremor asymmetry and a good response to a trial of levodopa therapy. Shoulder bursitis is a common early feature of IPD, perhaps reflecting reduced mobility (31). Essential tremor is frequently mistaken for IPD. However, it is kinetic and not present at rest.

Barbeau and Roy have suggested essential tremor to be a significant risk factor for developing IPD. Essential tremor–related PD affects 10% of IPD cases and is transmitted in an autosomal-dominant mode (32).

The onset of symptoms is insidious, frequently unilateral, with the patient complaining of a resting tremor as a symptom first seen in 70% of cases. Fatigue, minor clumsiness of an arm, or dragging of a leg may be present, and symptoms may remain unilateral for several years before spreading to the opposite side. A hemiparesis may be closely simulated; however, deep tendon reflexes are not exaggerated, results of the sensory examination are usually normal, and the plantar responses remain flexor. Although not specific to IPD, abnormal reflexes, including the palmomental, gag, snout, and sucking reflexes, as well as an exaggerated glabellar reflex (i.e., Myerson sign), also may be found. Specific joint limitation, chest expansion, equilibrium, and gait may need to be assessed, as well as the time that it takes to complete each individual task.

Motor speech in patients with IPD may be characterized by decreased volume with monopitch and prosodic insufficiency due to hypokinetic dysarthria.

Sabate et al., in a study of 58 patients with PD, found a high prevalence of obstructive airway disease and restrictive pulmonary disease (33). Patients with PD often lead sedentary lives. Sabate et al. found a higher degree of deterioration in ADL activities in patients with PD with ventilatory problems than in patients with normal pulmonary function (33). Shenkman and Butler have suggested that loss of musculoskeletal flexibility and kyphotic posture may cause ventilatory problems that may contribute to ADL difficulties (34).

High field strength (1.5 tesla) magnetic resonance imaging (MRI) may show abnormal signal hypodensity in the striatum on T2-weighted images in atypical parkinsonism. Striatal {^{18}F} 6-floro-L-dopa {FD} uptake measured by positron emission tomography (PET) is a good index of the nigrostriatal dopaminergic system (35). PET provides a unique opportunity to investigate the alterations of blood flow, energy metabolism, and neurotransmitter system in vivo in humans. It assists in the understanding of the pathophysiology of IPD, and it may improve the diagnostic accuracy of various forms of parkinsonism. PET can be used for preclinical or early detection of IPD. This may be important in the future, especially if treatment became available to arrest or slow down the progression of IPD or other forms of parkinsonism (36).

Response to levodopa may be helpful in differentiating between patients with IPD and patients with atypical parkinsonism because the former respond well, whereas the latter, due to degeneration of striatal or pallidal neurons, may not respond.

A correct diagnosis is important to provide accurate prognosis and appropriate medical management.

Course and Prognosis

In the majority of patients, IPD develops insidiously and progresses slowly. There are often long periods during which the progression is so slow that it appears to be in partial remission. Eventually, usually over 5 to 15 years, overall function diminishes, perhaps to the point of wheelchair and bed dependency.

In general, tremor is not as disabling as rigidity or bradykinesia. Patients with an early tremor have been shown to progress more slowly (37), whereas akinesia indicates a more rapidly progressing disease (38). Positive prognostic features include early tremor, rigidity, and family history. Negative prognostic features include bradykinesia, akinesia, postural instability and gait difficulties, cognitive deficits, and late age of onset. Current medical treatments and rehabilitation programs can significantly modify the course of the disease, but neuronal degeneration continues to progress and the patient's symptoms ultimately fail to respond. New frontiers in the research of PD are aimed at delaying neuronal degeneration, thereby halting the patient's progressive functional decline.

Although IPD is not lethal, there is an increase in morbidity and mortality even when it has been reduced dramatically with the introduction of levodopa (39). The symptom that is least responsive is the loss of postural reflexes, which can result in falls with hip fractures as a potential consequence. Mortality usually occurs secondary to the patient's debility, from aspiration pneumonia, urinary tract infections, and decubiti.

Symptomatic or Secondary Parkinsonism

Secondary parkinsonism can be due to various pathologic processes affecting basal ganglia, i.e., hemorrhage, trauma, tumor, hydrocephalus, or infectious diseases (Table 42-1). Drugs such as amiodarone and metoclopramide can cause parkinsonism and may be diagnosed by a history of drug exposure and improvement after drug withdrawal. In general, patients with symptomatic parkinsonism have symmetric symptoms and signs (the exception being parkinsonism secondary to focal head injury). Rest tremor is rarely seen in these cases. Perhaps the best diagnostic aid is the lack of response to levodopa, exceptions being some cases of MPTP and postencephalitic parkinsonism.

Progressive Supranuclear Palsy

This syndrome, an example of Parkinson's plus syndrome, was first described by Posey (40). It is a rare disorder characterized by a loss of vertical ocular gaze, rigidity of the neck and trunk muscles, dementia, and parkinsonian signs, usually with the absence of tremor. Onset is typically in the fifth to sixth decades of life, and men are affected more often than women. Impairment of gait is usually the first apparent clinical sign, with episodes of unsteadiness and falling. Bradykinesia, diplopia, dysphagia, bowel and bladder disturbances, and neurobehavioral features, including depression, withdrawal, forgetfulness, and irritability, are commonly seen. Sustained frontalis contraction, lid retraction, and infrequent eye blinking give the patient a characteristic surprised facial expression. The characteristic feature is loss of upward and downward gaze, followed by lateral gaze, with preservation of ocular movements on oculocephalic maneuvers (if eyes are fixed on a target and the head is turned, full movement can be obtained), indicating that the ocular palsy is supranuclear in nature (41). Because of the rigidity, the patient has difficulty flexing the neck to compensate for impaired ocular motion. The progressive course of Parkinson's plus syndrome is more rapid than that of IPD, with death usually occurring within 6 to 10 years. Histologic findings include neuronal degeneration within the brain stem and basal ganglia with neurofibrillary tangles.

Pharmacologic treatment includes the use of levodopa or dopaminergic agonists to alleviate the parkinsonian symptoms, but benefits are usually short lived. Anticholinergic medications for drooling and tricyclic antidepressants for depression and emotional disturbances may be used. Rehabilitation is similar to the management of the parkinson patient. Weighted walkers or wheelchairs were used in two cases to provide added stability as reported by Sosner et al. (42). Prism glasses and mirrors may help alleviate visual disturbances.

Treatment of Parkinsonism

The three methods of management include pharmacology, rehabilitation, and neurosurgical procedures.

Pharmacologic Management

A variety of medications (Table 42-3) are available to relieve PD symptomatology. Because the disease is attributed to a deficiency of DA with a relative excess of cholinergic activity, antiparkinsonian drugs are mainly dopaminergic or anticholinergic in nature.

DA itself does not cross the blood–brain barrier. However, levodopa can cross the blood–brain barrier and is decarboxylated to DA in the brain. It is combined with carbidopa, which is a peripheral decarboxylase inhibitor to provide excellent benefit without the side effects of nausea or vomiting (1). It also allows about a fourfold dose reduction of levodopa. Recent studies have shown no adverse consequences of early levodopa treatment. These studies also indicate that the decline in therapeutic response relates to disease progression rather than to treatment duration (39).

Levodopa-induced neuropsychiatric problems consist of confusion and hallucinations, which are more frequent in older patients and may reflect the fact that one third of the patients with PD develop dementia (43). These problems can be minimized by eliminating unnecessary sedative or psychoactive medications and using the lowest dose of levodopa/carbidopa to obtain relief. Treatment with levodopa has prolonged life expectancy and considerably improved the quality of life of patients with PD. The course of the

TABLE 42-3. *Medications used for Parkinson's disease*

Drug	Recommended dose	Mode of action	Indication	Side effects
Dopamine precursors				
Carbidopa/ levodopa standard	25/100 mg, 50/200 mg, start 1 tablet 3× daily 1 hr before meals and gradually increase to 2½ to 3 tablets 3× daily.	Levodopa activates D1 and D2 DA receptors in the brain. Carbidopa is a peripheral dopadecarboxylase inhibitor. It increases therapeutic potency and decreases gastrointestinal side effects of levodopa.	IPD	Motor fluctuations, dyskinesias, psychosis. 75% develop these after 5 years of treatment, although it may be due to the disease progression and not a drug side effect. Levodopa forms free radicals, which may cause progression of IPD.
Carbidopa/levodopa controlled release	25/100 mg, 50/200 mg, start 1 tablet 2× daily and then gradually increase to 2 or 3 tablets 2× daily.	Slow-release form allows smoothing out of the clinical fluctuations.	IPD	Longer half-life and lower peak plasma level of levodopa cause delay in response and may cause excessive response, resulting in sustained severe dyskinesias.
Dopamine agonists				
Bromocriptine	Bromocriptine initially 1.25 mg at bedtime for 3 days, thereafter switch to daytime for 3 days and then increase slowly. Usual dose 10–40 mg/day.	Bromocriptine eliminates hydroxyl free radicals and is neuroprotective in experiments.	Used as conjunctive therapy with levodopa to potentiate antiparkinsonism and to reduce the dosage needed for levodopa alone.	May cause orthostatic hypotension, especially when first started. Bromocriptine can cause more psychosis and confusion. May produce red inflamed skin (St. Anthony's fire), which is reversible on drug discontinuation.
Pergolide	Pergolide 0.05 mg at bedtime for 3 days, thereafter switch to daytime for 3 days and then increase by 0.25 mg/day every third day, titrating for optimal effects. Average daily dose 3 mg.	Pergolide acts on D1 and D2 DA receptors and has a longer half-life than bromocriptine.	Also may be used as monotherapy in early IPD. May be used to overcome some adverse side effects from long-term levodopa use.	Pergolide causes more dyskinesias.
Not available in the United States: lisuride, apomorphine, cabergoline, ropinirole				
Dopamine releaser				
Amantidine	100 mg twice daily	Augments DA release from storage sites, possibly blocks reuptake of DA in presynaptic terminals, mildly anticholinergic.	Early phase of IPD or in conjunction with levodopa and DA agonists in advanced IPD.	Livedo reticularis (reddish mottling of skin) around the knees, ankle edema, visual hallucinations.
Monoamine oxidase type B inhibitors (MAO-B inhibitors)				
Selegiline hydrochloride (Deprenyl or Eldepryl)	5 mg at breakfast and 5 mg at noon.	Considered neuroprotective. Rescues dopaminergic neurons by inducing changes in transcription with new protein synthesis and alteration in gene expression. May potentiate levodopa.	Some clinicians use it as monotherapy in early IPD. May delay the need for levodopa for about 9 months. Used with levodopa to potentiate its effects and reduce the dose of levodopa.	Hypertensive reactions may occur if taken with theophylline, ephedrine, carbidopa/levodopa and foods containing tyramine.

(continued)

TABLE 42-3. *Continued.*

Drug	Recommended dose	Mode of action	Indication	Side effects
Anticholinergics				
Trihexiphenydryl, benztropine, procyclidine, ethopropazine, cycrimine, biperiden	Trihexyphenidyl 2 mg 3× daily. May be increased to 6 mg 3× daily. Benztropine 2–3 mg/day	Cross the blood–brain barrier and blunt the cholinergic activity of the basal ganglia.	May improve parkinsonism in 20%. Useful if tremors not relieved by levodopa. May be used as monotherapy for tremor in early IPD.	Common, especially in people over 70 years of age. Adverse cerebral side effects include forgetfulness, decreased short-term memory, rarely hallucinations and psychosis. Peripheral side effects include blurring of vision, dry mouth, urinary difficulties.
Antihistamines				
Diphenhydramine, orphenadrine	50 mg 3× daily	Mildly anticholinergic	Tremor control and hypnosis used in older individuals who cannot take strong anticholinergics.	Similar to anticholinergics
Antipsychotics				
Clozapine	Start at 12.5 mg/day, then increase to 25–50 mg/day, up to 300–450 mg/day in severe cases.	Selective D4 receptor antagonist.	Used to treat levodopa-induced psychosis. Fewer extrapyramidal side effects.	Monitor white cell count to prevent agranulocytosis.

DA, dopamine; IPD, idiopathic Parkinson's disease.

disease is now marked with motor response fluctuations and drug-induced dyskinesias (44).

Dyskinesias may be choreiform or dystonic. The cause may be upregulation of DA receptors or postsynaptic changes due to IPD and exposure to levodopa. Motor response fluctuations consist of variation in response to a single dose of levodopa: when it may respond to the drug (on period) and when it will not (off period). It is postulated that both of these complications may have similar pathophysiologic mechanisms. It is also noted that both complications were more frequent in patients whose illness began at an early age. However, length of levodopa treatment has no influence on either complication (45).

Motor fluctuations may be due to a reduction in the IPD-affected brain's capacity to store DA because of the progressive loss of DA terminals.

DA agonists (e.g., bromocriptine and pergolide) have the capacity to stimulate DA receptors directly without requiring biochemical conversion (46). They have less antiparkinsonism effects but also have less side effects. Combining a low dose of DA agonist with levodopa early in the course of treatment diminishes side effects without losing antiparkinsonism effects (47).

Anticholinergic medications cross the blood–brain barrier and blunt the cholinergic activity of the basal ganglia. They are particularly effective for treatment of tremor. Anticholinergics such as trihexyphenidyl or benztropine may be used with levodopa in patients with early IPD who also have tremors. Use in older patients with IPD should be avoided due to the higher incidence of adverse mental effects. Antihistaminics and tricyclics with milder anticholinergic properties may be used in older patients.

Amantidine, an antiviral agent, is believed to increase DA release from certain striatal neurons and also act on DA sites. It is used as an adjunct to levodopa.

The monoamine oxidase-B (MAO-B) inhibitor selegiline hydrochloride (Deprenyl or Eldepryl [Somerset Pharmaceuticals, Tampa, FL]) is considered neuroprotective by delaying the symptoms of disability (48). Some believe that selegiline may have symptomatic effects that could mask rather than delay neurodegeneration (49).

It was shown recently by Tatton et al. that selegiline rescues dopaminergic neurons by inducing changes in transcription with new protein synthesis and alteration in gene expression (50). Selegiline mildly potentiates the levodopa response by blocking one avenue of DA breakdown. A few cases have been reported of hypertensive reactions occurring in patients on recommended doses of selegiline ingesting tyramine-containing foods (51).

Alpha tocopherol or vitamin E, an antioxidant, has been found to be of no use in the management of IPD.

Depression is an important concern in IPD. It is not clear if it is an inherent component of parkinsonism or is a reaction to the chronic progressive neurodegenerative disorder. Treatment of PD may reduce depression. If not, serotonin reuptake inhibitors such as fluoxetine or sertraline may be used. They have no anticholinergic actions but may interfere with levodopa's antiparkinsonism effects.

Rehabilitation and neurosurgical techniques common to movement disorders are discussed at the end of this chapter.

Other Disorders of Movement

Table 42-4 lists all major movement disorders other than parkinsonism that are encountered in clinical practice.

Chorea, Athetosis, and Ballismus

Chorea

Chorea, derived from the Greek word for dance, is an involuntary movement that is brief, rapid, forceful, and dysrhythmic. In general, choreic movements are discrete and purposeless and have a bizarre character. Its distinction from other movement disorders is not clear. It may resemble athetosis if it presents as a series of slow, confluent movements. When the involuntary movement involves the proximal limb muscles, it may be difficult to distinguish from ballismus. This has prompted some to consider chorea, athetosis, and ballismus as various manifestations of one type of movement disorder. The anatomic basis of chorea is uncertain, but it is believed that the contralateral subthalamic nucleus, caudate nucleus, and putamen may be responsible (52–55). Bilateral thalamic involvement has been described as well. Chorea, along with athetosis, dystonia, and other movement disorders, may present paroxysmally and are referred to as paroxysmal movement disorders or paroxysmal dyskinesias (56).

Several conditions are associated with choreic movements, among them Sydenham's chorea, hyperthyroidism, cerebral arteritis, polycythemia vera, systemic lupus erythematosus, and phenothiazine intake. Chorea is also a prominent feature of Huntington's disease (HD). This will be discussed in more detail because it is one neurologic condition for which physiatric expertise is valuable in disability evaluation and functional remediation.

HD is an inherited degenerative disorder that characteristically affects the basal ganglia (57). The HD gene, localized in the short arm of chromosome 4, is inherited in an autosomal-dominant manner (58). Symptoms typically begin in childhood and adolescence, and the illness lasts from 10 to 25 years. Some die from associated illness such as aspiration pneumonia, whereas others, experiencing depression, commit suicide (57).

TABLE 42-4. *Movement disorders other than parkinsonism*

Chorea
Brief, rapid, forceful, dysrhythmic, discrete, purposeless, flinging of limb
Athetosis
Slow, writhing movements and inability to maintain position of limb or body part
Ballismus
Large amplitude, flinging movement of limb (usually proximal)
Dystonia
Sustained muscle contraction that leads to repetitive twisting movements of variable speed and abnormal posture
Tremor
Rhythmic, oscillatory movements of a body part
Tic
Intermittent, repetitive, stereotypical, abrupt, jerky, typically affecting the face and head
Stereotypy
Purposeless, uniformly repetitive, voluntary, movement of whole body areas
Akathisia
Subjective restlessness, compulsion to move about
Myoclonus
Sudden, brief, irregular, contraction of a group of muscles
Posttraumatic
Drug induced (neuroleptics and others)
Psychogenic

Patients with HD display the triad of motor, emotional, and cognitive disturbances. Chorea is the most characteristic movement abnormality. Others include impaired manual dexterity, oculomotor abnormalities, gait ataxia, dysphasia, dysarthria, bradykinesia, spasticity, and rigidity, which may lead to devastating functional disability. Typical emotional and behavioral problems include depression, apathy, social withdrawal, suicidal behavior, irritability, aggression, anxiety and psychoticlike states. Impaired memory, disorientation, and dementia are among the cognitive and intellectual disturbances in HD (59).

The management of HD is directed toward the amelioration of specific emotional and cognitive symptoms and control of motor disorder. Nonpharmacologic measures are preferred for the initial treatment of chorea because drug side effects, such as neuroleptic-induced tardive dyskinesia, may worsen the original motor impairment. Exercises to maintain range of motion and strengthening should be performed to support proximal trunk stability and posture. Adaptive seating evaluation helps determine the seating system that will allow comfortable posture and stability. The chair and bed should be padded to guard against injury resulting from the sudden flinging of the limbs, and weights may be applied to the involved limbs to suppress chorea amplitude. Need for medications should be evaluated periodically because various symptoms predominate at different stages of HD.

Medications used to treat chorea include haloperidol, fluphenazine, reserpine, clonazepam, thioridazine, and tetrabenazine (59). Antiparkinsonian drugs such as amantadine, levo/carbidopa, and bromocriptine may be used to treat bradykinesia and rigidity (57,60). Baclofen and local botulinum toxin injections may be helpful in managing spasticity and certain forms of dystonia such as torticollis. Severe myoclonus may be relieved by clonazepam or valproic acid (60).

There is no effective pharmacologic intervention for the cognitive deterioration seen in HD. However, cognitive functioning must be maximized by strategies such as avoidance of medications with negative cognitive side effects (e.g., anticholinergics), development of compensatory techniques for memory loss (use of a memory notebook), and environmental management. Other HD-related problems that should be addressed include dysphasia, nutritional deficits, and dysarthria.

Athetosis

Athetosis is a movement disorder slower in nature than chorea. It is characterized by writhing movements and inability to maintain the position of fingers, wrists, toes, or any other body part. Although the limbs are commonly affected, the axial musculature may be involved as well. It may be seen in Wilson's disease, cerebral palsy, and basal ganglia disease. In some cases, athetosis is drug induced. When it appears with chorea, it is referred to as choreoathetosis.

Ballismus

In contrast to chorea, ballistic movements are of large amplitude and involve the proximal limbs. Because ballismus is frequently unilateral, it is also commonly referred to as hemiballismus. Involvement of the contralateral subthalamic nucleus has been suggested (53,61), but other subcortical structures may be involved as well (54). It is thought that a lesion in the contralateral subthalamic nucleus disrupts the inhibitory pathways to the globus pallidus, leading to DA hyperactivity in the striatum (62). Bilateral involvement (biballism) may be seen in bilateral basal ganglia disease (63). Ballismus also has been associated with metabolic abnormalities, such as hyperglycemia (64), neoplasms, systemic lupus erythematosus, and encephalitis (54).

Treatment of Chorea, Athetosis, and Ballismus

Antiepileptic drugs, such as phenobarbital and valproic acid, may be of benefit in chorea, athetosis, hemiballismus, or in any combination of these disorders (65,66). In hemiballismus, DA antagonists such as haloperidol and phenothiazines, and DA-depleting agents such as reserpine and tetrabenazine (67), may be helpful. Gamma-aminobutyric acid (GABA)-ergic drugs, such as clonazepam, also may ameliorate chorea because GABA appears to mediate the inhibitory action of the subthalamic nucleus (67). Stereotactic thalamotomy (68) may be considered in severe conditions refractory to drugs.

Dystonia

Sustained muscle contraction that causes repetitive, twisting movements of variable speed and leads to abnormal posture is referred to as dystonia. This disorder can be classified according to age of onset, etiology, and anatomic distribution (65). Infantile dystonia begins before 2 years of age; childhood dystonia between 2 and 12 years of age; juvenile dystonia at 13 to 20 years of age; and adult dystonia at over 20 years of age.

Classified based on etiology, dystonia may either be primary or secondary. Primary dystonia may have either a hereditary (autosomal dominant, X-linked recessive) or sporadic occurrence. In the autosomal-dominant pattern, chromosome 9q has been implicated. Secondary dystonia is associated with neurologic disorders such as Huntington's disease and parkinsonism. It also may be a sequela of brain injury, cerebral tumor, infections, and drugs such as phenothiazines.

Dystonia may be focal, segmental, multifocal, or generalized (65). Focal dystonia involves single body parts (e.g., blepharospasm, writer's cramp), whereas the segmental variety affects two or more contiguous regions (e.g., craniocervical). Multifocal dystonia consists of abnormalities in noncontiguous body parts. Generalized dystonia involves segmental crural dystonia and at least one other body part. Unilateral dystonia, usually associated with abnormalities in the contralateral basal ganglia, is also called hemidystonia. Regardless of anatomic distribution, dystonic contractions typically begin intermittently and become severe and persistent, leading to sustained abnormal postures.

Impairment of basal ganglia output is thought to play a role in the genesis of dystonia (69). Lesions in the putamen have been linked to hemidystonia (65), whereas bilateral putaminal involvement may be responsible for generalized dystonia. Torticollis and hand dystonia are thought to result from involvement of the head of the caudate nucleus and thalamus, respectively (70). Disease of the thalamus and subthalamus (71) and derangement of hypothalamic function (72) also have been suspected.

Dystonia may be a clinical manifestation of conditions such as Wilson's disease (hepatolenticular degeneration), hypoxic brain injury, traumatic brain injury, Hallervorden-Spatz disease, Huntington's disease, Leigh disease, lipid storage disease, and PD (65). Thus, in addition to a thorough history and physical examination, blood chemistries including liver function tests, ceruloplasmin and copper blood levels, MRI or computed tomography scan of the brain, slit-lamp eye examination for Kayser-Fleischer rings, and 24-hour urine copper analysis should be considered in the evaluation of dystonia.

Dystonia musculorum deformans, or torsion dystonia, is the term used to describe a generalized form of the disease that involves the trunk and limbs. The onset is usually before adolescence, presenting infrequently as abnormal movement of a limb after an activity. Later, it progresses in severity and frequency until it becomes a continuous spasm giving rise to body contortion. At first, rest relieves the spasms but as the disease progresses, level of activity and position have no effect. The shoulder, trunk, and pelvic muscles undergo spasmodic twisting, as do the limbs. The hands are seldom involved. Orofacial muscles also may be affected, leading to dysarthria and dysphagia (55).

The pathology of dystonia musculorum deformans is yet to be described. In some cases genetics appear to play a role. Autosomal-dominant and -recessive patterns of inheritance have been reported. A sex-linked form, associated with parkinsonism, has been described in the Philippines (73).

Cranial (Meige's) Dystonia/Oromandibular and Lingual Dystonia

Oromandibular, facial, and lingual dystonias are discussed together here because they may coexist. Cranial dystonia, also known as Meige's syndrome, is the most common form of the craniocervical dystonias (74). Women are more commonly affected and onset is in the sixth decade of life. The most common type involves forced jaw opening, lip retraction, tongue protrusion, and spasm of the platysma. In other cases, the lips purse and the jaw forcibly closes. Intermittent chewing, tongue curling, and pain in the temporomandibular joint area may occur as well. It may be associated with blepharospasm, spasmodic dysphonia, torticollis, and trunk and limb dystonia. Eating and talking may trigger a dystonic event.

Dental appliances have been used with limited success. Medications that have provided some relief include anticholinergics and benzodiazepines. Local botulinum toxin injection of the involved muscles (masseter, digastric, pterygoids, genioglossus, hypoglossus, temporalis) has yielded excellent results (75,76).

Hemifacial Spasm

Hemifacial spasm typically begins as a unilateral clonic twitching of the orbicularis oculi, later becoming sustained. As it progresses, it may spread to involve other facial muscles. This is a disease of adulthood with a predilection for women. Previously, this condition was treated with clonazepam, carbamazepine, baclofen (77), and facial nerve decompression (78) with some success. The current treatment of choice is local botulinum toxin injection of the involved facial muscles.

Cervical Dystonia

Cervical dystonia, the most common focal dystonia, involves the sternocleidomastoid, trapezius, and posterior cervical muscles. It gives rise to a patterned, repetitive, and spasmodic movement that causes the head to twist (rotational torticollis), extend (retrocollis), flex (anterocollis), or tilt toward the shoulder (laterocollis). One or more of these head movements may occur simultaneously. The onset is insidious, presenting as intermittent spasms of the neck muscles or abnormal head movement (79). Women are more commonly affected. Onset is between the fourth and fifth decades of life but may present earlier.

Like many other movement disorders, cervical dystonia was initially attributed to a psychiatric disturbance. Although some patients may be anxious or depressed, these symptoms usually result from the patient's distress and frustration with not being able to function well. No definite genetic marker has been identified, but hereditary factors have been considered based on reports of autosomal-dominant familial cervical dystonia (80,81) and the finding that up to 44% of patients have a family history of similar or other movement disorders (82). Because they play a role in maintaining normal head posture, the basal ganglia and the vestibulo-ocular reflex pathway have been implicated in the development of cervical dystonia (83,84). Disturbances of neurotransmitter systems also have been described in dystonias (85). Abnormalities in blink reflex recovery (86) suggest involvement of the brain stem. Earlier cervical and upper limb trauma also have been implicated (87,88).

Walking or standing worsens the condition, but the patient may be able to return the head to midline by placing the hand on the jaw or chin. The neck movement may be associated with blepharospasm, lip or chewing movements, and tremor. The patient should be evaluated at rest and while standing and walking. The head must be allowed to assume the abnormal posture, cervical range of motion in all planes determined, and the abnormally contracting muscles identified. Although the clinical presentation is obvious, the clinician should rule out treatable etiologies such as Wilson's disease, inflammation of cervical soft tissues, cervical disc disease, or fractures.

Limb Dystonia

Limb dystonia involves cramping and posturing of the hand and fingers, resulting in the inability to perform certain occupational tasks. Thus, it is also known as occupational cramp, writer's cramp, and graphospasm. This task-specific dystonia, manifesting as hyperextension or hyperflexion of the wrist and fingers, may be triggered by activities such as writing and attempting to play the piano or other musical instruments (89). Upon cessation of the task, the spasms disappear. Fifty-five different occupations in which individuals suffer from this condition have been described (90). Torticollis, tremor, and pain are accompanying symptoms, but it is usually the spasm that is limiting. Men and women are equally affected, and onset is during the second to fifth decades of life. Physical and neurologic examinations are typically unremarkable. A corresponding nervous system pathology has not been found, thus tempting some to label the condition as an occupational neurosis. Limb dystonia also may affect the lower limb, as in dystonia-parkinsonism syndrome (91).

Treatment of Various Dystonias

The current lack of knowledge of the exact pathophysiology of dystonia has made it difficult to define specific pharmacologic therapy.

Baclofen, benzodiazepines (e.g., clonazepam), anticholinergics (e.g., trihexyphenidyl), carbamazepine, and DA agonists or antagonists (92–95) also have been tried, but their side effects limit their use. Local injection of botulinum toxin into the offending muscles, typically the sternocleidomastoid, trapezius, and splenius capitis, has been successful and not associated with significant complications (96). In a few cases, dysphagia developed because of local spread of the toxin to neighboring pharyngeal and laryngeal muscles. Surgical techniques include myectomy, neurectomy, rhizotomy, cervical cord stimulation, and cryothalamotomy. Intrathecal baclofen therapy is another promising intervention. The efficacy of physical therapy techniques such as soft-tissue mobilization, cervical muscle strengthening and stretching, and orthotic intervention have not been well studied. Similarly, limited success has been achieved through behavioral modifications, including hypnosis, biofeedback, and relaxation techniques.

Tremors

Tremors are regular, oscillatory movements produced by alternating but synchronous contractions of antagonistic muscles. Its rhythmic quality distinguishes it from other involuntary movement disorders. In contradistinction to the unidirectional quality of clonus, tremors are bidirectional. They are usually associated with diseases of the basal ganglia and cerebellum.

Tremors may be physiologic or pathologic. As the name implies, physiologic tremor may be a normal finding. It is usually present in all muscle groups, and its amplitude may be too small to detect visually. Frequency ranges from 7 to 12 Hz (89,97). Pathologic tremors, on the other hand, are focal, with a frequency range of 4 to 7 Hz. Table 42-5 lists some tremor subtypes and clinical features.

Tremors also may be classified as the resting or action type. The former is usually associated with PD and is discussed in an earlier section. Action tremors are further classified into the postural and intention, or kinetic, types (98). Postural tremor sets in when one attempts to maintain a limb in a certain position. A variant of postural tremor is associated with multiple sclerosis due to involvement of cerebellar pathways (99). This type of tremor affects the axial and proximal limb muscles more commonly. Essential, enhanced physiologic and posttraumatic tremors are classified as action type, as are tremors related to neuropathy and alcohol withdrawal.

Essential tremor may be familial in some cases, with an autosomal-dominant inheritance pattern and a frequency range of 5.5 to 7 Hz, which is slower than the physiologic tremor (92). Lou and Jankovic (100) analyzed the clinical characteristics of 350 consecutive patients with essential tremors and found a bimodal age of onset with peaks in the second and sixth decades of life. They also noted that the hand was most frequently involved, followed by the head and voice. Roughly half of the patients had associated dystonia, and about 20% had parkinsonism. Senile tremor is a variant of essential tremor. Enhanced physiologic tremor is often aggravated by anxiety, fatigue, metabolic derangement (hypoglycemia), endocrine abnormality (hyperthyroidism), caffeine, and nicotine. Intention, or kinetic, tremor, as manifested in cerebellar disease states, presents as an irregular movement that disrupts the smooth progression of a goal-directed motor task. Clinically, this is commonly observed during finger-to-nose testing to uncover dysmetria. Some tremors are task specific. These are not related to maintenance of posture and manifest only during certain motor activities such as writing. Hysterical tremor also has been described (97).

Treatment of Various Tremors

Propranolol has been effective in controlling physiologic tremor and in some cases of action tremor. Clonidine, clonazepam, and antiepileptic drugs (primidone, carbamazepine, valproic acid) also may be of value (101–104). Essential tremor may improve with alcohol, propranolol, and primidone (100) administration. Local injection of botulinum toxin is a promising alternative (105). Tremor related to parkinsonism may be helped by thalamic stimulation or thalamotomy. Levodopa may alleviate rubral tremor related to multiple sclerosis. A biobehavioral rehabilitation approach involving functional analysis of behavior, neuromuscular reeducation, relaxation, and coping skills also has been recommended (106).

Tics, Stereotypy, and Akathisia

Tics

Tics are intermittent, stereotypical, repetitive, jerky movements. Although the individual is aware of such movements, he or she is unable to resist performing the action (107). Many tics are associated with purposeful tasks such as eye

TABLE 42-5. *Tremor subtypes and clinical features*

Tremor subtype	Clinical features	Pharmacologic treatment
Physiologic/enhanced physiologic	7–12 Hz; worsened by posture, improved with alcohol	Beta-adrenergic antagonists; alcohol; benzodiazepines
Essential	5.5–7 Hz; hand commonly involved; improved with alcohol; senile tremor is a variant	Beta-adrenergic antagonists, benzodiazepines, methazolamide
Parkinsonian	4–4.5 Hz; more prominent at rest; prominent with posture (rubral)	Dopaminergic agents, anticholinergic agents, beta-adrenergic antagonists
Cerebellar	2.5–4 Hz; may be intentional or postural; worsened by alcohol and beta agonists	Carbamazepine, isoniazid (intention tremor in multiple sclerosis)
Task specific	Irregular; occurs with specific tasks, such as writing	Local botulinum toxin injection

Adapted with permission from Findley L. Tremors: differential diagnosis and pharmacology. In: Jankovic J, Tolosa E, eds. *Parkinson's disease and movement disorders,* 2nd ed. Baltimore: Williams & Wilkins, 1993; 293–313; and Camicioli R. Movement disorders in geriatric rehabilitation. *Clin Geriatr Med* 1993; 9:756–781.

blinking and throat clearing. They generally do not interfere with willed voluntary movements and may be volitionally suppressed to some extent. Tics usually disappear during sleep and worsen during stressful situations. Tics may be simple, such as grimacing, or complex, as in Gilles de la Tourette syndrome. This distressing syndrome consists of multiple motor and vocal tics associated with coprolalia, palilalia, and aggressive behavior. It generally begins in the first two decades of life, and males are more commonly affected. Although the etiology in unknown, it has been suggested that childhood exposure to methylphenidate or amphetamine predisposes to this disorder (55,107). Tics may be helped by clonazepam and clonidine (89,108).

Stereotypy

Stereotypy is purposeless, uniformly repetitive, voluntary movement of whole body areas. Examples include head nodding, head banging, body rocking, and arm jerking, seen in individuals with mental retardation and amphetamine addiction (104,109). Haloperidol and clomipramine may suppress this movement abnormality.

Akathisia

Akathisia is defined as inner restlessness and compulsion to move about that is commonly mistaken for anxiety or agitation. Although akathisia is a subjective experience, it may manifest overtly as inability to stand or sit still, or as an urge to pace constantly. In some, the only finding is toe tapping or leg shaking. Akathisia is thought to result from DA blockade in the frontal area (110). Thus, antidopaminergic medications such as neuroleptics may induce this disorder. The DA agonists amantadine (111), clonidine (112), propranolol (113), piracetam (114), and clozapine (115) may be beneficial. Neuroleptic-induced akathisia may be treated with amantadine (111) but is best managed by reducing the dose or discontinuing the offending drug or substituting another medication.

Myoclonus

Myoclonus is a sudden, brief, and irregular contraction of a group of muscles that may occur at rest or with voluntary movement. It can be triggered by muscle activity (positive myoclonus) or cessation of muscle activity (negative myoclonus), and sensory stimulation. Clinically, myoclonus may present as a focal, multifocal, or generalized disorder. Subtypes of focal myoclonus include cortical myoclonus, which typically involves only a few distal, flexor limb muscles; palatal myoclonus, which may be accompanied by ocular, facial, cervical, and laryngeal movement; spinal myoclonus, which results from overactivity of spinal neurons; and peripheral myoclonus, which results from disease of the peripheral nervous system. Posthypoxic action myoclonus is associated with ataxia, dementia, seizures, and postural and gait disturbances and is thought to result from the disruption of inhibitory synapses in the brain stem reticular formation. Myoclonus has been described in human immunodeficiency virus infection (116). Persistent facial myoclonus has been described as a negative prognostic sign in patients with severe brain injury (117).

Unlike the other movement disorders, myoclonus does not appear to be related to abnormalities in the dopaminergic system. Instead, the cholinergic and GABA-ergic systems have been implicated based on therapeutic response to anticholinergic and GABA-enhancing medications (118). Antiepileptic agents (clonazepam, carbamazepine, phenytoin, valproic acid, primidone, piracetam [119], and fluoxetine) may be of benefit in alleviating the disorder. Anticholinergics in particular are helpful in palatal myoclonus. Biofeedback in conjunction with pharmacotherapy may help manage myoclonus secondary to anoxic encephalopathy (120).

Posttraumatic Movement Disorder

The contribution of central and peripheral trauma to the genesis of movement disorders has been suggested through the years (121,122). However, in the absence of unequivocal neuroanatomic and neurochemical correlates, this concept has been challenged because of unclear temporal relationship and lack of correlation between the severity of trauma and resultant movement disorder.

The exact incidence of posttraumatic movement disorders is not known. It appears to be more common after status epilepticus than after anoxic or traumatic brain insult (123). Focal peripheral nerve injuries may result in disruption of afferent input to the spinal cord and secondarily affect higher central nervous centers. Direct structural damage and ischemic and hemorrhagic changes are believed to be involved, along with secondary consequences such as alterations in the various neurochemical systems (124). Delayed sequelae including aberrant ephaptic transmission, inflammatory changes, and central synaptic reorganization all have been implicated, particularly in late-onset movement disorders (125). Progressive movement disorders also may occur after static brain lesions (126). Clinically, posttraumatic movement disorders may be indistinguishable from the various abnormalities described earlier. An interesting condition referred to as dementia pugilistica or punch-drunk syndrome presents with parkinsonian symptoms that result from the cumulative effects of brain injury due to boxing. Tremors, tics, dystonia, chorea, athetosis, ballismus, myoclonus, akathisia, progressive supranuclear palsy, and ataxia all have been described after traumatic brain injury (67,104,124,127–129).

The treatment of posttraumatic movement disorders is largely based on that of movement disorders not due to trauma. These management approaches are described elsewhere in this chapter. It can never be overemphasized that benefits of drug use must be weighed against risks, especially in traumatic brain injury survivors who are more susceptible to the cognitive and sedative side effects of various medications.

Psychogenic Movement Disorders

Psychogenic movement disorders (PMDs) result from various psychiatric conditions. They usually have an acute onset and static course characterized by spontaneous remissions. PMDs are worsened by attention and dampened by distraction. Typically, they are recalcitrant to medications but responsive to placebo.

Up to 9% of neurologic conditions are believed to have no organic basis (130,131). In a retrospective evaluation of 4,470 patients, 405 were found to have psychogenic disorders with motor disorders one of the more common symptoms (130). In another series of 842 patients with movement disorders, 3.3% were diagnosed as having clinically documented PMD (131). This frequency does not differ much from Fahn's report of 2.1% in 3,700 patients with idiopathic movement disorder (132). Common PMDs are tremor, dystonia, myoclonus, tics, chorea, hemiballismus and parkinsonism, and paralysis (133). Associated psychiatric diagnosis (usually depression), precipitating events, and secondary gain were obvious in up to 60% of cases (131).

Diagnosis of PMDs is difficult because many organic conditions lack specific diagnostic features. For instance, up to 52% of patients with idiopathic dystonia were diagnosed as having a psychiatric illness (134,135). To complicate matters further, PMDs also may be superimposed on an organic movement disorder (131,136). When a diagnosis of PMDs is entertained, attempts should be made in making a psychiatric diagnosis even if the diagnosis of PMD is based on neurologic examination. Common psychiatric diagnoses include malingering, somatoform disorder, factitious disorder, depression, and anxiety.

Fahn and Williams proposed a classification of psychogenic dystonia based on the level of diagnostic certainty (137). The four classes are (a) documented, (b) clinically established, (c) probable, and (d) possible. This classification also may be used for PMDs other than dystonia.

Drug-induced Movement Disorders

In determining the etiology of movement disorders, drugs and other substances should be included in the differential diagnosis. Extrapyramidal syndromes including akathisia, parkinsonism, dystonia, tardive dyskinesia, and neuroleptic malignant syndrome are among the most serious side effects of antipsychotic drug therapy and are believed to result from postsynaptic blockade of DA receptors. Acute extrapyramidal syndromes present within a few days after administration of neuroleptics and may persist days after withdrawal of the offending agent. Although considered different manifestations of the same underlying etiology, drug-induced akathisia, dystonia, and parkinsonism have unique distinguishing motor and mental symptoms (138). A less common extrapyramidal reaction to neuroleptics is acute laryngeal dystonia (139).

Tardive dyskinesia characterized by orofacial dyskinesia, dystonia, and choreoathetosis is thought to result from the hypersensitivity of DA receptors in the basal ganglia due to prolonged postsynaptic receptor blockade by neuroleptics. Advanced age, female gender, history of alcohol or substance abuse, diabetes, and smoking, are considered risk factors for tardive dyskinesia in older individuals (140,141). In contrast to tardive dyskinesia, the parkinsonian side effect is thought to arise from blockade of DA receptors in the striatum. In a study of 125 patients with neuroleptic-induced movement disorders, tardive dyskinesia was the most commonly observed abnormality followed by parkinsonism, dystonia, akathisia, and tremor (141).

In addition to neuroleptics, lithium, methyldopa, and metoclopramide (142) may bring about parkinsonism. Choreoathetosis may result from tricyclic antidepressants, oral contraceptives, and amphetamines. Diphenhydramine (143) and flecainide (144) have been implicated in dystonia, and asterixis has been blamed on carbamazepine. Phenytoin may cause choreoathetosis with or without orofacial dyskinesia, possibly by disrupting basal ganglia receptors (145). Tremor may result from administration of MAO inhibitors, tricyclic antidepressants, phenothiazines, lithium, caffeine, amphetamine, valproic acid, felbamate (146), ephedrine, and thyroid replacement drugs. Medications for PD such as levodopa may induce dyskinesias. Cocaine has been implicated in the causation and exacerbation of hyperkinetic disorders (147,148). In one report (149), isoniazid ameliorated levodopa-induced dyskinesias but worsened parkinsonian signs. Table 42-6 lists some drugs encountered in physiatric practice that may induce movement disorders.

Because tardive dyskinesia and the other disorders discussed in this section are iatrogenic, the most logical approach is prevention. This can be performed by using less potent drugs (141) or substituting novel medications with less extrapyramidal side effects such as clozapine (138) and risperidone, discontinuing unnecessary drugs, and prescribing the lowest therapeutic dose possible. Despite discontinuation of the offending drug, tardive dyskinesia may persist. Diphenhydramine is effective in the treatment of acute dystonic spasms. Antiparkinsonian drugs with anticholinergic properties (trihexyphenidyl, benztropine) may be helpful in parkinsonian syndrome, akathisia, and acute dystonia. They have no value in treating neuroleptic malignant syndrome, which may respond to dantrolene and bromocriptine. Propranolol may be useful in treating drug-induced tremor. Valproate-induced tremor may respond to acetazolamide (150).

Rehabilitation of Movement Disorders

A rehabilitation program may not reverse the progressive nature of the disease, but it teaches the patient compensatory mechanisms, helps prevent complications, and enhances the quality of the patient's life. Physiatric intervention is impor-

TABLE 42-6. *Some drugs that may induce movement disorders*

Dopamine antagonists
Haloperidol
Metoclopramide
Dopamine agonists
Levodopa
Antihypertensives
MAO inhibitors
Antiepileptics
Phenytoin
Carbamazepine
Valproic acid
Felbamate
Adrenergic agents
Amphetamines
Methylphenidate
Caffeine
Beta-agonists
Others
Antihistaminics
Tricyclic antidepressants
Buspirone
Lithium
Cimetidine
Oral contraceptives
Cocaine

tant to coordinate an interdisciplinary treatment program to allow the patient to be as functionally independent as possible, and to provide counseling to help the patient and family cope with the illness. Individualized treatment programs are prescribed based on the deficits that predominate in each patient. Guidelines for therapeutic prescriptions for a patient with IPD are listed in Table 42-7 and can be used in other movement disorders.

Medical and Nursing

The goal of medical and nursing intervention is to prevent morbidity due to IPD and other movement disorders. Skin care to prevent bedsores should be emphasized. Hospital beds with head-raising controls are beneficial for severely affected patients. Training in a rocking motion can help the patient rise from a chair, but the patient may ultimately require an electric chair lift.

Monitoring the patient's vital capacity and reinforcing incentive spirometry can help prevent atelectasis and pneumonia. A bowel program for gastrointestinal hypomobility, including the use of bulk-forming agents, stool softeners, and suppositories, may be required. Urologic dysfunction may be evaluated through urodynamic studies. Ditropan is often beneficial for patients with a hyperreflexic bladder. Eye care for lack of blinking is important. For postural hypotension, treatment initially requires the gradual changing of positions and evaluation of the patient's medications, but it may include the need for elastic stockings, an abdominal binder, sodium tablets, and possibly ephedrine and fludrocortisone. Patients with IPD may have poor dietary intake because of their tremor, depression, or dysphagia. A dietary consult may be helpful to monitor nutritional status and to train the patient's family to prepare a soft, high-residue, low-protein diet. A high-protein diet may decrease the patient's responsiveness to DA replacement therapy (151). Sexual dysfunction also should be approached and management individualized to meet the patient's needs (152).

Physical Therapy

The long-term benefit of physical therapy intervention has been controversial. There is a lack of rehabilitative techniques tailored to the pathophysiologic alterations specific to the disease, which in turn limits its effect or even results in negative results. Proprioceptive neuromuscular facilitation (PNF) or Bobath techniques have no therapeutic value. Other studies have shown benefits from continued therapy. Stefaniewski and Bilowit found that movement initiation and speed were improved in patients with IPD after training with sensory cues for 3 weeks (153). Szekely and colleagues, using exercises suggested by the American Parkinson's Disease Association, documented significant improvement in gait (154). Palmer and colleagues showed an improvement in gait, strength, and coordination and a general sense of well-being in patients participating in their exercise program (155). Formisano et al. have shown improvement in functional performance of patients with IPD who were placed on drug therapy and physical therapy consisting of active and passive mobilization exercise, postural control and equilibrium exercises, walking, and prevention of contractures (156). It has been shown that a supervised home exercise program resulted in significant improvement in recent memory, diminution of nausea, improved sucking ability, and less urinary retention and incontinence (157). Yekutiel et al. described a program emphasizing whole body movement and conscious strategies for overcoming obstacles to movement. Patients who participated in this program improved significantly (158). Morris et al. have concluded that regulation of stride length is the fundamental problem in gait hypokinesia and the relative increase in cadence as seen in PD is a compensatory mechanism. It suggests that visual cueing to focus patients' attention on the size of consecutive steps should help patients with PD achieve a more normal stride length (159). Training in a rhythmic pattern to music or with auditory cues such as clapping may help the patient in alternating motions required for activity, encouraging a more automatic pattern.

Handford has recommended that problems caused by the primary symptoms of PD (rigidity, tremor, bradykinesia, and impaired postural reflexes) be differentiated from symptoms caused by the aging process, movement adaptation, and deficits due to side effects of the disease (muscle weakness due to disease and contractures), and a therapeutic plan based on these factors should be developed (160). Gait disturbance in patients with IPD includes freezing when walking and

TABLE 42-7. *Therapeutic plan for patients with Parkinson's disease*

Medical and nursing
- Firm bed to decrease contractures and improve bed mobility
- Gradual changing of positions, elastic stockings, abdominal binder, sodium tablets, and possibly ephedrine and fludrocortisone for orthostasis
- Regular meals with proper diet (low protein); nutritional consultation
- Measure vital capacity and enforce incentive spirometry to prevent atelectasis and pneumonia
- Bowel program for GI hypomobility (stool softeners, bulk-forming agents, cisapride, and suppositories may be required)
- Bladder evaluation and urodynamics; ditropan for hyperreflexic bladder
- Artificial tears for lack of blinking
- Sexual dysfunction evaluation
- Anticholinergic medications before mealtime to help facilitate oral and pharyngeal movements

Physical therapy
- Relaxation techniques to decrease rigidity
- Slow rhythmic rotational movements
- Gentle ROM and stretching exercises to prevent contractures, quadriceps and hip extensor isometric exercises
- Neck and trunk rotation exercises
- Back extension exercises and pelvic tilt
- Proper sitting and postural control (static and dynamic) Emphasize whole body movements
- Breathing exercises stressing both the inspiratory and expiratory phase
- Functional mobility training, including bed mobility, transfer training, and learning to rise out of a chair by rocking; may require a chair lift
- Stationary bicycle to help train reciprocal movements
- Training in rhythmic pattern to music or with auditory cues such as clapping may help in alternating movements
- Standing or balancing in parallel bars (static and dynamic) with weight shifting, ball throwing
- Slowly progressive ambulation training (large steps using blocks to have patients lift legs, teaching proper heel-to-toe gait patterns, feet 12–15 inches apart, armswing; use inverted walking stick, colored squares, or stripes as visual aids)
- Use of assistive devices (may need a weighted walker)
- Aerobic conditioning (swimming, walking, cycling)
- Frequent rest periods
- Family training and home exercise program

Occupational therapy
- ROM activities of upper extremity with stretching
- Fine motor coordination and training, hand dexterity training using colored pegs or beads
- Hand cycling to help train reciprocal movements
- Rocking chair to help with mobilization
- Transfer training
- Safety skills
- Adaptive equipment evaluation, including Velcro closures, raised toilet, grab bars, eating utensils with built-up handles, and key holders
- Family training and home exercise program

Speech
- Deep breathing before talking
- Diaphragmatic breathing exercises
- Swallowing evaluation, including a modified barium swallow as needed; training including icing, supraglottal swallow, vibration of laryngopharyngeal muscles, and chin tuck
- Dysarthria training
- Facial, oral, and lingual muscle exercises

Psychology
- Psychological support
- Patient and family counseling
- Cognitive evaluation
- Group therapy

GI, gastrointestinal; ROM, range of motion.

gait initiation problems due to severe rigidity and poor posture. The treatment plan might include exercises and instructions for standing balance and improved posture and to ensure that the patient is standing on his heels and not on his toes as is seen in IPD festinating gait. Plantar flexion contractures may have to be countered by raising the heels of the shoes (160).

The disability and immobility that occur with IPD can contribute to cardiovascular deconditioning with decreased endurance. Although IPD influences extremity and spine musculature, not all areas are affected equally. Muscular rigidity affects proximally around the shoulders and neck and may spread to the face and extremities.

Turnbull has suggested that an aerobic training program would assist patients with PD in maintaining optimal physical function (161).

Canning et al. recently investigated the effect of respiratory and gait impairments on the exercise capacity of patients with PD. They concluded that mild to moderate patients with PD can maintain their exercise capacity with regular aerobic training despite gait and respiratory impairments (162).

Oxygen consumption (VO_2) and heart rate response to submaximal exercise are increased in patients with IPD when more affected extremities are used. Protas et al. have shown different exercise responses to the upper and lower extremity exercises with mildly involved patients with IPD showing higher metabolic demand for upper extremity exercises when compared with normals, whereas there was no difference in lower extremity exercises between mild IPD and controls. It is suggested that individuals with mild IPD can reach peak exercise using standard exercise testing protocols. Patients with IPD have been shown to have lower efficiency during exercise and need exercise conditioning to all four extremities (163).

The effect of a systemic program of physical therapy consisting of 69 repetitive exercises to improve range of motion, endurance, balance and gait, and fine motor dexterity provided for 1 hour, three times a week, for four consecutive weeks, was reported. Patients significantly improved in rigidity, bradykinesia, and ADL activities. However, no change was noted in action or rest tremor or mentation score. These improvements were not sustained when normal activity was resumed and regular exercises were not performed, suggesting the need for regular physical rehabilitation programs (164).

Relaxation techniques have been shown to be effective in decreasing rigidity (165) with slow, rhythmic rotational movements beginning with passive motion in distal extremities, progressing proximally, and then adding active motion. These activities are better achieved while sitting because rigidity may increase in the supine position. Gentle, prolonged passive stretching and flexibility exercises are used to increase the range of motion of joints, all levels of the spine, and the pectoral and chest wall muscles to prevent debilitating contractures and limitations to breathing.

Once a decrease in rigidity is achieved through relaxation, functional activity training can be initiated. This includes bed mobility, transfer training, and learning to rise from a chair. Postural control, including stabilization, balancing activities, and weight shifting to counter changes in the center of gravity and to elicit normal righting reflexes, is followed by progressive ambulation training. A tilt table may be required if the patient is orthostatic.

The patients are trained to walk with proper posture, look up, widen the base of the gait (i.e., feet 12 to 15 inches apart), use a high-step gait pattern (at times walking over boxes), and take long strides. Arm swinging is encouraged. Changes in direction, movement patterns, stopping, and starting are stressed. Lack of coordination may preclude the safe use of assistive devices because some patients tend to carry a cane rather than using it for balancing. For those patients who tend to fall backward, a cane may increase this posteriorly directed force. Rolling walkers may increase the festinating gait pattern.

PD leads to a breakdown in the execution of practiced skilled movement such as walking and handwriting. However, with practice patients with PD can improve their motor performance but they need more practice than controls (166).

The breakdown of movement control in IPD is related to alterations in the functional capacity of the basal ganglia and their major output regions, namely the premotor areas. The motor area in the medial wall of the frontal lobe drives internally willed movement, whereas those in the lateral wall regulate externally (sensory) cued movements. A PET study showed that in patients with IPD who had difficulty initiating movements, the medial wall motor areas failed to be activated when the patient performed free selection tasks. However, the patient with IPD can perform fluent movements in response to visual stimuli, and motor performance may suddenly decline if visual aids are removed. Stripes or rods stuck to the floor can be used to improve stride length. Inverted walking stick may be used to overcome akinetic freezing (167).

Sensory-enhanced physiotherapy consisting of execution of different tasks was coupled with sensory reinforcement (e.g., patients had to place their feet on colored squares or foot prints painted on the floor). Finger dexterity was improved by having patients assemble figures using colored pegs or string colored beads with different sized holes. Sensory-enhanced physiotherapy produced retained motor skills and increased abilities in ADLs, suggesting that motor learning is still possible in patients with IPD (168).

Corcos et al. have shown that withdrawal of antiparkinsonian medication produces muscle weakness, especially in extensor muscles in IPD. The cause of this weakness in due to reduced agonist muscle activation, resulting in increase in relaxation time. The phasic EMG burst is reduced in patients with IPD off medication. It is suggested that many patients with IPD may benefit from exercise programs designed to increase both muscle strength and muscle power (169).

An exercise bike, pulleys, and hand cycle can be used to achieve reciprocal motion and maintain mobility of the arms and legs. A general aerobic conditioning exercise program, including walking, swimming, and cycling, as well as coordination exercises (i.e., Frenkel's) also can be prescribed. These patients require frequent rest periods, and fatigue should be avoided. A home exercise program graded to the individual's capability and the training of family members are extremely important.

Occupational Therapy

Occupational therapy goals are similar to physical therapy goals. Fine motor upper extremity coordination is emphasized (170). ADL evaluation is crucial to allow maintenance of independence in self-care skills. The treatment for bed mobility might include trunk mobilization exercises, providing grab rails, firm mattresses, and loose bed clothes. Adaptive equipment for eating, built-up handles for hygiene, the use of Velcro closures rather than buttons, and bathroom equipment (e.g., grab bars, raised toilet seat) will assist the patient in basic self-care activities. Training in handwriting skills may influence vocational tasks.

There is a tendency for the patient to assume an ulnar deviated position with flexion at the metacarpophalangeal joints (i.e., striatal hand) and extension at the interphalangeal joints, resulting in reduced finger flexion. Specific exercises and positioning can help improve posture and retard the development of deformities. Radial neuropathy has been described in patients with IPD secondary to a combination of bradykinesia and improper positioning (171).

Patients with complaints of dysphagia or with a history of pneumonia should have a modified barium swallow to help identify the specific nature of their dysfunction. Treatment strategies can help prevent silent aspiration and decrease morbidity (22). Supraglottal swallow, vibration of laryngopharyngeal muscles, and chin tuck maneuvers can help protect the airway and prevent aspiration. Tongue exercises may improve chewing and swallowing (23). Eating smaller portions with proper textures and consistencies of food also can be helpful. Administration of medications before mealtime will help facilitate oral and pharyngeal movements.

Speech

The speech pathologist can train the patient in facial exercises (e.g., a series of alternating facial expressions including grimacing, frowning, smiling, blowing) to improve the masked faces. Smith et al. have shown that intensive speech therapy focusing on phonatory effort improves adduction of the vocal folds, which may help improve functional communication in patients with IPD (172).

Psychotherapy

Psychological support and counseling for the patient and family are an integral part of the treatment program (173). Antidepressant medications may be indicated. Depression should be considered when a sudden worsening of symptomatology occurs with little change in the physical examination. Cognitive evaluation may be required in some patients as the disease progresses. Patients with PD seem to perform better in group settings. This setting may help diminish the depression and lack of initiative often shown, as well as to serve as an extra support system for these patients. Family involvement is extremely important to help manage the patient and cope with the chronic progressive nature of the disease.

An example of a case history and management of the patient with IPD will provide a blueprint for management of all movement disorders discussed in this chapter.

CASE HISTORY AND MANAGEMENT OF A PATIENT WITH IPD

A 64-year-old banker developed difficulty in swallowing and speech in September 1990. A change in gait also was noted. He reported earlier episodes of drooling and voice changes. He had no tremor. His family history was significant in that his father had developed IPD in his 70s. He also had no tremor but had difficulty with speech and balance (174).

A diagnosis of early IPD was made, and the patient was placed on selegiline hydrochloride and levodopa/carbidopa. In June 1992, the patient was employed full time but had a low-volume voice and some decrease in cognitive function. He noted increasing pain in both shoulders with decreasing range, requiring surgery for bilateral rotator cuff tears in 1994. The patient retired after this surgery due to increasing disabling symptoms. At this time, he had drooling, decreased voice amplitudes, and some akinesia, and he had suffered several falls. He had restrictions of range of motion of both shoulders, hips, and knees and needed assistance in activities of daily living. He became depressed.

Medications were adjusted to levodopa/carbidopa 25/100 mg twice a day, selegiline hydrochloride 2.5 mg at 7 a.m. and 3 p.m., and sertraline hydrochloride 50 mg daily.

He was seen by a physiatrist, and a therapeutic plan was developed (2) (Table 42-7).

OTHER THERAPEUTIC INTERVENTIONS

Botulinum Toxin Injection

Local intramuscular injection of botulinum toxin is arguably the most important advancement in the nonsurgical management of dystonia and various movement disorders. The neurotoxin, derived from *Clostridium botulinum* serotype A, blocks neuromuscular transmission by inhibiting the release of acetylcholine, but not its synthesis or storage. Injected intramuscularly, the toxin results in partial denervation. Clinical effects are seen 24 to 72 hours after injection, and peak effects occur 4 to 6 weeks later, and the average duration of effect is 3 to 4 months. Injections are guided by surface anatomy, electromyography or electrical stimulation. The recommended maximum dose per session is 400 units. Early indications for treatment were blepharospasm and strabismus. Over the years, more disorders have been found to be successfully managed by this technique. Among these are the various dystonias and facial synkinesis complicating recovery from facial paralysis (175–180). Because it affects neuromuscular transmission, the toxin is contraindicated in disorders of neuromuscular junction such as myasthenia gravis and myasthenic syndrome. Possible adverse effects include excessive weakness in the injected and adjacent muscles. Flulike symptoms and allergic reactions have been described, but these have rarely occurred in our experience. Since the clinical effects wear off in 3 to 4 months, reinjection may be necessary. Readministration of the toxin within 3 months of the previous injection is discouraged in order to avoid potential development of antibodies.

Intrathecal Baclofen

Intrathecal baclofen has been found to be helpful in alleviating focal limb (181) and axial (182) dystonia. Although it is a neurosurgical procedure, physiatrists may participate in screening patients with movement disorders who may benefit from this procedure. Trained physiatrists also play a critical role in postimplantation rehabilitation care by monitoring response and complications and prescribing appropriate therapy interventions. This procedure is an alternative when oral medications are ineffective and their side effects are intolerable or when the severity of the condition requires more than the recommended dose of botulinum toxin. Patients who respond to a trial dose of baclofen are considered for surgical implantation of the infusion system. The pump with the drug reservoir is placed in the abdominal wall and connected to a catheter that has been introduced into the intrathecal space, usually at the lower thoracic level. An external programmer adjusts the dose, rate, and mode of drug delivery by radiotelemetry. The drug reservoir can be refilled through transcutaneous insertion of a Huber-type needle into the reservoir port.

Simple dose titration and safe concurrent use with oral medications and local botulinum toxin are among the advantages of intrathecal baclofen. Common adverse effects include drowsiness, weakness, and dizziness, which subside with dose reduction. Pump-related problems include catheter kinks, dislodgement, or disconnection, which are corrected surgically. Although it has been shown to be effective in various movement disorders (181,182), its efficacy has not been compared against oral medications, botulinum toxin, and other neurosurgical techniques.

Surgical Treatment

Although not considered part of the initial management of movement disorders, neurosurgical procedures have long been performed to alleviate these symptoms. Initially, rhizotomy, neurectomy, and myelotomy were used for spasticity, and stereotactic surgery was performed to treat Huntington's chorea. Later, other techniques were developed, including brain and spinal cord stimulator implantation. Currently, stereotactic and nonstereotactic procedures are being used to manage various movement disorders, including thalamotomy and pallidotomy.

Surgery is not considered for hemiballismus until it has stabilized for 2 to 3 months because this disorder is usually self-limited. Stereotactic thalamotomy and chronic thalamic stimulation should be considered in persistent cases and in those instances when ballism is violent and endangers the patient (68,183,184). Other conditions that may benefit from thalamotomy include dystonia musculorum deformans, Huntington's chorea, choreoathetosis, myoclonus, essential tremor, cerebellar tremor, writer's cramp, and PD (184–186). Caudatomy using a gamma knife is sometimes performed to reduce bradykinesia in PD (187).

Pallidotomy involves lesioning the anterodorsal globus pallidus and has not been of benefit in relieving the symptoms of PD, especially bradykinesia (186). Spinal cord stimulation may be used for spasticity and spasmodic torticollis and cerebellar stimulation for choreoathetosis. Success with chronic electrical stimulation of the ventralis intermedius nucleus of the thalamus in treating essential tremor has been described (186). In PD this procedure improved only tremor, not rigidity or bradykinesia. Other neurosurgical procedures include facial nerve decompression in hemifacial spasm, and rhizotomy and neurectomy for spasticity and spasmodic torticollis (188). Transplantation of fetal mesencephalic cells into the striatum (caudate nucleus and globus pallidus) is sometimes performed with the hope that transplants might synthesize and release DA within the striatum) (189).

REFERENCES

1. Carpenter MB, Sutin J. *Human neuroanatomy.* 8th ed. Baltimore: Williams & Wilkins, 1982.
2. Jain SS, Kirshblum SC. Movement disorders including tremors. In: DeLisa JA, Gans B, eds. *Rehabilitation medicine: principles and practice.* 2nd ed. Philadelphia: JB Lippincott, 1993; 700–713.
3. Chokroverty S. An approach to a patient with disorders of voluntary movements. In: Chokroverty S, ed. *Movement disorders.* Costa Mesa, CA: PMA Publishing Corporation, 1990; 1–43.
4. Weiner WJ, Lang AE. *Movement disorders: a comprehensive survey.* Mt. Kisco, NY: Futura Publishing, 1989; 1–22.
5. Hornykiewicz O. Metabolism of brain dopamine in human parkinsonism: neurochemical and clinical aspects. In: Costa E, Cote LT, Yahr MD, eds. *Biochemistry and pharmacology of the basal ganglia.* Hewlett, NY: Raven, 1966; 171–181.
6. Neafsey EJ, Hull CD, Buchwald NA. Preparation for movement in the cat. I: unit activity in the cerebral cortex. *Electroencephalogr Clin Neurophysiol* 1978; 44:706–713.
7. Neafsey EJ, Hull CD, Buchwald NA. Preparation for movement in the cat. II: unit activity in the basal ganglia and thalamus. *Electroencephalogr Clin Neurophysiol* 1978; 44:714–723.
8. Melnick ME, Hull CD, Buchwald NA. Activity of forebrain neurons during alternating movements in cats. *Electroencephalogr Clin Neurophysiol* 1984; 57:57–68.
9. Teuber HL. Complex functions of basal ganglia. In: Yahr MD, ed. *The basal ganglia.* New York: Raven, 1976; 151–168.
10. DeLong MR, Georgopoulos AP. Motor functions in the basal ganglia. In: Mountcastle VB, Brookhart JM, eds. *Handbook of physiology.* Section 1: Nervous system. Vol. II. Motor control, Part 2. Bethesda, MD: American Physiological Society, 1981; 1017–1061.
11. Oberg RGE, Divac E. Cognitive functions of the neostriatum. In: Divac I, Oberg RGE, eds. *Neostriatum.* Oxford, England: Pergamon, 1979; 291–313.
12. Parkinson J. *An essay on the shaking palsy.* London: Sherwood, Nealy & Jones, 1817.
13. Koller W. *Handbook of Parkinson's disease: diagnosis and treatment for practicing physicians.* New York: Marcel Dekker, 1987.
14. Marsden CD. Parkinson's disease. *J Neurol Neurosurg Psychiatry* 1994; 57:672–681.
15. Bennett DA, Beckett LA, Murray AM, et al. Prevalence of parkinsonian signs and associated mortality in a community population of older people. *N Engl J Med* 1996; 334:71–76.
16. Shahani BT, Young RR. Clinical electromyography. In: Baker AB, Joynt R, eds. *Clinical neurology.* Philadelphia: JB Lippincott, 1985; 39–47.
17. Lance JW, Schwab RS, Peterson EA. Action tremor and the cogwheel phenomenon in Parkinson's disease. *Brain* 1963; 86:95–110.
18. Milner-Brown HS, Fisher MA, Weiner WJ. Electrical properties of motor units in parkinsonism and a possible relationship with bradykinesia. *J Neurol Neurosurg Psychiatry* 1979; 42:35–41.
19. Cedarbaum JM, McDowell FH. Sixteen-year follow-up of 100 patients begun on levodopa in 1968: emerging problem. *Adv Neurol* 1987; 45:469–472.
20. Stern Y, Mayeux R, Rosen J, Ilson J. Perceptual mode dysfunction in Parkinson's disease, a deficit in sequential and predictive voluntary movement. *J Neurol Neurosurg Psychiatry* 1983; 46:145–151.
21. Mortimer JA, Pirozzolo FJ, Hansch EC, Webster DD. Relationship of motor symptoms to intellectual deficits in Parkinson disease. *Neurology* 1982; 32:133–137.
22. Bushmann M, Dobmeyer SM, Leeker L, Perlmutter JS. Swallowing abnormalities and their response to treatment in Parkinson's disease. *Neurology* 1989; 39:1309–1314.
23. Logemann JA, Blonsky ER, Boshes B. Lingual control in Parkinson's disease. *Trans Am Neurol Assoc* 1973; 98:276–278.
24. DeMichele G, Filla A, Volpe G, Gogliettino A, Ambrosio G, Campanella G. Etiology of Parkinson's disease. The role of environment and heredity. *Adv Neurol* 1996; 69:19–24.
25. Tanner CM, Langston JW. Do environmental factors cause Parkinson's disease? A critical review. *Neurology* 990; 40:17–30.
26. Jenner P, Schapira AH, Marsden CD. New insights into the cause of Parkinson's disease. *Neurology* 992; 42:2241–2250.
27. Kessler II, Diamond EL. Epidemiologic studies of Parkinson's disease. I. Smoking and Parkinson's disease: a survey and explanatory hypothesis. *Am J Epidemiol* 1978; 94:16–25.
28. Logroscino G, Marder K, Cote L, Tang MX, Shea S, Mayeux R. Dietary lipids and antioxidants in Parkinson's disease: a population-based, case-control study. *Ann Neurol* 1996; 39:89–94.
29. Olanow CM. Mechanism of cell death in Parkinson's disease. *J Neurol Transm Suppl* 1993; 91:161–180.
30. Bethlem J, Den Hartog Jager WA. The incidence and characteristics of Lewy bodies in idiopathic paralysis agitans (Parkinson's disease). *J Neurol Neurosurg Psychiatry* 1960; 23:74–80.
31. Riley D, Lang AE, Blair RDG, Birnbaum A, Reid B. Frozen shoulder

and other shoulder disturbances in Parkinson's disease. *J Neurol Neurosurg Psychiatry* 1989; 52:63–66.
32. Barbeau A, Roy M. Familial subsets in idiopathic Parkinson's disease. *Can J Neurol Sci* 1984; 11:144–150.
33. Sabate M, Rodriguez M, Mendez E, Enriquez E, Gonzalez I. Obstructive and restrictive pulmonary dysfunction increases disability in Parkinson's disease. *Arch Phys Med Rehabil* 1996; 77:29.
34. Schenkman M, Butler RB. A model for multisystem evaluation treatment of individuals with Parkinson's disease. *Physical Therapy* 1989; 69:932–943.
35. Shinotoh H, Calne DB. The use of PET in Parkinson's disease. *Brain Cogn* 1995; 28:297–310.
36. Snow BJ. Fluorodopa PET scanning in Parkinson's disease. *Adv Neurol* 1996; 69:449–457.
37. Pollock M, Hornabrook RW. The prevalence, natural history and dementia of Parkinson's disease. *Brain* 1966; 89:429–449.
38. Marttila RJ, Rinne UK. Disability and progression in Parkinson's disease. *Acta Neurol Scand* 1977; 56:159–169.
39. Hoehn MH, Yahr MD. Parkinsonism: onset, progression and mortality. *Neurology* 1967; 17:427–442.
40. Posey WC (cited in Jankovic J). Progressive supranuclear palsy: clinical and pharmacologic update. *Neurol Clin* 1984; 2:473–486.
41. Troost BT, Daroff RB. The ocular motor defects in progressive supranuclear palsy. *Ann Neurol* 1977; 2:397–403.
42. Sosner J, Wall GC, Sznajder J. Progressive supranuclear palsy; clinical presentation and rehabilitation of two patients. *Arch Phys Med Rehabil* 1993; 74:537–539.
43. Cederbaum JM, Gandy SE, McDowell FH. ''Early'' initiation of levodopa treatment does not promote the development of motor response fluctuations, dyskinesias, or dementia in Parkinson's disease. *Neurology* 1991; 41:622–629.
44. Lesser RP, Fahn S, Snider SR, Cote LJ, Isgreen WP, Barrett RE. Analysis of the clinical problems in parkinsonism and the complications of long-term levodopa therapy. *Neurology* 1979; 29:1253–1260.
45. DiRocco A, Molinari SP, Kollmeier D, Yahr MD. Parkinson's disease: progression and mortality in L-DOPA era. *Adv Neurol* 1996; 69:3–11.
46. Lieberman A. Dopamine agonists: new perspectives and trends. *Clin Neurol* 1988; 4:1–19.
47. Rinne UK. Combined bromocriptine-levodopa therapy early in Parkinson's disease. *Neurology* 1985; 35:1196–1198.
48. The Parkinson's Study Group. Effect of deprenyl on the progression of disability in early Parkinson's disease. *N Engl J Med* 1989; 321: 1364–1371.
49. Rinne JD, Roytta M, Paljarvi L, Rummukainen J, Rinne U. Selegiline (deprenyl) treatment and death of nigral neurons in Parkinson's disease. *Neurology* 1991; 41:859–861.
50. Tatton WG, Ju WYH, Wadia J, Tatton NA. Reduction of neuronal apoptosis by small molecules, promises for new approaches to neurological therapy. In: Olanow CM, Jenner P, Yondin MHB, eds. *Neurodegeneration and prospects of neuroprotection.* London: Academic (in press).
51. Lefebre H, Noblet C, Moore N, Wolf LM. Pseudo-phaeochromocytoma after multiple drug interactions involving the selective monoamine inhibitor selegiline. *Clin Endocrinol* 1995; 42:95–99.
52. Vonsattel JP, Myers RH, Stevens TJ, et al. Neuropathological classification of Huntington's disease. *J Neuropathol Exp Neurol* 1985; 44: 559–577.
53. McGeer PL, McGeer EG, Itagaki S, Mizukawa K. Anatomy and pathology of the basal ganglia. *Can J Neurol Sci* 1987; 14:363–372.
54. Dewey RB Jr, Jankovic J. Hemiballism-hemichorea. Clinical and pharmacologic findings in 21 patients. *Arch Neurol* 1989; 46: 862–867.
55. Adams RD, Victor M. *Principles of neurology*, 5th ed. New York: McGraw-Hill, 1993.
56. Shulman LM, Weiner WJ. Paroxysmal movement disorders. *Semin Neurol* 1995; 15:188–193.
57. Shoulson I. Huntington's disease: a decade of progress. *Neurol Clin* 1984; 2:515–526.
58. Gusella JF. Genetic linkage of the Huntington's disease gene to a DNA marker. *Can Neurol Sci* 1984; 11:421–425.
59. McDowell F, Cedarbaum J. The extrapyramidal system and disorders of movement. In: Joynt RJ, ed. *Clinical neurology*. Vol. 3. Philadelphia: Lippincott–Raven, 1991; 1–120.
60. Ranen NG, Peyser CE, Folstein SE. *A physician's guide to the management of Huntington's disease: pharmacologic and non-pharmacologic interventions.* New York: Huntington's Disease Society of America, 1993.
61. Provenzale JM, Glass JP. Hemiballisumus: CT and MR findings. *Comput Assist Tomogr* 1995; 19:537–540.
62. DeLong MR. Primate models of movement disorders of basal ganglia origin. *Trends Neurosci* 1990; 13:281–285.
63. Biary N, Singh B, Bahou Y, et al. Posttraumatic paroxysmal nocturnal hemidystonia. *Mov Disord* 1993; 1:98–99.
64. Lietz TE, Huff JS. Hemiballismus as a presenting sign of hyperglycemia. *Am J Emerg Med* 1995; 13:647–648.
65. Jankovic J, Fahn S. Dystonic disorders. In: Jankovic J, Tolosa E, ed. *Parkinson's disease and movement disorders*, 2nd ed. Baltimore: Williams & Wilkins, 1993; 337–374.
66. Robin JJ. Paroxysmal choreoathetosis following head injury. *Ann Neurol* 1977; 2:447–448.
67. Kant R, Zeiler D. Hemiballismus following closed head injury. *Brain Injury* 1996; 10:155–158.
68. Levesque MF, Markham C, Nakasato N. MR-guided ventral intermediate thalamotomy for posttraumatic hemiballismus. *Stereotact Funct Neurosurg* 1992; 58:88.
69. Marsden CD, Rothwell JC. The physiology of idiopathic dystonia. *Can J Neurol Sci* 1987; 14:521–527.
70. Obeso JA, Gimenez-Roldan S. Clinicopathological correlation in symptomatic dystonia. *Adv Neurol* 1988; 50:113–122.
71. Lee MS, Marsden CD. Movement disorders following lesions of the thalamus or subthalamic region. *Mov Disord* 1994; 9:493–507.
72. Sandyk R, Bamford CR. The hypothalamus in dystonic movement disorders. *Int J Neurosci* 1988; 40:41–44.
73. Lee LV, Kupke KG, Caballar-Gonzaga F, Hebron-Ortiz M, Muller U. The phenotype of X-linked dystonia-parkinsonism syndrome. An assessment of 42 cases in the Philippines. *Medicine* 1991; 70: 179–187.
74. Jankovic J. Cranial-cervical dyskinesias: an overview. *Adv Neurol* 1988; 49:1–13.
75. Jankovic J, Orman J. Botulinum A toxin for cranial-cervical dystonia: a double-blind, placebo-controlled study. *Neurology* 1987; 37: 616–623.
76. Blitzer A, Brin MF, Greene PE, Fahn, S. Botulinum toxin injection for the treatment of oromandibular dystonia. *Ann Otol Rhinol Laryngol* 1989; 98:93–97
77. Jankovic J, Ford J. Blepharospasm and orofacial-cervical dystonia: clinical and pharmacological findings in 100 patients. *Ann Neurol* 1983; 13:402–411.
78. Auger RG, Piepgras DG, Laws ER, Jr. Hemifacial spasm: results of microvascular decompression of the facial nerve in 54 patients. *Mayo Clin Proc* 1986; 61:640–644.
79. Weiner WJ, Lang AE. *Movement disorders: a comprehensive review.* New York: Futura, 1989; 391–418.
80. Rondot P, Marchand MP, Dellatolas G. Spasmodic torticollis—review of 220 patients. *Can J Neurol Sci* 1991; 18:143–151.
81. Chan J, Brin MF Fahn S. Idiopathic cervical dystonia: clinical characteristics. *Mov Disord* 1991; 6:119–126.
82. Jankovic J, Leder S, Warner D, Schwartz K. Cervical dystonia: clinical findings and associated movement disorders. *Neurology* 1991; 41: 1088–1091.
83. Huygen PL, Verhagen WI, Van Hoof JJ Horetink MW. Vestibular hyperractivity in patients with idiopathic spasmodic torticollis. *J Neurol Neurosurg Psychiatry* 1989; 52:782–785.
84. Rothwell JC, Obeso JA, Day BL, Marsden CD. Pathophysiology of dystonias. *Adv Neurol* 1983; 39:851–863.
85. Hornykiewicz O, Kish SJ, Becker LE, Farley I, Shannak K. Biochemical evidence for brain neurotransmitter changes in idiopathic torsion dystonia (dystonia musculorum deformans). *Adv Neurol* 1988; 50: 157–165.
86. Tolosa E, Montserrat L, Bayes A. Blink reflex studies in focal dystonias: enhanced excitability of brainstem interneurons in cranial dystonia and spasmodic torticollis. *Mov Disord* 1988; 3:61–69.
87. Jankovic J, Van der Linden C. Dystonia and tremor induced by peripheral trauma: predisposing factors. *J Neurol Neurosurg Psychiatry* 1988; 51:1512–1519.
88. Lowenstein DH, Aminoff MJ. The clinical course of spasmodic torticollis. *Neurology* 1988; 38:530–532.

89. Camicioli R. Movement disorders in geriatric rehabilitation. *Clin Geriatr Med* 1993; 9:756–781.
90. Jankovic J, Shale H. Dystonia in musicians. *Semin Neurol* 1989; 9: 131–135.
91. Hunter D. *The diseases of occupations*. London: Hodder & Stoughton, 1978.
92. LeWitt PA, Burns RS, Newman RP. Dystonia in untreated parkinsonism. *Clin Neuropharmacol* 1986; 9:293–297.
93. Sandyk R. Treatment of writer s cramp with sodium valproate and baclofen. A case report. *S Afr Med J* 1983; 63:702–703.
94. Seibel MO, Date ES, Zeiner H, Schwartz M. Rehabilitation of patients with Hallervorden-Spatz syndrome. *Arch Phys Med Rehabil* 1993; 74:328–329.
95. Truong DD, Sandroni P, van der Noort s, Matsumoto RR. Diphenhydramine is effective in the treatment of idiopathic dystonia. *Arch Neurol* 1995; 52:405–407.
96. Jankovic J. Botulinum toxin in the treatment of dystonic tics. *Mov Disord* 1994; 9:347–349.
97. Findley LJ. Tremors: differential diagnosis and pharmacology. In: Jankovic J, Tolosa E, eds. *Parkinson's disease and movement disorders*, 2nd ed. Baltimore: Williams & Wilkins, 1993; 293–313.
98. Jankovic J, Fahn S. Physiologic and pathologic tremors. Diagnosis, mechanism, and management. *Ann Intern Med* 1980; 93:460–465.
99. Tranchant C, Bhatia KP, Marsden CD. Movement disorders in multiple sclerosis. *Mov Disord* 1995; 10:418–423.
100. Lou JS, Jankovic J. Essential tremors: clinical correlates in 350 patients. *Neurology* 1991; 41:234–238.
101. Trelles L, Trelles JL, Castro C, Altamirano J, Benzaquen M. Successful treatment of two cases of intention tremor with clonazepam [Letter]. *Ann Neurol* 1984; 16:621.
102. Muenter MD, Daube JR, Caviness JN, Miller PM. Treatment of essential tremor with methazolamide. *Mayo Clin Proc* 1991; 66:991–997.
103. Sechi GP, Zuddas M, Piredda M, et al. Treatment of cerebellar tremors with carbamazepine: a controlled trial with long-term follow-up. *Neurology* 1989; 39:1113–1115.
104. Ivanhoe CB, Bontke CF. Movement disorders after traumatic brain injury. In: Horn L, Zasler ND, eds. *Medical rehabilitation of traumatic brain injury*. Philadelphia: Hanley-Belfus, 1995; 395–410.
105. Jankovic J, Schwartz K. Botulinum toxin treatment of tremors. *Neurology* 1991; 41:1185–1188.
106. Lundervold DA, Poppen R. Biobehavioral rehabilitation for older adults with essential tremor. *Gerontologist* 1995; 35:556–559.
107. Lees AJ, Tolosa E. Tics. In: Jankovic J, Tolosa E, eds. *Parkinson's disease and movement disorders*, 2nd ed. Baltimore: Williams & Wilkins, 1993; 329–335.
108. Koller WC, Wong GF, Lang A. Posttraumatic movement disorders: a review. *Mov Disord* 1989; 4:20–36.
109. Lewis MH, Bodfish JW, Powell SB, Golden RN. Clomipramine treatment for stereotypy and related repetitive movement disorders associated with mental retardation. *Am J Ment Retard* 1995; 100:299–312.
110. Stewart JT. Akathisia following traumatic brain injury: treatment with bromocriptine [Letter]. *J Neurol Neurosurg Psychiatry* 1989; 52: 1200–1201.
111. Borison RL. Amantadine in the management of extrapyramidal side effects. *Clin Neuropharmacol* 1983; 6(suppl 1):57–63.
112. Adler L, Angrist B, Peselow E, et al. A controlled assessment of propranolol in the treatment of neuroleptic-induced akathisia. *Br J Psychiatry* 1986; 149:42–45.
113. Lipinski JF, Zubenko GS, Barreira P, Cohen BN. Propranolol in the treatment of neuroleptic-induced akathisia. *Lancet* 1983; 2:685–686.
114. Kabes J, Sikora J, Pisvejc J, et al. Effect of piracetam on extrapyramidal side effects induced by neuroleptic drugs. *Int Pharmacopsychiatry* 1982; 17:185–192.
115. Wirshing WC, Phelan CK, Van Putten T, Marder SP, Engel J. Effects of clozapine on treatment-resistant akathisia and concomitant tardive dyskinesia [Letter]. *J Clin Psychopharmacol* 1990; 10:371–373.
116. Nath A, Jankovic J, Pettigrew LC. Movement disorders and AIDS. *Neurology* 1987; 37:37–41.
117. Sandel ME, O Dell MW. Persistent facial myoclonus: a negative prognostic sign in patients with severe brain injury. *Arch Phys Med Rehabil* 1993; 74:411–415.
118. Fahn S. Newer drugs for posthypoxic action myoclonus: observations from a well-studied case. In: Fahn S, Marsden CD, Van Woert M, eds. *Myoclonus*. New York: Raven, 1986; 197–199.
119. Obeso JA, Artieda J, Quinn N, et al. Piracetam in the treatment of different types of myoclonus. *Clin Neuropharmacol* 1988; 11: 529–536.
120. Duckett S, Kramer T. Managing myoclonus secondary to anoxic encephalopathy through EMG biofeedback. *Brain Inj* 1994; 8:185–188.
121. Haley SM, Cioffi MI, Lewin JE, Baryza MJ. Motor dysfunction in children and adolescents after traumatic brain injury. *J Head Trauma Rehabil* 1990; 5:77–90.
122. Schott GD. Induction of involuntary movements by peripheral trauma: an analogy with causalgia. *Lancet* 1986; 2:712–716.
123. Fowler WE, Kriel RL, Krach LE. Movement disorders after status epilepticus and other brain injuries. *Pediatr Neurol* 1992; 8:281–284.
124. Sandyk R, Iacono RP, Fisher H. Posttraumatic cerebellar syndrome: response to l-tryptophan. *Int J Neurosci* 1989; 47:301–302.
125. Anonymous. Trauma and dystonia. *Lancet* 1989; 1:759–760.
126. Scott BL, Jankovic J. Delayed-onset progressive movement disorders after static brain lesions. *Neurology* 1996; 46:68–74.
127. Katz DI. Movement disorders following traumatic head injury. J. *Head Trauma Rehabil* 1990; 5:86–90.
128. Goetz CG, Pappert EJ. Trauma and movement disorders. *Neurol Clin* 1992; 10:907–919.
129. Jankovic J. Post-traumatic movement disorders: central and peripheral mechanisms. *Neurology* 1994; 44:2006–2014.
130. Lempert T, Dieterich M, Huppert D, Brandt T. Psychogenic disorders in neurology: frequency and clinical spectrum. *Acta Neurol Scand* 1990; 82:335–340.
131. Factor SA, Podskalny GD, Molho ES. Psychogenic movement disorders: frequency, clinical profile, and characteristics. *J Neurol Neurosurg Psychiatry* 1995; 59:406–412.
132. Fahn S. Psychogenic movement disorders. In: Marsden CD, Fahn S, eds. *Movement disorders*. Oxford, England: Butterworth-Heinemann, 1994; 359–372.
133. Marjama J, Troster AI, Koller WC. Psychogenic movement disorders. *Neurol Clin* 1995; 13:283–297.
134. Cooper IS, Cullinan T, Riklan M. The natural history of dystonia. *Adv Neurol* 1976; 14:157–169.
135. Eldridge R, Tiklan M, Cooper IS. The limited role of psychotherapy in torsion dystonia: experience with 44 cases. *JAMA* 1969; 210:705–708.
136. Ranawaya R, Riley D, Lang A. Psychogenic dyskinesias with organic movement disorders. *Mov Disord* 1990; 5:127–133.
137. Fahn S, Williams D. Psychogenic dystonia. *Adv Neurol* 1988; 50: 431–455.
138. Casey DE. Motor and mental aspects of acute extra pyramidal syndromes. *Acta Psychiatr Scand Suppl* 1994; 380:14–20.
139. Koek RJ, Pi EH. Acute laryngeal dystonic reactions to neuroleptics. *Psychosomatics* 1989; 30:359–364.
140. Jeste DV, Caligiuri MP, Paulsen JS, et al. Risk of tardive dyskinesia in older patients: a prospective longitudinal study of 266 outpatients. *Arch Gen Psychiatry* 1995; 52:756–765.
141. Miller LG, Jankovic J. Neurologic approach to drug-induced movement disorders: a study of 125 patients. *South Med J* 1990; 83: 525–532.
142. Miller LG Jankovic J. Metoclopramide-induced movement disorders. Clinical findings with a review of the literature. *Arch Intern Med* 1989; 149:2486–2492.
143. Santora J, Rozek S, Samie MR. Diphenhydramine-induced dystonia [Letter]. *Clin Pharm* 1989; 8:471
144. Miller LG, Jankovic J. Persistent dystonia probably induced by flecainide. *Mov Disord* 1992; 7:62–63
145. Harrison MB, Lyons GR, Landow ER. Phenytoin and dyskinesias: a report of two cases and review of the literature. *Mov Disord* 1993; 8:19–27.
146. Kerrick JM, Kelley BJ, Maister BH, Graves NM, Leppik IE. Involuntary movement disorders associated with felbamate. *Neurology* 1995; 45:185–187.
147. Merab J. Acute dystonic reaction to cocaine [Letter]. *Am J Med* 1988; 84:564.
148. Cardoso FE, Jankovic J. Cocaine-related movement disorders. *Mov Disord* 1993; 8:175–178.
149. Gershanik OS, Luquin MR, Scipioni O, Obeso JA. Isoniazid therapy in Parkinson's disease. *Mov Disord* 1988; 3:133–139.
150. Lancman ME, Asconape JJ, Walker F. Acetazolamide appears effective in the management of valproate-induced tremor [Letter]. *Mov Disord* 1994; 9:369.

151. Cotzias GC. Protein intake in treatment of Parkinson's disease with levodopa. *N Engl J Med* 1975; 292:181–184.
152. Brown RG, Jahanshahi M, Quinn N, Marsden CD. Sexual function in patients with Parkinson's disease and their partners. *J Neurol Neurosurg Psychiatry* 1990; 53:480–486.
153. Stefaniwsky L, Bilowit DS. Parkinsonism: facilitation of motion by sensory stimulation. *Arch Phys Med Rehabil* 1973; 54:75–90.
154. Szekely BC, Kosanovich NN, Sheppard W. Adjunctive treatment in Parkinson's disease: physical therapy and comprehensive group therapy. *Rehabil Lit* 1982; 43:72–76.
155. Palmer SS, Mortimer JA, Webster DD, Bistevins R, Dickinson GL. Exercise therapy for Parkinson's disease. *Arch Phys Med Rehabil* 1986; 67:741–745.
156. Formisano R, Pratesi L, Modarelli FT, Bonifati V, Meco G. Rehabilitation and Parkinson's disease. *Scand J Rehabil Med* 1992; 24: 157–160.
157. Hurwitz A. The benefits of a home exercise regimen for ambulatory Parkinson's disease patients. *J Neurosci Nurs* 1989; 21:180–184.
158. Yekutiel MP, Pinhasov A, Shahar G, Sroka H. A clinical trial of the reduction of movement in patients with Parkinson's disease. *Clin Rehabil* 1991; 5:207–214.
159. Morris ME, Iansek R, Matyas TA, Summers JJ. The pathogenesis of gait hypokinesia in Parkinson's disease. *Brain* 1994; 117:1169–1181.
160. Handford F. Towards a rational basis for physiotherapy in Parkinson's disease. *Baillieres Clin Neurol* 1993; 2:141–158.
161. Turnbull G. The role of physiotherapy intervention. In: Turnbull G, ed. *Physical therapy management of Parkinson's disease.* New York: Churchill-Livingstone, 1992; 91–120.
162. Canning CG, Alison JA, Allen NE, Goeller H. Parkinson's disease: an investigation of exercise capacity, respiratory function and gait. *Arch Phys Med Rehabil* 1997; 78:199–207.
163. Protas EJ, Stanley RK, Jankovic J, MacNeill B. Cardiovascular and metabolic responses to upper- and lower-extremity exercise in men with idiopathic Parkinson's disease. *Phys Ther* 1996; 76:34–40.
164. Comella CL, Stebbins GT, Brown-Toms N, Goetz CG. Physical therapy and Parkinson's disease, a controlled clinical trial. *Neurology* 1994; 44:376–378.
165. Schenkman M, Donovan J, Tsubota J, Kluss M, Stebbins P, Butler RB. Management of individuals with Parkinson's disease: rationale and case studies. *Phys Ther* 1989; 69:944–955.
166. Soliveri P, Brown RG, Jahanshani M, Marsden CD. Effect of practice of performance of a skilled motor task in patients with Parkinson's disease. *J Neurol Neurosurg Psychiatry* 1993; 56:295–297.
167. Dietz MA, Goetz CG, Stebbins GT. Evaluation of a modified inverted walking stick as a treatment for parkinsonian freezing episodes. *Mov Disord* 1990; 5:243–247.
168. Dam M, Tonin P, Casson S, et al. Effect of conventional and sensory enhanced physiotherapy on disability of Parkinson's disease patients. *Adv Neurol* 1996; 69:551–555.
169. Corcos DM, Chen C-M, Quinn NP, McAuley J, Rothwell JC. Strength in Parkinson's disease: relationship to rate of force generation and clinical status. *Ann Neurol* 1996; 39:79–88.
170. Davis JC. Team management of Parkinson's disease. *Am J Occup Ther* 1977; 31:300–308.
171. Preston DN, Grimes JD. Radial compression neuropathy in advanced Parkinson's disease. *Arch Neurol* 1985; 42:695–696.
172. Smith ME, Ramig LO, Dromey C, Perez KS, Samandari R. Intensive voice treatment in Parkinson's disease laryngostroboscopic findings. *Voice* 1995; 9:453–459.
173. Diller L, Ricklen M. Psychosocial factors in Parkinson's disease. *J Am Geriatr Soc* 1956; 4:1291–1300.
174. Olanow CW. A 61-yr-old man with Parkinson's disease (clinical conference). *JAMA* 1996; 275:716–722.
175. Greene P, Kang U, Fahn S, et al. Double-blind, placebo-controlled trial of botulinum toxin injections for the treatment of spasmodic torticollis. *Neurology* 1990; 40:1213–1218.
176. Yoshimura DM, Aminoff MJ, Olney RK. Botulinum toxin therapy for limb dystonias. *Neurology* 1992; 42:627–630.
177. Jankovic J, Schwartz K, Donovan DT. Botulinum toxin treatment of cranial-cervical dystonia, spasmodic dysphonia, other focal dystonias and hemifacial spasm. *J Neurol Neurosurg Psychiatry* 1990; 53: 633–639.
178. Edwards LL, Normand MM, Wszolek ZK. Cervical dystonia: a review of the role of botulinum toxin. *Nebr Med J* 1995; 80:109–115.
179. Poungvarin N, Devahastin V, Viriyavejakul A. Treatment of various movement disorders with botulinum A toxin injection: an experience of 900 patients. *J Med Assoc Thai* 1995; 78:281–288.
180. Van den Bergh P, Francart J, Mourin S, Kollmann P, Latorre EC. Five-year experience in the treatment of focal movement disorders with low-dose Dysport botulinum toxin. *Muscle Nerve* 1995; 18: 720–729.
181. Penn RD, Gianino JM, York MM. Intrathecal baclofen for motor disorders. *Mov Disord* 1995; 10:675–677.
182. Narayan RK, Loubser PG, Jankovic J, Donovan WH, Bontke CF. Inrathecal baclofen for intractable axial dystonia. *Neurology* 1991; 41:1141–1142.
183. Benabid AL, Pollak P, Gao D, et al. Chronic electrical stimulation of the ventralis intermedius nucleus of the thalamus as a treatment of movement disorders. *J Neurosurg* 1996; 84:203–214.
184. Cardoso F, Jankovic J, Grossman RG, et al. Outcome after stereotactic thalamotomy for dystonia and hemiballismus. *Neurosurgery* 1995; 36:501–508.
185. Friehs GM, Ojakangas CL, Pachatz P, Schrottner O, Ott E, Pendl G. Thalamotomy and caudatotomy with the gamma knife as a treatment for parkinsonism with a comment on lesion sizes. *Stereotact Funct Neurosurg* 1995; 64(suppl 1):209–221.
186. Friedman JH, Epstein M, Sanes JN, et al. Gamma knife pallidotomy in advanced Parkinson's disease. *Ann Neurol* 1996; 39:535–538.
187. Tsubokawa T, Katayama Y, Yamamoto T. Control of persistent hemiballismus by chronic thalamic stimulation: report of two cases. *J Neurosurg* 1995; 82:501–505.
188. Auger RG, Piepgras DG, Laws ER. Hemifacial spasm: results of microvascular decompression of the facial nerve in 54 patients. *Mayo Clin Proc* 1986; 61:640.
189. Kelly PJ, Ahlskog JE, Van Heerden JA, Carmichael SW, Stoddard SL, Bell GN. Adrenal medullary autograft transplantation into the striatum of patients with Parkinson's disease. *Mayo Clin Proc* 1989; 64:282–290.

Rehabilitation Medicine: Principles and Practice, Third Edition,
edited by Joel A. DeLisa and Bruce M. Gans.
Lippincott–Raven Publishers, Philadelphia © 1998.

CHAPTER 43

Pressure Ulcers

Kevin C. O'Connor and Steven C. Kirshblum

Pressure ulcers have been challenging societies for centuries (1). Despite new understanding of wound causation and management, the pressure ulcer problem continues to be a significant health-care concern. The number of persons affected and costs in terms of dollars, productivity and life is enormous. Pressure ulcers increase a patient's length of hospital stay and delay return to home and work, and add to the risk of complications (2). As our health-care system becomes more cost conscious and result oriented, pressure ulcers must be viewed as preventable and not merely a complication of illness and immobility (1).

The Agency for Health Care Policy and Research (AHCPR) selected pressure ulcers as one of seven medical disorders for the development of clinical guidelines that were compiled in a 1992 report and identified them as a major preventable problem (3). This guideline recommended strategies for identifying at-risk individuals, implementing preventive measures and treatment of early pressure ulcers. In 1994, the AHCPR developed additional guidelines for clinicians on the treatment of pressure ulcers (4).

The purpose of this chapter is to review the etiology of pressure ulceration and to explore advances in the prevention and treatment of this clinically significant problem. It is noteworthy that over the past two decades there has been little new knowledge on pressure ulceration pathophysiology. More advancement has been made in the area of tissue biomechanics, and there has been extensive effort toward producing surfaces and products that prevent and help heal pressure ulceration.

K. C. O'Connor: Department of Physical Medicine and Rehabilitation, University of Medicine and Dentistry of New Jersey, New Jersey Medical School, Newark, New Jersey 07103; and Kessler Institute for Rehabilitation, West Orange, New Jersey 07052.

S. C. Kirshblum: Department of Physical Medicine and Rehabilitation, University of Medicine and Dentistry of New Jersey, New Jersey Medical School, Newark, New Jersey 07103; and Spinal Cord Injury Program, Kessler Institute for Rehabilitation, West Orange, New Jersey 07052.

Defining the Problem

The National Pressure Ulcer Advisory Panel (NPUAP), an independent organization formed in 1987 dedicated to the prevention, management, treatment, and research of pressure ulcers, defines a pressure ulcer as an area of unrelieved pressure over a defined area, usually over a bony prominence, resulting in ischemia, cell death, and tissue necrosis (5). The scope of pressure ulcers is difficult to define with the interchangeable nomenclature used for pressure ulcers, nonuniform standards used to describe ulcers, multitude of staging systems, and lack of reporting guidelines (5). Incidence and severity are difficult to quantitate because of lack of uniformity of staging criteria. This results in under- and overreporting (2,6).

Definition

Numerous terms have been used to describe the tissue necrosis that occurs as the end result of obstructed blood flow, including decubitus ulcers and bedsores. The terms "decubitus ulcers" and "bedsores" originated from the observation that sores or ulcers frequently occurred in people who were bedridden. The term "decubitus" is a Latin derivative meaning "to lie down" and implies that the ulcer is caused only by prolonged recumbence. Because pressure ulcers can occur from pressure in almost any prolonged maintained position, it is more accurate and useful to use a term that includes the etiology rather than the specific body position. The term "pressure ulcer" reflects the current belief that the etiology is excessive pressure, which causes ischemia and necrosis, eventually resulting in tissue ulceration (2,7).

STAGING OF PRESSURE ULCERS

The staging of an ulcer helps to objectify the depth of tissue destruction. The recommended classification system

TABLE 43-1. *Staging of pressure ulcers*

Staging I	Nonblachable erythema not resolved within 30 min; epidermus intact
Staging II	Partial-thickness loss of skin involving epidermus, possibly into dermis; may appear as blisters with erythema
Stage III	Full-thickness destruction through dermis into subcutaneous tissue
Stage IV	Deep tissue destruction through subcutaneous tissue to fascia, muscle, bone, or joint

Data from Panel for Prediction and Prevention of Pressure Ulcers in Adults. *Prediction and prevention.* Clinical Practic Guideline No. 3, AHCPR publication No. 92-0047, 1994. Rockville, MD: Agency for Health Care Policy and Research, Public Health Service, US Department of Health and Human Services, 1994.

for staging ulcers is a system that combines many of the other systems found in the literature. This system was drafted by members of the National Pressure Ulcer Advisory Panel in 1989. The descriptions that follow allow for recording only visually observed changes in the skin. In addition, numerical progression of stages does not necessarily imply progression in ulcer severity (Table 43-1).

Stage I: Nonblanchable erythema of intact skin, the heralding lesion of skin ulceration. In individuals with darker skin, discoloration of the skin, warmth, edema, induration, or hardness also MAY be indicators.

Stage II: Partial thickness skin loss involves the epidermis, dermis, or both. The ulcer is superficial and presents clinically as an abrasion, blister, or shallow crater.

Stage III: Full-thickness skin loss involving damage to or necrosis of subcutaneous tissue that may extend down to, but not through, underlying fascia. The ulcer presents clinically as a deep crater with or without undermining of adjacent tissue.

Stage IV: Full-thickness skin loss with extensive distraction, tissue necrosis, or damage to muscle, bone, or supporting structures (e.g., tendon, joint capsule).

Undermining and sinus tracts also may be associated with stage IV pressure ulcers. Other classifications exist, such as the use described by Daniel (8); however, the AHCPR recommends the above classification as the standard for all pressure ulcers.

ASSESSMENT AND EVALUATION OF PRESSURE ULCERS

There are two main outcome measures currently in use for pressure sores. They include the depth of tissue destruction or staging and size. Pressure ulcers are commonly classified according to grading or staging systems based on depth of tissue distruction. However, progression within as well as among stages has not been addressed, and the lack of refinement hinders assessment of specific criteria in the healing process (9). Preston (10) points out additional problems with staging systems. Accurate meaningful communication is difficult because each clinician may not have the experience necessary to recognize various tissue layers that identify the stage or grade. Many times ulcers caused by factors other than pressure are classified using the same systems, further confusing the issue. In research on pressure ulcers, reliability and validity are seldom mentioned or established in relation to staging systems.

Size and outcome measurements have their own set of problems. Area measurement is commonly used in clinical practice as an index of wound healing (11). Verhonick (12) noted that the first obvious measurable aspect to pressure sore healing is wound size. However, area measurements are not reliable and may not indicate the rate of wound healing (13,14). Wound depth may be judged by actual measurement of the deepest part of the wound. Casts or molds made of various substances (15) and the use of the Kundin measuring gauge (16) also have been used to measure wound depth. Linear measurements have not been shown to have reliability (14). Other methods of determining wound size include stereophotogrammetry (17), use of photographs and planimetry (11), acetate tracing of wounds subject to planimetry, and counting blocks on graph paper (18). Although these methods may have proven valuable for research, they may not be clinically useful. One common problem with using size as the only indicator of wound healing is in the case of a debrided wound. When a wound is debrided, the size generally increases, although overall the wound is improved. More sophisticated radiographic techniques such as sinus x-rays, computer tomography, and magnetic resonance imaging are too expensive for routine use (19). In response to the shortcomings of the current methods of evaluating pressure ulcers, numerous systems have been developed that incorporate further wound characteristics, including but not limited to wound edges, undermining necrotic tissue type and amount, exudate type and amount, skin color, edema and induration, granulation tissue and epithelization, in addition to size and depth as a means of evaluating wound healing and therapeutic interventions. A standardized system of measuring wounds in a reliable, valid, and clinically simple means has yet to be widely used. At this time, the most common method of monitoring the healing of pressure ulcers uses photography and diagrams (19).

Pressure Ulcer Risk Assessment Scales

The goal of risk assessment is to identify at risk individuals needing prevention methods and the specific factors placing them at risk. Risk assessment scales have been developed to identify which populations are most at risk to allow resources and efforts to be concentrated on that particular population. Risk assessment scales include factors of immobility, incontinence, nutritional factors such as dietary intake and impaired nutritional status, and altered levels of consciousness, which are thought to increase incidence and severity of pressure ulcers (3). In the scales, scoring of individuals should be performed upon admission and periodically during hospitalization and follow-up. The three most commonly used scales are the Norton Scale, the Gosnell Pressure Sore Risk Assessment Scale, and the Braden Scale.

Norton Scale

The Norton Scale (20) consists of five factors: physical condition, mental condition, activity, mobility, and incontinence. Each factor is rated 1 to 4, with total scores ranging from 5 to 20; the lower the score, the greater the risk. Norton reported in a survey of 250 geriatric patients using this rating scale that 48% of patients who scored less than 12 developed pressure ulcers. In contrast, there was only a 5% incidence rate for those with a score of 18 or greater. However, this scale does not have specific guidelines for rating, which may lead to interater reliability problems (2).

Gosnell Pressure Sore Risk Assessment Scale

The Gosnell Scale (21) was based on the initial work of Norton. The nutrition factor is substituted for physical conditioning, incontinence was renamed continence, and demographic data, medical diagnosis, admission, and discharge data were added. Additional items on the instrument included vital signs, height, weight, skin appearance, tone, sensation, medications, hydration status of the patient, and information as to whether a preventative device was being used. Like the Norton Scale, the range of scores is 5 to 20; however, a higher score indicates a higher risk. In a study of long-term care patients, Gosnell (21) found that although 57% of patients were rated as high risk for pressure sores, only two actually developed them. The Gosnell Scale also has been shown to have high inter- and intrarater reliability (22).

Braden Scale

The Braden Scale consists of six factors: mobility, activity, moisture, sensory perception, nutrition, and friction and shear. The subscales are rated 1 to 4, except for friction and shear, which are rated 1 to 3. A score of 4 to 23 is possible, with 16 or below being considered at risk. The Braden Scale was tested and validated in critical acute and long-term care settings and has shown high interrater validity (2,3,23).

The usefulness of risk assessment tools in the rehabilitation setting is not certain (24,25). The sensitivity of the tool may not predict the more at-risk rehabilitation client when many will be at high risk with impaired mobility and activity and impaired states of consciousness. Additional risk factors need to be understood, validated, and used to increase sensitivity of risk assessment scales for certain groups. Because of this, the risk assessment tools are useful in instituting early prevention and focusing care on the highest risk population but should not be used exclusively in monitoring at-risk populations or those affected (2).

The Norton and Braden Scales have been incorporated into the AHCPR Prevention Guidelines as the part of the risk assessment process (4). However, in addition to these assessment scales, identification of risk factors may provide better systematic risk assessment than can be accomplished by these scales.

EPIDEMOLOGY

Because prevalence requires only one observation, it is reported more frequently than incidence. In acute hospital settings, the prevalence of pressure ulcers is 15% to 18.3% (5,26). Meehan (27) surveyed 148 hospitals representing the most extensive study of acute care facilities and found that the prevalence of pressure ulcers was 9.2%. In long-term hospital admissions, the prevalence of pressure ulceration varies from 3.5% (28) to 29.5% (29). Among persons in skilled care facilities and nursing homes, the prevalence ranged from 2.4% (30) to 23% (31).

Several special subpopulations may be at higher risk than the general hospital population for pressure ulcer formation. Brandeis (32) conducted a large-scale longitudinal multicenter study of the elderly and found the prevalence of pressure ulcers to be 17.4%. Of these, 83.4% occurred in the group admitted from acute hospitals. The prevalence of pressure ulcer in patients with spinal cord injury (SCI) is reported from 25% to 40% (33–35). In 1992, Hunter (36) looked at the rehabilitation population and found a 25% prevalence rate; in this same population the incidence was 0% at that facility during the time of the study.

Incidence

The incidence of pressure ulcers varies widely by population and setting. From acute care settings, the incidence varies from 3% to 14% (5). Allman (6) found that at least 7.7% of hospitalized patients develop ulcers within 3 weeks of admission. In studies of specific populations, the geriatric and orthopedic groups had rates of 24% (6,29,37). In the SCI population, the incidence has a wide range, from 24% to 59% (38–40). Young and Burns (35) found the incidence rate in SCI patients to be 40% in their acute and rehabilitation hospital and 30% in each of the five follow-up years. Higher rates of incidence are found in patients with complete quadriplegia and paraplegia than in patients with incomplete injuries. In this study, a higher incidence also was reported in quadriplegic patients during acute and rehabilitation hospitalization, but not in follow-up. Recently Carlson (41) found a 29% incidence of pressure ulcers during the acute hospitalization of 125 SCI persons.

The incidence of pressure ulcers in persons cared for in the home with professional supervision is not completely clear. Clarke and Kadhom (42) reported an incidence of 20% in home care patients. A recent study of 326 home health care patients reported an incidence of 4.3% and a prevalence of 12.9% of pressure ulcers (43).

In summary, the incidence and prevalence of pressure ulcers are sufficiently high to warrant concern, yet determining these rates has been complicated because many studies were not sufficiently controlled for pressure ulcer classification and data acquisition. To help correct these problems, the AHCPR recommends that information about the incidence and prevalence of pressure ulcers take into account the stage of the lesion, the type of health-care facility, the specific diagnosis, the individual's level of mobility, and other risk factors so as to permit the allocation of services to those populations at risk.

Economic Impact

The economic impact of pressure ulcers is difficult to estimate because of underreporting of pressure ulcers. Miller and Delozier (44) estimate the costs of a primary diagnosis of pressure elcers at $836 million in 1992. As a secondary diagnosis, pressure ulcers cost an additional $500 million. Implementation of preventative measures and aggressive initial treatment of pressure ulcers may provide lower economic and human costs by reducing the need for high acuity care, expensive equipment, and surgical intervention.

ETIOLOGY

Pressure ulcers develop in response to a number of factors, the most important being pressure (45–49). These factors can be thought of as primary and secondary (7). Pressure, shear, and friction are the three primary factors; the secondary factors include mobility status, sensory-motor function, nutrition, age, hematopoietic changes, diabetes, circulatory dysfunction, fecal and urinary incontinence, medications, and psychosocial issues.

Pressure

The critical issue of pressure and its effect on tissue was defined by early researchers (48). Researchers agree that the risk of viceration is prolonged, uninterrupted mechanical loading of tissue (3,48). There are three important aspects of pressure: intensity, duration, and tissue tolerance to pressure (2). In experiments in dogs and cats, Kosiak (48) developed time–pressure relationships demonstrating the inverse relationship of pressure and time. Intense pressure applied for a short duration can be as damaging as lower intensity pressure for extended periods (47,48). In his studies, he found that 70 mm Hg of pressure applied continuously for 2 hours produced pathologic changes. He also demonstrated that tissues can tolerate much higher cyclic pressures than constant pressures. If pressure is relieved intermittently every 3 to 5 minutes, higher pressures can be tolerated (48). Pressure must be relieved frequently over time as well as reduced at the surface–skin interface. It is upon these studies that the clinical practice of weight shifting and the use of 2-hour minimum turning times in bed or frequent small position changes in bed to provide pressure relief were instituted (3,25,50).

The concept of tissue tolerance was initially described by Husain (51). The sensitivity of skin to pressure was studied by Daniel (45), and he found that muscle was more sensitive to the effects of pressure than skin. When muscle is damaged without skin breakdown, a second application of less pressure and less time result in an ulcer. This is clinically important in the need to relieve pressure at the first sign of skin impairment, or blanchable hyperemia, and allow time for superficial and deep tissue recovery.

Pressure is transmitted from the body surface to the underlying bone, and the greatest pressure is to the tissues overlying the bone. The pressure is distributed in a conelike fashion, with the base of the cone on the underlying body surface. This leads to an understanding of why the greatest damage is often seen at the muscle layer and not at the skin surface. Ulcer presentations often reflect this concept when they appear with a small skin defect and a large area undermining below the surface of the intact skin.

In 1930, Landis (52), by microinjection technique, determined 32 mm Hg to be the average capillary pressure at its arterial inflow, and thus capillary closing pressure. Lindan (53) demonstrated that pressure causes tissue damage by closure of blood vessels, resulting in tissue necrosis. The pressure of blood as it enters the capillaries at the arterial end is approximately 32 mm Hg, decreasing to about 12 mm Hg at the venous end (52). Therefore, the mean capillary blood pressure is thought to be approximately 20 mm Hg, which is much lower than the pressure of 85 to 100 mm Hg seen in the larger arteries (54). These early capillary blood flow studies were performed in the fingertips of young healthy men. However, more recent capillary closure studies have shown that much lower pressures are needed to collapse capillaries in elderly and debilitated individuals and that these pressures can vary over different sites on the body (2,55,56). There is some difficulty extrapolating these data to the skin–support surface interface pressure. Other ways of measuring skin–support pressures have been attempted. These include the use of a pressure transducer placed on the skin at the interface. This pressure is measured indirectly at the skin–support surface interface and may not accurately reflect blood flow through the deep capillaries (2). Clinically this led to searching for support surfaces to reduce skin–support surface pressure below 32 mm Hg.

The relationship between tissue compression and ischemia is well established. When examining the compression component more closely, both the intensity and the duration must be considered. Experimental studies in animals have established an inverse relationship between the amount of time and pressure necessary to produce pathologic tissue changes (48). This inverse pressure–time relationship is widely accepted as a valid theory to be applied to human tissue necrosis. Husian (51) believed that low pressure maintained for long periods produce more damage than high pressure for short periods. In the 1970s, Reswick and Rogers (57) developed a curve that has been used as a clinical guideline for maximum pressure–time application over bony prominences in seated individuals. If the pressure is relieved by shifting the body weight, blood flows back into the tissue again and the area becomes hyperemic (58). This phenomenon is called reactive hyperemia because a bright red flush appears as the body attempts to flood the starved tissue with oxygen. This protective mechanism of local vasodilatation is a naturally occurring compensatory response to temporary ischemia. If the pressure–time threshold has been exceeded, tissue damage continues to occur even after relief of the compression.

Shear

Shear occurs when the skin remains stationary and the underlying tissue shifts (3). These shearing forces are produced when adjacent surfaces slide over one another (2). Reichel (59) found that shearing forces cause perforating arteries to become angulated, disrupting the supply of blood. Shearing forces are said to account for the high incidence of sacral ulcers. When the head of the bed is elevated, a greater compressive force is placed on the posterior sacral tissues than when the bed is in the flat position. Although the sacral skin adheres by friction to the bed linen, the patient's skeletal frame slides downward toward the foot of the bed, which compromises the arteries that supply the skin from the underlying fascia and muscle. If the skin becomes ischemic by this process, the result would be a shear ulcer with a wide undermining around its base (2,60). Common causes of shearing include spasticity, poor sitting position, poor bed position, and sliding rather than lifting during transfers, etc. In relation to pressure ulcer etiology, the role of shear is less clear than the role of pressure. Although most authorities on pressure ulcers consider shear to be a major significant contributor to ulcer development, there is relatively little scientific data available on shear in the pressure ulcer literature.

Friction

Friction occurs when the skin moves against a support surface. It is the force of two surfaces moving across each other. In its mildest forms, friction produces skin tears and abrasions limited to the epidermal and dermal layers (2,3,61). In cases where pressure and shear are combined, friction contributes to extensive injury and can decrease the amount of external pressure required to produce a pressure sore (2,46).

Secondary Contributing Factors to Pressure Ulcer Development

In 1989, the Consensus Developing Conference of the National Pressure Ulcer Advisory Panel proposed secondary risk factors in the development of pressure ulcers. These are defined as identifiable intrinsic or external characteristics that increase a person's susceptibility to forces that induce pressure ulcers (5).

Mobility

The inability or decreased ability to change and/or control body position is the most frequently cited factor in the risk of pressure ulceration (7,19,20,21,23,62,63). The major conditions contributing to immobility are stroke, arthritis, multiple sclerosis, spinal cord trauma, head injury, oversedation, depression, weakness, and confusion. Individuals should be assisted to obtain and maintain the highest possible level of mobility and to use assistive devices that may enhance safe physical mobility.

Nutrition

Malnutrition may be second only to pressure in the etiology, pathogenesis, and lack of healing of pressure ulcers (6,64). Allman (6), Stotts (9), and Pinchocofsky-Devin (65) all reported low serum albumin levels to be highly associated with pressure ulcer development. Two prospective studies showed evidence of a poor diet as a causative factor in pressure ulcer formation (3,62). Lean mass is a good measure of adequate nutrition; weight or total mass is not. Adipose tissue, which is poorly vascularized, should not be equated with adequate nutrition (66). High caloric diets, rich in protein and carbohydrates, are recommended to provide a positive nitrogen balance and to meet the metabolic and nutritional requirements crucial to pressure sore prevention.

Age

With aging, there are changes that impair the ability to distribute pressure effectively, as well as changes in collagen synthesis that result in tissues with lowered mechanical strength and increased stiffness. These factors may lower resistance to interstitial fluid flow (54). As a person ages, the elastin content of the soft tissue decreases, which increases the mechanical load on the skin.

Moisture/Incontinence

Moisture is an important contributing factor to pressure ulcer development, and when uncontrolled it softens the skin. With softening of the epidermal tissue, there is a decrease in tensile strength, and it is easily macerated by compression and eroded by frictional forces. Excessive moisture may result from perspiration, wound drainage, and fecal or urinary incontinence. Norton showed incontinence to be the most reliable predictor for pressure ulcer formation (67). Bowel incontinence may be a more important risk factor than urinary incontinence as a predictor of pressure ulcer formation (6). In addition to the maceration associated with fecal incontinence, the exposure of the skin to the bacteria and toxins in the stool may be important in the pathogenesis of pressure ulcers.

Smoking

Lamid and Ghetit (68), in studying SCI patients, found smoking to correlate positively with pressure ulcers.

Elevated Temperature

Researchers have correlated increases in body temperature with increased risk of pressure ulceration. The elevated temperature may place increased demands on an already compromised area. It has been determined that an increase of 1°C in temperature causes a 10% increase in tissue metabolism and oxygen demand (69). If the soft tissue is already at risk for pressure-induced ischemia, it becomes even more susceptible to necrosis if the temperature of the skin is elevated. Temperature scanning devices have been used to monitor changes in the cutaneous circulation. Verhonick (12) reported the use of thermography in studying pressure ulcers with infrared imaging to measure the spectrum of energy emitted by the skin. If temperature is a factor in the etiology of pressure ulcers, attention should be given to clothing and support surfaces that either insulate or conduct heat away from the skin.

Education

Vidal and Sarrus (60) found lower educational level related positively with severity of ulcers. However, Carlson (41) did not find this to be a factor during acute rehabilitation, but it was strongly related to ulcer formation at the time of follow-up. In addition, knowledge of the increased risks of pressure ulcers can help guide prediction and prevention of the pressure ulcers through educational programs. Programs developed toward behavioral changes may enhance outcomes.

Psychosocial

Anderson and Andberg (70) found life satisfaction, self-esteem, and practice of responsibility to be important factors in both the initial development and recurrence of pressure ulcers.

Cognitive Status

Impairment of the ability to detect sensations that indicate a need for a change in position is critical to the development of pressure ulcers. Sensory perception is impaired in a variety of diseases and should alert the clinician to the increased risk of pressure ulcers (1).

Spinal Cord Injury

As previously mentioned, the incidence and prevalence of pressure ulcers in the SCI population is significant. Therefore, a great deal of research has been devoted to this patient population (71–76). Lloyd and Baker (71) found no relationship between severity of pressure ulcers and level of SCI. Young and Burns (72) found a higher incidence of pressure ulcers in quadriplegics than in paraplegics during initial hospitalization but not at follow-up. Carlson (41) found that the higher the level of injury during the acute care, the greater the incidence of pressure ulcer, but there was no associated significance between level of injury and rehabilitation follow-up phases. This study also found a significant relationship between complete lesions and increased incidence of pressure ulcers at follow-up. Those patients with complete lesions had a greater incidence of pressure ulcer during rehabilitation and follow-up. All those who developed pressure ulcers during rehabilitation had a complete injury on the Frankel Scale (41). Of major interest is that no subject who had any preserved function below the level of injury developed a pressure ulcer during rehabilitation and follow-up. It appears that even nonfunctional preserved motor activity reduces the risk of pressure ulcer (41). SCI patients have lower levels of hydroxylysine, a collagen specific amino acid, when injured more than 3 years and compared with those injured less than 3 years. The skin below the level of injury has lower concentrations of proline, lysine, and hydroxylysine than does skin above the level of injury, which has implications for the tensile strength of skin and its ability to withstand pressure (38).

COMMON SITES OF PRESSURE ULCERS

More then 95% of all pressure ulcers develop over a bony prominence on the lower half of the body. Sixty-seven percent of the ulcers occur around the hips and buttocks, and 29% occur on the lower limbs (30). The most common sites for pressure ulcers are the ischium, sacrum, greater trochanter of the femur, and the heel. Pressure ulcers will occur anywhere on the body where there is compression of soft tissue, including compression from splints, orthoses, and orthopedic immobilizers. In studies of the SCI population, the sacrum was found to be the most frequent site of severe pressure ulcers (41,73,74). As more time is spent in wheelchairs, the pressure ulcer incidence is reflected in increased frequency at the ischial tuberosities and feet. Carlson (41) found that 47% of all ulcers discovered in follow-up were on the foot. In a study of children 10 weeks to 13 years of age, Solis (75) found the occiput to be the site of greatest pressures, changing to the sacrum as the child aged. This is not surprising in consideration of the percentage of body weight that the child's head represents, and the child's positioning needs must be considered separately from the adult's.

PREVENTION OF PRESSURE ULCERATION

Prevention of pressure ulcers is based on an understanding of the etiology. Risk factors that may affect the quality of the patient's wound must be addressed. In addition to the risk factors described elsewhere in the chapter, hygiene and good skin care is of critical importance.

Preventive measures to provide relief from prolonged pressure cannot be overemphasized. Physical lifting and manual turning of immobile patients are the simplest and most frequently used methods of avoiding sustained pressure. For bedridden patients, a turning schedule of once every 2 hours is now widely accepted and applied. No turning schedule is absolute, and skin inspection must be an integral part of the turning procedure. Correct positioning is aimed at distributing the load over maximum surface area and avoiding weight loading on bony prominences (54,76). Difficulty in positioning can be exacerbated by obesity, spasticity, contractures, orthotic devices, traction, and pain.

These changes in position can be accomplished with schedules incorporating all four surfaces: supine, prone, and right and left lateral positioning. The prone position can be accomplished on standard surfaces with bridging techniques (3) or on a standard water mattress without bridging (24,25). The side-lying position should avoid direct positioning over the trochanteric area. Seiler (56) recommend a 30° laterally inclined position for side lying. Efforts should be made to keep bony prominences from being positioned over another body surface via the use of foam wedges and pillows. The heels have been shown in several studies to be particularly vulnerable to pressure even on pressure-reducing surfaces (3,77). Pillows can be used for this purpose, but often an insensate extremity will be inadvertently repositioned off the pillow and onto the mattress. A number of pressure relief devices are commercially available, such as foam or sheepskin boots. Heel protectors have not been shown to appreciably decrease or dissipate pressure. A device that elevates the foot totally from the support surface is most effective when pressure relief is needed (74,78). When transferring off the bed surface, patients need to be taught techniques that decrease the amount of friction and shearing on the body and extremities across the bed or chair surface.

Wheelchair positioning should assure maximal support over the available seated area. Foot plates should be set at a height that does not transfer weight to the ischium but allows this weight to be borne by the thighs (79). If lateral supports are required to maintain the trunk in alignment, they should not cause pressure problems in another location. In the wheelchair, position changes should ideally be performed at least every half hour. Weight relief while in the wheelchair can be accomplished in a variety of ways, including tilt back, anterior, lateral, and press-up weight shifts. Devices such as beeping chairpads, watches, and timers have not proved successful in assisting patients to remember weight shifts because patients have found them to be loud and bothersome (76). Power tilt or recline mechanism for high-level SCI patients are extremely helpful in allowing the patient to perform their weight shifts independently.

A systematic skin inspection needs to be performed at least twice daily, with particular attention to the quality of the skin integrity especially over bony prominences. Although there is no evidence that systematic, comprehensive and routine skin inspection decreases the incidence of pressure ulcers, it provides information for designing intervention as early as possible and standards to evaluate outcomes as well a means for the patient to make necessary changes based on skin inspection (3,80).

Support Surfaces

Support surfaces reduce interface pressure over a bony prominence by maximizing contact and redistributing weight over a larger surface area (54,81). Numerous investigators have measured the characteristics and properties of support surfaces. The AHCPR reviewed clinical studies and found evidence that pressure-reducing devices can decrease the incidence of pressure ulcers but that one type of pressure-reducing device is no more effective than another to prevent pressure ulcers (3). Because one support surface is not necessarily superior to another for reducing pressure ulcers, other factors must be considered when selecting a device. In evaluating these devices, cost as well as both patient and caregiver approval can assist as a guide (82). Support surfaces are available as overlays (support surface placed over the hospital mattress), replacement mattresses, and specialty beds (Table 43-2).

Overlays

Overlays are available as foam, water, gel, air or a combination of these materials.

Foam

Foam overlays should be at least 4 inches in height to provide some pressure relief. High-density foams can be contoured to meet individual postural needs; however, foam may be hot, increasing skin temperatures and local metabolic needs. In addition, foam cannot be washed in the event of incontinence and requires replacement after 6 months. Examples include eggerate (2-inch foam) and 4-inch foams.

Water

Water systems must be checked for proper inflation so that the person floats. If under- or overfilled, the support surface may increase the interface pressure. In addition, water systems have problems related to overweight patients and puncturing, and turning individuals on water surfaces may be more difficult.

Gel

Gel systems are usually combined with foam. The gel systems are easy to clean, low maintenance, and puncture resistant, and they do not have the disadvantages of the water overlays and difficulty of turning individuals (2). Disadvantages of gel systems include their weight and expense. The increased weight for the wheelchair cushion is of particular concern, as is the instability that may be created during transfers. In addition, some gels become harder in cold temperatures, making them less useful in cold climates (82).

TABLE 43-2. *Support surfaces*

Support services	Advantages	Disadvantages
Static surfaces (bed or cushion)		
Foam	Inexpensive, lightweight, versatile	Absorbs liquids, odors, short life span
Air	Lightweight, good pressure relief, easily cleaned	Puncture, monitoring for proper inflation, less stable, expensive
Flotation (gel/water)	Good pressure relief, adjusts to movement	Heavy, expensive, retains heat
Combination cushions (foam base with gel)	Good posture, pressure relief	Heavy, expensive
Mattresses/beds		
Dynamic overlays	Portable, easily cleaned moisture control	Power required, expensive, noisy
Low air loss bed/overlays	Good pressure relief, moisture control, may be portable (as overlays), reduced friction/shear	Expensive
Hospital replacement mattress	Built-in pressure relief, low maintenance	High initial cost
Air fluidized beds	Good pressure relief, bacteriostatic glass beads, fluid/moisture absorption	Expensive, difficult transfers, sensory deprivation, dehydration

Air

Air overlays are further subdivided into static air, alternating air, and low air loss systems.

Static Air

In a static air overlay, air is forced through interconnected bladders to provide proper pressure. Static air devices require skilled monitoring to check for proper inflation (2). These are usually low-maintenance systems but are easily punctured and expensive. Static air overlays are easily cleaned if there is incontinence.

Alternating Air

In an alternating air overlay, air is pumped through interconnecting tunnels with intervals of inflation and deflation. The device is promoted to reduce pressure and stimulate circulation through shifting of pressure from one area of the body to another as the system cycles through inflation and deflation. However, the alternating air system does not appear to provide additional pressure relief over that of the static air overlay (76).

Low Air Loss

In addition to filling channels with air, low air loss systems provide air movement around the skin. This feature reduces moisture and may help reduce friction and shear (2). As with the alternating air overlay, puncture problems and noise are major drawbacks.

Replacement Mattresses

Replacement mattresses have surface characteristics similar to those of the overlays, but they provide the pressure relief attained with those systems without the additional height problem of an overlay. Many hospitals are replacing their standard hospital mattresses with replacement mattresses. Although the initial cost of these mattresses may be greater than the standard mattress, the use of further overlays may be avoided while at the same time providing a measure of prevention of pressure ulceration for all patients.

Specialty Beds

Specialty beds replace the hospital bed and provide pressure relief as well as decreased shearing, friction, and moisture. Although these beds are expensive, they may be useful for assisting in wound care. They are available as air-fluidized beds, low air loss beds, and kinetic specialty beds.

Air-Fluidized Beds

In the air-fluidized bed, the individual floats on a bed of silicone-coated air-fluidized beads. In these beds, pressure relief is not absolute but still exists at the heels, necessitating additional prevention measures there. The air-fluidized bed is extremely helpful for patients after skin flap surgery, as well as for those with large amounts of drainage. Because the overlying nylon cover is permeable, wound drainage and body moisture is removed from the patient through the porous nylon cover. In addition, the silicone beads are bacteriostatic. Concerns for these specialty beds include dehydration, wound drying, client disorientation, and the extreme weight of the bed. In addition, transfers on and off the bed become more difficult because of the unstable surface as well as the height of the bed (77).

Low Air Loss

Low air loss beds consist of a series of interconnecting air-filled pillows. Each pillow is filled and calibrated for proper inflation and to provide air flow. The head of the bed can be elevated, and transfers are easier; however, the surface may be slippery. Like the air-fluidized bed, the bed decreases both shearing and pressure, and the circulating air may help with moisture.

Kinetic Beds

Kinetic beds provide continuous motion and may be combined with a low air loss feature. These are primarily used for the management of multiple problems of immobility, usually from trauma.

COMPLICATIONS OF PRESSURE ULCERS

The clinician treating a patient with a pressure ulcer must be aware of possible complications of pressure ulcers and of their treatment (Table 43-3). Many complications are infectious, including endocarditis (83), maggot infestation (84), meningitis (85), septic arthritis (86), and sinus tract or abscess formation (87). Computed tomography scanning was reported to be effective in detecting deep abscesses associated with pressure ulcers (88). Sinography was reported to be useful for defining the extent of sinus tracts underlying pressure ulcers (87,89). Heterotopic bone formation (90) as well as fistula formation (91), pseudoaneurysm (92), and squamous cell carcinoma in the ulcer (93) all have been reported as additional complications. The clinician also must be aware that some treatments for pressure ulcers may lead to other complications. For example, iodine-containing agents when applied topically may unmask subclinical hyperthyroidism (94) or result in iodine toxicity (95). In addition, Johnson (96) found that topical aminoglycoside treatment has been associated with hearing loss. The management of three other complications—osteomyelitis, bacteremia, and advancing cellulitis—are discussed in the following section.

TREATMENT OF PRESSURE ULCERS

Despite appropriate local and systemic treatment, failure to elucidate the cause of the pressure ulcer will result in a nonhealing wound. The use of dressings as well as specialty mattresses and cushions supports the wound; the healing comes from removing the cause and addressing systemic concerns.

TABLE 43-3. *Complications of pressure ulcers*

Amyloidosis
Maggot infection
Septic arthritis
Heterotopic bone formation
Sinus tract or abscess
Squamous cell carcinoma
Perineal-urethral fistula
Complications of treatment including hearing loss, iodine toxicity
Osteomyelitis
Bacteremia
Advancing cellulitis
Endocarditis
Pseudoaneurysm
Meningitis

Wound Cleansing

In a clean proliferating wound, the goal is to promote healthy tissue. The AHCPR recommends using normal saline with enough irrigation pressure to enhance wound cleansing without causing trauma to the wound bed. Antiseptic cleansers such as povidone-iodine, acetic acid, Dakin's solution, and hydrogen peroxide should not be used because of harmful effect on healing tissue (97). Wounds are to be cleansed initially and with each dressing change. Material on the wound surfaces such as foreign bodies, residual topical agents, dressing residue, wound exudate, and metabolic waste can be removed with careful wound cleansing (98,99).

Infected Wounds

Several bacteriologic studies found a direct correlation between high levels of bacteria in pressure ulcers and failure to heal (100–103). Colonization of a pressure ulcer as well as enhancement of its healing can be accomplished through effective wound cleansing and debridement. It is not recommended to use swab cultures to diagnose wound infection because all pressure ulcers are colonized. As recommended by the Center for Disease Control, documenting the presence of wound infection can be accomplished by the culture of fluid obtained by needle aspiration or biopsy of ulcer tissue (104).

If the pressure ulcer is clean and either continues to produce exudate or is not healing after 2 to 4 weeks of optimal care, the AHCPR recommends initiating a 2-week trial of topical antibiotics effective against gram-negative and positive organisms as well as anaerobic organisms (e.g., sulfadiazine, triple antibiotic ointment) (4). In addition, other studies have suggested that approximately 25% of nonhealing pressure ulcers have underlying osteomyelitis (6,105). The standard practice for diagnosing osteomyelitis is a bone biopsy, and numerous strategies for noninvasive diagnosis of osteomyelitis have been reported, including computed tomography and magnetic resonance imaging. Lewis and colleagues (106) reported that bone scans are rarely useful in practice because of their high false-positive rate. Their study suggested using a combination of three tests (white blood cell count, erythrocyte sedimentation rate, and plain x-ray) with a positive predicted value for osteomyelitis of 69% when all three tests were positive. In the event of bacteremia, sepsis, advancing cellulitis, and osteomyelitis, the AHCPR (4) recommends systemic antibiotics because systemic infections cannot be successfully treated with further cleansing or debridement.

Necrotic Wounds

Necrotic wounds require more aggressive cleansing. Debridement can be accomplished enzymatically, mechanically, or through sharp debridement. Removal of necrotic tissue speeds the healing process and is considered necessary for wound healing (105,107). Because these devitalized tissues are avascular, systemic antibiotics are of limited use.

Sharp Debridement

Sharp debridement involves the use of a scalpel, scissors, or other sharp instruments to remove devitalized tissue. Sharp debridement works best when necrotic tissue is clearly delineated and avascular tissue is grasped easily. Surgical laser debridement is now being used on an outpatient basis. It has superior qualities because of its instant homeostasis and sterilization of the wound.

Mechanical Debridement

Mechanical debridement includes the use of wet-to-dry dressings at prescribed intervals, hydrotherapy, wound irrigation, and dextranomers. One disadvantage of wet-to-dry dressings is that they are nonselective, removing both nonviable and viable tissues, and therefore may be potentially traumatic to granulation tissue (108–110).

Wound irrigation with a safe and effective device such as a syringe with a 19-gauge angiocatheter will provide enough force to remove eschar, common bacteria, and other debris (111). Dextranomers are beads that are placed in the wound bed to absorb exudate, bacteria, and other debris. One disadvantage of its use is that they may be difficult to apply if the patient cannot be positioned so that they can be poured into a wound. In addition, the beads are expensive. In one study with the use of dextranomers, healing time did not appear to decrease greatly (112).

Enzymatic Debridement

Enzymatic treatment uses a number of topical ointments (e.g., Avante [Biofactures, Lynbrook, NY] Travase [Knoll Laboratories, Mt. Olive, NJ], Santyl, Elase [Fujisawa, Deerfield, IL], Colagenase (Knoll Laboratories, Mt. Olive, NJ]). Enzymes can be used alone to break down an eschar, after sharp debridement, or in conjunction with mechanical debridement.

Exception to Debridement

An exception to debridement of necrotic tissue is heel ulcers. Stable heel ulcers with a protective eschar are considered an exception to the recommendation that all eschar be debrided. The eschar provides a natural protective cover and should not be debrided if ulcers do not have any edema, erythema, fluctuance, or drainage (4).

Wound Dressings

Pressure ulcers require wound coverings that enhance the nature environment and maintain their physiologic integrity. An ideal dressing should protect the wound, be biocompatible, and provide ideal hydration. Research from wound healing shows that wounds heal faster with a moist environment, allowing the natural factors in the wound exudate to promote healing of the wound (113,114). Although wounds heal better in a moist environment, excessive exudate can macerate surrounding tissue and should be absorbed away from the ulcer bed (115,116).

Ring cushions (donut) are noted to cause venous congestion and edema, although few studies have been performed to document their deleterious effects. In the study of at-risk patients, Crewe (117) found that ring cushions are more likely to cause pressure ulcers than to prevent them. They are not recommended.

Dressings must be chosen in order to support the wound at various states. More research is needed to compare dressing choice and wound outcome. Failure of a wound to improve could be due to infection, and new dressing methods may be necessary (Table 43-4).

Transparent Adhesive Dressing

Transparent adhesive films are a good choice for dry necrotic wounds requiring debridement. Thin film dressings were the first occlusive dressing devised to insulate, protect, and maintain the moist wound surface. Because they are occlusive, exudate can build up under the film.

Hydrocolloid Dressings

Hydrocolloid dressings insulate and protect the moist wound surface and absorb some exudate. These are also occlusive and do not permit oxygen to diffuse into the wound. The occlusion promotes wound healing, with growth

TABLE 43-4. *Topical treatments for pressure ulcers*

Wound cleansers
Protectants/creams
Antimicrobials/antiseptic agents
Topical circulatory stimulants
Enzymatic agents
Semipermeable dressings
Hydrocolloid dressings
Gels/hydrogels
Exudate absorbers
Calcium aliginote dressings
Foams
Composites
Nonadherent impregnated dressings
Gauzes
Wet to dry dressings
Moist saline dressings

factors allowed to proliferate beneath the dressings. These dressings are also contraindicated for infected wounds and wounds with large amounts of exudate or secretions. Examples include Comfeel (Coloplast, Marietta, GA) and DuoDerm (ConvaTec, Princeton, NJ).

Hydrogel

Hydrogel is available in sheets or granules to pour onto the wound and provides mild absorption. The dressing must be covered with a secondary dressing but can be used to fill in dead space while providing a moist wound environment. An example is Vigilon (C.R. Bardi, Murray Hill, NJ).

Foam

Foam dressings are nonadherent wafers used to promote moist wound healing and provide absorption. These dressings are highly adsorptive, and their hydrophobic surfaces repel contaminants. Because they are not adherent, they require additional taping or have been developed into an ''island dressing'' where the foam dressing is surrounded by an occlusive dressing such as a transparent film. An example is PolyMem (Capital Medical, Harrisburg, PA).

Exudate Absorbers

Exudate absorbers are powders or beads used to provide minimal debridement and maintain a moist wound bed. An example is Debrisan.

Calcium Alginates

Calcium alginates occur naturally in seaweed. They require a dressing on top, usually gauze. They are able to absorb large amounts of exudate and can be removed with irrigation. When dry, they resemble cotton but become a gel when absorbing exudate. An example is Sorbsan (Dow Pharmaceuticals Hickam, Sugar Land, TX).

Lubricating Spray

Lubricating sprays are convenient to use and maintain a moist wound bed. They can be sprayed on a gauze to wet the gauze before packing the wound. Lubricating sprays require a secondary dressing for absorption. An example is Granulex (Dow Hickam, Sugar Land, TX).

Wound Care Modalities

Therapeutic modalities may augment wound healing. Modalities that have been evaluated in wound healing include whirlpool, light, ultrasound, and electrical stimulation.

Whirlpool

Whirlpool may be used for cleansing pressure ulcers that contain thick exudate, slough, or necrotic tissue. Feedar and Kloth (118) recommend twice daily whirlpool cleansing to remove debris and residue. Whirlpool trauma should be discontinued when the ulcer is considered clean, because the benefits of wound cleansing are outweighed by the potential for trauma to regenerating tissue as a result of the agitating water (118).

Light

Ultraviolet (UV) light has been used clinically to treat a variety of skin conditions, including pressure sores (119). UV light rays with wave lengths of 253 nm have been reported effective in killing bacteria by destroying essential cellular components (120) or by producing toxic substances. Kelner (121) proposed that exposure to UV inhibits DNA synthesis, and Painter (122) implied that UV may affect RNA activity, thereby contributing to bacterial death. In addition, UV exposure has been reported to stimulate production of vitamin D.

Geronimus (123) found that UVB (wave lengths of 280 to 315 nm) at a dosage of 400 mJ/cm^2 or UVC (wave lengths of 180 to 280 nm) at a dosage of 135 mJ/cm^2 stimulated reepithelization in both exposed and nonexposed wounds on a pig model. These results suggested that UV may be capable of influencing wound healing at remote sites. Wills et al. (124) treated pressure sores twice weekly at 2.5 times the minimal erythema dose (second-degree erythema). Freytes (120) reported satisfactory results using UV on nonhealing ulcers.

UV should not be used on very fragile skin or in patients with excessive edema in periwound tissues. Other contraindications to UV include acute onset of psoriasis, lupus erythematosus, herpes simplex, acute eczema, small vessel disease, scleroderma, cardiac or renal failure, hyperthyroidism, tuberculosis, dermatitis, and patients taking a UV-sensitizing agent such as tetracycline or steroids.

Ultrasound

Therapeutic ultrasound has been found to accelerate wound healing by enhancing the inflammatory phase and therefore assisting the proliferative phase to occur earlier. Ultrasound using 3 mHz is indicated for treating superficial wounds and 1 mHz for deep wounds. If local circulation is compromised, it is recommended that pulsed ultrasound be used with a wattage for treating pressure sores of 0.8 W/cm^2 (125). In addition to the precautions and contraindications for using ultrasound, it should not be used on acutely infected wounds or with osteomyelitis. Ultrasound stimulates macrophages to release growth factors and chemotactic agents that are necessary for development of new connective tissue at the injury site (126). In chronic ischemic muscle, ultrasound can cause new capillaries to develop and circulation to be restored at an accelerated rate (127). Ultrasound-stimulated full-thickness wounds have been shown to be significantly stronger and possess greater elasticity than placebo-controlled wounds when treated immediately after injury (128). Increase in the strength of the treated scar tissue believed to be due to its increased collagen content and increased elasticity is related to a change in the collagen fiber pattern. As remodeling continues, it becomes more structurally and functionally similar to normal tissue. However, it never reaches preinjury strength nor does it develop original tensile properties.

Electrical Stimulation

Electrical stimulation for tissue repair has been used clinically to treat a variety of conditions and wound types, including pressure sores. The rationale for using electrical stimulation in chronic wound healing includes stimulation of endogenous bioelectric circuits, facilitating galvanotaxis, improving the transcutaneous partial pressure of oxygen, and increasing calcium uptake and adenosine triphosphate and protein synthesis, as well as for its bactericidal effects. Electrical stimulation is used with low-intensity direct current, high-voltage pulsating current, and monophasic pulsed current. Data from five clinical trials involving a total of 147 patients support the effectiveness of electrotherapy and enhancing the healing rate of pressure ulcers that have been unresponsive to conventional therapy (129–133). Adverse reactions in these studies were limited to minor uncomfortable tingling sensations in 15% of patients in one study.

It should be noted that the therapeutic efficiency of hyperbaric oxygen, infrared, UV, and low-energy laser radiation as well as ultrasound have not been sufficiently established for recommendation of these therapies for the treatment of pressure ulcers (4). Only electrical stimulation has had sufficient supporting evidence to warrant recommendation by the AHCPR (4) and should be considered for stage III and IV ulcers unresponsive to conventional therapy as well as for recalcitrant stage II ulcers.

Surgical Treatment

When wounds reach stage III to IV, surgical closure becomes an option (134). Early closure of the wound will decrease loss of fluid and nutrients and improve the patient's general health status as well as lead to earlier mobilization and re-entry into social structure (105). Surgical closure of chronic pressure ulcers allows patients to be mobilized quickly and to return to work, family, and school without the chronic loss of time to bedrest and threatened complications of immobility. In order of increasing complexity, operative procedures for pressure ulcers include direct closure, skin grafts, skin flaps, musculocutaneous flaps, and free flaps. Musculocutaneous flaps are usually the best choice for SCI patients or when the loss of muscle function does not contribute to comorbidity. Musculocutaneous flaps also can help heal osteomyelitis and limit the damage caused by shearing friction and pressure (135–137). Free flaps have not been described in the literature for closure of pressure ulcers.

At the time of surgical closure, the patient should be free of infection. Positioning during surgery should stimulate the position that places the ulcerated area under maximal tension such that there is adequate coverage and minimal tension on the flap. All contaminated tissue is removed, including bone if it is infected and all scar tissue is removed. Closed drainage is maintained to prevent seroma formation. Postoperatively, all pressure is kept off the area by proper positioning and use of specialty mattresses such as an air-fluidized bed. Mobility begins after 3 weeks with careful monitoring of the skin (2,138). Prophylactic ischectomy is not recommended for ischial ulcers because it often results in perineal ulcers and urethral fistulas, more difficult management problems than ischial ulcers (139).

Rehabilitation of the patient with flap surgery includes progressively longer periods of sitting with flap viability checked after each sitting period. The patients are taught to shift their body weight once they are bearing weight on the flap and inspect the skin twice daily using a mirror. Recurrence rates for pressure ulcers after operative repair range from 13% to 56% (140,141). Carelessness and noncompliance are important risk factors for recurrence (138,142). Recurrence rates may be reduced with the use of sensate flaps. However, it is more important to develop programs in ulcer prevention with an emphasis on patient education and adherence. The long-term preventative value of musculocutaneous flap coverage of pressure ulcers must be evaluated in large series of patients.

SUMMARY

Overall management of patients at risk for developing pressure ulcers include education about risk factors for patients and family, as well as early intervention for good nutritional support and use of proper surfaces and transfer techniques. Treatment options, aimed at wound care, mobilization and surgery, depend on good medical management and follow-up.

REFERENCES

1. Copeland-Fields LD, Hoshiko BR. Clinical validation of Braden and Bergstrom's conceptual schema of pressure sores risk factors. *Rehabil Nurs* 1989; 14:257–260.
2. Bryant R, Shannon ML, Pieper B, Braden B, Morris DJ. Pressure ulcers. In: Bryant R, ed. *Acute and chronic wounds: nursing management.* St. Louis: Mosby Year Book, 1992.
3. Panel for Prediction and Prevention of Pressure Ulcers in Adults. *Prediction and prevention.* Clinical Practice Guideline No. 3, AHCPR publication No. 92-0047, 1992. Rockville, MD: Agency for Health Care Policy and Research, Public Health Service, US Department of Health and Human Services, 1992.
4. Panel for Prediction and Prevention of Pressure Ulcers in Adults. *Prediction and prevention.* Clinical Practice Guideline No. 3, AHCPR

publication No. 92-0047, 1994. Rockville, MD: Agency for Health Care Policy and Research, Public Health Service, US Department of Health and Human Services, 1994.
5. National Pressure Ulcer Advisory Panel. Pressure ulcers prevalence, cost and risk assessment: consensus development conference statement. *Decubitus* 1989; 2:24–28.
6. Allman RM. Epidemiology of pressure sores in different populations. *Decubitus* 1989; 2:30–33.
7. Maklebust J. Pressure ulcers: etiology and prevention. *Nurs Clin North Am* 1987; 22:359–377.
8. Daniels R. Skin. Presented at the Workshop on the effects of mechanical stress on soft tissues. Dallas, Texas, November 1980; 5–6.
9. Stotts NA. Nutritional parameters at hospital admission as predictors of pressure ulcers in surgical patients. *Nurs Res* 1985; 34:383.
10. Preston KM. Dermal ulcers: simplifying a complex problem. *Rehabil Nurs* 1987; 12:17–21.
11. Thomas AC, Wysocki AB. The healing wound: a comparison of three clinically useful methods of measurements. *Decubitus* 1990; 3:18–25.
12. Verhonick PJ. Decubitus ulcer observations measured objectively. *Nurs Res* 1961; 10:211–214.
13. Gilman TH. Parameters for measurement of wound closure. *Wounds* 1990; 2:95–101.
14. Maklebust J, Sieggreen M. *Pressure ulcers: guidelines for prevention and nursing management.* West Dundee, IL: S-N Publications, 1991; 14–30.
15. Resch CS, Kermer E, Robson MC, et al. Pressure sore volume measurement. *J Am Geriatr Soc* 1988; 36:444–446.
16. Kundn J. A new way to size up a wound. *Am J Nurs* 1989; 89:206–207.
17. Bulstrode CJK, Goode AW, Scott PJ. Measurement and prediction of progress in delayed wound healing. *J R Soc Med* 1987; 80:210–212.
18. Bohannon RW, Pfaller BA. Documentation of wound surface area from tracings of wound perimeters. *Phys Ther* 1983; 63:1622–1624.
19. Yarkony GM. Pressure ulcers: a review. *Arch Phys Med Rehabil* 1994; 75:908–917.
20. Norton D. Calculating the risk: reflections on the Norton Scale. *Decubitus* 1989; 2:24–31.
21. Gosnell D. An assessment tool to identify pressure sores. *Nurs Res* 1973; 22:55–59.
22. Gosnell D. Assessment and evaluation of pressure sores. *Nurs Clin North Am* 1987; 22:399–416.
23. Bergstrom N, Demuth PJ, Braden BJ. A clinical trial of the Braden Scale for Predicting Pressure Sore Risk. *Nurs Clin North Am* 1987; 22:417–428.
24. La Mantia JG, Hirschwald JF, Goodman CI, Wooden VM, Delisser O, Staas WE. A program design to reduce chronic readmissions for pressure sores. *Rehabil Nurs* 1987; 12:22–25.
25. Staas WE Jr, Cioschi HM. Pressure sores: a multifaceted approach to prevention and treatment. *West J Med* 1991; 154:539.
26. Maklebust J, Mondoux L, Sieggreen M. Pressure relief characteristics of various support surfaces used in prevention and treatment of pressure ulcers enterostomal therapy. *J Enterostomal Ther* 1986; 13: 85–89.
27. Meehan M. Multisite pressure ulcer prevalence survey. *Decubitus* 1990; 3:14–7.
28. Shannon ML, Skorga P. Pressure ulcer prevalence in two general hospitals. *Decubitus* 1989; 2:38–43.
29. Oot-Giromini B, Bidwell FC, Heller NB, et al. Pressure ulcer prevention versus treatment, comparative product cost study. *Decubitus* 1989; 2:52–4.
30. Peterson NC, Bittmann S. The epidemiology of pressure sores. *Scand J Plast Reconstr Surg* 1971; 5:62–66.
31. Young L. Pressure ulcer prevalence and associated patient characteristics in one long-term care facility. *Decubitus* 1989; 2:52.
32. Brandeis GH, Morris JN, Nash DJ, Lipsitz LA. The epidemiology and natural history of pressure ulcers in elderly nursing home residents. *JAMA* 1990; 262:2905–2909.
33. McFarland GK, McFarland EA. *Nursing diagnosis and intervention,* 2nd ed. St. Louis: Mosby Yearbook, 1993.
34. Yetzer EA, Sullivan RL. The foot at risk: identification and prevention of skin breakdown. *Rehabil Nurs* 1992; 17:247–251.
35. Young EA, Burns PE. Pressure sores and the spinal cord injured. *Model Systems SCI Dig* 1981; 3:1981.
36. Hunter SM, Cathcart-Silberang TC, Langemo D, et al. Pressure ulcer prevalence and incidence in a rehabilitation hospital. *Rehabil Nurs* 1992; 17:239–242.
37. Yarkony GM, Roth EJ, Cybulski GR, Jaeger RJ. Neuromuscular stimulation in spinal cord injury. II. Prevention of secondary complications. *Arch Phys Med Rehabil* 1992; 73:195–200.
38. Mawson AR, Biundo JJ Jr, Neville P, Linares HA, Winchester Y, Lopez A. Risk factors for early occurring pressure ulcers following spinal cord injury. *Am J Phys Med Rehabil* 1988; 67:123–127.
39. Munro NH. Aging. In: Kinney JM, Jeejeebhoy KN, Hill G, Owen OE, eds. *Nutrition and metabolism in patient care.* Philadelphia: WB Saunders, 1988.
40. Richardson RR, Meyer PR. Prevalence and incidence of pressure sores in acute spinal cord injuries. *Paraplegia* 1981; 19:235–247.
41. Carlson CE, King RB, Kirk PM, Temple R, Heinemann A. Incidence and correlates of pressure ulcers development after spinal cord injury. *Rehabil Nurs Res* 1992; 1:34–40.
42. Clarke M, Kadhom HM. The nursing prevention of pressure sores in hospital and community patients. *J Adv Nurs* 1988; 13:365–373.
43. Hentziem B, Bergstrom N, Poxehl B. Prevalence and incidence of pressure ulcers and associated risk factors in a rural-based home health population. Poster presented at 17th Annual Midwest Nursing Research Society, Cleveland OH, March 28–30, 1993.
44. Miller H, Delozier J. *Cost implications of the pressure ulcer treatment guideline.* Contract No. 282-91-0070 p 17. Sponsored by the Agency for Health Care Policy and Research. Columbia, MD: Center for Health Policy Studies; 1994.
45. Daniel RK, Priest DL, Wheatley DC. Etiologic factors in pressure sores: an experimental model. *Arch Phys Med Rehabil* 1981; 62: 492–498.
46. Dinsdale SM. Decubitus ulcers: role of pressure and function in causation. *Arch Phys Med Rehabil* 1974; 55:146–152.
47. Kosiak M, Kubicek WG, Olson M, Danz JN, Kotlke FJ. Evaluation of pressure as a factor in the production of ischial ulcers. *Arch Phys Med Rehabil* 1958; 39:623–629.
48. Koziak M. Etiology and pathology of ischemic ulcers. *Arch Phys Med Rehabil* 1959; 40:62–69.
49. Langemo DK, Olson B, Hunter S, Hanson D, Burd C, Cathcart-Silberberg T. Incidence and prediction of pressure ulcers in five patient care settings. *Decubitus* 1991; 4:25–36.
50. Norton D, McCaren R, Exton-Smith AN. *An investigation of geriatric nursing problems in hospitals.* London: Churchill Livingstone, 1975.
51. Husain T. An experimental study of some pressure effects on tissues with reference to the bedsore problems. *J Pathol Bacteriol* 1953; 66: 347–382.
52. Landis EM. Micro-injection: studies of capillary blood pressure in human skin. *Heart* 1930; 15:209–228.
53. Lindan O. Etiology of decubitus ulcers: an experimental study. *Arch Phys Med Rehabil* 1961; 42:774–783.
54. Krouskop T, Noble PC, Garber SL, Spencer WA. The effectiveness of preventative management in reducing the occurrence of pressure sores. *J Rehabil Res Dev* 1983; 20:74–83.
55. Garber SL, Krouskop TA. Body build and its relationship to pressure distribution in the seated wheelchair patient. *Arch Phys Med Rehabil* 1982; 63:17–20.
56. Seiler WO, Allen S, Stahelin HB. Influence of the 30 degrees laterally included position and the ''super-soft'' 3-piece mattress on skin oxygen tension on areas of maximum pressure—implications for pressure sores prevention. *Gerontology* 1986; 32:158–166.
57. Reswick JB, Rogers JE. Experience at Rancho Los Amigos. Hospital with devices and techniques to prevent pressure sores. In: Kened RM, Conden JM, Scales JT, eds. *Bedsore biomechanics.* London: University Park Press, 1976; 300.
58. Daniel RK, Hall EJ, MacLeod MK. Pressure sores: a reappraisal. *Ann Plast Surg* 1979; 3:53–63.
59. Reichel S. shearing force as a factor in decubitus ulcers in paraplegics. *JAMA* 1958; 166:762–763.
60. Vidal J, Sarrias M. An analysis of the diverse factors concerned with the development of pressure sores on spinal cord patients. *Paraplegia* 1991; 29:261–267.
61. Luckman K, Sorensen K. *Medical surgical nursing—a psycho physiological approach.* Philadelphia: WB Saunders, 1980.
62. Bergstrom N, Braden B. A prospective study of pressure sore risk among the institutionalized elderly. *J Am Geriatr Soc* 1992; 40: 747–758.

63. Sieggren MY. Healing of physical wounds. *Nurs Clin North Am* 1987; 22:439–447.
64. Agarwal N, Del Guerico LRM, Lee B. The role of nutrition in the management of pressure sores. In: Lee BY, ed. *Chronic ulcers of the skin.* New York: McGraw-Hill, 1985.
65. Pinchocofsky-Devin G. Nutritional assessment and intervention. In: Krasner D, ed. *Chronic wound care.* King of Prussia, PA: Health Management Publications, 1990.
66. Natow AB. Nutrition in prevention and treatment of decutitus ulcers. *Top Clin Nurs* 1983; 5:32–44.
67. Powell JW. Increasing acuity of nursing home ptients and the prevalence of pressure ulcers: a ten year comparison. *Decubitus* 1989; 2: 56–58.
68. Lamid S, Ghatit AZ. Smoking spasticity and pressure sores in spinal cord injured patients. *Am J Phys Med Rehabil* 1983; 62:300–306.
69. Fisher BH. Topical hyperbaric oxygen treatment of pressure sores and skin ulcers. *Lancet* 1969; 2:405–409.
70. Anderson TP, Amdberg MM. Psychosocial factors associated with pressure sores. *Arch Phys Med Rehabil* 1979; 60:341–346.
71. Lloyd EE, Baker F. An examination of variables in spinal cord injury patients with pressure sores. *SCI Nurs* 1986; 3:219–222.
72. Young JS, Burns PE. Pressure sores and the spinal cord injured. *Model Systems SCI Dig* 1981; 3:9–18.
73. Richardson RR, Meyer PR. Prevalence and incidence of pressure sores in acute spinal cord injuries. *Paraplegia* 1981; 19:235–247.
74. Yetzer EA, Sullivan RL. The foot at risk: identification and prevention of skin breakdown. *Rehabil Nurs* 1992; 17:247–251.
75. Solis I, Krouskop T, Trainer N, Marbunger R. Spine interface pressure in children. *Arch Phys Med Rehabil* 1988; 69:524–526.
76. Krouskop TA, Garber SL. The role of technology in the prevention of pressure sores. *Ostomy Wound Management* 1987; 16:44–54.
77. Maklebust J, Sieggreen MY, Mondoux L. Pressure relief capabilities of the Sof-Care bed and the Clinitron bed. *Ostomy Wound Management* 1988; 32:36–41.
78. Pinzur MS, Schumacher D, Reddy N, Osterman H, Havey R, Patwardin A. Preventing heel ulcers: a comparison of prophylactic body support system. *Arch Phys Med Rehabil* 1991; 72:508–510.
79. Donovan W, Gargr S, Hamilton S, et al. Pressure ulcers in DeLisa JA, ed. *Rehabilitation medicine: principles and practices.* Philadelphia: JB Lippincott, 1988.
80. King RB, French ET. Procedures to maintain and restore tissue integrity. In: *Rehabilitation Institute of Chicago, Division of Nursing Rehabilitation procedures manual.* Rockville, MD: Aspen, 1990.
81. Hicks DJ. An incidence study of pressure sores following surgery. In: *ANA Clinical Sessions 1970.* New York: Appleton-Century-Crofts, 1971.
82. Conine TA, Choi AK, Lim R. The user friendliness of protective support surgaces in prevention of pressure sores. *Rehabil Nurs* 1989; 14:261–263.
83. Schwartz IS, Pervez N. Bacterial endocarditis associated with a permanent transvenous cardiac pacemaker. *JAMA* 1971; 218:736–737.
84. Roche S, Cross S, Burgess I, Pines C, Cayley AC. Cutaneous myiasis in an elderly debilitated patient. *Postgrad Med J* 1990; 66:776–777.
85. Soriano F, Aguado JM, Tormero J, Fernandez-Guerrero ML, Gomez-Garces JL. Bacteroides fragiles meningitis sucessfully treated with metronidazole after previous failure with thiamphenicol. *J Clin Microbiol* 1986; 24:472–473.
86. Klein NE, Moore T, Capen D, Green S. Sepsis of the hip paraplegic patients. *J Bone Joint Surg [Am]* 1988; 70:839–843.
87. Putnam T, Calenoff L, Betts HB, Rosen JS. Sinography in management of decubitus ulcers. *Arch Phys Med Rehabil* 1978; 59:243–245.
88. Firooznia H, Rafii M, Golimbu S, Sokolow J. Computerized temography in diagnosis of pelvic abscess in spinal cord injured patients. *Comput Radiol* 1983; 7:335–341.
89. Hooker EZ, Sibley P, Nemchusky B, Lopez E. A method for quantifying the area of closed pressure sores by senography and digitometry. *J Neurosci Nurs* 1988; 20:118–127.
90. Reuler JB, Cooney TG. The pressure sore: pathophysiology and principles of management. *Ann Intern Med* 1981; 94:661–666.
91. Hackler RH, Zampieri TA. Urethral complications following ischiectomy in spinal cord injury patients: a urethral pressure study. *J Urol* 1987; 137:253–255.
92. Wang TN, Lineaweaver WC, Scott T, Feldman R. Internal pudendal pseudo aneurysm complicatingan ischial pressure sore. *Ann Plast Surg* 1987; 19:381–383.
93. Berkwits L, Yarkony GM, Lewis V. Marjolin's ulcer complicating a pressure ulcer: case report and literature review. *Arch Phys Med Rehabil* 1986; 67:831–833.
94. Shetty KR, Duthie EH Jr. Thyrotoxicosis induced by topical iodine application. *Arch Intern Med* 1990; 150:2400–2401.
95. Aronoff GR, Friedman SJ, Doedems DJ, Lavelle KJ. Increased serum iodine concentration from iodine absorption through wounds treated topically with povidine-iodine. *Am J Med* Sci 1980; 279:173–176.
96. Johnson CA. Hearing loss following the application of topical meomycin. *J Burn Care* Rehabil 1988; 9:162–164.
97. Baxter C, Rodheaver G. Wound assessment and categorization. In: Eaglstein W, Baxter C, Mertz P, eds. *New directions in wound healing.* Princeton, NJ: ER Squibb, 1990.
98. Jones RC, Shires GT. Principles in the management of wounds. In: Schwartz SI, ed. *Principles of surgery.* New York: McGraw-Hill; 1974; 204.
99. Westaby S. *Wound care.* St. Louis: CV Mosby, 1987; 14.
100. Bendy RH Jr, Nuccio PA, Wolfe E, et al. Relationship of quantitative wound bacterial counts to healing of decubiti: effect of topical gentamicin. *Antimicrob Agents Chemother* 1964; 4:147–155.
101. Daltrey DC, Rhodes B, Chattwood JG. Investigation into the microbial flora of healing and non-healing ducubitus ulcers. *J Clin Pathol* 1981; 34:701–705.
102. Lyman IR, Tenry JH, Basson RP. Correlation between decrease in bacterial load and rate of wound healing. *Surg Gyncol Obstet* 1970; 130:616–621.
103. Sapico FL, Ginunas VJ, Thornhill-Joynes M, et al. Quantitative microbiology of pressure sores in different stages of healing. *Diagn Microbiol Infect Dis* 1986; 5:31–38.
104. Garner JS, Jarvis WR, Emori TG, Horan TC, Hughes JM. CDC definitions for nocosomial infections: guideline for handwashing and hospital environmental control, 1985. *Am J Infect Cont* 1986; 14:110–129.
105. Black JM, Black SB. Surgical management of pressure ulcers. *Nurs Clin North Am* 1987; 22:429–438.
106. Lewis VL Jr, Bailey MH, Pulawski G, King G, Basioum RW, Hendrix RW. The diagnosis of osteomyelitis in patients with pressure sores. *Plast Reconstr Surg* 1988; 81:229–232.
107. Boxer AM, Gottesman N, Bernstein H, Mandle I. Debridement of dermal ulcers and decubiti with collagenase. *Geriatrics* 1969; 24: 75–86.
108. Alverez OM, Mertz PM, Eaglstein WH. The effects of occlusive dressings on collagen synthesis and re-epithelization in superficial wounds. *J Surg Res* 1983; 35:142–148.
109. Longe RL. Current concepts in clinical therapeutic: pressure sores. *Clin Pharm* 1986; 5:669–681.
110. Torrance C. Pressure sores: what goes on? *Community Outlook* Nov 1983:332–340.
111. Stevenson TR, Thacker JG, Rodeheaver GT, Bacchetta C, Edgerton MT, Edlich RF. Cleaning the traumatic wound by high pressure syringe irrigation. *JACEP* 1976; 5:17–21.
112. Shand JE, McClement E. Recent advances in the treatment of pressure sores. *Paraplegia* 1979; 17:400–408.
113. Kurzuk-Howard G, Simpson L, Palmieri A. Decubitus ulcer care: a comparative study. *West J Nurs Res* 1985; 7:58–79.
114. Saydak SJ. A pilot test of two methods for the treatment of pressure ulcers. *J Enterostomal Ther* 1990; 17:139–142.
115. Gorse GJ, Messner RL. Improved pressure sore healing with hydrocelloid dressings. *Arch Dermatol* 1987; 123:766–771.
116. Xakellis GC, Chrischilles EA. Hydrocelloid versus saline gauge dressings in treating pressure ulcers: a cost-effectiveness analysis. *Arch Phys Med Rehabil* 1992; 73:463–469.
117. Crewe RA. Problems of rubber ring nursing cushions and a clinical survey of alternative cushions for ill patients. *Care Sci Pract* 1987; 5:9–11.
118. Feedar JA, Kloth LC. Conservative management of chronic wounds. In: Kloth LC, McCulloch JM, Feedar JA, eds. *Wound healing: alternatives in management.* Philadelphia: FA Davis, 1990.
119. Stillwell GK. Therapeutic heat and cold. In: Krusen FH, ed. *Handbook of physical medicine and rehabilitation,* 2nd ed. Philadelphia: WB Saunders, 1971.
120. Freytes HA, Fernandez B, Fleming WC. Ultraviolet light in the treatment of indolent ulcers. *South Med J* 1965; 58:223–226.

121. Kener J. Growth, respiration, and nuclear acid synthesis in ultravoilet-irradiated and in photoactivated *escherichia coli. J Bacteriol* 1953; 65:252–262.
122. Painter RB. The action of ultraviolet light on mammalian cells. In: Giese A, ed. *Photophysiology.* New York: Academic, 1970.
123. Geronemus R. The effect of UVC and UVB on epidermal wound healing. *Clin Res* 1982; 50:586.
124. Wills EE, Anderson TW, Beattie BL, Scott A. A randomized placebo-controlled trial of ultraviolet light in the treatment of superficial pressure sores. *J Am Geriatr Soc* 1983; 31:131.
125. McDiarmid T, Burns PN, Lewith GT, Machin D. Ultrasound and the treatment of pressure sores. *Physiotherapy* 1985; 71:66–70.
126. Clark RAF. Cutaneous tissue repair: basic biologic considerations. *J Am Inst Dermatol* 1965; 13:701.
127. Hogan RD, Burke KM, Franklin TD. The effect of ultrasound on miscrovascular hemodynamics in skeletal muscle: effects during ischemia. *Microvasc Res* 1982; 23:370–374.
128. Dyson M. The effect of ultrasound on the rate of wound healing and the quality of scar tissue. In: Mortimer A, Lee N, eds. *Proceedings of the International Symposium on Therapeutic Ultrasound.* Winnipeg, Manitoba: Canada Physiotherapy Association, 1981; 110–117.
129. Carley PJ, Wainapel SF. Electrotherapy for acceleration of wound healing: low intensity direct current. *Arch Phys Med Rehabil* 1985; 66:443–446.
130. Feedar JA, Kloth LC, Gentzkow GD. Chronic dermal ulcer healing enhanced with monophasic pulsed electrical stimulation. *Phys Ther* 1991; 71:639–649.
131. Gentzkow GD, Pollack SV, Kloth LC, Stubbs HA. Improved healing of pressure ulcers using dermapulse, a new electrical stimulation device. *Wounds* 1991; 3:158–170.
132. Griffen JW, Tooms RE, Mendius RA, Clifft JK, Vander Zwaag R, El-Zeky F. Efficacy of high voltage pulsed current for healing of pressure ulcers in patients with spinal cord injury. *Phys Ther* 1991; 71:443–442.
133. Kloth LC, Feeder JA. Acceleration of wound healing with high voltage, monophasic pulsed current. *Phys Ther* 1988; 68:503–508.
134. Linden RM, Morris D. The surgical management of pressure ulcers: a systematic approach based on staging. *Decubitus* 1990; 3:32–38.
135. Daniel RK, Faibisoff B. Muscle coverage of pressure points—the role of myocutaneous flaps. *Am Plast Surg* 1982; 6:446–452.
136. Mathes SJ, Feng LJ, Hunt TK. Coverage of the infected wound. *Am Surg* 1983; 198:420–429.
137. Vasconez LO, Schneider WJ, Trukiewicz MJ. Pressure sores. *Curr Prob Surg* 1977; 24:23.
138. Disa JJ, Carlton JM, Goldberg MH. Efficacy of operative cure in pressure sore patients. *Plast Reconstr Surg* 1992; 89:272–278.
139. Karaca AR, Binns JH, Blumenthal FA. Complications of total ischiectomy for the treatment of ischial pressure sores. *Plast Reconstr Surg* 1978; 62:96–99.
140. Mandrekas AD, Mastorakos DP. The management of decubitus ulcers by musculocutaneous flaps: a five year experience. *Ann Plast Surg* 1992; 28:167–174.
141. Relander M, Palmer B. Recurrence of surgically treated pressure sores. *Scand J Plast Reconstr Surg Hand Surg* 1988; 22:89–92.
142. Morgan JE. Recurrence of pressure ulcers: a study of the cases. *JAMA* 1976; 236:2430–2431.

Rehabilitation Medicine: Principles and Practice, Third Edition,
edited by Joel A. DeLisa and Bruce M. Gans.
Lippincott–Raven Publishers, Philadelphia © 1998.

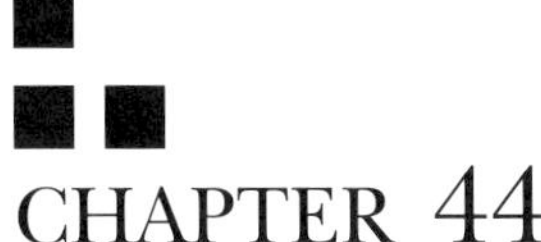

CHAPTER 44

Neurogenic Bladder and Bowel Dysfunction

Todd A. Linsenmeyer and James M. Stone

Voiding dysfunctions are commonly encountered in patients who are referred for rehabilitation. These voiding problems may result from medications, cognitive changes, physical impairments, or neurologic etiologies. Timely identification of voiding dysfunctions, treatment, and follow-up are important. This is particularly true in the rehabilitation setting, where voiding dysfunctions may cause patient embarrassment, interruption of therapy, and increased morbidity and ultimately make the difference between reintegration into the community and being confined to a home or nursing home.

ANATOMY AND PHYSIOLOGY OF THE UPPER AND LOWER URINARY TRACTS

Upper Urinary Tracts

The kidney can be thought of as two parts, the renal parenchyma, which secretes, concentrates, and excretes urine, and the collecting system, which drains urine from multiple renal calyces into a renal pelvis. The renal pelvis then narrows to become the ureter; this is known as the ureteropelvic junction (1).

The ureter is approximately 30 cm in length in the adult. It has three areas of physiological narrowing that take on clinical significance with respect to possible obstruction from stones. These areas are the ureteropelvic junction, the crossing over of the iliac artery, and the ureterovesical junction (2,3).

The ureterovesical junction is the place where the ureteral orifice opens up into the bladder. Its function is to allow urine to flow into the bladder but prevent reflux backward up into the ureter. This can be accomplished because the ureters traverse obliquely between the muscular and submucosal layers of the bladder wall for a distance of 1 to 2 cm before opening into the bladder (Fig. 44-1). Any increase in intravesical pressure simultaneously compresses the submucosal ureter and effectively creates a one-way valve (4). Presence of ureteral muscle in the submucosal segment also has been shown to be important in preventing reflux (5).

Normal Urine Transport from the Kidneys to the Bladder

Urine transport is the result of both passive and active forces. Passive forces are created by the filtration pressure of the kidneys. The normal proximal tubular pressure is 14 mm Hg, and the renal pelvis pressure is 6.5 mm Hg, which slightly exceeds resting ureteral and bladder pressures. Active forces are the result of peristalsis of the calyces, renal pelvis, and ureter. Peristalsis begins with the electrical activity of pacemaker cells at the proximal portion of the urinary collecting tract (6).

For the ureter to efficiently propel the bolus of urine, the contraction wave must completely coapt the ureteral walls (7). Ureteral dilation for any reason results in inefficient propulsion of the urine bolus, and this can delay drainage proximal to that point. This can result in further dilation and, over time, lead to hydronephrosis.

Lower Urinary Tracts

Anatomically, the bladder is divided into the detrusor and the trigone. The detrusor is composed of smooth muscle bundles that freely crisscross and interlace with each other. Near the bladder neck, the muscle fibers assume three distinct layers. The circular arrangement of the smooth muscles at the bladder neck allows them to act as a functional sphincter. The trigone is located at the inferior base of the bladder. It extends from the ureteral orifices to the bladder neck. The deep trigone is continuous with the detrusor smooth muscle;

T. A. Linsenmeyer: Departments of Physical Medicine and Rehabilitation and Surgery (Urology), University of Medicine and Dentistry of New Jersey, New Jersey Medical School, Newark, New Jersey 07103; and Department of Urology, Kessler Institute for Rehabilitation, West Orange, New Jersey 07052.

J. M. Stone: Northern California Surgical Group, Redding, California 96001.

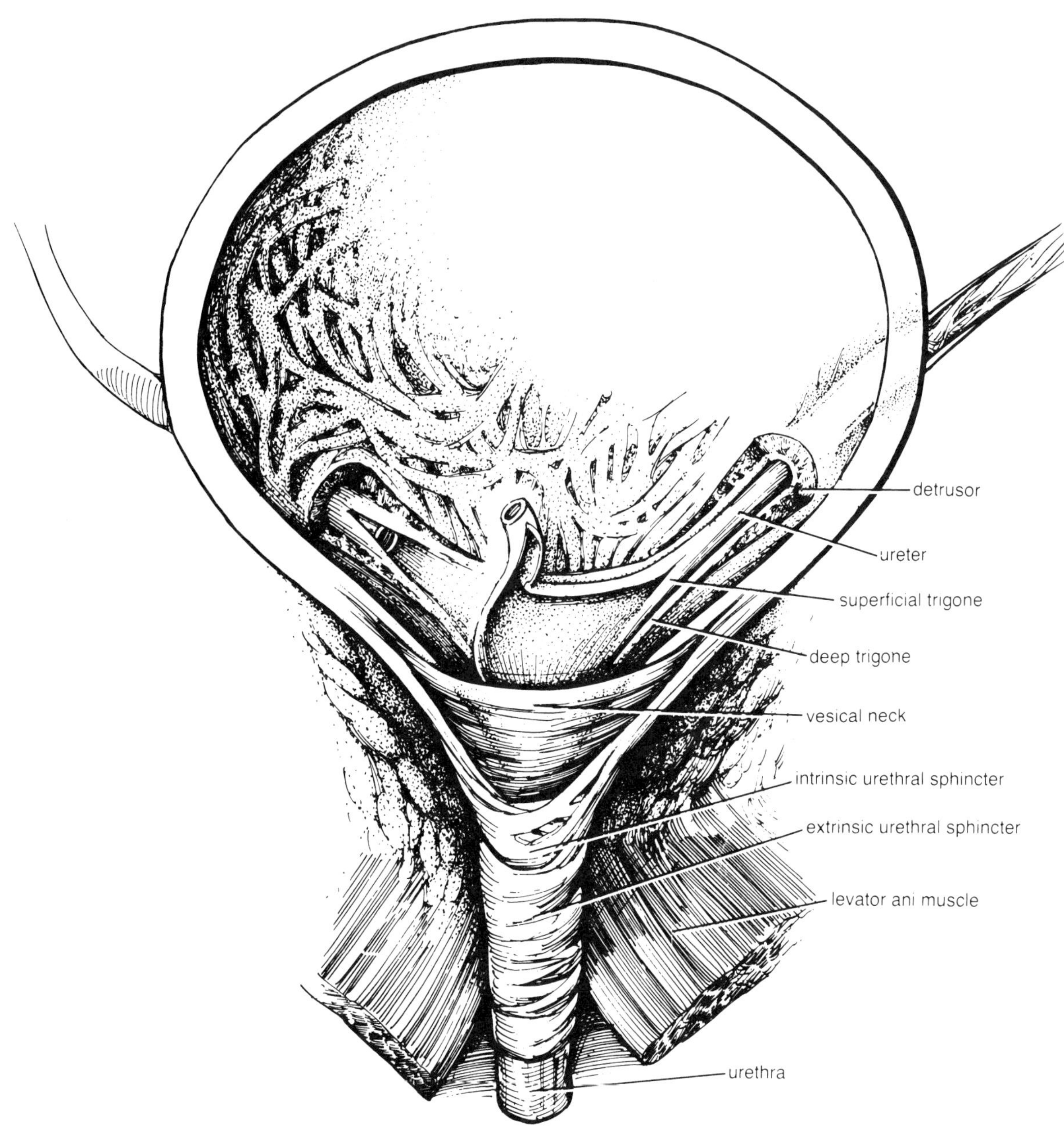

FIG. 44-1. Anatomy of the bladder and related structures in a woman. Note how the ureter tunnels for a distance through the bladder wall, helping to prevent vesicoureteral reflux. Also note that there is not a clear demarcation between the bladder neck and sphincter mechanism. (From Hinman F, Jr. Bladder repair. In: Hinman F, Jr., ed. *Urological surgery.* Philadelphia: WB Saunders, 1989; 433.)

the superficial trigone is an extension of the ureteral musculature (see Fig. 44-1) (4).

There is no clear demarcation of the musculature of the bladder neck and the beginning of the urethra in the man or woman. In the woman, the urethra contains an inner longitudinal and outer semicircular layer of smooth muscle. The circular muscle layer exerts a sphincteric effect along the entire length of the urethra, which is approximately 4 cm long.

In the man, the penis is made up of two corpora cavernosa that contain the spongy erectile tissue, and a corpora spongiosum that surrounds the urethra. The male urethra is divided into the posterior or prostatic urethra, extending from the bladder neck to the urogenital diaphragm, and the anterior urethra, which extends to the meatus. The junction between the anterior and posterior urethra is known as the membranous urethra.

Urinary Urethral Sphincters

Traditionally the urethra has been thought to have two distinct sphincters, the internal and the external or rhabdosphincter. The internal sphincter is not a true anatomic sphincter. Instead, in both men and women, the term refers to the junction of the bladder neck and proximal urethra, formed from the circular arrangement of connective tissue and smooth muscle smooth muscle fibers that extend from the bladder. This area is considered to be a functional sphincter because there is a progressive increase in tone with bladder filling so that the urethral pressure is greater than the intravesical pressure. These smooth muscle fibers also extend submucosally down the urethra and lie above the external rhabdosphincter (8).

In the man, the external or urethral rhabdosphincter often is diagrammatically illustrated as a thin circular band of striated muscle forming a diaphragm just distal to the prostatic urethra (i.e., membranous urethra). In an anatomic study, however, Myers and associates reconfirmed earlier studies showing that the urethral external striated sphincter does not form a circular band but has fibers that run up to the base of the bladder (8). The bulk of the fibers are found at the membranous urethra (9). This sphincter is under voluntary control. The striated muscular fibers in both the man and woman are thought to have a significant proportion of slow-twitch fibers with the capacity for steady tonic compression of the urethra. In the woman, striated skeletal muscle fibers circle the upper two-thirds of the urethra (9).

STRUCTURE AND FUNCTION OF THE MALE AND FEMALE CONTINENCE MECHANISM

In the man, the structures responsible for continence at the level of the membranous urethra include the mucosa, longitudinal smooth muscle of the urethra, striated sphincter, and levator ani musculature. Traditionally, the striated sphincter has been considered responsible for maintaining continence. However, experimental paralysis of the striated sphincter and levator ani following surgery for prostate outlet obstruction did not result in incontinence. This demonstrated the important role of the smooth muscle fibroelastic component of the membranous urethra. The increased tone at the bladder outlet (i.e., internal sphincter) also helps maintain continence (10).

In the woman, there are three important factors in maintaining continence:

1. Adequate pelvic floor support from the endopelvic fascia and anterior vagina.
2. Good sphincter function.
3. Maintenance of the intra-abdominal position of the proximal urethra.

During an increase in intra-abdominal pressure, continence is maintained by the downward-moving pelvic viscera compressing the urethra against the layer of endopelvic fascia and distribution of the increase of intra-abdominal pressure to the proximal intra-abdominal urethra. The urethral epithelium, which is sensitive to estrogen, is believed to help maintain continence by forming a mucosal seal (9).

NEUROANATOMY OF THE LOWER URINARY TRACT

Urine storage and emptying is a function of interactions among the peripheral parasympathetic, sympathetic, and somatic innervation of the lower urinary tract. Additionally, there is modulation from the central nervous system (CNS).

Bladder Neuroanatomy

Efferent System

The parasympathetic efferent supply originates from a distinct detrusor nucleus located in the intermediolateral gray matter of the sacral cord at S2 to S4. Sacral efferents emerge as preganglionic fibers in the ventral roots and travel through the pelvic nerves to ganglia immediately adjacent to or within the detrusor muscle to provide excitatory input to the bladder. After impulses arrive at the parasympathetic ganglia, they travel through short postganglionics to the smooth muscle cholinergic receptors. These receptors, called cholinergic because the primary postganglionic neurotransmitter is acetylcholine, are distributed through the bladder. Stimulation causes a bladder contraction (11,12).

The sympathetic efferent nerve supply to the bladder and urethra begins in the intermediolateral gray column from T11 through L2 and provide inhibitory imput to the bladder. Sympathetic impulses travel a relatively short distance to the lumbar sympathetic paravertebral ganglia. From here the sympathetic impulses travel along long postganglionic nerves in the hypogastric nerves to synapse at alpha- and beta-adrenergic receptors within the bladder and urethra. Variations in this anatomic arrangement do occur; sympathetic ganglia sometimes also are located near the bladder, and sympathetic efferent fibers may travel along the pelvic as well as the hypogastric nerves (Fig. 44-2) (11,12).

Sympathetic stimulation facilitates bladder storage because of the strategic location of the adrenergic receptors. Beta-adrenergic receptors predominate in the superior portion (i.e., body) of the bladder. Stimulation of beta receptors cause smooth muscle relaxation. Alpha receptors have a higher density near the base of the bladder and prostatic urethra; stimulation of these receptors causes smooth muscle contractions and therefore increases the outlet resistance of the bladder and prostatic urethra (Fig. 44-3) (11–13).

After spinal cord injury (SCI), several changes occur to the bladder receptors that alter bladder function. There is evidence that when smooth muscle is denervated, its sensitivity to a given amount of neurotransmitter increases (i.e., denervation supersensitivity). Therefore, smaller doses of various pharmacologic agents would be expected to have a much more pronounced effect in those with SCI as compared to those with nonneurogenic bladders (14).

A change in receptor location and density may also occur. Norlen and colleagues found that after complete denervation there was a change from a beta receptor predominance to an alpha receptor predominance (15). Because alpha receptors

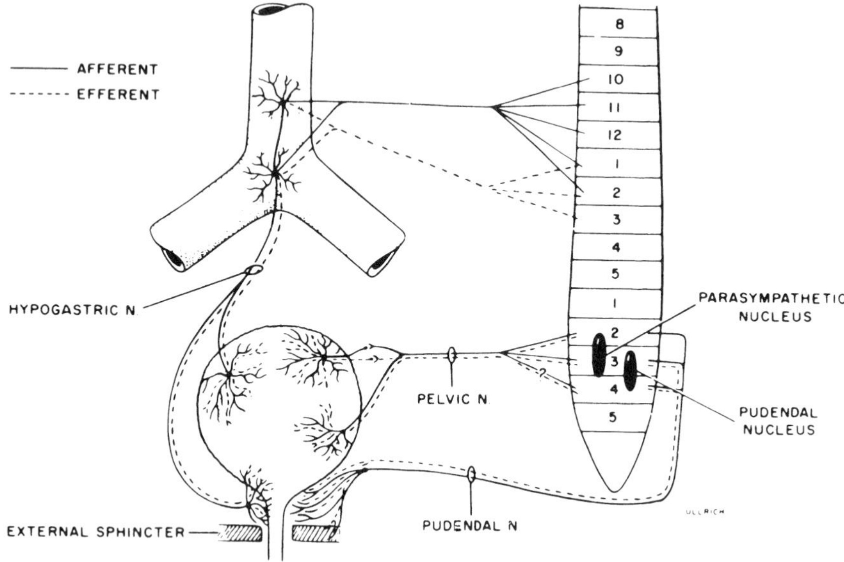

FIG. 44-2. Peripheral innervation of the bladder and urethra. Sympathetic stimulation responsible for storage travels through the hypogastric plexus. Parasympathetic stimulation causing bladder contractions travels through the pelvic nerve. (From Blaivas JG. Management of bladder dysfunction in multiple sclerosis. *Neurology* 1980; 30: 73.)

cause contraction of smooth muscle, a change in receptors may be one reason for some individuals to have poor compliance of the bladder after SCI.

Animal studies have revealed that, although the previously described long postganglionic neurons exist, there are ganglia close to the bladder and urethra in which there are both cholinergic and adrenergic fibers. This has been termed the urogenital short neuron system. These ganglia are composed of three cell types, adrenergic neurons, cholinergic neurons, and small intensely fluorescent (SIF) cells, which are believed to be responsible for this interganglionic modulation of the adrenergic and cholinergic neurons. Further work is needed to define this system in humans (16).

Afferent System

The most important afferents that stimulate voiding are those that pass to the sacral cord via the pelvic nerves. These afferents include two types of afferents, small myelinated A-delta and unmyelinated (C) fibers.

The small myelinated A-delta respond in a graded fashion to bladder distention and are essential for normal voiding. The unmyelinated (C) fibers have been termed "silent C-fibers" because they do not respond to bladder distention and therefore are not essential for normal voiding. However, these "silent C-fibers" do exhibit spontaneous firing when they are activated by chemical or cold temperature irritation at the bladder wall. Additionally, the unmyelinated (C) fi-

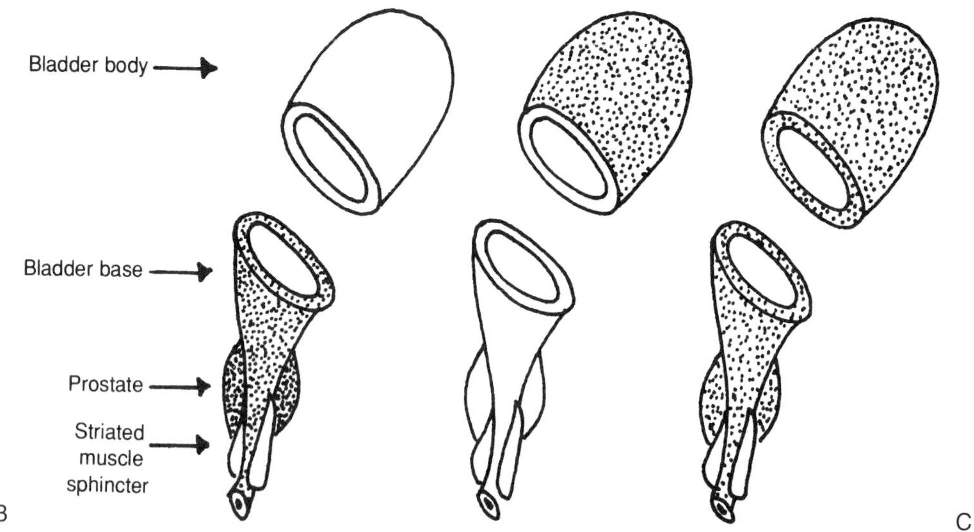

FIG. 44-3. Location of bladder receptors. Bladder storage is maintained by simultaneous sympathetic alpha-adrenergic receptor (contraction) **(A)** and beta-adrenergic receptor (relaxation) stimulation **(B)**. Bladder emptying occurs with parasympathetic cholinergic receptor stimulation **(C)**.

bers, rather than A-delta afferents, have been found to ''wake up'' and respond to distention and stimulate bladder contractions in animals with suprasacral SCI.

Increased C-fiber afferent activity after SCI has been experimentally demonstrated by systemic administration of capsaicin, a neurotoxin that is known to disrupt the function of C-fiber afferents. In non-SCI animals (with A-delta afferents), there was no blockage of bladder contractions with bladder distention. However, in SCI animals, capsaicin completely blocked rhythmic bladder contractions induced with bladder distention. These findings have important potential therapeutic implications. To date there has been some success at blocking uninhibited contractions with the use of intravesical capsacin in patients with neurogenic bladders. However, further work is needed to determine the optimal dosage and vehicle for intravesical instillation (18).

Bladder Neurotransmitters

It is known that there are more transmitters than acetylcholine and norepinephrine, including nitric oxide, vasoactive intestinal polypeptide (VIP), endogenous opioid peptides, and neuropeptide Y. These transmitters may work on their own or help modulate the classic neurotransmitters. Nitric oxide and VIP have smooth muscle relaxant effects. This helps to explain the concept of ''atropine resistance.'' It has been found that a single neurotransmitter blocking agent such as atropine fails to suppress 100% of the bladder or urethral activity (14,18). This explains why a combination of agents may be more effective than a higher dose of a single agent.

Urethral Sphincter Innervation

The external urethral sphincter classically has been described as having somatic innervation allowing the sphincter to be closed at will. Somatic efferents originate from a pudendal nucleus of sacral segments from S1 to S4. Somatic efferents then travel through the pudendal nerve to the neuromuscular junction of the striated muscle fibers in the external urethral sphincter.

The internal urethral sphincter has been described as being under control of the autonomic system. This area has a large number of sympathetic alpha receptors, which cause closure when stimulated. Animal studies have revealed that nitric oxide is an important parasympathetic neurotransmitter mediating relaxation of the urethral smooth muscle (8,18).

The distinction between the internal and external sphincter is, however, becoming less clear. Elbadawi and Schenk reported histochemical evidence of a triple innervation pattern of the external sphincter (i.e., rhabdosphincter) in five mammalian species, with dual sympathetic and parasympathetic autonomic components superimposed on the somatic component (17). Sundin and Dahlstrom demonstrated sprouting and increasing adrenergic terminals after parasympathetic denervation in cats (19). Crowe and associates reported a substantial invasion of adrenergic nerve fibers in smooth and striated muscle in the urethra in SCI patients with lower motor neuron lesions (20).

Influences of the Central Nervous System on the Lower Urinary Tract

Facilitation and inhibition of the autonomic nervous system are under control of the CNS. There are several theories of how this occurs. Denny-Brown and Robertson suggested that micturition was primarily mediated by a sacral micturition reflex (21). According to their theory, descending nervous system pathways modulate this micturition reflex (21). Barrington, Bradley, and de Groat thought that facilitative impulses to the bladder originated from a region of the anterior pons termed ''Barrington's center'' (22–24).

De Groat and associates additionally stressed the importance of the sympathetic nervous system in facilitating urine storage (24). Carlsson provided evidence that this pontine mesencephalic area also plays a role in coordinating detrusor and sphincter activity. Stimulation of Barrington's center significantly decreased electromyographic (EMG) activity in the periurethral striated sphincter while causing a bladder contraction (25).

Transection experiments in cats suggest that the net effect of the cerebral cortex on micturition is inhibitory. This also is true for the basal ganglia and corresponds to clinical findings of detrusor hyperreflexia in those with basal ganglia dysfunction (e.g., Parkinson's disease). The cerebellum is thought to maintain tone in the pelvis floor musculature and influence coordination between periurethral striated muscle relaxation and bladder emptying (15,25).

NORMAL VOIDING PHYSIOLOGY

Micturition should be considered as having two phases: the filling (storage) phase and the emptying (voiding) phase. The filling phase occurs when a person is not trying to void. The emptying phase occurs when a person is attempting to void or told to void.

During filling (filling or storage phase), there should be very little rise in bladder pressure. As filling continues, low intravesical pressure is maintained by a progressive increase in sympathetic stimulation of the beta receptors located in the body of the bladder that cause relaxation, and stimulation of the alpha receptors located at the base of the bladder and urethra that cause contraction. Sympathetic stimulation also inhibits excitatory parasympathetic ganglionic transmission, which helps supress bladder contractions. During the filling phase, there is a progressive increase in urethral sphincter EMG activity (26). Increased urethral sphincter activity also reflexly inhibits bladder contractions. When a bladder is full and has normal compliance, intravesical pressures are between 0 and 6 cm H_2O and should not rise above 15 cm H_2O. Filling continued past the limit of the viscoelastic properties of the bladder results in a steady progressive rise in intravesical pressure (27). This part of the filling curve usually is not seen in a person with normal bladder function, because this much filling would cause significant discomfort and not be tolerated.

When a patient is told to void (voiding or emptying phase), there should be cessation of urethral sphincter EMG activity and a drop in urethral sphincter pressure and funneling of the bladder neck. There is no longer reflex inhibition to the sacral micturition center from the sphincter mechanism. This is followed by a detrusor contraction. The urethral sphincter should remain open throughout voiding, and there should be no rises in intra-abdominal pressure during voiding. In younger individuals, there should be no postvoid residual (PVR), although PVRs may increase with aging (see Evaluation of Bladder Emptying—Postvoid Residual Urine Determinations).

GERIATIC VOIDING PHYSIOLOGY

Voiding physiology is often affected by the aging process. The kidneys undergo an age-related decrease in glomerular blood flow and renal blood flow (28). The elderly also experience a loss in concentrating ability and often excrete most of their fluid intake at night, even in the absence of medical conditions such as prostate outlet obstruction, diabetes, remobilization of lower extremity edema, and use of evening diuretics (29).

Detrusor overactivity (DO) has been reported as the most common type of voiding dysfunction in incontinent elderly men and women (29). This may be associated with a central nervous lesion (such as a stroke, head injury, cervical disk disease, etc.) and be called detrusor hyperreflexia. Alternatively, it may result from local changes in the bladder and be called detrusor instability. A replacement of normal muscle cell junctions by novel "protrusion junction cells" and ultraclose abutments, connecting cells into chains, which facilitates and increases spontaneous smooth muscle activity, has been found in incontinent elderly patients (30). There is often a combination of causes that results in DO. Detrusor hyperactivity may coexist with impaired contractility (DHIC) of the bladder wall, resulting in both incontinence and retention. This combination was found to be one of the most common urodynamic findings in the elderly incontinent nursing home population (29).

Outlet obstruction by prostatic hypertrophy is the second most common cause of incontinence in men, although most men with outlet obstruction do not have incontinence (29). Outlet obstruction results in a significant increase in collagen, leading to bladder trabeculation. This in turn can cause a decrease in the viscoelastic properties for storage as well as the ability to contract and may be one reason for increasing PVRs and decreasing bladder capacity with aging (31). It should be noted that outlet obstruction in women is rare; however, it may occur from various etiologies such as urethral stenosis or kinking from a large cystocele or a previous bladder neck suspension. A trabeculated bladder appearance in older women without obstruction usually results from a thinning of the bladder wall with more prominent muscle bundles rather than deposition of collagen (31).

Stress incontinence is the second most common cause of incontinence in elderly women (29). In younger women, stress incontinence frequently results from pelvic laxity; however, in elderly women, it is also caused by a decrease in urethral closure pressure. This decrease in urethral pressure has been attributed to a decrease in estrogen, which causes a loss of muscle bulk and atrophic changes of the urethra and vagina. This, in turn, can cause inflammation and friability of these tissues, decreased periurethral blood flow, further laxity of pelvic structures, and possible urethral prolapse (31).

Detrusor underactivity may also occur with aging. At a cellular level this has been characterized by widespread degenerative changes of both muscle cells and axons without accompanying regenerative changes (32). Ouslander and associates reported that approximately 25% of elderly patients evaluated had PVRs greater than 100 ml (33). Approximately 10% of geriatric incontinence has been attributed to overflow incontinence (29).

PEDIATRIC VOIDING PHYSIOLOGY

Voiding physiology also changes with age in children. In the newborn, the sacral micturition reflex is primarily responsible for voiding. Because the brainstem is intact, there is coordination of the bladder contraction with sphincter relaxation; however, there is little inhibition of the micturition reflex from the cerebral cortex. As the child grows, the voided volume increases, and voiding frequency decreases. By 3 years of age, most children have some voluntary control of voiding. This control usually is complete by the age of 4 years. There are some neurologically intact children, however, for whom complete control of voiding may take 5 or 6 years (34).

CLASSIFICATION OF VOIDING DYSFUNCTION

There are a wide variety of classifications to describe voiding dysfunctions. Ideally, the system should describe the type of neurologic lesion, clinical symptoms, urodynamic data, and treatment options. A single classification focusing on all of these factors does not exist. Current classifications have been based on neurologic lesion (e.g., Bors–Comarr, Bradley), urodynamic findings (e.g., Lapides, Krane–Siroky), functional classification (e.g., Wein), and combination of bladder and urethral function based on urodynamics (e.g., International Continence Society) (35–40).

Table 44-1 shows a combination of Wein's classification and possible urodynamic findings. Treatment then can be directed at the specific urodynamic findings.

TABLE 44-1. *Urodynamic and functional classification*

Incontinence
Caused by the bladder
Uninhibited contractions
Decreased capacity
Low compliance
Normal (cognitive/mobility issue)
Caused by the outlet
Decreased bladder neck pressure
Decreased external sphincter pressure
Retention
Caused by the bladder
Detrusor areflexia
Large capacity/high compliance
Normal (cognitive/mobility issue)
Caused by the outlet
High voiding pressure with low flow rate
Internal sphincter dyssynergia
External sphincter dyssynergia
Overactive sphincter mechanism (i.e., sphincter or pseudosphincter dyssynergia)
Retention and Incontinence
Caused by the bladder
Uninhibited contractions with underactive detrusor

VOIDING DYSFUNCTIONS FOUND IN COMMON NEUROLOGIC DISORDERS

Suprapontine Lesions

Any suprapontine lesion may affect voiding. Lesions may result from cerebrovascular disease, hydrocephalus, intracranial neoplasms, traumatic head injury, Parkinson's disease, and multiple sclerosis. It should be noted that multiple sclerosis is unique among the suprapontine lesions because it also affects the white matter of the spinal cord and often has a relapsing and remitting nature. The expected urodynamic finding following a suprapontine lesion is detrusor hyperreflexia without detrusor sphincter dyssynergia. As a result of various factors such as medications, prostate obstruction, and possible normal bladder function but poor cognition, however, the voiding dysfunctions may be very different from expectations. Voiding dysfunction following cerebrovascular accident (CVA), Parkinson's disease, and multiple sclerosis has been studied more extensively than those associated with other suprapontine lesions and is reviewed in the following discussion.

Cerebrovascular Accidents

After a CVA, some patients initially have acute urinary retention. The reason for this detrusor areflexia is unknown. Urinary incontinence, however, is the most common urologic problem following an acute CVA. Various series have reported that 49% to 60% of patients are incontinent 1 week post-CVA (41–43). In the inpatient rehabilitation setting, a 33% incidence of incontinence during the first 3 months post-CVA has been reported (44). It also has been well documented that this problem significantly improves or resolves in the majority of patients. At 1 month, the percentage of incontinent patients dropped to between 29% and 42%. By 6 months to 1 year post-CVA, 14% to 15% of patients still were incontinent, which is similar to the 15% to 30% incidence in the general geriatric population (41–43).

Detrusor hyperreflexia with uninhibited bladder contractions is the most common urodynamic finding following a stroke. It has been reported to occur 70% to 90% of the time (42,45,46). One hypothesis for this finding is the release of the spinal micturition reflexes from the inhibitory higher centers. Symptoms, however, often do not correlate with urodynamic findings. Linsenmeyer and Zorowitz evaluated 33 consecutive incontinent patients who were 1 to 3 months post-CVA. They found that whereas 82% of men had uninhibited contractions, 43% also had urodynamic evidence of outlet obstruction. Six percent of the incontinent group had no bladder contractions, and 12% had normal urodynamic findings (46). Voluntary sphincter contractions (i.e., pseudodyssynergia) to keep from voiding should not be misinterpreted as true detrusor sphincter dyssynergia. In a review of 550 patients, Blaivas reported that patients with CVAs do not develop true detrusor sphincter dyssynergia (47). Electromyographic studies by Siroky and Krane gave similar results (48).

Parkinson's Disease

Symptoms of bladder dysfunction have been reported in 37% to 72% of patients with Parkinson's disease. These symptoms may be frequency or urgency (57%), obstruction (23%), or a combination of the two (20%). Detrusor hyperreflexia with uninhibited bladder contractions has been the most common urodynamic finding (72% to 100%) (49–51). Detrusor hyperreflexia is thought to occur because of loss of the inhibitory input from the basal ganglia on the micturition reflexes; however, detrusor instability also has been associated with benign prostatic obstruction. Detrusor areflexia may result from bladder decompensation through a combination of bladder outlet obstruction and chronic use of anticholinergic and alpha-adrenergic medications (51).

Electromyographic studies of the external sphincter reveal that patients may have pseudodyssynergia or bradykinesia but not have true detrusor sphincter dyssynergia (49–51). The majority of patients (63% to 75%) have normal sphincter function (49,51).

Multiple Sclerosis

Only 6% of patients with multiple sclerosis first present with urologic complaints (52). Bemelmans and associates, however, reported that 50% of asymptomatic patients with early multiple sclerosis had urodynamic abnormalities that needed further follow-up, and 50% of these required therapeutic intervention (53). As the disease progresses, urologic symptoms become common, eventually affecting at least 50% of men and 80% of women (54). The type of voiding dysfunction often is difficult to predict because of the diffuse involvement and changing nature of the disease.

Goldstein and colleagues reported that in a series of 86 symptomatic patients, 49% had incontinence, 32% had urgency and frequency, and 19% had obstructive hesitancy and retention. They also documented that patients with similar neurologic findings may have different voiding dysfunctions and that urologic signs and symptoms do not accurately reflect the voiding dysfunction (55). Wheeler and associates found that 55% of patients who were followed had changes in their urodynamic picture. The urodynamic pattern varied from detrusor areflexia to detrusor hyperreflexia and vice versa (56).

Because suprapontine and suprasacral plaques occur most frequently, detrusor hyperreflexia is the most common urodynamic finding; however, up to 50% of patients have poorly sustained uninhibited bladder contractions with inefficient bladder emptying. Detrusor areflexia is found in approximately 20% of patients with urologic symptoms. This is believed to be a result of sacral plaque involvement (57).

True detrusor sphincter dyssynergia may occur in multiple sclerosis when there is involvement of the suprasacral spinal cord. Approximately 15% to 20% of patients develop detrusor sphincter dyssynergia. Blaivas reported that this was an ominous sign because of the potential for upper tract damage and development of reflux as a result of the increased intravesical pressures needed to force urine past the dyssynergic sphincter. Upper tract pathologic processes, including pyelonephritis, renal calculi, reflux, and hydronephrosis, have been reported to occur in 10% to 20% of patients with multiple sclerosis (58,59).

Suprasacral Spinal Cord Lesions

Traumatic SCI is the most common suprasacral lesion affecting voiding. Other suprasacral lesions include transverse myelitis, multiple sclerosis, and primary or metastatic spinal cord tumor.

Patients with suprasacral spinal cord lesions would be expected to have detrusor hyperreflexia with detrusor sphincter dyssynergia. However, in cases of partial lesions, occult lesions of the sacral cord, or persistent spinal shock, this is not always the case (60).

Traumatic suprasacral SCI results in an initial period of spinal shock, in which there is hyporeflexia of the somatic system below the level of injury and detrusor areflexia. During this phase, the bladder has no contractions, even with various maneuvers such as water filling, bethanechol supersensitivity testing, or suprapubic tapping. The neurophysiology of spinal shock and its recovery is not known. Recovery of bladder function usually follows recovery of skeletal muscle reflexes. Uninhibited bladder contractions gradually return after 6 to 8 weeks (61).

Clinically, a person with a traumatic suprasacral SCI may begin having episodes of urinary incontinence and various visceral sensations, such as tingling, flushing, increased lower extremity spasms, or autonomic dysreflexia with the onset of uninhibited contractions. As uninhibited bladder contractions become stronger, the PVRs decrease. Rudy and associates reported that voiding function appears optimal at 12 weeks postinjury (62). However, detrusor hyperreflexia has been reported to have a delayed onset up to 22 months postinjury. Eventually, all of these patients did develop uninhibited contractions (63). Bors and Comarr considered the bladder "balanced" when PVRs were less than 20% of the total bladder capacity in those with detrusor hyperreflexia (35). Graham reports that 50% to 70% of patients will develop balanced bladders without therapy (64). Unfortunately, high intravesical voiding pressures usually are required for the development of a balanced bladder. These high pressures may cause renal deterioration (see Hydronephrosis; Vesicoureteral Reflux).

Traditionally, it has been thought that there is decreased activity of the external urethral sphincter during acute spinal shock. However, Downie and Awad noted in dogs that with surgical transection between T2 and T8, there was no change in the activity of the periurethral striated musculature despite detrusor areflexia (65). In humans, Nanninga and Meyer found that in 44 patients in spinal shock with suprasacral lesions, all had a positive bulbocavernosus reflex, and 30 of 32 had sphincter activity despite detrusor areflexia within 72 hours of injury (66). Koyanagi and colleagues noted that external sphincter electrical activity was not affected during acute spinal shock but was likely to increase after recovery from spinal shock. This increase was more marked in those with high suprasacral lesions than in those with low suprasacral lesions (67).

Detrusor–external sphincter dyssynergia also commonly occurs following suprasacral lesions. Blaivas and associates noted that it occurred in 96% of patients with suprasacral lesions. They found several different patterns of striated sphincter dyssynergia (68). Rudy and associates proposed that detrusor–external sphincter dyssynergia is an exaggerated continence reflex. The continence reflex is the normal phenomenon of increasing urethral sphincter activity with bladder filling. They believed that the patterns described by Blaivas and colleagues represented variations of the single continence reflex (62).

In addition to the detrusor external sphincter dyssynergia, internal sphincter dyssynergia also has been reported, often occurring at the same time as detrusor external sphincter dyssynergia.

Sacral Lesions

There are a variety of lesions that may affect the sacral cord or roots. These include spinal trauma, herniated lumbar disk, primary or metastatic tumors, myelodysplasia, arteriovenous malformation, lumbar stenosis, and inflammatory process (e.g., arachnoiditis). In Pavlakis and associates' series, trauma was responsible for conus and cauda equina lesions over 50% of the time. The next most common cause was L4–L5 or L5–S1 intervertebral disk protrusion. The incidence of lumbar disk prolapse causing cauda equina syndrome is between 1% and 15% (69). Damage to the sacral cord or roots generally results in a highly compliant acontractile bladder; however, particularly in patients with partial injuries, the areflexia may be accompanied by decreased bladder compliance, resulting in progressive increases in intravesical pressure with filling (70). The exact mechanism by which sacral parasympathetic decentralization of the bladder causes decreased compliance is unknown (70,71).

It has been noted that the external sphincter is not affected to the same extent as the detrusor. This is because the pelvic nerve innervation to the bladder usually arises one segment higher than the pudendal nerve innervation to the sphincter (72). The nuclei also are located in different portions of the sacral cord, with the detrusor nuclei located in the intermediolateral cell column and the pudendal nuclei located in the ventral gray matter. This combination of detrusor areflexia and an intact sphincter helps contribute to bladder overdistention and decompensation.

Peripheral Lesions

There are multiple etiologies for peripheral lesions that could affect voiding. The most common lesion is a peripheral neuropathy secondary to diabetes mellitus. Other peripheral neuropathies that have been associated with voiding dysfunction include chronic alcoholism, herpes zoster, Guillain–Barré syndrome, and pelvic surgery (73,74). A sensory neuropathy is the most frequent finding in diabetes. Urodynamic findings, including decreased bladder sensation, chronic bladder overdistention, increased PVRs, and possible bladder decompensation, may result from bladder overdistention secondary to decreased sensation of fullness. Andersen and Bradley reported that in their series, mean bladder capacity was 635 ml, with a range of 200 to 1,150 ml (75). An autonomic neuropathy also may be responsible for decreased bladder contractility. Guillain–Barré syndrome and herpes zoster are predominantly motor neuropathies. Transient voiding symptoms, predominantly urinary retention, have been reported to occur in 0% to 40% of patients and are thought to represent involvement of the autonomic sacral parasympathetic nerves. Detrusor hyperreflexia occasionally has been found in those with Guillain–Barré syndrome (76). Voiding dysfunctions resulting from pelvic surgery or pelvic trauma usually involve both motor and sensory innervation of the bladder (75).

COMPREHENSIVE EVALUATION OF VOIDING DYSFUNCTION

Neurourologic History

A thorough patient history is required to identify the neurologic diagnosis, cognitive deficits, and associated medical problems. The urologic history should focus initially on the patient's voiding complaints. Symptoms related to urinary retention may include a decreased urinary stream, intermittent stream, feeling of the bladder not being empty, or having to strain to void. Symptoms of urinary incontinence may include frequency, urgency, and feeling of wetness. Information can be obtained in those who are poor historians by reviewing the nurses' notes, from family members, and from the patient's intake and output chart. Outpatients should be asked to record their intake and output and incontinent episodes for at least 48 hours. The history should establish whether the onset of the current symptoms is new, has become worse, or has remained unchanged since the neurologic insult. This will allow for more meaningful discussions when patients and family ask about ''returning to normal.'' A preexisting problem such as urinary frequency may cause incontinence from decreased mobility.

Despite the importance of getting a clear understanding of the patient's symptoms, it is important not to initiate treatment based on symptoms. It is well established that symptoms often correlate poorly with the actual voiding problem. Katz and Blaivas, in a prospective study of 425 consecutive patients, found that the clinical assessment based on symptoms did not correlate with the objective urodynamic findings in 45% of patients thought to have storage problems, in 25% believed to have emptying problems, and in 54% of those believed to have storage and emptying problems (77). Ouslander and associates found in the geriatric female population that presenting symptoms were predictive of the urodynamic diagnosis in only 55% of those with pure urge incontinence (78).

Significant past history includes additional medical problems that may contribute to present problems, such as diabetes, previous CVAs, hypertension, and use of diuretics. The past history also needs to focus on surgery that may affect voiding, such as previous transurethral resection of the prostate, surgery for stress incontinence, or pelvic surgery. Questions about past and present bowel and erectile function should be asked. Potentially reversible causes of voiding disorders need to be investigated. A helpful mnemonic coined by Resnick and Yalla to describe the reversible causes of incontinence in the elderly is *DIAPPERS* (79). These same factors also may be responsible for problems with retention. The mnemonic can be broken down as follows:

Delirium
Infection
Atrophic vaginitis, urethritis
Pharmaceuticals
Psychological
Endocrine
Reduced mobility
Stool impaction

The physiatric history that has particular significance for voiding dysfunction is hand function, dressing skills, sitting balance, ability to perform transfers, and ability to ambulate. These factors not only play a role in why a person may be incontinent (e.g., not being able to undress, get to the bathroom, or transfer to a commode) but also are important considerations in developing management strategies.

Neurourologic Examination

The neurourologic physical examination should focus on the abdomen, external genitalia, and perineal skin. In performing the rectal examination, it is important to note that it is not the overall size of the prostate but the amount of prostate growing inward that causes obstruction. Therefore, urodynamic study rather than rectal examination is needed to diagnose outflow obstruction objectively.

In the postmenopausal woman, the urethra and vaginal introitus should be examined for atrophic changes suggestive of estrogen deficiency. In women, the examination also should focus on the degree of pelvic support. A determination of masses producing extrinsic compression on the bladder should be made during the vaginal examination.

The mental status portion of the neurourologic examination should, as a minimum, evaluate the patient's level of consciousness, orientation, speech, long- and short-term memory, and comprehension. Voiding disorders may be secondary to or made worse by disorientation, inability to communicate the desire to void, or lack of understanding when the patient is told to void.

The sensory examination should focus on determining the level of injury in those with SCI. Especially important is establishing if the level of injury is above T6, which would make the patient prone to autonomic dysreflexia. Sacral sensation evaluates the afferent limb (i.e., pudendal nerve) of the sacral micturition center. Loss of pinprick and light touch sensation in the hands and feet is suggestive of a peripheral neuropathy.

The motor examination helps to establish the level of injury and degree of completeness in those with SCI. Hand function should be assessed to determine the ability to undress or possibly perform intermittent catheterization (IC). Upper and lower extremity spasticity, sitting, standing, and ambulating need to be evaluated. Anal sphincter tone also should be evaluated. Decreased or absent tone suggests a sacral or peripheral nerve lesion, whereas increased tone suggests a suprasacral lesion. Voluntary contraction of the anal sphincter tests sacral innervation, suprasacral integrity, and the ability to understand commands.

Cutaneous reflexes that are helpful to the neurourologic examination are the cremasteric (L1–L2), bulbocavernosus (S2–S4), and anal reflex (S2–S4). Absence of these cutaneous reflexes suggests pyramidal tract disease or a peripheral lesion. The bulbocavernosus reflex has been reported to be present only 70% to 85% of the time in neurologically intact people (80). A false negative often results from a person being nervous and already having his or her anal sphincter clamped down at the time of the examination. Muscle stretch reflexes also should be evaluated. A sudden increase in spasticity may indicate a urinary tract infection. In addition, pathologic reflexes (e.g., Babinski reflex) may help localize the neurologic lesion.

UROLOGIC ASSESSMENT OF THE UPPER AND LOWER URINARY TRACT

Indications for Testing

A variety of tests can be performed to evaluate the upper and lower urinary tract. The exact types of tests and follow-up depend on the disease process, the patient's clinical course, and any preexisting urologic problems needing further follow-up.

If the disease process is one that is not known generally to affect the upper tracts, such as a stroke, hip replacement with retention, or peripheral neuropathy, then the evaluation can be directed at the lower urinary tracts. Evaluation of the upper tracts should be undertaken if there is any suggestion of upper tract involvement such as an episode of fever or chills attributed to pyelonephritis or hematuria.

Patients with disease processes that occasionally affect the upper tracts, such as multiple sclerosis, should undergo baseline testing of the upper tracts and then periodic screening. Emphasis otherwise is directed primarily at the lower tract with the use of urine analysis (UA), culture and sensitivity (CS), PVR, and urodynamics. Testing usually is done annually, but may be needed more or less frequently depending on the patient's clinical course.

Spinal-cord-injured patients, particularly those with potential high intravesical voiding pressures, need constant surveillance of the upper tracts as well as lower tracts. There are no studies investigating the frequency with which these tests should be done. Institutions often will have SCI patients undergo a yearly evaluation for the first 5 to 10 years, and if their upper tracts are stable, then evaluations every other year. People with an indwelling suprapubic or Foley catheter, however, often will get yearly cystoscopy to rule out stones and bladder tumors.

Specific Upper and Lower Tract Tests

Tests designed to evaluate the upper tracts include an intravenous pyelogram (IVP), renal ultrasound, 24-hour urine creatinine clearance, and quantitative renal scan (81,82). The IVP traditionally has been used to visualize kidneys and ureters but has largely been replaced by ultrasound and renal scan. Reasons for not using IVPs to screen patients include potential allergic reactions, radiation exposure, and patient inconvenience, specifically getting an IVP laxative preparation the night before the test. Because an IVP with tomograms gives good anatomic detail, this test is often very helpful when there is a concern about possible kidney or ureteral tumors, possible ureteral stones, or equivocal ultrasound or renal scan findings.

The kidney ultrasound is helpful for detecting hydronephrosis and kidney stones (81). The major disadvantage of ultrasound is that it is user dependent and does not show renal function. Some institutions use renal ultrasound for initial screening, and many use renal ultrasound as an adjunctive study if there is a possible anatomic abnormality or stone noted on KUB, IVP, or renal scan. If further anatomic definition is needed, computerized tomography should be considered.

The quantitative renal scan is an excellent way to monitor renal function and drainage. Many institutions use this as the primary modality to evaluate renal function. Attempts should be made to obtain the glomerular filtration rate (GFR) or effective renal plasma flow (ERPF) (82). If the nuclear medicine department does not have the capability to obtain a GFR or ERPF, a renal scan and a 24-hour urine creatinine clearance can be used to follow year-to-year renal function quantitatively. Serum creatinine is not helpful for monitoring yearly kidney function because it may remain normal despite moderate to severe renal deterioration (83).

Tests to evaluate the lower tracts include cystogram, cystoscopy, and urodynamics. Because each of these involves instrumentation, it is best to obtain a urine CS and give antibiotics if positive before the testing.

Some indications for cystoscopy in those with voiding disorders include hematuria, recurrent symptomatic urinary tract infections, recurrent asymptomatic bacteriuria with a stone-forming organism (i.e., *Proteus mirabilis*), an episode of genitourinary sepsis, urinary retention, or incontinence, pieces of eggshell calculi obtained when irrigating a catheter, and long-term indwelling catheter. Cystoscopy also is indicated when one is removing an indwelling Foley catheter that has been in place 4 to 6 weeks or changing to a different type of management, such as IC or a balanced bladder. Cystoscopy can reveal a pubic hair or eggshell calculus that may be missed on radiography and serve as a nidus for bladder stones. Urodynamics provides objective information on voiding function (Table 44-2).

TABLE 44-2. *Common tests for neurourologic evaluation*

Upper tracts
Intravenous pyleogram
Quantitative renal scan
24-Hour urine creatinine clearance
Renal ultrasound
Lower tracts
Urine culture and sensitivity
Cystoscopy
Postvoid residual
Cystogram
Urodynamics

Urodynamics

Urodynamics is defined as the study of normal and abnormal factors in the storage, transport, and emptying of urine from the bladder and urethra by any appropriate method (40). When deciding on an appropriate urodynamic test, one needs to consider whether information is needed about the filling phase, emptying phase, or both phases of micturition.

The following are some of the more common indications for a urodynamics evaluation:

Recurrent urinary tract infections (UTIs) in a patient with neurogenic bladder
Urinary incontinence
Frequency
Large PVRs (i.e., retention)
Deterioration of the upper tracts
Monitoring of voiding pressures
Evaluation and monitoring of pharmacotherapy

The physician's presence is important to help direct the urodynamics study. Typical decisions include how much water to put in the bladder, whether to repeat the study, and whether to have the patient sit or stand to void. Observing the patient during urodynamics also will help in getting an idea of factors that might influence the test, such as patient anxiety or inability to understand when told to void. Blood pressure monitoring is particularly important in SCI patients prone to autonomic dysreflexia.

Evaluation of Bladder Filling (Storage Phase)

The bedside cystometrogram involves filling the bladder with water through a Foley catheter. It is often attached by means of a Y-connector to a manometer, which is used to measure the rise in water pressure. This test can be used to evaluate sensation, stability, and capacity, and as a screening test to determine if a SCI patient has come out of spinal shock. There are several limitations to the bedside cystometrogram, however. It is difficult to determine if small rises in the water column result from intra-abdominal pressure (i.e., straining) or a bladder contraction. An iatrogenic bladder contraction can be elicited if the tip of the Foley catheter rubs against the trigone pressure sensors, which can then trigger bladder contractions. Most important, the voiding phase cannot be evaluated.

The carbon dioxide urodynamics apparatus often has an additional channel to measure intraabdominal pressure, making it easier to interpret rises in the intravesical pressure. Although the gas is cleaner and neater to use than water, the major disadvantage is that the voiding phase of micturition cannot be evaluated.

Evaluation of Bladder Emptying

One of the easiest screening tests to evaluate bladder emptying is a PVR; however, it should not be used to characterize the specific type of voiding dysfunction. The PVRs can be determined with catheterization or bladder ultrasound. A younger person should have no PVR; however, an elderly person with no voiding complaints may have a PVR or 100 to 150 ml. A normal PVR does not rule out a voiding problem. For example, a PVR may be normal despite significant outflow obstruction (e.g., benign prostate hypertrophy, sphincter–detrusor dyssynergia) as a result of a compensatory increase in the strength of detrusor contractions or of absent bladder contractions in the presence of increasing intra-abdominal pressure (e.g., Valsalva maneuver, Crede maneuver). Caution also has to be taken in interpreting a large PVR. It may be abnormal because it was not taken immediately after voiding, because of poor patient understanding, or because of an abnormal voiding situation (e.g., the patient was given a bedpan at 2:00 a.m.).

A waterfill urodynamic study is necessary to measure both the filling and the emptying phase of micturition. More sophisticated urodynamic studies also may incorporate urethral pressure recordings, urethral sphincter or anal sphincter EMG, videofluoroscopy, and the use of various pharmacologic agents such as bethanechol (Fig. 44-4).

Normal Waterfill Urodynamics Study

A waterfill urodynamic study evaluates two distinct phases of bladder function. The first is the filling (storage) phase, during which water is being infused into the bladder. Urodynamic parameters that can be evaluated during this phase include bladder sensation, bladder capacity, bladder wall compliance, and bladder stability (whether or not there are uninhibited contractions). The second portion of the study is the voiding (emptying) phase. The voiding phase is considered to begin when a person is told to void. In those who have neurogenic bladders and reflexly void, the voiding phase is considered to begin when the person has an uninhibited contraction and voiding begins. Urodynamic parameters that can be evaluated during the voiding phase include opening or leak-point pressure (bladder pressure at which voiding begins), maximum voiding pressure, urethral sphincter activity (EMG or actual pressure), flow rate, voided volume, and postvoid residual. In those who have the potential for autonomic dysreflexia, changes in blood pressure before, during, and after voiding can also be evaluated.

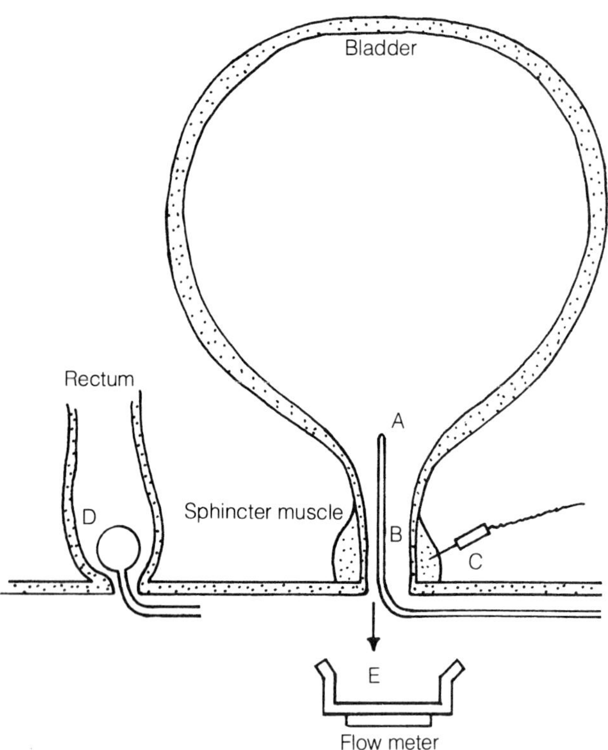

FIG. 44-4. Waterfill urodynamics setup. Simultaneous monitoring of various urodynamics parameters are shown. Intravesical pressure minus intra-abdominal pressure will produce the detrusor pressure (P_{det}). **A:** Intravesical pressure, P_{ves}. **B:** Urethral sphincter pressure, P_{ur}. **C:** Urethral sphincter electromyography. **D:** Intra-abdominal pressure, P_{abd}. **E:** Urine flow rate.

With an empty bladder, there should be no sensation of fluid within the bladder. During the filling phase, the first sensation of fullness usually occurs with 100 to 200 ml within the bladder. The sensation of fullness occurs around 300 to 400 ml, and the onset of urgency usually occurs between 400 to 500 ml. There is, however, variability in bladder capacity, which ranges between 400 and 750 ml in adults. There should be little to no rise in the intravesical pressure, which indicates normal bladder wall compliance. Additionally, there should be no involuntary bladder contractions during this part of the study.

During the voiding phase, the detrusor pressures usually are less than 30 cm H_2O in women and between 30 and 50 cm H_2O in men. A normal maximum flow rate is 15 to 20 ml/sec and should not be less than 10 ml/sec in any age group. The patient should have at least 150 ml in the bladder because the flow rate depends on the voided volume (44). The flow usually has a bell-shaped curve, progressively increasing to its maximum rate and then decreasing. The urethral sphincter should remain open throughout voiding, and there should be no rises in intra-abdominal pressure during voiding. As previously discussed, there should be no PVR, although PVRs increase with aging. A single elevated PVR during urodynamics should be interpreted with caution because the patient may be nervous and voluntarily stop the urine stream. Several catheterized or ultrasound PVR tests should be done to confirm an increased urodynamic PVR (Fig. 44-5). Urodynamics is able to characterize specific types of voiding patterns (Fig. 44-6).

Special Considerations in Children

At one time, urodynamic evaluation was delayed until a child was school aged and definitive corrective surgery was to be performed. However, reflux and renal deterioration often occur during the first 3 years of life. McGuire reported that there was a high incidence of renal deterioration in patients with urethral leak point pressures above 40 cm H_2O (85). Therefore, it is recommended that all myelodysplastic newborn children be evaluated as soon as possible (86).

It is difficult to obtain high-quality waterfill urodynamic

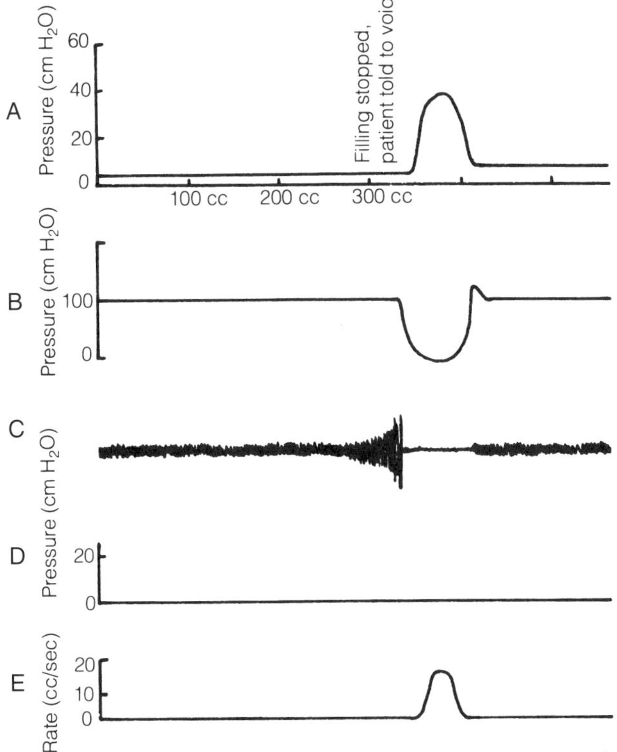

FIG. 44-5. Normal urodynamic findings. There is a minimal rise in intravesical pressure during the filling phase. The voiding phase is initiated with quieting of electromyographic activity, and relaxation of the external urethral sphincter is followed by a bladder contraction. **A:** Intravesical pressure (P_{ves}). **B:** Urethral sphincter pressure (P_{ur}). **C:** Urethral sphincter electromyography. **D:** Intra-abdominal pressure (P_{abd}). **E:** Urine flow rate.

studies on children younger than 4 or 5 years. In younger children, it sometimes is necessary to use sedation or general anesthesia. It is important that children feel comfortable with the physician, nurses, and test. As a general principle, the amount of additional information gained from insertion of EMG needles usually is not enough to warrant the risk of obtaining poor urodynamics results from a crying, fearful child. This is especially true if it is anticipated that the child will come back for follow-up studies.

Pharmacologic Testing

Pharmacologic testing sometimes is done in conjunction with this urodynamics test. Lapides and associates popularized the bethanechol supersensitivity test. A 15-cm rise in pressure of subcutaneous bethanechol is considered positive (87). Wheeler and colleagues have pointed out that false-positive tests may be caused by urinary tract infections, psychogenic stress, and azotemia (88). Therefore, when this test is used, it should be interpreted in light of the rest of the neurologic examination.

MANAGEMENT OF VOIDING DYSFUNCTIONS

A useful way to organize management of voiding dysfunctions is to base options on a modification of the Wein classification: incontinence caused by the bladder or by the outlet (e.g., bladder neck, sphincter, or prostate) or retention caused by the bladder or by the outlet. Management can be categorized as behavioral, pharmacologic, surgical, or supportive. Table 44-3 shows various treatment options. Often using a combination of management options is useful.

It is important to know the type of voiding dysfunction, particularly when considering pharmacologic and surgical options (see Table 44-3). Empirical pharmacotherapy should

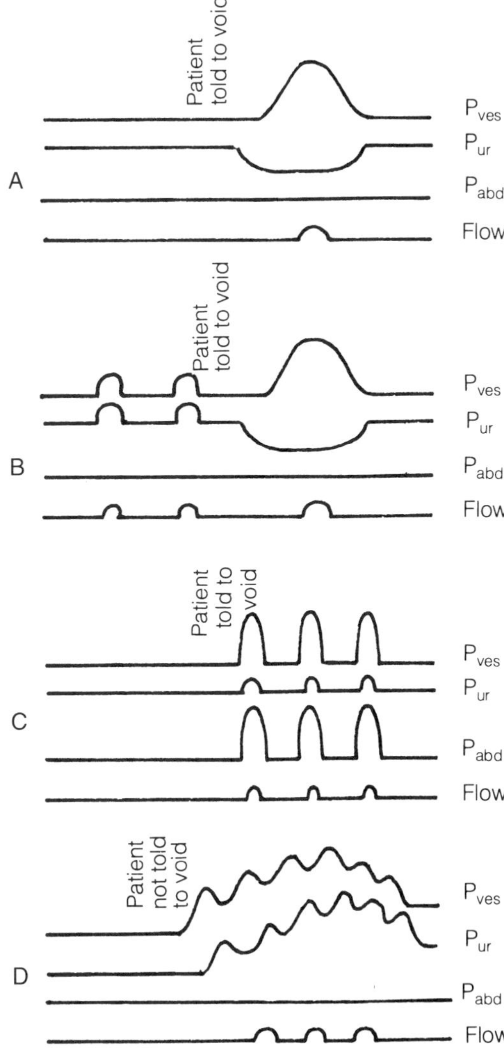

FIG. 44-6. Schematic representation of various voiding patterns. **A:** Normal. **B:** Uninhibited contractions occur with filling. The sphincter is attempting to inhibit contractions. Patient has a normal voiding phase. **C:** No bladder contractions. Rises in bladder pressure result from rises in abdominal pressure (i.e., Valsalva voiding). **D:** Uninhibited contractions occur with simultaneous sphincter contractions (i.e., detrusor sphincter dyssynergia). P_{abd}, intra-abdominal pressure; P_{ur}, urethral sphincter pressure; P_{ves}, intravesical pressure.

TABLE 44-3. *Treatment options for voiding disorders*

Incontinence caused by the bladder
- Behavioral: Scheduled voiding
- Pharmacologic: Anticholinergics, antispasmodics, tricyclic antidepressants, calcium antagonists,[a] prostaglandin inhibitors[a]
- Surgical: Augmentation cystoplasty, interruption of innervation, neurostimulation[a]
- Supportive: Diapers, external condom catheter, intermittent catheterization, indwelling catheter

Incontinence caused by the sphincter
- Behavioral: Scheduled voiding, pelvic floor exercises, biofeedback
- Pharmacologic: Alpha-adrenergic agonists, estrogen, injectable periurethral collagen[a]
- Surgical: Artificial sphincter, urethral suspension, neurostimulation[a]
- Supportive: Same as with bladder

Retention caused by the bladder
- Behavioral: Scheduled voiding combined with suprapubic tapping, Valsalva, Credé
- Pharmacologic: Cholinergic agonists, intravesical prostaglandin,[a] narcotic antagonists[a]
- Surgical: sphincterotomy, neurostimulation[a]
- Supportive: intermittent catheterization, indwelling catheter

Retention caused by the sphincter/outlet
- Behavioral: biofeedback, suprapubic tapping, anal stretch/scissoring
- Pharmacologic: alpha-adrenergic blockers, baclofen, diazepam, dantrolene
- Surgical: sphincterotomy, pudendal neurectomy, bladder outlet surgery, stents,[a] balloon dilation[a]
- Supportive: same as with bladder

[a] Investigational use.

be discouraged because there is a risk of potential side effects of drugs that may have no benefit or make the problem worse. In addition to the type of voiding dysfunction, the physician needs to consider the type of disease process (i.e., progressive, stable, or remitting), cognition, mobility, family support, and medical conditions when recommending a bladder management program.

The following are goals of management in patients with voiding dysfunctions:

- Prevent upper tract complications (e.g., deterioration of renal function, hydronephrosis, renal calculi, pyelonephritis).
- Prevent lower tract complications (e.g., cystitis, bladder stones, vesicoureteral reflux).
- Develop a bladder management program that will allow patient to reintegrate most easily back into the community.

Therapy for Incontinence Caused by the Bladder

Behavioral Treatment Options

Many patients with incontinence caused by the bladder benefit from a scheduled voiding regimen. Patients with incontinence resulting from poor cognition, aphasia, or poor mobility but normal bladder function often are helped by being placed on a commode or offered a urinal at set intervals (i.e., timed voiding). Patients who have uninhibited contractions also can have decreased incontinence by voiding by the clock rather than waiting for a sense of fullness. They are taught to void before reaching their full bladder capacity because uninhibited contractions often become more forceful and frequent as the bladder is reaching its full capacity.

Another type of behavioral intervention is bladder training. This is done by progressively increasing the time between voiding by 10 to 15 minutes every 2 to 5 days until a reasonable interval between voidings is obtained (89). Bladder training often is effective for a person who has recovered or is recovering from a neurologic lesion (e.g., head injury, stroke) with improved bladder function but is voiding frequently out of habit or from fear of incontinence based on past experience.

Pharmacologic Treatment Options

Pharmacologic treatment often is needed in addition to timed voiding in patients with incontinence caused by uninhibited contractions. There are a number of anticholinergic agents whose primary action is to block acetylcholine receptors competitively at the postganglionic autonomic receptor sites. Some agents such as oxybutynin also have a localized smooth muscle antispasmodic effect distal to the cholinergic receptor site and a local anesthetic effect on the bladder wall. It sometimes is helpful to combine an agent such as propantheline, with primarily anticholinergic effects, with one that also has local effects (90).

Tricyclic antidepressants sometimes are used alone or in combination with anticholinergic agents. These medications, of which imipramine has been used most extensively, are thought to have a peripheral anticholinergic effect and a central effect. They have been found to suppress uninhibited bladder contractions, increase bladder capacity, and increase urethral resistance (91). There have been several reports of severe autonomic dysreflexia in SCI patients secondary to overdistention of the bladder with urine (92).

Other medications that have been reported or are being investigated to improve storage include intravesical capsaicin, intrathecal baclofen, prostaglandin inhibitors, and intravesical instillations of anticholinergic medications (93–96). Desmopressin acetate has been found to decrease the number of episodes of nocturia in patients with multiple sclerosis. However, further studies are needed to determine its usefulness in the elderly because of the high prevalence of contraindications such as renal insufficiency, heart failure, and risks of inducing hyponatremia and fluid retention (29). Potential side effects and contraindications must be weighed against potential benefits when using any pharmacologic agents for treatment of incontinence caused by the bladder (90,91).

Surgical Treatment Options

Surgical treatment to improve bladder capacity in adult patients with neurogenic voiding disorders is sometimes needed. The usual indications for surgical intervention are severe detrusor hyperreflexia or poor bladder wall compliance, or continued upper tract deterioration despite aggressive pharmacotherapy and other types of management.

One technique to increase bladder capacity and lower intravesical pressures is an augmentation cystoplasty, in which a portion of the bladder is removed and a larger segment of bowel is attached to the remaining bladder. Mast and associates reviewed 28 of their patients with an augmentation who were refractory to prolonged conservative treatment. They reported a 70% success rate at stopping incontinence (mean length of follow-up 1½ years). This was increased to 85% with the addition of an artificial sphincter in those with low sphincter resistance. Complications included recurrent urinary tract infection (59%) and stone formation (22%). Complications led to the need for further surgery in 44% of the patients (97). Patients need to be well motivated and understand that inefficient bladder emptying may occur after surgery, requiring long-term clean intermittent catheterization (CIC). There also is increased mucus in the urine because of the bowel segment; this sometimes is annoying to the patient. Long-term consequences of bowel attached to bladder are unknown. There have been a few reports of patients who had an augmentation cystoplasty for more than 10 years developing adenocarcinoma in the bladder (98).

Surgical methods also have been designed to interrupt innervation to the bladder. This can be done centrally (e.g., subarachnoid block, cordectomy), peripherally (e.g., anterior or anteroposterior rhizotomy), or perivesically (e.g., extensive mobilization of the bladder) (99–101). Although there usually is a successful short-term outcome, decreased compliance or detrusor hyperreflexia may return. This may result from an increased sensitivity of receptors following decentralization (24). Impotence usually occurs after these procedures.

Neurostimulation still is investigational, but one of its uses is in the attempt to decrease uninhibited bladder contractions. Ohlsson and colleagues reported an average 49% increase in bladder capacity by stimulation of the pudendal nerve with anal and vaginal electrode plugs (102). Tanago has reported success at selective sacral root stimulation to increase sphincter tone, which in turn suppresses detrusor activity (103).

Supportive Treatment Options

Diapers often are helpful either as primary management or as back-up to management for timed voiding. Custom-fit diapers are much more cosmetic than in the past. Major drawbacks include expense, patient embarrassment, difficulty getting them on and off, and potential skin breakdowns if they are not changed within 2 to 4 hours after getting wet.

External condom catheters often are a good option for men with detrusor hyperreflexia or normal bladder function with incontinence secondary to mobility or cognitive factors. An advantage over diapers is that the condom catheter needs to be changed only once a day. Major drawbacks include wearing of a leg bag, potential for penile skin breakdown, condom catheter falling off, and slight increase in bladder infections.

IC, usually combined with anticholinergics, is another effective way to manage patients with detrusor hyperreflexia and incontinence. Guttman popularized sterile IC for SCI patients in the 1960s. He reported that in 476 SCI patients followed over 11 years on sterile IC, only 7.4% developed hydronephrosis, 4.4% had vesicoureteral reflux, 1.7% developed kidney stones, and 0.6% developed bladder stones (104). In the mid-1970s, Lapides reported on the effectiveness of CIC. He attributed the success of CIC to the ease of performing CIC compared to sterile technique so that patients were more likely to catheterize themselves and prevent bladder overdistention than with sterile technique (105). Maynard and Glass reported that 80% of patients on CICs followed for 60 months continued on IC, suggesting low morbidity and high patient acceptance (106). Although clean technique works well in the outpatient setting, Anderson reported that there was a high rate of significant bacteriuria despite antibiotic prophylaxis in the hospital setting and suggested that sterile technique may be preferred in the acute spinal cord center (107).

The important principles of IC are to restrict fluids to 2 liters a day and to catheterize frequently enough to keep the bladder from becoming overdistended (<400 ml). Use of prophylactic antibiotics is controversial (106,107). Relative contraindications to IC are women with significant adductor leg spasticity, patients with history of a urethral false passage, or those with poor hand–eye coordination, poor cognition, or poor motivation.

Because there is no satisfactory external collecting device for women, an indwelling catheter may be needed if diapers cannot be changed regularly and she is unable to perform IC. An indwelling catheter also may be an option for men who are unable to wear a condom catheter or have contraindications to performing IC.

Because an indwelling catheter can irritate the bladder, causing increased uninhibited contractions, high intravesical pressure, and decreased drainage from the upper tracts, use of an anticholinergic also should be considered, particularly in someone with urodynamic evidence of detrusor hyperreflexia. For discussion of management and complications of an indwelling catheter, see the section on supportive options for retention caused by the bladder.

Therapy for Incontinence Caused by the Outlet or Sphincter

Behavioral Treatment Options

Timed voiding sometimes is helpful in patients with mild incontinence who have normal bladder function but an underactive urethral sphincter mechanism. The object is to have the patient void before the bladder reaches full capacity. At full capacity, intravesical pressure is more likely to overcome the urethral pressure, resulting in leakage.

Pelvic floor (i.e., Kegel) exercises also may be tried in neurologically intact patients with mild to moderate stress incontinence caused by the sphincter (108). There is a great variation in the number of sets and repetitions described by various authors, with the total number of exercise contractions varying from eight to 160 per day (109). Exercises sometimes are combined with commercial biofeedback units (110). Patients have to be highly motivated, and effects may not be seen for 4 to 8 weeks.

Pharmacologic Treatment Options

Alpha-adrenergic agonists may be useful at improving minimal to moderate stress incontinence caused by the sphincter. Wyndaele has reported success at decreasing urinary leakage around the Foley catheter in incomplete SCI women with patulous urethras (92). Ephedrine and phenylpropanolamine are two commonly used agents. Ephedrine causes a release of norepinephrine as well as directly stimulating alpha and beta receptors. Phenylpropanolamine is pharmacologically similar to ephedrine but provides less CNS stimulation (111). Before these medications are used, it is essential that detrusor hyperreflexia or poor bladder compliance be ruled out with urodynamics; otherwise, increasing the urethral sphincter tone may increase intravesical pressures, which could result in poor drainage from the upper tracts.

A 4- to 6-week course of estrogen supplementation may be helpful in postmenopausal women with atrophy of the urethral epithelium or irritative symptoms from atrophic urethritis (112). Its beneficial effect may result from improving the local mucosal seal effect or increasing sensitivity or improving the number of alpha-adrenergic receptors (113). The risks of endometrial cancer, thrombosis, or withdrawal bleeding are negligible when estrogen supplementation is used topically for this short duration.

Potential side effects and contraindications need to be weighed against potential benefits of using any agents to treat incontinence caused by the sphincter (111).

Periurethral collagen injection therapy has recently received Food and Drug Administration (FDA) approval for those with intrinsic urethral sphincter deficiency. Although clinic trials have focused primarily on non-SCI individuals, this therapy appears to be a promising method to increase urethral resistance to the flow of urine. Appell reported that 80% of female patients treated by this method were continent after two treatments. The major contraindication in properly selected patients is an allergy to bovine collagen (114). This should also not be used in a person with forceful uninhibited bladder contractions, since obstructing the urethra could cause back pressure into the kidneys.

Surgical Treatment Options

In patients with a selective injury affecting just the sphincter mechanism, such as postprostatectomy or pelvic fracture, surgical implantation of an artificial urethral sphincter should be strongly considered. Surgery should be delayed at least 6 months to 1 year to make sure there is not going to be a return of sphincter function. Artificial sphincters are used infrequently in the adult SCI population, because they potentially can cause upper tract damage in those with detrusor hyperreflexia and high intravesical pressure. In addition, there is an increased risk of prosthesis infection or erosion of the cuff in SCI patients because of frequent episodes of bacteriuria. Light and Scott reported that 24% of their SCI patients developed infection requiring removal of the device (115). Artificial sphincters are better tolerated in children with myelodysplasia (116).

For women with stress incontinence caused by the sphincter, or intrinsic sphincter damage, such as from a long term indwelling catheter, a variety of surgeries have been developed to anatomically improve the urethral support and position. These procedures can be performed transabdominally, transvaginally, and even without surgical incisions. One- to three-year follow-up success rates have been reported to be 57% to 91% (117). A potential problem is that the operation works too well and causes retention. Patients therefore should be aware of the possibility of needing to perform postoperative IC. Other surgical options for those intrinsic sphincter damage, include surgical closure of the bladder neck followed by urinary diversion with an abdominal stoma which can be catheterized or the insertion of a suprapubic tube.

Supportive Treatment Options

Supportive options are similar to those for incontinence caused by the bladder. Specifically, these include diapers, external condom catheters, and indwelling catheters.

Therapy for Retention Caused by the Bladder

Behavioral Treatment Options

Timed voiding combined with increasing intravesical pressure either manually (i.e., Crede maneuver) or through increased intra-abdominal pressure (i.e., Valsalva voiding) may allow bladder emptying. In patients with weak uninhibited bladder contractions, suprapubic bladder tapping may be used to trigger a contraction. The goal for patients who use Crede or Valsalva maneuvers to void should be to become catheter-free. This goal can be reached through an organized program of bladder retraining consisting of fluid restriction and catheterization every 4 to 6 hours to check residual urine volumes. Catheterization is discontinued when the patient is maintaining regular (i.e., every 3 hours) and complete (i.e., $<$100 ml residual urine volume) emptying of the bladder (118).

Crede and Valsalva maneuvers may cause exacerbation of hemorrhoids, rectal prolapse, or hernia; they are best reserved for those who are unable to perform IC and have decreased urethral sphincter activity, such as elderly women or SCI men with lower motor lesions and sphincterotomy. Increasing intra-abdominal pressure in those with sphincter–detrusor dyssynergia often worsens the dyssynergia (119). Vesicoureteral reflux is a contraindication to this type of voiding.

Pharmacologic Treatment Options

Bethanechol chloride, which provides relatively selective stimulation of the bladder and bowel and is resistant to rapid hydrolysis by acetylcholinesterase, often is used to augment bladder contractions. A review of the literature shows that bethanechol is most useful in patients with bladder hypocontractility and coordinated sphincter function (120). Light and Scott reported that it failed to induce bladder contractions in SCI patients with detrusor areflexia (121). Sporer and associates found that bethanechol increased external sphincter pressures by 10 to 20 cm H_2O in SCI men (122). Therefore, it should not be used in those with sphincter–detrusor dyssynergia. It also is contraindicated in patients with bladder outlet obstruction. Potential side-effects and contraindications must be weighed against potential benefits when pharmacologic agents are used to improve emptying (123).

Two investigational agents to improve bladder emptying are prostaglandins and narcotic antagonists. Intravesical prostaglandin F2a was noted to increase detrusor pressures in SCI patients with suprasacral lesions (124). Narcotic antagonists are thought to block enkephalins, which are believed to inhibit the sacral micturition reflex (125).

Surgical Treatment Options

There have been reports of surgically reducing the size of the bladder to decrease the PVR; however, there is no effective way surgically to augment bladder contractions by operating on the bladder itself (126). Sphincterotomy has been reported in SCI men with detrusor areflexia, however this is generally not recommended since there is a high failure rate at decreasing PVRs (127).

Investigators continue to try to improve voiding through the use of neurostimulation. Techniques include placing electrodes on the bladder itself, the pelvic nerves, conus medullaris, sacral nerves and the sacral anterior roots. The largest experience is with surgically implanted Finetech-Brindley sacral afferent stimulator in which there have been an estimated 800 implants over fifteen years (128). Prerequisites for successful neurostimulation include an intact sacral reflex arc and a detrusor capable of contracting. Stimulation of the sacral afferent nerves causes reflex activation of the efferent nerves to the sphincter. However this reflex accommodates so that fatigue of the sphincter occurs and the pressure generated in the urethra is overcome by the bladder contraction. A posterior rhizotomy is often performed at the same time as the sacral implant. This is done to abolish uninhibited bladder contractions, abolish contractions of the sphincter and improve bladder wall compliance. The disadvantage of the posterior rhizotomy is the loss of reflex erections and reflex ejaculations, loss of perineal sensation, and loss of reflex bladder contractions (128). Kerrebroeck and colleagues reviewed the world wide experience with the Finetech-Brindley sacral stimulator. In 184 cases of whom 170 were using the stimulator, 95% had PVRS less than 60 ccs. There was no deterioration of the upper tracts. Two thirds of men reported stimulated erections, however only one third used these for coitus (129).

Supportive Treatment Options

One of the many important and successful methods for management of failure to empty caused by the bladder is CIC. In those unable to tolerate pharmacotherapy and unable to perform IC, an alternative is an indwelling catheter. Principles of management include an oral fluid intake of at least 2 liters a day, keeping the catheter taped up to the abdomen of men when they are lying down to decrease the risk of a penile scrotal fistula, cleaning the urethral meatus of incrustations with soap and water twice a day, preventing reflux of urine into the bladder by never raising the drainage bag above the level of the bladder, and changing the Foley catheter every 2 to 4 weeks. Before removing an indwelling Foley catheter, the authors believe it is important to obtain urine CS tests and to treat with an appropriate antibiotic for several days before and after catheter removal. This is to decrease the risk of bacteremia if the patient is unable to void and gets a distended bladder. If a Foley catheter has been in place for 4 to 6 weeks before switching a patient over to IC, cystoscopy is recommended to remove eggshell calculi and debris that may have collected in the bladder and have the potential of becoming a nidus for large bladder stones. Prophylactic antibiotics are not recommended for a patient with an indwelling catheter because of the risk of developing resistant organisms. Complications of indwelling catheter include the development of the following:

bladder stones
hematuria
bacteremia, especially if the catheter becomes obstructed
meatal erosions
penile scrotal fistulas
epididymitis

Therapy for Retention Caused by the Outlet or Sphincter

Behavioral Treatment Options

Timed voiding and biofeedback methods have not been reported as successful methods of treatment in patients with neurogenic sphincter–detrusor dyssynergia. Biofeedback has been reported to be successful in patients with voluntary pseudo-sphincter–detrusor dyssynergia. These patients, who often are children, voluntarily tighten their sphincters during voiding, resulting in large PVRs and urinary tract infections (130).

In SCI patients with detrusor hyperreflexia and detrusor sphincter dyssynergia, anal stretching or scissoring and suprapubic bladder tapping have been reported as ways temporarily to interrupt the dyssynergia and allow voiding (131).

Pharmacologic Treatment Options

In those with an intact sacral micturition reflex, reflex voiding into a condom catheter attached to a leg bag is a common method of bladder management in men with spinal cord injury. However, upper tract damage or elevated post void residuals can occur secondary to detrusor sphincter dyssynergia. Alpha-adrenergic blocking agents have been shown to be effective at improving bladder emptying in patients with sphincter–detrusor dyssynergia and prostate outlet obstruction (132,133). In those with prostate outlet obstruction, this is because the prostate smooth muscle is mediated by alpha-adrenergic stimulation (134). Placebo-controlled studies have shown both a clinical and statistically significant improvement in voiding in subjects taking phenoxybenzamine, prazosin, and more recently, terazosin (134, 135).

Alpha blocking agents may improve voiding in patients with sphincter dyssynergia secondary to a SCI caused by several factors. After denervation, a supersensitivity of the urethra to alpha-adrenergic stimulation can occur. In addition, there may be a conversion of the usual beta receptors to alpha receptors (24,26). Scott and Morrow found that phenoxybenzamine worked well at decreasing residual urine volume in patients with suprasacral SCI and autonomic dysreflexia, but had variable effect on those without dysreflexia (136). An added benefit of alpha blockers is their ability to blunt autonomic dysreflexia (137). When deciding which alpha blocker to use, it is important to know that the manufacturer of phenoxybenzamine has indicated a dose-related incidence of gastrointestinal tumors in rats. There have been no cases of gastrointestinal tumors linked to phenoxybenzamine in humans in over 30 years of use (138); however, the potential medicolegal issues of long-term use of phenoxybenzamine in young SCI patients should be considered.

Three drugs that have been used for striated external sphincter relaxation are baclofen, diazepam, and dantrolene. In the authors' experience, these agents are not as effective as alpha blocking agents and should not be used as the drugs of choice for external sphincter relaxation. Baclofen functions as an agonist for the inhibitory neurotransmitter gamma-aminobutyric acid (GABA), which blocks excitatory synaptic transmission, resulting in external sphincter relaxation. Diazepam is believed to cause external sphincter relaxation by increasing GABA inhibitory transmission in the spinal cord. Dantrolene acts peripherally by decreasing calcium release from the sarcoplasmic reticulum, thereby inhibiting excitation-contraction of the striated skeletal muscle fibers.

Potential side effects and contraindications must be weighed against potential benefits when using pharmacologic agents to improve emptying (137,139).

Surgical Treatment Options

Pudendal block or neurectomy was used in the past in SCI men with sphincter–detrusor dyssynergia (140). This procedure largely has been replaced by sphincterotomy. Pudendal block or neurectomy is being used to relax the sphincter mechanism by some investigators working at perfecting electrical stimulation for voiding (103). A unilateral neurectomy is recommended over a bilateral procedure to help decrease the risk of impotence and fecal incontinence (99).

Transurethral sphincterotomy is a well established treatment for SCI men with sphincter–detrusor dyssynergia. Indications include vesicoureteral reflux, high residuals with severe autonomic dysreflexia or recurrent urinary tract infections, upper tract changes with sustained high intravesical pressures, and poor compliance or side-effects from medications being used to relax the outlet. Perkash reported an over 90% success rate at relief of dysreflexic symptoms, decrease in residual urine, decrease in infected urine, and significant radiologic improvement. He stressed the importance of extending the incision to the bladder neck (141).

Longitudinal studies have shown a 25–50% sphincterotomy failure rate. This has been attributed to a variety of causes such as, poor patient selection, i.e., those with detrusor areflexia or bladder contractions less than 30 cm H_2O, recurrent detrusor sphincter dyssnergia, failure to recognize the need for a concomittent procedure such as bladder neck incision or prostate resection or new onset detrusor hypocontractility (142).

The major concerns of most SCI patients are that the procedure is irreversible, it is a surgical procedure, and they will have to wear a leg bag. The traditional electrocautery method of performing a sphincterotomy has been reported to at times be bloody with hemorrhage requiring blood transfusion varying from 5% to 26%. This risk of bleeding has been largely eliminated with the use of Nd:YAG contact laser sphincterotomy. Perkash reported that in 30 patients undergoing laser sphincterotomy blood loss was 150cc in one patient and less than 50 cc's in the other 29 patients (143). The major advantages to a sphincterotomy and reflex voiding are that there are no fluid restrictions, the procedure is effective for the previously mentioned problems, and it will decrease attendant care in those who had previously performed IC (141).

Another method of sphincter dyssynergia treatment is the stainless steel woven mesh stent (e.g., Urolume Endourethral Wallstent, American Medical Systems) which holds the sphincter mechanism open. With an experienced team, this can be done under local anesthesia. Since the sphincter is not cut the procedure is potentially reversible with removal of the stent. The stent becomes covered by epithelium in 3 to 6 months, preventing calcium encrustations. A multicenter study of 153 men with SCI revealed a significant decrease in voiding pressures and post void residual urine volumes up to two years. Hydronephrosis resolved in 22 of 28 patients (78.6%). There was no loss or erectile function. Complications included mild post operative hematuria in 10 patienta (7.1%), penile edema in 2 patients, incrustation of the stent in 3 patients, stent removal (usually caused by stent migration) in 10 patients, and subsequent operation for bladder neck obstruction in 13. Long-term follow-up studies are underway. This device has recently been approved by the FDA for the treatment of urethral strictures (144).

Another method under investigation to decrease urethral sphincter pressure is botulism toxin. Dykstra and colleagues reported decreased detrusor dyssynergia in 10 of 11 men with suprasacral SCI with injection of botulism toxin into the sphincter (145).

Supportive Treatment Options

Supportive treatment options for the outlet are the same as those for retention caused by the bladder—specifically, IC or indwelling catheters. Occasionally a person has so much sphincter spasticity that it is difficult to pass a catheter. Instillation of lidocaine jelly down the urethra 5 minutes before catheterization, administration of alpha-adrenergic blockers, or use of a coudé catheter often facilitates catheterization.

Pediatric Considerations

Children with incomplete emptying and sphincter dyssynergia caused by a nonneurogenic learned disorder have been treated successfully with biofeedback. This has involved looking at or listening to their sphincter EMG patterns during voiding. Sugar and Firlit reported that all 10 of their patients aged 6 to 16 years converted to a synergistic voiding pattern within 48 hours of therapy (146).

The same pharmacologic principles discussed under the general management section apply for children. The age of the child and decreased dosages need to be considered.

The same surgical procedures discussed under management can be used in children. In the past, children with vesicoureteral reflux were treated with urinary diversion, but because of long-term complications of urinary diversion and the excellent success of IC and ureteral reimplantation, this rarely if ever is used today. Surgical procedures for children with severe incontinence include an anterior fascial sling around the urethra, and artificial urinary sphincter (46). There have been reports of 90% long-term success rates with the use of the artificial sphincter in children (116). The Kropp procedure, in which a new urethra is formed from a portion of bladder and tunneled submucosally in the trigone, has been described and may be a good alternative to an artificial urinary sphincter (147).

Clean intermittent catheterization has been shown to be effective treatment for children with failure to empty. In those with incontinence caused by the bladder, an anticholinergic medication often is also required (oxybutynin, 1.0 mg/year of age twice daily). Parents often can learn IC in 1 day. It is thought that parents and children adjust to this program if it is started when the child is a newborn. There have been no reported cases of urethral injury, epididymitis, or urinary tract infections requiring hospitalizations caused by this procedure. Children usually can begin performing their own IC at age 5 years (46).

COMPLICATIONS OF VOIDING DYSFUNCTIONS

Urinary Tract Infections

Bacteriuria is a common problem in patients with voiding dysfunctions. Lloyd and associates followed 181 new SCI patients discharged from an acute SCI center initially with sterile urine and on a variety of bladder management programs for 1 year. At 1 year, 66.7% to 100% had at least one episode of bacteriuria, depending on their bladder management program (148). Maynard and Diokno reported on 50 new SCI inpatients on IC and found that 88% had one or more episodes of bacteriuria (i.e., any bacteria present) (149). Elderly patients often comprise a large part of the patient population in a rehabilitation hospital. Asymptomatic bacteriuria has been found to be present in 10% to 25% of community-dwelling and 25% to 40% of nursing home patients over 65 years of age (150). These numbers would be expected to be at least as high, if not higher, in those with a voiding disorder.

Traditionally, a urinary tract infection was defined as more than 100,000 organisms in a midstream urine sample (151). The probability increased from 80% to 90% if this was found in two separate specimens. There is increasing controversy, however, about what is the true definition of urinary tract infection. This is based on studies showing that symptomatic patients often have fewer than 100,000 organisms, uncertainty about the significance of asymptomatic bacteriuria and the presence or absence of pyuria, and the potential impact of other factors such as high voiding pressures, frequency of voiding, and PVRs. It has been found that 30% of able-bodied women with acute dysuria had less than 10,000 coliforms/ml, and many had less than 200/ml (152,153).

In SCI patients, Rhame and Perkash reported that any specimen with more than 1,000 coliforms/ml was significant (154). Donovan and associates thought that the appearance of any count of the same organism for two consecutive days was significant (155). The National Institute on Disability and Rehabilitation Research (NIDRR) UTI consensus conference based the definition of significant bacteria on the method of urine collection and colony count. Significant bacteria did not necessarily mean an infection but, rather, confidence that the bacteria cultured were from the bladder and not contamination. For those on intermittent catheterization, "significant" meant >102 colony-forming units (cfu)/ml; for those who did not use catheterization, >104 cfu/ml; and for those who used an indwelling catheter, any detectable pathogens (156). There is controversy as to whether significant bacteriuria should be regarded as a urinary tract infection or colonization.

With regard to pyuria, Stamm found that 96% of patients with symptomatic infections had ≥10 leukocytes/mm3 (153). Deresinski and associates reported that 79% of 70 SCI patients with symptoms and bacteriuria also had pyuria; however, 46% of asymptomatic patients also had significant pyuria (157). Anderson and Hsieh-ma also found that gram-negative bacteria caused significant pyuria, but that this was not true of *Staphylococcus epidermidis* or *Streptococcus faecalis* even in high numbers (158).

Signs and Symptoms

Signs and symptoms of a urinary tract infection involving the lower tract may include dysuria, frequency, urinary incontinence, and hematuria. Unless a person has had acute retention or urologic instrumentation, fever is less likely when the lower urinary tract is involved. Whereas many SCI patients have decreased or no bladder sensation, a lower urinary tract infection often will cause cloudy, strong-smelling urine, increased abdominal or lower extremity spasticity, new onset of urinary incontinence, occasionally retention from increased sphincter–detrusor dyssynergia, or autonomic dysreflexia in those with a lesion above T6.

Patients with acute upper tract involvement may present with any of the above signs and symptoms. They also usually will have fever and chills and an elevated serum white blood cell count. Those with sensation usually complain of costal vertebral angle tenderness. It should be noted in the elderly that signs and symptoms may be much more subtle and patients may present simply with confusion or lethargy. Urinary tract infections also should be considered in the differential diagnosis of new cognitive changes in a head-injured patient.

Treatment of Asymptomatic Urinary Tract Infection

Guidelines for treatment have been difficult to establish for asymptomatic bacteriuria because of controversy on whether this represents colonization rather than an infection. Ideally, the urine should be sterile; however, the side-effects of antibiotics and development of resistant organisms need to be taken into account. Kass and associates followed 225 children on CIC for 10 years and reported that in the absence of vesicoureteral reflux, bacilluria proved innocuous, with only 2.6% of subjects developing fresh renal damage. In high-grade reflux, however, 60% developed pyelonephritis (159).

Lewis and colleagues followed 52 acute SCI patients during their initial hospitalization. Seventy-eight percent of patients had greater than 100,000 organisms, but only 13% had symptoms and required antimicrobial therapy over 6 months. Of interest is that 35% of cultures changed weekly from positive to negative, negative to positive, or one organism to another, necessitating a short course of antibiotics (160).

An accurate characterization of voiding dysfunction such as voiding pressure, bladder compliance, and PVRs, along with accurate characterization of level and completeness of injury often are lacking in various studies discussing urinary tract infections in SCI patients. It is hoped that prospective evaluations considering these factors in relation to factors such as bacteriuria, pyuria, upper and lower tract anatomy, virulence of organisms, and types of bladder management will allow guidelines to be formulated for the treatment of asymptomatic bacteriuria. There is general agreement that asymptomatic bacteriuria in a patient with an indwelling Foley catheter should not be treated. Attempts should be made to eradicate asymptomatic bacteriuria in those with high-grade reflux, before urologic instrumentation, in hydronephrosis, or in the presence of urea-splitting organisms.

Treatment of Symptomatic Urinary Tract Infections

Once a urine culture has been obtained, empiric oral antibiotic treatment can be started for patients with minimal symptoms while waiting for the culture results. Patients usually do well with a 7-day course of antibiotics. In those with high fevers, dehydration, or autonomic dysreflexia, more aggressive therapy should be instituted. It is the authors' opinion that these patients should be hospitalized, closely monitored, hydrated, and given broad-spectrum antibiotics (e.g., gentamicin and ampicillin) while waiting for the culture results and for the fever to defervesce. It is important to have an indwelling Foley catheter in place during intravenous or oral fluid hydration to keep the bladder decompressed. The authors believe that it also is beneficial to give an anticholinergic medication while the Foley catheter is in place; this will decrease the intrinsic pressure within the detrusor, allowing relaxation of the ureterovesical junction and improving drainage of the kidneys. Tempkin and associates showed on renal scans that there was improved drainage of the upper tracts in SCI patients given anticholinergics (161). Patients with significant fever should be considered to have upper tract involvement (i.e., pyelonephritis) and therefore be continued on 2 to 3 weeks of oral antibiotics after the fever has resolved. In addition, these patients should undergo a urologic evaluation for cause of urosepsis. Acutely, this should consist of a plain abdominal radiograph to rule out an obvious stone, followed by a renal ultrasound. If there is a question of a stone, hydronephrosis, or persistent fever, an IVP should be performed. Once the patient has been treated, it is often necessary that he or she undergo a cystogram to evaluate for reflux, a cystoscopy to evaluate the bladder outlet and bladder, and urodynamics to evaluate voiding function.

Complications of Urinary Tract Infections

In addition to acute lower urinary tract infections (i.e., cystitis) and acute upper urinary tract infections (i.e., pyelonephritis) the physician should be aware of other potential problems. Those from lower urinary tract infections include epididymitis, prostatic or scrotal abscess, sepsis, or an ascending infection to the upper tracts. Complications that may occur from upper tract infections include chronic pyelonephritis, renal scarring, progressive renal deterioration, renal calculi if there is a urea-splitting organism such as Proteus, papillary necrosis, renal or retroperitoneal abscess, or bacteremia and sepsis.

Role of Prophylactic Antibiotics

There is controversy over the role of prophylactic antibiotics (107,149,162). Anderson reported a statistically significant difference in bacteriuria in SCI inpatients on a combination of oral nitrofurdantoin and neomycin/polymyxin B solution compared with controls (107). Merritt and colleagues reported a statistically significant decrease in bacteriuria with methenamine salt or co-trimoxazole compared with controls at 3 to 9 months but not at greater than 15 months (163). Maynard and Diokno reported that antibiotic prophylaxis significantly reduces the probability of a laboratory infection but not the probability of a clinical infection (149). Kuhlemeier and associates evaluated vitamin C and a number of antimicrobial agents as prophylactic agents and found no beneficial effect in SCI patients compared with controls (162). These studies seem to show that prophylactic agents do not have a long-term effect in decreasing bacteriuria compared with controls. The role of prophylactic antibiotics in patients with recurrent clinical infections, anatomic abnormalities such as vesicoureteral reflux, or hydronephrosis is not known. Prophylactic antibiotics should be considered before urologic tesing requiring instrumentation, particularily in those with bacteriuria.

Hydronephrosis

Ureteral dilation for any reason results in inefficient propulsion of the urine bolus caused by inability of the walls to coapt completely, as well as in decreased intraluminal pressure caused by the increased ureteral diameter. Over time, this may result in further distention of the ureter with eventual hydronephrosis (7,164). There are several causes for ureteral dilation. It can occur transiently from a brisk diuresis effectively overloading the ureters, not allowing enough time for individual boluses to travel down the ureter. Another cause may be a mechanical obstruction such as a stone or stricture. Those with poor bladder wall compliance, sphincter–detrusor dyssynergia, or outlet obstruction may develop a functional obstruction caused by high intravesical pressures. The elevated intravesical pressure increases the tension within the bladder wall, which in turn constricts the submucosal ureter as well as increasing the hydrostatic force within the bladder. Ureteral dilation will occur if ureteral peristalsis is unable to overcome these increased pressures (165).

McGuire and colleagues reported that 81% of myelodysplastic children with leak point pressures greater than 40 cm H_2O developed upper urinary tract changes, whereas only 11% with leak point pressures below 40 cm H_2O developed upper tract changes. Hydrostatic forces in the ureter and kidneys also may be increased by vesicoureteral reflux blocking the downward egress of urine (44). Teague and Boyarski have identified another potential cause of ureteral dilation. They found that *Citrobacter* sp. and *Escherichia coli* from human urine cultures injected into the lumen of dog ureters produced marked suppression of peristalsis and ureteral dilation lasting up to 2 hours (166).

Vesicoureteral Reflux

Prince and Kottke reported in an 8-year study that vesicoureteral reflux was one of the factors frequently associated with renal deterioration after SCI (167). Fellows and Silver found that there was a definite association of the degree of reflux and renal damage (168). Vesicoureteral reflux in children has been associated with a congenital shortening or absence of the submucosal ureter, absence of ureteral muscle in the submucosal segment, or association with a paraureteral diverticulum of the bladder (169). In people with neurogenic voiding dysfunctions, high intravesical pressures are thought to be a major cause of reflux. Recurrent cystitis and anatomic changes in the oblique course of the intravesical ureter caused by bladder thickening and trabeculation are believed to be other causes of reflux. Renal deterioration from reflux is thought to be secondary to recurrent pyelonephritis resulting in renal scars as well as back-pressure hydronephrosis.

The mainstay of treatment in those with reflux and voiding dysfunction is to lower intravesical pressures and eradicate infections. Ureteral reimplants are technically difficult to perform in a trabeculated bladder and have not been uniformly successful.

Renal Calculi

Approximately 8% of patients with SCI develop renal calculi (i.e., staghorn calculi or struvite stones) (170). Kuhlemeier and associates found that renal calculi were the single most important cause of renal deterioration (171). Without treatment, a patient with a staghorn calculus has a 50% chance of losing the involved kidney (172). DeVivo and Fine evaluated 25 SCI patients who developed calculi compared with 100 SCI patients who did not have calculi and found that those with calculi were more likely to have neuro-

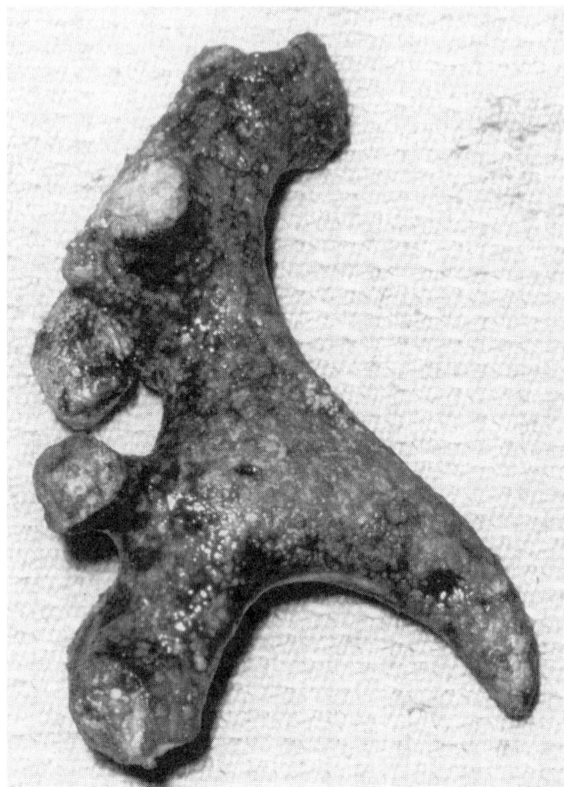

FIG. 44-7. Example of a surgically removed staghorn calculus. This calculus completely filled the renal pelvis and calyces and assumed their shape.

logically complete quadriplegia, have *Klebsiella* or *Serratia* infections, a history of bladder calculi, and high serum calcium values (170). Patients who present with persistent *Proteus* infections also should be monitored for renal calculi. Urea-splitting organisms form alkaline urine that in turn causes supersaturation and crystallization of magnesium ammonium phosphate.

Previously, a surgical pyelolithotomy or nephrolithotomy was performed to remove these stones (Fig. 44-7). Newer techniques, including percutaneous nephrolithotomy and extracorporeal shock wave lithotripsy, have largely replaced open surgical procedures (173). All of these procedures need to be combined with sterilization of the urinary tract of urea-splitting organisms. DeVivo and Fine reported a 72% recurrence rate within 2 years of the first kidney stone (170). Investigations are under way on the use of acetohydroxamic acid as a prophylactic agent; limitations of this agent are reported side effects and high cost (174).

Renal Deterioration

Renal failure previously was the leading cause of death following SCI. The death rate from renal causes was reported in the 1960s at between 37% and 76%. The use of IC and sphincterotomy have markedly reduced death from renal causes. Price and Kottke followed 280 patients for 8 years and reported 78% had good function, 13% mild deterioration, 4% moderate deterioration, and 5% severe deterioration (167). Factors most frequently associated with renal deterioration were vesicoureteral reflux, renal calculi, recurrent pyelonephritis, and recurrent decubitus ulcers. Kuhlemeier and colleagues evaluated 519 SCI patients with renal scans for up to 10 years. They found that factors associated with a statistically significant decreased ERPF were quadriplegia, renal stones, female patients over 30 years of age, and a history of chills and fever presumably caused by acute urinary tract infections. Renal calculi were the most important cause. Factors not found to be statistically significant included years since injury, presence of severe decubitus, bladder calculi, bacteriuria without reflux, and completeness of injury (171).

Bladder Cancer

Paraplegia patients have been found to have a 16 to 28 times higher risk for squamous cell bladder cancer than their able-bodied counterparts. These cancers seem to occur after a person has been injured for more than 10 years. Possible causes include chronic irritation from urinary tract infections, stasis of urine, and bladder stones. Kaufman and associates reported that 5 of 6 patients with squamous cell cancer had an indwelling Foley catheter in place for more than 15 to 30 years (average 21 years). Although only two of the six had an obvious tumor on cystoscopy, three had gross hematuria, one had known invasive squamous cell cancer of the urethra, and only one had no signs or symptoms (175). These studies suggest that yearly cystoscopy should be performed in people who have had indwelling catheters for more than 10 years. Most centers do perform yearly cystoscopy on those with an indwelling catheter, primarily to rule out bladder stones.

NEUROGENIC BOWEL DYSFUNCTION

Although for most purposes the urinary and gastrointestinal systems are considered distinct entities, it is traditional to combine the systems when discussing the effect of neurologic dysfunction. The rational basis for such a grouping is the striking similarity between the urinary bladder and the anorectum in terms of function, structure, and response to stimulation. There are, however, limits to this analogy. The anorectum makes up only a small portion of the gastrointestinal tract, and although urinary bladder function is not greatly influenced by the behavior of the proximal urinary tract, anorectal function is greatly dependent on the remainder of the gastrointestinal tract. Anorectal function therefore must be considered in the context of the complete gastrointestinal tract. Another important difference, which perhaps explains why neurogenic bowel is less well studied than neurogenic bladder, is that neurogenic bladder dysfunction has been a major cause of morbidity and premature death, whereas bowel dysfunction rarely shortens the life span. Although neurogenic bowel dysfunction only occasionally causes life-threatening problems, it often has profound effects on the quality of life.

Anatomic and Physiological Considerations

Colon

The lower gastrointestinal tract serves to transport the intestinal content from the ileum to the rectum, store fecal material, and then evacuate it completely at the appropriate time. Aside from its role as a transport and storage organ, the colon functions to absorb water and electrolytes. The colon normally reduces the approximately 1,500 ml of small intestinal content that is introduced into the the cecum to about 150 ml per day.

The transport of material through the colon depends on colonic motility. The term "motility" frequently is misused and misunderstood. With the colon, measurements of wall motion, intraluminal pressure, electrical events in the muscular colonic tube, or rate of transit of material may be used to describe motility. The interrelationships of these various measures of motility are not well understood. For example, it is not possible to deduce the movement of material through the colon by the measurement of electrical activity. Therefore, unqualified terms such as "increased motility" or "decreased motility" have little meaning. Furthermore, alterations in colonic transport function may be caused by events that occur outside of the colon, such as distal obstruction, proximal dilation caused by the intestinocolic inhibitory reflex, or severe dehydration. Although indices of motility may be abnormal in these settings, interventions directed solely at correcting the abnormal indices of colonic motility are doomed to failure.

The most clinically useful index of motility is colonic transit time, the amount of time required for content to pass from the cecum to the outside. Several techniques exist for measuring transit time; we follow radiopaque markers through the intestinal tract with serial abdominal radiographs for the sake of simplicity (176).

Anorectum

The anal canal provides the primary mechanism for fecal continence and is the barrier that must be traversed for evacuation to occur. The internal anal sphincter (IAS), the specialized continuation of the circular smooth muscle coat of the rectum, is in a continuous state of maximal contraction and is responsible for the majority of resting tone in the anal canal (177). Normal anal canal resting tones range from 50 to 100 cm H_2O. Resting tone is not altered after SCI (178). The external anal sphincter (EAS) is a striated muscle and is innervated by the pudendal nerves. The EAS, along with muscles of the pelvic floor, displays the unusual property of continuous electrical activity in both the waking and sleeping states (179). Presumably this special property allows the EAS and pelvic floor to maintain continence without conscious will and during sleep. Although the EAS plays a small role in the resting state, contraction of the EAS can double anal canal pressure for short periods of time. External sphincter function is felt to be important during events that are an acute threat to continence such as coughing, acute rectal contraction, or assuming an upright position.

The pelvic floor, in particular the puborectalis muscle, is responsible for maintenance of the anorectal angle. The puborectalis derives its origin from the back of the pubic symphysis in such a way that it loops around the anorectal junction. With contraction of the puborectalis, which is its normal resting state, the anorectal junction is pulled forward to create an angle between the rectum and anal canal, the anorectal angle. Although the exact function of the anorectal angle in maintaining continence is controversial, it is clear that straightening of the anorectal angle is associated with incontinence. Conversely, failure of the puborectalis to relax appropriately, with persistence of an acute anorectal angle, has been associated with inability to defecate (180). Patients with complete lesions of the sacral spinal cord will be incontinent on the basis of loss of the anorectal angle and low anal sphincter pressure.

There is an area of specialized mucosa at the proximal end of the anal canal that is rich in sensory receptors. Presumably it is this area that allows differentiation of liquid, solid, and gaseous material in the rectum. The rectoanal inhibitory or sampling reflex allows a sample of the rectal contents to come into contact with this sensory zone. The rectoanal inhibitory reflex consists of a transient relaxation of the IAS stimulated by a rise in rectal pressure. A simultaneous increase in EAS tone, the guarding reflex, occurs to preserve continence. The rectoanal inhibitory reflex occurs during sleep and throughout the day, usually at a subconscious level.

Regulation of Gastrointestinal Function

Most cells within the gastrointestinal tract possess intrinsic activities that give them a degree of autonomy. The activity of these cells is then modulated by regulatory systems both within and outside of the gut. The regulatory system of the gastrointestinal tract incorporates a complex, interrelated system of hormonal, neural, and luminal influences that control a broad range of secretory, absorptive, and motor functions.

Gastrointestinal Hormones

The gastrointestinal hormone system has important effects on all levels of gut function. The activities of the hormonal system are effected by blood-borne chemical messengers (i.e., endocrine action) as well as messengers that are released locally and traverse the interstitial space to reach a target cell (i.e., paracrine action). A third chemical messenger system, even more specific in its location of activity, is the neurocrine system. Neuropeptides are active only at the nerve terminals where they are released. The central role of neuropeptides in both neural and endocrine function illustrates the overlap and inseparability of these two systems.

Understanding of the physiological role of the gastrointestinal peptide hormones has increased dramatically in the past few years. Gastrointestinal hormones are involved in such widely disparate functions as stimulating, inhibiting, or coordinating gut motility, growth and maintenance of gut mass, stimulation and inhibition of secretions, controlling the release of other hormones, and the modulation of neural transmission. The effect of neurologic injury on the gastrointestinal hormone system is unstudied.

Intraluminal Content

The intraluminal content can affect gastrointestinal function through alteration of the physical characteristics of stool, bacterial action, or the effects of specific substances on mucosal receptors. The physical characteristics of the intraluminal content have an important effect on colonic motility and the ease of defecation. The typical Western diet, deficient in fiber, results in small, hard (i.e., scybalous) stool that is difficult for the colon to propel and the anorectum to evacuate. Addition of vegetable fiber to the diet increases the volume and water content of stool and speeds transit time (181). The effect of stool consistency on rectal evacuation has been well studied in able-bodied subjects (182,183). It is clear that small, hard stool is much less efficiently evacuated than bulky, soft stool. Although these studies have not been repeated in neurogenic bowel patients, it seems likely that the same effect of stool consistency on colonic transit and evacuation mechanics would obtain.

With increased dietary fiber, fecal microbial mass increases (184). Bacterial fermentation of indigestible fiber within the colon also generates short-chain fatty acids. These short-chain fatty acids are passively absorbed by colonic mucosa and may be oxidized as an important energy source (185). Bacteria also are important in the metabolism of bile salts. Bile salts stimulate colonic motility and may play a role in the hypermotility of patients with the irritable bowel syndrome (186).

The luminal content also can affect gastrointestinal function by stimulation of specific mucosal receptors. Five types of gastrointestinal sensory receptors are known to exist. These respond to mechanical, chemical, osmotic, thermal, or painful stimuli.

Intrinsic or Enteric Neural Regulation

The enteric nervous system is embedded in the wall of the gut and runs the length of the digestive tube, from the pharynx to the anus. The enteric nervous system is organized into three levels:

1. Afferent neurons, which gather sensory information and relay it to an array of interneurons
2. Interneurons, which process information locally, integrate the incoming sensory information, and form commands that are passed to efferent neurons
3. Efferent neurons, which exert their influence on target cells such as secretory, absorptive, or muscle cells

The function of the enteric nervous system is to integrate the uncontrolled and undirected intrinsic motor and secretory activity of the gut and convert it to directed, coordinated activity. Ablation of all enteric nervous activity by the neurotoxin tetrodotoxin causes the colon to contract, the rectum to undergo tonic and phasic contractions, and the IAS to contract tonically (187). Thus, it appears that the major effect of the enteric nervous system on the lower gastrointestinal tract is to provide an inhibitory influence.

Extrinsic or Extraintestinal Neural Regulation

Extrinsic neural influences provide overall coordination of intestinal reflexes as well as integration of the gastrointestinal tract with the whole organism. Sensory receptors in the gut may send afferents directly to the CNS, to prevertebral sympathetic ganglia, or to interneurons within the gut wall. The sensory information may be processed within the CNS, the prevertebral ganglia, or within the enteric nervous system (Fig. 44-8). The enteric nervous system contains a greater number of neurons than the spinal cord (188). This is not so surprising when the complexity and variety of gastrointestinal functions controlled by the enteric nervous system are considered. The important regulatory role of the enteric nervous system also is apparent in the organization of visceral efferents from the CNS. All efferents except those to striated muscle in the pharynx or EAS (i.e., alpha motor neurons) synapse with enteric interneurons before reaching an effector cell.

The extrinsic efferent nerves to the gastrointestinal tract are classified as parasympathetic or sympathetic. The function of the parasympathetic efferents is complex. Separate groups of vagal preganglionic fibers may innervate inhibitory or excitatory neurons in the same organ. Therefore, nerve stimulation may produce excitatory as well as inhibitory effects on the same organ. Transection of the vagus at the level of the lower esophagus (i.e., truncal vagotomy) frequently is done as treatment for peptic ulcer disease. Gastric acid secretion is diminished to a variable extent, and gastric motility is significantly impaired; however, small bowel and colonic motility are largely unaffected. Sacral parasympathetic injury may lead to impaired defecation and constipation (189). The function of the sympathetic nerves is generally to cause inhibition of motor and secretory activity and contraction of gastrointestinal sphincters. Sympathetic stimulation leads to adynamic ileus and decreased bowel activity. Surgical sympathectomy has little clinical effect on bowel function, although diarrhea has been reported in animal models (190).

The striated muscle of the pharynx and the EAS are inner-

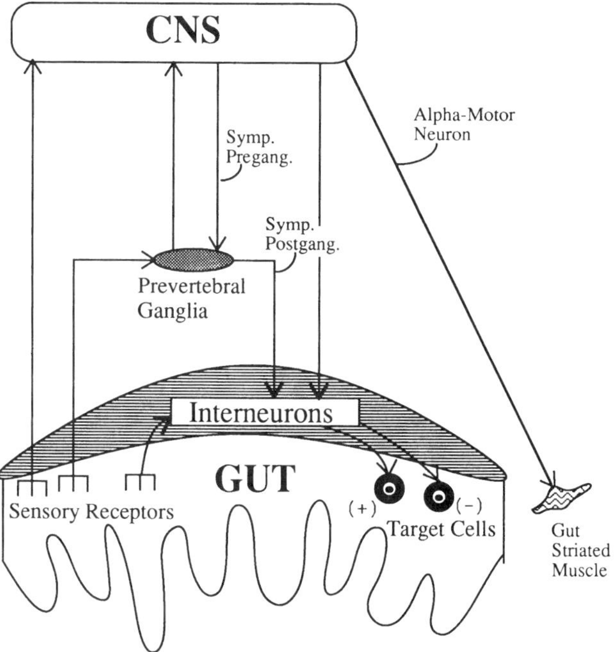

FIG. 44-8. General organization of the enteric nervous system. Sensory fibers in the gut send afferents to: the central nervous system (CNS), through the vagus nerve (cell bodies in nodose ganglia) or the sympathetic nerves (cell bodies in the dorsal root ganglia); prevertebral ganglia; and interneurons within the gut wall. Input may be processed and efferent fibers sent to effector cells at all three levels. The only efferent neurons that do not involve the enteric nervous system are the alpha-motor neurons that innervate the striated muscle at both ends of the gut (i.e., cricopharyngeus and external anal sphincter).

vated by alpha motor neurons directly from the CNS. The cell bodies of the alpha motor neurons to the EAS are located in the anterior horn cells of spinal segments S2 through S4. Their axons are carried in the pudendal nerve. Injuries to the pudendal nerves or the sacral cord produce flaccid paralysis of the external sphincter with fecal incontinence.

As can be inferred from the previous discussion, the regulatory mechanisms for gastrointestinal function are highly interdependent and frequently redundant. Loss of any individual component does not necessarily result in an identifiable syndrome. In fact, the inherent automaticity of the gut often allows it to function quite well in the absence of all extrinsic control. The effects of loss of extrinsic neural control (i.e., neurogenic bowel) are most apparent at the two ends of the gastrointestinal tract, where complex voluntary behaviors occur. The primary function lost with neurogenic bowel is voluntary control over defecation.

Colonic Motility

Studies of colonic transit time in people with SCI generally have shown a prolongation of total colonic transit time that is predominantly caused by slowing through the rectosigmoid segment (191,192). Interpretation of this finding is difficult because transit time studies cannot differentiate slow transit through the rectosigmoid because of altered colonic motility from slow transit because of infrequent or inefficient evacuation of the rectum. In our SCI population, bowel care was performed at a mean interval of approximately 2 days; the interval between bowel movements in a neurologically intact control group was 1 day. Because any movement in the rectosigmoid colon between bowel care days would not be expected, the difference between SCI and controls may simply be related to the frequency of bowel care and bowel movements. Furthermore, Kellow has demonstrated that distention of the rectum slows intestinal transit in both the fasting and fed states. Inhibition of contraction in one portion of the intestinal tract by distention of another (i.e., intestinointestinal, intestinocolic, and colocolic reflexes) was first reported 50 years ago (193). Interestingly, these reflexes are mediated in the prevertebral ganglia, not the spinal cord, so they likely would be unaffected by SCI (194).

Attempts to describe the effect of SCI on colonic motility by measurement of electrical or pressure events have yielded inconsistent results. Connell and associates, measuring intraluminal pressure waves, concluded that people with injury levels above T9 had decreased rectosigmoid motor activities, whereas those with lesions below T9 had increased motor activity (195). Aaronson and colleagues found an increase in rectal myoelectric activity in a disparate group of six people with SCI when compared with neurologically intact controls (196). Glick and colleagues found no change in myoelectric activity when nine people with SCI were compared with controls (197). Interpretation of these studies is plagued by many of the previously mentioned methodologic problems. The study groups were small and uncontrolled for important variables such as time after injury, age, level and completeness of injury, and presence of gastrointestinal symptoms. Even if a consistent pattern of motility disorder could be found, it could as easily be caused by the inability to evacuate as by a primary motility problem.

Fecal Continence

Fecal continence is the result of a series of anatomic and physiological barriers to the passage of stool through the anus. These barriers are removable to allow bowel evacuation to occur. The current state, continence or evacuation, depends on the balance between those forces that favor expulsion of stool and those that resist it (Fig. 44-9). Expulsive forces include intra-abdominal pressure, colorectal contraction, elastic forces, and gravity. Resistive forces include the anorectal angle, anal canal tone contributed by the IAS and EAS, and friction. Stool consistency is a pivotal factor that can shift the balance in either direction. Small, hard stool is evacuated less completely and with more difficulty than soft, bulky stool (183,182), whereas subjects with normal conti-

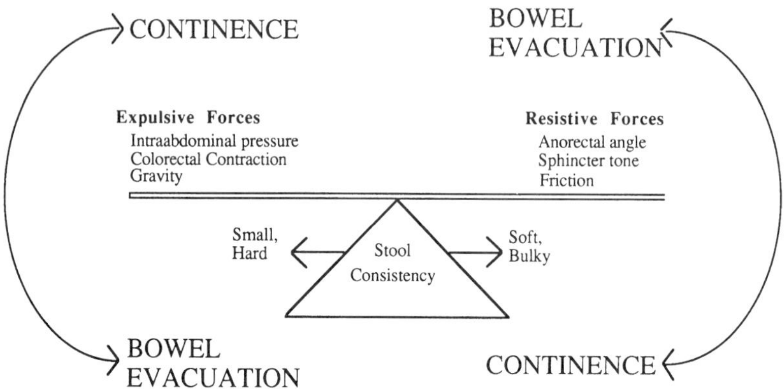

FIG. 44-9. Balance of forces favoring continence or bowel evacuation. Physical character of stool is the pivotal variable that can shift the balance in either direction. Small, hard stool shifts the fulcrum to the left, and more force is required to evacuate. Soft, bulky stool causes the fulcrum to shift the opposite way.

nence mechanisms may be incontinent when faced with large volumes of liquid stool during an acute diarrheal illness.

Clinical Evaluation

As with any patient, the evaluation begins with a complete history and physical examination. Although abdominal symptoms typically are vague, clues to their origin may be derived from a careful search for a relationship to exacerbating or remitting factors. The effect of body position, time of day, eating, bowel care, medications, and urinary function should be elicited. The presence of associated symptoms such as autonomic dysreflexia, abdominal wall spasticity, fever, and weight change should be noted. Events that occurred around the time of a symptom's onset such as a change in medication, bowel program, or living situation also should be elicited. A careful query of premorbid bowel function should be made, because neurologic lesions may alter the way that preexisting problems are manifest. Some sense of the impact of the symptom on the patient's ability to work, travel, interact with others, and carry out the activities of daily living is useful. Finally, the bowel program should be thoroughly evaluated. A history of the type of diet with special emphasis on fluid and fiber intake, use of laxatives, stool softeners, fiber supplements, and medications with anticholinergic properties should be obtained. The frequency, duration, and technique of bowel care are elicited as well as problems with stool consistency, lack of stool in the rectum at the time of stimulation, incontinence, and bleeding.

Rectodynamics

To better understand the effects of SCI on bowel evacuation, we designed a test to measure the opposing expulsive and resistive forces at work in the anorectum. We call the test rectodynamics because of its similarity to urodynamics, the study of bladder emptying (Fig. 44-10). Rectodynamics is performed by placing a triple-lumen catheter through the anus so that one pressure-measuring sideport is in the rectum and another is in the high-pressure zone of the anal canal. The third lumen is used to fill a balloon located in the rectum. A concentric EMG needle is placed in the EAS. Rectal and anal pressures, along with external sphincter EMG, are measured at rest and during stimulation of the anorectum by digital stimulation, the Valsalva maneuver, rapid rectal distention (i.e., air is rapidly injected and removed from rectal balloon to elicit the rectoanal inhibitory reflex), and slow, continuous filling of the rectal balloon with saline.

The typical features of rectodynamic study of an asymptomatic person with upper motor neuron SCI are illustrated in Figure 44-11*A*. During continuous filling of the rectal balloon, the intermittent rises in rectal pressure (i.e., rectal contractions) are invariably linked with decreases in anal canal pressure. When the rectal threshold pressure is reached (20 to 30 cm H_2O), the external sphincter EMG becomes silent, and anal pressure decreases toward zero. The rectal pressure rises slowly until the rectal reservoir capacity is

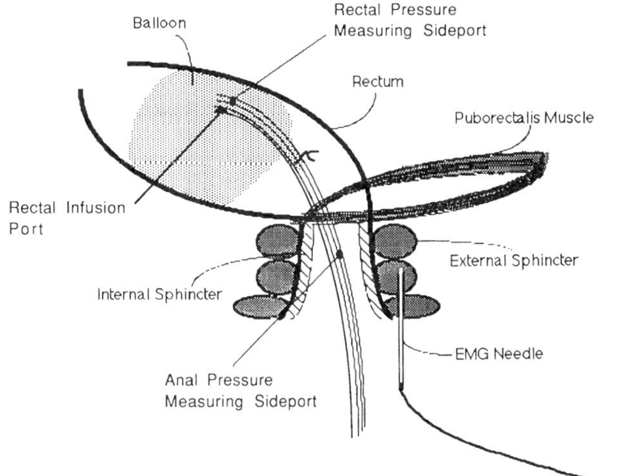

FIG. 44-10. Rectodynamics setup. Expulsive forces (e.g., intra-abdominal pressure, colorectal contraction, rectal elasticity) are reflected by the pressure in the balloon in the rectum. Resistive forces are measured by the anal sphincter pressure. The contribution of the external sphincter is reflected by the electromyographic activity. Pressures are measured at rest and during stimulation by anal stretch (i.e., digital stimulation); rapid rectal stretch (i.e., rectoanal inhibitory reflex); and continuous infusion of saline into the rectal balloon.

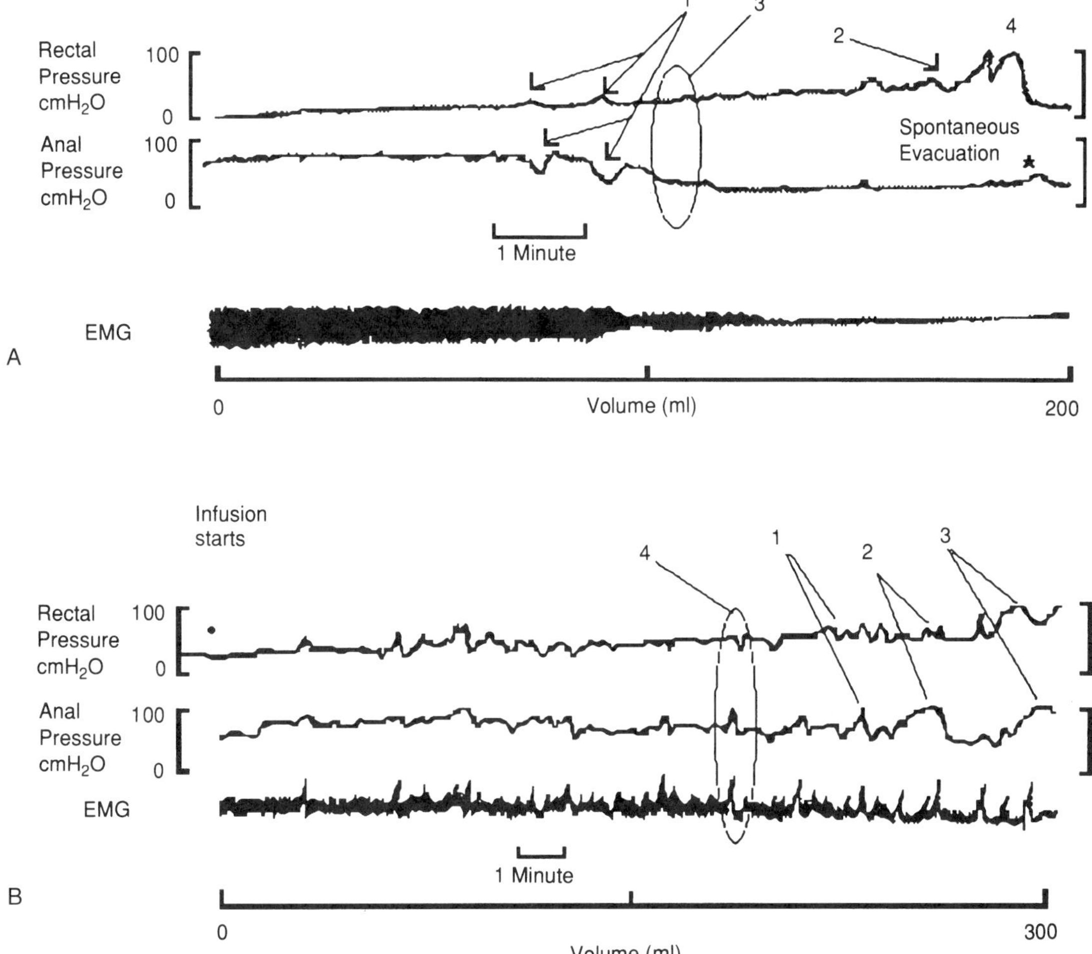

FIG. 44-11. Rectodynamics study. During the tracing, the balloon in the rectum is being filled with saline at a constant rate (20 ml/min). **A:** Normal evacuation pattern after SCI. *1*, Small rises in rectal pressure (i.e., rectal contractions) are invariably linked to anal pressure relaxation. Later contraction does not show linked relaxation because anal pressure cannot go below zero. *2*, Gradual rise in rectal pressure becomes rapid when rectal reservoir capacity is overcome (usually 150–300 ml). *3*, When rectal threshold pressure (20–30 cm H_2O) is reached, anal pressure goes to zero. *4*, Spontaneous evacuation of the balloon occurs when expulsive forces exceed resistive forces. **B:** Dyssynergia. *1*, Loss of normal anal relaxation with rectal contraction. In this patient there is total loss of coordination between the rectum and anus. *2*, Anal pressure fails to go to zero when the normal threshold (20–30 cm H_2O) of rectal pressure is reached. *3*, No spontaneous evacuation of the rectal balloon occurs despite rectal pressures of 100 cm H_2O. Anal pressures increase concomitantly. *4*, Spikes of electromyographic activity reflect contractions of the striated external anal sphincter. These contractions occur inappropriately and cause an elevation in anal pressure.

overcome (usually at 150 to 300 ml) and then rises rapidly until anal pressure is overcome and spontaneous evacuation of the balloon occurs.

Bowel Evacuation Mechanics

In neurologically intact people, the sequence of defecation begins with the perception of rectal fullness. Rectal distention may be perceived at volumes as low as 10 ml by stretch receptors in the rectal wall and the pelvic floor. Continued rectal distention triggers rectal contraction and the rectoanal inhibitory reflex (198). Freckner, studying a small group of SCI patients, found that distention of the rectum with small volumes caused increased activity of the EAS (i.e., guarding reflex), whereas distention with large amounts caused the EAS totally to cease its electrical activity (178). This cessation of EAS activity rarely is seen in neurologically intact subjects. We have found that the volume at which the cessation of EAS activity occurs is variable and probably related to rectal capacity but that the intrarectal pressure at which it occurs is quite constant (20 to 30 cm H_2O; see Fig. 44-11*A*). There is a subgroup of patients with upper motor neuron lesions in whom EAS activity is aberrantly linked to rectal pressure (see Fig. 44-11*B*). In these patients, the spikes in rectal pressure that occur during dynamic rectal filling are met by increases in anal pressure. There is a failure to "turn off" EAS sphincter activity despite the presence of rectal pressures greater than 100 cm H_2O. We call this pattern anorectal dyssynergia, by analogy with detrusor–sphincter dyssynergia of the bladder. These SCI patients usually have significant difficulty with bowel evacuation.

If the choice is made to defecate, the sitting position is assumed. Sitting makes the angle between the rectum and anal canal less acute (199). In the able-bodied, a rise in intra-abdominal and perhaps intrarectal pressure is generated, followed by relaxation of the IAS, EAS, and puborectalis muscle. Neurologically intact people often are able to increase intrarectal pressure by 100 cm H_2O or more with a Valsalva maneuver. Upper motor neuron SCI patients initiate bowel evacuation by digital stimulation (i.e., sphincter stretch). Digital stimulation results in the transient loss of approximately 75% of resting anal tone and presumably further straightens the anorectal angle. Contrary to popular belief, digital stimulation, performed by a variety of techniques in the empty and full rectum, does not cause rectal contraction. Expulsive force is added by performance of a Valsalva maneuver as well as the addition of external abdominal compression. The ability to elevate intra-abdominal pressure with the use of these techniques is closely related to the level and completeness of SCI. Patients with C5 to C6 level injuries rarely can generate intra-abdominal pressures greater than 10 cm H_2O.

The most common rectodynamic finding in patients with symptomatic difficulty with bowel evacuation is a failure to generate expulsive forces that are sufficient to overcome the residual tone of the normal, fully relaxed sphincter mechanism. These patients typically have long-standing cervical cord injuries, often with associated megacolon and megarectum. In these patients, the relationship between rectal pressure and anal relaxation remains intact, although it can take rectal volumes greater than 500 ml to generate enough rectal stretch to trigger anal relaxation. Rectal volumes of 100 to 150 ml usually are sufficient to turn off the anal sphincter mechanism.

Once evacuation is initiated, the entire left colon may empty by mass peristaltic action, or the fecal bolus may be passed bit by bit. The presence of an anocolic reflex (i.e., stool passing through the anus causes colonic contraction) has been postulated but not proven. Stool consistency is probably the major determinant of the pattern of defecation. Stool consistency is of even greater importance in SCI patients, in whom the balance between expulsive and resistive forces is so tenuous.

Neurogenic Bowel Function

Supraspinal bowel dysfunction occurs with lesions rostral to the pons. Voluntary defecation depends on an accurate perception of the need to evacuate as well as the necessary motor function to reach a bathroom and to initiate the complex motor activity of bowel evacuation. A failure to perceive rectal fullness is common in the elderly and may manifest as overflow incontinence around a fecal impaction. Although disorders of continence and bowel evacuation are not uncommon after stroke, few distinct syndromes have been described. One syndrome, frontal lobe incontinence, is caused by lesions involving the anterior cingulate gyri (200). Patients with frontal lobe incontinence are said to have no awareness of bladder or rectal fullness. A pontine defecation center, analogous to the pontine micturition center, has been postulated but not proven (201). Patients with Parkinson's disease and multiple sclerosis often have disordered bowel evacuation; however, it may be difficult to factor out the effects of immobility, diet, and medications in these cases.

Upper motor neuron bowel dysfunction occurs with lesions between the pons and the sacral spinal cord. This is the type of dysfunction most commonly seen in SCI patients. The most significant gastrointestinal consequence of SCI is loss of voluntary control over defecation. People with SCI, or their attendants, must be trained to stimulate a reflex evacuation, which can be referred to as bowel care. An overall plan that is designed to optimize stool volume and consistency while minimizing abdominal discomfort and attendant time is known as the bowel program. Through empirical manipulation of diet, hydration, medications, and stimulation techniques, a balance is maintained between continence and evacuation.

Using the rectodynamics technique, we have identified two patterns of bowel evacuation mechanics that are associated with an inability to undergo satisfactory reflex evacuation: anorectal dyssynergia and insufficient expulsive forces. In both situations, spontaneous evacuation of the saline-filled balloon rarely occurs. In asymptomatic patients, spontaneous evacuation at volumes of 150 to 300 ml is the rule. Patients with insufficient expulsive forces tend to be older and to have had their SCI longer than patients with anorectal dyssynergia. It is attractive to postulate that both patterns are different stages of the same process. Chronically obstructed evacuation from dyssynergia may result in an end-stage decompensated rectum that is unable to generate a sufficient expulsive force. Against this theory is the finding that many patients with the insufficient expulsive force pattern retain a normal linkage between rectal and anal pressures, albeit at much higher volumes. Because patients with insufficient expulsive force all have cervical injuries, it is tempting to implicate a specific neurophysiologic cause such as an overabundance of sympathetic input, although it is difficult to explain why the majority of patients with complete cervical injuries do not manifest this pattern. A more likely association with cervical injuries is that with denervation of the abdominal wall, only minimal increases in intra-abdominal pressure can be generated. Although these studies do not reveal the underlying pathophysiological process of neurogenic bowel, they do provide a practical basis for thinking about the management of patients with neurogenic bowel.

Gastrointestinal Problems After Spinal Cord Injury

It has long been clear to clinicians that gastrointestinal complaints are very common in the chronic phase after SCI. Glickman and Kamm evaluated 115 consecutive outpatients with chronic SCI. Eighty-nine were male, the mean duration of injury was 62 months, and the level of injury was categorized as 48% cervical, 47% thoracic, and 5% lumbar. In this group, 95% required at least one therapeutic method to initiate defecation, half were dependent on others for toileting, and 49% took more than 30 minutes to complete their bowel program (202). In a prospective study carried out by the Palo Alto Veterans Affairs Medical Center Spinal Cord Injury Service, chronic gastrointestinal problems that were severe enough to alter life style or require chronic treatment occurred in 27% of subjects. The limited way in which people with SCI can manifest symptoms resulted in complaints that were characteristically nonspecific. The most common problems were difficult bowel evacuation (20%) and poorly localized abdominal pain (14%). The term ''pain'' was used in its most general sense and was defined as a distressing sensation in a particular part of the body. Presumably, the pain sensation was carried to the brain by means of autonomic afferents (203).

Difficult bowel evacuation was said to be present in patients who required more than 60 minutes per day for their bowel care or needed manual disimpaction more than once a week. The term ''constipation'' is avoided because it is an imprecise term with different meanings for different people. The impact of problems with bowel evacuation on quality of life is formidable. In patients with difficult bowel evacuation, bowel care routinely occupies a significant part of the day, greatly restricted diets are adopted to minimize symptoms, and emergency trips to a physician for disimpaction are common. Episodes of dysreflexia, rectal bleeding, and incontinence from overtreatment with laxatives also occur frequently. Colostomy has been performed with good success in the subgroup of these patients with the most severe disability (204).

Incontinence was common in lesions of the cauda equina but uncommon in upper motor neuron SCI except during diarrheal illness or as a result of overtreatment for difficult bowel evacuation. Autonomic dysreflexia arising from the gastrointestinal tract occurred in almost one-half of the subjects with lesions above T6 at some time but was rarely a significant problem by itself. Fecal impaction was the most common precipitating cause of autonomic dysreflexia. Other, less common causes were massive abdominal distention and routine digital stimulation. Rectal bleeding during bowel care occurred in 74% of subjects. The majority of these patients were treated with hemorrhoidal bands or expectant management. Twelve percent eventually required operative hemorrhoidectomy. Esophageal reflux symptoms were present in 24% of subjects, and 10% of patients had a proven peptic ulcer. These rates are similar to those seen in the nondisabled population (203).

Gastrointestinal problems have special significance for people with SCI. Some problems, such as autonomic hyperreflexia and ventilatory insufficiency caused by massive abdominal distention, are life-threatening problems that are unique to SCI patients. Other problems are shared with the nondisabled population but are associated with disproportionate morbidity when they occur in people with SCI. Twenty-three percent of our patients required an admission to the hospital for evaluation or treatment of a chronic gastrointestinal problem. Absence of specific symptoms caused emergency operations to be the rule rather than the exception for problems such as peptic ulcers and gallstones.

Stone and associates noted that chronic gastrointestinal problems usually do not develop for several years after injury (203). This finding is particularly significant because it suggests that these problems potentially are preventable. The situation may be analogous to that of the urinary tract in years past, where improvement in chronic care protocols has greatly reduced morbidity. For example, if chronic rectal overdistention eventually impairs the ability to evacuate, techniques to reduce rectal distention such as more frequent bowel care may be of benefit. In this way, decompensation of the rectum may be analogous to detrusor decompensation from chronic bladder overdistention.

There is great heterogeneity of gastrointestinal function within the SCI population. Spinal-cord-injured patients differ not only in neurologic status and amount of time since injury but also in a myriad of factors such as age, premorbid gastrointestinal function, and quality of long-term care. This heterogeneity makes the results of previous studies that group all SCI patients together for comparison with neurologically intact controls, or compare small groups of unselected people with low cord lesions to people with high cord lesions, highly suspect. Future research into gastrointestinal function after SCI must control for this heterogeneity.

Management

People with SCI, particularly at the cervical or high thoracic level, have very little reserve in the balance between expulsive and resistive forces (see Fig. 44-9). Manipulations that may be trivial in the nondisabled population can shift the balance here. Stool consistency is the pivotal variable, although use of gravity (i.e., by sitting upright) and addition of external compression may be necessary.

Avoidance of colorectal overdistention is desirable because rectal distention is known to decrease intestinal transit by the colocolic reflex. Frequent bowel care (i.e., every 1 to 2 days) will avoid colonic distention with stool and may also enhance colonic transit by the hypothetical anocolic reflex. A high-fiber diet of at least 30 g of dietary fiber per day should be encouraged. Wheat bran and psyllium have been found to work by increasing the fecal water content (205).

The first step in initiating bowel evacuation is movement of the sigmoid contents into the rectum. This may be accomplished by timing bowel care with meals to take advantage of the gastrocolic reflex. Rectal suppositories and digital stimulation usually play important roles in the management of bowel evacuation. A suppository is first inserted as high as possible into the rectal vault. Suppositories containing bisacodyl are commonly used. Its major action is to stimulate the sensory nerve endings, resulting in increased peristalsis of the sigmoid colon. It generally takes 15 to 60 minutes for passage of the first flatus, which is followed shortly thereafter by stool flow. Steins reported a significant reduction in the duration of the bowel program using polyethylene glycol-based (PGB) bisacodyl compared to hydrogenated vegetable oil-based (HVB) bisacodyl. The time to first flatus was 10 minutes with the PGB suppository compared to 37 minutes with the HVB suppository. The average total bowel program time was 46 minutes with the PGB suppository compared to 85 minutes with the HVB suppository (206). Suppositories containing sodium bicarbonate and potassium bitartrate are sometimes used. With this suppository, there is a chemical reaction that releases carbon dioxide. The expansion from this reaction often initiates a rectal anal reflex. However, use of this type of suppository usually requires significant anal sphincter activity to prevent the carbon dioxide from being expelled without causing expansion within the recal vault. Glycerine suppositories are often used as a transition from bisacodyl suppositories to no suppositories. The effect of glycerine is to draw water into the stool.

Following an adequate time for the suppository to take effect, digital stimulation is attempted. If a person is having difficulty with autonomic dysreflexia during digital stimulation, pretreatment with topical application of viscous 2% lidocaine may be beneficial. If no stool is present in the rectal vault, stimulation may be repeated a few minutes later. If stool still is not present in the rectal vault, a small-volume saline enema may be given to lubricate the rectum and create acute rectal distention. If this is still unsuccessful, a small-volume bisacodyl enema may be helpful to stimulate colorectal activity.

Oral medications may also be used to facilitate defecation. Oral dioctyl sodium sulfosuccinate functions as a stool softener by having a detergent effect and increasing fluid accumulation in the bowel. Oral senna preparations are sometimes needed 6 to 12 hours before a bowel program. Its action is limited to the colon and felt to stimulate Auerbach's plexus. An oral bisacodyl preparation or a senna preparation approximately 6 to 12 hours before the bowel program is needed to augmented the suppository in some individuals (205).

In patients with difficult bowel evacuation, the first step is optimization of stool consistency with fluids, fiber, oral osmotic agents, or glycerin suppositories. If possible, anticholinergic agents such as oxybutinin are discontinued. If rectodynamic studies show anorectal dyssynergia, topical application of viscous 2% lidocaine occasionally is of benefit. Changing the stimulation technique to provide prolonged anal stretch also may be of benefit. If the rectodynamic study shows that a megarectum already exists, large-volume enemas (300 to 500 ml) may be necessary to provide the necessary rectal distention to raise rectal pressures and shut down anal sphincter activity. In those prone to autonomic dysreflexia, careful monitoring of blood pressure is necessary.

In patients who have failed all attempts to manage their bowel care, colostomy may provide remarkable relief (204). We currently reserve colostomy for patients with severe long-term disability, weight loss, and exhaustion of all nonsurgical options. Transit time studies are performed before colostomy. If markers accumulate in the rectosigmoid, a sigmoid colostomy is performed. If the entire colon is atonic, an ileostomy is performed.

Traumatic superficial mucosal erosion is by far the most common cause of bright red rectal bleeding after SCI. It usually is manifest as streaks of blood on the glove or stool. This should be distinguished from hemorrhoidal bleeding (i.e., bleeding from high-pressure vessels within hemorrhoids), which usually manifests as blood dripping into the commode, or passage of clots. Traumatic erosion usually is treated conservatively. Hemorrhoids need only be treated when they cause a symptom such as bleeding, mucus soilage, or difficulty with anal hygiene. A minimal evaluation for bright red rectal bleeding includes digital examination, anoscopy, and proctoscopy or flexible sigmoidoscopy.

Bright red rectal bleeding, when it occurs after SCI, tends to arise from circumferential mucosal excoriation rather than a discrete site on a hemorrhoid. Therefore, treatment of the entire circumference of the anal canal may be necessary to eliminate bleeding. We have had good success with rubber band ligation of bleeding hemorrhoids. Patients must be aware that the likelihood of recurrent bleeding is high, that multiple applications may be necessary, and that complications, although rare, do occur. Transient episodes of autonomic dysreflexia have occurred at the time of banding, although all have been brief and self-limited (203,204).

In patients with irreducible hemorrhoidal prolapse, blood loss sufficient to cause anemia, or failure of rubber band ligation, operative hemorrhoidectomy must be performed. A conventional surgical technique is used. To avoid manipulation of the fresh suture lines, however, we perform a full mechanical bowel preparation before surgery. No bowel care is performed for 4 days after operative hemorrhoidectomy.

The frequency with which rectal bleeding occurs makes screening for colorectal cancer by testing for occult blood of little value. We screen patients over 45 years old with flexible sigmoidoscopy. If polyps or tumors are seen, a full colonoscopy is performed (203,204).

REFERENCES

1. Grant JCB. *An atlas of anatomy, 6th ed.* Baltimore: Williams & Wilkins, 1972; 181–189.
2. Olsson CA. Anatomy of the upper urinary tract. In: Walsh PC, Gittes RF, Perlmutter AD, Stamey TA, eds. *Campbell's urology, 5th ed.* Philadelphia: WB Saunders, 1986; 12–29.
3. Kaye KW, Goldberg ME. Applied anatomy of the kidneys and ureters. *Urol Clin North Am* 1982; 9:3–13.

4. Tanago EA. Anatomy of the lower urinary tract. In: Walsh PC, Gittes RF, Perlmutter AD, Stamey TA, eds. *Campbell's urology, 5th ed.* Philadelphia: WB Saunders, 1986; 46–61.
5. Stephens FD, Lenaghan D. The anatomical basis and dynamics of vesicoureteral reflux. *J Urol* 1962; 87:669–680.
6. Gosling JA, Dixon JS. Species variation in the location of upper urinary tract pacemaker cells. *Invest Urol* 1974; 11:418–423.
7. Griffiths DJ, Notschaele C. Mechanics of urine transport in the upper urinary tract: 1. The dynamics of the isolated bolus. *Neurourol Urodyn* 1983; 2:155–166.
8. Myers RP, Goellner JR, Cahill DR. Prostate shape, external striated urethral sphincter and radical prostatectomy: the apical dissection. *J Urol* 1987; 138:543–547.
9. Delancey JO. Structure and function of the continence mechanism relative to stress incontinence. In: Leach GE, Paulson DF, eds. *Problems in urology, vol 1. Female urology.* Philadelphia: JB Lippincott, 1991; 1–9.
10. Myers RP. Male urethral sphincteric anatomy and radical prostatectomy. *Urol Clin North Am* 1991; 18:211–227.
11. Fletcher TF, Bradley WE. Neuroanatomy of the bladder-urethra. *J Urol* 1978; 119:153–160.
12. Benson GS, McConnell JA, Wood JG. Adrenergic innervation of the human bladder body. *J Urol* 1979; 122:189–191.
13. Elbadawi A. Autonomic muscular innervation of the vesical outlet and its role in micturition. In: Hinman F Jr, ed. *Benign prostatic hypertrophy.* New York: Springer Verlag, 1983; 330–348.
14. Burnstock G. The changing face of autonomic neurotransmission. *Acta Physiol Scand* 1986; 126:67–91.
15. Norlen L, Dahlstrom A, Sundin T, Svedmyr N. The adrenergic innervation and adrenergic receptor activity of the feline urinary bladder and urethra in the normal state and after hypogastric and/or parasympathetic denervation. *Scand J Urol Nephrol* 1976; 10:177–184.
16. Elbadawi A. Ultrastructure of vesicourethral innervation: III. axoaxonal synapses between postganglionic cholinergic axons and probably SIF-cell derived processes in feline lissosphincter. *J Urol* 1985; 133: 524–528.
17. Elbadawi A, Schenk EA. A new theory of the innervation of bladder musculature: part 4. Innervation of the vesicourethral junction and external urethral sphincter. *J Urol* 1974; 111:613–615.
18. de Groat WC. Mechanism underlying the recovery of lower urinary tract function following spinal cord injury. *Paraplegia* 1995; 33: 493–505.
19. Sundin T, Dahlstrom A. The sympathetic innervation of the urinary bladder and urethra in the normal state and after parasympathetic denervation at the spinal root level. *Scand J Urol Nephrol* 1973; 7: 131–149.
20. Crowe R, Burnstock G, Light JK. Adrenergic innervation of the striated muscle of the intrinsic external urethral sphincter from patients with lower motor spinal cord lesion. *J Urol* 1989; 141:47–49.
21. Denny-Brown D, Robertson EG. On the physiology of micturition. *Brain* 1933; 56:149–190.
22. Barrington FJF. The relation of the hindbrain to micturition. *Brain* 1921; 44:23–53.
23. Bradley WE. Physiology of the urinary bladder. In: Walsh PC, Gittes RF, Perlmutter AD, Stamey TA, eds. *Campbell's urology, 5th ed.* Philadelphia: WB Saunders, 1986; 129–185.
24. de Groat WC. Nervous control of the urinary bladder of the cat. *Brain Res* 1975; 87:201–211.
25. Carlsson CA. The supraspinal control of the urinary bladder. *Acta Pharmacol Toxicol* 1978; 43A(Suppl II):8–12.
26. Bradley WE, Teague CT. Spinal cord organization of micturitional reflex afferents. *Exp Neurol* 1968; 22:504–516.
27. Barrett DM, Wein AJ. Voiding dysfunction: diagnosis, classification and management. In: Gillenwater JY, Grayhack JT, Howards SS, Duckett JW, eds. *Adult and pediatric urology, 2nd ed.* St Louis: Mosby Year Book, 1991; 1001–1099.
28. Lewis WH Jr, Alving AS. Changes with age in the renal function in adult men. *Am J Physiol* 1938; 123:500–515.
29. Resnick NM. Geriatric incontinence. *Urol Clin North Am* 1996; 23(1): 55–74.
30. Elbadawi A, Yalla SV, Resnick NM. Structural basis of geriatric voiding. III. Detrusor overactivity. *J Urol* 1993; 150:1668–1680.
31. Staskin DR. Age-related physiologic and pathologic changes affecting lower urinary tract function. *Clin Geriatr Med* 1986; 2:701–710.
32. Elbadawi A, Yalla SV, Resnick NM. Structural basis of geriatric voiding. Methods of a correlative study and overview of findings. *J Urol* 1993; 150:1650–1656.
33. Ouslander JG, Hepps K, Raz S, Su HL. Genitourinary dysfunction in a geriatric outpatient population. *J Am Geriatr Soc* 1986; 34:507–514.
34. Kaplan GW, Brock WA. Voiding dysfunction in children. *Curr Probl Pediatr* 1980; 10(8):15–16.
35. Comarr AE. Diagnosis of the traumatic cord bladder. In: Boyarski S, ed. *The neurogenic bladder.* Baltimore: Williams & Wilkins, 1967; 147–152.
36. Bradley WE, Chou S, Markland C. Classifying neurologic dysfunction of the urinary bladder. In: Boyarsky S, ed. *The neurogenic bladder.* Baltimore: Williams & Wilkins, 1967; 139–146.
37. Lapides J. Neuromuscular vesical and ureteral dysfunction. In: Campbell MF, Harrison JH, eds. *Urology, 3rd ed.* Philadelphia: WB Saunders, 1970; 1343–1379.
38. Krane RJ, Siroky MB. Classification of neuro-urologic disorders. In: Krane RJ, Siroky MB, eds. *Clinical neuro-urology, 2nd ed.* Boston: Little, Brown & Co, 1979; 143–158.
39. Wein AJ. Classification of neurogenic voiding dysfunction. *J Urol* 1981; 125:605–609.
40. Abrams P, Blaivas JG, Stanton SL, Andersen JT. Standardization of terminology of lower urinary tract function. *Neurourol Urodyn* 1988; 7:403–427.
41. Barer DH. Continence after stroke: useful predictor or goal of therapy? *Age Ageing* 1989; 18:183–191.
42. Borrie MJ, Campbell AJ, Caradoc-Davies TH, Spears GF. Urinary incontinence after stroke: a prospective study. *Age Ageing* 1986; 15: 177–181.
43. Brocklehurst JC, Andrews K, Richards B, Laycock PJ. Incidence and correlates of incontinence in stroke patients. *J Am Geriatr Soc* 1985; 33:540–542.
44. Linsenmeyer TA. Characterization of voiding dysfunction following recent cerebrovascular accident. *Arch Phys Med Rehabil* 1990; 71: 778.
45. Tsuchida S, Noto H, Yamaguchi O, Itoh M. Urodynamic studies on hemiplegic patients after cerebrovascular accident. *Urology* 1983; 21: 315–318.
46. Linsenmeyer TA, Zorowitz RD. Urodynamic findings in patients with urinary incontinence after cerebrovascular accident. *Neuro Rehabil* 1992; 2(2):23–26.
47. Blaivas JG. The neurophysiology of micturition: a clinical study of 550 patients. *J Urol* 1982; 127:958–963.
48. Siroky MB, Krane RJ. Neurologic aspects of detrusor–sphincter dyssynergia with reference to the guarding reflex. *J Urol* 1982; 127: 953–957.
49. Staskin DR. Intracranial lesions that affect lower urinary tract function. In: Krane RJ, Siroky MB, eds. *Clinical neuro-urology, 2nd ed.* Boston: Little, Brown & Co, 1991; 345–451.
50. Pavlakis AJ, Siroky MB, Goldstein I, Krane RJ. Neurourologic findings in Parkinson's disease. *J Urol* 1983; 129:80–83.
51. Andersen JT. Detrusor hyperreflexia in benign infravesical obstruction. A cystometric study. *J Urol* 1976; 115:532.
52. Ivers RR, Goldstein NP. Multiple sclerosis: a current appraisal of symptoms and signs. *Proc Staff Meet Mayo Clin* 1963; 38:457–466.
53. Bemelmans BL, Hommes OR, Van Kerrebroeck PE, Lemmens WA, Doesburg WH, Debruyne FM. Evidence for early lower urinary tract dysfunction in clinically silent multiple sclerosis. *J Urol* 1991; 145: 1219–1224.
54. Miller H, Simpson CA, Yeates WK. Bladder dysfunction in multiple sclerosis. *Br Med J* 1965; 1:1265–1269.
55. Goldstein I, Siroky MB, Sax DS, Krane RJ. Neurourologic abnormalities in multiple sclerosis. *J Urol* 1982; 128:541–545.
56. Wheeler JS, Siroky MB, Pavlakis AJ, Goldstein I, Krane RJ. The changing neurourologic pattern of multiple sclerosis. *J Urol* 1983; 130:1123–1126.
57. Gonor SE, Carroll DJ, Metcalfe JB. Vesical dysfunction in multiple sclerosis. *Urology* 1985; 25:429–431.
58. Blaivas JG, Barbalias GA. Detrusor–external sphincter dyssynergia in men with multiple sclerosis: an ominous urologic condition. *J Urol* 1984; 131:91–94.
59. Wheeler JS. Multiple sclerosis. In: Krane RJ, Siroky MB, eds. *Clinical neuro-urology, 2nd ed.* Boston: Little, Brown & Co, 1991; 353–363.

60. Kaplan SA, Chancellor MB, Blaivas JG. Bladder and sphincter behavior in patients with spinal cord lesions. *J Urol* 1991; 146:113–117.
61. Yalla SV, Fam BA. Spinal cord injury. In: Krane RJ, Siroky MB, eds. *Clinical neuro-urology, 2nd ed.* Boston: Little, Brown & Co, 1991; 319–331.
62. Rudy DC, Awad SA, Downie JW. External sphincter dyssynergia: an abnormal continence reflex. *J Urol* 140:105–110.
63. Light JK, Faganel J, Beric A. Detrusor areflexia in suprasacral spinal cord injuries. *J Urol* 1985; 134:295–297.
64. Graham SD. Present urological treatment of spinal cord injury patients. *J Urol* 1981; 126:1–4.
65. Downie JW, Awad SA. The state of urethral musculature during the detrusor areflexia after spinal cord transection. *Invest Urol* 1979; 17: 55–59.
66. Nanninga JB, Meyer P. Urethral sphincter activity following acute spinal cord injury. *J Urol* 1980; 123:528–530.
67. Koyanagi T, Arikado K, Takamatsu T, Tsuji I. Experience with electromyography of the external urethral sphincter in spinal cord injury patients. *J Urol* 1982; 127:272–276.
68. Blaivas JG, Sinha HP, Zayed AAH, Labib KB. Detrusor–external sphincter dyssynergia. *J Urol* 1981; 125:542–544.
69. Pavlakis AJ, Siroky MB, Goldstein I, Krane RJ. Neurourologic findings in conus medullaris and cauda equina injury. *Arch Neurol* 1983; 40:570–573.
70. Sharr MM, Carfield JC, Jenkins JD. Lumbar spondylosis and neuropathic bladder investigations of 73 patients with chronic urinary symptoms. *Br Med J* 1976; 1:645.
71. Hackler RH, Hall MK, Zampieri TA. Bladder hypocompliance in the spinal cord injury population. *J Urol* 1989; 141:1390–1393.
72. Sislow JG, Mayo ME. Reduction in human bladder wall compliance following decentralization. *J Urol* 1990; 144:945–947.
73. Appell RA, Whiteside HV. Diabetes and other peripheral neuropathies affecting lower urinary tract function. In: Krane RJ, Siroky MG, eds. *Clinical neuro-urology, 2nd ed.* Boston: Little, Brown & Co, 1991; 365–373.
74. Bradley WE. Autonomic neuropathy and the genitourinary system. *J Urol* 1978; 119:299–302.
75. Andersen JT, Bradley WE. Abnormalities of bladder innervation in diabetes mellitus. *Urology* 1976; 7:442–448.
76. Wheeler JS Jr, Siroky MB, Pavlakis A, Krane RJ. The urodynamic aspects of the Guillain-Barré syndrome. *J Urol* 1984; 131:917–919.
77. Katz GP, Blaivas JG. A diagnostic dilemma: when urodynamic findings differ from the clinical impression. *J Urol* 1983; 129:1170–1174.
78. Ouslander J, Staskin D, Raz S, Su HL, Hepps K. Clinical versus urodynamic diagnosis in an incontinent geriatric female population. *J Urol* 1987; 137:68–71.
79. Resnick NM, Yalla SV. Management of urinary incontinence in the elderly. *N Engl J Med* 1985; 313:800–805.
80. Blaivas JG, Zayed AAH, Labib KB. The bulbocavernosus reflex in urology: a prospective study of 299 patients. *J Urol* 1981; 126: 197–199.
81. Rao KG, Hackler RH, Woodlief RM, Ozer MN, Fields WR. Real time renal sonography in spinal cord injury patients: prospective comparison with excretory urography. *J Urol* 1986; 135:72–77.
82. Lloyd LK, Dubovsky EV, Bueschen AJ, et al. Comprehensive renal scintillation procedures in spinal cord injury: comparison with excretory urography. *J Urol* 1981; 126:10–13.
83. Kuhlemeier KV, McEachran AB, Lloyd LK, Stover SL, Fine PR. Serum creatinine as an indicator of renal function after spinal cord injury. *Arch Phys Med Rehabil* 1984; 65:694–697.
84. Khanna OP. Cystometry: water. In: Barrett DM, Wein AJ, eds. *Controversies in neuro-urology.* New York: Churchill-Livingston, 1984; 11–12.
85. McGuire EJ, Woodside JR, Borden TA, Weiss RM. Prognostic value of urodynamic testing in myelodysplastic patients. *J Urol* 1981; 126: 205–209.
86. Bauer SB. Urologic management of the myelodysplastic child. *Probl Urol* 1989; 3:86–101.
87. Lapides J, Friend CR, Ajemian EP, Reus WF. A new test for neurogenic bladder. *J Urol* 1962; 88:245–247.
88. Wheeler JS Jr, Culkin DJ, Canning JR. Positive bethanechol supersensitivity test in neurologically normal patients. *Urology* 1988; 31: 86–89.
89. Burgio KL, Burgio LD. Behavior therapies for urinary incontinence in the elderly. *Clin Geriatr Med* 1986; 2:809–827.
90. Brown JH. Atropine, scopolamine and related antimuscarinic drugs. In: Gilman AG, Rall TW, Nies AS, Taylor P, eds. *Goodman and Gilman's the pharmacologic basis of therapeutics, 8th ed.* New York: Pergamon Press, 1990; 150–165.
91. Baldessarini RJ. Drugs and the treatment of psychiatric disorders. In: Gillman AG, Rall TW, Nies AS, Taylor P, eds. *Goodman and Gilman's the pharmacologic basis of therapeutics, 8th ed.* New York: Pergamon Press, 1990; 383–435.
92. Wyndaele JJ. Pharmacotherapy for urinary bladder dysfunction in spinal cord injury patients. *Paraplegia* 1990; 28:146–150.
93. Das A, Chancellor MB, Watanabe T, Sedor J, Rivas DA. Intravesical capsaicin in neurologic impaired patients with detrusor hyperreflexia. *J Sci Med* 1996; 19(3):190–193.
94. Nanniga JB, Frost F, Penn R. Effect of intrathecal baclofen on bladder and sphincter function. *J Urol* 1989; 142:101–105.
95. Cardozo LD, Stanton SL, Robinson H, Hole D. Evaluation of flurbiprofen in detrusor instability. *Br Med J* 1980; 280:281–282.
96. Brendler CB, Radebaugh LC, Mohler JL. Topical oxybutynin chloride for relaxation of dysfunctional bladder. *J Urol* 1989; 141:1350–1352.
97. Mast P, Hoebeke P, Wyndaele JJ, Oosterlinck W, Everaert K. Experience with augmentation cystoplasty. A review. *Paraplegia* 1995; 33: 560–564.
98. Golomb J, Klutke CG, Lewin KJ, Goodwin WE, deKernion JB, Raz S. Bladder neoplasms associated with augmentation cystoplasty: report of 2 cases and literature review. *J Urol* 1989; 142:377–380.
99. Misak SJ, Bunts RC, Ulmer JL, Eagles WM. Nerve interruption procedures in the urologic management of paraplegic patients. *J Urol* 1962; 88:392.
100. Leach GE, Goldman D, Raz S. Surgical treatment of detrusor hyperreflexia. In: Raz S, ed. *Female urology.* Philadelphia: WB Saunders, 1983; 326–334.
101. Hodgkinson CP, Drukker BH. Infravesical nerve resection for detrusor dyssynergia: the Ingelman-Sundberg operation. *Acta Obstet Gynecol Scand* 1977; 56:401–408.
102. Ohlsson BL, Frankenberg-Sommar S. Effects of external and direct pudendal nerve maximal electrical stimulation in the treatment of the uninhibited overactive bladder. *Br J Urol* 1989; 64:374–380.
103. Tanago EA. Concepts of Neuromodulation. *Neurourol Urodyn* 1993; 12:497–498.
104. Guttmann L, Frankel H. The value of intermittent catheterisation in the early management of traumatic paraplegia and tetraplegia. *Paraplegia* 1966/1967; 4:63–84.
105. Lapides J, Diokno AC, Silber SJ, Lowe BS. Clean, intermittent self catheterization in treatment of urinary tract disease. *J Urol* 1972; 107: 458–461.
106. Maynard FM, Glass J. Management of the neuropathic bladder by clean intermittent catheterisation: 5 year outcomes. *Paraplegia* 1987; 25:106–110.
107. Anderson RU. Non sterile intermittent catheterization with antibiotic prophylaxis in the acute spinal cord injured male patient. *J Urol* 1980; 124:392–394.
108. Kegel AH. Progressive resistance exercises in the functional restoration of the perineal muscles. *Am J Obstet Gynecol* 1948; 56:238–248.
109. Wells TJ, Brink CA, Diokno AC, Wolfe R, Gillis GL. Pelvic muscle exercise for stress urinary incontinence in elderly women. *J Am Geriatr Soc* 1991; 39:785–791.
110. Jeter KF. Pelvic muscle exercises with and without biofeedback for the treatment of urinary incontinence. *Probl Urol* 1991; 5:72–84.
111. Hoffman BB, Lefkowitz RJ. Catecholamines and sympathomimetic drugs. In: Gillman AG, Rall TW, Nies AS, Taylor P, eds. *Goodman and Gilman's the pharmacological basis of therapeutics, 8th ed.* New York: Pergamon Press, 1990:187–220.
112. Walter S, Wolf H, Barlebo H, Jensen HK. Urinary incontinence in post menopausal women treated with estrogens. *Urol Int* 1978; 33: 135.
113. Hodgson BJ, Dumas S, Bolling DR, Heesch CM. Effect of estrogen on sensitivity of rabbit bladder and urethra to phenylephrine. *Invest Urol* 1978; 16:67–69.
114. Appell RA. Periurethral collagen injection for female incontinence. *Probl Urol* 1991; 5:134–140.
115. Light JK, Scott FB. Use of the artificial urinary sphincter in spinal cord injury patients. *J Urol* 1983; 130:1127–1129.

116. Bosco PJ, Bauer SB, Colodny AH, Mandell J, Retik AB. The long term results of artificial sphincters in children. *J Urol* 1991; 146: 396–399.
117. Kelly MJ, Leach GE. Long term results of bladder neck suspension procedures. *Probl Urol* 1991; 5:94–105.
118. Opitz JL. Treatment of voiding dysfunction in spinal cord injured patients: bladder retraining. In: Barrett DM, Wein AJ, eds. *Controversies in neuro-urology.* New York: Churchill-Livingston, 1984; 437–451.
119. Barbalias GA, Klauber GT, Blaivas JG. Critical evaluation of the Crede maneuver: a urodynamic study of 207 patients. *J Urol* 1983; 130:720–723.
120. Finkbeiner AE. Is bethanechol chloride clinically effective in promoting bladder emptying? A literature review. *J Urol* 1985; 134:443–449.
121. Light KJ, Scott FB. Bethanechol chloride and the traumatic cord bladder. *J Urol* 1982; 128:85–87.
122. Sporer A, Leyson JFJ, Martin BF. Effects of bethanechol chloride on the external urethral sphincter in spinal cord injury patients. *J Urol* 1978; 120:62–66.
123. Taylor P. Cholinergic agonists. In: Gilman AC, Rall TW, Nies AS, Taylor P, eds. *Goodman and Gilman's the pharmacological basis of therapeutics, 8th ed.* New York: Pergamon Press, 1990; 122–130.
124. Vaidyanathan S, Rao MS, Mapa MK, et al. Study of intravesical instillation of 1A(*s*)-15 methy prostaglandin F_2 in patients with neurogenic bladder dysfunction. *J Urol* 1981; 126:81–85.
125. Booth AM, Hisamitsu T, Kawatani M, de Groat WC. Regulation of urinary bladder capacity by endogenous opioid peptides. *J Urol* 1985; 133:339–342.
126. Hanna MK. New concept in bladder remodeling. *Urology* 1982; 19:6.
127. Lockhart JL, Vorstman B, Weinstein D, Politano V. Sphincterotomy failure in neurogenic bladder disease. *J Urol* 1986; 135:86–89.
128. Creasey GH, Bodner DR. Review of sacral electrical stimulation in the management of the neurogenic bladder. *Neurorehabilitation* 1994; 4(4):266–274.
129. Van Kerrebroeck PEV. World wide experience with the Finetech-Brindley sacral anterior root stimulator. *Neurourol Urodyn* 1993; 12(5):497–503.
130. Maizels M, King LR, Firlit CR. Urodynamic biofeedback: a new approach to treat vesical sphincter dyssynergia. *J Urol* 1979; 122: 205–209.
131. Kiviat MD, Zimmermann TA, Donovan WH. Sphincter stretch: new technique resulting in continence and complete voiding in paraplegics. *J Urol* 1975; 114:895–897.
132. Lepor H. Alpha blockers for the treatment of benign prostatic hypertrophy. *Probl Urol* 1991; 5:419–429.
133. Scott MB, Morrow JW. Phenoxybenzamine in neurogenic bladder dysfunction after spinal cord injury: I. voiding dysfunction. *J Urol* 1978; 119:480–482.
134. Lepor H, Gup DI, Baumann M, Shapiro E. Laboratory assessment of terazosin and alpha 1 blockade in prostatic hyperplasia. *Urology* 1988; 32(Suppl 6):21–26.
136. Scott MB, Morrow JW. Phenoxybenzamine in neurogenic bladder dysfunction after spinal cord injury: II. autonomic dysreflexia. *J Urol* 1978; 119:483–484.
137. Hoffman BB, Lefkowitz RJ. Adrenergic receptor antagonists. In: Gilman AG, Rall TW, Nies AS, Taylor J, eds. *Goodman and Gilman's the pharmacological basis of therapeutics, 8th ed.* New York: Pergamon Press, 1990; 221–243.
138. Wein AJ. Prazosin in the treatment of prostatic obstruction: a placebo controlled study (editorial comment). *J Urol* 1989; 141:693.
139. Cedarbaum JM, Schleifer LS. Drugs for Parkinson's disease, spasticity and acute muscle spasms. In: Gilman AG, Rall TW, Nies AS, Taylor P, eds. *Goodman and Gilman's the pharmacological basis of therapeutics, 8th ed.* New York: Pergamon Press, 1990; 463–484.
140. Engel RME, Schirmer HKA. Pudendal neurectomy in neurogenic bladder. *J Urol* 1974; 112:57–59.
141. Perkash I. Modified approach to sphincterotomy in spinal cord injury patients. *Paraplegia* 1976; 13:247–260.
142. Yang CC, Mayo ME. External sphincterotomy; long term follow up. *Neurourol Urodynam* 1995; 14:25–31.
143. Perkash I. Contact laser transurethral external sphincterotomy; a perliminary report. *Neurorehabilitation* 1994; 4(4):249–254.
144. Chancellor MB, Rivas DA, Linsenmeyer T, Abdill CA, Ackman CFD, Appell RA, et al. Multicenter trial in North America of Urolume urinary sphincter prosthesis. *J Urol* 1994; 152:924–930.
145. Dykstra DD, Sidi AA, Scott AB, Pagel JM, Goldish GD. Effects of botulinum A toxin on detrusor sphincter dyssynergia in spinal cord injury patients. *J Urol* 1988; 139:919–922.
146. Sugar EC, Firlit CF. Urodynamic biofeedback: a new therapeutic approach for childhood incontinence/infection (vesical voluntary sphincter dyssynergia). *J Urol* 1982; 128:1253–1257.
147. Parres JA, Kropp KA. Urodynamic evaluation of the continence mechanism following urethral lengthening: reimplantation and enterocystoplasty. *J Urol* 1991; 146:535–538.
148. Lloyd LK, Kuhlemeier KV, Fine PR, Stover SL. Initial bladder management in spinal cord injury: does it make a difference? *J Urol* 1986; 135:523–527.
149. Maynard FM, Diokno AC. Urinary infection and complications during clean intermittent catheterization following spinal cord injury. *J Urol* 1984; 132:943–946.
150. Romano JM, Kaye D. UTI in the elderly: common yet atypical. *Geriatrics* 1981; 36(6):113–120.
151. Kass EH. The role of asymptomatic bacteriuria in the pathogenesis of pyelonephritis. In: Quinn EL, Kass EH, eds. *Biology of pyelonephritis.* Boston: Little, Brown & Co, 1960; 399–418.
152. Stamey TA. Recurrent urinary tract infections in female patients: an overview of management and treatment. *Rev Infect Dis* 1987; 9(Suppl 2):S195–S210.
153. Stamm WE, Counts GW, Running KR, Fihn S, Turck M, Holmes KK. Diagnosis of coliform infection in acutely dysuric women. *N Engl J Med* 1982; 307:463–468.
154. Rhame FS, Perkash I. Urinary tract infections occurring in recent spinal cord injury patients on intermittent catheterization. *J Urol* 1979; 122:669–673.
155. Donovan WH, Stolov WC, Clowers DE, Clowers MR. Bacteriuria during intermittent catheterization following spinal cord injury. *Arch Phys Med Rehabil* 1978; 59:351–357.
156. The prevention and management of urinary tract infections among people with spinal cord injuries; National Institute on Disabilities and Rehabilitation Research Consensus Conference Statement. January 27–29, 1992. *J Am Paraplegia Soc* 1992; 15:194–204.
157. Deresinski SC, Perkash I. Urinary tract infections in male spinal cord injured patients: part 2. Diagnostic value of symptoms and of quantitative urinalysis. *J Am Paraplegia Soc* 1985; 8:7–10.
158. Anderson RU, Hsieh-ma ST. Association of bacteriuria and pyuria during intermittent catheterization after spinal cord injury. *J Urol* 1983; 130:299–301.
159. Kass EJ, Koff SA, Diokno AC, Lapides J. The significance of bacilluria in children on long term intermittent catheterization. *J Urol* 1981; 126:223–225.
160. Lewis RI, Carrion HM, Lockhart JL, Politano VA. Significance of asymptomatic bacteriuria in neurogenic bladder disease. *Urology* 1984; 23:343–347.
161. Tempkin A, Sullivan G, Paldi J, Perkash I. Radioisotope renography in spinal cord injury. *J Urol* 1985; 133:228–230.
162. Kuhlemeier KV, Stover SL, Lloyd LK. Prophylactic antibacterial therapy for preventing urinary tract infections in spinal cord injury patients. *J Urol* 1985; 134:514–517.
163. Merritt JLM, Erickson RP, Opitz JL. Bacteriuria during follow up in patients with spinal cord injury: Part II. Efficacy of antimicrobial suppressants. *Arch Phys Med Rehabil* 1982; 63:413–415.
164. Gillenwater JY. Hydronephrosis. In: Gillenwater JY, Grayhack JT, Howards SS, Duckett JW, eds. *Adult and pediatric urology, 2nd ed.* St Louis: Mosby Year Book, 1991; 789–813.
165. Staskin DR. Hydroureteronephrosis after spinal cord injury. *Urol Clin North Am* 1991; 18:309–316.
166. Teague N, Boyarsky S. Further effects of coliform bacteria on ureteral peristalsis. *J Urol* 1968; 99:720–724.
167. Price M, Kottke FJ. Renal function in patients with spinal cord injury: the eighth year of a ten year continuing study. *Arch Phys Med Rehabil* 1975; 56:76–79.
168. Fellows GJ, Silver JR. Long term follow up of paraplegic patients with vesico-ureteric reflux. *Paraplegia* 1976; 14:130–134.
169. Winberg J. Urinary tract infections in infants and children. In: Walsh PC, Gittes RF, Perlmutter AD, Stamey TA, eds. *Campbell's urology, 5th ed.* Philadelphia: WB Saunders, 1986; 848–867.

170. DeVivo MJ, Fine PR. Predicting renal calculus occurrence in spinal cord injury patients. *Arch Phys Med Rehabil* 1986; 67:722–775.
171. Kuhlemeier KV, Lloyd LK, Stover SL. Long term followup of renal function after spinal cord injury. *J Urol* 1985; 134:510–513.
172. Singh M, Chapman R, Tresidder GC, Blandy J. Fate of unoperated staghorn calculus. *Br J Urol* 1973; 45:581–585.
173. Irwin PP, Evans C, Chawla JC, Matthews PN. Stone surgery in the spinal patient. *Paraplegia* 1991; 29:161–166.
174. Rodman JS, Williams JJ, Peterson CM. Partial dissolution of struvite calculus with oral acetohydroxamic acid. *Urology* 1983; 22:410–412.
175. Kaufman JM, Fam B, Jacobs SC, et al. Bladder cancer and squamous metaplasia in spinal cord injury patients. *J Urol* 1977; 118:967–971.
176. Arhan P, Devroede G, Jehannin B, et al. Segmental colonic transit time. *Dis Colon Rectum* 1981; 24:625–629.
177. Duthie HL, Watts JM. Contribution of the external anal sphincter to the pressure zone in the anal canal. *Gut* 1965; 6:64–68.
178. Frenckner B. Function of the anal sphincters in spinal man. *Gut* 1975; 16:638–644.
179. Parks AG, Porter NH, Melzack J. Experimental study of the reflex mechanism controlling the muscles of the pelvic floor. *Dis Colon Rectum* 1962; 5:407–414.
180. Wallace WC, Madden WM. Partial puborectalis resection: a new surgical technique for anorectal dysfunction. *South Med J* 1969; 62: 1121–1126.
181. Findlay JM, Smith AN, Mitchell WD, Anderson AJB, Eastwood MA. Effects of unprocessed bran on colon function in normal subjects and in diverticular disease. *Lancet* 1974; 1:146.
182. Bannister JJ, Gibbons C, Read NW. Preservation of faecal continence during rises in intraabdominal pressure: is there a role for the flap valve? *Gut* 1987; 28:1242–1245.
183. Ambroze WL, Bell AM, Pemberton JH, Brown AR, Zinsmeister AR. The effect of stool consistency on rectal and neorectal emptying. *Gastroenterology* 1989; 96(Suppl 5):A11.
184. Cummings JH. Constipation, dietary fibre and the control of large bowel function. *Postgrad Med J* 1984; 60:811–819.
185. Bond JH, Currier BE, Buchwald H, Levitt MD. Colonic conservation of malabsorbed carbohydrate. *J Gastroenterol* 1980; 78:444–449.
186. Flynn M, Hammond P, Darby C, Hyland J, Taylor I. Faecal bile acids and the irritable colon syndrome. *Digestion* 1981; 22:144–149.
187. Goyal RK, Crist JR. Neurology of the gut. In: Sleisenger MH, Fordtran JS, eds. *Gastrointestinal disease: pathophysiology, diagnosis, management, 4th ed.* Philadelphia: WB Saunders, 1989; 21–47.
188. Furness JB, Costa M. Types of nerves in the enteric nervous system. *Neuroscience* 1980; 5:1–20.
189. Devroede G, Arhan P, Duguay C, Tetreault L, Akoury H, Perey B. Traumatic constipation. *Gastroenterology* 1979; 77:1258–1267.
190. Graffner H, Ekelund M, Hakanson R, Oscarson J, Rosengren E, Sundler F. Effects of upper abdominal sympathectomy on gastric acid, serum gastrin, and catecholamines in the rat gut. *Scand J Gastroenterol* 1984; 19:711–716.
191. Menardo G, Bausano G, Corazziari E, et al. Large bowel transit in paraplegic patients. *Dis Colon Rectum* 1987; 30:924–928.
192. Nino-Murcia M, Stone JM, Chang PJ, Perkash I. Colonic transit in spinal cord injured patients. *Invest Radiol* 1990; 25:109–112.
193. Kellow JE, Gill RC, Wingate DL. Modulation of human upper gastrointestinal motility by rectal distention. *Gut* 1987; 28:864–868.
194. Kreulen DL, Szurszewski JH. Reflex pathways in the abdominal prevertebral ganglia: evidence for the colo-colonic inhibitory reflex. *J Physiol* 1979; 295:21–32.
195. Connell AM, Frankel H, Guttman L. The motility of the pelvic colon following complete lesions of the spinal cord. *Paraplegia* 1963; 1: 98–115.
196. Aaronson MJ, Freed MM, Burakoff R. Colonic myoelectric activity in persons with spinal cord injury. *Dig Dis Sci* 1985; 30:295–300.
197. Glick ME, Haldeman S, Meshkinpour H. The neurovisceral and electrodiagnostic evaluation of patients with thoracic spinal cord injury. *Paraplegia* 1986; 24:129–137.
198. Read NW, Timms JM. Defecation and the pathophysiology of constipation. *Clin Gastroenterol* 1986; 15:937–965.
199. Barkel DC, Pemberton JH, Pezim ME, Phillips SF, Kelly KA, Brown ML. Scintigraphic assessment of the anorectal angle in health and after ileal pouch-anal anastomosis. *Ann Surg* 1988; 208:42–49.
200. Adams RD, Victor M. Neurologic disorders caused by lesions in particular parts of the cerebrum. In: *Principles of neurology, 4th ed.* New York: McGraw-Hill, 1989; 347–376.
201. Weber J, Denis P, Mihout B, et al. Effect of brain-stem lesion on colonic and anorectal motility. Study of three patients. *Dig Dis Sci* 1985; 30:419–425.
202. Glickman S, Kamm MA. Bowel dysfunction in spinal cord injured patients. *Lancet* 1996; 347:1651–1653.
203. Stone JM, Nino-Murcia M, Wolfe VA, Perkash I. Chronic gastrointestinal problems in spinal cord injury patients: a prospective analysis. *Am J Gastroenterol* 1990; 85:1114–1149.
204. Stone JM, Wolfe VA, Nino-Murcia M, Perkash I. Colostomy as treatment for complications of spinal cord injury. *Arch Phys Med Rehabil* 1990; 71:514–518.
205. Weingarden SI. The gastrointestinal system and spinal cord injury. *Phys Med Rehabil Clin North Am* 1992; 3(4):765–773.
206. Steins SA. Reduction in bowel program duration with polyethylene glycol based bisacodyl suppositories. *Arch Phys Med Rehabil* 1995; 76:674–677.

Rehabilitation Medicine: Principles and Practice, Third Edition, edited by Joel A. DeLisa and Bruce M. Gans. Lippincott–Raven Publishers, Philadelphia © 1998.

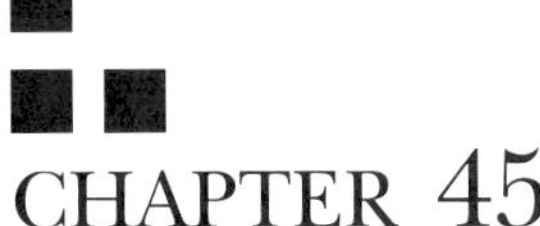

CHAPTER 45

Sexuality and Disability

Marca L. Sipski and Craig Alexander

Sexuality can be an important part of life from the time an individual is born until the time he or she dies. Moreover, it is an important means of expressing one's feelings towards self or others. Unfortunately, during medical crises and serious chronic illness, issues pertaining to sexuality and sexual functioning have lower priority. Furthermore, some physicians are uncomfortable speaking about their patients' sexual concerns, and this discomfort is communicated to the patient. Hence, the patient may have a concern about his or her sexuality or sexual functioning that he or she may not mention.

It is the goal of this chapter to provide the reader with an up-to-date understanding of sexual functioning in the able-bodied individual and how that can be affected by aging or medications. The general impact of disability on sexual functioning is then discussed, as is the method of performing a sexual history and physical examination. Specific disorders and their impact on sexual functioning are then reviewed, and wherever possible, specific research results are addressed. Finally, treatment of sexual dysfunctions is addressed.

THE SEXUAL RESPONSE CYCLE

Probably the most widely accepted model of sexual response is the four-stage model of Masters and Johnson (1). More recently, however, Kaplan (2,3) recommended that a three-phase model of sexual response was more appropriate in order to pay attention to the importance of desire as a component of sexual response. This latter model was incorporated into the *Diagnostic and Statistical Manual of Mental Disorders,* third edition.

M. L. Sipski: Department of Physical Medicine and Rehabilitation, University of Medicine and Dentistry of New Jersey, New Jersey Medical School, Newark, New Jersey 07103; and Kessler Rehabilitation Corporation, West Orange, New Jersey 07052.

C. Alexander: Department of Physical Medicine and Rehabilitation, University of Medicine and Dentistry of New Jersey, New Jersey Medical School, Newark, New Jersey 07103; and Kessler Institute for Rehabilitation, West Orange, New Jersey 07052.

The four phases of Masters and Johnson (1) model for sexual response include excitement, plateau, orgasm, and resolution. These phases were chosen on the basis of laboratory-based analysis of the sexual responses of over 600 able-bodied men and women. The male and female pathways were overall similar; however, men would have only one orgasm with each cycle, whereas women could achieve one or multiple orgasms. Moreover, it was noted that women could become ''stalled'' at the plateau phase of sexual response and then go straight down to a resolution period.

During the excitement phase of sexual response, men demonstrate engorgement of the corpora cavernosa of the penis, beginning testicular elevation, and scrotal skin flattening. In women there is clitoral enlargement in diameter, vaginal lubrication, constriction of the lower third of the vagina coupled with dilation of the upper two-thirds, and beginning uterine elevation out of the deep pelvis. Two-thirds of men and women develop nipple erection, and in women there is associated areolar enlargement and deepening in color. Myotonia also becomes obvious in both males and females late in the excitement phase of sexual arousal.

The plateau phase of sexual response of men is characterized by an increase in the diameter and color of the glans penis, an increase in testicular size of 50% to 100% over baseline and the potential for a drop of secretion from the Cowper's gland to appear at the urethral meatus. In women, as a result of continued vasocongestion, the orgasmic platform develops in the vagina with further ballooning out of the upper two-thirds while the clitoral shaft and glans retract. Furthermore, female breast size can increase up to 50%. In both sexes, increased muscle tone, heart rate, and respiratory rate are expected. Moreover, the sex flush, a measles-like rash over the chest, neck, and face, may occur.

Orgasm is characterized by further increases in heart rate, blood pressure, and respiratory rate. Furthermore, involuntary rhythmic contractions occur in the perineal musculature. In men, contraction of the seminal vesicles, vas deferens, and prostate occur, resulting in pooling of seminal fluid, which is followed by ejaculation. Concomitant closure of the bladder neck also occurs. In women, there is contraction of the uterus and fallopian tubes; moreover, one or more orgasms may occur.

The resolution phase is marked by general perspiration in conjunction with gradual reversal of the above-described anatomic and physical changes. Furthermore, in men there is a refractory period postejaculation for repeated ejaculation.

Critics of the Masters and Johnson four-stage model have indicated that there is an unnecessary separation of the plateau and orgasm phases of sexual response (4). Furthermore, the model does not consider factors associated with subjective arousal and does not offer an explanation for the pattern of neurologic components of sexual response (5). Kaplan's model of sexual response involves the phases of desire, excitement, and orgasm. By desire, Kaplan means "the experience of specific sensations that motivate the individual to initiate or become responsive to sexual stimulation" (5, p. 42), a process that is said to be under central neurophysiological control. According to Kaplan, the excitement phase is simply characterized by genital vasocongestion, and the orgasm phase consists of reflex muscle contractions in the pelvis. Furthermore, Kaplan indicates that these other two phases are associated with stimulation of peripheral reflex pathways of the spinal cord. Critics point out that Kaplan's model does not always hold true; for instance, desire is not always a necessary precursor to arousal or orgasm. Moreover, the latter two phases are spoken of as if they occurred via purely reflex mechanisms, and that may be too simplistic (5).

THE NEUROLOGIC PATHWAYS INVOLVED IN SEXUAL RESPONSE

The predominant model of the neurophysiology of male sexual arousal predicts a dual innervation, which in large part was derived from the studies of men with SCI (6). Innervation for reflex erectile function includes excitation of the dorsal penile nerve with resultant transmission of the impulse to the sacral cord via the pudendal nerve. Sacral parasympathetic excitation of the pelvic nerve is later followed by cavernosal nerve stimulation and resultant engorgement (7). Innervation for psychogenic function is mediated by impulses starting in the brain and then traveling down the lateral columns of the spinal cord near the pyramidal tracts and then connecting to thoracolumbar sympathetic and sacral parasympathetic pathways to produce erection (8).

Ejaculation involves two processes: emission and ejaculation. Emission is produced via thoracolumbar sympathetic stimulation, which results in prostatic, seminal vesicle, and vas deferens contractions. Ejaculation involves the forceful propulsion of semen from the urethra and relies on sacral parasympathetic and somatic efferent stimulation in addition to sympathetic stimulation to close the bladder neck (7).

Whereas the neurologic pathways for vaginal lubrication have not been well described, it can be hypothesized that these pathways are similar between men and women. If this is the case, reflex lubrication should be controlled via sacral parasympathetics and psychogenic via thoracolumbar sympathetics and sacral parasympathetics (9). A female equivalent for emission has been described as consisting of smooth-muscle contraction in the fallopian tubes, uterus, and paraurethral glands. These events are thought to be mediated by thoracolumbar sympathetics (10). The parallel of ejaculation includes contractions of striated pelvic floor and of perineal and anal sphincter muscles and is thought to be mediated by sacral parasympathetics and somatic efferents (9,10).

SEXUALITY AND AGING

Any discussion regarding sexuality must take into account the effects of age on sexual functioning. Age results in predictable changes in sexual response and psychological functioning, which must be considered in evaluating sexual functioning. Previously, it was thought that aging itself resulted in a great decrease in frequency of sexual activity (11). However, other surveys have not revealed a significant change in the frequency of sexual activity for elderly persons as compared to their youth (12,13).

With aging there are predictable changes in the sexual organs and sexual response. In women, menopause leads to a decrease in estrogen levels and resultant loss of labial fullness, thinning of pubic hair, and dryness, thinning, and increased friability of the vaginal mucosa (14). With regard to sexual response, Masters and Johnson (1) found that elderly women had less vaginal lubrication, and it took longer to present itself, than in younger women. Other changes during the excitement phase included smaller increases in breast size and a loss of the flattening, separation, and elevation of the major labia along with a decrease in the vasocongestive thickening of the genital organs during advanced excitement. During the plateau phase there was a decrease in the intensity of areolar engorgement, loss of the preorgasmic color change of the minor labia, and a decrease in the vasocongestion in the outer one-third of the vagina. Orgasm was characterized by an overall decrease in myotonia with less muscular tension during both voluntary and involuntary contractions. Rectal contractions also occurred less frequently, as did contractions of the orgasmic platform. It was further noted, however, that those women who were more sexually active did not have changes in their muscular contractions.

Elderly men were also studied (1). The time it takes to achieve an erection was found to be increased by two- to threefold. Furthermore, the older a man was, the longer it would take to achieve an erection, and if the erection was lost without ejaculation, it would take even longer to regain it. Scrotal vasocongestion was also found to be markedly reduced in older males. During the plateau phase, myotonia is diminished except in more sexually active men. Nipple rigidity is decreased, and the sex flush is lost. Testicular elevation occurs later and is decreased. Full erection may not occur, and erection may be maintained a long time without ejaculation. The decrease in myotonia continues during orgasm, along with less frequent contractions of the penis and rectal sphincter. Ejaculatory fluid is decreased and travels less than in the young. Resolution is remarkable for more rapid reversal of genital changes; however, there is an extended refractory period, which may last for days.

In addition to the physical changes associated with aging, there are psychological changes that occur. As people age, their bodies are less physically taut, and it is not uncommon to gain weight. Hair may gray or else be lost. These physical changes may contribute to a decrease in self-esteem, which can contribute to sexual problems. Moreover, changes in sexual responsiveness can cause further insecurities and sexual difficulties. The classic story is of the man who becomes emotionally disturbed about his declining erectile function (all normal and physically based) and therefore develops psychogenic erectile dysfunction. Through adequate education, it is hoped the person would be aware of the normal physical changes and subsequently not develop the psychological problems.

Other emotional changes that occur with aging include fears about illness and death, which can preclude an individual's interest in sex. Depression, which is more common in the elderly, may also cause a decrease in interest in sex. Moreover, elderly people may have lost their partners through death or divorce and may not feel that pursuing a new relationship is something they should do. Some aging individuals may also feel that sex is for procreation and the young, and therefore, it is something they should not be concerned about.

In addition to the expected physical and emotional changes accompanying aging, the elderly are also more prone to having medical problems that can impact on their sexual functioning. Diabetes and cardiac and pulmonary disease each can produce its own effects on sexual functioning and must be taken into account in evaluating the sexual functioning of the elderly person. Moreover, the elderly can suffer from a myriad of other diseases and disabilities that can impact on their sexual functioning by increasing their overall level of tiredness and fatigue and thereby decreasing their interest in sexual activity. Furthermore, as a result of the medical problems that elderly patients have, they may need to take medications, many of which may have a negative impact on sexual functioning.

One must not underestimate the impact medications can have on a person's sexual desire or response. Ignoring the effects that various medications have on a person's sexual function can result in unnecessary costly treatments being prescribed when a change in medication may be all that is necessary to regain the lost or altered function. For instance, in the male patient with a spinal cord injury (SCI), high doses of baclofen will cause a decrease in the ability to attain an erection. In this case, rather than prescribing injections or a pump the individual may best be treated by an alteration in the drugs he uses to treat spasticity.

Many types of medications can have an impact on sexuality and sexual functioning, and a complete discussion of this topic is beyond the scope of this chapter; therefore, we limit our discussion here to those medications most likely to be seen in a physiatric practice. Some of the more common classes of drugs include antihypertensives, anticholesterolemics, antidepressants, and antianxiety medications. Anticonvulsants, antiulcer medications, anticancer drugs, and medications used to treat prostate problems can also be problematic. Unfortunately, most research that has assessed the impact of medications on sexual functioning has relied on self-report information rather than laboratory based analysis, and thus, data are subject to bias. Moreover, the study of sexual functioning in men is far advanced over that in women.

Antihypertensive drugs are some of the most commonly prescribed medications, and sexual side effects are one of the main reasons for noncompliance with these drugs (15). Of the antihypertensives, two major classes have been strongly associated with adverse effects on sexual functions. These include the sympatholytic or adrenergic-inhibiting drugs and the diuretics (16). Hogan, Wallin, and Baer (17) noted that of 861 hypertensive men, 23% of those treated with propranolol and diuretics reported sexual dysfunction compared with 15% taking clonidine and 13% on methyldopa. Furthermore, they noted only 4% of untreated controls had sexual dysfunction. Croog et al. (18) also found a greater incidence of sexual dysfunction in patients on propranolol as compared with captopril and methyldopa. Thiazide diuretics were studied in a randomized placebo-controlled study of 176 men (19). Sex drive, erectile ability, and ejaculatory function were all adversely affected in the men on thiazides.

Other medications taken by patients with cardiac disease have also been associated with sexual dysfunction in males. The antihypercholesterol agent clofibrate has been associated with erectile dysfunction and low sexual desire (20–22). In contrast, the newer drugs pravastatin and lovastatin may result in slight improvements in sexual functioning (16). Digoxin has been shown to cause sexual dysfunction including decreased testosterone and luteinizing hormone in male patients in conjunction with increased estrogen (23). Moreover, another study found that men treated with digoxin for 2 years had diminished desire, arousal, and erectile functioning as compared to those receiving other treatments (24). The antiarrhythmic disopyramide has also been associated with erectile dysfunction (25,26).

PSYCHOTROPIC DRUGS

Many of the psychotropic drugs can cause sexual side effects; however, it is difficult to differentiate these drug-induced side effects from the effects of the disorder the patient has. For instance the tricyclic antidepressants can have a negative impact on sexual functioning; however, depression in and of itself will also cause a decline in sexual functioning. Therefore, the clinician must carefully perform the history in an attempt to determine which problem came first.

Among the antidepressants, imipramine has been shown to cause erectile or ejaculatory problems in about one-third of men (27). In contrast clomipramine has been associated with high rates of anorgasmia in both men and women (28), and other reports claim spontaneous orgasms and ejaculation have occurred in relation to clomipramine administration (29). Orgasmic problems have also been noted in both men and women taking imipramine, amoxapine, and MAO inhibitors (30–32).

Selective serotonin-specific reuptake inhibitors (SSRIs) have more recently been utilized for the treatment of depression. In a recent retrospective review of 596 men and women taking fluoxetine, sertraline, paroxetine, or venlafaxine, 16.3% of cases had sexual dysfunction. Anorgasmia and decreased sexual desire were most common and generally occurred within 1 to 2 months of taking the medications. Men (23.4%) were more likely than women (13.8%) to have sexual dysfunction (33). Antidotes for this SSRI sexual dysfunction have been tried, and one report revealed that 81% of patients responded positively to yohimbine. Other, newer antidepressant drugs may have fewer sexual side effects. These include bupropion, trazodone, and nefazodone (16).

The benzodiazepines diazepam, alprazolam, and clonazepam have been noted to cause sexual dysfunction including delayed orgasm or anorgasmia in women (34–37) and delayed ejaculation in men (38,39). Decreased sexual desire and arousal have also been reported (34,40). In contrast, buspirone has not been associated with negative sexual side effects.

Other commonly used drugs can cause sexual side effects. The anticonvulsants primidone and phenobarbital have been associated with erectile dysfunction and diminished sexual desire (41). In another study, 85 epileptic patients receiving carbamazepine, valproate, or phenytoin had a prevalence of sexual dysfunction similar to that in controls (42). Cimetidine, a histamine antagonist used to treat ulcer disease, has been shown to cause low libido and erectile dysfunction (43,44). Decreased sperm count has also been noted in men taking 1,200 mg/day of cimetidine (45). Ranitidine, another commonly used antiulcer drug has not been shown to have sexual side effects, and switching to ranitidine can resolve the symptoms caused by cimetidine (46).

PERFORMANCE OF THE SEXUAL HISTORY AND PHYSICAL EXAMINATION

Sexuality issues may be approached as primary or secondary concerns. In the former case it is appropriate to begin the discussion with sexual concerns, whereas in the latter, questions about sexual functioning may be associated with questions of bladder and bowel function.

Once the chief sexual complaint is obtained, the examiner should assess duration of the dysfunction, and its relationship to the overall disability or illness, what the predisability sexual functioning was, and how it differs from that at present.

A listing of the person's other medical problems and treatments must be obtained. Any history of sexually transmitted diseases should be elicited. Moreover, any history of radiation therapy or surgical procedures should be ascertained. Finally, any history of alcohol or illicit drug use should be determined.

For women, the presence and quality of their menstrual cycles should be elicited; furthermore, in those women who are peri- or postmenopausal, the circumstances surrounding these events should be ascertained. Method of birth control, if any, should be noted. A full obstetric history should also be obtained determining the number of pregnancies, miscarriages, abortions, and live births. With regard to sexual response, women should be queried about their ability to be sexually aroused and whether they are able to lubricate. Moreover, an attempt should be made to distinguish reflex from psychogenic lubrication. Adequacy of lubrication should be noted, as should the ability to achieve orgasm. Situational factors associated with arousal and orgasm should be sought, and any history of and timing of change in function should be elicited.

Men should be queried about the quality of their erections, both reflex and psychogenic. Their ability to sustain the erection should be noted, as should their ability to ejaculate in an anterograde fashion and achieve orgasm. Situational difficulties should be elicited, and any history of change in pattern of response should be noted. Furthermore, if there was a change in their response pattern when it happened and any associated events should be noted. Whether birth control is used and what type should be determined.

Finally, the person's psychosocial history should be taken. Sexual orientation, relationship, and family status should be noted. Any history of current or former psychiatric illness must be noted. Occupational status, ability to care for oneself, and living status should be discussed. Furthermore, any transportation difficulties should be addressed.

The sexual physical examination of the person with a disability is similar to the general physiatric examination; however, special attention must be paid to certain areas. Table 45-1 indicates those areas that could impact on sexual functioning and that should be evaluated as part of the routine examination.

UNIVERSAL ISSUES PSYCHOLOGICALLY

Trieschmann (47) has described a model of assessment of sexual functioning following disability that emphasizes the psychological along with the physical components affecting the desire for sex, the sexual act itself, and the broader concept of sexuality. Sexuality involves an interplay between the psychological and the physical. In fact, most sexual dysfunctions originate in reaction to psychological processes or are compounded by psychological reaction to organic pathology (48). Thus, in discussing sexuality, we must examine the emotional and physical elements involved.

The rate and manner in which a person adjusts to disability

TABLE 45-1. *Medications and sexual functioning*

Drug class	Impact on sexual function
Antihypertensives	Diminished sex drive, erectile ability, ejaculatory function
Anticholesterolemics	Erectile dysfunction, low sexual desire
Digoxin	Decreased testosterone and luteinizing hormone in conjunction with increased estrogen; decreased desire, arousal, and erectile function
Antiarrhythmics	Erectile dysfunction
Antidepressants	Erectile and ejaculatory dysfunction, anorgasmia, spontaneous orgasms and ejaculation, decreased sexual desire
Benzodiazepines	Delayed orgasm or anorgasmia in women, delayed ejaculation in men, decreased sexual desire and arousal
Anticonvulsants	Erectile dysfunction, diminished sexual desire
H_2 blockers	Decreased libido, erectile dysfunction, decreased sperm count

will affect his or her sense of sexuality. Emotional adjustment to disability, however, will vary. Although some theorists have advanced defined stages of adjustment, including depression as a necessary component, each person tends to adjust in his or her own way and own time. Disability is an insult to our innate sense of narcissism, resulting in a blow to self-esteem. The issue of self—how we think of ourselves, feel about ourselves, and perceive our ability to act and influence the world—must be addressed following disability. Failure to resolve these issues can result in emotional consequences affecting one's adjustment and sense of sexuality. As Taylor (49) points out, there are at least three issues that one must address following disability. First is the universal question of ''Why did this happen to me?'' Individuals wrestle with this question until it is somehow put to rest. Of course, there is no correct answer to this question. It is through the process of attempting to answer the question that the issue can become resolved. Second, one must attempt to regain a sense of control in life. This can be accomplished in a variety of ways from immersing oneself in the physical therapy process to practicing self-regulation techniques such as relaxation or meditation. Last but not least is the long-term process of self-enhancement, the feeling that one is a ''survivor'' and is a ''better'' person for what he or she has experienced.

Failure to adequately resolve or develop a functional method for addressing these issues can result in mood disorders such as depression or anxiety. On the other hand, for some people, mood depression and anxiety may be a ''normal'' part of the adjustment process and may not necessarily signal an ''abnormal'' reaction. These reactions, whether considered normal or abnormal, are painful. The individual must do the work necessary to resolve his or her depression in order to successfully work through the issue and become functional and achieve satisfaction. At times, however, the pain becomes too much, and the person is unable to stick it through to complete the work necessary for healing. Regardless, this process will likely interfere with one's energy level and sense of self, temporarily affecting one's sexual life.

The age at which one acquires a disability can significantly affect one's adjustment to the condition. Developmental psychologists have theorized various models involving critical stages of both psychological and sexual development. Typically, these theories hold that individuals progress through a prescribed sequence of stages of development. In each stage critical issues are addressed as the individual matures and develops. When traumatic events occur that interfere with the smooth progression through these developmental stages, emotional problems can ensue. Take, for example, the instance of a catastrophic injury leading to a disability. If a teenage boy sustains an SCI, its impact will be quite different than the same injury experienced by an elderly man. Because of the nature of spinal cord injuries, they tend to occur in more youthful and active individuals. It is understandable then that a high incidence of spinal cord injuries occurs in young active men, usually in their late teens or early adulthood. According to the late psychologist Erik Erikson, late adolescence and early adulthood is the critical time for one to resolve the developmental conflicts of ''identity versus role confusion'' as well as ''intimacy versus isolation'' (50). It is during this critical period of life that one struggles with answering the question ''Who am I?'' gains comfort with his or her physical and sexual development, achieves a sense of independence from family, and develops the skills necessary for sexual intimacy. We all can think back and relate to that time in our lives as teenagers when we looked forward with enthusiasm and excitement in search of our freedom and independence—the very aspects interfered with by the paralyzing effects of an SCI. The young victim of an SCI may struggle more than his able-bodied counterpart at developing a sense of self and identity and, along with it, a sense of self-esteem, self-image, and sense of intimacy acquired through productive relationships with peers of the same and opposite sex. Presumably, the elderly man will have already experienced and resolved these psychosocial developmental crises and will have moved on to other age-appropriate issues. Thus, the age of onset of a disability or chronic illness will affect the kinds of issues with which one must meet. Certainly, these psychological issues are closely linked to one's sense of sexuality.

Disability and illness affect both the patient and his or her partner. Thus, when we evaluate the patient's sexuality, we must assess the factors affecting the couple. Some of these issues may have existed before the onset of disability and illness and have become exacerbated, but in other instances the illness may have brought on an issue that did not previously exist. There is no question that disability and illness create stress, which can lead to increased conflict in a relationship. One must determine the degree of conflict that presently exists between the partners and to what extent it is related to the illness. Similarly, the amount of hostility in both the patient and partner must be assessed. Following illness or disability, there is the inevitable question of ''Why did this happen to me?'' Of course, there is usually no good answer to this question, which often leads to frustration and more anger on the patient's part. The partner too has similar questions and can be left feeling cheated and hostile about the changes in their life situation. Moreover, disability can disrupt the usual balance of power that exists within any relationship, leading to struggles to regain the homeostasis that is comfortable for both partners. The disabled person may feel particularly vulnerable and replete with fears. These fears may be rational or irrational but exist nonetheless. The disabled partner might harbor feelings of inadequacy—both as a person and as a sexual partner. These feelings can lead to an intense fear of disappointing his or her partner sexually or even a more broader fear of abandonment, that the partner will leave him or her for a more ''adequate,'' ''healthy,'' and ''worthy'' person. Disability and illness may have changed the couple's lives significantly to the point that their life goals, which were once compatible, may no longer be compatible.

Situational and cultural factors can also interfere with the couple's sexual relationship. Disability and illness can highlight some issues that existed previously but posed few problems. Differing attitudes and values regarding intimacy, religion, and roles within the family system can lead to conflict both within the individual and between the partners. A common scenario occurs when the traditional role played by the male (e.g., masculine, wage earner) is disrupted by disability, forcing a reversal of roles with his wife. Some cultures place a premium on maintaining the traditional masculine role, and any deviation from this can be a blow to the self-esteem, leading to a variety of insecurities and conflict. The economic impact of disability often is substantial, may have significant impact on self-esteem, and may be associated with role reversal within the family.

All of these issues underscore the need for healthy communication, mutual trust and openness, and a strong sense of commitment on the part of each partner. Of course, these issues are not unique to the disabled. However, because of the magnitude of the potential problems that may exist, these qualities are even more important for the satisfaction of the couple's relationship and sexual lives. It has been said that there is no greater test of love than disability. It is easy to see why this might be the case. However, with these problems and obstacles comes the opportunity through resolution for an even greater degree of intimacy and satisfaction for the couple.

DISABILITY-SPECIFIC ISSUES PERTAINING TO SEXUAL FUNCTIONING

Little is known about the impact of many specific disabilities on sexual functioning. Most research that has examined the impact of different disabilities on sexual functioning has relied on self-report methodology. Most studies lack control groups, and very few reports include any type of psychophysiological measures. In addition, there is a disproportionate amount of information examining the issues of men as compared to those of women. For this reason it may be helpful to consider specific groups of disabilities with similar pathology together in order to better understand their effects on sexual function. For instance, the individual with hemiparesis from a traumatic brain injury will have some similarities with an individual with hemiparesis from a cerebrovascular accident. Moreover, the individual with paraplegia related to multiple sclerosis will have some similarities with an individual with the same level and degree of paraplegia related to an SCI. Although all aspects of these disabilities will not be the same, their similarities can be equal to if not more important than their differences in determining their impact on sexual function.

Spinal Cord Injury

With regard to sexual function we probably understand more about SCI than any other disability. However, to understand its impact, we must first understand the natural history of sexual response after SCI. Furthermore, the best way to do this is to determine what the impact of the injury is, based on its level and severity.

In men with upper motor neuron complete spinal injuries affecting the sacral spinal segments, based on the neurologic pathways involved, we would anticipate that all men would be able to achieve reflex erections; however, no men would be able to have psychogenic erections. The literature reports that as many as 93% (51) to as few as 70% (52) of men with this pattern of injury have reflex erections, although none are reported to have psychogenic erections. With consideration for the neurologic pathways involved in the production of anterograde ejaculation we would anticipate this to be unlikely. Bors and Comarr (51) noted that 4% of patients with this type of injury reported they could achieve anterograde ejaculation.

In men with upper motor neuron incomplete spinal injuries, one would anticipate that reflex erection should remain intact and that psychogenic erection should be possible depending on where the neurologic damage occurred. Furthermore, it has been postulated that whether or not psychogenic erections will occur may be dependent on the integrity of the of the lateral columns of the spinal cord (8,9). Via self-report studies, Bors and Comarr (51) noted that 80% of men with this injury pattern should have an isolated reflex erection, whereas 19% of these men should have combined reflex and psychogenic erections. Comarr and Vigue (53) noted that 100% of these men would have some type of nonspecified type of erection. Because of the need to coordinate various neurologic impulses, one would anticipate the ability to achieve anterograde ejaculation to be diminished. This is consistent with the findings of Bors and Comarr (51), who reported that 32% of these patients were able to experience ejaculation, 72% following reflex erection and 26% following psychogenic erections.

With complete lower motor neuron injury affecting the sacral spinal segments, it follows that the ability to achieve psychogenic erection should remain based on the integrity of the lateral spinothalamic tracts, especially those in the thoracolumbar part of the spinal cord. Bors and Comarr noted that 26% of these patients could achieve psychogenic erection; however, none of these patients could achieve reflex erections. In contrast Comarr and Vigue (53) reported that 50% of these patients could achieve psychogenic erections. Perhaps the discrepancy in these figures arose in part from the fact that attention was not paid to the degree of remaining function these patients had in the thoracolumbar region. With regard to ejaculatory function, 18% of the men in Bors and Comarr's study had anterograde ejaculations, and it was noted that these occurred in conjunction with psychogenic erections.

With regard to incomplete lower motor neuron injuries, the ability to achieve psychogenic erections should theoretically be based on the integrity of the lateral spinothalamic tracts in the thoracolumbar region, while the ability to achieve reflex erections should be diminished in varying degrees. The ability to achieve these functions has not been examined through research studies; however, reports have noted that between 67% (53) and 95% (54) of these patients will have some type of erectile function remaining. With regard to ejaculation, Bors and Comarr (51) noted that 70% of these patients were able to ejaculate.

The impact of SCI on female sexual response has been postulated based on male sexual response (9,55). Furthermore, this issue has recently been systematically studied in a laboratory-based controlled setting. In women with complete upper motor neuron injuries affecting the sacral spinal segments, reflex lubrication should remain but not psychogenic lubrication (54,55). This hypothesis was recently tested in a laboratory-based study comparing the vaginal pulse amplitudes of 13 women with complete SCIs with those in eight able-bodied women. Of note, the able-bodied women demonstrated a significant increase in vaginal pulse amplitude coupled with a significant increase in their level of subjective sexual arousal in response to the viewing of an erotic videotape, whereas the women with complete SCIs had a significant increase in their level of arousal under the same conditions but did not have a significant increase in their vaginal pulse amplitudes. Furthermore, both the able-bodied women and the women with complete SCIs had significant increases in their vaginal pulse amplitudes when manual stimulation was added to the stimulation of the erotic videotape; however, only the able-bodied women had further increases in their level of arousal (56). Taken together these results support the aforementioned hypotheses about genital responses in women with complete SCIs.

It has been anecdotally stated that women with incomplete upper motor neuron injuries affecting the sacral spinal segments should retain the ability to achieve reflex lubrication (55). Furthermore, based on the location of the intermediolateral cell columns, it has been hypothesized that women with incomplete SCIs and upper motor neuron injuries affecting the sacral spinal segments who retained the capacity to feel the presence of pinprick sensation in the T11–L2 dermatomes would retain the capacity for psychogenic lubrication (14). This hypothesis was tested in 17 women with incomplete SCIs, ten with partial to normal pinprick sensation in the T11–L2 dermatomes and seven without any preservation of pinprick sensation in the T11–L2 dermatomes. Whereas subjective arousal during audiovisual erotic stimulation similarly increased in both groups of subjects, only those subjects with the ability to perceive T11–L2 pinprick sensation had concomitant increases in their level of vaginal pulse amplitude. Moreover, both groups of subjects showed similar increases in vaginal pulse amplitude when manual stimulation was added to the audiovisual stimulation; however, only those subjects with preserved pinprick sensation continued to demonstrate increases in their level of subjective arousal (14). These findings support the above-mentioned hypotheses that all women with incomplete SCIs and upper motor neuron injuries affecting the sacral segments will retain the capacity for reflex lubrication; however, they will only retain the capacity for psychogenic lubrication if they have the ability to perceive pinprick sensation in the T11–L2 dermatomes.

For women with complete lower motor neuron injuries affecting the sacral spinal segments it has been hypothesized that 25% of women should be able to achieve psychogenic lubrication and no women would retain the capacity for reflex lubrication (9). It follows that those women with T11–L2 pinprick sensation should be the ones to retain the capacity for psychogenic lubrication; however, this hypothesis still needs to be tested in a laboratory-based setting. In those women with incomplete lower motor neuron injuries affecting the sacral spinal segments 95% should have some type of combined lubrication (9). Whether these women are able to have psychogenic and reflex lubrication may be related to the preservation of pinprick sensation in the T11–L2 dermatomes and the degree of incompleteness of their injury; however, this must still be tested in a laboratory-based setting.

Based on self-report studies, orgasm is known to occur in men with SCIs. Recent reports revealed that 42% (57) to 47% (58) of men with SCIs reported the capacity to achieve orgasm. Similarly, recent questionnaire studies revealed that 44% (58) to 50% of women with SCIs (59) reported the ability to achieve orgasm. Self-report studies, however, are unable to allow characterization of the physiological responses accompanying orgasm. Therefore, Sipski et al. (56) conducted a laboratory-based assessment of 25 women with SCIs and nine able-bodied women during self-stimulation to orgasm. All able-bodied women achieved orgasm as compared to 52% of women with SCIs. There was not a significant relationship between the degree and type of SCI that women had and their ability to achieve orgasm. Women with no lower extremity strength took significantly longer than able-bodied women to achieve orgasm. Heart rate and respiratory rate significantly increased in both able-bodied and SCI subjects during orgasm, whereas systolic blood pressure increased significantly during orgasm only in women with SCIs. Furthermore, it was noted that those subjects who achieved orgasm scored higher on the sexual information and sex drive components of the Derogatis Sexual Function Inventory. Based on these results, the development of therapeutic programs to improve the capacity of women with SCIs to achieve orgasm should be explored.

Frequency of sexual activity, satisfaction, and which activities people participate in after SCI have been studied in both men and women. These concepts, however, are largely subjective and difficult to measure (60), which may be why there are many inconsistencies in the literature. Frequency of sexual activity has been reported to decrease in men and women after SCI (7,57,58,61); however, level or severity of injury has not been shown to be related to frequency (58). Satisfaction has also been shown to decrease in men (58,61,62) and women (63) after SCI. Except for a lower frequency of intercourse, the types of activities men engaged in were similar pre- and postinjury. Moreover, women did not demonstrate a significant difference in the types of activities they participated in post-SCI (64).

Reproductive Concerns

Fertility has been shown to be impaired in men with SCI. One reason for infertility is the inability of most men with SCIs to achieve an anterograde ejaculation (65). Furthermore, decreased number and motility of sperm are present (65). Possible reasons for decreased number and motility of sperm include recurrent urinary tract infections, stasis of fluid, lack of testicular temperature control, prolonged sitting in a wheelchair, long-term use of medications, and retrograde ejaculation causing sperm to come in contact with urine (65). Via laboratory-based analysis of Sprague–Dawley rats with SCIs, Linsenmeyer et al. (66) noted that testicular function and sperm degenerate in the first few weeks after injury and that partial recovery is not noted until 4 to 6 months postinjury. Based on these results, it is thought that a combination of factors result in the decline in semen quality after SCI (67).

Remediation of male infertility after SCI has been made possible through the development of electroejaculation and electrovibration, which are often successfully utilized in conjunction with assisted reproductive technologies. The technique of electroejaculation was first used in men with SCI in 1948 (68). It was not until 1975, however, that a live birth was reported (69).

Performance of an electroejaculation procedure begins with preparation. The urine is cultured and treated if infection is present; moreover, prophylactic antibiotics are administered if the urine is clear. The evening before the procedure, the patient performs his bowel program. The bladder is drained of urine just before the procedure and rinsed with a physiological solution in case of retrograde ejaculation. Prophylaxis for autonomic dysreflexia is then provided, followed by digital rectal examination and anoscopy to rule out any preexisting rectal lesions. Electrical stimulation is then performed via a rectal probe with the electrodes placed on the prostate until an ejaculate is obtained or the blood pressure elevation is too high. If unable to stimulate an ejaculate after 15 times, the procedure is aborted. Postejaculate, any anterograde ejaculate is collected, followed by catheterization to achieve any retrograde ejaculate. The rectum is examined to rule out any damage, and the semen is processed for insemination (67).

The electrovibration procedure is similar pre- and postejaculation to electroejaculation; however, there is no need to examine the rectum. The vibrator is applied on the underside of the penis near the glans, and vibration is applied until an ejaculate occurs or for up to 5 minutes. Autonomic dysreflexia is also a risk with this procedure; therefore, blood pressure monitoring and potentially prophylaxis is necessary (67).

Recent research pertaining to electroejaculation and electrovibration has targeted determination of success rates and ways for improvement. For electrovibration optimum stimulation parameters of 100-Hz frequency and 2.5-mm amplitude have been defined (70). Utilizing these parameters, Ohl, Menge, and Sonksen (71) found that of 34 men with SCIs undergoing electrovibration, 65% had anterograde ejaculation. Furthermore, sperm averaged 26% motility with counts of 968 million. Ohl et al. (72) also studied electroejaculation, noting that 44% of men with SCI using intermittent catheterization achieved pregnancy as compared to 7% of men using other bladder management techniques. Furthermore, the presence of sterile male urine improved the pregnancy rates from 10% to 30%.

In the woman with SCI, the outlook for successful childbirth is much more positive. Of 38 women with SCI (73) who were queried in depth about their menstrual cycle, 58% were found to have temporary amenorrhea of an average of 5 months' duration. Amount of flow was unchanged in 76% of women, duration remained unchanged in 60%, and cycle length remained the same in 68%. Menstrual pain was stable pre- and post-SCI in 56% of women, with the remainder being equally divided between increased and decreased pain.

With resumption of a regular ovulatory menstrual cycle, there should be no decrease in the potential for women with SCIs to be able to conceive. However, of 231 women with SCIs who were studied, the pregnancy rate postinjury was only 0.34 per person as compared to a preinjury rate of 1.3 per person (59). Furthermore, there was a lower pregnancy rate for those women with more significant impairments.

When a woman with an SCI does become pregnant, there can be unique problems because of her injury. Urinary tract infections, increased spasticity, and decubitus ulcers have all been noted (74–76). Whereas anemia has also been noted as a problem (77), Baker and Cardenas point out that anemia is also common in the able-bodied pregnant woman, and the outcomes of anemic women with SCIs should be correlated with specific blood levels (74). Other issues that must be monitored for in the pregnant woman with SCI include declining pulmonary function as the growing fetus takes up more room and autonomic dysreflexia in women with injuries around and above the level of T6. Care must be taken to differentiate autonomic dysreflexia from preeclampsia. Although various methods have been described for treating dysreflexia, continuous epidural anesthesia has been most commonly recommended (74).

Management of pregnancy in the woman with SCI must take into account the poor sensation that these women have. Labor is generally perceived through sympathetic symptoms including leg spasms, back pain, difficulty breathing, or symptoms of autonomic dysreflexia (78). Preterm labor may be slightly higher than the 5% to 10% rate in the general population. Therefore, Baker and Cardenas recommend that women with paraplegia be instructed in uterine palpation to detect preterm labor, and patients with sensation should have symptom-generated examinations in addition to routine pregnancy visits. Furthermore, consideration should be give to home uterine contraction monitoring in women who are unable to detect any symptoms of preterm labor (74).

Multiple Sclerosis

The impact of multiple sclerosis (MS) on a person's sexuality and sexual functioning can vary tremendously, just as the extent of the neurologic compromise can vary. Despite this fact, the incidence of sexual dysfunction associated with MS is generally considered high. In fact, over 50% of women with MS and 75% of men are thought to experience some type of sexual dysfunction at some point in time (79,80).

Because of the changing nature of MS, the sexual symptomatology associated with it can vary. Moreover, the affective and biological impacts of MS are highly interdependent and can influence sexual function separately or in concert. For patients with some patterns of MS, such as transverse myelitis with associated bladder and bowel incontinence and paraplegia, the changes that occur in sexual functioning may be similar to those occurring in men and women with SCIs. Alternatively, other people with MS may have neurologic deficits resembling those of a stroke or brain injury, and their sexual difficulties may approach those of persons with similar dysfunctions. Other issues associated with sexual dysfunction in persons with MS can include loss of the ability to achieve orgasm, fatigue, tremor, muscle weakness, and spasticity (81). Moreover, the cognitive changes and psychological impact of the disorder can result in anxiety, depression, poor self-image, and lack of interest in sex in both patient and partner.

Modifications of sexual activity may be useful to preserve the sexual relationships of persons with MS. Timing of activity so as to diminish the impact of fatigue may be helpful. Furthermore, assurance that sexual activity will not cause disease progression may help some couples adjust to the disorder. Appropriate education about management of bladder and bowel incontinence can make sexual activity more desirable. Finally, special attention to treating spasticity in the adductor muscles, both through range of motion and medical management, can help maintain the capacity for active participation in sexual activities.

Based on what is known about MS, it follows that some men will be unable to achieve erections or will have difficulty maintaining them. Moreover, other men will be unable to have anterograde ejaculations. If erectile or ejaculatory dysfunction is present in the man with MS, these can be treated in a similar fashion to men with SCIs or other disabilities (see SCI section for discussion of treatment of infertility). Sexual dysfunction in women with MS should be treated similarly to that in other disabilities.

Fertility is generally unimpaired in the woman with MS. For those women not wishing to conceive, birth control should be utilized. For those women who become pregnant, there are no contraindications associated with pregnancy. It has been noted that there is a decrease in exacerbations during pregnancy (82); however, the risk of aggravation of MS increases with childbirth. Three extensive studies have, however, found that, overall, pregnancy does not affect the long-term prognosis for women with MS (83–85). Therefore, women with MS should be appropriately counseled regarding their potential for childbirth, and consideration should be given to obtaining extra help at home during the postpartum period.

Stroke

Despite the high incidence and prevalence of stroke, surprisingly little is known about its effects on sexual functioning. Furthermore, most reports that have examined the impact of stroke on sexual functioning have relied on small numbers of subjects and have focused on the presence or absence of libido and patient's frequency of intercourse (86). Our understanding of the effect of stroke on sexuality is also clouded by the fact that most patients with stroke are elderly, suffer from concomitant medical problems that can impact their sexuality, and may take many medications.

Men who sustain strokes have been noted to have a decrease in libido (87). Erectile dysfunction has also been noted to be more common poststroke (88,89), and it has been noted that premature ejaculation is more common after stroke (87). Perhaps these various dysfunctions are part of the reason that multiple reports have found there is a decrease in the frequency of sexual activity poststroke (87,88,90).

Libido has also been noted to decrease in women who sustain strokes (91–93). With regard to sexual response, one study queried women about their ability to lubricate. Of 35 women 29% report normal lubrication poststroke as compared to 63% prestroke. Orgasm has also been noted to be less frequent in women who sustain strokes (87–89). Finally, the frequency of sexual activity has also been shown to decline in women who sustain strokes (87).

Traumatic Brain Injury

The effect of traumatic brain injury (TBI) on sexual functioning is even less well studied than that of other disabilities. Furthermore, because of the profound interpersonal and cognitive effects of TBI, research should take into account the distinct effects of the psychological and physiological effects of the injury. This is especially unfortunate because brain injuries occur most frequently between the ages of 15 and 24 (94), at a time when people are often just beginning to explore their sexual potential and develop sexual relationships.

The incidence of sexual dysfunction in men with TBI has been studied; however, results vary from 71% of a group of 100 male TBI survivors reporting erectile dysfunction (95) to 8.1% of a group of 739 male TBI survivors reporting erectile dysfunction (96). The incidence of sexual dysfunction in women with TBI has not been determined; however, one study examined 15 couples with partners affected by TBI, 11 with injured men and four with injured women (97). A decrease in the frequency of intercourse was noted, more so in those couples with injured men, and a decrease in the frequency of orgasm was also noted in able-bodied women.

The effects of various brain lesions on sexual responsiveness have been studied primarily in animals. Injury to the brainstem may decrease the general level of arousal, thereby impairing sexual functioning (98). Stimulation of the thalamus has been noted to cause erection in animals (99). Because the hypothalamus secretes gonadotropin-releasing hormone, it is involved in regulation of the menstrual cycle in female subjects and testosterone secretion in male animals. Hypothalamic injury as a child can therefore result in precocious puberty (100), whereas injury as an adult can lead to amenorrhea or sexual dysfunction. Lesions in the medial preoptic area of the hypothalamus result in reduced or eliminated copulatory behavior. Stimulation of the dorsomedial nucleus of the hypothalamus results in ejaculation in animals, whereas stimulation of the ventromedial nucleus is thought to play a role in female sexual behaviors (101). Damage to the limbic and paralimbic systems can cause hypersexual behaviors. Damage to the dorsolateral frontal lobes can cause impairments in libido and sexual assertiveness (101); furthermore, frontal lobe damage can result in an inability to fantasize (102). Erections have been produced via stimulation of the hippocampus, septal complex, and amygdala (103). The Kluver–Bucy syndrome results from lesions in the anterior temporal poles and leads to hypersexual and exploratory behaviors with hyperorality (104–106). Temporal lobe seizures can result in genital sensations and either hypo- or hypersexual behavior (101). Finally, stimulation of the hippocampus results in erection in animals, and damage may result in sexual dysfunction (99).

Research in 100 male TBI survivors has indicated that location and severity of injury are related to erectile functioning (95). Miller et al. (107) also studied eight TBI patients and noted that medial basal–frontal injury or diencephalic injury would result in hypersexuality and that limbic injury could result in changes in sexual preference. Sandel et al. (108) recently studied 52 persons with TBI and noted that those with frontal lobe lesions reported higher levels of sexual satisfaction and functioning and more sexual cognitions and fantasies than persons with brain injuries in other locations. Furthermore, persons with right hemisphere injuries had higher sexual arousal and more sexual experiences than did other brain injury survivors.

When working with couples or persons with TBI, it is important to take into account the effects of the brain injury on the person's cognitive status and personality. These psychological factors may impact significantly on the quality of their relationships. With regard to physical factors, the impact of paralysis, loss of sensation, altered mental status, and potential bladder and bowel dysfunction on sexual functioning must be taken into account. Spasticity, hypersensitivity, and the inability to transfer also may impact on the ability of person with TBI to engage in sexual activities.

Education is important in working with couples affected by TBI. The general effects of the injury should be discussed in addition to the potential impacts on sexual functioning. Issues surrounding positioning and problems with sexual functioning should be addressed. Most importantly, if necessary, appropriate psychological and sexual counseling should be pursued.

Neuromuscular Diseases

As a whole, the impact of neuromuscular diseases on sexuality and sexual functioning is primarily related to peripheral rather than genital dysfunction. These disorders have a wide span in the degree of illness and disability they cause, ranging from significant paralysis including loss of pulmonary capacity, which can result in as serious a consequence as death to as small a consequence as moderate degrees of loss of stamina and strength in peripheral musculature. These disorders also vary significantly in the time they manifest themselves, which can range from birth to the elderly. Because of these variables, the effects of neuromuscular diseases on sexual functioning can be quite different.

Treatment of sexual dysfunctioning in the person with a neuromuscular disease begins with educating the person regarding the impact of their disability on sexual functioning. Specific problems such as difficulties with positioning or difficulty achieving orgasm should be elicited, and specific suggestions provided to remediate the patient's concerns. These may include such things as showing the patient pictures regarding positioning with their degree of paralysis or recommending the use of a vibrator for persons with limited mobility in order to allow more effective genital stimulation. Psychological counseling or sex therapy may be necessary if significant depression or anxiety is detected or for couples issues.

Arthritis and Connective Tissue Diseases

The overall impact of arthritis on sexual functioning is primarily related to the associated pain, joint stiffness, and fatigue (109). Other factors can also cause sexual dysfunction, however, including loss of mobility, altered body image (110), and depression (111). Medications can also cause sexual dysfunctions, such as corticosteroids, which can cause a decrease in libido, and those used to decrease pain and improve sleep (112).

Rheumatoid arthritis (RA) is known to cause sexual dysfunction in both men and women. Of 31 men with RA queried about their sexual functioning, 33% reported periods of impotence, and 50% reported decreased libido while they suffered from active inflammatory periods (113). In another study of 91 married women with RA, over 50% noted a decrease in their desire for sex since their disease onset, and another 50% complained of arthralgia associated with intercourse. Furthermore, 22% of women noted their arthritis symptomatology was worsened the day after intercourse (114). Seventeen women with rheumatoid arthritis were grouped with six women with systemic lupus erythematosus (SLE) (115), and significant decreases were noted in sexual satisfaction, frequency of sexual intercourse, and desire for sexual intercourse 1 year after disease onset. The majority of women considered joint pain and fatigue as factors impacting on their sexual performance. In another report, 100 women with SLE were noted to more frequently abstain from sex, have less frequent sex, poorer sexual adjustment, and diminished vaginal lubrication as compared to a group of 71 controls (116).

Progressive systemic sclerosis (PSS) has also been noted to impact sexual functioning in both men and women. Sixty women with PSS were compared to an age- and disease-matched control group of women with RA and SLE (115). Decreased desire, sexual satisfaction, and frequency of sexual intercourse were noted with women with PSS. A greater frequency of vaginal dryness, dyspareunia, and perineal fissures and ulcerations were also noted since the onset of PSS; furthermore, these women reported a decrease in the number and intensity of their orgasms. One-third to one-half of men with PSS have also been noted to have erectile problems (117,118), which are thought to result from vascular changes limiting penile blood flow (119).

Treatment of sexual dysfunction in the patient with arthritis or other connective tissue disorders begins with assuring maximal overall physical functioning. Educating the patient and his or her partner about the impact of the disease on sexual functioning is also important. Pamphlets demonstrating proper positioning such as those available through the Arthritis Foundation may be useful aids for patients. During sexual activity, prolonged pressure on painful joints must be avoided. Premedication or the use of heat before sexual activity may also be useful (120). Lubricants may be useful, as may the use of adapted erotic aids such as vibrators for people with poor hand functioning. As with all disabilities, counseling should be utilized when appropriate.

Total Joint Replacement

A significant effect of joint disease can be its impact on sexual functioning. Furthermore, total hip replacement can substantially improve sexual functioning. In one survey, 57% of 121 patients (121) who underwent total hip replacements report some relief of sexual difficulties after surgery, and 34% had complete or considerable improvement. Another report noted that 65% of patients were free from sexual difficulties after hip replacement. Nevertheless, one study reported that 81% of surgeons did not discuss when to resume sexual activity with their patients (122).

Sexual intercourse should be able to be resumed within 1 to 2 months after total hip surgery. By this time significant healing should have taken place, reducing the risk of dislocation. Preferred positions include the missionary for men, as excess motion is eliminated at the hip joint, and side lying with the nonoperative side down and the operative side supported by pillows for women (123). Other joint replacements generally cause less impact on sexual activity; however, proper positioning to decrease stress across the operative joint should be practiced.

Diabetes

Approximately 16 million Americans have diabetes (124). Many of these patients develop secondary complications such as amputation or stroke, for which they may be seen by a physiatrist. Therefore, it is important to be aware of the sexual consequences of diabetes, and the subject deserves special mention.

The impact of diabetes on male sexual functioning has been extensively studied. Erectile dysfunction is known to occur in 50% of men with diabetes and is at least three to five times more prevalent among men with diabetes than in the general population. Timing is an important factor in determining the reversibility of impotence in the diabetic population. Impotence can occur when poor glycemic control results in temporary chemical changes in the autonomic nerves and resolves when the metabolic derangements are corrected. Alternatively, erectile dysfunction that develops more slowly is most likely related to permanent changes in the autonomic nerve fibers of the corpora cavernosa (125). Furthermore, erectile dysfunction has been shown to occur whenever there are other signs and symptoms of diabetic autonomic neuropathy (126–129). The effect of microangiopathy is less clear on sexual functioning. One histopathologic autopsy study of diabetic men found no correlation between erectile dysfunction and diabetic microangiopathy (130). In contrast, two larger studies of diabetic men noted a positive association between erectile dysfunction and microangiopathic changes (127,131).

The impact of diabetes on ejaculation and orgasm is less common than that on erectile dysfunction. One study of 80 diabetic men revealed that 27 had erectile dysfunction, whereas only five had any orgasmic dysfunction, and of these, three had premature ejaculation and two had retarded ejaculation (132). Retrograde ejaculation can also be a problem for diabetic men whose internal vesical sphincter does not close properly during ejaculation as a result of autonomic neuropathy (126).

The impact of diabetes on female sexual functioning has been studied much less than that on male sexual functioning. Conflicting reports have arisen as to whether there is an impact of diabetes on lubrication (132–135); however, the majority of reports were based upon questionnaire studies, which are notoriously inaccurate in assessing lubrication. Two small laboratory-based studies included one of ten women that utilized vaginal photoplethysmography to compare able-bodied and diabetic subjects' responses to erotic videos (136). This report did not eliminate women with autonomic neuropathy and revealed a decrease in vaginal responsiveness in diabetic women. In contrast, another study used labia minora temperatures to compare the responses of women with IDDM and able-bodied age-matched controls to erotic videos and revealed no significant differences between the two groups. Studies of orgasm in diabetic women have also been inconclusive as to whether there is (137–139) or is not (132,133,140) a decrease in their ability to achieve orgasm.

Fertility is affected in both men and women with diabetes. There is a lower than expected rate of pregnancy in the partners of diabetic men. Proposed reasons include erectile dysfunction, retrograde ejaculation, and endocrine abnormalities (125). Whereas the ability to conceive in a diabetic woman is only slightly decreased, the likelihood of a live birth occurring from pregnancy is decreased in diabetic women (141). Furthermore, preexisting and gestational diabetes can result in macrosomia and birth defects including congenital heart disease, kidney disease, poorly developed colon and central nervous system and spinal deformities (142).

Amputation

The effect of amputation on sexual functioning is primarily related to peripheral as opposed to genital causes. The loss of a limb and/or loss of range of motion may result in difficulties with positioning in sexual activity and require the individual to alter his or her patterns of sexual behavior. Preservation of the knee joint is helpful to maintain balance during coitus; however, for transfemoral amputees, positioning with pillows can help maintain stability (120). Those individuals with upper limb amputations may benefit from a side-lying position for intercourse, thereby permitting free movement of the intact arm.

Psychological issues are also important in the sexuality of persons with amputations. Depression in adults with amputation may persist for years (143). Amputees need to adjust to their altered body image. Furthermore, anxiety about disease progression can be a problem for nontraumatic amputees.

Cardiac Disease

A large body of literature exists concerning the impact of cardiac disease on sexual functioning. Although cardiac disease does not have a direct impact on genital sexual functioning, the psychological and peripheral effects on physical functioning are great. As with most other studies examining sexual functioning, there is a great imbalance in the attention paid to male as opposed to female sexual response.

Frequency of sexual activity has been shown to decrease in 40% to 70% of men after myocardial infarction (MI) (144). Of 130 women who suffered from MI (145), 44% reported decreased frequency of intercourse, and another 27% became completely abstinent. In another report of 100 male veterans surveyed 6 months after their MIs (146), common reasons for not resuming intercourse included erectile dysfunction (39%), chest pain (28%), deconditioning (28%), decreased libido (19%), anxiety about recurrence of MI (16%), boredom (15%) and depression (14%).

Denial, anxiety and depression have been noted as the psychological disturbances most commonly to occur after MI (147). Denial is usually the first response and does not impact upon sexual functioning. Anxiety, however, can become chronic after MI and can result in erectile dysfunction. Furthermore, anxiety is often inappropriately focused on the occurrence of MI during sexual activity. Of 858 patients with acute MIs who were sexually active in the previous year, only 3% reported sexual activity in the 2 hours preceding their MI; moreover, the risk of MI during sexual activity was no different in patients with or without a preexisting history of MI, and sexual activity was thought to contribute to the etiology of MI in only 0.9% of cases (148). Of the psychological impacts of MI, depression is felt to be the most clearly established cause for sexual dysfunction (149) and can result in decreased libido and erectile and orgasmic dysfunctions.

Physical consequences of cardiac disease on sexual functioning include diminished cardiac reserve, which can make the patient less physically able to perform (150), and angina (151). Notably, angina after MI is more frequent during the resolution phase of sexual response than during orgasm (152). Sternal incisional pain is common in the first 6 to 8 weeks after coronary artery bypass grafting (144) and can infrequently persist, causing long-term sexual difficulties. Most patients with cardiac disease are also on multiple medications, many of which can cause sexual dysfunctions.

The energy requirements during sexual activity have been studied. Orgasm requires 4 to 6 metabolic equivalents (METs) for 10 to 15 seconds, whereas the other phases of sexual response require 3 to 4 METs (153). Furthermore, in a study of middle-aged married men, requirements were generally noted not to exceed 4 METs (154). Walking on a treadmill at 3 miles/hr at 5% grade and climbing two flights of stairs at a rate of 20 steps in 10 seconds (155) are felt to require equivalent amounts of energy as sexual intercourse. Furthermore, the energy requirements for sexual intercourse are thought to be less for familiar positions than unfamiliar positions, regardless of what they may be (156).

The two-flight test has been used to determine safe return to sexual activity after MI; however, it has been noted that the test can be used only to make a rough estimate (157), and the test is unable to detect silent ischemia. One study of 88 men (158) undergoing ambulatory electrocardiogram (ECG) monitoring revealed that one-third of patients had ischemia during sexual activity, and silent ischemia was more common than symptomatic. Furthermore, they noted that a positive exercise stress test was noted in all patients with ischemia. Therefore, a true exercise stress test may be the best mechanism to determine safe return to sexual activity post-MI.

Treatment of the patient with cardiac disease and sexual difficulties begins with education and reassurance of the patient about the effects of cardiac disease on sexual functioning. The importance of a general conditioning program should also be emphasized, as one report noted that heart rate reduction and increased exercise tolerance should theoretically decrease ischemic episodes during sex (158). Timing of sexual activity when not fatigued (159,160) and possibly in the morning with rest periods before and after is important for patients with cardiac disease (161,162). Foreplay has also been noted to be particularly important in order to allow a gradual increase in heart rate (152). Sexual intercourse should be avoided after a heavy meal and for at least 3 hours after drinking alcohol (159,161,163,164). Sex should also be avoided during emotional stress or in association with anxiety-producing conditions (161,162,164). Positioning during sexual activity should stress comfort, ease, and familiarity.

Patients should also be counseled about what symptoms should be reported to their physicians (159). These include a rapid heart rate and/or breathing pattern persisting for 7 to 10 minutes after orgasm, angina, extreme fatigue after orgasm, or the development of other sexual difficulties. For those persons with angina, prophylactic nitroglycerin may be useful during sexual activity (163–168).

Pulmonary Disease

Patients with chronic pulmonary disease are likely to experience sexual dysfunction; however, little research has been done on this topic (169). Dyspnea leading to decreased activity tolerance can cause sexual difficulties in patients with chronic obstructive pulmonary disease (COPD) (170). Because respiratory rates of 40 to 60 per minute may be reached during sexual activity, the ability to achieve full exhalation may be diminished in COPD patients. Furthermore, if the patient is on the bottom, dyspnea can be exacerbated through the pressure of the partner on the chest (171). This can lead to anxiety and fear, beginning a vicious cycle that makes the sexual act even more difficult. Bronchospasm with resultant coughing can also diminish an erection (170), leading to further psychological and sexual difficulties.

An association has been demonstrated between COPD and impotence (172). Other potential causes of sexual dysfunction in the individual with pulmonary disease include side effects of medications such as corticosteroids, antihypertensives, digoxin, and antidepressants. Deconditioning can impair one's ability to participate in sexual activity. Furthermore, altered body image, depression, and general anxiety can cause sexual difficulties.

Patients with cystic fibrosis deserve special mention with regard to the impact of their disease on sexual functioning. Of 30 married male and female cystic fibrosis patients (173), 57% reported no or only occasional problems in sexual functioning; however, 30% complained of serious sexual problems. Men with cystic fibrosis are also noted routinely to have bilateral absence or atrophy of the vas deferens (174), and azoospermia is universal (175). Despite these abnormalities, successful pregnancies have resulted from microsurgical epididymal sperm aspiration followed by intracytoplasmic sperm injection (176).

Treatment of patients with pulmonary disease involves education about the impact of their pulmonary dysfunction on sexual activity. Patients should be encouraged to talk about anxieties associated with sexual functioning and may benefit from trying mutual masturbation rather than oral sex or intercourse as a form of sexual activity (171). Alternatively, agreeing not to have intercourse and just play around during sexual activity may decrease anxiety.

Patients should be instructed to plan their sexual activity (170). This includes getting a good night's rest before sex but avoiding sex on awakening because of accumulated secretions (171,177). One should wait 2 to 3 hours after meals before having sex (177) and avoid physical activity right before sex (170,171). A familiar, relaxing atmosphere should help keep anxiety down (177,178). Furthermore, some persons with pulmonary dysfunction may feel it is easier to have sex on firm surfaces, whereas other persons may feel that the surface of a waterbed is useful (170).

The use of an inhaler or cough drop just before sex can help prevent bronchospasm and coughing (170). Oxygen should also be used if helpful, but with adequate length and positioning of tubing. Restrictive clothing should be removed before sexual activity, and having a box of tissues nearby can help prevent interruptions during sexual activity. Avoiding prolonged kissing and oral sex before intercourse should be considered if they result in dyspnea. Finally, patients should adjust the rate and intensity of intercourse to their breathing needs (170), and positions for intercourse should avoid putting pressure on the chest (171). The side-lying position and the seated position are both considered good to make breathing easier (178).

Cancer

The emotional impact of a diagnosis of cancer can not be overestimated. Nevertheless, advances in treatment of persons with cancer have made extended survival and cure a realistic possibility in many cases. Therefore, issues pertaining to sexuality and sexual functioning are important. The physical impact of cancer on sexual functioning is in a large part determined by the location of the primary tumor. Furthermore, various treatments for cancer can often cause iatrogenically induced sexual dysfunction.

Prostate cancer is the most common form of cancer diagnosed in men, with an incidence of approximately 244,000 in l995 (179). All treatment options can cause sexual changes (180). Radical prostatectomy, an option for early-stage cancer that includes removal of the entire prostate, seminal vesicles, and vas deferens, results in permanent erectile dysfunction in 85% to 90% of men. Fortunately, nerve-sparing surgery will result in a 76% return of erectile ability if both neurovascular bundles are preserved and a 60% return of erectile capacity if only one neurovascular bundle is preserved (181). With radiation therapy sexual dysfunction is influenced by the size of the radiation field, whether there is damage to the pelvic vascular bed, sympathetic nerves, or testicles with resultant decreased testosterone levels (182). Erectile dysfunction and ejaculatory pain from a reduction in semen flow (183) can both result from radiation. With internal beam radiation therapy, 15% of men report subsequent erectile dysfunction (184). Hormonal manipulation is aimed at decreasing androgen availability to prevent tumor growth. Testosterone levels decrease 90% to 95%, with associated side effects including decreased libido, hot flashes, and erectile dysfunction. Furthermore, it is felt that the effect of hormonal therapy on sexual functioning may be greatest through its effect on the brain in decreasing desire and arousability (185).

Testicular cancer is the most common form of cancer in men between the ages of 15 and 35 (179). Retroperitoneal lymphadenectomy may be a necessary part of treatment, resulting in severance of para-aortic sympathetic nerves necessary for ejaculation. Retrograde ejaculation along with decreased semen volume occurs almost universally (186); therefore, nerve-sparing procedures are advocated when possible. Although desire, erection, and orgasm are usually unchanged physiologically, the psychological impact of testicular cancer may decrease a persons desire for sexual activity. Fertility will be impaired through both direct damage to the sperm and altered ejaculation, and sperm banking and assisted ejaculation procedures may need to be considered.

Penile carcinoma includes only 1% of male cancers, generally occurring after the age of 50 (187). Treatment can range from partial penectomy, radiation therapy, or topical chemotherapy for small lesions to total penectomy with perineal urethrostomy for more advanced disease (180). Despite changes in erectile functioning, the capacity for arousal to other erotically sensitive areas including the mons, scrotum, perineum, and anus and ejaculation and orgasm persists. For those individuals with complete penectomy, penile implants have been reported to result in satisfaction with function and appearance in 89% of patients and their mates (186).

Breast cancer is diagnosed in approximately 182,000 women in the United States annually (179). Administration of antiestrogens can result in temporary or permanent menopause, as can chemotherapy. Soreness, dryness, vaginal atrophy, hot flashes, and decreased sexual desire can result (188). Local estrogen cream may alleviate some of this symptomatology. In addition to the physical changes associated with treatment, the profound psychological impact of breast cancer results in orgasmic difficulties and reduced frequency of intercourse in up to 39% of women (189). These effects have been noted despite the attempts to preserve women's breasts through breast-saving surgery or reconstruction.

Ovarian cancer is the third most frequently diagnosed gynecologic malignancy (179). Sexual dysfunction including postcoital bleeding or pelvic pain can be the presenting symptom (189). Surgical removal of the ovaries results in the onset of menopause with the symptomatology mentioned above. In addition, the resultant infertility can be psychologically devastating. For advanced cancers total pelvic exenteration including surgical removal of the bladder, vagina, uterus, rectum and associated structures may be necessary, after which most women cease all sexual activity (190,191)

Women with cervical cancer may experience sexual dysfunction related to fibrosis, pain with penetration, decreased lubrication, and vaginal stenosis associated with radiation therapy (180). Vaginal dilators and lubricants may be useful to minimize these side effects. Furthermore, alternative positioning during intercourse may minimize discomfort.

Other gynecologic cancers are rare. Cancer of the vulva most often occurs in postmenopausal women (179). Treatment can include simple vulvectomy, after which sexual functioning and the capacity for orgasm may be preserved. However, removal of the clitoris results in more substantial impairment. Despite this, because adrenal androgens and ovarian hormone function are unaffected, some women retain the capacity for desire, arousal, and orgasm after radical vulvectomy. Furthermore, it is thought that psychological distress may be a factor in those women with an inability to achieve orgasm (180). Cancer of the vagina and associated treatments may result in shortening and narrowing of the vagina, dryness, and dyspareunia. For those women who undergo total vaginectomy, however, 30% to 70% of patients will have a return of orgasm provided the clitoris is left intact (192).

Colorectal cancer is the third most common cause of cancer in both sexes. Abdominoperineal resection can result in erectile dysfunction in 50% to 100% of patients (193) and ejaculatory dysfunction in 50% to 75% of patients after surgery. Furthermore, both sexes experience changes in self-image and sexuality as a result of colostomy.

Bladder cancer is usually treated by surgery followed by radiation. Radical cystectomy results in erectile dysfunction in nearly 100% of cases, and ejaculation is retrograde. However, orgasm and sexual desire remain unaffected. In women, total abdominal hysterectomy, bilateral oophorectomy, and removal of the anterior vaginal wall can result in numbness in the perineum and decreased estrogens with resultant decreases in vaginal size and lubrication and dyspareunia. The ability to achieve orgasm, however, should remain in women who successfully resume sexual activity (189). The use of an ileal conduit can also result in changes in self-image and resultant sexual dysfunction similar to those resulting from colostomy.

Other cancers, though primarily nongenital, can also have profound impacts on sexual functioning. Head and neck cancers and their associated treatments can result in profound disfigurement and change in self-image. Metastatic tumors to the brain or spinal cord can result in changes in sexual functioning due to neurologic dysfunction. Depression and anxiety will be associated with a diagnosis of cancer no matter where the primary tumor is and weakness and fatigue will occur regardless of the location of the primary tumor. Furthermore, treatments prescribed for cancer including chemotherapeutic agents, radiation therapy and hormonal manipulation can cause general side effects of fatigue and other medical problems in addition to specific sexual side effects regardless of the types of tumors they are treating.

Treatment of sexual dysfunction in the person with cancer should begin with giving them permission to talk about their concerns regarding sexuality and then providing them with basic information, tailored to their particular problem. Recommendations regarding timing for sexual activity when free from fatigue and positioning to decrease energy requirements may be useful. Treatment of specific dysfunctions is warranted as is referral for further psychological and sexual counseling, if appropriate.

Other Disorders

Discussion of the sexual problems associated with all potential physical disorders is beyond the scope of this chapter. However, the basic principles discussed here should be utilized when working with persons with other diagnoses. Determination of premorbid sexual dysfunction is important. Furthermore, the impact of medication use and other concomitant medical problems must be addressed. The psychologic status of the patient including evidence of depression and anxiety must be considered. Physical examination should look for signs previously discussed associated with changes in sexual functioning. For those disorders similar to another which we do have some understanding of sexuality, it may be useful to discuss the effects of the other disorder with the patient. Basic education should be provided regarding sexuality; furthermore, this should be supplemented by referral for further psychological and sexual counseling and/or treatment if appropriate.

TREATMENT STRATEGIES

Sexuality Counseling

Sexuality is a sensitive topic and one that many of us feel uncomfortable addressing with our patients. The reasons for this are at least twofold. First, few of us have received professional training in the area of sexuality. Second, the subject of sexuality is replete with our own personal values and biases based on our own upbringing and life experiences. For many, it is difficult to separate our own values and attitudes to address the issue objectively. It is not surprising therefore that the subject is either not approached with our patients, raised inappropriately, or simply dismissed when the patient raises the topic. Annon (194) has proposed a multilayered framework for sexual counseling incorporating all health care personnel working with the patient. The so-called *PLISSIT* model is an acronym for *p*ermission, *l*imited *i*nformation, *s*pecific *s*uggestions, and *i*ntensive *t*herapy. According to this model, all personnel working with the patient should feel comfortable enough with their own sexuality and knowledgeable enough to engage in the first two levels of this model. That is, professionals should feel comfortable raising the issue with the patient to "permit" discussion of the topic. In addition, the professional should possess enough knowledge about sexuality and the specific disability/illness to impart limited information. Moreover, they should possess enough information to know their limits or to "know what they do not know." In this case, they would move up to the next level of the model, which involves referring the patient to a more knowledgeable professional for specific suggestions and/or intensive therapy. Successful implementation of this model would require an ongoing institutional commitment to train all staff having contact with patients on basic sexuality issues. This model also argues for the existence of a standing multidisciplinary hospitalwide committee addressing sexuality issues including education of patients and staff along with ongoing ethical issues.

The need for sexual counseling has been reported differently depending on the population. Pauly and Goldstein (195) reported that 10% of the general population is in need of some sort of sexual counseling. Burnap and Golden (196) reported that 15% of their general medical practice needed sexual therapy, whereas Stuntz (197) stated that 50% of his gynecologic patients were in need of sexual counseling services. More recently, Alexander, Sipski, and Findley (58) and Sipski and Alexander (56) reported that 27% of their male and 20% of their female spinal-cord-injured subjects acknowledged poor sexual adjustment. Moreover, these same researchers reported that 74% of their male and 44% of their female spinal-cord-injured subjects claimed that their disability significantly and negatively affected the quality of their sexual relationships (58,63).

Schover (198) described a model for brief, problem-focused sexual counseling following chronic illness. According to her model, there are at least five criteria for counseling: (a) a sexual dysfunction that predated the illness or disability; (b) a relationship that is conflicted by the illness; (c) sexual dysfunction as a result of poor coping; (d) difficulty coping because of severe changes in sexual self-image; and (e) adjustment to medical or surgical procedures. The model calls for practical, realistic, and humane interventions with clear goals. When referring someone for sexual counseling, one must be sensitive to the emotional concerns of patients. When a patient is referred for sexual counseling he or she may react with disapproval because of fear that the problem is interpreted as emotional. However, a patient referred to the urologist with erectile dysfunction following illness or disability will probably be quite receptive to help. This situation, viewed as clearly medical, is less threatening and therefore more acceptable to the individual. Thus, one must use sensitivity in educating a patient to the role of both the emotional and physical aspects involved in sexual problems.

Schover (198) delineates five aspects to her model of brief sexual counseling: (a) sexual education; (b) changing maladaptive sexual attitudes; (c) helping couples resume sex; (d) overcoming the physical handicaps; and (e) decreasing any marital conflict. The issue of sexual education cannot be overstated. Couples must be educated about the normal sexual response cycle and the impact of their specific disability on the sexual response cycle. Couples must also be knowledgeable about the impact of medications, life-style changes, and the aging process on their sexuality. Chronic illness and disability often result in maladaptive attitudes (e.g., sex is unhealthy, sex must be spontaneous, intercourse is the only worthwhile form of sexual expression) that must be challenged and corrected (198). Not infrequently, couples will need assistance resuming their sexual activity. This can be accomplished through improving communication and self-esteem along with educating the couple on alternative methods of sexual expression and caring. This will help decrease any performance anxiety. Disability will usually present physical barriers that must be successfully hurdled. Issues such as diminished movement and sensation, bowel and bladder programs, and chronic pain must be addressed. Last, when marital conflict exists because of changes in roles, changes in the homeostasis of power in the relationship, or fear that the able-bodied partner will leave, it must be confronted and corrected. An all too common conflict arises when the spouse ends up serving in the dual role of lover as well as caretaker. This situation should be actively avoided whenever possible.

Sexuality involves an interplay between physiological and psychological components, and disability and illness impact each of these areas. As Trieschmann (47) has noted, the physiological and psychological contributions to the sexual act, the desire for sex, and the broader concept of sexuality must be assessed. All too often, when discussing sexuality we only focus on the narrow aspect of the sexual act and forget the more important global aspects of sexuality. The late and noted social worker Mary Romano (199) eloquently described female sexuality as the following: "Sexuality is more than the act of sexual intercourse. It involves for most women the whole business of relating to another person; the tenderness, the desire to give as well as take, the compliments, casual caresses, reciprocal concerns, tolerance, the forms of communication that both include and go beyond words. For women, sexuality includes a range of behaviors from smiling through orgasm; it is not just what happens between two people in bed" (199, p. 28). The goal in our work with couples in sexual counseling is to help them increase their personal definition of sexuality. To the extent that their personal definition is narrow, they will have more difficulties adjusting to disability. On the other hand, when their definition of sexuality is broad and encompassing, they will likely adjust more smoothly to the physical challenges in their lives.

Management of Erectile Dysfunction

Management of the patient with erectile dysfunction begins with a thorough history and physical examination designed to identify treatable causes of erectile dysfunction. For instance, review of medications may reveal that the patient is on medications that cause erectile dysfunction but may be substituted by other, less disruptive medications. Comprehensive evaluation should also include psychological evaluation and may also include determination of serum testosterone level, electrodiagnostic studies, penile Doppler, and nocturnal penile tumescence monitoring via Rigiscan (Dacomed, Minneapolis, MN). However, in many cases of disability such as a young man suffering from a decrease in the ability to sustain a reflex erection subsequent to a spinal cord injury, comprehensive testing may result in unnecessary cost without resultant change in treatment.

Topical and Intraurethral Therapies

Several different medications have been applied to the penis with a goal of improving erectile functioning. Topical nitroglycerin has been utilized to treat erectile dysfunction (200–202); however, only 21 of 53 men with erectile dysfunction of varying etiologies achieved satisfactory erections. Furthermore, negative side effects included headache and hypotension. Topical minoxidil was reported to be more effective than nitroglycerin or placebo in improving penile diameter and rigidity as measured by Rigiscan (203); however, two subsequent studies failed to demonstrate clinical efficacy (204,205). Intraurethral application of prostaglandin E_1 and E_2 (PGE_1 and PGE_2) has been tried to remediate erectile dysfunction. Of 20 subjects using a mixture of PGE_2, 70% responded to treatment, and 30% had erection with adequate rigidity for intercourse (206). In another report 1,511 men participated in a double-blind, placebo-controlled multicenter study of intraurethral pellets of varying doses of

PGE_1. Sixty-five percent of patients were able to engage in intercourse; however, 11% of subjects reported penile pain from the treatment. Further studies are examining the use of intraurethral medications to treat erectile dysfunction.

Oral Medications

Multiple oral medications have been tried to improve erectile functioning, with mixed results. Yohimbine, an alkaloid agent that blocks presynaptic alpha-2 adrenergic receptors, is thought to augment the physiological shunting of blood to the corporal bodies. Although some researchers (207) note there is inadequate evidence to support the use of yohimbine in persons whose erectile dysfunction is a result of altered shunting mechanisms or other etiologies, yohimbine was found to be useful in treating erectile dysfunction associated with the use of SSRIs (208). Oral phentolamine was noted to produce erection adequate for vaginal penetration in 42% of 100 men with erectile dysfunction (209). Effectiveness was greatest in men with nonspecific, psychogenic, or mild vascular impotence; however, side effects included dizziness, palpitations, and nasal congestion. Recent investigations have revealed that sildenifil, a selective inhibitor of type 5 cyclic guanosine monophosphate (cGMP), is effective in improving erectile function. Although it is not yet available for use in the United States, recent investigations noted that the drug is safe and effective in improving erectile duration and rigidity in 70% to 90% of patients (210–212). It is anticipated that this drug will have a major role in future therapeutic regimens for erectile dysfunction.

Vacuum-Assisted Erections

One of the least invasive means of achieving penile rigidity involves the use of a vacuum erection device (see Fig. 45-1). These devices, of which there are many, generally consist of a hard plastic cylindrical tube, at the end of which is a smaller, soft plastic tube leading to the pump. Depending on the individual's motoric capabilities, a manual or electrically powered pump can be used to generate the vacuum, which will result in engorgement of both corporeal and extracorporeal tissues. Finally, once the erection is attained, a constricting ring (see Fig. 45-2) must be placed on the base of the penis to maintain the erection.

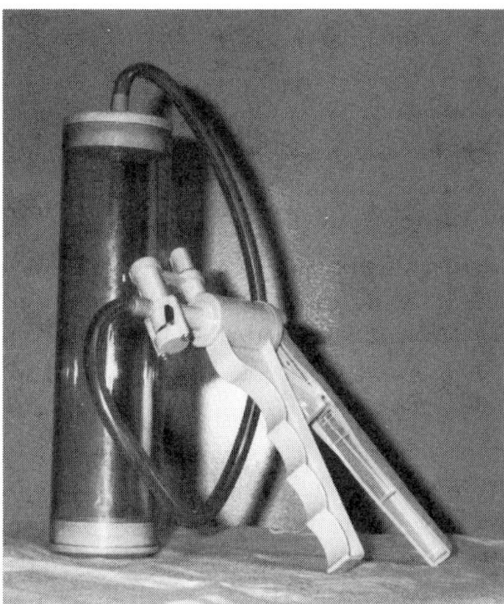

FIG. 45-1. Vacuum erection device (© Performance Medical, Sewell, NJ).

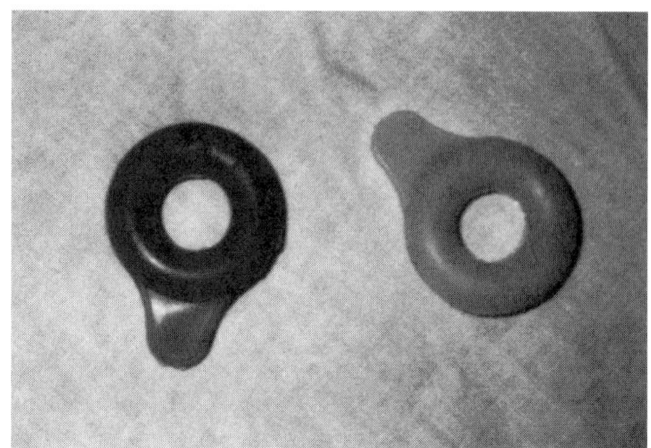

FIG. 45-2. Constriction ring. (© Performance Medical, Sewell, NJ).

Vacuum-assisted erections are less esthetically pleasing than those achieved through the use of medications. Because of the engorgement of the extracorporeal tissues, there will be superficial dilation of veins, and the penis will be wider than its usual diameter. Furthermore, there will be an abrupt lack of erection proximal to the constricting band. Although less invasive, vacuum erections are not without potential complications and must not be used in persons on anticoagulants because of the potential risk of hematoma. Most importantly, the maximum time the constricting band may remain in place is 30 minutes because of the potential development of necrosis of the penile skin and injury to the corporeal tissues, resulting in permanent penile deformity (213). For those men who are able to achieve an erection but unable to sustain it, the use of constricting bands may be adequate to remediate their erectile dysfunction; however, similar time precautions should be adhered to.

Injection Erections

Intracavernosal injection therapy is useful to treat most types of erectile dysfunction; however, it is less successful in men with impaired penile arterial blood flow. Relaxation of the sinusoidal smooth muscle by the medications enhances corporeal filling, with the duration of the erection being directly related to the dose of medication administered (214). Although various medications including papaverine and rigitine have been used for intracavernosal injections, Food and Drug Administration (FDA) approval has only recently been obtained, and solely for the use of PGE_1, which

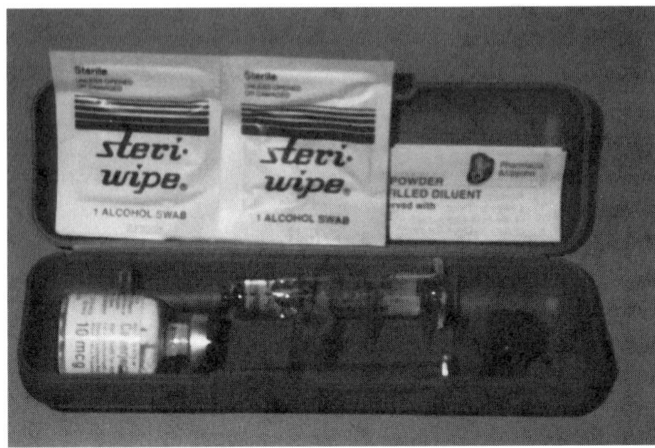

FIG. 45-3. Prostaglandin E_1 (Alprostadil, Pharmacia and Upjohn, Kalamazoo, MI).

is now available in a convenient package (see Fig. 45-3). The use of intracavernosal PGE_1 was studied in 683 men with varying types of erectile dysfunction (215). Erections were satisfactory for intercourse in 94% of injections, and 87% of men and 86% of their partners reported satisfaction with intercourse. Complications included penile pain in 11% of injections, prolonged erections in 5% but priapism in only 1%, penile fibrosis in 2%, and ecchymosis or hematoma in 8% (215).

Chronic administration of intracorporal mediations can result in scarring of the tunica albuginea with resultant permanent curvature in the erect penis (216). Priapism is also a realistic complication of this treatment and must be treated as a medical emergency. Blood must be aspirated from each corporal body, and an alpha-adrenergic agonist should be injected to promote contraction of the smooth muscle and restore venous drainage to the system (217).

The Penile Prosthesis

Before the development of the previously mentioned treatments for erectile dysfunction, the penile prosthesis was the mainstay of treatment. Unfortunately, it is the most invasive therapy available and often results in complications in persons with impaired genital sensation. These can include mechanical failures of the devices, infections, and extrusion of the devices.

Types of prostheses include the malleable prosthesis, which results in permanent erection, although the penis can be manipulated in order to hide it, and the inflatable penile prosthesis. Two erectile cylinders containing fluid reservoirs at the base, an inflation pump at the tip, and an expansile chamber in the middle are surgically implanted into the corporal bodies. Manual pumping of the device results in an erection without great increase in the diameter of the penis. Postcoitus, pressure on a relief valve causes detumescence (213).

Satisfaction rates approximate only 75% with an implantable inflatable prosthesis. Altered orgasm and ejaculation are reported in approximately 25% of patients, and up to 10% of patients report the erection is inadequate to enjoy intercourse (218). Additionally, as might be expected with such an invasive device, many potential complications exist. Internal scar formation can result in device dysfunction, failure of the device components can result in penile deformity, and extravasation of the internal fluid of the device can occur. Moreover, the rate of prosthesis infection can be as high as 16.5% (219) in patients with spinal cord injuries, and infection coupled with the risk of extrusion led to a 25% explantation rate in another study of men with SCIs and penile prostheses (220). Because of the invasiveness, cost, and potential complications associated with insertion of a penile prosthesis, all other means of treating erectile dysfunction should be tried before this type of therapy is undertaken.

Management of Hypoactive Sexual Desire

Hypoactive sexual desire disorder is a persistent or recurrent lack of sexual fantasies and desire for sexual activity that causes the individual marked personal or interpersonal distress (DSM-IV). Hypoactive sexual desire is one of the most common problems addressed in general sex therapy and is quite common, occurring in 15% to 34% of the able-bodied population (221). In addition to being primary and premorbid, decreased desire associated with disability or illness can also be related to depression or other psychological distress related to disability or illness or related to the use of medications or medical illness. Treatment involves discontinuing any medications that could be responsible for the dysfunction and referral for counseling.

Management of Premature Ejaculation

Premature ejaculation is one of the most common male sexual dysfunctions (222). Although the name remains premature ejaculation in the DSM-IV, practitioners have been notoriously unable to come to a consistent definition, and the use of the term *early ejaculation* has been recommended to be less pejorative and more accurate (223). Masters and Johnson's (48) definition for early ejaculation was that the male ejaculated before the female was orgasmic at least 50% of the time. However, because some women are unable to experience orgasm through genital intercourse, this definition has some pitfalls. Other researchers have utilized time, such as 1 or 2 minutes of intercourse thrusting, whereas others have noted the inability to maintain control with over 20 seconds of rapid thrusting (223). The DSM-IV defines premature ejaculation as "persistent or recurrent ejaculation with minimal sexual stimulation before, on, or shortly after penetration and before the person wishes it. The clinician must take into account factors that affect duration of the excitement phase . . ." (224). Furthermore, the disturbance must cause marked distress.

In men with disabilities, premature ejaculation is usually

premorbid (225). New diagnoses should prompt a workup for prostate or urinary infection (226) and may be easily treatable with antibiotics. For other cases, a cognitive–behavioral treatment model is used to treat early ejaculation. New attitudes and skills are taught to increase the man's pleasure and decrease the pressure to perform for the woman. Ejaculatory control is then relearned as a couple through progressively increasing stimulation and identifying the point of ejaculatory inevitability, at which point stimulation is stopped and then resumed. Furthermore, alternative intercourse positions and movements are added as control is achieved (223).

Recent research has also demonstrated that medical treatment may be appropriate to treat problems with early ejaculation. For those couples who have failed behavioral interventions, medical treatment with SSRIs may help improve ejaculatory latency. Fluoxetine and clomipramine have both been shown to have beneficial effects in this regard (222).

Management of Inhibited Ejaculation

Inhibited ejaculation is rare in the nondisabled population; however, it is extremely common in men with some neurologic disorders, particularly SCIs. In this population inhibited ejaculation may or may not be accompanied by anorgasmia. To date, treatments have relied on the restoration of ejaculatory function, solely for fertility purposes. As some men with complete SCIs still retain the ability to achieve orgasm, future research should include a focus on what can be done to improve orgasmic capabilities in men with SCIs and other neurologic disabilities.

Management of Female Sexual Arousal Disorder

The DSM-IV defines female sexual arousal disorder as the inability to attain or maintain the lubrication and swelling of sexual excitement until the completion of sexual activity. Furthermore, there is resultant distress. Inability to achieve lubrication can be primary, or it may be secondary to medications, other psychological dysfunction, or illness. Treatment in the person with disability must include assessment of whether the condition was premorbid, along with removal of any potential causative agents. The use of water-based lubricants is appropriate, as is education about the impact of the particular disability on their sexual functioning. Furthermore, the use of vibratory stimulation may increase arousal. Sexual counseling is appropriate in cases of premorbid disorders.

Inhibited Female Orgasm

Inhibited orgasm is the absence or delay in orgasm when desired, following sexual excitement. It should be noted that many women are unable to achieve orgasm through intercourse without added clitoral stimulation but may achieve it with clitoral stimulation with or without intercourse. This is not considered inhibited orgasm. In the general population, however, persistent or recurrent inhibited orgasm is present in 5% to 10% of women (221); thus, in working with women with disabilities, it is important to determine if the dysfunction was premorbid.

Treatment depends on whether the dysfunction is premorbid. For those women with primary anorgasmia, learning about their bodies through masturbation with gradual increasing stimulation until they reach orgasm is one treatment method. Sex therapy may also be beneficial. For those women with disabilities, scant laboratory-based research has examined the ability of women with various disabilities to achieved orgasm. However, recent results with women with complete SCIs indicates that neurologic dysfunction may not preclude orgasm (56). Therefore, we recommend that the liberal use of vibrators and other sexual aids to augment sexual response be tried in women with disabilities, and women should be taught to masturbate to learn what feels good to them now. Furthermore, future research should focus on improving the capabilities of women with disabilities to achieve orgasm.

Dyspareunia and Vaginismus

Dyspareunia is the occurrence of pain during intercourse. It may be caused by insufficient lubrication and resultant pain during intercourse. Recurrent dyspareunia can result in vaginismus or recurrent or persistent involuntary spasm of the outer third of the vagina, which interferes with sexual intercourse. Both dyspareunia and vaginismus can be primary or can be secondary to other psychological or sexual dysfunction or physiological effects of a medical condition. Treatment includes assurance of adequate vaginal lubrication in addition to relaxation training in conjunction with sex therapy. Furthermore, progressively larger well-lubricated dilators may be used by the patient to practice stimulation. Above all, it is important that the woman always be in charge of when and how penetration takes place (227).

REFERENCES

1. Masters WH, Johnson VE. *Human sexual response*. Boston: Little, Brown, 1966.
2. Kaplan HS. Hypoactive sexual desire. *J Sex Marital Ther* 1977; 3: 3–9.
3. Kaplan HS. *Disorders of sexual desire*. New York: Simon and Schuster, 1979.
4. Robinson P. *The modernization of sex*. New York: Harper & Row, 1976.
5. Rosen RC, Beck JG. *Patterns of sexual arousal: psychophysiological processes and clinical applications*. New York: Guilford Press, 1988.
6. Weiss HD. The physiology of human penile erection. *Ann Intern Med* 1972; 76:793.
7. Sipski ML, Alexander CJ. Sexual function and dysfunction after spinal cord injury. *Phys Med Rehab Clin North Am* 1992; 3:811–828.
8. Bennett CJ, Seager SW, Vasher EA, McGuire EJ. Sexual dysfunction and electroejaculation in men with spinal cord injury: review. *J Urol* 1988; 139:453–457.
9. Sipski ML. Spinal cord injury: what is the effect on sexual response? *J Am Paraplegia Soc* 1991; 14:40–43.

10. Griffith ER, Trieschmann RB. Sexual functioning in women with spinal cord injury. *Arch Phys Med Rehabil* 1975; 56:18–21.
11. Kleitsch EC, O'Donnell PD. Sex and aging. *Phys Med Rehabil State Art Rev.* 1990; 4:121–134.
12. Starr BD, Weiner MB. *The Starr-Weiner report on sex and sexuality in the mature years.* New York: McGraw-Hill, 1981.
13. Whitten P, Whiteside EJ. Can exercise make you sexier? *Psychol Today* 1989; April:42–44.
14. Sipski ML, Alexander CJ, eds. *Sexual function in people with disability and chronic illness: a health professional's guide.* Gaithersburg, MD: Aspen Publishers, 1997.
15. Breckenridge A. Angiotensin converting enzyme inhibitors and quality of life. *Am J Hypertens* 1991; 4:79S–82S.
16. Weiner DN, Rosen RC. Medications and their impact. In: Sipski ML, Alexander CJ, eds. *Sexual function in people with disability and chronic ilness: a health professional's guide.* Gaithersburg, MD: Aspen Publishers, 1997; 6:85–118.
17. Hogan MJ, Wallin JD, Baer RM. Antihypertensive therapy and male sexual dysfunction. *Psychosomatics* 1980; 21:235–237.
18. Croog SH, Levine S, Sudilovsky A, Baume RM, Clive J. Sexual symptoms in hypertensive patients: a clinical trial of antihypertensive medications. *Arch Intern Med* 1988; 148:788–794.
19. Chang SW, Fine R, Siegel D, et al. The impact of diuretic therapy on reported sexual function. *Arch Intern Med* 1991; 151:2402–2408.
20. Blane GF. Comparative toxicity and safety profile of fenofibrate and other fibric acid derivatives. *Am J Med* 1987; 83:26–36.
21. Coronary Drug Research Group. Clofibrate and niacin in coronary heart disease. *JAMA* 1975; 231:360–388.
22. Schneider J, Kaffarnik H. Impotence in patients treated with clofibrate. *Atherosclerosis* 1975; 21:455–475.
23. Stoffer SS, Hynes KM, Jiang NS, Ryan RJ. Digoxin and abnormal serum hormone levels. *JAMA* 1973; 225:1643–1644.
24. Neri A, Aygen M, Zuckerman Z, Bahary C. Subjective assessment of sexual dysfunction of patients on long-term administration of digoxin. *Arch Sex Behav* 1980; 9:343–347.
25. Amahd S. Disopyramide and impotence [Letter to the editor]. *South Med J* 1980; 73:958.
26. McHaffie DJ, Guz A, Johnston A. Impotence in a patient on disopyramide. *Lancet* 1977; 1:859.
27. Couper-Smartt JD, Rodham R. A technique for surveying side effects of tricyclic drugs with reference to reported side effects. *J Intern Med Res* 1973; 1:473–476.
28. Monteiro WO, Noshirvani HF, Marks IM, Lelliott PT. Anorgasmia from clomipramine in obsessive-compulsive disorder: a controlled trial. *Br J Psychiatry* 1987; 151:107–112.
29. McLean JD, Forsyth RG, Kapkin IA. Unusual side effects of clomipramine associated with yawning. *Can J Psychiatry* 1983:28: 569–570.
30. Sovner R. Anorgasmia associated with imipramine but not desipramine: case report. *J Clin Psychiatry* 1983; 44:345–346.
31. Shen WW. Female orgasmic inhibition by amoxapine. *Am J Psychiatry* 1982; 139:1220–1221.
32. Nurnberg HG, Levine PE. Spontaneous remission of MAOI-induced anorgasmia. *Am J Psychiatry* 1987; 144:805–807.
33. Ashton AK, Hamer R, Rosen RC. SSRI-induced sexual dysfunction and its treatment: a large-scale retrospective study of 596 psychiatric outpatients. (in press).
34. Nutt D, Hackman A, Hawton K. Increased sexual function in benzodiazepine withdrawal. *Lancet* 1986; 2:1101–1102.
35. Riley AJ, Riley EJ. Cyproheptadine and antidepressant-induced anorgasmia. *Br J Psychiatry* 1986; 148:217–218.
36. Sangal, R. Inhibited female orgasm as a side effect of alprazolam. *Am J Psychiatry* 1985; 142:1223–1224.
37. Uhde TW, Tancer ME, Shea CA. Sexual dysfunction related to alprazolam treatment of social phobia [Letter to the editor]. *Am J Psychiatry* 1988; 145:531–532.
38. Hughs JM. Failure to ejaculate with chlordiazepoxide. *Am J Psychiatry* 1964; 121:610–611.
39. Segraves RT. Treatment of premature ejaculation with lorazepam. *Am J Psychiatry* 1987; 144:1240.
40. Balon R, Ramesh C, Pohl R. Sexual dysfunction associated with diazepam but not clonazepam. *Can J Psychiatry* 1989; 34:947–948.
41. Mattson RH, Cramer JA, Collines JF, Smith DB, et al. Comparison of carbamazepine, phenobarbital, phenytoin, primidone in partial and secondary generalized tonic–clonic seizures. *N Engl J Med* 1985; 313: 145–151.
42. Jensen P, Jensen SB, Sorensen PS, Bjerre BD, Klysner R, Brinch K, Jespersen B, Nielsen H. Sexual dysfunction in male and female patients with epilepsy: a study of 86 outpatients. *Arch Sex Behav* 1990; 19:1–14.
43. Niv Y. Male sexual dysfunction due to cimetidine. *Ir Med J* 1986; 79:352.
44. Wolfe MM. Impotence of cimetidine therapy. *N Engl J Med* 1979; 300:94.
45. Van Thiel PH, Gavaler BS, Smith WI, Paul G. Hypothalamic–pituitary–gonadal dysfunction in men using cimetidine. *N Engl J Med* 1979; 300:1012–1015.
46. Peden N.R., Wormsley, K.G. Effect of cimetidine on gonadal function in man [Letter to the editor]. *Br J Clin Pharmacol* 1982; 14:565.
47. Trieschmann RB. *Spinal cord injuries: psychological, social and vocational adjustment, 2nd ed.* New York: Pergamon, 1988.
48. Masters WH, Johnson VE. *Human sexual inadequacy.* Boston: Little, Brown, 1970.
49. Taylor SE. Adjustment to threatening events: a theory of cognitive adaptation. *Am Psychologist* 1983; 38(11):1161–1173.
50. Erikson EH. *Identity: youth and crisis.* New York: Norton, 1968..
51. Bors E, Comarr AE. Neurological disturbances of sexual function with special reference to 529 patients with spinal cord injury. *Urol Surv* 1960; 110:191.
52. Talbot HS. The sexual function in paraplegia. *J Urol* 1955; 73:91.
53. Comarr AE, Vigue M. Sexual counseling among male and female patients with spinal cord injury and/or cauda equina injury. *Am J Phys Med* 1978; 57:107–122,216–227.
54. Geiger RC. Neurophysiology of sexual response in spinal cord injury. *Sex Disabil* 1979; 2(4):257–266.
55. Berard EJJ. The sexuality of spinal cord injured women: physiology and pathophysiology. A review. *Paraplegia* 1989; 27:99–112.
56. Sipski ML, Alexander CJ, Rosen RC. Physiologic parameters associated with psychogenic sexual arousal in women with complete spinal cord injuries. *Arch Phys Med Rehabil* 1995; 76:811–818.
57. Phelps G, Brown M, Chen J, et al. Sexual experience and plasma testosterone levels in male veterans after spinal cord injury. *Arch Phys Med Rehabil* 1983; 64:47–52.
58. Alexander CJ, Sipski ML, Findley TW. Sexual activities, desire, and satisfaction in males pre- and post-spinal cord injury. *Arch Sex Behav* 1993; 22(3):217–228.
59. Charlifue SW, Gerhart KA, Menter RR, Whiteneck GG, Manley MS. Sexual issues of women with spinal cord injuries. *Paraplegia* 1992; 30:192–199.
60. Willmuth ME. Sexuality after spinal cord injury: a critical review. *Clin Psychol Rev* 1987; 7:389–412.
61. Sjogren K and Egberg K. The sexual experience in younger males with complete spinal cord injury. *Scand J Rehabil Med [Suppl]* 1983; 9189–194.
62. Berkman AH, Weissman R, Frielich MH. Sexual adjustment of spinal cord injured veterans living in the community. *Arch Phys Med Rehabil* 1978; 59:29–33.
63. Sipski ML, Alexander CJ. Sexual activities, response and satisfaction in women pre- and post-spinal cord injury. *Arch Phys Med Rehabil* 1993; 74:1025–1029.
64. Alexander CJ, Sipski ML, Findley TW. Sexual activities, desire, and satisfaction in males pre- and post-spinal cord injury. *Arch Sex Behav* 1993; 22(3):217–228.
65. Linsenmeyer TA, Perkash I. Infertility in men with spinal cord injury. *Arch Phys Med Rehabil* 1991; 72:747–754.
66. Linsenmeyer TA, Pogach LM, Ottenweller JE, Huang HFS. Spermatogenesis and the pituitary–testicular hormone axis in rats during the acute phase of spinal cord injury. *J Urol* 1994; 152:1302–1307.
67. Linsenmeyer TA. Management of male infertility. In: Sipski ML, Alexander CJ, eds. *Sexual function in people with disability and chronic illness: a health professional's guide.* Gaithersburg, MD: Aspen Publishers, 1997; 24:487–509.
68. Horne HW, Paul DA, Munro D. Fertility studies in the human male with traumatic injuries of the spinal cord and cauda equina. *N Engl J Med* 1948; 239:959–951.
69. Thomas RJS, McLeish G, McDonald IA. Electroejaculation of the paraplegic male followed by pregnancy. *Med J Aust* 1975; 2:798–799.
70. Sonksen J, Biering-Sorensen F, Kristensen JK. Ejaculation induced

by penile vibratory stimulation in men with spinal cord injuries. The importance of the vibratory amplitude. *Paraplegia* 1994; 32:651–660.

71. Ohl DA, Menge AC, Sonksen J. Penile vibratory stimulation in spinal cord injured men: optimized vibration parameters and prognostic factors. *Arch Phys Med Rehabil* 1996; 77:903–905.
72. Ohl DA, Denil J, Fitzgerald-Shelton K, McCabe M, McGuire EJ, Menge AC, Randolph JF. Fertility of spinal cord injured males: effect of genitourinary infection and bladder management on results of electroejaculation. *J Am Paraplegia Soc* 1992; 15(2):53–59.
73. Axel SJ. Spinal cord injured women's concerns: menstruation and pregnancy. *Rehabil Nurs* 1982; 7(5):10–15.
74. Baker ER, Cardenas DD. Pregnancy in spinal cord injured women. *Arch Phys Med Rehabil* 1996; 77:501–507.
75. Feyi-Waboso PA. An audit of five years experience of pregnancy in spinal cord damaged women: a regional unit's experience and a review of the literature. *Paraplegia* 1992; 30:631–635.
76. Westgren N, Hultling C, Levi R, Westgren M. Pregnancy and delivery in women with a traumatic spinal cord injury in Sweden, 1980–1991. *Obstet Gynecol* 1993; 81:926–930.
77. Robertson DNS, Guttman L. The paraplegic patient in pregnancy and labour. *Proc R Soc Med* 1963; 56:381–387.
78. Wanner MB, Rageth CJ, Zach GA. Pregnancy and autonomic hyperreflexia in patients with spinal cord lesions. *Paraplegia* 1987; 25: 482–490.
79. Valleroy ML, Kraft G. Sexual dysfunction in multiple sclerosis. *Arch Phys Med Rehabil* 1984; 65:125–128.
80. Mattson DH, Petrie M, Srivastava DK, McDermott M. Multiple sclerosis—sexual dysfunction and its response to medications. *Arch Neurol* 1995; 52:862–868.
81. Smeltzer SC, Kelley LC. Multiple sclerosis. In: Sipski ML, Alexander CJ, eds. *Sexual function in people with disability and chronic illness: a health professional's guide.* Gaithersburg, MD: Aspen Publishers, 1997; 10:177–188.
82. Birk K, Rudick R. Pregnancy and multiple sclerosis. *Arch Neurol* 1986; 43:719–726.
83. Korn-Lubetzki I, Kahana E, Cooper G. Activity of multiple sclerosis during pregnancy and puerperium. *Ann Neurol* 1984; 16:229–231.
84. Thompson DS, Nelson LM, Burns A, Burks JS, Franklin GM. The effect of pregnancy in multiple sclerosis: a retrospective study. *Neurology* 1986; 36:1097–1099.
85. Weinshenker BG, Hader W, Carriere W, Baskerville J, Ebers GC. The influence of pregnancy on disability from multiple sclerosis: a population-based study in Middlesex County, Ontario. *Neurology* 1989; 39:1438–1440.
86. Monga TN, Kerrigan AJ. Cerebrovascular accidents. In: Sipski ML, Alexander CJ, eds. *Sexual function in people with disability and chronic illness: a health professional's guide*. Gaithersburg, MD: Aspen Publishers, 1997; 11:189–219.
87. Monga TN, Lawson JS, Inglis J. Sexual dysfunction in stroke patients. *Arch Phys Med Rehabil* 1986; 67(1):19–22.
88. Sjogren K, Damber JE, Liliequist B. Sexuality after stroke with hemiplegia. 1. Aspects of sexual function. *Scand J Rehabil Med* 1983; 15: 55–61.
89. Bray GP, DeFrank RS, Wolfe TL. Sexual functioning in stroke patients. *Arch Phys Med Rehabil* 1981; 62(6):286–288.
90. Boldrini P, Basaglia N, Calanca MC. Sexual changes in hemiparetic patients. *Arch Phys Med Rehabil* 1991; 72:202–207.
91. Aloni R, Ring H, Rozenthul N, Schwart J. Sexual function in male patients after stroke. A follow-up study. *Sex Disabil* 1993; 11(2): 121–128.
92. Kalliomaki JL, Markkanen TK, Mustonen VA. Sexual behavior after cerebral vascular accident: study on patients below age 60 years. *Fertil Steril* 1961; 12:156–158.
93. Kinsella GH, Duffy FD. Psychosocial readjustment in the spouses of aphasic patients: a comparative survey of 79 subjects. *Scand J Rehabil Med* 1979; 11(3):129–132.
94. Elovic E, Antoinette T. Epidemiology and primary prevention of traumatic brain injury. In: Horn LJ, Zasler ND, eds. *Medical rehabilitation of traumatic brain injury*. Philadelphia: Hanley and Belfus, 1996; 1–28.
95. Meyer JE. Die sexuellen storungen der hirnverletzten. *Arch Psychiatr Z Neurol* 1955; 193:449–469.
96. Walker AE, Jablon S. *A follow-up study of head wounds in World War II.* Washington, DC: Veterans Administration Medical Monograph, 1961.
97. Garden FH, Bonke CF, Hoffman M. Sexual functioning and marital adjustment after traumatic brain injury. *J Head Trauma Rehabil* 1990; 5:52–59.
98. Boller F, Frank E. *Sexual dysfunction in neurologic disorders: diagnosis, management and rehabilitation.* New York: Raven Press, 1982.
99. MacLean O. Brain mechanisms of primal sexual functions and related behavior. In: Sandler M, Gessa G, eds. *Sexual behavior: pharmacology and biochemistry.* New York: Raven Press, 1975.
100. Blendonohy P, Philip P. Precocious puberty in children after traumatic brain injury. *Brain Injury* 1991; 5:63–68.
101. Sandel ME. Traumatic brain injury. In: Sipski ML, Alexander CJ, eds. *Sexual function in people with disability and chronic illness: a health professional's guide.* Gaithersburg, MD: Aspen Publishers, 1997; 12:221–245.
102. Horn LJ, Zasler ND. Neuroanatomy and neurophysiology of sexual dysfunction. *J Head Trauma Rehabil* 1990; 5:1–13.
103. Heath RG. Pleasure response of human subjects to direct stimulation of the brain: physiologic and psycho-dynamic considerations. In: Heath RG, ed. *The role of pleasure in behavior.* New York: Harper & Row, 1964.
104. Kluver H, Bucy PC. Preliminary analysis of functions of temporal lobes in monkeys. *Arch Neurol Psychiatry* 1939; 42:979–1000.
105. Lilly R. The human Kluver-Bucy syndrome. *Neurology* 1983; 33: 1141.
106. Mesulum M. *Principles of behavioral neurology.* Philadelphia: FA Davis, 1985.
107. Miller B, Cummings J, McIntyre H, et al. Hypersexuality or altered sexual preference following brain injury. *J Neurol Neurosurg Psychiatry* 1986; 49:867–873.
108. Sandel ME, Williams KS, DellaPietra L, Derogatis LR. Sexual functioning following traumatic brain injury. *Brain Inj* 1996; 10:719–728.
109. Blake DJ, Maisiak R, Alarcon GS, Brown S. Sexual quality of life of patients with arthritis compared to arthritis-free controls. *J Rheumatol* 1987; 14:570–576.
110. Pigg JS, Schroeder PM. Frequently occurring problems of patients with rheumatic disease. The ANA outcome standards for rheumatology nursing practice. *Nurs Clin North Am* 1984; 19(4):697–708.
111. Lipe H, Longstreth WT, Bird TD, Linde M. Sexual function in married men with Parkinson's disease compared to married men with arthritis. *Neurology* 1990; 40:1347–1349.
112. Conine TA, Evans JH. Sexual reactivation of chronically ill and disabled adults. *J Allied Health* 1982; 11:261–270.
113. Gordon D, Beastall GH, Thomson JA, Sturrock RD. Androgenic status and sexual function in males with rheumatoid arthritis and ankylosing spondylitis. *Q J Med* 1986; 231:671–679.
114. Yoshino S, Uchida S. Sexual problems of women with rheumatoid arthritis. *Arch Phys Med Rehabil* 1981; 62:122–123.
115. Bhadauria S, Moser DK, Clements PJ, Singh RR, Lachenbruch PA, Pitkin RM, Weiner SR. Genital tract abnormalities and female sexual function impairment in systemic sclerosis. *Am J Obstet Gynecol* 1995; 172:580–587.
116. Curry SL, Levine SB, Conty E, Jones PK, Kurit DM. The impact of systemic lupus erythematosus on women's sexual functioning. *J Rheum* 1994; 21:2254–2260.
117. Lally EV, Jimenez SA. Erectile failure in systemic sclerosis. *N Engl J Med* 1990; 322:1398.
118. Simeon CP, Fonollosa V, Vilardell M, Ordi J, Solans R, Lima J. Impotence and Peyronie's disease in systemic sclerosis. *Clin Exp Rheumatol* 1994; 12:464.
119. Saad CS, Behrendt AE. Scleroderma and sexuality. *J Sex Res* 1996; 33:215–220.
120. Buckwalter KC, Wernimont T, Buckwalter JA. Musculoskeletal conditions and sexuality (Part I). *Sex Disabil* 1982; 4(3):131–142.
121. Currey HLF. Osteoarthritis of the hip joint and sexual activity. *Ann Rheum Dis* 1970; 29:488–493.
122. Stern SH, Fuchs MD, Ganz SB, Classi P, Sculco TP, Salvati EA. Sexual function after total hip arthroplasty. *Clin Orthop Rel Res* 1991; 269:228–235.
123. Nadler SN. Arthritis and other connective tissue diseases. In: Sipski ML, Alexander CJ, eds. *Sexual function in people with disability and chronic illness: a health professional's guide.* Gaithersburg, MD: Aspen Publishers, 1997; 14:261–278.

124. Karan JH, Forsham PH. Pancreatic hormones and diabetes mellitus. In: Greenspan FS, Baxter JD, eds. *Basic and clinical endocrinology.* Norwalk, CT: Appleton & Lange, 1994; 50.
125. Tilton MC. Diabetes and amputation. In: Sipski ML, Alexander CJ, eds. *Sexual function in people with disability and chronic illness: a health professional's guide.* Gaithersburg, MD: Aspen Publishers, 1997; 15:279–302.
126. Faerman I, Jadzinsky M, Podolsky S. Diabetic neuropathy and sexual dysfunction. In: Podolsky S, ed. *Clinical diabetes: modern management* New York: Appleton-Century-Crofts, 1980; 306–316.
127. McCulloch DK, Young RJ, Prescott RJ, Campbell IW, Clarke BF. The natural history of impotence in diabetic men. *Diabetologia* 1984; 26:437–440.
128. Melman A, Henry DP, Felten DL, O'Connor B. Effect of diabetes upon penile sympathetic nerves in impotent patients. *South Med J* 1980; 73(3):307–317.
129. Baum N, Neiman M, Lewis R. Evaluation and treatment of organic impotence in the male with diabetes mellitus. *Diabetes Educ* 1988; 14(2):123–129.
130. Faerman I, Glocer L, Fox D, Jadzinsky MN, Rapaport M. Impotence and diabetes: histological studies of the autonomic nervous fibers of the corpora cavernosa in impotent diabetic males. *Diabetes* 1974; 23(12):971–976.
131. Buvat J, Lemaire A, Buvat-Herbaut M, Guidu JD, Bailleul JP, Fossati P. Comparative investigations in 26 impotent and 26 nonimpotent diabetic patients. *J Urol* 1985; 133:34–38.
132. Jensen SB. Diabetic sexual dysfunction: a comparative study of 160 insulin treated diabetic men and women and an age-matched control group. *Arch Sex Behav* 1981; 10(6):493–504.
133. Tyrer G, Steel JM, Ewing DJ, Bancroft J, Werner P, Clarke BF. Sexual responsiveness in diabetic women. *Diabetologia* 1983; 24:166–171.
134. Whitley M, Berke P. Sexuality and diabetes. In: Woods NF, ed. *Human sexuality in health and illness.* St Louis: CV Mosby, 1984; 328–340.
135. Leedom L, Feldman M, Procci W, Zeidler A. Symptoms of sexual dysfunction and depression in diabetic women. *J Diabetic Complic* 1991; 5(1):38–41.
136. Albert A, Wincze JP. *Sexual arousal in diabetic females: a psychophysiological investigation.* Unpublished manuscript, Brown University, 1990.
137. Campbell LV, Redelman MJ, Borkman M, McLay JG, Chisholm DJ. Factors in sexual dysfunction in diabetic female volunteer subjects. *Med J Aust* 1989; 151:550–552.
138. Kolodny RC. Sexual dysfunction in diabetic females. *Diabetes* 1971; 20:557–559.
139. Zrustova M, Rostlaplil J, Kabrhelova A. Sexual disorders in diabetic women. *Csek Gynekol* 1978; 43:277–281.
140. Ellenberg M. Sexual aspects of the female diabetic. *Mt Sinai J Med* 1977; 44:495–499.
141. Williams RH. The endocrine pancreas and diabetes mellitus. In: Williams RH, ed. *Textbook of endocrinology.* Philadelphia: WB Saunders, 1981:831.
142. Hare JW. Diabetes and pregnancy. In: Kahn CR, Weir GC, eds. *Joslin's diabetes mellitus.* Philadelphia: Lea & Febiger, 1994; 889–899.
143. Rybarczyk B, Nyenhuis DL, Nicholas JJ, Cash SM, Kaiser J. Body image, perceived social stigma, the prediction of psychosocial adjustment to leg amputation. *Rehabil Psychol* 1995; 40(2):95–110.
144. Blocker WP Jr. Coronary heart disease and sexuality. In: *Physical medicine and rehabilitation: state of the art reviews, vol 9.* Philadelphia: Hanley and Belfus, 1995; 387.
145. Papadopoulos C, Beaumont C, Shelley SI, Larrimore P. Myocardial infarction and sexual activity of the female patient. *Arch Intern Med* 1983; 143:1528–1530.
146. Mehta J, Krop H. The effect of myocardial infarction on sexual functioning. *Sex Disabil* 1979; 2:115–121.
147. Blocker WP. Cardiac rehabilitation. In: Halstead L, Grabois M, eds. *Medical rehabilitation.* New York: Raven Press, 1985; 181–192.
148. Muller JE, Mittleman MA, Maclure M, Sherwood JB, Tofler GH. Triggering myocardial infarction by sexual activity: low absolute risk and prevention by regular physical exertion. *JAMA* 1996; 275: 1405–1409.
149. Cassem NH, Hackett TP. Physiological rehabilitation of myocardial infarction patients in the acute phase. *Heart Lung* 1973; 2:382–388.
150. Stitik TP, Benevento BT. Cardiac and pulmonary disease. In: Sipski ML, Alexander CJ, eds. *Sexual function in people with disability and chronic illness: a health professional's giude.* Gaithersburg, MD: Aspen Publishers, 1997; 16:303–335.
151. Hamilton GA, Seidman RN. A comparison of the recovery period for women and men after an acute myocardial infarction. *Heart Lung* 1993; 22:308–315.
152. Conine TA, Evans JH. Sexual reactivation of chronically ill and disabled adults. *J Allied Health* 1982; 264:261–270.
153. Cohen JA. Sexual counseling of the patient following myocardial infarction. *Crit Care Nurs* 1986; 6(6):18–29.
154. Skinner JB. Sexual relations and the cardiac patient. In: Pollock ML, Schmat DH, eds. *Heart disease and rehabilitation.* New York: John Wiley & Sons, 1986; 583–589.
155. Hellerstein HK, Friedman EH. Sexual activity and the postcoronary patient. *Med Aspects Hum Sexuality* 1969; 3(3):70–96.
156. Bohlen JG, Held JP, Sanderson MO, Patterson RP. Heart rate, rate pressure product and oxygen uptake during four sexual activities. *Arch Intern Med* 1984; 144:1745–1748.
157. Elster SE, Mansfield LW. Stair climbing as a test of readiness for resumption of sexual activity after a heart attack (abstracted). *Circulation* 1977; 55–56(Suppl III):102.
158. Drory Y, Shapira I, Fisman E, Pines A. Myocardial ischemia during sexual activity in patients with coronary artery disease. *Am J Cardiol* 1995; 75:835–837.
159. Scalzi CC. Sexual counseling and sexual therapy for patients after myocardial infarction. *Cardiovasc Nurs* 1982; 18:13–17.
160. McCauley K, Choromanski JD, Wallinger C, Liu K. Learning to live with controlled ventricular tachycardia: utilizing the Johnson model. *Heart Lung* 1984; 13(6):637.
161. Griffith GC. Sexuality and the cardiac patient. *Heart Lung* 1973; 2: 70–73.
162. Masur FT. Resumption of sexual activity following myocardial infarction. *Sex Disabil* 1979; 2:98–114.
163. Abbott MA, McWhirter DP. Resuming sexual activity after myocardial infarction. *Med Aspects Hum Sexuality* 1978; 12(6):18–28.
164. Semmler C, Semmler M. Counseling the coronary patient. *Am J Occup Ther* 1974; 28:609–614.
165. Eliot RS, Miles RR. Advising the cardiac patient about sexual intercourse. *Med Aspects Hum Sexuality* 1975; 9(6):49–50.
166. Friedman JM. Sexual adjustment of the postcoronary male. In: LoPicolo J, LoPicolo L, eds. *Handbook of sex therapy.* New York: Plenum Press, 1978.
167. Koller R, Kennedy KW, Butler JC, Wagner NN. Counseling the coronary patient on sexual activity. *Postgrad Med* 1972; 51(4):133–136.
168. Wagner NN. Sexual activity and the cardiac patient. In: Green R, ed. *Human sexuality: a health practitioner's text.* Baltimore: Williams & Wilkins, 1975; 173–179.
169. Plummer JK. Psychosocial factors in pulmonary rehabilitation. In: O'Ryan, Burns, eds. *Pulmonary rehabilitation from hospital to home.* Chicago: Year Book Medical Publishers, 1984.
170. Hahn K. Sexuality and COPD. *Rehabil Nurs* 1989; 14(4):191–195.
171. Rabinowitz B, Florian V. Chronic obstructive pulmonary disease—psychosocial issues and treatment goals. *Social Work Health Care* 1992; 16(4):60–86.
172. Fletcher EC, Martin R. Sexual dysfunction and erectile impotence in chronic obstructive pulmonary disease. *Chest* 1982; 81:4.
173. Levine SB, Stern RC. Sexual function in cystic fibrosis: relationship to overall health status and pulmonary disease severity in 30 married patients. *Chest* 1982; 81(4):422–428.
174. Kaplan E, Shwachman H, Perlmuter AD, Rule A, Khaw K-T, Holsclaw DS. Reproductive failure in males with cystic fibrosis. *N Engl J Med* 1968; 279:65–69.
175. Stern RC, Boat TF. Doershuk cystic fibrosis. Obstructive azoospermia as a diagnostic criterion for cystic fibrosis syndrome. *Lancet* 1983; 1:1401–1404.
176. Fogdestam I, Hamberger L, Ludin K, Sjogren A, Hjelte L, Strandvik B. Successful pregnancies after in vitro fertilization with sperm from men with cystic fibrosis. Paper presented at 19th European Cystic Fibrosis Conference, 1994.
177. Campbell M. Sexual dysfunction in the COPD patient. *Dimensions Crit Care Nurs* 1987; 6(2):70–74.
178. Thompson WL. Sexual problems in chronic respiratory disease: achieving and maintaining intimacy. *Postgrad Med* 1986; 79:41–52.

179. American Cancer Society. *Cancer facts & figures—1995*. New York: American Cancer Society, 1995.
180. Waldman TL, Eliasof B. Cancer. In: Sipski ML, Alexander CJ, eds. *Sexual function in people with disability and chronic illness: a health professional's guide*. Gaithersburg, MD: Aspen Publishers, 1997; 17: 337–354.
181. Brender C, Walsh P. Prostate cancer: evaluation and radiotherapeutic management. *CA Cancer J Clin* 1992; 42:223–240.
182. Perez CA, Fair WR, Ihde DC. Carcinoma of the prostate. In: DeVita VT, Hellman S, Rosenberg S, eds. *Cancer principles and practice of oncology, 3rd ed.* Boston: Jones & Bartlett, 1989; 1023–1058.
183. Heinrich-Rynning T. Prostatic cancer treatments and their effects on sexual function. *Oncol Nurs Forum* 1987; 14(6):37–41.
184. Porter A, Forman J. Prostate brachytherapy: an overview. *Cancer* 1993; 71(Suppl 3):953–958.
185. Taylor R. Endocrine therapy for advanced stage D prostate cancer. *Urol Nurs* 1991; 11(3):22–26.
186. Krebs LU. Sexual and reproductive dysfunction. In: Groenwald SL, Goodman M, Frogge MH, Yarbro CH, eds. *Cancer nursing: principles and practice*. Boston: Jones & Bartlett, 1993; 697–719.
187. Anderson BL, Lamb MA. Sexuality and cancer. In: *Textbook of clinical oncology*. 1995; 700–711.
188. Kaplan HS. A neglected issue: the sexual side effects of current treatments for breast cancer, *J Sex Marital Ther* 1992; 18(1):3–19.
189. Lamb M. Alterations in sexuality and sexual functioning. In: Baird SB, McCorkle R, Grant M, eds. *Cancer nursing: a comprehensive textbook*. Philadelphia: WB Saunders, 1991; 831–849.
190. Vera MI. Quality of life following pelvic exenteration. *Gynecol Oncol* 1981; 12; 355–366.
191. Auchincloss SS. Sexual dysfunction in cancer patients: issues in evaluation and treatment. In: Holland JC, Rowland JH, eds. *Handbook of psychooncology: psychological care of the patient with cancer*. New York: Oxford University Press, 1989; 383–413.
192. Hubbard JL, Shingleton HM. Sexual function of patients after cancer of the cervix treatment. *Clin Obstet Gynecol* 1985; 12:247–264.
193. Grunberg KJ. Sexual rehabilitation of the cancer patient undergoing ostomy surgery. *J Enterostom Ther* 1986; 13:148–152.
194. Annon J. *The behavioral treatment of sexual problems: brief therapy*. New York: Harper & Row, 1976.
195. Pauly IH, Goldstein SG. Prevalence of sexual dysfunction. *Med Aspects Hum Sexuality* 1970; 4:48–52.
196. Burnap DW, Golden JS. Sexual problems in medical practice. *J Med Educ* 1967; 42:673–680.
197. Stuntz RC. Assessment of organic factors in sexual dysfunctions. In Brown RA, Field JR, eds. *Treatment of sexual problems in individual and couples therapy*. Columbia, MD: PMA, 1988; 187–207.
198. Schover LR. Sexual problems in chronic illness. In Leiblum SR, Rosen RC, eds. *Principles and practice of sex therapy: update for the 1990s, 2nd ed.* New York: Guilford Press, 1989; 319–351.
199. Romano M. Sexuality and the disabled female. *Accent on Living* 1973; Winter:27–34.
200. Claes H, Baert L. Transcutaneous nitroglycerin therapy in the treatment of impotence. *Urol Int* 1989; 44:309–312.
201. Meyhoff HH, Rosenkilde P, Bodker A. Non-invasive management of impotence with transcutaneous nitroglycerin. *Br J Urol* 1992; 69: 88–90.
202. Sonksen J, Biering-Sorensen F. Transcutaneous nitroglycerin in the treatment of erectile dysfunction in spinal cord injured. *Paraplegia* 1992; 30:554–557.
203. Cavallini G. Minoxidil versus nitroglycerin: a prospective double-blind controlled trial in transcutaneous erection facilitation for organic impotence. *J Urol* 1991; 146:50–53.
204. Radomsky SB, Herschorn S, Rangaswamy S. Topical minoxidil in the treatment of male erectile dysfunction. *J Urol* 1994; 151:1225–1226.
205. Chancellor MB, Rivas DA, Panzer DE, Freedman MK, Staas WE. Prospective comparison of topical minoxidil to vacuum constriction device and intracorporal papaverine injection in the treatment of erectile dysfunction due to spinal cord injury. *Urology* 1994; 43:365–369.
206. Wolfson B, Pickett S, Scott NE, DeKernion JB, Rajfer J. Intraurethral prostaglandin E_2 cream: a possible alternative treatment for erectile dysfunction. *Urology* 1993; 42:73–75.
207. Smith EM, Bodner DR. Sexual dysfunction after spinal cord injury. *Urol Clinic North Am* 1993; 20:535–542.
208. Ashton AK, Hamer R, Rosen RC. SSRI-induced sexual dysfunction and its treatment: a large-scale retrospective study of 596 psychiatric outpatients. (in press).
209. Zorgniotti AW, Lizza AF. On demand oral drugs for erection on impotent men. *J Urol* 1993; 147:308A.
210. Eardley I, Morgan RJ, Dinsmore WW, Pearson J, Wulff MB, Boolell M. A new oral therapy for erectile dysfunction. A double-blind, placebo controlled trial with treatment taken as required. *J Urol* 1996; 155:495A.
211. Gingell JCJ, Jardin A, Olsson AM, Dinsmore WW, Osterloh IA, Kirkpatrick J, Cuddigan M, Multicenter Study Group. UK-92,480, A new oral treatment for erectile dysfunction: a double-blind, placebo controlled, once daily dosage response study. *J Urol* 1996; 155:495A.
212. Boolell M, Gepi-Attee S, Gingell C, Allen M. A new oral treatment for erectile dysfunction. A double-blind, placebo-controlled study demonstrating dose response with Rigiscan and efficacy with outpatient diary. *J Urol* 1996; 155:495A.
213. Rivas DA, Chancellor MB. Management of erective dysfunction. In: Sipski ML, Alexander CJ, eds. *Sexual function in people with disability and chronic illness: a health professional's guide*. Gaithersburg, MD: Aspen Publishers, 1997; 22:429–464.
214. Wein AJ, Malloy TR, Hanno PM. Intracavernosal injection programs—their place in management of erectile dysfunction. *Prob Urol* 1987; 1:496–506.
215. Linet OI, Ogrinc FG. Efficacy and safety of intracavernosal alprostadil in men with erectile dysfunction. *N Engl J Med* 1996; 334:873–877.
216. Lakin MM, Montague DR, Vanderbrug MS, Tesar L, Schover LR. Intracavernous injection therapy: analysis of results and complications. *J Urol* 1990; 143:1138–1141.
217. Lue TF, Tanagho EA. Physiology of erection and pharmacological management of impotence. *J Urol* 1987; 137:829–836.
218. Lewis RW. Long-term results of penile prosthetic implants. *Urol Clin North Am* 1995; 22:847–855.
219. Rossier AB, Fam BA. Indication and results of semirigid penile prostheses in spinal cord injury patients: long-term follow-up. *J Urol* 1984; 131:59–62.
220. Kabalin JN, Kessler R. Infectious complications of penile prosthesis surgery. *J Urol* 1988; 139:953–955.
221. Spector I, Carey M. Incidence and prevalence of the sexual dysfunctions. a critical review of the empirical literature. *Arch Sex Behav* 1990; 19:389–408.
222. Rosen RC, Leiblum SR. Treatment of sexual disorders in the 1990s: an integrated approach. *J Consult Clin Psychol* 1995; 63(6):877–890.
223. McCarthy BW. Cognitive-behavioral strategies and techniques in the treatment of early ejaculation. In: Leiblum SR, Rosen RC, eds. *Principles and practice of sex therapy*. New York: Guilford Press, 1989; 141–167.
224. American Psychiatric Association. *Diagnostic and statistical manual of mental disorders, 4th ed.* Washington, DC: American Psychiatric Association, 1994.
225. Ducharme S, Gill K. Management of other male sexual dysfunctions. In: Sipski ML, Alexander CJ, eds. *Sexual function in people with disability and chronic illness: a health professional's guide*. Gaithersburg, MD: Aspen Publishers, 1997; 23:465–485.
226. Tordjman G. A new therapeutic perspective for premature ejaculation disorder. *Cah Sexol Clin* 1993; 10:5–6.
227. Whipple B, McGreer KB. Management of female sexual dysfunction. In: Sipski ML, Alexander CJ, eds. *Sexual function in people with disability and chronic illness: a health professional's guide*. Gaithersburg, MD: Aspen Publishers, 1997; 25:511–536.

Rehabilitation Medicine: Principles and Practice, Third Edition, edited by Joel A. DeLisa and Bruce M. Gans. Lippincott–Raven Publishers, Philadelphia © 1998.

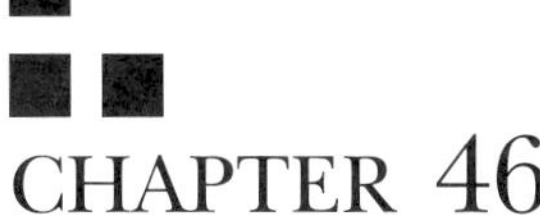

CHAPTER 46

Medical Emergencies in Rehabilitation Medicine

Keith M. Robinson, Eugenia L. Siegler, and Joel E. Streim

Dorland's Illustrated Medical Dictionary defines an emergency as "an un-looked for or sudden occasion; an accident; an urgent or pressing need" (1). This definition must be broadened within the context of rehabilitation, where medical emergencies include life-threatening events as well as events that interfere with rehabilitation interventions and functional progress.

MORE EMERGENCIES ARE EXPECTED IN REHABILITATION

Several demographic and epidemiologic observations support the expectation that medical emergencies occur commonly in rehabilitation settings:

More older people are participating in rehabilitation (2). Although the absolute life span of the population has not increased, more people are living over the age of 65 years. The fastest growing segment of the elderly is the group over the age of 85 years (3–5). Gerontologists have characterized usual anatomic and physiological aging as a linear decrease in reserve capacity of organ systems (6,7). The elderly have less adaptive resilience in response to stressors such as acute illness and rehabilitation interventions. The prevalence of comorbidity and associated functional disability increases with age (8,9). In addition, in the United States, older patients are not spared interventions that make use of highly technological life-saving procedures (10,11) despite increased vulnerability to undesirable complications in response to these interventions (12).

Sicker people are participating in rehabilitation. Rehabilitation personnel are expected to intervene when patients still are acutely ill. As highly technological interventions are saving lives of those who have sustained spinal cord injury, traumatic brain injury, and multiple trauma, so early rehabilitation is preventing secondary disability. In addition, early rehabilitation interventions during the course of an illness, such as cerebrovascular accident, may shorten length of hospital stay, promote improved functional outcome, and ultimately may contribute toward containing health care costs (13). Over the last 15 years, the prospective payment and managed care systems have created financial disincentives to provide prolonged acute care services in hospitals. As long as rehabilitation facilities continue their diagnostic-related group-exempt status from prospective payment formulas, physicians will be encouraged to discharge patients early from acute care hospitals to inpatient rehabilitation facilities or to community settings with home or outpatient rehabilitation services (14,15). Moreover, the impact of "managed care" systems of health services reimbursement have reinforced the financial disincentives for prolonged acute hospital-based care, including hospital-based rehabilitation. Sicker people, thus, are moving through acute medical/surgical and rehabilitation services at a more rapid pace, often continuing their rehabilitation programs in less intensive and less expensive settings such as skilled nursing facilities and at home (15–18).

More people with chronic diseases that are treated with highly technical surgical and medical interventions are participating in rehabilitation. Such patients include those who are immunocompromised from human immunodeficiency virus (HIV) or immune-suppressive therapies (19,20), those who have undergone organ transplantation (21–23), and those with end-stage or intractable medical problems such as

K. M. Robinson: Department of Rehabilitation Medicine, University of Pennsylvania Health System, Philadelphia, Pennsylvania 19104.

E. L. Siegler: Department of Medicine, New York University School of Medicine, Brooklyn Hospital Center, Brooklyn, New York 11201.

J. E. Streim: Departments of Psychiatry and Rehabilitation Medicine, Hospital of The University of Pennsylvania, Philadelphia, Pennsylvania 19104-2676.

renal failure (24,25), chronic obstructive pulmonary disease (26,27), or cardiomyopathies with low ejection fractions (28,29). In these patients, sophisticated medical and technological regimens must be integrated into the rehabilitation program, regardless of the setting provided.

Medicare has continued to reinforce the financial incentives for inpatient rehabilitation for more acutely ill patients, given its more liberal definition of the "3-hour rule." Patients in rehabilitation hospitals are expected to participate in at least 3 hours of rehabilitation services per day to qualify for this intensive and expensive level of services. Since 1990, the rule has become less focused on specific therapy services such as physical therapy and occupational therapy and instead embraces a broader constellation of rehabilitation services including medical services, physical therapy, occupational therapy, speech therapy, orthotics and prosthetics services, as well as rehabilitation nursing, social work, and psychological services (30).

This broader interpretation of the 3-hour rule supports the treatment of acute medical problems such as deep venous thrombosis (DVT), pneumonia, and bacteremia in inpatient rehabilitation settings, with the expectation that the progress and functional trajectory may be interrupted many times during the course of a rehabilitation hospital stay. The patient may not necessarily require readmission to the acute medical/surgical services unless in need of an intensive care unit, a major surgical procedure, or prolonged diagnostic investigation. Additionally, many "managed care" health insurance plans, as well as Medicare, will not pay for hospital-based inpatient rehabilitation programs unless medical justification explicitly can be defined to keep patients in a hospital setting. Thus, those patients expected to be medically unstable during their progression through functionally oriented therapeutic exercise programs merit hospital-based rehabilitation programs. Otherwise, less expensive settings for participating in rehabilitation programs are sought (15–17).

Cost-containment strategies, such as algorithmic application of critical pathways that intend to guide acute and rehabilitation treatments on a day-to-day basis, are presently being applied. These strategies typically do not consider acute or life-threatening complications that prolong hospital stay in patients participating in hospital-based rehabilitation programs. As experience grows using these strategies, there appears to be less incentive to treat these complications in hospital-based rehabilitation facilities because there is uncertain guarantee for being appropriately reimbursed; treating acute medical comorbid conditions will extend the rehabilitation stay beyond that initially predicated and contracted for. Thus, the pattern of future treatment of medical/surgical problems likely to interrupt inpatient rehabilitation programs in rehabilitation facilities remains unclear. The reimbursement process for rehabilitation will most likely continue to determine where these patients are treated.

Thus, demographic trends, the increased sophistication of medical and surgical interventions, and social policies directed toward cost containment are creating a rehabilitation population at greater risk for developing medical emergencies that may interfere with traditional rehabilitation interventions. Rehabilitation professionals are expected to prevent emergencies by anticipating the anatomic and pathophysiological impact of rehabilitation interventions in these high-risk patients.

THE ROLE OF THE PHYSIATRIST

Appropriate management of rehabilitation patients requires that physiatrists become the "gatekeepers" of medical and nonmedical services when patients are participating in rehabilitation (31,32). Promoted among the medical specialties of internal medicine, family practice, and pediatrics, the "gatekeeping" model requires that physiatrists become both the general coordinator of medical services and the medical specialist in disability. The physiatrist must provide primary medical care alone or in consultation with general medical and surgical health care providers in all rehabilitation settings (33). This role includes knowing when to request early consultation to prevent minor medical problems from developing into major ones.

Many of the mistakes made in requesting assistance from medical colleagues can be viewed as the failure to recognize that a problem is developing, or the failure to use consultants effectively. Goldman and colleagues described how to perform effective medical consultations (34). Physiatrists requesting medical consultation can obtain the best results by using the following guidelines:

- Ask specific questions.
- Evaluate the patient before the consultant does and have sufficient information (for example, vital signs, mental status examination) at hand to allow the consultant to determine urgency.
- Communicate over the phone or in person, not through the chart.
- Learn from the consultant. The consultation is both a management and an educational tool.
- Consult one physician at a time. It usually is best to begin with the general medical consultant, allowing her or him to serve as auxiliary "gatekeeper." For example, requesting advice on investigation of anemia simultaneously from medical, oncology, hematology, and gastrointestinal consultants is expensive, frustrating to the consultants, and guaranteed to lead to conflicting advice about patient management.

Both inside and outside the hospital setting, the physiatrist is the best medical specialist to prescribe, monitor, and revise rehabilitation services. Therapists who practice in hospital, outpatient, and home care settings seek collegial relationships with physiatrists because these physicians have the broadest understanding of the interactions between the medical and rehabilitation interventions as well as how to justify continuation of rehabilitation services beyond what originally is approved by managed care insurance plans.

In the "gatekeeping" role, the physiatrist must understand highly technological state-of-the-art interventions and be prepared to respond quickly to medical emergencies. He or she integrates this knowledge by specifying medical contraindications on therapy referrals and helping therapists to develop specific monitoring strategies to anticipate and prevent complications. Thus, the physiatrist coordinates medical and surgical subspecialists and nonmedical rehabilitation professionals for the anticipation, prevention, and treatment of medical emergencies. A competent "gatekeeper" will "troubleshoot" effectively.

COMORBIDITY IN REHABILITATION

As discussed previously, the likelihood of greater magnitude and high severity of comorbidity in rehabilitation patients predicts that medical emergencies will occur. If acquired impairments, such as cerebrovascular accidents, amputations, peripheral neuropathies, and spinal diseases are viewed as manifestations of end-stage disease processes, then medical problems should be expected. Some of these problems will manifest themselves as medical emergencies.

Death during inpatient rehabilitation is rare. The overall mortality rate on inpatient rehabilitation services is reported to be at most 3%. The rate of transfer back to acute medical/surgical services from inpatient rehabilitation is between 5% and 20% despite prescreening for obvious severe medical illnesses that would predispose to emergency situations (15,31,35–37). Two studies have characterized the quantity and severity of medical diagnoses in elderly rehabilitation patients. Both document a variety of medical problems, some of which are quite serious. Parry described 97 patients over the age of 85 years who were admitted to a rehabilitation unit (35). Fifty-eight percent had orthopedic problems, 18% had cerebrovascular accidents, 13% had general debility, and 2% were amputees. Complications included five urinary tract infections, four episodes of congestive heart failure, three episodes of thrombophlebitis, two new strokes, and one each of a variety of other problems, totaling 20 patients. Five percent were readmitted to a general hospital, and one died on the unit. In a similar survey, Felsenthal and colleagues characterized 82 patients admitted to a predominantly geriatric inpatient rehabilitation unit (31). A mean of 3.7 indications for medical intervention was reported. These medical interventions usually were straightforward and uncomplicated. That is, problems were easily handled by the physiatrist on this rehabilitation unit. One patient died of a cardiopulmonary arrest. Although these surveys document the extent of medical complications among rehabilitation patients who are elderly, they fail to correlate the impact of these medical complications on functional outcome.

Siegler and colleagues (38) reported the prevalence of serious medical complications occurring in a hospital-based rehabilitation program during a 7-year time period (1980–1986) that spanned the introduction of prospective payment reimbursement formulas that defined rehabilitation as exempt from these formulas. Of over 1,200 rehabilitation medicine service admissions, there were five (0.42%) deaths, four from cardiac causes and one from a pulmonary embolus (PE). Almost 90% of these patients in this tertiary care center-based rehabilitation unit had at least one medical complication during their rehabilitation stay, and about 13% of these patients required transfer back to acute medical/surgical services for treatment. Over half of the patients had complications that required their rehabilitation program to be interrupted. The average number of comorbid condition for this patient group was 1.8 per patient; more comorbid conditions and lower functional status were predictive of complications. These complications are summarized in Table 46-1. Surgical complications, especially wound infections with or without sepsis requiring intravenous antibiotics, were most common overall. Other infectious complications and cardiac and thromboembolic complications were also common. Excluding those patients who died, life-threatening complication occurred in eight (0.67%) patients.

Thus, based on these and other data reviewed above, life-threatening medical events appear to be unusual during rehabilitation, before and during the early years of acute care prospective payment reimbursement. Since the era of "managed care," there are empirical but not yet substantiated observations that still, even sicker patients are being provided rehabilitation in hospital-based programs and that high medical comorbidity is one of the major reasons to justify the high expense of these programs. Otherwise, patients treated in hospital-based programs during the 1980s are being provided rehabilitation in "subacute" or skilled nursing facility-based, that is, less expensive programs, during the 1990s. There are some data that report that life-threatening events requiring transfer back to acute medical/surgical

TABLE 46-1. *Medical/surgical complications during rehabilitation*

Type of complication	Incidence (%)	Reason for transfer back to an acute service (%)
Surgical	71 (19.8)	36 (22.8)
Infection/fever	62 (17.3)	27 (17.1)
General medical	39 (10.9)	10 (6.3)
Cardiac	34 (9.5)	20 (12.7)
Thromboembolic	33 (9.2)	26 (16.5)
Gastrointestinal/ genitourinary	31 (8.6)	12 (7.6)
Neurologic	31 (8.6)	14 (8.9)
Arthritic	12 (3.3)	0 (0.0)
Renal/electrolyte	12 (3.3)	5 (3.2)
Blood presure control	9 (2.5)	0 (0.0)
Other	9 (2.5)	0 (0.0)
Diabetes	8 (2.2)	3 (1.9)
Psychiatric	7 (2.0)	5 (3.2)
Details unknown	1 (0.3)	0 (0.0)
Total	359 (100)	158 (100)

Adapted from Siegler EL, Stineman MG, Maislin G. Development of complications during rehabilitation. *Arch Intern Med* 1994; 154(19): 2185–2190.

services are more common in subacute than in hospital-based rehabilitation programs, suggesting that the lower intensity of medical surveillance in subacute programs may be inadequate to address some medical problems appropriately during rehabilitation (37). Physiatrists should be able to treat most medical complications regardless of setting. Their role as ''gatekeeper'' is then emphasized in that this largely involves the goal of anticipatory medical problem solving, that is, preventing minor complications from evolving into life-threatening complications.

MEDICAL EMERGENCIES COMMONLY SEEN IN REHABILITATION

How does the rehabilitation patient differ from the typical medical/surgical patient? For any presenting clinical symptom or sign, the differential diagnostic approach remains the same, yet the order of likelihood of diagnostic possibilities is biased by the specific impairments. This will influence the clinician's problem solving in considering whether presenting symptoms or signs indicate a potentially life-threatening situation. For example, upper extremity pain in stroke patients may, as with any patient, be caused by osteoarthritis, bursitis, gout, trauma, or myocardial ischemia. Higher on the differential diagnostic list in these patients, however, will be other pathologic conditions such as glenohumeral shoulder subluxation, reflex sympathetic dystrophy, or imbalance of tone between anterior and posterior muscle groups, which are more prevalent among stroke patients.

In addition, because of underlying neurologic impairments, common diagnoses may not present in the usual fashion. Among rehabilitation patients in general, cognitive and sensory deficits may mask important clinical clues, so the practitioner may not be able to depend completely on history and physical examination to distinguish among the diagnostic possibilities. Deep venous thromboses, for example, may be more difficult to detect clinically in stroke patients because the patient may not feel lower extremity pain in the hemiparetic limb with sensory compromise. Moreover, dependent edema from muscle disuse may result in asymmetry between legs, potentially masking an evolving deep venous thrombosis or masquerading as one.

It is beyond the scope of this chapter to present the differential diagnoses and investigation for all of the major medical problems found on inpatient rehabilitation services. This material is discussed at the appropriate depth in major textbooks. An inpatient rehabilitation service should have a library of clinically relevant materials, and the staff should have access to them at all times. Texts must be current, and most will require replacement every 2 to 3 years.

Materials important to the emergency management of patients include:

- Standard textbooks of medicine, general surgery, orthopedic surgery, emergency medicine, and neurology
- A standard textbook of ambulatory medicine
- A standard textbook of geriatric medicine
- A drug information text
- A manual of easily accessible emergency treatments
- A training textbook of emergency intervention for cardiopulmonary arrests

A list of additional selected references is presented in Table 46-2. Access to the medical and rehabilitation litera-

TABLE 46-2. *Important texts for handling emergencies in rehabilitation*

Internal medicine
- Isselbacher KJ, Braunwald E, Wilson JD, et al. *Harrison's principles of internal medicine, 13th ed.* New York: McGraw-Hill, 1994.
- Kelly WN, editor-in-chief. *Textbook of internal medicine, 3rd ed.* Philadelphia: Lippincott–Raven, 1997.

Ambulatory medicine
- Barker LR, Burton JR, Zieve PD. *Principles of ambulatory medicine, 4th ed.* Baltimore: Williams & Wilkins, 1995.
- Noble J. *Textbook of primary care medicine, 2nd ed.* Boston: Little, Brown, 1996.

Geriatric medicine
- Hazzard WR, Andres R, Bierman EL, Blass JP. *Principles of geriatric medicine and gerontology, 3rd ed.* New York: McGraw-HIll, 1994.
- Abrams WB, Beer MH, Berkow R, eds. *The Merck manual of geriatrics, 2nd ed.* Rahway, NJ: Merck, Sharp & Dohme, 1995.

Neurology
- Adams RD, Victor M. *Principles of neurology, 6th ed.* New York: McGraw-Hill Information Sciences, 1997.
- Rowland LP, ed. *Merritt's textbook of neurology, 9th ed.* Philadelphia: Lea & Febiger, 1995.

Emergency medicine
- Rosen P, Baker FJ, Barker RM, Braen GR, Daily RH, Levy RC, eds. *Emergency medicine: concepts and clinical practice, 3rd ed.* St Louis: Mosby-Year Book, 1992.

Surgery
- Sabiston DC, ed. *Textbook of surgery, 15th ed.* Philadelphia: WB Saunders, 1997.
- Schwartz SI, editor-in-chief. *Principles of surgery, 6th ed.* New York: McGraw-Hill, 1994.

Orthopedic surgery
- Crenshaw AH, ed. *Campbell's operative orthopaedics, 8th ed.* St Louis: Mosby-Year Book, 1991.
- Rockwood CA, Green DP, Bucholz RW, eds. *Rockwood and Green's fractures in adults. Vols. 1 and 2, 4th ed.* Philadelphia: Lippincott–Raven, 1996.

Drug therapy
- *Physician's desk reference, 51st ed.* Oradell, NJ: Medical Economics, 1997.
- Skidmore-Roth L. *Mosby's 1997 nursing drug reference.* St Louis, CV Mosby, 1997.

Handbooks
- Ewald GA, McKenzie CR, eds. *Manual of medical therpapeutics, 28th ed.* Boston: Little, Brown, 1995.
- Jenkins JL, Loscalzo J, Braen GR. *Manual of emergency medicine, 3rd ed.* Boston: Little, Brown, 1995.
- Samuels MH. *Manual of neurological therapeutics, 5th ed.* Boston: Little, Brown, 1995.
- Cummins RO. *Textbook of advanced cardiac life support.* New York: Americal Heart Association, 1994.

ture through computerized data bases such as MedLine is also recommended.

Autonomic Dysreflexia

Autonomic dysreflexia in cervical or high thoracic spinal cord injury, when it presents in its most severe form as hypertensive crisis, is a prototype for a comorbid condition that must be treated as an emergency in rehabilitation. It often is preventable; yet it requires immediate intervention because of the potentially disastrous consequences of hypertensive crisis, such as stroke and seizures (39,40). The rehabilitation physician must thoroughly understand its pathophysiology as well as be fastidious in the performance of the physical examination in looking for causes during differential diagnosis (41). An algorithm can be applied to guide treatment systematically, from less invasive to more invasive interventions (Fig. 46-1).

Other comorbid medical problems in the spinal cord injury population can present either classically as in other patients or nonspecifically as autonomic dysreflexia. These include pneumonia, urinary tract infection, and deep venous thrombosis (42–45). Even with classic presentations, early recognition of these types of acute medical problems can be difficult in the spinal cord injury population because of the impairment to the neurologic system, especially the autonomic system, which controls such automatic responses to acute illnesses as fever, tachycardia, tachypnea, hypertension, and pain (46). Acute medical problems such as pneumonia, deep venous thrombosis, and urinary tract infection may not be recognized until they are so advanced that the patient is hemodynamically unstable. Sepsis and hypoxemia may be life-threatening, requiring emergent interventions such as systemic antibiotics, blood-pressure-altering intravenous medications, and mechanical ventilation. Further, during the prolonged hospital stay in the acute phase of rehabilitation, the spinal cord injury population is at risk for nosocomial infections with unusual and opportunistic organisms that require more aggressive antibacterial, antifungal, antiviral, and other supportive treatments (47,48).

Thromboembolic Diseases

The literature describing risk for thromboembolic disease in the stroke population is summarized in Table 46-3. From these data and the literature on thromboembolic disease in mixed major trauma and spinal-cord-injured populations (56–58), several conclusions can be drawn.

Clinical diagnosis alone will fail to identify many lower extremity DVTs. Similarly, other diagnoses, such as Baker cysts, heterotopic ossification, reflex sympathetic dystrophy, and cellulitis, can result in lower extremity swelling (59) and be incorrectly labeled as DVTs.

Various techniques are available to identify clinically silent or confirm clinically suspicious DVTs (59–62). They include venography, which is the gold standard, impedance plethysmography, Doppler, duplex ultrasound, and ^{125}I-fibrinogen scanning. Determining which technique to use depends on cost, dangers of the test (for example, venography has all the hazards of an intravenous dye load), and sensitivity and specificity of the technique in the hands of the technicians and clinicians who will be performing the tests at your institution.

In stroke patients, most DVTs occur in the paretic limb.

Heparinization of stroke patients reduces the risk of DVT and probably of PE as well. It should be noted, however, that the only definitive studies have been performed by McCarthy's group, with 5,000 units of calcium heparin every 8 hours, not 5,000 units every 12 hours (53,55). Gelmers showed a reduction using the latter dose, but the screening technique was physical examination (54).

The following, however, are not known and require additional study:

The usefulness of screening at-risk patients. It is not known whether identification and treatment of clinically silent DVTs outweigh the disadvantage of anticoagulating a rehabilitation patient who, by definition, is at greater risk for falling. For example, Meythaler and colleagues (63) prospectively screened both traumatic and acquired brain-injured patients for proximal DVT. They reported DVT screening as potentially cost-saving in these high-risk rehabilitation patient groups when using the projected expense of treating

TABLE 46-3. *Development of deep venous thrombosis in cerebrovascular accident*

First author	Number of patients	Detection method	Incidence	Heparin dose
Warlow (49)	76	^{125}I-Fibrinogen	53% Plegic limb 7% Normal limb	
Gibberd (50)	26	^{125}I-Fibrinogen	38% Plegic limb 12% Normal limb	
Miyamoto (51)	141	^{125}I-Fibrinogen	29%	
Sioson (52)	105	Impedance plethysmography	3%	
McCarthy (53)	32	^{125}I-Fibrinogen	75% Control 12.5% Heparin	 5,000 U q8h
Gelmers (54)	101	Physical examination	23% Control 2% Heparin	 5,000 U q12h
McCarthy (55)	305	^{125}I-Fibrinogen	72.7% Control 22.2% Heparin	 5,000 U q8h

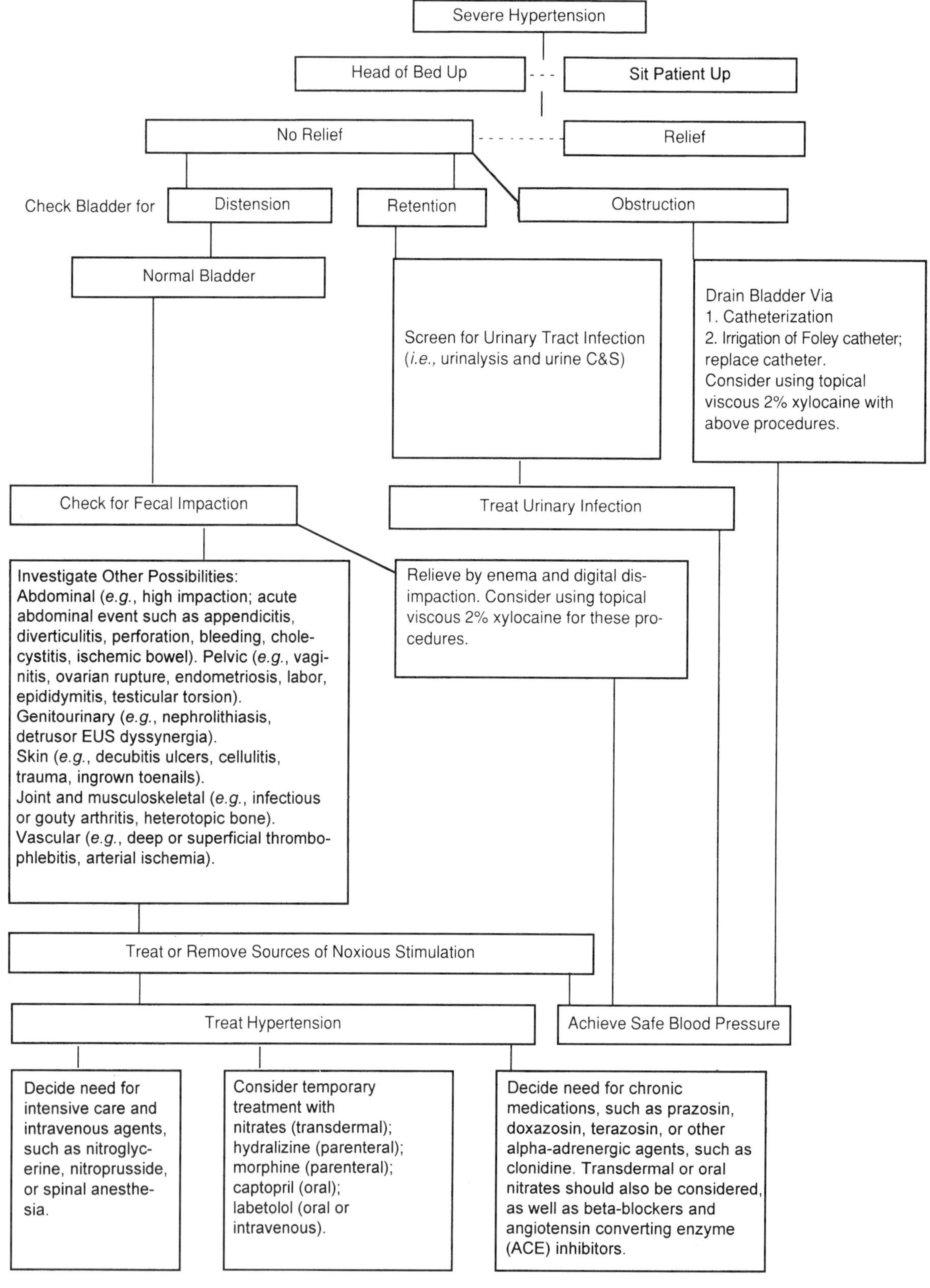

FIG. 46-1. Algorithm for managing severe hypertension in automatic dysreflexia in spinal cord injury. *C & S*, culture and sensitivity; *EUS*, external urethral sphincter. (Adapted from McGuire TJ, Kumar VN. Autonomic dysreflexia in the spinal cord injured. *Postgrad Med* 1986; 80:87–89; and Abdelwahab W, Frishman W, Landau A. Management of hypertensive urgencies and emergencies. *J Clin Pharm* 1995; 35:747–762.)

patients who did develop DVTs not detected earlier as comparison. Complications of anticoagulation based on screening, however, were not reported. Doppler and duplex ultrasound are presented as more promising than impedance plethysmography as a noninvasive screening technique, but this requires further investigation (63,64).

The appropriate dose of low-dose heparin for prophylaxis in this population. Is it effective at all? Is 5,000 units every 8 hours of subcutaneous heparin more effective prophylaxis than 5,000 units every 12 hours? For example, Pambianco and colleagues (65) reported that low-dose heparin prophylaxis was effective in preventing DVT in stroke patients. Moreover, when low-dose heparin was compared to intermittent pneumatic compression, their prophylactic efficacy was comparable. Importantly, in this study the dose of heparin was adjustable to achieve a partial thromboplastin time (PTT) between 30 and 39, starting at a dose of 8,000 units subcutaneously every 8 hours but requiring no more than 10,000 units subcutaneously every 8 hours to achieve this ''prophylactic'' range.

The practical efficacy of low-molecular-weight heparin (LMWH) for prophylaxis of DVT. The use of LMWH has been better studied in surgical than in stroke populations. For example, Leizorovicz and colleagues (66) performed a meta-analysis comparing LMWH administered once to twice daily, fixed low-dose heparin (5,000 units two to three times daily), intravenous dextran, and placebo. Both forms of heparin were similarly efficacious and safe and superior to dextran and placebo in mixed (including orthopedic) surgical patients for prevention of perioperative DVT. The LMWH was presented as potentially more efficacious than low-dose heparin, but adjustable low-dose heparin protocols were poorly represented in the studies analyzed. A study of major mixed trauma patients by Geerts and colleagues (56) again reported LMWH to be more beneficial than traditional heparin prophylaxis, but this study compared a twice-daily fixed dose of LMWH (30 mg enoxaparin) with twice-daily fixed low-dose heparin (5,000 units). Further, the superiority of LMWH over low-dose heparin as a prophylaxis has been disputed in general surgical patients but not in orthopedic patients in another meta-analysis (67). Thus, LMWH is becoming established as more effective than fixed low-dose heparin in orthopedic populations. Whether LMWH will have a clear superiority in other rehabilitation populations remains to be firmly established.

How long to continue prophylactic anticoagulation of at-risk patients. Should heparinization continue throughout hospitalization, or should it be discontinued once the patient can bear weight? For example, two studies using LMWH as DVT/PE prophylaxis, one in traumatic spinal cord injury and another in patients undergoing total hip replacement, suggest that prophylaxis should be continued beyond hospitalization (including rehabilitation): 8 weeks in spinal-cord-injury patients and 1 month in total hip replacement patients (68,69). The literature has not yet adequately addressed length of prophylaxis for stroke patients.

Questions that have not had answers considered in the recent literature include the following:

- What else might be added to or substituted for prophylactic heparin to reduce further the risk of thromboembolic disease in the stroke patient (for example, aspirin)?
- Can the data from research on rehabilitation patients with stroke be extrapolated to other impairments, and vice versa?

Ultimately, the clinician must decide how much heparin to use and for how long. Questions about the safety of prophylactic anticoagulation in unusual populations (for example, in patients after hemorrhagic stroke or recent eye surgery) should be referred to the appropriate specialist.

DVTs and PE still occur despite prophylactic anticoagulation. Identification requires both clinical vigilance and an understanding of the use of diagnostic tests (70). Patients with PE should be transferred to an acute care facility for treatment and observation. Deep venous thromboses can be treated in rehabilitation facilities, but the following are necessary for appropriate and safe management in this setting:

- Administration of therapeutic heparin doses and ongoing assessment of patients on heparin
- Access to daily phlebotomy and coagulation studies
- Facility with the principles of heparin and coumadin dosage adjustments
- Appropriate reimbursement for management of the problem on the rehabilitation service because skilled therapies will be interrupted for at least 3 days
- Willingness on the part of the staff to provide bedside skilled and preventive programs
- Willingness on the part of the staff to resume aggressive therapies in anticoagulated patients

Hull and colleagues presented data on the use of subcutaneous low-molecular-weight heparin as about as safe and efficacious as classic continuous intravenous heparin therapy in the treatment of acute proximal lower extremity venous thrombosis (71). The simplified dose for subcutaneous low-molecular-weight heparin given once or twice every 24 hours may preclude the need for transfer back from rehabilitation to an acute care setting for this problem. Finally, clinicians always should consult a pharmacist or internist about drug interactions with anticoagulants.

Cardiovascular Complications

Cardiovascular disease has a major deleterious impact on rehabilitation. In a stroke patient, for example, not only can cardiovascular events interrupt or abort rehabilitation efforts, but heart disease itself also impairs function.

Ben-Shlomo's group assessed the cardiac status of a general rehabilitation population by measuring blood pressures and using a screening device called a trendscriber to measure single-lead electrocardiogram (ECG) of patients during specific exercises (72). Although 63% of patients required further diagnostic investigation or alteration of medical therapy, physical therapy regimens were altered in only 38% of the patients. Six percent of the patients underwent an actual change in medical therapy. Most required only further medical testing such as a Holter monitor. This study illustrates how clinical observation with noninvasive diagnostic testing can be used to monitor and modify therapy interventions; it does not tell us whether the patients actually benefited from these interventions.

Siegler and colleagues used 24-hour ambulatory Holter monitoring to determine if silent ischemia was a useful predictor of cardiac complications in a general rehabilitation population (73). In this case, a strict definition of a complication was used: a condition that interrupted rehabilitation, caused transfer out of the rehabilitation service, or resulted in death. The authors believed that Holter monitor screening for silent ischemia was not a useful technique; low positive predictive value of the test was reported in this study.

Screening of any type for these purposes will most likely have poor positive predictive value. It is unlikely that an inpatient rehabilitation service whose patients have already been prescreened clinically for severe cardiac disease will have a population with a true cardiac complication rate of even 10%. The positive predictive value for tests of good sensitivity and specificity will be high enough to avoid large numbers of false positives only when incidence rates approach 15% to 20%.

Thus, no single effective test can identify patients at risk for cardiac complications in rehabilitation. It is most likely that some combination of history, physical examination, and laboratory data may provide the best warning that a patient is at risk for a cardiac event. Once a reliable method is found for identifying those at risk, more research will be needed to determine how to make rehabilitation safer for them.

Cardiac Disease and Amputation

The literature on dysvascular amputation is not as supportive as that in stroke for identifying increased cardiovascular complications. Overall, 75% of amputations occur in people over the age of 65 years, and 60% of these amputations are associated with peripheral vascular disease, according to Clark and associates' review of the demography of amputation (74). The rehabilitation literature supports the observations that the higher the level of amputation (that is, above-knee versus below-knee amputation), and the more extremities amputated (that is, bilateral versus unilateral amputations), the higher the cardiac energy consumption over distance traveled during ambulation (75,76). It has not been demonstrated that high-level amputees have more cardiovascular complications, however, despite increased energy use per unit distance. Patients with above-knee amputations tend to ambulate more slowly, and the amount of energy per unit time tends to approach controls, regardless of level (77). It is possible that cardiac disease may prevent optimal prosthetic use, however.

In Thornhill and associates' retrospective review of 18 patients with atherosclerosis as a cause of their bilateral amputations who failed to use bilateral prostheses, nine had "organic mental symptoms/psychosis," six had "diminished cardiovascular reserve" (no elaboration), three had cardiovascular accidents, and one had contractures too severe to permit prosthesis use (78). Finally, Steinberg and colleagues' retrospective study used a stricter definition of successful prosthesis use (79). Of those who were not fitted with artificial limbs (18/116), most had "poor effort tolerance" secondary to congestive heart failure. Three had previous strokes on the nonamputated side. Other causes of prosthetic failure were neuropathy, end-stage renal failure, and metastatic cancer. Age differences were not significant. These studies are case series; little is known about selection processes, types of interventions, and other issues implicit in the selection and rehabilitation processes (78,79).

Some studies have attempted to study amputees at risk for cardiac complications (80–82). Roth and colleagues screened 31 amputees during special physical therapy sessions. Seventeen patients showed ECG or blood pressure abnormalities (80). The range of abnormalities was broadly defined to include preexisting and insignificant S-T segment depression and asymptomatic ventricular ectopy. Cardiovascular complications were defined as significant only when a medication change was required (for example, extreme blood pressure elevations, angina, congestive heart failure, arrhythmia). The functional consequences of these abnormalities or complications were not considered. In this study, the authors report a positive predictive value of 33% for cardiac monitoring in these patients with amputations and a history of heart disease versus 31% for presence of a positive history alone. Confidence intervals were not reported, and it is doubtful that the difference was significant. The sensitivity of history alone, however, was better (83%) than that of monitoring plus history (67%).

Other investigators have modified existing exercise devices for screening purposes to make them suitable for use by amputees. Cruts's group used arm ergometry to assess cardiac risk of amputee patients (81). Twenty-nine of the 39 patients studied had cardiac problems that were broadly defined: atrial fibrillation, beta-blocker use, or myocardial infarction were most common. Eleven of 39 had S-T segment depressions during exercise testing, but all of these patients had ECG abnormalities at rest or as a digitalis effect. Despite the high prevalence of cardiac disease, 34 of the 39 patients were able to learn to use a prosthesis. Of the five who could not learn, one died, one had a myocardial infarction, two had poor wound healing, and one had dizziness. Patients with low peak workload were less likely to be able to walk without a walker. Statistical analysis was not performed in this study, and no attempt was made to correlate S-T segment changes with outcome.

Cardiac Disease and Cerebrovascular Accident

Cardiovascular disease as a complication in cerebrovascular accidents is well recognized. Overall, after carotid circulation cerebrovascular accidents, 17% of the patients will be dead in a month and 39% in 5 years from many causes, including cardiovascular (83). More specifically, acute myocardial infarction can lead to stroke, especially when the infarction is large or congestive heart failure is present (84). The reverse relationship also exists. Cerebrovascular accidents cause ECG changes, transient arrhythmias, and myocardial damage. Dimant and Grob documented this latter relationship in a prospective study of 100 consecutive patients admitted with strokes of all types (85). They compared the ECGs and enzyme changes of these stroke patients with colon cancer patients as controls. Ninety percent of stroke patients but only 50% of the colon cancer controls had ECG abnormalities, including S-T segment depression, prolonged Q-T intervals, inverted T waves, atrial fibrillation, conduction defects, premature ventricular contractions, and left ventricular hypertrophy. From this study, 29 patients had elevated cardiac enzymes, especially creatine phosphokinase (CPK). Only five of those 29 patients demonstrated ECG evidence of myocardial infarction. The authors presented evidence that an elevated CPK in the context of a stroke is associated with significantly increased risk of dying acutely, although not necessarily from a cardiac cause.

In another study of cardiac events immediately after stroke, Myers' group obtained 24-hour ECGs, cardiac enzymes, and plasma norepinephrine in 100 stroke patients admitted to a stroke intensive care unit and compared these results with 50 controls admitted with no stroke or transient ischemic attacks (86). Stroke patients had more serious arrhythmias (for example, ventricular tachycardia, couplets, or more than five ventricular premature beats per minute) than did the controls, even after controlling for age and coexisting heart disease. Patients with cerebral infarctions had more arrhythmias than those with brainstem infarctions, as well as higher and more frequent elevations in CPK. Isoenzymes were not analyzed in this study. Plasma norepinephrine also was elevated in stroke patients and compared with controls, but there was no correlation between level of norepinephrine and presence of arrhythmia. Norris (87) and Reinstein and colleagues (88) also found increased frequency of arrhythmias acutely after stroke, but they did not obtain any evidence that these changes affected outcome. Norris looked at CPK isoenzymes in 230 patients with stroke (87). One hundred one of these 230 patients had elevated CPK, but CPK-MB levels were elevated in only 25 of these 101 patients. The CPK-MB isoenzymes rose progressively until the fourth day, when the study authors had stopped measuring, rather than peaking within 2 days as is more typical for a myocardial infarction. In addition, the rise in isoenzymes was correlated with risk of arrhythmia. A myonecrosis phenomenon associated with sympathetic neurotransmitter release secondary to brain damage during stroke is postulated by these authors. This confirms the impression that increased norepinephrine level may be responsible for cardiac damage in stroke patients. Further, autopsy studies have reported focal myocytolysis in the hearts of patients dying soon after stroke.

Thus, it is likely that stroke itself can cause ECG changes or cardiac damage independently of coexisting heart disease. Most but not all studies show that acute mortality increases in groups with arrhythmias and elevated CPK. It may be important to distinguish ECG changes secondary to central nervous system damage from those reflecting coronary artery disease, because the prognosis should differ between the two etiologies. Although the effect of these changes on mortality and capacity for functional gains has not been assessed, it is possible that these patients are at risk for emergent cardiac events during the rehabilitation phase of care.

Some of the most intriguing studies have examined the role of heart disease on patient outcomes. Two major studies have examined comorbidities of stroke survivors (89,90). In a large Olmstead County population, the leading cause of death following stroke was cardiac disease (89). Cardiovascular disease also was the most frequent comorbidity, being symptomatic in 31% of patients at the time of their acute presentation of stroke. In this study, based at the Mayo Clinic, Dombovy's group found that only 12% of the original 292 patients with stroke were transferred to rehabilitation units. Twenty-nine percent of survivors were otherwise institutionalized at the beginning of the study, a rate that was reduced to 18% by 1 year. Unfortunately, it is not known what proportion of the decline in institutionalization rate was attrition through death and what proportion represented discharge of patients back to the community (89). The Framingham Study confirmed the significance of heart disease in the stroke population (90). The study noted hypertension in 67% of stroke patients, hypertensive heart disease in 53% of these patients, coronary artery disease in 32%, and congestive heart failure in 18% (90). The presence of heart disease in the stroke population was significantly higher than in controls matched for age and gender. More importantly, the Framingham Study documented that heart disease itself is associated with significant diminution of function. After controlling for functional deficits related to cardiac comorbidity in stroke patients and matched controls, the study found a much lower prevalence of functional deficits among stroke survivors, approaching the levels found in matched controls. Further, although numbers were small, stroke patients and these controls had similar levels of vocational function and socialization within the home as well as rates of institutionalization, after control of the functional deficits directly associated with comorbidities associated with cardiac disease. The Framingham Study implies that much disability of stroke patients is directly related to coexisting cardiovascular disease.

This correlation between the presence of heart disease and increased disability after stroke was recognized in another retrospective study. Roth and associates found that patients with coronary artery disease with and without congestive heart failure had a diminished ability to perform activities of daily living, compared to controls without coronary artery disease (91). The rate of institutionalization and the length of stay were no different among the three groups. Since this study did not control for admission functional status as a predictor of discharge functional status, it is possible that cases with coronary artery disease and congestive heart failure had more severe strokes to begin with, rather than a poorer outcome because of the comorbidity itself. Nonetheless, this study confirms the significant negative impact of coronary artery disease on stroke outcome that was observed in the Framingham data.

Not all studies, however, are in agreement with the above findings. Feigenson and associates' retrospective review failed to show any relationship among atherosclerotic heart disease, discharge disposition, length of stay, and discharge functional status (92). Only general descriptive statistical methods, however, were used in Feigenson and associates' study, and no attempt was made to sort out confounding variables. Anderson and colleagues used a multiple regression approach to examine what factors were predictive of stroke outcome in a population of 233 patients (93). Dependent variables were improvement at discharge and follow-up rather than absolute functional status. Nonetheless, in this study, heart disease failed to be a significant predictor of improvement or decline in functional status.

For the present time, patients with active heart disease are managed best by having consultants follow them throughout their rehabilitation stay. Plans for management of conditions such as chest pain or shortness of breath should be developed at the time of admission with the consultant: What is the patient's usual pattern, and when is deviation from the pattern serious enough to warrant further investigation, such as ECG or blood gas determination? When will symptoms warrant interruption of therapy? Monitoring heart rate, blood pressure, and hemoglobin oxygen arterial saturation noninvasively by pulse oximetry at rest and during therapies can be useful to guide progress of therapies in these patients. Roth's recently published two-part review of heart disease in stroke patients underscores the fact that managing cardiovascular diseases in this patient population is essential during the daily care of these patients (94,95).

In addition, the decision to put patients on cardiac precautions, and the attempt to determine exactly what those precautions are, should be made jointly by physiatrist, internist/cardiologist, and physical therapist. As a general guideline, all patients with a known history of cardiovascular diseases should have cardiac precautions defined as part of their therapy orders. These patients enter rehabilitation programs after variable periods of bed rest and with organ systems compromised with a variety of impairments, for example, hemiparesis, amputation, suboptimal pulmonary ventilation, and painful extremities during weight bearing or volitional movement. Thus, the increased cardiovascular demands of remobilization are obvious in these patients. Observation of their performance, including blood pressure and heart rate responses, during simple motor tasks on the physical examination (isometric contractions during manual muscle testing, bed mobility, sitting, standing, weight shifting, transfers, ambulation) becomes the informal exercise tolerance test to use as a basis for defining cardiac precautions.

The standard formulas for determining intensity of exercise are not useful in these patients in that many have a baseline tachycardia and are on medications that may damper autonomic responses to increasing activity. One pragmatic approach for defining cardiac precautions in these patients is to monitor baseline heart rate and blood pressure regularly and then, as a starting point, keep their heart rate within a range of resting plus 20 during initial therapy sessions while simultaneously monitoring changes in blood pressure during exercise. Definitions of baseline and exercise blood pressure precautions must also be individualized. Moreover, hypertension can be unmasked during monitored activity in otherwise normotensive patients at rest. The normal blood pressure response to progressive exercise can be used as a general guideline for what to expect and what type of blood pressure parameters to set: systolic pressure normally increases by 50 to 70 mm Hg, whereas diastolic pressures should remain unchanged or decrease by 4 to 8 mm Hg because of peripheral vasodilation. Sick, deconditioned patients may start exercise at variable baseline blood pressures, and they will respond variably depending on a number of factors including hydration, temperature, and medications on board. Thus, these guidelines should be considered maximal expected changes in sick rehabilitation patients. More specifically, exercised-induced increases in blood pressure consistently over 200 systolic and 90 diastolic should be monitored closely and potentially treated (96).

Aspiration

Aspiration pneumonia is a well-recognized and frequently life-threatening problem among hospitalized patients, leading to bacteremia, sepsis, respiratory arrest, and death (97). It is associated with swallowing dysfunction and upper gastrointestinal disorders secondary to central and peripheral neurologic diseases and peripheral mechanical and obstructive diseases (98–102). Aspiration pneumonia not only is an indication for enteral forms of nutritional support but also is recognized as a complication of these alternative forms of feeding (103–105). Aspiration pneumonia is viewed as potentially preventable by a clearer definition of the anatomy and pathophysiology of oropharyngeal and esophageal dysphagia through a bedside swallowing examination by a swallowing therapist combined with radiographic studies of the oropharynx, esophagus, and upper gastrointestinal tract (106–108). These assessment strategies can direct preventive management interventions and potentially prevent respiratory emergencies.

Aspiration involves a spectrum of situations from laryngeal penetration to frank aspiration pneumonia. Aspiration pneumonia can involve segmental or lobar areas of the lung and be associated with either more diffuse pulmonary inflammatory reaction or systemic effects with bacteremia, sepsis, and end-organ consequences of hypoxia (97,104).

Pennza presents an excellent discussion of the incidence, pathophysiology, natural history, and treatment of aspiration (97). He clarifies the difference between macroaspiration and microaspiration. Most macroaspirations involve bacterial and nonbacterial materials. Aspiration of gastric contents is associated with more diffuse respiratory and systemic findings, in comparison with aspiration of oropharyngeal secretions. Laryngeal penetration and microaspiration do not always lead to aspiration pneumonia but may be serious predisposing factors to an emergent event. Pingleton presents another excellent discussion of the pathophysiology of aspiration in relation to enteral nutrition (103). Enteral nutrition may alkalinize the gastric environment, leading to bacterial overgrowth. These bacteria are then transmitted to the oropharynx and trachea through reflux and aspiration.

Aspiration is associated with a broad range of diseases commonly encountered among rehabilitation patients. Aspiration can be categorized into three major mechanisms that encompass these diseases (104):

1. *Neuromuscular mechanisms.* Any impairment of the central and peripheral nervous systems, neuromuscular junction and muscles may result in aspiration because of dysphagia and/or reflux. For example, any structural, metabolic, traumatic, or infectious condition that compromises mental status will predispose to aspiration. The basic cognitive skills of selective attention and concentration for orally presented food and for handling secretions can be suppressed. Further, protective cough and gross gag reflexes can be suppressed. Diseases that commonly produce dysphagia include cerebrovascular accident, traumatic brain injury, brain tumors, central nervous system infections, demyelinating diseases such as multiple sclerosis, progressive neurologic diseases such as Parkinson's disease and dementia, peripheral neurologic diseases such as amyotrophic lateral sclerosis and Guillain–Barré syndrome, and muscular dystrophies such as oculopharyngeal muscular dystrophy (99,100,109–111). Additionally, dysmotility disorders of the esophagus and gastrointestinal tract producing gastrointestinal reflux include achalasia. Diabetes mellitus, and other diseases that result in gastric autonomic peripheral neuropathies, gastroesophageal reflux disease, and hiatal hernia may result in aspiration (101,112).

Among these disorders, dysphagia as a consequence of stroke has been best studied. Dysphagia is reported to occur in at least 50% of stroke survivors, and aspiration is reported to occur in up to 75% of these (113,114). "Silent" aspiration is demonstrable in about one-third to one-half of patients (99). Lesion site or bilaterality are not predictive of dysphagia, aspiration, or their related symptoms (116). The absence of a gag reflex is not predictive, and its presence is not protective of dysphagia and aspiration (116). The single best reported predictor of aspiration in dysphagic stroke patients is the presence of an involuntary cough while or for 1 minute after being challenged to drink and swallowing 3 ounces of water without interruption (117). An adequate voluntary cough, however, does not indicate an effective protective cough reflex. The absence of voluntary cough should preclude further oral intake until further clinical and/or radiographic investigation (116).

2. *Mechanical mechanisms.* Mechanical interruption of the swallowing mechanism may result in aspiration. This may have a variety of causes and be inflammatory (for example, retropharyngeal or submandibular infections), anatomic (for example, Zenker's diverticulum, tracheoesophageal fistula), traumatic (both blunt and penetrating), or cancer-related (for example, tumors of the tongue and floor of the mouth, pharyngeal and esophageal tumors) in origin (102,118).

3. *Iatrogenic mechanisms.* These include enteral feeding, endotracheal tubes and tracheostomies, general anesthesia, and head and neck cancer treatments. Sitzmann reported 15 (26.3%) aspiration pneumonias in a study of 57 enterally fed patients with dysphagia (119). These 15 incidents of aspiration occurred in patients fed with continuous infusion through nasoduodenal, gastrostomy, and jejunostomy tubes. A 30% mortality rate is reported in patients treated with nasoduodenal tubes, significantly higher than with gastrostomies and jejunostomies. Based on these findings, Sitzmann recommends that nasoenteric feeding should not be used in people who have pharyngeal or esophageal dysfunction as a cause of dysphagia, as documented by dynamic radiographic studies. This recommendation is reinforced by another series of studies. Flynn and associates report a 26.4% (14 patients) aspiration rate among 53 acutely ill adults with mixed diagnoses (age range 17 to 90 years) fed by enteral tubes in a tertiary care hospital (120). About two-thirds of the overall group were fed nasogastrically (66%), and others were fed by jejunostomy (17%), gastrostomy (9.4%), cervical esophagostomy (3.8%), or a combination (3.8%). Both continuous and intermittent feeding schedules were used. Among those who aspirated, 71.4% had an artificial airway. Neither tube size nor tube location was associated consistently with aspiration. Stroke was the major diagnosis represented in the group who aspirated (6/14). Pritchard reported 20 patients with central neurologic causes for dysphagia who were fed with nasogastric feeding tubes intermittently over a 6-month period: 70% (12/20) of the nasogastric feeding tube-associated respiratory tract infections were associated with the use of a large-bore feeding tube; 25% (5/20) of these respiratory infections were pneumonias associated with tube displacement or aspiration (121).

The iatrogenic risk of aspiration must also be considered when a patient is enterally fed by gastrostomy and jejunostomy. Llaneza and colleagues reported 73 patients who had percutaneous endoscopic gastrostomy (PEG) tube placement over a 27-month period (122). Approximately one-half of these patients had neurologic, oropharyngeal, or esophageal reasons for swallowing dysfunction. The others required long-term enteral alimentation because of malnutrition or chronic aspiration. Aspiration pneumonia was the major late complication (that is, 48 hours after tube placement) in 8.2%

(6/73) of patients. This compared with 13 of these patients in whom aspiration actually was the indication for PEG placement. Kaplan and associates reported 23 patients studied prospectively over a 2-year period who had percutaneous endoscopic jejunostomy (PEJ) placement: 5 of 23 (21.7%) episodes of aspiration pneumonia occurred in four patients (123). This is compared retrospectively to those in this same group who required nasogastric tube placement before PEJ: 13 of 23 (56.5%) episodes of aspiration were observed in six of the nasogastrically fed patients. When the PEJ tubes failed, and the patients were then converted to PEG tubes, 11 of 23 (47.8%) episodes of aspiration were reported in seven patients. Thus, the use of both gastrostomy and jejunostomy for enteral alimentation can result in aspiration, but the risk does not seem to be as high as with nasoenteral access.

Hicks and colleagues reported 158 patients over a 2-year period who had either PEG or PEJ tube placement (124). The indications for tube placement specific to a distal site were different in this study in that jejunostomy tubes were placed in patients with evidence of gastroesophageal reflux, aspiration, gastric atony, and partial gastric obstruction. Aspiration was not reported as a complication associated with the procedure itself. Aspiration or significant reflux was reported in only 5% (8/158) of these patients in both groups. Thus, it appears that when a specific rationale dictates the type of tube placement, the incidence of aspiration pneumonia can be minimized. Lazarus and associates reviewed 10 years of literature on aspiration associated with long-term gastric versus jejunal feeding (125). The relative risk of aspiration associated with either type of feeding could not be determined reliably because of methodologic problems with most of the studies. The majority of the studies involved gastric rather than jejunal feeding. This review gave little empiric evidence to support preferential use of either jejunal or gastric feeding in management of patients with neurogenic dysphagia.

Aspiration, in its full-blown form as pneumonitis, is a life-threatening and costly problem, sometimes requiring mechanical ventilation and intensive care unit stays. Up to a 40% mortality rate is reported in patients with aspiration pneumonitis, with over 50% of these patients requiring mechanical ventilation (126). Dysphagia is a common problem among patients participating in rehabilitation, especially those with central and peripheral neurologic disorders. Tracheostomies and enteral feeding tubes also are commonly encountered among rehabilitation patients; the latter are especially important to facilitate nutritional support during rehabilitation interventions at the time of the recovery phase of disease.

The assessment of dysphagia is a multidisciplinary effort. It is a problem that crosses boundaries among medical and rehabilitation specialists because of the range of diseases in which it is encountered and the need for multiple concurrent management interventions directed toward maintaining nutrition and preventing complications. Physiatrists, in their "gatekeeping" role, are instrumental in recognizing it as a problem and directing assessment and management interventions with other specialists (for example, radiologists, gastroenterologists, otorhinolaryngologists). Swallowing therapists, either speech therapists or occupational therapists, are emerging as experts in more focused clinical assessment and management strategies. Bedside clinical evaluation of swallowing, however, may miss up to 40% of aspirations seen radiographically in dysphagic patients (127). The most productive assessment approach is joint radiographic evaluation by the swallowing therapist and radiologist. With this approach, specific management interventions can be tested, such as different textures and consistencies of oral feedings, various head and neck positions during feeding, and specific oral and pharyngeal motor treatments. The swallowing therapist can advise nursing and nutritional support teams on level of supervision and body position required during oral feeding, specific oral dietary orders, the progression of oral feeding, and the oral caloric intake during concurrent enteral nutritional support (92,102,106,107). The physiatrist must synthesize information from multiple sources and make ongoing decisions for specific assessment and changes in feeding and dietary orders. Anticipation and prevention are the guiding principles. Further, a team enterprise is essential with the physiatrist as orchestrator for successful prevention of a life-threatening event.

Specific prevention and anticipation strategies for the physiatrist include:

- Knowledge of those disorders commonly associated with dysphagia.
- A thorough neurologic and functional history and physical examination to screen for feeding and swallowing problems. The history should include directed interviews with personnel who usually are present during feeding. Symptoms associated with dysphagia include drooling, nasal regurgitation, difficulty clearing phlegm, fatigue after eating or drinking, dysphonia with or without a "wet voice," and coughing or choking during eating or drinking.
- Allowing patients to be NPO temporarily until the swallowing mechanism is clinically and, if indicated, radiographically defined and then writing all feeding, dietary, and nutrition support orders.
- Consulting the swallowing therapist, either a speech or occupational therapist, for a clinical evaluation of the oral–pharyngeal mechanism.
- Integrating compensatory feeding and positioning strategies and supervision orders for nursing and dietary/nutrition personnel to be executed during progressive feeding programs and concurrent swallowing therapies.
- Referral to radiology for videofluoroscopic evaluation of the swallowing mechanism, ensuring that the swallowing therapist is present to allow radiographic evaluation under different conditions of varying food textures and head–neck positions.

- Referral to other medical specialists:
  - Otorhinolaryngologist for laryngoscopic visualization of the oropharynx to detect obstructive-mechanical lesions and vocal cord lesions and paralysis.
  - Gastroenterologist for endoscopic visualization and advice for further radiographic studies when esophageal disease and gastrointestinal reflux are implicated as predisposing factors.
  - Dietary and clinical nutrition consultants for assessment of nutritional status, advice on enteral nutritional support, and monitoring of caloric intake.
  - Gastroenterologist or surgeon when gastric or jejunal enteral feeding tubes, requiring either endoscopically guided percutaneous or open surgical placement, are needed. The physiatrist can direct the consultant on the type of enteral tube preferred for minimizing aspiration risk and minimizing interruption of the rehabilitation program.
- Directing advancement of oral intake and withdrawal of enteral support.
- Case management—ongoing rehabilitation team goal setting for feeding, diet, and nutrition.
- Assuring that the common-sense aspiration precautions are executed during enteral feeding; for example, feeding in an upright position (at least 30°) and maintaining this position for as long as 1 to 2 hours after feeding; monitoring for retention of gastric or intestinal materials during and after enteral feedings; checking for enteral tube placement with regular auscultation (105,121,128).

When enteral support is necessary, the choice of tube is not always straightforward. Treatment or prevention of malnutrition is the basic goal. The bowel must be intact and functional to handle enteral feedings; otherwise, parenteral support and its complications must be considered. The usual choices of feeding tube include nasogastric, nasoduodenal, gastrostomy, and jejunostomy. As previously discussed nasoenteric tubes have their own theoretical and observed risk of reflux and aspiration possibly related to the physical presence of a tube in the pharynx and across the gastroesophageal and pyloric sphincters. Radiographic guidance and verification of position of nasojejunal tubes is required, especially when continuous tube feedings are given.

When the choice between gastrostomy and jejunostomy is considered, the clinical risk/benefit ratio must be discussed. Percutaneous placement is less costly than surgical placement and does not require general anesthesia. Surgical placement is preferred in patients who have had previous bowel surgery that has caused adhesions or unusual gastrointestinal anatomy. Both types of procedures have complications, and it is unclear whether one procedure is safer than the other (122,129). Further, jejunostomy tubes are theoretically safer than gastrostomy tubes because there are two sphincters (that is, gastroesophageal and pyloric) protecting from reflux, but this has not been well studied clinically (125). Jejunostomy feeding requires continuous feeding regimens, but these are convenient in rehabilitation settings only if they can be given overnight, so gastrostomy feeding with intermittent bolus regimens sometimes is preferred. Smaller tubes are associated with less reflux and aspiration, but they more frequently become clogged, especially when elixir forms of medications are unavailable (105,121).

Changes in Mental Status

A variety of medical emergencies may present with changes in mental status. Abnormal neuropsychiatric behavior may be the predominant or sole manifestation of a serious underlying medical problem (130,131). Usual somatic symptoms may be minimal or absent, or the disabled patient may be unable to recognize or report the symptoms. Neuropsychiatric or behavioral presentations of medical emergencies should not be regarded as atypical. They are especially common in rehabilitation patients who are elderly or whose cognitive or sensory functions already are impaired (132,133).

Mental status changes include disturbances of cognition, perception, thought form and content, mood and affect, personality, and behavior (134).

Disturbances of cognition may present as impaired attention or ability to shift attention, concentration, short- and long-term memory, language, abstract thinking, and executive functions.

Disturbances of perception may include illusions, which are misperceptions or misinterpretations of real external sensory stimuli, or hallucinations, which are internal sensory experiences in the absence of external stimuli. Illusions and hallucinations may be visual, auditory, tactile, olfactory, or gustatory.

Disturbances of thinking may include disorganized, rambling, racing, irrelevant, disconnected, or bizarre thoughts. Thought content may be delusional, with misbeliefs or ideas that are not consistent with reality. Hallucinations and delusions are examples of psychotic symptoms. They do not accurately reflect real external stimuli, events, or relationships.

Disturbances of mood include extreme, persistent, or labile internal emotional states, such as dysphoria or depression, euphoria, anxiety, irritability, anger, or hostility. Affect is the constellation of observable outward manifestations of these internal mood states.

Disturbances in affect are displayed in facial expressions, eye contact, speech quality (for example, volume, rate, tone, prosody), social demeanor, body posture, psychomotor activity, gestures, and other behaviors. Sometimes, disturbances of affect are associated with an uncoupling of affect and mood, so that the manifest affect is incongruent with the underlying mood. Pseudobulbar affect is an example of this—patients' affect may be tearful, although the mood they experience is not sad.

Disturbances of personality may include exaggeration of premorbid defenses and traits or alterations in the patient's characteristic style of relating to the environment or other people. These styles or traits may be passive or dependent, histrionic, narcissistic, obsessional, antisocial, or aggressive. Often, combinations of such features are observed.

Disturbances of behavior entail changes in usual functional patterns of activity, including social activity or interpersonal behavior. Behavioral disturbances frequently are associated with other changes in mental status, such as cognitive impairment, mood lability, or personality disorder.

Changes in the patient's mental status may compound the disability (135). For example, cognitive dysfunction or maladaptive behavior may further disrupt the ability to interact effectively in the rehabilitation environment or with care providers and therapists. When such changes are disruptive, they appropriately become a focus of attention and clinical intervention. For example, disruptive or nonproductive behaviors seriously can threaten a patient s continued participation in rehabilitation unless they are understood and treated. Before responding to the management challenges posed for rehabilitation staff, however, it is important to determine the etiology of mental status changes, maintaining a high level of vigilance for those causes that represent medical emergencies.

Delirium

Although comorbid medical conditions can present with isolated changes in any aspect of mental status, they are often manifest as delirium. This is a syndrome defined by the DSM-IV diagnostic criteria outlined in Table 46-4 (130,136). The essential features of this syndrome are disturbances of consciousness and impairment in the ability of the patient to focus and maintain attention to external stimuli or to shift attention appropriately to new external stimuli. There may be perceptual disturbances such as illusions and hallucinations and impaired cognitive function with disorientation, confusion, and memory deficits. Patients with delirium also may develop disturbed sleep–wake cycles, and they may exhibit psychomotor agitation or retardation. Symptoms develop over a short period of time (that is, hours to days) and typically fluctuate over the course of a day (130). Delirium is a transient syndrome. Yet, resolution of symptoms may occur over weeks, slowing down learning in the context of rehabilitation but still allowing participation in structured therapy programs (132). Delirium is associated with decrements in performance of everyday life activities such that continued community life is seriously threatened unless it is immediately recognized and its causes clearly identified, with prompt, appropriate treatment and sufficient resolution of symptoms to ensure a safe community-based existence (137,138).

TABLE 46-4. *Diagnosis of delirium*

Disturbance of consciousness, that is, reduced clarity of awareness of the environment, with reduced ability to focus, sustain, or shift attention
A change in cognition, such as memory deficit, disorientation, or language disturbances, or the development of a perceptual disturbance that is not better accounted for by a preexisting, established, or evolving dementia
The disturbance develops over a short period of time (usually hours to days) and tends to fluctuate during the course of the day
There is evidence from the history, physical examination, or laboratory findings that the disturbance is caused by the direct physiological consequences of a general medical condition

Adapted from *Diagnostic and statistical manual of mental disorders, 4th ed. Primary care version.* Washington, D.C.: American Psychiatric Association, 1995; 79–81.

Estimates of the incidence of delirium vary, depending on the diagnostic criteria used, the setting, and the patient population. For example, studies on medical and surgical units of general hospitals suggest an incidence ranging from 10% to 15% (139) and up to 35% in geriatric patients (130,140–142). For example, one-third of patients who have open heart surgery and one-half of patients who have surgery for hip fracture fixation display delirium. Despite its frequent occurrence, delirium has not been well studied. Its incidence and prevalence in rehabilitation settings are not known. Numerous factors that predispose patients to delirium are becoming recognized, including structural brain lesions, degenerative brain diseases, impaired vision and hearing, reduced capacity for homeostatic regulation, age-related changes in pharmacokinetics and pharmacodynamics, sleep deprivation, pain, burden of chronic disease, and psychosocial stressors (143,144). These can also be viewed as common risk factors for delirium in the rehabilitation setting and are especially frequent in elderly rehabilitation patients.

Retrospective studies have shown that delirium often is unrecognized in acute hospital settings (139,145). To our knowledge, reliability of case ascertainment in rehabilitation settings has not been investigated. Delirium is associated with high morbidity and mortality, however, and its recognition is crucial in any setting (140,141,146–150). Once recognized, the presence of delirium should prompt a thorough diagnostic evaluation, including careful history with attention to the following:

- Environmental factors
- Review of systems for associated symptoms and signs
- Medication inventory including drugs taken on an as-needed basis, nonprescription drugs, and illicit drug or alcohol abuse
- Complete physical examination
- Mental status examination
- Selected laboratory and other diagnostic studies (139,150)

This evaluation should be directed to determine the cause or causes of the delirium. Table 46-5 lists the general categories of causes of delirium and gives examples, highlighting those that are considered potential medical emergencies. It should be noted that although some of these causes have an obvious direct relationship to central nervous system

TABLE 46-5. *Causes of delirium*

Category	Potential medical emergencies	Other causes
Intoxication	Medications, alcohol, drugs of abuse, poisons	Heavy metals
Withdrawal	Alcohol, sedatives, and hypnotics	
Metabolic	Hypoxia, acidosis, electrolyte imbalance, hyperosmolar state	Dehydration, alkalosis, renal or hepatic failure
Endocrine	Hypoglycemia, hypoadrenalism	Thyroid dysfunction, parathyroid dysfunction, hypopituitarism
Vitamin deficiency	Thiamine depletion	Folate, nicotinic acid, vitamin B_{12}, deficiency
Infection	Meningitis, septicemia, pneumonia	Urinary tract infection, encephalitis, any systemic infection
Cardiovascular/ cardiopulmonary	Shock, malignant hypertension, myocardial infarction, arrhythmia, pulmonary edema, pulmonary embolus	Hypotension, congestive heart failure
Neurologic	Cerebrovascular accident, transient ischemic attack, subdural hematoma, increased intracranial pressure, seizure	Vasculitis, tumor, cerebral edema, postictal state
Trauma	Head injury, hypothermia, hyperthermia, electrocution	Pain

function, many are factors that are several steps removed from the central nervous system and appear to exert their effects indirectly. For example, viral encephalitis can cause delirium, but so can urinary tract infection in the absence of direct central nervous system infection.

When patients develop delirium, the diagnostic evaluation should begin with a rapid screening for the most likely potential emergencies. For example, in patients who have had closed head injuries, the possibility of subdural hematoma, intracerebral hemorrhage, increased intracranial pressure, severe hypertension, cardiac arrhythmias, and seizures should be considered. Delirious patients who have had invasion of the central nervous system (for example, traumatic, diagnostic, surgical, therapeutic) should be evaluated for bacterial meningitis. Patients who have survived a stroke may become delirious from extension of the stroke, cerebral edema, intracerebral hemorrhage, or the resultant increase in intracranial pressure. Patients with brain tumors can develop delirium through similar mechanisms. Rehabilitation patients with vascular disease may become delirious from any condition that causes reduced cardiac output or results in cerebral hypoperfusion, such as cardiac arrhythmias, hypotension, myocardial ischemia with compromised left ventricular function or papillary muscle dysfunction, or other causes of congestive heart failure. Delirious patients with risk factors for DVT should be considered for possible PE. Of note, myocardial ischemia or infarction, or PEs, may present with delirium without chest pain or complaints of dyspnea or obvious signs of hemodynamic compromise. Moreover, hypotension and shock frequently are associated with delirium.

Any other condition associated with hypoxia can cause delirium, with airway obstruction and pneumonia on the list of potential medical emergencies. Rehabilitation patients with swallowing dysfunction should be suspected of aspiration if they develop delirium. Hypertensive crisis can be a cause of delirium (encephalopathy) in patients with spinal cord injury and autonomic instability. Rehabilitation patients with acute or chronic infections (for example, pneumonia, urinary tract infection, osteomyelitis) may develop delirium without infectious involvement of the central nervous system; however, sepsis, shock, and bacterial meningitis are complications that represent medical emergencies. Delirium is common in the context of hypoglycemia and adrenal insufficiency, and both conditions warrant prompt diagnosis and treatment. Finally, withdrawal from central nervous system depressants, especially alcohol, barbiturates, and benzodiazepines, often is associated with delirium. Recognition and prompt treatment are important to avert life-threatening withdrawal phenomena such as seizures.

Appropriate management of each case of delirium depends on identification of the likely causal, contributory, or aggravating factors. Management entails treatment, elimination, or modification of these underlying factors. In some cases this requires active medical or surgical treatment or change or discontinuation of medications (150,151). Restoration and maintenance of fluid and electrolyte balance, management of sleep deprivation, and provision of general comfort, including control of pain and other distressing symptoms, often are crucial components of successful treatment. Supportive measures include the following:

- Close nursing surveillance for changes in vital signs and mental status
- Adjusting the level of environmental stimulation to avoid extremes of sensory deprivation or overload
- Simple explanations and reassurance
- Frequent reorientation and clarification of perceptions
- Minimizing isolation
- Facilitating contact with familiar people and objects

Pharmacologic management should be directed at specific target symptoms that require treatment (for example, agitation, hallucinations) (150). Although we are not aware of any controlled trials of psychotropic drugs for treatment of delirium, low doses of neuroleptics, specifically haloperidol, may be useful to damper agitation and psychotic symptoms in that haloperidol is rapidly acting, nonsedating, and can be administered parenterally or orally (152). Benzodiazepines with short elimination half-lives may be useful to regulate sleep–wake cycles.

An acute mental status change not only may be a harbinger or manifestation of a medical emergency, it also may complicate the medical emergency. Patients with delirium, especially those with psychotic symptoms such as hallucinations or paranoid delusions, often exhibit behaviors that interfere with medical care. They may refuse diagnostic procedures or treatment, becoming combative when attempts are made to help them, or actively try to leave the hospital. When this occurs in the context of mental status changes, the patient's decision-making capacity should be assessed (153,154). If the cognitive impairment or psychosis renders the patient unable to recognize the presence and nature of their illness, disability, or other problem; understand the available options for treatment or assistance to meet their needs; and appreciate the consequences of their choice to accept or refuse treatment or assistance, then a proxy decision-maker should be identified. The proxy, who may be a family member, friend, or health care professional, makes decisions on behalf of the patient, who may then be treated involuntarily. In most states in this country, if a medical emergency exists, or if there is imminent danger to the patient or others, the patient may be detained involuntarily in the hospital and treated. Psychiatric consultation can be useful in these situations for diagnostic evaluation, clinical assessment of decision-making capacity, and advice on medicolegal issues regarding mental health and protective statutes. In some cases, consultation with hospital legal counsel is indicated.

Psychiatric Emergencies

Psychiatric emergencies commonly observed in rehabilitation settings include suicidal and self-neglectful behaviors, panic reactions, assaultive and aggressive behaviors, delirium presenting as severe agitation or psychosis (discussed previously), and psychosocial neglect and abuse. Some of these behaviors represent extreme reactions to the expected loss observed in disabled patients. They require immediate investigation and intervention when recognized because they will inevitably complicate the course of recovery and interrupt or prolong the need for rehabilitation services.

Severely depressed patients and those with known histories of depression with or without suicidal behaviors always must have their suicidal potential assessed and monitored. Previous alcohol use, antisocial behavior, chronic pain, and psychoses are other recognized risk factors for suicide. Articulation of suicidal intention or demonstration of self-injurious behaviors must be explored in terms of help-seeking versus actual plans to act. Lack of participation in a prescribed or recommended rehabilitation program should also be explored as a possible passive manifestation of self-injurious behavior. One-to-one nursing supervision often is essential in the suicidal patient until a treatment plan is clear. Psychiatric consultation is mandatory to verify such behavior and to define a plan of treatment, including acute psychiatric admission (155,156).

Panic reactions and other extreme manifestations of acute anxiety must initially be considered an expected and appropriate physiological response to cardiopulmonary compromise (myocardial ischemia, hypoxemia), as well as to other serious medical conditions such as thyrotoxicosis and noradrenergic secreting tumors. Visual and hearing impairment may interfere with comprehension and communication, resulting in extreme anxiety and disorganization when a patient is expected to demonstrate goal-directed behavior during rehabilitation treatments. These causes of panic and anxiety must be ruled out before interpreting and treating these behaviors as extreme and inappropriate situational reactions. Environmental or interpersonal precipitants must be identified. Appropriate use of antidepressant agents or anxiolytic agents in combination with organized behavioral management can be useful to minimize interference of these behaviors with progression through a rehabilitation program (157).

Violent, assaultive, or aggressive behaviors directed toward others cannot be tolerated and must be treated decisively and quickly during rehabilitation programs. The immediate environment must be stripped of items that could be injurious to the patient and to others. Temporary restraint by care providers sometimes is necessary until the patient can be secluded in a protected room and further restrained physically. In these situations, a care provider should never act alone. When possible, security personnel and other care providers—at least 5 people—should be recruited. Parenteral psychopharmacologic agents, such as benzodiazepines (lorazepam 1 to 2 mg intramuscularly), or neuroleptics (haloperidol 2 to 5 mg intramuscularly) should be administered in repeated doses as necessary until the patient is calm and physical restraints can be safely removed. During these episodes, the treating physician must direct the process of restraining the patient and attempt to explain to the patient the necessity of such action. Diagnostic investigation and further treatment must occur in a psychiatric setting. Behaviors that may warn rehabilitation personnel of impending violence include verbal threats, hyperactivity, mania, possession of weapons, autonomic arousal, nonprescribed substance use, paranoia, antisocial behaviors, panic reactions, and disinhibition. Needless to say, interventions that minimize physical and chemical restraints are preferred. A nonconfrontational, empathic, affectively neutral approach, reinforcing that the immediate environment is safe while not leaving the patient alone, can often diminish the potential for violence until urgent psychiatric consultation is obtained. Patients' fears, sense of helplessness, and loss of control must be explored as situational precipitants and then allowed to be expressed verbally by the patient. If possible, realistic suggestions to minimize these precipitants should be operationalized in an effort to minimize aggressive behaviors (155–157).

Psychosocial abuse or neglect among patients and informal (''family'') care providers often is not recognized until an explicit discharge or continuing care plan is defined. When family meetings and therapy education sessions are missed by potential future informal home care providers, this should warn the rehabilitation team that the family members are overwhelmed. Lack of followthrough with essential preventive/maintenance care by informal care providers may become evident. Substance abuse and mental illness within a household should prompt increased vigilance for an abusive or neglectful situation. Inability for an informal care provider to participate in or to learn a home-based personal care regimen should also cause worry about a potentially inadvertent neglectful situation. Medical and social service assessments should include exploration of the motivations (e.g., altruistic, financial) or lack thereof underpinning these relationships. Relationships that historically have inadvertently been difficult, and role reversals, should be reasons to invite the involved parties into formal and ongoing counseling, at least for preventive purposes. When possible, especially when personal financial or health insurance resources allow, skilled home services can serve monitoring and supportive purposes. Formal home care services increasingly are viewed as scarce and complementary to self- or family-directed care for disabled patients in this era of managed care. ''Family'' members considered potential informal care providers come from social connections that extend beyond traditional nuclear family relationships. The limits of an informal care provider's tolerance for disability must be made explicit. Time out via respite by formal services on a regular basis can help prevent abuse and neglect. Service reciprocity between a patient and an informal care provider often supports the ''balance of power'' for both parties, who may perceive these relationships in which no one has control.

REFERENCES

1. *Dorland's illustrated medical dictionary, 28th ed.* Philadelphia: WB Saunders, 1994; 544.
2. Hanks RA, Lichtenberg PA. Physical, psychological and social outcomes in geriatric rehabilitation patients. *Arch Phys Med Rehabil* 1996; 77:783–792.
3. Fries JF. Aging, natural death and the compression of morbidity. *N Engl J Med* 1980; 303:130–135.
4. Schneider EL, Brody JA. Aging, natural death and the compression of morbidity: another view. *N Engl J Med* 1983; 309:854–856.
5. Schneider EL, Reed JD. Life extension. *N Engl J Med* 1985; 312: 1159–1168.
6. Rowe JW. Health care of the elderly. *N Engl J Med* 1985; 312: 827–835.
7. Rowe JW, Warg S. The biology and physiology of aging. In: Rowe JW, Besdine RW, eds. *Geriatric medicine.* Boston: Little, Brown, 1988; 1–11.
8. National Center for Health Statistics, Dawson D, Hendershot G, Fulton J. *Aging in the eighties: functional limitations of individuals aged 65 and over. Advance data from vital health statistics, No. 133, DHHS publication No. (PHS) 87-1250.* Hyattsville, MD: US Public Health Service, 1987.
9. Williams TF. The aging process: biological and psychosocial considerations. In: Brody SJ, Ruff GE, eds. *Aging and rehabilitation.* New York: Springer-Verlag, 1986; 13–18.
10. Edmunds LH, Stephenson LW, Edie RN, Ratcliffe MB. Open heart surgery in octogenarians. *N Engl J Med* 1988; 319:131–136.
11. Patterson C, Crescenzi C, Steel K. Hospital use by the extremely elderly (nonagenarians): a two-year study. *J Am Geriatr Soc* 1984; 32:350–352.
12. Steel K. Iatrogenic disease on a medical service. *J Am Geriatr Soc* 1984; 32:445–449.
13. Hayes SH, Carroll SR. Early intervention care in the acute stroke patient. *Arch Phys Med Rehabil* 1986; 67:319–321.
14. Kane JT, Gallagher AJ, Davis DM, Cummings V. Diagnostic-related groups: their impact on an inpatient rehabilitation program. *Arch Phys Med Rehabil* 1987; 68:833—836.
15. Marcinaiak CM, Heinemann AW, Monga T. Changes in medical stability upon admission to a rehabilitation unit. *Arch Phys Med Rehabil* 1993; 74:1157–1160.
16. Keith RA, Wilson DB, Gutierrez P. Acute and subacute rehabilitation for stroke: a comparison. *Arch Phys Med Rehabil* 1995; 76:495–500.
17. Haffey WJ, Welsh JH. Subacute care: evolution in search of value. *Arch Phys Med Rehabil* 1995; 76:SC-2–SC-4.
18. Frederickson M, Cannon NL. The role of the rehabilitation physician in the postacute continuum. *Arch Phys Med Rehabil* 1995; 76:SC-5–SC-9.
19. Meythaler JM, Cross LL. Traumatic spinal cord injury complicated by AIDS-related complex. *Arch Phys Med Rehabil* 1988; 69:219–222.
20. Sliwa JH, Smith JC. Rehabilitation of neurologic disability related to human immunodeficiency virus. *Arch Phys Med Rehabil* 1991; 72: 759–762.
21. Sliwa HA, Blendonohy PM. Stroke rehabilitation in a patient with a history of heart transplantation. *Arch Phys Med Rehabil* 1988; 69: 973–975.
22. Nicholas JJ, Oleske D, Robinson LR, Switala JA, Tarter R. The quality of life after orthotopic liver transplantation: an analysis of 166 cases. *Arch Phys Med Rehabil* 1994; 75:431–435.
23. Rosenblum DS, Rosen ML, Pine ZM, Rosen SH, Borg-Stein J. Health status and quality of life following cardiac transplantation. *Arch Phys Med Rehabil* 1993; 74:490–493.
24. Kutner NG, Brogan DJ. Assisted survival, aging, and rehabilitation needs: comparison of older dialysis patients. *Arch Phys Med Rehabil* 1992; 73:309–315.
25. Cowen TD, Huang C-T, Lebow J, Devivo MJ, Hawkins LN. Functional outcomes after inpatient rehabilitation of patients with end-stage renal disease. *Arch Phys Med Rehabil* 1995; 76:355–359.
26. Hughes RL, Davison R. Limitations of exercise conditioning in chronic obstructive lung disease. *Chest* 1983; 83:241–249.
27. Braun NMT, Faulkner J, Hughes RL, Roussos C, Sahgal V. When should respiratory muscles be exercised? *Chest* 1984; 84:76–84.
28. Miers LJ, Arnold R. The cardiovascular response to exercise in the patient with congestive heart failure. *J Cardiovasc Nurs* 1990; 4: 47–58.
29. Sullivan MJ, Higginbothom MB, Cobb FR. Exercise training in patients with severe left ventricular dysfunction. *Circulation* 1988; 78: 506–515.
30. Health Care Financing Administration. *Medicare hospital manual, publication No. 10.* Washington, D.C.: US Government Printing Office, Revision 582, 1990.
31. Felsenthal G, Cohen S, Hilton B, Panagos AV, Aiken BM. The physiatrist as primary physician for patients on an in-patient rehabilitation unit. *Arch Phys Med Rehabil* 1984; 65:375–378.
32. Eisenberg JM. The internist as gatekeeper: preparing the general internist for a new role. *Ann Intern Med* 1985; 102:537–543.
33. Gans BM, Mann NR, Becker BE. Delivery of primary care to the physically challenged. *Arch Phys Med Rehabil* 1993; 74:S-15–S-19.
34. Goldman L, Lee T, Rudd P. Ten commandments for effective consultations. *Arch Intern Med* 1983; 143:1753–1755.
35. Parry F. Physical rehabilitation of the old patient. *J Am Geriatr Soc* 1983; 31:482–484.
36. Stineman MG, Brody SJ, Shelton B, Shin G. Severe medical complications during rehabilitation pre- and post-introduction of acute care prospective payment (abstract). *Arch Phys Med Rehabil* 1986; 67: 650.
37. Wright RE, Rao N, Smith RM, Harvey RF. Risk factors for death

and emergency transfer in acute and subacute inpatient rehabilitation. *Arch Phys Med Rehabil* 1996; 77:1049–1055.
38. Siegler EL, Stineman MG, Maislin G. Development of complications during rehabilitation. *Arch Intern Med* 1994; 54:2185–2190.
39. McGuire TJ, Kumar VN. Autonomic dysreflexia in the spinal cord injured. *Postgrad Med* 1986; 80:87–89.
40. Yarkony GM, Katz RT, Wu Y-C. Seizures secondary to autonomic dysreflexia. *Arch Phys Med Rehabil* 1986; 67:834–835.
41. Naftchi NE. Mechanism of autonomic dysreflexia: contributions of catecholamines and peptide neurotransmitters. *Ann NY Acad Sci* 1990; 579:133–148.
42. Fishburn MJ, Marino RJ, Ditunno JF. Atelectasis and pneumonia in acute spinal cord injury. *Arch Phys Med Rehabil* 1990; 71:197–200.
43. Stover SL, Lloyd K, Waites KB, Jackson AB. Urinary tract infection in spinal cord injury. *Arch Phys Med Rehabil* 1989; 70:47–54.
44. Peterson JR, Roth EJ. Fever, bacteriuria and pyuria in spinal cord injured patients with indwelling urethral catheters. *Arch Phys Med Rehabil* 1989; 70:839–841.
45. Weingarden ST, Weingarden DS, Belen J. Fever and thromboembolic disease in acute spinal cord injury. *Paraplegia* 1988; 26:35–42.
46. Mallory BS. Autonomic function in the isolated spinal cord. In: Downey JA, Myers SJ, Gonzalez EG, Lieberman JS, eds. *Physiological basis of rehabilitation medicine, 2nd ed.* Boston: Butterworth-Heinemann, 1994; 519–542.
47. Nicolle LE, Buffet L, Alfieri N, Tate R. Nosocomial infections on a rehabilitation unit in an acute care hospital. *Infect Control Hosp Epidemiol* 1988; 9:553–558.
48. Sandin KJ, Light K, Holzman M, Donovan WH. Candida pyelonephritis complicating traumatic C5 quadriplegia: diagnosis and management. *Arch Phys Med Rehabil* 1991; 72:243–246.
49. Warlow C, Ogston D, Douglas AS. Deep venous thrombosis of the legs after strokes. *Br Med J* 1976; 1:1178–1183.
50. Gibberd FB, Gould SR, Marks P. Incidence of deep vein thrombosis and leg oedema in patients with strokes. *J Neurol Neurosurg Psychiatry* 1976; 39:1222–1225.
51. Miyamoto AT, Miller LS. Pulmonary embolism in stroke: prevention by early heparinization of venous thrombosis detected by iodine-125 fibrinogen leg scans. *Arch Phys Med Rehabil* 1980; 61:584–587.
52. Sioson ER, Crowe WE, Dawson NV. Occult proximal deep vein thrombosis: its prevalence among patients admitted to a rehabilitation hospital. *Arch Phys Med Rehabil* 1988; 69:183–185.
53. McCarthy ST, Robertson D, Turner JJ, Hawkey CS, Macey OJ. Low-dose heparin as a prophylaxis against deep-vein thrombosis after acute stroke. *Lancet* 1977; 1:800–801.
54. Gelmers HJ. Effects of low-dose subcutaneous heparin on the occurrence of deep vein thrombosis in patients with ischemic stroke. *Acta Neurol Scand* 1980; 61:313–318.
55. McCarthy ST, Turner J. Low-dose subcutaneous heparin in the prevention of deep-vein thrombosis and pulmonary emboli following acute stroke. *Age Ageing* 1986; 15:84–88.
56. Geerts WH, Code KI, Jay RM, Chen E, Szalai JP. A prospective study of venous thromboembolism after major trauma. *N Engl J Med* 1994; 331:1601–1606.
57. Kim SW, Charallel JT, Park KW, Bauerle LC, Shang CC, Gordon SK, Bauman WA. Prevalence of deep venous thrombosis in patients with chronic spinal cord injuries. *Arch Phys Med Rehabil* 1994; 75: 965–968.
58. Dennis JW, Menawat S, Von Thron J, Fallon WF, et al. Efficacy of deep venous thrombosis prophylaxis in trauma patients and identification of high-risk groups. *J Trauma* 1993; 35:132–139.
59. White RH, McGahan JP, Daschback MM, Hartling RP. Diagnosis of deep-vein thrombosis using duplex ultrasound. *Ann Intern Med* 1989; 111:297–304.
60. Hull RD, Raskob GE, LeClerc JR, Jay RM, Hirsh J. The diagnosis of clinically suspected venous thrombosis. *Clin Chest Med* 1984; 5: 439–456.
61. Huisman MV, Wouter ten Cate J. Diagnosis of deep-vein thrombosis using an objective doppler method. *Ann Intern Med* 1990; 113:9–13.
62. Izzo KL, Aquino E. Deep venous thrombosis in high-risk hemiplegic patients: detection by impedance plethysmography. *Arch Phys Med Rehabil* 1986; 67:799–802.
63. Meythaler JM, DeVivo MJ, Hayne JB. Cost-effectiveness of routine screening for proximal deep venous thrombosis in acquired brain injury patients admitted to rehabilitation. *Arch Phys Med Rehabil* 1996; 77:1–5.
64. Katz RT, McCulla SrMM. Impedence plethysmography as a screening procedure for asymptomatic deep venous thrombosis in a rehabilitation hospital. *Arch Phys Med Rehabil* 1995; 76:833–839.
65. Pambianco G, Orchard T, Landau D. Deep venous thrombosis: prevention in stroke patients during rehabilitation. *Arch Phys Med Rehabil* 1995; 76:324–330.
66. Leizorovicz A, Haugh MC, Chapnis F-R, Samana MM, Boissel J-P. Low molecular weight heparin in prevention of perioperative thrombosis. *Br Med J* 1992; 305:913–920.
67. Routledge PA, West RR. Low molecular weight heparin. *Br Med J* 1992; 305:906.
68. Green D, Chen D, Chmiel JS, Olsen NK, et al. Prevention of thromboembolism in spinal cord injury: role of low molecular weight heparin. *Arch Phys Med Rehabil* 1994; 75:290–292.
69. Bergqvist D, Benoni G, Bjorgell O, Fredin A, et al. Low molecular weight heparin (enoxaparin) as prophylaxis against venous thromboembolism after total hip replacement. *N Engl J Med* 1996; 335: 696–700.
70. Kelley MA, Carson JL, Palevsky HI, Schwartz JS. Diagnosing pulmonary embolism: new facts and strategies. *Ann Intern Med* 1991; 114: 300–306.
71. Hull RD, Raskob GE, Pineo GF, Green D, et al. Subcutaneous low molecular-weight heparin compared with continuous intravenous heparin in the treatment of proximal-vein thrombosis. *N Engl J Med* 1992; 326:975–982.
72. Ben-Shlomo LS, Palaima MM, Leonardo JJ, Boudreau KA, LaRaia PJ. Cardiac evaluation during physical rehabilitation of the complex medical patient. *Arch Phys Med Rehabil* 1988; 69:932–936.
73. Siegler EL, Taylor L, Norris R, Jedrziewski K, Reichek N. Silent ischemia can be detected in rehabilitation patients, but it has limited clinical utility. *Arch Phys Med Rehabil* 1992; 73:730–734.
74. Clark GS, Blue B, Bearer JB. Rehabilitation of the elderly amputee. *J Am Geriatr Soc* 1983; 31:439–448.
75. Gonzalez EG, Corcoran PJ. Energy expenditure during ambulation. In: Myers SJ, Gonzalez EG, Lieberman JS, eds. *Physiological basis of rehabilitation medicine, 2nd ed.* Boston: Butterworth-Heinemann 1994; 413–336.
76. Fisher SV, Gullickson G. Energy cost of ambulation in health and disability: a literature review. *Arch Phys Med Rehabil* 1978; 59: 124–133.
77. Huang C-T, Jackson JR, Moore NB, et al. Amputation: energy costs of ambulation. *Arch Phys Med Rehabil* 1979; 60:18–24.
78. Thornhill HL, Jones GD, Brodski W, van Bockstaele P. Bilateral below-knee amputations: experience with 80 patients. *Arch Phys Med Rehabil* 1986; 67:159–163.
79. Steinberg FU, Sunwoo I, Roettger RF. Prosthetic rehabilitation of geriatric amputee patients: a follow-up study. *Arch Phys Med Rehabil* 1985; 66:742–745.
80. Roth EJ, Wiesner S, Green D, Wu Y. Dysvascular amputee rehabilitation the role of continuous noninvasive cardiovascular monitoring during physical therapy. *Am J Phys Med Rehabil* 1987; 69:16–22.
81. Cruts HEP, de Vries J, Zilvold G, Huisman K, can Alste JA, Boom HBK. Lower extremity amputees with peripheral vascular disease: graded exercise testing and results of prosthetic training. *Arch Phys Med Rehabil* 1987; 68:14–19.
82. Finestone H, Lampman R, Islam S, Westbury L, Schultz JS. Arm ergometry exercise testing in the dysvascular amputee: resting and dynamic electrocardiographic findings (abstract). *Arch Phys Med Rehabil* 1989; 70:A75.
83. Chambers BR, Norris JW, Shurvell BL, Hachinski V. Prognosis of acute stroke. *Neurology* 1987; 37:221–225.
84. Meltzer RS, Visser CA, Fuster V. Intracardiac thrombi and systemic embolization. *Ann Intern Med* 1986; 104:689–698.
85. Dimant J, Grob D. Electrocardiographic changes and myocardial damage in patients with acute cerebrovascular accidents. *Stroke* 1977; 8: 448–455.
86. Myers MS, Norris JW, Hachinski VC, Weingert ME, Sole MJ. Cardiac sequelae of acute stroke. *Stroke* 1982; 13:838–842.
87. Norris JW. Effects of cerebrovascular lesions on the heart. *Neurol Clin* 1983; 1:98–101.
88. Reinstein L, Purdue E, Haber C. Decreased need for diabetes medica-

tion during inpatient stroke and amputee rehabilitation (abstract). *Arch Phys Med Rehabil* 1982; 68:663.
89. Dombovy ML, Basford JR, Whisnant JP, Bergstralh EJ. Disability and use of rehabilitation services following stroke in Rochester, Minnesota 1975–1979. *Stroke* 1987; 18:830–836.
90. Gresham GE, Phillips TF, Wolf PA, Konnel WB, Dawber TR. The epidemiologic profile of long term stroke disability: the Framingham study. *Arch Phys Med Rehabil* 1978; 60:487–491.
91. Roth EJ, Mueller K, Green D. Stroke rehabilitation outcome: impact of coronary artery disease. *Stroke* 1988; 19:47–49.
92. Feigenson JS, McDowell FH, Meese P, McCarthy ML, Greenberg SD. Factors influencing outcome and length of stay in a stroke rehabilitation unit: part 1. *Stroke* 1977; 8:651–656.
93. Anderson TD, Bourestrom N, Greenberg FR, Hidyard VG. Predictive factors in stroke rehabilitation. *Arch Phys Med Rehabil* 1974; 55: 545–553.
94. Roth EJ. Heart disease in patients with stroke: incidence, impact, and implications for rehabilitation. Part I: classification and prevalence. *Arch Phys Med Rehabil* 1993; 74:752–760.
95. Roth EJ. Heart disease in patients with stroke. Part II: impact and implications for rehabilitation. *Arch Phys Med Rehabil* 1994; 75: 94–101.
96. Lim PO, MacFadyen RJ, Clarkson PBM, MacDonald TM. Impaired exercise tolerance in hypertensive patients. *Am Intern Med* 1996; 124: 41–55.
97. Pennza PT. Aspiration pneumonia, necrotizing pneumonia, and lung abscess. *Emerg Med Clin North Am* 1989; 7:279–307.
98. Lazarus C, Logemann JA. Swallowing disorders in closed head trauma patients. *Arch Phys Med Rehabil* 1987; 68:79–84.
99. Horner J, Massey EW. Silent aspiration following stroke. *Neurology* 1988; 38:317–319.
100. Janzen VD, Rae RE, Hudson AJ. Otolaryngologic manifestations of amyotrophic lateral sclerosis. *J Otolaryngol* 1988; 17:41–42.
101. Ogorek CP, Fisher RS. Detection and treatment of gastroesophageal reflux disease. *Gastroenterol Clin North Am* 1989; 18:293–313.
102. Muz, CL, Mathog RH, Nelson R, Jones LA Jr. Aspiration in patients with head and neck cancer and tracheostomy. *Am J Otolaryngol* 1989; 10:282–286.
103. Pingleton SK. Enteral nutrition as a risk factor for nosocomial pneumonia. *Eur J Clin Microbiol Infect Dis* 1989; 8:51–55.
104. Robinson KM, Zorowitz, RD. Mechanisms of aspiration disorders. In: Fishman AP, editor-in-chief, *Pulmonary diseases and disorders, 3rd ed.* New York: McGraw-Hill, 1998; 1211–1214.
105. Kohn CL, Keithley JK. Enteral nutrition: potential complications and patient monitoring. *Nurs Clin North Am* 1989; 23:339–342.
106. Logemann JA. The role of the speech language pathologist in the management of dysphagia. *Otolaryngol Clin North Am* 1988; 21: 783–788.
107. Muz J, Mathog RH, Miller PR, Rosen R, Borrero G. Detection and quantification of laryngotracheopulmonary aspiration with scintigraphy. *Laryngoscope* 1987; 97:1180–1185.
108. Bevan K, Griffiths MB. Chronic aspiration and laryngeal competence. *J Laryngol Otol* 1989; 103:196–199.
109. Bushman M, Dobmeyer SM, Leeker L, Perlmutter JS. Swallowing abnormalities and their response to treatment in Parkinson's disease. *Neurology* 1989; 39:1309–1314.
110. Horner J, Alberts MJ, Dawson DV, Cook GM. Swallowing in Alzheimer's disease. *Alzheimer Dis Assoc Disord* 1994; 8(3):177–189.
111. Eustace S, Gleeson C, Joyce M, Sullivan P. Oculopharyngeal muscular dystrophy in an Irish family. *Ir J Med Sci* 1989; 158:120.
112. Sauer L, Pellegrini CA, Way LW. The treatment of achalasia: a current perspective. *Arch Surg* 1989; 124:929–932.
113. Horner J, Massey EW, Riski JE, et al. Aspiration following stroke: clinical correlates and outcomes. *Neurology* 1988; 38:1359–1362.
114. Johnson ER, McKenzie SW, Sievers A. Aspiration pneumonia in stroke. *Arch Phys Med Rehabil* 1993; 74:973–976.
115. Alberts MJ, Horner J, Gray L, Brazer SR. Aspiration after stroke: lesion analysis by brain MRI. *Dysphagia* 1992; 7:170–173.
116. Pennington GR, Krutsch JA. Swallowing disorders: assessment and rehabilitation. *Br J Hosp Med* 1990; 44:17–20.
117. DePippo KL, Holas MA, Reding MJ. The Burke dysphagia screening test: validation of its use in patients with stroke. *Arch Phys Med Rehabil* 1994; 75:1284–1286.
118. Pezner RD, Archambeau JO, Lipsett JA, Kokal WA, Thayer W, Hill LR. Tube feeding enteral nutritional support in patients after receiving radiation therapy for advanced head and neck cancer. *Int J Radiat Oncol Biol Phys* 1987; 13:935–939.
119. Sitzmann JV. Nutritional support of the dysphagic patient: methods, risks and complications of therapy. *J Parent Ent Nutr* 1990; 14:60–63.
120. Flynn KT, Norton LC, Fisher RL. Enteral tube feeding: indications, practices and outcomes. *Image J Nurs Scholar* 1987; 19:16–19.
121. Pritchard B. Tube feeding: related pneumonias. *J Gerontol Nurs* 1988; 14:32–36.
122. Llaneza PP, Menendez AM, Roberts R, Dunn GD. Percutaneous endoscopic gastrostomy: clinical experience and follow-up. *South Med J* 1988; 81:321–324.
123. Kaplan DS, Murthy UK, Linscheer WG. Percutaneous endoscopic jejunostomy: long-term follow-up of 23 patients. *Gastrointest Endosc* 1989; 35:403–406.
124. Hicks ME, Surratt RS, Picus D, Marx MV, Lang EV. Fluoroscopically guided percutaneous gastrostomy and gastroenterostomy: analysis of 158 consecutive cases. *Am J Roentgenol* 1990; 154:725–728.
125. Lazarus BA, Murphy JB, Culpepper L. Aspiration associated with long-term gastric versus jejunal feeding: a critical analysis of the literature. *Arch Phys Med Rehabil* 1990; 71:46–53.
126. Cohen B, Malik N, Robinson KM. A multidisciplinary swallowing team for prevention of aspiration pneumonia (abstract). *Arch Phys Med Rehabil* 1991; 72:793.
127. Logemann JA. *Evaluation and treatment of swallowing disorders.* Austin, TX: Professional Education, 1983.
128. Pingleton SK. Aspiration of enteral feedings in mechanically ventilated patients: how do we monitor? *Crit Care Med* 1994; 22: 1524–1525.
129. Mamel JJ. Percutaneous endoscopic gastrostomy. *Am J Gastroenterol* 1989; 84:703–710.
130. Lipowski ZJ. Update on delirium. *Psychiatr Clin North Am* 1992; 15(2):335–346.
131. Hodkinson HM. *Common symptoms of disease in the elderly.* Oxford: Blackwell, 1976; 24.
132. Lerkoff SE, Evans DA, Liptzin B, Cleary PD, et al. Delirium. *Arch Intern Med* 1992; 152:334–340.
133. Schor JD, Lerkoff SE, Lipsitz LA, Reilly CH, Clearly PD, Rowe JW, Evans DA. Risk factors for delirium in hospitalized elderly. *JAMA* 1992; 267:827–831.
134. Kaplan HI, Freedman AM, Sadock BJ, eds. *Comprehensive textbook of psychiatry, 3rd ed.* Baltimore: Williams & Wilkins, 1981.
135. Kemp B. Psychosocial and mental health issues in rehabilitation of older persons. In: Brody SJ, Ruff GE, eds. *Aging and rehabilitation: advances in the state of the art.* New York: Springer-Verlag, 1986: 127–132.
136. *Diagnostic and statistical manual of mental disorders, 4th ed. Primary care version.* Washington, D.C.: American Psychiatric Association, 1995:79–81.
137. Murray AM, Lerkoff SE, Wetle TT, Beckett L, et al. Acute delirium and functional decline in hospital elderly patients. *J Gerontol* 1993; 48(5):M181–M186.
138. Francis J, Kapoor WN. Prognosis after hospital discharge of older medical patients with delirium. *J Am Geriatr Soc* 1992; 40:601–606.
139. Beresin EV. Delirium in the elderly. *J Geriatr Psychiatry Neurol* 1988; 1:127–143.
140. Hodkinson HM. Mental impairment in the elderly. *J R Coll Physicians Lond* 1973; 7:305–317.
141. Millar HR. Psychiatric morbidity in elderly surgical patients. *Br J Psychiatry* 1981; 138:17–20.
142. Lipowski ZJ. Transient cognitive disorders (delirium, acute confusional states) in the elderly. *Am J Psychiatry* 1983; 140:1426–1436.
143. Lipowski ZJ. Delirium in the elderly patient. *N Engl J Med* 1989; 320:578–582.
144. Levkoff SE, Besdine RW, Wetle T. Acute confusional states (delirium) in the hospitalized elderly. *Annu Rev Gerontol Geriatr* 1986; 6: 1–26.
145. McCartney JR, Palmateer LM. Assessment of cognitive deficits in geriatric patients: a study of physician behavior. *J Am Geriatr Soc* 1985; 33:467–471.
146. Liston EJ. Delirium in the aged. *Psychiatr Clin North Am* 1982; 5: 49–66.
147. Lipowski ZK. *Delirium: acute confusional states.* New York: Oxford University Press, 1990.

148. Francis J, Martin D, Kapoor WN. A prospective study on delirium in hospitalized elderly. *JAMA* 1990; 263:1097–1101.
149. Rabins P, Folstein MF. Delirium and dementia: diagnostic criteria and fatality rates. *Br J Psychiatry* 1982; 140:149–153.
150. Conn DK. Delirium and other organic mental disorder. In: Sadavoy J, Lazarus LW, Jarvik LF, eds. *Comprehensive review of geriatric psychiatry*. Washington, D.C.: American Psychiatric Press, 1991: 311–336.
151. Wise MG. Delirium. In: Hales RE, Yudofsky SC, eds. *Textbook of neuropsychiatry*. Washington, D.C.: American Psychiatric Press, 1987:89–103.
152. Seneff MG, Matthews RA. Use of haloperidol infusions to control delirium in critically ill adults. *Ann Pharm* 1995; 29:690–693.
153. Applebaum PS, Grisso T. Assessing patients' capacities to consent to treatment. *N Engl J Med* 1988; 319:1635–1638.
154. Applebaum PS, Roth LH. Clinical issues in the assessment of competency. *N Engl J Med* 1981; 138:1462–1426.
155. Kennedy GJ, Lowinger R. Pscyhogeriatric emergencies. *Clin Geriatr Med* 1993; 9(3):641–653.
156. Tueth MJ. Diagnosing psychiatric emergencies in the elderly. *Am J Emerg Med* 1994; 12:364–396.
157. Tueth MJ. Management of behavioral emergencies. *Am J Emerg Med* 1995; 13:344–350.

Rehabilitation Medicine: Principles and Practice, Third Edition,
edited by Joel A. DeLisa and Bruce M. Gans.
Lippincott–Raven Publishers, Philadelphia © 1998.

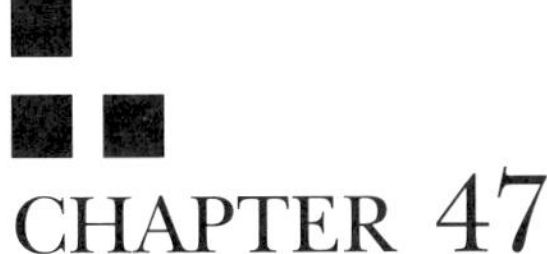

CHAPTER 47

Vocational Rehabilitation, Independent Living, and Consumerism

Denise G. Tate, Robert K. Heinrich, Liina Paasuke, and Don Anderson

Vocational rehabilitation (VR) services in the United States have traditionally emphasized the provision of services for persons with disabilities who have vocational potential. It was not until 1978 that services were also provided for those without vocational goals. Title VII, Comprehensive Services for Independent Living (IL), an amendment to the Rehabilitation Act of 1973, authorizes services for persons with severe disabilities. Severely disabled individuals are defined by law as those who require multiple services over an extended period of time and whose disability prevents them from working or disrupts other major life activities.

The VR services provided by public and private agencies include vocational evaluation, functional assessment, work hardening and reconditioning, work capacity evaluation, job site analysis, job accommodations, job-seeking skills, employer development, employment skill training, job placement, and follow-up services. The IL services are most often provided by a national network of Centers for Independent Living (CILs) across the country.

An independent living program can be defined as a community-based program with substantial consumer involvement that provides direct or indirect services (through referral) for persons with severe disabilities. These services are intended to increase self-determination and to minimize dependence on others. The IL services most often provided include housing, attendant care, reading and/or interpreting, and information about other necessary goods and services. They may also include transportation, peer counseling, advocacy or political action, training in independent living skills, equipment maintenance and repair, and social and recreational services (1). The IL programs are designed to address the needs of a population in one particular geographic community, as opposed to a region, state, or country. The programs depend on the people and resources in the community for direction and subsistence. Consumer involvement insures that programs do not lose touch with client needs and that they maintain their practical and down-to-earth characteristics.

Consumer sovereignty and empowerment have always been hallmarks of the independent living movement. Consumer sovereignty, sometimes referred as consumer involvement, asserts that persons with disabilities are the best judges of their own interests and should ultimately determine what services are provided to them. The current rise of consumerism directly challenges the traditional service delivery system. In both the VR and IL systems, professionals no longer have the final word in case planning. Instead, service provision plans are to be drawn up jointly by the client or person with the disability and the counselor. Because of the increased awareness created by advocacy skills training at CILs, many persons with disabilities are increasingly more informed about their benefits and the regulations of the agencies they must deal with (2).

The present chapter provides the reader with an overview of both the vocational rehabilitation and independent living programs. First, the authors review the legislative history and purpose of VR and IL service provision and discuss contrasts between the two. Program service settings and staff patterns are described. The processes and services that are utilized to reach individual goals are discussed for both types of programs. Current and future trends in rehabilitation affecting these services and programs are outlined. These include societal and economic trends such as cost containment

D. G. Tate: Department of Physical Medicine and Rehabilitation, University of Michigan Medical Center, Ann Arbor, Michigan 48109-0050.
R. K. Heinrich: McAuley Mental Health Services, St. Joseph Mercy Hospital, Ann Arbor, Michigan 48105.
L. Paasuke: Department of Rehabilitation Services, Michigan Jobs Commission, Ann Arbor, Michigan 48109-0050.
D. Anderson: Disability Rights and Education, Ann Arbor Center for Independent Living, Ann Arbor, Michigan 48104.

of health care, social disincentives to work, advances in technology, and trends toward consumer empowerment and self-care. Finally, conclusive remarks are offered.

HISTORY OF VOCATIONAL REHABILITATION AND INDEPENDENT LIVING SERVICES

Purpose and Characteristics of the Vocational Rehabilitation Service Delivery Process

The primary purpose of VR has been to assist and enable persons with disabilities to increase their productivity, usually through competitive employment. In recent years, greater emphasis has been put on assisting people with disabilities to live independently of institutional settings regardless of their vocational potential.

Vocational rehabilitation counselors, particularly those working within state VR agencies, work with consumers of services with a wide range of disabilities. These include physical characteristics, such as spinal cord injury, stroke, arthritis, multiple sclerosis, congenital or orthopedic difficulties, cumulative trauma or chronic pain disorders, amputations; cognitive characteristics, such as traumatic brain injury, organic brain syndromes, developmental and learning disabilities; and those with mental or emotional disorders. Vocational rehabilitation services are also provided to persons with serious alcohol and drug abuse problems. State agencies provide VR services at no cost to the consumer. Eligibility for these services is based on the extent to which a disability impedes a person's ability to obtain or maintain employment.

The VR process is focused on the person seeking assistance. The goal of VR is to identify a feasible employment goal and, then, outline the VR services needed to achieve this goal. The VR process generally involves (a) individual assessment and planning, which may include interviewing, paper-and-pencil tests, and performance evaluation in real or simulated work situations; (b) service provision, which may include counseling, education, skill training, medical restoration, and procurement of adaptive equipment; and (c) job placement, which may include trial work placements, job development, marketing, and placement in permanent employment.

The service provision plan is formalized with an Individualized Written Rehabilitation Plan, which is jointly developed by the consumer and counselor. Once job placement has been achieved, follow-up services are provided for a minimum of 60 days to provide support and consultation to the new employee and his or her employer. This helps to ensure that the employment situation is working out satisfactorily for all parties. As a result of the passage of the Technology-Related Assistance for Individuals with Disabilities Act of 1988, special emphasis has been placed on identifying the consumer's accommodation needs throughout the rehabilitation process. This enables the person with a disability to participate more fully in his or her vocational evaluation, training, and job placement processes as well as to maintain employment over time.

Legislative History

Vocational rehabilitation was formally inaugurated in the United States in 1918 with passage of the Soldiers Rehabilitation Act (Smith-Hughes; Public Law 65-178). The then-recently established Federal Board for Vocational Education was authorized to create vocational rehabilitation programs for disabled veterans. The U.S. Department of Labor was charged with locating jobs for these veterans. In part because of the enormity of this task and the priority given to returning servicemen, civilian rehabilitation did not begin until 1920 with passage of the Civilian Rehabilitation Act (Smith-Fess; PL 66-236). From the beginning, civilian rehabilitation was set up as a grant-in-aid program to encourage participation of the states. This was in contrast to the veterans' rehabilitation program, which was run solely by the federal government.

There was little preexisting knowledge about the VR process. This knowledge had to be gained through much trial and error. One of the important principles that emerged early on was that VR is an individualized process. Each person with a disability presents a somewhat different set of issues and characteristics. Consequently, a casework approach was generally adopted to address each person's needs. For example, issues of training, education, transportation, functional limitations, vocational interests and aptitudes, family, public stereotypes, work attitude, and market factors were seen to impact differentially on any given individual's ability to obtain suitable employment. This was in sharp contrast to the Worker's Compensation system, which was much more narrowly focused on obtaining a fair monetary settlement for an injured worker. This conceptual and fundamental difference has been largely responsible for the lack of coordination between these two large disability programs over the years.

Over the years, there were opponents to the provision of VR services by the government. Some felt the program to be too socialistic, outside the purview of the federal government, and questioned its constitutionality. The 1920 bill had to be reauthorized every few years. Thus, the program was frequently in danger of being discontinued. However, during the Depression years, a number of new economic security programs were instituted under the direction of President Roosevelt. The groundbreaking Social Security Act of 1935 included unemployment compensation, old age insurance, aid to dependent children, maternal and child health services, as well as other important programs. Lobbyists of the National Rehabilitation Association, founded in 1923, were able to have an amendment attached to this important legislation that permanently authorized annual VR grants to participating states. By 1939, $3.5 million a year was being given to the states for VR service provision. The program had developed solid support among the majority of federal legislators.

Like the veterans' rehabilitation program, federal oversight of civilian rehabilitation was the responsibility of the Federal Board for Vocational Education. Although there were several administrative shifts during the first 20 years, rehabilitation remained under the auspices of vocational education. Consequently, strong emphasis was put on education and training. Monies could not be spent on medical costs or on income maintenance for persons undergoing VR training. These were significant limitations.

World War II brought some major changes to both the veterans' and civilian rehabilitation systems. The Servicemen's Readjustment Act (PL 78-346) of 1944, called the GI Bill of Rights, guaranteed up to 4 years of tuition and a stipend for living expenses for returning veterans, whether disabled or not. Between 1943 and 1953, over 600,000 World War II veterans obtained VR services while another 8 million took advantage of the GI Bill. Civilian rehabilitation was significantly expanded with the Vocational Rehabilitation Act Amendments of 1943 (Barden-LaFollette; PL 78-113). Eligibility for VR services was broadened to include persons with emotional disturbances and mental retardation. In addition, medical services and income maintenance for trainees were authorized for the first time. Forty-four thousand disabled civilians were successfully helped to find employment in 1949 at an average cost of $150. At the same time, it was estimated that there were over 1.5 million vocationally disabled citizens (3).

The Vocational Rehabilitation Act Amendments of 1954 (PL 83-565) laid the groundwork for a tremendous expansion of the rehabilitation program. Important facets of this legislation included authorization for the use of federal funds to build and expand rehabilitation facilities, authorization of training grants to educational institutions for the preparation of new rehabilitation professionals, and extensive funding for research and demonstration projects to improve and disseminate rehabilitation methods. This legislation promoted the professionalization of vocational rehabilitation and ultimately led to its legitimacy as an academic discipline (4). However, increasing professionalism led to the alienation of many persons who became part of the disability rights movement of the 1970s and 1980s. Federal expenditures for vocational rehabilitation increased from $23 million in 1954 to $125 million in 1964. In 1967, VR was charged with applying its methods to assist persons who were disadvantaged by reason of educational attainment, ethnic or cultural factors, criminal history, or impoverishment (3). This VR expansion effort was discontinued under the Nixon administration of the early 1970s.

Between 1959 and 1971, there were several attempts in the U.S. Congress to pass legislation authorizing comprehensive rehabilitation services for those with severe disabilities without vocational potential. In 1959, a bill (HR 361) was introduced that contained the term "independent living services" for the first time. In 1961, other bills were introduced calling for the state VR agencies and other organizations to provide IL services. These bills failed to pass. In 1972, a new bill was written to replace existing VR legislation. The bill (HR 8395) was passed by Congress and included comprehensive rehabilitation services and independent living provisions. This legislation was vetoed by President Nixon, who believed that independent living would dilute the resources of the VR program. The bill was resubmitted in 1973 and once again vetoed. The President's advisors felt that the rehabilitation of persons without vocational potential was too expensive. In 1973, a compromise was reached, and the Rehabilitation Act was made law. Although the IL provisions were eliminated, an emphasis was placed on the delivery of VR services to clients with severe disabilities.

The Rehabilitation Act of 1973 (PL 93-112) had a major impact on VR programs. Additional important features of the 1973 Act were the creation of the IWRPs and client grievance procedures. These two innovative measures emphasized for the first time the notion of consumer empowerment with simultaneous changes in language from "client" to "consumer" (5,6). Perhaps the most significant feature of the 1973 Act was the inclusion of a civil rights clause (Section 504) that guaranteed nondiscrimination against persons with disabilities in any federally assisted program or activity. The law was interpreted to mean that employers or institutions receiving federal funds were required to make "reasonable accommodations" for otherwise qualified persons with handicaps. This provision in the legislation represented potential cost implications for educational institutions and public transportation systems in the years to follow. For employers, this meant job restructuring, workplace modifications, provision of specialized training, or ongoing support. Other sections of the Act provided for affirmative action programs for the employment of the "handicapped," for barrier-free work areas, and for the creation of the Architectural and Transportation Barrier Board.

In 1974, the Rehabilitation Act of 1973 was amended to include a broader definition of the term "handicapped individual." The new definition emphasized major life activities rather than vocational objectives. In 1978, several amendments were made to the Rehabilitation Act of 1973. The most important was Title VII: "Comprehensive Services for Independent Living." Its purpose was to authorize grants to states to provide services for severely disabled clients who had little potential for employment. However, these persons could benefit from services that would enable them to live and function independently.

A major limitation of the Rehabilitation Act was that nondiscrimination against persons with disabilities was limited to the federal sector or to organizations receiving federal funds. Furthermore, ". . . despite annual expenditures of $200 to $300 billion on direct subsidies and supports for people with disabilities, more than 70 percent of those who were capable of working and desired to work were still unemployed" (7). The Americans with Disabilities Act (ADA; PL 101-336) was passed in 1990 with extensive bipartisan support after 2 years of intensive lobbying by disability rights groups. This bill was to people with disabilities what the Civil Rights Act of 1964 was to African-Americans (8).

The ADA prohibits discrimination against people with disabilities in employment, public services, public transportation, places of public accommodation (e.g., hotels and restaurants), and telecommunications. Businesses with more than 15 employees were required to make reasonable accommodations for qualified candidates with disabilities unless such accommodations would impose undue hardship. Such accommodations might include improving worksite accessibility, equipment modification, work schedule modification, or provision of interpreters. The bill also spells out regulations for making public accommodations accessible. A distinction is made between existing facilities and newly created facilities, which have more stringent requirements. Accessibility to public transportation was hotly contested because of the potential expense. In the end, it was decided that modification of the transportation system would be phased in over a period of years. Because the bill is so broad and far-reaching, its application to specific circumstances requires some measure of interpretation. In fact, debate on this bill has continued, with some members of Congress still calling for repeal. Nevertheless, the ADA was a historic, landmark piece of legislation that guarantees civil rights for persons with disabilities. As President Bush said when signing this bill, ''Let the shameful wall of exclusion finally come tumbling down.''

Philosophy and Goals of the Independent Living and Disability Rights Movements

The IL and Disability Rights movements embody our national ideal of liberty and justice for all and are the latest expression of the historical processes that liberated African-Americans from slavery, extended to women the right to vote, safeguarded the rights of workers, and thereby ensured greater participation in our country's government. Since its conception, our nation's vocational rehabilitation system has been the vehicle that has carried people with disabilities from the dark corners of society's fears and prejudices toward the light of inclusion and self-sufficiency. Unfortunately, throughout most of its history, the VR system has been limited, as is all social policy, by societal stereotypes, attitudes, and beliefs about people with disabilities.

During our nation's colonial period, people with disabilities were noticeably excluded from social and political life. Many of the Articles of Incorporation that created the original U.S. colonies specified that individuals emigrating to the New World needed to be sound of wind and limb. The original prohibition excluding people with disabilities from colonial America was no doubt based on the physical and social requirements of living in a frontier society. Given the harsh realities of colonial life, the exclusion of people with disabilities made a certain amount of social and economic sense. However, it created a fertile ground for the fears and prejudices about disability in society at large. The belief that people with disabilities were evil, or just morally inferior, reached its zenith during the latter part of the 19th century when the majority of states enacted laws sanctioning the involuntary sterilization of people with disabilities. Another demonstration of the prejudices against people with disabilities manifested itself with the institution of compulsory education in 1860, which at the time included children with disabilities. However, the fears and stereotypes held by the parents of nondisabled children regarding people with disabilities gave rise to a movement to ban children with disabilities from our nation's classrooms. This policy remained in effect for over 100 years, until the passage of the Education of All Handicapped Children Act in 1975. Over time, with advances in the medical treatment of the causes of disability, government services for people with disabilities and protection of their civil rights have expanded.

With the emergence of the consumer (in contrast to clients or patients) movement in the early 1970s and its emphasis on self-help, responsible consumption, and self-direction, the stage was set for the emergence of the IL and Disability Rights movements. Pioneered by Ed Roberts and other individuals with severe disabilities during the early 1970s, the philosophy of IL asserted that individuals with severe disabilities were capable of managing and directing their own lives. Furthermore, the services and supports that people with disabilities need are best delivered by individuals who themselves have disabilities and whose knowledge about both disability and services is derived from first-hand experience.

Empowerment of Consumers

Since its beginning, the IL movement has placed a very high value on consumer control and direction, not only of the services needed by its individual constituents but of the institutions and organizations that house its activities and administer its resources. Thus, the 1992 Amendments to the Rehabilitation Act required that a majority of CIL staff, management, and directors must be individuals with disabilities.

Increasingly CILs distinguish themselves from traditional rehabilitation providers by their emphasis on teaching individuals with disabilities how to procure and direct services to meet their needs as they define them to be. This is in contrast to medically oriented rehabilitation programs, which rely on the diagnosis of a doctor or therapist to determine the need. Nowhere has consumer empowerment been more strongly embraced by CILs than in the area of advocacy. With the increasing emphasis placed on advocacy by the Rehabilitation Services Agency (federal), many CILs have shifted from active involvement in the process of removing barriers for their clients to teaching individuals with disabilities how to overcome obstacles, remove barriers, and advocate for change on their own.

Community Settings and Centers for Independent Living

The specific features of individual IL programs are determined by the needs of the consumers served, the availability of existing community resources, the physical and social make-up of the community, and the goals of the program itself. Independent living support services can be provided by a variety of community-based programs such as self-help and information referral centers, generic service providers, transitional programs, and residential programs. Between 1977 and 1988, the number of independent living programs in the United States grew from 52 to more than 400.

Although many independent living programs began within the traditional VR system, many quickly evolved into autonomous nonprofit organizations. This trend was accelerated by the inclusion of Part B of Title VII in the 1978 amendments, which authorized grants for the establishment of Centers for Independent Living. Traditional medically oriented rehabilitation programs see the problem of disability as a deficit or impairment that must be fixed. The CILs accept that disability is an inevitable aspect of the human experience and focus on assisting individuals to adapt themselves and their environment to that reality.

At a minimum, CIL services consist of peer counseling, information and referral, independent living skills training, and advocacy. These services are primarily provided by other individuals with disabilities, who may or may not have professional training in those areas but who have personal experience in living with a disability. Many CILs also offer such services as housing assistance, personal assistant training and referral, sign language interpreter referral, and community awareness programs. In addition, with the 1992 Amendments to the Rehabilitation Act, many CILs are currently placing greater emphasis on systems advocacy and consumer empowerment. Systems advocacy aims at inclusion of people with disabilities in the policy-making roles that regulate delivery of medical, social, rehabilitation, or other services. Systems advocacy may be focused at the local, state, regional, or national level depending on the nature of the underlying issue being addressed.

CONTRASTS AND CONCEPTUAL DIFFERENCES BETWEEN THE VOCATIONAL REHABILITATION AND THE INDEPENDENT LIVING PROGRAMS

Central to the IL concept is the belief that management of medically stabilized disabilities is primarily a personal matter and only secondarily a medical matter. The persistent involvement of trained professional medical or rehabilitation personnel in the life of a person with a disability fosters dependency and can hinder the achievement of rehabilitation and IL goals. The IL movement rejects the behavioral expectations created by both the sick role and its derivative, the impaired role. It presumes that a person with a disability does not want to be relieved of his or her familial, occupational, and civic responsibilities in exchange for complete dependency. In fact, the movement considers any such relief of responsibility tantamount to denying persons with disability their rights to participate in the life of the community and their right to full personhood.

DeJong argues that there are sufficient differences between the traditional medical/vocational rehabilitation and independent living to speak of two paradigms (3). According to the rehabilitation paradigm, individual problems are generally defined in terms of inadequate performance in activities of daily living (ADL) or in terms of inadequate preparation for gainful employment. In both instances, the problem is assumed to reside in the individual. Therefore, the individual needs to change behaviors, skills, or way of life. To overcome these problems, individuals receiving rehabilitation care are expected to follow the instructions of a physician, physical therapist, occupational therapist, nurse, psychologist, and/or vocational counselor and to assume the patient role. Success in traditional medical/VR rehabilitation is a reflection of one's compliance with the prescribed therapeutic regimen.

In contrast, according to the IL paradigm, the problem seldom resides in the individual but often in the solution offered by the rehabilitation paradigm. Primarily this refers to the dependency-inducing features of the relationship process, the physical environment, and the social control mechanisms of society at large. To cope with these barriers, individuals with disabilities need to exchange the patient and client roles for the consumer role. Advocacy, peer counseling, environmental barrier removal, self-help, and consumer control are the trademarks of the IL paradigm. Table 47-1 summarizes these contrasts.

TABLE 47-1. *A comparison of the rehabilitation and independent living paradigm*

Item	Rehabilitation paradigm	Independent living paradigm
Definition of problem	Physical impairment; lack of vocational skill; psychological maladjustment; lack of motivation and cooperation	Dependence on professionals, relatives, etc.; inadequate support services; architectural barriers; economic barriers
Locus of problem	In individual	In environment; in the rehabilitation process
Social roll	Patient/client	Consumer
Solution to problem	Professional intervention by physician, physical therapist, occupational therapist, vocational counselor, etc.	Peer counseling; advocacy; self-help; consumer control; removal of barriers and disincentives
Who controls	Professional	Consumer
Desired outcomes	Maximum ADL; gainful employment; psychological adjustment; improved motivation; completed treatment	Self-direction; least restrictive environment; social and economic productivity

ADL, activities of daily living.

From Crewe NM, Zola IK. *Independent living for physically disabled people.* San Francisco: Jossey-Bass, 1983; 23.

Moreover, the IL paradigm differs from the rehabilitation paradigm in defining and identifying desired outcomes. Medical rehabilitation stresses the value of self-care, mobility, and employment; IL emphasizes additional outcomes such as the importance of living arrangements, consumer assertiveness, outdoor mobility, environmental accessibility, and out-of-home activity (3,4). As explained by DeJong, the IL paradigm occasionally rejects self-care as an important outcome. To illustrate, a working person needing personal assistance to get dressed or fed may actually be more independent than someone who dresses him- or herself yet has no productive involvement in the community.

SERVICE NETWORKS AND STAFF PATTERNS

State Vocational Rehabilitation Agencies

Although many CILs require that those providing services have first-hand experience with disability, VR counselors hired by state agencies or private rehabilitation firms are specifically trained to provide employment counseling for persons with disabilities. Typically, the counselor has a Master's degree in guidance and counseling, rehabilitation counseling, or occasionally social work. A rehabilitation counselor may be certified through the Commission on Rehabilitation Counselor Certification or may be licensed through their state. Licensure or certification is not a standard requirement, however, particularly in state agencies.

Vocational rehabilitation services occur in multiple settings. The state agencies comprise the largest of these. State agencies work with multiple community partners, both to increase awareness of services to consumers as well as to implement services. These partners include school systems, CILs, community mental health agencies, hospitals and health care clinics, substance abuse centers, local support groups, other state and county employment programs, and a whole host of social service agencies. State or private rehabilitation providers may also contract with community private not-for-profit organizations, which may provide work evaluation, community work adjustment programs, sheltered or transitional employment, job coaching, or other specialized job placement services. It is required that these community rehabilitation facilities be accredited by the Commission on Association of Rehabilitation Facility (CARF). Many medical centers have also established work evaluation services and sometimes also provide VR counseling services as well.

Private Rehabilitation

In the late 1970s and 1980s, there was a tremendous growth in the number of private, for-profit rehabilitation firms. Likewise, graduates of rehabilitation counselor training programs were increasingly taking jobs in the private sector rather than within the state and federal VR system. Part of this was because of the lack of growth in the established VR system. Another important factor was the increasing attention that insurance companies were paying to controlling costs in an ever-growing medical care reimbursement system. Payers found that, in many cases, disability payments to injured or ill members could be minimized by contracting for vocational rehabilitation services relatively early in the return-to-work process. Private rehabilitation firms tend to be smaller, less bureaucratic, and more efficient in their approach to return to work than their state VR counterparts. Their services focus more intensely on vocational guidance and placement and are not as holistic in their approach to the consumer. Counselors working in the private sector need basic business skills, knowledge of the insurance business, an understanding of the worker's compensation system, expertise in legal and medical case management, and the ability to provide vocational expert testimony (9). Many rehabilitation counselors in the private sector are self-employed or co-owners of small firms (10). Private rehabilitation counselors often contract with insurance carriers to provide VR services to those who qualify for these services through workers compensation, auto no-fault, or long-term disability policies. These services are provided within the context of what the insurers will pay for and the specific legislation involved. Consequently, private rehabilitation firms are usually very responsive to the payers' goals and objectives.

Medical Center Settings and Partnerships with Centers for Independent Living

Custodial care facilities and primary medical care facilities are specifically excluded from the definition of an IL program (11). Generic IL service providers are organizations that provide discrete services that can increase an individual's ability or opportunity to live independently. For example, a medical rehabilitation facility may provide outpatient services designed to maintain the physical health of a person who lives independently in the community. However, if the center does not provide or coordinate a full set of services, including transportation, attendant care, and so forth, it is an IL service provider rather than an IL program. However, the provider's services may be used or coordinated by an IL program.

Both anecdotal and published evidence indicate that service relationships exist between medical rehabilitation programs and IL programs in many communities in the United States (12,13). Some relationships are limited to referring potential clients from one program to another. Others encompass formalized, long-standing arrangements involving reciprocal services or services aimed at a common goal. An example would be preparation for independent living after the onset of chronic illness or physical disability. In 1990, Fuhrer et al. conducted a survey of centers for independent living and medical rehabilitation programs with cooperative relationships. They found that the most frequently reported relationships were making referrals to or supplying information about medical rehabilitation programs, providing peer counseling services, and conducting training in daily living skills for medical rehabilitation patients (12).

In this survey, the three most frequently endorsed barriers to stronger relationships were conflicting approaches or styles of service delivery, funding of services, and conflicting program philosophies. The medical centers programs that were surveyed reported using CIL services more for patients with spinal cord injuries (SCI) than for any other condition including stroke. This finding suggests a preferred inclination to refer SCI patients to CILs. In most rehabilitation hospitals, patients with SCI are outnumbered by patients with other conditions, especially stroke. A national evaluation of CILs revealed that persons with SCI being served by CILs outnumbered those with strokes or head injuries (14). The deemphasis of services for persons with head injuries may reflect CILs' difficulties in serving persons with a limited capacity for self-management (15).

Some medical centers have played a role in founding CILs in their communities such as Access Living of metropolitan Chicago and Great Lakes CIL in Detroit. Others have collaborated to develop needed community resources, e.g., Allegheny Independence House and Hamarville Rehabilitation Hospital (16). The University of Michigan Medical Center has worked jointly with the Ann Arbor CIL to provide IL services and training that begins with acute care hospitalization, continuing through inpatient rehabilitation, and extending to community living. This collaborative relationship is being developed also by six other medical centers serving persons with SCI across the country (17,18).

These examples suggest that CILs and medical centers are indeed complementary in meeting the multiplicity of services needed by persons with disabilities. The medical center emphasis on restoring the individual's health and functional independence is complemented by the CIL focus on assisting persons with disabilities to maintain independent life styles and on improving their community environmnent (12).

THE VOCATIONAL REHABILITATION PROCESS

Vocational Evaluation and Functional Assessment

Vocational rehabilitation begins with assessment of the person's vocational interests, wishes, abilities, needs, and potentials. The purposes of assessment are to identify the person's relative strengths and weaknesses, set goals, and plan a course of action. Assessment is also used to determine eligibility for services and to make predictions about a person's potential to benefit from rehabilitation. Assessment initially involves gathering data from a variety of sources. Medical evaluation is essential to understanding a client's abilities and needs. The client's history provides information about educational attainment, specialized skills, past employment, financial expectations, and transportation needs. Paper-and-pencil tests can provide useful information about aptitudes, abilities, and vocational interests. Work samples, situational assessments, and on-the-job evaluations provide job-specific information.

Functional assessment is an important part of vocational evaluation. A diagnostic approach to assessment seeks to place a person in a category. In contrast, an assessment of function attempts to define what a person can and can't do. It is a broad concept that can be applied to various domains such as mobility, interpersonal communication, sensory awareness, emotional stability, learning ability, general stamina, and motivity, i.e., the capacity to initiate and control physical movements as required by specific task demands and situations. An adequate functional assessment combined with an adequate analysis of the demands of a specific occupation provide a major component in making decisions about the appropriateness or advisability of pursuing particular vocational objectives. There are several kinds of evaluations that may go into a complete functional assessment (19). Medical rehabilitation specialists will likely measure a person's capacity to perform ADLs, using instruments such as the Barthel Index and the Functional Independence Measure. A functional capacity evaluation (FCE) provides an objective, comprehensive measurement of a person's optimal work abilities. The work sample approach to measurement has been used most often. Historically, both simulated job work samples (e.g., VALPAR or Singer) and actual work samples (e.g., TOWER) were widely utilized (20). More recently, sophisticated systems designed to measure a wide range of physical capabilities have been developed. The most popular include the ERGOS Work Simulator, the BTE Work Simulator, KEY Functional Assessment, Isernhagen Work Systems, and the Blankenship FCE.

The multiplicity of FCE systems can make it difficult for professionals in different disciplines to communicate clearly about an individual's physical capacity for work. Comparability of research efforts has also been hampered. More significantly, there has been little research demonstrating a significant relationship between physical performance factors and actual return to work (21). A serious limitation of FCE is the lack of attention paid to the actual work environment. Even further, beyond the question of physical capacity, it must be asked, Does the person want to work? Is the work environment a place in which any reasonable person would have incentive to work? Is the work good for the person (22)?

Any personal limitation in functional ability becomes a handicap only when the environment fails to sufficiently accommodate individual differences. For example, purely environmental limitations, such as narrowed doorways, may keep a person from successful job opportunities. Stereotypes and social expectations may also impose limitations. For example, a person with a facial disfigurement may not be able to find work as a salesperson. The assessment process must include specific information about work environments and actual job demands in order to appropriately meet the needs of people with physical limitations. This assessment focus is particularly necessary in vocational rehabilitation planning for persons with severe physical disabilities.

Three general questions that the rehabilitation counselor tries to answer through the assessment process are: (a) Can the client return to his or her former occupation? Sometimes job accommodations can make this possible. (b) Which of the client's skills might be transferable to other occupations? For example, a surgeon with impaired hand function may be able to assist in the design of expert software systems involved in medical decision making. (c) What training or other services can contribute to successful reemployment? As data are gathered, hypotheses are developed concerning possible vocational objectives and needed services. The counselor attempts to make some predictions about how the client might respond to a particular work environment. Tentative ideas are tested against future observations.

The Individualized Written Rehabilitation Plan (IWRP)

As hypotheses about the client gain in substance, they become the basis for discussion between counselor and client. Naturally, the client has also been developing his or her own ideas during the assessment. Experience has shown that active client participation improves vocational success. More importantly, involvement of the client in the decision-making process is an important ethical principle and is required by federal law. Ultimately this dialectic process leads to a mutually agreed-on plan, formalized in the IWRP.

The IWRP, mandated by the Rehabilitation Act of 1973, must document (a) long-term vocational goal and intermediate objectives, (b) services to be provided, (c) financial responsibilities for the services to be provided, (d) counselor and client responsibilities, (e) criteria and procedures for evaluating progress, and (f) an annual review for as long as the case is open. Objectives in the plan might include (a) provision of services such as medical evaluation or treatment, training (e.g., college, on-the-job training, vocational schools), (b) developing individualized job placement strategies, and (c) the provision of specialized adaptive equipment or transportation.

If the client and counselor disagree about the IWRP, the dispute may be mediated by an ombudsman. Provision of this service is required by federal statute and is intended as a safeguard for consumer rights. There are several considerations in writing an effective IWRP. The barriers to rehabilitation and the steps needed to overcome them must be identified in the evaluation process. The evaluation is often a learning experience for the client, who may need help in understanding what the barriers are. On the other hand, the counselor is responsible for understanding the client's unmet needs, aspirations, and potentials. Finally, the development of a schedule of when and how services will be provided permits periodic evaluation of how the program is going. This enables adjustments to be made as necessary.

One of the hallmarks of the state–federal vocational rehabilitation system is its reliance on outside providers for testing, education, training, adaptive equipment, transportation, therapy, medical restoration, and other services. The VR counselor is often in the role of coordinator or case manager and frequently does not provide many direct services. It is the counselor's responsibility to make appropriate referrals for the client based on the services called for in the IWRP. Usually, the state VR agency has an established network of service providers to draw on. The services to be provided must be defined, a timetable agreed on, costs indicated, and a mechanism for evaluation must be put in place.

Achieving Employment Readiness

Once a vocational evaluation has been completed, vocational goals and objectives have been set, an IWRP has been formulated, and the agreed-on services have been provided, the counselor must determine that the client is ready to be placed in employment. In practice, there are usually intermediate points of evaluation tied to the sequence of services provided.

Several key dimensions must be assessed to determine job readiness. Medical stability is an important concern. Many impairments fluctuate over time, e.g., multiple sclerosis. This can interfere with the ability to maintain employment, especially when starting a new job. A related concern is the person's endurance. Are the requirements of the proposed job (e.g., full time) likely to overtax someone who, for instance, reports the need to take a nap every afternoon? In addition, the client's support systems are critical to employment success. This includes the cooperation of key family members. The availability of adequate attendant care may be essential to preparing for work. Transportation is an extremely important element in job success. Not being able to drive one's own vehicle is a significant obstacle to employment that is difficult to overcome. Public transportation can be hard to access and is often unreliable.

The person's psychological readiness to go to work must also be assessed. This includes motivation, self-confidence, interpersonal flexibility, coping resources, and realistic expectations about what it will be like. Often overlooked is some assessment of what the particular work environment has to offer to the client. Motivation to work is not simply a personal characteristic. It is a function of a person–environment interaction (22). People have needs beyond making money. For example, unmet needs for satisfying interpersonal contact, a sense of belonging, a sense of making a contribution, or creative expression may undermine a person's motivation for work.

Job Placement Strategies

Once the person is ready to seek employment in a new setting, he or she must develop the employment skills that will be required for success in the job search. These skills include identifying and following up on job leads, résumé writing, application completion, and interviewing skills. The disabled job seeker must ultimately accept responsibility for his or her own ability to obtain and maintain employment. The prospective employee must be able to convince the employer that he or she has the ability to be productive and an asset to the company (23).

Job placement activities can be viewed as a continuum ranging from self-placement to the counselor assuming all placement responsibility. The skills and personality traits of the job seeker, the nature of the disability, local market conditions, and even luck influence the extent of counselor involvement. In cases of severe disability, counselor involvement is likely to be greater. By taking ownership of the job search to whatever extent possible, the job seeker learns lifelong job search skills, which will always be useful. The IWRP will target the consumer's job goal, specify acceptable geographic and environmental criteria, consider the types of job accommodations that are likely to be needed, and specify follow-up and support services required.

A primary role of the VR counselor is to assist the consumer to develop employment skills using such tools as coaching, role playing, or video taping. The consumer needs to learn to effectively complete applications, cover letters, and other correspondence. He or she must also know what to do in response to questions about disability, either on an application or in an interview. The consumer will also need to know where to obtain business specific information needed to target their job search as well as to prepare for the interview and how to obtain job leads through formal and networking channels.

Legally, the only question that can be asked regarding disability is ''Do you have any condition or disability that would interfere with your ability to perform the tasks of this job?'' The description of the disability should focus on relevant functional limitations and avoid medical terminology. All communications or interactions with the employer need to remain focused on skills and abilities and not on disability issues. It is the consumer's responsibility to know what job accommodations are needed. The consumer needs to be able to take the initiative in discussing the disability, especially if it is visible. In taking the initiative, the applicant can better control the discussion, clear up any misconception, and address any employer concerns.

Job Analysis

A good job site assessment is critical to the success of the job placement process. It is the basis on which job accommodation recommendations are made. It may be done by the counselor or by an occupational therapist specialized in work assessment. The job must be analyzed for factors involved in the work environment, in the job tasks themselves, and for production expectations; i.e., How is it determined that the employee is performing adequately? An analysis of worksite physical factors may consider parking at the work site, restrooms, cafeteria, and building accessibility. Specific physical requirements must be assessed, such as lifting, grasping, standing, walking, sitting, talking, hearing, writing, and reading. For persons with cognitive or affective limitations, the critical factors might include work atmosphere, i.e., busy or relaxed, what type of memory is involved, how much abstract thinking or problem solving is required, etc. Worksite analysis is one of the most complex components of vocational rehabilitation. The rehabilitation professional must be knowledgeable about state and national standards for accessibility, occupational safety and health standards, business practices and organizational structure, roles of labor and management, along with employer needs in order to best represent the consumer (23).

Job Accommodations

Asking for job accommodations is another skill that needs to be developed. Again, it is the consumer's responsibility to know what accommodations are needed and to be knowledgeable about resources and relative cost. These issues can be thought through ahead of time per the vocational assessment and with the aid of a counselor if needed. The counselor can often act as a consultant to the employer and can help to negotiate accommodations. The accommodation should be presented as good business, not as charity or as a legal requirement. The consumer should use his or her own adaptive equipment whenever possible, and solutions should be kept as simple and cost effective as possible. If an employer has a clear idea of what is needed, why it is needed, and of what benefit it has for him as well as for the applicant, there will be less resistance. If architectural barriers are involved, the employer can be advised of tax credits that are available for this purpose. The employer is required to make reasonable accommodations; this term is not clearly defined in current legislation. Factors that are to be considered are the size of the employer and the nature and the cost of the accommodation. If a problem exists with the request for or the provision of accommodations, advocacy services can be obtained through CILs and VR agencies.

The Work Environment and Technology Committee of the President's Committee of Employment of the Handicapped indicates that there are generally four types of job accommodations: (a) accommodation to facilities and equipment, (b) job design, (c) training, and (d) ongoing support (23). The first addresses the need for modifications to the physical setting, such as a ramp or an ergonomically designed work station. At times, a redesign of the job is indicated. This might necessitate elimination of some job duties or establishing a flexible work schedules with longer break periods. Training focuses on development of personal skills related to job demands. Ongoing supports refers to assistance that the individual may need on an ongoing basis such as a reader for a visually impaired individual or obtaining supplies for an individual who cannot physically obtain them. Each accommodation is individualized to the specific needs of the consumer and the work environment. It is critical to remember that two people with the same medical diagnosis may have different degrees of limitations, different personal styles, preferences, and capabilities, and may benefit from different accommodations. The goal of the accommodation process is to enable a qualified individual to perform the required job duties of a position despite a limitation, thus contributing his or her skills to the organization.

Job Follow-Up Services

Follow-up services to both consumer and employer help to ensure a successful outcome when employment begins. Intervention may be needed to help solve problems the consumer may be having that affect work performance or work relationships (23). It needs to be ascertained that there is a good match between the consumer's capabilities and the job's requirements. The consumer needs to try out the accommodations provided to determine whether additional modifications are necessary. It is also essential that an employee who is not able to function successfully be removed from the job. It is not to the consumer's or employer's benefit to continue an employment situation when there is not a good match. The goal is to assist the consumer and the employer to have a successful experience.

Employer Development

In addition to developing specific jobs for consumers in the community, another role for the vocational rehabilitation professional is to market the concept itself within the employer community. Many employers still object to hiring disabled workers on what they believe are reasonable grounds and reflect concerns around increased cost or risk in the areas of insurance rates, physical modifications, safety, job performance, and job stability. They are defensive about having to assume the burden of proof when personal practices are questioned. Thus, a primary goal of the rehabilitation community continues to be to dispel employer misconceptions both of rehabilitation agencies and of disabled workers (23). It is essential for rehabilitation professionals to be visible and active in business organizations and to continue to build credibility within the community. Services that can be marketed include (a) recruitment services—referral of qualified applicants, (b) consultant services in the areas of affirmative action assistance, ADA compliance, job modification and accommodation, and accessibility and disability awareness training programs, (c) troubled employee assistance programming in which the rehabilitation agency works directly with an injured or disabled worker referred by the employer, and (d) support and follow-up services. If this groundwork is laid appropriately, the business climate will be greatly improved toward employment consideration of applicants with disabilities. In addition, if allies are cultivated in the business community, they can be very effective in advocating for the concept with their colleagues (23).

THE INDEPENDENT LIVING PROCESS AND PLAN OF SERVICES

The process of assisting individuals to adapt themselves and their environment to the reality of disability is less linear and more flexible than the VR process. Living independently with a severe disability in a physical and social world designed in every way by and for nondisabled people presents a lifetime of challenges. The IL process can be conceptualized as consisting of four phases: (a) assessment, (b) planning, (c) intervention, and (d) evaluation. However, it must be remembered that living with a disability is deeply embedded in the life-long process of human development. The same individual who may appear totally unhampered by his or her disability in one area of life, or during one stage of development, may at another time or under different circumstances be completely overwhelmed by any one of the myriad challenges presented by a severe disability. Although the VR process consistently remains focused on employment, the focus of the IL process changes with each individual at different points in time and with changing circumstances and interests.

Assessment

The IL process begins when an individual with a disability realizes that an obstacle exists as a result of that disability that prevents the realization of a desired goal. For some individuals, that realization may come with the acquisition of a disability, whereas for others, it may come after years of institutionalization. In other instances, the IL process may begin when an individual who has lived independently with a severe disability encounters new circumstances, such as a change in employment, housing, physical capacity, or relational status. Wherever the process begins, the need exists for an assessment of that individual's life skills and abilities to live independently.

For an individual with a developmental disability who may have lived all of his or her life in an institution and now wants to live in his or her own apartment, the IL assessment will need to be comprehensive. It will include such areas as personal hygiene, medication management, problem solving and decision making skills, social skills, housekeeping, menu planning, shopping, meal preparation, money management, bill-paying skills, money-handling skills, telephone skills, and emergency procedures. In contrast, for a middle-aged individual returning home after a spinal cord injury, the initial assessment would consist of a much simpler series of questions regarding his or her ability to perform a standard list of ADLs, need for social services, emotional concerns, feelings regarding the impact of his or her disability on personal relationships, and needs for home modification and personal assistance. In either case, the goal of the IL assessment is to identify the individual's goal and provide the IL counselor with the information necessary to assist that individual in developing a plan to achieve his or her goal.

Planning

One critical difference between the VR and IL processes is perhaps most evident during the planning phase. Whereas in the VR process, the rehabilitation counselor retains a great deal of control over the planning process, in the IL process, the counselor's role is to assist the consumer in creating his or her own plan.

The IL programs place a much stronger emphasis on the cognitive and emotional aspects of independence. Their approach emphasizes the peer role model, i.e., the person with a severe disability living independently who can provide motivation and counseling about dealing with the realities of living with a disability. As consumers are assisted in growing and adapting to disability, the IL program provides concurrent services directed at changing the environment by removing barriers to the realization of personal goals and by remediating discriminatory practices (24).

In the early days of the IL movement, programs generally started as service projects of grass roots consumer advocacy organizations or traditional service providers. Over the years, the tendency has been to separate from the parent organization. As the IL movement has expanded, there has been a corresponding rise of IL program networks. The National Council on Independent Living (NCIL) has grown to be an effective and respected vehicle for systems advocacy for persons with disabilities.

Recent efforts by the federal government to establish performance criteria for IL programs have identified minimum basic IL services to be information and referral, peer counseling, IL skills training, and advocacy. The IL programs can also offer housing assistance, attendant care training and referral, reader and interpreter referral, financial benefits counseling, and community awareness and barrier removal programs. Other services may include family counseling, vocational counseling, legal service counseling, health care or nutrition education, equipment maintenance and repair, and social–recreational programs.

Attendant care is one of the services most closely associated with the movement for IL, especially with respect to persons with severe physical disabilities for whom it is essential for living independently. The attendant care concept touches nearly all the themes considered important to the IL movement. The attendant care model assumes that the person with a disability is well informed of his or her own medical care needs and has the necessary skill and ability to direct and monitor his or her own personal care (25). The Medicaid program has become one of the main sources of funding for consumer-directed attendant care services. The CILs are responsible for educating consumers about their rights and benefits under Medicaid and about how to recruit and train their own attendants. Another important IL service is peer counseling. The person with a disability possessing the necessary personal qualifications can, with training, offer unique assistance to clients with a disability. In a survey of CILs conducted during the early 1980s, 89% of the respondents stated that peer counseling is of major importance in CILs, provided that the peer counselors had formal training. Specific areas in which peer counselors can provide help include management of personal care attendant services, equipment purchase, exploration of community resources, dealing with grief and anxiety, and self-advocacy. Peer counselors can also help in finding accessible transportation and accessible housing (26).

CONCLUSIONS

Independence in a medical setting entitles patients to make choices about their lives. Although much has been said about the need for independence, many traditional medical and VR programs often fail to encourage independence to the fullest extent. They often do not facilitate the development of a person's maximum potential for productivity, quality of life, and social participation after disability. Although philosophically they are at different ends of the continuum, the VR and IL paradigms also complement each other in many ways. The VR programs are goal oriented and provide persons with disabilities with resources and training needed to find employment or to further education, which can lead to vocational opportunities; VR also promotes an independence that can facilitate vocational options.

Goal setting is a sensitive issue for the IL movement. Although IL programs encourage goal setting, it is not as simple as it seems. Consumers of IL services are less likely to have a clear idea of their goals than VR consumers, and many have found the concept of goal setting to be unfamiliar if decisions had previously been made on their behalf by someone else. Often goal planning was an evolutionary process rather than a first step. Sometimes the establishment of goals is an outcome in and of itself (27).

In contrast to VR, IL programs promote a greater sense of inner control, self-reliance, and personal achievement. They offer options and encourage self-sufficiency and self-determination in the conduct of daily routines, establishment of social identity, and life choices. The role and nature of professional involvement comprise another major difference between the two models of service. The empowerment philosophy that embodies the IL approach to rehabilitation specifies that professionals can play only a facilitating role in the process. Professionals are seen as agents of change and facilitators to help persons with disabilities become as independent as possible. Their success in the rehabilitation process is based on their ability to assist consumers to achieve their own goals, which are not necessarily those of traditional rehabilitation programs. Once personal decisions have been made, the availability of training and other resources external to the individual as offered by traditional VR programs become more meaningful to persons with disabilities. The VR emphasis on restoring the individual's functional independence is complemented by the IL focus on assisting persons with disabilities to maintain independent life styles and on improving their community environment. These relationships can best be observed in actual partnerships or collaborations among IL and traditional rehabilitation programs.

The emphasis on outcomes selected from both programs accentuates differences between the VR and IL approach as well. Functional assessment is rapidly becoming the most recognized outcome of rehabilitation interventions. We discussed some of the functional measures used by VR in this chapter. The IL services focus on broader and more comprehensive outcomes that tend to be less quantifiable and concrete. The IL outcomes relate to improvement in one's overall quality of life and self-dignity. These more individualized outcomes are often more difficult to document as identifiable and immediate benefits to payors of rehabilitation services.

Technology is also an important issue for both VR and IL programs. Independence in the basic ADL is necessary before such activities as getting an education or gaining employment are possible. Technology can help to compensate for functional loss and increase physical and psychological independence. Assistive technology projects more recently being offered in conjunction with VR programs are vital to promote independence in the workplace and beyond. According to the IL philosophy, technology is key to the removal of barriers facing persons with disabilities in the areas of transportation, housing, self-care, and mobility. Independent living services, as discussed, promote further independence in these areas.

In summary, the delicate balance between competency and autonomy fostered by the VR and IL model of services need not to be viewed as exclusive of each other. Although most persons with disabilities are able to maintain the capacity to make decisions concerning their needs and life styles, they may need time to be educated and empowered about new roles and options in learning to cope with disability.

REFERENCES

1. Frieden L. Understanding alternative program models. In: Crewe NM, Zola IK, eds. *Independent living for physically disabled people.* San Francisco: Jossey-Bass, 1983; 62–72.
2. DeJong G. Defining and implementing the independent living concept. In: Crewe NM, Zola IK, eds. *Independent living for physically disabled people.* San Francisco: Jossey-Bass, 1983; 4–27.
3. Wright G. *Total rehabilitation.* New York: Little, Brown, 1980.
4. Berkowitz E. *Disabled policy: America's programs for the handicapped.* Cambridge: Cambridge University Press, 1987.
5. Nosek M. A response to Kenneth R. Thomas Commentary: Some observations on the use of the word consumer. *J Rehabil* 1993; 59:9–10.
6. Thomas K. Commentary: Some observations on the use of the word consumer. *J Rehabil* 1993; 59:6–8.
7. Anderson D. The ADA: Our next step toward liberty and justice for all. *Mich Munic Rev* 1994; 67:240–243.
8. Treanor RB. *We overcame: The story of civil rights for disabled people.* Falls Church, VA: Regal Direct Publishing, 1993.
9. Lynch RK, Martin T. Rehabilitation counseling in the private sector: A training needs survey. *J Rehabil* 1982; 48:51–53,73.
10. Matkin RE. Rehabilitation services offered in the private sector: A pilot investigation. *J Rehabil* 1982; 48:31–33.
11. Frieden L. Understanding alternative program models. In: Crewe NM, Zola IK, eds. *Independent living for physically disabled people.* San Francisco: Jossey-Bass, 1983; 62–72.
12. Fuhrer MJ, Rossi D, Gerken L, Nosek M, Richards L. Relationships between independent living centers and medical rehabilitation programs. *Arch Phys Med Rehabil* 1990; 71(6):519–522.
13. Rasmussen L, Tate D, Casaglos T, Maynard F, Cassidy C. *The Hospital to Community Program: A Collaborative Program Between the University of Michigan Medical Center and the Ann Arbor Center for Independent Living. Program manual.* Ann Arbor, MI: University of Michigan Department of Physical Medicine and Rehabilitation, 1990.
14. Berkeley Planning Associates. *Comprehensive evaluation of the title VI, part B of the Rehabilitation Act of 1973. Centers for Independent Living Programs: Final Report. Contract #300-84-0209.* Berkeley, CA: Berkeley Planning Associates, 1986.
15. Wilkerson DL. Disability due to traumatic brain injury: What are independent living centers doing to fill the gap? Paper presented at the National Conference on Independent Living 1987, May, 1987, Washington DC.
16. Krouskop A, Barricella J. Service relationships between the Hamarville Rehabilitation Center and the Three Rivers Center for Independent Living. Paper presented at the 64th Annual Session of the American Congress of Rehabilitation Medicine, October 23, 1987, Orlando, FL.
17. Groomes D, Tate D, Forchheimer M, et al. *Hospital to Community Independent Living Program Manual. A collaborative project between the University of Michigan Medical Center and the Ann Arbor Center for Independent Living.* Ann Arbor, MI: University of Michigan Department of Physical Medicine and Rehabilitation, 1996.
18. Tate D, Cole T. *The University of Michigan Model SCI Care System. Enhancing Community Reintegration: A Collaborative Project.* Ann Arbor, MI: University of Michigan Department of Physical Medicine and Rehabilitation, 1995.
19. Halern AS, Fuhrer MJ, eds. *Functional assessment in rehabilitation.* Baltimore: Paul H. Brookes, 1984.
20. Malzahn DE, Fernandez JE, Kattel BP. Design-oriented functional capacity evaluation: the Available Motions Inventory—a review. *Disabil Rehabil* 1996; 18:382–395.
21. Velozo CA. Work evaluations: Critique of the state of the art of functional assessment of work. *Am J Occup Ther* 1992; 47:203–209.
22. Kielhofner G. Functional assessment: toward a dialectical view of person-environment relations. *Am J Occup Ther* 1993; 47:248–251.
23. Davis DJ, Paasuke L. Vocational evaluation and rehabilitation. In: DeLisa JA, ed. *Rehabilitation medicine: principles and practice.* Philadelphia: JB Lippincott,1988 s–94.
24. Nosek MA, Zhu Y, Howland CA. The evolution of Independent Living programs. *Rehabil Couns Bull* 1992;35(3):174–189.
25. DeJong G, Wenker T. Attendant care. In: Crewe NM, Zola IK, eds. *Independent living for physically disabled people.* San Francisco: Jossey-Bass, 1983;157–170.
26. Saxton M. Peer counseling. In: Crewe NM, Zola IK, eds. *Independent living for physically disabled people.* San Francisco: Jossey-Bass, 1983; 171–186.
27. Nosek MA. Outcome analysis in independent living. In: Fuhrer MJ, ed. *Rehabilitation outcomes analysis and measurement.* Baltimore: Brook Publishing Co., 1981; 56.

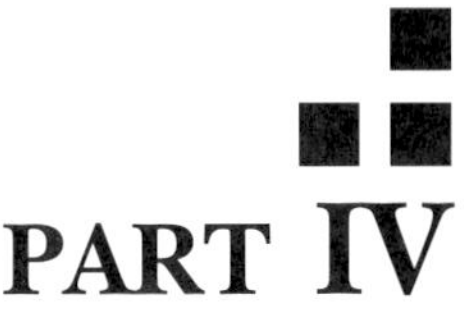

PART IV

Rehabilitation of Specific Disorders

Rehabilitation Medicine: Principles and Practice, Third Edition,
edited by Joel A. DeLisa and Bruce M. Gans.
Lippincott–Raven Publishers, Philadelphia © 1998.

CHAPTER 48

Stroke Rehabilitation

Murray E. Brandstater

DEFINITION

A stroke is a clinical syndrome characterized by the sudden development of a persisting focal neurologic deficit. *Stroke* is a useful clinical term, its abrupt or rapid onset implying its vascular pathogenesis. A clinical diagnosis of stroke excludes nonvascular causes of focal brain deficits such as seizure, brain tumor, encephalitis, abscess, trauma, or syncope, all of which represent important differential diagnoses of stroke. The expression *cerebrovascular accident* or *CVA* has been used interchangeably with the term stroke, but its use is discouraged. Both terms convey the same information, but "CVA" is often a source of confusion (does a R. CVA describe the lesion location or the clinical deficit?), and the lesion is not accidental. *Stroke* is a useful term for general description of events secondary to cerebrovascular disease, but, like CVA, it is not specific enough to use as a diagnosis. For individual patient description, a pathologic diagnosis should be made, such as cerebral infarction or cerebral hemorrhage.

The focal brain lesions encountered in patients with stroke produce a wide variety of neurologic deficits such as hemiplegia, hemisensory loss, aphasia, hemianopia, etc., the specific clinical signs in each case reflecting the anatomic site of the lesion. The size and extent of the lesion determine the severity of the deficits, which in rehabilitation medicine are referred to as impairments. The objectives of stroke rehabilitation are to reduce the impairments through therapy, achieve a maximum level of functional independence, minimize disability, successfully reintegrate back into home, family, and community, and reestablish a meaningful and gratifying life.

EPIDEMIOLOGY

Stroke is the most common serious neurologic disorder in the United States, comprising half of all patients admitted to hospital for a neurologic disease. It is the third leading cause of death after heart disease and cancer. The incidence of stroke in the 1960s was reported at around 200 per 100,000 population, or approximately 500,000 new cases per year in the United States. A decline in the overall incidence was noted late in the 1960s and 1970s, to levels around 115/100,000, but this decline flattened out in the 1980s. There may have been a small rise in incidence since then. Incidence is age related, being uncommon under age 50 but doubling each decade after age 55. Over the age of 80, the incidence of stroke may be as high as 2,500/100,000. The decline in incidence in the 1970s was probably attributable in most part to improved management of hypertension in the general population (1).

Most patients who die from acute stroke succumb in the first 30 days. The overall 30-day survival following a new stroke is reported to be 70% to 85%, survival being largely dependent on stroke type. The 30-day survival of patients with intracerebral hemorrhage is only about 20%, most of the deaths occurring in the first 3 days. The 30-day survival of patients with cerebral infarction is around 85%. Death during the first few days following onset is usually attributed to cerebral causes, especially transtentorial herniation, but pneumonia, pulmonary embolism, and cardiac conditions contribute to the 30-day mortality. After the initial 30 days, the death rate declines. The overall mortality from stroke is declining, reflecting better risk factor reduction and hence lower incidence and better medical management of patients during the acute phase. It should be noted that long-term survival poststroke is improving, so that despite reduced incidence, prevalence of stroke in the population has stayed the same or has increased.

RISK FACTORS AND PREVENTION

There is no successful medical treatment to reverse the neurologic sequelae of a completed stroke, and therefore, interventions aimed at stroke prevention are extremely important. The following is a summary of risk factors for stroke

M. E. Brandstater: Department of Physical Medicine and Rehabilitation, Loma Linda University Medical Center, Loma Linda, California 92354.

TABLE 48-1. *Modifiable risk factors for stroke*

Hypertension
Heart disease
Ischemic/hypertensive
Valvular
Arrhythmias
Smoking
Diabetes mellitus
Elevated fibrinogen
Erythrocytosis
Hyperlipidemia

and a description of opportunities for stroke prevention. Age, race, sex, and family history are all important biological indicators of enhanced stroke susceptibility, but these are inherent characteristics and cannot be altered. The following discussion focuses on those other risk factors that are modifiable, listed in Table 48-1.

Modifiable Risk Factors in Asymptomatic Patients

Hypertension is the most important risk factor. The degree of risk increases with higher levels of pressure and becomes particularly strong with levels over 160/95 mm Hg. Systolic hypertension and high mean arterial pressure represent parallel risks. In the Framingham Study, a sevenfold increased risk of cerebral infarction was observed in patients who were hypertensive (2). Hypertension increases the risk of thrombotic, lacunar, and hemorrhagic stroke and increases the likelihood of subarachnoid hemorrhage. Successful long-term treatment of hypertension greatly reduces the risk of these events. Every effort should be made to diagnose hypertension early and establish adequate blood pressure control before the secondary changes of hypertensive vascular disease develop. Treatment of late hypertension, e.g., after an individual has sustained a stroke, is much less effective in reducing risk of future events.

Heart disease is an important risk factor for stroke. To some degree this reflects the common underlying precursors of stroke and heart disease—hypertension and atherosclerosis. The risk of stroke is doubled in individuals who have coronary artery disease (3), and coronary artery disease accounts for the majority of subsequent deaths among stroke survivors. Atrial fibrillation and valvular heart disease increase the risk of cerebral infarction because both may cause cerebral emboli. In patients with chronic, stable atrial fibrillation, the risk of stroke is increased fivefold (4). When atrial fibrillation is a manifestation of rheumatic heart disease, the risk of embolic stroke is increased up to 17 times normal (4). Prevention of embolic stroke in these patients is best achieved by long-term anticoagulation with warfarin. Treatment carries the danger of intracranial hemorrhage, especially in elderly individuals and in those with impaired balance and who are likely to fall. When the risk of hemorrhage appears to be high, aspirin in a dose of 325 mg daily may be used as an alternative to warfarin in patients with nonvalvular atrial fibrillation, although aspirin is much less effective than warfarin in preventing embolism.

Diabetes doubles the risk of stroke. Unfortunately, good blood sugar control does not seem to halt the progression of cerebrovascular disease.

Smoking has been shown to increase the risk of stroke about 1.5 times (1.9 times for cerebral infarction) (5). There is clear evidence that smoking cessation reduces the risk of cerebral infarction in addition to reducing the risk of myocardial infarction and sudden death.

Hyperlipidemia poses only a small additional risk for stroke, mainly for individuals under the age of 55. Elevated fibrinogen levels correlate with higher risk of stroke, and it should be noted that fibrinogen levels are higher in individuals who smoke and have a high-cholesterol diet. A *raised hematocrit* increases the risk of stroke. It is unproven whether reducing the hematocrit lessens the risk for stroke.

Risk Factors in Symptomatic Patients

Transient ischemic attacks (TIAs) and minor stroke are important warning signals of an impending completed stroke. Patients with recent onset of TIAs should be treated in an attempt to prevent a stroke. The most widely accepted intervention is prescription of daily antiplatelet drugs such as aspirin (6). Several clinical trials have reported results using low- and high-dose daily aspirin. There is some controversy about the optimal dose of aspirin, but at present there is no evidence to indicate that a dose higher than 325 mg daily is more efficacious (6). Ticlopidine is an antiplatelet drug with a different action from aspirin, and it has comparable and perhaps slightly more beneficial effect on stroke risk reduction. However, it is expensive and has side effects (diarrhea, neutropenia), which may diminish its value compared to aspirin (6). Anticoagulants have been used to prevent stroke in patients with recent-onset TIAs, but no clinical trial has shown that treatment with warfarin is better than placebo. Warfarin is not recommended unless the patient has a major cardiac source of potential embolism.

Carotid endarterectomy has reduced the risk of stroke in those patients with single or multiple TIAs and with 70% or greater stenosis of the ipsilateral internal carotid artery (7). Patients with stenosis of 50% to 70% do not have a hemodynamically significant lesion but may be considered for surgery if symptomatic, i.e., they are having TIAs ipsilateral to the carotid lesion. Carotid endarterectomy has still not been proven superior to medical treatment in asymptomatic patients (8).

Risk Factors for Recurrent Stroke

The probability of stroke recurrence is highest in the postacute period. For survivors of an initial stroke, the annual risk of a second stroke is around 5% with a 5-year cumulative risk of recurrence around 25% (9,10), although it may be as high as 42% (9). Risk factors for initial stroke also increase the risk of recurrence, especially hypertension, heart disease, and diabetes mellitus (11,12). Heavy alcohol consumption is also a risk factor for recurrent stroke. As a risk factor, hypertension is more important for an initial than a recurrent stroke, probably because stroke occurrence depends more on the duration of elevated hypertension than on the current level of blood pressure. By the time a first stroke occurs, widespread hypertensive vascular damage is already present and will predispose to recurrent stroke even after blood pressure has been controlled. The beneficial effects of therapeutic blood pressure control are seen only after many years through delay or prevention of hypertensive vascular disease. Treatment of severe hypertension in patients who have had a stroke reduces rate of recurrence, but in patients with mild or moderate hypertension, treatment has little effect on rate of recurrent stroke. However, treatment of mild to moderate hypertension is still recommended because successful control reduces the incidence of cardiovascular complications such as congestive heart failure and myocardial infarction and therefore prolongs survival.

Many authors have reported on the high mortality of stroke survivors. Reported 5-year cumulative mortality rates depend on the presence of risk factors. Patients with a stroke who have hypertension and cardiac symptoms have only a 25% chance of surviving 5 years. Patients with one of these risk factors have a 50% chance of surviving 5 years, and those without heart disease and without hypertension have a 75% chance of surviving 5 years (10). Leonberg and Elliott (11) were able to achieve 16% reduction in stroke recurrence rate by an energetic and sustained program of control of multiple risk factors. Therefore, efforts should be made to reduce risk of recurrent stroke and mortality through controlling risk factors. The risk of recurrent embolism is reduced by anticoagulation in patients with atrial fibrillation or valvular disease.

CLINICAL PROFILES

Transient Ischemic Attacks

TIAs reflect focal areas of retinal or cerebral ischemia of sufficient duration to cause neurologic symptoms and signs. The ischemia is brief and does not persist long enough to develop a functionally significant cerebral infarction. The symptoms of a TIA begin abruptly, and they may persist for only a few seconds or minutes, finally resolving without any sequelae. By definition, all clinical features of a TIA resolve within 24 hours. A TIA may occur as an isolated event, or it may recur quite frequently, sometimes many times a day. The nature of the symptoms evoked by the TIA usually permits its localization into the distribution of the right or left carotid artery, or the vertebrobasilar system. Recurrent TIAs may be benign, and spontaneously stop, but in up to 30% of patients, a functionally significant stroke will develop within 5 years (6).

Usually TIAs are caused by microembolism of small platelet aggregates from ulcerated atherosclerotic plaques in large extracranial arteries, or from myocardium or cardiac valves. The small platelet emboli cause symptoms by occluding small blood vessels in the brain or retina before fragmenting enough to allow resumption of blood flow. Alternatively, a TIA may have a hemodynamic basis. Fluctuations in cardiac output or systemic arterial pressure may cause critical hypoperfusion distal to atherosclerotic stenosis of the large extracranial vessels. Cerebral hypoperfusion under these conditions would result in brief and self-limited neurologic symptoms and signs.

Cerebral Thrombosis

Thrombosis of the large extracranial and intracranial vessels occurs on the basis of atherosclerotic cerebrovascular disease, and accounts for about 30% of all cases of stroke (see Table 48-2) (12). Atherosclerotic plaques are particularly prominent in the large vessels of the neck and at the base of the brain. Occlusion of one of these large vessels, in the absence of good collateral channels, usually results in a large brain infarction. Atherosclerosis is accelerated by hypertension, diabetes and other risk factors. Following arterial thrombosis, the volume of infarcted brain depends on the rate at which the vessel becomes occluded, and the adequacy of the collateral circulation. A large vessel such as the internal carotid artery may slowly become stenotic and finally occlude without causing clinical signs or infarction if the slowly progressive stenosis had stimulated the development of sufficient collateral circulation prior to its occlusion.

A thrombotic occlusion occurs most commonly at night during sleep or during periods of inactivity. Often patients only become aware that they have weakness or other impairment when they attempt to get out of bed. The extent of the clinical deficit usually worsens over some hours or several days, then stabilizes, with clinical improvement generally beginning after 7 days post onset. Progression of neurologic deficits in the first several days following a thrombotic stroke is frequently observed and is due to several factors, particularly development of surrounding cerebral edema and alterations in perfusion and metabolism in tissue adjacent to the infarction. With large infarctions edema may be severe enough to cause brain displacement, herniation and death.

TABLE 48-2. *Causes of stroke*

Cause	%
Large vessel occlusion/infarction	32
Embolism	32
Small vessel occlusion, lacunar	18
Intracerebral hemorrhage	11
Subarachnoid hemorrhage	7

TABLE 48-3. *Sources of cerebral embolism*

Cardiac
- Atrial fibrillation, other arrhythmias
- Mural thrombus—recent MI, hypokinesis, cardiomyopathy
- Bacterial endocarditis
- Valve prosthesis
- Nonbacterial valve vegetations
- Atrial myxoma

Large artery
- Atherosclerosis of aorta and carotid arteries

Paradoxical
- Peripheral venous embolism with R-to-L cardiac shunt

Cerebral Embolism

Embolism is responsible for about 30% of all cases of stroke. Emboli may arise from thrombi in the heart, or on heart valves or the large extracranial arteries (Table 48-3). Thrombi develop at different sites such as the endocardium in the region of a recent myocardial infarction, an area of myocardial hypokinesis, the atrium associated with fibrillation or on diseased or prosthetic values. The clinical neurologic deficit from a cerebral embolus has an abrupt onset due to sudden loss of arterial perfusion to a focal area of the brain. The affected vessels tend to be small distal cortical branches of the middle cerebral artery, and their occlusion results in characteristic, wedge-shaped, superficial cortical infarctions seen on brain imaging studies. They are often multiple. However large vessel occlusions do occur and may involve the carotid or vertebrobasilar circulation.

Although emboli commonly affect the elderly, they represent an important cause of stroke in younger adults. It is important for the clinician to recognize that a cerebral infarction is due to embolism because the risk of recurrence can be greatly reduced by long-term anticoagulation. Diagnosis may be difficult in some cases e.g. when all of a mural cardiac thrombus embolizes, leaving no residual thrombus. The echocardiogram in such a case would not show a mural thrombus, although other features suggesting the possibility of thrombus may be present such as heart dilatation, hypokinetic myocardial segment, acute ischemic ECG changes, atrial fibrillation, etc.

Lacunar Stroke

Lacunar lesions constitute approximately 20% of all strokes. They are small, circumscribed lesions, at most 1.5 cm in diameter, and frequently much smaller. They represent occlusions in the deep penetrating branches of the large vessels which perfuse the subcortical structures including internal capsule, basal ganglia, thalamus, and brainstem. Small lacunar infarcts may produce major neurologic deficits if they are strategically located, but in general the associated deficits are less than those with a large vessel thrombosis, and lacunar infarctions may even occur without overt symptoms. Lacunar lesions are noteworthy because of their earlier, more rapid and greater degree of neurologic recovery.

The arteries involved in lacunar lesions are small-diameter branches of the middle cerebral artery called lenticulostriate arteries and comparably small penetrating branches of the anterior cerebral, posterior cerebral, and basilar arteries. The disease process affecting these small vessels may involve microatheroma, but very commonly the pathology is different, with progressive vessel wall thickening and fibrinoid necrosis, especially in patients with hypertension and diabetes. The clinical features associated with lacunar strokes are often mixed and difficult to distinguish, frequently because the lesions may be multiple. However, several characteristic lesions have been recognized, and these are described below.

Cerebral Hemorrhage

Intracerebral hemorrhage accounts for 11% of all cases of stroke. Spontaneous intracerebral hemorrhage most commonly occurs at the site of small, deep penetrating arteries, the same vessels responsible for lacunar stroke if they undergo occlusion rather than hemorrhage. It is thought that hemorrhage occurs through rupture of microaneurysms (Charcot–Bouchard aneurysms) that develop in these vessels in hypertensive patients. The majority of lesions occur in the putamen or thalamus, and in about 10% of patients the spontaneous hemorrhage occurs in the cerebellum.

The clinical onset of the hemorrhage is usually dramatic, with an otherwise fit patient abruptly developing a severe headache and major neurologic deficits within minutes. In many patients consciousness becomes progressively impaired, with coma developing rapidly. Brain displacement from the hematoma and cerebral edema may give rise to transtentorial herniation and death within the first 2 to 3 days. Mortality rates of patients with this type of clinical presentation are high, over 80%. The initial deficits may partially be secondary to edema and brain displacement rather than large volumes of tissue disruption from the arterial bleeding, and the degree of functional recovery may be surprisingly good.

Spontaneous intracerebral hemorrhage is a well-recognized complication of anticoagulant therapy, especially when prothrombin times are maintained at the upper level of the therapeutic range, or in a patient who falls and sustains a head injury. Other causes of intracerebral hemorrhage include trauma, vasculitis, and bleeding into a tumor (see Table 48-4). Patients with a bleeding diathesis, for example throm-

TABLE 48-4. *Causes of intracranial hemorrhage*

Primary intracerebral hemorrhage
Ruptured saccular aneurysm
Ruptured arteriovenous malformation
Trauma
Cerebral infarction
Brain tumor
Amyloid angiopathy
Hemorrhagic disorders: leukemia, thrombocytopenia, anticoagulant therapy

bocytopenia or coagulation disorders, may develop an intracranial hemorrhage. Cerebral amyloid angiopathy is an unusual cause of hemorrhage in the elderly. The lesions in this disorder tend to be superficial and recurrent.

Patients with acute hemorrhages in the cerebellum develop a sudden headache and inability to stand, along with nausea, vomiting, and vertigo. With large lesions the hematoma and edema may occlude cerebrospinal fluid (CSF) flow, causing acute hydrocephalus. Rapid death can be prevented by urgent evacuation of the hematoma in what is a true medical emergency. Patients who survive surgical evacuation of a cerebellar hemorrhage, or who have a less severe lesion, usually make a good functional recovery.

Subarachnoid Hemorrhage

In about 7% of all stroke patients, the lesion is a subarachnoid hemorrhage, usually resulting from rupture of an arterial aneurysm at the base of the brain, with bleeding into the subarachnoid space. Aneurysms develop from small defects in the wall of the arteries and slowly increase in size. Eventually they develop a tendency to bleed in midlife. Major rupture of an aneurysm may be preceded by headache from a small bleed or by localized cranial nerve lesions caused by direct pressure by the aneurysm. When rupture occurs, the clinical onset is usually dramatically abrupt. There is severe headache followed by vomiting and signs of meningeal irritation. Focal signs are usually not observed initially but may develop as a result of associated intracerebral bleeding or cerebral infarction occurring as a complication of arterial vasospasm. Coma frequently occurs, and up to a third of patients may die acutely. Rebleeding is unfortunately very common, especially in the first 2 to 3 weeks following the initial episode. Therefore, early surgical intervention has become routine with the objective of ligation of the aneurysm to prevent recurrent hemorrhage, which is usually fatal. Blood in the subarachnoid space may cause arterial vasospasm, leading to localized areas of cerebral infarction with associated focal neurologic deficits. Hydrocephalus may develop several weeks after the acute event as a result of arachnoiditis from blood in the CSF. Successful surgical clipping of an aneurysm is curative. If the patient has not developed focal deficits or an encephalopathy, there may be total clinical cure.

Subarachnoid hemorrhage may also result from bleeding from an arteriovenous malformation (AVM), which is a tangle of dilated vessels found on the surface of the brain or within the brain parenchyma. These lesions are congenital abnormalities and tend to bleed in childhood or young adulthood. In about half the cases, the hemorrhage is the first clinical indication of the lesion. In about a third of patients the AVM presents as a seizure disorder or with chronic headaches. In most patients the lesions eventually bleed. Most patients survive a single hemorrhagic event. The rate of rebleeding is about 6% in the first year and 2% to 3% per year thereafter. The treatment of choice is surgical excision of the AVM or neurovascular ablation through embolization. Irradiation with proton beam therapy to destroy the lesion has become an attractive alternative to surgery (13).

LESION LOCALIZATION

The pathology of the lesion can be surmised from an analysis of the temporal profile of the clinical presentation, i.e., the history, along with the progression and pattern of recovery of the lesion. Anatomic localization of a lesion can usually be established with reasonable accuracy based on a careful delineation of the neurologic deficits. A complete picture of the neurologic deficits may not be possible initially if the patient is confused and unable to cooperate fully with the examination. Therefore, repeat examinations of the patient in the early recovery phase help to further define the combination of deficits and assist in establishing the precise localization of the lesion. The following discussion describes in some detail the typical features observed in patients with commonly encountered focal stroke syndromes.

Internal Carotid Artery Syndrome

The most minor clinical deficits associated with internal carotid artery ischemia are TIAs caused by microembolic platelet aggregates carried peripherally from atherosclerotic plaques in the internal carotid or other large arteries. Transient occlusion of the retinal branches of an ophthalmic artery produces sudden, transient loss of vision in one eye, the amaurosis fugax syndrome. Cerebral TIAs take the form of brief motor, sensory, or language deficits.

The clinical consequences of complete occlusion of an internal carotid artery vary from no observable clinical deficit if there is good collateral circulation to massive cerebral infarction in the distribution of the anterior and middle cerebral arteries with rapid severe obtundation, with head and eyes turned toward the side of the lesion and dense contralateral motor and sensory deficits. There is often cerebral edema with transtentorial herniation and death. Less extensive infarctions result in partial or total lesions in the distribution of the middle cerebral artery. The anterior cerebral circulation may be preserved through flow from the opposite side via the anterior communicating artery. If there is inadequate collateral flow through the orbit from the external carotid artery, there may be ipsilateral blindness from retinal ischemia on the side of the lesion associated with contralateral hemiplegia.

Middle Cerebral Artery Syndromes

The middle cerebral artery (MCA) supplies the lateral aspect of the frontal, parietal, and temporal lobes and the underlying corona radiata, extending as deep as the putamen and the posterior limb of the internal capsule. Its first branch is the ophthalmic artery, and it then divides into the anterior and middle cerebral arteries. As the main stem of the middle cerebral artery passes out through the Sylvian fissure, it gives rise to a series of small branches called lenticulostriate arteries, which penetrate deeply into the subcortical portion of the brain and perfuse the basal ganglia and internal capsule. At the lateral surface of the hemisphere, the MCA divides into upper and lower divisions, which perfuse the lateral surface of the hemisphere. When the MCA is occluded at its origin, a large cerebral infarction develops involving all the structures mentioned above. Because of the cerebral edema that usually accompanies such a large lesion with brain displacement, the patient initially shows depressed consciousness, with head and eyes deviated to the side of the lesion, and there are contralateral hemiplegia, decreased sensation, and homonymous hemianopia. If the dominant hemisphere is involved, a global aphasia is usually present. As the patient's mental status improves, other features become evident, namely dysphagia, contralateral hemianopia, and, in patients with nondominant hemisphere lesions, perceptual deficits and neglect. Patients who survive the acute lesion regain control of head and eye movements, and normal level of consciousness is restored. However, severe deficits involving motor, visuospatial, and language function usually persist with only limited recovery.

Occlusion of the branches of the middle cerebral artery, except for the lenticulostriate, are almost always embolic in origin, and the associated infarctions are correspondingly smaller and more peripherally located. The superior division of the middle cerebral artery supplies the Rolandic and pre-Rolandic areas, and an infarction in this territory will result in a dense sensory–motor deficit on the contralateral face, arm, and leg, with less involvement of the leg. As recovery occurs, the patient is usually able to walk with a spastic, hemiparetic gait. Little recovery occurs in motor function of the arm. If the left hemisphere is involved, there is usually severe aphasia initially with eventual improvement in comprehension, although an expressive aphasia is likely to persist. Small focal infarctions from occlusions of branches of the superior division will produce more limited deficits such as pure motor weakness of the contralateral arm and face, apraxia, or expressive aphasia.

The inferior division of the middle cerebral artery supplies the parietal and temporal lobes, and lesions on the left side result in severe involvement of language comprehension. The optic radiation is usually involved, resulting in partial or complete homonymous hemianopia on the contralateral side. Lesions affecting the right hemisphere often result in neglect of the left side of the body. Initially, the patient may completely ignore the affected side and even assert that the arm on his left side belongs not to him but to somebody else. Such severe neglect seen initially often gradually improves but may be followed by a variety of persisting impairments such as constructional apraxia, dressing apraxia, and perceptual deficits.

The lenticulostriate arteries are branches arising from the main stem of the middle cerebral artery that penetrate into the subcortical region and perfuse the basal ganglia and posterior internal capsule. Several characteristic and rather common isolated syndromes have been described when discrete focal lesions occur. They are frequently referred to as lacunar strokes. The most common is a lesion in the internal capsule causing a pure motor hemiplegia. An anterior lesion in the internal capsule may cause dysarthria with hand clumsiness, and a lesion of the thalamus or adjacent internal capsule causes a contralateral sensory loss with or without weakness. The neurologic deficits in these lesions often show early and progressive recovery with good ultimate outcome.

Patients with hypertension and diabetes are at risk for recurrent lacunar strokes. Pseudobulbar palsy is a syndrome that develops when multiple small lesions affect the anterior limb of both internal capsules, including the corticobulbar pathways. This syndrome consists of excessive emotional lability and spastic bulbar (''pseudobulbar'') paralysis, i.e., dysarthria, dysphonia, dysphagia, and facial weakness. There are often sudden outbursts of inappropriate and uncontrolled crying and laughter, at times blending into each other, without corresponding emotional stimulus. Drooling is often prominent. The term ''pseudobulbar'' is applied to this syndrome to distinguish it as an upper motor neuron lesion in contrast to a lower motor neuron lesion in the medulla. More widespread and posterior subcortical lacunar infarctions will often produce a dementia, often called multi-infarct dementia.

Anterior Cerebral Artery Syndromes

Branches of the anterior cerebral arteries supply the median and paramedian regions of the frontal cortex and the strip of the lateral surface of the hemisphere along its upper border. There are deep penetrating branches that supply the head of the caudate nucleus and the anterior limb of the internal capsule. Occlusions of the anterior cerebral artery are not common, but when they occur, there is contralateral hemiparesis with relative sparing of the hand and face and greater weakness of the leg. There is associated sensory loss of the leg and foot. Lesions affecting the left side may produce a transcortical motor aphasia characterized by diminution of spontaneous speech but preserved ability to repeat words. A grasp reflex is often present along with a sucking reflex and paratonic rigidity (gegenhalten). Urinary incontinence is common. Large lesions of the frontal cortex often produce behavioral changes such as lack of spontaneity, distractibility, and tendency to perseverate. Patients may have diminished reasoning ability.

Vertebrobasilar Syndromes

The two vertebral arteries join at the junction of the medulla and pons to form the basilar artery. Together, the vertebral and basilar arteries supply the brainstem by paramedian and short circumferential branches and supply the cerebellum by long circumferential branches. The basilar artery terminates by bifurcating at the upper midbrain level to form the two posterior cerebral arteries. The posterior communicating arteries connect the middle to the posterior cerebral arteries, completing the circle of Willis.

Some general clinical features of lesions in the vertebrobasilar system should be noted. In contrast to lesions in the hemispheres, which are unilateral, lesions involving the pons and medulla often cross the midline and cause bilateral features. When motor impairments are present, they are often bilateral, with asymmetric corticospinal signs, and they are frequently accompanied by cerebellar signs. Cranial nerve lesions are very frequent and occur ipsilateral to the main lesion, producing contralateral corticospinal signs. There may be disassociated sensory loss (involvement of the spinothalamic pathway with preservation of the dorsal column pathway or vice versa), dysarthria, dysphagia, disequilibrium and vertigo, and Horner syndrome. Of particular note is absence of cortical deficits such as aphasia and cognitive impairments. Visual field loss and visuospatial deficits may occur if the posterior cerebral artery is involved, but not with brainstem lesions. Identification of a specific cranial nerve lesion allows precise anatomic localization of the lesion.

Lacunar infarcts are common in the vertebrobasilar distribution, arising from occlusion of small penetrating branches of the basilar artery or posterior cerebral artery. In contrast to cerebral lacunes, most brainstem lacunes produce clinical features. There are a variety of characteristic brainstem syndromes associated with lesions at various levels in the brainstem. The reader is referred to neurologic texts for a comprehensive discussion of these lesions. Three brainstem syndromes are not infrequently encountered in rehabilitation centers, and these are described in some detail.

The *lateral medullary syndrome* (Wallenberg syndrome) is produced by an infarction in the lateral wedge of the medulla. It may occur as an occlusion of the vertebral artery or the posterior inferior cerebellar artery. The clinical features of this syndrome, along with the corresponding anatomic structures involved, are impairment of contralateral pain and temperature (spinothalamic tract); ipsilateral Horner syndrome consisting of miosis, ptosis, and decreased facial sweating (descending sympathetic tract); dysphagia, dysarthria, and dysphonia (ipsilateral paralysis of the palate and vocal cords); nystagmus, vertigo, nausea, and vomiting (vestibular nucleus); ipsilateral limb ataxia (spinocerebellar fibers); ipsilateral impaired sensation of the face (sensory nucleus of the fifth nerve). Patients with this syndrome are frequently quite disabled initially because of vertigo, disequilibrium, and ataxia, but they often make a good functional recovery.

Occlusion of the basilar artery may result in severe deficits with complete motor and sensory loss and cranial nerve signs from which patients do not recover. Patients are often comatose. Less extensive lesions however are compatible with life, and a characteristic syndrome observed occasionally is the *locked-in syndrome*. The infarction in such cases affects the upper ventral pons, involving the bilateral corticospinal and corticobulbar pathways but sparing the reticular activating system and ascending sensory pathways. Patients have normal sensation and can see and hear but are unable to move or speak. Blinking and upward gaze are preserved, which provides a very limited but usable means for communication. The patient is alert, and fully oriented. Some patients do not survive, and those who do are severely disabled and dependent. Some slow progressive improvement and partial recovery may occur in this group of patients, justifying appropriate levels of rehabilitation intervention.

Focal infarctions may occur in the midbrain and affect the descending corticospinal pathway, sometimes also involving the third cranial nerve nucleus (Weber syndrome) resulting in ipsilateral third nerve palsy and paralysis of the contralateral arm and leg.

The posterior cerebral artery perfuses the thalamus through perforating arteries, as well as the temporal and occipital lobes with their subcortical structures including the optic radiation. An occipital lobe infarction will cause a partial or complete contralateral hemianopia, and when these visual deficits involve the dominant hemisphere, there may be associated difficulty in reading or in naming objects. When the thalamus is involved, there is contralateral hemisensory loss. A lesion involving the thalamus may cause a syndrome characterized by contralateral hemianesthesia and central pain, although only about 25% of cases of central pain in stroke are caused by lesions of the thalamus. Other lesion sites reported to be associated with central pain are the brainstem and parietal lobe projections from the thalamus. In the thalamic syndrome, patients complain of unremitting, unpleasant, burning pain affecting the opposite side of the body. The pain usually begins a few weeks after stroke onset and becomes intractable to conventional medication, including narcotics. It may be partly relieved with tricyclic antidepressants. Examination of the patient reveals contralateral impairment of all sensory modalities, often with dysesthesia. There may be involvement of adjacent structures such as the internal capsule (hemiparesis, ataxia) or basal ganglia (choreoathetosis).

STROKE DIAGNOSIS

The clinical diagnosis of stroke is often self-evident from the dramatic and abrupt onset of the clinical features, but other disorders may cause relatively sudden neurologic deficits and be mistaken for stroke. For example, a patient with hemiparesis and depressed level of consciousness may have a subdural hematoma from a fall, a cerebral abscess, a brain tumor, or be postictal. It is imperative, therefore, that the diagnosis of stroke be firmly established at the beginning of the patient's care. It is the responsibility of the rehabilitation physician to be sure that an adequate diagnostic evaluation has been completed.

Once a firm diagnosis of stroke has been made, the characteristics of the lesion need to be determined. This can be done by answering three questions: what is it (pathologic diagnosis), where is it (anatomic diagnosis), and why did it happen (etiologic diagnosis). The answers to these questions will influence acute and long-term medical management and will give insights to the rehabilitation team about prognosis and optimum therapeutic procedures.

Pathologic Diagnosis

The pathologic diagnosis—cerebral infarction, intracerebral hemorrhage, or subarachnoid hemorrhage—is suggested by the clinical presentation but is established by imaging studies, which should be done as early as possible. Computed tomography (CT) of the head will reveal acute hemorrhage but will often be negative for the first 1 to 2 days in patients with cerebral infarction. In such cases, with obvious clinical features of stroke, it is reasonable to conclude that a negative CT scan in the first 48 hours represents an infarction. Magnetic resonance imaging (MRI) shows changes of cerebral infarction as early as a few hours postonset, but CT is usually performed early because it is less expensive and because it reveals those structural lesions (hemorrhages, tumor, abscess) that may require surgical management. Within several days an infarction becomes apparent on the CT as a hypodense area. In the postacute phase, both CT and MRI show changes of cerebral infarction. However, MRI is more sensitive in detection of small lacunar strokes because of its greater resolution, and it is more sensitive than CT for detecting lesions in the brainstem and cerebellum. Magnetic resonance angiography is a technique for display of details of cerebrovascular anatomy and pathology without the risks of conventional angiography.

Anatomic Diagnosis

Anatomic localization of the lesion is determined by the neurologic examination, although sometimes the clinical deficits are inconclusive. For example, a patient with a pure motor hemiplegia may have a small embolic infarction involving the motor cortex from occlusion of a branch of the upper division of the MCA. Alternatively, a lacunar stroke affecting the internal capsule or brainstem may also result in a pure motor hemiplegia. Imaging studies are therefore very helpful in documenting the location of the structural lesion responsible for the patient's set of neurologic signs.

Etiologic Diagnosis

For many patients, a stroke, either infarction or hemorrhage, is a late event in the natural course of progressive cerebrovascular disease. Such patients will often have risk factors for stroke, such as age, a history of hypertension, diabetes and smoking, and features of generalized atherosclerosis, especially coronary artery disease and peripheral vascular disease. The etiology of the stroke in these patients is rarely in doubt. But in other patients with thrombotic infarctions, there may be no particular risk factors and no evidence of clinical atherosclerosis. Other less obvious causes of arterial occlusion should then be considered as possible reasons for the stroke. This is particularly important in younger patients who have not had time to develop advanced atherosclerosis. It is a useful strategy for the clinician to always consider the possibility of an alternative cause of arterial occlusion in patients under 55 years of age when there are no risk factors for atherosclerosis or lipohyalinosis. A list of important causes of arterial thrombosis is noted in Table 48-5.

TABLE 48-5. *Causes of arterial thrombosis*

Atherosclerosis (large vessels)
Lipohyalinosis (small vessels)
Arterial dissection (extracranial trauma)
Fibromuscular dysplasia
Vasculitis
Homocystinuria
Coagulopathy
Sickle-cell anemia
Plasma C-protein deficiency
Antithrombin-3 deficiency

In embolic infarction, the deficit occurs rapidly and may involve the carotid or the vertebrobasilar circulation. Sometimes the embolus will undergo lysis, with clearing of the arterial occlusion and rapid recovery of the neurologic deficit. The characteristic features of embolic infarctions as seen on CT scan or MRI are small wedge-shaped superficial cortical lesions. Hemorrhage may occur into the infarction, especially if it is large. When hemorrhage is observed in an infarction on CT or MRI, it can almost always be assumed that the basis for the infarction is embolic rather than thrombotic.

STROKE IN CHILDREN AND YOUNG ADULTS

Stroke is a recognized phenomenon in children and is relatively common in young adults. In a significant number of cases, 40% to 50%, no obvious risk factors such as sources of cardiogenic emboli and atherosclerosis are found. These patients should be thoroughly investigated for primary etiology of the stroke. A list of possible diagnoses is given in Table 48-6. Coagulation disorders may be inherited or acquired, but they may account for up to 20% of cases with thrombotic infarction in young adults. Deficiencies of antithrombin III, protein C, and protein S are among the most important coagulopathies, as each of these substances is part of the naturally occurring anticoagulant system. Each of these conditions requires long-term treatment with warfarin. There have been many reports of external trauma to the neck in children and adults causing thrombosis or dissection of the carotid artery and corresponding cerebral infarction. There are numerous reports of chiropractic manipulation of the cervical spine causing brainstem stroke from trauma and subsequent occlusion or dissection of the vertebral arteries.

Vasculitis may exist as a primary disorder or may occur as part of multisystem inflammatory disease such as juvenile rheumatoid arthritis, systemic lupus erythematosus, polyarteritis nodosa, or Takayasu disease. The pattern of clinical features includes both generalized encephalopathy and focal lesions such as hemiplegia (14).

The inherited disorder homocysteinuria predisposes individuals to early atherosclerosis, and stroke is a frequent occurrence in young adults with this disorder. Stroke has been reported as an occasional complication occurring during pregnancy or in the postpartum period.

ACUTE INTERVENTION

Once a diagnosis of stroke has been made, medical care is directed at prevention of further neurologic deterioration and prevention or treatment of general medical complications. In the past there was no proven method for favorably altering the course of the intracranial pathophysiology. Brain damage from cerebral hemorrhage or infarction followed a course consisting of acute resolution and subsequent slow progressive partial recovery with some restoration of some neurologic function. The severity of the deficit and extent of recovery appeared to be determined by the lesion, and there was no intervention that could alter the outcome. However, some specific therapeutic interventions have emerged recently to ameliorate the brain damage resulting from the stroke. These developments have led to the promotion of the concept of ''brain attack,'' with emphasis on rapid diagnosis and treatment in the intensive care setting as described below.

General Medical Treatment

Any patients who survive an acute stroke may subsequently die in the acute phase from systemic complications such as pneumonia or pulmonary embolism. Very careful attention to the general medical management of the patient is therefore important. This involves measures to preserve a good airway, assistance in clearing pulmonary secretions, and prevention of aspiration. Intermittent catheterization is preferable to prolonged indwelling bladder catheterization to minimize the chances of urinary tract infection. The risk of deep venous thrombosis is high, especially in patients with hemiplegia, and many peripheral thrombi appear within the first several days following the stroke. Every patient should therefore have some form of deep vein thrombosis (DVT) prophylaxis, either subcutaneous heparin or external pneumatic compression stockings, or both. There should be adequate hydration and nutrition. Many patients have cardiac arrythmia, and some have concomitant ischemic heart disease. Appropriate cardiac monitoring and intervention are therefore important.

Many patients with acute stroke are hypertensive on admission, often as a physiological response to the stroke. Blood pressure will gradually fall spontaneously during the first few days, and no specific treatment is necessary. Overenthusiastic reduction of blood pressure in the acute stage may be harmful through reducing perfusion in ischemic brain around the infarction, the ischemic penumbra. Ischemic tissue has impaired local autoregulation of blood flow, and therefore blood flow will passively follow systemic pressure. Maintaining a high mean arterial pressure is important in preservation of perfusion, especially in those patients who have a history of hypertension.

TABLE 48-6. *Causes of stroke in children and young adults*

Cerebral embolism
Trauma to extracranial arteries
Thromboembolic occlusion
Dissection
Subarachnoid hemorrhage
Aneurysm
AVM
Sickle-cell anemia
Vasculopathy
Moya moya disease
SLE
Drug induced
Vasculitis
Coagulopathy
Deficiency of antithrombin III
Deficiency of protein C
Deficiency of protein S
Homocystinuria
Oral contraceptives
Postpartum
Drug-induced

AVM, arteriovenous malformation; SLE, systemic lupus erythematosis.

Stroke Management

In the past a number of pharmacologic interventions have been tried in an effort to reverse the clinical effects of arterial occlusion and diminish neural injury. Most of the proposed regimens have not proven efficacious and have been abandoned, for example, hyperbaric oxygen therapy, carbon dioxide inhalation, infusion of dextran, cerebral vasodilators, overhydration, systemic steroids, and routine use of anticoagulants. Anticoagulants may be used in those patients with small embolic infarctions who have a high risk of recurrence. Recently there have been reports of improved outcome with intravenous infusions of thrombolytic agents such as streptokinase and tissue-type plasminogen activator (t-PA) (15). Studies reported to date have offered encouraging evidence that in selected patients treated very early within the first 3 hours poststroke, outcome can be improved. These agents are not effective if given later, and they do carry the risk of inducing cerebral hemorrhage. They are still under study to determine their optimal method of utilization.

Another class of agents for treatment of acute stroke are cytoprotective agents shown to be effective in animal experimental studies. There is an ''excitotoxic theory'' that holds that neuronal ischemia in the penumbra around an infarction triggers extracellular accumulation of excitatory amino acids, particularly glutamate, which activate cell membrane channels allowing toxic levels of calcium to accumulate inside the cells. There may be other sources of excessive intracellular calcium such as release from storage sites. The high level of intracellular calcium initiates an array of neurochemical changes within the neurons that eventually generate free radicals and progress to cell death. Clinical research has been started testing the value of glutamate receptor antagonists and free radical scavengers for acute stroke. In the future there is promise that effective treatments will evolve and that medical treatment of cerebral infarction will turn from a realm of fatalism to a field of therapeutic opportunity. For further reading see reviews by Dobkin (16) and Stein et al. (17).

Patients with cerebral hemorrhage have a high mortality because of the risk of progressive bleeding, raised intracranial pressure and herniation. In selected patients at risk for brain displacement and herniation, craniotomy and evacuation of the hematoma can be a life-saving procedure. This is particularly the case in patients with cerebellar hemorrhage in whom raised pressure in the posterior fossa can cause acute hydrocephalus and death. With surgical evacuation of the hematoma, these patients will survive and often have very good functional outcome.

Rehabilitation During the Acute Phase

Rehabilitation is not a distinctly separate phase of care, beginning after acute medical intervention. Rather, it is an integral part of medical management and continues longitudinally through acute care, post acute care and community reintegration. Although diagnosis and medical treatment are the principal focus of early treatment, rehabilitation measures should be offered concurrently. Many of these can be considered preventive in nature. For example patients who are paralyzed, lethargic, and have bladder incontinence are at high risk for developing pressure ulcers. Deliberate strategies should be followed to prevent skin breakdowns, including protection of skin from moisture such as urine, avoidance of undue pressure through use of heel-protecting pads, maintenance of proper position with frequent turning, and daily inspection and routine skin cleansing (18).

Many patients with acute stroke have dysphagia and are at risk for aspiration and pneumonia. Aspiration will usually result in coughing, but in up to 40% of patients with acute stroke, aspiration is silent, without coughing. Patients who are lethargic or have decreased arousal should not be fed orally. Even in alert patients, the ability to swallow should be assessed carefully before oral intake of fluids or food is begun. This is done with a bedside evaluation, and if any doubt exists about aspiration, a swallowing videofluoroscopy examination is performed. During the acute phase, nasogastric tube feeding is necessary. It should be noted that patients who are lying flat in bed are at significant risk for regurgitation and aspiration (19).

Impairment of bladder control is frequent following a stroke, which initially causes hypotonic bladder with overflow incontinence. If an indwelling catheter is used for drainage, this should be removed as soon as possible because reflex voiding returns quite quickly and retention is rarely a problem. The indwelling catheter may be useful in the first several days to monitor fluid balance, but it carries an increased risk of urinary tract infection. Regular intermittent catheterization is preferable to an indwelling catheter (20).

There is a strong belief that early mobilization is beneficial to patient outcome by reducing the risks of DVT, gastroesophageal regurgitation and aspiration pneumonia, contracture formation, skin breakdown, and orthostatic intolerance. Early activation is assumed to have a strong positive psychological benefit for the patient. Mobilization involves a set of physical activities that may be started passively but that quickly progress to active participation by the patient in the activity. Specific tasks include turning from side to side in bed and changing position, sitting up in bed, transferring to a wheelchair, standing, and walking. Mobilization also includes self-care activities such as self-feeding, grooming, and dressing. The timing of patient participation and progression in these activities depends on the patient's condition. The activities would be precluded by progressive neurologic signs, intracranial hemorrhage, coma, or cardiovascular instability. If the patient's condition is stable, however, active mobilization should begin as soon as possible, within 24 to 48 hours of admission (20).

Evaluation for Rehabilitation Program

Within several days of admission, once the patient appears to be neurologically and medically stable, the patient should be evaluated for admission to a comprehensive rehabilitation program. The criteria for admission into a postacute rehabilitation program are listed in Table 48-7. A comprehensive rehabilitation program involving multiple professionals is justified when the patient has identified disability affecting multiple areas of function. A patient with an isolated disability such as a partial aphasia, visual loss, or monoparesis may need rehabilitation, but for these cases, therapy can be provided by a therapist, one discipline only, usually in an outpatient setting. In the very early post-onset phase, it may not be possible to judge whether the patient has sufficient cognitive function or communicative ability to engage in the program or sufficient physical tolerance to participate fully.

TABLE 48-7. *Criteria for admission to a comprehensive rehabilitation program*

Stable neurologic status
Significant persisting neurologic deficit
Identified disability affecting at least two of the following: mobility, self-care activities, communication, bowel or bladder control, or swallowing
Sufficient cognitive function to learn
Sufficient communicative ability to engage with the therapists
Physical ability to tolerate the active program
Achievable therapeutic goals

It may be necessary in such cases to offer a short trial of therapy to observe the patient's true capacity and potential before deciding on candidacy.

Evaluation of the acute stroke patient should include information about the patient's general medical status, including the presence of important comorbidities. Equally important, the patient's psychosocial status influences the way the patient copes with the disability, impacts motivation and physical outcome, and forms the basis of discharge planning. It is important to establish at the outset the nature of the patient's family support, living situation, and postdischarge environment. Knowledge of all of these factors will assist the team in counseling the patient and family and in planning for discharge.

Medical stability has traditionally been required for admission of a patient to a specialized rehabilitation unit. However, hospitals are increasingly transferring patients from acute wards to rehabilitation units at earlier stages, often when they still have unresolved medical problems. This practice has forced rehabilitation centers to expand their resources to care for these more complex cases and to provide closer medical and nursing monitoring. Local institutional referral patterns and practices will usually determine the timing of transfer, but if earlier transfer to rehabilitation can be accomplished safely, patient care may be enhanced by earlier active participation of the patient in the rehabilitation program.

The rehabilitation program may be offered in different settings, such as an acute inpatient rehabilitation unit, a subacute rehabilitation inpatient unit, home care, or an outpatient center. The acute rehabilitation setting is appropriate for those patients who meet the admission criteria and are able to tolerate 3 hours or more of active therapy per day. An acute rehabilitation setting is preferred if the patient requires close medical and nursing monitoring of the medical status. If the patient's medical status is stable, but the patient is unable to tolerate more than 1 hour of therapy a day, a subacute rehabilitation setting is more appropriate. Other patients who require only minor degrees of assistance in self-care and mobility would be suitable for outpatient therapy or a home care program.

PRINCIPLES OF STROKE REHABILITATION

Although rehabilitation intervention is important during the acute phase of care, it is secondary to the activities involved in diagnosis and acute medical treatment. However, when a patient has a persisting major continuing impairment such as hemiplegia with disabilities, the rehabilitation components of care quickly become the main focus of management. The rehabilitation process for patients with complex problems requires a carefully planned and integrated program. Some general principles have evolved over time to form the basis of stroke rehabilitation. Some of these principles are based on conclusions from clinical trials, but many represent a general consensus based on clinical experience. They are:

1. There is a clear need for committed medical direction. The role of the physician includes provision of medical care. Many patients have ongoing associated medical problems that require appropriate monitoring and therapy. The physician must act as medical counselor, offering reasonable prognostication to patient and family along with guidance in stroke risk factor reduction and ongoing medical care. The physician must also give leadership to the team and assist in developing treatment protocols and setting treatment expectations.
2. The multiple problems of a patient require the active participation of a team of professionals. The treatment activities of the team members must be coordinated so that detailed evaluations are shared and goals and treatment interventions are agreed on.
3. Each of the professional therapists on the team should be knowledgeable regarding the appropriate interventions within his or her discipline for treating the disabilities of stroke patients.
4. The interventions should be directed at achieving specific therapeutic goals, which may be short-term, e.g., week to week, or longer-term, e.g., goals to be reached by discharge. Having achieved those goals, the patient moves on to the next phase of rehabilitation or is discharged home to continue treatment as an outpatient.
5. There is evidence from clinical trials that early initiation of therapy favorably influences the outcome. During delays in starting therapy, patients may develop secondary avoidable complications such as contractures and deconditioning.
6. Therapy should be directed at specific training of skills and functional training. Therapy should be given with sufficient intensity to promote skill acquisition.
7. Planning for discharge from the inpatient rehabilitation program should begin on admission.
8. Psychosocial issues are obviously very important. Numerous studies have reported on the influence of spouse, family, and the patient's own psychological adjustment and coping mechanisms in determining ultimate outcome. Family involvement is essential throughout the treatment program and in discharge planning.
9. There should be an emphasis on patient and family education about stroke, risk factor reduction, and strategies to maximize functional independence.
10. Rehabilitation requires a functional approach. When impairments cannot be altered, every effort should be made to assist patients to compensate for deficits and adapt with alternative methods to achieve optimal functional independence.
11. Discharge from hospital is often thought of as the end of rehabilitation, with the assumption that a good program prepares the patient for reintegration into home and community. However, hospital discharge should instead

be looked on as the end of the beginning of a new life in which the patient faces the challenge of adopting different roles and relationships and a search for new meaning in life. This will involve resuming as much as possible former roles in the family and with friends and finding ways to live a meaningful life in the community.

RECOVERY FROM STROKE

Numerous studies have described the patterns of improvement in neurologic deficits and in recovery of function after stroke. There is marked variation among patients in the time course of recovery and in its degree. An important objective of many of these studies has been identification of specific variables that would predict the course of recovery from neurologic impairments.

Recovery from Impairments

Hemiparesis and motor recovery have been the most studied of all stroke impairments. As many as 88% of patients with an acute stroke have hemiparesis (21). In a classic report, Twitchell (22) described in detail the pattern of motor recovery following stroke. At onset the arm is more involved than the leg, and eventual motor recovery in the arm is less than in the leg. The severity of arm weakness at onset and the timing of the return of movement in the hand are both important predictors of eventual motor recovery in the arm (23–25). The prognosis for return of useful hand function is poor when there is complete arm paralysis at onset or no measurable grasp strength by 4 weeks. However, even among those patients with severe arm weakness at onset, as many as 9% may gain good recovery of hand function. Some other generalizations can be made. For patients showing some motor recovery in the hand by 4 weeks, as many as 70% will make a full or good recovery. Full recovery, when it occurs, is usually complete within 3 months of onset. Bard and Hirshberg claim that "if no initial motion is noticed during the first 3 weeks, or if motion in one segment is not followed within a week by the appearance of motion in a second segment, the prognosis for recovery of full motion is poor" (23).

The course of motor recovery reaches a plateau after an early phase of progressive improvement. Most recovery takes place in the first 3 months, and only minor additional measurable improvement occurs after 6 months post-onset (26). However, in some patients who have significant partial return of voluntary movement, recovery may continue over a longer period of time.

About one-third of patients with acute stroke have clinical features of aphasia. Language function in many of these patients improves, and at 6 months or more after stroke, only 12% to 18% have identifiable aphasia (27,28). Skilbeck et al. (28) reported that patients with aphasia continue to show some late improvement in language function, even beyond 1 year after onset. Patients who would be initially classified as having Broca aphasia have a variable outcome. In patients with large hemisphere lesions, Broca aphasia persists with little recovery, but patients with smaller lesions confined to the posterior frontal lobe often show early progressive improvement, the impairment evolving into a milder form of aphasia with anomia and word-finding difficulty. Patients with global aphasia tend to progress slowly, with comprehension often improving more than expressive ability. Communicative ability of patients who initially have global aphasia improve over a longer period of time, up to a year or more post-onset. Patients with global aphasia associated with large lesions may show only minor recovery, but recovery may be quite good in those patients with smaller lesions. Language recovery in Wernicke's aphasia is variable.

About 20% of patients have a visual field defect. In general, the degree of visual improvement following stroke is not as impressive as recovery of motor and sensory function, and if the field defect persists beyond a few weeks, late recovery is less likely.

Mechanisms of Neurologic Recovery

In the early phase poststroke, there is prompt initial improvement in function as the pathologic processes in the ischemic penumbra—ischemia, metabolic injury, edema, hemorrhage, and pressure—resolve. The time frame for recovery of function in these reversibly injured neurons is relatively short and accounts for improvement in the first several weeks. The later, ongoing improvement in neurologic function occurs by a different set of mechanisms that allow structural and functional reorganization within the brain. The processes involved in this reorganization represent neuroplasticity and may continue for many months. There is restitution of partially damaged pathways and expansion of representational brain maps, implying recruitment of neurons not ordinarily involved in an activity. A key aspect of neuroplasticity that has important implications for rehabilitation is that the modifications in neuronal networks are use dependent. Animal experimental studies and clinical trials in humans have shown that forced use and functional training contribute to improved function. On the other hand, techniques that promote nonuse may inhibit recovery. It used to be taught that benefits from rehabilitation are primarily achieved through training patients in new techniques to compensate for impairments, e.g., using the uninvolved hand to achieve self-care independence. This approach avoided intense therapy on the weak upper limb. It is now recognized that repeated participation by patients in active physical therapeutic programs probably directly influences functional reorganization in the brain and enhances neurologic recovery. See Chapter 49 for more details about neuroplasticity.

IMPAIRMENT EVALUATION

The focal neurologic lesion that accompanies a stroke confers on the patient a set of neurologic deficits, which in

TABLE 48-8. *Medical diagnosis versus rehabilitation diagnosis*

Medical diagnosis
  Pathology (e.g., infarction) → Neurologic deficits (e.g., hemiplegia)
Rehabilitation diagnosis
  Impairments (e.g., hemiplegia) → Disability (e.g., inability to walk)

rehabilitation medicine are referred to as impairments. Evaluation of these impairments constitutes an essential first step in rehabilitation management of the patient. When the physician and therapist understand the nature of a patient's impairments, they can provide specific targeted therapy to optimize the rehabilitation program. The relationship between medical diagnosis and rehabilitation diagnosis is described in Table 48-8 (29). The initial clinical examination of a patient with an acute stroke includes a thorough, detailed neurologic examination. The neurologic findings are used by the rehabilitation team for prognostication, development of the specific details of the rehabilitation plan, and selection of the appropriate setting for rehabilitation. Reassessment of the patient during rehabilitation provides a means of monitoring progress and subsequently evaluating outcome. The initial rehabilitation assessment should begin immediately postonset, within 2 to 7 days, and then at repeated subsequent intervals.

The following sections summarize the important details of the neurologic impairments encountered in postacute stroke patients.

Higher Mental Function

Focal brain lesions associated with a stroke frequently produce measurable impairments in higher mental function. Even small lesions may significantly impair cognition, particularly when they are multiple. However, interpretation of test information must be made in the context of the clinical situation because other nonstroke factors may contribute to impaired mental status. Many patients are elderly and may have had some premorbid decline in mental status. Further, general medical disorders such as a fever, electrolyte disturbance, hypothyroidism, congestive heart failure, and reaction to medication may produce an encephalopathy. Such patients are often confused and may have a diminished level of consciousness; they have a generalized disturbance of mental status with abnormalities in most or all cognitive tests. The encephalopathy associated with these general medical problems is reversible following correction of the complicating disorder. Only when nonstroke factors have been excluded can changes in mental status be attributed to the focal lesion of the brain.

The cognitive impairments observed with focal lesions frequently show specific disturbances, for example, memory loss, neglect, or constructional apraxia. Disturbances such as these can usually be recognized at the bedside. Because cognitive impairments can have a significant influence on the rehabilitation program and on outcome, the bedside mental status examination should be an essential part of the assessment of every stroke patient. The components of the examination are shown in Table 48-9. For a more detailed description of this assessment see Strub and Black (30). The Mini-Mental State Examination developed by Folstein et al. (31) is a useful bedside tool that screens a variety of mental demands quickly and gives a well-validated measure of overall mental function. It requires less than 10 minutes to administer. Formal psychological tests may be used to establish global intellectual level and to reveal specific areas of diminished performance reflecting focal brain impairment. The Weschler Adult Intelligence Scale (WAIS) is commonly used in stroke patients.

Perceptual impairments are extremely important in stroke rehabilitation, and their recognition is an essential part of the higher mental function evaluation. A perceptual deficit is an impairment in the recognition and interpretation of sensory information when the sensory input system is intact. Impaired perception is caused by a lesion at the cortical level, almost always in the nondominant parietal lobe. The patient exhibits selective inattention, which can be detected by careful observation of his or her behavior. A patient with hemisensory loss or homonymous hemianopia will also ignore the affected side. However, inattention is only referred to as true neglect when the sensory and visual pathways are intact. Unilateral neglect may be visual, tactile, spatial, or auditory. Visual neglect is demonstrated at the bedside when the patient, on request, attempts to draw numbers on a clockface, draw a stick figure, or bisect a horizontal line on a piece of paper. The patient is inattentive to the affected side. Other bedside tests of perceptual function are failure to recognize palm writing (graphesthesia), inability to identify objects in the hand (astereognosis), and extinction of simultaneous bilateral stimulation.

The term *apraxia* describes the inability of a patient to execute a willed movement when motor and sensory function are apparently preserved. Apraxia may be detected when a patient is unable to carry out a task on command such as "comb your hair" or "wave goodbye" even though there is no paralysis. Patients with lesions of the nondominant

TABLE 48-9. *Mental status examination*

Level of consciousness
  Alertness, response to stimulation
Attention
Memory
  Orientation, new learning, remote memory
Cognition
  Fund of knowledge, calculation, problem solving, abstract thinking, judgment
Perception, constructional ability, apraxia
Affect and behavior

TABLE 48-10. *Classification of aphasia*

Classification	Fluency	Comprehension	Repetition	Naming
Global	Poor	Poor	Poor	Poor
Broca	Poor	Good	Variable	Poor
Isolation	Poor	Poor	Good	Poor
Transcortical motor	Poor	Good	Good	Poor
Wernicke	Good	Poor	Poor	Poor
Transcortical sensory	Good	Poor	Good	Poor
Conduction	Good	Good	Poor	Poor
Anomic	Good	Good	Good	Poor

parietal lobe may have apraxia of putting on their clothes and getting dressed.

Communication Disorders

Communication is a complex function involving reception, central processing, and sending of information (see Chapter 12). Communication occurs through the use of language and consists of a system of symbols that are combined to convey ideas, i.e., letters, words, or gestures. Impairment of language is called aphasia, and its presence reflects an abnormality in the dominant hemisphere. Speech, on the other hand, is a term that refers to the motor mechanism involved in the production of spoken words, namely breathing, phonation, and articulation. Dysphonia and dysarthria are disorders of speech.

Although there are many classifications for aphasia, certain identifiable groups of patients are observed with clinically similar disorders of communication. In the simplest classification, aphasia is divided into two main categories: motor aphasia (sometimes called expressive or anterior aphasia), characterized by nonfluent speech, and sensory aphasia (sometimes called receptive, posterior, or Wernicke's aphasia), characterized by fluent speech. A common system of classification of aphasia is listed in Table 48-10 (29). Use of simple bedside tests can allow the clinician to categorize the communication disorder according to this classification. During the evaluation of a patient, the clinician should avoid using nonverbal cues such as gestures. The questions addressed during the bedside assessment of aphasia are provided in Table 48-11.

TABLE 48-11. *The bedside test*

Questions	Clinical test
Does the patient understand?	Give verbal commands, ask patient to point to objects.
Is the patient able to talk?	Ask the patient to name objects, describe them, count. Listen for spontaneous speech.
Can the patient repeat?	Ask the patient to repeat words.
Can the patient read?	Give commands in writing.
Can the patient write?	Ask the patient to copy or to write dictated words.

Complete evaluations of patients can be performed using formal aphasia tests. Table 48-12 summarizes the more commonly used formal aphasia test instruments.

For assessment of dysarthria, clinicians subjectively rate the degree of impairment as a percentage intelligibility of speech.

Cranial Nerves

In patients with lesions involving the hemispheres, visual field defects may be present. Patients with hemianopia will often fail to detect objects on the affected side of the body, which confers significant disability. The precise nature of the defect can be characterized by confrontation testing. Extraocular palsies involving lesions of the midbrain or pons can produce characteristic dysfunction.

Dysphagia is a frequent impairment with unilateral hemisphere stroke, but it is much more pronounced in bilateral disease and in brainstem lesions. Other cranial nerve lesions may be identified in lesions involving the brainstem. The reader is referred to standard neurologic texts and to Chapter 12 for detailed descriptions.

TABLE 48-12. *Commonly used formal aphasia test*

- The Boston Diagnostic Aphasia Examination (32) produces a classification of the aphasic features observed in a particular patient. Besides classifying the aphasia, it also provides a score of the severity of the aphasia, which can be compared to aphasic patients in general.
- The Western Aphasia Battery (33) is somewhat similar to the Boston. It measures various parameters of spontaneous speech and examines comprehension, fluency, object naming, and repetition. It provides a total score called an aphasia quotient, which is a measure of the severity of the aphasia.
- The Porch Index of Communication Ability (PICA) is different from the other tests in that it evaluates verbal, gestural, and graphic responses. It is very structured in its format and must be given by a trained professional. It provides a useful statistical summary of the details of the language impairments and offers outcome prediction.
- The Functional Communication Profile (34) provides an overall rating of functional communication. It is not a diagnostic test. The score indicates severity and can be a useful indicator of recovery.

Motor Impairment

Paralysis is such a common feature among central nervous system impairments with stroke that the terms hemiplegia and stroke are often used interchangeably. Assessment of motor impairment includes an evaluation of tone, strength, coordination, and balance.

The most widely used scale to assess strength is the Medical Research Council (MRC) six-point scale, 0 to 5, in which 0 represents complete paralysis, 3 is the ability to fully move the joint against gravity, and 5 indicates normal strength. The test is insensitive in its upper range, where the examiner must assess strength by offering manual resistance to maximum muscle activation. The MRC scale is designed to assess the strength of individual muscles, and it is therefore most useful in grading strength in patients with lower motor neuron lesions. There are drawbacks to the use of this scale in patients with upper motor neuron lesions such as stroke. A patient recovering from hemiplegia may not be able to selectively activate a particular muscle in isolation and hence will be given a 0 grade on the MRC scale. However, the patient may be able to forcefully activate the muscle within a gross motor pattern in which groups of muscles contract together in synergy, for example, a flexor or extensor synergy pattern. Further, as tone increases during recovery, the capacity of the patient to move a joint may be restricted by spasticity in the antagonists. Cocontraction of agonists and antagonists can diminish the force of muscle contraction recorded externally. Despite these shortcomings, the MRC scale may be quite useful in the early phases following a stroke, before significant spasticity develops.

Brunnstrom (35) adopted a different approach for assessment of motor function in hemiplegic patients. She developed a test in which movement patterns are evaluated and motor function is rated according to stages of motor recovery. The clinician assesses the presence of flexor and extensor synergies and the degree of selective muscle activation from the synergy pattern (Table 48-13) (29). The rating can be performed very quickly, and although the scale defines recovery only in broad categories, these categories do correlate with progressive functional recovery (36).

TABLE 48-13. *Brunnstrom stages of motor recovery*

Stage	Characteristics
Stage 1	No activation of the limb
Stage 2	Spasticity appears, and weak basic flexor and extensor synergies are present
Stage 3	Spasticity is prominent; the patient voluntarily moves the limb, but muscle activation is all within the synergy patterns
Stage 4	The patient begins to activate muscles selectively outside the flexor and extensor synergies
Stage 5	Spasticity decreases; most muscle activation is selective and independent from the limb synergies
Stage 6	Isolated movements are performed in a smooth, phasic, well-coordinated manner

Rather than subjectively assess strength using the MRC scale, Bohannon advocated direct measurement of force with a dynamometer (37). Despite the limitations of assessing and interpreting muscle strength in patients with upper motor neuron lesions, strength does correlate with performance on functional tasks (38). Fugl-Meyer et al. (39) designed a more detailed and comprehensive motor scale in which 50 different movements and abilities were rated. The test evaluates strength, reflexes, and coordination, and a composite score is derived on a scale of 0 to 100. The Fugl-Meyer Scale is reliable, and repeat scores reflect motor recovery over time. It is quite useful and informative but has not been widely adopted by clinicians because it is time-consuming to complete each evaluation.

Muscle tone refers to the resistance felt when the examiner passively stretches a muscle by moving a joint. The rating is subjective and depends on the judgment of the examiner. Physiological conditions such as position of body segments and body posture strongly influence the level of muscle tone, and these must be controlled as much as possible. For example, tone will be increased if the patient is supine rather than prone, or standing rather than sitting. Tone in the leg muscles may be quite modest in a sitting hemiplegic patient but be very severe when the patient is standing. A high level of anxiety will also increase the degree of muscle tone. Quantitation of spasticity is difficult. The most widely used scale is the Ashworth Scale (see Chapter 40) (40).

Sensory Impairment

When sensory deficits exist as part of a clinical picture following a stroke, they frequently accompany motor impairment in the same anatomic distribution. Interpretation of sensory testing may be difficult in a confused or cognitively impaired patient. Clinical examination involves testing pain, temperature, touch, joint position, and vibration. Lesions of the thalamus may cause severe contralateral sensory loss. With lesions of the cortex, sensation, although preserved, is qualitatively and quantitatively reduced. Parietal lobe lesions cause perceptual deficits in which primary modalities of sensation may be intact. Typical tests to reveal the presence of perceptual impairment include: simultaneous bilateral stimulation for inattention, two-point discrimination, object recognition for stereognosis, and recognition of digits drawn in the palm.

Balance, Coordination, and Posture

Impaired balance may be caused by deficits in motor and sensory function, cerebellar lesions, and vestibular dysfunctions. Clinical testing involves assessing coordination using finger-to-nose pointing and rapid alternating movements. The ability of the patient to sit unsupported or, if able, to stand and walk provides important information. Ataxia caused by sensory impairment can be differentiated from ataxia resulting from cerebellar loss because performance of a motor task with the eyes closed is much poorer in sensory ataxia, when the patient has no vision to compensate for sensory loss.

Evaluation of the neurologic impairments should be made repeatedly during the course of the rehabilitation program. Ideally, evaluation should be made weekly in the early phases of rehabilitation, to allow monitoring of the recovery process and to guide the therapeutic intervention.

OUTCOME AND PROGNOSTICATION IN STROKE REHABILITATION

Prognostication regarding outcome for a stroke patient is often expressed in the simple question: "Is this patient a good candidate for rehabilitation?" The benefits of good prognostication are self-evident. Patients and family members need to know the prospects for survival, the degree of recovery that may be expected, and the extent of possible residual disability following rehabilitation. Professionals providing care need information with which to counsel patients and families. Knowledge of prognosis of individual patients can guide physicians and therapists in selection of specific therapies and appropriate intensities of therapies. Finally, good prognostication can help to reduce costs of care through reduction of misdirected therapy and optimal use of facilities and staff.

Accurate prognostication of the ultimate status of patients after recovery from stroke has proven to be elusive because of difficulties encountered in stroke outcome research. Some factors that have made conclusions about prognostication imprecise include the following. The effects of cerebrovascular disease are heterogeneous, and pathologies are different: some patients have only transient symptoms, whereas others have severe and lasting impairment. Many studies are not comparable; for example, it is difficult to compare studies that aggregate all patients regardless of pathology, lesion site, time interval since onset, and degree of impairment with those studies of selected subgroups of patients. A major limitation in interpretation of many early reports on prediction of stroke outcome has been poor definition of prognostic variables and outcome variables. Methodologic issues in stroke outcome research were reviewed in a symposium in 1989 (41,42). Important recommendations were made to standardize methodologies in outcome studies in stroke research, and in 1989 the World Health Organization (WHO) task force issued similar recommendations (43).

It is important to distinguish between prognostic and outcome variables. Prognostic variables influence the survival, recovery, and ultimate outcome of an individual who has sustained an acute stroke (Table 48-14) (44). These variables may be categorized into those that are patient related, those that are lesion related, those that are intervention and therapy related, and those that are psychosocial. Outcome variables, on the other hand describe different aspects of the status of the patient at a particular end point. Typical outcome variables of interest are listed in Table 48-15 (44).

TABLE 48-14. *Classification of prognostic variables*

Patient demographic variables
General medical characteristics
Examples: hypertension, heart disease, diabetes
Lesion-related variables
Pathology
Lesion site and size
Impairment characteristics
Coma at onset
Bladder and bowel continence
Specific therapy interventions
Nature of therapy
Time of initiating therapy
Intensity of therapy
Psychosocial variables
Socioeconomic status
Premorbid personality
Patient family role

Predicting Survival

Early death following a stroke is usually related to the underlying pathology and to the severity of the lesion. The 30-day survival for patients with cerebral infarction is 85%, but for patients with intracerebral hemorrhage, survival is reported to be only 20% to 52% (45,46). Better management of cardiac and respiratory disorders has decreased early mortality. Hypertension, heart disease, and diabetes, however, remain as risk factors for recurrence of stroke. Coma following a stroke onset indicates a poor prognosis, presumably because coma occurs frequently in cerebral hemorrhage, and when it occurs in relationship to cerebral infarction, it reflects a large lesion with cerebral edema.

Predicting Disability and Functional Status

The key outcomes from a rehabilitation perspective are those that describe the disability status of the patient. The central purpose of the rehabilitation program is to lessen ultimate disability; therefore, considerable attention has been

TABLE 48-15. *Outcome variables*

Survival
Impairment: neurologic deficit
Degree of paralysis
Aphasia
Visual field defect, neglect
Disability
Activities of daily living (ADL)
Ambulation
Social variables
Discharge destination
Living arrangements
Social integration

directed at the identification of factors that will predict the late functional status of the patient, especially with respect to walking and activities of daily living (ADL).

Most patients admitted to an inpatient stroke rehabilitation program in the postacute phase have hemiparesis of sufficient severity that walking is impossible. Some recovery of leg function almost always occurs, and improvement in mobility follows. By 3 months post-onset, 54% to 80% of patients are independent in walking (47,48). In a retrospective study of 248 patients with stroke treated at a rehabilitation center, Feigenson et al. (49) reported that 85% of patients were ambulatory at discharge. The degree of recovery in walking ability depends on motor recovery (36). As measured on the Brunnstrom Scale for stages of motor recovery, very few patients who remain in stage II (minimal voluntary movement) regain the ability to walk; however, most patients in stage III (active flexion and extension synergy through range of motion) do eventually walk. Data from the Framingham cohort reported by Gresham et al. (50) indicate that long-term survivors of stroke show good recovery of functional mobility, with 80% being independent in mobility.

Most patients with significant neurologic impairment who survive a stroke are dependent in basic ADL, that is, bathing, dressing, feeding, toileting, grooming, and transfers. The capacity of individuals to perform these activities is usually scored on disability rating scales such as the Functional Independent Measure (FIM) (see Chapter 7). Almost all patients show improved function in ADL as recovery occurs. Most improvement is noted in the first 6 months (51,52), although as many as 5% of patients show continued measurable improvement to 12 months post-onset. Other patients may show some functionally worthwhile improvement beyond 6 months, which the disability scales usually fail to detect because of their limited sensitivity at the upper end of the functional range. The levels of functional independence eventually reached by stroke patients after recovery as reported by different authors are variable. This probably reflects differences between study populations and differences in methods of treatment, follow-up, and data reporting. In most reports, between 47% and 76% of survivors achieve partial or total independence in ADL (49,51,52).

Most authors who have attempted to determine which factors predict ultimate ADL functional outcome have used multivariate analysis. Of many independent variables tested, those reported to have the most influence on outcome are listed in Table 48-16. Not all of these factors were shown in every study to statistically predict outcome status.

The effect of age on outcome may partly be related to more frequent coimpairments. If elderly patients are less functional prestroke, this alone could explain poorer outcomes following a stroke. Furthermore, elderly patients often do not receive as intensive therapy as younger patients, and they may be discharged from the rehabilitation program sooner. Some studies designed to examine age as an independent prognostic factor have not found a correlation between age and functional ADL outcome in 6 months (53). Coexisting heart disease and diabetes represent comorbidities that are likely to increase the chance of recurrent stroke and may limit a patient's full participation in an intensive program. These comorbidities affect survival, i.e., increase the likelihood of recurrence or death, but it is not known to what degree their presence influences functional recovery from stroke. Such measures of the severity of the stroke as reduced sitting balance, visuospatial impairment, mental changes, and incontinence all influence functional outcome. Intuitively, it would seem reasonable to assume that patients with more severe neurologic deficits would have worse functional outcomes, but this is not necessarily the case when isolated neurologic impairments are considered. For example, analyses of predictive variables have failed to show that patients with sensory deficits have a poorer ultimate outcome (54). The severity of the neurologic deficit is reflected in the overall ADL score, and most authors have reported that the initial ADL score is a good predictor of ultimate ADL function. Patients admitted for rehabilitation with lower ADL scores do not have as good a functional outcome as patients who initially had higher admission ADL scores.

TABLE 48-16. *Factors predicting poor ADL outcome*

Advanced age
Comorbidities
Myocardial infarction
Diabetes mellitus
Severity of stroke
Severe weakness
Poor sitting balance
Visuospatial deficits
Mental changes
Incontinence
Low initial ADL scores
Time interval: onset to rehabilitation

ADL, activities of daily living.

It is generally accepted that early initiation of therapies is desirable. Early rehabilitation minimizes secondary complications such as contractures and deconditioning and helps motivation. It is not known whether higher-intensity therapy as an independent variable improves ultimate functional recovery.

Social Variables

The discharge destination of a patient, home or institutional placement, living arrangements, and social integration are all important in reflecting the social status of patients following recovery. Patients most likely to require long-term institutional care are those with severe disabilities who need maximum physical assistance in ADL and who have bowel or bladder incontinence (49). However, psychosocial variables, especially prestroke family interaction (55) and the presence of an able spouse, also influence whether the patient returns home. A supportive family whose members are willing to provide significant physical care may be able to manage a severely disabled patient at home. By contrast, a patient with much less disability but no family support may require institutional care if not fully independent.

When a clinician is confronted with the challenge of evaluating an individual patient, guidelines for predicting functional outcome are useful but are not precise because multiple variables interact. A patient who might be judged as having a good prognosis for functional outcome may do poorly because of a negative psychosocial factor. The best estimate of prognosis can be made only after a thorough and comprehensive evaluation of the patient's medical, neurologic, functional, and psychosocial status. The clinician at the bedside is in the best position to formulate a prognosis and provide an answer to the question, "Is this patient a good candidate for rehabilitation?"

MEDICAL MANAGEMENT IN THE POSTACUTE PHASE

There is a high incidence of coexisting medical disorders among patients recovering from stroke, reflecting the age of the patient population and the fact that cerebrovascular disease is part of a generalized disease process. If severe, or if poorly managed, these disorders may interfere with the patient's participation in the rehabilitation program and may adversely affect outcome. It is imperative, therefore, that the attending physician assess the patient thoroughly and monitor the medical status closely, being prepared to intervene promptly when required. Some of the important and more frequent disorders are discussed briefly.

Medical Comorbidities

In a large majority of patients, a stroke is an acute event in the course of a systemic disease, e.g., atherosclerosis, hypertensive vascular disease, or cardiac embolism. These patients frequently exhibit other clinical features of the underlying systemic disorder, especially heart disease. Up to 75% of stroke patients may show evidence of coexisting cardiovascular disease, including hypertension (estimates range from 50% to 84%) (56) and coronary artery disease (up to 65%) (56). Another group of heart diseases cause a stroke through cardiogenic cerebral embolism. These diseases include atrial fibrillation and other arrhythmias from multiple causes, valvular disease, cardiomyopathy, endocarditis, recent myocardial infarction, and left atrial myxoma.

Concomitant heart disease has a negative impact on short-term and long-term survival and probably on functional outcome of stroke patients (57,58). Acute exacerbations of heart disease occur frequently during postacute stroke rehabilitation (57). Common problems include angina, uncontrolled hypertension, hypotension, myocardial infarction, congestive heart failure, atrial fibrillation, and ventricular arrhythmias. Development of one of these complications may have minimal or no impact on the patient's progress or outcome if the problem is promptly diagnosed and appropriately treated. However, these complications often do impact the patient's capacity to participate fully in the therapeutic program. Congestive heart failure and angina decrease exercise tolerance and reduce capacity to roll over in bed, transfer, and walk.

All patients should be monitored carefully during postacute rehabilitation for evidence of cardiac disease. The classical features of coronary artery disease and congestive heart failure may be present, but often they are not. Ischemia may be silent. The clinical clues to significant coexisting heart disease may be subtle, e.g., slower than expected progress, excessive fatigue, lethargy, or mental changes. Patients should undergo appropriate cardiac investigation with electrocardiography, Holter monitoring, echocardiography, etc. and should receive optimal therapy. These cardiac complications can be successfully treated and are not contraindications for rehabilitation.

The rehabilitation management of patients with identified cardiac complications should include formal clinical monitoring of pulse and blood pressure during physical activities. Brief electrocardiac monitoring during exercise can add more specific information. A useful set of cardiac precautions in patients undergoing rehabilitation was developed by Fletcher et al. (59) and are listed in Table 48-17. It should be noted that in deconditioned patients, the resting heart rate may be high, and in an elderly patient the estimated limit for heart rate based on 50% above resting may be too high. For patients on beta blockers, a reasonable limit might be a heart rate at around 20 beats above the resting level.

Medical Complications

Medical complications frequently occur during the postacute phase of rehabilitation, affecting up to 60% of patients and up to 94% of patients with severe lesions (60). Common medical and neurologic complications are listed in Table 48-18 (49–52).

Pulmonary Aspiration and Pneumonia

Dysphagia is a frequent and serious complication of stroke. It is a usual feature in brainstem lesions or bilateral

TABLE 48-17. *Cardiac precautions*

Activity should be terminated if any of the following develops:
1. New onset cardiopulmonary symptoms
2. Heart rate decreases >20% of baseline
3. Heart rate increases >50% of baseline
4. Systolic BP increases to 240 mm Hg
5. Systolic BP decreases ≥30 mm Hg from baseline or to <90 mm Hg
6. Diastolic BP increases to 120 mm Hg

BP, blood pressure.

From Fletcher BJ, Dunbar S, Coleman J, Jann B, Fletcher GF. Cardiac precautions for nonacute inpatient settings. *Am J Phys Med Rehabil* 1993; 72:140–143.

TABLE 48-18. *Medical complications during postacute stroke rehabilitation*

Complication	Frequency (%)
Medical	
Pulmonary aspiration, pneumonia	40
Urinary tract infection	40
Depression	30
Musculoskeletal pain, RSD	30
Falls	25
Malnutrition	16
Venous thromboembolism	6
Pressure ulcer	3
Neurologic	
Toxic or metabolic encephalopathy	10
Stroke progression	5
Seizure	4

RSD, reflex sympathetic dystrophy.

Data are from the following sources: Wade DT, Wood VA, Langton Hewer R. Recovery after stroke—the first 3 months. *J Neurol Neurosurg Psychiatry* 1985; 48:7–13; Feigenson JS, McDowell FH, Meese P, McCarthy ML, Greenberg SD. Factors influencing outcome and length of stay in a stroke rehabilitation unit Part 1. *Stroke* 1977; 8:651–656; Gresham GE, Fitzpatrick TE, Wolf PA, MacNamara PM, Kannel WB, Dawber TR. Residual disability in survivors of stroke: The Framingham Study. *N Engl J Med* 1975; 293:954–956; Wade DT, Langton Hewer R. Functional abilities after stroke: measurement, natural history and prognosis. *J Neurol Neurosurg Psychiatry* 1987; 50:177–182; and Dombovy ML, Basford JR, Whisnut JP, Bergstralh EJ. Disability and use of rehabilitation services following stroke in Rochester Minnesota, 1975–1979. *Stroke* 1987; 18:830–836.

hemisphere lesions (61), but it also occurs in patients with unilateral hemisphere lesions (19,62). Difficulty in swallowing may occur in the oral preparatory phase or in the pharyngeal phase. There is usually delay in or absence of the swallowing reflex. Evaluation of a patient includes observation of the muscles of the lips, tongue, cheeks, and jaw and elevation of the larynx during swallowing. Poor muscle control results in trickling of saliva or liquids into the valleculae or inability to handle solids. There is poor protection of the airway, with high risk for aspiration.

Aspiration usually causes coughing, but some studies report a significant number of patients with silent aspiration (63). Careful bedside evaluation should be performed in all patients before oral feeding is started. Muscles of the lips and tongue should be tested, and the patient observed when taking sips of water and during eating. If the patient has a poor cough response, or if there is any question about the safety of swallowing, a videofluoroscopy using a modified barium swallow should be performed to assess swallowing and to detect aspiration. Numerous therapeutic interventions can improve swallowing. Techniques include stimulation to increase arousal, sitting the patient upright in a chair with head forward, close supervision of the patient, modifying the consistency of food to pureed solids and thickened liquids, and exercise. If swallowing is not safe, a nasogastric (NG) tube is indicated for enteral feedings. It should be noted that patients fed via a NG tube are still at risk for aspiration because of gastroesophageal reflux, especially when lying flat in bed. Dysphagia rapidly improves in patients with unilateral stroke, and by 1 month post-onset, only about 2% of patients still have difficulty (64). Patients with brainstem lesions or bilateral hemisphere lesions may progress more slowly and hence require gastrostomy.

Urinary Tract Infection

Urinary tract infections are common because of the neurogenic bladder and need for catheterization in the acute phase. Immediately post-onset, the sacral reflexes mediating micturition are depressed, and the bladder will overdistend and, if not drained, empty by overflow incontinence. Overdistention is best avoided in the acute stage by intermittent catheterization every 4 or 6 hours, depending on the rate of urine flow. The objective is to prevent the bladder from filling beyond about 500 ml and to stimulate physiological emptying. There is a modest risk of urinary tract infection with catheterization, but the risk is greatly increased if an indwelling Foley catheter is used. Intermittent catheterization is preferred, especially as the need for catheter drainage may be very brief, for a few days or less. As soon as spontaneous voiding begins, the intermittent catheterization can be reduced in frequency and may be stopped when postvoid residual bladder volumes are below 100 to 150 ml. The patient can be helped to achieve better bladder control by using a posture that increases intra-abdominal pressure, namely, sitting on a commode or toilet or standing to use a urinal.

In the postacute phase of stroke rehabilitation, the problem is not one of bladder overdistention but one of uninhibited bladder with incontinence. The patient has a sense of urgency to micturate and cannot postpone voiding. Bladder volumes and voided volumes are often rather small. At least some improvement in bladder function during the day can be achieved through deliberate training or pharmacologically, using anticholinergics such as oxybutynin chloride (Ditropan) to inhibit bladder contraction. Tricyclic antidepressants such as imipramine may also be useful because they exhibit both peripheral anticholinergic and alpha-adrenergic agonist activity, relaxing the bladder and increasing urethral pressure and sphincter tone. Bladder infections must be promptly recognized and treated. Management of incontinence can be quite difficult and usually involves one or all of the following: intermittent catheterization (self-catheterization whenever possible), medication, fluid restriction, and use of special diapers.

Malnutrition

A surprising number of patients admitted for stroke rehabilitation are malnourished, and in one report, 22% of patients showed nutritional deficiencies (65). Elderly patients may be admitted to hospital following a stroke already in a marginal nutritional status, and their condition is exacerbated by the low calorie intake during the initial acute care. If not closely monitored during postacute rehabilitation, a patient's nutritional status may be further compromised because of dysphagia, reliance on others for oral or tube feedings, lack of interest in food, depression, and problems with communication. The risk of malnutrition and/or dehydration should be recognized, and the intake of fluid, protein, and total calories should be monitored closely in all patients. Oral nutritional supplements may have to be prescribed, and if a patient continues to have inadequate intake, enteral tube feeding may be necessary.

Musculoskeletal Pain and Reflex Sympathetic Dystrophy

Pain in the shoulder and arm is a frequent complaint of patients undergoing postacute stroke rehabilitation. It tends to develop early, several weeks to 6 months post-onset, and may affect up to 72% of individuals, especially those with more severe hemiplegia (66).

Although some patients may have preexisting shoulder problems such as rotator cuff tendinitis, most hemiplegic patients with shoulder pain have varying combinations of glenohumeral subluxation, spasticity, and contracture. The role of subluxation in generating a painful shoulder has been debated, but it often precedes and then accompanies a painful shoulder. Subluxation of the glenohumeral joint is a clinical diagnosis that can be quantified by x-ray. It occurs in 30% to 50% of patients and is probably caused by the weight of the arm pulling down the humerus at a stage when the supraspinatus and deltoid muscles are flaccid and weak and by weakness of the scapular muscles, which allow the glenoid cavity to rotate facing downward (67). The shoulder is best managed in the early phases of rehabilitation through proper positioning of the arm and hand and avoidance of pulling on the arm during assisted transfers. Whenever the patient is sitting, the arm should be supported in an arm trough or lapboard. Therapy should be directed at facilitating return of active movement at the shoulder and should include techniques such as stretching to minimize spasticity, especially in shoulder depressors and internal rotators. When spasticity becomes severe and cannot be controlled with stretching, consideration may be given to reducing the tone in the subscapularis muscle with intramuscular phenol neurolysis or with botulinum toxin (68).

The syndrome of reflex sympathetic dystrophy (RSD) occurs quite commonly in the hemiplegic arm (shoulder–hand syndrome). A clinical diagnosis was made in 12.5% of cases reported by Davis et al. (69) and in 25% of patients studied with a bone scan (70). The clinical features usually develop between 1 and 4 months post-onset and, once established, run a rather predictable, protracted course. Pain dominates the clinical picture. The hand is swollen, and contractures develop at the shoulder, wrist, and hand, and these will persist as permanent sequelae unless the syndrome is treated early and aggressively. Treatment is most effective when begun early and consists of medical and physical measures. Some authorities have reported good results with prompt resolution of the clinical features with a short course of relatively high-dose prednisone, tapering and discontinuing the drug over several weeks. A series of stellate ganglion blocks is also advocated in acute cases. The blocks are repeated every few days. Analgesics or nonsteroidal anti-inflammatory drugs (NSAIDs) are necessary for pain control. The most important intervention is therapy to the limb to maintain range of motion of all joints, reduce swelling, and desensitize the limb through physiological stimulation such as massage and hot and cold contrast baths.

Venous Thromboembolism

Immediately post-onset, stroke patients are at high risk for DVT, the risk being greater when the leg is paralyzed. The risk of DVT may be as high as 75% in untreated hemiplegic patients. The thrombosis begins early, sometimes as soon as the second day and usually within the first week, although some new DVT events are recorded weeks after onset in the postacute rehabilitation phase.

All patients with stroke should receive DVT prophylaxis. Low-dose subcutaneous heparin is effective in reducing the incidence of DVT and is given in doses of 5,000 units bid or tid. Larger doses are appropriate for heavier patients. External pneumatic compression stockings are an alternative to heparin when the risk of bleeding is high, e.g., patients with peptic ulcer disease or intracerebral hemorrhage. Prophylaxis should continue well into the postacute phase and preferably until the patient is walking, although there are no studies to indicate the optimal duration of DVT prophylaxis (71).

The clinical signs of DVT are not reliable, being absent in about 50% of cases with proven DVT (71). However, the development of clinical signs suggesting DVT should always prompt laboratory investigation. The test of choice for diagnosis of DVT is venous duplex scanning, which has a high degree of sensitivity and specificity in patients with clinical features suggesting DVT. A positive scan is sufficient to justify treatment for DVT with anticoagulation.

The diagnosis of a new-onset DVT is a medical emergency, and immediate full-dose anticoagulation should be started with heparin infusion. Warfarin can be started on day 1, and once the prothrombin time is therapeutic, usually within 5 days, the heparin infusion can be stopped. It is advisable to keep a patient with an acute DVT on bed rest for at least 24 hours and until the heparin is therapeutic with a partial thromboplastin time between 55 and 75 seconds. In patients who are at risk of hemorrhage, e.g., those with hemorrhagic stroke, DVT may be treated by installing a vena cava filter to prevent pulmonary embolism. The reader is referred to recent reviews on venous thromboembolism in stroke (71,72).

REHABILITATION MANAGEMENT

Therapy for Hemiplegia

Early Phase

In the early poststroke phase, the hemiplegic limbs are often paralyzed and flaccid. At this stage, which may last for a few hours to days, the limbs and joints are prone to development of contractures. Through poor positioning, a stuporous patient may develop nerve pressure palsies. If the patient sits up or stands with a flaccid weak arm, the weight of the arm may stretch the capsule of the shoulder joint, leading to development of subluxation and painful shoulder.

Therapy during this early phase should consist of proper positioning of the patient in bed and support of the arm in a wheelchair trough when sitting. Traction on the arm should be avoided when the patient is moved in bed or is transferred to a wheelchair. All joints of the affected limbs should be passively moved through a full range of motion at least once daily to prevent contractures. Within hours or a few days, muscle tone returns to the paralyzed limbs, and spasticity progressively increases. Different approaches are used by therapists during this phase of motor recovery. The most widely accepted method, the neurodevelopmental technique (NDT) advocated by Bobath (73), stresses exercises that tend to normalize muscle tone and prevent excessive spasticity. This is achieved through the use of special reflex-inhibiting postures and movements. If spasticity becomes severe, tone can be reduced by slow, sustained stretching, which neurophysiologically reduces Ia afferent discharge rate as the muscle spindles accommodate to their elongation. Vibration of an antagonist muscle will also reduce tone in a spastic muscle through reciprocal inhibition, although the effect does not persist after the vibration stops.

Development of Motor Control

Movements in a hemiparetic limb show typical features of an upper motor neuron (UMN) lesion. Muscles show increased tone and are weak. Initiation and termination of muscle activation are prolonged, and there is a variable degree of cocontraction of agonists and antagonists, making movements slow and clumsy. Studies of recruitment patterns of individual motor units in affected muscles show slower firing rates and impersistent firing; i.e., there are more gaps in long motor unit firing trains (74–76).

Conventional methods of rehabilitation to regain motor control consist of stretching and strengthening, attempting to retrain weak muscles through reeducation. Use of sensory feedback is often stressed to facilitate muscle activation, e.g., stroking the overlying skin, sudden stretching of the muscle, and vibration of the muscle or its tendon. Some of these latter facilitation techniques are incorporated into well-defined systems of therapy. The system developed by Rood involves superficial cutaneous stimulation using stroking, brushing, tapping, and icing, or muscle stimulation with vibration, to evoke voluntary muscle activation. Brunnstrom emphasized the synergistic patterns of movement that develop during recovery from hemiplegia. She encouraged the development of flexor and extensor synergies during early recovery, hoping that synergistic activation of muscle would, with training, transition into voluntary activation. Proprioceptive neuromuscular facilitation (PNF) was developed by Kabat, Knott, and Voss and relies on quick stretching and manual resistance of muscle activation of the limbs in functional directions, which often are spiral and diagonal. The PNF methods are more useful when muscle weakness is not due to UMN lesions. As described above, the NDT (Bobath) approach aims to inhibit spasticity and synergies, using inhibitory postures and movements, and to facilitate normal automatic responses that are involved in voluntary movement. For a review of these methods, see Lorish et al. (77). As yet no clinical trial has shown that application of any of these approaches improves patient outcome over conventional therapy.

Therapy for the Hemiparetic Arm

As outlined above, early intervention is important to support the arm, preserve joint range of motion, and maintain shoulder integrity. If the arm becomes quite spastic, frequent slow stretching can help to reduce tone. Spasticity usually dominates in the flexors and may hold the wrist and fingers in a constant position of excessive flexion. A static wrist–hand orthosis is often helpful in maintaining these joints in a functional position.

The challenge of poor function in the hemiparetic hand has prompted therapists to develop new forms of therapy. One approach that has undergone considerable study is focused neuromuscular reeducation supplemented by electromyogram (EMG) biofeedback. Results of trials have been mixed, some showing benefit but others no better results than control therapy. One review of clinical trials of biofeedback did appear to show that biofeedback was an effective treatment method (78). The EMG biofeedback involves recording surface EMG from the test muscle and using auditory and/or visual display of the EMG signal as feedback to the patient on the ongoing activity status of the muscle. The EMG signal supplements conventional reeducation given by the therapist. Another form of therapy uses functional electrical stimulation (FES) to provide sensory–motor reeducation. The most promising technique for the hemiparetic arm appears to be FES when it is initiated by the EMG signal of the test muscle (79). These techniques may be useful in individual patients. They should be viewed as supplemental to all the other forms of therapy given to the patient.

When severe weakness of the hemiparetic arm persists, attention of the therapist and patient is directed toward functional retraining, using the unaffected limb to achieve independence in self-care skills, etc. Several recent reports indicate that some individuals who begin to use the unaffected limb early and ignore the paretic limb succumb to what is called "learned nonuse" of the weak limb. These individuals have latent potential for improved motor function but do not improve because of failure to use the limb (80–82). Forcing patients to use the weak limb by repeated encouragement or even restraint of the unaffected hand produces measurable improvement in function in the weak hand. Trials have shown significant increases in speed and strength of contraction. These studies appear to confirm the belief that improved function may occur with vigorous and intensive therapy, strong motivation, and good cognition, providing some selective hand movement is present.

Therapy for Mobility

An important rehabilitation goal for a hemiplegic patient is to achieve independent ambulation. In the early stages of recovery, or if recovery is limited to weak synergy patterns only, walking will not be possible because of poor upright trunk control, inability to achieve single-limb support during stance, and inability to advance the leg during swing phase. Patients should receive initial therapy to develop gross trunk control and training in pregait activities such as posture, balance, and weight transfer to the hemiparetic leg. As recovery progresses, patients develop better gross motor skills and trunk balance and greater strength in the leg. At Brunnstrom stage 3 recovery (see above), characterized by strong synergies and spasticity but no selective muscle activation, most patients will walk, although many will require an ankle–foot orthrosis (AFO) and cane and will walk slowly. Ambulation improves as motor recovery provides for selective phasic activation of muscles during the gait cycle. For details on evaluation of hemiplegic gait and therapeutic interventions, see recent reviews (83,84).

There have been recent reports of the benefit of intensive gait training in hemiplegic patients who received gait training on a treadmill with body weight supported with a harness (85,86). It was found that with treadmill training, some nonambulatory hemiplegic patients learned to walk, and those who were already walking significantly increased their gait speed.

Communication Therapy

Language therapy is based on the detailed evaluation of the patient's cognitive and linguistic capabilities and deficits. Generally, speech pathologists attempt to improve communicative ability by circumventing or deblocking the language deficit or by helping the patient to compensate. In the early stages of rehabilitation it is important for the therapist to help the patient establish a reliable means for basic yes/no communication. The therapist then progresses to specific techniques based on the patient's deficits. Even though spontaneous recovery is responsible for early improvement, speech therapy plays an extremely important role in minimizing patient isolation and encouraging the patient to actively engage in the program. Although communication may be difficult, simple childish phrases or tasks should be avoided, as patients perceive them as infantile and may withdraw. Specific techniques have been described for improving comprehension, word or phoneme retrieval and gestures to supplement verbal communication. There have been reports of patients showing continued slow recovery between 6 and 12 months and beyond. It is difficult to predict which patients will show late recovery, but it seems quite justified to continue speech therapy while patients are showing measurable gains in communication.

Disorders of Cognition and Behavior

Cerebrovascular lesions produce a wide spectrum of cognitive and behavioral clinical features. At the extreme end is dementia, which may preclude functional recovery and render efforts at rehabilitation futile. Less severe impairments of higher-level function may be observed frequently in patients undergoing rehabilitation, e.g., poor attention, decreased memory, ignoring the food on one side of a plate, or bumping into one side of a doorway. Other more subtle changes may not be apparent until the patient returns home, and family members notice mild behavioral changes such as decreased judgment or insight. All of these conditions affect performance of functional activities, sometimes profoundly. Therefore, the professional should be able to recognize significant cognitive and behavioral disorders and anticipate how therapeutic strategies may be employed to ameliorate them.

Lesion and Cognition/Behavior

In general, the absolute size of a brain lesion determines the severity of behavioral and psychological changes poststroke. For example, large cortical lesions produce more psychological changes than smaller subcortical lesions. Behavioral and organic mental changes occur most often in association with frontal lesions and less often with parietal, temporal, or occipital lesions. Patients with multiple lesions, especially when bilateral, are more likely to show features of dementia (87). Numerous studies have shown that in patients with a history of stroke, those with more extensive white matter changes are at higher risk for dementia.

It has been reported that patients with left hemisphere lesions, especially when they are anterior, are more likely to be depressed, although this has been disputed. Patients with right hemisphere lesions are more likely to be unduly cheerful. Emotional lability occurs in up to 20% of patients poststroke, and is more common in patients with right hemisphere lesions. It is a typical feature of the syndrome of pseudobulbar palsy. The clinical features of emotional lability tend to improve with time and often respond to tricyclic antidepressants (88,89).

Unilateral Neglect

Many patients with a nondominant parietal lobe lesion have neglect and ignore the opposite side of the body or hemispace. Inattention also occurs with impaired sensation or homonymous hemianopia. Patients with persistent inattention perform functional tasks less well, and various therapies have been tried to remediate the inattention. Therapy is directed at retraining, with repetitive exercises or use of compensatory techniques, to teach new methods of task completion. These therapies include training patients to visually scan from side to side, offering stimuli to draw attention to the left hemispace, and environmental adaptations. An example of environmental adaptation is orientation of the patient's neglected hemispace toward the side most frequently stimulated, e.g., entrance to the room. Specific therapy is usually given to remediate visual neglect and/or hemianopia, which almost always includes visual scanning. Another strategy for improving vision in patients with complete hemianopia is the use of Fresnel prisms applied to eye glasses. These devices shift images in the affected hemivisual field toward the center of the retina and hence into the field of view (90).

Depression

Depression is very common following stroke and, depending on diagnostic criteria, has been reported in up to 50% of patients (91,92). Although there is some dispute about lesion location and depression, there is apparently a relationship between left frontal lesions and major depression (93), though this relationship may operate only in the early phase poststroke. It has been hypothesized that the depression in these cases may be induced by catecholamine depletion through lesion-induced damage to the frontal noradrenergic, dopaminergic, and serotonergic projections. Many authors have pointed out the important psychological factors that can lead to depression following stroke. These include psychological responses to the physical and personal losses caused by the stroke and the state of helplessness and loss of control that often accompanies severe disability.

The diagnosis of poststroke depression is often difficult because some of the diagnostic criteria used may simply reflect sequelae of the stroke, e.g., vegetative symptoms such as sleep disturbance, fatigue, and psychomotor retardation. Of particular importance in the diagnosis is depressed mood and loss of interest in participating in daily activities such as the rehabilitation program (94).

Persisting depression correlates with delayed recovery and poorer ultimate outcome. Active treatment should be considered for all patients with significant clinical depression. There is general acceptance of the importance of psychosocial intervention by all professional staff, with individual psychotherapy supplemented by positive reinforcement of the progress being made in rehabilitation. Many patients respond to drug therapy. Antidepressants improve depression in a majority of patients, desipramine or the SSRI group being favored because of fewer side effects. Some practitioners prescribe methylphenidate (Ritalin [CibaGeneva, Summit, New Jersey]) with the antidepressant, as this drug will often bring about an abrupt improvement in arousal and motivation to participate in the therapeutic program.

Sexuality

It has been well documented that the majority of elderly persons continue to enjoy active and satisfying sexual relationships. By contrast, however, there is considerable sexual dysfunction following stroke (95). Before-and-after studies have reported a marked decline in sexual activity, involving both men and women. There is a marked reduction in libido with a corresponding decrease in coital frequency. In one study (96), male patients reported that before the stroke 95% had erections, but only 38% reported normal erections poststroke, and 58% believed that after the stroke they had a sexual problem. These and most other poststroke sexual problems are related to emotional factors, such as fear, anxiety, or guilt regarding the stroke itself. Patients have a loss of self esteem, and they may fear rejection or abandonment by their partner. They are, therefore, reluctant to make emotional demands. Health care professionals should be sensitive to relationship issues and be prepared to ask questions about intimacy, sexual attitudes, needs, and behavior. Most will require supportive psychotherapy to provide them with better mechanisms to cope with the sequelae of the stroke.

Psychosocial Aspects

The psychological, social, and family aspects of stroke rehabilitation are extremely important. The abrupt change in the life situation of the stroke survivor impacts all phases of care. The patient fears loss of independence, and the disabilities reduce self-esteem and self-worth. Patients are often concerned about the capacity of their spouse to sustain them following discharge, and whether they will both be able to make the appropriate role adjustments. The response of some patients to the stroke may be catastrophic with subsequent maladaptive behavior. All members of the rehabilitation team should contribute to a positive and supportive milieu to promote appropriate coping strategies on the part of the patient and to assist the patient and family prepare for discharge and reintegration into the home and community. This will involve early discussions around planning for discharge, education about stroke and its consequences, and detailed discussions around potential problems and opportunities that patient and family will encounter in the future.

Late Rehabilitation Issues

There are important issues that make postdischarge follow-up mandatory. From a medical perspective the majority of patients have ongoing medical problems requiring monitoring and therapeutic intervention such as hypertension, heart disease, diabetes, etc. Appropriate management will reduce the risk of stroke recurrence and prolong survival. A seizure disorder develops in about 8% of stroke survivors, and this requires conventional monitoring and treatment.

There are also rehabilitation issues that are ongoing. The rehabilitation program does not finish when the patient leaves the hospital, and almost all patients benefit from continued therapy. There are many reports describing continued improvement over many months postdischarge, and many patients require formal therapy to achieve that continued progress. The physician overseeing the rehabilitation program should regularly reevaluate the patient to document physical progress and define ongoing therapeutic goals. Specific problems that may become prominent following discharge from hospital, during the outpatient therapy phase of care, include the following: psychological maladjustment and depression, reduced sexuality, poor role adjustment in the home and family, equipment needs, transportation and driving, and secondary physical problems such as excessive spasticity in the arm, reflex sympathetic dystrophy, changing pattern of ambulation, etc. Management of spasticity requires careful evaluation, goal setting, and selection of appropriate therapies (97). Dantrolene (Proctor & Gamble Pharmaceuticals, Cincinnati, Ohio) has been used for many years for pharmacologic treatment of hemiplegic spasticity caused by stroke (98), but early use of dantrolene did not improve function in a recent double-blind study (99). A small number of patients are bothered by spontaneous spasms occurring mostly at night in bed. These can usually be adequately controlled by small doses of diazepam before bedtime. For localized spasticity, such as forearm flexors of the calf muscles, intramuscular neurolysis with phenol or chemodenervation with intramuscular botulinum toxin injections can be very effective.

For all of these reasons, the rehabilitation physician should continue to monitor the progress of the patient as long as necessary to be satisfied that the patient has reached a stable, optimal level of function.

REFERENCES

1. Bonita R. Epidemiology of stroke. *Lancet* 1992; 339:342–344.
2. Kannel WB, Dawber TR, Sorlie P, Wolf PA. Components of blood pressure and risk of atherothrombotic brain infarction: The Framingham Study. *Stroke* 1976; 7:327–331.
3. Wolf PA, Kannel WB, Venter J. Current status of risk factors for stroke. *Neurol Clin* 1983; 1:317–343.
4. Wolf PA, Dawber TR, Thomas HE Jr, Kannel WB. Epidemiologic assessment of chronic atrial fibrillation and risk of stroke: The Framingham Study. *Neurology* 1978; 23:973–977.
5. Shinton R, Beevers G. Meta-analysis of relation between cigarette smoking and stroke. *Br Med J* 1989; 298:789–794.
6. Feinberg WM, Albers GW, Barnett HJM, et al. Guidelines for the management of transient ischemic attacks. *Stroke* 1994; 25:1320–1335.
7. North American Symptomatic Carotid Endarterectomy Trial Collaborators. Beneficial effect of carotid endarterectomy in symptomatic patients with high-grade carotid stenosis. *N Engl J Med* 1991; 325: 445–453.
8. Barnett HJM, Haines SJ. Carotid endarterectomy for asymptomatic carotid stenosis. *N Engl J Med* 1993; 328:276–279.
9. Sacco RL. Risk factors and outcomes for ischemic stroke. *Neurology* 1995; 45(Suppl 1):S10–S14.
10. Viitanen M, Eriksson S, Asplund K. Risk of recurrent stroke, myocardial infarction and epilepsy. *Eur Neurol* 1988; 28:227–231.
11. Leonberg SC, Elliott FA. Prevention of recurrent stroke. *Stroke* 1981; 12:731–735.
12. Mohr JP, Caplan LR, Melski JW, et al. The Harvard cooperative stroke registry; a prospective study. *Neurology* 1978; 28:754–762.
13. Steinberg GK, Fabrikant JI, Marks MP, Levy RP, Frankel KA, Phillips MH, Shuer LM, Silverberg GD. Stereotactic heavy-charged-particle Bragg-Peak radiation for intracranial arteriovenous malformations. *N Engl J Med* 1990; 323:96–101.
14. Ashwal S, Schneider S. Neurologic complications of vasculitic disorders of childhood, In: Swaiman KF, ed. *Pediatric neurology: principles and practice, 2nd ed.* St Louis: CV Mosby, 1994.
15. The National Institute of Neurological Disorders and Stroke rt-PA Stroke Study Group. Tissue plasminogen activator for acute ischemic stroke. *N Engl J Med* 1995; 333:1581–1587.
16. Dobkin BH. *Neurologic rehabilitation.* Philadelphia: FA Davis, 1966.
17. Stein DG, Brailowsky S, Will B. *Brain repair.* New York: Oxford University Press, 1995.
18. Roth EJ. Medical complications encountered in stroke rehabilitation. *Phys Med Rehab Clin North Am* 1991; 2(3):563–578.
19. Horner J, Massey EW, Riski JE, Lathrop DL, Chase KN. Aspiration following stroke: clinical correlates and outcomes. *Neurology* 1988; 38:1359–1362.
20. Gresham GE, Duncan PW, Stason WB, et al. *Post-Stroke Rehabilitation. Clinical Practice Guideline, No 16.* Rockville, MD: US Department of Health and Human Services, Public Health Service, Agency for Health Care Policy and Research. AHCPR Publication No. 95-0662, May, 1995.
21. Foulkes MA, Wolf PA, Price TR, Mohr JP, Hier DB. The Stroke Data Bank: design, methods and baseline characteristics. *Stroke* 1988; 19: 547–554.
22. Twitchell TE. The restoration of motor function following hemiplegia in man. *Brain* 1951; 74:443–480.
23. Bard G, Hirshberg CG. Recovery of voluntary motion in upper extremity following hemiplegia. *Arch Phys Med Rehabil* 1965; 46:567–572.
24. Gowland C. Management of hemiplegic upper limb. In: Brandstater ME, Basmajian J, eds. *Stroke rehabilitation.* Baltimore: Williams & Wilkins, 1987; 217–245.
25. Wade DT, Langton Hewer R, Wood VA, Skilbeck CE, Ismail HM. The hemiplegic arm after stroke: measurement and recovery. *J Neurol Neurosurg Psychiatry* 1983; 46:521–524.
26. Kelly-Hayes M, Wolf PA, Kase CS, Gresham GE, Kannel WB, D'Agostino RB. Time course of functional recovery after stroke: the Framingham Study. *J Neurol Rehabil* 1989; 3:65–70.
27. Wade DT, Langton Hewer R, David RM, Enderby PM. Aphasia after stroke: Natural history and associated deficits. *J Neurol Neurosurg Psychiatry* 1986; 49:11–16.
28. Skilbeck CE, Wade DT, Langton Hewer R, Wood VA. Recovery after stroke. *J Neurol Neurosurg Psychiatry* 1983; 46:5–8.
29. Brandstater ME. Basic aspects of impairment evaluation in stroke patients. In: Chino N, Melvin JL, eds. *Functional evaluation of stroke patients.* New York: Springer-Verlag, 1996; 9–18.
30. Strub R, Black F. *The Mental Status Examination in Neurology, 2nd ed.* Philadelphia: FA Davis, 1995.
31. Folstein MF, Folstein SF, McHugh PR. Mini-Mental State: a practical method for grading the cognitive state for the clinician. *J Psychiatr Res* 1975; 12:189–198.
32. Goodglass H, Kaplan E. *The assessment of aphasia and related disorders.* Philadelphia: Lea & Febiger, 1983.
33. Kertesz A. *Western Aphasia Battery.* New York: Grune & Stratton, 1982.
34. Sarno MT. *The Functional Communication Profile: Manual of directions. Rehabilitation monograph 42.* New York: Institute of Rehabilitation Medicine, 1969.
35. Brunnstrom S. *Movement therapy in hemiplegia: a neurophysiological approach.* New York: Harper & Row, 1970.
36. Brandstater ME, deBruin H, Gowland C, Clark B. Hemiplegic gait: analysis of temporal variables. *Arch Phys Med Rehabil* 1983; 64: 583–587.
37. Bohannon RW. Is the measurement of muscle strength appropriate in patients with brain lesions? *Phys Ther* 1989; 69:225–230.
38. Bohannon RW. Correlation of lower limb strengths and other variables with standing performance in stroke patients. *Physiother Can* 1989; 41:198–202.
39. Fugl-Meyer AR, Jaasko L, Leyman I, Olsson S, Steglind S. The post-stroke hemiplegic patient. I: A method for evaluation of physical performance. *Scand J Rehab Med* 1975; 7:13–31.
40. Bohannon RW, Smith MB. Interrater reliability of a modified Ashworth scale of muscle spasticity. *Phys Ther* 1987; 67:206–207.
41. Gresham GE. Past achievements and new directions in stroke outcome research. *Stroke* 1990; 21(Suppl II):II-1–II-2.
42. Jongbloed L. Problems of methodologic heterogeneity in studies predicting disability after stroke. *Stroke* 1990; 21(Suppl II):II-32–II-34.
43. World Health Organization (WHO). Recommendations on stroke prevention, diagnosis, and therapy: report of WHO Taskforce on Stroke and Other Cerebral Vascular Disorders. *Stroke* 1989; 20:1407–1431.
44. Brandstater ME. Prognostication in stroke rehabilitation. In: Chino N,

Melvin JL eds. *Functional evaluation of stroke patients.* New York: Springer-Verlag, 1996; 93–102.

45. Broderick JP, Phillips SJ, Whisnant JP, O'Fallon WM, Bergstralh EJ. Incidence rates of stroke in the eighties: the end of the decline in stroke. *Stroke* 1989; 20:577–582.
46. Sacco RL, Wolf PA, Kannel WB, MacNamara PM. Survival and recurrence following stroke: The Framingham Study. *Stroke* 1982; 13: 290–295.
47. Skilbeck CE, Wade DT, Langton Hewer R, Wood VA. Recovery after stroke. *J Neurol Neurosurg Psychiatry* 1983; 46:5–8.
48. Wade DT, Wood VA, Langton Hewer R. Recovery after stroke—the first 3 months. *J Neurol Neurosurg Psychiatry* 1985; 48:7–13.
49. Feigenson JS, McDowell FH, Meese P, McCarthy ML, Greenberg SD. Factors influencing outcome and length of stay in a stroke rehabilitation unit Part 1. *Stroke* 1977; 8:651–656.
50. Gresham GE, Fitzpatrick TE, Wolf PA, MacNamara PM, Kannel WB, Dawber TR. Residual disability in survivors of stroke: The Framingham Study. *N Engl J Med* 1975; 293:954–956.
51. Wade DT, Langton Hewer R. Functional abilities after stroke: measurement, natural history and prognosis. *J Neurol Neurosurg Psychiatry* 1987; 50:177–182.
52. Dombovy ML, Basford JR, Whisnut JP, Bergstralh EJ. Disability and use of rehabilitation services following stroke in Rochester Minnesota, 1975–1979. *Stroke* 1987; 18:830–836.
53. Wade DT, Langton Hewer R, Wood VA. Stroke: the influence of age on the outcome. *Age Ageing* 1984; 13:357–362.
54. Wade DT, Skilbeck CE, Langton Hewer R. Predicting Barthel ADL Score at 6 months after an acute stroke. *Arch Phys Med Rehabil* 1983; 64:24–28.
55. Evans RL, Bishop DS, Matlock AL, Stranahan S, Smith CG, Halar EM. Family interaction and treatment adherence after stroke. *Arch Phys Med Rehabil* 1987; 68:513–517.
56. Hertzer NR, Young JR, Beven EG, et al. Coronary angiography in 506 patients with extracranial cerebrovascular disease. *Arch Intern Med* 1985; 145:849–852.
57. Roth EJ, Mueller K, Green D. Stroke rehabilitation outcome: impact of coronary artery disease. *Stroke* 1988; 19:42–47.
58. Roth EJ. Heart disease in patients with stroke. Part II: impact and implications for rehabilitation. *Arch Phys Med Rehabil* 1994; 75: 94–101.
59. Fletcher BJ, Dunbar S, Coleman J, Jann B, Fletcher GF. Cardiac precautions for nonacute inpatient settings. *Am J Phys Med Rehabil* 1993; 72:140–143.
60. Kalra L, Yu G, Wilson K, Roots P. Medical complications during stroke rehabilitation. *Stroke* 1995; 26:990–994.
61. Horner J, Massey EW, Brazer SR. Aspiration in bilateral stroke patients. *Neurology* 1990; 40:1686–1688.
62. Teasell RW, Bach D, MacRae M. Prevalence and recovery of aspiration post-stroke: a retrospective analysis. *Dysphagia* 1994; 9:35–39.
63. Horner J, Massey EW. Silent aspiration following stroke. *Neurology* 1988; 38:317–319.
64. Blauer D. The natural history and functional consequences of dysphagia after hemispheric stroke. *J Neurol Neurosurg Psychiatry* 1989; 52: 236–241.
65. Axelsson K, Asplund K, Norberg A, Alafuzoff I. Nutritional status in patients with acute stroke. *Acta Med Scand* 1988; 224:217–224.
66. Van Onwenaller C, LaPlace PM, Chartraine A. Painful shoulder in hemiplegia. *Arch Phys Med Rehabil* 1985; 67:23–26.
67. Basmajian JV. *Muscles alive: their function revealed by electromyography, 4th ed.* Baltimore: Williams & Wilkins, 1978.
68. Hecht JS. Subscapular nerve block in the painful hemiplegic shoulder. *Arch Phys Med Rehabil* 1992; 73:1036–1039.
69. Davis SW, Petrillo CR, Eichberg RD, Chu DS. Shoulder–hand syndrome in a hemiplegic population: 5-year retrospective study. *Arch Phys Med Rehabil* 1977; 58:353–356.
70. Tepperman PS, Greyson ND, Hilbert L, Jiminez J, Williams JI. Reflex sympathetic dystrophy in hemiplegia. *Arch Phys Med Rehabil* 1984; 65:442–447.
71. Brandstater ME, Siebens H, Roth EJ. Venous thromboembolism in stroke: Part I. Literature review and implications for clinical practice. *Arch Phys Med Rehabil* 1992; 73:S379–S391.
72. Harvey RL, Green D. Deep venous thrombosis and pulmonary embolism in stroke. *Top Stroke Rehabil* 1996; 3(1):54–70.
73. Bobath B. *Adult hemiplegia: evaluation and treatment.* London: Heinemann, 1976.
74. Freund HJ, Hefter H, Homberg V. Motor unit activity in motor disorders. In: Shahani B, ed. *Electromyography in CNS disorders: Central EMG.* Boston: Butterworths, 1984; 29–44.
75. Kraft GH, Fitts SS, Hammond MC, et al. Motor unit activity in forearm muscles following cerebral vascular accident. *Arch Phys Med Rehabil* 1986; 67:673–674.
76. Hammond MC, Kraft GH, Fitts SS. Recruitment and termination of EMG activity in the hemiparetic forearm. *Arch Phys Med Rehabil* 1988; 69:106–110.
77. Lorish TR, Sandin KJ, Roth EJ, Noll SF. Stroke rehabilitation: 3, rehabilitation evaluation and management. *Arch Phys Med Rehabil* 1994; 75:S47–S51.
78. Schleenbaker RE, Mainous AG III. Electromyographic biofeedback for neuromuscular reeducation in the hemiplegic stroke patient: a meta-analysis. *Arch Phys Med Rehabil* 1993; 74:1301–1304.
79. Kraft GH, Fitts SS, Hammond MC. Techniques to improve function of the arm and hand in chronic hemiplegia. *Arch Phys Med Rehabil* 1992; 73:220–227.
80. Wolf SL, Lecraw DE, Barton LA, Jann FF. Forced use of hemiplegic upper extremities to reverse the effect of learned nonuse among chronic stroke and head injured patients. *Exp Neurol* 1989; 104:125–132.
81. Taub E, Miller NE, Novack TA, et al. A technique for improving chronic motor deficit after stroke. *Arch Phys Med Rehabil* 1993; 74: 347–354
82. Taub E, Wolf SL. Constraint induced movement techniques to facilitate upper extremity use in stroke patients. *Top Stroke Rehabil* 1997; 3(4): 38–61.
83. Perry J, Montgomery J. Gait of the stroke patient and orthotic indications. In: Brandstater ME, Basmajian JV, eds. *Stroke rehabilitation.* Baltimore: Williams & Wilkins, 1987.
84. Perry J. *Gait analysis: normal and pathological function.* Thorofare, NJ: Slack, 1992.
85. Hesse S, Bertelt C, Jahnke M, et al. Treadmill training with partial body weight support compared to physiotherapy in nonambulatory hemiparetic patients. *Stroke* 1995; 26:976–981.
86. Hesse S, Bertelt C, Schaffrin A, et al. Restoration of gait in nonambulatory hemiparetic patients by treadmill training with partial body weight support. *Arch Phys Med Rehabil* 1994; 75:1087–1093.
87. Adams RD, Victor M. *Principles of neurology, 4th ed.* New York: McGraw-Hill, 338, 1989.
88. Seliger G, Hornstein A, Flax J, et al. Fluoxetine improves emotional incontinence. *Brain Inj* 1991; 5:1–4.
89. Robinson RG, Parikh RM, Lipsey JR, Starkstein SE, Price TR. Pathological laughing and crying following stroke: validation of a measurement scale and a double-blind study. *Am J Psychiatry* 1993; 150: 286–293.
90. Rossi P, Kheyfets S, Reding M. Fresnel prisms improve visual perception in stroke patients with homonymous hemianopia or unilateral visual neglect. *Neurology* 1990; 40:1597–1599.
91. Robinson RG, Starr LB, Kubos K. A two-year longitudinal study of post-stroke mood disorders: findings during the initial evaluation. *Stroke* 1983; 14:736–741.
92. Coll P, Erickson RJ. Mood disorders associated with stroke. *Phys Med Rehabil State Art Rev* 1989; 3:619–628.
93. Robinson RG, Szetela B. Mood change following left hemisphere brain injury. *Ann Neurol* 1981; 9:447–53.
94. Lazarus LW, Moberg PJ, Langsley PR, Lingam VR. Methylphenidate and nortiptyline in the treatment of poststroke depression: a retrospective comparision. *Arch Phys Med Rehabil* 1994; 75:403–406.
95. Monga TN. Sexuality post stroke. *Phys Med Rehab: State Art Rev* 1993; 7:225–236.
96. Monga TN, Lawson JS, Inglis J. Sexual dysfunction in stroke patients. *Arch Phys Med Rehabil* 1986; 67:19–22.
97. O'Brien CF, Seeberger LC, Smith DB. Spasticity after stroke. Epidemiology and optimal treatment. *Drugs Aging* 1996; 9:332–340.
98. Chyatte SB, Bridsong JH, Bergman BA. the effects of dantrolene sodium on spasticity and motor performance in hemiplegia. *South Med* 1971; 64:180–185.
99. Katrak PH, Cole AMD, Poulos CM, McCauley JCK. Objective assessment of spasticity, strength, and function with early exhibition of dantrolene sodium after cerebrovascular accident: a randomized double-blind study. *Arch Phys Med Rehabil* 1992; 73:4–9.

Rehabilitation Medicine: Principles and Practice, Third Edition,
edited by Joel A. DeLisa and Bruce M. Gans.
Lippincott–Raven Publishers, Philadelphia © 1998.

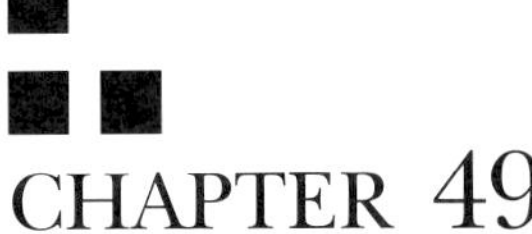

CHAPTER 49

Rehabilitation of the Patient with Traumatic Brain Injury

John Whyte, Tessa Hart, Andrea Laborde, and Mitchell Rosenthal

NATURE OF TRAUMATIC BRAIN INJURY

Traumatic brain injury (TBI) is a major health problem in the United States and other countries where vehicular accidents, sporting accidents, and interpersonal violence are commonplace. The systematic study of the residual effects of TBI can be traced to World War II and the work of Alexander Luria, Kurt Goldstein, and others (1,2). In this early work, much was learned about the deficits following penetrating injuries to the brain in soldiers with gunshot wounds. The pattern of residual dysfunction often corresponded to a focal lesion caused by the bullet passing through the brain. These focal deficits were similar to those observed in strokes.

The vast majority of peacetime TBIs seen in hospitals are classified as closed head injuries, wherein the skull is not actually penetrated. The nature of injury sustained in vehicular accidents (e.g., blunt impact, acceleration–deceleration) often results in multifocal lesions and diffuse brain damage with a variety of physical, cognitive, and neurobehavioral impairments that are unique to each person and pose a great challenge for the rehabilitation team and the patient's family.

Traumatic brain injury affects all age groups. However, additional complex issues are posed by children with TBI because the injury interacts with the processes of biological, psychological, and social development. The special problems of children with TBI are not treated in detail here, but there are excellent sources for additional information on this topic (e.g., 3–5).

J. Whyte: Department of Physical Medicine and Rehabilitation, Temple University School of Medicine, Philadelphia, Pennsylvania 19140; and Moss Rehabilitation Research Institute, MossRehab, Philadelphia, Pennsylvania 19141.

T. Hart: Drucker Brain Injury Center, Moss Rehabilitation Hospital, Philadelphia, Pennsylvania 19141.

A. Laborde: Department of Physical Medicine and Rehabilitation, Temple University School of Medicine, Philadelphia, Pennsylvania 19140; and Drucker Brain Injury Center, Moss Rehabilitation Research Institute, Philadelphia, Pennsylvania 19141.

M. Rosenthal: Department of Physical Medicine and Rehabilitation, Wayne State University, Rehabilitation Institute of Michigan, Detroit, Michigan 48201.

The Range of Outcomes: Death to Complete Recovery

The pattern and severity of injury and resultant outcome also are highly variable. In some injuries, commonly referred to as mild, the person may not suffer any loss of consciousness or only a very brief period of altered consciousness. In these cases, the person may be seen in a hospital emergency room, held for observation, and released several hours later. In the absence of any further medical complications, the person may return to normal activities within a few days. In other mild injuries, a posttraumatic syndrome consisting of headaches, vertigo, fatigability, memory disturbance, and emotional irritability may follow and cause a disruption of vocational activity up to 3 months postinjury (6). In a small percentage of cases, physical and psychosocial symptomatology may be reported for months and years after injury (7). Mild brain injuries constitute the vast majority of TBIs within the United States—approximately 290,000 hospital admissions per year (8).

Most rehabilitation efforts are focused on those with severe TBI (i.e., unconsciousness for 6 hours or longer). Approximately 50,000 to 75,000 people per year in the United States suffer severe TBI (9). Within this broad category, a variety of outcomes may be observed. Approximately one-third to one-half of those with severe brain injuries die (10–13). In the survivors, global outcome usually is defined by the categories of the Glasgow Outcome Scale (GOS) (14). Table 49-1 depicts the percentage of survivors in these categories at various time periods after injury. Even those who achieve a "good recovery" status according to the GOS, however, may have significant psychosocial impairments that preclude a return to premorbid level of function.

TABLE 49-1. *Outcome in survivors of severe head injury*

Outcome	3 Months (*n* = 534)	6 Months (*n* = 515)	12 Months (*n* = 376)
Vegetative state	7%	5%	3%
Severe disability	29%	19%	16%
Moderate disability	33%	34%	31%
Good recovery	31%	42%	50%
Moderate–good (combined)	64%	76%	81%

n, number of patients.

From Jennett B, Teasdale G. *Management of head injuries.* Philadelphia: FA Davis, 1981; 309

Measures of Injury Severity

Both *depth* and *duration* of coma have been considered to be indices of the severity of TBI. Clinical assessment of coma was made more precise and objective with the advent of the Glasgow Coma Scale (GCS) (15), a quantitative measure of the depth of unconsciousness (Table 49-2). Coma is defined as not opening the eyes, not obeying commands, and not uttering understandable words. A GCS score of 8 or less is operationally defined as a comatose state (16).

Duration of coma is often defined as the time to follow commands. Severe brain injury may be defined as coma lasting 6 hours or longer. Both duration of coma and initial GCS score have been reported to predict neurobehavioral outcome from TBI (17,18), varying with the outcome measures selected and the time since injury. Stein and Spettell (19) showed that when the GCS was modified slightly to include complications such as intracranial lesions, its predictive power was improved.

Russell was the first to suggest the duration of *posttraumatic amnesia* (PTA) as a measure of injury severity (20). During PTA, patients are out of coma but remain disoriented and amnesic for day-to-day events. Duration of PTA is measured from the onset of TBI to the resumption of ongoing memory; the duration of coma, if any, is thus included. Researchers have used PTA as an index of injury severity and an important predictor of outcome (21,22). Unfortunately, retrospective measurement of PTA from medical records often is unreliable. The Galveston Orientation and Amnesia Test (GOAT; Table 49-3) has provided an objective, reliable way of measuring PTA prospectively (23). A children's version has also been developed and validated (24,25). The GOAT has been criticized on the grounds that although it assesses orientation, it fails to capture the amnesia characteristic of PTA. A recent alternative, the Westmead PTA Scale, includes a measure of day-to-day memory as well as standard orientation questions (26). Duration of PTA, assessed prospectively with the Westmead, is a strong predictor of long-term outcome variables such as employment status (27). The predictive power of PTA duration is better for patients whose brain damage is caused primarily by diffuse axonal injury than for those with primarily contusions or other focal brain injury (28).

TABLE 49-2. *Glasgow Coma Scale*

Examiner's test	Patient's response	Assigned score
Eye opening		
Spontaneous	Opens eyes on own	4
Speech	Opens eyes when asked in a loud voice	3
Pain	Opens eyes when pinched	2
Pain	Does not open eyes	1
Best motor response		
Commands	Follows simple commands	6
Pain	Pulls examiner's hands away when pinched	5
Pain	Pulls a part of the body away when pinched	4
Pain	Flexes body inappropriately when pinched (decorticate posturing)	3
Pain	Body becomes rigid in an extended position when pinched (decerebrate posturing)	2
Pain	Has no motor response to pinch	1
Verbal response (talking)		
Speech	Carries on a conversation correctly and tells examiner where he or she is, month and year	5
Speech	Seems confused or disoriented	4
Speech	Talks so examiner can understand victim but makes no sense	3
Speech	Makes sounds that examiner cannot understand	2
Speech	Makes no noise	1

From Teasdale G, Jennett B. Assessment of coma and impaired consciousness. *Lancet* 1974; 2:81.

TABLE 49-3. *The Galveston Orientation and Amnesia Test*

Name ______	Date of test ______
Age ______ Sex M F	Day of the week S M T W T F S
Date of birth ______	Time A.M. P.M.
Diagnosis ______	Date of injury ______

	Error Points
1. What is your name? (2)	______
When were you born? (4)	______
Where do you live? (4)	______
2. Where are you now? (5) (City)	______
Hospital (5) (unnecessary to state name of hospital)	______
3. On what date were you admitted to this hospital? (5)	______
How did you get here? (5)	______
4. What is the first event you can remember after the injury? (5)	______
Can you describe in detail (e.g., date, time, companions) the first event you can recall after the injury? (5)	______
5. Can you describe the last event you recall before the accident? (5)	______
Can you describe in detail (e.g., date, time, companions) the last event you can recall before the injury? (5)	______
6. What time is it now? (1 for each half hour removed from current time to a maximum of 5 points)	______
7. What day of the week is it? (1 for each day removed from the correct one)	______
8. What day of the month is it? (1 for each day removed from the correct one to a maximum of 5 points)	______
9. What is the month? (5 for each month removed from the correct one to a maximum of 15 points)	______
10. What is the year? (10 for each year removed from the correct one to a maximum of 30 points)	______
Total error points	______
Total score (100 minus total error points)	______

EPIDEMIOLOGY OF TRAUMATIC BRAIN INJURY

The incidence of TBI requiring hospitalization is estimated to be approximately 200 to 225/100,000 population in the United States (9). In all, approximately 500,000 new cases of TBI occur annually in the United States (29). Precise measures of prevalence within the population are unknown; however, within the past 15 years, epidemiologic studies have shown great uniformity in the yearly incidence of TBI. Approximately 20/100,000, or 44,000 people per year, survive TBI with moderate to severe physical or neurobehavioral sequelae (30).

The age distribution is bimodal, with young adults (aged 15 to 24 years, 200 to 225/100,000) and the elderly (aged 65 to 75 years, 200/100,000) showing the highest incidence. The elderly population has the highest level of mortality (31). Elderly patients have a much slower and less certain recovery process, compared with the young adult population (32).

In all studies of TBI, men outnumber women by at least two to one. Further, male TBI mortalities are three to four times greater than those in the female population (9). Several studies have noted that TBI tends to occur with slightly greater frequency among minority groups (33).

About one-half of all TBI are transportation related. The other one-half are caused by falls, assaults, and other causes (9). With rising age, increasing numbers of TBI are caused by falls and suicide attempts, and the increasing mortality is correlated with a rising incidence of subdural hematomas (31,32). In the Traumatic Brain Injury Model Systems, the overall incidence of motor-vehicle-induced TBI was 47%, with interpersonal violence (32%), falls (12%), and pedestrian accidents (9%) as other important etiologies. However, the prevalence of these different etiologies was strongly age-dependent, with motor vehicle accidents accounting for 58% of injuries in those under 25, violence most common among those 36 to 45 (43% of their injuries), and pedestrian accidents quite common (21% of their injuries) in individuals over 65. Over three-quarters of all fall-related injuries occurred in those over the age of 55 (34).

A variety of risk factors have been identified as influential in determining who is likely to sustain a TBI. The most common factor cited is alcohol intake before the TBI (35). In the Model Systems data base, 51% of those injured were legally intoxicated at the time of injury (34). Other factors have been noted, such as preinjury personality disturbance, family discord, or antisocial behavior, but little systematic research has been done to relate these factors to risk of injury (36,37). Helmet use by both motorcyclists and bicyclists reduces the severity of injuries that occur (38,39), and both seatbelt use and helmet use remain uncommon among those who are seriously hurt, with only 24% using seatbelts and

16% wearing helmets (34). Automobile airbags, when used in conjunction with belt restraints, have been shown to reduce fatalities in high-speed crashes (40), and presumably a considerable proportion of the deaths prevented would have been from TBI.

The economic and social impact of TBI is considered enormous but has not been extensively researched to date. In a study based on 327,907 TBIs, Max and associates estimated that the total lifetime costs for all people who sustained TBI in 1985 in the United States was $37.8 billion (41). Charges simply for acute care and rehabilitation of individuals in the Model Systems data base averaged about $120,000 per patient, excluding physician charges (42). Estimates of return to work vary greatly, from 15% to 100%, depending on selection criteria for the vocational program under study (43,44). Traumatic brain injury creates significant disruption for family members, causes marital strain, affects role relationships, fosters economic hardship, and creates a great burden on the family (45). These issues are discussed further later in this chapter.

PATHOPHYSIOLOGY OF TRAUMATIC BRAIN INJURY

Primary Injury

Diffuse axonal injury (DAI) is the distinguishing feature of TBI. Acceleration–deceleration and rotational forces that commonly result from motor vehicle accidents produce diffuse axonal disruption. Depending on the severity of injury, such lesions may be microscopic, or they may coalesce into focal macroscopic lesions, with a preponderance in the midbrain and pons, corpus callosum, and white matter of the cerebral hemispheres (Fig. 49-1) (46–48). Diffuse axonal injury is primarily responsible for the initial loss of consciousness (49). The precise mechanism of axonal damage remains controversial but includes impairment of axoplasmic transport, which leads to swelling and disconnection (50). This pathologic condition in a subtle form is seen even after minor TBI and may be a risk factor for later dementia (51,52). Animal data suggest that some of the loss of axonal integrity may happen after a delay of some hours (53), allowing the possibility that preventive treatments may be developed.

Cerebral contusions are another form of primary injury. These cortical bruises occur at the crests of the gyri and extend to variable depths, depending on severity. Contusions occur primarily on the undersurface of the frontal lobes and at the temporal tips, regardless of the site of impact (Fig. 49-2). The lesions usually are bilateral but may be asymmetric (54). Cerebral contusions may produce focal cognitive and sensory motor deficits and are risk factors for seizure disorders but are not directly responsible for loss of consciousness. In contrast to DAI, contusions may result from relatively low-velocity impact such as blows and falls (55). A given patient's pattern of functional deficits may be more focal (e.g., from contusions) or diffuse (e.g., from DAI) or may include features of both. The balance of these two pathologic features influences the nature of deficits. Deficits related to DAI tend to recover gradually, with the pace of recovery inversely related to the duration of coma, whereas recovery from deficits related to cortical contusions depends more on the size and location of the focal injury rather than coma duration (28).

Secondary Injury and Initial Neurosurgical Management

The initial injury may set in motion a variety of pathologic processes that result in more severe and widespread brain

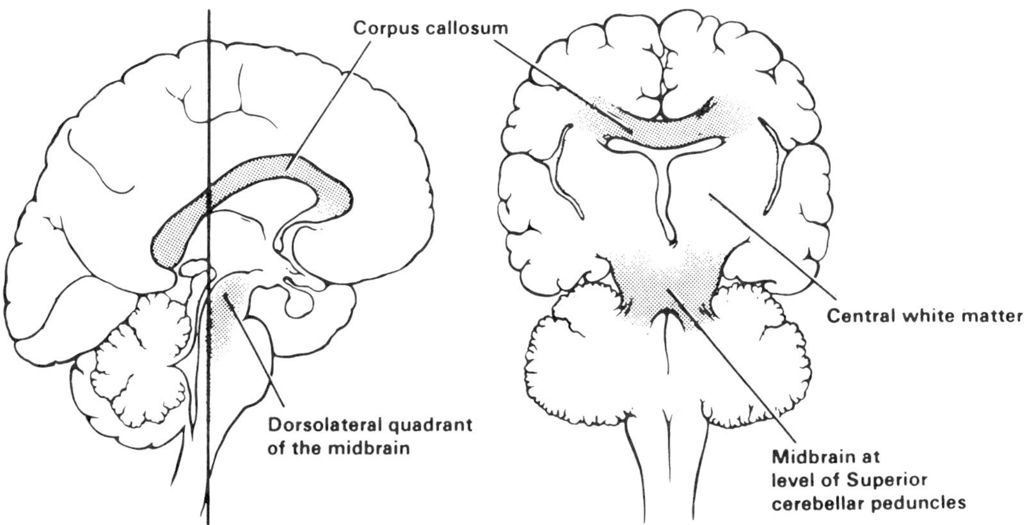

FIG. 49-1. Brain regions particularly involved by diffuse axonal injury include the corpus callosum and parasagittal white matter as well as the dorsolateral quadrants of the midbrain. (From Auerbach SH. Neuroanatomical correlates of attention and memory disorders in traumatic brain injury: an application of behavioral subtypes. *J Head Trauma Rehabil* 1986; 1:1–12. Reprinted with permission of Aspen Publishers, Inc. © 1986.)

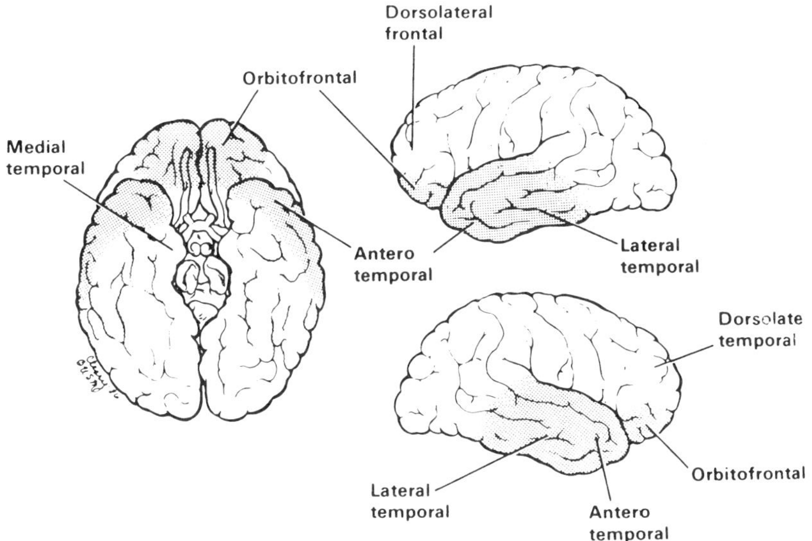

FIG. 49-2. Areas predominantly affected by cortical contusions. *Shading* represents more frequently involved areas. Anterotemporal and orbitofrontal regions are particularly involved. Note relative sparing of dorsolateral frontal lobe and medial temporal lobe. (Adapted from Courville CB. *Mythology of the central nervous system.* Mountain View, CA: Pacific Press, 1937; with permission.)

damage. Any factor that leads to increased intracranial pressure (ICP) can decrease cerebral perfusion pressure and cause ischemic damage. Expanding hematomas or acute hydrocephalus lead to dramatic pressure changes. However, increased blood volume is considered the major contributing factor leading to increased ICP (56). Vasogenic edema related to disruption of the blood–brain barrier can occur in tissue near areas of contusion (57). This edema may lead to compression of the cerebral vasculature that compromises perfusion, furthers cytotoxic edema, and creates a self-perpetuating cycle (56). Indeed, intermittent peaks in ICP during the first 24 hours are a risk factor for sustained increases in ICP (58).

In the past, intracranial pressure was routinely monitored in severe TBI. More recent guidelines recommend ICP monitoring in patients with severe head injury (GCS of 3 to 8) and an abnormal computed tomography (CT) scan (hematomas, contusions, edema, or compressed basal cisterns); or a normal CT scan and two out of three adverse features (age > 40, unilateral or bilateral motor posturing, or systolic blood pressure [BP] < 90 mm Hg) (59). Increased ICP is no longer treated in isolation but as a determinant of cerebral perfusion pressure (CPP), which is defined as the mean arterial pressure (MAP) minus ICP (60). Values of CPP below 70 mm Hg, whether caused by an increase in ICP, a decrease in BP, or both, appear to be associated with inadequate cerebral perfusion (61). If there is a CPP deficit in conjunction with increased ICP because of increased cerebral blood flow, it can be managed by elevating the head of the bed, providing MAP is stable. Aggressive hyperventilation and the use of barbiturate coma should be reserved for patients refractory to other methods of management (59). Treatment with glucocorticoids, although still common, has been shown to be ineffective (62). Bolus doses of mannitol may be employed for increased ICP secondary to edema, providing MAP is maintained through adequate fluid replacement (60). Optimal management of ICP in conjunction with CPP can lead to a reduction in ischemic injury, focal vascular occlusion, and tentorial herniation.

The initial DAI may initiate the release of excitatory neurotransmitters, which greatly increases the activity of certain brain regions at a time when such metabolic demand cannot be supported. Use of neuroprotective drugs has proved promising in animal models. The efficacy of neurotransmitter blockade in minimizing this type of secondary injury in humans is under investigation (63).

Systemic factors such as blood loss and hypotension, pulmonary injury, and cardiac or respiratory arrest also may contribute to secondary hypoxic/ischemic brain injury. Brain infection may occur from open skull fractures, cerebrospinal fluid rhinorrhea, or iatrogenically from ICP monitoring (64). Protracted seizures also can lead to deterioration through increased metabolic requirements, disruption of spontaneous respiration, and aspiration.

OUTCOME AFTER TRAUMATIC BRAIN INJURY

Types of Deficits

The majority of survivors of severe TBI emerge from coma and achieve remarkable progress toward regaining their preinjury functional abilities. In most cases, however, the person is left with a combination of physical and neurobehavioral impairments. These, in turn, interact to produce a broad array of disabilities and handicaps that may persist for many months or years after the injury. Each individual's specific pattern of deficits is a consequence of the severity of the injury, nature of brain damage, and medical complications, varying greatly from one person to the next. However, deficits in cognition are nearly ubiquitous after moderate or severe TBI. Some common cognitive impairments are listed in Table 49-4.

Changes in behavior, mood, and personality after TBI

TABLE 49-4. *Common cognitive impairments in traumatic brain injury*

Attention and arousal
- Lethargy and fatigue
- Psychomotor slowing
- Distractibility
- Deficits in selective, sustained, and divided attention

Memory
- Anterograde and retrograde amnesia
- Impaired episodic (day-to-day) recall
- Impaired orientation to time and/or place
- Slow inefficient learning
- Prospective memory deficits

Sensory/perceptual function
- Impaired visual/spatial perception
- Misperceptions of complex stimuli

Language and communication
- Dysnomia, impaired word finding
- Impaired organization of language
- Impaired pragmatics of communication

Intellect and executive function
- Concrete reasoning
- Cognitive rigidity
- Deficits in initiation, sequencing, and inhibition of action
- Poor planning and problem solving
- Impaired self-monitoring, self-regulation, and insight
- Poor or inconsistent allocation of cognitive resources, e.g., in divided attention, working memory, mental effort
- Impaired temporal continuity of behavior, e.g., in prospective actions, maintenance of goal states

have been documented by many investigators and are considered by clinicians to be among the most difficult disabilities to manage effectively (Table 49-5) (65–67). Behavior problems range from minor irritability or passivity to disinhibited, bizarre, or aggressive behavior. Many behavioral changes can be traced to specific patterns of neurologic damage (68). The severely brain-injured person often appears egocentric and regressed and may require a highly structured, consistent, positively reinforcing environment.

TABLE 49-5. *Common changes in behavior, mood, and personality*

- Apathy
- Impulsivity
- Irritability
- Aggressive behavior
- Anxiety
- Depression
- Emotional lability
- Silliness
- Poor self-image, reduced self-worth
- Denial of disability and its consequences
- Childlike behavior
- Bizarre ideation and behavior
- Loss of empathy and concern for others
- Dependency, passivity
- Indecision
- Slovenliness
- Sexual disturbances
- Substance abuse

From Rosenthal M, Griffith ER, Bond MR, et al. *Rehabilitation of the head-injured adult.* Philadelphia: FA Davis, 1983; 29.

Real-world tasks require the integrated operation of many different neurobehavioral and physical capacities. Thus, a patient who has several physical, cognitive, and behavioral *impairments* will likely experience *disabilities* as a result. For example, a patient with lower extremity weakness, ataxia, and impulsivety (i.e., impairments) may have difficulty climbing stairs safely (i.e., disability). A patient who has a memory deficit and poor self-monitoring may be repetitive and have difficulty conducting an appropriate conversation. These disabilities, in turn, may lead to *handicaps.* For example, a patient who has reduced mobility and inappropriate communication skills (i.e., disabilities) may have difficulty obtaining and retaining a job or developing intimate relationships (i.e., handicaps). Traumatic brain injury may produce a large number of physical and cognitive impairments, and the pattern of impairments varies greatly from patient to patient. Thus, it often is challenging for the clinician to determine what combination of impairments is responsible for the disabilities and handicaps that are observed. Handicaps are further affected by variations in the social and physical environments to which individuals with brain injury return. Thus, one individual may be employed in a supportive family business while another, less disabled person may be unable to secure a job in the competitive market.

Disability in the areas of self-care, toileting, mobility, communication, and feeding commonly occur in severe TBI. In those with less severe injuries, disability may not be revealed until more complex community-oriented skills are attempted, such as time and money management, community mobility, and school or vocational tasks. Handicaps in vocational, educational, and interpersonal functioning are widespread. There is frequently loss or diminution of friendships and intimate relationships and a devastating impact on the family system. The psychosocial disabilities that commonly follow TBI, and the cognitive and behavioral impairments that underlie them, are reviewed in greater detail later in this chapter.

Outcomes Measurement

The measurement and prediction of outcomes have taken on increased importance in health care generally and rehabilitation specifically. There are several distinct uses for outcomes measurement, with different implications for the types of outcomes measured and their interpretation. Outcomes data are Commission for the Accreditation of Rehabilitation Facilities (CARF) requirements for clinical program evaluation systems in brain injury rehabilitation, with the intent of ensuring that the types of functional outcomes achieved by each program are reasonable and in line with their programmatic missions. However, the quality of functional outcomes can be interpreted only in light of the characteristics of the clients entering the program, and the ability to adjust for the effects of these "case mix" variables (e.g., injury severity, etiology, time postinjury) is still rather primitive. Outcomes measurement can also be used simply to describe what is achieved in the course of treatment so that future program goals and services can be modified accordingly. For example, innovative vocational rehabilitation programs for individuals with TBI arose only when data showed poor vocational outcomes. Similarly, accurate outcomes data can help service providers or policy makers predict how many nursing home beds, personal care attendants, neurobehavioral programs, etc., will be required within a given region.

Outcomes measurement can also be useful in the pilot phases of research: by comparing innovative treatments to the standard system, one can get a sense of whether the new treatment is improving outcomes. Highly accurate outcomes prediction could also, in principle, guide individual treatment decisions. For example, if it could be predicted in the first few days postinjury that a patient would remain permanently vegetative, the physician and family might choose not to pursue aggressive treatment; if independent ambulation were predicted not to be possible, the energies of physical therapy could be redirected to other goals, and a definitive wheelchair could be prescribed earlier. For outcomes prediction to be used in this way, it would need to be highly accurate in projecting the specific outcomes of individual patients; unfortunately this has not been achieved.

In the past, large-group, multicenter studies have investigated a host of epidemiologic, demographic, medical, and other variables to determine how they correlate with outcome (69). Because the outcome categories used in these studies are global, it is rare that a true picture of an individual can be obtained. In contrast, detailed serial investigation of a single case can allow that person's outcome to be predicted more precisely but does not enable generalization to the larger population.

The outcome scale that has been used in most studies of acute TBI is the Glasgow Outcome Scale (GOS). As shown in Table 49-6, the GOS consists of five global categories ranging from good recovery to death. It has been demonstrated to have a high degree of interrater reliability in large, multicenter, international studies (69). It has been used to correlate early injury severity measures (e.g., GCS, length of PTA) and outcome at 6 months postinjury. Several major drawbacks in the utility of the scale for rehabilitation purposes have been identified:

- The categories are so broad that it is not a sensitive measure of progress during rehabilitation.
- The global categories do not provide a real indication of functional abilities.
- Cognitive and behavioral dysfunctions are poorly addressed in the outcome categories.

Despite these limitations, it continues to have widespread use for its intended purpose—to provide a quantitative, general way of describing outcome.

Several other outcome measurement scales have been developed to be more sensitive to functional changes that are of interest in rehabilitation. Some of these are brain-injury-specific, and others are general rehabilitation scales. The Disability Rating Scale (DRS) was developed specifically for TBI and is intended to assess changes "from coma to community" (70). This scale produces a quantitative index of disability across ten levels of severity. Interrater reliability is high, and this measure is considerably more sensitive to clinical change than is the GOS (71). The scale is more sensitive to changes at the severe end of the spectrum but has larger scoring gaps between self-care and ability to live

TABLE 49-6. *Glasgow Outcome Scale*

Score	Category	Definition
1	Death	As a direct result of brain trauma. Patient regained consciousness and died thereafter from secondary complications or other causes.
2	Persistent vegetative state	Patient remains unresponsive and speechless for an extended period of time. Patient may open the eyes and show sleep–wake cycles but an absence of function in the cerebral cortex judged behaviorally.
3	Severe disability (conscious but disabled)	Dependent for a daily support by reason of mental or physical disability, usually a combination of both. Severe mental disability may occasionally justify this classification in a patient with little or no physical disability.
4	Moderate (disabled but independent)	Can travel by public transport and work in a sheltered environment and can therefore be independent as far as daily life is concerned. The disabilities found include varying degrees of dysphasia, hemiparesis, or ataxia as well as intellectual and memory deficits and personality change. Independence is greater than simple ability to maintain self-care within the patient's home.
5	Good recovery	Resumption of normal life even though there may be minor neurologic and pathologic deficits.

From Jennett B, Bond MR. Assessment of outcome in severe brain damage: a practical scale. *Lancet* 1975; 1:480–484.

TABLE 49-7. *Rancho Los Amigos Levels of Cognitive Function Scale*

I.	No response
II.	Generalized response to stimulation
III.	Localized response to stimuli
IV.	Confused and agitated behavior
V.	Confused with inappropriate behavior (nonagitated)
VI.	Confused but appropriate behavior
VII.	Automatic and appropriate behavior
VIII.	Purposeful and appropriate behavior

From Hagen C, Malkmus D, Durham P. Levels of cognitive functions. In: *Rehabilitation of the head-injured adult: comprehensive physical management.* Downey, CA: Professional Staff Association, Rancho Los Amigos Hospital, 1979.

independently, and between independent living and employment (72).

The Rancho Los Amigos Levels of Cognitive Functioning Scale (Table 49-7) focuses on cognitive recovery after TBI. Each level is accompanied by a lengthy description of behaviors that meet the criteria for placement at that level (73). A comparison of this scale with the DRS revealed that it has slightly lower validity and reliability (74). The Rancho Scale is used primarily as a descriptive tool for charting the patient's level of awareness and capacity to interact appropriately and effectively with the environment. In addition, the scale has been used as a basis for planning specific therapeutic, educational, and vocational interventions as well as a means of categorizing groups of patients within large TBI facilities.

The Functional Independence Measure (FIM) has been advocated for widespread use in rehabilitation generally (75). The emphasis of this scale is on physical ability, however, which often is of less interest in TBI. Furthermore, it assesses whether individuals are capable of various skills rather than whether they actually perform those skills in daily life. One characteristic of people with severe TBI is that, although they may be able to perform tasks when specifically told to do so, they may fail to initiate and complete tasks on their own. Because of the relative insensitivity of the FIM to cognitive and behavioral deficits, the Functional Assessment Measure (FAM) was developed to supplement it with more cognitively oriented items. Interrater agreement for the FAM is lower (67%) than for the FIM (88%), and although it extends the range of difficulty somewhat compared to the FIM alone, its items are highly redundant with existing FIM items in terms of their scoring (72).

All of the outcome scales discussed above are well suited to measuring the changes that occur during acute rehabilitation, but none of them adequately addresses higher-level functions for those with mild injuries or for those with severe injuries who have been discharged into the community (76). Similarly, none of these scales is appropriate for measuring the small changes that occur in individuals emerging from the vegetative state.

Prediction of Outcome

The GCS is the most widely used measure of injury severity and is a primary basis for most predictions of outcome. The total coma score when taken at 2 to 3 or 4 to 7 days postinjury is highly predictive of outcome at 6 months, as measured by the GOS (12). Scores less than 8 are usually predictive of poor outcome. The Glasgow–Liege Score is a modification of the GCS that adds assessment of several brainstem reflexes to the examination. Use of this score has been reported to improve outcome classification (10,11). Duration of PTA also is highly correlated with ultimate outcome, with PTA greater than 14 days associated with greater likelihood of moderate or severe disability (12). The rate of early recovery, as reflected in serial DRS scores, is also predictive of final outcome (77).

Multimodality evoked potentials (MEP) also have been used as an early means of assessing neurologic status and predicting outcome. It appears that MEP do improve the prognostic value of the GCS and correlate with outcome measures such as the DRS (78). Somatosensory evoked potentials (SEP), in particular, have been shown to have good sensitivity and specificity (73% and 95%) in grossly predicting outcomes as favorable or unfavorable (13). Greenberg and colleagues found that maximal recovery occurs in approximately 3 months for patients with minimal EP abnormalities (79). Severe EP abnormalities, however, suggest that maximal recovery may extend to 12 months, if rehabilitation occurs during that time period.

Reactive pupils are associated with better outcomes than nonreactive pupils—50% of those with reactive pupils achieve the moderate disability or good recovery range, as opposed to 4% with nonreactive pupils (80). An absent oculovestibular response, elicited by injecting ice water into the ear of a comatose patient, is an indication of severe brainstem dysfunction and poorer outcome (81). The presence of an intracranial hematoma appears to increase the chance of a poor outcome when the patient is under 20 years of age (12). The level of creatine kinase (i.e., BB fraction) measured early after TBI also is a prognostic indicator because it reflects brain tissue destruction (11,82). Hyperglycemia and low levels of thyroid hormones have negative prognostic significance, presumably reflecting the severity of stress response (83,84).

In most studies reporting correlations between age and outcome, children and young adults appear to have a generally more positive prognosis than older adults. Children appear to have fewer physical and neurobehavioral sequelae after deep or prolonged coma. They also have accelerated recovery of physical and cognitive functions compared with the adult population. Children younger than 5 years of age and adults older than 65 years of age have the greatest mortality, however (29).

The research from Glasgow and other major TBI centers strongly suggests that the bulk of neurologic recovery from acute brain injury occurs within the first 6 months postinjury.

The maximal duration of the recovery period is more controversial. Some researchers affirm that neurologic recovery is virtually complete by 1 year, whereas others assert that recovery can extend 2 years or more postinjury (85). It is clear, however, that certain areas of dysfunction recover more quickly than others. For example, recovery of physical abilities and functional skills such as mobility occurs rapidly, often within 3 months after injury (86). The same is generally true for recovery of speech and language functions. The overlearned or "crystallized" verbal abilities measured by Verbal IQ scores recover rapidly and reach a plateau by 6 months postinjury, whereas more "fluid" problem-solving skills, as assessed by Performance IQ, do not reach a plateau until 12 months postinjury (87). However, neuropsychologists generally recognize that IQ scores do not provide a true indication of the presence or absence of residual cognitive deficits. Other neuropsychological measures, such as those used in the Traumatic Coma Data Bank study (88) and in the Model Traumatic Brain Injury Systems Project (89), appear to have greater sensitivity to the effects of TBI and to hold greater promise as measures of outcome.

Preinjury medical and psychological factors also may affect the prognosis. For example, the presence of a prior TBI or neurologic deficit before the injury is likely to slow the recovery process. Also, if cognitive or behavioral abnormalities existed before the injury, there is a greater likelihood of a slower and less complete recovery. Acquired brain damage is thought to exacerbate preexisting behavior disorders (90).

Finally, the prevalence of preinjury substance abuse has been documented to affect the recovery process. Sparadeo and Gill studied 102 patients admitted to a trauma center and found that 56% had a documentable blood alcohol level (91). Patients with TBI and an elevated blood alcohol level (>0.10) had a longer length of stay, longer duration of agitation, and lower cognitive status at discharge than those with TBI who were not intoxicated.

There probably is no final endpoint to the recovery process; rather, the pace of recovery slows, and its scope narrows. Even those with permanent cognitive and physical impairments can continue to learn new skills for solving particular functional problems, albeit slowly. Thus, neurologic and cognitive recovery merge imperceptibly into ongoing learning and adaptation.

POSSIBLE MECHANISMS OF FUNCTIONAL RECOVERY

Recovery from TBI often is incomplete. Reports have identified subtle but persistent deficits after even mild TBI (92,93). Yet many brain-injured people make tremendous gains from coma to the reemergence of a variety of complex skills. This recovery is believed to occur at multiple levels, from alterations in biochemical processes to changes in family structure (94). The precise mechanisms of these recovery processes are not entirely clear. Even less clear are the relative contributions of various types of recovery throughout the postinjury period. Some of the potential contributions to recovery are identified below.

Resolution of Temporary Factors

On impact, some brain tissue is irreparably damaged by gray matter contusion or axonal disruption. As noted earlier, a variety of secondary processes may also magnify the extent of functional impairment. Brain edema may depress metabolic activity of intact neurons and cause ischemia in intact neural structures. Associated pulmonary and cardiac problems may contribute to hypoxia and ischemia (95,96). Anticonvulsant administration may depress marginal neural activity (97). These and many other processes may impair the activity of relatively spared neural structures. Brain tissue that is functionally impaired but not destroyed may gradually resume function as medical status stabilizes and edema resolves. This recovery mechanism would be expected to operate in the first days to weeks after injury.

Neuronal Regeneration

There is evidence that central nervous system neurons in a variety of animal species are capable of dendritic and axonal sprouting after injury (98,99). This represents a potential mechanism for reestablishment of neural connections over time that could contribute to functional recovery. The importance of nerve fiber growth to the recovery process is unclear for several reasons, however:

- The degree of fiber sprouting may vary by species, with more extensive sprouting occurring in nonmammalian species.
- Fiber sprouting may be age dependent, occurring more readily in infancy during normal neural development.
- Fiber sprouting is likely to occur to different degrees in different brain systems. Phylogenetically old, unmyelinated fibers show more sprouting than newer myelinated systems.
- Fiber sprouting is more easily demonstrated over short distances. Reconnection of distant structures is more questionable and may be inhibited by intervening glial proliferation.
- The outcome of fiber sprouting may not be beneficial to the organism. New synaptic connections have been shown to enhance recovery of function, to contribute to unwanted symptoms, or to be "neutral," depending on the situation (100).

Recently, a number of substances have been studied for their effects on nerve fiber growth. Improved motor recovery in spinal cord injury has been demonstrated through the use of G_{M1} ganglioside, which is believed to enhance neuronal sprouting (101). Administration of G_{M1} has also been shown to mitigate the effects of brain injury in animals (102). Other substances, including nerve growth factor (103,104) and adrenocorticotropic hormone (ACTH) analogs (105), have been administered after experimental brain injury in animals, with promising results.

If neuronal regeneration plays a role in human functional recovery, it probably takes a relatively long period of time (i.e., weeks to months). Experience and training may play a role in promoting fiber sprouting or in selecting and perpetuating new, useful connections. This possibility is suggested by studies showing that enriched environments ameliorate the effects of brain injury and promote dendritic branching, even in adult animals (106).

Functional Reorganization

Even in areas of the central nervous system that are relatively "hard-wired" for sensory or motor functions, a striking degree of plasticity can occur in response to traumatic changes. In monkeys, for example, removal of peripheral inputs to the somatosensory cortex results in reorganization of the deafferented brain region such that it responds to input from different, intact peripheral receptors. Conversely, ablation of somatosensory cortical tissue is followed by "reassignment" of adjacent healthy cortex to the inputs formerly subserved by the lesioned area (107). Because these reorganizations can occur very quickly, it is speculated that they represent potentiation of existing (perhaps unused) connections rather than the effects of neuronal regeneration.

It is increasingly clear that training and experience play a major role in the neuronal representation of function, with or without trauma to the nervous system. For example, the area of monkey auditory cortex devoted to a specific frequency range enlarges when animals are trained to perform discriminations within that range (108). Following motor cortex ablations in monkeys, training and practice in fine motor skills appears to recruit adjacent cortex to assume the outflow representation of the nearby ablated tissue (109). In humans, increasingly sophisticated imaging techniques have allowed study of the plastic responses of intact cortex to practice and training. Functional magnetic resonance imaging (MRI), for instance, shows that the area of motor cortex activated by performing a motor sequence enlarges with repeated practice of that sequence (110). Furthermore, *mental* rehearsal of a movement sequence appears to potentiate new motor cortex outputs nearly as well as actual physical practice (111). Use of these experimental paradigms in brain-injured subjects may eventually help to uncover the physiological rationale for rehabilitation practices.

Synaptic Alterations

Central nervous system neurons depend on a variety of inputs for their ongoing activity. Sudden loss of stimulating inputs can lead to marked depression of undamaged structures (i.e., diaschisis) (112). For example, cerebral blood flow on the uninvolved side is markedly diminished following a cerebrovascular accident for as long as 1 month (113). Robinson and colleagues have shown that widespread changes in catecholamine neurotransmitter concentrations persist for several weeks after localized lesions in rats (114). It appears that a central nervous system lesion, therefore, potentially can disrupt not only functions served by that region but also those served by a variety of regions to which it projects.

Over time, alterations can occur in receptor sensitivity to remaining neurotransmitters. This process is analogous to denervation supersensitivity or tachyphylaxis occurring in the periphery. There is potential for partially disrupted neural connections to reexert normal levels of function if neurotransmitter receptor regulation leads to increased sensitivity to residual transmitter levels. There is considerable evidence in several animal species and some in humans that certain receptor agonists can hasten functional recovery, whereas doses of antagonists cause regression (115,116).

As yet there is limited application of this concept in TBI rehabilitation. Our knowledge of the many neurotransmitter systems and their interconnections is primitive, and the diffuse and multifocal nature of TBI limits the ability to apply existing knowledge of neurotransmitter localization. Furthermore, alterations in receptor sensitivity also could lead to disproportionate importance of particular neural inputs, producing dysfunctional results such as spasticity (116).

Functional Substitution

A person with a particular deficit may have difficulty accomplishing a task in the usual way. In theory, however, such an individual may discover another strategy for accomplishing the task that relies on remaining intact neural systems (117). It has been difficult to study systematically the role of functional substitution in human recovery because the alternate strategy itself can only be inferred from observing the outcome. The more successful the alternate strategy is in achieving the outcome, the more invisible the strategy becomes. Nevertheless, some possible examples and functional substitution strategies have been proposed:

- Reliance on a different sensory modality to guide behaviors formerly guided by another sensory-perceptual system that is damaged (118).
- Recoding verbal material into visual images or nonverbal material into verbal statements to maximize reliance on relatively spared cognitive systems (119).
- Discovery of existing motor synergy and reflex patterns that can be called on for certain movement goals (120).

The ability to develop broadly applicable alternate strategies is likely to vary with the neural system damaged. A highly specialized system may be less capable of functional replacement. Damage to multiple systems would be expected to complicate the development of alternate strategies by limiting the availability of systems capable of substituting function. Finally, the degree to which compensatory strategies can become generally applicable, spontaneous, and relatively automatic is unclear.

Learning of Specific Skills

Those with more severe deficits may find it difficult to learn general alternate strategies applicable to a broad range of circumstances. This need not, however, indicate an inability to learn specific useful skills. For example, an individual with an acquired reading disorder may not be able to reacquire the ability to sound out unfamiliar words but may be able to acquire a list of specific sight words useful in daily tasks. Similarly, someone with a significant verbal memory deficit may not be able to develop any general strategies for improving memory performance but may, through repetition, learn the names of caregivers and the locations of therapy activities. To maximize the usefulness of this recovery strategy, training must be tailored to the individual's anticipated environment and functional tasks. In contrast to the biological mechanisms previously discussed, this type of recovery need not be time limited because preserved learning capacities may be applied to specific tasks at any time.

Numerous avenues to functional recovery are theoretically possible after TBI. Much more research is needed to clarify the roles of these mechanisms in clinically important improvement. Furthermore, our ability to intervene is limited mainly to the more psychological and behavioral domains. In the future, systematic encouragement of neuronal reconnection and enhanced neurotransmitter function may be added to the rehabilitation armamentarium.

ASSESSMENT AND TREATMENT-PLANNING PROCESS

The rehabilitation needs of the survivor of severe TBI often begin at the roadside or site of emergency care but are not likely to end for many years (121). Although many medical conditions and physical deficits stabilize within 1 year after injury, the presence of long-term psychosocial disorders often necessitates a variety of interventions, including behavioral management and cognitive rehabilitation (122).

Treatment and Support Options

To help the person with brain injury achieve and sustain a reasonable quality of life, a broad spectrum of services are available that may be provided in hospital, community-based, or home settings, depending on the severity of injury and residual sequelae.

Initial management takes the form of aggressive neurosurgical intervention designed to evacuate hematomas, reduce brain edema, treat hydrocephalus, and monitor intracranial pressure and cerebral perfusion. When the patient stabilizes, the physiatrist may be called in as a consultant even when the patient is still in the ICU. The role of the physiatrist is to assist the acute care team in preventing complications such as contractures, decubitus ulcers, heterotopic ossification (HO), and bowel and bladder problems that may impede later rehabilitation of surviving patients. Such complications, if not prevented acutely, may consume resources that otherwise would be directed to functional training (123). In addition, the physiatrist may assist in choosing medications that minimize sedation of recovering patients. Following neurosurgical intensive care, a tremendous variety of treatment programs may be appropriate for a given individual at various points in the recovery process (124). Some of these are briefly described in the following section.

In the acute rehabilitation phase, the patient typically is medically stable and recovering consciousness. Such patients may have multiple medical and physical problems and display confusion, agitation, and PTA. Comprehensive interdisciplinary rehabilitation services are provided in an inpatient hospital setting. During this period, patients often regain a measure of physical mobility, capacity to perform routine activities of daily living (ADL), better recall of day-to-day events, improved communication skills, and increased awareness of their condition and the surrounding environment. This phase often lasts several weeks to months, until the patient is safe to live in a less intensive setting.

Subacute rehabilitation provides a less expensive and less intensive program. It may be designated for patients who are in a prolonged vegetative state or are slow to recover. Currently there are limited data to demonstrate that subacute or acute rehabilitation is more appropriate for this patient population. The goal of subacute care may be to improve the patient to a level where acute rehabilitation may be applied or to prepare the patient and family for long-term care should the patient plateau. Standards of care are currently being developed (125).

When the patient is ready to be discharged, several options are available for the postacute rehabilitation phase. These options depend on the expressed and perceived needs of the patient and family. If comprehensive daily rehabilitation still is required, but a slow rate of progress is expected, the individual may be referred to an extended care facility. These facilities often have categorical TBI programs and can provide rehabilitation services for many months or years, depending on reimbursement. In other cases, if a person can be managed at home but continues to display a variety of physical or neurobehavioral problems, a day treatment program may be recommended. This type of treatment often is conducted in a rehabilitation center and provides extensive cognitive rehabilitation, behavior management, daily life skills training, community activities, and prevocational activities (126,127).

Some brain-injured individuals display disinhibited, aggressive self-abusive or otherwise inappropriate behavior that cannot be managed effectively within the home. For this reason, residential behavioral management programs have been developed. In such programs, a primary objective is the modification of inappropriate behaviors and the teaching of more effective means of communication and social interaction. Often, these programs use a contingency management approach, frequently a token economy, along with other techniques (128). Other restorative and therapeutic services also are provided at these facilities.

When a brain-injured person has mastered basic skills and demonstrated the ability to learn and interact appropriately with others, community-based treatment alternatives may be considered. In the transitional living model, the brain-injured person lives in a supervised group home setting and is given instruction and progressively increasing responsibility in skills needed to live independently (e.g., cooking, cleaning, money management, community mobility, job seeking). After a 6- to 12-month period, brain-injured adults may be ready to graduate into their own apartment or into an unsupervised apartment with a roommate.

A final step in community reintegration is return to work. There are a number of vocational rehabilitation facilities in the United States that have programs designed for brain injury survivors. These programs provide intensive vocational assessment, work adjustment training, vocational training, and placement into a job in the community (often within a supported work context) or a sheltered work setting. Participation in these programs often is under the sponsorship of the state vocational rehabilitation agency. Many state vocational rehabilitation agencies were slow to recognize the unique needs of those with brain injuries, but increasingly, specialized vocational services for those with brain injury are found within state VR agencies. The vocational rehabilitation agency can provide a variety of vocational services and assistance in financial planning that can be valuable for many brain-injured clients.

Many clients may have difficulty applying knowledge gained in one setting to related problems or different environments. This limits the general benefit to be gained from transitional living training and vocational rehabilitation. In such instances, it is particularly important that the training be given in the actual community or on the actual job that the individual will be attempting.

During the long recovery process, a case manager may provide crucial coordination and social support. This role often is filled by a rehabilitation nurse, vocational counselor, social worker, or insurance rehabilitation specialist. The case manager serves as a liaison among the patient, family, and service providers and gathers medical records, arranges for medical visits, screens programs and facilities, and helps coordinate admission and discharge. The case manager often assists with financial and insurance matters, which are of critical importance in long-term planning.

With the advent of managed care, intensive case management may be even more crucial. In a report by Bryant and colleagues, outcomes comparable to national means could be achieved at costs significantly lower than average ranges for acute medical care, acute inpatient rehabilitation, and outpatient services through a managed care system with intensive case management. It was noted, however, that facilities providing the care were owned and operated by the health maintenence organization (HMO), thus significantly reducing total costs. Patients were restricted to a 60-day inpatient rehabilitation stay. Although this was sufficient for many of their members (provided appropriate outpatient services could be obtained), patients with severe brain injury were more problematic. For these patients, state funds, third-party liability, and workman's compensation needed to be utilized once HMO benefits were exhausted (129).

The continuum of services discussed above is not needed by all survivors of TBI. Rather, certain components of the continuum must be selected to meet the particular needs of each individual. However, with the rapidly evolving changes in healthcare financing, many individuals who could benefit from specific services will find that those services are not covered by their funding sources. This calls for creative financing strategies, assisted by case managers or social workers working with the patient, and advocacy efforts to expand the range of services accessible to individuals with TBI.

Patient Assessment and Treatment Planning

Rehabilitation services traditionally are organized on a team model to promote coordination and information sharing across disciplines. There is perhaps no disability group for which this interdisciplinary process is more critical than the brain-injured. The cognitive impairments are highly varied and unique to each patient. A specific cognitive impairment may interfere with the performance and retention of a mobility, communication, or ADL skill. Disruptive behaviors and lack of initiation cut across all therapy domains. Each of these problems requires the development of a unified team view of the patient's deficits and needs and the creation of a unified treatment plan.

When a patient enters a rehabilitation service, an initial assessment is needed to guide treatment planning. Typically, a member of each discipline conducts an individual assessment in his or her area of expertise. The goals of this assessment will vary with time since injury. A recently injured patient has the potential for considerable recovery. Therefore, assessment usually is aimed at defining broad functional areas in need of treatment (e.g., impaired mobility, memory deficits). As the pace of recovery slows, and discharge to home or another facility approaches, assessment must shift to identification of the specific skills and behaviors that will be prerequisites in the new environment (e.g., toilet transfers, learning a daily schedule). Assessment also depends on injury severity. It will be focused more on physical function and basic sensory processing in the severely impaired and on cognitive, social, and vocational function in the mildly impaired.

Discipline-specific assessments must be melded into a patient-oriented assessment for treatment-planning purposes (see Chapters 1 and 13). The different theoretical and clinical backgrounds of various disciplines may be an obstacle to this. A patient's inability to retain treatment instructions may be identified as a memory deficit by an occupational therapist, an attentional deficit by a neuropsychologist, and a language comprehension deficit by a speech pathologist unless group definitions have been developed.

Typically, severely injured patients have a large number of medical, physical, cognitive, and behavioral problems. Therefore, the team must develop priorities for treatment based on such factors as estimated length of stay, functional importance of each deficit, age and developmental stage, and prognosis for improvement.

Treatment priorities should be framed in terms of long- and short-term goals (see Chapter 13). Certainly this is important for accountability, but it also is very useful for clarifying the team's thinking. For example, the goal "the patient will demonstrate improved memory" has quite different implications from "the patient will remember where his room is with the help of a map." As time passes, the goals are likely to become more specific and functionally oriented, such that "the patient will have increased ROM in all joints" becomes "the patient will have adequate hip flexion for erect sitting throughout the day." Identification of the patient's physical and cognitive strengths can be very helpful in determining the best way to circumvent a specific deficit.

In general, once the problem and goal are identified, appropriate team members accept responsibility for carrying out each intervention. Complete division of labor, however, defeats the interdisciplinary purpose. A communication strategy designed by a speech pathologist, for example, should be carried out by nurses, other therapists, and family to promote generalization of the skill.

Treatment planning also must consider the hierarchy of impairment, disability, and handicap and must choose at which of these levels to intervene. For example, it may be concluded that a patient's ambulation *disability* is related to *impairments* in range of motion, tone, strength, balance, proprioception, and attention. Clinicians then must choose whether to try to address each of these impairments to improve ambulation, or whether to assess the patient's mobility skills in a motorized wheelchair instead, which would be a *disability*-level intervention. Decisions to focus treatment energy at the impairment level are most appropriate in the following situations:

- A single impairment appears to be the predominant cause of one or more disabilities.
- The patient is in a relatively acute phase, and many impairments are likely to improve.
- The impairment or impairments of concern are known to be responsive to treatment (e.g., contractures, paresis, hypertonia rather than paralysis, ataxia, amnesia).

In contrast, when there are numerous interacting impairments with a poor prognosis for improvement and uncertain relationship to disability, energy is better spent on task-level compensatory strategies or environmental modifications.

The neuropsychological assessment is important in identifying intact cognitive skills and clarifying cognitive mechanisms responsible for various behavior and skill deficits. In the severely impaired patient, formal testing may be impossible; however, the neuropsychologist's observation of the patient may still be helpful. Higher-level patients should receive formal testing of such core cognitive areas as attention, learning and remembering, language comprehension and production, visual perception, planning, reasoning, and organization. It should be kept in mind that the results of formal neuropsychological testing still have limited predictive ability for real-world function (130). Thus, patients' skills also should be assessed in naturalistic settings. The neuropsychologist also should conduct periodic problem-oriented assessment in response to clinical questions raised by other team members. In some postacute programs, the neuropsychologist is the primary coordinator of treatment planning.

Patient reassessment by the team should be conducted continuously on an informal basis and periodically in a more structured fashion. Such reassessment has several functions. It allows objective documentation of changes in status that should prompt rediscussion of treatment goals and plans. It provides program evaluation data with which to judge the success of a program's various treatment objectives. In addition, reassessment may lead to more appropriate distribution of resources to areas amenable to change or redesign of interventions to treat difficult problems more adequately.

Standards of Care

Since 1985, the Commission for the Accreditation of Rehabilitation Facilities (CARF) has promulgated standards of acceptable care for people with brain injury. These standards, developed by experts in brain injury rehabilitation, have been updated and modified several times to reflect changes in philosophy or methodology of treatment approach. It is important to note that CARF standards do not just define acceptable levels and types of medical and therapeutic services but also require documentation of the manner in which people with brain injuries and their families are a vital part of the treatment-planning and decision-making process. A program can receive accreditation in several categories: acute, postacute, or both acute and postacute (131). In many states CARF accreditation is important in determining whether a given facility is eligible to receive third-party reimbursement or if it appears on a listing of approved providers.

SPECIAL SUBPOPULATIONS

Coma and the Vegetative State

Initial coma is universal in patients with severe TBI. Up to one-half of patients in coma for longer than 6 hours die without ever regaining consciousness (10,12,13). About 10% of the total (20% of survivors) remain unresponsive 1 month after injury, with the remainder emerging from coma and gradually improving in function (132). Patients who remain unresponsive for more than 2 to 4 weeks evolve into the vegetative state, a state of wakeful unresponsiveness that is characterized by the presence of spontaneous sleep–wake cycles but absence of cortical activity as judged behaviorally (133).

Patients who are vegetative 1 month postinjury still may experience substantial recovery, but their chances of doing so diminish over time. Of patients who are vegetative at 1 month, there is approximately a 50% chance of regaining some degree of consciousness within a year and approximately a 28% chance of improving to a level of independence (134).

Patients continue to emerge from the vegetative state following trauma for at least a year and perhaps longer (little research is available for follow-up periods greater than a year), but nearly all are severely disabled if their emergence is this late. Emergence from the vegetative state following nontraumatic injuries (such as cardiac arrest) is far less likely overall, and very few patients emerge beyond 3 months postinjury (134). This suggests that patients with traumatic injuries complicated by substantial secondary anoxic injury are also likely to have a poorer prognosis than those with uncomplicated trauma.

The following factors have positive prognostic significance for emergence from unresponsiveness: young age, reactive pupils and conjugate eye movements, decorticate posturing rather than decerebrate or flaccid states, early spontaneous eye opening, and absence of ventilator dependence or hydrocephalus (132,135). Unfortunately, no set of prognostic variables is precise enough to guide early clinical decision making (132). The life expectancy of those who remain permanently vegetative is not precisely known, but one study of patients in vegetative states of mixed etiologies revealed that almost 75% had died within 5 years (136).

The term *persistent vegetative state* has been used extensively in the literature, but without consensus on its definition. Recently, it has been suggested that this term be abandoned because it confuses diagnosis (vegetative) with prognosis (persistent). However, recommendations have been made to add a new term to this topic area: minimally conscious state (137). This refers to individuals who show some evidence of awareness in the form of visual tracking and/or motor behavior that is nonreflexive and contingent on environmental events (e.g., intermittent following of simple commands, replicable pulling out of tubes) but who do not yet follow two-step commands or communicate intelligibly. The minimally conscious state, like the vegetative state, can be a transitional state on the way to greater recovery or can be the permanent functional plateau.

Initial coma in TBI probably reflects disruption of brainstem alerting mechanisms, often with relative preservation of higher brain structures. Brainstem alerting mechanisms tend to recover with time, however. Thus, a vegetative state of long duration generally includes extensive damage to subcortical white matter in higher brain regions, including the thalamus (138,139). Akinetic mutism and the locked-in syndrome may be confused with the vegetative state, but akinetic mutism generally involves damage to the medial frontal lobes, and hypertonia and posturing are absent. The locked-in syndrome generally results from a pontine stroke, and there is evidence of preserved consciousness and communication through eye movements (140,141).

Establishing the diagnosis of the vegetative state can be done clinically, by observing for volitional responses to the environment, such as following commands, orienting visually to salient objects, attempting to remove tubes and restraints, and the like. Essentially, any behavior that is nonstereotyped and that indicates some evaluation of environmental stimuli is evidence of emerging consciousness. A formal and quantitative assessment strategy is an absolute requirement in working with vegetative and minimally conscious patients; without this, team and family members will disagree about whether or not evidence of consciousness is present and whether improvement is occurring. Several standardized scales are available for objectively grading responsiveness in vegetative and minimally conscious patients (142–145). In addition, the principles of single-subject experimental design can be used to answer important clinical questions in individual patients, such as whether the patient can see (146), follow commands, or reliably use a yes/no signaling system; and whether he or she responds to therapeutic medications (147). Assessment should take place repeatedly and at various times of day because patients may respond inconsistently, particularly as they are first emerging from the vegetative state. When family members report observing volitional behavior that has not been witnessed by staff, individualized assessments of the relevant behaviors can be conducted. Family members may overinterpret reflexive or coincidental behaviors, but staff members may fail to elicit the patient's best performance. Definitive assessment of the vegetative state must await withdrawal of potentially sedating drugs and ruling out peripheral sensory deficits (e.g., blindness, deafness) (148,149).

Many treatments have been attempted in the vegetative state, but none has been subjected to an adequate controlled clinical trial. The pathologic heterogeneity of unresponsive states makes it unlikely that one treatment will help all affected people. Electrical stimulation of the mesencephalic reticular formation or nonspecific thalamic activating system with implanted electrodes has been reported to improve the electroencephalographic (EEG) spectrum and clinical status in some vegetative patients with stroke or TBI (150–153). However, these studies have used small samples of patients with vegetative states of varying intervals and of mixed etiologies. Thus, ruling out spontaneous recovery is difficult. Dopaminergic pharmacologic treatments, including L-dopa, bromocriptine, and amantadine, also have been reported to be of help (154–156). All of these treatments act primarily to augment ascending arousing influences. From a theoretical standpoint, this would seem unlikely to benefit patients with extensive cerebral lesions.

Coma stimulation treatment has been used widely in vegetative patients. This involves the systematic and frequent provision of sensory stimulation to all sensory modalities and is based on animal research that shows that enriched environments improve neurologic recovery (94). However, it should be noted that studies that show a role of experience in promoting neurologic recovery have involved active participation of the animal, not merely passive stimulation (157). Several small studies on coma stimulation have been done, but all suffer from serious methodologic flaws, which have been summarized in recent review articles (158,159). A large, multicenter clinical trial will be needed to settle this issue.

In the absence of definitive treatments to alter the prognosis in the vegetative state, the main goals for rehabilitation are to optimize medical stability, preserve bodily integrity, and objectively define the patient's current sensory and cognitive capacities with measures that can be monitored for change over time (148,149). This includes screening for adverse medical events such as undiagnosed seizures, hydrocephalus, and endocrine disorders. Attempts to optimize pulmonary hygiene and maintain skin integrity also are essential. Aggressive treatment of hypertonia and contractures is warranted early because they will predispose to skin breakdown and interfere with positioning. Much time and money can be saved for those patients who do recover by preventing the development of severe deformities. Finally, sedating medications should be avoided until the prognosis has declared itself. This includes a variety of antispasticity, anticonvulsant, antihypertensive, anticholinergic, and antihistaminic medications that may have subtle cognitive effects in susceptible patients (148).

Regular evaluation with a quantitative assessment scale should be carried out. This will reveal subtle improvement that should lead to updated treatment plans, deterioration that should lead to further diagnostic evaluation, or no change, which should lead to family counseling about prognosis and planning toward home or chronic care placement. When a patient remains permanently vegetative, or when a patient remains minimally conscious but has left a specific advance directive, the possibility of forgoing further medical treatments and even life-sustaining fluid and nutrition may be discussed with the family after careful review of local legal guidelines relevant to this area and any institutional policies and ethical guidelines relevant to end-of-life determinations.

Mild Traumatic Brain Injury

At the other end of the spectrum from unresponsive states is the patient with mild, or minor, traumatic brain injury (MTBI). This is generally defined as a TBI with the following characteristics:

- Loss of consciousness, if any, 30 minutes or less
- Posttraumatic amnesia 24 hours or less
- Initial GCS 13 to 15
- No focal neurologic deficit
- Negative CT and/or MRI

The etiology of MTBI involves either direct mechanical trauma or acceleration–deceleration forces only (e.g., whiplash) (160). The initial symptoms of the cerebral injury may be difficult to disentangle from those of the common coincident injuries to the scalp, neck, and peripheral vestibular apparatus (161). Acute complaints after MTBI typically fall into three symptom clusters (162):

- Cognitive: attention and concentration difficulties, memory impairment
- Affective: irritability, depression, anxiety
- Somatic: headache, dizziness, insomnia, fatigue, sensory impairments (163)

These symptoms clear within the first few weeks or months postinjury for the majority of patients. Group studies have generally revealed no decrement, or only modest or transient decrement, on neuropsychological measures for subjects with MTBI compared to uninjured controls (164–166). For some individuals, however, difficulties persist and are associated with social and vocational failure seemingly out of proportion to the severity of the neurologic insult. The etiology of these persistent complaints (often termed postconcussion syndrome, PCS) has been elusive and remains controversial. Premorbid factors such as substance abuse, psychiatric disorder, and age have been implicated but do not explain all cases of persistent disability. Similarly, the idea that pending litigation or financial gain accounts for PCS has not been confirmed (162). In a recent single photon emission CT (SPECT) study, MTBI patients with unusually persistent disability showed hypoperfusion in the anterior mesial regions of the temporal lobes (167). There is probably no one cause of PCS; premorbid variables, idiosyncratic neurologic vulnerability, and psychological reactions to acute symptoms may all be found to play roles.

The treatment of MTBI should include patient and family education about the typical symptoms and their time frame and guidance on how and when to resume preinjury activities. Patients with persistent symptoms may benefit from psychotherapy (168), pain management protocols (169), or holistic community reentry programs offering these components along with education, vocational counseling, and group support. Many of the somatic symptoms are responsive to interventions that can be provided through an experienced physical therapist in conjunction with judicious use of medications. Therapeutic interventions include vestibular habituation exercises (170), Rocabado exercises (171), myofascial release, trigger point injections, nonsteroidal anti-inflammatory medications, and muscle relaxants. For more extensive information, the reader is referred to more detailed publications on this aspect of brain injury (172–174).

MEDICAL PROBLEMS AFTER TRAUMATIC BRAIN INJURY

Neurodiagnostic Techniques

Many imaging and neurophysiological technologies are available to assist in TBI management. In the acute postinjury period, CT scanning can detect intracranial hematomas, brain swelling, hydrocephalus, and infarction (175). However, it is not sensitive in identifying small contusions and white matter injury (176). In the postacute phase, CT scanning is useful in evaluating the progress of hydrocephalus and cortical atrophy.

MRI has advantages over CT, including lack of x-ray exposure, greater resolution in the brainstem, better identification of isodense collections of blood, and detection of small white matter lesions (177). Even MRI may be normal in patients with mild TBI, however, despite a well-documented loss of consciousness (178).

Magnetic transfer and fluid-attenuated inversion recovery (FLAIR) are two pulse sequence techniques used to improve MRI sensitivity to white matter injury (179,180). Subtle midline shifts in the brain following trauma may be detected through use of a MRI computer registration program (181).

Positron emission tomography (PET) can provide information about brain function as well as anatomy. Labeled metabolic substrates or blood components are taken up by brain tissue in proportion to metabolic demand or blood flow. Thus, metabolically hypoactive but anatomically normal tissue may be identified. This method, though limited in availability, has the potential to correlate directly with neuropsychological performance by demonstrating metabolic hypoactivity in regions subserving specific cognitive functions, in the absence of gross structural change (182). SPECT scanning is more widely available and shares some of the beneficial functional features of PET scanning. We have found it useful in confirming organic pathologic conditions in patients with mild TBI who were thought to be malingering. Several studies show that SPECT scans are more sensitive than CT in detecting minor TBI and that they may indicate areas of impending hematoma enlargement that may require evacuation (183,184).

The standard EEG can provide gross information about the severity, location, and extent of brain damage. In addition, epileptiform activity may suggest seizure risk. Interictal EEGs have low sensitivity for seizure disorders, however, especially in areas distant from the cortical convexities (e.g., medial temporal lobes) (185). Sensitivity can be increased by sleep deprivation or prolonged monitoring with behavioral correlation. Electroencephalographic measures may at times be misleading, as in the case of improvement of a patient with an isoelectric EEG (186).

Quantitative EEG has potential advantages in providing information regarding the neurophysiology of brain injury. Because it is not automated or standardized, however, results vary depending on the technician. Obtaining normative data has been difficult, limiting its current role in mainstream management of brain injury (187).

Much research has been done on evoked potentials in brain trauma (see Chapter 16). In group studies it has been shown that MEPs add to the prognostic accuracy of the GCS score (188,189). Specifically, somatosensory evoked potentials (SSEP) can assess the gross outcome of acutely injured patients with positive predictive values greater than 80% (10). The ability to make accurate prognostications about individual patients remains more limited. For example, in the study described above, predictive accuracy was good only if one does not care about distinguishing among death, the vegetative state, and severe disability. The predictive value of MEP or SEP remains significant in chronic TBI but drops sharply in magnitude (190,191). Rappaport reports the use of MEP to allocate rehabilitation resources to patients with a potential to benefit. It remains to be demonstrated that this decision strategy is superior to allocation on clinical grounds.

The clinical utility of MEP for individual patients is clear in at least three situations. They may document organic pathologic processes in patients with minor TBI with otherwise negative evaluations (192); they may help localize the site of a neurologic deficit (193); and in patients who are unconscious or uncooperative, MEP provide a way of diagnosing somatosensory, hearing, or visual deficits that might interfere with rehabilitation treatments.

Standard nerve conduction and electromyography (EMG) play an important role in evaluation of patients with possible peripheral nerve, plexus, or root lesions. Because of the traumatic etiology of the brain injury, peripheral nerves may be stretched or damaged by fractures. Tone-related posturing may lead to pressure neuropathies at the ulnar groove and carpal tunnel.

Thus, patients who show focal muscle wasting, numbness, unexplained weakness, or flaccid extremities in the context of other upper motor neuron findings, should receive EMG evaluation.

Fractures

Many fractures are diagnosed in the acute injury period, but more subtle ones often are missed until transfer to rehabilitation, when the patient shows increased movement and responsiveness to pain. Any unexplained swelling, deformity, or pain response should prompt evaluation for occult fracture. Fractures in TBI predispose to HO. For example, despite appropriate operative management of 23 acetabular fractures, 61% had poor outcomes because of HO (194). In general, open reduction and internal fixation are used more aggressively in TBI to promote early mobilization, simplify patient care, and improve predictability of fracture outcome without adverse cerebral effects (195). Early fixation may reduce health care costs and delay in mobility, but effects on ultimate functional recovery need to be further explored (196). Although fractures may complicate the rehabilitation process by delaying mobility, they have little impact on the ultimate functional level.

Seizures

Posttraumatic epilepsy is common after significant TBI. The risk of ongoing seizures is related to injury severity, specifically depressed skull fracture, intracranial hematoma, early seizure, and prolonged disturbance of consciousness (9). The risk of seizure development is greatest in the first 2 years postinjury and gradually declines. Spontaneous resolution of a seizure disorder also occurs, indicating the need for periodic reevaluation.

Most seizures are diagnosed clinically on the basis of focal or generalized motor activity. Patients with muscle spasms or tremors may present diagnostic dilemmas. In such cases, a routine or sleep-deprived EEG may reveal epileptiform activity. More definitive is a 24-hour EEG correlated with observations of the suspicious activity. Seizures in limbic areas may lead only to altered behavior or states of consciousness, presenting further diagnostic challenges.

Long-term seizure prophylaxis is no longer recommended and has not been shown to be beneficial in preventing late-onset posttraumatic seizures (197,198). Treatment of patients with penetrating wounds or those at high risk for medical complications is more controversial and may need to be considered on a case-by-case basis, depending on overall severity of injury (199).

Carbamazepine and valproic acid have been found to be more cognitively benign than phenobarbital; their superiority over phenytoin is debated (148,200–202). Patients who have difficulties with compliance may benefit from Tegretol-oros, a slow-release form of carbamazepine. In patients with more refractory seizures, newer agents such as gabapentin and lamotrigine may be employed, with use of felbamate being reserved for patients who are unresponsive to all other medication regimens (because of risks of hepatotoxicity and aplastic anemia) (203). Fosphenytoin is a water-soluble phenytoin prodrug that can be rapidly infused (either intramuscularly or intravenously) without the side effects of intravenous phenytoin, improving the management of status epilepticus and potentially reducing its long-term effects on brain tissue (204).

There are no standard recommendations on duration of treatment. In view of the expense and potential toxicity of anticonvulsants, most clinicians withdraw medications after 1 to 2 seizure-free years. Of patients with previous seizure disorders of mixed etiologies who had been seizure-free for 2 years, 35% relapsed after tapering of their anticonvulsants (205).

Hydrocephalus

Ventricular dilation occurs in up to 40% of patients with severe TBI and usually begins to appear within 2 weeks of injury. In most instances, ventriculomegaly results from diffuse atrophy or focal infarction of brain tissue (i.e., hydrocephalus *ex vacuo*). Flattening of the cortical sulci and periventricular lucency tend to support the diagnosis of clinically important hydrocephalus (206).

Hydrocephalus in TBI is most often of the communicating or normal-pressure type. Unfortunately, the classic diagnostic triad of incontinence, gait disorder, and dementia is of little help in severely disabled patients. New-onset hypertension has been reported as a consequence of hydrocephalus in one patient and resolved with shunting (207). Failure to improve or deterioration of cognitive or behavioral function should prompt assessment with a CT scan. If the scan is equivocal, cisternography may be done; however, one study in idiopathic hydrocephalus suggested that the cisternogram does not add to clinical diagnostic accuracy (208). Pressure measurements during fluid infusion into the lumbar space (209) and behavioral changes in response to withdrawal of cerebrospinal fluid via lumbar puncture (the "tap test") (210) also have been reported to be of diagnostic value. Patients with ventricular shunts may experience shunt failure. Thus, a deterioration in such patients also should prompt a follow-up CT scan and a shunt flow study or pressure measurements. Even when a patient has definitive hydrocephalus, the prognosis from shunting is uncertain. This may be partly because the patient has other cognitive and motor deficits unrelated to hydrocephalus.

Frequently the patient's therapists and nurses are the best judges of subtle cognitive improvements and deteriorations. Hydrocephalus and shunt failure may not be identified through the standard neurologic examination, especially in a patient with an abnormal baseline examination. Hence, it is critical that consulting neurologists and neurosurgeons incorporate the entire team's assessments of cognitive and behavioral fluctuations into their evaluation.

Hypertension

Hypertension, tachycardia, and increased cardiac output in the acute postinjury period result from the increased release of epinephrine and norepinephrine (211). Therefore, beta blockers represent the most specific intervention in this patient group. Propranolol and methyldopa cause cognitive impairments in hypertensive patients (212). Consequently, use of highly polar beta blockers such as atenolol or nadolol may be preferable. These agents cross the blood–brain barrier very little in uninjured people (213,214), but this has not been studied in diffuse brain injury, where the blood–brain barrier may be disrupted.

In severe brain injury, hypertension may persist beyond the acute phase. This may be linked to injury to the brainstem, hypothalamus, and orbitofrontal regions, but there may be other contributing factors (215). Evaluation to rule out occult spinal cord injury, increased intracranial pressure, renal and adrenal abnormalities, or hypothyroidism should be considered (216).

Sustained hypertension is infrequent after TBI unless there was preexisting hypertension. Where hypertension does exist, angiotensin-converting enzyme (ACE) inhibitors, calcium channel blockers, and diuretics are least likely to cause cognitive impairment. If medication with central nervous system side effects must be used, it is wise to inform therapy staff so that subtle cognitive deterioration is noted and reported to the physiatrist.

Cardiopulmonary Disorders

Severe TBI can produce cardiorespiratory arrest or dysrhythmias. Such disturbances of cardiorespiratory control are indications of severe brain injury and causes of further hypoxic injury. Cardiac injury occurs as a result of blunt trauma to the right ventricle against the sternum. This results in early elevations of cardiac enzymes, cardiac wall motion abnormalities, and decreased cardiac output. Central sympathetic hyperactivity can lead to ongoing myocardial necrosis over the next few days (217). Although these injuries may result in lasting electrocardiogram changes (e.g., Q waves, S-T segment alterations), their relevance to the long-term cardiovascular health of survivors is unknown.

Multiple trauma often causes pneumothorax, pulmonary contusions, and lacerations. In addition, intense alpha-adrenergic outflow is believed to cause noncardiogenic pulmonary edema (218,219). These and other problems can further compromise cerebral oxygenation.

Many brain-injured patients require tracheostomies for ventilation and suctioning. Humidified air may be delivered through a tracheostomy collar to maintain moist secretions and prevent tracheitis, and frequent suctioning may be required (220). Thick, copious secretions may be managed with intratracheal instillation of 1-acetylcysteine (Mucomyst, Bristol-Myers Laboratories, Evansville, IN). Patients who initially require supplemental oxygen usually can be weaned from it by assessing pulse oximetry on oxygen and again after it has been stopped. If there is a concern about retention of carbon dioxide, arterial blood gas measurement may be conducted. Patients who require long-term tracheostomies but have begun to vocalize may benefit from one of the varieties of tubes that permit vocalization. Pneumonia in patients with tracheostomies is common, but prophylactic use of antibiotics is unwarranted (221).

Most TBI patients eventually can be decannulated. Indirect laryngoscopy screening can be used to check for adequate vocal cord abduction and to rule out subglottic stenosis (222). In some instances tracheal or subglottic stenosis will prevent decannulation and will require dilation or surgical management. If there is no sign of anatomic obstruction, a small-caliber tracheostomy tube will allow air to bypass the tube while it is plugged for progressive intervals. The patient is checked at the end of each interval or at any sign of distress with pulse oximetry. Once the patient has tolerated 24 hours of plugging without incident, decannulation can take place, and the tracheostomy stoma can be covered by a gauze pad or occlusive dressing until it heals. Some patients will have difficulty with decannulation because of the quantity of secretions and inability to cough them up into the pharynx. Thus, persistent suctioning is required. The tracheostomy tube itself may be an irritant that evokes secretions, however. To evaluate this possibility, a tracheal button (i.e., a small plug that keeps the stoma open) can replace the tube temporarily to see if the elimination of the tube allows patients to manage their own secretions; if not, the tube can be replaced (223). When a patient is nearly ready to be decannulated but is just beginning oral feeding, we usually choose to retain the tracheostomy until oral feeding function has been fully evaluated to have it available in the event of aspiration and to be able to perform diagnostic suctioning after feeding methylene blue-dyed food.

Long-term survivors of severe TBI have been reported to show decreased lung capacity, vital capacity, and forced expiratory volume. The etiology of these abnormalities is not entirely clear but appears to be a combination of muscle weakness and incoordination, decreased compliance, and deconditioning (224). The role of cardiopulmonary conditioning in TBI has not been systematically assessed.

Hypothalamic and Endocrine Dysfunction

Acute TBI causes numerous endocrine changes, including an outpouring of norepinephrine and epinephrine, a rise in aldosterone, glucose, and cortisol, and a drop in thyroid hormones, all of which are related to injury severity (225–227). Elevation of cortisol is related to increased ICP but only in the presence of an intact brainstem (228). The mechanism is unknown, since it is not associated with elevated ACTH secretion. In mildly to moderately injured patients, there is an inverse correlation between levels of epinephrine and norepinephrine and thyroid hormones, and it appears that the adrenergic hormones may directly inhibit thyroid hormone release. The administration of exogenous thyroid hormones in other stressed patient groups has not improved outcomes, however.

Chronic endocrine alterations also occur after TBI. An autopsy study of 100 brain-injured patients revealed a 62% incidence of pituitary injury (229). Hypothalamic injuries coexisted in some patients. Less is known about endocrine status in TBI survivors. Case reports document a variety of endocrine dysfunctions but no study has evaluated prevalence in a population with varying severity of injury, or longitudinally during recovery. Potentially, TBI may injure the pituitary directly or may impair hypothalamic excitatory or inhibitory control.

Traumatic brain injury may result either in diabetes insipidus or in the syndrome of inappropriate antidiuretic hormone secretion (SIADH) (230). Antidiuretic hormone is secreted from neuroendocrine cells in the posterior pituitary. The mechanism of traumatic SIADH is unknown, but may relate to the loss of cortical or limbic inhibition of the hypothalamus (231). Diabetes insipidus occurs as a result of impairment or necrosis of the posterior pituitary. It may appear as late as 1 month postinjury, perhaps because dying tissue can release stored ADH for that period (232). Both disorders can be managed acutely by controlling fluid and electrolyte intake and monitoring serum electrolytes and osmolality. Persistent or late appearance of diabetes insipidus usually is permanent and may be managed with a synthetic ADH analogue.

Anterior pituitary damage may range from panhypopituitarism to selective loss of gonadal stimulating hormones, thyrotropin, or ACTH (233,234). Clinical signs may be subtle and confounded with other causes of cognitive, behavioral, and physiological abnormalities. Hypotension or hypothermia or cognitive decline may be an indicator of endocrine dysfunction. Secondary amenorrhea in female patients is common and may predispose to osteoporosis. Ironically, precocious puberty after TBI has been reported in children (235).

Gynecomastia and galactorrhea occur from elevations in prolactin. In normal subjects, prolactin secretion is controlled by tonic hypothalamic inhibition. Brain injury frequently disrupts these inhibitory influences (236). Chest trauma and a number of medications also may result in galactorrhea.

Sexual dysfunction in brain-injured men is more common than can be accounted for on the basis of endocrine dysfunction but is related to other indices of injury severity, suggesting a psychosocial component (237).

In summary, it appears that endocrine dysfunction is common at least in the severely injured and may remit with neurologic recovery. Clinical evaluation may be difficult because of confounding deficits, so the clinician should have a high index of suspicion. Uncorrected endocrine disorders may limit cognitive and behavioral recovery and lead to serious physical sequelae.

PHYSICAL IMPAIRMENTS

Cranial Nerve Dysfunction

Olfactory nerve injuries commonly accompany significant head trauma because of the delicate anatomy of the fibers exiting the cribriform plate; they are particularly likely in association with cerebrospinal fluid rhinorrhea. The diagnosis may be missed by incomplete sensory testing. Objective testing of olfaction using a scratch-and-sniff odor panel is possible (238). Serial testing may reveal some degree of recovery. Olfactory deficits may play a role in altered feeding behavior.

Visual impairment may occur as spotty scotomata that differ in the two eyes, as homonymous hemianopia, or as complete blindness. Optic nerve lesions must be distinguished from hemi-inattention, cortical blindness, and visual agnosia. Early assessment can be done in gross terms through funduscopic examination, visual evoked response studies, and pupillary assessment. Vision and visual attention can be evaluated in severely impaired patients, using repeated presentations of colorful photographs and cards in each hemifield (146). Crude measurement of visual acuity can be performed with an optokinetic drum (239). When cooperation allows, more precise visual field and acuity testing should be performed. Neuropsychological assessment may clarify visual perceptual disorders. Information about field cuts and acuity should be shared with all team members to ensure that therapy stimuli are of appropriate size and placement.

Extraocular movements may be affected by damage to cranial nerves, their brainstem nuclei, or by impairment of coordinative structures in the midbrain and cerebellum (240,241). In addition, orbital fractures or damage to the extraocular muscles may produce disconjugate gaze. Neuro-ophthalmologic examination may help clarify the pathophysiology of the deficit. Alternating or unilateral eye patching can eliminate diplopia. Prisms and strabismus surgery require that the patient be capable of ocular fusion to achieve binocular vision, but surgery sometimes may be appropriate solely for cosmetic purposes. Many medications can exacerbate diplopia (242).

Temporal bone fractures may disrupt facial nerve function temporarily or permanently. This must be differentiated from cortical or subcortical central facial weakness. Early nerve conduction and EMG studies may clarify the prognosis for facial nerve recovery (243). Facial weakness, when combined with corneal insensitivity as a result of trigeminal lesions, can lead to corneal ulceration; corneal lubricants or tarsorrhaphy may be indicated.

Skull fractures also may disrupt the auditory or vestibular pathways (244). Ossicular dislocation can lead to conductive hearing loss. Brainstem auditory evoked responses can be helpful in assessment of auditory function in comatose or uncooperative patients; however, if no response is seen at normal intensity, hearing threshold should be evaluated with increasing intensities. Caloric testing can provide information about vestibular function. Later, standard audiologic evaluation, including speech perception, should be performed. Hearing aids or ossicular repair can be helpful in selected patients. The patient's auditory capabilities should be shared with the entire treatment team so that care can be taken to communicate in the environment and style that optimize comprehension.

Movements of the tongue, pharynx, and larynx often are impaired by severe TBI at various levels in the central nervous system (245). Evaluation of oral motor function including cough and gag reflexes and indirect laryngoscopy may help clarify the location and extent of the problem. Such disturbances will be relevant for safe oral feeding as well as vocal communication.

Sensory Deficits

Traumatic brain injury can produce disturbances of any of the sensory modalities. Depending on the location and severity of the damage, these may be disturbances of basic sensation (e.g., decreased visual activity) or of perceptual processing of that sensation (e.g., impaired visual spatial perception). Both forms of disturbance can be disabling.

Disorders of somesthetic sensation can result from damage to a variety of brain structures and may distort touch, pain, temperature, and position information. Pain syndromes may result from central injury to the thalamus, other cerebral structures, or from dynamic reverberation of corticothalamic loops (246,247).

Basic sensation can be assessed in each modality as soon as the patient is able to cooperate. Visual, auditory, and somesthetic sensation can be assessed grossly earlier with evoked potential studies. The presence of normal basic sensation, however, does not ensure that the patient can form the complex perceptions needed to recognize a visually presented object through tactile exploration, or identify a letter through stereognosis.

When patients fail at a task for which basic sensory input is intact, other causes of inability to perform can be explored. A patient recovering from cortical blindness, for example, may have full visual fields and functional acuity but may be unable to name visually presented objects. Neuropsychological assessment can help to differentiate among object-naming disorders, visual agnosias, scanning disorders, and disorders of complex visual perception (248).

There is no uniform strategy for coping with sensory deficits. Rather, treatment is planned around the severity of the deficit, strength of remaining sensory capabilities, and cognitive status of the patient. All team members should be involved in this planning because the patient's sensory, motor, and cognitive capacities all are relevant to the process.

Heterotopic Ossification

Heterotopic ossification (HO) occurs in 11% to 76% of severely injured patients, primarily in proximal joints of the upper and lower extremities (249). The etiology of HO in brain injury is unknown. Risk factors include prolonged coma, increased muscle tone in the involved extremity, and associated fractures (250).

A study using historical controls suggested that diphosphonates may have a role in prevention of HO after TBI (249). Garland has reported that patients who remain severely cognitively and physically impaired have a high rate of recurrent bone formation after surgical treatment (251). This may imply an ongoing stimulus for HO in such patients, raising questions about the efficiency of time-limited prophylaxis. More research is needed on the role of prophylaxis in various subgroups of TBI patients.

Heterotopic ossification may present with pain, warmth, swelling, and contracture formation but may be occult. Earliest diagnosis is possible with a bone scan, but ossification subsequently is visible on plain radiographs (252). Diphosphonates and nonsteroidal anti-inflammatory agents, particularly indomethacin, have been used in an attempt to arrest early HO or to prevent its postoperative recurrence, but their efficacy has not been adequately established (253–255). A recent study of patients with early and intermediate HO found that calcium deposition occurred in the early phase, inflammation in the intermediate phase, and appearance of osteoclasts and osteoblasts in the late phase (256). This suggests that diphosphonates may be beneficial early and anti-inflammatories at an intermediate time, but no controlled treatment comparisons have been performed to date. Radiation has been used to inhibit HO after total hip replacement, but concerns about neoplasia limit its application in younger patient groups (257). Range-of-motion exercises are indicated to prevent ankylosis. If ankylosis seems inevitable despite exercises, it should be encouraged to occur in the most functional position.

Surgery for removal of ectopic bone should be undertaken only for clear functional goals, such as improved standing posture or ambulation or independent dressing and feeding. In general, surgery is not undertaken earlier than 18 months after injury. More functional patients with normal alkaline phosphatase levels are less likely to experience recurrence (251).

Increased Muscle Tone and Contractures

Increased muscle tone following TBI may include true spasticity (i.e., increased phasic stretch reflexes). Dystonia, posturing in response to head position and cutaneous stimulation, and extrapyramidal syndromes also are common. The mere existence of abnormal tone is not an indication for treatment. Treatment should be based on functional considerations (Table 49-8). Physical modalities such as heat, cold, stretch, and inhibitory postures can be helpful in mild to moderate tone but are unlikely to provide lasting control of severe tone. Medications such as dantrolene sodium, baclofen, or diazepam may be used (258). It has been claimed that only dantrolene is effective in spasticity of cerebral origin (259), although this remains controversial (260,261). When dantrolene is used, hepatic function must be monitored closely (262). Dystonia, a severe functional problem, rarely responds dramatically to antispasticity drugs. Furthermore, all three agents produce sedation often enough to raise concerns about their effects on marginal cognitive function (263). Little research has been done on any of these medications specifically in TBI.

Phenol nerve and motor point blocks are an effective strategy in severe disorders of tone (264). Although their efficacy is best documented in true spasticity (265), we have found them effective to varying degrees in spasms, posturing, and dystonia. Multiple muscle groups may need to be blocked, and blocks may need to be repeated periodically. The advantage, however, is the effectiveness in severely increased tone

TABLE 49-8. *Indications for treatment of increased muscle tone*

Interference with active movement
Contracture formation or progression in a posturing limb
Interference with appropriate positioning or hygiene
Self-inflicted trauma during muscle spasms
Excessive pain on range-of-motion exercises or during muscle spasms
Excessive therapy time devoted to contracture prevention rather than functional activities

and the lack of cognitive side effects (266). Dynamic EMG may help identify which muscles have volitional activity and which exhibit the greatest hypertonia (267,268). In the postacute period, more definitive procedures such as myotendinous lengthening or release or neurosurgical interventions may be considered.

Botulinum toxin may be an effective alternative to phenol blocks in some cases (269). The effects of botulinum toxin last 3 to 4 months with a more complete return to baseline, making it more desirable for patients in the early stages of recovery. It may also be helpful when blocking of multiple muscle groups is desired. Disadvantages include delay in onset (up to 72 hours), making assessment and titration of effects difficult. Also, patients may become refractory to its effects with repeated injections as a result of development of antibodies (270).

Intrathecal baclofen has been approved for use in patients with spasticity secondary to cerebral causes. Early studies demonstrated improvements in seating position, posture, transfers, and, in some cases, ambulation (271). As with other interventions for spasticity, clear goals need to be established (either functional or hygienic).

Contractures after TBI usually result from increased tone or HO. Ideally, contractures should be prevented through range-of-motion exercises, splinting, and treatment of tone. The functional prognosis of patients cannot accurately be predicted early after injury. Therefore, at this point attempts should be made to treat all contractures by nonsurgical means such as ultrasound, traction, serial casting, and so forth. Contractures in patients with TBI in the more distant past should be treated only for clear functional goals such as improved hygiene, positioning, or active movement. Surgical treatment of contractures should be undertaken only for clear functional goals after conservative measures have failed.

Motor Disturbances

A variety of other motor disturbances result from TBI. The diffuse and multifocal nature of the neuropathologic condition often challenges a precise neurophysiological diagnosis. Disorders of muscle tone have been discussed previously. Additional deficits include paralysis or paresis involving isolated muscle groups, combinations of limbs, or the whole body.

Disorders of balance and coordination may result from damage to the cerebellum or its connections. Patients with good muscle strength may be unable to ambulate or even sit independently because of profound ataxia. Similarly, limb ataxia may preclude self-feeding, writing, and independent ADLs. Tremors, bradykinesia, and parkinsonism may accompany basal ganglia and substantia nigra lesions (272).

The patient's movement abilities should be assessed by the physiatrist, physical therapist, and occupational therapist (273). Weakness can be addressed through active assistive range-of-motion and progressive resistive exercises. Occult peripheral neuropathy is common in TBI, particularly in contracted limbs with HO (274). Therefore, focal weakness with atrophy should be evaluated by EMG, because the prognosis for recovery with surgical treatment is excellent.

Ataxia is notoriously difficult to treat. A weighted walker or wrist cuffs may be of modest benefit. If ataxia varies markedly from proximal to distal joints, selective splinting or strategies to stabilize the extremity may be useful.

An attempt should be made to diagnose tremors specifically with reference to their frequency, amplitude, and occurrence during action, rest, and sleep (275). L-Dopa and propranolol both have been used in movement disorders such as tremors and ataxia, but functional tests should be performed on and off medication to assess efficacy in individual patients (276). Some improvement in disability may be seen with botulinum toxin injections (277). Orthoses and adaptive devices may assist weak or ataxic patients in performing functional tasks. Dexterity exercises may be used to increase manual speed and coordination.

Slowed motor responses are among the most common deficits associated with TBI and may limit self-care and employment productivity. It appears, however, that much of this motor slowness can be attributed to central processing delays rather than a motor deficit *per se* (278). There is no consensus on how to treat this generalized slowness.

Dysarthria sometimes is noted after brain injury and may be the result of either peripheral or central nervous system damage affecting motor control of the speech mechanism. It has been found to occur in people with focal mass lesions of the left hemisphere (279) and in cases of diffuse injury (280). The dysarthric patient may receive oral motor strengthening and coordination exercises to improve articulation, a palatal lift for nasality, and breath support training to improve sustained volume.

Nutrition and Feeding

Traumatic brain injury can produce dramatic increases in basal metabolism, with catabolism, weight loss, and low serum albumin. These metabolic responses occur independently of steroid treatment (281). Thus, the acutely injured patient must have increased caloric and protein intake, but the need for invasive procedures and difficulty in achieving high rates of tube feeding may interfere.

The obtunded patient usually can be fed nasogastrically relatively soon after injury. There is no consensus on how soon to consider gastrostomy or jejunostomy placement in patients who remain obtunded or lack oral motor capability, but enterostomy improves cosmesis and lowers the risk of aspiration and sinusitis (282). Continuous feeding is less likely than bolus feeding to induce vomiting and aspiration. If done overnight, the feedings will not interfere with therapy activities, and the patient will not have a full stomach when engaging in gross motor activities, but regurgitation and aspiration may occur if the patient is fully supine. There is little known about the effect, if any, of nocturnal feeding on circadian rhythm.

Gastroesophageal reflux is common following brain injury even in those without nasogastric tubes (283). It may lead to aspiration and esophagitis. Antacids and acid suppressants may improve esophagitis. Metoclopramide increases gastroesophageal sphincter tone but it can cause sedation and extrapyramidal side effects (284). Cisapride may be a better choice because it lacks dopaminergic effects (285). Age, past medical history, dosage, and potential drug interactions should be carefully considered because of reports of associated cardiac abnormalities (286,287). Head elevation may reduce aspiration of regurgitated feedings.

In patients with recurrent pneumonia and possible aspiration, more distal placement of feeding tubes should be considered. This may be done by means of surgical jejunostomy or through fluoroscopic guidance of a tube through the gastrostomy site into the jejunum. The gastric source of the aspiration should be confirmed, however, because some patients may merely be aspirating oral secretions and will not benefit from jejunal tubes. Adding methylene blue or food coloring to gastrostomy tube feedings and suctioning from a tracheostomy or scanning the lungs for radioactive tracers introduced into the stomach are two useful alternatives.

Obstacles to oral feeding include both cognitive and oral motor deficits (288). Attempts at oral feeding generally begin with assessment of the reflexive and voluntary components of oral motor function by a speech, occupational, or physical therapist experienced in dysphagia treatment. This is followed, if necessary, by an oral motor facilitation treatment program to decrease the latency of the swallowing reflex and improve oral motor strength and coordination.

When appropriate, small quantities of pureed foods are introduced and increased in amount to build endurance. As performance improves, the variety of thickness and texture is increased until liquids can be handled safely. Failure to become a functional feeder is associated with persistently poor intraoral manipulation or cognitive levels below V on the Ranchos Los Amigos Scale.

Patients who appear to be candidates for oral feeding but who have frequent coughing or an episode of clinical aspiration may benefit from a videofluoroscopy performed collaboratively by an experienced feeding therapist and a radiologist (see Chapter 12) (289). By using different food textures and placements, it may be possible to determine a strategy to normalize swallowing. Videofluoroscopy as a screening test is not appropriate because its predictive validity for aspiration pneumonia is unknown.

When the patient has made maximal progress in terms of food quantity and texture, the patient or family and nursing staff should be trained in the optimal oral feeding methods.

Bowel and Bladder Dysfunction

Frontal lobe lesions, so common in TBI, can impair inhibitory control over bowel and bladder evacuation, leading to urgency and incontinence (290). Clinically, postvoid residuals seldom are elevated in incontinent brain-injured patients, suggesting that, if neurogenic bladder exists, it is usually of the uninhibited detrusor type. Detrusor–sphincter dyssynergia can occur, however, particularly with significant brainstem involvement below the pontine micturition center (291). Slowed mobility, poor communication, and impaired initiation also contribute to incontinence indirectly.

The presence of a neurogenic bladder can be assessed by noting the frequency and volume of individual voids and measuring the postvoid residual. Normal residuals with frequent small voids suggest an uninhibited detrusor reflex. The patient can be managed with frequent toileting. If the needed frequency is not feasible, anticholinergic medications may increase bladder capacity (292); however, the physician must be aware of the potential for urinary retention, sedation, and memory impairment.

Once a feasible voiding pattern is established, a behavioral toileting program designed around the patient's high-probability voiding times is instituted (293). When the patient is successful in this program, attempts should be made to teach initiation of toileting.

If a toileting program is unsuccessful, a cystometrogram (CMG) EMG may help clarify the patient's degree of sensation and voluntary control. If continence is not a feasible goal, a condom catheter is an option for men. Condom catheters carry an increased risk of urinary tract infection when used in agitated patients who manipulate or kink the tubing (294). Absorbent pads for women are less ideal but have a lower risk of infection than indwelling catheters.

Bowel management is similar to that in other neurologic disabilities. Regulation of stool consistency and induction of a regularly timed bowel movement will help the majority of patients remain continent.

COGNITIVE IMPAIRMENTS AFTER TRAUMATIC BRAIN INJURY

Traumatic brain injury is by nature a diffuse and multifocal insult. For this reason, there is great variability in the patterns of cognitive impairments, depending on the pattern and severity of focal gray and white matter lesions. Neuropsychological investigation of individual patients can be highly informative but generally should not be performed too early, when generalized confusion will produce invalid results. Administration of standardized batteries may be useful for research or medicolegal purposes or for documenting the pace of neurologic recovery or deterioration. For guiding treatment planning, however, focused assessment that attends to the *process* of cognitive performance rather than the quality of the end result is most useful because it may reveal the underlying cognitive mechanism of errors that are made.

Despite the variability in cognitive deficits, certain common patterns exist. This is most likely related to the common areas of gray matter injury (i.e., frontal and temporal poles) and white matter damage (i.e., midbrain and corpus callosum). Even mildly injured individuals may complain of difficulty with alertness, memory, and concentration (7). These same deficits appear in more severe forms in seriously injured patients who may have, in addition, significant disorders of perception, communication, and interpersonal behavior.

Impairments of Arousal and Attention

Deficits in arousal and attention are among the most widespread (278). The comatose patient suffers from profoundly impaired arousal, and many of the cognitive and emotional complaints in minor TBI are hypothesized to be attentional in nature (278). Arousal may be defined as the general state of responsiveness to environmental stimuli. Normally, arousal undergoes slow fluctuations in relation to diurnal rhythm, temperature, and activity level (i.e., tonic arousal). Arousal also can be modulated over brief intervals by demands in the environment (i.e., phasic arousal) (295). The reticular activating system (RAS) has a primary role in control of arousal, exerting its influence over diffuse cortical regions and receiving cortical inputs in return (296). Damage to the RAS plays a critical part in coma onset (49,118). In principle, a deficit in tonic arousal could lead to generalized impairments in responsiveness and profound slowing of information processing. Impaired phasic arousal could interfere with the ability to modify arousal to cope with cognitively demanding situations.

Attention may be considered to be the selective channeling of arousal. Attention (associated with conscious awareness) is directed to a particular set of internal or external stimuli out of the infinite set of possible targets of awareness. Attention is not a unitary phenomenon either in psychological or neurophysiological terms, and there is no precise agreement about how to divide up its component processes; at the least, the following phenomena can be distinguished (297,298):

- **Arousal**: the state of receptivity to sensory information and readiness to respond.
- **Selection** (sometimes referred to as focused attention): the ability to focus attention on particular stimuli or responses. Selection is often made on spatial grounds (i.e., selecting a stimulus in a certain location), and damage, particularly to right parietal or frontal lobes, can interfere with normal spatial selective attention (hemispatial neglect).
- **Strategic control**: the ability to sustain attention over time, inhibit disruption by distracting influences, shift attention in line with changing goals and priorities, manipulate information currently held in mind (referred to as working memory), and divide attention between 2 or more task demands.
- **Processing speed**: the speed at which information is transmitted within the nervous system to allow cognitive processing to occur.

Numerous brain regions appear to play a role in attentional processes. Research has particularly highlighted the roles of the right hemisphere and prefrontal regions in attentional function (299,300). Disorders of attention may impair learning and performance in several ways. Affected patients may have difficulty focusing on any task, may be easily distracted, or may show hemispatial neglect. Attention deficits can lead to secondary decreases in language comprehension or visuospatial processing because the patient's information processing is interrupted and disorganized. Inability to shift attention might be manifested, for example, in the inability to attend to task instructions and also monitor one's own performance. It has been suggested that PTA is most appropriately considered a confusional state related to attention deficit rather than a true memory disturbance (55). Similarly, frontal lobe disorders such as impulsivity and perseveration may be interpreted in attentional terms. These disorders may reflect a loss of goal-directed control over attention such that attention is easily pulled or dysfunctionally fixed on irrelevant aspects of a task (299).

Exactly which of these aspects of attention are disrupted in TBI remains a subject of some controversy. There is general agreement that processing speed is reduced in TBI, but the location of this slowing in the stream of information processing is still under debate. Recent laboratory research shows that patients with TBI have difficulties with sustained attention (301) but that phasic arousal to auditory stimuli is preserved even in severe injury (302). Moreover, when performing independent work in distracting environments, individuals with TBI have more off-task behavior than uninjured controls both in the presence of distractions and in their absence (303). On the basis of the many attentional studies in TBI, it appears that, other than slowed processing, most attentional complaints can be linked to strategic control of attention rather than basic arousal or selection. Strategic control, in turn, is believed to be dependent on prefrontal and limbic goals and motivations being linked to basic attentional mechanisms.

Arousal and attention are assessed best by a combination of formal neuropsychological tests such as line bisection (304), letter cancellation (305), digit span (306), and behavioral observation by all disciplines (298). It is critical to arrive at more precise diagnoses than "impaired attention" because impairments of different components of attention have different therapeutic implications. In general, treatment of these disorders can be grouped in terms of pharmacologic, behavioral, and compensatory strategies (Table 49-9).

Many medications used for other purposes have negative effects on arousal, attention, and general cognitive function. Anticonvulsants such as phenytoin and phenobarbital, antihypertensives such as methyldopa and propranolol, and antispasticity drugs such as diazepam, baclofen, and dantrolene all may impair cognitive performance (213,260, 264,307). Therefore, attempts should be made to withdraw such medications or replace them with less sedating alterna-

TABLE 49-9. *Treatment of disorders of arousal and attention*

Component	Pharmacologic[a]	Behavioral[a]	Compensatory strategy[a]
Tonic arousal	Methylphenidate[b] D-Amphetamine Pemoline Nonsedating tricyclics Amantadine Bromocriptine	Naps Upright position	Engage in tasks when most alert
Phasic arousal		Frequent task changes	Give alerting clues
Selective attention		Reinforce attention	Nondistracting environment
Hemispatial neglect	Bromocriptine	Graded training to attend to left	Position tasks to the patient's right
Strategic control		Training in hierarchic attention skills	Simplify decision making, provide supervision, train solutions to specific problems
Processing speed		Reinforce rapid performance	Allow adequate time for responding

[a] Note that most of these treatments are investigational.
[b] All of these medications may have uses beyond regulation of arousal and act on other components of the attentional network. Their respective roles are under investigation.

tives (e.g., carbamazepine, ACE inhibitors, phenol nerve blocks) (148,265).

The role of pharmacologic treatment remains controversial. Some studies have suggested attentional benefits from psychostimulants such as methylphenidate (308–310) but are subject to methodologic criticisms (small numbers of subjects, inadequate control for spontaneous recovery, and failure to specify which attentional components are being assessed). Although methylphenidate has been reported to increase seizure risk, this is not well documented, and research suggests that, on the contrary, it may have some anticonvulsant effect (311). Other dopaminergic drugs such as amantadine and bromocriptine have been reported to improve attentiveness or diminish hemispatial neglect (311–313). Selection of appropriate patients for drug treatment, however, has not been clarified. Therefore, it is recommended that, when a patient is being considered for pharmacologic therapy of attention deficits, individualized measures of the behaviors of interest be assessed both on and off the medication (314).

Behavioral retraining of attention has been advocated but is of uncertain efficacy. Some studies have suggested benefit from retraining of patients with neglect or distractibility (315–317), whereas others have failed to document changes (318–320). Few of the studies that demonstrate improvement have assessed generalization of benefits to the everyday environment. Even when the patient's attention deficit cannot be treated effectively, teaching strategies and the environment can be modified to help accommodate or compensate for attentional deficits.

In uninjured people, extensive practice of virtually any task leads to the ability to perform it with minimal attention (i.e., automatically) (321). This phenomenon has received little study in brain-damaged patients; however, it would seem possible to deal with some attentional impairments by practicing activities to such a degree that they no longer place much demand on disordered attentional processes.

One of the concerns in treatment is to ensure that strategies learned in a therapy environment are carried over into a variety of functional activities. Therefore, if a team member is training spatial attention in, for example, reading, interdisciplinary plans should be made to transfer the same protocol to other settings such as ambulation and ADL tasks.

Impairments of Learning and Memory

Memory impairments are among the most common, persistent, and handicapping of the cognitive complaints after TBI. All patients with moderate to severe injuries, and most with mild injuries, experience permanent amnesia for the events immediately preceding and following the injury. These intervals are referred to as retrograde and posttraumatic amnesias, respectively. As patients recover from the acute confusional state postinjury, retrograde amnesia typically "shrinks" toward the present (322). The final interval unaccounted for ranges from minutes to weeks or months, depending on the severity of the injury; retrograde amnesias covering several years are not unknown. PTA is the interval of permanently lost memory following the injury; it covers both coma and the acute confusional state and is nearly always longer than retrograde amnesia. As noted earlier, its duration is one of the best measures of injury severity.

These permanent gaps in memory are often emotionally disturbing to patients who must reconstruct the missing interval by obtaining reports from others. Retrograde and posttraumatic amnesias also have legal ramifications, particularly when injuries are caused by assaults or reckless driving; medical professionals may need to intervene with the legal system when patients are asked to testify about events they are unable to remember.

Most individuals with TBI suffer from ongoing deficits in anterograde memory, i.e., difficulty in storing and retrieving new information, well beyond the resolution of PTA. Traumatic brain injury has been associated with persistent impairments in the ability to learn and recall novel information on a variety of laboratory-type tasks (e.g., list learning, reproduction or recognition of visual stimuli, paragraph recall) (35,323). These impairments are correlated, although imperfectly, with the everyday memory complaints of patients and their caretakers (324). The substrate of memory deficits after TBI is not fully understood; however, memory test scores have been shown to correlate with the degree of posttraumatic atrophy of the hippocampus, a limbic structure thought to play an important role in new learning (325). Given the prevalence of attentional deficits in TBI, it is also plausible that some so-called memory impairment can be attributed to defective processing of information at the time of presentation (326,327). However, one recent study showed that challenging attentional resources at the time of stimulus encoding did not disproportionately affect the later recall of TBI patients (328). Among the other cognitive processes that affect memory performance, frontal executive function appears to play an important role. Frontal dysfunction may lead to defective use of strategies during encoding or storage of information and/or a disorganized mental search at the time of retrieval (326).

Executive dysfunction (see next section) may also underlie commonly seen impairments in prospective memory, which is the ability to remember to do something in the future. Although this may require memory for instructions using anterograde memory processes, it appears also to require participation of frontal processes that maintain an active goal state over time and provide "triggers" for action at the appropriate moment (329,330). Thus, TBI patients may be able to recall specifics of the tasks they were supposed to perform even though they fail to perform them at the necessary time.

Early research on memory impairments after TBI was concerned with documenting the types of tests or tasks that could quantify the deficit and with correlating memory test performance with injury variables such as severity or presence and laterality of mass lesions. More recent investigators have been inspired in part by newer models of normal memory, which distinguish between *explicit, effortful* learning—the conscious process needed to memorize a list of words, for example—and *implicit, automatic* learning, which can take place without conscious awareness. There is growing evidence that the latter type of process is spared after TBI relative to the former. For example, severely injured TBI patients are much better able to recall actions they have recently performed than to memorize a word list when the tasks are roughly equivalent in difficulty in other ways (331). It is thought that memory for actions is dependent on automatic, noneffortful memory processes. Similar results have been found using incidental learning of a repeated pattern (332) and long-term memory for naturalistic pictorial scenes (333). The performance of TBI patients is typically worse than normal on such tasks but superior to their performance on effortful memory tasks. Even patients in PTA, who are densely amnesic from day to day, improve with practice on skills or tasks that are not dependent on explicit memory (i.e., they demonstrate *procedural learning*) (334). Patients in PTA can also learn factual verbal information if it is presented in a format that capitalizes on their more intact implicit memory (335).

To date, the standardized tests of memory that are widely used in clinical settings have not reflected these conceptualizations of memory function. The most widely used test of memory, the Wechsler Memory Scale–Revised (336), tests only explicit, effortful learning over a limited exposure interval. An alternative battery, the Rivermead Behavioral Memory Test (337), includes a subtest of prospective memory and requires the subject to learn more functionally oriented material (e.g., name–face pairs instead of word pairs). There are many other well-normed tests of memory suitable for the evaluation of TBI that have been thoroughly reviewed (338). It is relatively uninformative to test memory in isolation, however, because of the probability that attentional deficits, executive dysfunction, and other cognitive disorders (e.g., limitations in language processing) will affect the results of memory tests as well as real-world memory performance. Evaluation of memory after TBI should not rely on testing alone. It should also include a functional assessment by the interdisciplinary team and the family or caretakers to identify the environmental situations in which the disorder disrupts function and the frequency with which real-world memory problems occur.

The remediation of memory deficits has received a great deal of attention in recent years. Despite the intuitive and popular appeal of "exercise" analogies, there is no convincing evidence that simply practicing memory tasks produces generalized improvement in memory function (337). Thus, the commercially available computerized memory games and drills appear to lack therapeutic value for TBI patients. The ability to use nonverbal memory to compensate for verbal memory deficits or vice versa has shown some promise in laboratory settings, but patients have not demonstrated spontaneous use of such strategies. This could be because the strategies require considerable conscious effort (339) and because their practical applications are limited. The teaching of specific strategies appears to be more effective than practice drills or no training at all, although the benefit appears to dissipate after training (340). In clinical settings, by far the most common remedial approach is to teach compensatory strategies for everyday use, such as writing in date books, diaries, organizers, etc. The success of these approaches, however, depends on an individual's awareness of memory deficits and acceptance of the need to use prosthetic devices, both of which may be problematic. Even if they use written strategies, individuals with TBI may not benefit from them as much as uninjured persons do (341). In addition, they may have difficulty with the executive demands of these strategies, i.e., knowing *what* to record *when*, remembering to do it consistently, and using recorded information prospectively. Schmitter-Edgecombe and colleagues used a structured training regimen to teach TBI patients how to use memory notebooks, with beneficial effects on measures of everyday memory function (342). Other devices have obviated executive demands with computerized prosthetics that, in essence, supply the executive functions of memory. Success has been reported with an interactive computer that cues and monitors vocational performance (343) and with a paging device that reminds the individual of specific tasks to be completed throughout the day (344).

Another approach to the rehabilitation of individuals with memory disorders is to use so-called *errorless learning*. As shown by Wilson and her colleagues (345,346), patients with severe learning and memory deficits learn new skills much more efficiently and show less forgetting when they are prevented from making errors during the learning process. Glisky (347) has used a similar approach to train factual job-related knowledge to amnesics, essentially preventing errors by providing many repetitions of material that is gradually "faded" as the patient learns it. For both skill-based and knowledge-based learning, the ability to benefit from a trial-and-error approach may take more explicit or effortful processing than is available to memory-impaired patients.

As yet there is little convincing evidence that memory can be enhanced pharmacologically after TBI. The controlled studies in this area have been reviewed by Wroblewski and Glenn (310).

For the rehabilitation setting the following summary points should be considered:

- Most TBI patients benefit more from hands-on training of procedural skills than from verbally based or didactic instruction.
- The learning of TBI patients should be judged more by changes in their performance than by their verbal self-report, as learning can take place of which patients are unaware.
- Errorless learning can be effective for patients with severe memory impairments. It may be necessary to provide hand-over-hand assistance (e.g., during the training of ADL) to prevent the patient from making errors. This assistance can be gradually faded as the patient begins to initiate more of the actions correctly.
- Memory notebooks are useful for many patients. They are most effective when the entire rehabilitation team focuses on teaching only one or two applications (e.g., scheduling appointments, recording phone calls). This allows the team to achieve more consistency in teaching "how and when to record what." As the patient masters the strategy, the team can add more applications (e.g., recording important daily events).

Impairments of Frontal Executive Function

The mark of intelligent behavior is the ability to adapt to change, solve unexpected problems, anticipate outcomes, and otherwise cope with situations that fall outside of one's routine. These abilities in turn require cognitive flexibility, self-monitoring, and self-adjustment of performance as well as simultaneous consideration of multiple alternatives and their probable consequences. From these alternatives an appropriate plan of action must be selected and the intention carried out over time. Complex abilities such as these, which are thought to provide superordinate controls for adaptive human behavior, have been termed *executive functions*. There is considerable evidence that executive functions, though they are surely subserved by more than one region of the brain, are highly dependent on the integrity of prefrontal cortex (299,329,348,349). Traumatic brain injury, which often involves damage to the frontal poles and orbitomesial cortex (350,351), commonly leads to disorders of reasoning, planning, and goal-directed behavior attributable to breakdowns in executive function. Depending on the nature and severity of the injury as well as premorbid factors, these impairments may appear clinically as disorganized speech and action, aimless behavior, or stimulus-boundedness (i.e., a tendency to be "pulled" by irrelevant stimuli), aberrant or inappropriate interpersonal or sexual behavior, and impulsive and/or perseverative thought and action (352). Lack of insight into these and other deficits and poor ability to profit from feedback are usually part of the clinical picture.

Most conceptualizations of executive function include the notion of attentional control, especially the balancing of internal and external inputs guiding behavior. Normal attention is externally controlled at times. For example, one attends to a loud noise or bright moving object. Attention is also normally modulated, however, in the service of one's intentions. For example, if the goal is to get to an appointment as rapidly as possible, one will be more likely to attend to street signs and less likely to attend to shop windows. For such modulation to occur, emotional and motivational states must be linked to perceptual and motor systems so that the appropriate aspects of the environment may be attended and acted on, and the irrelevant ones screened out. The breakdown of this linkage contributes to the distractibility and aimlessness of many TBI patients. There is growing evidence that failures in this attentional control of action can account for the disorganized ADL performances, including flagrant and bizarre misuse of objects, seen in many acute or severely injured TBI patients (353).

Another important aspect of executive function is control over one's responses to people and situations, such that some behaviors are inhibited in favor of others that are more appropriate to the context. For example, to meet certain interpersonal needs, one must judge, then select, which of many possible behaviors will achieve the goal and fit with the social milieu. Individuals with TBI often appear to lack this judgment, behaving in ways that appear inappropriate and short-sighted to others. Thus a patient may exhibit a sexually aggressive manner with a therapist to whom he is attracted, oblivious not only to her anger and discomfort but also to the certainty that his behaviors will not be rewarded.

These deficits are among the most difficult to address for several reasons. They remain poorly understood in terms of their neuropsychological and neurophysiological underpinnings. By virtue of late phylogenetic and ontological development, frontal executive functions may show more interindividual variation than relatively hard-wired functions (e.g. perception and language). Thus, two people could have identical prefrontal injuries yet display different patterns of executive dysfunction (352). Assessment of these abilities is also complicated by the fact that they are least obvious in highly structured and routine environments such as hospitals. Because executive disorders relate to the ability to deal with novelty and change, they are difficult to see within structured tasks but must be looked for in challenging or open-ended situations. Patients may do fairly well on traditional neuropsychological tests yet show profound life disruption from executive dysfunction. Recent attempts to capture these deficits with tests of planning and prioritizing have failed to show effects of frontal damage from TBI (354,355). Specially designed tests that rely on coordination and shifting of task goals have proved more sensitive (322,356). In addition, Varney and colleagues (357) developed an executive dysfunction interview for relatives of TBI patients that may be particularly sensitive to the effects of orbitofrontal injury.

Attempts to treat executive impairments have been based on one of three general perspectives (358). At one extreme, the clinician may conclude that the deficits are irremediable and that the physical and social environments will therefore need to be fully structured in order to guide every aspect of the patient's adaptive behavior. In this view, the treatment consists of determining and implementing the specific environmental conditions that will elicit and support the desired behaviors. A less "hopeless" view seeks to train specific behaviors that are disrupted by executive dysfunction, e.g., socially acceptable behaviors or the solution to a frequently occurring problem. Treatment is task- or behavior-specific and generalization to untrained situations is not expected. The third approach assumes that central processes such as cognitive flexibility and self-monitoring may be remediated, with the hope of improving the patient's response to a broad range of unanticipated circumstances.

There is, as yet, little controlled research on the efficacy of these treatment strategies and even less guidance as to how to select strategies for the individual case. Behavior modification strategies can been used to increase prosocial behavior and decrease inappropriate behavior after TBI (359), but generalization beyond the target behavior may not occur. There have been some attempts to develop training procedures that will have a broader impact on planning and problem solving. These programs teach skills such as how to break complex problems down into manageable units (360), and how to instruct oneself through a multiple step task (361). Encouraging results have been reported on specific measures of problem solving, but the impact on patients' everyday function has not yet been thoroughly studied.

Executive impairments are of profound functional significance for severely brain-injured patients and are major obstacles to independent living, employment and successful relationships. Until more information is available as to the effectiveness of general strategy training, it would seem prudent not to focus exclusively on retraining abstract capacities, but to include functional problems such as planning a meal, organizing transportation, and the like.

All team members are likely to be involved in addressing these problems. The neuropsychologist may be able to suggest treatment strategies applicable to all disciplines. In addition, each therapist can assist the patient in solving the specific problems faced within tasks. For example, the physical therapist may help the patient plan how to navigate an unfamiliar route, while the occupational therapist may help the patient learn strategies for organizing a menu.

Impairments of Language and Communication

Language disorders following TBI may take many forms, depending on the site and extent of the lesion or lesions. Unlike stroke, classic aphasic syndromes are not prominent after brain injury, unless there is a focal dominant hemisphere lesion. Sarno reported that 30% of her head-injured patients were clinically aphasic at 1 year postinjury (280). In many cases posttraumatic aphasia tends to resolve within the first 6 months. Dysnomia, a deficit in naming or word finding, is perhaps the most common aphasic disturbance seen in TBI. Levin and colleagues reported that anomic aphasia usually takes the form of semantic errors, circumlocution, and concretism (35). The neuroanatomic locus is considered to be the dominant parietal area, although a focal lesion is not necessary for production of the disorder. Dysnomia may be accompanied by elements of dysgraphia, dyslexia, and dyscalculia (362). Verbal fluency may be affected more generally by left frontal or bifrontal lesions (363). Classic alexia is infrequent after TBI, although reading can be impaired by a host of nonlanguage factors such as attentional deficits and eye movement disturbances.

A variety of nonaphasic communication problems also may be manifest after TBI, with major impact on social function. Prigatano found talkativeness in 16% of a sample of TBI survivors who were at least 16 months postinjury (127). He noted that this problem was accompanied by serious interpersonal difficulties and mood disturbance. Hagen reported that the tangential expression of ideas, reflective of fragmented thought processes, was also characteristic of many brain-injured patients (364). Coelho (365) reviewed the literature on discourse production (e.g., conversation or narrative story telling) after TBI. Cohesion of speech is consistently found to be impaired in these studies, as is the overall efficiency of communication (i.e., patients tend to impart less information in longer utterances). Peculiar phraseology, as when patients speak of themselves in the third person, also occurs. Dysprosodia, an impairment of the melody, affective coloring, and cadence of speech, may appear especially with nondominant hemisphere involvement (366).

Still other communication problems manifested after TBI relate to the pragmatics, or social rules, of communication. Patients may have extreme difficulty initiating conversation, participating in give-and-take, staying on topic, and using social cues emitted by the listener. They frequently rely on others to assume most of the burden of communication during an exchange (365). These types of deficits are poorly, if at all, detected by traditional tests of language function. It is helpful to supplement the evaluation of communication after TBI with scales designed to tap the logical structure and pragmatics of speech (367).

In the clinical setting it can be difficult to separate disorders of language and communication from the cognitive impairments that may appear concomitantly. For example, a patient may respond inappropriately to questions asked in a crowded, noisy room because of problems in auditory comprehension, complex information processing, and/or divided attention. For the majority of head-injured people, basic language skills will recover by 6 months postinjury so that they may appear functionally normal to the casual observer. In a more challenging environment such as school or work, however, or in grappling with the communication demands of intimate relationships, language difficulties may come to the fore and pose major obstacles to successful reentry.

The treatment of language impairments often is delegated to the speech–language pathologist on the rehabilitation team. In the case of aphasia, techniques such as visual–auditory cuing, gestures, and object-naming exercises are used. For the severely dysarthric patient who has limited speech but relatively intact comprehension, augmentative communication devices may be provided. Structured *in vivo* modeling and shaping techniques known as incidental teaching have been found effective in improving the completeness and intelligibility of utterances (368).

It is important to ensure that the strategies that optimize language are shared among all disciplines so that consistent demands are placed on the patient in all environments, and consistent cues are provided to maximize practice opportunities. Another critical part of treatment involves the education and counseling of family members. Speech–language pathologists, as well as other team members, provide specific information to families about the nature of language disorders, their relationship to the brain injury, prognosis for recovery, and ways in which family members can facilitate recovery of language skills or use compensatory techniques to circumvent fixed deficits. The role of the family in facilitating communication is very important. It can be intensely frustrating for both patients and family members when the patient cannot make his or her needs understood or when family members fail to adjust their own communications to accommodate the patient's limitations.

Pragmatic disorders of communication, such as tangentiality and overtalkativeness, can be treated within structured groups in which audiotape, videotape, and listener feedback is provided immediately. In addition, patients can benefit from modeling of good communication skills by other group members and group leaders.

Impairments of Visuospatial Perception and Construction

Visuospatial disorders are observed less commonly than other disorders after TBI, perhaps because the posterior areas of the brain are less often damaged than the frontal and temporal regions. A brain-injured patient may perform poorly on visually mediated or spatial activities because of deficits in attention, problem solving, organization, or motor deficits rather than visuospatial deficits *per se.*

Nevertheless, several types of visuospatial perception disorders can be identified. Prosopagnosia, the inability to recognize familiar faces, is an unusual disorder that has been studied extensively by Benton (369). The etiology of this condition is usually vascular, and it has been correlated with bilateral lesions, although the right inferior occipitotemporal region appears crucial (369,370). Levin and Peters reported a case of posttraumatic prosopagnosia that persisted for several months (371). In addition, TBI patients without clinical evidence of the disorder have difficulty discriminating unfamiliar faces (372). Deficits in the ability to interpret the emotions of others from their facial expressions can also occur, particularly with involvement of the nondominant hemisphere. Other visuospatial deficits include visual scanning disturbances, alterations in body schema, and impaired perception of form, spatial relations, color, and figure–ground relationships (373). Even if perception appears intact, patients may have difficulty organizing or reproducing complex visuospatial stimuli, e.g., in drawing or constructional tasks. Visuospatial disorders have functional consequences in many areas of daily life skills such as dressing, grooming, preparation of meals and eating, driving a vehicle, ambulating, writing, and performing manual assembly tasks (374).

A variety of tests can be used to determine the presence of visuospatial dysfunction and to differentiate perceptual from constructional disorders. Tests such as the Frostig, Rey-Osterreith Complex Figure, or Block Design can reveal difficulties in the visuospatial domains. The Motor Free Visual Perception Test may be used to ascertain whether a gross visuospatial problem exists independent of constructional abilities. In general, patients with nondominant hemisphere lesions will tend to display greater and more dramatic impairment in perceptual and constructional functions than those with dominant hemisphere lesions (375).

A variety of treatment techniques may be used to attempt to remediate or compensate for these problems. A mirror to provide visual feedback while dressing or walking may be used to treat disturbances of body schema. Reliance on verbal or written cues instead of gestures or environmental cues may help patients with generalized visuospatial problems when working on functional activities such as ambulation, transfers, or route finding. None of these treatment approaches has been validated extensively. Therefore, it is critical to document changes in performance objectively and to verify that they transfer to meaningful functional tasks.

Cognitive Remediation

In recent years, cognitive remediation has become a fundamental component of the treatment offered to brain-injured patients in the acute and postacute rehabilitation phases. Since the term was first used, there has been considerable debate over both its definition and its legitimacy. Whereas earlier definitions focused on the idea of remediating specific functions such as memory or perception (376), the recent trend is toward concepts that are more comprehensive and more functional. A position paper by the American Congress of Rehabilitation Medicine (ACRM) Interdisciplinary Special Interest Group in this area broadened the term to *cognitive rehabilitation* and defined it as "a systematic, functionally oriented service of therapeutic cognitive activities . . . directed to achieve functional changes by . . . reinforcing . . . previously learned patterns of behavior, or . . . establishing new patterns of cognitive activity or compensatory mechanisms for impaired neurological systems" (377). Most current definitions acknowledge two contrasting approaches to such rehabilitation: restorative, which seeks to improve directly the diminished function; and compensatory, which aims to teach ways of bypassing the impairment altogether (378). Tension between these differing models has helped to fuel the sometimes passionate debate about the most appropriate way to manage cognitive deficits.

Another aspect of the controversy has been the proliferation of methods or techniques, not always grounded in theory, that some felt were offered prematurely to consumers at an emotional as well as financial cost (130). Early cognitive remediation stressed the use of specialized computer software; however, computer-assisted treatment has not proved more effective than more traditional cognitive therapy (379). In fact, computers may have their greatest value as cognitive orthoses or sophisticated trainers for specific job-related skills (339,343,347,380). There has also been a trend to deemphasize rote exercises (reflecting the restorative model) in favor of a more naturalistic approach to devising compensations for cognitive deficits in the real-world, community environment (381,382). Of the numerous cognitive retraining approaches, only a few have generated any evidence of efficacy (316,317,339,342,383); others have been shown not to be effective (319,320), and many remain to be studied objectively. Some claims of efficacy are difficult to evaluate because the chosen outcome measures have a tenuous relationship with real-life function (e.g., test scores) and/or because subjects are not followed for more than a few weeks.

To date, programs with a more holistic approach to cognitive rehabilitation (i.e., combining skill-based interventions with individual and group psychotherapy, milieu treatment, vocational rehabilitation, family counseling, and awareness training) have been able to produce the most convincing outcome data (127,384,385). The term *neuropsychological rehabilitation* is sometimes used for these comprehensive programs, which include, but also go beyond, the attempted remediation of cognitive skills (386).

SOCIAL AND BEHAVIORAL DISABILITIES

Psychosocial problems are among the leading causes of prolonged disability in individuals with TBI and are a leading source of family stress, relationship failure, and vocational handicap. Such disabilities usually result from a combination of cognitive and behavioral regulation deficits, which interact in complex ways with one another, with mood states, and with idiosyncratic social and environmental variables. Thus, the approach to psychosocial and behavioral disability requires a careful analysis of each problem for the individual.

In the following sections we discuss the behavioral and social problems that face the rehabilitation team working with TBI patients. When thinking about these problems and how to treat them, the clinician should always bear in mind their potential relationships with constellations of cognitive deficits. Simply put, a problem labeled as "behavioral" could be but one manifestation of a compromise in cognitive abilities, and a problem called "social" could refer to one of the final outcomes of the interplay between them. In 20 years of experience with inpatient and outpatient brain injury rehabilitation, we have never evaluated or treated a patient (aside from the rare malingerer) who had injury-related behavioral problems in the absence of cognitive deficits. Some of the cognitive impairments especially predictive of behavioral disturbance, in our experience, are the following:

Deficits in attention, arousal, and information-processing speed can induce patients to act out in frustration when they reach overload. A "normal" level of hallway noise (which can easily be tuned out by staff members) is a culprit in many hospitals, where patients must be parked in the hallway to receive adequate supervision. The simple intervention of moving a patient to a quieter section of the hall can sometimes eliminate disruptive behavior (387). Similarly, patients can exhibit hostile behavior when they are unable to follow what is going on around them. One wife of a severely impaired patient reported that her husband's aggression at home had ceased when she enforced the rule that "only one person talks at a time."

Deficits in perception and communication can also be associated with extreme behavioral dysfunction. Patients may display frank paranoia and agitation as a result of misinterpreting facial expressions and voice tones of staff and family members. Paranoia and symptoms of extreme fear can also result from dominant temporal lesions that severely compromise the ability to decode the communications of others. Expressive dysprosodia has been associated with physical aggression; patients have reported that they felt they "had to take action" because others did not understand the feelings they were trying to communicate. Deficits in the perception of body position or relative distances can cause patients to act out in panic when they perceive themselves to be in danger of falling.

Memory deficits can give rise to a host of behavioral disturbances, including the conviction that others are stealing one's belongings (which are in fact being misplaced by the patient). Memory-impaired patients can become severely withdrawn as a consequence of forgetting the interactions and conversations that comprise the fabric of relationships. They can additionally be perceived as demanding or intrusive if they repeat the same requests or make the same phone calls over and over. Memory disorders also interact with behavioral problems by making it more difficult to design effective learning situations to overcome them.

As mentioned earlier in this chapter, executive dysfunction is nearly always manifested as some form of behavioral disturbance: sexually inappropriate behavior, impulsivity, bizarreness, and rigid "unreasonable" behavior related to concretism are relatively common. An inability to appreciate one's own errors and limitations contributes greatly to the argumentativeness and hostility of many patients with TBI.

We prefer to conceptualize the totality of deficits after TBI as *neurobehavioral,* which reminds us of the underpinnings of behavioral symptoms and avoids at least some of the arbitrary semantic distinctions among them.

Agitated, Aggressive, and Disinhibited Behavior

Behaviors such as thrashing, screaming, striking out, destroying property, and masturbating in public are common occurrences on the inpatient TBI unit. Such behaviors are typical of a generally agitated state as patients emerge from coma and posttraumatic amnesia. In a consecutive series of 100 severe TBI admissions, Brooke et al. (388) documented restlessness in 35 and agitation (defined as aggressive or threatening behaviors) in 11. The factors that predispose to agitation are not known; one study showed that acutely aggressive patients were likely to be older and more likely to be disoriented to both place and time (389). Posttraumatic agitation typically resolves within 2 to 3 weeks of its appearance (388). Its resolution is generally paralleled by improvement in orientation and other cognitive skills as the patient emerges from PTA, lending credence to the clinical view that agitation is a "stage of recovery" for some patients (390).

Medications may exacerbate these behaviors. Benzodiazepines and other sedatives can produce paradoxical agitation (391), perhaps by making the patient less able to process events in the environment and by further impairing inhibitory mechanisms. Psychostimulants given to improve alertness and attention may lead to excessive stimulation and agitation (392). Neuroleptics may produce akathisia that can mimic agitation (393), and they have been reported to produce paradoxical delusions (394).

As discussed in earlier sections of this chapter, some patients with TBI do not fully recover control over volatile or disinhibited behavior. The frontal regions so frequently damaged by TBI are believed to play an important role in inhibition of impulsive and inappropriate responses (90). Thus, in some brain-injured patients, even beyond the acute phase, a minimal provocation can lead to a dramatic outburst of verbal or physical aggression. In slightly milder form, this can present as a chronic irritability, forcing those around the patient to "walk on eggshells." Mood instability is often present, and the patient can sometimes be redirected or distracted following the outburst. However, insight into the consequences of such behavior is typically absent. Miller (395) contrasts this pattern of disinhibited behavior with the pattern that has been termed the *episodic dyscontrol syndrome,* which is thought to reflect not frontal but temporal lobe pathology. In episodic dyscontrol, the outburst can be completely unprovoked. It is typically short-lived, primitive and stereotyped, and not directed at a specific target; the patient commonly suffers deep remorse on becoming aware of the episode afterwards (395). It has been suggested that such outbursts reflect limbic seizure activity or temporal lobe epilepsy (396). In any case, the episodic dyscontrol syndrome is associated with an increased incidence of subtle neurologic signs such as nonlocalizing EEG abnormalities (397).

There are other sources of problematic behavior as well. Patients who are aware of their deficits may display reactive irritability and other behavioral symptoms of depression. Patients who have been institutionalized for some time may have been taught their maladaptive behaviors unintentionally. For example, they may have discovered that screaming or throwing objects receives the prompt attention of staff members. The role of preinjury behavior patterns cannot be discounted. The population of TBI patients includes disproportionate numbers of persons with long-standing problems such as personality disorder, impulsive behavior, and substance abuse.

Treatment of maladaptive behavior may include behavior modification, redirection techniques that help the patient shift attention from the source of the behavior (398), and psychoactive medications. The optimal combination of these elements has not been identified precisely, nor are there agreed-on guidelines for matching patients and treatments. A possible stepwise behavior management protocol is, however, outlined below:

- *Watchful waiting.* Recently injured patients may move rapidly through a stage of combative and agitated behavior (388). In such instances, the best strategy may be to provide intensive staffing, remove dangerous objects, and wait for the patient to calm spontaneously. Environmental conditions that promote calm behavior should be observed and implemented. Inadvertent reinforcement of maladaptive behavior should be avoided.
- *Baseline data.* Patients whose maladaptive behaviors persist require more active intervention. Sedatives and other behaviorally active medications should be withdrawn whenever possible to allow accurate baseline assessment

of the relevant behaviors. Staff members must be prepared for exacerbation but will be surprised by how often the behaviors improve or at least remain stable when sedatives are tapered. Baseline data should be collected by all disciplines using an agreed-on operational definition of the behavior. It is helpful to use quantitative measures developed for this purpose, such as the Agitated Behavior Scale (399) or the Overt Aggression Scale (400). Data should document frequency, duration, or intensity of the behavior, possible environmental factors that may have contributed to it (e.g., a difficult task, a late-arriving meal), and the consequences that followed it (e.g., a need was met, the patient was scolded).

- *Treatment planning.* The entire rehabilitation team should meet to share and analyze data for patterns. A mood disturbance may be revealed by occurrence of a behavior at times of family contact or by episodes of crying. Cognitive impairments may be implicated if the behavior occurs primarily when the patient is working on one content area or frustrated by attempts at communication. Plans should be made to compensate for these deficits by altering the difficulty of tasks or the method of giving instructions. Too often, planning revolves around what to do after a maladaptive behavior occurs. The emphasis should be shifted to prevention of the situations that trigger unwanted acts where possible, and to positive reinforcement and modeling of appropriate behaviors. This might include training patients in appropriate ways of expressing anger and frustration or meeting other needs. The reinforcements that can be used to strengthen these alternative behaviors include food, tokens, and rewards with special significance to the individual patient. Slifer and colleagues (401) reported dramatic increases in prosocial behavior and decreases in uncooperative behavior in acutely brain-injured adolescents using differential reinforcement of appropriate behavior (DRA). In this simple paradigm, social reinforcement (i.e., praise and attention) and other rewards are given for cooperative behaviors, while disruptive behaviors are socially ignored. Such behavior modification techniques do not appear to require explicit memory and thus can be used effectively with cognitively impaired patients (402). Environmental restructuring may also be indicated. For example, if aggression occurs primarily in large group activities, the patient can be treated in small groups and gradually reintroduced to larger groups as behavior improves. Consequences for the maladaptive behavior can range from simple nonreinforcement to timeout or loss of privileges. It is critical for these consequences to be planned by the team at a dispassionate moment, not invoked by angry staff members concerned with making the punishment fit the crime.
- *Reassessment.* It is crucial for the whole team to adopt a uniform treatment approach until reassessment takes place. Continued data collection may reveal dramatic improvement, partial response, or no improvement. Reanalysis may clarify the reasons and allow for modification of the treatment plan. Subjective assessment of change is notoriously unreliable and must be avoided (403). If behavioral analysis reveals partial response or no response, the interventions can be modified for another treatment period, or medications may be considered.
- *Medication trial.* Few guidelines exist for choosing behaviorally active medications, although helpful references have recently become available (404). The physician must select among several alternatives (Table 49-10) and monitor individual patients for efficacy through similar behavioral data collection methods as described above (314). It should be noted, however, that there is no medication effective specifically against, for example, "screaming." Therefore, a drug that decreases screaming also may decrease numerous other, more adaptive behaviors. Therapists should note unwanted changes. Deteriorating performance may also be revealed by repeated neuropsychological tests.

TABLE 49-10. *Psychoactive medications for behavioral management*

Psychostimulants, e.g., methylphenidate, dextroamphetamine, pemoline
Tricyclic antidepressants
Serotonergic agents (SSRIs, buspirone)
Carbamazepine
Valproic acid
Lithium carbonate
Beta blockers
Benzodiazepines[a]
Neuroleptics[a]

[a] Less recommended

We tend to rely on psychostimulants or tricyclic antidepressants to treat undirected restless agitation that occurs early after brain injury and fails to improve with behavioral or environmental measures (403,405). This is based on the theory that such behavior is a reflection of inadequate arousal or attention; in addition, the tricyclics can help to normalize the sleep cycle and to reduce pain that may trigger agitation. In a controlled study, propranolol reduced the intensity of acute TBI agitation, although the number of agitated episodes did not change (406). More alert patients who have episodes of aggression or agitation may benefit from carbamazepine, valproic acid, lithium carbonate, or high-dose beta blockers (407–410). We have also seen positive effects with serotonergic agonists, particularly trazodone, in hyperaroused verbally or physically aggressive patients. In many patients, neuroleptics have a nonspecific depressant effect on behavior. Thus, we reserve them for the relatively infrequent crisis situations when sedation is the overt treatment goal and less toxic drugs have proved inadequate. Occasional patients may benefit, with minimal sedation, from low doses of neuroleptics. This should be assessed on an individual basis, usually after other agents have failed. We rarely prescribe benzodiazepines except for sleep because the agitation of

TBI differs from true anxiety, and we have seen little evidence of efficacy.

The literature includes reports of medications that have been used for specific problem behaviors. For example, Emory and colleagues (411) used Depo-Provera (Upjohn, Kalamazoo, MI) for intractable hypersexuality in eight TBI patients. All problematic sexual behaviors ceased during a 6-month course of medication (combined with psychotherapy), and there were unexpected improvements in concentration and other cognitive functions. When drug therapy was stopped, some patients showed reappearance of the unwanted behaviors, but others remained symptom-free.

All psychoactive medications should be reassessed periodically by attempted tapering to determine their continued utility and lowest effective dose. We have found double-blind, placebo-controlled trials with behavioral ratings to be of great clinical value in determining drug efficacy for individual patients (403).

When acceptable behavior has been achieved in the controlled clinical environment, it should be generalized into home and community settings. Family members should be taught relevant interventions, including how to deal with behavioral regression when the patient is exposed to new people or environments. Careful attention to generalization of appropriate behavior has been shown to allow transition to less restrictive environments for severely impaired patients (128). There has recently been more acknowledgment of the critical role played by family members and other caretakers in the long-term maintenance of behavioral gains after severe TBI, and more explicit programming designed to train involved lay persons in basic behavior analysis and modification techniques (412).

Reduced Initiation

Some brain-injured patients simply fail to act without extensive cuing or structure imposed from without. In extreme cases, patients may be able to describe a course of action verbally, and express a sincere intention to carry it out, but still do nothing. This type of deficit may accompany particular patterns of neurologic damage that disrupt the linkage between limbic motivational inputs and the cognitive and motor components of action (413). Lesions of the mesial surface of the frontal cortex may be particularly disruptive to initiation of action based on internal states, whereas dorsolateral prefrontal injury may interfere with the ability to maintain an active goal state over time (414).

Impaired initiation is a difficult rehabilitation problem for a number of reasons. It may be difficult to differentiate from disorders of mood (i.e., depression) or impaired arousal. This may be a problem of differential diagnosis because there are shared behavioral characteristics among the three conditions. However, these common characteristics could point to some underlying neurophysiological mechanisms subserving mood, arousal, and initiation such that these are not completely independent phenomena. We have seen patients who demonstrate striking increases in initiation in response to psychostimulants or activating tricyclics such as protriptyline in the absence of overt signs of depression or lethargy. Both desipramine and amitriptyline have been used to improve arousal and initiation after very severe TBI, sometimes with dramatic results (415). Dopaminergic agonists such as Sinemet, bromocriptine, or pergolide may also be helpful in improving initiation. Marin and colleagues (416) report several cases of improvement in organically based apathetic behavior (i.e., diminished interest or initiation in the absence of depression) after treatment with methylphenidate, bupropion, and dopaminergic agonists.

Commonly used rehabilitative approaches to impaired initiation include physical, verbal, written, or pictorial cues for the steps involved in a task, with behavioral reinforcement for proceeding from one step to the next rather than for completion of the previous step. Structured time frames for task completion, enforced by timers and buzzers, may also be of help. We have successfully used "real-time" tape-recorded step-by-step instructions, in the patient's own voice, to help several patients with large right frontal lobe lesions to initiate and complete the steps of showering, dressing, and grooming without having to rely on a caretaker for these cues.

Difficulty is often encountered in generalizing to varied tasks. That is, the patient may learn to initiate a morning ADL sequence but show no improvement in starting homework independently. Development of prompting strategies that can be used across tasks may be of help. For example, if a patient learns to use a timer to prompt a dressing sequence, it may be possible to use the same device for other tasks with minimal new learning required. Obviously, this requires interdisciplinary treatment planning.

Disorders of initiation can have profound effects on independent living and psychosocial function. Whereas patients with severe physical disabilities often have the help of personal care attendants, little appreciation is given to the need for cueing or prompting by attendants. In some instances, individuals with TBI might be able to live semi-independently with the assistance of someone to check their progress periodically and prompt completion of necessary tasks. However, even if an individual can function with this level of assistance, he or she will probably still have difficulty with initiation beyond the bare necessities, e.g., leisure activities, new friendships, or new ideas for life goals. Family members require explicit education about these deficits, as otherwise they are prone to interpret such behavior as laziness or poor motivation.

Depression

Depression is very common after TBI and has a major impact on functional and psychosocial outcome. Studies of patients involved in TBI rehabilitation have found that well over half are significantly depressed or have been at some point since the injury (417–419). A prospective study of 66 unselected, consecutive admissions for acute TBI revealed that 28 met the criteria for major depressive disorder at some time during the first year (420). In most follow-up studies of TBI, depressed mood is reported by both client and family for years after the injury. In fact, Brooks and associates (21) reported that depression appeared to increase from 1 to 5 years postinjury, according to relatives' reports. Posttraumatic depression is often accompanied by other disturbances of emotional function, such as anxiety or lability of mood (421). Concomitant depression and anxiety in patients' spouses is also reported (418).

Depression after TBI probably results from both neurologic and psychosocial factors. The diffuse axonal injury of TBI induces acute disruption of neurotransmitter systems. It is plausible that neurotransmitter depletion, particularly in noradrenergic and serotonergic systems, could contribute to acute depressive symptomatology (421). Interestingly, in the prospective study cited above, Jorge and colleagues (420) found a subgroup of "transiently depressed" patients whose symptoms cleared within 3 months. Transient depression was most often associated with left frontal or subcortical lesions. This is reminiscent of the robust association between left hemisphere lesions and depression in stroke patients (422). However, other investigators have failed to find correlations between lesion site and depression after TBI, nor does severity of the injury appear to be a good predictor of mood disorder (127).

The development of depression after TBI may be influenced by pre- as well as postinjury psychosocial factors, although these remain poorly understood. Prior psychiatric disorder may predispose to posttraumatic depression (423), although some studies have shown negligible effects of both personal and familial psychiatric history (424).

Reactive depression appears to be the most common form of depression after TBI. Prigatano described depression reactive to TBI as a constellation of symptoms including "feelings of worthlessness, helplessness, loss of interest in work and family activities and decreased libido" (127). It may occur weeks, months, or years after the initial neurologic insult but often signals the individual's fuller recognition of the deficits and life changes caused by the injury. In some studies depression has been correlated with the degree of self-reported, as opposed to objectively measured, disability (424). It has also been reported that as organic unawareness of deficits begins to resolve, depression becomes more manifest (425).

The diagnosis of TBI-related depression can be complicated. Silver and Yudofsky (421) enumerate the issues that the physician must consider:

- Medications commonly administered to TBI patients can cause or exacerbate depression. These include anticonvulsants, narcotics, and benzodiazepines.
- Depression may predate the injury even if it has never been diagnosed. Premorbid alcohol abuse and injury circumstances that hint at self-destructive behavior are common indicators.
- As mentioned previously in this chapter, the behavioral appearance of depression can be confused with that of organic apathy, indifference, or impaired initiation.
- The vegetative signs of depression, such as insomnia or hypersomnia, or decreased appetite, may be present for other reasons after TBI in patients who are not depressed. However, one study showed that some vegetative signs do appear more frequently in TBI patients who also complain of depressed mood (426). The usual cognitive signs of depression (e.g., difficulty in concentrating) are useless for making the diagnosis following TBI.

Whatever the exact etiology of posttraumatic depression, it has a tremendous impact on rehabilitation outcomes, social functioning, and quality of life. Depression has been consistently linked to poor outcome following TBI (427). Depressed mood may be only one manifestation of a psychological reaction to the devastation of TBI that includes shock, anger, and emotional paralysis (428). The neurobehavioral sequelae of TBI further exacerbate these problems by making it difficult for victims to use accustomed emotional coping mechanisms (429) such as information seeking, reasoning through problems, and initiating requests for social support (430).

The incidence of suicide after TBI has not been studied systematically; unfortunately, every experienced clinician can cite at least a few cases. Of 111 patients followed by Klonoff and Lage (431), two committed suicide, and another two were hospitalized emergently to prevent self-injury. Interestingly, in a large sample of wartime (mostly penetrating) brain injuries, an almost identical percentage (1.4%) of patients committed suicide (432). In the Knonoff and Lage study, 14 patients reported suicidal ideation; however, half of these had sustained their TBI via self-destructive acts. These authors list risk factors for suicide and provide recommendations for staff training and other interventions. For example, it is important to counsel families to remove firearms from the homes of individuals who are both impulsive and depressed.

The treatment of depression usually requires persistent application of more than one therapeutic modality. Medication, psychotherapy, and community reentry programs are all effective, especially in combination. Group and individual psychotherapy can help survivors of TBI reestablish a sense of identity and self-worth. Comprehensive rehabilitation programs help by reestablishing active involvement in work, recreation, and social activities.

Silver and Yudofsky (421) provide guidelines for the use of tricyclic and serotonergic antidepressants in TBI. They point out that although TBI patients are more sensitive to side effects of all medications, antidepressants are worth trying because of studies showing their efficacy in this population. One reason to use caution with tricyclics, however, is their effects on seizure threshold (433). Dopaminergic agonists and other psychostimulants should also be kept in mind for their antidepressant effects, particularly if the clinical picture includes problems with attention and arousal and if the depression is not severe (434).

Awareness Deficits

It has been observed for over 100 years that some persons with acquired brain injury are unaware of their neurologic deficits. The term *anosognosia* was originally used to refer to unawareness of hemiplegia but has gained wider currency as a descriptor for unawareness of sensory loss, amnesia, and a host of other cognitive, physical, and behavioral problems. Although the phenomenon was first recorded in stroke patients with left neglect, it has since been noted for a number of diagnoses, including Wernicke's (fluent) aphasia, the dementias, and traumatic brain injury.

Brain-injured patients frequently seem to lack insight into obvious deficits and their implications. Patients who are disoriented, requiring staff to lead them from one room to another, may insist that there is nothing wrong and that they should be released from the hospital. In less severe cases patients may acknowledge residual problems with thinking or memory but maintain that they are nonetheless ready to return to a demanding job. This is a clinically difficult problem because without careful management, the vastly differing perspectives of staff vs. patient can lead to unproductive power struggles and alienation on both sides.

A number of studies on unawareness of deficit in TBI have revealed that it is not a unitary phenomenon; i.e., patients can be aware of some deficits and not others. Patients with TBI are usually less aware of cognitive or behavioral limitations than they are of physical deficits (435,436). Furthermore, unawareness is not all-or-none: patients may underestimate the severity of the problem or minimize its implications, even when the problem itself is acknowledged (437).

Unawareness of deficit may resolve somewhat over time as patients recover neurologically and gain more real-world experience of their limitations. Godfrey et al. (425) found that patients' estimation of their behavioral deficits became more realistic between 6 months and 1 year postinjury. An increase in emotional disturbance (anxiety, depression, and low self-esteem) occurred at the same time, suggesting that patients were reacting emotionally to a fuller realization of their impairments. Similarly, Gasquoine reported that emotional dysphoria was correlated with awareness of sensory and cognitive changes after TBI (438).

Unawareness of deficit is not the same as psychological denial, which is the conscious or unconscious refusal to admit to a problem of which one is (at some level) aware. However, it can be difficult to distinguish clinically between the two phenomena. Prigatano (417) suggests that the differentiation can be made by observing the patient's response to a clinician providing cautious feedback about his or her deficits. Unaware patients often respond openly and with curiosity, whereas patients in denial may "dig in their heels" or display emotional distress.

Whether it is neurologically or psychologically mediated, or both, the failure to appreciate deficits creates a significant obstacle to rehabilitation efforts. Unawareness of deficits after TBI predicts poor performance in rehabilitation and poor outcome (439). This may be because patients who are unaware of deficits may be unmotivated to practice therapy tasks and unwilling to consider changes in employment or educational plans. In extreme cases, they may see no purpose in, or need for, the entire rehabilitation effort.

Crosson and colleagues (440) described three different levels of awareness, each with its own characteristic signs. In intellectual awareness, the lowest level, the patient is aware in a general way that a function is impaired. In the next level, emergent awareness, the patient is able to recognize when a deficit is affecting performance. Anticipatory awareness, the highest level, means that deficits in performance can actually be predicted (and, presumably, prevented). According to the authors, each level has its most appropriate compensatory treatment strategies.

In our experience, it is crucial to address awareness issues at all phases of the rehabilitation process in order to avoid patient dropout and intense frustration on the part of both patients and staff. It can be helpful simply to remind staff that unawareness is a neurologic deficit and that expecting a brain-injured patient to recognize deficits may be as unreasonable as expecting sudden recovery in the ability to walk. We also begin the education process for patients very early, so that references to brain injury, injury-related problems, and their corresponding solutions will gradually be accepted as part of everyday parlance. An emphasis on tasks and content areas that are both familiar and important to the patient is also beneficial in promoting a patient's recognition of the need for further rehabilitation.

Social and Family Impact

For many severely brain-injured patients, the most obvious and disabling impairments are in the sphere of social behavior. Brain-injured adults may appear childlike and egocentric, show a lack of regard for social conventions, and have great difficulty maintaining preinjury relationships or establishing new ones. These behaviors are ultimately attributable to the interplay among neurobehavioral deficits, unique premorbid personalities, and postinjury coping responses. Deficits in frontal executive functions, communication, and behavioral control (described in previous sections of this chapter) may particularly predispose patients to longstanding social problems. Poor performance on tests of cognitive flexibility is predictive of social withdrawal (441), as is impaired initiation (430). Reviewing the literature on social disability after TBI, Morton and Wehman (442) pointed to four recurring themes:

- Decline in friendships and social supports, leading to isolation that does not improve spontaneously

- Lack of opportunity to make new social contacts because of a restricted range of activities (e.g., unemployment, inability to drive)
- Inability to engage in preinjury leisure activities
- Depression, which further reduces social initiative and increases isolation

Without intervention, these problems may persist over the individual's lifetime. Thomsen (443) followed 31 severely injured individuals more than 20 years postinjury; she found that 61% had no friends or acquaintances. Unfortunately, treatment of social behavior problems is seldom completely effective. Group therapy with modeling of appropriate behavior can be beneficial and is part of most comprehensive community reentry programs for TBI. Success has been reported using structured social skills training, with videotaped feedback, in postacute patients (444).

Only a few investigators have systematically examined the effects of TBI on leisure and recreational participation. Bond found that work and leisure activities were the most disrupted of all daily activities after TBI (65). Oddy and colleagues reported that the most severely injured in their sample of 50 young adults did not return to all of their leisure activities at 12 months postinjury (445). Clinicians working in rehabilitation settings recognize that residual physical and neurobehavioral sequelae prevent many brain-injured people from returning to their premorbid recreational pursuits. Because many do not return to work either, loss of leisure activity may be psychologically devastating. As specialized TBI units and community reentry programs have been developed, the recreational therapist has become an integral team member. He or she performs leisure skill assessments and develops both individual and group treatments to teach new ways of occupying leisure time or adaptive methods for performing favorite premorbid activities.

In recent years an innovative approach to the social isolation of persons with TBI has emerged as an alternative to long-term therapy-based programming. This approach, the Clubhouse model, has been described by Jacobs and DeMello (446). Clubhouse programs are organized around a work-ordered day (i.e., up to full-time participation). They are run by clients who have suffered TBI, with support and guidance from a limited number of carefully selected staff members. A productive social milieu with peer support and naturalistic learning and opportunities for both recreational and vocational activity are key features of such programs. Client strengths and contributions are stressed, in contrast to the ''deficit'' emphasis found in many therapy programs.

The effects of TBI on the family have attracted a great deal of interest and attention. Several thorough reviews of recent literature are available (447–449). Numerous studies have attested to the extreme stress placed by TBI on the family system. For example, Rosenbaum and Najenson (450) examined marital relationships 1 year postinjury in Israeli brain-injured veterans. They found interpersonal tension within the family; feelings of loneliness, depression, and isolation in the wives; lack of sexual contact with husbands because of loss of feelings of attractiveness and personality changes; and role changes within the family. American studies have amply replicated these findings (418,451–454). Furthermore, the stress and family disruption experienced by caretaking spouses may be worse than that experienced by parents in a comparable role (452,453). Presumably this is because the marital relationship has been radically altered, whereas for parents the caretaking role is not totally unfamiliar. Studies of the sources of family stress invariably find greater impact of cognitive and behavioral deficits than physical care needs (65,452). Childishness, irritability and aggression, lack of initiation, and lability of mood appear most problematic (448).

McKinlay and associates attempted to identify the major sources of psychosocial burden on 55 relatives of the brain-injured within 1 year postinjury (45). They identified several types of burdens: changes in the family's routine and financial status; posttraumatic symptoms and changes in the patient's behavior; and subjective stresses felt by the caregiver as a result. This last type of burden has been correlated with substance abuse and other health problems in caregivers (448,452). However, follow-up studies have found that caregiver stress may decrease after the first year postinjury as families develop new coping mechanisms (453). Kosciulek (455) identified five distinct and effective coping strategies used by families after TBI:

- Positive appraisal, which is commitment to seeking the positive while accepting things as they are
- Resource acquisition, or the tendency to seek help and guidance
- Family tension management, which involves open expression of feelings
- Head injury demand reduction, e.g., seeking support groups or becoming involved in advocacy
- Acquiring social support from friends and relatives

Inclusion of the family in rehabilitation programs has become standard practice within the past 15 years. Studies show that families of TBI patients feel strong needs for regular communication with staff, specific information about the injury, and honest answers to their questions (454). Perhaps in response to this, a great emphasis has been placed on individual or group family education (456). Other treatments include family counseling, family therapy, and support groups (457). Most commonly, the rehabilitation psychologist, neuropsychologist, and social worker are the members of the team who deliver these services. However, a coordinated approach to providing the family with education about TBI and training in how to care for the patient requires the participation of every team member.

Sexual Relationships

Disturbances in sexual function after TBI often have been noted by clinicians but have not been well studied. Sexual dysfunctions may include hypersexuality, hyposexuality, impotence, loss of feelings of attractiveness, inability to find appropriate partners, and incapacity to engage in intimate interpersonal relationships requiring the interpretation and expression of complex emotions (458,459). Staff members and relatives often are dismayed by the sexual dysfunctions after TBI and have difficulty in managing these problems effectively. Rehabilitation facilities have developed sexual reeducation programs for brain-injured patients in which specific information is provided about sexual function and basic social skills in interpersonal intimacy are taught (460).

Sexual behavior most often is perceived by staff as a problem when the patient engages in overtly inappropriate behavior, such as public masturbation or continual advances toward uninterested partners. In these cases, team members often are asked to intervene to help reeducate and redirect the patients toward more appropriate expression of their sexual drives.

Inadequate sexual function too often is neglected because it creates fewer problems for family and staff. Patients may have hormonal or neurologic disorders that interfere with sexual function and may lack the relevant psychosocial skills for forming intimate relationships. As with other patient groups, such information rarely is provided unless it is solicited. Furthermore, patients with memory impairments or lack of awareness of their disabilities may be unable accurately to report presence of erections, lubrication, orgasm, and so forth.

It is critical for the physician to provide information regarding safe sex practices and contraception to all patients. These include mutual disease screening if indicated and use of condoms and spermacides (461). However, education alone is often inadequate for individuals who have difficulties with impulse control and executive function and who may be vulnerable to manipulation by others. Therefore, sexual counseling should occur in the context of a full appreciation of the individual's neuropsychological and emotional status. Communication and intimacy may be enhanced for some patients and their partners through the use of educational literature. Several publications are available for the layperson (462,463). Some patients, particularly those with specific sexual disorders, may require the intervention of a sex therapist.

Substance Abuse

Substance abuse is a problem that complicates not only the acute recovery from TBI but also the inpatient and postacute rehabilitation process. The relationship between alcohol and TBI is illustrated by the fact that 35% to 50% of TBI patients are intoxicated at the time of injury; moreover, 50% to 70% of all people hospitalized for TBI have a history of alcohol or other drug abuse (464). Such history predicts a poorer overall outcome (464). Based on observations of greater brain atrophy in TBI patients with alcohol abuse histories, Bigler and colleagues (465) speculated that "the abused brain may be more susceptible to injury from TBI." After injury, continued substance abuse can exacerbate neurobehavioral deficits, further disrupt family relationships, and limit the likelihood of successful return to work. Kreutzer and colleagues (466) studied the pre- and postinjury drinking habits of a cumulative series of 327 outpatients with severe TBI at least 6 months after their injury. Contrary to their expectation of increased drinking after TBI, these investigators found that the proportion of abstinent persons doubled. There is no doubt, however, that substance abuse remains a significant problem for many persons following TBI and that rehabilitation facilities must be ready to help patients address the issue.

In 1988, the National Head Injury Foundation (now the Brain Injury Association) convened a task force to study the problems of substance abuse associated with TBI. Their findings, based in part on a substance abuse questionnaire sent to 75 head injury facilities throughout the United States (response rate 70%), suggested that few specialized head injury rehabilitation centers were organized to treat the dual diagnoses of TBI and substance abuse (467). There are published program descriptions, however, for centers wishing to learn how to deal with these problems more effectively. Corrigan and colleagues described a community-based demonstration project (part of the TBI Model Systems initiative) known as the TBI Network, which provides comprehensive substance abuse services (468). The principles of the model, for which outcome data have been encouraging (468,469), emphasize holistic treatment, client autonomy, community orientation, and acceptance of a variety of client attitudes toward alcohol. There are also published lists of suggestions for ways to adapt 12-step programs (i.e., Alcoholics Anonymous, Narcotics Anonymous) to meet the cognitive needs of TBI patients undergoing rehabilitation (470). Regardless of the model chosen, all facilities treating people with TBI need to have appropriate staff or referral mechanisms to deal with this serious problem.

Identification of the problem is a critical first step in any treatment setting. Although clinical interviews with the patient and family can often reveal the problem, more formalized measures such as the Brief Michigan Alcohol Screening Test, the Quantity–Frequency–Variability Index, and the General Health and History Questionnaire may be helpful in objectively documenting the extent and severity of substance abuse problems (471).

HANDICAPS IN EVERYDAY FUNCTION

Concept of Task Analysis

As already discussed, many different impairments may contribute to the defective performance of important skills and, in interaction with the physical and social environment, to the production of social and vocational handicaps. To understand which impairments are responsible for specific disabilities, a task analysis must be conducted. This involves

TABLE 49-11. *Some component processes relevant to mobility*

Component	Role in mobility
Range of motion	Must allow for required movements
Strength	Necessary for ambulation, wheelchair propulsion, or switch operation
Balance and postural reflexes	Necessary for safe ambulation and transfer and adjustment to sudden perturbations
Muscle tone	Must allow for effective use of strength
Visuospatial perception	Necessary for environmental navigation
Spatial attention	Necessary for awareness of both sides of space
Concentration	Necessary for maintenance of locomotion in presence of distractions
Memory	Necessary for using previous experience of routes and locations
Planning, organization, and reasoning skills	Necessary for mobility in unfamiliar environments and using public transportation
Initiation	Necessary for turning plans into action

considering the physical, cognitive, and social demands that different tasks place on the patient to clarify where task breakdown occurs. Ultimately, a clinician specializing in TBI rehabilitation must be as perceptive and knowledgeable about tasks as about patients. In Table 49-11, a simple task analysis has been done for a mobility skill, demonstrating that an ability that is often thought of as physical has important cognitive requirements as well. Once the task demands have been understood, there is a choice about whether to modify the task to be more accommodating to the patient, or to modify the patient to be more adept at the task. This choice will depend on time since injury, learning ability of the patient, flexibility of the task requirements, and many other factors.

Community Mobility

Community mobility may be limited for a variety of reasons, ranging from the purely physical to the purely cognitive (see Table 49-11). These interact with availability of transportation services, where the individual lives, presence of curb cuts, and so forth, in determining community mobility status. A physical assessment by the physiatrist, physical therapist, and occupational therapist will identify contractures and motor disturbances that limit mobility. Aggressive attempts should be made in the early months postinjury to improve these impairments. Purchase of permanent assistive devices should be postponed until the patient's ultimate level of physical function is relatively certain.

Before an electric or one-arm drive wheelchair is purchased for a patient of limited physical function, it is wise to assess the patient's spatial attention and motor planning abilities. Visuospatial and perceptual testing may contribute to this assessment, but a trial of the equipment with assessment by the relevant therapists will provide more definite information about the patient's ability to learn the chair's operation and navigate the environment.

Patients who can navigate safely on foot or in a wheelchair may nevertheless get lost or confused. In most cases this should be handled in some way other than by mobility restriction. The ability to be mobile, even aimlessly, in response to environmental stimuli may contribute to quality of life.

High-level patients may have all the physical prerequisites for mobility yet have difficulty learning routes and mastering bus schedules and mobility services. Such patients may benefit from maps, written sequences of instructions, training in reading of schedules, and use of the telephone to arrange mobility services, depending on their particular patterns of strengths and weaknesses. Many patients have difficulty transferring these strategies to a new environment. It therefore appears most useful to teach community mobility skills in the community where the individual will reside.

Many TBI patients lose the ability to drive because of epilepsy or visual, cognitive, or motor impairments (472). This severely limits community mobility, particularly in rural areas. Some patients may regain the ability to drive, but the criteria on which to base this judgment are controversial. Certain perceptual and motor tests may reveal impairments that preclude driving (473), but good performance does not guarantee safe driving. We rely on road testing supervised by a driver evaluator knowledgeable about TBI. In selected cases, we request multiple evaluations because performance may be variable. Preliminary research suggests that some poor drivers may benefit from specific retraining (474).

Self-Care Skills

As with mobility, ADL independence may be limited by a complex combination of physical and cognitive impairments. A similar process of interdisciplinary physical and cognitive assessment may lead to identification of particular component processes that are especially significant (see Chapter 7).

Basic ADL skills such as dressing, bathing, and feeding may be improved with a treatment program aimed at three components:

- Attempts to improve salient physical or cognitive deficits such as serial casting for contractures or stimulant medications for arousal deficits
- Attempts to compensate for salient physical or cognitive deficits such as provision of assistive devices for physical deficits, or written or pictorial cue cards for cognitive deficits
- Attempts to retrain a task without specific regard for the contributing deficits using behavioral training methods (e.g., breaking down into small steps, backwards chaining, errorless learning, reinforcement) (475)

Patients who master basic ADL skills may progress to home management skills such as cooking, shopping, budgeting, and cleaning. Similar treatment principles are involved, but these tasks place greater emphasis on the cognitive components in that they are less routine and require more planning and organization.

Skills at ADL may suffer when the patient returns to an environment where the stimuli are different and demands placed by family members differ from those experienced in the rehabilitation setting. This problem should be anticipated, and training should be provided to family members. Ideally, the patient should be phased into the home environment gradually, and communication with the therapy staff maintained to assist in the transition. This can be accomplished through the use of periodic home passes with follow-up communication between the family and team, by systematic home visits by team members, or by a transition from inpatient to full-time outpatient to part-time outpatient status.

Many patients who are capable of performing all of the routines of daily living fail to initiate them appropriately and integrate them into a daily pattern of activity (382). Such patients may benefit from a structured activity schedule and a cuing system to help them initiate the day's major activities.

Educational, Prevocational, and Vocational Function

The presence of disabling motor and cognitive deficits adversely affects the person's capacity to reenter the educational system, whether at an elementary, secondary, or postsecondary level. Although Public Law 94-142 guarantees educational opportunities for brain-injured children, as well as other disability groups, up to the age of 21 years, the implementation of special accommodations for them varies greatly, depending on the local school district's educational philosophy, available resources, and understanding of the nature of the problem. For the elementary and secondary school child, transition back into school can be traumatic. For this reason, it is advisable for school personnel, rehabilitation team members, and the family to help the school develop an individualized education plan. A variety of broad options must be considered:

- Tutoring at home or school
- Regular class placement
- Regular class placement with a variety of support services (e.g., speech therapy, physical therapy, counseling, adaptive physical education)
- Resource room services
- Self-contained classroom
- Full-time, 12-month residential program (476)

For the postsecondary adolescent or adult, further educational and vocational services may be required. A growing number of community colleges and universities offer educational programs tailored to individuals with brain injury. At these schools, remedial courses in basic skill areas such as reading or mathematics are provided. In other cases, supplemental tutoring may be made available. To assist with daily living needs, a group-living situation with assistance from a residential counselor sometimes is available. These modifications allow a higher-level brain-injured person to progress at a slower pace with a great deal of support and a far greater likelihood of academic success than in a typical college environment.

Vocational goals are important to many brain-injured people once they complete their acute rehabilitation. The major problem is that vocational goals may be based on their premorbid abilities or vocation and may be unrealistic. Some comprehensive rehabilitation programs include prevocational assessment and vocational training (477). After the patient completes a period of extensive cognitive rehabilitation, a vocational counselor designs a vocational program that usually involves work trials within the rehabilitation setting. Another model of vocational rehabilitation after brain injury has been the supported employment approach, as developed by Wehman and colleagues at the Medical College of Virginia (478–480). In this approach, the client may be placed directly into a competitive employment situation. A job coach provides daily on-the-job instruction and guidance, advises the employer as to potential job modifications needed to maximize the client's performance, and assists with other job-related issues such as transportation, housing, financial management, and substance abuse. The supported work model has been viewed as the most effective in returning brain-injured people to competitive employment, although long-term job retention remains an issue.

Every state has a Department of Vocational Rehabilitation. Brain-injured individuals are referred routinely to the state vocational rehabilitation agency by the rehabilitation team members. The vocational counselor meets with the client and family to determine what a feasible vocational goal might be and develops an Individualized Written Rehabilitation Plan. This plan may include any of a wide variety of services, including prevocational assessment, vocational assessment, work adjustment training, sheltered workshop training, or a supported work program. Vocational assessment, which is accomplished through the administration of standardized work samples, tests of ability and vocational interest, physical endurance, and work habits, forms the basis for much of the vocational planning. The neuropsychological assessment usually is requested by vocational counselors as an essential component on which to base the vocational plan.

FINANCIAL, ETHICAL, AND MEDICOLEGAL ISSUES

A TBI taxes not only the adaptive resources of the family but their financial resources as well. Programs have been developed that provide extended rehabilitation services for months and years after the injury, but these programs are costly. Cost is less of a problem for the few who have gained large settlements from personal injury litigation, have workers' compensation, or benefit from living in a no-fault insurance state. With the advent of managed care for most consumers, third-party reimbursement is ever more difficult to obtain, with shrinkage in the number of rehabilitation services covered and in the choice of providers. For the vast majority of survivors of severe TBI, third-party reimbursement and personal finances become exhausted within the first few months after injury. Federal and state programs, such as Medicare and Medicaid, generally do not support long-term treatments that meet all the needs of the TBI survivor. To achieve financial as well as psychosocial survival, many patients and their families must gain access to public welfare funds or social security disability or engage in private fund-raising efforts.

A variety of medicolegal issues can complicate the rehabilitation process. There is frequently the need to determine the competency of the brain-injured person to manage financial affairs, engage in vocational pursuits, or make medical decisions. Competency assessments after TBI can be complex, involving the contributions of many disciplines (481). If the court deems a brain-injured person to be incompetent, a conservator may need to be appointed to manage financial affairs or a guardian to make decisions for the person. Another issue for many is personal injury litigation, which often results from accident cases. In this circumstance, the brain-injured person tries to recoup financially for past medical expenses, pain and suffering, and past and future lost wages. Although a large settlement can be very beneficial for the patient, it often takes 5 years or longer for a case to be settled in the courts. This produces a severe stress on the patient and the family. Furthermore, brain-injured patients can be their own worst witnesses because of their memory impairments and normal physical appearance, and many achieve minimal financial gain (482).

A variety of professionals can assist brain-injured people and their families to deal with these complex financial and medicolegal problems. The social worker or case manager often is relied on to assist in financial planning, obtaining governmental benefits, and locating needed home health services after discharge from the hospital. A lawyer frequently is hired to represent the brain-injured person in various types of litigation. Unfortunately, most attorneys are not knowledgeable about TBI and must be educated by health professionals. All of the members of the rehabilitation team may be asked to assist in medicolegal cases, although typically the physician specialists (e.g., neurologist, neurosurgeon, physiatrist) and psychologist (e.g., neuropsychologist or rehabilitation psychologist) are those who are asked to provide detailed records and to testify in court.

Important ethical issues may present themselves anywhere from acute care to community reentry. As brain injury rehabilitation programs have multiplied in the past 20 years, so too have the issues of importance to practitioners seeking to provide not only the best care but care that preserves the dignity and rights of the patient and significant others.

Perhaps the most dramatic ethical issues have been raised about the treatment of patients in coma or the vegetative state. Clinicians, lawyers and theologians have debated the rights of family to withdraw life-sustaining nutrition for people in this state (483,484). Obtaining informed consent in the rehabilitation setting (485) for people with TBI (486) poses its own unique difficulties—as related to the use of behavioral or psychopharmacologic restrictive procedures (487), decision making about surgical interventions or transfer to a different type of treatment program, and rights to privacy (488).

In addition to these are complex issues about the use of treatment techniques of questionable efficacy with the brain-injured patient (489). Examples of such treatments may include coma stimulation and cognitive rehabilitation. Both of these treatments have become popular but continue to lack a clear theoretical foundation or body of empirical literature that attests to their value. Clinicians and researchers have become attuned to this problem and have started to develop and systematically use more objective test procedures to demonstrate effectiveness or the lack thereof. There has also been more attention paid to the need for ethical marketing practices (490).

Finally, as the spectrum of postacute rehabilitation options for the brain-injured person has expanded (e.g., day treatment, transitional living, residential care, supported employment, lifelong living programs), third-party payers have questioned the duration and cost-benefit outcomes for these often very expensive services (491). Providers must continue to analyze the costs versus benefits of their programs to ensure that intensive, extended services for brain-injured patients result in worthwhile functional outcomes and improved quality of life (492) and to ensure that the values and desired outcomes of clients with TBI are held paramount (493).

SUMMARY

Increased interest has been focused on TBI in recent years as more patients survive severe injury and as the long-term sequelae of all grades of injury become clearer. During this time, TBI rehabilitation has emerged as a subspecialty of interest to physiatrists, nurses, psychologists, and therapists.

The focused interest in TBI has led to a number of important advances in knowledge. The epidemiology, pathophysiology, and course of recovery have been substantially defined. Our ability to estimate prognosis has improved. The medical, physical, cognitive, and behavioral sequelae of TBI have been more clearly identified and classified.

Treatment advances also have occurred. The acute management of patients with TBI has benefited from advances in neurosurgical intensive care. Medical management of the complications of TBI also has improved. The physical sequelae of TBI such as paralysis, contractures, and HO have been lessened by the same treatments used in the rehabilitation of other physical and neurologic disabilities. Yet the neurobehavioral deficits of many brain-injured patients represent their most significant obstacles to community reintegration. It is in these cognitive and behavioral realms that our ability to improve function is least clearly defined.

Much research is in progress to refine our classification of these deficits, to clarify the extent to which they are remediable, and to identify the most effective remediation strategies. Because each brain-injured patient's pattern of deficits is unique, however, it will always remain a challenge to apply the knowledge gathered from group studies to the management of the individual patient. For this reason, a thoughtful interdisciplinary treatment-planning process that considers the complex interactions of the many physical, cognitive, and behavioral deficits is essential.

ACKNOWLEDGMENTS

Many thanks are due to Mary Czerniak for preparation of the manuscript.

REFERENCES

1. Goldstein K. *Aftereffects of brain injury in war.* New York: Grune & Stratton, 1942.
2. Luria AR. *Higher cortical functions in man.* New York: Basic Books, 1966.
3. Rosenthal M, Griffith ER, Bond MR, Miller ID, eds. *Rehabilitation of the adult and child with traumatic brain injury, 2nd ed.* Philadelphia: FA Davis, 1990.
4. Michaud L, ed. Pediatric brain injury. *J Head Trauma Rehabil* 1995; 10(5).
5. Massagli TL, Jaffe KM, Fay GC, Polissar NL, Liao S, Rivara JB. Neurobehavioral sequelae of pediatric traumatic brain injury: a cohort study. *Arch Phys Med Rehabil* 1996; 77(3):223–231.
6. Rimel RW, Giordini B, Barth JT, Boll TJ, Jane JA. Disability caused by minor head injury. *Neurosurgery* 1981; 9:221–228.
7. Ruff RM, Levin HS, Marshall L. Neurobehavioral methods of assessment and the study of outcome in minor head injury. *J Head Trauma Rehabil* 1986; 1(2):43–52.
8. Marshall L, Marshall S. Current clinical head injury research in the U.S. In: Becker DP, Povlishock JT, eds. *Central nervous system research status report.* Bethesda, MD: NINCDS, 1985.
9. Frankowski RF. The demography of head injury in the United States. In: Miner M, Wagner KA, eds. *Neurotrauma, vol 1.* Boston: Butterworths, 1986; 1–17.
10. Born JD, Albert A, Hans P, Bonnal J. Relative prognostic value of best motor response and brain stem reflexes in patients with severe head injury. *Neurosurgery* 1985; 16:595–600.
11. Hans P, Albert A, Franssen C, Born J. Improved outcome prediction based on CSF extrapolated creatine kinase BB isoenzyme activity and other risk factors in severe head injury. *J Neurosurg* 1989; 71:54–58.
12. Jennett B, Teasdale G. *Management of head injuries.* Philadelphia: FA Davis, 1981.
13. Judson JA, Cant BR, Shaw NA. Early prediction of outcome from cerebral trauma by somatosensory evoked potentials. *Crit Care Med* 1990; 18:363–368.
14. Jennett B, Bond MR. Assessment of outcome after severe brain damage: a practical scale. *Lancet* 1975; 1:480–484.
15. Teasdale G, Jennett B. Assessment of coma and impaired consciousness. *Lancet* 1974; 2:81–84.
16. Miller JD, Pentland B, Berrol S. Early evaluation and management. In: Rosenthal MR, Griffith ER, Bond MR, Miller JD, eds. *Rehabilitation of the adult and child with traumatic brain injury, 2nd ed.* Philadelphia: FA Davis, 1990; 21–51.
17. Dikmen S, Machamer JE. Neurobehavioral outcomes and their determinants. *J Head Trauma Rehabil* 1995; 10:74–86.
18. Dikmen SS, Ross BL, Machamer JE, Temkin NR. One year psychosocial outcome in head injury. *J Int Neuropsychiatr Soc* 1995; 1:67–77.
19. Stein SC, Spettell C. The Head Injury Severity Scale (HISS): a practical classification of closed-head injury. *Brain Injury* 1995; 9:437–444.
20. Russell WR. Cerebral involvement in head injury. *Brain* 1932; 35: 549–603.
21. Brooks N, Campsie L, Symington C, Beattie A, McKinlay W. The effects of severe head injury on patient and relative within seven years post injury. *J Head Trauma Rehabil* 1987; 2:1–13.
22. Bishara SN, Partridge FM, Godfrey HPD, Knight RG. posttraumatic amnesia and Glasgow Coma Scale related to outcome in survivors in a consecutive series of patients with severe closed-head injury. *Brain Injury* 1992; 6:373–380.
23. Levin HS, O'Donnell VM, Grossman RG. The Galveston orientation and amnesia test: a practical scale to assess cognition after head injury. *J Nerv Ment Dis* 1979; 167:675–684.
24. Ewing-Cobbs L, Levin HS, Fletcher JM. The Child's Orientation and Amnesia Test: relationship to severity of acute head injury and to recovery of memory. *Neurosurgery* 1990; 27:683–691.
25. McDonald CM, Jaffe KM, Fay GC, Polissar NL, Martin KM, Liao S, Rivara JB. Comparison of indices of traumatic brain injury severity as predictors of neurobehavioral outcome in children. *Arch Phys Med Rehabil* 1994; 75:328–337.
26. Shores EA, Marosszeky JE, Sandanam J, Batchelor J. Preliminary validation of a clinical scale for measuring the duration of posttraumatic amnesia. *Med J Aust* 1986; 144:569–572.
27. Ponsford JL, Oliver JH, Curran C, Ng K. Prediction of employment status 2 years after traumatic brain injury. *Brain Injury* 1995; 9:11–20.
28. Katz DI, Alexander MP. Traumatic brain injury: predicting course of recovery and outcome for patients admitted to rehabilitation. *Arch Neurol* 1994; 51:661–670.
29. Frankowski RF, Annegers JF, Whitman S. The descriptive epidemiology of head trauma in the United States. In: Becker DP, Povlishock JT, eds. *Central nervous system research status report.* Bethesda, MD: NINCDS, 1985; 33–43.
30. Kraus JF, Black MA, Hessol N, et al. The incidence of acute brain injury and serious impairment in a defined population. *Am J Epidemiol* 1984; 119:186–201.
31. Annegers JF, Grabow JD, Kurland LT. The incidence, causes and secular trends of head trauma in Olmstead County, Minnesota. *Neurology* 1980; 30:912–919.
32. Goldstein FC, Levin HS. Neurobehavioral outcome of traumatic brain injury in older adults: initial findings. *J Head Trauma Rehabil* 1995; 10(1):57–73.
33. Whitman S, Coonley-Hoyanson R, Desai BT. Comparative head trauma experiences in two socioeconomically different Chicago-area communities: a population study. *Am J Epidemiol* 1984; 119: 186–201.
34. Gordon WA, Mann N, Wilier B. Demographic and social characteristics of the traumatic brain injury model system database. *J Head Trauma Rehabil* 1993; 8(2):26–33.
35. Levin HS, Benton AL, Grossman RG. *Neurobehavioral consequences of closed head injury.* New York: Oxford University Press, 1982.
36. Brown G, Chadwick O, Shaffer D, Ratter M, Traub M. A prospective study of children with head injuries: III. Psychiatric sequelae. *Psychol Med* 1981; 11:63–78.
37. Tobis J, Pure K, Sheridan J. *Rehabilitation of the severely brain injured patient.* Paper presented at the American Congress of Rehabilitation Medicine, San Diego, California, November, 1976.
38. Sosin DM, Sacks JJ, Holmgreen P. Head injury-associated deaths from motorcycle crashes. Relationship to helmet use laws. *JAMA* 1990; 264:2395–2399.
39. Wasserman RC, Buccini RV. Helmet protection from head injuries among recreational bicyclists. *Am J Sports Med* 1990; 18:96–97.
40. Zador PL, Ciccone ME. Automobile driver fatalities in frontal impacts: airbags compared with manual belts. *Am J Public Health* 1993; 83(5):661–666.
41. Max W, MacKenzie EJ, Rice DP. Head injuries: costs and consequences. *J Head Trauma Rehabil* 1991; 6(2):76–91.
42. Lehmkuhl LD, Hall KM, Mann N, Gordon WA. Factors that influence costs and length of stay of persons with traumatic brain injury in acute care and inpatient rehabilitation. *J Head Trauma Rehabil* 1993; 8(2): 88–100.
43. Ben-Yishay Y, Silver S, Piasetsky E, Rattok J. Relationship between

employability and vocational outcome after intensive holistic cognitive rehabilitation. *J Head Trauma Rehabil* 1987; 2(1):35–48.
44. Haffey WJ, Abrams DL. Employment outcomes for participants in a brain injury work reentry program: preliminary findings. *J Head Trauma Rehabil* 1991; 6(3):24–34.
45. McKinlay WW, Brooks DN, Bond MR, Martinage DP, Marshall MM. The short-term outcome of severe blunt head injury as reported by relatives of the injured persons. *J Neurol Neurosurg Psychiatry* 1981; 44:527–533.
46. Adams JH, Doyle D, Ford I, Gennarelli TA, Graham DI, McLellan DR. Diffuse axonal injury in head injury: definition, diagnosis and grading. *Histopathology* 1989; 15:49–59.
47. Blumbergs PC, Scott G, Manavis J, Wainwright H, Simpson DA, McClean AJ. Topography of axonal injury as defined by amyloid precursor protein and the sector scoring method in mild and severe closed head injury. *J Neurotrauma* 1995; 12:565–572.
48. Sahuquillo J, Vilalta J, Lamarca J, et al. Diffuse axonal injury after severe head trauma. *Acta Neurochir* 1989; 101:149–58.
49. Denny-Brown D, Russell WR. Experimental cerebral concussion. *Brain* 1941; 64:93–164.
50. Povlishock JT, Christman CW. The pathobiology of traumatically induced axonal injury in animals and humans: a review of current thoughts. *J Neurotrauma* 1995; 12(4):55–64.
51. Povlishock JT, Becker DP, Cheng CLY, et al. Axonal change in minor head injury. *J Neuropathol Exp Neurol* 1983; 42:225–242.
52. Rasmussen DX, Brandt J, Martin DB, Folstein MF. Head injury as a risk factor in Alzheimer's disease. *Brain Injury* 1995; 9(3):213–219.
53. Povlishock JT. Structural aspects of brain injury. In: Bach-y-Rita P, ed. *Traumatic brain injury: comprehensive neurologic rehabilitation, vol 2.* New York: Demos Publications, 1989; 87–96.
54. Clifton GL, Grossman RG, Makela ME, Miner ME, Handel S, Sadhu V. Neurological course and correlated computerized tomography findings after severe closed head injury. *J Neurosurg* 1980; 52:611–624.
55. Auerbach SH. Neuroanatomical correlates of attention and memory disorders in traumatic brain injury: an application of behavioral subtypes. *J Head Trauma Rehabil* 1986; 1(3):1–12.
56. Marmarou A. Pathophysiology of intracranial pressure. In: Narayan RK, Wilberger JE, Povlishock JT, eds. *Neurotrauma.* New York: McGraw-Hill, 1996; 413–429.
57. Tornheim PA, Prioleau GR, McLaurin RL. Acute responses to experimental blunt head trauma: topography of cerebral cortical edema. *J Neurosurg* 1984; 60:473–480.
58. Klauber MR, Toutant SM, Marshall LF. A model for predicting delayed intracranial hypertension following severe head injury. *J Neurosurg* 1984; 61:695–699.
59. Bullock R, Chesnut RM, Clifton G, Ghajar J, Marion D, Narayan R, Newell D, Pitts LH, Rosner M, Wilberger J. *Guidelines for the management of severe head injury.* New York: Brain Trauma Foundation, 1995.
60. Rosner MJ, Daughton S. Cerebral perfusion pressure managment in head injury. *J Trauma* 1990; 30:933–941.
61. Chan K-H, Miller JD, Dearden NM, Andrews PJD, Midgley S. The effect of changes in cerebral perfusion pressure upon middle cerebral artery blood flow velocity and jugular bulb venous oxygen saturation after severe brain injury. *J Neurosurg* 1992; 77:55–61.
62. Kelly DF. Steroids in head injury. *New Horiz* 1995; 3(3):453–455.
63. Bullock R. Opportunities for neuroprotective drugs in clinical management of head injury. *J Emerg Med* 1993; 11(Suppl 1):23–30.
64. Kaufmann BA, Tunkel AR, Pryor JC, et al. Menigitis in the neurosurgical patient. *Infect Dis Clin North Am* 1990; 4:677–701.
65. Bond MR. Assessment of the psychosocial outcome of severe head injury. *Acta Neurochir* 1976; 34:57–70.
66. Lezak MD. Living with the characterologically altered brain injured patient. *J Clin Psychiatry* 1978; 39:592–598.
67. Lishman WA. Brain damage in relation to psychiatric disability after head injury. *Br J Psychiatry* 1968; 114:373–410.
68. Alexander MP. Traumatic brain injury. In: Benson DF, Blumer D, eds. *Psychiatric aspects of neurologic disease, vol 2.* New York: Grune & Stratton, 1982.
69. Jennett B, Snoek J, Bond MR, Brooks N. Disability after severe head injury: observations on the use of the Glasgow Outcome Scale. *J Neurol Neurosurg Psychiatry* 1981; 44:285–293.
70. Rappaport M, Hall KM, Hopkins K, Belleza T, Cope DN. Disability rating scale for severe head trauma: coma to community. *Arch Phys Med Rehabil* 1982; 63:118–123.
71. Hall KM, Cope DN, Rappaport M. Glasgow Outcome Scale and Disability Rating Scale: comparative usefulness in following recovery in traumatic brain injury. *Arch Phys Med Rehabil* 1985; 66:35–37.
72. Hall KM, Hamilton BB, Gordon WA, Zasler ND. Characteristics and comparisons of functional assessment indices: Disability Rating Scale, Functional Independence Measure, and Functional Assessment Measure. *J Head Trauma Rehabil* 1993; 8(2):60–74.
73. Hagen C, Malkmus D, Durham P. *Levels of cognitive functioning.* Downey, CA: Rancho Los Amigos Hospital, 1972.
74. Gouvier WD, Blanton PD, LaPorte KK, Nepomuceno C. Reliability and validity of the Disability Rating Scale and the Levels of Cognitive Functioning Scale in monitoring recovery from severe head injury. *Arch Phys Med Rehabil* 1987; 68:94–97.
75. Granger CV, Hamilton BB, Sherwin FS. *Guide for use of the uniform data set for medical rehabilitation.* Buffalo, NY: Research Foundation—State University of New York, 1986.
76. Hall KM, Johnston MV. Outcomes evaluation in TBI rehabilitation. Part II: measurement tools for a nationwide data system. *Arch Phys Med Rehabil* 1994; 75:SC10–SC18.
77. Fleming JM, Thy BO, Maas F. Prognosis of rehabilitation outcome in head injury using the Disability Rating Scale. *Arch Phys Med Rehabil* 1994; 75:156–163.
78. Rappaport M. Evoked potential and head injury in a rehabilitation setting. In: Miner M, Wagner K, eds. *Neurotrauma: treatment, rehabilitation and related issues.* Boston: Butterworths, 1986.
79. Greenberg RP, Becker DP, Miller JD, Mayer DJ. Evaluation of brain function in severe head trauma with multimodality evoked potentials: Part 2. Localization of brain dysfunction and correlation with posttraumatic neurological conditions. *J Neurosurg* 1977; 47:163–177.
80. Jennett B, Teasdale G, Braakman R, Minderhoud J, Heiden J, Kurze T. Prognosis in series of patients with severe head injury. *Neurosurgery* 1979; 4:283–289.
81. Miller JD. The neurologic evaluation. In: Rosenthal M, Griffith ER, Bond MR, Miller JD, eds. *Rehabilitation of the child and adult with traumatic brain injury, 2nd ed.* Philadelphia: FA Davis, 1990; 52–58.
82. Nordby HK, Urdal P. The diagnostic value of measuring creatine kinase BB activity in cerebrospinal fluid following acute head injury. *Acta Neurochir* 1982; 65:93–101.
83. Woolf PD, Lee LA, Hamill RW, McDonald JV. Thyroid test abnormalities in traumatic brain injury: correlation with neurologic impairment and sympathetic nervous system activation. *Am J Med* 1988; 84:201–208.
84. Young B, Ott L, Dempsey R, Haack D, Tibbs P. Relationship between admission hyperglycemia and neurologic outcomes of severely brain-injured patients. *Ann Surg* 1989; 210:466–473.
85. Najenson T, Mendelson L, Schechter I, David C, Mintz N, Groswasser Z. Rehabilitation after severe head injury. *Scand J Rehabil Med* 1974; 6:5–14.
86. Head Injury Rehabilitation Project. *Final report: severe head trauma-comprehensive medical approach. Project 13-P-59156/9.* San Jose, CA: Santa Clara Valley Medical Center, 1982.
87. Mandleberg IA. Cognitive recovery after severe brain injury: 3. WAIS verbal and performance IQs as a function of posttraumatic amnesia duration and time from injury. *J Neurol Neurosurg Psychiatry* 1975; 39:1001–1007.
88. Levin HS, Gary HE Jr, Eisenberg HM, et al. Neurobehavioral outcome one year after severe head injury: experience of the traumatic coma data bank. *J Neurosurg* 1990; 73:699–709.
89. Kreutzer JS. *A manual for the administration and scoring of neuropsychological tests.* Richmond, VA: Medical College of Virginia Rehabilitation Research and Training Center, 1991.
90. Bond MR. The psychiatry of closed head injury. In: Brooks N, ed. *Closed head injury: psychological, social and family consequences.* Oxford: Oxford University Press, 1984; 148–178.
91. Sparadeo F, Gill D. Effects of prior alcohol use on head injury recovery. *J Head Trauma Rehabil* 1989; 4:75–82.
92. Barth JT, Macciocchi S, Giordani B, Rimel R, Jane JA, Boll TJ. Neuropsychological sequelae after minor head injury. *Neurosurgery* 1983; 13:529–533.
93. McLean A Jr, Temkin N, Dikmen S, Wyler AR. The behavioral sequelae of head injury. *J Clin Neuropsychol* 1983; 5:361–376.
94. Whyte J. Mechanisms of recovery of function in the central nervous

system. In: Griffith ER, Rosenthal M, Bond MR, Miller JD, eds. *Rehabilitation of the child and adult with traumatic brain injury, 2nd ed.* Philadelphia: FA Davis, 1990; 79–88.
95. Frost EA. Respiratory problems associated with head trauma. *Neurosurgery* 1977; 1:300–306.
96. Sutherland GR, Amacher AL, Sibbald WJ, Driedger AL. Heart injury in head-injured adolescents. *Childs Nerv Syst* 1985; 1:219–222.
97. Rall TW, Schleifer LS. Drugs effective in the therapy of the epilepsies. In: Gilman AG, Rall TW, Nies AS, et al, eds. *Goodman and Gilman's the pharmacological basis of therapeutics, 8th ed.* New York: Pergamon Press, 1990; 436–462.
98. Field PM, Colman DE, Raisman G. Synapse formation after injury in the adult rat brain: preferential reinnervation of denervated sites by axons of the contralateral fimbria. *Brain Res* 1980; 189:103–113.
99. Marshall JF. Neural plasticity and recovery of function after brain injury. *Int Rev Neurobiol* 1985; 26:201–247.
100. Almli CR, Finger S. Brain injury and recovery of function: theories and mechanisms of functional reorganization. *J Head Trauma Rehabil* 1992; 7:70–77.
101. Geisler FH, Dorsey FC, Coleman WP. Recovery of motor function after spinal cord injury. A randomized placebo controlled trial with GM-1 gangliosides. *N Engl J Med* 1991; 324(26):1829–1838.
102. Dunbar GL, Lescaudron LL, Stein DG. Comparison of GM1 ganglioside, AGF2, and D-amphetamine as treatments for spatial reversal and place learning deficits following lesions of the neostriatum. *Behav Brain Res* 1993; 54:67–79.
103. Hart T, Chaimas N, Moore R, Stein DG. Effects of nerve growth factor on behavioral recovery following caudate nucleus lesions in rats. *Brain Res Bull* 1978; 3:245–250.
104. Janis LS, Glasier MM, Martin G, Stackman RW, Walsh TJ, Stein DG. A single intraseptal injection of nerve growth factor facilitates radial maze performance following damage to the medial septum in rats. *Brain Res* 1995; 679:99–109.
105. Stein DG, Glasier MM, Hoffman SW. Pharmacological treatments for brain-injury repair: progress and prognosis. *Neuropsychol Rehabil* 1994; 4:337–357.
106. Rosenzweig MR. Animal models for effects of brain lesions and for rehabilitation. In: Bach-y-Rita P, ed. *Recovery of function: theoretical considerations for brain injury rehabilitation.* Bern, Switzerland: Hans Huber, 1980; 127–172.
107. Kaas JH. Plasticity of sensory and motor maps in adult mammals. *Annu Rev Neurosci* 1991; 14:137–167.
108. Recanzone GH, Schreiner CE, Merzenich MM. Plasticity in the frequency representation of primary auditory cortex following discrimination training in adult owl monkeys. *J Neurosci* 1993; 13:87–103.
109. Nudo RJ, Wise BM, SiFuentes F, Milliken GW. Neural substrates for the effects of rehabilitative training on motor recovery after ischemic infarct. *Science* 1996; 272:1791–1794.
110. Karni A, Meyer G, Jezzard P, Adams MM, Turner R, Ungerleider LG. Functional MRI evidence for adult motor cortex plasticity during motor skill learning. *Nature* 1995; 377:155–158.
111. Pascual-Leone A, Dang N, Cohen LG, Brasil-Neto JP, Cammarota A, Hallett M. Modulation of muscle responses evoked by transcranial magnetic stimulation during the acquisition of new fine motor skills. *J Neurophysiol* 1995; 74:1037–1045.
112. Dail WG, Feeney DM, Murray HM, Linn RT, Boyeson MG. Responses to cortical injury: II. Widespread depression of the activity of an enzyme in cortex remote from a focal injury. *Brain Res* 1981; 211:79–89.
113. Meyer JS, Shinohara Y, Kanda T, Fukuuchi Y, Ericsson AD, Kok ND. Diaschisis resulting from acute unilateral cerebral infarction. *Arch Neurol* 1970; 23:241–247.
114. Robinson RG, Bloom FE, Battenberg ELF. A fluorescent histochemical study of changes in noradrenergic neurons following experimental cerebral infarction in the rat. *Brain Res* 1977; 132:259–272.
115. Feeney DM, Gonzalez A, Law WA. Amphetamine, haloperidol, and experience interact to affect the rate of recovery after motor cortex injury. *Science* 1982; 217:855–857.
116. Boyeson MG, Harmon RL. Acute and postacute drug-induced effects on rate of behavioral recovery after brain injury. *J Head Trauma Rehabil* 1994; 9(3):78–90.
117. Sperry RW. Effect of crossing nerves to antagonistic limb muscles in the monkey. *Arch Neurol Psychiatry* 1947; 58:452–473.
118. Finger S, Stein DG. *Brain damage and recovery.* New York: Academic Press, 1982.
119. Jones MK. Imagery as a mnemonic aid after left temporal lobectomy: contrast between material-specific and generalized memory disorders. *Neuropsychologia* 1974; 12:21–30.
120. Brunnstrom S. *Movement therapy in hemiplegia.* New York: Harper & Row, 1970; 44.
121. Thomsen IV. Late outcome of very severe blunt head trauma: a 10–15 year second follow-up. *J Neurol Neurosurg Psychiatry* 1984; 47: 260–268.
122. Brooks N, ed. *Closed head injury: psychological, social and family consequences.* Oxford: Oxford University Press, 1984.
123. Singer W, Giebler K, Feldman P, et al. *The cost of rehabilitating contractures.* Paper presented at the 3rd Annual Houston Conference on Neurotrauma, Houston, TX, February 1987; 25–27.
124. Cope DN. Traumatic closed head injury: status of rehabilitation treatment. *Semin Neurol* 1985; 5:212–220.
125. Bontke CF, Zasler ND, Boake C. Rehabilitation of the head-injured patient. In: Narayan RK, Wilberger JE, Povlishok JT. *Neurotrauma.* New York: McGraw-Hill, 1995; 841–858.
126. Ben-Yishay Y, Diller L. Cognitive remediation. In: Rosenthal M, Griffith ER, Bond MR, Miller JD, eds. *Rehabilitation of the brain injured adult.* Philadelphia: FA Davis, 1983; 367–380.
127. Prigatano GP. *Neuropsychological rehabilitation after brain injury.* Baltimore: Johns Hopkins Press, 1986.
128. Eames P, Wood R. Rehabilitation after severe brain injury: a follow-up study of a behaviour modification approach. *J Neurol Neurosurg Psychiatry* 1985; 48:613–619.
129. Bryant ET, Sundance P, Hobbs A, et al. Managing costs and outcome of patients with traumatic brain injury in an HMO setting. *J Head Trauma Rehabil* 1993; 8(4):15–29.
130. Hart T, Hayden ME. The ecological validity of neuropsychological assessment and remediation. In: Uzzell BP, Gross Y, eds. *Clinical neuropsychology of intervention.* Boston: Martinus Nijhoff, 1986; 21–50.
131. Commission for the Accreditation of Rehabilitation Facilities. *Standards manual.* Tucson, AZ: CARF, 1991.
132. Braakman R, Jennett WB, Minderhoud JM. Prognosis of the posttraumatic vegetative state. *Acta Neurochir* 1988; 95:49–52.
133. Jennett B, Plum F. Persistent vegetative state after brain damage: a syndrome in search of a name. *Lancet* 1972; 1:734–7.
134. The Multi-Society Task Force on PVS. Medical aspects of the persistent vegetative state (part 2). *N Engl J Med* 1994; 330(22):1572–1579.
135. Sazbon L, Fuchs C, Costeff H. Prognosis for recovery from prolonged posttraumatic unawareness: logistic analysis. *J Neurol Neurosurg Psychiatry* 1991; 54:49–52.
136. Higashi K, Hatano M, Abiko S, et al. Five-year follow-up study of patients with persistent vegetative state. *J Neurol Neurosurg Psychiatry* 1981; 44:552–554.
137. Aspen Neurobehavioral Conference. *Draft consensus statement.* Aspen, CO: Author, 1996.
138. Danze F, Brule JF, Haddad K. Chronic vegetative state after severe head injury: clinical study: electrophysiological investigations and CT scan in 15 cases. *Neurosurg Rev* 1989; 12(Suppl 1):477–499.
139. Kinney HC, Korein J, Panigrahy A, Dikkes P, Goode R. Neuropathological findings in the brain of Karen Ann Quinlan—the role of the thalamus in the persistent vegetative state. *N Engl J Med* 1994; 330: 1469–1475.
140. Nordgren RE, Markesbery WR, Fukunda K, Reeves AG. Seven cases of cerebromedullospinal disconnection: the "locked-in" syndrome. *Neurology* 1971; 21:1140–1148.
141. Giacino J, Zasler N, Whyte J, Katz D, Glen M, Andary M. Recommendations for use of uniform nomenclature pertinent to patients with severe alterations in consciousness. *Arch Phys Med Rehabil* 1995; 76(2):205–209.
142. Ansell BJ, Keenan JE. The Western Neuro Sensory Stimulation Profile: a tool for assessing slow-to-recover head-injured patients. *Arch Phys Med Rehabil* 1989; 70:104–108.
143. Giacino JT, Kezmarsky MA, DeLuca J, Cicerone KD. Monitoring rate of recovery to predict outcome in minimally-responsive patients. *Arch Phys Med Rehabil* 1991; 72:897–901.
144. Rader MA, Alston JB, Ellis DW. Sensory stimulation of severely brain injured patients. *Brain Injury* 1989; 3:141–147.

145. Rappaport M, Dougherty AM, Kelting DL. Evaluation of coma and vegetative states. *Arch Phys Med Rehabil* 1992; 73:628–634.
146. Whyte J, DiPasquale M. Assessment of vision and visual attention in minimally responsive brain injured patients. *Arch Phys Med Rehabil* 1995; 76(9):804–810.
147. Whyte J. Toward rational psychopharmacological treatment: integrating research and clinical practice. *J Head Trauma Rehabil* 1994; 9(3): 91–103.
148. Whyte J, Glenn MB. The care and rehabilitation of the patient in a persistent vegetative state. *J Head Trauma Rehabil* 1986; 1(1):39–53.
149. Whyte J, Laborde A, DiPasquale MC. Assessment and treatment of the vegetative and minimally conscious patient. In: Rosenthal M, Griffith ER, Kreutzer JS, Pentland B, eds. *Rehabilitation of the adult and child with traumatic brain injury, 3rd ed.* Philadelphia: FA Davis, (in press).
150. Kanno T, Kamei Y, Yokoyama T, Jain VK. Neurostimulation for patients in vegetative status. *PACE* 1987; 10:207–208.
151. Katayama Y, Tsubokawa T, Yamamoto T, Hirayama T, Miyazaki S, Koyama S. Characterization and modification of brain activity with deep brain stimulation in patients in a persistent vegetative state: pain-related late positive component of cerebral evoked potential. *PACE* 1991; 14:116–121.
152. Sturm V, Kuhner A, Schmitt HP, Assmus H, Stock G. Chronic electrical stimulation of the thalamic unspecific activating system in a patient with coma due to midbrain and upper brain stem infarction. *Acta Neurochir* 1979; 47:235–244.
153. Tsubokawa T, Yamamoto T, Katayama Y, Hirayama T, Maljima S, Moriya T. Deep-rain stimulation in a persistent vegetative state: follow-up results and criteria for selection of candidates. *Brain Injury* 1990; 4:315–327.
154. Di Rocco C, Maira G, Meglio M, Rossi GF. L-Dopa treatment of comatose states due to cerebral lesions. *J Neurosurg Sci* 1974; 18(3): 169–176.
155. Horiguchi J, Inami Y, Shoda T. Effects of long-term amantadine treatment on clinical symptoms and EEG of a patient in a vegetative state. *Clin Neuropharmacol* 1990; 13:84–88.
156. Ross ED, Stewart RM. Akinetic mutism from hypothalamic damage: successful treatment with dopamine agonists. *Neurology* 1981; 31: 1435–1439.
157. Recanzone GH, Merzenich MM, Schreiner CE. Changes in the distributed temporal response properties of SI cortical neurons reflect improvements in performance on a temporally based tactile discrimination task. *J Neurophysiol* 1992; 67(5):1071–1091.
158. Zasler ND, Kreutzer JS, Taylor D. Coma stimulation and coma recovery: a critical review. *Neurorehabil* 1991; 1(3):33–40.
159. Wilson SL, McMillan TM. A review of the evidence for the effectiveness of sensory stimulation treatment for coma and vegetative states. *Neuropsychol Rehabil* 1993; 3(2):149–160.
160. Ettlin TM, Kischka U, Reichmann S, Radii EW, Heim S, Wengen DA, Benson DF. Cerebral symptoms after whiplash injury of the neck: a prospective clinical and neuropsychological study of whiplash injury. *J Neurol Neurosurg Psychiatry* 1992; 55:943–948.
161. Alexander MP. Mild traumatic brain injury: pathophysiology, natural history, and clinical management. *Neurology* 1995; 45:1253–1260.
162. McAllister TW. Mild traumatic brain injury and the postconcussive syndrome. In: Silver JM, Yudofsky SC, Hales RE, eds. *Neuropsychiatry of traumatic brain injury.* Washington, D.C.: American Psychiatric Press, 1994; 357–392.
163. Zasler N. Neuromedical diagnosis and management of postconcussive disorders. In: Horn L, Zasler N, eds. *Medical rehabilitation of traumatic brain injury.* Philadelphia: Hanley & Belfus, 1996; 133–170.
164. Levin HS, Mattis S, Ruff RM, Eisenberg HM, Marshall LF, Tabaddor K, High WM, Frankowski RF. Neurobehavioral outcome following minor head injury: a three-center study. *J Neurosurg* 1987; 66: 234–243.
165. Newcombe F, Rabbitt P, Briggs M. Minor head injury: pathophysiological or iatrogenic sequelae? *J Neurol Neurosurg Psychiatry* 1994; 57:709–716.
166. Dikmen S, McLean A, Temkin N. Neuropsychological and psychosocial consequences of minor head injury. *J Neurol Neurosurg Psychiatry* 1986; 49:1227–1232.
167. Varney NR, Bushnell DL, Nathan M, Kahn D, Roberts R, Rezai K, Walker W, Kirchner P. NeuroSPECT correlates of disabling mild head injury: preliminary findings. *J Head Trauma Rehabil* 1995; 10: 18–28.
168. Cicerone KD. Psychotherapy after mild traumatic brain injury: relation to the nature and severity of subjective complaints. *J Head Trauma Rehabil* 1991; 6:30–43.
169. Richter KJ, Cowan DM, Kaschalk SM. A protocol for managing pain, sleep disorders, and associated psychological sequelae of presumed mild head injury. *J Head Trauma Rehabil* 1995; 10:7–15.
170. Schumway-Cook A, Horak FB. Rehabilitation strategies for patients with vestibular deficits. *Neurol Clin* 1990; 8:441–457.
171. Rocabado M, Johnson B, Blakney M. Physical therapy and dentistry: An overview. *J Craniomandib Pract* 1983; 1:46.
172. Barth JT, Macciocchi N, eds. Mild traumatic brain injury. *J Head Trauma Rehabil* 1993; 8(3):13–29.
173. Horn LJ, Zasler N, eds. Rehabilitation of post-concussive disorders. *Phys Med Rehabil* 1992; 6(1):69–78.
174. Rizzo M, Tranel D, eds. *Head injury and post-concussive syndrome.* New York: Churchill-Livingstone, 1995.
175. Kishore PR, Lipper MH, Girevendulis AK, Becker DP, Vines FS. posttraumatic hydrocephalus in patients with severe head injury. *Neuroradiology* 1978; 16:261–265.
176. Teasdale G, Mendelow D. Pathophysiology of head injuries. In: Brooks N, ed. *Closed head injury: psychological, social, and family consequences.* Oxford: Oxford University Press, 1984; 4–36.
177. Levin HS, Kalisky Z, Handel SF, et al. Magnetic resonance imaging in relation to the sequelae and rehabilitation of diffuse closed head injury: preliminary findings. *Semin Neurol* 1985; 5:221–232.
178. Jordan BD, Zimmerman RD. Magnetic resonance imaging in amateur boxers. *Arch Neurol* 1988; 45:1207–1208.
179. deSouza NM, Hajnal JV, Baudouin CJ. Potential for increasing conspicuity of short-T_1 lesions in the brain using magnetisation transfer imagining. *Neuroradiology* 1995; 37(4):278–283.
180. Noguchi K, Ogawa T, Inugami A. Acute subarachnoid hemorrhage: fluid-attenuated inversion recovery pulse sequences. *Radiology* 1995; 196:773–777.
181. Hajnal JV, Saeed N, Oatridged A, Williams EJ, et al. Detection of subtle brain changes using subvoxel registration and subtraction of serial MR images. *J CAT* 1995; 19(5):677–691.
182. Foster NL, Chase TN, Fedio P, Patronas NJ, Brooks RA, DiChiro G. Alzheimer's disease: focal cortical changes shown by positron emission tomography. *Neurology* 1983; 33:961–965.
183. Masdeu JC, Abdel-Dayem H, Van Heertum RL. Head trauma: use of SPECT. *J Neuroimag* 1995; 5(Suppl 1):S53–S57.
184. Choskey MS, Costa DC, Iannotti F, Ell PJ, Crockard HA. ^{99}TcM-HMPAO SPECT studies in traumatic intracerebral haematoma. *J Neurol Neurosurg Psychiatry* 1991; 54:6–11.
185. Riley TI. Electroencephalography in the management of epilepsy. In: Browne TR, Feldman RG, eds. *Epilepsy: diagnosis and management.* Boston: Little, Brown & Co, 1983.
186. Askenazy J-J, Sazbon L, Hackett P, Najenson T. The value of electroencephalography in prolonged coma: a comparative EEG-computed axial tomography study of two patients one year after trauma. *Resuscitation* 1980; 8:181–194.
187. Rodin EA. Some problems in the clinical use of topographic EEG analysis. *Clin Electroencephalogr* 1991; 22:23–29.
188. Rappaport M, Hall K, Hopkins HK, Belleza T. Evoked potentials and head injury: 1. Rating of evoked potential abnormality. *Clin Electroencephalogr* 1981; 12:154–166.
189. Rappaport M, Hopkins HK, Hall K, Belleza T. Evoked potentials after head injury: 2. Clinical applications. *Clin Electroencephalogr* 1981; 12:167–176.
190. Rappaport M, Hemmerle AV, Rappaport ML. Intermediate and long latency SEPs in relation to clinical disability in traumatic brain injury patients. *Clin Electroencephalogr* 1990; 21:188–191.
191. Shin DY, Ehrenberg B, Whyte J, Bach J, DeLisa JA. Evoked potential assessment: utility in prognosis of chronic head injury. *Arch Phys Med Rehabil* 1989; 70:189–193.
192. Rowe MJ III, Carlson C. Brainstem auditory evoked potentials in postconcussion dizziness. *Arch Neurol* 1980; 37:679–683.
193. Greenberg RP, Stablein DM, Becker DP. Noninvasive localization of brain-stem lesions in the cat with multimodality evoked potentials: correlation with human head-injury data. *J Neurosurg* 1981; 54: 740–750.
194. Webb LX, Bosse MJ, Mayo KA, Lange RH, Miller ME, Swiontkow-

ski MF. Results in patients with craniocerebral trauma and an operatively managed acetabular fracture. *J Orthop Trauma* 1990; 4: 376–382.
195. Poole GV, Miller JD, Agnew SG, Griswold JA. Lower extremity fracture fixation in head-injured patients. *J Trauma* 1992; 32(5): 654–659.
196. Schmeling GJ, Schwab JP. Polytrauma care. The effect of head injuries and timing of skeletal fixation. *Clin Orthop* 1995; 106–116.
197. Temkin NR, Dikmen SS, Wilensky AJ, et al. A randomized, double-blind study of phenytoin for the prevention of post traumatic seizures. *N Engl J Med* 1990; 323(8):497–502.
198. Yablon SA. Posttraumatic seizures. *Arch Phys Med Rehabil* 1993; 74:983–1001.
199. Reinhard DL, Yablon SA, Bontke CF. Anticonvulsant prophylaxis for the prevention of late posttraumatic epilepsy. *J Head Trauma Rehabil* 1993; 8(4):101–107.
200. Dikmen SS, Temkin NR, Miller B, Machamer J, Winn HR, Neurobehavioral effects of phenytoin prophylaxis of posttraumatic seizures. *JAMA* 1991; 265:1271–1278.
201. Meador KJ, Loring DW, Huh K, Gallagher BB, King DW. Comparative cognitive effects of anticonvulsants. *Neurology* 1990; 40: 391–394.
202. Trimble MR, Thompson PJ. Sodium valproate and cognitive function. *Epilepsia* 1984; 25(Suppl 1):60–64.
203. Dichter MA, Brodie MJ. New Antiepileptic drugs. *N Engl J Med* 1996; 354(24):1583–1590.
204. Allen FH, Runge Jw, Legarda S, et al. Multi-center, open label study on safety, tolerance and pharmacokinetics of intravenous fosphenytoin in status epilepticus. *Epilepsia* 1994; 35(Suppl 118):93.
205. Callaghan N, Garrett A, Goggin T. Withdrawal of anticonvulsant drugs in patients free of seizures for two years. *N Engl J Med* 1988; 318:942–946.
206. Bakay L, Glasauer FE. posttraumatic hydrocephalus. In: *Head injury.* Boston: Little, Brown & Co, 1980.
207. Mysiw WJ, Jackson RD. Relationship of new-onset systemic hypertension and normal pressure hydrocephalus. *Brain Injury* 1990; 4: 233–238.
208. Benzel EC, Pelletier AL, Levy PG. Communicating hydrocephalus in adults: prediction of outcome after ventricular shunting procedures. *Neurosurgery* 1990; 26:655–660.
209. Maksymowicz W, Czosnyka M, Koszewski W, Szymanska A, Tracezewski W. The role of cerebrospinal compensatory parameters in the estimation of functioning of implanted shunt system in patients with communicating hydrocephalus (preliminary report). *Acta Neurochir* 1989; 101:112–116.
210. Wikkelso C, Andersson H, Blomstrand C. Normal pressure hydrocephalus: predictive value of CSF tap test. *Acta Neurol Scand* 1983; 73:566.
211. Clifton GL, Robertson CS, Grossman RG. Cardiovascular and metabolic responses to severe head injury. *Neurosurg Rev* 1989; 12(Suppl 1):465–473.
212. Solomon S, Hotchkiss E, Saravay SM, Bayer C, Ramsey P, Blum RS. Impairment of memory function by antihypertensive medication. *Arch Gen Psychiatry* 1983; 40:1109–1112.
213. Cruikshank JM, Neil-Dwyer G. Beta-blocker brain concentrations in man. *Eur J Clin Pharmacol* 1985; 28(Suppl):21–23.
214. Nadolol (corgard)—a new beta-blocker. *Med Lett Drugs Ther* 1980; 22(8):33–34.
215. Sandel ME, Abrams PL, Horn LJ. Hypertension after brain injury: case report. *Arch Phys Med Rehabil* 1986; 67:469–472.
216. Manhem P, Hallengren B, Hansson B-G. Plasma noradrenaline and blood pressure in hypothyroid patients, effect of gradual thyroxine treatment. *Clin Endocrinol* 1984; 20:701–707.
217. Hackenberry LE, Miner ME, Rea GL, Woo J, Graham SH. Biochemical evidence of myocardial injury after severe head trauma. *Crit Care Med* 1982; 10:641–644.
218. Baigelman W, O'Brien JC. Pulmonary effects of head trauma. *Neurosurgery* 1981; 9:729–740.
219. Dettbarn CL, Davidson LJ. Pulmonary complications in the patient with acute head injury: neurogenic pulmonary edema. *Heart Lung* 1989; 18:583–589.
220. Ballenger JJ. *Diseases of the nose, throat, ear, head, and neck, 13th ed.* Philadelphia: Lea & Febiger, 1985; 404–405.
221. Goodpasture HC, Romig DA, Voth DW, Liu C, Brackett CE. A prospective study of tracheobronchial bacterial flora in acutely brain-injured patients with and without antibiotic prophylaxis. *J Neurosurg* 1977; 47:228–235.
222. Law JH, Barnhart K, Rowlett W, et al. Increased frequency of obstructive airway abnormalities with long-term tracheostomy. *Chest* 1993; 104:136–138.
223. Akers SM, Bartter TC, Pratter MR. Respiratory care. *State Art Rev Phys Med Rehabil* 1990; 4:527–542.
224. Becker E, Bar-Or O, Mendelson L, Najenson T. Pulmonary functions and responses to exercise of patients following craniocerebral injury. *Scand J Rehabil Med* 1978; 10:47–50.
225. Node Y, Nakazawa S, Tusuji Y, Hasegawa T. A study of changes in plasma aldosterone in patients with acute head injury. *Neurosurg Rev* 1989; 12(Suppl 1):389–392.
226. Woolf PD, Cox C, Kelly M, et al. The adrenocortical response to brain injury: correlation with the severity of neurologic dysfunction, effects of intoxication, and patient outcome. *Alcoholism* 1990; 14: 917–921.
227. Ziegler MG, Morrissey EC, Marshall LF. Catecholamine and thyroid hormones in traumatic injury. *Crit Care Med* 1990; 18:253–258.
228. Feibel J, Kelly M, Lee L, Woolf PD. Loss of adrenocortical suppression after acute brain injury: role of increased intracranial pressure and brainstem function. *J Clin Endocrinol Metab* 1983; 57:1245–1250.
229. Kornblum RN, Fisher RS. Pituitary lesions in craniocerebral injuries. *Arch Pathol* 1969; 88:242–248.
230. Hansen JR, Cook JS. Posttraumatic neuroendocrine disorders. *Phys Med Rehabil* 1993; 7:569–580.
231. Davis BP, Matukas VJ. Inappropriate secretion of antidiuretic hormone after cerebral injury. *J Oral Surg* 1976; 34:609–615.
232. Hadani M, Findler G, Shaked I, Sahar A. Unusual delayed onset of diabetes insipidus following closed head trauma. *J Neurosurg* 1985; 63:456–458.
233. Fleischer AS, Rudman DR, Payne NS, Tindall GT. Hypothalamic hypothyroidism and hypogonadism in prolonged traumatic coma. *J Neurosurg* 1978; 49:650–657.
234. Klingbell GE, Cline P. Anterior hypopituitarism: a consequence of head injury. *Arch Phys Med Rehabil* 1985; 66:44–46.
235. Sockalosky JJ, Kriel RL, Krach LE, Sheehan M. Precocious puberty after traumatic brain injury. *J Pediatr* 1987; 110:373–377.
236. de Leo R, Petruk KC, Crockford P. Galactorrhea after prolonged traumatic coma: a case report. *Neurosurgery* 1981; 9:177–178.
237. Kosteljanetz M, Jensen TS, Norgard B, Lunde I, Jensen PB, Johnsen SG. Sexual and hypothalamic dysfunction in postconcussional syndrome. *Acta Neurol Scand* 1981; 63:169–180.
238. Doty RL, Shaman P, Dann M. Development of the University of Pennsylvania Smell Identification Test: a standardized microencapsulated test of olfactory function. *Physiol Behav* 1984; 32:498–502.
239. Narayan RK, Gokaslan ZL, Bontke CF, Berrol S. Neurologic sequelae of head injury. In: Rosenthal MR, Griffith ER, Bond MR, Miller JD, eds. *Rehabilitation of the adult and child with traumatic brain injury, 2nd ed.* Philadelphia: FA Davis, 1990; 94–106.
240. Burde RM, Savino PJ, Trobe JD. *Clinical decisions in neuro-ophthalmology.* St. Louis: CV Mosby, 1985.
241. Richards BW, Jones FR, Younge BR. Causes and prognosis in 4,278 cases of paralysis of the oculomotor, trochlear, and abducens cranial nerves. *Am J Ophthamol* 1992; 113:489–496.
242. Leigh RJ, Zee DS. *The neurology of eye movements.* Philadelphia: FA Davis, 1983.
243. Goodgold J, Eberstein A. *Electrodiagnosis of neuromuscular diseases, 3rd ed.* Baltimore: Williams & Wilkins, 1983.
244. Keane JR, Baloh RW. posttraumatic cranial neuropathies. *Neurol Clin* 1992; 10:849–867.
245. Hammer AJ. Lower cranial nerve palsies: Potentially lethal in association with upper cervical fracture-dislocations. *Clin Orthop Rel Res* 1991; 266:64–69.
246. Griffith ER. Types of disability. In: Rosenthal M, Griffith ER, Bond MR, Miller JD, eds. *Rehabilitation of the brain injured adult.* Philadelphia: FA Davis, 1983; 23–32.
247. Canavero S. Dynamic reverberation. A unified mechanism for central and phantom pain. *Neurosurg Clin* 1994; 42(3):203–207.
248. Gouvier WD, Cubic B. Behavioral assessment and treatment of acquired visuoperceptual disorders. *Neuropsychol Rev* 1991; 2:3–28.
249. Glenn M, Rosenthal M. Rehabilitation following severe traumatic brain injury. *Semin Neurol* 1985; 5:233–246.

250. Spielman G, Gennarelli TA, Rogers CR. Disodium etidronate: its role in preventing heterotopic ossification in severe head injury. *Arch Phys Med Rehabil* 1983; 64:539–542.
251. Garland DE, Hanscom DA, Keenan MA, Smith C, Moore T. Resection of heterotopic ossification in the adult with head trauma. *J Bone Joint Surg [Am]* 1985; 67:1261–1269.
252. Freed MM. Traumatic and congenital lesions of the spinal cord. In: Kottke FJ, Stillwell GK, Lehmann JF, eds. *Krusen's handbook of physical medicine and rehabilitation, 3rd ed.* Philadelphia: WB Saunders, 1982; 643–673.
253. Mital MA, Garber JE, Stinson JT. Ectopic bone formation in children and adolescents with head injuries: its management. *J Pediatr Orthop* 1987; 7:83–90.
254. Ritter MA, Sieber JM. Prophylactic indomethacin for the prevention of heterotopic bone formation following total hip arthroplasty. *Clin Orthop* 1985; 196:217–225.
255. Stover SL, Hahn HA, Miller JM. Disodium etidronate in the prevention of heterotopic ossification following spinal cord injury. *Paraplegia* 1976; 14:146–156.
256. Keenan MA, Haider T. The formation of heterotopic ossification after traumatic brain injury: a biopsy study with ultrastructural analysis. *J Head Trauma Rehabil* 1996; 11(4):8–22.
257. Coventry MB, Scanlon PW. The use of radiation to discourage ectopic bone. *J Bone Joint Surg [Am]* 1981; 63:201–208.
258. Whyte J, Robinson K. Pharmacologic management. In: Glenn MB, Whyte J, eds. *The practical management of spasticity in children and adults.* Philadelphia: Lea & Febiger, 1990; 201–226.
259. Young RR, Delwaide PJ. Drug therapy: spasticity (part 1). *N Engl J Med* 1981; 304:28–33.
260. Kendall PH. The use of diazepam in hemiplegia. *Ann Phys Med* 1964; 7(6):225–228.
261. Pinto ODeS, Polikar M, Debono G. Results of international clinical trials with Lioresal. *Postgrad Med J* 1972; 48(Suppl 5):18–25.
262. Chan CH. Dantrolene sodium and hepatic injury. *Neurology* 1990; 40:1427–1432.
263. Young RR, Delwaide PJ. Drug therapy: spasticity (part 2). *N Engl J Med* 1981; 304:96–99.
264. Glenn MB. Nerve blocks. In: Glenn MB, Whyte J, eds. *The practical management of spasticity in children and adults.* Philadelphia: Lea & Febiger, 1990; 227–258.
265. Easton JKM, Ozel T, Halpern D. Intramuscular neurolysis for spasticity in children. Arch Phys Med Rehabil 1979; 60:155–158.
266. Glenn MB. Update on pharmacology: nerve blocks in the treatment of spasticity. *J Head Trauma Rehabil* 1986; 1(3):72–74.
267. Mayer NH, Esquenazi A, Keenan, MA. Analysis and management of spasticity, contracture and impaired motor control. In: Horn LJ, Zasler ND. *Medical rehabilitation of traumatic brain injury.* Philadelphia: Hartley & Belfus, 1995; 411–458.
268. Mayer NH, Esquenazi A, Wannstedt G. Surgical planning of upper motorneuron dysfunction: the role of motor control evaluation. *J Head Trauma Rehabil* 1996; 11(4):37–56.
269. Borg-Stein J, Stein J. Pharmacology of botulinum toxin and implications for use in disorders of muscle tone. *J Head Trauma Rehabil* 1993; 8(3):103–106.
270. Schwartz KS, Jankovic J. Predicting the response to botulinum toxin injections for the treatment of cervical dystonia. *Neurology* 1990; 40(Suppl 1):382.
271. Meythaler JM, DeVivo MJ, Hadley M. Prospective study on the use of bolus intrathecal baclofen for spastic hypertonia due to acquired brain injury. *Arch Phys Med Rehabil* 1996; 77:461–466.
272. Nayernouri T. Posttraumatic parkinsonism. *Surg Neurol* 1985; 24: 263–264.
273. Geurts AC, Ribber GM, Knoop JA, van Limbeek J. Identification of static and dynamic postural instability following traumatic brain injury. *Arch Phys Med Rehabil* 1996; 77(7):639–644.
274. Keenan MAE, Kauffman DL, Garland DE, Smith C. Late ulnar neuropathy in the brain-injured adult. *J Hand Surg [Am]* 1988; 13: 120–124.
275. Hallet M. Classification and treatment of tremor. *JAMA* 1991; 266: 1115–1117.
276. Ellison PA. Propranolol for severe head injury action tremor. *Neurology* 1978; 28:197–199.
277. Jankovic J. Botulinum toxin treatment of tremors. *Neurology* 1991; 41:1185–1188.
278. van Zomeren AH, Brower WH, Deelman BG. Attention deficits: the riddles of selectivity, speed, and alertness. In: Brooks N, ed. *Closed head injury: psychological, social, and family consequences.* Oxford: Oxford University Press, 1984; 74–107.
279. Thomsen IV. Evaluation and outcome of aphasia in patients with severe closed head trauma. *J Neurol Neurosurg Psychiatry* 1975; 38: 713–718.
280. Sarno MT. The nature of verbal impairment after closed head trauma. *J Nerv Ment Dis* 1980; 168:685–692.
281. Young B, Ott L, Norton J, et al. Metabolic and nutritional sequelae in the non-steroid treated head injury patient. *Neurosurgery* 1985; 17: 784–791.
282. Twomey PL, St John JN. The neurological patient. In: Rombeau JL, Caldwell MD, eds. *Clinical nutrition, vol 1. Enteral and tube feeding.* Philadelphia: WB Saunders, 1984; 292–302.
283. Vane DW, Shiffler M, Grosfeld JL, et al. Reduced lower esophageal sphincter (LES) pressure after acute and chronic brain injury. *J Pediatr Surg* 1982; 17:960–964.
284. Metoclopramide (Reglan) for gastroesophageal reflux. *Med Lett Drugs Ther* 1985; 27:21–22.
285. Cisapride for nocturnal heartburn. *Med Lett Drugs Ther* 1994; 36(915):11–13.
286. Bran S, Murray WA, Hirsch IB, Palmer JP. Long QT syndrome during high-dose cisapride. *Arch Intern Med* 1995; 155(7):765–768.
287. Wysowski DK, Bacsanyi J. Cisapride and fatal arythmia. *N Engl J Med* 1996; 335(4):290–291.
288. Winstein CJ. Neurogenic dysphagia: frequency, progression, and outcome in adults following head injury. *Phys Ther* 1983; 63:1992–1997.
289. Logemann J. *Evaluation and treatment of swallowing disorders.* San Diego, CA: College Hill Press, 1983.
290. Andrew J, Nathan PW. Lesions of the anterior frontal lobes and disturbances of micturition and defaecation. *Brain* 1964; 87:233–262.
291. Perkash I. Management of neurogenic dysfunction of the bladder and bowel. In: Kottke FJ, Stillwell GK, Lehmann JF, eds. *Krusen's handbook of physical medicine and rehabilitation, 3rd ed.* Philadelphia: WB Saunders, 1982; 724–745.
292. Brown JH. Atropine, scopolamine, and related antimuscarinic drugs. In: Gilman AG, Rail TW, Nies AS, et al, eds. *Goodman and Gilman's the pharmacologic basis of therapeutics, 8th ed.* New York: Pergamon Press, 1990; 150–165.
293. Garcia JG, Lam C. Treating urinary incontinence in a head-injured adult. *Brain Injury* 1990; 4:203–207.
294. Hirsh DD, Fainstein V, Musher DM. Do condom catheters cause urinary tract infections? *JAMA* 1979; 242:340–341.
295. Posner MI. *Chronometric explorations of mind.* New York: Oxford University Press, 1986.
296. Plum F, Posner JB. *The diagnosis of stupor and coma, 2nd ed.* Philadelphia: FA Davis, 1972.
297. Whyte J. Attention and arousal: basic science aspects. *Arch Phys Med Rehabil* 1992; 73:940–949.
298. Whyte J. Neurologic disorders of attention and arousal: assessment and treatment. *Arch Phys Med Rehabil* 1992; 73:1094–1103.
299. Damasio AR. The frontal lobes. In: Heilman KM, Valenstein E, eds. *Clinical neuropsychology, 2nd ed.* New York: Oxford University Press, 1985; 339–375.
300. Mesulam MM, Waxman SG, Geschwind N, Sabin TD. Acute confusional states with right middle cerebral artery infarctions. *J Neurol Neurosurg Psychiatry* 1976; 39:84–89.
301. Whyte J, Polansky M, Fleming M, Coslett HB, Cavallucci C. Sustained arousal and attention after traumatic brain injury. *Neuropsychologia* 1995; 33(7):797–813.
302. Whyte J, Fleming M, Polansky M, Cavallucci C, Coslett HB. Phasic arousal in response to auditory warnings after traumatic brain injury. *Neuropsychologia* 1997; 35:313–324.
303. Whyte J, Polansky M, Cavallucci C, Fleming M, Lhulier J, Coslett HB. Inattentive behavior after traumatic brain injury. *J Int Neuropsychol Soc* 1996; 2:274–281.
304. Heilman KM, Watson RT, Valenstein E. Neglect and related disorders. In: Heilman KM, Valenstein E, eds. *Clinical neuropsychology, 2nd ed.* New York: Oxford University Press, 1985; 243–293.
305. Mesulam MM. Attention, confusional states, and neglect. In: Mesulam MM, ed. *Principles of behavioral neurology.* Philadelphia: FA Davis, 1985; 125–168.

306. Wechsler D. A standardized memory scale for clinical use. *J Psychol* 1945; 19:87–95.
307. Thompson PJ, Trimble MR. Anticonvulsant drugs and cognitive functions. *Epilepsia* 1982; 23:531–544.
308. Kaelin DL, Cifu DX, Matthies B. Methylphenidate effect on attention deficit in the acutely brain-injured adult. *Arch Phys Med Rehabil* 1996; 77:6–9.
309. Plenger PM, Dixon CE, Castillo RM, Frankowski RF, Yablon SA, Levin HS. Subacute methylphenidate treatment for moderate to moderately severe traumatic brain injury: a preliminary double-blind placebo-controlled study. *Arch Phys Med Rehabil* 1996; 77:536–540.
310. Wroblewski BA, Glenn MB. Pharmacologic treatment of arousal and cognitive deficits. *J Head Trauma Rehabil* 1994; 9(3):19–42.
311. Wroblewski BA, Leary JM, Phelan AM, Whyte J, Manning K. Methylphenidate and seizure frequency in brain injured patients with seizure disorders. *J Clin Psychiatry* 1992; 53(3):86–89.
312. Fleet WS, Vallenstein E, Watson RT, et al. Dopamine agonist therapy for neglect in humans. *Neurology* 1987; 37:1765–1770.
313. Gualtieri T, Chandler M, Coons TB, Brown LT. Amantadine: a new clinical profile for traumatic brain injury. *Clin Neuropharmacol* 1989; 12:258–270.
314. Whyte J. Toward rational psychopharmacologic treatment: integrating research and clinical practice. *J Head Trauma Rehabil* 1994; 9(3): 91–103.
315. Gray JM, Robertson I. Remediation of attentional difficulties following brain injury: three experimental single case studies. *Brain Injury* 1989; 3:163–170.
316. Sohlberg MM, Mateer CA. Effectiveness of an attention-training program. *J Clin Exp Neuropsychol* 1987; 9:117–130.
317. Weinberg J, Diller L, Gordon W, Stubbs K. Visual scanning training effect on reading-related tasks in acquired brain damage. *Arch Phys Med Rehabil* 1977; 58:479–486.
318. Malec J, Jones R, Rao N, et al. Video game practice effects on sustained attention in patients with craniocerebral trauma. *Cognit Rehabil* 1984; 2(4):18–24.
319. Ponsford JL, Kinsella G. Evaluation of a remedial programme for attentional deficits following closed-head injury. *J Clin Exp Neuropsychol* 1988; 10:693–708.
320. Robertson IH, Gray JM, Pentland B, Waite LJ. Microcomputer-based rehabilitation for unilateral visual neglect: a randomized controlled trial. *Arch Phys Med Rehabil* 1990; 71:663–668.
321. Whyte J. *Automatization of a motor skill: practice makes perfect.* Doctoral dissertation. Philadelphia: University of Pennsylvania, August, 1981.
322. Russell WR, Nathan PW. Traumatic amnesia. *Brain* 1946; 69: 183–187.
323. Schacter DL, Crovitz HF. Memory function after closed head injury: a review of the quantitative research. *Cortex* 1977; 13:150–176.
324. Kinsella G, Murtagh D, Landry A, Homfray K, Hammond M, O'Beirne L, Dwyer L, Lamont M, Ponsford J. Everyday memory following traumatic brain injury. *Brain Injury* 1996; 10:499–507.
325. Bigler ED, Blatter DD, Gale SD, Ryser DK, Macnamara SE, Bailey BJ, Hopkins RO, Johnson SC, Anderson CV, Russo AA, Abildskov TJ. Traumatic brain injury and memory: the role of hippocampal atrophy. *Neuropsychology* 1996; 10:333–342.
326. Mack JL. Clinical assessment of disorders of attention and memory. *J Head Trauma Rehabil* 1986; 1:22–33.
327. Nissen MJ. Neuropsychology of attention and memory. *J Head Trauma Rehabil* 1986; 1:13–21.
328. Schmitter-Edgecombe M. Effects of divided attention on implicit and explicit memory performance following severe closed head injury. *Neuropsychology* 1996; 10:155–167.
329. Shallice T, Burgess PW. Deficits in strategy application following frontal lobe damage in man. *Brain* 1991; 114:727–741.
330. Cockburn J. Failure of prospective memory after acquired brain damage: preliminary investigation and suggestions for future directions. *J Clin Exp Neuropsychol* 1996; 18:304–309.
331. Cooke DL, Kausler DH. Content memory and temporal memory for actions in survivors of traumatic brain injury. *J Clin Exp Neuropsychol* 1995; 17:90–99.
332. Mutter SA, Howard JH, Howard DV. Serial pattern learning after head injury. *J Clin Exp Neuropsychol* 1994; 16:271–288.
333. Spikman JM, Berg IJ, Deelman BG. Spared recognition capacity in elderly and closed-head-injury subjects with clinical memory deficits. *J Clin Exp Neuropsychol* 1995; 17:29–34.
334. Ewert J, Levin HS, Watson MG, Kalisky Z. Procedural memory during posttraumatic amnesia in survivors of severe closed head injury. *Arch Neurol* 1989; 46:911–916.
335. Glisky EL, Delaney SM. Implicit memory and new semantic learning in posttraumatic amnesia. *J Head Trauma Rehabil* 1996; 11:31–42.
336. Wechsler D. *Wechsler Memory Scale-Revised Manual.* San Antonio, TX: Psych Corp, 1987.
337. Wilson BA, Cockburn J, Baddeley A. *The Rivermead Behavioral Memory Test.* Reading, England: Thames Valley Test Co, 1985.
338. Lezak MD. *Neuropsychological assessment, 3rd ed.* New York: Oxford University Press, 1995.
339. Glisky EL, Schacter DL. Remediation of organic memory disorders: current status and future prospects. *J Head Trauma Rehabil* 1986; 1(3):54–63.
340. Milders MV, Berg IJ, Deelman BG. Four-year follow-up of a controlled memory training study in closed head injured patients. *Neuropsychol Rehabil* 1995; 5:223–238.
341. Prigatano GP, Amin K, Jaramillo K. Memory performance and use of a compensation after traumatic brain injury. *Neuropsychol Rehabil* 1993; 3:53–62.
342. Schmitter-Edgecombe M, Fahy JF, Whelan JP, Long CJ. Memory remediation after severe closed head injury: notebook training versus supportive therapy. *J Consult Clin Psychol* 1995; 63:484–489.
343. Kirsch NL, Levine SP, Lajiness-O'Neill R, Schnyder M. Computer-assisted interactive task guidance: facilitating the performance of a simulated vocational task. *J Head Trauma Rehabil* 1992; 7:13–25.
344. Hersh N, Treadgold L. NeuroPage: the rehabilitation of memory dysfunction by prosthetic memory and cueing. *Neurorehabilitation* 1994; 4:187–197.
345. Wilson BA, Evans JJ. Error-free learning in the rehabilitation of people with memory impairments. *J Head Trauma Rehabil* 1996; 11: 54–64.
346. Wilson BA, Baddeley A, Evans J. Errorless learning in the rehabilitation of memory impaired people. *Neuropsychol Rehabil* 1994; 4: 307–326.
347. Glisky EL. Computer-assisted instruction for patients with traumatic brain injury: teaching of domain-specific knowledge. *J Head Trauma Rehabil* 1992; 7:1–12.
348. Freedman PE, Bleiberg J, Freedland K. Anticipatory behavior deficits in closed head injury. *J Neurol Neurosurg Psychiatry* 1987; 50: 398–401.
349. Mesulam MM. Frontal cortex and behavior. *Ann Neurol* 1986; 19: 320–324.
350. Mattson AJ, Levin HS. Frontal lobe dysfunction following closed head injury: a review of the literature. *J Nerv Ment Dis* 1990; 178: 282–291.
351. Levin HS, Kraus MF. The frontal lobes and traumatic brain injury. *J Neuropsychiatry Clin Sci* 1994; 6:443–454.
352. Hart T, Jacobs HE. Rehabilitation and management of behavioral disturbances following frontal lobe injury. *J Head Trauma Rehabil* 1993; 8:1–12.
353. Schwartz MF, Mayer NH, Fitzpatrick-DeSalme EJ, Montgomery MW. Cognitive theory and the study of everyday action disorders after brain damage. *J Head Trauma Rehabil* 1993; 8:59–72.
354. Cockburn J. Performance on the Tower of London test after severe head injury. *J Int Neuropsychiatr Soc* 1995; 1:537–544.
355. Todd JA, Anderson V, Lawrence JA. Planning skills in head-injured adolesents and their peers. Neuropsychol Rehabil 1996; 6:81–99.
356. Lezak MD. Newer contributions to the neuropsychological assessment of executive functions. *J Head Trauma Rehabil* 1993; 8:24–31.
357. Varney NR, Menefee L. Psychosocial and executive deficits following closed head injury: implications for orbital frontal cortex. *J Head Trauma Rehabil* 1993; 8:32–44.
358. Sohlberg MM, Mateer CA, Stuss DT. Contemporary approaches to the management of executive control dysfunction. *J Head Trauma Rehabil* 1993; 8:45–58.
359. Alderman N, Fry RK, Youngson HA. Improvement of self-monitoring skills, reduction of behaviour disturbance and the dysexecutive syndrome: comparison of response cost and a new programme of self-monitoring training. *Neuropsychol Rehabil* 1995; 5:193–221.
360. von Cramon DY, Matthes-von Cramon G. Frontal lobe dysfunctions in patients—therapeutical approaches. In: Wood RL, Fussey I, eds.

Cognitive rehabilitation in perspective. New York: Taylor and Francis, 1990; 164–179.

361. Cicerone KD, Giacino JT. Remediation of executive function deficits after traumatic brain injury. *Neurorehabilitation* 1992; 2:12–22.
362. Heilman KM, Safran A, Geschwind N. Closed head trauma and aphasia. *J Neurol Neurosurg Psychiatry* 1971; 34:265–269.
363. Benton AL. Differential behavioral effects of frontal lobe disease. *Neuropsychologia* 1968; 6:53–60.
364. Hagen C. Language disorders in head trauma. In: Holland AL, ed. *Language disorders in adults.* San Diego, CA: College Hill Press, 1984; 245–281.
365. Coelho CA. Discourse production deficits following traumatic brain injury: a critical review of the recent literature. *Aphasiology* 1995; 9: 409–429.
366. Burns MS, Halper AS, Mogil SI. *Clinical management of right hemisphere dysfunction.* Rockville, MD: Aspen, 1986.
367. Linscott RJ, Knight RG, Godfrey HPD. The Profile of Functional Impairment in Communication (PFIC): a measure of communication impairment for clinical use. *Brain Injury* 1996; 10:397–412.
368. Lennox DB, Brune P. Incidental teaching for training communication in individuals with traumatic brain injury. *Brain Injury* 1993; 7: 449–454.
369. Benton AL. Behavioral consequences of closed head injury. In: Odom GL, ed. *Central nervous system trauma research status report.* Washington, D.C.: NINCDS, 1979; 220–231.
370. Meadows JC. The anatomical basis of prosopagnosia. *J Neurol Neurosurg Psychiatry* 1974; 37:439–450.
371. Levin HS, Peters BH. Neuropsychological testing following head injuries: prosopagnosia without visual field defect. *Dis Nerv Syst* 1976; 68–71.
372. Levin HS, Grossman RG, Kelly PJ. Impairment of facial recognition after closed head injuries of varying severity. *Cortex* 1977; 13: 119–130.
373. Zoltan B. Remediation of visual-perceptual and perceptual motor deficits. In: Rosenthal MR, Griffith ER, Bond MR, Miller JD, eds. *Rehabilitation of the adult and child with traumatic brain injury, 2nd ed.* Philadelphia: FA Davis, 1990; 351–365.
374. Baum B, Hall KM. Relationship between constructional praxis and dressing in the brain injured adult. *Am J Occup Ther* 1981; 35: 438–442.
375. Lezak M. *Neuropsychological assessment, 2nd ed.* New York: Oxford University Press, 1983.
376. Gianutsos R, Gianutsos J. Rehabilitating the verbal recall of brain injured patients by mnemonic training: an experimental demonstration using single-case methodology. *J Clin Neuropsychol* 1979; 1: 117–135.
377. Head Injury Interdisciplinary Special Interest Group of the ACRM. Guidelines for cognitive rehabilitation. *Neurorehabilitation* 1992; 2: 62–67.
378. Ben-Yishay Y, Diller L. Cognitive remediation in traumatic brain injury: update and issues. *Arch Phys Med Rehabil* 1993; 74:204–213.
379. Batchelor J, Shores EA, Marosszeky JE, Sandanam J, Lovarini M. Cognitive rehabilitation of severely closed head-injured patients using computer-assisted and noncomputerized treatment techniques. *J Head Trauma Rehabil* 1988; 3(3):78–84.
380. Kirsh NL, Levine SP, Fallon-Krueger M, Jaros LA. The microcomputer as an ''orthotic'' device for patients with cognitive deficits. *J Head Trauma Rehabil* 1987; 2(4):77–86.
381. Kniepp S. Cognitive remediation within the context of a community reentry program. In: Kreutzer JS, Wehman PH, eds. *Cognitive rehabilitation for persons with traumatic brain injury: a functional approach.* Baltimore: Paul Brookes, 1991; 239–251.
382. Mayer NS, Keating DJ, Rapp D. Skills, routines and activity patterns of daily living: a functional nested approach. In: Uzzell B, Gross Y, eds. *Clinical neuropsychology of intervention.* Boston: Martinus Nijhoff, 1986; 205–222.
383. Wood RL. Rehabilitation of patients with disorders of attention. *J Head Trauma Rehabil* 1986; 1(3):43–53.
384. Prigatano GP, Klonoff PS, O'Brien KP, Altman IM, Amin K, Chiapello D, Shepherd J. Cunningham M, Mora M. Productivity after neuropsychologically oriented milieu rehabilitation. *J Head Trauma Rehabil* 1994; 9:91–102.
385. Rattok J, Ben-Yishay Y, Ezrachi O, Lakin P, Piasetsky E, Ross B, Silver S, Vakil E, Zide E, Diller L. Outcome of different treatment mixes in a multidimensional neuropsychological rehabilitation program. *Neuropsychology* 1992; 6:395–415.
386. Bergquist TF, Boll TJ, Corrigan JD, Harley JP, Malec JF, Millis SR, Schmidt MF. Neuropsychological rehabilitation: proceedings of a consensus conference. *J Head Trauma Rehabil* 1994; 9:50–61.
387. Jacobs HE, Hart T, Mory KD, Griffin C, Martin BA, Probst J. Single-subject evaluation designs in rehabilitation: case studies on inpatient units. *J Head Trauma Rehabil* 1996; 11:86–94.
388. Brooke MM, Questad KA, Patterson DR, Bushak KJ. Agitation and restlessness after closed head injury: a prospective study of 100 consecutive admissions. *Arch Phys Med Rehabil* 1992; 73:320–323.
389. Galski T, Palasz J, Bruno RL, Walker JE. Predicting physical and verbal aggression on a brain trauma unit. *Arch Phys Med Rehabil* 1994; 75:380–383.
390. Corrigan JD, Mysiw WJ. Agitation following traumatic brain injury: equivocal evidence for a discrete stage of cognitive recovery. *Arch Phys Med Rehabil* 1988; 69:487–492.
391. Rall TW. Hypnotics and sedatives: ethanol. In: Gilman AG, Rall TW, Nies AS, et al, eds. *Goodman and Gilman's the pharmacological basis of therapeutics, 8th ed.* New York: Pergamon Press, 1990; 345–382.
392. Hoffman BB, Lefkowitz, RJ. Catecholamines and sympathomimetic drugs. In: Gilman AG, Rall TW, Nies AS, et al, eds. *Goodman and Gilman's the pharmacological basis of therapeutics, 8th ed.* New York: Pergamon Press, 1990; 187–220.
393. Baldessarini RJ. Drugs and the treatment of psychiatric disorders. In: Gilman AG, Rall TW, Nies AS, et al, eds. *Goodman and Gilman's the pharmacological basic of therapeutics, 8th ed.* New York: Pergamon Press, 1990; 383–435.
394. Sandel ME, Olive DA, Rader MA. Chlorpromazine-induced psychosis after brain injury. *Brain Injury* 1993; 7:77–83.
395. Miller L. Traumatic brain injury and aggression. In: *The psychobiology of aggression.* Haworth Press, 1994; 91–103.
396. Wood RL. Behavior disorders following severe brain injury: their presentation and psychological management. In: Brooks N, ed. *Closed head injury: psychological, social and family consequences.* Oxford: Oxford University Press, 1984; 195–219.
397. Maletzky BM. The episodic dyscontrol syndrome. *Dis Nerv Syst* 1973; 34:178–185.
398. Yuen HK, Benzing P. Guiding of behavior through redirection in brain injury rehabilitation. *Brain Injury* 1996; 10:229–238.
399. Corrigan JD. Development of a scale for assessment of agitation following traumatic brain? injury. *J Clin Exp Neuropsychol* 1989; 11: 261–277.
400. Yudovsky SC, Silver JM, Jackson W. The Overt Aggression Scale for the objective rating of verbal and physical aggression. *Am J Psychiatry* 1986; 143:35–39.
401. Slifer KJ, Cataldo MD, Babbitt RL, Kane AC, Harrison KA, Cataldo MF. Behavior analysis and intervention during hospitalization for brain trauma rehabilitation. *Arch Phys Med Rehabil* 1993; 74: 810–817.
402. Lloyd LF, Cuvo AJ. Maintenance and generalization of behaviors after treatment of persons with traumatic brain injury. *Brain Injury* 1994; 8:529–540.
403. Whyte J. Clinical drug evaluation. *J Head Trauma Rehabil* 1988; 3(4):95–99.
404. Silver JM, Yudofsky SC, Hales RE, eds. *Neuropsychiatry of traumatic brain injury.* Washington, D.C.: American Psychiatric Press, 1994.
405. Mysiw WJ, Jackson RD, Corrigan JD. Amitriptyline for posttraumatic agitation. *Am J Phys Med Rehabil* 1988; 67:29–33.
406. Brooke MM, Patterson DR, Questad KA, Cardenas D, Farrel-Roberts L. The treatment of agitation duirng initial hospitalization after traumatic brain injury. *Arch Phys Med Rehabil* 1992; 73:917–921.
407. Cope DN, ed. Psychopharmacology. *J Head Trauma Rehabil* 1987; 2(4).
408. Greendyke RM, Kanter DR. Therapeutic effects of pindolol on behavioral disturbances associated with organic brain disease: a double-blind study. *J Clin Psychiatry* 1986; 47:423–426.
409. Glenn MB, Wroblewski B, Parziale J, Levine L, Whyte J, Rosenthal M. Lithium carbonate for aggressive behavior of affective instability in ten brain-injured patients. *Am J Phys Med Rehabil* 1989; 68(5): 221–226.
410. Hale MS, Donaldson JO. Lithium carbonate in the treatment of organic brain syndrome. *J Nerv Ment Dis* 1982; 170:362–365.
411. Emory LE, Cole CM, Meyer WJ. Use of Depo-Provera to control

sexual aggression in persons with traumatic brain injury. *J Head Trauma Rehabil* 1995; 10:47–58.
412. Carnevale GJ. Natural-setting behavior management for individuals with traumatic brain injury: results of a three-year caregiver training program. *J Head Trauma Rehabil* 1996; 11:27–38.
413. Naute WJH. *Some thoughts about thought and movement: an essay based on Hughlings Jackson's notions.* Paper presented at Frontiers of Neuroscience: Symposium in honor of WJH Naute, MIT, Cambridge, MA, 1986.
414. Fuster JM. *The prefrontal cortex: anatomy, physiology, and neuropsychology of the frontal lobe, 2nd ed.* New York: Raven Press, 1989.
415. Reinhard DL, Whyte J, Sandel ME. Improved arousal and initiation following tricyclic antidepressant use in severe brain injury. *Arch Phys Med Rehabil* 1996; 77:80–83.
416. Marin RS, Fogel BS, Hawkins J, Duffy J, Krupp B. Apathy: a treatable syndrome. *J Neuropsychiatry* 1995; 7:23–30.
417. Prigatano GP. Personality disturbances associated with traumatic brain injury. *J Consult Clin Psychol* 1992; 60:360–368.
418. Linn RT, Allen K, Wilier BS. Affective symptoms in the chronic stage of traumatic brain injury: a study of married couples. *Brain Injury* 1994; 8:135–148.
419. Varney NR, Martzke JS, Roberts RJ. Major depression in patients with closed head injury. *Neuropsychology* 1987; 1:7–9.
420. Jorge RE, Robinson RG, Arndt SV, Starkstein SE, Forrester AW, Geisler F. Depression following traumatic brain injury: a 1 year longitudinal study. *J Affect Dis* 1993; 27:233–243.
421. Silver JM, Yudofsky SC. Psychopharmacological approaches to the patient with affective and psychotic features. *J Head Trauma Rehabil* 1994; 9:61–77.
422. Robinson RG, Kubos KL, Starr LB. Mood disorders in stroke patients: importance of lesion location. *Brain* 1984; 107:81–93.
423. Fedoroff JP, Starkstein SE, Forrester AW, Geisler FH, Jorge RE, Arndt SV, Robinson RG. Depression in patients with acute traumatic brain injury. *Am J Psychiatry* 1992; 149:918–923.
424. Fann JR, Katon WJ, Uomoto JM, Esselman PC. Psychiatric disorders and functional disability in outpatients with traumatic brain injuries. *Am J Psychiatry* 1995; 152:1493–1499.
425. Godfrey HPD, Partridge FM, Knight RG, Bishara S. Course of insight disorder and emotional dysfunction following closed head injury: a controlled cross-sectional follow-up study. *J Clin Exp Neuropsychol* 1993; 15:503–515.
426. Jorge RE, Robinson RG, Arndt S. Are there symptoms that are specific for depressed mood in patients with traumatic brain injury? *J Nerv Ment Dis* 1993; 181:91–99.
427. Jorge RE, Robinson RG, Starkstein SE, Arndt SV. Influence of major depression on 1-year outcome in patients with traumatic brain injury. *J Neurosurg* 1994; 81:726–733.
428. Antonak RF, Livneh H, Antonak C. A review of research on psychosocial adjustment to impairment in persons with traumatic brain injury. *J Head Trauma Rehabil* 1993; 8:87–100.
429. Hayden ME, Hart T. Rehabilitation of cognitive and behavioral dysfunction in head injury. In: Peterson LG, O'Shanick GJ, eds. *Psychosomatic aspects of trauma.* Basel: Karger, 1986; 194–229.
430. Finset A, Dyrnes S, Krogstad JM, Berstad J. Self-reported social networks and interpersonal support 2 years after severe traumatic brain injury. *Brain Injury* 1995; 9:141–150.
431. Klonoff PS, Lage GA. Suicide in patients with traumatic brain injury: risk and prevention. *J Head Trauma Rehabil* 1995; 10:16–24.
432. Hilbom E. After effects of brain injuries. *Acta Psychiatr Neurol Scand* 1960; 142:107.
433. Wroblewski BA, McColgan K, Smith K, Whyte J, Singer WD. The incidence of seizures during tricyclic antidepressant drug treatment in a brain-injured population. *J Clin Psychopharmacol* 1990; 10: 124–128.
434. Joseph AB, Wroblewski B. Depression, antidepressants, and traumatic brain injury. *J Head Trauma Rehabil* 1995; 10:90–95.
435. Prigatano GP, Altman IM. Impaired awareness of behavioral limitations after traumatic brain injury. *Arch Phys Med Rehabil* 1990; 71: 1058–1064.
436. Prigatano GP, Altman IM, O'Brien KP. Behavioral limitations that brain injured patients tend to underestimate. *Clin Neuropsychologist* 1990; 4:163–176.
437. Prigatano GP, Pepping M, Klonoff P. Cognitive, personality and psychosocial factors in the neuropsychological assessment of brain-injured patients. In: Uzzell BP and Gross Y, eds. *The clinical neuropsychology of intervention.* Boston, Martinus Nijhoff, 1986; 135–166.
438. Gasquoine PG. Affective state and awareness of sensory and cognitive effects after closed head injury. *Neuropsychology* 1992; 6:187–196.
439. Lam CS, McMahon BT, Priddy DA, Gehred-Schultz A. Deficit awareness and treatment performance among traumatic head injury adults. *Brain Injury* 1988; 2:235–242.
440. Crosson B, Barco P, Velozo C, et al. Awareness and compensation in post-acute head injury rehabilitation. *J Head Trauma Rehabil* 1989; 4(3):46–54.
441. Vilkki J, Ahola K, Hoist P, Ohman J, Servo A, Heiskanen O. Prediction of psychosocial recovery after head injury with cognitive tests and neurobehavioral ratings. *J Clin Exp Neuropsychol* 1994; 16:325–338.
442. Morton MV, Wehman P. Psychosocial and emotional sequelae of individuals with traumatic brain injury: a literature review and recommendations. *Brain Injury* 1995; 9:81–92.
443. Thomsen IV. Late psychosocial outcome in severe traumatic brain injury. *Scand J Rehab Med Suppl* 1992; 26:142–152.
444. Brotherton FA, Thomas LL, Wisotzek IE, Milan MA. Social skills training in the rehabilitation of patients with traumatic closed head injury. *Arch Phys Med Rehabil* 1988; 69:827–832.
445. Oddy M, Humphrey M, Uttley D. Subjective impairment and social recovery after closed head injury. *J Neurol Neurosurg Psychiatry* 1978; 41:611–616.
446. Jacobs HE, DeMello C. The clubhouse model and employment following brain injury. *J Vocational Rehabil* (in press).
447. Sachs PR. *Treating families of brain injury survivors.* New York: Springer-Verlag, 1991.
448. Williams JM, Kay T. *Head injury: a family matter.* Baltimore: Paul Brookes, 1991.
449. Kreutzer JS, Marwitz JH, Kepler K. Traumatic brain injury: family response and outcome. *Arch Phys Med Rehabil* 1992; 73:771–778.
450. Rosenbaum M, Najenson T. Changes in life patterns and symptoms of low mood as reported by wives of severely brain injured soldiers. *J Consult Clin Psychol* 1976; 44:681–688.
451. Chwalisz K, Stark-Wroblewski K. The subjective experiences of spouse caregivers of persons with brain injuries: a qualitative analysis. *Appl Neuropsychol* 1996; 3:28–40.
452. Leathem J, Heath G, Woolley C. Relatives' perceptions of role change, social support and stress after traumatic brain injury. *Brain Injury* 1996; 10:27–38.
453. Hall KM, Karzmark P, Stevens M, Englander J, O'Hare P, Wright J. Family stressors in traumatic brain injury: a two-year follow-up. *Arch Phys Med Rehabil* 1994; 75:876–884.
454. Kreutzer JS, Serio CD, Bergquist S. Family needs after brain injury: a quantitative analysis. *J Head Trauma Rehabil* 1994; 9:104–115.
455. Kosciulek JF. Relationship of family coping with head injury to family adaptations. *Rehabil Psychol* 1994; 39:215–230.
456. Muir CA, Rosenthal M, Diehl L. Methods of family intervention. In: Rosenthal M, Griffith ER, Miller JD, eds. *Rehabilitation of the adult and child with traumatic brain injury, 2nd ed.* Philadelphia: FA Davis, 1990; 433–448.
457. Rosenthal M. Strategies for family intervention. In: Edelstein B, Couture E, eds. *Behavioral approaches to the traumatically brain damaged.* New York: Plenum Press, 1984; 227–246.
458. Griffith ER, Cole S, Cole TM. Sexuality and sexual dysfunction. In: Rosenthal M, Griffith ER, Bond MR, Miller JD, eds. *Rehabilitation of the adult and child with traumatic brain injury, 2nd ed.* Philadelphia: FA Davis, 1990; 206–224.
459. Sandel ME, Deregatis LR, Williams KS. Sexual functioning following traumatic brain injury (abstract). *Arch Phys Med Rehabil* 1993; 74: 1284.
460. Medler TM. Sexual counseling and traumatic brain injury. *Sex Disabil* 1993; 11:57–71.
461. Sandel ME. Sexuality and reproduction after traumatic brain injury. In: Horn LJ, Zasler ND. *Medical rehabilitation of traumatic brain injury.* Philadelphia: Hanley & Belfus, 1996; 557–572.
462. Griffith ER, Lemberg S. *Sexuality and the person with traumatic brain injury. A guide for families.* Philadelphia: FA Davis, 1993.
463. Kroll K, Levy Klein E. *Enabling romance: a guide to love, sex and relationships for the disabled.* New York: Harmony Books, 1992.
464. Corrigan JD. Substance abuse as a mediating factor in outcome from traumatic brain injury. *Arch Phys Med Rehabil* 1995; 76:302–309.
465. Bigler ED, Blatter DD, Johnson SC, Anderson CV, Russo AA, Gale

SD, Ryser DK, Macnamara SE, Bailey BJ. Traumatic brain injury, alcohol and quantitative neuroimaging: preliminary findings. *Brain Injury* 1996; 10:197–206.
466. Kreutzer JS, Marwitz JH, Witol AD. Interrelationships between crime, substance abuse, and aggressive behaviours among persons with traumatic brain injury. *Brain Injury* 1995; 9:757–768.
467. National Head Injury Foundation. *Substance Abuse Task Force white paper.* Framingham, MA: NHIF, 1988.
468. Corrigan JD, Lamb-Hart GL, Rust E. A program or intervention for substance abuse following traumatic brain injury. *Brain Injury* 1995; 9:221–236.
469. Corrigan JD, Rust E, Lamb-Hart GL. The nature and extent of substance abuse problems in persons with traumatic brain injury. *J Head Trauma Rehabil* 1995; 10:29–46.
470. Kramer TH, Hoisington D. Use of AA and NA in the treatment of chemical dependencies of traumatic brain injury survivors. *Brain Injury* 1992; 6:81–88.
471. Kreutzer JS, Doherty KR, Harris JA, Zasler ND. Alcohol use among persons with traumatic brain injury. *J Head Trauma Rehabil* 1990; 5(3):9–20.
472. van Zomeren AH, Brower WH, Minderhoud JM. Acquired brain damage and driving: a review. *Arch Phys Med Rehabil* 1987; 68:697–705.
473. Korteling JE. Perception–response speed and driving gapabilities of brain-damaged and older drivers. *Hum Factors* 1990; 32:95–108.
474. Kewman DG, Seigerman C, Kintner H, Chu S, Henson D, Reeder C. Simulation training of psychomotor skills: teaching the brain-injured to drive. *Rehabil Psychol* 1985; 30(1):11–27.
475. Giles GM, Shore M. A rapid method for teaching severely brain injured adults how to wash and dress. *Arch Phys Med Rehabil* 1989; 70:156–158.
476. National Head Injury Foundation. *An educator's manual.* Framingham, MA: NHIF, 1985.
477. Ben-Yishay Y. Neuropsychological rehabilitation: quest for a holistic approach. *Semin Neurol* 1985; 5:252–259.
478. Wehman P, Kreutzer JS, West M, et al. Employment outcomes of persons following traumatic brain injury: preinjury, post injury and supported employment. *Brain Injury* 1989; 3:397–412.
479. Wehman P, Kreutzer JS, West M, et al. Return to work for persons with traumatic brain injury: a supported employment approach. *Arch Phys Med Rehabil* 1990; 71:1047–1052.
480. Wehman PH, West MD, Kregel J, et al. Return to work for persons with severe traumatic brain injury: A data-based approach to program development. *J Head Trauma Rehabil* 1995; 10:27–39.
481. Hart T, Nagele D. The assessment of competency in traumatic brain injury. *Neurorehabilitation* 1996; 7:27–38.
482. Rosenthal M, Kolpan K. Head injury rehabilitation: psycholegal issues and roles for the rehabilitation psychologist. *Rehabil Psychol* 1986; 31:37–46.
483. Berrol S. Considerations for management of the persistent vegetative state. *Arch Phys Med Rehabil* 1986; 67:283–285.
484. Bontke CF, Dolan JM, Ivanhoe CB. Should we withhold food from persons in a persistent vegetative state? *J Head Trauma Rehabil* 1994; 9:62–69.
485. Caplan A. Informed consent and provider–patient relationships in rehabilitation medicine. *Arch Phys Med Rehabil*1988; 69:312–317.
486. Haffey W. The assessment of clinical competency to consent to medical rehabilitative interventions. *J Head Trauma Rehabil* 1989; 4(1): 43–56.
487. Cope DN. Legal and ethical issues in the psychopharmacologic treatment of traumatic brain injury. *J Head Trauma Rehabil* 1989; 4(1): 13–21.
488. Banja JD, Higgins P. Videotaping therapeutic sessions and the right of privacy. *J Head Trauma Rehabil* 1989; 4(1):65–74.
489. Banja JD. Ethics, fraud, and the misallocation of rehabilitation resources. *J Head Trauma Rehabil* 1992; 7:114–116.
490. Ulicny GR. Marketing brain injury rehabilitation services: toward a more ethical approach. *J Head Trauma Rehabil* 1994; 9:73–76.
491. Johnston MV. Outcomes of community re-entry programmes for brain injury survivors: Part 2. Further investigations. *Brain Injury* 1991; 5: 155–169.
492. Ashley MJ, Persel CS, Krych DK. Changes in reimbursement climate: relationship among outcome, cost, and payor type in the postacute rehabilitation environment. *J Head Trauma Rehabil* 1993; 8:30–47.
493. Banja J, Johnston MV. Ethical perspectives and social policy. *Arch Phys Med Rehabil* 1994; 75:19–26.

Rehabilitation Medicine: Principles and Practice, Third Edition,
edited by Joel A. DeLisa and Bruce M. Gans.
Lippincott–Raven Publishers, Philadelphia © 1998.

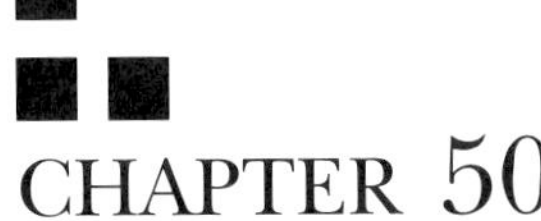

CHAPTER 50

Multiple Sclerosis

James A. Sliwa and Bruce A. Cohen

Individuals with multiple sclerosis (MS) provide a challenge to rehabilitation medicine because of the variable nature of the disease and the broad spectrum of impairments that can result in functional loss, including impairments of cognition, vision, speech, swallowing, weakness, spasticity, sensation, cerebellar and bowel and bladder function. The physiatrist must have not only a broad understanding of rehabilitation principles to provide management for the myriad of functional problems these patients encounter but also an understanding of the preventable secondary complications that can cause severe impairment in the multiple sclerosis patient. In many disabilities neurologic and functional deficits are fixed, and rehabilitation takes place following acute care treatment of static impairments. This is not the case in MS, where the disease can follow a variable course and be progressive in nature. For those in rehabilitation, this means adjusting treatment to changing or fluctuating impairments. Consequently, rehabilitation is an ongoing part of the medical care of the MS patient, with periodic review of functional status and impairments by the physiatrist. Rehabilitation intervention and setting of appropriate functional goals will depend on the pattern of the disease, the time course it follows, and the functional status of the patient at the time of intervention. An understanding of MS concepts is mandatory for optimal and efficient use of services for the individual impaired by MS. This chapter is an attempt to provide those treating these patients with an understanding of the disease, its treatment, and current rehabilitation management.

EPIDEMIOLOGY

Multiple sclerosis is a chronic disease of the central nervous system that represents a significant cause of disability affecting young and middle aged adults. It has been estimated that 250,000 to 350,000 Americans may be affected, and the National Multiple Sclerosis Society in the United States estimates that 8,800 new cases are diagnosed annually (1). A recent study for the World Federation of Multiple Sclerosis Societies estimates that 1.1 million people worldwide have the disease (2). The impact of this condition is highly variable and difficult to predict on an individual basis. For those with significant neurologic impairments, rehabilitative therapies are an important and continuing aspect of medical care contributing to the optimization of function and quality of life and mitigating the occurrence of secondary acute and chronic complications resulting from neurologic impairments. A detailed description of the pathophysiology, etiologic theories, and immunologically based therapies is beyond the scope of this chapter; however, the following provides a grounding in basic concepts of the disease and its course. The interested reader is referred to the cited reviews and texts on MS for more detailed information.

ETIOLOGY

The cause of multiple sclerosis is currently unknown; however, clues have been sought from its epidemiology. Zones of prevalence for the occurrence of MS in a North–South gradient have been described for Europe, North America, and Australia/New Zealand, which correspond to regions of temperate climate. Studies of migration suggest that risk of acquiring the disease is established by adolescence and that movement between areas of higher and lower prevalence has no impact after onset of adulthood. This pattern has suggested to some the possibility that exposure to an environmental agent or agents endemic to such regions is an important element in the occurrence of the disease (3,4). Additional support for an environmental factor may be drawn from clusters of cases described in areas of low prevalence or during defined time periods with increased frequency and from recognition of differing prevalence in

J. A. Sliwa: Department of Physical Medicine and Rehabilitation, Northwestern University Medical School, Rehabilitation Institute of Chicago, Chicago, Illinois 60611.
B. A. Cohen: Department of Neurology, Northwestern University Medical School, Chicago, Illinois 60611.

populations of similar ethnic origin residing in different geographic regions, although analysis of such patterns is complex. Another interpretation of the data that has been offered is the possibility that genetic characteristics carried by migrants might explain susceptibility to the disease. Failure to demonstrate increased occurrence in adopted children has been taken as additional evidence against a transmissible environmental factor (5,6).

The results of twin and family studies on increased risk have lent support to the concept of an inherited susceptibility to the acquisition of MS. Studies of twins reveal a concordance rate of about 25% to 30% in monozygotic twins compared to about 3% to 5% in dizygotic twins, essentially the same concordance in the latter as among siblings of differing age or other first-degree relatives (7,8). The investigators have noted that the difference in concordance rates between monozygotic and dizygotic twins is consistent with influence by multiple genes, and the relatively low concordance among monozygotic twins suggests activity of noninherited environmental factors in determining the occurrence of disease (8). Attention in genetic studies has focused to date on the mixed histocompatibility complex (MHC or HLA) region of chromosome 6 (9); however, other regions on different chromosomes may also prove to be important.

PATHOLOGY

Multiple sclerosis is characterized by multiple lesions occurring in the white matter of the brain and spinal cord. Plaques are more frequently found in white matter adjacent to the lateral ventricles and floor of the fourth ventricle, in the corpus callosum and periaqueductal region, in the optic nerves, chiasm, and tracts, in the corticomedullary junction, and in white matter tracts of the spinal cord (Fig. 50-1). Acute plaques are marked by an inflammatory reaction with perivascular lymphocytic cuffing, local disruption of the blood–brain barrier with edema, and migration of T lymphocytes and some plasma cells into the parenchyma, followed by macrophages, which appear foamy as they ingest fragmented myelin debris. Relative sparing of axons occurs, and surviving oligodendrocytes or differentiated oligodendrocyte precursors initiate a repair process resulting in shadow plaques characterized by diminished myelin staining. With recurrent attacks, increasing astrocytic gliosis and extension and coalescence of these plaques result in enlarged areas of demyelination. The chronic plaque is characterized by absent oligodendrocytes, sparse or absent macrophages and inflammatory cells, and secondary axonal damage marked by diminished size and numbers of fibers (10,11).

The process is presumed to reflect an autoimmune reaction against myelin antigens, though a specific antigenic target has not yet been identified and may vary among individuals or between attacks within the same individual. The process is believed dependent on activated T lymphocytes known as Th-1 cells moving across the endothelium, perhaps facilitated by adhesion molecules, into the affected central nervous system (CNS) region. There they form a trimolecular complex with an antigen presenting cell which may be a migrant macrophage or a microglial cell, and an antigen. This process is accompanied by release of cytokines such as gamma interferon, interleukin 2, and tumor necrosis factor alpha which upregulate and augment the inflammatory response and have been found in acute plaques. These proinflammatory cytokines are thought to be opposed, and their effects modulated by anti-inflammatory cytokines and other factors which down-regulate the inflammatory response including interleukins 4, 10, and 13, interferons alpha and beta, transforming growth factor beta and suppressor T lymphocytes (11,12).

The functional impairments which result from this pathologic process reflect the loss of the insulating properties of myelin resulting in passive ion leakage through exposed channels which degrades impulse strength between nodes of Ranvier. If the impulse arriving is of insufficient strength to

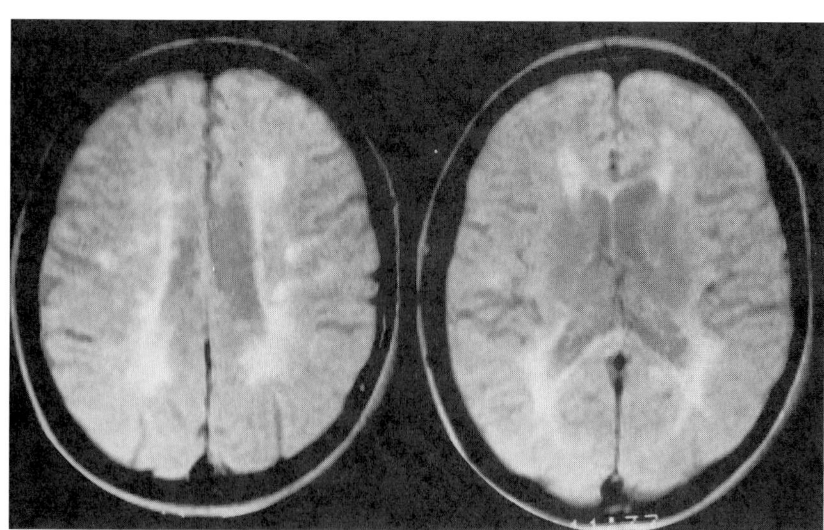

FIG. 50-1. Typical white matter changes of multiple sclerosis seen on MRI.

depolarize the node, conduction through affected fibers is blocked (13). Slowed or blocked impulse conduction in varying locations results in disruption of the precise synchronization and timing of neural signals and impairment of the related functions. Increased irritability of demyelinated fibers may also result in positive sensory or paroxysmal symptoms.

In patients with remitting disease, recovery is marked by thinner and shorter remyelinated segments. Function may return, to varying degree; however, physiological stresses such as fatigue, heat, or intercurrent illness may increase demands beyond the capacity of the impulse to be conducted through affected fibers, causing physiological conduction blocks that result in transient return of symptoms until resolution of the physiological stress (13). Recovery probably results from a combination of factors that restore conduction, including resolution of the acute inflammatory process, remyelination, and perhaps activation of collateral pathways and local reparative factors. Recurrent inflammation may underlie ultimate failure of remyelination and secondary axonal degeneration (14). As the disease enters a slow progressive phase, axonal degeneration may result in cumulative neurologic impairment in the absence of recurrent active inflammation.

CLINICAL PRESENTATIONS

The range of symptoms and signs encountered in MS patients reflects the diversity of function of the CNS. Individual symptoms are nonspecific, reflecting localization rather than causation. The single most common symptom may be paresthesias, though these are often ignored when they are brief and self-limited. Symptoms prompting medical consultation include visual impairments secondary to optic neuritis, oculomotor disturbances producing diplopia, limb weakness, dysequilibrium resulting in gait impairment or alteration of upper extremity fine motor coordination, sensory symptoms including paresthesisas, dysesthesias, and loss of sensation, symptoms of urinary bladder dysfunction, vertigo, bulbar symptoms such as dysarthria, facial or oral-lingual weakness or hypesthesia, fatigue, and, less commonly, cognitive complaints, paroxysmal symptoms, or neuralgic pain.

Neurologic examination may likewise disclose a wide variety of patient-recognized or occult abnormalities, including spasticity and weakness or ataxia of limbs, loss of sensation, which may be patchy or reflect spinal or cerebral levels, hyperactive stretch reflexes with pathologic reflexes such as Babinski signs, absent abdominal reflexes, optic disk pallor, abnormalities of pupillary responses, nystagmus, ophthalmoparesis, visual field deficits, cranial nerve abnormalities, or other less common manifestations (15). Cognitive impairments are uncommon as presenting complaints, but may be found in a substantial number of patients with clinically definite MS when sensitive neurocognitive testing is performed and may be related to lesion load on MRI (16,17).

DIAGNOSIS

Diagnosis of multiple sclerosis remains a clinical judgment at present, based on the satisfaction of three general criteria. Neurologic lesions must be shown to occur in differing locations within the CNS, at different points in time, and not be the result of another pathologic process. Evidence to satisfy these criteria may come from clinical evaluation, paraclinical measurements such as MRI and evoked potential studies, and demonstration of inflammatory proteins in the cerebrospinal fluid by laboratory evaluation. The degree to which these criteria are satisfied may be considered a probability estimate in the absence of rarely obtained tissue confirmation of the diagnosis. Consensus panels have established criteria for assigning the diagnostic probability for multicenter clinical trials, which may be adopted to clinical practice (18). Criteria for interpreting MRI results have also been recommended, emphasizing characteristic features of MS lesions including an ovoid appearance of the areas of high signal, size of the lesions, and location in both periventricular white matter and posterior fossa regions (19,20). None of the means of satisfying these diagnostic criteria provides results specific to multiple sclerosis, and reevaluation should be considered when subsequent events or atypical features of the disease course suggest the possibility of an alternate process. Even experienced MS clinicians in a tertiary setting may err as much as 9% of the time (21,22).

NATURAL HISTORY

The natural history of multiple sclerosis in an individual case is highly variable and difficult to predict. Studies of natural history may be hampered by difficulties in accurately determining disease onset, identifying cases with mild or very aggressive clinical courses, limitations of commonly used assessment measures, and the possibility that a number of different pathophysiological entities are currently grouped together as multiple sclerosis. Clinical descriptions of disease course have been based on identifiable relapses and remissions and accumulation of neurologic impairment; however, serial magnetic resonance imaging (MRI) studies have clearly shown occurrence of new lesions in the absence of perceived symptoms or detectable changes on neurologic examination in patients with relapsing disease (23). Commonly used descriptions of the clinical patterns include:

1. Relapsing–remitting MS, in which discrete attacks produce increased neurologic impairment, which subsequently improves or resolves over ensuing weeks to months (Fig. 50-2).
2. Secondary progressive MS, in which the course begins with relapses and remissions and then evolves into a gradually progressive accumulation of neurologic deficits (Fig. 50-3).
3. Primary progressive MS, in which gradual accumulation of neurologic deficit is present from the onset of the

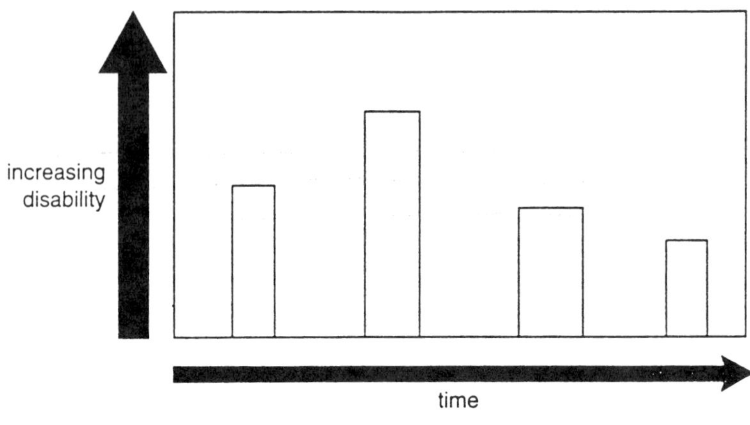

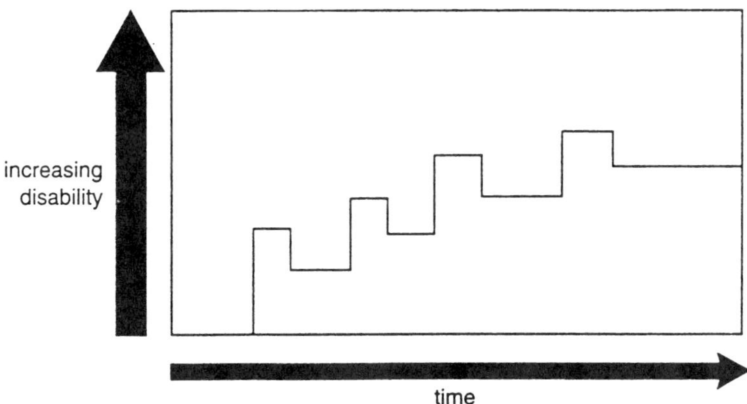

FIG. 50-2. Clinical patterns of MS: Relapsing and remitting MS. Characterized by clearly defined acute attacks with full recovery **(top)** or with sequelae and residual deficit on recovery **(bottom)**. Periods between disease relapses are characterized by a lack of disease progression.

disease course without superimposed relapses (Fig. 50-4).

4. Plateaued MS, in which the disease appears clinically quiescent without progressive neurologic deficit.

Some clinicians also use the terms:

5. Benign MS, in which individuals with initial relapses and remissions have little or no neurolgic deficit 10 years following disease onset. Some of these patients, however, may later go on to develop progressive disease.
6. Malignant MS, which is a particularly aggresive course of primary progressive MS leading to death from fulminunt disease or within 5 years of onset.

The most common standard for classifying MS patients has been the disability status scale (and currently the expanded version, EDSS) developed by Kurtzke (24–26). Limitations of the scales are that they weigh ambulation heavily, and steps between levels are not linear. Alternatives have been suggested to provide additional measures of neurologic and functional assessment (27).

Survival in MS approaches that of the general population overall, with some reduction because of increased mortality related to complications of severe disability. In a large population-based study from Rochester, MN, about three-fourths of patients were alive 25 years following diagnosis (28), whereas studies in European populations have reported median survivals of 25 to 42 years (29,30). European and Canadian studies have related survival to disability with mildly increased mortality in ambulatory patients and sharply increased rates in wheelchair dependent or less mobile individuals. Death in MS patients may result from complications of the disease, resulting infection, pulmonary embolism, malnutrition, or dehydration. About 50% to 60% of patients with multiple sclerosis die of such potentially related causes (29,31). A significant factor in mortality in some studies has been suicide, which accounted for over one-fourth of the deaths in a Canadian study but appears to vary among populations as it has not apparently been a factor in the Minnesota cohort (32).

The prognosis for disability has been evaluated by a number of longitudinal studies. Rates of benign MS, defined as minimal or no disability at 10 years, have ranged from 0% to 37% (33–35). On the other hand, 50% of a Canadian series reported by Weinshenker et al. (35) and a similar proportion of a Swedish group reported by Runmarker and Anderson (36) progressed to the point of requiring a cane for ambulation at 15 years. In the former group, 10% required a wheelchair at this point (35). Identifying which patients may go on to develop progressive disease has been an intense focus of recent investigation.

Most MS patients present with relapsing disease; only about 15% will have a primary progressive course. Attack rates range from about 0.5 to 1 per year but tend to decline over the duration of disease course. A number of environmental factors have been proposed to provoke attacks, but the only well-established relationship is a preceding or concurrent viral infection (37). Analysis of placebo groups from clinical trial reports has shown decreases of attack rate within as short a period as 3 years, though it is cautioned that this may reflect a selection bias among patients entering a clinical study (30). Weinshenker and colleagues identified the occurrence of moderate disability (EDSS 3 or more), residual pyramidal and cerebellar deficits persisting 6 months after an attack, older age at disease onset, and frequent early exacerbations, particularly with motor, cerebellar, and possibly brainstem manifestations, in decreasing importance as predictive of later development of a progressive course (38). The association between attack frequency and progression was the weakest factor and has not shown significance in some other studies (36,39). Current interest focuses on the use of cerebral imaging techniques as markers of prognosis; however, conventional MRI techniques have a limited correlation with disability at the present time and are not felt reliable enough to be used as primary outcome measures in definitive clinical trials of agents for the treatment of established multiple sclerosis (40). Studies evaluating the prognostic value of variation in rates of enhancing lesions and newer techniques such as magnetic transfer ratios and magnetic resonance spectroscopy may yield better prognostic markers in the future.

THERAPY

Therapy of multiple sclerosis may be divided into two broad complementary categories: disease-modifying therapies directed at the presumed pathophysiological processes and symptomatic and supportive therapies that seek to optimize functional capabilities and mitigate secondary complications that may result from irreversible neurologic impairment. The focus of this chapter is on the second aspect of MS treatment. A brief discussion of the basic issues in disease-modifying treatment follows.

For many years, the only treatment of established benefit in multiple sclerosis was the administration of corticosteroids. Studies using adrenal corticotropic hormone demonstrated a faster return of function compared to patients treated with placebo, but with disappearance of any differences between placebo and treated groups by 3 months (40). Currently, the use of high doses of methylprednisolone given intravenously is commonly used and has been shown to have

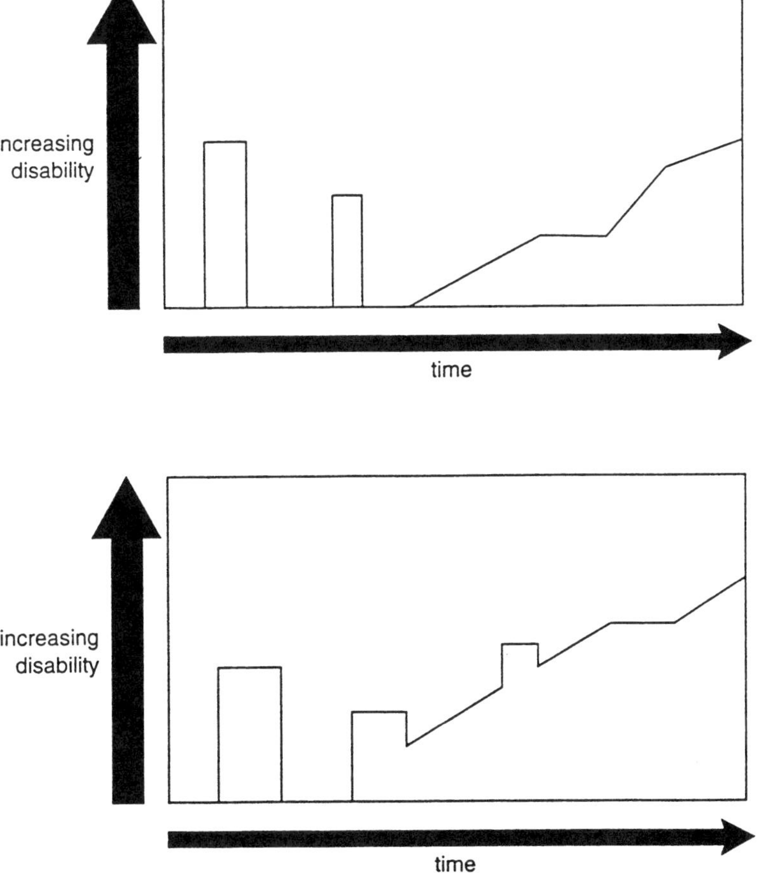

FIG. 50-3. Clinical patterns of MS: Secondary progressive MS. Begins with an initial relapsing–remitting disease course, followed by progression of variable rate **(top)**, which may also include occasional relapses and minor remissions and plateaus **(bottom)**.

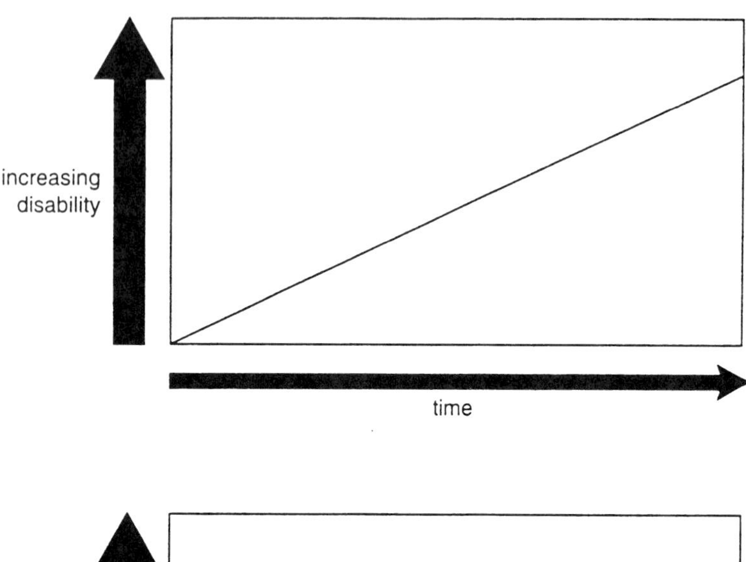

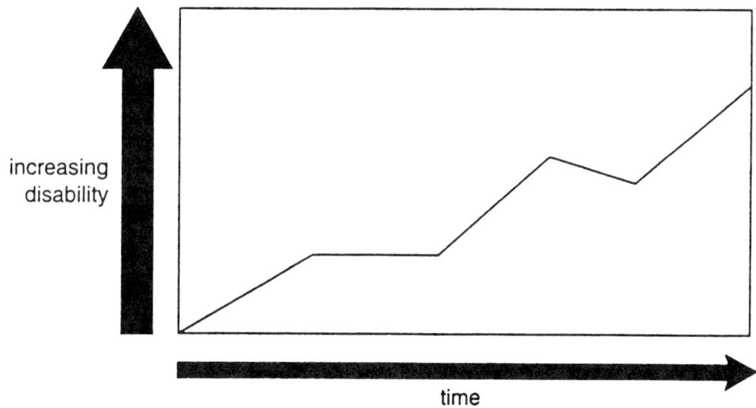

FIG. 50-4. Clinical patterns of MS: Primary progressive MS. Characterized by showing progression of disability from onset, without plateaus or remissions **(top)** or with occasional plateaus and temporary minor improvements **(bottom)**.

similar benefit (41,42). Other forms of steroid including oral prednisone and dexamethasone are also employed, and regimens differ among treating physicians with no optimal therapeutic regimen established at this time. In patients with isolated optic neuritis, oral prednisone was associated with an increased relapse rate compared to placebo or a combined intravenous methylprednisolone and tapering oral steroid regimen, but these results have not been shown to generalize to patients with multiple sclerosis (43). It is unclear by what mechanism steroids exert their effect, whether by anti-inflammatory or physiological influence.

Recently clinical trials have shown benefit of beta-interferon in reducing the frequency and severity of relapses in ambulatory patients with the relapsing form of multiple sclerosis having a relapse rate of at least one attack per year over a 2-year period before initiation of therapy. Serial MRI studies on participants showed a reduction in accumulated lesion burden in patients on active therapy compared to controls, and studies with one of two available formulations demonstrated a delay in disease progression of one EDSS grade in patients with mild impairment taking active drug and followed for at least 2 years compared to controls given placebo (44,45). Both agents may cause side effects including a flu-like syndrome, which usually attenuates on continued use, depression, increased spasticity, menstrual disorders, and injection site reactions. Neutralizing antibodies may form in almost 40% of patients and may adversely affect the efficacy of interferon beta-1b. Occasional elevation of liver transaminases or neutropenia occurred in the clinical trials of patients taking the latter drug, and recommendations for the use of both agents include serial monitoring for such side effects. Consensus panels recommend consideration of these agents for patients with definite multiple sclerosis having at least two relapses over a 2-year period (46,47). The value of beta-interferon in patients with progressive disease who do not have relapses is currently being studied and has not yet been established.

Another agent that appears efficacious in reducing the frequency of exacerbations in patients with relapsing multiple sclerosis is copolymer-1. When this agent is given on a daily basis by subcutaneous injection, side effects are mild and limited to local site reactions and a transient flushing and respiratory wheezing reaction, which is self-limited, in some individuals (48).

A variety of immunosuppressive therapeutic regimens have been tried in patients with progressive multiple sclerosis in hopes of retarding disease progression. Evidence for efficacy varies from conflicting reports to results of small exploratory trials and cannot be presently considered to be established for any of these treatments. Among the modalities currently being used are azathioprine, methotrexate, cyclophosphamide, cyclosporine, cladribine, sulfasalazine, mitoxantrone, plasmapheresis, and lymphoid irradiation. Studies evaluating the use of oral myelin to promote tolerance of the immune system for myelin antigens failed to show benefit. Monoclonal antibodies to lymphocyte antigens and T cell receptor peptide sequences are currently being evaluated. Most of the immunosuppressive therapies have potentially serious toxicities and should be reserved for patients with active severe disease progression. Patients on immunosuppressive regimens require regular hematologic, hepatic, and renal monitoring and alertness for opportunistic infections or other complications of therapy. A full discussion of such therapy is beyond the scope of this chapter, but a brief current review can be found in the reference by Thompson and Noseworthy (49).

TRAUMA

The association between trauma and either the development of MS or an exacerbation of the disease has been debated for years and may be of particular interest to the physiatrist who will be called on to provide rehabilitation care and set appropriate goals for MS patients who have lost function following fractures, non-MS-related surgeries, or other forms of physical trauma. Some authors have suggested that such trauma initiates a vascular change or an alteration in the blood–brain barrier responsible for initiation of the disease (50,51). Others have postulated that direct trauma to the spinal cord predisposes it to MS lesions (52). Most epidemiologic studies investigating the relationship between trauma and MS have shown no association between any form of mechanical trauma and the disease. In an 8-year study of mechanical trauma including dental procedures, surgery, burns, sprains, fractures, head injuries, and abrasions/lacerations/contusions on exacerbation rate and progression of MS, no form of mechanical trauma was associated with worsening of the disease with the exception of electrical injuries (53). More recently, a review of 223 cases of MS failed to show any association between head injury, spinal surgery, or skeletal fractures and MS onset or exacerbation (54). Although anecdotal reports have described the onset of MS or exacerbations of the disease following trauma and postulated theoretical pathophysiological relationships, controlled studies to date have failed to confirm this association.

INFECTIONS

Viral infections are well established as a precipitant of exacerbations (37). In one study, 27% of documented MS attacks were preceded or accompanied by viral infections, and more than 8% of infections were associated with exacerbations of the disease (37). More recently, as part of the beta-interferon study, Panitch prospectively looked at MS exacerbations during periods of risk, 1 week before to 5 weeks after onset of an infection (55). A strong correlation was found between upper respiratory tract infections (URIs) and MS exacerbations, with two-thirds of exacerbations occurring during periods of risk and one-third of infections accompanied or followed by attacks. Interestingly, there was a seasonal variation to the occurrence of URIs, but no such variation was noted in MS exacerbations, suggesting that the beta-interferon may have prevented some of the infections from triggering attacks. The authors concluded that mild infectious illnesses such as viral infections trigger the majority of exacerbations in early relapsing–remitting MS.

PREGNANCY

Multiple sclerosis has not been shown to affect a woman's fertility. The disease tends to be quiescent during pregnancy and has little impact on the outcome or course of gestation. Consideration of pregnancy in an MS patient is an important time in the care of the individual for a number of reasons. Several studies have shown an increased risk of exacerbation in the 6- to 9-month postpartum period (56–58). Shapiro reviewed 321 women with MS, 58 of whom experienced a pregnancy after the diagnosis. There was a 50% increase in relapses during the pregnancy years, with the majority of relapses occurring postpartum (57). Poser likewise showed twice as many relapses in the postpartum period than during the pregnancy (59). In a study of 515 women with MS, 130 of whom had one or more pregnancies, a total of 96 exacerbations occurred during 235 completed pregnancies. Of the 96 exacerbations, 27 occurred during the pregnancy, with 13 in the first trimester, seven in the second, two in the third, and six unspecified. Compared to the average relapse rate in nonpregnant MS patients of 0.28 relapses per person per year, there was a dramatic reduction in the third-trimester relapse rate at 0.03 and a significant increase postpartum at 0.71 relapses per person per year. There was no difference, however, between the total number of expected and observed relapses in the pregnant group (60).

Despite the increased rate of attacks following parturition in some studies, MS is not incompatible with pregnancy when physical capability allows for adequate child care. Pregnancy has not been shown to influence the long-term disease course. Although attacks of MS during pregnancy are reduced, the physiological changes that occur can alter functional status. The enlarging fetus, weight gain, and increasing fatigue can have a significant impact on functional skills, particularly mobility. This may be a period where assistive devices not previously necessary become required. Following delivery, when child care becomes a major functional activity, independence in these tasks may be an important therapy goal when attacks do occur in the postpartum period.

SEXUAL DYSFUNCTION

Sexual dysfunction is a common symptom in MS, with approximately 75% of men and 50% of women reporting symptoms (61). In some cases it can be the initial symptom of their disease. In men, the most common problem is difficulty in achieving an erection. Other frequent complaints include decreased sensation, difficulty in maintaining an erection, fatigue, and decreased libido (62). In women, decreased sensation, fatigue, decreased libido, diminished orgasms, anorgasmia, diminished arousal, and decreased lubrication are reported (61,62). Other common problems associated with MS can impact on sexual activity. For example, weakness, spasticity, contractures, and bladder dysfunction have all been cited as causes of decreased sexual activity (62).

No correlation has been found between sexual dysfunction and age at onset of disease, disease duration, or extent of physical impairment. However, a correlations between sexual dysfunction and both spasticity and disruption of bladder function have been reported (62). As a result of sexual dysfunction, there is a reduction in the frequency of sexual activity. Sixty-two percent of 217 MS patients who completed a questionnaire on sexuality reported a decrease in the frequency of intercourse after the diagnosis of MS (62).

Sexual dysfunction may not be reported by patients and thus is frequently overlooked by those providing care to the MS patient. Pacing and techniques to control fatigue, management of spasticity, and treatment of bowel and bladder function may be helpful. In men, techniques to improve erectile function, injections or mechanical devices, and vaginal lubrication in women can also improve the sexual function of many patients.

BLADDER DYSFUNCTION

The majority of individuals with MS will experience disruption of normal bladder function, with the prevalence of urologic symptoms in this population estimated to be as high as 79% (63). Although it is not common, bladder dysfunction has been reported as an initial symptom of the disease, and in 2% of cases it will be the only presenting symptom (63). Many studies have looked at urinary symptoms in MS patients and have universally found urgency, frequency, and urge incontinence to be most common (63). However, a broad range of symptoms may be seen that have been classified into two categories, irritative and obstructive. Urgency, frequency, nocturia, dysuria, and urge incontinence are considered irritative symptoms, whereas hesitancy, urinary retention, postvoid dribbling, and decreased force and caliber of the stream represent obstructive symptoms (64).

Urodynamic studies have helped clarify the nature of bladder dysfunction in MS. A spectrum of disturbances have been identified, including bladder areflexia, hyporeflexia, and hyperreflexia (65–69). An areflexic bladder will typically exhibit a large capacity, with large residual urines and no evidence of uninhibited contractions. The hyporeflexic bladder is characterized by moderate uninhibited contractions at large volumes whereas the hyperreflexic bladder exhibits high-amplitude uninhibited contractions at low volumes (67). Although bladder function can change as the disease progresses, most patients will have hyperreflexic small-capacity bladders.

Sphincter function has also been studied in MS patients. Bradley described three types of sphincter activity: volitional relaxation, uncontrollable or reflex relaxation, and sphincter dyssynergy (65). Blaivas has classified dyssynergy by the nature of the sphincter electrical activity during bladder contractions. He described type I dyssynergy as increasing sphincter EMG activity during the increase in bladder pressure with a relaxation of sphincter activity at maximum pressure. Type 2 dyssynergy is characterized by sporadic increases of EMG activity throughout the bladder contraction, and type 3 represents a crescendo–decrescendo pattern of electrical activity in the sphincter occurring concurrently with detrusor contractions (70).

Unlike a static disability, the variable and progressive nature of MS can result in changing bladder function. Frequent cystometric evaluation is not practical, and consequently some determination of urologic function from easily obtainable data is necessary for management decisions. Volumes of voided urine with postvoid residuals can provide necessary information to make some judgments about bladder functioning. With this information, the bladder can be classified as reflexic or areflexic, with or without sphincter dyssynergy, as outlined in Figure 50-5.

In the areflexic bladder, small amounts of urine overflow can occur with very large residual urines. Total bladder volumes, voided volume, and residual urine are very large and greater than normal bladder capacity. Bladder emptying becomes the goal of management. In the hyporeflexic bladder, small to moderate voiding volumes can occur with large postvoid residuals. Total bladder volume can be normal or larger than the expected, and treatment is directed at adequate emptying of the bladder. With a hyperreflexic bladder, strong bladder contractions occur at smaller volumes. Symptoms of frequency and urgency are common, and voided urine volumes may be small or moderate in amount. Residual urine volumes may vary from negligible to moderate amounts. Total bladder volumes are typically smaller than normal. Because total bladder volume is low, improving storage can be the management goal if the patient finds frequent voids disruptive. If postvoid residuals are significant because of sphincter dyssynergy, then bladder emptying is also a treatment goal.

Management is directed to the bladder dysfunction identified, either lack of emptying or diminished storage. Failure to empty can result from either diminished detrusor contractions or dyssynergy with outlet obstruction. If poor or absent bladder contractions are the etiology, then medications such as bethanecol can be tried to increase contractures. If dyssynergy with outlet obstruction is responsible, then striated muscle relaxers to decrease external sphincter contractions or alpha antagonists to diminish outlet obstruction could be tried. In both cases, intermittent catheterization to allow emptying of the bladder would be appropriate. Storage prob-

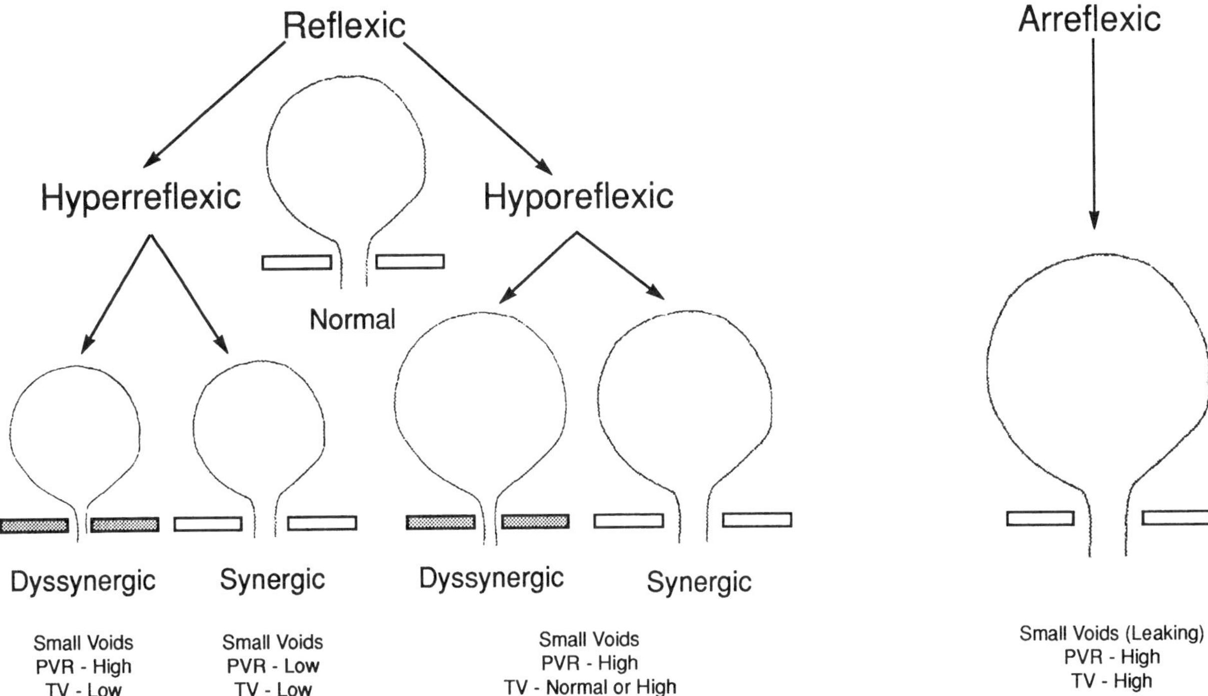

FIG. 50-5. Clinical determination of bladder dysfunction.

lems result from strong uninhibited contractions at small volumes. Anticholinergic medications or medications with anticholinergic properties can be used to increase storage capacity.

There is some controversy over the risk of upper tract abnormalities such as stones and hydronephrosis in MS patients with neurologenic bladder. Although some have reported no upper tract abnormalities (68,71), other studies have disagreed (12,73,74). Our own study of individuals with urinary symptoms referred for rehabilitation showed a prevalence of upper tract abnormalities of 21% (75).

COGNITIVE DYSFUNCTION

Cognitive impairment was appreciated as a consequence of multiple sclerosis early in the history of the disease. However, what once was thought to present as marked cognitive dysfunction in a small percentage of severely disabled individuals is now appreciated to occur at higher rates and in a spectrum of mild to severe cognitive involvement. The impact of such impairment, even if relatively mild, can have significant consequences on daily functioning, success in rehabilitation, and vocational goals (76).

Studies using neuropsychological evaluation have shown rates of cognitive impairments to range from 43% to 63% in individuals with MS (16,77,78). The nature of these impairments can be such that routine screening tests such as the Mini-Mental Status Exam will not be sensitive enough to identify these deficits (16). Despite the relatively high prevalence of cognitive dysfunction, not all functions are affected uniformly. In general, overall intellectual functioning is only mildly decreased when compared to controls; however, performance IQ appears to be more impaired than verbal IQ (79). Also consistently reported is a slowing of information processing (79) and consequently deficits in problem solving, as reported by Rao (16). Memory is the most frequently reported cognitive impairment in MS patients. The most extensive deficits are noted in recent memory, that is, with information presented within minutes to weeks, as opposed to immediate memory, information presented within seconds, and remote memory, information presented in the remote past (79).

It is not clear that cognitive decline follows a predictable pattern or is related to disease duration. It has been shown that individuals with more extensive brain lesions have more severe cognitive impairments, and total lesion area was a better predictor for measures of recent memory, abstraction, language, and visual-spatial skills, whereas callosal size was a better predictor of information processing (80). In a review of cognitive performance in MS, Beatty tentatively concluded that: (a) patients with large total lesion areas will show significant cognitive disturbances; (b) a broad range of cognitive disturbances are related to total lesion area; and (c) callosal size may be related to the degree of cognitive impairment in functions that require interhemispheric transfer of information (81).

Emotional disturbances are also frequently reported in MS. Euphoria associated with the disease is typically used to describe the persistent cheerfulness and optimism that patients will display despite significant disease or simply the lack of concern about their disabilities expressed to the clinician. Rabins (82) has shown that euphoria is associated with severe cognitive deficits, a progressive disease course, greater disability, and enlarged ventricles. The range of depression in the MS population is 27% to 54% (81). Patients with MS do have more episodes of depression than normal controls, patients with other neurologic disease, or patients with disabling conditions that do not affect the brain (82–84). Furthermore, MS patients with cerebral lesions have more episodes of depression than do those with primarily spinal lesions, supporting the belief that brain lesions play some role in their depression (82).

Cognitive dysfunction can impact on function, employment, and the rehabilitation process. However, assessment of the degree of cognitive impairment can be difficult. Routine screening may not be sensitive enough to identify patients with impairment, whereas formal testing can be time consuming and costly. Franklin described four factors that may predict cognitive impairment in MS: (a) chronic progressive disease course; (b) MRI-documented moderate to severe periventricular demyelination, ventricular enlargement, or collosal atrophy; (c) gait apraxia; and (d) affective disorder (81).

SPASTICITY

Spasticity can have a significant impact on function in MS patients. It can accompany weakness or interfere with function despite relatively normal strength. For some individuals spasticity can be useful and help in transfers and standing, but in others it can interfere with mobility, activities of daily living, and sexual activity. Because MS plaques can occur throughout the central nervous system, spasticity can result from spinal or supraspinal lesions.

Treatment should be initiated if spasticity results in a functional impairment, disturbance of gait, or pain. Three broad categories of intervention should be considered when the decision to treat spasticity is made. These include physical strategies, pharmacologic intervention, and surgical procedures (Fig. 50-6). Physical strategies include the prevention of noxious stimuli, a regular stretching program, spasticity-reducing postures, cold applications, and casting or splinting (85,86). When spasticity remains a problem despite these measures, pharmacologic intervention is indicated. The most common oral medications include baclofen, tizanidine, diazepam, dantrolene, and clonidine. The transdermal clonidine system is also useful. Whereas baclofen and diazepam work at the central nervous system level, baclofen providing

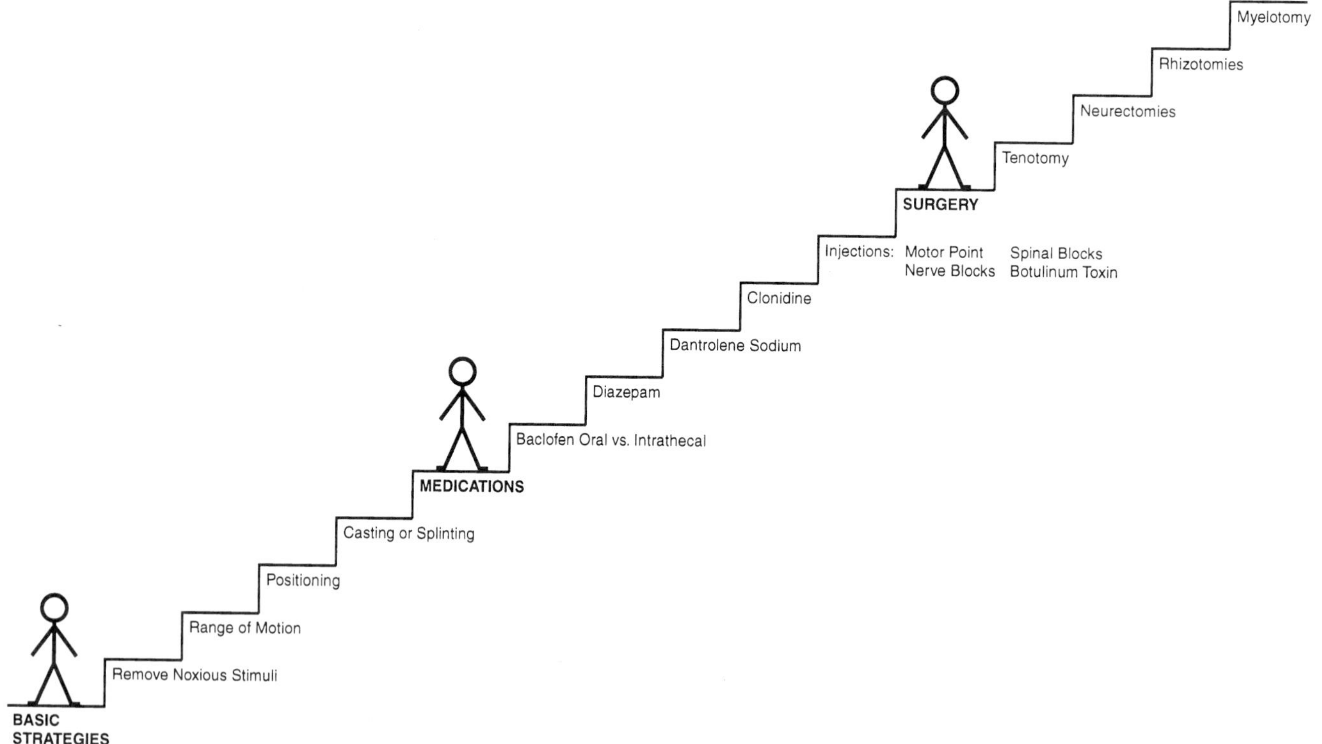

FIG. 50-6. Stepwise management of spasticity.

presynaptic inhibition and diazepam facilitating postsynaptic effects of GABA, dantrolene works at the muscular level, reducing the release of calcium into the sarcoplasmic reticulum (86). Tizanidine is an alpha noradrenergic agonist which decreases facilitory inputs from spinal polysynaptic pathways acting at brain and spinal levels.

All can have significant side effects, and baclofen and diazepam should be tapered rather than discontinued abruptly. When spasticity remains a problem, intrathecal baclofen administered by an implantable pump has been shown effective in the treatment of refractory spasticity (86). The direct instillation of baclofen into the spinal fluid allows for small doses and more precise titration to provide improvement. Nerve and motor point blocks can provide a local reduction of spasticity in a specific muscle or group of muscles that interfere with function. Results are temporary, depending on the agent injected. Spinal blocks, intrathecal injection of agents, can provide a more diffuse effect by affecting multiple spinal roots but result in bladder and bowel incontinence, weakness, and paresthesias (86). Finally, surgical procedures, including tenotomies, the release of a tendon, and neurectomies and rhizotomies, can be beneficial in select patients. The lesioning of nerves or nerve roots can improve function or make it easier for care to be given.

FATIGUE

Fatigue is ubiquitous to varying degrees in MS patients. Although most individuals have experienced fatigue and may be aware of the lack of energy associated with depression, the fatigue reported by individuals with MS appears to be a distinct clinical entity. Patients will frequently report that their fatigue occurs daily, worsens with heat, stress, and activity, and is severe enough to prevent physical activity (87). It is a common complaint reported in as many as 77% of MS patients and can have a significant impact on function (88,89). Frequently it is misunderstood by patients and family members (90).

Although one would expect worsening fatigue with increasing neurologic impairment this has not necessarily been the case. In a study of 115 MS patients with fatigue no correlation between degree of disability and fatigue was noted (91). Similiarly, depression has not necessarily been associated with symptoms of fatigue (90).

Treatment of MS fatigue has been largely pharmacologic in nature. In a randomized, double blind, placebo-controlled crossover trial, amantadine was shown to have an effect on fatigue severity and to decrease the effect of fatigue on activity (91). In a smaller crossover study, amantadine was shown to improve energy level, sense of well-being, perceived attention and memory, and problem-solving capability (92). Pemoline, a central nervous system stimulant, has also been investigated as a potential treatment of fatigue. Forty-one patients with clinically definite MS and severe fatigue were studied. Although the differences between pemoline and placebo for the relief of fatigue did not reach statistical significance, there was a trend in favor of pemoline. The authors concluded that pemoline may be an effective treatment option in MS-associated fatigue (93). However, neither drug has shown an effect on improving cognitive function, leading to the belief that fatigue may not affect cognitive function in MS patients (94).

Recently, Schwartz investigated the role of psychosocial and psychological factors in MS fatigue. She reported an association between a low sense of environmental mastery and both global fatigue and fatigue-related distress. Furthermore, reports of severe fatigue were associated with depression. Based on these findings, treatment options for MS-related fatigue might be broadened beyond just pharmacologic considerations to include techniques that would help individuals master their environment, such as pacing, energy conservation, work simplification, and time management (90). These techniques, which have been applied to other disabled populations, may also help in the symptom management of the MS patient.

EXERCISE

Weakness is a common finding in individuals with MS and a frequent cause of impairment. For years physicians felt exercise was contraindicated for MS patients because of the concern that overexertion could initiate exacerbations of the disease. It is now felt that appropriate exercise can be beneficial and prevent secondary disability. Exercise to improve strength and endurance is the cornerstone of many rehabilitation programs; however, the response to exercise in MS patients has not been completely elucidated.

Autonomic regulation of the cardiovascular response to exercise is important in determining exercise capabilities. Dysfunction of the autonomic system is common in patients with MS and typically appreciated as bowel and bladder dysfunction. Studies using heart rate and blood pressure response have investigated the cardiovascular influences to exercise in MS patients. The results have been quite variable, possibly because of the varying degrees of neurologic impairment among study groups (95). Although the cardiovascular response to exercise may be blunted, it has been shown adequate to improve exercise capacity (96). In a study of 25 MS patients divided into a more- (EDSS > 3.5) and a less-impaired (EDSS ≤ 3.5) group, Shapiro showed that both groups improved their exercise capacity relative to the non-exercising control group but that those in the less-impaired group were able to exercise longer, achieve a higher maximal exercise intensity, and showed overall greater improvement following an exercise program than did the more impaired group (96). Gehlsen studied ten MS patients who underwent a 10-week training program of swimming and/or calisthenics at an intensity of 60% to 75% of estimated maximal heart rate. Improvements in isokinetic peak torque of upper and lower extremities and improvements in lower extremity fatigability were noted (97).

It appears that training can have a positive affect on the fitness of persons with MS. The degree of neurologic impairment does appear to influence the maximum aerobic capacity of MS patients. Individuals who are less impaired are able to exercise for longer periods of time and achieve higher maximal exercise intensities and maximal oxygen uptake (95).

ATAXIA, DYSMETRIA, AND INCOORDINATION

Some of the most incapacitating problems seen in patients with MS results from a constellation of symptoms including incoordination, dysmetria, ataxia, and tremor. Symptoms can vary from minimal annoying movements with no functional impairment to severe loss of control resulting in an inability to use the upper extremities for functional tasks, an inability to sit unsupported, or declining ambulatory status. Worsening of symptoms over time will typically be described as increasing difficulty with fine motor tasks including the use of utensils for feeding, with the patient resorting to finger foods for independence in eating. With lower extremity involvement, patients will typically describe worsening balance during ambulation and the need to hold on to walls or furniture. During ambulation, patients will typically display a wide-base gait with worsening balance when initiating gait or changing directions.

Three treatment categories—medications, physical interventions, and compensating techniques—should be considered in addressing these problems. A number of medications have been tried to decrease the tremor seen in MS patients. Sabro (98) studied the benefits of isoniazid (INH) on the wide-amplitude postural tremor seen in four MS patients. All four patients had improvement in their tremor to the degree that functional status improved. Other studies with INH have shown either no benefit or only mild improvement in tremor with insignificant functional improvement (99–101). Primidone, an anticonvulsant drug, has been shown to be effective in reducing the amplitude of essential tremors (102). Henkin (103) described a reduction in the kinetic tremor of the two MS patients with the use of primidone. Other medications used to reduce tremors in the MS population include propranolol and clonazepam.

Physical interventions might include such interventions as strengthening of proximal or stabilizing muscles, balance training utilizing treatment sequences in appropriate functional tasks, and endurance training (104). Frankel exercises have long been reported in the treatment of ataxia. These exercises utilize other sensory organs, repetition of lost functions, and retraining of functional patterns to regain coordination. Although their original use was in patients with loss of proprioception, they have been described as helpful in cerebellar ataxia as seen in MS (105).

Compensatory techniques may also prove helpful in alleviating symptoms and improving function. Arm weights are commonly utilized; adaptive equipment including weighted utensils, walkers, or canes are sometimes beneficial in decreasing the tremor and improving function. Appropriate seating systems and other adaptations to improve trunk and proximal muscle stabilization can also be helpful in decreasing symptoms.

DYSPHAGIA AND DYSARTHRIA

Treatment of dysphagia and dysarthria is often difficult and unsuccessful. Swallowing difficulties are not uncommon and have been reported in 10% to 33% of patients with MS (106). The range of abnormalities that can be encountered is varied. Early symptoms typically present as occasional complaints of choking on food or liquids, particularly thin liquids. Such events will frequently occur when large amounts are ingested or the individual is distracted or inattentive during eating. Worsening of symptoms can occur and result in mild, moderate, or severe impairment requiring modifications of diet, swallowing precautions, and techniques to prevent aspiration or alternative forms of feeding (106). Reduced pharyngeal peristalsis and delayed swallowing reflex are the most commonly seen features of dysphagia in MS patients (106).

In early descriptions of the disease, Charcot described the classic triad of signs in multiple sclerosis: nystagmus, intention tremor, and dysarthria (107). Furthermore, he described the speech as slow and drawling, with pauses after each syllable, with the words sounding as if measured or scanned. Although spastic, ataxic, and spastic/ataxic dysarthria occur in MS, many other speech deviations are also noted in this population. In a study of 169 MS patients, evaluation revealed abnormal speech performance in 41% (107). The most frequent deviation was impairment of loudness control, followed by harsh voice quality, defective articulation impairing emphasis, impaired pitch control, and hypernasality, among others (107). Only 9% displayed articulation typical of ataxic dysarthria, and 14% displayed characteristics of scanning speech. In this study the severity of dysarthria was related to the severity of the neurologic involvement.

IMPAIRMENT RATING IN MULTIPLE SCLEROSIS

The unpredictable course of the disease and the variable nature of associated physical impairment have necessitated the development of a standardized system of profiling and communicating about patients with MS. It was with this purpose in mind that the Minimal Record of Disability (MRD) was developed (108). The MRD profiles the main dysfunctions associated with MS and consists of five parts: (a) demographic information, (b) the Kurtzke Functional Systems (FS), (c) the Kurtzke Expanded Disability Status Scale (EDSS), (d) the Incapacity Status Scale (ISS), and (e) the Environmental Status Scale (ESS) (108).

The ISS is a 16-item inventory of functional status based on the Pulses profile and the Barthel Index. The ESS is an assessment of social handicap and addresses such areas as work, financial/economic status, personal residence/home, required personal assistance, transportation, community ser-

TABLE 50-1. *Expanded Disability Status Scale (EDSS) of Kurtzke*

0 =	Normal neurologic exam (all grade 0 in Functional Systems [FS]; Cerebral grade 1 acceptable).
1.0 =	No disability, minimal signs in one FS (i.e., grade 1 excluding Cerebral grade 1).
1.5 =	No disability, minimal signs in more than one FS (more than one grade 1 excluding Cerebral grade 1).
2.0 =	Minimal disability in one FS (one FS grade 2, others 0 or 1).
2.5 =	Minimal disability in two FS (two FS grade 2, others 0 or 1).
3.0 =	Moderate disability in one FS (one FS grade 3, others 0 or 1), or mild disability in three or four FS (three/four FS grade 2, others 0 or 1) though fully ambulatory.
3.5 =	Fully ambulatory but with moderate disability in one FS (one grade 3) and one or two FS grade 2; or two FS grade 3; or five FS grade 2 (others 0 or 1).
4.0 =	Fully ambulatory without aid, self-sufficient, up and about some 12 hours a day despite relatively severe disability consisting of one FS grade 4 (others 0 or 1) or combinations of lesser grades exceeding limits of previous steps. Able to walk without aid or rest some 500 m.
4.5 =	Fully ambulatory without aid, up and about much of the day, able to work a full day, may otherwise have some limitation of full activity or require minimal assistance; characterized by relatively severe disability, usually consisting of one FS grade 4 (others 0 or 1) or combinations of lesser grades exceeding limits of previous steps. Able to walk without aid or rest for some 300 m.
5.0 =	Ambulatory without aid or rest for about 200 m; disability severe enough to impair full daily activities (e.g., to work full day without special provisions). Usual FS equivalents are one grade 5 alone, others 0 or 1; or combinations of lesser grades usually exceeding specifications for step 4.0.
5.5 =	Ambulatory without aid or rest for about 100 m; disability severe enough to preclude full daily activities. Usual FS equivalents are one grade 5 alone, others 0 or 1; or combinations of lesser grades usually exceeding those for step 4.0.
6.0 =	Intermittent or unilateral constant assistance (cane, crutch, or brace) required to walk about 100 m with or without resting. Usual FS equivalents are combinations with more than two FS grade 3+ .
6.5 =	Constant bilateral assistance (canes, crutches, or braces) required to walk about 20 m without resting. Usual FS equivalents are combinations with more than two FS grade 3+ .
7.0 =	Unable to walk beyond about 5 m even with aid, essentially restricted to wheelchair; wheels self in standard wheelchair and transfers alone; up and about in wheelchair some 12 hours a day. Usual FS equivalents are combinations with more than one FS grade 4+ ; very rarely, pyramidal grade 5 alone.
7.5 =	Unable to take more than a few steps; restricted to wheelchair; may need aid in transfer; wheels self but cannot carry on in standard wheelchair a full day; may require motorized wheelchair. Usual FS equivalents are combinations with more than one FS grade 4+ .
8.0 =	Essentially restricted to bed or chair or perambulated in wheelchair, but may be out of bed itself much of the day; retains many self-care functions; generally has effective use of arms. Usual FS equivalents are combinations, generally grade 4+ in several systems.
8.5 =	Essentially restricted to bed much of the day; has some effective use of arm(s); retains some self-care functions. Usual FS equivalents are combinations, generally 4+ in several systems.
9.0 =	Helpless bed patient; can communicate and eat. Usual FS equivalents are combinations, mostly grade 4+ .
9.5 =	Totally helpless bed patient; unable to communicate effectively or eat/swallow. Usual FS equivalents are combinations, almost all grade 4+ .
10 =	Death caused by MS.

vices, and social activity (108). The most frequently used rating scale for neurologic impairments is the EDSS of Kurtze (26). First described in 1955, the scale has undergone revisions resulting in its present format. The EDSS is a 10-point scale intended to measure maximal function and limitations resulting from neurologic deficits (Table 50-1). The EDSS is half of a two-part rating scale, the other part being the eight FS of Kurtzke, which represents the neurologic abnormalities that can be attributed to MS lesions (Table 50-2). The eight functional systems are pyramidal, cerebellar, brainstem, sensory, bowel and bladder, visual, cerebral, and miscellaneous functions. Mutually exclusive, these eight functional systems are give a numerical rating based on objective deficits, with greater dysfunction represented by higher numbers. The FS is not additive and can be compared over time only with itself.

The EDSS is used widely in the MS literature. It has been used to classify patients' levels of neurologic impairment in drug trials, in rehabilitation interventions, and in attempts to correlate many variables with severity of the disease. Because of its widespread use, a basic understanding of this scale is necessary for health care providers treating MS patients.

CONCLUSION

Multiple sclerosis is a relatively common progressive neurologic disease of young adults. Most patients will develop symptoms early in life and live a relatively normal life span. Consequently, many patients will experience chronic neurologic impairments and diminished functional status. Rehabilitation and optimization of functional status are important components of the medical care provided to MS patients. Little, however, has been written about rehabilitation, its benefits, cost effectiveness, or most appropriate setting in the MS population. Greenspun looked at 28 MS patients who underwent inpatient rehabilitation. A significant per-

TABLE 50-2. *Kurtzke functional systems*

Pyramidal functions
0. Normal
1. Abnormal signs without disability
2. Minimal disability
3. Mild or moderate paraparesis or hemiparesis; severe monoparesis
4. Marked paraparesis or hemiparesis; moderate quadriparesis; or monoplegia
5. Paraplegia, hemiplegia, or marked quadriparesis
6. Quadriplegia
V. Unknown

Cerebellar functions
0. Normal
1. Abnormal signs without disability
2. Mild ataxia
3. Moderate truncal or limb ataxia
4. Severe ataxia, all limbs
5. Unable to perform coordinated movements because of ataxia
V. Unknown
X. Is used throughout after each number when weakness (grade 3 or more on pyramidal) interferes with testing

Brainstem functions
0. Normal
1. Signs only
2. Moderate nystagmus or other mild disability
3. Severe nystagmus, marked extraocular weakness, or moderate disability of other cranial nerves
4. Marked dysarthria or other marked disability
5. Inability to speak or swallow
V. Unknown

Sensory functions (revised 1982)
0. Normal
1. Vibration or figure-writing decrease only, in one or two limbs
2. Mild decrease in touch or pain or position sense and/or moderate decrease in vibration in one or two limbs; or vibratory (c/s figure writing) decrease alone in three or four limbs
3. Moderate decrease in touch or pain or position sense, and/or essentially lost vibration in one or two limbs; or mild decrease in touch or pain and/or moderate decrease in all proprioceptive tests in three or four limbs
4. Marked decrease in touch or pain or loss of proprioception, alone or combined, in one or two limbs; or moderate decrease in touch or pain and/or severe proprioceptive decrease in more than two limbs
5. Loss (essentially) of sensation in one or two limbs; or moderate decrease in touch or pain and/or loss of proprioceptive for most of the body below the head
6. Sensation essentially lost below the head
V. Unknown

Bowel and bladder functions (revised 1982)
0. Normal
1. Mild urinary hesitancy, urgency, or retention
2. Moderate hesitancy, urgency, retention of bowel or bladder, or rare urinary incontinence
3. Frequent urinary incontinence
4. In need for almost constant catheterization
5. Loss of bladder function
6. Loss of bowel and bladder function
V. Unknown

Visual (or optic) functions
0. Normal
1. Scotoma with visual acuity (corrected) better than 20/30
2. Worse eye with scotoma with maximal visual acuity (corrected) of 20/30 to 20/59
3. Worse eye with large scotoma, or moderate decrease in fields, but with maximal visual acuity (corrected) of 20/60 to 20/99
4. Worse eye with marked decrease of fields and maximal visual acuity (corrected) of 20/100 to 20/200; grade 3 plus maximal acuity of better eye of 20/60 or less
5. Worse eye with maximal visual acuity (corrected) less than 20/200; grade 4 plus maximal acuity of better eye of 20/60 or less
6. Grade 5 plus maximal visual acuity of better eye of 20/60 or less
V. Unknown
X. Is added to grades 0 to 6 for presence of temporal pallor

Cerebral (or mental) functions
0. Normal
1. Mood alterations only (does not affect DSS score)
2. Mild decrease in mentation
3. Moderate decrease in mentation
4. Marked decrease in mentation (chronic brain syndrome, moderate)
5. Dementia or chronic brain syndrome—severe or incompetent
V. Unknown

Other functions
0. None
1. Any other neurologic findings attributed to MS (specify)
V. Unknown

centage of patients showed improvement to independent ambulation, transfers, stair climbing, dressing, bathing, and toileting (109). In a pilot study of 20 MS patients, Feigenson showed that intensive multidisciplinary therapy produced significant improvements in balance, self-care activities, mobility skills, and bladder control (110). Furthermore, a cost analysis of treatment and care needed to maintain individuals at home showed significant reductions in home care costs following rehabilitation and an overall saving during the year after rehabilitation. Bourdette et al. retrospectively evaluated the health care costs of 165 veterans with MS and attempted to correlate costs with measures of neurologic impairment and disability (111). The majority of costs incurred were VA benefits and home health costs. Overall costs rose precipitously with a Kurtzke EDSS score greater than 5.0. The EDSS score was the best predictor of VA benefit costs, and the incapacity scale was the best predictor of home health costs.

Some general conclusions can be drawn about the role of rehabilitation in MS. Functional status can be improved, but certain forms of impairment are more amenable to treatment than others. Patients with severe cerebellar symptoms make less improvement than those without severe tremor, ataxia, or dysmetria (110). Improvements in functional status can lower care-giving needs, and there is evidence to support the cost effectiveness of rehabilitation (110). Yet further research is needed to determine the effect of disease duration or disease pattern on rehabilitation outcome and level of rehabilitation care needed, acute or subacute, to improve function.

REFERENCES

1. Anderson DW, Ellenberg JH, Leventhal M, et al. Revised estimate of the prevalence of multiple sclerosis in the United States. *Ann Neurol* 1992; 31:333–336.
2. Dean G. How many people in the world have multiple sclerosis? *Neuroepidemiology* 1994; 13:1–7.
3. Kurtzke JF, Hyllested K. Multiple sclerosis in the Faroe Islands II. Clinical update, transmission and the nature of MS *Neurology* 1985; 35:307–328.
4. Martyn C. Epidemiology. In: Matthews WB, ed. *McAlpine's multiple sclerosis, 2nd ed.* Edinburgh: Churchill Livingstone, 1991; 3–35.
5. Weinshenker BG. Epidemiology of multiple sclerosis. *Neurol Clin* 1996; 14:291–308.
6. Rosati G. Descriptive epidemiology of multiple sclerosis in Europe in the 1980's: a critical overview. *Ann Neurol* 1994; 36(S2):S164–S174.
7. Mumford CJ, Wood NW, Kellar-Wood H, Thorpe JW, Miller DH, Compston DAS. The British Isles survey of multiple sclerosis in twins. *Neurology* 1994; 44:11–15.
8. Sadovnick AD, Armstrong H, Rice GP, et al. A Population-based study of multiple sclerosis in twins: update. *Ann Neurol* 1993; 33: 281–285.
9. Haegert DG, Marrosu MG. Genetic susceptibility to multiple sclerosis. *Ann Neurol* 1994; 36(S2):2S04–S210.
10. Prineas JW. Pathology of multiple sclerosis. In: Cook SD, ed. *Handbook of multiple sclerosis.* New York: Marcel Dekker, 1990; 187–218.
11. Sobel RA. The pathology of multiple sclerosis. *Neurol Clin* 1995; 13: 1–21.
12. Giovannoni G, Hartung HP. The immunopathogenesis of multiple sclerosis and Guillain–Barre sydrome. *Curr Opin Neurol* 1996; 9: 165–177.
13. Waxman SG. Pathophysiology of multiple sclerosis. In: Cook SD, ed. *Handbook of multiple sclerosis.* New York: Marcel Dekker, 1990; 219–249.
14. Prineas JW, Barnard RD, Revesz T, et al. Multiple sclerosis: pathology of recurrent lesions. *Brain* 1993; 116:681–693.
15. Matthews WB. Symptoms and signs. In: Matthews WB, ed. *McAlpine's multiple sclerosis, 2nd ed.* Edinburgh: Churchill Livingstone, 1991; 43–105.
16. Rao SM, Leo GJ, Bernadin L, Unverzagt F. Cognitive dysfunction in multiple sclerosis: frequency, patterns, and prediction. *Neurology* 1991; 41:685–691.
17. Krupp LB, Sliwinski M, Masur DM, Freidberg F, Coyle PK. Cognitive functioning and depression in patients with chronic fatigue syndrome and multiple sclerosis. *Arch Neurol* 1994; 51:705–710.
18. Poser CM, Paty DW, Scheinberg L, et al. New diagnostic criteria for multiple sclerosis: guidelines for research protocols. *Ann Neurol* 1983; 13:227–231.
19. Paty DW, Oger JJF, Kastrukoff LF, et al. MRI in the diagnosis of MS: a prospective study with comparison of clinical evaluation, evoked potentials, oligoclonal banding, and CT. *Neurology* 1988; 38: 180–185.
20. Offenbacher H, Fazekas F, Schmidt R, et al. Assessment of MRI criteria for a diagnosis of MS. *Neurology* 1993; 43:905–909.
21. Herndon RM, Brooks B. Misdiagnosis of multiple sclerosis. *Semin Neurol* 1985; 5:94–98.
22. Rudick RA, Schiffer RB, Schwetz KM, Herndon RM. Multiple sclerosis. The problem of misdiagnosis. *Arch Neurol* 1986; 43:578–583.
23. Willoughby EW, Grochowski E, Li DKB, Oger J, Kastrukoff LF, Paty DW. Serial magnetic resonance scanning in multiple sclerosis: a second prospective study in relapsing patients. *Ann Neurol* 1989; 25:43–49.
24. Kurtzke JF. A new scale for evaluating disability in multiple sclerosis. *Neurology* 1955; 5:580–583.
25. Kurtzke JF. Further notes on disability evaluation in multiple sclerosis with scale modifications. *Neurology* 1965; 15:654–661.
26. Kurtzke JF. Rating neurologic impairment in multiple sclerosis; and expanded disability status scale (EDSS). *Neurology* 1983; 33: 1444–1452.
27. Sipe JC, Knobler RL, Braheny SL, Rice GPA, Panitch HS, Oldstone MBA. A neurologic rating scale (NRS) for use in multiple sclerosis. *Neurology* 1984; 34:1368–1372.
28. Wynn DR, Rodriguez M, O'Fallon M, et al. A reappraisal of the epidemiology of multiple sclerosis in Olmstead County Minnesota. *Neurology* 1990; 40:780–786.
29. Phadke JG. Survival pattern and cause of death in patients with multiple sclerosis: results from an epidemiological survey in north east Scotland. *J Neurol Neurosurg Psychiatry* 1987; 50:523–531.
30. Poser S, Kurtzke JF, Poser W, Schlaf G. Survival in multiple sclerosis. *J Clin Epidemiol* 1989; 42:159–168.
31. Sadovnick AD, Ebers GC, Wilson RW, Paty DW. Life expectancy in patients attending multiple sclerosis clinics. *Neurology* 1992; 42: 991–994.
32. Weinshenker BG. Natural history of multiple sclerosis. *Ann Neurol* 1994; 36(s):S6–S11.
33. Phadke JG. Clinical aspects of multiple sclerosis in north east Scotland with particular reference to its course and prognosis. *Brain* 1990; 113: 1597–1628.
34. McAlphine D. The benign form of multiple sclerosis: results of a long term study. *Br Med J* 1964; 2:1029–1032.
35. Weinshenker BG, Bass B, Rice GPA, et al. The natural history of multiple sclerosis: a geographically based study. 1. Clinical course and disability. *Brain* 1989; 112:133–146.
36. Runmarker B, Anderson O. Prognostic factors in a multiple sclerosis incidence cohort with twenty-five years of follow-up. *Brain* 1993; 116:117–134.
37. Sibley WA, Bamford CR, Clark K. Clinical viral infections and multiple sclerosis. *Lancet* 1985; 1:1313–1315.
38. Weinshenker BG, Rice GPA, Noseworthy JH, et al. The natural history of multiple sclerosis; a geographically based study 3. Multivariate analysis of predictive factors and models of outcome. *Brain* 1991; 114:1045–1056.
39. Kurtzke JF, Beebe GW, Nagler B, Kurland LT, Auth TL. Studies on the natural history of multiple sclerosis. VIII: Early prognostic features of the later course of the illness. *J Chron Dis* 1977; 30:819–830.
40. Miller DH, Albert PS, Barkof F, et al. Guidelines for the use of magnetic resonance techniques in monitoring the treatment of multiple sclerosis. *Ann Neurol* 1996; 39:6–16.
41. Rose AS, Kuzma JW, Kurtzke JF, Namerow NS, Sibley WA, Tourtellotte WW. Cooperative study in the evaluation of therapy in multiple sclerosis; ACTH vs. placebo. *Neurology* 1970; 20:1–59.
42. Thompson AJ, Kennard C, Swash M, et al. Relative efficacy of intravenous methylprednisolone and ACTH in the treatment of acute relapse in MS. *Neurology* 1989; 39:969–971.
43. Beck RW, Cleary PA, Anderson MM Jr, et al. A randomized controlled trial of corticosteroids in the treatment of acute optic neuritis. *N Engl J Med* 1992; 326:581–588.
44. The IFNB multiple sclerosis study group and the University of British Columbia MS/MRI analysis group. Interferon beta-1b in the treatment of multiple sclerosis: final outcome of the randomized controlled trial. *Neurology* 1995; 45:1277–1285.
45. Jacobs LD, Cookfair DL, Rudick RA, et al. Intramuscular interferon beta-1a for disease progression in relapsing multiple sclerosis. *Ann Neurol* 1996; 39:285–294.

46. Report of the quality standards subcommittee of the American Academy of Neurology. Practice advisory on selection of patients with multiple sclerosis for treatment with Betaseron. *Neurology* 1994; 44: 1537–1540.
47. Lublin FD, Whitaker JN, Eidelman BH, Miller AE, Arnason BGW, Burks JS. Management of patients receiving interferon beta-1b for multiple sclerosis: report of a consensus conference. *Neurology* 1996; 46:12–18.
48. Johnson KP, Brooks BR, Cohen JA, et al. Copolymer-1 reduces relapse rate and improved disability in relapsing-remitting multiple sclerosis; results of a phase III multicenter, double-blind, placebo-controlled trial. *Neurology* 1995; 45:1268–1276.
49. Thompson AJ, Noseworthy JH. New treatments for multiple sclerosis: a clinical perspective. *Curr Opin Neurol* 1996; 9:187–198.
50. Miller H. Trauma and multiple sclerosis. *Lancet* 1964; 1:848–850.
51. Poser CM. Trauma and multiple sclerosis. A hypotheses. *J Neurol* 1987; 234:155–159.
52. Brain R, Wilkinson M. The association of cervical spondylosis and disseminated sclerosis. *Brain* 1957; 80:456–478.
53. Sibley WA, Bamford CR, Clark K, Smith MS, Laguna JF. A prospective study of physical trauma and multiple sclerosis. *J Neurol Neurosurg Psychiatry* 1991; 54:584–589.
54. Kurland LT. Trauma and multiple sclerosis. *Ann Neurol* 1994; 36: 533–537.
55. Panitch HS. Influence of infection on exacerbations of multiple sclerosis. *Ann Neurol* 1994; 36:525–528.
56. Millar JHD, Allison RS, Cheesimen EA. Pregnancy as a factor influencing relapse in disseminated sclerosis. *Brain* 1959; 82:417–426.
57. Shapiro K, Poskanzar DC, Newell DJ. Marriage, preganancy and multiple sclerosis. *Brain* 1966; 89:419–428.
58. Ghezzi A, Caputo D. Pregnancy: a factor influencing the course of multiple sclerosis. *Eur Neurol* 1981; 20:517–519.
59. Poser S, Poser W. Multiple sclerosis and gestation. *Neurology* 1983; 33:1422–1427.
60. Korn-Labetzki I, Khana E, Cooper G, Abramsky O. Activity of multiple sclerosis during pregnancy and puerperum. *Ann Neurol* 1984; 16: 229–231.
61. Stenager E, Stenager EN, Jensen K. Sexual aspects of multiple sclerosis. *Semin Neurology* 1992; 2:120–124.
62. Valleroy ML, Kraft G. Sexual dysfunction in multiple sclerosis. *Arch Phys Med Rehabil* 1984; 65:125–128.
63. Miller H, Simpson CA, Yeates WK. Bladder dysfunction in multiple sclerosis. *Br Med J* 1965; 1:1265–1269.
64. Blaivas JG. Management of bladder dysfunction in multiple sclerosis. *Neurology* 1980; 30:12–18.
65. Bradley WE, Logothetis JL, Timm GW. Cystometric and sphincter abnormalities in multiple sclerosis. *Neurology* 1973; 23:1131–1139.
66. Schoenberg HW, Gutrich J, Banno J. Urodynamic patterns in multiple sclerosis. *J Urol* 1979; 122:648–650.
67. Blaivas JG, Bhimani G, Labib KB. Vesicourethral dysfunction in multiple sclerosis. *J Urol* 1979; 122:324–327.
68. Schoenberg HW, Gutrich JM. Management of vesical dysfunction in multiple sclerosis. *Urology* 1980; 16:444–447.
69. Philp T, Read DJ, Higson RH. The urodynamic characteristics of multiple sclerosis. *Br J Urol* 1981; 53:672–675.
70. Blaivas JG, Barbolios GA. Detrusor–external sphincter dyssynergia in men with multiple sclerosis: An ominous urologic condition. *J Urol* 1984; 131:91–94.
71. Anderson JT, Bradley WE. Abnormalties of detrusor and sphincter function in multiple sclerosis. *Br J Urol* 1976; 48:193–198.
72. Samellas W, Rubin B. Management of upper tract complications in multiple sclerosis by means of urinary diversion to an ileal conduit. *J Urol* 1965; 93:548–552.
73. Jameson RM. Management of the bladder in non-traumatic paraplegia. *Paraplegia* 1974; 12:92–97.
74. Bradley WE. Urinary bladder dysfunction in multiple sclerosis. *Neurology* 1978; 28:52–58.
75. Sliwa JA, Bell HK, Mason KD, Gore RM, Nanninga J, Cohen B. Upper urinary tract abnormalities in multiple sclerosis patients with urinary symptoms. *Arch Phys Med Rehabil* 1996; 77:247–251.
76. Rao SM, Leo GJ, Ellington L, Nauertz T, Bernardin MS, Unverzagt F. Cognitive dysfunction in multiple sclerosis. II. Impact on employment and social functioning. *Neurology* 1991; 41:692–696.
77. Peyser JM, Edwards KR, Poser CM, Filskov SB. Cognitive function in patients with multiple sclerosis. *Arch Neurol* 1980; 37:577–579.
78. Rao SM, Hammeke TA, McQuillen MP, Khatri BO, Illoyd D. Memory disturbances in chronic progressive multiple sclerosis. *Arch Neurol* 1984; 41:625–631.
79. Heaton RK, Nelson LM, Thompson DS, Burks JS, Franklin GM. Neuropsychological findings in relapsing–remitting and chronic-progression multiple sclerosis. *J Consult Clin Psychol* 1985; 53:103–110.
80. Rao SM, Leo GJ, Haughton VM, St Aubin-Faubert P, Bernandin L. Correlation of magnetic resonance imaging with neuropsychological testing in multiple sclerosis. *Neurology* 1989; 39:161–166.
81. Beatty WW. Cognitive and emotional disturbances in multiple sclerosis. *Neurol Clin* 1993; 11:189–203.
82. Rabins PV, Brooks BR, O'Donnel P, et al. Structural brain correlates of emotional disorder in multiple sclerosis. *Brain* 1986; 109:587–597.
83. Minden SL, Orav J, Reich P. Depression in multiple sclerosis. *Gen Hosp Psychiatriy* 1987; 9:426–434.
84. Whitlock FA, Siskind MM. Depression as a major symptom in multiple sclerosis. *J Neurol Neurosurg Psychiatry* 1980; 43:861–865.
85. Erickson RP, Lie M, Wineinger MA. Rehabilitation in multiple sclerosis. *Mayo Clin Proc* 1989; 64:818–828.
86. Katz R. Management of spasticity. *Am J Phys Med Rehabil* 1988; 67: 108–116.
87. Krupp LB, Alvarez LA, LaRoccu NG, Schienberg LC. Fatigue in multiple sclerosis. *Arch Neurol* 1988; 45:435–437.
88. Murray TJ. Amantadine therapy for fatigue in multiple sclerosis. *Can J Neurol Sci* 1885; 12:251–254.
89. Freal JE, Kraft GH, Coryell JK. Symptomatic fatigue in multiple sclerosis. *Arch Phys Med Rehabil* 1984; 65:165–168.
90. Schwartz CE, Coulthard-Morris L, Zeng Q. Psychosocial correlates of fatigue in multiple sclerosis. *Arch Phys Med Rehabil* 1996; 77: 165–170.
91. The Canadian Research Group. A randomized controlled trial of amantadine in fatigue associated with multiple sclerosis. *Can J Neurol Sci* 1987; 14:273–278.
92. Cohen RA, Fisher M. Amantadine treatment of fatigue associated with multiple sclerosis. *Arch Neurol* 1989; 46:676–680.
93. Weinshenker BG, Penman M, Boss R, Ebers GC, Rice GPA. A double blind, randomized, crossover trial of pemoline in fatigue associated with multiple sclerosis. *Neurology* 1992; 42:1468–1471.
94. Geisler MW, Sliwinski M, Coyle PK, Masur DM, Dascher C, Krupp LB. The effects of amantadine and pemoline on cognitive functioning in multiple sclerosis. *Arch Neurol* 1996; 53:185–188.
95. Ponichtero-Mulcore JA. Exercise and multiple sclerosis. *Med Sci Sport Exerc* 1993; 25:451–465.
96. Shapiro RT, Petajan JH, Kasich D, Malk B, Feeney J. Role of cardiovascular fitness in multiple sclerosis. *J Neurol Rehabil* 1988; 2:43–49.
97. Gehlsen GM, Grigsby SA, Winant DM. Effects of an aquatic fitness program on the muscular strength and endurance of patients with multiple sclerosis. *Phys Ther* 1984; 64:653–657.
98. Sabro AF, Hallet M, Sudarsky L, Mullally W. Treatment of action tremor in multiple sclerosis with isoniazid. *Neurology* 1982; 32: 912–913.
99. Koller WC. Pharmacologic trials in the treatment of cerebellar tremor. *Arch Neurol* 1984; 41:280–281.
100. Duquette P, Pleines J, du Souich P. Isoniazid for tremor in multiple sclerosis: A controlled trial. *Neurology* 1985; 35:1772–1775.
101. Francis DA, Grundy D, Heron JR. The response to isoniazid of action tremor in multiple sclerosis and its assessment using polarized light goniometry. *J Neurol Neurosurg Psychiatry* 1986; 49:87–89.
102. Koller WC, Royses LC. Efficiacy of primidone in essential tremor. *Neurology* 1986; 36:121–124.
103. Henkin Y, Herishanu YO. Primidone as a treatment for cerebellar tremor in multiple sclerosis—two case reports. *Isr J Med Sci* 1989; 25:720–721.
104. Frankel D. Multiple sclerosis. In: Umphred DA, ed. *Neurological rehabilitation.* St Louis: Mosby-Year Book, 1995; 588–605.

105. Cailliet R. Exercise in multiple sclerosis. In: Basmajian JV, ed. *Therapeutic exercise.* Baltimore: Williams & Wilkins, 1978; 375–388.
106. Yorkston KM, Miller R, Strand E. *Management of speech and swallowing in degenerative disease.* Tucson: Communication Skill Builders, 1995.
107. Darley FL, Aronson AE, Brown JR. *Motor speech disorders.* Philadelphia: WB Saunders, 1975.
108. International Federation of Multiple Sclerosis Societies. *Minimal record of disability for multiple sclerosis.* National Multiple Sclerosis Society, 1985.
109. Greenspun B, Stineman M, Agri R. Multiple sclerosis and rehabilitation outcome. *Arch Phys Med Rehabil* 1987; 64:434–437.
110. Feigenson JS, Schienberg L, Catalano M, et al. The cost-effectiveness of multiple sclerosis rehabilitation: a model. *Neurology* 1981; 31: 1316–1322.
111. Bourdetta DN, Prochazka AV, Mitchel W, Licari P, Burks J. Health care costs of veterans with multiple sclerosis: implications for the rehabilitation of MS. *Arch Phys Med Rehabil* 1993; 74:26–31.

Rehabilitation Medicine: Principles and Practice, Third Edition,
edited by Joel A. DeLisa and Bruce M. Gans.
Lippincott–Raven Publishers, Philadelphia © 1998.

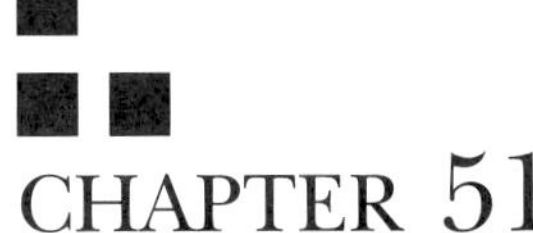

CHAPTER 51

Spinal Cord Injury and Spinal Cord Injury Medicine

William E. Staas, Jr., Christopher S. Formal, Mitchell K. Freedman, Guy W. Fried, and Mary E. Schmidt Read

Spinal cord injury (SCI) is a traumatic insult to the spinal cord that can result in alterations of normal motor, sensory, and autonomic function. Paraplegia involves the lower extremities. Tetraplegia involves all extremities. Optimal management of SCI requires an interdisciplinary team. The team members must be competent as individuals and familiar with each other's treatment approaches, and they must work within a system that promotes effective interaction. The rehabilitation principles presented here also apply to nontraumatic spinal cord disorders. Pediatric SCI is discussed in Chapter 37. Management of the ventilator-dependent patient is discussed in Chapter 55. Management of bowel and bladder problems is discussed in Chapter 44. Management of sexual problems is discussed in Chapter 45. Management of spasticity is discussed in Chapter 40. Management of pressure ulcers is discussed in Chapter 43.

MEDICAL ISSUES AFTER SPINAL CORD INJURY

Classification

There is more than one neurologic classification system for SCI. This chapter uses that of the American Spinal Injury Association (ASIA) (1,2). This system was most recently revised in 1996. Details of the examination are available in instructional materials produced by ASIA.

The standards involve the physical examination only. Imaging studies do not contribute. The basic examination involves motor and sensory function. When this basic information is collected, the level of injury can be determined and the degree of completeness can be specified.

Tetraplegia refers to SCI that involves the arms. *Paraplegia* refers to SCI occurring below the innervation of the arms. Tetraplegia is preferred over quadriplegia. The use of the term "-paresis" is discouraged; rather, the ASIA impairment scale specifies the degree of completeness. An incomplete injury is one in which there is sparing of perianal sensation, deep anal sensation, and sparing of voluntary function of the anal sphincter. Figure 51-1 summarizes the ASIA standards.

Motor Examination

Table 51-1 lists the motor grading scale. If a muscle receives a score of less than 5 but the examiner feels that it is actually fully innervated and that other factors such as pain must be considered, then the muscle can be given a grade of 5. Table 51-2 lists the key muscles. In addition to testing of the key muscles, the presence or absence of voluntary contraction of the anal sphincter is noted. Not all spinal segments have a key muscle. Muscles are always tested in the supine position, although this may differ from standard procedure in settings other than SCI.

Sensory Examination

The sensory grading scale is depicted in Table 51-3. Table 51-4 lists the key sensory points. Each dermatome is graded

W. E. Staas, Jr.: Department of Physical Medicine and Rehabilitation, Thomas Jefferson University; and Magee Rehabilitation Hospital, Philadelphia, Pennsylvania 19102.
C. S. Formal: Department of Rehabilitation Medicine, Thomas Jefferson University Hospital, Philadelphia, Pennsylvania 19102.
M. K. Freedman: Department of Physical Medicine and Rehabilitation, Magee Rehabilitation Hospital, Philadelphia, Pennsylvania 19102.
G. W. Fried: Department of Rehabilitation Medicine, Thomas Jefferson University Hospital; and Magee Rehabilitation Hospital, Philadelphia, Pennsylvania 19102.
M. E. Schmidt Read: Department of Physical Therapy and Spinal Cord Injury Program, Magee Rehabilitation Hospital; and Allegheny University of the Health Sciences, Philadelphia, Pennsylvania 19102.

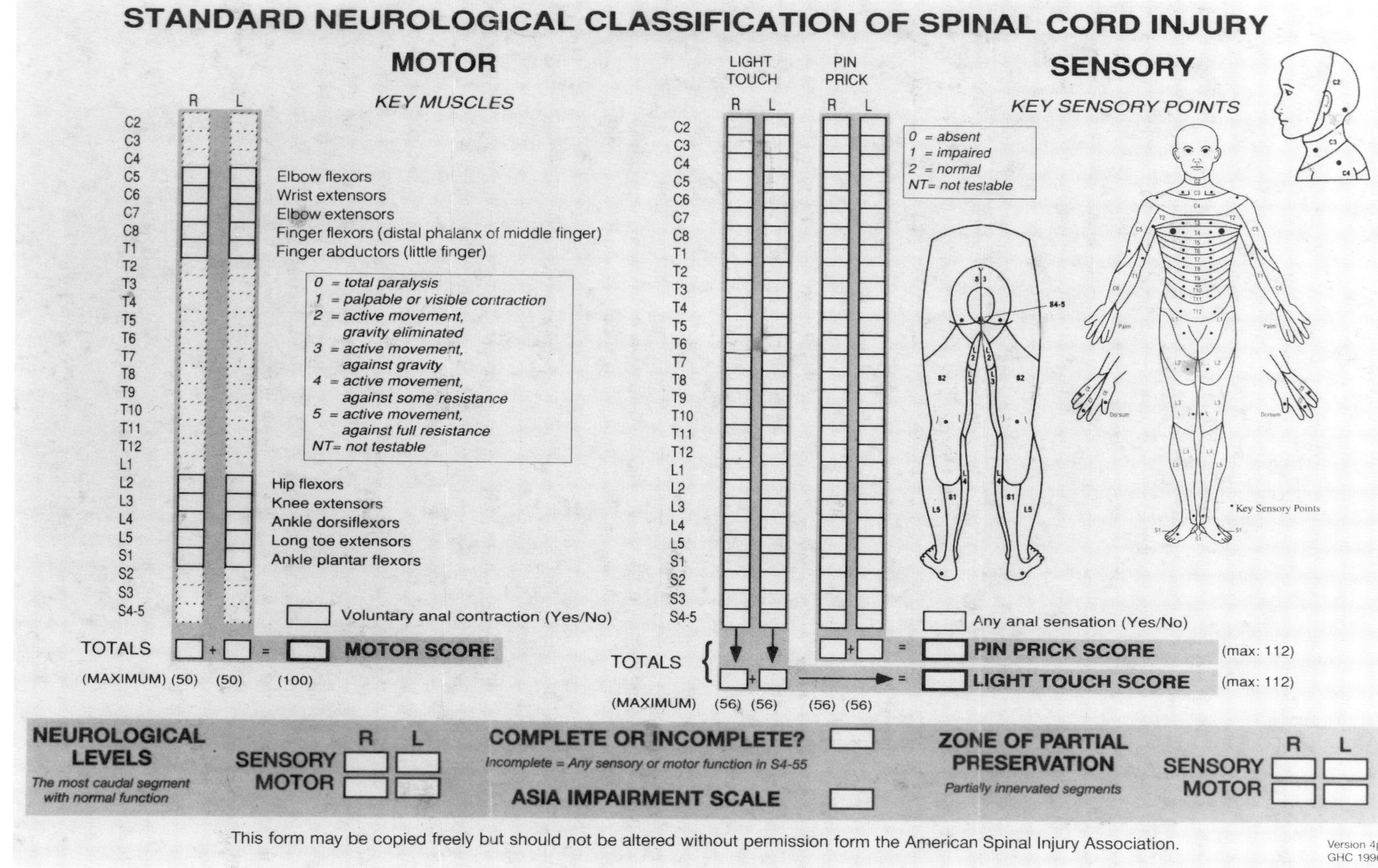

STANDARD NEUROLOGICAL CLASSIFICATION OF SPINAL CORD INJURY

MOTOR

KEY MUSCLES

R L

C2
C3
C4
C5 Elbow flexors
C6 Wrist extensors
C7 Elbow extensors
C8 Finger flexors (distal phalanx of middle finger)
T1 Finger abductors (little finger)
T2
T3
T4
T5
T6
T7
T8
T9
T10
T11
T12
L1
L2 Hip flexors
L3 Knee extensors
L4 Ankle dorsiflexors
L5 Long toe extensors
S1 Ankle plantar flexors
S2
S3
S4-5

0 = total paralysis
1 = palpable or visible contraction
2 = active movement, gravity eliminated
3 = active movement, against gravity
4 = active movement, against some resistance
5 = active movement, against full resistance
NT= not testable

Voluntary anal contraction (Yes/No)

TOTALS [ ] + [ ] = [ ] **MOTOR SCORE**

(MAXIMUM) (50) (50) (100)

SENSORY

KEY SENSORY POINTS

LIGHT TOUCH R L — PIN PRICK R L

C2, C3, C4, C5, C6, C7, C8, T1, T2, T3, T4, T5, T6, T7, T8, T9, T10, T11, T12, L1, L2, L3, L4, L5, S1, S2, S3, S4-5

0 = absent
1 = impaired
2 = normal
NT= not testable

Any anal sensation (Yes/No)

TOTALS [ ] + [ ] = **PIN PRICK SCORE** (max: 112)

[ ] + [ ] → = **LIGHT TOUCH SCORE** (max: 112)

(MAXIMUM) (56) (56) (56) (56)

• Key Sensory Points

NEUROLOGICAL LEVELS
The most caudal segment with normal function
R L
SENSORY
MOTOR

COMPLETE OR INCOMPLETE?
Incomplete = Any sensory or motor function in S4-55

ASIA IMPAIRMENT SCALE

ZONE OF PARTIAL PRESERVATION
Partially innervated segments
R L
SENSORY
MOTOR

This form may be copied freely but should not be altered without permission form the American Spinal Injury Association.

Version 4p
GHC 1996

FIG. 51-1. Summary sheet of International Standards for Neurological and Functional Classification of Spinal Cord Injury. (Reprinted with permission from the American Spinal Injury Association. *International standards for neurological and functional classification of spinal cord injury.* Chicago: American Spinal Injury Association, 1996.)

TABLE 51-1. *Scale for motor testing*

0:	Total paralysis
1:	Palpable or visible contraction
2:	Active movement, full ROM with gravity eliminated
3:	Active movement, full ROM against gravity
4:	Active movement, full ROM against moderate resistance
5:	(Normal) active movement, full ROM against full resistance
NT:	Not testable

Reprinted with permission from the American Spinal Injury Association. *International standards for neurological and functional classification of spinal cord injury.* Chicago: American Spinal Injury Association, 1996.

for both sharp and light touch sensation. Sharp sensation is tested using a disposable safety pin, and light touch with cotton. Hyperesthesia is graded as 1, not 2. When testing for sharp sensation, if the pin is perceived, but not as sharp, the grade is 0, not 1.

Determination of Level

In general the level is the segment just above the most rostral abnormal segment. If C5 is the most rostral abnormal segment, then the level is C4. One can derive a motor level, a sensory level, and a level for the right and the left. For purposes of determining level, a muscle that tests 3 or 4 can be considered normal, provided that the next most rostral muscle is 5. The rationale for this is that muscles are innervated by multiple roots. Thus, for example, the key muscle for L3 could be weak with injury to the L4 spinal segment.

Determination of Degree of Completeness

The ASIA impairment scale is depicted in Table 51-5. This scale closely parallels that of Frankel.

Epidemiology

Incidence and Prevalence

The national annual incidence of cases of SCI with hospitalization is 30 to 40 per million. The national prevalence is from 183,000 to 230,000 (3).

TABLE 51-2. *Key muscles*

C5:	Elbow flexors
C6:	Wrist extensors
C7:	Elbow extensors
C8:	Flexor digitorum profundus to the middle finger
T1:	Small finger abductors
L2:	Hip flexors
L3:	Knee extensors
L4:	Ankle dorsiflexors
L5:	Extensor hallucis longus
S1:	Ankle plantar flexors

Reprinted with permission from the American Spinal Injury Association. *International standards for neurological and functional classification of spinal cord injury.* Chicago: American Spinal Injury Association, 1996.

TABLE 51-3. *Scale for sensory testing*

0:	Absent
1:	Impaired (partial or altered sensation, including hyperesthesia)
2:	Normal
3:	Not testable

Reprinted with permission from the American Spinal Injury Association. *International standards for neurological and functional classification of spinal cord injury.* Chicago: American Spinal Injury Association, 1996.

Age and Gender

SCI occurs primarily in young adults, with more than half occurring in persons 16 to 30 years of age. Males account for about 80% of cases (3).

Causes

The four most common causes of traumatic SCI are motor vehicle crashes (44.5%), falls (18.1%), acts of violence

TABLE 51-4. *Key sensory points*

C2:	Occipital protuberance
C3:	Supraclavicular fossa
C4:	Top of the acromioclavicular joint
C5:	Lateral side of the antecubital fossa
C6:	Thumb
C7:	Middle finger
C8:	Little finger
T1:	Medial (ulnar) side of the antecubital fossa
T2:	Apex of the axilla
T3:	Third intercostal space
T4:	Fourth intercostal space (nipple line)
T5:	Fifth intercostal space (midway between T4 and T6)
T6:	Sixth intercostal space (level of xiphisternum)
T7:	Seventh intercostal space (midway between T6 and T8)
T8:	Eight intercostal space (midway between T10 and T12)
T9:	Ninth intercostal space (midway between T8 and T10)
T10:	Tenth intercostal space (umbilicus)
T11:	Eleventh intercostal space (midway between T10 and T12)
T12:	Inguinal ligament at mid-point
L1:	Half the distance between T12 and L2
L2:	Mid-anterior thigh
L3:	Medial femoral condyle
L4:	Medial malleolus
L5:	Dorsum of the foot at the third metatarsal phalangeal joint
S1:	Lateral heel
S2:	Popliteal fossa in the midline
S3:	Ischial tuberosity
S4–S5:	Perianal area

Reprinted with permission from the American Spinal Injury Association. *International standards for neurological and functional classification of spinal cord injury.* Chicago: American Spinal Injury Association, 1996.

TABLE 51-5. *ASIA Impairment Scale for Completeness*

A: Complete; no sensory or motor function in the sacral segments S4–S5
B: Incomplete; sensory but not motor function is preserved below the neurologic level and includes sacral segments S4–S5.
C: Incomplete; motor function is preserved below the neurologic level, and more than half of the key muscles below the neurologic level have a muscle grade less than 3
D: Incomplete; motor function is preserved below the neurologic level, and at least half of key muscles below the neurologic level have a muscle grade greater than or equal to 3
E: Normal; sensory and motor function are normal

ASIA, American Spinal Injury Association.

Modified from the Frankel scale with permission from the American Spinal Injury Association. *International standards for neurological and functional classification of spinal cord injury.* Chicago: American Spinal Injury Association, 1996.

(16.6%), and sports injuries (12.7%). For those injured after 45 years of age, falls are the most common cause. The most common sports activity causing SCI is diving (3).

Time

SCI is most common in July, and least common in February. The most common day of injury is Saturday (3).

Level and Degree of Completeness

The most common levels at the time of admission are C5, C4, and C6. For those with paraplegia, the most common levels are in the area of the thoracolumbar junction. The Frankel admission grade is A in 50.5%, B in 13.2%, C in 12.9%, and D in 21.6%. Over time, the percentage of incomplete injuries has increased (4).

Nontraumatic Diseases of the Spinal Cord

The epidemiology of nontraumatic spinal cord disease is not well examined. Cancer alone may be a more common cause of cord disease than trauma. Spondylosis is also a common cause. Traumatic injury is more common in persons under 40 years of age, whereas nontraumatic disease may be more common in persons over 40 years of age.

Acute Management

Goals of Acute Management

The major goal of management of spinal injury is to prevent or minimize any resulting neurologic deficit (5). This goal is pursued while simultaneously attending to associated injuries that can be serious and may pose a greater threat to life than the spinal injury. If spinal injury is apparent, the first rescuers on the scene should begin immoblization. All personnel should be alert to the possibility of occult spinal injury.

Occult Spinal and Spinal Cord Injuries

Spinal and spinal cord injury may not be obvious to treating personnel for a variety of reasons. The cervical spine is injured and unstable in 5% of victims of major trauma, often without any neurologic deficit (5). In such cases, other injuries may be more apparent. A person with a decreased level of conciousness, due to intoxication or head injury, may have no complaints referable to the spine. Although a head injury can cause neurologic changes, a coexisting SCI also could account for such signs. The coexistence of head and spinal injury is high (6).

Proof of a spinal injury at one level does not rule out a noncontiguous injury elsewhere; thus, films of the entire spine should be considered if a fracture is noted anywhere in the spine. In summary, spinal injury should be considered in victims of major trauma, in victims of minor trauma who have complaints referable to the spine or nervous system, and in those with a decreased level of conciousness after trauma (5).

Immobilization in the Field

Immobilization of the spine should begin even before extrication of an injured person from, for example, a swimming pool or crashed automobile. A variety of techniques are available (5,7). The cervical spine can be splinted with a rigid cervical collar, and the thoracolumbar spine with a short spine board, before extrication from a wrecked motor vehicle. A diver with cervical spine injury should be brought to the surface of the water with attention to the maintenance of straight spinal alignment. The patient should be maintained on the surface of the water until a spine board or an adequate number of rescuers are available for transfer out of the water. Transportation from the scene to the hospital should be on a spine board, with the head and neck immobilized by straps, with rolled towels or sandbags placed adjacent to the head. Transportation in the sitting or prone position should be avoided.

Associated Injuries

Associated injuries are common after traumatic SCI (5). Just as these injuries may direct attention away from SCI, SCI can eliminate the symptoms and signs of, for example, abdominal injury. When possible, the injured person should be completely undressed and observed for injuries not otherwise apparent.

Acute Medical Management

The ABCs—airway, breathing, circulation—are supported, with attention to spinal immobilization (7). Intubation, if required, can be nasotracheal, orotracheal, or, ideally, by fiberoptic bronchoscope, with avoidance of hyperflexion or extension of the neck. Supplemental oxygen should be administered. Hypoventilation may not be obvious but can be detected by blood gas measurements and measurement of vital capacity. A person with cervical SCI may initially ventilate adequately but may soon decompensate due to fatigue, aspiration, or pneumonia, and require mechanical ventilation. Loss of sympathetic tone may result in hypotension and bradycardia, which can be treated with intravenous fluids. A catheter should be placed to prevent overdistention of the paralyzed bladder. If no contraindication exists, a nasogastric tube can be passed to decrease abdominal distention and lower the risk of aspiration.

Pharmacotherapy of Acute SCI

Standard treatment of traumatic SCI, when the person is seen within 8 hours of injury, includes intravenous administration of 30 mg/kg of methylprednisolone over a 15-minute period, followed by a gap of 45 minutes, then 5.4 mg/kg/hr for 23 hours (8). Methylprednisolone treatment beginning after 8 hours has not been shown to be helpful and might be detrimental (9).

Spinal Stability

Definition

The concept of spinal stability is quite rich and is difficult to describe comprehensively. A stable spine can maintain the normal relationships of the vertebrae in the face of physiologic stresses. Damage to the vertebrae, ligaments, intervertebral disks, and muscles can result in loss of stability. The importance of this for the patient is the presence of, or potential for, deformity, pain, and loss of neurologic function (10).

Assessment

Stability can be assessed by observation of the movement of vertebrae using, for example, flexion and extension radiographs. This is most useful in a person with a long-standing injury. In an acute situation it is more commonly assessed from the history, physical examination, and static imaging studies. Several systems exist for assessing stability, but there is no single standard (10–13). Determination of stability is technical and is the responsibility of the treating surgeon. Stability can be relative. Assessment of stability is crucial to the rehabilitation process because it affects the timing of mobilization and restrictions upon mobilization, such as the need to use a spinal orthosis.

Information Taken from the History

The history can suggest a mechanism of injury, with implications for stability. A person who falls and strikes the chin, with subsequent tetraplegia, may have sustained an extension injury of the cervical spine. This often ruptures the anterior longitudinal ligament and causes a teardrop fracture of the vertebral body, without affecting the posterior elements. The injury would then be stable in the flexed position. A person falling backwards and striking the occiput can sustain a flexion injury, with a wedge compression fracture of the anterior vertebral body, and possible tension injury of the posterior ligaments. This might result in instability in flexion, but stability in extension, in which the anterior longitudinal ligament provides adequate support.

Information Taken from the Physical Examination

The physical examination also can provide information. A person rescued from a motor vehicle crash may demonstrate paraplegia and a palpable gap between the spinous processes of adjacent lumbar vertebrae. The gap may indicate a dislocation and an unstable injury. A person sustaining a blow to the head, with a consequent tilt and rotation of the head to one side, may have a contralateral ''locked'' facet joint, which may be unstable.

Information Taken from Imaging Studies

Imaging studies can demonstrate injury to various elements, with implications for stability. For example, destruction of posterior elements may place the person at risk for progressive kyphosis. Destruction of the posterior vertebral body, with retropulsion of fragments into the canal, and incomplete cord injury, may place the person at risk for neurologic decline if mobilization is injudicious. Horizontal translation of one vertebra upon another, or sagittal rotation of a vertebra relative to another, may signify destruction of multiple structures and instability. The number of ''columns'' in the spine that are injured, the degree of displacement of one vertebra upon another, the angulation of one vertebra upon another, the percentage loss of height of a vertebra, and the degree of canal compromise all can be assessed by imaging studies and can contribute to the assessment of stability.

External Spinal Stabilization

Overview

Devices to provide external spinal stabilization are used in the acute and rehabilitation phases of treatment after traumatic SCI. They can be used as the primary means of managing instability or can be used after a stabilization procedure. They may allow mobility out of bed, preventing the problems that might develop if traumatic spinal instability were treated with prolonged bed rest. Various orthoses are available for immobilizing different segments of the spine. They are grouped according to the segment of the spine that requires immobilization. This discussion will focus on the halo vest and the molded thoracolumbosacral orthosis.

Halo-Vest Orthosis

The halo-plaster body jacket for cervical immobilization was described in 1959 (14). It is useful in the management of cervical instability (15). The halo is a ring secured to the skull by four pins. The ring, in turn, is secured to the body jacket by two or four uprights. The cervical spine, situated between the ring and the jacket, is immobilized. However, immobilization is not absolute (16). Fixation of the jacket to the trunk is not complete, and the large number of vertebral segments involved can allow a ''snaking'' motion of the spine to occur. Modifications of the original design have been made over the years and include the development of plastic vests to replace the plaster body jacket. The plastic vests can be designed to provide rapid access to the chest in the event that cardiopulmonary resuscitation is required. Radiolucent and magnetic resonance imaging (MRI)-compatible substances have been substituted for some of the metal components. In some devices the ring is not continuous posteriorly, allowing better access to the occiput and upper cervical area.

The pins are threaded over the portion that passes through the ring, so that they are screwed into the ring. The pointed tip is not threaded. The pin is held in place by pressure, with counterforce provided by another pin diagonally across the skull.

The two anterior pins are applied 1 cm over the lateral aspect of the eyebrow. This positioning avoids placing the pin too medially, which would threaten the supraorbital and supratrochlear nerve and artery, while also avoiding lateral placement, which would pierce the temoralis muscle, causing painful mastication, and which would also locate the pin in a thin area of the skull. Placement of the pin too inferiorly could pierce the orbit, while placement too superiorly would locate the pin above the equator of the skull, which would make it more likely to cut out. The posterior pins are positioned roughly diagonally across from the anterior pins, at the 2:00 and 10:00 positions, with the occiput representing 12:00. The posterior pins should be below the equator of the skull but also should allow the ring to clear the pinna of the ear.

Halo maintenance on the rehabilitation unit should include regular cleansing of the pin sites and observation for signs of infection. The skin beneath the jacket should be inspected for pressure ulceration. Looseness of the pins at the pin–skull interface can present with a complaint of pain and a feeling of looseness at the site. In some cases there may be no pain, but there can be visible motion between the pin and the skull. A loose pin requires tightening or replacement. Tightening is performed by an experienced physician using a torque wrench, and only to a certain level, such as 8 lb-in, and only if resistance is met within the first two complete turns of the pin. Loosening of the jacket components can be resolved through use of the torque wrench supplied with the orthosis.

Molded Thoracolumbosacral Orthosis

A plastic custom-molded thoracolumbosacral orthosis is recommended for thoracic and lumbar spinal instability (15). This provides greater stability, including rotational stability, than other devices. Low lumbar instability may require extension of the orthosis across the hip joint. High thoracic instability may require an extension on the jacket to immobilize the cervical spine. The skin beneath the orthosis should be surveyed for pressure breakdown. The device must be long enough to provide adequate immobilization but should not impinge the axillae or unduly dig into the upper thigh while the patient is sitting. At the discretion of the treating surgeon, the device may be removed while the patient is in bed. The patient should then be turned using the log-rolling method.

Spinal Surgery after Trauma

Goals of Spinal Surgery after Trauma

The goals of spinal surgery after trauma include establishment of a properly aligned and stable spine and removal of any bone fragments that might be compressing the cord. In situations where both surgical and nonsurgical tratment could be followed, surgery may allow earlier mobilization, thus reducing the sequelae of immobilization, and hastening return to the community (10).

Emergency Spinal Surgery

In general, emergency surgery is not indicated. It should be condidered in cases in which there is ongoing neurologic decline and in patients with incomplete injuries and a spinal dislocation that cannot be reduced by nonsurgical measures (17). A rationale once offered for rapid decompressive laminectomy in acute traumatic SCI held that it could foster neurologic recovery. The line of thought was that the injured cord is swollen and compressed within the spinal canal and that surgery to remove the pressure on the cord could lead to a better neurologic outcome. This has never been proven and is felt to be untrue.

Overview of Spinal Surgery

A major goal of spinal surgery after trauma is to bring about a fusion of bone across the injury site. This is achieved by applying a bone graft, which can serve as a matrix through which the fusion can occur. The process of fusion requires months, during which some other means of immobilization is required. This can be accomplished via implanted metal fixation devices, external orthoses, or both. Once fusion is complete, any external orthosis can be discontinued. An implanted fixation device could be removed after the fusion is mature, but there usually is no reason to remove it. Surgery can be performed anteriorly or posteriorly, or both, depend-

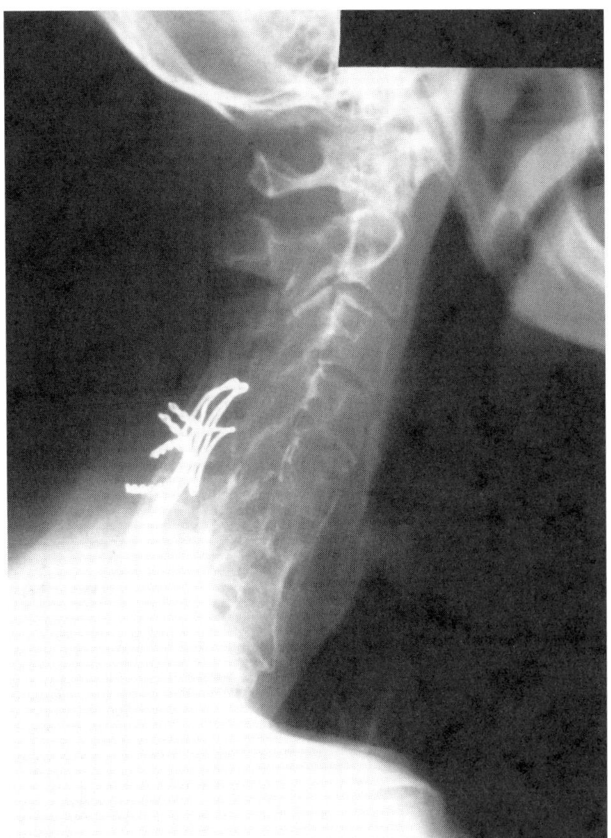

FIG. 51-2. Mature anterior and posterior cervical fusions, with posterior wiring.

ing on the mechanism of injury and the site of greatest instability (Fig. 51-2).

Bone Graft Harvesting

Autologous bone graft material can be harvested from iliac crest, tibia, fibula, or rib. Cancellous bone provides a collagen-mineral scaffolding for graft maturation and is rich in ostoeprogenitor cells, although these may not all survive transplantation. Cortical grafts are not as successful overall but may be useful when initial mechanical strength of the graft is important (18).

Bone Graft Application

A number of techniques are available (17). In general, an anteriorly applied graft is plugged into a cavity created in the injured vertebral body and extends to contact an adjacent veretebral body. Posterior grafts are positioned against the laminae or spinous processes and can be wired into place. Before application of the graft, bone of the fusion site is decorticated, in order to maximize exposure of osteoprogenitor cells to the graft.

Instrumentation

Metal fixation devices can be used with either anterior or posterior procedures. These span the injured segment and provide stability while the bone graft incorporates. They are held in place by screws, hooks, or wires (Figs. 51-3 and 51-4).

Postoperative Care

Postoperative care while on the rehabilitation unit includes surveillance for wound infection (including the bone graft donor site) and regular neurologic examination to detect any decline that could indicate a loss of stabilization. A sore throat or dysphagia after anterior fusion can sometimes indicate dislodgement of the bone graft. Surgical follow-up should be scheduled to determine the need to continue any spinal orthosis or movement restrictions.

Pulmonary Problems

A majority of patients admitted for SCI have pulmonary complications during acute care and initial rehabilitation. Atelectasis, pneumonia, and ventilatory failure are the most common problems (19). Disease of the respiratory system, particularly pneumonia, is the primary cause of death in patients with SCI (20). Three quarters of ventilator-dependent patients admitted to an SCI care system within 1 day of injury die within the first year, but those who survive the

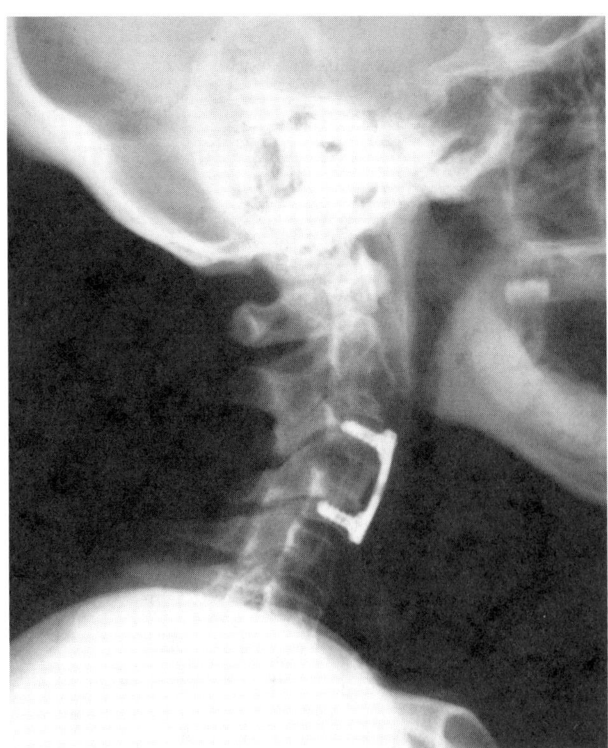

FIG. 51-3. Anterior fixation device with screws, and anterior bone graft.

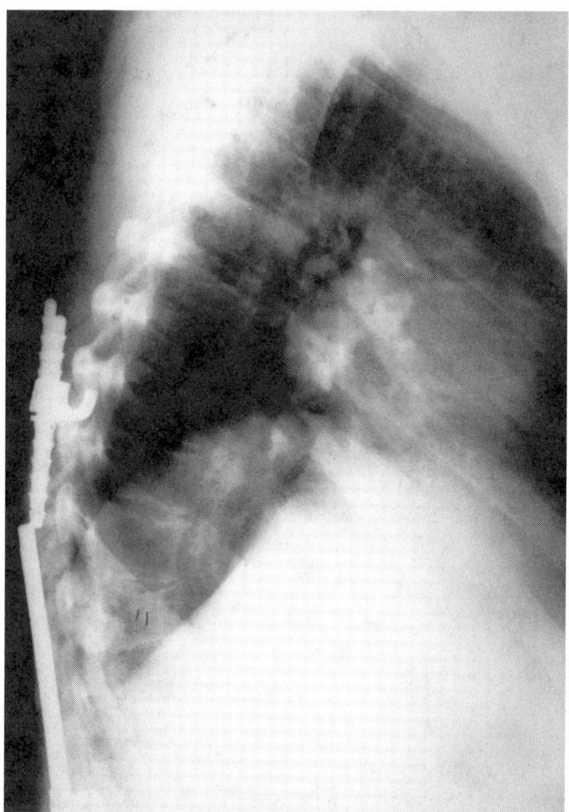

FIG. 51-4. Posterior fixation rods with hooks. The rods have broken. Without a solid boney fusion, such rods can eventually fail.

first year have a survival rate of 61% for the next 14 years (21). This subject area is also considered in Chapter 55.

Physiology

Four major muscle groups are involved in respiration. Proceeding according to the location of central nervous system innervation, these are the accessory neck muscles of respiration, the diaphragm, the muscles of the chest wall, and the abdominal muscles. The muscles of the mouth and throat constitute a potential fifth group, which has importance because of its relatively rostral innervation. Observation of breathing of a tetraplegic individual shows elevation of the abdomen during inspiration, as the diaphragm descends. This is accompanied by retraction of the chest wall, which is a passive response to the negative intrathoracic pressure generated by descent of the diaphragm. The retraction is counterproductive because it negates in part the inspiratory force developed by the diaphragm. This retraction is normally opposed by the muscles of the chest wall. The tetaplegic person with a paralyzed chest wall cannot splint against the retraction. If the person is instructed to expire forcefully, or to cough, little force is observed because of the paralyzed chest wall and the abdominal muscles. If spared, the clavicular portion of the pectoralis major can provide some active expiration in tetraplegia (22,23). Persons with high tetraplegia also can use glossopharyngeal breathing to provide brief respiratory support (24).

Respiratory failure is generally divided into problems of ventilation and problems of oxygenation. Immediately or soon after injury, a person with SCI can develop ventilatory failure secondary to weakness. Superimposed atelectasis and pneumonia can worsen the situation and can contribute to the development of oxygenation failure (25). Problems may be more likely in the left lung, which is more difficult to suction (26).

Vital capacity is generally diminished with higher neurologic levels. It is a useful indicator of overall ventilatory function. Ventilatory failure is better detected sooner than later. If vital capacity is decreasing, then mechanical ventilation may become necessary. Negative inspiratory pressure (NIP) and positive expiratory pressure (PIP) also may be useful parameters to follow (27).

Management

Pulmonary toilet includes chest physiotherapy (PT) and postural drainage, assisted (''quad'') coughs, and bronchodilator and/or mucolytic therapy via nebulizer. These measures mobilize and clear secretions and prevent atelectasis and pneumonia (28). Breathing parameters may improve in the supine position, compared with upright because when supine the abdominal viscera can substitute for the muscles of expiration (29). Infections must be treated aggressively with appropriate antibiotics and pulmonary toilet. Influenza vaccines should be considered in October of each year. Pneumococcal vaccination should be given soon after SCI.

Cardiac Problems

Heart disease is a leading cause of death after SCI (20). In addition, nonfatal cardiovascular problems can interfere with management, especially in the acute phase.

Changes in Physiology after SCI

SCI alters cardiovascular physiology. When a person with SCI exercises, there is an increase in heart rate and oxygen uptake, as in able-bodied subjects. However, the levels reached are lower than normal. The higher the neurologic level, the less the heart rate and oxygen uptake can increase with exercise (30). This may be due to less functioning muscle mass, poor venous return, and poor ventilatory dynamics. Persons with tetraplegia have an impaired autonomic response, which limits heart rate elevation, positive cardiac chronotropy and inotropy, catecholamine production, and thermoregulation. This results in lower physical work capacity (31,32). Decreased exercise capacity after SCI may contribute to a lower level of high-density lipoprotein (HDL) cholesterol, increasing the risk of cardiovascular disease. Exercise may favorably affect HDL levels in SCI patients (33).

Persons with SCI are prone to carbohydrate intolerance, secondary to insulin resistance. This also may increase the risk of cardiac disease (34).

Exercise

Persons with tetraplegia may benefit from endurance training with upper extremity ergometry. The effect may be limited by venous pooling in the lower extremities and abdomen, which can result in upper extremity ischemia. Cardiovascular improvement occurs secondary to physiologic changes that occur peripherally. Electrical stimulation leg cycle ergometry (ES-LCE) may result in improved exercise performance, secondary to central and peripheral adaptation.

Orthostatic Hypotension

Orthostatic hypotension is a sudden decrease in blood pressure caused by moving from a reclining to an upright position. It is usually associated with an increase in heart rate. It is commonly seen in persons with higher neurologic levels. It results in dizziness, lightheadedness, or sudden loss of consciousness. Persons with SCI frequently have low baseline blood pressure. They may become symptomatic with postural changes and transfer activities. Orthostasis most commonly develops as a result of blood pooling in the lower extremities and ineffective vasoconstriction secondary to altered autonomic response. Symptoms may develop on the basis of altered cerebral blood flow as opposed to a decrease in the absolute value of the blood pressure (35). Orthostasis may be exacerbated by medications such as alpha-adrenergic blockers, which are frequently used in bladder management after SCI. On occasion, patients develop orthostasis secondary to a posttraumatic cystic myelopathy (36).

Conservative treatment suffices for most cases. Care is taken to slowly elevate the head in bed in the morning, before the patient is moved to a sitting position. Elastic garments are used for the legs and abdomen. Elevated leg rests can be used. Progressive elevation in a recliner wheelchair or a tilt table may be beneficial. Liberal salt and fluid intake is encouraged. The patient is instructed to exercise if he or she recognizes the symptoms. Caregivers will generally give the patient a tilt-back in the wheelchair to restore adequate blood pressure. Medications that may be effective include sodium chloride tablets, ephedrine, and fludrocortisone (37). Biofeedback also has been found to be useful (38).

Bradyarrhythmias

Severe bradyarrhythmias progressing to cardiac arrest have been reported (39,40). This may occur after tracheal suction. The cause may be reflex vagal influence on the heart unopposed by sympathetics. Treatment involves atropine. On occasion, a pacemaker may be necessary (41,42).

Succinylcholine

Persons with SCI can develop hyperkalemia and cardiac arrest in response to the administration of succinylcholine and therefore should not receive the drug (43). The mechanism may involve an exagerrated sensitivity of muscle cell membranes.

Deep Venous Thrombosis and Pulmonary Embolus

Deep venous thrombosis (DVT) is highly prevalent after SCI (44,45). SCI greatly increases the risk of death from pulmonary embolus in the subsequent year (20). Attention to the possibility of DVT is one of the greatest medical issues during acute care and rehabilitation of those with SCI.

Pathophysiology

The high risk of DVT is likely related to venous stasis and hypercoagulability (44). An ideal prophylactic regimen should address each of these.

Detection

Regular physical examination of the legs should be performed. However, this is neither sensitive nor specific for DVT. Supplementary study should be considered. Ultrasound imaging is useful and can be performed as a screening test, as well as in response to a clinical finding (46). DVT can present as unexplained fever (47).

Prophylaxis

Prophylaxis should be considered for all persons with SCI. A typical regimen could include compression boots for 2 weeks and subcutaneous heparin for 3 months (48,49). Low molecular-weight heparin may also be used for prophylaxis (49a,49b). Insertion of a caval filter can be considered (49c,49d). Migration has occurred with quad coughing (50).

Gastrointestinal Problems

Clinical Evaluation

Clinical evaluation for abdominal disease in patients with SCI can be difficult. Specific symptoms may be lacking due to loss of sensation. During the acute phase of spinal shock, there may be no rigidity despite pathology, but conversely there may be absent bowel sounds when no disease is present. With chronic SCI, the most pronounced signs of abdominal pathology may be an increase in spasticity or autonomic dysreflexia (51).

Gastric Atony

Acute SCI is commonly accompanied by gastric atony, with the risk of aspiration. Stomach decompression by nasogastric tube should be considered. If gastroparesis is prolonged, cisapride or metoclopramide can be helpful (52). Metoclopramide can cause an acute dystonic reaction that could be disasterous with an unstable spine.

Gastrointestinal Bleeding

Gastrointestinal bleeding can occur early after SCI (53,54). Vagal tone unopposed by paralyzed sympathetic innervation may contribute. It is reasonable to administer prophylactic medications for a period after injury.

Superior Mesenteric Artery Syndrome

The superior mesenteric artery syndrome can cause recurrent vomiting in tetraplegia (55). It occurs when the third part of the duodenum is compressed between the underlying aorta and the overlying superior mesenteric artery. Predisposing factors include prolonged supine positioning and loss of retroperitoneal fat. The diagnosis is determined via upper gastrointestinal series, which show the cutoff. Symptoms can sometimes be relieved by positioning.

Hypercalemia

Immobilization hypercalcemia after SCI can present with abdominal complaints. Treatment can include mobilization, hydration, diuresis, and medications such as calcitonin and etidronate (56,57).

Heterotopic Ossification

Heterotopic ossification (HO) is the deposition of new bone around a joint. Its greatest clinical importance is the potential for loss of joint range. It can occur in several settings, including the person who is post-SCI, where it has been reported to be present in 16% to 53% (58). Most commonly the hip is involved, followed by the knee. Less frequently the shoulder and elbow are affected. HO has been reported only in the area of paralysis, unless another causative factor, such as head injury or burns, is present (59,60). It develops in persons with spastic or flaccid paralysis and complete or incomplete SCI. Typically, the HO is noted 1 to 4 months after injury, but it has occurred as early as 19 days and as late as several years after injury (61).

Etiology

The etiology of HO is poorly understood. Decreased tissue oxygenation or some unknown factor is believed to induce changes in multipotential connective tissue cells (62). The new bone forms in planes between connective tissue layers (63). Trauma to the involved area is a possibility, but this has not been borne out clinically (64).

Presentation

The early clinical findings of HO are swelling and heat. Fever also may be present. In the lower extremity, this may be mistaken for DVT (58). DVT and HO can coexist. Hematoma, infection, fracture, and tumor are other considerations. Over several days, the swelling becomes more firm and localized. Alternatively, this inflammatory phase may go undetected and the HO will present with decreasing range of motion (ROM) of a joint. The natural course of HO is to progress to mature bone. In a minority of patients, joint ankylosis will occur (60). Restriction of joint ROM of even a modest degree may impair function or interfere with hygiene.

Laboratory Studies

Roentgenograms show the process only after sufficient ossification has taken place. The third, or bone, phase of the bone scan correlates well and usually precedes roentgenographic findings by at least 7 to 10 days. During the active phase, an elevated alkaline phosphatase level also may be present (65). The combination of elevated serum alkaline phosphatase and phosphorus values may be suggestive (66).

Complications

HO can cause peripheral nerve entrapment (67). A pressure sore can occur as a secondary complication of HO. Increased pressure may occur indirectly from altered positioning related to HO of the hip, particularly beneath the contralateral ischial tuberosity (68). Patients with hips fused in extension may sit directly on the sacrum with hyperflexion of the lumbar spine and develop a sacral ulcer. HO overlying a bony prominence, such as trochanter or ischial tuberosity, will directly predispose to a pressure ulcer (69).

Management

Stretching exercises appear to limit the ultimate loss of ROM in cases of HO (64). Others have suggested that stretching may worsen HO (70).

Disodium etidronate has been shown to be effective in limiting the extent of the ossification, particularly if therapy is started early (59,71). A dose of 20 mg/kg is given daily for 2 weeks, followed by 10 mg/kg daily. The optimal length of treatment with this medication is not known; it may be longer than the manufacturer's suggestion of 12 weeks (72). Disodium etidronate also has been used prophylactically after SCI (59).

When HO is causing severely limited ROM or frank ankylosis that is impairing function, surgery is indicated. A wedge resection of the bone is usually performed. Surgery is best deferred until the HO is felt to be mature; otherwise, it may

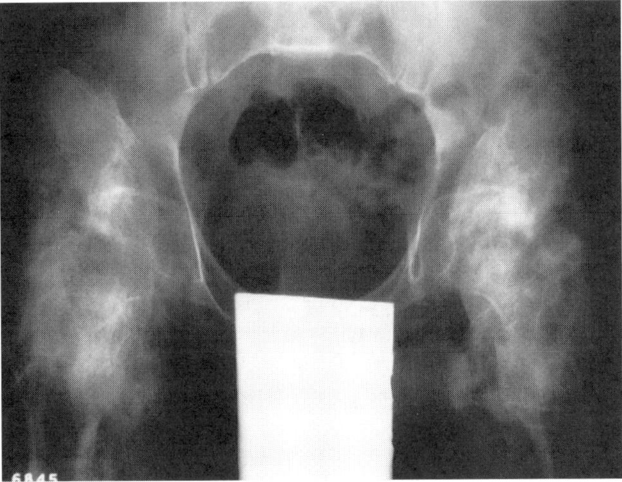

FIG. 51-5. Severe heterotopic ossification about the hips.

recur (Figs. 51-5 through 51-7). The length of time from the onset, a stable clinical examination, a stable roentgenographic appearance, an alkaline phosphatase level that has returned to normal, and declining activity on bone scan support maturity. Disodium etidronate may be useful in preventing recurrence of HO after surgery, but this is not certain (73). Radiation therapy and indomethacin have been re-

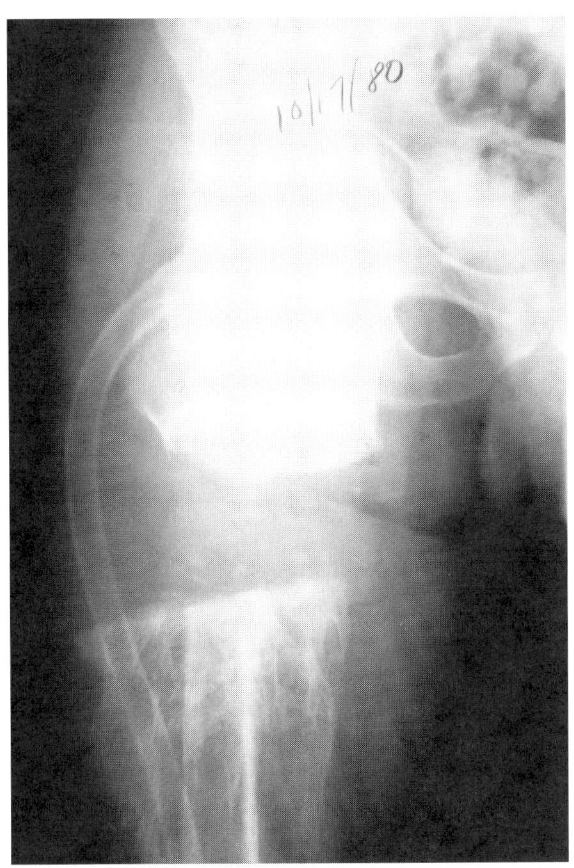

FIG. 51-6. Appearance after wedge resection.

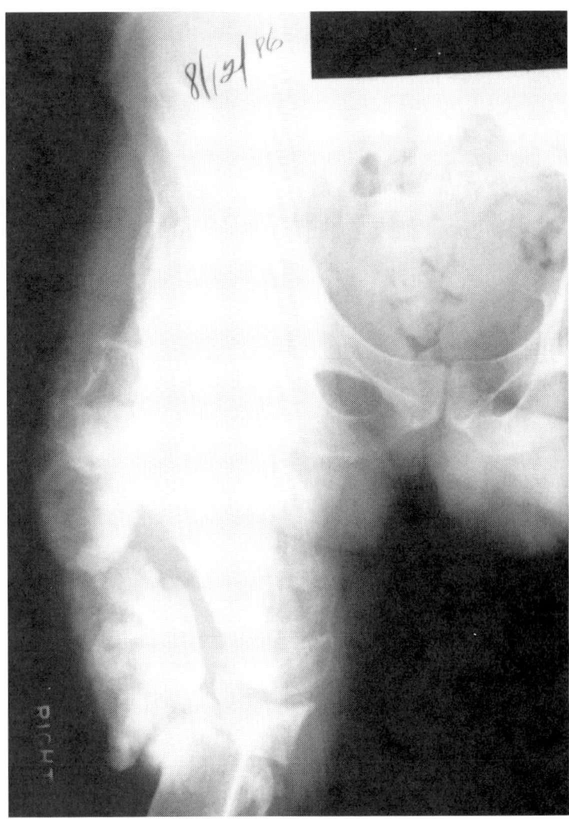

FIG. 51-7. Recurrence of heterotopic ossification after surgery.

ported to be useful in the postoperative prophylaxis of HO in situations other than SCI (74,75).

Pain

Pain has been reported to occur in 11% to 94% of persons with SCI. Central pain, characterized by diffuse dysesthetic pain below the level of the lesion, has been noted to be present in 13%. Pain most commonly presents within 6 months of injury. Patients describe pain as severe 25% of the time. Forty-four percent of those with SCI claim that pain interferes with daily activities (76–78).

Classification

There is no universally accepted classification system for pain after SCI. One system proposes the following types of pain:

1. Radicular or segmental pain, including radicular and/or end-zone pain
2. Central or diffuse pain
3. Visceral pain
4. Musculoskeletal
5. Psychogenic pain (79)

Other classification systems also have been proposed (76,78,80,81).

Central or Diffuse Pain

This is often called "spinal" pain. It is perceived below the level of SCI. The words most frequently chosen to describe central pain include cutting, burning, piercing, radiating, tight, cool, and nagging. The pain is often in a saddle distribution as well as in the lower extremities (81).

The cause of central pain is not known. It has been postulated that the pain generator is located at the lower brain stem level or thalamus, with dysesthesias resulting from central misinterpretation of dorsal column input. The misinterpretation is felt to be due to the absence of suppression from the spinal thalamic system (76). Another theory holds that the source of the pain is in the spinal cord and brain stem, with deafferentation causing abnormal activity in spinal and brain cells. These cells fire spontaneously and have frequent bursts of electrical activity (82).

Treatment of spinal pain always begins with consideration of the possibility that the pain is actually caused or exacerbated by a central problem (such as a syrinx) or peripheral pathology (such as a ureteral stone). Conservative treatment of central pain syndromes includes patient education, cognitive strategies of pain management, biofeedback and relaxation techniques, and hypnosis (83,84). Central pain most commonly responds to tricyclic antidepressants. This has never been proven in a controlled study. Amitriptyline and carbamazepine have been used effectively together (85). Intrathecal baclofen has been used to treat central pain (86). Narcotic usage in benign pain syndromes is controversial (87). Intrathecal morphine, alone and in combination with clonidine, has been used with some success (88). Patients with a history of substance abuse should probably not be treated with narcotics. In general, spinal cord stimulation does not decrease pain from central etiology (89). Patients who suffer from end-zone or radicular pain may benefit from a dosal root entry-zone ablation (90). Other ablative procedures, such as cordotomy, have not been proven to be beneficial.

Noncentral Pain after Spinal Cord Injury

Radicular pain is localized, often about the level of injury. It can be shooting, or can come in waves. It is often worse during inactivity. Because the pain is perceived in a relatively small area, measures such as desensitization, extremity ROM, TENS, and topical capsaicin are more practical than with central pain. Medications such as antidepressants and anticonvulsants are useful. As noted above, in certain patients with persistant pain over time, despite other measures, dorsal root entry zone ablation may be considered.

Visceral pain is perceived in the abdominal or pelvic area, in contrast to central pain, which is usually felt in the distal lower extremities and saddle areas. Its pathophysiology may involve transmission of signals through the autonomic nervous system. As described in the previously mentioned classification system, it is not due to visceral pathology, but rather is neuropathic. There is no specific treatment. Visceral pathology can present similarly, and diagnosis here is crucial so that specific therapy can be provided.

Musculoskeletal pain presents as aching or other pain, localized to musculoskeletal structures. It is exacerbated by activity and relieved by rest. After SCI, certain muscles can be overused, or used in a novel manner, or muscle function can become unbalanced. Wheelchair use may favor development of certain shoulder groups over others, and injury level of C5 may leave certain shoulder muscles strong, and others weak. Trunk muscle weakness may cause poor posture. Treatment includes typical measures for musculoskeletal pain, as well as treatment specific for problems of muscle imbalance and poor posture. The upper extremity can be rested through proper use of a power wheelchair.

Psychogenic pain is variable in presentation, and perhaps it does not exist in pure form, but rather in overlap with one of the other types of pain. The person's reaction to pain is maladaptive. Active organic pathology must be ruled out, and the patient's pain may benefit from this. Management can involve support, mobilization, exercise and other general health measures, intervention for psychological problems and an approach to stressors in the person's environment (79).

Syringomyelia

A syrinx is a fluid-filled cavity within the spinal cord. It can develop in several settings, including the person who is post-SCI. A posttraumatic syrinx, which is also referred to as posttraumatic syringomyelia or posttraumatic cystic myelopathy, develops in 0.3% to 3.2% of patients with chronic SCI, according to the older literature. With newer imaging, the reported frequency will increase (91–96).

Presentation

Typical presentation can involve ascending neurologic findings with sparing of dorsal column sensation, due to the superficial location of these pathways, and the fact that they do not cross within the spinal cord. Pain is the most common initial symptom. It may be located at the site of the original injury and radiate to the neck or upper limbs. On occasion, pain refers to the area below the injury. Symptoms may be exacerbated by strain, coughing, or sneezing. Asymmetric motor loss may occur in combination with loss of sensation. Loss of reflexes is common. Increased spasticity, hyperhidrosis, alternating Horner's syndrome, and increased incidence of autonomic dysreflexia have been reported (91,92,96). A person with paraplegia and an insidiously developing syrinx may present with a Charcot joint at the shoulder (97). MRI is the initial study of choice. Cavities are seen as regions of low signal intensity on T1-weighted images. Intraoperative sonography is superior to MRI in detecting septations and small additional cysts.

Pathogenesis

The pathogenesis is uncertain (91,95). The syrinx may begin from liquifaction of cord tissue or hematoma after SCI. Arachnoid adhesions may tether the cord. Motion of the spine may then result in, for example, movement of the posterior portion of the cord independent of the anterior portion, thus initiating a cavity by traction–distraction. Expansion of the syrinx may occur from "suck and slosh." This postulated mechanism involves pressure changes in the cerebrospinal fluid (CSF) in the presence of a partial subarachnoid block. For example, if the person coughs, the increase in adominal pressure may drive CSF from caudal to rostral, past the partial block. Upon relaxation, the block delays return of the CSF, and a negative pressure is thus present in the caudal area of the cord. This is the "suck." This negative pressure draws fluid downward in the syrinx (the "slosh"), causing expansion (91,95,96,98).

Management

Conservative treatment may include pain control, addressing functional deficits with appropriate rehabilitation, and avoidance of activities involving Valsalva maneuvers. Indications for surgery include neurologic deterioration and development of a pain syndrome. Surgical intervention can involve drainage of the cavity and placement of a shunt to a low-pressure system such as the subarachnoid space or the peritoneal cavity (91—93,96). The results are variable, and progression of the syrinx is not unusual. Shunt failure may occur secondary to blockage, which occurs more frequently at the cystic end of the tube. Septations within the cyst or multiple cysts also may result in inadequate results.

Osteoporosis and Pathologic Fracture

Location and Timing of Bone Loss

Bone mineral loss after SCI occurs throughout the entire skeleton except the skull. Loss occurs most rapidly during the first 4 months after injury. It is initially greatest in the pelvis and proximal femur. However, there is also initial bone loss in the upper extremities and trunk in patients with paraplegia and tetraplegia. Between 4 and 16 months postinjury, bone loss continues in the lower extremities. Maximal bone loss is reached at 16 months, and equilibrium is established. There is a decrease in bone marrow between 4 and 16 months postinjury. More rapid loss is noted in areas rich with trabecular bone, such as the upper tibia, which can suffer a total loss of 50% by 18 months. The femoral shaft loss levels off at 20% at 18 months. Those with partial neurologic recovery also develop lower extremity osteoporosis. Paraplegic patients with partial recovery have lost 30% of bone stock in the pelvis and 10% in the lower limbs at 1 year after injury (99,100).

Treatment of Osteoporosis after Spinal Cord Injury

Treatment of osteoporosis after SCI is largely empiric and unproven. Mobilization out of bed, standing, and electrical stimulation of lower extremity musculature are possible strategies. Tiludrinate, a biphosphonate, may be effective in reducing bone resorption (101).

Lower Extremity Fractures

Fractures are reported in about 4% of those with chronic SCI (102). The actual figure is probably somewhat higher because many fractures go unnoticed. Persons with SCI are at increased risk for fracture because of osteoporosis. Fractures may occur during ROM exercises or from falls during transfers. The majority of fractures are in the distal femur or proximal tibia (103). Lower extremity fractures that occur at the time of the acute injury are best treated according to the usual principles of fracture management. The trend is toward open reduction and internal fixation, which provides early stabilization and fewer complications (102,104,105). In persons with acute and chronic paraplegia or tetraplegia, angulation, shortening, and rotation are unacceptable in the upper limbs. Persons with chronic SCI generally receive conservative, closed treatment in lower extremity long-bone fractures (102,103). Fractures generally heal within 3 to 4 weeks. Fractures in the shaft of the femur, tibia, ankle, and foot generally heal with the use of soft splints. Traction should be avoided. Plastic splints and hard materials are potentially dangerous. Shortening and angulation in the lower limbs of healed fractures is acceptable in patients who sit. Rotational deformity is not acceptable in patients who are ambulatory, who should be treated in the same manner as those without paralysis. Mobilization should be rapid. Problematic fractures include those of the femoral neck and subtrochanteric regions. These areas often do not heal. Nonunion in a femoral neck fracture may be an acceptable result (103). However, rotational deformity is not acceptable, and in such a case open reduction and internal fixation may be considered (106).

Autonomic Hyperreflexia

Autonomic hyperreflexia, also known as autonomic dysreflexia, is a medical problem unique to persons with SCI. It develops quickly and can cause related morbidity and even mortality. It can be mimicked by other conditions.

Presentation

The presention includes excruciating headache, a feeling that something is suddenly wrong, and hypertension in a person with mid-thoracic or higher SCI (107–110). Other signs of autonomic change, such as nasal congestion, diaphoresis, piloerection, tachycardia or bradycardia, and flushing may be present. A differential diagnosis could include pheochromocytoma, intracranial pathology, and toxemia of pregnancy.

Pathophysiology

A noxious stimulus below the level of the lesion triggers an aberrant adrenergic response. It is thought that the response is aberrant due to the loss of descending control, as well as to hypersensitivity of adrenoreceptors below the injury. The reason autonomic dysreflexia affects those with lesions in the mid-thoracic region and higher is that lesions below this level do not affect the splanchnic vascular bed and the hemodynamic changes are not great enough to cause hypertension. When hypertension develops, the body attempts to respond with changes driven by the nervous system above the level of the lesion. Thus, flushing can occur in the face, and bradycardia may be noted.

Triggering Stimuli

The most typical inciting stimulus is a distended bladder. Other stimuli, including bowel impaction, abdominal or pelvic pathology, or extremity injury, also may be blamed. Occasionally simple hip stretching can cause the problem, and sometimes no cause can be determined.

Treatment

The patient should be placed in the sitting position in order to decrease cerebral blood pressure. A rapid search is made for an inciting cause, with particular attention to bladder drainage. Straightening a kinked catheter can resolve the problem. If a catheter must be passed, its tip can be coated with lidocaine jelly. If bowel impaction is suspected, vigorous manipulation must be avoided lest the hypertension be aggravated. In this circumstance, the episode may spontaneously resolve, or the episode can be controlled with medications, and then gentle disimpaction, with local application of an anesthetic jelly, can be performed. Numerous medications can be used to control the blood pressure. Topical nitroglycerin is rapid and effective. Beta blockers should be avoided because they will simply allow continued unopposed alpha stimulation.

Prophylaxis

An alpha blocker such as terazosin can be used as prophylaxis in individuals with recurrent episodes (111).

Other agents, such as guanethidine and mecamylamine, can be useful.

Upper Extremity Pain and Overuse

Persons with SCI are subject to overuse syndromes of the upper extremities. Able-bodied individuals use the upper extremities primarily for prehensile activities. Persons with SCI are forced to rely heavily on the upper extremities for wheelchair propulsion, transfers, weight shifts, ambulation, and pain can result (112). Upper extremity dysfunction has far greater functional ramifications in persons with SCI than in able-bodied individuals. Patients who depend on their upper extremities for mobility and self-care may be temporarily dependent. A power wheelchair may be needed, and a mechanical lift device may be required for transfers. This may be temporary or permanent and can result in loss of independence and placement into an institution.

Prevalence and Location

One study found that 55% of all tetraplegic patients reported pain in at least one region of the upper extremity. Forty-six percent had discomfort related to shoulder disorders. Disorders of the elbow, wrist, and hand occurred in 15% (112). Sixty-four percent of paraplegic patients reported upper extremity pain. Carpal tunnel symptoms were most frequently noted. The prevalence of carpal tunnel symptoms increased with time postinjury. Shoulders were reported as painful in 36% of paraplegic individuals, followed by elbow complaints in 16% and wrist complaints in 13%. Excluding carpal tunnel syndrome, prevalence of upper extremity pain tended to increase in patients 20 or more years postinjury relative to pain immediately postinjury. Patients with tetraplegia tended to report that pain limited function or required analgesic medication more frequently than in those with paraplegia. Another study found an incidence of shoulder pain in 51% of all persons with SCI (113).

Shoulder Pain

Shoulder pain is frequent in tetraplegia (112–114). Pain may develop secondary to cervical radiculopathy with radiation of pain to the shoulder. Trauma directly related to a shoulder injury is frequent. Cervical bracing and initial shoulder weakness without proper therapy will lead to cervical spine tightness and shoulder contracture. The trapezius might shorten because of weakness in the scapular depressors. Rotator cuff weakness can lead to biomechanical instability. If the cuff muscles are weak relative to the deltoid, shoulder impingement may result. Those with pre-existing shoulder dysfunction may be particularly prone to impingement secondary to anatomic changes in the subacromial arch as well as biomechanical instability from muscular weakness (114–116).

Initiation of ROM exercises within the first 2 weeks of SCI may prevent acute shoulder pain (116). Glenohumeral motion as well as scapular–thoracic motion must be promoted. Cervical ROM and strengthening should be addressed when not contraindicated. Proper seating in the wheelchair is important. Modalities including hot packs, ultrasound, ice, and electrical stimulation may be helpful. Heat generally should be avoided in areas with impaired sensation. Joint injections and nonsteroidal anti-inflammatories and/or analgesics can be used. Strengthening of the rotator cuff musculature is important whenever possible. When there is anatomic impingement, strengthening should be performed short of pain and within a pain-free ROM (114,115). Those with rotator cuff damage may benefit from surgery involving decompression and rotator cuff repair (117).

Paraplegia often results in overuse of the upper extremity for wheelchair propulsion. This may cause hypertrophy of the anterior deltoids relative to the posterior deltoids, causing shoulder instability, which might be treated by strengthening the shoulder extensors. Use of an overhead trapeze for transfers may cause impingement, and transfers with the hands held low and close to the body should be encouraged. Osteonecrosis of the humeral head has been reported (118).

Upper Extremity Compression Neuropathies

Upper extremity compressive neuropathies are common in paraplegia (112,119–121). Carpal tunnel syndrome has a prevalence of 49% to 73%. A recent study on wheelchair racers showed a 50% prevalence in median mononeuropathy. Ulnar and radial mononeuropathies were found in 25% and 16% of the racers, respectively (121). Bearing weight with the extended wrist may contribute to the development of carpal tunnel syndrome. Weight bearing on the knuckles, when possible, may be preferable.

Cure

The possibility of limiting or reversing SCI historically has been regarded with skepticism. This outlook has changed within recent years (122). As noted earlier, methylprednisolone is now generally considered to improve outcome when used in acute SCI. Other efforts can be broadly categorized as targeting either acute or chronic injury.

Acute Injury

Acute trauma to the cord is compounded by processes that occur within the cord in subsequent hours or days. These processes cause further damage, and therapy to block them would presumably improve outcome.

GM-1 ganglioside sodium salt, 100 mg intravenously per day for 18 to 32 days, beginning within 72 hours of injury, may be beneficial (123). Recovery of lower extremity function may be facilitated more than that of upper extremities, suggesting an effect on white matter. A large study is in progress. Tirilazad mesylate is a potent inhibitor of lipid peroxidation and has been shown to limit acute SCI in animals (124). It is under investigation in the third National Acute Spinal Cord Injury Study (125).

Chronic Injury

A number of treatments have been considered for chronic SCI. 4-aminopyridine may improve function in the presence of partial SCI by facilitating action potential propagation (126). Omental transposition does not appear helpful (127). Transplantation is under investigation (128). Peripheral nerve grafts to the spinal cord have functioned in rats (129).

Morbidity and Mortality

Morbidity

One large study of persons with SCI found that the most common morbidity was pressure ulceration (130). The overall annual incidence reported was 23%. The second most common problem was urinary tract infection. Musculoskeletal difficulties were particulary common in long-term survivors.

Early Mortality

Mortality after SCI can be considered according to when it occurs. Causes for mortality during the first year after injury differ somewhat from later causes. Causes of mortality can be considered in absolute terms, such as determining the most common cause of death. Causes also can be considered according to how they are affected by SCI, such as which cause is most increased by the fact that a person has sustained SCI.

For those surviving more than 24 hours but less than 1 year from injury the most common cause of death is pneumonia, followed by nonischemic heart disease and pulmonary embolus (20). The three etiologies whose frequencies are most increased by SCI are pulmonary embolus (by a factor of 210), sepsis, and pneumonia.

Late Mortality

For those surviving more than 5 years from injury, the three most common causes of death are pneumonia, nonishemic heart disease, and unintentional injury (20). The three specific causes most increased by SCI are sepsis (which is likely often due to urinary tract infection, pressure ulcers, or pneumonia), pneumonia, and urinary tract infection.

Overall Mortality

Overall the most common causes of death for those surviving more than 24 hours are pneumonia, nonischemic heart disease, and sepsis (20). If nonischemic and ishemic heart disease are considered together, then heart disease is the most common cause. Sepsis, pulmonary embolus, and pneumonia are the entities most increased by SCI.

Life Expectancy

Life expectancy for those with SCI has increased in recent decades but remains somewhat below normal (20). Life expectancy decreases with the severity of injury. Renal failure is no longer a major causes of death.

Neurologic Prognosis

The primary initial concern of most injured persons is the neurologic prognosis. Prognosis will change as the effectiveness of treatment for acute SCI increases. Indeed, the percentage of individuals with incomplete injuries has increased in recent decades (4). Functional prognosis is considered in later sections.

Prognosis for Change in ASIA Impairment Grade

This is probably the most important question involving neurologic prognosis. The Model Systems Database figures for the change in Frankel grade (which closely parallels ASIA impairment grade) are reported in Table 51-6 (4). The likelihood for improvement is low for those admitted with a grade of A, whereas prognosis is good for those admitted with a grade of D. Prognosis is less certain for admission grades of B and C. However, for those admitted with a grade of B, partial or complete preservation of pin sensation on admission has been associated with eventual ability to ambulate (131). For those admitted with a grade of C, recovery of quadriceps function (on at least one side) to greater than 3/5 at 2 months has been associated with eventual ability to ambulate (132).

Prognosis for Change in Level

The single neurologic level usually does not change between acute admission and discharge (4). However, this appears due to lack of improvement in the sensory level. Usually the sensory level is higher than the motor level and thus determines the single neurologic level. Evidence suggests that although the sensory level usually does not improve,

TABLE 51-6. *Relationship of admission and discharge Frankel grades*

	Admission Frankel grade		Discharge Frankel grade	
	A	B	C	D
A	89	5	3	3
B	5	49	16	28
C	2	1	41	53
D	1	1	1	90

Comparison of Frankel grade upon acute admission to that upon hospital discharge. The percentages are adapted from Ditunno JF Jr, Cohen ME, Formal C, Whiteneck GG. Functional outcomes. In: Stover SL, DeLisa JA, Whiteneck GG, eds. *Spinal cord injury*. Gaithersburg, MD: Aspen, 1995; 170–184. The rows and columns do not sum to 100 because data were incomplete in some cases, and cases involving a Frankel grade of E are not included.

the motor level commonly does. This is crucial, especially in tetraplegia, because the motor level is more important in determining function (133). Peripheral sprouting may be a mechanism for such motor recovery in those with ASIA grades A and B (134).

FUNCTIONAL ISSUES AFTER SPINAL CORD INJURY

Expected Levels of Function

The expected level of function after SCI depends heavily on neurologic impairment. Typical achievements for various neurologic levels are summarized in Table 51-7. Rigorously collected data are only available for certain levels (135,136). Motor level is a better predictor than the single neurologic level (133).

With the increased sophistication of acute management of SCI, the extent of injury has decreased. We are seeing more incomplete injuries, with the potential for some neurologic improvement for months or years after injury. Individuals with incomplete injuries present a new challenge to the rehabilitation team: to be creative and progressive in treatment approaches as well as up to date on the ever-changing medical interventions and technology to facilitate or enhance partial function.

Functional outcomes for the incomplete population are impossible to predict because they depend on such factors as extent of incompleteness, timing of return of function, level of spasticity, and so on. Rehabilitation programs for this group of individuals must remain flexible to maximize potential as change in neurologic function occurs.

The maximum functional level that any person with SCI can achieve will be modified by a variety of factors apart from the spinal impairment. Modifying factors include age, body proportions and weight distribution, spinal and extremity immobilization devices, spasticity, contractures, heterotopic bone, and associated injury such as head injury. Psychosocial influences include patient motivation, patient goals, the support system of family and/or significant others, living arrangements, and prior life-style. Financial support may be the major determinant in achievement of certain levels of function because of the expense of high-tech equipment, as well as most of the basic equipment. The equipment and services, such as home modifications and attendants, depend upon funding. For example, with C4 tetraplegia, a power wheelchair with an environmental control unit (ECU), purchased by the insurer or from personal resources, will significantly change the functional independence and quality of life achieved.

Acute Functional Intervention

Intervention in the very early stages of hospitalization includes prevention of complications. Problems that develop during this phase, such as contractures and pressure ulceration, can come to dominate subsequent rehabilitation management, and their prevention is paramount. Training in active exercise can prevent disuse weakness and provides the patient with a feeling of participating in management rather than simply being an object of management. The educational process of patient and family is begun. Discharge planning starts on the day of or the day after injury. Neurologic status is closely followed and documented.

Prevention of Contractures

Proper positioning of the trunk and extremities will help prevent joint contractures and pressure sores. Rotating beds that have positioning troughs for the arms and legs are an aid during the acute period when the person is immobilized and at bed rest. Shoulder positioning in abduction may decrease the later onset of shoulder contracture and pain (137). A person at bed rest with a level of C5 may be at particular risk of developing elbow flexion (and supination) contractures, as the elbow flexors are functioning, while the two main elbow extensors—the triceps and gravity—are inoperative. Mild contracture due to shortening of the finger flexors may be beneficial for the development of a tenodesis grasp. Hip extension can be maintained by periods of lying prone. Ankle plantar flexion contractures can be prevented by proper positioning splints, or high-top athletic shoes. A person with paraplegia may plan to pursue ambulation training at some point, only to find that fixed ankle plantar flexion contractures, or hip flexion contractures, prevent the required forward position of the hips. Loss of shoulder, elbow, hip (where rotation may be lost first), or knee range may signal the development of heterotopic bone. Heterotopic bone can develop above the level of spinal injury after SCI if the person has sustained a concomitant head injury. Chapter 41 contains other details about positioning and ROM exercises.

Range of Motion Exercises

For persons with paraplegia or tetraplegia, there are specific joints at which having greater or less than normal ROM is a distinct functional advantage. This is often referred to as selective stretch or selective tightness. These considerations should guide the ROM exercise program.

Selective stretch is important in certain muscle groups of the individual with an SCI for particular functional tasks. Selective stretch of the hamstrings will allow a straight-leg raise to approximate 120° from supine. This allows activities such as certain types of transfers and donning pants, socks, shoes, and possibly knee–ankle–foot orthoses. Sitting for long periods without adequate hamstring ROM can result in problems because of repeated lumbar hyperflexion. An overstretched low back due to inadequate hamstring ROM could in turn lead to sitting instabilities such as sacral sitting and poor postural alignment, especially for the person with tetraplegia. Selective stretch of the anterior pectoral muscles allows full shoulder extension for bed mobility, transfers, and wheelchair hooking tasks. Selective stretch of the hip flexors and plantar flexors is important for the individual using long leg braces for swing-through ambulation and standing stability.

Selective tightness is encouraged for certain muscle groups to enhance function and compensate for paralysis. Shortening of the finger flexors is important for the individual with C6 tetraplegia because it allows active wrist extension to power palmar grasp by the tenodesis mechanism. In tetraplegia and high paraplegia, tightness of the low back spinal extensors will facilitate a more stable trunk and erect sitting position without the use of upper extremity support. Overstretched trunk extensors could lead to the following problems:

1. Kyphosis, scoliosis, or both, with a resultant decrease in vital capacity and respiratory function
2. Sitting instability with possible compromise of upper extremity functioning or development of pressure sores
3. Transfer difficulties due to the passive lengthening of the spinal column during the push-up phase of the transfer

When allowing trunk musculature tightness, rib cage flexibility also must be maintained so that vital capacity is not compromised.

Muscle Substitution Patterns

A person with SCI can use a working muscle to perform an action of which it is capable but would not do under ordinary circumstances. This can substitute for a muscle whose function has been lost (138). For example, a person with a level of C5 could use shoulder abduction and external rotation to bring about elbow extension by gravity. An inattentive examiner might thus assign a muscle grade of 2/5 to a person with no triceps function. Abduction and internal rotation can bring about forearm pronation; external rotation leads to supination. Similar maneuvers can be used for wrist flexion and extension, with gravity providing the ultimate force for joint motion.

A paralyzed muscle that crosses two joints can be tightened by motion at one joint, bringing about motion at the second joint. For example, wrist extension by a person with a level of C6 can passively tighten the finger flexors, producing palmar grasp. This mechanism is called tenodesis and is facilitated by a modest contracture of the finger flexors.

When the hand is fixed to a supporting system, the upper extremity is in a closed kinetic chain. Muscles can then power joints that they do not cross. A person with C6 tetraplegia could use the anterior deltoid and pectoralis major for elbow extension (139,140).

Typical origin–insertion relationships can be reversed. A person with paraplegia relies on the action of latissimus dorsi upon the pelvis to assist with push-up weight shifts (141). Interestingly, such function avoids loading the shoulder

TABLE 51-7. *Typical functional outcomes for patients with complete SCIs*

Location of injury	Pressure relief	Wheelchair transfers	Wheelchair propulsion	Ambulation	Orthotic devices	Transportation	Communication
C3–C4	Independent in power recliner wheelchair; dependent in bed or manual wheelchair	Total dependence	Independent in pneumatic or chin control–driven power wheelchair with power recliner	Not applicable	Upper extremity externally powered orthosis, dorsal cock-up splint, BFOs	Dependent on others in accessible van with lift; unable to drive	Independent with adapted equipment for phone or typing
C5	Most require assistance	Assistance of one person with or without transfer board	Independent in powered wheelchair indoors and outdoors; short distances in manual wheelchair with adapted handrims indoors	Not applicable	As above	Independent driving in specially adapted van	As above
C6	Independent	Potentially independent with transfer board	Independent moderate distances with manual wheelchair with plastic rims or lugs indoors; assistance needed outdoors; independent in hand-driven wheelchair	Not applicable	Wrist-driven orthosis, universal cuff, writing devices, built-up handles	Independent in driving specially adapted van	Independent with adapted equipment for phone, typing, and writing; independent in turning pages
C7	Independent	Independent with or without transfer board including car, except to or from floor with assistance	Independent in manual wheelchair indoors and outdoors, except stairs	Not applicable	None	Independent driving car with hand controls or specially adapted van; independent placement of wheelchair into car	Independent with adapted equipment for phone, typing, and writing; independent in turning pages
C8–T1	Independent	Independent, including to and from floor and car	Independent in manual wheelchair indoors and outdoors; with curbs, escalators; assistance on stairs	Exercise only (not functional with orthoses); requires physical assistance or guarding	None	As above	Independent
T2–T10	Independent	Independent	Independent	Exercise only (not functional with orthoses); may not require assistance	Knee–ankle–foot orthoses with forearm crutches or walker	As above	Independent
T11–L2	Independent	Independent	Independent	Functional ambulation indoors with orthoses; stairs using railing	Knee–ankle–foot orthoses or ankle–foot orthoses with forearm crutches	As above	Independent
L3–S3	Independent	Independent	Independent	Community ambulation; independent indoors and outdoors with orthoses	Ankle–foot orthoses with forearm crutches or canes	As above	Independent

TABLE 51-7. *Continued*

Location of injury	Pulmonary hygiene	Feeding	Grooming	Dressing	Bathing	Bowel and bladder routine	Bed mobility
C3–C4	Totally assisted cough	May be unable to feed self; use of BFOs with universal cuff and adapted utensils indicated; drinks with long straw after set-up	Total dependence	Total dependence	Total dependence	Total dependence	Total dependence
C5	Assisted cough	Independent with specially adapted equipment for feeding after set-up	Independent with adapted equipment	Assistance with upper extremity dressing; dependent for lower extremity dressing	Total dependence	Total dependence	Assisted by others and by equipment
C6	Some assistance required in supine position; independent in sitting postion	Independent with equipment; drinks from glass	Independent with equipment	Independent with upper extremity dressing; assistance needed for lower extremity dressing	Independent in upper and lower extremity bathing with equipment	Independent for bowel routine; assistance needed with bladder routing	Independent with equipment
C7	As above	Independent	Independent	Potential for independence in upper and lower extremity dressing with equipment	Independent with equipment	Independent	Independent
C8–T1	As above	Independent	Independent	Independent	Independent	Independent	Independent
T2–T10	T2–T6 as above; T6–T10 independent	Independent	Independent	Independent	Independent	Independent	Independent
T11–L2	Not applicable	Independent	Independent	Independent	Independent	Independent	Independent
L3–S3	Not applicable	Independent	Independent	Independent	Independent	Independent	Independent

BFO, balanced forearm orthosis.

joint. In another example, pectoralis major can generate some active expiration in a person with tetraplegia (142).

Hand Function

Maintenance of adequate ROM is vital to increased hand function. Particular attention is given to the metacarpophalangeal joints, the proximal interphalangeal joints, and the web space. Static splints that are regularly used include the volar resting hand splint, dorsal wrist supports with web space straps, wrist cock-up splints, and long and short opponens splints. These splints may incorporate C-bars to maintain the web space and metacarpophalangeal extension stops when needed.

In tetraplegia, much treatment time will be spent in maximizing hand function. Care is taken to allow the finger flexors to develop the tightness needed for a functional tenodesis grasp. Persons with active wrist extension are taught how to use tenodesis pinch and gravity-assisted wrist flexion for release during functional tasks. Patients without active wrist extension may be taught how to use a manually operated ratchet wrist orthosis to achieve pinch. Powered prehension orthoses also may be considered. Patients may consider such devices too cumbersome.

These orthotic devices can be made with thermoplastic materials for temporary training purposes. The patient can practice using the specific device in various graded grasp–release activities. Level of motivation and acceptance can be assessed. A permanent orthosis can then be fabricated from metal or plastic.

Other devices that can be used to compensate for decreased hand function are listed as follows:

1. Universal cuff—a leather or webbing cuff that has a palm pouch that holds such things as eating utensils, toothbrushes, razors, and typing sticks
2. Commercially available writing devices that attach to the hand to stabilize a pen or pencil
3. Built-up or cuff-type handles that can be adapted to many hygiene, grooming, and household items

In high-level tetraplegia, additional adaptive equipment is needed to aid in upper extremity function, particularly for prepositioning the shoulder in preparation for functional use of the hand. Overhead suspension slings, counterbalance slings, and mobile arm supports are the most commonly used devices. Each device supports the upper extremity in a more functional position. The overhead sling and the counterbalance sling eliminate the force of gravity; the mobile arm supports allow gravity to assist the weakest muscles to move in one direction while the patient exerts his or her own muscle power to move in the opposite direction.

Activities of Daily Living

Tetraplegia

Training in activities of daily living (ADLs) is especially significant when treating the person with tetraplegia with varying degrees of involvement in the trunk and upper extremities. Self-care activities such as eating, grooming, and upper extremity dressing can be performed while in bed and can then progress to a wheelchair level. When possible, lower extremity dressing is accomplished while in the bed. Bathing needs require assistance and are successfully completed while in bed or with the use of a shower chair. Adaptive devices are used to compensate for functional deficits and mobility limitations (143).

Examples of various pieces of adaptive equipment are listed as follows:

- Feeding
  - Universal cuffs
  - Built-up utensil handles
  - Long, flexible straws
  - Angled or swiveled utensils
  - Scoop dishes/plate guards
- Bathing
  - Wash mitt
  - Soap on a rope
  - Tub bench
  - Hand-held shower
  - Shower chair
  - Long-handled sponges
- Dressing (144)
  - "Quad" handle dressing stick
  - Loops on socks
  - Zipper loops
  - Button hooks with universal cuff
- Grooming and hygiene
  - Cuff handles on razors and brushes
  - Dispensers for toothpaste and deodorant
  - Long-handled self-inspection mirrors
- Mouthsticks (145,146)
  - Static, with wooden or other lightweight shaft
  - Dynamic, including tongue-activated pincer type

Paraplegia

A person with paraplegia can perform most grooming and hygiene tasks independently—in bed at first, then from the wheelchair. These independent tasks include hair brushing, combing, shaving, applying makeup, oral hygiene, nail care, and applying deodorant. Bathing is done from the bed initially, with assistance for the back, perineum, and lower extremities. The patient progresses to use of a shower chair and tub bench for independent bathing.

The patient becomes more independent in dressing skills as balance improves. Early on, lower extremity dressing may need to be performed with the use of adaptive equipment. The most frequently used equipment includes reachers, dressing sticks, adapted shoe laces or an alternate closure system, and leg-lifting straps.

Wheelchair Use

Wheelchair prescription is complex (147). The task requires knowledge of current models and their advantages and disadvantages. Each available model has different standard and optional accessories. The components of a wheelchair can make the ultimate difference in an individual's independence level for transfers, locomotion over distances, and management of different surfaces. The wheelchair affects balance and can determine the availability of the upper extremities for functional tasks. Wheelchairs are also considered in Chapter 30.

In prescribing the wheelchair, the input of the entire team is needed, including patient, family, and insurance provider. Some of the important considerations in wheelchair prescription are listed as follows:

- Primary and secondary diagnoses
- Prognosis
- Age
- Expected functional level and type of activities
- Home and work environment
- Funding
- Medical complications
- Psychosocial considerations
- Body proportions
- Weight of person and wheelchair
- Durability
- Maintenance
- Transportation

The seating system, which consists of a cushion and any postural adjuncts, must be considered before the rest of the wheelchair prescription. The seating support may then direct the type of chair, its dimensions, and the individual's needs for accessories.

Once this information is gathered, selection of the chair by manufacturer, model, and accessories (e.g., frame style, weight, upholstery, size and dimension specifications, armrests, footrest–legrest assembly, wheels, tires, rims) may be completed.

For the person with high-level tetraplegia, powered wheelchairs may be the only functional mode of mobility (148). There must be a thorough hands-on evaluation to determine the most appropriate system. The durable medical equipment vendor should be used to obtain trial power systems to evaluate with individual users. Physical, functional, environmental, financial, and cosmetic factors must be addressed before the procurement of the definitive system. Examples of these needs may include weight, posture, strength, endurance, skin integrity, ROM, maintenance of the system, terrain over which the system will be used, environmental and architectural barriers, transportability and van conversion, long or short distance use of the system, primary and secondary use of the wheelchair (i.e., school, work), insurance reimbursement, comfort, color, size, and type of seating system required. When prescribing power mobility, a manual wheelchair should always be provided as a backup.

There are two tiers of power chair controls. The higher level of control—which includes determining what the chair will respond to and how it will respond—is governed by a microprocessor-based controller. This allows adjustment of the characteristics of the chair in response to the needs of the individual user.

The lower level of controls involve the moment-to-moment determination of chair activity, including basic functions, such as its speed, direction, and acceleration, and more advanced functions such as pressure relief, and operation of lights and horns. Input from the user can be through several controls or switches; for the user with limited options for input, all the input can be channeled through a single, integrated device. The response of the chair can be proportional or on-off. For example, an operator with excellent hand control might wish to have proportional control of the chair speed. With this type of control, the further the control device (such as a joystick) is pressed, the faster the chair goes. An operator with less precise capabilities might prefer a system in which activation of a switch causes the chair to locomote at a preset speed, without further input from the operator.

Power chairs can be belt drive, direct drive, or friction drive. Belt drive is used on traditional power chairs and performs well indoors. A direct-drive chair can be more responsive. Direct-drive motors are availabe on powered bases upon which a separate seating unit can be attached. A friction drive can be used as an add-on to a manual chair, when the user anticipates having to traverse long distances.

In addition to wheelchair controls, ECUs can be interfaced into the power wheelchair control mechanism to increase the system's overall function and the individual's independence.

Functional Mobility

Training for functional mobility activities (e.g., bed mobility, wheelchair propulsion, transfers) is performed concomitantly with the general exercise program. Selection of which activities can be performed independently, with supervision, or with assistance or dependence is made in accordance with physical capacity projections (Table 51-7). A spinal stabilization device can delay training in certain activities. Training uses some of the following basic principles:

1. Sequence the skill from simple to complex.
2. Break the whole task down into simpler units and then recombine units into the whole.
3. Use the momentum of nonparalyzed parts of the body (such as the head and shoulders) and muscle substitutions to augment weakened or paralyzed muscles. For example, swinging the arms side to side can assist in achieving rolling from supine to side-lying for a person with weak or paralyzed thoracic and abdominal muscles.
4. When possible, use the body weight as the resistance during exercise. Exercises will need to be performed supine, side-lying, long-sitting, short-sitting, semireclining, and in the wheelchair.
5. Muscle groups should be exercised in the position in which they are used functionally (138).

Functional mobility training includes a broad variety of activities, such as the following:

1. Bed mobility: rolling, moving between supine and sitting, transferring the legs on and off bed, and moving across the bed side to side or top to bottom.
2. Bed transfers: transfers from either the long-sit or short-sit position, with or without a transfer board.
3. Advanced transfers: transfers between floor and wheelchair, car transfers, negotiation of steps without wheelchair use, placement of the wheelchair into a car.
4. General wheelchair mobility skills: indoor and outdoor propulsion, skills on uneven terrain, curbs, ramps, escalators, ascending and descending stairs using the wheelchair.

The individual's ability to achieve various levels of independence in these tasks is directly related to such issues as strength, ROM, spasticity, body proportions, completeness of injury, level, judgment, and assistance available from others.

If the patient will not be independent, training is given on two levels: to the patient, who must be competent to instruct another person in the safe accomplishment of that particular activity, and to the significant other, family members, or attendant, who must offer assistance on a daily basis. Family involvement occurs as early as is allowed by the physical and emotional status of the patient and family.

Ambulation

The first question of most people with SCI is, "Will I walk?" This is not surprising because humans develop the ability to walk before bowel control, bladder control, and other self-care abilities. Some become so focused on walking that assumption of other functional skills or resumption of life-style, vocation, or education in the community is deferred.

Definitions

The term ''ambulation'' can cover an enormous range of capability. The rehabilitation team may be pleased with the progress of a person with SCI using an ambulation aid, only to hear from the person, ''But this isn't walking!'' Communication regarding ambulation, whether between professionals or between a professional and a patient, must be precise.

In most centers specializing in spinal cord management, four levels of ambulation are identified:

1. Standing only.
2. Therapeutic ambulation. Use of ambulation for exercise only. Walking for short distances with the assistance of another for any or all of the following: donning/removal of orthoses, sit-to-stand transfers, balance, assistance while ambulating, assistance from floor to chair, assistance standing after a fall.
3. Indoor/functional ambulation. Walks full or part time in orthoses within the home, has the ability to don and remove orthoses, can transfer from sitting to standing and from floor to chair or to standing independently, uses wheelchair mostly outdoors for long-distance mobility.
4. Community ambulation. Is completely independent at the ambulatory level and does not use the wheelchair for the majority of mobility.

Any of these levels may constitute a worthwhile goal for ambulation training, depending on the individual's circumstances and motivation. Orthotic prescription should be considered when there is a specific need or barrier in the environment and the use of orthoses and ambulatory aids will resolve the problem. Orthoses have been successfully used for many patients who use a chair at all times except when access to an otherwise inaccessible part of the home, school, or office or a particular work or homemaking activity requires just standing or minimal ambulation.

Timing of Training

For those individuals with incomplete injuries, ambulation training becomes part of the therapeutic program as neuromuscular function evolves. There is controversy over whether and when an individual with a complete injury should be afforded the opportunity to attempt ambulation. One approach is to begin ambulation training during the initial phase; another is to complete initial rehabilitation at a wheelchair level, revisiting the issue of ambulation after several months of adjusting to life in the community when the person may have a broader perspective. In any case, a trial training program with defined mutually agreed upon goals has advantages. This program should define specific levels of performance that must be achieved before orthotic prescription is completed. It allows the therapist, physician, and patient to assess the effect of such factors as spasticity, limitations of ROM, spinal hypermobility or stiffness, upper extremity strength, and endurance. It affords the individual the opportunity to exhibit that he or she has the motivation and perseverance to succeed in the activity and allows him or her to assess the advantages and drawbacks of everyday brace use. A complete ambulation program includes the following skills: donning and doffing braces, transfers, level surface ambulation, rising from the floor, and navigation of stairs, ramps, curbs, sidewalks, and uneven terrain.

Prediction of Ability to Ambulate

Prediction of ability to ambulate must always be individual. Exceptional motivation may cause a patient to exceed prediction; fixed ankle contractures may make any ambulation impossible. Table 51-8 lists data regarding prediction of future ambulatory capacity as a function of neurologic impairment.

Specific Systems

For those individuals who choose to pursue standing only, several options exist, including mechanical or power standup wheelchairs or power/manual/hydraulic standing frames. A simple standing frame, with ankle, knee, and hip straps to prevent buckling, and a surface upon which to rest the arms, can often be assembled in a home workshop. For those using long leg braces, options include metal or metal/plastic conventional design orthoses, Scott Craig design orthoses, or the reciprocating gait orthoses (152). The use of molded plastic orthoses for an individual with sensory loss requires education regarding the risk of pressure injury. For those with lower-level paraplegia or incomplete injuries, a variety of ankle–foot orthoses exist, depending on the patient's neuromuscular needs.

Energy Consumption

A number of studies have evaluated the energy consumption of paraplegic gait, and various bracing systems have been considered. The energy consumption is consistently significantly elevated above that of normal gait and to levels that could not be sustained over long distances. The increased energy consumption and decreased speed associated with ambulation in paraplegia compare unfavorably with the relatively normal energy expenditure and velocity of wheelchair use.

Homemaking and Community Skills

The ability to function independently in household tasks is addressed before discharge. This may involve a combination of individual and group sessions. Areas discussed and practiced are meal preparation, food purchase, cooking, serv-

TABLE 51-8. *Early predictors of later ambulation status*

Source	Population	Relationship	Definition of ambulation
Penrod, 1990 (149)	Symmetrical incomplete tetraplegia with some motor return	29 of 30 subjects <50 yr of age ambulated, compared with seven of 17 subjects ≥50	Amulation of 50 ft
Crozier, 1991 (131)	Persons admitted with Frankel B injuries	Eight of nine subjects who had initial appreciation of pin sense below the level of injury could later ambulate, vs. two of 18 subjects without initial pin appreciation	Ability to walk independently with reciprocal gait for 200 ft
Crozier, 1992 (132)	C4–T10, Frankel C injuries with initial quadriceps strength ≤2/5 bilaterally	Nine of nine subjects who achieved a quadriceps grade of >3/5 on one side by 2 mo could ambulate at 6 mo, compared with two of eight who did not achieve such quadriceps recovery at 2 mo	Able to ambulate in the home with relative independence
Waters, 1994 (150)	Persons with incomplete paraplegia 1 mo after injury	41 of 54 could ambulate with reciprocal gait at follow-up; 29 of 29 subjects with an LEMS of 10 at 1 mo could ambulate at 1 yr; those with a hip flexor or knee extensor grade of 2 at 1 mo could ambulate at 1 yr	Ability to get out of a wheelchair and walk reasonable distances in and out of the home, with devices but without another person to assist
Waters, 1994 (151)	Persons with incomplete tetraplegia 1 mo after injury	23 of 50 could ambulate in the community at 1 yr; none of 13 with an LEMS of 0 at 1 mo could ambulate at 1 yr; 15 of 15 with an LEMS 20 could ambulate at 1 yr	Ability to ambulate in the community with a reciprocal gait and devices

ASIA, American Spinal Injury Association; LEMS, lower extremity motor score. Frankel grade closely approximates ASIA grade. LEMS is the sum of the motor scores for the ASIA key lower extremity muscles; the maximum score for these five pairs of muscles is 50.

ing, laundry, house cleaning (e.g. dusting, vacuuming), and making beds. At this time, other functional tasks, such as use of the telephone and operating light switches, stereo, door locks, tape recorder, and similar items, are practiced and adapted as needed.

To better prepare for reintegration into the community, many rehabilitation facilities offer community skills group therapy. Typical outings include use of public transportation, accessing and using a shopping mall, going to the movies, grocery shopping, banking and using automatic teller machines, going to health spas, and eating in restaurants. Planning for and learning from these outings is emphasized to reinforce successful reintegration into the community.

Home Visits, Home Modifications, and Environmental Access

Part of a comprehensive rehabilitation program involves the assessment of a person's home environment and the ability of the person to function within that environment. Home visits are designed to evaluate accessibility and safety, recommend modifications, assist patient and family in recognizing potential problems, gather specific information regarding the home situation (e.g., measurements), and test for functional skills within the home environment.

In making recommendations, the home visit team takes four basic areas into consideration:

1. The patient's needs
2. The family's needs
3. Architectural needs and limitations
4. Financial resources

The process of solving identified problems is usually handled by discussion among family members, staff, the patient, and the insurance representative. Usually both short- and long-term solutions are presented so as not to overwhelm or complicate the situation. Additionally, the team will try to make the recommendations as simple as possible.

Architectural adaptations that minimize barriers and improve access range from the simple to the complex and from the economical to the expensive. Simple adaptations include ramps and door widening, whereas the complex or expensive include wheelchair elevators, stair glides, remodeling of the bathroom to include a roll-in shower, or construction of an entirely accessible home (153). Adaptations should not be confined solely to the home environment. Adaptations to the school or work setting permit the resumption of a productive life-style.

Returning some measure of control over one's environment is a priority for the person with high level tetraplegia. One way to restore control is through the use of an ECU. An ECU is a system of electronic components that remotely controls lights, telephones, sound equipment, television, radio, appliances, intercoms, doors, and other items that are powered electrically in a home and office. The systems available today vary greatly in cost and complexity.

A critical component of the system is the interface with the operator. Switches for controlling the system include hand controls with specific modifications, mouthsticks, tongue switches, pneumatic switches and brow switches, and a rocking lever that can be operated with the head, hand, or foot.

Choices must be made regarding the complexity of the system. Some individuals require only a remote control unit, which is portable and operates without special wiring. This is most appropriate for those needing to control only light switches and appliances. Others will need to operate special built-in telephones, electric beds, televisions, window drapes, and doors. These units require complex electrical connections and are more costly and used on a more permanent basis. This subject is also considered in Chapter 29.

Motor Vehicle Transportation

Both operating and riding in a motor vehicle present problems for those with SCI. These are addressed by driver education programs for the disabled. There is also the Association of Driver Educators for the Disabled, which conducts conferences for professionals.

A complete program consists of three parts. The predriving screening includes assessment of visual acuity, reaction response, field of vision, depth perception, color perception, visual accommodation, judgment, attention, problem solving, sequencing, memory, recognition of signs and symbols, number recognition, upper and lower extremity mobility skills, hand function, and transfer skills. The results of the evaluation provide the basis for determining the person's capabilities and specific needs for driving. A driving simulator can be used for parts of the evaluation.

Once the person is deemed eligible, the next step is the selection of the appropriate vehicle with the necessary modifications or adaptive equipment (154,155). A wide variety of such equipment is commercially available, ranging from steering wheel attachments, power seats, console controls, and hand controls for throttle and brake to completely converted vans with hydraulic lifts. In making these decisions, the professional takes into consideration the person's goals and life-style, wheelchair type, functional abilities, safety, and financial resources.

Prescription of a vehicle requires specification of a mode of entrance and exit, arrangements for seating within the vehicle, and, in some cases, modifications to allow the disabled individual to drive the vehicle. Vendors are a source of detailed information about various products.

If the person is to use a conventional sedan, a two-door model is preferable because of greater ease of entry. The chair can either be pulled in behind the person, or stored in a specialized carrier on the roof. A van can be entered via a lift, or by a ramp. Lowering the floor of the vehicle facilitates ramp entrance. Entrance can either be from the right side of the vehicle or from the back. A lowered floor or raised roof allows clearance of the head while entering. Once the van has been entered, the person can either remain sitting in the wheelchair, which must be fixed to the floor of the van, or can transfer to an appropriate seat. For long trips, a bed may be useful for pressure relief and hygiene tasks. Driver controls vary with the level of injury. ECU technology has been adapted to facilitate certain operations, such as operating the lights or horn, without diverting the use of the upper extremities.

The final step is the behind-the-wheel training. This requires that the person have a valid license or learner's permit. Those who are not yet ready to drive may receive an abbreviated evaluation aimed at determining the appropriate vehicle or safety equipment needed to be a passenger.

Recreation and Sports

Recreation, constructive use of leisure time, and participation in sports enhance quality of life. Disability does not obviate the right to involvement in leisure activities as an integral part of life-style.

The use of leisure time is often perceived by the newly injured person as a problem. Mobility limitations can be obstacles for returning to previous leisure activities. Thus, the overall program should include the following:

1. Education in the community's recreational resources
2. Adaptations for previous leisure skills and interests
3. Learning of new leisure skills
4. Refinement of functional abilities related to specific leisure activities

Community skills groups feature both discussions and trips to develop the skills, planning, and participation necessary to take an active role in recreational opportunities.

Wheelchair sports for both recreational and competitive purposes are widely available. These allow the individual with SCI to increase his or her activity level, improve strength and endurance, and promote good health. Wheelchair sports also provide the opportunity to compete aggressively with people at the same functional level and provide an arena for achievement of athletic excellence as well as for camaraderie and sportsmanship. Examples of sports activities successfully participated in by SCI men and women include rugby, archery, boating, football, camping, hunting, flying, golf, scuba diving, swimming, basketball, table tennis, weight lifting, tennis, horseback riding, distance racing, track and field events, and skiing (156,157). A person with tetraplegia and an interest in contact team sports might consider ''quad'' rugby; a person with paraplegia could pursue wheelchair basketball. Many sports and recreational activities in which a person participated before injury can be adapted for participation after injury. In some instances, the disabled can compete with their able-bodied counterparts. In addition to sports activities, some health spas and fitness centers have incorporated the needs of the disabled into their programs. Wheelchair atheltics are increasingly visible in the lay press, and are closely reported in periodicals such as *Sports 'n' Spokes*.

The participation in sports and a general fitness program is viewed by many as an expression of well-being and a step toward improved general health (158,159). Secondary gains include a more positive self-image, often resulting in better interpersonal relationships and a decrease in secondary medical complications associated with inactivity.

The learning of appropriate leisure skills and the incorporation of these activities into the individual's life-style will have long-lasting effects. A person who can use leisure time constructively is less likely to become depressed (160). As in all aspects of rehabilitation, the choice belongs to the person, who must take an active role in deciding what direction to take. The discovery and development of quality in life-style has its beginning in the discovery that many sources of self-satisfaction and participation with society remain open.

Upper Extremity Reconstructive Surgery

Upper extremity reconstructive surgery can offer certain persons with tetraplegia the opportunity to increase elbow and wrist control, as well as to perform pinch and grasp, and release (161–163). Analogous procedures for the lower extremity are not available. "Tendon transfer" is a shorthand descriptor for this type of surgery.

In general such surgery is not considered until at least 1 year after injury. This allows time for most neurologic improvement to occur. Candidates must be aware of the specific benefits expected, which may not be dramatic. They also must be tolerant of postoperative immobilization, which will temporarily halt gains made during initial rehabilitation. A loss of strength may be noted in the motion normally served by the involved muscle.

Initial screening involves detailed assessment of joint ROM and muscle function. Two-point discrimination over the pulp of the thumb indicates the usefulness of cutaneous afferents; less than 10 mm is favorable.

A muscle used for transfer should have strength of at least 4/5. A spastic muscle may be unsuitable for transfer, due to the difficulty of re-education. If both surgery for elbow control and surgery for wrist–hand function are planned, surgery for elbow control is performed first. If surgery on both upper extremities is planned, the stronger is usually reconstructed first; if they are of equal strength, the dominant is reconstructed first. If afferent input is deficient in both upper extremities, then surgery may only be indicated for one because the candidate will have to rely on visual information and can only look at one extremity at a time.

Several procedures are available; four will be described. A person with a level of C5 may have good shoulder control and elbow flexion. Although gravity can normally be used to accomplish elbow extension, this is not possible with overhead activities, during which the elbow can collapse into flexion. Such a person may benefit from transfer of the posterior deltoid to triceps via a free tendon graft harvested from the lower extremity. This allows overhead activities and may increase the ability of the upper extremity to assist with sitting (164). Improvement may not be sufficient to restore push-up and transfer ability, especially because other crucial muscles, such as latissimus dorsi, may remain weak. A majority who undergo the procedure report functional improvement (165).

A person with a level of C6 may have strong wrist extension, but no active pinch. Lateral or key pinch, between the distal thumb and the middle phalanx of the index finger, can occur when the wrist is extended, via passive tightening of the tendon of the flexor pollicis longus (FPL). This tenodesis mechanism requires a contracture of the FPL. The effect can be mimicked by dividing the FPL tendon and attaching the proximal end of the distal segment to the distal radius, with wrist extension then causing lateral pinch (166). The interphalangeal joint of the thumb may require surgical stabilization. Lateral pinch is easier to obtain than three jaw chuck because less precision is required in positioning the digits. The majority of patients who undergo the procedure are pleased with the results (167).

Lateral pinch also can be restored by transfer of a muscle, such as the brachioradialis, to the FPL. This allows more freedom of wrist postition than tenodesis-driven pinch, which requires wrist extension (168).

A person with a level of C6 may have strong wrist extensors, elbow flexors, and pronator teres. However, active grasp between fingers and palm is lacking. This can be restored by attachment of an active motor to the flexor digitorum profundus (169,170). Functional improvement and patient satisfaction are reported.

Postoperative management involves immobilization, with positioning to eliminate any tension on sutured tendons. Over time, ROM is restored, and muscle re-education for functional activities is performed.

Biofeedback

Biofeedback involves the use of artificial sensors to provide an individual with information about motor or autonomic function. It is considered in Chapter 21. The greatest role of biofeedback in the management of individuals with SCI is as an adjunct to motor retraining (171). Electromyographic biofeedback uses surface electrodes and converts the input from muscle into a visual or auditory signal, which is used by the patient to guide muscle exercise. Subjects can increase the biofeedback signal from affected muscles when provided with biofeedback within an operant conditioning sytem (172). It may allow the patient to increase either the number or the firing rate of motor units already under voluntary control (173). It also may allow optimal performance of exercises to increase muscle fiber strength. In certain circumstances it may be useful to decrease cocontraction of muscles. Although persons with SCI can increase strength while using a biofeedback program, it is not proven that biofeedback offers an advantage over conventional exercise programs (174,175). Biofeedback also may be useful in the management of autonomic problems associated with SCI, such as orthostatic hypotension, uninhibited sweating, control of skin temperature, or incontinence retraining (38).

Neuromuscular Stimulation

Electrical stimulation of muscle, either through nerve or through stimulation of the muscle itself, can be used for therapeutic purposes. This is considered in Chapter 24. In persons with SCI, muscles paralyzed by upper motor neuron injury are usually involved, and the actual stimulation is of a peripheral nerve, hence the term ''neuromuscular stimulation'' (NMS) (176,177). It can be used to combat some of the deleterious effects of immobilization, and it can be used to produce extremity motions for functional activities. This latter use is termed ''functional neuromuscular stimulation'' (FNS). The balance of benefits versus the financial costs and practical difficulties is such that FNS is not used by the majority of those with SCI. As the technology improves, it is likely that use will become more widespread. Electrical stimulation can be deleterious in lower motor neuron injury, and therefore should be avoided in muscles around the level of injury.

SCI predisposes to the development of DVT. NMS of paralyzed calf muscles can decrease the risk (178). This use is demanding and is much less common than the use of pneumatic compression devices. Osteoporosis develops in paralyzed extremities after SCI. A study of persons with chronic SCI failed to find an effect of NMS exercise on bone mineral density (179). Maximal exercise capacity is lowered after SCI, which results in cardiovascular deconditioning (30). NMS can be used to provide a cardiovascular conditioning program (180–182). It is uncertain whether this provides an advantage over arm crank exercise (176). The bulk of muscle and its strength and endurance in response to NMS can be increased (183). NMS can strengthen paretic muscle after incomplete SCI if the individual can tolerate the stimulation (174).

FNS can produce lower extremity motion for functional activities, including standing and ambulation (176). Systems vary in several ways. Stimulation electrodes can be surface, percutaneous, or implanted. Surface electrodes must be applied before each individual session but lack the risk of infection. The power source can be external, or, in specialized centers, implanted. The system can be open loop, in which the stimulation is applied in a predetermined manner, or closed loop, in which some variable, such as joint angle, is used to affect stimulation. A closed loop system provides a more modulated response but is more demanding to design. A system can exclusively use muscle contractions brought about directly by FNS or can incorporate reflex responses elicited by stimulation. Hybrid systems use FNS in combination with orthoses. FNS systems are not adequate to replace a wheelchair.

The Parastep I(TM) system (Sigmedics, Inc., Northfield, IL) is commercially available for ambulation for persons with paraplegia (184). It uses external electrodes applied to the quadriceps and to the peroneal nerve at the fibular head. The latter electrode produces stepping by eliciting a triple flexion response. In one version the glutei and/or paraspinal muscles are also stimulated. Power is provided by an external battery. Stimulation is open loop and is controlled by the subject through switches mounted on a walker. Ankle–foot orthoses are commonly used.

Upper extremity FNS is also under investigation for those with SCI. Commercial units were recently made available. Generally the systems are applied to distal upper extremity function, such as lateral (key) and palmar prehension, rather than to proximal upper limb muscles (185). Movement of the contralateral shoulder can be used to control stimulation. Upper extremity FNS can be combined with reconstructive surgery (186).

PSYCHOSOCIAL ISSUES AFTER SPINAL CORD INJURY

Scientific and technologic advances in recent decades have significantly improved the survival rate and life expectancy for the person with SCI. However, attention to quality-of-life issues has lagged behind advances in quantity of life. The impact of this often catastrophic injury influences the individual and the family for a lifetime and affects every aspect of their lives. The individual, family, and rehabilitation professionals share responsibility for rebuilding a different life. This new life will obviously retain many aspects of the preinjury life, but new skills and new coping strategies must be incorporated.

Individual and Family Adjustment

Adjustment to Disability

Rehabilitation professionals are concerned with a patient's ''adjustment to disability,'' but a single definition is lacking. Adjustment is usually felt to have cognitive, affective, and behavioral components. An adjusted individual (whether a person with SCI, a family member, or a caretaker) understands diagnosis and prognosis, maintains a positive outlook, and behaves in a manner conducive to health and productivity. The injury neither destroys the sense of personhood nor dominates the person's life. The topic is considered in Chapter 9.

In evaluating adjustment issues, consideration also must be given to the family and the patient's broader support system. Friends and other peer systems must be included as an integral part of the individual's support network, particularly for adolescents. In many respects, the entire family structure and extended support system must adjust to the disability. The impact on the family is not only emotional but also often physical and economic. The roles and responsibilities previously assumed by the person with the disability must be temporarily or permanently assumed by other family members. In addition, new responsibilities for the physical care of the disabled person may be assumed by family members. The family must be an integral part of any treatment program for they will need assistance in coping with the disability and their response to the disabled person and in dealing with their own increased responsibilities and pressures.

Past Views of Adjustment after Spinal Cord Injury

Past views have held that adjustment after SCI occurred in stages. Depression was identified as one of those stages and therefore was an expected and not unwelcome occurrence (187). Although this may be true for certain individuals, it does not appear to be generally applicable.

Depression after Spinal Cord Injury

The *Diagnostic and Statistical Manual of Mental Disorders,* 3rd revised edition (DSM-IIIR), provides criteria for defining depression, but the relevance of some of these is uncertain in the population with SCI. Rehabilitation professionals may not be very accurate judges of depression in their patients and can overestimate its presence (188). Studies regarding depression after SCI are difficult to compare due to a variation in definitions. One study noted that immediately after discharge from rehabilitation, individuals with SCI were more depressed than control subjects, but the difference diminished to statistically insignificant levels within 3 months (189). Another author noted a rate of depression for a group of individuals with SCI as 13%, or more than double the estimated rate for major and minor depression in the U.S. population (190). The figure is still substantially below that for stroke (191). Whether depression after SCI should be treated differently from depression in the general population is not known.

Coming from a different direction is research regarding subjective quality of life, objective quality of life, and life satisfaction after SCI. Life satisfaction after SCI is lower than that of the general population (192). However, most of those injured for a long period of time still rate their quality of life as ''good'' or ''excellent'' (130).

Relative Importance of Impairment, Disability, and Handicap

The relationship between impairment, disability, and handicap on the one hand and depression, quality of life, and life satisfaction on the other hand is fascinating, important, and unsettled. Our ability to influence impairment after SCI is limited compared with the capacity to improve handicap; therefore, a relatively higher contribution of handicap would be welcome. Several studies do suggest the higher influence of handicap compared with impairment and disability (192,193). Other studies have found greater disability to be associated with a lesser quality of life (194).

Suicide after Spinal Cord Injury

Research involving suicide after SCI is difficult because some deaths due to sepsis and pressure ulcers, for example, may reflect ''indirect suicide'' (195). About 6% of deaths after SCI are clearly related to suicide. This is several times the rate for the general population.

Marital Status after Spinal Cord Injury

Those who are married at the time of injury appear to have an increased rate of divorce in the years after injury, but most married at the time of injury are still married at the fifth anniversary of injury (195). Whether marriages occurring after SCI are more or less resilient than those occurring before injury is uncertain. Those single at the time of injury have a decreased rate of marriage in subsequent years; between 10% and 30% will marry by the 15th anniversary.

Independent Living

Although the disabled individual must make certain adaptations and accommodations, these changes lose meaning unless society affords the opportunity for participation in community life. The Independent Living Movement, which gained momentum in the 1970s, started from the premise that the person with a disability should have the same life choices as the nondisabled person, including where to live, how to live, how to travel, and what recreational or social activities to pursue.

The political activism of the disabled population, as well as a more enlightened attitude among some legislators, has brought about changes. The 1973 Rehabilitation Act and the 1978 amendments are examples. Finally, on July 26, 1990, the Americans with Disability Act was signed into law. This legislation ensures civil rights for individuals with disability. However, as with any civil rights legislation, considerable effort must now be expended to ensure meaningful regulations and full compliance.

At present more than 90% of individuals admitted to hospitals with SCI are discharged to private residences in the community. Nursing homes account for 4% of discharges.

Debates are continuing on legislation to provide personal care assistance. Affordable, accessible housing for families remains a critical issue. Accessible transportation is a problem in many urban areas and in most rural and suburban areas.

Independent living centers have emerged as a focal point of services and advocacy for individuals with disability. However, until attitudinal and architectural barriers are eliminated, the disabled person will continue to confront obstacles in the struggle to reintegrate into the community. Because the person with a disability also must master skills in system management and advocacy to reach the goal of independent living, these must be taught in the rehabilitation program.

Education

Persons with SCI often improve their educational level after injury (195). More than 15% advance their grade level. The extent of injury correlates with achievement because those with tetraplegia achieve a higher educational level than do those with paraplegia, and persons with complete injuries reach a higher level than persons with incomplete injuries. Interestingly, at 5 years after injury, persons with SCI have an educational level below the national average, but at 10 and 15 years after injury the situation has reversed and the educational level for those with SCI exceeds the national average. This may reflect adaptation to economic pressures because persons with SCI presumably require a higher educational level to compete for employment.

Vocational Issues

For many individuals, the attainment of self-sufficiency and independence means a return to work or to training or education leading to return to work. The vocational process should begin early after injury, with a discussion of work history and job skills or interests, an introduction of work expectation, and an opportunity for return to work when this is an appropriate goal. Vocational rehabilitation is considered in Chapter 47.

The vocational process must incorporate two parallel processes: one takes place within the person with the disability, and the second occurs within the business community. Because of the severity of SCI and the average age at onset, many individuals are faced with the need to both define and redefine vocational options and opportunities. Even an experienced worker with a salable realistic job skill may need to learn new skills in resumé writing and interviewing to compensate for the limitations imposed by the disability.

Education of and technical assistance for employers can be powerful tools in enhancing vocational opportunities for people with disabilities. Many employers are unaware of the person's capabilities or are afraid and unsure of their ability to accommodate a disabled employee. Businesses are unsure of what adaptations may be needed for their physical plant and envision expensive and disruptive modifications. Other employers are reluctant to raise concerns about physical capabilities and ability to perform certain job tasks, and there are also colleague and union concerns. Supervisors may have difficulty in coping with disability-related issues and may believe that they need to change standards to accommodate a disabled employee. Specific information may need to be transmitted, technical assistance offered, and myths and prejudices dispelled before an employer is comfortable with hiring a person with a disability. Business advisory groups and federally funded programs, such as Projects with Industry, have been effective in opening dialogue between rehabilitation professionals, disabled employees, and the business community. These efforts have enhanced employment opportunities for individuals with disability.

About 60% of persons with SCI were working before injury (195). This decreases sharply in the years immediately after injury but increases to a peak of about 30% approximately 10 years after injury. In contrast to educational achievement, likelihood of employment correlates inversely with severity of injury. Completion of a vocational rehabilitation program correlates with subsequent employment. Of those who were homemakers at the time of injury, about half return to that role by the first anniversary of injury; more than half of those who were students are again students at 1 year after injury. Increased knowledge regarding disincentives to work and more creative interventions are required to enable a larger portion of individuals with SCI to reach the goal of economic self-sufficiency.

SYSTEMS OF CARE FOR SPINAL CORD INJURY

History

The outlook for individuals with SCI has improved dramatically since early in this century, when mortality was high (196). Effective modern management began with the establishment of systems of care, by Sir Ludwig Guttmann at Stoke Mandeville Hospital in England, and Donald Munro in the United States (197). In 1970, the first federally designated model system for SCI care was implemented in the United States. At present, 18 such centers exist, designated and sponsored by the National Institute on Disability and Rehabilitation Research (NIDDR). The centers collaborate in data collection and research.

Characteristics of a System

An SCI system of care should provide a continuum from retrieval through lifetime follow-up. This includes several phases, such as acute care, inpatient rehabilitation, and outpatient follow-up, through which the person with SCI flows, meeting multiple medical specialists and other professionals. Ideally the flow is in one direction, but set-backs are unavoidable, and may require, for example, transfer from inpatient rehabilitation back to an acute setting. An efficient system, in which the various professionals involved have confidence in each other, allows expeditious movement of the patient between the different phases. The physiatrist is the professional best suited to follow the patient through all of these various settings.

Outpatient Follow-up

Medical, functional, and psychosocial issues arise after discharge home and must be met by the outpatient follow-up system. The system must work in synergy with the patient's primary care physician, if one exists, serving as a resource for SCI-related problems. Follow-up visits are conducted by the physiatrist and include consultation as needed with other members of the rehabilitation team and other medical specialists. Routine follow-up should occur on an annual basis, at which point medical and neurologic status, functional issues, and psychosocial situation should be reviewed. In particular urologic status should be considered annually, and studies to assess the upper tracts (such as a renal nuclear scan) and lower tract (such as a cystogram) are often indicated. Occasionally, patients require readmission for management of new problems or development of new potential. Scheduled follow-up visits serve primarily for problem identification. Problem solving frequently occurs during the interim between scheduled visits.

System Benefits

Early admission to a system of care has been associated with benefits such as decreased risk of pressure ulcer and contracture (198). Mortality may be less. There is a higher rate of discharge to private residences in the community.

THE FUTURE OF SPINAL CORD INJURY MEDICINE

Those caring for spinal cord injured persons will be under increasing pressure to practice efficiently as the influence of managed care increases. Clinicians will be called upon to demostrate that interventions, such as intensive inpatient rehabilitation, provide cost savings in areas such as the development of medical complications, and the need for assistance in mobility and activities of daily living.

Spinal cord injured persons have highly specialized needs. This has resulted in the development of the Spinal Cord Injury Medicine, as a subspecialty of Physical Medicine and Rehabilitation (PM&R). Fellowship training in this area can also be pursued by physicians with training in other specialties. Spinal Cord Injury Medicine is concerned with persons with traumatic SCI, as well as persons with problems such as multiple sclerosis, amyotrophic lateral sclerosis, and spinal bifida.

PM&R is the specialty most concerned with outcome after SCI, and with care in the postacute phase. The logical progression of this involvement will be increased activity in research involving intervention to decrease the chronic neurologic deficits after SCI.

ACKNOWLEDGMENT

This work was supported in part by the Regional Spinal Cord Injury Center of Delaware Valley Model SCI Systems grant to Thomas Jefferson University from the National Institute for Disability Research and Rehabilitation (grant no. H133N50021). The authors would like to thank Kimberly McNamara and Paul Carmine for their assistance.

REFERENCES

1. American Spinal Injury Association. *International standards for neurological and functional classification of spinal cord injury*. Chicago: American Spinal Injury Associaton, 1996.
2. Ditunno JF Jr, Young W, Donovan WH, Creasey G. The international standards booklet for neurological and functional classification of spinal cord injury. *Paraplegia* 1994; 32:70–80.
3. Go BK, DeVivo MJ, Richards JS. The epidemiology of spinal cord injury. In: Stover SL, DeLisa JA, Whiteneck GG, eds. *Spinal cord injury*. Gaithersburg, MD: Aspen, 1995; 21–55.
4. Ditunno JF Jr, Cohen ME, Formal C, Whiteneck GG. Functional outcomes. In: Stover SL, DeLisa JA, Whiteneck GG, eds. *Spinal cord injury*. Gaithersburg, MD: Aspen, 1995; 170–184.
5. Chiles BW III, Cooper P. Acute spinal injury. *N Engl J Med* 1996; 334:514–520.
6. Bailes JE, Cerullo LJ, Engelhard HH. Neurologic assessment and management of head injuries. In: Meyer PR Jr, ed. *Surgery of spine trauma*. New York: Churchill-Livingstone, 1989; 137–156.
7. Meyer PR Jr. Acute injury retrieval and splinting techniques: onsite care. In: Meyer PR Jr, ed. *Surgery of spine trauma*. New York: Churchill-Livingstone, 1989; 1–21.
8. Bracken MB, Shepard MJ, Collins WF Jr, et al. A randomized, controlled trial of methylprednisolone or naloxone in the treatment of acute spinal-cord injury: results of the second National Acute Spinal Cord Injury Study. *N Engl J Med* 1990; 322:1405–1411.
9. Bracken MB, Shepard MJ, Collins WF Jr, et al. Methylprednisolone or naloxone treatment after acute spinal cord injury: 1-year follow-up data. *J Neurosurg* 1992; 76:23–31.
10. Donovan WH. Operative and nonoperative management of spinal cord injury. A review. *Paraplegia* 1994; 32:375–388.
11. Holdsworth F. Fractures, dislocations, and fracture–dislocations of the spine. *J Bone Joint Surg [Am]* 1970; 52:1534–1551.
12. White A, Southwick WO, Panjabai MM. Clinical instability in the lower cervical spine: a review of past and current concepts. *Spine* 1976; 1:15–27.
13. Denis F. Spine instability as defined by the three column spine concept in acute spinal trauma. *Clin Orthop* 1984; 189:65–76.
14. Perry J, Nickel V. Total cervical spine fusion for neck paralysis. *J Bone Joint Surg [Am]* 1959; 41:37–60.
15. Lavernia CJ, Botte MJ, Garfin SR. Spinal orthoses for traumatic and degenerative disease. In: Rothman RH, Simeone FA, eds. *The spine,* 3rd ed. Philadelphia: WB Saunders, 1992; 1197–1224.
16. Glaser JA, Whitehill R, Stamp WG, Jane JA. Complications associated with the halo vest. *J Neurosurg* 1986; 65:762–769.
17. Meyer PR Jr, ed. *Surgery of spine trauma*. New York: Churchill-Livingstone, 1989.
18. Lane JM, Muschler GF. Principles of bone fusion. In: Rothman RJ, Simeone FA, eds. *The Spine,* 3rd ed. Philadelphia: WB Saunders, 1992; 1739–1755.
19. Jackson AB, Groomes TE. Incidence of respiratory complications following spinal cord injury. *Arch Phys Med Rehabil* 1994; 75: 270–275.
20. DeVivo MJ, Stover SL. Long-term survival and causes of death. In: Stover SL, DeLisa JA, Whiteneck GG, eds. *Spinal cord injury*. Gaithersburg, MD: Aspen, 1995; 289–316.
21. DeVivo, MJ, Ivie CS. Life expectancy of ventilator-dependent persons with spinal cord injuries. *Chest* 1995; 108:226–232.
22. De Troyer A, Estenne M, Heilporn A. Mechanism of active expiration in tetraplegic subjects. *N Engl J Med* 1986;314:740–744.
23. Estenne M, De Troyer A. Cough in tetraplegic subjects: an active process. *Ann Intern Med* 1990; 112:22–28.
24. Clough P. Glossopharyngeal breathing: its application with a traumatic quadriplegic patient. *Arch Phys Med Rehabil* 1983; 64: 384–385.
25. Slack, RS, Shucart W. Respiratory dysfunction associated with traumatic injury to the central nervous system. *Clin Chest Med* 1994; 15: 739–749.
26. Fishburn MJ, Marino RJ, Ditunno JF Jr. Atelectasis and pneumonia in acute spinal cord injury. *Arch Phys Med Rehabil* 1991; 71:197–200.
27. Roth EJ, Nussbaum SB, Berkowitz M, et al. Pulmonary function testing in spinal cord injury: correlation with vital capacity. *Paraplegia* 1995; 454–457.
28. Cohn JR. Pulmonary management of the patient with spinal cord injury. *Trauma Q* 1993; 9:65–71.
29. Huang C, Kuhlemeier KV, Ratanaubol U, McEachran AB, DeVivo MJ, Fine PR. Cardiopulmonary response in spinal cord injury patients: effect of pneumatic compressive devices. *Arch Phys Med Rehabil* 1983; 64:101–106.

30. Coutts KD, Rhodes EC, McKenzie DC. Maximal exercise responses of tetraplegics and paraplegics. *J Appl Physiol* 1983; 55:479–482.
31. Drory Y, Ohry A, Brooks ME, Dolphin D, Kellermann JJ. Arm crank ergometry in chronic spinal cord injured patients. *Arch Phys Med Rehabil* 1990; 71:389–392.
32. Figoni SF, Dayton OH. Exercise responses and quadriplegia. *Med Sci Sports Exerc* 1993; 25:433–441.
33. Brenes F, Dearwater S, Shapera R, LaPorte RE, Collins E. High density lipoprotein cholesterol concentrations in physically active and sedentary spinal cord injured patients. *Arch Phys Med Rehabil* 1986; 67:445–50.
34. Bauman W, Spungen A. Disorders of carbohydrate and lipid metabolism in veterans with paraplegia or quadriplegia: a model of premature aging. *Metabolism* 1994; 43:749–756.
35. Gonzalez F, Chang JY, Banovac K, Messina D, Martinez-Arizala A, Kelly RE. Autoregulation of cerebral blood flow in patients with orthostatic hypotension after spinal cord injury. *Paraplegia* 1991; 29: 1–7.
36. Maynard FM. Post-traumatic cystic myelopathy in motor incomplete quadriplegia presenting as progressive orthostasis. *Arch Phys Med Rehabil* 1984; 65:30–32.
37. Groomes TE, Chi-Tsou H. Orthostatic hypotension after spinal cord injury: treatment with fludrocortisone and ergotamine. *Arch Phys Med Rehabil* 1991; 72:56–58.
38. Brucker, BS, Ince LP. Biofeedback as an experimental treatment for postural hypotension in a patient with a spinal cord lesion. *Arch Phys Med Rehabil* 1977; 58:49–53.
39. Frankel HL, Mathias CJ, Spalding JMK. Mechanisms of reflex cardiac arrest in tetraplegic patients. *Lancet* 1975; 2:1183–1185.
40. Mathias CJ. Bradycardia and cardiac arrest during tracheal suction mechanisms in tetraplegic patients. *Eur J Intens Care Med* 1976; 2: 147–156.
41. Kay MM, Kranz JM. External transcutaneous pacemaker for profound bradycardia associated with spinal cord trauma. *Surg Neurol* 1984; 22:344–346.
42. Gilgoff IS, Davidson Ward SL, Hohn AR. Cardiac pacemaker in high spinal cord injury. *Arch Phys Med Rehabil* 1991; 72:601–603.
43. Brooke MM, Donovan WH, Stolov WC. Paraplegia: succinylcholine-induced hyperkalemia and cardiac arrest. *Arch Phys Rehabil* 1978; 59:306–309.
44. Merli GJ, Crabbe S, Palluzzi RG, Fritz D. Etiology, incidence, and prevention of deep vein thrombois in acute spinal cord injury. *Arch Phys Med Rehabil* 1993; 74:1199–1205.
45. Geerts WH, Code KI, Jay RM, Chen E, Szalai JP. A prospective study of venous thromboembolism after major trauma. *N Engl J Med* 1994; 331:1601–1606.
46. Weinmann EE, Salzman EW. Deep vein thrombosis. *N Engl J Med* 1994; 331:1630–1641.
47. Weingarden DS, Weingarden SI, Belen J. Thromboembolic disease presenting as fever in spinal cord injury. *Arch Phys Med Rehabil* 1987; 68:176–177.
48. Merli GJ, Crabbe S, Doyle L, Ditunno JF, Herbison GJ. Mechanical plus pharmacological prophylaxis for deep vein thrombosis in acute spinal cord injury. *Paraplegia* 1992; 30:558–562.
49. Green D, Hull RD, Mammen EF, Merli GJ, Weingarden SI, Yao JST. Deep venous thrombosis in spinal cord injury. *Chest* 1992; 102: 633S–635S.
49a. Green d, Chen D, Chmiel JS, et al. Prevention of thromboembolism in spinal cord injury: role of low molecular weight heparin. *Arch Phys Med Rehabil* 1994; 75:290–292.
49b. Geerts WH, Jay RM, Code KI, et al. A comparison of low-dose heparin with low-molecular-weight heparin as prophylaxis against venous thromboembolism after major trauma. *N Engl J Med* 1996; 335: 701–707.
49c. Rogers FB, Shackford SR, Ricci MA, Wilson JT, Parsons S. Routine prophylactic vena cava insertion in severely injured trauma patients decreases the incidence of pulmonary embolism. *J Am Coll Surg* 1995; 180:641–647.
49d. Ginsberg JS. Management of venous thromboembolism. *N Engl J Med* 1996; 335:1816–1828.
50. Merli GJ. Management of deep vein thrombosis in spinal cord injury. *Chest* 1992; 102(suppl):652–657.
51. Juler GL, Eltorai IM. The acute abdomen in spinal cord injury patients. *Paraplegia* 1985; 23:118–123.
52. Miller F, Fenzi TC. Prolonged ileus with acute spinal cord injury responding to metaclopramide. *Paraplegia* 1981; 19:43–45.
53. Berlly MH, Wilmot CB. Acute abdominal emergencies during the first four weeks after spinal cord injury. *Arch Phys Med Rehabil* 1984; 65:687–690.
54. Kewalramani LS. Neurogenic gastroduodenal ulceration and bleeding associated with spinal cord injuries. *J Trauma* 1979; 19:259–265.
55. Roth EJ, Fenton LL, Gaebler-Spira DJ, Frost FS, Yarkony GM. Superior mesenteric artery syndrome in acute traumatic quadriplegia: case reports and literature review. *Arch Phys Med Rehabil* 1991; 72: 417–420.
56. Maynard FM. Immobilization hypercalcemia following spinal cord injury. *Arch Phys Med Rehabil* 1986;67:441–44.
57. Merli GJ, McElwain GE, Adler AG, et al. Immobilization hypercalcemia in acute spinal cord injury treated with etidronate. *Arch Intern Med* 1984; 144:1286–1288.
58. Venier LH, Ditunno JF Jr. Heterotopic ossification in the paraplegic patient. *Arch Phys Med Rehabil* 1971; 52:475–479.
59. Stover SL, Hahn HR, Miller JM III. Disodium etidronate in the prevention of heterotopic ossification following spinal cord injury (preliminary report). *Parplegia* 1976; 14:146–156.
60. Wharton GW, Morgan TH. Anklyosis in the paralyzed patient. *J Bone Joint Surg [Am]* 1970; 52:105–112.
61. Hardy S, Dickson J. Pathologic ossification in traumatic paraplegia. *J Bone Joint Surg [Br]* 1963; 45:76–87.
62. Chantraine A, Minaire P. Para-osteoarthropathies. *Scand J Rehabil Med* 1981; 13:31–37.
63. Freehafer AA, Yurish R, Mast WA. Para-articular ossification in spinal cord injury. *Med Serv J Can* 1966; 22:471–478.
64. Stover SL, Hataway CG, Zerger HE. Heterotopic ossification in spinal cord impaired patients. *Arch Phys Med Rehabil* 1975; 56:199–204.
65. Freed JH, Hahn H, Menter R, Dillon T. The use of the three-phase bone scan in the early diagnosis of heterotopic ossification and in the evaluation of Didronel therapy. *Paraplegia* 1982; 13:208–216.
66. Kim SW, Charter RA, Chai CJ, Kim SK, Kim ES. Serum alkaline phosphatase and inorganic phosphorus values in spinal cord injury patients with heterotopic ossification. *Paraplegia* 1990; 28:441–447.
67. Brooke MM, Heard DL, de Lateur BJ, Moeller DA, Alquist AD. Heterotopic ossification and peripheral nerve entrapment: early diagnosis and excision. *Arch Phys Med Rehabil* 1991; 72:425–429.
68. Hassard GH. Heterotopic bone formation about the hip and unilateral decubitus ulcers in spinal cord injury. *Arch Phys Med Rehabil* 1975; 56:355–358.
69. Damanski J. Heterotopic ossification in paraplegia. *J Bone Joint Surg [Br]* 1961; 43:286–299.
70. Daub O, Sett P, Burr RG, Silver JR. The relationship of heterotopic ossification to passive movements in paraplegic patients. *Disabil Rehabil* 1993; 15:114–118.
71. Stover SL, Neimann KM, Miller JM III. Disodium etidronate in the prevention of post-operative recurrence of heterotopic ossification in spinal cord injury patients. *J Bone Joint Surg [Am]* 1976; 58:683–688.
72. Garland DE, Betzabe A, Venos KG, Vogt JC. Diphosphonate treatment for heterotopic ossification in spinal cord injury patients. *Clin Orthop* 1983; 176:197–200.
73. Stover SL, Niemann Tulloss JR. Experience with surgical resection of heterotopic bone in spinal cord injury patients. *Clin Orthop* 1991; 263:71–77.
74. Ayers DG, Evarts CM, Parkinson JR. The prevention of heterotopic ossification in high risk patients by low dose radiation therapy after total hip arthroplasty. *J Bone Joint Surg [Am]* 1986; 68:1423–1430.
75. Schmidt SA, Kjaersgaard-Anderson P, Pedersen NW, et al. The use of indomethacin to prevent the formation of heterotopic bone after total hip replacement. *J Bone Joint Surg [Am]* 1988; 70:834–838.
76. Beric A, Dimitrijevic M, Lindblom U. Central dysesthesia syndrome in spinal cord injury patients. *Pain* 1988; 34:109–116.
77. Nepomuceno C, Fine PR, Richards JS, et al. Pain in patients with spinal cord injury. *Arch Phys Med Rehabil* 1979; 60:605–609.
78. Anke AG, Stanghelle JK. Pain and life quality within two years of spinal cord injury. *Paraplegia* 1995; 33:555–559.
79. Donovan WH, Dimitrijevic MR. Neurophysiological approaches to chronic pain following spinal cord injury. *Paraplegia* 1982; 20: 135–146.
80. Frisbie JH, Aguilera EJ. Chronic pain after spinal cord injury: an expedient diagnostic approach. *Paraplegia* 1990; 28:460–456.

81. Davidoff G, Roth E, Guarracini M, Sliwa J, Yarkony G. Function-limiting dysethestic pain sydrome among spinal cord injury patients: a cross-sectional study. *Pain* 1987; 29:39–48.
82. Melzack R, Loseser J. Phantom body pain in paraplegics: evidence for a central pattern generating mechanism for pain. *Pain* 1978; 9: 195–210.
83. Balazy TE. Clinical management of chronic pain in spinal cord injury. *Clin J Pain* 1992; 8:102–110.
84. Umlauf RL. Psychological intervention for chronic pain following spinal cord injury. *Clin J Pain* 1992; 8:111–118.
85. Sanford PR, Lindbloom LB, Haddox JD. Amitriptyline and carbamazepine in the treatment of dysesthetic pain in spinal cord injury. *Arch Phys Med Rehabil* 1992; 73:300–301.
86. Herman, RM, D'Luzansky SC. Intrathecal baclofen supresses central pain in patients with spinal lesions. *Clin J Pain* 1992; 8:338–345.
87. Dunbar SA, Katz NP. Chronic opioid therapy for non-malignant pain in patients with history of substance abuse: reports of twenty cases. *J Pain Symptom Manage* 1996; 11:163–171.
88. Siddall PJ, Gray M, Rutkowski S, Cousins MJ. Intrathecal morphine and clonidine in the management of spinal cord injury pain: a case report. *Pain* 1994; 59:147–148.
89. Cole JD, Illis LS, Sedgwick EM. Intractable central pain in spinal cord injury is not relieved by spinal cord stimulation. *Paraplegia* 1991; 29:167–172.
90. Friedman AH, Nashold BS Jr. DREZ lesions for relief of pain related to spinal cord injury. *J Neurosurg* 1986; 65:465–469.
91. Biyani A, Masry WS. Post-traumatic syringomyelia: A review of the literature. *Paraplegia* 1994; 32:723–731.
92. Edgar R, Quail P. Progressive post-traumatic cystic and noncystic myelopathy. *Br J Neurosurg* 1994; 8:7–22.
93. Wiart L, Dautheribes M, Pointillart V, Petit H, Barat. Mean term follow-up of a series of post-traumatic syringomyelia patients after syringo-peritoneal shunting. *Paraplegia* 1995; 33:241–245.
94. Hilda K, Iwasaki Y. Post-traumatic syringomyelia: its characteristic MRI findings and surgical management. *Neurosurgery* 1994; 35: 886–891.
95. Dworkin GE, Staas WE Jr. Post-traumatic syringomyelia. *Arch Phys Med Rehabil* 1985; 66:329–331.
96. Schurch B, Wickman W, Rossier A. A prospective study of 449 patients with spinal cord injury. *J Neurol Neurosurg Psychiatry* 1996; 60:61–67.
97. Ken S, Lewis MM, Main WK, Hermann G, Abdelwahab IF. Neuropathic arthropathy of the shoulder mimicking soft tissue sarcoma. *Orthopedics* 1993; 16:133–136.
98. Sgouros S, Williams B. Management and outcome of posttraumatic syringomyelia. *J Neurosurg* 1996; 85:197–205.
99. Garland DE, Stewart CA, Adkins RH, et al. Osteoporosis after spinal cord injury. *J Orthop Res* 1992; 10:371–378.
100. Wilmet E, Ismail AA, Heilporn A, Welraeds D, Bergmann P. Longitudinal study of the bone mineral content and of soft tissue composition after spinal cord section. *Paraplegia* 1995; 33:674–677.
101. Chappard D, Minaire P, Privat C, et al. Effects of tiludronate on bone loss in paraplegic patients. *J Bone Miner Res* 1995; 10:112–118.
102. Ragnarsson KT, Sell GH. Lower extremity fractures after spinal cord injury: a retrospective study. *Arch Phys Med Rehabil* 1981; 62: 418–423.
103. Freehafer A. Limb fractures in patients with spinal cord injury. *Arch Phys Med Rehabil* 1995; 76:823–827.
104. Sobel M, Lyden J. Long bone fracture in a spinal cord injured patient: complication of treatment—a case report and review of the literature. *J Trauma* 1991; 31:1440–1444.
105. Garland DE, Reiser TV, Singer DI. Treatment of femoral shaft fractures associated with acute spinal cord injuries. *Clin Orthop* 1985; 197:191–195.
106. McMaster W, Stauffer E. The management of long bone fracture in the spinal cord injury patient. *Clin Orthop* 1975; 112:44–52.
107. Colachis SC III. Autonomic hyperreflexia with spinal cord injury. *J Spinal Cord Med* 1992; 15:171–186.
108. Erickson RP. Autonomic hyperreflexia: pathophysiology and medical management. *Arch Phys Med Rehabil* 1980; 61:4431–440.
109. Lee BY, Karmakar MG, Herz BL, Sturgill RA. Autonomic dysreflexia revisited. *J Spinal Cord Med* 1995; 18:75–87.
110. Trop CS, Bennett CJ. Autonomic dysreflexia and its urological implications: a review. *J Urol* 1991; 146:1461–1469.
111. Chancellor MB, Erhard MJ, Hirsch IH, Staas WE Jr. Prospective evaluation of terazosin for the treatment of autonomic dysreflexia. *J Urol* 1994; 151:111–113.
112. Sie IH, Waters RL, Adkins RH, Gellman H. Upper extremity pain in the postrehabilitation spinal cord injured patient. *Arch Phys Med Rehabil* 1992; 73:44–48.
113. Nicholas P, Norman P, Ennis P. Wheelchair users' shoulder. *Scand J Rehabil Med* 1979; 11:29–32.
114. Silfverskiold J, Waters RL. Shoulder pain and functional disability in spinal cord injury patients. *Clin Orth* 1991; 272:141–145.
115. Campbell C, Koris M. Etiologies of shoulder pain in cervical spinal cord injury. *Clin Orth* 1996; 322:140–145.
116. Waring WP, Maynard FM. Shoulder pain in acute traumatic quadriplegia. *Paraplegia* 1991; 29:37–42.
117. Robinson MD, Hussey RW, Ha CY. Surgical decompression of impingement in the weightbearing shoulder. *Arch Phys Med Rehabil* 1993; 74:324–327.
118. Barber, DB, Gall NG. Osteonecrosis: an overuse injury of the shoulder in paraplegia: case report. *Paraplegia* 1991; 29:423–426.
119. Aljure J, Eltorai I, Bradley WE, Lin JE, Johnson B. Carpal tunnel syndrome in paraplegic patients. *Paraplegia* 1985; 23:182–186.
120. Davidoff G, Werner R, Waring W. Compressive mononeuropathies of the upper extremity in chronic paraplegia. *Paraplegia* 1991; 28: 17–24.
121. Boninger ML, Robertson RN, Wolff M, Cooper RA. Upper extremity nerve entrapments in elite wheelchair racers. *Am J Phys Med* 1996; 75:170–175.
122. Harper GP, Banyard PJ, Sharpe PC. The International Spinal Research Trust's strategic approach to the development of strategies for the repair of spinal cord injury. *Paraplegia* 1996; 34:449–459.
123. Geisler FH, Dorsey FC, Coleman WP. Recovery of motor function after spinal-cord injury—a randomized, placebo-controlled trial with GM-1 ganglioside. *N Engl J Med* 1991; 324:1829–1838.
124. Francel PC, Long BA, Malik JM, Tribble C, Jane JA, Kron IL. Limiting ischemic spinal cord injury using a free radical scavenger 21-aminosteroid and/or cerebrospinal fluid drainage. *J Neurosurg* 1993; 79:742–751.
125. Bracken MB. Pharmacological treatment of acute spinal cord injury: current status and future projects. *J Emerg Med* 1993; 11:43–48.
126. Hayes KC, Blight AR, Potter PJ, et al. Preclinical trial of 4-aminopyridine in patients with chronic spinal cord injury. *Paraplegia* 1993; 31: 216–224.
127. Clifton GL, Donovan WH, Dimitrijevic MM, et al. Omental transposition in chronic spinal cord injury. *Paraplegia* 1996; 34:193–203.
128. Reier PJ, Anderson DK, Young W, Michel ME, Fessler R. Workshop on intraspinal transplantation and clinical application. *J Neurotrauma* 1994; 11:369–377.
129. Cheng H, Cao Y, Olson L. Spinal cord repair in adult paraplegic rats: partial restoration of hind limb function. *Science* 1996; 273:510–513.
130. Whiteneck GG, Charlifue SW, Frankel HL. Mortality, morbidity, and psychosocial outcomes of persons spinal cord injured more than 10 years ago. *Paraplegia* 1992; 30:617–630.
131. Crozier KS, Graziani V, Ditunno JF Jr, Herbison GH. Spinal cord injury: prognosis for ambulation based on sensory examination in patients who are initially motor complete. *Arch Phys Med Rehabil* 1991; 72:119–121.
132. Crozier KS, Cheng LL, Graziani V, Zorn G, Herbison G, Ditunno JF Jr. Spinal cord injury: prognosis for ambulation based on quadriceps recovery. *Paraplegia* 1992; 30:762–767.
133. Marino RJ, Rider-Foster D, Maissel G, Ditunno JF Jr. Superiority of motor level over single neurological level in categorizing tetraplegia. *Paraplegia* 1995; 33:510–513.
134. Marino RJ, Herbison GJ, Ditunno JF Jr. Peripheral sprouting as a mechanism for recovery in the zone of injury in acute quadriplegia: a single-fiber emg study. *Muscle Nerve* 1994; 17:1466–1468.
135. Yarkony GM, Roth EJ, Heinemann AW, Lovell L. Rehabilitation outcomes in C6 tetraplegia. *Paraplegia* 1988; 26:177–185.
136. Yarkony GM, Roth EJ, Heinemann WA, Katz RT, Wu Y. Rehabilitation outcomes in complete C5 quadriplegia. *Am J Phys Med Rehabil* 1988; 67:73–76.
137. Scott JA, Donovan WH. The prevention of shoulder pain and contracture in the acute tetraplegic patient. *Paraplegia* 1981; 19:313–319.
138. Somers MF. *Spinal cord injury: functional rehabilitation*. Norwalk, CT: Appleton & Lange, 1992.

139. Marciello MA, Herbison GJ, Cohen ME, Schmidt R. Elbow extension using anterior deltoids and upper pectorals in spinal cord-injured subjects. *Arch Phys Med Rehabil* 1995; 76:426–432.
140. Zerby SA, Herbison GJ, Marino RJ, Cohen ME, Schmidt RR. Elbow extension using anterior deltoid and upper pectorals. *Muscle Nerve* 1994; 17:1472–1474.
141. Reyes ML, Gronley JK, Newsam CJ, Mulroy SJ, Perry J. Electromyographic analysis of shoulder muscles of men with low level paraplegia during a weight relief raise. *Arch Phys Med Rehabil* 1995; 76: 433–439.
142. De Troyer A, Estenne M. Review article: the expiratory muscles in tetraplegia. *Paraplegia* 1993; 29:359–363.
143. Formal C, Smith J. Upper extremity function in spinal cord injury. *Top Spinal Cord Inj Rehabil* 1996; 1:1–14.
144. Runge M. Self-dressing techniques for patients with spinal cord injury. *Am J Occup Ther* 1967; 21:367–375.
145. Stow RW. Grasping mouthstick. *Arch Phys Med Rehabil* 1966; 47: 31–33.
146. Garcia S, Greenfield J. Dynamic protractible mouthstick. *Am J Occup Ther* 1981; 35:529–30.
147. Kreutz D. Manual wheelchairs: prescribing for function. *Top Spinal Cord Inj Rehabil* 1995; 1:1–16.
148. Taylor SJ. Powered mobility evaluation and technology. *Top Spinal Cord Inj Rehabil* 1995; 1:23–36.
149. Penrod LE, Hegde SK, Ditunno JF Jr. Age effect on prognosis for functional recovery in acute, traumatic central cord syndrome. *Arch Phys Med Rehabil* 1990; 71:963–968.
150. Waters RL, Adkins RH, Yakura JS, Sie I. Motor and sensory recovery following incomplete paraplegia. *Arch Phys Med Rehabil* 1994; 75: 67–72.
151. Waters RL, Adkins RH, Yakura JS, Sie I. Motor and sensory recovery following incomplete tetraplegia. *Arch Phys Med Rehabil* 1994; 75: 306–311.
152. Nene AV, Hermens HJ, Zilvold G. Paraplegic locomotion: a review. *Paraplegia* 1996; 34:507–524.
153. Jackson RH. Home modifications for people with disabilities. In: Yarkony GM, ed. *Spinal cord injury*. Gaithersburg, MD: Aspen, 1994; 183–203.
154. Kohlmeyer KM, Rom C. Driver assessment. In: Yarkony GM, ed. *Spinal cord injury*. Gaithersburg, MD: Aspen, 1994; 205–215.
155. Garber SL, Lathem P. Adaptive driving: mobility and community integration for persons with spinal cord injury. *Top Spinal Cord Inj Rehabil* 1995; 1:59–65.
156. Kelley JD, Frieden L. *Go for it!* Chicago: Harcourt Brace, 1989.
157. Paralyzed Veterans of America. *A guide to wheelchair sports and recreation,* 2nd ed. Washington, D.C.: Paralyzed Veterans of America.
158. Curtis KA, Hall KM, McClanahan S, Dillon D, Brown KF. Health, vocational, and functional status in spinal cord injured athletes and nonathletes. *Arch Phys Med Rehabil* 1986; 67:862–865.
159. Stotts KM. Health maintenance: paraplegic athletes and non-athletes. *Arch Phys Med Rehabil* 1986; 67:109–114.
160. Horvat M, French R, Henschen K. A comparison of the psychological characteristics of male and female able-bodied and wheelchair athletes. *Paraplegia* 1986; 24:115–122.
161. Moberg E. The present state of surgical rehabilitation of the upper limb in tetraplgia. *Paraplegia* 1987; 25:351–356.
162. Johnstone BR, Jordan CJ, Buntine JA. A review of surgical rehabilitation of the upper limb in quadriplegia. *Paraplegia* 1988; 26:317–339.
163. Waters RL, Sie IH, Gellman H, Tognella M. Functional hand surgery following tetraplegia. *Arch Phys Med Rehabil* 1996; 77:86–94.
164. Moberg E. Surgical treatment of absent single-hand grip and elbow extension in quadriplegia: principles and preliminary experience. *J Bone Joint Surg [Am]* 1975; 75:196–206.
165. Raczka R. Posterior deltoid to triceps transfer: a review of the experience at Rancho Los Amigos Hospital. *Paraplegia* 1984; 22:45–54.
166. Moberg E. *The upper limb in tetraplegia*. New York: Thieme Stratton, 1978.
167. Colyer R, Kappelman B. Flexor pollicis longus tenodesis in tetraplegia at the sixth cervical level. *J Bone Joint Surg [Am]* 1981: 63:376–379.
168. Waters R, Moore KR, Graboff SR, Paris K. Brachioradialis to flexor pollicis longus tendon transfer for active lateral pinch in the tetraplegic. *J Hand Surg [Am]* 1985; 10:385–391.
169. Lamb DW, Chan KM. Surgical reconstruction of the upper limb in traumatic tetraplegia. *J Bone Joint Surg [Br]* 1983: 65:291–298.
170. Gansel J, Waters RL, Gellman H. Pronator teres to flexor digitorum profundus transfer in quadriplegia. *J Bone Joint Surg [Am]* 1990; 72: 427–432.
171. Goldsmith MF. Computerized biofeedback training aids in spinal injury rehabilitation. *JAMA* 1985; 253:1097–1099.
172. Brucker BS, Bulaeva NV. Biofeedback effect on electromyography responses in patients with spinal cord injury. *Arch Phys Med Rehabil* 1996; 77:133–137.
173. Stein RB, Brucker BS, Ayyar DR. Motor units in incomplete spinal cord injury: electrical activity, contractile properties and the effects of biofeedback. *J Neurol Neurosurg Psychiatry* 1990; 53:880–885.
174. Klose KJ, Schmidt DL, Needham BM, Brucker BS, Green BA, Ayyar DR. Rehabilitation therapy for patients with long-term spinal cord injuries. *Arch Phys Med Rehabil* 1990; 71:659–662.
175. Klose KJ, Needhan BM, Schmidt D, Broton JG, Green BA. An assessment of the contribution of electromyographic biofeedback as an adjunct therapy in the physical training of spinal cord injured persons. *Arch Phys Med Rehabil* 1993; 74:453–456.
176. Yarkony GM, Roth EJ, Cybulski G, Jaeger RJ. Neuromuscular stimulation in spinal cord injury. I. Restoration of functional movement of the extremities. *Arch Phys Med Rehabil* 1992; 73:78–86.
177. Yarkony GM, Roth EJ, Cybulski G, Jaeger RJ. Neuromuscular stimulation in spinal cord injury. II. Prevention of secondary complications. *Arch Phys Med Rehabil* 1992; 73:195–200.
178. Merli GJ, Herbison GJ, Ditunno JF, et al. Deep vein thrombosis: prophylaxis in acute spinal cord injured patients. *Arch Phys Med Rehabil* 1988; 69:661–664.
179. Leeds EM, Klose KJ, Ganz W, Serafini A, Green BA. Bone mineral density after bicycle ergometry training. *Arch Phys Med Rehabil* 1990; 71:207–209.
180. Hooker SP, Figoni SF, Glaser RM, Rodgers MM, Enzenwa BN, Faghri PD. Physiologic responses to prolonged electrically stimulated leg-cycle exercises in the spinal cord injured. *Arch Phys Med Rehabil* 1990; 71:863–869.
181. Arnold PB, McVey PP, Farrell WJ, Deurloo TM, Grasso AR. Functional electrical stimulation: its efficacy and safety in improving pulmonary function and musculoskeletal fitness. *Arch Phys Med Rehabil* 1992; 73:665–668.
182. Faghri PD, Glaser RM, Figoni SF. Functional electrical stimulation leg cycle ergometer exercise: training effects on cardiorespiratory responses of spinal cord injured subjects at rest and during submaximal exercise. *Arch Phys Med Rehabil* 1992; 73:1085–1093.
183. Ragnarsson KT, Pollack S, O'Daniel W, Edgar R, Petrofsky J, Nash MS. Clinical evaluation of computerized functional electrical stimulation after spinal cord injury: a multicenter pilot study. *Arch Phys Med Rehabil* 1988; 69:672–677.
184. Chaplin E. Functional neuromuscular stimulation for mobility in people with spinal cord injuries. The Parastep I system. *J Spinal Cord Med* 1996; 19:99–105.
185. Keith MW, Peckham PH, Thrope GB, Buckett JR, Stroh KC, Menger V. Functional neuromuscular stimulation neuroprostheses for the tetraplegic hand. *Clin Orthop* 1988; 233:25–33.
186. Triolo RJ, Betz RR, Mulcahey MJ, Gardner ER. Application of functional neuromuscular stimulation to children with spinal cord injuries: candidate selection for upper and lower extremity research. *Paraplegia* 1994; 32:824–843.
187. Elliot TR, Frank RG. Depression following spinal cord injury. *Arch Phys Med Rehabil* 1996; 77:816–823.
188. Dijkers M, Cushman LA. Differences between rehabilitation disciplines in views of depression in spinal cord injury patients. *Parplegia* 1990; 28:380–391.
189. Richards JS. Psychological adjustment to spinal cord injury during the first post-discharge year. *Arch Phys Med Rehabil* 1986; 67:362–365.
190. MacDonald MR, Nielson WR, Cameron MG. Depression and activity patterns of spinal cord injured persons living in the community. *Arch Phys Med Rehabil* 1987; 68:339–343.
191. Robinson RB, Starr LB, Kubos KL, Price TR. A two-year longitudinal study of post-stroke mood disorders: findings during the initial evaluation. *Stroke* 1983; 14:736–741.
192. Fuhrer MJ, Rintala DH, Hart KA, Clearman R, Young ME. Relationship of life satisfaction to impairment, disability, and handicap among

persons with spinal cord injury living in the community. *Arch Phys Med Rehabil* 1992; 73:552–557.
193. Fuhrer MJ, Rintala DH, Hart KA, Clearman R, Young ME. Depressive symptomatology in persons with spinal cord injury who reside in the community. *Arch Phys Med Rehabil* 1993; 74:255–260.
194. Clayton KS, Chubon RA. Factors associated with the quality of life of long-term spinal cord injured persons. *Arch Phys Med Rehabil* 1994; 75:633–638.
195. Dijkers MP, Abela MB, Gans BM, Gordon WA. The aftermath of spinal cord injury. In: Stover SL, DeLisa JA, Whiteneck GG, eds. *Spinal cord injury*. Gaithersburg, MD: Aspen, 1995; 185–212.
196. Ditunno JF Jr, Formal CS. Chronic spinal cord injury. *N Engl J Med* 1994; 330:550–556.
197. Staas WE Jr, Ditunno JF Jr. A system of spinal cord injury care. *Phys Med Rehabil Clin North Am* 1992; 3:893–902.
198. Stover SL, Hall KM, DeLisa JA, Donovan WH. System benefits. In: Stover SL, Hall KM, DeLisa JA, Donovan WH, eds. *Spinal cord injury*. Gaithersburg, MD: Aspen, 1995; 317–326.

Rehabilitation Medicine: Principles and Practice, Third Edition,
edited by Joel A. DeLisa and Bruce M. Gans.
Lippincott–Raven Publishers, Philadelphia 1998.

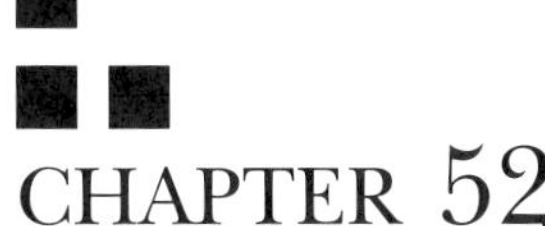

CHAPTER 52

Rehabilitation for Patients with Cancer Diagnoses

Lynn H. Gerber and Mary Vargo

GENERAL ASPECT OF REHABILITATION AND MODELS OF CARE FOR CANCER PATIENTS

Patients with cancer diagnoses are living longer, in part because of early detection, a broader selection of cancer treatment options, and better general medical management. The 5-year relative survival rates for a variety of tumors is presented in Table 52-1 (1,2). It is clear that some tumors—notably stomach, esophagus, hepatic, pancreas, lung, nervous system, and leukemias/myeloma—have a low 5-year survival rate. Others—breast, larynx, prostate, and kidney, among others—have a much better prognosis. Historically, rehabilitation interventions were rarely considered for the former group of tumors because of the poor prognosis. Traditionally, rehabilitation specialists were an afterthought for this population and were only contacted for patients who needed an orthosis or prosthesis, gait aides, or adaptive equipment. Patients did not survive long enough to warrant rehabilitation or to justify the expense. Many received only acute or postoperative care.

One large survey of the needs of cancer patients identified 438 of 805 patients who had physical medicine problems (3). These problems occurred with all tumor types; and for those with central nervous system (CNS), breast, lung, or head and neck tumors, they were present in over 70%. Psychological problems were found in 335 patients. There was a large gap between the identified rehabilitation needs and the services delivered to this population, which improved dramatically after initiating a program for patient education, automatic screening of patients for their rehabilitation needs, and introducing a physiatrist into the clinical oncology team.

This chapter will outline the contributions that rehabilitation can make to help meet the needs of cancer patients. There has been a shift in thinking about what these patients need and who can provide it for them. There is consensus that cancer patients frequently require treatment for the following general problems: pain, problems of mobility and self-care, fatigue, and weakness. Problems more specific to tumor types include dysphagia, cognitive impairment, lymphedema, neuropathy, and soft-tissue or bony excision. These are situations in which the rehabilitation professions are able to make significant contributions.

As the treatment options have broadened, rehabilitation is considered more than the "third wave of medicine." Not only can supportive care be provided, but prevention and restoration of function have become expectations for this population. Rehabilitation professionals are often introduced into staging and treatment decision making, especially when this involves the musculoskeletal system and when limb surgeries are involved. The rehabilitation team is well organized to evaluate functional needs and deliver functionally based care. Several functional outcome measures developed for cancer patients (4–6) have demonstrated clinical efficacy of these interventions (6–8) (Table 52-2). These indices have helped demonstrate that when treatments are selected that are associated with less morbidity, a more desired outcome and better quality of life are achieved, even if life is not prolonged (6). This has influenced the primary treatment of cancer, including development of surgical procedures that are designed to spare a limb or breast from amputation. Data suggest that the biopsychosocial aspects of cancer are important to survival and tumor recurrence. Higher levels of coping and enhancement of active behavioral coping over time are predictive of lower rates of recurrence and death (9).

L. H. Gerber: Department of Rehabilitation Medicine, National Institutes of Health, Bethesda, Maryland 20892-1604; and Department of Rheumatology, Georgetown University Medical Center, Washington, D.C. 20057; and Department of Internal Medicine, George Washington University Medical Center, Washington, D.C. 20037.

M. Vargo: MetroHealth Medical Center, Cleveland, Ohio 44109.

TABLE 52-1. *Summary of changes in cancer incidence and mortality (1950–1991) and 5-year relative survival rates (1950–1990)[a]*

	All races		Whites					
			Percent change 1950–1990				5-Year relative survival rates (percentage)	
			Incidence		U.S. mortality			
Primary site	Estimated cancer cases in 1991	Actual cancer in 1991	Total	EAPC	Total	EAPC	1950–1954	1983–1990
Oral cavity and pharynx	30,800	8,277	−31.0	−0.6	−28.8	−0.7	46	47.5
Esophagus	10,999	9,967	−9.8	−0.1	10.9	0.2	4	10.5
Stomach	23,888	14,225	−75.1	−2.9	−76.7	−3.7	12	17.5
Colon and rectum	157,500	56,776	7.6	0.3	−29.5	−0.8	36	59.7
Colon	112,000	49,132	23.7	0.6	−13.0	−0.2	41	60.9
Rectum	45,500	7,644	−18.8	−0.4	−66.9	−3.0	40	58.4
Liver and intrahepatic	15,000	8,847	100.9	1.5	19.7	0.4	1	6.6
Pancreas	28,200	25,534	10.5	0.1	17.8	0.2	1	3.0
Larynx	12,500	3,986	50.7	0.9	−8.4	−0.2	52	69.1
Lung and bronchus	161,000	143,620	261.3	3.0	264.6	3.3	6	13.7
Males	101,000	91,600	208.0	2.4	222.2	2.9	5	12.1
Females	60,000	52,020	548.7	5.0	555.9	5.6	9	16.2
Melanomas of skin	32,000	6,451	3,467	4.2	157.0	2.4	49	85.3
Breast (females)	175,000	43,582	54.9	1.3	2.8	0.1	60	81.6
Cervix uteri	13,000	4,514	−75.7	−3.4	−73.7	−3.9	59	69.9
Corpus and uterus, NOS	33,000	5,925	−2.3	−0.6	−66.8	−2.5	72	84.9
Ovary	20,700	13,028	9.1	0.2	2.2	−0.2	30	41.6
Prostate	122,000	33,563	189.9	2.5	20.6	0.3	43	81.3
Testis	6,100	366	119.9	2.2	−70.2	−3.0	57	93.6
Urinary bladder	50,200	10,406	54.1	1.2	−34.7	−1.1	53	80.7
Kidney and renal pelvis	25,300	10,270	117.4	2.0	35.3	0.6	34	56.9
Brain and other nervous	16,700	11,952	74.4	1.3	51.0	0.8	21	26.7
Thyroid	12,400	1,026	107.4	1.6	−50.6	−2.1	80	94.7
Hodgkin's disease	7,400	1,625	24.4	0.4	−67.4	−3.3	30	79.4
Non-Hodgkin's lymphomas	37,200	19,582	183.7	2.9	118.5	1.6	33	54.4
Multiple myeloma	12,300	9,268	205.4	2.3	194.6	2.4	6	27.4
Leukemias	28,000	19,103	3.2	0.1	−2.2	−0.3	10	39.5
Childhood (0–14 yr)	7,800	1,709	−8.0	0.4	−60.6	−2.6	21	70.8
All sites, excluding lungs and bronchus	939,000	371,016	35.6	0.7	−14.5	−0.4	37	60.2
All sites	1,100,000	514,636	49.3	1.0	10.1	0.2	35	53.2

[a] Males and females, by primary cancer site.

Good symptom management is associated with good physical and mental functioning (10).

Options for effective treatment have been broadened with the introduction of newer lightweight orthotics and prosthetics. A better understanding of the mechanisms by which tissue is influenced by radiation and chemotherapy. The influence of exercise on the immune system has resulted in a broader, more effective treatment armamentarium. Patients with head and neck tumors who have had laryngectomy use communication devices that synthesize voice, can record phrases and store them in memory for recall, and are small enough for a pocket. Long-life batteries have extended the range that wheelchairs can travel.

Legislation, including the Rehabilitation Act of 1973 and the Americans with Disability Act (ADA), has helped establish standards for accessibility for all disabled. These regulations also have assured that acts of discrimination against those who are otherwise qualified are against the law and will be remedied with back pay and reinstatement. The Equal Employment Commission (1-800 872-3362) is responsible for enforcement of the employee's rights under ADA.

Cancer remains the second leading cause of death in the United States and is associated with significant morbidity and disability. The incidence of tumors has increased during the interval 1973–1991 in all tumors except uterus/cervix, leukemias, Hodgkin's disease, oral cavity, pancreas, and stomach. However, the incidence by age has been decreasing for the younger age groups and increasing for those over 55 years of age. The 5-year relative survival rate has increased since 1983 for most tumors, and the average increase is 53.2% (1). Notably, 5-year survival rates for individuals with cancers of the stomach, esophagus, liver, pancreas, lung and bronchus, brain, and multiple myeloma remain below 30%. Knowledge of these statistics is important for decision making because clinical judgment must be exercised in delivering comprehensive services to those with a significantly reduced life expectancy. Not all patients stand to benefit from care. Hence, it is extremely likely that the physiatrist will

TABLE 52-2. *Karnofsky Scale*

Able to carry on normal activity; no special care is needed.	
10	Normal; no complaints, no evidence of disease
9	Able to carry on normal activity; minor signs or symptons of disease
8	Normal activity with effort; some signs or symptoms of disease
Unable to work; able to live at home; cares for most personal needs; varying amounts of assistance is needed.	
7	Cares for self; unable to carry on normal activity or do active work
6	Requires occasional assistance, but is able to care for most of own needs
5	Requires considerable assistance and frequent medical care
Unable to care for self; requires equivalent of institutional or hospital care; disease may be progressing rapidly.	
4	Disabled; requires special care and assistance
3	Severly disabled; hospitalization is indicated, although death is not imminent
2	Very sick; hospitalization necessary; active supportive treatment necessary
1	Moribund; fatal process progressing rapidly
0	Dead

be consulted in the care of the cancer patient and that this patient is likely to be older and may have comorbidities and reduced tolerance to cancer treatment.

Options for Delivering Rehabilitation Services

Cancer rehabilitation care can be provided under various models, including inpatient rehabilitation hospital setting, consultative care, while patients are receiving their primary oncologic treatment, and during their outpatient status (including home care). Table 52-3 presents a scheme for those settings that are most appropriate for meeting the rehabilitation needs of this patient population. The physiatrist is in a strong position to provide concrete strategies that will improve functional status and overall quality of life, often anticipating needs through many stages of cancer. Thus, strong doctor–patient relationships are forged. In the authors' experience, individuals with cancer do benefit from rehabilitation strategies and are, as a whole, a highly receptive, motivated, and grateful population.

Close communication with other physicians and care providers is essential. Cancer has become a chronic illness and for those patients who have sustained a long-term disabling effect from their malignancy or its treatment, the physiatrist may in fact be the primary provider for care over the long term. Patients in whom the cancer progresses may need different interventions. The rehabilitation interventions from which the patient initially benefited may no longer be appropriate, and in terminal stages of the condition there may indeed be little to offer. This may present a significant challenge to the physician because one must avoid abandoning the patient while at the same time not offering false hope.

The ability to provide support and treatments throughout the various stages of cancer management can be shared, for the physiatrist rarely works alone and is frequently responsible for coordinating interventions from a group of professionals, including occupational therapists (OTs), physical therapists (PTs), recreation therapists (RTs), and speech language pathologists (SLPs). Vocational counselors are consulted, as needed. Each one has unique contributions to offer the cancer patient. Typically, the OT is responsible for those activities that pertain to self-care, require adaptive equipment and address issues of bathroom safety. They help with problems concerning feeding and swallowing. The PT is usually concerned with issues of mobility and limb/vertebral column stability and trains patients in the use of orthotics and gait aids. The PT is also frequently involved with management of pain and edema. The RT provides support and guidance for leisure time activity and while in the hospital helps patients develop positive attitudes by producing products (e.g., crafts) and constructively participating in social activities. The SLP helps in the diagnosis and treatment of dysphagia and provides speech therapy for the cognitively impaired. SLPs are highly integrated into programs in which head and neck tumors are frequently seen. They also provide substantial support in the provision of communication devices.

Inpatient Rehabilitation

There is increasing evidence that patients treated for cancer on an inpatient basis can do well. Cancer patients make

TABLE 52-3. *Settings for rehabilitation of cancer patients*

Problems	Treatment	Setting[a]
Confusion/lack of information about process	Education/support	O, C
Fatigue	Aerobic conditioning, strengthening	I, O
Pain	Modalities heat/cold, electricity	I, O, C
Mobility/self-care	Strengthening, adaptive aides	I, O, C
SCI	Comprehensive rehabilitation orthotics, devices	I, C
Cognitive deficits/communication	Comprehensive rehabilitation communication	I, C
Dysphagia	Swallowing strategies	C
Peripheral neuropathy	Orthoses	O, C
Bladder, bowel, stoma	Training	C

SCI, spinal cord injury.
[a] C, consult; I, inpatient; O, outpatient.

comparable gains in function, as measured by Functional Independence Measure (FIM) scores, as do other noncancer patients receiving inpatient rehabilitation. However, the incidence of an interrupted rehabilitation course is higher: 33% versus 12% (11) and 24% in another series (12). Chemotherapy, radiation therapy, and specific tumor type have not been shown to adversely affect rehabilitation outcome (11). Length of stay and number of patients discharged home are comparable with other diagnostic categories (12). A retrospective review of patients admitted for rehabilitation due to neoplastic spinal cord injury found that functional improvements were made and maintained at 3 months postdischarge.

In approaching inpatients undergoing cancer treatment, it is particularly important to be alert for intercurrent medical problems, which are often related to the treatment regimen. Particularly important are infection as a result of myelosuppression, CNS complications of chemotherapy, and inanition. Their problems may necessitate transfer from rehabilitation back to acute medical care.

Chemotherapy side effects are outlined in Table 52-4. Complications of chemotherapeutic agents are listed in Table 52-5. Effects such as myelosuppression, nausea, and vomiting are widespread among these agents and therefore not included.

The physiatrist should routinely check for the following conditions, which when present will have a substantial impact on the ability of the patient to tolerate some rehabilitation services safely (13). For example, the use of modalities of heat, therapeutic pool, and exercise may have to be discontinued if the following are present:

1. Hematologic profile: hemoglobin <7.5 g, platelets <50,000; white blood cell count <3,000.
2. Metastatic bone disease with involvement of long bones (femur, tibia, humerus) such that there is more than 50% of the cortex involved, cortical bone erosion approaching the diameter of the bone, and more than 3 cm lesion in the femur.
3. Compression of a hollow viscus (bowel, bladder, or ureter), vessel, or spinal cord.
4. Fluid accumulation in the pleura, pericardium, abdomen, or retroperitoneum associated with persistent pain, dyspnea, or problems with mobility.
5. CNS depression or coma or increased intracranial pressure.
6. Hypo-/hyperkalemia, hyponatremia, or hypo-/hypercalcemia.
7. Orthostatic hypotension, blood pressure in excess of 160/100 mm Hg.
8. Heart rate in excess of 110 beats/min or ventricular arrhythmia (14).

Despite favorable outcome data, the prospect of rehabilitating patients with cancer in an inpatient setting still may be met with skepticism. A patient's long-term prognosis may be uncertain, complicating decision making about allocating rehabilitation resources. Pain, weakness, fatigue, and inanition (often major causes of disability in this population) are rarely ''allowable'' problems for admission to acute rehabilitation under existing funding sources. Cancer patients do have other factors that complicate their course, or at least their schedules, such as radiation therapy, chemotherapy, or wound or drain care, so that medical supervision and nursing expertise is needed. Such factors may interrupt the rehabilitation schedule, but when combined with the rehabilitation needs, they may provide additional justification for rehabilitation in an acute rather than subacute setting. Close communication with both medical oncologists and nursing specialists should be available.

Prognosis must of course be weighed in the decision for inpatient rehabilitation, although poor long-term survival should not preclude inpatient rehabilitation if substantial functional gains are likely to be made even in the short or intermediate term.

Coordinated therapy programs can offer some benefit even for the terminally ill in a hospice setting, where improved mobility scores were demonstrated after 1 month of an individualized physical therapy program (15).

Outpatient Rehabilitation

Outpatient care most commonly addresses specific musculoskeletal or soft-tissue problems, such as lymphedema, contracture, mobility, self-care, and pain. Patients must be mobile enough to be easily transported and should be medically stable. Pain syndromes most amenable to physiatric intervention in outpatient settings include those due to bony metastatic disease and to peripheral polyneuropathy, where pharmacologic strategies will intersect with nonpharmacologic treatments. Treatment that is likely to be ongoing, such as supervised exercise, mobility training, proper use of orthotic devices, and other adaptive and ambulatory aides, are best provided in the outpatient setting so that staff can determine how the patient is doing in his or her home environment. The ultimate goal of the treatments is improved performance. Monitoring how and what the patient is actually doing is best done over time in the outpatient setting. Home health care may need to be prescribed if mobility is a significant obstacle to treatment.

Consultation During Acute Care

Patients in the acute care setting—being staged for their tumors, receiving definitive oncologic treatment, or admitted for complications of tumor or its treatment—are often in need of rehabilitation services. The problems may be tumor specific or general. Consultative services that are most frequently requested include evaluation and treatment of mobility and self-care needs, as well as assessment of cognitive status, communication, and swallowing skills. Consultative services that address issues of pain control and the provision of orthotic/prosthetic devices are also requested.

TABLE 52-4. *Chemotherapeutic agents and side effects*

Cytoxan
- Hemorrhagic cystitis
- Bladder fibrosis
- Bladder carcinoma
- Cardiac necrosis (massive doses)
- Stomatitis

Nitrogen mustard
- Skin necrosis if extravasated
- Dermatitis
- Neurologic toxicity (rare)

Nitrosoureas
- Stomatitis
- Lung fibrosis
- Ataxia
- Organic brain syndrome
- Optic neuritis

Platinum complexes
- Nephrotoxicity
- Ototoxicity
- Peripheral neuropathy
- Loss of taste
- Seizures

5 Azacytidine
- Hepatic dysfunction
- Rhabdomyolysis
- Lethargy
- Weakness
- Confusion
- Fever
- Skin rashes
- Stomatitis
- Phlebitis
- Hypotension

Cytarabine
- Arachnoiditis with intrathecal administration
- Stomatitis
- Esophagitis
- Hepatic dysfunction (mild, reversible)
- Thrombophlebitis

Fluorouracil
- Diarrhea
- Stomatitis
- Esophagitis
- Intestinal bleeding
- Dermatitis
- Photosensitivity
- Loss of nails or dark band on nails
- "Black hairy tongue"
- Lacrimation, lacrimal duct stenosis
- Cerebellar ataxia
- Myocardial ischemia

Mercaptopurine
- Cholestasis
- Stomatitis
- Diarrhea
- Dermatitis
- Fever
- Hematuria
- Budd-Chiari–like syndrome

Methotrexate
- Stomatitis
- Diarrhea (intestinal hemorrhagic, ulceration, perforation)
- Renal tubular necrosis
- Liver cirrhosis
- Osteoporosis (in children)
- Dermatitis
- Furunculosis
- Fever
- Headache
- Pneumonitis
- Intrathecal: arachnoiditis with radicular syndrome, myelitis, seizures
- Previously irradiated areas: skin erythema, pulmonary fibrosis, transverse myelitis, cerebritis

Thioguanine
- Cholestasis

Actinomycin D
- Stomatitis
- Cheilitis
- Glossitis
- Proctitis
- Diarrhea
- Skin erythema, desquamation, hyperpigmentation
- Necrosis with SQ injection

Bleomycin
- Shaking chills, fever
- Anaphylaxislike reaction with hypotension, fever, delirium, bronchospasm in lymphoma patients
- Severe pneumonitis
- Pulmonary fibrosis
- Skin hyperpigmentation, hardening
- Loss of fingernails
- Erythroderma
- Desquamation

Doxorubicin (Adriamycin), Daunorubicin, Adriamycin
- Cardiomyopathy
- Stomatitis
- Extravasation: severe ulceration and necrosis
- Erythema, desquamation in previously irradiated skin areas
- Diarrhea

Mitomycin C
- Necrosis with SQ injection
- Stomatitis
- Rash
- Pulmonary fibrosis
- Hepatic and renal dysfunction

Vinblastine
- Local vesicant if injected SQ
- Stomatitis
- Glossitis
- Neurologic toxicities similar to vincristine

Vincristine
- Peripheral polyneuropathy with severe paresthesias
- Parelytic ileus
- Abdominal pain
- Local vesicant if injected SQ

Vindesine
- Neurotoxicity as per vincristine, but less severe

VP-16-213 (etoposide, VP-16)
- Orthostatic hypotension with rapid infusion

L-Asparaginase
- Allergic reactions
- Hepatitis (<50%)
- Pancreatitis (5%)
- Coagulation defects
- CNS depression
- Glucose intolerance

Dacarbazine (DTIC)
- Local irritant if injected SQ
- Flulike syndrome
- Hepatotoxicity
- Diarrhea
- Cerebral dysfunction

Hexamethylmelamine (HMM)
- Rash
- Neurotoxicity

Hydroxyurea
- Stomatitis
- Rash
- Headaches
- Increased BUN

Mitotane
- Diarrhea
- Depression
- Lethargy
- Dermatitis
- Permanent cerebral dysfunction (rare)

Procarbazine
- Lethargy
- Depression
- Muscle cramps
- Arthralgia
- Sensitization of tissue to radiation
- Peripheral neuropathy
- Vertigo
- Headache
- Seizures
- Dermatitis, hyperpigmentation
- Stomatitis
- Dysphagia
- Diarrhea

Streptozocin
- Nephrotoxicity
- Renal tubular acidosis
- Renal failure
- Hepatotoxicity
- Diarrhea

Adrenocorticosteroids
- Peptic ulcer disease
- Na retention
- Hypertension
- K^+ wasting
- Glucose intolerance
- Weight gain
- Proximal myopathy
- Psychologic effects: euphoria, depression, psychosis
- Osteoporosis
- Avascular hip necrosis
- Skin fragility
- Susceptibility to infection

Androgens
- Virilization
- Fluid retention
- Hepatotoxicity

Estrogens
- Fluid retention
- Feminization
- Uterine bleeding
- Hypercalcemic flare (breast cancer)

Progestins
- Mild fluid retention

Taxol
- Hypersensitivity reactions
- Peripheral polyneuropathy
- Myalgias, arthralgias
- Bradycardia

Suramin
- Peripheral polyneuropathy
- Coagulopathy
- Adrenal insufficiency
- Renal toxicity

BUN, blood urea nitrogen; SQ, subcutaneous.

Reprinted with permission from Casciato DA, Lowitz BB. *Manual of bedside oncology,* 1st ed. Boston: Little, Brown, 1986.

TABLE 52-5. *Complications of chemotherapeutic agents*

Soft-tissue necrosis with extravasation	Encephalopathy
Doxorubicin	Methotrexate (arachnoiditis)
Daunorubicin	Hexamethylmelamine
Dactinomycin	5-Fluorouracil (acute cerebellar syndrome)
Dacarbazine	L-asparaginase (acute and delayed forms possible)
Bisantrene	Procarbazine
Amsacrine	Nitrogen mustard (supratherapeutic doses only)
Nitrogen mustard	BCNU (with intra-arterial infusion)
Mitomycin C	Chlorambucil (supratherapeutic doses only)
Vincristine	Cytarabine/ARA-C (arachnoiditis)
Vinblastine	
5-Azacytidine	
Vindesine	

SIGNIFICANT PROBLEMS FACED BY CANCER PATIENTS

Pain Patterns and Their Treatment in Cancer Patients

It is estimated that 70% of patients with cancer have cancer-related pain that will need treatment during the course of their illness (16). Distinguishing between acute pain and chronic pain syndromes is important for proper selection of pharmacologic and nonmedicinal treatment. Evaluation should include location, severity and quality of pain, a determination of its impact on sleep, and the ability to perform usual daily routines. Acute or chronic pain may be the result of interventions, treatments, or intercurrent medical problems. Treatment guidelines for the management of acute pain recently have been published by the Agency for Health Care Policy and Research (1,17), which builds on the World Health Organization (WHO) analgesic ladder (18), which matches the intensity of pain to the treatment recommended. The first line of treatment is the nonopioid analgesics (aspirin, acetaminophen, and nonsteroidal anti-inflammatories, etc.). Should these fail to control the pain, then an opioid (propoxyphene, codeine, oxycodone, morphine, fentanyl, methodone etc.) should be added. Dosing depends on the severity of symptoms. The prescribed route of administration depends on whether the patient can consume medication by mouth and whether the severity of the pain can be adequately controlled using oral medication, as well as on the ease of administration. Adjuvant pain medication may be added, if needed, for better control and includes the addition of antidepressants, benzodiazepines, psychostimulants, corticosteroids, and clonidine. Nerve blocks, epidural injections, and surgical ablation also may be useful in the treatment of acute cancer pain. Modalities of heat, cold, electricity, and nontraditional therapy (acupuncture) all have been shown to be helpful in relieving acute pain in patients with cancer diagnoses (2,19).

The likelihood of cancer pain being chronic is high (20). The WHO has strongly urged use of pain management strategies that are designed to totally relieve symptoms, and the efficacy of the analgesic ladder described above has been demonstrated to be effective (21). Detailed and systematic assessment of pain must be performed both initially and at regular intervals. Chronic pain in this population is either visceral (poorly localized, cramping, or deep aching), somatic (well localized to discreet anatomic areas, often sharp or stabbing), or neuropathic (burning, tingling, throbbing in the peripheral or central nervous system).

There are four key principles to effective pharmacologic pain management. These include choosing a medication, selecting a route for administration, picking the proper dosage, and recognizing and mitigating side effects or toxicities (Table 52-6). In general, dosing should be advanced to the level at which pain is controlled or at which toxicities preclude higher dosing. Adjuvant pain control should be provided for those patients in whom control is inadequate. Typically these diverse medications are used in treating somatic pain. Neuropathic pain and musculoskeletal pain are responsive to this approach (Table 52-7).

Among the nonpharmacologic approaches are somatic and sympathetic nerve blocks. Intraspinal opioids also have been used successfully (22). Ablative procedures such as cordotomy, dorsal column stimulators, and local stimulators such as transcutaneous electrical nerve stimulation (TENS) also have been used effectively. Comprehensive pain treatment centers offer cognitive and behavioral management strategies as adjuvant treatment for cancer-related pain. These techniques include relaxation training, hypnotherapy, and biofeedback. Controlled trials demonstrating efficacy in treating this population have not been undertaken.

Bony Metastatic Disease

Bony metastatic disease can occur with most types of malignancies but is especially common in tumors involving the prostate, breast, lung, kidney, and thyroid (23–25). Additionally, hematologic malignancies such as multiple myeloma, the lymphomas, and leukemia are often associated with widespread bony infiltration by tumor. Bone is the third most common site for metastases, and the vertebrae, pelvis, femur, ribs, and skull are most frequently involved (26). Bony metastatic lesions usually affect multiple sites, 20% of which are in the upper extremities (27).

Bony metastatic disease can produce pain, instability with risk of pathologic fracture, and, in the case of spine or skull metastasis, compromise of adjacent neurologic structures. About 10% of patients with known bone metastases will sustain a fracture (28). One must suspect bony metastatic disease when bone pain is present. Most patients with high-risk conditions for bone metastasis are also followed serially with bone scans to detect occult metastasis because not all

TABLE 52-6. *Pharmacologic management of pain*

Analgesic	Route	Duration of analgesic	Dose	Side effects
Aspirin	Oral	4–6 hr	650 mg every 4 hr	Gastritis, tinnitus
Acetominophen	Oral	4–6 hr	650–1,000 mg every 4 hr	Sedation, nausea
Naproxen	Oral	8–12 hr	250–500 mg every 8 hr	Gastritis, headache
Diffunisal	Oral	8–12 hr	500–1,000 mg every 12 hr	Gastritis, somnolence
Morphine	Oral	2–4 hr	30–60 mg	Sedation, respiratory depression, constipation, confusion
Delayed-release MS	Parenteral	2–4 hr	10 mg	
Contin, Roxanol	Oral	3–4 hr	30 mg	Sedation, respiratory depression, constipation, confusion
Methadone	Oral	4–8 hr	20 mg	Sedation, respiratory depression
	Parenteral	4–8 hr	10 mg	Constipation, confusion
Oxycodone	Oral	3–6 hr	30 mg	Sedation, respiratory depression, constipation, confusion
Hydromorphone	Oral	2–4 hr	1.5 mg	Sedation, respiratory depression
	Parenteral	2–4 hr	7.5 mg	Constipation, confusion
Meperidine	Oral	2–4 hr	300 mg	Sedation, respiratory depression
	Parenteral	2–4 hr	75 mg	Constipation, confusion
Hydrocodone	Oral	3–5 hr	200 mg	Sedation, respiratory depression, constipation, confusion
Fentanyl TTS	Patch	48–72 hr	50 mg/hr, equivalent to 1 mg/hr morphine	

lesions are painful. It remains controversial as to whether most large lesions with impending pathologic fracture are painful. Other potential effects of metastatic bone disease include hematopoietic suppression and hypercalcemia (29).

In assessing bony stability, one relies on factors such as size, location, and type of metastasis (lytic versus blastic) (30). When a patient presents with a symptomatic bony lesion, one must investigate whether lesions are present at other sites because more widespread lesions may further impact weight-bearing recommendations.

Size criteria for pathologic fracture risk in long bone include lesions measuring more than 2.5 cm in lower extremity long bones (more than 3.0 cm in upper extremity lesions) (31–34), involvement of more than 50% of the bony cortex, intramedullary lesions with greater than 50% to 60% (35–37) cross-sectional diameter, involvement of a length of cortex equal to or greater than the cross-sectional diameter of the bone, or, in the femoral neck, cortical destruction greater than 1.3 cm in axial length (Table 52-8). Another method of assessing fracture risk involves multiplying the quotient of the diameter of the lesion and the bone by 100 to obtain the percentage probability of fracture (38) (e.g., lesion diameter 2 cm ÷ bone width 5 cm × 100 = 40% chance of fracture). Unfortunately, in practice it is often difficult to gauge the size of bony lesions, especially lytic ones, which may be irregular, permeative, and difficult to distinguish from surrounding osteopenia (39).

In the spine, there are not validated criteria for assessing fracture risk. The three-column model of Denis (40) is often used, with the spine considered to have anterior, middle, and posterior columns. The anterior column includes the anterior longitudinal ligament and anterior wall of the vertebral body, disk, and annulus; the middle column the posterior wall of those structures and the posterior longitudinal ligament; and the posterior column the posterior elements and associated ligaments and facet capsules. If two or more of these col-

TABLE 52-7. *Adjuvant used in cancer pain management*

Type of pain	Anticonvulsant	Adjuvant antidepressant	Antispasticity	Steroids	Local anesthetics	Other
Neuropathic (chronic throbbing)	0	+ + +	0	+	+ +	Clonidine
Neuropathic lancinating stabbing	+ +	+	+ (baclofen)	0	+ +	Clonazepam
Bone	0	+	0	+ +	+	NSAID, bisphosphonates, calcitonin
Soft-tissue	0	+ +	0	+ +	+ +	NSAID

NSAID, nonsteroidal anti-inflammatory drug.

TABLE 52-8. *Fracture risk*

	Points assigned		
	1	2	3
Anatomic site	Upper extremity	Lower extremity	Trochanter
Lesion type	Blastic	Blastic/lytic	Lytic
Lesion size	<1/3 diameter of femur	>1/3, <2/3	>2/3
Intensity of pain	Mild	Moderate	Severe

umns are involved, or the middle column alone is involved, the lesion is considered unstable. A refinement of this model, described for spine tumors, divides the spine into six columns: anterior, middle and posterior as per the Denis (40) model, with left and right components. The spine is considered stable if fewer than three columns are destroyed, unstable if three or four columns are destroyed, and markedly unstable if five or six columns are destroyed. The spine is also considered unstable if greater than 20° of angulation is present (41). Pal and Sherk (42) described a somewhat different three-column model in the cervical spine, with one anterior column (vertebral bodies and disks; 36% load) and two posterior columns on either side (articular processes forming the neural arch; 32% load each).

Location of a metastatic lesion is also important in assessing stability. One must consider whether weight-bearing bone is involved. In the case of the spine, thoracic lesions are afforded some inherent stability due to the rib cage, whereas lesions in the more flexible cervical and lumbar spine are more prone to instability.

In general, lytic lesions are considered more prone to fracture than blastic ones, although blastic lesions are not immune to fracture. Lytic lesions typically occur in tumors of the breast, lung, kidney, thyroid, gastrointestinal tumors, neuroblastoma, lymphoma, and melanoma. Breast cancer is responsible for 30% to 50% of all long bone pathologic fractures, more than half of those in the proximal femur (39). Renal cell tumors produce large lytic lesions and are at especially high risk for fracture.

In evaluating bony stability, plain x-rays are the most useful tool, especially in long bones. In the spine, flexion extension views also should be obtained. Lesions measuring less than 1 cm are not reliably seen on plain films. In the spine, computed tomography (CT) or magnetic resonance imaging (MRI) is also often indicated to quantify the extent of tumor infiltration, including any extension into the spinal cord (41). MRI is especially useful in this regard. CT is better for bony detail, given its better spatial resolution, and is useful in elucidating subtle cortical erosions or fractures (43). Both studies are useful in distinguishing osteoporotic vertebral collapse from pathologic fracture. Total body bone scan is indicated to define the range of bony neoplastic involvement. It is highly sensitive (95% to 97%) but not highly specific for tumor (44). False-negative results can occur in the setting of bone destruction without significant ongoing repair, as can occur in multiple myeloma, the leukemias, and lymphomas.

When an unstable lesion is suspected, surgical referral should be placed and the patient made non–weight bearing to the affected structure. Surgical procedures should include the use of methylmethacrylate (28). Often surgical stabilization is followed by radiation therapy to reduce tumor mass, thereby facilitating pain control and eventual regrowth of normal bone (45). In borderline cases, radiation therapy alone may be applied, especially for radiosensitive tumors such as breast cancer, lung cancer, or multiple myeloma (27). Hormonal treatment in responsive tumor types such as breast or prostate may reduce bone pain, as can chemotherapy; and radiation therapy alone is often highly effective in controlling pain. Fracture risk may actually increase over the first 6 to 8 weeks due to tumor necrosis and softening of bone (46).

It is important to remember that although bony metastatic disease is a finding of progressive malignancy usually without hope of cure, survival often can be expected for a period of years, especially in breast, prostate, and thyroid malignancies (27).

Depending on the severity of the lesion, mobility recommendations may range from complete non–weight bearing of an affected limb to no precautions whatsoever. Bed rest should be avoided because additional functional loss will occur, and hypercalcemia and thromboembolic disease may complicate the course (28). A walker or crutches will be needed for complete non–weight bearing of a lower limb (30). A single cane can be used in cases of smaller, but painful lesions, or, for somewhat larger or more symptomatic lesions, a forearm crutch that permits about 25% more force transmission than a conventional cane (47). In the spine, Jewett bracing or a custom-molded thoracolumbar orthosis (TLSO) in a two-piece clam shell design (Fig. 52-1) can be used in cases of anterior or middle column involvement. Often patients are resistant to the use of spine orthotics due to poor skin tolerance, perceived discomfort, and lack of a clear end point. In such cases a thoracolumbar corset can provide limited support and pain relief. Use in combination with gait aids such as a walker will minimize torque across the spine.

For the cervical spine, a Philadelphia collar, sternal occipital mandibular immobilizer (SOMI), or even a halo orthotic

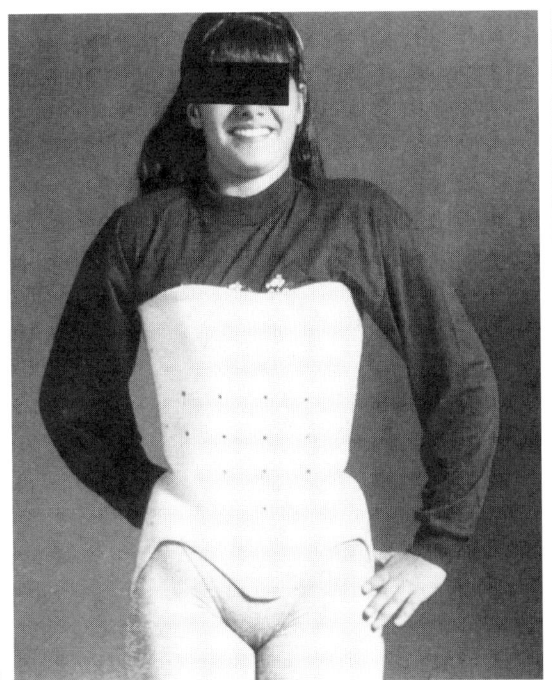
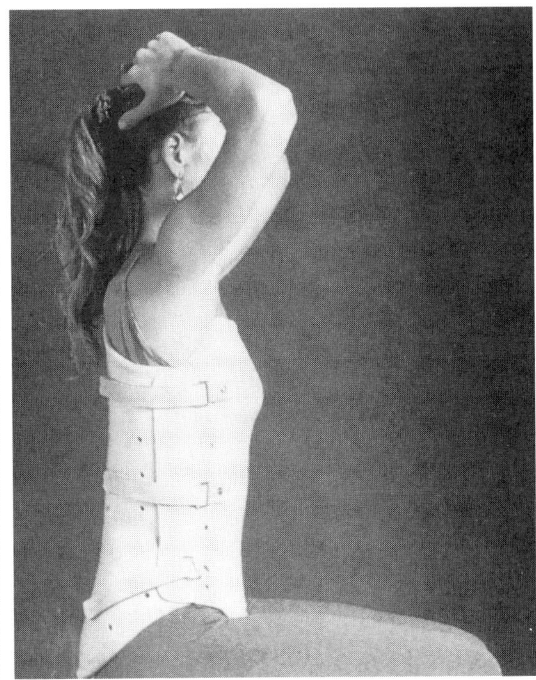

A B

FIG. 52-1. Custom-molded body jacket. Front **(A)** and side **(B)** views.

can be used depending on the severity of the findings (i.e., whether mechanical excursion is seen on plain films or progressing neurologic deficits are present). For cervicothoracic junction lesions, a thoracic extension can be added to a SOMI or Philadelphia collar (Fig. 52-2). One should wear the neck orthosis at all times, especially in the car.

Activity recommendations should focus on exercise that promotes strength and stamina but minimizes bony impact, such as isometric strengthening, isotonic nonresistive exercise, and aerobic exercise such as swimming, riding a stationary bike, or walking. Climbing steps using a step-to pattern rather than a step-over-step pattern will minimize the period of single limb support (48). Further guidance should focus on attention to proper body mechanics (in particular avoiding sudden spine or limb torsions) and on fall prevention strategies (including environmental modifications) and should address possible influence of medication on balance and orthostatic hypotension.

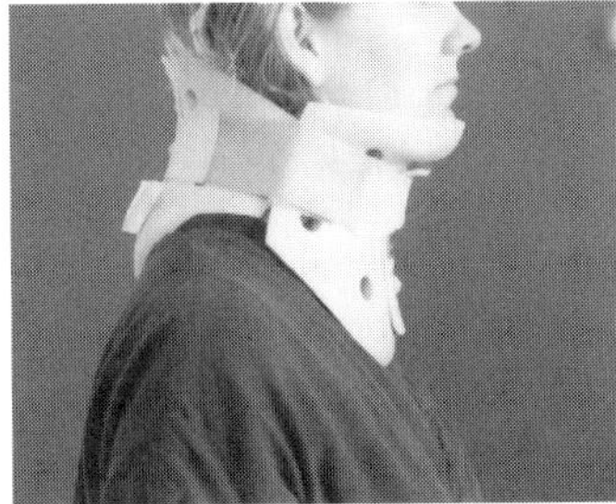

FIG. 52-2. Philadelphia collar.

Brain Metastasis

Brain metastasis occurs in about 20% of patients with cancer and may be intracerebral (77% of cases) or leptomeningeal (40% of cases) (49). The most common primary tumors that metastasize to the brain are lung, breast, and melanoma. Tumors of hematologic origin and genitourinary tract sites also metastasize to the brain. Uterine, cervical, and prostatic carcinoma rarely spread to the brain (49).

The clinical presentation may be insidious or sudden in onset. Headache is often present, followed by focal neurologic signs, especially hemiparesis (50). Seizure may also be a presenting feature. Contrast-enhanced MRI or CT is the best diagnostic test. Treatment for the acute condition includes steroids and radiation therapy. Whole-brain irradiation is standard treatment, 2,000 to 4,000 rad given over 5 days to 4 weeks. Steroids will be needed to control edema and should be continued until the completion of radiation therapy (50). Brain irradiation is frequently completed during inpatient rehabilitation, and it is important to remember not to taper the steroids too soon, or neurologic decline can result. Occasionally, chemotherapeutic agents are used concomitantly. Excision of brain metastasis may be indicated, especially if the metastasis is single, the cancer otherwise well controlled, and the brain metastasis appears to be the major factor limiting survival (50).

Relatively favorable prognostic factors are solitary brain lesion and ambulatory status. Presence of headache, visual disturbance, or impaired consciousness at presentation are poor prognostic factors (51).

Leptomeningeal involvement is most common at the base of the brain, the major brain fissures, and the cauda equina. Lymphomas, leukemias (especially acute), lung (especially small cell), breast, melanoma, and gastric carcinoma most commonly metastasize to the leptomeninges.

Clinically, these patients present with deficits of cranial nerves and spinal nerve roots (52). Treatment consists of radiation therapy and intrathecal chemotherapy, but prognosis is poor (52).

Spinal Cord Metastasis

Cancer-related spinal cord involvement may be due to compression by tumor or to bony instability in patients with metastatic bone disease, both ocologic emergencies, or to radiation fibrosis. Spinal metastatic involvement can affect the thoracic spine (70%), lumbosacral spine (20%), and cervical spine (10%) (53,54). About 5% of patients with cancer eventually develop clinical evidence of cord compression (54).

The most commonly seen primary tumors that cause cord compression are lung (15%), breast (10%), prostate (10%), unknown (10%), lymphomas (10%), and myeloma (10%) (53,54). Ninety-five percent of cases are due to epidural extension of tumor (53). Infarction of vertebral blood supply may occur in hematologic malignancies.

Pain is the first symptom of cord compression and may persist for months before other features develop, especially in patients with breast cancer or lymphoma. Pain can either be local, radicular, or referred. The quality of the pain is different in each case. Local pain in usually aching and constant. Referred pain may be aching or sharp and is remote from the site involved. Radicular pain is usually sharp, shooting pain. Local vertebral tenderness is present in about a third of cases (55). Once neurologic abnormalities develop, progression is often rapid. Epidural metastases characteristically are associated with pain when supine, exacerbated by coughing or the Valsalva maneuver (55). Stretching is usually poorly tolerated (such as neck and back flexion).

In addition to pain, myelopathy is common at the time of diagnosis of spine metastases. Seventy-six percent complain of weakness, 87% are weak on examination, 57% have autonomic dysfunction, and 78% have sensory deficits (55). Motor abnormalities usually precede sensory abnormalities due to epidural extension, preferentially affecting the anterior spinal cord, and recovery occurs in the reverse order. Perineal hypesthesia may be the first sign of a cauda equina syndrome. Sphincter incontinence is a very poor prognostic sign, as is rapid (less than 72 hours) evolution of symptoms (fewer than 5% recover). Complete paraplegia is not reversible (54).

Spine films are 80% sensitive in detecting metastatic lesions (54). CT is indicated if plain films are negative, but MRI is the evaluation of choice in patients with myelopathy.

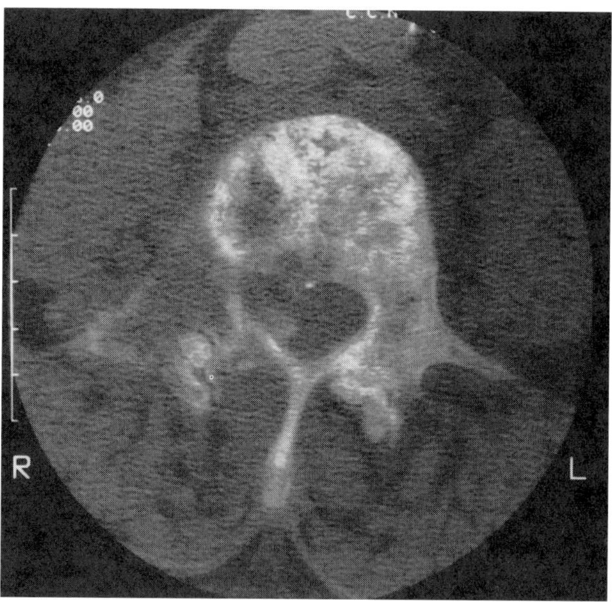

FIG. 52-3. Spinal metastasis involving posterior column.

Because 1-year survival rates are better in those who remain ambulatory (66% versus 10%) (56), early intervention is appropriate. Treatment algorithms have been developed for management of back pain (Fig. 52-3).

Treatment includes dexamethasone 100 mg daily tapered over 2 to 3 weeks, laminectomy (surgical results best with tumors located posterior or lateral) in selected cases, and radiation therapy (in virtually all cases). Favorable prognostic factors are primary diagnosis of lymphoma, myeloma, or breast cancer, early or slowly progressing neurologic signs and ambulatory status at time of diagnosis of cord compression (54,55). A dosage of 3,000 to 4,000 rad over 2 to 4 weeks is typically given. Adjuvant chemotherapy may be considered in certain cases.

Paraneoplastic Neuromuscular Syndromes

Paraneoplastic syndromes include subacute cerebellar degeneration, peripheral neuropathies, myopathies, and neuromuscular junction disorders. Organic dementias may occur (54). Reflex sympathetic dystrophy has been described with local or recurrent tumor (57). Many combinations of motor and sensory neuropathies may occur (see discussion under Peripheral Neuropathy).

The ataxia associated with cerebellar degeneration may antedate the diagnosis of tumor, as seen with lung, breast, and ovarian carcinomas (58). The syndrome may be associated with organic dementia. Ataxia also may be induced by cytotoxic drugs, such as fluorouracil, procarbazine, and nitrosureas, as well as by brain metastases. Treatment of the underlying disease may halt the progression, but neurologic improvement of paraneoplastic cerebellar degeneration is rare. However, sustained functional benefit has been reported after comprehensive inpatient rehabilitation (59).

Shy-Drager syndrome may occur as a paraneoplastic syndrome in small cell lung cancer. Treatment is administered in the form of indomethacin, salt loading, fludrocortisone, and compressive stockings. Proximal myopathies that may occur include inflammatory myopathies, carcinoid myopathy, steroid myopathy, and weakness from cachexia. Treatment of tumor may result in improvement of the myopathy, especially carcinoid and, less consistently, inflammatory forms (60). Isometric exercises in combination with stretching, mobility aides, and adaptive devices to maintain functional independence are indicated for myopathic conditions.

Myasthenia gravis may occur in association with thymoma, and antibodies to thymus are usually present. Myasthenic syndrome occurs in association with small cell lung cancer. The condition may improve with treatment of the underlying cancer and with guanidine hydrochloride (60).

Devastating paraneoplastic neurologic complications include acute necrotizing myopathy and ascending hemorrhagic myelonecrosis. It is unclear whether amyotrophic lateral sclerosis occurs as a paraneoplastic syndrome.

Peripheral Polyneuropathy

Peripheral neuropathy can occur as a remote effect of tumor. Carcinomatous neuromyopathy, occurring most notably in lung cancer, is a distal peripheral polyneuropathy with associated proximal muscle weakness (61), type II fiber atrophy (62), weight loss (63), and variable electromyographic changes of proximal myopathy (61). The myopathic changes may be attributable to abnormalities in the intramuscular segments of axons, seen on electron microscopy (64).

Peripheral polyneuropathy has been described in various types of lung cancer (small cell, adenocarcinoma, undifferentiated) (61) as well as in multiple myeloma, breast, and colon malignancies (61). Subacute sensory neuropathy has been reported with carcinoma of the lung, breast, ovary, esophagus, uterus, with Hodgkin's disease, and sarcoma (65,66). Polyneuropathy is associated pathologic findings of widespread degeneration of the dorsal root ganglia and as an inflammatory response. Pain, paresthesias, and numbness predominate, with unsteady gait. Face, bowel, and bladder are usually spared. Abnormal muscle findings such as fibrillations or polyphasic motor unit potentials can be seen on electromyography (EMG). Hematogenous metastases to the dorsal root ganglia also can occur, described with oat cell carcinoma and poorly differentiated colon cancer (67). Subacute motor neuropathy occurs with lymphomas, especially Hodgkin's disease. Anterior horn cells degenerate, resulting in progressive weakness, followed by stabilization and subsequent improvement (60). Direct infiltration of roots and peripheral nerves is more likely to occur with lymphomas than with carcinoma (68,69).

Paraproteinemic neuropathies with monoclonal serum protein occur in association with multiple myeloma, osteosclerotic myeloma, Waldenstrom's macroglobulinemia, amyloidosis, gamma heavy chain disease, and, most commonly, idiopathic cause. Typically the neuropathy is distal, mixed sensory and motor, with axonal loss and segmental demyelination. Amyloidosis often is characterized by autonomic involvement, infiltrative myopathy, and superimposed carpal tunnel syndrome. Compared with other paraproteinemic neuropathies, the neuropathy of osteosclerotic myeloma is most likely to respond to treatment of the underlying condition.

One of the most frequently seen causes of peripheral neuropathy in this population is chemotherapy. Many agents have impact on the peripheral nervous system, which already may be at increased risk because of poor nutrition or prior radiation therapy. A description of the peripheral neuropathies, as well as the tumors or chemotherapies causing them, are presented in Table 52-9.

Treatment includes therapy for the underlying malignancy, and medication to treat pain or cramping includes carbamazepine, quinidine, or tricyclic agents (62). Attention should be directed to appropriate nonconstrictive footwear to minimize the likelihood of ulceration resulting from poor sensory feedback. Other measures include exercise to maintain strength and range of motion, appropriate prescription of orthotics, assistive and adaptive devices, and energy conservation strategies.

Radiation Therapy

Radiation therapy can be applied for curative or palliative intent. Used alone, it can be curative for certain carcinomas of the face, scalp, head and neck, upper esophagus, breast, genitourinary system, nervous system, or hematologic system. It is often used in combination with surgery (head and neck, breast, lung, gastrointestinal, genitourinary, nervous system, and sarcomas) or chemotherapy (small cell carcinoma, Ewing's sarcoma, hematologic malignancies), or both (Wilms' tumor, rhabdomyosarcoma, and neuroblastoma) for curative intent (54). Use for palliation is indicated for symptom control or prevention, as in the case of pain, brain metastasis, or to prevent complications such as pathologic fracture or superior vena cava syndrome (54).

Acute adverse effects of radiation therapy include fatigue, desquamation, oral cavity changes (decreased salivation, mucositis, loss of taste), nausea, vomiting, anorexia, esophagitis, proctitis, urinary cystitis, decreased libido, sterility, amenorrhea, leukopenia, and thrombocytopenia. Subacute or late effects can include soft-tissue fibrosis with contracture, skin atrophy or ulceration, xerostomia, auditory or visual changes, Meniere's syndrome, osteonecrosis (with more than 6,000 rad), pulmonary fibrosis, gastrointestinal strictures, chronic cystitis or nephritis, impotence, sterility, endocrine insufficiencies, brain necrosis, transverse myelitis, lymphedema, and late malignancies including sarcoma, skin cancers, and leukemia (54). Patients receiving combined chemotherapy and radiation therapy are at risk for additive toxicities.

After radiation therapy of 3,000 to 5,000 rad to bony meta-

TABLE 52-9. *Peripheral polyneuropathy in cancer*

	Tumor	Chemotherapy (severe)	Chemotherapy (mild)
Distal sensorimotor axonal	Lung (all histologies) Multiple myeloma (with or without amyloidosis) Leukemia, lymphoma (infiltrative) Prostate, (vasculitic) Testes Kidney, (vasculitic)	Taxol Hexamethylmelamine (HMM)	Procarbazine Etoposide Hexamethylmelamine
Sensory predominant	Lung Breast Ovary Hodgkin's disease Gastrointestinal sites Kidney Testes Penis	Cisplatin Cytarabine (ARA-C)	Platinum (DDP)
Motor predominant	Lung Leukemia (CML) Penis	Vincristine (may progress to quadriparesis, involve cranial nerves, produce dysautonomia)	Vinblastine
Subacute or chronic demyelinating	Lymphoma (especially Hodgkin's disease) Osteosclerotic myeloma Small cell	Suramin	
Mononeuropathy multiplex (vasculitic)	Small cell Lymphoma		
Mononeuropathies	Small cell Multiple myeloma with amyloidosis Lymphoma and leukemia (especially cranial nerve involvement)	Platinum (DDP) hearing loss	
Proximal motor (myopathic)	Lung Breast Leukemia Stomach Ovary Sarcoma Head and neck		

static lesions, remineralization is noted within 2 months and maximal at 3 months, and remodeling is completed at 6 months to 1 year (70). If the epiphysis is irradiated, growth will be arrested.

CNS effects include early delayed encephalopathy, presenting in the first 8 months due to demyelination. This may be distinguished from tumor by its response to steroids (71). Chronic and delayed radiation encephalopathy (rare with a total dose of less than 5,600 rad) begins a year or two after treatment and causes coagulative necrosis of white matter, sparing the cortex. Response to corticosteroids is unpredictable. Memory loss or cognitive dysfunction may result from brain atrophy after whole-brain irradiation (72).

Radiation to the spinal cord can produce Lhermitte's syndrome (onset 1 to 4 months, lasting weeks to months), which can be seen in patients undergoing radiation for head and neck tumors. Transverse myelitis or delayed radiation myelopathy usually has its onset at 9 to 18 months, usually after more than 5,000 rad, often presenting as a Brown-Sequard syndrome or with radicular pain. For the latter, deficits usually progress slowly, then stabilize without improvement (72). Sphincter dysfunction is common with an upper motor neuron presentation, but rare with lower motor neuron picture. Radiation-induced plexopathies occur and are late findings, seen months to years after completion of treatment (54).

Nutrition

Cancer and its treatment can impede optimal nutrition. The malignancy itself can lead to cachexia. Weight loss may result from an increase in energy requirements. An increase in cytokines such as tumor necrosis factor (also known as cachectin) may induce anaerobic glycolysis, fever, amino acid release from muscle, hepatic lipid secretion, and reduced albumin synthesis (73,74). Abnormalities in the regulation of anabolic hormones such as insulin, growth hormone, and somatostatin also may contribute to cachexia (74). Dysphagia is a common accompaniment of gastrointestinal and head and neck tumors.

Surgical therapies can interfere with the ability to eat (especially in patients with head and neck tumors), or in those with stomach or bowel tumors, producing malabsorption states with resulting nutritional depletion. Megaloblastic anemia can result from gastric resection due to loss of intrinsic factor for binding vitamin B_{12}. Bowel resection can produce deficiencies of vitamins B_{12}, D, B, and A, as well as water and electrolyte imbalance (73). Increased nutrition is needed to allow healing after major surgical procedures.

Radiation to the head and neck can alter taste and salivation and can interfere with swallowing (75). Radiation to the stomach or small intestine may produce nausea, vomiting, and the sensation of fullness. Over the long term, intestinal obstruction, perforation, bleeding, malabsorption, or fistulas may occur. Bowel rest and total parenteral nutrition may be needed in cases of severe radiation enteritis.

Chemotherapy commonly produces nausea, vomiting, and anorexia, as well as oral problems such as stomatitis, glossitis, pharyngitis, and mucosal ulceration. Prolonged vomiting can cause vitamin B_1 deficiency. Folic acid deficiency, common with methotrexate, can produce stomatitis, pharyngitis, gastroenteritis, and proctitis with malabsorption (73). Antimetabolites such as 5-fluorouracil and 6-mercaptopurine result in thymine deficiency, producing lip and oral cavity changes. Other common deficiencies are of vitamins B_2 and K. Edema may result from hypoproteinemia (73).

Measures should be taken to maximize intake by the oral route. Often antiemetics such as Compazine (SmithKline Beecham, Philadelphia, PA), Tigan (Roberts, Eatontown, NJ), or Ondansetron are needed. Oral supplements may be more easily ingested or tolerated than solid foods. Learned food aversions are common, a conditioned response from associating consumption of a food with subsequent gastrointestinal symptoms. To avoid developing aversion to familiar or preferred food items, one might avoid consuming those in the 24 hours before receiving the therapy that produces nausea. Meats, vegetables, and caffeinated beverages in particular often produce food aversions. In patients with dumping syndrome after gastric surgery, small frequent meals should be taken. For hyposalivation, dry mouth products are available in many forms: gum, toothpaste, rinses, etc.

Medications such as pilocarpine or bromhexine can promote increased salivary flow (73). Medications with anticholinergic side effects should be avoided.

Use of total parenteral nutrition is thought to reduce morbidity and mortality in surgical patients but has not been found to benefit patients undergoing chemotherapy and may be associated with increased complications such as infection or increase in tumor growth (74). Nutritional counseling is often of benefit to advise patients on strategies for maximizing oral intake. Patients need to be made aware not to rely on appetite alone because this will be insufficient. Patient's may have strong opinions, often complete misconceptions or based on no factual data, about the role of specific foods in being causative or curative of their malignancy. They may be taking toxic doses of nutritional supplements such as fat-soluble vitamins (73).

Caution should be used during this period to assure that patients are well hydrated before beginning or resuming exercise. Many patients report that exercise is an appetite suppressant, although many find it a stimulant. Individual treatments should be planned around individual patient responses. An attempt to build lean mass, when possible, is beneficial for patients.

Sexual Function

Sexual dysfunction may occur as a primary effect of malignancy, but more commonly occurs as a side effect of treatment. Sexual function can be affected by disturbance at many levels, including psychologic, central or peripheral nervous system, endocrine, pelvic vascular, and local effects on gonadal structures. Physical changes may interfere with the patient's concept of his or her sexual attractiveness. Depression may result in low sexual drive. Psychologic distress with impact on sexual function may be more common in younger adults with cancer than in older individuals (76).

Endocrine effects occur in men with prostate cancer treated with orchiectomy or with hormonal regimens to reduce serum testosterone. Sexual desire and function is reduced but is preserved in a minority of cases.

In men, chemotherapy can have adverse effects on spermatogenesis and testosterone production. Neuropathies, including dysautonomia, can impact sexual function, including the emission phase of male orgasm. Common complications of chemotherapy in men include low sexual desire, erectile dysfunction, dry orgasm, and reduced pleasure with orgasm (76). Less is known about the effects of chemotherapy on female sexual function, but alkylating agents have the most gonadal toxicity. Permanent menopause may occur with combination chemotherapy, accompanied by menopausal symptoms such as hot flashes. Vaginal mucosal changes can lead to dyspareunia (76).

Radiation therapy to the prostate or testicles can produce erectile dysfunction, possibly due to acceleration of pre-existing atherosclerosis from postradiation fibrotic changes. In women, radiation therapy to the pelvis produces premature menopause, with a dose of as low as 600 to 1,000 rad permanently destroying ovarian function. Radiation also produces damage to the vaginal epithelium, and the fibrotic process can continue over years. The result can be dyspareunia, postcoital bleeding, even vaginal ulcers. After local radiation therapy for cervical cancer, stenosis of the upper vagina can occur. Vaginal dilators can preserve the integrity of the vagina. Estrogen therapy also may be of some benefit, as well as vaginal lubricants (76).

Radical prostatectomy has a high rate of erectile dysfunction, although newer surgical procedures sparing the neurovascular bundles permits gradual (up to 1 year) recovery of erectile function (77). Radical prostatectomy typically does not affect desire, sensation, or orgasm (except that no semen is produced). More rarely, urinary incontinence occurs. Similar problems may occur after radical cystectomy and abdominoperineal resection of gastrointestinal tumors (78) (lesser incidence of erectile dysfunction after low anterior resection) (77). Sperm banking before surgery should be considered due to incidence of reduced emission secondary to sympathetic plexus dissection. Options to restore erectile function, including surgical implants, use of a vacuum erection device, or papaverine injections, can be considered. Generally one waits about 6 months after treatment before considering surgery for a penile prosthesis because erectile dysfunction may gradually improve on its own. No specific measures can improve sexual desire, penile sensation, or ability to reach orgasm (76).

Radical hysterectomy, where there is removal of the uterus, cervix, upper portion of the vagina, and one ovary, does not usually produce changes in sexual function or desire. Radical cystectomy, which includes removal of the bladder, urethra, uterus, cervix, ovaries, and anterior vaginal wall, with vaginal reconstruction, is associated with initial dyspareunia, which can gradually improve over time. Abdominoperineal resection, with loss of cushioning of the posterior vagina, and postoperative pelvic adhesions, can produce dyspareunia and loss of sexual desire (76).

Total pelvic exenteration involves removal of the uterus, fallopian tubes, ovaries, cervix, vagina, urethra, bladder, and rectum, with urinary and bowel diversions created. A vagina is constructed from myocutaneous gracilis flaps, with normal skin rather than mucosa forming the vaginal walls. A water-based lubricant is needed during intercourse, as is regular douching to avoid odor (77).

Radical vulvectomy leads to dyspareunia and reduced genital sensation and desire due to removal of the clitoris and scar tissue formation at the introitus. Nevertheless, the capacity for orgasm may be regained in about half the cases, with psychologic factors in the relationship the major variable (76).

For women, specific surgical reconstructive measures may be indicated, such as reconstruction of the vagina or labia via myocutaneous flap or split-thickness skin grafting to repair stenosis of the vaginal introitus. Hormonal replacement therapy should be considered in cases of premature menopause for its benefit in preventing osteoporosis and cardiovascular disease. Vaginal relaxation exercises, vaginal dilators, and water-based lubricants also may be helpful (77,79). In general, greasy lubricants such as petroleum jelly should be avoided because they may block the urethral opening (78).

Counseling is an important technique in treating sexual disorders in cancer patients because despite the often profound physiologic or anatomic changes, psychologic adjustment has been found to be a more important determinant of sexual satisfaction (79). Counseling is usually short-term and optimally includes both partners. Disease or treatment-specific effects on sexual function should be discussed with the patient, including the use of drawings or diagrams when appropriate (78).

Timing of resumption of sexual activity can be an important factor for patients with fatigue, ostomies or significant psychological trauma associated with their cancer diagnosis. Peer support through ostomy groups can be of benefit (78). Patients should be encouraged to maintain a healthy body through fitness and other strategies, as well as a good personal image. The American Cancer Society's Look Good, Feel Better and Reach to Recovery programs can be very helpful (79). Regardless of whether formal counseling is pursued, patients should be encouraged to pursue and not avoid physical closeness and intimacy. The varied aspects of an intimate relationship should be encouraged, rather than focusing attention solely on coitus (79).

Exercise and Cancer

Moderate exercise is thought to be beneficial for individuals with cancer. In establishing exercise precautions, one needs to consider hematologic, cardiac, pulmonary, and skeletal factors (80). Depression and fatigue may limit exercise participation, and fever will reduce exercise tolerance.

Most hematologic parameters for exercise are empiric. In a study of acute leukemia patients (81), grossly visible hemorrhage was rare with a platelet count greater than 20,000, and no intracranial hemorrhage occurred with a platelet count greater than 10,000. The risk of hemorrhage correlates with the platelet count but is mitigated by other systemic factors, such that a safe threshold level cannot be ascertained. The concern with exercise in the thrombocytopenic state lies in the potential for increased blood pressure, which occurs most dramatically with isometric exercise, to result in intracranial hemorrhage (80), and high-impact activities to result in muscular or intra-articular hemorrhage (82). In general, unrestricted exercise can be pursued with platelet counts greater than about 30,000 to 50,000 Aerobic, but not resistive, activities can be considered with platelet counts greater than 10,000 to 20,000. Active therapy is not advocated with platelet counts less than 10,000 (80). Exercise is also not recommended with fever greater than 40°C (104°F) due to poor tolerance, increased respiratory and heart rates, and increased platelet consumption (82). No specific precautions exist regarding white blood cell count, but exercise can produce transient increases in the white blood cell count, so that patients might be counseled to avoid intense exercise before routine laboratory monitoring (83).

Exercise programs have been developed for bone marrow transplant recipients to counteract the debility occurring with medical morbidity and prolonged hospitalization, as well as to counteract other factors such as depression and social isolation (80). Supine or sitting exercise is generally well tolerated, but standing exercise should be attempted at least for brief periods to minimize gastroc-soleus tightness. Supine exercise may be most comfortably performed with the head of the bed slightly elevated. Exercise programs emphasize range of motion, aerobic activity such as use of a bedside stationary bicycle or jogging in place, light resistive exercise with 2 to 4 pound weights or manual resistance, and deep breathing to prevent atelectasis and pneumonia. In patients who develop hepatic veno-occlusive disease, supine exercise or abdominal exercises should be avoided because they may aggravate abdominal pain. In those with graft-versus-host disease, skin erythema and rash may occur, and protective padding will prevent pain and skin irritation during exercise, especially over the soles of the feet (80). Active assisted range of motion should be performed to prevent contractures in this setting, as well as nighttime orthotic devices to preserve functional positioning of the hands and feet. Often patients will need encouragement to engage in the exercise regimen, but even limited treatment such as passive range of motion or massage can build patients' trust and future compliance (82).

Cancer patients treated with cardiotoxic agents such as arthracyclines can sustain permanent cardiac damage that affects physical performance. Patients treated with significant doses of these agents (greater than 100 mg/m^2) can have reduced exercise time, reduced maximal oxygen uptake, abnormal heart rate response, ST- and T-wave changes, and exercise-induced hypotension (84). However, such patients undergoing a conditioning program can improve exercise time (by about 10%), peak oxygen uptake, and ventilatory anaerobic threshold. Exercise heart rate and stroke volume do not increase with a 12-week, 24-session aerobic program (84).

A 10-week, thrice weekly aerobic training program in women undergoing treatment for breast cancer found 40% improvement in functional capacity, with longer work periods and higher intensity workload attainable at posttest than for placebo or controls. Such gain was comparable with that seen with other medical conditions such as end-stage renal disease or pulmonary or cardiac disease (85).

Fatigue and anemia pose limitations to exercise performance. Endogenous tumor necrosis factor, or that administered exogenously as antineoplastic therapy, can reduce skeletal muscle protein stores. The resulting muscle wasting can predispose to fatigue with exercise because the reduced cross-sectional area of muscle results in less force production. Increased effort will be needed by the patient to do the same work. A moderate intensity of exercise, which relies mainly on type I muscle fibers, which are fatigue resistant, should be encouraged (83). Exercise that produces marked fatigue is probably too intense. Patients receiving tumor necrosis factor as therapy might delay exercise a few days to allow muscle regeneration. Those with marked cachexia, possibly tumor necrosis factor alpha–mediated, might not tolerate exercise at all, and rehabilitation efforts might focus on routes other than aerobic conditioning to achieve functional goals (83).

Rehabilitation of Patients with Breast Cancer

One in eight women in the United States has a lifetime risk of being diagnosed with breast cancer, and one in 28 will die from it (2). The 5-year survival rates was 82% for white women and 66% for black women in the United States. Half of the whites and only one third of the blacks were diagnosed at the localized stage. The most significant risk factor for breast cancer is age (relative risk 17), and residency in North America or Europe (relative risk 4 to 5) (86).

The rehabilitation for women with breast cancer should be divided into two groups: those with local disease and disability and those with systemic illness and disability. The general goals for both groups is to help the patient reach her desired level of function when possible. This process is accomplished via education and building a therapeutic alliance that addresses the like problems and complications the patient may face. Patients with primary breast cancer are likely to experience limitation of shoulder motion postoperatively and incisional pain of the chest wall (and axillary region for those undergoing mastectomy), and 20% may develop lymphedema (87,88). Patients with recurrent regional disease are likely to have shoulder and arm symptoms, not unlike the primary breast cancer patients, and development of lymphedema is likely. Those with distant and metastatic disease are likely to have spread to bone, lung, and liver. However, the patient referred to the physiatrist is most likely to complain of local back pain without radiculopathy or long bone pain with referred pain to the adjacent joints (e.g., shoulder, hip, knee). There is likely to be negative impact on mobility and stamina.

Definitive surgical treatment for breast cancer depends on the classification of the tumor and the preference of the patient for breast-conserving therapy or not. The modified radical mastectomy removes all breast tissue and a sampling of axillary nodes. Usually, the pectoralis minor is preserved. In the lumpectomy treatment, only tumor and a margin of breast tissue is removed, and an axillary sampling is taken. The chest is subsequently radiated, as is the axilla when more than three nodes are positive for tumor. The decision to irradiate the supraclavicular region is dependent on the extent of the surgery. Complications of mastectomy include wound complications, phantom breast sensations, and arm edema; those that occur after radiation include chest wall pain, shoulder stiffness, and arm edema.

We developed a comprehensive evaluation and treatment plan for patients undergoing breast surgery for treatment of cancer (89). Shoulder mobility and strength are negatively influenced by the extent of surgery, radiation dose and schedule of delivery, and amount of postoperative pain (90–92). Pain should be treated with adequate analgesia and use of heat or cold and early, but not immediate, mobilization. Active motion only should be performed until the drains are out. The recommended range includes internal/external rotation to tolerance from the first postoperative day onward. Until day 4, 40 to 45,° of flexion and abduction are permitted. From days 4 to 6 flexion should be advanced from 45° to 90°, but abduction should remain at 45°. Thereafter, flexion, abduction, and rotation should be performed to tolerance. Immediate mobilization through range has been associated with more lymph drainage and wound complications (93–95). Once healing has occurred, there is no need to restrict functional and customary activity.

The use of the overhead pulley helps restore range of motion. However, performing exercises in recumbency is also useful to provide scapular support, especially if there has been damage to the serratus anterior. Transient muscle weakness of the shoulder girdle muscles also may occur (89). Isometric exercise, using resistive elastic bands and gradually progressing to isotonic exercise, is recommended. Recovery is usually complete.

Lymphedema or a sense of fullness in the arm even without circumferential changes of more than 2 cm are frequently reported by patients undergoing mastectomy or lumpectomy. Many patients do not report this symptom to the physician. It tends to develop over a protracted period of time, and the median interval between treatment and follow-up is 39 months (88). Risk factors for lymphedema include extent of surgery, receipt of axillary radiation, obesity, and possibly surgical technique (88,92). Prevention of lymphedema depends on two factors: (a) not interfering with lymph outflow, hence not constricting the arm and protecting from infection, scarring, and burns, and (b) limiting lymph production by using compression garments when exercising and avoiding vasodilation through heat exposure (sun, sauna, and steam). Raising the arm against gravity is useful. Use of a compression garment that uses 30 to 50 mm Hg also is effective. Compression therapy is useful. There is a major controversy in the literature about the usefulness of compression pumps, either single or multi-channel machines. Some efficacy has been shown for this approach (96,97). Currently manual lymph drainage has been shown effective. The technique requires training in the use of a special manual drainage using a delicate massage technique, compression bandaging, and a series of exercises (Fig. 52-4) (98). Several reports have surfaced indicating efficacy of the use of benzopyrones in the treatment of chronic lymphedema (99). Efficacy of surgical treatments for this problem is not yet proven.

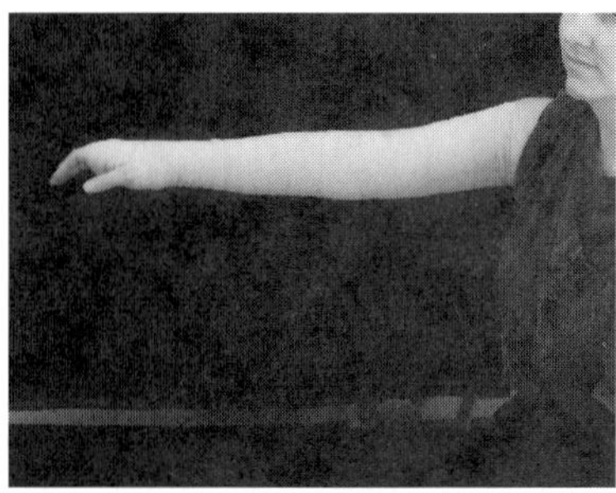

FIG. 52-4. Compressive bandage for lymphedema.

Involvement of the skeleton, lungs or pleura, and CNS presents a significant problem to the rehabilitation team. Metastatic disease is often accompanied by significant pain, fatigue, mobility, and self-care deficits as well as depression. It is also a period of resumption of treatment, often including radiation, surgery, and chemotherapies. For some patients, newer experimental treatments are also used. It is a period of great uncertainty, and anxiety and sleep disruption are common. The major goals for the rehabilitation professionals at this stage of the disease are (a) to achieve good pain relief and comfort, (b) to enable self-care and as near normal social and vocational activities as possible, (c) to assure bony stability of the skeleton and long bones, (d) to maintain stamina and strength, and (e) to provide education and support while being realistically hopeful.

The sites for bone metastases in breast cancer are those bones rich in marrow: vertebrae, pelvis, ribs, and proximal long bones. The medical consequences of this involvement include fracture, neurologic compromise (spinal cord or peripheral motor/neuropathy,) or metabolic complications. Often the patient presents with dull pain, nocturnal and often not relieved with rest. Lytic changes with some sclerotic foci are the most characteristic radiographic findings of metastatic breast cancer. Bone scan remains one of the most frequently used techniques for identifying the extent of bony involvement but is inadequate for quantifying the extent of the lesion. MRI and CT are used for better lesion quantification. Plain films are somewhat useful in identifying which lesions are likely to result in fracture, but their usefulness is limited by the lack of sensitivity (bone loss of 30% to 50% must occur before the radiograph is positive) (100). A critical review of the predictors of fracture of the proximal femur was performed in breast cancer patients (39), and the criteria did not distinguish those patients who did from those who did not fracture. Other assessment schemes have been proposed that assign points for site, level of pain, type, and size of lesion (Table 52-8). Scores of 9 or more points have a 33% risk of fracture. Surgical intervention is suggested for impending fracture, and fracture should be treated with surgical stabilization. Fracture fixation is associated with good return to ambulation status and improved survival (100). The responsibilities of the rehabilitation professionals are to identify those who are at risk for fracture and refer them to orthopedics and to provide gait aids for those in need of protective ambulation. Those with impending fracture should be on non–weight-bearing status. Those with upper extremity lesions should be treated with a sling or a light-weight humeral cuff and instructed in activities designed to reduce loads. It becomes quite important to assess the status of the upper and lower extremities: commonly the use of crutches or canes may be proscribed because of an upper extremity lesion.

The evaluation of the vertebral column starts with bone scan and plain radiographs. Those patients in whom there is vertebral body compression of more than 50% should be assessed via MRI or CT. The degree of involvement can be scored as follows:

I. No significant neurologic involvement
II. Bone involvement without instability/collapse
III. Major neurologic involvement without bone involvement
IV. Bony collapse without neurologic compromise
V. Major neurologic compromise and vertebral collapse (101)

Those in category I–III can benefit from rehabilitation treatment designed to relieve pain and promote function. These patients benefit from lightweight, easily donned corsets, which offer pain relief, as does the use of superficial heat and TENS units. Patients who have stage IV and V involvement, when not responsive to radiation and chemotherapy for their bony or neurologic problems, require surgical stabilization. Patients with significant bony instability and cord compromise should not be treated with rigid corsets because the goal of management is to prevent, or stabilize, cord compromise.

Plexopathy due to tumor invasion is reported in 4% to 5% of patients attending a cancer pain center (102).

The most frequent presenting symptom is pain, which is usually antecedent to paresthesias or focal weakness (103). Pain is usually moderately severe and originates in the shoulder girdle with radiation to the elbow, medial forearm, and fingers. Because 75% of patients have sensory involvement of the lower plexus (104) and 25% have involvement of the entire plexus, sensation in the fourth and fifth fingers is more commonly affected (C7–C8, T1) than thumb and index (C5–C6).

Differentiation between tumor infiltration and radiation-induced plexopathy is often difficult. Spread of tumor through lymphatics will cause lower trunk involvement because of the proximity of the lymph nodes to the lower trunk. Few nodes are adjacent to the upper trunk. Radiation-induced fibrosis occurs, on average, 5.5 years from therapy (103). Paresthesias occur most commonly, and pain is less common and less severe than in tumor-induced plexpathy. The upper trunk is more frequently involved.

The diagnosis of tumor or radiation-induced plexopathy may require MRI to distinguish soft-tissue changes. EMG will show fibrillation potentials and positive waves. Median somatosensory evoked potentials may aid in identifying root involvement. The presence of myokymic discharges suggest radiation-induced changes (105).

Head and Neck Cancer

Head and neck cancer and its treatment can result in major effects on communication, nutrition, swallowing, dental health, and musculoskeletal function. Most head and neck malignancies are squamous cell carcinomas. Lesions usually arise at the surface but may invade muscle and spread along muscle or fascial planes. Bone or cartilage invasion usually does not occur until later in the disease process. Perineural spread may occur and may track along a nerve to the base of the skull, or less commonly, peripherally. Lymphatic spread commonly occurs, and distant metastasis is less common, occurring in about 10% to 12% overall (106). Surgery and radiation therapy are the only curative treatment options. Depending on the location, size, and degree of extension of the lesion, either radiation or surgery may be used as the initial option and may or may not need to be followed by the other. Medically, comorbidity such as alcohol and tobacco abuse, poor nutritional state, diabetes, and pulmonary and cardiovascular disease are common.

Radical neck dissection involves removal of the sternocleidomastoid muscle, internal and external jugular veins, spinal accessory nerve, and submandibular gland as a single unit. Deep to the dissection in the posterior triangle lie the nerves to the rhomboids, the long thoracic nerve, brachial plexus (trunk level), subclavian vessels, and phrenic nerve. This area has been referred to as the danger zone and is not routinely included in the dissection (107). In recent years, less drastic procedures have been used in selected cases, including sparing of the spinal accessory nerve when possible. The functional neck dissection involves selective removal of only the superficial and deep cervical fascia and its nodes.

Complications of radical neck dissection include lymphedema, wound infection and dehiscence, injury to cranial nerves VII, X, and XII, and carotid injury. Asymmetric neck motion results from removal of the sternocleidomastoid, platysmus, and other muscles, and shoulder dysfunction from sacrifice of the spinal accessory nerve (108). Loss of trapezius function results in shoulder depression and protraction, and this malalignment produces incomplete and painful active excursion of the shoulder, often with range of abduction of less than 90°. The rhomboids and levator scapula become overstretched, and the pectoralis major shortened (108). The sternoclavicular joint bears the weight of the arm, leading to clavicle subluxation and arthritic changes (109).

Rehabilitation treatment is directed toward preventing or correcting the above deformities. Passive neck range of motion, emphasizing flexion and rotation, is begun when sutures are removed to the limits of graft or suture line stretch, progressing to active range of motion and isometric strengthening by week 4 (108). Neck exercise is contraindicated if there is felt to be significant risk of carotid rupture, and prolonged coughing also should be discouraged in this setting to avoid increased intrathoracic pressure (110). Some patients with chronic obstructive pulmonary disease may use the sternocleidomastoid and platysmus for accessory respiration and may become transiently more dyspneic after this muscle function is lost. Energy conservation measures and breathing exercises can be taught (110). In the setting of radiation therapy, which produces soft-tissue fibrosis and contracture, especially in higher doses, the patient should receive instruction in neck range of motion pretreatment and perform the exercises throughout the radiation course and for an indefinite period thereafter.

The shoulder program includes strengthening, especially of scapular stabilizers such as the serratus anterior, rhomboids, and levator scapula, and stretching of the protractors (109). Internal rotation, which results in protraction, should be avoided. The patient should not do strenuous activities such as lifting heavy objects with the affected side (108). An orthotic may improve shoulder alignment and reduce pain (111). Spinal accessory nerve grafting may be an option. In the case of neurapraxic lesions, functional electrical stimulation can be considered to maintain the contractile elements as reinnervation occurs (108).

In addition to soft-tissue fibrosis in the neck, radiation therapy may induce dental and salivary abnormalities, limited jaw motion, and laryngeal edema with voice changes. Voice changes such as change in quality or reduced volume may be most prominent at the end of the day.

Radiation-induced dental disease is due largely to greater salivary acidity and decreased (106) salivary flow and to a lesser extent to a direct effect on the teeth and surrounding soft tissues. Saliva becomes sticky (108) and mastication painful (106), with the patient converting to a soft, high-carbohydrate diet that promotes dental caries and plaque. Routine dental hygiene also becomes more painful. Diligent dental follow-up is important to minimize extent of dental caries. Artificial saliva products are recommended (108). A sodium fluoride gel should be used daily, and dilute peroxide or saline rinses can be used during the course of treatment to cleanse the mouth. Sugarless gum or lozenges may stimulate salivation (108). Diet should emphasize fluids, moist foods, and high-calorie supplements. For edentulous patients, one should wait 6 months after radiation therapy before replacing dentures secondary to gingival shrinking and remodeling (108).

Techniques for improving jaw motion include active stretching exercises, mechanical stretching progressively with tongue blades or other devices (such as Therabite, Therabite Corp, Newton Sq, PA), and continuous passive motion devices (112).

Drooling or microstomia may result after excision of lip lesions. Mandibulectomy can affect cosmesis and the ability to chew, especially anterior mandible (arch) resections. Reconstructive procedures may be considered. After unilateral mandibular resections, strengthening of masticatory muscles is needed to prevent drift to the nonsurgical side (108).

Tongue lesions will affect speech and swallowing, especially if extensive muscle infiltration has occurred. Palsy of the hypoglossal nerve rarely occurs from direct invasion in posterior tongue lesions, or postirradiation or surgery (106). Irradiation is often selected as initial therapy for base of tongue malignancies because surgical approaches impair speech and swallow more frequently (106). Glossectomy is performed initially if the lesion is advanced at presentation. Enunciation difficulties result if the tongue is bound down by scarring. Radiation therapy produces tongue sensitivity, which is temporary, reduced taste sensation, which usually improves over time, and dry mouth. Fibrosis of the base of the tongue postradiation therapy produces dysphagia, but aspiration is rare (106). Local and systemic pain management strategies for painful soft-tissue necrosis may be needed (106). After glossectomy, the patient should be instructed in strengthening and range of motion of residual tongue tissue, especially if radiation therapy is to follow. The program usually begins 10 to 14 days after surgery. Compensatory strategies such as forward or backward head tilts, strengthening of buccal musculature, and even use of an intraoral appliance may facilitate deglutition. Oral transit can be achieved with use of a syringe or pusher spoon (108).

Buccal mucosa and tonsillar lesions often refer pain to the ear. Trismus may result from posterior extension to the buccinator or masseter muscles or from high radiation doses to these muscles (106). Soft palate lesions when advanced can cause dysphagia and voice change. If soft-tissue destruction occurs, material may be regurgitated into the nasopharynx. Local extension may lead to trismus, headache, and cranial nerve involvement (106). After soft palate resection, a prosthesis is needed to restore velopharyngeal competence.

Strategies for improved communication include use of good eye contact and appropriate gestures, oral exercises for articulation, and any necessary modification of pitch, loudness, and voice quality (113).

Laryngeal lesions are divided into supraglottic, glottic, and subglottic sites. Glottic tumors usually present early with hoarseness, and lymphatic spread is rare due to a sparse lymphatic network. Supraglottic lesions most commonly involve the epiglottis but may affect the aryepiglottic fold and false vocal cord and are more likely to undergo lymphatic spread. Common symptoms include dysphagia, throat irritation, hoarseness, odynophagia, and otalgia. The subglottic area extends from about 5 mm below the vocal cords to the inferior border of the cricoid cartilage. Lesions in this area are uncommon. Among laryngeal tumors, true vocal cord lesions are the most curable, followed by false cord, epiglottic, aryepiglottic fold, pyriform sinus, and hypopharyngeal lesions (106).

Surgical options include vocal cord stripping, hemilaryngectomy and supraglottic laryngectomy (which preserve the voice), and total laryngectomy. With the latter, a permanent tracheostomy is placed, and the pharynx is sutured to the base of the tongue (106). Patients may learn esophageal speech or may use electronic devices for speech. Trancheoesophageal puncture, in which exhaled air is channeled through a voice prosthesis into the esophagus, can result in a more natural sounding voice. During speech, the tracheostomy is occluded with a finger or one-way valve (114).

Patients with pre-existing pulmonary impairment, specifically low forced expiratory volume in one second/forced vital capacity (FEV_1/FVC) ratio are more likely to have intractable aspiration after supraglottic laryngectomy (115). Other risk factors for long-term dysphagia include bilateral supraglottic laryngectomy, bilateral superior laryngeal nerve excision (116), sacrifice of the tongue base (106), and possibly combined treatment with radiation therapy (116). Many patients experience postoperative dysphagia that is transient, with up to 85% of supraglottic laryngectomy patients attaining a functional swallow (improved from only 39% in the early postoperative period) (115). Techniques such as breath holding during the swallow and throat clear afterward may prevent or minimize aspiration (108). When feasible, occluding the trachestomy decreases frequency and amount of aspiration (117).

Pharyngeal tumors most commonly involve the pyriform sinus. The recurrent laryngeal nerve may be involved. Extensive regional infiltration is common. Initial symptoms are often unilateral. Partial or total laryngopharyngectomy may be indicated. Total laryngopharyngectomy may be combined with reconstruction from a pectoralis myocutaneous flap. Either of these procedures may be complicated by fistula, and in the case of the partial laryngopharyngectomy, by dysphagia and aspiration (106). For posterior pharyngeal lesions, radiation therapy is generally the preferred treatment, but carotid rupture and radiation myelitis are risks (106).

Nasopharyngeal tumors have a high incidence, about 25%, of associated cranial nerve symptoms. Cavernous sinus invasion affects cranial nerves II through VI, and extension from the lateral pharyngeal space laterally can involve nerves IX through XII and the sympathetic chain. Facial neuralgia may result from trigeminal nerve involvement. Proptosis, epistaxis, and otitis media may occur (106). Surgical resection is often not feasible. Radiation therapy complications can include radiation encephalopathy, especially involving the hypothalamus, pituitary, and frontal and temporal lobes; recovery usually occurs (106). Radiation myelitis of the cervical cord or brain stem can be more severe. Radiation fibrosis involving the pterygoid muscles causes trismus, and involvement of the lateral pharyngeal space can cause palsy of cranial nerves IX through XII as a delayed complication (106).

Nasal cavity and paranasal sinus tumors typically present with sinusitis-type symptoms, including discharge, aching, intermittent headache or tooth pain, epistaxis, proptosis, or diplopia. Excision can be deforming but is appropriate for smaller lesions. Complications of radiation therapy can involve the CNS, including radiation-induced CNS disease, cerebrospinal fluid leak, meningitis, brain abscess, and a delayed, transient vertiginous syndrome (106).

Salivary gland tumors often present with a palpable mass. Facial nerve involvement may occur. More rare is involvement of cranial nerves IX through XII and the sympathetic chain, as well as the mandibular branch of cranial nerve V. Postoperatively, facial nerve palsy often occurs but usually recovers over a few months (106). Xerostomia and trismus may occur postradiation therapy.

Hematologic Malignancies

Hematologic malignancies include tumors involving the lymphatics and hematopoietic system. Lymphomas include Hodgkin's disease, non-Hodgkin's lymphomas, mycosis fungoides, and Burkitt's lymphomas. Bone marrow disorders include acute and chronic leukemias and myeloproliferative disorders such as polycythemia vera, myelofibrosis, and primary thrombocytopenia. Immunoproliferative diseases include multiple myeloma and Waldenstrom's macroglobulinemia (54).

Lymphomas characteristically invade lymphatics but can readily invade any tissue. They are frequently associated with pain, due to painful lytic or blastic invasion of bone. Neuritic pain may result from nerve root infiltration, spinal cord compression, or herpes zoster. Lymphomas have been associated with acute inflammatory demyelinating polyneuropathy. Lymphedema can result from lymphatic obstruction, and thrombophlebitis from extrinsic compression on adjacent veins. Depressed cell-mediated immunity in Hodgkin's disease results in increased risk of opportunistic infection, and herpes zoster is common, especially in patients treated with radiation therapy. Standard chemotherapy with MOPP (mechlorethamine, vincristine, prednisone, and procarbazine) may result in peripheral polyneuropathy (54).

Thoracic (mantle) radiation therapy may be complicated by radiation pneumonitis, cardiac abnormalities (constrictive pericarditis, cardiomyopathy), and hypothyroidism. Aseptic necrosis of the femoral heads is described in 10% of long-term survivors of inverted y-field (abdominopelvic) irradiation and MOPP (54,118).

Non-Hodgkin's lymphoma is likely to be widely disseminated and involve bone marrow at the time of presentation. Nodular and diffuse lymphomas have a more favorable prognosis than lymphoblastic or undifferentiated tumors. Advanced disease is treated with multiple agent chemotherapy such as cyclophosphamide, doxorubicin, vincristine, prednisone (CHOP) or bleomycin, doxorubicin, cyclophosphamide, vincristine, prednisone (BACOP) (54).

Mycosis fungoides is a cutaneous T-cell lymphoma involving helper T-lymphocytes. Patients have significant itching and skin management problems with this lymphoma. Whirlpool treatment may be of benefit for the intractable pruritus and widespread skin scaling that can occur.

Burkitt's lymphoma typically presents in childhood and is rapidly progressive and disseminating. Facial bones and long bones are often involved, as are retroperitoneal soft tissues and the CNS. Whole brain irradiation is performed for CNS involvement (54).

Immunoproliferative diseases such as multiple myeloma and Waldenstrom's macroglobulinemia occur in older individuals (average age 60 years at diagnosis). With multiple myeloma, multiple lytic lesions are seen in about 70% of patients, single osteolytic lesions or diffuse osteoporosis in 15%, and normal x-rays in 15%. The skull, vertebrae, ribs, pelvis, and proximal long bones are the most common sites of involvement (54). The lytic lesions occur due to production of osteoclast activating factor by tumor. Bone scans are of limited usefulness and are only positive in areas of fracture or arthritis, or areas of perilesional osteoblastic activity. Osteoblastic lesions are rare (incidence of less than 2%) and often occur with neuropathy (54). Painful pathologic frac-

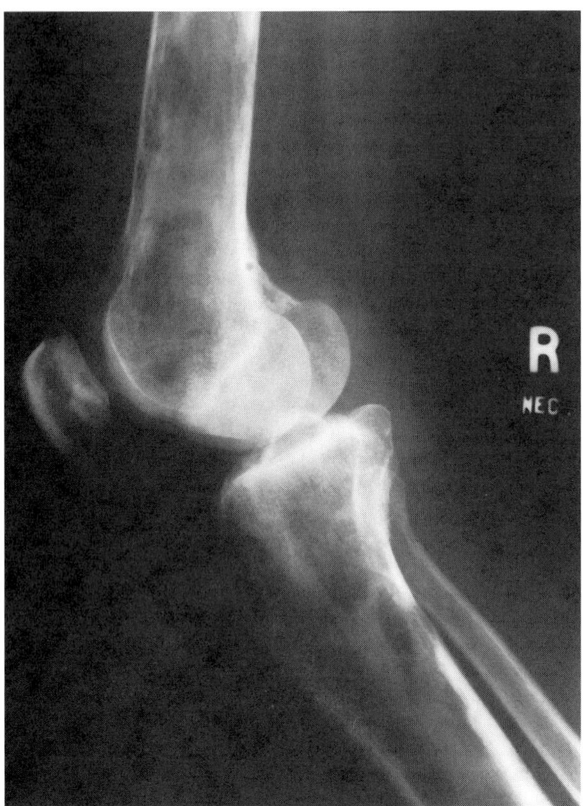

FIG. 52-5. Leukemic infiltrates involving femur, with significant cortical involvement.

tures are common. Neurologic dysfunction is common, including spinal cord or nerve root compression from epidural plasmacytoma, amyloidosis, or vertebral body collapse. Cranial nerve palsies occur from tumor-occluding calvarial foramina and focal peripheral neuropathies, such as carpal tunnel syndrome, from soft-tissue amyloid infiltration. Fatigue, weakness, and weight loss are common. Bone lesions are responsive to radiation therapy, which can be used for pain control and to shrink a bone mass before fracture occurs. Alkylating agents with or without prednisone are also used (Fig. 52-5). Ambulation should be encouraged, with bracing or assistive devices as needed to control pain.

Waldenstrom's macroglobulinemia may produce neurologic symptoms on the basis of hyperviscosity, such as malaise, stroke, and coma (54).

The leukemias produce fatigue. Bone pain may result from leukemic masses in the bone marrow (54). Leukostasis can produce severe CNS abnormalities, when the white blood count is more than 100,000, especially in the later acute stage of chronic myelogenous leukemia. Cerebrospinal fluid involvement may occur, producing leukemic meningitis with associated cranial nerve palsy and mental status changes (118,110). In children, the skeleton is often the first body system to manifest abnormality, and acute leukemia must be included in the differential diagnosis of unexplained musculoskeletal pain or bony pathology (119).

Rehabilitation intervention for leukemias and lymphomas involves active exercise, including walking, to maintain stamina during the treatment course, which is often protracted. Precautions surround the risk of bleeding in thrombocytopenic patients (see Exercise and Cancer), pressure palsies, especially in patients receiving neurotoxic drugs or with severe immobilization, and orthostasis, especially in those on fluid restriction (e.g., due to treatment with Ara-C) or with poor nutritional state (118). Restricted weight bearing is advised for bony extensive infiltration or aseptic necrosis.

Bone marrow transplant recipients have additional needs. High-dose steroids are needed to counteract graft-versus-host disease, with potential complications including steroid myopathy, aseptic necrosis, and osteoporosis. The exercise program should include proximal muscle strengthening, back extension, and upper extremity weight bearing (118) (see "Exercise and Cancer" section for further discussion of exercise for bone marrow transplant recipients).

Lung Cancer

Lung malignancies remain very common and are challenging for the physiatrist. Cure is possible in some cases, especially when the disease is detected early and in an operable location, but generally the prognosis remains poor. Often even short or intermediate-term prognosis is poor, so a traditional inpatient rehabilitation admission is often both a poor use of resources and a poor way for the patient to spend his or her remaining days. This often poses a dilemma for the physiatrist because lung cancer produces the fatigue and deconditioning that occur with virtually any chronic illness, as well as myriad potential neurologic complications. These include peripheral polyneuropathy, mixed sensory-motor axonal in type, and, more rarely, a sensory polyneuropathy due to dorsal root ganglionitis. Myasthenic syndrome is linked to small cell carcinoma and may or may not respond to treatment of the underlying malignancy. Nerve root infiltration may occur, producing pain and weakness. Vertebral bony involvement can produce extradural spinal cord compression, and brain metastasis is common, resulting in severe neurologic impairment. Apical lung tumors, such as Pancoast tumor, can invade the brachial plexus or lower cervical nerve roots by direct extensions, producing pain as an early symptom that is often referred to the shoulder, and appropriate diagnosis may be delayed while the patient is treated for a nonexistent musculoskeletal shoulder problem. Eventually a full blown brachial plexopathy occurs, with paresthesias, weakness, and numbness, characteristically involving the lower fibers more than upper fibers.

The neurologic complications often occur early in the clinical course and may even be the presenting feature. Thus, the patient and family are coping with the new diagnosis and with the functional impact of the neurologic complications simultaneously. Often the family is willing but ill equipped to care for the patient at home. In selected cases, a short rehabilitation admission is appropriate to train the patient and family in safe mobility strategies and to assess for appropriate adaptive equipment.

Strategies for pain management using modalities of heat and cold, as well as education about pulmonary hygiene and breathing techniques, may be useful. Patients treated with surgical resection (either lobectomy or pneumonectomy) should be instructed in techniques to promote maximal chest expansion, including coughing, pursed-lip diaphagmatic breathing, and segmental breathing exercises. Trunk mobility should be taught to avoid splinting the operative side. Early progressive ambulation is recommended (120).

Gastrointestinal Malignancies

Gastrointestinal malignancies vary hugely in prognosis and in rapidity of clinical deterioration when cure does not occur. Pancreatic cancer remains among the most refractory to cure of all malignancies, and favorable prognostic indicators have not been delineated (121). Esophageal carcinoma also carries a poor prognosis, although improvements in survival with multimodality approaches (122,123) and in palliation for nutrition, using dilatation laser curettage (124), esophageal stents, or photodynamic therapy, have occurred in recent years (125). Liver and stomach malignancies (126,127) also carry a poor prognosis. Colon cancer is curable when caught early, and 5-year survival rates have increased to over 50% (128). In general, when liver metastasis occurs, the clinical state deteriorates rapidly (this is also true for nongastrointestinal malignancies).

Gastrointestinal malignancies are low to intermediate in risk for metastasis to bone and neurologic structures. Most often, rehabilitation is indicated for deconditioning, often occurring after extensive abdominal surgical procedures. In selected cases, a short rehabilitation course before return home is beneficial. Tolerance to active therapy and overall medical stability will determine whether this is done on an acute or subacute level. In postsurgical cases, close communication with the referring surgeon is important for management of drains and potential complications.

Brain Tumors

Brain tumors have increased in incidence since the mid-1960s, primarily in the elderly (129). Brain tumors vary widely in aggressiveness and in prognosis. However, unlike most other regions in the body, even a benign or relatively low-grade lesion may have severe functional consequences depending on location and the extent to which excision is feasible. Brain stem lesions in particular can have a profound impact on motor function, cranial nerves, swallowing, and coordination. In patients who have undergone resection, communication with the referring surgeon as to which structures have been sacrificed will be important in advising the patient about recovery of neurologic function.

In adults, meningiomas are the most common benign brain tumor, comprising about 15% of all primary brain tumors. Their growth may have a hormonal component, and increased incidence is seen in breast cancer patients (52). Other benign tumors include pituitary adenomas, acoustic neuromas, craniopharyngiomas, epidermoid tumors, colloid cysts of the third ventricle, and hemangioblastomas associated with Von-Hippel-Lindau disease. Pituitary adenomas present with features of hormonal hypersecretion, bitemporal visual field loss, or headache (52). Variants include prolactinomas, growth hormone–producing adenomas causing acromegaly, and corticotrophin-secreting adenomas producing Cushing's disease. Most are resectable. Acoustic neuromas grow on the nerve sheath of the vestibular nerve and may occur sporadically or with neurofibromatosis. Patients can develop hearing loss, vertigo, facial palsy, dysphagia, facial numbness, and even hydrocephalus. Results of microsurgery are generally good, especially with tumors measuring less than 2 cm (52). Craniopharyngiomas arise from pharyngeal epithelium, presenting with growth failure in children and sexual dysfunction or visual loss in adults. After treatment, deficits in memory, behavior, appetite, and endocrine function are common. Adjunctive radiation therapy is often used, with great improvement in the 10-year survival rate (52).

More than 90% of primary brain malignancies are malignant gliomas (129), subdivided into astrocytoma, anaplastic astrocytoma, and glioblastoma multiforme, each carrying a progressively poorer prognosis (52). Low-grade astrocytomas of the cerebral hemispheres may be resectable, but deeper lesions are more difficult to resect, and radiation therapy may be used. With the higher grade lesions, aggressive surgical excision is performed, except for diffuse pontine, hypothalamic, and deep frontal lesions. Adjunctive radiation therapy prolongs survival, either external beam irradiation or interstitial radiation with iodine 125 or iridium 192. External beam radiation typically consists of 5,000 to 6,000 rad and may be delivered to a limited field rather than the whole brain. Chemotherapy also shows promise in prolonging survival, and trials of immunotherapy are underway (52). Favorable prognostic features are younger age (130), high performance rating at diagnosis (8), and favorable histology (52).

Medulloblastomas comprise only about 5% of adult brain tumors, usually presenting in the cerebellar hemispheres, as opposed to the cerebral vermis in children. Primary cerebral lymphomas are increasing in incidence due to their association with the human immunodeficiency virus. Multiple tumor deposits are often present (131), and median survival is less than 1 year (52). Surgical removal does not improve outcome (132).

In children, brain malignancies are the most common type of solid tumor, comprising about a quarter of all childhood malignancies (54) and of all childhood cancer deaths (129). The most frequent tumors are of glial origin (including astrocytomas, oligodendroglioma, and ependymoma). However, the most common malignant tumor is medulloblastoma, which produces parenchymal invasion and leptomeningeal dissemination (133). Primitive neuroectodermal tumors are highly malignant and may seed the neuraxis (52). Tumors may be associated with underlying diseases such as neurofibromatosis, tuberous sclerosis, and Von Hippel-Lindau disease. Germinomas typically present during the first two decades of life and have a relatively favorable prognosis. Typically, they extend from the suprasellar or pineal region, producing endocrine, visual field, autonomic, cognitive, and behavioral disturbance (134). The lesions are highly radiosensitive. Stereotactic surgery also may be of benefit (134).

In patients 2 to 12 years of age, the majority of tumors are infratentorial (133), and the most common age of presentation is 4 to 8 years (135). Low-grade astrocytomas have a more than 90% 5-year survival rate if they can be surgically excised (54). Surgically accessible low-grade tumors include cerebellar astrocytoma, choroid plexus papilloma, and meningioma (133). In general, more superficial tumors are less likely to be malignant (135). Surgery is also a component of treatment for malignant or anatomically unresectable masses, augmented by radiation therapy. Chemotherapy can be life prolonging but seldom curative (133). It may have an increasing role in very young children (under 3 years of age) for whom radiation therapy has the most complications.

Long-term complications of brain tumor and its treatment can include intellectual, psychological, and endocrine deficits (133). Rehabilitation decisions are guided by the patient's neurologic status and clinical course. A patient whose neurologic status is actively worsening will likely not benefit from intensive rehabilitation, whereas, for example, a younger patient with anaplastic astrocytoma and median anticipated survival of over 3 years may benefit (130).

Rehabilitation interventions depend in part on the symptoms with which the patient presents. For the bed-bound patient, frequent turning, proper mattresses, sensory stimulation, and socialization are critical for supportive care. For those with mobility or potential for mobility, the use of orthotic devices and ambulation aides, including wheelchairs for those with significant balance difficulties, must be considered. Patients in whom weakness is the predominant concern may have a restorative option, and physical and occupational therapists should be consulted for activities of daily living assessment and provision of adaptive equipment and strengthening exercises. The cognitive, linguistic, and communicative ability should be assessed. Identifying the presence of cognitive deficits may be extremely helpful to frustrated family members. Treatment options may be available that can significantly improve the quality of life and socialization for this population.

Sarcomas of Bone and Soft Tissue

Sarcoma represents 1% of the total adult malignancies in the United States. These include osteosarcoma, Ewing's sarcoma, chondrosarcoma, giant cell sarcoma of bone, and soft-tissue sarcoma (muscle, fat, fibrous tissue, neuroectoderm). There is a 1.5:1 male to female ratio, and 45% of the tumors involve the lower extremity, 40% the head, neck, or trunk, and 15% the upper extremity (136). Management of sarcoma of the soft tissue or bone presents a substantial challenge to rehabilitation specialists. The key to successful oncologic management and ultimate functional outcome is good local control. This implies that the initial biopsy was performed carefully, tissue planes were not violated, and adequate margins of uninvolved tissue were obtained. Early detection and treatment are essential if individuals are to have a limb-sparing option. Most patients with soft-tissue sarcoma undergo a pretreatment staging, surgery that may consist of wide local excision, and chemotherapy. Many have additional radiation to the primary tumor site. Limb salvage surgery is possible for those who can achieve good local control without amputation. These patients must have a neurovascular bundle that is not compromised by tumor, have no pathologic fracture, have little extraosseous extension of tumor (for osteosarcoma group), have no distant spread of tumor, and have a high probability for good cosmetic and fucntional outcome. Patients must be informed of the possibility of subsequent need for amputation in the face of infection, fracture, or continued prosthetic loosening in the athletic population. The conversion rate may approach 15% to 20% in some series (137,138).

The pretreatment phase of sarcoma provides the rehabilitation team an opportunity to educate family and patient about what to expect, begin a program aimed at strength and stamina building, and introduce the patient to the use of ambulation devices and bathroom safety. The amputee is treated similarly to patients undergoing amputation for any reason. The cancer amputee, however, is likely to have relatively shorter residual limb because of the need to achieve adequate tumor-free margins. The concomitant use of chemotherapy and/or radiation may prolong the interval between surgery and delivery of a definitive prosthesis. Wound healing may be delayed, and residual limb volume shifts may interfere with weight stabilization. Socket adaptations can be made by adding and subtracting stump socks, using a series of flexible sockets, or padding the lining to adapt the fit. Meticulous wound care may be needed for those who have had irradiation to the stump. Details of postamputation management and prosthetic fitting are presented in Chapter 27.

Rehabilitation after limb-sparing surgery depends on the extent of soft tissue and bony structural excision. Patients with proximal tibia or distal femur lesions may be eligible for en bloc resection and use of a prosthetic knee (139). An internal hemipelvectomy may be possible for those with proximal femur lesions. Postoperatively, 1 to 2 weeks (and occasionally longer) of bed rest is needed to promote wound healing, reduce edema, and maintain alignment. Barring complications, quadriceps and gluteal sets, active assisted straight leg raises, and ankle pumps may be started 1 to 2 weeks postoperatively. Upright activity progresses from non–weight bearing to partial and full weight bearing based on muscle strength and wound healing (139).

Other limb-sparing procedures that are frequently undertaken in this population include the removal of portions of muscle. Muscles typically removed include the adductors, quadriceps, hamstrings, and gastrocnemius. Patients undergoing these procedures will need a period of bed rest until wound drainage stops. Leg elevation, compression garments, and active range of motion should be instituted as part of the rehabilitation process. Patients with quadriceps excision will need a knee immobilizer postoperatively and will need to ambulate with an ankle–foot orthrosis (AFO) that keeps the foot plantarflexed and blocks out dorsiflexion to create an extension moment at the knee. Some patients are able to develop a gait pattern substituting hip flexors, such that they have a stable knee and will not require an orthotic device (140). Adductor muscle group and hamstring excision rarely require assistive aides or orthotic device use. However, if there is sciatic nerve excision, an AFO will be needed to provide toe clearance. When the gastrocnemius is excised, a rocker sole needs to be added to the sole of the shoe to promote push-off. Achilles tendon stretching should be performed regularly to maintain ankle range of motion (140).

Prostate Cancer

Prostate cancer has a proclivity for metastasis to bone, but survival may be quite prolonged even after onset of bony metastatic disease. Metastatic lesions are typically blastic, and although it has been stated in the literature that blastic metastasis produces less risk of fracture than lytic lesions, in the experience of the authors pathologic fracture in prostate cancer is quite common. Often there is surrounding or generalized osteopenia, and this may be the basis or at least contributory to the fracture risk.

Patients also have genitourinary and sexual issues, especially those treated with radical prostatectomy. Inguinal or pelvic lymphadenopathy can result in lymphedema or deep venous thrombosis.

The rehabilitation problems of this population includes bone pain (for those who have metastatic lesions), fracture, and impaired mobility (see Bony Metastatic Disease section). Men who have undergone radical prostatectomy, radiation, and have antiandrogen therapy have impotence or sexual dysfunction (see section on Sexual Dysfunction). In addition, antiandrogen therapy is often associated with loss of muscle mass, strength, and endurance. These patients are frequently fatigued. Early intervention with strengthening and aerobic conditioning exercise may help mitigate the impact of this treatment.

CONCLUSION

The focus of rehabilitation interventions for this population is on pain relief, preservation or restoration of function, and education about planning and prioritizing life activities to assure quality. The rehabilitation team is in the unique position of being able to recommend practical suggestions to improve function and preserve independence, thereby offering patients some degree of hopefulness throughout the course of their illness.

REFERENCES

1. Boring CC, Squires TS, Tong T, Montgomery S. Cancer statistics 1994. *CA Cancer J Clin* 1994; 44:7–26.
2. Ries LAG, Miller BA, Hankey BF, et al. SEER cancer statistics review 1973-1991.
3. Lehmann J, DeLisa JA, Waarren CG, et al. Cancer rehabilitation assessment of need development and education of a model of care. *Arch Phys Med Rehabil* 1978; 59:410.
4. DeRogatis L, Abeloff M, Melisaratos N. Psychological coping mechanisms and survival time in metastatic breast cancer. *JAMA* 1979; 242: 1504.
5. Bergner M, Bobbitt R, Carter W, Gibson B. The sickness impact profile: development and final revision of a health status measure. *Med Care* 1981; 19:787.
6. Ganz PA. Long range effect of clinical trial interventions on quality of life. *Cancer* 1994; 74(suppl 9):2620–2624.
7. Osoba D. Lessons learned from measuring health-related quality of life in oncology. *J Clin Oncol* 1994; 12:608–616.
8. Karnofsky DA, Abelmann WH, Craver LF, Burchenal, JH. The use of the nitrogen mustards in palliative treatment of carcinoma. *Cancer* 1948; 1:634–656.
9. Fawzy FI, Fawzy NW, Hyun CS, Elashoff R, et al. Malignant melanoma: effects of an early structured psychiatric intervention, coping and affective state on recurrence and survival 6 years laters. *Arch Gen Psych* 1993; 50:681–689.
10. Given CW, Given BA, Stommel M. The impact of age, treatment and symptoms on the physical and mental health of cancer patients: a longitudinal perspective. *Cancer* 1994; 74(suppl 7):2128–2138.
11. Marciniak CM, Sliwa JA, Spill G, Heinemann AW, Semik PE. Functional outcome following rehabilitation of the cancer patient. *Arch Phys Med Rehabil* 1996; 77:54–57.
12. O'Toole DM, Golden AM. Evaluating cancer patients for rehabilitation potential. *West J Med* 1991; 155:3847–3847.
13. Mellette SJ. The evolving role of cancer rehabilitation in cancer care. *Rehabil Oncol* 1995; 13:25.
14. McKinley WO, Conti-Wyneken AR, Vokac CW, Cifu DX. Rehabilitative functional outcome of patients with neoplastic spinal cord compression. *Arch Phys Med Rehabil* 1996; 77:892–895.
15. Yoshioka H. Rehabilitation for the terminal cancer patient. *Am J Phys Med Rehabil* 1994; 73:199–206.
16. Portenoy RK. Cancer pain pathophysiology and syndromes. *Lancet* 1992; 339:1026.
17. Acute pain management guideline panel. *Acute pain management: operative or medical procedures and trauma.* Rockville, MD: AHCPR, PHS, US Department of Health and Human Services 1992; 145 (Clinical Practice Guideline, AHCPR Publication No. 92-0032).
18. World Health Organization. *Cancer pain and relief and palliative care.* Geneva, Switzerland: World Health Organization, 1990; 75.
19. Management of cancer pain guideline panel. *Management of cancer pain.* Clinical practice guideline no. 9. U.S. Department of Health and Human Services, PHS, Agency for Health Care Policy and Research. AHCPR Pub. No. 94-0592, 1994; 75–88.
20. Cherny NI, Portenoy RK. Cancer pain: principles of assessment and syndromes. In: Wall PO, Melzack R, eds. *Textbook of pain,* 3rd ed. London: Churchill-Livingstone, 1994; 782.
21. Ventafridda V, Tamburini M, Caraceni A, et al. A validation study of the WHO method for cancer pain relief. *Cancer* 1987; 59:850–856.
22. Cousins MJ, Bridenbough PO, eds. *Neural blockade in clinical anesthesia and management of pain,* 2nd ed. Philadelphia: JB Lippincott, 1988; 1171.
23. Abrams HL, Spiro R, Goldstein N. Metastases in carcinoma: analysis of 1,000 autopsied cases. *Cancer* 1950; Jan:74–85.
24. Sherry HS, Levy RN, Siffert RS. Metastatic disease of bone in orthopedic surgery. *Clin Orthop Rel Res* 1982; 169:44–52.
25. Tubiana-Hulin M. Incidence, prevalence and distribution of bone metastases. *Bone* 1991; 12(suppl 1):9–10.

26. Bhalla SK. Metastatic disease of the spine. *Clin Orthop* 1970; 73: 52–60.
27. Brage ME, Simon MA. Evaluation, prognosis and medical treatment considerations of metastatic bone tumors. *Orthopedics* 1992; 15: 589–595.
28. Boland PJ, Billings J, Healey JH. The management of pathologic fractures. *J Back Musculoskel Rehabil* 1993; 3:27–34.
29. Sim FH. Metastatic bone disease: philosophy of treatment. *Orthopedics* 1992; 15:541–544.
30. Vargo MM. Orthopedic management of malignant bone lesions. *PM&R State Art Rev* 1994; 8:363–391.
31. Beals R, Lawton GD, Snell W. Prophylactic internal fixation of the femur in metastatic breast cancer. *Cancer* 1971; 28:1350–1354.
32. Behr JT, Dobozi WR, Badrinath K. The treatment of pathologic and impending pathologic fractures of the proximal femur in the elderly. *Clin Orthop Rel Res* 1985; 198:173–178.
33. Harrington KD. New trends in the management of lower extremity metastases. *Clin Orthop* 1982; 169:53–61.
34. Thompson RC. Impending fracture associated with bone destruction. *Orthopedics* 1992; 15:547–550.
35. Habermann ET, Sachs R, Stern RE, Hirsh DM, Anderson WJ. The pathology and treatment of metastatic disease of the femur. *Clin Orthop* 1982; 169:70–82.
36. Lane JM, Sculco TP, Zolan S. Treatment of pathological fractures of the hip by endoprosthetic replacement. *J Bone Joint Surgery [Am]* 1980; 62:954–959.
37. Menck H, Schulze S, Larsen E. Metastasis size in pathologic femoral fractures. *Acta Orthop Scand* 1988; 59:151–154.
38. Mandi A, Szepesi K, Morocz I. Surgical treatment of pathologic fractures from metastatic tumors of long bones. *Orthop Surg Hungary* 1991; 14:43–49.
39. Keene JS, Sellinger DS, McBeath AA, Engber WD. Metastatic breast cancer in the femur: a search for the lesions at risk of fracture. *Clin Orthop* 1986; 203:282–288.
40. Denis F. Spinal instability as defined by the three-column spine concept in acute spinal trauma. *Clin Orthop* 1984; 189:65–76.
41. O'Connor MI, Currier BL. Metastatic disease of the spine. *Orthopedics* 1992; 15:611–620.
42. Pal GP, Sherk HH. The vertical stability of the cervical spine. *Spine* 1988; 13:447–449.
43. Richardson ML, Kilcoyne RF, Gillespy T, Helms CA, Genant HK. Magnetic resonance imaging of musculoskeletal neoplasms. *Radiol Clin North Am* 1986; 24:259–267.
44. Citrin DL, Bessent RG, Greig WR. A comparison of the sensitivity and accuracy of the phosphate bone scan and skeletal radiograph in the diagnosis of bone metastases. *Clin Radiol* 1977; 28:107–117.
45. Garmatis CJ, Ghu FCH. The effectiveness of radiation therapy in the treatment of bone metastases from breast cancer. *Radiology* 1978; 126:235–237.
46. Blake DD. Radiation treatment of metastatic bone disease. *Clin Orthop* 1970; 73:89–100.
47. Robinson HS. Cane for measurement and recording of stress. *Arch Phys Med Rehabil* 1969; 50:457–459.
48. McDonnell ME, Shea BD. The role of physical therapy in patients with metastatic disease to bone. *J Back Musculoskel Rehabil* 1993; 3:78–84.
49. Posner JB, Chernik NL. Intracranial metastases from systemic cancer. *Adv Neurol* 1978; 19:579–592.
50. Patchell RA. Brain metastases: neurologic complications of systemic cancer. *Neurol Clin* 1991; 9:817–824.
51. Zimm S, Wampler GL, Stablein D, Hazra T, Young HF. Intracerebral metastases in solid tumor patient: natural history and results of treatment. *Cancer* 1981; 48:384–394.
52. Black P. Medical progress: brain tumors. *N Engl J Med* 1991; 324: 1471–1476; 1555–1564.
53. Schlicht LA, Smelz JK. Metastatic spinal cord compression. *PM&R State Art Rev* 1994; 8:345–361.
54. Casciato DA, Lowitz BB. *Manual of bedside oncology,* 1st ed. Boston: Little, Brown, 1986.
55. Gilbert RW, Kim JH, Posner JB. Epidural spinal cord comperssion from metastatic tumor: diagnosis and treatment. *Ann Neurol* 1978; 3: 40–51.
56. Hill ME, Richards MA, Gregory WM, et al. Spinal cord compression in breast cancer: a review of 70 cases. *Br J Cancer* 1993; 68:969.
57. Ku A, Lachmann E, Tunkel R, Nagler W. Upper limb reflex sympathetic dystrophy associated with occult malignancy. *Arch Phys Med Rehabil* 1996; 77:726–728.
58. Hammack JE, Kimmel DW, O'Neill BP, Lennon Va. Paraneoplastic cerebellar degeneration: a clinical comparison of patients with and without Purkinje cell cytoplasmic antibodies. *Mayo Clin Proc* 1990; 65:1423–1431.
59. Sliwa JA, Thatcher S, Jet J. Paraneoplastic subacute cerebellar degeneration: functional improvement and the role of rehabilitation. *Arch Phys Med Rehabil* 1994; 75:355–357.
60. Stubgen JP. Neuromuscular disorders in systemic malignancy and its treatment. *Muscle Nerve* 1995; 18:636–648.
61. Campbell MJ, Paty DW. Carcinomatous neuromyopathy: electrophysiological studies—an electrophysiological and immunological study of patients with carcinoma of the lung. *J Neurol Neurosurg Psychiatry* 1974; 37:131–141.
62. Forman A. Peripheral neuropathy in cancer patients: incidence, features, and pathophysiology. Part 1. *Oncology* 1990; 4:57–62.
63. Hawley RJ, Cohen MH, Saini N, Armbrustmacher VW. The carcinomatous neuromyopathy of oat cell lung cancer. *Ann Neurol* 1980; 7:65–72.
64. Barron SA, Heffer RR. Weakness in malignancy: evidence for a remote effect of tumor on distal axons. *Ann Neurol* 1978; 4:268–274.
65. Horwich MS, Cho L, Porro RS, Posner JB. Subactue sensory neuropathy a remote effect of carcinoma. *Ann Neurol* 1977; 2:7–19.
66. Pourmand R, Maybury BG. AAEM case report #31: paraneoplastic sensory neuronopathy. *Muscle Nerve* 1996; 19:1517–1522.
67. Johnson PC. Hematogenous metastases of carcinoma to dorsal root ganglia. *Acta Neuropathol* 1977; 38:171–172.
68. McLeod JF, Walsh JC. Peripheral neuropathy associated with lymphomas and other reticuloses. In: Dyck PJ, ed. *Peripheral neuropathy.* Philadelphia: WB Saunders, 1984; 2192–2203.
69. Kelly JJ. Peripheral neuropathies associated with plasma cell dyscrasias. In: Brown WF, Bolton CF, eds. *Clinical electromyography.* Boston: Butterworths, 1986.
70. Matsubayashi T, Koga H, Nishiyama Y, Shinicki T, Sawanda T. The reparative process of metastatic bone lesions after radiotherapy. *Jpn J Clin Oncol Suppl* 1981; 11:253–264.
71. Watne K, Hager B, Heier M, Hirschberg H. Reversible edema and necrosis after irradiation of the brain. *Acta Oncol* 1990; 29:891–895.
72. DeLattre JY, Posner JB. Neurological complications of chemotherapy and radiation therapy. In: Aminoff MJ, ed. *Neurology and general medicine.* New York: Churchill-Livingstone, 1989; 365–387.
73. Spence R. Nutritional concerns in cancer patients. *PM&R State Art Rev* 1994; 8:404.
74. Daly JM, Torosian MH. Nutritional support. In: DeVita VT, Hellman S, Rosenberg SA, eds. *Cancer: principles and practice of oncology,* 4th ed. Philadelphia: JB Lippincott, 1993; 2480–2501.
75. Sonis ST. Oral complications of cancer therapy. In: DeVita VT, Hellman S, Rosenberg SA, eds. *Cancer: principles and practice of oncology,* 4th ed. Philadelphia: JB Lippincott, 1993; 2385–2394.
76. Schover LR, Montague DK, Schain W. Sexual problems. In: DeVita VT, Helllman S, Rosenberg SA, eds. *Cancer: principles and practice of oncology,* 4th ed. Philadelphia: JB Lippincott, 1993; 2464–2480.
77. Schover LR. Sexual rehabilitation after treatment for prostrate cancer. *Cancer Suppl* 1993; 71:1024–1030.
78. Glasgow M, Halfin V, Althausen AF. Sexual response and cancer. *CA Cancer J Clin* 1987; 37:322–333.
79. Gerraughty SM. Sexual function in cancer patients. *PM&R State Art Rev* 1994; 8:251–260.
80. Smelz JK, Schlicht LA. Rehabilitation of the cancer patient after bone marrow transplantation. *PM&R State Art Rev* 1994; 8:321–323.
81. Gaydos LA, Freireich EJ, Mantel N. The quantitative relation between platelet count and hemorrhage in patients with acute leukemia. *N Engl J Med* 1962; 226:905–909.
82. James MC. Physical therapy for patients after bone marrow transplantation. *Phys Ther* 1987; 67:946–952.
83. St. Pierre BA, Kasper CE, Lindsey AM. Fatigue mechanisms in patients with cancer: effects of tumor necrosis factor and exercise on skeletal muscle. *Oncol Nurs Forum* 1991; 19:419–425.
84. Sharkey AM, Carey AB, Heise CT, Barber G. Cardiac rehabilitation after cancer therapy in children and young adults. *Am J Cardiol* 1993; 71:1488–1490.
85. MacVicar MG, Winningham ML, Nickel JL. Effects of aerobic interval training on cancer patients functional capacity. *Nurs Res* 1989; 38:348–351.
86. Bruzzi P, Green SB, Byar DP, et al. Estimating the population attribut-

able risk for multiple risk factors using case-control data. *Am J Epidemiol* 1985; 122:904.

87. Kissin MW, dellaRovere QG, Easton D, et al. Risk of lymphedema following the treatment of breast cancer. *Br J Surg* 1986; 7:580.
88. Werner RS, McCormick B, Petrek JA, et al. Arm edema in conservatively managed breast cancer: obesity is a major predictive factor. *Radiology* 1991; 180:177.
89. Gerber LH. Rehabilitation management for women with breast cancer: maximizing functional outcomes. In: Harris JR, Lippman MG, Morrow M, Hellman S, eds. *Diseases of the breast.* Philadelphia: Lippincott-Raven, 1996; 939–947.
90. Atkins H, Hayward JL, Klugman DJ, et al. Treatment of early breast cancer: a report after 10 years of a clinical trial. *Br Med J* 1972; 2: 423.
91. Pollard K, Callum KG, Altman DG, et al. Shoulder movement following mastectomy. *Clin Oncol* 1976; 2:343.
92. Aitken RJ, Gaze MN, Rodger A, et al. Arm morbidity within a trial of mastectomy and either nodal sample with selective radiotherapy or axillary clearance. *Br J Surg* 1989; 76:568.
93. Lotze MT, Duncan MA, Gerber LH, et al. Early vs delayed shoulder motion following axillary dissection. *Ann Surg* 1981; 193:288.
94. Jansen RF, van Geel AN, de Groot HG, et al. Immediate versus delayed shoulder exercises after axillary lymph node dissection. *Am J Surg* 1990; 160:481.
95. Dawson I, Stan K, Heslinga JM, et al. Effect of shoulder immobilization on wound seroma and shoulder dysfunction following modified radical mastectomy: a randomized prospective clinical trial. *Br J Surg* 1989; 76:311.
96. Zelikovski A, Deutsch A, Reiss R. The sequential pneumatic compression device in surgery for lymphedema of the limbs. *J Cardiovasc Surg* 1983; 24:18.
97. Bastien MR, Goldstein BG, Lesher JL Jr, et al. Treatment of lymphedema with a multicompartmental pneumatic compression device. *J Am Acad Dermatol* 1989; 20:853.
98. Foeldi E, Foeldi M, Weissleder H. Conservative treatment of lymphedema of the limbs. *Angiol J Vasc Dis* 1985; 36:171.
99. Casley-Smith JR, Morgan RG, Piller NB. Treatment of lymphedema of the arms and legs with 5,6-benzo-[alpha]-pyrone. *N Engl J Med* 1993; 16:329.
100. Harrington KD. *Orthopaedic management of metastatic bone disease.* St. Louis: CV Mosby, 1988; 7.
101. Harrington KD. Metastatic disease of the spine. *J Bone Joint Surg [Am]* 1986; 68:1110.
102. Gonzales GR, Elliiot KJ, Portenoy RK, et al. The impact of a comprehensive evaluation in the management of cancer pain. *Pain* 1991; 47: 141.
103. Kori SH, Foley KM, Posner JB, et al. Brachial plexus lesions in patients with cancer 100 cases. *Neurology* 1981; 31:45.
104. Bagley FH, Walsh JW, Cady B, et al. Carcinomatous versus radiation induced brachial plexus neuropathy in breast cancer. *Cancer* 1978; 41:2154.
105. Lederman RJ, Wilbourn AJ. Brachial plexopathy, recurrent cancer or radiation? *Neurology* 1984; 34:1331.
106. Million RR, Cassisi NJ, Clark JR. Cancer of the head and neck. In: DevVita VT, Hellman S, Rosenberg SA, eds. *Cancer: principles and practice of oncology,* 3rd ed. Philadelphia: JB Lippincott, 1989; 488–590.
107. Beahrs OH. Surgical anatomy and technique of radical neck dissection. *Surg Clin North Am* 1977; 57:663–700.
108. Dudgeon BJ, DeLisa JA, Miller RM. Head and neck cancer: rehabilitation approach. *Am J Occup Ther* 1980; 34:243–251.
109. Saunders WH, Johnson EW. Rehabilitation of the shoulder after radical neck dissection. *Ann Otol* 1975; 84:812–816.
110. Roberts WL. Rehabilitation of the head and neck cancers patient. In: McGarvey CL, ed. *Physical therapy for the cancer patient.* New York: Churchill-Livingstone, 1990.
111. Villanueva R. Orthosis to correct shoulder pain and deformity after trapezius palsy. *Arch Phys Med Rehabil* 1977; 58:30–34.
112. Buchbinder D, Currivan RB, Kaplan AJ, Urken ML. Mobilization regimens for the prevention of jaw hypomobility in the radiated patient. *J Oral Maxillofac Surg* 1993; 51:863–867.
113. LaBlance GR, Kraus K, Karen FS. Rehabilitation of swallowing and communication following glossectomy. *Rehabil Nurs* 1991; 16: 266–269.
114. Lockhart JS, Bryce J. Restoring speech and tracheoesophageal puncture. *Nursing* 1993; 23:59–61.
115. Beckhardt RN, Murray JG, Ford CH, Grossman JE, Brandenburg JH. Factors influencing functional outcome in supraglottic laryngectomy. *Head Neck* 1994; 16:232–239.
116. Weaver AW, Fleming SM. Partial laryngectomy: analysis of associated swallowing disorders. *Am J Surg* 1978; 136:486–489.
117. Muz J, Hamlet S, Mathog R, Farris R. Scintigraphic assessment of aspiration in head and neck cancer patients with tracheostomy. *Head Neck* 1994; 16:17–20.
118. Holtzman L, Chesey K. Rehabilitation of the leukemia/lymphoma patient. In: McGarvey CL, ed. *Physical therapy for the cancer patient.* New York: Churchill-Livingstone, 1990; 85–110.
119. Gallagher D, Heinrich SD, Craver R, Ward K, Warrier R. Skeletal manifestations of acute leukemia in childhood. *Orthopedics* 1991; 14: 485–492.
120. Shea BD, Vlad G. Rehabilitation of the lung cancer patient. In: McGarvey CL, ed. *Physical therapy for the cancer patient.* New York: Churchill-Livingstone, 1990; 29–45.
121. Gudjonsson B. Cancer of the pancreas: 50 years of surgery. *Cancer* 1987; 60:2284–2303.
122. Roth JA, Ajani JA, Rich TA. Multidisciplinary therapy for esophageal cancer. *Adv Surg* 1990; 23:239–260.
123. Ellis FH. Treatment of carcinoma of the esophagus or cardia. *Mayo Clin Proc* 1989; 64:945–955.
124. Lundell L, Leth R, Lind T, Lonroth H, Sjovall M, Olbe L. Palliative endoscopic dilatation of the esophagus and esophagogastric junction. *Acta Chir Scand* 1989; 155:179–184.
125. Boyce GA. Palliation of malignant esophageal obstruciton. *Dysphagia* 1990; 5:220–226.
126. Meyers WC, Damiano RJ, Rotolo FS, Postlethwait RW. Adenocarcinoma of the stomach: changing patterns over the last 4 decades. *Ann Surg* 1987; 205:1–7.
127. Baba H, Korenaga D, Okamura T, Saito A, Sugimachi K. Prognostic factor in gastric cancer with serosal invasion. *Arch Surg* 1989; 124: 1061–1064.
128. Cohen AM, Minsky BD, Schilsky RL. Colon cancer. In: DeVita VT, Hellman S, Rosenberg SA, eds. *Cancer: principles and practice of oncology,* 4th ed. Philadelphia: JB Lippincott, 1993; 929–930.
129. Bondy ML, Wrensch M. Perspective in prevention: update on brain cancer epidemiology. *Cancer Bull* 1993; 45:365–369.
130. Silverstein MD, Cascino TL, Harmsen WS, et al. High grade astrocytomas: resource use, clinical outcomes and cost care. *Mayo Clin Proc* 1996; 71:936–944.
131. Remick SC, Diamond C, Migliozzi JA, Solis O, et al. Primary central nervous system lymphoma in patients with and without the acquired immune deficiency syndrome. *Medicine* 1990; 69:345–360.
132. O Neill BP, Illig JJ. Primary central nervous system lymphoma. *Mayo Clin Proc* 1989; 64:1005–1020.
133. Friedman HS, Horowitz M, Oakes WJ. Tumors of the central nervous system: improvement in outcome through a multimodality approach. *Pediatr Clin North Am* 1991; 38:381–391.
134. Horowitz MB, Hall WA. Central nervous system germinomas. *Arch Neurol* 1991; 48:652–657.
135. Hardwood-Nash DC. Primary neoplasms of the central nervous system in children. *Cancer* 1991; 67:1223–1228.
136. Sondak V, Economow J, Eilber F. Soft tissue sarcoma of the extremity and retroperitoneum: advances in management. *Adv Surg* 1991; 24: 241.
137. Quill G, Gitelis S, Morton T. Complications associated with limb salvage for extremity sarcomas and their management. *Clin Orthop Rel Res* 1990; 260:242.
138. Murray JA, Jessup K, Romsdahl M, et al. Limb salvage study in osteosarcoma: early experience at M.D. Anderson Hospital and Tumor Institute. *Cancer Treat Symp* 1985; 3:131.
139. Meyer WH, Malawer MM. Osteosarcoma clinical features and evolving surgical and chemotherapeutic strategies. *Pediatr Clin North Am* 1991; 38:317–341.
140. Siegel KL, Stanhope SJ, Caldwell GE. Kinematic and kinetic adaptations in the lower limb during stance in gait of unilateral femoral neuropathy patients. *Clin Biomech* 1993; 8:147–155.
141. Lampert M, Gahagen C. Rehabilitation of the sarcoma patient. In: McGarvey CL, ed. *Physical therapy for the cancer patient.* New York: Churchill-Livingstone, 1990; 111–135.

Rehabilitation Medicine: Principles and Practice, Third Edition,
edited by Joel A. DeLisa and Bruce M. Gans.
Lippincott–Raven Publishers, Philadelphia © 1998.

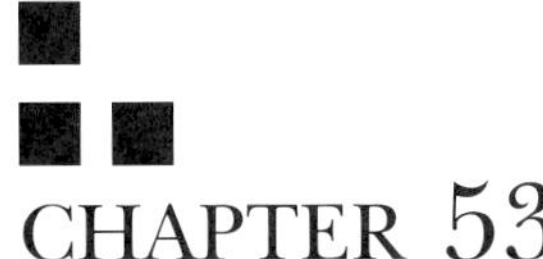

CHAPTER 53

Rehabilitation of the Individual with Human Immunodeficiency Virus

Stephen F. Levinson and Steven M. Fine

The quest for effective treatment, prevention, and cure of the acquired immunodeficiency syndrome (AIDS) has resulted in one of the most concentrated research efforts in the history of medicine. Since its discovery in the early 1980s, the human immunodeficiency virus (HIV) has become one of the most studied of human pathogens. Although an outright cure for AIDS still seems to be a distant dream, developments in recent years have been breathtaking, and, at the time of this writing, the possibility of controlling the progression of HIV infection and of ultimately preventing the usual decline in immune function that leads to AIDS may be within grasp. Although much is known about the pathogenesis of HIV type I (HIV-I), the most prevalent form of the virus, and about the mechanisms leading to immune dysfunction, the prevalence of disability is far less well known.

HIV is important to the field of rehabilitation for two reasons: because of its occurrence in traditional rehabilitation patients and because it can, in and of itself, cause disability. If nothing else, all rehabilitation professionals should recognize the potential for any of their patients to carry HIV and other blood-borne pathogens, and they should stringently apply universal precautions. Equally important, however, is the need to recognize that HIV is among the differential diagnosis of many disorders commonly seen in rehabilitation settings. In patients with known HIV infection, rehabilitation professionals need to be familiar with the many chemotherapeutic agents commonly used for treatment and with their side effects and drug interactions. This last task is particularly daunting given the accelerated process for U.S. Food and Drug Administration (FDA) review and approval of new treatments.

This chapter emphasizes the nature of HIV and the many ways that it can cause disability. Current medical treatment strategies are also discussed. However, the discussion is not intended to be comprehensive, and interested readers are urged to follow the literature closely. Specific rehabilitation strategies used to manage functional impairments typical of those found in association with HIV, such as spinal cord injury, brain injury, neuropathies, and rheumatologic disorders, are discussed elsewhere in this book.

HIV-RELATED DISABILITY

The full extent of disability resulting from HIV is unknown. One of the earliest studies attempting to evaluate this, the National Institutes of Health retrospective study, looked only at individuals with AIDS who were involved in research protocols and were referred for various rehabilitation interventions (1). Because the study did not include a representative cross-section of the HIV-seropositive population, however, the results must be interpreted with caution. A more comprehensive prospective study of disability in a population of men with HIV was obtained as part of the AIDS Time-oriented Health Outcome Study (ATHOS). This study longitudinally followed four groups: a high-risk seronegative group, a group of HIV-seropositive individuals without symptoms of immune deficiency, a seropositive group with symptoms, and a group with AIDS. An interim analysis was obtained from a self-reporting questionnaire in 1990 (2). The results of this survey are shown graphically in Figure 53-1.

Of those individuals with AIDS, more than 50% reported difficulty with one or more instrumental activities of daily living (ADLs), nearly 30% with basic ADLs, and more than

S. F. Levinson: Department of Physical Medicine and Rehabilitation, University of Rochester School of Medicine and Dentistry, Rochester, New York 14642.

S. M. Fine: Department of Medicine—Infectious Diseases Unit, University of Rochester School of Medicine and Dentistry, Rochester, New York 14642.

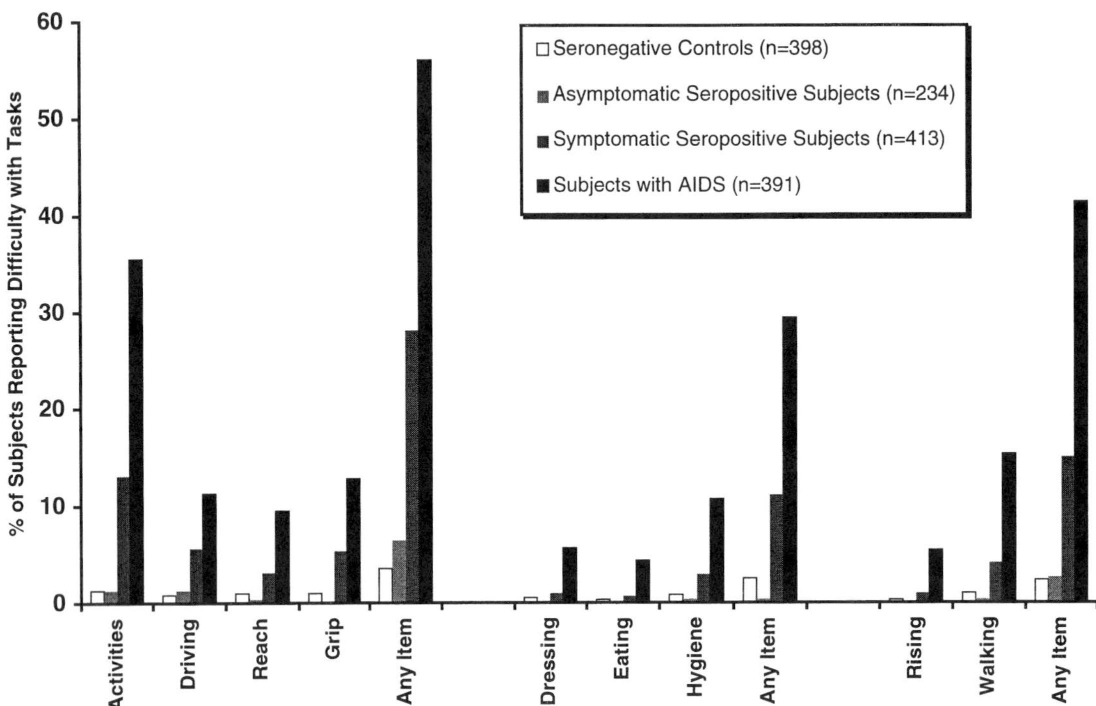

FIG. 53-1. The incidence of functional impairment seen in association with HIV (the AIDS Time-oriented Health Outcome Study [ATHOS]).

40% with basic mobility. Even among symptomatic seropositive individuals, nearly 30% reported difficulties with instrumental ADLs, more than 10% with basic ADLs, and 15% with basic mobility. However, seropositive individuals who were asymptomatic did not experience functional deficits to a significantly greater degree than those who were seronegative. These data underscore the need for rehabilitation interventions in those with AIDS and, to some extent, in those with HIV in general.

TRANSMISSION OF HIV

Classification

It cannot be overemphasized that AIDS and infection with HIV are not equivalent, nor does infection automatically lead to AIDS. Indeed, a small number of individuals with documented infection for 10 years or more have never developed AIDS. The Centers for Disease Control and Prevention (CDC) has developed a revised classification scheme based on the development of signs and symptoms and the CD4 lymphocyte count (3). Group A patients are seropositive but essentially symptom free. Group C patients have one or more AIDS-indicator illnesses. A comprehensive list of AIDS-indicator conditions is beyond the scope of this chapter, but suffice it to say that they include most opportunistic infections and malignancies, HIV dementia, and the AIDS wasting syndrome. Group B patients have early symptoms of immune deficiency in the absence of an AIDS-indicator condition. Patients are further subdivided into categories 1, 2, and 3, corresponding to CD4 counts of 500/mm^3 or above, 200 to 499, and less than 200, respectively. Patients falling into either group C or category 3 are classified as having AIDS.

Demographics

The World Health Organization (WHO) estimates that 18 million adults and 1.5 million children worldwide have been infected with HIV-1 (4). An estimated 41,930 United States residents died of HIV-1 infection in 1994, and AIDS was the leading cause of death among all Americans 25 to 44 years of age (5). Of the 247,741 cases reported from 1993 to 1995, 18% were female, 43% were white, 38% were black, and 18% were Hispanic, reflecting a significant shift to minority populations in recent years.

Documented Routes of Transmission

Documented routes of transmission include sexual contact with infected individuals, percutaneous or mucous membrane exposure to infected blood or body fluids, or transplacental, perinatal, or breast milk transmission from mother to infant. In 1995, intravenous drug use was the second most frequently reported risk behavior in the United States (6). HIV-1 is not transmitted by casual skin contact, airborne routes, or contact with saliva or sweat.

Occupational Exposure and Universal Precautions

Occupational exposure to HIV-1 among health-care workers has been extensively studied, and an excess number of cases beyond that detected in the general population has not been found (7). The risk of HIV-1 infection is estimated to be 0.3% after percutaneous injury involving infected blood (8) and 0.1% after mucous membrane exposure (9). Universal precautions should be used at all times that contact with blood or body fluids may be anticipated. These include the use of gloves to prevent potential exposure to infectious body fluids or broken skin during procedures such as wound care and electromyography (EMG), and the use of a gown, goggles, and a mask during procedures in which spattering of blood is possible.

Postexposure prophylaxis is recommended for percutaneous or mucous membrane exposure. In a case control study, postexposure zidovudine (AZT) decreased HIV-1 infection by 79% (10). The CDC currently recommends the following regimens for high-risk exposures: zidovudine 200 mg three times daily, plus lamivudine 150 mg twice daily and indinavir 800 mg three times daily. Prophylaxis should start within 12 to 24 hours of exposure and preferably within 1 to 2 hours. Baseline complete blood count (CBC) and hepatic enzymes should be drawn and repeated in 2 weeks. A medical evaluation, counseling, and follow-up by an experienced physician should be provided (11).

Prevention of Transmission among the Disabled

One of the most significant things rehabilitation professionals can do to stop the spread of HIV is to educate their patients as to the modes of transmission and means of preventing transmission. High-risk behaviors must be strongly discouraged, and education in safer sex practices should be included as part of all discussions on sexuality. Although no sexual technique is foolproof, safer sex practices are highly effective if used 100% of the time.

The most effective protective measure is the use of a barrier device whenever contact with infectious fluids is anticipated. This includes the use of condoms, the dental dam for oral sex, and gloves or a finger cot for digital anal penetration. Safe touching should be substituted for scratching, biting, and abrading activities that might lead to inadvertent fluid exposures. Water-soluble lubricants should be used particularly in insensate areas to reduce the likelihood of inadvertent abrasion. Mutual masturbation may be suggested as an activity that is virtually risk free. Patients should be reminded to clean and disinfect all enrichment aids (sex toys) using a solution such as 3% hydrogen peroxide.

When patients experience direct exposure to infectious fluids, prophylaxis should be offered as it is to health-care workers. Because about a fourth of children delivered vaginally to infected mothers will also be infected, prophylaxis also should be used to reduce vertical transmission. A prospective trial showed that pregnant women who took zidovudine could decrease the risk of perinatal transmission by 67% (12,13). Prevention of transmission in the adolescent patient demands particular attention (14). The avoidance of HIV transmission among patients who lack the capacity to modify their behavior, such as brain-injured individuals with impaired impulse control, remains a difficult area without clear-cut solutions (15,16).

CLINICAL EVALUATION OF HIV

Pathogenesis

HIV-1 infection results in the destruction of CD4-positive lymphocytes, leading to a decline in their numbers. In acute primary infection, HIV-1 replicates briskly and viral titer increases rapidly (17–20). Within 1 week of onset, 10^4 to 10^5 infectious particles per microliter of plasma can be measured (21–23). Fifty percent to 70% of patients experience a clinical syndrome that may include fever, rash, sore throat, lymphadenopathy, splenomegaly, myalgias, arthritis, and, rarely, meningitis (22,24,25).

Within a few weeks to months, seroconversion occurs and HIV-1 antibodies can be measured by the enzyme-linked immunosorbent assay (ELISA) or Western blot tests. Rapid viral replication persists, however, in the bloodstream, lymphoid tissue, and central nervous system (CNS), leading to a high turnover of infected cells (20,26–28). A steady state of plasma HIV ribonucleic acid (RNA) level is established within 6 to 12 months of seroconversion, and measurements of the viral load are felt to be prognostic (29–31). Levels of 10^6 HIV-1 RNA copies per microliter of blood or greater correlate with rapid progression over a few years, 10^3 to 10^5 with progression in 8 to 10 years, and less than 10^3 with long-term nonprogression (32). Unfortunately, rapid viral turnover and mutation leads to the appearance of resistant strains once antiretroviral therapy has begun (21,33–37).

Serologic Testing

The mainstay of HIV-1 testing involves screening for anti–HIV-1 antibodies with the ELISA, with the Western blot test used for confirmation. Serologic testing can only detect infection after seroconversion has occurred, which may take up to 6 months after acute infection. When ELISA screening and confirmatory Western blot testing are used, the false-positive rate is negligible. Pre- and posttest counseling are advisable to educate patients about the need for repeat testing, as well as modification of high-risk behaviors and, in the event of a positive test, the need to seek medical care. Home test kits, in which samples of saliva, blood, or urine can be collected by the patient at home or in a doctor's office and sent directly to testing laboratories, recently have become available.

Evaluation of the Seropositive Patient

With the benefit of early interventions in HIV infection now apparent, the need to identify seropositive individuals has become particularly acute. For individuals with unexplained sweats, fevers, or weight loss, skin lesions characteristic of opportunistic infections or malignancy, dyspnea unrelated to intrinsic cardiac or pulmonary disease, or altered neurologic function not attributable to a specific lesion, injury, or toxin, HIV infection must be considered in the differential diagnosis. The presence of other sexually transmitted diseases (STDs) also should be considered an indication for HIV testing. Even the presence of diseases seen occasionally in conjunction with HIV, such as tuberculosis (TB), should be considered an indication for testing.

The physical examination should focus on findings often seen in association with HIV. The skin and oral cavity should be carefully examined for mucocutaneous lesions, particularly those associated with Kaposi's sarcoma (KS). The presence of lymphadenopathy or hepatosplenomegaly are also important indicators. Because of the propensity of HIV to involve the nervous system, a detailed neurologic examination is essential. Peripheral neuropathies, cognitive disorders, myelopathy, and focal CNS dysfunction all may be seen in association with HIV. Although cognitive dysfunction is not common before the development of AIDS, a neuropsychologic evaluation is helpful to establish a baseline.

The laboratory evaluation should include routine chemistries and a complete blood count. A mild increase in transaminases may be seen, along with an elevated erythrocyte sedimentation rate, anemia, and general cytopenias. Serum protein electrophoresis may demonstrate an increase in immunoglobulins. Lymphocyte evaluation may demonstrate a decrease in CD4-positive lymphocytes or a reversal in the CD4/CD8 ratio. Viral load tests such as the polymerase chain reaction (PCR) or branched deoxyribonucleic acid (DNA) are important for establishing prognosis and for evaluating the effectiveness of antiretroviral treatments.

TREATMENT STRATEGIES IN AIDS

Because clinically latent stages of HIV-1 infection involve rapid viral replication, strategies now aim to decrease steady-state viral RNA levels. Asymptomatic individuals should be treated early in the course of disease with a combination of antiretroviral agents. A summary of recommendations has recently been published (38). Appropriate antimicrobial agents are used to control the effects of concomitant opportunistic infections. Medications commonly used in HIV along with their indications and side effects are summarized in Table 53-1. Numerous important side effects and drug interactions may occur that may limit effectiveness or tolerability of therapy, or may result in dangerous iatrogenic complications (39–42).

Antiretroviral Agents

Dideoxynucleosides

In 1987, zidovudine (AZT), a nucleoside analog reverse transcriptase inhibitor, was approved by the FDA. Subsequently approved were other nucleoside analogs, including didanosine (ddI), zalcitabine (ddC), stavudine (d4T), and lamivudine (3TC), which is synergistic with zidovudine and

TABLE 53-1. *Common drugs used in human immunodeficiency virus*

Drug	Common usage	Side effects	Drug interactions
Antiretrovirals (nucleoside analog reverse transcriptase inhibitors)			
Zidovudine (AZT)	First-line antiretroviral	Nausea, headache, fatigue, anemia, neutropenia, myopathy	Increased hematotoxicity of amphotericin B, ganciclovir
Didanosine (ddI)	First-line antiretroviral	Painful neuropathy, pancreatitis	May decrease absorption of other drugs
Zalcitabine (ddC)	Second-line antiretroviral	Painful neuropathy, pancreatitis, oral ulcers, granulocytopenia, rash, fever, hepatitis	Increased toxicity with foscarnet and valproic acid; alcohol may increase risk of pancreatitis
Lamivudine (3TC)	First-line antiretroviral	GI intolerance	
Stavudine (d4T)	Second-line antiretroviral	Painful neuropathy, hepatic dysfunction	
Antiretrovirals (non-nucleoside reverse transcriptase inhibitors)			
Nevirapine	Used in combination	Rash	May decrease protease inhibitor levels
Delavirdine	Used in combination	Rash	May decrease didanosine levels

TABLE 53-1. *Continued.*

Drug	Common usage	Side effects	Drug interactions
Antiretrovirals (protease inhibitors)			
Saquinavir	Used in combination	GI distress, elevated LFTs	Increased bioavailability of Ca channel blockers
Indinavir	Used in combination	Hepatotoxicity, nephrolithiasis	As above, plus ↑ desipramine and rifabutin levels; prolonged sedation with midazolam and triazolam; decreased OCP effectiveness; fatal arrhythmias with astemizole and cisapride
Ritonavir	Used in combination	GI upset, perioral paresthesias, alteration of taste, headache, elevated LFTs	Similar to indinavir, but may be more pronounced, failure of oral contraception
Nelfinavir	Used in combination	Diarrhea	Similar to ritonavir
Prophylactic agents			
Trimethoprim/sulfamethoxazole	PCP prophylaxis and treatment	Rash, fever, neutropenia, thrombocytopenia, hepatitis, headache, meningitis, hyperkalemia	Potentiation of coumadin, oral hypoglycemics, and phenytoin; decreased effectiveness of cyclosporine
Dapsone	PCP prophylaxis	Rash, fever, hemolysis in G6PD deficiency	ddl decreases absorption; decreased effectiveness of oral contraceptives
Pentamidine	PCP prophylaxis and treatment	Aerosol: bronchospasm. IV: nephritis, pancreatitis, hypo- or hyperglycemia, rash, neutropenia	Renal failure with amphotericin B; hypocalcemia with foscarnet
Rifabutin	MAC prophylaxis	GI, auditory, iritis	Decreases levels of quinidine, oral contraceptives, phenytoin, methadone, digoxin, cyclosporine, azoles, corticosteroids, beta blockers
Common treatments			
Acyclovir	Herpes simplex, zoster	Diarrhea, phlebitis (IV)	
Ganciclovir	CMV	Neutropenia, GI upset	Increased nephrotoxicity with cyclosporine
Foscarnet	CMV	Nephrotoxicity, seizure, nausea, hypomagnesemia, hypocalcemia and hyponatremia, nephrotoxicity, headache	Hypocalcemia with pentamidine
Cidofovir	CMV	Nephrotoxicity	
Fluconazole	Antifungal: candida and cryptococcus	Hepatotoxicity, nausea, rash	Decreased absorption with cimetidine; decreased levels with carbamazepine and rifampin; increases phenytoin levels
Ketoconazole	Antifungal: candida	GI upset, pruritis, headache, rash	Fatal arrhythmias with terfenadine, astemizole, and cisapride; decreases rifampin; potentiates coumadin
Itraconazole	Antifungal histoplasmosis, aspergillis	Hepatitis, GI upset, rash, headache	Fatal arrhythmias with terfenadine, astemizole, and cisapride; decreased levels with carbamazepine; increased sedation with midazolam
Amphotericin B	Antifungal: serious fungal infections	Nephrotoxicity, fever, chills, hypomagnesemia, hypocalcemia	Dosage must be adjusted in renal failure

CMV, cytomegalovirus; IV, intravenous; LFT, liver function test; MAC, *Mycobacterium avium* complex; OCP, oral contraceptive pill; PCP, *Pneumocystis carinii* pneumonia.

active against zidovudine-resistant isolates (39,40,43). Numerous clinical trials have suggested that the effectiveness of monotherapy is limited by the emergence of resistant strains (44–46). Combinations including zidovudine and didanosine, zalcitabine, or lamivudine are superior to the use of zidovudine alone (39,47–49).

Protease Inhibitors

As of this writing, four protease inhibitors have been approved by the FDA: saquinavir (50), indinavir, ritonavir, and nelfinavir. These result in the production of immature, noninfectious HIV-1 particles by blocking the cleavage of HIV-1 poly-proteins into component proteins. Combinations of protease inhibitors and reverse transcriptase inhibitors have been shown to reduce plasma HIV-1 RNA levels below detectable levels and to reduce morbidity and mortality (33,34,41,42,51,52).

Other Agents

Numerous other antiretroviral agents and vaccines are undergoing clinical trials and are at various stages of FDA approval. Two non-nucleoside analog reverse transcriptase inhibitors, nevirapine and delavirdine, recently were approved.

Immune Stimulants

The use of cytokines to stimulate production of CD4 cells has been used in clinical trials with inconclusive results (53). Although interleukin-2 can stimulate CD4 cell production, it may increase virus production as well. The use of stimulating cytokines in conjunction with potent antiretroviral combinations to inhibit viral production appears promising.

COMMON CAUSES OF DEBILITY

Although HIV itself is felt to be responsible for many forms of functional compromise, particularly in the CNS, a large number of disabling syndromes are associated with opportunistic infections and malignancies. The relative rates vary, depending on the population and the use of prophylaxis. Statistics from an urban United States HIV-1 clinic showed, per 100 patient years, 13.3 occurrences of *Candida* esophagitis; between five and nine each of *Pneumocystis carinii* pneumonia (PCP), *Mycobacterium avium* complex (MAC), cytomegalovirus (CMV), and dementia; two to four occurrences each of toxoplasmosis, cryptococcus, herpes zoster, HIV-1–associated wasting, and KS; and one to two occurrences each of non-Hodgkin's lymphoma, *Mycobacterium tuberculosis* (mTB), and progressive multifocal leukoencephalopathy (PML) (54). A summary of the types and causes of functional impairment seen in association with HIV is listed in Table 53-2.

Pneumonias and Disseminated Infections

Pneumocystis carinii *Pneumonia*

Pneumocystis carinii is a funguslike pathogen that causes PCP, the most common AIDS-defining illness in the United States, accounting for about 18% of cases (55–57). Symptoms may develop gradually and include dyspnea on exertion, shortness of breath, cough, weight loss, fevers, and night sweats. Chest x-ray may show a diffuse alveolar infiltrate and serum lactate dehydrogenase (LDH) may be elevated. Diagnosis is most often made by identification of *Pneumocystis* organisms in expectorated sputum or from bronchoscopic specimens.

A room air arterial blood gas with PaO_2 less than or equal to 70 mm Hg indicates severe disease, which is treated with intravenous trimethoprim/sulfa or pentamidine for 21 days, plus steroids. Trimetrexate plus dapsone also may be used. Atovaquone suspension can be used for mild to moderate PCP. Prophylaxis with trimethoprim/sulfa is a mainstay of AIDS treatment when CD4 counts are less than 200.

Mycobacterium Tuberculosis

Tuberculosis caused by mTB is common and severe in AIDS patients, most often occurring at CD4 counts above 200 cells/μl (58,59). Symptoms may be more subtle than in non–HIV-infected individuals. TB may disseminate to a wide variety of other organs, including the brain and spine. Guidelines for the diagnosis, treatment, and prophylaxis of infectious TB have been detailed by the CDC (60,61). Of concern, however, are outbreaks of multidrug-resistant TB (62,63).

Mycobacterium Avium Complex

MAC, an atypical mycobacterial infection, is one of the most common opportunistic infections in AIDS patients in the United States, with an incidence of 18% to 43% (64). It may be present as a nonpathogenic colonizer or may cause disease in the bone marrow, lungs, liver, colon, and, rarely, the CNS. The course may be indolent with fevers, night sweats, weight loss and wasting, cough, diarrhea, abdominal pains, lymphadenopathy, and lymph node pain.

The most effective drug combinations for treatment of MAC include clarithromycin as the drug of first choice at a dose of 500 mg twice a day, with ethambutol as the second choice. Rifabutin, clofazamine, ethambutol, and ciprofloxacin also have been used, and azithromycin and aminoglycosides (amikacin) are under study (65). Clarithromycin has been shown to be effective in preventing disseminated MAC (66). Primary prophylaxis against MAC with rifabutin is

TABLE 53-2. *Common functional impairment syndromes in HIV*

Cause of Impairment	When seen	Features	Prognosis	Management
Respiratory compromise and disseminated infection				
PCP	Throughout AIDS	Nonspecific fever, cough, etc.	Good except in late AIDS	TMPX, dapsone, pentamadine; prophylaxis in all AIDS
mTB	Early AIDS	Nonspecific fever, cough, etc.	Fair	Antituberculin therapy
MAC	Late AIDS	Fever, night sweats, weight loss, etc.	Poor	Clarithromycin, ethambutol, etc; prophylaxis when CD4 count is <50–75
Pathogenic fungi	Pre-AIDS and AIDS	Wasting, fevers, etc.	Benign or fulminate	Antifungal agents
GI compromise and swallowing disorders				
Candidiasis	Pre-AIDS and AIDS	Oral plaques, dysphagia	Good with treatment	Topical antifungal agents; systemic agents in severe cases
Intestinal parasites	Late AIDS	Diarrhea	Good if diagnosed	Antiparasitic agents
Kaposi's sarcoma	Throughout AIDS	Characteristic lesions	Slow progression	Appropriate chemotherapy
Sicca syndrome		Impaired lacrimation and salivation	Benign course	Symptomatic treatment (artificial tears, oral lubricants, etc.)
Neurogenic swallowing disorders	Throughout AIDS, especially late	Related to underlying neurologic disorder	Related to underlying disorder	Video-fluoroscopy, modified swallow, parenteral nutrition
Weakness and fatigue				
Myopathy (polymyositis)	Any stage of HIV	Proximal weakness	Good	Steroids, exercise as tolerated
Fibromyalgia	Any stage of HIV	Pain and fatigue	Good	Standard measures (NSAIDs, etc.)
Chronic fatigue	Pre-AIDS and AIDS	Many causes	Fair	Energy conservation and pacing
AIDS wasting syndrome	Late AIDS	Proximal weakness	Poor	Supportive care, anabolic steroids
Pain syndromes and neuropathies				
Arthritis and arthralgias		Psoriasis associated, Reiter's syndrome, reactive and HIV	Similar to idiopathic varieties	Similar to idiopathic varieties (NSAIDs, injections, joint preservation etc.)
Distal symmetric neuropathy	Increased with decreased CD4 count	Distal numbness, pain, and decreased strength	Responds to symptomatic therapy	Tricyclics, neuroleptics, heat/cold, gait aids, orthotics
Segmental neuropathies	Early or late	Zoster, mononeuritis simplex/multiplex, vasculitis, etc.	Variable	Similar to that in non-HIV patients
Drug-induced neuropathies, vitamin deficiencies	Related to drugs	Didanosine, zalcitabine, stavudine, vincristine, dapsone, rifampin, isoniazide, ethambutol	Good	Cessation or alterations of medications, vitamin supplementation, symptomatic management
Plantar Kaposi's sarcoma	Throughout AIDS	Characteristic lesions	Good	Radiation, custom insoles, etc.
Cognitive dysfunction				
HIV dementia	Late AIDS, but occasionally seen at presentation	Decreased memory, dysphagia, associated myelopathy	Poor	Antiretrovirals, memory book, adaptive strategies, decreased stimulation, etc.

(continued)

TABLE 53-2. *Continued.*

Cause of Impairment	When seen	Features	Prognosis	Management
Cognitive dysfunction				
Cryptococcal meningitis	Throughout AIDS	Fever, headache, meningismus, etc.	About 50% respond to treatment	Amphotericin B, followed by lifetime fluconazole
Neurosyphilis	Throughout AIDS	Nonspecific CNS	Fair, frequent relapse	High-dose PCN
Encephalitis (herpesviruses)	Throughout AIDS	Headache, seizure, altered consciousness, focal signs	May be self-limited, fair to good with antiviral treatment	Acyclovir for HSV, ganciclovir or foscarnet for CMV
Focal lesions (see below)	Throughout AIDS	Focal signs	Lesion specific	See below
Metabolic/iatrogenic dementia	Throughout HIV	Nonspecific CNS	Good	Proper diagnosis and correction of underlying problem
Focal brain disorders				
CMV retinitis	Advanced AIDS	Visual field loss	Progressive	Ganciclovir and foscarnet
Cerebral toxoplasmosis	Throughout AIDS	Focal signs, altered consciousness, ring-enhancing lesions	Good with treatment	Pyrimethamine and folinic acid, plus sulfadiazine or clindamycin; prophylaxis when CD4 count is <100
PML	Advanced AIDS	Focal signs, altered consciousness	Very poor except in rare cases	High-dose cytarabine, cidofovir and antiretrovirals
Primary CNS lymphoma	Advanced AIDS	Similar to above, occasional paraneoplastic signs	Extremely poor	Palliative radiation extends both quality and quantity of life
Other metastatic disease	Throughout AIDS	Similar to above	Lesion-specific	Appropriate to lesion
CNS abscesses	Throughout AIDS	Similar to above	Lesion-specific	Drainage of abscess, antimicrobials, antituberculin agents
Myelopathy/ascending paralysis				
Vacuolar myelopathy	Late AIDS	Progressive paraparesis	Poor for recovery	As in other forms of SCI
Other myelitis	Throughout AIDS	Tropical spastic paraparesis (HTLV-1), herpesviruses, meningitis, Pott's disease	Poor	As in other forms of SCI
Inflammatory demyelinating polyneuropathies	Early in HIV	Gullian-Barré, CIDP	Very good	Same as in idiopathic forms
CMV polyradiculopathy	Late AIDS	Flaccid paralysis	Arrested if treatment started quickly	Ganciclovir, foscarnet, rehabilitative interventions as in SCI
Pediatric HIV				
LIP	Common throughout AIDS	Nonspecific with variable course	Usually benign	Corticosteroids, symptomatic management for exacerbations
HIV encephalopathy	Common and progressive with AIDS	Static, progressive, or progressive/plateau	Variable	Rehabilitative interventions similar to spastic diplegic cerebral palsy

AIDS, acquired immunodeficiency syndrome; CIDP,chronic inflammatory demyelinating polyneuropathy; CMV, cytomegalovirus; CNS, central nervous system; HIV, human immunodeficiency virus; HSV, herpes simplex virus; HTLV, human T-cell lymphotrophic virus; LIP, lymphoid interstitial pneumonitis; MAC, *Mycobacterium avium* complex; mTB, *Mycobacterium tuberculosis*; NSAIDs, nonsteroidal anti-inflammatory drugs; PCN, penicillin; PCP, *Pneumocystis carinii* pneumonia; PML, primary multifocal leukoencephalopathy; SCI, spinal cord injury; TMPX, trimethoprim/sulfamethoxazole.

recommended for those with CD4 counts less than 50 to 75 cells/μl. Azithromycin is also effective for prophylaxis (67).

Pathogenic Fungi

Endemic pathogenic fungi such as histoplasma capsulatum, blastomyces dermatidis, and coccidioides immitis can cause disease in normal hosts (68), particularly in those with AIDS. Endemic areas for histoplasmosis occur along the Ohio, Mississippi, and Missouri river valleys (69). Patients often present with slowly progressive wasting, fevers, weight loss, or ulcerations of skin. Bone marrow dysfunction may occur. Occasionally disseminated intravascular coagulation and death may occur. The chest x-ray may be normal or show a progressive infiltrate (70). The serum test for histoplasma polysaccharide is specific and sensitive. Treatment consists of induction with amphotericin B and maintenance with itraconazole (71,72).

Gastrointestinal Disorders

Gastrointestinal disease in AIDS is common and presents with diarrhea, weight loss, biliary disorders, abdominal pain, dysphagia, and oral disease. A wide range of causes including infections with CMV, herpes simplex virus (HSV), MAC, intestinal parasites, and malignancies such as KS and non-Hodgkin's lymphoma were seen in one series (73). Drug reactions are also a frequent cause. Dysphagia is due to a treatable cause in 90% of cases and is most often caused by *Candida albicans,* HSV, or CMV esophagitis (73,74). Other causes include hairy leukoplakia, KS, human papilloma virus infection, and neurogenic causes. Colitis often presents with abdominal pain and bloody or mucous diarrhea and is most often caused by CMV, which responds to treatment with ganciclovir (73–75). *Clostridium difficile, Campylobacter jejuni, Entamoeba histolytica,* and *Shigella flexneri* are also seen in colitis in AIDS patients (73).

Candidiasis

Oral candidiasis (thrush) occurs in 43% to 93% of AIDS patients (76). It most often appears as creamy white, yellow, or erythematous patches on the palate, tongue, and buccal mucosa and causes angular cheilitis and fissures at the corners of the mouth. With more severe immunodeficiency, *Candida* may extend into the pharynx and esophagus (77,78). It presents more often in patients with CD4 counts under 200 cells/μl but can occur at higher counts as well. Candidiasis may be treated with oral nystatin suspension, clotrimazole troche, or fluconazole or other azoles.

Intestinal Parasites

Cryptosporidium parvum is an intracellular protozoan responsible for 1% of AIDS indicator diseases and about 1% of AIDS deaths (73). Disease ranges from mild and self-limited to life-threatening diarrhea with severe wasting, most often in patients with CD4 counts below 200. Oral paromomycin or azithromycin may be effective in decreasing diarrhea and stabilizing body weight (79,80). Microsporidiosis causes similar symptoms and may be treated with albendazole (81,82). *Isospora belli* is a protozoan parasite that is less common in the United States and generally causes less severe disease (83). Other intestinal parasites include *Entamoeba histolytica* and *Giardia lamblia.*

Kaposi's Sarcoma

KS is a highly vascular malignant lesion containing endothelial cells and spindle-shaped mesenchymal cells. It can involve the skin, oral mucosa, and visceral organs and often appears as dark blue or purple papules or nodules. Although initially seen in 25% to 30% of homosexual men (84–86), its incidence seems to be decreasing. Cosmetically, lesions can be treated by laser bleaching and spot radiation. More severe disease has been treated with antiretrovirals and drugs such as foscarnet (87), localized radiation, immunotherapy with interferon alpha, cytotoxic chemotherapy (53,88), and liposomal doxorubicin (89,90). Intralesional human chorionic gonadotropin also has been effective (91). Associated edema may be controlled with the use of compressive garments, and painful lesions in the feet may be managed with the use of soft insoles and by unweighting the affected extremity.

HIV-Related Cardiac Disease

Although the mechanisms involved are not clear, HIV-related cardiomyopathy is common, although almost always asymptomatic, being seen in up to 95% of cases (92). Other causes of cardiac dysfunction include pericardial disease, infectious and noninfectious endocarditis, metastatic KS, and lymphoma. When symptomatic, management is similar to that of congestive heart failure of other causes, with the use of vasodilators, diuretics, and digitalis preparations. Exercise is instituted as tolerated in a similar fashion.

HIV Nephropathy

An HIV-related nephropathy has been described (93). It is characterized by fluid and electrolyte abnormalities, acid-base imbalance, and protienuria. Acute renal failure is usually the result of hypovolemia and ischemia or iatrogenic factors from the toxic effects of diagnostic agents and medications.

Rheumatologic Disorders

Arthritic Disorders

Arthralgias arising from a variety of ill-defined causes are common in association with HIV (94). Arthritis is also relatively frequent, with psoriasis-associated arthritis, Reiter's syndrome, and reactive arthritis all being described (95). An HIV-associated arthritis also has been described that may be chronic or transient and generally has a preponderance of lower limb involvement (96). However, septic arthritis is a fairly rare complication of AIDS. The prognosis and management is comparable with that of idiopathic arthritides.

Myopathies

HIV myopathy may present at any stage of infection, usually as proximal muscle weakness most prominently in the thighs, particularly after exertion (97). Myalgia occurs in 25% to 50% of cases (98,99). Weight loss is common. Creatinine kinase is usually elevated, and EMG demonstrates abundant spontaneous activity with short-duration, low-amplitude polyphasic motor unit action potentials (100). Confirmation can usually be obtained from muscle biopsy, which demonstrates focal necrosis with regeneration. Prednisone has been reported to improve strength (101). The role of exercise is thought to be similar to that in non–HIV-associated myopathies.

Nemaline myopathy also has been described and is clinically and electrophysiologically indistinguishable from HIV myopathy. Other myopathies may be toxic, autoimmune, or related to coxsackievirus or human T-cell lymphotrophic virus type I (HTLV-I) co-infection. These must be distinguished from the AIDS wasting syndrome, which presents insidiously late in the course of disease with symmetrical proximal muscle weakness.

Other Rheumatologic Disorders

Vasculitis is an unusual finding in HIV, with a reported incidence of 0.4% to 1% (102). Unfortunately, the prognosis is generally poor. The sicca syndrome, seen often in association with lymphadenopathy, may be treated symptomatically with increased fluids, artificial tears, and careful attention to oral hygiene. Fibromyalgia is commonly seen, and the response to traditional measures is generally good.

Chronic Fatigue in HIV

Persons with HIV are often fatigued for a variety of reasons, including fibromyalgia, pulmonary dysfunction, anemia, encephalopathy, endocrine dysfunction, myopathies, cardiomyopathy, psychiatric disorders, and depression. Fatigue also may result from the effects of antiretroviral therapy. The importance of preventative measures cannot be overemphasized with this population, including the use of light exercise to tolerance, early mobilization after an acute illness, and other measures to prevent common complications of immobility.

NEUROLOGIC IMPAIRMENT IN HIV

Disorders of Peripheral Nerve

Distal Symmetric Neuropathy

Peripheral neuropathies are frequently seen in HIV, with a distal symmetrical polyneuropathy being demonstrable on EMG in 35% of AIDS cases (103). Symptomatic in about 18% of patients with AIDS, its incidence increases with decreasing CD4 count, and pathologic evidence can be found in nearly all cases on sural nerve biopsy or at autopsy. It remains essential, however, to rule out treatable causes of neuropathy.

On biopsy, a ''dying back'' of distal fibers is seen, with loss of both myelinated and nonmyelinated fibers. In some cases, perivascular mononuclear inflammatory infiltrates are seen. Electromyographically, sensory nerve action potentials are reduced in amplitude initially and F waves are abnormal. In time, denervation potentials become evident in distal muscle groups and long duration polyphasic motor unit action potentials, decreased recruitment, and increased amplitude may be seen (100).

Other Sensorimotor Neuropathies

Drug-induced neuropathies commonly result from the antiretroviral drugs didanosine, zalcitabine, and stavudine. Other drugs commonly used in AIDS patients that can cause neuropathies include vincristine, dapsone, rifampin, isoniazid, and ethambutol (104).

Mononeuropathy simplex and multiplex may occur early in HIV as a limited peripheral neuropathy that must be distinguished from segmental herpes zoster, also a common cause of painful neuropathy (103). A multifocal neuropathy associated with severe weakness and disability, and often with fever and cachexia, also may be seen in advanced AIDS. EMG is consistent with both axonal loss and demyelination (100). Motor neuron disease has rarely been reported in patients with HIV, and there is little direct evidence of an association between the two (97).

Inflammatory Demyelinating Neuropathies

HIV is a major cause of inflammatory demyelinating polyneuropathies and must always be considered in the differential (105–107). Guillain-Barré syndrome or acute inflammatory demyelinating polyneuropathy (AIDP), occurs early, often around the time of seroconversion, and is clinically and histopathologically indistinguishable from the idiopathic form. It is managed similarly. In some cases, chronic inflammatory demyelinating polyneuropathy (CIDP) or relapsing polyneuropathy may be seen.

Nerve conduction studies are significant for prolonged sensory and motor latencies with patchy slowing to less than 60% to 70% of normal (100). Marked reduction in motor action potential amplitude or even motor conduction block may be indicative of focal demyelination. F wave and H reflexes are often markedly delayed or absent. The EMG needle examination usually fails to show abnormal spontaneous activity, although denervation potentials with diminished recruitment may sometimes be seen in weak distal muscles.

CMV Polyradiculopathy

CMV causes a common and debilitating peripheral neuropathy in which CMV infects the nerve roots and ganglia (103,108). Patients present with back and lower extremity sensory changes and weakness that may rapidly progress to flaccid paralysis (109,110). It can be rapidly fatal unless treatment is started within the first 24 to 48 hours (110–112). Treatment is effective in halting progression, although patients are often left with severe deficits that may require rehabilitation.

Findings include loss of lower extremity deep tendon reflexes, saddle anesthesia, and urinary retention, whereas upper extremity strength is preserved. Diffuse spontaneous activity is seen on EMG, with decreased recruitment but near normal conduction velocities (100). The cerebrospinal fluid (CSF) often has a pleocytosis with neutrophils and may show elevated protein and inclusion cells that may stain positive for CMV antigens (103,109). Improvement upon treatment with ganciclovir has been described (109,111, 113,114). Foscarnet also can be effective.

Autonomic Neuropathy

Autonomic neuropathy is commonly found in association with HIV infection, particularly in advanced AIDS (97). Patients may experience orthostatic hypotension, syncope, impotence, decreased sweating, and diarrhea. As always, it is important to rule out iatrogenic causes from the use of common medications.

Diffuse Involvement of the Brain in HIV

Except in iatrogenic cases, cognitive dysfunction is usually a relatively late finding in AIDS; therefore, the rehabilitation management should be adjusted accordingly. Memory assistance and coping strategies should be implemented so that the individual can be maintained in the community as long as possible.

HIV Dementia

The most common cause of cognitive dysfunction is HIV dementia, also known as the AIDS dementia complex, subacute encephalitis, and HIV encephalopathy (107). Although it is usually not seen until advanced disease, it may be present in 3% to 7% of cases at the time of diagnosis (115) and can be found in up to 90% of cases at autopsy (116). Although electrophysiologic abnormalities can be demonstrated on evoked potential testing in a majority of individuals with HIV, cognitive dysfunction does not usually become evident before the development of AIDS (117–120). An associated vacuolar myelopathy is usual in advanced disease.

Cryptococcal Meningitis

Cryptococcus is an important fungal pathogen in patients with CD4 counts under 200 cells/μl. Infection most often presents with meningitis, and symptoms include fever, headache, neck stiffness, and memory loss. Patients may show signs of lethargy, confusion, meningismis, or cranial nerve palsies. Signs and symptoms in AIDS patients, however, are often mild (121). Cryptococcal antigen may be detected in the CSF or serum for diagnosis. Initial treatment is with amphotericin B or fluconazole followed by lifetime fluconazole maintenance (122).

Other Causes of Cognitive Dysfunction

Treponema pallidum may cause chronic meningitis, neuropathy, or dementia when infecting the CNS of AIDS patients (i.e., neurosyphilis) (122,123). CSF pleocytosis is often seen, and a CSF Venereal Disease Research Laboratory test (VDRL) may be positive, but sensitivity is low. Treatment is usually with 10 days of 12 to 24 million units/day of intravenous penicillin G, but relapses are common.

Varicella zoster, a common cause of pneumonia and skin eruptions in AIDS patients, also results in a variety of neurologic syndromes, including painful nerve palsies, transverse myelitis, ascending myelitis, encephalitis, and leukoencephalopathy (124). In contrast to HSV encephalitis, herpes zoster encephalitis rarely causes focal neurologic signs, deep alterations in consciousness, or seizures. The usual duration of neurologic symptoms is around 16 days, and the outcome is generally better than that with the other CNS infections. Acute mononucleosis caused by Epstein-Barr virus is also common, often leading to encephalitis, acute cerebellar syndrome, transverse or ascending myelitis, or acute psychosis (125).

Other causes of cognitive dysfunction include CMV encephalitis, aseptic meningitis, and cerebral vasculitis (104,107,115,124,126–130). Cognitive dysfunction also may result from disorders that cause focal CNS syndromes. As always, with any dementia workup it is essential to rule out iatrogenic and other potentially treatable causes.

Focal Brain Lesions Found in HIV

The focal deficits seen in association with AIDS are related directly to the areas of the brain affected and may include blindness, hemiparesis, ataxia, aphasia, dysarthria, and cranial nerve deficits (104,129–136). Movement disorders, including hemichorea-ballismus, segmental myoclonus, postural tremor, parkinsonism, and dystonia, also may be found. Knowledge of the prognosis is essential to the design of appropriate rehabilitation strategies, which are otherwise similar to those used in other focal brain disorders.

CMV Retinopathy

CMV is one of the most common pathogens in AIDS patients, affecting 21.4% of patients in one series, with CD4 counts of less than 100 cells/μl (137). About 85% of CMV disease in AIDS patients presents as retinitis, which usually affects those with CD4 counts less than 50 cells/μl. Productive infection of the retina can cause full-thickness necrosis, although patients may be asymptomatic and gradual visual loss may be unnoticed until vision is significantly impaired. Ophthalmologic examination shows characteristic perivascular yellow–white lesions that are frequently associated with retinal hemorrhage (138). These must be distinguished from cotton-wool spots, which are white, fluffy, superficial infarcts of the nerve fiber layer that usually spontaneously regress and do not lead to blindness.

The mainstays of treatment have been ganciclovir, a nucleoside analog, and foscarnet, a pyrophosphate analog (139). Both are used with a 2- to 3-week intravenous induction phase followed by a lifelong daily maintenance dose. Cidofovir, a newer nucleoside analog, has a long half-life and can suppress CMV up to 3 weeks after a single administration. Intravitreal injection of ganciclovir and cidofovir as well as intraocular implants of timed-release devices with ganciclovir or foscarnet also have been used with success (140–142). Complications are common with all of these drugs (Table 53-1). Eventual progression to blindness remains common, making early institution of visual retraining and blind rehabilitation particularly important.

Toxoplasmosis

Cerebral toxoplasmosis is the most common CNS mass lesion in AIDS, occurring in 3% to 40% of cases (104,143). Without prophylaxis, 30% of previously toxoplasma-seropositive AIDS patients may develop toxoplasmosis, and 40% of CNS lesions in AIDS patients are due to toxoplasmosis. Most patients present with focal or nonfocal neurologic signs produced by space-occupying lesions in the brain. Headaches, confusion, lethargy, and seizures are common. Sixty-nine percent of patients have focal signs such as hemiparesis, ataxia, and cranial nerve palsies (144). Contrast-enhanced computed tomography or magnetic resonance imaging (MRI) of the head shows single or multiple ring-enhancing lesions that may be distinguished from lymphoma by biopsy or radiolabeled thallium uptake (145).

A common diagnostic strategy is to initiate antitoxoplasma therapy and observe for clinical response, which is often dramatic. Treatment regimens include pyrimethamine and folinic acid plus either sulfadiazine or clindamycin. Patients with a positive antitoxoplasmosis immunoglobulin G antibody should take prophylaxis when their CD4 count is less than 100 cells/μl (146). Trimethoprim/sulfa, often used for PCP prophylaxis, is effective, as is clindamycin plus pyremethamine.

Progressive Multifocal Leukoencephalopathy

PML is a white matter disease associated with infection by the JC virus. It occurs in approximately 4% of AIDS patients (147). Single or multifocal lesions confined to the white matter without the presence of a mass effect or contrast enhancement may be seen on MRI. Diagnosis can be made based on radiographic appearance or more definitively by biopsy (148). The median survival is on the order of 2 to 4 months, although in approximately 10% of cases a more benign course is seen, and spontaneous remissions may even occur (131). High-dose cytarabine has been effective in some cases.

CNS Lymphoma

CNS lymphoma is associated with late-stage AIDS and CD4 counts of less than 100 cells/μl (149). It may present as a mass lesion with confusion, headache, memory loss, or focal neurologic signs (136). Untreated, it usually progresses to death in 1 month or less. Palliative radiation can temporarily improve symptoms and extend survival, with an increased quality of life in 75% of cases (150). Associated paraneoplastic syndromes are common. Rarely, metastatic lesions may be seen in the brain from other malignancies, particularly KS.

Other Causes of Focal CNS Syndromes

HSV-I may infect the brain in AIDS patients, causing an encephalitis characterized by the acute onset of headache, behavioral changes with focal neurologic signs, seizures, and coma. Although an increased incidence of thromboembolic cerebrovascular events has been reported (151,152), in one study the incidence of stroke was not found to be greater than in age-matched controls (153). This is in contrast to cerebral vasculitis, which does have an association with AIDS. Primary CNS angiitis is a rare and usually fatal disorder. It has a predilection for small cortical vessels (102,154).

There have been a few reports of fulminate multiple sclerosis in AIDS patients, although the numbers have been too small to establish a causal relationship (155). Bacterial and fungal abscesses also may cause focal neurologic deficits. TB is of particular concern and may require biopsy for diagnosis. Antituberculin therapy is often initiated in those with a positive PPD and a new focal lesion when the diagnosis is uncertain.

Spinal Cord Dysfunction

Vacuolar myelopathy is the most common cause of spinal cord dysfunction in HIV, being found in 11% to 22% of AIDS cases and demonstrable in up to 40% of cases at autopsy (107). It is strongly associated with HIV dementia and shares a virtually identical histopathology. Patients present with progressive paraparesis, ataxia, posterior column sensory loss, spasticity, and neurogenic bowel and bladder (129).

Spinal cord dysfunction also may result from viral myelitis secondary to varicella zoster virus, HSV, CMV, and HTLV-I. Spinal cord disorders also may be seen with tuberculin involvement (Pott's disease), multiple sclerosis, and aseptic, cryptococcal, and lymphomatous meningitis.

PEDIATRIC HIV

Pediatric cases of HIV differ significantly from their adult counterparts (156–159). More than 80% of cases of HIV infection in children are the result of perinatal transmission, with transmission from blood products being less frequent (160). The most effective strategy to minimize vertical transmission is prophylactic treatment of the mother (161,162). Because of transplacental transmission of antibodies, however, most infants of HIV-positive mothers will initially be seropositive at birth, with signs of infection developing in approximately 80% of those with disease at a median age of 5 months (163). Approximately 50% of children with perinatally acquired HIV are alive at 9 years of age.

Opportunistic Infections

In contrast to adults, opportunistic infections of the nervous system are extremely uncommon (163). AIDS-defining criteria in children include recurrent bacterial infections, opportunistic infections, lymphoid interstitial pneumonitis (LIP), malignancies, cardiomyopathies, hepatitis, nephropathy, and encephalopathy. Infants with AIDS often present with hepatosplenomegaly, lymphadenopathy, diarrhea, oral candidiasis, parotid enlargement, delayed developmental milestones, and failure to thrive.

Over 80% of HIV-infected children eventually develop either acute or chronic lung diseases (164). Although most are acute infectious processes, chronic diseases such as LIP may occur in 30% to 50% (165). The etiology and natural history of LIP are incompletely understood. Although some patients are asymptomatic with infiltrates on chest x-ray, others experience a slowly progressive course with exacerbations caused by lung infections, and some may progress to chronic respiratory decompensation and hypoxemia. HIV-infected children with LIP are believed to have a better long-term prognosis than those with other pulmonary infections (164). Corticosteroids are used to suppress the lymphocytic infiltrate.

HIV Encephalopathy

The most common neurologic disorder seen in children is HIV encephalopathy. This may be static, progressive, or progressive with a plateau (163,166–171). Static encephalopathy is characterized by delayed acquisition of developmental skills and is seen in 25% of those with CNS deficits. With progressive encephalopathy, on the other hand, the pace of development becomes progressively slower and may halt altogether, or show signs of regression. The clinical picture is not unlike that of spastic diplegic cerebral palsy, but with progressive deficits.

Other children may demonstrate more subtle neurodevelopmental deficits, including easy fatigability, mild depression, expressive language deficits, and mild regression in school performance (166,168). The response to antiretroviral therapies has been reported to be good (171). Uncommon neurologic disorders that may be encountered in children include CNS lymphoma, corticospinal tract degeneration, and, rarely, myelopathy, myopathy, and peripheral neuropathy.

PSYCHOSOCIAL AND VOCATIONAL ISSUES

HIV remains one of the most stigmatized diseases of our time. As in oncologic rehabilitation, patients may be faced with issues of death and dying and, perhaps surprisingly, hope and survival. Discrimination remains a particular problem due to the infectious nature of the disease and to public misperceptions and prejudice. The health of the caregiver, if there is one, is of particular concern when developing rehabilitation strategies. As always, rehabilitation professionals must deal with the patient in the context of their surroundings and their external support network.

Before the onset of symptoms, 70% to 90% of people with HIV are still employed (172). Even in the first year after the onset of symptoms, fewer than one third leave the work force. People with HIV commonly experience workplace discrimination and, with advancing symptoms, may experience a diminished work capacity. Significant controversy exists regarding persons with HIV in the health-care field. Those who are forced to leave the work force face a potential loss of health insurance. In all other respects, vocational rehabilitation of the HIV patient is similar to that of the patient with cancer or multiple sclerosis.

THE FUTURE OF HIV REHABILITATION

The management of HIV is one of the most rapidly changing fields of medicine, with entirely new treatment strategies often becoming available in a period of months rather than years. By the time this is published, it is likely that new medications not discussed here will be in common usage. The complexion of HIV rehabilitation could potentially change overnight, and the future of HIV rehabilitation is thus largely unknown. Because a cure does not seem to be imminent, however, it is reasonable to expect a need for rehabilitation interventions for the foreseeable future.

Most HIV strategists see HIV as eventually being managed as a chronic disease similar to diabetes mellitus. Although not curable, its progression will be held in check by medical therapies. This comparison with diabetes may be particularly apt in the case of rehabilitation. Although the most serious morbidity and mortality of diabetes is avoidable, even with stringent control of blood glucose, amputation, blindness, and peripheral neuropathy remain common sequellae that often respond to rehabilitation interventions. The extent to which new HIV treatment strategies will arrest the development of functional impairments and disability remains to be seen.

Although this discussion is highly speculative, rehabilitation professionals must face the possibility that a large segment of their future patient population may consist of otherwise healthy individuals with HIV and a variety of disabling conditions such as Guillian-Barré syndrome, polymyositis, distal symmetric polyneuropathy, HIV dementia, and vacuolar myelopathy. The role of rehabilitation may be critical in keeping these people functional in their communities.

REFERENCES

1. O'Connell PG, Levinson SF. Experience with rehabilitation in the acquired immunodeficiency system. *Am J Phys Med Rehabil* 1991; 70:195–200.
2. O'Dell MW. The epidemiology of HIV-related physical disability. In: O'Dell MW, ed. *HIV-related disability: assessment and management.* Philadelphia: Hanley & Belfus, 1993; S29–S42.
3. Centers for Disease Control and Prevention. 1993 revised classification system for HIV infection and expanded surveillance case definition for AIDS among adolescents and adults. *MMWR* 1992;41: RR-17.
4. World Health Organization. *The current global situation of the HIV-AIDS pandemic.* Geneva, Switzerland: WHO, 1995.
5. Centers for Disease Control and Prevention. Update: mortality attributable to HIV infection among persons aged 25–44 years—United States, 1994. *MMWR* 1995; 45:121–124.
6. Centers for Disease Control and Prevention. AIDS associated with injecting-drug use—United States, 1995. *MMWR* 1996; 45:392–398.
7. Tokars JI, Chamberland ME, Schable CA, et al. A survey of occupational blood contact and HIV infection among orthopedic surgeons. The American Academy of Orthopedic Surgeons Serosurvey Study Committee. *JAMA* 1992; 268:489–494.
8. Tokars JI, Marcus R, Culver DH, et al. Surveillance of HIV infection and zidovudine use among health care workers after occupational exposure to HIV-infected blood. the CDC Cooperative Needlestick Surveillance Group [see comments]. *Ann Intern Med* 1993; 118: 913–919.
9. Gerberding JL. Management of occupational exposures to blood-borne viruses. *N Engl J Med* 1995; 332:444–451.
10. Centers for Disease Control and Prevention. Case-control study of HIV seroconversion in health-care workers after percutaneous exposure to HIV-infected blood—France, United Kingdom, and United States, January 1988–August 1994. *MMWR* 1995; 44:929–933.
11. Centers for Disease Control and Prevention. Update: provisional Public Health Service recommendations for chemoprophylaxis after occupational exposure to HIV. *MMWR* 1996; 45:468–480.
12. Connor EM, Sperling RS, Gelber R, et al. Reduction of maternal—infant transmission of human immunodeficiency virus type 1 with zidu-vudine treatment. Pediatric AIDS Clinical Trial Group Protocol 076 Study Group. *N Engl J Med* 1994; 331:1173–1180.
13. Mauskopf JA, Paul JE, Wichman DS, White AD, Tilson HH. Economic impact of treatment of HIV-positive pregnant women and their newborns with zidovudine. *JAMA* 1996; 276:132–138.
14. Rotheram-Borus MJ, Mahler KA, Rosario M. AIDS prevention with adolescents [Review]. *AIDS Educ Prev* 1995; 7:320–336.
15. Auerbach V, Jann B. Neurorehabilitation and HIV infection: clinical dilemmas. *J Head Trauma Rehabil* 1989; 4:23–31.
16. Boccellari A, Zeifert P. Management of neurobehavioral impairment in HIV-1 infection [Review]. *Psych Clin North Am* 1994; 17:183–203.
17. Fauci AS, Pantanleo G, Stanley S, Weissman D. Immunopathogenic mechanisms of HIV infection [Review]. *Ann Intern Med* 1996; 124: 654–663.
18. Fox CH, Tenner-Racz K, Racz P, Firpo A, Pizzo PA, Fauci AS. Lymphoid germinal centers are reserviors of human immunodeficiency virus type 1 RNA. *J Infect Dis* 1991; 164:1051–1057.
19. Pantoleo G, Graziosi C, Fauci AS. New concepts in the immunopathogenesis of human immunodeficiency virus infection [Review]. *N Engl J Med* 1993; 328:327–335.
20. Pantoleo G, Graziosi C, Demarest JF, et al. HIV infection is active and progressive in lymphoid tissue during the clinically latent stage of disease. *Nature* 1993; 362:355–358.
21. Havlir DV, Richman DD. Viral dynamics of HIV: implications for drug development and therapeutic strategies. *Ann Intern Med* 1996; 124:984–994.
22. Clark SJ, Saag MS, Decker WD, et al. High titers of cytopathic virus in plasma of patients with symptomatic primary HIV-1 infection. *N Engl J Med* 1991; 324:954–960.
23. Koup RA, Safrit JT, Cao Y, et al. Temporal association of cellular immune responses with the initial control of viremia in primary human immunodeficiency virus type 1 syndrome. *J Virol* 1994; 68: 4650—4655.
24. Daar ES, Moudgil T, Meyer RD, Ho DD. Transient high levels of viremia in patients with primary human immunodeficiency virus type 1 infection. *N Engl J Med* 1991; 324:961–964.
25. Tindall B, Cooper DA. Primary HIV infection: host responses and intervention strategies [Editorial]. *AIDS* 1995; 5:1–14.
26. Jackson JB, Kwok SY, Sninsky JJ, et al. Human immunodeficiency virus type 1 detected in all seropositive symptomatic and asymptomatic individuals. *J Clin Microbiol* 1990; 28:16–19.
27. Hollander H, Levy JA. Neurologic abnormalities and recovery of human immunodeficiency virus from cerebrospinal fluid. *Ann Intern Med* 1987; 106:692–695.
28. Embretson J, Zupancic M, Ribas JL, et al. Massive covert infection of helper T lymphocytes and macrophages by HIV during the incubation period of AIDS. *Nature* 1993; 362:359–362.
29. Paitak MJ, Saag MS, Yang LC, et al. High levels of HIV-1 in plasma during all stages of infection determined by competitive PCR. *Science* 1993; 259:1749–1754.
30. Mellors JW, Kingsley LA, Rinaldo CRJ, et al. Quantitation of HIV-1 RNA in plasma predict outcome after seroconversion. *Ann Intern Med* 1995; 122:573–579.
31. Henrad DR, Phillips JF, Muenz LR, et al. Natural history of HIV-1 cell-free viremia. *JAMA* 1995; 274:554–558.
32. O'Brien TR, Blattner WA, Waters D, et al. Serum HIV-1 RNA levels and time to development of AIDS in the multicenter hemophilia cohort study. *JAMA* 1996; 276:105–110.
33. Ho DD, Neumann AU, Perelson AS, Chen W, Leonard JM, Markowitz M. Rapid turnover of plasma virions and CD4 lymphocytes in HIV-1 infection. *Nature* 1995; 373:117–122.
34. Wei X, Ghosh SK, Taylor ME, et al. Viral dynamics in human immunodeficiency virus type 1 infection. *Nature* 1995; 373:117–122.
35. Perelson AS, Neumann AU, Markowitz M, Leonard JM, Ho DD. HIV-1 dynamics in vivo: virion clearance rate, infected cell lifetime, and viral generation time. *Science* 1996; 271:1582–1586.
36. Najera I, Richman DD, Olivares I, et al. Natural occurrence of drug resistance mutations in the reverse transcriptase of human immunodeficiency virus type 1 isolates. *AIDS Res Hum Retrovir* 1994; 10: 1479–1488.
37. Najera I, Holquin A, Quinones-Mateu ME, et al. Pol gene quasispecies of human immunodeficiency virus: mutations associated with drug resistance in virus from patients undergoing no drug therapy. *J Virol* 1995; 69:23–31.
38. Carpenter CCJ, Fischl M, Hammer SM, et al. Antiretroviral therapy for HIV infection in 1996. Recommendations of an International Panel. *JAMA* 1996; 276:146–154.
39. Bartlett JA, Benoit SL, Johnson VA, et al. Lamivudine plus zidovudine compared with zalcitabine plus zidovudine in patients with HIV infection. *Ann Intern Med* 1996; 125:161–172.
40. Katlama C, Ingrand D, Loveday C, et al. Safety and efficacy of lamivudine-zidovudine combination therapy in antiretroviral-naive patients. A randomized controlled comparison with ziduvudine monotherapy. *JAMA* 1996; 276:118–125.
41. Schapiro JM, Winters MA, Stewart F, et al. The effect of high-dose

saquinavir on viral load and CD4+ T-cell counts in HIV-infected patients. *Ann Intern Med* 1996; 124:1039–1050.

42. Markowitz M, Saag M, Powderly WG, et al. A preliminary study of ritonavir, an inhibitor of HIV-1 protease, to treat HIV-1 infection. *N Engl J Med* 1995; 333:1534–1539.
43. Coates A, Cammack N, Jenkinson HJ, et al. (−)-2′deoxy-3′thiacytidine is a potent, highly selective inhibitor of human immunodeficiency virus type 1 and type 2 replication in vitro. *Antimicrob Agents Chemother* 1992; 36:733–739.
44. Concord Coordinating Committee. Concorde: MRC/ANS randomised double-blind controlled trial of immediate and deferred zidovudine in symptom-free HIV-infection. *Lancet* 1994; 343:871–881.
45. Volberding PA, Lagakos SW, Grimes JM, et al. The duration of zidovudine benefit in persons with asymptomatic HIV infection. Prolonged evalation of protocol 019 of the AIDS clinical Trials Group. *JAMA* 1994; 272:437–442.
46. Hammer S, Katzenstein D, Hughes M, et al. Nucleoside monotherapy vs. combination therapy in HIV-infected adults: a randomized, double-blind, placebo-controlled trial in persons with CD4 cell counts 200–500 per cubic millimeter. *N Engl J Med* 1996; 335:1081–1090.
47. Meng TC, Fischl MA, Boota AM, et al. Combination therapy with zidovudine and dideoxycytidine in patients with advanced human immunodeficiency virus infection. A phase I/II study. *Ann Intern Med* 1992; 116:13–20.
48. Collier AC, Coombs RW, Fischl MA, et al. Combination therapy with zidovidine and didanosine compared with zidovudine alone in HIV-1 infection. *Ann Intern Med* 1993; 119:786–793.
49. Fischl AM, Stanley K, Collier AC, et al. Combination and monotherapy with zidovudine and zalcitabine in patients with advanced HIV disease. The NIAID AIDS Clinical Trials Group. *Ann Intern Med* 1995; 122:24–32.
50. Kitchen VS, Skinner C, Ariyoshi K, et al. Safety and activity of saquinavir in HIV infection. *Lancet* 1996; 345:952–955.
51. Ho DD, Toyoshima T, Mo H, et al. Characterization of human immunodeficiency virus type 1 variants with increased resistance to a C2-symmetric protease inhibitor. *J Virol* 1994; 68:2016–2020.
52. Danner SA, Carr A, Leonard JM, et al. A short-term study of the safety, pharmacokinetics, and efficacy of ritonavir, an inhibitor of HIV-1 protease. European-Australian Collaborative Ritonavir Study Group. *N Engl J Med* 1995; 333:1528–1533.
53. Kovacs JA, Deyton L, Davey R, et al. Combined zidovudine and interferon-alpha therapy in patients with Kaposi's sarcoma and acquired immunodeficiency syndrome (AIDS). *Ann Intern Med* 1989; 111:280–287.
54. Moore RD, Chaisson RE. Natural history of opportunistic disease in an HIV-infected urban clinical cohort. *Ann Intern Med* 1996; 124:633–642.
55. Centers for Disease Control and Prevention. Recommendations for prophylaxis against PCP for adults and adolescents infected with HIV. *MMWR* 1992; 41:1–11.
56. Centers for Disease Control and Prevention. USPHS/IDSA guidelines for the prevention of opportunistic infections in persons infected with HIV. A summary. *MMWR* 1994; 44:1–39.
57. Centers for Disease Control and Prevention. *HIV/AIDS surveillance report Atlanta.* U.S. Department of Health and Human Services, Center for Disease Control and Prevention, National Center of Infectious Diseases, Division of HIV/AIDS, Atlanta, Georgia: CDC National Clearinghouse, 1994; 1–36.
58. Chaisson RE, Schecter GF, Theuer CP, et al. Tuberculosis-acquired immunodeficiency syndrome: clinical feature, response to therapy, and survival. *Am Rev Respir Dis* 1987; 136:570–574.
59. Selwyn PA, Hartel D, Lewis VA, et al. A prospective study of risk of tuberculosis among intravenous drug users with human immunodeficiency virus infection. *N Engl J Med* 1989; 320:545–550.
60. Centers for Disease Control and Prevention. Tuberculosis and human immunodeficiency viral infection: recommendations of the advisory committee for the elimination of tuberculosis (ACET). *MMWR* 1989; 38:236–238, 243–250.
61. Centers for Disease Control and Prevention. Guidelines for preventing the transmission of *Mycobacterium tuberculosis* in health-care facilities. *MMWR* 1994; 43:1–132.
62. Kent JH. The epidemiology of multidrug-resistant tuberculosis in the United States. *Med Clin North Am* 1993; 77:1391–1409.
63. Centers for Disease Control and Prevention. Multidrug-resistant tuberculosis outbreak on an HIV ward—Madrid, Spain, 1991–1995. *MMWR* 1996; 45:330–333.
64. Masur H. Recommendations on prophylaxis and therapy for disseminated *Mycobacterium avium* complex disease in patients infected with the human immunodeficiency virus. Public Health Service Task Force on Prophylaxis for *Mycobacterium avium* Complex [Comments]. *N Engl J Med* 1993; 329:898–904.
65. Shafran SD, Singer J, Zarowny DP, et al. A comparison of two regimens for the treatment of *Mycobacterium avuim* complex bacteremia in AIDS: rifabutin, ethambutol, and clarithromycin versus rifampin, ethambutol, clofazimine and ciprofloxacin. *N Engl J Med* 1996; 335:377–383.
66. Peirce M, Crampton S, Henry D, et al. A randomized trial of clarithromycin as prophylaxis against disseminated *Mycobacteruim avium* complex infection in patients with advanced acquired immunodeficiency syndrome. *N Engl J Med* 1996; 335:384–391.
67. Havlir DV, Dube MP, Sattler FR, et al. Prophylaxis against disseminated *Mycobacterium avium* complex with weekly azithromycin, daily rifabutin or both. *N Engl J Med* 1996; 335:392–398.
68. Schaffner A, Davis CE, Schaffer T, et al. In vitro susceptibility of fungi to killing neutrophil granulocytes discriminates between primary pathogenesis and opportunism. *J Clin Invest* 1986; 78:511–524.
69. Sarosi GA, Johnson PC. Disseminated histoplasmosis in patients infected with human immunodeficiency virus. *Clin Infect Dis* 1992; 14(suppl):60–67.
70. Wheat LJ, Connolly-Stringfield PA, Baker RL, et al. Disseminated histoplasmosis in the acquired immunodeficiency syndrome: clinical findings, diagnosis, and review of the literature. *Medicine* 1990; 69:361–374.
71. Wheat LJ, Hafner R, Wulfsohn M, et al. Prevention of relapse of histoplasmosis with itraconazole in patients with the acquired immunodeficiency syndrome. *Ann Intern Med* 1993; 118:610–616.
72. Wheat LJ, Hafner RE, Korzun AH, et al. Itraconozole treatment of disseminated histoplasmosis in patients with acquired immunodeficiency syndrome. *Am J Med* 1995; 98:336–343.
73. Edwards P, Wodak A, Cooper DA, Thompson IL, Penny R. The gastrointestinal manifestation of AIDS. *Aust NZ J Med* 1990; 20:141–148.
74. Parente F, Cernuschi M, Rizzardini G, Lazzarin A, Balsechhi L, Bianchi Porro G. Opportunistic infection of the esophagus not responding to oral systemic antifungals in patients with AIDS: their frequency and treatment. *Am J Gastroenterol* 1991; 86:1729–1734.
75. Deiterich DT, et al. Ganciclovir treatment of cytomegalovirus colitis in AIDS: a randomized double-blind, placebo controlled multicenter study. *J Infect Dis* 1993; 167:278–282.
76. Sangeorzan JA, Bradley SF, He X, et al. Epidemiology of oral candidiasis in HIV-infected patients: colonization, infection, treatment, and emergence of fluconazole resistance. *Am J Med* 1994; 97:339–346.
77. Bonacini M, Young T, Liane L. The causes of esophageal symptoms in human immunodeficiency virus infection. A prospective study of 110 patients. *Arch Intern Med* 1991; 151:1567–1572.
78. Connolly GM, Hawkins D, Harcourt-Webster JN, Parsons PA, Husain OA, Gazzard BG. Oesophageal symptoms, their causes, treatment, and prognosis in patients with the acquired immunodeficiency syndrome. *Gut* 1989; 30:1033–1039.
79. Fichtenbaum CJ, Ritchie DJ, Powderly WG. Use of paromomycin for treatment of cryptosporidiosis in patients with AIDS. *Clin Infect Dis* 1993; 16:298–300.
80. White AC, Chappell CL, Hayat CS, Kimball KT, Flanigan TP, Goodgame RW. Paromomycin for cryptosporidiosis in AIDS—a prospective double-blind trial. *J Infect Dis* 1994; 70:419–424.
81. Blanshard C, Ellis DS, Tovey DG, Dowell S, Gazzard BG. Treatment of intestinal microsporidiosis with albendazole in patients with AIDS. *AIDS* 1992; 6:311–313.
82. Weber R, Bryan RT. Microsporidial infections in immunodeficient and immunocompetent patients. *Clin Infect Dis* 1994; 19:517–521.
83. Benator DA, French AL, Beaudet LM, Levy CS, Orenstein JM. Isospora belli infection associated with acalculous cholecystitis in a patient with AIDS. *Ann Intern Med* 1994; 121:663–664.
84. Klatt EC, Nichols L, Noguchi TT. Evolving trends revealed by autopsies of patients with the acquired immunodeficiency syndrome, Los Angeles, California, 1992–3. *Arch Pathol Lab Med* 1994; 118:884–890.
85. Katz MH, Hessol NA, Buchbinder SP, et al. Temporal trends of oppor-

tunistic infections and malignancies in homosexual men with AIDS. *J Infect Dis* 1994; 170:198–202.

86. Safai B, Johnson KG, Myskowski P, et al. The natural history of Kaposi's sarcoma in the acquired immunodeficiency syndrome. *Ann Intern Med* 1985; 103:744–750.
87. Morfeldt L, Torssander J. Long-term remission of Kaposi's sarcoma following foscarnet treatment in HIV-infected patients. *Scand J Infect Dis* 1994; 26:749–752.
88. Krown SE, Gold JW, Niedwiecki D, et al. Interferon-alpha with zidovudine-safety, tolerance and clinical and virologic effects in patients with Kaposi's sarcoma associated with the acquired immunodeficiency syndrome (AIDS). *Ann Intern Med* 1990; 112:812–821.
89. Gill PS, Espina BM, Muggia F, et al. Phase I/II clinical and pharmacokinet evaluation of liposomal daunorubicin. *J Clin Oncol* 1995; 13: 996–1003.
90. Bogner JR, Kronawitter U, Rolinski B, et al. Liposomal doxorubicin in the treatment of advanced AIDS-related Kaposi's sarcoma. *J AIDS Hum Retrovir* 1994; 7:463–468.
91. Gill PS, Laudadi-Iskandar Y, Louie S, et al. The effects of preparation of human chorionic gonadotropin on AIDS-related Kaposi's sarcoma. *N Engl J Med* 1996; 335:1261–1269.
92. Lubeck DP, Nobunaga AI, Williams CA, O'Dell MW. Rehabilitation of selected nonneurologic disability. In: O'Dell MW, ed. *HIV-related disability: assessment and management.* Philadelphia: Hanley & Belfus, 1993; S131–S153.
93. Strauss J, Zilleruelo G, Abitbol C, Montane B, Pardo V. Human immunodeficiency virus nephropathy [Review]. *Pediatr Nephrol* 1993; 7: 220–225.
94. Berman A, Espinoza LR, Diaz JD, et al. Rheumatic manifestations of human immunodeficiency virus infection. *Am J Med* 1988; 85: 59–64.
95. Espinoza LR, Aguilar JL, Berman A, Gutierrez F, Vasey FB, Germain BF. Rheumatic manifestations associated with human immunodeficiency virus infection. *Arthritis Rheum* 1989; 32:1615–1622.
96. Rynes RI, Goldenberg DL, DiGiacomo R, Olson R, Hussain M, Veazy J. Acquired immune deficiency syndrome-associated arthritis. *Am J Med* 1988; 84:810–816.
97. Simpson DM. Neuromuscular complications of human immunodeficiency virus infection. *Semin Neurol* 1992; 12:34–42.
98. Simpson DM, Bender AN. Human immunodeficiency virus-associated myopathy: analysis of 11 patients. *Ann Neurol* 1988; 24:79–84.
99. Simpson DM, Citak KA, Godfrey E, Godbold J, Wolfe DE. Myopathies associated with human immunodeficiency virus and zidovudine: can their effects be distinguished? *Neurology* 1993; 43:971–976.
100. Ma DM. Electrodiagnosis of neuromuscular disease in HIV infection. In: O'Dell MW, ed. *HIV-related disability: assessment and management.* Philadelphia: Hanley & Belfus, 1993; S73–S82.
101. Hassett J, Tagliati M, Godbold J, Godfrey E, Feinstein R, Simpson D. A placebo-controlled study of prednisone in HIV-associated myopathy [Abstract]. *Neurology* 1994; 44(suppl 2):A250.
102. Calabrese LH. Vasculitis and infection with the human immunodeficiency virus. *Rheum Dis Clin North Am* 1991; 17:131–147.
103. Simpson DM, Olney RK. Peripheral neuropathies associated with human immunodeficiency virus infection. *Neurol Clin* 1992; 10: 685–711.
104. Simpson DM, Tagliati M. Neurologic manifestations of HIV infections [Review]. *Ann Intern Med* 1994; 121:769–785 [erratum *Ann Intern Med* 1995; 122:317].
105. Cornblatt DR, McArthur JC, Kennedy PG, Witte AS, Griffin JW. Inflammatory demyelinating peripheral neuropathy associated with human T-cell lymphotrophic virus type III infection. *Ann Neurol* 1987; 21:32–40.
106. Miller RG. Neuromuscular complications of human immunodeficiency virus infection and antiretroviral therapy [Review]. *West J Med* 1994; 160:447–452.
107. Simpson DM, Tagliati M, Ramcharitar S. Neurologic complications of AIDS: new concepts and treatments [Review]. *Mt Sinai J Med* 1994; 61:484–491.
108. Eidelberg D, Sortel A, Vogel H, et al. Progressive polyradiculopathy in acquired immune deficiency syndorme. *Neurology* 1986; 36: 912–916.
109. So YT, Olney RK. Acute lumbosacral polyradiculopathy in acquired immunodefiency syndrome: experience in 23 patients. *Ann Neurol* 1994; 35:53–58.
110. Cohen BA, McArthur JC, Grohman W, et al. Neurologic prognosis of cytomegalovirus polyradiculopathy in AIDS. *Neurology* 1993; 43: 493–499.
111. Fuller GN, Gill SK, Guiloff RJ, et al. Ganciclovir for lumbosacral polyradiculopathy in AIDS. *Lancet* 1990; 335:48–49.
112. Fuller GN. Cytomegalovirus and the peripheral nervous system in AIDS [Review]. *J AIDS* 1992; 5(suppl 1):533–536.
113. de Gans J, Portegies P, Tiessesns G, et al. Therapy for cytomegalovirus polyradiculomyelitis in patients with AIDS: treatment with ganciclovir. *AIDS* 1990; 4:421–425.
114. Miller RG, Storey JR, Greco CM. Ganciclovir in the treatment of progressive AIDS-related polyradiculopathy. *Neurology* 1990; 40: 569–574.
115. Janssen RS. Epidemiology of human immunodeficiency virus infection and the neurologic complications of the infection. *Neurology* 1992; 41:10–17.
116. McArthur JC. Neurologic manifestations of AIDS. *Medicine* 1987; 66:407–437.
117. Janssen RS, Saykin AJ, Cannon L, et al. Neurological and neuropsychological manifestations of HIV-1 infection: association with AIDS-related complex but not asymptomatic HIV-1 infection. *Ann Neurol* 1989; 26:592–600.
118. Miller EN. Selnes OA, McArthur JC, et al. Neuropsychological performance in HIV-1-infected homosexual men: the multicenter AIDS cohort study (MACS). *Neurology* 1990; 40:197–203.
119. Perdices M, Cooper DA. Neuropsychological investigation of patients with AIDS and ARC. *J AIDS* 1990; 3:555–564.
120. Selnes OA, Miller E, McArthur J, et al. HIV-1 infection: no evidence of cognitive decline during the asymptomatic stages. *Neurology* 1990; 40:204–208.
121. Powderly WG. Cryptococcal meningitis and AIDS. *Clin Infect Dis* 1993; 17:837–842.
122. Musher DM, Hamill RJ, Baughn RE. The effect of human immunodeficiency virus (HIV) infection on the course of syphilis and on the response to treatment. *Ann Intern Med* 1990; 113:872–881.
123. Johns DR. Tierne M, Flesenstein D. Alteration in the natural history of neurosyphilis by concurrent infection with the human immunodeficiency virus. *N Engl J Med* 1987; 316:1569–1572.
124. Clifford D, Campbell JW. Management of neurologic opportunistic disorders in human immunodeficiency virus infection. *Semin Neurol* 1992; 12:28–33.
125. Dix RD, Bredesen DE. Opportunistic viral infections in acquired immunodeficiency syndrome. In: Rosenblum ML, Levy RM, Bredesen DE, eds. *AIDS and the nervous system.* New York: Raven, 1988; 221–261.
126. Portegies P, Brew BJ. Update on HIV-related neurological illness [Review]. *AIDS* 1991; 5(suppl 2):S211–S217.
127. Berger JR, Levy JA. The human immunodeficiency virus, type 1: the virus and its role in neurologic disease [Review]. *Semin Neurol* 1992; 12:1–9.
128. Robertson KR, Hall CD. Human immunodeficiency virus-related cognitive impairment and the acquired immunodeficiency syndrome dementia complex [Review]. *Semin Neurol* 1992; 12:18–27.
129. Berger JR, Levy RM. The neurologic complications of human immunodeficiency virus infection [Review]. *Med Clin North Am* 1993; 77: 1–23.
130. Newton HB. Common neurologic complications of HIV-1 infection and AIDS [Review]. *Am Fam Physician* 1995; 51:387–398.
131. Gillespie SM, Chang Y, Limp G, et al. Progressive multifocal leukoencephalopathy in persons infected with human immunodeficiency virus: San Francisco 1981–1989. *Ann Neurol* 1991; 30:597–604.
132. Grant JW, Isaacson PG. Primary central nervous system lymphoma [Review]. *Brain Pathol* 1992; 2:97–109.
133. Noel S, Guillaume MP, Telerman-Toppet N, Cogan E. Movement disorders due to cerebral toxoplasma gondii infection in patients with the acquired immunodeficiency syndrome (AIDS) [Review]. *Acta Neurol Belg* 1992; 92:148–156.
134. Royal W III, Updike M, Selnes OA, et al. HIV-1 infection and nervous system abnormalities among a cohort of intravenous drug users. *Neurology* 1991; 41:1905–1910.
135. Simpson DM, Tagliati M. Neurologic manifestations of HIV infection. *Ann Intern Med* 1996; 121:769–785.
136. So YT, Beckstead JH, Davis RL. Primary central nervous system

lymphoma in acquired immune deficiency syndrome: a clinical and pathological study. *Ann Neurol* 1986; 20:566–572.

137. Gallant JE, Moore RD, Richman DD, Keruly J, Chaisson RE, Zidovudine Epidemiology Study Group. Incidence and natural history of cytomegalovirus disease in patients with advanced human immunodeficiency virus treated with zidovudine. *J Infect Dis* 1992; 166: 1223–1227.
138. Bloom JN, Palestine AG. The diagnosis of cytomegalovirus retinitis. *Ann Intern Med* 1988; 109:963–969.
139. Studies of the Ocular Complication of AIDS Research Group in Collaboration with the AIDS Clinical Trials Group. Mortality in patients with the acquired immunodeficiency syndrome treated with either foscarnet or ganciclovir for cytomegalovirus retinitis. *N Engl J Med* 1992; 326:213–220.
140. Martin DF, Parks DJ, Mellow SD, et al. Treatment of cytomegalovirus retinitis with an intraocular sustained-release ganciclovir implant: a randomized controlled clinical trial. *Arch Ophthalmol* 1994; 112: 1531–1539.
141. Rahhal FM, Arevalo JF, Chavez de la Paz E, Manguia D, Azen SP, Freeman WR. Treatment of cytomegalovirus retinitis with intravitreous codifovir in patients with AIDS. A preliminary report. *Ann Intern Med* 1996; 125:98–103.
142. Jabs DA. Treatment of cytomegalovirus retinitis in patients with AIDS. *Ann Intern Med* 1996; 125:144–145.
143. Luft BJ, Remington JS. Toxoplasmic encephalitis in AIDS [Review]. *Clin Infect Dis* 1992; 15:211–222.
144. Porter SB, Sande MA. Toxoplasmosis of the central nervous system in the acquired immunodeficiency syndrome. *N Engl J Med* 1992; 327:1643–1648.
145. Borggreve F, Dierckx RA, Crols R, et al. Repeat thalluim-210 SPECT in cerebral lymphoma. *Funct Neurol* 1993; 8:95–101.
146. Carr A, Tindall B, Brew BJ, et al. Low dose trimethoprim-sulfamethoxazole prophylaxis for toxoplasmic encephalitis in patients with AIDS. *Antimicrob Agents Chemother* 1991; 34:2049–2052.
147. Berger JR, Kaszovitz B, Post JD, Dickinson G. Progressive multifocal leukoencephalopathy associated with human immunodeficiency virus infection. A review of the literature with a report of sixteen cases. *Ann Intern Med* 1987; 107:78–87.
148. von Einsiedal RW, Fife TD, Aksamit AJ, et al. Progressive multifocal leukoencephalopathy in AIDS: a clinicopathological study and review of the literature. *J Neurol* 1993; 240:391–406.
149. Pluda JM, Yarchoan R, Jaffe ES, et al. Development of non-Hodgkin lymphoma in a cohort of patients with severe human immunodeficiency virus (HIV) infection on long-term antiretroviral therapy. *Ann Intern Med* 1990; 113:276–282.
150. Nisce LZ, Kaufmann T, Metroda C. Radiation therapy in patients with AIDS-related central nervous system lymphomas. *JAMA* 1992; 267: 1921–1922.
151. Levy RM, Bredesen DE, Rosenblum ML. Neurological manifestations of the acquired immunodeficiency syndrome (AIDS). Experience at UCSF and review of the literature. *J Neurosurg* 1985; 62:475–495.
152. Engstrom JW, Lowenstein DH, Bredesen DE. Cerebral infarctions and transient neurologic deficits associated with acquired immunodeficiency syndrome. *Am J Med* 1989; 86:528–532.
153. Berger JR, Harris JO, Gergorios J, Norenberg M. Cerebrovascular disease in AIDS: a case control study. *AIDS* 1990; 4:239–244.
154. Calabrese LH, Furlan AJ, Gragg LA, Ropos TJ. Primary angiitis of the central nervous system: diagnostic criteria and clinical approach [Review]. *Cleve Clin J Med* 1992; 59:293–306.
155. Gray F, Chimelli L, Mohr M, Clavelou P, Scaravilli F, Poirier J. Fulminating multiple sclerosis-like leukoencephalopathy revealing human immunodeficiency virus infection. *Neurology* 1991; 41: 105–109.
156. Ammann AJ. Human immunodeficiency virus/AIDS in children: the next decade [Review]. *Pediatrics* 1994; 93:930–935.
157. Brady MT. Management of children with human immunodeficiency virus infection [Review]. *Comprehens Ther* 1995; 21:139–147.
158. Chadwick EG, Yogev R. Pediatric AIDS [Review]. *Pediatr Clin North Am* 1995; 42:969–992.
159. Krasinski K. Antiretroviral therapy for children [Review]. *Acta Paediatr Suppl* 1994; 400:63–69.
160. Jones DS, Byers RH, Bush TJ, et al. Epidemiology of transfusion-associated acquired immunodeficiency syndrome. *Pediatrics* 1992; 89:123–127.
161. Kovelesky Ra, Minor JR. Antiretroviral therapy during pregnancy [Review]. *Am J Hosp Pharm* 1994; 51:2187–2189.
162. Minkoff H, Mofenson LM. The role of obstetric interventions in the prevention of pediatric human immunodeficiency virus infection [see comments] [Review]. *Am J Obstet Gynecol* 1994; 171:1167–1175.
163. Pavlakis SG, Frank Y, Nocyze M, Porricolo M, Prohovnik I, Wiznia A. Acquired immunodeficiency syndrome and the developing nervous system [Review]. *Adv Pediatr* 1994; 41:427–451.
164. Pitt J. Lymphocytic interstitial pneumonia. *Pediatr Clin North Am* 1991; 38:89–95.
165. Connor EM, Andiman WA. Lymphoid interstitial pneumonitis. In: Pizzo PA, Wilfert CM, ed. *Pediatric AIDS.* Baltimore: Williams & Wilkins, 1994; 467–481.
166. Armstrong FD. Seidel JF, Swales TP. Pediatric HIV infection: a neuropsychological and educational challenge [Review]. *J Learn Disabil* 1993; 26:92–103.
167. Belman AL. Acquired immunodeficiency syndrome and the child's nervous system [Review]. *Pediatr Clin North Am* 1992; 39:691–714.
168. Binder H, Castagnino M. Rehabilitation considerations in pediatric HIV infection. In: O'Dell MW, ed. *HIV-related disability: assessment and management.* Philadelphia: Hanley & Belfus, 1993; S175–S187.
169. Burns DK. The neuropathology of pediatric acquired immunodeficiency syndrome [Review]. *J Child Neurol* 1992; 7:332–346.
170. Dowe DA, Heitzman ER, Larkin JJ. Human immunodeficiency virus infection in children [Review]. *Clin Imaging* 1992; 16:145–151.
171. Mintz M, Epstein LG. Neurologic manifestation of pediatric acquired immunodeficiency syndrome: clinical features and therapeutic approaches [Review]. *Semin Neurol* 1992; 12:51–56.
172. Vachon RA. Employment assistance and vocational rehabilitation for people with HIV or AIDS: policy, practice, and prospects. In: O'Dell MW, ed. *HIV-related disability: assessment and management.* Philadelphia: Hanley & Belfus, 1993; S189–201.

Rehabilitation Medicine: Principles and Practice, Third Edition,
edited by Joel A. DeLisa and Bruce M. Gans.
Lippincott–Raven Publishers, Philadelphia © 1998.

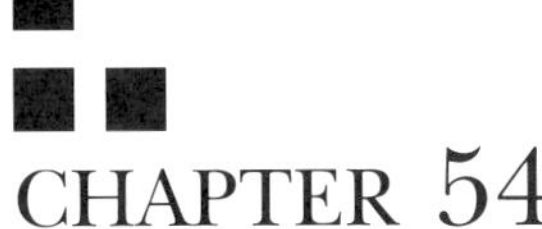

CHAPTER 54

Rehabilitation of the Cardiac Patient

Angeles M. Flores and Lenore R. Zohman

This chapter reviews the theory and practice of cardiac rehabilitation and the aspects of exercise stress testing that are important to the physiatrist. The principles of cardiovascular conditioning are translated into clinically applicable exercise conditioning programs. The recent use of exercises that were formerly considered to be contraindicated for cardiac patients is explored.

How to assess a patient's progress on an exercise program is also covered, including how to recognize peripheral training effects as well as determining whether exercise has benefited the myocardium. The rehabilitation of special groups of patients is also discussed—women, the elderly, heart transplant patients, and the physically impaired person with cardiac disease.

Because of space constraints, regretfully only brief mention can be made of the role of health-related staff in facilitating the psychological and social well-being of the patient, as well as their valuable assistance in returning patients to a healthy lifestyle. This chapter is limited to what physicians can contribute in programming and in prognosticating and preventing present and future problems.

CARDIAC REHABILITATION: A GROWING DISCIPLINE

Cardiac rehabilitation is the process of restoring an individual with a cardiac problem to the maximum level of activity compatible with the functional capacity of his or her heart. Traditionally, cardiac rehabilitation programs involved patients with coronary artery disease and were begun at the time of their acute myocardial infarction (MI) (1–4).

In the past two decades, cardiac rehabilitation has been broadened to include patients with other types of cardiovascular disease (5), as well as those recovering from coronary angioplasty (6,7) or heart surgery (5,8). Patients are referred for rehabilitation after coronary artery bypass grafting (CABG) (9–12), heart valve replacement (13,14), ventricular aneurysmectomy (15), and heart transplantation (16,17). Age and medical complexity are not necessarily limiting factors (18).

The 1996–1997 Cardiopulmonary Rehabilitation Program Directory published by the American Association of Cardiovascular and Pulmonary Rehabilitation (AACVPR) in 1996 lists 1,191 programs. Of these, 511 provide cardiac rehabilitation, 584 programs provide both cardiac and pulmonary services, and 96 are for pulmonary rehabilitation (19). In the first *Directory of Exercise Programs for Cardiacs,* which was published in 1970 as a joint effort by the President's Council on Physical Fitness and Sports and the American Heart Association, there were only 83 cardiac rehabilitation programs, with three programs also providing additional services such as pulmonary function testing and dietary management (20).

PROGRAM SUPERVISION: CARDIOLOGIST OR PHYSIATRIST

Cardiac rehabilitation programs can be supervised by either a cardiologist or a physiatrist. The nonsupervising discipline should be available to consult on complicated cases (e.g., if the physiatrist directed the program, cardiology consultation would be needed for cases requiring frequent medication adjustment, or those with changing medical problems needing ongoing diagnostic workup).

Conversely, if the cardiologist directed the program, physiatric consultation would be indicated for patients with multisystem problems such as stroke or lower extremity vascular obstructive disease in addition to coronary disease. Of the patients with both acute stroke and acute MI, either they had both on admission or the stroke occurred after admission

A. M. Flores: Department of Physical Medicine and Rehabilitation, University of Medicine and Dentistry of New Jersey, New Jersey Medical School, Newark, New Jersey 07103; and Veterans Administration Medical Center, East Orange, New Jersey 07018.
L. R. Zohman: Cardiac Rehabilitation Service, Department of Physical Medicine and Rehabilitation, Montefiore Medical Center, Bronx, New York 10467.

(2% of 750 cases admitted for acute MI) within the first 4 weeks, with the highest occurrence rate (77%) within the first week (21–23).

Among patients with lower extremity obstructive vascular disease, myocardial ischemia on exercise stress testing is frequent (24), and myocardial ischemia and infarction are the most frequent complications of vascular reconstructive surgery (25,26). In lower extremity amputations, the most significant factors complicating the rehabilitation of these patients are cardiopulmonary problems (27,28).

Physiatrists contemplating directing a complete cardiac rehabilitation program should be knowledgeable in the following areas:

- Recording and interpreting 12-lead exercise electrocardiograms (ECGs)
- Performing and interpreting standard ECG exercise stress tests; understanding nuclear imaging techniques and interpretation although may not have performed these personally
- Exercise ECG monitoring by on-line or transtelephone telemetry
- Cardiac medications such as digitalis, beta-adrenergic, and calcium channel blockers, angiotensin converting enzyme (ACE) inhibitors, coronary vasodilators, antiarrhythmic medications, anticoagulants, and lipid-lowering drugs including maintenance therapy
- Familiarity with techniques, meaning and implications of data from cardiac catheterization, angiography, stress echocardiography, programmed electrical stimulation, Holter monitoring, etc.
- Understanding of concepts of thrombolysis, coronary angioplasty, stenting, atherectomy, endarterectomy
- Expertise in cardiac exercise prescription, progression, and long-term follow-up (aerobic as well as strength-building exercise)
- Dietary intervention procedures in broad terms, role of the dietician and diabetes educator
- Vocational assessment: procedures and implications of various impairments for disability evaluation
- Familiarity with the possible contributions of occupational and physical therapists, social workers, vocational counselors, psychologists, holistic nurses, among others to a cardiac rehabilitation program if these individuals are available to the program
- Basic and advanced life support
- Communication techniques to inform colleagues of the expectations, outcomes, and methods of cardiac rehabilitation

DOES CARDIAC REHABILITATION DO MORE THAN MAKE PATIENTS FEEL GOOD?

The aim of cardiac rehabilitation is not only to improve cardiovascular functional capacity, hence improving the quality of life, but also to control coronary risk factors, minimizing the chance of recurrence and decreasing morbidity and mortality. Both a scientific and a layman's summary of the benefits of cardiac rehabilitation have been published by the National Heart, Lung and Blood Institute with the cooperation of the American Association of Cardiovascular and Pulmonary Rehabilitation.

The most clearly established favorable outcome of exercise training is its beneficial effect on exercise tolerance (18). Although almost 100% of patients report subjective benefits from exercise training programs, including enhanced well-being and self-esteem, less fatigue, less angina, less depression, and better sleep, the process is labor intensive, costly, and not entirely without risk.

Peripheral Training Effects

The objective benefits derived from exercise by patients who have had MI include both peripheral training effects and myocardial benefits. Peripheral or skeletal muscle adaptations to training include the following:

Increased oxygen extraction and a wider arteriovenous oxygen difference. Skeletal muscles take up more oxygen from the entering blood supply so that the venous return carries less back to the heart. The heart is thus doing less work to bring adequate oxygen to the tissues (29).

Improved utilization of oxygen by active muscle, resulting from the increase in oxidative enzymes in the muscle that occurs as a result of training (30).

Increased maximal oxygen consumption and physical work capacity. Maximal oxygen uptake may improve by 11% to 56% after acute MI patients are trained, and 14% to 66% when post–coronary bypass patients have trained for 3 to 6 months. The lower the initial maximun oxygen consumption ($\dot{V}O_{2max}$), the greater the improvement (31). Although cardiac patients do not have a particular need to increase peak performance *per se*, an increased capacity means that activities of daily living (ADL) are carried out at a lower percentage of peak performance. Endurance is enhanced and there is less fatigue.

The conditioned patient generally has a slower pulse, lower blood pressure, and lower rate-pressure product (RPP = heart rate × systolic blood pressure) after exercise training. Because RPP is a good indicator of myocardial oxygen demand, the trained cardiac patient functions at a lower myocardial oxygen demand—albeit for peripheral adaptation reasons. Thus, an angina patient may be below the angina threshold in daily life and may be able to perform certain activities without angina or silent ischemia, identified by Holter monitoring, that he or she could not do before beginning the exercise training program. Training in this respect produces symptomatic improvement by the same mechanism as beta-blockade.

All of the above can be accomplished as a result of improvement in skeletal muscle efficiency.

Myocardial Training Effects

Among 169 patients followed for 7 years before 1976, all felt subjectively improved by the rehabilitation program,

85% demonstrated a peripheral training effect, and only 8.9% seemed to show a "myocardial training effect" (32). The latter group showed consistently at least 1.0 mm less ST depression at the same RPP that had caused ST depression before training. All of the patients who demonstrated this lesser ST depression at the same RPP had been training at least 2 years without new disease and without a change in medication, because either change could have resulted in such findings.

The elusive search for confirmation of myocardial benefit has continued to date. Improvement in ventricular contractile function has been shown by Ehsani and colleagues when cardiac patients added bouts of high-intensity exercise at 85% to 90% of maximal heart rate to their training regimens (33–35). Froehlicher and colleagues (36) and Jensen and associates (37) have reported improved ventricular function, and Sebrechts et al. (38) and Goodman and associates (39) have reported improved myocardial perfusion on thallium scan after training, but there is only limited direct evidence in humans that exercise stimulates the growth of new collateral vessels within the myocardium (40,41).

In animals such as the dog, monkey, and pig, however, exercise training does indeed increase myocardial vascularity and may enlarge the main coronary vessels. The study of Kramsch and colleagues is of special interest in that those monkeys that he had placed on an atherogenic diet and required to run on treadmills had significantly less coronary atherosclerosis and wider coronary arteries than did the group on the atherogenic diet that did not exercise (42). Although of great interest, these results cannot be extrapolated to humans, despite pathologic observations that men who have performed lifelong heavy physical labor have larger coronary arteries (43). Figure 54-1*A* and *B* depicts work load, heart rate, blood pressure, and amount of ECG ischemia for a patient when he was not trained (preprogram), when he had trained his periphery, and when he began to have a myocardial training effect.

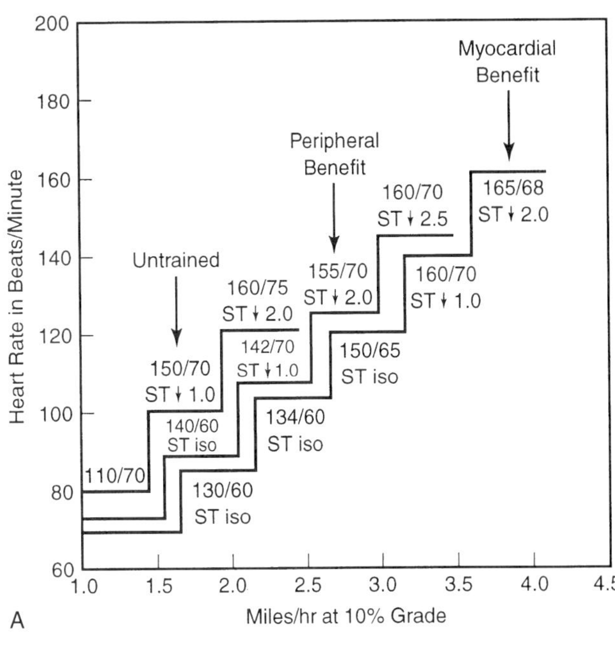

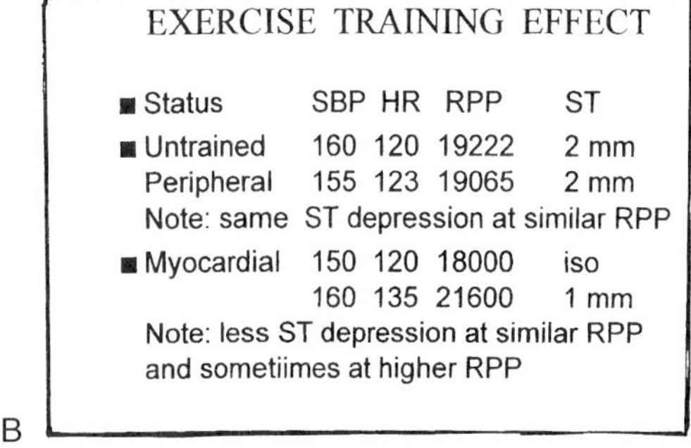

EXERCISE TRAINING EFFECT

Status	SBP	HR	RPP	ST
■ Untrained	160	120	19222	2 mm
Peripheral	155	123	19065	2 mm
Note: same ST depression at similar RPP				
■ Myocardial	150	120	18000	iso
	160	135	21600	1 mm
Note: less ST depression at similar RPP and sometiimes at higher RPP				

B

FIG. 54-1. A, B: Peripheral and myocardial benefits resulting from the effects of exercise training on heart rate, blood pressure and ECG ischemia.

Mortality and Morbidity

Individual randomized trials of cardiac rehabilitation exercise after MI have not demonstrated a statistically significant lower mortality rate among the cardiac rehabilitation groups. However, by pooling data from the various randomized trials and conducting various meta-analyses, a significant benefit is demonstrated on overall mortality over at least a 3-year period after infarction. May and colleagues showed a 19% reduction in total mortality for the exercise group (44), Shephard reported a 29% reduction in the 3-year mortality rate (45), Collins and associates estimated a 20% reduction (46), Oldridge and colleagues reported a 24% reduction in all causes of mortality and a 25% reduction in cardiovascular death (47), and O'Connor and associates found a 20% reduction in overall mortality in the cardiac rehabilitation group (48). Although there is this reported decrease in mortality, particularly sudden death during the first year after infarction, there does not seem to be a difference in nonfatal reinfarction rates between the rehabilitation groups and the controls (48). Van Hees et al. in their work on peak oxygen consumption (VO_2) after physical training found that cardiovascular mortality decreased more with greater increase in peak VO_2 after physical training, noting that the prognostic value of peak VO_2 was higher after training than before. This was true for both post-MI and post-CABG patients (49).

Reduction of Risk Factors for Coronary Disease

Reduction in coronary risk factors is important in retarding the progress of coronary atherosclerosis (50,51); in addition, continued reduction of these risk factors after coronary bypass graft surgery may help prolong the patency of these grafts (52). Exercise training is known to promote weight loss (53), increase high-density lipoprotein (HDL) cholesterol (54), decrease low-density lipoprotein (LDL) and triglycerides (55), exert a beneficial effect on blood pressure, and improve glucose utilization and insulin resistance (56). In hypertension, physical training has a beneficial effect in lowering both systolic and diastolic pressure, but this has to involve intensive exercise training (57,58) and is just for a short-term period, lasting only a few months after cessation of training.

CARDIAC REHABILITATION AND COST CONTAINMENT

A comprehensive cardiac rehabilitation program involves the total care of the patient, including the medical aspects of the case as well as psychological, social, and vocational services. The team approach to the cardiac patient, advocated in the 1960s and 1970s, is no longer compatible with the need to cut health-care costs. Fortunately, in rehabilitation medicine departments that retain a health team with the primary purpose of rehabilitation of the disabled (e.g., physician, nurse, physical and occupational therapists, dietician, psychologist, social worker, vocational rehabilitation specialist), that same team can provide therapy and guidance to the cardiac patient. The multidisciplinary structure of a rehabilitation medicine practice or service is often able to provide comprehensive management to cardiac patients not available through cardiology services, which cannot serve this dual function.

Furthermore, because of the shortened hospital stay of cardiac patients under diagnosis-related groups, cardiac rehabilitation can barely be begun and often is not even discussed when the patient is in the hospital. The special training of the physiatrist in the holistic approach to patient care and his or her familiarity with the expertise of various rehabilitation team members make it important for the physiatrist or his or her representative to maintain a presence on the cardiac service. He or she should be there to answer questions, describe available services, and provide guidance and information to busy cardiologists who may not be aware of benefits of cardiac rehabilitation.

INPATIENT CARDIAC REHABILITATION

In many busy private or teaching hospitals, the patients started on inpatient programs are probably somewhat more impaired and sicker than those who have rapid transit through the hospital system. If patients are stable and have the luxury of a few days of comprehensive care, or if they are in a less acute step-down facility, cardiac rehabilitation consisting of progressive physical activity and education may be begun. Patients are usually post-MI, post–heart surgery, or have acute coronary insufficiency without MI. Those who benefit most, however, are those who have had a prolonged hospital course due to a variety of complications and are markedly debilitated or deconditioned.

The exercises provided are in the form of either progressive range-of-motion exercises, from passive to active to low-level resistive exercises with the use of 1- to 2-pound weights (3,5,8), or calisthenics (12,59). Calisthenics are preferable because they involve not only motion of the extremities but also the neck and trunk, and they simulate the movements used in self-care and ADLs. The calisthenics designed by Karpovich and Weiss (60) are explained by means of simple pictures that are easy for patients to follow. The energy cost of each exercise is listed, as is the metronome count, which assures that the exercise is performed at the appropriate tempo.

Early ambulation begins as soon as the patient is out of the coronary/intensive care unit, using the patient's room, then in the hospital corridors. Walking as an early exercise also may be started on a treadmill. Treadmill ambulation progresses from 0% grade at 1 mph for 10 to 15 minutes to 3 mph on the level treadmill as the patient's endurance improves. Early treadmill walking exercise should not produce heart rates above 70% of age-predicted maximum and should not cause symptoms, ischemia, or arrhythmia. Blood pressure is measured after the first 3 minutes and before progressing to a higher speed. It should not increase more than 20 mm Hg at this stage, and exercise should be discontinued if blood pressure begins to decrease (59).

Occupational therapy can work with the patient at this time so that a progressive activity program might enhance development of endurance for self-care and ADLs.

During the hospitalization period, patient education focuses on the anatomy and physiology of the cardiac disease, the purpose of medications, cessation of smoking, heart-healthy diet, and the rehabilitation process and its goals. Initial sessions should be short (5 to 15 minutes) and involve the family if possible. Groups of patients may continue for 30 to 50 minutes if the interaction among patients and staff is helpful. Inpatient education sessions are usually conducted by the nursing staff with the assistance of representatives from rehabilitation medicine (e.g., therapists, exercise physiologists, physiatrists, fellows, or residents) as well as the dietician, the social worker, and possibly the psychologist.

When a cardiac rehabilitation team is not available, the physiatrist or cardiologist should provide guidance in control of risk factors through other means. This usually cannot be done through personal patient contact because of the time-consuming nature of these interactions and the general lack of expertise among physicians in detailed dietary assessment, techniques to help patients discontinue smoking, sex counseling, and providing specific exercise recommendations. Some alternatives are:

Refer the patient to a full-service local cardiac rehabilitation program. Listings are available through the local chapters of the American Heart Association.

Have the patient keep a 3-day dietary record (i.e., 2 weekdays and 1 weekend day), including type of food eaten and portion size, and evaluate this record for calories from fat, percentage saturated and unsaturated fat, and total calories. The American Heart Association recommends less than 30% of total calories from fat, with less than 10% from saturated fat.

Refer the patient to a registered dietician with experience in counseling, not just any nutritionist. The American Dietetic Association will provide the names of qualified individuals in your area. Third-party payers generally do not reimburse for nutritional counseling, but a single evaluation by a dietician of what the patient is eating certainly should be affordable even when ongoing counseling is not.

Computer programs are available for dietary analysis in the office or in a hospital setting.

Encourage patients to make a written contract with you about a target date to stop smoking. Have patients keep a list of the circumstances under which they smoke each cigarette so that some of the addicting circumstances can be avoided.

Encourage attendance at commercial smoking cessation programs, hypnosis, or acupuncture. Nicorette gum (Smith Kline Beecham, Pittsburgh, PA) and clonidine patches to suppress cigarette craving are helpful for some patients.

Predischarge Stress Testing of Inpatients

It has become common practice to administer inpatient predischarge stress tests, which is preferable to discharging patients without one and having them inadvertently perform their own tests outside the hospital as they climb the steps to their homes or drive their cars.

Exercise testing is performed before hospital discharge, primarily for risk stratification and as a guide to subsequent medical management (61). It also serves as clearance for ADLs but is not suitable as the basis for the exercise prescription because the predischarge test does not proceed to a high enough work load.

Testing may be conducted as early as day 5 or 6 after the cardiac episode. The test can be an ECG exercise test or a thallium exercise and reperfusion scan. The level attained is usually arbitrarily limited to one of the following:

- 70% of maximal age-predicted heart rate (Fig. 54-2).
- A heart rate of 140 beats/min or seven METs for patients no more than 40 years of age and 130 beats/min or 5 METs for those 40 years of age and older (62). (1 MET = multiple of resting oxygen consumption).
- Patients on beta-blockade can be tested on the treadmill to 2.5 mph, 10% grade (6 METs) on the Kattus protocol if younger than 50 years of age and to 2.0 mph, 10% grade (5 METs) if 50 years or older. These work loads represent approximately 60% of the maximal predicted oxygen consumption for age. Sixty percent of the maximal oxygen consumption, which should not be affected by beta-blockade, occurs at approximately 70% of maximal heart rate in an unblocked patient (63).
- Symptom-limited tests, rather than stress tests arbitrarily stopped at a certain heart rate or work load, are performed by some groups (64) and may even be preferable (65), but their use is not usual. These tests have been associated with greater ST depression or angina, and their safety requires further study (66).

EARLY CONVALESCENT CARDIAC REHABILITATION

After discharge from the hospital, walking is the most popular exercise prescribed because patients can walk every day either outdoors or in a covered mall, progressively increasing the duration of walking from 15 to 30 minutes, then gradually increasing the speed of walking as tolerated (67). Between 4 and 8 weeks after the acute episode, depending on the extent of myocardial damage, the age of the patient, the urgency of return to work, and the philosophy of the physician, the patient should have an exercise stress test to maximal effort and start on a more vigorous conditioning program to improve cardiovascular functional capacity and endurance.

Patient education during this period is directed toward additional behavior modification (5). Previous smokers who develop a health-conscious lifestyle and adhere to a regular exercise training program are more likely to remain abstinent once they discontinue smoking. Conversely, exercise programs alone do not always foster psychosocial benefits, such as in areas of self-esteem, confidence, depression, and domestic activities (68,69). It is important to include family members or the significant other in patient education because adherence to behavior modification may be influenced by the expectations of the significant other (70). Family counseling is important at this point to avoid treating the patient as an invalid (71).

At the end of this convalescent period, a functional exercise test is performed, as opposed to a diagnostic type of test. The functional test is done to evaluate physical work capacity and cardiovascular function, once the diagnosis is known. Functional tests proceed to maximal effort, whereas diagnostic tests may be terminated once significant ST depression provides diagnostic information. Functional tests are performed on medication, whereas diagnostic information may be masked or confounded by medication. The results of the functional stress test are then used for decision making concerning return to work, exercise, and sexual activity. Functional tests are also useful in assessing the effects of treatment, whether medical, angioplasty, or revascularization.

ELECTROCARDIOGRAPHIC EXERCISE STRESS TESTING

Five Test Questions

Before performing a stress test for a patient, the physician should answer the following five questions:

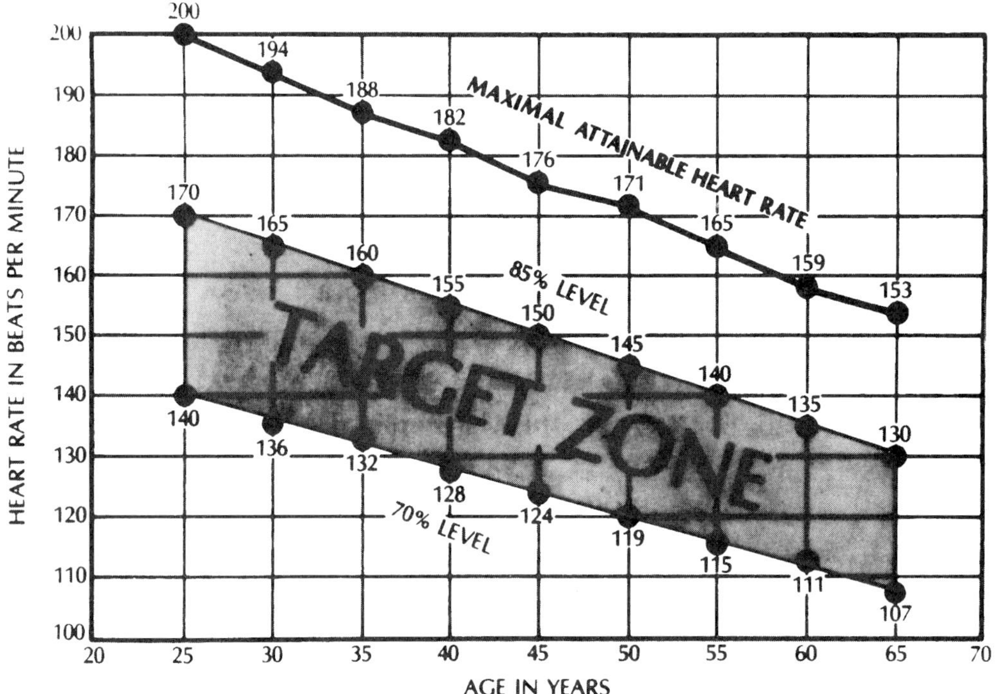

FIG. 54-2. Optimal level of exercise intensity based on the predicted age-adjusted maximal heart rate. (Reprinted with permission from Zohman LR. *Beyond diet—exercise your way to fitness and heart health.* Englewood Cliffs, NJ: CPC International, 1974; 15.)

1. Which modality should be used to present the exercise challenge to this patient? Cycle? Treadmill? Arm ergometer? Arm–leg ergometer?
2. Which exercise pattern (i.e., protocol) shall I select for this particular patient?
3. Should the test be submaximal or proceed to maximal effort? How will I recognize maximal effort in this patient? Is a submaximal test safer than a maximal stress test?
4. Are there any contraindications to testing this patient? While testing this person, what observations would alert me that continuing the test is contraindicated?
5. Are there any additional procedures I should perform as part of this stress test to answer the questions for which the test is being done?

Modalities

Although stress tests in Scandinavian countries are usually performed on a cycle, treadmill testing is more common in the United States. However, the cycle ergometer is still useful in many situations. Individuals with balance or gait problems may be too unsteady to walk on a treadmill without holding onto the handrail, which is not permissible. Obese individuals whose weight exceeds the weight limit of the treadmill (usually 350 pounds) may damage the equipment. Patients with calf claudication may be stopped by leg pain on the treadmill before an adequate cardiovascular challenge occurs, although they may be able to exercise on a cycle. Very agitated or fearful people may jump off the treadmill with resultant injury. In each of these cases, the cycle ergometer is a better choice.

The physician should not automatically exclude some seemingly unlikely candidates for use of the treadmill. A very slow protocol with rest periods on the treadmill may be easier for a frail 85-year-old woman than the cycle. An amputee can walk on a treadmill provided he or she has sufficient ankle motion to accommodate some slope, and provided the speed selected allows for swing-through.

Cycle ergometers are a good choice for testing someone who plans to train with a stationary cycle or a rolling bicycle. Cycles are also best if another procedure is to be performed that requires limited chest motion (e.g., exercise echocardiography or radionuclide ventriculography, which may be performed with either supine or erect cycling). Testing obese patients on cycles may require a larger cycle seat. Testing hemiplegics with one-legged cycling requires that the paretic extremity be secured to the pedal and that the patient have sufficient trunk stability to be able to maintain balance sitting on the cycle.

The upper extremity cycle ergometer is usually used for patients with lower extremity impairment, for those going back to heavy manual labor, or for persons who will be exercising mainly with their upper extremities. Because swimming is mainly an upper extremity activity, actual tethered swimming or arm ergometry is probably the best preparticipation test for swimmers (72). There are conflicting re-

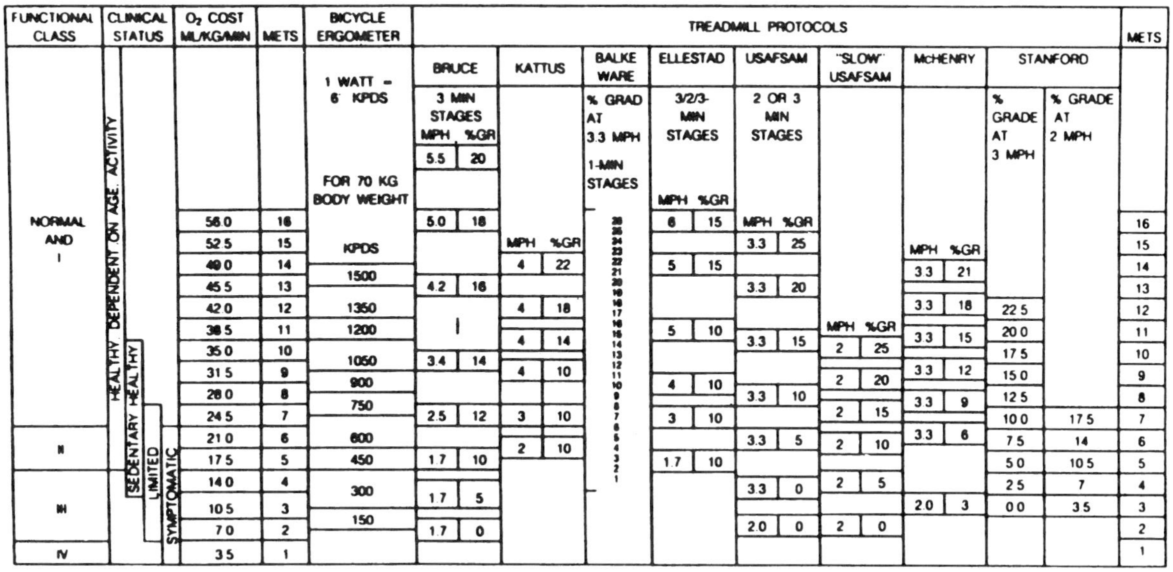

FUNCTIONAL CLASS	CLINICAL STATUS	O₂ COST ML/KG/MIN	METS	BICYCLE ERGOMETER	TREADMILL PROTOCOLS																METS
				1 WATT = 6 KPDS; FOR 70 KG BODY WEIGHT	BRUCE		KATTUS		BALKE WARE	ELLESTAD		USAFSAM		"SLOW" USAFSAM		McHENRY		STANFORD			
					3 MIN STAGES				% GRAD AT 3.3 MPH; 1-MIN STAGES	3/2/3-MIN STAGES		2 OR 3 MIN STAGES						% GRADE AT 3 MPH	% GRADE AT 2 MPH		
					MPH	%GR				MPH	%GR										
					5.5	20															
NORMAL AND I	HEALTHY, DEPENDENT ON AGE, ACTIVITY	56.0	16		5.0	18			26 25	6	15	MPH	%GR								16
		52.5	15	KPDS			MPH	%GR	24 23			3.3	25			MPH	%GR				15
		49.0	14	1500			4	22	22 21	5	15					3.3	21				14
		45.5	13		4.2	16			20 19			3.3	20								13
		42.0	12	1350			4	18	18 17							3.3	18	22.5			12
		38.5	11	1200	|				16 15	5	10	3.3	15	MPH	%GR	3.3	15	20.0			11
	SEDENTARY HEALTHY	35.0	10	1050	3.4	14	4	14	14 13					2	25			17.5			10
		31.5	9	900			4	10	12 11					2	20	3.3	12	15.0			9
	LIMITED	28.0	8	750					10 9	4	10	3.3	10			3.3	9	12.5			8
	SYMPTOMATIC	24.5	7		2.5	12	3	10	8 7	3	10			2	15			10.0	17.5		7
II		21.0	6	600			2	10	6 5 4			3.3	5	2	10	3.3	6	7.5	14		6
		17.5	5	450	1.7	10			3 2	1.7	10							5.0	10.5		5
III		14.0	4	300					1			3.3	0	2	5			2.5	7		4
		10.5	3	150	1.7	5										2.0	3	0.0	3.5		3
		7.0	2		1.7	0						2.0	0	2	0						2
IV		3.5	1																		1

FIG. 54-3. Stress test protocols, with their corresponding energy cost, correlated to the cardiac functional class. (Reprinted with permission from Fletcher GF, Froelicher VF, Hartley, et al. *Exercise standards—a statement for health professionals.* American Heart Association, 1991; 2289.)

ports on whether treadmill testing is useful as the basis for exercise prescription in swimmers.

The arm–leg ergometer has the advantage of spreading the work load over a greater muscle mass (73). Perceived exertion is less, and angina patients and heart failure patients can do more work before becoming symptomatic on such a device.

Protocols

Graded exercise tests are usually conducted in a continuous manner without a rest period between stages. Each work level is performed for a minimum of 3 minutes so that a steady state is reached in every stage. For the deconditioned patient, the test can be performed discontinuously, with a rest period following each stage. The discontinuous test or intermittent test is particularly useful for elderly patients who can do a surprising amount of exercise if allowed rest periods. Any protocol can be performed intermittently.

Figure 54-3 defines some of the treadmill protocols in terms of speed, grade, and duration of each stage. These patterns are shown side by side at equivalent MET levels so that a test performed on a patient using one protocol can be compared with a subsequent test performed using another protocol. At Montefiore Medical Center, we use a Bruce test or Kattus test for individuals who we surmise will have a good performance capacity so that the exercise can be completed in less than 15 minutes.

For patients who may have some degree of impairment, we prefer a slower version of the Kattus treadmill test in which the slope of the treadmill is held at 10% grade and the speed is raised 0.5 mph every 3 minutes. The work levels are therefore 1.5 mph at 10% grade (4 METs), 2.0 mph at 10% (5 METs), 2.5 mph at 10% (6 METs), 3.0 mph at 10% (7 METs), 3.5 mph at 10% (8 METs), and 4.0 mph at 10% (9 METs). This is entirely a walking test so that ECG recordings are of high quality (56).

For early testing post–acute coronary event, an alternative to the Kattus protocol is a modified Bruce protocol starting at 1.7 mph level treadmill and proceeding to 1.7 mph 5% grade before entering the traditional protocol speeds and grades. The recommended protocol for low-level testing is one that starts at a low work level and has gradually increasing intensity (74–76). The Naughton/Balke protocol is one that meets these criteria and is used at the East Orange Veterans Administration Medical Center Cardiac Rehabilitation Unit. The test starts at 2 METs and increases in 1-MET increments. As noted earlier, a MET is the multiple of the resting oxygen consumption with the resting energy cost, given the equivalent unit of 1 MET. The slow protocols are also useful for deconditioned or older individuals who are starting on an exercise program for the first time.

Maximal or Submaximal

Testing to physiologic maximum is evidenced by failure of heart rate, blood pressure, or oxygen consumption, or all three, to increase despite increasing work loads (77). Exercise to this level is usually possible for normal healthy people or athletes who are involved in vigorous competitive sports. The cardiac patient is usually limited by either disease or deconditioning so that attaining physiologic maximum is generally not possible. Patients are tested to their clinical maximum or peak effort, which is usually the point of symptoms, or significant ischemia, arrhythmia, or abnormal hemodynamic responses. Patients should not be encouraged to proceed beyond clinical maximum even if they are willing to try to do so.

It is important in both functional and diagnostic testing to be sure that patients proceed to at least 85% of their predicted maximal heart rate, because half of the abnormalities will be missed if patients are not challenged to at least this level (78). Patients on pulse-lowering medication (e.g., beta-blockers) should be tested to an external work load that would incur oxygen consumption of 80% of maximum VO_2, which in turn would be approximately equivalent to 85% of maximal heart rate if there were no heart rate suppression.

Submaximal testing is usually performed by nonphysicians who are testing apparently healthy people. These tests proceed to a level above the level of a planned exercise program in a gym but remain below 85% of maximum heart rate. Although ECGs may be used in these tests for more accurate heart rate counts, these testers are not permitted to interpret the exercise ECG because that would be practicing medicine without a medical license. Submaximal tests are usually stopped with the appearance of any abnormality. In our opinion submaximal testing is generally not useful for patients. National statistics on morbidity and mortality from stress tests are the same for submaximal and maximal testing, with one death and 2.4 serious cardiac events per 10,000 stress tests. These cardiac events include nonfatal MI, serious dysrhythmias, syncope, respiratory arrest, and so on (79).

TABLE 54-1. *Absolute and relative contraindications to exercise testing*

Absolute contraindications	Relative contraindications[a]
Acute myocardial infarction or recent change on resting ECG	Less serious noncardiac disorder
Active unstable angina	Significant arterial or pulmonary hypertension
Serious cardiac arrhythmias	Tachyarrhythmias or bradyarrhythmias
Acute pericarditis	Moderate valvular or myocardial heart disease
Endocarditis	Drug effect or electrolyte abnormalities
Severe aortic stenosis	Left main coronary obstructive or its equivalent
Severe left ventricular dysfunction	Hypertrophic cardiomyopathy
Acute pulmonary embolus or pulmonary infarction	Psychiatric disease
Acute or serious noncardiac disorder	
Severe physical handicap or disability	

[a] Under certain circumstances and with appropriate precautions, relative contraindications can be superceded.

Reprinted with permission from Fletcher GF, Froelicher VF, Hartley, et al. *Exercise standards: a statement for health professionals.* American Heart Association, 1991; 2289. Reproduced with permission from the American Heart Association.

Contraindications

Any clinical condition that can be aggravated by vigorous exercise is a contraindication to functional exercise stress testing (Table 54-1) (80). Acute cardiac conditions such as acute or impending MI, acute myocarditis or pericarditis, and unstable angina are absolute contraindications because of the danger of precipitating MI; any other acute systemic illnesses are contraindications as well (81). Stable congestive heart failure *per se* is not. It is the presence of acute heart failure or worsening chronic heart failure that contraindicates testing (82,83). Severe aortic stenosis, uncontrolled severe hypertension, left main coronary artery stenosis, and hypertrophic obstructive cardiomyopathy with a history of syncope are also considered contraindications (76,82).

Sometimes seeming contraindications turn out not to be contraindications. For example, although severe hypertension is a contraindication to stress testing, in our facilities we have often begun a test with elevated baseline resting blood pressures (e.g., 250/115 mm Hg) without untoward complications. In most patients who were hypertensive because of anxiety at the start of the test, blood pressure remained the same or decreased to appropriate levels during the first two to three stages, without any accompanying signs of circulatory failure or abnormal ECG changes, and increased normally thereafter as anxiety abated with exercise. Testing should not proceed, however, if during the early stages of exercise the pressure increases further.

Occasionally, testing in the presence of a contraindication is safer than not testing at all. In a patient with severe aortic stenosis who has neither dizziness nor syncope and who insists on doing vigorous exercises, it would be acceptable to do a functional stress test to determine the level of safety.

Similarly, although hypertrophic cardiomyopathy is a major cause of fatality in strenuous exercise and has been found to be the most common cause of sudden death in young competitive athletes (62,84), not all idiopathic hypertrophic subaortic stenosis (IHSS) is lethal. Although echocardiography may demonstrate the presence of a disproportionately thick interventricular septum, exercise echo may show that the abnormality does not obstruct outflow significantly. Exercise stress testing to determine functional capacity would probably not be contraindicated in such situations. Conversely, physiatrists involved in sports medicine should be aware that significantly obstructive IHSS can be asymptomatic with a seemingly functional murmur or no murmur at rest, the murmur becoming characteristic only on auscultation after exercise. Tests that become abnormal in asymptomatic young people should be aborted, auscultation performed immediately, and further cardiac evaluation sought. Idiopathic hypertrophic subaortic stenosis can be suspected when symptoms such as chest pain, exertional dyspnea, palpitations, and syncope are present in young individuals, especially when the ECG shows left ventricular hypertrophy (85). Stress testing should wait until other cardiac workup has been completed in such cases.

Although rapid ventricular or atrial arrhythmias are contraindications to stress testing (86), the presence of dysrhythmias at rest is not necessarily a contraindication to exercise testing. Extrasystoles, or bigeminy, often abates as exercise proceeds. A long cool-down period after the stress test is important, however, because the pretest dysrhythmia will probably return in recovery as the heart rate slows. In fact, in patients with baseline dysrhythmia, stress testing is important before prescribing exercise to determine whether the dysrhythmia remains the same, is rate suppressed, or increases to dangerous levels during exercise. When dysrhythmia increases with exercise in coronary exercisers, premedication with nitroglycerin before a stress test may be helpful in deciding whether the dysrhythmia is indeed an ischemic response.

Both the subjective and objective criteria for terminating an exercise test are delineated in Table 54-2. The principal endpoints are primarily signs and symptoms of ischemia affecting various organ systems: angina, arrhythmia, or signs of circulatory insufficiency in cardiac ischemia; clumsiness or dizziness in central nervous system ischemia; nausea or vomiting in gastrointestinal ischemia; and leg pain or discomfort in ischemic peripheral vascular disease. Other endpoints are occurrences that are not necessarily dangerous but would preclude accurate interpretation of the test results, including the appearance of conduction abnormalities or rapid tachycardia, which might shorten diastole, impair coronary filling, and cause ischemia unrelated to coronary obstructive disease.

TABLE 54-2. *Criteria to stop exercise test*

Clinical
Fatigue, or dyspnea, or both, beyond that experienced after a heavy activity in daily life
Chest pain of 3+ or greater severity
Other induced symptoms of dizziness, unsteadiness, clumsiness, nausea, or vomiting
Leg disconfort or pain that increases as exercise is continued
Sign of peripheral circulatory insufficiency
Pallor
Clammy skin
Decrease in blood pressure
ECG changes
Exercise ST segment deviation (3 mm or more)
Ventricular tachycardia
PVCs precipitated or aggravated by exercise (over 25% of heartbeats)
Ectopic supraventicular tachycardia
Intracardiac block not present at rest
Patient wants to stop

PVC, premature ventricular contraindications.

Adapted form Sheffield LT. Exercise stress testing. In: Brunwald E, ed. *Heart disease: a textbook of cardiovascular medicine.* Philadelphia: WB Saunders, 1988; 239.

Competent stress testing involves both recognizing abnormalities such as ischemia even before the patient perceives them (i.e., some patients may have silent ischemia) and avoiding overinterpretation of nonsignificant findings as ischemia. Also, danger signals of imminent peripheral circulatory collapse, such as pallor, clammy skin, or decrease in blood pressure, may not necessarily be perceived by the patient. Conversely, a single low blood pressure reading, not accompanied by signs or symptoms, should be repeated and the test discontinued only if there is a consistent downward trend.

Nonstandard Testing

There are four additions to the functional stress test that can provide information useful in planning a patient's exercise program: walk-through testing, second-effort testing, the nitroglycerin exercise test, and nonstandard monitoring. The first three test the patient's ability to adapt to exercise in progress. Nonstandard monitoring can be performed when patients are not able to perform a standard stress test, or it can be used as a supplement to stress testing in a more convenient setting.

If the patient gives a history of being able to "walk through" his or her angina and continue to do the same activity without angina thereafter, this observation can be verified by a walk-through test. The patient exercises on the treadmill until he or she perceives mild but constant angina and then continues to walk at the same speed and grade of the treadmill during the angina. Within 10 minutes of walking, if he or she has true walk-through angina, the discomfort will subside. He or she may then be able to proceed to even higher work loads without angina. If the angina continues beyond 10 minutes or worsens during this test, the procedure should be discontinued.

Second-effort testing is similar to walk-through testing. The patient exercises until mild, constant angina is felt, and then stops and rests for 10 to 15 minutes. He or she repeats the performance, and if the previous work level is surpassed without angina, he or she has shown adaptive capacity. Such ability has been found to predict trainability and may imply the slow opening of collateral vessels or at least emphasize the importance of a long warm-up for that particular patient (87).

The nitroglycerin exercise test can also provide information useful for the cardiac rehabilitation exercise program. If a previous stress test was terminated because of angina or ischemic ST changes, a patient can be retested to the point of mild but constant angina. During uninterrupted exercise, nitroglycerin can be administered and the exercise continued for up to 10 minutes, provided angina does not worsen. If ST depression or angina, or both, lessens and the patient can proceed to higher work levels, nitroglycerin can be prescribed before exercise classes, making it possible for the patient to exercise above the previous angina threshold. It is important not to stop the patient's exercise to administer the nitroglycerin in the test situation because the rest itself may decrease the angina. The use of nitroglycerin before the exercise class is of particular importance in the debilitated or deconditioned patient with angina pectoris, making it possible to exercise at a higher intensity to increase the strength of the peripheral musculature, and then to proceed to improving endurance and the level of physical fitness.

Nonstandard Monitoring

The Holter monitor or ECG telemetry can be used when evaluating the effects of physical activity that is different from the exercise used in standard exercise stress tests. This type of assessment is particularly useful in evaluating the cardiac demands of rehabilitation training of the physically disabled, such as hemiplegics, paraplegics, and lower extremity amputees. Nonstandard monitoring also can be performed using a simple office ECG machine by wiring the patient with the ECG cable and plugging the cable into the ECG recorder immediately after the activity to be evaluated. If the postexercise ECG is taken within 10 seconds after completion of exercise, it will show essentially the same findings as if it had been taken during the exercise (88).

Recent advances in surveillance of cardiac rehabilitation service is by means of transtelephone telemetry monitoring in settings outside a structured, supervised program (59,89). For example, patients can be monitored via two-channel ECG and voice telemetry during each exercise session at home. Or they can be monitored by phone from a community cardiac maintenance exercise program periodically.

NUCLEAR EXERCISE STRESS TESTING

The two nuclear imaging techniques used with exercise stress testing are the multigated acquisition (MUGA) and the thallium scan. The MUGA scan or radionuclide ventriculogram requires labeling of the blood pool with technetium 99m and creation of a cine (i.e., movie) during supine cycling. The radioactivity counts are picked up by the computerized gamma camera, which packages them into systolic and diastolic components. The test is used mainly to determine left ventricular dysfunction through evaluation of regional and global wall motion and ejection fraction. Ischemic or infarcted areas contract slower or less forcefully on exercise than normal areas (i.e, hypokinetic), may not contract at all (i.e., akinetic), or may bulge (i.e., dyskinetic). Ejection fraction should increase at least 5% on exercise compared with rest.

Thallium 201 injected intravenously at peak treadmill exercise passes through the myocardial capillary network and accumulates intracellularly within the wall of the left ventricle to the extent that the area is perfused. Computerized still images result from acquisition of radioactive counts by the gamma camera immediately after the exercise and 3 hours later, at which time perfusion deficits due to ischemia will have received enough thallium via the bloodstream to appear normal, whereas infarcted areas will show a persistent deficit. The newer isonitrils (i.e., perfusion imaging agents such as sestaMIBI and teboroxine) are now being used in dual acquisition studies along with thallium, providing higher quality images without exessive radiation to the patient, as well as more information about myocardial viability.

For the physiatrist who performs functional ECG stress testing, there are also times when other means of stress testing may be indicated. Nuclear stress tests are useful when the exercise ECG cannot be evaluated for ischemia to the desired degree (e.g., patient with conduction abnormalities or on digitalis, positive test in the asymptomatic patient, equivocal results in a symptomatic patient). Nuclear tests are no more useful than ECG stress tests when the exercise capacity of the patient is limited, such as the markedly debilitated individual, or in the presence of congestive heart failure where the radioisotope may be picked up by the lungs. Multigated acquisitions cannot be performed on patients with an irregular cardiac rhythm because of the ECG gating requirement.

In patients with neuromusculoskeletal impairments that preclude lower extremity exercise, or in the presence of obstructive arterial disease when claudication limits the extent of the exercise, a pharmacologic stress test with dipyridamole infusion, without any or with only minimal exercise, can be ordered. The exercise can be performed in a tilt position, sitting up, using a handgrip with a dynamometer, or by walking slowly. Dipyridamole increases myocardial blood flow by inducing maximal coronary vasodilation. The obstructed artery dilates less, resulting in a steal phenomenon from the obstructed to the patent (i.e., dilated) vessels.

ECHOCARDIOGRAPHIC STRESS TESTING

Exercise stress testing with echocardiographic assessment of ventricular wall motion and ejection fraction at rest and immediately following exercise is another way to detect exercise-induced myocardial ischemia. Exercise echo can be performed with either a cycle ergometer or a treadmill. Or, echocardiograms can be recorded after dipyridamole infusion. Although exercise echo is technically more difficult than nuclear imaging, it can detect wall motion abnormalities—and therefore ischemia—at different exercise levels, information that is more useful to the physiatrist developing an exercise prescription than merely knowing ventricular function or wall perfusion at maximal effort. There is also no radioactive substance used with echocardiography, and the procedure can be repeated frequently.

CARDIOVASCULAR PHYSICAL CONDITIONING

After a maximal functional stress test, patients can participate in a cardiovascular physical conditioning program in either a monitored and supervised, supervised but unmonitored, or unsupervised setting. Not all patients need to be treated in expensive cardiac rehabilitation facilities monitored by nurses and supervised by exercise physiologists or physical therapists—even if third-party payers would pay the entire bill—because some medical situations do not warrant such intensive rehabilitation. Some cardiologists, internists, and family medicine physicians provide excellent assessment and exercise recommendations, whereas others lose interest as soon as the angioplasty catheter is removed or staunchly refuse to refer any of their cardiac patients to physiatrists, certain that their own meager recommendations are all that is needed.

Monitored Rehabilitation, Supervised Rehabilitation, or Both?

The recent report on Cardiac Rehabilitation from AACVPR and the National Institutes of Health (Publication 96-0672, 10/95) points out that the safety and effectiveness of unsupervised cardiac rehabilitation exercise must be determined for various populations of coronary patients because economic constraints and logistics often limit the availability of supervised training.

There has never been a formal randomized study showing that monitored cardiac rehabilitation exercise programs are safer than unmonitored programs. VanCamp and Petersen, from survey data, suggest that unmonitored programs have the same mortality and morbidity as monitored programs (90). Work of Vong Vanich and Merz showed that 11% of patients had alteration of their care (4% based on telemetry) in supervised exercise programs (91). In the Montefiore supervised community exercise program at the Manhattan Beach Jewish Center in Brooklyn, New York, there were three resuscitated cardiac arrests and one death in 25 years in an unmonitored setting (92). It is therefore controversial as to which patients need a supervised, monitored program. We suggest the following candidates for monitoring:

Those with severely depressed left ventricular function (less than 25% left ventricular ejection fraction [LVEF]) after very severe/complicated MI

Individuals who have ischemia on ECG during the exercise program

Angina or anginal-equivalent patients

Individuals who are arrhythmic during exercise or recovery

Those less than 6 months post–heart attack, angioplasty, or heart surgery, especially if they have had a complicated hospital course

Very deconditioned patients who will be exercising at high intensity

Patients who require monitoring of more than heart rate or cannot count their own heart rates

Patients who also have other major diseases in addition to the cardiac problem (e.g., diabetics, stroke amputees, etc.)

Those who need the services of other cardiac rehabilitation disciplines as well

Patients who have completed monitored programs would probably do well to remain in a supervised setting if they continue to be symptomatic on exertion or if their exercise ECGs are ischemic or arrhythmic. Others can be guided to establish continuation programs in convenient exercise facilities near work or home or at home. However, a recovered cardiac patient probably should not exercise completely alone in an environment where no immediate help is available in case of emergency.

For the low-risk coronary patient, medically prescribed home exercise, unsupervised, can be prescribed (93). Exercise testing of such patients also may be conducted by exercise physiologists (94). These programs should include nutritional guidance, smoking cessation, and lipid-lowering therapy, and have been found efficacious under a managed care system.

PRINCIPLES OF CARDIOVASCULAR CONDITIONING

Physical training is the performance of repetitive exercise to increase physical work capacity, and to induce physical conditioning, it must be of considerable energy cost relative to the individual's level of fitness and performed regularly for an extended period of time. Cardiovascular conditioning involves physical training to improve cardiovascular functional capacity and endurance.

To achieve significant benefit from physical training, one should follow the four principles of physiologic conditioning (95).

1. Principle of overloading: an exercise, to be effective in augmenting conditioning, must be at a work level greater than that at which the individual usually performs. This can be accomplished by manipulating the intensity, duration, and frequency of the exercise, with intensity as the most important component.
2. Principle of specificity: each type of exercise brings about a specific metabolic and physiologic adaptation resulting in a specific training effect. Power training using isometric exercises results in an increase in strength but may not increase endurance. Aerobic training is the type of exercise that leads to improvement in endurance, and, provided it includes exercise of large muscle masses, it can improve cardiovascular functional capacity. All these types of training are important in rehabilitation to improve ADL and job-related performance.
3. Principle of individual variation: training should be individualized according to the person's capacities and needs. Although some cardiac patients can run marathons, for example, the functional capacities of most cardiac patients will not permit this to be accomplished, regardless of the amount of training that the cardiac patient is willing to perform.
4. Principle of reversibility: the beneficial effects of train-

TABLE 54-3. *Exercise prescription*

Drug prescription	Exercise prescription
Name of drug	Type of exercise
Strength of drug	Exercise intensity
Dose	Duration of each session
Frequency	Frequency

ing are not permanent. The improvements attained begin to disappear only 2 weeks after cessation of exercise (96), and half of the gains may be lost in only 5 weeks. When a patient on an exercise program goes on vacation, that patient should continue to exercise in a format similar to the exercise program or should plan other similar activities to be continued during the vacation.

EXERCISE PRESCRIPTION

Exercise for the cardiac patient must be prescribed in a manner similar to, and with as much care as, a drug prescription. The prescription should specify the type of exercise, intensity, duration, and frequency (Table 54-3).

Types of Exercise

Exercise for cardiovascular conditioning should be isotonic, rhythmic, and aerobic; should use large muscle masses; and should not involve a large isometric component. The most popular exercises are the walk-jog-run group, stationary or moving cycling, and swimming. Skipping rope can be substituted for jogging or running (97) but may be contraindicated in individuals with moderate to marked osteoporosis because of the danger of fractures from impact shock or accident. In recent years, strength training (isometric, resistive training exercises) and circuit weight training (CWT) are being added to ongoing aerobic training and have been found to be a low risk for patients with good left ventricular function (71,98–103). However, patients with impaired left ventricular function may decompensate on resistive exercises so these exercises are not prescribed for them or for those with uncontrolled arrhythmias or unstable angina. The resultant improvement in muscular strength and local muscular endurance in addition to improvement of cardiovascular functional capacity has been particularly important to individuals who are returning to jobs requiring moving heavy work loads, to those involved in high-intensity sports, and to the elderly who sustain fewer hip fractures if muscles are stronger. In addition, improved muscle strength in the combined CWT/aerobic training programs not only improves the patient's ability to perform physical tasks in daily life but enhances self-image (98).

Intensity of Exercise

Exercise intensity may be prescribed in accordance with one of five methods:

1. American Heart Association method: a target heart rate of 70% to 85% of the maximum attainable heart rate (Fig. 54-2) determined on a stress test or derived for normal young adults by subtracting the exerciser's age from 220.
2. Karvonen method: heart rate range is calculated as peak heart rate attained on a stress test, minus resting heart rate. Then 40% to 60% of the heart rate range is added to the resting heart rate to give a target heart rate zone for exercise.
3. Oxygen consumption method: 67% to 80% of maximal oxygen consumption is an appropriate intensity and can be expressed in terms of heart rate using the stress test as a template if expired gases were measured.
4. Work load methods (104)
   a. Training sessions should be at two thirds of the maximal MET (1 MET = 3.5 ml/kg/min O_2 consumed) level attained on the stress test, or
   b. 150 KPM (25 watts) lower than the maximal level attained on the cycle ergometer stress test, or
   c. use the highest speed reached at 10% grade on the treadmill test as the speed for walking on flat terrain.
5. Perceived exertion method
   a. Borg RPE scale: Ratings of 11 to 15 on the Borg scale (105) usually correspond to an appropriate training intensity.
   b. Conversational exercise level: Patients should be able to talk while exercising (talk test) but probably would be too breathless to sing while exercising (54,62,104–106) (Fig. 54-4).

The Borg scale used ratings of 6 to 20, which correlated linearly with heart rate, ventilation, O_2 consumption, and

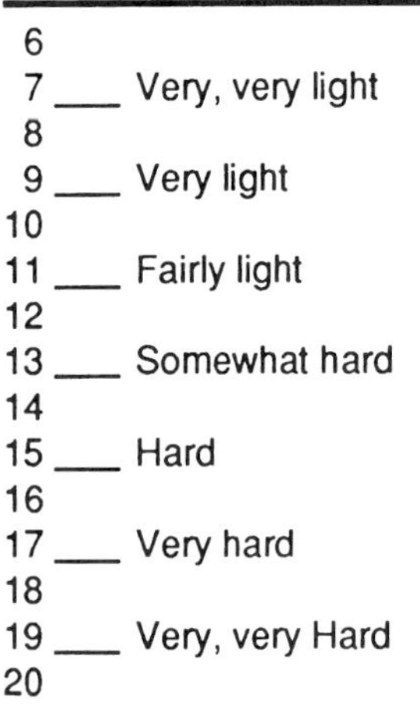

FIG. 54-4. Borg's Rating of Perceived Exertion (RPE) Scale. This linear scale of ratings is used to indicate the degree of perceived physical exertion in a patient performing an exercise. (Reprinted with permission from Borg G. Perceived exertion as an indicator of somatic stress. *Scand J Rehabil Med* 1970; 2–3:92–98.)

lactate levels (62,107,108). A newer Borg scale uses numbers up to 10, but it is less popular than the older version.

For patients on heart rate–altering medication, exercise training at 85% of symptom-limited heart rate (109) or 70% to 90% of maximum work load (110,111), attained on exercise stress testing, resulted in significant beneficial physiologic changes with a decrease in heart rate and an increase in stroke volume, cardiac output, and oxygen uptake comparable with individuals not on beta-blockers. These physical conditioning effects occur whether the beta-blockade therapy is selective or nonselective (112).

Duration and Frequency of Exercise

Improvement can be achieved while exercising for varying lengths of time per session, the duration depending on the level of fitness of the individual and the intensity of the exercise. The usual duration when exercise is at 70% of maximum heart rate is 20 to 30 minutes at conditioning level. In the poorly conditioned individual, daily exercises for 3 to 5 minutes can bring about improvement. For the conditioned individual who prefers to exercise at higher intensities, duration of exercise may be reduced to 10 to 15 minutes.

All studies agree on the importance of training frequency to bring about cardiovascular improvement; some studies show that these improvements were no different whether training frequencies were 2 or 5 days per week (96). But the most consistent benefits appears to occur with frequencies of three times per week for 12 weeks or more (18). There is no contraindication to exercising every day, but as the number of sessions increases, the likelihood of musculoskeletal injury increases (113).

FORMAT OF AN EXERCISE SESSION

The training sessions of an exercise program should follow a specific format. There should be a warm-up phase before, and a cool-down phase after, the period of training (i.e., stimulus phase) where the exercise is performed at the prescribed intensity and duration that induce a training effect. The warm-up period is usually at the lower intensity levels of exercise to be performed, gradually increasing to the prescribed intensity, or it may be in the form of limbering-up exercise. The purpose is to increase joint readiness, theoretically to open up existing collateral circulation, and prevent sudden changes in peripheral resistance before the maximum contraction of the skeletal muscles required by the exercise. At the cool-down period there is a gradual reduction in exercise intensity to allow the gradual redistribution of blood from the extremities to other tissues and to prevent the sudden reduction in venous return, thereby reducing the possibility of postexercise hypotension or even syncope. Cool-down also reduces the development of stiffness or soreness of joints and muscles.

MAINTENANCE PROGRAMS

After completion of formal exercise training in a cardiac rehabilitation program, which is now approximately 12 weeks, with performance safely up to 7 to 8 METs verifiable by stress test, exercisers should continue their physical conditioning in order to maintain the level of fitness that was attained. They can continue the same exercise at the same work level as their last exercise prescription using target pulse rate, conversational exercise level, or Borg RPE as a guideline to avoid overexertion. The exercise can be performed at the YMCA or YWCA, at a private club, at home, or even at the individual's place of employment. The American Medical Association's Committee on Exercise and Physical Fitness has established guidelines for physical fitness programs in business and industry, and many corporations have established their own physical fitness programs, not just for the executives but for all levels of employees (114). To encourage the patient's continued physical training, exercise should become part of the individual's recreational lifestyle.

Sports activities can be incorporated into the cardiovascular conditioning program and may be used as the exercise for maintenance but should not exceed the safe heart rate and symptomatic guidelines previously established. Sports that require bursts of heavy activity, especially if highly competitive, should probably be avoided (e.g., racquetball). If tennis is used to maintain conditioning, it is important to play against an opponent of comparable skill, fostering a more continuous rather than intermittent game. Ice or roller skating, canoeing, or rowing a boat also can be used to maintain conditioning. Other types of sports may be pursued to improve the quality of life but may not be used as the conditioning exercise because the energy cost may be too low or the activity may be too intermittent to retain fitness. Examples of these are bowling, golf played with use of a golf cart rather than walking, group volleyball, etc.

EXERCISE TRAINING FOR SPECIAL GROUPS OF PATIENTS

Exercise Conditioning after Heart Surgery

The cardiac rehabilitation program for the patient who has undergone heart surgery such as CABG or valve replacement is essentially the same as the program for the patient who has sustained an acute MI. The control of coronary risk factors continues to be important after CABG for secondary prevention and to try to avoid graft closure (52). Surgery has provided the coronary patient with a stay of execution but not a pardon from his disease.

With the presence of pain in the operated sites (i.e., the split sternum and the sites of vein harvesting in the legs), the inpatient exercise program should be started soon after surgery to maintain the functional range of motion of the shoulders in particular and prevent contractures, as well as to minimize the development of peripheral edema in the lower extremities. However, high-intensity arm exercise should be avoided for 3 to 6 months after a sternum-splitting incision. Respiratory and chest physical therapy are equally important in the immediate postoperative period, as they are in other types of chest surgery.

Exercise Postangioplasty

There is no reliable information as to whether exercise training after percutaneous transluminal angioplasty, atherectomy, or stenting decreases the incidence of restenosis; however, exercise tolerance does improve irrespective of exercise programming (89).

Exercise Training for Heart Transplant Patients

Medically prescribed exercise training as part of the cardiac rehabilitation of the heart transplant patient has been found to be beneficial, with an effective increase in aerobic capacity and peripheral muscle strength. There is no evidence of any adverse effect (16,115,116).

In training the orthotopic transplant patient with his new heart, we are working with a denervated heart in which heart rate changes occur by humoral regulation through changes in circulatory catecholamines (117). The heart rate response to exercise in the denervated heart compared with the intact heart is a slower increase at the start of the exercise, a lower peak rate, and a more gradual return to the preexercise level after cessation of the exercise (16,118). In addition, the left ventricular ejection fraction, cardiac output, maximum oxygen uptake, and anaerobic threshold are lower (16).

When a patient has a heterotopic cardiac transplant (the diseased heart is not removed and the new heart is implanted in the chest parallel to it), the transplanted heart shows training responses similar to those of the orthotopic heart, whereas the innervated but diseased heart that remains will develop a training bradycardia and reduction in ventricular ectopy (115).

In prescribing exercise for these patients, the heart rate is not used in monitoring exercise intensity (16,119). Instead, the Borg RPE scale (16,116) and expired air measurements, particularly the anaerobic threshold (16), have been found most useful in determining the exercise intensity level.

Patients with Severe Left Ventricular Dysfunction

Impaired LVEF has been considered a contraindication to cardiac rehabilitation exercise based on the assumption that increased exertion would precipitate acute heart failure or death. In the past decade, this approach has changed as studies have shown that exercise stress testing can be performed safely in patients with left ventricular dysfunction (83,120–122). Surprisingly, the functional capacity of the heart failure patient may have no relationship to resting left ventricular ejection fraction (121,122). At times, heart failure patients may achieve physical work capacities similar to those of subjects with normal resting ejection fractions (122).

Among patients tested by Tavazzi and colleagues, 21% with LVEFs of less than 30% had normal hemodynamics, and 28% attained a work capacity of 100 watts. In the patients with LVEFs of more than 45%, there were abnormal hemodynamic responses in 33%, and 12% to 37% had a lower work capacity of 50 to 75 watts, lower than those with a low ejection fraction (83). It is thus evident that performance capacity among those with left ventricular dysfunction is dependent not only on myocardial function but also on peripheral adaptations. In our own experience with a young, trained person, performance capacity may approach normal even with a left ventricular ejection fraction of only 15% to 20%. In patients with extensive anterior transmural MI, it is controversial whether these patients are included in, or excluded from, early exercise training before the complete healing of the infarct (123,124). The initial reports mandating exclusion have been tempered by further long-term data (18).

For selected patients with severe left ventricular dysfunction who are clinically stable with no signs of acute heart failure, a conditioning program may be performed safely under carefully supervised conditions. Although the training effects after physical conditioning are probably all peripheral rather than myocardial, they include a decrease in heart rate at rest and at submaximal work levels, increased maximal oxygen consumption, and improved exercise performance (125–127), as in patients without left ventricular dysfunction. Cardiac rehabilitation also may help these patients return to productive employment (128). For the hospitalized individual with left ventricular dysfunction, it is very important to evaluate self-care activities and other ADLs and to provide training in deficient areas. This is useful in making discharge plans and may make the difference between returning home and being placed in a nursing home.

Cardiac Rehabilitation of Women

Each year, approximately 250,000 women die of coronary heart disease and 100,000 of other forms of cardiac disease. Heart disease is the leading cause of death among women, and heart disease (38%) is more common than breast cancer (4%) as a cause of death in women. Women are more likely to present with angina rather than MI and are more likely to have heart failure and cardiac rupture than are men. They are less likely to lose their angina after bypass or angioplasty. The operative mortality for women is 2.7 times higher than that for men. The rehabilitation challenge women present have not received adequate attention because research studies in this area are generally conducted on men. Some of the relevant observations concerning the differences between coronary disease in men and women are listed as follows:

1. Symptoms that might represent cardiac disease seem to be taken less seriously if they occur in women than in

men, so women receive more complicated testing later than they should and as a group are "sicker" than coronary men. This is described as "sex bias" by Tobin and colleagues (129).

2. Although there may be more false-positive ECG stress test results among women than among men, and an overlying breast shadow may confound thallium scans, probability tables that give the likelihood of disease based on age, gender, symptoms, and ECG findings indicate that stress testing is still useful in women.
3. Male standards may not hold for women. For example, if ejection fraction on MUGA stays the same or decreases on exercise compared with the resting value in men, that would be abnormal. Thirty percent of normal women demonstrate no change in LVEF on exercise.
4. The American Heart Association diet for reducing cholesterol levels may be less effective in women than in men. In men, the diet reduces LDL 24% to 26% and HDL 0% to 12%. Although a similar reduction in LDL occurs in women, the HDL is reduced 16% to 20%.
5. Among women, the relationship between heart rate response and anaerobic threshold differs from that in men. In the work of Coplan and associates (130), at 85% predicted maximum heart rate, 73% of the men have exceeded their anaerobic threshold, whereas only 44% of women have (130). Thus, if the target zone for exercise training is to be set at 70% to 85% of maximal heart rate, this heart rate zone would bring most men above anaerobic threshold, but not most women.
6. Women are more likely to drop out of exercise programs than are men. Women who do participate obtain the same beneficial training effects as their male counterparts (131,132). Physical conditioning also can be provided through forms of activity that women enjoy, such as dancing. Traditional female household activities also can be appropriately used as the physical activity for cardiovascular fitness when properly planned according to the warm-up–stimulus–cool-down format of an exercise training session (133).

Exercise Conditioning for the Elderly Cardiac Patient

The number of persons 65 years and older in the United States is increasing at a growth rate twice that of the total population. The "oldest old" (i.e., more than 85 years of age) already are the fastest growing age group (134), with approximately half of this entire group having some cardiac disorder (135).

Aging is accompanied by a gradual decline in physiologic functions with an accelerated decline in cardiovascular function and muscle strength, due to deconditioning from decreasing physical activity (136–138). The decline is about 25% less by maintaining a physically active lifestyle (81). Sedentary older persons can increase their aerobic capacity and muscle strength by exercise training (136,137), but older persons have a lesser degree of improvement when they begin their physical conditioning at an older age as compared with the young (96).

For the hospitalized elderly individual, early gradual mobilization is important to prevent further deconditioning. The more debilitated the patient, the less exercise is needed to bring about improvement. One can start just by increasing duration and frequency of sitting, then doing standing balance exercises at bedside, followed by ambulation as tolerated, and increasing self-care activities. The best exercise for the elderly is walking.

Exercise stress testing to determine the functional capacity of an older individual before an exercise program is important. Patients who do not have enough endurance to perform the treadmill test continuously can be tested with a discontinuous protocol, or they can be tested on a cycle ergometer. Hardwire ECG or ECG telemetric monitoring of a patient while walking at his own pace, to his or her level of tolerance or after two 6- to 12-minute walk test protocols, may be sufficient as a pre-exercise stress test for a debilitated individual. It was also found that a 600-foot walk (three times back and forth in a 100-foot hospital corridor) brings the patient's heart rate to the target heart zone for exercise training as determined from a treadmill stress test on the same patient (139).

The absence of chest pain as an indicator of ischemia is not reliable among the elderly. Dyspnea may represent an anginal equivalent rather than a breathing problem. Among the "old old" (i.e., more than 70 years of age), over 70% have abnormal stress test results, often with silent ischemia (139).

Of particular importance to the elderly are limbering-up exercises that increase flexibility of joints and improve agility. There may be an increasing need to rely on the upper extremities to maintain independence in locomotion by the use of ambulatory aids, or even just for transfer activities, so strengthening exercises to the upper extremities are important. Patient education should include the importance of regular physical activity. Also, because of reduced cardiac reserve and decreased ability to sweat efficiently (135), the need for rest periods during physical activity and avoidance of exercise and other moderate work during hot, humid weather must be emphasized.

Pacemakers

Patients with pacemakers are not to be excluded from a cardiac exercise program. In the demand type, which are the pacemakers in current use, after the pacing rate is overridden, the same principles are followed as in the nonpaced hearts, although after a period of pacing, nonischemic ST segment depression may temporarily occur.

RESUMPTION OF A NORMAL LIFE

Sexual Activity

Resumption of sexual activity is one of the major concerns of the patient who has had an acute coronary event, whether it was MI or heart surgery. There are two indirect tests that can be performed to determine if the patient is ready to resume sexual activity. One is the "two-flight" test, during which the patient is monitored while rapidly ascending and descending two flights of stairs (140,141). Larsen and colleagues (142) recommend that stair climbing be preceded by several minutes of rapid walking.

Other guidelines can be provided by the stress test. If the patient can complete the 5- to 6-MET level, he should have the physical capacity for sex based on data that sexual intercourse between normal, middle-aged couples is about 3 to 4 METs, and at the point of orgasm is 4 to 5 METs (143,144).

Sexual activity between long-married spouses generally does not incur heart rates above 117 beats per minute and may cause less ST depression or ischemia than other ADLs: watching an exciting sport on television, driving, or working at the office. Extramarital, clandestine sex preceded by heavy eating and drinking may place excessive demands on a damaged myocardium, however, leading to the declaration that the cardiac patient may return to lovemaking with his wife in 6 weeks and his mistress in 6 months. Other useful advice appears in this poem by Dr. D. Kritchevsky (145):

Couplets on Cardiac Coupling
Coronary have a care
Think before that new affair
Dr. Zohman studied swingers
And her facts are really zingers
Sex domestic, also straight
Hardly makes you palpitate
Heart beats stay at normal rate
When one beds with legal mate
And the dangers that it bears
Loom like—well, two sets of stairs
But roosting in another's nest
Flirts with cardiac arrest
End result of evening's sport is
Very often rigor mortis
So seduction's needs are three
Soft lights, music, EKG.

Frohlicher et al. (146) found that although patients usually returned to sexual activity (as well as driving and outdoor activities) by 12 weeks, over 50% returned to these activities within 3 weeks after acute MI. Drory et al. (147) found that recovered cardiacs who did not have ischemia on the exercise stress test had none during intercourse (by Holter), but those with positive stress test results might also be ischemic or have unduly high heart rates during sex. The latter group deserves counseling and might require additional medication. Ectopic activity was present during intercourse in 11% of the 88 patients in an Israeli study, but it was usually simple and similar to that present in daily activities (148).

In addition, cardiac rehabilitation exercise training after MI can make sexual activity less physically demanding. Hellerstein and Friedman showed there was an average 5.5% decrease in peak coital heart rate after exercise training, whereas the control group did not show any significant changes (143,149). Another study showed that trained cardiacs had less decrease in frequency of coitus as compared with the untrained patients (143,150). Those who reported decreased sexual activity had poorer attendance and showed less training effect. (151).

Return to Employment

Evaluation to determine the capacity to return to gainful employment should involve assessment of the clinical status of the patient as well as the type of work required on the job. The cardiovascular functional classification by the New York Heart Association and Canadian Cardiovascular Society correlated with the corresponding level of metabolic cost of work allowable is useful in matching the patient's capacities to the job requirements (152,153).

The level of performance attained on the exercise stress test is also predictive of whether a job is too strenuous for a patient. In the United States, individuals who can perform 7 METs or higher without any limitations or abnormal responses should be able to return to most jobs, except those of a heavy industrial nature. Those who can exercise at 5 METs or greater but less than 7 METs can perform sedentary work and most household chores, whereas those who perform at the 3- or 4-MET level may not be suited to return to employment (154). When the reason for the low peak work load attained is a low level of physical fitness, a cardiovascular conditioning program can help. Cardiac patients in the 5-MET or greater range can increase their capacity by 15% to as much as 50% after 2 to 3 months of reconditioning (154).

To be able to match the patient's clinical status and cardiovascular functional capacity to the requirements of the job, a thorough evaluation of the job should include a detailed pen and paper analysis of the energy cost of the walking, climbing, and lifting done and the duration of these activities during the 8-hour workday. Not only the routine tasks performed at work but also the peak activity and duration of this activity should be determined. In an exercise test for work evaluation, one can simulate this peak level of activity by a spurt of increased exercise intensity during the exercise test. The environmental conditions in the area, the mode of transportation to and from work, and the household chores needed to be done after work are equally important considerations.

Unfortunately, despite our best predictions of work capacity, job demands, patient education, counseling, and behavioral interventions, return to work has not improved because of the social and policy issues involved (18).

REHABILITATION OF PHYSICALLY DISABLED PATIENTS WITH A CARDIAC COMPLICATION

At times patients with recent neuromusculoskeletal impairment, such as hemiplegics or amputees, referred to the rehabilitation service have a concomitant acute cardiac disorder occurring just before, at the time of, or shortly after the physical impairment was sustained. This requires that

TABLE 54-4. *Correlation of the energy cost of crutch ambulation (weight bearing on only one extremity) to the work level of the upper extremity exercise stress test*

UE stress test work level (KGM)	Weight of individual (kg)	MET
150	50–70	3.5
225	70–80	4.0
300	80–120	5.0

both conditions be addressed simultaneously so that the rehabilitation process can proceed without delay. The dipyridamole thallium scan stress test discussed earlier in the chapter is helpful in determining the integrity of the coronary circulation and the myocardium before beginning rehabilitation.

The two most common physical disabilities associated with coronary artery disease (CAD) are stroke and lower extremity dysvascular amputation. Their etiologies are the same. The cardiac capacity to respond to the metabolic functional needs of ambulation training is a major question in this group of patients. The initial evaluation and the start of ambulation training usually are the most stressful periods because the patient is most anxious and most inefficient at this time. Furthermore, some patients who appear medically stable may decompensate when they perform higher levels of physical activity. Monitoring the patient's initial performance by ECG telemetry may be very useful in guiding therapy. If expensive ECG telemetry is not available, even a simple office ECG machine is enough to permit monitoring by wiring the patient with the ECG cable and then plugging it into the recorder only for a baseline tracing and a postactivity tracing.

In the cardiac amputee, before starting preprosthetic ambulation training, the cardiac capacity to walk on only one extremity can be assessed by upper extremity ergometry. By knowing the weight of the individual, one can test the patient to a specific work stage (155) (Table 54-4) (i.e., for a 50- to 70-kg person, one can test the patient to more than 150 KGM, the 70- to 81-kg person to 225 KGM, 80- to 120-kg person to 300 KGM, etc.). Prosthetic ambulation, even in the trained indivudal, is a high energy cost physical activity (Table 54-5). Compared with the average energy cost of normal ambulation at 3 METs, prosthetic ambulation requires a 9% to 28% increase in the unilateral below-the-knee amputee, a 40% to 65% increase in the unilateral above-knee amputee, a 125% increase in the hemipelvectomy patient, and a 280% increase in the bilateral above-the-knee amputee (156–158). Knowing the New York Heart Association functional class of the amputee, one can get an estimate of cardiac functional capacity and the patient's ability to ambulate with a prosthesis (Table 54-6). Except for some unilateral below-the-knee amputees, class III patients usually have to function from a wheelchair level, class II may have the capacity to walk with a prosthesis, except for the bilateral above-the-knee amputee, who must be class I and physically fit to be able to tolerate a prosthesis.

TABLE 54-5. *Energy cost of amputee ambulation (based on percentage increase above cost of normal [3 METs])*

	Increase (%)	MET
No prosthesis, with crutches	50	4.5
Unilateral BK with prosthesis	9–28	3.3–3.8
Unilateral AK with prosthesis	40–65	4.2–5.8
Bilateral BK with prostheses	41–100	4.2–6.0
BK plus AK with prostheses	75	5.3
Bilateral AK with prostheses	280	11.4
Unilateral hip disarticulation with prosthesis	82	5.5
Hemipelvectomy with prosthesis	125	6.75

AK, above-the-knee amputation; BK, below-the-knee amputation.

TABLE 54-6. *Correlation of the energy cost of ambulation according to the level of amputation with the estimated work capacity according to cardiac functional class*

Cardiac class	MET	Amputee ambulation	MET
Class IV	<2	—	—
Class III	<2 to <5	Wheelchair	2.0–3.0
		Unilateral BK with prosthesis	3.3–3.8
Class II	>5 to <7	No prosthesis with crutches	4.5
		Unilateral AK with prosthesis	4.2–5.0
		Bilateral AK with prostheses	4.2–6.0
		BK plus AK with prostheses	5.3
		Hip disarticulation with prosthesis	5.5
		Hemipelvectomy with prosthesis	6.75
Class I	>7	Bilateral AK with prostheses	11.4

AK, above-the-knee amputation; BK, below-the-knee amputation.

In the stroke patient, the trained independently ambulatory hemiplegic, with or without lower extremity orthosis, walks at a speed 40% to 45% slower than the normal individual, yet the energy cost of hemiplegic ambulation is 50% to 65% higher (159).

Negotiating stairs is another activity that is of high intensity, so monitoring may be important to determine safety during the period of training and for discharge home. Other physical rehabilitation training activities where monitoring will be of value are the use of ambulatory aids, wheelchair activities, and upper extremity strengthening exercises. Monitoring could also be a way of convincing a patient with a lower extremity amputation that it is safe to proceed with prosthetic training, or that prosthetic training is contraindicated and that functioning at the wheelchair level is all that is within his or her cardiac capacity.

Cardiovascular Conditioning

The principles of training in the physical conditioning of the physically impaired individual are the same as for the able-bodied person. The problem is the performance of an exercise stress test to evaluate the individual's initial functional cardiovascular capacity.

For the individual with lower extremity impairment but normal upper extremities, the hand-cranked cycle ergometer is most commonly used. For the hemiparetic patient, the lower extremity cycle ergometer may be used by strapping the paretic extremities to the handlebars and the foot pedal and scaling down the intensity of the work by halving the resistance for each stage.

Various modifications of exercise equipment or adaptive devices have been successfully used for exercise tolerance testing of the disabled, such as the supine bicycle ergometer, modified arm–leg bicycle, wheelchair on rollers, and wheelchair connected to a cycle ergometer (160). The same modified equipment can then be used as the modality for the exercise activity.

The Schwinn Air-Dyne arm–leg cycle is a useful exercise testing device for the disabled. It is also useful as a training modality for individuals with lower extremity weakness because part of the work load is distributed to the upper extremities, reducing the work intensity of the lower extremity without reducing the total work load needed to induce a cardiovascular training effect.

The presence of a physical impairment should not be a deterrent to the rehabilitation of a cardiac patient. The physiatrist can use special exercise stress tests and can modify cardiovascular conditioning equipment, adapting it to accommodate the patient's type of physical impairment.

REFERENCES

1. Cain HD, Frasher WG Jr, Stivelman R. Graded activity program for safe return to self-care after acute myocardial infarction. *JAMA* 1961; 177:111.
2. Newman LB, Wasserman RR, Borden C. Productive living for those with heart disease—the role of physical medicine and rehabilitation. *Arch Phys Med Rehabil* 1956; 37:137.
3. Tobis JS, Zohman LR. A rehabilitation program for inpatients with recent myocardial infarction. *Arch Phys Med Rehabil* 1968; 49:443.
4. Torkelson LD. Rehabilitation of the patient with acute myocardial infarction. *J Chronic Dis* 1964; 17:685.
5. Fardy PS, Yanowitz FG, Wilson PK. *Cardiac rehabilitation—adult fitness and exercise testing.* Philadelphia: Lea & Febiger, 1988; 171–175, 200, 303–321, 365–376.
6. Cantwell JD. Cardiac rehabilitation in the mid-1980s. *Phys Sports Med* 1986; 14:89.
7. Hoffmeister JM, Gruntzig AR, Wenger NK. Longterm management of patients following successful percutaneous transluminal coronary angioplasty and coronary artery bypass grafting. *Cardiology* 1986; 73:323–332.
8. Wilson PK, Edgett JW, Porter GA. Rehabilitation of the cardiac patient—program organization. In: Pollock ML, Schmidt DH, eds. *Heart diseases and rehabilitation,* 2nd ed. New York: Wiley, 1986; 390–395.
9. Meyer CP, Pollock ML, Graves JE. Exercise prescription for the coronary artery bypass graft surgery patient. *J Cardiac Rehabil* 1986; 6: 85.
10. Oberman A, Kouchoukos NT. Role of exercise after coronary artery surgery. In: Wenger NK, ed. *Exercise and the heart.* Philadelphia: FA Davis, 1978; 155–172.
11. Robinson G, Froelicher VF, Utley JR. Rehabilitation of the coronary artery bypass graft surgery patient. *J Cardiac Rehabil* 1984; 4:74.
12. Wenger NK. Early ambulation physical activity—myocardial infarction and coronary artery bypass surgery. *Heart Lung* 1984; 13:14–18.
13. Newell JP, Kappagoda CT, Stoker JB, et al. Physical training after heart valve replacement. *Br Heart J* 1980; 44:638–649.
14. Wingate S. Rehabilitation of the patient with valvular heart disease. *J Cardiovasc Nurs* 1987; 1:52–64.
15. Lampman RM, Stewart JR, Collins JA, et al. Exercise training soon after left ventricular aneurysectomy and endocardial resection. *J Cardiac Rehabil* 1982; 2:134.
16. Squires RW. Cardiac rehabilitation issues for heart transplantation patients. *J Cardiopul Rehabil* 1990; 10:159–168.
17. Squires RW, Arthur PR, Gau GT, et al. Exercise after cardiac transplantation—a report of two cases. *J Cardiac Rehabil* 1983; 3: 570–574.
18. Wenger NK, Froelicker ES, Smith LK, et al. *Cardiac rehabilitation—clinical practice.* Washington, D.C.: U.S. Department of Health and Human Services, 1995; 9–26, 27–47, 100–102, 121–128.
19. *Membership and cardiopulmonary rehabilitation programs directory.* Middleton, WI: Association of Cardiopulmonary Rehabilitation Programs, 1996; 1–95.
20. American Heart Association, New York City; The President's Council on Physical Fitness and Sports, Washington, D.C.; Department of Rehabilitation Medicine, Montefiore Hospital, Bronx, NY. *Directory: exercise programs for cardiacs.* New York: American Heart Association, 1970.
21. Komrad MS, Coffey E, Coffey KS, et al. Myocardial infarction and stroke. *Neurology* 1989; 34:1403–1409.
22. O'Connor CM, Califf RM, Massey EW, et al. Stroke and acute myocardial infarction in the thrombolytic era—clinical correlates and long term prognosis. *J Am Coll Cardiol* 1990; 16:533–540.
23. Thompson PL, Robinson JS. Stroke after acute myocardial infarction—relation to infarct size. *Br Med J* 1978; 2:457–459.
24. Arous EJ, Baum PL, Cutler BS. The ischemic exercise test in patients with peripheral vascular disease. *Arch Surg* 1984; 119:780–783.
25. Cutler BS. Prevention of cardiac complications in peripheral vascular surgery. *Surg Clin North Am* 1986; 66:281–292.
26. McCann RL, Clements FM. Silent myocardial ischemia in patients undergoing peripheral vascular surgery—incidence and association with perioperative cardiac morbidity and mortality. *J Vasc Surg* 1989; 9:583–587.
27. Kerstein MD, Zimmer H, Dugdale FE, et al. Amputations of the lower extremity—a study of 194 cases. *Arch Phys Med Rehabil* 1974; 55: 454–459.
28. Sterling HM. Influence of cardiac status on rehabilitation of lower-extremity amputees. *Arch Phys Med Rehabil* 1970; 51:588–591.
29. Detry J, Rousseau M, Vandenbroucke G, et al. Increased arteriovenous oxygen difference after physical training in coronary heart disease. *Circulation* 1971; 44:109–118.
30. Holloszy JO. Biochemical and muscular effects of training. In: Cohen LS, Mock MB, Ringgvist I, eds. *Physical conditioning and cardiovascular rehabilitation.* New York: Wiley, 1981:175.
31. Leon AS. Scientific evidence of value of cardiac rehabilitation services with emphasis on patients following MI—Section I. Exercise conditioning component. Position paper of the American Association of Cardiac and Pulmonary Rehabilitation. *J Cardiopul Rehabil* 1990; 10:79–87.
32. Zohman LR, Kattus AA, eds. Ten years of exercise programming for cardiacs. In: *Cardiac rehabilitation for the practicing physician.* New York: Stratton Intercontinental, 1979;45–62.
33. Ehsani AA, Biello DR, Schultz J, et al. Improvement of left ventricular contractile function by exercise training in patients with coronary artery disease. *Circulation* 1986; 74:350–366.
34. Ehsani AA, Heath GG, Hagberg JM, et al. Effects of 12 months of intense exercise training on ischemic ST-segment depression in patients with coronary artery disease. *Circulation* 1981; 64:1116–1124.
35. Ehsani AA, Martin WH, Heath GG, et al. Cardiac effects of prolonged and intense exercise training in patients with coronary artery disease. *Am J Cardiol* 1982;50:246–254.
36. Froelicher V, Jensen D, Genter F, et al. A randomized trial of training in patients with coronary heart disease. *JAMA* 1984; 252:1291–1297.

37. Jensen D, Atwood JE, Froelicher V, et al. Improvement in ventricular function during exercise studied with radionuclide ventriculography after cardiac rehabilitation. *Am J Cardiol* 1980; 46:770–775.
38. Sebrechts CP, Klein JL, Ahnue S, et al. Myocardial perfusion changes following 1 year of exercise training assessed by thallium 201 circumferential count profiles. *Am Heart J* 1986; 112:1217–1225.
39. Goodman LS, McKenzie DC, Nath CR, et al. Central adaptations in aerobic circuit versus walking/jogging trained cardiac patients. *Can J Appl Physiol* 1995; 20:178–197.
40. Ferguson RJ, Petticlerc R, Choquette G, et al. Effect of physical training on treadmill exercise capacity, collateral circulation and progression of coronary disease. *Am J Cardiol* 1974; 34:764–769.
41. Connor JF, LaCamera R Jr, Swanick EJ, et al. Effects of exercise on coronary collateralization—angiographic studies of six patients in a supervised exercise program. *Med Sci Sports Exerc* 1976; 8:145–151.
42. Kramsch DM, Aspen AJ, Abramowitz BM. Reduction of coronary atherosclerosis by moderate conditioning exercise in monkeys on a diet. *N Engl J Med* 1981; 305:1483–1488.
43. Rose G, Prineas R, Rhell JRA. Myocardial infarction and the intrinsic calibre of the coronary arteries. *Br Med J* 1986; 29:548–552.
44. May GS, Eberlein KA, Furberg CD, Passamani ER, DeMets DL. Secondary prevention after myocardial infarction: a view of long-term trials. *Prog Cardiovasc Dis* 1983; 34:331–352.
45. Shephard RJ. The value of exercise in ischemic heart disease: a cumulative analysis. *J Cardiac Rehabil* 1983; 3:294–298.
46. Collins R, Yusuf S, Peto R. Exercise after myocardial infarction reduces mortality: evidence from randomized controlled trials (RCTs) [Abstract]. *J Am Coll Cardiol* 1984; 3:622.
47. Oldridge NB, Guyatt GH, Fischer ME, et al. Cardiac rehabilitation after myocardial infarction: combined experience of randomized clinical trials. *JAMA* 1988; 260:945–950.
48. O'Connor GT, Buring JE, Yusuf S, et al. An overview of randomized trials of rehabilitation with exercise after myocardial infarction. *Circulation* 1989; 80:234–244.
49. Van Hees L, Fagard R, Thijs R, et al. Prognostic value of training induced changes in peak exercise capacity in patients with coronary bypass surgery. *Am J Cardiol* 1995; 76:104–109.
50. Selwyn AP, Braunwald E. Ischemic heart disease. In: Wilson JD, Braunwald E, Isselbacker KJ, et al., eds. *Harrison's principles of internal medicine.* New York: McGraw-Hill, 1991; 967.
51. Haskell WL, Alderman EL, Fair JN, et al. Effects of intensive multiple risk factor reduction on coronary atherosclerosis and clinical cardiac events in men and women with coronary artery disease. The Stanford Coronary Risk Prevention Program (SCRIP). *Circulation* 1994; 89: 975–990.
52. Virmani R, Atkinson JB, Forman MB. Aortocoronary saphenous vein bypass grafts. *Cardiovasc Clin* 1988; 18:41.
53. Garrow JS. Effects of exercise on obesity. *Acta Med Scand* 1986; 711(suppl):67–74.
54. Haskell WL. The influence of exercise training on plasma lipids and lipoproteins in health and disease. *Acta Med Scand* 1986; 711(suppl): 25–38.
55. Lavie CH, Milani RV. Factors predicting improvements in lipid values following cardiac rehabilitation and exercise training. *Arch Int Med* 1993; 153:982–988.
56. Holloszy JO, Schultz J, Kusnierkiewicz J, et al. Glucose tolerance and insulin resistance. *Acta Med Scand* 1986; 711(suppl):67–73.
57. Filipovsky J, Simon J, Chrastek J, et al. Changes in blood pressure and lipid pattern during a physical training in hypertensive subjects. *Cardiology* 1991; 78:31–38.
58. Blumenthal JA, Thyrum ET, Gulette ED, et al. Do exercise and weight loss reduce blood pressure in patients with hypertension? *N C Med J* 1995; 56:92–95.
59. Flores AM, Zohman LR, Rehabilitation of the cardiac patient. In: DeLisa JA, ed. *Rehabilitation medicine principles and practice,* 2nd ed. Philadelphia: JB Lippincott, 1993; 934–951.
60. Weiss RA, Karpovich PV. Energy cost of exercise in convalescents. *Arch Phys Med* 1947; 28:447.
61. DeBusk RF. Techniques of exercise testing. In: Hurst JW, ed. *The heart, arteries and veins.* New York: McGraw-Hill, 1990; 1828–1830.
62. Froelicher VF. *Exercise and the heart.* Chicago: Yearbook Medical Publishers, 1987; 16, 89, 200, 409.
63. Zohman LR, Young JL, Kattus AA. Treadmill walking protocol for the diagnostic evaluation and exercise programming of cardiac patients. *Am J Cardiol* 1983; 51:1081.
64. DeBusk RF, Haskell W. Symptom-limited versus heart rate-limited exercise testing soon after myocardial infarction. *Circulation* 1980; 61:738–743.
65. Starling MR, Crawford MH, O'Rourke RA. Superiority of selected treadmill exercise protocols predischarge and six weeks post-infarction for detecting ischemic abnormalities. *Am Heart J* 1982; 104: 1054–1060.
66. Chaitman B. Exercise stress testing. In: Braunwald E, ed. *Heart disease—a textbook of cardiovascular medicine,* 4th ed. Philadelphia: WB Saunders, 1992; 172–173.
67. Flores AM. Hospital-based cardiac rehabilitation. *Phys Med Rehabil Clin North Am* 1995; 6:243–259.
68. Greenland P. Efficacy of supervised cardiac rehabilitation programs for coronary patients—update 1986 to 1990. *J Cardiopul Rehabil* 1991; 11:197–203.
69. Stern MJ, Cleary P. The national exercise and heart disease project—longterm psychosocial outcome. *Arch Intern Med* 1982; 142:1093–1097.
70. McMahon M, Miller P, Wikoff R. Life situations, health beliefs, and medical regimen adherence of patients with myocardial infarction. *Heart Lung* 1986; 15:82–86.
71. Wenger NK. Rehabilitation of the patient with coronary heart disease. In: Sclant RG, Alexander RW, eds. *The heart, arteries and veins,* 8th ed. New York: McGraw-Hill, 1994; 1223–1237.
72. Magel JR, Foglia GR, McArdle WD. Specificity of swim training on maximum oxygen uptake. *J Appl Physiol* 1974; 38:151–155.
73. Mostardi RA, Gandee RN, Norris WA. Exercise training using arms and legs versus legs alone. *Arch Phys Med Rehabil* 1981; 62:332–341.
74. DeBusk R. Early exercise testing after myocardial infarction. In: Wenger NK, ed. *Exercise and the heart.* Philadelphia: FA Davis, 1976; 135.
75. DeBusk R. The value of exercise testing. *JAMA* 1975; 232:956–958.
76. Sheffield LT. Exercise stress testing. In: Braunwald L, ed. *Heart disease—a textbook of cardiovascular medicine.* Philadelphia: WB Saunders, 1988; 228, 238.
77. Mitchell JH, Blomqvist G. Maximal oxygen uptake. *N Engl J Med* 1971; 284:1018–1022.
78. Cumming G. Yield of ischemic exercise electrocardiograms in relation to exercise intensity in a normal population. *Br Heart J* 1972; 34: 919–923.
79. Rochmis P, Blackburn H. Exercise tests: a survey of procedures, safety litigation experience in approximately 170,000 tests. *JAMA* 1971; 217: 1061–1066.
80. Fletcher GF, Froelicher VF, Hartley H, et al. Exercise standards—a statement for health professionals. New York: American Heart Association, 1991; 2289.
81. Council on Scientific Affairs-American Medical Association. Indications for exercise testing. *JAMA* 1981; 246:1015–1018.
82. Crawford MH. Non-invasive techniques. In: Stein JH, ed. *Internal medicine.* Boston: Little, Brown, 1987; 348.
83. Tavazzi L, Ignone G, Giordano A, et al. Cardiac rehabilitation in patients with recent myocardial infarction and left ventricular dysfunction. *Adv Cardiol* 1986; 34:156–169.
84. Wynns J, Braunwald E. The cardiomyopathies and myocarditis. In: Braunwald E, ed. *Heart disease—a textbook of cardiovascular medicine.* Philadelphia: WB Saunders, 1988; 1429.
85. Goss JE, Shadoff N. Sudden cardiac death in sports. In: Appenzeller O, ed. Sports medicine—fitness, training, injuries. Baltimore: Urban & Schwarzenberg, 1988; 212–213.
86. Ellestad MH, Stewart RJ. Exercise stress testing—principles and clinical application. In: Parmley WW, Chatterjee K, eds. *Cardiology.* Vol. 1. Philadelphia: JB Lippincott, 1990; 5.
87. Kattus AA, MacAlpin RN. Role of exercise in discovery, evaluation, and management of ischemic heart disease. *Cardiovasc Clin* 1969; 1:255–279.
88. Cotton FS, Dill DB. On the relation between the heart rate during exercise and that of the immediate post-exercise period. *Am J Physiol* 1935; 256:554.
89. Wenger NK, Froelicher ES, Smith LK, et al. *Cardiac rehabilitation as secondary prevention.* Washington, D.C.: U.S. Department of Health and Human Services, 1995; 20.

90. VanCamp SP, Petersen RA. Cardiovascular complications of outpatient cardiac rehabilitation programs. *JAMA* 1986; 256:1160–1163.
91. VongVanich P, Merz CND. Supervised exercises at electrocardiographic monitoring during cardiac rehabilitation. *J Cardiopul Rehabil* 1996; 16:233–238.
92. Zohman LR, DiMattia D, Peimer L. Twenty five years of inexpensive community-based cardiac rehabilitation. *Curr Sci* 1991; 2:409–414.
93. DeBusk RF, Miller NH, Superko HR, et al. A case-management system for coronary risk factor modification after acute myocardial infarction. *Ann Intern Med* 1994; 120:721–729.
94. Knight JA, Laubach CA Jr, Butcher RJ, et al. Supervision of clinical exercise testing by exercise physiologists. *Am J Cardiol* 1995; 75: 390.
95. Katch FI, McArdle WD. *Nutrition, weight control, and exercise.* Philadelphia: Lea & Febiger, 1988; 194–196, 240–241.
96. McArdle WD, Katch FI, Katch VL. *Exercise physiology—energy, nutrition and human performance.* Philadelphia: WB Saunders, 1988; 355–361, 375–376, 568.
97. Baker JA. Comparison of rope skipping and jogging as a method of improving cardiovascular efficiency of college men. *Res Q* 1966; 39: 240.
98. Stewart KJ. Weight training in coronary artery disease and hypertension. *Prog Cardiovasc Dis* 1992; 35:159–168.
99. Faigenbaum AD, Skrinar GS, Cesare WF, et al. Physiologic and symptomatic response of cardiac patients to resistance exercise. *Arch Phys Med Rehabil* 1990; 71:395–398.
100. Haennel RG, Quinney HA, Kappagoda CT. Effects of hydraulic circuit training following coronary artery bypass surgery. *Med Sci Sports Exerc* 1991; 23:158–165.
101. Kelemen MH, Stewart JK. Circuit weight training—a new direction for cardiac rehabilitation. *Sports Med* 1985; 2:385–388.
102. Sparling PB, Cantwell JD, Dolan CM, Niederman RK. Strength training in a cardiac rehabilitation program—six month follow up. *Arch Phys Med Rehabil* 1990; 7:148–152.
103. Lillegard NA, Terrio JD. Appropriate strength training. *Med Clin North Am* 1994; 78:457–477.
104. Zohman LR. Practical aspects of vigorous exercise programming for coronary patients. *Adv Cardiol* 1982; 31:205–211.
105. Nobel SJ. Clinical application of perceived exertion. *Med Sci Sports Exerc* 1982; 14:406–411.
106. Pollock ML, Pils AE, Foster C, et al. Exercise prescription for rehabilitation of the cardiac patient. In: Pollock ML, Schmidt DH, eds. *Heart disease and rehabilitation.* New York: Wiley, 1986; 483–485.
107. Borg GA. Psychological bases of perceived exertion. *Med Sci Sports Exerc* 1982; 14:377–381.
108. Borg GA. Subjective effort in relation to physical performance and working capacity. In: Pick HL Jr, ed. *Psychology from research to practice.* New York: Plenum, 1978; 357–358.
109. Gordon NF, Kruger PE, Cilliers JF. Improved exercise ventilatory responses after training in coronary heart disease during long-term beta-adrenergic blockade. *Am J Cardiol* 1983; 51:755–758.
110. Laslett LJ, Paumer L, Scott-Baier P, et al. Efficacy of exercise training in patients with coronary artery disease who are taking propranolol. *Circulation* 1983; 68:1029–1034.
111. Vanhees L, Fagard R, Amery A. Influence of beta-adrenergic blockade on the hemodynamic effects of physical training in patients with ischemic heart disease. *Am Heart J* 1984; 108:270–275.
112. Sweeney ME, Fletcher BJ, Fletcher GF. Exercise testing and training with beta-adrenergic blockade—role of the drug washout period in "unmasking" training effect. *Am Heart J* 1989; 118:941–946.
113. Pollock ML, Gettman LR, Milesis CA, et al. Effects of frequency and duration of training on attrition and incidence of injury. *Med Sci Sports* 1977; 9:31–36.
114. Swengvos G. Industrial physical fitness programs. In: Wilson PK, ed. *Adult fitness and cardiac rehabilitation.* Baltimore: University Park Press, 1975; 227–232.
115. Kavanagh T, Yacoub MH, Mertena D, et al. Exercise rehabilitation after heterotopic cardiac transplantation. *J Cardiopul Rehabil* 1989; 9:303–310.
116. Keteyian S, Ehrman J, Fedel F, Rhoads K. Heart rate perceived exertion relationship during exercise in orthotopic heart transplant patients. *J Cardiopul Rehabil* 1990; 10:287–293.
117. Savin WM, Haskell WL, Schroeder JS, et al. Cardiorespiratory response of cardiac transplant patients to graded, symptom-limited exercise. *Circulation* 1980; 62:55–60.
118. Thompson ML, Dummer JS, Griffith BP. Cardiac and cardiopulmonary transplantation. In: Parmley WW, Chatterjee K, eds. *Cardiology.* Vol. 2. Philadelphia: JB Lippincott, 1989; 7.
119. Golding LA, Granger BC. Competing in varsity athletics after cardiac transplantation. *J Cardiopul Rehabil* 1989; 9:486–491.
120. Borer JS, Bradni-Pifano S, Puigbo JJ, et al. Rehabilitation of patients with left ventricular dysfunction and heart failure. *Adv Cardiol* 1986; 33:160–169.
121. Shabetai R. Beneficial effects of exercise training in compensated heart failure. *Circulation* 1988; 78:775–776.
122. Williams RS. Exercise training of patients with left ventricular dysfunction and heart failure. *Cardiovasc Clin* 1985; 15:219–231.
123. Fishman EZ, Kellerman JJ. Does exercise training deteriorate ventricular function? *J Am Coll Cardiol* 1989; 14:263–264.
124. Jugdutt BI, Michorowski BL, Kappagoda CT. Exercise training after anterior Q wave myocardial infarction—importance of regional left ventricular function and topography. *J Am Coll Cardiol* 1988; 12: 362–372.
125. Coats AJS, Adamopoulos S, Meyer TE, et al. Effects of physical training in chronic heart failure. *Lancet* 1990; 335:63–66.
126. Conn EH, Williams RH, Wallace AG. Exercise responses before and after physical conditioning in patients with severely depressed left ventricular function. *Am J Cardiol* 1982; 49:296–300.
127. Sullivan MJ, Higginbotham MB, Cobb FR. Exercise training in patients with severe left ventricular dysfunction. *Circulation* 1988; 78: 506–515.
128. Squires RW, Lavis J, Brandt TR, et al. Cardiac rehabilitation in patients with severe ischemic left ventricular dysfunction. *Mayo Clin Proc* 1987; 62:997–1002.
129. Tobin JN, Wassertheil-Smoller S, Wexler JP, et al. Sex bias in considering coronary bypass surgery. *Ann Intern Med* 1987; 107:19–25.
130. Coplan N, Eskenazzi M, Stachenfeld N, et al. Gender differences and the endpoint for exercise testing [Abstract]. *J Am Coll Cardiol* 1991; 17:81.
131. Cannistra LB, Balady J, O'Malley CJ, et al. Clinical profile and outcome of women compared to men in phase II-III cardiac rehabilitation [Abstract]. *J Am Coll Cardiol* 1991; 17:296.
132. Hanson JS, Medle WH. Longterm physical training effect in sedentary females. *J Appl Physiol* 1974; 37:112–116.
133. Zohman LR, Kattus AA, Softness DG. *The cardiologist's guide to fitness and health through exercise.* New York: Simon & Schuster, 1979; 187–191.
134. Soldo BJ, Manton KG. Demography characteristics and implications of an aging population. In: Rowe JW, Besline RW, eds. *Geriatrics medicine.* Boston: Little, Brown, 1988; 12–14.
135. Wenger NK. Specific cardiac disorders. In: Williams TF, ed. *Rehabilitation in the aging.* New York: Raven, 1984; 265.
136. Fleg JL, Goldberg AP. Exercise in older people—cardiovascular and metabolic adaptations. In: Hazzard WR, Anders R, Bierman EL, Blass JP, eds. *Principles of geriatric medicine and gerontology.* New York: McGraw-Hill, 1990; 85–92.
137. Jones RH. Physiological bases of rehabilitation therapy. In: Williams TF, ed. *Rehabilitation in the aging.* New York: Raven, 1984:105.
138. Oh-Park M, Zohman LR, Abrahams C. A simple walk test for exercise programming of elderly cardiac patients. 1996 (personal communication).
139. Strandell T. Electrocardiographic findings at rest, during and after exercise in healthy old men compared with young men. *Acta Med Scand* 1963; 174:479.
140. Zohman LR, Tobis JS. *Cardiac rehabilitation.* New York: Grune & Stratton, 1970; 195–205.
141. Bartlett RG, Bohr VC. Physiologic response during coitus in the human [Abstract]. *Fed Proc* 1956; 15:10.
142. Larsen JL, McNaughton MW, Kennedy JW, et al. Heartrate and blood pressure response to sexual activity and a stair-climbing test. *Heart Lung* 1980; 9:1025–1030.
143. Hellerstein HK, Friedman EH. Sexual activity and the post-coronary patient. *Arch Intern Med* 1970; 125:987–999.
144. Skinner JS. Sexual relations and the cardiac patient. In: Pollock ML, Schmidt DH, eds. *Heart disease and rehabilitation.* New York: Wiley, 1986; 591–592.

145. Kritchevsky D. Couplets on cardiac coupling. *Med Tribune* 1972; 13: 6.
146. Froelicher ES, Keell, Henton KM, et al. Return to work, sexual activity and other activities after acute myocardial infarction. *Heart Lung* 1994:20; 423–435.
147. Drory Y, Shapira J, Fisman E, et al. Myocardial ischemia during sexual activity in patients with coronary artery disease. *Am J Cardiol* 1995; 75:835–837
148. Drory Y, Fishman EZ, Shapira Y, et al. Ventricular araythmia during sexual activity in patients with coronary artery disease. *Chest* 1996; 109:922–924.
149. Stein RA. The effect of exercise training in the post myocardial infarction patient. *Circulation* 1977; 55:738–740.
150. Johnston B, Cantwell JD, Watt EW, et al. Sexual activity in exercising patients after myocardial infarction and revascularization. *Heart Lung* 1978; 7:1026–1031.
151. Kavanagh T, Shephard RJ. Sexual activity after myocardial infarction. *Can Med Assoc J* 1973; 116:1250–1253.
152. Goldman L, Hasbimato B, Cook EF, Loscalzo A. Comparative reproducibility and validity of systems for assessing functional class—advantages of a new specific activity score. *Circulation* 1981; 64: 1227–1234.
153. Smith TW. Approach to the patient with cardiovascular disease. In: Wyngaaden JB, Smith CH Jr, eds. *Textbook of medicine*. Philadelphia: WB Saunders, 1988; 179.
154. Naughton J. The President's Committee on Employment of the Handicapped. Proceedings of the Cardiac Seminar, Washington, DC, February 6–7, 1975; 18–19.
155. Malanga GA, Dubov WE, Flores AM. Correlation of energy cost of upper extremity testing and crutch walking [Abstract]. *Arch Phys Med Rehabil* 1992; 73:960.
156. Fisher SV, Gullickson G Jr. Energy cost of ambulation in health and disability—a literature review. *Arch Phys Med Rehabil* 1978; 59: 124–133.
157. Huang CT, Judson Jr, Moor MB, et al. Amputation-energy cost of ambulation. *Arch Phys Med Rehabil* 1979; 60:18–24.
158. Nowroozi F, Islanneli ML, Gerber LH. Energy expenditure of hip disarticulation and hemipelvectomy amputees. *Arch Phys Med Rehabil* 1983; 6:300–303.
159. Corcoran PJ, Jebsen RH, Brengelmann GL, Simons BC. Effects of plastic and metal leg braces on speed and energy cost of hemiparetic ambulation. *Arch Phys Med Rehabil* 1970; 51:69–77.
160. Moldover JR, Daum MD, Downey JA. Cardiac stress testing of hemiplegic patients with a supine bicycle ergometer—preliminary study. *Arch Phys Med Rehabil* 1984; 65:470–473.

Rehabilitation Medicine: Principles and Practice, Third Edition,
edited by Joel A. DeLisa and Bruce M. Gans.
Lippincott–Raven Publishers, Philadelphia © 1998.

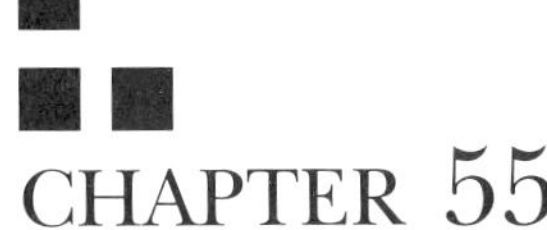

CHAPTER 55

Rehabilitation of the Patient with Respiratory Dysfunction

John R. Bach

A classical description of breathing exercises dates to 2500 B.C., and therapeutic respiratory exercises date to Tissot's work in 1781 (1). Historically speaking, pulmonary rehabilitation has been the cornerstone of the field of rehabilitation medicine. The first institutions dedicated to holistic and comprehensive rehabilitation in the United States and elsewhere were created in the late 1940s and early 1950s. They were dedicated to the postacute rehabilitation of both patients with intrinsic lung disease (i.e., tuberculosis) or patients with neuromuscular respiratory paralysis (i.e., poliomyelitis). With the subsequent decreased prevalence of these conditions, the institutions evolved into general rehabilitation facilities, but they have retained wide-ranging pulmonary rehabilitation programs. Of late, the greatly increasing incidence of conditions analogous to tuberculosis and poliomyelitis, such as chronic obstructive pulmonary disease (COPD) and neuromuscular and spinal cord diseases, again demand an ever-increasing commitment of pulmonary rehabilitation services.

At a recent National Institutes of Health workshop, pulmonary rehabilitation was redefined as "a multidimensional continuum of services directed to persons with pulmonary disease and their families, usually by an interdisciplinary team of specialists, with the goal of achieving and maintaining the individual's maximum level of independence and functioning in the community" (2). The goals of pulmonary rehabilitation are listed in Table 55-1. Although these principles and goals for the most part have been applied only to individuals with obstructive and intrinsic pulmonary diseases, they also can be applied to patients with neuromuscular and restrictive conditions. Indeed, the most useful techniques for managing neuromuscular patients, including ventilatory support via the mouth, nose, and oronasal interfaces, glossopharyngeal breathing, and the rocking bed have historically been described, developed, or initially adapted by physiatrists in the United States (3–8) and elsewhere (9), and should be more widely applied by other members of our field.

Physiatric management principles also can be applied to a third clinical situation, that of patients with sleep-disordered breathing. When severe, these patients may present and need to be managed in a manner similar to that of patients with purely restrictive pulmonary conditions (10). Sleep-disordered breathing also can complicate obstructive or restrictive conditions and is most common in the elderly.

Finally, pulmonary dysfunction often complicates a variety of musculoskeletal, medical, and central nervous system disorders, including traumatic brain injury, stroke, multiple sclerosis, and autoimmune deficiency syndrome. It is a frequent cause of morbidity and mortality and can hamper the rehabilitation of patients with these and other disorders. This latter situation has been little explored in the medical literature.

Although there may be significant overlap, particularly in the elderly, in the four clinical situations just noted, the respiratory pathology can be categorized as intrinsic versus mechanical, or obstructive versus restrictive. Patients with intrinsic or obstructive disease have significant ventilation–perfusion mismatching, which results primarily in impaired oxygenation of the blood. These patients are normally eucapnic or hypocapnic, often despite severe hypoxia. Significant hypercapnia occurs only during episodes of acute respiratory failure or with end-stage disease. On the other hand, patients with principally mechanical dysfunction of the lungs or chest wall have respiratory muscle dysfunction that results in impaired lung ventilation. For these patients, hypercapnia usually precedes significant hypoxia or oxyhe-

J. R. Bach: Department of Physical Medicine and Rehabilitation, University of Medicine and Dentistry of New Jersey, New Jersey Medical School, Newark, New Jersey 07103.

TABLE 55-1. *Pulmonary rehabilitation goals*

1. An improvement in cardiopulmonary function
2. The prevention and treatment of complications
3. The recognition and treatment of stress and depression, which often can interfere with coping mechanisms and independence
4. The facilitation of coping mechanisms to overcome any sense of loss, loss of control of personal and social relationships, self-esteem, or sense of self-worth
5. The promotion of increasing patient responsibility for his or her own care and well-being including acceptance of and compliance with optimum medical care with the goal of reducing numbers of exacerbations, emergency room visits, and hospitalizations
6. An increased understanding of the disease and the disease process so that the patient and family can confront it realistically
7. A return to work and/or a more active, productive, and emotionally satisfying life for the patient and his family

Adapted from Haas F, Axen K. *Pulmonary therapy and rehabilitation: principles and practice.* Baltimore: Williams & Wilkins, 1991.

moglobin desaturation (SaO_2). Therefore, ventilatory dysfunction causes the abnormality in blood oxygenation.

Although some medical and rehabilitation techniques pertain equally to both patients with impairment of oxygenation or ventilation, there is a common mistaken tendency to manage the latter as the former. Common errors in managing ventilatory dysfunction include the administration of oxygen, intermittent positive pressure breathing (IPPB) treatments at inadequate pressures to significantly assist inspiratory muscle function, and overmedication, especially during respiratory tract infections. Patients with obesity hypoventilation or neuromuscular ventilatory dysfunction are often ineffectively managed by continuous positive airway pressure (CPAP) or bi-level positive airway pressure (BPAP) when intermittent positive pressure ventilation (IPPV) is indicated. Indeed, for patients with impaired oxygenation or ventilatory dysfunction, effective noninvasive methods of respiratory muscle rest and airway secretion clearance are underused, as are other rehabilitation methods and resources in general. For both patient groups this leads to unnecessary dyspnea and hospitalizations, overreliance on intubation and tracheostomy, excessive physical deconditioning, and restriction in activities of daily living (ADL).

This chapter will consider the clinical situations and the two basic management constructs in which the application of pulmonary rehabilitation and physical medicine principles can benefit both quality and duration of life. It will highlight physiatrist diagnostic and management interventions.

REHABILITATION OF PATIENTS WITH OBSTRUCTIVE LUNG DISEASE

COPD affects 10% to 40% of all Americans and is the fifth leading cause of death in the United States. Its incidence is increasing rapidly, and it is likely to become increasingly prevalent with the increasing life expectancy of the general population. Fifty percent of patients have activity limitations, and 25% are bed disabled (11). It is the fourth largest cause of major activity limitation.

PATHOPHYSIOLOGY

Chronic bronchitis, emphysema, asthmatic bronchitis, and cystic fibrosis (CF) are the most common causes of COPD. These conditions usually have significant elements of both airway obstruction and parenchymal lung disease. COPD often results from a combination of genetic predisposition and environmental factors in which allergic diatheses (e.g., asthma), respiratory infections (e.g., bronchopneumonitis), chemical inflammation (cigarette smoke, asbestosis), and possibly metabolic abnormalities (e.g., $alpha_1$ antitrypsin deficiency) play a role.

Cigarette smoking is the most frequent cause of chronic bronchitis–emphysema. Smokers are 3.5 to 25 times more likely (depending on the amounts smoked) to die of COPD than nonsmokers (12). All one-pack-a-day smokers would eventually develop emphysema. One in 15 will succumb to lung cancer. On the average, patients 30 to 35 years of age who smoke 10 to 20 cigarettes per day die 5 years sooner than nonsmokers. One- to two-pack-a-day smokers of the same age die 6.5 years sooner (13). Smoking cessation has been associated with improvement in symptoms (14), pulmonary function (15), decreased risk of respiratory tract infection (16), and a long-term decreased reduction in rate of loss of forced expiratory volumes (17).

Emphysema is characterized by distention of air spaces distal to terminal nonrespiratory bronchioles with destruction of alveolar walls. This occurs because of the unimpeded action of neutrophil-derived elastase. This enzyme is present in polymorphonuclear leukocytes, which occur in large numbers at the bases of normal human lungs. The neutrophil-derived elastase is extremely proteolytic and punches holes in biologic membranes, allowing neutrophil entry. $Alpha_1$-antiprotease, which primarily inactivates neutrophil-derived elastase, normally protects the lungs but is destroyed by cigarette smoke and other toxins, which also cause chronic inflammation and impair mucociliary clearance (18). Ultimately, there is loss of lung recoil, excessive airway collapse on exhalation, and chronic airflow obstruction. Chronic bronchitis and CF are characterized by enlargement of tracheobronchial mucous glands and chronic mucous hypersecretion and chest infections. Chronic bronchitis is distinguished from asthmatic bronchitis by its irreversibility, lack of bronchial hyperreactivity, lack of responsiveness to bronchodilators, and distinctive abnormalities in ventilation–perfusion (19). Mucous hypersecretion occurs, blocks airways, and sets the stage for recurrent infection, airway and alveolar damage, and irreversible airflow obstruction. Asthmatics develop hypertrophy of bronchial muscle, mucosal edema, infiltration with mononuclear cells and eosinophils, and changes in basement membrane. Chronic bronchitis can develop from asthma.

The gas exchange surface of the lung, which under normal circumstances is effective to a 20-fold range of metabolic demand and maintains normal arterial blood gases, is greatly reduced in patients with intrinsic lung disease. Gas exchange is dependent on ventilation, perfusion, and diffusion, all of which are commonly affected. Oxygen and carbon dioxide diffusion across the respiratory exchange membrane of the lung is a function of the gas partial pressures, the respiratory exchange membrane area, and is inversely related to membrane thickness (20). Exchange normally takes place in one third of the pulmonary capillary blood transit time. With decreased diffusion or increased blood flow, arterial partial pressure of oxygen (pO_2) is significantly lower than alveolar pO_2. Arterial pO_2 decreases before there is an observed increase in partial pressure of carbon dioxide (pCO_2) because of the greater rate of diffusion of CO_2. Thus, hypoxia in the presence of normal or hyperventilation (pCO_2 less than 45 mm Hg) is characteristic of intrinsic lung disease. Such patients may develop overt respiratory failure with or without hypercapnia. Pulmonary vascular resistance increases in the presence of generalized or local pulmonary tissue hypoxia, especially in the presence of acidosis. Widespread alveolar hypoventilation leads to severe pulmonary artery hypertension and right ventricular failure.

Peripheral chemoreceptors in the aortic and carotid bodies sense pO_2, pCO_2, and pH. Central receptors on the surface of the medulla respond to hydrogen ion levels in the cerebrospinal fluid (20). Response to pCO_2 is reduced by drugs, heavy mechanical loads, and elevated bicarbonate levels. Hypercapnia is caused by the resort to shallow breathing to avoid respiratory muscle fatigue (21). Hypercapnic COPD patients also have weaker respiratory muscles than eucapnic patients (22,23).

PATIENT EVALUATION

The patient's family history should be explored for the presence of pulmonary diseases. The medical history should focus on the rate of progression of symptoms, their impact on the patient's functional activities, and on any factors—medical, physical, financial, or psychological—that might interfere with a rehabilitation program. Various dyspnea assessment surveys can be used to objectively evaluate the effects of rehabilitation (24–27). In addition, the presence of any coughing, wheezing, chest pains, neurologic or psychological disturbances, allergies, previous communicable diseases, injuries, and hospitalizations should be explored. Dyspnea and exacerbations of respiratory insufficiency associated with respiratory tract infections are the most frequent reasons for hospital admission. Hospitalization rates, morbidity, and mortality correlate with the extent of hypercapnia (28).

Poor nutrition is characterized by low protein values. Serum albumin level is a good indicator of visceral protein depletion, correlates better with hypoxia than does spirometric values, and is a good predictor of rehabilitation potential (29). Hypophosphatemia is common in critically ill COPD patients (30). Significant improvement of respiratory muscle weakness has been well documented in patients on mechanical ventilation for respiratory failure after correction of hypophosphatemia (31). In addition, intracellular phosphate shifts may occur with correction of acute respiratory acidosis (32). Hypomagnesemia, hypocalcemia, and hypokalemia also may cause respiratory muscle weakness that is reversible after replacement (33). Past and present medications are explored, as is the use of tobacco and alcohol. Social, educational, and vocational histories and any relevant environmental factors are explored (34).

On physical examination the typical emphysema patient is asthenic with a hyperresonant, ''barrel'' chest and poor breath sounds. Cardiac sounds are dull. The chest radiograph demonstrates a low, flattened diaphragm, a long, narrow heart shadow, increased retrosternal translucency on the lateral film, and narrowing of peripheral pulmonary vessels. These patients have decreased gas diffusion capacities. Arterial blood gases may be normal at rest but abnormal during exercise. Early on, resting hypoxemia is absent, but ventilation is high with low or normal pCO_2 so the classical emphysema patient has no cyanosis (''pink puffer'').

The chronic bronchitic patient often has a plethoric complexion with a wet cough, wheeze, basal rales, and sputum production with infective exacerbations. Characteristically there is greater than 100 ml of sputum production per day for over 3 months for at least 2 consecutive years. When first visiting a physician, the chronic bronchitic patient usually has severe airways obstruction with a maximum voluntary ventilation of 50% or less, and age-, height-, and sex-adjusted forced expiratory volume in 1 second (FEV_1) less than 65% of predicted normal, or an FEV_1/forced vital capacity (FVC) ratio less than 70% of predicted (19). The diffusion capacity is not impaired. There is an increase in PaO_2 and $PaCO_2$ with exercise, the former due to improvement in ventilation perfusion ratios. There is a tendency to develop polycythemia, edema, and finally cor pulmonale (''blue bloater''). The majority of COPD patients have elements of both bronchitis and emphysema, and about 10% of COPD patients have a component of reversible bronchospasm.

Asthma is characterized by episodic widespread narrowing of airways and paroxysms of nocturnal expiratory dyspnea. Half the cases begin before the patient is 10 years of age, but asthma may begin at any age. The male:female incidence is 2:1, but there is equal male:female ratio after 30 years of age. Allergic asthma usually occurs in children with a family history of hay fever, urticaria, eczema, positive skin test to many antigens, elevated immunoglobulin (Ig)E in blood, and eosinophils in sputum. Infective asthma occurs in adult life. In this condition there is generally continuous bronchial constriction, worsening with respiratory infections, fatigue, and dehydration. The sputum contains few eosinophils. Skin tests are negative. There is hypertrophy of bronchial muscle, mucosal edema, and infiltration with mononuclear cells and eosinophils, and changes in basement membrane and chronic bronchitis may result. Obstruction must be extremely severe before hypercapnia develops. Pulmonary function studies indicate obstruction and occasionally only hyperinflation (12,19).

The pulmonary function studies of COPD patients demonstrate air trapping, low maximum mid-expiratory flow rates and increased mid-expiratory times, normal or increased lung compliance, and increased flow work. Residual volume and total lung capacity are generally increased. Exertional dyspnea tends to occur when the FEV_1 is less than 1,500 ml. FEV_1 decreases by 45 to 75 ml per year for COPD patients (35,36), a rate up to three times normal. Arterial oxygen tensions may be posturally related, significantly decreased with the patient supine (37), and desaturation may be episodically severe during sleep (38). The patient is assessed during sleep for blood gas alterations when daytime hypercapnia is present or there are symptoms suggestive of nocturnal hypercapnia.

Thirty percent of COPD patients with FEV_1 less than 750 ml die within 1 year and 50% within 3 years (35). However, pulmonary function impairment does not predict the overall extent of the patient's functional impairment. Clinical exercise testing, on the other hand, measures the functional reserve of all mechanisms taking part in oxygen and carbon dioxide transport and yields information regarding the capacity to perform exercise, the factors that limit exercise, the reasons for exercise-related symptoms, and the diagnosis (39). It permits the clinician to determine whether the primary disability is pulmonary, cardiac, or related to exercise-induced bronchospasm (40). The latter two diagnoses, and even the presence of purely restrictive pulmonary syndromes are commonly mistaken for COPD and, therefore, may be mismanaged. Clinical exercise testing also can be useful for documenting patient progress when performed both before and after the rehabilitation program.

Clinical exercise testing, whether by using a treadmill, stationary bicycle, or upper extremity ergometer, includes monitoring of the following: vital signs, electrocardiography, oxygen consumption, carbon dioxide production, the respiratory quotient, the ventilatory equivalent, minute ventilation, and metabolic rate. The respiratory quotient is the ratio of carbon dioxide produced divided by the oxygen consumed. The ventilatory equivalent is equal to the volume of air breathed for 1 L of oxygen consumed. A metabolic equivalent (MET) is the resting metabolic rate per kilogram of body weight (i.e., 1 MET = 3.5 ml 0_2/kg/min). Other useful measures for noninvasively assessing cardiac function include the oxygen pulse, a measure of the oxygen consumed per heart beat (40). A clinical exercise test should advance until oxygen consumption fails to increase or maximum allowable heart rate for age is reached (usually 220 − age in years), or when electrocardiographic change, chest pain, severe dyspnea, or intolerable fatigue occurs. A minute ventilation 37.5 times the patient's FEV_1 is the goal. Arterial blood gas analyses and oximetry are performed to determine the need for supplemental oxygen therapy to maintain an SaO_2 greater than 90% during reconditioning exercise or greater than 60 mm Hg long-term (41). When energy cost studies are not available, maximum exercise tolerance may be estimated from pulmonary function data (42). A 3-, 6-, or 12-minute walk test also can provide useful information. The patient is instructed to gradually increase walking speed and duration on subsequent walking tests. The test is simple and may be performed daily in the hospital or at home (43).

Any motivated COPD patient who has respiratory symptoms that limit ADL and who has adequate medical, neuromusculoskeletal, financial, and psychosocial status to permit active participation is a candidate for rehabilitation. Active patients who are still able to walk several blocks but who have noted yearly decreases in exercise tolerance or who have recently begun to require ongoing medical attention for pulmonary symptoms or complications are ideal candidates.

ORGANIZATION OF A COMPREHENSIVE REHABILITATION PROGRAM

The pulmonary rehabilitation multidisciplinary team can consist of a physiatrist and pulmonologist, respiratory, physical, and occupational therapists, an exercise physiologist, a psychiatrist or psychologist, a social worker, vocational counselor, and dietician. However, in the present fiscal environment, an effective small program may have only one specifically trained therapist or nurse under physician supervision. Well-designed small programs appear to be as effective as programs involving greater resources for the majority of patients (44,45), especially ambulatory patients with only mild to moderate disease. Other potential team members can be consulted on an individual basis for patients with difficult-to-address nutritional, psychological, emotional, physical, or equipment training problems. Because there is no evidence that inpatient programs are more effective than outpatient programs (44), the former should be reserved for severely debilitated patients, for ventilator weaning, or for optimizing the ventilatory aid regimen while initiating other aspects of comprehensive rehabilitation. Table 55-2 is a sample therapeutic prescription for an ambulatory moderately affected COPD patient.

THERAPEUTIC INTERVENTIONS

Medications

The patient's medical regimen is optimized before undertaking the program. Pharmacologic management of reversible bronchospasm may include the use of methylxanthines (46), adrenergics (preferably $beta_2$ agonists), and anticholinergics. Most of these medications can be delivered orally or as aerosolized solutions. Orally administered beta agonists are used when aerosolized medications are ineffective or when metered dose inhalers cannot be efficiently used. Theophylline can act as a bronchodilator, and it appears to allevi-

TABLE 55-2. *A sample therapeutic prescription for a patient with chronic obstructive pulmonary disease*

Diagnosis
- Chronic obstructive pulmonary disease

Prognosis
- Favorable, patient on stable self-medication program

Goals
- Improve endurance and efficiency
- Optimize oxygen needs and control of secretions
- Increase independence in ambulation and self-care activities
- Reduce anxiety and improve self-esteem through enhanced body awareness

Precautions
- Supplemental oxygen needed during exercise
- Discontinue and notify physician if patient becomes severely dyspneic with exercise or develops ventricular premature beats of more than 6 per min
- Patient to self-monitor heart rate and maintain less than 120 beats/min

Respiratory therapy
- Conduct ear oximetry at rest and during exercise to determine portable oxygen flow rate needed to maintain oxygen saturation of at least 90% at all times
- Instruct patient in diaphragmatic and pursed-lip breathing
- Instruct patient and family in postural drainage techniques
- Instruct patient and family on home portable oxygen use
- Instruct in use of metered-dose inhaler before exercise

Physical therapy
- Assess baseline endurance using 12-minute walk test
- Begin incremental exercise program to improve endurance through ambulation and stair climbing. Begin with 5-min sessions, followed by rest periods between sessions. When patient tolerates 20 min of total exercise per day, begin consolidating the sessions.
- Initial treatments on daily basis during weeks 1 and 2, taper to three times per week over weeks 3 and 4, and then taper to home program with self-monitoring over weeks 5 and 6
- Review proper body mechanics and coordinate with breathing patterns, using diaphragmatic and pursed-lip breathing when appropriate

Occupational therapy
- Assess upper extremity mobility, strength, and endurance
- Evaluate basic and advanced self-care activities and provide adaptive aids to improve independence with dressing, hygiene, bathing, cooking, and other chores
- Train the patient in energy conservation and work simplification techniques
- Evaluate home environment and make recommendations for workspace modifications and equipment to improve safety, efficiency, and independence
- Provide relaxation exercise training with visual imagery techniques

ate diaphragm fatigue (47), increases cardiac output, inhibits mast cell degranulation, and enhances mucociliary clearance for COPD patients. Greater than 20% improvement in FEV_1 is significant with bronchodilator use, but many physicians use bronchodilators with no apparent effect on FEV_1. Mast cell membrane stabilizing medications can prevent release of bronchoconstrictor substances for some patients.

Medications that can impair respiratory function are considered, e.g., nonselective beta-blocker antihypertensive agents. Systemic glucocorticoid use is discontinued in favor of the use of synthetic steroid inhalers if at all possible. The synthetic beclomethasone diproprionate has little or no systemic steroid effects in therapeutic dosages. Other medications such as expectorants, mucolytics, and antibiotics are used along with humidification, ample fluid intake, and facilitated airway secretion elimination as warranted. Low flow nasal supplemental oxygen can be provided to decrease dyspnea, enhance performance, and exert a cardioprotective effect on patients with coronary artery disease. Early medical attention is important during intercurrent respiratory tract infections (48).

Counseling and General Medical Care

Dyspnea often causes fear and panic. This may worsen tachypnea while increasing dead space ventilation, the work of breathing, hyperinflation, and air trapping, and may cause further shortness of breath. Relaxation exercises such as Jacobson exercises and biofeedback may be used to decrease tension and anxiety (49,50). Diaphragmatic and pursed-lip breathing also aid in relaxation.

Life quality is perceived to be impaired by COPD patients. Depression has been reported in 50% of patients, and there is often severe reduction in social interaction (51). Integrating psychosocial support with multimodal pulmonary rehabilitation optimizes intervention (52). Loss of employment and physical independence also may need to be addressed.

Numerous strategies, including the use of nicotine-impregnated gum and skin patches, scare tactics, ''rapid smoking,'' acupuncture, and programmed reduction, have been used to initiate and sustain smoking cessation (53). It is unclear which strategies are most effective. Although health professionals rank ''not smoking'' as the most important action to protect one's health, ''not smoking'' is ranked only 10th by the general public (53). Thus, physicians must play key political and educational roles for the general public as well as make continued abstinence from smoking a necessary component of any pulmonary rehabilitation program.

COPD patients tend to overuse medications during periods of respiratory distress and underuse them otherwise. They are counseled on adhering to their medication regimens (54) and on avoiding atmospheric or vocational pollutants and other aggravating factors such as pollen, aerosols, excessive humidity, stress, and respiratory tract pathogens. Yearly flu vaccinations are recommended, and pneumococcal vaccines are used one time or every 6 years for high-risk cases. High-altitude travel may require additional supplemental oxygen administration for those already requiring supplemental oxygen; otherwise, oxygen therapy generally need not be used only for short flights (55). Good hydration should be maintained with ample fluid intake.

Nutrition

Significant weight loss occurs in 19% to 71% of COPD patients (33). In one study, 30 of 50 consecutive COPD patients presenting with acute respiratory failure had evidence of significant undernutrition using a multiparameter nutritional index, and impaired nutritional status was more prevalent in those patients requiring mechanical ventilation (74% versus 43%) (56). Undernutrition complicating COPD has been associated with increased morbidity and mortality. It has been associated with an increased susceptibility to infection due in part to impaired cell-mediated immunity, reduced secretory IgA, depressed pulmonary alveolar macrophage function, and increased colonization and adherence of bacteria in the upper and lower airways. Patients with significant nutritional impairment are more frequently colonized by *Pseudomonas* species (57,58). In addition, malnutrition also can adversely affect lung repair, surfactant synthesis, control of ventilation and response to hypoxia, respiratory muscle function and lung mechanics (59), and water homeostasis. It can lead to respiratory muscle atrophy and decreased exercise capacity, cor pulmonale, increased rate of hospitalization for pulmonary-related problems, hypercapnic respiratory failure, and difficulty in weaning from mechanical ventilation (56,60,61). Likewise, inappropriate nutrition such as increasing carbohydrate intake can exacerbate hypercapnia.

Short-term refeeding of malnourished patients can lead to improved respiratory muscle endurance and to increases in respiratory muscle strength in the absence of demonstrable changes in skeletal muscle function (62). Bloating and abdominal distention is common and in the presence of an already low diaphragm may increase dyspnea (63). Patients are advised to take smaller mouthfuls of food, eat more slowly, and take smaller and more frequent meals. SaO_2 can be evaluated while eating. If desaturation occurs, supplemental oxygen is used or increased.

Inhalers

Over 60% of COPD patients use their metered-dose inhalers incorrectly (64). Training in the proper use of inhalers, ''spacers,'' nebulizers, and ventilatory equipment is critical; otherwise, medications are often largely deposited uselessly on the tongue.

Breathing Retraining

Shallow rapid breathing is commonly seen in anxious and often dyspneic patients. This increases dead space ventilation and airflow through narrowed airways, thus increasing the flow work of breathing. Patients with chronic airflow obstruction also have an altered pattern of ventilatory muscle recruitment in which the most effective ventilatory pressure is generated by the rib cage inspiratory muscles rather than by the diaphragm, with significant contribution by expiratory muscles (65). Diaphragmatic breathing and pursed lip exhalation can help to reverse these tendencies. These techniques are usually initiated in the supine or 15% to 25% head down position. Deep, essentially diaphragmatic breathing is guided by having the patient place one hand over the abdomen and the other on the thorax just below the clavicle. He or she should breathe deeply through the nose while distending the abdomen forward as appreciated by movement of the hand on the abdomen. Movement of the rib cage and, thus, the hand on the thorax should be kept to a minimum. Small weights can be placed on the abdomen to provide some resistance training and enhance the patient's focus. During exhalation the abdominal muscles and the hand on the abdomen should compress the abdominal contents and exhalation should be via pursed lips (66). Classically, a lighted candle is put several feet in front of the patient and the patient flickers the flame while exhaling. This equalizes pleural and bronchial pressures, thus preventing collapse of smaller bronchi and decreasing air trapping. The combination of diaphragmatic and pursed lip breathing decreases the respiratory rate and coordinates the breathing pattern, and can improve blood gases (67). It should be used often, particularly during routine ADL. When used correctly, it should help maintain the cadence of breathing during exercise. It also may improve exercise performance by relaxing accessory muscles and improving breathing efficiency.

Air shifting techniques may be useful to decrease microatelectasis. Air shifting involves taking a deep inspiration that is held with the glottis closed for 5 seconds during which time the air shifts to lesser ventilated areas of the lung. The subsequent expiration is via pursed lips. This technique may be most beneficial when performed several times per hour.

Airway Secretion Elimination

Airway secretion clearance is crucial. The patient's cough may be weak, and frequent bouts of coughing are fatiguing. The high expulsive pressures generated during coughing attempts can exacerbate air trapping and secretion retention. ''Huffing,'' or frequent short expulsive bursts following a deep breath, is often an effective and more comfortable alternative to coughing. Chest percussion and postural drainage can be useful for patients with chronic bronchitis or others with greater than 30 ml of sputum production per day (68), although caution must be taken to increase oxygen delivery as necessary during treatment.

Autogenic drainage involves breathing with low tidal volumes between the functional residual capacity and residual volume to mobilize secretions in small airways. This is followed by taking increasingly larger tidal volumes and forced expirations to transport mucus to the mouth (69).

Application of positive expiratory pressure (PEP) breathing is based on the theory that mucus in small airways is more effectively mobilized by coughing or forced expirations if alveolar pressure and volume behind mucous plugs are increased. PEP is applied by breathing through a face mask or mouth piece with an inspiratory tube containing a one-way valve, and an expiratory tube containing a variable expiratory resistance. Expiratory pressures of 10 to 20 cm H_2O are maintained throughout expiration. PEP increases functional residual capacity, reducing resistance to airflow in collateral and small airways (70,71). The results of studies on the effect of PEP breathing have been inconclusive (72) for both CF (73–77) and COPD (77–79).

Flutter breathing is a combination of PEP and oscillation applied at the mouth. The patient expires through a small pipe. A small stainless-steel ball rests on the expiratory end of the pipe; it is pushed upward during expiration, producing PEP, and falls downward again, interrupting flow. The mucus-mobilizing effect is thought to be due to widening of the airways because of the increased expiratory pressure and the airflow oscillations due to the oscillating ball (80). For this too, however, the results of clinical trials have been conflicting (81). Pryor and colleagues (82), in fact, found that use of the active cycle of breathing technique resulted in a significantly greater amount of expectorated mucus than flutter breathing in a study of CF patients. Use of the Flutter mucus clearance device (Scandipharm, Inc., Birmingham, AL) is demanding and it cannot be easily used by patients with severe disease. Controlled studies need to be done before widely recommending this technique.

With currently available technology, mechanical vibration or oscillation can be mechanically applied to the thorax or directly to the airway to facilitate airway secretion elimination. Vibration is possible at frequencies up to 170 Hz applied under a soft plastic shell to the thorax and abdomen (Hayek Oscillator, Breasy Medical Equipment Inc., Stamford, CT). Another device delivers rapid burst airflows at up to 25 Hz under a vest covering the chest and upper abdomen (THAIRapy System, American Biosystems, Inc., St. Paul, MN). The effects of mechanical chest percussion and vibration appear to be frequency dependent (83–85). In most animal studies, frequencies between 10 to 15 Hz appear to best facilitate mucus transport (83,85,86), especially the transport of a thicker mucous layer (87). Warwick and Hansen (88) found long-term increases in forced vital capacity and forced expiratory flows for CF patients treated with high-frequency chest wall compression as compared with receiving chest percussion alone. Others have reported improvement in pulmonary function (89) and in gas exchange during high-frequency oscillation (89–92); Sibuya et al. (92) found that chest wall vibration decreased dyspnea. Most studies on COPD and CF patients, however, have failed to demonstrate objective clinical benefits from percussion or vibration on mucus transport (93–96). Side effects of percussion and vibration can include increasing obstruction to airflow for some patients with COPD (97,98). In an animal model, the application of vibration and percussion also was associated with the development of atelectasis (99).

The Percussionator (Percussionaire Corp., Sandpoint, ID) can deliver aerosolized medications while providing high-flow percussive mini-bursts of air directly to the airways at rates of 2.5 to 5 Hz. This intrapulmonary percussive ventilation also has been reported to be more effective than chest percussion and postural drainage in the treatment of postoperative atelectasis and secretion mobilization in COPD patients (100,101). Although there have been no controlled studies, in one study, the majority of patients using the technique have felt that it was helpful (102).

Patterson and coworkers (103) found in a 10-year study of CF patients that good patient compliance with methods to assist in mobilizing airway secretions was associated with a slower rate of loss of pulmonary function. Patient compliance with mucus-mobilizing interventions is generally poor, however (104–106). There is greater patient compliance for the use of simpler methods that can be used independently. Some expensive mechanical oscillators are difficult to use independently, and little has been documented concerning long-term safety and efficacy. Thus, they should only be used when there is convincing evidence of clinical benefit. Although promising, it is reasonable to conclude that there is not enough evidence to justify the routine use of expensive percussion, vibration, or oscillation techniques.

Mechanical insufflation–exsufflation (MI-E) involves the use of a blower motor to provide about 10 L/sec of expiratory flow directly to the airways (In-Exsufflator, J.H. Emerson Co., Cambridge, MA). It can be applied via an oronasal interface, mouth piece, or directly via an endotracheal or tracheostomy tube with an inflated cuff. Its application for patients with restrictive pulmonary syndromes is discussed elsewhere in this text. Part of the benefit of MI-E for COPD patients was explained by the fact that high expiratory flows occur with lower intrathoracic pressures than autonomous coughing (107). It was suggested that COPD patients and others with severe intrinsic lung disease practice passive MI-E (108). Its effectiveness has been suggested but not documented for COPD or CF, and its use also should be compared with that of other mechanical methods that facilitate secretion elimination.

Inspiratory Resistive Exercises

Inspiratory resistive exercises, including maximum sustained ventilation, inspiratory resistive loading, and inspiratory threshold loading, can improve the endurance of respiratory muscles (109,110). Typically, patients breathe through these devices for a total of 30 minutes daily for 8 to 10 weeks. The settings of the devices are adjusted to increase difficulty as patients improve and the program advances. Levine and associates conducted an evaluation of the isocapnic hyperpnea method and determined that no more benefits could be derived from it than could be achieved using periodic intermittent positive pressure breathing treatments, a regimen that was considered equivalent to placebo (111). However, Ries et al. randomly assigned 18 patients to either a home isocapnic hyperventilation training program or a walking program and found that the former led to improvements in ventilatory muscle endurance and exercise performance and significant improvements in VO_2max, whereas walking exercise improved exercise endurance but did not improve ventilatory muscle endurance (112).

Twenty-one controlled studies of inspiratory resistive loading involving 259 COPD patients documented significant improvements in inspiratory muscle strength and endurance (113). The mean increase in strength (increase in maximum inspiratory pressure) was 19%. However, it recently became apparent that many of the subjects of inspiratory resistive training consciously or unconsciously reduced their inspiratory flow rates and lengthened their inspiratory time to reduce the severity of the imposed loads. Consequently, targeted or threshold inspiratory muscle training has been recommended over the simpler flow-resistive training to assure adequate intensity of inspiratory muscle activity during training.

With targeted training, the subject is provided feedback regarding the inspiratory flow rates through the resistor or the inspiratory pressure generated by flow through the resistor; with threshold training, the subject is unable to generate flow through the device until a predetermined pressure is achieved. Six of the nine controlled studies of the use of targeted or threshold resistor devices in COPD reported significantly greater improvements in inspiratory muscle function in the subjects than in the controls (113). In three of the six studies in which it was assessed, exercise tolerance was greater for trained subjects than for controls. In one controlled study comparing exercise reconditioning plus threshold inspiratory muscle training with exercise reconditioning alone, the former resulted in significantly greater increases in inspiratory muscle strength and endurance and in exercise tolerance (114). Exercise tolerance seemed to be improved, particularly for those with electromyographic changes indicating inspiratory muscle fatigue with exercise (115). One controlled, well-designed but small study of threshold inspiratory exercise for CF patients demonstrated significant improvements in inspiratory muscle strength, FVC, total lung capacity (TLC), and exercise tolerance in the experimental group (116). In another controlled study of patients taking corticosteroids, inspiratory muscle training appeared to prevent the weakness that would have otherwise resulted from the steroid use (117). In general, improvements in inspiratory muscle function and in exercise tolerance were greater for the targeted and threshold studies than for the flow resistor studies.

When COPD patients failed to demonstrate significantly greater improvements from inspiratory muscle training than did untrained or sham-trained subjects, it may have been because of lack of cooperation with such a tedious and uncomfortable exercise, the presence of chronic inspiratory muscle fatigue, inadequate nutritional status, or concomitant drug therapy (corticosteroids or beta-adrenergic blocking agents or agonists) which could prevent or diminish a positive response to a training regimen (113). A recent 6-month controlled study of inspiratory muscle training for asthmatics indicated not only improved inspiratory muscle strength and endurance but also improvement in asthma symptoms, hospitalization and emergency department contact rates, school or work attendance, and medication consumption (118).

Despite the generally positive results of inspiratory training programs on inspiratory muscle strength and endurance, the positive effects have not been shown to translate into fewer COPD exacerbations or in decreased risk of pulmonary complications or mortality. It is also not clear which regimen of inspiratory resistance training offers the best results or whether the benefits are long term. Thus, although controlled trials of inspiratory muscle training have thus far failed to demonstrate a major benefit in a broad range of patients, highly motivated and adequately nourished patients do appear to benefit from training. Improvements are consistently observed and readily demonstrable, and training is inexpensive and lends itself well to home-based exercise programs and the logging of daily results.

Respiratory Muscle Rest

Relatively minor changes in the pattern of breathing or respiratory muscle loading can place many patients in the critical zone for developing acute respiratory muscle fatigue and failure. Interspersing periods of exercise and muscle rest is a basic principle of rehabilitation. Hypercapnia is an indication of limited reserve before the appearance of overt fatigue and may indicate the need for periods of respiratory muscle assistance or rest before using strengthening exercise (119). Diaphragm rest can be achieved by assisted ventilation using either body ventilators or mouth or nasal IPPV.

Despite high ventilation rates in COPD, ventilatory response to both hypercapnia and hypoxia may be reduced. This is often exacerbated during sleep. The increase in pulmonary vascular resistance that occurs in the presence of pulmonary tissue hypoxia is exacerbated by acidosis, and when severe leads to right ventricular failure. The use of oxygen therapy alone may exacerbate CO_2 retention and acidosis. Several studies have suggested better prognosis for hypercapnic COPD patients since 1975, when long term home tracheostomy IPPV became more widespread (120–122).

Two groups of patients may be suited to ventilatory assistance at home. The first and smaller group includes those who require aid around the clock, usually by tracheostomy, but who are medically and psychologically stable. However, these patients tend to require frequent hospital readmission and to have a poorer prognosis than ventilator-assisted individuals with neuromuscular disease. The second group may benefit from nocturnal assistance alone.

There have been numerous reports of the success of various regimens of daytime or nocturnal negative pressure body ventilator (NPBV) use in normalizing arterial blood gases, increasing maximum inspiratory and expiratory pressures (123–127), maximal transdiaphragmatic pressure, quality of life, 12-minute walking distance (125), respiratory muscle endurance, and decreasing dyspnea (124). NPBVs (128) have even been used as alternatives to intubation and tracheostomy for patients with acute respiratory failure. Rochester and Martin suggested that daily NPBV use should be considered for patients with a maximal inspiratory force of less than 50 cm H_2O, an FEV_1 of less than 25% of predicted, a $PaCO_2$ greater than 45 mm Hg, a respiratory rate greater than 30 breaths/min, or chest/abdomen dyssynchrony (129). Although several controlled studies have disaffirmed these positive results, these studies were marred by difficulties with subject compliance, short periods of NPBV use (under 4 to 5 hours a day), reliance on the patient's historical statements regarding hours of NPBV use, and use on few patients with significant hypercapnia (130). Other studies have suggested that the tendency of the upper airway to collapse accompanied by periods of oxyhemoglobin desaturation during sleep with NPBV use may negate potentially beneficial effects of respiratory muscle rest (131,132).

More recently, a controlled study of the use of CPAP (133) was reported to result in similar benefits to those reported with NPBVs. It therefore seemed reasonable to evaluate the use of noninvasive IPPV and bilevel positive airway pressure as a means to rest respiratory muscles, maintain airway patency, and support alveolar ventilation. Belman reported greater diaphragm relaxation by nasal IPPV than by use of NPBVs (134). Marino demonstrated reversal of nocturnal ventilatory insufficiency for COPD patients using nasal IPPV (135), and others have used IPPV via oronasal interfaces as an alternative to intubation and tracheostomy for COPD patients in acute exacerbation (136). Noninvasive IPPV not only assists ventilation but acts as a pneumatic splint to prevent airway collapse. These techniques may play larger roles as alternative ventilatory assistance techniques for COPD patients in the future.

Supplemental Oxygen Therapy

Supplemental oxygen therapy is indicated for patients with pO_2 continuously less than 55 to 60 mm Hg (41). Home oxygen therapy can decrease pulmonary hypertension, polycythemia, and perception of effort during exercise, and it can prolong life (137,138). In addition, cognitive function can be improved, and hospital needs reduced.

An international consensus on the current status and indications for long-term oxygen therapy recently suggested that the prescription be based on the following elements (139):

1. An appropriately documented diagnosis
2. Concurrent optimal use of other rehabilitative approaches such as pharmacotherapy, smoking abstinence, and exercise training
3. Properly documented chronic hypoxemia

Oxygen therapy should be given with caution to hypercapnic patients whether or not they are using noninvasive IPPV (140).

There is also a possible need for supplemental oxygen during exercise. Many patients exhibit exercise hypoxemia. Often the decrease in SaO_2 occurs within the first minute, after which SaO_2 stabilizes; but occasionally there is a progressive decline in SaO_2 with exercise. In a study of 38 subjects in whom the mean resting SaO_2 was 93 $\pm$ 3%, a decrease in SaO_2 of 4.7 $\pm$ 3.6% (range 1% to 18%) was observed during submaximal exercise (141). Decreases in SaO_2 are noted at physical activity levels comparable with those necessary to perform ADL.

In a crossover study of 12 subjects with severe COPD (142), four patients more than doubled their duration of exercise while receiving 40% oxygen but in only two of these was desaturation observed in the absence of oxygen. Bradley et al. (143) reported that in subjects with mild hypoxemia and exercise desaturation, supplemental oxygen by nasal prongs did not influence maximum work rate but did influence endurance. Davidson noted that oxygen increased mean walking endurance time by 59% and 6-minute walking distance by 17%. Moreover, submaximal cycle time at a constant workload was increased by 51% at a flow rate of 2 L/min and by 88% at 4 L/min, suggesting a dose-response curve (144). The exercise response to oxygen could not be predicted from the degree of desaturation, resting pulmonary function tests, echocardiographic measurements of right ventricular systolic pressure, or other clinical parameters (142). Marcus et al. also reported significantly greater exercise tolerance in CF patients receiving oxygen (145).

The most widely accepted guideline for prescribing oxygen use during exercise is that of exercise-induced SaO_2 below 90%. However, it seems reasonable to recommend that measurements of dyspnea and exercise tolerance be undertaken with and without supplemental oxygen to determine which individuals are less short of breath or walk farther (have greater exercise tolerance) when given supplemental oxygen. Certainly, exercise-induced decreases in SaO_2 below 90% when combined with increased exercise tolerance with oxygen therapy warrants the prescription of oxygen therapy during exercise.

Inspiratory phase or pulsed oxygen therapy, especially when delivered transtracheally, avoids waste and decreases discomfort and drying of mucous membranes. Oxygen flow delivery is 0.25 to 0.4 L/min compared with 2 to 4 L/min when delivered via nasal cannulas or face masks (146,147). Oxygen therapy should be used in combination with mechanical ventilation for patients with concomitant carbon dioxide retention.

Reconditioning Exercise

Because of decreased efficiency of gas exchange, there is an abnormally high ventilatory requirement and a rapid increase in breathing frequency by comparison with tidal volume during exercise. The COPD patient's maximal exercise ventilation (VEmax) is close to or exceeds maximum voluntary ventilation. Cardiac output increases normally with exercise, but exercise ceases at relatively low heart rates because of the ventilatory limitation associated with dyspnea. Hypoxia (148) and, in severely limited patients, hypercapnia may occur with exercise. Thus, most patients cannot attain the 60% to 70% of predicted maximum heart rate nor the minute oxygen consumption needed for cardiac or aerobic exercise training. Maximum oxygen consumption at anaerobic thresholds, reliable guides to aerobic capacity in normal subjects, is thus of limited usefulness in these dyspneic patients (149). Maximum symptom-limited oxygen consumption does, however, correlate with the ability to perform ADL and this can be significantly increased with exercise training (150).

Although exercise may be limited by pain, fatigue, dyspnea, or lightheadedness in these deconditioned individuals, exercise intensity can be guided by parameters of clinical exercise testing, e.g., heart rate at ventilation levels of 37.5 times the FEV_1. Walking, stair climbing, calisthenics, bicycling, and pool activities may be effective. Upper extremity reconditioning is also part of any comprehensive program. The patient is made responsible for a progressive program. We recommend the purchase of a stationary bicycle for the patient's home and its daily use. A daily 12-minute walk is recommended, as are daily 15 minute sessions of inspiratory muscle training. A daily log of time and distance walked and bicycled and of the inspiratory resistance tolerated during 15-minute inspiratory training sessions provides feedback to both the patient and physician. In general, the pulse should increase at least 20% to 30% and return to baseline 5 to 10 minutes after exercise. Increased endurance for exercise can occur independently of changes in ventilatory muscle endurance. The program should consist of weekly reevaluations for 10 to 12 weeks, during which time the patient logs are reviewed and exercise parameters modified; educational and peer group sessions reinforce the activities. Such a program is inexpensive and minimally intrusive and optimizes the chances for continued independent adherence to the protocol after the 10- to 12-week program.

Upper Extremity Exercise

Many arm and shoulder muscles are also accessory muscles of respiration and, as such, are very active for patients with COPD. The overlap in function explains why COPD patients are particularly short of breath when performing upper extremity ADL. However, because only muscles that are trained respond to the training, no carry-over of benefit to upper extremity function has been demonstrated from lower extremity exercise. Belman and Kendregan demonstrated a significant increase in arm cycle endurance for an arm-trained group and leg cycle endurance for a leg-trained group, without cross-over effect (151). Since then, several other studies have demonstrated benefits in gas exchange, strength, endurance, and performance in ADL when arm cranking is added to leg exercise as part of comprehensive programs of rehabilitation (152–155). Training of the upper extremities in COPD patients reduces the increased metabolic demand and ventilation associated with arm elevation and reduces dyspnea (154). Although upper extremity training increases endurance for arm exercise, no apparent effects have been demonstrated on ADL (156). However, further studies on upper extremity exercise training are required before firm conclusions can be drawn concerning ADL performance.

Unsupported upper extremity activities range from typing, lifting, reaching, and carrying to athletic activities and personal daily care (eating, grooming, cleaning). Unsupported arm exercise shifts work to the diaphragm, leading to earlier fatigue (152). In a randomized controlled trial comparing supported arm exercise with unsupported arm exercise in a general rehabilitation program for COPD patients, the group performing the unsupported upper extremity exercise demonstrated significantly greater improvements and decreases in oxygen consumption during upper extremity exercise than the supported upper extremity exercise group (153). Five other studies have recently substantiated the greater benefits to be derived from unsupported rather than supported upper extremity exercise (152).

THE RESULTS OF PULMONARY REHABILITATION

In a recent review of 48 pulmonary rehabilitation studies that included exercise reconditioning, exercise tolerance improved significantly in all 48 studies, including 14 controlled studies (44). It improved equally significantly (proportionally) in patients with mild or advanced (hypercapnic) disease (157). Consistent improvements included decreases in the ventilatory equivalent or the ventilation/oxygen consumption ratio, increases in work efficiency (external work per unit of oxygen consumed), and, thus, in exercise tolerance, ambulation capacity, general well-being, and dyspnea tolerance. The patients developed better performance strategies and greater confidence in performing the tests. In many programs decreases in blood lactate levels were also observed in combination with higher maximum oxygen consumption (VO_2max), implying a physiologic training effect or, at least, improved motivation and effort. Maximum tolerated intensity exercise regimens yielded better results than low-intensity exercise for proportionally longer periods (158,159). In general, peak performance appeared to be reached in 26 to 51 weeks (158–161). The use of specific physiologic parameters to guide the exercise regimens did not result in better outcomes. Quality of life measures, hospitalization rates, and physical functioning were likewise reported to be significantly improved in the majority of both the controlled and the repetitive measure studies (44). Outcomes were equivalent for inpatient and outpatient programs, although many of the outpatient programs were predominantly home based. Pulmonary function parameters, such as FEV_1, did not significantly improve in 31 of 35 studies (44).

Thus, all studies indicated that pulmonary rehabilitation including exercise training results in significant increases in ambulation capacity and exercise endurance for COPD patients as well as for many patients with other intrinsic lung pathology (162). The often reported decreased resting oxygen consumption and carbon dioxide production may, at least in part, account for the significant decrease in perception of dyspnea, the general increase in functional performance, and the often found improved sense of well-being.

One study of 120 advanced hypercapnic COPD patients, 117 of whom with FEV_1 less than 1 liter demonstrated significant increases in PaO_2, vital capacity (VC), FEV_1, maximum inspiratory pressures, and ambulation tolerance with pulmonary rehabilitation including exercise reconditioning. Maximum expiratory pressures did not change significantly. The higher the initial $PaCO_2$, the more $PaCO_2$ decreased and PaO_2 increased during the rehabilitation program. The patients' improvement in ADL performance correlated with increased walking distance. Thus, hypercapnia is not a contraindication to intensive rehabilitation, and the use of rigorous reconditioning exercise does not precipitate respiratory muscle fatigue in this population (157). Indeed, because improvements in both physiologic and psychologic parameters are not directly related to lung function, the benefits of rehabilitation can extend to all patients with COPD, regardless of the severity of pre-existing pulmonary disease (150).

After the acute rehabilitation period, continued surveillance and attention to abstinence from smoking, bronchial hygiene, breathing retraining, physical reconditioning, oxygen therapy, and airway secretion mobilization have been shown to reduce hospital admissions, length of hospital stays, and cost (163). The benefits of pulmonary rehabilitation on exercise performance and quality of life persist for up to 4 years after rehabilitation and peak at 12 to 18 months (158,164–167).

REHABILITATION OF PATIENTS WITH RESTRICTIVE PULMONARY IMPAIRMENT AND SLEEP-DISORDERED BREATHING

Pathophysiology

Patients with severe back deformity and conditions associated with bulbar or generalized muscle dysfunction often have severe restrictive pulmonary syndromes. Respiratory complications are the most common causes of death when these conditions are advanced.

The four pathophysiologic presentations of restrictive pulmonary impairment are (a) primary parenchymal disease, (b) surgical removal of lung tissue, (c) diseases of pleura and chest wall, (d) and reduced generation of respiratory muscle force (168). Of these, ventilatory dysfunction characterizes the last three, and only the first represents a combination of oxygenation impairment and ventilatory dysfunction.

Restrictive pulmonary syndromes are characterized by low VC, reduced TLC, tachypnea, shallow breathing, reduced pulmonary compliance, and increased elastic work of breathing. The VC is directly related to respiratory muscle strength and pulmonary compliance (169). The VC normally plateaus at 19 years of age, then decreases by about 1% per year throughout life (170). Although restriction in pulmonary function is generally defined by a reduction in all lung volumes, spinal cord injured patients often have increased residual volume at the expense of decreased expiratory reserve volume. Lung volumes and ventilatory capacity also can be very different when measured with the patient in sitting, recumbent, or side-lying positions, particularly for patients with kyphoscoliosis, non-Duchenne myopathies (171), postpoliomyelitis, or spinal cord injury. For example, in spinal cord–injured individuals, the strength of the diaphragm relative to the weak abdominal wall tends to allow abdominal contents to sag, thus decreasing diaphragm excursion and VC in the sitting position.

Mechanical factors involving the chest wall and lungs include thoracic deformities, obesity, hypopharyngeal collapse during sleep with obstructive apneas (171), and any complicating conditions that decrease lung or chest wall expansion, including intercurrent pulmonary infiltrations or pleural disease. Severe carbon dioxide retention itself has been demonstrated to independently decrease muscle strength (61). Pulmonary deterioration is exacerbated by acute respiratory tract infections, which can lead to repeated pneumonias and lung scarring. Patients with restrictive pulmonary syndromes invariably worsen with aging or disease progression. For instance, for individuals with Duchenne muscular dystrophy, the VC plateaus between 1,100 and 2,800 ml (mean 1,800 ml) (172) between 10 and 15 years of age. With or without severe concomitant chest wall deformity, VC is then lost at a rate of 200 to 250 ml per year, with the rate of loss tapering off below 400 ml (170,173). Patients with amyotrophic lateral sclerosis may lose VC at a rate of 1,000 ml or more per year, whereas patients with postpoliomyelitis can lose about 1.8% of VC per year (174).

The maximum insufflation capacity (MIC) is a measure of the maximum volume of air that can be held with a closed glottis and then expelled. The MIC is obtained by some combination of the air stacking of mechanically delivered insufflations (retaining consecutive insufflations with a closed glottis) and glossopharyngeal breathing (GPB). It is a function of pulmonary compliance and strength of oropharyngeal and laryngeal muscles. With the loss of VC comes the inability to take deep breaths. Without access to regular deep mechanically assisted insufflations, the MIC diminishes, pulmonary compliance decreases, and patients develop chronic microatelectasis (175). Increased elastic work of breathing becomes necessary to overcome the decreased elasticity of the lungs and, eventually, the chest wall. In the long term, microatelectasis results in permanent loss of lung and chest wall elasticity and rib cage mobility (176–178). Thus, decreased pulmonary compliance results initially from microatelectasis and ultimately from increased stiffness of the chest wall and lung tissues themselves (179).

The first significant blood gas abnormality with restrictive disease is hypercapnia (180) and hypoxia during rapid eye movement (REM) sleep. The ventilatory responses to hypoxia and hypercapnia are diminished during sleep (181), and with the increased work of breathing, central respiratory control mechanisms accommodate worsening blood gases. Hypercapnia and hypoxia gradually extend throughout most of the night before they occur with the patient awake (182,183). Unless treated, this results in cor pulmonale and cardiac arrhythmias. Wake hypercapnia occurs when the VC decreases below 40% (184) to 55% (169) of predicted normal. When wake carbon dioxide levels exceed 50 mm Hg, nocturnal oxyhemoglobin desaturations can be severe (185). Increasing $PaCO_2$ and decreasing PaO_2 levels intersect at about 60 mm Hg, a point at which it is a tempting mistake to provide supplemental oxygen.

Medications including calcium channel blockers, aminoglycosides, corticosteroids, benzodiazepines and other sedatives can further reduce the ventilatory response to hypercapnia and hypoxia and exacerbate chronic alveolar hypoventilation. Malnutrition, acidosis, electrolyte disturbances, cachexia, infection, fatigue, supplemental oxygen administration, and muscle disuse or overuse also can worsen ventilatory insufficiency or increase hypercapnia.

Sleep-disordered breathing refers to the occurrence of apneas and hypopneas, which may be centrally derived or result from upper airway obstruction. Obstruction is most commonly due to hypopharyngeal collapse from a transluminal pressure gradient across the airway and failure of airway dilator muscles that are normally reflexly activated at the onset of inspiration. Overt obstructive sleep apnea syndrome (OSAS) occurs in at least 3% of the general population, and its incidence may be greater for patients with generalized neuromuscular disorders due to weakened pharyngeal musculature and a higher incidence of complicating obesity. Cardiovascular and neuropsychiatric sequelae of OSAS are common. Obstructive apneas also occur in patients using electrophrenic pacing or NPBVs (131,132).

Inspiratory muscle dysfunction and ventilatory insufficiency progresses insidiously. Patients with restrictive pulmonary syndromes also often have greater weakness of expiratory than of inspiratory muscles (169,186). These patients have difficulty clearing secretions, particularly during respiratory infections. Weak oropharyngeal musculature increases this difficulty. Chronic mucous plugging of the airway can cause ventilation–perfusion imbalance, atelectasis, pulmonary infiltrates, further loss of lung compliance, cor pulmonale, and eventually cardiopulmonary arrest. The cough reflex is suppressed during sleep, when mucous plugs may be more likely to cause sudden hypoxia. Patients with cardiomyopathies may be especially susceptible to hypoxia-triggered arrhythmia and cardiac decompensation.

PATIENT EVALUATION

Patients able to walk chiefly complain of exertional dyspnea, but headaches, fatigue, sleep disturbances, hypersomnolence, and difficulty with concentration are also common complaints (171). For wheelchair users, symptoms may be minimal except during intercurrent respiratory infections that cause profuse airway secretion. Dyspnea, anxiety, and sleep impairment usually occur only for patients with very rapidly evolving conditions such as amyotrophic lateral sclerosis during respiratory tract infections, or occasionally with very advanced disease. Other symptoms may include difficulty in controlling airway secretions and drooling because of chronic fatigue, nausea and retching, headache, impairment of intellectual function, nightmares, depression, and weight loss (171). There also may be a history of repeated hospitalizations for respiratory difficulties.

The patient is observed for increased rate, decreased depth, or irregularity of breathing. Purely diaphragmatic breathing or asymmetric movement of the abdomen or thorax are often present. Inability to count to more than 15 with one breath, reduced capacity for blowing and coughing, nasal alae flaring, use of auxiliary respiratory musculature, peribuccale or generalized cyanosis with or without polycythemia, flushing or pallor, hypertension, drooling and difficulty controlling airway secretions, dysphagia, regurgitation of fluids through the nose, nasality of speech, cor pulmonale, confusion, and fluid retention all may be signs of ventilatory insufficiency.

Maximum inspiratory and expiratory pressures generated at the mouth correlate best with inspiratory and expiratory muscle strength. The maximum voluntary ventilation measures respiratory muscle endurance. The VC gives an indication of both of these parameters and is simple, easy to measure, objective, and very reproducible. Because hypoventilation is often worse during sleep and patients prefer to sleep recumbent, the supine VC is often an earlier indication of ventilatory dysfunction. The VC is evaluated with patients wearing thoracolumbar orthotics when applicable. Spirometry is also useful for monitoring progress with GPB and air stacking. A lip seal can be used to splint weak oral muscles to increase air stacking (Fig. 55-1). With the glottis closed for a few seconds, the stacked air shifts to underventilated areas of the lungs (187). An MIC of at least 500 ml is necessary to achieve adequate peak cough flows (PCFs) during attempts at manually assisted coughing (188) to prevent mucous plugging, atelectasis, and pneumonia during respiratory tract infections. The lower the MIC, the greater the need for mechanically assisted coughing.

Because impaired clearance of airway secretions is the major cause of acute respiratory failure for these individuals, PCFs are measured using a peak flow meter (Access Peak Flow Meter, Healthscan Products Inc., Cedar Grove, NJ). PCFs of 160 L/min are the minimum needed to eliminate airway secretions (189), and this is the best indicator for tracheostomy tube removal irrespective of remaining pulmonary function (190). Patients with VCs less than 1,500 ml and PCFs less than 300 L/min learn air stacking and manually assisted coughing techniques, and assisted PCFs are measured using these techniques.

For the stable patient without intrinsic pulmonary disease, arterial blood gas sampling is unnecessary. Besides the technical difficulty involved in obtaining an accurate sample from many of these patients, 25% of patients either hyperventilate or hypoventilate due to anxiety or pain during the procedure, thus decreasing the accuracy of the test (104). Noninvasive continuous blood gas monitoring including capnography, transcutaneous blood gas monitoring, and ox-

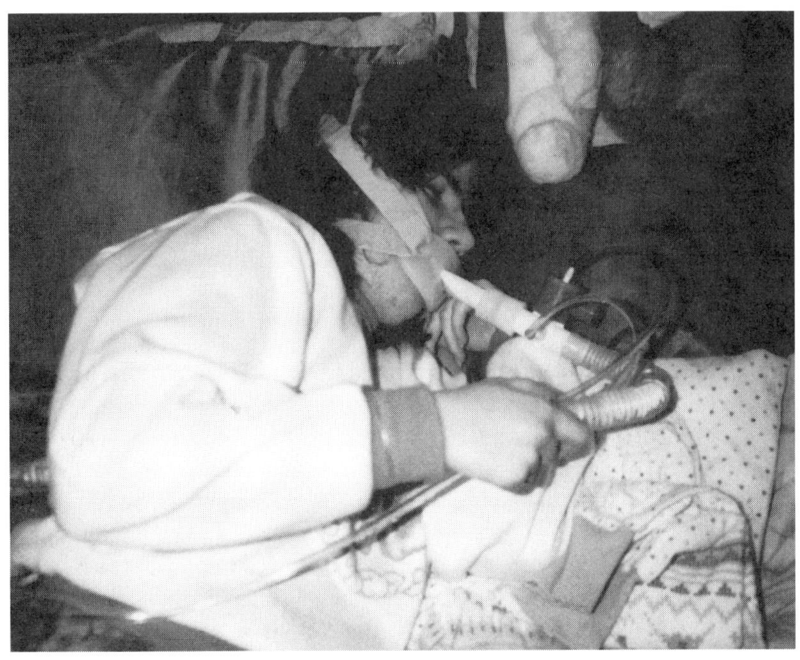

FIG. 55-1. Mouth IPPV for nocturnal ventilatory support with a lip seal retained mouthpiece. For individuals with weak oropharyngeal musculature air stacking of insufflations can be maximized and the maximum insufflation capacity increased by applying mild hand pressure to the lip seal during insufflations.

imetry yield more useful information, particularly during sleep.

Nocturnal noninvasive blood gas monitoring may be performed yearly for patients with supine VC less than 40% of predicted normal, especially for those with rapidly evolving conditions and loss of VC. The oximeter, as well as the capnograph, which measures end-tidal pCO_2, must be capable of summarizing and printing out the data (171). These studies are most conveniently performed on an ambulatory basis. Any SaO_2 below 95% is evaluated and the artifact ruled out (191). Any symptomatic patient with a VC less than 50% of predicted normal, mean nocturnal SaO_2 less than 95%, and maximum $PaCO_2$ greater than 50 mm Hg has significant nocturnal hypoventilation and requires treatment.

For symptomatic patients with greater than 60% of predicted VC, an unclear pattern of oxyhemoglobin desaturation, and no apparently significant carbon dioxide retention, sleep disordered breathing is suspected. This is particularly true when loud, high-pitched snoring, interrupted breathing, obesity, and hypersomnolence dominate the picture (192). These patients should undergo polysomnography.

When concurrent obstructive or interstitial lung disease is documented by pulmonary function studies, capnography is correlated to $PaCO_2$. With severely disturbed pulmonary gas exchange and PaO_2 less than 60 mm Hg in the presence of eucapnia or hypocapnia, supplemental oxygen administration is indicated, and neither oximetry nor capnography can adequately gauge alveolar ventilation.

TREATMENT

Counseling

The use of physical medicine interventions can prevent respiratory tract infections from developing into pneumonia, acute respiratory failure, and the need for hospitalizations and tracheal intubations. Besides explaining the various therapeutic options, the patient is cautioned to avoid oxygen therapy, obesity, heavy meals, extremes of temperature, humidity, excessive fatigue, crowded areas or exposure to respiratory tract pathogens, and sedatives, especially at bedtime. The need for flu and bacterial vaccinations and possibly the use of antiviral agents such as amantadine are considered (193,194). An abdominal binder may be useful to increase diaphragmatic excursion and VC for seated spinal cord–injured patients. Because treated patients with progressive neuromuscular diseases can have greatly prolonged survival, they are encouraged to undertake goal-oriented activities and plan for their futures.

Medical Options

Good hydration, nutrition, and electrolyte status are important. For example, patients with Duchenne muscular dystrophy have decreased muscle potassium content, decreased total body potassium, and a treatable predilection for hypokalemia, which is exacerbated during acute illnesses and which may exacerbate respiratory muscle insufficiency (195).

No medical intervention has been shown to improve respiratory muscle function for these patients (196), and the risk of pulmonary complications may be increased by the nocturnal oxygen administration used to give the "patient a comfortable night's rest" (105,197). Although SaO_2 can be improved by oxygen therapy, central ventilatory drive can be suppressed, carbon dioxide retention exacerbated, and the risk of acute respiratory failure increased (44). With the increase in hypercapnia, central nervous system–mediated reflex muscle activity needed for noninvasive IPPV to be effective during sleep also appears to be suppressed (171).

Oxygen therapy has been shown to prolong hypopneas and apneas by 33% during REM sleep and 19% otherwise, even in individuals with mild neuromuscular disease (198). Hypercapnic hypoxia is treated by assisted ventilation rather than by oxygen administration.

Maintenance of Respiratory Muscle Strength and Endurance

In the few studies of respiratory muscle exercise performed on neuromuscular disease patients, short daily sessions of inspiratory resistive exercise alone were reported to have no effect on spirometry or maximum inspiratory or expiratory pressures (199–201) but did improve respiratory muscle endurance (149,199,200). However, the degree of improvement in endurance correlated significantly with the level of VC and maximum inspiratory pressure at the outset of training, and no patient with less than 30% of predicted VC improved (199). This is the level of VC at which point patients often require nocturnal ventilatory aid and have considerable difficulty during respiratory tract infections (171). There is also no evidence that beginning an exercise program earlier would preserve more muscle function for the time when the patient requires aid nor that the improvement in endurance for relatively strong patients (mean VC 54% to 59% in the patients studied) delays the occurrence of pulmonary complications as suggested (199). Indeed, there is some evidence to the contrary. Mildly affected amyotrophic lateral sclerosis patients were reported to respond to a respiratory muscle resistive exercise program with a decrease in VC and inspiratory pressures (202). There also may be a greater subsequent rate of loss of muscle strength in any temporarily strengthened muscles. The training itself may be hazardous for patients in an advanced stage of disease. Thus, for those most likely to have respiratory complications, the use of resistance exercise is likely to be of little or no value. Interestingly, however, the combination of interspersing respiratory muscle rest by ventilatory assistance and inspiratory muscle training has been reported to improve the respiratory muscle strength and endurance of neuromuscular patients during ventilator weaning (203).

Deep Breathing and Insufflation

The use of range of motion exercises for hypomobile tissues is a basic rehabilitation principle and may be even more important to apply to the lungs and chest walls of these patients. Alveolar multiplication ceases at 8 years of age, but alveoli continue to grow through adolescence (204). Frequent deep breaths or insufflations are necessary for this to proceed as well as for normal development of the rib cage and thorax. Regular deep insufflations delivered via anesthesia masks and later via mouthpieces or nasal interfaces to 100 children with spinal muscular atrophy from 18 months of age have been reported to have ameliorated this problem (204,205).

Although short periods of mechanical hyperinflation (10,206) can briefly increase dynamic pulmonary compliance and reverse acute atelectasis (207–209), multiple daily periods of mechanical hyperinflations of up to 30 cm H_2O pressure have not been shown to improve static compliance in adults (210). It is not yet known whether more aggressive treatments or treatments introduced before lung compliance is greatly reduced would be of benefit (176). At the very latest, hyperinflation treatments may be indicated before the VC has declined to 50% to 60% of normal.

Regular, maximum tolerated insufflations can be conveniently delivered in the home via manual resuscitators, portable ventilators, mechanical insufflator–exsufflators, or GPB. Incentive spirometry cannot substitute for insufflation. Maximum insufflations are usually most conveniently delivered via a mouthpiece. However, if oral and buccal musculature is weak and the patient experiences difficulty in grasping a mouthpiece or if greater volumes can be insufflated via a nose piece, then this interface is used. With weak oropharyngeal musculature, a mouthpiece also may be used with a lip seal flange. With mild hand pressure applied to a lip seal, air leakage is reduced, and the depth of insufflation increased. For small children or adults with less than 1,000 ml of MIC via oral or nasal interfaces, an oronasal mask is used.

A program is undertaken of air stacking hyperinflations two to four times a day to increasingly higher volumes to approach the predicted inspiratory capacity. In addition to preventing atelectasis, there is some evidence that regular lung hyperinflation can have a beneficial effect on VC (211,212). For traumatic quadriplegics (213), the use of combining hyperinflation with inspiratory muscle training may be more useful than either method alone.

Glossopharyngeal Breathing

Glossopharyngeal breathing is a method for providing maximal insufflations and as a noninvasive method for supporting ventilation. It is an excellent back-up in the event of ventilator equipment failure. The patient is instructed to take a deep breath and then augments it by GPB. The tongue and pharyngeal muscles project boluses of air past the vocal cords. The vocal cords close with each "gulp." One breath consists of six to nine gulps of 60 to 200 ml each. During the training period the efficiency of GPB is monitored by spirometrically measuring the number of milliliters of air per gulp, gulps per breath, and breaths per minute. A training manual and video are available (6,214). A GPB rate of 12 to 14 per minute can provide patients with little or no VC with normal tidal volumes, minute ventilation, and hours of ventilator-free time (Fig. 55-2) (215). GPB can normalize the volume and rhythm of speech and permit the patient to shout and cough more effectively.

The use of GPB is dependent on oropharyngeal muscle integrity such that the maximum glossopharyngeal single

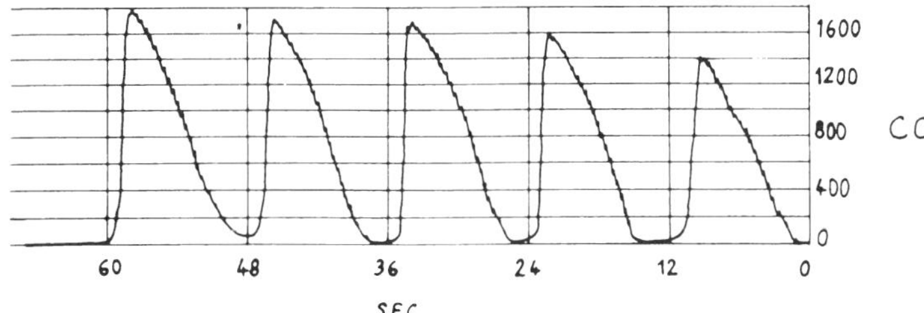

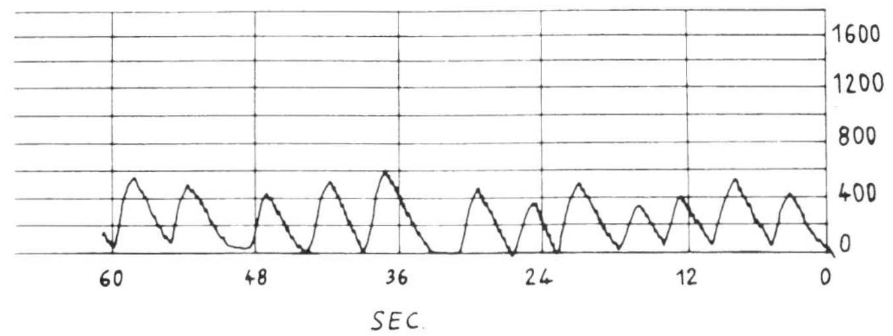

FIG. 55-2. Normal minute ventilation (60 to 90 ml per gulp, six to eight gulps per breath, 12 breaths per minute) throughout daytime hours by GPB for an individual with no measurable vital capacity otherwise. Maximum glossopharyngeal single breath capacities can exceed 3,000 ml for such individuals.

breath capacity (215) approximates the MIC. Despite severely affected bulbar musculature, however, two ventilator-assisted Duchenne muscular dystrophy patients were reported to be very successful using GPB for ventilator-free time (216). We have seen four Duchenne types and many others with non-Duchenne myopathies and spinal muscular atrophies who also used GPB for hours of ventilator-free time. A tracheostomy virtually precludes successful training in and use of GPB, because even with the tube plugged, gulped air leaks around the tube and out the tracheostomy site.

Airway Secretion Clearance

Patients with respiratory muscle dysfunction and especially ventilator users are often unable to generate the 160 L/min of PCF necessary to eliminate airway secretions. Thus, airway secretions can precipitate life-threatening bronchial mucous plugging and acute respiratory failure. This is also true for intubated or tracheostomized patients who cannot close their glotti to generate expiratory pressures. Airway secretions are especially profuse and hazardous after the translaryngeal extubation of patients.

There is overreliance on airway suctioning. Airway suctioning via the nose or mouth is ineffective and poorly tolerated. Suctioning via an endotracheal tube does not mobilize deep secretions and has many potential complications. In adults, the suction catheter also usually fails to enter the left main stem bronchus (217). It irritates airway membranes (exacerbating secretions and inflammatory changes), induces airway edema and wheezing, and necessitates further bronchial suctioning and cleansing of the tracheostomy site itself. Mucous plugs that adhere to the cuff or the wall of a tube cannot be suctioned and may eventually plug a bronchus, causing atelectasis and airway collapse.

The requirements for effective airway clearance are intact mucociliary clearance mechanisms, including normal ciliary and alveolar macrophage activity and generation of optimal PCF. Intubation and tracheostomy tubes incapacitate these systems. Chronic bacterial colonization and chronic inflammatory changes impair mucociliary clearance, an effect exacerbated by malnutrition (57). Swallowing (218) and verbal communication, which is crucial for timely management of airway secretions, is precluded by the presence of an endotracheal tube and also may be impaired by the presence of a tracheostomy. The generation of adequate intrathoracic pressures for the explosive decompression of coughing is also impossible when receiving IPPV via an endotracheal tube.

Methods used to facilitate airway secretion elimination for patients with intrinsic lung or airways diseases are commonly used for patients with paralytic conditions, even though these patients have the capacity for adequate generation of PCF to effectively eliminate secretions. Chest percussion and postural drainage are most widely prescribed, but no controlled studies have demonstrated that they shorten hospital stays, reduce morbidity, lessen the number of exacerbations, or decrease mortality (68,96,219,220). Likewise, the other previously described methods of applying rapid pressure changes and oscillating the chest or airways have not been shown to be useful in this population.

On the other hand, the 12 described methods of manually assisted coughing are effective but underused (221). After a breath or deep insufflation, optimally to greater than 1,500 ml, some combination of anterior chest and abdominal compression can usually provide PCF of 300 to 400 L/min (Fig. 55-3). However, like chest physical therapy, these techniques can be effort intensive and must be applied frequently. They are inadequate for patients with scoliosis or

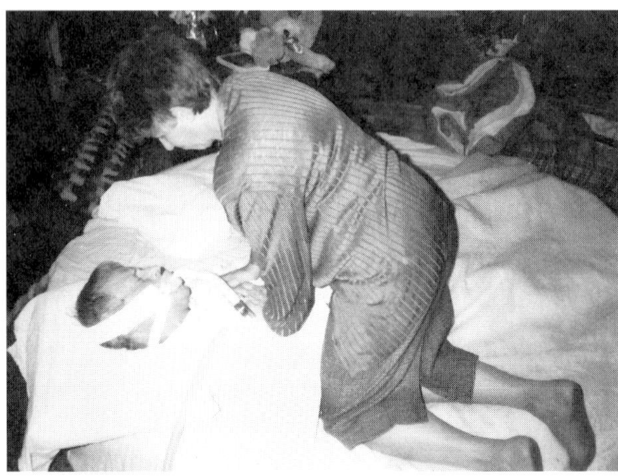

FIG. 55-3. A tussive squeeze to the chest to increase cough flows to eliminate airway secretions. This patient also uses lip seal ventilation in a regimen of 24-hour mouthpiece IPPV.

severely impaired function of the glottis and cannot be used on a full stomach. When inadequate to eliminate secretions and maintain normal SaO_2, mechanically assisted coughing is indicated.

The mechanical insufflator–exsufflator (J.H. Emerson Inc., Cambridge, MA) (Fig. 55-4) is the most effective mechanical aid for airway secretion clearance for patients with paralytic conditions. It delivers an independently adjusted positive pressure insufflation followed by an independently adjusted negative pressure exsufflation via an anesthesia mask. When used through a facial interface, an abdominal thrust is applied during the exsufflation phase unless the patient has recently eaten and the stomach is not empty. It is also very effective when applied through endotracheal or tracheostomy tubes. The pressure decrease desired by the patient is usually about 80 cm H_2O. It occurs instantaneously and may be sustained for 2 or 3 seconds. This creates flows of up to 10 L/sec that carry secretions, mucous plugs, and any other debris into the mouth, anesthesia mask, or tube, from which they can be easily suctioned. The mechanical exsufflator can reliably provide airway secretion clearance during respiratory tract infections without the need for intubation. It can immediately increase pulmonary volumes and SaO_2 as secretions and plugs are cleared (222). Its use can be instrumental in allowing continued ventilatory support without a tracheostomy (223–227). No complications have been reported in 43 years and thousands of applications (10,224,225–227).

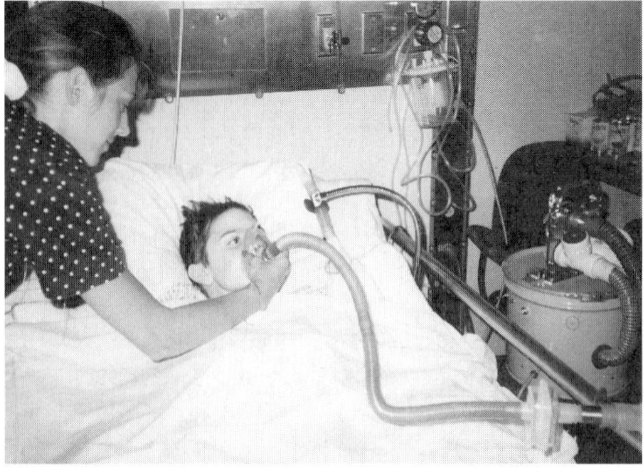

FIG. 55-4. Mechanical insufflation–exsufflation to eliminate airway secretions postoperative scoliosis surgery for a Duchenne muscular dystrophy patient who requires 24-hour noninvasive IPPV.

Noninvasive Ventilatory Support by IPPV

IPPV can be provided via oral (174,215,223,224, 228–233), nasal (7,171,224,232,234–236), or oronasal (7,233,237,238) interfaces. All varieties can be custom fabricated (7,237,239). Mouthpiece IPPV or use of an intermittent abdominal pressure ventilator (IAPV) is the method of choice for daytime ventilatory support and nasal IPPV for nocturnal support. During sleep, both mouthpiece and nasal IPPV are effective because of central nervous system–mediated reflex muscle activity that prevents excessive air leakage and oxyhemoglobin desaturation (240). Improvement in SaO_2 and carbon dioxide levels by noninvasive IPPV exceed those obtained by body ventilator use (171). There also may be less hypercapnia and fewer REM-associated desaturations and sleep disturbances or arousals (241). Patients for whom normal ventilation is maintained during daytime hours and who, therefore, do not have depressed ventilatory drive, often maintain normal SaO_2 and $PaCO_2$ during sleep using these methods despite having no measurable VC (171).

Mouthpiece IPPV

Mouthpiece IPPV, which is ventilatory support via a mouthpiece, has been used by many patients with little or no autonomous breathing ability for long-term 24-hour ventilatory support (174,215,223,224,230,233). For daytime use, a small flexed mouthpiece is either kept in the mouth or is fixed onto the motorized wheelchair controls adjacent to the patient's mouth for assisted breaths as needed (Fig. 55-5) (215). The mouthpiece has the advantages of being simple, inexpensive, and commercially available. The rate, rhythm, and volume of speech is more normal, and eating is less compromised than for patients using tracheostomy IPPV. Mouth stick activities are also unhindered by mouthpiece IPPV unless the patient has little or no significant ventilator-free time, in which case the intermittent abdominal pressure ventilator (IAPV) is often preferred for daytime aid.

Mouthpiece IPPV also has been used for nocturnal ventilatory support since 1964 (242). To avoid potentially severe oxyhemoglobin desaturation, it is recommended that a lip seal flange be used during sleep (Fig. 55-1). A soft flexible scuba mouthpiece or a mouthpiece that accommodates bite

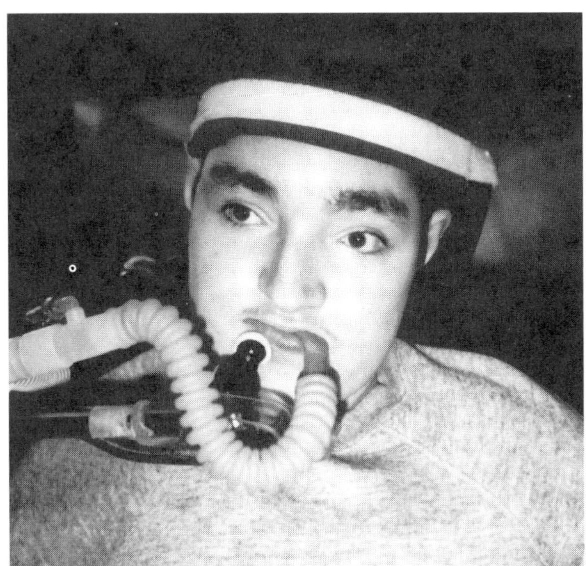

FIG. 55-5. A Duchenne muscular dystrophy patient who has required ventilatory support 24 hours a day using mouthpiece IPPV for 15 years. The mouthpiece is fixed adajacent to the chin controls of the motorized wheelchair to deliver IPPV for daytime ventilatory support.

may be substituted for the mouthpiece in the lip seal for additional comfort and relief of orthodontic pressure.

For the occasional patient with periods of excessive nasal leakage during sleep, cotton pledgets can be placed into the nostrils and sealed in place by adhesive tape, or nose clips can be used for an air-tight oronasal seal. Patients who require pressures exceeding 45 cm H_2O or who do not have reliable attendant care to aid in placement of a strap retention system can use a custom-molded acrylic mouthpiece with bite plate retention and an acrylic lip seal (7). This interface can be easily removed by tongue thrust. Because mouthpiece IPPV can safely and effectively ventilate patients both day and night, is safe, and is associated with few complications (174,188), it is of paramount importance for the conversion of patients from tracheostomy to noninvasive aid and also can be used for patient weaning (243).

Nasal IPPV

In 1984, Delaubier (9) described nasal IPPV. In 1987, Bach (244) reported its utility as a means of assisting ventilation up to 24 hours a day for a patient with no autonomous breathing ability. Commercially available CPAP masks are now being used as nasal interfaces for IPPV. All are held in place by a head gear or strap assembly. They are simple, inexpensive, durable, and readily available. Because all were designed to provide a leakage-free interface for CPAPs, which are generally less than 15 cm H_2O, they are not always adequate for providing nasal IPPV at pressures that must invariably exceed 18 cm H_2O. Thus, custom-molded interfaces are constructed for many patients using nasal IPPV (171).

Custom nasal IPPV interfaces increase comfort, decrease insufflation leakage, and provide better appearance. SEFAM assembly kits can be used to make several styles of nasal interfaces (available from Respironics Inc., Murrysville, PA) (232). They contain elastic strap sets, small plastic housing, and sufficient silicone putty to make three to six interfaces. The putty is mixed and molded by the patient or caregiver into interfaces. The interfaces are strap retained and require refabrication every few months. Firm, durable custom acrylic nasal interfaces also have been described (7). Nasal IPPV is the preferred and most practical ventilatory aid for nocturnal support (171). Although it also can be used for daytime aid, it is preferable to mouthpiece IPPV only for the patient who is too weak to rotate the neck and grasp a mouthpiece.

IPPV via Oronasal Interfaces

A custom-molded strapless oronasal interface was designed for the nocturnal ventilatory support of patients who are uncomfortable or inadequately ventilated by other techniques or unable to reliably don a strap-retained interface (7). It consists of an acrylic bite plate with metal clasps for retention to the teeth. The bite plate is fixed to an extraoral mask shell, which is connected to a respirator hose. It may be open to both nose and mouth, allowing concurrent nasal and mouth IPPV. This interface provides an essentially air-tight system. It can be thrust out by tongue movement alone. The greatest impediment to its use is the lack of adequate and stable dentition seen in pediatric patients and some adults.

Ventilator Equipment

Both volume-cycled, and pressure-cycled ventilators that deliver bilevel positive airway pressure are available to deliver air through the interfaces, but only the former can deliver sufficient volumes for effective coughing and should therefore be used (245,246). The assist-control mode is used when the patient is able to trigger the machine. Otherwise control modes are used.

Although volume-cycled ventilator volumes of less than 900 ml are useful for introducing mouthpiece or nasal IPPV, these may be increased gradually to 1,500 ml or more to permit the user to optimally vary insufflation volumes by volitionally leaking air. A closed system with an air-tight seal of both nose and mouth also can be used (7). Continuous nocturnal SaO_2 monitoring is an adequate gauge of assisted alveolar ventilation provided that no supplemental oxygen is used.

Body Ventilators

Body ventilators can be categorized by the way in which they assist the patient's ventilation. There are those that act directly on the body to produce diaphragmatic movement such as the IAPV (229,247,248) and the rocking bed (249), and there are NPBVs (4,8,228) that induce air movement by creating subatmospheric pressure in a chamber covering the chest wall and abdomen.

Intermittent Abdominal Pressure Ventilator

The IAPV is the ventilator preferred for daytime ventilatory support by the majority of wheelchair users with less than 1 hour of ventilator-free breathing time and is a key reason for effectively (surgically) preventing the development of significant scoliosis (229). It is a convenient mode of assisted ventilation, optimizes patient appearance, and frees the mouth for mouth stick and other activities. It is only effective when the user is in the sitting position, and it may not be effective for patients with scoliosis or extremes of body weight. About 250-ml (229) to 1,200-ml (224) tidal volumes can be provided by IAPV action. These volumes can be supplemented by diaphragm action when present as well as by GPB. Although the IAPV has been used for daytime support by individuals who receive tracheostomy IPPV overnight (247,248), the greatest benefit is derived when it is used during daytime hours and complements nocturnal mouthpiece or nasal IPPV without an indwelling tracheostomy.

The Rocking Bed

The rocking bed rocks the patient from 15° to 30° from the horizontal and moves the abdominal contents against the diaphragm to assist ventilation. It is the least effective of the body ventilators but can be adequate for patients with good pulmonary compliance. Its main advantages include ease of application, weight shifting for skin protection, benefits on bowel motility (249), and energy conservation for sleeping with significant others (250).

Negative Pressure Body Ventilators

The Emerson iron lungs with the motor-driven bellows developed in 1931 were the main devices used to provide 24-hour long-term ventilatory support, and in particular, nocturnal ventilatory support, for patients with paralytic respiratory failure, until 1952. They are extremely dependable and continue to be used by many individuals (8,228). The Porta-lung is a smaller and lighter counterpart of an iron lung. The negative chamber pressure is created by the action of a negative pressure generator (ventilator) that is separate from the chamber itself. It can achieve negative pressures and ventilatory volumes that equal those of the iron lung.

The cuirass or chest shell ventilator consists of an easy-to-don firm shell that covers the anterior chest and abdomen and a negative pressure ventilator that creates the subatmospheric pressure under the shell. Although less effective than tank ventilators, they are adequate for most patients provided that there is no significant back deformity, intrinsic lung disease, or impairment of pulmonary compliance (206). Unlike other NPBVs, the chest shell also can be used for daytime ventilatory aid in the seated position, although the IAPV and mouthpiece IPPV are invariably preferred. Because of its convenience and simplicity, when effective, it is the method of choice for ventilatory assistance during tracheostomy site closure or during extubation for patients being converted from IPPV via endotracheal intubation to noninvasive IPPV.

The "wrap ventilators" work on the same principle as the chest shell, but they provide greater volumes when carefully placed and correctly used. However, they are time consuming to don. They consist of a firm plastic grid covering the thorax and abdomen which may be applied to a rigid backplate that optimizes effectiveness. The grid and the body under it may be covered by a variety of wraps made of various materials in several forms. A popular design is made of wind-proof nylon or Gortex cloth (W.C. Gore & Assoc. Inc, Elkton, MD) in the style of a poncho or one-piece suit (206). Gortex makes a cooler, more flexible wrap than plastic or cloth and increases both comfort and expense. The wrap is sealed around the patient's wrists, neck, and abdomen or lower extremities depending on the style. Despite its inconvenience for donning, wrap ventilators continue to be a popular option for nocturnal assisted ventilation.

The majority of individuals using NPBVs or the rocking bed have significant obstructive apneas and oxyhemoglobin desaturations during sleep (131). Much of this activity occurs during REM sleep (241). This can cause patient fatigue and other symptoms of hypoventilation, particularly for patients using little or no aid during daytime hours. Baydur et al. reported an increased association of recurrent aspiration with body ventilator use (216). The use of mechanical exsufflation or manually assisted airway secretion clearance also may be less convenient during body ventilator use. Because most patients are better ventilated by and prefer noninvasive IPPV methods and because mouthpiece and nasal IPPV are more convenient, they have become the methods of choice for long-term ventilatory support.

Oximetry Monitoring and Feedback

For a patient with chronic alveolar hypoventilation who has not been using ventilatory support, or the patient being weaned from tracheostomy IPPV, introduction to and use of mouthpiece or nasal IPPV is facilitated by oximetry feedback. An SaO_2 alarm may be set from 93% to 94%. The patient sees that by taking slightly deeper breaths SaO_2 will exceed 95% within seconds. He or she is instructed to maintain SaO_2 above 94% all day. This can be achieved by unassisted breathing for a period of time and, once tiring, by mouthpiece or nasal IPPV. With time the patient requires increasing periods of IPPV to maintain adequate ventilation (SaO_2 greater than 94%). In this manner an oximeter may may help to reset central ventilatory drive.

Oximetry feedback is also particularly useful during the management of respiratory tract infections. Patients at risk for acute respiratory failure undergo continuous SaO_2 monitoring and are taught that any dip in SaO_2 below 95% is due either to underventilation or bronchial mucous plugging, and if these two causes are not quickly addressed, lead to atelectasis or pneumonia. Patients are instructed to use noninvasive IPPV to maintain normal ventilation and manually or mechanically assisted coughing to reverse mucous plug-associated oxyhemoglobin desaturations. In this way most episodes that would otherwise cause acute respiratory failure are successfully managed at home.

TREATMENT OF SLEEP-DISORDERED BREATHING

Significant weight reduction can improve or completely resolve the OSAS for many obese patients (251). Unfortunately, this is frequently only a temporary effect. CPAP can be effective for many patients but is not adequate for most who have restricted pulmonary volumes and hypercapnia. Mask discomfort and air leakage into the eyes can make the use of CPAP via CPAP masks intolerable for about 35% of patients (252).

Independently varying inspiratory positive airway pressures (IPAP) and expiratory positive airway pressures (EPAP) with the newly available bilevel positive airway pressure machines increases effectiveness, comfort, and cost. The greater the pulse pressure difference (i.e., the difference between the IPAP and EPAP), the greater the inspiratory muscle assistance. Often 20 cm H_2O IPAP and minimum EPAP are most effective (10). Custom-molded nasal interfaces also should be used for patients who require greater comfort and better fit than can be accorded by commercially available CPAP masks (7). Portable volume ventilators are used instead of BPAP to deliver nasal IPPV for hypercapnic morbidly obese patients who require greater inspiratory muscle assist at higher peak ventilator pressures than can be provided by BPAP.

Another convenient long-term solution, effective for many OSAS patients, is the use of an orthodontic splint that brings the mandible and tongue forward, thus helping to splint open the hypopharynx (253). Preventing supine positioning during sleep, perhaps by sewing a tennis ball to the back of his pajama shirt, also may be helpful. Uvulopalatopharyngoplasty and mandibular advancement procedures also have been used but are often ineffective. These options and the use of nasopharyngeal or tracheostomy tubes should be used only as a last resort (254–256).

INVASIVE VENTILATORY SUPPORT

The maintenance of an indwelling tracheostomy is indicated only when the use of noninvasive aids are contraindicated by the presence of any of the following: depressed cognitive function, orthopedic conditions interfering with the application of noninvasive IPPV interfaces and exsufflation techniques, inadequate oropharyngeal muscle strength for functional articulation of speech and swallowing, severe intrinsic pulmonary disease necessitating high FiO_2, uncontrolled seizures or substance abuse, or assisted PCF not exceeding 160 L/min (189,257). Also, the presence of a nasogastric tube can hamper the fitting of a nasal interface and the use of mouthpiece or nasal IPPV by interfering with both soft palate closure of the pharynx and seal at the nose. Although tracheostomy IPPV can greatly extend survival for patients with neuromuscular ventilatory failure (245), morbidity and mortality outcomes are not as favorable as by management via strictly noninvasive approaches (258).

When tracheostomy IPPV is continued for any reason and oropharyngeal muscles are sufficiently intact for swallowing and speaking, either cuffless tubes or tracheostomy cuff deflation are used up to 24 hours a day (106). Delivered air volumes are increased to compensate leak and support speech and one-way valves used to further facilitate verbal communication (103). Tracheostomy buttons are useful to optimize air passage through the upper airway for autonomous breathing as well as during transition from tracheostomy to noninvasive IPPV (224).

The use of pacemakers for electrophrenic respiration has been an option for assisting the ventilation of patients with intact phrenic nerves and diaphragms. However, the initial equipment, surgery, and training expenses exceed $300,000 in the United States and can be much greater when it takes more than 1 month to condition the nerves and diaphragm to function adequately with stimulation. Conditioning, in fact, often requires 6 months or more (259). Costs can be reduced somewhat if the conditioning period takes place in lower cost, generally $1,500/day, ventilator units of rehabilitation hospitals.

Despite the cost and the new pacing methods to more evenly distribute the electrical impulses to the nerves (260), pacing can be used for full-time ventilatory support in less than 40% of patients (261,243); and, with the availability of less expensive, noninvasive inspiratory aids, it is not indicated for spinal cord–injured adolescents and adults unless full-time support is required and neck and facial muscles are too weak for use of noninvasive IPPV (224,262–264). An indwelling tracheostomy tube is also retained for over 90% of these patients because of pacer-induced upper airway collapse during sleep and the possibility of sudden pacer failure. Thus, the local and pulmonary complications associated with long-term tracheostomy are also a liability (261). In addition, there are numerous associated complications and a high incidence of both short and long-term damage to both diaphragm and phrenic nerves (265,266). It may be for these reasons that, although the VC can increase and the patient can wean from ventilator use up to 8 years after spinal cord injury (224,267), increased pulmonary functioning and late ventilator weaning has not been reported in phrenic pacemaker users. Patients given the choice between electrophrenic pacing and noninvasive IPPV without an indwelling tracheostomy tube invariably choose the latter (268).

QUALITY OF LIFE

Misconceptions about the undesirability of '''going on a respirator' have far-reaching negative effects for persons now happily being supported on a respirator and mitigate the positive effects it could have for some types of chronically impaired persons whose quality of life also could be enhanced by the use of a ventilator'' (269). Although it would seem that intelligent, self-directed individuals should be fully informed about therapeutic options, in the frenzy of seeking a less expensive health-care delivery system, some physicians have suggested eliminating the patient from the decision-making process. As recently as 1989 it was recommended that a physician's assessment of patients' quality of life be conducted ''independent of the patient's feelings'' to guide the clinician in whether to institute mechanical ventilation (270).

Poor quality of life is usually given as the reason for withholding ventilator use (271). However, no quality of life criteria can be appropriately applied to all individuals. Life satisfaction depends rather on personal preferences (272) and on subjective satisfaction in physical, mental, and social situations, even though these may be deficient in some manner. Thus, not quality of life but potential satisfaction with life should be considered. It is particularly appropriate that the life satisfaction of individuals who are living the consequences of having chosen to use ventilators be considered when deciding about such ethically and financially complex matters as ventilator use for others. Interestingly, data indicate that severely disabled long-term postpoliomyelitis, Duchenne muscular dystrophy (DMD), and spinal cord–injured ventilator users (271) generally have very positive views of their lives and life satisfaction. These individuals find quality of life in interpersonal activities and they are very significantly more satisfied with life than health-care professional estimates suggest (271). Crucial for this is often the availability of personal attendant care services. Thus, in the face of calls to limit entitlement spending, it should be noted that a society willing to provide free room, board, health care, legal and educational services, vocational training, and cable television for murders, rapists, drug dealers, and other felons at exorbitant cost has the ethical responsibility to provide attentant care services to those in need, some of whom are crime victims themselves.

As noted, the use of noninvasive respiratory muscle aids was largely developed by physiatrists (273). Besides preventing acute pulmonary morbidity, hospitalization, intubation, premature death, and the undue expense associated with tracheostomy and specialized nursing care, the use of these methods eliminates the ethical consideration concerning suicide by withdrawal of ventilatory support because users are not passively attached to a respirator but actively control their alveolar ventilation. The individual's personal sense of controlling his or her life is also enhanced in this manner.

Our specialty needs to do more than instruct the patients and their families; it must advocate for them to assure that they have access to appropriate community resources. We especially need to advocate for our patients against those who would detract from their personal freedom, even when that freedom incurs reasonable risk. ''The Bush administration estimated that America spends more than $200 billion annually to keep people dependent (institutionalized) . . . that amounts to about $50,000 a person each year. But personal attendant services can serve as many as five people for the same amount while providing the individual with the opportunity to live an independent, productive, and meaningful life'' (274).

REFERENCES

1. Haas F, Haas A. History of pulmonary rehabilitation, or, the more things change, the more they remain the same. In: Haas F, Axen K, eds. *Pulmonary therapy and rehabilitation: principles and practice,* 2nd ed. Philadelphia: Williams & Wilkins, 1991; 179–195.
2. Fishman AP. The chest physician and physiatrist: perspectives on the scientific basis of pulmonary rehabilitation and related research. In: Bach JR, ed. *Pulmonary rehabilitation: the obstructive and paralytic conditions.* Philadelphia: Hanley & Belfus, 1996; 1–12.
3. Alberion G, Alba A, Lee M, Solomon M. Pulmonary care of Duchenne type of dystrophy. *N Y State J Med* 1973; 73:1206–1207.
4. Alexander MA, Johnson EW, Petty J, Stauch D. Mechanical ventilation of patients with late stage Duchenne muscular dystrophy: management in the home. *Arch Phys Med Rehabil* 1979; 60:289–292.
5. Curran FJ, Colbert AP. Night ventilation by body respirators for patients in chronic respiratory failure due to late stage Duchenne muscular dystrophy. *Arch Phys Med Rehabil* 1981; 62:270–274.
6. Dail C, Rodgers M, Guess V, Adkins HV. *Glossopharyngeal breathing manual.* Downey, CA: Professional Staff Association of Rancho Los Amigos Hospital, 1979.
7. McDermott I, Bach JR, Parker C, Sortor S. Custom-fabricated interfaces for intermittent positive pressure ventilation. *Int J Prosthodont* 1989; 2:224–233.
8. Splaingard ML, Frates RC, Jefferson LS, Rosen CL, Harrison GM. Home negative pressure ventilation: report of 20 years of experience in patients with neuromuscular disease. *Arch Phys Med Rehabil* 1985; 66:239–242.
9. Delaubier A. Traitement de l'insuffisance respiratoire chronique dans les dystrophies musculaires. In: *Memoires de certificat d'etudes superieures de reeducation et readaptation fonctionnelles.* Paris: Universite R Descarte, 1984; 1–124.
10. Bach JR. Mechanical insufflation-exsufflation: comparison of peak expiratory flows with manually assisted and unassisted coughing techniques. *Chest* 1993; 104:1553–1562.
11. Higgins ITT. Epidemiology of bronchitis and emphysema. In: Fishman AP, ed. *Pulmonary diseases and disorders,* 2nd ed. New York: McGraw-Hill, 1988; 70–90.
12. Fishman AP. The spectrum of chronic obstructive disease of the airways. In: Fishman AP, ed. *Pulmonary diseases and disorders.* New York: McGraw-Hill, 1988; 1159–1171.
13. Department of Health Education and Welfare. *Smoking and health: a report of the Surgeon General.* DHEW Publication No. (PHS) 79-50066. Washington, DC: DHEW, 1979.
14. Leeder SR, Colley JRT, Corkhill R, et al. Change in respiratory symptom prevalence in adults who alter their smoking habits. *Am J Epidemiol* 1977; 105:522–529.
15. Buist AS, Nagy JM, Sexton GJ. The effect of smoking cessation on pulmonary function: a 30-month follow-up of two smoking cessation clinics. *Am Rev Respir Dis* 1979; 120:953–957.
16. Kark JD, Leguish M, Rannon L. Cigarette smoking as a risk factor for epidemic A (HI,NI) influenza in young men. *N Engl J Med* 1982; 307:1042–1046.
17. Bosse R, Sparrow D, Rose CL, et al. Longitudinal effect of age and smoking cessation on pulmonary function. *Am Rev Respir Dis* 1981; 123:378–381.
18. Hillberg RE. Chronic obstructive pulmonary disease: causes and clinicopathologic considerations. In: Bach JR, ed. *Pulmonary rehabilitation: the obstructive and paralytic conditions.* Philadelphia: Hanley & Belfus, 1996:27–38.
19. Tager IB. Chronic bronchitis. In: Fishman AP, ed. *Pulmonary diseases and disorders.* New York: McGraw-Hill, 1988; 1543–1551.
20. Slonim NB, Hamilton LH, eds. *Respiratory physiology,* 5th ed. St. Louis: CV Mosby, 1987.

21. Begin P, Grassino A. Inspiratory muscle dysfunction and chronic hypercapnia in chronic obstructive pulmonary disease. *Am Rev Respir Dis* 1991; 143:905–912.
22. Rochester DF, Braun NMT. Determinants of maximal inspiratory pressure in chronic obstructive pulmonary disease. *Am Rev Respir Dis* 1985; 132:42–47.
23. Stubbing DG, Pengelly LD, Morse JLC, Jones NL. Pulmonary mechanics during exercise in subjects with chronic airflow obstruction. *J Appl Physiol* 1980; 49:511–515.
24. Holden DA, Stelmach KD, Curtis PS, Beck GJ, Stoller JK. The impact of a rehabilitation program on functional status of patients with chronic lung disease. *Respir Care* 1990; 35:332–341.
25. Mahler DA, Weinberg DH, Wells CK, Feinstein AR. The measurement of dyspnea: contents, interobserver agreement, and physiologic correlates of two new clinical indexes. *Chest* 1984; 85:751–758.
26. Moser K, Bokinsky G, Savage R, et al. Results of a comprehensive rehabilitation program. Physiologic and functional effects on patients with chronic obstructive pulmonary disease. *Arch Intern Med* 1980; 140:1596–1601.
27. Stoller JK, Ferranti R, Feinstein AR. Further specification and evaluation of a new clinical index for dyspnea. *Am Rev Respir Dis* 1986; 134:1129–1134.
28. Boushy SF, Thompson HK Jr, North LB, Beale AR, Snow TR. Prognosis in chronic obstructive pulmonary disease. *Am Rev Respir Dis* 1973; 108:1373–1383.
29. Ferranti RD, Roberto M, Brown C Jr, Cohelo C. Oral intake, oxygen, dyspnea, dysphagia and other considerations for the COPD patient. In: Ferranti RD, Ranpulla C, Fracchia C, Ambrosino N, eds. *Current topics in rehabilitation.* Verona, Italy: Bi & Gi, 1992; 181–190.
30. Fiaccadori E, Coffrini E, Ronda N, et al. Hypophosphatemia in the course of chronic obstructive pulmonary disease: prevalence, mechanisms, and relationships with skeletal muscle phosphorus content. *Chest* 1990; 97:857–868.
31. Aubier M, Murciano D, Lecocguic Y, et al. Effect of hypophosphatemia on diaphragmatic contractility in patients with acute respiratory failure. *N Engl J Med* 1985; 313:420–442.
32. Laaban JP, Grateau G, Psychoyos I, Vuong TK, Kouchakji B, Rochmaure J. Hypophosphatemia induced by mechanical ventilation in COPD patients [Abstract]. *Am Rev Respir Dis* 1988; 137:61.
33. Lewis MI. Nutrition and chronic obstructive pulmonary disease: a clinical overview. In: Bach JR, ed. *Pulmonary rehabilitation: the obstructive and paralytic conditions.* Philadelphia: Hanley & Belfus, 1996; 156–172.
34. Haas A, Pineda H, Haas F, Axen K. *Pulmonary therapy and rehabilitation: principles and practice.* Baltimore: Williams & Wilkens, 1979; 57–69.
35. Burrows B. Course and prognosis in advanced disease. In: Petty T, ed. *Chronic obstructive pulmonary disease,* 2nd ed. New York: Marcel Dekker, 1985.
36. Burrows B. An overview of obstructive lung diseases. *Med Clin North Am* 1981; 65:455–471.
37. Stokes DC, Wohl MEB, Khaw KT, Strieder DJ. Postural hypoxemia in cystic fibrosis. *Chest* 1985; 87:785–791.
38. Flick MR, Block AJ. Continuous in-vivo monitoring of arterial oxygenation in chronic obstructive lung disease. *Ann Intern Med* 1977; 86:725–730.
39. Jones NL. Current concepts: new tests to assess lung function. *N Engl J Med* 1975; 293:541–544.
40. Jones NL, Campbell EJM. *Clinical exercise testing,* 2nd ed. Philadelphia: WB Saunders, 1982; 158.
41. Goldstein RS. Supplemental oxygen in chronic respiratory disease. In: Bach JR, ed. *Pulmonary rehabilitation: the obstructive and paralytic conditions.* Philadelphia: Hanley & Belfus, 1996; 55–84.
42. Carlson DJ, Ries AL, Kaplan RM. Prediction of maximum exercise tolerance in patients with COPD. *Chest* 1991; 100:307–311.
43. Guyatt GH, Thompson PJ, Berman LB, et al. How should we measure function in patients with chronic heart and lung disease? *J Chron Dis* 1985; 38:517–524.
44. Bach JR. The effectiveness of pulmonary rehabilitation. Report to the Office of Civilian Health and Medical Programs for the Uniform Services, Washington, DC, 1995.
45. Reina-Rosenbaum R, Bach JR, Penek J. The cost/benefits of outpatient based pulmonary rehabilitation. *Arch Phys Med Rehabil* 1997; 78:240–244.
46. Murciano D, Aubier M, Lecocguic Y, Pariente R. Effects of theophylline on diaphragmatic strength and fatigue in patients with chronic obstructive pulmonary disease. *N Engl J Med* 1984; 311:349–353.
47. Vitres N, Aubier M, Musciano D, et al. Effects of aminophylline on diaphragmatic fatigue during acute respiratory failure. *Am Rev Respir Dis* 1984; 129:396–402.
48. Nicotra MB, Rivera M, Awe RJ. Antibiotic therapy of acute exacerbations of chronic bronchitis: a controlled study using tetracycline. *Ann Intern Med* 1982; 97:18–21.
49. Haas A, Pineda H, Haas F, Axen K. *Pulmonary therapy and rehabilitation: principles and practice.* Baltimore: Williams & Wilkins, 1979; 124–125.
50. Kahn AU. Effectiveness of biofeedback and counter conditioning in the treatment of bronchial asthma. *J Psychosom Res* 1977; 21:97–104.
51. Light RW, Marrill EJ, Despars JA, Gordon GH, Mutalipacsi LR. Prevalence of depression and anxiety in patients with COPD: relationships to functional capacity. *Chest* 1985; 87:35–38.
52. Dudley DL, Glaser EM, Jorgenson BN, et al. Psychosocial concomitants in chronic obstructive pulmonary disease II: psychosocial treatment. *Chest* 1980; 77:544–551.
53. Fisher EB Jr, Rost K. Smoking cessation: a practical guide for the physician. *Clin Chest Med* 1986; 7:551–565.
54. Dolce JJ, Crisp C, Manzella B, Richards JM, Hardin JM, Bailey WC. Medication adherence patterns in chronic obstructive pulmonary disease. *Chest* 1991; 99:837–841.
55. Stoller JK. Travel for the technology-dependent individual. *Respir Care* 1994; 39:347–362.
56. Laaban J-P, Kouchakji B, Dore M-F, Orvoen-Frija E, David P, Rochemaure J. Nutritional status of patients with chronic obstructive pulmonary disease and acute respiratory failure. *Chest* 1993; 103: 1362–1368.
57. Mohsenin V, Ferranti R, Loke JS. Nutrition for the respiratory insufficient patient. *Eur Respir J* 1989; 2(suppl):663–665.
58. Niederman MS, Merrill WW, Ferranti RD, Pagano KM, Palmer LB, Reynolds HY. Nutritional status and bacterial binding in the lower respiratory tract in patients with chronic tracheostomy. *Ann Intern Med* 1984; 100:795–800.
59. Frankfort JD, Fischer CE, Stansbury DW, McArthur DL, Brown SE, Light RW. Effects of high- and low-carbohydrate meals on maximum exercise performance in chronic airflow obstruction. *Chest* 1991; 100: 792–795.
60. Memsic L, Silberman AW, Silberman H. Malnutrition and respiratory distress: who's at risk. *J Respir Dis* 1990; 11:529–535.
61. Juan G, Calverley P, Talamo C. Effect of carbon dioxide on diaphragmatic function in human beings. *N Engl J Med* 1984; 310:874–877.
62. Whittaker JS, Ryan CR, Buckley PA, Road JD. The effects of refeeding on peripheral and respiratory muscle function in malnourished chronic obstructive pulmonary disease patients. *Am Rev Respir Dis* 1990; 142:283–288.
63. Wilson DO, Rogers RM, Openbrier D. Nutritional aspects of chronic obstructive pulmonary disease. *Clin Chest Med* 1986; 7:643–656.
64. De Blaquiere P, Christensen DB, Carter WB, Martin TR. Use and misuse of metered-dose inhalers by patients with chronic lung disease. *Am Rev Respir Dis* 1989; 140:910–916.
65. Fartinez FJ, Couser JI, Celli BR. Factors influencing ventilatory muscle recruitment in patients with chronic airflow obstruction. *Am Rev Respir Dis* 1990; 142:276–282.
66. Haas A, Pineda H, Haas F, Axen K. *Pulmonary therapy and rehabilitation: principles and practice.* Baltimore: Williams & Wilkins, 1979; 128–131.
67. Mueller RE, Petty TL, Filley GF. Ventilation and arterial blood gas changes induced by pursed-lip breathing. *J Appl Physiol* 1970; 28: 784–789.
68. Kirilloff LH, Owens GR, Rogers RM, Mazzocco MC. Does chest physical therapy work. *Chest* 1985; 88:436–444.
69. Schoni MH. Autogenic drainage: a modern approach to physiotherapy in cystic fibrosis. *J R Soc Med* 1989; 82(suppl 16):32–37.
70. Menkes HA, Traystman RJ: State of the art. Collateral ventilation. *Am Rev Respir Dis* 1977; 116:287–309.
71. Peters RM. Pulmonary physiologic studies of the perioperative period. *Chest* 1979; 76:576–584.
72. Falk M, Kelstrup M, Andersen JB, et al. Improving the ketchup bottle method with positive expiratory pressure, PEP. A controlled study in patients with cystic fibrosis. *Eur J Respir Dis* 1984; 65:57–66.

73. Hofmeyer JL, Webber BA, Hodson ME. Evaluation of positive expiratory pressure as an adjunct to chest physiotherapy in the treatment of cystic fibrosis. *Thorax* 1986; 41:951–954.
74. Mortensen J, Falk M, Groth S, Jensen C. The effects of postural drainage and positive expiratory pressure physiotherapy on tracheobronchial clearance in cystic fibrosis. *Chest* 1991; 100:1350–1357.
75. Tyrrell JC, Hiller EJ, Martin J. Face mask physiotherapy in cystic fibrosis. *Arch Dis Child* 1986; 61:598–611.
76. van Asperen PP, Jackson L, Hennessy P, Brown J. Comparison of positive expiratory pressure (PEP) mask with postural drainage in patients with cystic fibrosis. *Aust Paediatr J* 1987; 23:283–284.
77. van der Schans CP, van der Mark ThW, de Vries G, et al. Effect of positive expiratory pressure breathing in patients with cystic fibrosis. *Thorax* 1991; 46:252–256.
78. van Hengstum M, Festen J, Beurskens C, et al. The effect of positive expiratory pressure versus forced expiration technique on tracheobronchial clearance in chronic bronchitis. *Scand J Gastrenterol* 1988; 23(suppl 143):114–118.
79. Olséni L, Midgren B, Honblad Y, Wollmer P. Chest physiotherapy in chronic obstructive pulmonary disease: forced expiratory technique combined with either postural drainage or positive expiratory pressure breathing. *Respir Med* 1994; 88:435–440.
80. Schibler A, Casaulta C, Kraemer R. Rational of oscillatory breathing in patients with cystic fibrosis. *Paediatr Pulmonol* 1992; 8(suppl): 301.
81. Konstan MW, Stern RC, Doershuk CF. Efficacy of the Flutter device for airway mucus clearance in patients with cystic fibrosis. *J Pediatr* 1994; 124:689–693.
82. Pryor JA, Webber BA, Hodson ME, Warner JO. The Flutter VRP1 as an adjunct to chest physiotherapy in cystic fibrosis. *Respir Med* 1994; 88:677–681.
83. King M, Phillips DM, Gross D, Vartian V, Chang HK, Zidulka A. Enhanced tracheal mucus clearance with high frequency chest wall compression. *Am Rev Respir Dis* 1983; 128:511–515.
84. Radford R, Barutt J, Billingsley JG, Hill W, Lawson WH, Willich W. A rational basis for percussion augmented mucociliary clearance. *Respir Care* 1982; 27:556–563.
85. Rubin EM, Scantlen GE, Chapman GA, Eldridge M, Menendez R, Wanner A. Effect of chest wall oscillation on mucus clearance: comparison of two vibrators. *Pediatr Pulmonol* 1989; 6:123–127.
86. Flower KA, Eden RI, Lomax L, Mann NM, Burgess J. New mechanical aid to physiotherapy in cystic fibrosis. *Br Med J* 1979; 2:630–631.
87. Chang HK, Weber ME, King M. Mucus transport by high frequency nonsymmetrical airflow. *J Appl Physiol* 1988; 65:1203–1209.
88. Warwick WJ, Hansen LG. The long-term effect of high-frequency chest compression therapy on pulmonary complications of cystic fibrosis. *Pediatr Pulmonol* 1991; 11:265–271.
89. Christensen EF, Nedergaard, Dahl R. Long-term treatment of chronic bronchitis with positive expiratory pressure mask and chest physiotherapy. *Chest* 1990; 97:645–650.
90. Holody B, Goldberg HS. The effect of mechanical vibration physiotherapy on arterial oxygenation in acutely ill patients with atelectasis or pneumonia. *Am Rev Respir Dis* 1981; 124:372–375.
91. Piquet J, Brochard L, Isabey D, et al. High frequency chest wall oscillation in patients with chronic air-flow obstruction. *Am Rev Respir Dis* 1987; 136:1355–1359.
92. Sibuya M, Yamada M, Kanamaru A, et al. Effect of chest wall vibration on dyspnea in patients with chronic respiratory disease. *Am J Respir Crit Care Med* 1994; 149:1235–1240.
93. Pryor JA, Parker RA, Webber BA. A comparison of mechanical and manual percussion as adjuncts to postural drainage in the treatment of cystic fibrosis in adolescents and adults. *Physiotherapy* 1981; 6: 140–141.
94. Sutton PP, Parker RA, Webber BA, et al. Assessment of the forced expiration technique, postural drainage and directed coughing in chest physiotherapy. *Eur J Respir Dis* 1983; 64:62–68.
95. van Hengstum M, Festen J, Beurskens C, Hankel M, van den Broek W, Corstens F. No effect of oral high frequency oscillation combined with forced expiration maneuvers on tracheobronchial clearance in chronic bronchitis. *Eur Respir J* 1990; 3:14–18.
96. van der Schans CP, Piers DA, Postma DS. Effect of manual percussion on tracheobronchial clearance in patients with chronic airflow obstruction and excessive tracheobronchial secretions. *Thorax* 1986; 41: 448–452.
97. Campbell AH, O'Connell JM, Wilson F. The effect of chest physiotherapy upon the FEV1 in chronic bronchitis. *Med J Aust* 1975; 1: 33–35.
98. Zapletal A, Stefanova J, Horak J, Vavrova V, Samanek M. Chest physiotherapy and airway obstruction in patients with cystic fibrosis—a negative report. Eur J Respir Dis 1983; 64:426–433.
99. Zidulka A, Chrome JF, Wight DW, Burnett S, Bonnier L, Fraser R. Clapping or percussion causes atelectasis in dogs and influences gas exchange. *J Appl Physiol* 1989; 66:2833–2838.
100. Toussaint M, De Win H, Steens M, Soudon P. A new technique in secretion clearance by the percussionaire for patients with neuromuscular disease [Abstract]. In: *Programme des Journes Internationales de Ventilation Domicile.* Lyon, France: Hopital de la Croix Rousse, 1993; 27.
101. Thangathuria D, Holm AP, Mikhail M, Fox D, Escajeda D, Pancho L. HFV in management of a patient with severe bronchorrhea. *Respir Management* 1988; 1:31–33.
102. McInturff SL, Shaw LI, Hodgkin JE, Rumble L, Bird FM. Intrapulmonary percussive ventilation in the treatment of COPD. *Respir Care* 1985; 30:885.
103. Passy V. Passy-Muir tracheostomy speaking valve. *Otolaryngol Head Neck Surg* 1986; 95:247–248.
104. Cinel D, Markwell K, Lee R, Szidon P. Variability of the respiratory gas exchange ratio during arterial puncture. *Am Rev Respir Dis* 1991; 143:217–218.
105. Siegel IM. Update on Duchenne muscular dystrophy. *Compr Ther* 1989; 15:45–52.
106. Bach JR, Alba AS. Tracheostomy ventilation: a study of efficacy with deflated cuffs and cuffless tubes. *Chest* 1990; 97:679–683.
107. Barach AL, Beck GJ. Exsufflation with negative pressure: physiologic and clinical studies in poliomyelitis, bronchial asthma, pulmonary emphysema and bronchiectasis. *Arch Intern Med* 1954; 93:25–41.
108. Barach AL. The application of pressure, including exsufflation, in pulmonary emphysema. *Am J Surg* 1955; 89:372–382.
109. Pardy RL, Reid WD, Belman MJ. Respiratory muscle training. *Clin Chest Med* 1989; 9:287–295.
110. Belman MJ. Exercise in chronic obstructive pulmonary disease. *Clin Chest Med* 1986; 7:585–597.
111. Levine S, Weiser P, Gillen J. Evaluation of a ventilatory muscle endurance training program in the rehabilitation of patients with chronic obstructive pulmonary disease. *Am Rev Respir Dis* 1986; 133: 400–406.
112. Ries AL, Moser KM. Comparison of isocapnic hyperventilation and walking exercise training at home in pulmonary rehabilitation. *Chest* 1986; 90:285–289.
113. Aldrich TK. Inspiratory muscle training in COPD. In: Bach JR, ed. *Pulmonary rehabilitation: the obstructive and paralytic conditions.* Philadelphia: Hanley & Belfus, 1996; 285–301.
114. Weiner P, Azgad Y, Ganam R. Inspiratory muscle training combined with general exercise reconditioning in patients with COPD. *Chest* 1992; 102:1351–1356.
115. Pardy RL, Rivington RM, Despas PJ, Macklem PT. Effects of inspiratory muscle training on exercise performance in chronic airflow limitation. *Am Rev Respir Dis* 1981; 123:426–433.
116. Sawyer EH, Clanton TL. Improved pulmonary function and exercise tolerance with inspiratory muscle conditioning in children with cystic fibrosis. *Chest* 1993; 104:490–497.
117. Weiner P, Azgad Y, Weiner M. Inspiratory muscle training during treatment with corticosteroids in humans. *Chest* 1995; 107: 1041–1044.
118. Weiner P, Azgad Y, Ganam R, Weiner M. Inspiratory muscle training in patients with bronchial asthma. *Chest* 1992; 102:1357–1361.
119. Braun NMT, Faulkner J, Hughes RL, et al. When should respiratory muscles be exercised. *Chest* 1983; 84:76–83.
120. Hudson LD. Immediate and long term sequelae of ARF. *Respir Care* 1983; 28:663–667.
121. Petty TL. *Intensive and rehabilitative respiratory care,* 3rd ed. Philadelphia: Lea & Febiger, 1982; 238.
122. Vanderbergh E, van de Woestijne KP, Gyseline A. Conservative treatment of ARF in patients with COLD. *Am Rev Respir Dis* 1968; 98: 60–69.
123. Braun NMT, Marino WD. Effect of daily intermittent rest on respiratory muscles in patients with chronic airflow limitation. *Chest* 1984; 85:595–605.

124. Cropp A, Dimarco AF. Effects of intermittent negative pressure ventilation on respiratory muscle function in patients with severe chronic obstructive pulmonary disease. *Am Rev Respir Dis* 1987; 135: 1056–1061.
125. Gutierrez M, Beroiza T, Contreras G, et al. Weekly cuirass ventilation improves blood gases and inspiratory muscle strength in patients with chronic air-flow limitation and hypercarbia. *Am Rev Respir Dis* 1988; 138:617–623.
126. Nava S, Ambrosino N, Zocchi L, Rampulla C. Diaphragmatic rest during negative pressure ventilation by pneumowrap: assessment in normal and COPD patients. *Chest* 1990; 98:857–865.
127. Scano G, Gigliotti F, Duranti R, Spinelli A, Gorini M, Schiavina M. Changes in ventilatory muscle function with negative pressure ventilation in patients with severe COPD. *Chest* 1990; 97:322–327.
128. Sauret JM, Guitart AC, Rodriguez-Frojan G, Cornudella R. Intermittent short-term negative pressure ventilation and increased oxygenation in COPD patients with severe hypercapnic respiratory failure. *Chest* 1991; 100:455–459.
129. Rochester D, Martin LL. Respiratory muscle rest. In: Roussos C, Macklem B, eds. *The thorax*. New York: Marcel Dekker, 1985; 1303–1328.
130. Shapiro SH, Ernst P, Gray-Donald K. Effect of negative pressure ventilation in severe chronic obstructive pulmonary disease. *Lancet* 1992; 340:1425–1429.
131. Bach JR, Penek J. Obstructive sleep apnea complicating negative pressure ventilatory support in patients with chronic paralytic/restrictive ventilatory dysfunction. *Chest* 1991; 99:1386–1393.
132. Levy RD, Bradley TD, Newman SL, Macklem PT, Martin JG. Negative pressure ventilation: effects on ventilation during sleep in normal subjects. *Chest* 1989; 65:95–99.
133. Mezzanotte WS, Tangel DJ, Fox AM, Ballard RD, White DP. Nocturnal nasal continuous positive airway pressure in patients with chronic obstructive pulmonary disease: influence on waking respiratory muscle function. *Chest* 1994; 106:1100–1108.
134. Belman MJ, Soo Hoo GW, Kuei JH, Shadmehr R. Efficacy of positive vs negative pressure ventilation in unloading the respiratory muscles. *Chest* 1990; 98:850–856.
135. Marino W. Intermittent volume cycled mechanical ventilation via nasal mask in patients with respiratory failure due to COPD. *Chest* 1991; 99:681–684.
136. Meduri GU, Abou-Shala N, Fox RC, Jones CB, Leeper KV, Wunderink RG. Noninvasive face mask mechanical ventilation in patients with acute hypercapnic respiratory failure. *Chest* 1991; 100:445–454.
137. Anthonisen NR. Home oxygen therapy in chronic obstructive pulmonary disease. *Clin Chest Med* 1986; 7:673–677.
138. Nixon PA, Orenstein DM, Curtis SE, Ross EA. Oxygen supplementation during exercise in cystic fibrosis. *Am Rev Respir Dis* 1990; 142: 807–811.
139. Pierson DJ. Current status of home oxygen in the U.S.A. In: Kira S, Petty TL, eds. *Progress in domiciliary respiratory care—current status and perspective*. New York: Elsevier Science, 1994; 93–98.
140. Sassoon CSH, Hassell KT, Mahutte CK. Hyperoxic-induced hypercapnia in stable chronic obstructive pulmonary disease. *Am Rev Respir Dis* 1987; 135:907–911.
141. D'Urzo AD, Mateika J, Bradley TD, Li D, Contreras MA, Goldstein RS. Correlates of arterial oxygenation during exercise in severe chronic obstructive pulmonary disease. *Chest* 1989; 95:13–17.
142. Dean NC, Brown JK, Himelman RB, Doherty JJ, Gold WM, Stulbarg MS. Oxygen may improve dyspnea and endurance in patients with chronic obstructive pulmonary disease and only mild hypoxemia. *Am Rev Respir Dis* 1992; 146:941–945.
143. Bradley BL, Garner AE, Billiu D, Mestas JM, Forma J. Oxygen assisted exercise in chronic obstructive lung disease: the effect on exercise capacity and arterial blood gas tensions. *Am Rev Respir Dis* 1978; 118:239–243.
144. Davidson AC, Leach R, George RJD, Geddes DM. Supplemental oxygen and exercise ability in chronic obstructive airways disease. *Thorax* 1988; 43:965–971.
145. Marcus CL, Bader D, Stabile MW, Wang CI, Osher AB, Keens TG. Supplemental oxygen and exercise performance in patients with cystic fibrosis with severe pulmonary disease. *Chest* 1992; 101:52–57.
146. O'Donohue WJ. The future of home oxygen therapy. *Respir Care* 1988; 33:1125–1130.
147. Tiep BL, Christopher KL, Spofford BT, Goodman JR, Worley PD, Macy SL. Pulsed nasal and transtracheal oxygen delivery. *Chest* 1990; 97:364–368.
148. Dantzker DR, D'Alonzo GE. The effect of exercise on pulmonary gas exchange in patients with severe chronic obstructive pulmonary disease. *Am Rev Respir Dis* 1986; 134:1135–1139.
149. Smith PEM, Coakley JH, Edwards RHT. Respiratory muscle training in Duchenne muscular dystrophy [Letter]. *Muscle Nerve* 1988; 11: 784–785.
150. Niederman MS, Clemente PH, Fein AM, et al. Benefits of a multidisciplinary pulmonary rehabilitation program: improvements are independent of lung function. *Chest* 1991; 99:798–804.
151. Belman M, Kendregan BA. Exercise training fails to increase skeletal muscle enzymes in patients with chronic obstructive pulmonary disease. *Am Rev Respir Dis* 1981; 36:256–261.
152. Celli B, Gotlief S. Biofeedback and upper extremity exercise in COPD. In: Bach JR, ed. *Pulmonary rehabilitation: the obstructive and paralytic/restrictive pulmonary syndromes*. Philadelphia: Hanley & Belfus, 1996; 285–301.
153. Martinez FJ, Vogel PD, Dupont DN, Stanopoulos I, Gray A, Beamis JF. Supported arm exercise vs. unsupported arm exercise in the rehabilitation of patients with severe chronic airflow obstruction. *Chest* 1993; 103:1397–1402.
154. Couser J, Martinez F, Celli BR. Pulmonary rehabilitation that includes arm exercise reduces metabolic and ventilatory requirements for simple arm elevation. *Chest* 1993; 103:37–41.
155. Lake FR, Herndersen K, Briffa T. Upper limb and lower limb exercise training in patients with chronic airflow obstruction. *Chest* 1990; 97: 1077–1082.
156. Make BJ, Glenn K. Outcomes of pulmonary rehabilitation. In: Bach JR, ed. *Pulmonary rehabilitation: the obstructive and paralytic/restrictive pulmonary syndromes*. Philadelphia: Hanley & Belfus, 1996; 173–191.
157. Foster S, Lopez D, Thomas HM. Pulmonary rehabilitation in COPD patients with elevated pCO_2. *Am Rev Respir Dis* 1988; 138: 1519–1523.
158. Ries AL, Kaplan RM, Limberg TM, Prewitt LM. Effects of pulmonary rehabilitation on physiologic and psychosocial outcomes in patients with chronic obstructive pulmonary disease. *Ann Intern Med* 1995; 122:823–832.
159. Casaburi R, Patessio A, Ioli F, Zanaboni S, Donner CF, Wasserman K. Reductions in exercise lactic acidosis and ventilation as a result of exercise training in patients with obstructive lung disease. *Am Rev Respir Dis* 1991; 143:9–18.
160. Wijkstra PJ, TenVergert EM, van Altena R, et al. Long term benefits of rehabilitation at home on quality of life and exercise tolerance in patients with chronic obstructive pulmonary disease. *Thorax* 1995; 50:824–828.
161. Tydeman DE, Chandler AR, Graveling BM, Culot A, Harrison BDW. An investigation into the effects of exercise tolerance training of patients with chronic airways obstruction. *Physiotherapy* 1984; 70: 261–264.
162. de Jong W, Grevink RG, Roorda RJ, Kaptein AA, van der Schans CP. Effect of a home exercise training program in patients with cystic fibrosis. *Chest* 1994; 105:463–468.
163. Roselle S, D'Amico FJ. The effect of home respiratory therapy on hospital re-admission rates of patients with chronic obstructive pulmonary disease. *Respir Care* 1990; 35:1208–1213.
164. Holle RHO, Williams DV, Vandree JC, Starks GL, Schoene RB. Increased muscle efficiency and sustained benefits in an outpatient community hospital-based pulmonary rehabilitation program. *Chest* 1988; 94:1161–1168.
165. Ilowite J, Niederman M, Fein A, Feinsilver S, Kivana G, Bernstein M. Can benefits seen in pulmonary rehabilitation be sustained long term? *Chest* 1991; 100:182.
166. Mall RW, Medieros M. Objective evaluation of results of a pulmonary rehabilitation program in a community hospital. *Chest* 1988; 94: 1156–1160.
167. Vale F, Reardon J, ZuWallack R. Is improvement sustained following pulmonary rehabilitation? *Chest* 1991; 100(suppl):56.
168. Grippi MA, Metzger LF, Krupinski AV, Fishman AP. Pulmonary function testing. In: Fishman AP, ed. *Pulmonary diseases and disorders*. New York: McGraw-Hill, 1988; 2469–2521.
169. Braun NMT, Arora NS, Rochester DF. Respiratory muscle and pulmo-

nary function in polymyositis and other proximal myopathies. *Thorax* 1983; 38:616–623.
170. Bach JR. Pulmonary assessment and management of the aging and older patient. In: Felsenthal G, Garrison SJ, Steinberg FU, eds. *Rehabilitation of the aging and elderly patient.* Baltimore: Williams & Wilkins, 1993; 263–273.
171. Bach JR, Alba AS. Management of chronic alveolar hypoventilation by nasal ventilation. *Chest* 1990; 97:52–57.
172. Delaubier A, Guillou C, Renardel A. Prolongation de la duree de vie: prise en charge de l'insuffisance respiratoire. *Cah Kinesiother* 1988; 133:64–72.
173. Bach J, Alba A, Pilkington LA, Lee M. Long-term rehabilitation in advanced stage of childhood onset, rapidly progressive muscular dystrophy. *Arch Phys Med Rehabil* 1981; 62:328–331.
174. Bach JR, Alba AS, Bohatiuk G, Saporito L, Lee M. Mouth intermittent positive pressure ventilation in the management of post-polio respiratory insufficiency. *Chest* 1987; 91:859–864.
175. Miller WF. Rehabilitation of patients with chronic obstructive lung disease. *Med Clin North Am* 1967; 51:349–361.
176. De Troyer A, Deisser P. The effects of intermittent positive pressure breathing on patients with respiratory muscle weakness. *Am Rev Respir Dis* 1981; 124:132–137.
177. De Troyer A, Borenstein S, Cordier R. Analysis of lung volume restriction in patients with respiratory muscle weakness. *Thorax* 1980; 35:603–610.
178. Gibson GJ, Pride NB, Newsom-Davis J, Loh LC. Pulmonary mechanics in patients with respiratory muscle weakness. *Am Rev Respir Dis* 1977; 115:389–395.
179. Estenne M, De Troyer A. The effects of tetraplegia on chest wall statics. *Am Rev Respir Dis* 1986; 134:121–124.
180. Redding GJ, Okamoto GA, Guthrie RD, Rollevson D, Milstein JM. Sleep patterns in nonambulatory boys with Duchenne muscular dystrophy. *Arch Phys Med Rehabil* 1985; 66:818–821.
181. Shneerson J. *Disorders of ventilation.* Boston: Blackwell Scientific, 1988; 43.
182. Smith PEM, Edwards RHT, Calverley PMA. Ventilation and breathing pattern during sleep in Duchenne muscular dystrophy. *Chest* 1989; 96:1346–1351.
183. Soudon P. Ventilation assistee au long cours dans les maladies neuromusculaire: exprience actuelle. *Readaptation Revalidatie* 1987; 3: 45–65.
184. Canny GJ, Szeinberg A, Koreska J, Levison H. Hypercapnia in relation to pulmonary function in Duchenne muscular dystrophy. *Pediatr Pulmonol* 1989; 6:169–171.
185. Ohtake S. Nocturnal blood gas disturbances and treatment of patients with Duchenne muscular dystrophy. *Kokyu To Junkan* 1990; 38: 463–469.
186. Griggs RG, Donohoe KM, Utell MJ, Goldblatt D, Moxley TR. Evaluation of pulmonary function in neuromuscular disease. *Arch Neurol* 1981; 38:9–12.
187. Alvarez SE, Peterson M, Lunsford BR. Respiratory treatment of the adult patient with spinal cord injury. *Phys Ther* 1981; 61:1737–1745.
188. Bach JR. Pulmonary rehabilitation considerations for Duchenne muscular dystrophy: the prolongation of life by respiratory muscle aids. *Crit Rev Phys Rehabil Med* 1992; 3:239–269.
189. Bach JR. Amyotrophic lateral sclerosis: predictors for prolongation of life by noninvasive respiratory aids. *Arch Phys Med Rehabil* 1995; 76:828–832.
190. Bach JR, Saporito LR. Indications and criteria for decannulation and transition from invasive to noninvasive long-term ventilatory support. *Respir Care* 1994; 39:515–531.
191. Welch JR, DeCesare R, Hess D. Pulse oximetry: instrumentation and clinical applications. *Respir Care* 1990; 35:584–594.
192. Williams AJ, Yu G, Santiago S, Stein M. Screening for sleep apnea using pulse oximetry and a clinical score. *Chest* 1991; 100:631–635.
193. Centers for Disease Control. Recommendations for the prevention and control of influenza. *Ann Intern Med* 1986; 105:399–404.
194. Centers for Disease Control. Update: Pneumococcal polysaccharide vaccine usage—United States. *Ann Intern Med* 1984; 101:348–350.
195. McDonald B, Rosenthal SA. Hypokalemia complicating Duchenne muscular dystrophy. *Yale J Biol Med* 1987; 60:405–408.
196. Bach JR. Pulmonary rehabilitation. In: DeLisa JD, ed. *Rehabilitation medicine: principles and practice.* Philadelphia: JB Lippincott, 1993; 952–972.
197. Brooke MH. *A clinician's view of neuromuscular diseases,* 2nd ed. Baltimore: Williams & Wilkins, 1986; 117.
198. Smith PEM, Edwards RHT, Calverley PMA. Oxygen treatment of sleep hypoxaemia in Duchenne muscular dystrophy. *Thorax* 1989; 44:997–1001.
199. DiMarco AF, Kelling JS, DiMarco MS, Jacobs I, Shields R, Altose MD. The effects of inspiratory resistive training on respiratory muscle function in patients with muscular dystrophy. *Muscle Nerve* 1985:8: 284–290.
200. Martin AJ, Stern L, Yeates J, Lepp D, Little J. Respiratory muscle training in Duchenne muscular dystrophy. *Dev Med Child Neurol* 1986; 28:314–318.
201. Rodillo E, Noble-Jamieson CM, Aber V, Heckmatt JZ, Muntoni F, Dubowitz. Respiratory muscle training in Duchenne muscular dystrophy. *Arch Dis Child* 1989; 64:736–738.
202. Schiffman PL, Belsh JM. Effect of inspiratory resistance and theophylline on respiratory muscle strength in patients with amyotrophic lateral sclerosis. *Am Rev Respir Dis* 1989; 139:1418–1423.
203. Aldrich JK, Karpel JP, Uhrlass RM, Sparapani MA, Eramo D, Ferranti R. Weaning from mechanical ventilation: adjunctive use of inspiratory muscle resistive training. *Crit Care Med* 1989; 17:143–147.
204. Barois A, Bataille J, Estournet B. La ventilation a domicile par voie buccale chez l'enfant dans les maladies neuromusculaires. *Agressologie* 1985; 26:645–649.
205. Barois A, Estournet B, Duval-Beaupere G, Bataille J, Leclair-Richard D. Amyotrophie spinale infantile. *Rev Neurol (Paris)* 1989; 145: 299–304.
206. Bach JR. Update and perspectives on noninvasive respiratory muscle aids: part 1—the inspiratory muscle aids. *Chest* 1994; 105: 1230–1240.
207. Egberg LD, Laver MB, Bendixen HH. Intermittent deep breaths and compliance during anesthesia in man. *Anesthesiology* 1963:24:57–59.
208. Mead J, Collier C. Relation of volume history of lungs to respiratory mechanics in anesthetized dogs. *J Appl Physiol* 1959; 14:669–678.
209. O'Donohue W. Maximum volume IPPB for the management of pulmonary atelectasis. *Chest* 1976; 76:683–687.
210. McCool FD, Mayewski RF, Shayne DS, Gibson CJ, Griggs RC, Hyde RW. Intermittent positive pressure breathing in patients with respiratory muscle weakness: alterations in total respiratory system compliance. *Chest* 1986; 90:546–552.
211. Adams MA, Chandler LS. Effects of physical therapy program on vital capacity of patients with muscular dystrophy. *Phys Ther* 1974; 54:494–496.
212. Houser CR, Johnson DM. Breathing exercises for children with pseudohypertrophic muscular dystrophy. *Phys Ther* 1971; 51:751–759.
213. Huldtgren AC, Fugl-Meyer AR, Jonasson E, Bake B. Ventilatory dysfunction and respiratory rehabilitation in post-traumatic quadriplegia. *Eur J Respir Dis* 1980; 61:347–356.
214. Dail CW, Affeldt JE. *Glossopharyngeal breathing* (video). Los Angeles: Los Angeles Department of Visual Education, College of Medical Evangelists, 1954.
215. Bach JR, Alba AS, Bodofsky E, Curran FJ, Schultheiss M. Glossopharyngeal breathing and non-invasive aids in the management of post-polio respiratory insufficiency. *Birth Defects* 1987; 23:99–113.
216. Baydur A, Gilgoff I, Prentice W, Carlson M, Fischer A. Decline in respiratory function and experience with long-term assisted ventilation in advanced Duchenne's muscular dystrophy. *Chest* 1990; 97: 884–889.
217. Fishburn MJ, Marino RJ, Ditunno JF Jr. Atelectasis and pneumonia in acute spinal cord injury. *Arch Phys Med Rehabil* 1990; 71:197–200.
218. Leonard C, Criner GJ. Swallowing function in patients with tracheostomy receiving prolonged mechanical ventilation. In: *International Conference on Pulmonary Rehabilitation and Home Ventilation Abstracts.* Denver, CO, 1991; 58.
219. Graham WGB, Bradley DA. Efficacy of chest physiotherapy and intermittent positive-pressure breathing in the resolution of pneumonia. *N Engl J Med* 1978; 299:624–627.
220. Make B. Pulmonary rehabilitation: myth or reality? *Clin Chest Med* 1986; 7:519–540.
221. Massery M. Manual breathing and coughing aids. *Phys Med Rehabil Clin North Am* 1996; 7:407–422.
222. Bach JR. Update and perspectives on noninvasive respiratory muscle aids: part 2—the expiratory muscle aids. *Chest* 1994; 105:1538–1544.
223. Bach JR, O'Brien J, Krotenberg R, Alba A. Management of end stage

respiratory failure in Duchenne muscular dystrophy. *Muscle Nerve* 1987; 10:177–182.

224. Bach JR, Alba AS. Noninvasive options for ventilatory support of the traumatic high level quadriplegic. *Chest* 1990; 98:613–619.
225. Barach AL, Beck GJ, Bickerman HA, Seanor HE. Physical methods simulating cough mechanisms. *JAMA* 1952; 150:1380–1385.
226. Barach AL, Beck GJ, Smith RH. Mechanical production of expiratory flow rates surpassing the capacity of human coughing. *Am J Med Sci* 1953; 226:241–248.
227. Barach AL, Beck GJ. Exsufflation with negative pressure: physiological studies in poliomyelitis, bronchial asthma, pulmonary emphysema, and bronchiectasis. *Arch Intern Med* 1954; 93:825–841.
228. Curran FJ, Colbert AP. Ventilator management in Duchenne muscular dystrophy and postpoliomyelitis syndrome: twelve years' experience. *Arch Phys Med Rehabil* 1989:70; 180–185.
229. Bach JR, Alba AS. Total ventilatory support by the intermittent abdominal pressure ventilator. *Chest* 1991; 99:630–636.
230. Bach JR, Zaniewski R, Lee H. Cardiac arrhythmias from a malpositioned Greenfield filter in a traumatic quadriplegic. *Am J Phys Med Rehabil* 1990; 69:251–253.
231. Bockenek W, Bach JR, Alba AS, Cravioto A. Cartilagenous emboli to the spinal cord: a case study. *Arch Phys Med Rehabil* 1990; 71: 754–757.
232. Leger P, Jennequin J, Gerard M, Robert D. Home positive pressure ventilation via nasal mask for patients with neuromuscular weakness or restrictive lung or chest-wall disease. *Respir Care* 1989; 34:73–79.
233. Viroslav J, Sortor S, Rosenblatt R. Alternatives to tracheostomy ventilation in high level SCI [Abstract]. *J Am Paraplegia Soc* 1991; 14: 87.
234. Carroll N, Branthwaite MA. Control of nocturnal hypoventilation by nasal intermittent positive pressure ventilation. *Thorax* 1988; 43: 349–353.
235. Ellis ER, Bye PTP, Bruderer JW, Sullivan CE. Treatment of respiratory failure during sleep in patients with neuromuscular disease, positive-pressure ventilation through a nose mask. *Am Rev Respir Dis* 1987; 135:148–152.
236. Kerby GR, Mayer LS, Pingleton SK. Nocturnal positive pressure ventilation via nasal mask. *Am Rev Respir Dis* 1987; 135:738–740.
237. Bach JR, McDermott I. Strapless oral-nasal interfaces for positive pressure ventilation. *Arch Phys Med Rehabil* 1990; 71:908–911.
238. Ratzka A. Uberdruckbeatmung durch Mundstuck. In: Frehse U, ed. *Spatfolgen nach Poliomyelitis: Chronische Unterbeatmung und Moglichkeiten selbstbestimmter Lebensfuhrung Schwerbehinderter.* Munich: Pfennigparade eV, 1989; 149.
239. Blitzer B. *Directory of sources for ventilation face masks.* St. Louis: Gazette International Networking Institute Press, 1991.
240. Bach JR, Robert D, Leger P, Langevin B. Sleep fragmentation in kyphoscoliotic individuals with alveolar hypoventilation treated by nasal IPPV. *Chest* 1995; 107:1552–1558.
241. Goldstein RS, Avendano MA. Long-term mechanical ventilation as elective therapy: clinical status and future prospects. *Respir Care* 1991; 36:297–304.
242. Bach JR. A historical perspective on the use of noninvasive ventilatory support alternatives. *Respir Clin North Am* 1996; 2:161–181.
243. Bach JR. Alternative methods of ventilatory support for the patient with ventilatory failure due to spinal cord injury. *J Am Paraplegia Soc* 1991; 14:158–174.
244. Bach JR, Alba AS, Mosher R, Delaubier A. Intermittent positive pressure ventilation via nasal access in the management of respiratory insufficiency. *Chest* 1987; 92:168–170.
245. Bach JR. Conventional approaches to managing neuromuscular ventilatory failure. In: Bach JR, ed. *Pulmonary rehabilitation: the obstructive and paralytic conditions.* Philadelphia: Hanley & Belfus, 1996; 285–301.
246. Bach JR. Prevention of morbidity and mortality with the use of physical medicine aids. In: Bach JR, ed. *Pulmonary rehabilitation: the obstructive and paralytic conditions.* Philadelphia: Hanley & Belfus, 1996; 303–329.
247. Milane J, Bertrand P, Montredon C, Jonquet O, Bertrand A. Intérêt de l'assistance ventilatoire abdomino-diaphragmatique dans la réadaptation des grands handicapés respiratoires. *Actualités Rééducation Fonctionnelle Réadaptation* 1990; 1:71–76.
248. Miller HJ, Thomas E, Wilmot CB. Pneumobelt use among high quadriplegic population. *Arch Phys Med Rehabil* 1988; 69:369–372.
249. Goldstein RS, Molotiu N, Skrastins R, Long S, Contreras M. Assisting ventilation in respiratory failure by negative pressure ventilation and by rocking bed. *Chest* 1987; 92:470–474.
250. Bach JR, Bardach JL. Neuromuscular diseases. In: Sipski ML, Alexander CJ, eds. *Sexual function in people with disability and chronic illness: a health practitioner's guide.* Gaithersburg, MD: Aspen, 1997; 147–160.
251. Lombard R Jr, Zwillich CW. Medical therapy of obstructive sleep apnea. *Med Clin North Am* 1985; 69:1317–1335.
252. Waldhorn RE, Herrick TW, Nguyen MC, O'Donnell AE, Sodero J, Potolicchio SJ. Long-term compliance with nasal continuous positive airway pressure therapy of obstructive sleep apnea. *Chest* 1990; 97: 33–38.
253. Clark GT, Nakano M. Dental appliances for the treatment of obstructive sleep apnea. *J Am Dent Assoc* 1989; 118:611–619.
254. Katsantonis GP, Walsh JK, Schweitzer PK, Friedman WH. Further evaluation of uvulopalatopharyngoplasty in the treatment of obstructive sleep apnea syndrome. *Otolaryngol Head Neck Surg* 1985; 93: 244–250.
255. Riley RW, Powell NB, Guilleminault C, Mino-Murcia G. Maxillary, mandibular, and hyoid advancement: an alternative to tracheostomy in obstructive sleep apnea syndrome. *Otolaryngol Head Neck Surg* 1986; 94:584–588.
256. Thawley SE. Surgical treatment of obstructive sleep apnea. *Med Clin North Am* 1985; 69:1337–1358.
257. Bach JR, Saporito LR. Criteria for extubation and tracheostomy tube removal for patients with ventilatory failure: a different approach to weaning. *Chest* 1996; 110: 1566–1571.
258. Bach JR, Rajaraman R, Ballanger F, Tzeng AC, Ishikawa Y, Kulessa R, Bansal T. Neuromuscular ventilatory insufficiency: the effect of home mechanical ventilator use vs. oxygen therapy on pneumonia and hospitalization rates. *Am J Phys Med Rehabil* 1998; 77:8–19.
259. Baer GA, Talonen PP, Hakkinen V, Exner G, Yrjola H. Phrenic nerve stimulation in tetraplegia. *Scand J Rehabil Med* 1990; 22:107–111.
260. Baer GA, Talonen PP, Shneerson JM, Markkula H, Exner G, Wells FC. Phrenic nerve stimulation for central ventilatory failure with bipolar and four-pole electrode systems. *PACE* 1990; 13:1061–1072.
261. Bach JR, O'Connor K. Electrophrenic ventilation: a different perspective. *J Am Paraplegia Soc* 1991; 14:9–17.
262. Bach JR. New approaches in the rehabilitation of the traumatic high level quadriplegic. *Am J Phys Med Rehabil* 1991; 70:13–20.
263. Viroslav J, Rosenblatt R, Morris-Tomazevic S. Respiratory management, survival, and quality of life for high-level traumatic tetraplegics. *Respir Care Clin North Am* 1996; 2:313–322.
264. Moxham J, Shneerson JM. Diaphragmatic pacing. *Am Rev Respir Dis* 1993; 148:533–536.
265. Creasey G, Elefteriades J, DiMarco A, et al. Electrical stimulation to restore respiration. *J Rehabil Res Develop* 1996; 33:123–312.
266. Chervin RD, Guilleminault C. Diaphragm pacing: review and reassessment. *Sleep* 1994; 17:176–187.
267. Bach JR. Inappropriate weaning and late onset ventilatory failure of individuals with traumatic quadriplegia. *Paraplegia* 1993; 31: 430–438.
268. Bach JR. A comparison of long-term ventilatory support alternatives from the perspective of the patient and care giver. *Chest* 1993; 104: 1702–1706.
269. Purtilo RB. Ethical Issues in the treatment of chronic ventilator-dependent patients. *Arch Phys Med Rehabil* 1986; 67:718–721.
270. Dracup K, Raffin T. Withholding and withdrawing mechanical ventilation: assessing quality of life. *Am Rev Respir Dis* 1989; 140: S44–S46.
271. Bach JR, Barnett V. Psychosocial, vocational, quality of life and ethical issues. In: Bach JR, ed. *Pulmonary rehabilitation: the obstructive and paralytic conditions.* Philadelphia: Hanley & Belfus, 1996; 395–411.
272. Jonsen R, Siegler M, Winslade WJ. *Clinical ethics: a practical approach to ethical decisions in clinical medicine.* New York: Macmillan, 1982.
273. Bach JR. The role of the physiatrist in the management of neuromuscular disease. *Am J Phys Med Rehabil* 1996; 75:239–241.
274. Starkloff M. Disabled and despondent. *Rehabil Gazette* 1993; 33:7–8.

Rehabilitation Medicine: Principles and Practice, Third Edition,
edited by Joel A. DeLisa and Bruce M. Gans.
Lippincott–Raven Publishers, Philadelphia © 1998.

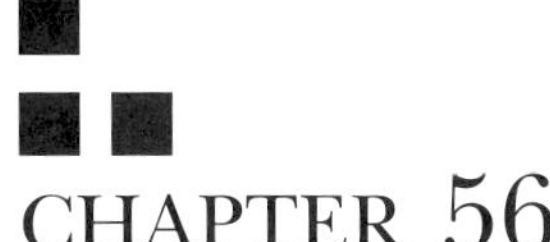

CHAPTER 56

Treatment of the Patient with Chronic Pain

Nicolas E. Walsh, Daniel Dumitru, Lawrence S. Schoenfeld, and Somayaji Ramamurthy

Pain is purely subjective, difficult to define, and often difficult to describe or interpret. It is currently defined as an unpleasant sensory and emotional response to a stimulus associated with actual or potential tissue damage (1,2). However, pain has never been shown to be a simple function of the amount of physical injury; it is extensively influenced by anxiety, depression, expectation, and other psychological variables. It is a multifaceted experience, an interweaving of the physical characteristics of the stimulus with the motivational, affective, and cognitive functions of the individual. The result is behavior based on an interpretation of the event, influenced by present and past experiences.

Acute pain is a biologic symptom of an apparent nociceptive stimulus, such as tissue damage due to disease or trauma. The pain may be highly localized and may radiate. It is generally sharp and persists only as long as the tissue pathology itself persists. Acute pain is generally self-limiting, and as the nociceptive stimulus lessens, the pain decreases. Acute pain usually lasts less than 3 months (2). If it is not effectively treated, it may progress to a chronic form.

Chronic pain is a disease process. Differing significantly from acute pain, it is defined as pain lasting longer than the usual course of an acute disease or injury. The pain may be associated with continued pathology or may persist after recovery from a disease or injury. As with acute pain, treatable chronic pain due to organic disease is managed by effectively treating the underlying disorder. Chronic pain is often poorly localized and tends to be dull, aching, and constant. The associated signs of autonomic nervous system response may be absent, and the patient may appear exhausted, listless, depressed, and withdrawn.

Proper management of pain requires an understanding of its complexity and a knowledge of the non-neurologic factors that determine its individual expression. The treatment of pain with physical modalities is as ancient as the history of humanity, but the use of interdisciplinary rehabilitation techniques has gained acceptance only within the past few decades.

N. E. Walsh and D. Dumitru: Department of Rehabilitation Medicine, University of Texas Health Science Center at San Antonio, San Antonio, Texas 78284-7798.

L. S. Schoenfeld: Department of Psychiatry, University of Texas Health Science Center at San Antonio, San Antonio, Texas 78284-7792.

S. Ramamurthy: Department of Anesthesiology, University of Texas Health Science Center at San Antonio, San Antonio, Texas 78284-7838.

EPIDEMIOLOGY

Nearly everyone experiences acute pain. Its incidence approximates the cumulative total of all acute diseases, trauma, and surgical procedures.

Chronic pain is less frequently experienced but is reaching epidemic proportions in the United States. There are more than 36 million individuals with arthritis, 70 million with episodic back pain, 20 million with migraine headaches, and additional millions with pain due to gout, myofascial pain syndromes, phantom limb pain, and reflex sympathetic dystrophies (RSDs) (3). The pain resulting from cancer afflicts approximately 1 million Americans and 20 million individuals worldwide. Moderate to severe pain occurs in about 40% of patients with intermediate stage cancer and in 60% to 80% of patients with advanced cancer (4–6). Back pain, as a general condition, episodically affects nearly 75% of the population in most industrialized nations. It is estimated that at least 10% to 15% of the working population of industrialized nations are affected by back pain each year (7,8).

In studies of the general population, patients have identified the head and lower extremities as the most common sites of acute pain and have identified the back as the most common site of chronic pain (9).

ETIOLOGY

Chronic pain is not merely a physical sensation. In the affective component of chronic pain, most patients show a degree of depression resulting from anger, jealousy, and anxiety. For many individuals, depression is the primary factor in the perception or experience of pain. Fifty percent to 70% of patients with chronic pain have either a primary depression or a depression secondary to their pain syndrome. Chronic pain, with accompanying depression, often leads to extensive periods of limited productivity and prolonged inactivity (10). Prolonged immobility and inactivity alter cardiovascular function, impair musculoskeletal flexibility, and cause abnormal joint function (11–13). Prevention involves the encouragement of patient activity as soon as it is reasonable.

The motivational component is concerned with the vocational, economic, and interpersonal reinforcement contingencies that contribute to the learning of pain behavior and the maintenance of chronic pain. Over 75% of patients with chronic pain display behavioral characteristics, including difficulties with job or housework, leisure activities, sexual function, and vocational endeavors (14). The patient also may have significant functional limitations due to multiple previous surgeries with little success and prolonged convalescence, disuse/physical deconditioning syndrome, or narcotic medication (15).

The cognitive component is involved with how patients think and the part that pain plays in their belief systems and views of self. The more the patient views pain as a signal, which mandates a reduction of activity and protection of the affected part, the more difficult it is for the physician to achieve compliance with exercise, stretching, and other elements of the treatment program. Pain is often the result of sensory input, affective state, cognition, and motivational factors, which requires a multidimensional evaluation process with treatment interventions directed at those components most responsible for the pain experience (16).

Pain Pathways

Pain is a central perception of multiple primary sensory modalities. This interpretive function is complex, involving psychological, neuroanatomic, neurochemical, and neurophysiologic factors of both the pain stimulus and the memory of past pain experiences. The peripheral mechanisms for sensing and modulating pain have been extensively studied during the past 20 years. The pathways for pain sensation, from the initial stimulus of the nociceptors to the central nervous system, are summarized in Figure 56-1 (17–21). There appear to be several descending systems which play a role in control of the modification of the ascending pain pathways, which are summarized in Figure 56-2 (18,21–25).

Polymodal nociceptors respond to stimuli that damage tissue. This stimulation results in impulses ascending in the A-delta or C fibers to the marginal layers of the dorsal horn of the spinal cord. The A-delta fibers primarily synapse in laminae I and V, whereas C fibers synapse primarily in laminae II. Deeper regions of the dorsal horn may be polysynaptically involved in the processing of noxious stimuli.

The major ascending nociceptive pathways are the spinothalamic and spinoreticular tracts. The ascending pain pathways involve both oligosynaptic and polysynaptic neurons. The oligosynaptic pathways are fast conducting with discrete somatotopic organization resulting in rapid transmission of nociceptive information regarding site, intensity, and duration of stimulus. The oligosynaptic tracts provide somatic information by way of the posterior ventral nuclei of the thalamus to the postcentral cortex. The sensory discriminatory characteristics are delineated from the neospinothalamic portion of the lateral spinothalamic tract and the nonproprioceptive portion of the dorsal columns.

Polysynaptic pathways are slow conducting with a lack of somatotopic organization resulting in poor localization,

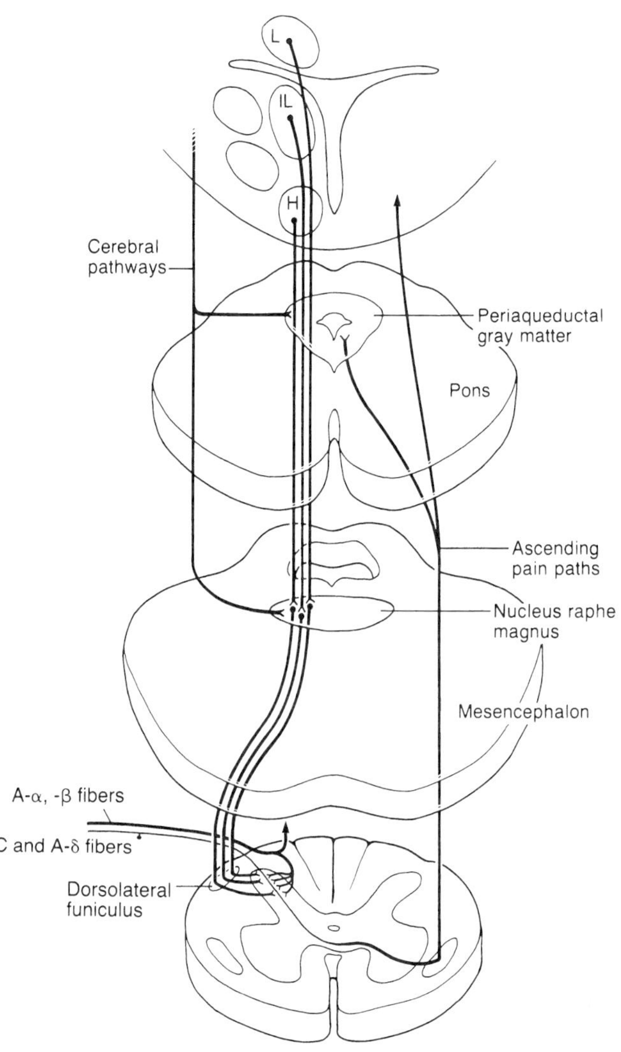

FIG. 56-1. Central nervous system structures that modify ascending pain pathways. *H,* hypothamamus; *IL,* intralaminar thalamic nuclei; *L,* limbic system.

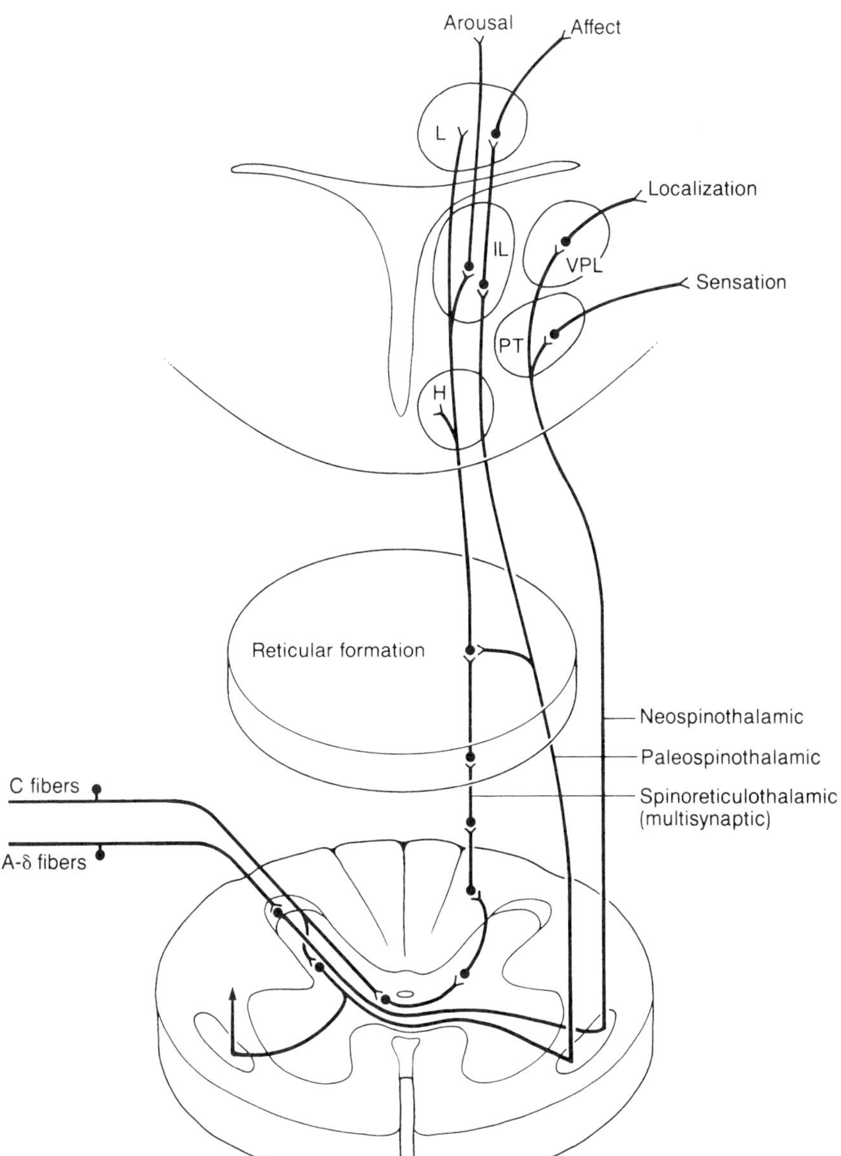

FIG. 56-2. Ascending pathways for pain sensation from nociceptors to the central nervous system. *H*, hypothalamus; *IL*, intralaminar thalamic nuclei; *L*, limbic system; *PT*, posterior thalamic nuclei; *VPL*, ventral posterolateral thalamic nuclei.

dull aching, and burning sensations. The nociceptive impulses transmitted through this system result in suprasegmental reflex responses related to ventilation, circulation, and endocrine function. Pathways contributing to this slow conducting system are the paleospinothalamic tract, spinoreticular tract, spinocollicular tract, and the dorsal intercornual tract, as well as the spinomesencephalic tract. The polysynaptic tracts form the brain stem reticular activating system with projections to the medial and interlaminar nuclei of the thalamus. From these nuclei diffuse radiation occurs to the cerebral cortex, limbic system, and basal ganglia.

There are multiple levels of processing and convergence of nociceptive information in its ascending transmission to the cerebral cortex. In addition, there appear to be several descending pain control systems that play a role in the control and modification of the ascending pain pathways. The most complete studies have been of the periaqueductal gray region of the mid-brain (PAG). Stimulation of the PAG neurons and the subsequent descending impulses result in release of endogenous opioids at the nucleus raphe magnus (NRM) and nucleus locus ceruleus (NLC). Endogenous opioids activate the serotonergic cells in the NRM and norepinergic neurons in the NLC. The axons of both of these monoaminergic neurons descend in the dorsolateral tract to interneurons, predominately in laminae I, II, and V. These monoamines activate opioid-secreting interneurons. The morphinelike transmitter released may vary, depending on what type of receptor in the periphery has been activated. Both A-delta and C afferent fibers are inhibited by descending influences in the dorsal horn. The opioid inhibitory interneurons may be influenced by intersegmental and descending pathways, but the intersegmental and segmental mechanisms have not been established. These interneurons may function neither by presynaptic inhibition on the terminals with the primary nociceptive afferents preventing the release of substance P or by postsynaptic inhibition on second-order neurons. Cells in the raphe magnus are activated by ascending sensory pathways transmitted to the reticular formation as well as by descending input from cells in the periaqueductal gray region.

Other descending monoamine systems include locus ceruleus to the dorsal horn; interneurons, nucleus reticularis, magnicellularis to the dorsal horn interneurons; and the mesencephalic lateral reticular formation to the dorsal horn interneurons. It has been suggested that monoamines are involved with supraspinal and spinal nociceptive mechanisms. Hormonally based descending pathways have been described but are poorly understood.

Resolution of Pain

Acute pain is frequently the result of tissue damage in which the initial pain leads to an increase in anxiety, which magnifies the pain experience. The amount of anxiety generated (and pain) seems to be more influenced by the setting in which the pain develops than by personality variables. With the healing process comes a reduction or termination of the anxiety and acute pain perception. When acute pain, which functions as a warning signal, fails to respond to treatment with conventional medical therapies, illness behavior and chronic pain develops. The anxiety characteristic of acute pain is replaced by hopelessness, helplessness, and despair. When pain relief fails, physical activities decrease, and suffering and depression increase.

Acute pain usually resolves when the source of nociperception is removed or cured. Acute pain, by definition, resolves quickly and is often readily treated by a single modality. The cause of acute pain can be documented by the findings on physical examination and diagnostic procedures. When indicated, appropriate operative intervention can be performed on the basis of these findings. A short course of analgesic medication usually controls postoperative pain, and a return to full painless function can be anticipated in a matter of weeks. Acute pain control requires the administration of an efficacious analgesic dosage. Too little analgesia promotes suffering and anxiety, thus defeating the purpose of prescribing medication, but fear or drug addiction contributes to the underutilization of analgesic medication, and physicians tend to undermedicate in terms of frequency and dosage of pain medications (26,27). By prescribing low oral doses of narcotics at infrequent intervals, physicians inadvertently force patients to adopt pain behavior in order to obtain adequate narcotic analgesia. Pain behavior is characterized by high verbalization of pain, dependency, and the inability to work. Addiction in the acute pain situation is extraordinarily rare, probably less than 0.1% (28,29).

Unfortunately a significant minority of acute pain patients continue to experience pain, which may progress into a more complex disease entity. Pain, a symptom of physiologic malfunction, now becomes the disease itself. Chronic pain represents a complex interaction of physical, psychological, and social factors in which the pain complaint is a socially acceptable manifestation of the disease. The etiology of chronic pain may be persistent nociceptive input, such as arthritis or terminal cancer; psychological disorders, such an anxiety, depression, and learned behavior; or social factors, such as job loss, divorce, and secondary gain.

The optimal treatment for chronic pain is prevention. Once the disease state of chronic pain commences, reinforcers such as monetary compensation, presence of job-related problems, manipulation of the environment to satisfy unmet needs, and retirement from the competitive world obstruct resolution of the disease. Therapies designed for acute pain are often contraindicated for chronic pain.

Prevention of chronic pain requires identifying contributing factors and resolving them early in the acute stage. Aspects worthy of attention include psychological stress, drug or alcohol abuse, and poor posture or muscle tone, as well as significant psychological and operant pain mechanisms. Physicians should set a reasonable time frame for the resolution of the acute pain process. Patients should be advised when the pain medication will no longer be needed. The patient's attention should be directed to a gradual return of full activity on a prescribed schedule. Follow-up appointments should be planned at specified intervals so the patient does not need to justify a visit. Work intolerance should be resolved.

Pain-Reinforcing Factors

Chronic pain syndrome is a learned behavior pattern reinforced by multiple factors. These behaviors are frequently found in individuals who are depressed and inactive and who lack the skills or opportunity to compete in the community. These environmental factors promote pain behavior, regardless of the etiology of the pain that distinguishes the patient with chronic pain from the population at large. Patients often develop a new self-image and see themselves as disabled by their pain. This self-perceived disability justifies their inactivity, their manipulation of others, and their attempts to collect compensation from society. The typical patient often has been unemployed or on sick leave for long periods of time (30). Our data indicate that individuals who have been removed from the labor market due to pain for less than 6 months have a 90% chance of returning to full employment; those removed from the labor force due to pain for more than 1 year have less than a 10% chance of returning (31).

Individuals with chronic pain syndrome receive gains from their pain behavior; hence, they continue pain behavior to maintain those positive reinforcers. Physicians reinforce the pain behaviors by lacking knowledge of this chronic disease process, failing to identify the chronic pain behavior, and prolonging prescription of inappropriate medications, inactivity, and work limitations. The physician's failure to acknowledge and direct the patient toward recovery tends to validate the chronic pain syndrome by providing an undiagnosable and untreatable problem. Family members also frequently reinforce the chronic pain behavior. They allow the individual to become inactive and cater to the patient's requests and needs over prolonged periods of time. In some instances, patients with chronic pain provide role models for pain or disability behavior for other family members (32,33).

Worker's Compensation

In 1911, worker's compensation laws were enacted in the United States that required employers to assume the cost of occupational disability without regard to fault. These laws have dramatically influenced the recovery from injury. In many instances they have become counterproductive; financial compensation may discourage return to work, the appeal process may increase disability, an open claim may inhibit return to work, and recovering patients may be unable to return to work. Often the accident and resulting symptoms represent the patient's solution to life's problems (34). The pain literature suggests an enhanced pain experience and reduced treatment efficacy in patients with chronic pain who are receiving financial compensation (35,36).

Litigation

Disability, along with pain and suffering, greatly determines the amount of compensation awarded in worker's compensation cases. The patient/client's pain behavior may be reinforced, maximized, and groomed with the hope of a large cash settlement. As a result of this reinforcement, the pain behavior develops into a learned response. The pain also becomes the disability for which the patient/client is seeking compensation. Therefore, a learned behavior becomes a determining factor in the amount of compensation awarded (37,38).

Alteration of the disability laws could decrease the number of acute pain patients who develop the behavioral disease of chronic pain syndrome. Changes that might discourage the development of chronic pain include allowing an injured worker to continue working at a job he or she is physically able to accomplish during the recuperation period, rapid adjudication of disability and compensation claims, and physicians restricting the patient's use of addicting and depressant medication to less than 1 month. The extensive use of conservative intervention to include physical therapy and stress management early in treatment also could prevent the emergence of chronic pain syndrome (39,40). For additional information on disability determination and mediolegal aspects, the reader is referred to Chapters 10 and 11.

Complications of Chronic Pain

Chronic pain is an elusive disease complicated by iatrogenic, idiopathic, and psychosocial factors. These complications encompass physical, psychological, and environmental issues.

Physical

The patient with chronic pain often develops secondary pain loci due to inactivity. Decreased range of motion, myofascial pain, and weakness due to disuse also may develop (41).

Medically induced drug addiction and dependence are particularly serious problems for both patients with chronic pain and their physicians (42,43). It has been estimated that 30% to 50% of patients with chronic nonmalignant pain have a significant drug dependency problem (44,45). Substance abuse, dependence, and addiction are negative prognostic factors in outcome studies (46). Treatment of the drug impairment is essential and results in a greater overall improvement in functioning (47).

Psychological

Depression is a common complication noted with chronic pain (48). These patients often manipulate family, friends, and co-workers to achieve secondary gain. Chronic pain causes considerable distress to spouses and family members (49); sexual dysfunctions (50) are common. Twenty-five percent of spouses report clinical depression, and over 35% rate their marriage as maladjusted (51).

Environmental

Nearly one third of the American population has persistent or recurrent chronic pain. One half to two thirds of these individuals are partly or totally disabled for varying lengths of time. Bonica estimates $70 billion a year is spent on medical needs, lost working days, and compensation (52). Data compiled in 1982 suggest that lost wages and social support systems cost the taxpayer $15,000 to $24,000 per chronic pain patient per year (53).

CURRENT THEORIES OF PAIN

Gate Control Theory

The gate control theory of pain was developed by Melzack and Wall to account for mechanisms by which other cutaneous stimuli and emotional states alter the level of pain (54). They suggested that within the substantia gelatinosa of the dorsal horn there are interneurons that presynaptically inhibit transmission of nociceptive information to the ascending tracts. These interneurons are activated by large-diameter afferents and inhibited by small-diameter afferents. In addition, they suggested that the brain exerted descending control on this system, relying on the fact that cognitive factors are known to influence pain behavior.

Several studies have failed to provide support for the gate

control theory. It remains significant, although incorrect in detail. The gate control theory of pain has altered the concept of pain as solely an afferent sensory experience, broadening the concept to include the affective and motivational factors involved in the human pain experience (55). The gate control theory has been modified extensively during the past 30 years (56). It still represents the first attempt to describe a pain modulating system that responds to input by noxious stimuli, innocuous afferent impulses, and descending control.

Biochemical Theory

The biochemical theory of pain has evolved since the discovery of the endorphins. The endogenous opioid system consists of three families of opioid peptides: beta endorphin, enkephalin, and dynorphin/neoendorphin. The beta endorphins are primarily concentrated in the pituitary and the basal hypothalamus. The other endogenous opioids are distributed extensively in the central nervous system. The dynorphins/neoendorphins and enkephalins are found in the caudate nucleus, amygdala, periaqueductal gray matter, locus ceruleus, and dorsal horn of the spinal cord. In addition, the enkephalins are found in the nucleus raphe magnus and the thalamic periventricular nuclei. The dynorphins/neoendorphins are found in the hypothalamus and substantia nigra (22).

The endogenous opioids are involved in analgesia, as well as multiple other clinical events. There are at least seven different opiate receptors, of which the mu, delta, and kappa appear to be involved in analgesia (57). The others are associated with such functions as respiration, appetite, hallucinations, dysphoria, immune function, temperature regulation, memory, and blood pressure control. The beta endorphins may function in the modulation of local blood flow and immune function (58). The discovery of multiple opiate receptors and multiple endogenous opioid compounds provides an explanation for the multiple effects of the endogenous opioids. Within the peripheral and central nervous systems the enkephalins act as neurotransmitters and the beta endorphins act predominately as hormones. Endogenous opioids are only one part of a complex modulatory system involved in the collating, processing, and filtering of information concerning tissue damage (59). Other possible neural peptides having analgesia or antinociceptive properties are calcitonin, cholecystokinin, somatostatin, and neurotensin (51,58,60).

Chronic Pain Theory

The chronic pain theory encompasses many of the physical, motivational, cognitive, and affective components of pain. The anatomic pain pathways are relatively clear and represent a mechanism for nociceptive pain in the animal model. Multiple pain mechanisms exist in the human model due to the complex integration of nociceptive stimuli, conceptual and judgmental factors, sociocultural influences, and the motivational and emotional states of the individual. Pain mechanisms include nociceptive pain, central pain, psychogenic, and operant pain. The human perception and reaction to pain are a blending of these mechanisms. The nociceptive pain mechanism is detailed in the pain pathways, as previously described, and represents pain originating from tissue damage such as pain from cancer, degenerative joint disease, myofascial pain, and trauma. Central pain originates from denervation occurring after a cerebrovascular accident, spinal cord injury, or amputation. This pain may be due to a loss of the peripheral modulating influences on the central nervous system resulting in an unmodulated activity of afferent A-delta and C fibers.

Psychosis is the interpretation of emotional distress as aversive and unpleasant sensation and its description in terms of pain language and behavior. The psychological states that are interpreted in this manner include anxiety, neurosis, hysteria, and depression. This mechanism of pain is often overlooked in patients with chronic pain.

Operant or learned pain behavior is often a major factor in chronic pain. Although the initial precipitating event causing the pain may be quite minor, the pain behavior is often long lasting, owing to reinforcement by environmental influences. Pain behavior may be directly reinforced by family and physician attention or the delivery of medication. Indirect reinforcement (physical or psychological demands) occurs with avoidance of aversive consequences, which would have to be met if there were no pain. Operant pain behavior is also reinforced through a punishment cycle, when an injured party is overprotected and "punished" by outside factors if he or she begins to function more independently.

ANATOMY OF PAIN

Knowledge of the peripheral anatomy of the human body is essential in evaluating the complex problems found in a patient with pain. The clinical problem is often reduced to the simple question, "Is the pain in an area supplied by a single nerve root, a single peripheral nerve, or a branch of a peripheral nerve?" A physical examination to evaluate pain, weakness, and their distribution often leads the clinician to better localize the nerves involved in the patient's pain complaint.

Somatic Innervation

A difficulty encountered in diagnosis is secondary to the overlap of cutaneous fields of segmental and peripheral nerves as well as the overlapping innervation of muscle. Single cutaneous nerves innervate sharply defined regions with little overlap, but these fibers regroup in the peripheral nerve and are again redistributed in the plexus such that it is impossible to follow individual fibers from the dorsal roots to the areas innervated by the individual cutaneous nerve. Adjacent cutaneous nerves may be fibers from more than one spinal nerve (Fig. 56-3) (61). Anatomists and physicians have attempted to define areas of the skin,

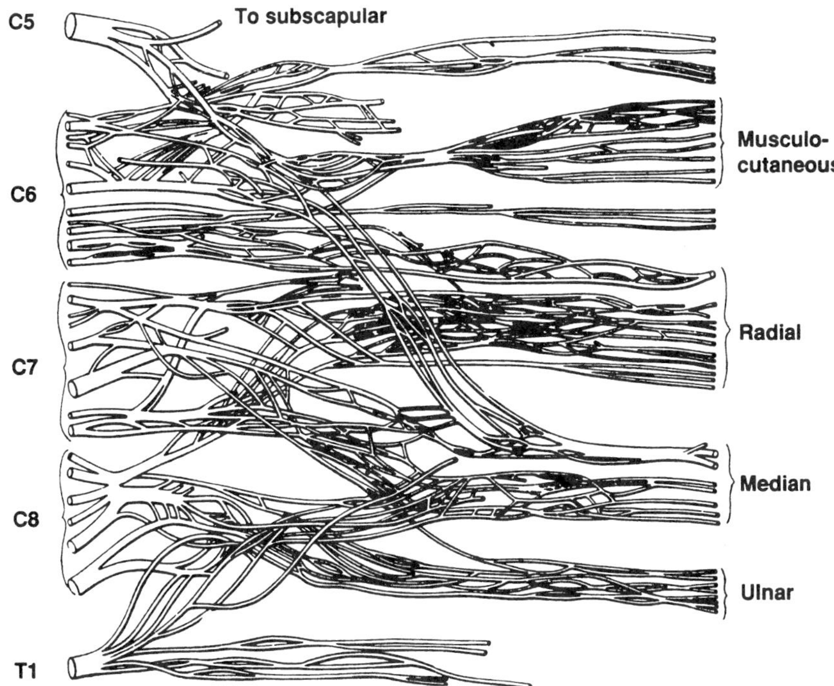

FIG. 56-3. The connections and interchanges of the funiculi in the brachial plexus.

muscle, and bone that are of the exclusive domain of a single spinal cord root, as well as the areas of overlap. The size of these areas varies from nerve to nerve and from individual to individual. As with all knowledge of the human body, anatomy of sensation and pain rests on a foundation of original work performed by investigators too numerous to list. The figures in this chapter have taken some of the best work in the field and compiled it into a comprehensive review (Figs. 56-4 through 56-17). In delving into the literature in this area of anatomy, one cannot help but feel that they are standing on the shoulders of giants without whose work the figures in this chapter would not be possible.[1]

Dermatomes

Different techniques were used in determining the site and extent of innervation. Foerster's (62) data were based on remaining sensibility of the skin innervated by an intact posterior root isolated by severing several nerve roots above and below. In determining the field of unaltered sensation, Foerster demonstrated considerable overlap of contiguous nerve roots. Similar techniques were used by Bing (63), the Armed Forces Institute of Pathology, and Haymaker and Woodall (64). Keagan and Garrett (65) used hyposensitivity to pin scratch in cases of herniated innervertebral disc, which resulted in the most extensive dermatome map. Keagan and Garrett contended that no sensory overlap exists between dermatomes, which is contrary to most investigators' experience. Victor and Woodruff used the electrical skin resistance method (66) over sympathectomized areas of the skin. It is noted that dermatomes of almost all cutaneous nerves are beyond the anatomic boundaries noted on gross disection. Clinical data suggest that areas of sensory deficit extend further proximally than mapped by Foerster, but not as far proximally as suggested by Keagan and Garrett. For this reason the dermatomes used in the figures are derived from an interpolation of areas determined by personal experience and multiple other authors (62–70).

Myotomal Innervation

The determination of muscular innervation is the result of the analysis by many observers of traumatic and surgical outcomes evaluated during the postoperative and recovery periods (64,70–75). The results of these analyses are provided in detail in Tables 56-1 and 56-2. The dermatomes used in these drawings are derived from the experience of multiple clinicians.

Sclerotomes

Areas of segmental innervation of bone (sclerotomes) are closely linked with muscle innervation. Injury to bone, ligament, tendon, fascia, and other mesodermal structures of the body may result in pain referred in distribution of the sclerotomes (64,76). Notable references for peripheral nerve innervation of the skeleton include Haymaker and Woodall

[1] "I say with Didacus Stella, a dwarf standing on the shoulders of a giant may see farther than a giant himself."—Robert Burton, 1577–1640

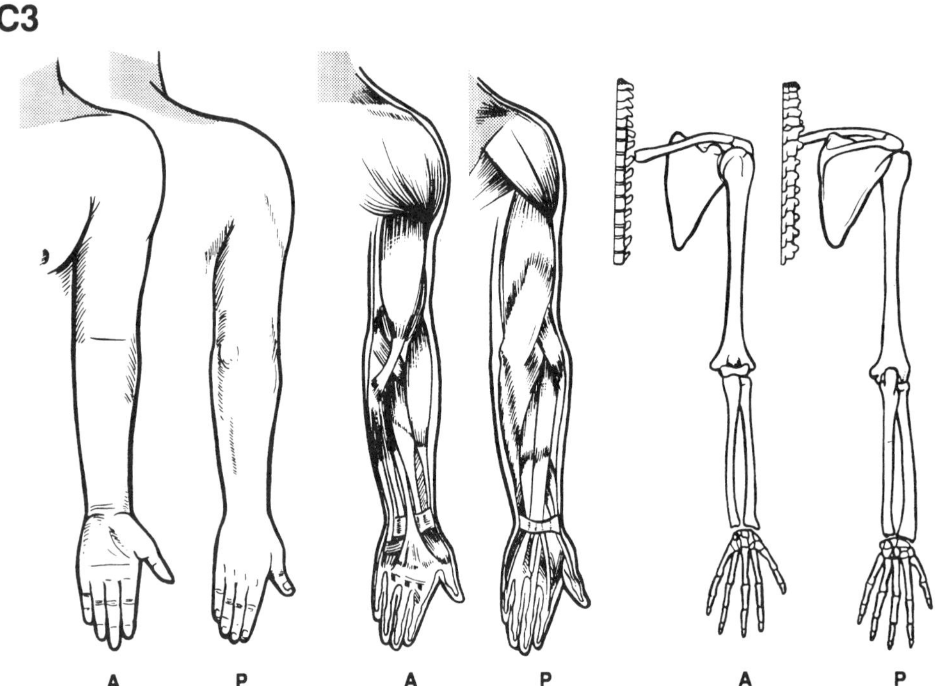

FIG. 56-4. Dermatome, myotome, and sclerotome distribution for C3. *Dermatome*: neck. *Myotome*: paraspinals, trapezius, and diaphragm. *Sclerotome*: bones—vertebra and periosteum; joints—facet; ligaments—longitudinal, ligamentum flavum, and interspinous.

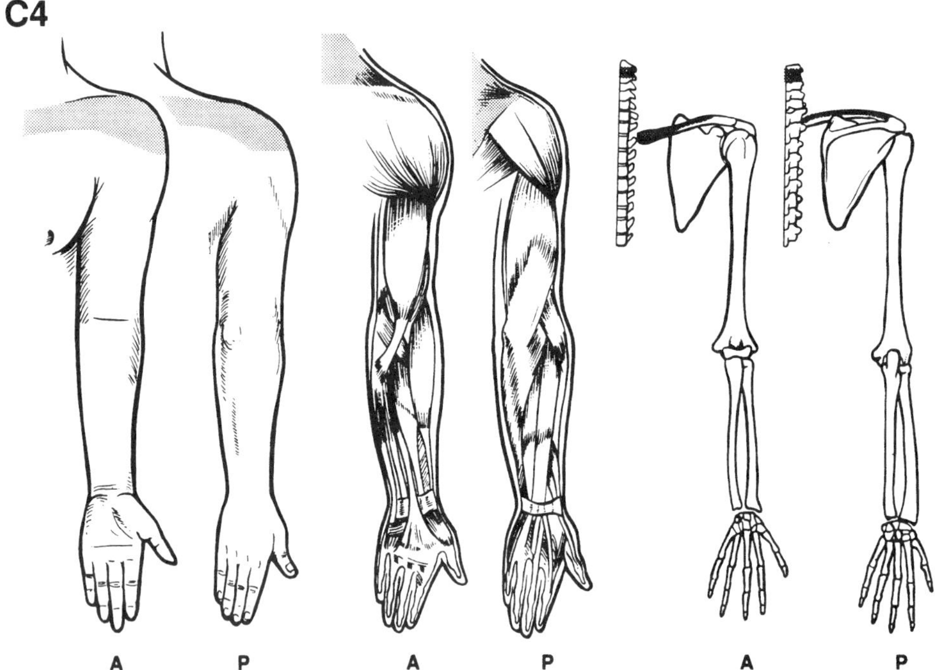

FIG. 56-5. Dermatome, myotome, and sclerotome distribution for C4. *Dermatome*: shoulder. *Myotome*: paraspinals, trapezius, diaphragm, scapular abductors. *Sclerotome*: bones—vertebra, periosteum, and clavical; joints—facet; ligaments—longitudinal, ligamentum flavum, and interspinous.

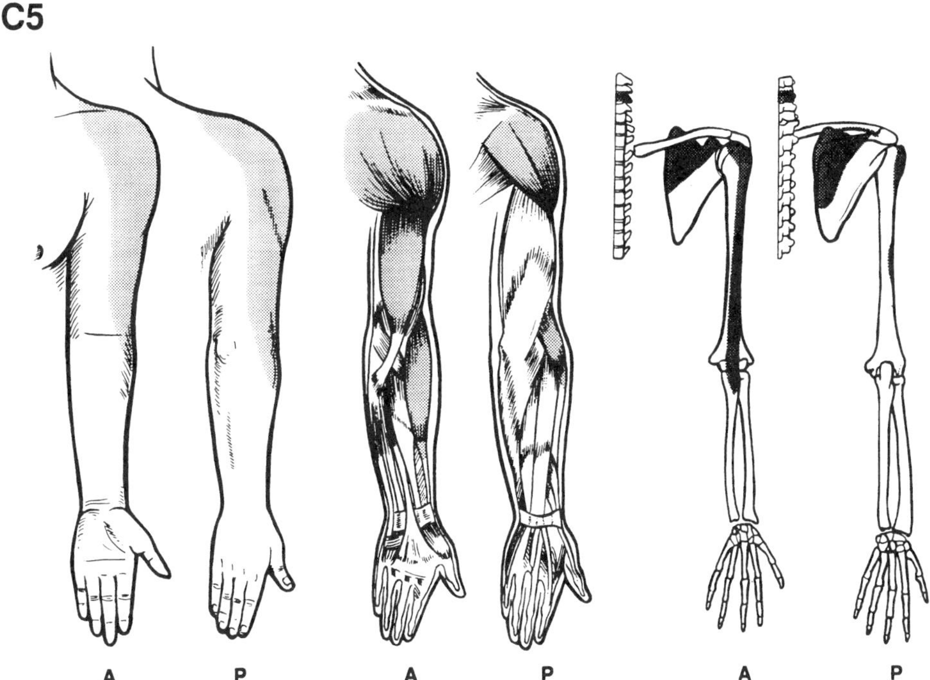

FIG. 56-6. Dermatome, myotome, and sclerotome distribution for C5. *Dermatome*: lateral shoulder and lateral arm. *Myotome*: paraspinals, scapular abductors, scapular elevators, shoulder extensors, shoulder rotators, and elbow flexors. *Sclerotome*: bones—vertebra and periosteum, scapula, and humerus; joints—facet; ligaments—rotator cuff, longitudinal, ligamentum flavum, and interspinous.

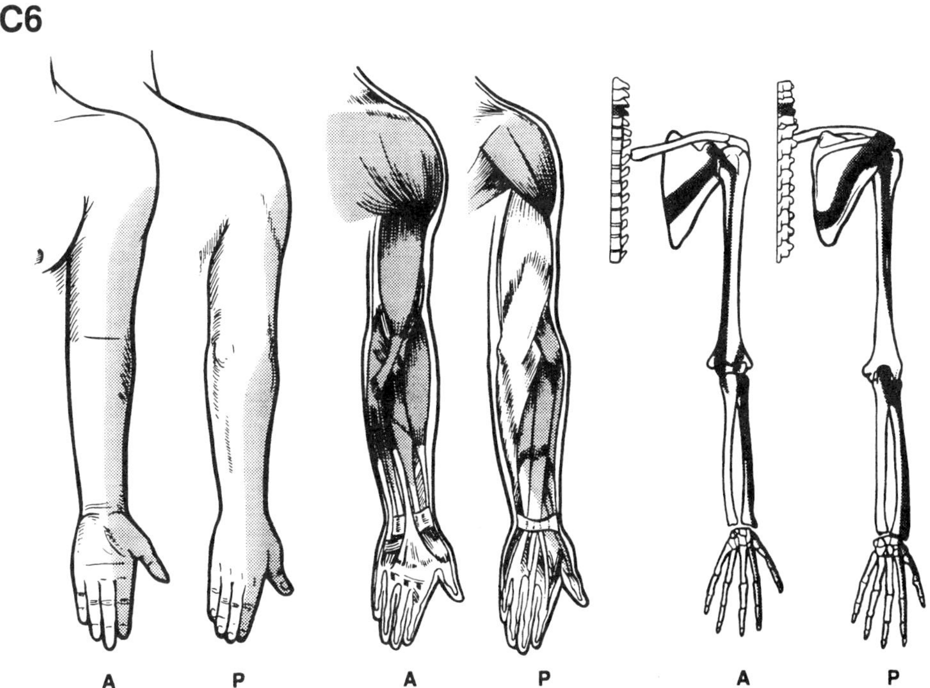

FIG. 56-7. Dermatome, myotome, and sclerotome distribution for C6. *Dermatome*: lateral arm, lateral forearm, and lateral hand. *Myotome*: paraspinals, shoulder adductors, elbow flexors, forearm pronators, forearm supinators, and wrist flexors. *Sclerotome*: bones--scapula, humerus, radius, and lateral fingers; joints—facet, shoulder, and elbow; ligaments—longitudinal, ligamentum flavum, and interspinous.

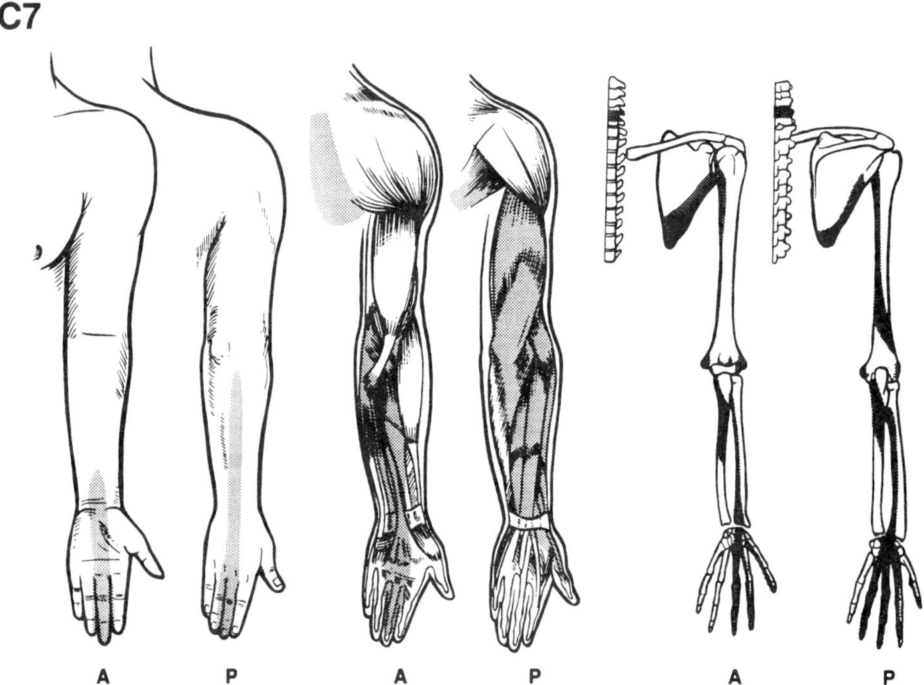

FIG. 56-8. Dermatome, myotome, and sclerotome distribution for C7. *Dermatome*: mid-hand and middle finger. *Myotome*: paraspinals, elbow extensors, forearm pronators, and wrist extensors. *Sclerotome*: bones—scapula, humerus, radius, ulna, and middle fingers; joints—facet and wrist; ligaments—longitudinal, ligamentum flavum, and interspinous.

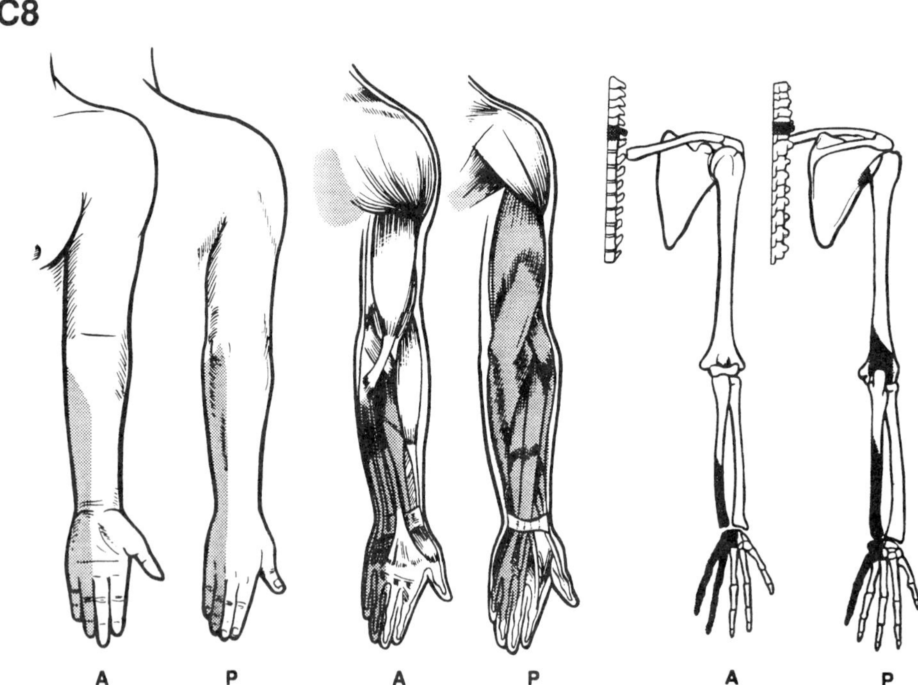

FIG. 56-9. Dermatome, myotome, and sclerotome distribution for C8. *Dermatome*: medial forearm and medial hand. *Myotome*: paraspinals, elbow extensors, wrist flexors, grip, finger abduction, finger flexion, finger adduction, finger opposition, and finger extension. *Sclerotome*: bones—vertebra and periosteum, ulna, and medial fingers; joints—facet and wrist; ligaments—longitudinal, ligamentum flavum, and interspinous.

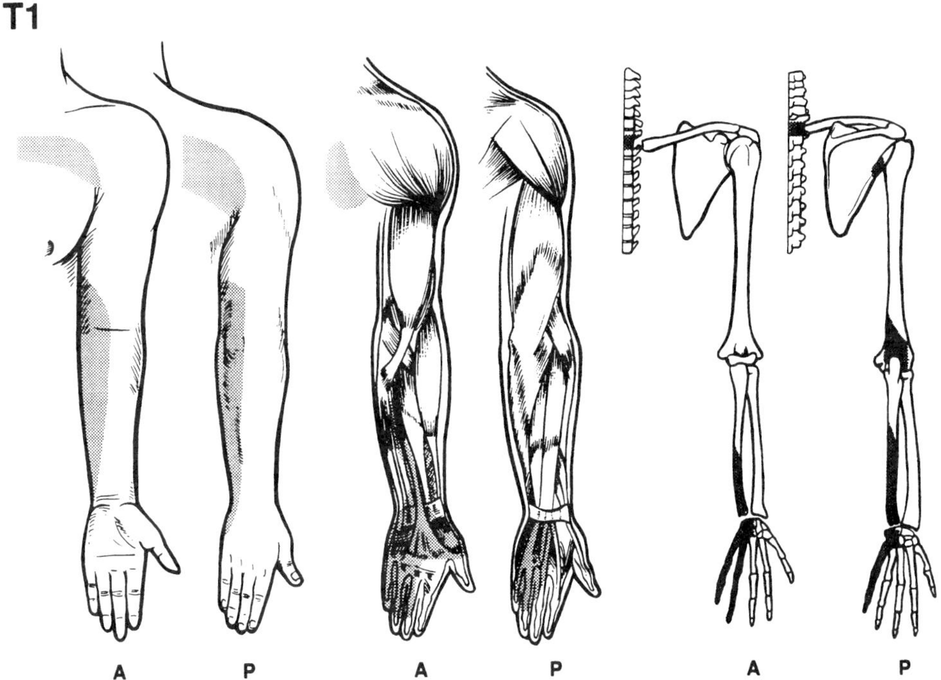

FIG. 56-10. Dermatome, myotome, and sclerotome distribution for T1. *Dermatome*: medial arm and medial forearm. *Myotome*: paraspinals, finger adduction, finger flexion, finger abduction, finger opposition, and finger extension. *Sclerotome*: bones—vertebra and periosteum, ulna, and medial fingers; joints—facet; ligaments—longitudinal, ligamentum flavum, and interspinous.

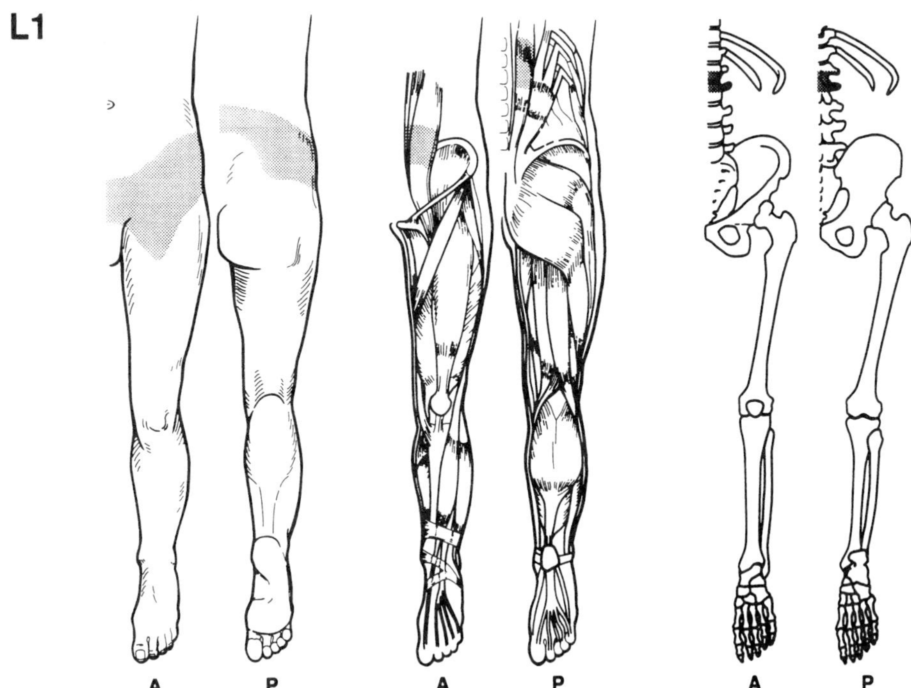

FIG. 56-11. Dermatome, myotome, and sclerotome distribution for L1. *Dermatome*: groin and flank. *Myotome*: paraspinals, hip flexors, spine extensors, and spine rotators. *Sclerotome*: bones—vertebra and periosteum; joints—facet; ligaments—longitudinal, ligamentum flavum, interspinous. *Serosal service*: abdominal wall. *Viscera*: large intestine, kidney, ureter, suprarenal, prostate, and uterus.

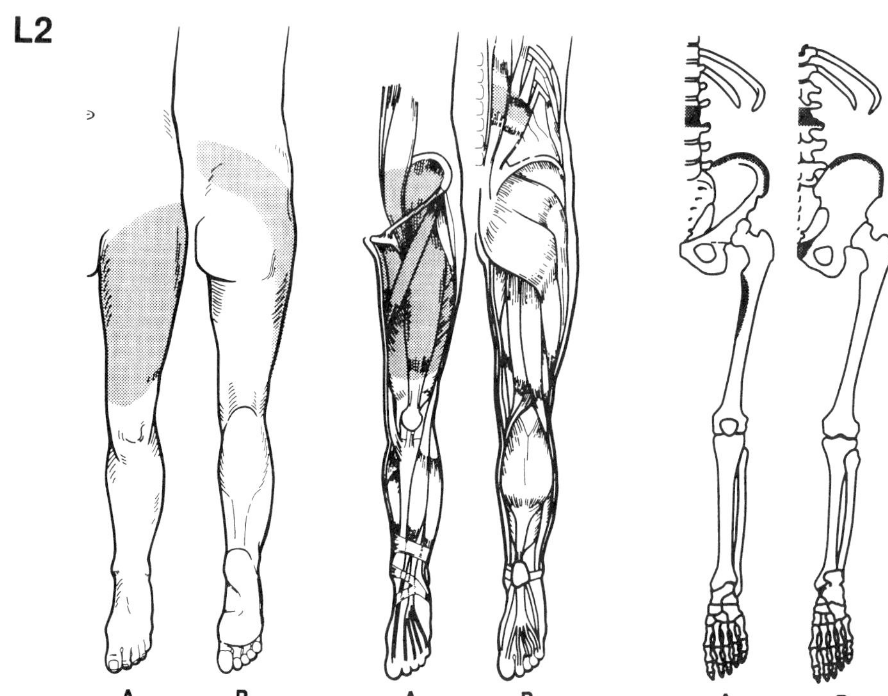

FIG. 56-12. Dermatome, myotome, and sclerotome distribution for L2. *Dermatome*: thigh and upper buttock. *Myotome*: paraspinals, hip flexors, and hip adductors. *Sclerotome*: bones—vertebra and periosteum, iliac crest, and medial femur; joints—facet; ligaments—longitudinal, ligamentum flavum, and interspinous. *Serosal Surface*: posterior abdominal wall, descending large intestine, ureter, bladder, and abdominal aorta.

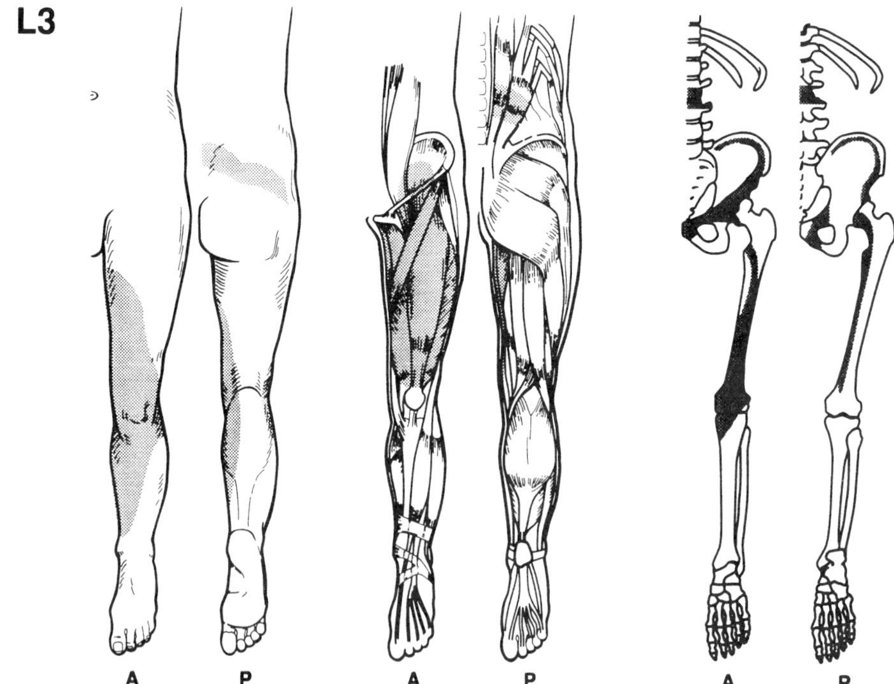

FIG. 56-13. Dermatome, myotome, and sclerotome distribution for L3. *Dermatome*: upper buttock, medial thigh, knee, and medial calf. *Myotome*: paraspinals, hip flexors, hip adductors, and knee extensors. *Sclerotome*: bones—iliac crest, ischium, femur, patella, and proximal tibia; joints—facet, hip, and knee; ligaments—longitudinal, ligamentum flavum, and interspinous. *Serosal surface*: posterior abdominal wall. *Viscera*: abdominal aorta.

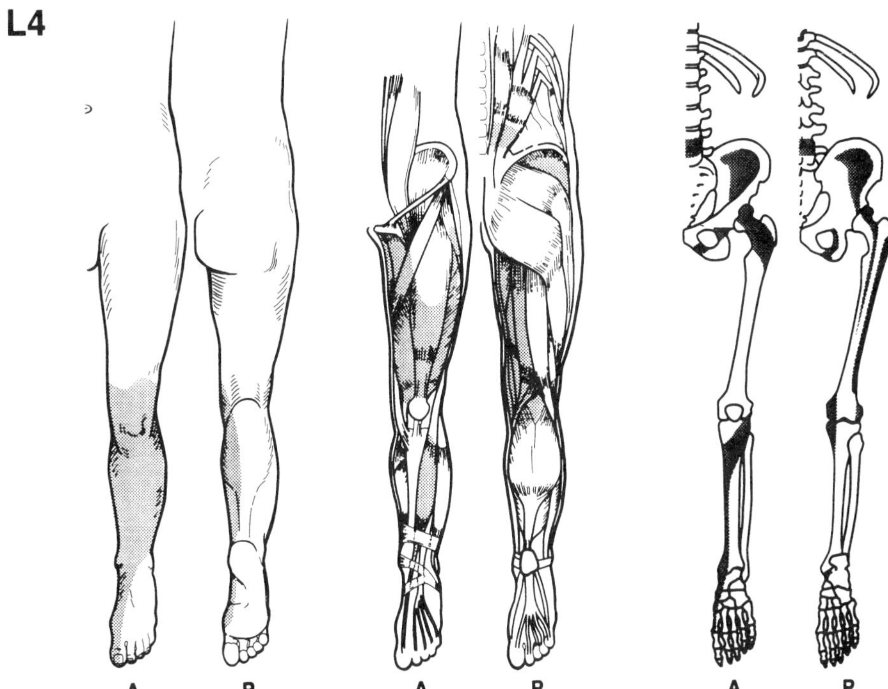

FIG. 56-14. Dermatome, myotome, and sclerotome distribution for L4. *Dermatome*: knee, anterior lower leg, and medial foot. *Myotome*: hip adductors, hip extensors, knee extensors, ankle dorsiflexors, and ankle invertors. *Sclerotome*: bones—vertebra and periosteum, iliac wing, femur, tibia, and medial foot; joints—facet, hip, and knee; ligaments—longitudinal, ligamentum flavum, and interspinous. *Serosal surface*: posterior abdominal wall. *Viscera*: abdominal aorta.

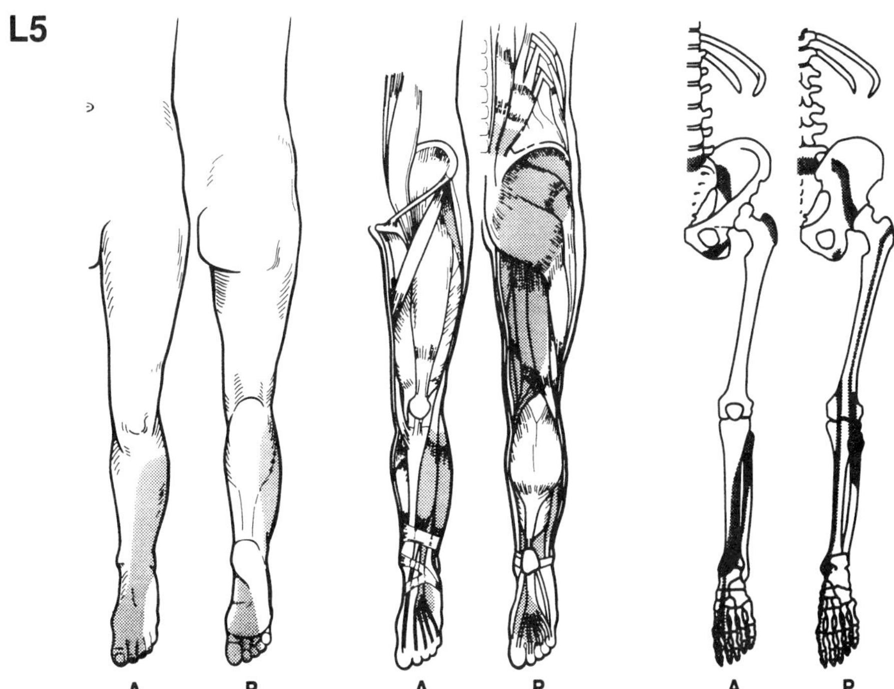

FIG. 56-15. Dermatome, myotome, and sclerotome distribution for L5. *Dermatome*: lateral lower leg, medial foot. *Myotome*: paraspinals, hip extension, knee flexion, ankle eversion, ankle inversion, and big toe extension. *Sclerotome*: bones—vertebra and periosteum, iliac wing, femur, tibia, proximal fibula, and medial foot; joints—facet, sacroiliac, hip, knee, ankle, and large toe; ligaments—longitudinal, ligamentum flavum, and interspinous.

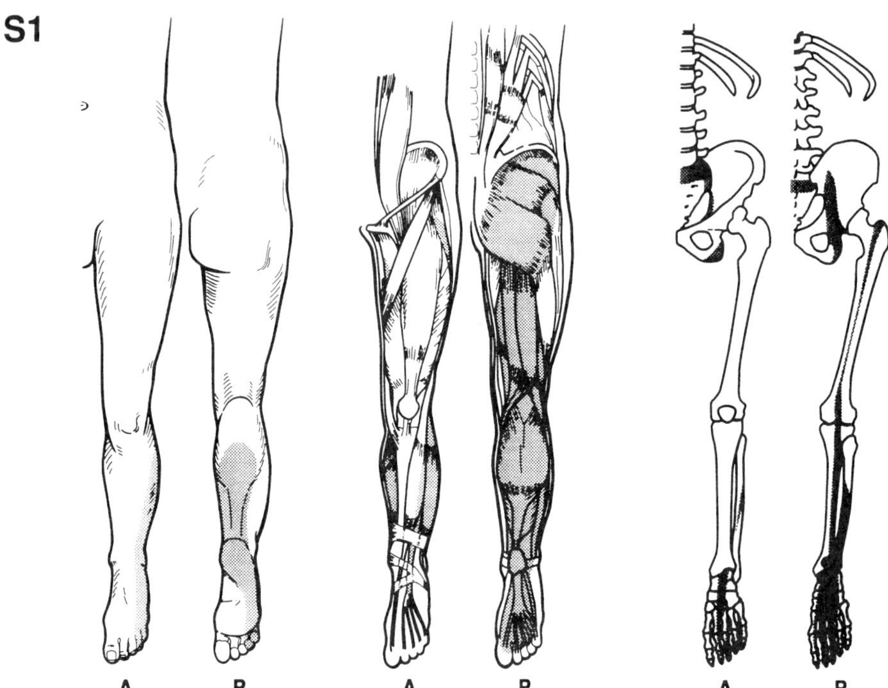

FIG. 56-16. Dermatome, myotome, and sclerotome distribution for S1. *Dermatome*: posterior lower leg, lateral lower leg, and lateral foot. *Myotome*: hip extensors, hip abductors, knee flexors, ankle evertors, ankle plantar flexors, and toe dorsiflexors. *Sclerotome*: bones—vertebra and periosteum, sacrum, ischium, femur, tibia, and mid-foot; joints—sacroiliac, hip, knee, ankle, and large toe; ligaments—longitudinal, ligamentum flavum, and interspinous.

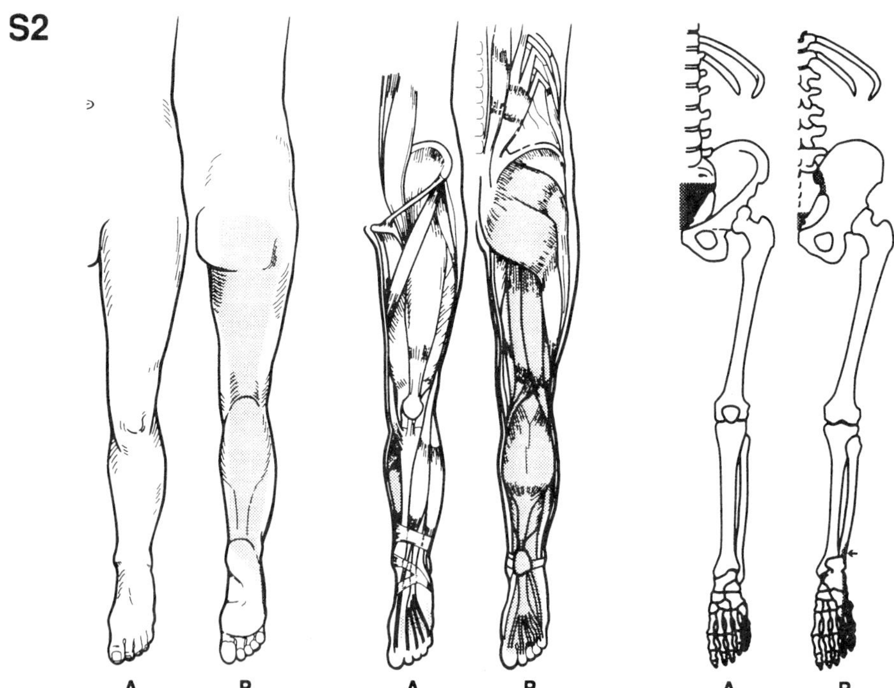

FIG. 56-17. Dermatome, myotome, and sclerotome distribution for S2. *Dermatome*: posterior upper leg and posterior lower leg. *Myotome*: knee flexors, ankle plantar flexors, toe dorsiflexors, toe abduction, and toe adduction. *Sclerotome*: bones—sacrum, coccyx, distal fibula and lateral foot; joints—sacroiliac, ankle, and toes; ligaments—longitudinal, ligamentum flavum, and interspinous.

TABLE 56-1. *Upper extremity muscle innervation*

Muscle	Peripheral nerve	Spinal segment
Levator scapulae	Trapezius	**C3,C4**
Serratus anterior	Long thoracic nerve	**C3,C4**,C5,**C6,C7**
Rhomboid major/minor	Dorsal scapular	(C4),**C5**
Supraspinatus	Suprascapular	**C5**,C6
Infraspinatus	Suprascapular	**C5,C6**
Latissimus dorsi	Thoracodorsal	**C6,C7,C8**
Teres major	Lower subscapular	C5,**C6**,C7
Teres minor	Axillary	**C5,C6**
Pectoralis major (clavicular)	Lateral pectoral	C5,**C6**,C7
Pectoralis major (sternal)	Lateral/medial pectoral	C6,**C7,C8**,T1
Deltoid	Axillary	**C5,C6**
Coracobrachialis	Musculocutaneous	**C6,C7**
Biceps brachii	Musculocutaneous	**C5,C6**
Brachialis	Musculocutaneous[a]	**C5,C6**
Triceps	Radial	C6,**C7,C8**
Anconeus	Radial	C6,**C7,C8**
Brachioradialis	Radial	**C5,C6**
Extensor carpi radialis longus	Radial	**C6,C7**
Supinator	Radial	C5,**C6**,(C7)
Extensor digitorum communis	Radial	**C7**,C8
Extensor digiti minimi	Radial	**C7,C8**
Extensor carpi ulnaris	Radial	**C7,C8**
Abductor pollicis longus	Radial	**C7,C8**
Extensor pollicis brevis	Radial	**C7,C8**
Extensor pollicis longus	Radial	**C7,C8**
Extensor indicis	Radial	**C7,C8**
Pronator teres	Median	**C6,C7**
Flexor carpi radialis	Median	**C6,C7**,C8
Palmaris longus	Median	**C7,C8**,T1
Flexor digitorum superficialis	Median	**C7,C8,T1**
Flexor digitorum profundus I and II	Median	C7,**C8,T1**
Flexor pollicus brevis	Median	
Flexor pollicis longus	Median	C7,**C8,T1**
Pronator quadratus	Median	**C8,T1**
Abductor pollicis brevis	Median	**C8,T1**
Opponens pollicis	Median	**C8,T1**
Lumbrical I and II	Median	**C8,T1**
Flexor carpi ulnaris	Ulnar	C7,**C8**,T1
Flexor digitorum profundus III and IV	Ulnar	C7,**C8,T1**
Abductor digiti minimi	Ulnar	**C8,T1**
Palmar/dorsal interossei	Ulnar	**C8,T1**
Lumbrical III and IV	Ulnar	**C8,T1**
Adductor pollicis	Ulnar	**C8,T1**

Spinal segments in parentheses signify those that are occasionally present; those in boldface are the major segments supplying the muscle designated. Segments not in boldface are usually present but to a minor degree.

[a] The small branch from the radial nerve also innervates the brachialis muscle.

(64), Dejerine (77), Foerster (78), and Brash (74). The peripheral nervous system of the skeleton is closely linked to muscle innervation. Most of the bones of the skeleton receive their innervation from nerve twigs of the attached muscles. Some parts of the skeleton, especially the joints, receive branches directly from nerve trunks (65).

Autonomic Innervation

The peripheral component of the autonomic nervous system is concerned with the innervation of the visceral glands, blood vessels, and nonstriated muscle. The relationship to pain has been confined to the visceral components in this section (70,75,79–81).

DIAGNOSTIC AND CLINICAL EVALUATION

Physical Examination

In establishing the etiology of pain, it is essential to consider its characteristics, its chronology, the limitations it imposes on the patient, and the results of previous therapy. This is accomplished by a thorough pain evaluation, including a detailed history, a comprehensive physical examination, and

TABLE 56-2. *Lower extremity muscle innervation*

Muscle	Peripheral nerve	Spinal segment
Psoas major	Lumbar plexus	L1,**L2,L3**
Iliacus	Femoral	**L2,L3**,L4
Sartorius	Femoral	**L2,L3**,L4
Quadriceps femoris	Femoral	**L2,L3,L4**
Adductor longus	Obturator	**L2,L3**,L4
Adductor brevis	Obturator	**L2,L3,L4**
Gracilis	Obturator	**L2,L3,L4**
Adductor magnus	Obturator and sciatic	L2,**L3,L4**,L5,S1
Gluteus medius	Superior gluteal	(L4),**L5,S1**
Gluteus minimus	Superior gluteal	(L4),**L5,S1**
Tensor fascia lata	Superior gluteal	(L4),**L5,S1**
Gluteus maximus	Inferior gluteal	**L5,S1**,S2
Biceps femoris (long head)	Sciatic (tibial div)	L5,**S1,S2**
Semitendinosus	Sciatic (tibial div)	**L5,S1**,S2
Semimembranosus	Sciatic (tibial div)	L4,**L5,S1,S2**
Biceps femoris (short head)	Sciatic (peroneal div)	L5,**S1**,S2
Tibialis anterior	Peroneal	**L4,L5**,S1
Extensor hallucis longus	Peroneal	L4,**L5**,S1
Extensor digitorum longus	Peroneal	L4,**L5,S1**
Peroneus tertius	Peroneal	L4,**L5,S1**
Extensor digitorum brevis	Peroneal	**L5,S1**
Peroneus longus	Peroneal	(L4),**L5**,S1
Peroneus brevis	Peroneal	L4,**L5,S1**
Gastrocnemius (medial head)	Tibial	L5,**S1,S2**
Gastrocnemius (lateral head)	Tibial	**L5,S1**
Soleus	Tibial	(L5),**S1,S2**
Tibialis posterior	Tibial	(L4),**L5**,S1
Flexor digitorum longus	Tibial	**L5,S1**
Flexor hallucis longus	Tibial	**L5,S1**,S2
Abductor hallucis	Tibial	(L5),**S1,S2**
Abductor digiti minimi	Tibial	**S1,S2**
Plantar/dorsal interossei	Tibial	**S1, S2**

Spinal segments in parentheses signify those that are occasionally present; those in boldface are the major segments supplying the muscle designated. Segments not in boldface are usually present but to a minor degree.

appropriate tests. Most pain patients present a complex array of physical, motivational, cognitive, and affective manifestations and therefore require detailed psychological and social evaluations.

A detailed history of the pain complaint identifies the pain in terms of its location of origin, radiation, quality, severity, and time intensity attributes, as well as mode of onset, duration, time of occurrence, and factors that aggravate and relieve it. Previous treatments for pain should be noted, including comments regarding usefulness in the reduction of pain. Medications currently being taken, as well as those used in the past, should be recorded, along with the patient's perceptions as to the results achieved by each. The details of physical therapy, including types of modalities, exercise, and effective regimes, should be recorded. An inquiry as to the patient's attempts at biofeedback, relaxation, and hypnosis are also helpful. Information regarding associated findings including sensory deficits, muscle weakness, and altered body function should be obtained. It should be determined whether compensation is involved and if the patient is working; if not, the employment history should be obtained. The physical examination and related diagnostic studies should be directed toward evaluating the site of pain and related regions. This process is useful in acquiring objective data to substantiate the clinical history.

Physical examination begins when the patient is first seen and continues through every contact made with the patient. This provides the opportunity for the physician to evaluate how the pain affects motion and activities. Physical examination always includes examination of related components of the spine and musculoskeletal system, as well as a neurologic evaluation. Painful regions need to be compared with normal areas on the contralateral side of the patient for sensation, temperature, and sensitivity to palpation.

Functional evaluation measures the appropriateness of the patient's functional capabilities for the level of impairment. Objective, quantitative measurements give a baseline with which to evaluate progress and long-term outcome.

Diagnostic Procedures

Laboratory Tests

Laboratory findings in acute and chronic pain usually have no features distinct from those found with a primary disease.

Drug screening tests of the blood and urine may provide valuable information as to the variety and type of pain medications being ingested. Serum drug level testing provides data to determine the bioavailability of medications being taken by the patient.

Radiology

Radiographic procedures are extensively used in the evaluation of pain. Spinal radiography has minimal value in the evaluation of most low back pain conditions because of the equal prevalence of abnormalities in symptomatic and asymptomatic populations, that is, low specificity and predictive value (82,83). In a specific diagnosis of low back pain in sciatica due to herniated nucleus pulposus, plain radiography has been shown to have no value (84,85).

Radiography, computed tomography (CT), and magnetic resonance imaging (MRI) demonstrate anatomic or structural disorders, which account for a low percentage of functional abnormalities. However, CT, myelography, and MRI are well established in the diagnosis of disk herniation and provide significant false-positive results in subjects with no history of back pain. Asymptomatic individuals are diagnosed as having abnormalities (24% to 50%) on myelography (86), discography (87), CT (88), and MRI (89). The clinical usage of diagnostic tests requires a careful correlation between clinical signs, symptoms, and test results. For additional information on imaging studies, the reader is referred to Chapter 19.

Psychological Evaluation

The assessment of psychological issues in the overall evaluation and treatment of patients with chronic pain is an important component of any pain management program (90). Psychological evaluation often involves the use of questionnaires, inventories, and the clinical interview. Psychophysical methods of pain assessment (91) (tourniquet test, cold pressor test, and visual analog scales) often augment the psychological evaluation.

The *McGill Pain Questionnaire* (92) is an often-used instrument designed to measure three dimensions of the pain experience: sensory, affective, and evaluative. The *Minnesota Multiphasic Personality Inventory* (MMPI or MMPI-2) has been used in the United States perhaps more than any other psychological instrument in the assessment of personality factors contributing to the experience of chronic pain (48). The typical *Minnesota Multiphasic Personality Inventory* profile for a patient with chronic pain denotes increased levels of hypochondriasis, depression, and hysteria. Numerous MMPI typologies based on clustering algorithms have been proposed. A combination of 10 investigations resulted in four types (P-A-I-N) appearing to have clinical and demographic correlates (93). The clinical interview helps to identify the affective, motivational, cognitive, and personality components of the patient with chronic pain. The emphasis of this evaluation is on the patient's behavioral response to pain, adjustments to impairment/disability, primary/secondary gain, and motivation. The psychological evaluation will help clarify affective, cognitive, and motivational components of the chronic pain. In conjunction with pentothal and amytal challenges, the psychological evaluation is helpful in differentiating patients with significant somatic/peripheral pain from somatoform pain disorders and conscience exaggerators (94).

Electrodiagnosis

Electrodiagnosis is an objective neurophysiologic extension of the physical examination. It typically includes the determination of nerve conduction velocities (NCV) and needle electromyographic (EMG) studies of individual muscles. In addition, a relatively new technique known as somatosensory evoked potentials (SSEP) has expanded the armamentarium of the electromyographer in evaluating the peripheral and central nervous system (95–97). For additional information on electrodiagnostic evaluation, the reader is referred to Chapters 15 and 16. EMG and evoked potential studies demonstrate the pathophysiologic changes associated with or due to structural abnormalities. The documentation of existing pathology is vitally important to the comprehensive management of complex painful conditions. Careful clinical correlation is essential when interpreting all tests related to chronic pain (98).

Anesthetic Procedures

The subsequent response of the body and mind to pain results in sympathetic nervous system and psychogenic responses. Although clinical examination and appropriate investigations can help in delineating the contribution of the various mechanisms in an individual patient, many patients do not exhibit clearcut mechanisms of pain. In these patients, differential diagnostic blocks may be valuable. Clinicians using the differential blocks are frequently impressed by their usefulness in pointing to mechanisms not suspected when considering the results of previous clinical examinations and laboratory workup (99–101).

Thiobarbiturates such as pentothal and sodium amytal are useful in differentiating the patients who have somatic pain from those who have psychogenic or malingering pain (102,103).

Thermography

Thermography is a new and controversial method of evaluating pain. This procedure uses measurements of infrared radiation from the body for diagnostic purposes. The infrared energy emissions from one area of the skin, representing skin temperature, are recorded for comparison with patterns from adjacent skin areas. Thermal patterns that are bilaterally symmetrical are considered normal.

Thermography is based on the hypothesis that localized irritation of sympathetic nerves results in sympathetic nervous system stimulation. The increased output of the autonomic nervous system constricts the small arterioles in the skin, producing diminished temperature in the area that the sympathetic nerves innervate. The nerve topography of the vessels in the sympathetic chain are different from those of the somatasensory nervous system (104,105). Thermography is reported to provide objective evidence of physiologic dysfunction in pain patients (106). However, it has not yet been shown to be a valid assessment of pain other than of that due to neurovascular compression syndromes and autonomic nervous system etiology (107,108).

The diagnostic reliability of thermography is still unknown. The studies to date have failed to use a carefully selected control population, or the observers were not blinded and, therefore, were subject to observer bias. In the absence of carefully controlled experiments with a large sample size, the accuracy of thermography in the diagnosis of the evaluation of back pain, spinal lesions, and similar pain syndromes is still speculative (107,109–111).

CLINICAL MANAGEMENT

The primary goals of treating a patient with pain are alleviating the pain and enhancing the patient's quality of life and functional capabilities. The management of acute pain is based on pharmacologic, psychological, medical, and surgical innovations or advancements within the past century. And yet, the management of chronic pain has been recognized as a major health-care problem only in the past 25 years. It remains unclear why some people become patients with chronic pain and others resolve their acute pain without significant difficulty.

Multidisciplinary Approach

The chronic pain problem is multifaceted. No single physician has the resources to care comprehensively for the complex psychological, social, legal, medical, and physical problems involved in chronic pain. Therefore, the multidisciplinary team approach is necessary. Using an interdisciplinary approach does not mean the patient is referred from one specialist to another because this tends to result in conflicting and overlapping treatment and a loss of hope of treatment in the patient. Ideally, the team should work together to provide a unified explanation of the illness and a comprehensive treatment program. The multidisciplinary pain service has the advantage of offering a variety of coherent treatment approaches to the patient. This type of program recognizes that a multifaceted problem requires a multifaceted approach, as well as continuity of care in which the patient is an active participant (112).

The core group for the multidisciplinary treatment service includes a physiatrist, an anesthesiologist, and a clinical psychologist or psychiatrist. This group may vary considerably according to local needs, resources, and available expertise. However, the team must have the knowledge to manage the psychological and social problems with optimal medical and anesthetic treatments. They must also have a thorough understanding of physical treatments and the rehabilitation process.

The multidisciplinary pain approach begins with a complete clinical evaluation. Comprehensive medical and psychosocial evaluations with particular emphasis on functional capabilities and behavioral responses to pain are essential. The somatic, affective, cognitive, and emotional components of the chronic pain experience are explored. All previous medical records are needed to avoid repeating appropriately performed studies and unsuccessful treatment approaches. This comprehensive clinical evaluation also includes functional capabilities to determine impairment level. The psychosocial evaluation focuses on the behavioral response to pain, adjustments to the physical impairment, and degree of motivation (113). The MMPI-2 and other written tests are often used for generalized screening.

The multidisciplinary team functions at several levels within the treatment process. They attempt to identify and resolve documentable organic problems when present and to improve the patient's ability to cope with the pain through medication, psychological intervention, and patient education. In addition, considerable effort is devoted to improving the patient's functional outcome as measured by increased activity time, improved activities of daily living, increased distance walked, and increased tolerance for specific homemaking or vocational activities. To accomplish these objectives, the multidisciplinary team must use many skills. In many cases, the patient with chronic pain is so entrenched in pain behavior that a behavior modification approach is essential. These patients are often characterized by low levels of activities of daily living, high demand for medication accompanied by physical and psychological dependency, high verbalization of pain, and the inability to work.

Pain Treatment Centers

The organization and operation of the multidisciplinary pain clinic have been discussed by Grabois (114). Many behavior modification programs use the Fordyce model (48,115). This approach uses the general principles of interruption of the pain behavior reinforcement cycle, reward of healthy behavior, appropriate goals that the patient must achieve, measurement of improvement by functional assessment as well as pain level, and psychosocial adjustment. Particular emphasis is placed on detoxification and medication reduction, pain reduction, increased activity, and modification of pain behavior.

If the patient is on pain medications and determined to be physically or psychologically dependent, he or she must be detoxified. This is routinely accomplished by establishing the equivalent dosage of each medication type (e.g., narcotics, benzodiazepines, barbiturates, alcohol). Narcotic medications are replaced with methadone, and long-acting barbiturates are replaced with phenobarbital or pentobarbital. Medication equivalents are placed in orange juice or in capsulated form and decreased at a rate of 5% to 10% per day. The medication is then given on an around-the-clock basis at fixed intervals. Gradual reduction of the pain ingredients occurs without significant side effects of withdrawal. The patient is not aware of the timing of the decrease but has been informed of the concept before starting the program. Nonsteroidal anti-inflammatory drugs (NSAIDs) and tricyclic or selective serotonin reuptake inhibitor (SSRI) antidepressants are routinely integrated as long-term medications. The pain management program is designed to reduce rather than eliminate pain, while increasing the patient's functional capabilities.

The patient with chronic pain usually exhibits a decreased activity level, which results in a disuse syndrome. The exercise programs are based on the initial specific and general exercise that the individual can perform. The exercise regimen is progressive, with the goals rising along with the patient's ability. Rewards for accomplishing tasks are a mainstay of this program with no reinforcement given for pain behavior. The achievable goals provide success and confidence and allow for frequent reinforcement when they are met. Cooperation by all staff members is essential; they must consistently ignore pain complaints and encourage improved function. Psychological intervention is used as indicated. The chronic pain behavior modification programs report short-term success rates in medication reduction, increased activity, and more productive behavior patterns (116,117). Statistics suggest 60% to 80% improvement in patients with chronic pain without major psychosocial components, 30% to 50% in patients with significant psychosocial components, and approximately 20% in patients with major psychiatric components or secondary gains (114,118–120).

Multidisciplinary chronic pain treatment is a focused unified approach to the chronic pain syndrome. In this country, pain treatment centers differ widely in organization and emphasis. They are generally multidisciplinary centers that use some combination of anesthesiologists, clinical psychologists, dentists, neurologists, orthopedists, pharmacists, physiatrists, and psychiatrists. The goals of these centers are to diminish, if not eliminate, chronic pain; increase the patient's functional capabilities to allow for a more active life; and decrease the patient's dependence on drugs for pain control.

Physical Modalities

Physical modalities are valuable adjuncts to the successful management of acute and chronic pain. Therapeutic heat and cryotherapy are time-honored interventions in treating musculoskeletal pain. More recent clinical evaluation of transcutaneous electrical nerve stimulation (TENS), acupuncture, and cold laser have questioned the efficacy of these methods available to the physician in alleviating discomfort (121). For additional information on physical agents, the reader is referred to Chapter 20.

Pain arising from the musculoskeletal system is often caused by muscle spasm (89). Heat and cold applications are primarily directed at reducing spasmodic muscle shortening (122). The shortened muscle may be a result of direct muscular trauma or underlying primary neurologic or skeletal disease. Investigators have studied the muscle spindle and its firing rate in relation to thermal changes (123,124). Direct and indirect effects on the muscle spindle are detected from both heat and cold applications (125). The return of the muscle to its normal resting length is also believed to promote the reduction and resolution of pain (126), but precisely how muscle spasm is relieved is not completely understood.

Cryotherapy

Therapeutic cold has four distinct applications in medicine: stop or slow bleeding; induce hypothermia; decrease spasticity; and relieve pain (127). It may be applied as a solid, liquid, or gas. Ice is a common solid form of direct cold therapy and is usually rubbed in a circular fashion over the localized painful area. Immersing a body part in water combined with ice chips may provide pain relief. Cold applied directly to an injured area in acute musculoskeletal trauma serves to reduce hemorrhage and vasodilation, blunts the local inflammatory response, decreases edema production, and reduces pain perception. The so-called PRICE (protection, rest, ice, compression, and elevation) method is commonly prescribed for acute sports-related injuries (128).

In addition to acute musculoskeletal injuries, cryotherapy has been shown to benefit chronic painful conditions. Pain may be alleviated by direct or indirect mechanisms (129). The direct effect is the decrease in temperature of the affected area. Reduced pain sensation is presumed to result through an indirect effect on the nerve fibers and sensory end organs. Additionally, the decreased temperature reduces the firing rate of the muscle spindle and decreases the painful muscle tone (124,129).

The direct application of ice massage has been shown to be therapeutically efficacious in several clinical trials. Grant demonstrated the beneficial effects of direct ice application on a large population of young individuals sustaining acute and chronic musculoskeletal trauma (130). Pegg demonstrated that chronic inflammatory joint disease improved clinically with cold in regard to pain, stiffness, and range of motion (131). Patients with low back pain also responded well to controlled clinical trials using cryotherapy (132).

The application of cold as a vapocoolant spray was popularized by Travell in treating myofascial pain syndromes (133,134). A counterirritant effect is presumed to provide the mechanism of muscle spasm relief and pain alleviation. The combination of vapocoolant spray, stretching, and trigger point injection has been reported to provide significant pain relief in the myofascial pain syndromes (134,135). The mechanism of this pain relief remains unclear.

Adverse effects also have been reported with the use of cold (129). The major reaction is hypersensitivity. Patients with Raynaud's and peripheral vascular disease should not have their limbs exposed to cold temperatures because this produces vasoconstriction. In addition, patients who display a marked cold pressor response are poor candidates for cryotherapy.

Heat Therapy

Heat application is a common form of pain treatment. It is generally accepted that therapeutic heat is best tolerated in the subacute and chronic phases of a disease process. The physiologic responses produced by heat are increased collagen extensibility, increased blood flow and metabolic rate, and inflammation resolution. Decreased joint stiffness, muscle spasm, and pain are also beneficial effects of heat.

Therapeutic heat is believed to have direct and indirect effects on the muscle spindle. Local elevated temperatures have been shown to directly decrease the spindle sensitivity (136), and superficial heating of the skin has been demonstrated to indirectly reduce spindle excitability (125). This mechanism is similar to that proposed for decreased muscle spindle activity with the application of cold. It is also believed that the pain threshold may be raised by the direct and indirect actions of heat.

Pain associated with numerous conditions has been successfully treated with therapeutic heat application. Musculoskeletal contractures respond well to deep heat used in association with prolonged stretch (137). Joint stiffness associated with chronic inflammatory diseases, particularly those affecting the limbs, responds to superficial heating with decreased pain and increased range of motion and function. Subacute and chronic bursitis, tenosynovitis, and epicondylitis also may respond to heat with decreased pain and symptom resolution.

TENS Therapy

The use of electrical currents dates back to the Greeks, who applied torpedo fish to individuals suffering from pain (138). Electricity eventually fell into disrepute until Melzak and Wall proposed the gate control theory of pain (54). This gate control model provided the theoretical basis for the use of electrical current in pain control. They found that the preferential activation of large afferent fibers (using TENS) would inhibit the transmission of painful impulses. The exact physiologic basis by which TENS produces pain control is unknown.

Available equipment can produce a variety of specific wave forms, and the most effective one has not yet been determined (139). Therefore, it is clinically efficacious to try different wave forms when a particular one fails to achieve optimal pain suppression.

Electrode placement for a TENS unit must be based on a knowledge of anatomic and physiologic principles. The painful area is often initially chosen as the site for electrode placement. The actual landmarks for the electrode may be a dermatome, peripheral nerve, motor point, or acupuncture point. Electrode arrangement over the painful area may be linear, triangular, or criss-cross. Occasionally electrodes also may be placed on nonpainful areas (140).

The conventional short-duration, high-frequency TENS has been applied with a current of low frequency and long duration (acupuncturelike TENS). It appears that TENS may achieve pain relief by stimulating large sensory afferent fibers and inhibiting pain perception, or by enhancing the production of endogenous opioids.

TENS also has been used extensively to manage chronic pain. The results have been less promising and more variable than those in acute pain trials. Rigorous controlled trials suggest that TENS is no better than placebo in the management of chronic low back pain (1,141). Patients with RSD, phantom limb pain, and peripheral nerve injury all have demonstrated pain control with TENS (142–144). The most efficacious use of TENS appears to be in the control of selected acute pain conditions such as postoperative incisional pain.

There are relatively few side effects related to TENS. The major problem is one of skin irritation related to the conducting paste or tape that secures the electrodes. Currently, the use of TENS in patients with demand cardiac pacemakers is inadvisable (144).

Acupuncture

Acupuncture (originating from the Latin *acus* or "sharp point" and *punctura,* "to puncture") is an ancient Chinese therapy practiced for more than 2,500 years to cure disease or relieve pain. Thin metal needles are inserted into specific body sites and slowly twisted manually or stimulated electrically. Various sensations may be produced, ranging from a dull ache or warmth, to that of a pinprick. The Chinese believe that acupuncture achieves its beneficial results by restoring the balance between *yang* (spirit) and *yin* (blood), which flow in 14 channels or meridians containing 361 acupuncture sites.

Researchers have considered acupuncture to be a form of neuromodulation. Two theories have been proposed for its use in pain control. First, acupuncture may stimulate large sensory afferent fibers and suppress pain perception as explained by the gate control theory of pain. Second, the needle insertion may act as a noxious stimulus and induce endogenous production of opiatelike substances to effect pain control (145).

It has been demonstrated that there is a significant overlap between traditional acupuncture sites, myofascial trigger points, and muscular motor points (146). The sensation induced by the application of an acupuncture needle is very similar to the dull ache often experienced by the patient when a trigger point is injected. The insertion of a needle, regardless of the substance injected, appears to produce the beneficial pain relief and is termed the *needle effect.* The injection of trigger points may share not only similar areas of needle insertion, but also associated mechanisms of pain control.

Acupuncture has been used in a wide variety of painful conditions. The insertion of a needle is considered an invasive procedure, and many states require a physician to perform or supervise the treatment. Uniform agreement does not yet exist as to the preferred time necessary for an adequate trial of acupuncture. The efficacy of acupuncture has not been scientifically demonstrated (88,147).

Reported side effects of acupuncture include localized hyperemia occurring frequently following needle insertion. Infrequently, syncopal episodes, hematoma formation, and pneumothorax also have been reported. Caution is suggested in the use of electrical acupuncture with patients who have cardiac pacemakers (148).

Laser Treatment

Light amplification by stimulated emission of radiation (LASER), which can result in tissue destruction (hot laser), is an accepted form of treatment in many surgical procedures (149). Cold laser therapy is reportedly incapable of tissue destruction and has been used empirically on a variety of painful conditions (150). The effectiveness of this technique has not been demonstrated scientifically, and its mode of action, if any, remains speculative. Therefore, it is advisable to use cold laser therapy cautiously. More controlled studies are needed to determine its scientific credibility, mode of action, and efficacy (151–154).

Therapeutic Exercise

During acute injuries to the musculoskeletal system, a muscle may shorten as a protective reaction to pain. Treatment typically consists of immobilization combined with compression and cryotherapy. As the pain subsides, mobility is restored gradually. If normal range of motion is not achieved, the muscle may become chronically shortened and result in additional pain.

Prolonged muscle shortening will add to the painful condition by producing contracted soft-tissue structures. In the chronic phase of pain, the optimal treatment methodology combines graded stretching movements, strengthening exercises, heat or cold, and massage. The patient is also educated regarding proper body mechanics and the need to continue the prescribed therapeutic exercise regimen outside of formal therapy sessions.

Therapeutic exercise, prescribed to correct a specific abnormal condition, is often used to treat chronic painful conditions. The primary goal is to aid the patient in achieving pain control. This may be accomplished through the restoration of normal muscle tone, length, strength, and optimal joint range of motion. Finally, the patient is urged to continue a home program after formal therapy sessions have ceased (155).

Therapeutic exercise consists of passive movements, active-assistive exercises, active exercises, stretching, and relaxing exercises. Each may be used alone or in combination to achieve the desired effect (119,156–158). Therapeutic stretching exercises, similar to the YMCA program developed by Kraus, are effective in the management of chronic low back pain (1). For additional information on therapeutic exercise, the reader is referred to Chapter 28.

Behavioral Treatment Modalities

Among the treatment goals of pain management are the decrease in illness behavior (reduced drug use and visits to physicians) and the increase in well behavior (increased physical activities, mobility, and return to gainful employment). This may be accomplished by blocking noxious sensory input, decreasing tension and depression, rearranging reinforcement contingencies, or assisting in the learning of new behaviors (159). Biofeedback, cognitive behavior modification, operant approaches, hypnosis, operant pain hypnosis, and relaxation training can assist in the treatment of chronic pain behavior (160).

Biofeedback (161) has found some use in the treatment of chronic pain (162,163). Typically biofeedback teaches muscle relaxation (through EMG) or temperature control. The instrumentation is reported to be somewhat useful, although clinical experience suggests that relaxation without instrumentation is of equal value. Through biofeedback training the patient learns self-regulation of pain.

Cognitive behavior modification helps the patient learn self-coping statements and problem-solving cognitions (164) in order to alter the cognitive structures (schemata, beliefs) and cognitive process (automatic thoughts, images, and internal dialogue) associated with the pain experience. Cognitive strategies of imaginative inattention, imaginative transformation of pain, focused attention, and somatization in a dissociation manner have been found helpful.

The operant approach involves the identification of behaviors to be produced, increased, maintained, or eliminated. Reinforcement is then regulated to achieve the desired outcome. Activity and walking programs are followed to the prescribed level, not to discomfort. All medication is prescribed by schedule. Family and friends are instructed to avoid reinforcing all pain behavior.

Relaxation methods (165,166) to reduce tension may include deep muscle relaxation, deep diaphragmatic breathing, meditation, yoga, and autogenic training. Patients also may be taught self-hypnosis (161). Hypnosis has the advantage of providing relief without unpleasant side effects, with no reduction of normal functioning and no development of tolerance. Hypnotic strategies can suggest analgesia or anesthesia, substitute another feeling for pain, move the pain perception to a smaller or less vulnerable area, alter the meaning of pain, increase tolerance to pain, or, in some individuals, dissociate the perception of body from the patient's awareness.

Pharmacologic Intervention

Two groups of patients are encountered in the clinical management of chronic pain. The first group includes individuals with acute and recurrent pain due to chronic medical illness such as rheumatoid arthritis, cancer, and burn injuries. Primary therapy is usually directed at the underlying cause of pain. When the therapy is successful, the pain treatment is successful. Treatment commonly includes NSAIDs. Narcotic analgesics are used sparingly, on a limited basis, using time duration regimens to limit the development of psychological dependence.

The second group of patients consists of individuals who have chronic pain without organic etiology. Pharmacologic intervention is the most common means of treatment for chronic pain. Substances may be divided into three categories: NSAIDs, narcotics, and adjuvant drugs.

Nonsteroidal antiinflammatory analgesics include aspirin, acetaminophen, and the newer NSAIDs. These drugs are peripherally active analgesics that do not inhibit nociception or alter the perception of the pain input. They are best considered remittent agents that alter the pathologic processes which generate pain. Aspirin and other NSAIDs reduce pain by interfering with prostaglandin (PG) sensitization of nociceptors and inhibiting the synthesis of prostaglandins. Additional NSAID actions include inhibition of tissue reaction to bradykinin, suppressed release of histamine, and decreased vascular permeability. This improves the environment of the nociceptor, increasing pain control by decreasing sensitivity. With the exception of acetaminophen, the NSAIDs also possess anti-inflammatory effects that reduce local heat, swelling, and stiffness. These drugs are used to treat patients with acute and chronic pain of low to moderate severity.

NSAIDs are often chosen over narcotics because they have fewer side effects, including no constipation, very little sedation, no psychological or physical dependence, and no development of tolerance. The mainstays of non-narcotic analgesic therapy are aspirin and acetaminophen. Acetaminophen is an excellent alternative to aspirin in patients who are unable to tolerate other NSAID medication. All NSAIDs have ceiling effects, but the ceilings for some of these drugs are higher than that of aspirin (167).

Although aspirin, acetaminophen, and other NSAID compounds are available over the counter, they all have potential side effects. The most common complication, involving the gastrointestinal tract, is seen in 5% to 10% of patients. These drugs produce in varying degrees gastrointestinal, hematologic, renal, and hepatic toxicities. The side effects from prolonged use of all NSAIDs are similar to those occurring with aspirin, but there are significant differences in the potential for side effects. Aspirin, in the nonsalicylated salsalate form (Disalcid, 3M Pharmaceuticals, St. Paul, MN), remains the preferred drug for the patient with chronic pain. The newer NSAIDs have not been proven to offer any major advantage over aspirin, although their cost is much greater (88). Notable exceptions are patients unable to tolerate acetylsalicylic acid or who demonstrate difficulty with compliance.

Narcotic medication is useful and appropriate in the treatment of acute, recurrent, or cancer pain. Acute and recurrent pain are usually best managed by diagnosis and treatment of the underlying cause of the pain. The narcotic medication is used as an adjunct to provide relief during a period of temporary, excruciating pain. Narcotic analgesics are also preferred for relief of intractible pain due to cancer. The greatest obstacle to treating postoperative pain, pain related to cancer, acute pain, and recurrent pain due to chronic disease is the excessive concern of the physician regarding addiction. Repeated studies report that a high percentage of house officers tend to overestimate their patient's potential for addiction and, consequently, undermedicate them (168). Ironically, undermedication may increase the potential for addiction due to the operant conditioning, anxiety, and dependent behavior created by inadequate pain relief. Psychological dependence has not been a major problem in patients with acute pain or cancer pain who receive appropriately dosed narcotic analgesics for moderate to severe pain (169).

Narcotic medications should be avoided in the treatment of patients with chronic pain. There is almost no justification for the use of narcotic drugs in the patient with chronic pain having no organic etiology. The long-term use of narcotic drugs with these patients often produces behavioral complications that are more difficult to manage than the initial pain problem. The hazards of tolerance, physical dependence, and psychological dependence present major problems in the long-term management of this patient group. Deficits of cognition and motor function, as well as the masking of psychological disorders, are common. The indiscriminate use of narcotic medications in an attempt to control chronic pain only enhances chronic pain behavior.

Morphine is the prototype of the narcotic drugs and is commonly prescribed by many clinicians (3). Pain relief is often obtained by titrating the dose to the patient's needs. At equianalgesic doses there is no significant pharmacologic evidence to suggest the choice of one narcotic over another (170), but there are significant differences in their action times, equianalgesic dose, and parenteral/oral ratio (see Table 56-5 later in this chapter). Inappropriate drug dosing often occurs because of a lack of knowledge or attention to equianalgesic doses, resulting in inadequate pain relief.

All clinically useful narcotics produce similar side effects in equianalgesic doses. The undesirable side effects of narcotics on the central nervous system include unwanted sedation, mental clouding, inability to concentrate, lethargy, impairment of mental and physical performance, constipation, nausea and vomiting, tolerance, physical dependence, psychological dependence, and impaired respiration. These side effects inhibit the patient with chronic pain whose goal is to maintain a normal life-style.

Oral administration of medication is preferred in the treatment of all pain. A time-contingent round-the-clock schedule for pain medications is superior to an as-needed schedule.

This form of administration minimizes alterations in plasma levels and provides optimal pain control. The schedule should be based on such variables as potency, duration of the analgesic effect, and efficacy of the analgesic medication. A regularly scheduled dosage optimizes the reduction of pain by minimizing the peaks and valleys of pain intensity. Generally it is better to begin the initial dose of medication too high rather than too low. Starting suboptimally and titrating upward results in the patient's experiencing anxiety due to a lack of adequate analgesic.

The as-needed, or PRN, schedule does not have a place in the control of chronic pain. Such a schedule results in operant conditioning, craving, a sense of dependence, and anxiety about the drug wearing off. In chronic pain management, the drugs with longer duration of action are usually preferred. There is considerable patient-to-patient variation with respect to effective analgesic dosage (171,172).

The adjuvant analgesic drugs produce or potentiate analgesia by mechanisms not directly mediated through the opiate receptor system. This group includes a wide variety of compounds with no proven specific analgesic properties: tricyclic antidepressants, anticonvulsants, and antispasmodics. The use of these drugs is often based on anecdotal data, clinical surveys, or limited drug trials.

Tricyclic antidepressants, such as amitriptyline (Elavil, Zeneca Pharmaceuticals, Wilmington, DE), doxepin (Sinequan, Roerig, New York, NY), and imipramine (Tofranil, CibaGeneva, Summit, NJ), have been used in the treatment of chronic pain syndromes. One of the primary mechanisms of tricyclic compounds is to block the reuptake of the neurotransmitter serotonin in the central nervous system. This enhances pain inhibition by way of the dorsolateral pathway (22,173). In addition, amitriptyline is a potent sedative drug, which may be used as a sleeping medication in patients with chronic pain. The combination of antidepressant effect, enhanced cortical serotonergic mechanism, and improved sleep contributes to these medications being one of the most commonly used group of psychotropic agents in pain management (174–176).

Anticonvulsants such as phenytoin (Dilantin, Parke-Davis, Morris Plains, NJ) and carbamazepine (Tegretol, CibaGeneva, Summit, NJ) have been used in the management of pain syndromes affecting the central nervous system. Their applications include trigeminal neuralgia, postherpetic neuralgia, causalgia, and phantom pain syndromes. Although the mechanism is unclear, they appear to have a stabilizing effect on excitable cell membranes, which decreases afferent and deafferent second-order neuron activity. Carbamazepine may have a central serotonin action similar to that of amitriptyline (177).

Other anticonvulsants suggested for pain usage are valproic acid (Depakene, Abbott Laboratories, North Chicago, IL) and clonazepam (Klonopin, Roche Laboratories, Nutley, NJ). They increase the effectiveness of gamma amino butyric acid (GABA)-induced inhibition in the pre- and postsynaptic systems. These drugs appear to be most effective in the treatment of neuralgias and neuropathies.

Antispasmodics such as baclofen (Lioresal, CibaGeneva, Summit, NJ) are presumed to act by inhibiting gamma transaminases and their reuptake at gamma receptor sites. Valproic acid and clonazepam act in a similar fashion (178,179).

In addition to these medications, a number of other adjuvant medications have been used. These include methotrimeprazine, chlorpromazine, and fluphenazine. Butyrophenones are anecdotal in the management of pain disorders, with haloperidol being the most often reported. Antihistamines, amphetamines, steroids, and cannabinoids are also reported anecdotally. Steroids such as prednisone and dexamethasone are thought to interfere with prostaglandin sensitization of nociceptors. Selective serotonin reuptake inhibitors are being used for multiple pain conditions (180,181). Serotonin antagonists such as ergot alkaloids, the beta-blocking agents such as propranolol, and the antihistamines such as hydroxyzine all function by antagonizing transmitters that directly activate nociceptors. These medications have been used extensively in the treatment of migraine and cluster headaches. Lithium and calcium blocking agents have been proposed as drugs to interfere with the release of transmitters involved in the pain process (58).

Benzodiazepines and barbiturates are two groups that have little or no place as adjuvant drugs in chronic pain management. Long-term use of these medications may result in psychological and physical dependence as well as interference with cognition and motor function. Benzodiazepines, because of their claimed muscle relaxant properties, are often prescribed to patients with pain. However, their role as muscle relaxants is questionable in clinical studies. In addition to the adverse effects of dependency, it has been suggested that these medications adversely affect the serotonin system. These medications are depressants that, with long-term use, lower pain tolerance and tend to induce clinical depression as well as psychological and physical dependence. Due to their sedative effects, depressants often act as potent reinforcers of pain in drug-seeking behaviors. Chronic use of these medications may result in physical and mental incapacitation, emotional instability, and the inability to deal with initial physiologic or psychological problems. Benzodiazepines deplete serotonin, alter sleep patterns, and increase pain perception. It is recommended that these two groups of medications should not be part of the long-term management of chronic pain. The only possible indication for these sedatives or for antianxiety agents is for the short-term (less than 1 month) treatment of a self-limited crisis unrelated to the particular pain problem, or as an adjunct when detoxifying a patient from narcotic medication.

Anesthetic Procedures

Blocking the nerve with a local anesthetic agent is one of the most common procedures in the management of chronic pain. Nerve block by itself, however, is not effective in relieving pain completely for a long period in the majority of patients. Therefore, nerve blocks should be considered as only one of the therapeutic modalities used in the multidisciplinary pain clinic. Other factors, such as psychological problems and associated muscle tightness and weakness, should be treated by using other appropriate modalities. Nerve blocks are helpful in many patients by interrupting the pain process. It is the experience of many clinicians that when pain is temporarily interrupted by a local anesthetic block, often the patient's pain is permanently relieved. Nerve blocks are also useful in delineating the pain mechanisms and in blocking the pain when the patients are required to take part in physical therapy to mobilize the muscles and joints. Patients who have a nerve block followed by appropriate physical therapy display excellent results (182). The best results have been shown in patients requiring manipulation and mobilization of the knee and other joints. There are various nerve block techniques used in pain clinics; the most common and useful include epidural use of a local anesthetic or narcotic, and peripheral nerve block (98,183). For more information on injection techniques, the reader is referred to Chapter 23.

Administration of local anesthetic or narcotic can provide prolonged relief by placement of a catheter in the epidural space, which can be left in place for several days to a few weeks. A local anesthetic or narcotic can be administered intermittently or by continuous infusion, providing somatic and sympathetic block and analgesia for physical therapy. This is the most commonly applied technique in patients who have low back and lower extremity pain while they undergo physical therapy and mobilization (182).

Peripheral nerve block, such as suprascapular nerve block, is very useful in patients who have shoulder discomfort, frozen shoulder, or shoulder pain of other etiology. Patients can tolerate stretching and physical therapy after a suprascapular block with local anesthetic. In the upper extremities, brachial plexus blocks, especially continuous blocks performed by axillary or supraclavicular route, are of great value in patients requiring physical therapy. Other peripheral blocks, such as the lateral femoral cutaneous nerve block for patients with meralgia parasthetica, the femoral nerve block for patients with thigh and knee pain, and sciatic nerve and intercostal blocks, have been extremely useful in managing patients with chronic pain.

Depo- types of steroids, injected into the epidural space, have been extremely useful in relieving nerve root irritation and inflammation in patients who have a herniated disk. They also have been effective in patients who have nerve root irritation secondary to radiation or a malignancy. The steroid preparations commonly used are Depo-Medrol (Upjohn, Kalamazoo, MI) (40 to 80 mg) and Aristospan intralesional (Fujisawa USA, Deerfield, IL) (25 to 50 mg). Although steroid preparations may be used to produce anti-inflammatory action, the steroid preparations contain various preservatives such as benzyl alcohol, which may produce serious side effects, including paralysis. Only Depo-Medrol and Aristospan have been extensively used without producing significant neurologic damage (184).

The steroids are injected into the epidural space close to the involved root. These injections can be performed at any level, including cervical, thoracic, or lumbar. The steroid preparations stay in the epidural space for 2 to 3 weeks. Repeat injections, if necessary, are given a minimum of 2 to 4 weeks apart. Many clinicians give a series of three injections regardless of successful response after the first injection. The preferred procedure is to administer one injection and wait 2 weeks in order to assess the patient's response. If the patient is significantly pain free, no further injections are administered. If the patient does not respond to two or three injections of epidural steroid, steroid treatment is discontinued. If the patient receives only short-term pain relief, steroid injections are discontinued. Frequent injections of epidural steroid can produce problems related to chronic steroid administration as well as a remote possibility of infection.

Many clinicians combine the steroid injections with the administration of a local anesthetic agent. When this is done, the patient needs to be observed because the sympathetic block may produce postural hypotension and the patient may become unable to ambulate. No single technique has been proven to be more successful than another. Many clinicians use the caudal approach, using large volumes of local anesthetic agent or saline mixed with the steroid. This gives a 60% success rate as opposed to an 80% or higher success rate with a lumbar epidural technique because caudally administered agents may not reach the site of pathology at L4–L5 or L5–S1 levels in significant concentration, owing to the leakage through the sacral foraminae. Epidural steroid injection is also a useful technique in patients who have neural irritation. In addition, steroids may be injected into the subarachnoid space, especially in patients who have had multiple surgeries and in whom the epidural space has been obliterated. These patients, especially those with arachnoiditis, show significant pain relief. Epidural steroids can produce an initial increase in pain for 8 to 24 hours (182).

Clinical Research in Chronic Pain Treatment

There is a paucity of rigorous scientific research on most aspects of chronic pain, including natural history, etiology, diagnosis, therapy, and the cost effectiveness of treatment. Determining the efficacy of treatment of pain from the medical literature is difficult because there are few studies that meet basic scientific standards for internal validity and applicability of their results. Most research has been based on a collection of anecdotal or highly selected cases from which the true outcome of treatment is impossible to extrapolate. Multiple reports have been published critiquing clinical research in pain (106,155,185–187).

Some suggest that researchers neglect factors in chronic pain treatment. Outcome studies that include the brief duration of follow-up periods, vague criteria used for establishing the success of the therapeutic intervention, and other factors cast doubt on the applicability of the results to the general population. These include the high selection factors of patients in pain clinics, medical exclusion criteria, financial exclusion criteria, patient refusal to accept treatment, and patient attrition (188). In examining the significance of intervention in outcome studies, it is important to consider the limiting factors imposed by the methodology.

Previous research has resulted in little consensus regarding the appropriate diagnosis and treatment of chronic pain syndromes. Unorthodox therapies continue to proliferate, with few standard treatments having been shown to be more effective than the outcome without medical intervention or placebo. For progress to be made in the management of chronic pain, reasonable research design must be incorporated into the evaluation of treatment efficacy.

COMMON PAIN SYNDROMES: DETECTION AND TREATMENT

Myofascial Pain

Myofascial pain syndromes are commonly seen when evaluating and treating patients for chronic pain. Trigger points are characterized by pain originating from small circumscribed areas of local hyperirritability and myofascial structures, resulting in local and referred pain (133). The pain is aggravated by stretching the affected area, cooling, and compression, often giving rise to a characteristic pattern of referred pain (134,135). Although the exact pathophysiology of the trigger point phenomenon has not been identified, myofascial pain syndromes appear to be initiated by trauma, tension, inflammation, and other unidentified factors. The trigger point acts as a source of chronic nociception. The resultant muscle dysfunction and altered mechanics lead to the referred pain and associated phenomenon.

Trigger points may occur in any muscle or muscle group of the body. They are commonly found in muscle groups that are routinely overstressed or those that do not undergo full contraction and relaxation cycles. In the upper body, the group of muscles involved commonly include the trapezius, levator scapulae, and infraspinatus. In the lower body they include the gluteus group, tensor fasciae latae, quadratus lumborum, and gastrocnemius muscles.

Trigger points are best located by deep palpation of the affected muscle, which reproduces the patient's pain complaint both locally and in a referred zone. Trigger points are usually a sharply circumscribed spot of exquisite tenderness. When they are present, passive or active stretching of the affected muscle routinely increases the pain. The muscle in the immediate vicinity of the trigger point is often described as ropy, tense, or having a palpable band. Compared with equivalent pressure in palpation to normal muscle, the trigger point region displays isolated bands, increased tenderness, and referred pain.

The most reliable method of treating trigger points consists of routine, regular stretching to restore the normal resting length of the muscle. Methods to interrupt the pain cycle include injection or needle stimulation of the hypersensitive trigger points (189–193), coolant sprays (133), relaxation therapy, and pressure techniques (192). Recently, botulinum toxin type A injection has been reported to provide prolonged pain relief (194). After interrupting the pain cycle, the treatment is directed at restoring the normal resting muscle length with a regular routine stretching program of the involved muscle groups. This may be accomplished with physical modalities including heat, cold, and correction of poor body mechanics. Psychological intervention may be necessary if long-standing stress and tension are the underlying cause of the problem.

A long-term home modality and stretching program is essential in the management of patients with myofascial pain. Attention to body mechanics, stress, and daily routines may significantly alter their functional capabilities.

Cumulative Trauma Disorders

A new entity or type of disorder identifies repetitive overuse as a causative factor of many industrial injuries. This is a common problem seen in the rehabilitative industrial practice referred to as repetitive motion disorders, occupational overuse injuries, or repetitive strain injuries. Cumulative trauma disorders now account for greater than 50% of all worker's compensation claims (195). Upper extremity cumulative trauma disorders are far more common than lower extremity trauma disorders.

Etiology of cumulative trauma disorders appears to be repetitive motion and stress resulting in microtrauma primarily to the muscle and tendon. Less often, this microtrauma involves the ligaments, joints, cartilage, bones, and musculoskeletal structures. Presenting symptoms may include tendonitis, muscle strain, ligamentous injury, bursitis, myofascial pain, compression neuropathies, and intravertebral disc disease.

Treatment of cumulative trauma disorders often require aggressive intervention and adaptation of the workplace. If a patient's problem fails to resolve, careful screening as to the aspects of repetitive motion need to be assessed and careful discussion with the patient's supervisor/employer need to determine an adaptive environment to bring about satisfactory resolution of the problem. An altered work environment should be designed for the worker to perform different or rotating work tasks, using different muscle groups that in turn will minimize cumulative trauma disorders. For more information on cumulative trauma disorders, the reader is referred to Chapter 65 (196,197).

Peripheral Neuropathy

Pain is a common feature of peripheral neuropathy due to diabetes, amyloidosis, alcoholism, polyarteritis, Guillain-Barré syndrome, brachial neuritis, autoimmune deficiency

(AIDs), porphyria, and riboflavin deficiency. This pain may be of either a constant or intermittent nature and is often described as burning, aching, or lancinating. It may occur with or without signs of sensory loss, muscle weakness, atrophy, or reflex loss.

There are few placebo-controlled, double-blind, crossover studies concerning the effectiveness of medications in alleviating the pain of peripheral neuropathy. It is often suggested that rehabilitative interventions include exercise, desensitization training, TENS, and medications (198). Medications to control pain in diabetic neuropathy include amitriptyline (199), imipramine (200), paroxetine (201), carbamazepine (93,202), mexiletine (203), pyridoxine (204), and fluoxetine (205). NSAIDs are often used in association with the above adjunctive agents and simple physical measures (198). Pain resulting from alcoholic neuropathy is resolved after the correction of nutritional deficiencies. Pain resulting from polyarteritis may resolve after corticosteroid treatment, whereas pain secondary to cryoglobulinemia may resolve with plasmapheresis, and pain from brachial neuritis and other self-limiting conditions resolves spontaneously in weeks to months. Pain secondary to diabetic neuropathies rarely resolves completely. Drugs that induce painful peripheral neuropathies include isoniazid (Laniazid) and hydralazine (Hydralyn), which cause a decrease in tissue levels of pyridoxal phosphate, as well as nitrofurantoin (Furadantin, Dura Pharmaceuticals, San Diego, CA), which has neurotoxic effects.

The patient with chronic painful peripheral neuropathy has many of the associated problems of chronic pain, including depression, inactivity, disuse syndrome, and significant alteration of life-style. Psychological intervention and physical therapy are important aspects of treatment in these patients. Conventional physical therapy modalities, TENS, and general conditioning programs are often helpful, as are psychological programs and other nonpharmacologic methods of pain control.

Reflex Sympathetic Dystrophy and Causalgia

A contributing factor in many chronic pain syndromes is overactivity of the sympathetic nervous system. This is often reported as continuous burning pain in an extremity after trauma. *Causalgia* refers to partial injury to a major nerve followed by the symptoms of sympathetic system overactivity. *RSD* refers to cases of minor injury or no injury, with resulting overactivity of the sympathetic nervous system. Examples include shoulder–hand syndrome, posttraumatic edema, Sudeck's atrophy, and various other syndromes in which sympathetic overactivity seems to be the primary etiologic factor. Involvement of sympathetic nervous system is by no means proven (206,207).

The etiology of the sympathalgia is not distinct. The most common aspect of a sympathalgia is burning pain. Associated with hyperpathia are hypersensitivity to touch and relief of pain with an appropriate sympathetic nerve block. The patient also may show evidence of overactivity of the sympathetic nervous system, including hyperhydrosis and vasoconstriction. These symptoms result in cooling the extremity. When accompanied by disuse, this may produce trophic changes, including shiny thin skin, loss of hair, and demineralization of bone (208).

Diagnosis of sympathetic dystrophies is difficult. The patient's pain is usually diffuse and does not correspond to dermatomal or peripheral nerve patterns. Thus, these patients are often diagnosed as having psychogenic pain. Anatomic or pharmacologic nerve blocks may establish the diagnosis. Psychogalvanic reflex tests and thermography may be useful in documenting sympathetic nervous system hyperactivity. Technetium diphosphonate bone scans (static image 3 hours postinjection) have been used as a sensitive and specific test to objectively collaborate the presence of RSD (208,209).

The most effective treatment of a sympathetic dystrophy consists of an appropriate sympathetic nerve block using a local anesthetic agent (184). Phenoxybenzamine has been reported effective in the treatment causalgia (210). If the problem originates in the head, neck, upper extremity, or upper thorax, a stellate ganglion or a cervical sympathetic block at the C6 level may be used (211). If the pain is in the upper abdominal area, sympathetic blockade denervation can be achieved using the celiac plexus block. Pain originating in the lower extremities requires a lumbar paravertebral sympathetic block at the L2 level (183). Patients with a history of long-standing pain may receive only temporary pain relief from the local anesthetic blocks. These patients may require intravenous regional guanethidine or reserpine when the nerve block ceases to provide pain relief. Guanethidine and reserpine for intravenous (IV) use are not available in the United States. In a randomized double blind study, IV regional guanethidine did not provide any better relief of RSD symptoms compared with placebo (212). IV regional bretylium has been reported to provide statistically significant decrease in RSD symptoms (213). This technique can be applied to extremities and is useful when local anesthetic blocks are contraindicated (214,215).

If the patient does not receive pain relief from sympathetic blocks or the IV regional technique, then permanent interruption of the sympathetic pathways should be considered. This can be accomplished by a neurolytic injection of the sympathetic trunk or surgical sympathectomy.

Patients with neuropathic pain may benefit from spinal cord stimulation. The system can be implanted if a trial stimulation is successful (216).

In conjunction with sympathetic blocks or bretylium injection, physical therapy should be instituted. Often the patient receives relief of rest pain with the sympathetic block, but when the extremity is moved during physical therapy the patient experiences significant pain. This pain is secondary to tight muscles or stiffness of the joint, where the noxious input is carried through somatic fibers. These patients may be aided in the performance of physical therapy by somatic blocks, such as brachial plexus block or an epidural block.

When treating a patient with long-standing pain due to sympathetic dystrophy, it is important to consider the psychological aspects. Patients who develop RSD are usually overly tense. Their enhanced sympathetic pain, secondary to psychological tension, may be a contributing factor to this condition. Appropriate psychological and psychiatric consultation for relaxation training and biofeedback, in addition to other treatment modalities, is important.

Phantom Limb Pain

Phantom limb pain involves an amputated portion of the body. The etiology of phantom pain appears to be related to deafferentation of neurons and their spontaneous and evoked hyperexcitability. Pain may be continuous, in character with intermittent exacerbations. It is often reported by patients as cramping, aching, or burning, with occasional superimposed electriclike components. Studies have suggested that 50% to 85% of amputees have phantom limb pain (217,218). The current data do not suggest a predisposition for phantom pain among traumatic amputees, elderly amputees, those with pain in the amputated limb before amputation, or poor preamputation interpersonal relationships (218). Phantom limb pain does not appear to be correlated with amount of time after amputation or use of a prosthesis.

Multiple modalities, adjuvant medications, and anesthetic and surgical procedures have been used in the treatment of phantom limb pain with varying long-term success. Although at least 68 methods of treating phantom limb syndromes have been identified, successful treatment of persistent types is not commonly reported (219–221). Transcutaneous nerve stimulation (222), tricyclic antidepressants (223), anticonvulsants (224), calcitonin (225), and mexilitine (226) have been used with varying success. Chemical sympathectomy or neurosurgical procedures also have had variable success. Treatments yielding a temporary decrease in pain include analgesics, anesthetic procedures, stump desensitization, physical modalities, and sedative/hypnotic medication. One survey reported that treatments reducing stump problems also resulted in decreased phantom pain (218,227). Therapeutic regimens have had up to a 70% long-term efficacy in the treatment of phantom limb pain.

Phantom limb pain is reported to be more frequent in patients with stump pain. *Stump pain* is pain at the site of the extremity amputation. In the early evaluation of phantom limb pain, it is important that stump pain due to a neuroma is ruled out as the etiology of the pain complaints. This sharp, often jabbing, pain in the stump is usually aggravated by pressure or by infection in the stump. Pain is often elicited by tapping over a neuroma in a transected nerve. The increased sensitivity of sprouts from cut peripheral nerves to noradrenaline and adrenaline may partially explain why adrenergic-influenced emotional states (i.e., stress or anxiety) occasionally provoke attacks of phantom limb pain. For additional information on prosthetics, the reader is referred to Chapter 27.

Neuroma and Scar Pain

Injury to the nerve with a resulting neuroma or entrapment of the branches of the nerve in scar tissue can produce disabling pain. Neuromas are suspected when numbness appears in the distribution of a particular nerve and when pain is produced by palpation of the neuroma. It has been shown that the nerve fibers in the neuroma develop alpha receptors, which respond to catecholamines with spontaneous firing and pain production. Painful neuromas are difficult to treat; many patients continue to have pain despite multiple attempts at surgical excision of the neuroma. Suspected scar pain can be evaluated by picking up the scar from the deeper tissues with two fingers and palpating. If this does not reproduce the patient's pain, the pain is probably not originating in the scar tissue. Pain due to neuroma or scar tissue can be associated with RSD. Diagnosis can be established by infiltration of the scar or the neuroma with a local anesthetic agent, resulting in complete pain relief (100).

Repeated injection of a local anesthetic agent has proven to be an extremely useful technique. This should be followed by appropriate physical therapy to the scar, usually ultrasound followed by stretching or deep massage of the scar. This type of treatment has provided permanent or prolonged pain relief for longer than 6 months in many patients. When the local anesthetics, with or without steroids, do not provide prolonged relief, other methods should be considered. Cryoanalgesia using a cryoprobe and freezing the neuroma for 1 minute at −20°C has been used with good success (228). The advantage of using a cryoprobe lies in the fact that it is a physical method of blocking the nerve without producing further neuroma or neuritis. Neurolytic agents such as phenol or alcohol have been used to relieve neuroma and scar pain. Incomplete block with these agents can result in neuritis producing severe pain. These neurolytic techniques should be used only after repeated injections of local anesthetics produce consistent pain relief proportional to the duration of action of the local anesthetic agent. Although surgical revision of the scar is often considered, it is not very successful when the scar cannot be stretched out and there is significant nerve entrapment.

Cancer Pain

Pain is one of the greatest fears and a major source of morbidity for patients with cancer (202,229,230). Clinical experience suggests that patients with cancer pain are treated most effectively with a multidisciplinary approach, including multiple modalities, appropriate analgesic drugs, neurosurgical and anesthetic procedures, psychological intervention, and supportive care (4–6). The goals of pain therapy for cancer patients are a significant relief of pain to maintain the functional status they choose, a reasonable quality of life, and a death relatively free of pain.

Noninvasive treatment measures are often used singularly for mild to moderate pain and in combination with drug therapy for moderate or severe pain. Commonly used noninvasive measures include cutaneous stimulation, thermal modalities, and behavioral intervention. Their advantages include low risk of complications, low cost, and few serious side effects.

Non-narcotic, narcotic, and adjuvant analgesic drugs are the primary therapy for patients with cancer pain. Anesthetic, psychiatric, behavioral, and occasionally neurosurgical approaches are commonly used with pharmacologic intervention. This combination of treatment is estimated to provide adequate pain relief in at least 90% of the patients with cancer pain.

The World Health Organization has recommended a systematic approach for the selection of pharmacologic agents for treating patients with cancer pain (140) (Tables 56-3 through 56-5). Their protocol is based on the premise that

TABLE 56-3. *Step 1: nonopioid analgesics for mild to moderate pain*

Drug	Plasma half-life (hr)	Peak effect (hr)	Duration of analgesia (hr)	Usual dose (mg)[a]	Maximum recommended dose (mg/day)[b]	Comments
Aspirin	4–16	2	4–6	650 every 4–6 hr	6,000	Standard of comparison for non-narcotics.[c] Irreversible effect on platelet aggregation.
Acetaminophen (Tylenol, McNeil Consumer, Fort Washington, PA)	1–4	3	1–4	650 every 4–6 hr	6,000	No effect on gastric mucosa, platelet aggregation, or anti-inflammatory response. Increased hepatic toxicity of >4 g/day.
Didafenac (Voltaren, CibaGeneva, Summit, NJ)	6–8	2–4	10–12	50–75 every 12 hr	150	Decreased GI toxicity.
Difunisal (Dolobid, Merck & Co., West Point, PA)	8–12	2–3	8–12	500 every 12 hr	1,500	No effect on platelet aggregation of <1 g/day, descreased GI toxicity.
Indomethacin (Indocin, Merck & Co., West Point, PA)	4–5	1–2	4	25–50 every 8 hr	200	Not routinely used due to greater incidence of GI toxicity and CNS side effects.
Ibuprofen (Motrin, McNeil Consumer, Fort Washington, PA)	2–4	1–2	4–6	400–800 every 6–8 hr	3,200	Rapid onset of action. Side effects include nephotoxicity, tinnitus, CNS, and cardiovascular problem.
Naproxen (Naprosyn, Roche Laboratories, Nutley, NJ)	12–15	2–3	8–12	250–500 every 12 h	1,500	Available in liquid suspension.
Piroxicam (Feldene, Pratt Pharmaceuticals, New York, NY)	50	3–5	12	20 every 24 hr	40	Not recommended with liver or kidney dysfunction. Higher incidence of side effects at a dosage of 40 mg over 3 wk.
Salsalate (Disalcid, 3M Pharmaceuticals, St. Paul, MN)	4–16	2	4–12	1,000 every 8 hr	6,000	No effect on platelet aggregation. Lowest GI side effects of NSAIDs.
Sulindac (Clinoril, Merck & Co., West Point, PA)	14–16	3–4	8–12	150 every 12 hr	400	Decreased renal toxicity.
Ketoralac (Toradol, Roche Laboratories, Nutley, NJ)				10 every 4–6 hr	40	Limited to short-term therapy (for not more than 5 days).
Flurbiprofen (Ansaid, Upjohn, Kalamazoo, MI)				50 every 4–6 hr	300	
Relafen (SmithKline Beecham Pharmaceuticals, Philadelphia, PA)				500 mg orally twice daily		
Cholin magnesium trisalicyate (Trilisate, Purdue Frederick, Norwalk, CT)				1,000–1,500 mg every 12 hr	4,000	No effect on platelet aggregation. Decreased GI toxicity.

CNS, central nervous system; GI, gastrointestinal; NSAIDs, nonsteroidal anti-inflammatory drugs.

The authors will not assume liability for this table. No medication should be given until the complete prescribing recommendations, drug use indications, and potential side effects that are listed in the package insert with the product or contained in a drug reference manual are reviewed and understood thoroughly by the physician and patient. Drug dosages may need to be modified for the elderly.

[a] Dosage should be adjusted in elderly patients, patients on multiple medications, and patients with renal insufficiency or hepatic failure. Doses may be increased at weekly intervals if pain relief is inadequate and dosage is tolerated. Doses and intervals titrated to effect.

[b] The patient should be evaluated routinely for hepatic toxicity. Patients receiving NSAIDs also should be evaluated for renal toxicity and fecal blood loss due to gastrointestinal irritation. It is recommended that patients who develop visual complaints during treatment undergo ophthalmic evaluation. Gastrointestinal disturbance may be reduced if taken with milk, on a full stomach, or with antacids.

[c] A dose of 10 mg morphine orally is approximately equianalgesic to 650 mg aspirin orally.

TABLE 56-4. *Step 2: opioid analgesics for moderate pain*

Drug	Equianalgesic dosage: Aspirin orally[b]	Equianalgesic dosage: Morphine IM[c]	Equianalgesic dosage: Morphine orally[c]	Action time[a] Drug: Half-life (hr)	Action time[a] Drug: Peak effect (hr)	Action time[a] Drug: Duration of analgesic (hr)	Usual initial dose (mg)	Comments
Codeine	32	120	200	3	1–2	2–4	32–65 every 3–4 hr	Weak, short-acting; as dose increases, nausea, vomiting, and constipation occur more frequently.
Hydrocodone (Vicodin, Knoll Laboratories, Mount Olive, NJ)	2.5	15	30	3–4	½–1	3–5	5–10 every 3–4 hr	Combined with acetaminophen or NSAIDs.
Meperidine (Demerol, Sanofi Winthrop, New York, NY)	50	90	300	3–4	½–1	2–4	50–100 every 3 hr	Short-acting, risk of accumulation in patients with impaired renal function.
Oxycodone (Percocet, DuPont, Wilmington, DE)	2.5	15	30	3–4	½–1	2–4	5–10 every 3 hr	Fast-acting. Combined with acetaminophen or NSAIDs.
Pentazocine (Talwin, Sanofi Winthrop, New York, NY)	30	60	180	2–3	½–1	2–3	50–100 every 4 hr	Not standard for cancer pain.
Propxyphene (Darvocet, Eli Lilly, Indianapolis, IN)	100–200	—	300	2–3	1–2	3–6	100–200 every 4 hr	Not standard for cancer pain.

IM, intramuscularly; NSAIDS, nonsteroidal anti-inflammatory drugs.

The authors will not assume liability for this table. No medication should be given until the complete prescribing recommendations, drug use indications, and potential side effects that are listed in the package insert with the product or contained in a drug reference manual are reviewed and understood thoroughly by the physician and patient. Drug dosages may need to be modified for the elderly.

[a] Varies with route of administration.

[b] Dose providing analgesic equivalent to 650 mg aspirin orally.

[c] Dose providing analgesic equivalent to a single dose of 10 mg morphine IM.

doctors and health-care professionals should know how to use a few simple drugs well. A three-step analgesic ladder is the scheme that is used for analgesic selection and is summarized as follows:

1. Those patients who have mild to moderate pain should be initially treated with a nonopioid analgesic (Table 56-3) such as aspirin or one of the other NSAIDs and adjuvant analgesic (Table 56-6) if indicated.
2. Patients who have moderate to severe pain or are not able to achieve adequate relief with step 1 should be started on a weak oral opioid (Table 56-4), such as codeine, along with a nonopioid and an adjuvant analgesic if indicated. Pain secondary to soft tissue and bone metastases usually has a limited response to opioids. In these situations, NSAIDs are indicated at all levels of treatment.
3. Patients who have very severe pain or do not achieve adequate relief on step 2, the regimen should include treatment with a potent opioid such as morphine (Table 56-5) with or without the nonopioid, or with an adjuvant analgesic if indicated (231).

Narcotic analgesics are the drugs of choice for relief of intractable pain due to cancer (4,5). Slow-release morphine is an extremely useful analgesic in the treatment of cancer pain. The object is to titrate the level of analgesic to the optimal dose that prevents the recurrence of pain. Oral medications should be used whenever possible because they facilitate ambulatory care, encourage greater independence, and do not represent heroic intervention to the patient. It is important to remember that the maximum recommended dosages of narcotic medications were derived mainly from postoperative parenteral single-dose studies and are not applicable to administration by mouth in the long-term treatment of pain in advanced cancer. Dependency and respiratory depression should not be feared because they are seldom a problem. The most serious side effects of drug therapy,

TABLE 56-5. *Step 3: opioid analgesics for severe pain*

Drug	Equianalgesic dosage[a]			Action time[b]			Usual initial dose (mg)[c]	Comments[d]
	IM	orally	IV	Half-life (hr)	Peak effect (hr)	Duration of analgesia (hr)		
Hydromorphone (Dilaudid, Knoll Laboratories, Mount Olive, NJ)	3[e]	7.5	3[e]	2–3	½–1½	2–4	4–8 every 3–4 hr	Fast acting.
Levorphanol (Levo-Dromoran, Roche Laboratories, Nutley, NJ)	2	4	1	12–16	1–2	4–5	2–4 every 4–6 hr	Increased sedation with repeated doses.
Methadone (Dolophine, Roxane, Columbus, OH)	10	20		15–57	1-2	6–8	5–10 every 6–8 hr	Avoid in patients with significant respiratory, hepatic, or renal failure.
Morphine	10	30[f]	5	2–4	½–1½	4–6	5–10 every 4 hr	
Standard of comparison for narcotics.								
Controlled-release morphine		30[f]		2–4	—	8–12	30 mg every 8–12 hr	
Oxymorphone (Numorphan, DuPont, Wilmington, DE)	1	—	0.5	2–3	30–90	4–6		10 mg rectal suppository available (1).

IM, intramuscularly.

The authors will not assume liability for this table. No medication should be given until the complete prescribing recommendations, drug use indications, and potential side effects that are listed in the package insert with the product or contained in a drug reference manual are reviewed and understood thoroughly by the physician and patient. Drug dosages may need to be modified for the elderly.

[a] Dose providing analgesic equivalent to a single dose of 10 mg morphine IM.

[b] Varies with route of administration.

[c] Dosage varies considerably, titrate to control pain.

[d] Most common side effects of opioid drugs include constipation, nausea, and sedation. Less common side effects include urinary retention, bladder spasm, respiratory depression, and intermittent vomiting. Rare side effects include psychotic symptoms, pruritis, orthostatic hypotension, bronchoconstriction, and biliary colic. The dosage should be adjusted in elderly patients and patients with impaired ventilation, increased intracranial pressure, liver failure, or bronchial asthma.

[e] For chronic dosing only. For single dose use 1.5 mg.

[f] For chronic dosing only. For single dose use 60 mg.

which should be prevented or treated, include constipation and nausea.

Supportive care is designed to maintain the cancer patient in an outpatient setting, with pain a common cause for readmission to the hospital. Nerve blocks and neurolytic procedures are most often used to provide pain relief in the thoracic and abdominal regions (98,184). These procedures are often performed in the outpatient setting and often provide pain relief for up to 6 months. Supportive care may involve a hospice, hospital-based care teams, visiting nurses, and social services. The primary goal of the physician is to maintain the quality of life for the cancer patient to the end, allowing the patient a death with dignity.

It is essential that, during a cancer patient's hospitalization, outpatient treatment, and everyday activities they maintain their functional skills, strength, and mobility. Progressive immobilization is an insidious aspect of this disease and is often iatrogenic. Although radiation and chemotherapy may transiently render a patient unable to perform activities, the patient needs to be consistently evaluated and involved in active physical, occupational, corrective, and recreational therapy programs. The physiatrist may offer multiple methods of combating immobility and its morbidity. For additional information on cancer rehabilitation, the reader is referred to Chapter 52.

There are multiple invasive measures to control cancer pain. The most common is the surgical removal of all or part of the tumor in the hope of relieving pain and effecting a cure. Radiotherapy or chemotherapy also may relieve pain by shrinking the tumor. Common invasive anesthetic proce-

TABLE 56-6. *Adjuvant analgesics*

Drug class	Preferred drugs	Dosing schedule	Starting dose (mg)	Comments
Tricyclic-type antidepressants	Amitriptyline Doxepin Imipramine Nortriptyline Trazadone	Every night (or divide dose two or three times daily)	25 30 20 50 50	For neuropathic deafferentation pain or pain complicated by insomnia or depression. If daytime somnolence is a problem, give dose earlier in the evening.
Anticonvulsants	Carbamazepine (Tegretol, CibaGeneva, Summit, NJ)	Every 6–8 hr	200	For neuropathic deafferentation pain with shooting or lancinating quality; may need to follow blood levels.
	Phenytoin (Dilantin, Parke-Davis, Morris Plains, NJ)	Every night	300	
	Clonazepam (Klonopin, Roche Laboratories, Nutley, NJ)	Every 12 hr	0.5	
Neuroleptics	Fluphenazine (Prolixin)	Every 8 hr	2	For refractory deafferentation pain and pain complicated by nausea or delirium.
	Haloperidol (Haldol, Ortho-McNeil, Raritan, NJ)	Every 6–12 hr	2	
Antihistamines	Hydroxyzine (Vistaril, Pfizer, New York, NY)	Every 6–8 hr	25–75	Pain complicated by anxiety, nausea, or insomina.
	Diphenhydramine (Benadryl, Warner-Lambert Consumer, Morris Plains, NJ)	Every 4–6 hr	25–50	
Miscellaneous	Dexamethasone (Decadron, Merck & Co., West Point, PA)	Loading dose four times daily	16–20	For refractory bone and deafferentation pain.

The authors will not assume liability for this table. No medication should be given until the complete prescribing recommendations, drug use indications, and potential side effects that are listed in the package insert with the product or contained in a drug reference manual are reviewed and understood thoroughly by the physician and patient. Drug dosages may need to be modified for the elderly.

dures include trigger point injections and nerve blocks. Myofascial pain syndromes are often the result of inactivity and disuse and are commonly found in the cancer patient. Patients who have side effects with large doses of opioids may derive long-term benefit with chronically implanted epidural catheter or an intrathecal catheter and pump to administer opioids and/or clonidine (232,233). Multiple neurosurgical procedures have been used for the control of cancer pain (234,235).

Herpetic Neuralgia

Herpes zoster (shingles) is a reactivation of the varicella (chicken pox) virus, which has remained latent. The viral inflammation of the dorsal nerve root and ganglion causes vesicle formation and severe burning, aching, and lancinating pain in a radicular distribution. During the acute stage, NSAIDs and sympathetic blocks provide excellent pain relief. The majority of patients recover from the acute episode in approximately 2 weeks without sequelae. However, some patients develop postherpetic neuralgia. It is uncommon in patients under 40 years of age but occurs in over 50% of patients over 60 years of age.

Multiple reports indicate that postherpetic neuralgia may be prevented if the patient is treated with a sympathetic block within 1 month after the onset of herpes zoster (99). Postherpetic neuralgia is, thus, a preventable syndrome, but it is a difficult problem once established. A significant number of patients experience pain relief with sympathetic blocks. If the syndrome is allowed to progress untreated for 3 months to a year, it becomes more difficult to treat (179).

The most effective treatment for the management of established postherpetic neuralgia is the use of a tricyclic antidepressant such as amitriptyline (Elavil, Zeneca Pharmaceuticals, Wilmington, DE) in small doses (179). Most patients obtain pain relief with 25 to 75 mg administered at bedtime. If the patient does not get complete pain relief with administration of tricyclics alone, fluphenazine (Prolixin, Bristol-Myers Squibb, Princeton, NJ) may be added, beginning with 1 mg at bedtime and progressing as needed to a maximum dosage of 1 mg three times a day. Anticonvulsants, such as dilantin and carbamezapine, also have been administered with variable results (183). Pain reduction has been reported with topical lidocaine (236) and capsaicin (237). Peripheral nerve blocks and destructive neurosurgical procedures have not proved useful in treating established postherpetic neuralgia.

Pain in Spinal Cord Injury

The precise etiology underlying pain in spinal cord injuries is not known, but recent evidence suggests that trauma-induced alterations of the pain pathways are primarily involved (238–241). Hypersensitivity of the structures in the ascending pathway may play a role. Studies indicate that 50% of all spinal cord–injured patients have pain that is mild to moderate in severity; approximately 20% experience severe pain (242,243). Patients describe their pain as having one or more of the following components: burning in body parts below the injury, deep aching sensation over and around the site of injury, and radicular with lancinating characteristics. Burning pain in spinal cord–injured patients may be a variation of deafferentated pain occurring as a result of loss of inhibitory or augmentation of excitatory influences. The most effective treatments of this type of pain include tricyclic antidepressants and neuroaugmentive techniques (244).

Spinal fracture site pain results from an alteration of body mechanics causing pain-sensitive structures to be stretched or compressed. This mechanical pain may be the result of vertebral end-plate fractures, annulus fibrosus tears, or internal disk herniation after a spinal fracture (245). Fracture site pain or mechanical pain is often exacerbated by activity. NSAIDs, trigger point injections, TENS, cognitive/behavioral techniques, and adjuvant medication may be used. Orthotics also may be used to decrease the mechanical stress and alleviate the underlying etiology (246,247).

Radicular pain in these patients may be secondary to compression of nerve roots by a herniated nucleus pulposus, fracture fragment, dislocated vertebra, or the results of traumatic arachnoiditis. This type of pain is most effectively treated with anticonvulsants, with TENS used as a useful adjuvant (248). For additional information on spinal cord injury, the reader is referred to Chapter 51.

Pain in Multiple Sclerosis

Multiple sclerosis is a chronic remitting and relapsing disease characterized by multiple foci of demyelination that are randomly distributed in the white matter of the central nervous system. These patients often present initially with paroxismal lancinating and intense burning pain that primarily effects the face, shoulder region, or pelvic girdle. These painful paresthesias have been reported in 13% to 64% of patients with multiple sclerosis (249). Treatment of pain resulting from multiple sclerosis has been limited. Minimal response has been shown to tricyclic antidepressants, carbamazepine, and phenytoin. For additional information on multiple sclerosis, the reader is referred to Chapter 50.

Poststroke Pain

Pain after a cerebral vascular accident may be secondary to multiple etiologies, including central pain, RSD, pain due to spasticity, and pain from dysfunction of the affected extremities. Central pain due to thalamic infarction is often characterized as an agonizing burning pain on the side contralateral to that of the lesion. Pain to minimal cutaneous stimulation as well as aggravation by emotional stress and fatigue are characteristic findings. Sensory alteration is variable in these patients with minimal findings of motor weakness. Central pain due to lesions involving central thalamic spinal tracts may be manifest in pain distributed to the level of the tract involved. This results in loss of pain and temperature perception on the contralateral side at the level below the injury. Central pain of tract origin is similar to pain of thalamic origin but is usually less intense. This pain may be described as burning, pulling, or swelling. Information on central pain syndromes is scarce with treatment proven useful (250). Treatment options include sympathetic blockade (251), multiple medication (252), and TENS (253).

Spasticity secondary to stroke may result in pain. This may be treated with medication or nerve blocks (99). Studies have suggested that patients with spasticity and pain in the hemiplegic upper limb may benefit from selective posterior rhizotomy in the dorsal root entry zone (254). Poststroke pain due to dysfunction of the affected extremities is most often manifest in the upper extremity. This pain may be the result of shoulder subluxation, decreased range of motion due to adhesive capsulitis, or brachial plexis injury (185).

Other factors of affected limb dysfunction include bicipital tendonitis, arthritis, fracture, heteotopic ossification, and knee/ankle instability. Appropriate use of modalities as well as orthotics and assistive devices are indicated in the resolution if some of these problems are contributing to the patients pain (99,255). For additional information on stroke rehabilitation, the reader is referred to Chapter 48.

Low Back Pain

Low back pain episodically affects nearly 75% of the population in most industrial nations. It is estimated that 15% of this work force is affected by back pain each year (7,8). It is estimated that 90% of these incidences of back pain resolve in 12 weeks or less. It is estimated that the 10% of these workers who develop chronic low back pain (remaining off work for 3 months or longer) are responsible for 80% of the cost (lost wages, compensation, medical expenses, etc.) (256,257).

Strategies to prevent acute low back pain from progressing to chronic low back pain include use of conservative intervention, return to work as soon as possible, or continue working at a job the worker is physically able to accomplish during the recuperation period and rapid adjudication of disabilities/compensation claims (39,40). Comprehensive prevention and diagnostic programs have been identified (155,258). An extensive review of randomized control trials in industrial low back pain showed methodologic limitations for interventions (88,141,155,186,259–261). For additional information on rehabilitation of the patient with spinal pain, the reader is referred to Chapter 57.

REFERENCES

1. Deyo RA, Walsh NE, Martin DC, Schoenfeld LS, Ramamurthy S. A controlled trial of transcutaneous electrical nerve stimulation (TENS) and exercise for chronic low back pain. *N Engl J Med* 1990; 322: 1627–1634.
2. Merskey H, ed. Classification of chronic pain—descriptions of chronic pain syndromes and definitions of pain terms. *Pain* 1986; 3(suppl):1–225.
3. Bonica JJ. History of pain concepts and therapies. In: Bonica JJ, ed. *The management of pain,* 2nd ed. Philadelphia: Lea & Febiger, 1990; 2–17.
4. Bonica JJ. Cancer pain. In: Bonica JJ, ed. *The management of pain,* 2nd ed. Philadelphia: Lea & Febiger, 1990; 400–460.
5. Foley KM. The treatment of cancer pain. *N Engl J Med* 1985; 313: 84–95.
6. Twycross RG, Lack SA. *Symptom control and far advanced cancer: pain relief.* London: Pitman, 1984.
7. Cavanaugh JM, Weinstein JN. Low back pain: epidemiology, anatomy, and neurophysiology. In: Wall PD, Melzack R, eds. *Textbook of pain,* 3rd ed. New York: Churchill-Livingstone, 1994; 441–455.
8. Steinberg GG. Epidemiology of low back pain. In: Stanton-Hicks M, Boas R, eds. *Chronic low back pain.* New York: Raven, 1982:1–13.
9. Crook J. The prevalence of pain complaints in a general population. *Pain* 1984; 18:299–314.
10. Cailliet R. Disuse syndrome—fibrocytic and degenerative changes. In: Brena SF, Chapman SL, eds. *Management of patients with chronic pain.* New York: Sectrum, 1983; 63–71.
11. Browse NL. *The physiology and pathology of bed rest.* Springfield, IL: Charles C Thomas, 1965; 1–221.
12. Granger C, ed. *Functional assessment in rehabilitation.* Baltimore: Williams & Wilkins, 1984.
13. Powers JH. The abuse of rest as a therapeutic measure in surgery. *JAMA* 125:1079, 1944.
14. Snow BR, Pinter I, Gusmorino P, et al. Incidence of physical and psychosocial disabilities in chronic pain patients: initial report. *Bull Hosp Joint Dis Orthop Inst* 1986; 46:22–30.
15. Guck TP, Meilman PW, Skultety FM, Dowd ET. Prediction of long-term outcome of multidisciplinary pain treatment. *Arch Phys Med Rehabil* 1986; 67:293–296.
16. Chaplin ER. Chronic pain: a sociobiological problem. *Phys Med Rehabil Stars* 1991; 5:1–48.
17. Bishop B. Pain: its physiology and rationale for management. Part I. Neuroanatomical substrate for pain. *Phys Ther* 1980; 60:13–37.
18. Bonica JJ. Anatomic and physiologic basis of nocioception and pain. In: Bonica JJ, ed. *The management of pain,* 2nd ed. Philadelphia: Lea & Febiger, 1990; 28–94.
19. Edmeads J. The physiology of pain: a review. *Prog Neuropsychopharmacol Biol Psychiatry* 1983; 7:413–419.
20. Zimmerman M. The somatovisceral sensory system. In: Schmidt RF, Thews G, eds. *Human physiology,* 3rd ed. New York: Springer-Verlag, 1989; 224–233.
21. Schmidt RF. Nocioception and pain. In: Schmidt RF, Thews G, eds. *Human physiology,* 3rd ed. New York: Springer-Verlag, 1989; 223–236.
22. Basbaum AI, Fields HL. Endogenous pain control mechanisms—brainstem spinal pathways and endorphin circuitry. *Ann Rev Neurosci* 1984;7:309–38.
23. Kruger L, Mantyh P. Changing concepts in the anatomy of pain. *Semin Anesth* 1985; 4:209–217.
24. Liebeskind J, Sherman J, Cannon JT, Terman G. Neural and neurochemical mechanisms of pain inhibition. *Semin Anesth* 1985; 4: 218–222.
25. Snyder SH. Opiate receptors and internal opiates. *Sci Am* 1977; 236: 44–56.
26. Houde RW. The use and misuse of narcotics in the treatment of chronic pain. *Adv Neurol* 1974; 4:527–536.
27. Sharap AD. The knowledge, attitudes, and experience of medical personnel treating pain in the terminally ill. *Mt Sinai J Med* 1978; 45: 561–580.
28. Andrews IC. Management of postoperative pain. *Int Anesth Clin* 1983; 21:31–42.
29. Torda TA. Management of acute and post-operative pain. *Int Anesth Clin* 1983; 21:27–47.
30. Weinstein SM, Herring SA, Shelton JL. The injured worker: assessment and treatment. *Phys Med Rehabil Stars* 1990; 4:361–377.
31. Waddell G. Biopsychosocial analysis of low back pain. *Baillieres Clin Rheumatol* 1992; 6:523–557.
32. Fordyce WE. Learned pain: pain as a behavior. In: Bonica J, ed. *The management of pain,* 2nd ed. Philadelphia: Lea & Febiger, 1990; 291–299.
33. Fordyce W, McMahon R, Rainwater G. Pain complaint—exercise performance, relationship and chronic pain. *Pain* 1981; 10:311–321.
34. Behan RC, Hirschfeld AH. The accident process—toward more rational treatment of industrial injuries. *JAMA* 1963; 186:300–306.
35. Rohling ML, Binder LM, Langhinrichsen-Rohling J. Money matters: a meta-analytic review of the association between financial compensation and the experience and treatment of chronic pain. *Health Psychol* 1995; 14:537–547.
36. Loeser J. Back pain in the workplace II. *Pain* 1996; 65:2–8.
37. Beals RK. Compensation and recovery from injury. *West J Med* 1984; 140:233–237.
38. Walsh NE, Dumitru D. Compensation in low back pain. *Phys Med Rehabil Stars* 1991; 5:223–236.
39. Seres JS, Newman RI. Negative influence of the disability compensation system—perspectives for the clinician. *Semin Neurol* 1983; 3: 360–369.
40. Strang JP. Chronic disability syndrome. In: Aronoff GM, ed. *Evaluation and treatment of chronic pain,* 2nd ed. Baltimore: Urban & Schwarzenberg, 1992; 603–624.
31. Steinberg FU. *The immobilized patient—functional pathology and management.* New York: Plenum, 1980.
42. Portnow JM, Strassman HD. Medically induced drug addiction. *Int J Addiction* 1985; 20:605–611.
43. Stimmel B. Pain, analgesia, and addiction: an approach to the pharmacologic management of pain. *Clin J Pain* 1985; 1:14–22, 1985.
44. Halpern L. Substitution-detoxification and its role in the management of chronic benign pain. *J Clin Psychiatry* 1982; 43:10–14.
45. O'Brien CP. Drug addiction and drug abuse. In: Hardman JG, Goodman Gilman A, Limbird LE, eds. *The pharmacological basis of therapeutics.* New York: McGraw-Hill, 1996; 557–577.
46. Maruta T, Swanson DW, Finlayson RE. Drug abuse and dependency in patients with chronic pain. *Mayo Clin Proc* 1979; 54:241–244.
47. Finlayson RE, Maruta T, Morse RM. Substance dependence and chronic pain: experience with treatment and follow-up results. *Pain* 1986; 26:175–180.
48. Fordyce WE. *Behavioral methods for chronic pain and illness.* St. Louis: CV Mosby, 1976; 41–221.
49. Rowat KM, Knafl KA. Living with chronic pain: the spouse's perspective. *Pain* 1985; 23:259–271.
50. Infante M. Sexual dysfunction in the patient with chronic back pain. *Sex Disabil* 1981; 4:173–178.
51. Ahern D, Adams AE, Follick MJ. Emotional and marital disturbances in spouses of chronic low back pain patients. *Clin J Pain* 1985; 1: 69–74.
52. Bonica JJ. General considerations of chronic pain. In: Bonica JJ, ed. *The management of pain,* 2nd ed. Philadelphia: Lea & Febiger, 1990; 180–196
53. Brena SF, Chapman SL, Decker R. Chronic pain as a learned experience. In: Ng LKY, ed. *New approaches to treatment of chronic pain.* Washington, DC: U.S. Department of Health and Human Services, 1981; 76–83.
54. Melzack R, Wall PD. Pain mechanisms: a new theory. *Science* 1965; 150:971–977.
55. Jessell TM, Kelly DD. Pain and analgesia. In: Kandel ER, Schwartz JH, Jessell TM, eds. *Principles of neural science,* 3rd ed. New York: Elsevier/North Holland, 1991; 385–399.
56. Wall PD. Comments after 30 years of the gate control theory. *Pain Forum* 1996; 5:12–22.
57. Sjolund BH, Eriksson MBE. Endorphins and analgesia produced by peripheral conditioning stimulation. In: Bonica JJ, Abe-Fessard D, Liebeskind JC, eds. *Advances in pain research and therapy,* 3rd ed. New York: Raven, 1979; 587–599.
58. Morely GK, Erickson DL, Morley JE. The neurology of pain. In:

Baker AB, Joynt RJ, eds. *Clinical neurology.* Philadephia: Harper & Row, 1996; 1–95.
59. Watkins LR, Mayer DJ. Organization of endogenous opiate and non-opiate pain control systems. *Science* 1982; 216:11–85.
60. Smith G, Covino BG. *Acute pain.* London: Butterworth, 1985.
61. Kerr AT. The brachial plexus of hnerves in man, the variations in its formation, and branches. *Am J Anat* 1918; 23:285–395.
62. Foerster O. Dermatomes in man. *Brain* 1933; 56:1–39.
63. Bing R. *Compendium of regional diagnosis in the lesions of the brain and spinal cord,* 11th ed. [Translated and edited by W. Haymaker.] St. Louis: CV Mosby, 1940.
64. Haymaker W, Woodhall B. *Peripheral nerve injuries—principles of diagnosis,* 2nd ed. Philadelphia: WB Saunders, 1953.
65. Keagan JJ, Garrett FD. The segmental distribution of the cutaneous nerves in the limbs of man. *Anat Rec* 1948; 102:409–438.
66. Guttmamn L. Topographic studies of disturbances of sweat secretion after complete lesions of peripheral nerves. *J Neurol Psychiatry* 1940; 3:197–210.
67. Richter CP, Woodruff PG. Lumbar dermatomes in man determined by electrical skin resistance method. *J Electrophysiol* 1945; 8:323–338.
68. Low PA, Stevens JC, Swarez GA, Windebank AJ, Smith BE. Diseases of peripheral nerves. In: Joynt RJ, ed. *Clinical neurology.* Philadelphia: Lippincott-Raven, 1995; 1–193.
69. Patten J. *Neurological differential diagnosis.* New York: Springer-Verlag, 1977.
70. Levin KH. Cervical radiculopathies: comparison of surgical and EMG localization of simple-root lesions. *Neurology* 1996; 46:1022–1025.
71. Kendall FP, McCreary EK. *Muscles—testing and function,* 3rd ed. Baltimore: Williams & Wilkins, 1983.
72. Liguori R, Krurup C, Joberg T, Rojaborg W. Determining the segmental sensory and motor innervation of the lumbosacral spinal nerve. *Brain* 1992; 115:915–944.
73. Wilbourn AJ. The diabetic neuropathies. In: Brown WF, Bolton CF, eds. *Clinical electromyography.* Boston: Butterworths, 1987; 329–364.
74. Brash JC, ed. *Cunningham's textbook of anatomy,* 9th ed. London: Oxford University Press, 1951.
75. Warwick R, Williams PL. *Gray's anatomy,* 35th British edition. Philadelphia: WB Saunders, 1973; 994–1083.
76. Inman VT, Saunders JB. Referred pain from skeletal structures. *J Nerv Mental Disord* 1944; 99:660–667.
77. Dejerine J. *Semiologie des affections du systeme nerveux.* Paris: Masson & Cie, 1914.
78. Foerster O. Die Symptomatologie and Therapie der Kriegsverletzungen der Peripheren Nerven. *Dtsch Z Nervenh* 1918; 59:32–172.
79. Mitchell GAG. *Anatomy of the autonomic nervous system.* Edinburgh: Worthingstone, 1953.
80. Sheehan D. *Arch Neurol Psychiatry* 1936; 35:1081–1115.
81. Johnson RH, Lambie DG, Spalding JMK. The autonomic nervous system. In: Joynt RJ, ed. *Clinical neurology.* Philadelphia: Lippincott-Raven, 1986; 1–94.
82. Frymoyer JW, Newberg A, Pope MH. Spine radiographs in patient with low back pain. *J Bone Joint Surg [Am]* 1984; 66:1048–1055.
83. Horal J. The clinical appearance of low back disorders in the city of Gothenburg, Sweden. *Acta Orthop Scand Suppl* 1969; 118:8–73.
84. Scavone JG, Latshaw RF, Rohrer GV. The use of lumbar spine films—statistical evaluation at a university teaching hospital. *JAMA* 1981; 246:1105–1108.
85. Spangfort E. The lumbar disk herniation—a computer aided analysis of 2,504 operations. *Acta Orthop Scand* 1972; 142:1–95.
86. Hitselberger WE, Witten RM. Abnormal myelograms in asymptomatic patients. *J Neurosurg* 1968; 28:204–206.
87. Holt EP. The question of lumbar discography. *J Bone Joint Surg [Am]* 1968; 50:720–726.
88. Wiesel SW, Tsourmas N, Feffer H. A study of computer assisted thermography—the incidence of postive CAT scans in an asymptomatic group of patients. *Spine* 1984; 9:549–551.
89. Jensen MC, Brant-Zawadzki MN, Abuchowski N, Modic MT, Malkasian D, Rosa JS. Magnetic resonance imaging of the lumbar spine in people without back pain. *N Engl J Med* 1994; 331:69–73.
90. Duckno PW, Margolis R, Tait RC. Psychological assessment in chronic pain. *J Clin Psychol* 1985; 41:499–504.
91. Melzack R, Katy J. Pain management in persons in pain. In: Wall PD, Melzack R, eds. *Textbook of pain,* 3rd ed. New York: Churchill-Livingstone, 1994; 337–351.
92. Chapman CR, Casey KL, Dubner R, et al. Pain measurement: an overview. *Pain* 1985; 22:1–31.
93. Costello RM, Hulsey TL, Schoenfeld LS, Ramamurthy S. P-A-I-N: a four cluster MMPI typology for chronic pain. *Pain* 1987; 30:199–209.
94. Ramamurthy S, Rogers JN. *Decision making in pain management.* St. Louis: BC Decker, 1993.
95. American Association of Electromyography and Electrodiagnosis. *Guidelines in electrodiagnostic medicine.* Rochester, NY: American Association of Electromyography and Electrodiagnosis, 1984.
96. Kimura J. *Electrodiagnosis in diseases of nerve and muscle: principles and practice.* Philadelphia: FA Davis, 1983.
97. Dumitru D. *Electrodiagnostic medicine.* Philadelphia: Hanley & Belfus, 1995.
98. Dumitru D. Electrophysiologic evaluation of the pain patient. *Phys Med Rehabil Stars* 1991; 5:187–208.
99. Bonica JJ, Butter SH. Local anesthesia and regional blocks. In: Wall PD, Melzack R, eds. *Textbook of pain,* 3rd ed. Edinburgh: Churchill-Livingstone, 1994; 997–1024.
100. Raj PP, Ramamurthy S. Differential nerve block studies. In: Raj PP, ed. *Practical management of pain,* 2nd ed. Chicago: Year Book Medical, 1986; 173–177.
101. Ramamurthy S, Winnie AP. Diagnostic maneuvers in painful syndromes. In: Stein JM, Warfield CA, eds. *International Anesthesiology Clinics, Pain Management.* Boston: Little, Brown, 1983; 47–50.
102. Ellis JS, Schoenfeld LS, Ramamurthy S. Nonsomatic pain. *Phys Med Rehabil Stars* 1991; 5:103–132.
103. Shoichet R. Sodium amytal in the diagnosis of chronic pain. *Can Psychiatr J* 1978; 23:219–228.
104. Ash CJ, Shealy CN, Young PA, Van Beaumont W. Thermography and the sensory dermatome. *Skel Radiol* 1986; 15:40–46.
105. Gross D. Pain and autonomic nervous system. *Adv Neurol* 1974; 4: 93–104.
106. Chafetz N, Wexler CE, Kaiser JA. Thermography of the lumbar spine with CT correlation—a blinded study. *Radiology* 1985; 157:178.
107. Hoffman RM, Kent DL, Deyo RA. Diagnostic accuracy and clinical utility of thermography for lumbar radiculopathy: a meta-analysis. *Spine* 1991; 16:623–628.
108. Sherman R, Karstetter K, Damiano M, Evans C. Stability of temperature asymmetries in RSD over time, with treatment, and changes in pain. *Clin J Pain* 1994; 10:71–77.
109. Edeiken J, Shaber G. Thermography: a reevaluation. *Skel Radiol* 1986; 15:545–548.
110. Paul R. Thermography in the diagnosis of low back pain. *Neurosurg Clin North Am* 1991; 2:839–50.
111. Mills GH, Davids GH, Getty CJM, Conway J. The evaluation of liquid crystal thermography in the investigation of nerve root compression due to lumbosacral lateral spinal stenosis. *Spine* 1986; 11:427–432.
112. Loeser JD, Seres JL, Newman RI. Interdisciplinary, multimodal management of chronic pain. In: Bonica JJ, ed. *The management of pain,* 2nd ed. Philadelphia: Lea & Febiger, 1990; 2107–2120.
113. King JC, Kelleher WJ. The chronic pain syndrome: the in-patient interdisciplinary rehabilitative behavioral modification approach. *Phys Med Rehabil Stars* 1991; 5:165–186.
114. Grabois M. Pain clinics—role in the rehabilitation of patients with chronic pain. *Ann Acad Med* 1983; 12:428–433.
115. Kroening RJ. Pain clinics structure and function. *Semin Anesth* 1985; 4:231–236.
116. Deardorff WW, Rubin HS, Scott DW. Comprehensive multi-disciplinary treatment of chornic pain: a follow-up study of treated and non-treated groups. *Pain* 1991; 45:35–43.
117. Kames LD, Rapkin AJ, Naliboff BD, Afifi S, Ferrer-Brechner T. Effectiveness of interdisciplinary pain management program for the treatment of chronic pelvic pain. *Pain* 1990; 41:41–46.
118. Chapman SL, Brena SF, Bradford LA. Treatment outcome in a chronic pain rehabilitation program. *Pain* 1981; 11:255–268.
119. Maruta T, Swanson DW, McHardy MJ. Three-year follow-up of patients with chronic pain and were treated in multi-disciplinary pain management center. *Pain* 1990; 41:47–53.
120. Peters JL, Large RG. A randomized control trial evaluating in- and out-patient pain control programs. *Pain* 1990; 41:283–293.
121. Tunks E, Crook J. Persistent pain. In: Basmajian JV, Banerjee SN,

eds. *Clinical decision making in rehabilitation.* New York: Churchill-Livingstone, 1996; 93–118.

122. Lehmann JF, DeLateur BJ. Ultrasound, shortwave, superficial heat and cold in the treatment of pain. In: Wall PD, Melzack R, eds. *Textbook of pain,* 3rd ed. New York: Churchill-Livingstone, 1994; 1237–1250.
123. Eldred E, Lindsley DF, Buchwald JS. The effect of cooling on mammalian muscle spindles. *Exp Neurol* 1960; 2:144–157.
124. Ottoson D. The effects of temperature on the isolated muscle spindle. *J Physiol* 1965; 180:636–648.
125. Fischer E, Solomon S. Physiological responses to heat and cold. In: Licht S, ed. *Therapeutic heat and cold,* 2nd ed. Baltimore: Waverly, 1965; 126–169.
126. Kendall HO, Kendall FP, Boynton DA. *Posture and pain.* New York: Robert E Krieger, 1952.
127. Mennell JM. The therapeutic use of cold. *JAMA* 1975; 74:1146–1157.
128. Nicholos JA, Hershman EB. *The lower extremity and spine in sports medicine.* St. Louis: CV Mosby, 1986.
129. Lehmann JF, DeLateur RJ. *Therapeutic heat and cold,* 4th ed. Baltimore: Williams & Wilkins, 1990.
130. Grant AE. Massage with ice in the treatment of painful conditions of the musculoskeletal system. *Arch Phys Med Rehabil* 1964; 45: 233–238.
131. Pegg SMG, Littler TR, Littler EN. A trial of ice therapy and exercise in chronic arthritis. *Physiotherapy* 1969; 55:51–56.
132. Landen BR. Heat or cold for the relief of low back pain? *Phys Ther* 1967; 47:1126–1128.
133. Travell J. Ethyl chloride spray for painful muscle spasm. *Arch Phys Med Rehabil* 1952; 33:291–298.
134. Travell JG, Simons DG. *Myofascial pain and dysfunction—the trigger point manual.* Vol. 1. The Upper Extemities. Baltimore: Williams & Wilkins, 1983.
135. Travell JG, Simons DG. *Myofascial pain and dysfunction—the trigger point manual.* Vol. 2. The lower extremities. Baltimore: Williams & Wilkins, 1992.
136. Mense S. Effects of temperature on the discharge of muscle spindles and tendon organs. *Pflugers Arch* 1978; 375:159–166.
137. Kottke FJ, Pauley DL, Rudolph PA. The rational for prolonged stretching for correction of shortening of connective tissue. *Arch Phys Med Rehabil* 1966; 47:345–352.
138. Taub A, Kane K. A history of local analgesia. *Pain* 1975; 1:125–138.
139. World Health Organization. *Cancer pain relief.* Geneva, Switzerland: World Health Organization, 1982.
140. Mannheimer JS, Lampe GN. *Clinical transcutaneous electrical nerve stimulation.* Philadelphia: FA Davis, 1984.
141. Banerjee SN. Nonsurgical treatment of acute low back pain. In: Basmajian JV, Banerjee SN, eds. *Clinical decision making in rehabilitation.* New York: Churchill-Livingstone, 1996; 68–92.
142. Canthen JC, Renner EJ. Transcutaneous and peripheral nerve for chronic pain states. *Surg Neurol* 1975; 11:102–104.
143. Meyer GA, Fields HL. Causalgia treated by selective large fiber stimulation of peripheral nerve. *Brain* 1972; 95:163–168.
144. Woolf CF, Thompson JW. Stimulation fibre-induced analgesia: transcutanous electrical nerve stimulation (TENS) and vibration. In: Wall PD, Melzack R, eds. *Textbook of pain,* 3rd ed. New York: Churchill-Livingstone, 1994; 1191–1208.
145. Melzack R. Folk medicine and the sensory modulation of pain. In: Wall PD, Melzack R, eds. *Textbook of pain,* 3rd ed. New York: Churchill-Livingstone, 1994; 1209–1218.
146. Melzack R, Stillwell DM, Fox EJ. Trigger points and acupuncture points for pain: correlations and implications. *Pain* 1977; 3:3–23.
147. Ter Riet G, Kleijnen J, Knipschild P. Acupuncture and chronic pain: a criteria based meta-analysis. *J Clin Epidemiol* 1990; 43:1191–1199.
148. Lorenz KY. Acupuncture: a neuromodulation technique for pain control. In: Aronoff GM, ed. *Evaluation and treatment in chronic pain,* 2nd ed. Baltimore: Urban & Schwarttenberg, 1992; 539–547.
149. Council on Scientific Affairs. Lasers in medicine and surgery. *JAMA* 1986; 256:900–907.
150. Brasford JR. Low energy laser treatment of pain and wounds: hype, hope, or hokum? *Mayo Clin Proc* 1986; 61:671–678.
151. Ysla R, McAvley R. Effects of low power infra-red laser stimulation on carpal tunnel syndrome: a double-blind study. *Arch Phys Med Rehabil* 1985; 66:577.
152. Basford JR, Sheffield CG, Mair SD, Ilstrup DM. Low-energy helium-neon laser treatments of thumb osteoarthritis. *Arch Phys Med Rehabil* 1987; 68:794–797.
153. Haker EHK, Lundeberg TCM. Lateral epicondylogia: report of non-effective mid-laser treatment. *Arch Phys Med Rehabil* 1991; 72: 984–988.
154. Lehman JF, de Lateur BF. Ultrasound, shortwave, microwave, laser, superficial heat and cold in the treatment of pain. In: Wall PD, Melzack R, eds. *Textbook of pain,* 3rd ed. New York: Churchill-Livingstone, 1994; 1237–1249.
155. Bigos SJ, Bowyer OR, Braen GR, et al. *Acute low back problems in adults.* Clinical practice guideline number 14. Rockville, MD: U.S. Department of Health and Human Services, 1994.
156. Basmajian JV, Wolf SL. *Therapeutic exercise,* 5th ed. Baltimore: Williams & Wilkins, 1990.
157. Kraus H. *Therapeutic exercise,* 2nd ed. Springfield, IL: Charles C Thomas, 1963.
158. Wells P, Lessard E. Movement education and limitation of movement. In: Wall PD, Melzack R, eds. *Textbook of pain,* 3rd ed. New York: Churchill-Livingstone, 1994; 1263–1278.
159. Fulton WM. Psychological strategies and techniques in pain management. *Semin Anesth* 1985; 4:247–254.
160. Malone MD, Strube MJ. Meta-analysis of non-medical treatments for chronic pain. *Pain* 1988; 34:231–244.
161. Barber J, Adrian C, eds. *Psychological approaches to the management of pain.* New York: Brunner/Mazel, 1982.
162. Chapman S. A review and clinical perspective on the use of EMG and thermal biofeedback for chronic headaches. *Pain* 1986; 27:1–43.
163. Flor H, Haag G, Turk D. Long-term efficacy of EMG biofeedback for chronic rheumatic back pain. *Pain* 1986; 27:195–202.
164. Fernandez E. A classification system of cognitive coping strategies for pain. *Pain* 1986; 26:141–151.
165. Edmonston W Jr. *Hypnosis and relaxation.* New York: Wiley, 1981.
166. Smith J. *Relaxation dynamics.* Chicago, IL: Research Press, 1985.
167. Houde RW, Wallenstein SL, Beaver WT. Evaluation of analgesics in patients with cancer pain. In: Lasagna L, ed. *International encyclopedia of pharmacology and therapeutics.* New York: Pergamon, 1966.
168. Marks RW, Sacher EJ. Undertreatment of medical patients with narcotic analgesia. *Ann Intern Med* 1973; 78:173–181.
169. Kanner RM, Foley KM. Patterns of narcotic drug use in cancer pain clinic. *NY Acad Sci* 1981; 362:161–172.
170. Huber SL, Hill CS. Pharmacologic management of cancer pain. *Cancer Bull* 1980; 32:183–185.
171. Moertel CG. Relief of pain with oral medications. *Aust NZ J Med* 1976; 6:1–8.
172. White PF. Patient-controlled analgesia: a new approach to the management of postoperative pain. *Semin Anesth* 1985; 4:255–266.
173. Walsh PD. Antidepressants in chronic pain. *Clin Neuropharmacol* 1983; 6:271–295.
174. Aronoff GM, Evans WO. Doxipam as an adjuvant in the treatment of chronic pain. *J Clin Psychol* 1982; 43:42–47.
175. McQuay HJ, Tramer M, Nye BA, Carroll D, Wiffer PJ, Moore RA. A systematic review of antidepressants in neuropathic pain. *Pain* 1997; 68:217–228.
176. Anghena P, van Houdenkove B. Antidepressant-induced analgesia in chronic non-malignant pain: a meta-analysis of 39 placebo controlled studies. *Headache* 1994; 34:44–49.
177. McNamara JO. Drugs effective in the therapy of epilepsies. In: Hardman JG, Goodman Gilman A, Limbird LE, eds. *The pharmacological basis of therapeutics,* 9th ed. New York: McGraw-Hill, 1996; 201–226.
178. Ramamurthy S, Winnie AP. Regional anesthetic techniques for pain relief. *Semin Anesth* 1985; 4:237–245.
179. Raferty A. The management of postherpetic pain using sodium valproate and amitriptyline. *Irish Med J* 1979; 72:399–401.
180. Manna V, Bolino F, De Cicco L. Chronic tension-type headache, mood depression, and serotonin: therapeutic effects of fluvoxamine and mianserine. *Headache* 1994; 34:44–49.
181. Sindrup SH, Gram LF, Brosen K, Eshj O, Mogenson EF. The selective serotonin reuptake inhibitor paroxetine is effective in the treatment of diabetic neuropathy symptoms. *Pain* 1990; 42:135–144.
182. Swerdlow M. Anticonvulsant drugs in chronic pain. *Clin Neuropharmacol* 1984; 7:51–82.
183. Rowlingson JC, Chalkley J. Common pain syndromes—diagnosis and management. *Semin Anesth* 1985; 4:223–230.

184. Walsh NE, Ramamurthy S. Neck and upper extremity pain. In: Raj PP, ed. *Practical management of pain,* 2nd ed. Chicago: Year Book Medical, 1992; 272–295, 1992.
185. Deyo RA. Clinical research methods in low back pain. *Phys Med Rehabil Stars* 1991; 5:209–222.
186. Quebec Task Force on Spinal Disorders. Scientific approach to the assessment and management of activity related spinal disorders: a monograph for clinicians. *Spine* 1987; 12(suppl 7):22–30.
187. Deyo RA. Measuring the functional status of patients with low back pain. *Arch Phys Med Rehabil* 1988; 69:1044–1053.
188. Turk DC, Rudy TE. Neglected factors in chronic pain treatment outcome studies—referral patterns, failure to enter treatment, and attrition. *Pain* 1990; 43:7–25.
189. Bonica JJ. Managment of myofascial pain syndromes in general practice. *JAMA* 1957; 164:732–738.
190. Gunn CC, Milbrandt WE, Little AS, Mason KE. Dry needling of muscle motor points for chronic low back pain. *Spine* 1980; 5: 279–290.
191. Kraus H. Triggerpoints. *NY State J Med* 1973; 73:1310–1314.
192. Ready LB, Kozody R, Barsa JE, Murphy TM. Trigger point injections versus jet injection in the treatment of myofascial pain. *Pain* 1983; 15:201–206.
193. McCain GA. Fibromyalgia and myofascial pain syndromes. In: Wall PD, Melzack R, eds. *Textbook of pain,* 3rd ed. New York: Churchill-Livingstone, 1994; 475–493.
194. Cheshire WP, Abashian SW, Mann JD. Botulinum toxin in the treatment of myofascial pain syndrome. *Pain* 1994; 59:65–69.
195. Rempel DM, Harrison RJ, Barnhart S. Work-related cumulative trauma disorders of the upper extremity. *JAMA* 1992; 267:838–842.
196. Erdil M, Dickerson OB, Glackin E. Cumulative trauma disorders of the upper extremity. In: Zenz C, Dickerson OB, Orvath EP, eds. *Occupational medicine,* 3rd ed. St. Louis: Mosby Yearbook, 1994; 48–64.
197. Rogers SH, Kenworthy DA, Ingleton EM. *Ergonomic design for people at work.* Vol. 3. New York: Van Nostrand Reinhold, 1994.
198. Dumitru D, Gershkoff AM, Walsh NE. Peripheral nervous and muscular system. In: Felsenthal G, Garrison SJ, Steinberg FU, eds. *Rehabilitation of the aging and elderly patient.* Baltimore: Williams & Wilkins, 1994; 227–242.
199. Max MB, Culname M, Schafer SC, et al. Association of pain relief with drug side effects in postherpetic neuralgia: a single-dose study of clonidine, codeine, ibuprofen, and placebo. *Clin Pharmacol Ther* 1988; 43:363–371.
200. Kvinesdal B, Molin J, Froland A, Gram LF. Imipramine treatment of painful diabetic neuropathy. *JAMA* 1984; 251:1727–1730.
201. Sindrup SH, Gram LF, Brosen K, et al. The selective serotonin reuptake inhibitor paroxetine is effective in the treatment of diabetic neuropathy symptoms. *Pain* 1990; 42:135–144.
202. Peteet J, Tay V, Cohen G, MacIntyre J. Pain characteristics treatment in an outpatient cancer population. *Cancer* 1986; 57:1259–1265.
203. Dejgard A, Peterson P, Kastrup J. Mexiletine for treatment of chronic painful diabetic neuropathy. *Lancet* 1988; 1:9–11.
204. Byers CM, DeLisa JA, Frankel DL, Kraft GH. Pyridoxine metabolism in carpal tunnel syndrome with and without peripheral neuropathy. *Arch Phys Med Rehabil* 1984; 65:712–716.
205. Max MB, Lynch SA, Muir J, Shoaf SE, Smaller B, Dubner R. Effects of desipramine, amitriptyline, and fluoxetine on pain in diabetic neuropathy. *N Engl J Med* 1992; 326:1250–1256.
206. Ramamurthy S, Hoffman J, Guanethidine Study Group. Intravenous gegional guanethidine in the treatment of reflex sympathetic dystrophy/causalgia: a randomized double-blind study. *Anesth Analg* 1995; 81:718–723.
207. Verdugo RJ, Ochoa JL. Sympathetically maintained pain: I. Plentolamine block questions the concept. *Neurology* 1994; 44:1003–1010.
208. Dumitru D. Reflex sympathetic dystrophy. *Phys Med Rehabil Stars* 1991; 5:89–102.
209. Davidoff G, Werner R, Cremer S. Predictive value of the three-phase technetium bone scan and diagnosis of reflex sympathetic dystrophy syndrome. *Arch Phys Med Rehabil* 1989; 70:135–137.
210. Ghostine SY, Comair YG, Turner DM, et al. Phenoxybenzamine in the treatment of causalgia—report of 40 cases. *J Neurosurg* 1984; 60:1263–1268.
211. Lewis R Jr, Racz G, Fabian G. Therapeutic approaches to reflex sympathetic dystrophy of the upper extremity. *Clin Iss Reg Anesth* 1985; 1:1–6.
212. Ramamurthy S, Hoffman J, et al. Intravenous regional guanethidine in the treatment of reflex sympathetic dystrophy and causalgia: a randomized, double-blind study. *Anesth Analg* 1995; 81:718–23.
213. Ford SR, Forrest WH, Eltherington L. Treatment of reflex sympathetic dystrophy with intravenous regional bretylium. *Anesthesiology* 1988; 68:137–140.
214. Benzon HT, Chomka CM, Brunner EA. Treatment of reflex sympathetic dystrophy with regional intravenous reserpine. *Anesth Analg* 1980; 59:500–502.
215. Hannington-Kiff JG. Intravenous regional sympathetic block with guanethidine. *Lancet* 1974; 1:1019–1020.
216. North RB, Long DM. Spinal cord stimulation for intractable pain: eight year followup. *Pain* 1994; 29(suppl 2):79.
217. Sherman RA, Sherman CJ. Prevalence and characteristics of chronic phantom limb pain among American veterans. *Am J Phys Med* 1983; 62:227–238.
218. Jensen TS, Krebs B, Nielsen J, Rasmussen P. Immediate and long term phantom limb pain in amputees—incidence, clinical characteristics, and relationship to preamputation limb pain. *Pain* 1985; 21: 267–278.
219. Banerjee SN. Lower extremity amputations. In: Basmajian JO, Banerjee SN, eds. *Clinical decision making in rehabilitation.* New York: Churchill-Livingstone, 1996; 153–170.
220. Sherman R, Sherman C, Gall N. A survey of current phantom limb treatment in the United States. *Pain* 1980; 8:85–99.
221. Sherman RA, Sherman CJ, Parker L. Chronic phantom and stump pain among American veterans—result of a survey. *Pain* 1984; 18: 83–95.
222. Finsen V, Person L, Lovlien M, et al. Transcutaneous electrical nerve stimulation after major amputation. *J Bone Joint Surg [Br]* 1988; 70: 109–112.
223. Panerai AE, Monza G, Movilia, Bianchi M, Francucci BM, Tiehgo M. A randomized with inpatient crossover, placebo controlled trial on the efficacy and tolerability of the tricyclic antidepressant chlorimipramine and mortriphyline in central pain. *Acta Neurol Scand* 1990; 82:34–38.
224. Patterson JF. Carbamazepine in the treatment of phantom limb pain. *South Med J* 1988; 81:1100–1102.
225. Jaeger H, Maier C. Calcitonin in phantom limb pain: a double-blind study. *Pain* 1992; 48:21–27.
226. Davis RW. Successful treatment of phantom limb pain. *Orthopaedics* 1993; 16:691–695.
227. Cleeland C. The impact of pain on the patient with cancer. *Cancer* 1984; 54:2635–2641.
228. Ramamurthy S, Walsh NE, Schoenfeld LS, Hoffman J. Evaluation of neurolytic blocks using phenol and cryogenic block in the management of chronic pain. *J Pain Sympt Mgt* 1989; 4:72–75.
229. McGivney WT, Crooks GM. The case of patients with severe chronic pain in terminal illness. *JAMA* 1984; 251:1182–1188.
230. Black P. Management of cancer pain—an overview. *Neurosurgery* 1979; 5:507–518.
231. Jacox A, Carr D, Payne R, et al. *Management of cancer pain. Clinical practice guidelines*, No. 9. AHCPR 94-0592, Rockville, MD: Agency for Health Care Policy and Research, U.S., Department of Health and Human Services, Public Health Service, March 1994.
232. Cousins J, Mather L. Intrathecal and epidural administration of opiates. *Anesthesiology* 1984; 61:276–310.
233. Eisenach J, Rauck R, Buzzanell C, Lysak C. Epidural clonidine analgesia for intractable cancer pain: phase I. *Anesthesiology* 1989; 71: 647–652.
234. Freidberg SR. Neurosurgical treatment of pain caused by cancer. *Med Clin North Am* 1975; 59:481–485.
235. Epstein E. Intralesional triamcinolone therapy in herpes zoster and post herpetic neuralgia. *Ear Nose Throat Mon* 1973; 52:416.
236. Rowbotham MC, Fields HL. Topical lidocaine reduces pain in postherpetic neuralgia. *Pain* 1989; 38:297–302.
237. Bernstein JE, Korman NJ, Bickers DR, et al. Topical capsaicin treatment of chronic postherpetic neuralgia. *J Am Acad Dermatol* 1989; 21:265–270.
238. Pagni CA. Central pain due to spinal cord and brain stem damage. In: Wall PD, Melzack R, eds. *Textbook of pain.* London: Churchill-Livingstone, 1984; 481–495.
239. Yel C, Gonyea M, Lemke J, Volpe M. Physical therapy: evaluation and treatments of chronic pain. In: Aronoff GM, ed. *Evaluation and*

treatment of chronic pain, 2nd ed. Baltimore: Urban & Schwarzenberg, 1992; 251–261.

240. Young PA. The anatomy of the spinal cord pain paths—a review. *J Am Paraplegia Soc* 1986; 9:28–38.
241. Lamid S, Chia JK, Kohli A, Cid E. Chronic pain in spinal cord injury: comparison between inpatients and outpatients. *Arch Phys Med Rehabil* 1985; 66:777–778.
242. Woolsey RM. Chronic pain following spinal cord injury. *J Am Paraplegia Soc* 1986; 9:51–53.
243. Donovan WH, Dimitrijevic MR, Dahm L. Neurophysiological approaches to chronic pain following spinal cord injury. *Paraplegia* 1982; 20:135–246.
244. O'Brien JP. Mechanisms of spinal pain. In: Wall PD, Melzack R, eds. *Textbook of pain,* 3rd ed. New York: Churchill-Livingstone, 1994; 240–251.
245. Yezierki RP. Pain following spinal cord injury: the clinical problem and experimental studies. *Pain* 1997; 68:185–194.
246. Farkash AE, Portenoy RK. The pharmacological management of chronic pain in the paraplegic patient. *J Am Paraplegia Soc* 1986; 9: 41–50.
247. Britell CW, Mariano AJ. Chronic pain in spinal cord injury. *Phys Med Rehabil Stars* 1991; 5:71–82.
248. Hachen HA. Psychological, neuropsychological, and therapeutic aspects of chronic pain—preliminary results with transcutaneous electrical stimulation. *Paraplegia* 1977; 15:357–367.
249. Kassirer MR, Osterberger DH. Pain and chronic multiple sclerosis. *J Pain Sympt Mgmt* 1987; 2:95–97.
250. Martin JJ. Thalamic syndromes. In: Vinken PJ, Bruyne GW, eds. *Handbook of clinical neurology. Vol. 2. Localization in clinical neurology.* Amsterdam: North Holland Publishing, 1962; 469–496.
251. Stanton-Hicks M, Abram SE, Nolte H. Sympathetic blocks. In: Raj PP, ed. *Practical management of pain.* Chicago: Year Book Medical, 1986; 661–681.
252. Garrison SJ. Post-stroke pain. *Phys Med Rehabil Stars* 1991; 5:83–88.
253. Leijon G, Boivie J. Central post-stroke pain—the effect of high and low frequency TENS. *Pain* 1989; 38:187–191.
254. Sindow M, Mifsud JJ, Boisson D, Goutelle A. Selected posterior rhizotomy in the dorsal route entry zone for treatment of hyper-spasticity in pain in the hemiplegic upper limb. *Neurosurgery* 1986; 18: 587–595.
255. Tasker RR. Pain resulting from central nervous system pathology (central pain). In: Bonica JJ, ed. *The management of pain,* 2nd ed. Philadelphia: Lea & Febiger, 1990; 264–283.
256. Andersson GBJ, Pope MH, Frymoyer JW, Snook S. Epidemiology and cost. In: Pope MH, Andersson GBJ, Frymoyer JW, Chaffin DB, eds. *Occupational low back pain: assessment, treatment, and prevention.* St. Louis: CV Mosby, 1991; 95–113.
257. Biggos SJ, Spengler DM, Martin NA, et al. Back injuries in industry: employee related factors. *Spine* 1986; 3:252–256.
258. Borenstein DG, Wiesel SW. *Low back pain: medical diagnosis and comprehensive management.* Philadelphia: WB Saunders, 1989.
259. Scheer SJ, Radack KL, O'Brien DR. Randomized controlled trials in industrial low back pain. Part I. Acute interventions. *Arch Phys Med Rehabil* 1995; 76:966–973.
260. Scheer SJ, Radack KL, O'Brien DR. Randomized controlled trials in industrial low back pain relating to return to work. Part II. Discogenic back pain. *Arch Phys Med Rehabil* 1996; 77:1189–1197.
261. Scheer SJ, Radack KL, O'Brien DR. Randomized controlled trials in industrial low back pain. Part III. Subacute/chronic pain interventions. *Arch Phys Med Rehabil* 1997;78:414–423.

Rehabilitation Medicine: Principles and Practice, Third Edition,
edited by Joel A. DeLisa and Bruce M. Gans.
Lippincott–Raven Publishers, Philadelphia © 1998.

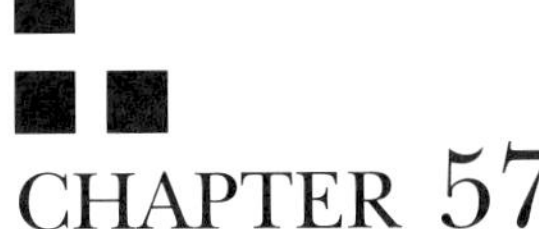

CHAPTER 57

Rehabilitation of the Patient with Spinal Pain

Stuart M. Weinstein, Stanley A. Herring, and Andrew J. Cole

The rehabilitation of patients with spinal pain requires the integration of a comprehensive knowledge of anatomy, physiology, and function. Similar to some other medical conditions, such as coronary artery and inflammatory bowel disease, the endpoint of treatment of a patient with spinal pain is reached when the patient is able to independently manage even with an impairment. Maximizing function—at home, at the workplace, and in the athletic arena—is equally important to resolving the symptoms related to the problem, which is often manifested by pain. It is critical to understand that the resolution of symptoms alone does not usually constitute satisfactory rehabilitation nor does it likely result in stable functional recovery. The classical description of the natural history of spinal pain and related syndromes (mostly described for low back pain) suggests a predictable and self-limited course, thus supporting the tenets of treatment minimalists. Even if this observation has merit, which recent data have questioned, the potential impact on one's quality of life and productivity, during the acute and subacute stages of spinal disorders, deserves recognition and should warrant reactive treatment. Successful rehabilitation in turn leads to proactive prehabilitation programs with the goal of prevention of pain and disability.

WHY TO REHABILITATE: FACTS AND AMBIGUITIES

Epidemiology

Epidemiologic data for spinal disorders has most commonly been reported for low back pain. Regardless of the diagnosis and cause, low back pain occurs commonly, with a 50% to 70% lifetime prevalence and 5% annual incidence (1,2). The prevalence and incidence of cervical and thoracic pain in the general population has been less frequently reported, with one study suggesting the prevalence of chronic neck pain in the general population to be approximately 14% (3). The annual incidence of neck pain after whiplash injury, based on review of the literature, has been described as approximately 0.1% (4). Spinal injury is universal in athletics. Low back pain is the most frequent site of injury in gymnastics, football, weightlifting, wrestling, rowing, swimming, amateur golf, and ballet; the second most frequent site of injury in professional golf and aerobic dance; and common in tennis, baseball, jogging, cycling, basketball, and the general dance population (5). The incidence of neck pain and noncatastrophic neck injury in athletes is less well known. However, catastrophic neck injury, by definition resulting in incomplete neurologic recovery, was 0.56 and 1.54 per 100,000, respectively, for high school and college football players (6). In the worker's compensation category, review of data from one jurisdiction identified that back and neck claims accounted for 20% of all claims and 45% of all claims with time lost from work of over 120 days (see Chapter 10).

S. M. Weinstein: Department of Rehabilitation Medicine, University of Washington, Seattle, Washington 98195; and Puget Sound Sports and Spine Physicians, Seattle, Washington 98122.
S. A. Herring: Departments of Rehabilitation Medicine and Orthopaedics, University of Washington, Seattle, Washington 98195; and Puget Sound Sports and Spine Physicians, Seattle, Washington 98122.
A. J. Cole: Puget Sound Sports and Spine Physicians, Seattle, Washington 98122.

Natural History

Spontaneous recovery from an episode of back pain has been ingrained in medical teaching: 90% of cases of low back pain resolve without medical attention in 6 to 12 weeks; 50% resolve within 1 week; and even 75% of people with sciatica are asymptomatic at 6 months. Furthermore, it is commonly expected that most people sustaining ''soft-tissue'' whiplash injury should recover relatively quickly. Despite this seemingly favorable natural history, a less optimistic prognosis for the absolute resolution of spinal pain may be more realistic. A more recent study on the natural history of back pain suggests that although a single episode of back pain is likely to improve, back pain is usually a recurrent condition and occasionally enters a chronic phase (7). The statistics for whiplash injury also indicate significant, chronic neck pain, ranging from 14% to 42%, and approximately 10% have constant, severe pain (8).

This so-called self-limited disease process is also the leading cause of disability in people under 45 years of age and the third cause of disability in those over 45 years of age (9). Furthermore, low back pain remains a leading reason for patient visits to a general practitioner's office (10), and although hospitalization rates have consistently decreased for low back pain, the rate of spinal surgery is 40% higher in the United States than any other country (11), and between 1979 and 1990, the rate of lumbar fusion surgery doubled (12). These statistics are compounded by the observation that lifetime return to work rates decrease to 50% if the injured worker is off work for 6 months, 25% if off work for 1 year, and nearly 0% if the worker has not returned to work by 2 years (13,14). Finally, the economic impact on society for the tangible expenditures (i.e., medical care and indemnity payments) and the intangible costs (e.g., production loss, employee retraining, administrative expenses, increased consumer costs, and litigation) may be well over $50 billion by the end of the century (1,15).

Historical Perspective

Manual therapy principles for low back pain may have their roots with Hippocrates, but classical manipulative therapy was not synthesized until the late nineteenth century. The historical challenge of treating spinal pain is loosely exemplified by the legacy of Saint Lawrence, one of the most honored martyrs of the Roman Church. He was said to have been executed in 258 A.D. for his patronage of the poor, notwithstanding his patronage against lumbago (16). Throughout modern history, innumerable "modalities" have been championed for the treatment of spinal pain, and although any rehabilitation tool may have a role in individual treatment, it cannot be overemphasized that fanatical application of any single technique does not have a place in proper rehabilitation. Indeed, a narrow and naive approach toward the treatment of spinal pain can promote disability.

Given the complexity of the biopsychosocial model of low back pain (Fig. 57-1) (17,18), it has been suggested that the physiatrist may have the best functional understanding of how to apply rehabilitation principles to the spinal–injured patient (19). However, all of the so-called support systems—medical team, employer, and family—have a responsibility for managing the spinal–injured patient. The team concept was never better supported than in the treatment of acute, subacute, and especially chronic low back pain. Individual practitioners, like isolated treatments, are destined to fail without adequate support mechanisms. With the proper application of rehabilitation techniques, minimization of recurrences and prevention of long-term disability should be possible. The improvement in quality of life and the ultimate financial savings to society warrant a critical appraisal and comprehensive approach to the evaluation and treatment of spinal pain.

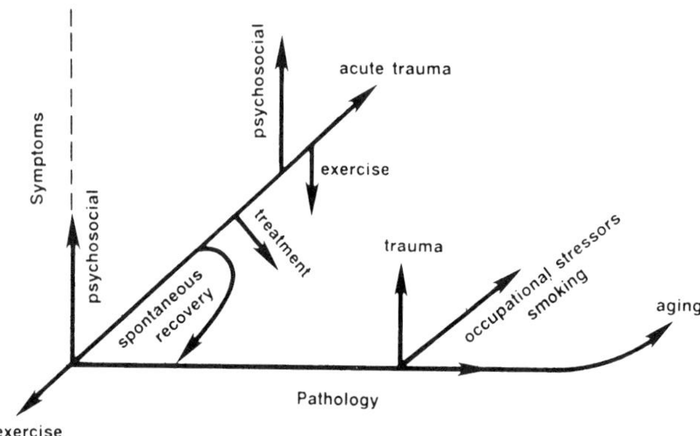

FIG. 57-1. Factors affecting the classical pathology model of low back pain. (Reprinted with permission from Haldeman S. Presidential address. North American Spine Society: failure of the pathology model to predict back pain. *Spine* 1990; 15:722.)

Ambiguous Nomenclature

A common nomenclature is critical for the effective communication between members of the treatment team, ultimately yielding effective treatment of the focal player on the team, the patient. However, terminology and concepts in the field of spinal medicine are often confusing and ambiguous for those involved. The following are some common examples.

Degenerative Disc Disease. Disc degeneration is a defined anatomic alteration that is sometimes associated with a recognizable etiology and consistent symptoms and signs, and thus by strict definition is probably a disease entity. However, the implication for the patient is that this condition is unalterable, with or without treatment, ultimately leading to chronic pain and disability. Furthermore, if such a vast majority of people experience back pain in their lifetimes and because imaging evidence for disc degeneration is so common (even in asymptomatic people) (20–23), should practitioners continue to label this condition a disease versus degenerative changes due to aging among other potential factors? This should not dissuade the physician from concluding that the disc may be the source of a patient's pain, but rather to label the problem in a less threatening manner. It is often the first words that are spoken to a patient that leave the greatest intellectual and emotional impact.

Disc Herniation and Radiculopathy. A variety of terms have been used interchangeably to describe disc herniation and nerve root abnormalities. The following are well-accepted definitions for these entities:

Disc herniation: focal extension of the disc beyond the vertebral end plate

Disc protrusion: contained by the outer annulus fibrosis with an intact posterior longitudinal ligament

Disc extrusion: noncontained and through the posterior longitudinal ligament
Disc fragment (sequestered): free fragment no longer in contact with parent disc
Disc bulge: nonfocal or circumferential, symmetric extension of disc beyond the margin of the vertebral end plate
Radiculopathy: radicular pain in a dermatomal distribution and/or neurologic symptoms (i.e., numbness or paresthesias) or signs (i.e., weakness in a myotomal distribution)
Radiculitis: radicular pain and/or radicular symptoms or signs in the absence of an obvious compressive lesion

Subjective Versus Objective. More often than not this distinction is an administrative requirement of a specific insurance system and frequently leads to ambiguities. For example, the rules and regulations of many worker's compensation programs do not require an objective abnormality (i.e., measurable pathology in the absence of a patient's verbal report) to allow opening of an injury claim, but will require objectivity to allow continued treatment beyond a given point. Often the identification of degenerative disc changes on advanced imaging studies are not readily accepted as objective substantiation of subjective complaints (i.e., a patient's verbal report of symptoms). Disallowing further intervention due to subjective complaints only may be interpreted by the patient as an invalidation of his problem. Ambiguity exists for the physician as well, whether acting as a treating physician or an independent examiner, being asked to interpret the same medical information for distinctly different purposes.

Physiologic Versus Psychologic. Especially in the framework of chronic pain, with the attendant psychosocial behavioral manifestations such as exaggerated pain behavior and depression, a psychological label or diagnosis tends to shift the burden and blame for the problem on the patient, divesting the practitioner or the system for any further responsibility. However, psychosocial issues often cannot be adequately separated from the spinal pathology in determining causation and need for further treatment. Inattention to these factors may in fact promote disability.

Operative Versus Nonoperative Management of Disc Herniations

The classic paper by Mixter and Barr (24) popularized the role of surgery for the management of the herniated disc with radiculopathy in the mid-twentieth century. However, in the past several years, numerous papers reporting on sequential imaging studies have demonstrated that the natural clinical course of disc herniation (both lumbar and cervical) is one of spontaneous resolution (25–34). The length of time for follow-up imaging examination ranged from 9 to 25 months. One study examined at least one portion of the cohort group every 3 months, finding that within 1 month, regression of disk material can be seen (30). Various mechanisms have been postulated to account for this spontaneous improvement, including an inflammatory reaction that is triggered by nuclear material that enters the epidural space, aggressive granulation into the disc fragment with subsequent phagocytosis and dehydration of the extruded fragment. Interestingly, the largest fragments that would have been considered surgically desirable demonstrated the greatest resolution in size in most of these studies. The success of nonoperative management in most of these studies was predicated on a combination of epidural corticosteroid injection and exercise, although none were controlled studies. Whether clinical improvement would have matched the resolution of disc herniation without any concurrent treatment is probably a study design that is not feasible.

This is not to imply that surgical care should never be considered for the treatment of disc herniations. In fact, conservative care does not always equate to nonoperative treatment. In certain clinical scenarios, early surgical intervention is more appropriate, and even essential, than comprehensive nonoperative rehabilitation. These include cervical myelopathy or lumbar cauda equina syndrome, rapidly progressive motor weakness due to single level radiculopathy, and intractable radicular pain in the acutely injured patient. The surgical management of these conditions will usually be a discectomy (in the lumbar spine, but variably a discectomy and fusion would be required in the cervical spine), which is a relatively minimally invasive procedure. The surgical approach to treating primarily axial pain without neurologic symptoms or signs would typically invoke the consideration of a fusion, the discussion of which is beyond the scope of this chapter.

There are certainly other issues in determining operative versus nonoperative management of radicular syndromes due to disc herniations. One of the prime considerations is quality of life as affected by pain and resultant disability. In the acute or subacute stages, surgery has been demonstrated to more quickly resolve radicular pain than other treatment modalities, but over a period of time (greater than 1 year), the benefits of operative versus nonoperative treatment equalized regarding functional outcome (35,36). Surgery also may allow a relatively accelerated return to activity pathway, which may be critical for an elite athlete. However, discetomy has not been demonstrated to resolve nonprogressive motor weakness any quicker than nonoperative measures; thus, nonprogressive weakness is only a relative indication for surgical intervention (36).

Without question, these ambiguities directly impact the assessment and treatment of spinal disorders. The results of a national survey of physician biases about treating low back pain demonstrated an overwhelming lack of consensus (37). A variety of theories were stated to explain this phenomenon: the absence of clear evidence-based clinical guidelines; ignorance or rejection of existing scientific evidence; excessive commitment to a particular mode of therapy; or a tendency to discount the efficacy of competing treatments. [These results regarding treatment mirrored a previous study on the variation of diagnostic tests ordered by different specialties (38)]. Physiatrists were the greatest opponents of deactivating treatments, including centrally acting medication and bed rest, and the greatest proponents for exercise and physical therapy. In fact, the literature is seriously lacking in adequately performed randomized clinical trials on the efficacy of commonly used interventions for spinal pain (39). Short of this, therefore, the rehabilitation principles and concepts presented in this chapter are based on generally accepted principles for the treatment of musculoskeletal disorders, noncontrolled clinical experience and the literature as it exists to date.

WHAT TO REHABILITATE

Functional Anatomy and Biomechanics (40–43)

Spinal Mobility

Gross spinal range of motion does not adequately reflect the complex spinal mechanism. Range of motion as observed in the clinical environment represents a summation of segmental motion. Except for the unique anatomic arrangement of the upper cervical spine (from the occiput to C2), each motion segment of the spinal axis is defined by the three joint complex—the single discovertebral joint anteriorly and the paired zygapophyseal joints (z joints) posteriorly. The cardinal planes of segmental motion are flexion and extension, and torsion and lateral flexion, and are all a combination of rotation in a specific plane (i.e., sagittal, axial, and coronal, respectively) plus translation in that same plane. Gross range of motion may be perceived as ''normal'' despite the presence of underlying segmental motion abnormalities, including hypo- and hypermobilities. Furthermore, segmental motion usually occurs as so-called coupled motion; that is, movement that occurs in one axis is consistently associated with motion that occurs about a second axis.

The cervical spine is the most mobile part of the spinal axis. The upper cervical segments (i.e., occiput [C0]–C1, C1–C2) are unique to the rest of the spinal axis in that there does not exist an intervertebral disc. All planes of range of motion are available in the cervical spine, and coupled motion patterns are well developed, particularly between axial rotation and lateral bending, probably due to the oblique orientation of the cervical zygapophyseal joints. Due to coupled motion, pure rotation does not occur at any segment, and the proportion of rotation to lateral bending increases more rostrally in the cervical spine. The following are generally accepted levels of maximal motion: head nodding at C0–C1; rotation at C1–C2 (accounts for 50% of total available rotation); lateral bending at C3–C4; and flexion–extension at C5–C6. Rotation and lateral bending are least at the C0–C1 articulation, representing a protective mechanism for the vertebral artery as it enters the cranium.

The thoracic spine with the rib cage is the stiffest and least mobile part of the spine and is vital for erect posture. The two main directions of segmental motion within the thoracic spine are sagittal flexion and extension and axial rotation, the latter more evident in the upper thoracic spine from approximately T1 to T6 and the former more typical of the lower thoracic segments. Above T9 the thoracic spine acts more like the cervical spine, and below this level it demonstrates motion more typical of the lumbar spine. Coupling patterns in the thoracic spine are much weaker than in the cervical region.

When considering the lumbar spine, observed motion is the additive effect of each motion segment from the thoracolumbar junction through the lumbosacral segment, plus lumbopelvic rhythm of the hip joint. The optimal lumbar mechanism provides risk-limited mobility, with the lower lumbar spine generally being the most mobile, but also subject to the greatest loads. All cardinal planes of motion occur in the lumbar spine, with associated coupling characteristics, including a strong coupling pattern between axial rotation and lateral flexion. The generally accepted levels of maximal motion are lateral flexion in the upper lumbar spine; flexion–extension at the L4–L5 and L5–S1 segments; and limited axial rotation (as a protective mechanism for the intervertebral disc) variably at all levels.

Spinal Stability

Throughout the spinal axis, various anatomic components variably contribute to spinal segmental stability, including the intervertebral disc, joints, ligaments, and muscles. Similar to the glenohumeral joint, the instantaneous center of rotation (ICR) principle applies to the three-joint complex as well. The ICR can be defined as a single pivot point around which movement occurs, the location of which can vary through the entire range of motion, but is consistent from time to time and at each instant. Maintenance of the ICR provides the most efficient motion with no symptom production and limits shear stresses across the three-joint complex, which in turn limits the tendency for acute injury or chronic degenerative changes to develop. However, the natural aging process, habitual postural alterations, and spinal injury all can lead to alterations in the ICR (i.e., segmental hypomobilities and hypermobilities) at any segmental level and often at a combination of levels simultaneously.

In the cervical spine, the ligamentous contribution to stability is probably greater than in the thoracic or lumbar spine. These ligaments provide the main restraint in the upper cervical spine complex, where neurovascular protection is vital, fixing the occiput to C2, the occiput to C1, and C1 to C2. In the middle to lower cervical spine, the posterior longitudinal ligament is well developed, serving to reinforce the posterior disc margin, thus protecting the spinal cord. The ligamentum flavum reinforces the z-joint capsule, and a combination of the interspinous, supraspinous, and nuchal ligaments provide posterior segmental stability, limiting excessive anterior translation.

The zygapophyseal joints of the cervical spine contribute little to stability and, in fact, are oriented to maximize mobility. Conversely, the uncovertebral joints provide stability,

TABLE 57-1. *Muscles controlling head and neck motion*

Flexors	Extensors
Head	
Rectus capitis anterior[a]	Rectus capitis posterior[a]
Rectus capitis lateralis	Obliquus capitis[a,b]
Longus capitis[a]	Splenius capitis[a,b]
Longus colli[a,b]	Longissimus capitis[a,b]
	Semispinalis capitis
Neck	
Sternocleidomastoid[a,b]	Upper trapezius[a,b]
Scalenes (anterior)[a,b]	Splenius cervicis[a,b]
Longus colli[a,b]	Erector spinae group
	Iliocostalis cervicis[b]
	Longissimus cervicis
	Spinalis cervicis
	Semispinalis cervicis[a]
	Multifidi[a]
	Rotatores[a]
	Interspinales[a]
	Intertransversarii[a]

[a] Also contributes to axial rotation.
[b] Also contributes to lateral flexion.

particularly to the posterolateral aspects of the intervertebral discs and also guide motion in the flexion–extension plane. These uncovertebral joints are synovial joints, present from C3 to C7, and develop postnatally. Uncovertebral joint arthropathy probably contributes to segmental motion abnormalities.

Multiple muscles act on the head and neck to provide stability and generate motion (Table 57-1). The main action of any muscle is proportional to the length of its lever arm, with shorter muscles acting mainly as segmental stabilizers and longer muscles as prime movers. In general, there is a balance between anterior and posterior muscular activity, with muscle strength and flexibility imbalances contributing to postural alterations. In the cervical spine, a normal lordosis places the C5–C6 segment anterior to and furthest from the center of gravity.

Thoracic spine stability is afforded primarily through the rib cage, which stiffens and strengthens the spine via the costovertebral joints and ligaments and by effectively increasing the transverse diameter of the spine, thus increasing its resistance to motion in any plane. At the costovertebral joints, the head of the rib articulates with the vertebral body at the same level and one rostral. Also, the rib tubercle articulates with the transverse process at the same level. Both articulations are synovial joints with ligamentous support from the radiate and costotransverse ligaments, respectively. The zygapophyseal joint and capsule also add to segmental stability. The joints of the upper thoracic levels protect primarily against anterior translation, and the joints of the lower levels protect against axial rotation. Due to the strong intrinsic stability of these joints, the muscular contributions of most thoracic muscles are as prime movers for movement of the trunk on the pelvis as opposed to segmental stabilizers.

In the lumbar spine, there are multiple factors providing segmental stability, including muscles, ligaments, intervertebral disc, and z joints, with the muscular contribution proportionally the most important in protecting the three-joint complex against excessive shear. The ligamentous structures include the midline ligaments, composed of the supraspinous ligament, interspinous ligament, posterior longitudinal ligament, ligamentum flavum, z-joint capsule, anterior longitudinal ligament, and iliolumbar ligament. The midline structures form a passive restraint system that is engaged with forward bending. The anterior longitudinal ligament and the iliolumbar ligament act to maintain the lumbar lordosis. The lumbar lordosis is an ideal posture for axial load bearing, with the ligaments and z joints assisting in unloading the intervertebral disc.

The ability of the z joint to contribute to lumbar stability is proportional to its geometry. Articulatory facets that are oriented perpendicular to the sagittal plane resist forward displacement and shear as the superior facet contacts the inferior facet. The shape of the facet (i.e., flat or curved) further determines how much surface area of contact between facets will occur. Resistance against segmental rotation is afforded by facets that are oriented parallel to the sagittal plane. It is this latter facet orientation that restricts axial rotation in the lumbar spine to typically no more than 3°. Greater axial rotation in the lumbar segments may result in annular deterioration.

An intact lumbar intervertebral disc functions in weight bearing (axial load), bending, and rotation to maintain lumbar stability. The intervertebral disc consists of the central nucleus pulposus (i.e., a fibrogelatinous mass composed of 80% to 90% water, collagen, and a mucopolysaccharide matrix) and the peripheral annulus fibrosis (formed by the concentric alternating lamellae of obliquely oriented collagenous fibers). Brief axial loads are resisted by the mass of the annular fibers, whereas with sustained loads, the nucleus pulposus transmits radial pressure to the annulus fibrosis and pressure to the endplates. Depending on the intactness of the annulus and endplate, these forces will be effectively resisted. The annulus is the primary disc structure that resists rotational force through the orientation of the lamellae. The resistance to forward bending is derived from the relatively greater thickness of the posterior lamellae and the greater cross-sectional surface area of the annulus fibrosis posteriorly due to its concave configuration.

The increase in intradiscal pressure with bending and lifting is due primarily to muscular compressive force and is proportional to the distance of the load being lifted from the body. With forward bending, the posterior annulus stretches and the nucleus pulposus is displaced posteriorly, which is an at-risk posture. The most disc-compromised posture is forward bending, rotation, and lifting a load away from the body. Given the great load demands on the lumbar three-joint complex, which can exceed the intrinsic capacity of these joints, ligaments, and discs, a large muscle contribution is necessary to provide dynamic stability.

The muscular components can be divided into posterior

TABLE 57-2. *Muscles controlling trunk motion*

Flexors	Extensors
External oblique[a]	Intrinsic
Internal oblique[a]	Deep (unisegmental)
Transversus abdominus	Interspinalis
Illopsoas[b]	Intertransversarii[a]
	Rotatores[a]
	Intermediate (multisegmental)
	Semispinalis[a]
	Multifidi[a]
	Superficial (polysegmental)
	Erector spinae
	Iliocostalis[a,b]
	Longissimus[a,b]
	Spinalis[a,b]
	Extrinsic
	Latissimus dorsi
	Quadratus lumborum
	Hip extensors
	Gluteus maximus
	Hamstrings

[a] Also contributes to axial rotation.
[b] Also contributes to lateral flexion.

muscles—intrinsic and extrinsic—and prevertebral muscles (Table 57-2). Some muscle groups do provide passive stability as well, such as the erector spinae and hip extensors. At approximately 90% of maximal lumbar flexion and 60% of hip flexion, the passive force generated in these muscles is fivefold greater than the ligamentous tension generated in the midline ligamentous structures. Dynamically, the contribution of these various muscles changes depending on the activity-standing posture, extension, lateral flexion, forward flexion, recovery phase (with or without load), and torsion. With upright posture, little muscle activity occurs because the lumbar spine is stabilized primarily by ligaments and the z joints. In approximately 75% of people, the line of gravity passes in front of the L4 vertebral body, thus the multifidi, owing to their force vectors, provide an extension moment. Extension of the lumbar spine from an upright posture is initiated by the shorter segmental lumbar muscles, but with increasing load, the longer lever arm erector spinae group is recruited. With lateral flexion, ipsilateral muscular activity initiates the motion, but gravity and bilateral lumbar and trunk muscle activity guides and controls motion. During trunk flexion, both lumbar segmental and hip joint motion occur. With the first 60° of forward bending, the lumbar segments flex with the hip extensors (i.e., gluteus maximus and hamstrings) acting eccentrically to ''lock'' the pelvis in extension, which maintains tension in the thoracolumbar fascia (TLF), and the erector spinae and multifidi act eccentrically, proportional to the angle of flexion. The next 25° is accomplished primarily by hip joint flexion. Recovery phase from a forward bent position is essentially a reversal in sequence of forward bending with the hip extensors, erector spinae, and multifidi all acting concentrically. The act of lifting a weight is basically recovery phase with a load. To accomplish this with minimal shear across the lumbar segments, the abdominal mechanism via the thoracolumbar fascia is one mechanism that is recruited. The thoracolumbar fascia is a broad soft-tissue structure with superficial and deep layers attaching to the spinous processes in the midline, the rib cage superiorly, the pelvis (including the fascia of the gluteus maximus) inferiorly, and the free edge to the internal oblique, transversus abdominous, and latissimus dorsi laterally (Fig. 57-2). The fibers of the thoracolumbar fascia are organized such that tension that is generated within this structure provides an extension moment to the spine with little shear. The attachment of the thoracolumbar fascia to the latissimus dorsi, which is a strong shoulder internal rotator, provides kinesiologic evidence of the kinetic chain impact of the lumbar spine on upper extremity function. Additionally, with lifting, tension generated within the TLF is transmitted directly to the erector spinae muscles via the hydraulic amplifier mechanism. Finally, torsion results from the synergistic effect between the multifidi and the internal oblique because there is no pure trunk or spine rotator. The internal oblique flexes and rotates the trunk, but as previously noted, the multifidi provide an extension moment only, thereby counterbalancing the flexion moment of the internal oblique, resulting in ''pure'' trunk rotation.

Specificity of Diagnosis

The reference to ''nonspecific'' spinal pain is commonly encountered in the literature. The ambiguity of this term is apparent. Does this imply that there is no easily identifiable source of pain or is the implication that there is no pathology? It has been demonstrated that offering a specific label (i.e., disc injury) to an acutely injured worker may be more likely to lead to chronic symptoms than providing a nonspecific label (i.e., strain or sprain) (44). The interpretation and correlation of advanced imaging test results also must be made carefully because a relatively large proportion of disc abnormalities, including degenerative changes and disc protrusions, have been demonstrated in asymptomatic people (20–23). Conversely, overt or covert suggestions to the patient that there is not a physiologic problem also may result in slow progression through the health-care system. The decision to communicate to a patient a specific or nonspecific label is dependent on a balance between the physician's confidence in determining a diagnosis and the needs of the patient in order to develop a trustful physician–patient relationship. This often requires a great deal of finesse.

Algorithms have been developed to assist with diagnosis (45,46). These cookbook approaches to spinal pain are particularly useful in establishing a diagnosis of a nonmechanical etiology (e.g., tumor or infection) or in identifying surgical emergencies (e.g., cauda equina syndrome) but unfortunately fall short in evaluating disorders of the three-joint complex. Labels of sprain and strain, especially after 4 to 6 weeks, provide little insight into the pathophysiology of the spinal motion segment.

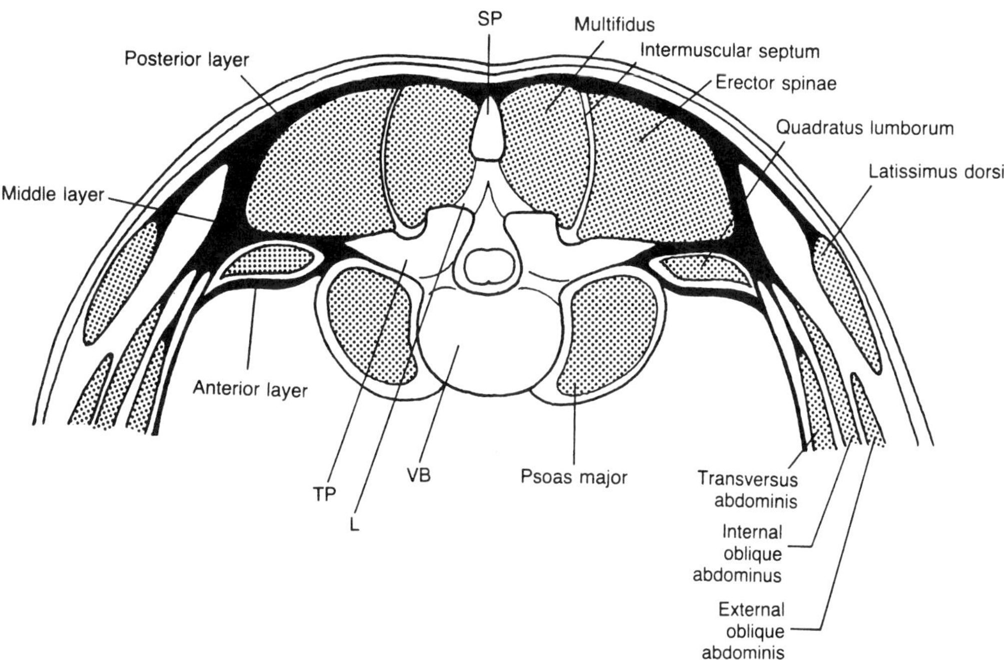

FIG. 57-2. Transverse section of the lumbar spine showing the layers of the thoracolumbar fascia (posterior, middle, and anterior) and the muscles attached to it and contained within it. *SP*, spinous process; *TP*, transverse process; *VB*, vertebral body; *L*, lamina. (Reprinted with permission from Porterfield JA, DeRosa C. *Mechanical low back pain. Perspectives in functional anatomy.* Philadelphia: WB Saunders, 1991; 56.)

There are many arbitrary ways of categorizing disorders of the spine (e.g., biomechanical and biochemical, surgical and nonsurgical, acquired and congenital), and clearly ruling out serious medical problems is of paramount importance. Whether an absolute diagnosis for mechanical spinal pain is required is debatable and may not even be obtainable despite the expertise of the medical provider. Nevertheless, functional categorization of the patient's symptoms and signs should be valuable for the initiation of reasonable treatment (see section on How to Rehabilitate). For example, if upon examination acute pain (spine or extremity) is consistently reproduced with a specific direction of motion, it is not necessary to document the responsible anatomic pathology or segmental dysfunctions in order to prescribe an initial range of motion program (e.g., flexion versus extension). Furthermore, this functional categorization allows a reference point by which to assess outcome, especially if no formal diagnostic tests (e.g., imaging studies) are eventually obtained. Because outcome studies are difficult to develop if no definitive diagnosis is sought or objectively determinable, this functional classification at least provides a frame of reference in which to monitor recovery.

An adequate assessment of spinal pain in general requires an intrinsic knowledge of functional anatomy and biomechanics, the degenerative cascade (see below); biochemistry; integration and proper interpretation of imaging and electrophysiologic studies (see Chapter 15); and a healthy index of suspicion for both missed diagnoses and the signs and symptoms of disability and nonorganicity. Early psychologic evaluations in patients with overwhelming subjective symptoms and minimal objective signs may yield insight into psychosocial barriers to recovery. Functional assessment of vocational and avocational activities completes the comprehensive evaluation. Preprepared spinal questionnaires regarding impairment of functional activities of daily living (e.g., sitting, standing, and walking tolerance; impact on social and sexual activities), and carefully worded questions and diagrams referring to nonorganicity can be extremely helpful in revealing characteristics of pain syndrome.

The functional diagnostic classification system of Kirkaldy-Willis (47) is intuitively sound and clinically correlatable. Separating the three-joint complex into its component parts, namely, discogenic and posterior joints, allows appreciation of different clinical presentations in the various phases of degeneration (Fig. 57-3) (i.e., dysfunction, instability, stabilization) and also allows an understanding of the interaction of the individual components leading to the various types of spinal stenosis. It should be noted that the initial presentation of symptoms can occur anywhere along this continuum, implying that sub–pain threshold degenerative changes occur throughout life. Also, degenerative changes in one motion segment may predispose to a similar process in adjacent segments. Different phases of the degenerative cascade can be found in different motion segments of the spine in one individual, so that dysfunctional or hypomobile segments might occur adjacent to a hypermobile segment.

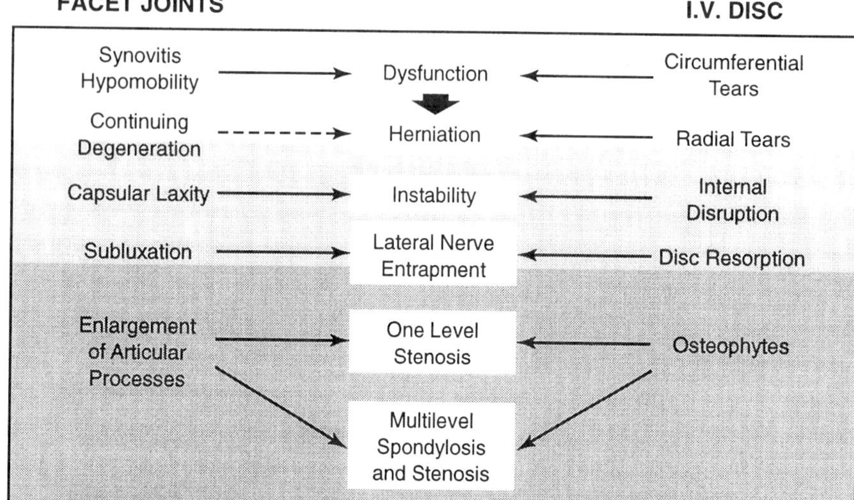

FIG. 57-3. Degenerative cascade. Interaction of facet joint and disc changes. Changes in facet joints appear on the left and changes in the disc on the right. Lesions that occur as a result of interaction of these changes are seen in the center. (Reprinted with permission from Kirkaldy-Willis WH, Burton CV. *Managing low back pain,* 3rd ed. New York: Churchill-Livingstone, 1992; 63.)

Lastly, the aging process does not always correlate with the clinical phase of degeneration.

The following discussion of the degenerative cascade was originally described for the lumbar spine motion segments. A similar schema has not been derived for the cervical spine. Some of these principles can be extrapolated to the cervical spine motion segments, but intrinsic variations in the anatomy of these two regions and the differences in physical demands placed on the cervical spine and upper quadrants does not allow direct application of these clinical correlates. Whereas the lumbar spine provides load-bearing support, the cervical spine is a more mobile structure and thus more sensitive to postural changes. Understanding the characteristics of typical postural dysfunction allows the development of proper rehabilitation program and will be discussed after a review of the lumbar degenerative cascade.

The Lumbar Spine Degenerative Cascade

Phase I of the degenerative cascade is segmental dysfunction, a state of abnormally reduced movement of the motion segment. The initial clinical presentation in this phase usually reflects joint dysfunction as opposed to disc herniation. Zygapophyseal joint dysfunction can include reactive synovitis and articular cartilage degeneration, resulting in joint pain, inflammation, and hypomobility. Abnormally sustained muscle contraction, especially of the short segmental extensors and rotators, can contribute to limited joint motion. The clinical presentation may be one of the often stated sprain–strain syndrome. Acute low back pain may be worse with static standing, walking, extension, or extension combined with rotation and somewhat relieved with flexion, although these findings are not pathognomonic, especially in the presence of chronic pain (see section on Biochemistry of Pain Generation and Perception). However, even flexion may irritate a restricted joint capsule or inflexible musculotendinous unit in spasm. Local tenderness and muscle spasm, limited range of motion, and normal neurologic examination are usual findings. Typically, posterior element dysfunction results in either nonradiating low back pain or referred pain to the buttock or proximal thigh. Mooney and Robertson suggested that "facet syndrome" can be associated with sclerotomal pain referral patterns in the distal lower extremity (48). Critical review of their study, however, showed that volumes of injected material (including contrast dye, hypertonic saline, and anesthetic) were a minimum of 3 ml and as much as 8 ml. A subsequent volume-controlled study of facet injection (49) found that the facet joint capsule can accommodate only up to 2 ml; therefore, Mooney and Robertson's results may have represented extravasation of potentially irritating substances into the epidural space or around nerve roots, or both. Pain radiating below the knee is negatively correlated with facet syndrome (50). Other syndromes have been postulated to describe the referred pain patterns that are nonradicular. For example, lumbar dorsal ramus syndrome is mediated solely through the primary posterior rami, which have been previously shown to innervate the z joint, posterior neural arch, and some musculoligamentous structures in the dorsal aspect of the three-joint complex (51). Referred pain patterns in this phase of segmental dysfunction also reflect the coexistence of mechanical dysfunction of the disc, joint, and nerve, as well as biochemical alterations. Residual low back pain after successful discectomy may reflect previously unrecognized posterior element pain and dysfunction.

Disc degeneration, including annular fiber tears, occurs in this first phase. Joint dysfunction may not allow adequate load bearing, thus transferring increased stress across the intervertebral disc. Radial tears are more likely to result in disc protrusion or herniation in the latter stages of dysfunction, but circumferential tears also may be painful due to the innervation of the outer annulus (see section on Biochemistry of Pain Generation and Perception). Classical discogenic radiculopathy can occur acutely, however, especially with a sudden, dynamic overload. Interestingly, lumbar disc herniation, previously considered to be a disease of adults, has been demonstrated in adolescents (52–55). Clearly disc degeneration and disc herniation occur in very young people and can be initiated without painful episodes.

The typical presentation of discogenic low back pain is pain exacerbated by flexion activities, activities that increase shear stress across the annulus (e.g., twisting), and activities that cause a Valsalva-type maneuver (e.g., coughing, sneezing). The disc protrusion or herniation usually occurs in a posterolateral direction, where the annular fibers are not well protected by the posterior longitudinal ligament and where shear forces are greatest with forward and lateral bending. This clinical picture is not always present, however, and experience has shown that atypical discogenic pain can be seen especially in young athletic individuals and people with central disc protrusions or herniations. The low back pain associated with disc protrusions or central herniations may be intense, possibly because of the large number of free nerve endings in the posterior longitudinal ligament. The ratio of back to lower extremity pain varies, but with an extruded or free fragment resulting in radiculopathy, low back pain may be minimal or absent. Occasionally, both low back and lower extremity pain can diminish in the presence of a disc extrusion when weakness is the predominant clinical feature.

Certain clinical examination findings may assist with prognosticating successful nonsurgical outcome with lumbar disc herniation. These include lower extremity pain (56), straight leg raise (i.e., Lasegue's sign) (57), and crossed straight leg raise (58). The process of centralizing pain from the lower extremity to the low back follows the extension principles of McKenzie (59). Schnebel and colleagues have demonstrated in vitro that compressive forces on the L5 nerve root due to an L4–L5 disc herniation increase with flexion of the L4–L5 motion segment and are compounded by increasing tension in the nerve root (60). Extension decreases the compressive force. Persistent peripheralization of pain despite properly performed McKenzie exercises has been discussed as a poor prognostic indicator, suggesting the need for surgical intervention (56). A positive crossed straight leg raise (i.e., pain in the symptomatic leg worsened by raising the contralateral lower extremity) suggests an extruded or sequestered disc fragment, which also may require surgical excision (57,58). A positive straight leg raise implies impairment of nerve root extensibility most commonly due to tethering over a herniated disc. The fifth lumbar and sacral nerve roots are maximally tightened between 30° and 70°, although in the presence of an extruded fragment, positive dural tension can be demonstrated at less than 30° (61). Variability between examiners may limit the usefulness of the straight leg raise sign, and a positive finding does not necessarily indicate the size or location of the herniation. A small herniation that tethers the nerve in the lateral recess can be extremely symptomatic and yield a positive test at early degrees of motion. Passive raising of the lower limb beyond 70° stretches muscles, ligaments, and joints but does not add to nerve tension. An important exception, however, is in certain athletes (e.g., gymnasts, dancers) in whom there exists an extreme of flexibility, a positive straight leg raise may not be obtained until well over 70°. A reverse straight leg raise, which is performed in a prone position, is necessary to document tension in the upper lumbar nerve roots (L2–L4) secondary to less common upper lumbar disc herniations. Straight leg raise testing may be positive or negative in the presence of lumbar disc herniation at the L4–L5 or L5–S1 levels, including far lateral disc herniations.

The far lateral disc herniation implies nerve root impingement at the foraminal exit zone or extraforaminal nerve root impingement. The radiculopathy therefore involves the root from the level above (i.e., a far lateral disc herniation at L4–L5 affects the L4 nerve root). Our experience and that of others (62,63) suggests that far lateral disc herniations occur in the older patient in whom disc herniations are relatively uncommon. This may reflect degenerative changes and calcification of the posterior disc margins. Clinically, far lateral herniations do not usually result in low back pain, but rather lower extremity pain, sensory disturbance, and weakness in an L3, L4, or L5 distribution. Radiculopathy of the S1 nerve root cannot occur from a far lateral disc herniation unless an S1–S2 disc is congenitally present. Symptoms are frequently worse with standing or walking and occasionally better with sitting. Straight leg raise or reverse straight leg raise testing is typically negative or minimally positive despite severe symptoms. This problem may actually fit in phase III because this lesion acts as much like stenosis as it does like discogenic pain.

Phase II refers to a condition of excessive segmental motion and, occasionally, frank segmental instability. This is a phase that is clinically more difficult to conceptualize. Because the border between phases I and II is somewhat arbitrary, a patient who has never had discogenic low back pain and has never been symptomatic may enter phase II. Abnormalities of the z joints include capsular laxity and joint hypermobility. Such movement may not be detectable by standard lateral flexion and extension x-rays because no translation may occur, but the instantaneous center of rotation may move abnormally (64) (Fig. 57-4). This relates to our clinical impression that the quality of motion is more representative of pathology than is the quantity. Gross range of motion evaluates soft-tissue extensibility and monitors the effects of treatment but does not provide information about segmental motion that could be obtained by a skilled manual examination. Observing dysrhythmia, a catching sensation or painful arc with recovery phase from forward bending, can be indicative of hypermobility. Tenderness, spasm, or both elicited by applying a torsional stress across a specific segment (i.e., lateral springing on the spinous process) is also a sign of a hypermobile segment. On the other hand, instability may be present without symptoms. Flexion and extension x-rays may be abnormal in asymptomatic people (65). This finding also implies that a combination of

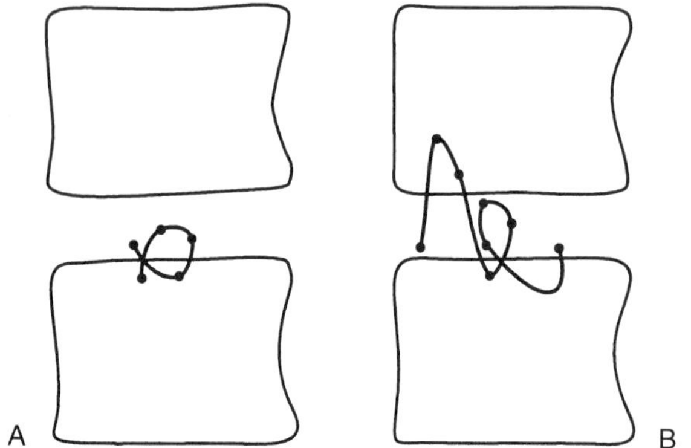

FIG. 57-4. A: The centrodes of normal cadaveric intervertebral joints are short and tightly clustered. **B:** Degenerative specimens exhibit longer, displaced, and seemingly erratic centrodes. (Reprinted with permission from Bogduk N, Twomey LT. *Clinical anatomy of the lumbar spine,* 2nd ed. Melbourne: Churchill-Livingstone, 1991; 81.)

disc and joint abnormalities, with an inflammatory trigger, is necessary for symptom production in this instability phase.

Disc-related abnormalities in phase II include internal disc disruption and narrowing of the intervertebral space. Internal disc disruption evolves as the process of degeneration progresses. Multiple annular tears allow random distribution of nuclear material throughout the disc, and an internally disrupted disc may be a pain generator. The pain may be from hyperexcitable annular nociceptive fibers or biochemical factors. In this phase, the disc is less tolerant of torsional stress. Typically, torsional and compressive loads occur simultaneously and the compressive force stabilizes the three-joint complex by loading the annular fibers (66). As the annular fibers become less competent, torsional load results in a greater degree of motion and potentially greater symptoms. The reduction in disc space height promotes z-joint laxity and narrows the intervertebral foramen and the lateral recess. Radiculopathy can occur secondary to direct impingement on the lumbar or sacral nerve roots from a herniated disc, dynamic lateral entrapment due to narrowing of the lateral recess, and radiculitis due to biochemical factors associated with an internally disrupted disc.

This less stable spinal segment allows excessive mechanical stimulation of the dorsal root ganglion and initiation of a degradative enzymatic cascade resulting in the production of inflammagens and other chemical mediators of pain (see section on Biochemistry of Pain Generation and Perception) (Fig. 57-5). Dynamic lateral entrapment occurs as the lax z-joint capsule allows to-and-fro migration of the superior facet (i.e., superior process of the inferior vertebra) in the sagittal plane with axial rotation, or flexion and extension of the motion segment. In the absence of back pain, hip (i.e., buttock, trochanteric area, or both), thigh, or leg pain may be precipitated through a number of dynamic clinical tests that cause forward displacement of the superior articular facet toward the vertebral body, thus narrowing the lateral recess. Dynamic lateral entrapment also can occur after discectomy and chemonucleolysis, usually within the first 2 years, before fixed bony or degenerative changes ensue.

In phase III, the process of segmental stabilization occurs over time. The z joints become fibrosed, enlarged, and arthrosed. The intervertebral disc becomes increasingly degenerated and desiccated, allowing approximation of the vertebral end-plates and osteophyte formation. This combination of anterior and posterior changes can manifest in ankylosis of the motion segment, although lesser degrees of spondylosis are common. Limited range of motion and

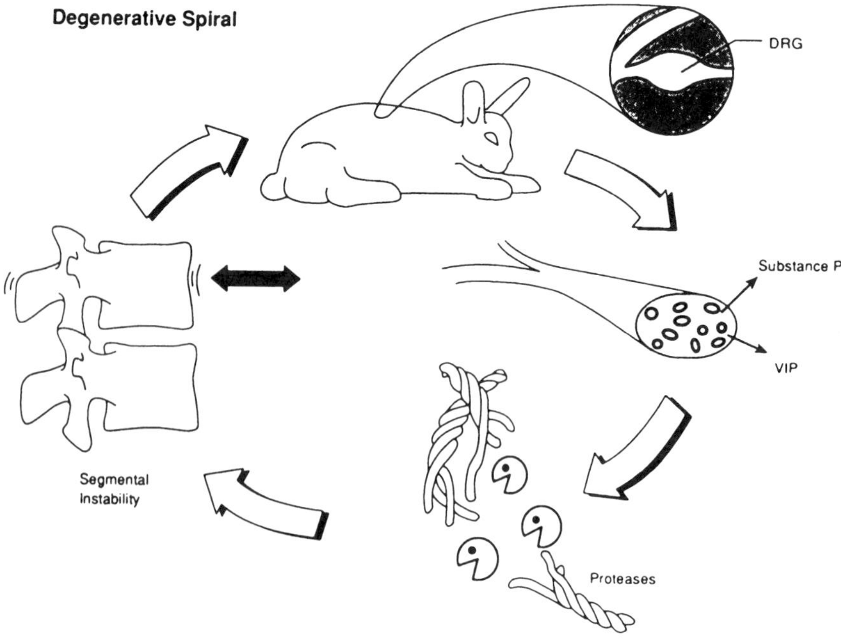

FIG. 57-5. Degenerative spiral. The functional spinal unit may undergo degeneration as a result of the interaction of mechanical and chemical stimuli seen in an injured or environmentally stimulated functional spinal unit. (Reprinted with permission from Weinstein JN. Recent advances in the neurophysiology of pain. *Phys Med Rehabil State Art Rev* 1990; 4:215.)

stiffness may become the predominant features, not unlike those observed in the dysfunctional stage. Low back pain may no longer be prominent, although severe degenerative changes may not permit this process of autofusion and, therefore, continuation of symptoms can occur. Symptomatic degenerative z joints usually cause low-grade, aching low back pain, which is sometimes bilateral and multilevel.

Spinal nerve root entrapment is relatively common in this phase because of fixed lateral stenosis, central stenosis, and degenerative spondylolisthesis. Fixed lateral stenosis can occur because medial z-joint osteophytes narrow the lateral recess or because forward subluxation of the superior facet persists. Degenerative spondylolisthesis occurs because erosion of the superior articular facet allows forward displacement of the upper vertebral body on the lower body, trapping the nerve root that exits one level below between the inferior facet and the back of the vertebral body (67). Such slips are usually isolated to one segment, typically L4–L5, impinging on the L5 nerve root. Symptomatic central stenosis of bony etiology is more controversial. A congenitally small spinal canal with acquired degeneration may become symptomatic with bilateral and multilevel radiculopathy. Analysis of the anatomic organization of the cauda equina may explain the clinical presentation of a skipped level (68) (i.e., S1 radiculopathy with central stenosis at L4–L5). This is consistent with the concept that central stenosis is due to medial hypertrophy of the inferior facet (67). Central and lateral stenosis can coexist at the same or different levels.

Neurogenic claudication or pseudoclaudication is the typical presentation of lumbar radiculopathy in this phase (69,70). Dermatomal symptoms of paresthesias and dysesthesias and myotomal distribution of muscle cramping and weakness consistently occur with erect postures or exercise. Typically, symptoms resolve with flexion maneuvers such as bending forward or sitting. The mechanism may be venous engorgement of the cauda equina. Differentiation from true vascular claudication is possible by exercising the lower extremities while the spine is in a flexed posture. Unlike radiculopathy associated with disc herniation, straight leg raising is usually unremarkable and may be a clinical sign to differentiate spinal stenosis from the more unusual disc herniation in this phase. The prevalence of disc herniations diminishes in people over 55 years of age (71), and these are typically far lateral herniations reflecting biochemical alterations of the disc, reduction in elasticity, and degenerative bony constraints.

Cervical Postural Dysfunction: The Forward Head Postural Attitude

One of the most common dysfunctional postures is depicted by the forward head position on the trunk, which is defined by certain segmental motion and myofascial abnormalities. It is noteworthy that most postural changes occur over time, thus allowing tissue accommodation without symptom manifestation. However, after any traumatic event (e.g. whiplash), this equilibrium is breached and a variety of symptoms may be generated.

The following is a description of the specific anatomic abnormalities that are identified with the forward head postural attitude: hyperextension of the upper cervical segments (C0–C1 and C1–C2), resulting in hypomobility; hyperflexion of the lower cervical and upper thoracic segments, resulting in hypomobility; slackening of the nuchal ligament which allows excessive shear through the mid-cervical spine, promoting hypermobility; a decrease in the size of the intervertebral foramen, potentially leading to radicular symptoms and/or signs; an increase in the weight-bearing load of the z joints, resulting in synovitis and ultimately degenerative arthropathy; excessive protraction of the scapulae, contributing to the increased thoracic kyphosis and impaired scapular stabilization; and myofascial flexibility and strength imbalances (Table 57-3). The first rib becomes elevated and fixed as the scalenes shorten and contract. This combined with pectoralis minor contraction may cause irritation of the brachial plexus (often the lower trunk) and thus contributes to the often observed upper extremity pain pattern described as thoracic outlet syndrome. It is quite uncommon to observe frank vascular or neurogenic compromise; thus, the connotation ''nonspecific thoracic outlet syndrome'' may be a more appropriate label for this symptom pattern. As the head is positioned more anteriorly, the distance from the C5–C6 segment to the center of gravity increases, with concomitant increases in the contractile demand on the posterior cervical musculature by as much as 200%, which in turn abnormally loads both the disc and the posterior elements.

Biochemistry of Pain Generation and Perception

Numerous biochemical substances have been identified as mediators of pain and inflammation, which can directly stimulate tissue nociceptors, sensitize peripheral nociceptors to other chemicals, lower the response threshold to mechanical stimuli, generate ectopic neuronal discharges, and sensitize the central nervous system via the dorsal horn of the spinal cord at the level of the substantia gelatinosa (72).

TABLE 57-3. *Forward head postural dysfunction: muscular imbalances*

Shortened (and weakened)	Lengthened (and weakened)
Neck	Neck
Capital extensors	Capital flexors
Sternocleidomastoid	Cervical extensors
Anterior and middle scalenes	Shoulder girdle
Shoulder girdle	Middle and lower trapezius
Upper trapezius	Rhomboids
Levator scapula	Latissumus dorsi
Pectoralis minor	Thoracic extensors
Subscapularis	
Serratus anterior	
Anterior deltoid	

These substances include inflammogens (immunologic and nonimmunologically induced) and neurogenic mediators. The former group includes the cytokines, nitric oxide, bradykinin, serotonin, histamine, and phospholipase A2; the latter group is composed primarily of the neuropeptides, including substance P, vasoactive intestinal peptide (VIP), calcitonin-generated peptide (CGRP), and somatostatin (73). The neuropeptides are produced primarily within the dorsal root ganglion (the cell bodies of primary afferent neurons), are released in response to noxious stimuli, act as neuromodulators at the level of the dorsal horn and activate inflammatory cells (e.g., stimulate release of histamine and leukotrienes from mast cells), and sensitize peripheral nociceptors. Vibratory frequencies typical of motorized, industrial machinery promote synthesis and release of substance P from the dorsal root ganglion (74,75). Substance P release is also enhanced by mechanical compression of the dorsal root ganglion via either bony stenosis or disc herniation (76).

It is the sensory innervation of a spinal structure that allows it to be a potential pain generator, and the advent of immunohistochemical staining techniques has greatly enhanced the understanding of the sensory innervation of the spine. Various elements of the three-joint complex have been demonstrated to be innervated, including the intervertebral disc, z joint, ligamentous structures, myofascial structures, and neurovascular structures. Details of the innervation of the disc and joints will follow (Fig. 57-6).

Lumbar z joints receive nerve supply from up to three different segmental levels via the medial branches of the dorsal primary rami (77–79). In an animal model, the lumbar z joints have been shown to contain both high-threshold mechanosensitive afferents serving primarily as nociceptors and low-threshold afferent fibers that modulate proprioceptive feedback (80). The joint capsule is richly innervated as well as in border regions within the ligamentum flavum, muscle, and tendon (81). Substance P receptors have been demonstrated within the capsule, subchondral bone, and erosion channels of degenerative cartilage of lumbar z joints (82,83). As previously discussed, Mooney and Robertson's report of facet syndrome generating lower extremity pain may be questioned due to excessive volume of injectate; theoretically, however, another potential explanation would be central sensitization over polysegmental pathways after prolonged substance P nociceptor excitability. In a double block paradigm, performing intra-articular z-joint injection or medial branch block technique, using differing duration local anesthetics, Schwarzer et al. determined that the prevalence of z joint–mediated pain was 15% and that no consistent clinical features, including lumbar extension and rotation, predicted a positive response (84). This lack of clinically reliable signs was also demonstrated by Revel et al. (85).

It is now well accepted that the outer annulus of the intervertebral disc is innervated, whereas the remainder of the annulus and the nucleus pulposus are not (86–88). Neuropeptide receptors also have been found in the outer annulus (89,90). The posterior aspect of the disc and posterior longitudinal ligament are supplied by the sinuvertebral nerve, formed by a branch of the ventral rami, which is somatic, and by a branch of the gray ramus communicans, which is

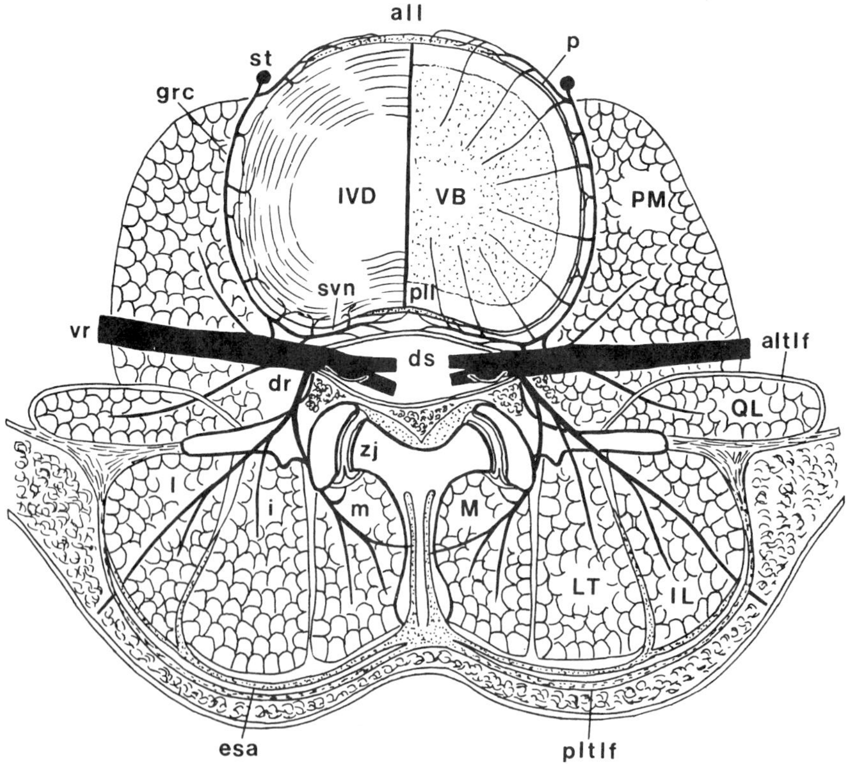

FIG. 57-6. Innervation of the lumbar spine. A cross-sectional view incorporating the level of the vertebral body *(VB)* and its periosteum *(p)* on the right and the intervertebral disc *(IVD)* on the left. *PM*, psoas major; *QL*, quadratus lumborum; *IL*, iliocostalis lumborum; *LT*, longissimus thoracis; *M*, multifidus; *altlf*, anterior layer of thoracolumbar fascia; *pltlf*, posterior layer of thoracolumbar fascia; *esa*, erector spinae aponeurosis; *ds*, dural sac; *zj*, zygapophysial joint; *pll*, posterior longitudinal ligament; *all*, anterior longitudinal ligament; *vr*, ventral ramus; *dr*, dorsal ramus; *m*, medial branch; *i*, intermediate branch; *l*, lateral branch; *svn*, sinuvertebral nerve; *grc*, gray ramus communicans; *st*, sympathertic trunk. (Reprinted with permission from Bogduk N, Twomey LT. *Clinical anatomy of the lumbar spine,* 2nd ed. Melbourne: Churchill-Livingstone, 1991; 119.)

autonomic. The sinuvertebral nerve transmits nociceptive, proprioceptive, vasomotor, and vasosensory modalities (78). The role of the sympathetic mediation of lumbar discogenic pain is unclear but the evidence is provocative: sympathetic afferents can transmit pain (91); low back pain has been eliminated by lumbar sympathetic blockade (92); low back pain often has a vague, visceral quality to it similar to other autonomically mediated pains; injection of local anesthetic around the L2 spinal nerve provided significant pain relief in patients with a diagnosis of discogenic pain (93); and stimulation of any of the lower lumbar intervertebral discs has led to plasma extravasation in the L2 dermatome, which is an autonomic reflex (94).

The anterior and lateral portions of the annulus fibrosis, including the anterior longitudinal ligament, receive innervation from the gray ramus communicans and ventral rami. The erector spinae and multifidi muscles receive innervation from lateral, intermediate, and medial branches of the dorsal primary rami.

The Role of Inflammation in Radicular Pain

Clinical observations support the postulate that mechanical compression is not always the sole cause of radicular pain. This includes the demonstration that radicular symptoms and signs can develop without significant nerve root compression (95,96) and conversely, radicular findings may not occur or even resolve despite the persistence of focal compressive disc lesions (20,21,97,98). Compression of normal spinal nerve results in neurologic symptoms such as paresthesias and motor loss (99), but pain is absent unless an inflammatory response also occurs (100). Furthermore, in patients with lumbar disc herniation, a beneficial response to epidural corticosteroid can occur without significant changes in pathoanatomy.

Inflammatory responses can be immunologically (i.e., T-cell and B-cell) or nonimmunologically mediated. In the 1960s, reports of antigenicity of nucleus pulposus in animal models was described (101,102). Marshall and colleagues postulated that chemical radiculitis might explain nerve root–mediated pain independent of the mechanical effects of edema and demyelination (103). Other more recent studies also have demonstrated an immunologic basis for the inflammatory reaction due to nucleus pulposus material, including the identification of immunoglobulins and cytokines (104–111).

Saal has reviewed inflammation as it relates to lumbar pain (112). Alterations in the enzymatic homeostasis within a lumbar disc (113), possibly related to a lowering of the pH after injury (114,115), may represent altered chondrocyte expression within the nucleus. Chondrocytes are capable of producing phospholipase A2, an enzyme that liberates arachidonic acid from cell membranes leading to the production of prostaglandins and leukotrienes (116). High titers of PLA2 have been identified in surgical herniated disc specimens (112,117). PLA2 may enter the epidural space via annular tears and may act directly on neural membranes, increasing the production of prostaglandins, leukotrienes, and neuropeptides (118–121). As shown by Weinstein, neuropeptides may act in a "degenerative spiral" (Fig. 57-5), promoting breakdown of the three-joint complex and facilitating the aforementioned enzymatic deregulation of collagenases and proteases (122). Breakdown of the outer annular fibers in turn allows PLA2 to leak into the epidural space. Weakening of the motion segment increases its susceptibility to vibrational and physical overload, resulting in further stimulation of the dorsal root ganglion and release of these neurogenic mediators of pain, intertwining the neurogenic and nonneurogenic mediators of spinal pain (Fig. 57-7).

Chronic Pain

Recognition of the spinal pain patient who is at risk for delayed recovery may allow interventional measures for prevention of long-term disability. Chronic pain syndrome is not a pathologic diagnosis but rather a diagnosis of impaired function. Nociception may begin with a specific tissue injury, but observable pain behaviors exceed the apparent physical impairment. Physical problems may contribute only 40% to the disability state (18) because psychological distress and social interactions reinforce illness behavior. Depression and somatic preoccupation are typical features. The combination of these can yield a firmly disabled state, often preventing usual activities (Fig. 57-8).

One of the best measures of future behavior is review of the history. A history of protracted spinal pain and disability, lack of response to treatment, escalating symptoms without progression of objective signs, and use of emotional words to describe symptoms is suspicious for the development of pain syndrome.

Chronic pain behavior has common physical examination findings of nonorganic signs suggesting symptom magnification and psychological distress, possibly an expression of suffering (123,124). These Waddell signs include superficial or nonanatomic distribution of tenderness, nonanatomic motor or sensory impairment, excessive verbalization of pain or gesturing (e.g., facial grimacing, tremors), production of pain complaints by tests that only simulate a specific movement (e.g., low back pain with axial loading on the crown of the head), and inconsistent reports of pain when the same movement is performed in different positions (e.g., straight leg raise in a seated versus supine position). Care must be taken not to overinterpret these signs, especially the latter, because pelvic tilt can alter testing responses. Objective clinical signs also may be present (e.g., impaired segmental motion, dural tension signs, even frank neurologic deficits) but do not exclude the possibility of coexistent chronic pain syndrome.

The pain psychologist, who usually has a Ph.D. and subspecialty training, is a crucial component of the diagnostic process. Before the psychological referral, the physician can glean valuable information from pain drawings (125,126),

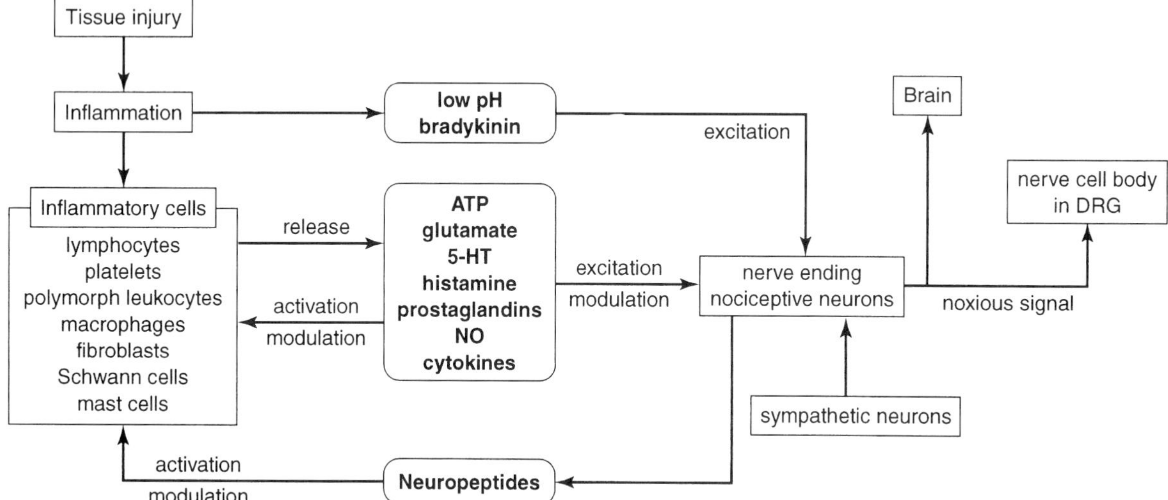

FIG. 57-7. Schematic diagram of the interaction between peripheral tissue injury and the central neurogenic components. This scheme demonstrates how neurogenic mediators can affect nonneurogenic (chemical) mediators through the stimulation of inflammatory cells. *ATP*, adenosine triphosphate; *5-HT*, 5-hydroxytryptamine; *NO*, nitric oxide; *DRG*, dorsal root ganglion. (Reprinted with permission from Kawakami M, Weinstein JN. Associated neurogenic and nonneurogenic pain mediators that probably are activated and responsible for nociceptive input. In: Weinstein JN, Gordon SL, eds. *Low back pain: a scientific and clinical overview.* Rosemont, IL: American Academy of Orthopedic Surgeons, 1996; 270.)

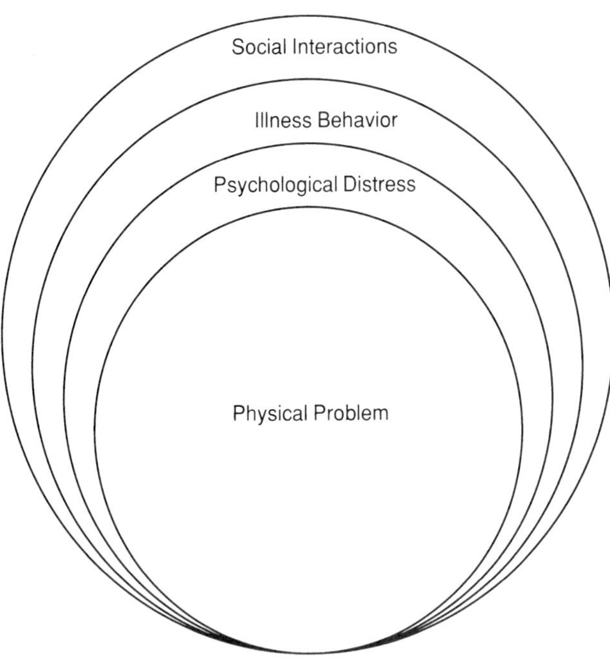

FIG. 57-8. The concept of illness: a visual representation based on the analysis of disability in chronic low back pain. (Reprinted with permission from Waddell G, Main CJ, Morris EW, et al. Chronic low back pain, psychological distress, and illness behavior. *Spine* 1984; 9:212.)

the visual analog pain scale, and disability indices such as the Vanderbilt Pain Management Inventory, Roland-Morris Functional Disability Scale, and Oswestry Disability Scales (127,128). Pain drawings including entire body markings, nonanatomic drawings, extracorporeal pain markings, and additional writing may indicate somatic preoccupation, depression, or hysterical features.

The referral to the pain psychologist should be approached in a nonthreatening manner, with the patient assured that his or her pain complaints are not disbelieved. Discussing the psychology of recovery often assists with referral acceptance. Any situation in which progress has been minimal, delayed, or regressive without an obvious cause should indicate referral to the pain psychologist.

Using available research and incorporating our own experience, we have summarized a number of variables that have predictive value for delayed recovery (Table 57-4) (127,129–134). Recognizing these factors, especially in the early stages of an injury, can thus help direct treatment to prevent disability. Interestingly, the occupational factors may play a larger role than psychosocial or medical issues. Occupational risk factors include both employee and employer variables. Job satisfaction can be inversely related to time loss, injury risk, and risk for delayed recovery. Employers' unwillingness or inability to provide transitional work is detrimental to the recovery process. A real or perceived mismatch between the physical demands of a particular job and the worker's physical capacities also delays recovery. Lastly, time off work has a negative correlation with return to work rates.

TABLE 57-4. *High risk factors for delayed recovery*

Occupational
Time off work
Job dissatisfaction
Patient's perception of heavy work
Job availability, including light or modified
Psychosocial
Poor English proficiency
Spouse disabled
Anger at system; excessive fault finding
Litigation or compensation
Physician's conviction of extreme high-risk status
Medical
History of previous injury
History of substance abuse

Selective Spinal Injections

Selective spinal injections, including epidural (e.g. caudal, translaminar, and transforaminal [nerve block]), zygapophyseal, and sacroiliac joint, provide both diagnostic and potentially therapeutic value. Theoretically, placement of local anesthetic and corticosteroid proximate to a suspected site of pathology and pain, maximizes diagnostic and therapeutic responses, respectively. Reduction in pain concordant with the pharmacokinetics of the specific anesthetic used, as opposed to solely pain provocation, indicates a particular anatomic site as a clinically relevant pain generator. The corticosteroid benefit is probably due to inhibition of inflammatory mediators rather than immunosuppresant action (135).

The literature is replete with noncontrolled reports of the benefits of epidural corticosteroid injections, but very few controlled, randomized studies have been undertaken. The well-designed studies that are available do show a significantly positive pain-reducing benefit. A detailed discussion and review of these studies are available (136–138). Furthermore, a meta-analysis of the efficacy of epidural steroid injection in the treatment of low back syndromes concluded that a small but statistically significant benefit exists (139). The results suggest that 14% of individuals who would not have otherwise improved would do so with an epidural steroid injection. No controlled studies regarding cervical epidural corticosteroid injections have been reported. The lack of prospective, randomized studies in the literature regarding epidural steroid injections in general may reflect ethical challenges; physicians and patients alike are unwilling to be randomized to the presumed "nontreatment" group when severe radicular pain is the primary, presenting symptom (140).

Clinically, epidural corticosteroid injections have potential benefit in the following syndromes: axial pain due to a focal disc herniation or annular tear; radiculopathy due to compressive lesion such as a herniated nucleus pulposus or spinal stenosis; and radiculitis due to noncompressive, inflammatory reactions. Selective injection should always be combined with a comprehensive rehabilitation prescription for maximal therapeutic gain. Injections are often performed to progress a rehabilitation program that has plateaued due to persistent pain.

The goal of diagnostic selective blocks is to differentiate the qualitative and quantitative contribution of posterior element, discogenic, or radicular pain. The concurrent use of local anesthetic may provide diagnostic value in the setting of multisegmental disease, as demonstrated by imaging studies or electrophysiologic testing, in situations with no objectively identified anatomic abnormalities and with suspected chemically mediated symptoms, or in postoperative cases where anatomic boundaries are disrupted and imaging studies are more difficult to interpret. Of paramount importance in determining a specific pain generator is precise needle localization. The technical difficulty in performing such procedures blindly demands the use of fluoroscopy and nonionic contrast agents (141–153). Ideally, an epidurogram (which should be confirmed with lateral imaging with cervical and lumbar translaminar procedures) or an epiradiculogram or neurogram (with transforaminal procedures) should be demonstrated. Epidural injections are frequently performed without radiographic guidance, but incorrect needle placement can occur up to 25% of the time, including subcutaneous, intraligamentous, intravenous, and intrathecal locations.

Lumbar epidural steroid injections can be performed in patients without previous imaging studies as long as the history and examination does not suggest a malignant, infectious, or nonspinal source of low back or lower extremity pain. Usually in patients over 50 years of age, an imaging study is required. Because L5 or S1 radiculitis/radiculopathy are most common, clinical symptoms and signs suggesting radicular involvement rostral to the L4–L5 segment should also lead to an imaging study before injection not only to yield a specific diagnosis, but to identify the presence of an adequate epidural space for injection. For the same technical reason, the performance of a cervical epidural steroid injection does require prior imaging to avoid the albeit remote possibility of spinal cord injection. Without advanced imaging, the caudal approach is the least risky and would access most pathology at the L4–L5 and L5–S1 levels. Before additional injections, lack of improvement after a single injection performed without previous imaging should lead to appropriate testing.

The injection should be directed as close to the presumed site of pathology as possible. Central or posterolateral disc herniations in the lumbar spine and central disc herniations or uncovertebral arthropathy in the cervical spine can be managed with a translaminar epidural injection at or adjacent to that segmental level, directed ipsilaterally. A caudal lumbar approach via the sacral hiatus can typically treat pathology at L4–L5 or L5–S1. Persistent radiculopathy after a technically proficient translaminar injection, especially in the presence of foraminal stenosis or lateral disc herniation, warrants a transforaminal injection at the level of pathology before abandoning injection therapy.

Detailed and explicit informed consent is required, which may be best managed with a standard form that the patient must read and sign. Risks of the procedure should be discussed in understandable terms, including but not limited to the more common side effects such as vasovagal reaction, nausea, flushing, insomnia, low-grade fever, nonpositional headache, transient increase in spinal and/or extremity pain, and the more uncommon risks such as intrathecal injection (154), spinal headache, allergic reaction, infection (155), elevated blood sugar (more common in diabetics), Cushing's syndrome (156), and neurologic compromise (including the potential for spinal nerve and spinal cord injury). Premedication should be considered in a patient with a history of prior vasovagal reaction or extreme anxiety. Oral anxiolytics (e.g., lorazepam or diazepam) may be used if planned ahead. Intravenous agents such as midazolam (Versed, Roche Laboratories, Nutley, NJ) and atropine along with intravenous hydration may be used, especially with cervical procedures. With adequate explanation and preparation, most patients are able to tolerate the procedure with little or no sedation. Because careful attention to any modification in symptoms post injection is important, any sedation used should be short acting. Cardiovascular monitoring and intravenous access are typically reserved for those patients receiving intravenous sedation.

The controversy regarding the existence of ''lumbar facet syndrome'' has already been discussed, and the principles and technical aspects of zygapophyseal joint injection have been thoroughly reviewed elsewhere (157). Only two controlled studies of lumbar z-joint intra-articular corticosteroid are present in the literature (158,159), both of which have methodologic flaws that have been clearly described by Dreyfuss et al. (153). Based on their comprehensive review of the literature, these authors concluded that the primary role of z-joint injections (intra-articular or medial branch block) is diagnostic, as described by Schwarzer (84) and the therapeutic benefit of z-joint injection remains controversial.

There are no controlled diagnostic or therapeutic studies in the literature regarding cervical z-joint injections. However, several factors would tend to support the existence of cervical z-joint syndrome, including documented sclerotomal pain referral patterns after single-level z-joint injection (160); reduction in pain after anesthetic blockade of a z joint suspected as a pain generator (161,162); cadaver studies in postwhiplash injury demonstrating intra-articular joint derangement (4); and the intrinsically greater segmental mobility of the cervical spine as opposed to the lumbar spine. Clinical experience of the authors suggests that the potential therapeutic benefit of z-joint corticosteroid injection is greater in the cervical than the lumbar spine. The positive response rate is increased if an abnormal level is documented by advanced imaging such as single-photon emission computed tomography (SPECT) bone scan and computed tomography (CT). Furthermore, a positive response to intra-articular anesthetic administration or medial branch block in the cervical spine may be a better prognostic sign regarding outcome from surgical fusion than described for the lumbar spine (163).

The type, amount, and concentration of the anesthetic agent should allow for partial anesthesia but should not result in a significant motor or sympathetic block. With epidural injection, this can be accomplished with volumes of 8 to 10 ml of 0.5% lidocaine administered via the sacral hiatus, or 3 to 4 ml via a translaminar approach. A longer-acting anesthetic such as bupivacaine 0.50 to 0.75% (0.5 to 1.0 ml) is used for transforaminal procedures. Comparison of pain levels pre- and postinjection by verbal report or visual analog scale is critical in gauging the response to the anesthetic. Provocative maneuvers such as evaluating spinal range of motion, straight leg raise, and ambulatory capabilities pre- and postinjection assist in determining the contribution of that particular structure as a pain generator. Persistent crossed straight leg raise immediately after a technically well-performed epidural steroid injection is a poor prognostic sign.

Usually the corticosteroid is administered simultaneously with the anesthetic agent to avoid the need for a repeat injection after the initial procedure. The proposed action of corticosteroids are several, including inhibition of prostaglandin synthesis by stabilizing membranes and blocking PLA2 action; impairment of cell-mediated, immunologic responses; inhibition of neuropeptide synthesis or action; and possibly exerting an anestheticlike action blocking c-fiber conduction (164). The duration of response varies from weeks to months, with permanent cures rarely occurring. Up to four epidural injections may be administered in a given year, usually administered in a 2- to 3-month period, depending on the degree of improvement after each injection. Lack of response to any injection demands a re-evaluation of the clinical diagnosis.

Diagnostic Imaging Techniques

A thorough review of the imaging techniques of spinal pain syndromes is beyond the scope of this chapter and can be found elsewhere (165). No single imaging study can effectively evaluate all components of the spinal motion segment; therefore, a knowledge of the relative specificity and sensitivity of the various available techniques is essential. As previously discussed, anatomic imaging abnormalities have been identified in asymptomatic people. Ultimately, the results of the studies must be interpreted in the context of clinical relevance. In general, magnetic resonance imaging (MRI) is ideal for soft-tissue pathology, which in the spine mainly refers to the intervertebral disc and neurologic contents of the spinal canal. Computed tomography (CT) and nuclear bone scanning are best suited for evaluating bony pathology, including the anterior and posterior elements. The following is a brief review of the best test of choice for four specific clinical entities: fracture, arthropathy, disc herniation, and stenosis.

Although the mechanism of fracture has not been discussed in this chapter, acute dynamic overload or chronic repetitive exertion can result in fracture of the vertebral body or posterior elements. Plain radiographs are always indicated if fracture is suspected. With lumbar compression fracture, special attention is required to rule out a burst fracture (a potentially unstable condition), necessitating in most cases either CT or MRI (the latter because compression of the spinal canal components can be easily demonstrated). If a posterior element fracture, either in the cervical or lumbar spine is suspected (e.g., spinous process, z joint, pars interarticularis), plain radiographs, followed by SPECT bone scan imaging (166) and limited CT, are indicated. Bone scanning is performed if the x-rays do not allow adequate localization of a specific level because this will not only confirm a serious bony injury, but will negate the need for screening CT imaging of multiple segmental levels. SPECT scanning provides twice the sensitivity of planar scanning and has become the standard for bone scan imaging of the spinal axis. This is particularly true when evaluating a young athlete for the possibility of spondylolysis (pars interarticularis fracture). The SPECT scan also can assist in determining if an obvious pars defect on plain radiograph is a potential source of symptoms. A normal SPECT scan essentially rules out an acute fracture. The evaluation of joint arthropathy (e.g., z joint, uncovertebral joint) follows a similar pathway.

The test of choice for evaluating a disc herniation is an MRI. The advantages over a noncontrast CT are listed as follows:

- No ionizing radiation
- Ability to assess the internal architecture and hydration of the disc
- Ability to evaluate for high-intensity zones in the posterior annulus fibrosis, which are indicative of annular tears (167,168)
- Ability to better define where the posterior disc margin ends and the thecal sac begins
- Ability to assess the spinal cord

Contrast-enhanced CT (i.e., a myelogram with CT) also clearly differentiates disc material from nerve tissue but cannot address these other issues. However, this test is equally as effective as MRI in evaluating spinal stenosis.

Possibly a more important question to ask is whether any imaging study is necessary in the acute clinical setting of discogenic/radicular syndromes. There certainly is no absolute answer to this question, but advanced imaging is probably not critical if certain conditions exist:

- The patient is a young, healthy adult.
- The onset/mechanism of injury is consistent with a disc injury.
- The clinical symptoms and/or signs indicate that only one segmental level is involved.
- The neurologic examination is stable (even in the presence of mild neurologic deficits).
- The pain is not incapacitating.

However, lack of improvement with appropriate treatment warrants further investigation. Clearly, every clinical situation is unique and early imaging should be the rule whenever there is any doubt.

Discography will be presented only to indicate that it is a controversial test, relying in large part on subjective reporting of concordant (familiar) pain provocation upon instillation of a contrast agent within the nucleus pulposus. Postdiscogram CT enhances the anatomic assessment of the intactness of the nucleus pulposus and annulus fibrosis. Although discography may be performed for purely diagnostic purposes (i.e., to determine whether a degenerative disc is painful), the test is almost always performed to address the potential benefit of a surgical fusion, therein lying the controversy (169). A recent report by Schellhas et al. demonstrated that with discography in the cervical spine, concordant pain provocation frequently occurred in normal-appearing discs on MRI, not the presumed degenerative discs; thus, in these cases discography was used to dissuade a fusion because too many levels would have to have been included in the surgical construct (170).

HOW TO REHABILITATE

The growth of managed care with the associated demand for outcome data has led some to critically review the available literature for proof of the purported benefits of various rehabilitation interventions (39). Prospective, randomized, single-intervention studies have traditionally been considered the ideal method to assess efficacy. However, although these studies may provide the most objective research design, the defined methodologies often have limited clinical applicability. In clinical practice, therapeutic intervention is usually multimodal and is likely to remain so. The premise that statistical analysis is superior, rather than complementary, to other forms of medical knowledge has been challenged (171). Furthermore, recent criticism of the methodologic quality of published randomized clinical trials on the treatment efficacy of low back pain (172) speaks against the narrow-visioned adherence to the use of only these studies in the development of reasonable parameters for the management of spinal disorders. Finally, the absence of proof should not indicate the proof of absence.

The rehabilitation principles and methods discussed below have been derived through a synthesis of the available literature; integration of functional anatomy and newer biochemical concepts; extensive clinical experience; and the primary physiatric postulate of functional progression. These principles can be applied to all spinal disorders in the acute, subacute, and chronic stages, as well as in both nonoperative and postsurgical patients. As discussed previously, disc herniations, including large extruded fragments, have been demonstrated to resolve without surgery, and resolution of signs and symptoms can occur even if disc material remains in the spinal canal. Invariably, changes in soft-tissue and articular mobility and loss of strength and overall fitness occur in cases of disc herniation and with other spinal problems.

Much of the literature regarding objective assessment of spinal strength and flexibility deficits regards the lumbar spine. Intuitively, however, similar changes must occur in the cervical spine as well. In the cervical and upper thoracic spine, postural dysfunction plays a key role in the onset and perpetuation of pain states. The forward head postural attitude (as discussed above) lends itself to a clearer understanding of the rehabilitation principles in the upper spinal region.

In both operative and nonoperative patients, absence of symptoms does not imply normal function. Correction of soft-tissue inflexibility and re-establishment of proper spinal segmental motion are necessary. Assessment and treatment of the entire kinetic chain is required. Normal trunk and lower extremity strength, endurance, and power should be combined with education and training for posture, body mechanics, and proprioception to allow successful and sustained return to activity (173).

In this section, the following topics will be addressed: goals of the acute and subacute phases of spinal rehabilitation; a review of the role of manual therapy for the treatment of spinal pain based on theoretical constructs, the literature, and clinical experience; the role of rest and exercise for the treatment and prevention of spinal injuries; discussion of specific exercise programs, including flexion, extension, and stabilization techniques; and, finally, a brief review of alternative movement therapies. The use of selective spinal injections, particularly epidural steroid and z-joint injections in the management (and diagnosis) of spinal disorders.

Goals of Spinal Rehabilitation

The acute phase goals of a spinal rehabilitation program are listed as follows:

1. Education and protection of the injured tissue
2. Control of pain and reduction of inflammation
3. Early mobilization and physiologic loading of joint and soft-tissue structures
4. Implementation of therapeutic exercise

The subacute phase goals of a spinal rehabilitation program are listed as follows:

1. Full pain-free range of motion of the injured and adjacent segments, as well as other spinal, hip/shoulder girdle, and lower/upper extremity structures that influence the spine (i.e., the entire kinetic chain)
2. Optimal strength, endurance, and coordination of the neuromuscular system affecting the spine
3. Return to normal activity
4. Prevention of further injury and recurrences

The Role of Manual Therapy: Mobilization and Manipulation

Regaining soft-tissue flexibility and segmental motion can be accomplished through a variety of manual therapy techniques, including myofascial release (174), joint mobilization or manipulation (175,176), muscle energy techniques (174), and stretching.

The myofascial system is a functional joint that must be addressed because of its ability to restrict motion and generate pain when in a dysfunctional state. The functions of the fascia are to separate and support muscles allowing for independent function while joining them into a functional unit, to absorb shock, to transmit mechanical force, and to exchange metabolites from fibrous elements to the circulatory and lymphatic systems. Immobility can result in dysfunction of the fascial system. This can result from an injury with associated pain, swelling, and adhesions; from treatment such as postoperative immobilization; and from avoidance behaviors and altered posture or body mechanics.

The fascia is connective tissue consisting of layers of collagen and elastin in a water-based ground substance matrix. The fascial sheaths are continuous and interwoven, enveloping all structures from the dermis to the periosteum. The superficial elements are thinner and more delicate, allowing freedom of movement of the skin, whereas the deeper layers are thicker and stronger, designed for structure and support. With immobility, the fascia desiccates, loses elasticity, and fails to maintain critical fiber distance. The layers of fascia are then glued together by cross-linking fibers and impede movement. Decreased mobility in the myofascial system can lead to decreased spinal segmental mobility and extremity flexibility. Myofascial releasing techniques are designed to apply pressure and shearing forces to the layers of fascia, loosening and separating them. Restoration of fluidity, nutrition, elasticity, and freedom of movement results.

Assessing spinal segmental motion and restoring motion to restricted or hypomobile segments again demands precisely applied manual techniques (175–177). Hypomobility can result from impairment of soft-tissue supporting structures (e.g., muscle hypertonus, fascial restriction) or from the intrinsic components of the three-joint complex (e.g., disc degeneration, z-joint dysfunction). The latter includes internal joint derangement, capsular fibrosis, and periarticular scarring. Adjacent hypomobile segments can cause increased stress on injured segments, and injured segments may cause hypermobilities at adjacent noninjured joints. As noted before, hypermobility is frequently associated with symptom production.

Standard grades of mobilization can be used for pain control or to generate motion (Fig. 57-9). Grades I and II, often referred to as oscillations, are low-velocity forces applied repetitively within resistance-free range of motion of a joint, most commonly used for pain control. Grades III and IV are stronger forces that move the joint into its restricted range and are useful for producing motion. In contrast, grade V mobilizations, often referred to as a manipulation, involves a small-amplitude, high-velocity thrust at or just beyond the normal physiologic range of the joint without exceeding its anatomic integrity. The crack or pop that frequently accompanies a manipulation is due to liberation of gas from the

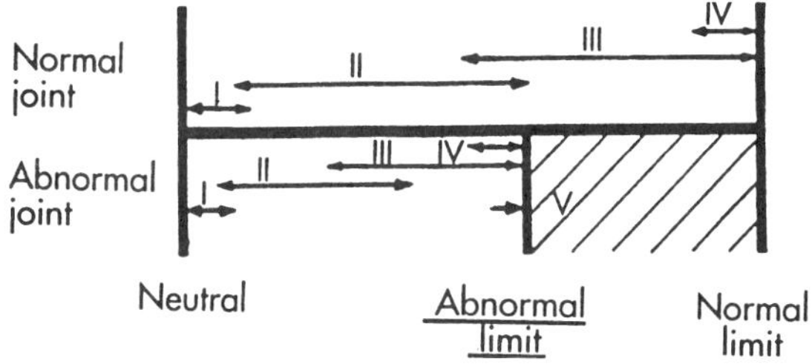

FIG. 57-9. Grades of mobilization for normal and abnormal joints. Movements of abnormal joints are usually, but not invariably, limited, and because the available excursion of movement is reduced, the grades of treatment are proportionately reduced. (Reprinted with permission from Grieve GP. *Mobilization of the spine,* 3rd ed. New York: Churchill-Livingstone, 1979.)

synovial fluid as a sudden negative pressure is generated with distraction of the joint.

The key to mobilization is to direct energy at a specific level only. Mobilization and manipulation in a healthy motion segment do not affect vertebral joint alignment *per se* as much as the smoothness and glide of joint motion (178). Gross rotatory manipulations that may affect multiple levels regardless of joint hypermobilities are not indicated. Mobilization techniques do not provide long-term relief to painful segments due primarily to discogenic abnormalities and do not reduce disc herniations. However, temporary pain relief may occur from mechanoreceptor stimulation, stretch of adhesions, or restoration of shortened muscle length. Muscle energy techniques can be used with mobilization to improve segmental mobility (174). These techniques use the patient's own isometric muscle contraction to relax hypertonic muscles by resetting the gamma gain in the muscle spindles. The isometric contraction also can be used to mobilize a joint and may be less painful than passive mobilizations.

Several comprehensive reviews of the randomized, prospective studies on this subject can be found in the literature (179–182). Generally, it appears that manual therapy, particularly manipulation, is beneficial in selective patient populations. Shekelle has suggested that those patients who are most likely to benefit from spinal manipulation presented with acute low back pain of less than three weeks' duration, with either minor or absent lower extremity neurologic signs and no evidence for dural tension signs (179). This is similar to the patient profile developed by DiFablo identified through 14 studies that met the criteria for a meta-analysis (180). These findings are in agreement with Agency for Health Care Policy and Research practice guidelines that state that acute low back pain without radiculopathy is the condition most likely to respond to manipulation.

Koes et al. published a prospective, randomized, placebo-controlled clinical trial that compared the efficacy of manual therapy to other treatments (including physiotherapy, defined as massage, exercise, and modalities; medication and education by the primary care provider; and sham treatment–inactive diathermy) (183). Symptoms were present for at least 6 weeks, and patients with suspected disc herniations were excluded. At 3 weeks' follow-up, the physiotherapy and manipulation group showed a significant decrease in the severity of complaints, but the authors attributed this improvement to nonspecific effects. In a recent, extensive review of spinal manipulation, Koes et al. identified that the efficacy of spinal manipulation for patients with acute or chronic low back pain has not been clearly demonstrated with sound randomized clinical trials, although the best methodologic studies appeared to conclude that small subgroups of back pain patients—mostly acute low back pain of 2 to 4 weeks' duration—may benefit from manipulation (182).

Rest and Exercise

Rest

Prolonged immobility results in a wide range of deleterious effects (184), including reduction in aerobic capacity; loss of muscle strength; impaired muscle and connective tissue flexibility; promotion of bone demineralization; increased segmental stiffness; impaired disc nutrition; and promotion of the illness role. Immobility has been clearly shown to result in strength deficits: 1% to 3%/day and 10% to 15%/week after complete bed rest (185); up to 70% loss in sagittal plane trunk strength 6 months after the onset of lumbosacral pain (186); and 30% loss of trunk strength for multiple parameters 1 year status post–lumbar diskectomy (187).

In the not too distant past, medical hospitalizations for bed rest after the acute onset of low back pain was the normaly prescribed course. Prolonged bed rest as a treatment option for this group is essentially obsolete due to the prospective, randomized study of Deyo et al. (188). Comparing 2 days with 7 days of bed rest, the study concluded that at 3 weeks and 3 months follow-up, the 2-day group missed significantly fewer days of work. The authors themselves indicated that there was an inability to conduct a truly randomized study in that 74% of the 7-day group did not adhere to the prescribed duration of bedrest. Compliance was also difficult to assess in the randomized, prospective study by Gilbert et al., in which it was shown that the bed rest group took 42% longer to achieve a normal level of activity as compared with those patients undertaking exercise or education but no rest (189). Other prospective randomized studies also have demonstrated no benefit of bed rest as compared with other forms of treatment during the acute phase of rehabilitation (190,191).

There are significant methodologic flaws with the bed rest studies, including noncompliance and lack of diagnoses (no physical examination or imaging data presented). Nevertheless, the available literature suggests that limiting bed rest to a short time period is not detrimental to most patients, even those with some radicular symptoms. There is no controlled data as to the efficacy of bed rest in patients with documented disc herniation with or without radiculopathy.

Exercise

Exercise has become a standard for the management of spinal pain. However, various parameters can be used to define the term "exercise," including strength (maximal force produced from a single effort), endurance (capacity to sustain submaximal work), aerobic fitness (as measured by VO_2 max), flexibility, and coordination training. Furthermore, exercise can be passive or active and supervised or unsupervised. It is illogical to assume that one exercise regimen will be effective in all patients with spinal pain. Furthermore, nonspecific exercise for a nonspecific diagnosis is destined to be unsuccessful. The following section highlights some of the strengths and deficits of the literature regarding exercise for the treatment and prevention of low back pain, after which some practical exercise programs are discussed.

Several prospective studies assess the role of aerobic fitness for the prevention of low back pain (192–196). The most commonly quoted study applauding aerobic fitness is that of Cady et al., which was a prospective, observational design. In this initial study (195), a fitness profile of firefighters was used that included cardiovascular fitness, as well as strength and flexibility. The firefighters with the highest fitness scores experienced the least number of back injuries at work. However, these were also the youngest workers, and the individual effect of cardiovascular fitness alone could not be determined. In a subsequent study by Cady et al. (196), assessment of individual fitness variables within a group of firefighters of similar age indicated that those firefighters with the lowest cardiovascular fitness as measured by a physical work capacity test, incurred a higher proportion of cost. Only work-related lumbar injury was reported, not complaints of low back pain.

Aerobic training may help to decrease acute pain by elevating endorphin levels and mechanoreceptor stimulation, provide biomechanical stress to promote tissue healing, and increase endurance and coordination of the neuromuscular system. However, there is no conclusive evidence in the literature that aerobic exercise prevents the development of or hastens recovery from an episode of acute low back pain. At best, aerobic fitness may be mildly protective against low back injury and low back pain. Low back pain may lead to reduced activity and concomitant reduction in aerobic fitness, which may be a more significant problem in chronic or recurrent situations. The loss of aerobic conditioning may have adverse consequences in terms of cardiovascular risk factors and decreased work capacity. This may be a basis to recommend aerobic exercise as a component of a spine rehabilitation program.

The goal of exercise for the treatment of acute back pain is pain control, not strength gains because acutely this does not physiologically occur. Several randomized, prospective studies have failed to demonstrate a benefit for exercise over placebo treatment in acute low back pain (189,190,197–201). However, methodologic flaws, including lack of physical examination and imaging data and institution of a standard exercise program (emphasizing either flexion or extension postures), irrespective of the clinical features, leave these conclusions suspect.

As stated earlier in this chapter, an absolute diagnosis is not necessary to initiate an exercise program that is based on dynamic assessment of the patient. One of the consistent failures of the above studies is randomization of patients to an exercise group without assessment of which direction of motion either increased or reduced pain. When direction of motion is selected based on symptoms, more positive results can be demonstrated from an exercise intervention (202,203). Initial exercises, movement into flexion or extension, depend on which activity centralizes low back pain (i.e., less radicular pain) or does not exacerbate low back pain.

Usually extension exercises are begun with prone lying with support under the stomach to maintain a neutral position. These are progressed as tolerated to prone lying unsupported, support under the chest, prone on elbows, and press-ups (59,203–205). Lateral trunk shifts must be corrected before initiating extension exercises. Patients can be instructed in self-correction techniques. Theoretically, extension exercises may be effective in reducing pain by decreasing tension in the posterior annular fibers, increasing mechanoreceptor input activating the gate mechanism (206), decreasing tension on the nerve root (60), changing intradiscal pressure (207), and allowing anterior migration of the nucleus pulposus (204). Repeated extension posturing in standing, for use after sitting or forward bending activities, should be taught. Contraindications to extension exercises include segmental hypermobility or instability, large or uncontained herniation, bilateral sensory or motor signs, significant increase in low back pain unless associated with concomitant reduction in radicular pain, and increase in radicular sensory disturbance. If hypermobility exists at a segment adjacent to a disc herniation, manual blocking of extension at that level can be applied by the therapist, and patients can be taught to generally reduce motion at the lower lumbar segments. Care must be taken to prevent secondary hypermobility at the thoracolumbar segment, however, which also can occur if extension exercises are emphasized in a patient with lumbar segmental hypomobility.

The classic Williams flexion exercises (208) are theoretically effective by decreasing z-joint compressive forces, stretching hip flexors and lumbar extensors, strengthening abdominal and gluteal muscles decreasing the compressive load to the posterior disc, and opening the intervertebral foramen. This explains its long history of use in acute disc presentations. Flexion exercises may be better tolerated in central disc herniations, but acute dural tension is likely to be aggravated by flexion.

Pelvic tilts should be performed in multiple positions, including bent knees, straight legs, and standing. Posterior pelvic tilt unloads the z joint and aids in pelvic awareness. Single knee-to-chest maneuvers help stretch the contralateral hip flexors and ipsilateral extensors, and double knee-to-chest positions promote stretching of the lumbar and hip extensors. Partial sit-ups strengthen the abdominal muscles. Contraindications to flexion exercises include segmental hypermobility or instability, increase in low back pain, and peripheralization of pain into the lower extremity.

Once the acute pain subsides, the focus of the rehabilitation program is to improve function. Strengthening exercises have long been considered an integral part of this process. There is some prospective data that support the position that improved trunk strength and/or endurance is protective from developing low back pain or injury, but the literature is certainly not conclusive regarding this subject (209–215). Exercises to improve the function of the spinal muscles are generally known as spinal stabilization (216–218).

Stability of the lumbar spine is provided by bony architecture, disc mechanics, ligamentous support, and muscular strength, endurance, and coordination. Optimal muscle strength can protect the spinal motion segment from chronic repetitive shear stress or acute dynamic overload. The concept of spine stabilization implies a muscle fusion. The various abdominal, pelvic, and trunk muscles that attach to the TLF flex, extend, and rotate the spine, thus acting as an abdominal corset (Fig. 57-2). Increased intra-abdominal pressure does not appear to be the mechanism of stabilizing the disc and joint because the force needed would compress the aorta and possibly cause a flexion moment of the lumbar spine. Rather, reduction of shear forces across the three-joint complex is accomplished by abdominal cocontraction and tension generation in the TLF and midline ligaments. The muscular stabilizers of the lumbar spine are identified in Table 57-2.

There has been controversy regarding the role of the smaller intersegmental muscles in stabilizing the lumbar spine (219,220). The multifidi span only two to four segments and lie very close to the midline and center of rotation of the motion segment. This implies poor mechanical advantage as a prime mover; indeed, these muscles are not efficient prime movers. The force vectors of the multifidi indicate that they can generate posterior rotation in a sagittal plane. Because contraction of the abdominal oblique muscles results in combined motion into flexion and rotation, the multifidi are recruited to cocontract with the internal oblique, counterbalancing the forward shear force, stabilizing the segment, and allowing pure axial rotation. Thus, the multifidi are effective as stabilizers, can balance shear forces, and seemingly produce rotation, although not as primary rotators. The multifidi also secondarily maintain the lumbar lordosis by the nature of the force vector posterior to the vertebral bodies. The multisegmental muscles of the spine have been shown to be more efficient prime movers, with the greatest efficiency occurring with those muscles originating from the pelvis, spanning the most segments, and located most laterally from the midline (219).

The stabilization sequence includes strengthening of the segmental muscles, neutral spine stabilization, and finally strengthening of the prime movers. The intersegmental muscles act as tonic or postural stabilizers of the spine, tending to fatigue first and atrophy first after spinal injury. Therefore, initial stabilization exercises are directed toward these muscles, which can control individual segmental mobility. These are typically manually resisted exercises of the trunk limited to short arcs performed in rotation, flexion, extension, and side-bending. The next phase of stability training involves direct and indirect strengthening of muscle groups through a variety of exercises performed in a neutral spine posture. Neutral spine is defined as the midpoint of available range between anterior and posterior pelvic tilt, not the absence of lordosis (Fig. 57-10). Neutral positioning has the following advantages:

- It is a loose-packed position that decreases tension on ligaments and joints
- It allows more balanced segmental force distribution between the disc and z joints
- It is close to the center of reaction, allowing movement into flexion or extension quickly
- It provides the greatest functional stability with axial loading
- It is usually the position of greatest comfort

Training begins with exercises designed to help locate the neutral spine in a variety of body positions—such as prone lying, standing, sitting, and jumping—which increases awareness of lumbar and pelvic motion. This is followed by exercises of the extremities while maintaining neutral spine and later with addition of resistance to the extremities, either manually or with weights. These exercises are performed slowly, with the emphasis on precise pelvic control. This

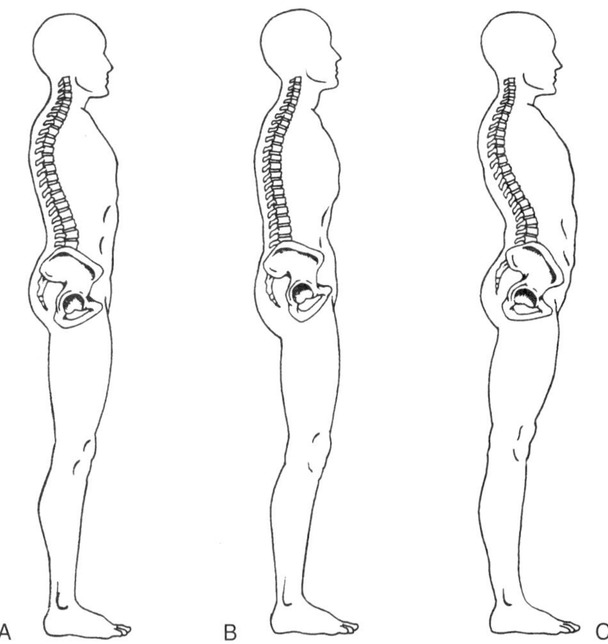

FIG. 57-10. Neutral spine posture. **A:** Neutral pelvis–pelvic bracing. **B:** Excessive posterior pelvic tilt–hypolordosis. **C:** Excessive anterior tilt–hyperlordosis. (Reprinted with permission from Herring SA, Weinstein SM. Assessment and management of athletic low back injury. In: Nicholas JA, Hershman EB, eds. *The lower extremity and spine in sports medicine.* Vol. 2. 2nd ed. St. Louis: CV Mosby, 1995; 1190.)

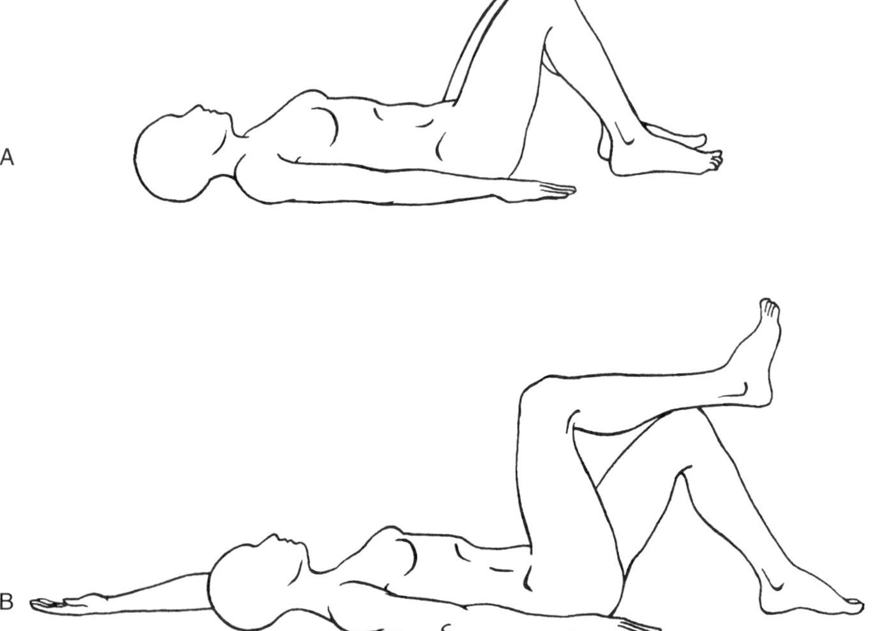

FIG. 57-11. Stabilization exercises. **A:** Supine pelvic bracing. **B:** Supine pelvic bracing with alternating arm and leg raises (dead bug). (Reprinted with permission from Herring SA, Weinstein SM. Assessment and management of athletic low back injury. In: Nicholas JA, Hershman EB, eds. *The lower extremity and spine in sports medicine.* Vol. 2. 2nd ed. St. Louis: CV Mosby, 1995; 1190.)

will facilitate neuromuscular coordination and enhance endurance and strength gains. These neutral spine-stabilizing exercises also emphasize the smaller postural stabilizers. Examples of these exercises include supine pelvic bracing (Fig. 57-11A); supine pelvic bracing with alternating arm and leg raises (''dead bug'') (Fig. 57-11B); bridging (progressing from the basic position) (Fig. 57-12) to balancing on a gymnastic ball with various lower extremity positions (Fig. 57-13) and resistance; and quadraped pelvic bracing with alternating arm and leg raises (Fig. 57-14) with and without resistance.

Ultimately, strengthening of prime movers, including abdominals, erector spinae, and latissimus dorsi, is required. The longer lever arms of these muscles provides for their efficiency and strength. Abdominal exercises have been historically emphasized as part of a low back exercise program, especially sit-ups. Sagittal plane sit-ups are used in the stabilization routine but are limited to partial curl-ups, lifting the head and upper body only. During this initial phase, the obliques and rectus abdominus are activated, whereas in the second half of a full sit-up, the iliacus and rectus femoris provide the main muscular force. Lower extremity strength is necessary because these muscles work in a coordinated manner with the trunk, especially during lifting, where the gluteal and hamstring muscles are the prime posterior rotators of the pelvis and trunk. Quadriceps strengthening is very important for support of body weight during squatting.

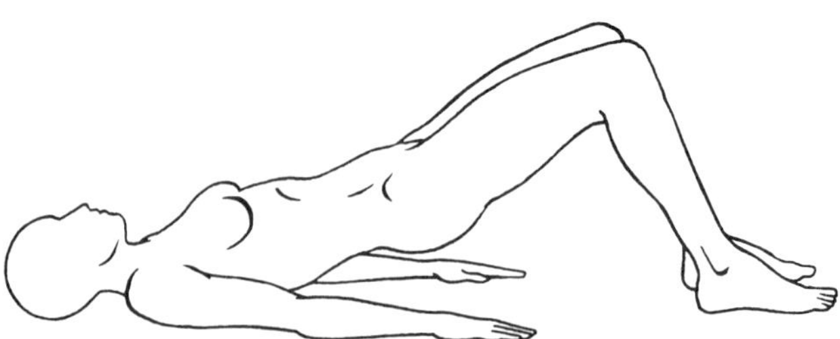

FIG. 57-12. Stabilization exercises. Basic position of bridging. (Reprinted with permission from Herring SA, Weinstein SM. Assessment and management of athletic low back injury. In: Nicholas JA, Hershman EB, eds. *The lower extremity and spine in sports medicine.* Vol. 2. 2nd ed. St. Louis: CV Mosby, 1995; 1191.)

Maximizing lower extremity muscular flexibility is also important for allowing normal lumbar motion. Because of their attachments to the pelvis, the hip flexors and extensors have a great influence on positioning of the lumbar spine. Adequate hip muscle flexibility allows for hip joint motion independent of lumbar segmental motion and is essential for the use of proper body mechanics and posture. Poor flexibility will cause excessive stress to be transmitted to the lumbar motion segments and sacroiliac joints. Two typical patterns of lower extremity inflexibility include hamstring, gluteus maximus, and gastrocnemius-soleus tightness, or hip flexor, tensor fascia lata, and quadriceps tightness. The later combination is most common in ballet dancers and runners. Tight hip flexors (i.e., iliopsoas) and quadriceps (i.e., rectus femoris) often cause extension and rotation hypermobilities in the lumbar spine. If the iliopsoas is contracted in a shortened position, the pelvis is maintained in excessive anterior tilt, placing the hip extensors (i.e., gluteus maximus and hamstrings) at a mechanical disadvantage. Therefore, early recruitment of lumbar extensor muscles (i.e., erector spinae) is necessary, resulting in excessive shear or torsion stress to the intervertebral disc. Self-stretching techniques should be

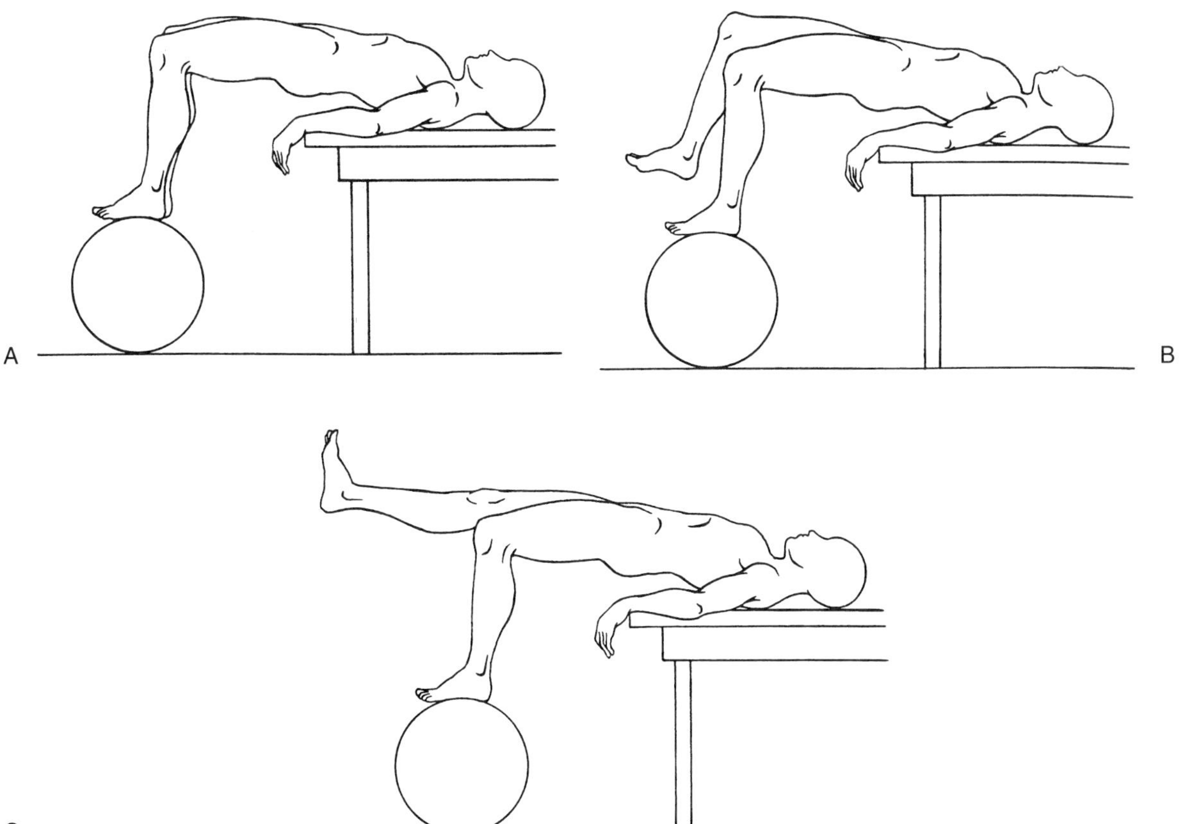

FIG. 57-13. Stabilization exercises. Gymnastic ball exercises. Degree of difficulty increases from A to C. (Reprinted with permission from Herring SA, Weinstein SM. Assessment and management of athletic low back injury. In: Nicholas JA, Hershman EB, eds. *The lower extremity and spine in sports medicine.* Vol. 2. 2nd ed. St. Louis: CV Mosby, 1995; 1192.)

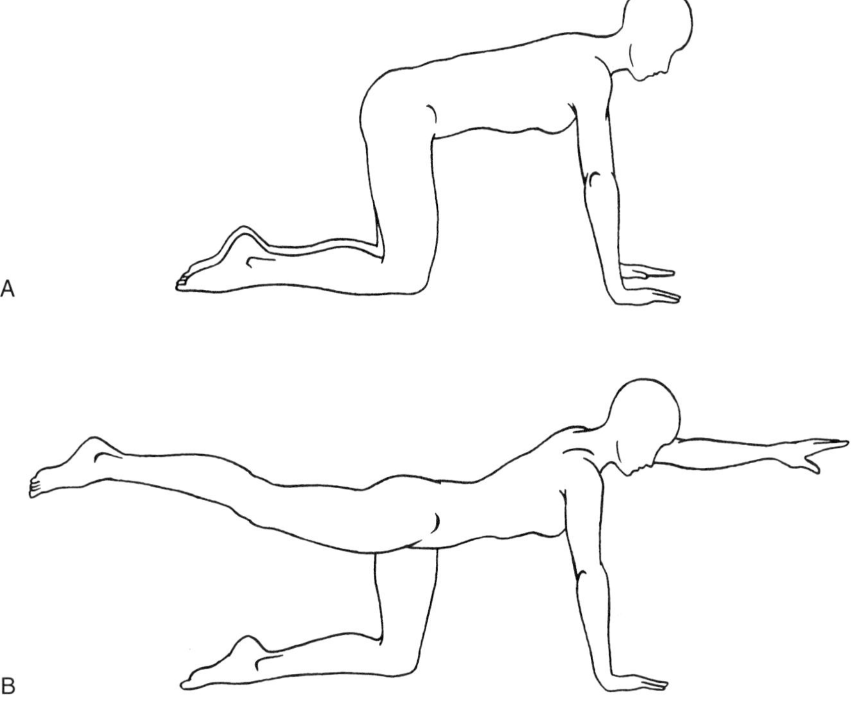

FIG. 57-14. Stabilization exercises. **A:** Quadruped position with pelvic bracing. **B:** Quadruped position with pelvic bracing and alternating arm and leg raises. (Reprinted with permission from Herring SA, Weinstein SM. Assessment and management of athletic low back injury. In: Nicholas JA, Hershman EB, eds. *The lower extremity and spine in sports medicine.* Vol. 2. 2nd ed. St. Louis: CV Mosby, 1995; 1191.)

taught as early as possible to allow active involvement in the rehabilitation program. It is essential to stretch with as neutral a pelvic position as possible because excessive anterior or posterior pelvic tilt will diminish the benefits of these flexibility exercises.

Because the trunk is the platform for the cervical spine and head, proper strength and stability of the lumbar spine is critical for obtaining and maintaining the position of optimal function of the cervical spine. Before postural strengthening exercises, the various segmental and myofascial abnormalities discussed earlier must be corrected as much as possible. Opening of the thoracic outlet through aggressive manual and active soft-tissue stretching exercises (emphasizing the anterior shoulder girdle and cervical spine), and mobilization of the stiff, hypomobile segments (avoiding the mid-cervical hypermobility) prepares the individual for a comprehensive cervicothoracic stabilization program.

The sequencing of strengthening begins with isometrics, initially with the head supported in a neutral position, varying positions relative to gravity and gradually progressing out of neutral positioning. This is followed by isotonic exercises, emphasizing concentric strengthening of the lengthened and weakened muscles (Table 57-3). Positions that may compromise the spinal nerves, such as extreme flexion or extension, are avoided, The exercise positions are varied from gravity eliminated to antigravity to place the maximal demands on these muscles. The scapular stabilizers and thoracic extensor muscles are emphasized, coupling cocontraction of these axial muscles with upper limb strengthening to simulate the physical demands of daily activities. Ultimately, complex, multiplane movements are incorporated to further prepare the injured individual for return to regular activities of daily living—at home, at work, and recreationally.

Adjunctive Therapies

Aquatic Rehabilitation

Properly designed aquatic programs can help rehabilitate patients with lumbar spine injuries (221). Aquatic stabilization techniques and swimming programs can be used with aggressive, comprehensive, land-based spine stabilization programs or as the only rehabilitative method. The success or failure of aquatic therapy is not determined by swimming skills alone, because swim stroke proficiency is not a model for successful treatment.

Aquatic spine programs offer advantages that are directly related to the intrinsic properties of water: buoyancy, resistance, viscosity, hydrostatic pressure, temperature, turbulence, and refraction. Graded elimination of gravitational forces through buoyancy allows training with controlled load through the lumbar spine. In essence, water increases the safety margin of postural dysfunction by decreasing the compressive and shear forces on the spine. The motion velocity can be controlled by water resistance, viscosity, buoyancy, and training devices. Buoyancy increases the range of training positions. Many believe that pain attenuation takes place in the water because of the "sensory overload" generated by hydrostatic pressure, temperature, and turbulence. The psychological outlook of athletes may be enhanced because rehabilitation occurs in their competitive environment.

Accurate diagnosis of a patient's spinal injuries and/or observation of his initial responses to land-based or aquatic stabilization programs helps determine further treatment. A transition from dry to wet exercise conditions is beneficial in that it eliminates dry-land risks; establishes a supportive training environment; provides a new therapeutic activity; decreases the risk of peripheral joint injury; and allows a return to prior activity. Moving from dry to wet environments also should be considered if a patient cannot tolerate axial or gravitational loads; increased support in the presence of a strength or proprioceptive deficit is required; or there is a risk of a compression fracture. Remaining in a water-supported environment is appropriate if a dry environment exacerbates symptoms or if the patient prefers water. Transition from a wet to a dry environment should occur if the exercise program is progressing in the water, but the patient must return to land to most efficiently achieve his or her functional goals. A detailed description of aquatic rehabilitation can be found in Chapter 35.

Somatic Physical Therapy Techniques

Alternative somatic physical therapy techniques are increasingly being integrated into traditional treatment programs (222). Somatic therapeutic treatment strategies can be integrated into an eclectic physical therapy approach to address disorders of the locomotor system, including those caused by spinal pain. The Alexander Technique, the Feldenkrais Method, Rolfing (structural integration), and Aston Patterning are types of alternative somatic physical therapy programs. These techniques emphasize the study of human movement and treatment through subjective experience.

Developed around the turn of the century by an Australian named F.M. Alexander, the Alexander Technique is a method of psychophysical education allowing for more graceful and fluid posture and movement. Although the emphasis of this technique is education rather than training, it often yields therapeutic benefit because improved posture and movement frequently help lumbar spine pain and dysfunction resolve. The essence of this technique is the difficult-to-define concept of "use." Use includes all aspects of human action. The technique teaches that movement must be preceded by conscious attention rather than unconscious action in response to a given stimulus. Verbal cues in conjunction with tactile feedback from the instructor provides kinesthetic awareness, helping patients achieve a sense of effortless poise and balance throughout their entire bodies.

The Feldenkrais Method was developed by an Israeli physicist, Moshe Feldenkrais. This method also helps patients improve their kinesthetic awareness to achieve better sensory-motor integration and learning. Two integrated formats are used: functional integration and awareness through movement. Functional Integration incorporates a one-on-one treatment format in which the practitioner's tactile input is used to facilitate a change in a patient's neuromuscular organization to produce efficient (non–energy-wasting) movement. The treatment approaches a dancelike style. Awareness through movement occurs in a group setting and incorporates repetitive, nonstrenuous active movements performed in a planned sequence. Verbal cues are provided to advance patients through a structured sequence of simple movements that are then integrated into complex movement patterns.

Rolfing, also known as structural integration, is another type of somatic therapy. It was developed by Ida Rolf, a biochemist and physiologist. This approach seeks to improve a patient's "vertical alignment" by deep manipulation of fascia, resulting in collagen realignment, restoration of soft-tissue mobility, and, theoretically, restoration of skeletal alignment and movement. Deep pressure is applied through the therapist's fingers, knuckles, or elbows to mechanically deform the connective tissue. Patients are told to move a specified area while the Rolfer maintains and directs pressure so that the patient's active movement synergistically complements the Rolfer's pressure. The applied forces are then functionally directed to optimally reorient and free the fascia in the desired direction. Symptomatic areas are not primarily addressed; rather, treatment focuses on the fascial tissues that support a given dysfunctional structure as well as all secondary sites of tissue dysfunction. Symptoms are decreased or eliminated as normal function is restored. Rolfing is not intended to treat acute lumbar spine pain. It is best reserved for chronic spine pain in which significant fascial restrictions are present.

Aston Patterning was developed by Judith Aston, an ergonomic product designer. Aston Patterning is considered unique among the somatic therapies because of its completeness. It is an integrated system of movement education, three-dimensional soft-tissue body work, environmental modification, and fitness training. It includes a comprehensive evaluation, manual therapy techniques, movement education, exercise programs, and a wide variety of fundamental concepts that allow it to have a large scope of application. The evaluation includes viewing the body structurally while at rest and then performing simple functional movements or a movement specific to Aston Patterning. Aston Patterning uses three different manual techniques—functional massage, myokinetics, and arthrokinetics—to progressively apply deeper tissue massage. Manual techniques are then used to facilitate movement education. Movements are broken down into their component parts ("units of work"), and patients are taught how to learn and integrate principles of movement into each component. Finally, all components are reassembled into the final full motion. The adroit application of both verbal and nonverbal (tactile and kinesthetic) communication is essential to the success of movement education. Aston Fitness exercise training is customized to meet each patient's individual training goals and includes horizontal loosening (lying on the floor) using weight in motion, vertical loosening (standing) using weight transfer, stretching, toning (using weights and a device called a toning platform to facilitate alignment), and cardiovascular conditioning. The level of integration of body work, movement education, and environmental modification, the recognition of and respect for asymmetry in structure and movement, and customized problem-solving make Aston Patterning unique within the somatic disciplines. Aston Patterning is appropriate for treating patients with either acute or chronic lumbar spine pain.

Hellerwork is a somatic therapy that developed as an offshoot of both Rolfing and Aston Patterning. It was created by Joseph Heller, a past president of the Rolf Institute. It is similar to Rolfing with the addition of intellectually emphasizing the holistic nature of the process. Each session also includes movement education and specific, purposeful verbal dialog. Hellerwork integrates verbal dialog, movement education, and deep connective tissue body work.

Each of these somatic therapies has a holistic orientation that emphasizes the fact that no structure or function exists in isolation. Thus, the treatment of spinal pain not only addresses the site of tissue injury, but also all secondary sites of dysfunction as well as the patient's emotional response to their pain. These techniques integrate refined manual therapy and movement education and differ to some degree from traditional manual therapeutic approaches by placing much greater emphasis on proprioceptive sensations to help change neuromuscular function.

REFERENCES

1. Frymoyer JW. Epidemiology. Magnitude of the problem. In: Weinstein JN, Wiesel SW, eds. *The lumbar spine: The International Society for the Study of the Lumbar Spine*. Philadelphia: WB Saunders, 1990; 32–38.
2. Biering-Sorenson F. Low back trouble in a general population of 30-, 40-, 50-, and 60-year-old men and women. Study design, representativeness and basic results. *Dan Med Bull* 1982; 29:289–299.
3. Bovim G, Schrader H, Sand T. Neck pain in the general population. *Spine* 1994; 19:1307–1309.
4. Barnsley L, Lord S, Bogduk N. Clinical review. Whiplash injury. *Pain* 1994; 58:283–307.
5. Herring SA, Weinstein SM. Assessment and management of athletic low back injury. In: Nicholas JA, Hershman EB, eds. *The lower extremity and spine in sports medicine*, 2nd ed. St. Louis: CV Mosby, 1995; 1171–1197.
6. Mueller FO, Cantu RC. *Annual survey of catastrophic football injuries, 1977–1995.* Chapel Hill, NC: National Center for Catastrophic Sports Injury Research, University of North Carolina, 1996.
7. Von Korff M. Studying the natural history of back pain. *Spine* 1994; 19(suppl):2041–2046.
8. Barnsley L, Lord S, Bogduk N. The pathophysiology of whiplash. *Spine State Art Rev* 1993; 7:329–353.
9. Andersson GBJ. The epidemiology of spinal disorders. In: Frymoyer JW, ed. *The adult spine: principles and practice*, 2nd ed. Philadelphia: Lippincott-Raven, 1997; 93–141.
10. Hart LG, Deyo RA, Cherkin DC. Physician office visits for low back pain. *Spine* 1995; 20:11–19.
11. Cherkin DC, Deyo RA, Loeser JD, Bush T, Waddell G. An international comparison of back surgery rates. *Spine* 1994; 19:1201–1206.
12. Taylor VM, Deyo RA, Cherkin DC, Kreuter W. Low back pain hospitalization. *Spine* 1994; 19:1207–1213.

13. McGill CM. Industrial back problems. A control program. *J Occup Med* 1968; 10:174–178.
14. Waddell G. Epidemiology. A new clinical model for the treatment of low back pain. In: Weinstein JN, Wiesel SW, eds. *The lumbar spine: The International Society for the Study of the Lumbar Spine*. Philadelphia: WB Saunders, 1990; 38–56.
15. Frymoyer JW, Cats-Baril WL. An overview of the incidences and costs of low back pain. *Orthop Clin North Am* 1991; 22:263–271.
16. Holweck FG. *A biographical dictionary of the saints*. St. Louis: B Herder, 1924; 594.
17. Haldeman S. Presidential address, North American Spine Society: failure of the pathology model to predict back pain. *Spine* 1990; 15: 718–724.
18. Waddell G, Main CJ, Morris EW, DiPaola M, Gray ICM. Chronic low-back pain, psychologic distress, and illness behavior. *Spine* 1984; 9:209–213.
19. Herring SA. The physiatrist as the primary care specialist. *Phys Med Rehabil Clin North Am* 1991; 2:1–5.
20. Boden SD, Davis DO, Dina TS, Patronas N, Wiesel S. Abnormal magnetic-resonance scans of the lumbar spine in asymptomatic subjects: a prospective investigation. *J Bone Joint Surg [Am]* 1990; 72: 403–408.
21. Boden SD, McCowin PR, Davis DO, Dina TS, Mark AS, Wiesel S. Abnormal magnetic-resonance scans of the cervical spine in asymptomatic subjects. *J Bone Joint Surg [Am]* 1990; 72:1178–1184.
22. Wiesel SW, Tsourmas N, Feffer HL, Citrin CM, Patronas N. A study of computer-assisted tomography I. The incidence of positive CAT scans in an asymptomatic group of patients. *Spine* 1984; 9:549–551.
23. Jensen MC, Brant-Zawadzki MN, Obuchowski N, Modic MT, Malkasian D, Ross JS. Magnetic resonance imaging of the lumbar spine in people without back pain. *N Engl J Med* 1994; 331:69–73.
24. Mixter WJ, Barr JS. Rupture of the intervertebral disc with involvement of the spinal canal. *N Engl J Med* 1934; 211:210–215.
25. Bozzao A, Gallucci M, Masciocchi C, Aprile I, Barile A, Passariello R. Lumbar disk herniation: MR imaging assessment of natural history in patients treated without surgery. *Radiology* 1992; 185:135–141.
26. Bush K, Cowan N, Katz DE, Gishen P. The natural history of sciatica associated with disc pathology: a prospective study with clinical and independent radiologic follow-up. *Spine* 1992; 17:1205–1212.
27. DeLauche-Cavallier M-C, Budet C, Laredo J-D, et al. Lumbar disc herniation: Computed tomography scan changes after conservative treatment of nerve root compression. *Spine* 1992; 17:927–933.
28. Didry C, Lopez P, Baixas P, Simon L. Medically treated lumbar disc herniation. Clinical and computed tomographic follow-up. *Presse Med* 1991; 20:299–302.
29. Ellenberg MR, Ross ML, Honet JC, Schwartz M, Chodoroff G, Enochs S. Prospective evaluation of the course of disc herniations in patients with proven radiculopathy. *Arch Phys Med Rehabil* 1993; 74: 3–8.
30. Maigne J-Y, Rime B, Deligne B. Computed tomographic follow-up study of forty-eight cases of nonoperatively treated lumbar intervertebral disc herniation. *Spine* 1992; 17:1071–1074.
31. Saal JA, Saal JS, Herzog RJ. The natural history of lumbar intervertebral disc extrusions treated nonoperatively. *Spine* 1990; 15:683–686.
32. Teplick JG, Haskin ME. Spontaneous regression of herniated nucleus pulposus. *AJR* 1985; 145:371–375.
33. Maigne J-Y, Deligne L. Computed tomographic follow-up study of 21 cases of nonoperatively treated cervical intervertebral soft disc herniation. *Spine* 1994; 19:189–191.
34. Bush K, Chaudhuri R, Hillier S, Penny J. The pathomorphologic changes that accompany the resolution of cervical radiculopathy: a prospective study with repeat magnetic resonance imaging. *Spine* 1997; 22:183–187.
35. Postacchini F. Spine update: results of surgery compared with conservative management for lumbar disc herniations. *Spine* 1996; 21: 1383–1387.
36. Weber H. Lumbar disc herniation: a controlled, prospective study with ten years of observation. *Spine* 1983; 8:131–140.
37. Cherkin DC, Deyo RA, Wheeler K, Ciol MA. Physician views about treating low back pain: the results of a national survey. *Spine* 1995; 20:1–9.
38. Cherkin DC, Deyo RA, Wheeler K, Ciol M. Physician variation in diagnostic testing for low back pain: who you see is what you get. *Arthritis Rheum* 1994; 37:15–22.
39. Agency for Health Care Policy and Research Publication. *Acute low back problems in adults: assessment and treatment.* Washington, D.C.: U.S. Department of Health and Human Services, December 1994.
40. Bogduk N, Twomey LT. *Clinical anatomy of the lumbar spine*, 2nd ed. Melbourne: Churchill-Livingstone, 1991.
41. White AA, Panjabi MM. *Clinical biomechanics of the spine*, 2nd ed. Philadelphia: JB Lippincott, 1990.
42. Gracovetsky S, Kary M, Levy S, et al. Analysis of spinal and muscular activity during flexion/extension and free lifts. *Spine* 1990; 15: 1333–1339.
43. Gracovetsky S, Farfan H, Helleur C. The abdominal mechanism. *Spine* 1985; 10:317–324.
44. Abenhaim L, Rossignol M, Gobeille D, Bonvalot Y, Fines P, Scott S. The prognostic consequences in making of the initial medical diagnosis of work-related back injuries. *Spine* 1995; 20:791–795.
45. Deyo RA. Early diagnostic evaluation of low back pain. *J Gen Intern Med* 1986; 1:328–338.
46. Wiesel SW, Feffer HL, Rothman RH. Industrial low-back pain. A prospective evaluation of a standardized diagnostic and treatment protocol. *Spine* 1984; 9:199–203.
47. Kirkaldy-Willis WH. Pathology and pathogenesis of low back pain. In: Kirkaldy-Willis WH, Burton CV eds. *Managing low back pain*, 3rd ed. New York: Churchill-Livingstone, 1992; 49–79.
48. Mooney V, Robertson J. The facet syndrome. *Clin Orthop* 1976; 115: 149–156.
49. Raymond J, Dumas JM. Intraarticular facet block: diagnostic test or therapeutic procedure? *Radiology* 1984; 151:333–336.
50. Helbig T, Lee CK. The lumbar facet syndrome. *Spine* 1988; 13:61–64.
51. Bogduk N. Lumbar dorsal ramus syndrome. *Med J Aust* 1980; 2: 537–541.
52. Gibson MJ, Szypryt EP, Buckley JH, et al. Magnetic resonance imaging of adolescent disc herniation. *J Bone Joint Surg [Br]* 1987; 69: 699–703.
53. Kujala UM, Taimela S, Erkintalo M, Salminen JJ, Kaprio J. Low-back pain in adolescent athletes. *Med Sci Sports Exerc* 1996; 28: 165–170.
54. Erkintalo M, Salminen JJ, Alanen A, Paajanen H, Kormano M. Development of degenrative changes in the lumbar intervertebral disc: results of a prospective MR imaging study in adolescents with and without low-back pain. *Radiology* 1995; 196:529–533.
55. Kurihara A, Kataoka O. Lumbar disc herniation in children and adolescents. A review of 70 operated cases and their minimum 5-year follow-up studies. *Spine* 1980; 5:443–451.
56. Donelson R, Silva G, Murphy K. Centralization phenomenon. Its usefulness in evaluating and treating referred pain. *Spine* 1990; 15: 211–213.
57. Kosteljanetz M, Bank F, Schmidt-Olsen S. The clinical significance of straight-leg raising (Lasgue's sign) in the diagnosis of prolapsed lumbar disc. Interobserver variation and correlation with surgical finding. *Spine* 1988; 13:393–395.
58. Khuffash B, Porter RW. Cross leg pain and trunk list. *Spine* 1989; 14:602–603.
59. McKenzie RA. Prophylaxis in recurrent low back pain. *N Z Med J* 1979; 89:22–23.
60. Schnebel BE, Watkins RG, Dillin W. The role of spinal flexion and extension in changing nerve root compression in disc herniations. *Spine* 1989; 14:835–837.
61. Jonsson B, Stromqvist B. The straight leg raising test and the severity of symptoms in lumbar disc herniation: a prospective and postoperative evaluation. *Spine* 1995; 20:27–30.
62. Jackson RP, Glah JJ. Foraminal and extraforaminal lumbar disc herniation: diagnosis and treatment. *Spine* 1987; 12:577–585.
63. Kornberg M. Extreme lateral lumbar disc herniations. Clinical syndrome and computed tomography recognition. *Spine* 1987; 12: 586–589.
64. Gertzbein SD, Seligman J, Holtby R, et al. Centrode patterns and segmental instability in degenerative disc disease. *Spine* 1985; 10: 257–261.
65. Hayes MA, Howard TC, Gruel CR, et al. Roentgenographic evaluation of lumbar spine flexion-extension in asymptomatic individuals. *Spine* 1989; 14:327–331.
66. Farfan HF, Gracovetsky S. The nature of instability. *Spine* 1984; 9: 714–719.

67. Kirkaldy-Willis WH, Wedge JH, Yong-Hing K, Reily J. Pathology and pathogenesis of lumbar spondylosis and stenosis. *Spine* 1978; 3: 319–328.
68. Wall EJ, Cohen MS, Massie JB, Rydevik B, Garfin SR. Cauda equina anatomy I: Intrathecal nerve root organization. *Spine* 1990; 15: 1244–1247.
69. Takahashi K, Kagechika K, Takino T, Matsui T, Miyazaki T, Shima I. Changes in epidural pressure during walking in patients with lumbar spinal stenosis. *Spine* 1995; 20:2746–2749.
70. Porter RW. Spinal stenosis and neurogenic claudication. *Spine* 1996; 21:2046–2052.
71. Vanharanta H. Etiology, epidemiology and natural history of lumbar disc disease. *Spine State Art Rev* 1989; 3:1–12.
72. Cavanaugh JM. Neural mechanisms of idiopathic low back pain. In: Weinstein JN, Gordon SL, eds. *Low back pain: a scientific and clinical overview*. Rosemont, IL: American Academy of Orthopedic Surgeons, 1996; 583–605.
73. Kawakami M, Weinstein JN. Associated neurogenic and nonneurogenic pain mediators that probably are activated and responsible for nociceptive input. In: Weinstein JN, Gordon SL, eds. *Low back pain: a scientific and clinical overview*. Rosemont, IL: American Academy of Orthopedic Surgeons, 1996; 265–273.
74. Badalamente MA, Dee R, Ghillani R, Chien P-F, Daniels K. Mechanical stimulation of dorsal root ganglion induces increased production of substance P: a mechanism for pain following nerve root compromise? *Spine* 1987; 12:552–555.
75. Weinstein J, Pope M, Schmidt R, Seroussi R. Neuropharmacologic effects of vibration on the dorsal root ganglion. An animal model. *Spine* 1988; 13:521–525.
76. Pedrini-Mille A, Weinstein JN, Found EM, Chung CB, Goel VK. Stimulation of the dorsal root ganglion and degradation of rabbit annulus fibrosis. *Spine* 1990; 15:1252–1256.
77. Bogduk N. The innervation of the lumbar spine. *Spine* 1983; 8: 286–293.
78. Pedersen HE, Blunck CFJ, Gardner E. The anatomy of lumbosacral posterior rami and meningeal branches of spinal nerves (sinu-vertebral nerves): with an experimental study of their functions. *J Bone Joint Surg [Am]* 1956; 38:377–391.
79. Giles L, Harvey A. Immunohistochemical demonstration of nociceptors in the capsule and synovial folds of human zygapophyseal joints. *Br J Rheumatol* 1987; 26:362–364.
80. Yamashita T, Cavanaugh JM, El-Bohy AA, Getchell TV, King AI. Mechanosensitive afferent units in the lumbar facet joint. *J Bone Joint Surg [Am]* 1990; 72:865–870.
81. Ozaktay AC, Yamashita T, Cavanaugh JM, King AI. Fine nerve fibers and endings in the fibrous capsule of the lumbar facet joint. *Trans Orthop Res Soc* 1991; 16:353.
82. Beaman DN, Graziano GP, Glover RA, Wojtys EM, Chang V. Substance P innervation of lumbar spine facet joints. *Spine* 1993;18: 1044–1049.
83. El-Bohy A, Cavanaugh JM, Getchell ML, et al. Localization of substance P and neurofilament immunoreactive fibers in the lumbar facet joint capsule and supraspinous ligament of the rabbit. *Brain Res* 1992; 10:72–78.
84. Schwarzer AC, Aprill CN, Derby R, Fortin J, Kine G, Bogduk N. Clinical features of patients with pain stemming from the lumbar zygapophysial joints: Is the lumbar facet syndrome a clinical entity? *Spine* 1994; 19:1132–1137.
85. Revel ME, Listrat VM, Chevalier XJ, et al. Facet joint block for low back pain: identifying predictors of a good response. *Arch Phys Med Rehabil* 1992; 73:824–828.
86. Bogduk N. The innervation of the lumbar spine. *Spine* 1983; 8: 286–293.
87. Bogduk N, Tynan W, Wilson AS. The nerve supply to the human lumbar intervertebral disc. *J Anat* 1981; 132:39–56.
88. Yoshizawa H, O'Brien JP, Smith W, et al. The neuropathology of intervertebral discs removed for low-back pain. *J Pathol* 1980; 132: 95–104.
89. Ashton IK, Roberts S, Jaffray DC, et al. Neuropeptides in the human intervertebral disc. *J Orthop Res* 1994; 12:186–192.
90. Konttinen YT, Gronblad M, Antti-Poiks I, et al. Neuroimmuno-histochemical analysis of peridiscal nociceptive neural elements. *Spine* 1990; 15:383–386.
91. Echlin F. Pain responses on stimulation of the lumbar sympathetic chain under local anesthesia. *J Neurosurg* 1949:6:530–533.
92. Brena SF, Wolf SL, Chapman SL, Hammonds WD. Chronic back pain: Electromyographic, motion and behavioral assessments following sympathetic nerve blocks and placebos. *Pain* 1980; 8:1–10.
93. Nakamura SI, Takahashi K, Takahashi Y, Yamagata M, Moriya H. The afferent pathways of discogenic low back pain. *J Bone Joint Surg [Br]* 1996; 78:606–611.
94. Takahashi Y, Nakajima Y, Moriya H, Takahashi K. Capsaicin applied to rat lumbar intervertebral disc causes extravasation in the groin skin: a possible mechanism of referred pain of the intervertebral disc. *Neurosci Lett* 1993; 161:1–3.
95. Thelander U, Fagerlund M, Friberg S, Larsson F. Straight leg raising test vs. Radiologic size, shape and position of lumbar disc herniations. *Spine* 1992; 17:395–399.
96. Jaffrey D, O'Brien JA. Isolated intervertebral disc resorption: a source of mechanical and inflammatory back pain. *Spine* 1986; 11:397–401.
97. Garfin SR, Rydevik BL, Brown RA, Saratoris DJ. Compressive neuropathy of spinal nerve roots. A mechanical or biological problem? *Spine* 1991; 16:162–166.
98. Hitselberger WE, Witten PM. Abnormal myelogram in asymptomatic patients. *J Neurosurg* 1986; 28:204–206.
99. Rydevik B, Brown M, Lundborg G. Pathoanatomy and pathophysiology of nerve compression. *Spine* 1984; 9:7–15.
100. Garfin SR, Rydevik B, Lind B, Massie J. Spinal nerve root compression. *Spine* 1995; 20:1810–1820.
101. Bobechko WP, Hirsch C. Autoimmune response to nucleus pulposus in the rabbit *J Bone Joint Surg [Br]* 1965; 47:574–580.
102. Pankovich AM, Korngold LA. A comparison of the antigen properties or nucleus pulposus and cartilage protein polysaccharide complexes. *J Immunol* 1967; 99:431–437.
103. Marshall LL, Trethewie ER, Curtain CC. Chemical radiculitis. A clinical, physiological and immunological study. *Clin Orthop* 1979; 129: 61–67.
104. McCarron RF, Wimpee MW, Hudkins PG, Laros GS. The inflammatory effect of nucleus pulposus. A possible element in the pathogenesis of low-back pain. *Spine* 1987; 12:760–764.
105. Habtemariam A, Gronblad M, Virri J, Seitsalo S, Ruuskanen M, Karaharju E. Immunocytochemical localization of immunoglobulins in disc herniations. *Spine* 1996; 21:1864–1869.
106. Doita M, Kanatani T, Harada T, Mizuno K. Immunohistologic study of the ruptured intervertebral disc of the lumbar spine. *Spine* 1996; 21:235–241.
107. Haro H, Shimomiya K, Komori H, et al. Upregulated expression of chemokines in herniated nucleus pulposus resorption. *Spine* 1996; 21: 1647–1652.
108. Gronblad M, Virri J, Tolonen J, et al. A controlled immunohistochemical study of inflammatory cells in disc herniation tissue. *Spine* 1994; 19:2744–2751.
109. Olmarker D, Byrod G, Cornefjord M, Nordborg C, Rydevik B. Effects of methylprednisolone on nucleus pulposus induced nerve root injury. *Spine* 1994; 19:1803–1808.
110. Olmarker K, Rydevik B, Nordborg C. Autologous nucleus pulposus induces neurophysiologic and histologic changes in porcine cauda equina nerve roots. *Spine* 1993; 18:1425–1432.
111. Takahashi H, Suguro T, Okazima Y, Motegi M, Okada Y, Kakiuchi T. Inflammatory cytokines in the herniated disc of the lumbar spine. *Spine* 1996; 21:218–224.
112. Saal JS. The role of inflammation in lumbar pain. *Spine* 1995; 20: 1821–1827.
113. Ng SCS, Weiss JB, Quennel R, Jayson MIV. Abnormal connective tissue degrading enzyme patterns in prolapsed intervertebral discs. *Spine* 1986; 11:695–701.
114. Nachemson A. Intradiscal measurements of pH in patients with lumbar rhizopathies. *Acta Orthop Scand* 1969; 40:23–32.
115. Weinstein J, Claverie W, Gibson S. The pain of discography. *Spine* 1988; 13:1344–1348.
116. Franson RC, Saal JS, Saal JA. Human disc phospholipase A2 is inflammatory. *Spine* 1992; 17(suppl):129–132.
117. Saal JS, Franson RC, Dobrow R, Saal JA, White AH, Goldthwaite N. High levels of inflammatory phospholipase A2 activity in lumbar spine disc herniations. *Spine* 1990; 15:674–678.
118. Gronblad M, Virri J, Ronkko S, et al. A controlled biochemical and immunohistochemical study of human synovial-type (group II) phos-

pholipase A2 and inflammatory cells in macroscopically normal, degenerated, and herniated human lumbar disc tissues. *Spine* 1996; 21: 2531–2538.
119. Ozaktay AC, Cavanaugh JM, Blagoev DC, King AI. Phospholipase A2-induced electrophysiologic and histologic changes in rabbit dirsal lumbar spine tissues. *Spine* 1995; 20:2659–2668.
120. Robertson J, Huffmon G, Thomas LB, Leffler CW, Gunter BC, White RP. Prostaglandin production after experimental discectomy. *Spine* 1996; 21:1731–1736.
121. Kang JD, Georgescu HI, McIntyre-Larkin L, Stefanovic-Racic M, Evans CH. Herniated cervical intervertebral discs spontaneously produce matirx metalloproteinases, nitric oxide, interleukin-6, and prostaglandin E2. *Spine* 1995; 20:2373–2378.
122. Weinstein JN. Recent advances in the neurophysiology of pain. *Phys Med Rehabil State Art Rev* 1990; 4:201–219.
123. Waddell G, McCulloch JA, Kummel E, Venner RM. Nonorganic physical signs in low-back pain. *Spine* 1980; 5:117–125.
124. Maruta T, Goldman S, Chan CW, Ilstrup DM, Kunselman AR, Colligan RC. Waddell's nonorganic signs and Minnesota Mutliphasic Personality Inventory profiles in patients with chronic low back pain. *Spine* 1997; 22:72–75.
125. Ransford AD, Cairns D, Mooney V. The pain drawing as an aid to the psychologic evaluation of patients with low back pain. *Spine* 1976; 1:127–134.
126. Ohlund C, Eek C, Palmblad S, Areskoug B, Nachemson A. Quantified pain drawing in subacute low back pain: validation in a nonselected outpatient industrial sample. *Spine* 1996; 21:1021–1031.
127. Shelton JL, Robinson JP. Psychological aspects of chronic back pain. *Phys Med Rehabil Clin North Am* 1991; 2:127–144.
128. Leclaire R, Blier F, Fortin L, Proulx R. A cross-sectional study comparing the Oswestry and Roland-Morris functional disability scales in two populations of patients with low back pain of different levels of severity. *Spine* 1997; 22:68–71.
129. Bigos SJ, Spengler DM, Martin NA, Zeh J, Fisher L, Nachemson A. Back injuries in industry: a retrospective study. III. Employee-related factors. *Spine* 1986; 11:252–256.
130. Carron H, DeGood DE, Tait R. A comparison of low back pain patients in the United States and New Zealand: psychosocial and economic factors affecting severity of disability. *Pain* 1985; 21:77–89.
131. Cats-Baril W, Frymoyer JW. Identifying patients at risk of becoming disabled because of low-back pain. The Vermont Rehabilitation Engineering Center predictive model. *Spine* 1991; 16:605–607.
132. Derebery VJ, Tullis WH. Delayed recovery in the patient with a work compensable injury. *J Occup Med* 1983; 25:829–835.
133. Frymoyer J, Cats-Baril W. Predictors of low back pain disability. *Clin Orthop* 1987; 221:89–98.
134. Walsh NE, Dumitru D. The influence of compensation on recovery from low back pain. *Spine State Art Rev* 1987; 2:109–121.
135. Robinson JP, Brown PB, Fisk JD. Pathophysiology of lumbar radiculopathies and the pharmacology of epidural corticosteroids and local anesthetics. *Phys Med Rehabil Clin North Am* 1995; 6:671–690.
136. Weinstein SM, Herring SA, Derby R. Contemporary concepts in spine care. Epidural steroid injections. *Spine* 1995; 20:1842–1846.
137. Woodward JL, Weinstein SM. Epidural injections for the diagnosis and management of axial and radicular pain syndromes. *Phys Med Rehabil Clin North Am* 1995; 6:691–714.
138. Bogduk N, Christophidis N, Cherry D, et al. *Epidural steroids in the management of back pain and sciatica of spinal origin. Report of the Working Party on epidural use of steroids in the management of back pain.* Canberra, Australia: National Health and Medical Research Council, 1993.
139. Rapp SE, Haselkorn JK, Elam K, Deyo R, Ciol MA. Epidural steroid injection in the treatment of low back pain: a meta-analysis [Abstract]. *Anesthesiology* 1994; 78:923.
140. Warfield CA. Correspondence. *J Bone Joint Surg [Am]* 1985; 67: 980–981.
141. Derby R. Diagnostic block procedures. Use in pain localization. *Spine State Art Rev* 1986; 1:47–64.
142. Destouet JM. Lumbar facet syndrome: diagnosis and treatment. *Surg Rounds Orthop* 1988; February:22–27.
143. Dooley JF, McBroom RJ, Taguchi T, Macnab I. Nerve root infiltration in the diagnosis of radicular pain. *Spine* 1988; 13:79–83.
144. Jeffries B. Epidural steroid injections. *Spine State Art Rev* 1988; 2: 419–26.
145. Jeffries B. Facet steroid injections. *Spine State Art Rev* 1988; 2: 409–417.
146. Krempen JF, Smith BS, DeFreest LJ. Selective nerve root infiltration for the evaluation of sciatica. *Orthop Clin North Am* 1975; 6:311–314.
147. Derby R, Bogduk N, Kine G. Precision percutaneous blocking procedures for localizing spinal pain. Part 2. The lumbar neuroaxial compartment. *Pain Dig* 1993; 3:175–188.
148. El-Khoury GY, Ehara S, Weinstein JN, Montgomery WJ, Kathol MH. Epidural steroid injection: a procedure ideally performed under fluoroscopic control. *Radiology* 1988; 168:554–557.
149. Mehta M, Salmon N. Extradural block. Confirmation of the injection site by x-ray monitoring. *Anesthesia* 1985; 40:1009–1012.
150. Renfrew DL, Moore TE, Kathol MH, El-Khoury GY, Lemke JH, Walker CW. Correct placement of epidural steroid injection: fluoroscopic guidance and contrast administration. *Am J Neuroradiol* 1991; 12:1003–1007.
151. White AH, Derby R, Wynne G. Epidural injection for the diagnosis and treatment of low-back pain. *Spine* 1980; 5:78–82.
152. White AH. Injection technique for the diagnosis and treatment of low back pain. *Orthop Clin North Am* 1983; 14:553–567.
153. Dreyfuss PH, Dreyer SJ, Herring SA. Contemporary concepts in spine care. Lumbar zygapophysial (facet) joint injections. *Spine* 1995; 20: 2040–2047.
154. Nelson DA. Dangers from methylprednisolone acetate therapy by intraspinal injection. *Arch Neurol* 1988; 45:804–806.
155. Rustin MHA, Flynn MD, Coomes EN. Acute sacral epidural abscess following local anesthetic injection. *Postgrad Med J* 1983; 59: 399–400.
156. Tuel SM, Meythalert JM, Cross LL. Cushing's syndrome from epidural methylprednisolone. *Pain* 1990; 40:81–84.
157. Dreyer SJ, Dreyfuss P, Cole AJ. Zygapophysial (facet) joint injection. Intra-articular and medial branch block techniques. *Phys Med Rehabil Clin North Am* 1995; 6:715–741.
158. Lilius G, Laasonen EM, Myllynen P, Harilainen A, Gronlund G. Lumbar facet joint syndorme: a randomized clinical trial. *J Bone Joint Surg [Br]* 1989; 71:681–684.
159. Carette S, Marcoux S, Truchon R, et al. A controlled trial of corticosteroid injections into the facet joints for chronic low back pain. *N Engl J Med* 1991; 325:1002–1007.
160. Dwyer A, Aprill C, Bogduk N. Cervical zygapophyseal joint pain patterns I: a study of normal volunteers. *Spine* 1990; 15:453–457.
161. Aprill C, Dwyer A, Bogduk N. Cervical zygapophyseal joint pain patterns II: a clinical evaluation. *Spine* 1990; 15:458–461.
162. Bogduk N, Marsland A. The cervical zygapophysial joints as source of neck pain. *Spine* 1988; 13:610–617.
163. Esses SI, Moro JK. The value of facet joint blocks in patient selection for lumbar fusion. *Spine* 1993; 18:185–190.
164. Johansson A, Hao J, Sjolund B. Local corticosteroid application blocks transmission in normal nociceptor C-fibres. *Acta Anaesthesiol Scand* 1990; 34:335–338.
165. Weinstein SM, Herring SA. Principles and practice of imaging athletic injuries to the cervical, thoracic and lumbar spine. In: Halpern B, Herring SA, Altchek D, Herzog R, eds. *Imaging in musculoskeletal sports medicine.* Cambridge, MA: Blackwell Science, 1997; 58–81.
166. Bodner RJ, Heyman S, Drummond DS, Gregg JR. The use of single photon emission computed tomography (SPECT) in the diagnosis of low-back pain in young patients. *Spine* 1988; 13:1155–1160.
167. Aprill C, Bogduk N. High-intensity zone: a diagnostic sign of painful lumbar disc on magnetic resonance imaging. *Br J Radiol* 1992; 65: 361–369.
168. Schellhas KP, Pollei SR, Gundry CR, Heithoff KB. Lumbar disc high-intensity zone: correlation of magnetic resonance imaging and discography. *Spine* 1996; 21:79–85.
169. Bogduk N, Modic MT. Lumbar discography. *Spine* 1996; 21: 402–404.
170. Schellhas KP, Smith MD, Gundry CR, Pollei SR. Cervical discogenic pain: prospective correlation of magnetic resonance imaging and discography in asymptomatic subjects and pain sufferers. *Spine* 1996; 21:300–310.
171. Tanenbaum SJ. What physcians know. *N Engl J Med* 1993; 329: 1268–1271.
172. Koes BW, Bouter LM, van der Heijden GJMG. Methodological quality of randomized clinical trials on treatment efficacy in low back pain. *Spine* 1995; 20:228–235.

173. Herring SA. Sports medicine early care. In: Mayer TG, Mooney V, Gatchel RJ, eds. *Contemporary conservative care for painful spinal disorders*. Philadelphia: Lea & Febiger, 1991; 235–244.
174. Greenman PE *Principles of manual medicines*. Baltimore: Williams & Wilkins, 1989.
175. Maitland GD. *Vertebral manipulation*, 5th ed. London: Butterworths, 1986.
176. Paris SV. Manipulation of the lumbar spine. In: Weinstein JN, Weisel SW, eds. *The lumbar spine*. Philadelphia: WB Saunders, 1990; 805–811.
177. Van Hoesen L. Mobilization and manipulation techniques for the lumbar spine. In: Grieve GP, ed. *Modern manual therapy of the vertebral column*. New York: Churchill-Livingstone, 1986.
178. McFadden KD, Taylor JR. Axial rotation in the lumbar spine and gaping of the zygapophyseal joints. *Spine* 1990; 15:295–299.
179. Shekelle PG. Spine update. Spinal manipulation. *Spine* 1994; 19: 858–861.
180. DiFablo RP. Efficacy of manual therapy. *Phys Ther* 1992; 72: 853–864.
181. Twomey L, Taylor J. Spine update. Exercise and spinal manipulation in the treatment of low back pain. *Spine* 1995; 20:615–619.
182. Koes BW, Assendelft WJJ, van der Heijden GJMG, Bouter LM. Spinal manipulation for low back pain: an updated systemic review of randomized clinical trials. *Spine* 1996; 21:2860–2870.
183. Koes BW, Bouter LM, vanMameren H, et al. The effectiveness of manual therapy, physiotherapy, and treatment by the general practitioner for nonspecific back and neck complaints. A randomized clinical trial. *Spine* 1992; 17:28–35.
184. Convertino VA, Bloomfield SA, Greenleaf JE. Symposium: physiological effects of bed rest and restricted physical activity: an update. *Med Sci Sports Exerc* 1997; 29:187–206.
185. Muller EA. Influence of training and of inactivity on muscle strength. *Arch Phys Med Rehabil* 1970; 51:449–462.
186. Mayer T, Smith S, Keeley J, Mooney V. Quantification of lumbar function. Part 2: sagittal plane strength in chronic low back pain patients. *Spine* 1985; 10:765–772.
187. Kahanovitz W, Viola K, Gallagher M. Long-term strength assessment of postoperative diskectomy patients. *Spine* 1989; 14:402–403.
188. Deyo RA, Diehl Ak, Rosenthal M. How many days of bed rest for acute low back pain? A randomized clinical trial. *N Engl J Med* 1986; 315:1064–1070.
189. Gilbert JR, Taylor DW, Hildebrand A, Evans C. Clinical trial of common treatments for low back pain in family practice. *Br Med J* 1985; 291:789–794.
190. Malmivaara A, Hakkinen U, Aro T, et al. The treatment of acute low back pain-bed rest, exercises, or ordinary activity? *N Engl J Med* 1995; 332:351–355.
191. Postachini F, Facchini M, Palleri T. Efficacy of various forms of conservative treatment in low back pain. A comparative study. *Neuro-orthopedics* 1988; 6:28–35.
192. Linton SJ, Bradley LA, Jensen I, Spangfort E, Sundell L. The secondary prevention of low back pain. *Pain* 1989; 36:197–207.
193. Kellet KM, Kellet DA, Nordholm LA. Effects of an exercise program on sick leave due to low back pain. *Phys Ther* 1991; 4:283–293.
194. Dehlin O, Berg S, Hedenrud B, Andersson GBJ, Grimby G. Effect of physical training and ergonomic counseling on the psychological perception of work and the subjective assessment of low back insufficiency. *Scand J Rehabil Med* 1981; 13:1–9.
195. Cady LD, Thomas PC, O Connell ER, Thomas PC, Sallan JH. Strength and fitness and subsequent back injury in firefighters. *J Occup Med* 1979; 21:269–272.
196. Cady LD, Thomas PC, Karwasky RJ. Program for increasing health and physical fitness of firefighters, *J Occup Med* 1985; 27:110–114.
197. Koes BW, Bouter LM, Beckerman H, van der Heijden GJMG, Knipschild PG. Physiotherapy exercises and back pain: a blinded review. *Br Med J* 1991; 302:1572–1576.
198. Coxhead CE, Meade TW, Inskip H, North WRS. Multicentre trial of physiotherapy in the management of sciatic symptoms. *Lancet* 1981; 229:1065–1068.
199. Evans C, Gilbert JR, Taylor W, Hildebarnd A. A randomized controlled trial of flexion exercises, education, and bed rest for patients with acute low back pain. *Physiother Can* 1987; 39:96–101.
200. Faas A, Chavanes AW, van Eijk JThM, Gubbels JW. A randomized, placebo-controlled trial of exercise therapy in patients with acute low back pain. *Spine* 1993; 18:1388–1395.
201. Dettori JR, Bullock SH, Sutlive TG, Franklin RJ, Patience T. The effects of spinal flexion and extension exercises and their associated postures in patients with acute low back pain. *Spine* 1995; 20: 2302–2312.
202. Donelson R, Grant W, Kamps C, Medcalf R. Pain response to sagittal end-range spinal motion. A prospective, randomized, multicentered trial. *Spine* 1991; 16:S206–S212.
203. Stankovic R, Johnell O. Conservative treatment of acute low-back pain. A prospective randomized trial: McKenzie method of treatment versus patient education in mini back school. *Spine* 1990; 15:120–123.
204. McKenzie RA. *The lumbar spine. Mechanical diagnosis and therapy*. Waikance, New Zealand: Spinal Publications, 1981.
205. Ponte DJ, Jensen GJ, Kent BE. A preliminary report on the use of the McKenzie protocol versus Williams protocol in the treatment of low back pain. *J Orthop Sports Phys Ther* 1984; 6:130–139.
206. Melzack R, Wall PD. Pain mechanisms: a new theory. *Science* 1965; 150:971–979.
207. Nachemson A, Elfstrom G. Intravital dynamic pressure measurements in lumbar discs: a study of common movements, maneuvers and exercises. *Scand J Rehabil Med* 1970; 1(suppl):1–40.
208. Williams P. *Low back and neck pain: causes and conservative treatment*, 3rd ed. Springfield, IL: Charles C Thomas, 1974.
209. Biering-Sorensen F. Physical measurements as risk indicators for low back trouble over a one-year period. *Spine* 1984; 9:106–119.
210. Battie MC, Bigos SJ, Fisher LD, et al. A prospective study of the role of cardiovascular risk factors and fitness in industrial back pain complaints. *Spine* 1989; 14:141–147.
211. Donchin M, Woolf O, Kaplan L, Floman Y. Secondary prevention of low-back pain: a clinical trial. *Spine* 1990; 15:1317–1320.
212. Gundewall B, Liljeqvist M, Hansson T. Primary prevention of back symptoms and absence from work. *Spine* 1993; 18:587–594.
213. Lahad A, Malter AD, Berg AO, Deyo RA. The effectiveness of four interventions for the prevention of low back pain. *JAMA* 1994; 272: 1286–1290.
214. Plowman SA. Physical activity, physical fitness, and low back pain. *Exerc Sports Sci Rev* 1992; 20:221–242.
215. Troup JDG, Foreman TK, Baxter CE, Brown D. The perception of back pain and the role of psychophysical tests of lifting capacity. *Spine* 1987; 12:645–657.
216. Porterfield JA. Dynamic stabilization of the trunk. *J Orthop Sports Phys Ther* 1985; 6:271–277.
217. Saal JA. Dynamic muscular stabilization in the nonoperative treatment of lumbar pain syndromes. *Orthop Rev* 1990; 19:691–700.
218. Sweeney T, Prentice C, Saal JA, Saal JS. Cervicothoracic muscular stabilization techniques. *Phys Med Rehabil State Art Rev* 1990; 4: 335–359.
219. Crisco JJ, Panjabi MM. The intersegmental and multisegmental muscles of the lumbar spine. A biomechanical model comparing lateral stabilizing potential. *Spine* 1991; 16:793–799.
220. Panjabi MM, Abumi K, Duranceay J, Oxland T. Spinal stability and intersegmental muscle forces. A biomechanical model. *Spine* 1989; 14:194–200.
221. Cole AJ, Moschetti ML, Eagleston RE. Spine pain: aquatic rehabilitation strategies. *J Back Musculoskel Rehabil* 1994; 4:273–286.
222. Miller B. Alternative somatic therapies. In: White AH, Anderson R, eds. *Conservative care of low back pain*. Baltimore: Williams & Wilkins, 1991; 120–133.

Rehabilitation Medicine: Principles and Practice, Third Edition,
edited by Joel A. DeLisa and Bruce M. Gans.
Lippincott–Raven Publishers, Philadelphia © 1998.

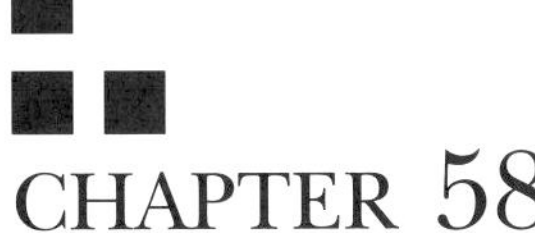

CHAPTER 58

Osteoporosis

Francis J. Bonner, Jr., Charles H. Chesnut III, Amy Fitzsimmons, and Robert Lindsay

Osteoporosis is a disease that occurs commonly in the rehabilitation patient population in its' primary and secondary forms. Over 60% of patients admitted from acute hospitalization to in-patient rehabilitation have been shown to have severe osteoporosis (1). Despite its prevalence, the disease continues to be under-recognized and hence not treated even after fractures have occurred. Large numbers of individuals are subjected to disability and chronic pain as a result. These numbers are increasing daily and are expected to reach epidemic proportions by the turn of the century. The predominant consequences of this chronic and progressive disease are fracture and disability, and because there are no warning signs, relatively few people are diagnosed in time for effective therapy to be administered in the preclinical phase. The majority of long bone fractures are associated with falls, and it is therefore the combination of reduced quantity and quality of bone, relative neuromuscular instability, and environmental hazards that the physiatrist must address not only in efforts to treat this disease but also to prevent it and its consequences (Fig. 58-1).

DEFINITION

Osteoporosis is a disease characterized by low bone mass and deterioration of microarchitecture of bone tissue, which leads to increased bone fragility with a resulting increase in fracture risk (Fig. 58-2). Fractures occur when applied loads are in excess of the capacity of the bone. This capacity is dependent on the degree of mineralization of the bone and its architecture. As osteoporosis progresses, both the mineralization and internal architecture deteriorate, increasing the risk that a given load will result in fracture. Although the bone mass is reduced in osteoporosis, the remaining bone demonstrates the normal composition of both organic (40%) and mineral components (60%).

The World Health Organization (WHO) endorses a definition of osteoporosis based on a bone mass measurement (2) of more than 2.5 standard deviations (SD) below the mean of normal young adults. ''Normal'' is considered a bone density within 1 SD of the mean and ''low bone mass'' is considered as an appropriate designation for those with bone density 1.0 to 2.5 SD below the mean for young adults. It is important to bear in mind that the diagnosis of this disease is not dependent on a fracture having occurred, but rather laboratory or clinical evidence of substantially increased risk for fracture because of reduced bone mass (2).

General osteoporosis is commonly seen in association with other diseases, (secondary osteoporosis). It is the most common of the metabolic bone diseases and does occur as a primary medical condition. When it occurs without association with other conditions, it is referred to as involutional osteoporosis, which is postmenopausal osteoporosis in women (type I) and senile osteoporosis (type II) in men. These two conditions have generalized osteopenia (bone mass reduction) and increased risk for fracture in common. Secondary osteoporosis occurs in association with other diseases (e.g., Cushing's disease) or medications (e.g., heparin), as well as physiologic aberration (e.g., disuse) (3). Localized osteoporosis is a condition manifested by anatomically discrete regions of bone mass reduction. In its primary form, it is seen in reflex sympathetic dystrophy and transient regional osteoporosis (Table 58-1).

F. J. Bonner, Jr.: Department of Physical Medicine and Rehabilitation, Allegheny Graduate Hospital, Philadelphia Pennsylvania 19146.
C. H. Chesnut III: Departments of Medicine, Radiology, and Orthopaedics, University of Washington Medical Center, Seattle, Washington 98112.
A. Fitzsimmons: Department of Physical Medicine and Rehabilitation, Graduate Hospital, Philadelphia, Pennsylvania 19146.
R. Lindsay: Department of Medicine, Columbia University, New York, New York 10027; and Department of Medicine, Helen Hayes Hospital, West Haverstraw, New York 10993.

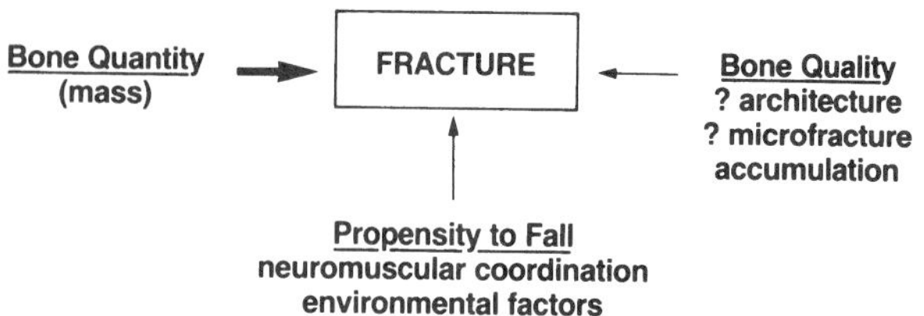

FIG. 58-1. Determinants of osteoporotic fracture, including bone quality, bone quantity, and propensity to fall.

EPIDEMIOLOGY

Osteoporosis has become a public health problem of epidemic proportions, affecting an estimated 75 million people in the United States, Europe, and Japan, including one out of three postmenopausal women and a majority of the elderly, including men. More than 1.2 million fractures per year in the United States are directly related to osteoporosis. Seventy percent of fractures in people over 45 years of age are attributable to osteoporosis (4). One third of women over 65 years of age will have a vertebral fracture. By 80 years of age, one of every three women and one of every six men will have sustained a hip fracture (5). The lifetime risk of hip, wrist, or vertebral fracture is about 40% for white women and 13% for white men. As life expectancy increases, osteoporosis will be more prevalent in men and women. Its importance as a public health problem is underscored by the fact that the lifetime risk of hip fracture in women is larger than the sum of lifetime risks of having breast, endometrial, and ovarian cancer. The lifetime risk of hip fracture in men is greater than that of prostate cancer (4).

Osteoporosis is an important clinical and public health problem for men. Whereas this disease in the past has been largely neglected in men, it is now recognized that hip fractures in men are approximately one third as prevalent as in women. Although women lose bone mass rapidly in the years after menopause, by 65 to 70 years of age, calcium absorption decreases in both sexes, resulting in an equal rate of bone loss for men and women. It is now recognized that osteoporosis is a disease that significantly affects men, resulting in 1.5 million American men with this disease in

TABLE 58-1. *Classification of osteoporosis*

A. Primary osteoporosis basic etiology unknown, no associated disease
   1. Postmenopausal osteoporosis: elderly women
   2. Senile osteoporosis: elderly men
B. Secondary osteoporosis: secondary to inherited or acquired abnormalities/diseases or to physiologic aberrations
   1. Hyperparathyroidism
   2. Cushing's disease
   3. Multiple myeloma
   4. Hyperthyroidism (endogenous and iatrogenic)
   5. Idiopathic hypercalciuria
      a. Due to renal calcium leak
      b. Due to renal phosphate leak
   6. Malabsorption (including partial gastrectomy)
   7. 25-OH vitamin D deficiency
      a. Due to chronic liver disease
      b. Due to chronic anticonvulsant therapy (phenytoin, barbiturates)
   8. 1,25$(OH)_2$ vitamin D deficiency due to lack of renal synthesis
      a. Due to chronic renal failure
   9. Adult hypophosphatasia
   10. Osteogenesis imperfecta tarda
   11. Male hypogonadism (Klinefelter's syndrome)
   12. Female hypogonadism (Turner's syndrome)
   13. Conditions consistent with hypoestrogenism secondary to anorexia and/or exercise
      a. Anorexia nervosa
      b. Exercise-induced amenorrhea
   14. Conditions associated with disuse
      a. Paraplegia/hemiplegia
      b. Immobilization
      c. Prolonged bed rest (?)
   15. Alcoholism
   16. Diabetes mellitus (?)
   17. Rheumatoid arthritis
   18. Chronic obstructive pulmonary disease
   19. Systemic mastocytosis
   20. Conditions associated with the use of medications
      a. Corticosteroids
      b. Heparin
      c. Anticonvulsants
      d. Excess thyroid hormone
   21. Malignancy

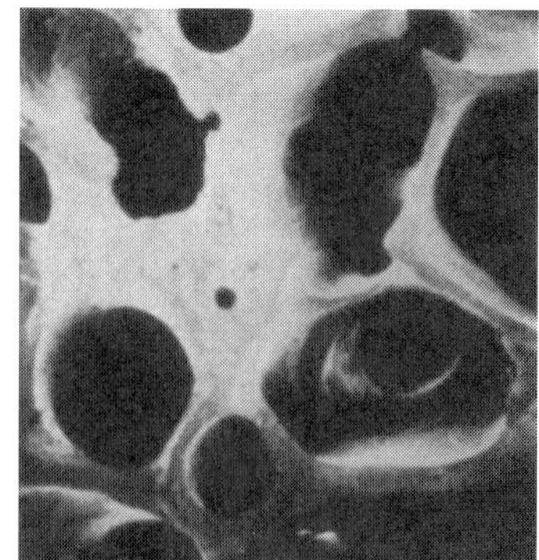
A

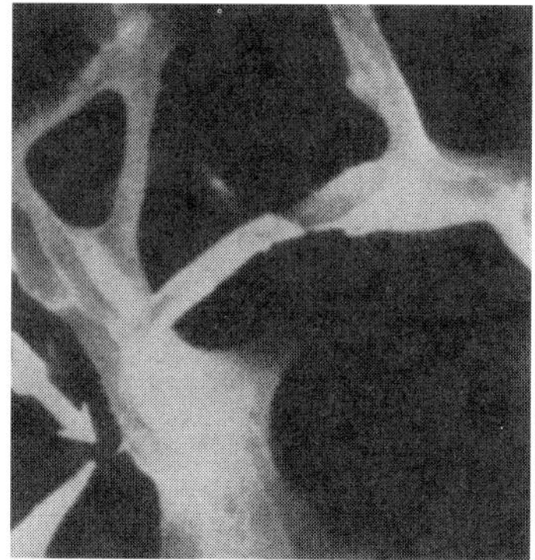
B

FIG. 58-2. Micrographs of biopsy specimens of normal **(A)** and osteoporotic **(B)** bone. **A:** From a 75-year-old normal woman. **B:** From a 47-year-old woman who had multiple vertebral compression fractures.

1997. Approximately 3.5 million men are at risk for this disease, and over the age of 75 years, osteoporosis effects half the population, men and women equally. Before the age of 90 years, 6% of all men will sustain an osteoporosis-related hip fracture. About one fifth to one third of all hip fractures occur in men, and symptomatic vertebral fractures occur about half as often in men as in women (6).

The morbidity associated with osteoporotic fractures is high. In 1986 there were 321,909 hospitalizations of women 45 years of age and older (7). Hip fractures were responsible for 167,421 admissions to hospitals, and 35,106 were admitted for vertebral fractures. At that time, the direct cost of osteoporosis was estimated at $5 billion to $6 billion annually in the United States (8). By 1994, these expenditures had increased to an estimated $13.3 billion in direct and indirect cost (9). The combined cost of care for 2.3 million osteoporosis fractures occurring in the United States and Europe is more than $23 billion. The majority of the social and economic burden is due to hip fracture (4).

Usually these fractures result in temporary disability, with most patients recovering function to near prefracture levels. However, many patients suffer consequences of fracture resulting in deformity, loss of function, dependence, and institutionalization. About 50% of all women who fracture their hips are admitted to a nursing home, and 14% of these patients are in a nursing home after 1 year. The Office of Technology Assessment of the United States has estimated that only one third of hip fracture patients regain their prefracture level of function. Activities of daily living (ADLs) for self-care are compromised in 60% of patients, and 80% were unable to perform at least one instrumental ADL, such as shopping or driving (10).

Fractures of the vertebra are common and are largely responsible for the "Dowagers hump" deformity. These fractures when severe may cause chronic back pain (11) and disturbed balance. There are subjective estimates (12) that 5% of patients with vertebral fractures have some dependency in ADLs and 2% of patients with wrist fractures have similar residual dependency. The National Osteoporosis Foundation (NOF) has looked at how osteoporotic fractures impact a person's life by determining the quality-adjusted life year (QALY) associated with these fractures (13). Perfect health for 1 year is assigned a QALY of 1. Death is assigned a QALY of 0. A disability that reduces a person's self-assessed quality of life by half, compared with perfect health, is assigned a QALY of 0.5. The NOF estimated the loss of QALYs associated with various outcomes based on the available published studies, their personal values, and their experience with patients. A focus group of postmenopausal women generally agreed with determinations made by the NOF Committee. Estimates of the effectiveness of various pharmacologic treatments in preventing fractures and their consequences were based on available evidence from randomized controlled trials. Effectiveness of rehabilitation strategies were not reviewed. However, the assumptions of effectiveness coupled with costs enable the calculation of the expected cost per QALY for any interventional strategy. This methodology allows a determination of whether any particular strategy is appropriate from a societal perspective. Table 58-2 references the NOF Committee's determination relative to various events and the QALYs associated with those events. Table 58-3 indicates cost associated with the event based on an assigned dollar value per QALY of $30,000 (13).

ETIOLOGY AND RISK FACTORS

Risk of developing an osteoporotic-related fracture is dependent on an individual peak bone mass and strength of bone achieved in one's lifetime and the subsequent rate of bone loss. However, there are specific identified risk factors and causes of low bone mass and osteoporosis. In secondary

TABLE 58-2. *National Osteoporosis Foundation Committee determinations*

Event	QALYs lost due to event	Rationale
Hip fracture		
Acute event	0.0833	Complete loss of quality of life for 1 mo (= 1/12)
Rehabilitation or short-stay hospital (9 days)	0.0247	Complete loss of quality for 9 days (= 9/365)
Readmitted (8 days)	0.0219	Complete loss of quality for 8 days (= 8/365)
Home care services (6 mo)	0.25	Quality of life reduced by 0.5 for 6 mo (= 0.5 × 6/12)
Nonmedical home care (6 mo)	0.25	Quality of life reduced by 0.5 for 6 mo (= 0.5 × 6/12)
Posthospital physician visits	0.011	Quality of life reduced by 0.5 for 8 days (= 0.5 × 8/365)
ER, ambulance	0.0027	Complete loss of quality for 1 day (= 1/365)
Wrist fracture, acute event	0.0404	Quality reduced by 0.3 for 7 wk (= 0.3 × 7/52)
Vertebral fracture, acute event	0.0324	33%: clinically silent with no loss of quality 57%: quality of life reduced by 0.5 for 1 mo 10%: complete loss of quality for 1 wk, and then loss of quality by 0.5 for an additional 7 wk {= (0.57 × 0.5) + (0.1 × (1 × 1/52) + (0.5 × 7/25)}

ER, emergency room

Data from the National Osteoporosis Foundation.

TABLE 58-3. *Cost evaluations*

Event	Probability of event	Cost of event[a]	QALYs lost due to event
Hip fractures			
Probability of hip fracture	Varies with age, BMD, and risk factors (see Table 1)		
Consequences of hip fracture			
Acute care			
50–64	1	$11,337	0.0833
≥65	1	$9,322	0.0833
Death	0.06	$4,00	1.0000
Discharge to nursing home, stay <1 yr	0.2772	$6,810	0.3000
Discharge to nursing home, stay ≥1 yr	0.1426	$27,516	0.800
Discharge to home, then to nursing home, stay <1 yr	0.06	$22,930	0.6000
Rehabilitation or short stay hospital (9 days)	0.12	$6,183	0.02457
Readmitted (average 8 days)	0.08	$5,496	0.0219
Home care services (average 6 mo)	0.3	$1,518	0.2500
Nonmedical home care	0.17	$1,935	0.2500
Posthospitalization doctor visits (average eight visits)			
50–64	1	$712	0.0110
≥65	1	$536	0.0110
ER, ambulance			
50–64	1	$459	0.0027
≥65	1	$289	0.0027
Total expected cost and QALYs for 1st yr events			
50–64		$28,242	0.6183
≥65		$26,227	0.6183
Prefracture ADL and IADL per year	0.33	$0	0.0500
Some disability (cane or walker), per year	0.27	$600	0.1000
Moderate disability, per year	0.26	$2,400	0.3000
Nursing home, per year	0.07	$27,516	0.6000
Wrist fractures			
Probability of wrist fracture	Varies with age, BMD, and risk factors (see Table 1)		
Consequences of wrist fracture			
Acute treatment	1	$1,000	0.0404
Dependency, per year	0.02	$2,400	0.3000
Vertebral fractures			
Probability of vertebral fracture	Varies with age, BMD, and risk factors (see Table 1)		
Consequences of vertebral fracture			
Acute treatment	1	$1,000	0.0324
Pain, not very often or very severe	0.035	$0	0.500
Pain, very often or daily	0.03	$0	0.2000
Pain, severe or very severe	0.02	$0	0.5000
Dependency, per year	0.05	$2,400	0.3000
Mild deformity, per year	0.06	$0	0.1000
Moderate deformity, per year	0.08	$0	0.2500
Severe deformity, per year	0.02	$0	0.4000
Other fractures[b]			
Probability of other fracture		Varies with age	
Consequences of other fractures			
Acute treatment	1	$3,266	0.0604
Chronic consequences	Calculated from hip, wrist and vertebral fractures[b]		
Dollar value of QALY		$30,000	

ADL, activities of daily living; BMD, bone mineral density; IADL, instrumental activities of daily living; MD, medical doctor; QALY, quality-adjusted life year.

[a] 1992 dollars

[b] Costs and QALYs for "other" fracture estimated on assumptions that 5% are similar to hip fractures, 15% are similar to spine fractures, 42% are similar to wrist fractures, and 30% are half as severe as wrist fractures.

Data from the National Osteoporosis Foundation, Washington, D.C., 1998.

osteoporosis, specific etiologies are easily defined; in involutional osteoporosis, however, multiple etiologic factors may act independently or in combination in an individual patient to produce diminished bone mass. The presence of one or more of these factors in the elderly increases the risk of accelerated bone loss and subsequent fracture; the ''weighting'' of each of these risk factors in terms of relative importance as an etiologic factor is undefined, although estrogen depletion, calcium, vitamin D and testosterone deficiency, smoking, advanced age, positive family history, diminished peak bone mass, and diminished physical activity and history of previous fractures are important. Corticosteroid use is an important risk factor, as are such factors as excessive alcohol intake, cigarette smoking, use of antiseizure medication, and inappropriate thyroxine replacement.

Glucocorticoids reduce bone mass directly by inhibiting bone formation and indirectly by inhibiting the secretion of androgen in the pituitary–gonadal and adrenal systems. Additionally, a secondary hyperparathyroidism results from the induced limitation of calcium absorption by the intestine and calcium reabsorption in the renal tubule. Glucocorticoids are well known as a cause of osteoporosis, and their use should be carefully monitored, regardless of the method of administration. In senile osteoporosis in men, alcoholism and testosterone depletion must be considered as significant risk factors; unfortunately, however, the specific etiology of osteopenia and osteoporosis in men is difficult to delineate (14). Although there are no randomized tests showing that smoking cessation increases bone mineral density (BMD), smoking doubles a woman's risk of hip or vertebral fractures.

PATHOGENESIS

Osteoporosis is a heterogeneous disease with multiple causes. Although the pathogenesis of bone mass loss in secondary osteoporosis may be readily apparent (e.g., corticosteroid excess in Cushing's disease or the lack of muscle effect on bone with subsequent negative bone remodeling in paraplegia and disuse osteoporosis) (15–18), the exact pathogenesis of primary osteoporosis may be more difficult to define. However, the pathogenesis of primary osteoporosis may be approached from the standpoint of low bone mass and osteoporosis. Low bone mass may be due to multiple causes, including failure to achieve adequate bone mass at skeletal maturity (age 13 to 25 for women) and/or subsequent age-related and postmenopausal bone loss (19–21). Although low bone mass is principally associated with fracture, other determinants of fracture include the quality of the bone (trabecular architecture [21]), its ability to heal trabecular microfractures (22), and the propensity to fall. The latter determinant consists of the decreased neuromuscular coordination of the elderly (resulting in their inability to break a fall's impact) and such environmental factors as confusion and dizziness due to medications, the use of ''throw rugs'' with subsequent increased slips and falls, and so on. The propensity to fall in the elderly population may be of equal importance as bone quantity, owing to the increased number and severity of falls in this age group (23,24). To date, no studies have examined the differences in frequency, mechanism, or risk factors for falling between men and women.

The pathogenetic basis of inadequate bone mass, particularly in the elderly, also may be considered from the standpoint of cellular, hormonal, and tissue abnormalities.

CELLULAR ABNORMALITIES

Conclusive evidence of cellular abnormalities contributing to the pathogenesis of osteoporosis is lacking, principally owing to an inability to define abnormalities of bone cells (osteoblast, osteoclast, or osteocyte) specific for osteoporosis and separate from abnormalities of bone cells occurring with aging alone. For instance, it may be that failure of the osteoblast (the cell responsible for bone formation), due to either decreased cell number or decreased cell activity, may accompany advancing age but is not specific for osteoporosis.

HORMONAL ABNORMALITIES

Many hormonal agents may affect bone cell function and bone mass; however, although there are numerous age- and menopause-related alterations in the physiology of these hormones, a specific pathogenetic hormonal abnormality in osteoporosis (excluding the osteopenia associated with hypercorticism and hyperparathyroidism) has not been conclusively defined. However, estrogen deficiency is most frequently incriminated in the pathogenesis of postmenopausal osteoporosis in women, and testosterone deficiency is considered a major factor in men.

Indeed, estrogen deficiency of whatever etiology (including early oophorectomy (25) and a functional hypogonadism associated with strenuous exercise) (4,26) may be considered a prime risk factor for bone mass loss. The specific mechanism of estrogen's effect on bone is unclear. A reasonable hypothesis for estrogen's effect may be apparent in its ability to decrease bone resorption via a decrease in the responsiveness of the osteoclast (the bone cell primarily responsible for bone resorption) to endogenous circulating parathyroid hormone. Estrogen deficiency from any cause would therefore result in increased skeletal responsiveness to parathyroid hormone and increased bone resorption, a transient increase in the serum calcium level, and a resultant decrease in parathyroid hormone secretion. With such a decrease, a reduced production of the active form of vitamin D, $1,25(OH)_2$ cholecalciferol, would be expected, with a consequent decrease in calcium absorption (19). A number of these hormonal perturbations are demonstrated in osteoporotic populations; however, estrogen deficiency alone is an incomplete pathogenetic explanation for osteoporosis because all postmenopausal women are relatively estrogen deficient but not all develop osteoporosis. The serum level of immunoreactive parathyroid hormone increases with aging (27), and it is also increased in about 10% of postmenopausal osteoporotic women; in the latter group this increase in parathyroid hormone may be related causally to bone loss. However, in the majority of postmenopausal osteoporotic women, parathyroid hormone is normal or low compared with that of normal elderly women via the mechanisms noted previously, and in these patients the pathogenetic contribution to osteoporosis is unclear.

A number of vitamin D abnormalities occur with aging, although an abnormality specific for osteoporosis (rather than simply aging) has not been defined. Decreased levels of 1,25(HO_2) vitamin D are noted with increasing age. A postulated defect in the osteoporotic elderly person of the renal 25(OH)D 1a-hydroxylase enzyme in response to parathyroid hormone has not been conclusively proven (28,29). Nevertheless, calcium absorption does decrease with advancing age and is even lower in postmenopausal osteoporotic women.

A deficiency of the hormone calcitonin also could contribute to ongoing bone loss. Calcitonin inhibits the production and activity of osteoclast and thus decreases osteoclastic bone resorption. Serum levels of immunoreactive calcitonin are indeed lower in women than in men and also decrease with age; in addition, a decreased calcitonin secretion in response to calcium stimulation has been noted in some, but not all, osteoporotic populations (30,31). However, it is unlikely that calcitonin deficiency exerts a major pathogenetic effect in osteoporosis.

TISSUE ABNORMALITIES

Although cellular and hormonal abnormalities undoubtedly contribute to osteopenia and osteoporosis, the basic abnormality in all types of osteoporosis is a disturbance of the normal bone remodeling sequence at the tissue level. Therefore, to fully understand the pathogenesis of osteoporosis, knowledge of bone remodeling is necessary.

Bone is constantly turning over (remodeling); the skeleton is a reservoir for calcium, and remodeling provides calcium to the organism without sacrificing the skeleton. In addition, remodeling allows bone mass to respond to increased and decreased muscle activity (e.g., bone mass is increased in a tennis player's dominant arm). As noted in Figure 58-3, the initial event in bone remodeling with normal bone turnover is an increase in bone resorption, as mediated by the osteoclast. This event is typically followed within 40 to 60 days with an increase in bone formation, as mediated by the osteoblast. Bone resorption and formation are normally presumably homoeostatically "coupled": an increase or decrease in resorption produces a corresponding increase or decrease in formation, so that the net change in bone mass is zero. In postmenopausal osteoporosis, and possibly in senile osteoporosis as well (Fig. 58-3), bone resorption is thought to be increased over normal resorption levels, without a corresponding increase in bone formation, leading to a net loss in bone mass. In this case, bone remodeling is described as "negatively uncoupled." In other forms of osteoporosis, particularly that associated with corticosteroid-induced osteoporosis, a primary decrease in bone formation may occur (Fig. 58-3); the end result is the same in either situation, that is, a net loss of bone mass and presumably an increased risk for fracture. Abnormalities of bone remodeling at the tissue level will therefore contribute to the pathogenesis of the disease.

Genetic Abnormalities

Whether a genetic abnormality may contribute to low bone mass at various skeletal sites is currently unproven. An abnormality of the vitamin D receptor has been described, but not universally found in all studies (32). Several studies have investigated the importance of genetic factors for both peak bone mass and subsequent development of osteoporosis (33). Multiple genes are likely to be involved in both the attainment of bone mass and possible control of bone turnover (32–36).

DIAGNOSIS

The first clinical indication of osteoporosis, either primary or secondary, will usually be a fracture. Fractures of the proximal femur and the distal forearm will usually follow a

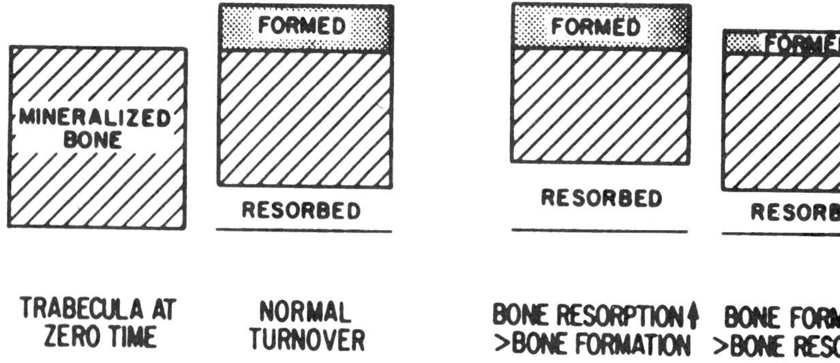

FIG. 58-3. Osteoporosis due to disruption of normal bone remodeling sequences.

fall or other significant trauma; patients will present with pain, and subsequent roentgenographic studies will confirm a fracture at these sites. Fractures of the vertebrae, however, may be associated with minimal trauma, and although usually associated with significant pain, they may occasionally be asymptomatic (see section on Management of Spinal Fracture).

An absolute diagnosis of osteoporosis is usually made when an atraumatic fracture occurs in the presence of low bone mass (most typically of the spine, femur, and/or distal ulna or radius). However, it is obviously of value from the standpoint of patient management to evaluate the patient at risk for fracture before a fracture occurs, as well as to determine the cause of the fracture in patients in whom a fracture has occurred. The diagnosis of osteoporosis is therefore approached from the standpoint of evaluating patients' potential risk of fracture based on low bone mass, as well as evaluating the patient who already has fractures. Diagnostic procedures, most frequently the radionuclide bone scan also may be used in evaluating the pain complex of osteoporosis.

Before describing such diagnostic evaluations, a brief outline of the noninvasive quantitation of bone mass is indicated. Because the amount of bone mass present is the principal determinant of fracture, a noninvasive technique for quantitating bone mass would consequently be of value not only in the diagnosis of osteoporosis, but in following a response to therapy.

Quantitating Bone Mass

There are a number of clinical parameters that positively correlate with bone mass; for example, paraspinal muscle strength in postmenopausal women and grip strength in premenopausal women and men. Whereas these are useful methods, they do not substitute for precise quantitation. A number of noninvasive procedures have been developed over the past 25–30 years to quantitate bone mass (bone density), including single- and dual-photon absorptiometry (SPA and DPA, respectively), quantitated computed tomography (QCT), and the current procedure of greatest clinical utility, dual-energy x-ray absorptiometry (DXA). Measurements of the peripheral skeleton (pDXA and pQCT) and technology using ultrasound (US) promise to be of value in this area as well. Such techniques quantitate bone mass at the spine, wrist, and hip, the principal areas usually involved in osteoporosis. In addition, DXA provides assessment of bone mass throughout the entire skeleton. The axial and appendicular sites noted above exhibit varying proportions of cortical (compact) and trabecular (cancellous) bone; it should be remembered that trabecular bone is metabolically more active than cortical bone. Trabecular bone appears to be preferentially altered in osteoporosis and is the type of bone most affected by medications used in treatment of osteoporosis. It also should be kept in mind that roentgenograms of the spine are relatively insensitive in quantitating bone mass because 30% to 35% of bone mass must be lost before roentgenographic demineralization is detected.

Attenuation or absorption of ionizing radiation by bone is the basic principle used in the majority of the noninvasive techniques (excepting US). A generally linear relationship exists between bone mass and radiation attenuation: the greater the amount of bone present, the greater the attenuation of ionizing radiation, and subsequently the less radiation quantitated in a detector.

The ideal noninvasive technique quantitates primarily trabecular bone at the spine and hip with an acceptable precision and accuracy; such procedures should be of reasonable cost and should be associated with low radiation exposure. Such techniques should be logistically simple to perform and, most importantly, should predict which patients are at risk for subsequent fracture, and should be readily applicable to assessing therapeutic response. The DXA technique currently satisfies these requirements to the greatest degree, as bone density measurements can be obtained within 30 seconds to 2 minutes with radiation exposure of approximately 10 millirads; one sixth the exposure of a chest x-ray with a 99% precision and approximate 97% accuracy. The Medicare reimbursement for this procedure in 1997 is approximately \$126. CT measurements of the spine are unique in their ability to provide an assessment of exclusively trabecular bone, but CT utilization is compromised by high radiation exposure and quality assurance difficulties. Peripheral measurements of bone density at the wrist, os calcis, and so forth (SPA, pDXA, pQCT) do measure primarily trabecular bone, but measure bone at skeletal sites that are subject to mechanical stresses and loading forces, as well as local hormonal interactions, which are quite different from those encountered at the spine and hip sites. Consequently, these peripheral measurements may have less clinical utility than axial (hip and spine) measurements. There is a consensus that this technology provides structural information in addition to density and has a sensitivity in prediction of hip fracture similar to hip BMD measured with DXA and superior to BMD of spine measured with DXA (37). Because of its low cost and lack of radiation exposure, it has great promise for clinical use.

When used appropriately, the noninvasive techniques (particularly DXA) are of definite value in the clinical evaluation of the osteopenic or osteoporotic patient. The clinical situations in which they may be used are as follows:

1. In selected perimenopausal and postmenopausal patients in defining their risk for subsequent fracture, when combined with the assessment and presence of historical risk factors (Table 58-4).
2. In screening for significant bone loss in conditions in which osteopenia is an accompanying manifestation, such as steroid-induced osteopenia, exercise-induced amenorrhea, eating disorders, and conditions causing chronic local or generalized immobilization.
3. In following response to treatment.

TABLE 58-4. *Etiologic factors contributing to the risk of osteopenia/osteoporosis*

1. Estrogen depletion
   a. Postmenopausal state (natural or artificial)
   b. Exercise-induced amenorrhea, anorexia nervosa
2. Calcium deficiency
   a. Inadequate calcium intake
   b. Malabsorption
   c. Lactose intolerance
3. Diminished peak bone mass at skeletal maturity; varies with sex (men > women), race (blacks > whites), and heredity
4. Diminished physical activity
5. Testosterone depletion
6. Aging (age >65 in men)
7. Leanness (adipose tissue is the major source of extragonadal estrogen production postmenopausally)
8. Alcoholism, smoking
9. Excessive coffee intake (>4–6 cups daily) and excessive dietary protein intake; increased calcium loss in the urine
10. Medications: corticosteroids, thyroid hormone, heparin

Data from the National Osteoporosis Foundation.

4. In research endeavors such as epidemiologic studies and clinical therapy trials.
5. In testosterone-deficient men.

Bone Markers

Serum and urine markers of bone resorption and formation are currently under evaluation as inexpensive diagnostic modalities to predict future risk of fracture, as well as to monitor therapy. In this sense the markers may be complementary to bone density assessment. The components of bone remodeling, bone resorption (BR), and bone formation (BF), can now be assessed with such urinary markers as pyridinaline/deoxypyridinal and n- and c-telepepticks (crosslinks for type I collagen), as well as such serum markers as estrocalcin and bone-specific alkaline phosphatase (BF). Early reports (38) suggest definite clinical utility of such markers of bone resorption as the n-telopeptide of type I collagen (NTX) for management of the patient with osteoporosis.

Diagnostic Evaluation of the Patient at Risk for Osteoporosis

The patient at risk (most typically the immediately postmenopausal woman concerned about her future risk for osteoporosis) requires a relatively brief evaluation, consisting of the following elements:

1. A brief history is taken to determine the presence of the risk factors noted in Table 58-4 and to exclude medical conditions resulting in the secondary osteoporoses noted in Table 58-1.
2. A brief physical examination is performed to exclude the secondary osteoporoses.
3. A minimal laboratory evaluation in this group (Table 58-5) might include determination of calcium, phosphorus, and alkaline phosphatase levels, plus a 2-hour spot urine (second morning void) for the n-telopeptide of collagen (NTX). However, the overall cost-benefit ratio of even these minimal procedures is unproven. In primary osteoporosis, results of laboratory tests typically are normal; the role of blood and urine tests (with the exception of the urinary NTX) is to exclude other diseases, and this can frequently be accomplished by the history and physical examination.
4. A measurement, noninvasively, of bone mass, usually at the spine (DXA), will be of value in the individual patient with positive risk factors. If such a bone mass measurement is low, more aggressive prophylactic therapy (i.e., estrogen) may be indicated; if a bone mass measurement at the spine is normal, activity and increased calcium intake may be sufficient.

Diagnostic Evaluation of the Patient with Osteoporosis (Fractures)

The patient with osteoporosis, who is most frequently female and in her late 50s or 60s, may present with one to five or six vertebral fractures and require a more thorough evaluation:

1. A complete history is obtained, again to determine the presence of risk factors and specifically to exclude medical conditions resulting in the secondary osteoporoses. This latter evaluation is most important because multiple myeloma, hyperparathyroidism, and hyperthyroidism are not uncommon in this elderly age group.
2. A more thorough physical examination is performed, but again primarily to exclude the secondary osteoporoses. Signs of hyperthyroidism or hyperparathyroidism; alveolar ridge resorption resulting in dental osteopenia

TABLE 58-5. *Laboratory evaluation in the diagnosis of osteoporosis*

Minimal	Maximal
Serum calcium Phosphorus Alkaline phosphatase (total)	The minimal tests plus the following: Ionized calcium iPTH 25-OH vitamin D $1,25(OH)_2$ vitamin D Protein electrophoresis Thyroid function tests SMA-12 studies (renal electrolytes, liver functions) Complete blood cell count Serum and urine markers of bone resorption and formation (urinary pyridinolines, telopeptides; serum bone specific alkaline phosphatase, osteocalcin) Iliac crest bone biopsy with tetracycline labeling

Data from the National Osteoporosis Foundation.

and missing teeth and dentures; proximal muscle weakness and discomfort in osteomalacia; and steroid excess should be kept in mind.

3. As noted in Table 58-5, a maximal laboratory evaluation in this group may be indicated; again, laboratory test results are frequently normal in primary osteoporosis, and the main function of the laboratory evaluations noted are to exclude other diseases, such as primary hyperparathyroidism with determination of ionized and total calcium, parathyroid hormone, and phosphorus values; multiple myeloma with protein electrophoresis and complete blood cell count; and possible vitamin D abnormalities with the vitamin D congeners noted. The urinary NTX measurements, and a 24-hour urine collection for calcium, normalized for creatinine, remains a mainstay of the evaluation of the patient with osteoporosis; a general assessment of dietary calcium adequacy and dietary calcium gut absorption and the exclusion of idiopathic hypercalciuria can be accomplished with this parameter. If the urinary calcium value is low, either inadequate calcium intake or absorption or a vitamin D abnormality must be considered; if the value is high, either dietary calcium excess or idiopathic hypercalciuria is a possibility. Lastly, the iliac crest bone biopsy is used primarily to exclude osteomalacia or other metabolic bone diseases, although such biopsies also can be used to define high and low bone turnover.
4. A noninvasive measurement of spine and hip bone mass will be of value as a baseline measurement to monitor response to therapy over time and to predict the future risk of fracture.

PHARMACOLOGIC TREATMENT OF BONE MASS DEFICIENCY (SKELETAL OSTEOPENIA/OSTEOPOROSIS)

Treatment of osteoporosis is directed at preservation or improvement of bone mass at the specific target sites. Because bone mass is the principal, although not the only, determinant of fracture, such preservation or improvement of bone mass is associated with a reduced risk of fracture.

To understand the rationale of the various therapeutic agents available for preserving or improving bone mass density or bone mass, some knowledge of bone remodeling is necessary. The cells responsible for bone resorption and bone formation are, respectively, the osteoclast and the osteoblast. Bone is constantly remodeling, with increase in bone resorption, typically followed within 30–45 days by the process of bone formation. With normal bone remodeling there is no net change in the amount of bone mass present.

In most forms of osteoporosis, however, a perturbation of bone remodeling occurs. Bone resorption increases over the normal levels, and bone formation does not compensate normally for this increase, with a net loss of bone mass overall.

The therapeutic agents available for the treatment and prevention of osteoporosis are those that can either decrease bone resorption or stimulate bone formation. The end result of each is the same: to preserve or improve bone mass, and thereby prevent fractures (Fig. 58-4).

As noted in Table 58-6, a number of U.S. Food and Drug Administration (FDA)-approved therapeutic agents are available to decrease bone resorption (antibone resorbers). There are also a number of therapeutic agents that increase bone formation (positive bone formers). As noted in Table

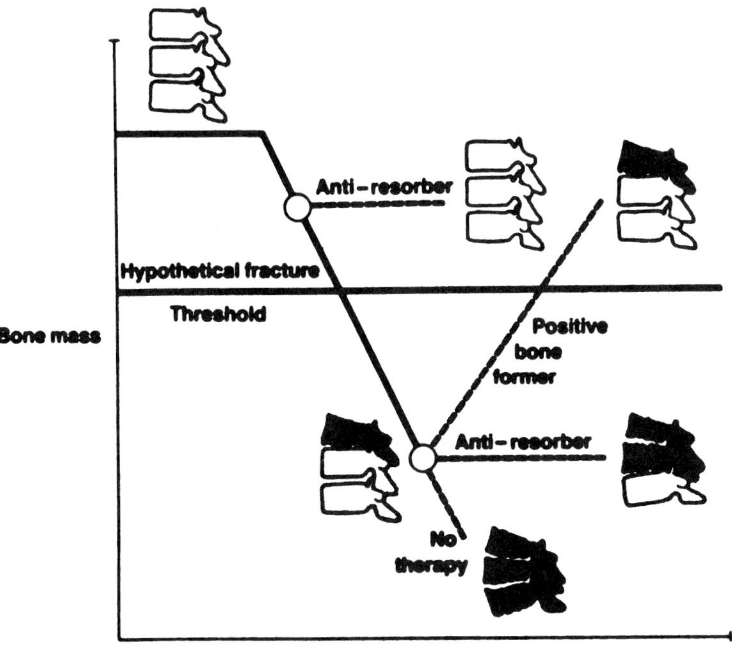

FIG. 58-4. Therapy for osteoporosis based on bone mass; darker vertebrae represent compression fractures. (Reprinted with permission from Chesnut CH. Treatment of postmenopausal osteoporosis. *Compr Ther* 1984; 10:41–47.)

TABLE 58-6. *Mode of action of specific osteoporosis therapies*

Decreased bone resorption ("anti-bone resorbers")
Calcium
Estrogen and selective estrogen receptor modulators (SERMs)
Calcitonin
Bisphosphonates
Increased bone formation ("positive bone formers")
Sodium fluoride[a]
Testosterone[a]
Anabolic steroids[a]
? 1,25 $(OH)_2$, Vitamin D[a]
Parathyroid hormone analogues[a]
? Exercise
Other
Thiazides (urinary calcium)[a]

[a] Experimental.

Data from the National Osteoporosis Foundation.

58-1, each of these agents remains experimental with the exception of exercise.

SPECIFIC THERAPIES (TABLE 58-7)

Calcium

Calcium is a mainstay of osteoporosis prevention and treatment; it is reasonable to recommend a minimal calcium intake of 1,000 to 1,500 mg/day in all perimenopausal and postmenopausal women. The calcium intake for men would presumably be 800 to 1,000 mg/day, although data supporting the benefit of such intake is unproven. Calcium is generally safe (in the absence of a history of previous kidney stones, or of idiopathic hypercalciuria), comparatively inexpensive, and logistically simple to ingest. Milk and dairy products and calcium supplements are acceptable sources of calcium.

The physiatrist should be mindful that immobilization occurring with hemiplegia and paraplegia, if coupled with excessive calcium intake, may result in elevated urinary calcium levels. A predisposition for kidney stones and nephrolithiasis may then be seen; in general, a urinary calcium excretion of up to 250 mg per 24 hours is acceptable in individuals without a history of kidney stones (39–43).

Vitamin D

Four hundred to 800 IU of vitamin D, administered in a multivitamin form, is reasonable treatment for osteoporosis; whether the active forms of vitamin D such as calcitriol are beneficial in osteoporosis is unproven. These agents all function to increase calcium absorption at the gut level, and use of such potent vitamin D analogs as calcitriol may result in increased risk for kidney stones or for hypercalciuria, nephrolithiasis, or even nephrocalcinosis. We must be mindful that many institutionalized and house-bound elderly patients are deficient in vitamin D and can benefit from its administration (42–46).

Estrogens

Estrogens are the mainstay of osteoporosis treatment in women. Data exist to indicate estrogens may preserve bone mass at multiple skeletal sites and prevent fracture. In addition, estrogens may prevent vasomotor symptoms as well as have a cardioprotective effect mediated through an effect on cholesterol and lipids and effects promoting relaxation of blood vessel walls. However, due to their potential for side effects (endometrial cancer if administered without progestational agents, and an apparent association with breast cancer if administered for a prolonged period after the menopause), compliance is disappointing despite the potential value of

TABLE 58-7. *Available therapies for osteoporosis*

Medication	Usual dosage[a]	Side-effects
Calcium	1,000–2,000 mg/day	Increased urinary calcium
Multivitamin with D_2 or D_3	400–800 IV/day	
Estrogen	0.625 mg/day (Premarin or equivalent) cycled 21/30 days with or without progesterone	Endometrial carcinoma, ?breast cancer, thromboembolic disease
Calcitonin (salmon)	200 MRC units/day nasal spray (Miacalcin)	Nasal irritation (rare)
Bisphosphonates (EHDP)[b]	(alendronate 5–10 mg/day; Fosamax)	Esophageal irritation
Selective estrogen receptor modulators	(raloxifene 60 mg/day; Evista)	Hot flashes, leg cramps

[a] Oral unless otherwise specified.

[b] Experimental therapy, not approved for use by the FDA.

Data from the National Osteoporosis Foundation.

TABLE 58-8. *Cost/benefit of pharmacologic treatment*

Scenario	Treatment	Annual cost[a]	HIp	Effectiveness[b] vertebra	Wrist	Other
1	Calcium + vitamin D	$50	≥10%	≥10%	≥10%	≥10%
2	Bisphosphonates	$740	50%	50%	50%	0
3	Calcitonin	$740	0	75%	0	0
4	HRT first 5 yr of treatment	$430	25%	50%	25%	25%
5	≥10 yr of therapy	$430	75%	75%	75%	75%

HRT, hormone replacement therapy.
[a]Includes office visits and any required tests.
[b]Reduction in fracture rate.
Data from the National Osteoporosis Foundation.

estrogens in preventing skeletal and cardiac disease. Research with newer "designer estrogens" offer promise of beneficial effects without the detrimental side effects.

Calcitonin

Calcitonin studies do indicate its ability to preserve bone density, and possibly to prevent fractures. It is currently available as not only an injectable therapeutic agent, but also by nasal spray. One of its benefits is its potential ability to decrease pain after acute compression fracture in the spine, presumably through a stimulation of beta-endorphins. Calcitonin has few side effects of significance (47–49).

Bisphosphonates

Available data suggest that bisphosphonates have the ability to preserve and increase bone mass at the spine and hip, as well as to prevent fractures at each of these skeletal sites. Spinal BMD increased by 6% to 8%, and femoral BMD demonstrated a 4% increase after 3 years of treatment. It is speculated that improvements in BMD achieved with short-term treatment will be maintained after treatment is stopped. Additionally, their use is also indicated as a preventive measure. Alendranate (Fosamax, Merck & Co., West Point, PA) accumulates and persists in bone, and the long-term effects of this are unknown. Alendranate must be taken at least half an hour before any food or drink in the morning, and the patient must maintain an upright position for that time to avoid the risk of esophageal ulceration. This effect is considered to be uncommon.

Etidronate, a second bisphosphonate, is considered to have a beneficial effect on bone mass. It is also used in hetertopic ossification. It may also be a value in the treatment of bone loss associated with paraplegia (Table 58-8).

Sodium Fluoride

Current data suggest that high-dosage sodium fluoride, which is a positive bone former, may actually worsen osteoporosis by increasing the risk of nonspinal fracture. Whether sodium fluoride in newer formulations, including a low-dose sustained-release preparation, will prove of benefit is unclear. Sodium fluoride must be viewed as an experimental therapy with some concerns regarding its overall benefit on osteoporosis (50–52).

Anabolic Steroids

These currently experimental agents may actually have a beneficial effect on bone mass; their side effects include liver toxicity, masculinization, and an increased cholesterol level. These side effects generally prohibit their overall usage in osteoporosis.

Testosterone

Testosterone may be of value in the treatment of osteoporosis in elderly men, particularly those with hypogonadism. Prostate and cholesterol status should always be checked when using testosterone.

Parathyroid Hormone

Parathyroid hormone, or fragments of the intact peptide molecule (e.g., the 1–34 fragment) may be of value in osteoporosis when administered parenterally. Such a usage is based on a presumed anabolic effect of parathyroid hormone when administered as a fragment, and it may be of value in established osteoporosis in terms of stimulating bone formation. However, the dosage remains to be defined.

Other Experimental Therapies

Estrogen agonist or antagonists such as reloxifene, tamoxifen, idoxifene, and droloxifene may have value in preserving bone mass in osteoporosis.

In theory, a number of cytokines may function as growth factors with potential benefit in osteoporosis (transforming growth factor beta, insulinlike growth factor, etc). However, their benefits as established by clinical trials are lacking at this time.

General Recommendations for Osteoporosis Therapy

The above pharmacology should be complemented by avoidance of life-styles known to result in bone loss, including cigarette smoking, excessive alcohol intake, a lack of exercise, a lack of calcium intake, and so forth.

The use of calcium, a multiple vitamin with vitamin D, and a consideration of the approved forms of therapy for osteoporosis (hormone replacement, a bisphosphonate such as alendronate, or nasal spray calcitonin) may definitely be of value in preventing progression of disease.

Patient Assessment for Rehabilitation

Rehabilitation management of the patient with osteoporosis depends on accurate diagnosis of the degree of bone loss, as well as a determination of the degree of frailty and propensity of the patient to fall. Osteoporosis is a disease that progresses from minimal impairment of the skeleton to bear stress to a disease characterized by frailty, deformity, chronic pain, and handicap. Individuals may therefore present to the physician with a spectrum of complaints warranting different degrees of investigation and intervention. Patients may be categorized into four groups (Fig. 58-5) ranging from those only requiring a prevention program to those requiring a comprehensive intervention program. Individuals presenting with risk factors, but without reduced bone mass, require education on osteoporosis prevention with an emphasis on reduction of risk factors and maintenance of bone mass. Others present with decline in bone mass and require diagnostic evaluation. These patients, who are most typically immediately postmenopausal women, require a full history to determine the number of risk factors as noted in Table 58-4 and to exclude medical conditions resulting in secondary osteoporosis noted in Table 58-1. Physical examination should focus on signs of secondary osteoporosis.

A laboratory evaluation in this group may include determination of calcium, phosphorus, and alkaline phosphatase levels plus a 24-hour urinary calcium-creatinine value; however, the overall cost-benefit ratio of even these minimal procedures is unproven. In primary osteoporosis, results of laboratory tests typically are normal; the role of blood and urine tests (with the exception of the urinary calcium value) is to exclude other diseases, and this can frequently be accomplished by the history and physical examination.

A noninvasive measurement of bone mass in the patient with positive risk factors is indicated. If bone mass measurement is low, more aggressive prophylactic therapy may be indicated; if a bone mass measurement at the spine is normal, activity and increased calcium intake may be sufficient, and specific exercise programs with proven osteogenic benefit should be initiated (53).

More commonly patients will present with significant risk factors, low bone mass, and fractures with acute or chronic disability. The first clinical presentation of osteoporosis, either primary or secondary, will usually be fracture. The pain associated with these fractures is usually severe but self-limiting. These fractures occur in one of three common sites: distal radius, proximal femur, and/or vertebra. Roentgenographic studies will confirm a fracture at these sites.

Progressive resistance exercises targeted to areas most commonly fractured can increase bone formation at those

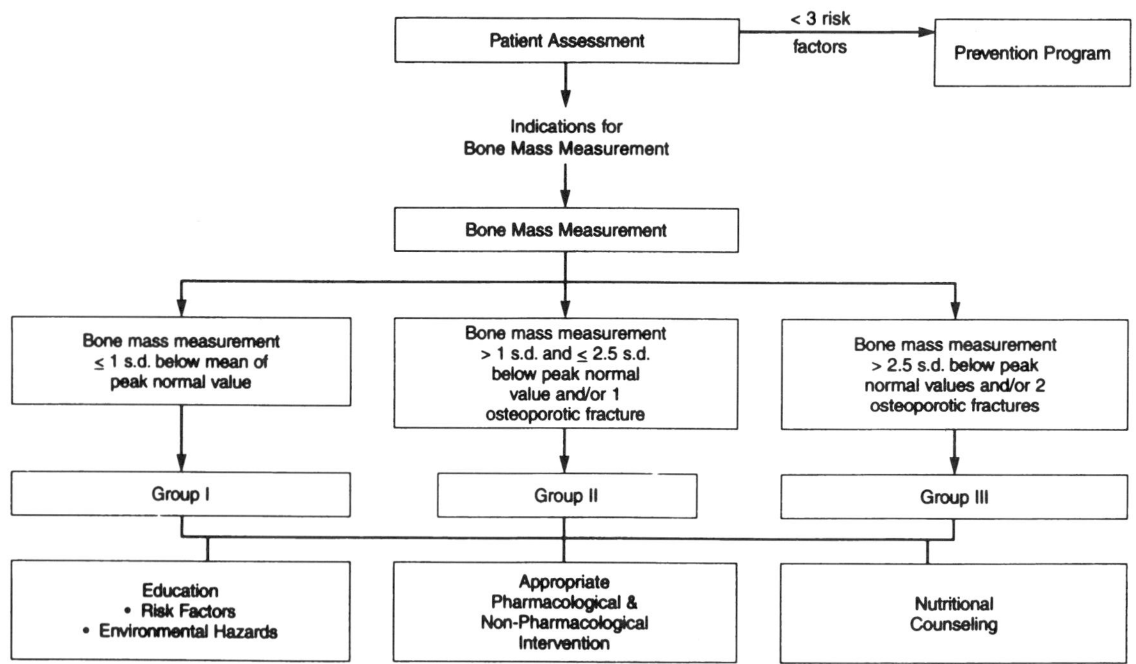

FIG. 58-5. Rehabilitation of the female patient with osteoporosis.

TABLE 58-9. *Physical medicine program for patients with osteoporosis*[a]

Group I	Group II	Group III
Stretching		
Pectoral	Same as group I	Same as group I
Shoulders abducted to 90° and hands behind head, hold for 30 sec, repeat 15×; increase time up to 1 min. Overhead extension incorporated—deep breathing.		
Manual stretching for soft tissue restriction		
Back extension strengthening		
Initially—done prone or sitting in a chair	Initially—sitting in a chair; may progress to prone position	Demonstration by professional
May continue on resistive equipment. Initially demonstrated by a trained professional	May continue on resistive equipment—supervised by a trained professional with a slow progression	May progress to supervised light resistance with slow progression
Instructed in daily home program or 3–5×/wk program on resistive equipment	Daily home program or 3–5×/wk of resistive equipment	Progress to daily home program
Isometric abdominal strengthening		
Lie supine with both knees bent, lift both legs to 90° of hip flexion and knee flexion, then lower, keeping back flat throughout. With hips and knees at 90°, lower and straighten legs, keeping back flat.	Lie supine with one knee bent and the opposite leg straight. Lift the straight leg 4 inches, hold 10 sec, do 15×. May sit or stand and contract abdominal and pelvic muscles.	Sit or stand and contract abdominal and pelvic muscles, hold 30 sec, repeat 15×. May lie supine as above if medically appropriate. Pelvic tilt
Upper extremity strengthening		
Theraband—2–4 lbs, moderate resistance (red, green). Shoulder—overhead extension Push-ups	Medium resistive exercise with 1–2 lbs or yellow Theraband. Wall push-offs (minimal impact) Putty hand exercises	Assistive range of motion exercises, progress to yellow Theraband. Monitored resistance wand exercise Putty hand exercise for postural hypotension
Weight bearing and lower extremity strengthening		
Walking Jogging/running Cross country ski machine Low-impact aerobics, step aerobics 30 min 3–5×/wk Leg presses	Acute—pool therapy Walking Nordic Track Low-impact aerobics, step aerobics 30 min 3–5×/wk Isometric quadraceps exercise and ankle pumps for isometric hypotension	Pool therapy Walking 30 min, 3–5×/wk Isometric quadraceps exercise and ankle pumps for postural hypotension
Balance training and transfer techniques		
Demonstrate unsupported standing balance Unsupported single limb stand for >30 sec Frenkel's exercise Fall prevention program	Same as group I Instruct on proper transfer activity Consider hip protectors Gait training with appropriate assistive device if needed	Same as group I, but goal for single limb stand to 15 sec Gait training with appropriate assistive device is needed Monitor transfer activity—bed, chair, toilet, tub, etc. Consider hip protectors
Proper lifting techniques		
All weight held close into body Use legs to lift, not back Avoid spinal flexion Ergonomics—work, home	Same as group I Precautuion with loads over 10 lbs	Same as group I Avoid loads over 10 lbs
Posture correction		
Self-correction—flat back exercises Wall stretch, chin tucks, shoulder rolls Manual stretching for soft tissue restriction	Same as group I, but may benefit from corset or PTS	Same as group II, but may require TLSO or molded body jacket
Pain control		
	Rest Hot packs, cold packs, TENS May benefit from PTS Abdominal corset or TLSO Pharmacologic Psychological support	Same as group II, may require facet and/or intercostal nerve block

PTS, posture training support; TENS, transcutaneous electrical nerve stimulation; TLSO, thoracolumbosacral orthosis.
[a] Commenced after stabilization of fracture. Precaution with comorbidity. © Francis J. Bonner, Jr.

sites (Table 58-9) but should be initiated only after consideration of the general fragility of the skeleton.

The evaluation of patients with low bone mass and fractures is more complex. Typically these patients are women in their late 50s or 60s, and they may present with more than one fracture. The history is an important part of the evaluation. The purpose of the history and physical examination is to exclude risk factors not only for osteoporosis but also for falling and medical conditions resulting in secondary osteoporoses. The later evaluation is most important because multiple myeloma, hyperparathyroidism, and hyperthyroidism are not uncommon in this elderly age group. There should be special focus on calcium intake, exercise, menopause, history of back pain, fractures, and a family history of osteoporosis. The amount of alcohol intake and smoking are both positively correlated with bone loss and should be noted (54). Bowel and bladder difficulties should be reviewed. Past medical history may show previous thyroid disorder, rheumatoid arthritis, diabetes mellitus, seizures, or liver disease. A review of current medications, especially antihypertensives, psychotropics, sedatives, analgesics, antihistamines, diuretics, and steroids should be included. The importance of the social history cannot be overemphasized, especially in the elderly woman who may require assistance in her living environment or nursing home placement.

A general physical examination should incorporate documentation of height and weight, station, posture, gait, and balance. Changes in height may be assessed by measuring arm span, which is usually within 1.5 inches of height. This measurement can provide a useful indication of progressive disease. Proprioception and general mobility of spine and joints of upper and lower extremities and an assessment of abdominal and spinal muscular strength should be made. The amount of kyphosis, chest expansion, and relationship of the lower ribs to the iliac crest should be recorded. Screening for vision and hearing are an important part of this examination (55,56).

As noted in Table 58-5, a maximal laboratory evaluation in this group may be indicated; again, laboratory test results are frequently normal in primary osteoporosis and the main function of the laboratory evaluations noted are to exclude other diseases, such as primary hyperparathyroidism with determination of ionized and total calcium, parathyroid hormone, and phosphorus values; multiple myeloma with protein electrophoresis and complete blood cell count; and possible vitamin D abnormalities with the vitamin D congeners noted. The 24-hour urine collection for calcium, normalized for creatinine, remains a mainstay of the evaluation of the patient with osteoporosis; a general assessment of dietary calcium and dietary calcium gut absorption and the exclusion of idiopathic hypercalciuria can be accomplished with this parameter; if the urinary calcium value is low, either inadequate calcium intake or absorption or a vitamin D abnormality must be considered; if the value is high, either dietary calcium excess or idiopathic hypercalciuria is a possibility. The urinary hydroxyproline and GLA (y-carboxyglutamic acid or osteocalcin, a noncollagenous bone protein measurable in serum) protein levels can monitor possible states of high bone remodeling, which may respond more to antiresorptive therapeutic agents; low remodeling as measured by a low GLA protein and urinary hydroxyproline would indicate an inactive and senescent bone, and such a condition may respond more favorably to bone-forming agents. Lastly, the iliac crest bone biopsy is used primarily to exclude osteomalacia or other metabolic bone diseases, although such biopsies can also be used to define high and low bone turnover.

These patients require imaging of symptomatic skeletal sites to ascertain the presence and degree of deformity associated with fractures. Magnetic resonance imaging is indicated if neurologic involvement is suspected. In severe vertebral collapse, retropulsed bone fragments may compromise neurologic function and cause increased pain. Bone mass measurement will be of value in determining the goals and intensity of the therapeutic exercise program. Additionally, this measurement will provide a baseline to monitor response to treatment over time.

Management of Osteoporosis-Related Disability

Osteoporotic fractures occur in virtually any bone. The loss of function resulting from these fracture can be severe, affecting mobility and ADLs, leading to loss of independence and institutionalization.

Patients with disability should be investigated for causes of osteoporosis and comprehensive treatment urgently initiated. Special attention should be directed to the possibility of calcium and vitamin D deficiency in the elderly, particularly those elderly residing in an institutional setting.

Psychological issues have been noted to contribute significantly to disability in the osteoporotic patient postfracture. Depression is the most common psychological problem identified in these patients. Anxiety, fear, and other emotional reactions are other psychological conditions affecting postfracture outcome. In a study of 200 women recovering from hip fractures, those with high depression scores postsurgery were more likely to experience poorer recovery of function (57). In another study of 100 women with osteoporosis-induced vertebral fracture, the women noted emotions as having greater importance than physical functioning, leisure and social activities, and ADLs (58). In this group, most reported fear of falling, fear of new fractures, frustration, anger, and feeling overwhelmed. Many of these patients suffered loss of self-esteem, isolation, vulnerability, and embarrassment related to physical appearance (59). Treatment should be directed at comorbidities, such as depression, as well as loss of bone mass.

Therapeutic exercise is an essential element of the rehabilitation program for patients with osteoporosis and should be tailored to the patient's level of fitness and anticipated propensity to fracture (Table 58-9). Objective measures such as bone density and manual muscle testing can provide some rationale to the assignment of a given patient to an entry level on a clinical pathway. Patients may be grouped according to the degree of impairment with or without disability. The beneficial effects of exercise are sought to attenuate bone loss and to increase strength and balance to prevent falls and avoid fracture.

The following five general principles should be considered when recommending therapeutic exercise (60):

1. *Principle of specificity*: Exercise should stress the specific physiologic system being trained. Activities selected should stress sites most at risk for fracture in patients without low bone mass. Patients with very low bone mass and multiple fractures need skeletal protection while building strength and increasing balance and flexibility. Activities involving spinal flexion should be avoided in this group of patients (61). Kerr has shown that the effects of exercise are site specific and result from progressive resistance exercise with maximum loading as opposed to an endurance regimen (62). Specifically, trochanteric and intratrochanteric bone mass was elevated by resistive hip exercise without an effect on the femoral neck. Exercise for osteogenesis may be prescribed for purposes of prevention of osteoporosis even for those with minimal reduction in bone mass. The goal of building bone through an exercise program is worthy but not applicable to all patients. Passive standing of spinal cord–injured patients has been a rehabilitative strategy to prevent bone loss as a result of mechanical loading. This strategy has been supported by clinical testing (60). There are those who not only have significantly reduced bone mass, but also muscle weakness and impaired balance yet remain quite functional. Many of the changes associated with aging have profound physical and clinical consequences. Age-related loss of skeletal muscle is referred to as sarcopenia (62a). This muscle loss may be reversed by exercise as shown by Fiatrone et al. (62b). Hence the necessity of differentiating goals of an exercise program for increasing bone mass and one for increasing muscle strength to prevent falls (62c).
2. *Principle of progression*: There must be a progressive increase in the intensity of the exercise for continued improvement. Applied loads must be within the capacity of the bone to sustain mechanical stress. Progression in resistance is important for goals of bone health and improved functional capacity (59,62).
3. *Principle of reversibility*: The positive effect of exercise will slowly be lost if the program is discontinued.
4. *Principle of initial values*: Those who initially have low capacity will have the greatest functional improvement from a given program (62a).
5. *Principle of diminishing returns*: There is a biologic ceiling to exercise-induced improvements in function. As this ceiling is approached, greater effort is needed to achieve minimal gain.

The program should incorporate both short and long-term goals, which are reviewed with the patient. Patient education concerning proper posture, body mechanics, increasing strength, and aerobic capacity are an essential component of short-term intervention. The patient needs to understand that osteoporosis is a disease that is progressive and if unchecked can cause severe disability. Prevention of falls and fractures through an ongoing program that maintains proper nutrition, strength, and aerobic capacity is coupled with adequate support for the spine, pain management, and psychological support as objectives for long-term goals.

Vertebral Fracture

The osteoporotic patient may have acute or chronic back pain related to recent compression fractures or to mechanical derangement of the spine such as kyphosis, paraspinal muscle spasm, spinal arthritis, or costal–iliac impingement syndrome. Signs and symptoms of vertebral fracture may be mimicked by neoplasm, herpes zoster, polymyalgia rheumatica, pancreatic disorders, and abdominal aortic aneurysm. It is important to investigate and treat the pain complaint promptly. As the patient experiences pain over prolonged periods, they may suffer consequences such as depression, sleep disturbance, and functional decline.

Acute vertebral fracture may occur with little discomfort and poor localization of pain with only complaints of generalized lumbosacral ache. Usually the pain is severe and most intense at the fracture level. It often follows a minor injury or physical activity such as coughing or sneezing that ordinarily would not be expected to cause a fracture (59). These fractures may occasionally be asymptomatic but are usually associated with sharp pain that increases with movement and is alleviated with bed rest. Severe and frequently disabling pain may persist for 2 to 3 weeks and then continue with decreased severity for 6–8 weeks, usually subsiding at this time until the next fracture occurs. The persistence of pain beyond 6 months at the site of a previous vertebral fracture should suggest causes other than osteoporotic fracture as a reason for the pain complaint, and the etiology of back pain in this group should be reconsidered.

Clusters of fractures may occur in patients ranging in age from 50 to 65 years of age in which there is a rapid progression from one to six spinal fractures. The cause of this most aggressive form of osteoporosis is unclear but may be associated with an accelerated trabecular bone loss soon after menopause.

It is unlikely that osteoporosis produces acute severe pain in the absence of a fracture, although it is possible that painful vertebral microfractures of individual trabeculae may develop. Such microfractures may not be visible on a roentgenogen but may be noted on a radionuclide bone scan.

After a number of fracture events in the spine, the collapsed and/or anteriorly wedged vertebrae may lead to deformity of the back, with subsequent kyphosis (the typical "dowager's hump" deformity), loss of height, and a chronic back pain in either the mid-thoracic or lumbosacral area, which is undoubtedly secondary to mechanical deformity and paraspinal muscle spasm. This chronic back pain is typically of lesser intensity than the pain associated with the acute fracture event; it radiates laterally, is associated with exertion, and is relieved to a certain extent with rest. In addition, with the progressive spinal deformity and height loss, an abdominal protuberance and resultant gastrointestinal discomfort (bloating and constipation) may occur, as well as some degree of pulmonary insufficiency secondary to thoracic cage deformity. In some severely affected patients, the spinal kyphosis may be sufficient to produce a painful rubbing of the lower ribs on the iliac crest.

Although chronic back pain is a common complaint of the elderly, the extent to which osteoporosis contributes to this pain is questionable. In a study involving 242 women 55 years of age, 30% had complaints of back pain, but there was no relationship between this pain and spinal curvature. In a group of older women (60–79 years of age), back pain affected a similar 30% but was twice as likely to occur in women with kyphosis or a loss in height exceeding 4 cm (64). There is not an absolute relationship, however, between osteoporosis and kyphosis. It is recognized that kyphosis may be secondary to chronic poor posture and age-related changes in muscle, ligaments, and intervertebral discs. Seventy percent of women over 60 years of age may demonstrate kyphosis without evidence of vertebral deformity. With aging, there is a progression of kyphosis (65), but back pain does not appear to be associated with the kyphosis unless vertebral deformity is such that there is a reduction in the height of the vertebral body greater than 4 standard deviations (SD) from normal (66).

Investigations into causes of back pain using bone scintigraphy showed a high incidence of facet joint disease in osteoporotic women with previous vertebral fracture. Abnormalities were noted in association with collapsed vertebral bodies in a majority of these women, but few showed evidence of degenerative disc disease. The most prominent abnormalities were noted in the facet joint at the level of the vertebral collapse. Smaller lesions were commonly found in the facets above and below the level of collapse (67).

Complaints of back pain in the patient with previous osteoporotic vertebral fractures may be associated with or due to other causes unrelated to osteoporosis. Back pain with neurologic symptoms in the lower extremities may occur when vertebral fracture results in retropulsed fragments (67).

Loss of height resulting from vertebral collapse may cause the lower ribs to impinge on the iliac crest (68), leading to pain from mechanical irritation. This pain may be located in the lower back and may radiate into the leg. Known as the costal–iliac impingement syndrome, its diagnosis may be made by palpating the lower ribs and the iliac crest. Lateral bending and rotation elicit pain and confirm the diagnosis. Injection of lidocaine into the margin of the iliac crest and lower ribs allows for performance of these maneuvers with markedly decreased pain and serves to readily confirm the diagnosis. Further injections into these areas with sclerosing material may give more prolonged relief (53). The use of a wide, soft belt has been reported as beneficial in relieving symptoms by allowing the ribs to avoid contact with the iliac crest by sinking into the pelvic cavity. In severe cases, resection of the lower ribs has been beneficial (69).

Again, the history and physical examination is essential to the evaluation of the patient with vertebral fracture. Standard radiographs of the spine are indicated, and other imaging studies may be warranted. The radionuclide bone scan can be used in the diagnostic evaluation of back pain, as well as in determining the current metabolic activity of the disease. Increased radionuclide accretion at the site of a recent fracture (usually a vertebral body, but also the hip) indicates ongoing bone formation and bone healing; normal radionuclide accretion indicates that healing is complete and that the metabolic activity of the disease at that site is normal. A positive scan correlates well with the presence of acute pain, indicating the need for continued aggressive therapy.

The osteoporotic patient complaining of acute pain resulting from vertebral fracture should be managed with rest, immobilization of fracture site, and analgesic agents. Because these vertebral fractures generally heal well, management is directed at pain control and providing adequate rest and immobilization of the fracture site. The unwanted side effects associated with analgesic agents may complicate treatment. Pharmacologic interventions used for acute fractures consist of codeine, morphine, and other narcoticlike analgesics. Within 1 to 2 weeks, other analgesic agents such as salicylates and acetaminophen should be used in conjunction with other pain therapies (70,70a). These compounds are to be used sparingly and with extreme caution. Pain management incorporating rest, orthoses, and physical agents should be used primarily, with pharmacologic agents serving as adjunctive therapy. Activities that aggravate the pain should be avoided. The use of a sheepskin, egg crate, or gel flotation pad on the mattress frequently enhances patient comfort. During the initial treatment involving bed rest, a stool softener and laxative will help prevent straining during defecation. Use of a bedside commode may prove easier than a bed pan and requires less energy expenditure. With the initiation of bed rest, a program of progressive activity is indicated. Graduated bed activities progressing to sitting in bed, bedside sitting, and progressive ambulation should be provided by the therapist.

Pain management of chronic back pain associated with osteoporotic vertebral fracture should include a program of strengthening paravertebral, abdominal, and gluteal muscles and programs to improve balance, flexibility, and provide postural correction. Relief of stress on the spine through use of proper body mechanics is encouraged. In severe cases, an orthosis can be of benefit. An assessment of ADLs may lead to the use of other techniques and devices that can help the patient to avoid situations that aggravate pain. The strategic placement of a pillow or towel roll behind the back frequently increases sitting tolerance in patients with kyphosis.

Physical agents such as heat, ice, transcutaneous electrical nerve stimulation, and acupuncture can be of benefit. Nonnarcotic agents such as ibuprofen, acetaminophen, and aspirin should be used sparingly and with knowledge of potential side effects. Calcitonin has been reported to be of benefit in the treatment of bone pain resulting from osteoporotic fractures (71,72). Hypnosis, behavioral modification, biofeedback, and counseling have been of benefit in treatment of chronic pain. When vertebral fractures are associated with significant deformity, injection of sclerosing agents into the facet joint at the fracture site, as well as into the joints above and below, may be of additional benefit.

A multidisciplinary team approach is beneficial to ensuring maintenance of function in this population. Nonpharmacologic interventions should be preferentially used to manage chronic back pain. Chronic back pain in the osteoporotic patient is managed by having the patient assume adequate recumbent bed rest for periods of 20 to 30 minutes twice daily. This program is supplemented by encouraging adjustments in life-style, medications, physical agents, orthoses, and other therapies considered useful for chronic pain. These interventions are used after ruling out other causes of back pain in the elderly and after assessment of the degree that depression is contributing to the symptoms.

HIP FRACTURE

Hip fractures may be divided into three categories according to the anatomic area in which they occur. Intracapusular fractures are located distal to the femoral head but proximal to the greater and lesser trochanters. These fractures frequently disrupt the blood supply to the femoral head and are therefore associated with nonunion and osteonecrosis of the femoral head (73). Fractures occurring between the greater and lesser trochanter are not associated with the complications seen in the intracapsular region. However, they are associated with malunion and shortening of the leg as a result of osteoporotic bone and the deforming forces exerted on this area of the proximal femur. Subtrochanteric fractures occur just below the lesser trochanter and are responsible for only 5% to 10% of all hip fractures. Intertrochanteric and femoral neck fractures occur about equally and together account for 90% of hip fractures. Because most of these fractures result from a fall, radiographs also should exclude fracture of the pubic ramus, acetabulum, and greater trochanter. The pain also may be due to or aggravated by a trochanteric bursitis. Most of these patients will require operative management. However, nonambulatory, institutionalized patients with dementia and minimal discomfort may be more suitable for nonoperative management. This is particularly true when considering the goal of treatment to return the patient, pain free, to his or her previous level of mobility.

Rehabilitation should begin on the first day after surgery with a progressive ambulation program. Special precautions to prevent deep venous thrombosis should be taken. Early mobilization beginning with moving from bed to chair is appropriate. Specific medication to prevent venous thrombosis is indicated. Most patients may begin walking on the first or second postoperative day. Walking with an assistive device should be promoted early with as much weight bearing as possible. In cases where the stability of the fixation is questionable, weight bearing may be modified to minimize the possibility of fixation failure.

The risk of death after a hip fracture is increased for the first 6 to 12 months after the fracture (74–76). The morbidity rate after 1 year ranges from 14% to 36% (77,78). The increased morbidity is associated with elderly men with psychiatric problems (79), institutionalization, surgical intervention before stabilization of coexisting medical conditions, poorly controlled systemic disorders, and complications of surgery (80).

The proportion of patients discharged to home after hip fracture ranges from 40% to 90% (81,82). However, there are many who remain institutionalized. Factors associated with permanent institutionalization are needed for assistance with ADLs; age greater than 80 years; lack of involvement of family members; and insufficient physical therapy at a skilled nursing facility (81). From our experience with a hospital-based comprehensive rehabilitation unit, over 90% of these patients are discharged to home. This has clearly been influenced by the selection process, but is directly related to the scope and intensity of rehabilitation services and the ability to manage acute exacerbation of comorbidities because of the close geographic relationship with an acute medical–surgical hospital. Factors associated with discharge to home are the presence of another person in the home, ability to walk independently before the fracture, the ability to perform ADLs (81,82). Of these, ADLs can be most influenced by a rehabilitation program, and the best predictors of this outcome are absence of pre-existing dementia, being of younger age, and being involved in a social network (83).

Recent trends in health-care delivery have challenged resources and have made rehabilitation strategies difficult to implement. The emphasis on shortened hospital stays has had a negative effect on patients with hip fractures. The number of patients remaining in a nursing home after 1 year is now much higher than before the initiation of the prospective payment system (75,82). There are increased cost to insurers and to patients as a result of the acceleration of patients through a system of care that does not account for patients individuality, degree of impairment or disability, existing comorbidities, and social resources. The largest cost to the patient is their loss of independence as a direct result of denial of access to the proper scope and intensity of rehabilitative services.

These patients require the care of a physiatrist, physical therapist, and occupational therapist, as well as of nurses and social workers (84–85). The benefits of the multi-disciplinary approach have been documented as resulting in fewer transfers for acute emergencies, fewer postoperative complications, improved ambulation at the time of discharge, and fewer discharges to nursing homes (81–83).

WRIST FRACTURES

Fractures of the wrist are the most common type of fractures in women before 75 years of age. These fractures increase in number after menopause, and although they usually occur in relatively healthy active women, they may be the first sign of an underlying problem such as low bone mass. The primary goal of treatment is return of pain-free, normal function of the hand and wrist. Initial casting usually extends above the elbow and restricts movement of both elbow and wrist. During the period of immobilization, usually 6 to 8 weeks, strength and flexibility should be maintained in the upper extremities. Active and passive range of motion exercises should be provided for the fingers and shoulder on the affected side.

These exercises to hand, wrist, forearm, elbow, and shoulder should be continued after cast removal. At this time, a local wrist splint may be used to support and protect the wrist. As a result of the wrist fracture, particularly on the dominant side, the patient may require assistance with ADLs such as getting dressed, combing hair, and brushing teeth.

BACK SUPPORTS AND BRACING IN OSTEOPOROSIS

The degree and types of skeletal pain and disability among patients with osteoporosis presents a complicated challenge to provide adequate mechanical support for the spine (87). When many solutions are available to answer a given problem, it usually means that there is no single good solution. Such is the case with mechanical supports for the osteoporotic spine. These orthoses may be used for pain relief and stabilization of the spine for both the acute fracture and long-term care. The use of an orthosis in the treatment of acute spine fracture may reduce pain and immobilize the spine, thereby promoting healing. Use in the long-term treatment of the osteoporotic spine may assist weakened spinal musculature, alleviate chronic pain, and prevent further fracture. Additionally, orthoses may be prescribed for special situations where it is anticipated that vertebral loads may be increased.

The success of spinal bracing in accomplishing the desired result depends on the goals of treatment. When prescribing a brace or a corset one must possess a general understanding of the principals of bracing as well as a clear understanding of the indications and hazards associated with the use of that particular orthotic device. One also must possess a healthy understanding of the types and causes of vertebral fractures as well as the areas most at risk for further fractures.

Vertebral compression fractures associated with osteoporosis most commonly occur in the lower thoracic and upper lumbar vertebrae (88). They involve the anterior portion of the spine, the vertebral body. This portion of the spine is made of predominantly cancellous bone (65% to 75% trabecular and 25% to 35% cortical). This differs from other parts of the body, for example, the mid-radius, which is about 95% cortical bone in content. Osteoporosis of aging preferentially decreases the density of trabecular bone by about 40% by 75 years of age (89).

It is also important to remember the function of the low thoracic and upper lumbar spine. The articulation of the thoracic vertebrae with the ribs as well as the overlapping of the spinous processes significantly limit the mobility of the spine in flexion and extension. However, rotation is relatively free in the thoracic spine. The lumbar spine has quite limited lateral flexion and axial rotation secondary to the relatively vertical orientation of the facet joints. In this region of the spine, flexion and extension account for the majority of movement. One must also understand the kinematic function or "coupling" that occurs in the thoracolumbar spine (90). While remembering these functions of the spine, it is important to remember that movements which cause loading of the vertebral bodies will most likely lead to fracture if the density is such that it will not support the increase in forces placed upon it. Hence, bracing to help prevent this additional loading of the vertebral bodies must restrict flexion, which is known to load the anterior bodies. This addresses one goal of bracing. Additional goals of bracing are to decrease pain, increase function, and prevent soft-tissue shortening, which may contribute to deformity.

There are several commonly used orthoses for stable, osteoporotic vertebral fractures. They are a postural training support (a weighted kypho-orthosis), a thoracolumbar support, and a lumbosacral or thoracolumbosacral orthosis (TLSO). It should be noted that all orthoses work on a principle of a three-point force system. It is generally accepted that the more rigid orthoses are used for acute thoracolumbar fractures, whereas nonrigid orthoses have been used more commonly in management of stable fractures and painful conditions. All of the orthoses described may not adequately prevent gravity-related axial compression, which may ultimately result in fracture.

The posture training support (PTS) has been described as an inexpensive, unobtrusive device that promotes improvement in posture and decreases back pain whether by producing a force posteriorly below the inferior angles of the scapulae or by acting as a proprioceptive reinforcement (91). A TLSO is a long spinal orthosis that provides virtual fixation from the pelvis through the shoulders. The lumbosacral region of the spine is thought of as one of the most difficult areas of the body to immobilize. Therefore, it is felt that the lumbosacral orthoses should not be relied upon to immobilize this area. Although the TLSO affords the greatest immobility, it is cumbersome and hot, and there is a great deal of noncompliance associated with its use. Custom-fitted TLSOs are also more expensive than the PTS. Something as simple and inexpensive as an abdominal corset has been used to help decrease pain and increase function after an acutely painful vertebral fracture. This is thought to work by increasing the intra-abdominal pressure and thereby placing an anteriorly directed force on the vertebral bodies. Again this can be hot, but it is not as bulky as a TLSO and can be worn under clothing.

Kaplan et al. recently conducted a pilot study to compare the effects of back supports on back strength (92). Women at least 40 years of age with a diagnosis of osteopenia or osteoporosis were recruited for this study. They were randomly assigned to one of three groups: postural exercises alone, postural exercises and a conventional thoracolumbar support, and postural exercise and the use of the PTS. It was found that compliance was poor among the group that wore the conventional thoracolumbar support. Both the group that wore the PTS and the group that did only the exercises increased their back strength significantly. This would imply that the more rigid orthosis, the conventional thoracolumbar orthosis, inhibited strengthening of this area. This is a known complication of rigid bracing across any joint.

Lumbosacral orthoses are frequently prescribed for low back pain from a variety of causes, including those stemming from vertebral fractures. The etiology of this decrease in pain is thought to be from restricting movement via both mechanical and sensory feedback, and it also may generate heat, pressure, or a massagelike effect that may be soothing for muscles that are in spasms. Some people also may experience a placebo or psychological effect. The use of corsets may relieve pain by increasing hydrostatic support of the spine through increased intra-abdominal pressure.

Continued use of spinal orthotics is generally discouraged because of the increased likelihood of weakening or atrophy of the trunk muscles. There is also reduced spinal mobility noted in long-term wearers. Continued orthotic use may in time lead to an increased likelihood of fracturing of the vertebral bodies secondary to the weakness of the supporting musculature caused by inactivity.

In summary, bracing will be of value at certain times and in certain conditions associated with osteoporotic fractures. When able, it is best to utilize one's own muscles to support the skeleton. However, bracing is extremely useful to aide the patient who is in too much pain to function without support and is also helpful to prevent soft-tissue deformity and excessive loading of the vertebral bodies.

Fall and Fracture

In the past, much attention has been directed to the degree of mineralization of bone as a risk factor for fracture. And it is likely that the degree of mineralization does predict risk of fracture. It is further likely that most of these fractures occur from the trauma of a fall. Nonetheless, supported antecdotal reports of spontaneous fracture are common when discussions arise concerning mechanisms of hip fracture (93). One study demonstrated that out of 11% spontaneous fractures, 25% occurred as patient's were getting up or sitting down and 60% occurred during simple ambulation (94). In another survey, 24% of patients reported falling as a result of the leg giving out (95). These studies support the position that fractures of the proximal femur can be the result of muscle forces acting on the hip exceeding the mechanical ability of the femur to withstand stress. It should be obvious that these hip fractures have multifactorial causes, and interventions must address not only increasing bone mineral density at the hips but also include increasing muscular strength, balance, and flexibility and reducing the forces of impact when a fall occurs (63). Of the utmost importance in the success of such a program is the educational component focusing on reduction of risk factors for falling. A fall prevention program consists of these elements together with an educational component focusing on reduction of risk factors for falling.

Given the enormous attention to methods of increasing bone density, there has been relatively little in the scientific literature that fully examines the mechanisms of the fall. The work of Hayes and Cummings has contributed much to the understanding of these mechanism (93,96–99). The severity of the fall is itself an independent risk factor for hip fracture (100) and is related to many factors, including the direction of the fall and the specific anatomic location of major impact (98). Whereas young adults tend to fall to the side or backwards, the elderly tend to fall sideways or drop in place. This is especially true in individuals with unsteady gaits (96). It is these falls to the side that result in major impact forces that greatly exceed the mechanical strength of the proximal femur and therefore result in fracture. The direction of a fall is a major risk factor for fracture, and these falls that cause impact to the hip raise the fracture risk considerably, but our own experience shows that some falls will cause fracture regardless of the degree of mineralization of the hip.

In a study of 336 elderly community dwellers, about 10% of falls occurred during acute illness but also occurred in the presence of environmental hazards (101). The risk of falling appears to increase linearly with the number of risk factors present. Risk factors for falling include decreased vision, sedative use, polypharmacy, cognitive impairment, lower extremity disability, palomental reflex, foot problems, peripheral neuropathy, and balance and gait abnormalities (101,102). Sedative use, particularly polypharmacy, is associated with falling independent of other risk factors. Benzodiazepines, phenothiazine, and antidepressants are used frequently in the elderly for dementia and depression, and their use is associated with increased falling. This is particularly true of the longer acting medications. Other medication such as diuretics and antihypertensive agents are also associated with increased risk of falling, possibly due to postural hypotensive effects.

The elderly populations have a general awareness and fear of falling. They are particularly fearful of not being able to get up after a fall (103). Comparing fallers who were able to get up with those who were not, Tinitti found that those unable to get up were more likely to suffer permanent decline in ADLs. This group was more likely to be hospitalized and had a higher mortality rate. The characteristics of those unable to get up included age of over 80 years, depression, and problems with balance and gait (103). In a separate study of fall intervention, 13 of 36 patients sustained fractures over a period of 1 year. It therefore seems reasonable that the elderly should be fearful of falling. Up to 20% of elderly avoid certain activities because of this fear.

For a fall to result in hip fracture, there must be impact

near the hip that is not reduced by body mechanisms or absorbed by soft-tissue structures. The fall itself may be divided into four phases: (99,104):

1. Instability phase, where balance is loss
2. Descent phase
3. Impact phase
4. Postimpact phase

A fall prevention program should address these four phases of a fall and present interventions at each level (104). General conditioning exercises, appropriate provision of assistive devices, adequate shoe wear, modification of medications, and attention to other risk factors for falling are targeted at preventing the instability that results in loss of balance (104a). Recently, a mobility system in which the patient is secured in a suspended harness has been used with some success in preventing falls (105). Tinnetti et al. have demonstrated the effective though costly benefit of a multifactorial risk factor abatement strategy resulting in 12% fewer falls at a cost of around $12,000 per individual in 1995 (103). There is ample other evidence of the benefit of osteogenic exercise programs for the purposes of building bones. However, these programs must be maintained for continued benefit to accrue to bone mass and muscle strength (106). There are several important determinants that govern the forces applied to the femur as the result of falling. These include the person's weight, thickness of subcutaneous tissue, height of the fall, configuration of the body during the fall, velocity at which the hip strikes the impact surface, and nature of the impact surface. Falling to the side raises the risk of hip fracture approximately sixfold compared with the threefold increase in relative risk associated with a decrease of 1 SD in hip bone mineral density (93,95–98). It is likely that contraction of the quadriceps and other muscles of the lower limb are a very effective means of reducing velocity at impact and reducing force at the proximal femur in falls to the side. Exercise programs aimed at increasing lower extremity strength may therefore prevent hip fracture by reducing fall severity (54–56,62,102,103,105–110). Low body weight and low body mass index are associated with an increased risk of hip fracture in elderly men and women (105, 107,108,111). Body weight and bone mass are positively correlated, as is body weight with increased subcutaneous tissue. The impact force most closely correlated with the individual's weight. However, the velocity on impact is most associated with height. So even though an individual may be heavier and the resultant force of impact may be more, that individual may well have more padding over the trochanter and stronger bone, thereby preventing fracture.

Recognition that increases in soft-tissue thickness around the hip substantially reduces peak force to the trochanter has led to the development of padding for the hip. Fractures have been prevented in women wearing hip protectors, and Lauritzin concludes that the use of hip protectors could reduce fracture by 53% (109). Problems with hip protectors relate to patient compliance, which was reported at 25% and to problems related to the design of the protector. These pads have been designed in two primary configuration. First is a simple pad that covers the trochanter and reduces impact force by absorbing energy in the pad material. The second form of pad is based on shunting energy from the fall away from the trochanter (110). This pad is designed in an inverted U shape and is filled with a colloidal-like substance that hardens on impact, thereby shunting forces away from the trochanter. This particular pad demonstrates a 68% reduction in peak force delivered to the hip with impact. Pads tested to date provide some degree of protection, even though some do not reduce femoral impact force to below fracture threshold.

Architectural modification of the flooring surface offers an approach to impact reduction that seems worth exploring, particularly in residential health-care facilities and housing projects for the elderly (54). Because protection is automatic, their use does not require changes in individual behavior. When compared with linoleum flooring, a thick pile carpet with underpad can reduce impact from a fall by 23%. This solution does seem impractical in light of the difficulties in ambulation presented by rugs of this design. Other flooring systems that provide impact reduction without presenting an obstacle to ambulation are being investigated.

SUMMARY

Physical medicine and rehabilitation strategies can be of value in the management of the osteoporotic patient and are currently underused. These strategies are used to reduce disability resulting from impairments in bone mass and structure, muscle strength, and coordination.

Osteoporosis is a disease that is defined by an intermediate outcome (BMD) as opposed to a health outcome (fracture). In this regard, it is similar to conditions such as hypertension, diabetes mellitus, hypercholesterolemia, and osteosclerosis. The decision to test for BMD should be based on an individual's risk factors and treatments being considered. It is important to ensure that adults receive between 100 and 1,500 mg of calcium per day and that those at risk receive 400 IU to 800 IU of vitamin D daily. Exercise can help prevent osteoporotic fractures through its osteogenic effects and prevention of frailty, which leads to falls.

Most hip fractures are associated with falls. It has been shown that interventions can reduce the risk of falling and the incidence of hip fracture. These interventions consist of exercise programs, padding of the hip, ensuring proper foot wear, appropriate environmental adaptation, and adjustment of medications contributing to polypharmacy, particularly sedatives, antidepressants, diuretics, and antihypertensive agents. Although not proven by clinical trials, clinical practice has shown the benefits of assistive devices, such as canes, walkers, and wheelchairs, for those with disturbed balance or deficits in gait.

The deformity associated with kyphosis is apparent, and when the kyphosis is the result of vertebral fractures, pain might contribute to disability. Various physical medicine and rehabilitation strategies are used to treat these conditions. Other devices, such as corsets and assists (PTS) are useful in unloading forces from vertebral fracture sites, immobilizing the recently fractured spine, and promoting extension of the thoracic spine. These devices have specific indications and are associated with varying compliance. However, they are widely used and considered part of the armamentarium in the treatment of vertebral fractures and deformity associated with osteoporosis. Education of patients regarding risk factors, particularly smoking, can help reduce the disabling consequences of this disease.

REFERENCES

1. Fitzsimmons A, Bonner F, Lindsay R. Failure to diagnose osteoporosis. *Am J Phys Med Rehabil* 1995; 74:240–242.
2. World Health Organization. *Assessment of fracture risk and its application to screening for postmenopausal osteoporosis.* WHO Technical report series 843. Geneva, Switzerland: WHO, 1994.
3. Abramson AS, Delagi EF. Influence of weight-bearing and muscle contraction on disuse osteoporosis. *Arch Phys Med Rehabil* 1961; 42: 147–151.
4. European Foundation for Osteoporosis and Bone Disease and the National Osteoporosis Foundation of USA. Consensus Development Statement. Who are candidates for prevention and treatment of osteoporosis? *Osteoporosis Int* 1997; 7:1–6.
5. Melton LJ III, Riggs BL. Epidemiology of age-related fractures. In: Avioli LV, ed. *The osteoporotic syndrome.* New York: Grune & Straton, 1983; 45–72.
6. National Osteoporosis Foundation. *1996–2015 Osteoporosis prevalence figures state by state report.* Washington, D.C.: NOF, 1997.
7. Phillips S, Fox N, Jacobs J, Wright WE. The direct medical costs of osteoporosis for American women aged 45 and older, 1986. *Bone* 1988; 9:271–279.
8. Holbrook TL, Grazier K, Kelsey JL, Stauffer RN. *The frequency of occurrence, impact and cost of selected musculoskeletal conditions in the United States.* Chicago: American Academy of Orthopedic Surgeons, 1984.
9. Ray NF, Chan JK, Thaemer M, Melton LJ III. Medical expenditures for the treatment of osteoporotic fractures in the United States in 1994. *J Bone Miner Res* 1997; 12:24–35.
10. U.S. Congress Office of Technology Assessment. *Effectiveness and costs of osteoporosis screening and hormone replacement therapy.* Vol. 1. Cost effectiveness analysis. OTA-BP-H-160. Washington, DC: U.S. Government Printing Office, August 1995A.
11. Ettinger B, Black DM, Nevitt MC, et al. Contribution of vertebral deformities to chronic back pain and disability. The study of osteoporotic fractures research group. *J Bone Miner Res* 1992; 7:449–456.
12. Chrischilles EA, Butler CD, Davis CS, Wallace RB. A model of lifetime osteoporosis impact. *Arch Intern Med* 1991; 151:2026–2032.
13. Guideline for the prevention, diagnosis, and treatment of osteoporosis: cost-effectiveness analysis and review of the evidence. Washington, D.C.: NOF, 1998.
14. Orwoll ES, Meier DE. Alterations in Calcium, vitamin D, and parathyroid hormone physiology in normal men with aging: relationship to the development of senile osteopenia. *J Clin Endocrinol Metab* 1986; 63:1262–1269.
15. Gross M, Roberts JG, Foster J, Shankardass K, Webber CE. Calcaneal bone density reduction in patients with restricted mobility. *Arch Phys Med Rehabil* 1987; 68:158–161.
16. del Puente A, Pappone N, Mandes MG, Mantova D, Scarpa R, Oriente P. Determinants of bone mineral density in immobilization: a study on hemiplegic patients. *Osteo Int* 1996; 6:50–54.
17. Minaire P, Meunier P, Edouard C, Bernard J, Courpron P, Bourret J. Quantitative histological data on disuse osteoporosis: comparison with biological data. *Calcif Tissue Res* 1974; 17:57–73.
18. Uhthoff HK, Jaworski ZFG, et al. Bone loss in response to long-term immobilization. *J Bone Joint Surg [Br]* 1978; 60:420–428.
19. Gallagher JC, Riggs BL, DeLuca HF. Effect of estrogen on calcium absorption and serum vitamin D metabolites in postmenopausal osteoporosis. *J Clin Endocrinol Metab* 1980; 51:1359–1365.
20. Smith DM, Khairi MRA, Johnston CC. The loss of bone mineral with aging and its relationship to risk of fracture. *J Clin Invest* 1975; 56: 311–318.
21. Parfitt AM, Matthews CHE, Villaneuva AR, et al. Relationships between surface, volume, and thickness of iliac trabecular bone in aging and in osteoporosis. *J Clin Invest* 1983; 72:1396–1409.
22. Frost HM. The Pathomechanics of osteoporoses. *Clin Orthop Rel Res* 1985; 200:198–226.
23. Baker SP, Harvey AH. Fall injuries in the elderly: symposium on falls in the elderly: biological aspects and behavioral aspects. *Clin Geriatr Med* 1985; 1:501–508.
24. Melton LJ, Riggs B. Risk factors for injury after a fall. *Clin Geriatr Med* 1985; 1:525–539.
25. Richelson LS, Wahner HW, Melton LJ, Riggs BL. Relative contributions of aging and estrogen deficiency to postmenopausal bone loss. *N Engl J Med* 1984; 311:1273–1275.
26. Drinkwater BL, Nilson K, Chestnut CH, et al. Bone mineral content of amenorrheic athletes. *N Engl J Med* 1984; 311:277–281.
27. Marcus R, Madvig P, Young G. Age-related changes in parathyroid hormone and parathyroid hormone action in normal humans. *J Clin Endocrinol Metab* 1984; 58:223–230.
28. Riggs BL, Hamstra A, DeLuca HF. Assessment of 25-hydroxy vitamin D α-hydroxylase reserve in postmenopausal osteoporosis by administration of parathyroid extract. *J Clin Endocrinol Metab* 1981; 53:833–835.
29. Slovik DM, Adams JS, Neer RM, et al. Deficient production of 1,25 dihydroxyvitamin D in elderly osteoporotic patients. *N Engl J Med* 1981; 25:372–374.
30. Taggart HM, Chesnut CH, Ivey JL, et al. Deficient calcitonin response to calcium stimulation in post-menopausal osteoporosis? *Lancet* 1982; 2:475–477.
31. Tiegs RD, Body JJ, Wahner HW, et al. Calcitonin secretion in postmenopausal osteoporosis. *N Engl J Med* 1985; 12:1097–1100.
32. Spotila LD, Colige A, Sereda L, et al. Mutation analysis of coding sequences for type I procollagen in individuals with low bone density. *J Bone Miner Res* 1994; 9; 6:923–932.
33. Slemenda CW, Christian JC, Williams CJ, Norton JA, Johnston CC Jr. Genetic determinants of bone mass in adult women; a revaluation of the model and the potential importance of gene interaction on heritability estimates. *J Bone Miner Res* 1991; 6:561–7.
34. Morrison NA, Qi JC, Tokita A, et al. Prediction of bone density from vitamin D receptor alleles. *Nature* 1994; 367:284–287.
35. Morrison NA, Yeoman R, Kelly PJ, Eisman JA. Contribution of transacting factor alleles to normal physiological varability: vitamin D receptor gene polymorphisms and circulating osteocalcin. *Proc Natl Acad Sci USA* 1992; 89:6665–6669.
36. Kobayashi S, Inoue S, Hoso T, Ouchi Y, Shiraki M, Orimo H. Association of bone minoral density with polymorphism of the estrogen receptor gene. *J Bone Miner Res* 1996; 11:306–311.
37. Njeh CF, boivin CM, Langton CM. The role of ultrasound in assessment of osteoporosis: a review. *Osteoporosis Int* 1997; 7:7–22.
38. Chesnut CH 3d, Bell NH, Clark GS, et al. Hormone replacement therapy in post menopausal women: urinary n-telepaptide of type I collagen monitors therapeutic affect and predicts response of bone marrow density. *Am J Med* 1997; 102:29–37.
39. Reid IR, Ames RW, Evans MC, Gamble GD, Sharpe SJ. Long-term effects of calcium suplementation on bone loss and fractures in postmenopausal women: a randomized controlled trial. *Am J Med* 1995; 98:331–335.
40. Orimo H, Shiraki M, Hayashi T, Nakamura T. Reduced occurrence of vertebral crush fractures in senile osteoporosis treated with 1δ-hydroxyvitamin D_3. *J Bone Miner Res* 1987; 3:47–52.
41. Chevalley T, Rizzoli R, Nydegger V, et al. Effects of calcium supplements on femoral bone mineral density and vertebral fracture rate in vitamin D replete elderly patients. *Osteoporosis Int* 1994; 4:245–252.
42. Chapuy MC, Arlot ME, Duboeuf F, et al. Vitamin D_3 and calcium to prevent hip fractures in elderly women. *N Engl J Med* 1992; 327: 1637–1642.
43. Chapuy MC, Arlot ME, Delmas PD, Meunier PJ. Effect of calcium and cholecalciferol treatment for three years on hip fractures in elderly women. *Br Med J* 1994; 308:1081–1082.

44. NIH Consensus Conference. Optimal calcium intake. NIH Consensus Development Panel on Optimal Calcium Intake. *JAMA* 1994; 272: 1942–1948.
45. Dawson-Hughes B, Harris SS, Krall EA, Dallal GE, Falconer G, Green CL. Rates of bone loss in postmenopausal women randomly assigned to one of two dosages of vitamin D_{1-4}. *Am J Clin Nutr* 1995; 61:1140–1150.
46. Ooms ME, Roos JC, Bezemer PD, VanDerVijgh WJF, Bouter LM, Lips P. Prevention of bone loss by vitamin D supplementation in elderly women: a randomized double-blind trial. *J Clin Endocrinol Metab* 1995; 80:1052–1058.
47. Overgaard K, Hansen MA, Jensen SB, Christiansen C. Effect of salcatonin given intranasally on bone mass and fracture rates in established osteoporosis. A dose-response study. *Br Med J* 1992; 305:556–561.
48. MacIntyre I, Stevenson JC, Whitehead MI, Wimalawansa SJ, Banks LM, Healy MJ. Calcitonin for prevention of postmenopausal bone loss. *Lancet* 1988; 1:900–902.
49. Gennari C, Chierichetti SM, Bigazzi S, et al. Comparative effects on bone mineral content or calcium and calcium plus salmon calcitonin given in two different regimens in postmenopausal osteoporosis. *Curr Ther Res* 1985; 38:455–464.
50. Kleerekoper M, Peterson EL, Nelson DA, et al. A randomized trial of sodium fluoride as a treatment ofor postmenopausal osteoporosis. *Osteoporosis Int* 1991; 1:155–161.
51. Pak CYC, Sakhaee K, Adams-Huet B, Piziak V, Peterson RD, Poindexter JR. Treatment of postmenopausal osteoporosis with slow-release sodium fluoride: final report of a randomized controlled trial. *Ann Intern Med* 1995; 123:401–408.
52. Riggs BL, Hodgson SF, O'Fallon WM, et al. Effect of fluoride treatment on the fracture rate in postmenopausal women with osteoporosis. *N Engl J Med* 1990; 332:802–809.
53. Kallings P. Nonsteroidal anti-inflammatory drugs. *Vet Clin North Am Equine Pract* 1993; 9:523–541.
54. Maki BE, Fernie GR. Impact attenuation of floor coverings in simulated falling accidents. *Appl Argo* 1990; 107–114.
55. Williams AR, Weiss NS, Ure CL, et al. Effect of weight, smoking, and estrogen use on the risk of hip and forearm fractures in postmenopausal women. *Obstet Gynecol* 1982; 60:695–699.
56. Tinetti M. Performance oriented assessment of mobility problems in elderly patients. *J Am Geriatr Soc* 1986; 34:119–126.
57. Mossey JM, Mutran E, Knoh K, Craik R. Determinants of recovery 12 months after hip fracture: the importance of psychological factors. *Am J Public Health* 1989; 79:279–286.
58. Cook DJ, Gugatt GH, Adachi JD, et al. Quality of life issues in women with vertebral fratures due to osteoporosis. *Arthritis Rheum* 1993; 36: 750–756.
59. Paier GS. Specter of the crone: the experience of vertebral fracture. *Adv Nurs Sci* 1996; 18:27–36.
60. National Osteoporosis Foundation. Scientific Advisory Board. Position paper on exercise and osteoporosis. 1991.
61. Sinaki M, Mikkelsen BA. Post-menopausal spinal osteoporosis: flexion versus extension exercises. *Arch Physical Med Rehabil* 1984; 65: 593–596.
62. Kerr D, Morton A, Dick I, Prince R. Exercise effects on bone mass in postmenopausal women are site-specific and load dependent. *J Bone Miner Res* 1996; 11:218–225.
62a. Evans W, Campbell W. Sacopenia and age-related changes in body composition and functional capacity. *J Nutr* 1993; 123:465–468.
62b. Fiatarone M, O'Neill E, Doyle N, et al. The Boston Ficsit study: the effects of resistance training and nutritional supplementation on physical fraility in the oldest old. *J Am Geriatr Soc* 1993; 41:333–337.
62c. Sinaki M, Wahner HW, Bergstrall EJ, et al. Three year controlled, randomized trial of the effect of dose-specified loading and strengthening exercises on bone mineral density of spine and femur in nonathletic, physically active women. *Bone* 1996; 19:233–244.
63. Felson DT, Anderson JJ, Hannan MT, et al. Impaired vision and hip fracture. *J Am Geriatr Soc* 1989; 37:495–500.
64. Ettinger B, Black DM, Palermo L, Nevitt MC, Melnikoff S, Cummings SR. Kyphosis in older women and its relation to back pain, disability and osteopenia: the study of osteoporosis fractures. *Osteoporosis Int* 1994; 4:55–60.
65. Gandy S, Payne R. Back pain in the elderly: updated diagnosis and management. *Geriatrics* 1986; 41:59–72.
66. Ettinger B, Black DM, Nevitt MC, et al. and the Study of Osteoporotic Fractures Research Group. Contribution of vertebral deformities to chronic back pain and disability. *J Bone Miner Res* 1992; 7:449–456.
67. Ryan PJ, Evans P, Gibson T, Fogelman I. Osteoporosis and chronic back pain: a study with single-photon emmission computed tomography bone scintigraphy. *J Bone Miner Res* 1992; 7:455–460.
68. Wynne AT, Nelson MA, Nordin BEC. Costoiliac impingement syndrome. *Br Edit Soc Bone Joint Surg* 1985; 67:124–125.
69. Hirschberg GG, Williams KA, Byrd JG. Medical management of iliocostal pain. *Geriatrics* 1992; 47:62–66.
70. Ferrell BA, Ferrell BR. Principles of pain management in older people. *Comprehens Ther* 1991; 17:53–58.
70a. Lukert BP. Vertebral compression fractures: how to manage pain, avoid disability. *Geriatrics* 1994; 49:22–26.
71. Rifat SF, Kiningham RB, Peggs JF. Calcitonin in the treatment of osteoporotic bone pain. *J Family Pract* 1992; 35:9393–9396.
72. Gennari C, Agnusdci D, Camporeale C. Use of calcitonin in the treatment of bone pain associated with osteoporosis. *Calcif Tissue Int* 1991; 49(suppl):9–13.
73. Goemaere S, Laere MV, DeNeve P, Kaufman JM. Bone mineral status in paraplegic patients who do or do not perform standing. *Osteoporosis Int* 1994; 4:138–143.
74. Ceder L, Thorngren KG, Walden B. Prognostic indicators and early home rehabilitation in elderly patients with hip fratures. *Clin Orthop* 1980; 152:173–184.
75. Magaziner J, Simonsick EM, Keshner TM, Hebel JR, Kenzora JE. Predictors of functional recovery one year following hospital discharge for hip fracture. *Zh Nrtonyol* 1990; 45:M101–M107.
76. Fitzgerald JF, Fogon LF, Tierney WM, Dittus RS. Changing patterns of hip fratures care before and after implementation of the prospective payment system. *JAMA* 1987; 258:218–221.
77. Barnes R, Brown JT, Garden RS, Nicoll EA. Subcapitol fratures of the femur: a prospective review. *J Bone Joint Surg [Br]* 1976; 58: 2–24.
78. Cummings SR, Kelsey JL, Nevitt MC, O'Dowel KJ. Epedemiology of osteoporosis and osteoperotic fratures. *Epidemiol Rev* 1985; 7: 178–208.
79. Magaziner J, Simonsick EM, Keshner TM, Hebel JR, Kenyora JF. Survival experience of aged hip fracture patients. *Am J Public Health* 1989; 79:274–278.
80. Kenyor JE, McCarthy RE, Lowell JD, Sledge CB. Hip frature mortality: relation to age, treatment, preoperative illness, time of surgery and complications. *Clin Orthop* 1984; 186:45–56.
81. White BL, Fisher WD, Lauriss CA. Rate of mortality for elderly patients after frature of the hip in the 1980's. *J Bone Joint Surg [Am]* 1987; 69:1335–1340.
82. Zuckerman JD, Sakales SR, Fabrien DR, Frankel VH. Hip fratures in geriatric patients: results of an interdisciplinary hospital care program. *Clin Orthop* 1992; 274:213–225.
83. Fitzgerald JF, Moore PS, Dittus RS. The case of elderly patients with hip frature: changes since implementation of the prospective pagment system. *N Engl J Med* 1988; 319:1392–1397.
84. Boncor SK, Tinetti ME, Spechley M, Ceonig LM. Factors associated with short-versus long-term skilled nursing facility placement among community living hip fracture patients. *J Am Geriatr Soc* 1990; 38: 1139–1144.
85. Pryor GA, Nyles JW, Williams DR, Amand JK. Team management of the elderly patient with hip frature. *Lancet* 1988; 1:401–403.
86. Ogilvie-Harris DJ, Botsford DJ, Hunter RW. Elderly patients with hip fratures: improved outcome with the use of care maps with high quality medical and nursing protocols. *J Orthop Trauma* 1993; 7: 428–437.
87. Frost HM. Managing the skeletal pain and disability of osteoporosis. *Orthop Clin North Am* 1972; 3:561–570.
88. Goltzman D. *L'actualite therapoatiquie.* Vol. 2. Basel, Switzerland: Sandoz, 1985.
89. Remagen W. *Osteoporosis.* Basel, Switzerland: Sandoz, 1991.
90. Stillo JV, Stein AB, Ragnarson KT. Low back orthoses. *Phys Med Rehabil Clin North Am* 1992; 3:57–94.
91. Kaplan RS, Sinaki M. Posture training support: preliminary report on a series of patients with diminished symptomatic complications of osteoporosis. *Mayo Clin Proc* 1993; 68:1171–1176.
92. Kaplan RS, Sinaki M, Hameister MD. Effect of back supports on back strength in patients with osteoporosis; a pilot study. *Mayo Clin Proc* 1996; 71:235–241.

93. Sloan J, Holloway O. Fractured neck of the femur: the cause of the fall? *Inj Br J Accident Surg* 1981; 13:230–232.
94. Yang K, Shen K, Demetroponlos C, King A, Lavine R, Fitzgerald R. The relationship between muscle contraction and fracture of the proximal femur. *Trans 41st ORS* 1995; 16:238.
95. Dep J. An analysis of the nature of injury in fractures of the neck of the femor. *Age Ageing* 1987; 16:373–377.
96. Cumming S, Klineberg R. Fall frequency and characteristics and the risk of hip fractures. *J Am Geriatr Soc* 1994; 42:774–778.
97. Lotz JC, Cheal EJ, Hayes WC. Stress distributions within the proximal femur during gait and falls: implications for osteoporotic fracture. *Osteoporosis Int* 1995; 5:252–261.
98. Ford CM, Keaveny TM, Hayes WC. The effect of impact direction on the structural capacity of the proximal femur during falls. *J Bone Miner Res* 1996; 11; 3:322–383.
99. Kroonenberg AJ, Hayes WC, McMahon TA. Dynamic models for sideways falls from standing height. *J Biomed Eng* 1995; 117: 309–318.
100. Greenspan SL, Myers ER, Maitland LA, Resnick NM, Hayes WC. Fall severity and bone mineral density as risk factors for hip fracture in ambulatory elderly. *JAMA* 1994; 271:128–133.
101. Tinetti ME, Speechley M, Ginter SF. Risk factors for falls among elderly persons living in the community. *N Engl J Med* 1988; 319: 1701–1707.
102. Tinetti ME, Speechley M. Prevention of falls among the elderly. *N Engl J Med* 1989; 320:1055–1059.
103. Tinetti ME, Liu WL, Claus EB. Predictors and prognosis of inability to get up after falls among elderly persons. *JAMA* 1993; 269:65–70.
104. Hayes WC, Myers ER, Robinovitch SN, Kroonenberg AV, Courtney AC. Etiology and prevention of age-related hip fractures. *Bone* 1996; 18(suppl):77–86.
104a. Tinetti ME, Baker D, Garrett P, Gottschalk C, Koch M, Horwitz R. Yale: risk factor abatement strategy for fall prevention. *J Am Geriatr Soc* 1993; 41:315-370.
105. Felson D, Zhang Y, Hannan M, Anderson J. Effects of weight and body mass index on bone mineral density in men and women: the Framingham study. *J Bone Miner Res* 1993; 8:567–573.
106. Tinetti ME, Baker DI, McAvay G, et al. A multifactorial intervention to reduce the risk of falling among elderly people living in the community. *N Engl J Med* 1994; 331:821–827.
107. Farmer ME, Harris T, Madans JH, Wallace RB, Coroni-Huntley J, White LR. Anthropometric indicators and hip fracture: the NHANES I epidemiologic follow-up study. *J Am Geriatr Soc* 1989; 37:9–16.
108. Perez Cano R, Galan F, Disen G. Risk factors for hip fracture in Spanish and Turkish women. *Bone* 1993; 14(suppl):69–72.
109. Lauritzen JS. Protection against hip fractures by energy absorption. *Dan Med Bull* 192; 39:91–93.
110. Robinovitch SN, Hayes WC, McHahan TA. Energy-shunting hip padding system attenuates femoral impact force in a simulated fall. *J Biomech Eng* 1995; 117:409–413.
111. Greenspan SL, Myers ER, Maitland LA, Resnick NM, Hayes WC. Fall severity and bone mineral density as risk factors for hip fracture in ambulatory elderly. *JAMA* 1994; 271:128–133.

Rehabilitation Medicine: Principles and Practice, Third Edition,
edited by Joel A. DeLisa and Bruce M. Gans.
Lippincott–Raven Publishers, Philadelphia 1998.

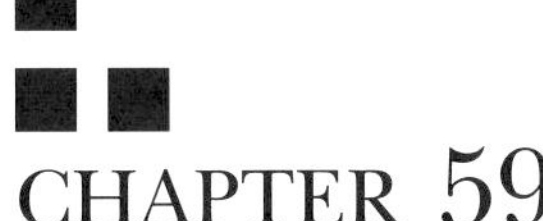

CHAPTER 59

Rehabilitation of the Patient With Arthritis and Connective Tissue Disease

Jeanne E. Hicks and Lynn H. Gerber

During the past decade, there has been increased interest in which measures are available for preventive and restorative goals to patients with rheumatic disease and increased awareness of significant improvements that have resulted from rehabilitation interventions (1). Whereas rheumatology is dedicated to the understanding and control of disease activity, rehabilitation medicine aims to maintain or restore function or prevent dysfunction by the use of physical modalities and techniques, exercise, orthotics, assistive and adaptive devices, energy conservation and joint protection education, and vocational planning. Rheumatic disease often impacts both articular and nonarticular structures. This chapter is confined mainly to articular disorders.

Arthritis involves a joint or joints and periarticular structures in an inflammatory or a noninflammatory mechanical, degenerative process. It may affect one or many joints, may be an acute process that completely resolves (e.g., septic joint), or may be a chronic event (e.g., rheumatoid arthritis [RA]). Arthritis may involve all the joint structures: synovium, cartilage, tendons, capsule, bone, and surrounding muscle. It is often part of a systemic rheumatic disease (i.e., connective tissue disease) such as RA, juvenile rheumatoid arthritis (JRA), systemic lupus erythematosus (SLE), polymyositis (PM), or progressive systemic sclerosis (PSS).

J. E. Hicks: Department of Rehabilitation Medicine, National Institutes of Health, Bethesda, Maryland 20892-1604; and Department of Internal Medicine, George Washington University Medical Center, Washington, D.C. 20037; and Department of Orthopedic Surgery, Georgetown University Medical Center, Washington, D.C. 20057; and Department of Internal Medicine, Uniformed Armed Services Institutes, Bethesda, Maryland 20814.

L. H. Gerber: Department of Rehabilitation Medicine, National Institutes of Health, Bethesda, Maryland 20892-1604; and Department of Rheumatology, Georgetown University Medical Center, Washington, D.C. 20057; and Department of Internal Medicine, George Washington University Medical Center, Washington, D.C. 20037.

These diseases are usually chronic, remitting, and relapsing; they are variable in their course and affect multiple organ systems in addition to joints. They require long-term treatments with drugs, which may have a significant impact on appearance, sleep, psychological function, and reproductive ability. The physiatrist directing the rehabilitation team must bear all these issues in mind when evaluating and devising a treatment plan.

This chapter emphasizes the importance of a good initial evaluation and periodic re-evaluation of the arthritis patient and the rational and stage-specific manner in which rehabilitative treatments are applied to the problems of patients with rheumatic diseases.

Equally important is to stress the critical importance of engaging the patient in his or her own treatment (2,3).

ARTHRITIC DISEASES

Classification

The important determinants in classifying arthritis are whether the disorder is inflammatory or noninflammatory, symmetrical or asymmetrical, or accompanied by systemic and extraarticular manifestations (Fig. 59-1).

A good history and physical examination and appropriate laboratory and x-ray studies will often allow a specific diagnosis to be made. Clinical features that suggest inflammatory rather than noninflammatory disease include acute painful onset, fever, erythema of the skin over the joint or joints involved, warmth of the joint or joints, and tenderness that usually parallels the degree of inflammation.

Laboratory and x-ray findings that suggest an inflammatory process include an increased peripheral white blood cell count with left shift, an elevated erythrocyte sedimentation rate, a group II joint fluid (Table 59-1), and x-ray demonstra-

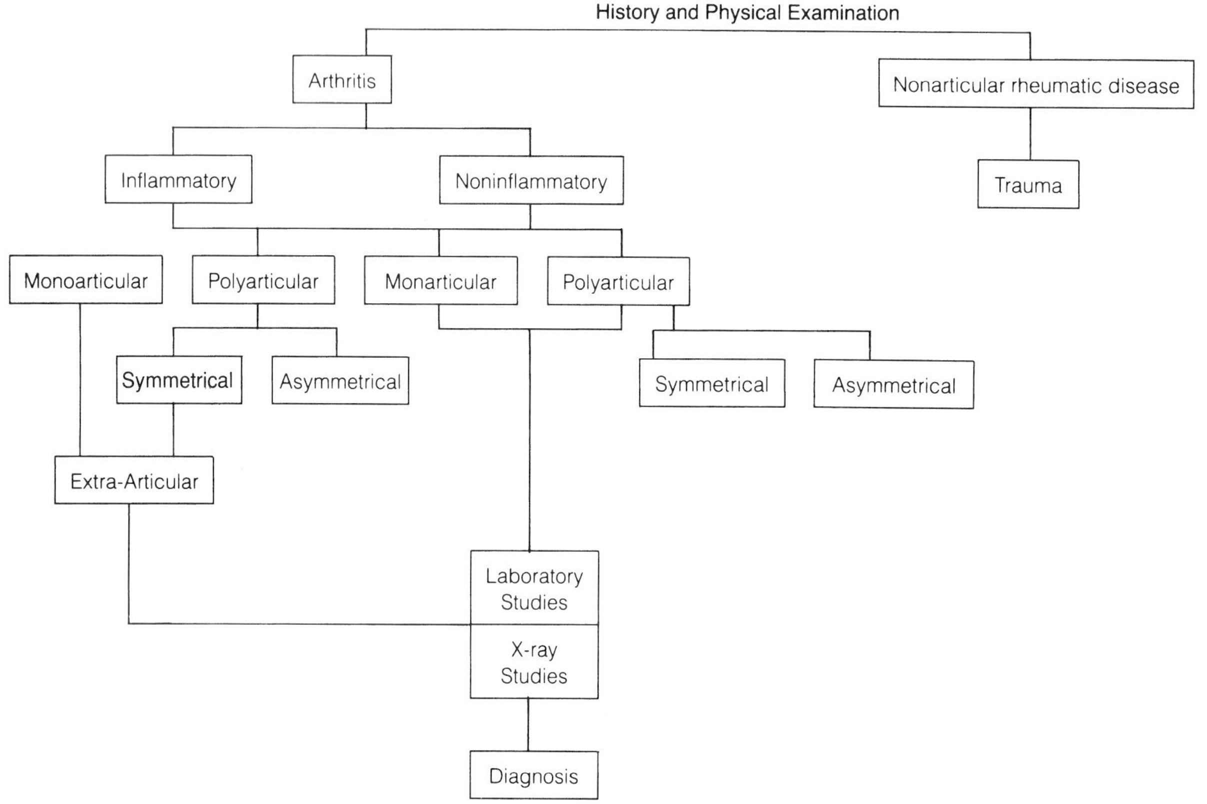

FIG. 59-1. Steps in the classification and diagnosis of rheumatic disease.

tion of soft-tissue swelling, periostitis, bony erosions, or uniform cartilage loss (Table 59-2).

Inflammatory arthritis falls into four different groups:

1. Inflammatory connective tissue disease (e.g., RA, JRA, SLE, dermatomyositis-polymyositis [DM-PM], mixed connective tissue disease)
2. Inflammatory crystal-induced disease (e.g., gout, pseudogout)
3. Inflammation induced by infectious agents (e.g., bacterial, viral, tuberculous, and fungal arthritis)
4. Seronegative spondyloarthropathies (e.g., ankylosing spondylitis [AS], psoriatic arthritis [PSA], Reiter's disease, inflammatory bowel disease [IBD])

Noninflammatory arthritis may be classified as degenerative (e.g., osteoarthritis [OA], posttraumatizing aseptic necrosis [AN]) or metabolic (e.g., lipid storage disease, hem-

TABLE 59-1. *Synovial fluid analysis*

Fluid group	Color	Clarity	Viscosity	Mucin clot	Cells/mm³	Percentage of white blood cells that are polymorphonuclear leukocytes
Normal	Pale yellow	Transparent	High	Good <200	<25%	
Group I (non inflammatory)	Yellow or straw	Transparent	High	Good	<2,000	<25%
Group II (moderatley inflammatory)	Yellow or straw	Transparent to opaque, slightly cloudy	Variably decreased	Fair to poor	3,000–50,000	>70%
Group III (highly inflammatory, septic)	Variable; yellow-gray, purulent	Opaque, cloudy	Low	Poor	50,000–100,000 (usually 100,000 or more)	>75%, usually close to 100%
Group IV (hemorrhagic)	Red	Opaque	High	Good	Up to normal count in blood	May be the same as normal blood

TABLE 59-2. *Radiographic findings in rheumatic diseases*

Disease	Anatomic distribution	Types of changes seen
Rheumatiod arthritis	Symmetrical: Most frequent: MCP, MTP, wrist, PIP Often: Knee, hip, ankle, shoulder, C-spine	Juxta-articular osteoporosis, soft-tissue swelling Marginal erosion Subluxation Late: bony eburnation
Osteoarthritis	Assymetrical: Most frequent: Hip, knee, DIP, 1st CMC, C-spine Less frequent: Ankle, shoulder	Joint space narrowing Marginal osteophyte Cortical sclerosis and cyst
Spondylarthropathies AS Reiter's PSA	Assymetrical: Most frequent: Sacroiliac joint, heel Vertebral column, hip, shoulder Knee, ankle MCP, PIP, DIP, MTP	Soft-tissue swelling, sausage fingers (i.e., Reiter's. PSA) New bone formation, fluffy periosteal bone, and syndesmophytes Enthesopathic ossification or erosion or both Bony anklyosis
Septic	Assymetrical: Knee, ankle, wrist, hip, small joints	Soft-tissue swelling Joint space enlargment Periosteal elevation Late: bony destruction
Gout	Assymetrical: 1st MTP, small joint, knee	Soft-tissue swelling Soft-tissue speckled calcification, gouty tophi Erosion of bone with marginal overhangs
Pseudogout	Symmetrical: Knee, wrist, hip	Chondrocalcinosis Subchondral cysts
SLE	Symmetrical: Small joints of hands, feet, wrists Articular osteonecrosis: Hip, knee, shoulder, ankle	Subchondral lucency (i.e., crescent sign) Subchondral sclerosis Subchondral collapse and remodeling of bone Late: joint space loss
PSS	Symmetrical: Small joints of hands and feet	Acro-osteolysis (i.e., bone resorption) Soft-tissue calcification Sausage digits

AS, ankylosing sponditis; CMC, carpometacarpal; DIP, distal interphalangeal; MCP, metacarpophalangeal; PIP, proximal interphalangeal; PSA, psoriatic arthritis; PSS, progressive systemic sclerosis; SLE, systemic lupus erythematosus.

ochromatosis, ochronosis, hypogammaglobulinemia, hemoglobinopathies) (4,5).

A number of diseases have systemic manifestations (Table 59-3), many of which need the attention of the rehabilitation physician in addition to treatment of the arthritis itself. The rehabilitation physician must be aware of the impact of a chronic, unpredictable illness on various life stages. For example, systemic disease may influence a young mother quite differently than a postmenopausal woman. In some diseases (e.g., RA, SLE, JRA, gout, AS), a number of set criteria delineated by the American College of Rheumatology must be fulfilled before a definite or probable diagnosis can be made. Preliminary criteria have been developed for PSS, Reiter's syndrome, and AS.

Demographics

Many types of arthritis tend to have specific distribution in terms of age, gender, race, and geographic appearance. Severity of disease may vary with age and gender. Genetics and occupation also may be influencing factors. It is helpful to be familiar with those portions of the population that are more susceptible to certain diseases (Table 59-4) (6).

Osteoarthritis

Osteoarthritis is the most common form of arthritis. Its prevalence increases with age. In radiologic studies of the hands, 7% of men and 2% of women 18 to 24 years of age showed evidence of OA; by 75 to 79 years of age, virtually

TABLE 59-3. *Systemic manifestations of rheumatic diseases*

System	Disease
Skin	Juvenile rheumatoid arthritis (Still's variety) Psoriatic arthritis Reiter's syndrome Colitic arthritis Sarcoid arthritis Septic arthritis (especially *Neisseria gonorrhoeae* and *meningitidis*) Hyperlipoproteinemia Systemic lupus erythematosus Amyloidosis
Nasopharynx and ear	Reiter's syndrome Rheumatoid arthritis
Eye	Juvenile rheumatoid arthritis Reiter's syndrome Rheumatoid arthritis Sarcoid arthritis
Gastrointestinal tract	Colitic arthritis Scleroderma Whipple's disease
Heart and circulation	Amyloidosis Polymyositis Juvenile rheumatoid arthritis Reiter's syndrome Ankylosing spondylitis
Respiratory tract	Sarcoidosis Polymyositis Rheumatoid arthritis
Nervous system	Systemic lupus erthematosus Rheumatoid arthritis
Renal system	Amyloidosis Gout Systemic lupus erythematosus Rheumatoid arthritis
Hematologic system	Rheumatoid arthritis Systemic lupus erythematosus

all had evidence of OA. When younger than 45 years of age, men are affected more often than women. When older than 45 years of age, women are affected more often and tend to have more severe disease than men (7–9). Women more commonly have OA of the distal interphalangeal (DIP), proximal interphalangeal (PIP), first carpometacarpal (CMC), and first metatarsophalangeal (MTP) joints; men more often have hip involvement. Knee involvement is seen equally in the two genders from 55 to 64 years of age (10). Severe OA of the knee is seen more commonly in women 65 to 74 years of age (6.9% versus 2%). At 55 to 64 years of age, hip involvement is twice as common in women (1.6% versus 0.79%). Hip involvement in men increases and becomes more common than in women from 65 to 74 years of age (2.3% versus 1.2%) (11).

Rheumatoid Arthritis

Rheumatoid arthritis is universal and found in all populations, but some populations and ethnic groups have a lower incidence rate. There is a low prevalence among African blacks (0.1% definite RA; 0.8% probable RA) (12), a medium-high prevalence in Israeli men (0.5% to 1.3%) and women (1.2% to 3.1%) (13), and a high prevalence in rural Germany (men 5.7%; women 3.0%) (14). Prevalence rates are influenced according to which set of criteria are used to diagnose RA and whether the RA is definite or probable.

There is a limited concordance of the disease in twins and a twofold increase among first-degree relatives of patients with RA, but there is no specific pattern of inheritance (15).

Systemic Lupus Erythematosus

SLE is one of the most frequent serious disorders of young women. It is more common in black women (16), North American Indians (17), and Chinese populations (18). It occurs in relatives of patients with the disease with a frequency between 0.4% and 5%, which is a several-hundred-fold increase over that of the general population (19,20). Monozygotic twins have a 50% chance of being concordant for SLE.

Progressive Systemic Sclerosis

Progressive systemic sclerosis occurs rarely and is more common in black women. There is no evidence of geographic preference or genetic inheritance (21).

Juvenile Rheumatoid Arthritis

Juvenile rheumatoid arthritis (or juvenile chronic arthritis) is the most common arthritis found in childhood. It has a prevalence rate of 0.16 to 1.1 per 1,000 population. Systemic onset JRA begins at any age during childhood and affects boys and girls equally. Occasionally it may have an adult onset. Rheumatoid factor–negative polyarthritis begins at any age during childhood with a female preponderance. Rheumatoid factor–positive polyarthritis begins after 8 years of age. Pauciarticular arthritis usually begins before 5 years of age and occurs mainly in women. The peak onset is between 1 and 3 years of age. Studies have indicated a hereditary predisposition to JRA among first-degree relatives and a 40% concordance among monozygotic twins (22).

Adult Stills Disease

This is a rare disease found worldwide. It occurs in young adults 16 to 35 years of age. Inconsistant associations with human leukocyte antigen (HLA) typing occur (23).

Polymyositis

Polymyositis has a worldwide distribution. It is basically a rare disease with five to 10 new cases per million population per year. It has a 2.5:1 ratio in favor of women, with a higher incidence in black women. In childhood myositis and that associated with malignancy it is 1:1. Two peaks occur: one in childhood (5 to 15 years of age) and one in adulthood (45 to 64 years of age) (24).

Spondyloarthropathies

Spondyloarthropathies include a spectrum of diseases (e.g., AS, Reiter's, psoriasis, IBD), all of which are relatively rare; the incidence is one case per 1,000 population for each type. The conditions present between the ages of 15 and 45 years. The incidence of Reiter's is higher in men than in women (60:1), as is the incidence of AS (3:1). Psoriasis and IBD have an equal incidence in men and women (25).

Etiology and Pathophysiology

Because the designation "rheumatic disease" includes such a broad spectrum of processes and syndromes, a classification system (Fig. 59-1) that groups arthritides to some extent by etiology may be useful.

Rheumatoid Arthritis

The etiology of RA remains unclear, although much has been learned in the past two decades about the inflammatory process, its relationship to the immune system, and molecular genetic regulation. Of the two hypotheses in vogue, one suggests that RA is an autoimmune disorder; the other proposes that specific external agents initiate the response, which then is perpetuated or amplified by the immune host response. Data in support of the first hypothesis are derived from the fact that antibodies against autologous immunoglobulin G are present in many patients with RA, which may represent a primary abnormality in the regulation of cells that control immunoglobulin synthesis (26). This primary defect may alter the control mechanisms, so that stimulation and control of these events are unbalanced and the response to endogenous immune products goes awry (27).

A more likely explanation for the etiology of RA is that specific external agents initiate an inflammation response, and in the susceptible host, the inflammation leads to continual disease activity. Infectious agents can cause synovitis. Some replicate in the joint space (e.g., *Mycobacterium, Staphylococcus*), and some enter the joint space and cause synovitis through initiating a local immune response (e.g., rubella, spirochete). Another type of arthritis follows gastrointestinal (GI) disease (e.g., *Shigella, Salmonella, Yersinia*). No organism is recovered from the joint, although a reactive arthritis occurs, and the inflammatory process is initiated by a remote infection. Recent data have supported the hypothesis that chlamydia trachomata and pneumonia have been identified in synovial biopsy samples of patients with reactive arthritis (28).

TABLE 59-4. *Demographic data on rheumatic diseases*

	Prevalence rate	Peak age (yr)	Gender	Race	Geographic preference
Osteoarthritis (primary)	4% (age 20–30), 80% (>age 60)	Men before 45; women after 45	Equal	None	
Rheumatoid arthritis	1%–2%	25–55	Two to three times higher in women	Higher in whites; lower in Japanese	
Systemic lupus erythematosus	1:1,000; 1:700 in white women; 1:245 in black women	15–25	90% female	Three times higher in blacks[a]	New Zealand; Rochester, MN; San Francisco; Oahu, HI
Scleroderma	Rare (5:1,000,000)	30–40	Three times higher in women	Three times higher in blacks	None
Juvenile rheumatoid arthritis	0.16–1.1:1,000	1–3 (2:1 women)		None	
		8–12			
Spondyloarthropathies					
Ankylosing spondylitis	1:1,000	15–45	3:1 men		
Reiter's syndrome	1:1,000	15–45	60:1 men	None	None
Psoriasis	1:1,000	15–45			
Inflammatory bowel disease	1:1,000	15–45			
Polymyositis	Uncommon (5–10:1,000,000)	(Bimodal)[b] 5–15 45–65	Two times higher in women; 10.8:4.6 black women to black men; 2.7:3.7 white women to white men	Three times higher in blacks	None

[a] Data from Kelley W, Harris ED, Ruddy S, Sledge CB. *Textbook of rheumatology*. Philadelphia: WB Saunders, 1985.
[b] Data from Shulman LR. *Epidemiology of the rheumatic diseases*. New York: Gower, 1984; 1–293.

Putting the pieces of the puzzle together in a coherent picture that conforms to Koch's postulates is not yet possible. Several components need to be acknowledged in the understanding of this process: an inciting agent, most likely exogenous and possibly a wide range of antigens; a genetic susceptibility; and an abnormality in the host immune response (29).

The mechanism of tissue injury in RA has been demonstrated to include the following components of the immune system and its associated mediators of inflammation (30). In the affected host, a stimulus initiates an inflammatory response directed against self or nonself, which sets into motion complement, leukocyte phagocytosis, lysosomal enzyme release, and several small mediators that initiate clotting and fibrolysis. In the joint, the local reactions are helper T-cell mediators that are attracted to macrophages and dendritic cells. Antibody synthesis is initiated, thus perpetuating the immunologic activities already begun. Some of the joint mononuclear cells can produce proteinases, prostaglandins (PG), and other small mediators of inflammation.

As the high-intensity inflammation subsides, repair takes place, often with the proliferation of fibroblasts and scar tissue. Although it is unclear what triggers all this, once the process is in place it often continues for a longer period than would be expected to successfully clear antigen. Hence, the host immunoregulatory system, which is genetically controlled, must be abnormal.

Osteoarthritis

In marked contrast to RA, OA seems to be a local phenomenon. The etiology of OA remains obscure, but the pathologic processes have been well described. Cartilage degeneration is the hallmark of the disease. The cause of the degeneration is unknown, but the possibilities include collagen framework damage secondary to fatigue or abrasion, changes in the synthesis of proteoglycan or its degradation, and defects in synovial fluid and chondrocyte function (31).

Other factors play an important role in the progression of OA. The location of the OA lesion determines progression. A cartilage lesion at the apex of the femoral head will undergo significant osteoarthritic changes, but lesions inferior to the fovea will not. Medial lesions of the patella are less likely to develop OA than lateral or central lesions, suggesting that local topographic variations exist. Bony resilience and the amount of cartilage loading may be factors in developing OA (32).

In some patients, OA is secondary to a pre-existing joint abnormality such as RA, congenital hip dislocation, Legg-Calve-Perthes disease, and avascular necrosis of bone. Some possible risk factors include age, weight, participation in sports that may result in repetitive microfractures (33), and repetitive occupational activities.

Regardless of the cause or initiating event, OA is associated with a progressive destruction of articular cartilage, which leads to fibrillation, abrasion, and shearing. The underlying exposed bone is damaged and attempts repair by formation of a new bone.

Spondyloarthropathies

Spondyloarthropathies are polyarticular disorders that involve the vertebral column. These arthritides share a number of additional features, including mucocutaneous lesions, sacroiliitis, heel pain, and the B27 antigen. Antecedent GI infection, caused by *Salmonella, Shigella,* and *Yersinia,* has stimulated interest that these diseases may be caused by a Gram-negative organism. The most convincing data in support of this came from the well-documented *Shigella* epidemics, in which Reiter's syndrome occurred in 344 of 150,000 infected persons in one study (34), and in nine of 602 in another study (35). No case occurred in anyone who was not infected. Arthritis with some additional features of Reiter's syndrome has followed *Salmonella* (36) and *Yersinia* infections (37). In PSA and AS, the data are less convincing, but evidence has linked the development of guttate psoriasis and streptococcal infection. The presence of B27 antigen appears to be the crucial link in expression of the disease. Antecedent urethritis has also been associated with acute arthritis, and chlamydia is the organism most frequently identified.

The pathology occurs at the entheses (insertion of tendon to bone). The axial spine may fuse, but if the peripheral joints are involved, there is erosion and often bony reaction and periosteal new bone growth. Usually, there is no periarticular osteoporosis.

The etiology of spondyloarthropathies is most likely to be an infective agent, possibly Gram-negative bacteria, that interacts with a susceptible gene host: B27 in AS and Reiter's, and perhaps B27, B38, and C6 in PSA.

Systemic Lupus Erythematosus

SLE is a multisystemic disease that is associated with abnormalities of immune regulation and immune complex–mediated tissue injury. It has been called a classic autoimmune disease, due to an abundance of autoantibodies generated against cytoplasmic and nuclear cellular components. The etiology of SLE is obscure, but viral inclusion bodies have been implicated because of electron microscopic observations made in lymphocytes and vessel walls (38). Virus has never been isolated in patients with SLE; even those diseases with documented infectious etiologies are often multifactorial. Family members with SLE are more likely to have immunologic abnormalities than are controls (39,40). Hormonal influences are important in the expression of SLE, and women in the child-bearing years appear to be at greater risk (41). Women taking progestational oral contraceptives are at higher risk than those taking estrogen-based oral contraceptives (42).

The pathogenesis of SLE depends on abnormalities in humoral and cellular immunity. Lymphopenia is common and is inversely related to disease activity. B-lymphocytes are normal in number but are hyperactive. T-lymphocytes are often decreased, most markedly in the T-suppressor lymphocyte subpopulation. Natural killer cell activity is diminished, but there is an increased number of lymphocytotoxic antibodies (43).

Progressive Systemic Sclerosis

PSS is a progressive disorder in which microvascular obliterative lesions in multiple organs terminate in fibrosis and atrophy. Patients with PSS have capillary abnormalities and small artery lesions, which appear late with organ involvement. The pathogenesis of organ involvement is most likely due to injury to the endothelial cell lining of vessels. Disturbing the lining activates the clotting system, with the release of vasoactive peptides. These factors stimulate smooth muscle cells to migrate in, proliferate, and deposit connective tissue, which results in the proliferative vascular lesion of PSS. The etiologic agent is obscure, and no strong hypotheses exist as to its nature.

Dermatomyositis–Polymyositis

Dermatomyositis–polymyositis is an inflammatory disease of muscle and skin often associated with profound weakness of all skeletal muscle, including the heart. There are six types, each of which may have a different etiology (44):

Group 1: primary idiopathic PM
Group 2: primary idiopathic DM
Group 3: DM-PM associated with neoplasia
Group 4: DM-PM associated with vasculitis
Group 5: DM-PM associated with collagen vascular disease
Group 6: inclusion body myositis (45)

Two leading hypotheses may explain the etiology of DM-PM: viral infection and abnormal recognition of self. Immunoglobulins have been demonstrated in vessel walls, especially in intramuscular blood vessels, suggesting that these deposits are immune complexes to muscle. These deposits are seen in a variety of muscle-wasting conditions and may be nonspecific. Cellular immunity is abnormal with DM-PM, as demonstrated by myotoxic activity of the lymphocytes in patients with DM-PM. Skeletal muscle antigens cause lymphocytes of patients with DM-PM to proliferate, suggesting that the lymphocytes are inappropriately responding to these antigens.

Crystal-Induced Synovitis

Crystal-induced synovitis can be caused by uric acid, calcium pyrophosphate, hydroxyapatite, and cholesterol crystals. Best understood is gout, a familial disorder in which there is a deficiency of hypoxanthine-guanine phosphotransferase, resulting in an overproduction of uric acid. Hyperuricemia results, and as the concentration of urate in the blood increases, monosodium urate crystals precipitate in the tissue. It has been shown that injecting urate crystals subcutaneously will cause tophus formation, and when urate is injected into joints, gouty attacks will ensue. Other factors involved in the pathogenesis of the gouty attack include elevated temperature, which increases joint urate concentration; lowered pH, which may precipitate an attack; and trauma and aging, which are thought to increase the likelihood of an attack.

Pseudogout, or calcium pyrophosphate dihydrate deposition (CPPD), can be hereditary or sporadic. The etiologic agent is the calcium pyrophosphate crystal, which is formed secondary to a disorder of local pyrophosphate metabolism. The crystals adhere to leukocytes, and often immunoglobulin is absorbed, which stimulates phagocytosis and the perpetuation of inflammatory arthritis.

Infectious Arthritis

A wide variety of infectious agents can cause arthritis secondary to the infection itself or as a consequence of the host's immunologic response. The organisms can be viral (e.g., hepatitis, rubella, mumps, herpes); bacterial (e.g., Gram-positive *Staphylococcus, Streptococcus,* and *Pneumococcus*; Gram-negative *Neisseria* and *Haemophilus influenzae*; *Pseudomonas*), or fungal. Recently, interest has developed in the role of hepatitis C and the development of an RA-like arthritis (28).

PATIENT EVALUATION

The physical examination and laboratory and x-ray findings are essential to the proper diagnosis and treatment of rheumatic diseases. Many schemes have been developed in an attempt to construct an organized approach to the classification of rheumatic diseases, including algorithms that sort signs and symptoms around the presence or absence of inflammation, symmetry, and number of involved joints. However, these categories are not very helpful in sorting out the underlying pathophysiologic processes that need therapeutic intervention.

A practical approach is suggested by James Fries, in which eight specific types of musculoskeletal pathology are distinguished (46). Patients can have more than one type of pathology; for example, enthesopathy and synovitis present in patients with PSA (Table 59-5).

Biomechanics

Evaluation of mobility can be performed with visual analysis or automated measures. The former has been standardized, and the latter have been significantly advanced with video-based high-speed systems. There is an increased ability to reliably measure motion in three dimensions in real time, ground reaction forces, and pressures on the bottoms

TABLE 59-5. *Evaluation of rheumatic diseases*

Pathology	Examples	Laboratory tests	Other organs involved
Synovitis	Rheumatoid arthritis	Latex, x-rays	Lung, heart, skin nodules
	Psoriatic arthritis/Reiter's syndrome	X-rays	Skin
Enthesopathy	Ankylosing spondylitis	HLA-B27, sacroiliac joint x-rays	Heart
	Psoriatic arthritis/Reiter's syndrome		Skin, mucous membranes
Cartilage degeneration	Osteoarthritis	X-rays	
Crystal arthritis	Gout	Serum uric acid, joint fluid	Skin, kidney
	Pseudogount	Joint fluid	
Joint infection	Bacterial	Joint culture	Vaginal infection
	Viral		Bacteremia
	Fungal		Hepatitis
Joint effusion	Trauma	Joint fluid	
	Reactive arthritis		
	Metabolic/endocrine disorders		Thyroid livers
Vasculitis	Scleroderma	Muscle biopsy, EMG	Any organ
	DM-PM	Antinuclear antibody	Heart
	SLE	Erythrocyte sedimentation rate	Any organ
	Polymyalgia rheumatica		
Tissue conditions			
Local	Tendinitis		
	Muscle spasm		
Generalized	Fibrositis		

DM-PM, dermatomyositis–polymyositis; EMG, electromyography; SLE, systemic lupus erythematosus.

of the feet, and an increased ability to calculate moments of force at various joints, and these procedures are being performed fairly frequently. In addition, newer instrumentation has been developed to describe foot pressure profiles and describe forces and their influences on the foot (47).

Data are published describing the gait abnormalities typical of patients with RA involving the feet (48). This gait has been termed "apropulsive" because of the absence of push-off from the ball of the foot. Similarly, studies of differences in gait before and after surgical procedures have been reported that describe which biomechanical changes occur as a result (49).

Laboratory Tests

The laboratory evaluation of blood, urine, and synovial fluid, coupled with radiographic evaluations, can usually establish a proper diagnosis. The following initial determinations are made: complete blood count, sedimentation rate, SMA-12 (sequential multiple analyzer), rheumatoid factor (RF), and antinuclear antibody. An HLA-B27 determination is performed if spondylitis is suspected.

Joint fluid is easy to obtain in the presence of effusion. Analysis of fluid is essential in the diagnosis of crystal-induced arthritis and joint infection, and it is helpful in differentiating traumatic and inflammatory arthritis. However, rarely will the diagnosis of RA, OA, PSA, or AS be made on the basis of joint fluid alone; rather, the fluid is confirmatory of these diagnoses. Joint taps must be done when a question of infection is raised and should be made before injecting steroid or other material into the joint. Classification of joint fluid into categories will help differentiate inflammatory, noninflammatory, septic, and hemorrhagic arthritis (Table 59-1).

Radiographic Assessment

Radiography is often the most valuable technique for differentiating among arthritides (50). Marginal erosion of bone with juxta-articular osteoporosis is the hallmark of RA. Nonuniform joint space loss in association with bony sclerosis and marginal osteophytes are the characteristic changes in OA. Spondyloarthropathies classically have involvement of the sacroiliac joints, either symmetrical, as in AS, or asymmetrical, as in Reiter's and PSA. Bony changes include periosteal new bone formation and ankylosis. Gout and pseudogout often involve only a few joints. In gout there are soft-tissue tophaceous deposits and marginal erosion with large bony overhangs, and in pseudogout there is calcinosis in fibrocartilage. Early in joint infection, the x-ray films may be negative, or there may be some joint space widening. If the process continues and osteomyelitis develops, periosteal reaction can occur, indicating bony destruction. Typical radiographic findings in patients with rheumatic diseases are presented in Table 59-2.

Functional Assessment

Rehabilitation assessment for patients with rheumatic diseases includes both process and outcome measures. Goniometry, the measurement of joint range of motion (ROM), is standardized and widely used, as is manual muscle testing (MMT). A new 10-point MMT has been devised and offers more sensitivity in the range that is most important to know for assessment of capability for independence (51). Quantifiable measures of spine motion are particularly useful for patients with rheumatic diseases (52). They can help chart progressive loss of spinal mobility, which prompts interventions designed to preserve posture as well as chest expansion programs, as in the management of patients with spondyloarthropathy.

Patients with arthritis often have stiffness rather than pain that limits function. Both symptoms are difficult to measure. However, duration of morning stiffness may be quantified. Pain can be measured in terms of severity in a descriptive way (e.g., mild, moderate, severe) or by use of a visual analog scale (53), which is quite reliable.

Fatigue is a frequent problem for patients with rheumatic disease. Its cause is multifactorial: medication, chronic inflammation, abnormal posture and gait that are energy inefficient, abnormalities of the sleep cycle, and atrophy of muscle secondary to disease or chronic pain. Fatigue is difficult to quantify because it can mean a decrease in stamina, true muscle weakness, and lack of motivation, all resulting in an inability to complete tasks. A visual analog of fatigue has been used with some success, but it has an imprecise reference. The multidimensional assessment of fatigue (Belza) has been devised and validated this population.

The Human Activity Profile is an instrument designed to measure activity and determine its energy requirements. It also has a dyspnea scale. These measures are helpful in quantifying activity and assisting the effort needed for performance (54).

Despite reliable, sensitive indices of strength, ROM, and grip strength, other measures are needed for evaluation of patients with rheumatic disease. The American Rheumatism Association in 1949 devised a functional scale for patients with RA (55). This scale was a simple, global assessment that rated patients' functional status as independent (i.e., class I), able to perform with pain (i.e., class II), able to do some activities (i.e., class III), and unable to perform (i.e., class IV). This scale was revised in 1992 (56).

Two generations of functional assessments have been used in evaluating patients with rheumatic disease. The first set looked primarily at performance of patients in ambulation, self-care, and other activities of daily living (ADL) (57–59). Most had some testing of reliability and validity and were relatively easy to use. The problem with them was that they defined function very narrowly and excluded psychological, social, and vocational functions. The newer functional indices are more comprehensive and offer a broader view of patients' functioning. They also have demonstrated validity and reliability (60–62).

When rheumatologists were asked which functional measures were important to use in evaluation of patients with rheumatic diseases, the consensus was mobility, pain, self-care, and role-activity (63). The evaluations needed may vary, because some rheumatic diseases involve only joints (e.g., OA), others primarily kidneys, skin, and central nervous system (e.g., SLE), and others still different organ systems. Other useful scales include The Wisconsin Brief Pain Questionnaire (64). The Sickness Impact Profile (65), and a multifaceted assessment of fatigue (66). Table 59-6 identifies standard functional measures likely to be needed for each of the rheumatic diseases.

Compliance

Sackett and Hayes have identified six key elements that influence compliance (67):

1. Demographic features
2. Nature of the disease
3. Therapeutic regimens
4. Setting in which treatment is given
5. Patient–doctor relationship
6. Sociobehavioral features of the patient

Good patient–physician communication leads to better compliance (68), and those diseases that require long-term treatment and multiple or frequent dosing are likely to result

TABLE 59-6. *Functional measures for rheumatic diseases*

	MMT	Range of motion	Pain	Fatigue	ADLs	Ambulation	Cognition	Role/social interaction
OA		+ + +	+ +		+	+ +		
RA	+	+ +	+ +	+ + +	+ +	+ +		+ + + +
Spondyloarthropathies		+ + +	+ +		+	+		+ +
DM-PM	+ +			+ + +	+ +	+ +		+ + + +
PSS		+ +	+ +	+	+ +			+ +
SLE	+			+ + +	+	+	+ +	+ + + +
Gout (crystals)			+ + +			+ +		
Fibromyalgia			+ + +	+ + +				+ + + +

+ , possibly useful evaluation; + +, recommended evaluation; + + +, strongly recommended; + + + +, must evaluate.

MMT, manual muscle test; OA, osteoarthritis; PSS, progressive systemic sclerosis; RA, rheumatoid arthritis.

in lower levels of compliance. These studies indicate that patients with rheumatic disease who have chronic illness and require long-term, multimodality interventions have a lower level of compliance than those with acute, short-term needs. Sackett and Hayes state that compliance is dependent in large measure on the individual patient's health beliefs, including the importance of the treatment goal, how likely the treatment is to achieve the goal or to reduce the disability, and the physical, psychological, and financial barriers to treatment (67).

Specifically, rehabilitation programs have been associated with improved function (69,70). Compliance with the use of splints (64) was 40% to 78% and was lower (71–73) in those patients with arthritis whose families did not expect them to use the devices. Compliance with exercise programs was 55% in one study (74) and 40% in another, but 90% in a study with visual feedback.

In view of this information, it is generally believed that good doctor–patient communication is important and that the treatment regimen must be clearly spelled out and agreed upon to improve patient compliance (75,76). Educating the patient is also recommended. The treatment should be as simple as possible, with one type of intervention planned and additional ones added after goal achievement is met or nearly met.

TREATMENT

Pharmacologic Management

Pharmacologic management of rheumatic diseases often requires the use of a variety of drugs, the pharmacology and pharmacokinetics of which may influence physical and psychological functioning.

Aspirin

Aspirin, or acetylsalicylic acid (ASA), is the foundation of management of rheumatic conditions and the symptoms of pain, fever, and inflammation. It has been shown to block the synthesis of PG in the anterior hypothalamus (77), which is responsible for the antipyretic effect. The analgesic effect of ASA is not entirely understood. Musculoskeletal pain may be mediated by bradykinin, a synthesizer of PG, which sensitizes nerves to painful stimuli. Aspirin blocks PG synthesis. At doses higher than those used for analgesia (e.g., 5.3 g/day), ASA reduces joint inflammation and swelling (78). The mechanisms for this action are multifactorial. Aspirin affects leukocyte migration and vascular permeability, both of which may be influenced by PG synthesis (79). The toxicities of ASA include allergy, tinnitus and hearing loss, GI blood loss, ulcer, chemical hepatitis, and reduced glomerular filtration rate. For patients who have clinically significant GI symptoms, enteric-coated preparations (e.g., Ecotrin [SmithKline Beecham Consumer, Pittsburgh, PA]), are usually well tolerated. Other forms of salicylate can be used that are often less GI toxic (e.g., choline salicylate).

Nonsteroidal Anti-inflammatory Drugs

Newer agents in use form the group of drugs called nonsteroidal anti-inflammatory drugs (NSAIDs). These drugs also suppress inflammation through the inhibition of synthesis of PG. They inhibit the cyclo-oxygenase effect on platelets and effects on leukocyte migration. Toxicities include GI bleeding, pancreatitis, hepatotoxicity, decreased renal blood flow, and allergic interstitial nephritis. Some have more GI toxicity than others and cause more sodium retention. A review of the comparative NSAID toxicities is available (80).

Nonsteroidal anti-inflammatory drugs are widely used as first-line drugs in the treatment of RA, JRA, OA, and spondyloarthritis. Only Tolectin (Ortho-McNeil Pharmaceutical, Raritan, NJ) and Naprosyn, (Roche Laboratories, Nutley, NJ) have been approved for use in children by the U.S. Food and Drug Administration. A list of those NSAIDs used in the United States is provided in Table 59-7.

Aspirin and NSAIDs are likely to provide significant clinical relief for patients with OA, RA, JRA, and spondyloarthritis. These drugs are not usually effective by themselves in controlling RA and vasculitic syndromes.

Antimalarials

Antimalarials are effective in discoid lupus erythematosus (81) and SLE (82) with improvement in skin involvement, as well as in RA (83,84). The arthritis and arthralgias associated with SLE also are improved. One study showed improvement in the course of glomerulonephritis (85). Patients with RA improved in joint count, grip strength, walk time, and sedimentation rate. The antimalarials are slow acting, taking 4 to 6 weeks before a therapeutic effect is observed. They are as effective as other slow-acting antirheumatic drugs (86).

TABLE 59-7. *NSAIDs in use*

Indole derivatives
Indomethacin (Indocin, Merck & Co., West Point, PA)
Sulindac (Clinoril, Merck & Co., West Point, PA)
Tolmetin (Tolectin, Ortho-McNeil Pharmaceuticals, Raritan, NJ)
Zomepirac (Zomax)
Pyrazolones
Phenylbutazone (Butazolidin)
Phenylpropionic Acids
Ibuprofen (Motrin, McNeil Consumer, Fort Washington, PA)
Naproxen (Naprosyn, Roche Laboratories, Nutley, NJ)
Fenoprofen (Nalfon, Dista, Indianapolis, IN)
Fenamates
Mefenamic acid (Ponstel, Parke-Davis, Morris Plains, NJ)
Meclofenamate (Meclomen, MyLan Pharmaceuticals, Morgantown, WV)
Oxicam
Piroxicam (Feldene, Pfizer, New York, NY)

The mechanism of action of these drugs is varied. They have been shown to impair enzymatic reactions, including phospholipase, cholinesterase-hyaluronidase, and proliferation of lymphocytes. They seem to block depolymerization by DNAase and interfere with DNA replication. The incidence of side effects and toxicities varies widely. Gastrointestinal disturbance is quite common, and retinopathy is infrequent but of greatest concern; it rarely occurs before a cumulative dose of 300 g is reached, specifically in chloroquine, but routine ophthalmologic examinations should be performed.

Gold

Parenteral gold, more recently oral gold, has been used in the treatment of synovitis in patients with RA. Gold is thought to work by inhibiting lysosomal enzymes or by inhibiting phagocytic activity in macrophages and polymorphonuclear leukocytes. It also inhibits aggregation of human gamma globulin in vitro, a phenomenon that is thought to be an inflammatory antigenic stimulus in RA. These events have been observed when parenteral gold is used. The oral preparation alters all mediated immunity, inhibits DNA synthesis in vitro, and suppresses humoral immunity (87).

Adverse effects of gold compounds include rash, stomatitis, proteinuria, and hematologic disorders (e.g., leukopenia, thrombocytopenia). This drug is not used in patients with SLE, partly because it may flare the skin involvement. The literature suggests that it may be useful in treating patients with peripheral arthritis associated with psoriasis (88). Gold is not contraindicated in treating patients with Felty's syndrome.

D-Penicillamine

D-penicillamine has been effective in the treatment of seronegative or seropositive RA (89). The patterns of response to penicillamine are similar to those observed with gold. Toxicities include leukopenia, thrombocytopenia, proteinuria, skin rash, stomatitis, GI upset, and a variety of autoimmune syndromes, including Goodpasture's disease, PM, and SLE. The mechanism of action is unknown, but it is neither cytotoxic nor anti-inflammatory.

Steroids

Glucocorticoids and therapeutics for rheumatic diseases are inseparable and probably have been tried in every rheumatic disease either systemically or locally. Exogenous glucocorticoids influence leukocyte movement, leukocyte function, and humoral factors; inhibit recruitment of neutrophils and monocytes into inflammatory sites (90); cause lymphocytopenia by inducing margination or redistribution of lymphocytes out of the circulation; modify the increased capillary and membrane permeability that occurs at an inflammatory site, reducing edema and antagonizing histamine-induced vasodilation; and inhibit PG synthesis.

Daily steroid use stimulates Cushing's syndrome, in which hypertension, hirsutism, acne, striae, obesity, psychiatric symptoms, and wound-healing problems occur. With exogenous steroid use, there is an increased incidence of glaucoma, cataracts, avascular necrosis, osteoporosis, and pancreatitis. The side effects are in part dependent on the particular glucocorticoid used and the dose. Alternate-day steroids are associated with fewer untoward effects. The oral route is usually selected for ease of administration, but glucocorticoids can safely be given intramuscularly or intravenously. They can be used intra-articularly and are best delivered in a suspension that is not water soluble.

Low-dose glucocorticoids are traditionally used in treating patients with RA (less than 15 mg orally every day). Higher doses are used in treating patients with SLE, vasculitis, and DM-PM (up to 100 mg prednisone every day). Benefit of steroid therapy to patients with AS, PSS, and PSA has not been shown.

Antihyperuricemic Agents

Pain and inflammation of crystal-induced arthritis are frequently adequately controlled with NSAIDs. Although these drugs are effective in controlling symptoms, they do not alter the metabolism of the substances forming crystals, nor do they influence their excretion. Probenecid competes with the tubular transport mechanism for uric acid, reduces the reabsorption of uric acid, and hence increases its excretion (91). Many other drugs have a uricosuric effect in humans. Their use is widespread, and their toxicities are well known, including nephrolithiasis, which is preventable if the urine is alkalinized and fluids increased. Acute gout can be precipitated as the uric acid levels are lowered; GI symptoms are not infrequently seen. A second approach toward controlling serum urate levels is that of regulating production of uric acid by inhibiting xanthine oxidase. This is done by using allopurinol as an analog of hypoxanthine. It, too, can precipitate an acute attack of gout and can cause xanthine renal stones. Side effects include rash and, rarely, blood dyscrasia. Allopurinol should not be used with azathioprine.

Cytotoxic Drugs

Immunoregulatory drugs have been used in the management of rheumatic diseases in an attempt to restore a balanced immune response by eliminating certain cell subsets. None of these drugs has cured patients with rheumatic diseases, but they have produced control and long-term remissions (92a). Three general classes of cytotoxic agents are used:

1. Alkylating agents (e.g., cyclophosphamide, chlorambucil) that cross-link DNA, preventing replication
2. Purine analogs (e.g., azathioprine), which incorporate

into cellular DNA, leading to inhibition of nucleic acid synthesis

3. Folate antagonists (e.g., methotrexate), which cause intracellular deficiency of folate

These drugs all cause marrow suppression and GI intolerance. Cytoxan causes alopecia, hemorrhagic cystitis, and gonadal suppression. Methotrexate causes cirrhosis and is highly teratogenic; it can also cause severe mucosal ulceration. Azathioprine is associated with an increased incidence of infection, and oncogenesis is usually of the lymphoid variety. A review of the therapeutic application of these drugs is presented in Table 59-8. Other types of immunoregulatory drugs are called immune enhancers, such as levamisole, which augments the effector phase of the inflammatory response.

Alternative Medicine

Patients with arthritis, particularly those with chronic arthritis that has been refractory to traditional medical care, often seek alternative treatment. These include acupuncture, relaxation therapy, massage, herbal remedies, diet adjustments, and various other modalities. The practitioner should be knowledgeable in these areas so that he or she can answer patients' questions. Many patients have reported treatment benefit from use of these treatment options, but good controlled trials are sparse in this area (92b).

Experimental Treatment

Experimental techniques such as total nodal lymphoid irradiation, therapeutic apheresis and photopheresis, and antilymphocyte serum have all been used with some success in patients with rheumatic diseases, primarily RA and SLE.

Cyclosporine A, an antifungal agent, has been shown to have suppressive effects on T-helper lymphocytes. Because of this mechanism, it has been used in the treatment of RA and PSA.

Biologic substances also have been used in treating rheumatic diseases. These include interleukins and interferons. Vitamin A derivatives (e.g., isotretinoin and etretinate) also have been used in RA and PSA.

TABLE 59-8. *Therapeutic application of drugs in rheumatic diseases*

Diseases	Recommended medications	Probable mechanisms	Precautions
OA	ASA NSAID	Inhibition of PG synthetase	Allergy bleeding Bleeding diathesis Renal failure
RA ASA, NSAID	As above	As above	As above
	Antimalarials	Block lysosomal enzymes	Retinal toxicity, psoriasis
	Gold	Inhibits phagocytic activity of macrophages	Nephritis, rash, marrow suppression
	D-penicillamine	Unknown	
	Steroids	Interfere with lymphocytic migration; decreases intra-articular membrane permeability	Nephritis, SLE, PM
	Azathioprine	Inhibits DNA synthesis	Lymphoid tumors Not used with allopurinol
	Methotrexate	Causes intracellular folate deficiency	Cirrhosis, leukopenia
	Cyclophopshamide	Prevents DNA replication	Ovarian cystitis
Spondyloarthritis	ASA, NSAID	As above	As above
	Gold	As above	As above
	Methotrexate	As above	As above
Gout	NSAID		
	Uricosurics	Increases excretion of uric acid	Often need to alkanize urine
	Allopurinol	Inhibits xanthine oxidase	Do not use with azathioprine
	Colchicine	Inhibits microtubular assembly and inhibits lysosomal-enyme release	
SLE	NSAID	As above	As above
	Steroids	As above	As above
	Antimalarials	As above	As above
	Azathioprine	As above	As above
PSS	D penicillamine	Unknown	As above
	Colchicine	As above	As above
DM-PM	Steriods	As above	As above
	Azathioprine	As above	As above
	Methotrexate	As above	As above

ASA, aspirin; DM—PM, dermatomyositis—polymyositis; DNA, deoxyribonucleic acid; NSAID, nonsteroidal anti-inflammatory drug; OA, osteoarthritis; PG, prostaglandin; PM, polymyositis; RA, rheumatoid arthritis; SLE, systemic lupus erythematosus.

Surgery: Soft-Tissue and Reconstructive Procedures

The surgical procedures relevant for arthritis include synovectomy, arthrodesis, tendon repair and realignment, osteotomy, and arthroplasty. Each of these procedures has specific indications. Much has been written about the degree of success of these procedures and the attendant complication rates.

Synovectomies

Synovectomies were first performed by Volkmann in 1877 for tuberculosis of the knee. Today they are sometimes performed on RA patients, most commonly to relieve pain and inflammation associated with chronic swelling uncontrolled by medication; to retard the progression of joint destruction, which is a controversial issue; and to prevent and retard tendon rupture. Other indications include the alleviation of decreased ROM caused by very hypertrophied synovial tissue and denervation effect.

Synovectomies are usually performed on the knee, wrist, and metacarpophalangeal joint. Tenosynovectomy is most frequently performed in extensor–flexor tendons of the hand and in the tibialis anterior. Regrowth of synovium commonly occurs postoperatively, so the procedure is not a curative one.

The major contraindications for synovectomy are very active polyarticular disease, which is controversial; poor general medical condition; poor motivation of the patient; and stage IV joint destruction (93). Synovectomy may be performed through an arthroscope.

Arthrodesis

Arthrodesis is performed less often today than in the past because of the popularity and success of joint replacement. It may still be the best procedure to eradicate resistant infection that has destroyed significant bone. The stability provided by an arthrodesis should be permanent. Adolescents and young adults with many more years of activity might well be considered for an arthrodesis in selected instances rather than a joint replacement, which often does not stand the stress placed on it by a young, vigorous patient. Arthrodesis for patients with arthritis is usually limited to the wrist, interphalangeal (IP) joints of the hand, CMC joint, ankle and subtalar joints, and vertebral bodies. Ankle and wrist fusing are often preferred to replacement.

Common indications for arthrodesis of a joint are to relieve persistent pain, to provide stability where there is mechanical destruction of a joint, and to halt progress of the disease (e.g., infection, RA). Joints should be fused in optimal functional position (94a,94b).

Contraindications for arthrodesis include significant bilateral joint disease—joint replacement is indicated more in this instance—and arthrodesis of the same joint on the contralateral side.

Tendon Surgery

Tendon surgery is common in RA for the following conditions:

- Ruptured extensor tendons in the fingers
- Ruptured central slip tendon of the extensor expansion of the extensor digitorum communis in the fourth and fifth digits (correction of boutonniere deformity)
- Long extensor tendon of the thumb
- Flexor tendon rupture in digits (surgery performed less commonly)
- Extensor tendon realignment when tendons have slipped in an ulnar direction over the metacarpophalangeal joints in the hand; commonly combined with synovectomy (95)
- Ruptured Achilles and patellar tendons in SLE
- Release of contracted tendons (e.g., intrinsic muscles of the hand)

Osteotomies

Osteotomy is most commonly performed on the knee in unicompartmental OA to help correct varus and valgus deformities, and it is used to help correct valgus deformity in JRA (96).

Joint Replacements

Patients with RA, JRA, OA, and AN in SLE may require joint replacement. Common indications for replacement are persistent pain despite adequate medical and rehabilitative management, loss of critical motion in the involved joint, and loss of functional status.

The main contraindications for joint replacement are inadequate bone stock and periarticular support, serious medical risk factors, and the presence of significant infection. Other contraindications include lack of patient motivation to cooperate in a postoperative rehabilitation program, and inability of the procedure to increase the patient's total functional level (97–102).

The three most frequently replaced joints are the hip, the knee, and the metacarpophalangeal joints. Other joints for which replacements are performed are the wrist, shoulder, elbow, MTP joints, and ankle. The latter has not been very successful. Joint replacements of the small joints in the hand are usually silastic (Swanson) implants. Those of the lower extremity include vitallium and polyethylene, hydroxyapatite-coated, and porous-coated that stimulate bony ingrowth.

Common complications of joint replacement include loosening, early or late infection, dislocation, fracture of bone adjacent to component, and wearing out of component parts. Other complications are nerve injury, heterotopic ossification, and pulmonary embolus. Infections are more common in patients with RA or SLE and in those taking steroids or immunosuppressive medication (98–102).

Preoperative Rehabilitation Management

To maximize postoperative gains, preoperative rehabilitation interventions are desirable. These interventions include teaching the patient crutch walking with the appropriate type of crutch for the patient; weight reduction for the obese patient; and strengthening of the quadriceps before knee replacement and the hip abductors before hip surgery (97).

Postoperative Rehabilitation Management

The rehabilitation management goals of a total joint replacement program are to relieve pain, to redevelop comfortable musculoskeletal function, and to develop joint protection techniques to avoid overstressing the prosthetic joint.

The postoperative management of hip replacement includes the following procedures:

Refer the patient for rehabilitation on the third to fifth postoperative day.
Perform active-assistive ROM exercises of the hip in all directions, while guarding against excessive flexion or internal rotation (IR) and adduction.
Use a tilt table.
Progress to parallel bars as hypotension is overcome.
Practice swing and stance in place, then take consecutive steps; stop if fatigued.
Progress outside of parallel bars with crutches using the three-point gait for unilateral replacement and the four-point gait for bilateral replacement.
Perform bilateral quadriceps exercises.
Restrict hip flexion to 90° for 3 months.
Provide written home instruction and adaptive devices to compensate for limited flexion of hip (e.g., elevated toilet seat).
When pain free, use isometric exercises to increase hip muscle strength.

The postoperative management of knee replacement includes the following procedures:

Refer the patient to rehabilitation on the third to fifth postoperative day.
Perform active-assistive ROM exercises of the knee. If the knee was immobilized in flexion, the goal is to regain full extension to facilitate maximal quadriceps muscle function.
Use gentle prolonged stretching without eliciting cocontraction in the third postoperative week if necessary to achieve knee extension.
Provide gait training as outlined for hip arthroplasty.
With porous-coated total knee replacements, touch weight bearing only should be done for 4 to 6 weeks or until good bone growth is confirmed (97).

The extent of rotator cuff repair influences the rehabilitation program, but the postoperative management of total shoulder replacement includes the following procedures:

Immobilize the shoulder for 2 to 8 weeks in an airplane splint with the shoulder in 80° of flexion, 70° of abduction, and 5° of IR.
Perform passive motion above the splint level in the supine position.
At 8 to 10 days, perform active-assistive shoulder exercise in the sitting position to 110° of flexion and 20° of external rotation (ER).
Six weeks after the operation, perform active normal range exercises and restrict lifting to 10 pounds (97).

Although the extent of soft tissue and tendon repair dictates the onset of a strengthening program, the postoperative management of elbow joint replacement includes the following procedures:

Refer the patient for rehabilitation on the third to fifth postoperative day.
Allow no varus and valgus strain for the first 6 to 8 weeks.
Six weeks after the operation, perform motion exercise for porous-coated prosthesis.

The postoperative management of total metacarpophalangeal joint replacement includes the following procedures:

Refer the patient for rehabilitation on the third to fifth postoperative day.
Construct static and dynamic splints.
Instruct the patient on monitoring antiedema measures.
Perform an initial exercise program of active-assistive ROM exercises with control of the arc of motion.

Rehabilitation Interventions

Rehabilitation treatment plans must be individualized for the patient's needs; they should be practical, economical, and valued by the patient to enhance compliance. Treatment is best begun early in the disease process so that the patient identifies this as part of the overall management plan. There is scientific and clinical rationale for the use of many specific rehabilitation treatments; others are based on clinical judgment. Rehabilitative rheumatology treatments and techniques must be monitored carefully, and periodic re-evaluation of the patient with adjustments in treatment should be made.

Rest

Three forms of rest can be provided for arthritic persons: local rest of a joint or joints provided by casts or splints, total bed rest, and short rest periods dispersed throughout the day. Although the literature supports the statement that all three forms of rest are beneficial for the arthritic patient (103–110), short rest periods are becoming more widely used. Both local rest and systemic bed rest may have deleterious effects.

Local Rest

Local rest of inflamed joints reduces pain and inflammation and may help to prevent contracture (103–105). Immobilization of the wrist for painful periarticular syndromes (e.g., de Quervain syndrome, carpal tunnel syndrome) is useful for pain relief. Rest for joints of 2 weeks' duration is not noted to cause adverse loss of motion.

Systemic Rest

When comprehensive outpatient rehabilitation management along with appropriate anti-inflammatory medication fails to relieve patients with RA and multiple inflamed joints, hospitalization for rest is appropriate for up to 4 weeks. Studies have verified benefits with this treatment, including a decrease in the number of inflamed joints, a decreased sedimentation rate, and decreased joint stiffness (107–109). Patients with acute PM benefit from bed rest during the acute phases of their illness. It is felt that this treatment may retard muscle destruction and creatine phosphokinase (CPK) elevation.

Short Rest Periods

Patients with RA who participated in a new workbook-based program of energy conservation have been shown to have increased physical activity level capacity when compared with a control group of patients who received standard occupational therapy (110). This workbook approach requires patients to interrupt daily activities lasting more than 30 continuous minutes to take short rest periods. The type of daily activities performed and the joint discomfort and fatigue experienced during them are recorded. Patients are taught how to recognize activities that cause them pain and fatigue and how to modify them to lessen these symptoms. In addition, the workbook includes instructions on behavior modification and health education strategies. This short rest period approach seems to be a cost-effective treatment strategy that can improve the activity level of RA patients.

Exercise

Arthritis commonly produces decreased biomechanical integrity of joints and their surrounding structures, which results in the following:

Decreased joint motion
Muscle atrophy
Weakness
Joint effusion
Pain
Instability
Energy-inefficient gait patterns
Altered joint-loading responses (111–113)

Arthritis patients may lose muscle strength and bulk because of inactivity (114). A muscle can lose 30% of its bulk in a week and up to 5% of its strength a day when maintained at strict bed rest (115,116). Other factors contributing to loss of strength are myositis, myopathy secondary to steroids (117), inhibition of muscle contraction due to joint effusion (118), and direct effects of the disease itself on muscle. For example, in RA, some destruction of muscle fibers occurs as well as intermuscular and perimuscular adhesions, which may impair blood flow. Muscle fascicles adhere to one another, and the entire muscle may adhere to the intermuscular septum and perimuscular fascia, causing inhibition of muscle contraction and normal movement. Myositis of muscle can occur with RA, PM, SLE, and PSS, causing weak, painful, and easily fatigable muscle. Reduced strength as determined by isometric testing has been documented in the quadriceps in RA (119,120), OA (120), PM (121), and JRA (122). Isokinetic strength testing has shown deficits in the quadriceps in RA (119), DM-PM (123), and OA (124). Patients with RA, OA, SLE, and DM have been found to have decreased aerobic capacity (125–127).

The biomechanical advantage of joints is compromised by the weak muscles. Normally, muscles function to provide postural stability and distribute forces of impact and stress across joints during activity. Normal joint function requires that muscles contract and relax synchronously. Atrophic muscles around joints do not coordinate well and are deficient in both static endurance and strength. If the quadriceps is atrophied, the hamstring may exert an overpull, causing excess flexion at the knee. A muscle with normal tone is in slight contraction all the time, and there is no slack in the muscle tendon apparatus, allowing it to be optimally ready for function. There is decreased tone and increased spasm in muscle surrounding arthritic joints, resulting in less coordinated motion of the joint (128).

Exercise programs for patients with arthritis are known to perform the following functions:

Increase and maintain ROM (128)
Re-educate and strengthen muscles (129)
Increase static and dynamic endurance (125,126,129–133)
Decrease the number of swollen joints (133)
Enable joints to function better biomechanically
Increase bone density (134,135)
Increase the patient's overall function and well-being (136)
Increase aerobic capacity (129–133)

Exercise prescriptions must take into account the degree of joint inflammation, mechanical derangement, and joint effusion in each of the joints to be treated; the condition of surrounding muscles; the patient's overall level of endurance; and the condition of the cardiorespiratory system. Programs need to be periodically re-evaluated and adjusted according to the disease activity and stage of the joints at any given time. Physicians should be specific when prescribing exercise programs for arthritis patients. Prescriptions should specify the joints with limited motion, the muscles that need strengthening, the type and duration of exercise to be used, and the specific precautions (113,137–139). It is helpful and generally felt to improve compliance if the patient is provided with a written exercise program that can be performed at home. The patient or family, or both, should be told the purpose of the exercises.

An exercise program should be progressive. It should start with relieving pain of the involved joints with appropriate modalities, and then progress to increasing ROM, if necessary, by stretching and an active or active-assistive ROM program; increasing muscle tone by muscle re-education (i.e., increasing the ability of the patient to relax and contract the muscle completely in a synchronous manner); increasing the static strength and endurance of the muscle by isometric exercise; introduction of an isotonic exercise program for endurance and for strengthening if joints permit; and allow recreational exercise (113).

Passive Exercise

Passive exercise is beneficial for patients with severe muscle weakness due to PM or neuropathic disease associated with stroke, peripheral neuropathy, and vasculitis. However, it should be avoided as much as possible in an acutely inflamed joint, because both Merritt and Hunder (140) and Agudelo and colleagues (141) found that it caused increased inflammation in dogs with urate-induced arthropathy. Passive exercise also increases intra-articular pressure in the presence of joint effusion and has been associated with rupture of the joint capsule (142)

Active Exercise

Active exercise uses three types of muscle contraction (143):

1. Isometric or static contraction: highly suited for arthritis patients with acute joints
2. Isotonic or dynamic contraction: most suited for patients without acutely inflamed or biomechanically deranged joints, because it stresses the joint throughout its range
3. Isokinetic contraction, which in most cases is not recommended for arthritis patients but is used after the acute phase of sports injuries of the knee to rebuild an atrophied quadriceps muscle

Strengthening Exercise

Strengthening of a muscle may be achieved via isometric, isotonic, or isokinetic exercise, but not all of these forms of exercise are appropriate for the arthritic patient.

Isometric (i.e., static) exercise is ideally suited for restoring and maintaining strength in patients with muscle atrophy from rheumatic diseases, as well as for the recovery phase of DM-PM (144). Muller and Rhomert (116,145) and Liberson (146) demonstrated that as little as two thirds of maximal contraction held for 1 to 6 seconds daily can increase strength. Repetitive contractions of 6 seconds each increase static endurance of muscle. Machover and Sapecky demonstrated a significant increase (27%) in quadriceps strength in patients with RA on an isometric strengthening program (129). This program consisted of three maximal contractions held for 6 seconds, with 20 seconds of rest between each, daily. The knee was in 90° of flexion. The opposite quadriceps had a crossover effect with a 17% increase in strength.

An advantage of isometrics is that maximal muscle tension can be generated with minimal work, muscle fatigue, and joint stress. Forceful, repetitive resistive exercise through full joint range is associated with increased joint inflammation, intra-articular pressures, and juxta-articular bone destruction (147). Merritt and Hunder demonstrated that in white rats with uric acid synovitis, isometric exercise of the knee did not increase the joint temperature or joint fluid white count (140). However, one study by Gnootveld and associates in adults indicates that isometric quadriceps exercise of inflamed knee joints in RA yields increased oxidative damage to hyaluronate and glucose, determined by analyzing synovial fluid 1 hour postexercise (148). Therefore, isometric exercise in an inflamed joint is not recommended. However, Ansell has recommended a few isometric contractions a day in children because loss of strength can be rapid around inflamed joints (149). Relaxation of tight muscle around joints is also facilitated by isometrics.

De Lateur and colleagues have shown that strength obtained by isometric training is not fully transferable to isotonic tasks (150); therefore, the addition of isotonic exercise into the arthritic program is warranted where appropriate. DeLorme progressive resistive exercises of isotonic high intensity, high resistance (i.e., high weight), and low repetition build strength but are time consuming and put much stress across joints. De Lateur and associates have shown that low-weight, low-intensity prolonged exercise can build strength as well as static endurance of muscle if carried to the point of fatigue (151). The de Lateur method with low weights is suited to patients with noninflamed joints, few ligamentous problems, and minimal x-ray changes. To further decrease the stress across the joint, the arc of motion is reduced. Isotonic exercise also can be performed in a pool setting.

Dynamic isotonic high-resistive exercise often causes exacerbation of inflammation in general, increases muscle fatigue and joint pain, and secondarily decreases joint ROM (152). Progressive resistive isotonic exercise and isokinetic exercise in general are not recommended for persons with arthritis. In addition, de Lateur and colleagues have found that the strength gains with isokinetic exercise do not exceed those obtained with a low-weight, isotonic strengthening program (153).

A recent study in patients with OA of the knees noted that progressive resistive isotonic exercise (with 4.5 pounds for women and up to 8 pounds for men) when added to a progressive program of isometric isotonic and aerobic exercise increases strength and function and decreases pain (154). An isotonic machine exercise program in RA patients increased strength without exacerbating disease (155).

Isokinetic testing of strength has been done in a 1990 study of RA patients with mild joint disease (119) and in PM patients (123) without deleterious effects. An isokinetic strengthening program used in RA patients increased strength. Complications included several joint flares and a ruptured Baker cyst (156). A 1994 study on a small group of RA patients showed that isokinetic strength training at four speeds for 3 weeks significantly increased strength without joint flares (157). An isokinetic program with medium (120 to 180 deg/sec) velocity is most likely safe in mild OA and RA patients. Low velocities (30 to 90 deg/sec) produce high torque around joints and are best avoided. Isokinetic exercise should not be used in arthritic patients with joint effusion, Baker cyst, ligamentous laxity, acute joints, or joint replacements. A recent study of isokinetic exercise in six PM-DM patients demonstrated a significant increase in strength without significant CPK increases (158).

Endurance

Patients with systemic rheumatic disease have overall limited endurance, and their ability to continue static or dynamic tasks is impaired. Endurance exercise can lead to an increased functional level in RA patients (159,160).

Dynamic endurance exercise for arthritis has proven usefulness. Ekblom and colleagues in 1975 reported a study of stage II and III RA patients who were trained for 6 weeks with bicycle ergometer and quadriceps strengthening exercises (161). They showed that improved mobility and cardiovascular function occurred, in comparison with the control group, without joint flares. This also was seen at 6-month follow-up (159).

Further studies showed an increased size in type I and II quadriceps muscle fibers without joint flares with both short-term training (132) and with longer 7-month training on ergometer cycles (130). In 1981, Nordemar described RA patients who were trained 4 to 8 years on a bicycle ergometer at home and a self-suited exercise program consisting of jogging, skiing, swimming, and cycling (131). He found improved ADL performance in the exercised group as well as less progression of x-ray changes in arthritis, more improvement in hamstring strength, and less sick leave. Harkcom and colleagues (162) also reported benefit from aerobic exercise in RA patients. Minor and colleagues showed that aerobic exercises increase aerobic capacity in both RA and OA patients. Decreased joint counts for pain and swelling also have been associated with aerobic programs for RA patient (130,133,160,162). Exercise programs using different combinations of ROM and strengthening and aerobic exercises on land and in the pool have been beneficial in RA (163). Nicholson demonstrated that SLE patients have decreased aerobic capacity and are able to increase it by 20% on an aerobic exercise program (126). Patients with JRA (164) and PM (165) have been shown to have decreased aerobic capacity and may therefore benefit from aerobic programs.

Bone mineralization is thought to be partially dependent on muscle contraction. Exercise has been shown to have a positive effect on bone mineralization in postmenopausal women (134) Exercise may increase bone mass and may be useful in the management of senile osteopenia (166). Patients with rheumatic disease develop osteopenia from disuse, medication, and calcium and collagen metabolism abnormalities (167). Most studies that support the positive effects of exercise in these areas cite the use of isotonic and some resistive exercises (166). Sinaki and Grubbs showed in a study that back extensor exercise can increase spinal bone density in postmenopausal women (135). This type of exercise may be useful for rheumatic disease patients.

Stretching Exercises

Stretching may be used to prevent contractures and maintain or restore ROM by breaking capsular adhesions. These exercises must be graded according to the degree of inflammation, pain present, and pain tolerance of the patient. Heat to increase collagen extensibility and cold to decrease pain may be used before stretching exercises.

Passive stretching to preserve or increase ROM should not be performed if there is acute inflammation, because it may increase it. It may be used for mechanically deranged joints in which active stretching should be avoided.

Active-assistive stretching can be used for maintaining or increasing ROM when the problem is subacute and pain is decreased. The patient initiates muscle contraction, and the therapist or an assistive device serves as an aid. Forceful stretching should be avoided in the presence of a large joint effusion because capsular rupture may occur.

Active stretching is performed in the absence of pain and inflammation to maintain ROM. It may be facilitated by the use of pulleys. Active stretching exercises in a pool are excellent. Devices may be needed to facilitate stretching for hip flexion contractures in JRA, knee flexion contractures in RA (168), and hemophiliac arthropathy (169). In adhesive capsulitis, traction with overhead pulleys combined with transcutaneous electrical nerve stimulation (TENS) can be used (170). Passive stretching has been found useful in increasing hip and shoulder motion in AS patients (171).

Aquatic Therapy

Aquatic therapy refers to an exercise pool program supervised by a medical professional or physical therapist. The patient is evaluated before the program, and specific exercise goals are set. The goals may include increasing or maintaining joint motion, strength, or endurance.

The benefits of performing exercise in a pool include elimination of gravity and the positive effect of water buoyancy, which may result in decreased joint compression and pain (172). This may further result in increased muscle relaxation. In addition, a greater level of aerobic exercise may be tolerated in the water than on land. Therefore, therapeutic pool therapy may be most useful for those persons with moderate to severe arthritis, post–joint replacement patients with AS, and those with any cardiopulmonary compromise.

Specifically, Danneskiold-Samsoe and colleagues have shown in a study on RA patients that isometric and isokinetic quadriceps strength can be increased by 38% and 16%, respectively, by adhering to a 2-month pool exercise program when compared with pretreatment values. A significant increase in aerobic capacity also can be obtained in RA patients on a pool program (125,173). Ankylosing spondylitis patients with low vital capacity (700–1,500 cm^3) have been shown capable of undergoing pool therapy programs without untoward effect (174). Exercise tolerance appears related to pulmonary function in these patients (175).

Recreational Exercise

Patients with rheumatic diseases often want to participate in recreational exercise programs. Care must be taken to advise the patient which activities or programs would be beneficial for him or her and to relate use of recreational exercise with the condition of the joints (i.e., inflamed, subacute, chronic, mechanical derangement problems). The use of preset rate-limited devices at high torque speeds (e.g., Biodex, Shirley, NY) or of muscle contraction against high resistive forces on Nautilus (Nautilus Corp., Huntersville, NC) machines should be avoided. Light weights and minimal repetitions on the Nautilus machines are permitted for patients with OA and RA with no inflammation, minimal x-ray changes, and no ligamentous laxity. If isotonic weight lifting is performed, it should be with light weights, minimal repetitions, and a short arc of motion. Swimming is an excellent form of isotonic exercise for arthritis patients because gravity is eliminated and ROM of the joints is less painful. ROM and stretching exercises and pool jogging or walking are good. Local chapters of the Arthritis Foundation have aquatic courses for arthritic patients and often make heated pools available. The YMCA also has special pool exercise programs.

Adaptive devices and special hand grips are available to help patients in specific sports (e.g., table tennis, golf, gardening, bowling).

Dance

Dance has now become a popular recreational activity for patients with arthritis. It can help increase joint motion, muscle strength, and aerobic capacity. Van Deusen and Harlowe describe the efficacy of a ROM dance program for adults with RA (176). Other more formal and therapeutic programs, such as Educize by Sue Pearlman, have formally shown increased strength, flexibility, and aerobic capacity along with decreased joint pain and depression (160). Low-impact aerobics are often suitable for arthritis patients. Patients should discuss the feasibility of a dance program with their physician.

Jogging

Jogging itself has not been implicated in causing premature OA of lower extremity joints (177). Running also has been shown to be associated with greater bone density (178).

Dry land jogging, which involves repetitive joint motion and offers little chance for increase in strength, is not recommended if arthritis of the knee or hip is present. If osteophytes appear on knee films with no joint narrowing and no pain, jogging can be permitted.

It is a good rule that a patient should be made as strong as possible by isometrics, and strength and local muscle endurance increased by light isotonic exercises, before recreational exercise is begun.

Indications of excess therapeutic and recreational exercise include postexercise pain at 2 or more hours, undue fatigue, increased weakness, decreased ROM, and joint swelling. If these occur, the program should be adjusted.

Treatment with Heat and Cold Modalities

Therapeutic heat can be applied with a number of devices and techniques (103). The effect on the tissue, location, surface area, depth of the tissue, and acuteness or chronicity of the arthritis must be considered in the selection of modalities.

Most investigations on the use of superficial and deep heat and cold modalities have produced conflicting data. Recent data have helped clarify some dilemas in this area. We now have enough knowledge of the effects of these various modalities on skin, muscle and joint temperature, pain threshold, elasticity of the tendon, relaxation of spasticity in muscle, and synovial fluid enzyme activity, cell count, and volume. With use of these data, plus clinical observation, recommendations can be made as to the appropriate use of heat and cold for acute or chronic arthritis.

Heat

The use of superficial heat for pain relief in patients with arthritis is well known. Patients report that warm baths, heated pools, hot packs, and warm mineral springs provide relief of pain and decrease the stiffness in their joints. Normal intra-articular temperature is reported to be lower than body temperature (179). Skin and joint temperature is increased by 34°C to 37.5°C in patients with active arthritis (180). Superficial moist heat applied for 3 minutes causes elevation of the soft-tissue temperature in normal individuals by 3°C to a depth of 1 cm (181). The old reports of Hollander in 1949 indicate that in inflamed knee joints, the joint temperature is decreased by 2.2°F with application of superficial heat hot packs and increased by paraffin packs (182). On the other hand, microwave application of deep heat to the knee increases the temperature by 8.4°F, and shortwave diathermy by 9.8°F. Lehmann and colleagues demonstrated that ultrasound elevated the temperature in the pig hip joint by 4°C more than did the application of microwave or shortwave diathermy (183). Hence the paradox of the past 45 years that some forms of superficial heat lower joint temperature while other forms and deep heat increase it. A recent study (184) urges us to discard the old heat pack Hollander data. These recent data indicate that superficial heat applied to patients with arthritis increases both skin and joint temperature in inflammatory arthritis. Painful stimuli, apprehension, alarm, or smoking lowers skin temperature and elevates knee joint temperature, as do active and passive exercise.

When joint temperature is increased from 30.5°C to 36°C, as it is in active RA, the collagenase enzyme from a rheumatoid synovium is four times as active with lysis of cartilage (185). Increasing joint temperatures could contribute to perpetuating inflammation and joint destruction. Ultrasound as a deep-heating modality has the capability of increasing joint temperature to this level in superficial and deep normal joints. Microwave increases intra-articular temperature in RA (182).

Dorwart and colleagues (186) showed that prolonged superficial heat (i.e., 4 hours) elevates the volume and white count of joint fluid in acute crystalline-induced arthritis. A temperature increase of 5°C increases the enzymes in urate-induced synovitis. There are no studies to indicate if superficial heat applied for a clinically acceptable time of 20 minutes causes the same phenomena or if the same effect is seen in RA as in crystalline disease. Mainardi and associates (187) found no increase in joint destruction and inflammatory activity in the hand in RA with the use of superficial heat.

Warren and co-workers (188) noted that rat tail tendon distended more when heated to 45°C than when heated to 39°C, and prolonged stretching could produce longer lasting and greater deformation of rat tail collagen when heated (189). Deep heat affects the viscoelastic properties of collagen. As tension is applied, stretch is effected, and an increase of creep (i.e., the plastic stretch of ligamentous structures placed under tension) occurs. Heat may enhance the efficacy of stretching if applied to appropriately chosen joints.

Both superficial and deep heat can raise the threshold for pain after application (190). They produce sedation and analgesia by acting on free nerve endings of both peripheral nerves and gamma fibers of muscle spindles (191).

Cold

Cold modalities decrease skin and muscle temperature (192). However, Hollander and Horvath found that cold packs elevated knee joint temperature (182). The application of cold to rheumatoid joints may therefore inhibit collagenase activity in the synovium (185). Recent studies indicate that cold air and ice decrease joint temperature in inflammatory arthritis patients (184).

Some clinical studies have shown more relief of pain with ice in patients with RA than with deep heat by diathermy. The pain threshold of the shoulder as measured with an algesimeter was higher immediately after and 30 minutes after treatment with ice than it was with shortwave diathermy (193). Ice also causes more prolonged relief of pain then superficial heat in RA patients (194).

Other investigations found the increase of knee joint ROM to be the same with either ice or superficial heat applied daily for 5 days, with a 9-day interval between the two treatments (195).

Cold decreases muscle spasticity (196) and muscle spindle activity and raises the pain threshold. Cold should not be used in patients with Raynaud's phenomenon, cold hypersensitivity, cryoglobulinemia, or paroxysmal cold hemoglobinuria (197). The abrupt application of cold causes discomfort and produces a stressful response (197).

One study indicated that cold significantly decreases joint stiffness and increases function in OA (198).

Controlled clinical trials in the use of modalities are still lacking. At best, information can be gleaned from noncontrolled studies and clinical observation to choose the appropriate modalities in treating patients with arthritis (199a,199b).

In treating the acutely inflamed or early subacute joint, the goal is pain relief. One is careful not to use interventions that may perpetuate inflammation. The use of cold seems most logical because it can decrease the pain threshold, can relax surrounding spastic muscles, and is associated with decreased joint temperature, collagenase, and cell count in the joint fluid.

Later in the subacute period, when inflammatory pain is subsiding and stiffness is present, and the patient may have lost some ROM, either cold or superficial heat with TENS is appropriate before starting active-assistive ROM and isometric exercise. When inflammation has fully subsided, superficial heat for pain is appropriate. If tight periarticular structures remain, ultrasound or cold and TENS followed by stretching to increase joint ROM is suitable. Transcutaneous electrical nerve stimulation has been reported to relieve joint pain in RA (200,201) and pain in RA neuropathy (103).

Orthotics

Splints and orthotics are used to unweight joints, stabilize joints, decrease joint motion, or support joints in a position of maximal function and increase joint motion (i.e., dynamic splint). Splints may be prefabricated but are best when molded to fit the individual patient (see Chapters 25 and 26) (202).

Upper Extremities

Orthotics for the upper extremities are mainly confined to the wrist and hand and include resting splints, functional wrist splints, thumb post splints, ring splints, and dynamic splints. Resting splints immobilize the hand and wrist and are used at night for patients with active RA, carpal tunnel syndrome, or extensor tendinitis. The role of splints in preventing deformity in RA has not yet been scientifically proven. The clinical recommendation is to use both resting and functional splints in early RA; in JRA they probably

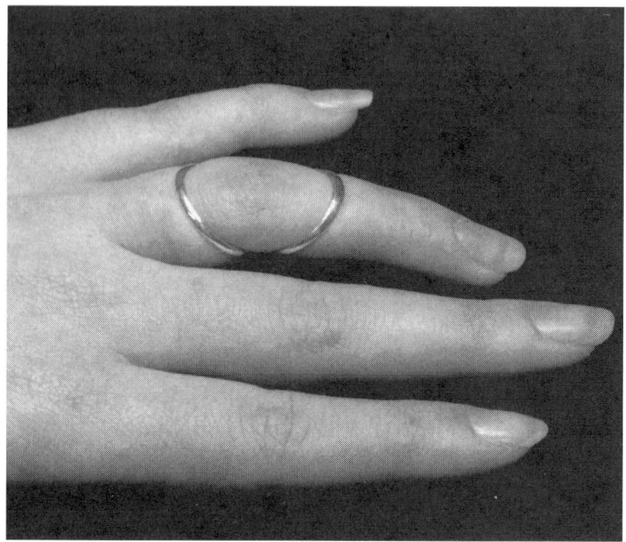

FIG. 59-2. Swan neck ring splint.

help in delaying ulnar deviation and in reducing pain, synovitis, and edema. Functional wrist splints extend to the midpalmar crease, permit finger function, block wrist flexion, and are used for activities during periods of inflammation. They provide wrist and ligament support. A functional thumb post splint may be used to relieve CMC and IP pain associated with OA. The same type of splint with a longer wrist extension is useful for de Quervain extensor tendinitis of the thumb. A functional wrist cock-up splint can help relieve pain in carpal tunnel syndrome.

Small ring splints (e.g., Bunnell orthoses, boutonniere orthoses) can reduce swan neck or boutonniere deformity. Cosmetic splints constructed of silver or gold and highlighted with semiprecious stones are available (Fig. 59-2).

For patients who have had MCP replacements or who have a radial nerve neurapraxia, a dynamic outrigger splint pulls the fingers into extension, from which patients must actively work to pull into flexion. They provide gentle stretch through limited range while supporting the wrist and MTPs. Splints that realign digits to help reduce ulnar deviation are also available (Fig. 59-3).

Elbow orthotics are rarely used. They may be useful in children with JRA and PM. Resting night splints may help to contain the advancement of an elbow flexion contracture. Braces with dial locks are used to increase extension during the day.

Compliance with splints has been assessed in a number of studies (71,203,204). Compliance is best when family members expect the patient to be compliant and when the patient uses splints to relieve pain. Cosmesis is a major factor for nonuse, as is fear of discrimination in the workplace.

Lower Extremities

The most useful orthotics in arthritis are those for the foot and ankle. Those for the knee have been less successful, and there are none generally used for the hip.

Foot–Ankle. Excess pronation at the subtalar joint, loss of the medial arch, and subtalar movement commonly seen in RA (205) can cause pain, contribute to tarsal tunnel syndrome, and cause strain on the knee and hip. Control of pronation by bringing the calcaneus perpendicular to the floor often relieves pain and helps to balance the weight-bearing column. The first step toward control is to fit the patient with a shoe with a good heel counter and a soft or rigid orthotic insert lined with Spenco (AliMed, Dedham, MA). The sole should not be too soft. This will minimize the flotation effect on heel-strike and stance during gait and decrease stress, hypermobility, or instability at the ankle or a higher joint level. If pronation is not controlled by a shoe, a hindfoot orthotic has been shown to improve gait and reduce pain (Fig. 59-4) (206). A beveled heel that makes a 20° angle with the floor can decrease ankle motion and pain (207). For the very painful or arthritically involved ankle from traumatic OA postfracture or RA, a short-leg patellar tendon–bearing orthosis that shifts weight away from the ankle to the patellar tendon is useful (208). Fasciitis of the heel may be relieved with a cup insert or an insert with a depression in the area of the tender fascia.

Appropriate wide-toe-box shoes should be used to accommodate a wide forefoot, cocked toes, and hallux valgus seen in RA or JRA, as well as the hallux valgus deformity seen in OA. A soft insert is added, as are metatarsal reliefs, whether in the form of a cookie inside the shoe or an external bar on the sole of the shoe. We prefer the former because we believe it to be safer. A rocker bottom shoe can facilitate rollover in the presence of a painful ankle (209).

Knee. Bracing for the knee may be for pain, instability caused by ligamentous laxity, significant quadriceps weakness, or excess recurvatum (210–212). A useful brace for quadriceps weakness is a double upright Klenzak (Pel Supply, Cleveland, OH) set at 5° plantar flexion at the ankle to put the knee in extension during heel-strike and stance (213).

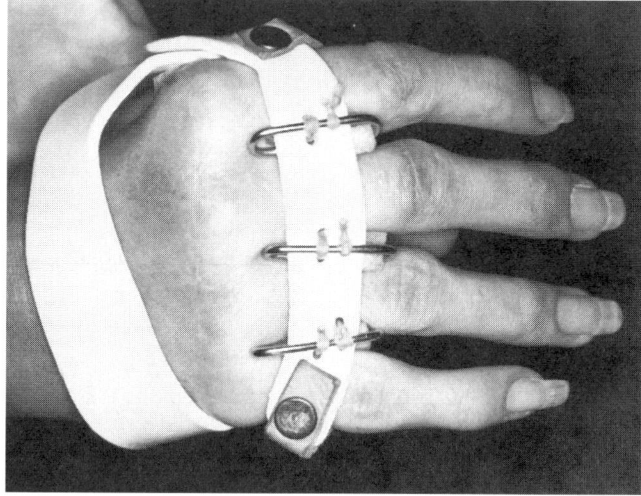

FIG. 59-3. Dynamic ulnar deviation splint with metacarpophalangeal hinge.

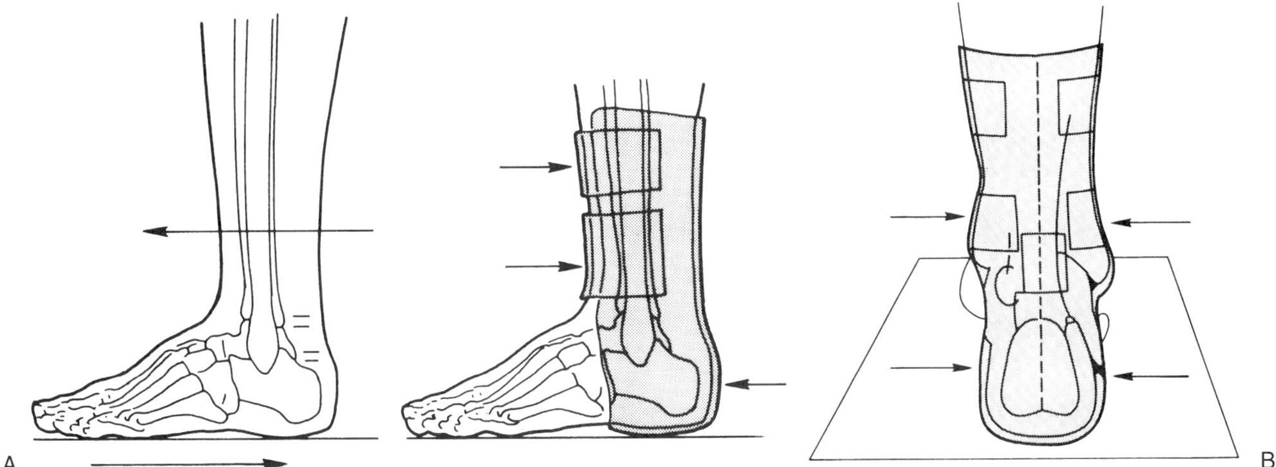

FIG. 59-4. A: A hindfoot orthotic. **B:** Rear view. On the braced limb, the arrows represent the resistive forces. On the unbraced limb, the arrows represent the direction of motion of the limb.

The Klenzak can be used for a unilateral problem or for the weaker side when the problem is bilateral, as in PM. Success also can be achieved with a plastic molded AFO cast in 5° plantar flexion with a small added 3/8-inch heel incorporated into the orthosis provided the patient is not overweight. A Lenox Hill orthosis (3-M, Long Island, NY) may be used to control mediolateral or rotational instability. These braces are rarely used in RA but are used for younger athletic individuals.

A knee–ankle–foot orthosis (KAFO) with ischial weight bearing and dial lock at the knee can be used to reduce knee pressure and may be adjusted to relieve medial or lateral compartmental stresses in OA or RA. This orthosis is difficult to fit with severe valgus deformities and in the obese patient. Compliance in the use of KAFOs is poor.

Smaller knee orthoses, such as hinged orthoses, the Swedish knee cage, or Lerhman orthoses (Pel Supply, Cleveland, OH), may be used to help control sagittal and frontal knee plane motion. A knee orthosis to help prevent dislocation of the patella is available and often effective. A shoe with a beveled heel at 20° also decreases knee flexion and promotes a more stable extended knee (207). Orthoses with a dial lock turned 1 or 2° daily can be used to reduce knee flexion contracture. Elasticized knee supports may help control swelling and often provide patients with a sense of control of the quadriceps.

Spinal Orthoses

Spinal orthoses are used primarily to relieve pain, limit motion, or support an unstable spine. A lumbar spinal orthosis or thoracic orthosis with mold and form insert will often relieve a painful back due to compression fracture or disc disease. This type of orthosis may reduce lordosis, reinforce abdominal muscles, and unload the spine (214,215). For thoracic compression fractures prone to gibbous deformity or an unstable lumbar or thoracic spine, a Jewett orthosis (Florida Brace, Winter Park, FL) or a molded polypropylene body jacket is required.

A lumbosacral corset does not limit motion but provides some abdominal support and relieves painful lower lumbar musculature.

The cervical spine is involved in RA, OA, JRA, and spondyloarthropathies. A variety of collars provide different levels of support (216). A soft cervical collar only minimally limits motion but provides some pain relief. A Philadelphia collar (Pel Supply, Cleveland, OH) offers slightly more support and some limitation of extension. A two-poster, four-poster, or sterno-occipital mandibular immobilizer collar substantially limits flexion and extension, particularly at C1–C2, but also at C4–C6 (217). A halo is needed to completely control C1–C2 instability.

Assistive Devices and Adaptive Aids

These aids and devices compensate for limited ROM and pain and help promote independence for arthritic patients. To help ensure patient acceptance, the appliance should be affordable, be easy to use, and improve patient function.

Ambulation and transfer skills are extremely important for persons with arthritis, and gait aids and devices may be needed.

Gait Aids

If joint pain is a problem, secondary to loss of cartilage, effusion, or active synovitis, the painful joint needs to be unloaded. Weight reduction is encouraged, because a 1-kg weight loss results in a 3- to 4-kg decrease in load across the hip joint (218). A straight cane or quad cane is good for balance but is not very efficient in unloading the limb, but a forearm crutch is. The elbow should be in 30° of flexion when such a device is in use.

Custom hand grip pieces can be made by making a mold

of the patient's hand in a functional position of weight bearing, or commercially made hand pieces on canes are available. Platform crutches distribute weight on the forearm, reducing the need for wrist extension. Forearm attachments for walkers and wheelchairs are available.

For significant loss of strength or endurance, a small, lightweight wheelchair is recommended. There are also small motorized scooters, such as the sporty Amigo Chair (Amego Mobility Intl. Inc., Bridgeport, MI).

Adaptive Devices for Transfer

Chronic hip or knee pain, limited motion, and proximal muscle weakness make transfers from low-level chairs, toilets, and beds difficult. Upper extremities may be needed for push-off, but when these are incapacitated by RA, such simple motion becomes impossible. Independence in making transfers can be restored by elevating the seat with a cushion or placing 3- or 4-inch blocks under each leg of chairs, tables, and beds (Fig. 59-5). Chairs with motorized seats, elevated toilet seats, and clamp-on tub seats are helpful.

Transfers in and out of the car are facilitated by the use of an extra-thick seat cushion and a mounted grab bar to increase leverage. In the car, use of the side, rearview, and wide-angle mirrors for patients with limited cervical ROM due to OA and spondyloarthropathies becomes essential. A spinner bar for the steering wheel and a large-handled door opener and ignition piece are adaptations for the patient with significant hand problems. Patients with back pain benefit from a firm seat and back cushion, such as a PCP Champion Sacro cushion (OTC Professional Appliances, Ripley, OH); those with neck pain need adjustable neck supports or pillows.

Self-Care

Dressing, undressing, and other daily self-care activities can be time- and energy-consuming tasks for persons with RA, SLE, and PM. Adaptive and self-care aids such as long-handled reachers, shoehorns, elastic shoelaces, long-handled sponges, brushes and toothbrushes, Stirex scissors (North Coast Medical, San Jose, CA), button hooks, zipper hooks, toilet paper holders, and large-handled items are all helpful devices that also conserve energy. Clothing made with elastic and Velcro is easier to don than that with buttons and hooks. Wrinkle-resistant fabrics that do not require ironing and lightweight fabrics and wools (e.g., mohair, alpaca) are useful. Large buttons and partial zippering before putting on the garment may facilitate dressing, as will stretch straps and waists, garments with large raglan sleeves, and those with smooth linings. Capes, ponchos, and down jackets are easy to put on, warm, and lightweight.

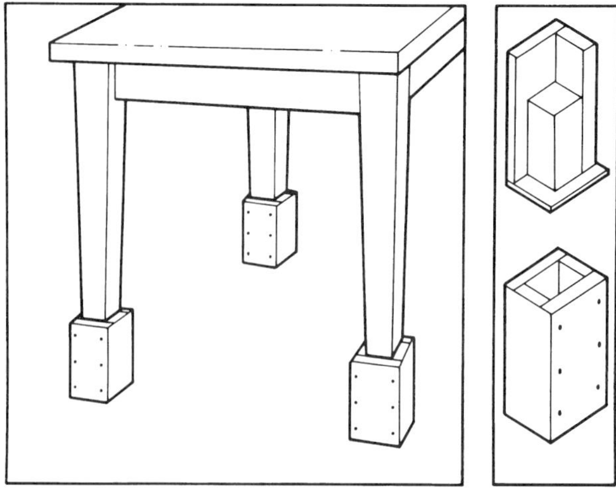

FIG. 59-5. Blocks for elevating chair or table legs.

Devices in the Kitchen

Useful kitchen devices include food processors, long-handled reachers, built-up handles on utensils, electric knives, mounted wedge-shaped jar openers, and lightweight aluminum pans. Lining pans with aluminum foil saves scrubbing. Bringing together items involved in a work area (e.g., kitchen stove, work area, sink, refrigerator) is helpful. A microwave oven cuts down on food preparation time. A kitchen cart loaded with often-used utensils cuts down on walking.

Environmental Design

Slopes, stairs with deep steps, high curbs, and buses or cars may be difficult to negotiate for someone with disease of the hips and knees. Appropriate placement of steps, lowered curbs, suitably graded inclines, and ramps are helpful. Buses that kneel to accept passengers are available in many communities. Indoors, thick carpets increase friction and are difficult to walk on or negotiate in a wheelchair. In the bathroom, guard rails are best for safety. The bathtub should have nonskid strips or an entire nonskid surface. Door openings should be wide enough to accept a wheelchair. Chest-high storage cabinets and waist-high work surfaces are best; special door handles are available. For those patients in wheelchairs, proper positioning of doorknobs, light switches, and kitchen equipment is necessary. Large-handled pencils and eating utensils are helpful. Devices to help with spray cans are available. The Arthritis Foundation provides a catalog of available assistive devices (219).

Education

Patient education should include a discussion about the natural history of the disease and the likely impact that it will have on life-style, job, and leisure activities. Many systemic rheumatic diseases are chronic and have periods of remission and exacerbation that affect function.

A good rapport between physician and patient must exist in discussing these problems. The physician must take a comprehensive approach to the patient to assist him or her in habilitation or adjustment to the chronic disease process. In addition, educational groups consisting of arthritis patients who gather to hear experts in the field and talk about aspects of medical and rehabilitative management are very informational and supportive. These groups are sponsored by hospitals, the YMCA, and the Arthritis Foundation.

Some studies relate that education increases patient compliance, whereas others report that it provides increased knowledge about the disease process, enhanced communication with physician and family, and improved coping ability (220–222). Other studies have deduced no knowledge differences (223,224).

Distinction between the psyche and the soma, and which role each plays in the expression of rheumatic disease, is being hotly debated. Some data support the idea that patients who are more educated about their illness and who become more active participants in the management of their disease function better. These patients experience less distress, pain, and sleep disturbance (2,225).

Joint Protection

In 1965, Cordery observed that arthritic patients change their life-style and habits to protect their joints and use devices that make work easier rather than persist with activity that causes pain (226). Melvin also has described practical suggestions about joint preservation (227).

Elements in a program of joint protection for arthritic patients include the following:

Avoid prolonged periods in the same position.
Minimize stress on particular joints by promoting good posture.
Maintain ROM, strength, and good joint alignment.
Reduce pain.
Unload the joint when very painful.
Avoid overuse during acute periods of pain.
Use appropriate adaptive equipment and splints when necessary.
Modify tasks to decrease joint stress.

Joint protection and its companion, energy conservation, are based on data that suggest that use exacerbates joint inflammation, and rest diminishes inflammation.

Energy Conservation

In systemic rheumatic disease accompanied by fatigue, conserving energy to maximize function is an important part of the arthritic patient's life-style. Some of the mechanisms for conserving energy are listed as follows:

Maximize biomechanical function of joints by use of proper orthotics and assistive devices to effect energy-efficient ambulation and hand function.
Use appropriate adaptive aids and clothing.
Provide proper environmental design.
Have rest periods throughout the day.
Maintain ROM and strength.
Maintain proper posture.

Good body posture, whether sitting or standing, balances the weight of the head and limbs on the body framework so that gravity helps to maintain joint position with minimal muscle activity. Significant changes in posture cause muscles to exert more energy to pull against the force of gravity. For example, standing takes 25% more energy than sitting to perform activities. Ideal posture cannot be maintained unless care is taken to preserve ROM and strength of muscles around the joints (228).

Psychosocial Interventions

Rheumatic disease has a major impact on the patient's mobility, ADLs, general life-style, self-image, family life, sexuality, and work. Major patient reactions ranging from denial and repression to depression occur, as do other components of chronic illness, such as anger, bargaining, and acceptance. The belief that there is a particular personality type prone to developing RA has been dropped. However, premorbid personality is an important determinant of the patient's reaction to illness. Patients with arthritis, in addition to coping with pain, may have to deal with losses in function and losses in physical attractiveness due to the disease and medication side effects, and they will have to deal with the reactions of friends, spouse, and family. The unpredictability of systemic disease complicates the coping process (229).

Some families adjust well, maintaining good communication, support, and flexibility in family routines. Other families are not able to reorganize and adjust to the needs of a person with arthritis. Psychiatric support for both patient and family is often needed. Group therapy including discussion about body image, job status, family relationships, and coping mechanisms is effective and has been used for a variety of arthritic groups (230,231).

Sexual Adjustment

About 50% of normal, well-educated, financially successful, and maritally stable U.S. adults admit to sexual dysfunction or difficulties (98). According to Ehrlich, "sexual orientation of the person who has a musculoskeletal disorder is not necessarily very different from that of someone who does not. However, arthritis may impose certain limitations or alterations that influence the sexual life as they do other activities of daily living" (232).

Particular sexual problems in the arthritic patient arise as a result of mechanical problems associated with decreased ROM, pain, and stiffness; depression, with decreased self-image and interest; drug therapy resulting in decreased libido; psychosocial problems in the family unit related to the patient's arthritis; and fatigue (233).

Mechanical Problems. Arthritic involvement of the hips, knees, lumbar spine, hands, and shoulders commonly causes mechanical or painful problems that interfere with sexual performance. Sixty-seven percent to 75% of all patients with arthritic hips have some mechanical sexual disability (234). Analgesics and warm baths before intercourse may help. In women with more advanced disease, a posterior approach by the man for intercourse may be successful. With severe limitation of motion, either unilateral or bilateral hip replacements may be requisite to achieve intercourse. After hip surgery, intercourse should not be resumed at all for 6 weeks, and hip flexion over 90° should be avoided (235). Neither pain, nor stiffness, nor limitation of motion of the knees should mechanically limit intercourse, but a change in position may be required for more comfort. For those patients with back pain (e.g., OA, spondyloarthropathies, disc disease), a lateral position for both the man and the woman is preferable.

Significant problems in the joints of the hands and arms, as in RA, are more restrictive for the man than for the woman, and a side-lying position may alleviate this. In both men and women, arthritis of these joints may interfere with the early stages of lovemaking involving caressing and manual stimulation (236).

Self-Image. Often arthritic patients experience a decrease in self-image, a feeling of helplessness, and ultimately depression, which in turn is associated with decreased libido. Chronic pain may reduce a woman's efforts to make herself more attractive for her partner, and it is difficult to reassure the woman who has significant joint deformities that she is still physically attractive. A man may abstain from sexual relations rather than cause his arthritic spouse pain, and the spontaneity is reduced. Appropriate counseling may help alleviate these problems.

Medications. Certain medications are associated with decreased libido (e.g., Aldomet [Merck & Co., West Point, PA], steroids). High-dose steroids used in SLE and DM-PM may affect physical appearance and contribute to decreased self-image or acceptance by one's spouse. Immunosuppressive medications may interfere with conception.

Psychosocial Problems. Psychosocial problems in the family unit may lead to decreased sexual relationships between husband and wife. Such problems include inability to work, inadequate finances, limited acceptance by friends, and limited participation in social or recreational events. Misunderstanding and anxieties of the children about the chronic disease of the parents also contribute to tension and adversely influence sexual relationships.

Fatigue. Fatigue associated with systemic diseases can be a major factor in limiting sexual activities. Energy conservation is essential.

Successful treatment of musculoskeletal disease does not necessarily serve as a sexual restorative; rather, understanding, counseling, alterations in sexual positions, or appropriate joint replacements are necessary.

Vocational Aspects

A vocational assessment should be part of the workup for rheumatic disease patients and should cover educational level, work history and achievements, physical functional level, and social and psychological adjustment. Musculoskeletal conditions rank second to disease of the circulatory system in restricting activities, make up 41% of persons referred to vocational rehabilitation, and are the second most frequent cause of work disability (237).

The arthritic patient's ability to remain in the work setting depends on the stage of arthritis and the concomitant functional limitations imposed by it; the duration of the disease; the use of the proper medical and rehabilitation treatment to ensure a maximal functional level; the type of job the person has; and the willingness of the employer to allow for modifications in the job or to make environmental changes (238). Rehabilitation with a team approach has been associated with improved functional level in terms of ADL, mobility, and economic independence (69,70).

The more flexibility or control over work conditions that a person has, the more likely he or she is to maintain a job (238). This is called locus of control. The first step in vocational counseling is to see if adjustments can be made in the job setting so that the patient can continue working. If changes cannot be made, then the patient may have to receive training for another vocation. Remaining in the work force or being a homemaker is an important goal for the person with arthritis, and rehabilitative care and the support of the family help ensure success.

Specific Diseases

Osteoarthritis

Osteoarthritis, the most common type of arthritis, is an asymmetrical noninflammatory disease that has no systemic component. Most frequently it becomes clinically significant after retirement. There are three types of OA:

1. Primary
2. Secondary
3. Erosive inflammatory

In primary OA, the joints that develop OA in order of decreasing frequency are the knees, first MTP joints, DIP joints, CMC joints, hips, cervical spine, and lumbar spine. It spares the elbows and shoulders, except if it is secondary OA caused by an injury, fracture, or occupation-related task. In a population of mill workers in North Carolina, Hadler relates specific tasks to the development of secondary OA as measured by x-ray films (239).

In OA, the main impact on function results from involvement of large weight-bearing joints, which can cause pain and limit mobility. Back involvement ranks next. Osteoarthritis of the hands (i.e., CMC, PIP, DIP joints) is generally not associated with significant impairment of function in daily activities, except significant CMC arthritis, which can cause difficulty at work with repetitive or manual labor tasks. Middle-aged women who have a clinical syndrome, inflammatory erosive OA described by Ehrlich (240), have painful swelling and redness of the PIPs and DIPs resembling RA in appearance and interfering with ADL. It often burns out in 5 years, with no long-term disability.

A 1983 study by Kramer and colleagues showed that 26% of patients with significant OA still worked full time, even though 44% indicated that they were always symptomatic (241). The mean number of bed days for a person with OA was 12.2 per year.

The course of OA is slow and variable. In one study, the mean time from onset of hip pain to severe loss of motion was 8 years (range 18 months to 23 years) (242). In some people, the disease stabilizes (243) and does not progress. Osteoarthritis of the knee has a worse prognosis than that of the hip (244), and varus deformity and early development of pain appear to be unfavorable prognostic factors.

Assessment

Rehabilitative assessment includes evaluating the biomechanical joint deficits as they relate to joint function as well as studying the impact of the joint defect on contiguous joints and the patient's comfort and independence.

Because OA is basically a degenerative process, pain is usually local and results from altered biomechanics of the involved joint, and stress and strain on periarticular structures (e.g., tendons, muscles, nerves), which may result in radiating pain to other sites. Specifically, pain can be caused by periosteal elevation by spurs, trabecular microfractures, and capsular distension with fluid accumulation and associated crystal deposition disease (i.e., pseudogout).

Many people with OA by radiography are clinically asymptomatic; most studies show 25% to 30% having no symptoms (245). However, the severity of symptoms when they occur seems to correlate with the extent of x-ray findings (8). In a recent study of quadriceps strength, age and degree of knee pain were more important determinants of functional impairment in OA in the elderly than severity of x-ray changes (246). Joint stiffness in the morning and after periods of inactivity is common. Limited joint motion occurs as the OA progresses and may be compounded by poor positioning of joints, particularly at night.

Treatment plans should include methods to decrease pain, preserve and restore ROM and strength, reduce joint loads, prevent or reduce contractures, and preserve joint alignment. Although vigorous exercise with normal joints does not appear to cause OA, its use when OA is present may accelerate it (247). However, appropriate exercise has been shown to increase strength and aerobic capacity and to decrease pain (125). Less disability also has been reported by OA patients after exercise programs (248).

Problems of Specific Joints

Hip. Osteophytes on x-ray are often an indication of the presence of OA; subchondral cysts, sclerosis, and joint-space narrowing usually follow. Hip pain, usually located around the greater trochanter, can be confused with trochanteric bursitis; it may radiate to the groin, the anterior thigh, the knee, and the sacroiliac joints. Unilateral hip disease has a high association with increased leg length on the affected side (249). A lift for the opposite shoe is indicated if there is more than a 0.25-inch discrepancy.

An important goal is to maintain at least 20° to 30° of hip flexion to assume normal gait. Osteoarthritis of the hip is associated with loss of motion in all planes and weakness of the abductors and extensors of the hip. Hip effusion may cause inhibition of contraction of the gluteus medius. Lurching to the same side or a Trendelenburg gait may be seen.

The patient should maintain hip extension by lying in the prone position for 30 to 40 minutes twice daily. For tight hip flexors unresponsive to active stretching exercise, prolonged stretching of the hip flexors may be effected in the supine position with a pillow under the affected buttocks and a 10- to 20-pound weight supported by a sling from the knee. Isometric exercise should emphasize both the abductors and the extensors.

Knee. In contradistinction to the hip, osteophytes on a knee joint x-ray without any other changes (e.g., joint space narrowing, cysts) are not usually an indication of OA, but are associated with the aging process in individuals over 40 years of age. Knee problems may be uni-, bi-, or tricompartmental. Pain in the knee with OA may be due to several conditions:

- Loss of cartilage
- Mechanical compression of the medial knee compartment with varus deformity or the lateral compartment with valgus deformity
- Stretch on the medial and lateral collateral ligament
- Microfractures and subchondral fractures
- Capsular distension by effusion
- Associated syndromes such as anserine bursitis or prepatellar bursitis
- Chondromalacia patellae
- PPD, which is seen in 28% of OA patients by 80 years of age (136)

Pain can be referred medially from the hip. As much as possible, identification of the mechanism of the pain should be determined before treatment. Moderate or large effusions should be tapped and the fluid should be checked for CPPD crystals. Steroid and lidocaine should be instilled if no indication of infection is present. Effusion can inhibit voluntary contraction of the quadriceps (250) and contribute to atrophy and is associated with instability and valgus or varus deformity. Range of motion of the knee in the presence of joint effusion increases intra-articular pressure.

Pain and swelling of the knee led to restricted ROM and contractures of the joint capsule and hamstrings. If the knee cannot fully extend, it depends on the weakened quadriceps for stability, causing increased mechanical stresses and further joint dysfunction. Deep knee bends may increase intra-articular pressure and thus should be avoided (251). The amount of valgus or varus deformity of the knee can be reduced with a medial or lateral wedge and a flare of the sole of the shoe.

The patient should avoid the use of a pillow under the knee at night because this encourages knee and hip flexion contracture, plantar flexion at the ankle, and venous obstruction in the popliteal area. A functionally important goal is to maintain extension. More than 10° of flexion contracture results in less than optimal knee biomechanics and increased stress with weight bearing.

Recent studies demonstrated that both the quadriceps and hamstring muscles show decreased strength on isometric and isokinetic testing (252). For strengthening, non–weight-bearing quadriceps and hamstring isometric exercises should be performed twice daily by all patients with OA of the knee. With patellofemoral disorders, quadriceps isometrics with the knee extended are best to avoid patellofemoral compression. A more comprehensive graded exercise program with isometrics, isotonic resistive and aerobic exercise for OA of the knee has been shown to result in increased quadriceps and hamstring strength and increased ability to perform chair rises, walking, and stair climbing (154).

Foot. Fifty percent of patients with OA have significant foot problems (251). The most commonly encountered problems are hallux valgus with or without bunions, hallux rigidus with cocked toes, metatarsal head calluses, and abrasions on the dorsum of the toes.

Ensuring properly fitting shoes is essential (see section on Foot–Ankle Orthotics). If hallux rigidus or painful first MTP is present, mobility at the toe-off portion of the gait cycle will be decreased; a rocker sole will help facilitate toe-off. The physician must be sure that the problem is a foot problem and not compensation for a more proximal problem (e.g., rotation of the tibia or hip).

Carpometacarpal Joint. The CMC is frequently affected by OA. The use of a thumb post splint to immobilize the thumb in a functional abducted position will relieve pain and allow for performance of functional activities. In severe OA, fusion in a functional position may be necessary.

Rheumatoid Arthritis

Rheumatoid arthritis is a systemic rheumatic disease that primarily affects the synovial lining of diarthrodial joints. It can affect almost any and all of the peripheral joints with relative sparing of the axial spine, except for the upper cervical (i.e., atlantoaxial) joints. However, degenerative change frequently accompanies it and involves C4–C5 and C5–C6. The end result of the process is joint pain, swelling, and malfunction. The muscles that surround the swollen, inflammed joints or biomechanically compromised joints are painful and are often atrophied or myositic. Ankylosis may occur, but subluxation is more common. Malalignment and pain result in increased problems with ADLs, mobility, and energy expenditure. Pain and deformity may cause problems with self-image and sexual activity (253).

Fatigue is a hallmark of RA. Its causes are varied and include pain, sleep disorder, depression, cardiorespiratory problems, and muscle weakness. Involvement of the cardiorespiratory system leads to further compromise of endurance. Involvement of the skin can lead to poorly healing ulcers of the lower extremity. Neuritis and vasculitis can impair mobility and function. Side effects from the chronic use of anti-inflammatory medications can cause GI tract disturbance, muscle atrophy, and sleep disruption.

Prognosis and Management

Clinically, 80% of those initially diagnosed as having possible or probable RA are misdiagnosed or experience complete remission. Definite or classical RA may take three courses:

1. Intermittent mild disease with partial or complete periods of remission lasting 1 month to 1 year or more (about 30% of patients)
2. Long clinical remission of 12 to 30 years
3. Progressive disease with either rapid or slow, but relentless, deterioration

There are two subgroups: those who respond to medical therapy and those who do not (i.e., less than 3% of those with definite or classical RA). It is these two subgroups that experience the greatest adverse impact on function that the disease may impose (254).

When we speak of prognosis in RA, we tend to refer to morbidity and disability. The morbidity is increased in patients in whom the disease has an insidious onset, who are seropositive, who have radiographic evidence of erosive disease, and who have persistent synovitis. The disease is hard to control in this group, and they need more medical services. Recent studies indicate that early use of immunosuppressive drugs such as methotrexate even during the first year of the disease in those patients who present with very active disease reduces the degree of disability (255).

Radiographic evaluation adds information about mechanical function. For example, if a patient is a functional class III and has only grade 2 radiographic scale changes, it is likely that aggressive rehabilitation with attention to joint and systemic problems will improve function to that of a class II.

In terms of work performance, Yellin and colleagues found that patients in class I or II had a 0.44 probability of disability from work, whereas in class III or IV the probability increased to 0.72. In those with class I or II disease of less than 5 years, the probability of disability was 0.33, compared with 0.7 in those with disease of greater than 5 years' duration (256). Women have more disability than men with RA, as do those over 45 years of age.

Although antirheumatic drugs have not been shown to definitely reverse the radiologic abnormalities of RA, it is our clinical impression that patients being treated today have a much better functional outcome than they did 20 years ago. This is probably due to several factors:

Prompt specialty care
Improved anti-inflammatory medications with restricted use of steroids
Exercise to improve joint ROM, strength, and endurance
Appropriate and timely joint replacements

Rehabilitation of patients with RA requires a team of health-care professionals and a significant time commitment and effort on the part of the patient and family. The disease may result in changes in life roles: homemakers need assistance, and those working may need to make significant adaptations in the work setting or change their vocational status. Techniques of energy conservation and joint protection are essential. Flexibility in the workplace is more likely to result in a person remaining on the job. The self-employed patient who is able to tailor his or her schedule to individual needs is likely to remain employed.

Comprehensive management of the RA patient has been said to be associated with better control of the activity of the disease. Thus, since 1965, emphasis has been placed on prevention of disability by early diagnosis and aggressive medical and rehabilitative management. Some studies indicate that outpatients with class II and III RA who had comprehensive rehabilitation suffered 50% less deterioration in their ADL and in the clinical manifestation of their disease and enjoyed a 25% improvement in economic status compared with a control group receiving conventional treatment (70).

Particular attention must be directedto the following elements of RA:

Physical effects of the disease
Degree of inflammatory involvement in the joints
Degree of integrity of the joints radiologically and clinically
State of the capsule, ligaments, and tendinous structures surrounding the joints
Condition and function of the key muscles surrounding the joints and skin
State of the cardiopulmonary system

Similarly, the psychosocial, sexual, and work impact of the disease needs assessment.

The specific main goals in the management of RA center around the following principles:

Pain control
Improvement of altered biomechanics
Improvement and maintenance of strength, endurance, and ROM of joints
Improvement of self-image and adjustment to disability

Joint-Specific Problems

Shoulder. Glenohumeral arthritis is associated with pain in the shoulder girdle, which is referred to the neck, back, and upper arm. Decreased motion of the joint, soft-tissue contracture, and muscle atrophy follow.

Limitation of IR is seen early. Proximal subluxation of the humeral head occurs late in the disease. Weakness of the rotator cuff may cause superior subluxation in about 33% of RA patients; about 21% of patients develop rotator cuff tears; and an additional 24% have fraying of the tendons (257). The insertion of the rotator cuff tendon into the greater tuberosity makes it vulnerable to erosion by synovitis (258). Adhesive capsulitis, subcromial and subdeltoid bursitis, and bicipital tendinitis are associated problems.

In addition to pain control with heat and cold, local steroid injection into the specific affected area is often useful. A ROM program to increase and prevent loss of mobility is crucial. For functional activities, the shoulder must have 30° to 45° of flexion and 10° of IR. Care must be taken to assess the degree of radiographic involvement and joint stability when prescribing mobilization so as not to injure a compromised joint. When pain and inflammation subside, Codman exercises and the use of a cane or wand can increase flexion and IR and ER. Wall walking is good for chronic capsulitis. In the presence of adhesive capsulitis, a technique of abduction-ER-flexion traction for 1 hour a day in conjunction with TENS has been successful in decreasing pain and increasing ROM (170). Isometric strengthening should first focus on the deltoid with the shoulder adducted, then wrist-restricted isometrics in IR and ER and finally triceps and biceps isometrics are added.

Instruction in joint protection is essential to avoid overusing the shoulder. Arthroplasty should be considered before end-stage erosion and soft-tissue contraction occur.

Elbow. Elbow involvement is common in RA (20% to 65%) (259), with loss of full extension an early problem. Preservation of flexion is needed for ADLs. In severe disease, lateral stability may be lost, which may cause significant pain and disability in ADL function. Olecranon bursitis and accumulation of RA nodules that may break down easily are annoying to the patient.

Bursitis may be caused by *Staphylococcus* infection, and care must be taken not to inject the bursae of the elbow with steroid before a culture is performed. Wearing a padded Heelbo (Heelbo, Niles, IL) is useful to relieve pressure.

Lateral and medial epicondylitis is common. Acute epicondylitis is managed with modalities. Steroid injection may be necessary. Stretching exercise should not be forceful because articular damage may occur easily in the arthritic elbow.

Hand and Wrist. The hand and wrist function as a unit. With weakness of the extensor carpi ulnaris, the carpal bones rotate (i.e., the proximal row in an ulnar direction and the distal ones radially), resulting in ulnar deviation of the MCPs (260). A power grasp (261) and weakened intrinsics (262) accentuate these problems.

Synovial proliferation increases pressures in the wrist joint, so that ligaments, tendons, and cartilage may begin to be destroyed. When the ulnar collateral ligament is stretched or ruptures, the ulnar head springs up. Synovium can cause median nerve compression. In advanced disease, the carpus becomes significantly compacted.

In the hand, muscle weakness and contraction occur and grip strength decreases. Swan neck deformity—flexion of the DIP and MCP with hyperextension of the PIP—occurs. Boutonniere deformity results when the extensor hood of the PIP is stretched, causing the PIP to pop up in flexion and the IP joint to hyperextend. With incomplete profundus contraction, limitation of full flexion occurs at the DIP joints. Similarly, tight intrinsics prevent full flexion of the PIP joints with the MCPs in extension.

Three types of deformity occur at the thumb (263):

Type I: a boutonniere type deformity at the IP joint (i.e., Nalebuff)
Type II: volar subluxation at the CMC joint during adduction
Type III: in severe disease, exaggerated adduction of the first carpometacarpal joint and flexion at the MCP, and hyperextension at the DIP joint

Flexor tenosynovitis and de Quervain thumb extensor synovitis are common.

Rehabilitative hand care involves stretching of tight intrinsics, use of functional wrist splints, and finger ring type splints to help reduce hyperextension or fixed flexion deformities, joint protection techniques, and postoperative care. These splints may help decrease synovitis, relieve pain and edema, and, when worn, reduce deformity and possibly retard its progression.

Hip. About 50% of patients with RA have radiographic hip involvement (264). Synovitis of the hip can cause pain radiating to the groin, whereas trochanteric bursitis causes pain radiating over the lateral thigh. Collapse of the femoral head and remodeling of the acetabulum, which is pushed medially (i.e., protrusio), occur in 5% of RA patients. Reduction in IR is an early finding with hip involvement. Synovial cysts can develop around the hip joint and communicate with the trochanteric bursae. Hip effusion can inhibit contraction of the gluteus medius muscle.

ROM are important first to maintain at least the crucial 30° of hip flexion. A tight tensor fascia lata should be stretched. Stretching in abduction helps to relieve pain. Stretching of the internal and external rotators, extensors, and abductors should be followed by isometric strengthening exercise for the hip abductors and extensors.

Ultrasound is best avoided in RA of the hip because it is somewhat difficult to assess the state of the inflammatory process in this deep joint. Because ultrasound increases joint temperature, it may aggrevate an acute or subacute process.

Knee. The knees are commonly involved in RA, and synovial inflammation and proliferation and effusion are easily seen. Quadriceps atrophy occurs within weeks of the onset of the disease and leads to increased forces through the patella to the femoral surface. Loss of full knee extension also occurs early, and fixed contractions may ensue (265).

Knee flexion in excess of 20° is associated with increased articular pressure, and caution must be observed in performing ROM exercises on a knee with significant fluid. Outpouching of the posterior joint space may occur, creating a popliteal or Baker cyst. Fluid from this popliteal portion does not readily return to the anterior joint space, but rather adds increased pressure to the popliteal space. There may be uncomfortable fullness or pain in the popliteal space, and rupture into the calf may simulate thrombophlebitis. If rupture occurs, a hematoma may be seen below the malleoli. Observe the patient from the rear while he or she is standing to check for a popliteal cyst.

Meniscal cartilage and cruciate ligaments can be easily destroyed by proliferative synovitis. Collateral ligaments become stretched. Tests for knee stability are always indicated in an examination. X-rays should be taken in the standing position to assess the cartilage and joint space.

Treatment is directed to the particular focal intra- or periarticular problem. The patient should be instructed in early ROM exercise to preserve knee extension and flexion. Ninety degrees of knee flexion is needed to kneel and 100 degrees is needed to climb stairs. A pillow under the knee at night is to be avoided because this will encourage a knee flexion contracture. Stretching of the hamstrings is important. Strengthening of the quadriceps mechanism by isometrics in 30° flexion, if performed early in the disease process, helps to maintain the biomechanical advantage of the knee. Isotonic exercise should follow for the noninflamed joint.

Moderate to large effusions that inhibit contraction of the quadriceps and contribute to knee pain are best removed. Deweighting the knee is indicated with acute flares. Bracing the knee for instability is possible (see section on Orthotics).

Inflamed periarticular or articular structures respond favorably to ice massage. When the joint is subacute or chronic, moist hot packs and TENS can be used.

Ankle and Foot. Ankles are less frequently involved than knees. Ankle involvement is usually present in severe RA. Synovial involvement can be prominent and is seen anterior and posterior to the malleoli. In acute disease, stretching and erosion of collateral ligaments around the ankle occur, resulting in incongruity and usually pronation of the hindfoot. Subtalar joint involvement is common, and patients experience more pain walking on uneven ground (266). About 50% of patients with RA have forefoot problems, such as widening at the metatarsal area, prominent MTP joints due to subluxed metatarsal heads, hammer toe deformities, and hallux valgus of the great toe. Areas of skin breakdown are common on the dorsum of the toes (i.e., hammer toes), and callus is seen under the MTP heads. Plantar fasciitis and sub-Achilles bursitis may occur. Gait is typically flat-footed with little heel-strike or toe-off and a shuffling type of gait. Pronation of the hindfoot can be prominent. Appropriate footware is extremely important.

Polymyositis

Polymyositis is a systemic rheumatic disease that affects skeletal muscle. The clinical picture is predominantly one of profound weakness of the shoulder and hip girdle muscle, as well as of the neck and pharynx. In severe cases the diaphragm, intercostals, and abdominal muscles are involved. Ten percent of patients also have distal muscle weakness, and some have weakness of the respiratory muscles. The muscle weakness is often compounded by steroid myopathy and atrophy of disease; a fair amount of muscle pain may be experienced when the inflammation is active. There may be complete remission of the disease or episodic periods of remission and exacerbation, which are often unpredictable and pose problems with functional activities and maintaining work status.

Survival and Prognosis

The heterogenicity of the disease makes predicting prognosis and responses to medical and rehabilitative management difficult (253). Before the introduction of steroid treatment in 1940, there was a 50% mortality rate (267). Good nursing, medical, and rehabilitation care has improved disease survival. Excluding cases with malignancy, the current overall survival at 5 years is 95%.

General factors associated with poor survival are listed as follows:

- Older age
- Malignancy
- Delayed initiation of corticosteroid therapy
- Myocardial involvement
- Pharyngeal dysphagia with aspiration pneumonia
- Steroid and immunosuppressive drug complications
- Gastrointestinal vasculitis (children)

Newer studies have found that clinical and autoantibody subsets can determine 5-year survival. For instance:

Clinical subsets
- Cancer-associated myositis (55%)
- Dermatomyositis (80%)
- Inclusion body myositis (95%)
- Connective tissue–related myositis (85%)

Autoantibody subsets
- Anti-SRP (30%)
- Antisynthetase group (65%)
- Anti–M-2 (95%)

These subsets also predict response to treatment (268).

The prognosis and particular functional problems seen with this disease depend on the type or subtype of DM-PM. There are six types and three clinical subtypes.

Type I: insidious onset, beginning in the pelvic girdle and later progressing to the shoulder girdle and neck muscles. Weakened posterior pharyngeal and laryngeal muscles result in dysphagia and dysphonia. Remission and exacerbations are quite common. Moderate to severe arthritis as well as Raynaud's phenomenon may be present. The skin over the knuckles and elbows is often atrophic.

Type II: acute onset. Proximal muscle weakness and an erythematous heliotropic rash on the skin of the eyelids and the dorsum of the hands are seen. Muscle tenderness is encountered in 25% of cases; subacute joint findings are common, as are systemic manifestations of malaise, fever, and weight loss.

Type III: associated with malignancy and most common in men over 40 years of age. Often, muscle weakness precedes the diagnosis of malignancy by 1 to 2 years. The muscle weakness is usually progressive and does not respond well to steroids. Dysphagia and respiratory muscle weakness are common events. The mortality rate is high, and death is often the result of respiratory failure and pneumonia.

Type IV: involves children. The muscle weakness is rapidly progressive, and problems with dysphagia, dysphonia, and respiratory weakness are quite common. It is important to remember that late exacerbations occur after 7 years of remission. The propensity for the development of severe joint contractures and muscle atrophy is high. Skin problems in the form of calcinosis universalis (i.e., cutaneous and muscle calcification), particularly over bony prominences, contribute to skin breakdown, draining lesions, and joint contracture.

Type V: associated with other collagen vascular diseases, namely, RA, SLE, and PSS. The functional problems associated with the individual collagen disease often dominate the clinical picture.

Type VI: most commonly involves men over 40 years of age and has a slowly progressive course of muscle weakness. In addition to proximal weakness, 50% of patients have significant distal weakness.

Subtypes based on autoantibody status present with a different set of problems (268).

Antisynthetase syndrome consists of interstitial lung diseases, fever, arthritis, Raynaud's phenomenon, and mechanic's hands. The disease often has a rapid onset and aggressive course. The arthritis can affect the hands, knees, elbows, and shoulders and be chronic and deforming. The lung disease can be severe and substantially limit ADLs and mobility.

Anti-SRP syndrome is associated with initial severe muscle weakness, myalgias, and cardiac involvement that significantly impacts on function.

Anti-M2 presents with the rash of dermatomyositis and cuticular overgrowth and responds well to treatment.

Rehabilitation intervention must be tailored to suit the needs of each patient depending on the disease type. Patients with type V PM and associated collagen vascular disease (e.g., PSS, RA, SLE) have muscle weakness plus the added problems of the additional disease, which needs to be addressed from a rehabilitation standpoint.

Adults with type I and II disease can recover completely or be left with residual muscle weakness and fatigue, which can respond to rehabilitation management. Patients with PM and associated incurable malignancy are not expected to recover from the disease. The rehabilitation goals are short-term. Ambulation mobility and self-care functions progressively decline. Preserving ROM and strength will aid in keeping the person functional as long as possible. Not being able to continue in the work force for long is difficult for a middle-aged person to accept. Disability support payments and community support efforts need to be mobilized early on. Psychological support in coping with a chronic illness is needed. Good medical backup to contend with the problems of respiratory compromise and infection will be needed. Children with type IV disease need to be watched carefully for contractures.

Patients with type IV inclusion body myositis (IBM) have a slow, progressive course of proximal and distal weakness. Significant atrophy of the deltoid and quadriceps muscles is seen. Patients often have frequent falls resulting in fractures. The ability to increase the strength of significantly atrophied muscle has been shown to be poor (121). Lower extremity bracing to support a weak quadriceps mechanism is often needed.

Problems and Interventions

The functional problems that arise depend on the muscle groups involved and the extent of the weakness. For example, weakness of the pelvic girdle muscles is associated with difficulty in rising from a chair or a prone position, difficulty going up stairs, difficulty getting in and out of a bathtub, frequent falls with difficulty returning to the standing position, waddling gait, and toe walking caused by heel cord tightness, which is common in children. Shoulder girdle weakness causes functional problems with dressing (e.g., difficulty pulling on shirt, hooking a bra) and grooming (e.g., combing hair, showering, shaving, brushing teeth), difficulty picking up heavy objects on a shelf, and difficulty eating. Neck weakness causes difficulty lifting and holding the head off a pillow and holding the head up while in a sitting position. Respiratory muscle weakness (e.g., intercostals, diaphragm) results in difficulty with respiration, causing shallow and sometimes inefficient respiration. Distal muscle weakness (seen in 10% to 50%) may cause footdrop and related ambulation problems and difficulties with hand function and activities (269).

Rehabilitation goals in the acute phase consist of maintaining ROM of the joints and preventing joint contractures. In the recovery phase, the goals are to increase and regain muscle strength, maintain ROM, return to functional ADL and ambulatory activities, and restore previous life-style activities as much as possible.

Joint contractures are prevented by active and passive ROM exercise and proper positioning and splint use when the patient is confined to bed. If contractures are already present, other techniques are necessary to restore joint ROM. Contractures of the ankle, hip, and knee are common in childhood dermatomyositis and make ambulation difficult. Likewise, they may occur in the upper extremity (e.g., shoulder, elbow, wrist) and make ADLs difficult. Static or isometric exercises are recommended initially when enzymes have decreased because they cause the least amount of fatigue. Isotonic resistive exercises with low 1- to 2-pound weights are needed when CPK values are normal or near normal. Swimming and stationery bike exercises are then added. If the patient is falling owing to quadriceps weakness, a short leg brace in 5° plantar flexion may be used to create a stabilizing hyperextension moment at the knee. Appropriate assistive and adaptive devices and ambulatory aids are needed.

If pharyngeal and laryngeal weakness is present, referral to a speech pathologist to teach the patient techniques to avoid aspiration of food and prevent respiratory infection is needed. Neck flexor muscle weakness has been shown to directly correlate with swallowing dysfunction in patients with DM-PM, and its presence may cue the clinician to obtain a speech and language consult (270). If respiratory muscle weakness is present, chest physical therapy breathing techniques, proper positioning, suctioning, postural drainage, and breathing exercises, if the patient is not in the acute stage, are indicated. Tidal volume should be checked daily with a bedside spirometer. A collar may be provided to support the neck when neck flexor or extensor weakness is present.

For muscle pain, gentle muscle massage may produce a sedative relaxing effect on the muscle. The use of heat therapy is poorly described in the literature. Microwave therapy, which heats superficial and deep muscle, is described as being useful.

Most patients with polymyositis do not have arthritis. Polymyositis associated with anti-JO-1 antibody is characterized by arthritis that may become chronic and deforming without bone erosions. It occurs in the wrists, hands, elbows, knees, and shoulders. DM-PM with associated rheumatic disease (e.g., RA, SLE, PSS) is frequently associated with arthritis, which can be deforming; therefore, the use of modalities, splints, and joint conservation techniques is needed.

Iatrogenic steroid problems cause vertebral compression fractures in the thoracic and lumbar spine, resulting in back pain and muscle spasm. Interventions include a corset to decrease spinal mobility, heat modalities to relieve pain, and a long-handled reacher and shoehorn. If AN of the femoral head causes pain in the hip and groin on weight bearing, unweighting the hip is indicated. Deep heat (i.e., ultrasound) to the hip may relieve pain.

Steroid myopathy presents with atrophy of muscle and increased muscle weakness. Repeated enzyme tests, electromyography (EMG), and muscle biopsy should be performed. If the enzymes have remained normal, the EMG will show no increased acute activity, and the biopsy no increased active inflammation; the steroid should be reduced and the exercise program continued.

A number of problems can occur with the respiratory system. In addition to respiratory insufficiency, aspiration pneumonia may result because of weak pharyngeal and laryngeal muscles. Patients with the myositisspecific antibodies (MAS) anti-JO-1 commonly have interstitial lung disease.

Primary interstitial fibrosis (271) in JO-1 patients with PM associated with SLE, RA, and PSS may have lung disease associated with these diseases. Pulmonary rehabilitation may be indicated.

Cardiovascular complications with DM-PM include congestive heart failure (3.3%), cardiomyopathy (1.3%), cor pulmonale (0.7%), and electrocardiogram abnormalities (50%) (272). They are most common in type I and type V disease. Rehabilitation includes cardiac precautions, energy conservation techniques, and an endurance program.

Dermatologic problems include pressure sores over bony prominences (e.g., sacrum, elbows, heels). Extensive calcinosis seen in childhood DM-PM causes breakdown of the skin over bony prominences of joints with drainage of calcium oxalate. Vasculitis with ulcerations of the fingertips and toes may occur in the overlap syndromes. Preventive measures include proper positioning, good nutrition with adequate protein intake, use of an eggcrate mattress pad or waterbed, and padded support over elbows, knees, and heels. Restoration measures include appropriate treatment if deep pressure sores are present.

Raynaud's syndrome precipitated by cold and stress is usually mild when it occurs, unless associated with collagen vascular disease. Symptoms include painful cold fingers and color changes from white to blue. Wearing gloves and using biofeedback have been useful.

Systemic Lupus Erythematosus

SLE is a chronic inflammatory disease that can affect any organ in the body. The most frequently involved sites are the skin, joints, pleuropericardium, kidneys, and central nervous system. Its course is varied in severity and duration.

The rehabilitation team is often consulted with respect to a number of functional problems. Fatigue is a common problem and is partly due to the chronic inflammatory process, but it also can be secondary to a disturbed sleep–wake process or myositis. The use of prednisone influences this also. Treatment may include an energy conservation training program teaching that physical activity is interrupted by rest. Naps are taken during the day, and sleep can be promoted by the use of relaxation tapes.

Pain is common in the small joints of the hands and feet because of arthralgias and arthritis. Joint pain also can result from avascular necrosis of bone. Joint deformity is also seen. Control of joint pain has been successful with acupuncture and acupressure techniques, heat, cold, and TENS (273). These techniques are more effective in treating arthralgias than in treating avascular necrosis, which requires unweighting of the lower extremity, which, when unsuccessful, requires joint replacement to control symptoms.

The rashes of lupus are usually not responsive to nonpharmacologic treatments, but the skin ulceration that can occur as a result of active Raynaud's syndrome responds to hand-warming techniques (274). Temperature biofeedback has been used to relieve vasospastic disease.

Patients with renal disease often have diminished stamina and fatigue. Improvement will occur with good blood pressure control and management of edema. In patients with nephrotic syndrome and significant edema, care must be taken to position the limb in the most functional position to minimize contracture; compression pumps and garments can be used to help with and maintain the reduction of limb edema. Precautions must be taken for patients with cardiac failure. They must be compressed slowly or not at all because they may not tolerate any additional fluid load resulting from compression.

Patients with SLE have been shown to have decreased aerobic capacity. An aerobic exercise program has been shown to increase endurance by 20% (126).

One of the major challenges to the rehabilitation team is the request to evaluate and treat patients with central nervous system involvement. Stroke, psychosis, depression, and memory deficits all have a significant impact on function. Treatment is aimed at the underlying problem. An uncommon but well-described problem is transverse myelitis. Management may require mobility aides, including wheelchair. Re-education in self-care skills and exercise to help promote stamina are needed. Spasticity may be controlled with baclofen (Lioresal Ciba Geigy Corp., Summit, NJ, and Geneva Pharmaceuticals, Bloomfield, CO) or diazepam (Valium, Roche Products, Manati, Puerto Rico) or local motor point blocks. Treatment of flaccidity with braces or adaptive equipment should be offered. Speech therapy can provide strategies to enhance memory with the use of lists and cues.

The patient with SLE has to overcome major obstacles to successfully cope with this multifaceted illness. Support groups and family have been shown to be helpful in increasing compliance and are an essential component in the rehabilitation process.

Progressive Systemic Sclerosis

PSS gets its name from the fibrosislike changes that occur in skin and epithelial tissues of affected organs. In addition, heart, lung, kidney, GI tract, and small vessels also can be involved. Although there is no cure, treatment is thought to prolong life (275). The rehabilitation management depends on the extent and severity of the involvement.

Skin involvement occurs in 90% of patients and is often accompanied by Raynaud's syndrome, a condition in which there is vasospasm of the digital arteries often leading to ulceration of the fingertips. Impact of the skin involvement produces characteristic effects. There is an early painless edematous phase, during which ROM may be limited but pain and weakness are not a problem. In a subsequent phase, the skin becomes tight and bound to deeper structures, the dermis becomes thin, and there is hair loss and decreased sweating. This period is associated with significant morbidity, with loss of joint motion, itching of the skin, and an overall decrease in functional level.

Rehabilitation interventions are directed at maintaining ROM, increasing skin elasticity, and preserving or increasing function. The techniques for accomplishing this include heat, paraffin, or ultrasound (191). The management of Raynaud's syndrome may require nothing more than education about hand protection in the cold and the use of warm mittens. For those who are significantly affected, there is evidence that temperature biofeedback is helpful in controlling vasospasm, although it has proved most effective in laboratory settings and less so in daily use. However, patients report feeling that they are more in control of their environment.

Exercise to maintain ROM is essential and should be performed daily or twice daily. Strengthening exercise should be prescribed with caution and only after inflammatory myositis with abnormal levels of muscle enzymes has been ruled out. A variant of PSS, eosinophilic fasciitis, a syndrome that has tight skin as one of its features, may be precipitated by unusually strenuous exercise, reinforcing the concern that strengthening exercise should be used with caution and properly supervised.

Pulmonary involvement takes the form of pleuritis, interstitial fibrosis, and pulmonary hypertension. Symptoms include chest wall pain, pleurisy, and dyspnea. Educating the patient about breathing mechanics and practicing chest wall expansion may help improve ventilation. Transcutaneous electrical nerve stimulation may relieve chest wall pain. Energy conservation training and the use of adaptive equipment may increase functional independence.

Weight loss, constipation, and dysphagia are GI symptoms that accompany PSS. The speech pathologist or occupational therapist may be helpful in demonstrating techniques that can improve mastication and swallowing.

The course of PSS is variable. All rehabilitation intervention must be on an individual basis and frequently reviewed to evaluate goal achievement. Supportive measures to preserve mobility and independence should be included as rehabilitation goals.

Spondyloarthropathies

The spondyloarthropathies encompass a number of diseases: AS, PSA, Reiter's syndrome, and arthritis of IBD. AS has a propensity for axial skeletal involvement but also affects such large joints as the hips and shoulders. Psoriatic arthritis and Reiter's syndrome are predominantly peripheral arthropathies with less frequent sacroiliitis and spondylitis (20%). Peripheral joint involvement is seen in 20% of IBD patients and axial involvement is seen in 10%.

With axial involvement, a number of rehabilitation problems occur, including limitation of motion of the cervical and lumbar spines, paravertebral muscle spasm, and decreased chest expansion due to thoracic and costovertebral involvement. Loss of both cervical extension and lumbar lordosis is common. Visual impairment is associated with the former (276). Functional disability is proportional to loss of axial motion in the cervical region.

In addition to back pain, which is frequently seen in this syndrome, feet and ankles are often the most symptomatic anatomic regions affected by arthritis. The entheses, including Achilles and posterior tibialis tendons, are involved. Reiter's syndrome is associated with fusion of the tarsal and metatarsal joints and Achilles tendon shortening (277). Key elements in a rehabilitation program include maintaining critical ROM, posture, and strength; relieving pain; and providing appropriate orthotics.

A ROM program to maintain at least critical joint motion is prescribed (e.g., maintaining at least 75° of shoulder abduction, 110° of elbow flexion, 90° of wrist supination, 15° of hip flexion, 30° of knee flexion, and the ability to obtain neutral position at the ankle and functional grasp at the hand) (278). In addition, encouraging good posture is extremely important, and a firm mattress or bed board should be recommended. The patient should rest in the prone position to encourage extension of the spine. Lying on the side is to be avoided because this encourages cervical and thoracic kyphosis. Use of good postural habits in walking and sitting is requisite.

Exercise studies in patients with AS have indicated benefit in terms of increased ROM and strength, and some studies have claimed long-term benefits provided that exercises are continued (171,279,280). Appropriate exercise should be prescribed to promote spinal extension and ROM of the neck, shoulders, and hips. Swimming is excellent for isotonic ROM and aerobic exercise and may require use of a mask and snorkel.

Mirror devices for the car or prism glasses for reading are helpful for patients with limited neck motion, as are long-handled reachers and shoehorns. All preventive and restorative rehabilitation strategies help ensure maximal function and psychological and vocational adjustment (281,282).

Pediatric Arthritides

The two rheumatic diseases that primarily affect the pediatric age group are JRA and type-IV DM-PM. Others include SLE, PSS, and vasculitis (283).

Juvenile Rheumatoid Arthritis

Juvenile rheumatoid arthritis is a systemic disease. It is manifested by three disease types, and the outcome depends on the type. In general, there is some similarity to RA in terms of joint and systemic involvement. However, there are also specific differences in both functional problems and the psychosocial impact of the disease on the child.

Early identification of the disease, advances in drug therapy, appropriate and well-timed surgical intervention, and active ongoing rehabilitation programs have contributed to better functional outcome. Many patients who in the past were wheelchair bound are now functionally ambulatory (149).

Manifesting Disease Types

There are three main ways for JRA to present, the most frequent of which is a pauciarticular arthritis involving four or fewer joints, the knee is the most commonly involved joint, followed by the ankle. Pauciarticular arthritis is usually subdivided further into that which has an early age of onset (before the age of 5 years), ANA positivity, particularly affects girls, and has a high risk of chronic iridocyclitis and that affecting boys over 9 years of age, who tend to belong to the spondylitis group with positive HLA-B27. In this latter group, ankles and feet tend to stiffen quickly. A third group presents at any age and often develops psoriasis later in life. Pauciarticular onset accounts for 55% to 75% of all cases of JRA.

The second type of JRA is polyarticular, in which more than four joints are involved during the first few months of the disease. This group is further divided into those patients who have a positive immunoglobulin-M RF and are usually older, with an adultlike seropositive disease, and those patients who are seronegative. Polyarticular disease has the greatest risk for chronic, severe arthritis. It accounts for 15% to 25% of all cases.

The final and rarest type of JRA is systemic. In this type, the child is acutely ill with fever, rash, lymphadenopathy, and at times pericarditis, myocarditis, and liver dysfunction. Initially, symptoms may only include arthralgia, but ultimately arthritis develops in varying severity, from a mild form affecting wrists, knees, and ankles, to an extremely severe form affecting all the joints. With persistently active arthritis, hip involvement is common (283). This is asymptomatic initially and manifested merely by loss of movement. It accounts for 10% to 20% of all cases.

Special problem areas exist that deserve the attention of the rehabilitation specialist. Growth retardation, in general, may limit full stature. Abnormalities in growth related to specific joints result in a number of problems: short toes and fingers, leg length discrepancies, and micrognathia (i.e., small mandible). These abnormalities are due to premature closure of epiphyseal plates caused by intra-articular inflammation disturbing the development of the growth plate. Iritis and blindness are other major problems with which to contend. It is important to remember that joint contractures and loss of ROM strength occur rapidly in JRA and must be managed quickly and efficiently (284). Decreased aerobic capacity also is present early in the course of the disease (122).

Specific Problems

Much information is available about specific management of JRA-related problems (285–287).

Upper Limbs. The wrist is often involved in JRA, and wrist flexion contracture can occur rapidly. A cock-up resting splint should be used at night. If the wrist is inflamed or forearm muscles are weak, contributing to wrist flexion, a functional splint should be used for activities. If a wrist flexion contracture is present, serial casting may be needed.

If there is PIP involvement, the resting splint should include the hand as well as the wrist. With IP joint contractures, a dynamic outrigger splint should be used during the day.

If the elbow is acute, an adjustable hinge splint can be used. ROM exercises to maintain extension, pronation, and supination are important. If a contracture exists, serial casting can be performed.

Neck. Every effort should be made to avoid flexion contracture at the neck. Proper positioning at night with the use of a single thin pillow, like a pediatric Wal-Pil-O (Roloke, Culver City, CA), is recommended. When there is acute pain, a soft cervical collar is worn. Sometimes torticollis becomes a problem, and a firmer plastazote collar may help. A collar is recommended for desk work. A desk with a tilt top may reduce pain and help maintain more ideal spinal posture.

Lower Limbs. Knee involvement should be managed promptly. If the joint is acute, a posterior resting splint should be used at night to prevent flexion contracture. If contracture already exists, a posterior splint may increase the danger of tibial subluxation and should not be used. Rather, the contracture should be reduced with a skin traction device or by serial casting. Occasionally soft-tissue release is necessary.

Valgus deformity frequently occurs, and a supracondylar osteotomy may be needed to achieve realignment if conservative measures fail. A hip flexion deformity contributes to knee flexion problems, and care must be taken to maintain hip extension. In severe disease knee joint replacement can be considered if pain management and function cannot be achieved by medical and rehabilitative means.

An acute hip joint is most often associated with acute muscle spasm and rapid formation of a flexion contracture. Often, skin traction is used during acute hip pain to prevent contracture, with the patient lying supine in bed; 1 kg of weight for each 10 kg of body weight is used. In the child with a tendency toward knee flexion contracture, use of light hip traction during the night reduces the chance of the formation of hip and knee contractures. There should be periods of lying prone during the day to encourage maintenance of hip extension. A prone lying board also may be used in bed. If hip contracture is not responsive to conservative treatment, a soft tissue release may be needed. Joint replacement may be needed in severe disease (288) and is usually performed before 16 years of age.

Ankle–Foot. Particular attention should be directed to management of the foot. Use of the proper shoe type and orthoses, as well as ROM exercise, is important (289). Leg length discrepancy should be corrected with a shoe insert or built-up shoe if a greater than 3/8-inch correction is needed.

Spine. Significant loss of motion, particularly in extension, can occur. The use of a small Wal-Pil-O while the child is supine at night gives support without causing unwanted flexion.

Compliance. Both the parents and the child should understand treatment regimens to ensure compliance. Many treatments are performed at home with parents supervising.

Psychosocial. The disease has an impact on the child's self-image, socialization, sexuality, and integration into school activities (290). Efforts should be made to keep acute admissions to hospitals at a minimum so the child can participate as fully as possible in school, family, and social activities. He or she should be allowed to participate as much as desired but should be given clear guidelines about limitations. Particular advice should be given in regard to sports activities. Body contact and high-impact sports are to be avoided (football, soccer, running, and ballet jumps); cycling and swimming are to be encouraged. Guidance and support are needed during adolescence to deal with issues of vocation and sexuality.

Geriatric Arthridites

The elderly are often subject to multiple pathologies. It is most unusual for the aged to have no limitations on health or function other than arthritis. Anyone treating the elderly arthritic patient must take this into consideration. Additionally, age is not always the best predictor of response to therapeutic intervention, and the physician does the patient a disservice by assuming that he or she has no rehabilitation potential simply because he or she is elderly (291).

Several considerations should be added to the traditional rehabilitation evaluation of the elderly with arthritis:

Does the patient look older/younger than the stated age? This may be a predictor of less or greater rehabilitation potential.

Does the patient have other illnesses or take medications that might affect cardiopulmonary performance, or neurologic or mental status?

Is there strong family support for rehabilitation and for achieving rehabilitation goals posthospitalization?

As the body ages, muscle power declines but is still quite functional. The ability to sustain a maximal contraction as well as to quickly change direction of motion diminishes. Proprioception and spatial orientation decrease, and difficulty is experienced in balancing and righting oneself. Falls are more common. Any exercise program must take this into account.

Those elderly who age normally and are active in the community are quite functional. The late-stage arthropathic problems seen in some elderly are usually the end-stage, fixed-deformity type of OA or RA associated with minimal pain at rest and more pain during physical activity. Attempts to stretch out contractures in the elderly are usually unsuccessful, and straightening joints with passive stretch is often painful. Surgical interventions and occasionally serial casting may help. Relief of pain may be achieved with analgesia, heat, and TENS. Most of the rehabilitation interventions should be performed early in the course of the disease, and attempts to prevent contracture and preserve strength are the desired approaches (292–295). Patients should be taught proper posture and adaptation of furniture and toilet.

If the therapeutic goals are realistic and the patient is committed, success is likely. Self-care activity is often the first goal and needs to be approached with adaptive aids and a maintenance program to support the required levels of strength and motion. Pain relief is critical if the patient is to perform a series of movements. The physician should select a modality not likely to be hazardous. Hydrotherapy or pool use is very effective in enhancing total body movement and in providing a relaxing environment. The elderly must be well supervised in this setting to ensure that the temperature is not unduly stressful to the cardiac status and that no anxiety or panic reactions occur while in the water.

Foot problems are very common in the arthritic patient and even more common in the elderly. Proper footwear should provide adequate depth to clear tops of toes and cushioning of the heels and metatarsals. Foot hygiene and prompt care of skin breakdown are essential to prevent infection in a patient with possible vascular compromise of the lower extremity.

REFERENCES

1. Robinson HS, Haldeman J, Imrie J, Neubauer P. Evaluation of a province wide physiotherapy monitoring service in an arthritis control program. *J Rheumatol* 1980; 7:387–389.
2. Lorig K, Lubeck D, Kraines RG, et al. Outcomes of self-help education for patients with arthritis. *Arthritis Rheum* 1985; 28:680–685.
3. Goeppinger J, Arthur MW, Baglioni AJ Jr, et al. A re-examination of the effectiveness of self-care education for patients with arthritis. *Arthritis Rheum* 1989; 32:706–716.
4. Sergent J. Polyarticular arthritis. In: Kelly W, Harris ED, Ruddy S, Sledge CB, eds. *Textbook of rheumatology,* 4th ed. Philadelphia: WB Saunders, 1993; 381–388.
5. McCune JW. Monoarticular arthritis. In: Kelley WN, Harris ED, Ruddy S, Sledge CB, eds. *Textbook of rheumatology,* 4th ed. Philadelphia: WB Saunders, 1993; 368–380.
6. Gordis L. Keynote address. *The role of epidemiology in the study of rheumatic disease.* New York: Gower, 1984; 6–15.
7. Acheson RM, Collart AB. New Haven survey of joint disease XVII. Relationship between some systemic characteristics and osteoarthrosis in a general population. *Ann Rheum Dis* 1975; 34: 379–387.
8. Lawrence JS, Bremmer JM, Boer F. Osteo-arthrosis. Prevalence in the population and relationship between symptoms and x-ray changes. *Ann Rheum Dis* 1966; 25:1–24.
9. *Osteoarthritis in adults by selected demographic characteristics.* Washington, DC: U.S. National Center for Health Statistics, 1966.
10. Kellgren JH, Lawrence JS. Osteoarthrosis and disk degeneration in an urban population. *Ann Rheum Dis* 1958; 17:388–397.
11. Mikkelsen WM, Duff IF, Dodge HJ. Age-sex specific prevalence of radiographic abnormalities of the joints of the hands, wrists, and cervical spine of adult residents of the Tecumseh, Michigan, community health study area, 1962–65. *J Chronic Dis* 1970; 23:151–159.
12. Solomon L, Beighton P, Valkenburg HA, et al. Rheumatic disorders in the South African Negro: Part I. Rheumatoid arthritis and ankylosing spondylitis. *S Afr Med J* 1975; 49:1292–1296.
13. Abramson JH, Adler E, Ben-hader S, Elkan Z, Gabrel KR, Wahl M. Studying the epidemiology of rheumatoid arthritis in Israel: methodological considerations. *Arthritis Rheum* 1964; 7:153–160.
14. Behrend T, Lawrence JS. Prevalence of rheumatoid arthritis in rural Germany. *Int J Epidemiol* 1972; 1:153.
15. Shulman L, Lawrence R. Current topics in rheumatology. In: Lawrence R, Shulman L, eds. *Epidemiology of rheumatic diseases.* New York: Gower, 1984.
16. Fessel WJ. Systemic lupus erythematosus in the community. *Arch Intern Med* 1974; 134:1027–1035.
17. Morton RO, Steinberg AD, Gershwin ME, Brady C. The incidence

of systemic lupus erythematosus in North American Indians. *J Rheumatol* 1976; 3:186–190.

18. Serdula MK, Rhoads GG. Frequency of systemic lupus erythematosus in different ethnic groups in Hawaii. *Arthritis Rheum* 1979; 22: 328–333.
19. Lehmann TJA, Hamsan V, Singyon BH, et al. Serum complement abnormalities in the antinuclear antibody positive relatives of children with systemic lupus erythematosis. *Arthritis Rheum* 1979; 22:954.
20. Leonhardt T. Family studies in systemic lupus erythematosus. *Acta Med Scand* 1964; 176(suppl 416):51.
21. Stallone R. The epidemiology of systemic sclerosis. In: Lawrence R, Shulman L, eds. *Epidemiology of the rheumatic diseases.* New York: Gower, 1984; 169–174.
22. Hochberg MC. The epidemiology of juvenile rheumatoid arthritis: review of current status and approaches for future research. In: Lawrence R, Shulman L, eds. *Epidemiology of the rheumatic diseases.* New York: Gower, 1984; 220–233.
23. Esdaile M. In: Klipple J, Dieppe PA, eds. *Adult stills disease in rheumatology.* New York: CV Mosby, 1994; 21.1–21.8.
24. Medsger TA, Oddis CV. In: Klipple J, Dieppe PA, eds. *Inflammatory muscle disease—clinical features.* New York: CV Mosby, 1994; 12.1–12.14
25. Calin A. *The epidemiology of ankylosing spondylitis: a clinician's point of view.* New York: Gower, 1984; 51–60.
26. Sites DP, Stabo JD, Fudenberg HH, et al. *Basic and clinical immunology,* 4th ed. Los Altos, CA: Lange Medical Publications, 1982.
27. Gershon RK, Eardley DD, Durum S, et al. Contrasuppression. A novel immunoregulatory activity. *J Exp Med* 1981; 153:1533–1546.
28. Branigan PJ, Gerard HC, Hudson AP, et al. Conparison of synovial tissue and synovial fluid as a source of nucleic acids for defection of chlamydia trachomatis by polymerase chain reaction. *Arthritis Rheum* 1996; 39:1740–1746.
29. Bennett JD. The infectious etiology of rheumatoid arthritis: new considerations. *Arthritis Rheum* 1978; 21:531–538.
30. Harris ED. Pathogenesis of RA. In: Kelly W, Harris ED, Ruddy S, Sledge CB, eds. *Textbook of rheumatology,* 4th ed. Philadelphia: WB Saunders, 1993; 833–873.
31. Meachim G, Brooke G. Pathology of OA. In: Moskowitz R, et al., eds. *Osteoarthritis: diagnosis and management.* Philadelphia: WB Saunders, 1992; 29–34.
32. Pedley RB, Meachim G. Topographical variation in patellar subarticular calcified tissue density. *J Anat* 1979; 128:737–745.
33. Lane NE, Bloch DA, Jones HH, et al. Long distance running, bone density and osteoarthritis. *JAMA* 1986; 225:1147–1152.
34. Paronen I. Reiter's disease; a study of 344 cases observed in Finland. *Acta Med Scand* 1948; 131(suppl 212):1.
35. Noer HR. An "experimental" epidemic of Reiter's syndrome. *JAMA* 1966; 198:693–698.
36. Warren CPW. Arthritis associated with *Salmonella* infections. *Ann Rheum Dis* 1970; 29:483–487.
37. Aho K, Ahvonen P, Lassus A, Slevers K, Tiilikginen A. HLA-27 in reactive arthritis. A study of Yersinia arthritis and Reiter's disease. *Arthritis Rheum* 1974; 17:521–526.
38. Fresco R. Virus-like particles in systemic lupus erythematosis. *N Engl J Med* 1970; 283:1231.
39. Block SR, Winfield JB, Lockshin, DiAngelo WA, Christian CL. Studies of twins with SLE. A review of the literature presentation of 12 additional sets. *Am J Med* 1975; 59:533–552.
40. Winchester RJ, Nunez-Roldon A. Some genetic aspects of systemic lupus erythematosus. *Arthritis Rheum* 1982; 25:833–837.
41. Maddock RK. Incidence of systemic lupus erythematosis by age and sex. *JAMA* 1965; 191:137–138.
42. Jungers P, Dongodos M, Pelissier C, et al. Influence of oral contraceptive therapy on the activity of systemic lupus erythematosis. *Arch Phys Med Rehabil* 1982; 25:618–623.
43. Woods VL. Pathogenesis of SLE. In: Kelly W, Harris ED, Ruddy S, Sledge CB, eds. *Textbook of rheumatology,* 4th ed. Philadelphia: WB Saunders, 1993; 999–1016.
44. Plotz PH, Miller FW. Inflammatory muscle disease—etiology and pathogenesis. In: Klipple J, Dieppe PA, eds. *Rheumatology,* St. Louis: CV Mosby, 1994; 13.1–13.10.
45. Dalakas M. Polymyositis, dermatomyositis and inclusion body myositis. *N Engl J Med* 1991; 325:1487–1498.
46. Fries JF. Assessment of the patients with rheumatic disease. In: Kelly W, Harris ED, Ruddy S, Sledge CB, eds. *Textbook of rheumatology,* 3rd ed. Philadelphia: WB Saunders, 1989; 361–365.
47. Siegel KL, Kepple TM, O'Connell P, et al. A technique to evaluate foot function during the stance phase of gait. *Foot Ankle* 1995; 16: 764–770.
48. Marshall RN, Myers DB, Palmer DG. Disturbance of gait due to rheumatoid disease. *J Rheumatol* 1980; 7:617–623.
49. Mazur JM, Schwartz E, Simon SR. Ankle arthrodesis: long term follow-up with gait analysis. *J Bone Joint Surg [Am]* 1979; 61:964–975.
50. Resnick D, Niwayama G. *Diagnosis of bone and joint disorders.* Philadelphia: WB Saunders, 1988.
51. Kendall FP, Lower extremity strength tests. In: Kendall FP, Kendall EM, Provance PG eds. *Muscles: testing function,* 4th ed. Baltimore: Williams & Wilkins, 1993; 179–191.
52. Merritt JL, McLean TJ, Erickson RP, Offord KP. Measurement of trunk flexibility in normal subjects: reproducibility of three clinical methods. *Mayo Clin Proc* 1986; 61:192–197.
53. Huskisson EC, Jones J, Scott PJ. Application of visual analog scales to the measurement of functional capacity. *Rheumatol Rehabil* 1976; 15:185–187.
54. Fixx AJ, Daughton DM. *Human study profile professional manual.* Odessa, FL: PAR Psychological Assessment Resources Inc., 1988.
55. Steinbrocker O, Tiraeger CH, Batterman RC. Therapeutic criteria in rheumatoid arthritis. *JAMA* 1949; 140:659–662.
56. Hochberg MC, Chang RW, Dwosh I, et al: The American College of Rheumatology 1991 revised criteria for the classification of global functional status in rheumatoid arthritis. *Arthritis Rheum* 1992; 35: 498–502.
57. Convery RF, Minteer MA, Amiel D, Connett KL. Polyarticular disability: a functional assessment. *Arch Phys Med Rehabil* 1977; 58: 494–499.
58. Ebert DR, Fasching V, Rahlfs V, Schleyer I, Wolf R. Repeatability and objectivity of various measurements in rheumatoid arthritis: a comparative study. *Arthritis Rheum* 1976; 19:1278–1286.
59. Katz S, Downs TD, Cash HR, et al. Progress in development of the index of ADL. *Gerontologist* 1970; 4:274.
60. Fries JF, Spitz P, Kraines RG, et al. Measurement of patient outcome in arthritis. *Arthritis Rheum* 1980; 23:137–145.
61. Jette AM. Functional capacity evaluation: an empirical approach. *Arch Phys Med Rehabil* 1980; 61:85–89.
62. Meenan RF, Gertman PM, Mason JH. Measuring health status in arthritis: the arthritis impact measurement scales. *Arthritis Rheum* 1980; 23:146–152.
63. Bombardier C, Tugwell P, Sinclair A, Dok C, Anderson G, Buchanon WW. Preference for end point measures in clinical trials: results of structured worshops. *J Rheumatol* 1982; 9:798.
64. Dart RL, Cleeland CS, Flanery RC. Development of the Wisconsin Brief Pain Questionnaire to assess pain in cancer and other diseases. *Pain* 1983; 17:197–210.
65. Bergner M, Bobbitt RA, Pollard WE, et al. The Sickness Impact Profile: validation of a health status measure. *Med Care* 1976; 14:57–67.
66. Belza BL, Henke CJ, Yelin EH, et al. Correlates of fatigue in older adults with rheumatoid arthritis. *Nurs Res* 1993; 42:93–99.
67. Sackett OH, Hayes RB. *Compliance with therapeutic regimens.* Baltimore: Johns Hopkins University Press, 1976.
68. Gerstein HR. Patient non-compliance within the context of seeking medical care for arthritis. *J Chronic Dis* 1973; 26:689–698.
69. Duff IE, Carpenter JO, Neukom JE. Comprehensive management of patients with rheumatoid arthritis: some results of the regional arthritis control program in Michigan. *Arthritis Rheum* 1974; 5:535–645.
70. Katz S, Vignos PJ, Moskowitz RN, et al. Comprehensive outpatient care in rheumatoid arthritis: a controlled study. *JAMA* 1968; 206: 1249–1254.
71. Fienberg J, Brandt K. Use of resting splints by patients with rheumatoid arthritis. *J Occup Ther* 1978; 35:173–178.
72. Oakes TW, Ward JR, Gray RM, Klauber MR, Moody PM. Family expectations and arthritis patient compliance to a hand resting splint regimen. *J Chronic Dis* 1970; 22:757–764.
73. Treuish FV, Krusen F. Physical therapy applied at home for arthritis. *Arch Intern Med* 1943; 72:231–238.
74. Carpenter JO. Medical recommendations followed or ignored? Factors influencing compliance in arthritis. *Arch Phys Med Rehabil* 1976; 57: 241–246.

75. Hicks JE. Compliance: a major factor in the successful treatment of patients with rheumatic disease. *Compr Ther* 1985;11:31–37.
76. Hicks J. Compliance a major factor in the management of rheumatic diseases. In: Hicks J, Nicholas J, Swezey R, eds. *Handbook of rehabilitative rheumatology.* Bayville, NY: Contact Associates, 1988; 133–149.
77. Avery DD, Penn PE. Blockade of pyrogen induced fever by intrahypothalamic injections of salicylate in the rat. *Neuropharmacology* 1974; 13:1179.
78. Boardman PL, Hart FD. Clinical measurements of the anti-inflammatory effects of salicilates in rheumatoid arthritis. *Br Med J* 1967; 4: 264–268.
79. Kaley G, Weiner R. Prostaglandin E, a potential mediator of the inflammatory response. *Ann N Y Acad Sci* 1971; 180:338–350.
80. Clements PJ, Paulus HE. Non-steroidal anti-inflammatory drugs. In: Kelly WN, Harris ED, Ruddy S, Sledge CB. *Textbook of rheumatology,* 4th ed. Philadelphia: WB Saunders, 1993; 700–730.
81. Davidson AM, Birt AR. Quinine bisulfate as a desensitizing agent in the treatment of lupus erythematosus. *Arch Dermatol* 1938; 37: 247–253.
82. Dubois EL. Quinacrine (Atabrine) in treatment of systemic and discoid lupus erythematosus. *Arch Intern Med* 1954; 94:131–144.
83. Bagnall AW. The value of chloroquine in rheumatoid arthritis—a four year study of continuous therapy. *Can Med Assoc J* 1957; 77: 182–194.
84. Freedman A, Bach F. Mepacrine and rheumatoid arthritis. *Lancet* 1952; 2:321.
85. Conte JJ, Mignon-Conte MA, Fournie GJ. La nephropathie loprove: tratement par l'association indometacine-hydroxchloraquine et comparison avec les corticoides. *Presse Med* 1975; 4:91–95.
86. Dwosh IL, Stein HB, Urowitz MB, Smythe HA, Hunter T, Ogryzlo MA. Azathioprine in early rheumatoid arthritis. Comparison with gold and chloroquine. *Arthritis Rheum* 1977; 20:685–692.
87. Horton RJ. Comparative safety and efficacy of Auranofin and parenteral gold compounds: a review. *Scand J Rheumatol* 1983; 51(suppl): 100–110.
88. Dorwart BB, Gall EP, Schumacher HR, Krauser RE. Chrysotherapy in psoriatic arthritis. *Arthritis Rheum* 1978; 21:513–515.
89. Hill HFH. Treatment of rheumatoid arthritis with penicillamine. *Semin Arthritis Rheum* 1977; 6:361–388.
90. Kirwan JR, Systemic corticosteriods in rheumatology. In: Klipple JH, Dieppe PA. eds. *Rheumatology,* 1st ed. St. Louis: CV Mosby 1993; 8:11–16.
91. Wallace SL, Singer JZ. Therapy in gout. *Rheum Dis Clin North Am* 1988; 14:441–447.
92a. Gerber NL, Steinberg AD. Clinical use of immuno-suppressive drugs. *Drugs* 1976; 11:90.
92b. Gerber L, Hicks J. Surgical rehabilitation options in the treatment of the rheumatoid arthritis patient resistant to pharmacologic agents. *Rheum Dis Clin North Am* 1995; 21:19–39.
93. Newman Alan P. Synovectomy. In: Kelly W, Harris ED, Ruddy S, Sledge CB, eds. *Textbook of rheumatology,* 4th ed. Philadelphia: WB Saunders, 1993;649–670.
94a. Carnesale PG. Arthrodesis of the ankle, knee and hip. In: Crenshaw AH, ed. *Campbell's operative orthopaedics,* 8th ed. St. Louis: CV Mosby, 1992; 317–352.
94b. Justus JE. Arthrodesis of the shoulder, elbow and wrist. In: Crenshaw AH, ed. *Campbell's operative orthopaedics,* 8th ed. St. Louis: CV Mosby, 1992; 353–370.
95. Simmons BP, Millender LH, Nalebuff EA. Reconstructive surgery and rehabilitation of the hand. In: Kelly W, Harris ED, Ruddy S, Sledge CB, eds. *Textbook of rheumatology,* 4th ed. Philadelphia: WB Saunders, 1993; 1752–1777.
96. Windsor RE, Insall JN. The knee. In: Kelly W, Harris ED, Ruddy S, Sledge CB, eds. *Textbook of rheumatology,* 4th ed. Philadelphia: WB Saunders, 1993; 1836–1854.
97. Gross EL. Rehabilitation following total joint replacement. In: Hicks J, Nicholas J, Swezey R, eds. *Handbook of rehabilitative rheumatology.* Bayville, NY: Contact Associates, 1988.
98. Morrey BF. The elbow. In: Kelly W, Harris ED, Ruddy S, Sledge CB, eds. *Textbook of rheumatology,* 4th ed. Philadelphia: WB Saunders, 1993; 1778–1797.
99. Neer CS. The shoulder. In: Kelly W, Harris ED, Ruddy S, Sledge CB, eds. *Textbook of rheumatology,* 4th ed. Philadelphia: WB Saunders, 1993; 1808–1822.
100. Tsahakis PJ, Brick GW, Poss R. The hip. In: Kelly W, Harris ED, Ruddy S, Sledge CB, eds. *Textbook of rheumatology.* Philadelphia: WB Saunders, 1993; 1823–1835.
101. Scott RD, Sledge CB. Surgical management of juvenile rheumatoid arthritis. In: Kelly W, Harris ED, Ruddy S, Sledge CB, eds. *Textbook of rheumatology,* 4th ed. Philadelphia: WB Saunders, 1993; 1873–1880.
102. Saltzman CL, Johnson KA. The ankle and foot. In: Kelly W, Harris ED, Ruddy S, Sledge CB, eds. *Textbook of rheumatology,* 4th ed. Philadelphia: WB Saunders, 1993; 1855–1872.
103. Hicks JE, Nicholas JJ. Treatment utilized in rehabilitative rheumatology. In: Hicks JE, Nicholas JJ, Swezey RL, eds. *Handbook of rehabilitative rheumatology.* Bayville, NY: Contact Associates, 1988; 31.
104. Gault SJ, Spyker JM. Beneficial effect of immobilization of joints in rheumatoid arthritides: a splint study using sequential analysis. *Arthritis Rheum* 1969; 12:34–44.
105. Harris R, Copp EP. Immobilization of the knee joint in rheumatoid arthritis. *Ann Rheum Dis* 1962; 21:353–359.
106. Alexander GJM, Girtas C, Bacon PA. Bed rest, activity and the inflammation of rheumatoid arthritis. *Br J Rheumatol* 1983; 22:134–140.
107. Lee P, Kennedy AC, Anderson J, Buchanan WW. Benefits of hospitalization in rheumatoid arthritis. *Q J Med* 1974; 43(new series): 205–214.
108. Mills JA, Pinals RS, Ropes MW, Short CL, Sutcliffe J. Value of bed rest in patients with rheumatoid arthritis. *N Engl J Med* 1971; 284: 453–458.
109. Partridge REH, Duthie JJR. Controlled trial of the effect of complete immobilization of the joints in rheumatoid arthritis. *Ann Rheum Dis* 1963; 22:91–99.
110. Gerber L, Furst G, Shulman B, et al. Patient education program to teach energy conservation behaviors to patients with rheumatoid arthritis: a pilot study. *Arch Phys Med Rehabil* 1987; 68:442–445.
111. Herbison GJ, Ditunno JF, Jaweed MM. Muscle atrophy in rheumatoid arthritis. *J Rheumatol* 1987; 14(suppl 15):78–81.
112. Hicks JE. Rehabilitation and biomechanics. *Curr Opin Rheumatol* 1990; 2:320–326.
113. Hicks J. Exercise in patients with inflammatory arthritis. *Rheum Dis Clin North Am* 1990; 16:845–870.
114. Booth FW. Physiologic and biochemical effects of immobilization on muscle. *Clin Orthop* 1987; 219:15–20.
115. Kohke F. The effects of limitation of activity upon the human body. *JAMA* 1966; 196:825–830.
116. Muller EA. Influence of training and activity on muscle strength. *Arch Phys Med* 1970; 51:449–462.
117. Danneskiold-Samsoe B, Grimby G. The relationship between the leg muscle strength and physical capacity in patients with rheumatoid arthritis, with reference to the influence of corticosteroids. *Clin Rheumatol* 1986; 5:468–474.
118. Fahrer H, Rentsch HU, Gerber NJ, et al. Knee effusion and reflex inhibition of the quadriceps: a bar to effective retraining. *J Bone Joint Surg [Br]* 1988; 70:635.
119. Hsieh LF, Didenko B, Schumacher HR. Isokinetic and isometric testing of knee musculature in patients with rheumatoid arthritis with mild knee involvement. *Arch Phys Med Rehabil* 1987; 68:294–297.
120. Nordesjo L, Nordgren B, Wigren A, Kolstok K. Isometric strength and endurance in patients with severe rheumatoid arthritis or osteoarthritis in the knee joints. *Scand J Rheumatol* 1983; 12:152–156.
121. Hicks JE, Muller F, Poltz P, et al. Strength improvement without CPK elevation in a polymyositis patient on an isometric exercise program [Abstract]. *Arthritis Rheum* 1988; 31(suppl 4):559.
122. Lindehammar H, Backman E. Muscle function in juvenile chronic arthritis. *J Rheumatol* 1995; 22:1159–1165.
123. Hicks JE, Fromherz W, Miller F, et al. Cybex II strength and endurance testing in normals and polymyositis patients [Abstract]. *Arthritis Rheum* 1988; 31(suppl 4):559.
124. Tan J, Balci N, Sepici V, et al. Isokinetic and isometric strength in osteoarthritis of the knee, a comparative study with healthy women. *Am J Phys Med Rehabil* 1995; 74:364–369.
125. Minor MA, Hewett JE, Webel RS, Anderson SK, Kay DR. Efficacy of physical conditioning exercise in patients with rheumatoid arthritis and osteoarthritis. *Arthritis Rheum* 1989; 32:1396–1405.
126. Nicholson CR, Daltroy L, Easton BSN, et al. Effects of aerobic condi-

tioning in lupus fatigue: a pilot study. *Br J Rheumatol* 1989; 28: 500–505.
127. Gerber L, Furst G, Drinkard B, Dale J, Straus S. Assessment of fatigue in patients with rheumatoid arthritis, polymyositis and chronic fatigue syndrome. *Arthritis Rheum* 1996; 39(suppl):176.
128. Banwell BF. Exercise and mobility in arthritis. *Nurs Clin North Am* 1984; 19:605–616.
129. Machover S, Sapecky AJ. Effect of isometric exercise on the quadriceps muscle in patients with rheumatoid arthritis. *Arch Phys Med Rehabil* 1966; 47:737–741.
130. Nordemar R, Berg U, Ekblom B, Edstrom L. Changes in muscle fibre size after physical performance in patients with rheumatoid arthritis after 7 months' physical training. *Scand J Rheumatol* 1976; 5: 233–238.
131. Nordemar R. Physical training in rheumatoid arthritis: a controlled long term study. II. Functional capacity and general attitudes. *Scand J Rheumatol* 1981; 10:25–30.
132. Nordemar R, Edstrom L, Ekblom B. Changes in muscle fibre size and physical performance in patients with rheumatoid arthritis after short-term physical training. *Scand J Rheumatol* 1976; 5:70–76.
133. Lyngberg K, Danneskiold-Samsoe B, Halskov. The effect of physical training on patients with rheumatoid arthritis: changes in disease activity, muscle strength and aerobic capacity: clinically controlled minimized cross-over study. *Clin Exp Rheumatol* 1988; 6:253–260.
134. Aloia JF, Cohn SH, Ostuni JA, Care C, Ellis K. Prevention of involutional bone loss by exercise. *Ann Intern Med* 1978; 89:356–358.
135. Sinaki M, Grubbs N. Back strengthening exercises: quantitative evaluation of their efficacy in women aged 40 to 60 years. *Arch Phys Med Rehabil* 1989; 70:16–20.
136. Minor M, Hewett J, Webel R, et al. efficacy of physical conditioning exercise in patients with RA and OA. *Arthritis Rheum* 1989; 32:1396.
137. Hicks JE. Exercise programs for patients with inflammatory arthritis. *J Musculoskel Med* 1989; 6:40–55.
138. Gerber L, Hicks J. Exercise in the rheumatic disease. In: Basmajian JV, Wolf SL, eds. *Therapeutic exercise,* 5th ed. Baltimore: Williams & Wilkins, 1990; 333.
139. Gerber L, Hicks J. Rehabilitative management of rheumatic diseases. In: Hicks JE, Nicholas JJ, Swezey RL, eds. *Handbook of rehabilitative rheumatology.* Bayville, NY: Contact Associates, 1988; 82.
140. Merritt JL, Hunder GG. Passive range of motion, not isometric exercise, amplifies acute urate synovitis. *Arch Phys Med Rehabil* 1983; 64:130–131.
141. Agudelo CA, Schumacher HR, Phelps P. Effect of exercise on urate crystal-induced inflammation in canine joints. *Arthritis Rheum* 1972; 15:609–616.
142. Jayson MIV, Dixon ASJ. Intra-articular pressure in rheumatoid arthritis of the knee. III: Pressure changes during joint use. *Ann Rheum Dis* 1970; 29:401–408.
143. de Lateur BJ. Exercise for strength and endurance. In: Basmajian JV, ed. *Therapeutic exercise,* 4th ed. Baltimore: Williams & Wilkins, 1984; 90–92.
144. Hicks JE. Comprehensive rehabilitative management of patients with polymyositis. In: Dalakas M, ed. *Polymyositis.* London: Butterworth, 1988.
145. Muller EA, Rhomert W. Die Geschwindigkeit der Muskelkraft-Zunahme bei isometrischem Training. *Int Z Angewandte Phys* 1963; 19: 403–419.
146. Liberson WT. Brief isometric exercises. In: Basmajian JV, ed. *Therapeutic exercise,* 4th ed. Baltimore: Williams & Wilkins, 1984; 236–256.
147. Jayson MIX, Rubenstein D, Dixon AS. Intra-articular pressure and rheumatoid geodes (bone "cysts"). *Ann Rheum Dis* 1970; 29: 496–502.
148. Gnootveld M, Henderson EB, Farrell A, et al. Oxidative damage to hyaluronate and glucose in synovial fluid during exercise of the inflamed rheumatoid joint. *Biochem J* 1991; 273:459–467.
149. Ansell B. Pediatric rehabilitative rheumatology. In: Hicks J, Nicholas J, Swezey R, eds. *Handbook of rehabilitative rheumatology.* Bayville, NY: Contact Associates, 1988; 167–183.
150. deLateur B, Lehman NJ, Stonebridge J, Warren CG. Isotonic versus isometric exercise: a double-shift transfer-of-training study. *Arch Phys Med Rehabil* 1972; 53:212–226.
151. deLateur BJ, Lehman NJF, Fordyce WE. A test of the DeLorme axion. *Arch Phys Med Rehabil* 1968; 49:245–248.
152. Castello BA, El Sallab RA, Scott JT. Physical activity, cystic erosions and osteoporosis in rheumatoid arthritis. *Ann Rheum Dis* 1965; 24: 522–527.
153. de Lateur BJ, Lehmann JF, Warren CG, et al. Comparison of effectiveness of isokinetic and isotonic exercise in quadriceps strengthening. *Arch Phys Med Rehabil* 1972; 53:60–64.
154. Fisher NM, Gresham GE, Abrams M, et al. Quantitative effects of physical therapy on muscular and functional performance in subjects with osteoarthritis of the knees. *Arch Phys Med Rehabil* 1993; 74: 840–847.
155. Rall LC, Maydone SN, Kehaylas JJ, et al. The effect of progressive resistance training in rheumatoid arthritis increased strength without changes in energy balance or body composition. *Arthritis Rheum* 1996; 39:415–426.
156. Leventhal L, Ganjei A, Hirsch D, Katchen K, Bomer F, Schumaker HR. Isokinetic strength training in patients with rheumatoid arthritis [Abstract]. *Arthritis Rheum* 1990; 33(suppl):123.
157. Lynberg KK, Ramsing BU, Nawrocke A. Safe and effective isokinetic knee extension training in rheumatoid arthritis. *Arthritis Rheum* 1994; 37:623–629.
158. Escalante A, Miller L, Beardmore TD. An N-of-1 trial of resistive versus non-resistive exercise in inflammatory muscle disease (IMD) [Abstract]. *Arthritis Rheum* 1991; 34(suppl):173.
159. Ekblom B, Lovgren O, Alderin M, et al. Effect of short-term physical training on patients with rheumatoid arthritis. II. *Scand J Rheumatol* 1975; 41:87–91.
160. Perlman SG, Connell KJ, Clark A, Robinson MS, et al. Dance based aerobic exercise for rheumatoid arthritis. *Arthritis Care Res* 1990; 3: 29–35.
161. Elkblom B, Lovgren O, Alderin M, et al. Effect of short-term training on patients with rheumatoid arthritis. *Scand J Rheumatol* 1975; 41: 80–86.
162. Harkcom TM, Lampman RM, Banwell BF, Castor CW. Therapeutic value of graded aerobic exercise training in rheumatoid arthritis. *Arthritis Rheum* 1985; 28:32–39.
163. Hicks JE. Exercise in rheumatoid arthritis. *Phys Med Rehabil Clin North Am* 1994; 5:701–728.
164. Klipper SE, Giannini MJ. Physical conditioning in children with arthritis assessment and guidelines for exercise prescription. *Arthritis Care Res* 1994; 7:226–236.
165. Herbert CA, Byrnes TJ, Baethge A, et al. Exercise limitation in patients with polymyositis. *Chest* 1990; 98:352–357.
166. Aloia JF, Cohn SH, Babu T, Abesamis C, Kalici N, Ellis K. Skeletal mass and body composition in marathon runners. *Metabolism* 1978; 27:1793–1796.
167. Hahn TJ, Hahn BH. Osteopenia in patients with rheumatic diseases: principles and diagnosis of therapy. *Semin Arthritis Rheum* 1975; 6: 165.
168. Fried DM. Splints for arthritis. In: Licht S, ed. *Arthritis and physical medicine.* New Haven, CT: E Licht, 1969; 285–314.
169. Stein H, Dickson RA. Reversed dynamic slings for knee flexion contractures in the hemophiliac. *J Bone Joint Surg [Am]* 1975; 51:282.
170. Rizk TE, Christopher RP, Pinals RS, et al. Adhesive capsulitis (frozen shoulder): a new approach to its management. *Arch Phys Med Rehabil* 1983; 64:29–33.
171. Bulstrode SJ, Barefoot J, Harrison RA, Clarke AK. The role of passive stretching in the treatment of ankylosing spondylitis. *Br J Rheumatol* 1987; 26:40–42.
172. McNeal RL. Aquatic therapy for patients with rheumatic disease. *Rheum Dis Clin North Am Exerc Arthritis* 1990; 16:915–929.
173. Danneskiold-Samsoe B, Lyngberg K, Risum T, Telleng M. The effect of water exercise therapy given to patients with rheumatoid arthritis. *Scand J Rehabil Med* 1987; 19:31–35.
174. Harrison RA. Tolerance of pool therapy by ankylosing spondylitis patients with low vital capacities. *Physiotherapy* 1981; 67:296–297.
175. Fisher LR, Cawley MID, Holgate ST. Relations between chest expansion, pulmonary function and exercise tolerance in patients with ankylosing spondylitis. *Ann Rheum Dis* 1990; 49:921–925.
176. Van Deusen J, Harlowe D. The efficacy of the ROM dance program for adults with rheumatoid arthritis. *Am J Occup Ther* 1987; 41:90.
177. Konradsen L, Hansen BE, Sondergard L. Long distance running and osteoarthritis. *Am J Sports Med* 1990; 18:379–381.
178. Lane NE, Bloch DA, Hubert HB, et al. Running, osteoarthritis and

bone density: initial 2-year longitudinal study. *Am J Med* 1990; 88: 452–459.
179. Hollander JL, Stoner EK, Brown EM, DeMoor P. Joint temperature measurement in the evaluation of anti-arthritic agents. *J Clin Invest* 1951; 30:701–706.
180. Horvath SM, Hollander SL. Intra-articular temperature as a measure of joint reaction. *J Clin Invest* 1949; 28:469–473.
181. Lehmann JF, Silverman DR, Baum BA, Kirk NL, Johnston VC. Temperature distributions in the human thigh, produced by infrared, hot pack and microwave applications. *Arch Phys Med Rehabil* 1966; 47: 291–299.
182. Hollander JL, Horvath SM. Changes in joint temperature produced by diseases and by physical therapy. *Arch Phys Med* 1949; 30:437–440.
183. Lehmann JF, McMillan JA, Brunner GD, Blumberg JB. Comparative study of the efficiency of short-wave microwave and ultrasonic diathermy in heating the hip joint. *Arch Phys Med Rehabil* 1959; 40: 510–512.
184. Oosterveld FG, Rasker JJ. Effects of local heat and cold treatment on the surface articular temperature of arthritic knees. *Arthritis Rheum* 1994; 37:1578–1582.
185. Harris ED Jr, McCroskery PA. The influence of temperature and fibril stability on degradation of cartilage collagen by rheumatoid synovial collagenase. *N Engl J Med* 1974; 290:1–6.
186. Dorwart BB, Hansell JR, Schumacher HR Jr. Effects of cold and heat on urate crystal-induced synovitis in the dog. *Arthritis Rheum* 1974; 17:563–571.
187. Mainardi CL, Walter CM, Spiegel PK, Goldkamp OG, Harris ED. Rheumatoid arthritis: failure of daily heat to affect its progression. *Arch Phys Med Rehabil* 1979; 60:390–393.
188. Warren CG, Lehmann JF, Koblanski JN. Elongation of rat tail tendon: effect of load and temperature. *Arch Phys Med Rehabil* 1977; 52: 465–474.
189. Warren CG, Lehmann JF, Koblanski JN. Heat and stretch procedures: evaluation using rat tail tendon. *Arch Phys Med Rehabil* 1976; 57: 122–126.
190. Lehmann JF, Brunner GD, Stow RW. Pain threshold measurements after therapeutic application of ultrasound, microwaves, and infrared. *Arch Phys Med Rehabil* 1958; 39:560–565.
191. Fischer E, Solomon S. Physiological responses to heat and cold. In: Licht S, Kamenetz HL, eds. *Therapeutic heat and cold.* New Haven, CT: E Licht, 1965; 126–169.
192. Knutsson E, Mattson E. Effects of local cooling on monosynaptic reflexes in man. *Scand J Rehabil Med* 1969; 1:126–132.
193. Benson TB, Copp EP. The effects of therapeutic forms of heat and ice on the pain threshold of the normal shoulder. *Rheumatol Rehabil* 1974; 13:101–105.
194. Curkovi B, Vituli V, Nagle D, et al. The influence of heat and cold on the pain threshold in rheumatoid arthritis. *Z Rheumatol* 1993; 52: 289–291.
195. Kirk JA, Kersley GD. Heat and cold in the physical treatment of rheumatoid arthritis of the knee—a controlled clinical trial. *Arch Phys Med* 1968; 9:270–274.
196. Miglietta O. Action of cold on spasticity. *Am J Phys Med* 1973; 52: 198–202.
197. Olson JE, Stravino VD. A review of cryotherapy. *Phys Ther* 1972; 52:840–853.
198. Clarke GR, Willis LA, Stenner L, et al. Evaluation of physiotherapy in the treatment of osteo-arthrosis of the knee. *Rheumatol Rehabil* 1974; 13:190–197.
199a. Oosterveld FG, Rasker JJ. *Semin Arthritis Rheum* 1994; 24:82–90.
199b. Nicholas JJ. Physical modalities in rheumatological rehabilitation. *Arch Phys Med Rehabil* 1994; 75:994–1001.
200. Mannheimer C, Carlsson CA. The analgesic effect of transcutaneous electrical nerve stimulation (TNS) in patients with rheumatoid arthritis. A comparative study of different patterns. *Pain* 1979; 6:329–334.
201. Mannheimer C, Lund S, Carlsson CA. The effect of transcutaneous electrical nerve stimulation (TENS) on joint pain in patients with rheumatoid arthritis. *Scand J Rheumatol* 1978; 7:13.
202. Hicks JE. Prosthetics, orthotics and assistive devices. General concepts of orthotics and prosthetic devices. *Arch Phys Med Rehabil* 1989; 70(suppl):5195–5201.
203. Moon MH. Compliance in splint-wearing behavior of patients with rheumatoid arthritis. *N Z Med J* 1976; 12:392–394.
204. Nicholas JJ, Gwen H. Splinting in rheumatoid arthritis. I. Factors affecting patient compliance. *Arch Phys Med Rehabil* 1982:63; 92–94.
205. Gerber L, Hunt G. Evaluation and treatment of the rheumatoid foot. *Bull N Y Acad Med* 1985; 61:359–368.
206. Gerber L, Hunt G. Ankle orthosis for rheumatoid disease. *Arthritis Rheum* 1985; 28:547.
207. Weist DR, Waters RL, Bontrager EL, et al. The influence of heel design on a rigid ankle foot orthosis. *Orthotics Prosthetics* 1979; 33:3.
208. Swezey RL. Below-knee weight-bearing brace for the arthritic foot. *Arch Phys Med Rehabil* 1978; 56:176–179.
209. Demopoulous JT. Orthotic and prosthetic management of foot disorders. In: Jahss MH, ed. *Disorders of the foot.* Philadelphia: WB Saunders, 1982; 1785.
210. Cassuan A, Wunder KE, Fultonberg DM. Orthotic management of the unstable knee. *Arch Phys Med Rehabil* 1977; 58:487–491.
211. Rubin G, Dixon M, Danisi M. VAPC prescription procedures for knee orthosis and knee-ankle-foot orthosis. *Orthotics Prosthetics* 1977; 31: 9–25.
212. Smith EM, Juvinoll RC, Corell EB, Nyboer KJ. Bracing the unstable arthritic knee. *Arch Phys Med Rehabil* 1970; 51:22–28.
213. Sugarbaker PH, Lampert MH. Excision of quadriceps muscle group. *Surgery* 1983; 93:462–466.
214. Bunch WH, Keagy RD. The spine. In: Bunch WH, Keagy RD, eds. *Principles of orthotic treatment.* St. Louis: CV Mosby, 1976; 84–90.
215. Norton PL, Brown T. The immobilizing efficiency of back braces. Their effect on the posture and motion of the lumbosacral spine. *J Bone Joint Surg [Am]* 1957; 39:111–139.
216. Hartman JT, Palumbo F, Hill BJ. Cineradiography of braced normal cervical spine: comparative study of five commonly used cervical orthoses. *Clin Orthop* 1975; 109:97–102.
217. Colachis SC Jr, Strohm BS, Ganter EL. Cervical spine motion in normal women: radiographic study of the effect of cervical collars. *Arch Phys Med Rehabil* 1973; 54:161–169.
218. Blount WP. Don't throw away the cane. *J Bone Joint Surg [Am]* 1956; 2:695–698.
219. *Guide to Independant Living for People with Arthritis.* Atlanta: Arthritis Foundation, 1988.
220. Schmitt A, McBriar W. Assessing the quality of education provided to rheumatoid arthritis patients in a suburban-rural setting. Presented at the 14th Scientific Meeting of Allied Health Professions, Section of the Arthritis Foundation. Denver, Colorado, 1979.
221. Stross JK, Mikkelsen WM. Educating patients with osteoarthritis. *J Rheumatol* 1977; 4:313–316.
222. Vignos P, Parker W, Thompson H. Evaluation of clinic education program for patients with rheumatoid arthritis. *J Rheumatol* 1976; 3: 155–165.
223. Holsten DJ, Morris AD, Moeschberger M. Effects of an organized educational program on patient understanding of rheumatoid arthritis and compliance with medical treatment. Presented at the 12th Scientific Meeting of the Allied Health Professions Section of the Arthritis Foundation, Miami Beach, Florida, December 1976.
224. Moll JMH, Wright V, Jeffrey MR, et al. The cartoon in doctor-patient communication: further study of the Arthritis and Rheumatism Council handbook on gout. *Ann Rheum Dis* 1977; 36:225–231.
225. Parker JC, Frank RG, Beck NC, et al. Pain management in rheumatoid arthritis patients. A cognitive-behavioral approach. *Arthritis Rheum* 1988; 31:593–601.
226. Cordery JC. Joint protection: a responsibility of the occupational therapist. *Am J Occup Ther* 1965; 19:285–294.
227. Melvin JL. *Rheumatic disease occupational therapy and rehabilitation,* 3rd ed. Philadelphia: FA Davis, 1982.
228. Furst G, Gerber L, Smith C. *Rehabilitation through learning: energy conservation and joint protection.* Baltimore: National Institutes of Health, 1982.
229. Barem J. A review of the psychological aspects of rheumatic diseases. *Semin Arthritis Rheum* 1981; 11:352–361.
230. Cobb S. Contained hostility in rheumatoid arthritis. *Arthritis Rheum* 1959; 2:419–425.

231. Spergel P, Ehrlich G, Glass D. The rheumatoid arthritic personality. *Psychosomatics* 1978; 19:79–86.
232. Potts MA. *Psychosocial aspects of rheumatic disease.* Boston: Butterworth, 1984; 309–319.
233. Swinburne WR. *Clinics in rheumatic disease: sexual counseling for the arthritic.* Philadelphia: WB Saunders, 1976; 639–651.
234. Currey HLF. Osteoarthrosis of the hip joint and sexual activity. *Ann Rheum Dis* 1970; 29:488–493.
235. Baldursson H, Brattstrom H. Sexual difficulties and total hip replacement in rheumatoid arthritis. *Scand J Rheumatol* 1979; 8:214–216.
236. Yoshino S. Sexual problems of women with rheumatoid arthritis. *Arch Phys Med Rehabil* 1981; 62:122–123.
237. U.S. Department of Health, Education, and Welfare. *Acute conditions: incidence and associated disability, US, 1974–1975.* Washington, DC: Vital Health Statistics, USDHEW Publication No. HRA, 1977; 77-1541.
238. Hicks JE. *Arthritis: impact of function in the work setting and comprehensive rehabilitation management.* Special report of the President's Committee on the Handicapped: impact of musculoskeletal problems on employment, May 4, 1984. Washington, DC: U.S. Government Printing Office, 1984.
239. Hadler N, Gillings D, Imbus H, et al. Hand structure and function in an industrial setting. *Arthritis Rheum* 1978; 21:210–220.
240. Ehrlich GE. Inflammatory osteoarthritis. The clinical syndrome. *J Chronic Dis* 1972; 25:317–328.
241. Kramer JS, Yellin EH, Epstein WV. Social and economic impacts of four musculoskeletal conditions. A study using commonly based data. *Arthritis Rheum* 1983; 26:901–907.
242. Pearson JR, Riddel DM. Idiopathic osteoarthritis of the hip. *Ann Rheum Dis* 1962; 21:31–39.
243. Perry GH, Smith MJ. Spontaneous recovery of the joint space in degenerative hip disease. *Ann Rheum Dis* 1972; 31:440–448.
244. Hernborg JS, Nilsson BE. The natural course of untreated osteoarthritis of the knee. *Clin Orthop* 1977; 123:130–137.
245. Cobb S, Merchant WR, Rubin T. The relation of symptoms to osteoarthritis. *J Chronic Dis* 1957:5:197–204.
246. McAlindon TE, Cooper C, Kerwan JR, et al. Determinants of disability in osteoarthritis of the knee. *Ann Rheum Dis* 1993; 52:258–262.
247. Panush RS, Lane NE. Exercise and the musculoskeletal system. *Baillieres Clin Rheumatol* 1994; 8:79–102.
248. Ettinger WH, Afable RF. Physical disability from knee osteoarthritis: the role of exercise as an intervention. *Med Sci Sports Exerc* 1994; 26:1435–1440.
249. Gofton JP. Studies in osteoarthritis of the hip. Part IV: Biomechanics and clinical consideration. *Can Med Assoc J* 1971; 104:1007–1011.
250. Nichols PIR. *Rehabilitation medicine.* London: Butterworth, 1980; 118–127.
251. Hicks J, Gerber L. Rehabilitation in the management of patients with osteoarthritis. In: Moskowitz R, Howell DS, Goldberg VR, Manalan H, eds. *Osteoarthritis.* Philadelphia: WB Saunders, 1992.
252. Madsen OR, Bliddal H, Egsmose C, et al. Isometric and isokinetic quadriceps strength in gonarthrosis; inter-relations between quadriceps strength, walking ability, radiology, subchondral bone density and pain. *Clin Rheumatol* 1995; 14:308–314.
253. Gerber L, Hicks JE. The scope of rehabilitative interventions in the treatment of patients with systemic rheumatic diseases. In: Hadler N, ed. *Arthritis in society.* London: Butterworth, 1985; 230–251.
254. Harris ED. The clinical features of rheumatoid arthritis. In: Kelley WN, Harris ED, Ruddy S, Sledge CB, eds. *Textbook of rheumatology,* 3rd ed. Philadelphia: WB Saunders, 1993; 874–911.
255. Fries JF, Williams CA, Morfeld D, et al. Reduction in long term disability in patients with rheumatoid arthritis treated with disease modifying antirheumatic drug based treatment strategies. *Arthritis Rheum* 1996; 39:616–623.
256. Yellin E, Meenan R, Nevitt M, Epstein W. Work disability in rheumatoid arthritis: effects of disease, social and work factors. *Ann Intern Med* 1980; 93:551–556.
257. Ennevaara K. Painful shoulder joint in rheumatoid arthritis. *Acta Rheumatol Scand* 1967; 11(suppl):1–116.
258. Weiss JJ, Thompson GR, Doust V, Burgener F. Rotator cuff tears in rheumatoid arthritis. *Arch Intern Med* 1975; 135:521.
259. Laine V, Vainio K. *The elbow in rheumatoid arthritis.* Amsterdam: Excerpta Medica, 1969; 112.
260. Shapiro JS. A new factor in the etiology of ulnar drift. *Clin Orthop* 1970; 68:32–43.
261. Inglis AE. Rheumatoid arthritis in the hand. *Am J Surg* 1965; 109: 368–741.
262. Swezey RL, Fiegenberg DS. Inappropriate intrinsic muscle action in the rheumatoid hand. *Ann Rheum Dis* 1972; 30:619–625.
263. Nalebuff EA. Diagnosis, classification and management of rheumatoid thumb deformities. *Bull Hosp Joint Dis* 1968; 24:119.
264. Duthie R, Harris C. A radiographic and clinical survey of the hip joints in sero-positive rheumatoid arthritis. *Acta Orthop Scand* 1969; 40:346.
265. Gupta PT. Physical examination of the arthritis patient. *Bull Rheum Dis* 1970; 20:596.
266. Dixon L. The rheumatoid foot. In: Hill AGS, ed. *Modern trends in rheumatology.* London: Butterworth, 1971; 158–173.
267. O'Leary PA, Waisman M. Dermatomyositis. A study of forty cases. *Arch Dermatol* 1940; 41:1001–1019.
268. Joffe MM, Love LA, Leff RL, et al. Drug therapy of the idiopathic inflammatory myopathies: predictors of response to prednisone azathiaprine and methotrexate and a comparison of their efficacy. *Am J Med* 1993; 94:379–387.
269. Dalakas MC. Clinical immunopathologic and therapeutic considerations of inflammatory myopathies. *Clin Neuropharmacol* 1992; 15: 327–351.
270. Hicks J, Richardson D, Sonies B. Correlation of neck flexor weakness and swallowing dysfunction in polymyositis patients. *Arthritis Rheum* 1990; 33(suppl):123.
271. Duncan PE, Griffin JP, Garcia A, Kaplan SB. Fibrosing alveolitis in polymyositis. A review of histologically confirmed cases. *Am J Med* 1974; 57:621–626.
272. Bohan A, Peter JB, Bowman RL, Pearson CM. A computer assisted analysis of 153 patients with polymyositis and dermatomyositis. *Medicine* 1977; 56:255–286.
273. Mann SC, Buragar FD. Preliminary study of acupuncture in rheumatoid arthritis. *J Rheumatol* 1974; 1:126.
274. Gerber LH, Smith C, Novick A, et al. Autogenic training in the treatment of Raynaud's phenomenon [Abstract]. *Arch Phys Med Rehabil* 1978; 59:522.
275. Siebold JR. Scleroderma systemic sclerosis—clinical features. In: Klipple JH, Dieppe PA, eds. *Rheumatology,* 1st ed. St. Louis: CV Mosby, 1993; 1–14.
276. Arnett F. Spondyloarthropathies. In: Gall E, Riggs G, eds. Rheumatic diseases, rehabilitation and management. London: Butterworth, 1984; 429–437.
277. Fox R, Calin A, Gerber RC, Gibson D. The chronicity of symptoms in Reiter's syndrome. *Ann Intern Med* 1979; 91:190–193.
278. Gerber L. Psoriatic arthritis: pharmacologic, surgical and rehabilitative management. In: Gerber L, Espinozal L, eds. *Psoriatic arthritis.* Orlando: Grune & Stratton, 1985; 147–165.
279. Viitanen JV, Lehtinen K, Suni J, et al. Fifteen months followup of intensive inpatient physiotherapy and exercise in ankylosing spondylitis. *Clin Rheumatol* 1995; 14:413–419.
280. Hidding A, Vander Linden S, Gielen X, et al. Continuation of group physical therapy is necessary in spondylitis: results of a randomized controlled trial. *Arthritis Care Res* 1994; 7:90–96.
281. Calin A. *Spondyloarthropathies.* Orlando: Grune & Stratton, 1984.
282. Gross M, Brandt KD. Educational support groups for patients with ankylosing spondylitis: a preliminary report. *Patient Counsel Health Educ* 1981; 3:6–12.
283. Cassidy JE. Juvenile rheumatoid arthritis. In: Kelly W, Harris ED, Ruddy S, Sledge CB, eds. *Textbook of rheumatology,* 3rd ed. Philadelphia: WB Saunders, 1993; 1189–1208.
284. Ansell BM, Unlu M. Hip involvement in juvenile chronic polyarthritis [Abstract]. *Ann Rheum Dis* 1970; 29:687–688.
285. Ansell BM. Joint manifestation in children with juvenile chronic polyarthritis. *Arthritis Rheum* 1977; 20:204.
286. Ansell BM. Rehabilitation in juvenile chronic arthritis. *Arthritis Rheumatol Rehabil* 1979; 20(suppl):74–76.
287. Rennebohm R, Correll JK. Comprehensive management of juvenile rheumatoid arthritis. *Nurs Clin North Am* 1984; 19:647–662.

288. Singsen BH, Isaacson AS, Bernstein BH, et al. Total hip replacement in children with arthritis. *Arthritis Rheum* 1978; 21:401–406.
289. Dhanedraw M, Hutton WC, Klenerman L, et al. Foot function in juvenile chronic arthritis. *Rheum Rehabil* 1980; 19:20–24.
290. Henoch MJ, Batson JW, Baum J. Psychosocial factors in juvenile rheumatoid arthritis. *Arthritis Rheum* 1978; 21:229–233.
291. Hicks JE. *Rehabilitative management of rheumatic diseases in the elderly. Elderly rehabilitation as art and science.* Cleveland: Springer, 1990.
292. Agate J. Physiotherapy problems and practice in the elderly: a critical evaluation. In: Wright V, ed. *Bone and joint disease in the elderly.* London: Churchill-Livingstone, 1983; 237–255.
293. Boum J. Rehabilitation aspects of aging in the elderly. In: Williams TF, ed. *Rehabilitation in the aging.* New York: Raven, 1984; 177–197.
294. Chamberlain A. Mobility in the elderly arthritic. In: Wright V, ed. *Bone and joint disease in the elderly.* London: Churchill-Livingstone, 1983; 222–236.
295. Gerber L. Aids and appliances. In: Wright V, ed. *Bone and joint disease in the elderly.* London: Churchill-Livingstone, 1983; 256–274.

Rehabilitation Medicine: Principles and Practice, Third Edition,
edited by Joel A. DeLisa and Bruce M. Gans.
Lippincott–Raven Publishers, Philadelphia © 1998.

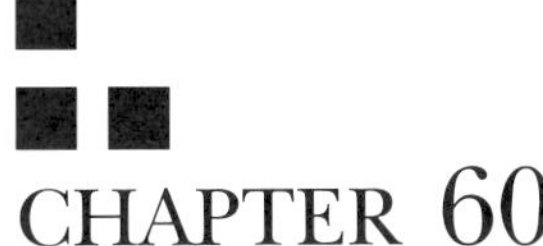

CHAPTER 60

Rehabilitation of the Patient with Peripheral Vascular Disease and Diabetic Foot Problems

Geetha Pandian, Farrukh Hamid, and Margaret C. Hammond

Preventing disability and achieving and maintaining a high functional level are goals of rehabilitation medicine. The vascular diseases and diabetic foot problems discussed in this chapter may cause significant acute and chronic functional impairment. Early diagnosis and prevention of complications, along with patient education, risk reduction, and proper medical management, reduce disability and improve disease prognosis.

PERIPHERAL VASCULAR DISEASE

History

William Harvey in 1620 demonstrated that there must be connections for blood flow from the arterial to venous systems. In 1661, Malpighi, with the help of lenses, demonstrated the capillaries. Leeuwenhoek in 1674 confirmed Malpighi's findings and observed the movement of red cells through the capillaries (1). Since those discoveries, our knowledge of anatomy, histology, and physiology of the peripheral vascular system has expanded, giving us a better understanding of pathophysiologic processes that cause disease and ways to prevent and treat it.

Physiology

In recent years, researchers have focused on complex local events that regulate blood flow. From the time when Barcroft in 1943 demonstrated that human skeletal muscles have sympathetic vasoconstrictor nerves (2), and Von Euler in 1948 showed that sympathetic nerves cause vasoconstriction by releasing norepinephrine (3), detailed mechanisms of action of the alpha and beta receptors and their regulation have since been described.

Positioned between the layers of endothelial cells and perivascular nerves are the smooth muscle cells responsible for the control of arterial and venous tone and distribution of blood flow throughout the body (4). The connections between the arteries and veins can be divided into the resistance vessels (arterioles), exchange vessels (capillaries), and capacitance vessels (venules). The regulatory mechanism in the above components involves humoral and nervous mechanisms, with complex interactions between smooth muscle cells, perivascular nerves, and endothelium and the local metabolic products. The smooth muscle cells form circular layers around the vessels and are innervated by perivascular nerve fibers. Transmitters released by these fibers activate receptors on the vascular smooth muscle cell membrane with resultant vasoconstriction or vasodilatation. These transmitters are not just adrenergic or cholinergic as described by Lagercrantz (5). A wide variety of peptides are present in the perivascular nerve. The exact function of some of these peptides is not understood, and a detailed discussion of them is beyond the scope of this chapter. However, the major neurologic control of blood vessel tone is accomplished by sympathetic nerves, and norepinephrine is the principle neurotransmitter that causes vasoconstriction via alpha adrenoreceptors, along with receptor-operated calcium channels. The amount of neurotransmitter release depends on the degree of activation of the sympathetic fibers and the presence of local metabolic (adenosine, CO_2, hydrogen ions, lactic acid, and potassium) and circulating vasoactive substances (acetylcholine, histamine, serotonin, and angiotensin II) as well as autoregulation (6).

Newer research has shown the role of endothelial cells in the regulation of blood flow. Endothelial cells respond to various stimuli regulating the tone in the smooth muscle cells (7). These stimuli include substances such as endothelium-derived relaxing factor, prostacyclin, endothelium-derived contracting factor, and angiotensin II, which effect platelet aggregation, platelet adhesion, and smooth muscle proliferation.

G. Pandian and F. Hamid: Department of Physical Medicine and Rehabilitation, University of Texas—Southwestern Medical Center at Dallas, Dallas, Texas 75235-9055.
M. C. Hammond: Department of Physical Medicine and Rehabilitation, University of Washington, Seattle, Washington 98195.

In order to develop strategies for prevention and treatment of vascular diseases, it is imperative to understand how vascular smooth muscle cells contract and relax in response to physical and chemical stimulation, the role that endothelium plays in this complex process, and the pathophysiology of the disease processes that disturb the fine balance in this regulation.

Pathophysiology

Congenital or acquired defects in endothelial cell function could lead to imbalance between relaxing and contracting factors, which is one of the major factors leading to pathophysiologic changes in the function of blood vessel walls. Endothelial dysfunction has been demonstrated in several diseases of the peripheral blood vessels, including hypertension, diabetes, atherosclerosis, hyperlipidemia, and vasospasm.

Changes in the morphology and histology of the vascular system may range from thickening of capillary basement membrane, a decrease in density of the microvessels, endothelial cell degeneration, and increased platelet adhesion and aggregation in diabetes mellitus, to endothelial injury, endothelial fat accumulation with fatty streak formation, and smooth muscle proliferation in atherosclerosis.

ATHEROSCLEROSIS

Atherosclerosis of the arteries in the lower limbs is one of the strongest indicators of atherosclerosis in other vessels in the body, such as the coronary and cerebral blood vessels (8). In the lower extremities it involves mostly the large and medium sized arteries. Lesions tend to develop at major arterial bifurcations and sites of acute vessel angulation. The disease does not affect all arteries to the same extent but shows a predilection for coronary arteries, carotid bifurcation, aortoiliac, and lower extremity vessels. The lower extremity site most commonly affected is the arterial segment between the superficial femoral and popliteal arteries in Hunter's canal. In nondiabetics, aortoiliac disease is the second most likely location, whereas in diabetics, popliteal and tibial disease are more likely to follow femoral disease (9).

Epidemiology

Symptomatic atherosclerosis predominates in men 50 to 70 years of age. Based on symptoms and clinical examination, the incidence was 0.9%, 3.6%, and 7.5% for men 40 to 44, 50 to 54, and 60 to 64 years of age, respectively (9). In a later review of the literature on patients with chronic leg ischemia, it was concluded that 1.5% of men under 50 years of age and 5% of men over 55 years of age develop symptomatic leg ischemia (10). These numbers most likely underestimate the true occurrence of obliterative arterial disease in the lower limbs (8). Using a battery of noninvasive tests, 11.7% of a population with a mean age of 66 years was found to have large vessel occlusive disease. Less than one fifth of them experienced intermittent claudication (11).

Dormandy in 1989 reported that progressive deterioration of intermittent claudication to rest pain or gangrene occurs in about 15% to 20% of patients (10). In two general population demographic studies, only 1.6% and 1.8% of claudicant patients ultimately underwent amputations (9,12).

The overall survival rate for patients with intermittent claudication is 73% at 5 years, in contrast to 93% at 5 years for normal age-matched controls (13). Patients are at greater risk for mortality from other vascular diseases, especially cerebral or cardiac arterial disease, than for morbidity associated with limb loss (14).

Risk Factors

A number of factors predispose to the development or acceleration of atherosclerosis:

1. Clinical and experimental studies have established that elevated plasma concentration of lipoproteins, particularly low-density lipoproteins, increase the risk and rate of progression of atherosclerosis (15,16). Cholesterol is a major constituent of advanced lesions (17). In patients with significant atherosclerosis, the mean plasma cholesterol was found to be more than 50 mg/dl higher than in controls (13,18).
2. Smoking is described as the single most powerful risk factor for peripheral vascular disease (13,19,20). Relative risk of smoking in the development of leg arterial disease ranges from 1.4 to more than 10 times depending on age, sex, definition of a smoker, and methods of evaluation of arterial disease. Three quarters of cases of intermittent claudication could eventually be attributable to smoking (21).
3. Hypertension exacerbates atherosclerosis with each incremental increase in pressure, directly increasing the risk of coronary artery disease (22). Systolic blood pressure appears to be a better predictor of arterial disease than diastolic blood pressure. Hypertension was found in 25% of patients with symptomatic disease of the aortoiliac and femoral popliteal arteries, but was found in only 9% of age-matched controls (13). The mechanism appears to be related to endothelial injury from hypertensive pressure or hemodynamic shearing.
4. Diabetes mellitus is associated with an earlier onset of atherosclerosis and a more rapid disease progression (23). The obstructive disease of the large arteries in diabetes, usually designated as macroangiopathy, is commonly held as indistinguishable from atherosclerosis in nondiabetes (24). In diabetes, distal vessels are more involved than are aortoiliac vessels; proposed mechanisms include disturbance of normal platelet, endothelial, and smooth muscle cell function, secondary to hyperglycemia, causing vasoconstriction and smooth muscle proliferation (25).

5. Other risk factors for generalized atherosclerosis include obesity, hyperuricemia, sedentary life-style, and a positive family history.

Clinical Presentations

In 1931 Lewis and Colleagues showed that claudication pain was not a consequence of vasoconstriction developing during exercise and concluded that it was due to a chemical or physicochemical stimulus that develops in the muscle during exercise, but even today the exact nature and mechanism of this stimulus is unknown.

Blood flow through the muscles can be hindered mechanically during exercise, depending on the strength of contraction. As a result, metabolites accumulate, activating afferent nerves in the contracted muscles, causing increased sympathetic outflow that increases the arterial blood pressure and tries to improve the blood flow to the muscles. In patients with occlusive arterial disease there is limited blood flow, causing an excessive increase in muscle metabolites. A comparison of calf blood flow after exercise in normal subjects and patients with occlusive vascular disease demonstrates different patterns. In normal subjects there is high initial flow and a rapid decrease to the resting levels. In patients with claudication, two patterns were found. In those with less severe lesions, the blood flow immediately after the exercise was less than that of normal subjects and declined more gradually to the resting level. In more severe cases, immediate postexercise flow was less than the prior resting value and gradually increased to reach the maximum that was much less than the normal 1 to 14 minutes after the exercise ended (26).

This difference can be explained by the vascular steal phenomenon; that is, the limited blood supply goes first to the dilated vascular bed of the thigh muscles, and only after the metabolic debt of these muscles is repaid does the blood flow to the calf begin to increase. This also explains the absence of blood flow to the foot immediately after exercise in these patients.

In the presence of obliterative disease, perfusion of capillaries depends on local hemodynamics and metabolic needs. Several compensatory mechanisms try to avoid local ischemia. Oxygen extraction increases and muscle metabolism adapts. Reflex increase in sympathetic activity increases the blood pressure. Obviously, the efficacy of these compensatory mechanisms depends on the extent of the metabolic needs. Time can play a critical role in these events. Therefore, even in severe stenosis, blood flow can often be maintained at a normal level in resting conditions. However, with exercise the blood flow requirements cannot be met, resulting in a decrease in perfusion pressure.

Intermittent claudication is the most common symptom of obliterative arterial disease of the leg. Fontaine classified the evolution of atherosclerosis of lower limb arteries into four stages (2):

1. Pathologic changes in arteries without any clinical symptoms
2. Presence of intermittent claudication
3. Rest pain
4. Trophic lesions

The symptoms of intermittent claudication—aching of the muscles in the lower limbs, more typically at the calf, occurring with walking and steadily increasing to a point where the patient has to stop because of intolerable pain—should be carefully analyzed and differentiated from other causes of pain, such as that caused by venous disease, peripheral nerve disease, or orthopedic disorders (Table 60-1).

Physical Examination

Findings on physical examination include arterial pulses that are decreased or absent to palpation, sometimes associated with bruits, delayed capillary filling and rubor, and pallor upon leg elevation. Palpation of arterial pulsations and auscultation of the bruit can locate the most important site of the lesion and provide an indication of the degree of stenosis. Sharply decreased amplitude of the pulse, along with a loud bruit over that vessel, indicates the presence of a stenosis of about 70%; an almost unpalpable pulsation with a soft bruit is a strong indication of a 90% stenosis. With complete occlusion, no pulsation and bruit are present (except for bruit due to collateral flow) (8). Ischemia-related findings may include trophic skin changes (thin, shiny, hairless appearance, paresthesias, and skin ulcerations), dependent rubor (an erythematous dusky color), and decreased temperature. The site of claudication may roughly indicate the level of occlusion (27). Occlusion at or above the ankle may cause claudication in the arch of the foot. Calf claudication suggests occlusion at or above the calf. Buttock pain or sexual dysfunction generally is associated with aortoiliac disease.

Table 60-1. *Differential diagnosis of intermittent claudication*

Neurospinal disorders
Spinal stenosis
Herniated lumbar disc
Spinal claudication or pseudoclaudication
Neuropathic disorders
Diabetic
Ischemic
Other peripheral entrapment (e.g., tarsal tunnel syndrome)
Plantar neuroma
Musculoskeletal disorders
Arthritis (e.g., of the hip, knee)
Popliteal cyst
Osteoporosis
Miscellaneous
McArdle disease

Reprinted with permission from Hammond MC, Merli GJ, Zierler RE. Rehabilitation of the patient with peripheral vascular disease of the lower extremity. In: DeLisa JA, ed. *Rehabilitation medicine: principles and practice,* 2nd ed. Philadelphia: JB Lippincott, 1993; 1083.

Diagnosis

Supplementing a careful history and physical examination, diagnostic tests serve to establish the diagnosis, document the location and severity of stenosis or occlusion, evaluate the relative importance of multilevel disease, and assess the presence of collateral vessels or vasospasm. They also provide a baseline from which to assess disease progression, therapeutic results, or the degree of functional impairment.

Noninvasive diagnostic procedures do not cause discomfort and permit quantitative assessment. The test to be used depends on the symptom. In general, techniques can be divided into those that look at the anatomic and those that look at the functional changes. How these tests are performed depends on the specific technology options available and on the particular questions that need to be answered. Testing may be needed for the following reasons:

1. To establish a diagnosis (e.g., to determine if claudication rather than pseudo-claudication is present)
2. To determine the severity of the disease (e.g., to assess a hemodynamically significant lesion for appropriate intervention)
3. To confirm failure or success of treatment (e.g., based on the therapeutic intervention)
4. To document the disease process (e.g., for disability evaluation/impairment rating or medicolegal reasons)

Diagnostic Testing

Diagnostic tests can assess blood flow or pressure. Patients with mild to moderate atherosclerosis and claudication have arterial occlusive disease that is sufficiently severe to produce symptoms during exercise but not while the patient is at rest; therefore, the total limb blood flow is usually normal at rest due to compensatory distal vasodilation. Noninvasive studies in this setting are indicated to determine the location, severity, and functional impairment caused by the disease. The initial laboratory evaluation of patients with claudication is performed at rest. The standard methods that may be used to obtain baseline information are listed as follows:

1. Continuous-wave Doppler: Using a hand-held duplex device, wave forms are determined from arteries from the lower extremities. The lesion is localized by interpreting the changes in wave form.
2. Segmental pressure: Arterial pressure is recorded from different segments of the lower extremity arterial tree and referenced against brachial pressure to create a pressure index. The ankle–brachial index is the most commonly used. This study provides both localization and quantitative information about the severity of the disease. An index of 0.9 or greater is considered normal, whereas an index of 0.7 to 0.9 indicates mild disease, 0.4 to 0.6 moderate to severe disease, and less than 0.4 severe disease. With an index greater than 0.5, occlusion of a single vessel is likely (28). In patients with calcified noncompressible vessels, the arterial pressures are falsely elevated, giving a high index, even in the presence of arterial occlusive disease.
3. Pulse volume recording: This technique uses arterial pulse as an index of vessel patency and is most useful as a back-up test for evaluation of noncompressible vessels.
4. Duplex scanning: Real-time echo Doppler ultrasound imaging (duplex scanning) is another standard measure for peripheral arterial circulation assessment (29). Besides providing information about the location and type of arterial lesion and pressure grading across any given lesion (30), duplex scanning also helps detect fistulae, aneurysms, and other structural problems.
5. Exercise studies: With isotonic exercise, peripheral vasodilatation and a decrease in resistance occurs in response to the metabolic demands of exercising muscle. Whereas exercise results in a markedly increased flow rate in a normal extremity, the corresponding increase in a limb with atherosclerosis is much less. This failure to increase flow during exercise is the physiologic basis of intermittent claudication. Creating temporary limb ischemia with a pneumatic cuff, and resultant reactive hyperemia, is another method of inducing maximal rest dilation.

   Exercise studies have been performed by recording ABI and common femoral cutaneous wave Doppler velocity profiles after a standard exercise protocol. (Treadmill walk at 2 miles per hour on a 10% incline for a maximum of 5 minutes in the Mayo Clinic laboratories). The disease severity is estimated from recovery of ABI at 1-, 3-, 5-, 10-, and 20-minute intervals using Clement guidelines (31).
6. Arteriography: Arteriography is an adequate method for the full characterization of the whole arterial supply of the leg. It should be considered an emergency procedure in patients when there is threat of spreading gangrene. Appropriate management decisions are made based on the results of arteriography, and serious complications can be prevented.

Other noninvasive flow studies include regional flow assessment with venous occlusion plethysmography (which according to a recent study is 75% sensitive and 93% specific, yielding an overall performance of 85%) (31) and indirect testing through calorimetry and thermography. Whereas the previously described tests measure regional blood flow, other techniques assess local tissue perfusion. Transcutaneous measurement of oxygen tension with the help of Clark-type oxygen-sensing recording and reference electrodes assesses skin oxygen content.

Assessment of ischemia is similar to that of claudication, using determination of temperature, segmental pressure, pulse, volume, and Doppler wave forms. These determina-

TABLE 60-2. *Severity of cutaneous ischemia based upon transcutaneous oxygen ($TcPO_2$) measurement*[a]

Severity of hypoperfusion	Supine $TcPO_2$ (mm Hg)	Elevated $TcPO_2$ (mm Hg)[b]	Effect on skin healing potential
None or mild	>40	—	Healing likely to occur
Moderate	20–40	$TcPO_2$ decreases by ≤10 mm Hg	Healing likely to occur
	20–40	$TcPO_2$ decreases by >10 mm Hg	Healing not likely to occur
Severe	<20	—	Healing not likely to occur

[a] Electrode temperature 45°C equilibrated for 20 min or until a steady state is achieved.
[b] For limbs with a supine $TcPO_2$ of 20 to 40 mm Hg, the limbs are elevated to 30° for 3 to 5 min and the decrease in $TcPo_2$ is determined.

Reprinted with permission from Clement DL, Shepherd JT, eds. *Vascular diseases in the limb.* St. Louis: Mosby Year Book, 1993;108.

tions help localize and quantify the severity of the disease process. Other specific means to measure the severity of ischemia include venous occlusion plethysmography, which is considered the method of choice for this purpose (29). However, there is no better method than transcutaneous oximetry for evaluating the cutaneous ischemia (Table 60-2) (32,33).

CRITICAL LEG ISCHEMIA

Critical leg ischemia as initially defined by Rutherford included patients with ischemic ulcers or rest pain whose ankle systolic pressure was below 40 to 60 mm Hg (34). However, many patients with ischemic ulcers or rest pain had ankle pressures above the defined limits. Chronic critical leg ischemia has been defined by the second European consensus document (1992) as follows (35).

Chronic critical leg ischemia in both diabetic and nondiabetic patients is defined by either of the following two criteria:

1. Persistently recurring ischemic rest pain requiring regular adequate analgesia for at least 2 weeks, with an ankle systolic pressure no more than 50 mm Hg and/or a toe systolic pressure no more than 30 mm Hg; or
2. Ulceration or gangrene of the foot or toes, with an ankle systolic pressure of no more than 50 mm Hg or toe systolic pressure of no more than 30 mm Hg (35).

In contrast to the pathophysiology of intermittent claudication, where there is atherosclerosis of the major supplying arteries but no detectable changes at the microcirculatory level, in critical leg ischemia there are permanent microcirculatory changes distal to the arterial lesion (35).

MANAGEMENT

Management depends on the severity of the arterial disease and the ability of the patient to tolerate certain treatment options. Patients with mild to moderate disease and only symptoms of claudication, patients with recent onset of disease who do not have fully developed collaterals, and patients who have failed vascular reconstruction or are high surgical risks are candidates for medical management.

Education

The patient must be educated about his or her disease to improve understanding and compliance with treatment and alleviate the fear of amputation.

Risk Reduction

Smoking is a major contributing factor, both in terms of operative risk and promotion of disease progression. Patients must stop smoking. Hypertension should be controlled. It should be remembered that the onset of intermittent claudication or exacerbation can occur if antihypertensive treatment is too aggressive. Reduction in calories and possibly cholesterol intake to control body weight is also important.

Treatment of Associated Disease

Associated diseases that exacerbate atherosclerosis require attention. Congestive heart failure must be treated to maximize cardiac function and lessen peripheral edema. Arterial oxygenation can be improved with treatment of chronic obstructive pulmonary disease or anemia. Diabetes must be controlled because of the association of arterial disease progression and neuropathy.

Foot Care

The entire lower extremities, especially the feet, require special attention. Overall the tissue oxygen demand should be decreased by avoiding trauma, inflammation, and heat. Meticulous foot care is essential. Patients should inspect and wash their feet daily and avoid prolonged soaking. Professional nail care, treatment of fungal infection, ingrown toenails, and daily lanolin application to maintain skin pliability are recommended. Shoes should be inspected before wearing, looking for items such as gravel or torn linings. Walking barefoot and in wet shoes, prolonged soaking in water, exposure to cold, and hot pads on feet should be avoided to prevent mechanical, chemical, or thermal injury.

Edema Control

Edema can decrease arterial perfusion. Elevating the head of the bed 6 to 8 inches may allow pain-free sleep with minimal edema formation (36). Vascular stockings that are not too tight and constricting also help resolve edema.

Medical Management

The goal of treatment is restoration of function and relief of pain, along with the treatment of any treatable associated disease. The long-term goal is to prevent disease progression and promote regression. Analgesic medications such as acetaminophen reduce pain. Antiplatelet agents (e.g., aspirin) have the added advantage of reducing platelet aggregation and are effective in low doses (37). Ticlopidine has been proven to increase cutaneous temperature and transcutaneous partial pressure of oxygen (38). Hemorrheologic agents (e.g., pentoxifylline, a methylxanthine derivative) affect red blood cell flexibility and have been associated with significant increase in walking distances in a double-blinded study of patients with intermittent claudication (39). The role of vasodilators in peripheral obstructive vascular disease remains questionable (40). In cases of critical leg ischemia, both the local and general factors should be considered. Optimization of cardiac output alone is sometimes sufficient to reverse critical ischemia. Subcutaneous catheter techniques and arterial reconstructive procedures are still the mainstay of treatment. If amputation is inevitable, it should be performed without wasting time.

In managing the ischemic leg, dependent positioning for the leg is beneficial because it increases the profusion pressure. It should be maintained except when edema starts to develop. Ambulation is also beneficial to the patient provided it is pain free and trauma can be avoided. Aspirin or ticlopidine should be administered. Even if a reversal of the ischemia is not achieved, these measures may be sufficient to stabilize the ischemia and make it safe to try a course of pharmacotherapy to improve critical ischemia. However, if the ischemia is deteriorating, reopening procedures should be attempted without delay. Pharmacotherapy has been accepted as a viable option for management of intermittent claudication, where the problem is intermittent reversible ischemia of skeletal muscle. However, the favorable results of pharmacotherapy cannot be extrapolated to patients with critical leg ischemia, where the pathologic changes are in the skin microcirculation (8).

Prostanoids (PGI_2, PGE_1, or the stable prostacyclin analog Iloprost) have been successfully used in critical leg ischemia in the form of infusion (41,42). Prostanoids are a reasonable treatment option for patients who are not candidates for reopening procedures (43). Acute thrombosis or acute arterial embolus is best managed with an initial course of heparin followed by arteriography to define the lesion. The surgical option is chosen based on the response to heparin therapy and the results of arteriography. Should an ischemic ulcer develop (Fig. 60-1), the patient should avoid weight bearing and protect the involved foot with lamb's wool separation of the toes, hydrotherapy, routine wound dressing, and antibiotics as indicated. Ambulation may be allowed as long as gangrene is dry and edema absent. Range of motion (ROM) exercises for joints of the lower extremities should be performed to prevent contractures.

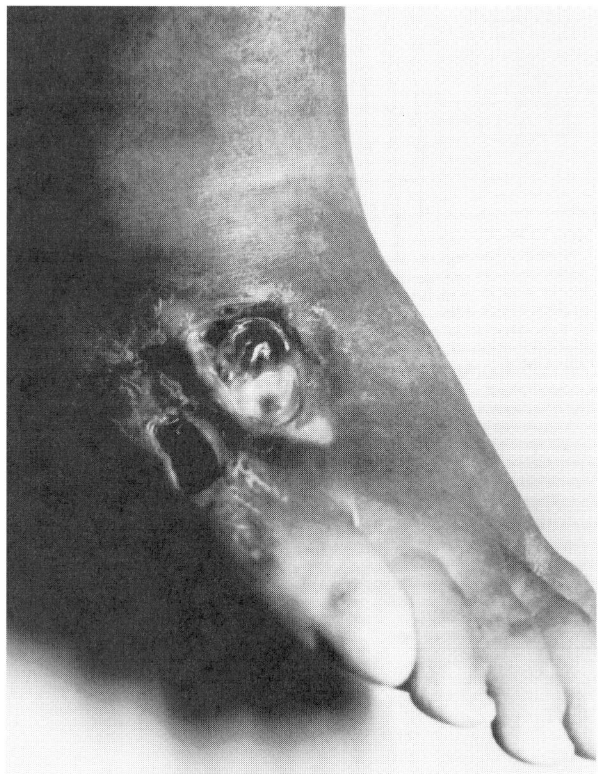

FIG. 60-1. Dorsal foot ischemic ulcer.

Surgical Management

Indications for surgical intervention include intractable ischemic pain, severe ischemia with a nonhealing ulcer or gangrene, and increasing disability. The following surgical options may be exercised:

1. Reopening procedures: Angioplasty is indicated for focal stenosis or short segmental occlusion with relatively disease-free adjacent vessels. Advantages of this procedure include short inpatient stay, low incidence of morbidity, and fairly successful long-term results (44).
2. Limb salvage procedures: Bypass surgery uses prosthetic materials such as Taylor patch or Miller cuff or distal arterial venous bypass graft (45,46). These procedures are indicated for diffuse arterial disease of a segment with an ABI less than 0.4 or a forefoot transcutane-

ous partial pressure of oxygen ($TcPO_2$) of less than 30 mm Hg (47). The standard procedures, depending on the location of the lesion, include aortobifemoral, femoral–femoral, iliofemoral, femoral–popliteal, or dorsalis pedis bypass. The last one has been especially beneficial for patients with diabetes whose occlusive disease frequently involves the tibial and peroneal vessels and spares the inframalleolar circulation (48,49).

3. Amputation: Primary amputation is indicated in patients with failed bypass surgery or spreading infection or toxemia. Delayed elective amputation is performed in later stages of the disease to achieve a more pain-free functional status after careful review of risk-to-benefit and cost-to-benefit ratios.

PHYSICAL REHABILITATION

Exercise

This is important at all stages of the disease. A number of studies support the use of exercise in the presence of intermittent claudication (50,51). The mechanisms behind the beneficial effect may include improved peripheral utilization of oxygen, increased patency of collateral circulation, and improved oxidative and glycolytic capacity (51–53). Multiple factors affect the exercise capacity of patients with intermittent claudication. Sorlie found a two- to 10-fold increase in lower leg blood flow in subjects with atherosclerosis, at maximum exercise, compared with a 20-fold increase in normal (54). In addition, a greater oxygen extraction in claudicant patients persists into the postexercise period (55). This may be due to increased red blood cell passage time as a consequence of decreased flow, or it may be due to increased tissue oxygenative capacity (56).

Exercise therapy is contraindicated in the presence of an ischemic ulcer or rest pain. A baseline treadmill exercise test should be performed in the absence of contraindications. Training may consist of walking, jogging, bicycling, or swimming; the upright exercise posture is preferable to the horizontal because it improves lower extremity perfusion (54). Walking programs should be individualized considering the precautions and contraindications in each case. Standard prescription includes a gradual increase in duration from 30 to 60 minutes three to five times per week at 2 miles per hour (44,50), as tolerated, with the provision of rest when claudication develops (47,53). In a program of group therapy three times per week with each session including walking, jogging, leg stretching, and leg relaxation, the patients doubled their walking distance after 3 months. Additional but less significant improvement was noted for another 6 months (56). Patients with aortoiliac disease respond as well as those with femoral popliteal disease (50). If exercise is limited to walking, the patient should walk three to five times per day to just beyond the onset of claudication. In patients with superficial femoral artery occlusion, symptomatic improvement can be expected in those with an ankle arm ratio greater than 0.6 (14). Low-level pain-free endurance training is also effective in increasing walking distance, exercise time, and energy expenditure.

Proper Shoe Wear

Proper shoe wear should be prescribed as needed. New shoes should be broken in slowly and carefully.

Orthotics

Although infrequently used, an ankle–foot orthosis may decrease plantar flexion activity and work during push off, contributing to subjective improvement and increase in walking distances (57). Occasionally a patient who refuses amputation for ischemic ulcers may ambulate safely with a patellar tendon-bearing orthosis (58).

VASOSPASTIC DISORDERS

Raynaud's phenomenon is a vascular spasm of unknown etiology. Raynaud described the attack of digital ischemia in women that results from cold exposure and emotional stress (59). Specific hypotheses for the etiology include abnormal sympathetic activity, abnormal digital vessels, or an immunologic process (60,61).

It is important to distinguish between primary and secondary causes of Raynaud's phenomenon. Primary disease is diagnosed after secondary causes have been ruled out (62). Raynaud's disease is more common in women, who constitute 70% to 90% of this patient population.

Diagnosis

In 1932, Allen and Brown outlined the following minimal diagnostic requirements:

1. Vasospasm precipitated by cold and emotional stress
2. Symptoms for more than 2 years
3. Bilateral involvement
4. Minimal or absent gangrene of finger tips
5. Absence of other diseases associated with vasospastic attacks (63)

Physical Examination

Clinically, the skin of the fingers changes color in response to cold. A classic triad presents as digital or occasionally proximal hand pallor with numbness, which persist for the duration of the cold stimulus. Cyanosis then develops after 10 to 30 minutes of warmth as a small amount of flowing blood desaturates. Lastly, a reactive hyperemia and rubor of the skin develops. Severe pain is rarely associated with the process, and gangrene of the tips is rare. In severe cases, atrophic changes consisting of atrophy of the skin, wasting of the tissues in the finger pads, and irregular nail growth may occur in the fingers. In about 40% of patients, the toes also may be involved (65). With time, the attacks become more prolonged, and the appearance of redness does not necessarily mean the spasm has subsided (66). In women 15 to 40 years of age, the disease is considered benign, provided there is no history of other underlying diseases or exposure to vasospastic agents, and physical examinations and laboratory tests are normal.

Laboratory Tests

Diagnosis can be frequently confirmed via an ice-water immersion test and serial digital pulp temperature measurements. Complete blood count (CBC), erythrocyte sedimentation rate (ESR), urinalysis, chest film, electrophoresis, antinuclear antibodies, and cryoglobulin are some of the tests that are indicated to rule out diseases such as scleroderma, lupus erythematosus, thromboangiitis obliterans, rheumatoid arthritis, polymyositis and dermatomyositis, and Sjögren's syndrome, which are known causes of secondary Raynaud's disease.

Treatment

Treatment is directed primarily at symptom relief. For a majority of patients with primary Raynaud's, maintaining local and general body warmth is adequate. Avoidance of cold, nicotine, and exacerbating drugs is essential. The use of gloves markedly reduces the frequency of attacks (67). Pharmacologic treatments include calcium channel blockers such as nifedipine, which frequently results in symptomatic improvement (64). Serotonin antagonists (e.g., Ketansarin, Janssen Pharmaceutica, Beerse, Belgium) have been shown to improve symptoms and decrease the frequency of vasospastic episodes. The use of prazosin, an alpha-adrenoceptor blocker, have shown a moderate benefit in decreasing the frequency of attacks (68). Other agents tested for topical application include prostaglandin, nitroglycerin, and minoxodil, without evidence of benefit.

Surgical sympathectomy has been used in the past but is ineffective in maintaining the blood flow and is now rarely considered a treatment option for Raynaud's disease (69,70). Biofeedback benefits some individuals by teaching them to warm their hands or dilate the blood vessels. Additional measures include relaxation training and stress management if stress is the inciting factor.

LYMPHEDEMA

Lymphedema is the increase in girth of an extremity or other body part due to disorder of transcapillary fluid exchange resulting from impaired function of lymphatic channels. It is characterized by overaccumulation of fluid in interstitial tissues and fibrotic changes in the soft tissue. These changes start in the subcutaneous fatty tissue and generally extend superficially to involve the skin and deep to involve the fascial sheets of the muscle.

The overall incidence is uncertain. A female:male ratio of 10:1 has been described (71). The peak incidence of onset is in the first decade after menarche.

Pathophysiology

There are three structural defects in lymphedema that result from or cause overaccumulation of protein-enriched interstitial fluid.

1. Obstruction of superficial and deep lymphatic with fibrosis of regional lymph nodes (72,73).
2. Increase in subcutaneous fatty tissue with fibrosis of interlobular septa.
3. Thickening of deep fascia.

Physiologically four factors influence the accumulation/inadequate removal of the fluid from the interstitial space. The plasma protein in the blood and interstitial pressure promote the reabsorption of fluid, whereas the capillary blood pressure and the plasma protein in interstitial fluid keep the fluid in the interstitium. Lymphedema develops when the compensatory mechanisms (e.g. the proteolytic activity of macrophages and the lymphatic collateral circulation) are exhausted and the transfer capacity of the lymphatic system is still inadequate to handle the lymphatic load.

Lymphedema can be classified as primary due to primary abnormalities of the lymphatic channels (congenital or hereditary) and secondary due to another pathology or disease process (infectious, malignant, traumatic, iatrogenic).

Diagnosis

History can help classify lymphedema as the primary or secondary variety with either family history as in Milroy's disease, or no family history as in congenital simple lymphedema. Other examples of primary disease are lymphedema praecox or tarda, where edema appears spontaneously later in life without an apparent etiology.

In secondary lymphedema there is history of either infection (e.g. filariasis, tuberculosis), malignancy (prostate in males and lymphoma in females) (71), radiation, or surgery.

Clinically the swelling is usually unilateral and if bilateral, not symmetrical. In fully developed edema, a specific feature of swelling of lymphatic origin is the involvement of the dorsum of the foot and toes with sparing of the metatarsophalangeal joints (Fig. 60-2). Edema is poorly responsive to bed rest and is usually nonpitting. Differential diagnosis includes venous disease and conditions that can cause secondary lymphedema. Evaluation includes exclusion of malignancy and metastatic disease. Computerized tomography (CT) or magnetic resonance imaging (MRI) is used to exclude pathologic processes in the inguinal, pelvic, and periaortic lymph nodes. Duplex scanning is the investigative method of choice for evaluation of venous disease. Lymphangiography has been replaced by lymphoscintigraphy for evaluation of the lymphatic system (74).

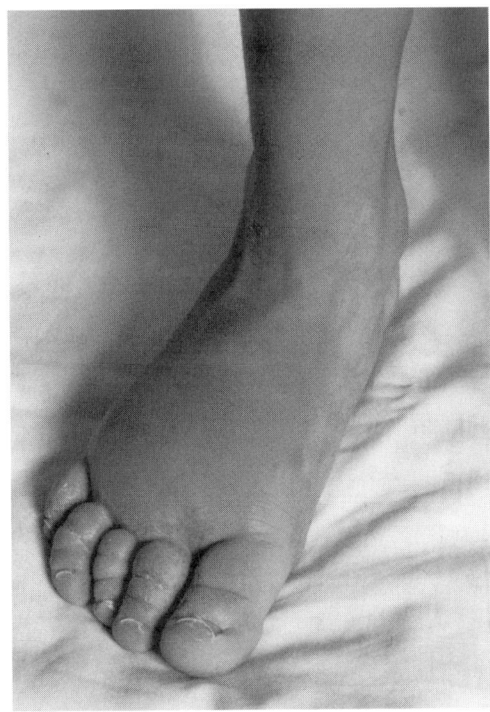

FIG. 60-2. Lymphema of the foot and toe with sparing of metatarsophalangeal joints.

Management

The general aim of treatment is mobilization of fluid, reduction of girth, and prevention of complications. Etiology should be determined before starting the treatment. Conservative treatment includes external compression in the form of manual massage, intermittent compression, and graded pressure garments.

Intermittent compression of 80 to 120 mm Hg as tolerated is applied preferably twice a day for 40 to 45 minutes each time and should be used with the extremity elevated, followed by manual massage and therapy repeated over 4 to 6 days until the volume is stabilized. The patient is then placed in interim pressure garments between therapy sessions and while a custom pressure graded garment is made. The patient is then placed in the definitive garment for long-term management. Ideally these garments should be worn all day, taken off only for bathing and cleaning of garment, and before going to bed with the extremity elevated. The average life of the garment is about 4 months. The patient should be re-evaluated monthly or more frequently if complications are present.

Education and use of the garment, isometric exercises, and elevation are important to help improve compliance and results (75). The patient also should be educated in skin and nail care to avoid infection. ROM exercises to prevent contracture and mobilize edema are also important. Weight reduction and a generalized conditioning program is also helpful.

Medical Management

Severe cases may need hospitalization. To avoid cardiopulmonary complications from rapid mobilization of fluid, diuretics may be indicated; otherwise, diuretics are rarely used to mobilize fluid. Infection is a common complication and needs immediate attention. Skin is the most common portal of infection. Penicillin, cephalosporin, and erythmyocin are appropriate antibiotic choices. Benzopyrones, although not available in the United States, are reported to be beneficial for stimulating proteolysis. The degradation of excess proteins facilitates their removal and minimizes the retention of water caused by interstitial proteins (76).

Surgical Management

Indications for surgery include failure of conservative management or treatment of a secondary disease process. The aim is to improve the drainage (e.g., lymphatic-to-lymphatic or lymphatic-to-venous anastomosis) or reduce the swelling (e.g., eradication of excess subcutaneous tissue) (77,78). The available literature does not show promising results with these surgical procedures (74).

VENOUS DISEASE

Venous disease affects as much as a quarter of the population in the United States. The morbidity associated with the venous disorders may result in life-style changes, loss of work, and frequent hospitalizations. The following sections review the anatomy, physiology, pathophysiology, clinical findings, diagnosis, and management of acute venous thrombosis and chronic venous insufficiency (CVI).

Anatomy

Veins are thin-walled capacitance vessels that carry blood from the periphery back to the heart. The vein wall is composed of three layers: the intima, media, and adventitia. Active changes in the vein wall diameter are produced by the media. Veins contain valves that ensure the unidirectional flow of blood. Valves are generally bivalved, strong, and able to resist pressures of up to 400 mm Hg. The presence of a sinus adjacent to the valve leaflet prevents them from coming into contact with the vein walls and facilitates rapid closure when pressure is reversed (Fig. 60-3) (79).

Veins of the lower extremity are divided into the superficial and deep groups. Greater and lesser saphenous veins are the principle superficial veins of the lower limb. The former run on the medial aspect of the leg and thigh to join the femoral vein, whereas the latter run behind the lateral malleolus and posterior leg and join the popliteal vein. Communicating veins connect the superficial and deep veins. The deep veins of the leg are three in number: anterior, posterior tibial, and peroneal. The calf veins converge toward the knee, gen-

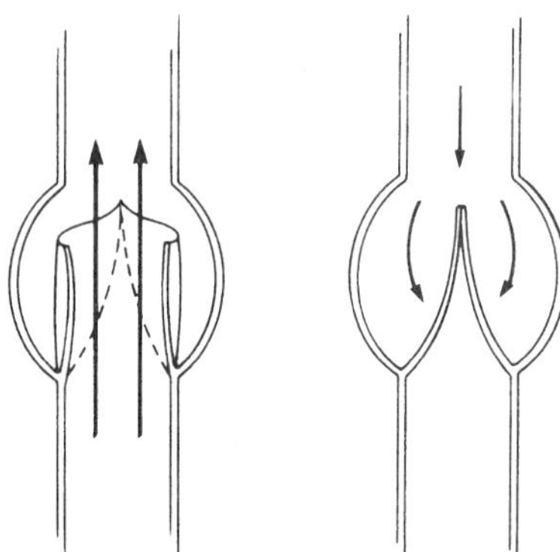

FIG. 60-3. Longitudinal section through a venous valve shows the open and closed position.

erally forming a single popliteal vein that continues as the superficial femoral vein (Fig. 60-4).

Physiology

Deep vein valves perform their antireflux role at different phases of the gait cycle. During walking or running, contractions of muscle groups increase the pressure in the deep veins and push blood centrally. The calf muscles are the most significant of these. During ambulation, contraction of the calf muscles compress the blood contained within the venous sinuses and deep calf veins, thereby pumping the blood toward the heart. Valves in the communicating veins prevent the reflux of blood and transmission of intramusculature pressure into the superficial veins during calf pump contraction (80).

CHRONIC VENOUS INSUFFICIENCY

Pathophysiology

The basic underlying pathophysiologic mechanism in CVI is increased pressure in the deep venous system. This venous hypertension is caused either by blocking of outflow (obstruction), inefficient or insufficient outflow or backflow (reflux), or a combination of these (80).

Venous obstruction can be due to thrombosis, pelvic and abdominal masses, pregnancy, or intraluminal obstruction (e.g., webs or tumors). Reflux is the result of valvular dysfunction; from congenital agenesis of the iliofemoral valve, defective valves of the greater and lesser saphenous veins, or ankle perforating veins to valves scarred or destroyed by thrombi (80). The incompetence of valves in the perforating veins permits the higher pressure generated in the deep venous system during contraction of calf muscle pump to be transmitted to the superficial veins, subcutaneous tissue, and skin.

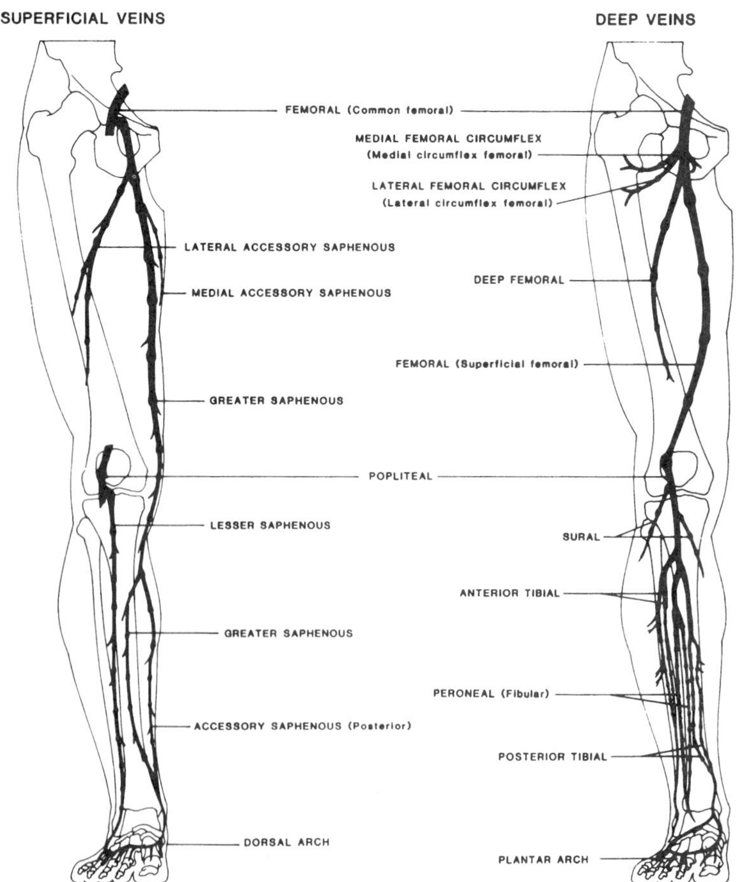

FIG. 60-4. Radiographic anatomy of the major vessels of the lower limb.

Clinical Findings

The chief clinical manifestations of CVI are dilated leg veins, edema, leg pain, skin pigmentation, subcutaneous fibrosis, dermatitis, and ulceration. Venous dilation is the most common initial sign and is most apparent along the dependent portion of the limb such as the lower, medial aspect of the calf or underneath the medial malleolus, the so-called ankle flare (80). With further progression of CVI, the veins become larger and tortuous and will begin to be seen in the proximal portions of the limb.

Edema is initially mild and is limited to the perimalleoler area and usually resolves with bed rest. The edema initially may be pitting, but in chronic stages it may fail to pit secondary to the occurrence of subcutaneous fibrosis. This fibrosis is probably related to the deposition of protein within subcutaneous tissue and the subsequent inflammatory process.

Although not all patients with CVI experience leg pain, several distinct types of pain are described. The most frequent type is the limb heaviness or ache that occurs with prolonged standing. The pain is usually localized to the calf area and is relieved by walking and lying down with the leg elevated. Some patients may experience pain along the dilated varicose veins after prolonged standing. Patients with obstruction of the deep venous system may experience venous claudication, a mild aching sensation at rest that becomes an intense cramping type sensation in the calf with ambulation (80). The patient may have to stop and allow venous congestion to resolve. Patients with valvular incompetence in the deep venous system also may note sudden development of leg heaviness with standing, which may increase to bursting type heaviness in the calf with further standing.

Cutaneous manifestations of CVI are characterized by brownish hemosiderin deposits in the skin. The secondary pruritus that occurs may induce scratching, eventually leading to development of eczematous stasis dermatitis.

The signs of CVI can be grouped into three stages depending on the severity of the disease (81) (Table 60-3). This classification directs the degree and intensity of care. Ultrasound scanning may be indicated for patients who are surgical candidates to assess both superficial and deep venous system and to locate incompetent perforating veins.

TABLE 60-3. *Chronic venous insufficiency*

Stage	Symptoms	Physical findings
I	Pain Heaviness Mild swelling	Superficial varicosities Edema along perimalleolar area
II	Heaviness Varicosities Pigmentation, pruritis Moderate to severe swelling	Moderate varicosities Pigmentation Dermatitis Moderate to severe edema
III	Ulceration Severe swelling Calf pain with or without venous claudication	Multiple varicositis Marked skin pigmentation Ulceration Severe edema

TABLE 60-4. *Conservative therapy for chronic venous insufficiency*

Stage I
- Custom-fitted elastic compression stockings
- Ace wrap or variant
- Circ-aid (legging [Shaw Therapeutics Inc., Rumson, New Jersey])
- Intermittent external pneumatic compression
- Skin care

Stage II
- Custom-fitted elastic compression stockings
- Skin care with water-based lotion
- Topical steroids for dermatitis
- Surgical consultation

Stage III
- Ulcer care
- Wet to dry saline dressings
- Duoderm
- Unna boot (Bayer Corporation, Connecticut)

Four-layer high compression bandage
- Custom fitted elastic compression stockings

Management

Nonsurgical treatment of CVI includes reduction of ambulatory superficial venous hypertension, improvement of skin nutrition, and wound care (80). Approach to treatment depends on the severity of disease as noted on the clinical examination and by the system involved as suggested by the noninvasive objective measurements (Table 60-4).

Patients with stage 1 disease are treated by nonsurgical methods, unless involvement of the superficial venous systems has produced cosmetically displeasing varicosities to the patient. Use of external compressive devices such as compressive wraps, elastic stockings, and intermittent pneumatic compression are the mainstay of treatment in stage 1 disease:

1. Compression bandages such as ace wraps are the simplest and least expensive form of external compression. Frequent problems noted are difficulty in wrapping, loss of elasticity with washing, and problems in maintaining the wrap in the correct position. Despite these disadvantages, ace wrap bandages are useful in elderly patients, who cannot pull on tight stockings and have abnormally contoured limbs.
2. Below-the-knee custom-fitted graduated elastic compression stockings are the standard for treatment of CVI. Above-the-knee stockings are not indicated because high pressure is needed primarily around the ankle and not above the knee; and thigh-high and above-the-knee stockings tend to bind around the popliteal area. Compression stockings reduce superficial venous volume and prevent transcapillary leakage of fluid into the interstitium. These stockings should be put on before

getting out of bed when there is maximal edema reduction. Companies such as Jobst, Sigvaris, Juzo, and Barton Carey custom make these stockings with several gradients of compression. For stage 1 disease, 20 to 30 mm Hg stocking pressure is recommended; for stage II and III, 40 to 50 mm Hg stocking pressure is recommended. These stockings maintain pressure for 4 to 6 months. Off-the-shelf stockings that provide 20 to 30 mm Hg are also available from some companies. The major disadvantage of graduated compression elastic stockings is difficulty pulling them on. The use of zippered stockings or rubber kitchen gloves to pull them on is helpful.

3. Intermittent compression devices have been shown to improve microcirculatory changes seen in CVI and improve ulcer healing. Multi-cell sequential inflation devices with at least three chambers are preferred.
4. Circ-aid (Shaw Therapeutics, Inc., Rumson, New Jersey) is a custom-fitted device composed of a series of Velcro straps from ankle to below knee and can be used as an alternative approach to elastic compression stockings. Advantages of this device are ease of application for an abnormally contoured leg and easier dressing changes.

In stage II disease, there is retrograde pressure from incompetent valves with resultant varicosities and their sequelae. Gradient elastic stockings are the principle treatment. Patients usually complain of pruritus from the eczematous skin changes associated with advanced stage II disease. Judicious use of topical steroid cream is helpful in reducing the pruritus and in preventing conversion from stage II to stage III disease caused by scratching. Acute infections should be treated vigorously with penicillin or erythromycin to prevent damage to lymphatics. Patients should be educated to observe for infection, avoid trauma, and encouraged to use water-based soluble skin cream or lotion to improve skin nutrition.

Ulceration is the disabling complication of stage III disease (Fig. 60-5). External compression is essential as in other stages to decrease transmural venous pressure and promote ulcer healing. Elastic compression bandages, stockings, or Circ-Aid may be used. These may be supplemented by either nightly or 2 to 4 hours of daytime use of pneumatic compression devices. McCullouch et al. have shown that the use of pneumatic devices twice weekly, even for 1 hour each session, promotes wound healing (82).

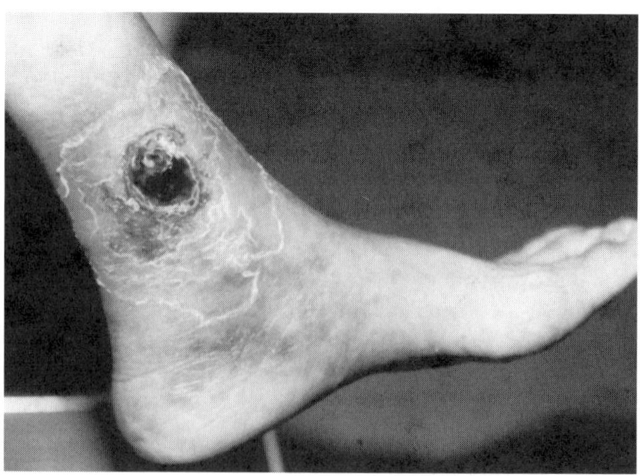

FIG. 60-5. Venous stasis ulcer with surrounding dermatitis.

Treatment of venous leg ulcers begins with treatment of cellulitis with appropriate antibiotics. Eczematous areas are treated with topical corticosteroids applied lightly two or three times a day. For ulcers with exudate, calcium alginate dressing, wet to dry saline, or Dakin's or Burrow's soaks are used with frequent changes (83). Bio-occlusive dressings such as Duoderm (ConvaTec—Division of E. R. Squibb and Sons, Inc., Princeton, New Jersey) also can be used. Hydrotherapy at 100°F is used for mechanical debridement of the wound. When there is no inflammation or cellulitis, impregnated bandages such as Unna boot dressings are used for management. They can be applied directly over the ulcer next to the skin. Unna Boot dressings are further covered with a layer of dry gauze and/or stockinette and an ace type elastic bandage. This combination generates approximately 30 mm Hg of mean pressure below the malleolus that decreases to 6 mm Hg below the knee. Advantages of Unna boot dressings are that wound care and external compressive devices are contained in one unit, they can be changed twice weekly, and they prevent the patient from scratching and causing further damage. Dockery recommends a four-layer high compression bandage system (Profore; Smith & Nephew United, Largo, FL) as a more efficient system than Unna boot dressings (83). The technique involves sequential application of orthopedic wool wrap, cotton crepe, elastic wrap bandage, and cohesive bandages with weekly dressing changes. This system creates 40 mm Hg of mean pressure at the ankle, which decreases to 17 mm Hg below the knee. Surgical treatment with skin grafting may be needed for ulcers that are large and do not heal. Once healing occurs, pressure gradient compression stockings are fitted and applied each morning to prevent recurrence.

Deep Vein Thrombosis

The pathogenesis of deep vein thrombosis (DVT) is related to Virchow's triad of venous stasis, vessel wall damage, and increased activation of clotting factors (hypercoagulability) (84).

1. Stasis or altered blood flow in the lower limb deep veins results from immobility, paralysis, or surgery. The stasis contributes to venous thrombosis by preventing the activated coagulation factors from being diluted by nonactivated blood, preventing clearance and mixing with naturally occurring inhibitors.
2. Injury to the vessel wall has been suggested to be the strongest risk factor for venous thrombosis. The intact endothelium is normally thromboresistant by eliminating contact between platelets and subendothelial colla-

gen. Once there is damage to the vessel wall, the exposed subendothelium leads to platelet adhesion, aggregation, and platelet release, with activation of components of both intrinsic and extrinsic pathways of coagulation.

3. Hypercoagulability results in imbalance between thrombosis and hemorrhage.
4. Other predisposing risk factors that are known to increase susceptibility to thrombosis include immobilization, surgery, trauma, increasing age, patients with neoplasm of gastrointestinal tract or breast, intracranial tumors, heart failure, previous venous thrombosis, obesity, pregnancy, and oral contraceptive pills. All of these risk factors contribute in varying degrees to formation of acute DVT.

Clinical Diagnosis

The accuracy of clinical evaluation for acute DVT is notoriously unreliable. Clinical findings of pain, edema, and venous distention are not always present; various nonthrombotic disorders can cause similar symptoms. Homan's sign, which is pain in the upper calf during passive dorsiflexion of the foot, is very nonspecific and insensitive. Objective diagnostic tests that can be used in diagnosis of DVT are venography, impedance plethysmography, and duplex ultrasonography.

Venography has been the standard for diagnosis of venous thrombosis. But it is not used routinely for fear of complications such as pain at injection site, superficial phlebitis or DVT, renal failure, hypersensitivity to the dye, and local skin and tissue necrosis if the dye is extravasated at the injection site. Noninvasive testing such as impedance plethysmography or duplex ultrasonography are preferable. However, impedance plethysmography does not allow localization of thrombosis and does not detect calf thrombi. Duplex ultrasonography has now been proven to be the superior method. In experienced hands, it has a sensitivity and specificity of 95% for proximal vein thrombosis and allows localization of thrombosis (84).

Prevention of Deep Venous Thrombosis and Pulmonary Embolism

Prevention of DVT and pulmonary embolism (PE) should be one of the primary directives in patients who are undergoing surgery, have had multiple trauma, and have sustained neurologic injury. The selection of prophylactic agents is based on their ability to prevent one or more components of Virchow's triad. Various prophylactic strategies are used depending on the risk groups; in many patients, multiple risk factors may be present, and the risks are cumulative.

Orthopedic patients, specifically those undergoing hip and knee joint replacement, are the most frequently seen high-risk population in rehabilitation practice. The incidence of DVT is 40% to 50% in patients undergoing total hip replacement and 72% in patients undergoing total knee replacement (85). These patients should receive low molecular weight heparin, adjusted-dose heparin, or oral anticoagulation (86). Enoxaparin sodium injection is given at a dosage of 30 mg subcutaneously every 12 hours; the starting dosage of adjusted-dose heparin is 3,500 U subcutaneously three times daily, and then it is adjusted up or down to prolong activated partial thromboplastin time (APTT) to the upper limit of normal. Warfarin is usually used for oral anticoagulation. There are two different ways by which warfarin is given for this purpose. The first is to start warfarin a number of days preoperatively and adjust the dose to prolong prothrombin time to reach the international normalized ratio (INR) of approximately 1.5 at the time of surgery, and then increase warfarin to reach an INR of 2 to 2.5 in the postoperative period. The second method is to start warfarin on the day before or the first postoperative day in doses that will result in an INR of 2.0 to 2.5 by the fourth to fifth postoperative day. Intermittent pneumatic leg compression devices can be used in conjunction with the above prophylactic regimen in these patients, especially those undergoing total knee joint replacement (86).

Patients undergoing neurosurgical procedures have a 19% to 32% incidence of DVT/PE (85). These patients and those undergoing eye, spine, or prostate surgery should receive intermittent pneumatic leg compression devices for prevention of DVT. The incidence of DVT after stroke has been reported to be 60% in the first 2 weeks after the cerebrovascular insult (87). Prophylaxis with low-dose heparin at 5,000 U subcutaneously every 8 to 12 hours or an external pneumatic leg compression device is important.

Patients with spinal cord injury have been reported to have a 47% to 60% incidence of DVT in the first 2 weeks after injury in motor complete and motor nonfunctional patients (88). Prophylaxis with low-dose heparin, external pneumatic leg compression devices, and elastic stockings are recommended. All of these provide inadequate protection against DVT when used alone but appear to be beneficial when used in combination.

Rehabilitation patients not in the above categories, general medical and surgical patients should receive prophylaxis with low dose heparin and/or external pneumatic compression devices if they are not fully ambulatory.

Treatment of Acute Deep Venous Thrombosis and Pulmonary Embolism

After DVT is confirmed by diagnostic studies, therapy is initiated with heparin or thrombolytic agents. Before initiating therapy with heparin, check for contraindications and obtain baseline APTT, prothrombin time (PT), and a complete blood count. Current guidelines for anticoagulation for DVT/PE are to begin heparin with a bolus of 5,000 to 10,000 U intravenously followed by a continuous infusion of 1,000 to 1,300 U/hr. APTT is assessed at 6 hours, and the heparin dose is adjusted up or down to maintain the value of APTT between 1.5 and 2.5 times the patient's baseline APTT. A platelet count is performed daily. Oral anticoagulation with warfarin is started on day 1 at 5 to 10 mg, and then it is administered daily at an established maintenance dose to maintain the PT in the therapeutic range of 1.3 to 1.5 times the laboratory control value or international normalized ratio of 2 to 3. Heparin therapy is discontinued after 4 to 7 days of combined therapy, when an INR of 2 to 3 is reached. Treatment is continued for 3 months, longer in high-risk patients (89).

Thrombolytic therapy with streptokinase, urokinase, or tissue plasminogen activator is reserved for PE with compromised cardiopulmonary status or DVT with threatened limb viability. Vena cava interruption using a Greenfield filter is indicated for patients who have contraindication to anticoagulation therapy, those with recurrent PE despite anticoagulation, those undergoing pulmonary embolectomy, and those with chronic recurrent PE (80). Some investigators include elderly patients at risk of falling, mentally unstable patients, patients with a free-floating proximal thrombus, patients with low cardiopulmonary reserve, or patients with pulmonary hypertension and massive PE among those for whom placement of a Greenfield filter would be recommended.

Patients with calf vein thrombosis are confined to bed for 72 hours, followed by gradual mobilization. Patients with proximal venous thrombosis require 4 to 7 days of bed rest with gradual mobilization when pain and swelling has subsided. All patients wear gradient elastic stockings when they are mobilized.

REHABILITATION OF DIABETIC FOOT PROBLEMS

Cause for Concern

Diabetes mellitus affects approximately 13 million individuals in the United States. One of the most feared complications of diabetes is loss of a leg or foot. About 51% of all nontraumatic amputations occur in diabetics due to diabetic-related complications. The economic impact of diabetic foot complications is enormous. Reiber reports that treatment of diabetic foot ulcerations accounted for $150 million (in 1986), and the average health-care cost for a diabetic patient undergoing amputation was $24,700 (90). Obviously, the cost has increased since then. Apart from the economic impact, the toll on loss of function and life is substantial. After amputation of a leg, 55% of the patients require amputation of the contralateral leg within 2 to 3 years; two thirds of diabetics die within 5 years after initial leg amputation. These data show that prevention of amputation has not been stressed (91). Fortunately, we are beginning to see development of multidisciplinary clinics whose primary goal is to identify and treat at-risk patients. These clinics have achieved an impressive 44% to 85% decrease in amputation rates (92).

ETIOPATHOGENESIS OF DIABETIC FOOT ULCERS

Diabetic foot ulcers are often caused by a combination of causes rather than a single cause. Pecoraro et al. described several potential causal pathways that lead to most amputations. These include neuropathy, minor trauma, cutaneous ulceration, infection, ischemia, faulty wound healing, and gangrene (93). Mechanical stress also has been implicated as causing foot ulcerations. Removal of one of these causes could theoretically break the causal chain and eliminate the need for amputation. Among these etiologies, neuropathy, ischemia, infection, and mechanical stress have been described as the most prevalent. Each of these factors are described below.

NEUROPATHY

Neuropathy is present in 12% of patients at the time of diagnosis, with a prevalence rate of 42% to 80% for individuals with less than 5 years and greater than 15 years duration of diabetes, respectively (94). The most common types of diabetic neuropathies are distal symmetric sensory motor neuropathy (with mainly sensory involvement) and autonomic neuropathy.

Sensory Motor Neuropathy

Boulton and Edmonds have implicated neuropathy as the major etiologic factor in 62% to 87% of patients who present with new foot ulcers (95). The lack of protective sensation allows the patient to tolerate poorly fitting shoes and makes them prone to unrecognized trauma, fracture, and neuropathic joint disease. Associated motor neuropathy causes intrinsic foot muscle dysfunction, resulting in deformities such as claw and hammer toes and metatarsophalangeal joint subluxation. These deformities lead to areas of abnormal foot pressure, particularly underneath the metatarsal head and tips and tops of the deformed toes. Calluses and corns are frequently formed over areas of abnormal pressure. Calluses are not painful in insensate patients and therefore do not limit ambulation, eventually causing ulceration due to the abnormal foot pressure. Sensory neuropathy allows the patient to wear tight shoes for prolonged periods of time without pain or discomfort. This results in local blockage of capillary blood flow with resultant tissue ischemia, causing ulceration. These ulcers tend to occur on the dorsal surfaces of toes and the medial and lateral borders of the feet.

Autonomic Neuropathy

Autonomic neuropathy in diabetic patients leads to impaired sweat and sebaceous gland secretion with resultant dry, cracked skin with fissures. These can become portals of entry for bacteria. The associated arteriovenous shunt that occurs as a consequence of the autonomic dysfunction is also strongly reported to be associated with ulceration and Charcot's arthropathy.

VASCULAR DISEASE

Vascular disease is the second major cause of diabetic foot lesions. In diabetic macroangiopathy, the popliteal, tibial, peroneal, and superficial femoral arteries are most frequently affected. Ischemic ulcers tend to occur more commonly along the toes and dorsal aspect of the foot rather than on the plantar surface of the foot. Lithner et al. noted that 64% of ischemic lesions occur on digits, 16% on heels, 10% on the dorsum of the foot, and 10% along the metatarsal head (96).

INFECTION

It is estimated that 25% of all diabetes-related hospital admissions are for the treatment of infected foot lesions and gangrene (97). Diabetic foot ulcers are inherently susceptible to infection due to defective leukocytosis with impaired intracellular bacterial killing and poor antibiotic perfusion of the infected area secondary to ischemia.

MECHANICAL STRESS

Brand identified three different types of mechanical stress that can result in foot ulcerations (98). One type of stress is a high-pressure penetrating injury that occurs when a person steps on a nail or piece of glass. Those with insensate feet will walk with the object embedded in their foot, causing repetitive injury and inflammation at the site. A second type of mechanical stress is from low pressure applied for a prolonged period of time. Skin breakdown is from the unrelenting low pressure (2 to 8 lb/in^2) applied to the tissues for an extended period (12 to 16 hours). This injury can occur when a person wears poorly fitting shoes (99). The third and most common type of injury results from repetitive stress of walking. This usually develops when tissues are subjected to higher levels of stress either by walking fast or longer distances. Walking generates 20 to 80 lb/in^2 pressure along the foot. A person with insensitive feet lacks the perception of discomfort and thus does not alter or limit ambulation. This continued stress with each step can result in tissue breakdown and inflammation. Areas vulnerable to repetitive stress from walking are the great toe and metatarsal heads (Table 60-5).

GENERAL GUIDELINES FOR PATIENT ASSESSMENT

Obtaining an accurate patient history and performing a careful clinical examination are the first steps in correctly diagnosing and managing these patients.

Patient History

Factors to be considered in history taking are diabetes control, current foot care, footwear practices, history of previous ulceration, and/or amputation and the events leading up to them. The clinician should record symptoms of claudication, cramps, paresthesia, shooting or burning pains. Finally it is important to ascertain the patient's understanding of the disease process as related to foot care.

CLINICAL EXAMINATION

Neurologic Evaluation

The role of neuropathy as a mediator of diabetic-related foot problems cannot be over emphasized. It is important to remember that neuropathy may be present even in the absence of subjective symptoms of numbness and paresthesia. Normal electrodiagnostic testing does not rule out the presence of a neuropathy. Neurologic examination should include evaluation of deep tendon reflexes, sensory testing, and a complete motor examination. Use of Semmes-Weinstein monofilaments provides reliable information about the presence of protective sensation (100). The monofilament is applied to various parts of the foot with just enough force

TABLE 60-5. *Risk factors for foot ulceration in diabetics*

Neuropathy	Thick mycotic nails
Sensorimotor (abnormal protective sensation)	Previous ulcers and amputation
Autonomic (dry, cracked skin)	Soft-tissue atrophy and fat pad displacement
Vascular disease	Poor hygiene
Abnormal plantar pressure (elevated in neuropathy even in absence of deformity)	Inappropriate Footwear
Abnormal gait in elderly living alone	Blind or partially sighted
Degenerative joint diseases of hip and knee	Elevated activity profile
Muscle weakness	Lack of education/poor
Heel cord tightness	Foot deformities
Pronation, supination deformities of the foot	Claw toes, hammer toes
Toe contractures	Hallux valgus and rigidus
	Deformities secondary to Charcot arthropathy

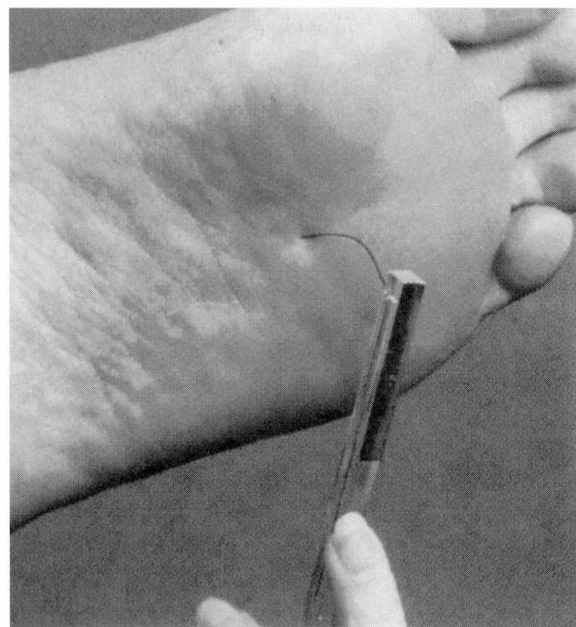

FIG. 60-6. Use of Semmes-Weinstein monofilament to determine the presence of protective sensation in the foot.

to barely buckle the nylon (Fig. 60-6). Those who can consistently perceive the 5.07 monofilament have enough protective sensation and are unlikely to sustain major foot injuries. Use of cotton swabs or pin prick does not provide such quantifiable information about the presence or absence of protective sensation. A tuning fork or biothesiometer (an electrical vibrating machine) can be used to assess large fiber function. Use of a 128-cycle tuning fork is more practical and should be used to test along both the first and fifth metatarsal phalangeal joints of both feet. An impairment is present if the patient perceives the vibratory endpoint 10 seconds or more before the examiner perceives the endpoint (101). Impaired vibratory perception is a significant risk factor for amputation.

Vascular Assessment

Signs and symptoms of peripheral vascular disease include intermittent claudication, nocturnal and rest pain relieved with dependency, shiny skin, hair loss on the feet and toes, blanching with limb elevation, and dependent rubor. Normal venous and capillary filling time is less than 15 seconds. It can be prolonged to minutes in patients with severe ischemia. Subcutaneous tissue atrophy often gives the overlying skin a "baked potato skin" feel. Dorsalis pedis and posterior tibialis pulses should be palpated. The temperature of the limb can be assessed using the dorsal hand and is compared side to side and proximal to distal.

If pedal pulses are weak or absent, Doppler ultrasound or other quantitative studies should be considered. Satisfactory healing can be predicted if flow is pulsatile and ankle pressure index is over 0.45. However, in the presence of vascular calcification, the ankle pressure index may be falsely elevated due to vessel incompressibility. In these patients, $TcPO_2$ values or photoplethysmography toe pressure measurements can be used to determine adequacy of blood flow. It is generally accepted that healing is likely to occur if $TcPO_2$ and absolute toe pressure are above 35 to 40 mm Hg (102).

Musculoskeletal Examination

A comprehensive musculoskeletal system examination must include evaluation for trunk deviation, leg length discrepancy, restricted hip movement (e.g., degenerative arthritis or total hip replacement), and knee deformities. Obviously all of the above can affect stance and gait and cause abnormal pressure distribution on the foot. For example, a patient with genu valgus deformity may walk on the medial side of the foot, whereas a patient with genu varus deformity may walk on the lateral side of the foot, thus causing excessive pressure along the medial or lateral border of the foot.

Diabetics often have limited ROM of the foot and ankle and have feet that are rigid. Intrinsic muscle atrophy caused by motor neuropathy results in clawing of toes, prominent metatarsal heads, and plantar fascia contractures. In addition, when the toes become clawed, the submetatarsal fat pad, which is closely invested in the flexor tendons, becomes displaced anteriorly, leaving heads of the metatarsals covered by only a thin layer of skin. Peroneal nerve compromise seen frequently in diabetics results in an unbalanced foot with weakness of dorsiflexors, evertors, and toe extensors. Functionally, the foot assumes a plantar flexed and inverted position resulting in unequal pressure distribution along the plantar forefoot, especially the fifth metatarsal head. Because of these reasons, metatarsal heads should always be palpated in a neuropathic patient; if they are found prominent, special footwear should be prescribed.

A metabolic reason for limitation of joint mobility is the impaired degradation of collagen, leading to changes in the mechanical properties of the skin and subcutaneous tissue, making them stiffer and less able to transmit the shear to the deeper tissues (103). Restricted joint mobility impairs the foot's ability to adapt and absorb shock during walking, thereby increasing the risk of plantar ulceration. Ideally patients should have 10° of dorsiflexion of ankle above neutral with knee extended and about 30° of subtalar joint ROM (104). With heel cord contractures, the patient will create the necessary movement from heel strike to mid-stance through excessive pronation, thus placing greater stress on tarsal and mid-tarsal joints. This may result in hyperostosis or acute Charcot collapse.

Charcot's neuroarthropathy causes the more obvious and the most devastating deformity of the diabetic foot. The foot may be completely immobile with subluxation of joints, particularly in the mid-foot area. The resultant rocker bottom deformity results in the entire body weight being concentrated on a few square centimeters of tissue, making the foot very prone to ulcerations.

It is important to be aware of the foot pressure changes that occur after amputations in the foot because these deviations often lead to subsequent amputations. Mann et al. found that the lateral shift that occurs after hallux amputations causes callus formation under the second and third metatarsal heads (105). Individual lesser toe amputations usually do not result in functional disturbance in gait. However a toe filler may be mandatory after a second toe amputation to avoid rapid development of hallux valgus. In first and fifth ray amputations, there is a high incidence of subsequent ulceration. The medial weight shift that occurs after first ray amputations, along with the loss of a portion of the plantar fascia and intrinsics to the hallux, leads to the collapse of the medial arch with subsequent ptosis of the navicular bone and ulcer formation (106). Fifth ray amputation causes supination of the foot due to loss of peroneus brevis insertion, with increased pressure over the fourth metatarsal and the potential for tissue breakdown. Thus, it is important to look for preulcerous changes in persons with amputations in the foot.

PREVENTION OF DIABETIC FOOT PROBLEMS

Patient education is the prerequisite for prevention of diabetic foot problems. The aim is to help the patient understand the risk of being injured by walking on the unprotected insensitive feet. Education needs to be conveyed at every patient contact and reinforced with printed materials. The patient should be educated about the importance of proper glucose control, routine foot care, adverse effects of smoking on the vascular system, and importance of using appropriate footwear in the presence of insensitive feet with decreased circulation. Patients should be provided with a list of "do's and don'ts" on how to take care of their feet (Table 60-6). Dialog should be encouraged during each follow-up visit to determine the patient's understanding of his or her disease process.

Routine Foot Care

If protective sensation is decreased, callus and nail trimming should be performed by a health professional on a routine basis. Calluses are shaved flush with the skin after the foot is cleansed with soap and water. Removal of a callus from a bony prominence reduces plantar pressure by 29% (107). Hemorrhagic calluses may be hiding an ulcer underneath, and once the callus is shaved, it deroofs the ulcer (Fig. 60-7). Areas of dry skin, cracks, and fissures should be lightly sanded. Toenails should be regularly trimmed and thick, and mycotic toenails are sanded to a smooth surface. The foot should be patted dry after cleaning and a lubricant applied to the skin, except between the toes. Mercurochrome can be lightly painted between the toes if there are any areas of maceration. Silopad digital pads (Silopos) can be used to prevent pressure- and friction-induced lesions along hammer toes and corns. Lamb's wool placed between toes alleviates pressure along soft corns. Instruction is given on mobility exercises and appropriate footwear. It is best for patients with insensitive feet to avoid wearing pressure stockings with open toes (e.g., Anti-Embolism Stockings [T.E.D.] hose) because they

TABLE 60-6. *Foot care instructions*

1. Wash your feet every day with a mild soap and warm water. Check the water temperature with your elbow. Use a soft wash cloth to clean.
2. Dry them with a soft towel by blotting or patting; dry thoroughly between the toes.
3. Inspect daily for redness, blisters, or cuts, change in temperature (hot or cool), and swelling or loss of feeling. If you cannot see to do this yourself, have another member of the family inspect your feet or use a mirror.
4. Clean dirt out from under the toenails; never use a knife or anything sharp. An orange stick or nail file should be used. Cut toe nails straight across. Use sandpaper or a fine emery board to rub down corns and callouses after soaking.
5. Never use corn remedies. Corn pads should be used only on doctor's advice.
6. Do not use inserts or pads without medical advice. Do not wear shoes without socks.
7. Use a lotion on feet and legs daily; do not use between the toes.
8. Never walk barefooted at home or on hot surfaces such as beaches or swimming pools.
9. Protect your feet with warm cotton or woolen socks in cold weather.
10. Inspect shoes daily for cracks in the soles, wrinkles in the lining, and bunching up of construction material. Wear shoes that fit properly with plenty of room for toes.
11. Avoid pointed or open-toed shoes. Sandals or thongs also may cause problems.
12. New shoes should always be broken in slowly. Start by wearing them for 1 hour on the first day, increasing by 1 hour each day. Gradually build up to a full day.
13. Wear leather or canvas shoes that permit moisture to evaporate and absorb perspiration better. Allow time for foot wear to air and dry between wearing.
14. Remove shoes whenever possible. Take frequent rest periods during the day and elevate your feet. Change your shoes every 5 hours.
15. Purchase shoes in the afternoon, when feet are the largest due to swelling.
16. Never use hot water bottles, compresses, heating pads or lamps near your feet.
17. Avoid elastic socks, garters, girdles, and socks that have holes, mends, seams, or edges. Do not tie your stockings.
18. To avoid nerve pressure injury, do not cross legs while sitting.
19. Loosen bed clothing at the bottom of the bed to reduce pressure on the toes.
20. Do not smoke.
21. Have your physician examine your feet at each visit.
22. Be sure that anyone caring for your feet knows that you are a diabetic. This includes the shoe salesman.
23. REMEMBER—THE FEET YOU SAVE ARE YOURS!

Reprinted with permission from the *Dallas Medical Journal* 1994:80; 502, Copyright 1994. Dallas County Medical Society.

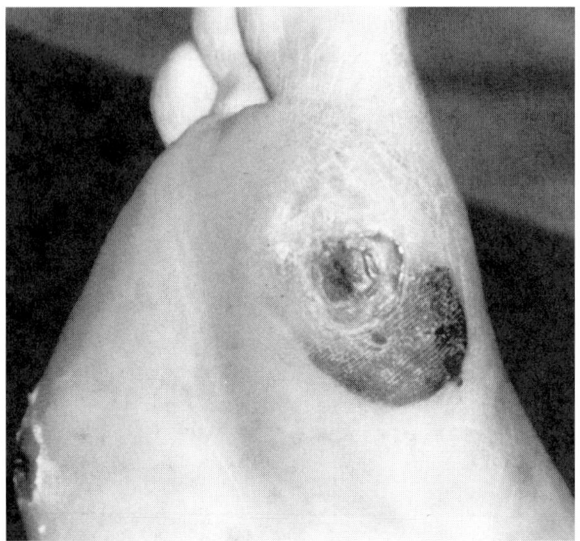

FIG. 60-7. Hemorrhagic callus, revealing a small underlying ulcer after debridement.

run a risk of causing constriction around the toes with resultant pressure ulceration and ischemic changes.

MANAGEMENT

Diabetic patients can be categorized into different risk categories such as those of the Hansen's Disease Center in Carville, Louisiana (108).

Risk Category 0

Patients in this category have a disease process, such as diabetes, that has the potential to cause sensory loss. However, they have not yet lost their protective sensation and have no present risk. These patients should have annual visits to check for loss of protective sensation. Patient education should focus on diabetes control, cessation of smoking, and proper footwear selection. However an overemphasis on proper footwear at this time may cause patients to resist footwear changes later, when the risk may be greater.

Risk Category I

Patients in this category have loss of protective sensation but have not had a plantar ulcer. These patients are followed every 6 months. They must be educated on daily foot inspection, foot care, and gradual break-in of new shoes. Their shoes must be examined for adequate room; shoe shape should be compared with foot shape for appropriate fit. A thin insole may be recommended to help protect the bottom of the feet.

Risk Category II

These patients have loss of protective sensation and may have deformity or limited mobility, which places them at higher risk for tissue breakdown. These patients ideally are followed every 3 months. Most of these patients require prescription footwear (extra-depth shoes) and molded insoles, except for those with minimal foot deformities, who might do well in athletic shoes (e.g., Nike, New Balance). Patients must be given guidelines on appropriate shoe fit. A shoe with correct length will allow ½ to ⅝ inch between the end of the shoe and the longest toe (109). The shoe should allow adequate room across the forefoot with the widest part corresponding to the metatarsal heads and should be snug around the heel. Encourage patients to buy shoes in the latter part of the afternoon when their foot is the largest (due to swelling) and to evaluate the new shoe fit when standing. Patients are taught to perform regular foot mobility exercises (109). Surgical correction of the deformities may be recommended in selected patients to stop callus formation and to ultimately prevent ulceration (110).

Risk Category III

Patients in this category have loss of protective sensation, have a history of prior ulceration, and are at the highest risk for recurrent ulceration. Frequent visits to foot clinics are required (every 1 to 2 months) to ensure that an ulcer is not emerging and the patient is continuing to wear proper footwear at all times. Medicare patients with or at risk for diabetic foot problems are eligible to obtain one pair of extra-depth shoes plus three pairs of inserts per year. The reimbursement is limited to 80% of the approved amount. A patient may substitute modifications of the prescription footwear such as rocker sole instead of obtaining one pair of the molded insoles. A certificate of medical necessity and a statement that the patient is in a comprehensive diabetes treatment program needs to be submitted for reimbursement.

Treatment of Diabetic Foot Ulcers

Despite all the precautions, diabetics may develop foot ulceration. Wagner's classification of foot lesions can be used to provide a rational approach to plan treatment and to help predict the healing potential of an ulcer (111). This classification is based on the depth of penetration of the deeper tissues and extent of the tissue necrosis and is detailed below:

Grade 0: Intact skin (may have bony deformities, limited mobility)
Grade 1: Localized superficial ulcer of the skin
Grade 2: Deep ulcer extending to tendon, bone, ligament, or joint
Grade 3: Deep abscess or osteomyelitis
Grade 4: Gangrene of one or more toes or forefoot
Grade 5: Gangrene of whole foot

When an ulcer is found it is classified according to the above classification. The circumference, depth, and size are recorded. The ulcer is probed looking for fistulas or sinus tracts. Grade 1 to 3 ulcers predominately are neuropathic and grades 4 to 5 mainly vascular. Grade 5 lesions with extensive gangrene require hospitalization and probable amputation. Grade 4 lesions with localized gangrene require urgent vascular consultation for assessment of peripheral circulation. Vascular reconstructive surgery or angioplasty may be needed to prevent amputation. Grade 3 ulcers with underlying osteomyelitis, joint involvement, and a deep abscess will probably require hospital admissions for debridement and intravenous antibiotics. Grade 1 and 2 lesions may or may not be infected. Infection is usually evidenced by purulent drainage, warmth, erythema, and swelling. Fever, chills, and leukocytosis may be absent in two thirds of patients, even with severe infection; however, hyperglycemia is usually present in limb- or life-threatening infections.

Infected ulcers are usually colonized by multiple organisms, but the most commonly isolated organisms are *Staphylococcus aureus* or streptococci (100). Superficial swab cultures are not usually performed because colonization from surface organisms makes them unreliable. When cultures are required, the specimen is obtained from deeper parts of the ulcer after debridement (100). Localized non–limb-threatening infections can be treated with cephalexin, clindamycin, dicloxacillin, or amoxicillin-clavulanate.

If osteomyelitis is suspected, plain radiographs should be ordered. Frank bony destruction or progression of periosteal changes if present indicates the presence of osteomyelitis. However, the presence of periosteal resorption and/or osteolysis on x-ray does not necessarily indicate osteomyelitis. If clinical suspicion remains high, a three-phase technetium bone scan should be ordered. If it is negative, acute or chronic osteomyelitis is essentially excluded. If it is positive, there is lack of consensus as to the next step to differentiate osteomyelitis from diabetic Charcot's arthropathy. Twenty-four hour indium 111–labeled leukocyte scanning is currently recommended as the most accurate radionucleotide study to diagnose osteomyelitis but is too expensive and difficult to interpret in the presence of soft-tissue infection (112). The key is to do both indium and technetium scans at the same time and compare the areas of positive uptake in both studies. If the location and size of the positive area of both scans are the same, it represents osteomyelitis. If the area of uptake in the indium scan is in soft tissue or superficial to the area of uptake of the technetium scan, then osteomyelitis is not present. The role of CT and MRI in diagnosing osteomyelitis accurately is still being debated (113). However, surgeons may use MRI preoperatively to assess the extent of the disease and to decide on the degree of surgical resection required (114).

According to current recommendations, if plain x-rays are negative and bone cannot be detected by advancing a sterile probe in the wound, the patient should be treated with a course of broad-spectrum antibiotics for soft-tissue infection (100). However, x-rays should be repeated every 2 weeks. If the diagnosis of osteomyelitis is confirmed with use of any of the above techniques, surgical debridement, limited amputation, or removal of infected bony prominence is recommended (100). In some patients with less serious infections, a 10- to 12-week course of antibiotics may be tried because this has been shown to cure pedal osteomyelitis without the need for bony debridement in some studies (100,115).

Plantar ulcers with adequate blood supply without evidence of osteomyelitis or acute infection can be managed with total-contact casting (Fig. 60-8) (116,117). If a patient presents with warmth, edema and localized infection, treatment with limb elevation, oral broad spectrum antibiotics, and non–weight-bearing ambulation with assistive aids should be commenced. After about 3 to 5 days, patients can be successfully treated with total-contact casting. Before casting, and in between each cast change, patients undergo hydrotherapy followed by debridement of necrotic tissue and local wound care; the wound is dressed with dry dressings. Generally it is best to apply the cast in the morning, when edema is less. Casting reduces the edema dramatically, causing the cast to loosen and rub, eventually causing the skin to break down. Therefore, the initial cast must be removed in 2 to 7 days, depending on the amount of edema that was present when the cast was applied. If a good fit is maintained, subsequent casts can be changed every 10 to 14 days (116,117). Ulcers best treated with total-contact casting are located on the plantar aspect of the foot and medial and lateral borders of the foot (Table 60-7) (116–118). Slow-healing foot amputation sites also can be effectively treated with total-contact casting.

Problems that may be encountered when using total-contact casting are fungal infection, skin abrasion, low back pain, muscle atrophy, osteoporosis, and joint stiffness (119,120). Use of a topical antifungal cream such as Lotrimin (Schering, Kenilworth, NJ) usually clears the fungal

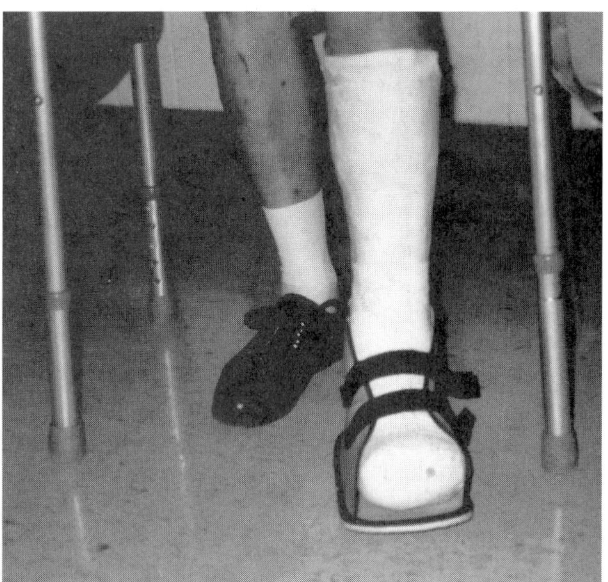

FIG. 60-8. Total-contact cast.

TABLE 60-7. *Advantages of total-contact casting*

1. Distributes weight-bearing stresses
2. Reduces focal areas of excessive pressure
3. Reduces pedal and lower leg edema
4. Protects foot from further trauma
5. Maintains weight-bearing ambulation
6. Helps localize and prevent spread of infection
7. Minimum patient compliance needed

TABLE 60-8. *Contraindications for the use of total-contact cast*

1. Active infection
2. Osteomyelitis
3. Excessively fragile skin
4. Excessive edema that is fluctuating
5. Noncompliance with follow-up visits for cast changes
6. Ischemic ulcer
7. Ulcer that is deeper than it is wide

infection once casting is discontinued. Skin abrasions usually occur along non–weight-bearing surfaces and heal quickly (Table 60-8).

Once the ulcer is healed, total-contact casts should be continued for another 10 to 14 days. This or use of a total-contact sandal (Fig. 60-9) allows time for the fragile newly healed scar to mature. The patient should then make a gradual transition into therapeutic footwear with molded insoles for ambulation at all times. Wearing time of the shoes and ambulation should be initially limited to prevent ulcer recurrence (120). Wearing two pairs of socks also may decrease the shear stress along the newly healed areas and reduce recurrence.

Healing Time and Ulcer Recurrence

Several studies have demonstrated the effectiveness of total-contact casting and reported the average healing time to be 30.6 to 42 days (118). Helm et al. studied 51 patients to observe the healing rate of ulcers after casting. Mean duration of ulcers in this study was 8 to 9 months, with a range of 3 days to 54 months. Average healing time for forefoot ulcers was 30.6 days; nonforefoot ulcers took longer to heal, about 42.1 days.

Studies conducted on ulcer recurrence indicates that reulceration is high within the first 6 months and typically occurs within the first 3 to 4 weeks after initial healing. The overall average recurrence rate is estimated to be 19.2% to 32% (121). Usual causes for ulcer recurrence are failure to comply with use of appropriate footwear, presence of biomechanical faults, osteomyelitis, and Charcot's joint (121).

Alternatives to total-contact walking casts include molded double rocker plantar shoes, scotch cast boots, walking splints, prefabricated total-contact posterior ankle–foot orthoses, and, for small ulcers, total-contact sandals (109). Platelet-derived wound healing factors and hyperbaric oxygen therapy are other forms of treatment of nonhealing ulcers (122). Generally it is best to reserve these options for patients in whom total-contact casting is contraindicated because healing rates are slower with these techniques (100,122).

Wound Care Options

Wound care for foot ulcerations can be conducted on an outpatient basis. Whirlpool treatments with water temperature at 97°F to 98°F for 10 to 15 minutes are used for cleansing and mechanical debridement of the wound. The entire foot and ulcer is scrubbed using Hibiclens (Zeneca, Wilmington, DE) soaked gauze. If there is swelling, the leg is elevated after whirlpool. Necrotic and devitalized tissue is debrided. Use of hydrogen peroxide or Betadine directly on the wound as wound dressing will disrupt the healing process (Table 60-9).

Diabetic Neuropathic Osteoarthropathy: Charcot's Foot

Diabetes is the most common cause of Charcot's arthropathy. The incidence has been reported to be 0.08% to 7.5% (123). Both sexes are equally affected. Bilateral involvement has been reported to be around 5.9% to 39.3%. Affected

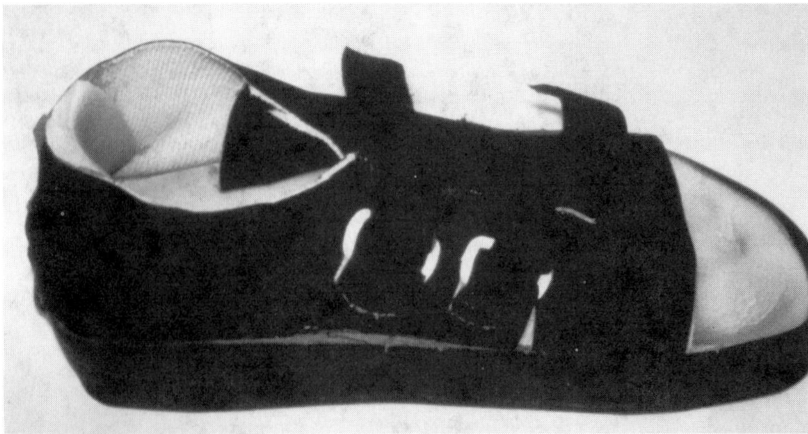

FIG. 60-9. Total-contact sandal.

TABLE 60-9. *Wound care options*

Agent	Indication
Silver nitrate applicators (silver nitrate 75%, potassium nitrate 25%)	Flattens/cauterizes hypergranulation tissue
Silver nitrate solution 0.4%	Protects/stimulates granulation tissue
Normal saline wet to dry	Facilitates debridement of necrotic tissue
Enzymatic debriders (Elase, Fujisawa USA, Deerfield, IL)	Debrides adherent eschar
Ultra-thin duoderm	Moistens dry, avascular wounds
Alginate dressings	Dries wounds with moderate exudate
Sorbsan	
Kaltostat	
Collagen	Stimulates growth of granulation tissue in wounds with mild exudate and good vascular bed
Kollagen sheets/or particles	
Dry coarse mesh patches	Stimulates growth of granulation tissue
Silvadene	Removes dry necrotic debris on wound—use only for a brief period
Iodoform or plain packing gauze	Used for gently packing areas that are undermined or where there is a tract

patients usually have had diabetes for 10 to 15 years and in many cases under poor control.

Charcot's arthropathy can cause a devastating deformity with joint instability, fracture, and dislocation with resultant high-pressure areas along the plantar foot, resulting in ulceration. The key to management is making an early accurate diagnosis. The classic presentation is a foot that is swollen, erythematous, and warm, with good pedal pulses (Fig. 60-10) (104). A history of antecedent minor trauma may or may not be present, and the patient may experience vague, poorly localized pain. Frequently these individuals are hospitalized with a presumed diagnosis of cellulitis or thrombophlebitis, and x-rays may not be ordered. Radiographs may be initially normal or show a stress fracture, dislocation, or bony fragmentation. Frequently the radiographic changes are interpreted to be degenerative changes or osteomyelitis. There is a clinical trick one can use to distinguish between erythema of cellulitis and dependent rubor of Charcot's joint. The dependent rubor of Charcot's arthropathy will recede after 5 minutes of elevation of the affected foot to above the heart level when the patient is supine, whereas the erythema of cellulitis will not (124). This is helpful when there are no discernable changes in the x-ray. If the problem is misdiagnosed and the patient is allowed to continue ambulation, bone destruction and deformity worsen and can become irreversible. In some patients, the neuroarthropathy may be caused by ligamentous lesions, causing spontaneous dislocation. The practitioner needs to have a high index of suspicion of a Charcot's foot when a diabetic patient presents with an increase in skin temperature of the foot of greater than 2°C without any open wounds or lymphangitis (104).

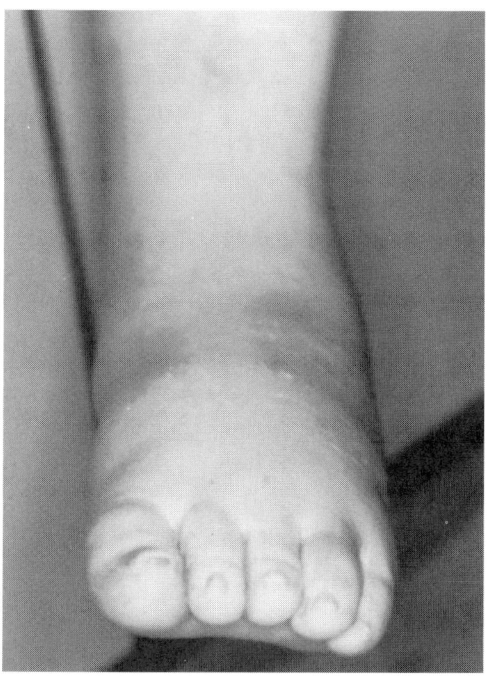

FIG. 60-10. Initial presentation of charcot arthropathy: warm, swollen, erythematous foot without any open areas.

Eichenholliz has divided the disease process into three radiographically distinct stages (123–125):

I. Stage of development: acute destructive period characterized by joint effusion, soft-tissue edema, subluxation, fragmentation of bone, intra-articular fractures, and formation of bone and cartilage debris (Fig. 60-11).
II. Stage of coalescence: period of healing with decreasing edema, absorption of debris, and healing of fractures (Fig. 60-12).
III. Stage of reconstruction: further repair and remodeling of bone with increased bone density and sclerosis with improved joint stability (Fig. 60-13).

CONSERVATIVE MANAGEMENT

Any patient with either confirmed or suspected Charcot's arthropathy should have the affected foot immediately immobilized and weight bearing eliminated. This can be done

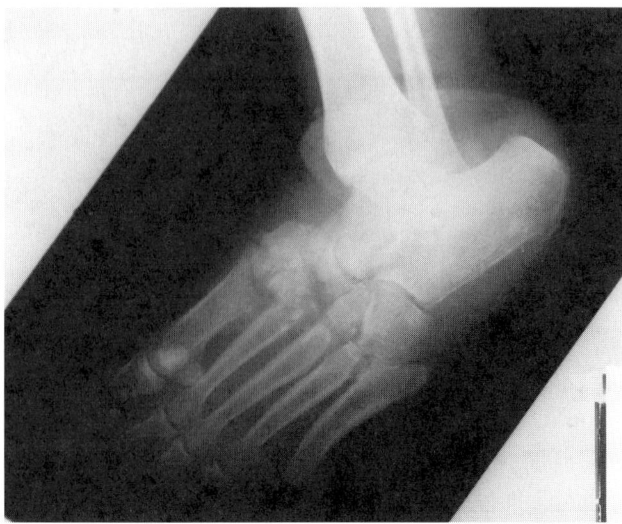

FIG. 60-11. Stage I Charcot arthropathy with x-ray evidence of fragmentation of first metatarsal and cuneiforms. Previous amputation of lateral three toes.

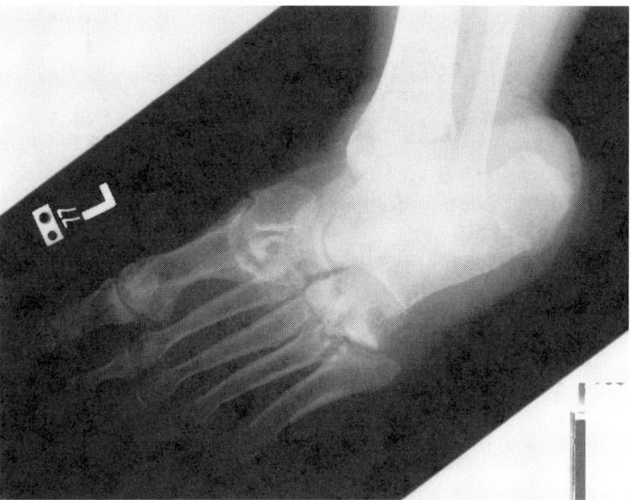

FIG. 60-13. Stage III Charcot arthopathy with increased bone density and sclerosis.

with total-contact casting and non–weight bearing with assistive aids. However, this may place the contralateral limb at increased risk for fracture–dislocation, which may become evident after about 4.5 months (123). For this reason, temporary use of a wheelchair may be indicated in some patients (104). A majority of Charcot's joints can and should be treated primarily by nonsurgical means. Surgical reconstruction even when correctly indicated does not speed the healing process and may even temporarily delay healing (124).

Casting and non–weight bearing are continued until all clinical signs of inflammation resolve. Erythema and swelling are the first to resolve. Warmth will be the last to resolve. Banks has advocated weight bearing in the cast only after the temperature of the two extremities becomes symmetrical (104). This total process may take 3 to 6 months. Sanders and Frykberg have recommended non–weight-bearing cast immobilization for 3 months (123).

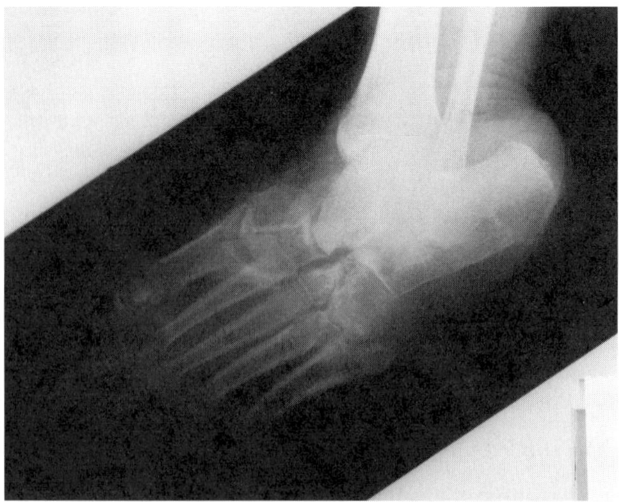

FIG. 60-12. Stage II Charcot arthropathy with x-ray evidence of healing fractures and sclerosis.

Various methods have been used to judge the onset of stage II. These include water displacement measurements of foot volume, measuring temperature with an infrared thermometer, or simply examining for decrease in swelling and warmth. The exact timing of advancement to the second stage of treatment is not that critical. Brodsky recommends progression to the second stage of treatment when there is reduction of acute erythema and warmth and a substantial reduction in the daily fluctuation of swelling (124). Because the bones may become osteoporotic from prolonged non–weight bearing, the immediate return to weight bearing without external support may cause further fracture and dislocation. For this reason, a bivalve ankle–foot orthosis is used (Fig. 60-14) (123). The patient is not allowed to bear weight without the orthosis for another few months.

When radiographic evidence of increased bone density and sclerosis along with stabilization of involved joints are seen, the patient can be graduated into a posterior shell ankle–foot orthosis and prescription footwear (104,123,125). A patellar tendon–bearing orthosis with prescription footwear also may be used (123). A few patients may need an exostosectomy of the bony prominence, which may have developed along the plantar aspect of foot, despite the appropriate conservative management (104,124). This is performed to prevent problems with chronic ulceration.

DIABETIC NEUROPATHIC PAIN

Approximately 10% of diabetics develop problems with painful neuropathy. This may occur early in the course of the disease and may be correlated with the institution of antidiabetic medications. It is often associated with precipi-

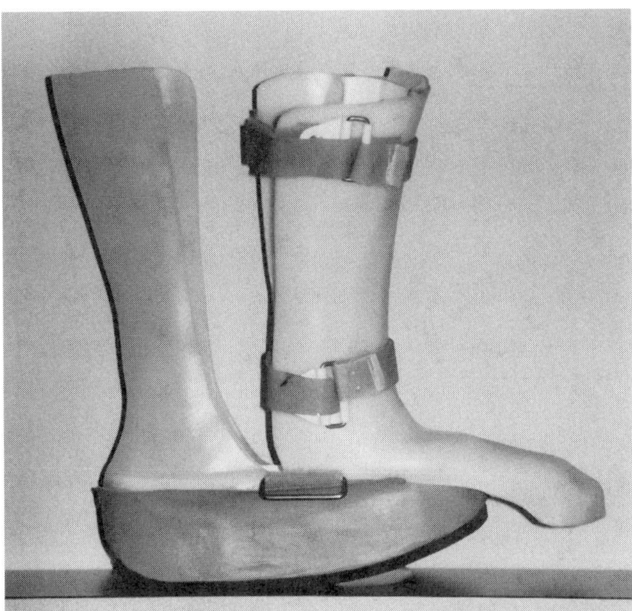

FIG. 60-14. Bivalve ankle foot orthosis.

tous weight loss. Generally two types of pain are seen (108,126):

1. The pain may occur in the form of significant superficial hyperesthesia with a burning laminating, dysesthetic component (epicritic type). Often the pain is worse at night and produces insomnia. Usually the neuropathy is limited to small myelinated fibers. Therefore, objective signs may be minimal or absent on clinical as well as electrodiagnostic examination. Spontaneous resolution of the pain can occur in several months. Reassurance may help the patient better cope with the pain.
2. The second type of pain may appear a few years after the diagnosis of diabetes. The pain is described as being a deep, gnawing, toothache type of pain (protopathic) with feelings of cold feet (108). Objectively the patient may show evidence of abnormal sensation, mild motor weakness, and autonomic dysfunction.

Treatment

Every effort should be made to optimize glycemic control. Simple measures such as a warm bath, soaking feet in cold water for a short period of time, or a transcutaneous electrical nerve stimulation unit may be tried. When patients have epicritic pain, use of a topical preparation such as capsaicin 0.075% cream applied to the painful area three to four times daily may be helpful.

Analgesics

Both types of pain may respond to simple analgesics such as Motrin (McNeil Consumer, Fort Washington, PA) 600 mg four times daily or sulindac 200 mg twice daily (108,126).

Tricyclics

Several studies have demonstrated significant benefits of tricyclic antidepressants, especially amitriptyline. Amitriptyline is started at a low dose of 10 to 25 mg at night and increased gradually until pain control is achieved or limiting side effects occurs. Pain relief may take days to several weeks and may require doses as high as 150 mg/day. Amitriptyline is contraindicated in patients with heart block, orthostatic hypotension, and urinary tract obstruction. Nortriptyline may be tried in patients who have problems with orthostatic hypotension. When tricyclics alone are not helpful, combinations of fluphenazine 1 to 6 mg/day or clonazepam 0.5 to 3.0 mg/day with tricyclics such as nortriptyline may be tried. Clonazepam is useful in patients who are experiencing lancinating or shooting pains (126).

Anticonvulsants

Anticonvulsants such as carbamazepine 400 to 1,200 mg/day in divided doses with an initial dose of 100 mg twice daily or phenytoin also may be tried. Although they have been shown to be effective in uncontrolled studies, they have not been proven to be effective in controlled clinical trials. In addition, because of the potential toxicity of anticonvulsants, use is limited to those who failed tricyclic therapy.

Clonidine

The beneficial effect of clonidine in patients with causalgia has prompted its use in the treatment of diabetic neuropathy. The clinician should start the patient with small doses of 75 to 100 μg at night to avoid hypotension and sleepiness and then gradually increase the dose as needed (126).

Mexiletine

An oral antidysrhythmic drug structurally similar to lidocaine has been shown to be effective in relieving both lancinating and chronic dysesthesic pain in diabetics. The recommended dosage is 10 mg/kg daily (108,126). The dosage is gradually increased over the first week to minimize gasterointestional side effects and dizziness. This drug is contraindicated in patients with pre-existing atrioventricular heart block.

There have been small short-term trials with aldose reductase inhibitors and myoinositol supplementation with conflicting results in treatment of polyneuropathy.

CUTANEOUS MANIFESTATIONS OF THE EXTREMITIES

The increased susceptibility of diabetic skin to injuries from unrecognized trauma and altered microvasculature in the dermis and subcutaneous tissue warrants a review of skin problems. Only the most common disorders are discussed.

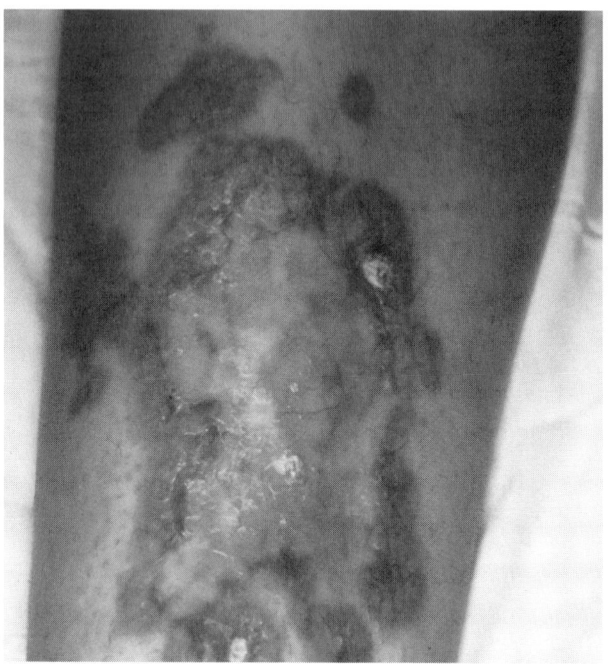

FIG. 60-15. Necrobiosis lipidica diabeticorum with typical yellowish atrophic telangiectatic center with raised peripheral borders.

Necrobiosis Lipidica Diabeticorum

Necrobiosis lipidica diabeticorum (NBLD) occurs in 0.3% of diabetics. Lesions can be solitary or multiple and are three times more common in women. These lesions frequently occur on the anterior aspect of the lower leg (along the tibial crest) and ankles but also can affect the thighs, arms, hands, abdomen, and back. Lesions appear initially as circumscribed, erythematous papules. Evolving lesions demonstrate atrophic telangiectatic centers, with a hard depressed yellow-brown surface with erythematous raised peripheral borders (Fig. 60-15). The pathophysiology of NBLD is not well understood. Intralesional injections of corticosteroids or topical applications of steroids seem to help. Patients with these lesions should be cautioned about dangers of trauma and ulcerations (127–129).

Diabetic Dermopathy (Shin Spots)

These occur on thin skinned areas such as the crest of the tibia and in nondiabetics as well as diabetics (Fig. 60-16). Lesions are 5 to 12 mm in diameter, atrophic, red-brown, sharply circumscribed, and often arranged in a linear fashion. These are asymptomatic, and no treatment is required.

Lipodystrophy

These are atrophic plaques that occur at the sites of insulin injections due to loss of adipose tissue. Treatment is to shift insulin injection sites.

Diabetic Hand Syndrome/Thick Skin

This occurs in 30% of insulin-dependent diabetics and presents as thick, waxy skin over the dorsal aspect of the hands and proximal interphalangeal joints, limiting joint mobility. Patients are usually unable to flatten their hands against a flat surface (127,128). Other joints such as wrists, elbows, ankles, and feet can be affected. Abnormalities in collagen metabolism may be the cause. Patients may require physical and/or occupational therapy to help them regain or maintain functional capabilities.

Diabetic Bullae

These occur in patients with insulin-dependent and non–insulin-dependent diabetes. Most patients have neuropathy and long-standing diabetes. Bullae are characterized as rapid in onset, 0.5 to 3 cm in size, occurring most commonly along plantar surface of the toes and soles, and the lateral aspect of the feet, heels, legs, and fingers. The blisters are not usually painful and heal within 2 to 6 weeks. Unrecognized trauma may be the cause. Treatment is usually reassurance, advice on appropriate shoes, and wearing gloves while working (127–129).

Nail Problems

Onychomycosis of the toenails is common in diabetics. The etiology is not clear. Diabetic neuropathy may make the toenails susceptible to nail trauma, with subsequent subungual hemorrhage, increasing the chance for fungal infections (127). The nail usually becomes multilayered and disorganized and may separate from the nail bed distally. Any nail can be affected, but the hallux is the most common. As the nail thickens, trauma from the shoe increases, with resultant

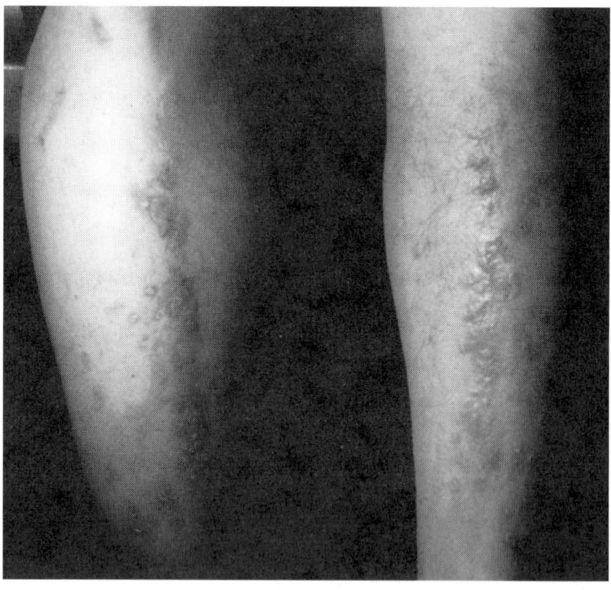

FIG. 60-16. Shin shots along the crest of the tibia.

TABLE 60-10. *Topical antifungals for onychomycosis*

1. Amorolfine (MT-861) nail lacquer 2% or 5%. Apply twice weekly to affected nail.
2. Naftifine Hydrochloride (Naftin, Allergan, Irvine, CA) 1% gel. Apply twice daily to affected nail.
3. Ciclopiroxolamine (Loprox, Hoechst Marion Roussel, Kansas City, MO) 1% cream. Apply two to three times daily to affected nail.
4. Fungoid tincture (triacetin, sodium propionate, benzalkonium chloride, chloroxylenol). Apply twice daily to affected nail.
5. Bifonazole 1% with urea (Mycosporonychoset, Bayer, Germany). Apply twice daily to affected nail and with occlusion at night.
6. Ketoconazole cream 2% (Nizoral, Janssen, Titusville, NJ). Apply daily to affected nail.
7. Terbinafine cream 1% (Lamisil, Novartis, East Hanover, NJ). Apply to nail plate daily.

From Topical treatment of onychomycosis. *Clin Podiatr Med Surg* 1995;12:249–53.

subungual hematoma and secondary bacterial infections. Periodic nail care on a routine basis can prevent these from becoming a major problem. Mycotic nails should be cut and sanded down as thin as possible to prevent injury and secondary infections. Many topical medications are available that may help improve or in some cases eradicate the fungal infection. Oral antifungals such as griseofulvin may be tried in patients without liver disease. Treatment should be continued for 6 to 12 months. The value of using Griseofulvin should be weighed against the risk of hepatitis. Newer agents such as oral itraconazole and oral terbinafine are able to increase cure rates, while shortening treatment duration to as brief as 12 weeks (Table 60-10).

Plantar Xerosis (Dry Skin)

Xerosis is common in diabetics due to the anhydrosis caused by diabetic autonomic neuropathy. When xerosis is present for a long time, fissures may occur, leading to ulceration. If these occur, silver nitrate is used to cauterize the base, followed by application of a mixture of a 20% urea cream as a keratolytic agent and hydrocortisone applied at night under an occlusive dressing. Once fissuring is resolved, use of emollient creams prophylactically after bathing, applied once or twice a day, will control the xerosis.

DIABETIC FOOTWEAR

Properly fitting footwear plays a key role in preventing injuries to insensate feet. Thus physicians who plan to manage diabetic feet should familiarize themselves with the basics of shoe prescriptions, design, and fitting. In-depth or extra-depth shoes are often prescribed. These provide the extra volume needed to accommodate common foot deformities seen in diabetics and the custom-molded insoles. The custom-molded insoles distribute plantar pressure over an enlarged contact area, thus reducing the abnormal peak pressures that may have been present along the plantar surface of the foot. Extra-depth shoes are usually blucher style, light weight, with shock-absorbing soles and strong counters (Figs. 60-17 and 60-18). San Antonio Shoes Free-time style for women and Time-out for men are good shoes for patients with mild to moderate toe and foot deformities. Shoes can be modified in a variety of ways for various clinical conditions (Table 60-11) (130).

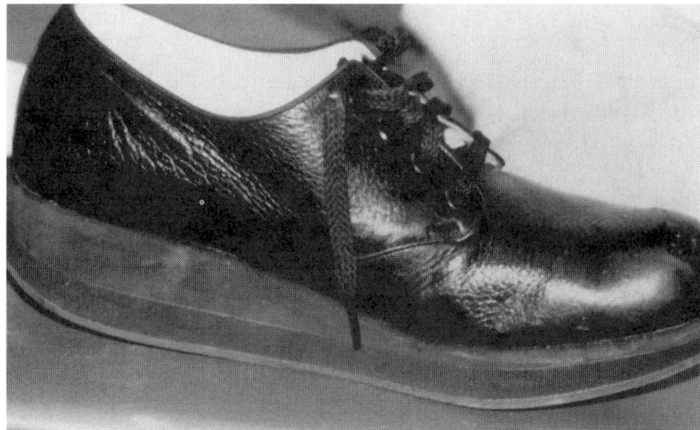

FIG. 60-17. Shoe with mild rocker sole.

SUMMARY

The current literature emphasizes the importance of (a) team approach, (b) patient education, and (c) prevention in the management of diabetic foot patients. More and more multidisciplinary foot clinics are developing to identify at-risk patients, provide appropriate education about foot care, and offer comprehensive management when problems occur. As physical medicine and rehabilitation physicians, we are uniquely positioned to treat these patients because we are already providing rehabilitation for diabetic-related problems. An organized approach for providing foot care already has been shown to be effective in lowering amputation rates. Runyan reported a 68% reduction in hospital days and amputation over a 2-year period by using a coordinated multidisciplinary approach (131). The goal of the American Diabetic Association (ADA), Centers for Disease Control (CDC), Na-

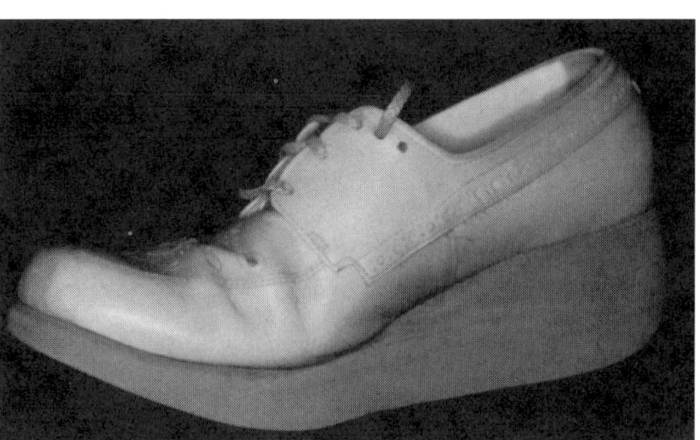

FIG. 60-18. Shoe with rocker sole.

TABLE 60-11. *Shoe modifications*

Modifications	Indication	Goal
Mild rocker sole (Fig. 60-17) (seen in athletic shoes)	Forefoot ulcers, callouses	Relieves pressure on metatarsal (MT) heads
Heel to toe rocker sole (rocker at heel and toe)	Rigid claw toes, hammer toes, calcaneal ulcer	Aids in toe off, decreases heel strike forces
Toe only rocker sole	Hallux rigidus, metatarsal and distal toe ulcers	Reduces forefoot stresses on toe off
Rocker sole (Fig. 60-18)	Metatarsal head ulcers	Reduces weight-bearing stresses anterior to MT head
Negative heel rocker sole (seen in healing shoes)	Fixed dorsiflexion at ankle, prominent MT head and distal tip callus and ulcers	Relieves forefoot pressure shifts weight to mid- and hindfoot
Double rocker sole (mild rocker with a section of sole removed in mid-foot area)	Rocker bottom feet (Charcot foot deformity)	Relieves pressure from mid-foot
Medial heel flare	Fixed valgus heel	Reduces eversion
Stabilizer (medial or lateral; always add to a broken-in shoe)	Medially or laterally collapsed Charcot foot	Provides extensive stabilization
Extended steel shank (combined usually with rocker sole)	Hallux rigidus, decreased ankle motion, proximal foot amputation	Aids in toe off, limits toe and mid-foot movement
Cushion heel	Calcaneal ulcer, rigid ankle and hindfoot	Maximum shock absorption
Medial wedge	Excessive pronation	Decreases pressure along medial aspect of foot
Lateral wedge	Ankle instability, varus heel deformity	Decreases pressure along lateral aspect of foot
Customized upper	Localized foot deformity	For accommodation of deformity, less expensive than custom shoes
Custom shoes	Foot deformity	
Extended steel shank Rocker sole, molded insole with filler	Major, toe, ray or distal transmetatarsal amputations	Aids toe off

Data from Dockery GL, Crawford ME. *Cutaneous disorders of the lower extremity.* Philadelphia: WB Saunders, 1997;176–200.

tional Diabetes Advisory Board, and state health departments is to decrease the amputation rate by 20% by 1996 and 50% by the year 2000. We can help reach this goal by providing comprehensive care for diabetic foot patients using the guidelines outlined in this chapter.

REFERENCES

1. Shepherd JT. Historical aspects. In: Clement DL, Shepherd JT, eds. *Vascular diseases in the limb.* St. Louis: Mosby Year Book, 1993; 1–10.
2. Shepherd JT. *Physiology of circulation in human limbs in health and disease.* Philadelphia: WB Saunders, 1963.
3. Von Euler US. *Noradrenaline: chemistry, physiology, pharmacology, and clinical aspects.* Springfield, IL: Charles C Thomas, 1956.
4. Berne RM, Levy MN, eds. *Physiology.* St. Louis: CV Mosby, 1988.
5. Lagercrantz H. Composition and function of large dense corded vesicles in sympathetic nerves. *Neuroscience* 1976; 1:81–92.
6. Shepherd JT, Vanhoutte PM. Local modulation of adrenergic neurotransmission in blood vessels. *J Cardiovasc Pharmacol* 1985; 7(suppl 3):167–178.
7. Furchgott RF, Vanhocitte PM. Endothelium-derived relaxing and contracting factors. *FASEB J* 1989; 3:2007–2019.
8. Clement DL, Verhaeghe R. Atherosclerosis and other occlusive arterial diseases. In: Clement DL, Shepherd JT, eds. *Vascular diseases in the limb.* St. Louis: Mosby Year Book, 1993; 71–89.
9. Widmer LK, Greensher A, Kannel WB. Occlusion of peripheral arteries: a study of 6,400 working subjects. *Circulation* 1964; 30:836–842.
10. Dormandy J, Mahir M, Ascady G. Fate of the patient with chronic leg ischemia. *J Cardiovasc Surg* 1989; 30:50–57.
11. Crigui MH, Fronek A, Garrett-Connor E. The prevalence of peripheral arterial disease in a defined population. *Circulation* 1985; 71: 510–515.
12. Rosenbloom MS, Flanigan DP, Schuler JJ. Risk factors affecting the natural history of intermittent claudication. *Arch Surg* 1988; 123: 867–870.
13. Juergens JL, Barker NW, Hines EA Jr. Arteriosclerosis obliterans: review of 520 cases with special reference to pathogenic and prognostic factors. *Circulation* 1960; 21:188–195.
14. Wilson SE, Schwartz I, Williams RA, Owens ML. Occlusion of the superficial femoral artery. What happens without operation. *Am J Surg* 1980; 140:112–116.
15. Ginsberg HN. Lipoprotein physiology in its relationship to atherogenesis, *Endocrinol Metab Clin North Am* 1990; 19:211–218.
16. Pownall HJ, Gotto Am Jr. Lipid metabolism and the plasma lipoproteins. In: Fozzard HA, Jennings RB Haber E, eds. *The heart and cardiovascular system.* New York: Raven, 1992.
17. Kovanen PT. Atheroma formation: defective control in the intimal round-trip of cholesterol. *Eur Heart J* 1990; 11(suppl E):238–246.
18. Juergens JL, Bernaatz PE. Atherosclerosis of the extremities. In: Juergens JL, Spittell JA Jr, Fairbairm II, eds. *Peripheral vascular diseases,* 5th ed. Philadelphia: WB Saunders, 1980; 253–273.
19. Hughson WG, Mann JI, Garrod A. Intermittent claudication: prevalence risk factors. *Br Med J* 1978; 1:1379–1381.
20. Strong JP, Richards ML. Cigarette smoking and atherosclerosis in autopsied men. *Atherosclerosis* 1973; 23:451–476.
21. Fowkes FGR. Epidemiology of atherosclerotic arterial disease in the lower limbs. *Eur J Vasc Surg* 1988; 18:614–618.
22. Fuchs JA. Medical management of atherosclerosis. In: Rutherford RB, ed. *Vascular surgery.* 2nd ed. Philadelphia: WB Saunders, 1984; 313–327.
23. Gruggenheim W, Koch G, Adams AP. Femoral and popliteal occlusive vascular disease. A report on 143 diabetic patients. *Diabetes* 1969; 18:428–433.

24. Ledet J, Heikendorff L, Rasmussen LM. Pathology of macrovascular disease. *Baillieres Clin Endocrinol Metab* 1988; 2:391–405.
25. Colwell JA, Lopes-Virella MF. A review of the development of large vessel disease in diabetes mellitus. *Am J Med* 1988; 85(suppl 5A): 113–118.
26. Shepherd JT. Evaluation of treatment in intermittent claudication. *Br Med J* 1950; 2:1413–1425.
27. Juergens JL, Spittell JA Jr, Fairbairn JF II. *Peripheral vascular disease*, 5th ed. Philadelphia: WB Saunders, 1980.
28. Strandness DE. Diagnostic considerations in occlusive arterial disease. *Vasc Surg* 1977; 11:271–277.
29. Moneta GL, Strandness DE Jr. Peripheral arterial duplex scanning. *J Clin Ultrasound* 1987; 15:645–651.
30. Kohler TR, Nicholls SC, Zierler RE. Assessment of pressure gradient by Doppler ultrasound: experimental and clinical observations. *J Vasc Surg* 1987; 6:460–469.
31. Clement DL, Van Maele GO, De Pue NY. Critical evaluation of venous occlusion plethysmography in the diagnosis of occlusive arterial diseases in the lower limbs. *Int Angiol* 1985; 4:69–74.
32. Spence VA, Walker WF. Tissue oxygen tension in normal and ischemic human skin. *Cardiovasc Res* 1984; 18:140–144.
33. Rooke TW, Osmundson PJ. The influence of age, sex, smoking, and diabetes on lower limb transcutaneous oxygen tension in patients with arterial occlusive disease. *Arch Intern Med* 1990; 150:129–132.
34. Rutherford RB, Preston Flanigan D, Gupta SK. Suggested standards of reports dealing with lower extremity ischemia. *J Vasc Surg* 1986; 4:80–94.
35. Second European consensus document on chronic critical leg ischemia. *Circulation* 1991; 84(suppl):4.
36. Lippmann HI. Medical management of trophic ulcers in chronic arterial occlusive disease. *Angiology* 1979; 29:683–690.
37. Hennekens CH, Buring JE, Sandercock P. Aspirin and other antiplatelet agents in the secondary and primary prevention of cardiovascular disease, *Circulation* 1989; 80:749–756.
38. Oian S, Iwai T. Effects of ticlopidine on the cutaneous circulation in peripheral vascular disease, *Angiology* 1993; 44:627–631.
39. Porter JM, Cutter BS, Lee BY et al. Pentoxifylline efficacy in the treatment of intermittent claudication: multi center controlled double blind trial with objective assessment of chronic occlusive arterial disease patients. *Am Heart J* 1982; 104:66–72.
40. Coffman JD. Vasodilator drugs in peripheral vascular disease. *N Engl J Med* 1979; 300:713.
41. Nizankowski R, Krolikowski W, Beilatowicz J, Szezeklik A. Prostocyclin for ischemic ulcers in peripheral arterial disease: a random-assignment, placebo controlled study. *Thromb Res* 1985; 37:21–28.
42. Belch JJF, Mckay A, Mcardle B, et al. Epoprostenol (Prostacyclin) and severe arterial disease: a double-blind trial. *Lancet* 1983; 1: 315–317.
43. Norgen L, Alwmark A, Angqvist KA, et al. A stable prostacyclin (iloprost) in the treatment of ischemic ulcers of the lower limb: a Scandinavian-Polish placebo-controlled, randomized multi center study, *Eur J Vasc Surg* 1990; 4:463–467.
44. Creasy TS, Mcmillan PJ, Fletcher EW, et al. Is percutaneous transluminal angioplasty better than exercise for claudication? Preliminary results from a prospective randomized trial. *Eur J Vasc Surg* 1990; 4:135.
45. Tyrrell M, Wolfe J. Vein collars make femorocrural PTFE grafts worth while. In: Greenhalg RM, Hollier LH, eds. *The maintenance of arterial reconstruction*. London: WB Saunders, 1990.
46. Rutherford RB, Jones DN, Bergentz SE, et al. Factors affecting the patency of infrainguinal bypass. *J Vasc Surg* 1988; 8:236–246.
47. Ernst CB, Stanley JC, ed. *Therapy in vascular surgery*. 2nd ed. Philadelphia: BC Decker, 1991.
48. Gibbons GW, Maraccio EJ Jr, Burgess AM, et al. Improved quality of diabetic foot care, 1984 vs 1990. *Arch Surg* 1993; 128:576.
49. Pomposelli FB Jr, Jepsen SJ, Gibbons GW, et al. Efficacy of the dorsal pedal bypass for limb salvage in diabetic patients: short-term observations. *J Vasc Surg* 1990; 11:745.
50. Ekroth R, Dahllof AG, Gundevall B, et al. Physical training of patients with intermittent claudication: indications, methods and results. *Surgery* 1978; 84:640.
51. Jonason T, Jonzon B, Ringqvist I, et al. Effects of physical training on different categories of patients with intermittent claudication. *Acta Med Scand* 1979; 206:253.
52. Zetterquist S. The effects of active training on the nutritive blood flow in exercising ischemic legs. *Scand J Clin Lab Invest* 1970; 25: 101–111.
53. Abramson DI. Physiologic basis for the use of physical agents in peripheral vascular disorders. *Arch Phys Med Rehabil* 1965; 46:216.
54. Sorlie D, Myhre K. Lower leg blood flow in intermittent claudication. *Scand J Clin Lab Invest* 1978; 38:171–179.
55. Sorlie D, Myhre K, Mjos OD. Exercise and post-exercise metabolism of the lower leg in patients with peripheral arterial insufficiency. *Scand J Clin Lab Invest* 1978; 38:635–642.
56. Cornenwett JL, Warner KG, Zelenock GB, et al. Intermittent claudication. Current results of nonoperative management. *Arch Surg* 1984; 119:430–436.
57. Honet JC, Strandness DE Jr, Stolov WC, et al. Short-leg bracing for intermittent claudication of the calf. *Arch Phys Med Rehabil* 1968; 49:578.
58. Friedmann LW. Selecting the therapeutic alternative for rehabilitating patients with occlusive arterial disease. *Vasc Surg* 1977; 11:321–332.
59. Raynaud M. *De l'asphyxie locale et de la gangrene symetrique des extremities*. Paris: Leclere, 1862.
60. Raynaud AGM. *New researches on the nature and treatment of local asphyxia of the extremities*. London: New Sydenham Society, 1888.
61. Lewis T. Experiments relating to the peripheral mechanisms involved in spasmodic arrest of the circulation to the fingers, a variety of Raynaud's disease. *Heart* 1929; 15:7–102.
62. Cohen RA, Coffman JD. Digital vasospasm: the pathophysiology of Raynaud's phenomenon. *Int Angiol* 1984; 3:47–55.
63. Allen EV, Brown GE. Raynaud's disease: a critical review of minimal requisites for diagnosis. *Am J Med Sci* 1932; 183:187–200.
64. Coffman JD. The enigma of Raynaud's disease. *Circulation* 1989; 80:1089–1090.
65. Coffman JD. *Raynaud's phenomenon*. New York: Oxford University Press, 1989.
66. Shepherd JT. *Physiology of circulation in human limbs in health and disease*. Philadelphia: WB Saunders, 1963.
67. Roath S. Management of Raynaud's phenomenon: focus on newer treatments. *Drugs* 1989; 37:700–712.
68. Wollersheim H, Thien T, Fennis J, et al. Double blind placebo-controlled study of prazosin in Raynaud's phenomenon. *Clin Pharmacol Ther* 1986; 40:219–225.
69. Barcroft H, Hamilton GTC. Further observations on the results of sympathectomy in the upper limb. *Lancet* 1948; 2:770–771.
70. Barcroft H, Walker AJ. Return of tone to blood vessels of the upper limb after sympathectomy. *Lancet* 1949; 1:1036–1039.
71. Schirger A, Harrison EG Jr, Jones JM. Idiopathic lymphedema: review of 131 cases. *JAMA* 1962; 182:14–22.
72. Cooke JP, Rooke TW. Lymphatic disorders. In: Loscalzo J, Creager MA, Dzau VJ, eds. *Vascular medicine*, 1st ed. Boston: Little, Brown and Company, 1994;1105–1107.
73. Wolfe JHN. The prognosis and possible cause of severe primary lymphoedema. *Ann R Coll Surg Engl* 1984; 66:251–257.
74. Pflug JJ, Schirger A. Chronic peripheral lymphedema. In: Clement DL, Shepherd JT, eds. *Vascular diseases in the limbs*. St. Louis: Mosby Year Book, 1993.
75. Stillwell GK, Redford JWB. Physical treatment of postmastectomy lymphedema. *Proc Staff Meet Mayo Clin* 1958; 33:1.
76. Casley-Smith JR, Morgan RG, Piller NB. Treatment of lymphedema of the arms and legs with 5,6-benza-[ac]-Pyrone. *N Engl J Med* 1993; 329:1158.
77. Ernst CV, Stanley JC, eds. *Therapy in vascular surgery*, 2nd ed. Philadelphia: BC Decker, 1991.
78. Watson J. Chronic lymphedema of the extremities and its management. *Br J Surg* 1953; 41:31–39.
79. Sumner DS. Applied physiology in venous problems. In: Bergan JJ, Yao JST, eds. *Surgery of the veins*. New York: Harcourt Brace Jovanovich, 1985; 3–23.
80. O'Donnell TF, Welch HJ. Chronic venous insufficiency and varicose veins. In: Young JR, Olin JW, Bartholomew JR, eds. *Peripheral vascular disease,* 2nd ed. St. Louis: CV Mosby, 1996;491–521.
81. Reporting standards in venous disease-venous subcommittee. Prepared by the Subcommittee on Reporting Standards in Venous Disease, Ad Hoc Committee on Reporting Standards, Society for Vascular Surgery/North American Chapter, International Society for Cardiovascular Surgery. *J Vasc Surg* 1988; 8:182–183.

82. McCullouch JM, Marler KC, Neal MB, Phifer TJ. Intermittent pneumatic compression improves venous ulcer healing. *Adv Wound Care* 1994; 7:22–24, 26.
83. Dockery GL, Crawford ME. Peripheral vascular disease and related disorders. In: *Cutaneous disorders of the lower extremity*. Philadelphia: WB Saunders, 1997; 102–131.
84. Nararro F, Bartholomew JR, Young JR, Olin JW. In: *Deep vein thrombosis in peripheral vascular diseases,* 2nd ed. St. Louis: CV Mosby, 1996; 451–467.
85. Merli G, Martinez J. Prophylaxis for deep vein thrombosis and pulmonary embolism in the surgical patient. *Med Clin North Am* 1987; 71: 377–397.
86. Agnelli G. Anticoagulation in the prevention and therapy of pulmonary embolism. *Chest* 1995; 107(suppl):1.
87. Warlow C, Ogsten D, Douglas A. Venous thrombosis following strokes. *Lancet* 1972; 1:1305.
88. Merli G, Herbison G, Ditunno J, et al. Deep vein thrombosis: prophylaxis in acute spinal cord injured patients. *Arch Phys Med Rehabil* 1988; 69:661–664.
89. Hyers TM, Hull RD, Weg JG. Antethrombotic therapy for venous thromboembolic disease. *Chest* 1995; 108(suppl):335.
90. Williams DRR. The size of the problem epidemiological and economic aspects of foot problems in diabetes. In: Boulton AJM, Connor H, Cavangh PR, eds. *The foot in diabetes,* 2nd ed. New York: Wiley 1994; 15–24.
91. Levin ME. Pathogenesis and management of diabetic foot lesions. In: Levin ME, O Neal LW, Bowker JH, eds. *The diabetic foot*. St. Louis: CV Mosby 1993; 17–60.
92. Grunfeld C. Diabetic foot ulcers: etiology, treatment and prevention. *Adv Intern Med* 1991; 37:103–124.
93. Pecoraro RE, Reiber GE, Burgers EM. Pathways to diabetic limb amputation: basis for prevention. *Diabetes Care* 1990; 13:513–521.
94. Vinik AI, Holland MT, LeBeau JM, Luzzi JF, Stanberry KB, Colen LB. Diabetic neuropathies. *Diabetes Care* 1992; 15:1927–1975.
95. Boulton AJM. The pathway to ulceration: etiopathogenesis. In: Boulton AJM, Connor H, Cavangh PR, eds. *The foot in diabetes*. New York: Wiley, 1994; 37–48.
96. Lithner I, Tomblom N. Gangrene localized to the feet in diabetic patients. *Acta Med Scand* 1984; 215:75–79.
97. Frykberg RG. Diabetic foot ulcerations. In: Frykberg RG, ed. *The high risk foot in diabetes mellitus*. New York: Churchill-Livingstone, 1991; 151–195.
98. Brand PW. The insensitive foot. In: Jahss MH, ed. *Disorders of the foot*, 2nd ed. Vol. 3. Philadelphia: WB Saunders, 1991.
99. Brand PW. Pressure sores: the problem. In: Kenedi RM, Cowden JM, Scales JT, eds. *Bedsore biomechanics*. London: MacMillan, 1976.
100. Caputo GM, Cavanagh PR, Ulbracht JS, Gibons GW, Karchmer A. Assessment and management of foot disease in patients with diabetes. *N Engl J Med* 1994; 29:854–860.
101. Harkless LB, Higgins KR. Evaluation of diabetic foot and leg. In: Fryklberg RG, ed. *The high risk foot in diabetes mellitus*. New York: Churchill-Livingstone, 1991; 61–77.
102. Giordano JM. Non-invasive vascular testing. In: Kominsky SJ, ed. *Medical and surgical management of the diabetic foot*. St. Louis: CV Mosby, 1994; 55–70.
103. Delbridge L, Ellis CS, Robertson K. Nonenzymatic glycosylation of keratin from the stratum corneum of diabetes mellitus foot. *Br J Dermatol* 1988; 122:547–554.
104. Banks AS. A clinical guide to the Charcot foot. In: Kominsky SJ, ed. *Medical and surgical management of the diabetic foot*. St. Louis: CV Mosby, 1994; 115–143.
105. Mann R, Poppen N, O'Konshi M. Amputations of the great toe: a clinical biomechanical study. *Clin Orthop* 1988; 226:197.
106. Schoenhaus HD, Wernick E, Cohen RS. Biomechanics of the diabetic foot. In: Frykberg RG, ed. *The high risk foot in diabetes mellitus*. New York: Churchill-Livingstone, 1991; 125–137.
107. Cavanagh PR, Ulbrocht JS. Biomechanics of the foot in diabetes mellitus. In: Levin ME, O Neal LN, Bowker JH, eds. *The diabetic foot*. St. Louis: CV Mosby, 1993; 199–232.
108. Coleman WC. Foot care and lower extremity problems of diabetes mellitus. In: Joshu DH, ed. *Management of diabetes mellitus*. St. Louis: CV Mosby, 1996; 309–332.
109. Coleman WC. Foot wear considerations. In: Frykberg RG, ed. *The high risk foot in diabetes mellitus*. New York: Churchill-Livingstone, 1991; 487–512.
110. Thompson FJ, Veves A, Ashe H, et al. The team approach to diabetic foot care—the Manchester experience. *Foot* 1991; 2:75–82.
111. Mooney V, Wagner FW. Neurocirculatory disorders of the foot. *Clin Orthop* 1977; 122:53.
112. Newman LG, Waller J, Palestro CJ, et al. Unsuspected osteomyelitis in diabetic foot ulcers—diagnosis and monitoring by leukocyte scanning with indium In III oxyquinoline. *JAMA* 1991; 266:1246–1251.
113. McEnery KW, Gilula LA, Hardy DC, Staple TW. Imaging of diabetic foot. In: Levin EM, O'Neal WL, Bowker JH, eds. *The diabetic foot*. St. Louis: CV Mosby, 1993; 341–364.
114. Jelinek J, Levy E. Radiologic considerations for the diabetic extremity. In: Kominsky S, ed. *Medical and surgical management of the diabetic foot*. St. Louis: CV Mosby, 1994; 145–160.
115. Peterson LR, Lissock LM, Canter K, et al. Therapy of lower extremity infections with Ciprofloxacin in patients with diabetes mellitus, peripheral vascular disease or both. *Am J Med* 1989; 86:801–808.
116. Helm PA, Walker SC, Pullium G. Total contact casting in diabetic patients with neuropathic foot ulcerations. *Arch Phys Med Rehabil* 1994; 65:691–693.
117. Birke JA, Novick A, Graham S, Coleman WC, Brasseaux DM. Methods of treating plantar ulcers. *Phys Ther* 1991; 71:116–122.
118. Walker SC, Helm PA, Pullium G. Total contact casting and chronic diabetic neuropathic foot ulcerations—healing rates by wound location. *Arch Phys Med Rehabil* 1987; 68:217–221.
119. Sinacore DR, Mueller MJ. Total contact casting in the treatment of neuropathic ulcers. In: Levin ME, O'Neal LW, Bowker JH, eds. *The diabetic foot*. St. Louis: CV Mosby, 1993; 283–304.
120. Kominsky SJ. The ambulatory total contact cast. In: Frykberg RG, ed. *The high risk foot in diabetes mellitus*. New York: Churchill-Livingstone, 1991; 449–461.
121. Helm PA, Walker SC, Pullium G. Recurrance of neuropathic ulceration following healing in a total contact cast. *Arch Phys Med Rehabil*. 1991; 72:967–970.
122. Knighton DR, Fiegel VD. Growth factors and repair of diabetic wounds. In: Levin ME, O Neal LW, Bowker JH, eds. *The diabetic foot*. St. Louis: CV Mosby, 1993; 247–257.
123. Sanders LJ, Frykberg RG. Charcot foot. In: Levin EM, O'Neal WL, Bowker JH, eds. *The diabetic foot*. St. Louis: CV Mosby, 1991; 149–180.
124. Brodsky JW. The diabetic foot. In: Mann RA, Coughlin MJ, eds. *Surgery of the foot and ankle,* 6th ed. St. Louis: CV Mosby, 1993; 877–958.
125. Helm PA, Pandian G. Prevention of amputation. In: Esquenazi A, ed. *Prosthetics—state of the art reviews. PM&R*. Philadelphia: Hanley & Belfus 1994; 9–24.
126. Vinik AI, et al. Diabetic neuropathies. *Diabetes Care* 1992; 15: 1926–1975.
127. McCarthy DJ. Cutaneous manifestations of the lower extremities in diabetes mellitus. In: Kominsky SJ, ed. *Medical and surgical management of the diabetic foot*. St. Louis: CV Mosby, 1994; 191–222.
128. Jelinek JE. Dermatology. In: Levin EM, O'Neal WL, Bowker JH, eds. *The diabetic foot*. St. Louis: CV Mosby, 1993; 61–77.
129. Dockery GL, Crawford ME. *Cutaneous disorders of the lower extremity*. Philadelphia: WB Saunders, 1997; 176–200.
130. Janisse DJ. Pedorthic care of the diabetic foot. In: Levin ME, O'Neal LW, Bowker JH. *The diabetic foot*. St. Louis: CV Mosby, 1993; 549–576.
131. Runyan JW. The Memphis chronic disease program. Comparisons in outcome and the nurse's extended role. *JAMA* 1975; 231:264–267.

Rehabilitation Medicine: Principles and Practice, Third Edition,
edited by Joel A. DeLisa and Bruce M. Gans.
Lippincott–Raven Publishers, Philadelphia © 1998.

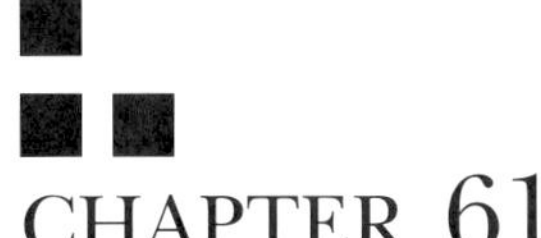

CHAPTER 61

Rehabilitation of the Patient with Diseases of the Motor Unit

Mark A. Thomas, Avital Fast, and John R. Bach

The diseases of the motor unit are a collection of genetic, infectious, autoimmune, inflammatory, toxic, or idiopathic disorders that result in the dysfunction of their final common expression: purposeful, controlled muscle contraction. The purpose of this section is to provide detailed information on diseases affecting the motor unit that are encountered in physiatric practice. The physiatrist may be called on to manage these conditions and at times may be required to diagnose them in patients presenting with new complaints of weakness, cramps, or functional difficulties. When medical intervention is considered or rehabilitation is planned, the identification of the disease process and knowledge of the natural history of that disease allows realistic treatment goals to be defined.

In order to develop a conception of the diseases of the motor unit as a spectrum of pathology with shared pathology and clinical expression, a brief review of the normal motor unit axis is helpful. The motor unit encompasses the anterior horn cell, the peripheral nerve, the myoneural junction, and muscle (see Fig. 61-1).

ANATOMY AND HISTOLOGY

The spinal gray anterior horn cell is the terminus for descending corticospinal impulses. This is the site where descending or modulating interneurons contribute to the common motor outflow. The resting potential of the anterior horn cell (central excitatory state) is affected by multiple impulses, which make discharge a higher- or lower-probability event. The anterior horn cell can be considered to be a switch that governs all subsequent activity in the motor unit (see Fig. 61-2).

The axon of the anterior horn cell acquires protective connective tissue (epineurium, perineurium) and forms the peripheral motor nerve. Each cell axon branches many times within a muscle, and the nerve fibers each innervate between a dozen and several thousand individual extrafusal muscle fibers. The number of muscle fibers innervated by one motor unit relates to the degree of muscle control. Muscles with fine motor function require substantially more anterior horn cells per unit volume of muscle than do muscles responsible for coarser movement (1).

The next segment to be considered along the axis of the motor unit is the peripheral nerve (see Fig. 61-3). This is formed by the axon of the anterior horn cell. Exiting the spinal cord, the nerve root or proximal portion of the axon is covered only by endoneurium. Thus, this is one site where the axon is vulnerable to trauma. The axon gains protective perineurium and epineurium layers and is enveloped by myelin. Myelin, elaborated by covering Schwann cells, is responsible for the saltatory conduction between the nodes of Ranvier. The resultant conduction velocity of the peripheral nerve is approximately 55 m/sec. The peripheral nerve branches multiple times within a muscle (about 20 to 100 times) (2) to end at the motor end plate of the myoneural junction.

The myoneural junction is the point where energy is transferred from a peripheral nerve to a muscle fiber (see Fig. 61-4). The peripheral nerve ends in close proximity to the muscle end plate. The presynaptic terminus of the peripheral nerve packages and releases the neurotransmitter, acetylcholine. The acetylcholine binds with receptors in the muscle at the postsynaptic surface, which are located in folds of the

M. A. Thomas and A. Fast: Department of Rehabilitation Medicine, Montefiore Medical Center, Albert Einstein College of Medicine, Bronx, New York 10467.

J. R. Bach: Department of Physical Medicine and Rehabilitation, University of Medicine and Dentistry of New Jersey, New Jersey Medical School, Newark, New Jersey 07103.

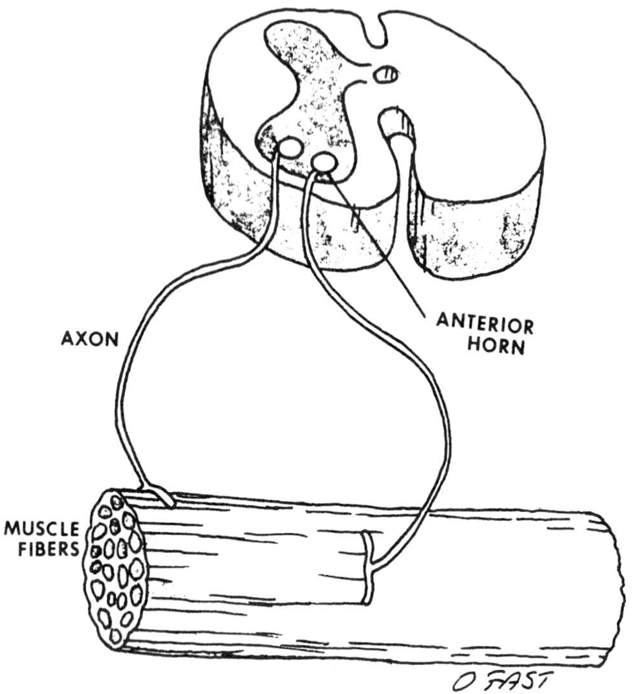

FIG. 61-1. The normal motor unit.

muscle membrane. This binding results in depolarization, transferring energy to the muscle's conduction system. The acetylcholine is subsequently degraded by acetylcholinesterase, which is stored on the postsynaptic surface. The constituents are recycled into the packaged quanta of neurotransmitter on the presynaptic surface.

Skeletal muscle is the final point in the motor unit. Muscle fibers of various types (see Table 61-1) are surrounded by an endomysial membrane, bundled into fibrils, which are each surrounded by epimysium, and the fibrils are collectively enveloped by the perimysium (see Fig. 61-5). The fibers themselves are the dynamic portion of a muscle and contract when membrane depolarization occurs. The proteins responsible for contraction include the thick filament myosin (heavy and light meromyosin components) and thin filament actin, tropomyosin, and troponin. Connective tissue and noncontractile proteins (C-protein, alpha- and beta-actinin, calsequestrin, dystrophin, parvalbumin, and myoglobin) constitute the static, noncontractile portion of the muscle. The noncontractile elements contribute to regulation of ion flux (calcium), structural support, or oxygen storage.

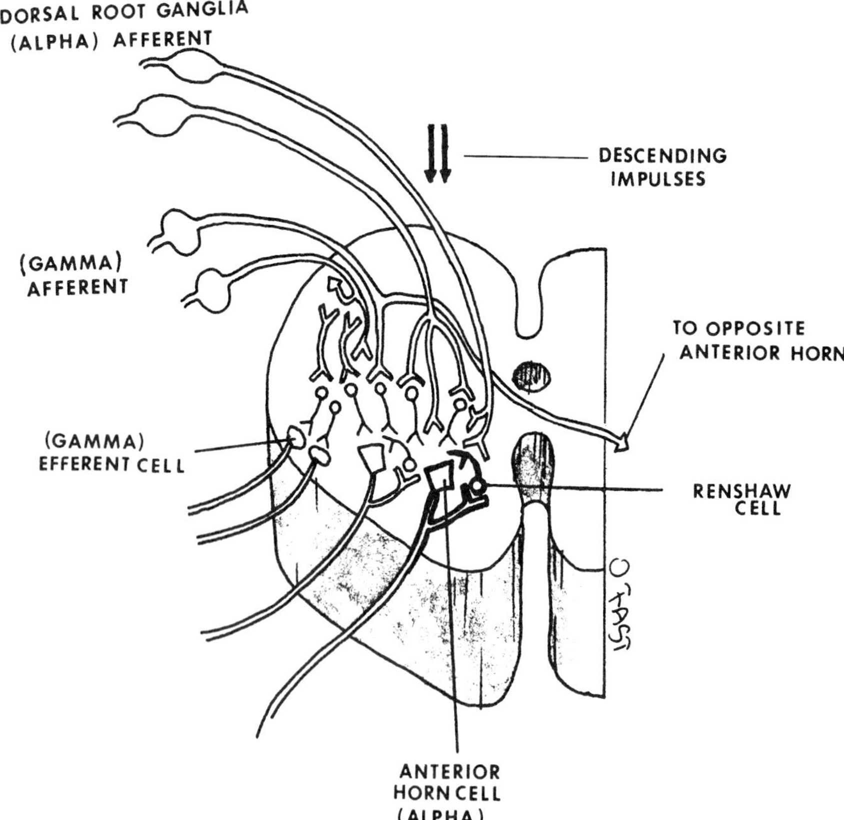

FIG. 61-2. The anterior horn cell: synaptic activity and axonal outflow.

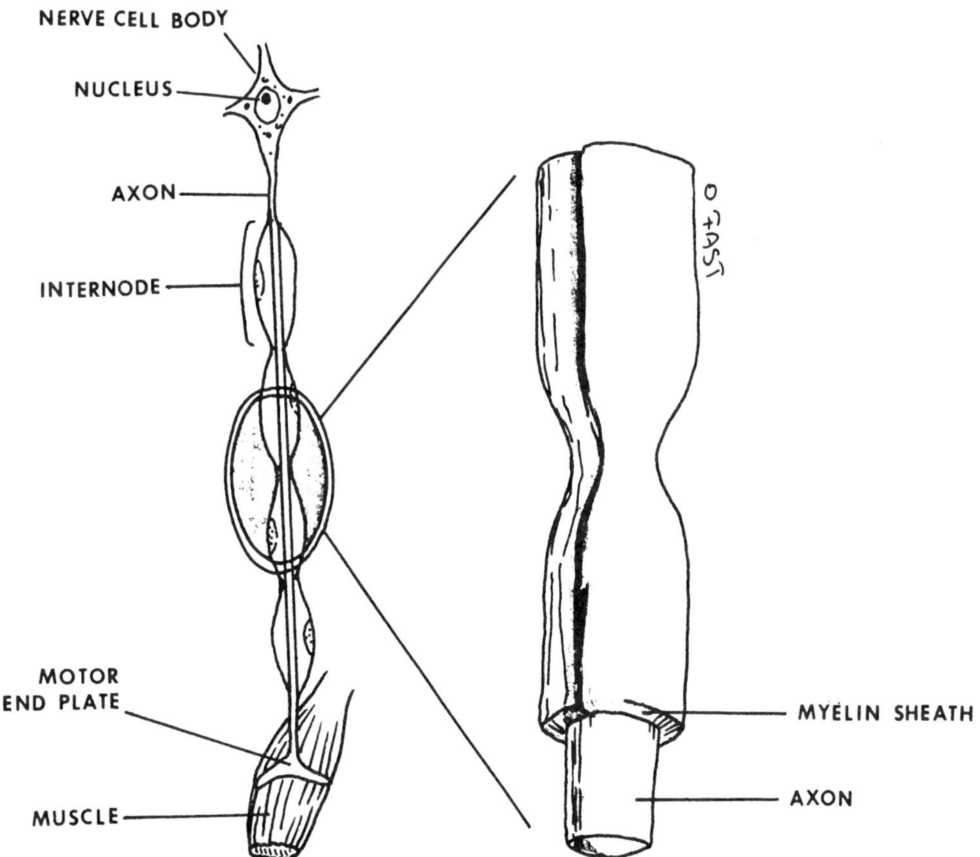

FIG. 61-3. Peripheral motor nerve.

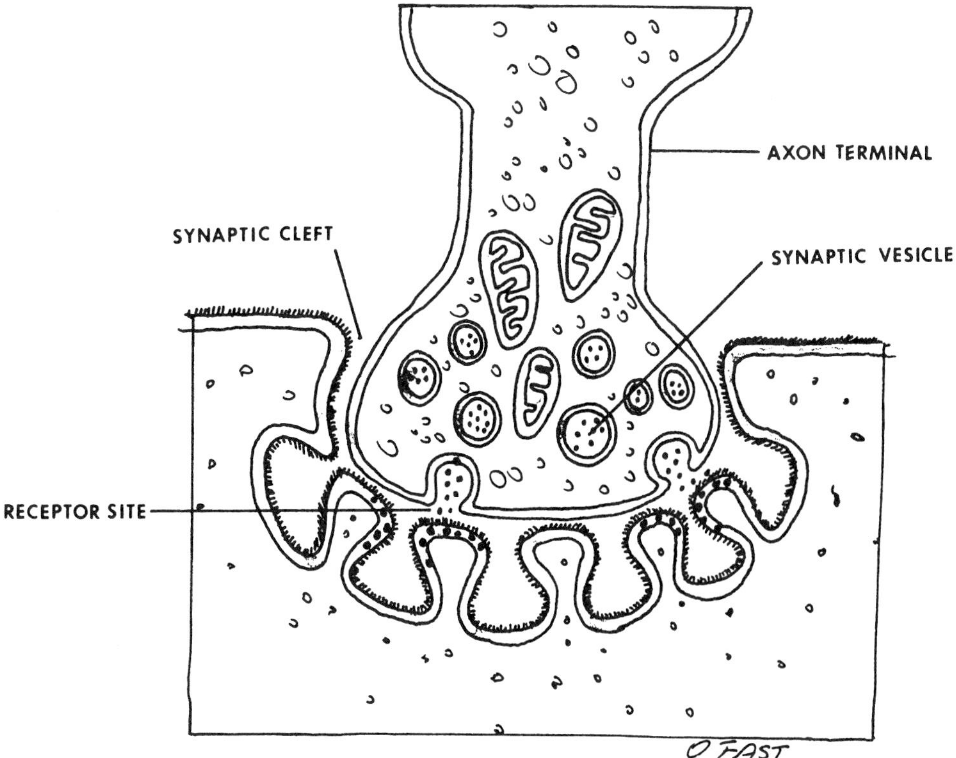

FIG. 61-4. Neuromuscular junction.

TABLE 61-1. *Muscle fibers*

Muscle fiber type	Color	Myoglobin content, vascular supply	Enzyme bias	Contraction type	Fatigue resistance
Type I	Red	High	Oxidative	Slow	High
Type IIA	Red	High	Phosphorylase > oxidative	Fast	High
Type IIB	White	Low	Phosphorylase	Fast	Low
Type IIC	—	—	Phosphorylase	Fast	Intermediate

PHYSIOLOGY

Direct feedback control of resting muscle length/tension and readiness to contract is supplied by the intrafusal muscle fibers (the muscle spindle) (see Fig. 61-6). The muscle tone, its resistance to passive stretch, is influenced by discharge of the spindles' static and dynamic response elements. The muscle spindle-mediated contraction response to quick stretch and elongation response to sustained stretch are mediated through the gamma and alpha motor systems.

It is important to note that as a normal consequence of aging there is loss of both anterior horn cells and muscle fibers. This significant diminution in reserve for the aging individual may eventually result in progression of the clinical deficits in a person affected with a motor-unit disease.

DISEASES OF THE MOTOR UNIT—GENERAL PRINCIPLES

Disease of the motor unit (see Table 61-2) disrupts neuromuscular anatomic or functional integrity with impairment of normal controlled muscle contraction. This has several clinical expressions, which are shared to varying extent by all the diseases considered in this chapter. Muscle weakness, loss of endurance, atrophy, joint and soft tissue contracture, postural abnormalities of the axial or appendicular skeleton (particularly equinovarus, kyphosis, and scoliosis), cardiovascular complications, and psychosocial problems constitute the basis for disability and handicap related to neuromuscular disease. Less common than weakness and contracture, disordered function of the motor unit may result in hyperactive muscle contracture in conditions such as myotonia or the stiff man syndrome. Because diseases of the motor unit vary more widely in their etiologic and pathophysiological elements than in their clinical expression, effective rehabilitation can be provided through many interventions that are common to the whole disease spectrum (see Table 61-3). These shared elements of physiatric care are supplemented by disease-specific treatment and individualized according to patient-specific goals.

Medical treatment of these diseases is based on their etiology and pathophysiology, whereas the rehabilitation treatment options are more determined by the stage of the disease. For example, treatment during the ambulatory stage versus the stage of wheelchair dependence versus the stage of prolonged survival is similar for patients with Duchenne muscular dystrophy, amyotrophic lateral sclerosis, or spinal muscular atrophy. The timing may differ, but the clinical problems that result in disability or handicap are similar.

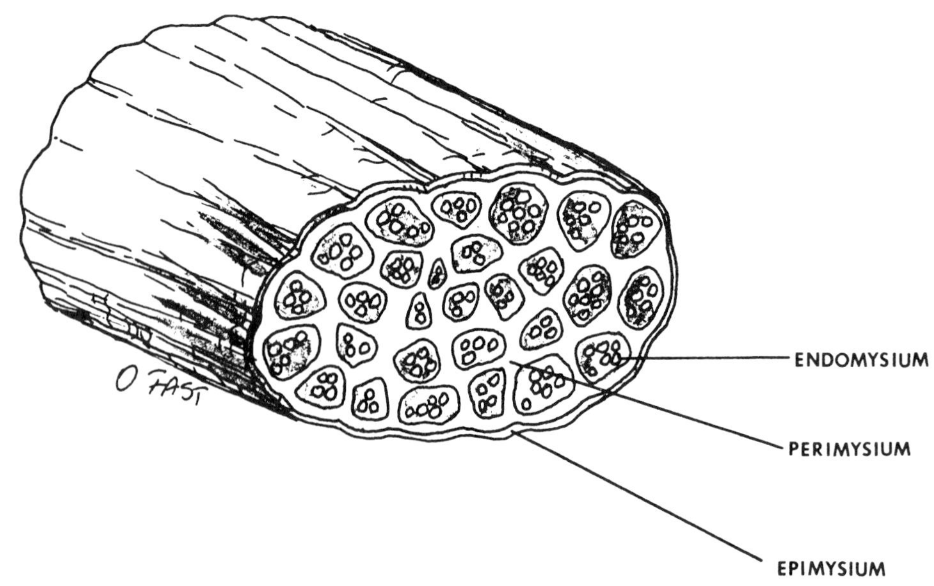

FIG. 61-5. Muscle: gross organization of fibers.

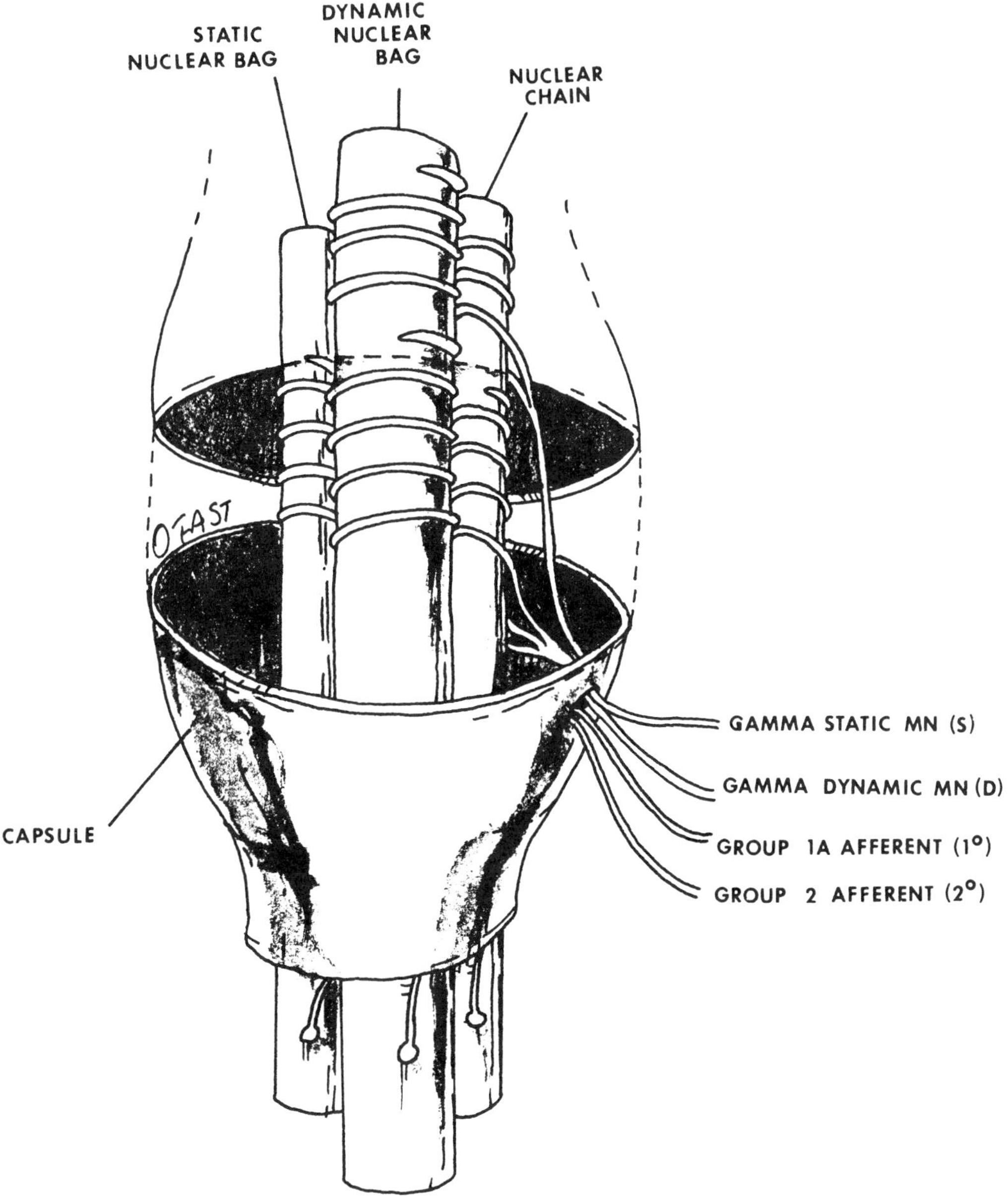

FIG. 61-6. The muscle spindle.

TABLE 61-2. *Motor unit diseases*

Site of lesion	Disease	Etiology
Anterior horn cell	Amyotrophic lateral sclerosis	
	Poliomyelitis	Infectious
	Spinal muscular atrophy	Genetic
Peripheral nerve	Motor neuropathy (various etiologies)	Toxic, infectious, inflammatory, autoimmune
	Mixed nerve neuropathy (various etiologies)	Genetic, autoimmune, toxic, metabolic
Neuromuscular junction	Myasthenia gravis	Autoimmune
	Eaton-Lambert syndrome	Autoimmune
	Botulism	Toxic
	Tick paralysis	Toxic
Muscle	Myopathy (all types, including muscular dystrophy)	Genetic, infectious, autoimmune, toxic, metabolic, inflammatory, idiopathic

TABLE 61-3. *Management principles for neuromuscular diseases*

Ambulatory stage	1. Establish the diagnosis and provide genetic counseling. 2. Provide early and informed counseling and psychological support to prevent counterproductive family psychodynamics. Encourage goal-oriented activities and prepare the patient and family for current and future therapeutic interventions. The advantages of early intervention during each stage should be stressed. 3. Manage and prevent musculotendinous contracture and decreased pulmonary compliance. 4. Use appropriate supportive physical and occupational therapy, including splinting and therapeutic exercise. 5. Prolong ambulation by the above, plus surgery (musculotendinous release or transfer, spinal stabilization) plus lower extremity bracing as indicated. 6. Monitor for, and prevent, cardiac complications. 7. Manage dysphagia and nutritional concerns.
Wheelchair-dependent stage	1. Enhance ADL independence with assistive devices. 2. Prevent or correct spine deformity. 3. Monitor for and manage cardiac insufficiency. 4. Maintain pulmonary compliance and alveolar ventilation. 5. Manage dysphagia and nutritional concerns as appropriate.
The stage of prolonged survival	1. Educate the patient and encourage taking responsibility for management decisions and directing caregivers. 2. Facilitate ADL independence with assistive devices. 3. Introduce noninvasive respiratory muscle aids to assist alveolar ventilation and clear airway secretions. 4. Manage dysphagia and nutritional concerns as appropriate.

ADL, activities of daily living.

Clinical Course

In order to determine the best plan of care, it is important to understand the etiology and natural history of the disease. Identifying the pattern of inheritance for genetic disorders such as muscular dystrophy or spinal muscular atrophy is important. Diseases with autosomal or X-linked recessive patterns of inheritance carry a worse prognosis in general and are typically complicated by more severe respiratory disease.

Motor unit disease may be progressive, static, or transient. It is also important to note the rate of recovery or of disease progression when setting goals or prescribing exercise and equipment. Additional issues to consider in planning rehabilitation intervention focus on the differences between myopathic and neuropathic disease and the distribution of clinical findings. Generally contractures caused by neurogenic disease that affects the distal limbs are less disabling than those caused by more proximal patterns of involvement. Proximal weakness and contracture are more severely disabling at an earlier point in the disease course. Myopathies often affect function of the lower extremities more significantly than upper extremities because of the effect of weakness on muscles with relatively higher strength demands for usual activities of daily living (ADL).

Rehabilitation

An aggressive approach to the patient with disease of the motor unit is essential. Rehabilitation treatment may be anticipatory, symptomatic, or restorative. Anticipatory care, particularly the prevention of contracture and functional decline, should be provided to a patient in the early stage of disease. Contractures are problematic because they limit motion, alter the center of gravity, and accentuate weakness by limiting the potential tension a residual muscle can produce (3). Contractures thus lead to rapid muscle fatigue and restrict ADL performance. Maintenance, or symptomatic care, addresses problems that already exist, such as contracture or ADL deficits. Restorative care, with the return of a patient to a higher level of function, is reasonable when a disease is transient or when it becomes possible to augment function with equipment or assistive devices. Restorative therapy is also appropriate to reverse the complications of concomitant acute or chronic illness or any adverse effects of treatment.

The rehabilitation of the patient with neuromuscular disease involves establishing the disability diagnosis and, within the constraints of disease prognosis, defining treatment goals, providing rehabilitation intervention, and coordinating appropriate medical and surgical care. Treatment goals must be agreed on by the entire treatment team, including the patient and family. Rehabilitation interventions are summarized in Table 61-4.

Exercise by patients with motor unit disease must be considered carefully and prescribed prudently. There is evidence that an increased functional demand may damage immature muscle and that dystrophic muscles are unable to sustain any overloading (4). Serum creatine kinase (CK) levels increase more following exercise in dystrophic patients than they do in normal subjects. Studies that compare the strength of dominant upper (5) and lower (6) limbs of dystrophic individuals with the strength of the opposite extremity demonstrate more

TABLE 61-4. *Rehabilitation intervention for diseases of the motor unit*

Problem/complication	Intervention
Weakness (decreased strength)	Exercise; early submaximal resistive or high-repetition aerobic exercise (139), particularly of deconditioned, uninvolved muscle
Proximal	Stand 2 to 3 hours per day; walk or swim
Distal: hand/feet intrinsic muscle	Time activities for strongest periods
Isolated	High seats, rails, home and workstation modification for easy reach; scapula-fixing orthoses
Decreased endurance/fatigue	Conditioning exercise
	Rest breaks/timed activities
Loss of fine motor control	Build-up tool handles; dampen response of electronic controls for wheelchair or communication devices
Impaired coordination	Weight extremities; biofeedback
Myotonia, stiffness, cramps	Membrane stabilizers, especially phenytoin (Dilantin); avoid cold temperatures
Muscle substitutions	Brace; adaptive equipment; EMG biofeedback
Immobilization	Standing table, parallel bar "therapeutic standing"
Structural changes	
Contracture/tightness:	Stretching program (see text), passive/active range-of-motion exercise, positioning and seating systems
Neck flexors	
Shoulder abductors	
Elbow flexors	
Pronators	
Web space	Splints
MP extension	
Hip flexors	Firm seating surface; avoid "hammock configuration"
Knee flexors	
Rectus femoris	
Tensor fascia lata	Surgical release; transfer; arthrodesis
Triceps surae	
Joint contracture	Serial casting; dynamic bracing; splinting
Equinovarus	
Postural changes	Lumbar extension support for facet stabilization, rigid seating, appropriate arm support, shoes, splints, etc.
Scoliosis	
Kyphosis	
Physiological changes	
Bone/osteoporosis	Weight bearing (standing table, bars)
Blood flow	Compression hose
Cardiovascular reflex	Tilt table
Cognitive changes	
Decubitus ulcers	Preventive measures, adequate nutrition, patient education, local care
Constipation	Stool softeners, laxatives, regular bowel routine
Impaired mobility	Grab bars, tub transfer seats, lightweight wheelchairs, motorized wheelchairs, motorized scooters, transfer (sliding) boards, mechanical lifts (Hoyer, etc.), elevated chairs/toilet seats; tape all wires and loose rugs, fill stair risers, assure adequate lighting
Ambulation	
Wheelchair mobility	
Standing transfer	Ramp (1/12 rise), guard rail, nonstick treads
Seated treansfer	Address obesity
Bed mobility	
BADL deficits	Long-handled combs and brushes, sponges, toilet paper holders, shoe horns, flexible shower hoses, tub chair or bench, bedside commode chairs, hospital beds, dressing and kitchen aids
Feeding	
Bathing	Zipper rings, ring pulls, elastic laces, larger sock size, velcro closures on clothing
Grooming	
Toileting	
Dressing	
IADL deficits	Environmental control systems with blink-activated eye switch (infrared limbus–pupil reflection) or electro-ocular switches
Housekeeping	
Shopping	
Instrument use	Home health aide; "hands-free" telephone headset
Cosmetic deformity	Plastic surgery
Pain	Membrane-stabilizing agents
Myogenic	Analgesics (TCAs)
Neurogenic	
Other	
Psychosocial deficits	Peer support (MDA, Easter Seal Society, etc.), patient/family counseling, plastic surgery, enhance function/mobility, antidepressant medication
Self-esteem	
Depression	
Discrimination	
Substance abuse	
Malnutrition	Follow body weight, serum protein; adapt cutlery, BFO, light wide-handled cutlery, modify food textures, restore normal blood gases by assisted ventilation
Respiratory compromise	Vaccinations (flu, pneumonia)
CAH	Noninvasive inspiratory and expiratory muscle aids
Respiratory failure	
Growth spurts	Monitor scoliosis, update bracing, wheelchair, other appliances in a timely manner
Communication deficits	Personal computer with keyboard emulator software to drive a voice synthesizer and printer
Aphonia	
Vocation	Training and ergonomic aids
Avocation	Refer to peer group
Transportation	Adapted van, hand controls/modifications

BADL, basic activities of daily living; BFO, balanced forearm orthosis; CAH, chronic alveolar hypoventilation; EMG, electromyography; IADL, instrumental activities of daily living; MDA, Muscular Dystrophy Association; TCAs, tricyclic antidepressants.

weakness in the dominant limb. This suggests that greater use results in overuse weakness. The possibility exists that overexercise may accelerate the dystrophic process, particularly if it is performed over an extended time period. Even routine ADL may cause overuse atrophy in patients with advanced muscle degeneration. In contrast to this, de Lateur found that strengthening or endurance training, when begun early in the course of Duchenne muscular dystrophy (DMD), can improve strength and slow disease progression (7). Resistance exercise may increase strength up to 50% in the antigravity and stronger musculature. Milner-Brown studied patients with fascioscapulohumeral, myotonic, Becker, and limb-girdle muscular dystrophies, spinal muscular atrophy, and polyneuropathies. The results of this study indicate that exercise increases strength and work tolerance and decreases fatigue if the initial strength of a patient is greater than 15% to 20% of normal. Thus, dynamic high-resistance exercise training can be beneficial and result in strength gain if the degree of weakness is not severe, the rate of disease progression is relative slow, the rate of exercise progression is slow, and the daily exercise period is limited. The timing and intensity of an exercise program also must take into account the usual pattern of daily physical activity (8). Unfortunately, it seems clear that exercise programs cannot benefit the weakest patients or the weakest muscles.

Disuse atrophy occurs when the force of muscle contraction is consistently less than 20% of maximal voluntary contraction. Such loss of strength can proceed at a rate up to 3% per day. This disuse weakening contributes to disability in patients with motor unit disease, but patients can usually partially or fully recover from this additional loss of strength. The return of a patient to premorbid strength is an appropriate goal after acute illness or surgery. This is achieved by daily active exercise at an intensity greater than 35% of maximal voluntary contraction (9).

One normal consequence of aging is the loss of muscle and anterior horn cells. By the sixth decade, only 50% of motor units remain in normal subjects (9). This emphasizes how problematic strengthening may be for the aging neuromuscular patient, particularly for those with anterior horn cell disease. Even with a static disease such as poliomyelitis, the aging patient may become weaker despite all efforts to maintain strength.

The best general conditioning exercise is 2 to 3 hours of standing, walking, or swimming daily (9). Standing tables, bracing, or other strategies may be needed to accomplish this. Submaximal resistive strengthening and high-repetition aerobic exercise are valuable when such exercise can be performed by a patient (10).

Stretching is a central component of the rehabilitation prescription for diseases of the motor unit. Lower extremity contractures may preclude independent ambulation. Upper extremity contractures may interfere with both ambulation and ADL. An elbow flexion contracture of 15°, for example, renders crutch use difficult, and this becomes impossible when the contracture exceeds 30°. When the elbow contracture is beyond 60°, dressing and other basic ADL skills are impaired. Although the shoulders usually retain a functional active range of motion, tightness does occur at this joint in limb girdle muscular dystrophy and acid maltase myopathy. A sustained passive stretch for 15 to 20 seconds ten times daily should be recommended for all joints. Stretching should focus on the iliotibial band, hamstrings, triceps surae, wrist flexors, and intrinsic muscles (hands, feet) as well as any specific tightening identified on physical examination.

Surgical interventions, including various lower extremity tenotomies and fasciotomies (for heel cord, hamstring, iliotibial band) can be valuable in the muscular dystrophies and congenital myopathies. Transfer of the posterior tibial tendon to the third cuneiform is another possible procedure when hindfoot varus is a problem and the dorsiflexors are very weak. Surgery can be relatively late, as soon as the patient becomes unable to ambulate. Orthotics are then required to restore standing and some ambulatory ability for an additional 2 to 5 years, particularly in patients with DMD (11–13). On the other hand, surgery can be performed early, before significant ambulation difficulties develop. This allows standing and ambulation to be retained without resorting to orthotics or extensive physical therapy (see Table 61-3).

MOTOR UNIT DISEASES

Abnormal function of the anterior horn cell may result from disease of the anterior horn cell, from a change in central excitatory state secondary to imbalance between facilitation and inhibition by interneurons, or as a result of a neurotransmitter abnormality. Diseases that most frequently affect the anterior horn cell include poliomyelitis, amyotrophic lateral sclerosis, spinal muscle atrophy, myelitis, and spinal cord injury.

Diseases of the peripheral nerve alter nerve structure and conduction. Both motor and mixed nerves may be affected. The disease involves the axon, its myelin sheath, or both. Functional lesions of the peripheral nerve include neurapraxia, axonotmesis, and neuronotmesis. Neurapraxia is the loss of nerve conduction without a change in nerve structure. Demyelination may or may not occur in this instance. Axonotmesis is the loss of axonal continuity. Because of this disruption, Wallerian degeneration of the distal nerve segment follows injury. The remaining category of nerve injury is neuronotmesis. This is defined as the complete loss of nerve integrity and separation of nerve segments. Peripheral neuropathies may be caused by metabolic/endocrine, organic or inorganic toxic, immune-mediated, or traumatic (compression, division) insults. They are characterized as motor, sensory, or mixed nerve dysfunctions. The spatial distribution may be proximal or distal, focal or generalized, and symmetric or asymmetric.

The peripheral nerve terminus of the myoneural junction is subject to disease in which a failure to package, store, or release acetylcholine quanta may occur. There also may be disordered anatomy and function of the muscle motor end plate, with abnormal receptor activity. Diseases of the myoneural junction include myasthenia gravis and the myasthenic syndromes such as Eaton-Lambert syndrome, botulism, and tick paralysis. The primary distinction guiding treatment is whether the dysfunction occurs at the pre- or postsynaptic surface.

Muscle may be affected by a host of diseases that interfere with normal anatomy, fiber proportion, or function. Weakness and reduced muscle tone are characteristic of myopathy, including the muscular dystrophies. Reduced tone is expressed as a decreased resistance to passive stretch. Myokymia, the involuntary continuous or regular contraction of muscle fibers, may be present. Cramps, painful involuntary contractions of the entire muscle, also occur in many muscle diseases.

SPECIFIC DISEASES OF THE MOTOR UNIT

Amyotrophic Lateral Sclerosis

Motor neuron diseases result in progressive degeneration and loss of motor neurons in the spinal cord, brainstem motor nuclei, and the motor cortex. The clinical manifestation of these diseases is determined by the extent and location of motor neuron loss.

Amyotrophic lateral sclerosis (ALS) usually occurs as a sporadic event. The disease is familial in 5% of cases. Inheritance is seen in an autosomal dominant pattern. The distribution of ALS is worldwide and without racial or ethnic predisposition, although geographic clustering of cases has been reported. It affects both genders but is more common in men.

Symptoms of ALS appear in middle and late life in most instances. Ten percent of patients become symptomatic before the age of 40 years. ALS is a progressive disease that invariably leads to death within a few years. The course of ALS tends to be slower, with longer survival, in male patients who are affected at a younger age.

The pathogenesis of ALS remains obscure and debated. It is thought to be a degenerative disease whose clinical expression results from premature motor neuron death. Possible triggering mechanisms that lead to motor neuron loss remain obscure. Theories about the pathogenesis of sporadically occurring ALS focus on environmental factors, viruses, metal intoxication by lead and mercury, glutamate toxicity, autoimmune mechanisms, and genetic susceptibility. Occasionally the disease appears in association with certain malignancies. Recently, autoimmune dysfunction with alteration of calcium channel function has been linked to ALS. About 20% of the familial cases show a significant reduction in Cu/Zn superoxide dismutase enzyme content/function. The gene related to this enzyme is located at chromosome 21 (14–16). Such a multiplicity of theories attests to the fact that the pathogenesis of ALS remains an enigma.

The diagnosis of ALS is made on the basis of a detailed history followed by a comprehensive clinical examination. The diagnosis can be confirmed by electrodiagnostic studies. These reveal diffuse denervation in at least three extremities in the presence of relatively normal motor and sensory response latencies and normal conduction velocity.

Asymmetric painless weakness may appear in the upper or lower extremities. The extraocular muscles are only rarely affected. The patient displays difficulties with activities that require fine motor coordination. Alternately, the patient may complain of subtle onset gait dysfunction and may begin to trip over his or her own feet or develop a foot drop. A spastic gait may develop. In a small number of patients, the presenting symptom may be difficulty with swallowing. Fasciculations occasionally appear before any other neurologic abnormality is observed. The disease course is relentless. The weakness is progressive and involves wider areas. The patient becomes increasingly dependent. When all the extremities are involved, the patient may become totally immobile.

In the late stages of ALS, the intercostal muscles and the diaphragm are affected, and the patient develops difficulty breathing. Respiratory muscle weakness may progress to the point of ventilator dependency. When pharyngeal muscles are affected, the patient becomes dysphagic. Emotional lability, expressed by inappropriate laughter or crying, may also develop. This is a manifestation of pseudobulbar palsy.

Diffuse fasciculations, muscle atrophy, and occasional cramps develop. Fasciculation of the tongue may be seen even when speech remains unaffected. Typically, the sensory system and sphincter muscles are spared. Minor sensory abnormalities such as paresthesia, decreased vibratory sensation, and pain can occur (17). Deep tendon reflexes are normal, increased, or decreased, and a combination of these findings can be seen. Occasionally a patient may lose the tendon reflexes in the lower extremities and have an upgoing toe on plantar stimulation.

Several clinical features help to differentiate between familial and sporadic ALS victims. In the familial variety of the disease, weakness usually starts in the legs, dementia is more prevalent, there is equal gender representation, and survival from symptom onset is shorter (17).

For most patients, the disease progresses relentlessly, and they succumb to recurrent pneumonia, sepsis, or pulmonary embolism. These complications are a direct consequence of complete immobility. Most patients succumb to the disease within 5 years of diagnosis. At some point many patients become ventilator dependent. Noninvasive respiratory muscle aids such as intermittent positive-pressure ventilation (IPPV) and intermittent abdominal pressure ventilation (IAPV) should be considered (see Chapter 55). These respiratory aids may prolong life while providing an acceptable quality of living (18).

Every effort should be made to exclude other, more benign conditions when the diagnosis is entertained. Included in the differential diagnosis are *cervical myelopathy, multifocal motor neuropathy, mutliple sclerosis, primary lateral sclerosis, and other motor unit diseases.*

Cervical myelopathy is a common condition that affects the elderly. In this condition, patients present with a slowly progressive gait dysfunction and difficulty with tasks that require fine motor coordination. The initial physical findings are subtle and found only by meticulous neurologic examination. The gait is typically wide based and occasionally jerky. The reflexes in the lower extremities may or may not be hyperactive, and the toes upgoing. Atrophy of small muscles takes place in the upper extremities (19). Patients may be gradually robbed of their functional independence by hand clumsiness and gait dysfunction. Unlike ALS patients, patients with cervical myelopathy complain of prominent sensory symptoms, such as numbness, tingling, and dysesthesia in the hands (20,21). Physical examination may disclose loss of proprioception, temperature, and pain sensation. There is a notable absence of muscle atrophy in the extremities. No fasciculations are observed in the tongue or the lower extremities. Cervical spine neuroimaging studies help to confirm this clinical diagnosis.

Multifocal motor neuropathy with conduction block (MMN) is another condition that should be included in the differential diagnosis of ALS. This rare condition mimics ALS but has a better outcome, as it responds to treatment with immunosuppressive drugs and intravenous immunoglobulin administration (22). MMN occurs more commonly in men.

MMN is characterized by progressive, asymmetric weakness in the distal limbs. Atrophy is prominent. No sensory involvement is seen. The patient may present with a painless foot or wrist drop. At times, the presenting symptom is grip weakness. Weakness may gradually involve all the extremities, and areflexic quadriparesis can occur. Bulbar and axial musculature is generally spared (23).

The diagnosis of MMN is confirmed by electrodiagnostic testing. Multifocal and incomplete motor conduction blocks are observed, typically at sites that are not prone to compressive neuropathy. The amplitude and negative peak area of the evoked response to proximal stimulation is reduced by at least 50%. There is less than a 15% change in the negative peak duration. The motor conduction velocity is slowed across affected nerve segments. There is a corresponding prolongation of F wave latencies in the involved nerves. At times the distal latency of nerves that do not show evidence of focal neuropathy is prolonged (24). Although minor abnormalities may be present, sensory nerve conduction studies most commonly remain normal.

Multiple sclerosis (MS) can clinically resemble ALS. Patients with MS may have pseudobulbar palsy and progressive weakness. The clinical course and ocular symptoms and findings distinguish MS from ALS. In addition, cerebrospinal fluid analysis and neuroimaging studies differentiate between the two conditions.

Primary lateral sclerosis (PLS) is a rare upper motor neuron disorder that should be distinguished from ALS. Unlike ALS, PLS presents with exclusively upper motor neuron findings. It affects both genders equally. The mean age at presentation is 50 years.

Patients with PLS develop a spastic gait in one or both lower extremities. The disease progresses slowly, sometimes over several decades, and the weakness and spasticity may involve all the extremities. Eventually the patient may become immobile as a result of extreme spasticity. Some patients develop the emotional lability typical of a pseudobulbar affective response. Some patients develop urinary incontinence (25,26).

Electrodiagnostic studies in PLS fail to provide evidence of denervation. Increased insertional activity and a few fibrillation potentials are sometimes found in the late stages of the disease. Peripheral motor and sensory nerve conduction studies remain normal. Magnetic resonance imaging studies disclose focal atrophy of the precentral gyrus (25,26).

Postpolio syndrome, monomelic amyotrophy (a benign condition affecting young men and usually limited to one extremity), *myasthenia gravis, tropical spastic paraparesis, vitamin* B_{12} *deficiency, and other diseases of the motor unit* should also be included in the differential diagnosis of ALS.

Unfortunately, ALS remains a progressive disease. The role of the physiatrist is to keep the patient at the highest possible level of function given the constraints of severe disability (27). Range-of-motion exercise should be provided to prevent contractures and maintain function. Strengthening exercise should be prescribed specifically for unaffected muscles that have weakened from disuse (27). Assistive devices are provided to enhance function, and ambulation aids and orthoses to delay wheelchair dependence. Communication devices may improve a patient's quality of life. Noninvasive respiratory muscle aids can delay or eliminate the need for tracheostomy and, at times, prolong life (28). More detailed information on physiatric pulmonary intervention is presented in the chapter on pulmonary rehabilitation (Chapter 55). A recently introduced neuroprotective drug, riluzole, appears to prolong survival in patients with ALS. One hundred milligrams daily seems to retard disease progression. The neuroprotective mechanism of riluzole is not fully understood (29,30).

Poliomyelitis and Postpolio Syndrome

The last poliomyelitis epidemic occurred in the 1950s, leaving behind a large number of patients. These patients have had to struggle with the sequelae of the disease. In the acute stage of infection, the polio virus attacks the motor neurons in the spinal cord and brainstem nuclei. In most cases the disease remains subclinical. In other instances, the disease leads to weakness or paralysis, depending on the number and distribution of motor neurons affected and the number of nerve cells that survive viral attack.

Many polio survivors who have exhibited stable, permanent impairments and loss of function begin to complain of symptoms similar to those experienced in the acute stage of infection. This is the postpolio syndrome (PPS), and it is estimated that between 22% and 28% of poliomyelitis patients develop the PPS (31,32).

The risk factors for the development of PPS are not fully established. Several factors associated with the original viral attack seem to confer a high risk for the subsequent development of PPS. Significant risk factors include involvement of all four extremities, prolonged hospitalization at the time of acute infection, significant respiratory involvement, and disease onset after age 10 years. Patients with severe and extensive poliomyelitis seem to develop PPS earlier than individuals who suffered only mild involvement (31–33).

The pathogenesis of PPS is probably multifactorial and remains unclear. It seems unlikely that the pathogenesis is directly related to the normal decrease in the number of anterior horn cells that is observed with aging because most PPS patients become symptomatic in their fourth or fifth decade (9). Several theories attempt to explain the occurrence of PPS. The most likely include premature attrition and death of unaffected motor neurons and death of motor neurons that were infected by the polio virus but survived. Early neuronal death may result from chronic and excessive metabolic demands such as those imposed by an increased motor unit size. Other possible, but less likely, pathogenetic factors include acquired vulnerability as a result of the viral attack, genetic predisposition, persistent chronic viral infection, metabolic muscular abnormalities, neuromuscular junction transmission defects, progressive terminal axonal loss, and immune-mediated syndromes (34–39).

The symptoms of PPS typically appear after a 25- to 35-year period of functional stability. The patient complains of increasing fatigue, diminished endurance, low energy levels, cold intolerance, and muscle and joint pain. The fatigue may be such that simple activities result in exhaustion. Gait difficulties begin to occur, and the patient is unable to cover the same distances as previously. Fatigue improves with rest, decreased activity, or sleep. The increase in muscle weakness may also interfere with ADL. Progressive weakness and atrophy may be observed in muscles that were initially affected by the polio virus or in muscles that were clinically spared. Atrophy and new weakness may appear bilaterally, but muscles tend to be affected at random, in an asymmetric distribution (40). Upper motor neuron signs may be observed in a small number of patients. These include increased deep tendon reflexes, an abnormal plantar response (upgoing toes), and, rarely, increased tone (41). Atrophy may occur in muscles that were previously unaffected as well as in partially denervated muscle. Fasciculations can be observed in these muscles. Fasciculations in PPS, however, appear much less frequently than they do in ALS.

Bulbar muscle deterioration may occur. The patient then complains of swallowing difficulties or a change in vocal quality. Fluoroscopic studies will show impaired tongue movement and a delay in pharyngeal contraction on swallowing. Deterioration of pulmonary function may result from further weakening of the respiratory muscles in patients who had decreased respiratory reserve after the initial infection. At times, the patient requires mechanical respiratory support.

Histologic studies show that following recovery from acute poliomyelitis, several different populations of neurons can be identified. In areas remote from viral attack, normal, unaffected neurons are usual. At the affected sites, the surviving neurons are reduced in size. These neurons have a decreased metabolic reserve and a short life span. Next to these, scarred neurons may be seen. Scarred neurons have only partially recovered from the initial infection and have a limited functional capacity (42).

Based on electrodiagnostic studies and muscle biopsy findings, it is believed that the recovery process commonly seen following poliomyelitis is a consequence of peripheral axonal sprouting. In this process, axons that belong to normal, intact or surviving neurons reinnervate the denervated muscle fibers. This eventually results in the electromyographic findings of high-voltage, long-duration polyphasic motor unit potentials and an increase in fiber density. Abnormal jitter and blocking may be found in some patients, particularly in those who have lived with polio for several decades (43–45). Electromyographic abnormalities are seen not only in weakened muscle but also in muscle that appears clinically normal.

Muscle biopsy specimens show fiber type grouping and small angular muscle fibers. This is indicative of chronic and active denervation, respectively (35). These changes appear in both affected and clinically unaffected muscles of patients with PPS or asymptomatic old polio.

The diagnosis of PPS is based on the history, physical examination, and exclusion of other disease. The accepted clinical criteria for PPS include:

1. Documented previous poliomyelitis with partial recovery.
2. A latency period of 20 to 25 years since original infection.
3. New onset weakness and fatigue (41).

Neuroimaging studies and electrodiagnostic testing are of paramount importance in order to exclude other conditions that compromise the motor unit. Normal blood panels are commonly seen, although at times the creatine kinase level is elevated. *Amyotrophic lateral sclerosis, spinal stenosis, spinal cord tumors, and peripheral neuropathies* are the principal differential diagnoses for PPS.

The management of PPS requires a good appreciation for a patient's attitude toward the disease and awareness of the resulting functional deficits. The patient must be educated about the natural history of the disease and reassured as much as possible. The importance of short rest periods interspersed between daily activities should be stressed (46). An early referral to occupational therapy for training in energy conservation techniques and adaptive equipment is important. The adverse effects and risks of decreasing levels of activity with attendant deconditioning must also be emphasized. Patients with PPS should also be referred to physical therapy. The goal of treatment is to strengthen weakened muscle and increase endurance. Physical therapists who have experience with PPS patients should be sought. A therapy program provided by athletic trainers in a sports medicine facility is bound to fail.

It is unclear whether new onset weakness results from overuse or disuse and what results can be expected from strength training. Studies that incorporate objective strength measurement can provide guidelines to the best therapeutic approach (47). Einarsson et al. conducted a study using isometric and isokinetic dynamometer measurements (Cybex II) and demonstrated that short-term (6 weeks) resistance exercise can increase knee extension peak torque by 29% for isometric strength and 24% for concentric isokinetic strength. No change was observed in the unexercised knee flexors over the study period. The study by Einarrson further demonstrated that the increase in strength translates to improved functional ability lasting up to 1 year, despite a significant increase in the fatigue index and loss of endurance over that same time period (48). The benefits of exercise were also observed in a long-term (up to 2-year follow-up) study of PPS patients placed on a regular schedule of nonfatiguing resistance exercise. In this study, muscles with a strength of grade 3/5 or more were exercised. Seventeen of 18 patients demonstrated a significant increase in strength (49). Similar benefits were observed in patients who exercised at home in a supervised program. After 12 weeks of exercise, the subjects were able to lift heavier loads, had improved endurance, and described a subjective increase in their work capacity (50). Jones et al., in a well-controlled study, demonstrated the beneficial effects of an aerobic exercise program for PPS patients. The subjects exercised three times per week for a period of 16 weeks on a stationary bicycle. Subjects exercised for 2 to 5 minutes at 70% of maximal heart rate. One-minute rest periods were provided between exercise bouts. Subjective and objective improvement was noted in the exercising subjects (51). These results have been confirmed by other researchers (47,52–54).

There is no doubt that properly prescribed and supervised exercise is of extreme importance and can lead to a substantial improvement in the quality of life for the PPS patient. *Strengthening programs should be prescribed with a focus on weak muscles with greater than fair (3/5) strength. Muscles with less than 3/5 strength should not be stressed.* An exercise program should be combined with an evaluation of, and appropriate changes in, life style. Patients should be advised to refrain from exercise at an intensity that produces muscle or joint pain or causes prolonged or excessive fatigue, and they should routinely schedule brief rest periods throughout the day.

Spinal Muscular Atrophy

Spinal muscular atrophy (SMA) is an inherited disorder resulting in the degeneration of anterior horn cells. The disease causes progressive weakness, paralysis, and muscle atrophy (55). There are several clinical expressions of the etiologic genetic deletions (see Table 61-5). These are SMA type I (Werdnig-Hoffman disease), SMA type II (intermediate or Werdnig-Hoffman disease), and SMA type III (Kugelberg-Welander disease). Some authors recognize an adult form of SMA, type IV (56).

The SMAs are inherited as autosomal recessive disorders. The probable involved chromosome is 5q11.2-13.3, between the D5S6 and MAP1B loci (57,58). The extent of gene deletion correlates with disease severity (59). The SMA type I is catastrophic. The chronic forms, type II and type III, are also severely disabling, but less rapidly so.

The ability of muscle fibers to regenerate is low in all types of SMA (59). In type I and type II SMA, denervation occurs very early, probably *in utero.* This severely impairs muscle fiber maturation. The degenerative process begins much later in type III SMA, allowing maturation of muscle fibers. Evidence for this difference between SMA type III and types I and II is the presence of developmental elements (neural cell adhesion molecule, developmental heavy-chain myosin, and the cytoskeletal components desmin and vimentin) in SMA types I and II. These are not present in type III SMA (59).

The incidence of SMA is about 20 per 100,000. The clinical expression of the disease ranges from severe generalized paralysis requiring ventilatory support at birth (type I) to mild, slowly progressive weakness presenting during the second or third decade (types III, IV) (see Table 61-5). Werdnig-Hoffman disease includes the infantile (type I) and chronic infantile (type II) SMAs. Type I SMA onset is between birth and 6 months of age. Rolling, sitting, and walk-

TABLE 61-5. *Spinal muscular atrophy*

Disease	Onset	Clinical features
SMA type I, infantile Werdnig-Hoffman	Early: birth (*in utero*) to 6 months	Contracture, generalized paralysis, early severe disability, respiratory compromise, scoliosis
SMA type II, chronic infantile Werdnig-Hoffman	Early: birth to 6 months	Contracture, scoliosis, late-onset severe disability
SMA type III, Kugelberg-Welander	Late: 2 to 17 years	Weakness in the second/third decade, late-onset severe disability
SMA type IV	Adult	Weakness in the second/third decade

SMA, spinal muscular atrophy.

ing are not achieved. In SMA type III, Kugelberg-Welander disease, the onset is between 2 and 17 years of age. Weakness begins in the distal musculature and ascends in a symmetric manner. Eighty percent of children lose ambulation before adulthood. Patients usually retain sufficient oropharyngeal muscle strength for speech, swallowing, and respiratory muscle supplementation. Intelligence is usually normal.

Although all ADL is dependent, it is possible to operate a wheelchair or environmental control equipment by joy stick, sip and puff, chin control, or infrared eye control.

The diagnosis of SMA is established by clinical presentation, deoxyribonucleic acid (DNA) testing, and electrodiagnosis. Direct DNA testing of patients for SMA is highly reliable (55). Standard electromyography (EMG) methods are often not helpful in establishing the diagnosis. Single-fiber EMG shows a marked increase in jitter and is helpful in differentiating SMA type III/IV from amyotrophic lateral sclerosis (56).

Rehabilitation during the early stages of disease includes focused stretching of the wrist flexors and intrinsic hand muscles, hip external rotators, and hip abductors. Strengthening of the wrist extensors should be done as possible. Musculotendinous contractures and scoliosis are universal in SMA types I and II. The contractures involve both upper and lower extremities.

Scoliosis (multiplanar with significant rotation) usually develops early in patients with SMA. Scoliosis may be severe in the child with the Werdnig-Hoffman variety and is usually mild early in the course of Kugelberg-Welander (type III) disease. Scoliosis may not become problematic for these patients with type III disease until adolescence. A body jacket thoracolumbar-sacral orthosis (TLSO) may be provided. When the deformity becomes too severe to manage with a TLSO, scoliosis in small children with SMA I is best managed with contoured seating systems. Because a TLSO can compromise breathing in this group of patients, a cutout over the abdomen is provided. The vital capacity is then checked with the brace both on and off. A TLSO allows more normal early vertebral growth by containing the spinal deformity until instrumentation and fusion can be done after age 6 years (60–62). Pommels and other seating modifications are inconvenient and inadequate. They do not prevent the pain, radiculopathy, ischial discomfort, or skin breakdown that occur in relation to scoliosis. Further, they may restrict sitting and leaning forward.

Patients with SMA III are provided with a TLSO while ambulatory, and surgical correction/stabilization of the curve is done once the individual becomes wheelchair bound. A rigid wheelchair molded spinal support system is often poorly tolerated as well, given the progressive nature of scoliosis. A large variety of commercially available compliant custom spinal support systems are available (63). With related pelvic obliquity, a Jay cushion provides a stable surface while accommodating the deformity, and a contoured seat with integrated arm, foot, and head rests can enhance patient comfort (64).

Pulmonary hypertension occurs and may affect the heart. Right ventricular overload occurs in about 37% of patients (65). Correct respiratory assistance and control of spinal deformity are essential to prevent pulmonary hypertension and right ventricular overload. Acute ventilatory failure can almost always be avoided for SMA types II through IV patients (see Chapter 55).

Peripheral Neuropathy

Peripheral neuropathies have many causes. It is important to identify the etiology of the disease, the pattern of peripheral nerve involvement, and the natural history of the disease. Etiologic mechanisms of peripheral nerve injury include *compression, trauma, infection, and genetic or autoimmune dysfunction*. The spatial pattern may be *generalized, proximal, distal, symmetric, or asymmetric. Sensory, motor, or mixed nerves* may be affected. Onset of the disease and temporal patterns may be *acute, chronic, or variable*. The lesion pattern involves *axon, myelin,* or the disruption of structure and function of both of these neural elements. The axon is particularly susceptible to toxic, metabolic, endocrine, or traumatic (section, traction, or compression) insults. The myelin sheath is subject to disease related to trauma and autoimmune or genetic disorders as well as to toxic or metabolic disease. Some of the diseases that affect the peripheral nerve portion of the motor unit include diabetes mellitus, HIV/AIDS, the vasculitides (nerve infarct), polyarteritis nodosa, rheumatoid arthritis, SLE, Lyme disease, Sjogren disease, cryoglobulinemia, temporal arteritis, scleroderma, sarcoidosis, leprosy, and hepatitis A.

Hereditary Peripheral Neuropathies

Hereditary peripheral neuropathies include the hereditary sensorimotor neuropathies (HSMN) (Charcot-Marie-Tooth disease [HSMN type I and II]; Dejerine-Sotas disease [HSMN type III]; Refsum disease [HSMN type IV]; HSMN types V–VII), Friedreich's ataxia, pressure-sensitive hereditary neuropathy, and various syndromes that impair structure or function of the peripheral nerve (acute intermittent porphyria, Roussy-Levy syndrome, Riley-Day syndrome, Fabry disease, Pelizaeus-Merzbacher disease).

The hereditary sensorimotor neuropathies are characterized by segmental demyelination and remyelination in the peripheral nerves. This results in marked slowing of nerve conduction. The diseases are inherited and progressive, usually at a slow rate. Large myelinated motor fibers are the most severely affected. Myelin degeneration progresses from distal to proximal segments of the involved nerve (66). This results in the clinical hallmark of these diseases: peroneal and distal leg muscle atrophy and weakness accompanied by sensory loss and areflexia (66). Atrophy and weakness occurring in the upper extremities is less striking. The different types of HSMN are all characterized by weakness, with a residual muscle force between 20% and 40%

less than normal (67). Pulmonary and cardiac abnormalities, significant spinal deformity, and severe joint contractures are unusual. Intellectual function and neuropsychological profiles are usually unremarkable (68).

Inheritance of the HSMNs may be either autosomal dominant or autosomal recessive. As with other genetic disorders, the autosomal recessive forms of the disease often carry a worse prognosis. Although most cases of HSMN type I/II are autosomal dominant, there is variable penetrance, resulting in a wide range of clinical severity. Classification of the different HMSN types is increasingly based on DNA testing. The mutations that occur affect the genes that encode myelin proteins. Several abnormalities have been identified to date. Duplication of chromosome 17p11.2 results in abnormalities of peripheral myelin protein 22 (68,69). Deletion of the same 17p11.2 chromosome results in a hereditary neuropathy with susceptibility to pressure palsies (70). Point mutation of the PO gene and defects of the connexin 32 gene (which encodes a gap junction protein) occur in X-linked forms of HSMN (71). Autosomal and X-linked dominant forms of HSMN include the HSMNs types I and II (Charcot-Marie-Tooth disease). HSMN type I may be further divided into subtypes on the basis of the genetic error: HMSN type Ia (chromosome 17), HSMN type Ib (chromosome 1) (68). Recessive forms of HSMN include HSMN type I with basal laminar onion bulbs and type I with focal myelin folds (68). HSMN type II inheritance is more heterogeneous, with a wide range of phenotype variation. Type II disease is less "hypertrophic," with more neuronal or axonal involvement than the HSMN type I (68,69,72,73).

HSMN type III, Dejerine-Sotas disease, is another inherited hypertrophic neuropathy with prominent demyelination and remyelination. "Congenital hypomyelination" of the peripheral nerve occurs, and a variable degree of neuropraxia is typical of the disease (73). Refsum disease, HSMN type IV, is characterized by altered mitochondria within the Schwann cells, and there is evidence for a similar mitochondrial abnormality in other HSMN types (74). HSMN type V is associated with spinocerebellar degeneration. HSMN type VI is associated with optic atrophy, and type VII with retinitis pigmentosa.

The HSMN types I and II (Charcot-Marie-Tooth) are the most common forms of HSMN. The prevalence of the disease is about 10 to 20 per 100,000 (75–77). The phenotypic expression is variable, and the disease is slowly progressive. As a rule the level of disability is mild.

The slowly progressive weakness is symmetric and more pronounced in the distal musculature than in proximal muscles. The distribution of sensory loss parallels that of weakness. Ankle deformities, including equinovarus, calcaneovarus, calcaneovalgus, and pes cavus, are the most common significant contractures that develop. Mild scoliosis is common, with a prevalence greater than that in the general population. Serial assessment of the curve is important, but intervention is not necessary in most cases.

HSMN type II has a particularly wide range of clinical expression, from very mild to severely disabling. In addition to the hallmark weakness, diaphragm, vocal cord, and intercostal muscle paresis has also been reported (78).

Because of the pattern of weakness and contracture, ambulation is affected and frequently complicated by falls. Rehabilitation efforts focus on maintaining a safe, effective gait. Bracing, particularly ankle–foot orthoses (AFOs), may provide sufficient improvement for restoring safe ambulation. If contracture requires surgical release, postoperative bracing with an AFO is essential. Weakness and contracture also result in equinus/cavus deformity of the feet. Adequate attention to footwear is important beyond bracing needs. A comfortable, protective shoe with adequate depth and support is essential in order to prevent pain, breakdown, and further compromise of gait by foot deformity.

Exercise in patients with HSMN is less controversial than in those with anterior horn cell or muscle disease. The possibility of over-exercise with exacerbation of the disease has not been demonstrated as it has with poliomyelitis (79). Strength training can be effective, particularly for the proximal muscles of the lower extremities.

Autoimmune Peripheral Neuropathies

Acute inflammatory demyelinating polyneuropathy (AIDP, Guillain-Barré syndrome) is a postinfections demyelination of the peripheral nerve. There is breakdown of the blood–nerve barrier and segmental, macrophage-mediated (cell mediated and humoral immune reactions) damage to the myelin sheath. Inflammation and subsequent demyelination also result in varying degrees of axonal degeneration. Conduction block (neuropraxia) is prominent.

Sixty-seven percent of patients with Guillain-Barré syndrome have a history of preceding viral infection, immunization, surgery, or a disease affecting the immune system (80). The clinical presentation of AIDP is that of acute onset weakness, hypotonia, and areflexia (81). The weakness is progressive and involves the extremities. Bulbar and facial musculature may also be affected. Autonomic dysfunction and sensory symptoms are usually mild (80), although primary sensory forms of the disease have been described. Autonomic dysfunction and respiratory failure may occur. Respiratory failure is noted in up to 20% or 30% of cases by 1 to 2 weeks following disease onset. Recovery usually occurs within 3 to 6 months but may take up to 12 to 18 months. Residual weakness, which is usually mild, is common.

A more benign variant of AIDP, the *Miller-Fisher syndrome*, is managed in the same manner as Guillain-Barré syndrome (82). The natural history of AIDP in children is also more benign, with a more rapid recovery, than adult Guillain-Barré syndrome (83). One-quarter of children lose the ability to walk, and 16% will require ventilatory support. The median time to recovery for children is 17 days for the start of clinical improvement. There is a median time of 37 days to independent ambulation and 66 days to full recovery. The best prognostic indicator is the degree to which the child is disabled at the height of illness (83).

Severe slowing of nerve conduction is present in AIDP. Electrodiagnostic studies, including evoked potentials and F waves, are valuable. Nerve conduction studies of the motor nerve show prolongation of the distal latency and negative peak duration. Temporal dispersion is a prominent feature of nerve conduction studies (84). Analysis of the cerebrospinal fluid (CSF) is important for establishing the diagnosis. The CSF protein is increased, and the cellular content is minimal.

The medical management of AIDP includes high-dose immunoglobulins and plasmapheresis (85–87). Plasmapheresis is especially helpful to reduce the duration of paralysis and intubation in severe cases (86). The CSF filtration of antibody complexes has been reported as useful in cases that are unresponsive to IgG or plasmapheresis (85). Steroids have no proven efficacy.

Rehabilitation management of AIDP is geared to the prevention of contractures, skin breakdown, pneumonia, and depression. During the acute phase of the disease, communication devices and means to facilitate bed mobility, such as a trapeze or bed rails, are helpful.

Because AIDP presents with evolving weakness, strengthening, bracing, adaptive equipment and vocational retraining are not appropriate until the clinical findings have stabilized and there is a static motor deficit. Retraining for ADLs and wheelchair or ambulation training may or may not be necessary, depending on the residual impairment and disability.

Chronic inflammatory demyelinating polyneuropathy (CIDP) is a T-cell-mediated autoimmune peripheral neuropathy. It involves motor and sensory nerves, with the most significant disability resulting from weakness.

Demyelination results in weakness or plegia. Deep tendon reflexes are absent, delayed, or prolonged (88). Cramps and fasciculations, commonly in the upper extremities, may be the primary expression of the disease (89).

Chronic, asymmetric, multifocal nerve conduction blocks are prominent on nerve conduction studies. These are very characteristic of CIDP (89,90). The differential diagnosis of CIDP includes *hereditary sensorimotor neuropathy and amyotrophic lateral sclerosis*. The differentiating histologic changes characteristic of CIDP include mononuclear cell infiltrates, prominent endoneurial edema, and wide interfascicle variability. This neuropathy may be associated with malignancy, particularly with melanoma. This association most likely relates to shared immunoreactivity with common surface antigens present in the melanoma and in the myelin sheath (91).

The medical treatment of CIDP includes high-dose intravenous immunoglobulins or immunosuppressive drugs. Treatment with steroids is probably not effective (86,92). Rehabilitation interventions relate to the clinical deficits and are necessarily patient specific.

Critical illness polyneuropathy (CIP) is a frequent cause of failure to wean from mechanical ventilator support (93,94). Up to 70% of patients will develop a polyneuropathy of motor or mixed nerves following sepsis, multisystem organ failure, the systemic inflammatory response syndrome, or high fever (93,95–100). Of these patients, about 30% will be symptomatic. The clinical findings in CIP are often confused by the primary medical condition, the use of steroids or neuromuscular blocking agents, or concomitant compression neuropathies. For this reason, electrodiagnostic studies are key in the diagnosis of CIP. The differential diagnosis also includes critical illness-associated transient neuromuscular blockade, thick-filament myopathy, or necrotizing myopathy (95).

The pathogenesis of CIP is poorly understood, but the pathology is well described. There is chronic nerve injury characterized by noninflammatory axonal degeneration and resulting neurogenic atrophy of muscle (93). This process occurs predominantly in distal motor fibers (100), although there is often striking weakness of the proximal musculature (93). Sensory fibers are usually uninvolved or minimally affected (95,101).

There is some suggestion that monitoring repetitive nerve conduction studies may be useful in order to titrate the dose of neuromuscular blocking agents and avoid overdosing and iatrogenic weakness (102). High-dose intravenous steroids have also been implicated in the production of the polyneuropathy and myopathy associated with critical illness.

The most common presentation of CIP is failure to wean from mechanical ventilation. Physical examination reveals generalized, moderate to severe weakness in all limbs, with notable muscle atrophy. Paraspinal and facial muscles may also be affected. Weakness is most striking in the proximal limb muscles, although if there is residual weakness after recovery, it is most common in a peroneal nerve distribution (93). Changes in deep tendon reflexes are inconsistent and may be normal, increased, or decreased. Serum creatine kinase levels are also helpful in following the course of the disease.

There is a relatively wide range of reported recovery times from CIP. Rapid recovery, recovery in 3 to 6 weeks, and recovery in 4 to 6 months have been reported in the literature (99,101). The prognosis is good, providing the patient survives the precipitating critical illness.

Rehabilitation efforts for patients with CIP focus on monitoring the evolution of the polyneuropathy and preventing decubitus ulceration, contractures, and compression neuropathies. Strengthening exercise, mobility, and ADL retraining, and provision of orthotics and adaptive equipment should be provided at appropriate stages of recovery.

Other diseases that affect the function of peripheral nerves include benign monoclonal gammopathy (IgG, IgA, or IgM), chronic liver or pulmonary disease, cryoglobulinemia, giant-cell arteritis, gout, necrotizing angiopathy, and various malignancies such as lymphoma, multiple myeloma, bronchogenic carcinoma, ovarian, testicular, penile, gastric, oral cavity, or meningeal cancer, oat-cell carcinoma, and osteosclerotic myeloma.

Metabolic/Endocrine Peripheral Neuropathies

Metabolic disease may result in peripheral neuropathy. Nutritional deficiencies, endocrine disease, and toxin exposure preferentially affect the peripheral nerve axon. Nutritional deficiencies such as *beriberi or pellagra* (B_1, *thiamine*), *riboflavin* (B_2), *pyridoxine* (B_6), *pernicious anemia* (B_{12}), *and protein or calorie deficiency* result in axonal dysfunction. *Diabetes mellitus and thyroid and parathyroid disease* also result in axonal derangement. Toxic causes of peripheral neuropathy include organic and inorganic toxins and heavy metals.

Many metabolic and toxic peripheral neuropathies resolve with appropriate treatment. It is important to identify and remove the inciting agent or to correct a nutritional deficiency. Many therapeutic drugs, environmental pollutants, industrial solvents, and other workplace chemicals are neurotoxic. Peripheral neuropathy is one of the most common responses of the nervous system to chemical attack (103). Most toxins produce distal axonal degeneration in long peripheral nerves and spinal tracts. Several toxic agents damage the nerve directly or induce primary demyelination (103). Therapeutic drugs may provoke a peripheral neuropathy. Amiodarone, chloramphenicol, corticosteroids, dapsone, diphenylhydantoin (phenytoin), disulfiram, nitrofurantoin, pyridoxine, sodium cyanate, tetanus toxoid, and thalidomide have been reported to be neurotoxic. Organic compounds that are toxic to the peripheral nerve include acrylamide, carbon disulfide, dichlorophenoxyacetic acid, ethyl alcohol, ethylene oxide, methylbutyl ketone, and triorthocresyl phosphate. Heavy metals that can damage the motor unit include antimony, arsenic, gold, lead, mercury, and thallium.

Toxic peripheral neuropathies typically present with a glove and stocking distribution of sensory loss. This is followed by weakness in the same distribution. The disease becomes evident within weeks of exposure to a toxin, although the presentation may be protracted and insidious for neuropathy caused by nutritional deficiency or endocrinopathy. Recovery often occurs over the subsequent several months to years following appropriate treatment (103).

Diabetic neuropathy may be expressed as a mononeuropathy/mononeuritis multiplex, a distal symmetric or proximal symmetric neuropathy, polyrodiculopathy autonomic neuropathy, or a painful peripheral neuropathy. Diabetic neuropathy affects 5% to 50% of diabetics in the United States. The incidence of the peripheral neuropathy increases with increasing age, duration of diabetes, and mean serum glucose (104). There is evidence that endoneurial and epineurial lymphocyte infiltration contributes to the pathogenesis of diabetic neuropathy (105).

Strict control of serum glucose will limit the development or progression of diabetic neuropathy. There is also increasing evidence that antioxidant therapy, aldose reductase inhibitors, and gamma-linolenic acid may also play a role in ameliorating, preventing, or halting progression of this diabetic complication (106).

The most common symptoms of diabetic neuropathy include paresthesias, in the feet, ankles, and calves. These are usually described as tingling or burning sensations. The involvement of motor nerves results in a shift in the locus of postural control from the ankle to the hip (107). Autonomic neuropathy causes arteriovenous shunting and tissue hypoxia in the feet as well as other organ systems (106). Pain, restless leg syndrome, skin breakdown, ulceration, and amputation are other complications of diabetic peripheral neuropathy.

It is essential to thoroughly educate the patient regarding footwear, foot care, and the need to maintain adequate control of serum glucose. Shoes should be wide and deep and oxford (Blucher) style. Shoe orthotics may be added if foot deformity or dynamic insufficiency caused by intrinsic muscle weakness is present. Pain may be managed with tricyclic antidepressants, topical application of capsaicin, and, less commonly, membrane-stabilizing agents, counter-irritants, transcutaneous nerve stimulation, antihistamines, and other analgesics.

Infectious Peripheral Neuropathy

The peripheral nerve portion of the motor unit is susceptible to damage following infection. The most common diseases that can involve the motor unit by peripheral nerve derangement include infection with *human immunodeficiency virus (HIV), cytomegalovirus, herpes zoster, diphtheria, leprosy, and rabies.*

HIV-related peripheral neuropathies are becoming better described and understood. Patterns of peripheral nerve involvement include *AIDP, CIDP, mononeuritis multiplex, lumbar polyradiculopathy, and lymphomatous neuropathy.* Other forms of peripheral nerve dysfunction occur that do not directly involve the motor unit (*autonomic, distal sensory, and ataxic neuropathies*) (108).

Treatment of the infectious neuropathies requires treatment of the concurrent infection. Appropriate antibiotic or antiviral agents should be prescribed. Hyperbaric O_2 has been proposed as an effective intervention to salvage peripheral nerve fibers from ischemic degeneration (109) following toxic or antibody-mediated damage.

Rehabilitation management is directed toward disease remission, improving or compensating for weakness, and maintaining independent function. Thus, depending on the constellation of clinical findings, exercise (including progressive resistance isotonic, isokinetic, or isoinertial strengthening), and stretching, splinting, and/or adaptive equipment may be components of the rehabilitation prescription.

Entrapment Neuropathies

Compressive lesions of a peripheral nerve affect the function of the corresponding motor units. These lesions are discussed in greater detail elsewhere in this text. Common sites of entrapment include the carpal tunnel, pronator teres, and ligament of Struthers for the median nerve; the olecranon groove/cubital tunnel, or Guyon's canal (ulnar nerve); humeral groove (radial nerve); and, in the lower extremities, at the lanciniate ligament (tarsal tunnel–tibial nerve) or fibular head (peroneal nerve). Compression neuropathy is less often recognized in the lower extremities but may be common (110) (see Fig. 61-7A–D).

Many disease states affect the fluid volume and pressure in fascial compartments. The compliance of compartment ''walls'' may also be affected by disease, generally becoming more rigid. Problems that predispose a peripheral nerve to entrapment include greater pressure within a contained site (for example, fluid retention before menses), rigid containment (carpal tunnel borders, tendon thickening/edema from overuse), a pathologic increase in nerve caliber (edema or hypertrophic remyelination), or the presence of anomalous objects in a common, confined space (foreign body, accessory muscle, orthopedic hardware, callus, or bone spur). In these instances, surgical release/removal is indicated when symptoms fail to respond to conservative care. Relative rest (splinting, positioning, taping), nonsteroidal antiinflammatory medication, massage (edema-reducing or fascial release), icing, and local injection of steroid are among the conservative treatment options for entrapment neuropathies.

Diseases of the Myoneural Junction

The most common diseases that affect the neuromuscular junction include myasthenia gravis, Eaton-Lambert syndrome, botulism, and tick paralysis. Pathologic mechanisms for these disorders include autoimmune disease, chromosomal defects, and exposure to such agents as organophosphates or botulinum toxin. The clinical presentation of the disease relates to the pathophysiology of the disease. It is important to distinguish presynaptic dysfunction in acetylcholine packaging and release from postsynaptic dysfunction in which there are impaired or insufficient acetylcholine receptors. Recognizing the site of lesion identifies the pathophysiology, and this is the first step in setting goals and determining medical and rehabilitation management (111).

Weakness and fatigue that fluctuate in relation to activity are the prominent symptoms. Diagnostic studies are useful to supplement the clinical examination. The most appropriate tests include single-fiber EMG, repetitive motor nerve stimulation, and biopsy with cytochemical studies of the neuromuscular junction.

Medical intervention is directed to the normalization of neurotransmission at the motor end plate. Identification and treatment of any associated malignancy or disease process is important.

Rehabilitation strategies focus on patient education and self-management. Energy conservation, including motion economy and posture optimization, are important. Adaptive equipment, particularly assistive devices for ADL activities and mobility aids such as a motorized scooter, may prove helpful. Appropriate timing of activities is important, as there is often a predictable temporal pattern of fatigue for many of these patients.

These diseases are frequently severely disabling or life threatening without intervention. Fortunately, at this time, most are treatable (112).

Myasthenia Gravis

Myasthenia gravis is a chronic autoimmune disease. The course of the disease begins with a transient inflammatory phase. This is followed by the degeneration of the neuromuscular junction (113). Myasthenic antibodies are produced which target the postsynaptic receptors. This results in the loss of active motor endplate receptor sites. Receptor inactivation leads to a compensatory increase in acetylcholine release (114), although this is insufficient to normalize neuromuscular junction transmission.

The prevalence of myasthenia gravis is about 1/10,000 (115). Women are affected twice as often as men. The disease usually presents with sudden weakness, but the onset may be insidious. Postexertional muscle weakness is the clinical hallmark of myasthenia. Weakness follows repetitive movement, prolonged static muscle tension, or forceful gross movement. Strength fluctuations that correspond to the time of day may be observed. Severe bulbar/respiratory muscle weakness may occur, as can ocular myasthenia. Following rest, neuromuscular transmission recovers.

The diagnosis of myasthenia gravis is often delayed up to 2 years and is most often confirmed around the age of 20 years (115). In the generalized and bulbar forms of the disease, interleukin-2 receptor titers are significantly increased. This is not the case for ocular myasthenia. The increase in interleukin-2 receptor levels seems to correspond to progression of the disease. Anti-acetylcholine receptor antibodies can also be isolated, but these do not correspond to disease activity (116). Electrodiagnostic studies show characteristic jitter and decremental amplitude response on repetitive stimulation of the nerve. The amplitude of the motor response during repetitive supramaximal stimulation will fall more than 20% within a train of five stimulations.

A good scale for evaluating disability and the daily frequency of symptoms in myasthenia gravis was developed by D'Alessandro et al. (117). This scale is useful for rehabilitation assessment and to follow treatment response. The D'Alessandro scale identifies significant functional impairment and temporal patterns of activity and weakness.

Myasthenia gravis responds well to corticosteroid therapy, immunosuppressive drugs, anticholinesterase administration, and plasmapheresis. Pulsed intravenous steroid infusion and intravenous administration of immunoglobulins are most frequently used, often in combination therapy (118). Combination therapy should be instituted during respiratory crisis, when preparing for thymectomy or postthymectomy, and during old age when a crisis-prone state is common (118). Treatment with ephedrine may provide a transient improvement in muscle strength from enhanced arousal (119). Patients who fail to respond to other interventions may be treated by immunoadsorption therapy. This de-

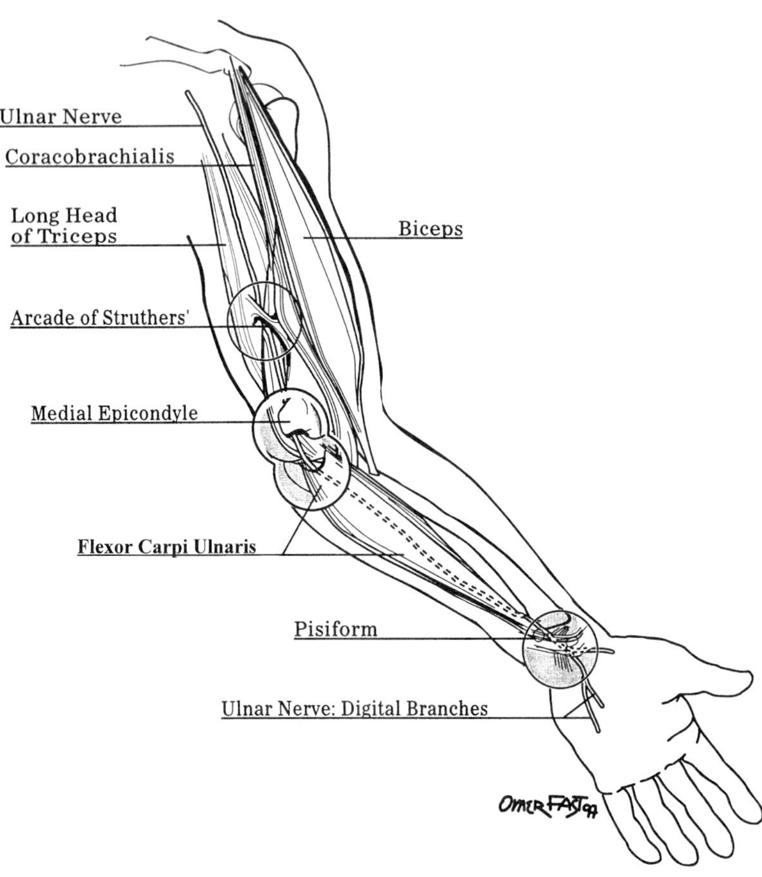

FIG. 61-7. A–D: Peripheral nerve entrapments: **A:** sites of ulnar nerve entrapment.

creases circulating acetylcholine receptor antibodies (120) and has been reported to be successful in recalcitrant cases.

Prompt attention to any change in respiratory function is a critical part of the myasthenic patient's care. Immunization against influenza and pneumococcus should be provided on a routine basis. Aggressive treatment of upper respiratory tract infections is important. Note that erythromycin and azithromycin have been reported to exacerbate myasthenia gravis (121).

Rehabilitation strategies emphasize patient education, timing activity, and providing adaptive equipment and assistive devices. Exercise is not useful. Patients generally do well with minimal equipment if adequate medical treatment of the disease is provided.

Eaton-Lambert syndrome, which is a presynaptic disease, frequently occurs in association with malignancy. Rehabilitation in these patients with weakness often requires identification, treatment, and rehabilitation of the associated condition.

In botulism there is a presynaptic failure to release acetylcholine following exposure to one of seven botulinum neurotoxin serotypes. Hypotonia and weakness occur, but botulism has a highly variable course. One-third of cases fall into each of the mild, moderate, or severe categories of disease state. Botulism is rarely fatal (122).

The clostridial neurotoxin blocks neurotransmitter release. The toxin is a metalloprotease that prevents the zinc-dependent protein cleavage needed for neuroexocytosis of the packaged acetylcholine (123). An experimental vaccine, suitable for human protection against botulism, has recently been developed (124).

Clostridium botulinum, the organism responsible for elaborating the neurotoxin, has been isolated from foods that cause botulism outbreaks. Recently this has included canned peppers, roasted eggplant, beef stew, home-cured ham, and sausage (122).

Tick paralysis remains primarily a veterinary disease but has been reported in humans living in the United States from Long Island to Washington State (125). Tick paralysis is an acute ascending (flaccid) motor paralysis directly resulting from toxin exposure. It is not caused by *Borrelia burgdorferi* as is Lyme disease. Tick species that have been reported to cause paralysis include *Ixodes brunneus, rubicundus,* and *scapularis.* Identification and removal of the tick are essential for successful management of the disease. Recovery is generally complete, and rehabilitation focuses on regaining strength and endurance.

The differential diagnosis of tick paralysis includes AIDP, botulism, and myasthenia gravis or myasthenic syndromes such as Eaton-Lambert.

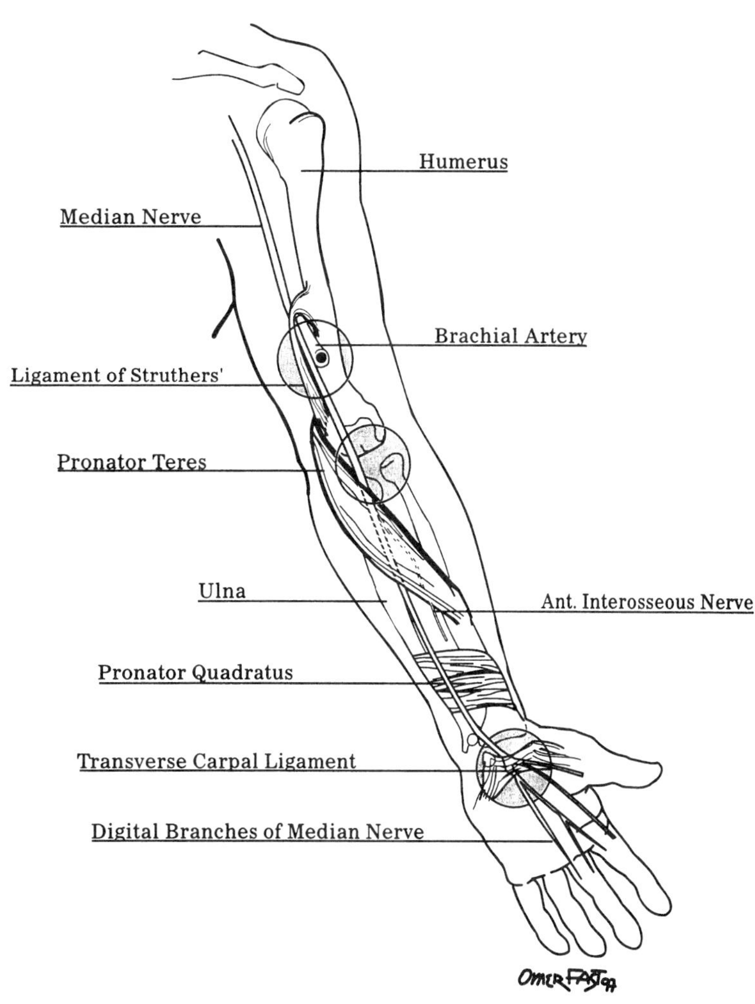

FIG. 61-7. *Continued.* **B:** Sites of median nerve entrapment.

Myopathy

Myopathy results from any biochemical, electrical, or other pathologic change occurring in muscle fibers or the connective tissue of muscle. Further, the pathology is not a result of nervous system dysfunction (126). Myopathy may result from a genetic abnormality (the muscular dystrophies, metabolic myopathies, other congenital myopathies), infection, autoimmune disease, or exposure to a toxic agent (see Table 61-6).

Fiber type disproportion (type II muscle fiber predominance) and nemaline rod and myotubular or centronuclear myopathies are congenital. They are inherited by both autosomal dominant and recessive means. Affected infants present at birth as a ''floppy baby.'' Congenital myopathies are characterized by generalized weakness, and a mild scoliosis may be evident.

Metabolic myopathies are autosomal recessive. They result from the absence or abnormal function of a specific enzyme system. These diseases include the *glycogen storage diseases, myopathy resulting from biochemical defects in carbohydrate or lipid metabolism, and mitochondrial abnormalities* that result in muscle dysfunction. Patients present with fatigue, muscle cramps, and weakness. Exercise intolerance is frequently noted. Contractures are rare. Associated findings include hemolysis, gout, jaundice, reticulocytosis, nausea/vomiting (phosphofructokinase deficiency), hepatomegaly (debranching enzyme deficiency), and myoglobinuria (McArdle's disease).

Laboratory studies are consistent with abnormal muscle metabolism. Serum creatine kinase (CK) is elevated, and myoglobinuria may be present. Electromyography reveals a characteristic ''myopathic'' pattern of low amplitude, early recruitment, and a full interference pattern on maximal contraction. The definitive diagnosis is established by muscle biopsy.

Endocrine myopathies typically present with proximal weakness. Generally shoulder weakness presents before hip muscle weakness except for myopathy secondary to steroid medications or hyperparathyroidism. In these instances, the hip muscle weakness may precede the weakness of the shoulder musculature. A diagnosis is made on the basis of history, findings on physical examination that are associated with

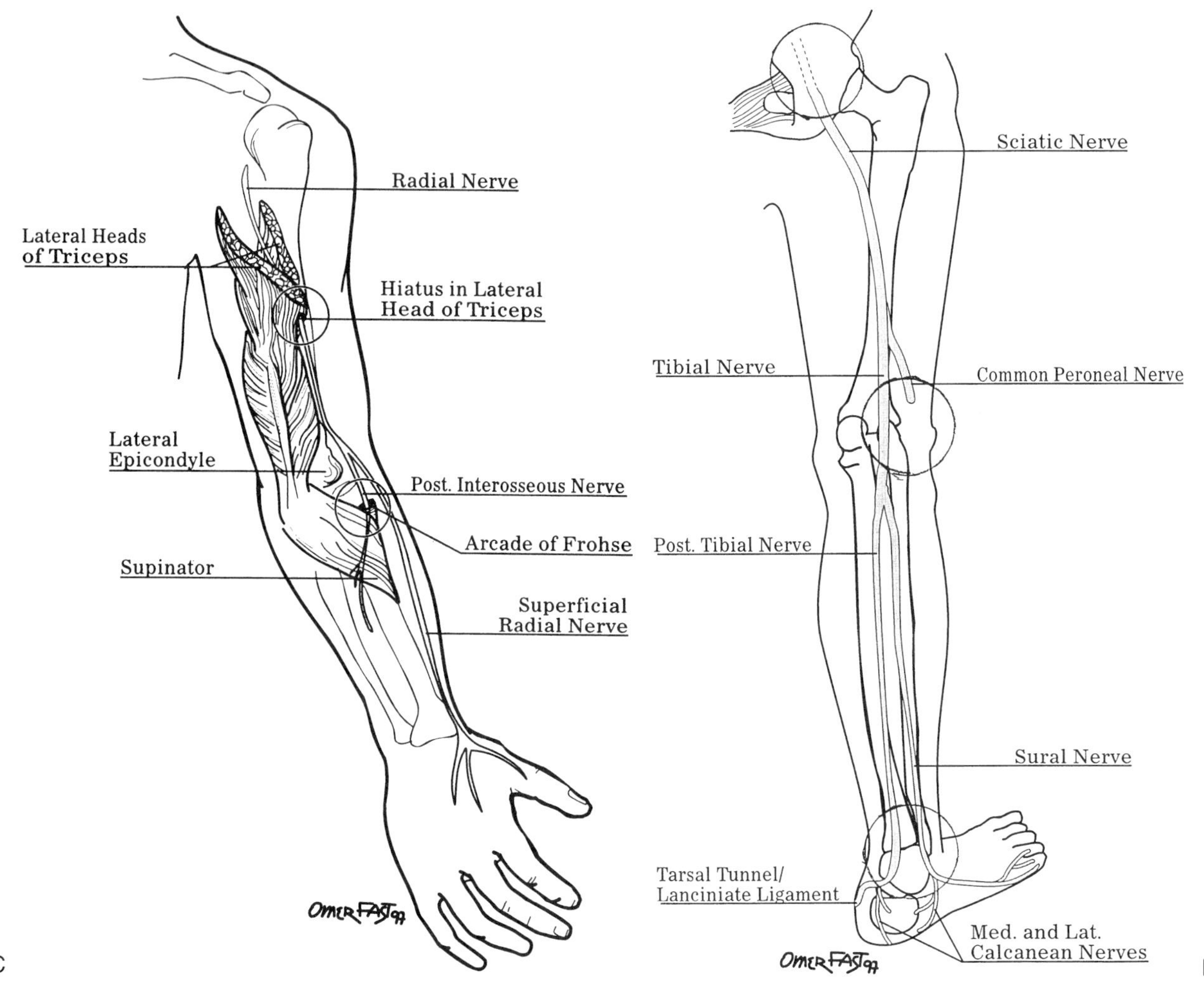

FIG. 61-7. *Continued.* **C:** Sites of radial nerve entrapment. **D:** Sites of peripheral nerve entrapment in the lower extremes.

the specific endocrinopathy, a ''myopathic pattern'' on electromyography, and abnormal blood chemistries.

Inflammatory Myopathy

Polymyositis is the most common form of inflammatory myopathy. It is more common in women than men. The progression of the disease may be rapid, but when slowly progressive it must be differentiated from limb-girdle muscular dystrophy (127). Spontaneous remission may occur. Neck and symmetric proximal muscle weakness is the clinical hallmark of the disease. Muscle atrophy is not severe. Skin abnormalities or other evidence of collagen vascular disease is generally present. Serum CK levels are elevated while the disease is active. Electromyographic evidence of myopathy, as well as fibrillation potentials, positive sharp waves, and high-frequency discharges are noted.

Dermatomyositis-related myopathy is essentially indistinguishable from the myopathy related to polymyositis. The course may be acute or subacute, and there is a somewhat higher association with neoplasm, vasculitis, or other collagen vascular disorder, than is the case with polymyositis.

The usual treatment for dermatomyositis or polymyositis myopathy is corticosteroid therapy and/or immunosuppressive agents. Such treatment may halt and even reverse the muscle weakness.

Muscular Dystrophy

The muscular dystrophies are inherited diseases characterized by progressive myopathy. Ongoing muscle degeneration and regeneration can be observed in biopsy specimens (127).

The Xp21-linked muscular dystrophies are Duchenne (DMD) and Becker (BMD) muscular dystrophy. These sex-linked recessive disorders result from a deletion in the p21 region of the short arm of the X chromosome (128,129). One-third of cases are caused by spontaneous mutation, two-thirds are born to carriers, and one-third of cases have an affected family member. The involved gene encodes the protein dystrophin. Dystrophin is located on the inner surface of the muscle cell membrane in close association with sarcolemmal glycoproteins (130). Skeletal and cardiac muscle normally contain significant quantities of dystrophin. This protein is also usually present to a lesser extent in smooth muscle, brain, lung, and skin fibroblasts (131). Dystrophin deficiency is associated with breaks in the sarcolemma and affects stretch-activated cation channels. This causes intracellular calcium accumulation (132). The deficiency most prominently impairs fast muscle fiber (type IIB) function (133,134).

Duchenne muscular dystrophy has an incidence between 25 and 33 per 100,000 male births (135–138). The diagnosis of DMD is often delayed. It is made on the basis of clinical presentation, family history, and carrier analysis. Seventy percent of carriers have serum muscle enzyme elevation between two and five times normal (139). Up to 8% of carriers have physical evidence of muscular dystrophy or cardiomyopathy (139,140). Appropriate enzyme assays for suspected patients and carriers include carbonic anhydrase II, pyruvate kinase, and lactate dehydrogenase (139,141). Other diagnostic testing includes quantitative EMG (142,143), electrocardiography, vectorcardiography (144), and DNA analysis. DNA analysis is the procedure of choice for detecting carriers or for establishing a prenatal diagnosis of DMD (145).

Children with DMD present before the age of 4 with clumsiness, poor walking, and frequent falls because of weakness. Significant muscle mass is lost by the age of 4 to 5 years, with a significant corresponding functional loss by age 7.5 years. After this age, 75% of children experience a measurable decline in function each subsequent year (146,147). There is calf pseudohypertrophy from fatty infiltration of the muscle. Weakness, atrophy, and joint contracture occur in a symmetric pattern.

Thirty-five percent of children walk by age 15 months, and 50% ambulate by age 18 months (148). There is no correlation between late walking and the speed at which disease progression occurs, although there is a correlation between the duration of independent function and the quantity of dystrophin present in muscle (149). Gower's sign, where children "climb" up their thighs and hips in order to compensate for quadriceps muscle weakness in order to stand, is invariably present. Gait is characterized by loss of heel-to-toe progression. Children with DMD are unable to run. Without aggressive intervention, the average age of wheelchair dependence is 8.6 to 9.5 years (150–154).

There are a wide range of abnormalities evident in DMD and BMD because of the systemic distribution of dystrophin. Reduced or dysfunctional dystrophin results in impaired cellular adhesiveness and metabolic and membrane abnormalities. Systemic involvement in DMD is evidenced by *increased head circumference* (155), *growth retardation and short stature* (156), *central nervous system neuropathology* (157–159), *cognitive impairment* (including IQ deficit and difficulties with abstraction, orientation, and spatial manipulation) (46,158), *decreased gastrointestinal motility* (160), and *abnormal blood flow patterns* as a result of abnormalities in vascular endothelial cells and platelet function (161).

Thirty percent of children with DMD develop scoliosis while they are still ambulatory. Scoliosis becomes much more problematic following wheelchair confinement. Unless treated, 90% of children will have a progressive scoliotic curve, which often exceeds 50° by the age of 16 years (162,163). Severe scoliosis may further compromise already impaired pulmonary and cardiac function, and it certainly contributes to cosmetic and psychosocial morbidity. Unfortunately, correction of the spinal curvature results in fixation of the rib cage, which further decreases vital capacity. Vital capacity decreases 4% for each 10° of thoracic scoliosis for patients with idiopathic scoliosis, and it decreases by 5% to 10% each year from the vital capacity plateau for patients with DMD (164). Wheelchair seating modification or thoracolumbar bracing does not affect the ultimate degree of curvature and should be avoided (165–168). Their use postpones effective surgical intervention (Luque instrumentation

TABLE 61-6. *Classification of myopathies by etiology*

Etiology	Myopathy
Endocrine	Hyperthyroidism Hypothyroid myopathy Hyperparathyroidism Corticosteroid myopathy
Inflammatory myopathy	Polymyositis Dermatomyositis Sarcoidosis
Infectious myopathy	Trichinosis Cysticercosis HIV/AIDS
Toxic myopathies	Alcoholic myopathy, acute and chronic forms Medication-related
Congenital	
Muscular dystrophy	Xp21-linked Duchenne muscular dystrophy Becker muscular dystrophy) Limb-girdle muscular dystrophy Fascioscapulohumeral muscular dystrophy Myotonic muscular dystrophy Emery-Dreifuss muscular dystrophy
Structural myopathies	Central core disease Nemaline rod myopathy Myotubular (centronuclear) myopathy Congenital fiber disproportion
Metabolic myopathies	Glycogenoses Muscle phosphorylase deficiency (type V, McArdle disease) Phosphofructokinase deficiency (type VII) Acid maltase deficiency (type II, infantile, Pompe disease) Debranching enzyme deficiency (type II)

HIV/AIDS, human immunodeficiency virus/ acquired immunodeficiency syndrome.

and variations of segmental wiring) (168), possibly to the point at which pulmonary function may no longer be adequate. The vital capacity should be evaluated every 6 months, and surgical intervention is recommended for even mild curves when there is a consistently low plateau vital capacity (169–172). Some investigators recommend prophylactic surgical fixation of the spine for all DMD patients (173). All DMD patients who have a vital capacity consistently below 1,500 ml should undergo surgical correction of scoliosis soon after they become wheelchair dependent. When vital capacity plateaus between 1,500 and 1,800 ml, a curve of 20° to 40° is an indication for surgery. When the vital capacity is consistently better than 1,800 ml, surgical intervention can be delayed until the curve reaches or exceeds 40°. New and safer surgical methods and hardware are continuously being developed, with a decrease in the incidence of hardware failure and other postoperative complications.

Fifty-five to ninety percent of patients with DMD die from complications of restrictive pulmonary syndrome and chronic alveolar hypoventilation (CAH). Chronic alveolar hypoventilation with resultant hypercarbia causes irritability, daytime somnolence, morning headaches, nausea, restless sleep, palpitations, dysphoria, and decreased energy. Death in patients with DMD usually occurs between the ages of 16.2 and 19 years (174–176). Recurrent pneumonia, intubation, and tracheostomy are common (177) despite being preventable.

Another significant cause of morbidity and death in patients with muscular dystrophy and other myopathies is cardiomyopathy (178). There is little correlation between the variables of severity of cardiac involvement, skeletal muscle weakness, and the degree of vital capacity and respiratory status impairment (179). Cardiac function in patients with DMD should be assessed with echocardiography or a MUGA scan and Holter monitor testing on a regular basis (180). A trial of captopril or hydralazine to treat congestive heart failure and/or severely decreased ventricular function (ejection fraction 20%) may allow some improvement in cardiac function and activity endurance. Patients with severe left ventricular function may develop mural thrombus and embolic complications. This is managed with anticoagulation. In addition, cor pulmonale and right ventricular failure are common (178,181).

Patients with DMD have delayed gastric emptying, up to three times longer than normal (182). This can result in complaints of malaise, anxiety, epigastric pain, and effortless vomiting. Acute episodes of gastric and intestinal distension, abdominal tenderness, vomiting, diarrhea, and tachycardia occur. There may be resultant dehydration, poor diaphragmatic excursion, and ventilatory compromise. Ultimately this can lead to acute congestive heart failure (183–186). Intestinal obstruction, malabsorption, and volvulus can also result in shock and cardiopulmonary arrest (187). Complaints of difficulty swallowing, choking, and heartburn increase in frequency as the patient with DMD ages (188). Dysphagia may result from orthodontic deformities, masticatory and pharyngeal muscle weakness, or a delay in bolus transit at the esophagogastric junction. Hypocontractility of the gallbladder may lead to cholelithiasis (189).

Most children with DMD are developmentally delayed in locomotor and language areas (190). Deficits include verbal comprehension, expressive language, and locomotor function (191–193). The resulting dyslexic pattern of developmental delay is significant in about one-half of all children with DMD (192). Another cognitive problem that may occur in patients with DMD is short-term memory impairment (193).

Rehabilitation intervention should be very aggressive. The focus of treatment is to maintain mobility, minimize contracture, and prolong the stage of independent function. Exercise may be appropriate, but the exercise prescription must explicitly avoid the possibly of overwork weakness.

Management of the pulmonary system includes education in glossopharyngeal breathing, intermittent positive-pressure breathing, and manually and mechanically assisted coughing. Prevention of chronic alveolar hypoventilation with the use of inspiratory muscle aids will prevent or correct hypercarbia and can reverse cor pulmonale and right ventricular failure. Assistance is provided when the patient becomes symptomatic from hypercarbia or demonstrates airway congestion during respiratory infections. Positive-pressure ventilation may be provided by an exsufflation belt or intermittent positive-pressure ventilation through mouth, nasal, or tracheostomy access. Note that intermittent abdominal pressure ventilation can effectively ventilate patients with little or no vital capacity, but it is not effective in the presence of significant scoliosis (194). Negative-pressure ventilators can also be used. These include the iron lung, portalung, negative-pressure wrap, rocking bed, and cuirass. The importance of supplementing respiratory muscle function is underscored by the correlation between vital capacity and life span. Vaccination in order to avoid infections by *Hemophilus influenzae* and pneumococcus should be a routine part of the care of DMD patients.

Becker muscular dystrophy occurs with an incidence of 4/100,000. It is usually diagnosed between the ages of 5 and 25 years. The genetics, evaluation, and management principles are similar to those for the patient with DMD but must appropriately correspond to the significantly milder course of the disease. Ambulation is not lost until about 20 years after clinical onset of weakness. Significant contracture, scoliosis, and ventilatory failure are uncommon among patients with BMD. The life span is usually normal unless severe cardiomyopathy is present.

The limb-girdle dystrophies include Landouzy-Dejerine disease, fascioscapulohumeral, scapuloperoneal, hereditary distal, and quadriceps muscular dystrophies. Limb-girdle muscular dystrophy is usually inherited as an autosomal recessive disease. The most frequent onset of symptoms is seen in the second or third decade. The disease does not appear before the age of 6 years. There is a wide variation in severity, but the clinical hallmark of the disease is shoulder and pelvic girdle muscular weakness. True calf hypertrophy can occur. Severe disability relating to weakness, muscular contracture, and skeletal deformities is commonly present 20 years after onset. Life span is shortened unless aggressive cardiopulmonary management is provided.

The proximal muscle weakness in the limb girdle muscular dystrophies makes moving the shoulder and elbow difficult. Patients tend to use trunk flexion to substitute for weak shoulder agonists. Many will use stationary surfaces or objects as levers for the forearm or use fingers to ''crawl'' up the opposite arm in order to effect movement at the elbow or shoulder.

If elbow flexor strength is at least poor, the use of overhead slings, counterweights, and motorized systems of arm suspension (195), or the use of a ball-bearing forearm orthosis or mobile arm support (196), will facilitate self-feeding and other ADL activities (195,196).

Fascioscapulohumeral dystrophy (FSH) may be inherited through an autosomal recessive or autosomal dominant mechanism. There are adult, juvenile, and infantile forms of FSH (197). Muscular hypertrophy and skeletal deformity are relatively rare and relate to the degree of weakness. The distribution of affected muscles is similar to that in other limb-girdle dystrophies except for the equal involvement of facial muscles. Patients may become unable to close their eyes. Speech may be indistinct, and smiling or whistling impossible. Anterior tibial muscle weakness is common.

Further rehabilitation of the patient with FSH dystrophy includes the provision of assistive devices to facilitate eating and drinking. Saline eye drops to combat scleral drying from weak eye closure should also be provided.

Surgical management for FSH or limb-girdle muscular dystrophy is directed toward improvement in mouth function and scapular stabilization to improve glenohumeral abduction. Patients with FSH can also use scapular fixing orthoses to prevent winging. This permits arm abduction and flexion beyond 90°. Note that for all patients with motor unit disease characterized by shoulder weakness, assistance in transfers should not be provided by lifting at the axillae or shoulders. A transfer board may be useful if the patient's residual strength is adequate.

Emery-Dreifuss is an X-linked recessive disorder with an incidence of approximately 1/100,000. It is characterized by flexion contracture of the elbows, ankle equinus, and limited neck flexion. There is a slow progression of weakness and atrophy in a humeroperoneal distribution. Elbow muscles are often weaker than scapular muscles. Distal muscles in the lower extremity are affected earlier than proximal muscles. Cardiac arrhythmias are common and life-threatening. A patient may present with syncopal episodes and atrial arrest (198). Survival to middle age is usual.

Treatment includes appropriately timed (early) placement of a cardiac pacemaker. Stretching, splinting, and dynamic bracing at the elbow, metacarpal joints, and ankle are part of the rehabilitation intervention.

General Principles of Rehabilitation Management in Muscular Dystrophy

When muscular dystrophy results in hip extensor weakness, there is an associated anterior pelvic tilt, hip flexor contracture, and increased lumbar lordosis in order to keep the weight line posterior to the hip. Iliotibial band tightness increases torque on the femur, flexing the knee, and eventually prevents adequate hip and spine hyperextension. Tensor fascia lata and iliotibial band contracture lead to a wide-based gait. Increasing quadriceps weakness causes the patient to move the weight line anterior to the knee. Strong plantar flexors encourage toe walking and lead to equinus deformity and minimal knee stabilization. Asymmetric heel cord shortening (which occurs in up to two-thirds of patients with DMD) is particularly problematic (141,195). This results in standing preferentially over the less contracted foot. With knee flexion contracture, it becomes impossible to keep the center of gravity behind the hip and in front of the knee. Once the flexion contracture exceeds 15°, stability of the knee joint is marginal and further compromised by quadriceps weakness. With imbalance of foot evertor strength, the tibialis posterior destabilizes the subtalar joint. Eventually, the patient falls on uneven and, subsequently, all surfaces.

In order to preserve ambulation, the rehabilitation program includes passive stretching of the lower extremities, regular walking or standing for 2 to 3 hours per day (199–202), appropriate positioning of the hip, knee, and ankle when seated or lying down, and prudent strengthening of lower extremity agonists. Stretching should focus on the gastrocnemius–soleus, hamstrings, and iliotibial bands, but not ignore the quadriceps or hip rotators. A stretch should be held for about 15 seconds and repeated ten times per session. Contracting the appropriate muscle during a stretch may also be helpful. The stretch is done slowly in order to prevent triggering of the opposing stretch reflex. Lying prone or sitting with the legs extended should also be encouraged. Just as the weakest patients are the worst candidates for exercise, the most severely contracted show the least improvement with stretch. This underscores the importance of early, aggressive stretching and early and regular submaximal strengthening exercise.

Lower extremity splinting and passive stretching reduces the rate of contracture and may prolong ambulation (199–201). Effective stretching programs can be supplemented by nocturnal splinting. Compliance with splint use is generally poor but can be improved through adequate patient/family education and motivation. The patient and family with DMD should be aware that an aggressive stretching/splinting program may prolong ambulation for these patients to a mean age of 10.3 years (202).

Therapeutic strengthening exercise should be performed at a submaximal level of intensity and duration in order to avoid overuse weakness. Aerobic high-repetition activities are encouraged when tolerated by a patient. The use of electrical stimulation in order to maintain or facilitate muscle strength may be considered, but there is no clear evidence supporting its usefulness in either improving strength or slowing the progression of weakness.

Contoured seating systems with arm rests or a lap tray of proper height are useful for the muscular dystrophy patient who is wheelchair confined. A standard wheelchair should be lightweight and folding, with desk or full-length arms and swing-away, removable leg rests. Offset foot plates with toe and heel loops are also useful if foot and ankle deformities are present. Head rests and a seat belt are needed if head and trunk control are poor. The patient should sit squarely on a firm seat or cushion, avoiding an oblique pelvic posturing that would hasten contracture. Wedges can assist in maintaining pelvic and lower extremity alignment and can be removed to permit urinal use. Although a flexible backrest with a posterior inclination is good for spinal alignment, it limits wheelchair propulsion and other upper extremity function and is usually poorly tolerated.

Wheelchair-mountable, programmable robotic arms (201), finger control motorized wheelchairs, and environmental control systems may be useful. Robot manipulators can permit the severely paretic patient to continue independent feeding and other upper extremity activities. Robot manipulators can be inexpensive and mounted by a layman, or they can be expensive and extremely sophisticated (203–206). If adequate upper extremity function and trunk stability are present, a motorized scooter is desirable. Otherwise a motorized wheelchair can provide a significant improvement in independent mobility. Any needed trays for a ventilator and batteries should be included in the wheelchair prescription when external respiratory assistance is necessary.

Surgical intervention for patients with muscular dystrophy typically includes heel cord lengthening, iliotibial band fasciotomy, and tibialis posterior transfer onto the third cuneiform. When performed late, surgery must be followed by rapid mobilization and bracing. When performed early, simple appropriate surgical procedures eliminate the need for any lower extremity bracing (207–209). The use of swivel walkers can sometimes be an alternative to surgery and TKAFOs for continued mobility and standing when the patient can longer ambulate safely (210).

Myotonic dystrophy is characterized by a delay in muscle fiber relaxation after contraction. It has an incidence of 13/100,000 (211). Myotonic dystrophy is inherited through a defective gene located on chromosome 19 (212). Myotonic dystrophy presents between age 20 and 50 years with myotonia, hand weakness, gait abnormalities, poor vision, ptosis, weight loss, impotence, and/or hypertrichoses. Muscular weakness is especially pronounced in the distal muscles. Atrophy is seen in facial, jaw, anterior neck, and distal limb musculature. Velar muscle weakness results in hypernasality. Complaints of muscle stiffness and cramps are common. The myotonia may be aggravated by exposure to cold temperatures.

Systemic manifestations of the disease include cataracts, gonadal atrophy, endocrine anomalies, cardiomyopathy (213), chronic alveolar hypoventilation (214), esophageal dilation, changes in bone composition, male frontal baldness, and dysarthria. Cognitive deficits include mental retardation and abnormalities of recall, abstraction, orientation, and spatial manipulation. In addition to identifying abnormalities of serum immunoglobulins, which are commonly present, appropriate laboratory investigation for myotonic dystrophy includes electromyography, where characteristic myotonic (''dive-bomber'') discharges are noted.

The medical management of myotonia relies on membrane-stabilizing agents such as phenytoin, carbamazepine, or procainamide. The use of tricyclic antidepressants has also been proposed as a means of addressing any cognitive slowing.

Rehabilitation of the patient with myotonic dystrophy requires patient and family education. Avoidance of cold ambient temperatures and appropriate use of medication are encouraged. Chronic alveolar hypoventilation and symptoms of hypercarbia should be addressed as previously noted. Dysphagia from esophageal dilation may improve with a change in bolus consistency. A soft palate orthosis may improve vocal tone if hypernasality is prominent. Effective exercise strategies that address the weakness and myotonia have not been described.

Other diseases of the motor unit that are characterized by myotonia include myotonia congenita (Thomsen disease), paramyotonia congenita, myotonia acquisita (following pesticide exposure, poisoning, trauma, or shock), and the Schwartz-Jampel syndrome (congenital chondrodystrophic myotonia).

Rarely diagnosed hyperactive states of the motor unit include the stiff man syndrome and Isaac syndrome. The stiff man syndrome affects the trunk, shoulder, neck, and to a lesser extent the feet and hands. Stimuli, such as a sudden noise or fright, leads to muscle spasm in the affected area. The facial muscles are usually spared, but laryngeal or respiratory muscle may be affected and result in stridor and significant anxiety. Treatment with diazepam or baclofen is usually adequate to control the symptoms of the disease (215).

Isaac syndrome is characterized by continuous muscle fiber contraction despite otherwise normal motor unit activity. This occurs even at rest or during sleep. The patient complains of pain and stiffness in the hands and feet, generalized muscle stiffness, and excessive sweating. Fasciculations, distal muscle atrophy and weakness, poor fine motor control, and gait abnormalities are observed on examination. The pathophysiology of Isaac syndrome is still unclear but seems to involve the terminal network of affected motor nerves. The onset of the disease is usually during the second or third decade, but symptoms may appear at any age. The severity and course of the disease are variable. The use of phenytoin often provides significant clinical improvement (215).

REFERENCES

1. Myers SJ, Lovelace RE. The motor unit and muscle action potential. In: Downey JA, Myers SJ, Gonzalez EG, Lieberman JS, eds. *The physiologic basis of rehabilitation medicine, 2nd ed.* Stoneham, MA: Butterworth-Heinemann, 1994; 244.
2. Myers SJ, Lovelace RE: The motor unit and muscle action potential. In: Downey JA, Myers SJ, Gonzalez EG, Lieberman JS, eds. *The physiologic basis of rehabilitation medicine, 2nd ed.* Stoneham, MA: Butterworth-Heinemann, 1994; 243–244.
3. Sutherland DH, Olsen R, Cooper L, et al. The pathomechanics of gait in Duchenne's muscular dystrophy. *Dev Med Child Neurol* 1981; 23: 3–22.
4. Dangain J, Vrbova G. Response of normal and dystrophic muscles to increased function demand. *Exp Neurol* 1986; 94:796–801.
5. Johnson EW, Braddom R. Over-work weakness in facioscapulohumeral muscular dystrophy. *Arch Phys Med Rehabil* 1971; 52:333–336.
6. Belanger AY, Noel G, Cote C. A comparison of contractile properties in the preferred and non-preferred leg in a mixed sample of dystrophic patients. *Am J Phys Med Rehabil* 1991; 70:201–205.
7. deLateur BJ, Giaconi RM. Effect on maximal strength of submaximal exercise in Duchenne muscular dystrophy. *Am J Phys Med* 1979; 58: 26–36.
8. Siegel IM. Update on Duchenne muscular dystrophy. *Compr Ther* 1989; 15:45–52.
9. Tomlinson BE, Irving D. The number of limb motor neurons in the human lumbosacral cord throughout life. *J Neurol Sci* 1977; 34: 213–219.
10. Hoffman EP, Fischbeck KJ, Brown RH, et al. Characterization of dystrophin in muscle biopsy specimens from patients with Duchenne's or Becker's muscular dystrophy. *N Engl J Med* 1988; 318:1363–1368.
11. Gardner-Medwin D, Bundey S, Green S. Early diagnosis of Duchenne muscular dystrophy. *Scand J Rehabil Med* 1989; 21:27–31.
12. Heckmatt J, Rodillo E, Dubowitz V. Management of children: pharmacological and physical. *Br Med Bull* 1989; 45:788–801.
13. Brooke MH, Fenichel GM, Griggs RC, et al. Duchenne muscular dystrophy: patterns of clinical progression and effects of supportive therapy. *Neurology* 1989; 39:475–480.
14. Appel SH, Smith RB, Engelhardt JI, Stefani E. Evidence for autoimmunity in amyotrophic lateral sclerosis. *J Neurol Sci* 1993; 118: 169–174.
15. Eisen A. Amyotrophic lateral sclerosis is a multifactorial disease. *Muscle Nerve* 1995; 18:741–752.
16. Al-Chalabi A, Powell FJ, Leigh PN. Neurofilaments, free radicals, excitotoxins, and amyotrophic lateral sclerosis. *Muscle Nerve* 1995; 18:540–545.
17. Rowland LP. Hereditary and acquired motor neuron diseases. In: Rowland LP, ed. *Merritt's textbook of neurology, 9th ed.* Baltimore: Williams & Wilkins, 1995; 742–750.
18. Bach JR. Amyotrophic lateral sclerosis. Communication status and survival with ventilatory support. *Am J Phys Med Rehabil* 1993; 72: 343–349.
19. Bernhardt M, Hynes RA, Blume HB, White AA. Cervical spondylotic myelopathy. *J Bone Joint Surg* 1993; 75-A:119–128.
20. Good DC, Couch JR, Wacaser L. "Numb clumsy hands" and high cervical spondylosis. *Surg Neurol* 1984; 22:285–291.
21. Voskuhl RR, Hinton RC. Sensory impairment in the hands secondary to spondylotic compression of the cervical spinal cord. *Arch Neurol* 1990; 47:309–311.
22. Nobile-Orazio E, Meucci N, Barbieri S, Carpo M, Scarlato G. High-dose intravenous immunoglobulin therapy in multifocal motor neuropathy. *Neurology* 1993; 43:537–544.
23. Van den Bergh P, Logigian EL, Kelly JJ. Motor neuropathy with multifocal conduction blocks. *Muscle Nerve* 1989; 11:26–31.
24. Chaudhry V, Corse AM, Cornblath DR, Kuncl RW, Freimer M, Griffin JW. Mutlifocal motor neuropathy: electrodiagnostic features. *Muscle Nerve* 1994; 17:198–205.
25. Pringle CE, Hudson AJ, Munoz DG, Kiernan JA, Brown WF, Ebers GC. Primary lateral sclerosis. Clinical features, neuropathology and diagnostic criteria. *Brain* 1992; 115:495–520.
26. Hudson AJ, Kiernan JA, Munoz DG, Pringle CE, Brown WF, Ebers GC. Clinicopathological features of primary lateral sclerosis are different from amyotrophic lateral sclerosis. *Brain Res Bull* 1993; 30: 359–364.
27. Sinaki M. Physical therapy and rehabilitation techniques for patients with amyotrophic lateral sclerosis. *Adv Exp Med Biol* 1987; 209: 239–252.
28. Bach JR. Amyotrophic lateral sclerosis: predictors for prolongation of life by noninvasive respiratory aids. *Arch Phys Med Rehabil* 1995; 76:828–832.
29. Lacomblez L, Bensimon G, Leigh PN, et al. Dose-ranging study of riluzole in amyotrophic lateral sclerosis. *Lancet* 1996; 347: 1425–1431.
30. Bensimon G, Lacomblez L, Meininger V. A controlled trial of riluzole in amyotrophic lateral sclerosis. *N Engl J Med* 1994; 330:580–591.
31. Birk T. Poliomyelitis and the post-polio syndrome: Exercise capacities and adaptation—current research, future directions, and widespread applicability. *Med Sci Sports Exerc* 1993; 25:466–472.
32. Ramlow J, Alexander M, LaPorte R, Kaufman C, Kuller L. Epidemiology of the post-polio syndrome. *Am J Epidemiol* 1992; 136:769–786.
33. Halstead LS, Rossi CD. Post-polio syndrome: Clinical experience with 132 consecutive outpatients. In: Halstead LS, Wiechers DO, eds. Research and clinical aspects of the late effects of poliomyelitis. *Birth Defects* 1987; 23:12–26.
34. Jubelt B, Cashman NR. Neurological manifestation of the post-polio syndrome. *Crit Rev Neurobiol* 1987; 3:199–220.
35. Dalakas MC, Sever JL, Madden DL, Papadopoulos NM, Shekarchi IC, Albrecht P, Krezlewicz A. Late poliomyelitis muscular atrophy; Clinical, virologic and immunologic studies. *Rev Infect Dis* 1984; 6(Suppl 2):S562.
36. Sivakumar K, Sinnwell T, Yildiz E, McLauchlin A, Dalakas MC. Study of fatigue in muscles of patients with post-polio syndrome by *in vivo* (^{31}P) magnetic resonance spectroscopy. *Ann NY Acad Sci* 1995; 753:397–401.
37. Miller DC. Post-polio syndrome spinal cord pathology. Case report with immunopathology. *Ann NY Acad Sci* 1955; 753:186–193.
38. Trojan DA, Gendron D, Cashman NR. Anti-cholinesterase responsive neuromuscular junction transmission defects in post-poliomyelitis fatigue. *J Neurol Sci* 1993; 114:170–177.
39. Maselli RA, Wollman R, Roos R. Function and ultrastructure of the neuromuscular junction in post-polio syndrome. *Ann NY Acad Sci* 1995; 753:129–137.
40. Dalakas M, Illa I. Post-polio syndrome: Concepts in clinical diagnosis, pathogenesis, and etiology. *Adv Neurol* 1995; 56:495–511.
41. Jubelt B, Drucker J. Post-polio syndrome: An update. *Semin Neurol* 1993; 13:283–290.
42. Dalakas M. Pathogenetic mechanisms of post-polio syndrome: Morphological, electrophysiological, virological, and immunological correlations. *Ann NY Acad Sci* 1995; 753:138–150.
43. Cashman NR, Trojan DA. Correlation of electrophysiology with pathology, pathogenesis, and anticholinesterase therapy in post-polio syndrome. *Ann NY Acad Sci* 1995; 753:138–150.
44. Dalakas M, Illa I. Post-polio syndrome: Concepts in clinical diagnosis, pathogenesis, and etiology. *Adv Neurol* 1995; 56:495–511.
45. Wiechers DO, Hubbell SL. Late changes in the motor unit after acute poliomyelitis. *Muscle Nerve* 1981; 4:524.
46. Spector SA, Gordon PL, Feuerstein IM, Sivakumar K, Hurley BF, Dalakas MC. Strength gains without muscle injury after strength training in patients with post-polio muscular atrophy. *Muscle Nerve* 1996; 19:1282–1290.
47. Grimby G, Einarsson G. Post-polio management. *CRC Crit Rev Phys Med Rehabil* 1991; 2:189–200.
48. Einarsson G. Muscle conditioning in late poliomyelitis. *Arch Phys Med Rehabil* 1991; 72:11–14.
49. Fillyaw MJ, Badger GD, Goodwin WG, Bradley TJ, Tries TJ, Shukla A. The effects of long-term non-fatiguing resistance exercise in subjects with post-polio syndrome. *Orthopedics* 1991; 14:1253–1256.
50. Agre JC. The role of exercise in the patient with post-polio syndrome. *Ann NY Acad Sci* 1995; 753:321–334.
51. Jones DR, Speier J, Canine K, Owen R, Stull A. Cardiorespiratory responses to aerobic training by patients with postpoliomyelitis sequelae. *JAMA* 1989; 261:3255–3258.
52. Agre JC, Rogriques AA. Intermittent isometric activity: Its effects on muscle fatigue in postpolio subjects. *Arch Phys Med Rehabil* 1991; 72:971–975.
53. Dean E, Ross J. Modified aerobic walking program: Effect on patients with postpolio syndrome symptoms. *Arch Phys Med Rehabil* 1988; 69:1033–1038.

54. Feldman RM, Soskolne CL. The use of nonfatiguing strengthening exercises in post-polio syndrome. *Birth Defects* 1987; 23:335–341.
55. Spiegel R, Hagmann A, Boltshauser E, Moser H. Molecular genetic diagnosis and deletion analysis in Type I–III spinal muscular atrophy. *Schweiz Med Wochenschr* 1996; 126(21):907–914.
56. Bartousek J, Hlustik P, Grenarova O, Beranova M. Advanced EMG techniques in diagnostics of spinal muscular atrophies and motor neuron disease—magnetic stimulation, single fiber EMG and macro EMG. *Acta Univ Palacki Olomuc Fac Med* 1993; 1336:37–39.
57. Whittle MR, Zatz M, Reinach FC. The use of chromosome 5q markers for confirming the diagnosis of proximal spinal muscular atrophy. *Braz J Med Biol Res* 1993; 26(11):1157–1173.
58. Brzustowicz LM, Merette C, Kleyn PW, et al. Assessment of nonallelic genetic heterogeneity of chronic (type II and II) spinal muscular atrophy. *Hum Hered* 1993; 43(6):380–387.
59. Soubrillard C, Pellissier JF, Lepidi H, Mancini J, Rougon G, Figarella-Branger D. Expression of developmentally regulated cytoskeleton and cell surface proteins in childhood spinal muscular atrophies. *J Neurol Sci* 1995; 133(1–2):155–163.
60. Brown JC, Zeller JL, Swank SM, Furumasu J, Warath SL. Surgical and functional results of spine fusion in spinal muscular atrophy. *Spine* 1989; 14:763–770.
61. Merlini L, Granata C, Bonfiglioli S, Marini ML, Cervellati S, Savini R. Scoliosis in spinal muscular atrophy: natural history and management. *Dev Med Child Neurol* 1989; 31:501–508.
62. Brown JC, Zeller JL, Swank SM, Furumasu J, Warath SL. Surgical and functional results of spine fusion in spinal muscular atrophy. *Spine* 1989; 14:763–770.
63. Silverman M. Commercial options for positioning the client with muscular dystrophy. *Clin Prosthet Orthot* 1986; 10:159–170.
64. Gibson DA, Albisser AM, Koreska J. Role of the wheelchair in the management of the muscular dystrophy patient. *Can Med Assoc J* 1975; 113:964–967.
65. DiStefano G, Sciacca P, Parisi MG, et al. Heart involvement in progressive spinal muscular atrophy. A review of the literature and case histories in childhood. *Pediatr Med Chir* 1994; 16(2):125–128.
66. Hahn AF. Hereditary motor and sensory neuropathy: HMSN type II (neuronal type) and X-linked HMSN. *Brain Pathol* 1993; 3(2): 147–155.
67. Carter GT, Abresch RT, Fowler WM Jr, Johnson ER, Kilmer DD, MacDonald CM. Profiles of neuromuscular diseases. Hereditary motor and sensory neuropathy, types I and II. *Am J Phys Med Rehabil* 1995; 74(5 Suppl):S140–S149.
68. Gabreels Festen A, Gabreels F. Hereditary demyelinating motor and sensory neuropathy. *Brain Pathol* 1993; 3(2):135–146.
69. Sghrilanzoni A, Pareyson D, Marazzi R, et al. Homozygous hypertrophic hereditary motor and sensory neuropathies. *Ital J Neurol Sci* 1994; 15(1):5–14.
70. Uncini A, DiGuglielmo G, Di Muzio A, et al. Differential electrophysiological features of neuropathies associated with 17p11.2 deletion and duplication. *Muscle Nerve* 1995; 18(6):628–635.
71. Harding AF. From the syndrome of Charcot, Marie and Tooth to disorders of peripheral myelin proteins. *Brain* 1995; 118(Pt 3): 809–818.
72. Gabreels-Festen AA, Bareels FJ, Hoogendijk JE, et al. Chronic inflammatory demyelinating polyneuropathy or hereditary motor and sensory neuropathy? Diagnostic value of morphological criteria. *Acta Neuropathol* 1993; 86(6):630–635.
73. Gabreels-Festen AA, Gabreels FJ, Jennekens FG, Janssen-van Kempen TW. The status of HMSN type III. *Neuromusc Dis* 1994; 4(1): 63–69.
74. Schroder JM. Neuropathy associated with mitochondrial disorders. *Brain Pathol* 1993; 3(2):177–190.
75. Mostacciuolo ML, Schiavon F, Angelini C, et al. Frequency of duplication at 17p11.2 in families of northeast Italy with Charcot-Marie-Tooth disease type 1. *Neuroepidemiology* 1995; 14(2):49–53.
76. MacMillen JC, Harper PS. The Charcot-Marie-Tooth syndrome: clinical aspects from a population study in South Wales, UK. *Clin Genet* 1994; 45(3):128–134.
77. Holmberg BH. Charcot-Marie-Tooth disease in northern Sweden: an epidemiological and clinical study. *Acta Neurol Scand* 1993; 87(5): 416–422.
78. Dyck PJ, Litchy WJ, Minnerath S, et al. Hereditary motor and sensory neuropathy with diaphragm and vocal cord paresis. *Ann Neurol* 1994; 35(5):608–615.
79. Lindemann E, Leffers P, Spaans F, et al. Strength training in patients with myotonic dystrophy and hereditary motor and sensory neuropathy: a randomized clinical trial. *Arch Phys Med Rehabil* 1995; 76(7): 612–620.
80. Lisak RP. The immunology of neuromuscular disease. In: Walton JN, ed. *Disorders of voluntary muscle, ed. 5*. London: Churchill Livingstone, 1988; 628–665.
81. Karlsen B, Vedeler C: Guillain-Barre syndrome. Variation on the theme. *Tidsskr Nor Laegeforen* 1996; 116(2):242–245.
82. Arakawa Y, Yoshimura M, Kobayashi S, et al. The use of intravenous immunoglobulin in Miller Fisher syndrome. *Brain Dev* 1993; 15(3): 231–233.
83. Korinthenberg R, Monting JS. Natural history and treatment effects in Guillain-Barre syndrome: a multicentre study. *Arch Dis Child* 1996; 74(4):281–287.
84. Clouston PD, Kiers L, Zuniga G, Cros D. Quantitative analysis of the compound muscle action potential in early acute inflammatory demyelinating polyneuropathy. *Electroencephalogr Clin Neurophysiol* 1994; 93(4):245–254.
85. Wollinsky KH, Hulser PJ, Brinkmeier H, et al. Filtration of cerebrospinal fluid in acute inflammatory demyelinating polyneuropathy (Guillain-Barre syndrome). *Ann Med Interne* 1994; 145(7):451–458.
86. Rostami AM. Pathogenesis of immune-mediated neuropathies. *Pediatr Res* 1993; 33(1 Suppl):S90–S94.
87. van der Meche FG, van Doorn PA, Jacobs BC. Inflammatory neuropathies—pathogenesis and the role of intravenous immune globulin. *J Clin Immunol* 1995; 15(6 Suppl):63S–69S.
88. Kuruoglie HR, Oh SJ. Tendon-reflex testing in chronic demyelinating polyneuropathy. *Muscle Nerve* 1994; 17(2):145–150.
89. Bouche P, Moulonguet A, Younes-Chennoufi AB, et al. Multifocal motor neuropathy with conduction block: a study of 24 patients. *J Neurol Neurosurg Psychiatry* 1995; 59(1):38–44.
90. Leger JM. Multifocal motor neuropathy and chronic inflammatory demyelinating polyradiculoneuropathy. *Curr Opin Neurol* 1995; 8(5): 359–363.
91. Bird SJ, Brown MJ, Shy ME, Scherer SS. Chronic inflammatory demyelinating polyneuropathy associated with malignant melanoma. *Neurology* 1996; 46(3):822–824.
92. Parry GJ. AAEM case report #30: multifocal motor neuropathy. *Muscle Nerve* 1996; 19(3):269–276.
93. Hund EF, Fogel W, Krieger D, et al. Critical illness polyneuropathy: clinical findings and outcomes of a frequent cause of neuromuscular weaning failure. *Crit Care Med* 1996; 24(8):1328–1333.
94. Alhan HC, Cakalagaoglu C, Hanci M, et al. Critcal-illness polyneuropathy complicating cardiac operation. *Ann Thorac Surg* 1996; 61(4): 1237–1239.
95. Sheth RD, Bolton CF. Neuromuscular complications of sepsis in children. *J Child Neurol* 1995; 10(5):346–352.
96. Souron V, Chollet S, Ordronneau JR, et al. Secondary neuromuscular deficiencies in critical care patients. *Ann Fr Anesth Reanim* 1995; 14(2):213–217.
97. Young GB. Neurologic complications of systemic critical illness. *Neurol Clin* 1995; 13(3):645–658.
98. Wilmshurst PT, Treacher DF, Lantos PL, et al. Critical illness polyneuropathy following severe hyperpyrexia. *Q J Med* 1995; 88(5): 351–355.
99. Wijdicks EF, Litchy WJ, Harrison BA, et al. The clinical spectrum of critical illness polyneuropathy. *Mayo Clin Proc* 1994; 69(10): 955–959.
100. Bolton CF, Young GB, Zochodne DW. The neurological complications of sepsis. *Ann Neurol* 1993; 33(1):94–100.
101. Gorson KC, Ropper AH. Acute respiratory failure neuropathy: a variant of critical illness polyneuropathy. *Crit Care Med* 1993; 21(2): 367–371.
102. Gopal S, Fishman L. Personal communication of ongoing research, April 21, 1997.
103. Ludolph AC, Spencer PS. Toxic neuropathies and their treatment. *Baillieres Clin Neurol* 1995; 4(3):505–527.
104. Calissi PT, Jaber LA. Peripheral diabetic neuropathy: current concepts in treatment. *Ann Pharmacother* 1995; 29(7–8):769–777.

105. Yonger DS, Rosoklija G, Hays AP, et al. Diabetic peripheral neuropathy: a clinicopathologic and immunohistochemical analysis of sural nerve biopsies. *Muscle Nerve* 1996; 19(6):722–727.
106. Veves A, Sarnow MR. Diagnosis, classification and treatment of diabetic peripheral neuropathy. *Clin Podiatr Med Surg* 1995; 12(1): 19–30.
107. Menzinger G, Uccioli L. Postural rearrangement in IDDM patients with peripheral neuropathy. *Diabetes Care* 1996; 19(4):372–374.
108. Harrison MJ, McArthur JC. *AIDS and neurology*. Edinburgh: Churchill Livingston, 1990; 87.
109. Kihara M, McManis PG, Schmelzer JD, et al. Experimental ischemic neuropathy: salvage with hyperbaric oxygenation. *Ann Neurol* 1995; 37(1):89–94.
110. Sanmarco GJ, Chalk DE, Feibel JH. Tarsal tunnel syndrome and additional nerve lesions in the same limb. *Foot Ankle* 1993; 14(2):71–77.
111. Kunzer T, Pedrazzi P. Myasthenia-like syndromes: current and future treatments. *Schweiz Rundsch Med Prax* 1995; 84(38):1042–1049.
112. Sahashi K, Ibi T. Pathophysiology on the the disorder of neuromuscular transmission defects. *Rinsho Byori* 1995; 43(9):902–909.
113. Maselli RA. Pathophysiology of myasthenia gravis and Lambert-Eaton syndrome. *Neurol Clin* 1994; 12(2):285–303.
114. Plomp JJ, Van Kempen GT, De Baets MG, et al. Acetylcholine release in myasthenia gravis: regulation at single end-plate level. *Ann Neurol* 1995; 37(5):627–636.
115. Simpson JA. Myasthenia gravis and myasthenic syndromes. In: Walton JN, ed. *Disorders of voluntary muscle, ed. 5*. London: Churchill Livingstone, 1988; 628–65.
116. Confalonieri P, Antozzi C, Cornelio F, et al. Immune activation in myasthenia gravis: soluble interleukin-2 receptor, interferon-gamma and tumor necrosis factor-alpha levels in patients' serum. *J Neuroimmunol* 1993; 48(1):33–36.
117. D'Alessandro J, Casmiro M, Benassi G, et al. Reliable disability scale for myasthenia gravis sensitive to clinical changes. *Acta Neurol Scand* 1995; 92(1):77–82.
118. Fornadi L, Horvath R, Bardosi Z, Szobor A. Myasthenia gravis: effect of immunoactive therapies. *Acta Med Hung* 1994; 50(1–2):83–92.
119. Molenaar PC, Biewenga JE, Van Kempen GT, De Priester JA. Effect of ephedrine on muscle weakness in a model of myasthenia gravis in rats. *Neuropharmacology* 1993; 32(4):373–376.
120. Shibuya N, Sato T, Osame M, et al. Immunoadsorption therapy for myasthenia gravis. *J Neurol Neurosurg Psychiatry* 1994; 57(5): 578–581.
121. Cadish R, Streit E, Hartmann K. Exacerbation of pseudoparalytic myasthenia gravis following azithromycin. *Schweiz Med Wochenschr* 1996; 126(8):308–310.
122. Oczko-Grzesik B, Adamek B, Kepa L. Poisoning after eating sausage in observations from I Clinic of Infectious Diseases of the Slask Academy of Medicine in 1985–1992. *Przegl Epidemiol* 1993; 47(3): 285–288.
123. Montecucco C, Schiavo G. Mechanism of action of tetanus and botulinum neurotoxins. *Mol Microbiol* 1994; 13(1):1–8.
124. Clayton MA, Clayton JM, Brown DR, Middlebrook JL. Protective vaccination with a recombinant fragment of *Clostridium botulinum* neurotoxin serotype A expressed from a synthetic gene in *Escherichia coli. Infect Immun* 1995; 63(7):2738–2742.
125. Tick paralysis—Washington, 1995. *Morbid Mortal Week Rep* 1996; 45(16):325–326.
126. Walton JN, Gardner-Medwin D. Progressive muscular dystrophy and the myotonic disorders. In: Walton J, ed. *Disorders of voluntary muscle, ed 3.* London: Churchill Livingstone, 1974; 561–613.
127. Fowler WM, Nayak NN. Slowly progressive proximal weakness: limb-girdle syndromes. *Arch Phys Med Rehabil* 1983; 64:527–538.
128. Davis KE, Pearson PL, Harper PS, Murray JM, O'Brian D, Sarafarzi M, Williamson R. Linkage analysis of two clone DNA sequences flanking the Duchenne muscular dystrophy loci on the short arm of the X chromosome. *Nucl Acids Res* 1983; 11:2303–2312.
129. Murray JM, Davies KE, Harper PS, Meredith C, Mueller C, Williamson R. Linkage relationship of a cloned DNA sequence on the short arm of the X chromosome to Duchenne muscular dystrophy. *Nature* 1982; 300:69–71.
130. Zubrzycka-Gaarn EE, Bulman DE, Karpati G, et al. The Duchenne muscular dystrophy gene product is localized in sarcolemma of human skeletal muscle. *Nature* 1988; 33:466–469.
131. Duncan CJ. Dystrophin and the integrity of the sarcolemma in Duchenne muscular dystrophy. *Experientia* 1989; 45:175–177.
132. Fong P, Turner PR, Denetclaw WF, Steinhardt RA. Increased activity of calcium leak channels in myotubes of Duchenne human and mdx mouse origin. *Science* 1990; 250:673–676.
133. Chelly J, Kaplan JC, Maire P, et al. Transcription of the dystrophin gene in human muscle and non-muscle tissues. *Nature* 1988; 333: 858–860.
134. Webster C, Silberstein L, Hays AP, Blau HM. Fast muscle fibers are preferentially affected in Duchenne muscular dystrophy. *Cell* 1988; 52:503–513.
135. Emery AEH. Duchenne muscular dystrophy: genetic aspects, carrier detection and antenatal diagnosis. *Br Med Bull* 1980; 36:117–122.
136. Bundey S. A genetic study of Duchenne muscular dystrophy in the West Midlands. *J Med Genet* 1981; 18:1–7.
137. Monckton G, Hoskin V, Warren S. Prevalence and incidence of muscular dystrophy in Alberta, Canada. *Clin Genet* 1982; 21:19–24.
138. Tansrud SE, Salvorsen S. Child neuromuscular disease in southern Norway, the prevalence and incidence of Duchenne muscular dystrophy. *Acta Paediatr Scand* 1989; 78:100–103.
139. Pearce JMS, Pennington RJT, Walton JN. Serum enzyme studies in muscle disease part II: serum creatine kinase activity in relatives of patients with Duchenne type of muscular dystrophy. *J Neurol Neurosurg Psychiatry* 1964; 27:181–185.
140. Mingo PU, Romero JT, Barbero JLT, Jalon EI. Miocardiopatia dilatada en una mujer portadora de la enfermedad de Duchenne de Boulogne. *Rev Clin Esp* 1987; 181:468.
141. Eiholzer U, Boltshauser E, Frey D, Molinari L, Zachmann M. Short stature: a common feature in Duchenne muscular dystrophy. *Eur J Pediatr* 1988; 147:602–605.
142. Preising BM, Hull ML, Taylor RG, Shumway RH. Carrier detection of Duchenne dystrophy by frequency analysis of the electromyogram. *J Biomed Eng* 1988; 10:417–425.
143. Moosa A, Brown BH, Dubowitz, V. Quantitative electromyography: carrier detection in Duchenne type muscular dystrophy using a new automatic technique. *J Neurol Neurosurg Psychiatry* 1972; 35: 841–844.
144. Seccgu MB, Wu SC, Obbiassi M, Oltrona L, Folli G. Etude electrovectodcardiographique dans la dystrophie musculaire progressive de Duchenne de Boulogne. *Arch Mal Coeur* 1982; 75:1297– 1301.
145. Emery AEH. Prevention of Duchenne muscular dystorphy and recombinant DNA technology. In: Serratrice G, Desnuelle C, Pellissier J, Cros D, Gastaut J, Pouget J, Schiano A, eds. *Neuromuscular diseases.* New York: Raven Press, 1984:25–28.
146. McDonald CM, Abresch RT, Carter GT, et al. Profiles of neuromuscular diseases. Duchenne muscular dystrophy. *Am J Phys Med Rehabil* 1995; 74:S70–92.
147. Hinge HF, Hein-Sorensen O, Reske-Nielsen E. X-linked Duchenne muscular dystrophy. *Scand J Rehab Med* 1989; 21:27–31.
148. Gardner-Medwin D, Bundey S, Green S. Early diagnosis of Duchenne muscular dystrophy. *Lancet* 1978; 1:1102.
149. Hoffman EP, Fischbeck KH, Brown RH, et al. Characterization of dystrophin in muscle-biopsy specimens from patients with Duchenne's or Becker's muscular dystrophy. *N Engl J Med* 1988; 318: 1363–1368.
150. Brooke MH, Fenichel GM, Griggs RC, et al. Clinical investigation in Duchenne dystrophy: 2. determination of the ''power'' of therapeutic trials based on the natural history. *Muscle Nerve* 1983; 6:91–103.
151. Demos J. Early diagnosis and treatment of rapidly developing Duchenne de Boulogne type myopathy. *Am J Phys Med* 1971; 50: 271–284.
152. Roland LP, Laycer RB. The X-linked muscular dystrophies. In: Vinken PJ, Gruyn GW, eds. *Handbook of clinical neurology, vol 40.* New York: North Holland, 1979; 349–414.
153. Glorion B, Burgot D, Bonnard C. Myopathie Duchenne de Boulogne et chirugie des membres inferieurs: 60 cas operes. *Readapt Revalid* 1987; 3:8–13.
154. Gardner-Medwin D. Clinical features and classification of the muscular dystrophies. *Br Med Bull* 1980; 36:109–115.
155. Schmidt B, Watters GV, Rosenblatt B, Silver K. Increased head circumference in patients with Duchenne muscular dystrophy. *Ann Neurol* 1985; 17:620–621.

156. Eiholzer U, Boltshauser E, Frey D, Molinari L, Zachmann M. Short stature: a common feature in Duchenne muscular dystrophy. *Eur J Pediatr* 1988; 147:602–605.
157. Jagadha V, Becker LE. Brain morphology in Duchenne muscular dystrophy: a Golgi study. *Pediatr Neurol* 1989; 4:87–92.
158. Yoshioka M, Okuno T, Honda Y, Nakano Y. Central nervous system involvement in progressive muscular dystrophy. *Arch Dis Child* 1980; 55:589–594.
159. Hirase T, Araki S. Cerebrospinal fluid proteins in muscular dystrophy patients. *Brain Dev* 1984; 6:10–16.
160. Miyatake M, Miike T, Zhao J, Yoshioka K, Uchino M, Usuku G. Possible systemic smooth muscle layer dysfunction due to a deficiency of dystrophin in Duchenne muscular dystrophy. *J Neurol Sci* 1989; 93:11–17.
161. Miike T, Sugino S, Ohtani Y, Taku K, Yoshioka K. Vascular endothelial cell injury and platelet embolism in Duchenne muscular dystrophy at the preclinical stage. *J Neurol Sci* 1987; 83:67–80.
162. Miller F, Moseley C, Koreska J. *Treatment of spinal deformity in Duchenne muscular dystrophy.* Paper reported in proceedings of the Scoliosis Research Society, Orlando, FL, 1984; 99.
163. Lord J, Behrman B, Varzos N, Cooper D, Lieberman JS, Fowler WM. Scoliosis associated with Duchenne muscular dystrophy. *Arch Phys Med Rehabil* 1990; 71:13–17.
164. Kurz LT, Mubarak SJ, Schultz P, Park SM, Leach J. Correlation of scoliosis and pulmonary function in Duchenne muscular dystrophy. *J Pediatr Orthop* 1983; 3:347–353.
165. Hsu JD, Hall VM, Swank S, et al. *Control of spine curvature in the Duchenne muscular dystrophy.* Paper presented at Scoliosis Research Society, 25th annual meeting, Denver, CO, October 1982; 108.
166. Seeger BR, Sutherland DA, Clark MS. Orthotic management of scoliosis in Duchenne muscular dystrophy. *Arch Phys Med Rehabil* 1984; 65:83–86.
167. Colbert AP, Craig C. Scoliosis management in Duchenne muscular dystrophy. *Arch Phys Med Rehabil* 1987; 68:302–304.
168. Luque ER. Segmental spinal instrumentation for correction of scoliosis. *Clin Orthop Relat Res* 1982; 163:192–198.
169. Susman MD. Advantage of early spinal stabilization and fusion in patients with Duchenne muscular dystrophy. *J Pediatr Orthop* 1984; 4:532–537.
170. Jenkins JG, Bohn D, Edmonds JF, Levison H, Barker GA. Evaluation of pulmonary function in muscular dystrophy patients requiring spinal surgery. *Crit Care Med* 1982; 10:645–649.
171. Kumano K, Tsuyama N. Pulmonary function before and surgical correction of scoliosis. *J Bone Joint Surg* 1982; 64A:242–248.
172. Cambridge W, Drennan JL. Scoliosis associated with Duchenne muscular dystrophy. *J Pediatr Orthop* 1987; 7:436–440.
173. Smith AD, Koreska J, Moseley CF. Progression of scoliosis in Duchenne muscular dystrophy. *J Bone Joint Surg* 1989; 71A:1066–1074.
174. Duport G, Gayet E, Pries P, Thirault C, Rehardel-Irani A, Fons N, Bach JR, Rideau Y. Spinal deformities and wheelchair seating in Duchenne muscular dystrophy: twenty years of research and clinical experience. *Semin Neurol* 1995; 15:29–37.
175. Rideau Y, Gatin G, Bach J, Gines G. Prolongation of life in Duchenne muscular dystorphy. *Acta Neurol* 1983; 5:118–124.
176. Vignos PJ. Respiratory function and pulmonary infection in Duchenne muscular dystrophy. *Isr J Med Sci* 1977; 13:207–214.
177. Inkley SR, Oldenberg FC, Vignos PJ. Pulmonary function in Duchenne muscular dystrophy related to stage of disease. *Am J Med* 1974; 56:297–306.
178. Tanaka H, Nishi S, Katanasako H. Natural course of cardiomyopathy in Duchenne muscular dystrophy. *Jpn Circ J* 1979; 43:974–984.
179. Nigro G, Comi LI, Limongelli FM, et al. Prospective study of X-linked progressive muscular dystrophy in Campania. *Muscle Nerve* 1983; 6:253–262.
180. Stewart CA, Gilgoff I, Baydur A, Prentice W, Applebaum D. Gated radionuclide ventriculography in the evaluation of cardiac function in Duchenne's muscular dystrophy. *Chest* 1988; 94:1245–1248.
181. Gardner-Medwin D. Clinical features and classification of the muscular dystrophies. *Br Med Bull* 1980; 36:109–115.
182. Barohn RJ, Levine EJ, Olson JO, Mendell JR. Gastric hypomotility in Duchenne's muscular dystrophy. *N Engl J Med* 1988; 319:15–18.
183. Robin GC, Falewski de Leon GH. Acute gastric dilatation in progressive muscular dystrophy. *Lancet* 1963; 2:171–172.
184. Schliephake E. Der Kardio-intestinale Symptomenkomplex bei der progressiven Muskeldystrophie. II. Graphische Untersuchungen. *Z Kinderheilkund* 1929; 47:85–93.
185. Berblinger W, Duken J. Der Kardio-intestinale Symptomenkomplex bei der progressiven Muskeldytrophie. I. Mitteilung: klinische und pathologischanatomische Beobachtungen. *Z Kinderheilkund* 1929; 47:1–26.
186. Siegel IM. Update on Duchenne muscular dystrophy. *Compr Ther* 1989; 15:45–52.
187. Jaffe KM, McDonald CM, Ingman E, Haas J. Symptoms of upper gastrointestinal dysfunction in Duchenne muscular dystrophy: case control study. *Arch Phys Med Rehabil* 1990; 71:742–744.
188. Bach JR, Tippett DC, McCrary MM. Bulbar dysfunction and associated cardiopulmonary considerations in polio and neuromuscular disease. *J Neurol Rehabil* 1992; 6:113–119.
189. Smith RA, Sibert JR, Wallace SJ, Harper PS. Early diagnosis and secondary prevention of Duchenne muscular dystrophy. *Arch Dis Child* 1989; 64:787–790.
190. Kaplan LC, Osborne P, Elias E. The diagnosis of muscular dystrophy in patients referred for language delay. *J Child Psychol Psychiatry* 1986; 27:545–549.
191. Marsh GM, Munsat LM. Evidence for early impairment of verbal intelligence in Duchenne muscular dystrophy. *Arch Dis Child* 1974; 49:118–122.
192. Dorman C, Hurley AD, d'Avignon J. Language and learning disorders of older boys with Duchenne muscular dystrophy. *Dev Med Child Neurol* 1988; 30:316–327.
193. Anderson SW, Routh DK, Ionasescu VV. Serial position memory of boys with Duchenne muscular dystrophy. *Dev Med Child Neurol* 1988; 30:328–333.
194. Bach JR, Alba AS. Total ventilatory support by the intermittent abdominal pressure ventilator. *Chest* 1991; 99:630–636.
195. Lord J, Behrman B, Varzos N, Cooper D, Lieberman JS, Fowler WM. Scoliosis associated with Duchenne muscular dystorphy. *Arch Phys Med Rehabil* 1990; 71:13–17.
196. Miller F, Moseley C, Koreska J. Treatment of spinal deformity in Duchenne muscular dystrophy. Paper presented in proceedings of Scoliosis Research Society, Orlando FL, 1984; 99.
197. Barohn RJ, Levine EJ, Olson JO, Mendell JR. Gastric hypomotility in Duchenne's muscular dystorphy. *N Engl J Med* 1988; 319:15–18.
198. Lazzeroni E, Favaro L, Botti G. Dilated cardiomyopathy with regional myocardial hypoperfusion in Becker's muscular dystrophy. *Int J Cardiol* 1989; 22:126–129.
199. Harris SE, Cherry DB. Childhood progressive muscular dystrophy and the role of physical therapy. *Phys Ther* 1974; 54:4–12.
200. Scott OM, Hyde SA, Goddard C, Dubowitz V. Prevention of deformity in Duchenne muscular dystrophy. A prospective study of passive stretching and splinting. *Physiotherapy* 1981; 67:177–180.
201. Seeger BR, Caudrey DJ, Little JD. Progression of equinus deformity in Duchenne muscular dystorphy. *Arch Phys Med Rehabil* 1985; 66: 286–288.
202. Rideau Y, Bach J. Efficacite therapeutique dans la dystorphie musculaire de Duchenne. *J Readapt Med* 1982; 2:96–100.
203. Bach JR, Zeelenberg A, Winter C. Wheelchair mounted robot manipulators: long term use by patients with Duchenne muscular dystrophy. *Am J Phys Med Rehabil* 1990; 69:55–59.
204. Shramowiat M, Bach JR, Bocobo C. The functional enhancement of patients with Duchenne muscular dystrophy with the use of robot-manipulator trainer arms. *J Neuro Rehab* 1989; 3:129–132.
205. Kwee HH, Duimel JJ, Smits JJ, Tuinhof de Moed AA, van Woerden JA, Kolk LW. *The Manus wheelchair-mounted manipulator: system review and first results.* Paper presented at the second International Workshop on Robotic Applications in Medical and Health Care, Newcastle Upon Tyne, England, September 1989; 1–11.
206. Kwee HH. Spartacus and Manus: telethesis developments in France and in the Netherlands. In: Foulds R, ed. *Interactive robotic aids—one option for independent living: an international perspective.* Monograph 37, New York: World Rehabilitation Fund, 1986; 7–17.
207. Eyring EJ, Johnson EW, Burnett C. Surgery in muscular dystrophy. *JAMA* 1972; 222:1056–1058.

208. Rideau Y, Duport G, Delaubier A, Guillou C, Renardel-Irani A, Bach JR. Early treatment to preserve quality of locomotion for children with Duchenne muscular dystrophy. *Semin Neurol* 1995; 14:9–17.
209. Bach JR, McKeon J. Orthopedic surgery and rehabilitation for the prolongation of brace-free ambulation of patients with Duchenne muscular dystrophy. *Am J Phys Med Rehabil* 1991; 70:323–331.
210. Sibert JR, Williams V, Burkinshaw R, Sibert S. Swivel walkers in Duchenne muscular dystrophy. *Arch Dis Child* 1987; 62:741–742.
211. Brooke MH. *A clinician's view of neuromuscular diseases, ed. 2.* Baltimore: Williams and Wilkins, 1986:194–212.
212. Aslanidis C, Jansen G, Amemiya C, et al. Cloning of the essential myotonic dystrophy region and mapping of the putative defect. *Nature* 1992; 355:548–551.
213. Church SC. The heart in myotonia atrophica. *Arch Intern Med* 1967; 119:176–181.
214. Begin R, Bureau MA, Lupien L, Lemieux B. Control and modulation of respiration in Steinert's myotonic dystrophy. *Am Rev Respir Dis* 1980; 121:281–289.
215. Fowler WJ, ed. Advances in the rehabilitation of neuromuscular diseases. *STAR (Phys Med Rehabil)* 1988(Nov); 2(4).

Rehabilitation Medicine: Principles and Practice, Third Edition,
edited by Joel A. DeLisa and Bruce M. Gans.
Lippincott–Raven Publishers, Philadelphia © 1998.

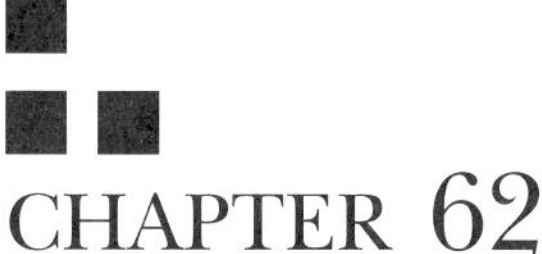

CHAPTER 62

Burn Injury Rehabilitation

Phala A. Helm, Steven V. Fisher, and G. Fred Cromes, Jr.

Of the 1.5 to 2.0 million persons who sustain burn injury annually in the United States, 70 to 100 thousand require hospitalization, and 35 to 50 thousand have temporary or permanent disability (1). The head and neck and upper extremities are the most frequently involved body parts. Injuries to these areas may cause functional and cosmetic deficits that result in impairment and disability (2).

Historically, three developments have significantly affected treatment of burn injury. In the 1960s, resuscitation formulas were developed that resulted in increased survival of persons with burn injury. These formulas counteracted the major fluid loss that is the most important factor in burn mortality. Deaths from burn injury decreased from 12,000 annually in 1970 to 6,000 in 1985 (3). In the mid-1960s, 50% total body surface area (TBSA) burn injuries had a 50% mortality rate. The mortality rate in the same injury is now about 10%, and survival of 70% TBSA injury is now about 50% at major burn centers (4). Increased survival created the demand to develop methods to reduce impairment and disability and improve quality of life.

The second important development addressed infection that could begin localized to the burn wound, become systemic, and result in death. Topical antimicrobial agents that significantly enhanced infection control were discovered and continue to be used extensively.

The third major development affected functional and cosmetic sequelae of burn injury. In the early 1970s it was learned that sustained stretching minimized contracture over major joints and counteracted abnormal collagen formation during healing. It was also discovered that scars under splints were less discolored and flatter (5). These findings led to the use of stretching and pressure becoming the core of burn rehabilitation treatment for hypertrophic scarring and contracture in major burn centers.

P. A. Helm and G. F. Cromes, Jr.: Department of Physical Medicine and Rehabilitation, University of Texas—Southwestern Medical Center at Dallas, Dallas, Texas 75235-9055.

S. V. Fisher: Department of Physical Medicine and Rehabilitation, University of Minnesota Medical School, Hennepin County Medicine Center, Minneapolis, Minnesota 55415.

Rehabilitation of burn injury begins as soon after hospital admission as feasible, continues up to 1 to 2 years depending on the severity of injury, and encourages an interdisciplinary approach (6). Extended rehabilitation time is required by the dynamic nature of scar healing and compliance difficulties because of pain/discomfort and other psychological factors. Interdisciplinary rehabilitation treatment with specialized personnel is the standard in 80% to 90% of major burn centers (7).

Classification of the burn injury is important for planning the patient's treatment regimen. Burns may be classified by causative agent, depth, and percentage of total body surface area burned (Table 62-1; Fig. 62-1). Other factors considered are body part burned, age of patient, preexisting illnesses, and associated injuries such as smoke inhalation and fractures (8).

PATHOPHYSIOLOGY

Normal Skin

The epidermis and dermis constitute the two layers of skin. Epidermal cells begin in the basal layer and gradually move to the surface. As the cells approach the surface, they undergo keratinization and flatten, leaving a thin layer of keratin fiber on the surface that provides a protective barrier to bacterial invasion and fluid loss. The epidermal cells line not only the basal layer of the epidermis but also the hair follicles and sweat glands, which are deep in the dermis. The dermis consists of vascular connective tissue that supports and provides nutrition to the epidermis and skin appendages and the sweat glands, hair follicles, and sebaceous glands. The dermis gives the skin strength and elasticity by an interlacing of collagen and elastic fibers. The skin thickness varies with age and body location, with thicker skin over the back and posterior neck and thinner skin over the medial aspect of the arms and legs.

TABLE 62-1. *Burn classification*

Causative agent
1. Thermal
   a. Heat
   b. Cold
2. Electrical
3. Chemical
4. Radiation

Depth of burn
1. Older Terminology
   a. 1st degree; epidermis injured
   b. 2nd degree; dermis partially damaged
   c. 3rd degree; all dermis destroyed
   d. 4th degree; muscle muscle, nerve and bone damaged
2. Newer terminology
   a. Superficial partial thickness; epidermis and upper part of dermis injured
   b. Deep partial thickness; epidermis and large upper portion of dermis injured
   c. Full thickness; all skin destroyed

Size of burn: rule of nines
1. Head = 9% BSA
2. Each upper extremity = 9% BSA
3. Each lower extremity = 18% BSA
4. Anterior trunk = 18% BSA
5. Posterior trunk = 18% BSA
6. Perineum = 1% BSA

American Burn Board classification
1. Minor
   a. <15% BSA partial thickness (10% in child)
   b. <2% BSA full thickness (not involving eyes, ears, face, or perineum)
2. Moderate[a]
   a. 15% to 20% BSA (10% to 20% in child)
   b. 2% to 10% BSA full thickness (not involving eyes, ears, face, or perineum)
3. Major[a]
   a. >25% BSA partial thickness (20% in child); ≥10% BSA full thickness
   b. All burns to eyes, ears, face, and perineum
   c. All electrical
   d. All inhalation
   e. All burns with fracture or major tissue trauma
   f. All with poor risk secondary to age or illness

[a] Most moderate and all major burns should be hospitalized; BSA, body surface area.

Local Effects of Heat Injury

Thermal destruction of the skin causes a chain of events that may be classified as local and systemic. The amount of tissue destroyed depends on local and systemic reactions to heat damage, the duration and intensity of thermal exposure, and the characteristics of the area burned. In children the rete pegs are not well developed in most body areas, and in the elderly they have become thin and atrophic, thus increasing the damage with burn injury because of fewer protective layers of epithelium (9).

It is very difficult, even for the most experienced, to determine with certainty the depth of burn for 3 to 5 days postburn. Shortly after the burn injury, histamine is released into the local area, causing intense vasoconstriction, and within a few hours there is vasodilation and increased capillary permeability, which permits plasma to escape into the wound. Damaged cells swell. Platelets and leukocytes aggregate, causing thrombotic ischemia and further damage.

Second- and third-degree burns impair the body's defenses against infection and cause loss of massive amounts of body fluids through open wounds. The evaporative loss results in a heat loss and a large caloric drain on the patient. Bacterial contamination of the burn wound may occur immediately, and local burn wound sepsis results.

Systemic Effects of Heat Injury

Some of the major systemic effects of burns include acute hypovolemia, with loss of fluid into the extravascular compartment and subsequent burn shock; pulmonary changes with hyperventilation; and markedly increased oxygen consumption. The high incidence of upper airway obstruction probably is related to direct damage by inhalation of noxious gases, and because of this, the patients are subject to pneumonia. Blood viscosity increases, and platelets increase their adhesiveness. Acute gastric dilation and gastrointestinal ileus commonly occur in the first 3 days postburn. Immunologic competence is depressed for many reasons, including depression of immunoglobulin (9).

Skin Regeneration and Scarring

Healing and regeneration of skin in partial-thickness burns arise from the epithelial linings, including the hair follicles and sweat glands. Depending on the depth, healing is completed within 14 to 21 days. The new skin again becomes active as a temperature regulator and a barrier against bacteria. After epithelialization, there is continued healing with regeneration of the peripheral nerves, sometimes associated with symptoms of pain and itching. It should be noted that split-thickness autografts have no dermal appendages. Although epithelium covers the wound, dermal scarring occurs in the burn wound on a continuous basis for several months after injury. The healing process is ongoing from 6 months to 2 years until the skin is mature. By that point, the vascularity of the wound has returned to near normal, and there is no further collagen deposition in the wound.

PATIENT MANAGEMENT

Acute Phase

Resuscitation

An immediate estimate of the total percentage of surface area burned is a priority in management to determine if intravenous fluid therapy is needed to prevent or treat burn shock. A shift of body fluids to involved areas can cause intravascular hypovolemia and massive edema of both injured and uninjured tissues. If treatment is inadequate, acute renal failure and death can occur. Several formulas are available for calibrating

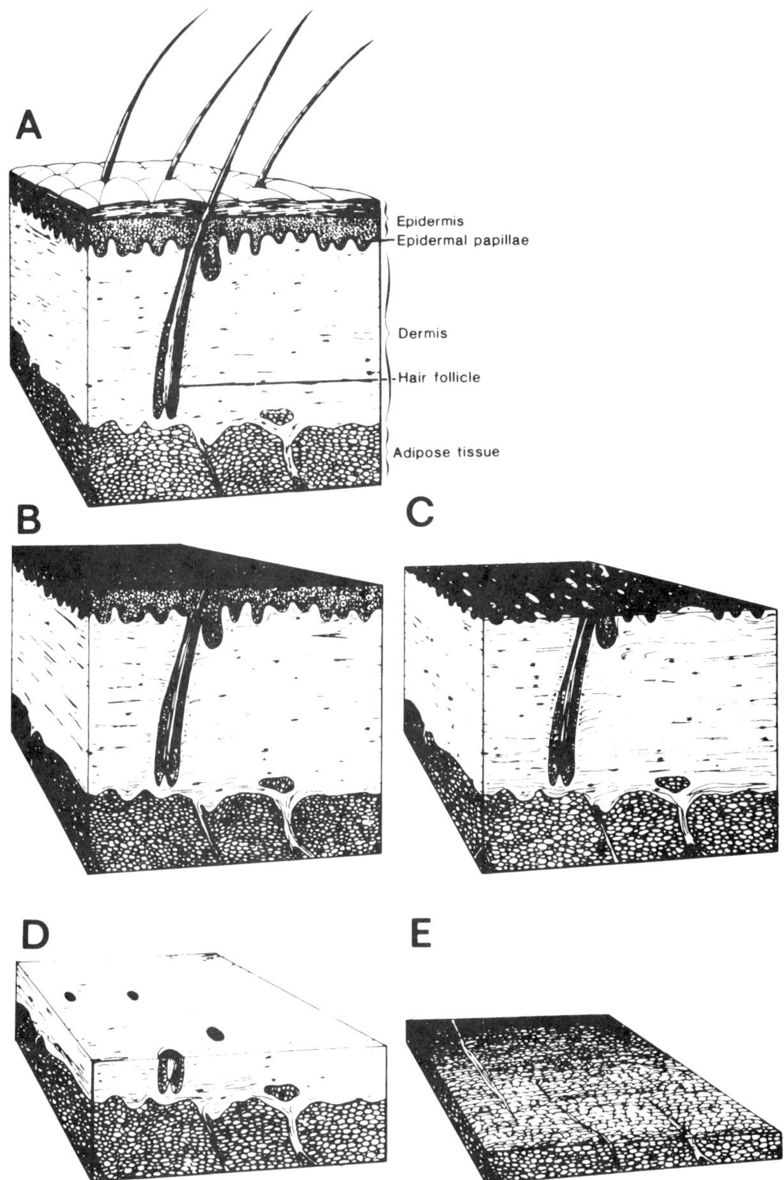

FIG. 62-1. Depth of burns. **A:** Normal skin. **B:** Superficial partial thickness (first degree). **C:** Superficial partial thickness (second degree). **D:** Deep partial thickness (second degree). **E:** Full thickness (third degree).

fluid requirements (e.g., Brooke, Evans, and Baxter formulas); however, the formulas serve only as guidelines, and individual adjustments must be made based on the patient's response. It is important that the fluids contain sodium and that fluid replacement be completed within 48 hours.

Escharotomy

An escharotomy is an incision through the burned tissue to relieve increased tissue pressure (Fig. 62-2). Massive edema of the extremities can cause neurovascular compromise, which could result in amputation. To prevent compartment syndromes, fasciotomies are recommended. Early assessment of blood flow is essential. This can be evaluated by physical examination, Doppler studies, and by measuring tissue pressures with a wick catheter. If tissue pressure is used as a guide, escharotomy is indicated when tissue pressure exceeds 40 mm Hg. Escharotomies are done on other parts of the body, such as the chest when chest expansion is limited and interferes with breathing.

Wound Coverage

Topical Antibacterial Agents. After resuscitation, the burn wound is cleaned, devitalized tissue is removed, and a topical antibacterial agent is applied. There are a number of effective topical agents used for the prevention of burn wound sepsis. Among the various agents available are mafenide, silver nitrate, gentamicin, povidone-iodine, and silver sulfadiazine, which is in widest use because of its comfort and fewer side effects. There is no single agent universally effective, and no one agent is superior to another in terms of patient survival.

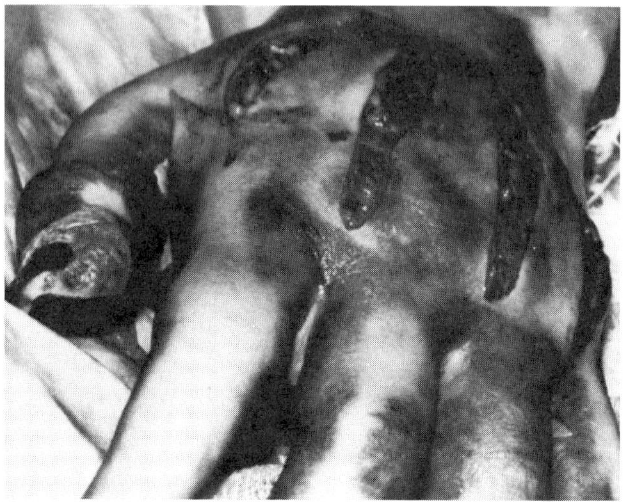

FIG. 62-2. Escharotomies on the dorsum of the hand.

Biological Dressings. A biological dressing is a skin substitute used for temporary coverage of the burn wound. These skin substitutes are skin grafts from cadavers, human fetal membranes (i.e., homografts or allografts), and skin grafts from pigs (i.e., heterografts or xenografts). The recommended uses for these dressings are for immediate coverage of a superficial partial-thickness burn; wound debridement; as a test dressing (i.e., if it adheres, the wound bed is ready for autografting); and for wound coverage after excision of burn eschar. In addition, closing a wound with a biological dressing prevents fluid loss, decreases pain, inhibits bacterial growth on clean wounds, and encourages growth of granulation tissue. The biological dressing should be changed every several days until the wound is healed or ready for autografting. If left in place too long, it becomes incorporated into the burn wound, making removal extremely difficult. It also can become dry and adhere to the wound, restricting range of motion.

Synthetic Dressings. Synthetic skin substitutes were developed to cover open wounds until the wound healed or until it could be autografted. They are used in place of xenografts or homografts. For the synthetic skin to be an effective replacement for certain biological dressings, it had to meet certain criteria. A product was needed that was readily available, nonallergenic, relatively inexpensive, easily removable, and that had a permeable membrane. One additional criterion was that it come in large sheets that would conform to various tissue planes. A product that met these criteria, and which is widely used, is Biobrane (Dow B. Hickam, Sugarland, TX). It has a bilaminar structure with silicone on the outside and nylon bonded to the bottom, which is covered with collagen (10). Opsite (Smith & Nephew Roylan, Menomonee Falls, WI) is another synthetic skin composed of a thin, transparent, elastic, adhesive-coated polyurethane film that is permeable to water vapor.

Artificial Skin. Over the past decade, techniques have been developed to cover an excised wound immediately after injury with artificial skin. This artificial skin has a dermal and epidermal layer; the dermal layer is a porous collagen fibrous matrix on which the patient's own fibroblasts and epidermal cells are seeded and grow into an epidermal replacement. The result is a permanent skin replacement with functioning dermis and epidermis. This procedure is primarily employed in cases of very large, full-thickness or deep partial-thickness injuries with minimal donor sites for grafting available. A drawback to this procedure is the requirement for immobility of the body part involved for 3 weeks, which increses risk of contractures. In addition, scarring has been observed to be worse (11).

Surgical Management

Debridement

Debridement is the removal of devitalized tissue (i.e., eschar) down to a viable tissue level to prepare the wound bed for definitive coverage. Removal of eschar aids in healing by preventing bacterial proliferation. Types of debridement include the following: mechanical with scissors and forceps (Fig. 62-3) and wet to dry dressings; enzymatic; and surgical (tangential, fascial, and full-thickness excisions).

Mechanical Debridement. Mechanical debridement is best accomplished either during hydrotherapy or immediately following. Removal of dressings when they are dry is effective in debridement of dead tissue because it adheres to the dressing. All areas should be cleaned gently to remove topical agents so that the wound is completely visible before sharp debridement begins. Hydrotherapy without wound care is poor patient management.

Wet-to-dry dressings also can be very effective in removal of eschar or exudate. Coarse mesh gauze, soaked in warmed antibacterial solution or normal saline, is applied to the wound and left to dry. With this technique the eschar softens, sticks to the dressing, and then is debrided as the dressing is removed.

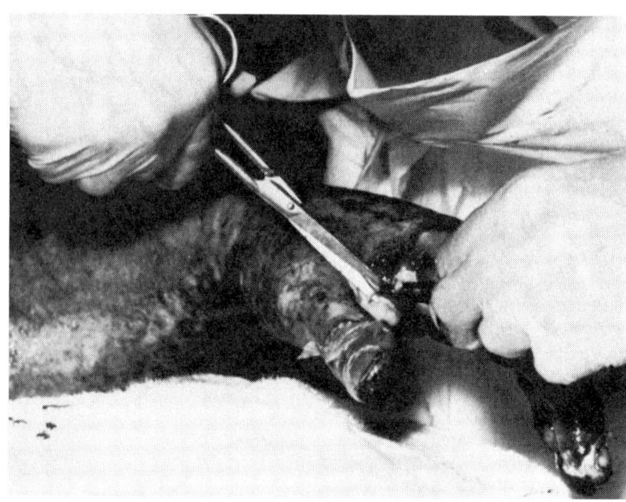

FIG. 62-3. Mechanical debridement.

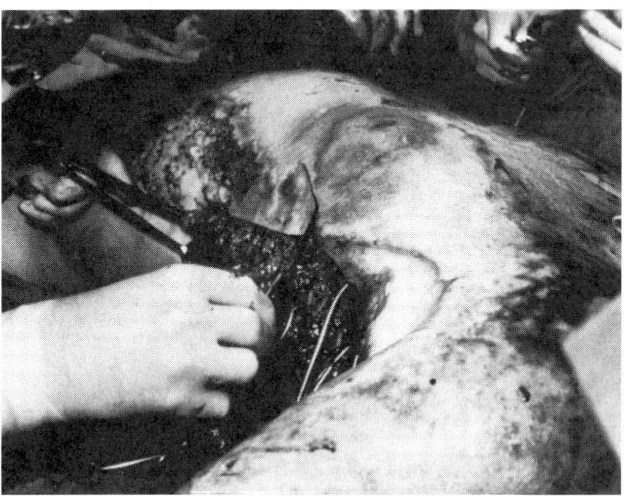

FIG. 62-4. Surgical debridement by excision.

Enzymatic Debridement. An enzymatic debriding agent such as sutilains (Travase, Flint Laboratories, Deerfield, IL) will selectively digest necrotic tissue without harming viable tissue. Because there is increased fluid drainage through the wound with enzymatic debridement, no more than 20% of the body surface area should be treated at one time. Other side effects include bleeding, body temperature elevation, and pain. The enzyme should not be used in conjunction with hexachlorophene or iodine preparations because enzyme activity will be impaired (12).

Surgical Debridement. The two primary surgical techniques used for wound debridement are fascial and tangential (i.e., sequential) excision (Figs. 62-4 and 62-5). Fascial excision removes nonviable burn tissue and a variable amount of viable tissue and is reserved for patients with very deep burns. It is believed that skin grafts adhere much better to fascia than to fat. The problem with fascial excision is that fat does not regenerate; this can cause severe cosmetic deformities.

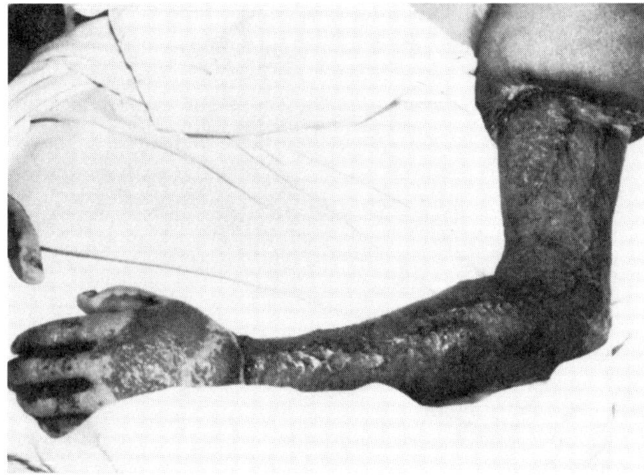

FIG. 62-5. Patient's arm after surgical debridement by fascial excision.

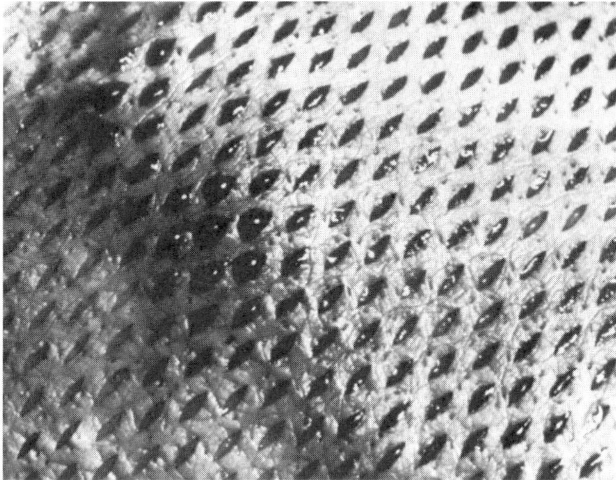

FIG. 62-6. Tanner mesh split-thickness skin graft.

The most widely used technique in surgical debridement is eschar removal by tangential excision, usually performed at 1 to 10 days postburn. The principle of tangential excision is to shave thin layers of burn eschar sequentially until viable tissue is apparent. There can be a significant amount of blood loss, and different methods are used to control this. Tourniquets are used for the extremities by the more experienced surgeon because there is the danger of sacrificing normal tissue by excising too deeply. Some surgeons control bleeding with microcrystalline collagen, thrombin, epinephrine, and electrocautery. Heimbeck reports that early excision and grafting, compared with the standard nonoperative treatment, has led to a decreased hospital stay, a slight fall in overall patient mortality, a decrease in systemic sepsis, and fewer deaths from burn wound sepsis (13).

Skin Grafting

With the exception of small wounds, all full-thickness wounds require skin grafting. Deep partial-thickness wounds that are slow to heal also may require skin grafting. Some investigators believe that grafting of deep partial-thickness wounds prevents the development of thick scar tissue. Autografting is the removal of skin from one part of the body and its transfer to another part. Split-thickness skin grafts are used primarily, whereas full-thickness grafts are used more for reconstructive procedures.

There are a variety of split-thickness skin grafts, each with different indications for use. The Tanner mesh graft is expandable skin that can be used to cover large wounds (Fig. 62-6). Expansion of the skin can be varied, with better cosmetic results with 1.5:1 expansion than, for example, with 6:1. Postage-stamp grafting is the application of squares or rectangles of various dimensions spread evenly over the wound. This type of grafting often leaves a poor cosmetic result because of hypertrophic scarring of the uncovered areas. Sheet grafting is another method used and involves using a piece of split-thickness skin without meshing or cutting it into small squares. This method is used on smaller burn wounds and on the face, neck, and hands for better cosmetic results. The part grafted should be immobilized for at least 3 days.

Rehabilitation

Wound Care

Wound care, debridement, and subsequent skin care are extremely important considerations for functional and cosmetic outcome, and therefore have a direct bearing on rehabilitation. Aggressive wound care is important to delineate wounds before early surgical intervention, to protect and promote good granulation tissue until grafting, or to promote rapid healing in moderate to deep partial-thickness wounds, which tend to have prolonged healing times and subsequently increased scarring (14). The goals of wound care are to prevent or control infection; to preserve as much tissue as possible; and to prepare the wound for earliest possible closure by primary healing or grafting.

Cleaning techniques include local care, spray or nonsubmersion hydrotherapy, and submersion with or without agitation of the water. The choice depends on the depth of injury, extent and location of the wound, and the overall condition of the patient. All areas should be scrubbed gently but thoroughly. When manual debridement is indicated, it should be done after the cleaning process. Daily wound care, which must be aggressive and vigorous, should always be done with as little trauma as possible to the wound and granulation tissue.

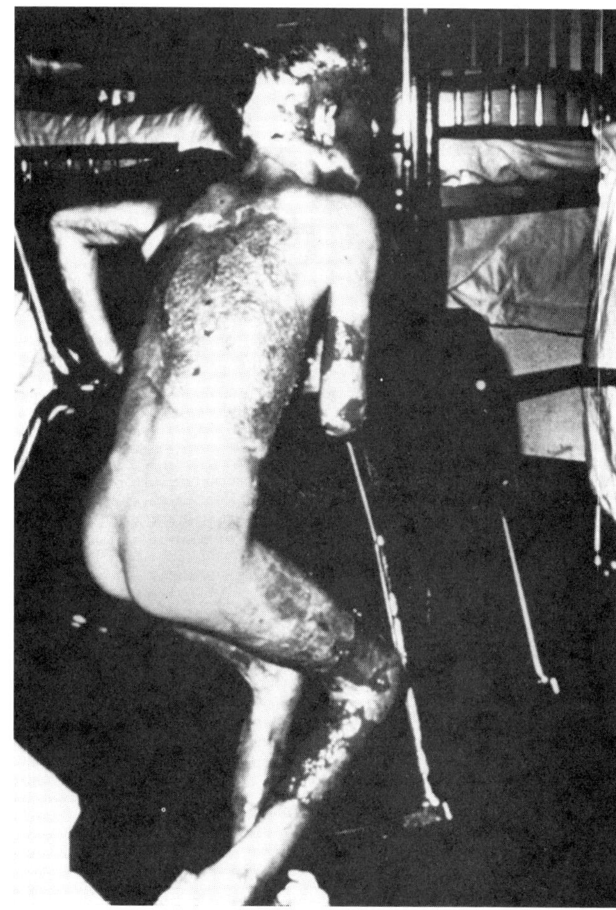

FIG. 62-7. Deformities will develop if the patient is allowed to remain in the position of comfort.

Positioning

In the acute care period, contracture prevention by proper positioning is fundamental to the overall program. The burn patient obviously is extremely uncomfortable and seeks relief by moving the extremities and trunk into a relaxed position to remove the stretch from the burned tissue. To do so he or she primarily flexes and adducts the extremities into a position of comfort (Fig. 62-7). Because contractures develop rapidly in these patients, antideformity positioning should begin immediately. It is only logical to stress abduction and extension (Fig. 62-8). The alternating of positions so that opposing deformities or pain problems are not created by trying to prevent these flexion–adduction contractures is often forgotten. To aid in positioning, the addition of orthopedic frames and shoulder boards to the bed allows for innovative techniques.

Another salient issue in positioning is the type of bed used. Often, air-fluidized beds are used on burn units for relief of pressure in decubitus prevention and for more even distribution of pressure over wounds and grafts. Although the pressure is better distributed, contractures can be encouraged because the patient sinks into the bed or often assumes a fetal position. The Roho mattress can be as effective as an air-fluidized bed for pressure distribution and is superior in preventing contractures.

Splinting

If voluntary positioning becomes a problem, as with the elderly, the noncompliant, and children, splinting becomes an important adjunct to care. If normal range of motion is maintained, there is no need to apply splints, with two major exceptions. Exposed tendons should be splinted in a slack position in an attempt to prevent rupture, whereas exposed joints should be splinted for protection. Opposite deformities can be created by prolonged immobilization with splinting; therefore, frequent assessments of joint range of motion are necessary. The major splints used in the acute phase are as follows:

- Resting hand splints
- Dorsiflexion splints to the ankles for tight heelcords and peroneal nerve palsies
- Knee-extension dorsiflexion splints to prevent "frog leg" position, particularly in children
- Elbow extension splints for limited elbow extension with the precaution that the patient should have close to full elbow flexion

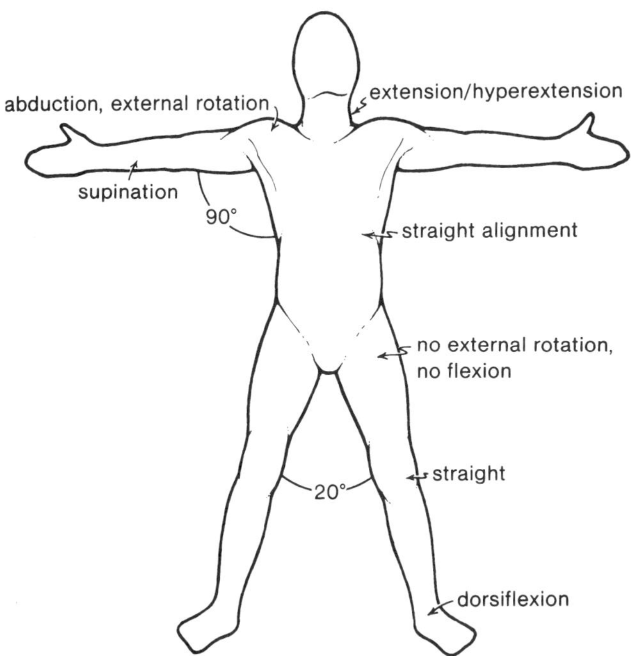

FIG. 62-8. Therapeutic positioning. (From Helm PA, Kevorkian GC, Lushbaugh MS, et al. Burn injury: rehabilitation management in 1982. *Arch Phys Med Rehabil* 1982; 63:6–16.)

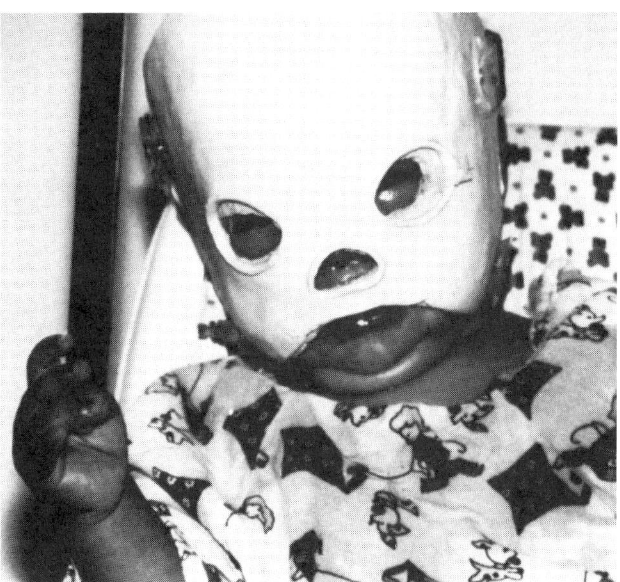

FIG. 62-9. Silicone face mask.

Serial plaster of Paris casting is an alternative to splinting, especially for children and the noncompliant adult. In a study of 35 refractory contractures in which casting was used for a mean total of 13 days, with casts changed every 3.3 days, range of motion increased from a mean of 56% of normal to a mean of 86% of normal. Full range of motion was attained in nine of 15 elbows and seven of ten knees. Improvement in ankle and wrist range of motion was not as successful (15).

The transparent face mask frequently is applied early in the acute phase. The plastic mask is made from a plaster model of the face and is applied over new grafts and over newly healed skin. Its advantages include conforming well to the contours of the face, transparency to allow viewing of the skin to verify appropriate pressure distribution, and, when worn properly, preventing severe cosmetic deformities. Many centers also are using silicone face masks immediately postgrafting and before application of the transparent face mask (Fig. 62-9).

Exercise and Ambulation

Throughout convalescence, gentle, sustained stretch is more effective than multiple repetitive movements in stretching burned tissue. Before the therapist begins an exercise program, the area to receive treatment must be viewed after cleaning; otherwise, an unrecognized injury to vital structures could be compounded by the exercise program. Exercise programs may be indicated three to four times daily to more involved areas, and without exception the patient should exercise independently between therapy sessions. Active exercises to the lower extremities, whether burned or not, assist in the prevention of thrombophlebitis. Range-of-motion exercises while the patient is anesthetized in the surgical suite permit evaluation of the true range of motion because of lack of patient's resistance (16). Escharotomies, heterografts, synthetic dressings, and tangential excisions are not contraindications for exercise; however, exercises should be discontinued for 3 days in joints proximal and distal to autografted and, sometimes, homografted areas.

In the acute period trunk mobilization is needed to prevent the robot-type posture that frequently occurs. Burns to the anterior trunk can cause rounding of the shoulders with a sunken chest and shoulder elevation as well as limited trunk rotary movements. To counteract these problems, vigorous trunk flexion–extension and rotation exercises and bilateral shoulder horizontal abduction exercises are necessary (Fig. 62-10). Every part of the body that has received a burn should be exercised in some manner.

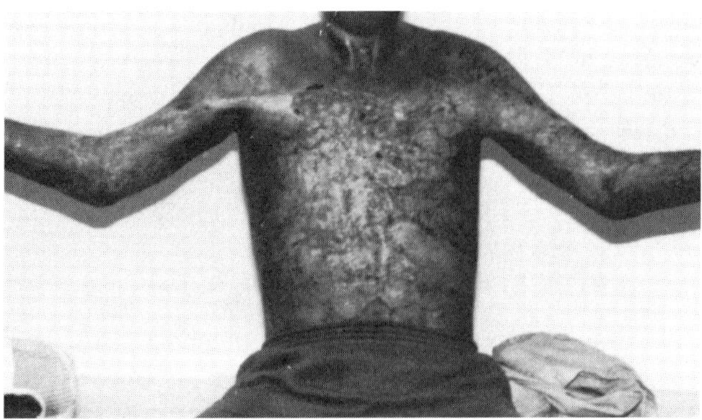

FIG. 62-10. Position for bilateral shoulder horizontal abduction exercise.

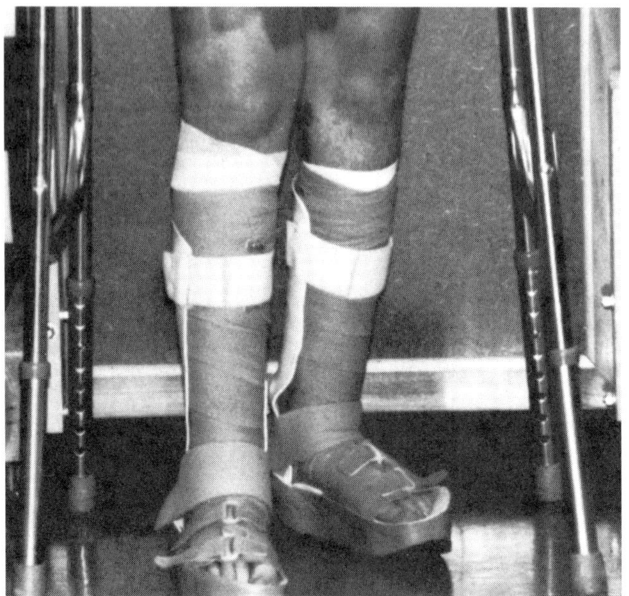

FIG. 62-11. Ambulation assistive devices.

Assistive devices, if needed to get the patient ambulatory or to keep him or her ambulatory, should be used (Fig. 62-11). A wheeled walker with an adjustable overhead attached bar can be used for patients with upper extremity burns to help stretch and increase range of motion of shoulders and elbows as well as reduce edema in the arms. Ambulatory patients have fewer problems with lower extremity contractures and endurance. Patients with burns to the feet requiring deep excision or partial foot amputations should be fitted early with extra-depth shoes, molded insoles, or inserts. Early application of proper footwear prevents later secondary complications of knee, hip, and back pain.

The historical consensus has been that 1 to 2 weeks of bed rest is necessary after lower extremity grafting. This protocol was concluded to be expensive and to contribute to deconditioning and weakness in a study of early ambulation after lower extremity grafting (17). In this study, 100 consecutive lower extremity burn admissions were excised and grafted. A dome paste boot (Unna boot) was applied within 24 hours, and ambulation was initiated 4 hours later with full weight bearing. Excellent to satisfactory graft take occurred in 96% of cases, and independent ambulation was achieved in 1 ± 1 days. Similar results were obtained by Burnsworth and associates (18). Thus, early ambulation (within 1 day with Unna boot) after lower extremity grafting facilitates functional outcome without risk to graft take.

HAND BURNS

Burn injuries to the hands have a profound effect on the patient's return to normal function; therefore, hand therapy is stressed during both acute and postacute phases. A comprehensive medical/surgical and hand treatment protocol including splinting, postgraft immobilization, web spacers, compression gloves, and exercise in warm water or silicone gel produced good functional recovery and reduced need for reconstructure surgery (19). A similar protocol was described by Sheridan and associates with good functional results if tendon, joint capsule, or bone involvement was absent (20).

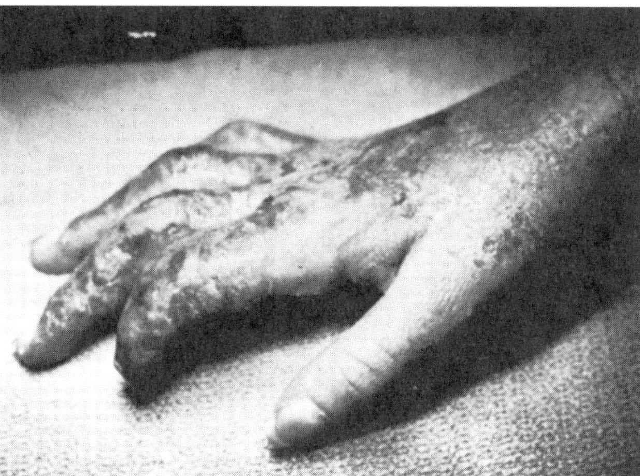

FIG. 62-12. Edematous "clawed" hand.

Edema

Edema is a major cause of the typical clawed burned hand with hyperextension of the metacarpophalangeal (MCP) joints, flexion of the proximal and distal interphalangeal (IP) joints, and the thumb in adduction and external rotation (Fig. 62-12). The protein-rich edema fluid appears to form a gel after about 12 hours, leading to obstruction of local lymphatic vessels and impairing edema clearance. Antideformity positioning is best achieved with a resting hand splint, positioning the wrist in slight extension (see Fig. 62-23*A,B*), the MCP joints in 60° to 90° flexion, the proximal and distal IP joints in full extension, and the thumb in palmar abduction. It may be necessary to wear the splints continuously until edema resolves and the patient is actively using his or her hands. Edema also is treated through elevation and active exercise. Immediately postinjury, the arms may be elevated with Robert Jones skeletal traction, with bedside troughs or nighttime stands.

A complication of the pneumatic tourniquet with prolonged application, as reported by Bruner, is the adverse effects on tissues of the hand, called the postischemic hand syndrome. Bruner's findings of puffiness of the hand and fingers, stiffness of the hand and finger joints, color changes in the hand (e.g., congested in the dependent position), subjective sensations of numbness, and objective evidence of weakness without real paralysis are frequently encountered in the postoperative burn patient (21).

Exposed Tendons and Joints

Exposed tendons in the hand can be a serious problem because they have a tendency to dehydrate rapidly, denature,

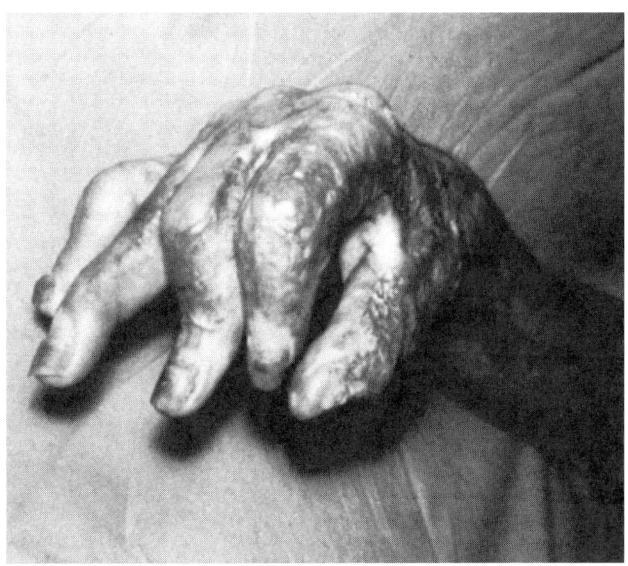

FIG. 62-13. Boutonniere deformity.

and subsequently rupture. Exposed tendons should therefore be covered with a moist dressing to prevent drying. Continuous splinting should be used to maintain the tendon in a slack position until permanent wound closure is obtained. Tendons that appear denatured or charred may ultimately revascularize and should not be debrided prematurely. If the dorsal hood mechanism is exposed, the IP joints should be splinted in extension until wound closure. Only then can gentle active range of motion begin. If the dorsal hood ruptures, the typical boutonniere deformity develops (Fig. 62-13). Immediately after rupture, immobilization of the finger for 6 weeks in extension may allow scar tissue to form across the extensor surface and provide a substitute for the destroyed extensor mechanism (Fig. 62-14). Active motion can then be started (22).

If joint capsules are exposed but not open, they may be gently exercised actively and protectively splinted. If the joint is open or draining, it will probably undergo spontaneous ankylosis; therefore, functional positioning should be encouraged.

Exercise

Primary considerations in exercising the burned hand include intrinsic muscle stretching by mobilizing the metacarpals and stretching the intrinsic muscles by hyperextension of the MCP joint in combination with flexion of the proximal IP joint. Traction applied to the joints with passive movement allows for additional ligamentous stretch.

Splinting

It is not unusual for the burned hand to require customized splinting. Dynamic, as well as static, splinting is used. Custom-conforming splints are used primarily on the flexor surfaces of the hand in patients who have developed contractures or banding over the palmar aspect. The pressure of the splint produces softening, flattening, and lengthening of the scar band. Splints may be used for serial splinting, with the splint being applied at maximum tension and constant pressure; as the contracture improves, the splint is remodeled.

Dynamic splinting can be effective in correcting contractures. Nail hooks, leather loops over the phalanges, flexion wrap, or a flexion glove may be used for dynamic stretch in extension contractures (see Fig. 62-23*F,G* later in this chapter). A custom-made elastomer foam insert placed at the first web space is helpful in maintaining the space and in decreasing an adduction contracture of the thumb.

Successful splinting of the hand requires therapist innovation as well as significant patient cooperation. Rehabilitation of a child's hand is different from that of the adult's and bears special mention. The child's hand is small, making it difficult to fabricate properly fitting hand orthoses, and children have a tendency to flex the hand, causing splint movement and thus producing pressure ulcers. Unfortunately, the young child cannot express pain complaints appropriately. For dorsal hand burns, it may be necessary to position the MCP as well as the IP joints in extension. In the uncooperative child, serial casting is very beneficial, and passive range-of-motion exercises are critical. Play activities become a much more important feature of the exercise program (23).

ELECTRICAL INJURIES

Mechanism of Injury

Electrical injuries constitute only a small number of most burn unit admissions; however, they probably represent the most devastating type of thermal injury. These injuries are arbitrarily divided into low voltage, those no greater than 500 to 1,000 volts, and high voltage, those greater than 1,000 volts. Home injuries usually involve 110 to 220 volts with 60-cycle current and cause little cutaneous and very rare deep muscle damage. These low-voltage accidents, however, can be associated with cardiac standstill or rhythm irregularities. The most common low-voltage burn injury is in the child who bites an electrical cord and sustains a burn of the commissure of the lips.

Generally, the greater the voltage, the greater the amperage, and, consequently, the more severe the injury. As current flows through the body, electrical energy is converted to heat, expressed as Joule's law:

$$\text{Power} = \text{Amperage}^2 \times \text{Resistance}$$

It is therefore apparent that amperage is of greater importance in causing tissue destruction than voltage. Damage is related primarily to tissue resistance and sensitivity to heat. The most resistant or nonconductive tissue is bone, followed by cartilage, tendon, skin, muscle, blood, and nerve. Blood vessels and nerves offer little resistance, which produces

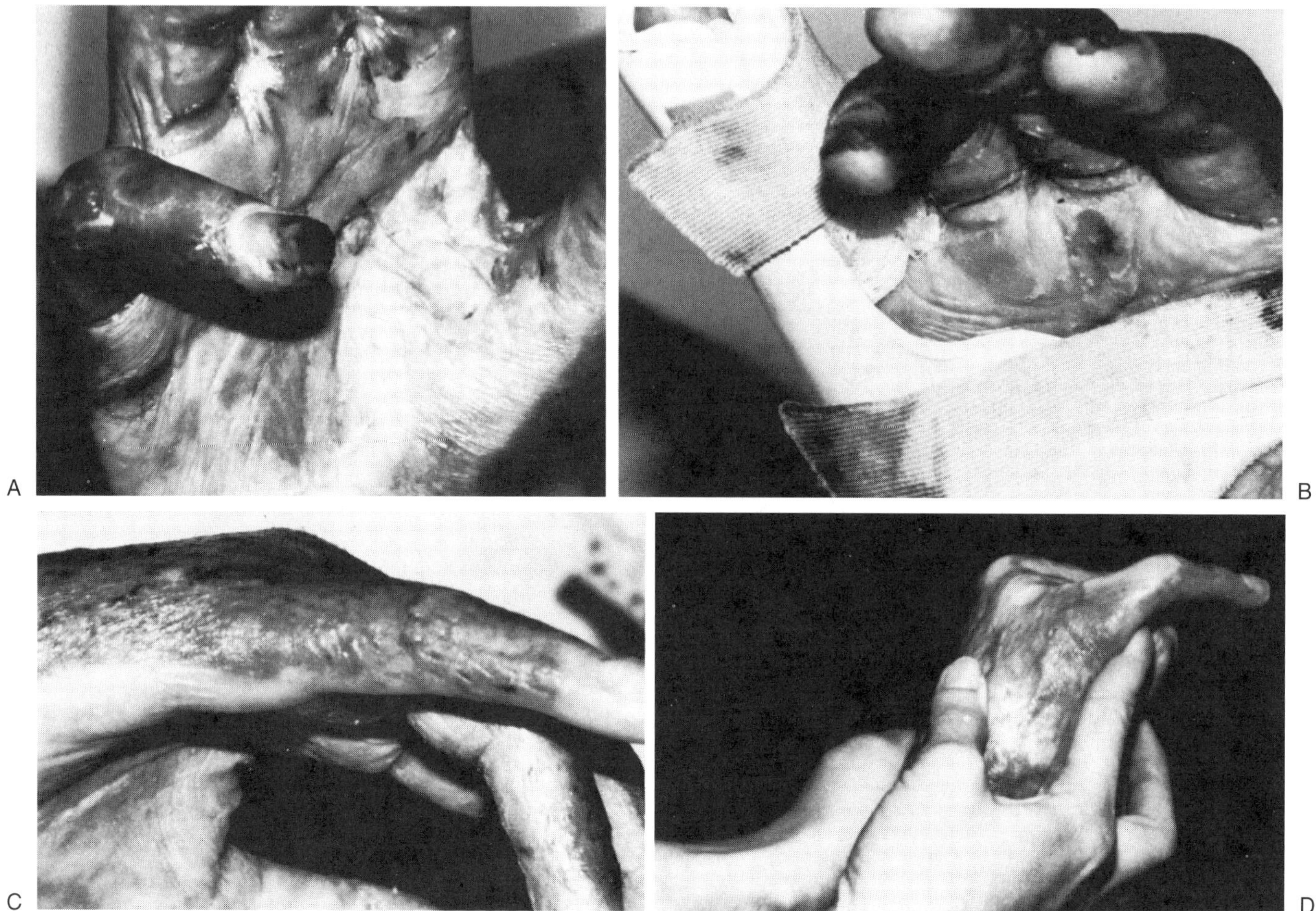

FIG. 62-14. A: Rupture of extensor hood. **B:** Finger splinted in full extension. **C:** Active extension of finger after 6 weeks. **D:** Active flexion of finger after 6 weeks.

higher current flow. These structures also seem to be particularly sensitive to heat damage and sustain injury despite their low resistance (24–26).

Soft Tissue and Bone Damage

Tissue destruction is always greatest in areas of the body with small volume such as fingers, toes, wrists, or ankles. The physician must therefore be knowledgeable about this iceberg-type injury, in which the cutaneous injury may give no indication of the possible underlying muscle, bone, and nerve damage.

The acute surgical treatment is early diagnosis and debridement of necrotic tissue. In all burn patients, the greatest number of amputations occur from electrical injuries (27). Bone that is exposed must be covered with moist dressings to prevent desiccation of the periosteum. Some surgeons drill burr holes in exposed bone to stimulate granulation tissue formation for eventual bone coverage (Fig. 62-15).

Localized Nerve and Central Nervous System Injury

Localized neuropathies may occur both in tissues that are directly burned and in tissue through which electrical energy passes. Radiculopathies as a result of neck hyperextension as the current flows through the body may appear immediately postinjury or later in the convalescent period. Patients who have had current pass through their legs often complain of weakness manifested by inability to stand on the feet for long periods of time and general lack of stamina. Electrodiagnostic tests are worthwhile to diagnose subtle peripheral neuropathies.

Central nervous system damage may result in memory loss, personality changes, and spinal cord pathology. Symptoms of central nervous system injury may not be evident for up to 2 years postinjury; therefore, long-term patient follow-up is needed.

Cataracts

Electrical contact on the head or shoulders may predispose a patient to cataract formation. Cataracts may form within 1 month or as late as 3 years postinjury. Therefore, serial eye examinations should be performed for at least 3 years postinjury.

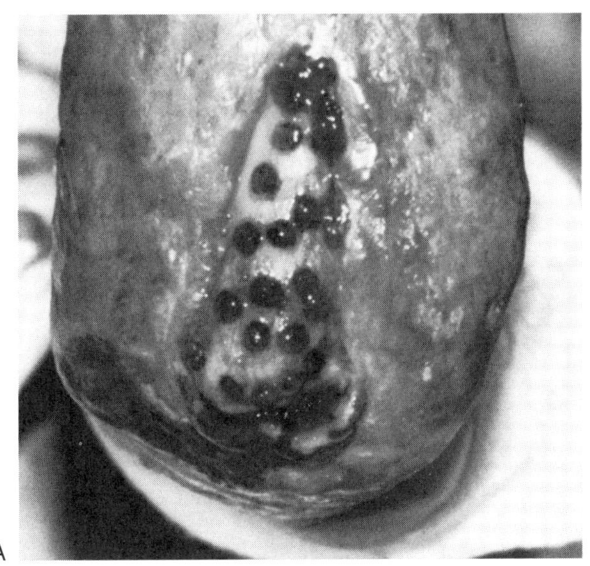

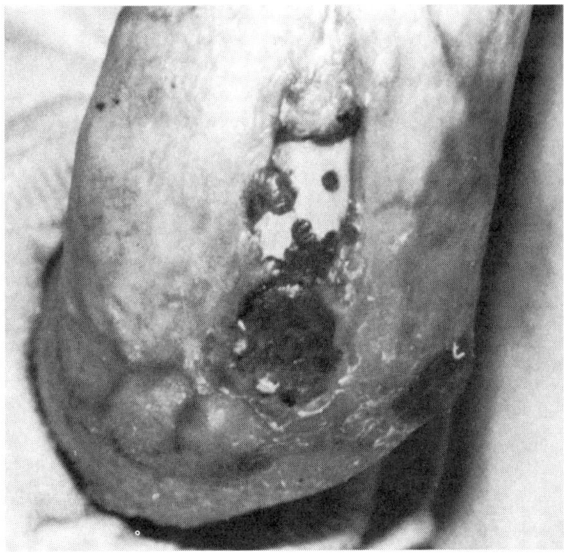

A B

FIG. 62-15. A: Burr holes with protruding granulation tissue. **B:** Wound coverage 4 weeks later.

NEUROLOGIC INJURIES

Localized Neuropathies

Peripheral neurologic complications in the burn patient are not uncommon; however, they frequently are undiagnosed because neurologic assessments are difficult in patients with multiple concurrent problems. To a great extent, the majority of nerve injuries are preventable, and therefore, a clear understanding of their etiology is essential. Certain patients are predisposed to peripheral nerve compromise because their nerves are diseased, as seen in diabetics and alcoholics. Elderly patients develop neuropathies because their peripheral nerves do not tolerate pressure well and because they are less mobile; therefore, they maintain prolonged positions that place their nerves at risk (28,29).

Brachial Plexus

There are several bed positions the burn patient may assume, and intraoperative positions in which he or she is placed, that put the brachial plexus at risk. In conjunction with these at-risk positions, loss of muscle tone in the anesthetized patient and immobility of the patient in bed add to the problem of positioning risks. Possible mechanisms of injury to the plexus during anesthesia have been reported by several authors. Jackson and Keats reported that plexus stretch injury could occur in patients positioned supine with shoulders abducted 90° or more and externally rotated. In addition, if the upper arm is posteriorly displaced (i.e., hung below table level), added tension is placed on the plexus.

The mechanism creating the injury is compression of the plexus between the clavicle and first rib, causing tension and stretch with these particular shoulder and arm movements (30). Ewing wrote that when the humerus is abducted in external rotation, its head forms a prominence in the axilla where the nerve trunks pass; the nerves may become angulated with resultant stretching. The nerve trunks to the upper extremity are anchored at the vertebral column and by fascial attachments in the axilla; they pass under a tendinous arch formed by the insertion of the pectoralis minor. Even though nerves are extensible, there is a limit to their stretch (31). Dhuner reported that a brachial plexus injury occured in as little as 40 minutes in the operating room. Other at-risk positions are prone and side-lying. In the prone position, the patient lies with arms abducted 90° or more and externally rotated (32). Patients positioned on one side with the opposite arm abducted, elbow extended, and then suspended from an intravenous pole or overhead frame can develop a traction injury to the brachial plexus. This position may be used in the surgical suite for grafting of the axilla or lateral chest wall, for bed positioning to decrease edema of the extremity, or to prevent axillary contractures.

In order to prevent compression or stretch injury to the brachial plexus, it has been recommended that the supine patient be positioned in 15° of arm horizontal adduction, lifting the clavicle off the first rib. One or two pillows under the chest of the prone-lying patient will adduct the extremities and lift the clavicle off the first rib.

One additional problem that can occur is a stretch injury of the plexus after an axillary contracture release, particularly if the contracture has been long-standing. All structures can become tight with prolonged limited mobility; therefore, the surgeon often chooses to do staged releases to try to prevent a stretch injury from occurring. In a stretch injury, the upper trunk (i.e., C5 and C6) of the brachial plexus is involved primarily; generally the patient recovers completely, but it may take several months.

Suprascapular Nerve

Injury to the suprascapular nerve often is overlooked because function is not markedly impaired and the burn usually

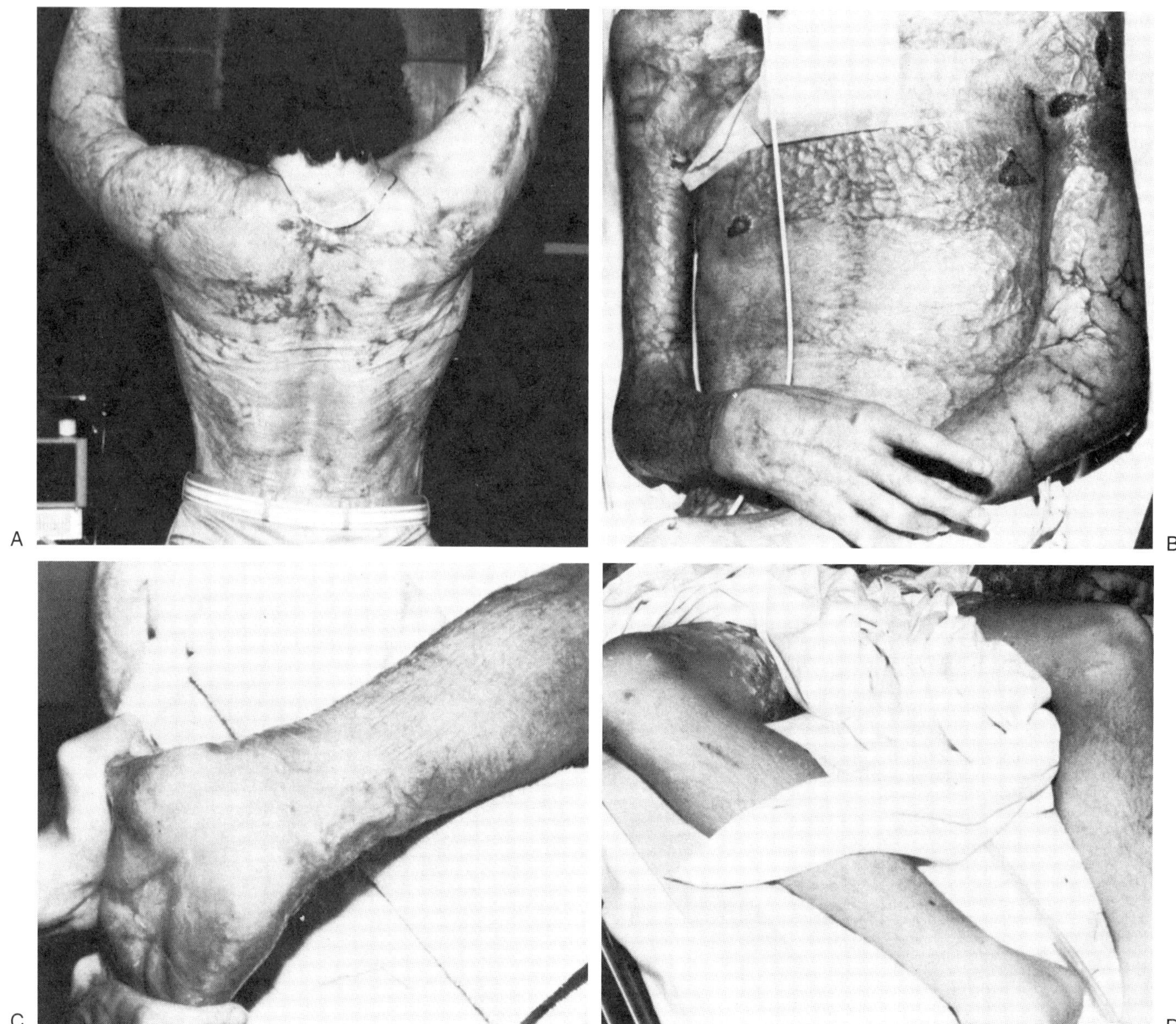

FIG. 62-16. A: Suprascapular nerve injury has occurred on the patient's right. **B:** At-risk position for ulnar nerve injury. **C:** At-risk position for median nerve injury. **D:** At-risk position for peroneal nerve injury.

involves the posterior shoulder girdle on the side of injury (Fig. 62-16*A*). The suprascapular nerve passes through a fibro-osseous tunnel of the suprascapular notch to innervate the supraspinatus and infraspinatus. As reported by Rask, hyperprotraction of the shoulder overstretches the nerve, with resultant swelling and unrelenting pain in the shoulder region. A hyperprotracted position can occur when the patient tries to stretch the skin in the posterior shoulder girdle by forward flexion and horizontal adduction of the arm. Injury can be prevented by stabilizing the scapula (33).

Ulnar Nerve

The primary area of involvement of the ulnar nerve in the burn patient is at the elbow in the cubital tunnel. The roof of the tunnel is the arcuate ligament, which extends from a fixed point on the medial epicondyle to a movable attachment on the olecranon. The floor of the tunnel is formed by the medial ligament of the elbow. Wadsworth reports that the capacity of the tunnel is maximal with elbow extension when the arcuate ligament is slack (34). When the elbow is flexed to 90°, the arcuate ligament becomes taut, and the medial ligament bulges, decreasing the capacity of the tunnel and putting the nerve at risk (Fig. 62-16*B*). He also noted that pronation of the forearm could cause surface contact with the cubital tunnel, whereas supination of the forearm lifts the tunnel containing the ulnar nerve away from the surface. Unfortunately, many burn patients assume the position of elbow flexion and forearm pronation in the supine and prone positions, causing elbow flexion–pronation contractures; this probably accounts for the majority of ulnar neuropathies. In the operating suite, the patient frequently is positioned in the same manner. An injury at this level usually spares the flexor carpi ulnaris and ulnar half of the flexor digitorum profundus because the fibers to these muscles are located deep in the central part of the nerve (34). Another circumstance predisposing a patient to an ulnar neuropathy is subluxation of the ulnar nerve onto the medial epicondyle, thereby essentially leaving it unprotected from pressure. In cases of heterotopic bone at the elbow, entrapment of the ulnar nerve in an osseous tunnel has been reported (35).

Radial Nerve

The radial nerve is involved most frequently in the burn patient by compression in the spiral groove, where the nerve winds around the humerus and virtually lies on bone. Compression injuries at this level may be secondary to the arm resting on the side rails of the bed, hanging over the edge of the operating table, or slipping off the edge of an arm board. In these cases, the triceps muscle usually is spared because it is innervated at a higher level. Restraints at the distal forearm–wrist level can injure the superficial cutaneous branch of the radial nerve, causing paresthesia of the dorsum of the hand and thumb.

Median Nerve

Most injuries to the median nerve occur at the wrist level and usually are caused by extremes of positioning used to gain range of motion (Fig. 62-16*C*). Prolonged or repeated hyperextension of the wrist compresses the nerve at the carpal tunnel, which can cause paresthesia in the thumb, index, middle, and ring fingers and weakness of the thenar muscles. Sustained stretch to the wrist in a hyperextended position, either with splints or in exercise programs, should be performed with caution.

Femoral Nerve

Femoral nerve dysfunction in the burn patient is uncommon; however, the femoral nerve has been known to be injured in the femoral triangle after hematoma formation, secondary to obtaining femoral blood samples. Femoral blood withdrawal often is necessary in the extensively burned patient.

The nerve also is susceptible to injury in patients on anticoagulant therapy who have had a retroperitoneal hemorrhage. Mant and colleagues studied 76 patients receiving heparin anticoagulation for venous thromboembolism and found a 7% incidence of retroperitoneal hemorrhage (36). Reinstein and associates studied femoral nerve dysfunction after retroperitoneal hemorrhage with computed tomography and were able to localize the hematoma. They found that localization of the hematoma within the tight iliacus muscle compartment could produce femoral nerve injury by compressing the nerve against the taut psoas tendon. It is reported that 75% of the patients experience complete recovery of nerve function with conservative management (37).

Peroneal Nerve

The peroneal nerve has several peculiarities that make it vulnerable to injury. Studies of the nerve by Berry and Richardson showed that the nerve is applied to the periosteum of the fibula for a total of 10 cm, is exposed over the bony prominence for about 4 cm, covered only by skin and fascia, and has limited longitudinal mobility of about 0.5 cm (38). Although compression injuries of the peroneal nerve are notoriously associated with the lateral decubitus position, metal stirrups, and leg straps, less attention is given to positions of the leg that cause stretch injuries. When a patient maintains a position of externally rotated hips, flexion of the knees, and inverted feet (i.e., frog leg; either because the bed is too short, because a urinal is placed between the thighs for men, or when there are tender medial thigh or perineum burns), the peroneal nerve is placed on a stretch and can be injured in a matter of hours because of its limited longitudinal mobility (Fig. 62-16*D*). This type of injury usually involves the common peroneal nerve, and moderate-to-good recovery is reported at about 3 months (38).

Another source of injury that cannot be ignored is pressure at the fibular head from heavy, bulky dressings. Windowing of the dressings over the fibular head helps relieve pressure.

Occasionally patients with deep burns on the dorsum of the feet and ankles complain of numbness between the great and second toes. On examination, extensor digitorum brevis atrophy may be noted; otherwise, there is no weakness in the common peroneal distribution. The distal deep peroneal nerve at the anterior tarsal tunnel may be compressed, causing these signs and symptoms.

Tourniquet Paralysis

Most articles on tourniquet paralysis usually state that since the pneumatic tourniquet has been employed, it has virtually eliminated the danger of nerve palsy. However, the pneumatic tourniquet used to establish a bloodless field has not prevented this complication to the extent reported. Aho and colleagues report that faulty gauges on pneumatic tourniquets can sometimes be the cause of the problem (39). Tourniquet inflation to 500 mm Hg instead of the intended 250 mm Hg can cause direct pressure injury of the nerve at the cuff edge. The radial nerve is most vulnerable, but ulnar and median nerves also can be damaged. It is reported by Sunderland that the nerve lesions heal in 3 to 6 months and are only exceptionally permanently damaged (40). In cases of paralysis, the tourniquet time has varied from 28 minutes to 2 hours and 40 minutes (21,39).

Peripheral Neuropathy

Generalized peripheral neuropathy is the most common peripheral neurologic disorder seen in the burn patient. It usually occurs in patients with burns of more than 20% of the total body surface area, with the exception of electrical injuries, in which the total body surface burn may be less. The incidence ranges from 15%, as determined by Henderson, Koepke, and Feller, to 29%, as reported by Helm and associates (28,41,42). The etiology of peripheral neuropathies is uncertain; however, metabolic complications and neurotoxic drugs have been implicated. The patient may have symptoms of paresthesia and signs of mild to moderate weakness in the muscles of the distal extremities. On manual muscle testing, most patients eventually appear to recover their strength, although they complain of lack of endurance and easy fatigability for years postburn (28,41,42).

Multiple mononeuropathy was found in 9 of 121 persons with more than 40% TBSA burn injury (43). Multiple mononeuropathy is defined as an asymmetric neuropathy that involves two or more nerves that results from multiple crush syndrome. Multiple crush syndrome represents the summation of the effects of neurotoxins, metabolic factors, and/or compression. At 1 year, lower extremity multiple mononeuropathies achieved good functional recovery; upper extremity results were less satisfactory. The intervention utilized with these persons included sensory education, range of motion exercise, and splinting.

BONE AND JOINT CHANGES

Bone Growth

Growth disturbances in burns may result from premature fusion of the entire epiphyseal plate or only a portion of the plate and subsequent growth arrest. Premature fusion of the epiphyseal plate can cause bone shortening and should be a consideration in children who have scar tissue crossing joints, or especially who have persistent joint contractures. Partial epiphyseal plate fusion may cause bone deviation and deformity (44). Pressure treatment of scar tissue as reported by Leung and colleagues can cause regressed skeletal growth in the chin and thoracic cage from wearing a face mask and body suit. The face was noted to be "birdlike" because of the slow-growing mandible and the thoracic cage developing a roundish appearance (45). Shortened legs, hands, and feet have occurred (Fig. 62-17).

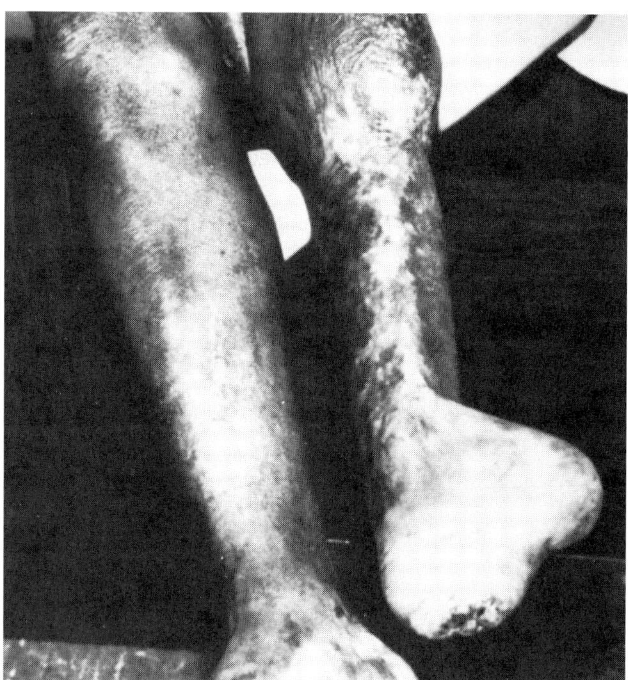

FIG. 62-17. Growth disturbance in a 56-year-old patient who was burned at 6 years of age.

Growth stimulation also has been found by some investigators and is described as growth spurts in children and increased shoe size in adults. It is postulated that skeletal growth is stimulated through stasis or passive hyperemia or a chronic inflammatory process.

Osteophytes

Evans and Smith report that osteophytes are the most frequently observed skeletal alteration in adult burn patients. They are most often seen at the elbow and occur along the articular margins of the olecranon or coronoid process (46,47).

New Bone Formation

Heterotopic Ossification

New bone formation begins as heterotopic calcification and is seen on plain film as a fluffy shadow. In at least 50% of patients this calcification will be absorbed; in the remainder it can ossify. Calcification and ossification have been reported to occur as early as 5 to 6 weeks postburn but usually develop in 3 to 4 months. Teperman and associates reported that bone scans assist in making early diagnosis; in one patient the positive bone scan preceded positive radiologic findings by 3 weeks. Rarely are there any detectable chemical changes by laboratory tests. One of the earliest signs of heterotopic ossification is loss of joint range of motion; this change can precede radiologic findings by 5 days (48). The most common site involved is the elbow, followed by the hip in children and the shoulder in adults.

Patients who are predisposed to the development of heterotopic ossification are those with full-thickness burns to the upper extremities of more than 20% total body surface area. Other commonalities for development are immobility, repeated minor trauma, and pressure, particularly over the medial epicondyle. Incidence of true heterotopic ossification probably ranges between 0.1% and 3.1% (48).

Once the diagnosis of heterotopic ossification has been made, forceful passive movements of the extremity are contraindicated because this type of exercise can make the condition worse. Only gentle movement within the patient's active range should be performed. Operative treatment is indicated if there is no spontaneous resolution of the heterotopic calcification. Most surgeons will not operate until the bone is mature, which can take 12 to 18 months. A retrospective review of 1,478 burn admissions indicated that 18 developed heterotopic ossification; ten of these recovered full range of motion with the above treatment protocol within 6 months of diagnosis. The remaining eight received surgery followed by rehabilitation, and all developed functional range of motion with no recurrence after 3 years (49).

Bony Changes in Electrical Burns

New bone formation at amputation sites in the electrical burn has been reported to involve long bones, or more specifically, above-elbow, below-elbow, above-knee, and below-knee residual limbs (Fig. 62-18). Helm and colleagues reported that 23 of 28 long-bone amputations (82%) developed new bone at the amputation site (22). Of the 61 amputations studied, 78% of upper extremity and 90% of lower extremity long-bone amputations had new bone formation. The average time from amputation to diagnosis of new bone was 38 weeks. Five patients (11.6%) required surgical revision of the stump, and an additional three patients (7%) required replacement of their prosthesis secondary to new bone formation. The cause of this high rate of new bone formation in the electrical amputee has not been determined; however, it has been postulated that perhaps the effect of high voltage on bone is similar to long-term low-voltage/amperage stimulation for promoting callus formation at fracture sites (50).

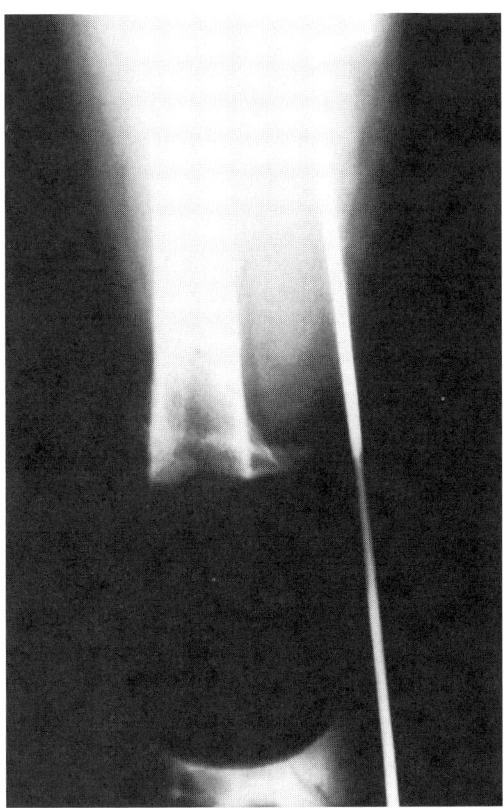

FIG. 62-18. Bone spur in an electrical burn in an above-knee amputee.

Vrabec and Kolar studied bone changes in the electrical burn and described bony changes directly related to the action of the passage of electric current as bone splitting, bone pearls from the melting of bone minerals, bony necrosis, and periosteal new bone caused by inflammatory reaction as a result of avulsion of the periosteum. Other authors have reported lucent holes in the bone and bone swelling (51).

Scoliosis and Kyphosis

Asymmetric burns of the trunk, hips, and shoulder girdle can cause the patient to favor the side of the body burned and shift weight to the same side. A functional scoliosis can develop because of the pain in maintaining correct posture, and the functional scoliosis can change to a structural scoliosis with vertebral wedging if a child has a growth spurt before this is corrected (52). Burns on the anterior neck, shoulders, and chest wall may produce a rounding of the shoulders and sunken chest. This is caused by burn scar shortening and by the patient assuming a protective posture. The result can be a kyphotic thoracic spine if not corrected with proper exercise and positioning programs. Surgical excision of adherent scar tissue to the anterior chest wall usually is not successful for correcting this abnormality.

Septic Arthritis

Septic arthritis can be overlooked easily in the severe burn patient. Inability to make the diagnosis results from lack of the usual clinical signs and symptoms. Some septic joints are pain-free, and some are covered with burn wounds that mask the usual fusiform swelling and local tenderness.

The two primary causes of a septic joint in burns are penetrating burns into joints and bacteremia. Septic arthritis may cause gross dislocation because of capsular laxity or cartilage and bone destruction (46), or it may result in severe restriction of movement or ankylosis. It occurs most frequently in the hips, knees, wrists, and joints of the hands.

Subluxations and Dislocations

Joint subluxation in the hands and feet is seen commonly in burn patients. Generally the burn is over the dorsal aspect of the part, and as the burn wound contracts, it pulls the joint into hyperextension. If this is allowed to persist, the joint will subluxate. This is more commonly seen in the MCP and metatarsophalangeal (MTP) joints. An ulnar neuropathy can accentuate the problem in the fourth and fifth digits (Fig.

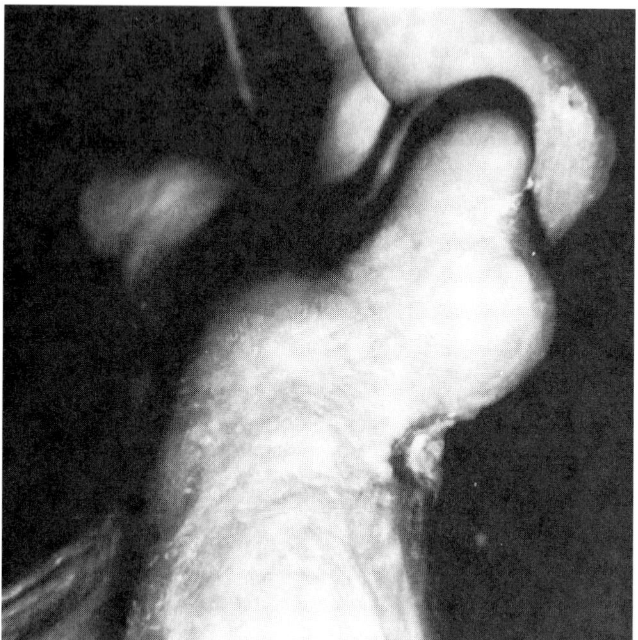

FIG. 62-19. Severe subluxation of the fifth metacarpal joint.

62-19). A hyperextended thumb at the MCP joint also can easily subluxate. Prevention in the hand begins in the acute phase of treatment by splinting the MCP joints in flexion to approximately 60° to 90°, thereby keeping the collateral ligament on a stretch. This is done in conjunction with an exercise program stressing joint flexion. The MTP joints of the toes become more of a problem posthealing as the burn scar contracts. Simple application of surgical high-top shoes with a metatarsal bar worn 24 hours a day keeps the toes in an antideformity position.

Hip dislocation can be a problem in children if the hip is allowed to remain in an adducted and flexed position. Shoulder dislocations are reported to occur in extreme positions of abduction and extension.

LONG-TERM REHABILITATION

The postacute rehabilitative phase of treatment can be five to ten times longer than the acute phase of treatment, and it is during this period that the patient undergoes a multitude of physical and emotional changes. It is usually during this time that the patient and family realize how devastating this insult has been to the body. They frequently react in adverse ways that can affect outcome if proper support is not available. The physicians and therapists assume a new role when rehabilitation, rather than survival, is the primary issue.

Skin and Wound Care

Rarely does the patient leave the hospital with completely healed wounds and donor sites; therefore, continuation of the wound care program with hydrotherapy, debridement, and dressing changes is necessary. Once the wounds are healed, or there are only spotty areas open, hydrotherapy should be discontinued because of the ultimate drying effect on the skin. This will, in turn, cause the skin to crack and make it more susceptible to bacteria invasion.

Additional problems can occur posthealing, such as skin breakdown, blistering, ulceration, and allergic reactions. Newly formed skin is especially fragile, and even the slightest trauma, as from stretching exercises, pressure from splints and garments, or from minor bumps, can cause abrasions and blisters (Fig. 62-20). Blisters can be drained with a sterile needle and flattened with a dressing. If denuded areas are created by large blisters, mercurochrome is excellent for treatment. These areas usually will dry, crust, and heal. All open wounds, however, should be gently cleaned with a mild soap. Ulcerations or chronic open wounds have a tendency to develop in tight bands of scar tissue in the axilla and cubital and popliteal fossae. These wounds generally are deep, and repeated splitting of the wounds with exercise prolongs healing and causes increased scarring. If the wound is clean, application of a biological dressing and placing the part at rest will speed the healing process.

Allergic reactions posthealing that produce moist, weeping wounds can be frustrating because finding the irritating agent is sometimes difficult. The most common agents that cause these reactions have been skin lubricants, particularly those products with mineral oil; pressure garments; and various soaps used to cleanse the skin. All of these agents should be discontinued for 2 to 4 days before beginning substitution with different products, one at a time.

The healed burn skin often lacks normal lubrication and suppleness. Dryness and decreased elasticity contribute to skin problems such as cracking, pruritus, and skin breakdown. Patients who are treated in settings where there is no hands-on technique suffer from hypersensitive skin and scars. Skin lubrication helps alleviate some of these problems and should be considered an essential part of the overall treatment program performed by the therapists. Massage of healed burn wounds can accomplish skin lubrication, de-

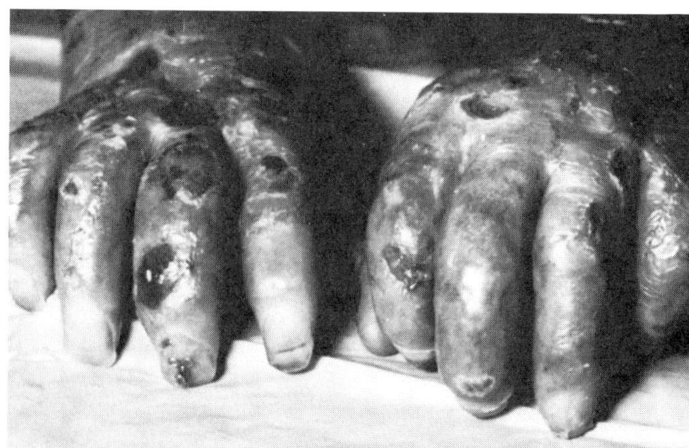

FIG. 62-20. Fragile skin with multiple open wounds.

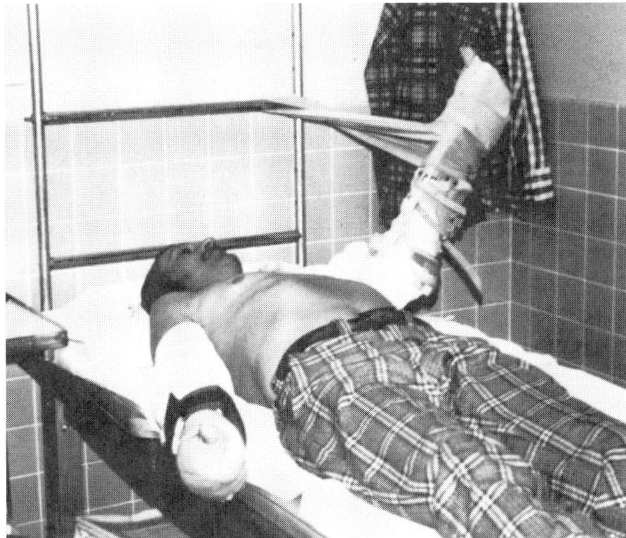

FIG. 62-21. Sustained stretch to gain range of motion.

crease skin hypersensitivity, and increase skin pliability. A variety of lotions have been found to be nonirritating, such as aloe vera moisturizers, vitamin E ointment, cocoa butter, and Corrective Concepts moisturizers (Pattee Products, Dallas, TX). Pruritic symptoms frequently require oral antihistamine medication as well as pressure garments to make the patient more comfortable (14).

Exercise

Techniques

Maintaining range of motion of a joint posthealing or postgrafting is more difficult than in the acute phase. Burn scars contract, form bands, and thicken, and joint range of motion is affected. Remolding of the burn scar is possible while the scar is actively undergoing internal changes, such as collagen degradation and deposition and myofibroblastic activity. Once the burn scar matures, stretching of skin contracture is of less benefit.

By far the most effective stretching technique for skin contractures is slow, sustained stretch. The part being stretched should be visible and should be palpated along the line of pull to ensure that the skin does not rupture. Stretching can be done manually with weights, traction, and serial casting. The technique of applying paraffin to the part being mobilized and allowing 30 minutes of sustained stretch has been very rewarding in gaining range of motion; at the same time it decreases joint discomfort and lubricates the skin (Fig. 62-21). The paraffin temperature must be lowered to 116°F to 118°F to prevent burning of hyperesthetic skin (53).

Another important principle in the exercise program is to put the entire length of a burn scar on a total stretch (Fig. 62-22). In other words, if a scar crosses multiple joints, all involved joints are stretched simultaneously. A joint does not have full range of motion unless full range is obtained in combined movements.

Finally, all patients should be on a generalized strengthening program for reconditioning after prolonged inactivity. Resistive exercises of opposing muscle groups also are beneficial in contracture prevention and treatment. Exercises for endurance and coordination frequently are overlooked in burn rehabilitation but are an essential aspect of the total program.

Specialized Splinting

Without the benefit of custom-made splints, exercise programs would be in vain. A joint contracture may be stretched to full range, but maintaining that range depends in part on static and dynamic positioning accomplished with splinting (Fig. 62-23). Hence, the mistake often is made to splint joints in full extension for prolonged periods because the patient looks anatomically correct; however, function is sacrificed. This unfortunately is true especially for elbows, which often are placed in extension.

Experienced therapists are able to make splints that control more than one joint and, at the same time, apply pressure over thick bands of scar tissue. Major areas of concern in the convalescent period are hands. Difficult areas requiring specialized splints include:

- Palmar contractures (Fig. 62-23*C*,*D*)
- Cupping of the palm (Fig. 62-23*E*)
- Fifth-digit flexion contracture (Fig. 62-23*H*)
- Tight thumb–index web space (Fig. 62-23*I*)
- Ruptured extensor hood mechanism
- Neck flexion contracture
- Hip flexion–abduction external rotation in children
- Ankle-dorsiflexion contractures.

There is another area of major concern for which no effec-

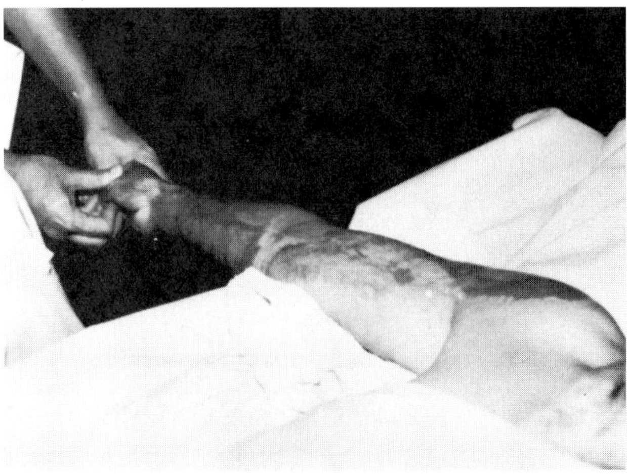

FIG. 62-22. The total length of the burn scar is involved in the stretch.

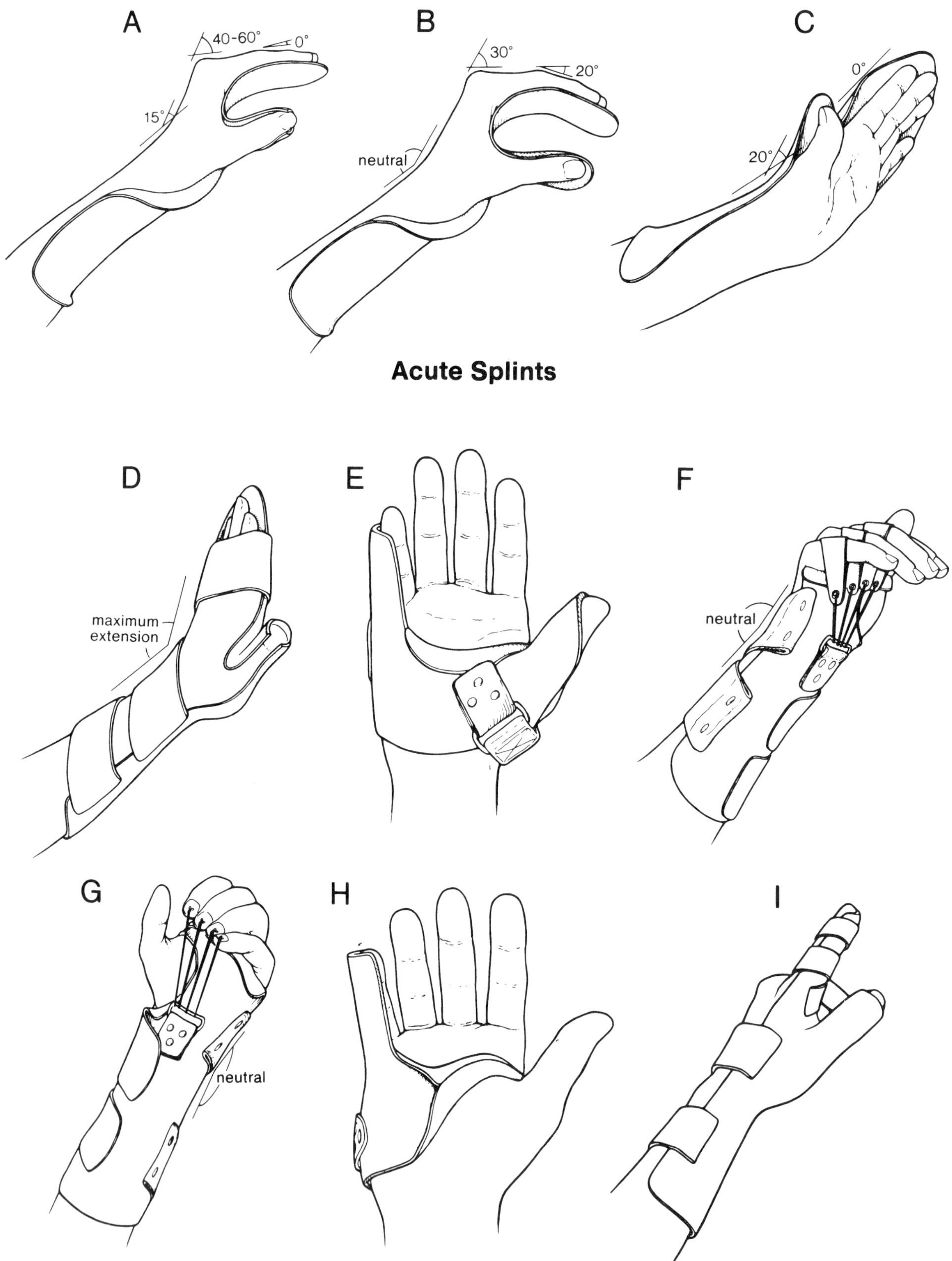

FIG. 62-23. A–I: Common hand splints. (From Helm PA, Kevorkian GC, Lushbaugh MS, et al. Burn injury: rehabilitation management in 1982. *Arch Phys Med Rehabil* 1982; 63:6–16.)

tive splint has yet been devised, and that is for pronation contractures of the forearm. As mentioned earlier, serial casting or serial splinting can be extremely effective in reducing contractures. The more common splints need not be addressed because their indications are obvious.

Modalities

There are certain modalities commonly used in rehabilitation medicine clinics that have been found useful in treating specific burn complications. Electrical stimulation, using an alternating current, is helpful in treating tendon adherence to underlying scar tissue. Bipolar, pulsed, or surged alternating current helps reduce edema and increases joint range of motion. The transcutaneous electrical stimulator is useful for treatment of various pain problems, particularly those involving the shoulder from prolonged or faulty positioning.

Ultrasound has been used to treat painful joints and facilitate better tolerance of range-of-motion exercise. It has also been applied along with ice massage to decrease hypertrophic scar pain. In a prospective randomized double-blind study, the effectiveness of ultrasound with passive stretching versus placebo ultrasound with passive stretching was investigated. The results indicated no difference in range of motion or perceived pain between these two groups. This suggests that although widely used, ultrasound may not have an effect on functional improvement of contractures (54).

Intermittent compression units or similar devices are valuable in reducing edema in extremities, primarily the edematous hand. Posthealing hand edema secondary to circumferential burns of the forearm, hands with reflex sympathetic dystrophy, and hands with postischemic hand syndrome usually respond well with elevation and compression. Persistent edema can be devastating if allowed to persist, because it can result in a ''frozen hand.''

Continuous passive motion (CPM) machines can never take the place of the hands-on exercises by the therapists. Occasionally CPM is indicated when the patient is resistant to the exercise program from fear of pain, in children who seem to relax better with CPM, and in those who need additional range-of-motion treatments for exceptionally tight areas.

Burn Sequelae

Hypertrophic Scarring

It is well known that hypertrophic scar and scar contracture can result from deep partial- and full-thickness burns. Many factors contribute to the severity of hypertrophic scarring: depth of burn, healing time, grafting, age of patient, and skin character. An excellent review on hypertrophic scarring and the effects of pressure was done by Jensen and Parshley (55). They reported on areas of the skin affected by the scar, noting that the epidermis was not thickened and did not contribute to the depth of the hypertrophic scar. They also reported, ''the regenerated epidermis lacks rete pegs and interconnections that attach it to the dermis; hence, it is cosmetically abnormal with respect to color, texture, and friability and is prone to abrasion with minor trauma (55). They noted that changes in the dermis involving fibroblasts, myofibroblasts, mast cells, collagen, mucopolysaccharides, and vasculature cause a metabolically active abnormal mass of thick tissue. In hypertrophic scars, collagen forms large nodules rather than loose wavy bundles as seen in normal dermis. In granulation tissue and hypertrophic scars, capillaries proliferate and are thought to have a mediating effect on hypertrophic scar formation. The mechanism for contraction of hypertrophic scar is thought to be the myofibroblast (55).

It has been known for years that external pressure in the form of special garments that provide at least 25 mm Hg or more of pressure (i.e., above capillary pressure) can flatten scar tissue if worn continuously until the scars lose redness and soften. It is postulated that pressure inhibits blood flow with occlusion of vessels in the scar, affecting fibroblastic activity and reducing tissue water content, thereby reducing the amount of ground substance. Prolonged pressure also may have detrimental effects, and the therapist should therefore be certain there are indications for its use. Burn scars that lose their redness within 8 to 10 weeks may not become hypertrophic.

In a study of 100 persons with burn injury to determine factors associated with risk of hypertrophic scar development, 38 persons developed hypertrophic scars in 63 of 245 anatomic areas. Incidence was greater in African-Americans, especially if healing required more than 10 days. Healing time also predicted scar formation; i.e., 33% scarred if healing required 14 to 21 days, whereas 78% scarred if healing required more than 21 days. These authors proposed the following treatment protocol based on these findings (56):

1. *No* pressure if healing within 10 days.
2. *Mandatory* pressure for African-Americans if healing requires 14 to 21 days.
3. *Recommended* pressure for all persons if healing requires 14 to 21 days.
4. *Mandatory* pressure for all persons if healing requires more than 21 days.
5. *Recommended* surgery if healing requires more than 21 days.

Silicone gel sheeting has been reported to assist in scar treatment without pressure assistance. To investigate the effectiveness of silicone gel, a sample of ten adults with 14 scarred areas was studied. Each was its own control, as one scarred area on each person was treated with silicone gel and another scarred area was treated without silicone, both for a period of 8 weeks. Based on elastometry, skin biopsy, texture, color, thickness, durability, and itching, the silicone-treated areas were more improved at 4 weeks, 8 weeks, and 4 weeks after treatment was stopped than the control scars

(57). This suggests that this silicone gel may be an effective intervention for hypertrophic scars.

Other Residual Defects

After the surgeon has completed all of the reconstructive procedures and the patient is, from a medical standpoint, totally rehabilitated, there are certain residual defects that affect the remainder of the burn patient's life (Table 62-2). These range from sensory impairment, cold intolerance, and calloused feet (Fig. 62-24), to social and psychological problems.

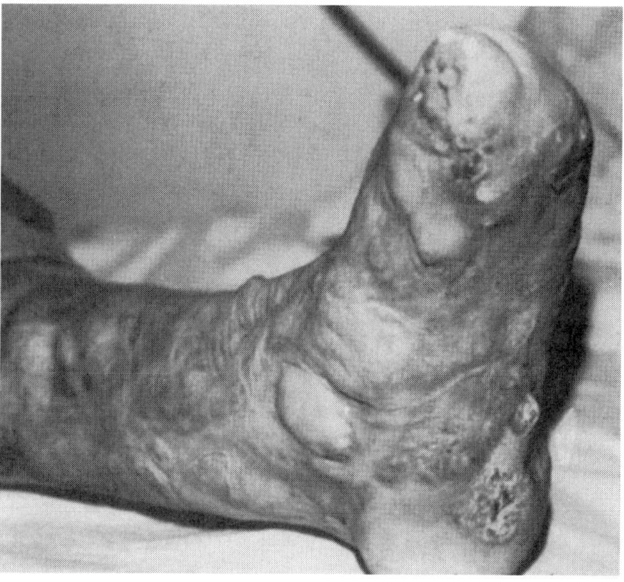

FIG. 62-24. Calloused foot.

Disability Determination

The rating of permanent impairment is a physician's function and is an appraisal of the nature and extent of the patient's illness or injury as it affects performance. Permanent disability is not purely a medical condition, but is based on a person's impairment and multiple psychosocial and economic factors. The evaluation of disability is much more complex, and factors such as age, gender, education, economics, and social relationships are involved.

The evaluation of the burn victim requires the physician to consider such unique factors as the following:

Heat and cold intolerance
Sensitivity to sunlight
Pain
Chemical sensitivity
Changes in apocrine function
Decreased coordination
Decreased sensation
Decreased strength
Contractures

If scars affect sweat glands, hair growth, nail growth, or range of motion, they may affect performance and cause impairment. Every state as well as private and governmental agencies have different criteria on which to base impairment ratings. By using the generally accepted methods of evaluating impairment, however, as well as by considering the burn patient's unique factors, the physician may, with relative objectivity, establish an impairment rating (58).

The physician has the ultimate responsibility in deciding when the burn patient is medically capable of returning to work, and some unique factors must be considered in this. Open wounds in employees involved in food handling should not be allowed. In other management areas, open wounds can be aggravated by irritants and dirt or constant friction or pressure on the skin, and the employee should refrain from any duties that inhibit wound closure. New immature skin is delicate and fragile, and laborers, especially those with hand burns, can easily reinjure freshly burned skin. Cold intolerance is a very common problem after thermal injury, and employees working in cold climates or re-

TABLE 62-2. *Burn sequelae*

Defect	Cause
Hypopigmentation, hyperpigmentation	Melanin abnormality and donor site choice
Sensory impairment	Sensory nerve fibers fail to penetrate thick scar tissue Damaged in full-thickness burns
Abnormal skin lubrication	Loss of sebaceous glands because of depth of burns Unable to penetrate heavy scar tissue
Abnormal hair growth	Hair follicle damage Unable to penetrate heavy scar
Abnormal sweating, heat intolerance	Loss of sweat glands as a result of depth of burn
Cold intolerance	Abnormal vasomotor response
Pruritus	Dry skin from lack of lubrication
Fragile skin	Loss of normal elasticity; thin
Ingrown hairs, pustules	Hair cannot penetrate thick scar and becomes infected
Permanent tanning	If exposed to direct sunlight before 12 to 18 months postburn
Marjolin ulcer	Chronic recurring ulcers Poorly nourished scar tissue
Calloused feet (Fig. 62-24)	Deep excision of feet Skin adherence to bone Bony abnormality
Cosmesis	Permanent scarring Flattened facies Body part amputated
Joint pain	Repeated minor trauma to hands and knees Joint pinning
Psychological, social	All of the above
Fatigability	
Lack of endurance	

frigerated areas may be unable to tolerate the discomfort and perform job responsibilities (59).

PSYCHOSOCIAL ISSUES IN BURN REHABILITATION

A major burn injury results in psychological/emotional difficulties as well as physical impairment/disability. There is a significant psychological shock/stress reaction to the initial injury and hospital experiences. In many cases, individuals do not remember ICU activities and early painful wound care and debridement. Gradually, the impact of the situation becomes apparent, and emotional problems can emerge. Among these psychological/emotional problems are anxiety, depression, and/or anger/frustration, which are reactions to functional and/or cosmetic factors, family integrity, sexual functioning, ability to return to work, and/or resumption of valued recreational activities. Phobia-like fear of the work place or other situations that may be a reminder of the burn injury circumstances can occur. Posttraumatic stress disorder is another problem that has been documented. Disrupted sleep, itching, and pain while performing therapy or other daily activities are also factors in these emotional difficulties.

The frequency of emotional problems as a result of burn injury is not clearly understood. In a review of long-term follow-up studies of the prevalence of psychosocial problems, it was found that the reported incidence varied from 28% to 76% (60). In another study it was reported that 10% of 340 adults manifested emotional difficulties up to 12 years postburn (61). This latter study also found that these problems were related to unemployment, reduced ocupational status, situation avoidance, and reduced recreational activities. Other research has attempted to relate emotional difficulty with burn-related factors. Burn severity (major burn injury) and face and/or hands being burned have been found to be related to long-term quality-of-life problems and emotional difficulty (62,63). However, other studies have found nonsignificant relationships between percentage TBSA burn injury or body parts burned and long-term emotional sequelae (61,64–66).

Posttraumatic stress disorder (PTSD) in persons who have been burned has also been studied. In one survey, 30% of patients met the full criteria for PTSD during hospitalization, but none did at discharge (67). Another study reported that PTSD increases after discharge from the hospital (68). Both PTSD and other significant emotional problems have also been found to be more prevalent in electrical burn injuries (69). It is clear that PTSD is a possible problem related to burn injury, but its persistence and long-term effect on quality of life are not well documented. It should also be considered that this symptom picture may be more consistent with an acute stress disorder diagnosis if duration is less than 4 weeks (70).

Return to work after burn injury has been studied extensively. Eight-five percent of a group of 115 hospitalized work-related burn injuries returned to work; the remaining 15% were permanently disabled, largely (about 80%) by electrical injury (71). The mean time to return to work in this study was 58 days, but some persons have extremely long return-to-work intervals. Other reports indicate a mean 19 weeks off work after burn injury (72), a 63-day return-to-work interval in 155 patients (73), and 17 weeks to return to work in 65 patients with a mean 25% TBSA burn injury (74). Although these results vary, it can be concluded that 70% to 80% of working persons who are burned return to work in an average 10 to 20 weeks and that size, depth, and location (hands) are factors that affect time to return to work.

CONCLUSION

The basic components of an interdisciplinary burn rehabilitation program are wound care, stretching and pressure, splinting, conditioning and strengthening, psychological assessment and intervention, and long-term medical rehabilitation follow-up. The effectiveness of this approach to burn injury has been indirectly demonstrated by the significant reduction in reconstruction surgery admissions from 1970 through 1985, despite no change in burn severity and greater survival rates (75). The following is a synopsis of burn rehabilitation planning during both acute and postdischarge phases of treatment.

Inpatient rehabilitation begins on the day of admission or within the first 24 hours. The rehabilitation burn team normally consists of a physician, physical therapist, occupational therapist, social worker, and psychologist and/or psychiatrist. The patient is generally seen once or twice daily, 6 days per week, by both the physical and occupational therapist. The typical inpatient treatment should involve:

1. Positioning with special devices in bed and chair.
2. Passive, active, and active assistive exercises.
3. Casting and splinting of body parts to prevent contractures.
4. Range of motion under anesthesia as indicated.
5. Transfer activities.
6. Ambulation/assistive devices.
7. Early application of pressure.

Patients are then discharged to a rehabilitation facility (usually those with larger debilitating burns) or to an outpatient clinic for follow-up therapy. Problems that require outpatient treatment include open wounds, contracture, fragile hypersensitive skin, early hypertrophic scarring, itching, pain, weakness and deconditioning, and possible psychological/emotional reactions. A typical rehabilitation program for a 25% burn injury to the upper and lower extremities would be treatment for 5 days per week for 5 to 6 hours per day and would include:

1. Hydrotherapy, wound care, and dressing change.
2. Paraffin and sustained stretch to all healed areas over joints with tightness.

3. Active and active assistive exercises to all joints involved.
4. Serial casting or splinting of major contractures.
5. Massage to healed skin to loosen scar tissue and desensitize skin.
6. Evaluate activities of daily living and modify with assistive devices as needed.
7. Conditioning program consisting of treadmill, upper body ergometer, and bike.
8. Individualized strengthening programs for mononeuropathies.
9. Fit with compression garments to control scarring (two sets). Order new garments every 3 to 4 months as they tend to wear out or become loose and ineffective.
10. Silicon gel sheeting.
11. Prescription for prosthetic or orthotic devices where needed.

This program could last anywhere from 4 to 6 months; it would decrease in number of days treated per week as the patient improves; it could last for a year or more if the burn injury is more severe. Rechecks by the physician prescribing treatment should occur every 2 weeks and less frequently as progress occurs.

The psychological/emotional needs of individuals with burn injury also require attention. Problems identified during acute hospitalization should be properly addressed. These problems may take on greater significance after discharge, when the individual is faced with beginning the process of community reentry. Because burn injury results in documented psychological sequelae that can be disruptive of functional independence and compliance with treatment, it is recommended that individuals with burn injury be evaluated after discharge and at longer-term follow-up to identify if problems exist. If they do exist, short-term psychotherapy (5–15 sessions) is suggested, and relaxation training/biofeedback can be used adjunctively for sleep, pain, or other stress-related problems.

Follow-up rehabilitation is required after reconstructive procedures such as contracture release. Wound care and range-of-motion exercises are usually restarted to assist with wound closure and prevent contracture recurrence. Specialized splinting or casting may be necessary to maintain proper positioning at night. In most cases this postreconstructive surgery rehabilitation period is much shorter, e.g., 5 to 6 weeks.

REFERENCES

1. Rice DP, MacKenzie EJ. *Cost of injury in the United States: A report to Congress.* Atlanta, GA: Centers for Disease Control, 1989.
2. Demling RH. Preface. In: LaLonde C, ed. *Burn trauma.* New York: Thieme, 1989; x.
3. Choctaw WF, Eisner ME, Wachtel TL. Causes, prevention, prehospital care, evaluation, emergency treatment, and prognosis. In: Achaver BM, ed. *Management of the burn patient.* Los Altos, CA: Appleton & Lange, 1987; 4–5.
4. Feller IJ. Introduction—statement of the problem. In: Fisher SV, Helm PA, eds. *Comprehensive rehabillitation of burns.* Baltimore: William & Wilkins, 1984; 4.
5. Larson DL, Abston S, Evans EB, Dobrkovsky M, Linares HA. Techniques for decreasing scar formation and contractures in the burned patient. *J Trauma* 1971; 10:807–823.
6. American Burn Association. Hospital and pre-hospital resources for optimal care of patients with burn injury: guidelines for development and operation of burn centers. *J Burn Care Rehabil* 1990; 11(2): 98–104.
7. Cromes GF, Helm PA. The status of burn rehabilitation services in the United States: results of a national survey. *J Burn Care Rehabil* 1992; 13(6):656--662.
8. Solem ID. Classification. In: Fisher SV, Helm PA, eds. *Comprehensive rehabilitation of burns.* Baltimore: Williams & Wilkins, 1984; 9–15.
9. Dimick AR. Pathophysiology. In: Fisher SV, Helm PA, eds. *Comprehensive rehabilitation of burns.* Baltimore: Williams & Wilkins, 1984; 16–27.
10. Robson M. Synthetic burn dressings: round table discussion. *J Burn Care Rehabil* 1985; 66:66–73.
11. Tompkins RG, Burke JF. Progress in burn treatment and the use of artificial skin. *World J Surg* 1990; 14(6):819–824.
12. Dimick AR. Debridement: surgical, mechanical, and biochemical. In: Dimick AR, ed. *Practical approaches to burn management.* Deerfield, IL: Flint Laboratories, Division of Travenol Laboratories, 1977; 21–26.
13. Heimbach DM, Engrav LH. Surgical management of the burn wound. New York: Raven Press, 1984.
14. Head MD. Wound and skin care. In: Fisher SV, Helm PA, eds. *Comrehensive rehabilitation of burns.* Baltimore: Williams & Wilkins, 1984; 148–176.
15. Bennett GB, Helm PA, Purdue GF, Hunt JL. Serial casting: a method for treating burn contractures. *J Burn Care Rehabil* 1989; 6:543–545.
16. Blassingame WM, Bennett GB, Helm PA, Purdue GF, Hunt JL. Range of motion of the shoulder performed while patient is anesthetized. *J Burn Care Rehabil* 1989; 10(6):539–542.
17. Grube BJ, Engrav LH, Heimbach DM. Early ambulation and discharge in 100 patients with burns of the foot treated by grafts. *J Trauma* 1992; 13(5):662–664.
18. Burnsworth B, Krob MJ, Langer-Schnepp M. Immediate ambulation of patients with lower-extremity grafts. *J Burn Care Rehabil* 1992; 1: 89–92.
19. Pegg SP, Cavaye D, Fowler D, Jones M. Results of early excision and grafting in hand burns. *Burns* 1984; 11(2):99–103.
20. Sheridan RL, Hurley J, Smith MA, Ryan CM, Bondoc CC, Quinby WC Jr, Tompkins RG, Burke JF. The acutely burned hand: management and outcome based on a ten-year experience with 1047 acute hand burns. *J Trauma* 1995; 38(3):406–411.
21. Bruner JM. Safety factors in the use of the pneumatic tourniquet for hemostasis in surgery of the hand. *J Bone Joint Surg* 1951; 33A: 221–224.
22. Helm PA, Kevorkian GC, Lushbaugh MS, Pullium G, Head M, Cromes GF. Burn injury rehabilitation management in 1982. *Arch Phys Med Rehabil* 1982; 63:6–16.
23. Pullium GF. Splinting and positioning. In: Fisher SV, Helm PA, eds. *Comprehensive rehabilitation of burns.* Baltimore: Williams & Wilkins, 1984; 64–95.
24. Artz CP. Electrical injury. In: Artz CP, Moncrief J, Pruitt BA Jr, eds. *Burns: a team approach.* Philadelphia: WB Saunders, 1979; 351–362.
25. Hunt JL. Electrical injuries. In: Fisher SV, Helm PA, eds. *Comprehensive rehabilitation of burns.* Baltimore: Williams & Wilkins, 1984; 249–266.
26. Hunt JL, Mason AD, Masterson TS, Pruitt BA. The pathophysiology of acute electrical injuries. *J Trauma* 1976; 16:335–340.
27. Meier RH III. Amputation and prosthetic fitting. In: Fisher SV, Helm PA, eds. *Comprehensive rehabilitation of burns.* Baltimore: Williams & Wilkins, 1984; 267–310.
28. Helm PA, Johnson ER, Carlton AM. Peripheral neurological problems in the acute burn patient. *Burns* 1977; 3:123–125.
29. Helm PA, Pandian G, Heck E. Neuromuscular problems in the burn patient: cause and prevention. *Arch Phys Med Rehabil* 1985; 66: 451–453.
30. Jackson L, Keats AS. Mechanism of brachial plexus palsy following anesthesia. *Anesthesiology* 1965; 26:190–194.
31. Ewing MR. Postoperative paralysis in the upper extremity: report of five cases. *Lancet* 1950; 1:99–103.

32. Dhuner KG. Nerve injuries following operations: a survey of cases occurring during a six year period. *Anesthesiology* 1950; 11:289–293.
33. Rask MR. Suprascapular nerve entrapment: a report of two cases treated with suprascapular notch resection. *Clin Orthop* 1977; 123:73–75.
34. Wadsworth TG. The external compression syndrome of the ulnar nerve at the cubital tunnel. *Clin Orthop* 1977; 124:189–204.
35. Edlich RF, Horowitz JH, Rheuban KS, et al. Heteropic calcification and ossification in burn patients. *Curr Concepts Trauma Care* 1985; 8:4–9.
36. Mant MJ, O'Brien BD, Thong KL, et al. Haemorrhagic complications of heparin therapy. *Lancet* 1977; 1:1133–1135.
37. Reinstein L, Alevizatos AC, Twardzik FG, DeMarco SJ. Femoral nerve dysfunction after retroperitoneal hemorrhage: pathophysiology revealed by computed tomography. *Arch Phys Med Rehabil* 1984; 65: 37–40.
38. Berry H, Richardson PM. Common peroneal nerve palsy: a clinical and electrophysiological review. *J Neurol Neurosurg Psychiatry* 1976; 39:1162–1171.
39. Aho K, Sainio K, Kianta M, Varpanen F. Pneumatic tourniquet paralysis: case report. *J Bone Joint Surg* 1983; 65B:441–443.
40. Sunderland S. Nerves and nerve injuries. Edinburgh: F & S Livingstone, 1968.
41. Helm PA. Neuromuscular considerations. In: Fisher SV, Helm PA, eds. *Comprehensive rehabilitation of burns.* Baltimore: Williams & Wilkins, 1984; 235–241.
42. Henderson B, Koepke GH, Feller I. Peripheral polyneuropathy among patients with burns. *Arch Phys Med Rehabil* 1971; 52:149–151.
43. Dagum AB, Eng BS, Peters WJ, Neligan PC, Douglas LG. Severe multiple mononeuropathy in patients with major thermal burns. *J Burn Care Rehabil* 1993; 14(4):440–445.
44. Jackson DM. Destructive burns: some orthopaedic complications. *Burns* 1980; 7:105–122.
45. Leung KS, Cheng JCY, Ma GFY, et al. Complications of pressure therapy for post-burn hypertrophic scars: biochemical analysis based on 5 patients. *Burns* 1984; 10:434–438.
46. Evans EB. Bone and joint changes secondary to burns. In: Lewis SR, ed. *Symposium on the treatment of burns.* St Louis: CV Mosby, 1973; 76–78.
47. Evans EB, Smith JR. Bone and joint changes following burns: a roentgenographic study—preliminary report. *J Bone Joint Surg* 1959; 41A: 785–799.
48. Teperman PS, Hilbert L, Peters WJ, Pritzker KPH. Heterotopic ossifications in burns. *J Burn Care Rehabil* 1984; 5:283–287.
49. Crawford CM, Varghese G, Mani MM, Neff JR. Heterotopic Ossification: Are range of motion exercises contraindicated? *J Burn Care Rehabil* 1986; 7(4):323–327.
50. Helm PA, Walker SC. New bone formation at amputation sites in electrically burn-injured patients. *Arch Phys Med Rehabil* 1987; 68: 284–286.
51. Vrabec R, Kolar J. Bone changes caused by electric current. In: *Transactions of the Fourth International Congress of Plastic and Reconstructive Surgery, Rome, 1967.* Amsterdam: Excerpta Medica, 1969; 215–217.
52. Evans EB. Scoliosis and kyphosis. In: Feller I, Crabb WC, eds. *Reconstruction and rehabilitation of the burned patient.* Ann Arbor, MI: National Institute for Burn Medicine, 1979; 264.
53. Head M, Helm P. Paraffin and sustained stretching in the treatment of burn contracture. *Burns* 1977; 4:136–139.
54. Ward RS, Hayes-Lundy C, Reddy R, Brockway C, Mells P, Saffle JR. Evaluation of topical therapeutic ultrasound to improve response to physical therapy and lessen scar contracture after burn injury. *J Burn Care Rehabil* 1994; 15(1):74–79.
55. Jensen LL, Parshley PF. Postburn scar contractures: histology and effects of pressure treatment. *J Burn Care Rehabil* 1984; 5:119–123.
56. Deitch EA, Wheelahan TM, Rose MP, Clothier J, Cotter J. Hypertrophic burn scars: Analysis of variables. *J Trauma* 1983; 10:895–898.
57. Ahn ST, Monafo WW, Mustoe TA. Topical silicone gel: a new treatment for hypertrophic scars. *Surgery* 1989; 4:781–787.
58. Engelberg AL, ed. *Guides to the evaluation of permanent impairment, 3rd ed.* Chicago: American Medical Association, 1988.
59. Fisher SV. Disability determination. In: Fisher SV, Helm PA, eds. *Comprehensive rehabilitation of burns.* Baltimore: Williams & Wilkins, 1984; 401–411.
60. Malt U. Long-term psychosocial follow-up studies of burned adults: review of the literature. *Burns* 1980; 6(3):190–197.
61. Browne G, Byrne C, Brown B, Pennock M, Streiner D, Roberts R, Eyles P, Truscott D, Dabbs R. Psychosocial adjustment of burn survivors. *Burns Incl Therm Injury* 1985; 12:28–35.
62. Cobb N, Maxwell G, Silverstein P. Patient perception of quality of life after burn injury-results of an eleven-year survey. *J Burn Care Rehabil* 1990; 10:251–257.
63. Chang FC, Herzog B. Burn morbidity: A follow-up study of physical and psychological disability. *Ann Surg* 1976; 183:34–37.
64. Orr DA, Reznikoff M, Smith GM. Body image, self esteem, and depression in burn-injured adolescents and young adults. *J Burn Care Rehabil* 1989; 10:454–461.
65. Sheffield CG, Irons GB, Mucha P Jr, Malec JF, Ilstrup DM, Stonnington HH. Physical and psychological outcome after burns. *J Burn Care Rehabil* 1988; 9:172–177.
66. Ward HW, Moss RL, Darko DF, Berry CC, Anderson J, Kolman P, Green A, Nielsen J, Klauber M, Wachtel TL. Prevalence of postburn depression following burn injury. *J Burn Care Rehabil* 1987; 8: 294–298.
67. Patterson DR, Carrigan L, Questad KA, Robinson R. Post-traumatic stress disorder in hospitalized patients with burn injuries. *J Burn Care Rehabil* 1990; 11:181–184.
68. Tucker P. Psychosocial problems among adult burn victims. *Burns Incl Therm Injury* 1987; 13:7–14.
69. Mancusi-Ungaro HR, Tarbox AR, Wainwright DJ. Post-traumatic stress disorder in electric burn patients. *J Burn Care Rehabil* 1986; 7: 521–525.
70. American Psychiatric Association. *Diagnostic and statistical manual of mental disorders, 4th ed.* Washington, D.C.: American Psychiatric Association, 1994.
71. Inancsi W, Guidotti TL. Return to work after occupation related burns: an exploratory study. *Can J Rehabil* 1989; 2:169–174.
72. Engrav LH, Covey MH, Dutcher KD, Heimbach DM, Walkinshaw MD, Marvin JA. Impairment, time out of schoool, and time off from work after burns. *Plast Reconstr Surg* 1987; 79:927–934.
73. Bowden ML, Thomson PD, Prasad JK. Factors influencing return to employment after a burn injury. *Arch Phys Med Rehabil* 1989; 70: 772–774.
74. Helm PA, Walker SC. Return to work after burn injury. *J Burn Care Rehabil* 1992; 13:53–57.
75. Prasad JK, Bowden ML, Thompson PD. A review of reconstructive surgery needs of 3167 survivors of burn injury. *Burns* 1991; 17: 302–305.

Rehabilitation Medicine: Principles and Practice, Third Edition,
edited by Joel A. DeLisa and Bruce M. Gans.
Lippincott–Raven Publishers, Philadelphia © 1998.

CHAPTER 63

The Physiatric Approach to Sports Medicine

Jeffrey L. Young, Brian A. Casazza, and Joel M. Press

THE HISTORY OF SPORTS AND SPORTS MEDICINE

"Sports" and "sports medicine" are far from 20th century terms. Evidence of development of the sport of wrestling dates as far back as 2500 B.C., and most ancient civilizations had some forms of loosely organized recreational activities (1). The first Olympic games were held over 2,500 years ago, with the games of 776 B.C. featuring wrestling, chariot racing, boxing, pentathlon, and running events (1). Swimming was utilized during military warfare; Assyrian warriors used animal bladders as swimming aides around this time (1). Alpine sports may have had their origin earlier than 600 B.C.—King Sennacherib of Assyria (705 to 681 B.C.) recreationally climbed mountains (1). The world's first famous athlete, Milo of Crotona, was crowned six times for winning the all-Greece championships during the sixth century B.C. (2). The Greek and Roman periods saw the growth of Olympic-type sports, with participants actually involved in athletic training in preparation for the games.

Sports events unrelated to the olympics or the military began to take place after the 10th century. Horse racing began in England in the 1170s (1). The precursor to modern tennis was played in England as far back as the 1350s (1). Cricket was first played by Edward VI of England in the late 1540s (1). Shortly thereafter, St. Andrew's golf club was founded. The 18th and 19th centuries saw the growth of boxing, cricket, rowing, and horse racing in England as well as the development of Rugby football. Skiing became a competitive sport in addition to a mode of transport in Europe during the middle of the 19th century.

The 19th century saw the birth of new sports in the United States. Abner Doubleday is credited with drawing up the rules for baseball in 1839. By 1845 the New York Knickerbocker Baseball Club was formed, and in 1869, the first professional baseball club, the Cincinnati Red Stockings, was founded (2). Around the same time, the first intercollegiate football game was played between Rutgers and Princeton (1). Just before the turn of the 20th century, basketball was developed as a collegiate recreational activity at Smith College in Massachusetts. Probably one of the more significant events that took place in Europe during this era was the formulation of the Queensberry rules (drawn up by the eighth Marquis of Queensberry) to establish a fair-play code for boxing in 1860s (1,3). The "modern" Olympic games organizing committee was established by Baron de Coubertin at the end of the 19th century.

The first half of the 20th century saw the first Tour de France bicycle race, the growth of the international Olympic movement, and the development of professional basketball and football in the United States. The latter half of the 20th century has seen sports evolve into a world-wide multimillion-dollar industry with advertising and media promotion of professional, amateur, and recreational sports on a daily basis. This massive interest in sports has brought sports medicine (and sports physicians) into the public eye as well.

The growth and development of sports has not been problem-free. The Emperor Theodosius of the Roman Empire banned the Olympic games in the latter portion of the fourth century (1). The Puritans objected to the playing of sports in the early 1600s (1). No less a figure than Oliver Cromwell, Lord Protector of the Commonwealth, was denounced for his participation in cricket (1). It was not until the 1740s that cricket was deemed a "legal" sport that all respectable citizens could participate in. Colonial America was slow to embrace sports as well—Princeton College banned "ball

J. L. Young: Department of Physical Medicine and Rehabilitation, Albert Einstein College of Medicine of Yeshiva University; and Department of Spine and Sports Rehabilitation, Beth Israel Medical Center, New York, New York 10003.

B. A. Casazza: Department of Physical Medicine and Rehabilitation, Division of Spine and Sports Care, University of Virginia Health System, Charlottesville, Virginia 22903.

J. M. Press: Department of Physical Medicine and Rehabilitation, Northwestern University, Chicago, Illinois 60611.

playing'' in the 1780s, describing the activity as ''low and unbecoming gentle-men students'' (2).

Women and minorities have struggled for equality in organized sports. Women were not even permitted to be spectators at the early Olympic games. Their ability to participate in events such as the Olympic marathon was denied until the latter portion of this century. Prize money for professional tournament play still lags behind the remuneration male athletes receive for participating in the same events. Although professional baseball is over 100 years old, it is only 50 years since the ''color barrier'' was broken when Jackie Robinson became the first African-American to participate in major league baseball. Despite the passage of the Americans with Disabilities Act, physically challenged athletes still do not have equal access to sports medicine services and receive far less media attention for their triumphs than do able-bodied athletes.

The gymnastes of the Greek period were the first sports physicians. Gymnastes were interested in all aspects of the athlete's training and supervised the masseurs and servants of the athletes (4). Herodicus, the most famous of the gymnastes, saw exercise not only as a component of training but as a means of physical rehabilitation for numerous maladies as well (4). More significant advances in medical care were implemented by Galen, who was appointed physician to the gladiators in the midsecond century. His dedication to one specific group of athletes essentially made him the first team physician in recorded history. Galen advanced our understanding of anatomy, physiology, and biomechanics through his observations regarding muscular, vascular, and nervous function. Galen is also credited with the utilization of plant juice extracts for healing purposes, giving trainers and physicians more options than just the use blood letting or topical salves (1).

Interest in the value of exercise as a therapeutic tool continued beyond the centuries of the first millennium. Avicenna of Persia (circa A.D. 1000) advocated moderate exercise as beneficial for health but warned against more vigorous exercise, noting the potential for dehydration (4). Maimonides (12th century) similarly believed in exercise in moderation. The Renaissance period gave rise to numerous physicians and scientists who viewed exercise as an important component of health. Vittorino da Feltre included exercise and sports as components of the curriculum school-aged children followed in a school he established (4). Exercises were practiced by the children daily and were ''prescribed'' on an individual basis. In the middle of the 16th century, Gerolamo Mercuriale published the illustrated text, *Six Books on the Art of Gymnastics,* which, among other issues, distinguished preventive from therapeutic exercises (4). The French physician Ambroise Paré encouraged exercise following the immobilization period from treatment of fractures. From this, it is obvious that ''sports rehabilitation'' had its origins long before contemporary sports medicine.

America's introduction to sports medicine occurred in the 19th century. Edward Hitchcock, an instructor in physical education at Amherst College, is considered America's first sports physician (5). At that time, sports physicians were professionals who interacted with athletes but who did not have a significant scientific basis for their injury management. Analysis of exercise performance and the physiological makeup of elite athletes was implemented by Dr. D.B. Hill and his associates at Harvard in the 1920s. As interest in the exercise sciences grew, more and more professionals began to focus on factors that impaired or enhanced athletic performance and on ways to prevent and treat athletic injury. Following the Second World War, sports and recreation became an important factor in the rehabilitation of injured soldiers as well.

The second half of the 20th century has seen the organization of sports medicine in the United States. In 1954, the American College of Sports Medicine (ACSM), a multidisciplinary organization of basic scientists and clinicians dedicated to sports medicine, was formed. The American Orthopedic Society for Sports Medicine was formed by the American Academy of Orthopedic Surgery in 1972. Other medical academies began to follow suit, and within this decade, the American Academy of Physical Medicine and Rehabilitation developed a Physiatric Association for Spine, Sports and Occupational Rehabilitation (PASSOR). Fellowship training in sports medicine is now available in many areas of medicine including pediatrics, internal medicine, emergency medicine, family practice, orthopedic surgery, and physical medicine and rehabilitation. Advances in technology, such as the development of magnetic resonance imaging (MRI) and advent of arthroscopic surgical techniques, have increased the precision with which clinicians are able to diagnose and treat sports injuries.

What, then, is the current scope of sports medicine practice? There is prevention of injury, education and training of athletes, and sideline coverage of athletic events. There is treatment of exercise-induced bronchospasm and management of glucoregulation in athletes with diabetes. There is psychological counseling for the injured athlete suddenly finding him- or herself unable to compete and for the amenorrheic runner presenting with fatigue, endocrine dysfunction, and stress fractures. There is the management of acute macrotraumatic injuries (e.g., fractures, dislocations, and ligamentous tears) and those associated with chronic microtrauma (e.g., lateral epicondylitis, iliotibial band syndrome, and plantar fasciitis). The list could go on and on.

Physiatric sports medicine is the delivery of comprehensive health services to individuals for whom vocational or avocational physical activity is an important component of life. This includes treatment of competitive and recreational athletes, from young to elderly, the able-bodied and disabled. It includes providing medical coverage at athletic events, preparticipation physical examination screening for the presence of conditions that jeopardize safe participation in athletics, and educational programs geared toward injury prevention. In addition to being knowledgeable in all the other aspects of rehabilitation medicine, the competent sports physiatrist has a solid understanding of anatomy and biomechanics, is able to apply the principles of exercise physiology across a broad array of health conditions, and has a firm grasp of the physiological and musculoskeletal demands that various sports place on the athlete's body. The ability to lead and work with a team of other physicians, trainers, therapists, coaches, athletes, and their families is essential.

It is beyond the scope of this chapter to cover all aspects of sports medicine. Instead, this section provides an overview of four topics—basic elements of exercise training, a model for analysis of musculotendinous overload injuries, an approach to rehabilitation of specific common musculoskeletal conditions, and development of a sports rehabilitation program.

BASIC ELEMENTS OF EXERCISE TRAINING

Appropriate application of exercise training principles enables injured athletes to recover from injury and prepares healthy athletes for higher levels of sports performance. This section focuses on basic physiological principles of sports rehabilitation.

Types of Muscular Contraction

Depending on the external resistance applied to the musculotendinous unit and the specific demands of the athletic activity, muscular contraction may be described in a number of ways.

Concentric. During this type of contraction, the muscular force generated is able to overcome an applied external resistance, and the whole muscle length is reduced (6). As a result, at least one of the two limb segments spanned by the contracting muscle moves, with the assigned origin and insertion being brought closer to one another. For example, the combined concentric contractions of the middle deltoid and rotator cuff muscles produce elevation (abduction) of the humerus. Concentric contractions are also important because they are utilized to accelerate the more distal link segments in the kinetic chain. Combined concentric contractions of the pectoralis major and the latissimus dorsi enable a quarterback to rapidly accelerate, in sequence, the upper arm, the lower arm and wrist, and the football. Healthy muscle and, for that matter, the entire musculotendinous unit is not usually injured when contracting in a concentric manner. This may be because the muscle length is moving toward a protected (shortened) state and the muscle is both at a lower absolute tension and at a lower point on the force–tension curve. Muscle that is acutely injured or that has been repeatedly injured but not rehabilitated may also demonstrate a smaller load to failure and break down under high-resistance concentric contraction conditions.

Eccentric. A contraction is considered to be eccentric when development of increased muscle tension is accompanied by muscle lengthening (6). Motion occurs, but the assigned origin and insertion move away from one another. The slow lowering of abducted humerus to the side of the body is an example of an eccentric contraction.

Muscles are capable of generating greater forces under eccentric conditions than either isometric (see following) or concentric conditions, and more isometrically than concentrically (7–10). Thus, it is easier to hold a weighted barbell still than to actually lift it, and it is even easier to gradually lower the barbell than to hold it still. This relationship is further modified by the speed of muscle contraction. Rapid eccentric contractions generate more force than slow ones (slower eccentric work approximates isometric), and slower concentric contractions generate more force than rapid ones (7,8,11). Eccentric contractions are also more efficient than concentric contractions (i.e., require less oxygen) at the same tension and contraction velocity (12,13). The time to reach peak tension is also faster during eccentric contractions than during concentric contractions (13,14).

Eccentric contractions are essential for deceleration of kinetic link segments that have acquired large amounts of kinetic energy. Once a quarterback's arm has accelerated forward and the football is released, the eccentric firing of scapular stabilizer muscles and rotator cuff muscles are necessary to retain normal glenohumeral relationships and prevent the humerus from flying toward the receiver with the ball. The large tensile forces that typically occur with sudden eccentric contractions in sports (i.e., the football defensive back who has to rapidly stop running toward the line of scrimmage and reverse direction because he had mistakenly read "run" instead of "pass"), or the microtraumatic tensile forces that occur with repetitive eccentric contractions (such as those within the gastrocnemius–soleus complex of an ultramarathon runner), both render muscle vulnerable to injury. Eccentric muscle overload can be associated with both early and delayed-onset muscle soreness (6). Muscle that is unprepared for eccentric work is injured more readily both because the absolute tension is higher and because the muscle–tendon length is closer to the load for tensile failure. Traditional athletic and sports rehabilitation programs have often omitted eccentric training as the final preparation before resumption of sport. Although no definitive study exists supporting the premise that eccentric training is a prerequisite for safe resumption of activity, the authors would suggest that, given the growing body of literature indicating the vulnerability of the musculotendinous unit under eccentric contraction conditions and the nature of skeletal muscle's response to overload (see section related to prescription of exercise), it is only logical to incorporate this type of exercise into a functionally based sports rehabilitation program.

Isometric. Under this condition, the length of the whole muscle is unchanged, and there is no net movement of the link segments spanned by the contracting muscles (6). While a gymnast holds himself in an "L" position on the parallel bars, the shoulder depressors, pectoralis major, latissimus dorsi, and triceps contract isometrically to stabilize the upper body while the abdominal muscles, hip flexors, and knee extensors contract isometrically to maintain the 90° angle between the legs and the torso. Although the forces generated during isometric contractions are potentially greater than during concentric work, muscles are rarely injured during isometric contractions. This is presumably because of the lack of change in muscle length, so that although the absolute tension is higher, the muscle does not move any closer to its failure length. Furthermore, if there are multiple muscles about a joint that are isometrically contracting together, there may be less chance of injury because the multimuscle cocontraction serves to stabilize the joint. Isometric exercises are often utilized during the early phases of rehabilitating musculotendinous injury because the intensity of contraction and the muscle length at which it contracts can be controlled.

Isotonic versus Dynamic. When originally used, the term isotonic encompassed contractions of both the eccentric and concentric type (11). This term implies that either the tension within the muscle or the torque generated by the muscle is constant throughout the arc of motion. This is an imprecise term at best because muscle tension changes constantly with alteration of joint angle, even when the speed of the contraction is kept constant (10,11,15). Therefore, it is more appropriate to use the term ''dynamic'' when categorizing contractions as those associated with limb motion.

Isokinetic. Literally taken, this is a contraction that takes place at a constant velocity (6). Computerized machines that can calculate external torque generation by a muscle group within a predetermined arc of motion and at a predetermined velocity are necessary to evaluate isokinetic strength. Although it is common for therapists, trainers, and researchers to utilize isokinetic data when evaluating strength and performance, it is important to recognize that isokinetic contractions do not occur in real life, making extrapolation from isokinetic data to clinical situations rather limited. Furthermore, training athletes on isokinetic equipment should probably be reserved for the injured or postsurgical athlete whose range of motion or exercise intensity needs to more carefully monitored.

Plyometric. This type of exercise is designed to utilize the viscoelastic properties of the whole muscle to produce greater forces than by sarcomere shortening alone (9). A rapid overload (prestretch) is placed on the muscle immediately before a concentric contraction. This both stretches the connective tissue (tendon as well as muscle) and places an eccentric load on the muscle, which facilitates subsequent concentric force generation (9,10,16). Plyometric exercises emphasize ''explosive''-type motions and are a valuable component of skill and agility training. They are also among the most ''sports—specific'' of all the types of contractions mentioned in this section. For example, high jumpers first lower their bodies toward the ground, placing prestretch on the gastrocnemius–soleus complex, quadriceps, upper hamstrings, and gluteal muscles before the shortening contractions of these muscles that propel them up and over the bar.

Closed Versus Open Kinetic Chain Exercises. The difference between closed kinetic chain (CKC) and open kinetic chain (OKC) exercises is an important one. If, for instance, during knee extension or flexion, the foot is allowed to move freely through space, the system is called open (17–20). In an OKC system, the hamstrings are predominant in knee flexion, whereas extension is dominated by the quadriceps. During CKC exercises for the lower limbs, the foot is kept immobile or maintains contact with a ground-reactive force, and there is creation of a multiarticular closed chain (17–20). Rather than the near isolation of the large muscle groups seen during OKC exercises, performance of CKC knee flexion and extension results in ''coactivation'' of both hamstrings and quadriceps groups (17,18). An example of a CKC lower limb exercise (leg press) is shown in Figure 63-1. Both agonists and antagonists are simultaneously strengthened via

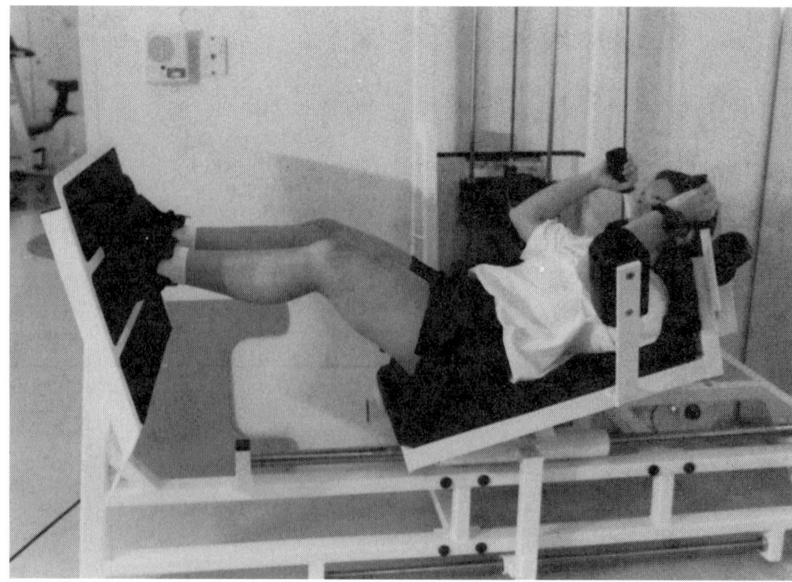

FIG. 63-1. Example of a closed kinetic chain knee extension.

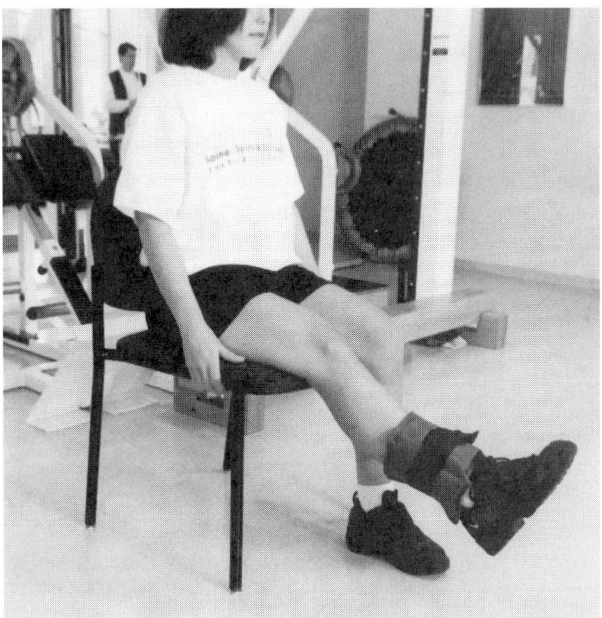

FIG. 63-2. Example of an open kinetic chain knee extension.

cocontraction and are more physiological for lower limb sports such as running. An OKC knee extension is depicted in Figure 63-2. Both CKC and OKC conditions exist for the upper limbs as well. The CKC upper limb exercises are particularly useful during the early recovery period from shoulder surgery, as less shear force is imparted across the glenoid labrum while multiple muscles about the scapula and glenohumeral joint can be simultaneously activated (19). An example of a rehabilitation technique that involves alternating between OKC and CKC exercise for the upper limbs is shown in Figure 63-3.

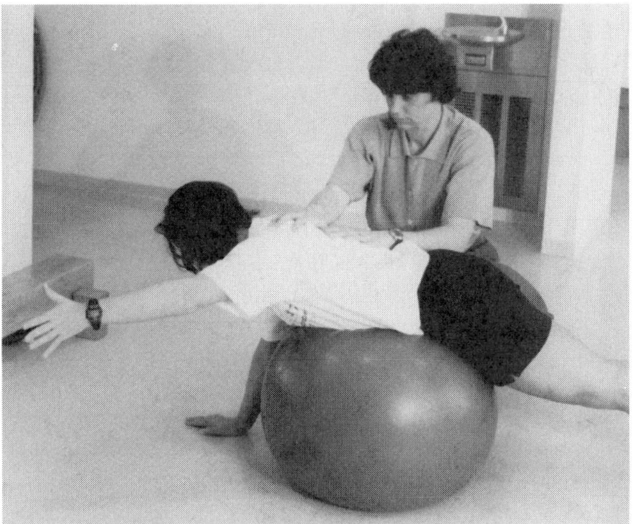

FIG. 63-3. Combination of open kinetic chain condition for the athlete's left upper limb and closed kinetic chain for the right upper limb. Note that the therapist is able to incorporate truncal control training as well.

Prescription of Exercise

The prescription of exercise for development of strength, power, or endurance is based on a relatively simple principle. The SAID (specific adaptation to imposed demand) principle recognizes that the human body will respond to given demands with specific and predictable adaptation (21). An important corollary of this is that although muscle is extremely adaptable and can "learn" to do many different things, it can probably do only one thing best. Although one can improve in more than one area of fitness at a time (i.e., "cross-training"), one cannot attain maximal gains in both strength and marathon-type endurance at the same time (7,22–24). This implies that in designing conditioning programs, it becomes important to identify what the goals of that program are and then select exercises that maximize the likelihood that the desired training effect will be achieved. The basic components of the exercise prescription are described below.

Intensity. Essentially, this describes how difficult the exercise is. For aerobic training, the exercise should be carried out at 40% to 85% maximal aerobic power ($\dot{V}O_{2max}$) or 55% to 90% of maximal heart rate (25). Lower intensities may promote a training effect, but they must be carried out for lengthy periods of time to do so (7,16,25). For recreational exercisers, use of the rating of perceived exertion (RPE) scale may be a convenient method of ensuring that approximately the same intensity is selected on a day-to-day basis (26,27). However, one must keep in mind that RPE is also related to the "familiarity" the athlete has with the given type of exercise and that an RPE of "14" on one mode of exercise does not necessarily equate to the same power output or caloric expenditure on another. For example, a recreational exerciser who only runs will perceive bicycle exercise of an equivalent oxygen uptake demand to be more intense. This sense of increased effort will be accompanied by a greater heart rate and metabolic response as well.

For sprint or anaerobic training, the absolute work intensity needs to be "supramaximal"; i.e., the athlete must exercise at work rates in excess of that necessary to elicit $\dot{V}O_2$max during a progressive exercise test (7,25,28). Intensities that promote endurance training effects do not have an effect on anaerobic capacity (28). However, if one employs Fartlek ("speed play")-type training, in which short fast bursts of running are interspersed within the running workout, there may be development of some anaerobic qualities as well (29).

Duration. This indicates how long the session is. Exercise should be carried out for between 15 and 60 minutes to develop an aerobic training effect and may be done continuously or discontinuously (25). Continuous-type training can have different outcomes, depending on the exercise intensity selected. Specificity dictates that if the athlete trains at high intensities for shorter periods of time, a tolerance for lactate will be built up, and $\dot{V}O_2$max will be likely to improve (7,10,28). If exercise is carried out near the intensity of the lactate threshold, then this is the parameter most influenced

(28,30). Exercise at lower intensities carried out for upward of 1 hour allows for large total energy expenditure without exposure to high levels of stress and promotes more efficient utilization of free fatty acid (FFA) stores (6,7,16). In general, there is an inverse relationship between the intensity of exercise and the length of time it can be sustained.

Interval training is a method of discontinuous training with alternating "work" and "relief" periods (7). The work interval typically consists of exercise that is a very high percentage of maximum for a short period of time, followed by the relief period that is of low intensity. The relief interval allows for resynthesis of phosphagens and decreases the need for glycolytic metabolism when the high-intensity work interval is started over again (7,10). When the cumulative exercise time is examined, it becomes apparent that this scheme potentially enables the individual to work for long periods at an intensity which would normally cause fatigue in a few minutes (7,10). Daniels recommends that a 1:1 work:relief ratio be used, with the work bouts kept less than 5 minutes for aerobic-type training (29).

Frequency. Frequency denotes how often the exercise is performed. This is typically 3 to 5 days per week for the majority of recreational exercisers (25). Competitive athletes' training schedules will vary depending on whether it is "preseason," during competition, or "off-season." During preseason training, high-level athletes may train up to 6 or 7 days per week and for more than one session on any given day. The nature of these workouts is varied, as the athlete may need to improve endurance, strength, and skill all at the same time. During competitive season, the number of formal workouts per week often drops. In contact sports such as football, days may be taken off to recover from acute and subacute musculotendinous injury. In sports such as tennis, a three- or five-set singles match may more than substitute for a session on a treadmill or bike ergometer.

Mode of exercise. The key issue to remember here is that if improvement in fitness is of interest, the athlete should be tested in a manner that resembles the mode of training as much as possible. A bicycle-trained athlete should be tested on a bike, a runner on a treadmill, and a swimmer in a flume. Failure to do so will often result in underprediction of the training effect. From a general conditioning standpoint, varying mode of exercise from session to session can be extremely useful by potentially increasing the number of muscle groups trained, reducing the likelihood of musculotendinous overload without adequate time for tissue healing and repair, and deceasing likelihood of boredom.

Muscular Overwork and Overtraining

Exercise that is too intense or that involves a significant amount of eccentric overload may induce excessive postexercise muscular soreness, reflecting a condition of acute muscular overwork. In general, if exercise results in elevation of blood levels of creatine phosphokinase (CPK), lactate dehydrogenase (LDH), or myoglobin, some level of rhabdomyolysis has occurred (31). This is apparent within 24 hours of exercise. Extremes of either intensity or duration are capable of producing these enzymatic changes, although intensity appears to be the more critical factor (31,32).

Intense eccentric exercise is associated with numerous disturbances of muscle ultrastructure. Forced lengthening of contracted muscle produces damage that includes sarcolemmal rupturing, degeneration and disorganization of myofibrils, and increased numbers of inflammatory cells (12,33–35). Eccentric exercise that induces delayed-onset muscle soreness (24 to 72 hours postexercise) is also associated with decreased ability to resynthesize glycogen during this time frame (33,36). Despite a more than 50-fold greater tensile strength than muscle, tendon, which represents the conduit between muscle and bone, can also become deformed and injured with either sudden high force or repetitive eccentric loads (7). If the athlete is not allowed adequate recovery following eccentric overload, microscopic breakdown will occur, and the nidus of both the tissue injury and tissue overload complexes (see later discussion) is created. This increases the likelihood that a maladaptive response to exercise will occur, with ultimate worsening of performance or injury.

Overtraining is the product of an imbalance between overload (training) and recovery. The individual who overtrains exhibits symptoms and findings of muscular and systemic breakdown (maladaptation), which are, unfortunately, frequently overlooked until athletic performance begins to suffer. From a subjective standpoint, the person who is overtraining may complain of feeling "stale," of not being as motivated, or of being generally fatigued (37). Sleep patterns may be disturbed, and the athlete may report that he or she is always tired on arising in the morning. The school-aged or college-aged athlete may admit having a difficult time keeping up in classes or receiving poorer grades. Teammates or family members may note that the athlete is more irritable or difficult to talk to. Loss of appetite is common (38). Complaints of pain and soreness of muscles and joints, often in the absence of overt cause, is another clue that the person is overtraining, and a "chronic athletic fatigue" syndrome is present (38).

Objective findings include elevation of the morning resting heart rate by more than 5 beats per minute, immune suppression with an increased frequency of respiratory illnesses, and weight loss (7,38,39). Testosterone levels tend to drop, whereas cortisol levels tend to rise, suggesting hypothalamic dysfunction (37,40). Glycogen depletion, which can be caused by repeated heavy bouts of exercise accompanied by inadequate ingestion of carbohydrates, may also contribute to muscular fatigue (38). Certain muscle enzyme concentrations (CPK, LDH, transaminase) and myoglobin rise rather dramatically following single bouts of heavy exertion, signifying muscle damage, but in and of themselves are not reliable markers of chronic overtraining (31,32,38). Recurrent stress fractures, at the very least, indicate some repetitive biomechanical overload. Although full discussion of this issue is beyond the scope of this chapter, when stress fractures are discovered in a lean female athlete, the athlete's dietary habits and menstrual history should be investigated. Consultation with a sports psychologist and formal endocrinologic evaluation may be required as well.

Ultimately, prevention of overtraining is more critical than its detection and treatment. Prudent recommendations include ensuring that the athlete matches energy expenditure with caloric intake, allowing the athlete to obtain adequate sleep every night, and increasing training frequency, duration, or intensity by small increments. Periodization of training (i.e., varying the volume and intensity of training sessions) at different times of the year so that the athlete "peaks" near competitions but does not have to maintain peak form year round is critical. Tapering the volume of training in the weeks before competition allows for reduction of muscular soreness, recovery from injury, and restoration of metabolic stores (16).

THE APPLICATION OF PHYSIOLOGICAL PRINCIPLES TO SPORT-SPECIFIC TRAINING

An understanding of the relative contributions of the different energy systems combined with recognition of the muscular demands of a given athletic activity enables the sports medicine professional to create a meaningful sport-specific training program. An excellent method of characterizing different sports in this manner is provided by Kibler (41). For each activity, five critical parameters (flexibility, strength, power, anaerobic endurance, aerobic endurance) are rated on the basis of how critical they are for performance of that sport. A rating of 1 indicates the parameter is minimally needed; a rating of 2 implies that it is necessary for injury reduction; a rating of 3 identifies the parameter as being synergistic for optimum performance; and a rating of 4 designates the parameter as being maximally required for optimum performance (41). A few profiles are outlined below.

Basketball. Players may be on the court for just a few seconds or for as much as 40 minutes per game. Although there are many breaks, the action is high intensity, with running, jumping, and quick changes of direction. The participant needs an aerobic base with superimposed anaerobic power and endurance. This sport has been rated as flexibility 3, strength 3, power 4, anaerobic endurance 4, and aerobic endurance 4 (41). From this profile, it is clear that this is a demanding sport in many areas. It is also clear that one cannot train for all these during the course of the season and play ball as well. Therefore, implementation of a vigorous aerobic training program out of season is essential. The $V\text{O}_2$max, if to be assessed, should also be evaluated during the off season as well. Strength and flexibility can be actively pursued during the season. Regular participation in the sport, augmented by additional preseason conditioning, will facilitate development of anaerobic endurance and power. If testing of anaerobic power and endurance is desired, the Wingate Test may be used (7,10).

Long-Distance Running. This is somewhat more straightforward, as the most important quality, by far, is aerobic endurance. The profile is flexibility 3, strength 2, power 2, anaerobic endurance 2, and aerobic endurance 4 (41). Beyond having to remember to stretch out appropriate muscle groups, this athlete can spend almost all training time in one area. Were this a "middle-distance runner," anaerobic work (or at least high-intensity aerobic work) and strength training would be encouraged. Measurement of $V\text{O}_2$max and the ventilatory breakpoint (work intensity during incremental exercise at which minute ventilation increases disproportionately to oxygen consumption but not to carbon dioxide production) or the onset of peripheral blood lactate accumulation during an incremental treadmill exercise test may be beneficial (6).

Similar profiles can be established for other sports (6). Montgomery analyzed ice hockey and found that the on-ice heart rate (HR) was 85% to 90% HRmax, and on-ice oxygen consumption 70% to 80% $V\text{O}_2$max with bursts in excess of 90% maximum for both parameters (42). Given the fast pace of the sport and the need for upper body strength, the need for development of power, strength, and anaerobic endurance was identified. The $V\text{O}_2$max values for forward were between 55 and 60 ml/kg per minute, indicative of the need for an aerobic base (42). Therefore, a battery of tests, including a skating $V\text{O}_2$max test would be appropriate. Interestingly, it was reported that an on-ice training program during the season did not induce an increase in $V\text{O}_2$max in the professional skaters (42). This further emphasizes the need for preseason conditioning programs to improve aerobic fitness in a skill sport. In the above system, hockey can be rated as flexibility 3, strength 3, power 4, anaerobic endurance 3, and aerobic endurance 3 or 4, depending on position (e.g., goalie versus forward) requirements (6).

ANALYSIS OF MUSCULOSKELETAL INJURIES

The overwhelming majority of musculoskeletal injuries can be treated nonsurgically. However, in order for rehabilitation to be successful, the physician must have a thorough understanding of applied anatomy, biomechanics, and the "kinetic chain." The effects of a musculoskeletal injury are rarely, if ever, confined to a single joint, and rehabilitation programs must consider the alterations in anatomy and biomechanics that have occurred proximal, distal, and contralateral to the site of acute injury. The physician must also be able to recognize the adaptations that have occurred in response to errors of training, particularly those maladaptations induced by musculotendinous overload. This section details a template for analysis and rehabilitation of injuries caused by musculotendinous overload. Application of this scheme to a select number of injuries is made in a later section of this chapter.

Step 1: Establish an Accurate Diagnosis. Inherent to this task is recognizing how muscle overload injuries and tendon injuries may present. The vicious cycle model for analysis of musculotendinous injury induced by repetitive overload is presented in Figure 63-4. To aid those unfamiliar with this model, some clarification of the terminology is provided:

Tissue injury complex: the area of actual tissue disruption (43–47)
Clinical symptom complex: the symptoms associated with the dysfunction and injury (43–47)
Tissue overload complex: the tissue group being subjected to tensile overload (43–47)
Functional biomechanical deficit: inflexibilities and/or muscle strength imbalances that create altered mechanics (43–47)
Subclinical adaptation complex: functional substitutions used by the patient in order to try to maintain activity (43–47)

When the musculotendinous unit is subjected to tensile overload, damage occurs at a cellular level. This typically produces symptoms of pain, dysfunction, and instability and also impairs athletic performance (44–47). If the extent of that overload is small (microtear), and nutrition and healing time are adequate, activities may be safely resumed. However, if the injury is not adequately treated and is allowed to progress (macrotear), healing is accompanied by development of scar tissue, with the development of subclinical adaptations such as loss of flexibility and loss of strength or strength imbalances (44–47). This leads to further decrements in performance and to biomechanical substitutions that perpetuate this ''negative feedback vicious cycle'' (Fig. 63-4*B*), creating the chance for more overload and injury (43–47). Musculotendinous injury therefore presents as acute or chronic injury, as exacerbation of a chronic injury, or as a subclinical injury (43,47). Muscle ''strain''-type injuries typically manifest themselves microscopically as a zone of myonecrosis confined to within 500 μm of the musculotendinous junction (48). Tendon injuries present as either an acute inflammatory process superimposed on acute or chronic injury (tendinitis) or as a product of maladaptation and intratendinous degeneration unaccompanied by mediators of inflammation (tendinosis) (43,46,49). In tendinitis, the immediate treatment goal is relief of symptoms, whereas in tendinosis, the immediate goal is restoration of function (46,47). Identification of the components of musculotendinous injury within the vicious cycle facilitates understanding the functional consequences of the injury that need to be addressed in the rehabilitation program.

Step 2. Acute Management. Efforts are directed toward minimizing the effects of inflammation and controlling pain. The PRICE principle (protection, relative rest, ice, compression, and elevation) is followed. Use of a cold compressive cuff to control the swelling from an acute knee injury is shown in Figure 63-5. This is usually a period for judicious

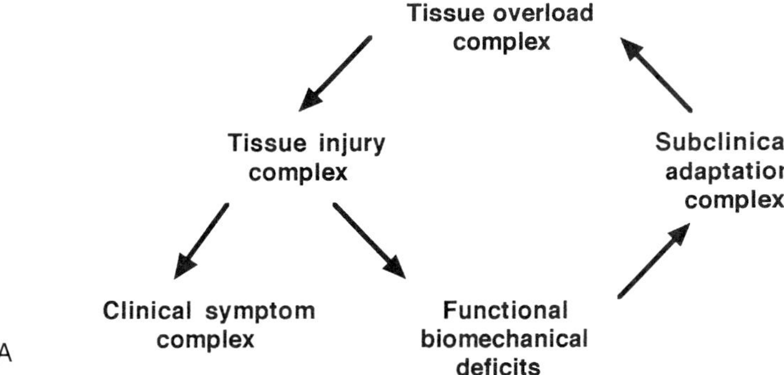

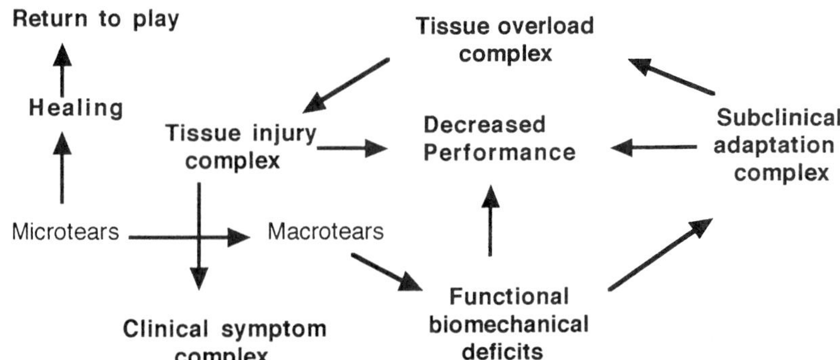

FIG. 63-4. A,B: Model for vicious cycle of musculotendinous overload. (See text for details.)

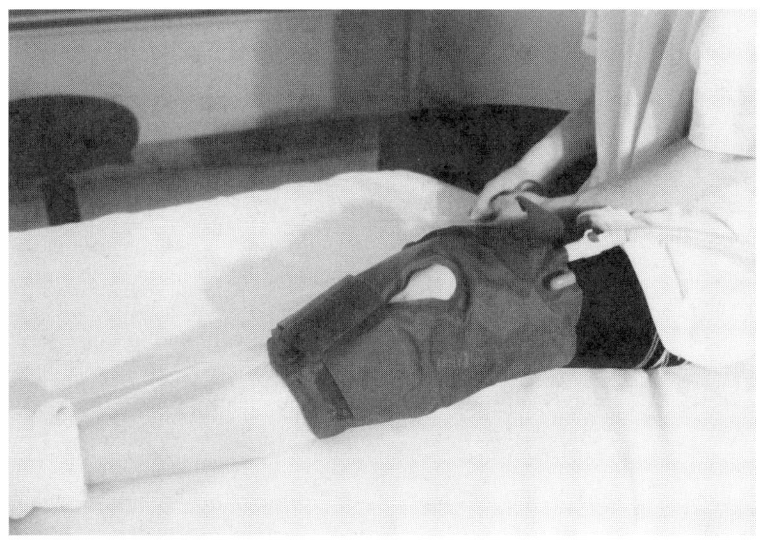

FIG. 63-5. Combination of cryotherapy and compression for control of acute knee swelling. Cold fluid is circulated through the compressive cuff.

use of anti-inflammatory medications and pain-relieving modalities (46,47,50–52). This may also be a key time to enlist the assistance of a counselor or psychologist to facilitate the development of coping skills and to assist with focusing on rehabilitation.

Step 3: Initial Rehabilitation. This phase continues to focus on promotion of proper healing. Restoration of motion helps to reduce the effects of immobilization, with controlled tensile loading promoting ordered collagen growth and alignment. Identification of correctable biomechanical imbalances is initiated. Rehabilitation programs typically fail by not progressing beyond this step (20,47,50).

Step 4: Correction of Imbalances. Development of symmetric motion and symmetric strength are goals. When the patient is pain-free, and when nearly full concentric strength has been achieved, it is essential that an eccentric strengthening program be initiated. This is a critical step in developing a musculotendinous unit that is less likely to fail in the face of future tensile stresses (20,47). Identification of flaws in exercise technique and training practices are initiated if the patient is capable of full weight bearing under controlled conditions. Alternative aerobic conditioning exercises are encouraged. Other than local icing, modalities are rarely indicated during this phase (20,47).

Step 5: Return to Normal Function. Cross-training, aqua training, and the use of alternative conditioning schemes give way to a gradual increase in activity-specific training and eventual resumption of full activity. Endurance performance, power, and agility should be restored to baseline.

THE SPORTS REHABILITATION HISTORY

A careful history is required to identify the diagnosis and mechanism of injury. The following represents an overview of basic questions that need to be asked of the injured athlete.

Chronology of the Injury. When did the pain first appear? Was the onset of pain sudden or gradual? Has this injury occurred before?

Mechanism of Injury. Was trauma involved? For the lower limb, was the foot planted or in the air at the time of injury? Did the foot invert or evert? Was there sudden inability to bear weight? Was there a valgus or varus moment at the knee? Did the athlete feel or hear a "pop" or a "snap" at the time of injury? An athlete who reports having sustained a noncontact knee injury with his foot planted, accompanied by a valgus moment, rotation, and a "pop" provides a classic history for disruption of his anterior cruciate ligament (20,47). The novice tennis player who reports medial elbow pain after practicing serving and forehand volleys probably has medial epicondylitis from repetitive overload of the forearm flexor–pronator muscle groups.

Nature of the Pain. Is the pain constant or intermittent? What makes it more tolerable, and what exacerbates it? Is it associated with weight bearing, and how soon does the pain appear after the onset of activity? Is the pain highly localized, or does it extend to or from another area? Is the pain associated with inflammation? Pain from a fracture is present at rest or provoked by minimal activity. Pain associated with a compartment syndrome is often less apparent at rest and at the onset of exercise but becomes worse after a relatively consistent amount of activity. Achy anterior knee pain worsened by squatting or prolonged sitting (i.e., "theater sign") alerts the clinician to patellofemoral joint dysfunction, whereas anterior knee pain aggravated by maintaining full knee extension suggests infrapatellar fat pad irritation (20,53,54). Tendinitis is accompanied by the cardinal signs of inflammation (redness, swelling, and increased warmth) within a painful tendon (49). Tendinosis is described as painful but lacks the signs of inflammation (49). Gradual-onset shoulder pain during nine innings of baseball pitching reflects musculotendinous overload of the rotator cuff, whereas shoulder pain that is unassociated with exertion but worsened by ipsilateral neck side-bending and relieved by elevating the painful side arm overhead suggests cervical radiculopathy.

Injury Inventory. How many other injuries have been sustained? What were the locations? Were they managed nonsurgically or surgically? A prior injury to the same area may not have undergone proper rehabilitation.

Age Considerations. The differential diagnosis of distal Achilles tendon pain in the skeletally immature runner must include calcaneal apophysitis (Sever's disease), whereas the elderly runner is much more likely to have pathology within the tendon itself (55,56). Hip pain in the young athlete should raise suspicion of femoral stress fracture or traction apophysitis, but the same symptoms in the elderly runner can indicate fracture or symptomatic spinal stenosis (55–57). Elbow pain from repetitive valgus overload in the throwing athlete can be from medial collateral ligament injury in athletes of all ages, but concern regarding the development of osteochondritis dissecans (localized avascular necrosis with subsequent articular surface softening and subchondral collapse) of the capitellum is much greater in the young athlete (58).

Exercise Habits. How much does the athlete exercise? What intensity is maintained? Does the athlete take days off? Has there been a sudden increase in frequency, intensity, or duration of workouts? Does the athlete routinely stretch before and/or after exercising? Which muscle groups are stretched? For seasonal athletes such as baseball pitchers, what is their "off season" exercise regimen? The athlete who trains intensely every day of the week without varying the muscle groups exercised and who does not stretch is a candidate for both musculotendinous overload and overtraining.

Equipment. What type of shoes does the athlete use? How often are new pairs purchased and old pairs discarded? Has the patient recently started wearing a new style of shoe? Are orthoses used? When were they originally constructed, and for what purpose? These questions help provide insight into potential errors of training and biomechanical imbalances. Shoes or inserts that have broken down and no longer serve their original intent are common and easily corrected sources of problems. Orthotic devices are especially useful to correct biomechanical imbalances that are not correctable by specific stretching and strengthening programs. In one survey study of 347 symptomatic runners, whose average training was approximately 40 miles per week, 75% reported marked improvement or resolution of their symptoms with the use of the shoe inserts (59). Subotnick and Newell have provided excellent reviews of the role of foot orthoses (60,61). Are the young football player's helmet and shoulder pads the appropriate size? The status of a contact sport athlete's equipment must be checked for fit and state of repair before every practice and competition.

Exercise Environment. Where does the athlete typically run? Does the runner train on a level dirt path, on a banked concrete surface, on a treadmill at a health club, or on a flat circular track? Have any of these factors changed recently? Poor running course selection may create imbalances at the level of the foot and ankle that are transmitted up the biomechanical chain to the more proximal structures. For example, running on a banked surface causes "uphill" foot pronation, which stresses the medial ankle and creates a knee valgus force, hip abduction, and elevation of that hemipelvis, while the "downhill" foot supinates more, stressing the lateral ankle, and creating a knee varus force, hip adduction, and lowering of that hemipelvis (51,57,62). Are field conditions safe? High school football and soccer fields must be inspected to ensure that there is no increased risk of injury from the field itself. Are environmental conditions safe for athletic competition? Exercise under conditions of excessive heat (above 30°C) or high relative humidity (over 80%) can induce heat illness or death if adequate medical precautions are not taken (63).

Review of Systems. Is there a nonmusculoskeletal process contributing to the current problem? Is the young female runner who presents with stress fractures and amenorrhea exhibiting signs of disordered body image? What medications are being used? Are anabolic steroids being taken? Does the athlete have two functioning kidneys? Is there a history of exercise-induced asthma or cardiac dysrhythmia? For physicians supervising preparticipation examinations, it is imperative that other factors that impinge on the athlete's overall health be identified.

Coping skills. Can this athlete emotionally tolerate relative or complete rest? How will this athlete react if total rest is required for an undetermined amount of time? As part of a holistic approach to the injured athlete, input from a sports psychologist or psychiatrist may be essential to successful rehabilitation.

THE SPORTS REHABILITATION PHYSICAL EXAMINATION

Establishing a diagnosis-specific rehabilitation program is not possible without performing a thorough physical examination. This in turn requires adherence to the concept of the kinetic chain and recognition that biomechanical dysfunction in one body region is capable of causing "injury at a distance." Thus, it should be routine to examine the low back, hip, knee, and ankle regions in all patients presenting with lower limb complaints, and examine the wrist, elbow, and shoulder regions along with the cervical and thoracic spine for upper limb problems.

The patient is first evaluated at rest. This helps identify such entities as cervicothoracic kyphosis with head-forward posture, scapular asymmetry, excessive lumbar lordosis, scoliosis, pelvic asymmetry, limb length discrepancy, genu varum or valgum, tibial torsion, side-to-side differences in muscle bulk, static ankle–foot deformities, blisters and calluses, and visible evidence of inflammation (20,47,64).

The patient is then asked to ambulate. The walking examination can reveal signs of foot pronation or supination, early heel rise from a tight gastrocnemius–soleus complex, increased knee valgum or varum and hip abductor weakness (Trendelenburg sign). More subtle gluteus medius weakness can be discerned by having the patient walk with hands on hips and watching the rise and fall of the elbows. The elbow contralateral to the weaker gluteus medius will dip more during midstance (57).

The greatest insight is achieved with direct visualization of the sports activity itself. Treadmill evaluations provide excellent insight into running injuries. Analysis of video recordings of the runner at varying speeds with and without shoes and with and without orthotics is recommended. Observation of the baseball pitcher's motion at slow as well as at normal speeds allows for isolating phases of the pitching motion. This enables the clinician to identify more subtle biomechanical imbalances as well as flaws in style. In this regard, video recordings are not only a useful diagnostic aid but also a vehicle for patient education. The recording and projecting system should be capable of high resolution when played at normal, fast forward, or slow motion speeds.

At the level of the ankle and foot, the following examination is felt to be the minimum: palpation of the Achilles tendon and origin and insertions of the plantar fascia; assessment of talar, subtalar, and midtarsal joint motion; and evaluation of laxity of the lateral and medial ligaments of the ankle. Goniometric measurement of the subtalar joint to check for deviation from the normal 2:1 ratio of inversion to eversion through a 45° range and evaluation of the forefoot for varus/valgus also aid in detecting areas of tightness that need stretching or regions of connective tissue laxity that might benefit from an orthosis (60). In cases where a specific problem such as excessive pronation is identified, maneuvers such as the *navicular drop test* are added. If the measured vertical descent of the navicular exceeds 1.5 cm when going from a position in which the entire foot is just touching the floor to one of full weight bearing on that side, there is felt to be excessive pronation (65).

At the level of the knee, range-of-motion testing is followed by evaluation of patellar position, patellar mobility, patellar tracking, and retropatellar pain. The Q angle (the angle formed between straight lines drawn from the anterior superior iliac spine [ASIS] to the distal femur and from the tibial tuberosity through the middle of the patella) is considered to be excessive if over 20° (51,62,66,67). Hypermobility of the patella, external tibial torsion, increased Q angle, femoral neck anteversion, a broad pelvis, and pes planus with pronation together form the "malalignment syndrome," which is associated with medial knee pain (51,68–70). Assessment of the collateral and cruciate ligaments and menisci is also routine. Ober's test is used to evaluate tightness of the tensor fascia lata. In instances in which an iliotibial band (ITB) friction syndrome is suspected, the ITB (Noble) compression test can be used. After positioning the knee in 90° of flexion, the examiner presses on or just proximal to the lateral condyle. The knee is then gradually extended. Pain occurring at about 30° (as the ITB crosses the bony prominence) is a positive finding (71). In cases of anterior knee pain, the exam focuses on patellar orientation (internal versus external rotation, the presence of a high- [alta] or low [baja]-riding patella), defects in the medial or lateral retinacula, increased laxity or pain with patellar mobilization, patellar apprehension, evidence of poor patellar tracking within the trochlea, retropatellar crepitus, and presence of vastus medialis obliquus (VMO) atrophy (20).

The hip and pelvic region must be evaluated for the presence of tight hip flexors, hip extensors, and adductors, as loss of mobility in this region may be a factor in development of an athlete's injury (72,73). The Thomas test consists of having the patient bring both knees up to the chest and then trying to let one leg descend to a flat lying position on the exam table. If the leg cannot assume this position, or if the spine must be arched to do so, it indicates hip flexor tightness (74). Stabilizing the pelvis with one hand while attempting a straight leg raise with the other gives a sense of hamstring tightness; retrotilting of the pelvis begins to occur as "maximum" length is approached. External rotator tightness can be checked by internally rotating the hip with the knee flexed with the patient lying prone. Placing the hip in flexion plus abduction and external rotation (Patrick's test) stresses the hip joint itself. Various maneuvers such as Gaenslen's maneuver (Fig. 63-6) and the Extension test (Fig. 63-7) may be used to nonspecifically stress the sacroiliac joint. Certain bony prominences and landmarks should be assessed for tenderness—the greater trochanter, posterior superior iliac spine (PSIS), ASIS, and posterior inferior iliac spine (PIIS). They also need to be checked for symmetry in the evaluation of malrotation of the sacroiliac joint or pelvis. In addition, the ASIS is a fixed landmark typically used in limb length measurement. Limb length inequalities have been estimated to have three times as much of an effect on a runner as on a walker (57).

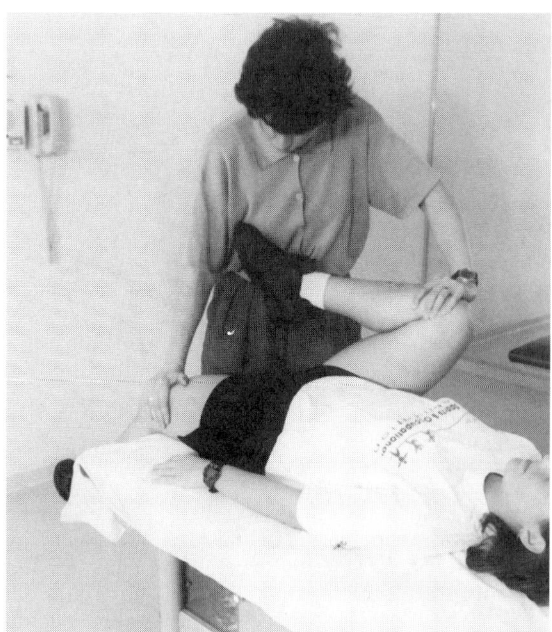

FIG. 63-6. Gaenslen's maneuver is used to stress the left sacroiliac joint. Note that the examiner's right hand is pressing downward on the athlete's left thigh to extend the left hip.

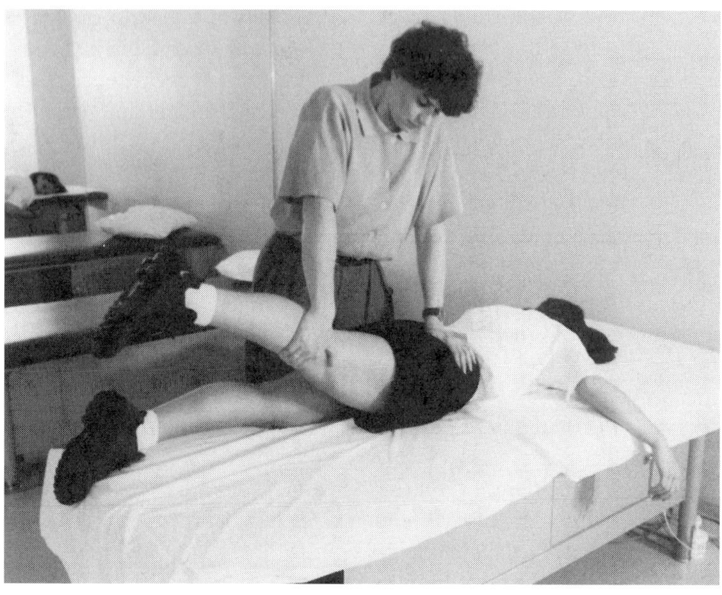

FIG. 63-7. The extension test is used to stress the right sacroiliac joint. Note that the examiner's right hand is pulling the athlete's thigh up into extension while the left hand pushes down over the iliac crest.

The examination of the upper limbs begins with the cervical region. Myofascial restrictions associated with inflexibilities of the scalenes, sternocleidomastoid, longus coli, levator scapula, and trapezius and elevation of the first rib may interfere with both neck and shoulder motion (64). Poor cervicothoracic posture is associated with rounded shoulders, tight pectoral muscles, and forward carriage of the head that also adversely affect the quality of shoulder motion. For the baseball pitcher, it is critical to be able to achieve 180° external rotation of the shoulder (as measured in Fig. 63-8) at the end of the arm-cocking phase so to maximize pitch velocity. Stiffness of the thoracic spine, limited or dyskinetic scapulothoracic motion, and inflexibility of the latissimus dorsi all

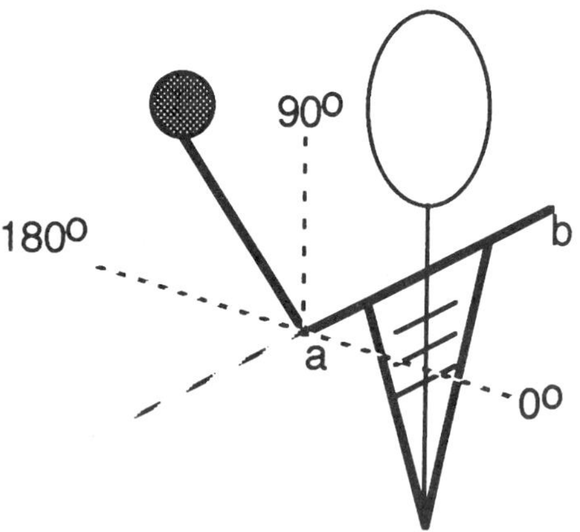

FIG. 63-8. Measurement of shoulder external rotation during the pitching motion. *Line ab* represents the shoulder–elbow axis. Rotation is measured in the sagittal plane and is described as a function of rotation of the forearm relative to an axis defined by the upright spine. When measured in this manner, 180° of external rotation represents the combined effects of pure glenohumeral joint external rotation plus scapulothoracic motion and spine extension.

impair pitching motion by preventing this functional position from occurring externally (75). The quality of scapular motion is statically estimated via the "lateral scapular slide," as described by Kibler (76). The distance between the medial border of the scapula and the thoracic spine is measured (in centimeters) on both the right and left sides in each of three positions. In position 1, the athlete stands with arms at sides. Positions 2 and 3 are shown in Figures 63-9*A* and 63-9*B*. A difference greater than 1.5 cm between sides is considered significant and indicative of weakness of the serratus anterior, rhomboids, or lower and middle trapezei (76). Range of motion of the glenohumeral joint proper should always be performed with the scapula stabilized. Throwing and overhead sport athletes typically have restricted internal rotation and posterior capsular tightness on their dominant side (45). Motion should be checked at the sternoclavicular and acromioclavicular joints. Adducting the humerus in a horizontal plane is often painful in acromioclavicular joint pathology. Description of all of the tests for laxity of the glenohumeral joint, labral injury, and impingement of the rotator cuff tendons is beyond the scope of this chapter. The reader is referred to the texts by Brukner and Khan (53) and Nicholas and Hershman (77). The bulk of the infraspinatus and supraspinatus must be examined. If both of these muscles are of diminished bulk, it may reflect cervical radiculopathy or suprascapular neuropathy at the level of the suprascapular notch. If only the infraspinatus is affected, the possibility of a paralabral cyst (at the level of the spinoglenoid notch) must be considered. Tests for clinical thoracic outlet syndrome should be included. Although true neurogenic and vascular thoracic syndromes are rare entities, clinical thoracic outlet syndrome is quite common (78).

At the level of the elbow and forearm, measurement of flexion and extension and assessment of laxity or pain with varus and valgus stress should be performed. Many throwing

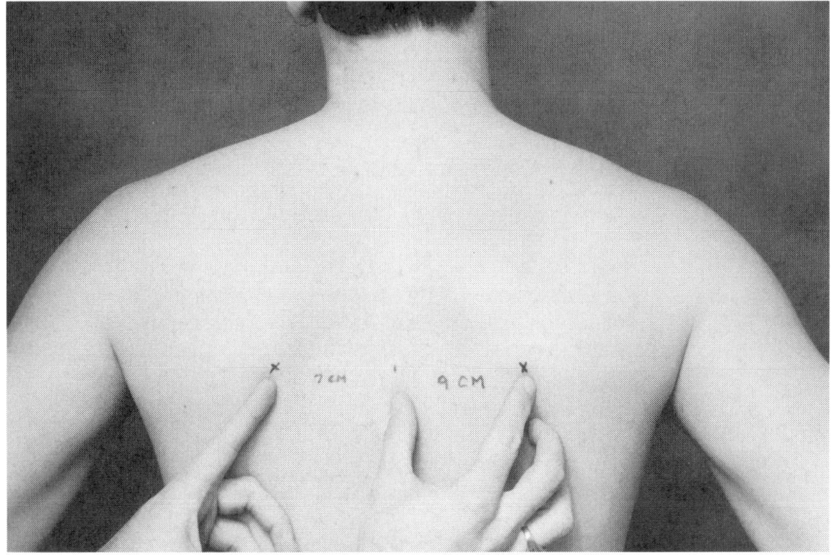

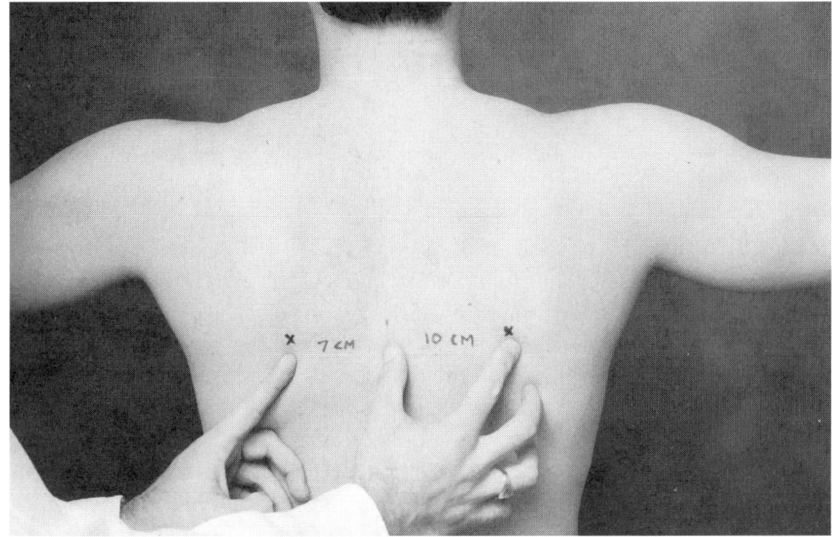

FIG. 63-9. The lateral scapular slide. Position 1 (not shown): the athlete stands with arms at his sides. Position 2 **(top):** the athlete's arms are placed on the iliac crests, and the distance between the medial scapular border and a spinous process of the thoracic spine is measured on each side. Position 3 **(bottom):** the athlete's arms are elevated in abduction at 90° from the body. This athlete has a "positive" lateral slide test on the right side in both of the above positions. (See text for further details.)

athletes have reduced elbow extension from capsular restrictions and musculotendinous contracture; many will exhibit medial joint line opening because of laxity of the medial collateral ligament. Athletes with pain over the lateral epicondylar region need to be assessed for worsening of pain with resisted extensor carpi radialis brevis and extensor digitorum comminus contraction. Mobility of the ulnar nerve and assessment for painful subluxation during repetitive elbow flexion–extension should be included as well. Crepitation within an oarsman's distal radial forearm and exacerbation of pain with resisted thenar extension and wrist radial deviation signify the presence of "intersection syndrome," or injury at the crossing of the abductor pollicis longus (APL) and extensor pollicis brevis (EPB) over the radial wrist extensors (79). This is in distinction to Finkelstein's test, which is sensitive for detection of tenosynovitis of the EPB and APL tendons in DeQuervain syndrome. The examination of the wrist includes checking of motion in all planes, palpation of the scaphoid in the anatomic snuff box, the capitate and lunate dorsally, the pisiform and hook of hamate volarly, and palpation of the distal radius and ulna. The reader is again referred to the text edited by Nicholas and Hershman for a review of tests of carpal instability (77).

A quick but effective screen of the back incorporates all the observations from the upper and lower body segments, as, once again, the concept of the kinetic chain must not be overlooked. Lumbosacral spine motion is intimately related to motion at the level of the hip and pelvis. Tightness of lower limb muscles attaching to the pelvis can interfere with the normally smooth combination of spine flexion–pelvic rotation and spine extension–pelvic derotation (lumbopelvic rhythm) observed during trunk flexion and extension (80). During spine flexion and extension, it is essential to identify which are the major motion segments—80% to 90% of the motion in the lumbosacral spine should be at L4–L5 and L5–S1 (80). Migration of the motion up toward the thoracolumbar junction, altered tone of the paraspinal muscles, and lack of a "springing sensation" in the lower spine during anterior glides (placement and release of pressure along the spine while the patient is in a relaxed prone-lying position) suggests spinal segmental dysfunction. Abdominal muscle weakness and weakness of the thoracolumbar fascia further indicates that the spine is in need of conditioning (81). Many individuals who appear to be otherwise highly fit from constant aerobic exercise fail to perform regular exercise that promotes conditioning of the supportive musculature of their spine. In the young runner with back pain, provocative tests such as extending the spine while standing on one leg help identify active posterior element irritation and/or symptomatic spondylolysis.

A brief neurologic exam is recommended. The elderly patient with "hip pain" may have unrecognized foraminal spinal stenosis with L5 nerve root compromise. The football running back with a chronic "hamstring strain" may have an unrecognized S1 radiculopathy (82). The volleyball player with new-onset shoulder weakness may have either cervical radiculopathy or suprascapular nerve entrapment. Dural stretch maneuvers (e.g., "slump sit"), foraminal compression tests, (e.g., Spurling maneuver), must be performed. Cutaneous nerve injuries need to be considered as well. Careful evaluation of a persistently painful ankle that appears to have healed from an inversion sprain may reveal ongoing irritation of the superficial peroneal nerve. Persistent medial foreleg pain in the presence of a negative bone scan may be related to saphenous nerve irritation rather than medial tibial stress syndrome.

Finally, the equipment, such as running shoes, should be inspected for signs of breakdown. Excessive lateral or medial wear may reflect excessive dynamic supination or pronation, respectively. In general, pronation control is achieved better with a straight board-lasted shoe with good rearfoot control, whereas the supinator does better with a flexible and curve-lasted shoe (57,59,62).

ANALYSIS OF ROTATOR CUFF INJURY IN THE THROWING OR OVERHEAD SPORT ATHLETE

The athlete's shoulder girdle can be afflicted by a variety of injuries (Table 63-1). The overhead throwing athlete is at particular risk for injury because of the repetitive, high-velocity mechanical stress placed on the shoulder. Phenomenally high angular velocities (over 7,000°/sec during the transition from external to internal rotation, going from arm cocking through the acceleration phase) and large forces (anterior translation forces of up to 40% body weight during acceleration, and distraction forces near 90% body weight during deceleration) have commonly been reported at the glenohumeral joint during baseball pitching (44,83,84). The shoulder is the most dynamic force transfer link in the kinetic chain. The price for this mobility is a lack of bony constraint within the glenohumeral joint. Therefore, stability is provided by a complex interaction of the dynamic stabilizers (muscles) and the static stabilizers (ligaments) (85). When these supporting structures are subjected to the high stresses of throwing, the fine balance between functional mobility and stability can be disrupted. This can lead to overload injuries of the glenohumeral ligament complex, the glenoid labrum, and the rotator cuff.

TABLE 63-1. *Shoulder problems in sports medicine practice*

Common	
Rotator cuff tendinitis	Subacromial bursitis
Partial rotator cuff tear	ACJ sprain
ACJ separation	Glenohumeral joint instability
Clavicular fracture	Glenohumeral joint separation
Cervical radiculopathy	Clinical thoracic outlet syndrome
Less Common	
Bankart lesion	Suprascapular nerve injury
Hill Sachs's lesion	Axillary nerve injury
SLAP lesion	Musculocutaneous nerve injury
Long thoracic nerve injury	Osteoarthritis
Uncommon	
Humeral stress fractures	Osteolysis of the distal clavicle
"Dead arm" syndrome	Axillary artery aneurysm
Axillary vein thrombosis	Pectoralis major muscle tear
Neurogenic thoracic outlet syndrome	

ACJ, acromiclavicular joint; SLAP, superior labral anterior to posterior.

The glenohumeral joint (GHJ) instant center of rotation is the most important biomechanical reference point for shoulder stability (44,45,76). In midranges of motion, the instant center does not vary more than 1 to 2 mm. However, 5 to 10 mm of anterior–posterior and 4 to 5 mm of superior–inferior translation can occur at extreme ranges of GHJ motion (86,87). Control of this motion is primarily provided by the muscular constraint system. It does this by means of force couples, muscles acting in a cocontraction pattern to maintain position. Rotator cuff muscle activity is essential to this process. For example, the supraspinatus, a humeral head depressor, and the deltoid, a humeral head elevator, fire together to achieve abduction and rotation of the humeral head in the glenoid with minimal translation. The rotator cuff muscles, as well as extrinsic shoulder muscles, also contract eccentrically in the follow-through phase of throwing to limit joint excursion (88). Through the contraction of large extrinsic muscles, muscle activity also helps to generate forces as well as maintain the important positioning of the scapula. The scapula must protract and retract (up to 15 cm) and rotate (through an arc of approximately 65°) on the thorax during the overhead throwing or serving motion so that the glenoid fossa can follow the humeral head through its arc of motion (76). The scapula (and in particular the acromion) must be elevated adequately during abduction and rotation of the humerus to avoid mechanical impingement. As previously noted, dynamic positioning of the scapula is a function of spine motion and morphology and the activation patterns of the trapezius, rhomboids, serratus anterior, levator scapula, and pectoralis minor.

Biomechanical analysis of the baseball throw and tennis

serve has helped us understand how such phenomenally high torques and velocities occur at the glenohumeral joint (44,83,84). It is important to recognize that the forces necessary to achieve such velocities are not exclusively developed in the shoulder. The lower limbs and spine are responsible for generating the majority of these forces (75). The spine and its associated musculature are also largely responsible for attenuation of these forces in the deceleration phase of throwing (75).

For the reasons stated above, evaluation and rehabilitation of the injured shoulder in a throwing athlete must involve a complete assessment of each segment link of the kinetic chain. A knowledge of the mechanics of the sport is also essential to identify all possible deficits and adaptations. For analysis of rotator cuff injury, the template described previously will be utilized.

The *clinical symptom complex* for rotator cuff injury consists of anterolateral shoulder pain, particularly with throwing or other overhead activities. Pain may extend into the lateral aspect of the arm. Nocturnal or rest pain may be indicative of rotator cuff tear (89). Pain with shoulder weakness or fatigue may indicate other or concomitant GHJ injury or neurologic injury. *The tissue injury complex* consists of myotendinous injury within of any of the rotator cuff muscles (most commonly supraspinatus), tears of the glenoid labrum or glenohumeral capsule, and bursal inflammation.

The *tissue overload complex* consists of those tissues that have been subjected to repetitive tensile overload with subtle pathologic change. At the shoulder, these structures would include the posterior rotator cuff muscles with inflexibility and weakness (because of eccentric overload during follow-through phase), the scapular stabilizers (rhomboids, serratus, middle and lower trapezei), and the suprascapular and long thoracic nerves from tensile overload and traction. Along the kinetic chain, overload can occur at any single or all segments of the cervical, thoracic, and lumbar spine regions as well as the hips (44,75,83,84,90).

The *functional biomechanical deficits* can be seen at any level where overload exists. At the shoulder, loss of glenohumeral internal rotation is common from posterior capsular tightness. A positive lateral scapular slide signifying weakness of the scapular stabilizing musculature and weakness of the external rotators, particularly in humeral abduction, is typical as well (76). Pectoralis minor tightness produces antetilting of the glenoid via its pull on the coracoid. Latissimus dorsi tightness prevents external rotation of the shoulder without assumption of lumbar spine lordosis. At the cervical spine, inflexibilities and weakness of the sternocleidomastoid, upper trapezius, and cervical flexors lead to restriction of rotation and lateral flexion, which interferes with the pitcher's ability to maintain view of the catcher's mitt (''target acquisition'') throughout the stride and acceleration phases (75). Loss of thoracic extension and reduced thoracic rotation lead to reduced ''external rotation.'' Weakness of the abdominal, lumbar spine extensor, and gluteal musculature create loss of truncal control and induce excessive or ill-timed lumbar lordosis (75,91). Loss of bilateral hip internal range of motion can also lead to increased lumbar lordosis (75). Tightness of the hip flexors and hamstrings shorten the pitcher's stride length, which also increases the stress on the pitcher's arm.

The throwing athlete will adopt *subclinical adaptations* to maintain performance despite the above biomechanical deficits. Failure at the level of the shoulder can lead to ''short arming'' the ball, in which the athlete will decrease the arc of shoulder motion in order to avoid excessive glenohumeral displacement. Excessive ''wrist snap'' may occur to compensate for loss of force transfer to the distal segment. Deficits at the level of the spine (lack of rotation and/or increased lumbar lordosis) and hips (loss of rotation) can lead to ''opening up'' too soon or ''throwing across the body'' (75,91). In ''opening up'' too soon, the throwing shoulder lags behind the body and spine, elbow position is not maintained, and pitching performance suffers (75,91).

The rehabilitation program begins with the acute management phase, addressing the clinical symptoms complex and the tissue injury complex. The goals of this phase are to control pain, inflammation, and irritation. It is also important to reestablish a nonpainful range of motion and neuromuscular control of the scapula in a neutral glenohumeral position and to prevent upper limb muscle atrophy (44–46). Nonsteroidals and modalities are helpful in decreasing pain and inflammation. Steroid injections should be avoided in most cases. Manual techniques can be useful to increase range of motion along with Codman or pendulum exercises. Ropes and pulleys may also be beneficial. Reestablishment of neuromuscular control of the shoulder girdle is begun with scapular muscle-strengthening and shoulder-closed kinetic chain exercises. Aerobic conditioning must be maintained throughout the rehabilitation process with running or biking.

When full passive shoulder range of motion, significant decreased pain, and good scapular control can be demonstrated, the athlete advances to the recovery phase to address the above functional biomechanical deficits and adaptations. First, the athlete must regain and improve entire upper limb muscle strength with full strengthening of the scapular stabilizers. Strengthening of the rotator cuff muscles may be accomplished with ''isolation'' exercises or, in a more protective fashion, in multimuscle group tasks (45,47,89). Inflexibilities must be addressed at all levels of the spine and hips during this stage. Spinal segmental dysfunction should be addressed by removing myofascial restrictions, reestablishing proper segmental motion, and then developing a neutral spine stabilization program. Alternating OKC and CKC exercises, utilizing two-handed and one-handed ball toss techniques, and incorporating trunk-stabilizing exercises while performing throwing-type motions (Figs. 63-10 and 63-11) are all important parts of the progression of this portion of the rehabilitation program.

Before the patient returns to play, power and endurance must be increased in the upper limb and the entire kinetic chain. Plyometrics, including wall push-ups and alternating

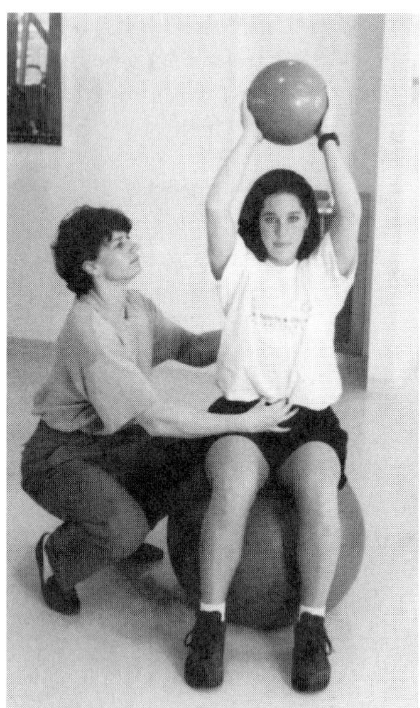

FIG. 63-10. Shoulder rehabilitation. The athlete works on truncal control and utilizes a two-handed ball toss as part of a functional progression

medicine ball catches and tosses are used to improve upper limb power and endurance (44–47). Aggressive proprioceptive neuromuscular facilitation and dynamic challenges are made to the athlete's ability to maintain a neutral spine under sport-specific conditions. The athlete then progresses to throwing with long-toss–short-toss program with eventual advancement to pitching activity. Analysis of the athlete's pitching motion at this point should reveal better overall pitching mechanics. When strength is near normal with a negative clinical examination and good progression through the entire clinical program, the athlete may return to full pitching activity.

SHOULDER DYSFUNCTION IN A PHYSICALLY CHALLENGED ATHLETE

The physically challenged athlete who competes in overhead sports from a wheelchair presents a different set of challenges for the sports physiatrist. Wheelchair use alters demands placed on the upper limbs and spine, and overload injuries reflect the alteration of the kinetic chain. Furthermore, depending on the athlete's particular impairments, certain muscles may not be available for rehabilitation. Thus, the sports physician must be creative both in injury analysis and in formulation of rehabilitation schemes.

A wheelchair tennis player is shown in Figures 63-12 and 63-13. In distinction from the athletes described in the previous section, this athlete cannot utilize a ground reaction force as part of his preparation to accelerate the racquet and strike the ball. At best, he has a "chair-reactive force," which he can only make use of if he grabs the chair with his nondominant hand. Grasping the chair or elevating the nonracquet side arm away from his body is also used to stabilize the upper torso and keep the athlete in the chair. The thoracic spine must be rapidly rotated (if mechanically or neurologically possible) to provide momentum for rotational acceleration of the humerus, and the muscles attaching to the cervical

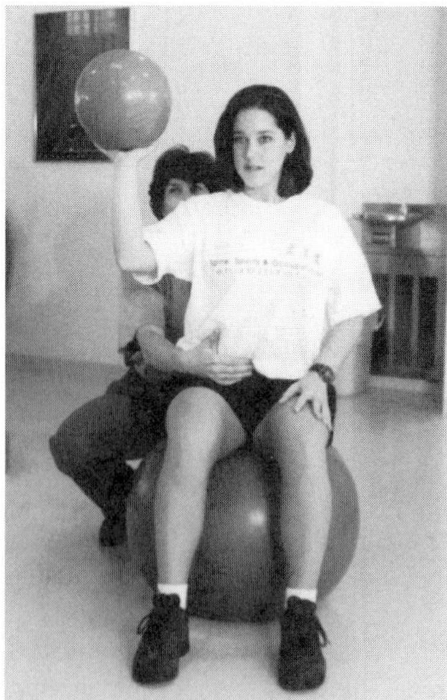

FIG. 63-11. Shoulder rehabilitation. The athlete places more stress on the scapular stabilizers and shoulder girdle muscles of the throwing arm side with this one-handed ball-toss exercise.

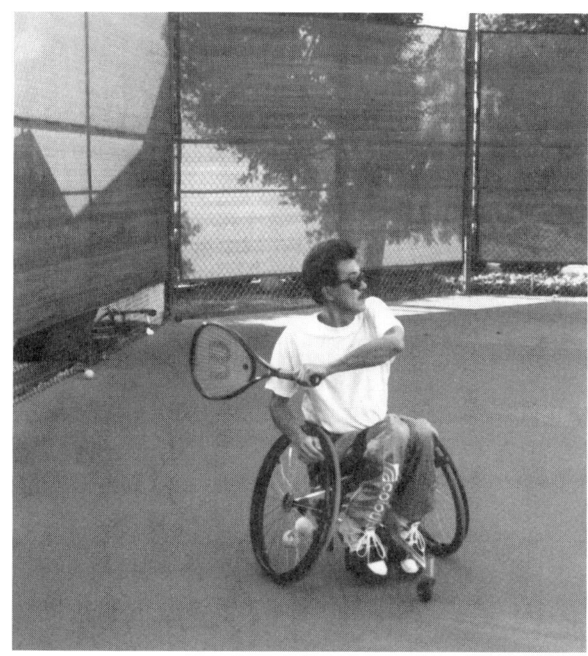

FIG. 63-12. Wheelchair tennis player: backhand stroke preparation. (See text for further details.)

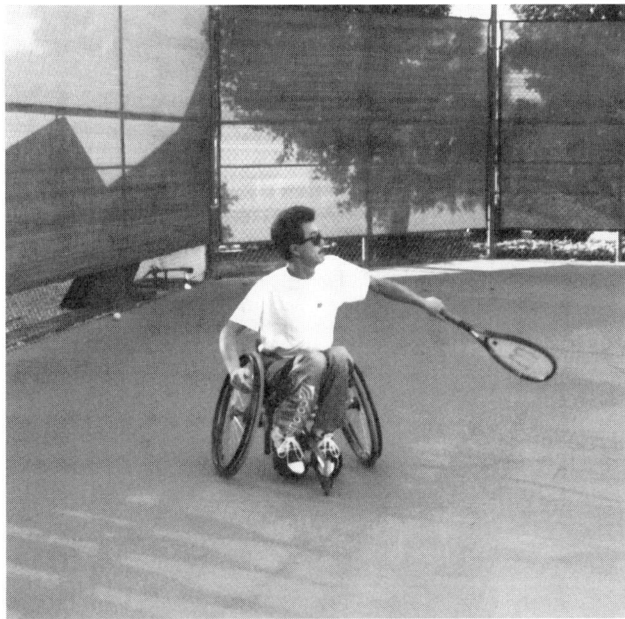

FIG. 63-13. Wheelchair tennis player: backhand stroke follow-through. (See text for further details.)

dorsal fascia (e.g., upper trapezius and sternocleidomastoid) must be utilized to elevate the shoulder girdle. Kinetic chain disruption is also apparent when one considers how the athlete reached the correct court position to strike the ball. The act of wheelchair propulsion turns upper limb muscles such as the rotator cuff, which normally only has to stabilize the GHJ, into a prime mover and kinetic chain link segments such as the wrist, which are typically at the terminus of the chain, into force generators. Propulsion of the chair also creates alternating upper limb CKC (hand in contact with the push rim) and OKC (hand releases the push rim) conditions. If the athlete cannot reach the intended court site in time, then he must lunge to hit the ball, which places even more stress on the shoulder girdle. Finally, the wheelchair tennis player is closer to the height of the net than the ambulatory athlete and must utilize a slightly different shot trajectory to ensure that the stroked ball remains in the court of play.

The *clinical symptom complex* and *tissue injury complex* are the same for both the wheelchair tennis player and the ambulatory athlete. The *tissue overload complex* in the wheelchair athlete includes the scapular stabilizers, rotator cuff, glenoid labrum, and cervical and thoracic spine. *Functional biomechanical deficits* include accentuated cervical lordosis with weak cervical flexors, reduced cervical spine side bending, loss of glenohumeral internal rotation, a lateral scapular slide, tightness of the pectoralis major and minor, and reduced thoracic extension. *Subclinical adaptations* include increased contralateral side bending in the thoracolumbar spine to compensate for reduced humeral abduction, "short arming" of serves and forehand strokes, and increased use of the pectoralis major to accelerate the humerus.

Rehabilitation of the wheelchair tennis player follows the same sequence as in the ambulatory athlete. Relative rest consists of halting sports participation with the understanding that this athlete will still be working the rotator cuff regularly in performance of daily wheelchair propulsion and transfers. If the athlete's symptoms are severe, use of an arm-crank-propelled "tricycle" may prove beneficial. Depending on the extent of the athlete's limitations, adaptive weight lifting equipment may be required. The reader is referred to the works of Laskowski (92,93) for further discussion of adaptive exercise equipment.

ANALYSIS OF PATELLOFEMORAL JOINT INJURY

Many types of knee injuries are seen in outpatient musculoskeletal practice (see Table 63-2) Patellofemoral pain syndrome is one of the most common knee injury patterns. It has been cited as the most common knee problem in runners (94). The etiology is believed to be abnormal stress resulting from patellofemoral malalignment rather than from primary articular cartilage damage (95). The patellofemoral joint is predominantly a soft-tissue joint lacking bony constraint. It relies on a proper balance of numerous muscular and fascial structures to maintain stability. Anteriorly, the knee extensor mechanism consists of the quadriceps group, the quadriceps tendon, the patellar tendon, and the patella. The posterior hamstrings act as antagonists to these anterior structures. The iliotibial tract, lateral retinaculum, and patellofemoral ligaments provide a laterally directed pull on the patella, while the VMO, medial retinaculum, and the medial patellofemoral ligaments pull medially. These stabilizing forces, by compressing the patella against the femur, create a patellofemoral joint reaction force (PFJRF). The PFJRF becomes greater with increases in quadriceps tension and with in-

TABLE 63-2. *Knee problems in sports medicine practice*

Common	
Patellofemoral pain	Anterior cruciate ligament sprain
Patellar tendinitis	Collateral ligament sprain
Meniscal strains	Iliotibial band friction syndrome
Pes anserine bursitis	Patellar subluxation
Osteoarthritis	
Less Common	
Posterior cruciate ligament tear	Hamstring tendinitis
Posterolateral corner injury	Osgood-Schlatter disease
Patellar fracture	Stress fracture of femur
Fat pad impingement	Stress fracture of tibia
Bakers cyst	Tibial plateau fracture
Uncommon	
Plica syndrome	Discoid meniscus
Fibular head dislocation	Saphenous nerve injury
Osteochondral lesion of medial femoral condyle	
Sinding-Larsen-Johansson syndrome	
Legg Calve Perthes' disease (referred pain)	
Slipped capital femoral epiphysis (referred pain)	

creased knee flexion. At near full extension, PFJRF equals zero, but at 90° of flexion, PRJRF is about 2.5 to 3.0 times body weight. The approximate PFJRFs for walking, ascending stairs, and squatting are 0.5, 3.3, and 6 to 7 times body weight, respectively (96). The patellofemoral joint reaction stress (PFJRS) refers to the PFJRF per unit contact area. A large PFJRF distributed over a large contact area produces a relatively smaller degree of articular stress. A large PFJRF over a smaller area yields high articular stresses and heightens the chances of subchondral degeneration occurring.

The amount of patellofemoral contact area changes with knee flexion. From full extension through the first 10° to 20° of flexion, little contact occurs. Trochlear engagement then begins, with the inferior margin of both medial and lateral facets sharing the load (96). Between 20° and 90° of flexion, there is increased proximal patellar and lateral edge contact, and over 90° the odd facet makes contact (97). The patellofemoral contact areas are the greatest in the midrange (30° to 90°) with maximal loading at 40° to 60° of flexion. Therefore, pain often occurs with loading in this range, and rehabilitation of patellofemoral dysfunction in the 60° to 90° and the 0° to 40° range is most desirable.

The *tissue injury complex* consists of injury at the patellar cartilage, the synovium, and the insertion site of the patellar tendon on the patella. Clinical symptoms complex consists of peripatellar pain, crepitation, and, occasionally, mild swelling. The pain, often located along the medial or lateral patellofemoral joint and retinaculum, is worsened with prolonged knee flexion and increased PFJRF during activities such as descending stairs and prolonged sitting, i.e., "the theater sign." Occasionally, there may be complaints of the "knee giving way," possibly related to reflex inhibition of the knee extensor mechanism (98). Pain with terminal knee extension should alert the clinician to the possibility of infrapatellar fat pad impingement between the inferior pole of the patella and the femoral condyle. Symptoms often gradually increase or may increase abruptly in response to an altered training pattern. The *tissue overload complex* consists of an inflamed patellar tendon, the undersurface of the patella, the medial retinaculum, and the superficial and deep lateral retinaculum.

Factors that predispose individuals to patellofemoral pain and abnormal tracking include the presence of patella alta, increased *Q* angle, femoral anteversion, a shallow intercondylar groove, and excessive pronation at the foot–ankle complex. The clinician should not only look for all of these but should mobilize the patella superiorly, inferiorly, medially, and laterally as well as observe patellar tilt, glide, and position. The *functional biomechanical deficits* that lead to patellofemoral injury include all factors above and below the knee joint that contribute to abnormal tracking. One of the most important factors affecting dynamic patella alignment is felt to be the balance between the medial and lateral structures. Insufficiency of the medial quadriceps (especially the vastus medialis obliquus) with inflexibility of the lateral retinaculum, vastus lateralis, and iliotibial band (ITB) will lead to lateral displacement of the patella, especially when the patella disengages from the femoral trochlear groove in the last 20° of extension (99). Inflexibility of the hamstrings and the gastrocnemius–soleus complex will effectively increase knee flexion. Hip external rotator weakness leads to increased medial rotation of the femur during midstance. This, in conjunction with gastrocnemius–soleus tightness creates excessive functional pronation at the ankle–foot, which increases the valgus vector at the knee and shear stress at the patellofemoral joint. Imbalance of hip internal and external rotators with tight internal rotators lead to increased torque at the knee. Functional adaptations (*Subclinical Adaptation Complex*) include altered stride to avoid full loading of the knee and avoidance of full-effort jumping activities.

The rehabilitation program again begins with the acute management phase, addressing the clinical symptoms complex and the tissue injury complex. The goals of this phase are to control pain, inflammation, and irritation and to prevent muscle atrophy while maintaining aerobic fitness. To decrease pain and inflammation, the use of cryotherapy (ice), electrical stimulation, and other modalities such as massage is indicated. Nonsteroidal anti-inflammatory medication can also be helpful, especially if an effusion is present. Activities such as jumping, squatting, hill running, cycling, excessive stair climbing, or prolonged sitting with the knees flexed greater than 40° should be avoided. A transition to aqua running with the use of a flotation device may be necessary if even minimal land running is painful (100).

Following acute management, the functional biomechanical deficits as described above, including all flexibility and strength deficits throughout the kinetic chain, should be corrected. Rehabilitation must continue beyond the resolution of the athlete's symptoms. Medial stabilization of the patella is initiated through abductor magnus–VMO complex strengthening. Strengthening of the quadriceps mechanism is typically performed in the last 30° of knee extension, but the selectivity of strengthening only the VMO is debatable (101). Most likely, a general quadriceps strengthening occurs with a subsequent restoration of VMO force production. The best method to strengthen the quadriceps group while incurring the smallest PFJRFs and PFJRS may be via short-arc (between 45° flexion and extension) closed kinetic chain exercises via the leg press (102). The CKC exercises such as a leg press provide greater protection of the patellofemoral joint and provide for more realistic proprioceptive feedback than do OKC knee extensions and curls (19,102). Adductor squeezes and closed kinetic chain short-arc knee extension exercises also help with VMO training. Leg extension exercises in which the foot is free to move should be avoided. These open kinetic chain exercises cause a greater PFJRF and can provoke an increase in the patient's symptoms. Increased flexibility in the hamstrings, gastrocnemius–soleus complex, and iliotibial band is essential. Proprioceptive neu-

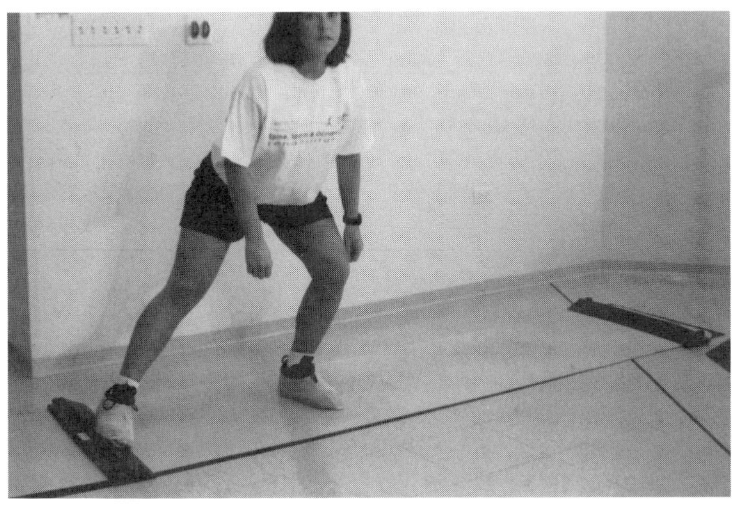

FIG. 63-14. Dynamic rehabilitation exercise utilizing a slideboard. This technique is excellent for training hip abductors and truncal control while providing proprioceptive feedback to the athlete.

romuscular facilitation techniques with reflex inhibition and contract–relax can be helpful to establish proper musculotendinous length. Mobilization and passive stretching of the lateral structures may also be necessary. Dynamic strengthening of the hip and pelvic stabilizers, especially the hip external rotators (gluteus medius), should be started. Slide board exercises, as shown in Figure 63-14, provide a functional technique for strengthening as well as enhancing proprioceptive feedback.

Consideration should also be given for bracing, orthoses, and taping. Patellar stabilizing braces may be appropriate but should not be the first plan of attack. Foot orthoses to correct pronation may also be used, but only if biomechanical deficits persist after achieving full flexibility of the gastrocnemius–soleus complex, hamstrings, iliotibial band, and VMO strengthening has occurred. Taping of the patella to simulate proper patellar alignment accompanied by neuromuscular reeducation of the knee musculature (McConnell technique) may be beneficial (103). McConnell has reported improvement rates of better than 90% with her technique (103). Taping, in the McConnell program, is a transitional step that allows patients to perform strengthening exercise pain-free. Figure 63-15 demonstrates the use of patellar taping in conjunction with performance of a kinetic chain strengthening exercise. Critics of her program point to the lack of radiographic change in patellar position, but the clinically observed improvement rates and reduction in pain scales ratings even among those without radiologic improvement are far more compelling. Also, the taping may dynamically control patellar motion, which would remain undetected by a static radiograph. A recent prospective study evaluating patellar taping versus nontaping revealed no difference in subjective pain complaints or strength pre- and posttherapy (104). However, no mention was made as to whether taping allowed pain-free exercise in those who had pain with exercise (the ultimate goal of McConnell taping), and no attention was paid to pathomechanics or rehabilitation about the hip or ankle joints.

Sport-specific training is reintroduced and maintained as long as the athlete remains pain-free while incorporating the dynamic demands of the particular sport. Return to sport occurs when the athlete has fully addressed the biomechanical deficits and associated functional adaptations and is pain-free with full athletic activity and has regained full aerobic conditioning.

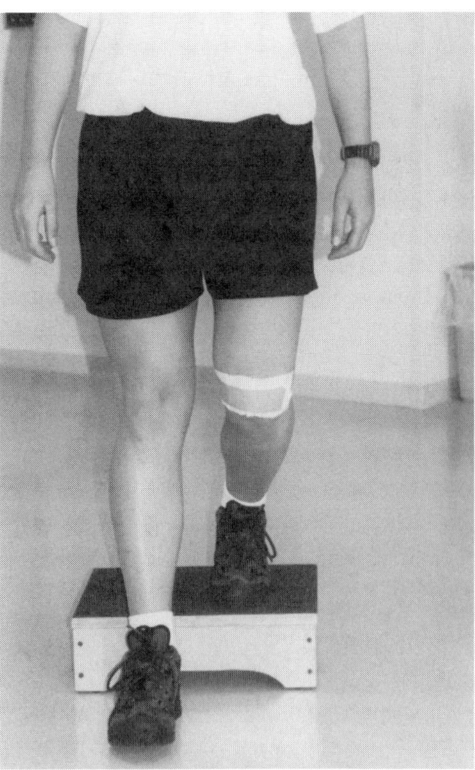

FIG. 63-15. Patellofemoral rehabilitation. McConnell taping of the athlete's knee is combined with dynamic gluteal and adductor stengthening as the athlete slowly steps down.

ANALYSIS OF ANKLE SPRAIN

Ankle injuries are probably the most common sports-related injury and one of the most frequently seen musculoskeletal problems presenting to the outpatient physiatrist's office. Table 63-3 outlines ankle injuries seen in a typical sports rehabilitation clinic. Inversion sprains alone account for at least 85% of the isolated ankle injuries (54,105,106). As with many of the entities previously discussed, without appropriate rehabilitation there is great likelihood for recurrent injury.

The ankle may be described as a hinge joint with a mortise (the tibia and fibula) and tenon (talus). The distal tibia forms the medial maleolus while the fibula, which extends further distally, forms the lateral maleolus. There are approximately 20° of dorsiflexion and 50° of available plantar flexion under normal conditions. Both the talar and tibiofibular joint are widest anteriorly, so the joint has its maximum osteologic stability in dorsiflexion (when the wide portion of the talus becomes wedged into the narrower portion of the mortise) and minimal osteologic stability in plantar flexion. The joint is obliquely placed relative to the knee joint axis and the line of progression, creating an external tibial torsion of approximately 20°. The subtalar (talocalcaneal) and midtarsal (talonavicular and calcaneocuboid) joints both permit the additional motions of inversion and eversion and influence hindfoot-to-midfoot load transfer. The critical ligamentous structures on the lateral side include the posterior talofibular ligament (PTFL), anterior talofibular ligament (ATFL), and the calcaneofibular ligament (CFL). Of the three lateral ligaments, the PTFL is the strongest, and the ATFL is the weakest. On the medial side is the deltoid ligament with its component parts, the anterior tibiotalar, posterior tibiotalar, tibionavicular, and tibiocalcaneal ligaments. Somewhat anterolaterally, between the fibula and the tibia, is the tibiofibular syndesmosis. The lateral ligaments tend to check inversion and stabilize against posterior talar displacement, while the medial complex guards against eversion injuries. The hinge motion of the talar joint has a direct effect on the tautness of the lateral collateral ligaments. Dorsiflexion promotes ATFL laxity but CFL tautness, whereas plantar flexion results in ATFL tautness and CFL laxity. The PTFL is the restraint against posterior displacement. Inversion sprains typically occur when the ankle is plantar flexed, so the ATFL is the most vulnerable of the lateral ligaments. The broadness of the medial maleolus, the angle of the mortise, and the toughness of the deltoid complex provide much greater restriction to extremes of eversion than do the lateral structures to extremes of inversion, so medial injuries are far less frequent. Muscular structures about the ankle that provide additional support include the peroneus longus and brevis laterally, the tibialis anterior dorsally, the posterior tibialis, flexor digitorum longus, and flexor hallucis longus medially, and the gastrocnemius–soleus complex posteriorly. Peripheral nerves vulnerable to injury in this region include the sural (laterally), deep and superficial peroneals (dorsolaterally), and saphenous (dorsomedially). The distal tibial nerve may be damaged with medial ankle injury or compressed in the region of the tarsal tunnel.

TABLE 63-3. *Ankle problems in sports medicine practice*

Most common	Less common
Ligamentous sprains–lateral complex	Deltoid ligament sprain
Uncommon	Stress fracture of fibula
Reflex sympathetic dystrophy	Subluxing peroneal tendon
Anterior tarsal tunnel syndrome	Fractures of tibia
Always consider	Fractures of fibula
Osteochondral lesions of talus	Metatarsal fractures
Syndesmosis injury	Fractures of talus
	Os trigonum
	Growth plate fracture
	Fracture/dislocation
	Superficial peroneal nerve injury
	Sural nerve injury

Ankle sprains typically occur at the time of foot–ground articulation with the foot and ankle in a position of minimum osteologic stability. The ATFL is generally the first structure injured with a combined inversion–plantar flexion stress, and the CFL will be the second structure injured as the inversion stress increases. For the PTFL to become injured, inversion must continue further, or some posterior displacement of the talus must occur (107). Inversion in neutral stresses the CFL. The deltoid ligament is injured with eversion stress. Addition of any rotatory stress to the above, or inversion in dorsiflexion leads to syndesmosis injury (51,107).

When ligaments endure injury, the most common site along the ligament tends to be within the midsubstance of the ligament (107). Tears that occur closer to the insertion are often accompanied by avulsion fractures. Each ligament is graded separately. The following system combines the categorization of numerous authors (107–110):

Grade I (mild): minor ligamentous disruption (essentially a stretch) with maintenance of integrity and no signs of instability.

Grade II (moderate): near-complete disruption with macroscopic tearing and swelling. There is a moderate amount of functional loss such as difficulty toe walking, and there is mild or moderate instability.

Grade III (severe): complete ligamentous rupture with obvious swelling, discoloration, and tenderness. There is significant functional loss with limited range of motion as a result of swelling, limited weight bearing tolerance because of pain, and reduced stability from the ligamentous disruption.

The mechanism and consequences of the acute ankle injury are reliably obtained from the history and physical examination. Sensation of a "tear" or "pop" with a "rolling over" the ankle are highly suggestive of an ATFL or CFL tear, whereas anteriorly based pain and inability to bear weight following the patient's foot "getting stuck" while the leg continued to rotate suggests syndesmosis injury.

The anterior drawer test is the hallmark test for integrity of the ATFL. The patient's calf muscles should be relaxed, and the foot should be in approximately 10° of plantar flexion. The calcaneus is grasped firmly and drawn forward while the tibia is pushed posteriorly with the other hand. Under normal conditions, the translation of the talus is no more than 4 mm (20,51,107). A "drawer" of more than 8 mm is indicative of, at least, an ATFL tear (20,51,107).

The talar tilt (inversion) test is more sensitive for CFL tears. The lower leg is held firmly by one hand while an inversion stress is applied to the talus and calcaneus with the other hand. Separation of the surface of the talus from the tibia (i.e., a tilting) is considered a positive test. The ankle should be kept in neutral during this maneuver; plantar flexion will lead to stressing of the ATFL.

The clunk (side to side) test is a gross assessment of mortise widening, as when there is a tibiofibular ligament complex injury. Grasping the calcaneus with one hand and surrounding the distal third of the tibia and fibula with the other, the examiner attempts to move the talus from side to side. A "clunk" or "thud" is felt as the talus hits the tibia or fibula. Care must be taken not to allow inversion or eversion to occur during this maneuver, or a false-positive result will ensue.

When there is true tibiofibular diastasis as a result of complete syndesmosis injury, the squeeze test may be helpful. Proximal compression of the tibia and fibula together produces pain at the level of the interosseous membrane (107,110,111). Diastasis compromises load bearing at the ankle joint severely and requires surgical consultation.

The eversion test assesses the integrity of the deltoid ligament complex. The lower tibia is grasped in one hand, and the heel in the other. If the tibiotalar joint widens medially with eversion stress, the test is positive.

If a sprain is felt to be grade 2 or more, x-rays should be obtained to rule out a coexisting fracture. Standard views include an A–P, a lateral, and a "mortise" view, taken with the lower leg in 20° of internal rotation. The mortise view is necessary to fully evaluate the talar dome surface as well as to adequately examine the distal tibial and fibular surfaces. If the mortise is not disrupted, the distances between the lateral talus and fibula and between the medial talus and the tibia are equal (107). A medial clear space (the distance between the medial tibia border and the talus border) greater than 5 mm suggests deltoid ligament injury, whereas a 5-mm or larger distance between the medial fibular cortex and the incisura fibularis of the talus indicates syndesmosis tear (107).

When examining radiographs of the ankle it is important to remember the "ring concept" (20,107). When the mortise is viewed directly (as in Fig. 63-16), the medial maleolus, the tibial plafond superiorly, the lateral maleolus, and the talus inferiorly form a ring that is held together by the lateral and medial ligaments and the syndesmosis (112). Disruption

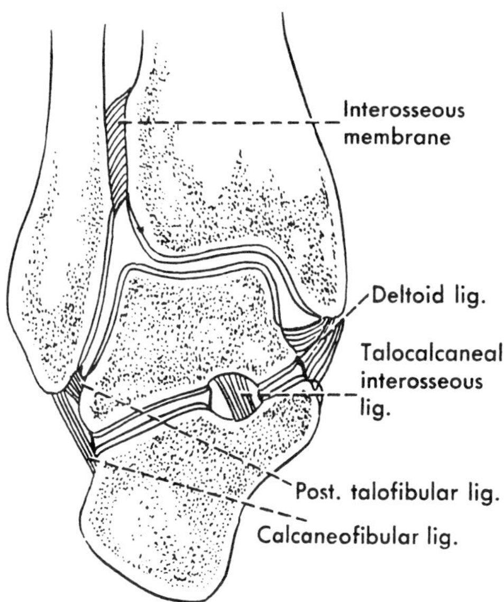

FIG. 63-16. The ring of the ankle. (From Hollinshead WH, Jenkins DB. *Functional anatomy of the limbs and back, 5th ed.* Philadelphia: WB Saunders, 1981. See text for further details.)

of any of these support structures will tend to alter the shape of the ring. Furthermore, if the ring is deformed on one side (i.e., a distal fibular fracture), one must always look for a coexisting injury somewhere else along the ring (i.e., a deltoid ligament injury with widening of the medial mortise).

Occasionally, "stress views" of the ankle are performed. These may be helpful in determining completeness of a ligamentous tear or, more importantly, determining the presence of avulsed fragments of bone. Traction forces are applied to the ankle to promote a tilt or drawer effect, and comparisons are made between injured and uninjured sides for asymmetry. For the "tilt stress," the angle between the talar dome and tibial plafond is measured. Although controversy exists as to the exact angle constituting a significant widening, lateral opening of more than 10° suggests either a CFL or ATFL injury, and more than 20° is highly suggestive of a combined CFL and ATFL injury (51,54,107).

There are many types of fractures associated with ankle sprains, and it is beyond the scope of this chapter to discuss them all. The *spiral fracture of the distal fibula* is one of the most common fractures of the ankle region. When this is seen, the proximal fibula end must also be examined, as forces may have been transmitted up the interosseous membrane. The *avulsion fracture* at the base of the fifth metatarsal associated with inversion sprain and the pulling of the peroneus brevis is also relatively common. This needs to be distinguished from the *Jones fracture,* which is a fracture of the proximal diaphysis of the fifth metatarsal. Whereas the avulsion fracture at the base of the fifth metatarsal can typically be treated with early immobilization (predominantly for pain relief) followed by a progressive rehabilitation program, the Jones fracture may need internal fixation for healing to take place. *Osteochondral talar dome fractures* may follow almost any type of ankle injury and should be considered in "slow healing" cases and where the region over the talus is tender. *Mortise disruption* follows syndesmosis and/or deltoid ligament injuries; the ring of the mortise should immediately be inspected for evidence of bimalleolar (or trimalleolar) fractures (51,54,67,107). With the exception of the nondisplaced Jones fracture, all of these problems may require surgical consultation.

In an ATFL sprain, the clinical symptom complex consists of pain and swelling over the anterolateral ankle with decreased weight-bearing tolerance. The tissue injury complex and tissue overload complex consist of the ATFL, joint capsule, and surrounding soft tissue structures. In higher-grade sprains, the fibula, talus, and syndesmosis are overloaded as well. Functional biomechanical deficits typically include tightness of the gastrocnemius–soleus complex, weakness of the ankle evertors, and weakness of the hip abductors. Clinical substitution patterns include decreased weight bearing, hesitancy to jump or land on the injured side and avoidance of lateral body motion.

Acute treatment of all sprains includes icing and compressive wrapping of the injured site. Cryocuffs are particularly helpful in minimizing the amount of postinjury swelling, which will facilitate the rehabilitation process. Early mobilization of the nonfractured ankle is the preferred treatment, and the ankle should be protected with elastic support, air stirrup splints, lace-up braces, or plastic molded supports. Casting of the uncomplicated sprain actually slows recovery, even in grade 3 sprains (110,113). Crutches are used only when gait is affected enough to increase the chance of further injury or pain precludes full weight bearing. Ankle pumping, "writing the alphabet" with the feet, and stretching of the gastrocnemius–soleus complex (Fig. 63-17) may all be started during this period. During the next phase, strengthening of the evertors, invertors, and plantar and dorsiflexors can be performed dynamically with elastic tubing and then via heel raises and partial squats. Hip muscle strengthening must be included as well. Balance boards and minitrampoline exercises (Figs. 63-18 and 63-19) are an essential part of the rehabilitation, as these help with proprioceptive retraining as well as strengthening. Bicycle exercise is a safe way to maintain or increase endurance without subjecting the ankle to excessive stress. As the individual progresses, more dynamic training is introduced such as slide board, figure of 8 running drills, hexagon drills, and carioca drills. Good functional tests to determine readiness to return to activity include "shuttle runs" and single-leg hopping tests, where side-to-side comparisons for hop height or time to cover a given distance can be made. In our experience, the majority of sprains treated in this manner are ready to return to activity within 1 to 3 weeks. The use of postrehabilitation

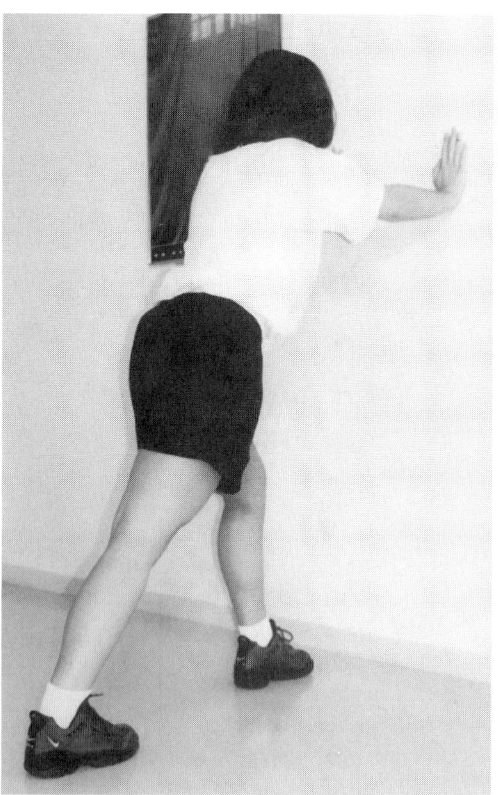
A

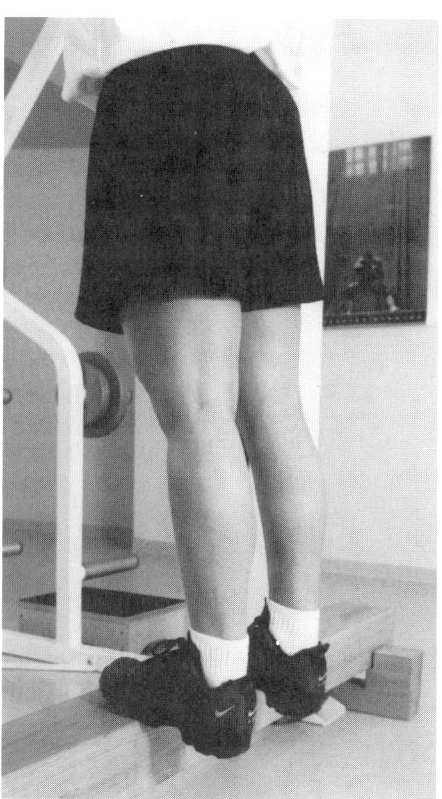
B

FIG. 63-17. A: Stretching of the right gastrocnemius–soleus complex in a standing position. Note that the athlete maintains good pelvic and truncal control while keeping the right heel on the ground. **B:** Bilateral gravity-assisted gastrocnemius–soleus stretching.

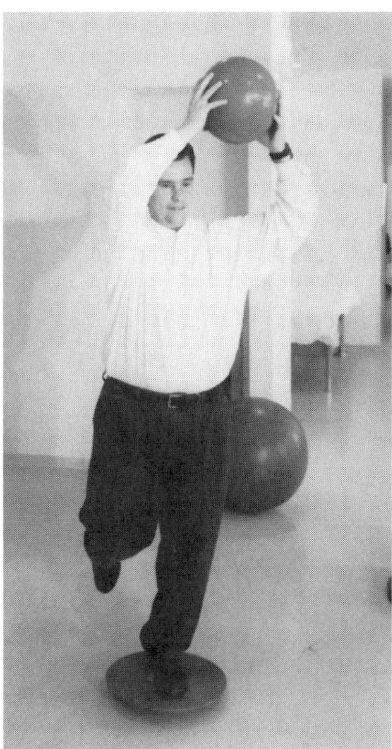

FIG. 63-18. Dynamic ankle rehabilitation utilizing a balance board. The athlete tries to maintain balance while moving the ball in different directions about his body.

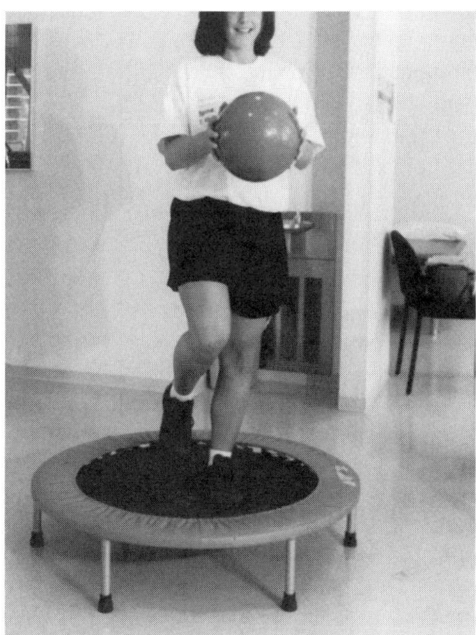

FIG. 63-19. Dynamic ankle rehabilitation utilizing a minitrampoline. The athlete tries to maintain balance while catching and tossing the ball.

bracing is not mandatory; athletes in "higher-risk" sports such as basketball, soccer, and football may elect to use high-top shoes, lace-up braces, or taping for injury prophylaxis.

ALTERNATIVE CONDITIONING DURING RECOVERY FROM INJURY

Maintaining fitness during periods of athletic injury is a major concern for athletes and sports medicine professionals alike. In this section, we provide examples of alternative conditioning exercises we have used successfully during rehabilitation of our injured athletes.

Inversion Ankle Sprain. The key is to prevent another inversion event while allowing weight bearing as tolerated. The stationary bicycle ergometer may be used early on without difficulty. Aqua jogging eliminates the weight-bearing concerns but can aggravate symptoms in grade 3 sprains as the water resistance forces the foot and ankle into inversion. In these instances, preexercise taping of the ankle into a neutral position facilitates comfortable water-based exercise. As weight-bearing tolerance improves, stair climbers can be added. Stationary ski machines are relatively safe to use, but the ankle dorsiflexion that occurs when the hip goes into extension may be painful if the ankle is still swollen. Tolerance for rowing machines is often dependent on the extent of ankle swelling and whether or not the foot straps cross over a tender portion of the ankle.

Patellofemoral Pain. This is a particularly frustrating problem for the endurance athlete, as the length of time required to resolve all the typical biomechanical deficits is quite variable. Running and bicycling (during which both excessive pronation and poor control of the hip and femur can occur), rowing machines and stair climbers (both of which can induce deep knee flexion) can all exacerbate symptoms until the athlete has adequate hip muscle control. Aqua jogging and free-style swimming usually do not evoke symptoms. Of the dry land activities, stationary ski machines generally work well.

If the athlete is coordinated enough, prolonged sessions on a slide board can be used; this activity has the additional bonus of strengthening the gluteal muscles, which are typically weak in patellofemoral tracking disorders.

Hamstring Tear. With grade 2 or higher higher tears, it is unlikely that the injured leg can be incorporated into the aerobic program during the acute rehabilitation phase. Options include trilimbed exercise on bicycle ergometers that offer both leg and arm work and swimming with a pull buoy held between the legs to lessen the need for leg work. As the athlete progresses, one of the first exercises to add is cycling, but without toe clips to lessen hamstring activation. Rowing ergometers can be utilized, but care must be taken to avoid excessive favoring of the injured side with development of mechanical flaws that could lead to further injury. Stair climbers and aqua jogging are helpful in the final preparatory phases for return to running. Stationary skiers can be used as well, but ski resistance must be increased cautiously lest reinjury occur.

Hip Adductor Injury. Fewer options exist than with the hamstring injury described above. Trilimb exercise can be used early on. However, swimming with a pull buoy between the legs will exacerbate symptoms in most cases. The bicycle and rower appear to be among the safest modes of exercise, as there is relatively little adductor activation; stair climbers may be used in the maintenance phase. Ski machines, aqua jogging, slide board, and treadmill walking all place too much demand on the adductor muscles to be used safely until the maintenance phase.

Rotator Cuff Injury in a Swimmer. For most swimmers, the initial response is to run, as this confers a good general cardiovascular training stimulus while resting the injured shoulder. The swimmer may elect to remain aquatic-based in his or her training and aqua jog. Land-based options that include upper body work include the rowing ergometer, arm ergometers (provided that the axis of the crank shaft is adjusted so that the humerus never enters the athlete's painful arc), and stationary skiers (as long as the arm work stays below 70° to 80° of elevation). Rowing machines and ski machines have the additional benefit of distributing the exercise over the entire body, as does swimming.

Acromioclavicular Joint Sprain in a Kayaker. As with the swimmer, most lower body exercises will be tolerated easily. Grade 1 sprains present no problem in this regard. However, with acute grade 2 sprains or greater, running becomes uncomfortable (and awkward if a sling is being used) and should not be encouraged unless the athlete is pain-free for the activity. Aqua jogging should be introduced cautiously—if the athlete is uncoordinated while in the water, excessive flailing of the arms may aggravate the injury. Rowing machines and stationary skiers appear to be relatively well tolerated after the immobilization period for the higher-grade sprains. Unlike rotator cuff injuries, arm ergometers place more stress on the injured A–C joint as the athlete pushes outward and consequently are not recommended.

SPORTS REHABILITATION PROGRAM DEVELOPMENT

Many professionals would like to incorporate sports medicine into their outpatient practices but have not had sufficient experience in this regard. This section provides some guidance for those planning to develop their own sports rehabilitation program (114).

Determining a community's need for and ability to support a sports rehabilitation program is an important first step. Questions include: (a) Who else is providing sports medicine services? (b) Are you proposing to duplicate services already in existence? (c) Who constitutes your major referral sources? (d) Who will be your philosophical and financial supporters at your institution? (e) Once the program is established, what will be its potential for growth?

In most communities, the physiatrist-directed sports rehabilitation program is a relatively new entity. Traditionally, the majority of sports medicine services, at a physician level, have been provided by orthopedic surgeons and family practitioners. Because the philosophy of physical medicine and rehabilitation differs from those of the other two specialties, the product offered will be different as well. This is particularly true if spine care and industrial injury rehabilitation are part of the package. Physical therapists and athletic trainers have also provided sports medicine services either independently or in concert with physician groups or institutions.

Establishing a reliable referral base is of paramount importance. The most important and dedicated source is comprised of former patients who are satisfied with the care they received. Every patient must be treated with courtesy, seen in a timely manner, and given the opportunity to ask questions about his or her condition. Patients need to know that telephone messages will be returned by some member of the office staff within 24 hours (preferably by the end of the same calendar day) and that there is provision for emergency after-hours care. Patients who are enthused about their prior treatment will go out of their way to return. Furthermore, remember that even the "difficult" patient has friends who are potential future patients for the practice. Other practice policies that attract patients include offering "urgent care" or "immediate care" clinics for acute or subacute musculoskeletal injuries, providing coverage for athletic events, and offering services during evening hours or weekends (114).

Cultivating referrals from athletic trainers, therapists, and physicians is the next step. Do not assume that other health professionals will automatically refer their patients to you just because you are all part of the same HMO or PPO. Call or write to thank them for the opportunity to participate in *their* patient's care, send copies of your assessment to them, and inform them about any new services you are capable of delivering. Inform athletic trainers of changes in an athlete's condition that may affect the athlete's training regimen or ability to compete the day the athlete is seen. Last, but not least, it is also critical to let these other professionals know when you are not capable of treating a particular patient's problem, or when you do not wish to manage certain types of problems (e.g., immediate postoperative orthopedic care, chronic pain). This promotes practice growth in the intended directions.

Perhaps one of the most overlooked referral sources of patients is one's own institution. Co-workers must know what you do so that they can promote your program as well. Be sure to advertise from within, making administrators and board members aware of the program and how the success of the program is something that they should be interested or invested in. Offer tours of your facility, lunchtime lectures or inservices, and attend board/institutional functions. Programmatic success is highly dependent upon the philosophical and financial support of the leaders of your institution. Future growth of the program and acquisition of more space (the "final frontier" in most buildings), is more readily accomplished if the leaders of the institution have the same felt need for expansion as you (114).

Promotion of a program requires marketing, which can be accomplished at many levels. Shirts, hats, magnets, and drinking bottles with your program's logo can be given to "graduates" of the program, or as gifts. Giving free educational lectures to community groups, health clubs, and businesses is often effective. Never forget to carry several business cards for distribution. Providing medical coverage for local sports events (while wearing clothing with your logo) reinforces your program's presence in the community. Publishing original research or writing articles for various journals is also an effective way of making your presence known.

Utilization of media to promote the practice has its advantages and disadvantages. Advertising on television or radio can be costly (and viewed as garish in certain communities). Advertising your services in certain magazines or newspapers and the telephone directory is almost universally acceptable. Occasionally one is fortunate enough to have local media select you for an interview regarding a topic that you may be familiar with. Although this has the potential to provide you instant credibility and brand you as an "expert," it can also lead to alteration of the issues you wanted to emphasize during the editorial process. Never give an interview or try to pass yourself off as an expert within an area you do not feel comfortable discussing.

A difficult task for the organizers of a sports rehabilitation program is to determine which services their program will provide in addition to traditional sports medicine. Many professionals fail to realize that the majority of programs selling only sports have a limited potential for economic growth unless the program is the only one selling sports medicine in the community (rare) or is so famous that patients are lining up at the door (rarer still). Furthermore, many of the activities that sports professionals are involved in to promote the practice are money losers. Little revenue, if any, is generated from athletic event coverage or community service. Thus, incorporation of other rehabilitation services and creation of specialty clinics becomes a key to survival. Seeing patients with industrial injuries, development of work hardening and spine rehabilitation, and offering electrodiagnostic (EMG) services can enhance revenue generation significantly. An industrial rehabilitation program requires the combined efforts of appropriately trained occupational and physical therapists and physicians. If staff members do not have the necessary skills, provision for continuing education should be made. When assembling a staff, recognize that therapists are more valuable to the growth of the practice if they have exceptional spine rehabilitation skills, which are more transferable across many types of patients than the "sports only" skills, which are more limited. On the other hand, therapists, trainers, and physicians with a great interest or substantial experience in a select area can become the basis for creation of a highly successful niche. Examples of specialty services that can be established with the right people include clinics for golfers (one must understand the biomechanics of golf), runners (you should have treadmills, video equipment, and the ability to arrange for fabrication and modification of foot orthoses), or clinics for fitness and performance testing (which requires expensive metabolic testing equipment). Physiatrists can become well known for their EMG skills and can market these as part of their ability to analyze mechanisms and consequences of sports-related and industrial injuries as well (114).

No matter what the marketing strategy employed, credibility is dependent on the ability to deliver what is promised. Offering acute care without access to radiology services, crutches, braces, or staff to provide immediate care is destined to fail, as it will leave patients and referring physicians frustrated and angry. Offering comprehensive spine care without a good working relationship between your center and the radiologists at the local MRI or CAT scan center is also unwise. Offering specialty clinics (for runners, golfers, dancers, etc.) without the ability to assess the kinetic chain and determine correctable biomechanical flaws leads to professional embarrassment and a poor reputation in the community.

Two extremely important issues are quality assurance and cost containment, factors that go a long way in determining the effectiveness of a program. It is not enough to deliver a good product, it must be rendered within a certain time frame for the providers, consumers, and third-party payers to be satisfied. This is particularly important in the era of managed care because for many provider plans, the more treatments a patient receives, the less the provider will be paid per unit time. Rehabilitation sessions that feature passive modes of treatment and excessive therapeutic modality use need to be replaced with sessions geared toward education so that patients can learn effective home exercise programs. All sports professionals should be able to tell third-party payers and patients approximately how many sessions of physical therapy or occupational therapy will be needed for rehabilitation of uncomplicated patellofemoral pain or rotator cuff tendinitis, for example.

The final pertinent element is the development of physiatric resident education. Isolated rotations in "sports" or participation in outpatient clinics where a smattering of musculoskeletal problems is seen but aggressive nonoperative care of acute and subacute injury is not emphasized do not adequately prepare residents for sports rehabilitation practice. PASSOR has developed educational objectives for physiatric residents that should serve as the starting point for musculoskeletal education. Journal clubs focusing on various aspects of operative and nonoperative care, sessions on anatomy, biomechanics, and exercise physiology, and radiology conferences need to be incorporated into the core curriculum. Participation in major interdisciplinary conferences and courses, such as those sponsored by the ACSM and the American Medical Society of Sports Medicine (AMSSM), are valuable ways to interact with professionals from other sports medicine groups and learn "cutting edge" information.

SUMMARY

Sports medicine has evolved considerably from the days of merely applying ice packs and ace wraps and allowing return to activity once the pain and swelling disappeared. The mission of sports *rehabilitation* is to rehabilitate the athlete beyond the resolution of symptoms. Sports rehabilitation emphasizes patient education, injury prevention, and, when injuries occur, restoration of optimal function before the return to sport. This cannot be accomplished without an understanding of anatomy, biomechanics, pathophysiology, and sports-specific knowledge. The physiatrist's training in basic and applied sciences, understanding of injury prevention and rehabilitation, ability to interact successfully with professionals from other disciplines, and advocacy for the physically challenged athlete makes the physiatrist ideally suited to pursue sports medicine practice.

REFERENCES

1. Grun B. *The timetables of history.* New York: Simon & Schuster, 1982.
2. Ward GC, Burns K. *Baseball.* New York: Alfred A. Knopf, 1994.
3. Voy RO. A history of boxing. In: *USA/ABF ringside physician's certificate manual.* Colorado Springs: USA Amateur Boxing Federation, 1990; 107–109.
4. Ryan AJ, Allman FL, eds. *Sports medicine.* New York: Academic Press, 1974.
5. Press JM, Young JL. The past, present, and future of sports medicine. *Chicago Med* 1994; 97(18):12–16.
6. Young JL, Press JM. The physiologic basis of sports rehabilitation. *Phys Med Rehabil Clin North Am* 1994; 5(1):9–36.
7. Astrand PO, Rodahl K. *Textbook of work physiology.* New York: McGraw-Hill, 1986.
8. Guyton AC. *Textbook of medical physiology, 8th ed.* Philadelphia: WB Saunders, 1991.
9. Komi PV, ed. *Strength and power in sport.* London: Blackwell Scientific Publications, 1992.
10. McArdle WD, Katch FI, Katch VL. *Exercise physiology: Energy, nutrition and human performance, 3rd ed.* Philadelphia: Lea & Febiger, 1991.
11. Lehmkuhl LD, Smith LK. *Brunnstrom's clinical kinesiology, 4th ed.* Philadelphia: FA Davis, 1985.
12. Friden J, Sjostrom M, Ekblom B. Myofibrillar damage following intense eccentric exercise in man. *Int J Sports Med* 1983; 4:170–176.
13. Knuttgen HG, Bonde Petersen F, Klausen K. Oxygen uptake and heart rate responses to exercise performed with concentric and eccentric contractions. *Med Sci Sports* 1971; 3:1–5.
14. Cavanagh PR, Komi PV. Electromechanical delay in human skeletal muscle under concentric and eccentric contractions. *Eur J Appl Physiol* 1979; 42:159–163.
15. DiNubile N. Strength training. *Clin Sports Med* 1991; 10(1):33–62.
16. Sharkey BJ. Training for sport. In: Cantu RC, Michelli LJ, eds. *ACSM's guidelines for the team physician.* Philadelphia: Lea & Febiger, 1991; 34–47.
17. Draganich LF, Jaeger RJ, Kralj AR. Coactivation of the hamstrings and quadriceps during extension of the knee. *J Bone Joint Surg* 1989; 71A(7):1075–1081.
18. Shelbourne KD, Wilckens JH, Mollabashy A, et al. Accelerated rehabilitation after acute anterior cruciate ligament reconstruction. *Am J Sports Med* 1990; 18:292–299.
19. Sobel J, Pettrone FA, Nirschl RP. Prevention and rehabilitation of racquet sports injuries. In: Nicholas JA, Hershman EB, eds. *The upper extremity in sports medicine.* St Louis, Mosby Yearbook, 1995; 805–823.
20. Young JL, Olsen NK, Press JM. Musculoskeletal disorders of the lower limbs. In: Braddom RL, ed. *Physical medicine and rehabilitation.* Philadelphia: WB Saunders, 1995; 783–812.
21. Allman FL. Exercise in sports medicine. In: Basmajian JV, ed. *Therapeutic exercise, 9th ed.* Baltimore: Williams & Wilkins, 1984.
22. Dudley GA, Djamil R. Incompatibility of endurance- and strength-training modes of exercise. *J Appl Physiol* 1985; 59(5):1446–1451.
23. Hickson RC. Interference of strength development by simultaneously training for strength and endurance. *Eur J Appl Physiol Occup Physiol* 1980; 45:255–263.
24. Sale DG, MacDougall JD, Jacobs I, et al. Interaction between concurrent strength and endurance training. *J Appl Physiol* 1990; 68(1): 260–270.
25. American College of Sports Medicine. *Guidelines for exercise testing and prescription, 4th ed.* Philadelphia: Lea & Febiger, 1991.
26. Borg GAV, Linderholm H. Perceived exertion and pulse rate during graded exercise in various age groups. *Acta Med Scand [Suppl]* 1967; 472:194–210.
27. Ceci R, Hassmen P. Self monitored exercise at three different RPE intensities in treadmill vs field running. *Med Sci Sports Exerc* 1991; 23(6):732–738.
27. Medbo JI, Burgers S. Effect of training on the anaerobic capacity. *Med Sci Sports Exerc* 1990; 22(4):501–507.
29. Daniels J. Training distance runners—a primer. *Sports Sci Exch* 1989; 1(11).
30. Pate RR, Branch JD. Training for endurance sport. *Med Sci Sports Exerc* 1992; 24(9):S340–S343.
31. Evans WJ. Exercise-induced skeletal muscle damage. *Physician Sports Med* 1987; 15(1):89–100.
32. Tiidus PM, Ianuzzo CD. Effects of intensity and duration of muscular exercise on delayed soreness and serum enzyme activities. *Med Sci Sports Exerc* 1983; 15(6):461–465.
33. Costill DL, Pascoe DD, Fink WJ, et al. Impaired muscle glycogen resynthesis after eccentric exercise. *J Appl Physiol* 1990; 69(1):46–50.
34. Russell B, Dix DJ, Haller DL, et al. Repair of injured skeletal muscle: a molecular approach. *Med Sci Sports Exerc* 1992; 24(2):189–196.
35. Waterman-Storer CM. The cytoskeleton of skeletal muscle: is it affected by exercise? A brief review. *Med Sci Sports Exerc* 1991; 23(11): 1240–1249.
36. O'Reilly KP, Warhol MJ, Fielding RA, et al. Eccentric exercise-induced muscle damage impairs glycogen repletion. *J Appl Physiol* 1987; 63(2):252–256.
37. Barron GL, Noakes TD, Levy W, et al. Hypothalamic dysfunction in overtrained athletes. *J Clin Endocrinol Metab* 1985; 60(4):803–806.
38. Sherman WS, Maglischo EW. Minimizing chronic athletic fatigue among swimmers: special emphasis on nutrition. *Sports Sci Exch* 1991:4(35).
39. Keast D, Cameron K, Morton AR. Exercise and the immune response. *Sports Med* 1988; 5:248–267.
40. O'Connor PJ, Morgan WP, Raglin JS, et al. Selected pseudoendocrine responses to overtraining. *Med Sci Sports Exerc* 1989; 21(2):S50.
41. Kibler WB. *The sport preparticipation fitness examination.* Champaign, IL: Human Kinetics Books, 1990.
42. Montgomery DL. Physiology of ice hockey. *Sports Med* 1988; 5: 99–126.
43. Kibler WB. Clinical aspects of muscle injury. *Med Sci Sports Exerc* 1990; 22(4):450–452.
44. Kibler WB. Evaluation of sports demands as a diagnostic tool in shoulder disorders. In: Matsen FR, Fu FH, Hawkins RT, eds. *The shoulder: A balance of mobility and stability.* Rosemont, IL: American Academy of Orthopedic Surgeons, 1993; 379–395.
45. Kibler WB, Chandler TJ. Racquet sports. In: Fu FH, Stone D, eds. *Sports injuries—mechanisms, prevention and treatment.* Baltimore: Williams & Wilkins, 1994.
46. Kibler WB, Chandler TJ, Pace BK. Principles of rehabilitation after chronic tendon injuries. *Clin Sports Med* 1992; 11:661–673.
47. Press JM, Herring SA, Kibler WB. *Rehabilitation of muculoskeletal disorders.* Washington, D.C.: United States Army Publication (in press).
48. Reddy AS, Reedy MK, Seaber AV, et al. Restriction of the injury response following an acute muscle strain. *Med Sci Sports Exerc* 1993; 25(3):321–327.
49. Leadbetter WB. Cell-matrix response in tendon injury. *Clin Sports Med* 1992; 11(3):533–578.
50. Herring SA. Rehabilitation from muscle injury. *Med Sci Sports Exerc* 1990; 22(4):453–456.
51. Roy S, Irvin R. *Sports medicine: Prevention, evaluation, management*

and rehabilitation. Englewood Cliffs, NJ: Prentice-Hall, 1983; 299–305.

52. Young JL, Laskowski ER, Rock M. Thigh injuries in athletes. *Mayo Clin Proc* 1993; 68(11):1099–1106.
53. Brukner P, Khan K. *Clinical sports medicine.* Sydney: McGraw-Hill, 1993.
54. Cox JS. Patellofemoral problems in runners. *Clin Sports Med* 1985; 4(4):699–715.
55. Apple DF Jr. Adolescent runners. *Clin Sports Med* 1985; 4:641–655.
56. Apple DF Jr. End stage running problems. *Clin Sports Med* 1985; 5: 657–670.
57. Young JL, Press JM. Rehabilitation of running injuries. In: Buschbacher R, Braddom RL, eds. *Sports medicine and rehabilitation: A sports specific approach.* Philadelphia: Hanley & Belfus, 1994; 123–134.
58. Cordasco FA, Parkes JC. Overuse injuries of the elbow. In: Nicholas JA, Hershman EB, eds. *The upper extremity in sports medicine.* St Louis: Mosby-Year Book, 1995; 317–330.
59. Gross ML, Dalvin LB, Evanski PM. Effectiveness of orthotic shoe inserts in the long distance runner. *Am J Sports Med* 1991; 19(4): 409–412.
60. Newell SG. Functional neutral orthoses and shoe modifications. *Phys Med Rehab Clin North Am* 1992; 3(1):193–222.
61. Subotnick SI. The biomechanics of running. *Sports Med* 1985; 2: 144–153.
62. Brody DM. Running injuries. *Clin Symp* 1987; 39(3):2–36.
63. Raven PB. Environmental physiology and medicine. In: Cantu RC, Micheli LJ, eds. *ACSM's guidelines for the team physician.* Philadelphia: Lea & Febiger, 1991; 101–117.
64. Cole AJ, Farrell JP, Stratton SA. Cervical spine injuries: a pain in the neck. *Phys Med Rehabil Clin North Am* 1994; 5(1):37–68.
65. Shuster R. Children's foot survey. *J Podiatr Soc NY* 1956; 17:13.
66. Bourne MH, Hazel WA, Scott SG, et al. Anterior knee pain. *Mayo Clin Proc* 1988; 63:482–491.
67. Kuland DN. *The injured athlete, 2nd ed.* Philadelphia: Lippincott, 1988; 428–453.
68. Bradley J, Dandy DJ. Osteochondritis dissecans and other lesions of the femoral condyles. *J Bone Joint Surg [Am]* 1983; 65:193–199.
69. James SL, Bates BT, Osterning LR. Injuries to runners. *Am J Sports Med* 1978; 6:40–50.
70. Lutter LD. The knee and running. *Clin Sports Med* 1985; 4(4): 685–698.
71. Noble CA. Iliotibial band friction syndrome in runners. *Am J Sports Med* 1980; 8:232–234.
72. O'Toole ML. Prevention and treatment of injuries to runners. *Med Sci Sports Exerc* 1992; 24(9):S360–S363.
73. Van Mechelen W, Hlobil H, Zijlstra WP, de Ridder M, Kemper HCG. Is range of motion at the hip and ankle joint related to running injuries? *Int J Sports Med* 1992; 13(8):605–610.
74. Hoppenfeld S. *Physical examination of the spine and extremities.* Norwalk, CT: Appelton-Century-Crofts, 1976.
75. Young JL, Herring SA, Press JM, Casazza BA. The influence of the spine on the shoulder in the throwing athlete. *J Back Musculoskel Rehabil* 1996; 7(1):5–17.
76. Kibler WB. The role of the scapula in the overhead throwing motion. *Contemp Orthop* 1991; 22:525–532.
77. Nicholas JA, Hershman EB, eds. *The upper extremity in sports medicine.* St Louis: Mosby-Yearbook, 1995.
78. Press JM, Young JL. Vague upper extremity symptoms? Consider thoracic outlet syndrome. *Physician Sports Med* 1994; 22(7):57–64.
79. Yates AJ Jr, Wilgis EFS. Wrist pain. In: Nicholas JA, Hershman EB, eds. *The upper extremity in sports medicine.* St Louis: Mosby-Yearbook, 1995; 471–482.
80. Cailliet R. *Low back pain syndrome.* Philadelphia: FA Davis, 1989.
81. Saal JA. Rehabilitation of sports related lumbar spine injuries. *Phys Med Rehabil State Art Rev* 1987; 1:613–638.
82. Bach DK, Green DS, Jensen GM, et al. A comparison of muscular tightness in runners and nonrunners and the relation of muscular tightness to low back pain in runners. *J Orthop Sports Phys Ther* 1985; 6:315–323.
83. Fleisig GS, Andrews JR, Dillman CJ, Escamilla RF. Kinetics of baseball pitching with implications about injury mechanisms. *Am J Sports Med* 1995; 23(2):233–239.
84. Pappas AM, Zawacki RM, Sullivan TJ. Biomechanics of baseball pitching. A preliminary report. *Am J Sports Med* 1985; 13:216–222.
85. Ticker JB, Fealy S, Fu FH. Instability and impingement in the athlete's shoulder. *Sports Med* 1995; 19(6):418–426.
86. Harryman DT, Sidles JA, Clark JM, et al. Translation of the humeral head on the glenoid with passive glenohumeral motions. *J Bone Joint Surg* 1990; 72A:1334–1343.
87. Howell SM, Galinat BJ, Renzi AJ, et al. Normal and abnormal mechanics of the glenohumeral joint in the horizontal plane. *J Bone Joint Surg* 1988; 70A:227–232.
88. Warner JJP, Caborn DNM, Berger R, et al. Dynamic capsuloligamentous anatomy of the glenohumeral joint. *J Shoulder Elbow Surg* 1993; 2:115–133.
89. Jobe FW, Bradley JP. The diagnosis and nonoperative treatment of shoulder injuries in athletes. *Clin Sports Med* 1989; 8(3):419–438.
90. Pappas AM, Zawacki RM, McCarthy CF. Rehabilitation of the pitching shoulder. *Am J Sports Med* 1985; 13(4):223–235.
91. Watkins RG, Dennis S, Dillin WH, Schnebel B, et al. Dynamic EMG analysis of torque transfer in professional baseball pitchers. *Spine* 1989; 14(4):404–408.
92. Laskowski ER. Snow skiing injuries in physically disabled skiiers. *Am J Sports Med* 1992; 20(5):553.
93. Laskowski ER. Rehabilitation of the physically challenged athlete. *Phys Med Rehabil Clin North Am* 1994; 5(1):215–233.
94. Putnam CA, Kozey JW. Substantive issue in running. In: Vaughn CL, ed. *Biomechanics of sport.* Boca Raton, FL: CRC Press, 1989; 2–33.
95. Insall J. Chondromalacia patellae: patellar malalignment syndrome. *Orthop Clin North Am* 1979; 10:117–127.
96. Ficat RP, Hungerford D. *Disorders of the patellofemoral joint.* Baltimore: Williams & Wilkins, 1977.
97. Hungerford DS, Barry M. Biomechanics of the patellofemoral joint. *Clin Orthop Rel Res* 1979; 144:9–15.
98. Fredericson M. Patellofemoral pain in runners. *J Back Musculoskel Rehabil* 1995; 5:305–316.
99. Bose K, Kanagasuntherum R, Osman M. Vastus medialis oblique: an anatomical and physiologic study. *Orthopedics* 1980; 3:880–883.
100. Wilder RP, Brennan DK. Fundamental and techniques of aqua running for athletic rehabilitation. *J Back Musculoskel Rehabil* 1994; 4(4): 287–296.
101. Grabiner MD, Koh TJ, Draganich LF. Neuromechanics of the patellofemoral joint. *Med Sci Sports Exerc* 1994; 26(1):10–21.
102. Steinkamp LA, Dillingham MF, Markel MD, et al. Biomechanical considerations in patellofemoral joint rehabilitation. *Am J Sports Med* 1993; 21(3):438–444.
103. McConnell J. The management of chondromalacia patellae: a long term solution. *Aust J Phys* 1986; 32(4):215–219.
104. Kowell MG, Kolk G, Nuber GW, et al. Patellar taping in the treatment of patellofemoral pain. *Am J Sports Med* 1996; 24(1):61–66.
105. Buschbacher R. The use and abuse of ankle supports in sports injuries. *J Back Musculoskel Rehabil* 1993; 3(3):57–68.
106. Stormont DM, Morrey B, An K, et al. Stability of the loaded ankle. *Am J Sports Med* 1985; 13:295–303.
107. Renstrom PAFH, Kannus P. Injuries of the foot and ankle. In: DeLee JC, Drez D Jr, eds. *Orthopedic sports medicine.* Philadelphia: WB Saunders, 1994; 1705–1767.
108. Balduni FC, Vegso JJ, Torg JS, et al. Management and rehabilitation of ligamentous injuries to the ankle. *Sports Med* 1987; 4:364–380.
109. Chapman MW. Part II. Sprains of the ankle. In: *Instructional Course Lectures, The American Academy of Orthopedic Surgeons, vol 24.* St Louis: CV Mosby, 1975; 294–308.
110. Kannus P, Renstrom P. Treatment for acute tears of the lateral ligaments of the ankle. *J Bone Joint Surg [Am]* 1991; 73(2):305–312.
111. Hopkinson WJ, St Pierre P, Ryan JB, et al. Syndesmosis sprains of the ankle. *Foot Ankle* 1990; 10:325–330.
112. Hollinshead WH, Jenkins DB. *Functional anatomy of the limbs and back, 5th ed.* Philadelphia: WB Saunders, 1981.
113. Jackson DW, Ashley RL, Powell JW. Ankle sprains in young athletes. Relation of severity and disability. *Clin Orthop* 1974; 101:201–215.
114. Young JL, Press JM. Creating a sports medicine product line. *Rehab Manage* 1995; 8(6):43–48.

Rehabilitation Medicine: Principles and Practice, Third Edition,
edited by Joel A. DeLisa and Bruce M. Gans.
Lippincott–Raven Publishers, Philadelphia © 1998.

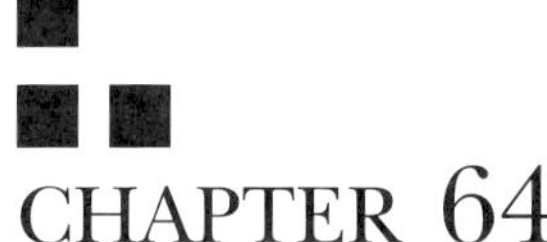

CHAPTER 64

Performing Artists' Occupational Disorders and Related Therapies

Fadi J. Bejjani, Glenn M. Kaye, and Joseph W. Cheu

MUSICIANS' OCCUPATIONAL DISORDERS

Anyone doubting the prevalence of injury in musicians need only hear the list of performance-related syndromes, which include cymbal player's shoulder; pianist's, violinist's, and harpist's cramp; English horn player's thumb; and even cellist's dermatitis (1).

As if to summarize the entire problem in one sentence, Ziporyn states in another passage: "Like athletes, musicians perform for the public; and like professional athletes, they can lose their jobs if they don't perform. But only athletes work with physicians and trainers almost daily" (1).

In general, musculoskeletal occupational disorders of musicians are similar to those encountered in other occupational groups and could be attributed to static loading, highly repetitive light loading on the joints and muscles, or cumulative trauma (2–4). Diagnosis, management, and treatment of these disorders, however, are much more complex in musicians and require special attention (5), precisely because of their specific ergonomic conditions and risk factors (6).

Characteristic Ergonomic Factors

The most characteristic factor for musicians may be their very early start on the instrument. In their studies, Bejjani and colleagues found that 39.4% started at age 6 years or before, 46.5% between ages 7 and 13 years, and only 12.7% at age 13 years or after (2,3) Thus, the overwhelming majority of professional musicians start playing their initial or final instrument long before final growth has occurred in their musculoskeletal system. Hence, one cannot help wondering about the effect of the instrument on their growth (7).

Musicians have to deal with a highly competitive environment and a limited number of secure jobs. They also have to face the puritanical assumption that because music making is a pleasurable activity, it also is unnecessary. "The general public perception is that musicians are doing what they want to be doing and therefore should put up with their problems" (1). This fact certainly helps explain musicians' lack of enthusiasm in seeking medical help as well as the paucity of federal grants allocated for research in this field.

Musicians also have an irregular schedule of auditions, competitions, and performances, which subjects them to unusual stress conditions such as abrupt increases in practice time or in intensity of practice and changes in technique or in instrument. Occasionally, for example, a professional musician may have to switch from violin to viola to fit the needs of a particular job or change repertoire for a recital or concert (e.g., a pianist abruptly undertaking a piece involving a lot of arpeggios and trills). It is also common knowledge that it is easier to play a Chopin etude than Rachmaninoff or that musicians who try to play Paganini get hurt because he wrote pieces only he could play. Performance stress can be aggravated by switching to a new teacher who advises major changes in technique or by working with a new conductor who imposes additional demands and new requirements.

These sources of physical stress obviously are compounded by added psychological stress. As early as 1932, Singer found nervousness to be the most frequent disorder of professional musicians (5). Its symptoms (e.g., increased irritability, quick fatigue, headache, trembling, insomnia) are thought to result from a disturbance of energy capacity in

F. J. Bejjani: Atlantic Occupational Orthopaedic Centers, Belleville, New Jersey 07109.

G. M. Kaye: Department of Otolaryngology—Head and Neck Surgery, McGill University, Montreal, Quebec, H3G 1Y6 Canada.

J. W. Cheu: Department of Physical Medicine and Rehabilitation, University of Medicine and Dentistry of New Jersey, New Jersey Medical School, Newark, New Jersey 07103.

the performer's constitution, in which the balance between absorption and release of energy is disrupted. Performance anxiety is well known among musicians (8). It can produce, among other effects, a decrease in hand temperature to a point that musculoskeletal performance is impaired (9,10). The famous pianist Glenn Gould was known to play with fingerless gloves because of cold hands.

Perhaps the most peculiar characteristic of musicians is their tendency to play through pain, sometimes under the romantic delusion that they are paying their dues, or because this would make their art better, as advocated by certain schools and teachers. Some string players have been known to practice passages over and over until their fingers bleed (1). This practice often results in a delay in seeking help or noncompliance with the rehabilitative or preventive treatment prescribed.

Musculoskeletal Adaptation to the Instrument

According to Benati (11) and Smith (12), Paganini showed anatomic abnormalities that made him particularly fit for the violin (e.g., very thin fingers, hyperlaxity of the left distal interphalangeal joints allowing lateral motion, left shoulder 1 inch higher than the right, hyperlaxity of the shoulders enhancing lateral motion). David pointed out that criteria for an ideal pianist's hand have changed a great deal since Chopin's time and that a virtuoso does not owe his or her talent only to the anatomy of his or her hand (13).

Does the hand make the pianist or does the piano make the pianist's hand? Priest and Nagel attempted to answer a similar question for athletes when they described a depression or droop of the dominant shoulder in tennis players—especially those who started as early as 8 years of age—associated with apparent scoliosis, which they called "tennis shoulder" and attributed to the increased mass of the hypertrophied racquet-holding extremity pulling on the shoulder (14). They also noted that this could be the reason why more than 50% of tennis players had shoulder problems at some point in their career—a finding recognized as a predisposing factor for thoracic outlet syndrome (14).

The asymmetric loads involved in music playing are somewhat comparable to those in tennis playing, as are anatomic changes. Bejjani and colleagues showed that symptoms first appeared before 10 years of playing in 18% of the musicians examined, between 10 and 20 years in 36%, between 20 and 30 years in 20.5%, and after 30 years in 25% (2,3). The earlier a musician started, the later symptoms seemed to appear. This suggests that musculoskeletal changes, when they occur in musicians, could be adaptive. Bejjani et al. compared musicians to controls and found musculoskeletal changes related to playing (7). They found decreased internal rotation of the left shoulder in 9% of violinists and 15% of bassists. In violinists the left shoulder was higher than the right, and the right upper extremity longer than the left. Cellists had a more elongated left hand, and violists a longer left middle finger. Harpists in general displayed a narrower first web in both hands. Mild functional spinal deformities were found in 56%, including increased or decreased thoracic kyphosis and scapular prominence (45%) or scoliotic curvatures (11%). The latter were lumbar, thoracic, or thoracolumbar, with left convexities for violinists, cellists, and guitarists and right or left convexities for harpists and pianists. Harpists had the highest incidence of scoliotic curvatures (29%).

Psychological Profile

Studies using the Profile of Mood States (POMS) questionnaire demonstrated that musicians as a group show the "iceberg profile" of below-average tension, depression, anger, fatigue, and confusion scores (i.e., below the 50th percentile) and above-average vigor scores (i.e., 66th percentile) (17). This iceberg profile had been described in earlier studies among Olympic-class athletes such as oarsmen, runners, and wrestlers. Musicians also were asked to answer a Millon Behavioral Health Inventory questionnaire. The scores of the latter self-reported stress scales were compared between musicians with the iceberg profile and those without. Musicians with the profile reported significantly less inhibition, stress, and anxiety than musicians without the profile. The iceberg profile is suggested as a useful screening tool to identify those musicians who respond to psychophysiological stressors with minimum levels of behavioral upset and minimum risk of injury thereafter. "There is no question that the more emotionally tense the player, the more likely a physical injury. Any sort of psychological conflict can make a performer more injury-prone" (1). Comparison of musicians' POMS scores with a data base of college students and psychiatric outpatients showed a much higher score for the positive trait of vigor in musicians and much lower scores in all the negative traits of tension, fatigue, anger, depression, and confusion.

Musicians are similar to the general population in their coping styles except in introversion, sociability, and confidence, where they score higher (Table 64-1). In the category of psychological stress factors, musicians show more self-imposed pressure than the general population and less exogenous pressure, premorbid pessimism, hopelessness, social alienation, and hypochondriasis. The level of psychological

TABLE 64-1. *Coping styles in 67 musicians, measured with the Millon Behavioral Health Inventory*

Coping styles	Mean score (total, %)	Coefficient of variation (%)
Introverted	56.2	24.0
Inhibited	46.9	24.7
Cooperative	51.3	20.3
Sociable	69.6	26.6
Confident	67.6	22.0
Forceful	45.9	20.2
Respectful	52.0	22.0
Sensitive	48.3	24.7

TABLE 64-2. *Psychological stressors in 67 musicians, measured with the Millon Behavioral Health Inventory*

Psychological stressors	Mean score (total, %)	Coefficient of variation (%)
Considerable self-imposed pressure	58.2	20.7
Considerable exogenous pressure	38.6	23.2
Premorbid pessimism	28.6	24.5
Hopelessness	34.1	25.8
Social alienation	32.8	25.2
Hypochondriasis	36.1	25.5
Psychological participation in pain	45.2	25.0

participation in pain also is slightly lower (Table 64-2). In self-assessed occupation-related psychophysiological stressors (Table 64-3) tested with the Stellman Job Satisfaction questionnaire (18), musicians score as high as high-risk occupational groups.

A task designed by Raynor and Smith involving setting and readjusting goals revealed differences in goal-setting tendencies among players of different instruments (19). Harpists tended to set goals that they could meet easily, whereas guitarists and pianists set goals that they generally could not meet. String players fell in between. Such differences in goal setting among musicians could help explain the high levels of self-imposed pressure encountered in some, and the willingness to play through pain encountered in others, both ultimately leading to overuse-related disorders.

The POMS questionnaire also was used to establish a relationship between increased tension and decreased finger temperature in musicians during performance (9). Since 1939, it has been shown that emotional conversations produce hand temperature decreases in people with Raynaud's disease or ''cold hands'' (20). Crawford and associates also showed that cognitively induced anxiety decreases hand temperature significantly (10). Cold also is known to impair manual performance through various processes such as loss of cutaneous sensitivity, changes in the characteristics of synovial fluid in the joints, and loss of muscle strength (21–23). Moreover, finger dexterity tasks show a greater impairment than manual dexterity tasks because there is an increased dependence on sensory feedback from joint articulation as the manipulated object becomes smaller (22). More specifically, McCloskey and Grandevia showed that control of thumb and index finger flexion was altered by cold (24). Parry found that the effect of cold was more marked on finger extension than finger flexion (25).

TABLE 64-3. *Incidence of self-assessed psychophysiological stressors in 67 musicians, measured by the Stellman and Associates Work Characteristics Questionnaire*

Psychophysiological stressors (self-assessed)	Mean score (total, %)
Hardship	92.6
Repetitivity	81.9
High speed	80.8
Exertion	77.9
Awkward motions	53.0

In addition to its relationship to mood states, finger temperature in musicians also is related to muscle tension. In the same study, the authors showed that the warm-up or practicing period had the apparently paradoxic effect of decreasing average finger temperature in musicians (9). Previous studies had found that an increase in forearm muscle electromyographic (EMG) activity produced a decrease in index finger temperature (26). This relationship among mood state, muscle tension, and hand temperature could be used to improve performance conditions and prevent injuries in musicians (e.g., through biofeedback regulation).

Nature and Prevalence of Injuries

One of the first attempts to compile and classify diseases of music professionals was made by Singer (5). Anecdotally, venereal diseases ranked first in those days. Both Singer (5) and Wittaker (27) stressed the importance of psychological factors in musicians' occupational disorders. They classified these disorders as occupational neuroses, based on the rationale that ''correctly guided movements during practice could act as reflex-irritation upon the brain and could arrest the coordination of the nerves and muscles through a real cramp'' (5).

By analyzing the role of occupational and industrial medicine in musicians' care, Schwander and colleagues performed one of the first systematic and epidemiologic studies focusing on the organic character of musicians' occupational disorders (28). Later, sporadic cases pertaining to various instrument groups were reported in the literature: phalangeal tuft fractures (8,29) or traumatic synovitis (30) in guitar players; first common digital nerve neuropathy in a flutist (31); and numbness of the thumb in horn players (32). In a report of six cases (two pianists, two guitarists, one clarinetist, and one violinist), Crabb attempted to understand the etiology of the symptoms in relation to the demands of the instrument (33).

A survey of musculoskeletal and neurologic occupation-related disorders among musicians, including primarily pianists (75 of 100 musicians), found the most common to be inflammatory disorders of tendons or joints (45%) or disorders of motor control (24%) (34). In a slightly smaller (71 musicians) but more evenly distributed series (i.e., violin, viola, cello, bass, piano, harp, and guitar), the authors found a 77.5% prevalence of upper extremity disorders serious enough to impair performance significantly or to cause the musician to stop playing at least temporarily (2,3). Sixty-two percent complained of back disorders, and 24% of neck disorders. All bassists examined had a history of upper extremity disorders; the lowest prevalence was among violinists (Fig. 64-1*A*). Inflammatory disorders such as tendinitis and bursitis ranked first among these disorders (36.6% of all musicians; Fig. 64-1*B*). Handedness of the musicians had no effect, and neither did their regular involvement in other hand activities (e.g., typing, tennis).

Cellists (75%) and harpists (73%) showed the highest prevalence of back disorders such as low back pain or functional deformities (Fig. 64-2). Pianists (38%) and harpists (36%) had the highest prevalence of neck disorders (Fig. 64-3). Musicians with neck disorders had a higher prevalence

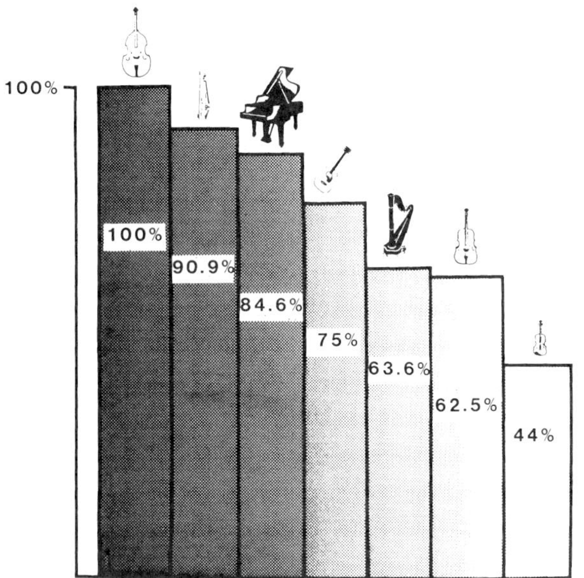

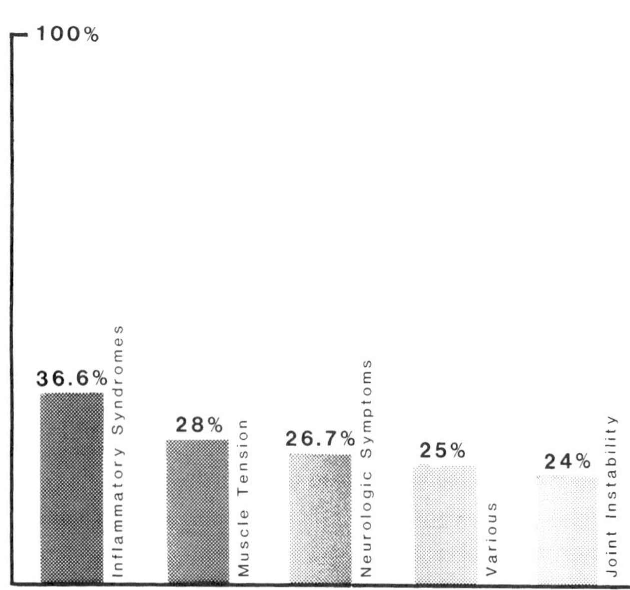

FIG. 64-1. A: Prevalence of upper extremity disorders in (from left to right) bassists, violists, pianists, guitarists, harpists, cellists, and violinists. **B:** Nature and prevalence of upper extremity disorders in musicians examined by the author.

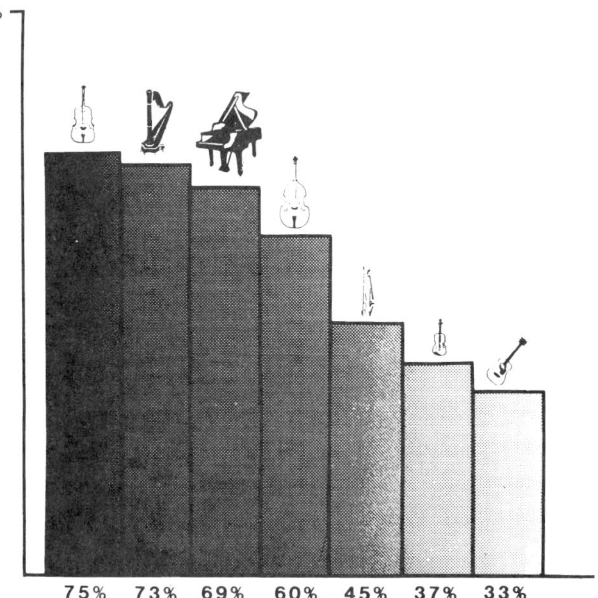

FIG. 64-2. Prevalence of back disorders in (from left to right) cellists, harpists, pianists, bassists, violists, violinists, and guitarists.

of upper extremity disorders, and vice versa. This fact demonstrates the role of compensatory mechanisms in transferring the loads from one body segment to an adjacent one in case of discomfort. If allowed to settle in, these compensatory mechanisms can follow a pace of their own and make treatment and rehabilitation much more difficult.

Ziporyn reported that the 128 string players responding to the Cleveland Clinic's survey complained primarily of stiffness, tension, pain, soreness, spasms, or numbness in shoulders, fingers, hands, neck, jaw, back, and wrist (1). In his series of 485 musicians, Fry noted the most common site of overuse syndrome to be the hand and wrist (41%), then the neck (38%), then the shoulder (35%) (35). Overuse syndrome was defined as an injury caused by the stressing, through overloading or through repetition of some movement or movements too frequently or too fast, of a particular structure or tissue beyond its anatomic and physiological limits. These limits vary from one musician to another, and several predisposing factors such as genetic or structural limitations, inadequate strength and flexibility, and inadequate conditioning may come into play. Conditioning, in particular, has not been a part of the usual training of a musician, although it has been much more a part of the dancer's curriculum, for example. In another study, Fry reported that the highest incidence of overuse syndrome of the upper limb among 379 musicians was in string players (48%) (36).

Overuse Syndrome, Myofascial Pain, and Inflammatory Disorders

The most prevalent medical problems among musicians are related to overuse or misuse stemming from the repetitive movements of playing, together with the prolonged muscular

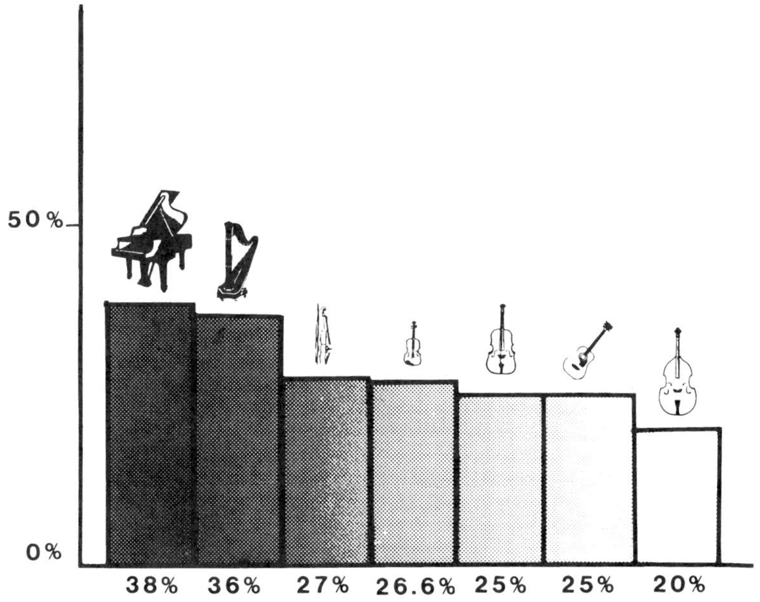

FIG. 64-3. Prevalence of neck disorders in (from left to right) pianists, harpists, violists, violinists, cellists, guitarists, and bassists.

effort required to bear the weight of the instrument, often in awkward positions (37). Overuse syndrome is described by Fry as a painful condition brought about by long, hard use of a limb that is excessive for the individual affected, taking the tissues beyond their biological tolerance and causing some subsequent change (38,39), or caused by tissues being stressed beyond their anatomical and physiological limits (40,41). Notwithstanding Fry's terminology and specificity, the term overuse syndrome is often used generically to mean disuse or misuse or to refer to all manner of tendinitis, tenosynovitis, dystonia, and related conditions (42). It can also mean different etiologies to different specialists, i.e., electrolyte imbalance to dietitians versus chronic compartment syndrome to sports medicine providers (43).

In Fry's overuse syndrome, the muscles are primarily affected, but some ligaments that take high loading may become involved (44). The predominant symptom is pain, which may be diffuse, and tenderness in a particular muscle group (42). There may be swelling, which will be localized to the muscle rather than tendon. There is electromyographic evidence that site-specific muscle hyperreactivity may play a role in the development and maintenance of the condition, but the cause-and-effect relationships are not known (45). It is prevalent in as many as 50% of professional symphony orchestra musicians (46), up to 21% of music students (47), and accounts for 50% to 80% of consultations (48–50).

Lambert described the regional pain syndrome, which is similar to what is commonly referred to as overuse syndrome but is not proven to be caused by overuse or misuse (51). As in overuse syndrome, it is usually triggered by changes in repertoire, technique, instrument, or an increase in daily playing time. The condition usually presents with localized pain and tenderness and sometimes fullness of the musculotendinous unit. Easy fatigability may be present. The importance of examining the patient while playing is stressed. Treatment includes complete rest until pain and tenderness are gone, followed by gentle physical therapy to restore tone and then gradually followed by short playing sessions. Technical faults should be identified and corrected, and static loads reduced.

Entrapment Neuropathies

Musicians not only are at high risk for these conditions but also are particularly sensitive to mild deficits. Predisposing factors include compression by hypertrophied muscles in the forearm compartments, anoxia secondary to venous congestion caused by pressure, traction on neural tissue from an awkward playing posture, or friction trauma from repetitive motion. In a group of musicians with hand problems studied by Hochberg et al., 15% showed evidence of nerve entrapment (48). In a series by Lederman of 226 instrumentalists with playing-related symptoms, 13% were diagnosed with entrapment neuropathies (52). Diagnosis may be difficult because the symptoms may be mild and only occur with playing. The EMG is probably the most sensitive way of confirming mild denervation, as there have been cases in whom nerve conduction studies (NCS) were repeatedly normal, yet surgery confirmed nerve compression and relieved symptoms (53,54).

The most common entrapment neuropathy in musicians is carpal tunnel syndrome (48). Other sites where the median nerve or its branches can become entrapped include the pronator teres or the fibrous arch forming the proximal edge of flexor digitorum superficialis (pronator syndrome), especially in musicians because of the frequent pronation required (53). Anterior interosseous compression can occur by overdeveloped forearm musculature. Median digital nerve compression may occur on the radial side of the left index finger of flute players (55), and other digital nerves may be compressed by gripping the bow too tightly (53).

The second most common entrapment syndrome in musicians is ulnar neuropathy (53). The nerve can be damaged by repeated flexion and extension of the elbow as it passes through the two heads of flexor carpii ulnaris in the cubital tunnel. This is most often encountered in the bowing arm of string players (54). Distal ulnar nerve damage may occur as it passes through Guyon's canal, often seen in flute players who maintain their left wrist in dorsiflexion and radial deviation (56). The radial nerve itself is rarely damaged, but involvement of the posterior cutaneous branch as a result of elbow extension in drummers is documented (57). The posterior interosseous branch may become entrapped beneath the arcade of Frohse, causing symptoms in the left extensor forearm of violinists (58). Repeated forced supination may also compress the (sensory) recurrent epicondylar branch of the radial nerve as well as the deep branch, resulting in a syndrome appearing as lateral epicondylitis with wrist drop (59).

Focal Motor Dystonias

Also known as painless focal dystonias, these consist of abnormal muscle spasms or posturing of isolated muscle groups. The signs of involuntary muscular contraction become apparent only during playing. They account for only a few percent of the upper limb problems of musicians but can be the most devastating. Hochberg et al. report a prevalence of 1.4% in a group of 1,000 patients seen in the Music Clinic at the Massachusetts General Hospital (60), but estimates vary (61). The pathogenesis is unknown. Some authors believed it to be of central origin (62), but others have associated it with different types of prior injury (61,63–66). The condition, once established, evolves very slowly over many years (67). Patients sometimes find that by producing a sensory input, such as stroking the skin, they are able to achieve temporary relief (51). Early electrophysiological research revealed concurrent contraction of agonist and antagonist muscle groups and abnormalities in the normal reflex inhibition of antagonist muscles (68,69). Newmark and Hochberg studied 57 musicians with focal dystonias (64).

There is currently no definitively successful treatment for focal dystonia. Prolonged rest, psychotherapy, steroids, injections, tricyclics, bromocriptine, other drugs, and surgery have all had no significant effect (39,41,64). Biofeedback has had only anecdotal success (70). So far, the most promising improvement has been found with botulinum toxin injections (71).

Joint Hypermobility

Excessive joint laxity results in lateral instability of a loaded joint and can contribute to the development of traumatic synovitis in instrumentalists. In musicians this most often occurs at the metacarpophalangeal (MCP), interphalangeal (IP), and wrist joints. Capsular laxity can lead to recurrent joint subluxation, which is disruptive to performance. This is common at the temporomandibular joint (TMJ) of hypermobile violinists and violists (72). Hyperextensibility of the wrist and elbow may contribute to neuropathy at these sites by exacerbating traction damage. Other studies demonstrated that the incidence of joint laxity was similar between musicians and nonmusicians, as measured by several tests on the whole body (15,16). More specifically, those musicians (21%) with abnormal laxity of one or more joints of the hand all presented with technical problems of some sort, thus casting some real doubt on the possible advantage Paganini may have had.

The prognosis for a good playing career despite this condition is good. Increasing muscle tone with a carefully designed exercise program will improve articular stability. Customized dynamic splinting to prevent gross instability or dislocation may be indicated in some cases but should not be viewed as a substitute for improving muscular tone. In severe cases of painful instability, surgical reconstruction of the ulnar collateral ligament of the first metacarpophalangeal (MCP) joint using a palmaris longus graft or plastic reconstruction of the carpometacarpal (CMC) basal ligament may be indicated (73).

Diagnostic Methodology

It is obvious that conventional clinical diagnostic tests have their place in musicians' health care because many of their symptoms belong to well-recognized pathologic entities such as carpal tunnel syndrome or epicondylitis, to mention just two. Diagnosis of the less-well-defined entities such as overuse syndrome or muscle tension, or rarer syndromes unique to this population, usually requires more specific and tailored methods of evaluation. Take the example of the illustrious composer Robert Schumann, whose hand dysfunction remains unexplained. Indeed, Schumann's hand injury still raises a great deal of controversy in the literature as to its etiology and diagnosis. Sams describes it as a weakness caused by mercury, a common treatment then for syphilis, a disease from which Schumann suffered most of his life (74). According to Ballantyne, it was more likely to be a posterior interosseous nerve injury at the elbow (75). Mather suggests that grueling finger-stretching exercises might have caused the injury (76). Walker describes the torturous machine that the composer built to help strengthen the fingers of his right hand; with it, he would draw up one of his fingers in a sling when practicing (77). Tragically, the device only aggravated the weakness, and Schumann's hand enigma still is unsolved.

An objective musculoskeletal performance evaluation aiming to optimize motion is needed all the more because training and level of experience are of paramount importance in this population. "Distributed excitation is the rule in the motor system, due to co-motions and secondary motions. The more intense the contraction, the farther it is propagated from its focus" (Meyer laws) (11). Lundervold found that adequate relaxation of antagonists is a feature of skilled repetitive movements and that training reduces the amount of EMG activity present in a muscle between its periods of contraction (78). Polnauer emphasized the importance of the least possible involvement of antagonists in violin playing (11).

In 1972, Basmajian and White studied the embouchure of brass instrumentalists, which is the control of the firmness and vibration of the lips in relation to each other and to the mouthpiece (79). They found that both register and intensity positively affect embouchure muscle activity, with register having a greater effect than intensity. Advanced trumpeters have more activity in the muscles surrounding the lips than in those in the lips; less advanced trumpeters show no difference. The latter demonstrate more muscle activity in the upper lip than in the lower lip, whereas advanced trumpeters show a smaller ratio of upper lip to lower muscle activity. These findings illustrate the effect of training on muscle activity in brass instrumentalists.

In her study on string instrument vibrato, Schlapp noted that after a vibrato run is stopped, there is a persistence of EMG activity in flexor, extensor, and dorsal interosseous muscles, with longer persistence in more strongly contracted muscles (80). Furthermore, when attempting to slow their vibrato rate, subjects with less technical training showed more loss of regularity in their muscle activity (i.e., smooth flexor–extensor alternation) than the better-trained musicians.

Thus, there seems to be a consensus on the effect of training on muscle activity in musicians. The better trained and, perhaps, the less injury prone use their muscles more efficiently and are less likely to produce untoward or excessive muscle contractions. Rolland summarized this fact as follows: "The ultimate goal is a beautiful sound, produced by efficient motion patterns and with the least possible effort" (81).

The principle of least muscle effort could be seen as the biological equivalent of the principle of conservation of energy. In evaluating musicians' performance, therefore, a thorough measurement of muscle activity is needed as well as a measurement of the output produced, be it motion or sound. This constitutes the basis for the biomechanical profile.

Biomechanical Profiles

The biomechanical profile is a task- and instrument-specific musculoskeletal performance evaluation tool that attempts to establish the normal ranges of the motions and activities of the various joints and muscles involved in a well-defined musical task such as bowing or a subtask such as vibrato. Various kinematic and kinetic parameters can be measured, depending on the instrument studied and the task. It is obvious that only experienced professional musicians should be tested to establish these norms. As in many routinely measured biological parameters and in gait analysis, the biomechanical parameters obtained for a given musician presenting with a relevant musculoskeletal disorder could be compared to the respective normal ranges established. Noninvasive and eminently objective and reproducible, this type of testing also can be performed preventively, as in sports, to assess a novice musician's efficiency and appropriate use of his or her music-making machine, thus attempting to enhance performance and prevent latent injuries.

Violin

Surface EMG activity of the left deltoid, extensor digitorum, pronator teres, biceps brachii, and flexor group was measured in 14 healthy professional violinists (seven men and seven women; average age 31.3 years; average experience 24.3 years) synchronously with the sound produced during the performance of four vibrato tasks, one for each finger, of comparable frequencies for 3 seconds each (82–84).

The sound signal obtained was periodic, simulating the actual vibrato motion. Vibrato rate ranged from 4.84 to 6.75 Hz and was significantly different between subjects, confirming the findings of previous studies (82). Flexor and extensor muscles followed a pattern similar to the sound in all cases; pronator and biceps did in most cases. This may mean that the former muscles are more dependent than the latter on the violinist's level of experience. The deltoid was mostly nonperiodic, which was to be expected because it acts primarily as a shoulder support muscle in this task. Electromyographic parameters or rise, fall, and peak-to-peak times were significantly intercorrelated, suggesting a normally distributed surface EMG signal, as described in the literature. These parameters, especially peak-to-peak time, showed little variability from cycle to cycle in all signals, confirming the issue of regularity in a vibrato played by experienced violinists. Peak-to-peak time also was strongly correlated between the sound and each of the muscles, giving a physiological origin to this regularity.

All subjects and all fingers followed the same muscle firing sequence: flexor–extensor/biceps–pronator/sound. The flexor–extensor complex seems to be most directly responsible for sound production, whereas the biceps–pronator complex primarily stabilizes the elbow in pronosupination (Fig. 64-4). Flexor and extensor energies also were found to be the most often correlated with the acoustic energy produced, but never simultaneously.

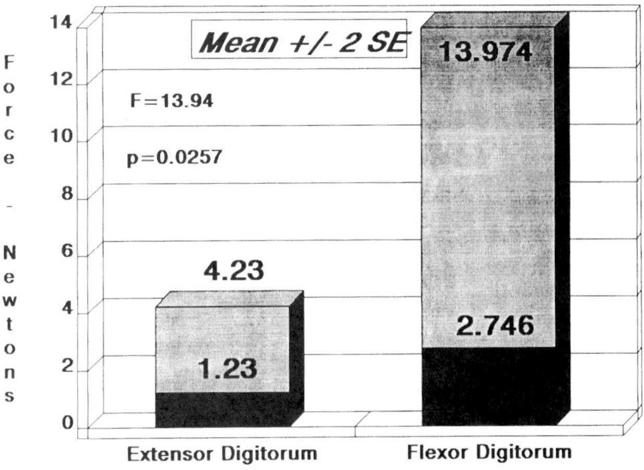

FIG. 64-4. Dynamic surface electromyographic activity of various upper extremity muscles during the performance of a violin vibrato task.

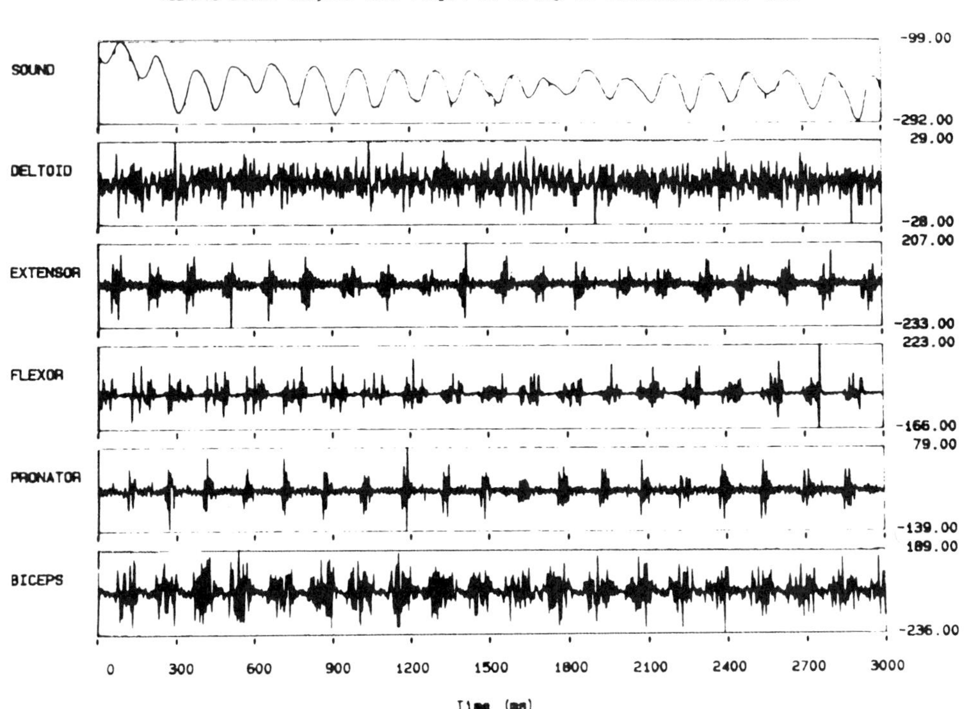

FIG. 64-5. Upper extremity flexor and extensor force requirements in violin vibrato (mean ± 2 SE). *F* and *p* values pertain to statistical significance of difference.

In another group of violinists (84), EMG–force calibration curves and regression equations were available from previous studies (85). Thus, force measurements of flexor and extensor groups during violin vibrato were derived from their respective dynamic EMG signals (Fig. 64-5). Extensor and flexor forces were found to be significantly different statistically.

Harp

Harp subtasks (e.g., arpeggios) were analyzed using three-dimensional video and synchronous EMG while varying tempo and loudness, to assess motion of the upper extremity joints involved: shoulder, elbow, wrist, and hand, for both sides alternately (Fig. 64-6) (3). Two major harp techniques, Grandjany and Salzedo, also were compared using the same model. Qualitative evaluation of the stick figures obtained was performed by harp teachers and provided insight and feedback for their students.

For harpists, tuning the instrument can be a considerable source of muscle tension. This is especially dangerous when followed immediately by playing. The traditional tuning key was not ergonomically designed. Besides being too small for efficient gripping and using the narrower diameter of the hand, the T-shaped handle forces the wrist into ulnar and radial deviation. Wrist position can be all the more awkward because the square hole fits the tuning pin only every 90° (Fig. 64-7*A*). An ergonomic key was designed by the author with a larger L-shaped handle and an eight-point double-square hole (Fig. 64-7*C*). Most of the lateral motion of the wrist is thus transformed into elbow flexion and extension (Fig. 64-7*B*). Preliminary trials of the new key, in comparison to the old one, show a significant decrease in flexor EMG activity with the former (Fig. 64-8).

Trumpet

A photographic postural study of 16 virtuoso trumpeters showed that they have to bend their knees and straighten their lumbar lordosis as they are trying to reach for higher notes (86–88). This postural change was maximal as they were sustaining a high F note above C (Fig. 64-9). Its magnitude was directly related to the trumpeter's anthropometry. This postural change can be explained by the increased need for downward diaphragmatic excursion to sustain expiration. Neck position remained constant from the low to the high notes, as did horn angle. The angle was found to be significantly correlated with the degree of upper jaw overbite of the trumpeter (i.e., the larger the overbite, the lower the horn; Figs. 64-10 and 64-11). This finding is all the more significant because novice trumpeters usually are dictated an arbitrary horn angle by their teachers based solely on their beliefs and traditions. An inadequate horn angle can throw the entire kinematic chain out of balance, potentially causing undue stress and subsequent degenerative changes in the temporomandibular joints. Also, the cervical spine would have to go

HARP - TECHNIQUE Side: Right Tempo: 60 Name: BEA
Type: ARPEGGIOS down Octaves: 2, 3 Loudness: forte

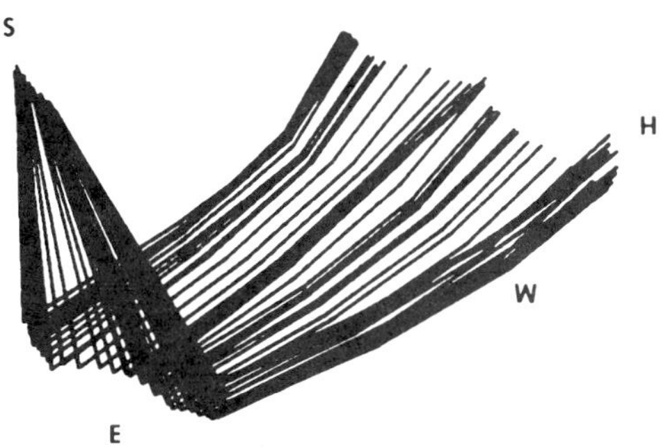

A

HARP - TECHNIQUE Side: Right Tempo: 60 Name: BEA
Type: ARPEGGIOS down Octaves: 2, 3, 4 Loudness: forte

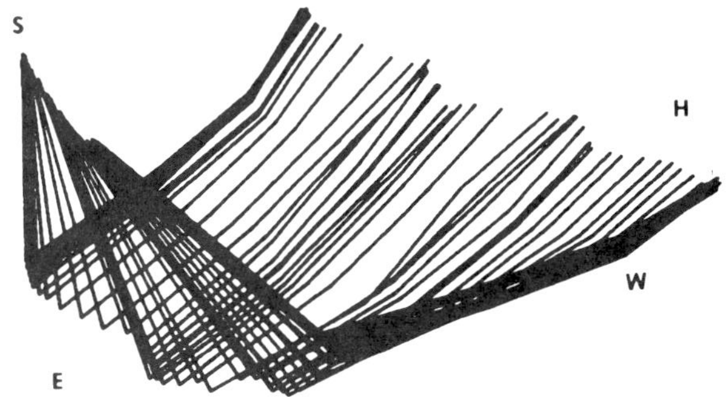

B

FIG. 64-6. Typical stick figures obtained from the video analysis of a harpist performing loud arpeggios of the second and third octaves with her right hand. Compare **(A)** the slow performance to **(B)** the fast one (*H*, hand; *W*, wrist; *E*, elbow; *S*, shoulder).

A

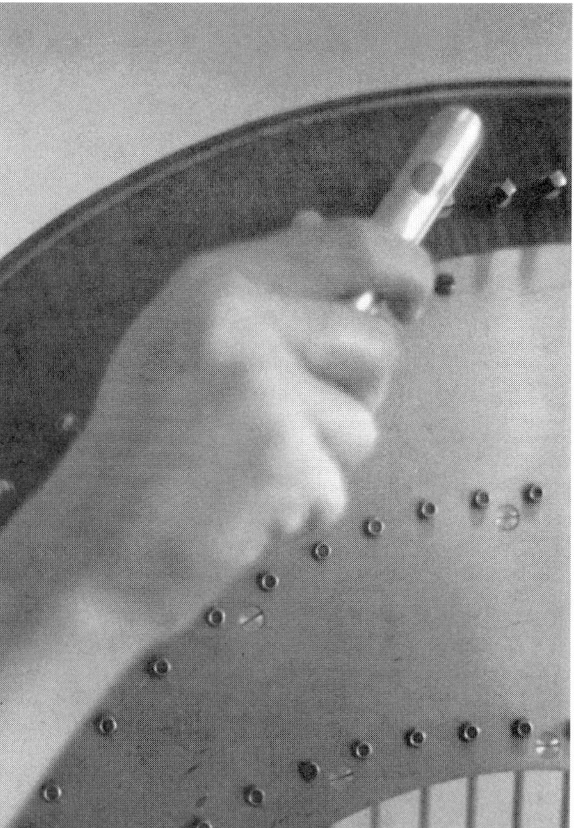

C

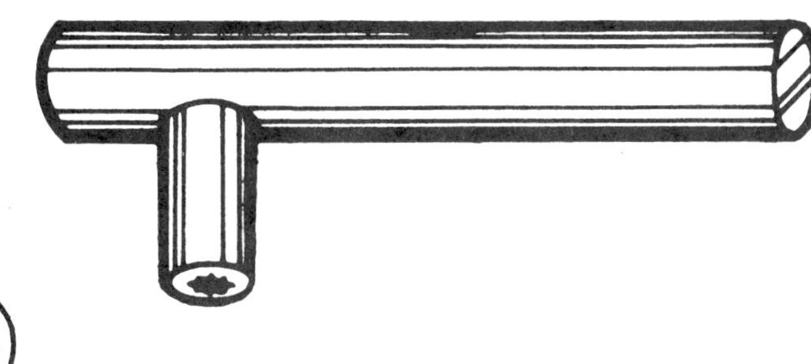

B

FIG. 64-7. A: BA, a professional harpist, using the traditional tuning key. Notice the awkward grip. **B:** Ergonomic tuning key with cross section of the eight-point double-square hole. **C:** BA, using the ergonomic tuning key. Note the typical cylindrical power grip.

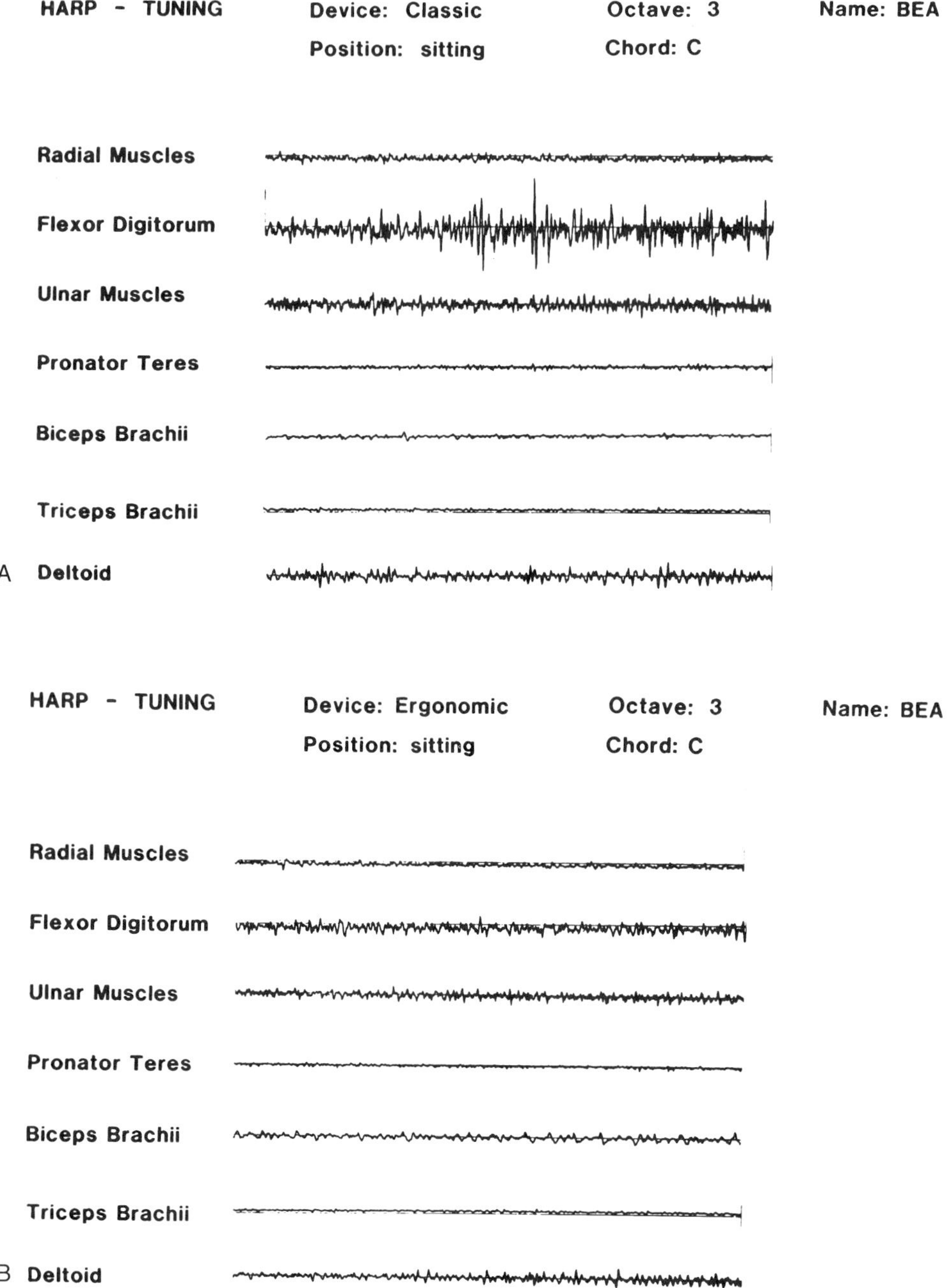

FIG. 64-8. Raw signal charts of the electromyographic activity of seven right upper extremity muscle groups of harpist BA, during tuning with the **(A)** traditional and **(B)** ergonomic tuning keys. Notice the difference in muscle activity.

into extension to accommodate, thus creating areas of less resistance in the anterior muscular wall of the neck and opening the way for pharyngeal herniation under the tremendous pressures involved.

Piano

An objective and reproducible model for comparison of commonly used piano techniques was established (89,90). Three basic, well known piano methods were delineated and followed for a professional pianist to perform with his right hand alone: method A, flat hand and extended fingers; method B, arched hand with rounded fingers and slightly palmarflexed wrist; and method C, quasi-right-angle flexion at the knuckles and slightly ulnarly deviated wrist (Fig. 64-12). The pianist played a 5-second arpeggiated chord task four times, with each of the three methods, in random order. Sound was collected with microphone, and three-dimensional video yielded the kinematics of the right fifth MCP joint, all three long-finger joints, wrist, elbow, and shoulder.

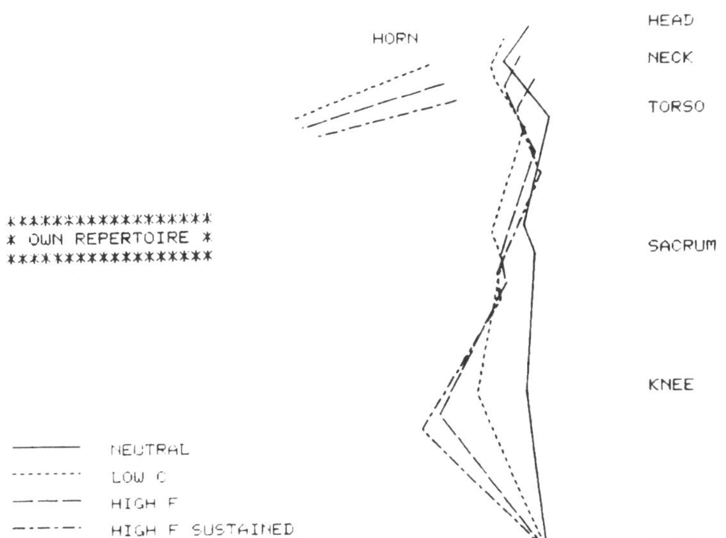

FIG. 64-9. Typical silhouette diagram of a trumpeter performing his own repertoire. Notice the changes in posture between neutral, low C, high F, and high F sustained.

Sound was found to be highly reproducible between tests, thus establishing the validity of the results: the motion of the distal interphalangeal and MCP joints of the middle finger was significantly less for method A in all tasks of the demonstration musical piece and was significantly greater using method C. Method C showed significantly more ulnar and less radial deviation of the wrist than methods A and B in all tasks (Fig. 64-13).

The following has been mathematically demonstrated:

To optimize the energy cost of a movement, the velocity as a function of time must be minimized.

To optimize the force cost in the movement, the acceleration must be minimized.

To obtain a smooth pattern of movement, the jerk function, defined as the third derivative of displacement, must be minimized.

The associated velocity, acceleration, and jerk (i.e., smoothness of motion) of each of the three piano methods are summarized in Figure 64-14. Energy, force, and jerk in general were optimized in method A or B. In practice, the professional pianist can alternate efficiently, accurately, and rapidly between these different postures. It would appear

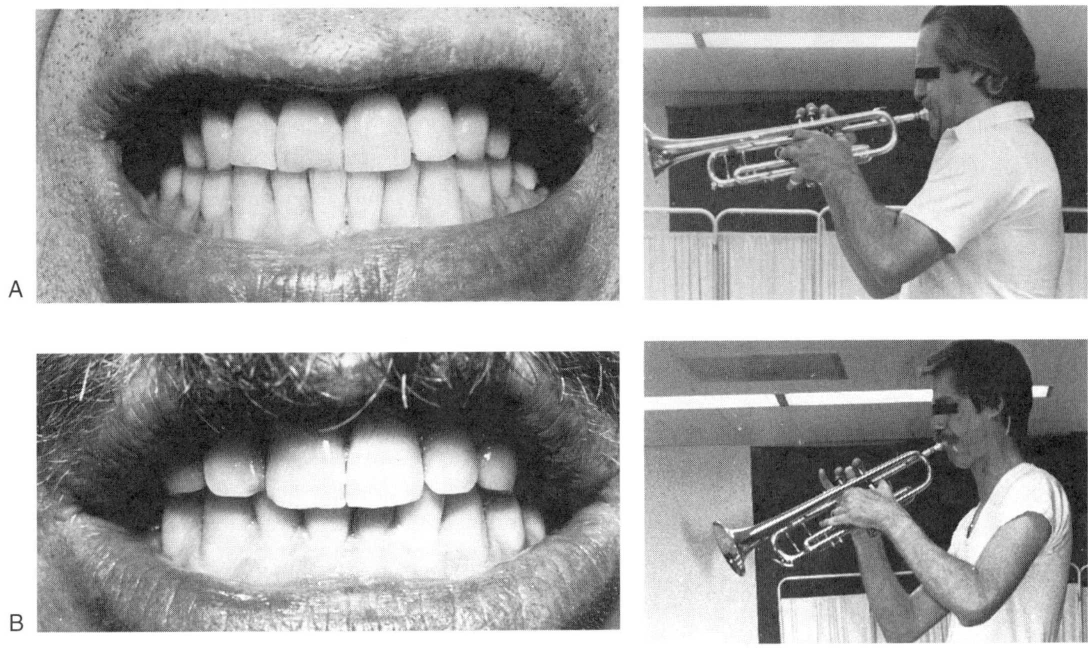

FIG. 64-10. Dental overbite and the trumpet angle of two players. **A:** The player with a small overbite has only a slight horn inclination. **B:** The player with the larger overbite has a larger horn inclination.

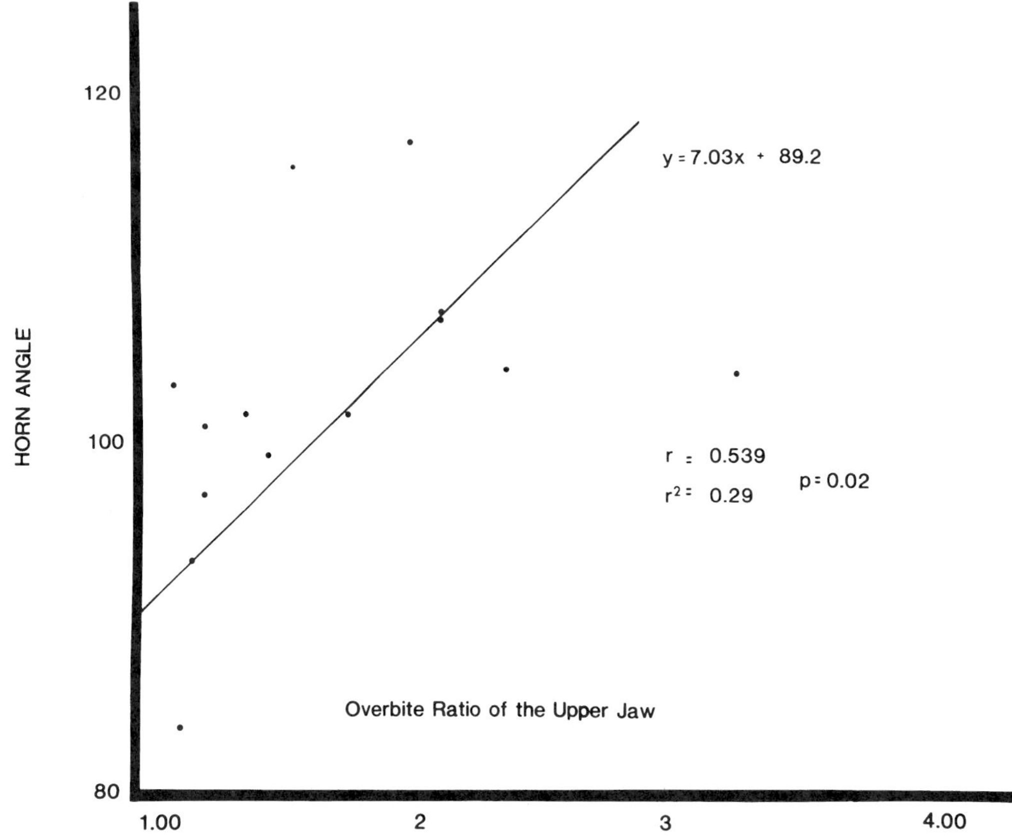

FIG. 64-11. Horn angle as a function of dental overbite ratio.

from the foregoing, however, that the energy and force requirements, and thus perhaps the risk of cumulative trauma injury, might be greatest for posture C.

Specific Solutions and Treatment Modalities

"When an ideal strength-economy is reached, there is no fatigue, there are no feelings of dislike in the peripheral organs—then also there are no diseases of profession . . . " (5). This view might seem slightly simplistic and idealistic; however, an optimal work–rest timetable was emphasized by several authors and may be one of the answers for the overuse disorders that often are reported (36,43,74). Based on a working period of 2 hours, Singer proposes the following timetable: 40 minutes of work, then a 2-minute pause, then 80 minutes of work, followed by a 4-minute pause (5). Flesch advised the following practice rule for violin: 1 hour of general technique (i.e., etudes, scales, and bowing); 1.5 hours of applied technique (i.e., repertoire, parts of compositions); 1.5 hours of purely artistic playing (i.e., style and finished performance); and 15 minutes of absolute rest every 2 hours (92).

Firmly believing that "use affects functioning (93)," Alexander started a technique based on whole-body relaxation, the principles of which can be summarized as follows:

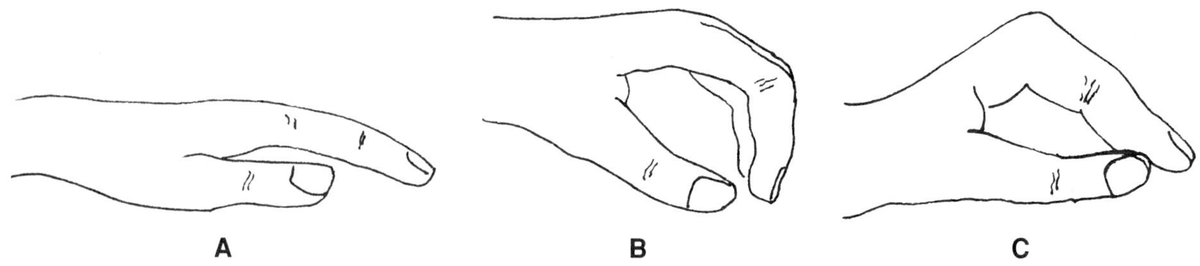

FIG. 64-12. Diagrams of the three piano methods. **A:** Flat hand and extended fingers. **B:** Arched hand with rounded fingers and slightly flexed wrist. **C:** Quasi-right-angle flexion at the metacarpophalangeal joints and slightly ulnarly deviated wrist.

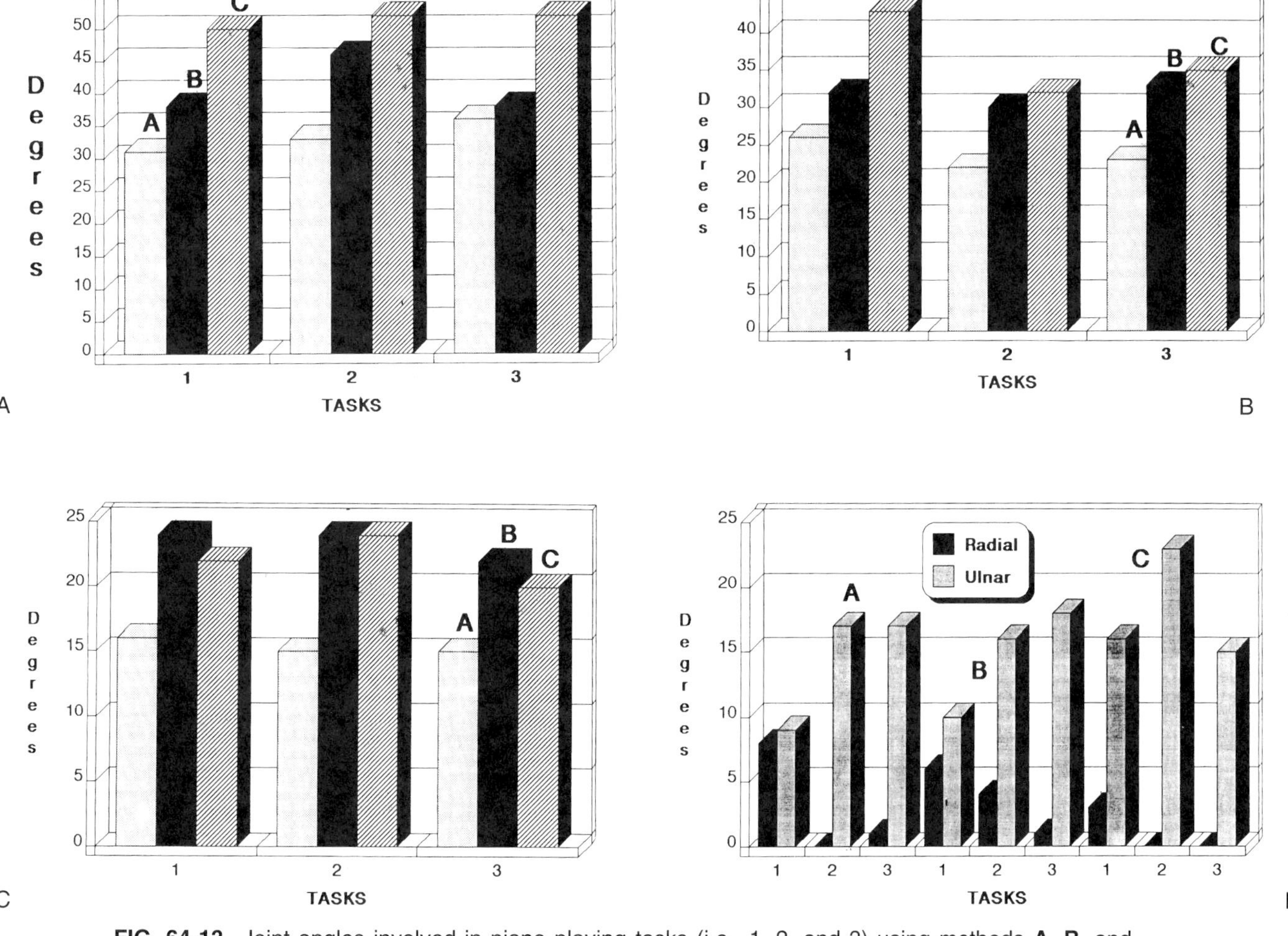

FIG. 64-13. Joint angles involved in piano playing tasks (i.e., 1, 2, and 3) using methods **A**, **B**, and **C** (see Fig. 64-12.) **A:** Distal interphalangeal joint flexion-extension. **B:** Metacarpophalangeal flexion-extension. **C:** Metacarpophalangeal abduction–adduction. **D:** Wrist radial–ulnar deviation.

- Keep the neck free
- Ensure symmetry and awareness of one's posture
- Perform relaxed and deep breathing, using both intercostal muscles and diaphragm (94)

In her method, Samama designed direct implementations of Alexander's principles for the various instrument groups (95). Bejjani and Halpern performed an extensive review of the various methods of music education, emphasizing their ergonomic risk factors as well as more controversial issues such as laterality and speed (96). They stressed the importance of early musculoskeletal awareness in music education, through enhancement of sensory feedback, whole-body involvement with least muscle effort and avoidance of static work, and adequate breathing and relaxation techniques.

Decreasing muscle tension seems to improve performance (97). Cratty showed that the less complex tasks usually are facilitated by tension, whereas the more complex ones usually are inhibited (98). A musician's daily activities include both kinds of tasks. The former tasks often are not familiar to the general public, including physicians, because they are done behind the scenes (e.g., preparing reeds for a clarinetist, carrying or tuning the harp for a harpist). These ancillary activities often can be the cause of the occupational disorder, either directly or indirectly by building up muscle tension to the point that subsequent playing would be mechanically impaired, leading to injury.

Electromyographic biofeedback training was shown to improve significantly the performance of a fine motor skill (99). It also was shown to reduce the muscle tension induced by a novel motor skill. In a woodwind musician, EMG biofeedback resulted in dramatic reductions in tension levels of the throat and facial muscles along with increased proficiency as a musician and in psychological functioning (100). Using EMG biofeedback on the left arm extensors of string players, Morasky and associates noted that biofeedback did facilitate significant decreases in EMG activity (101). These reductions persisted in a no-feedback situation, but generalization from extensors to flexors did not occur. These studies all were performed with one-channel biofeedback. Use of dual-channel EMG biofeedback, in a ratio mode, is sug-

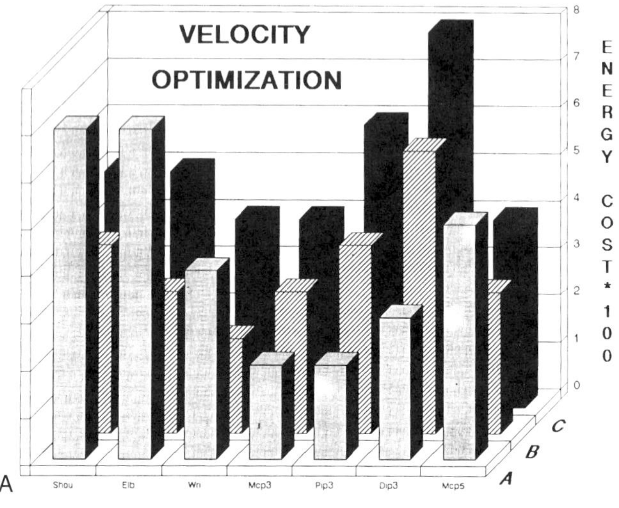

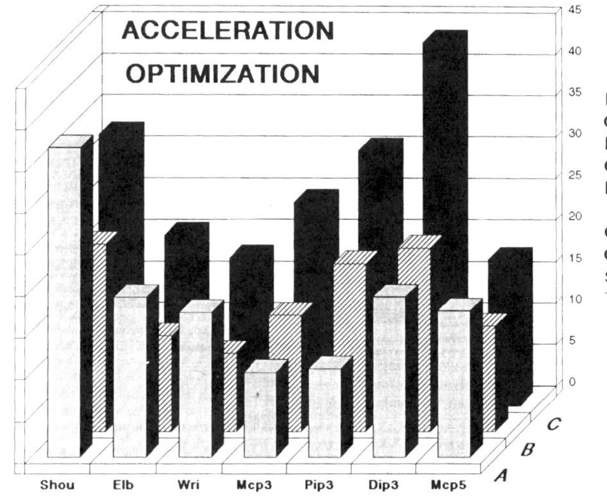

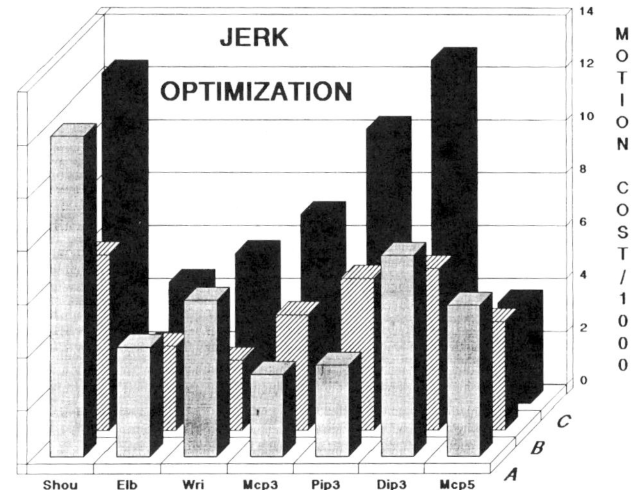

FIG. 64-14. Velocity **(A),** acceleration **(B),** and jerk **(C)** of various upper extremity joints in piano playing using methods **A**, **B**, and **C** (see Fig. 64-12).

gested to improve coordination between intrinsics, between intrinsics and extrinsics, and between agonists and antagonists, in musicians' hands.

Because cold impairs manual performance, and because forearm muscle tension is accompanied by decreased finger temperature, use of skin temperature biofeedback to warm hands may be useful. Biofeedback was shown to increase hand and skin temperature independently of the general somatic activity by a number of authors (102–107). Hand temperature also can be raised under hypnosis and suggestion, and the magnitude of the changes is large enough to account for the psychosomatic symptoms observed in clinical settings (104,108).

Visual postural feedback is recommended in cases in which the patient performs awkward motions or sustains awkward positions of which he or she is not aware. Merely showing some visual documentation of these positions (e.g., photos, video, or slides) to the patient, or having him or her play in front of a mirror, as dancers do, often can generate the necessary feedback to induce the correction. In more complex cases, where the process has been going on for too long or is compounded by untoward treatments, the use of multichannel electric muscle stimulation to cause involuntary movement can be used.

A more radical mode of treatment for pianists' hands was designed in 1857 by a Philadelphia surgeon, William S. Forbes (109). It consisted of surgically sectioning the junctura tendinae that bind the ring finger extensor to its neighbors. This operation arose from the nineteenth-century belief that a perfect independence of the fingers might enhance the bravura style of playing. This rather invasive practice fell from fashion in 1900; however, it unfortunately still is used in sporadic cases.

Surgery is indicated for the following conditions: nerve entrapment syndromes, trigger fingers, intractable rotator cuff tendinitis or tear, and similar injuries. Regardless of the indications, any intervention must be tailored to the unique needs of each instrumentalist (110). In view of the fact that surgery could mean the end of a musician's career because of its inherent morbidity and possible physical and psychological trauma, every effort should be made toward prevention and use of the less invasive and more conservative methods first.

Because "asking a serious musician to give up his or

her instrument (even temporarily) is like asking an Olympic runner to give up sprinting, a clergyman to give up preaching, or even a physician to give up doctoring'' (1), rehabilitation techniques should be aimed at preserving the musician's playing ability. As surely as a marathon runner should not be asked to stop running completely but to cut down on his or her mileage, as soon as the acute phase wears off, a professional musician almost never should be asked to give up his or her instrument completely but to adjust practice schedule and repertoire when possible.

DANCERS' OCCUPATIONAL DISORDERS

Patterns of injury in dance, particularly in ballet, tend to be related to age and skill, with knee or hip problems more characteristic of the young and novice and leg, ankle, and foot problems more frequently encountered in the older or professional dancer (111,112). There are, however, many exceptions to this rule. Back injuries, for example, may occur at any age or level of skill. They occur in both male and female dancers, with a somewhat higher prevalence in the former. Because male dancers are taller and heavier than their female counterparts and leap higher, osteoarthritis of the hip can be a significant problem with the dancer in his fourth or fifth decade. These factors contribute to making the male dancer retire about 10 years earlier than the female. The man's career is also made shorter by a later start (i.e., approximately 16 years of age) than that of the woman (i.e., approximately 6 years of age). Ongoing studies on aging dancers (mean age 56 years) performed at the Corps de Ballet in Oslo, Stockholm, Gothenburg, and Malmo, show a much higher incidence of first metatarsophalangeal (MTP) joint, hip, and knee osteoarthrosis in this group than in the general population.

The career of a ballet dancer, male or female, can end prematurely for other reasons as well. It is virtually impossible, for example, to return to major dancing after an Achilles tendon rupture. A progressing hallux rigidus spells an end to a career, particularly if first MTP dorsiflexion is already less than 45° at the age of about 18 years. When a hallux valgus develops later in a dancer's life, no surgery should be undertaken before retirement. Any major operation (i.e., a Keller arthroplasty) is not compatible with the continuation of a career as a dancer.

Epidemiology

Musculoskeletal injuries represent 85% of ballet dancers' occupational diseases; however, the documentation of these diseases began just one or two decades ago (Table 64-4). Documentation of similar injuries in athletic activities is now well advanced.

The injury rate is 25% lower in female ballet dancers than in males. Over a 15-year period, the Australian Ballet reported an injury rate of about 3.5 per dancer, all ages included (111,112).

The most common hip, thigh, and groin injuries in dancers are clicking hip and iliopsoas tendinitis. Muscle strains constitute more than one-third of all injuries in dancers. In dancers' lower extremities, hamstring strains top the list, along with calf muscle and foot intrinsics.

Among knee injuries, the most common in dancers are patellar chondromalacia, followed by jumper's knee, internal derangement, and subluxing patella. Meniscal tears are relatively rare. As for leg injuries, calf muscle strains and shin splints are the most common. Shin splints of the lower leg usually are posteromedial in runners and anterolateral in dancers.

Among ankle injuries, sprains and Achilles tendinitis are the most common in dancers. In an early study, osteoarthrosis of the tibiotalar joint was observed in all ballet dancers who had been dancing for more than 8 years. Posterior impingement syndrome and damage to the flexor hallucis longus are frequent in dancers. Flexor hallucis longus tendinitis often is mistaken for Achilles tendinitis. Partial as well as bilateral tears can be encountered.

Pathologic foot conditions are numerous in dancers. Deformities such as hallux valgus, hammer toes, and claw toes are most common. In a Bulgarian study, talonavicular arthrosis was found in 29% of ballet dancers, peritendinous calcium deposits in 25%, and various aseptic necroses of the foot in 14% of female dancers (111,112).

Although muscle (29%), tendon (17%), and ligament (15%) together account for 61% of all injuries in ballet dan-

TABLE 64-4. *Relative percentage of injuries by site in various dance groups*

Site	Ballet (*n* = 747; %)	Theatrical dance (%)	Theatrical dance students (*n* = 185; %)	Flamenco (*n* = 29; %)
Head/neck		1–5		26.8
Back	8.5–13	6–12	17.6	28.6
Upper limb	4	6–10		17.8
Hip	8.6	7	14.2	
Thigh/groin	4.3			
Knee	17.3–39	14–34	14.5	14.3
Leg	8.5	14	5.4	
Ankle	12–22.3	13–21	22.2	12.5
Foot	12–20.1	10–21	14.8	10

TABLE 64-5. *Comparative incidence of spondylolysis*

Population	Incidence (%)
General	
White women	2.3
White men	5–7
Eskimos	27.4
Ainu Japanese	41.3
Ballet dancers	11–20
Athletes	
Swimmers	23.7
Wrestlers	23.8
Football linemen	24
Gymnasts	11–32
Contortionists	25
Pole jumpers	26.3
Weightlifters	30
Javelin throwers	40–47.4

cers, stress fractures also are seen and account for 1.1% of all injuries. The most common sites for stress fractures in dancers are the femoral neck and the tibia. March and Jones fractures are uncommon in this population.

Spondylolysis is an intriguing pathologic entity in terms of occupational biomechanics. Although its incidence ranges from 25% to 41% in certain ethnic groups such as Eskimos and Ainu Japanese, its relationship to certain occupations is undeniable. The incidence in ballet dancers, for example, is about four times the incidence in the general white population (Table 64-5).

Functional Anatomy and Kinematics

In all five foot positions of ballet, the feet are turned out 180° to each other. Turnout is the very foundation of ballet. Three major factors at the hip determine the external rotation possible for each dancer:

1. Anteversion angle
2. Neck shaft angle
3. Degree of tightness of the Y ligament of Bigelow.

At age 8 years, femoral anteversion has reduced to about 15°, allowing for about 80° of external rotation at the hip. The child who is unable to externally rotate the hips beyond 45° should not plan to become a ballet dancer. In the ideal turnout position, the weight should fall from the body to the thigh and directly through the center of rotation of the knee and ankle. Following the kinematic chain theory, this distribution of weight can be achieved only if the external rotation of the lower extremities occurs at the hip.

Following the same theory, alignment of the toes without breaking at the MTPs as a straight line through the ankle to the knee provides the best support for pointe work. There also is more skeletal stability on pointe than on demipointe. Approximately 3 to 3.5 years of dancing in ballet shoes (i.e., soft-toed dance slippers) is required to develop the strength, balance, and style that permit a dancer to dance on pointe. No child today is permitted to dance on pointe before the age of 11.5 years. Also, because the female pelvis is cylindrical and wider than the male pelvis, a slightly knock-kneed shape is not uncommon in young ballet students, and subluxation of the patella can occur.

Anatomic variations play an often overlooked but very important role in the etiology of injuries, that is, of muscle and tendon strains. It is known, for example, that a peasant foot with a squared ankle, a sturdy arch, a broad forefoot, and the first three toes of nearly equal length is best fit for dancing in toe shoes. On the other hand, a short first ray, whether the shortening is in the first metatarsal or in the great toe itself, poses great problems with stability. If the first metatarsal is short, it is not effective for weight transmission, and the dancer must try to maintain stability over the second and third metatarsals. Sickling will occur if the weight is carried too medially in an attempt to get the first metatarsal head satisfactorily down to the ground, and damage will follow—sometimes as proximally as in the trunk.

Musculoskeletal Changes

Most hypertrophic changes of the osseous system observed in the growing ballet dancer are stable. These changes have been described by several Eastern European authors. About 50% of ballet dancers show hypertrophy of the femur, tibia, and foot bones (111). This figure rises to 79% in another survey (111). In the foot, these changes consist primarily of endosteal and periosteal hypertrophy in the second and third metatarsal diaphyses, with narrowing of the medullary canal. A German study pointed out that unlike ballet dancers, modern dancers all presented flat feet, splay feet, and even hallux valgus. This was thought to be related to the absence of forefoot support in the shoe, which does not occur in ballet (112).

Flexibility and Range of Motion

Flexibility of the spine, hips, and ankles is, of course, the hallmark of the ballet dancer, and the presence of hypermobility of these joints would be attributable to training. Training, however, is not directed to hyperextending knees, elbows, and fingers because this leads to unesthetic postures and usually is carefully avoided by dancers. The presence of hypermobility in these joints, therefore, is likely to be hereditary rather than acquired. In the same study, ballet students did show generalized joint hypermobility as compared to a control group of nurses (111).

Range-of-motion data on the spine and lower extremities, measured by regular goniometer, three-dimensional electromagnetic motion analyzer, Leighton flexometer, or two inclinometers, were compared among female ballet dancers, flamenco dancers, and a control group (Tables 64-6 and 64-

TABLE 64-6. *Comparative mean and standard deviation of hip and knee ranges of motion in dance groups*

Range of motion	Ballerinas (n = 25)	Flamencas (n = 10)	Controls
Hip			
Flexion–extension	198° (22°)	158° (8°)	
Abduction–adduction	80° (12°)		61° (6°)
Rotation	82° (11°)		70° (9°)
Knee			
Flexion–extension	177° (9°)	160° (9°)	144°

7) (111). Ballerinas have the widest range of spine flexion–extension, and flamencas a slightly wider range of lateral bending. All ranges of hip and knee motion are wider in ballerinas. Ankle range of motion is wider in ballerinas and flamencas than in the control group (112). In over 100 dancers with plantar fascia strain and Achilles tendinitis, 60% lacked full ankle dorsiflexion in the first exercise at the barre, demiplie (i.e., bending the knee without moving the heel from the floor). Flamencas had a wider range of subtalar and first MTP motion than did the control group (112).

Kinetics

Back Strength

Loads on the lumbosacral disk of male ballet dancers while lifting their female partners are considerable. They can reach a force of 15 times the body weight of the lifted dancer, especially if performed inadequately (i.e., excessive lumbar lordosis). Besides these acute overloads, dancing involves lighter but repetitive spinal loads related to posture or technique. These are particularly obvious in flamenco dancing.

Knee Strength

Development of inner thigh muscles and stretching of the hamstrings play an important role in lifting the body off the toes in pointe work in ballet. Failure to do so can cause hamstring strains. Strength imbalance in knee muscles also has been proposed as a leading cause of hamstring strains in athletes. A desirable ratio of hamstring to quadriceps maximum torque is thought to be 2:3.

TABLE 64-7. *Comparative mean and standard deviation of spine range of motion as measured by Leighton flexometer in ballerinas and flamencas, as measured by three-dimensional electromagnetic motion analyzer in controls*

Spine motion	Ballerinas (n = 25)	Flamencas (n = 10)	Controls (n = 101)
Flexion–extension	246° (20°)	141° (24°)	122° (14°)
Lateral bending	110° (8°)	121° (25°)	97° (8°)

To verify these theories, a comparative knee isokinetic study was performed. Data were compiled from the literature for athletes, ballet dancers, and a control group and were collected with a dynamometer for flamenco dancers. In women, knee extension was strongest in athletes and weakest in nonathletes. Dancers fell in between, with flamenco dancers being stronger than ballerinas. Strength decreased as the speed increased in all groups. Proportional flexion–extension ratios increased as the speed increased in all groups. They were slightly weaker for nonathletes. In men, knee extension was strongest in athletes and at low speeds. A similar pattern was seen in knee flexion. Proportional ratios increased at higher speeds. Ballet dancers had the highest ratio at low speed (111).

At peak season, the relative strength ratio (i.e., quadriceps:body weight) is 98% for male ballet dancers and 70% for female dancers, as measured with isokinetic equipment. Values for male dancers are comparable to those for male athletes, whereas female dancers are weaker than female athletes (Fig. 64-15). The balance ratio (i.e., right quadriceps:left quadriceps) usually is close to 1 in athletes, ballet dancers, and flamenco dancers (111).

Ankle Strength

The strength required to dance on pointe in ballet makes maximum demands on all intrinsic and extrinsic foot and ankle muscles. Isokinetic ankle torques are much higher in plantarflexion than dorsiflexion in general. They also are much higher in men than in women and at lower speeds than at higher speeds. Female ballet dancers and female jumpers have comparable plantarflexion torques.

Flamenco Dancing. Using the electrodynogram and skin-mounted accelerometers, foot pressure as well as hip and knee vibration transients were recorded in 10 female dancers after a thorough clinical evaluation (113–116). A health questionnaire also was distributed to 29 dancers. Foot pressure and acceleration data reveal the unique percussive nature of the dance form. Some clinical findings such as calluses are related to pressure distribution. Urogenital disorders were unusually frequent in this group. It is hypothesized that these disorders, and perhaps some of the low back and neck symptoms, could be vibration related. Indeed, the vibration frequencies measured were well comparable to the resonance frequencies of the abdominal viscera and the spine. Nonetheless, the hip joint seems to absorb most of the impact during dancing.

Vibration–pressure diagrams were obtained, plotting foot pressure in parallel with accelerometry data. A walking test displayed an obvious slow periodic pattern for all signals. In a relatively slow *allegria* step and fast *escudero redoble* step, vibration–pressure relationships were not as clearly defined but highly reproducible in this format, making this a useful tool for evaluating a dancer's biomechanical behavior as well as the effect of floors and footwear on this behavior.

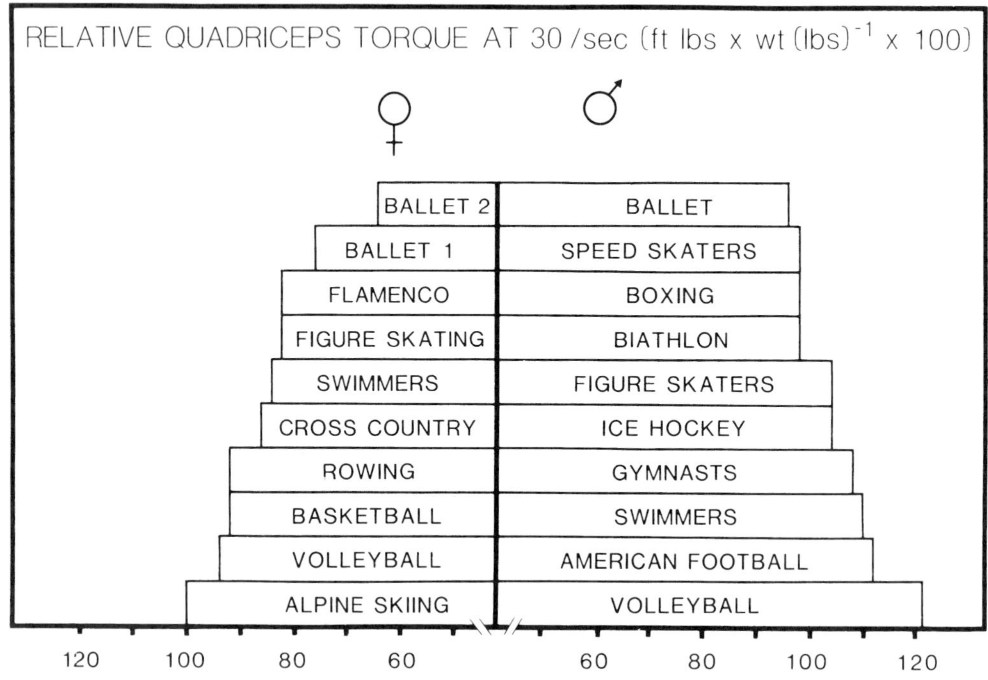

FIG. 64-15. Comparative graph of quadriceps muscle torque at 30°/sec, between men and women of various athletic and dance disciplines, including two different series of ballerinas.

Isometric and isokinetic spinal torques were measured seated, using a dynamometer. Discrete spinal range of motion also was measured with an electromagnetic three-dimensional motion analyzer and compared to the continuous range of motion during dancing both *zapateado* footsteps and backsteps such as *zambra* and *romba.* A larger-than-normal spinal extension range and larger isometric extension torques suggest an adaptation to the task. Sustained spinal position close to the functional limits during dancing backsteps may be responsible for some of the back symptoms reported.

Pathomechanics

The most common risk factors for overuse injuries in dance have been summarized as follows:

Training errors, including abrupt changes in intensity, duration, or frequency of training

Musculotendinous imbalance affecting strength, flexibility, or both

Anatomic malalignment of the lower extremity, including leg length discrepancy, rotation abnormalities of the hips, position of the kneecap, bow legs, knock-knees, or flat feet

Improper fit of shoewear and inadequate shock-absorbing material

Hard, nonresilient floor surface

Associated disease state of the lower extremity, including arthritis, poor circulation, old fracture, or other injury

Growth, in particular the growth spurt, because of the fast and often transiently uneven and asymmetric changes occurring in the musculoskeletal system.

Technique- and Training-Related Injuries in Ballet Dancers

Hip Snapping or Clicking. Most commonly affected is the iliacus muscle with pain on flexion, abduction, and external rotation of the hip during the *developpe* step at the barre (i.e., the hip and leg are brought from the first position upward and outward in external rotation and then returned to the first position). In landing from a leap, as in *entrechat* (i.e., jumping straight up, beating and changing the feet beneath her), the dancer may cause snapping of the tensor fascia lata backward across the greater trochanter, permitting the pelvis to rotate forward into lordosis. The dancer usually keeps producing the click voluntarily just to see if it is still present, then after a while does so automatically. Sometimes, the dancer even asserts that she has to click the hip to free it before dancing. Bursitis over the greater trochanter or the anterior hip also can occur as a result of lack of activity during periods of laying off, inadequate warm-up, or poor technique. Symptoms are exacerbated during performance of a grand plie.

Tendinitis. Tendinitis of the origin of the hamstrings presents with pain when landing from a leap and during other quick steps such as *tours en l'air* (i.e., turns in the air).

Avulsion. Avulsion or strain of the sartorius origin occurs primarily because the take-off for a leap takes place with the knee in maximum extension and the limb in external rotation. An injury with a similar mechanism can occur in the hamstrings in runners and in the rectus femoris in sprinters.

Partial Avulsion. Partial avulsion of the vastus medialis muscle at the superior aspect of the patella occurs in dancers who are improperly trained. This injury generally is uncommon in young athletes.

Jumper's Knee. During jumping, the knee is snapped into extension. If the ligaments are taut, this could lead to stretching of the medial collateral ligament and capsule and thereafter to jumper's syndrome and degenerative changes about the knee. Laxity of the knee ligaments is seen particularly in late starters who are forcing turnout, and especially in male dancers.

Retropatellar Irritation. Retropatellar irritation can happen when students are repeatedly asked to pull up on their thighs to give the appearance of a mildly hyperextended knee.

Screwing the Knee. Screwing the knee occurs when the dancer attempts, before being properly warmed up, position V, in which the hips and feet are turned out and the lateral side of one foot lies against the medial side of the other. To gain more turnout, the dancer would then assume a demiplie position (i.e., one-half knee bend), allowing the 180°-positioning of the feet to be achieved first at the floor and then straighten the knees without moving the feet. This puts a great deal of torque on the knee and can produce medial knee strain and patellar subluxation.

Shin Splints. Shin splints seem to occur more often in dancers with a faulty jumping technique, including too much double heel strike (i.e., heel rise between landing and pushing off).

Rolling of the Foot. Rolling of the foot consists of increased calcaneal eversion with apparent collapse of the arch, subtalar joint pronation, and disengagement of the locking mechanism of the Chopart joint. This usually is associated with the dancer trying to force turnout at the feet without controlling it at the hip. Posterior tibial tendinitis and bunions can occur.

Sickling of the Foot. Sickling of the foot is a common fault that affects dance posture both when standing on pointe or on demipointe. Sickling in occurs with the heel pointed inward and the forefoot in varus. Sickling out occurs with the forefoot pointed outward. The most common causes are poor training and beginning dance after the foot has matured, when the adult foot has stiffened.

Plantar Fasciitis. Plantar fasciitis results from repetitive jumps, especially in dancers with an inelastic arch. It also can be the result of poor training habits, neglecting to perform a flexibility program during long periods of inactivity, and a vigorous rehearsal schedule after a vacation.

Knuckling Down. Knuckling down is a collapsing of the toes inside the pointe shoes. Instead of dancing on her pointes in the hard-pointe shoe, the dancer dances on the interphalangeal joint of the hallux. This often happens when the child dances on pointe before her young body has the training and ability required to perform such steps. This prevents the development of proper technique and throws the ankle, knee, hip, and spine out of balance. Epiphyseal fractures of the phalanges and Freiberg infarction of the metatarsal heads can occur.

Gripping the Floor. Gripping the floor is a sustained plantarflexion of the digits to attain stability during dance. This activity provides continuous stress on the flexor hallucis longus, flexor digitorum longus, and plantar intrinsic musculature.

Ankle Sprains. Ankle sprains are rare in full plantarflexion or pointe position because of the locking that occurs between the posterior lip of the tibia and the os calcis. Lesser degrees of plantarflexion, however, are potentially unstable because of the anatomy of this joint; therefore, the toe–heel gait, known as feeling the floor, that ballet dancers are taught to do, even in simple walking, is a potential cause of sprains. Certain choreographies and certain steps are particularly dangerous, such as the *entrechat* six for women and the double *saut de basque* for men.

Tibiotalar Impingement Syndromes. As a result of repetitive extreme plantarflexion, especially in ankles with unfused os trigonum (7%), posterior compression or block can occur, leading to exostosis or stenosing tenosynovitis of the flexor hallucis longus with or without triggering. Similarly, because of repetitive extreme dorsiflexion, anterior impingement can occur, especially in young dancers with long, slender, flexible feet and with exostosis formation at the medial malleolus tip and the talar neck.

Lisfranc Joint Injuries. The hyperflexed position of the forefoot puts the foot at greatest risk for injury through this joint. Unlike the usual anatomic configuration in the plantigrade foot, in which the foot and leg act as separate levers with the ankle acting as an interposing articulation, in full plantarflexion the distal leg and hindfoot form one long lever with stress concentration at the tarsometatarsal junction. In running, the flexor hallucis longus is important for push-off; in ballet, it is the Achilles tendon of the foot when the dancer is on pointe. In addition, the Lisfranc joint serves as the locking mechanism for the entire tarsometatarsal complex, mainly because of the rigid socket formed by the medial and lateral cuneiforms around the second metatarsal base. This special anatomy appears to predispose it to injury.

Stress Fractures

The following sequential general scheme has been proposed to explain stress fracture occurrence:

- Increased muscular forces and increased rate of remodeling
- Resorption and rarefaction
- Focal trabecular microfractures
- Periosteal or endosteal response
- Linear stress fracture

Many predisposing factors such as forefoot varus and limited subtalar motion have been postulated. In general, however, the combination of a less-than-optimum shape with a high level of motivation and a relatively undisciplined method of training seems to set the stage for stress fracture.

Mechanisms might differ between age groups. In the femoral neck, for example, compression stress fracture is the most common in young people, whereas the more serious transverse fracture is more common in older people. In the middle tibia, distraction may be more important than compression in starting a fatigue fracture and therefore in determining the orientation of an infarction. The upper one-third of the tibia is the most frequently involved site in children and adolescents because it is in this site that the thinnest segment of tibial cortex is noted. In teenagers, this is entirely osteonal bone.

Shin splints can be considered as a special case of stress fractures. Several theories have been proposed to explain this pathologic process: damage of soft tissue—muscles, tendons, and ligaments; stress fractures or periosteal irritation, or both; and vascular compromise secondary to increased compartment pressure. A recent theory that ties together all of these theories suggests that shin splints represent a continuum of injury that begins with stress overload (111). The undue stress leads to muscle fatigue and muscle injury. The weakness of the soft tissue supporting mechanism results in loss of shock absorption. This, in turn, can lead to periostitis, stress fracture, or even a complete fracture. Any point of this continuum represents a shin splint injury.

Spondylolysis

The following hypotheses have been raised on the etiology of spondylolysis:

- Separate ossification centers
- Birth fracture
- Fracture during postnatal life
- Stress fracture
- Increased lumbar lordosis
- Impingement of the articular process on the pars articularis
- Weakness of supporting structures (e.g., fascia, spinal ligaments, intervertebral disks)
- Pathologic changes in the pars articularis
- Dysplasia of the pars interarticularis

Most authors agree, however, that mechanical factors are the cause or at least the trigger of the development of spondylolysis, especially when congenital abnormalities are present. In some cases, axial loading of only about 3,000 N (600 lb) is sufficient to produce a fracture in the isthmus of the neural arch if the spine is maintained in hyperlordosis. Torsion of the spinal column combined with hyperlordosis and repetitive axial loading further encourages propagation of this fracture. Another study showed that pars interarticularis are those elements of the lumbar vertebra most likely to fail because of loads produced during normal motion activity such as forward bending and lifting.

In ballet dancers, at least two predisposing factors can be pointed out, usually related to lifting technique: a too-small weight difference between male and female partners (i.e., <35 lb) and a hyperlordotic posture. With regard to the latter, it is known anatomically that tilting the pelvis backward allows increased external rotation at the hip because the acetabular shelf is much deeper posterosuperiorly than it is posteroinferiorly. Unfortunately, many dancers, especially young ones, use this trick to obtain a few more degrees of turnout at the hips.

MUSIC THERAPY IN PHYSICAL MEDICINE AND REHABILITATION

Music therapy (117,139) is defined as a systematic process of intervention wherein the therapist helps the client to achieve health, using musical experiences and the relationships that develop through them as dynamic forces of change.

Much of the music therapy that was done in the early years of this field was done with adults in psychiatric hospitals and with children with special needs. In more recent years, music therapy has become more accepted in general hospitals, and its uses in medical and dental work have been explored. Many of the applications of music therapy in occupational musculoskeletal medicine are derived from work in these related fields.

With recent awareness of the connections between the mind and the body, the ability of music to engage the whole person has made it a natural tool for healing.

Music therapy as a profession developed following World War II. During the war, musicians assisted in psychiatric hospitals, and therapeutic effects of the music were observed. The National Association for Music Therapy, Inc. (NAMT) was formed in 1950, and educational requirements for training music therapists were formalized. In the intervening years, an additional association, the American Association for Music Therapy (AAMT), has been formed, codes of ethics have been developed, and certification requirements have been established by the Certification Board for Music Therapists (CBMT).

Music therapy may be applied to the following areas in the treatment of musculoskeletal disorders: supplementing physical therapy and movement, pain relief, relaxation and stress reduction, and working through emotional areas that may be contributing to the disorder.

Much of the literature in music therapy with physical rehabilitation is in the area of supplementing physical therapy and movement. As documented in Staum's reviews of music therapy literature in this area, a number of these techniques have been experimentally validated (118,119). One experimental study used audioanalgesia as an adjunct to mobilization of the chronic frozen shoulder and found better results with regard to improvement of range of motion, rate of regaining motion, and the length of time required to achieve the results among the audioanalgesia group (120).

Recent research by Thaut and his colleagues has been on the use of auditory rhythm superimposed on physical movement and supports the relationship between rhythm and human motion (121–125). The results of this research suggest that using rhythmic repetition accompanied by an external beat may help people with Parkinson's disease and those who have had strokes and traumatic brain injury work on flexion–extension patterns, grasp-and-hold patterns, and exercises for range of motion, strength, and endurance.

Effects of Music on Pain

Researchers agree that two main factors influence the pain experience. The first is the organic sensory component, and the second is the affective component, including cognitive processes such as anxiety, attention, and anticipation (126). The latter component is sometimes labeled as the reactive or emotional component (127). Long and Johnson suggest that because anxiety contributes to pain enhancement, the relief of anxiety should be one of the methods of pain reduction (128). Music acts as a diverting or distracting stimulus to a patient suffering from pain in that it redirects the attention given to pain onto something more pleasing. Auditory stimulation has a positive effect on the body that can be related to the gate control theory of pain (127). This theory states that the stimuli's passage through the neocortical and central nervous system inhibits the release of neurotransmitters by the production of specific hormones (129). This, in effect, causes closure of the gate, and thus, diversion from the attention of pain decreases the nature of the stimulus.

A controlled experiment conducted by Zimmerman et al. indicated that listening to music with a positive suggestion of pain reduction has an effect on cancer patients' pain (127). Analysis tools included the Visual Analog Scale (VAS) and the McGill Pain Questionnaire (MPQ). Those patients who did listen, in the dark, to 30 minutes of personally selected "relaxing" music significantly lowered their pretest MPQ and VAS scores.

In a controlled study, Schorr investigated the use of music as a transformative means of altering the perception of chronic pain among women with rheumatoid arthritis (130). The two subject groups showed a statistically significant drop ($F = 32.67, p < 0.001$) in their Pain Rating Intensity scale of the MPQ. This study indicated that the pain perception threshold increased while the patient listened to music and that patients, at least for the duration of the intervention, were able to move beyond their joint pain limitations.

In Wolfe's controlled experiment, music was utilized as treatment for patients experiencing chronic pain, with focus on verbal interaction within a group setting, thus refocusing the attention/perception of pain (126). Patient data were collected for 2 weeks regarding activity level and verbal behavior (the response to a set of 12 questions concerning the patients well-being). A typical patient response showed increased positive verbalization and decreased negative responses, and physical activity increased by the end of the second week.

Barker presented a controlled study to show the effect of music, in addition to relaxation techniques, on the reduction of pain during debridement in burn victims (131). Variables such as perceived pain, heart rate, and behavioral responses to pain were recorded and evaluated. Five patients, who served as their own controls, had burns that covered from 5% to 48.5% of their body surface. Music and Progressive Muscle Relaxation (PMR) were administered at every other treatment period for 2 weeks. Results of the Wilcoxon Matched Pair Signed Rank Test for computed heart rates—considered an indicator of pain, stress, and tension—showed that there was a significant increase after debridement without music (critical value 83, $a = 0.01$), while the use of music and PMR functioned to maintain heart rate at the predebridement levels (critical value 91, $a = 0.01$). For the Behavioral Indicator of Pain Chart, a chi-square test showed a significant difference between pain and no pain, and levels of pain decreased in conditions with music ($a = 0.05$, 1 *df*).

Effect of Music on Gait

Various controlled experiments have involved music, specifically rhythmic auditory stimuli, as a superimposed structure in facilitating proprioceptive control of rhythmic gait. One study performed by Staum involved subjects who would listen to individually determined music and rhythmic percussive sounds and attempt to match their footsteps to the stimuli (132). As rhythmic control increased, stimulus conditions were gradually faded, and independence of the motor gain was established. Subjects were children with various gait disorders who listened to two groups of tapes, one with five musical selections and one with rhythmic pulses.

Overall results indicated that all subjects experienced an increase in rhythmic, even walking and/or consistency in speed. Dependent measures included cadence inconsistencies counted in consecutive 10-second intervals and cumulative timed deviations between footfalls in hundredths of a second. Additionally, observational ratings of improvement of randomly arranged videotape segments of baseline and treatment conditions were recorded. A special rating grid was used with 15 gait parameters including balance, rhythm, width between feet, amount of foot contact, foot elevation, speed, and stride length.

Specific results included a gain of rhythmic balance in 45% of patients. Forty-one percent of the subjects improved with only a 2- to 3-second deviation between footfalls. Arrhythmic walking demonstrated a slight increase at the end of fading for 32% and continuous improvement over time for an additional 52%. Consistency in speed improved for 68%, whereas 12% did not improve. Proprioceptive control of rhythmic walking was best facilitated in hemiparetic stroke patients, spastic disorders, and painful arthritic or scoliotic conditions.

In a controlled design, Eni used music, through its sensory effects, to lead to autonomic and physiological reactions in patients suffering from Parkinson's disease, specifically with a gait disorder in knee joint flexion (133). His basis for the use of music as a rehabilitative therapy is that the problem for a patient confronted with Parkinson's disease is primarily failure to call-up the appropriate anticipatory postural reflex. Patients with Parkinson's disease had been observed to achieve more spontaneous movements with musical accompaniment than without. Two groups of four patients, fitted with an electrogoniometer at the left knee, walked with and without music along a 60-m walkway for five trials. There was a significant effect of music on knee flexion, as subjects performed better in the music group (cross trials average of 62 of knee flexion) than in the no-music group (cross trials average of 47 of knee flexion). There was a significant effect for the interaction between the group factor and the music factor at the $p = 0.05$ level.

In a controlled experiment, Thaut and Rice investigated the effect of musical rhythm on temporal parameters of the stride cycle and EMG activity in gait of stroke victims (134). Ten subjects were used in three trials that consisted of a baseline walk without rhythm and a walk with rhythm matched to the cadence of the baseline walk. The data were recorded by two parameters, a surface EMG in the gastrocnemius muscle and pressure-sensitive voltage-coded switch mats on the dual walkway. The percentage change scores from no-rhythm to rhythm conditions showed several significant changes ($p = 0.05$). Variables of improvement included stride symmetry, decreased EMG activity on the affected side, decreased variability of integrated amplitude ratios, and increased muscle activation during the midstance push-off phase of the affected side. The specificity of changes in muscle activation and improvement in temporal gait parameters suggest a strong effect of auditory rhythmic cues on temporal gait control in stroke patients.

Effect of Music on Physiological and Psychological Stress Indicators

During the past 12 years, Spintge and Droh have conducted various controlled studies that utilized music as nonverbal communicative means for preventing patients from experiencing stress in a perioperative environment (135). Approximately 8,000 patients were studied, and the clinical follow-up of 62,000 patients was recorded. Five categories of music could be chosen according to the patient's preference. In addition to the pre- and postoperative questionnaires, interviews, State–Trait Anxiety Inventory (STAI), mean arterial blood pressure (MABP), heart rate, and plasma levels of stress hormones, e.g., norepinephrine and adrenocorticotropic (ACTH), were recorded. The music group showed significantly lowered plasma levels of norepinephrine, thus suggesting less perioperative stress.

Steelman studied the effects of tranquil intraoperative music on blood pressure in a group of patients undergoing surgery (136). The changes in systolic and diastolic blood pressure from pre- to postoperative status were analyzed using paired t-tests. Mean change in systolic pressure in the control group was not statistically significant ($M = -0.27$ mm Hg, $t = -0.10$, $p = 0.46$). In the experimental group there was a significant decrease in systolic blood pressure ($M = 6.48$ mm Hg, $t = 2.098$, $p = 0.024$). For diastolic pressure, there was a nonsignificant increase between pre- and postoperative measurements for the control group ($M = 1.41$ mm Hg, $t = -0.76$, $p = 0.27$). There was a statistically significant decrease in diastolic pressure for the experimental group ($M = 5.24$ mm Hg, $t = 2.79$, $p < 0.01$).

Kaempf and Amodei evaluated the effect of music on the anxiety of patients in the operating room holding area (137). Two groups of 15 patients each, randomly selected, comprised the experimental and control groups. The experimental group listened to classical music for 20 minutes while in the holding area preceding surgery. After 20 minutes, each patient group completed the anxiety state portion of the STAI in addition to having their blood pressure, pulse rate, and respiration recorded. An independent t-test compared the control group to the experimental group with respect to the variables measured when they arrived at the waiting room area. For the experimental group, there was a marginally significant difference at the $p < 0.05$ level for systolic blood pressure between the pre- and postoperative measurements ($M = 3.12$ mm Hg, $t = 1.69$, $p = 0.055$). Additionally, there was a statistically significant reduction for the experimental group in respiratory rate at $p < 0.05$ ($M = 15.2$, $t = 3.22$, $p = 0.002$).

Biederman attempted to isolate the effects of musical tempo and entrainment on listeners' heart rates (138). The controlled experimental design comprised three different conditions of 6 minutes each, under which the heart rate responses of 19 adult nonmusicians were recorded and compared. The three conditions were randomly presented following a 3-minute baseline period. The first condition used music "entrained" at a tempo setting first equal to the initial heart rate of the listener and then eventually decreased. The second condition utilized the same music at a tempo setting equal to 10 beats per minute below the listener's initial heart rate. The third was a control condition of silence. The dependent measures were heart rate and a preference survey for the music.

Correlation testing was used to analyze the significance of heart-rate changes, averaged across each 1 minute of treatment, from baseline levels. The heart rate decreased significantly from baseline levels during two 1-minute intervals within both music conditions, i.e., entrained ($m = 67.70$, $p < 0.05$) and slow ($m = 68.00$, $p < 0.05$). The greatest decreases in heart rate from baseline levels occurred during the entrained condition during the third minute ($m = 67.25$, $p < 0.01$). There was no significant difference, however, in heart-rate responses among the three overall treatment conditions as determined by a one-way analysis of variance and ANOVA. The entrainment procedure using music may offer a mechanism for decreasing listener heart rate. Additional research is necessary in order to yield these levels statistically differentiated from other treatment conditions.

OTHER CREATIVE ARTS THERAPIES

In addition to music therapy, other arts have been used as media for therapy. Art, dance/movement, drama, and poetry have each become the basis for an approach to therapy. Each is represented by a professional association, and each has its own literature.

Although few applications in the literature are specifically to occupational musculoskeletal disorders, see *Current Research in Arts Medicine* edited by Bejjani (139), *The Expressive Arts Therapies* by Feder and Feder (140), and *The Arts in Therapy* by Fleshman and Fryrear (141) as well as *The Arts in Psychotherapy,* a journal, and the professional journals in each field, for applications of these therapies.

SELECTED CASE REPORTS

Case 1

JF, 40 years old, is a male professional pianist. After a sudden change in repertoire, he started feeling pain and swelling in the thenar area of his right hand. Physical examination showed the presence of an anatomic variation consisting of a connection between the flexor pollicis longus and the flexor indicis longus, such that extreme flexion of the thumb forced the distal interphalangeal joint of the index into flexion (Fig. 64-16). This anatomic variation was first described by Lundborg (110). When sudden and sustained overexertion occurs, the presence of this abnormal connection was thought to cause symptoms of increased pressure and ischemia in the thenar muscles, associated with compartment syndrome. Surgical release of the connection and fasciotomy of the thenar muscles was performed; relief of symptoms was obtained.

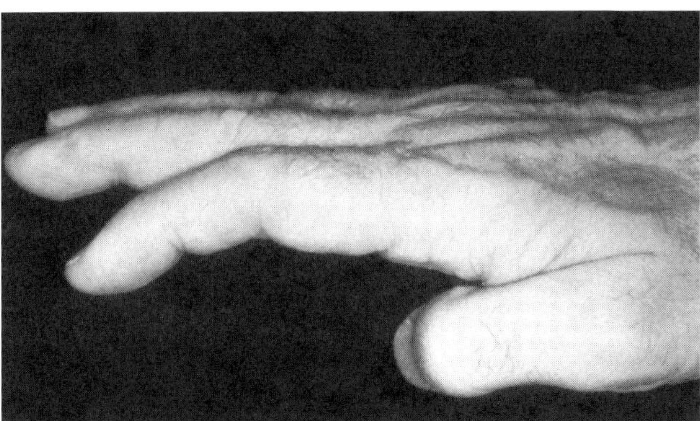

FIG. 64-16. JF, a 40-year-old man who is a professional pianist. The right hand demonstrates the effect of the Lundborg connection between the thumb and index flexor tendons.

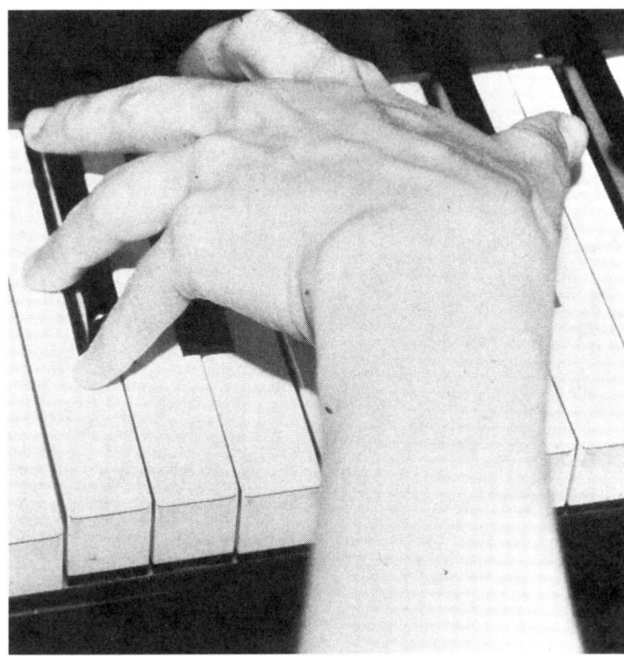

FIG. 64-17. KM, a 31-year-old woman who is a professional pianist, has flexor carpi ulnaris tendinitis of the left wrist. Notice the excessive ulnar deviation and the strain in the finger extensors.

Case 2

KM, 31 years old, is a female professional pianist. She presented with chronic flexor carpi ulnaris tendinitis of the left wrist. During playing, she was using excessive ulnar deviation of her wrist (Fig. 64-17). Visual postural feedback was used, and correction of the wrist technique obtained the relief of symptoms.

Case 3

PM, 29 years old, is a female professional pianist. She presented with a 7-year history of curling and loss of control of the right ring and small fingers (Fig. 64-18). She had been seen by many physicians, and the last one had performed two consecutive operations 2 years before her visit: a release of the junctura tendinae of the ring finger, then an intrinsic fasciotomy on same. These only aggravated her loss of stability and control of the fourth and fifth MCP joints; moreover, her wrist had to fall into excessive palmarflexion to attempt to stabilize them during playing (see Fig. 64-18). An orthosis was designed to limit fifth MCP extension and eventually generate some scarring of the palmar structures (Fig. 64-19). This was found to simulate the effect of a Zancolli palmar plate advancement procedure, but without the surgical morbidity. Bilateral intermittent electrical muscle stimulation of her wrist extensors also was used during playing to correct wrist position through modification of the proprioceptive sensory feedback (Fig. 64-20). The results were very encouraging, and the patient is back to concertizing.

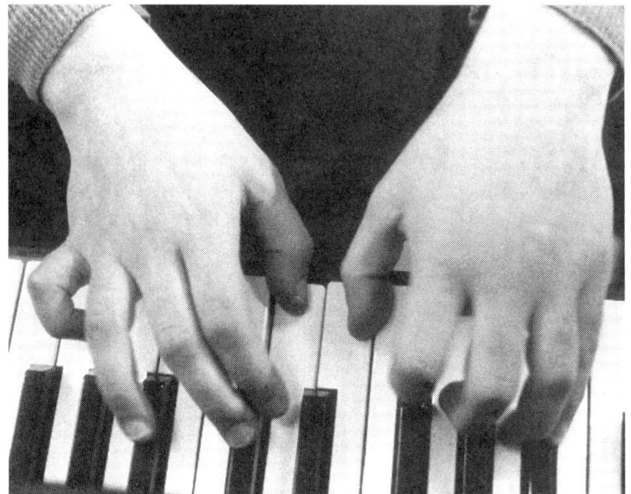

FIG. 64-18. PM, a 29-year-old woman who is a professional pianist. Notice the drooping of the wrists and the curling of the right ring and smaller fingers.

Case 4

LC, 22 years old, is a female professional violinist. She could play for barely 10 minutes before pain on the dorsum of the left fourth and fifth MCPs would stop her. Physical examination showed tenderness in this area, along with severe bilateral hyperlaxity of the joints of the hand. In particular, a loose fourth web and hyperextensibility of the fifth MCP joint were interfering with her ability to perform a vibrato of the fourth (Fig. 64-21*A*). The diagnosis was interosseous overuse syndrome secondary to hyperlaxity. LC was placed on an individualized hand exercise program using EMG biofeedback. Visual postural feedback also was used to position her elbow in slight abduction while playing, such that her fifth MCP joint would remain flexed and the small finger would fall naturally on the string (Fig. 64-21*B*). A year later, LC is pain-free, and she has been able to pursue her career and expand her repertoire considerably.

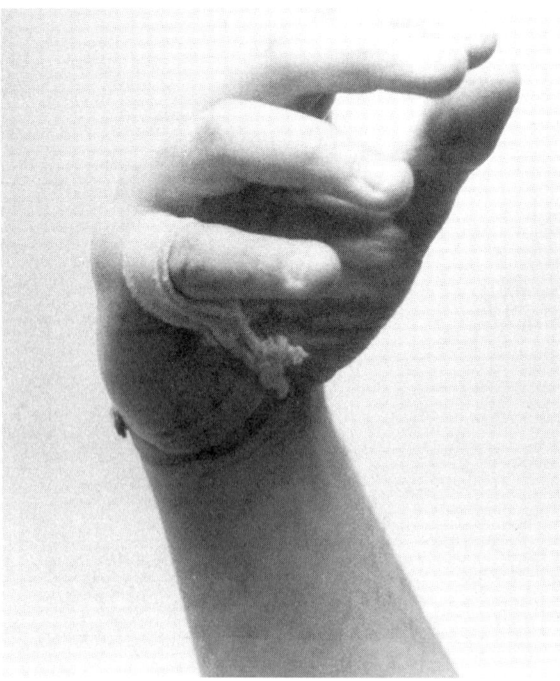

FIG. 64-19. An orthotic device to limit extension, consisting of a cloth sling around the small finger connected to a bracelet by an elastic band.

Case 5

SP, 32 years old, is a female professional cellist. She complained of intermittent pain in the base of her left thumb. In the high register, her first MCP joint would go into hyperextension (20°), and the first ray into a zig-zag position, known to generate stress concentration (Fig. 64-22). Visual postural feedback was used, and SP progressively corrected her thumb position, obtaining relief of symptoms.

Case 6

JL, 62 years old, is a male professional bassist. He presented with a lifelong history of inability to form calluses at his left fingertips. He had been performing as principal bassist in a major orchestra with leather fingertips (Fig. 64-23). He admitted that when he started playing his instrument, the pain was intolerable, and his family suggested he protect his fingers in this fashion rather than tolerate the discomfort until calluses eventually formed. This went on for more than 40 years, and he now is totally incapable of playing without his leather fingers. Examination of the middle, ring, and small fingertips showed hypoesthesia and trophic changes such as paper-thin skin and atrophy of the fat pads.

Case 7

ET, 23 years old, is a female student bassist. She presented with intermittent pain and paresthesias of her left medial elbow, radiating to the ulnar side of the hand. Symptoms were consistent with paroxystic ulnar tunnel syndrome. During playing, she was found to place her left elbow in extreme flexion (160°), possibly impinging the ulnar nerve when this position was sustained (Fig. 64-24*A*). Further assessment showed a marked discrepancy between the size of her instrument and the height of the pin, and her anthropometry (Fig. 64-24*B*). Visual postural feedback was used, attempting to modify pin height and musician-instrument contact, and ET was advised to try a smaller-sized instrument.

Case 8

DMW, 22 years old, is a female professional violinist. She presented with a chronically sore left shoulder. Physical examination was positive for mild subacromial bursitis with early subscapularis tendinitis. DMW routinely was using a

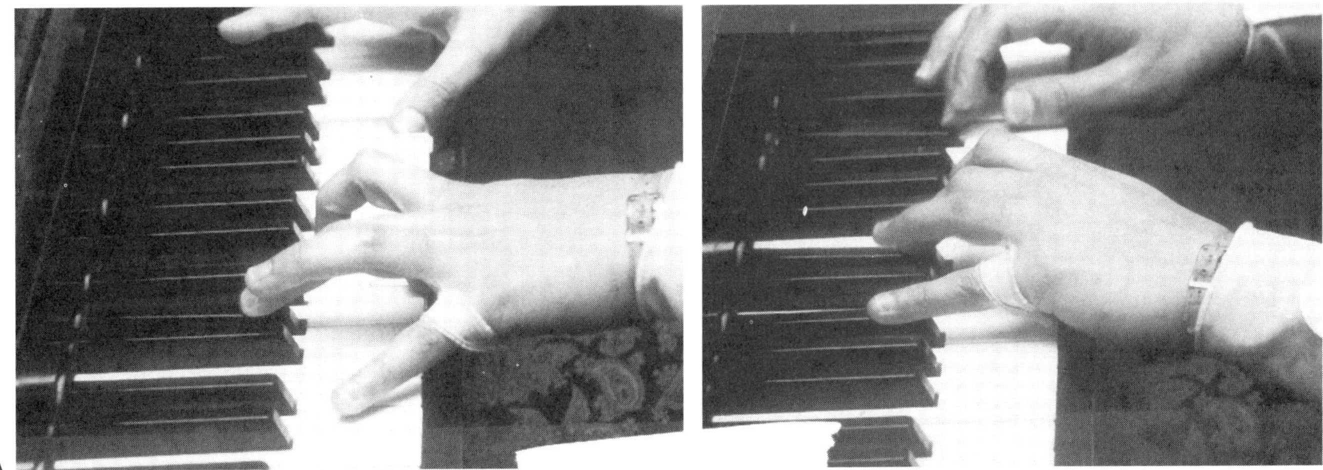

FIG. 64-20. PM, a professional pianist, with the orthosis (see Fig. 64-19) on her small finger, which is hooked to the dual-channel electric muscle stimulation (EMS) device. **A:** When the EMS is off, the left wrist droops, and the ring finger tends to curl. **B:** When the EMS is on, the wrist is slightly extended and the arches of the hand are normal.

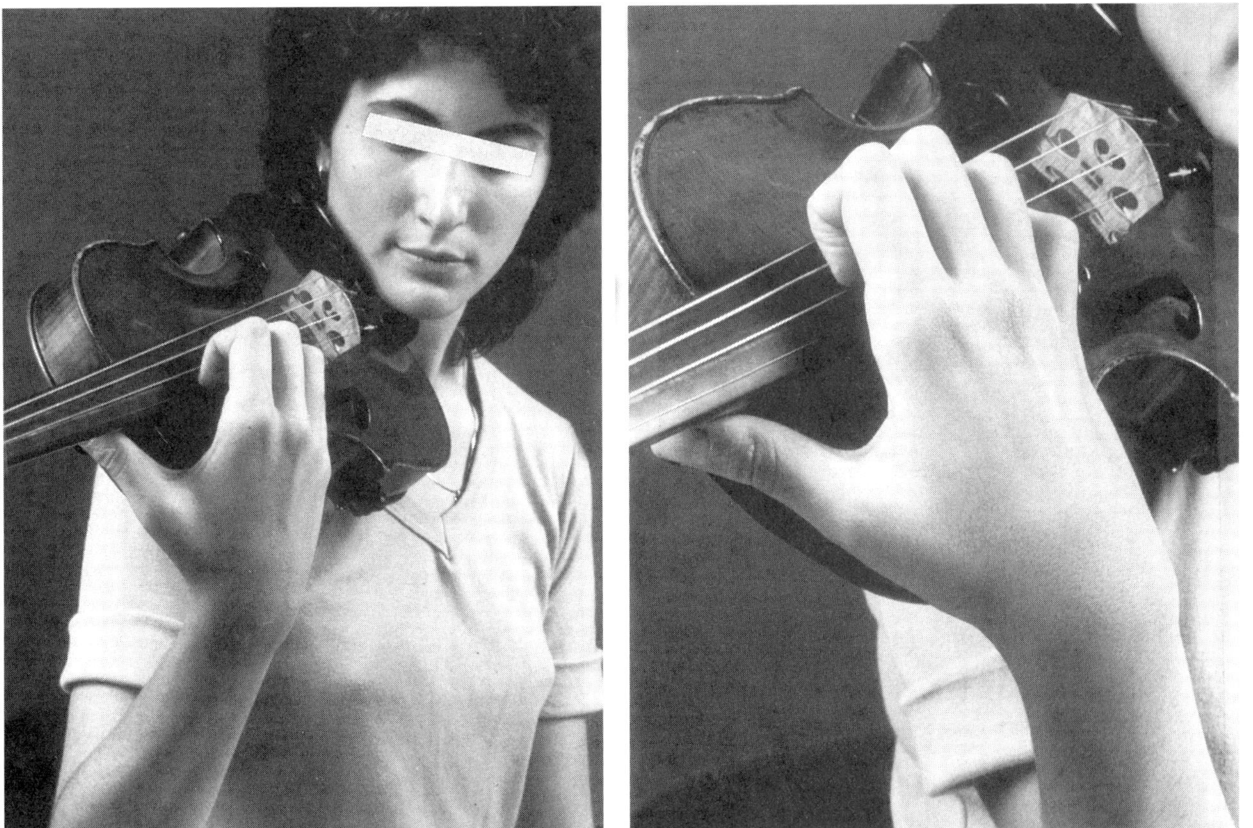

FIG. 64-21. **A:** LC, a 22-year-old woman who is a professional violinist. Notice the hyperextension of the small finger metacarpophalangeal joint. **B:** Slight abduction of the left shoulder allows the small finger to fall naturally on the string by reducing metacarpophalangeal extension.

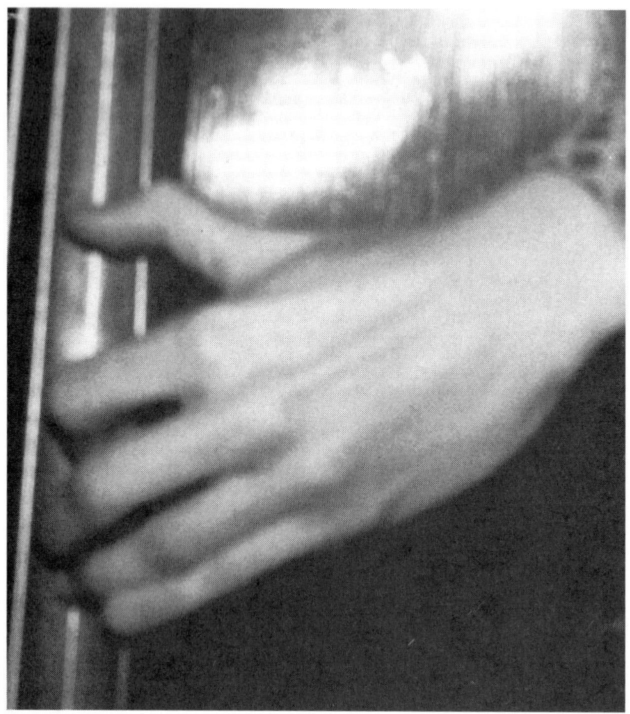

FIG. 64-22. SP, a 32-year-old woman who is a professional cellist. Notice the hyperextension of the first metacarpophalangeal joint in the high register.

double-thickness foam, connected to the violin with a rubber band, as a shoulder rest (Fig. 64-25*A*). This was replaced with a one-third-inch thick, moldable neoprene adjustable shoulder rest available on the market (Fig. 64-25*C*). The device was made to conform to the patient's shoulder anatomy, such that pressure was more evenly distributed. It also was hoped that the increased friction thus created would offset some of the weight of the instrument and decrease the antigravitational load on the shoulder muscles (Fig. 64-25*B*). It took several readjustments and 6 weeks to acclimate the patient to this new shoulder rest. Her shoulder symptoms gradually subsided.

Case 9

EMV, 48 years old, is a female professional harpist. She presented with radicular pain in the left upper extremity, exacerbated by performing. Physical examination pointed to a mild left C6 radiculopathy that was later confirmed by needle EMG. Cervical radiography showed degenerative changes in the C5-6 disk. Observation of harpists' performance shows a universal tendency to left neck rotation and slight flexion to read the music score placed on the stand as they play (Fig. 64-26). As in the case of EMV, this posture can be accentuated by shortsightedness and inadequate eyeglasses. This sustained quasistatic asymmetric neck position was believed to be responsible for the symptoms described.

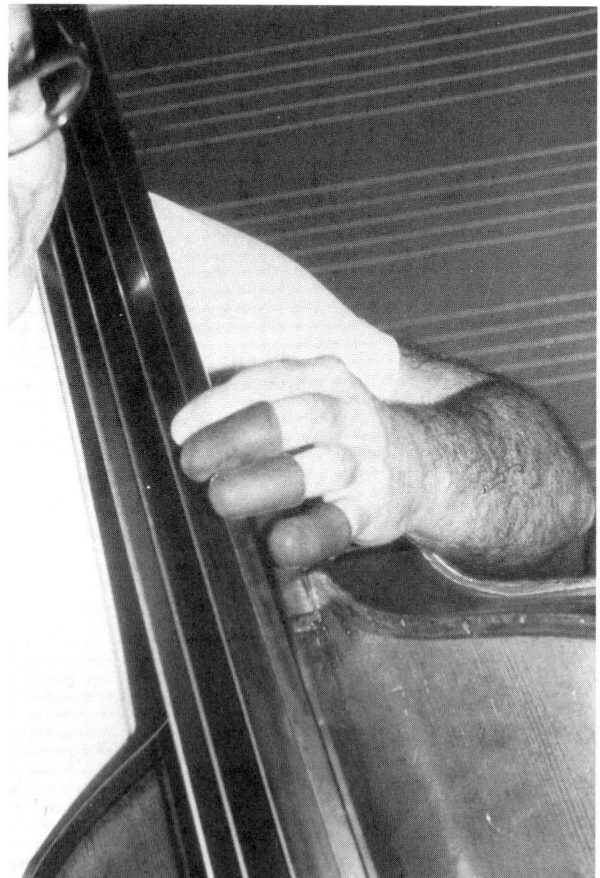

A

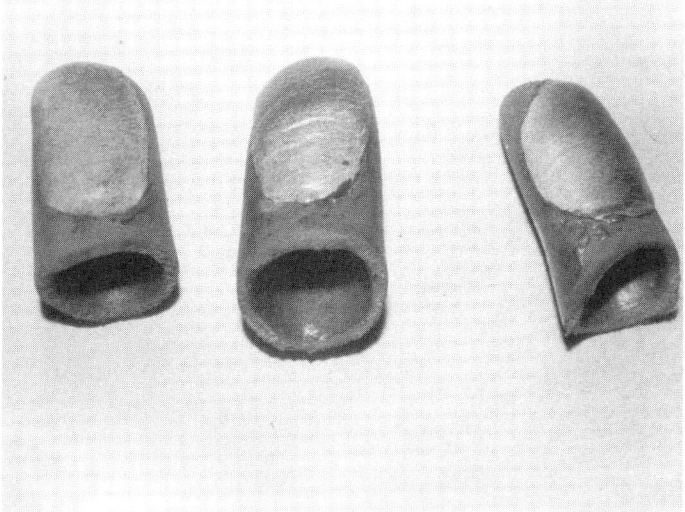

B

FIG. 64-23. A: JL, a 62-year-old man who is a professional bassist, plays with leather protection on his left small, ring, and middle finger tips. **B:** JL's leather fingers.

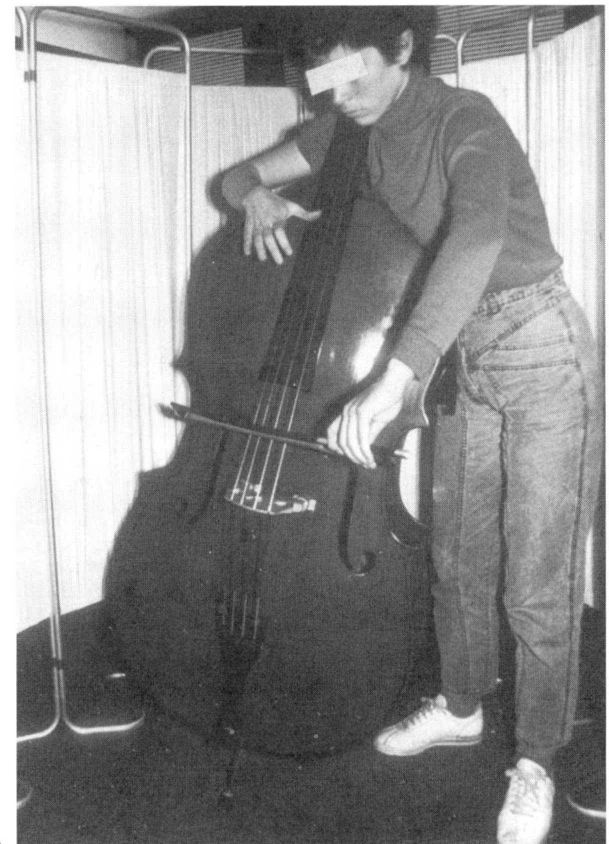
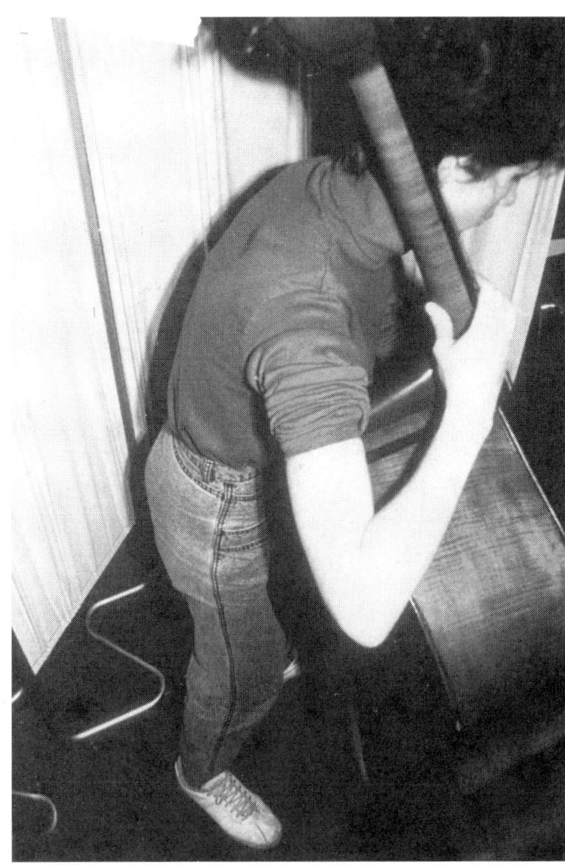

A B

FIG. 64-24. A: ET, a 23-year-old woman who is a student bassist. Notice the excessive flexion of the left elbow. **B:** The pin height is excessive, and there is a discrepancy between the musician's and instrument's sizes.

The patient was prescribed frequent neck range-of-motion and stretching exercises before, during, and after playing. Memorizing scores as much as possible and moving the music stand to the right side of the harp were also recommended. Nonsteroidal antiinflammatory drugs (NSAIDs) also were prescribed intermittently to help alleviate the pain during busy performance periods.

Case 10

SRD, 33 years old, is a male professional guitarist. He presented with a 6-month history of mild tremor and loss of coordination of his left middle finger. Physical examination showed a mild radial instability of the left third MCP joint as compared to the right. This was believed to be the sequela of a mild radial collateral ligament sprain. When he played chords, a slightly exaggerated spread of the second web was noticed (Fig. 64-27). The patient was prescribed specific hand-strengthening exercises with putties of incremental strength. Symptoms subsided after 3 months.

Case 11

LP, 25 years old, is a female semiprofessional rock guitarist. She presented with a 6-month history of left neck pain shooting down to the left radial fingers, which started abruptly while she was playing the guitar. Physical therapy and NSAIDs did not relieve the symptoms. A specially designed guitar strap (Spins International, Williamsburg, PA) was prescribed because it has the following ergonomic features: breadth of strap almost double that of ordinary straps, which is likely to decrease pressure on the shoulder by increasing the contact area; nature and thickness of the strap material, which is likely to decrease pressure further by absorbing some of the weight of the guitar (i.e., 8 lb in this case); right shoulder position instead of the usual left shoulder position, to increase the mechanical advantage of the neck muscles in counteracting the torque created by the weight of the guitar by reducing the lever arm; and direct attachment to the center-of-gravity area of the guitar instead of the usual two-point attachment, to better balance the instrument and divide its weight evenly between the two sides of the strap (Fig. 64-28). After 6 months of using this strap, LP was symptom-free. She has increased her practicing and rehearsal time considerably and is in the process of making a recording with her group. Research is under way to verify *in vivo,* using dynamic EMG, the theoretical advantages of the strap described above. It is forseeable that similar straps could be beneficial with other instruments, such as saxophone, bassoon, and oboe.

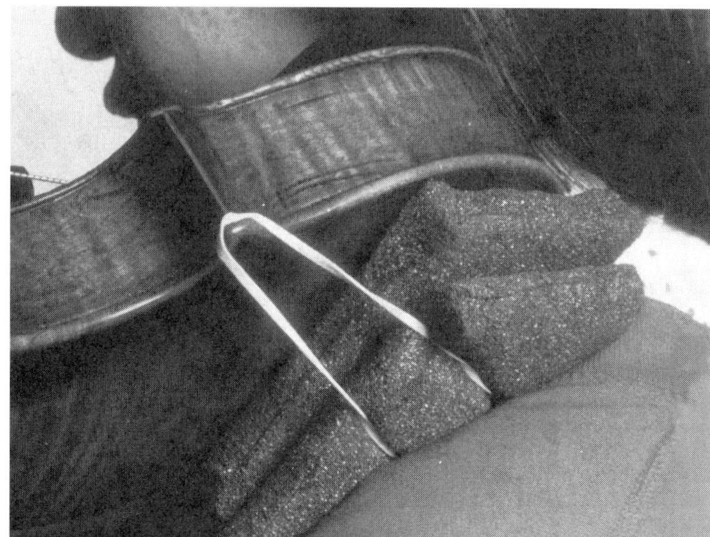

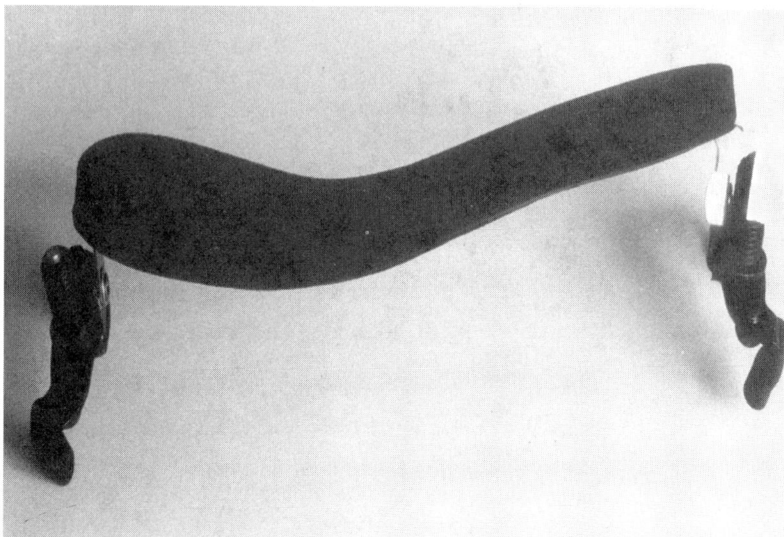

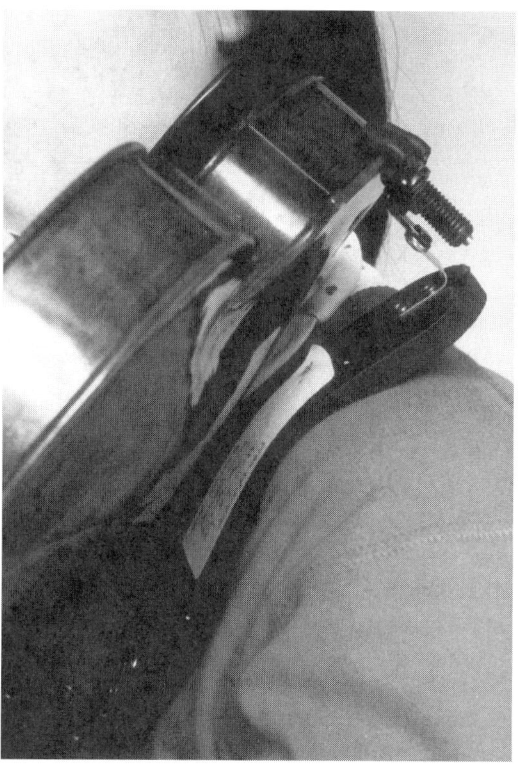

FIG. 64-25. A: DW, a professional violinist using two layers of sponges and a rubber band for shoulder rest. Notice the uneven load distribution and instability of the device. **B:** Thick, rigid foam, moldable shoulder rest. **C:** DW using the rigid foam, anatomically moldable shoulder rest.

Case 12

This 44-year-old professional man was seen for two sessions (117). He was referred for help dealing with stress that contributed to severe back and leg pain, which he had had for 6 months. He said that he had fallen 2 years earlier and that his back pain was related to a disk problem.

He arrived at the first appointment carrying a large pillow that he used to decrease his pain as he sat and required a special chair in which to sit. He reported that his entire life revolved around his pain and how to cope with it, which created many restrictions. He said that although he enjoyed listening to music, he generally listened to talk radio. Cognitively, it was noted that he seemed to feel that he could not change certain aspects of himself, including those that contributed to his stress. For example, he spoke of working very hard in a stressful job, but with no awareness that his attitudes and behavior contributed to the stress.

In the first session, this patient was first encouraged to utilize music to help relieve his stress by listening to relaxing, enjoyable music rather than talk radio while driving. Second, he was shown progressive relaxation and imagery techniques and encouraged to use them in conjunction with relaxing music. In the session, progressive relaxation was demonstrated as he tensed and then released parts of his body, in sequence from his feet to his head and then back to his feet. The use of imagery was demonstrated as he was told to image being in an outdoor place in which he could relax. Third, the importance of his cognitions in dealing with stress was discussed. He was encouraged to see how his attitudes and the messages that he gave himself perpetuated and increased his stress. He was going on a vacation and was encouraged to utilize these techniques, with relaxing music as a cue, while he was gone.

He returned for his second and final session a month later. He entered without the pillow and said that he could sit on any chair. He reported having utilized the techniques, particularly the progressive relaxation and imagery with relaxing music, and was feeling much better. Much of the pain seemed to have gone, and he was creating a more relaxed environment for himself. The session was spent discussing these changes and how to generalize them to other situations, followed by imagery with autogenic relaxation techniques, again utilizing relaxing music as a cue for relaxation. The autogenic relaxation techniques involved having him visualize various parts of his body as heavy and relaxed.

This patient, who had only two sessions, seemed able to utilize these techniques on his own to continue the reduction of stress and the back and leg pain that the stress was exacerbating. The therapy appeared to have been successful in helping him to learn some techniques for changing the way that he viewed and dealt with stress in his life.

Case 13[1]

History. The patient is a 19-year-old professional ballet dancer. He was struck by an automobile while crossing the street as a pedestrian. The resulting injuries were: fracture

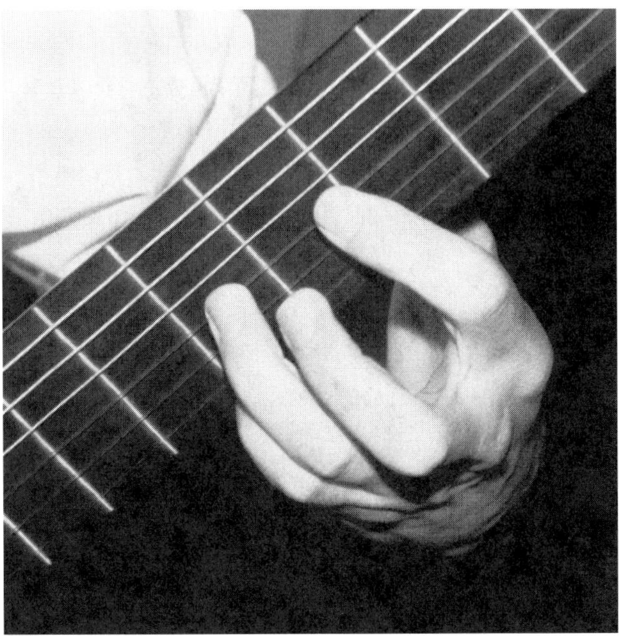

FIG. 64-27. SRD, a 33-year-old man who is a professional guitarist. When the left hand plays a chord, there is abnormal spread of the second web.

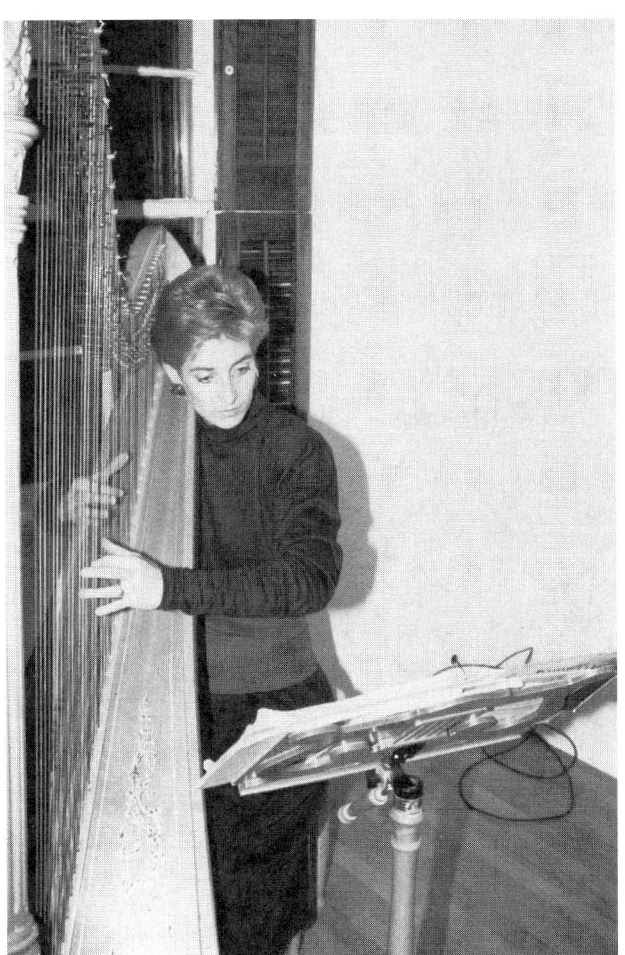

FIG. 64-26. Harpist playing while reading the score on the music stand.

of the left tibia/fibula, mild left peroneal nerve injury, left ankle lateral collateral ligament sprain and lumbar sprain/strain. The tibia was reduced surgically, and an IM rod was implanted. Four months post surgery, the question of returning to dance was considered. The patient was anxious to return to her profession. The surgeon was skeptical about safe return. To answer this delicate question, a performance analysis was ordered that included both the ballet positions one through five and a standard gait analysis, as well as an illustration of the ground reaction force vectors via force plate.

Study. Gait analysis confirmed a left limping pattern with a shortened step length and reduced stance phase. Kinematic analysis revealed a slight left knee terminal extension deficiency of 2° to 3°. Force platform analysis revealed a deficient weight translation from heel strike to forefoot push-off (Fig. 64-29).

The patient was asked to attempt various ballet positions, while standing on the force platform. The object of analysis was to determine if she could obtain and sustain a balanced left to right posture for each position. The analysis method utilized was Center of Pressure (COP) (Fig. 64-30).

Analysis revealed the patient was unable to hold or maintain any of the five positions in a center balance posture (Fig. 64-31*A,B*). Note the COP force vector of the uninjured leg is centered at the heel while the COP force vector of the injured subject is skewed more to the lateral side of the right foot.

Impression. The kinematic gait analysis confirmed continued gait asymmetry and left limb dysfunction. Kinetic balance posturogram during execution of standard ballet ex-

[1] The Ballet Dancer Case Study—Courtesy of Kinematic Consultants, Inc., Point Pleasant, NJ.

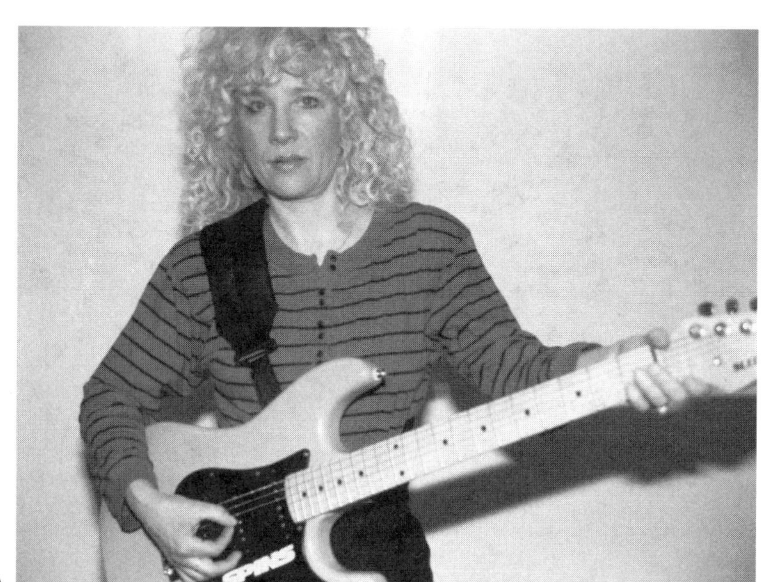

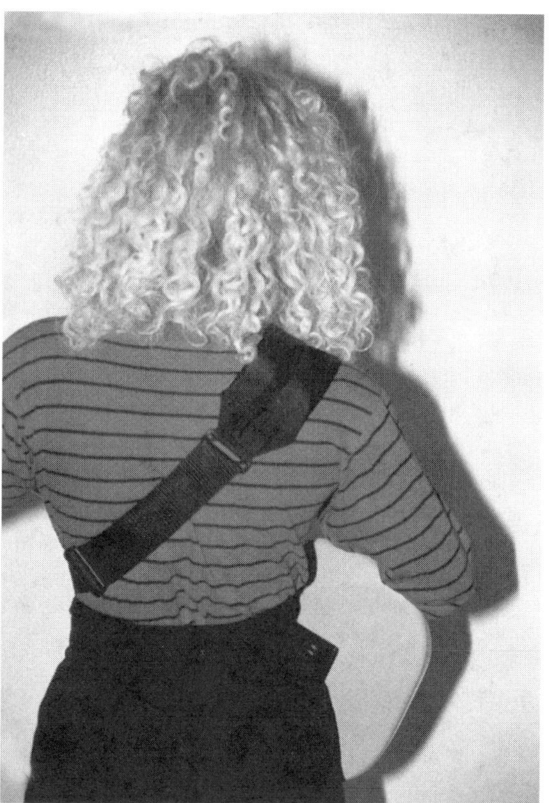

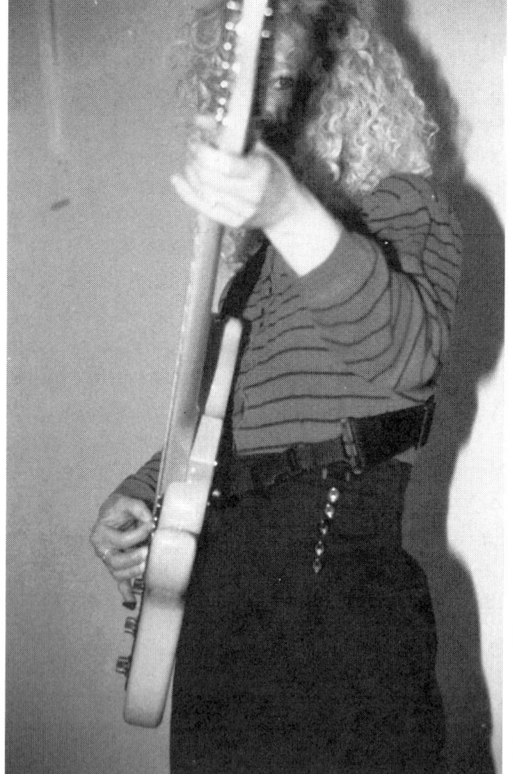

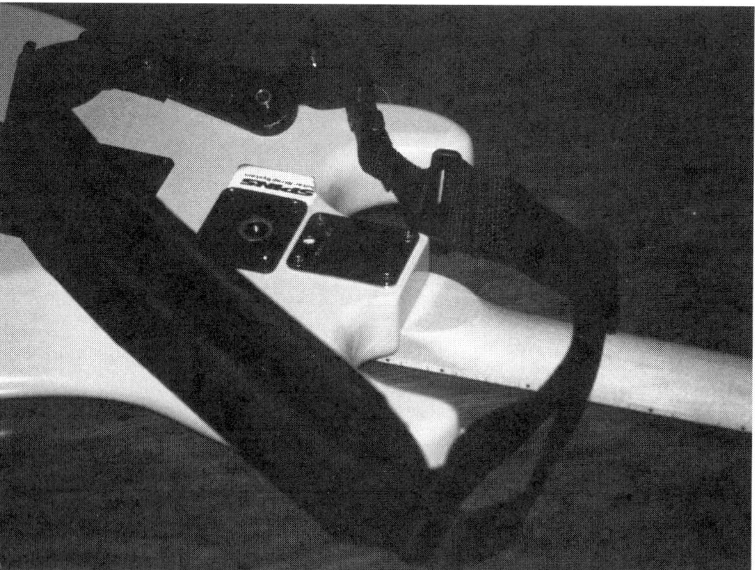

FIG. 64-28. LP, a 25-year-old woman who is a semiprofessional rock guitarist, using the Spins guitar strap. **A:** Front view. Note the position of the right shoulder and the breadth of the strap. **B:** Rear view. **C:** Left side view. Note the strap's attachment to the guitar and adjustability. **D:** Back of guitar with detached strap. Note the custom-applied attachment plate in the center-of-gravity area of the guitar and the thickness of strap material.

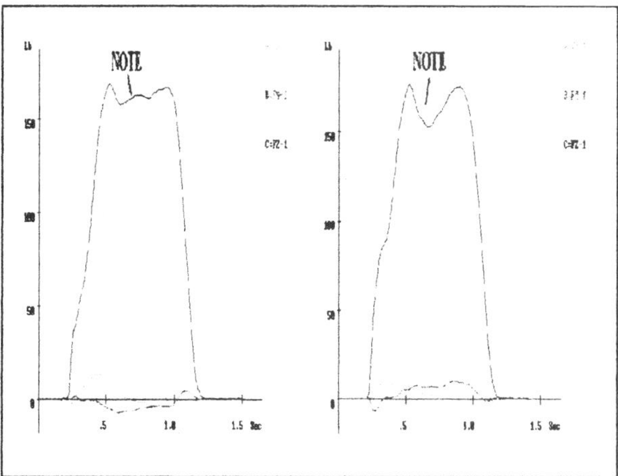

FIG. 64-29. Left vs. right stance ground reaction forces.

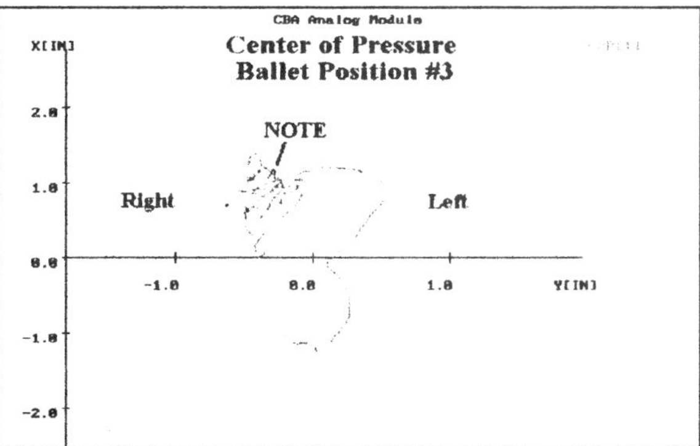

FIG. 64-30. COP posturogram—ballet position 3.

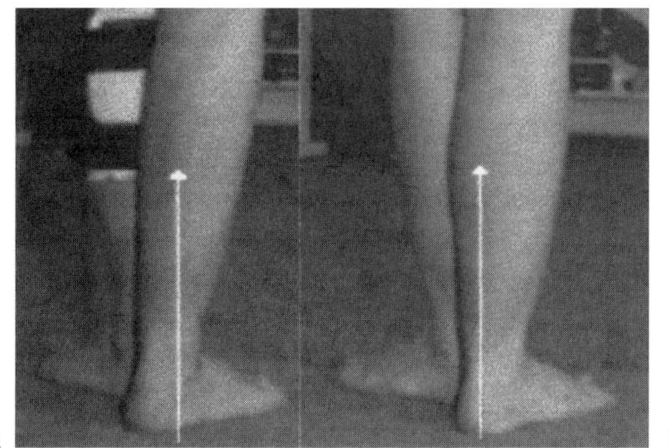

A B

FIG. 64-31. A: Injured ballet position 4. **B:** Normal ballet position 4.

ercise positions 1–5, confirmed the patient was unable to perform any ballet position in a center balanced posture. All five positions proved to be consistently skewed to the right

Outcome. The patient was unable to return to safe ballet training at that time. The patient needed to continue rehabilitation until balance and gait were symmetrical. Return to dance was postponed until a later date.

REFERENCES

1. Ziporyn T. Pianist's cramp to stage fright: the medical side of music-making. *JAMA* 1984; 252:985–989.
2. Bejjani FJ, Gross M, Brown P. Occupational hand disorders in musicians. *J Hand Surg [Am]* 1984; 9:295.
3. Bejjani FJ, Stuchin S, Brown P. Occupational disorders of string players, pianists, harpists and guitarists. *Orthop Trans* 1984; 8(1):133.
4. Bejjani FJ, Gross MS, Brown P. Occupational hand disorders in musicians. *Orthop Trans* 1984; 8:24.
5. Singer K. *Diseases of the musical profession: a systematic presentation of their causes, symptoms and methods of treatment.* Lakond V, trans. New York: Greenberg Publishers, 1932.
6. Bejjani FJ, Stuchin S. Structures and functions of an orthopaedic center for the arts. *Mediguide Orthop* 1984; 5(2):1.
7. Bejjani FJ, Nilsson B, Kella J. Effect of the instrument on the musician's musculoskeletal system. In: Atwood DA, McCann C, eds. *Proceedings of the 1984 International Conference on Occupational Ergonomics, 1.* Toronto: Human Factors Conference, 1984; 247–251.
8. Fry HJ. Music making and overuse injuries. *J Int Soc Study Tens Perform* 1986; 3:41–50.
9. Bejjani F, Cothier P, Schwartz M, Snow B. Hand temperature changes and effect of mood profile in musicians during performance. In: Karwowski W, ed. *Trends in ergonomics/human factors III, A.* Amsterdam: Elsevier, 1986; 397–406.
10. Crawford DG, Friesen DD, Tomlinson-Keasey C. Effects of cognitively induced anxiety on hand temperature. *Biofeedback Self Regul* 1977; 2:139–146.
11. Polnauer F. *Senso-motor study and its application to violin playing, 2nd ed.* Urbana, IL: American String Teachers Association, 1964.
12. Smith RD. Paganini's hand. *Arthritis Rheum* 1982; 25:1385–1386.
13. David A. A propos de la "main du virtuose." *Presse Med* 1970; 78: 100.
14. Priest JD, Nagel DA. Tennis shoulder. *Am J Sports Med* 1976; 4: 28–42.
15. Bejjani FJ, Stuchin S, Winchester R. The effect of joint laxity on musicians' occupational disorders. *Clin Res* 1983; 32:660.
16. Bejjani FJ. Joint laxity in performing musicians proven not beneficial. *Rheumatol News Int* 1984; 12(2):3.
17. Bejjani FJ, Snow BS. Use of mood scores as indices of athletic character and stress reactivity among musicians. *Med Probl Perf Art* 1990; 5(1):45–48.
18. Stellman JM, Klitzman S, Gordon GC, Snow BR. Air quality and ergonomics in the office: survey results and methodologic issues. *Am Ind Hyg Assoc J* 1985; 46:286–293.
19. Raynor JO, Smith CP. Achievement related motives and risk taking in games of skill and chance. *J Pers* 1966; 34:176–198.
20. Mittelmann B, Wolff HG. Affective states and skin temperature: experimental study of subjects with "cold hands" and Raynaud's syndrome. *Psychosom Med* 1939; 1:271–293.
21. Hunter J, Kerr EH, Williams MG. The relation between joint stiffness upon exposure to the cold and the characteristics of synovial fluid. *J Med Sci* 1952; 30:367–371.
22. Lokhart JM, Kiess HO, Clegg TI. Effect of rate of lowered finger surface temperature on manual performance. *J Appl Psychol* 1975; 60:106–113.
23. Mackworth NM. Finger numbness in very cold winds. *J Appl Physiol* 1953; 5:538–543.
24. McCloskey DI, Gandevia SC. Role of inputs from skin, joints and muscles and of corollary discharges in human discriminatory tasks. In: Gordon G, ed. *Active touch.* New York: Pergamon Press, 1978; 177–188.
25. Parry M. Skin temperature and motorcyclists' braking performance. *Percept Mot Skills* 1982; 54:1291–1296.
26. Rattenbury C, Donald MW. Forearm tension and change in finger temperature. *Percept Mot Skills* 1982; 55:1071–1075.
27. Wittaker AH. Occupational diseases of musicians. In: Schulman DM, Schoen M, eds. *Music and medicine.* New York: Henry Schulman, 1948; 87–92.
28. Schwander WD, Loock F, Lorenz M. The role of occupational and industrial medicine in the medical care of artists in the Berlin theatres, orchestras and ensembles. *Z Ges Hyg* 1976; 22:367–370.
29. Young RS, Bryk D, Ratner H. Selective phalangeal tuft fractures in a guitar player. *Br J Radiol* 1977; 50:147–148.

30. Bird HA, Wright V. Traumatic synovitis in a classical guitarist: a study of joint laxity. *Ann Rheum Dis* 1981; 40:161–163.
31. Cynamon KB. Flutist's neuropathy. *N Engl J Med* 1982; 305:961.
32. Shulman IA, Milberg P. Player's thumb (letter). *J Hand Surg [Am]* 1982; 7:424.
33. Crabb DJM. Hand injuries in professional musicians: a report of six cases. *Hand* 1980; 12:200–208.
34. Hochberg FH, Leffert RD, Hellner M, Merriman L. Hand difficulties among musicians. *JAMA* 1983; 249:1869–1872.
35. Fry HJ. Overuse syndrome of the upper limb in musicians. *Med J Aust* 1986; 144:182–185.
36. Fry HJ. Incidence of overuse syndrome in the symphony orchestra. *Med Probl Perf Art* 1986; 1(2):51–55.
37. Bejjani FJ, Kaye GM, Benham M. Musculoskeletal and neuromuscular conditions of instrumental musicians. *Arch Phys Med Rehabil* 1996; 77:406–413.
38. Fry HJH. Overuse syndrome of the upper limb in musicians. *Med J Aust* 1986; 144:182–185.
39. Fry HJH. The treatment of overuse injury syndrome. *Maryland Med J* 1993; 42:3; 277–282.
40. Hoppman RA, Patrone NA. A review of musculoskeletal problems in instrumental musicians. *Semin Arthritis Rheum* 1989; 19:117–126.
41. Lederman FJ, Calabrese LH. Overuse syndromes in instrumentalists. *Med Probl Perform Art* 1986; 1:7–11.
42. Fry HJH. Overuse syndrome, alias tenosynovitis/tendinitis: the terminological hoax. *Plast Reconstruct Surg* 1986; 78(3):414–417.
43. Bejjani FJ. Letter to the editor. *Med J Aust* 1987; 146:393.
44. Fry HJH. Occupational maladies of musicians: their cause and prevention. *Int J Music Ed* 1984; 12:63.
45. Moulton B, Spence SH. Site-specific muscle hyper-reactivity in musicians with occupational upper limb pain. *Behav Res Ther* 1992; 30(4): 375–386.
46. Fry HJH. Incidence of overuse syndrome in the symphony orchestra. *Med Probl Perform Art* 1986; 1:51–55.
47. Fry HJH. Prevalence of overuse (injury) syndrome in Australian music schools. *Br J Ind Med* 1987; 44:35–40.
48. Hochberg FH, Leffert RD, Hellner M, Merriman L. Hand difficulties among musicians. *JAMA* 1983; 249:1869–1872.
49. Caldron PH, Calabrese LH, Clough JD, Lederman RJ, Leatherman WG. A survey of musculoskeletal problems encountered in high level musicians. *Med Probl Perform Art* 1986; 1:136–139.
50. Dawson HJ. Hand and upper extremity problems in musicians; epidemiology and diagnosis. *Med Probl Perform Art* 1988; 3:19–22.
51. Lambert CM. Hand and upper limb problems of instrumental musicians. *Br J Rheumatol* 1992; 31:265–271.
52. Lederman RJ. Peripheral nerve disorders in instrumentalists. *Ann Neurol* 1989; 26:640–646.
53. Lederman RJ. Nerve entrapment syndromes in instrumental musicians. *Med Probl Perform Art* 1986; 1:45–48.
54. Charness ME, Parry GJ, Markison RE, et al. Entrapment neuropathies in musicians. *Neurology* 1985; 35(suppl 1):74.
55. Deleted in proof.
56. Wainapel SF, Cole JL. The not so magic flute: two cases of distal ulnar nerve entrapment. *Med Probl Perform Art* 1988; 3:63–65.
57. Makin GJV, Brown WF. Entrapment of the posterior cutaneous nerve of the arm. *Neurology* 1985; 5:1677–1678.
58. Maffulli N, Maffulli F. Transient entrpment neuropathy of the posterior interosseous nerve in violin players. *J Neurol Neurosurg Psychiatry* 1991; 54:65–67.
59. Sandin KJ. The neuromusculoskeletal problems of instrumental musicians: a review. *Curr Concepts Rehabil Med* 1989; 5(1):22–29.
60. Hochberg FH, Lavin P, Portney R, et al. Topical therapy of localized inflammation in musicians: a clinical evaluation of Aspercreme versus placebo. *Med Probl Perform Art* 1988; 3:9–14.
61. Lederman RJ. Occupational cramp in instrumental musicians. *Med Probl Perform Art* 1988; 3:45–51.
62. Bruce AN, ed. *Neurology*. London: Edward Arnold, 1940.
63. Lockwood AH, Lindsay ML. Reflex sympathetic dystrophy after overuse: the possible relationship to focal dystonia. *Med Probl Perform Art* 1989; 4(9)114–117.
64. Newmark J, Hochberg FH. Isolated painless manual incoordination in 57 musicians. *J Neurol Neurosurg Psychiatry* 1987; 50:291–295.
65. Schott GD. Induction of involuntary movements by peripheral trauma: an analogy with causalgia. *Lancet* 1986; 2:712–716.
66. Marsden CD, Obeso JA, Traub MM, Rothwell JC, Kranz H, La Cruz F. Muscle spasms associated with Sudeck's atrophy after injury. *Br Med J* 1984; 288:173–176.
67. Bejjani FJ. Performing artists occupational disorders. In: DeLisa JA, Gans BM, eds. *Rehabilitation medicine*. Philadelphia: JB Lippincott, 1993; 1165–1190.
68. Cohen LG, Hallett M. Hand cramps: clinical features and electromyographic patterns in a focal dystonia. *Neurology* 1988; 38:1005–1012.
69. Marsden CD, Rothwell JC. The physiology of idiopathic dystonia. *Can J Neurol Sci* 1987; 14(Suppl 3): 521–527.
70. LeVine WR. Behavioral and biofeedback therapy for a functionally impaired musician: a case report. *Biofeedback Self-Regul* 1983; 8(1): 101–107.
71. Cohen L, Hallett M, Geller B, et al. Treatment of focal dystonia of the hand with botulinum toxin injection. *Neurology* 1987; 37(Suppl 1):123–124.
72. Sataloff RT, Brandfonbrener AC, Lederman RJ, eds. *Textbook of performing arts medicine*. New York: Raven Press, 1990.
73. Nolan WB. Surgical treatment of acquired hand problems. In: Bejjani FJ, ed. *Current research in arts medicine*. Chicago: A Capella Books, 1993; 319–322.
74. Sams E. Schumann's hand injury: some further evidence. *Musical Times* 1972; 133:456.
75. Ballantyne J. Schumann's hand injury. *Br Med J* 1978; 1:1142.
76. Mather H. Schumann's hand injury. *Br Med J* 1978; 1:1281.
77. Walker A. Schumann's hand injury. *Br Med J* 1978; 1:1420.
78. Lundervold AJS. Electromyographic investigation of position and manner of working in typewriting. *Acta Physiol Scand* 1951; 24(Suppl 84).
79. Basmajian JV, White ER. Neuromuscular control of trumpeters' lips. *Nature* 1972; 241:70.
80. Schlapp M. Observations on a voluntary tremor: violinist's vibrato. *Q J Exp Physiol* 1973; 58:357–368.
81. Rolland P. *The teaching of action in string playing: developmental and remedial techniques: violin and viola*. Urbana, IL: String Research Associates, 1974.
82. Bejjani FJ, Ferrara L, Pavlidis L. A comparative electromyographic and acoustic analysis of violin vibrato: an electroymographic and sound analysis. *Med Probl Perform Art* 1989; 4(4):168–175.
83. Bejjani FJ, Pavlidis L. Kinetics of violin vibrato. *J Biomech* 1990; 23(7):30.
84. Titiloye VM, Bejjani FJ, Xu N, Tomaino CM. Upper extremity force requirements in violin vibrato: a dynamic electromyographic study. In: Anderson PA, Hobart DJ, Danoff JV, eds. *Electromyographical kinesiology*. Amsterdam: Elsevier Science, 1991; 477–480.
85. Xu N, Bejjani FJ, Titiloye VM, Lei L, Tomaino CM, Lockett R. Conversion of forearm surface EMG into force: experimental design and pilot study. In: Anderson PA, Hobart DJ, Danoff JV, eds. *Electromyographical kinesiology*. Amsterdam: Elsevier Science, 1991; 115–118.
86. Bejjani FJ, Halpern N, Lewis E. Standing postures of trumpeters. In: Oborne DJ, ed. *Contemporary ergonomics 1986*. London: Taylor & Francis, 1986; 217–221.
87. Bejjani FJ, Halpern N. Postural kinematics of trumpeters: a photographic and anthropometric study. *J Biomech* 1989; 22:439–446.
88. Halpern N, Bejjani FJ. Postural kinematics of trumpet playing. In: *Proceedings of the North American congress on biomechanics, 1*. Montreal: NACB, 1986; 57–58.
89. Bejjani FJ, Ferrara L, Tomaino CM, et al. Comparison of three piano techniques as an implementation of a proposed experimental design. *Med Probl Perform Art* 1989; 4(3):109–113.
90. Bejjani FJ, Xu N, Parnianpour M, Pavlidis L. Optimizing kinematics and kinetics of piano performance. *J Biomech* 1990; 23:730.
91. Deleted in proof.
92. Flesch C. *The art of violin playing, vol 2. Artistic realization and instruction*. Marten FH, trans. New York: Carl Fisher, 1930.
93. Alexander FM. *The use of the self: its conscious direction in relation to diagnosis, functioning and the control of reaction*. New York: EP Dutton, 1932.
94. Jones FP. *Body awareness in action: the Alexander technique*. New York: Schocken Books, 1976.
95. Samama A. *Muscle control for musicians*. Utrecht: Scheletema & Holkema, 1978.

96. Bejjani FJ, Halpern N. Music education of children: comparative review and principles of musculoskeletal awareness. *Early Child Educ* 1986/1987; 20(1):3–6.
97. Martens R. Anxiety and motor behavior: a review. *J Motor Behav* 1971; 3:151–179.
98. Cratty BJ. *Movement behavior and motor learning, 3rd ed.* Philadelphia: Lea & Febiger, 1973.
99. French SN. Electromyographic biofeedback for tension control during fine motor skill acquisition. *Biofeedback Self-Regul* 1980; 5:221–228.
100. Levee JR, Cohen MJ, Rickles WH. Electromyographic biofeedback for relief of tension in the facial and throat muscles of a woodwind musician. *Biofeedback Self-Regul* 1976; 1:113–120.
101. Morasky RL, Reynolds C, Clark G. Using biofeedback to reduce left arm extensor EMG of string players during musical performance. *Biofeedback Self Regul* 1981; 6:565–572.
102. Donald MW, Hovmand J. Autoregulation of skin temperature with feedback-assisted relaxation of the target limb and controlled variation in local temperature. *Percept Mot Skills* 1981; 53:799–809.
103. Surwit RS, Fenton CH. Feedback and instructions in the control of digital skin temperature. *Psychophysiology* 1983; 17:129–132.
104. Grabert JC, Bregman NJ, McAllister HA. Skin temperature regulation: the effect of suggestion and feedback. *Int J Neurosci* 1980; 10: 217–221.
105. Keefe FJ. Conditioning changes in differential skin temperature. *Percept Mot Skills* 1975; 40:283–288.
106. Sargent JD, Green EE, Walkers ED. Preliminary report of the use of autogenic feedback training in the treatment of migraine and tension headaches. *Psychosom Med* 1973; 35:129–135.
107. Surwit RS, Shapiro D, Feld JL. Digital temperature autoregulation and associated cardiovascular changes. *Psychophysiology* 1976; 13: 242–248.
108. Roberts A, Kewman DG, MacDonald H. Voluntary control of skin temperature unilateral changes using hypnosis and feedback. *J Abnorm Psychol* 1973; 82:163–168.
109. Parrott JR. Surgically dividing pianists' hands. *J Hand Surg [Am]* 1980; 5:619.
110. Lundborg G. The vascularization of the human flexor pollicis longus tendon. *The Hand* 1979; 11(1):28–33.
111. Bejjani FJ. Occupational biomechanics of athletes and dancers: a comparative approach. *Clin Podiatr Med Surg* 1987; 4:671–711.
112. Bejjani FJ. Occupational biomechanics. In: Jahss M, ed. *Disorders of the foot and ankle.* Philadelphia: WB Saunders, 1990; 583–599.
113. Bejjani FJ, Halpern N, Pio A, Dominguez R, Voloshin A, Frankel VH. Musculoskeletal demands on flamenco dancers: a clinical and biomechanical study. *Foot Ankle* 1988; 8(5):254–263.
114. Bejjani FJ, Halpern N, Nordin M, et al. Spinal motion and strength measurements of flamenco dancers, using 3D motion analyzer and Cybex II dynamometer. In: *Biomechanics XI.* Amsterdam: Vu Boekhandel Publishers, 1988; 925–930.
115. Voloshin A, Bejjani FJ, Halpern N, Frankel V. Dynamic loading in flamenco dancers: a biomechanical study. *Hum Move Sci* 1989; 8: 503–513.
116. Bejjani FJ, Halpern N, Pavlidis L. Spinal motion and strength measurements in flamenco dancers. *Med Probl Perform Art* 1990; 5(3): 121–124.
117. Wheeler B. Personal communications.
118. Staum MJ. Music for physical rehabilitation: an analysis of the literature from 1950–1993 and applications for rehabilitation settings. In: Furman CE, ed. *Effectiveness of music therapy procedures: documentation of research and clinical practice, rev. ed.* Silver Spring, MD: National Association for Music Therapy (in press).
119. Staum MJ. Music for physical rehabilitation: An analysis of the literature from 1950–1986 and applications for rehabilitation settings. In: Furman CE, ed. *Effectiveness of music therapy procedures: documentation of research and clinical practice.* Washington, D.C.: National Association for Music Therapy, 1988; 65.
120. Echternach JL. Audioanalgesia as an adjunct to mobilization of the chronic frozen shoulder. *J Am Phys Ther Assoc* 1966; 46:839.
121. Brown SH, Thaut MH, Benjamin J, Cooke JD. Effects of rhythmic auditory cuing on temporal sequencing of complex arm movements. *Proc Soc Neurosci* 1993; 227.2.
122. McIntosh GC, Thaut MH, Rice RR, Miller RA. Stride frequency modulation in Parkinsonian gait using rhythmic auditory stimulation. *Ann Neurol* 1994; 36:316.
123. Thaut MH, McIntosh GC, Prassas, SG, Rice RR. Effects of auditory cuing on temporal stride parameters and EMG patterns in hemiplegic gait of stroke patients. *J Neurol Rehabil* 1993; 7:9.
124. Thaut MH, McIntosh GC, Prassas, SG, Rice RR. Effects of auditory cuing on temporal stride parameters and EMG patterns in normal gait. *J Neurol Rehabil* 1992; 6:185.
125. Thaut M, Schleiffers S, Davis W. Analysis of EMG activity in biceps and triceps muscle in an upper extremity gross motor task under the influence of auditory rhythm. *J Music Ther* 1991; 28:64.
126. Wolfe D. Pain rehabilitation and music therapy. *J Music Ther* 1978; 14(4):162–178.
127. Zimmerman L. Effects of music in patients who had chronic cancer pain. *West J Nurs Res* 1989; 11(3):298–309.
128. Long L, Johnson J. Using music to aid relaxation and relieve pain. *Dent Surv* 1978; 54:35–38.
129. Melzack R, Wall PD. Pain mechanism: a new theory. *Science* 1965; 150:979.
130. Schorr J. Music and pattern change in chronic pain. *Adv Nurs Sci* 1993; 15(4):27–36.
131. Barker L. The use of music and relaxation techniques to reduce pain of burn patients during daily debridement. In: Maranto C, ed. *Applications of music in medicine.* Washington, D.C.: National Association for Music Therapy, 1991.
132. Staum M. Music and rhythmic stimuli in the rehabilitation of gait disorders. *J Music Ther* 1983; 20(2):69–87.
133. Eni G. Gait improvement in parkinsonism: The use of rhythmic music. *Int J Rehab Res* 1988; 11(3):272–274.
134. Thaut M, Rice R. The effect of auditory rhythmic cueing on stride and EMG patterns in hemiparetic gait of stroke patients. *Phys Ther* 1993; 73(6):S107.
135. Spintge R, Droh R. Ergonomic approach to treatment of patient's perioperative stress. *Can J Anaesth* 1988; 35(3 pt 2):S104–S106.
136. Steelman V. Intraoperative music therapy: effects on anxiety and blood pressure. *AORN J* 1990; 52(5):1026–1034.
137. Kaempf G, Amodei M. The effect of music on anxiety. *AORN J* 1989; 50(1):112–118.
138. Biederman B. Synchronizing music to heart-rate. In: Bejjani FJ, ed. *Current research in arts medicine.* Chicago: A Cappella Books, 1993.
139. Bejjani FJ, ed. *Current research in arts medicine.* Chicago: A Capella Books, 1993.
140. Feder E, Feder B. *The expressive arts therapies.* Englewood Cliffs, NJ: Prentice Hall, 1981.
141. Fleshman B, Fryrear JL. *The arts in therapy.* Chicago: Nelson-Hall, 1981.

Rehabilitation Medicine: Principles and Practice, Third Edition,
edited by Joel A. DeLisa and Bruce M. Gans.
Lippincott–Raven Publishers, Philadelphia © 1998.

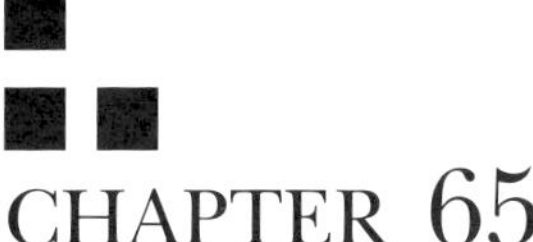

CHAPTER 65

Cumulative Trauma Disorders

Scott Nadler and Jodi Weiss Nadler

Cumulative trauma disorder (CTD) has been variously termed repetitive overuse disorder and repetitive strain disorder. These injuries first became prominent with the advent of the industrial revolution, as jobs evolved from being task oriented to being time dependent. Speed, efficiency, and productivity came to be valued more than a safe, employee-friendly work environment. Arndt suggested that a heightened work pace may produce job pressures that lead to increased muscular tension in the hands and arms when repetitive work is performed (1). Furthermore, this tension accelerates muscular overload and increases biomechanical stress on tendons, synovial membranes, joints, and nerves. Increased electromyographic activity of muscles has been documented in industrial settings with increased work speed (2). Other factors implicated in the generation of CTD include the use of wage incentives to increase productivity and psychological components such as stress or depression (3,4).

Over the past several decades, a major retooling of industry has been undertaken to make the work environment more employee friendly. Ergonomics is the science behind the design and operation of machines within the work environment (5). The proper management of CTD requires a thorough understanding of ergonomics, as the causes of CTD usually have contributing ergonomic factors. Treating the symptoms without modifying the workplace is the primary reason for recurrence of CTD, and magnifies the overall economic burden caused by these disorders.

ECONOMIC IMPACT

Musculoskeletal disorders are the leading cause of disability within the working population (6). Injuries to the hand and wrist have continued to grow in number. Holbrook estimated approximately 4 million physician visits in 1984 secondary to injuries of the upper extremity, costing an estimated $65 billion (7). In a telecommunications company in Australia employing 9,000 workers, more than $15 million was spent on "repetitive strain disorders" from 1981 to 1985 (8). Masear et al. reported more than $1 million spent on lost days from work and worker's compensation claims from carpal tunnel syndrome in a meat-packing plant from 1978 to 1983 (9). Low back pain is the most common and costly musculoskeletal problem affecting workers, costing approximately $16 billion in 1984 (7,10). The total cost of worker's compensation was estimated at $50 billion in 1990, with back care alone consuming $30 billion (11). The growing costs of managing CTD in industry will place a significant economic burden on the employer that will secondarily impact the consumer.

ERGONOMICS

Ergonomics, defined as the study of the individual within the work environment, is now a common term in the industrial setting. It requires an understanding of human abilities and the limitations imposed by the work environment, machines, tools, and specific job tasks (12,13). Ergonomics has received significant attention as the prevalence of CTD has risen in the workplace. Cumulative trauma disorders have been shown to be costly to employers and employees, as they contribute to time lost from work, decreases in productivity, and poor employee morale, all of which are factors in disability (14,15).

Several elements contribute to occupational CTD, including forceful exertions, repetitiveness of a work task, biomechanical postures, vibration, temperature, localized contact stress, and tool use and design (13,15,16).

Forceful Exertions

Forceful exertions in the workplace directly or indirectly cause CTD in combination with such environmental factors

S. Nadler: Department of Physical Medicine and Rehabilitation, University of Medicine and Dentistry of New Jersey, New Jersey Medical School, Newark, New Jersey 07103.

J. Weiss Nadler: Department of Occupational Therapy, Kessler Institute for Rehabilitation—Welkind Facility, Chester, New Jersey 07930.

as friction, equipment issues, gravity, and inertia (12,13). Force requirements may increase depending on the condition of a hand tool (sharpness versus dullness), poor body mechanics, high torque or speed of power tools, and friction between objects and the worker (16,17). Wearing gloves may also increase the force needed during certain activities. Using poor-quality or improperly fitted gloves may be detrimental by blunting sensory feedback, reducing friction between an object and the hand, and reducing strength (16,18).

High force requirements, in combination with other occupational factors (especially repetition), are reported to be responsible for the greatest frequency of CTD of the upper extremity. The incidence of carpal tunnel syndrome and tendinitis has been shown to increase with activities of food processing, carpentry, and secretarial work, where forceful buffing, polishing, cutting, and typing may be required (19).

Repetitiveness or Prolonged Activities

Repetitiveness is also commonly cited as an occupational factor leading to CTD of the upper extremity (15,20). Repetition may be defined as: (a) repeated motions requiring the same muscles and joints or (b) prolonged posture within a job task (13,15). After variable periods of time, repetitive work activities may lead to impairment secondary to CTD. Compromise of soft tissue function may produce inflammation of tendons within the upper extremity, leading to pain and/or loss of motion. It may also lead to compression of peripheral nerves, causing pain, numbness, and weakness in the involved nerve distribution. During muscle contraction, blood flow locally can be decreased by as much as 40%. If a contraction is maintained, the oxygen supply to the area is quickly diminished while metabolite levels increase, causing muscle fatigue and soreness (13).

Safe levels of repetitiveness have not been documented; workplace modifications should therefore be integrated as problems are identified. These modifications may include: avoiding repeated gripping motions, maintaining pinching force requirements under 7 lb, alternating among work tasks with a 5-minute break every hour (16), restructuring of work tasks to encourage a synergistic rather than isolated muscle activity, and using machinery to complete portions of tasks while rotating workers among tasks (13).

Posture

Improper postural mechanics during the performance of a task is an important causative risk factor for CTD. Sustained wrist and forearm flexion–extension or radial–ulnar deviation may induce friction between tendons and adjacent anatomic surfaces. Carpal tunnel syndrome and tenosynovitis of the flexor and extensor tendons of the wrist may be directly associated with sustained wrist or hand position (21–25). This is often seen in jobs that require a significant amount of typing, cashiering, or playing a musical instrument such as the violin (21). Positioning the wrist in radial or ulnar deviation has been associated with deQuervain tenosynovitis (25–28). Other problematic postures commonly cited include those for using pliers, knives, and other household items such as a vacuum cleaner (15). Common awkward postures during work tasks may include extreme elbow flexion–extension, pronation–supination, excessive shoulder elevation, and pinch grips (16,29).

To optimally control awkward postures during work tasks, either the work station should be redesigned or equipment modification (such as the use of bent-handled tools) should be considered to improve body position and alignment.

Localized Contact Stress

Contact stresses are produced when soft tissues of the body come in contact with an object or tool. Compression or shearing of soft tissue structures between bone and tool are the most common forms of contact stress (12). Activities that require the worker to rest the forearms on a work surface for long periods of time or to grip a sharp-edged tool may be causative (15). A very common injury from contact stress is trigger finger, caused by pressure to the A-1 anular pulley (Fig. 65-1). When the distal phalanx is used to control a tool's trigger release, stress is applied to the retinacular ligaments (16). Stress can be ameliorated by adjusting the trigger design so that flexion of the middle phalanx occurs before flexion of the distal phalanx. Another adapation may include the use of soft rubber-coated handles (13,16). Local contact stress may also cause compression of the distal nerves in the digits of the hand. Improper design or use of hand tools is commonly the cause of these stresses. In order to decrease local stress on specific anatomic strucures, one must consider handle shape and size. Handles should be as large as possible for a given task, and sharp edges should be avoided (12).

Temperature

Cold temperature in the workplace may also be a precipitating cause of CTD. It has been well documented that temperatures below 20°C cause reductions in tactile sensitivity, manual dexterity, and circulation (30,31). Exposure may originate from contact with cold tool handles, cold exhaust from air tools, or ambient air (31). Armstrong reported that workers in a cold environment must exert more force on tools or objects to prevent them from dropping out of their hands (32). Workers in normal temperature conditions exert approximately 4 lb of pressure per square inch to grip a hammer handle. Workers simulating cold environment conditions exert as much as 16 lb of pressure per square inch to complete the same task (32). The hands may be protected from the cold by the use of gloves; however, as discussed previously, glove usage may itself increase the grip force requirement to complete a task.

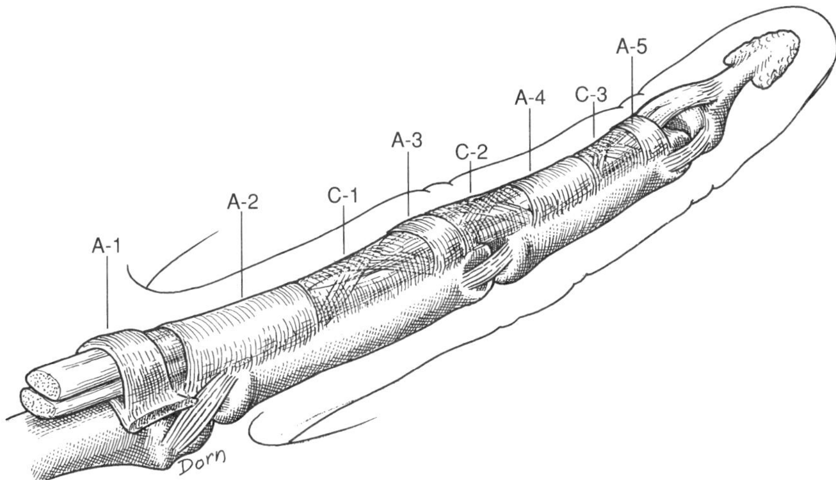

FIG. 65-1. Flexor tendon sheath pulley system. (From Aston SJ, Beasley RH, Thorne CHM. *Grabb & Smith's plastic surgery, 5th ed.* Philadelphia: Lippincott–Raven, 1997.)

Vibration

Another frequently mentioned risk factor in CTD is vibration (33,34). Exposure to vibration may occur with the use of power tools, maintaining a hold on a powered machine, or holding an object as it is processed in a machine (e.g., wood in a power saw). Vibration may also occur with the use of percussion tools, including hammers (32,35).

Raynaud phenomenon stems from reduced blood supply in the fingers. This is caused by constriction of the digital arteries secondary to vibration-induced vasospasm. Activities contributing to this may include using a chain saw or jackhammer (15). Vibration exposure may be difficult to modify, as heavy machinery is the likely culprit. The use of properly fitted antivibration gloves may help, but ultimately, avoidance or a change in tool design is the only curative factor. Unless a worker is exposed to very high-intensity vibration or exposed for very long periods of time, vibration may be a secondary factor after repetitiveness, contact stress, posture, and low temperature (12).

CUMULATIVE TRAUMA DISORDERS

As the various CTD of the upper extremity and spine are discussed (Table 65-1), emphasis is placed on anatomy, pathophysiology, incidence, clinical diagnosis, and management. Low back pain is the most common CTD but is discussed briefly, as a comprehensive review of this topic is outside the scope of this chapter (see Chapter 57).

TABLE 65-1. *Cumulative trauma disorders*

Trigger finger
Ganglion cyst
Raynaud phenomenon
DeQuervain's tenosynovitis
Epicondylitis
Shoulder impingement
Cervical myofascial pain
Low back pain
Nerve entrapments:
Carpal tunnel syndrome
Pronator syndrome
Ulnar nerve at Guyon's canal
Cubital tunnel syndrome
Thoracic outlet syndrome

Trigger Finger

The flexor tendons of the hand are enclosed by a synovial sheath that extends from the metacarpal bones to the distal interphalangeal joint. The pattern for the thumb is slightly different but extends similarly from the region of the radial styloid to the interphalangeal joint. There are a series of fibrous ''pulleys'' that tether the flexor tendons to the interphalangeal joints, providing for frictionless finger flexion. The pulleys are arranged in series along the flexor surface of the digits, from the A-1 pulley at the metacarpal–phalangeal joint to the A-5 pulley at the distal interphalangeal joint (Figs. 65-1 and 65-2).

Triggering of the digits of the hand is a result of an enlargement of the tendon or a thickening of the pulley, most commonly the proximal A-1 pulley (36). This thickening can be up to three to four times normal, and as a result, smooth gliding of the tendon is compromised. Histologically, fibrocartilaginous metaplasia and synovial proliferation are noted in and about the tendon and pulley (36).

The presenting symptom reported by a patient with trigger finger varies from pain to slight triggering to occasional frank locking (37). Triggering is more common in flexion, although it may occur in extension. On physical examination, pain is appreciated over the volar aspect of the metacarpal head. This pain has been previously attributed to a stenosing tenosynovitis of the flexor tendon, although this has not been confirmed histologically (36,38). A palpable thickening or prominence of the flexor tendon is noted. Passive range of motion may be painful but usually does not precipitate triggering, whereas active flexion of the digits will reproduce the triggering phenomenon.

Triggering of the digits is most commonly a multimodal process. A combination of degenerative changes, inflamma-

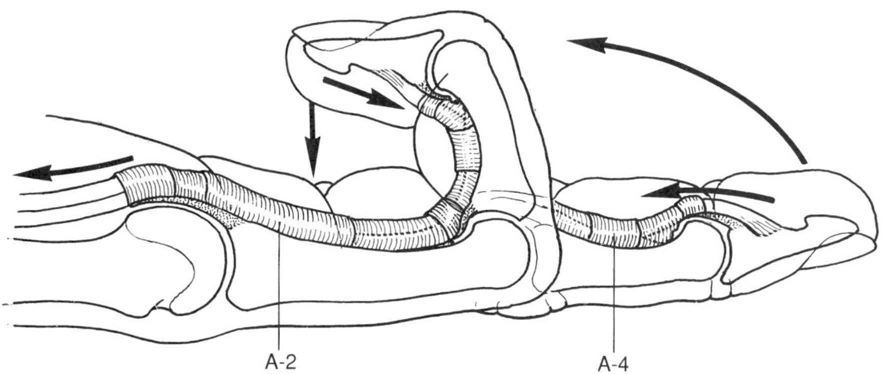

FIG. 65-2. The pulley system in motion with flexion. (From Aston SJ, Beasley RH, Thorne CHM. *Grabb & Smith's plastic surgery, 5th ed.* Philadelphia: Lippincott–Raven, 1997.)

tion, local trauma, and heredity has been implicated (36,39,40). When trauma is involved, it most commonly takes the form of direct pressure over the metacarpal–phalangeal joint region or in occupations requiring an excessively wide grip so that the distal joint is flexed and the interphalangeal and metacarpal–phalangeal joints are extended. Those in whose occupations trigger finger has been described include homemakers, manual laborers, sewing machine operators, welders, and processing plant workers (36,41).

The goal of treatment of the trigger finger is to restore the normal gliding of the tendon through the pulley system within the synovial sheath. The management of this syndrome is threefold: reduce inflammation, decrease local pressure, and make appropriate worksite changes. Local steroid injection into the synovial sheath at the level of the A-1 pulley may decrease inflammation and edema within the pulley and the flexor tendon. The steroid injections may be repeated up to three times over a several-month time frame. Success has been variable with this approach. Quinell reported that 47% of patients treated required no further treatment (42). Marks et al. demonstrated an 84% cure rate with one injection, which improved to 91% with a second steroid injection (43). Splinting is encouraged to reduce pressure and tension on the flexor tendon, maintaining the metacarpophalangeal joint at 0° of extension while allowing active interphalangeal joint motion. Evans reported improvement in 73% of patients with splinting alone (37). Finally, ergonomic changes—for example, decreasing grip size of equipment, decreasing pressure requirement of equipment, padding squared edges, or the use of modified gloves—can reduce local contact pressure (Fig. 65-3). Surgery is used for refractory cases of trigger finger.

Ganglion Cysts

Ganglia are common soft tissue lesions that are more prevalent in women (3:1), with 70% occurring between the second and fourth decades (44). The ganglion is a region of myxoid degeneration arising from tendons, ligaments, or joint capsules. The fluid within the ganglion is a highly viscous mucin containing glucosamine, albumin, globulin, and hyaluronic acid. The two most common areas of occurrence are from the scapholunate ligament dorsally and between the flexor carpi radialis and abductor pollicis longus tendons ventrally (45). Ganglia are thought to be caused by acute trauma or repetitive overuse of the wrist and hand; between 65% and 70% are symptomatic with pain, pressure, or loss of motion in the involved region (44). Ganglia are common in any occupation that requires excessive wrist movement or pressure over the hand or wrist, including jobs requiring polishing, sanding, sawing, or cutting (15). English noted an incidence of 18.8% of ganglia in 580 workers, with a significant association in machine operators and hairdressers (46). No treatment of ganglia may be needed if there are no symptoms. In symptomatic patients, aspiration of cyst material with local instillation of steroid may be curative. This may be repeated up to two additional times, and should it recur, surgical resection of the involved cyst and associated capsular tissue should be considered.

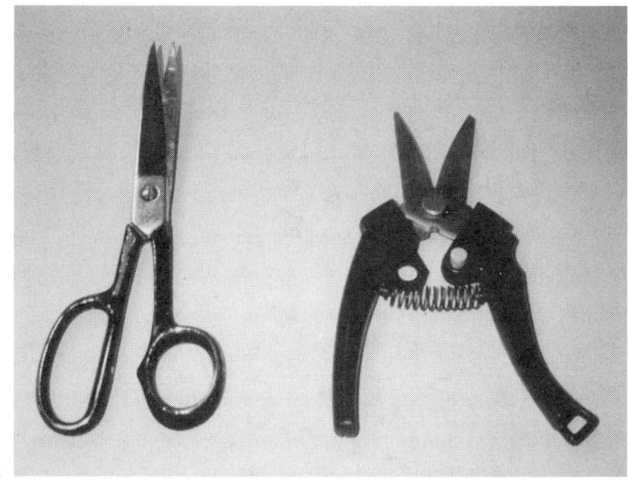

FIG. 65-3. A: Normal scissors. **B:** Ergonomic design to reduce pressure and stress.

Raynaud Phenomenon

Raynaud phenomenon is a vasospastic disorder most commonly associated with connective tissue diseases (scleroderma, rheumatoid arthritis, systemic lupus erythematosus) but also with medications for migraine headaches (ergotamine), cold temperatures, and stress. Vibration was implicated as cause for Raynaud with the advent of heavy machinery (47). Initially described in rock drillers in 1918, Raynaud was referred to as ''vibration white finger'' or ''dead man's hand'' (47). The pathophysiology behind Raynaud is not purely vascular in nature but may involve a sympathetic nerve hyperactivity, proximal obstruction of the neurovascular bundle, or blood hyperviscosity (48,49). Clinically, a classic triphasic color change may occur, though some patients may not have all phases. Pallor (white) is usually the presenting discoloration indicative of ischemia. Cyanosis (blue) follows as blood remains pooled in the digits without outflow. This is followed by hyperemia (red), indicative of the reopening of small arterioles. Patients may also complain of severe pain secondary to ischemic conditions within the digits. In addition to rock drillers, grinders, riveters, and pneumatic hammer and jackhammer operators are also susceptible to Raynaud (50–54). Treatment may initially consist of using antivibration gloves and coated tool handles to reduce vibration. Medications such as alpha blockers, vasodilators, calcium channel blockers, and nonsteroidal anti-inflammatory medications may help reduce symptoms. Without significant tool redesign, elimination of vibration exposure is the only measure likely to be useful (55).

DeQuervain Tenosynovitis

The extensor tendons of the wrist are divided into six compartments. The first dorsal compartment contains of the extensor pollicis brevis (EPB) and abductor pollicis longus (APL) tendons. These parallel the lateral aspect of the distal radius, coursing over the prominence of the radial styloid, prior to insertion in the thumb. The tendons share a common synovial lined sheath within an osseofibrous canal. The angulation of the tendons as they pass over the radial styloid places great stress on the first compartment and predisposes to stenosing tenosynovitis (56).

Inflammation within the first compartment is precipitated by repetitive wrist motion, especially ulnar deviation of the wrist (27,57). Other causes of the tenosynovitis include a direct blow or an acute strain with lifting (58,59). Stenosis of the tendons is precipitated by repeated bouts of inflammation leading to scarring and eventual narrowing of the tendon sheath. DeQuervain disorder is very common in women, who are affected up to ten times more frequently than men (38,60). Initially described as ''washer woman's sprain,'' it is often considered a condition of middle-aged women (61,62). DeQuervain is more common in jobs requiring repetitive wrist motion, especially radial-to-ulnar deviations. Typical activities that may precipitate the condition include buffing, grinding, polishing, sanding, sawing, cutting, and screwdriver use (15). DeQuervain has been described in waitresses, nurses, garment workers, machine operators, and domestic cleaners (63–65).

The patient with DeQuervain will typically complain of pain and swelling about the region of the radial styloid. Pain is precipitated by passive ulnar deviation of the wrist. The Finkelstein test, whereby the thumb is flexed into the palm and the wrist is then passively ulnar deviated, is a useful clinical maneuver (57). A positive test is marked by significant discomfort in the region of the radial styloid. Another useful clinical test is resisted thumb extension at the MCP joint with the wrist maintained in radial deviation, also resulting in lateral wrist pain (66). In chronic DeQuervain, there is a palpable fibrous thickening that occasionally is associated with a ganglion cyst (57).

The mainstay of treatment involves activity modification, especially of those activities that place great shear force on the first dorsal compartment. A thumb spica splint may be needed to further limit motion and rest the APL and EPB tendons. Steroid injection into the tendon sheath of the first dorsal compartment may be a useful adjunct during the acute inflammation stage to quiet the tenosynovitis. In chronic cases, steroid injection may be difficult because of stenosis in the tendon sheath. Up to three injections may be performed and should be combined with splint immobilization.

McKenzie reported an improvement in 90% of symptomatic patients treated by one to three injections of hydrocortisone into the tendon sheath at 18-month follow-up (67). In severe refractory cases, surgical decompression of the first dorsal compartment may be helpful or even curative.

Epicondylitis

The lateral and medial epicondyles serve as the origins of the musculature for the forearm and wrist. Lateral epicondylitis, also termed ''tennis elbow,'' and ''medial epicondylitis,'' also termed ''golfer's elbow,'' are overuse syndromes of these muscles. Lateral epicondylitis most commonly involves the origin of the extensor carpi radialis brevis and less commonly the extensor carpi radialis longus, extensor digitorum communis, or extensor carpi ulnaris. Medial epicondylitis typically involves the pronator teres and flexors carpi radialis and ulnaris.

Epicondylitis begins as an inflammatory reaction within the tendinous origin and progresses to microtears that heal through fibrosis and granulation tissue production. Mucinoid degeneration of the tendon structures and resultant tissue failure result. It is most typically an overuse syndrome precipitated by repetitive concentric contractions or eccentric overload (68). Epicondylitis is associated with an imbalance created by muscle weakness, impairing the ability to absorb significant forces of torque, and tissue inflexibility leading to tissue failure. An example is inflexibility and weakness of the wrist extensors (69). Cumulative trauma may occur in jobs that require repetitive contraction of the wrist flexors/

extensors or pronators/supinators. Epicondylitis is common in all industries where repetitive/strenuous tasks are required. Kurpper et al. demonstrated epicondylitis occurring in 1% of employees in nonstrenuous jobs in a meat-processing factory, 18% of female packers/sausage makers, and 6.4% of male meat cutters (70). Epicondylitis was found in 14.5% of employees in the fish-processing industry and 23% in pork-processing (71,72). Occupations requiring small parts assembly, turning screws, or hammering also have a causal role in the development of epicondylitis (15).

The patient with epicondylitis typically will report a history of focal elbow discomfort. Lateral epicondylitis will present with weakness of grip (secondary to muscle fatigue and discomfort), pain with resisted wrist extension, and a dull aching in the lateral epicondylar region. On physical examination, resisted wrist extension, resisted middle finger extension, or passive elbow extension with the wrist fully flexed will precipitate symptoms. Palpation reveals tenderness over the lateral epicondyle and the proximal wrist extensor unit. Medial epicondylitis presents with deep aching pain in the flexor/pronator musculature along with a perceived weakness of grip. On physical examination, pain will be reproduced with resisted wrist flexion or forearm pronation with the elbow extended. Palpation will reveal tenderness over the medial epicondyle and the proximal flexor compartment. The clinician must be aware of conditions that may mimic epicondylitis. Roles and Maudsley described entrapment of the posterior interosseous nerve as a cause for resistant "tennis elbow" (73). Gunn and Millbrandt reported cervical radiculopathy as another cause of lateral elbow discomfort (74). At the medial side of the elbow, Harrelson and Newman described ulnar neuropathy caused by hypertrophy of the flexor carpi ulnaris (75).

The primary component of treatment is to address underlying occupational causes such as tool design and repetitiveness of task. The medical care for epicondylitis begins with inflammation reduction via medication, icing, or steroid injection. A pain-free range of motion for wrist flexion/extension and pronation/supination should be obtained prior to beginning progressive strengthening exercises. Strengthening should begin with light concentric exercises for all motions about the wrist and forearm, including grip strength (Fig. 65-4). The program is then advanced to include some eccentric exercises as well as more work-specific activities (Fig. 65-5). Return to restricted work can be attempted when strength is 80% of that in the noninvolved side; work volume should not increase by more than 5% per day (76).

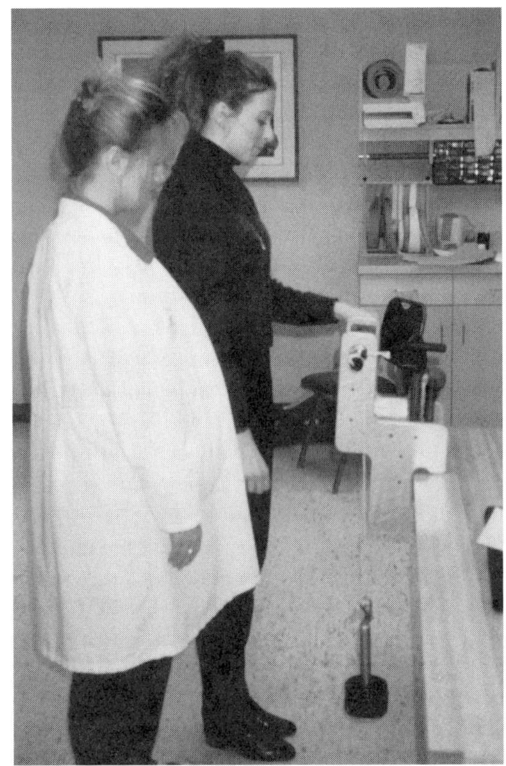

FIG. 65-4. Strengthening exercises for forearm musculature.

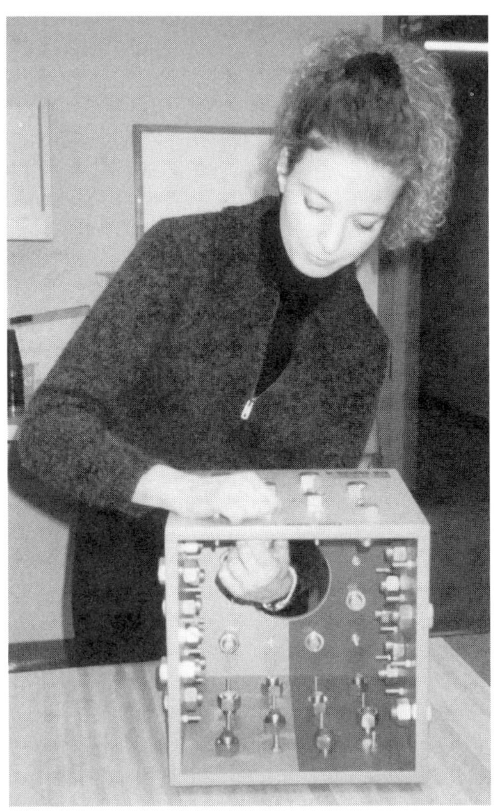

FIG. 65-5. Work-specific training.

Shoulder Impingement

The shoulder is a complex structure that affords the joint great mobility at the expense of stability. What stability is present has both static and dynamic components. Statically, the bony glenoid, cartilaginous labrum, glenohumeral ligaments, and joint capsule provide moderate stability. The rotator cuff (supraspinatus, infraspinatus, teres minor, and subscapularis) and the biceps tendon function dynamically to assist with stability. The rotator cuff plays a key role, especially with the arm in overhead elevation, where it must tonically contract to keep the humeral head anchored in the shallow glenoid fossa (77). The rotator cuff rests in the subacromial space, defined by the acromion, subacromial bursa, and coracoacromial ligament above, the coracoid process at the medial border, and the humeral head below. Numerous anatomic and pathophysiological factors may lead to a narrowing of the space and predisposition to rotator cuff impingement. Bicipital tendinitis may occur in concert with rotator cuff tendinitis as the biceps tendon passes underneath the subscapularis and supraspinatus tendons.

The impingement syndrome has been well described as a progression of changes to the rotator cuff eventually leading to a tearing of the tendons (78). The causes of rotator cuff impingement can be classified as intrinsic or extrinsic (79). Intrinsic causes include trauma or degeneration of the rotator cuff with instability or laxity of the shoulder complex. Extrinsic causes include bony changes to the acromion, coracoid, acromioclavicular joint or greater tuberosity, cervical nerve root compression, and other systemic conditions including rheumatic disorders (80). Morrison and Bigliani reported the relationship between acromial morphology (type I flat, type II curved, type III hooked) and rotator cuff impingement. Individuals with a hooked acromion were most likely to develop rotator cuff abnormality (81). The positioning of the rotator cuff has also been reported as having a relationship to rotator cuff pathology. Rathbun and MacNab reported the "wringing out" phenomenon, whereby a hypovascular region in the supraspinatus tendon was created with the arm held in adduction (82). Glenohumeral instability has been described as an inciting cause, with rotator cuff impingement occurring secondary to increased humeral motion (83). The torque placed on the rotator cuff is greatest at arm elevation of 90°, which may predispose to overuse injury in the overhead position (84). Loss of scapular motion, or asynchrony between the scapulothoracic and glenohumeral musculature, may also predispose to impingement.

Rotator cuff injury was the third most common diagnosis encountered in workers, accounting for 8.3% of cases (46). In a fish processing plant, shoulder girdle pain was encountered in 30.9% of workers, and was more prevalent in workers who performed both repetitive and forceful movements of their upper limbs during work (71). Among electricians, 29% reported shoulder symptoms that occurred at least three times or lasted greater than one week (85). Shoulder pain was also reported in 37% of construction workers, 19.6% of garment workers, and 8.8% of hospital workers (64,65,86). Herberts et al. reported 18% of shipyard welders and 16% of steel plate workers had shoulder pain (87). Welch noted a prevalence of 32% for rotator cuff injury in sheet metal workers, with most occurring from overhead duct work (4). Rotator cuff injury is more common overall in individuals who perform forceful overhead activities, or who require internal rotation of the shoulder, awkward or static postures; lack of rest and vibration may predispose to rotator cuff inflammation as well (29,88).

The individual with rotator cuff tendinitis or the impingement syndrome will report pain deep within the shoulder or posteriorly, with referral to the deltoid muscle insertion region. There may also be loss of strength and motion secondary to the pain. The discomfort is worsened by activities at shoulder level or above. Pain will occasionally occur at night while resting on the involved shoulder, perhaps from a concomitant subacromial bursitis. On physical examination, pain may be reproduced with palpation within the subacromial space or over the biceps tendon. There are several methods used to reproduce impingement of the rotator cuff (impingement signs). Hawkins described a method in which the arm is forward flexed 90° and with the elbow bent 90° the arm is forcibly internally rotated (89). Neer described forced forward flexion of the arm, maintaining pressure on the acromion, so as to impinge the humeral head under the acromion (78) (Fig. 65-6).

The impingement test was described as a method of obtaining pain relief from rotator cuff impingement (90). This test is performed by injection of lidocaine into the subacromial space and is described as positive, if there is return of strength and improved range after infiltration of the space. Strength testing of the rotator cuff should be performed, with weakness and pain of the supraspinatus and external shoulder rotators most apparent. A complete neurologic examination should also be performed to rule out the presence of cervical radiculopathy. The use of x-ray, magnetic resonance imaging (MRI), and electrodiagnosis is discussed elsewhere in other chapters within this text.

In the industrial setting, rehabilitation of shoulder impingement emphasizes decreasing overhead work, particularly on activities that promote internal rotation of the shoulder. Acute intervention emphasizes pain reduction, including

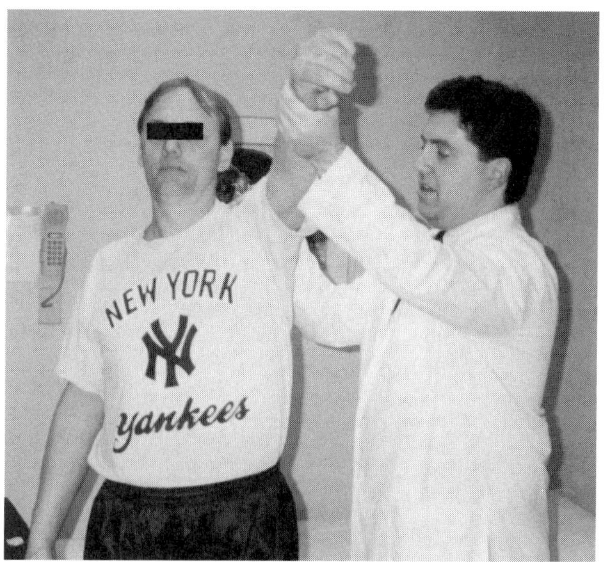

FIG. 65-6. Neer's impingement sign.

nonsteroidal anti-inflammatories, ice, and occasionally, injection of steroid into the subacromial space. Range of motion of both the glenohumeral and scapulothoracic articulations will decrease the likelihood of asynchronous motion leading to impingement. Finally, strengthening of the glenohumeral and scapulothoracic musculature concentrically and eccentrically will help to prevent future injury. Strengthening of the scapular stabilizers should be started immediately; the remainder of the strengthening program, i.e., of the cuff itself, is prescribed when such activity no longer reproduces much pain.

Neck Pain

The cervical spine is a complex structure consisting of eight individual motion segments, beginning with the articulation of the occiput on C1 (atlas) and ending with the articulation between C7 and T1. Individual nerve roots exit at subsequent levels from C1 to C8, innervating the corresponding myotomes and dermatomes of the head, neck, and arms. The musculature about the neck allows control of the head but at the same time helps to provide stability. Overwork of the musculature or impingement of the nerve roots account for most of the pathology about the neck.

Neck pain is commonly encountered in jobs requiring prolonged posturing of the neck, poor neck alignment (forward head), or sustained overhead work, especially with the neck forced into hyperextension. Neck pain in industrial settings is most commonly a result of fatigue of the musculature secondary to overuse, leading to tenderness within the trapezius and levator scapula (91). Nerve root compression can be induced by intrinsic factors such as dural sheath swelling or more common extrinsic factors such as cervical disk pathology or spondylosis.

Neck pain is commonly encountered in jobs requiring prolonged posturing either at a desk or on an assembly line (91–93). It may also occur with sustained overhead work (15). Neck symptoms were reported in 62% of dental hygienists and 66% of sewing machine operators with more than 15 years of experience (92,93). Tender points within the trapezius and levator scapula were much more prevalent in female office employees with neck and shoulder symptoms than in controls with occasional discomfort (91). Significant symptoms related to the neck have also been reported in dentists, meat carriers, miners, heavy labor workers, iron foundry workers, and civil servants (94). The most significant factor associated with neck discomfort appears to be posture Figure 65-7. Watson and Trott found a significant association between forward head posture and headaches (95). Mayoux-Benhamou and Revel demonstrated improved neck muscle efficiency with neutral head position as compared to the flexed or extended position (96). Improper neck positioning may thus influence the early development of neck muscle fatigue. Increased neck extension has also been reported to increase pressure significantly within the intervertebral foramina, predisposing to nerve root impingement (97).

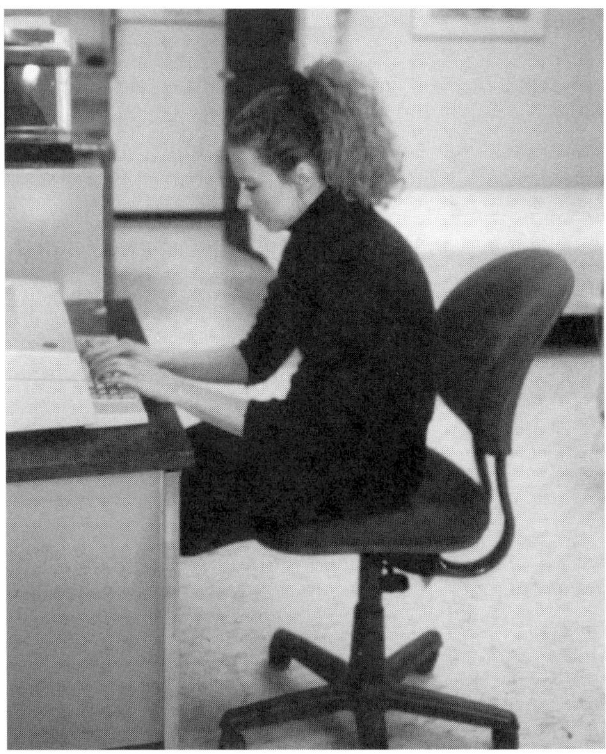

FIG. 65-7. Poor posture at the worksite.

The individual with neck tension syndrome complains of aching discomfort in the base of the neck and upper back. Headaches are common, especially with involvement of the suboccipital and trapezius musculature. Muscle irritation may cause referred pain not only to the head but also into the upper extremities, elbows, forearms, and hands (98). Occasionally, the nerve roots themselves may be inflamed, causing numbness, tingling, or pain to be referred in a specific dermatomal pattern, weakness localized in a myotomal distribution, and corresponding reflex diminution. Skilled palpatory examination will help localize areas of muscle hypertonicity and can precipitate a referred pain pattern beyond the site of palpation.

Postural biomechanics will be the mainstay in management of neck tension syndrome as well as nerve root irritation. The main goal will be to change postures causing excessive neck extension or head-forward position (Figs. 65-8 and 65-9). The individual should be instructed in neck retraction exercises along with stretching of the anterior shoulder capsule/pectoralis muscles and strengthening of the middle trapezius/rhomboids. Strengthening and stretching of the musculature required for good neck posture will decrease pressure on the posterior spine structures and improve overall efficiency of neck musculature (96,97). Making the appropriate changes to the work environment to reduce undue stress and postural overload is of paramount importance.

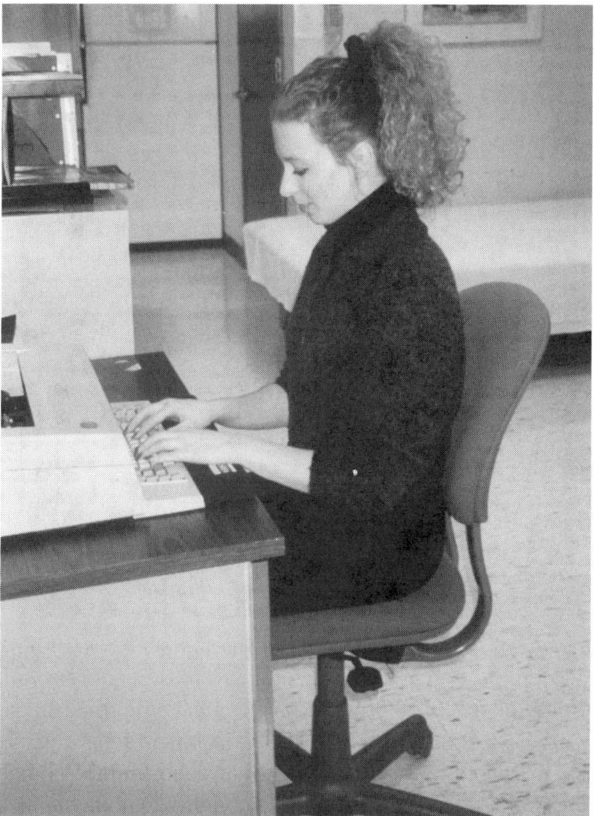

FIG. 65-8. Proper posture for work activities.

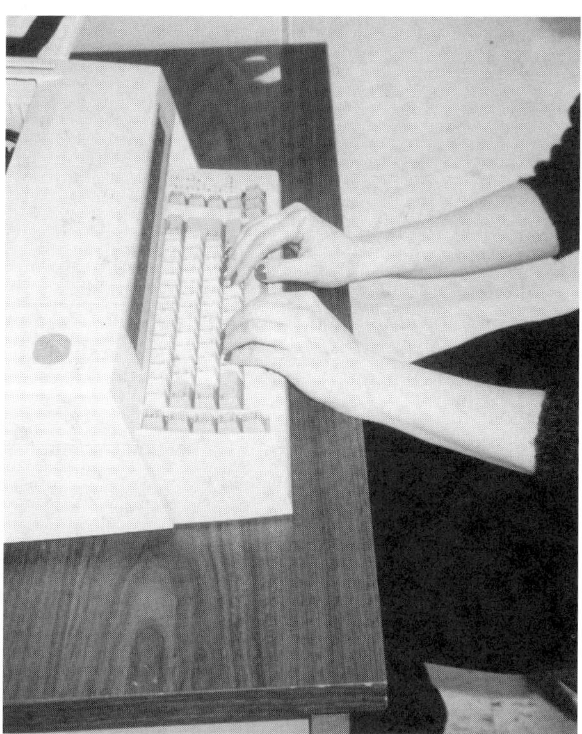

FIG. 65-9. Improper wrist positioning for typing.

Low Back Pain

Low back pain is one of the most common cumulative trauma disorders encountered in industry. Snook reported that truck driving was the occupation with the highest rate of compensable back injuries, followed by material handlers, nurses, and nurse aides (99). Heliovarra reported similar relationships, with a high incidence in truck drivers and industrial workers, especially metal or machine workers (100). Low back pain in those two studies was attributed to heavy manual work (99,100). Lifting in particular may precipitate low back pain, depending on the amount of weight, the frequency of lifts, the amount of twisting or asymmetric lifts, and poor postural biomechanics (26,99). Improved overall fitness has been demonstrated to decrease the incidence of back pain in firefighters, so lack of fitness may be more likely to predispose to back pain via increased intradiscal pressure or as yet unknown factors (101,102). Vibration to the spine has been implicated as the likely cause in truck drivers, forklift drivers, and crane operators (103–105). Vibration may promote development of back pain via involvement of the intervertebral disk, muscles, or ligaments (54). Psychosocial issues are extremely important in industry as a factor in the development of disabling low back pain (106). Low back pain pathophysiology, diagnosis, and management are discussed elsewhere in the text (Chapter 57).

Nerve Entrapment Syndromes

Carpal Tunnel Syndrome

The carpal tunnel is an enclosed space running from the radially situated scaphoid and trapezium bones toward the pisiform and hamate bones at the ulnar border. The transverse carpal ligament is tethered ventrally across the carpal bones, enclosing the space. Within the tunnel lie the four tendons of both flexors digitorum superficialis and profundus, the tendon of the flexor pollicis longus, and the median nerve.

The carpal tunnel syndrome (CTS) is one of the most common cumulative trauma disorders noted in clinical practice. Median nerve compression within the carpal tunnel occurs secondary to many factors, among them vibration, awkward positioning of the wrist and hand, local pressure at the base of the palm, and forceful hand motions (107,108). Symptoms are produced not by local nerve compression but by intraneural ischemia, although pressures within the enclosed tunnel may be a significant factor in development of ischemia (109). Gelberman et al. demonstrated normal pressures within the canal to be 2.5 mm Hg at 90° of wrist flexion or extension. In those with CTS, pressure was 32 mm Hg in neutral position and increased to 94 mm Hg at 90° of wrist flexion and to 110 mm Hg with 90° of wrist extension (110). Pressures greater than 30 mm Hg applied to peripheral nerves will rapidly result in slowing of intraneural blood flow (111).

English et al. demonstrated CTS to be the most common

disorder present in 580 occupational injuries, comprising 29.5% of cases (46). Carpal tunnel syndrome occurred in 64% and 57% of garment and hospital workers, respectively (64,65). It has also been noted in rock drillers, cashiers, secretaries, assemblers, packers, sheet metal workers, and housewives (4,112,113). There are myriad causes for carpal tunnel syndrome, including high-force, high-repetition jobs, prolonged posturing, and vibration (114).

The earliest symptoms in CTS include numbness and tingling of the thumb, index, middle, and radial half of the ring finger. Symptoms worsen during the night, which may be related to increased edema secondary to a nocturnal increase in tissue pressures (115). A flick sign, in which the patient vigorously shakes the hand to relieve symptoms, is reported in 93% of those with CTS (116). Weakness will follow sensory symptoms after a variable amount of time and may lead to thenar muscle atrophy (117). The common clinical provocative tests used to diagnose CTS, the Tinel and Phalen tests, have been shown to be positive in 60% to 70% and 80%, respectively, in classic cases (22,118). Heller demonstrated Tinel and Phalen sensitivity to be 60% to 67%, and their specificity to be 59% to 77% (119). The carpal compression test, whereby the examiner presses over the tunnel for 30 seconds, recreates symptoms in up to 90% of patients with classic CTS (120). Semmes-Weinstein monofilament testing for pressure threshold, vibration at 256 Hz, and two-point discrimination are also used to assess CTS. Szalbo et al. compared vibration and two-point sensation; the former was abnormal in 87% of CTS patients, the latter in 22% (121). Grip strength can also be used as a screening test, with data from symptomatic patients compared to normative data (122). Electrodiagnostic testing for CTS is discussed elsewhere in this text.

The cornerstone in management of CTS is making the appropriate changes to those workplace factors that may have precipitated the condition (123). Simple keyboard pads may decrease pressure and change wrist inclination for typists and keyboard entry workers (Fig. 65-10). In industry, increasing attention is paid to reducing the repetitiveness of tasks and limiting "wrist intensive" duties. Beyond these workplace issues, a decision must be made regarding nonoperative versus surgical care.

Factors proposed to favor nonoperative management include: (a) symptoms less than 1 year, (b) no thenar weakness or atrophy, (c) lack of denervation on needle electromyography, and (d) prolongation of evoked median sensory distal latency by less than 1 msec relative to the opposite side (124). Characteristics predictive of poor outcome from nonoperative treatment include: (a) symptoms greater than 1 year, (b) constant numbness in digits 1, 2, and 3, (c) objective weakness of the abductor pollicis brevis, (d) thenar atrophy, (e) two-point discrimination greater than 6 mm, (f) median motor latency greater than 6 ms, and (g) electromyographic evidence of fibrillation potentials in the median supplied thenar muscles (125). Nonsurgical management consists of nighttime splinting (during the day as well, if the splint does not interfere with usual activities), nonsteroidal anti-inflammatories, tendon/nerve gliding exercises, and local steroid injections. Goodman reported 67% of 51 patients treated with splinting alone being free of symptoms after 6 to 30 months of follow-up (126,127). Gianini et al. reported relief of symptoms in 90% of CTS patients within 45 days, and in 93% after 6 months, in those who received steroid injection (128). Gelberman et al. had less favorable results with steroid injection: after 18 months, only 40% remained symptom-free (129). Open or endoscopic division of the transverse carpal ligament is performed in severe or refractory cases.

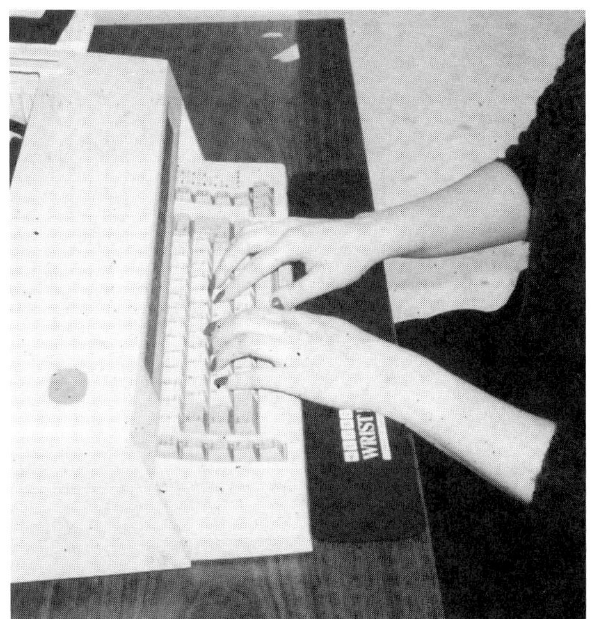

FIG. 65-10. Use of a wrist support to improve positioning.

Pronator Syndrome

The median nerve exits the upper arm and enters the forearm by passing under the bicipital aponeurosis between the two heads of the pronator teres. Entrapment of the nerve can occur at four points: under the ligament of Struthers in the medial distal arm, under the lacertus fibrosus (a thickened aponeurosis from the biceps tendon to the flexor forearm mass), under the pronator teres, or under a thickened or fibrous portion of the flexor digitorum superficialis. The four entrapment areas can be differentiated on physical examination. Entrapment at the ligament of Struthers and at the lacertus fibrosis can be accentuated by resisted full elbow flexion or resisted supination. Entrapment at the pronator teres and flexor digitorum superficialis can be accentuated by resisted forearm pronation and resisted middle finger flexion respectively (130–132). Symptoms of the pronator teres syndrome include hyperesthesia and/or paresthesias of the hand in a median nerve distribution, weakness of median innervated muscles distal to the entrapment, and pain and tenderness at the proximal forearm (130,131,133). The pronator syndrome is far less common than CTS but may occur in the workplace, especially from jobs requiring repeated pronation or supination, lifting, carrying, or placing heavy objects (130). It is also encountered in individuals performing repetitive hammering, buffing, grinding, or cleaning fish (15,134). Treatment begins with modification of duties, along with relative rest to decrease repetitive overuse injury. Anti-inflammatory medication can be used to decrease pain, along with occupational/physical therapy techniques to stretch and strengthen the involved area. Should nonoperative treatment fail, surgical resection of fascial bands, tendinous arches, or an involved ligament of Struthers may be considered.

Ulnar Neuropathy

The ulnar nerve becomes superficial between the biceps and triceps in the medial arm and then passes behind the medial epicondyle in the ulnar groove and enters the forearm between the two heads of the flexor carpi ulnaris (FCU). The cubital tunnel is formed just distal to the ulnar groove as the ulnar nerve passes underneath the FCU. The roof of the tunnel is formed by the triangular arcuate ligament, which bridges across the two heads of the FCU; the floor is the FCU itself. The ulnar nerve traverses the forearm lying beneath the FCU. It gives off the dorsal and palmar cutaneous branches before passing through the Guyon canal, which is defined by the pisiform and hamate bones and the overlying transverse carpal ligament.

Entrapment or compression of the ulnar nerve within the cubital tunnel is the second most common compression neuropathy in the upper limb, after CTS (117). Normal motion of the elbow potentially places great pressure on the ulnar nerve. Elbow flexion causes the arcuate ligament to become taut, the FCU to tighten, and the ulnar collateral ligament of the elbow to buckle and encroach into the tunnel (135,136). Apfelberg and Larson demonstrated a 55% narrowing of the cubital tunnel during elbow flexion (137). Repetitive flexion and extension of the elbow itself may chronically irritate the nerve or result in hypertrophy of the arcuate ligament, leading to further compression (138). The second most common site for ulnar nerve compression is in the region of the Guyon canal (139). Chronic focal compression, ganglion cysts within the canal, ulnar artery thrombosis, or acute blunt trauma to the region may lead to a distal ulnar neuropathy (136,140).

The patient with cubital tunnel syndrome will present with numbness, tingling, or paresthesias of the fourth and fifth digits, weakness of grip strength, wasting of ulnar innervated hand intrinsics, and, later, a "clawing" of the hand from muscle imbalance. The elbow flexion test, maintaining the fully flexed elbow for 1 minute, will provoke paresthesias in an ulnar distribution (141). Applying pressure to the ulnar nerve with the elbow fully flexed has been identified as a sensitive measure of cubital tunnel syndrome (142). Compression of the ulnar nerve at Guyon canal may cause variable clinical findings, depending on where within the canal the nerve is injured. Sensory, motor, or both sensory and motor loss may be noted. Focal pressure applied between the pisiform and the hook of the hamate may induce symptoms.

Cubital tunnel syndrome is commonly encountered in industry. Because of the inherent flexed elbow posture, it has been noted in computer operators and truck drivers (139). Direct compression at the cubital tunnel secondary to resting the elbows on a work station occurs in sewing machine operators (143). Cubital tunnel syndrome has also been noted in assembly line workers because of repetitive elbow flexion and extension (144). Ulnar nerve entrapment at the Guyon canal was first identified in gold polishers in 1896 (145) and has also been reported in boot makers, secretaries/typists, machine operators, meat packers, pipe cutters, mechanics, and long-distance cyclists (93,146–149).

In the industrial setting, the first step in management is to reduce extrinsic compression of the ulnar nerve via avoidance or padding. In jobs requiring repeated elbow flexion, modification of duties may be necessary. Additional measures include anti-inflammatory medication and splinting of the elbow at night to prevent elbow flexion greater than 60°. Seror demonstrated 100% subjective improvement in 22 patients with cubital tunnel syndrome using a night splint preventing flexion beyond 60° for 6 months. Nerve conduction velocity across the elbow measured at a mean follow-up of 11.3 months was improved by 6.5 m/sec in motor nerve conduction and 9.5 m/sec in sensory nerve conduction in 16 of 17 patients (150).

Thoracic Outlet Syndrome

Thoracic outlet syndrome (TOS) comprises several subsets of conditions that all lead to compression of the brachial plexus or subclavian vessels along the costoclavicular passages. Varieties of TOS include scalenus anticus, costoclavicular, and the hyperabduction syndromes. In the neck, the subclavian vein passes between the subclavius and anterior scalene muscles, and the subclavian artery and lower trunk of the brachial plexus pass between the anterior and middle scalene muscles. The neurovascular bundle then travels between the clavicle and first rib and underneath the pectoralis minor muscle as it reaches the arm. Compression is theorized to occur at any of these anatomic sites (Fig. 65-11).

Clinically, the patient will complain variably of paresthesias in the fourth and fifth digits, vascular changes including Raynaud phenomenon, hand weakness, and production or exacerbation of symptoms with various postures or arm positions. On physical examination, sensory abnormalities may be apparent in the C8-T1 dermatomes. Cyanosis or loss of pulse may be precipitated with the Adson maneuver, the costoclavicular test, or Wright hyperabduction test, although the specificity of these tests in only fair (151,152).

Physiological narrowing of the costoclavicular space occurs during habitual weightlifting and with sustained activi-

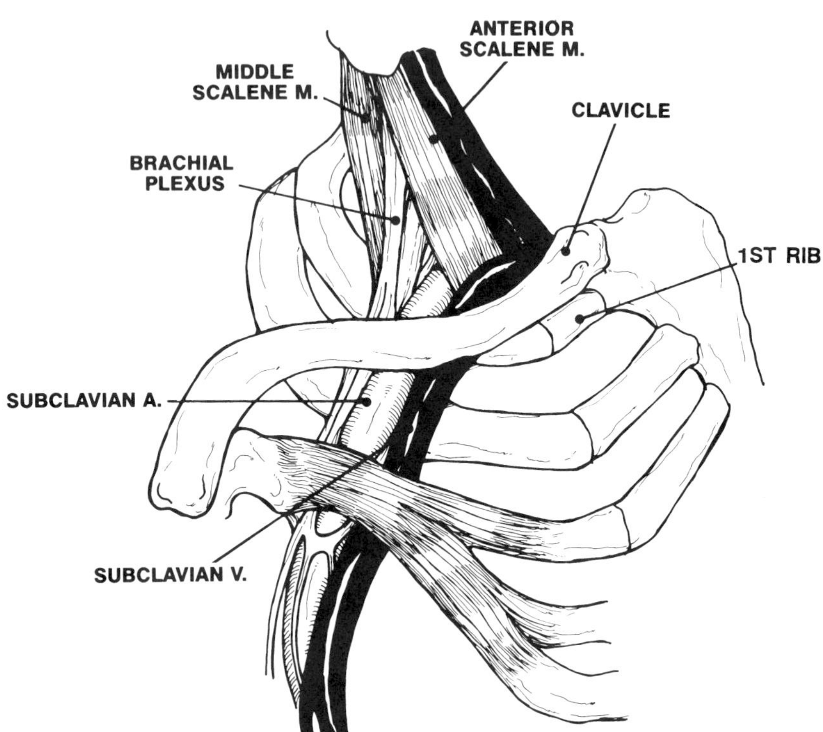

FIG. 65-11. The anatomy of the thoracic outlet.

ties requiring hyperabduction of the arms, drooping of the shoulders, and contractions of the scalene muscles with flexion or rotation of the cervical spine, in individuals with excessive muscular development (80). This narrowing also occurs during overhead work or lifting, including assembly, painting, auto repair, material handling, and mail sorting. Individuals whose occupations require prolonged posturing of the neck are at risk, e.g., secretaries, cashiers, some machine operators, surgeons, and truck drivers (3,15,153).

Initial management consists of a coordinated program to ameliorate occupationally induced factors, along with physical therapy to stretch implicated muscles (scalenes, pectoralis minor, trapezius, and levator scapula). In addition, strengthening of scapular elevators and stabilizers, such as the upper/middle trapezius and rhomboid muscles, is used to improve posture and increase the area within the costoclavicular space (154). Postural biomechanics must be emphasized, as this likely underlies most cases of mild to moderate TOS. Surgery for resection of anomalous fibrous bands, thickened musculature, or an incidental first rib is reserved for refractory cases thought to be caused by those anatomic factors.

ERGONOMIC CONSIDERATIONS IN THE WORKPLACE

Prevention of CTD may begin with a professional evaluation of the individual's work station, along with appropriate recommendations for redesign, as occupationally induced CTDs are much easier to prevent than to treat. Although an in-depth discussion of ergonomic evaluation and management is beyond the scope of this chapter, some general considerations follow.

Positioning/Movements

The following postures should be avoided:

- Maintenance of the elbow in the overhead position during repetitive or sustained activities.
- Extreme flexion of the elbow.
- Sustained supination or pronation of the forearm.
- Extreme flexion or extension of the wrist.
- Repetitive radial or ulnar deviation of the wrist.
- Sustained grip or pinch.

Seated Work Station

The arrangement of a work station should follow several guidelines. The top of the computer monitor should be in line with the worker's eyes, allowing for a natural downward gaze angle of 15° toward the middle of the screen. This position also allows the worker to maintain the normal lordotic curve of the cervical spine, avoiding the forward head position. The optimum distance from the monitor is 12 to 28 inches. If the monitor is too close, the worker will experience eye strain, whereas if it is too far away, the worker is forced to slouch forward, increasing stress throughout the entire spine. The worker should also be directly in front of the screen to decrease excessive cervical rotation or coupled sidebending.

The worker should maintain neutral postures of the wrist

and forearm. During repetitive work (e.g., typing), the upper extremities should be relaxed at the sides, with the elbows flexed no more than 70° to 90°. The height of the work station is a very important component in the overall design, as small changes in height alone may influence the positioning of the neck, shoulders, elbows, and wrists. If a desk area is too high, the worker is forced either to abduct or elevate the shoulders, forcing increased sustained muscle contraction along with compensatory ulnar deviation at the wrists.

Chair Positioning

Height. The chair height should allow good clearance under the desk/work area while the feet are comfortably placed on the floor or foot rest. The knees should be maintained at an angle between 90° and 105°. If the seat is too low, the result may be increased pressure under the ischial tuberosities. A low seat may also lead to increased elbow flexion and wrist extension as the worker reaches for the keyboard. An excessively high seat will force the worker to sit forward in the chair without lumbar support, increasing compressive forces on the lumbar spine.

Seat Depth. This should allow 1 to 4 inches between the popliteal angle and the front edge of the seat. A shorter depth seat will require the buttocks and upper thighs to sustain excessive pressures, whereas a longer seat depth may impede circulation behind the knees.

Back Rest. This important component helps to reduce fatigue by decreasing the sustained contraction of the back muscles as they maintain an unsupported seated posture. A back rest should be deep enough to support the lumbar curve while maintaining the thoracic spine in contact with the chair back.

In general, a seated work station is recommended when:

1. Items to be handled are no more than 10 lb.
2. Writing or other fine motor tasks predominate the work.
3. The task does not require the hands to be more than 6 inches from the work surface.
4. All work items are within reach from the seated position.

Standing Work Station

Standing work station considerations are similar to those in seated positions for the upper extremity, with additional generalizations for work height, station reorganization, and lifting assists. A standing work station is best used when the worker must handle objects over 10 lb, when extended reaches are required, when the worker must frequently move between stations, or when downward forces are exerted (155).

Workstation Redesign

Reorganization of a workstation pertains to changes in the physical layout of components of the work task. A common layout for the transfer of items is to have the points of origin and destination within an arm's reach of the worker. This encourages employees to maintain their feet in one place while twisting the trunk, placing increased stress on the spine. A small change in the origin or destination location may allow the worker to utilize a smaller motion, reducing excessive stress.

Height Adjustments

Following proper height guidelines during work activities may also help reduce stress on the back. Recommended heights are as follows:

For precision work in the upright position, the surface should be between 95 and 105 cm high for a woman and between 100 and 110 cm for a man. This would allow the work to be completed approximately 7 to 10 cm above the waistline, with the forearms maintained parallel with the floor.

Light work should be completed at a level between 85 and 90 cm for a woman and between 90 and 95 cm for a man. Those heights allow activities to be completed approximately 5 cm below the waistline. Heavy work is completed on the lowest work height, between 70 and 85 cm for women and between 75 and 90 cm for men (155). Workstation redesign and maintaining the proper height of the workstation may help reduce stress throughout the entire body in the upright position. Optimizing worksite considerations enhances the worker's ability to function most efficiently.

CONCLUSION

Cumulative trauma disorders are common in our society. The prevalence of industry- and computer-based occupations may lead to continuing proliferation of these conditions if we are not careful. Multiple correlational as well as interventional research studies have been performed that enhance our knowledge of the causes and management of these conditions.

The clinician treating CTDs should be skilled in understanding the pathophysiology and biomechanics at the core of the problem, performing the appropriate diagnostic regimen, and coordinating the comprehensive treatment program. Above all, the mainstay of treatment should be based on correcting the underlying causative factors, which may encompass equipment, technique, and postural issues or basic musculoskeletal overuse.

REFERENCES

1. Arndt R. Work pace, stress and cumulative trauma disorder. *J Hand Surg* 1987; 12A(5):866–869.
2. Laville A. Cadence de travail et posture. *Trav Humain* 1968; 31:1–2.
3. Maeda K. Occupational cervicobrachial and its causative factors. *J Hum Ergol* 1977; 6(2):193–202.
4. Welch LS, Hunting KL, Kellogg J. Work-related musculoskeletal

symptoms among sheet metal workers. *Am J Ind Med* 1995; 27: 783–791.

5. Steadman TL. *Steadman's medical dictionary, 24th ed.* Baltimore: Williams & Wilkins, 1982; 482.
6. Miller JD. Summary of proposed national strategies for the prevention of leading work-related diseases and injuries Part I. *Am J Ind Med* 1988; 13:223–240.
7. Holbrook TL, Grazier K, Kelsey JL, Stauffer RN. The frequency of occurrence, impact and cost of selected musculoskeletal conditions in the United States. *Am Acad Orthop Surg* 1984; 1–87,154–156.
8. Hocking B. Epidemiological aspects of repetition strain injury: in Telecom Australia. *Med J Aust* 1987; 147:218–222.
9. Masear VR, Hayes JM, Hyde AG. An industrial cause of carpal tunnel syndrome. *J Hand Surg* 1986; 11A:222.
10. Andersson GBJ, Pope MH, Frymoyer JW. Epidemiology. In: Pope MH, Frymoyer JW, Andersson GBJ, eds. *Occupational low back pain.* New York: Praeger, 1984; 104–114.
11. Burton CV, Cassidy JD. Economics, epidemiology and risk factors. In: Kirkcaldy-Willis WH, Burton CV, eds. *Managing low back pain.* New York: Churchill Livingstone, 1992; 3.
12. Armstrong TJ, Ulin SS. Analysis and design of jobs for control of work related upper limb disorders. In: Hunter JM, Mackin EJ, Callahan AD, eds. *Rehabilitation of the hand: Surgery and therapy.* St Louis: Mosby, 1995; 1705.
13. Armstrong TJ. Ergonomics and cumulative trauma disorders. *Hand Clin* 1986; 2(3):553–565.
14. Pederson DM, White GL, Murdock RT, Richarson GE, Trunnel EP. Identifying workers risk of cumulative trauma disorders. *J Am Acad Physician Assist* 1989; 4:280–288.
15. Williams R, Westmorland M. Occupational cumulative trauma disorders of the upper extremity. *Am J Occup Ther* 1994; 48(5):411–442.
16. Johnson SL. Ergonomic hand tool design. *Hand Clin* 1993; 9(2): 299–311.
17. Radwin RG, Armstrong TJ, Chaffin DB. Power hand tool vibration effects on grip exertion. *Ergonomics* 1987; 30:833.
18. Helzberg T. Some contributions of applied physical anthrometry to human engineering. *Ann NY Acad Sci* 1955; 63:616–629.
19. Weinstein SM, Scheer SJ. Industrial rehabilitation medicine. 2. Assessment of the problem, pathology, and risk factors for disability. *Arch Phys Med Rehabil* 1992; 73(5-S):S360–S365.
20. Keyserling WM, Armstrong TJ, Punnett L. Ergonomic job analysis: a structured approach for identifying risk factors associated with overexertion injuries and disorders. *Appl Occup Eviron Hyg* 1991; 6: 353–363.
21. Armstrong TJ, Castelli W, Evans F, et al. Some histological changes in carpal tunnel contents and their biomechanical implications. *J Occup Med* 1984; 26:197–201.
22. Phalen G. The carpal tunnel syndrome; clinical evaluation of 598 hands. *Clin Orthop* 1972; 83:29–40.
23. Robbins H. Anatomical study of the median nerve in the carpal tunnel and etiologies of the carpal tunnel syndrome. *J Bone Joint Surg* 1963; 45A:953–966.
24. Tanzer R. The carpal tunnel syndrome. *J Bone Joint Surg* 1959; 41A: 626–634.
25. Tichauer E. Some aspects of stress on the forearm and hand in industry. *J Occup Med* 1966; 8:63–71.
26. Kelsey JL, Githens PB. White AA III, et al. An epidemiologic study of lifting and twisting on the job and risk for acute prolapsed lumbar intervertebral disc. *J Orthop Res* 1984; 2:61.
27. Muckart R. Stenosing tenosynovitis of the abductor pollicis longus and extensor pollicis brevis at the radial styloid. *Clin Orthop* 1964; 33:201–208.
28. Thompson A, Plewes L, Shaw Z. Peritendonitis crepitans and simple tenosynovitis: A clinical study of 544 cases in industry. *Br J Ind Med* 1951; 8:150–160.
29. Sommerich CM, McGlotrin JD, Marras WS. Occupational risk factors associated with soft tissue disorders of the shoulder: a review of recent investigations in the literature. *Ergonomics* 1993; 36:697–717.
30. Clark R. The limiting hand skin temperature unaffected manual performance in the cold. *J Appl Psychol* 1961; 45:193.
31. Williamson D, Chrenko F, Hanley Z. A study of exposure to cold in stores. *Appl Ergonomic* 1984; 15:25.
32. Armstrong TJ. Cumulative trauma disorders of the upper limb and identification of work related factors. In: Millender LH, Louis DS, Simmons BP, eds. *Occupational disorders of the upper extremities.* New York: Churchill Livingstone, 1992; 19–45.
33. Armstrong TJ. Ergonomics and the effect of vibration in hand intensive work. *Scand J Work Environ Health* 1987; 13:286.
34. Lucas E. Lesion of the peripheral nervous system due to vibration. *Scand J Work Environ Health* 1970; 7:67.
35. Falkenburg RE, Kok R, Lewis MI, Meese GB. Finger skin temperature and manual dexterity; some intergroup differences. *Appl Ergonomics* 1984; 15:135–141.
36. Fahey JJ, Bollinger JA. Trigger finger in adults and children. *J Bone Joint Surg* 1954; 36A:1200–1218.
37. Evans RB, Hunter JM, Burkhalter WE. Conservative management of the trigger finger: a new approach. *J Hand Ther* 1988; 1:59–68.
38. Lipscomb PR. Tenosynovitis of the hand and wrist: carpal tunnel syndrome, deQuervain's disease, trigger digit. *Clin Orthop* 1959; 13: 164–180.
39. Bonnici AV, Spencer JD. A survey of trigger fingers in adults. *J Hand Surg* 1965; 13B:202–203.
40. Gerster JC, Lazier R. Upper limb pyrophosphate tenosynovitis outside the carpal tunnel. *Ann Rheum Dis* 1989; 48:689–691.
41. Lapidus PW. Stenosing tenovaginitis. *Surg Clin North Am* 1953; 33: 1317–1347.
42. Quinnell RC. Conservative management of trigger finger. *Practitioner* 1980; 224:187–190.
43. Marks MR, Gunther SF. Efficacy of cortisone injection in treatment of trigger fingers and thumbs. *J Hand Surg* 1989; 14A:722–727.
44. Dick HM. Tumors of the hand and wrist. In: Dee R, Mango E, Hurst LC, eds. *Principles of orthopaedic practice.* New York: McGraw-Hill, 1989; 767–768.
45. Angelides AC, Wallace PF. The dorsal ganglion of the wrist. *J Hand Surg* 1976; 1:228–235.
46. English CJ, Maclaren WM, Court-Brown C, et al. Relations between upper limb soft tissue disorders and repetitive movement at work. *Am J Ind Med* 1995; 27:75–90.
47. Hamilton A. *A study of spastic anemia in the hands of stone cutters.* Washington, D.C.: US Bureau of Labor Statistics, 1918; 236–253.
48. Raynaud M. *On local asphyxia and symmetrical gangrene of the extremities,* Barlow T, Transl. London: New Syndenheim Society, 1888; 121:1.
49. Tara JS, Lemel MS, Nathan R. Vascular disorders of the upper extremity. In: Hunter JM, et al, eds. *Rehabilitation of the hand: Surgery and therapy.* St Louis: CV Mosby, 1995; 972.
50. Agate JN, Druett HA, Tombleson JBL. Raynaud's phenomenon in grinders of small metal casting. *Br J Indocin Med* 1946; 3:157–174.
51. Hunter D, McLaughlin AK, Perry KMA. Effects of the use of pneumatic tools. *Br J Indocin Med* 1945; 2:10.
52. Greenstein D, Kent PJ, Wilkinson D, Kester RC. Raynaud's phenomenon of occupational origin. *J Hand Surg [Br]* 1991; 16:370.
53. Suzuki H. Vibration syndrome of vibrating tool users in a factory of a steel foundry. *Jpn J Ind Health* 1978; 20:261.
54. Wilder DG. The biomechanics of vibration and low back pain. *Am J Ind Med* 1993; 23:577–588.
55. Cherniak MG. Raynaud's phenomenon of occupational origin. *Arch Intern Med* 1990; 150:519–522.
56. Leao L. DeQuervain's disease. *J Bone Joint Surg* 1958; 40A(5):1063.
57. Finkelstein H. Stenosing tendovaginitis at the radial styloid process. *J Bone Joint Surg* 1930; 12:509.
58. Kirkpatrick WH, Lisser S. Soft tissue conditions: Trigger fingers and DeQuervain's. In: Hunter JM, et al, eds. *Rehabilitation of the hand: surgery and therapy, Vol II.* St Louis: CV Mosby, 1995; 1007–1033.
59. Kelly A, Jacoban H. Hand disability due to tenosynovitis. *Ind J Med Surg* 1964; 33:570–574.
60. Hall CL. Chronic stenosing tenovaginitis of the wrist. *J Int Coll Surg* 1950; 14(1):48.
61. DeQuervain F. Uber eine form von chronicher tenovaginitis. *Correspondeg-Blatt F Schweizer Aerzte* 1895; 25:389.
62. Lipscomb PR. Stenosing tenosynovitis at the radial styloid process. *Ann Surg* 1951; 134:110.
63. Chipman JR, Kasdan ML, Camacho DG. Tendinitis of the upper extremity. In: Kasdan ML, ed. *Occupational hand and upper extremity injuries and diseases.* Philadelphia: Hanley & Belfus, 8; 1991, 403–421.
64. Punnett L, Robins JM, Wegman DH, Keyserling WM. Soft tissue

disorders in the upper limbs of female garment workers. *Scand J Work Environ Health* 1985; 11:417–425.

65. Punnett L. Upper extremity musculoskeletal disorders in hospital workers. *J Hand Surg* 1987; 12A(5):858–863.
66. Cooney WPI. Sports injuries to the upper extremity. *Postgrad Med* 1984; 76(4):45–50.
67. McKenzie JMM. Conservative treatment of deQuervain's disease. *Br Med J* 1972; 4:659.
68. Nirschl RP. Elbow tendinosis/tennis elbow. *Clin Sport Med* 1992; 11: 851–870.
69. Kibler WB. Pathophysiology of overload injuries around the elbow. *Clin Sport Med* 1995; 14(2):447–457.
70. Kurppa K, Viikari-Juntura E, Kuosma E, et al. Incidence of tenosynovitis or peritendinitis and epicondylitis in a meat processing factory. *Scand J Work Environ Health* 1991; 17(1):32–37.
71. Chiang HC, Ko YC, Chen SS, Yu HS, et al. Prevalence of shoulder and upper limb disorders among workers in the fish processing industry. *Scand J Work Environ Health* 1993; 19(2):126–131.
72. Moore JS, Gang A. Upper extremity disorders in a pork processing plant: relationship between job risk factors and morbidity. *Am Ind Hyg Assoc J* 1994; 55(8):703–715.
73. Roles NC, Maudsley RH. Radial tunnel syndrome: Resistant tennis elbow as a nerve entrapment. *J Bone Joint Surg* 1972; 54(B):499–508.
74. Gunn CC, Millbrandt WE. Tennis elbow and the cervical spine. *Clin Med Assoc J* 1976; 114:803–809.
75. Harrelson JM, Newman M. Hypertrophy of the flexor carpi ulnaris as a cause of ulnar nerve compression. *J Bone Joint Surg* 1975; 57(4): 554–555.
76. Thomas DR, Plancher KD, Hawkins RJ. Prevention and rehabilitation of overuse injuries of the elbow. *Clin Sport Med* 1995; 14:459–477.
77. Silliman JF, Hawkins RJ. Current concepts and recent advances in the athlete's shoulder. *Clin Sport Med* 1991; 10(4):693–705.
78. Neer CS. Impingement lesions. *Clin Orthop* 1973; 173:70–77.
79. Uhthoff HK, Sarkar K. Classification and definition of tendinopathies. *Clin Sport Med* 1991; 10(4):707–720.
80. Urschel HC, Paulson DL, McNamara JJ. Thoracic outlet syndrome. *Ann Thorac Surg* 1986; 6:1–10.
81. Morrison DS, Bigliani LU. The clinical significance of variations in acromial morphology. *Orthop Trans* 1987; 11:234.
82. Rathbun JB, MacNab I. The microvascular pattern of the rotator cuff. *J Bone Joint Surg* 1970; 52B:540–553.
83. Jobe FW, Kvitne RS. Shoulder pain in the overhand or throwing athlete. *Orthop Rev* 1989; 18:963–975.
84. Perry J, Glousman RE. Biomechanics of throwing. In: Nicholas JA, Hershman EB, eds. *The upper extremity in sports medicine.* St Louis: CV Mosby, 1995; 697–720.
85. Hunting KL, Welch LS, Cuccherini BA, Seiger LA. Musculoskeletal symptoms among electricians. *Am J Ind Med* 1994; 25:149–163.
86. Holmstrom EB, Lindell J, Moritz U. Low back and neck/shoulder pain in construction; occupational workload and psychosocial risk factors. Part 2: Relationship to neck and shoulder pain. *Spine* 1992; 17:672–677.
87. Herberts P, Kadefors R, Hogfors C, Sigholm G. Shoulder pain and heavy manual labor. *Clin Orthop* 1984; 191:166.
88. Stenlund B, Goldie I, Hagberg M, Hogstedt C. Shoulder tendinitis and its relations to heavy manual work and exposure to vibration. *Scand J Work Environ Health* 1993; 19(1):43–49.
89. Hawkins RJ, Kennedy JC. Impingement syndromes in athletes. *Am J Sports Med* 1980; 8:151–158.
90. Neer CS, Welsh RP. The shoulder in sports. *Orthop Clin North Am* 1977; 8:583–591.
91. Levorka S. Manual palpation and pain threshold in female office employees with and without neck–shoulder symptoms. *Clin J Pain* 1993; 9(4):236–241.
92. Anderson JH, Gaardboe O. Musculoskeletal disorders of the neck and upper limb among sewing machine operators: a clinical investigation. *Am J Ind Med* 1993; 24(6):689–700.
93. Oberg T, Oberg U. Musculoskeletal complaints in dental hygiene: A survey study from a Swedish country. *J Dent Hyg* 1993; 67(5): 257–261.
94. Hagberg M, Wegman DH. Prevalence and odds ratios of shoulder–neck diseases in different occupational groups. *Br J Ind Med* 1987; 44(9):602–610.
95. Watson DH, Trott PH. Cervical headache: an investigation of neutral head posture and upper cervical flexor muscle performance. *Cephalgia* 1993; 13(4):272–284.
96. Mayoux-Benhamou MA, Revel M. Influence of head position on dorsal neck muscle efficiency. *Electromyogr Clin Neurophysiol* 1993; 33(3):161–166.
97. Farmer JC, Wisneski RJ. Cervical spine root compression: An analysis of neuroforaminal pressures with varying head and arm positions. *Spine* 1994; 19(16):1850–1855.
98. Travell JG, Simmons DG. *Myofascial pain and dysfunction: the trigger point manual.* Baltimore: Williams & Wilkins, 1983; 45–102.
99. Snook SH. Low back pain in industry. In: White AA, Gordon SSL, eds. *American Academy of Orthopedic Surgery Symposium on Idiopathic Low Back Pain.* St Louis: CV Mosby, 1982; 23.
100. Heliovaara M. Occupation and risk of herniated lumbar intervertebral disc or sciatica leading to hospitalization. *J Chron Dis* 1987; 40:259.
101. Andersson GBJ. Epidemiologic aspects of low back pain in industry. *Spine* 1981; 6:53.
102. Cady LD, Bischoff DP, O'Connell ER, et al. Strength and subsequent back injuries in firefighters. *J Occup Med* 1979; 21:269.
103. Bongers PM, Boshaizen HC, Hulshof CTJ, et al. Back disorders in crane operators exposed to whole-body vibration. *Int Arch Occup Environ Health* 1988; 60:129.
104. Brendstrup T, Biering-Sorensen F. Effect of forklift driving on low back trouble. *Scand J Work Environ Health* 1987; 13:445.
105. Kelsey JL, Hardy RJ. Driving of motor vehicles as a risk factor for herniated lumbar intervertebral disc. *Am J Epidemiol* 1975; 102:63.
106. Bigos SJ, Spengler DM, Martin NA, et al. Back injuries in industry: A retrospective study III employee related factors. *Spine* 1986; 11: 252.
107. Ekenvall G, Gemne, Tegne R. Correspondence between neurological symptoms and outcomes of quantitative sensory testing in hand–arm vibration syndrome. *Br J Ind Med* 1989; 46:570–574.
108. Koskimes K, Farkila M, Pyykko I, et al. Carpal tunnel syndrome in vibration disease. *Br J Ind Med* 1990; 47:411–416.
109. Lundborg G, Gelberman GH, Minteer-Convery M, et al. Median nerve compression in the carpal tunnel functional response to experimentally induced controlled pressures. *J Hand Surg* 1982; 7:252.
110. Gelberman RH, Hergenroeder PT, Hargens AR, et al. The carpal tunnel syndrome: a study of carpal canal pressures. *J Bone Joint Surg* 1981; 36A:380.
111. Rydevik B, Lundborg G, Bagge U. Effects of graded compression on intraneural blood flow. *J Hand Surg* 1981; 6:3.
112. Birkbeck MQ, Beer TC. Occupation in relation to the carpal tunnel syndrome. *Rheum Rehabil* 1975; 14:218–221.
113. Chatterjee DS, Barwick DD, Petrie A. Exploratory electromyography in the study of vibration-induced white finger in rock drillers. *Br J Intern Med* 1982; 39:89.
114. Silverstein BA, Fine LJ, Armstrong TJ. Occupational factors and carpal tunnel syndrome. *Am J Ind Med* 1987; 11:343–358.
115. Sunderland S. The nerve lesion in the carpal tunnel syndrome. *J Neurol Neurosurg Psychiatry* 1976; 39:615.
116. Pryse-Phillips W. Validation of a diagnostic sign in CTS. *J Neurol Neurosurg Psychiatry* 1984; 47:870–872.
117. Nakano KK. Entrapement neuropathies. *Muscle Nerve* 1978; 1: 264–279.
118. Gellman H, Gelberman RH, Tan AM, et al. Carpal tunnel syndrome: evaluation of the provocative diagnostic tests. *J Bone Joint Surg* 1986; 68A:735.
119. Heller L, Ring H, Costeff H, Solzi P. Evaluation of Tinel's and Phalen's signs in diagnosis of the carpal tunnel syndrome. *Eur Neurol* 1986; 25(1):40–42.
120. Durkam JA. New diagnostic test for CTS. *J Bone Joint Surg* 1991; 73A:535–538.
121. Szalbo RM, Gelberman RH, Dimick MP. Sensibility testing in patients with carpal tunnel syndrome. *J Bone Joint Surg* 1984; 66A:60.
122. Mathiowitz VM, Kashman N, Volland G, Weber K, et al. Grip and pinch strength: normative data for adults. *Arch Phys Med Rehabil* 1985; 66:69–74.
123. Nakano KK. Peripheral nerve entrapment, repetitive strain disorder and occupation related syndromes. *Curr Opinion Rheumatol* 1990; 2: 253–269.
124. McGrath M. Local steroid therapy in the hand. *J Hand Surg* 1984; 9(A):915–921.

125. Gelberman RH, Aronson D, Weisman MH. Carpal tunnel syndrome. *J Bone Joint Surg* 1980; 62A:1181–1184.
126. Goodman HV, Gilliat RW. The effect of treatment on median nerve conduction in patients with the carpal tunnel syndrome. *Ann Phys Med* 1961; 6:137–155.
127. Goodman HV, Foster JB. Effect of local corticosteroid injection on median nerve conduction in carpal tunnel syndrome. *Ann Phys Med* 1962; 6:287–294.
128. Gianini F, Passero S, Cioni R, Paradiso C, et al. Electrophysiologic evaluation of local steroid injection in carpal tunnel syndrome. *Arch Phys Med Rehabil* 1991; 72:738–742.
129. Gelberman RH, Aronson D, Weisman MH. Carpal tunnel syndrome: results of a prospective trial of steroid injection and splinting. *J Bone Joint Surg* 1980; 62:1181–1184.
130. Eversmann WW. Proximal median nerve compression. *Hand Clin* 1992; 8(2):307–315.
131. Hartz CR, Linscheid RL, Gramse RR, Daube JR. Pronator teres syndrome: compressive neuropathy of the median nerve. *J Bone Joint Surg* 1981; 63(A):885–890.
132. Martinelli P, Gambellini A, Poppi M Gallassi R, Pozzati E. Pronator syndrome due to thickened bicipital aponeurosis. *J Neurol Neurosurg Psychiatry* 1982; 45:181–182.
133. Morris HH, Peters BH. Pronator syndrome clinical and electrophysiological features in seven cases. *J Neurol Neurosurg Psychiatry* 1976; 39:461–464.
134. Dawson DM, Hallet M, Millender LH. *Peripheral entrapment: Ulnar nerve entrapment at the wrist.* Boston: Little, Brown, 1983; 123–140.
135. Feindel W, Stratford J. The role of the cubital tunnel in tardy ulnar palsy. *Clin J Surg* 1958; 1:287–300.
136. Vanderpool SW, Chalmers J, Lamb DW, et al. Peripheral compression lesions of the ulnar nerve. *J Bone Joint Surg* 1968; 50B:792–803.
137. Apfelberg DB, Larson SJ. Dynamic anatomy of the ulnar nerve at the elbow. *Plast Reconstruct Surg* 1973; 51:76–81.
138. Miller RG. The cubital tunnel syndrome: diagnosis and precise localization. *Ann Neurol* 1979; 6:56–59.
139. Dumitru D. *Electrodiagnostic medicine: focal peripheral neuropathies.* Philadelphia: Hanley & Belfus, 1994; 851–927.
140. Moneim MS. Ulnar nerve compression at the wrist: ulnar tunnel syndrome. *Hand Clin* 1992; 8(2):337–344.
141. Rayam GM, Jensen C, Duke J. Elbow flexion test in the normal population. *J Hand Surg* 1992; 17A:86–89.
142. Novak CB, Lee GW, Mackinnon SE, Lay L. Provocative testing for cubital tunnel syndrome. *J Hand Surg* 1994; 19(5A):817–820.
143. Agnesi R, Dal Vecchio L, Todros A, Sparta S, Valenti F. Ulnar neuropathy at the elbow in workers using column sewing machines: case reports and follow-up. *Med Lavoro* 1993; 84(2):147–161.
144. Rayam GM. Proximal ulnar nerve compression cubital tunnel syndrome. *Hand Clin* 1992; 8(2):325–326.
145. Gessler H. Eine eigenartige form von progressive muskelatrophie bei goldpoliererinnen medsche kon. *Bl Wurtt Arzte Landesver* 1896; 66: 281.
146. Dawson DM, Hallett M, Millender LH. Entrapment neuropathies. Boston: Little, Brown, 1983; 61–86.
147. Streib EW. Distal ulnar neuropathy as a cause of finger tremor: a case report. *Neurology* 1990; 40(1):153–154.
148. Streib EW, Sun SF. Distal ulnar neuropathy in meat packers: an occupational disease? *J Occup Med* 1984; 26:842–843.
149. Noth J, Dietz V, Mauritz KH. Cyclist's palsy. *J Neurol Sci* 1980; 47: 111.
150. Seror P. Treatment of ulnar nerve palsy at the elbow with a night splint. *J Bone Joint Surg* 1993; 75(B):322–327.
151. Adson AW. Symptoms, differential diagnosis for section of the insertion of the scalenus anticus muscle. *J Int Coll Surg* 1951; 16:546.
152. Wright IS. The neurovascular syndrome produced by hyperabduction of the arms. *Am Heart* 1945; 29:1.
153. Lindgren KA, Leino E, Lepantalo M, Paukker P. Recurrent thoracic outlet syndrome after first rib resection. *Arch Phys Med Rehabil* 1991; 72(3):208–210.
154. Cuetter AC, Bartosek DM. The thoracic outlet syndrome: controversies, overdiagnosis, overtreatment, and recommendations for management. *Muscle Nerve* 1989; 12:410–419.
155. Grandjean E. Fitting the task to the man. New York: Taylor & Francis, 1969.

Rehabilitation Medicine: Principles and Practice, Third Edition, edited by Joel A. DeLisa and Bruce M. Gans.
Lippincott–Raven Publishers, Philadelphia © 1998.

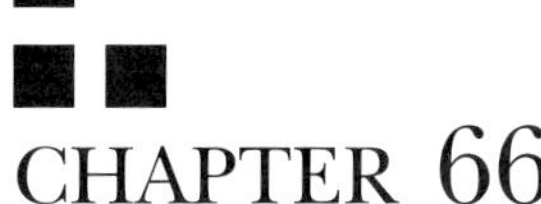

CHAPTER 66

Rehabilitation of Total Hip and Total Knee Replacements

Jerald R. Zimmerman

Total hip arthroplasty (THA) and total knee arthroplasty (TKA) are among the most common operative procedures performed in the United States (1). Over the past 35 years, the use of these procedures has grown dramatically, providing relief from pain and improving the quality of life for millions of patients. During this time, the role of therapy has been emphasized as an integral part of the postoperative management of the patient. Instead of spending days in bed waiting for tissues to heal (2,3), patients now begin functional activities as early as the first postoperative day (4–6). A recent NIH Consensus Conference on total hip replacements identified patient education and rehabilitation as areas deserving further independent study (7).

Rehabilitation services are now provided in various settings, depending on such factors as level of function, social situation, and insurance coverage. Although most patients are able to return home after total joint replacement (TJR), others are unable to be safely discharged. According to a review of Medicare discharge data from 1988, 15% of patients were discharged to a short-term facility (8) providing either acute or subacute rehabilitation services. Providers of care are still searching for the optimum conditions under which to deliver the postoperative care that will help patients regain strength, endurance, and function while minimizing long-term nursing home placement. In this chapter, information pertinent to the care of patients undergoing THA or TKA is presented, providing a scientific basis to maximize function and minimize postoperative complications. Because of the similarities to THA, hemiarthroplasties of the hip, used for the treatment of femoral neck fractures, are also discussed.

J. R. Zimmerman: Department of Rehabilitation Medicine, Englewood Hospital and Medical Center, Englewood, New Jersey 07631.

HISTORY

Surgical attempts to treat the painful hip date back to at least 1826, when Barton described the first osteotomy on an ankylosed hip (9). A number of interpositional materials, such as soft tissue, wood, and gold foil, were unsuccessful (9). Replacement of just the femoral head was first described by Moore in 1952 (10). Although this procedure was not successful for the pain of osteoarthritis, it remains useful as a standard treatment option for femoral neck fractures in the elderly (11). The first attempt at replacing both articular surfaces of the hip, called a total hip arthroplasty, was performed by Wiles in 1938 (9,12). Fixation of the components remained a major problem until Charnley (2) reported two major developments: (a) the concept of low-friction arthroplasty with a metal femoral head articulating in a plastic socket, and (b) the use of acrylic cement to improve the mechanical bond between the prosthesis and the bone. Initially, Charnley used Teflon for the acetabular component. However, because of excessive wear of the Teflon, he soon changed to high-density polyethylene, which, with some minor modifications, remains in use today. The appropriateness of his choice of materials was borne out by the 96% success rate he reported in his 10-year follow-up study (13) (Fig. 66-1).

The first attempts at designing a total knee arthroplasty began in the 1950s with a hinged design by Walldius (14). As with the hip, early successes were tempered by high failure rates. The first unlinked design, using the same materials as Charnley, was reported by Gunston in 1971 (15). This approach was too simplistic and was soon replaced by designs that attempted to duplicate the anatomy and biomechanics of the knee, which is much more complicated than the hip. These anatomic designs, including replacement of the patellofemoral articulation, are now the standard for the majority of total knee replacements, with clinical results equal

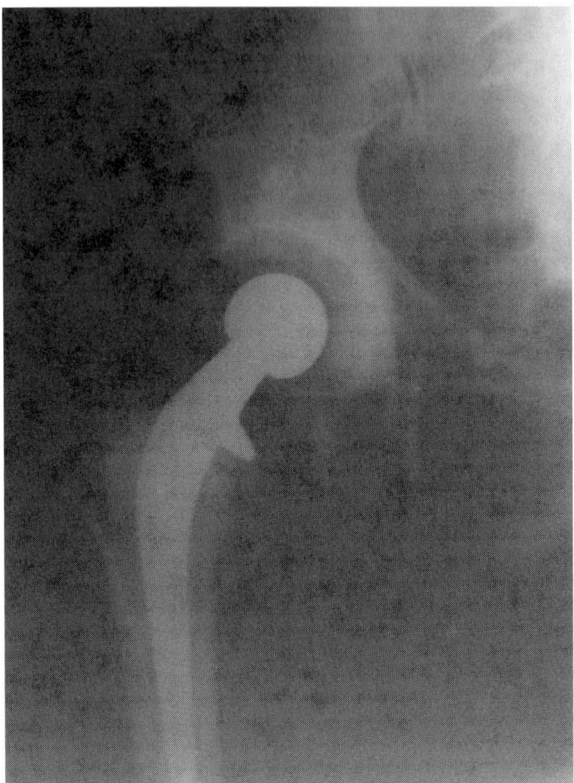

FIG. 66-1. Anteroposterior radiograph of a cemented total hip arthroplasty. Note the metal femoral component and the radiolucent acetabular component made of ultrahigh-molecular-weight polyethylene. The polymethylmethacrylate cement, which is normally a clear acrylic, is made with barium so that it will appear radiodense on the radiographs.

to or better than those reported for total hip replacements (16–19) (Fig. 66-2).

EPIDEMIOLOGY

The total number of THA and TKA performed annually has grown dramatically over the past 20 years. The estimated number of procedures performed annually in the United States grew from 80,000 THA and 40,000 TKA in 1976 to 125,000 THA and 179,000 TKA in 1993 (1,20). The utilization rate of these procedures per 100,000 persons per year is similar to rates from Scandinavian countries (21–23). Levy estimated that 300,000 to 400,000 THAs were performed worldwide in 1985 (24).

The greatest incidence of THA and TKA is in patients between the ages of 65 and 79 (21–25). Variations in usage exist by geographic location, age, sex, and race (8). The highest rates of utilization were found in the Northwest and Midwest, and the lowest rates were in the East and South. Approximately 65% of recipients are female. There is also a higher prevalence of these procedures in Caucasians and in those with a higher income.

INDICATIONS AND CONTRAINDICATIONS

Both THA and TKA are indicated for those patients who have severe disabling pain as a result of destruction of the joint and either have not responded to nonoperative management or are not candidates for less aggressive procedures (e.g., synovectomy). Common causes of joint destruction include osteoarthritis, rheumatoid arthritis, avascular necrosis, traumatic arthritis, Legg-Calve-Perthes' disease, slipped capital femoral epiphysis, and a failed previous operation (19,25–29). Nonoperative management could include, but not be limited to, the use of nonsteroidal anti-inflammatory drugs or acetaminophen, weight reduction, physical therapy to maintain range of motion and improve muscle strength about the affected joint, modification of activities, and the use of a cane (7,18,30). Patients with pain from inflammatory arthritis should first attempt a comprehensive medical management program. Both THA and TKA are elective procedures whose goals are to provide relief of pain with a return of function (2,18).

Although THA and TKA are elective procedures, the use of hemiarthroplasties, in which only the femoral head is replaced, has gained wide acceptance as a treatment option for patients with intracapsular (femoral neck) fractures of the hip (11,31). The most commonly used design has been similar to the prosthesis described by Moore (32). Because there is a single articulation between the metal head and the acetabular cartilage, it has also been called a unipolar design (Fig. 66-3). The bipolar design has an inner bearing of ultrahigh-molecular-weight polyethylene (Fig. 66-4). With a low-friction surface incorporated into the system, the complications of loosening, acetabular erosion, and dislocation seen with the Austin Moore design should be reduced. However, the benefit of one design over the other has not yet been proven. In patients with pre-existing osteoarthritis, placement of a THA may be indicated (33,34). The choice of a device for a femoral neck fracture should depend on the age, life expectancy, degree of osteoporosis, and functional demands of the patient.

The only absolute contraindication to elective total joint replacement is active sepsis, local or systemic (17,35). Several relative contraindications have been described, including younger age and obesity as well as the presence of severe muscle weakness or paralysis about the joint, as may be seen with polio. However, age (36) and obesity (37–39) have not been shown to have an adverse effect on outcome. Finally, the patient must be psychologically prepared to be an active participant in the postoperative rehabilitation program, or a suboptimal result could occur.

METHODS OF FIXATION

Firm fixation of the prosthetic components to the surrounding bone is essential for a pain-free joint. Although micromotion, on the order of microns, may be tolerated without adverse results, greater motion, associated with pain in the joint, is indicative of aseptic loosening, the most common complication of total joint replacements. Revision surgery is often necessary, which can be more difficult to perform (40,41), more costly (42), and produce less satisfactory results than primary arthroplasty (43–45). There are four primary methods of fixation (see Table 66-1). Each one may be used alone, and some may be used in combination with each other. It is important to understand how these materials affect both the short-term postoperative management of the patient (e.g., weight-bearing status) as well as the long-term clinical results.

Polymethylmethacrylate (Bone Cement)

The introduction of polymethylmethacrylate (PMMA) in 1961 by Charnley (2) signified a breakthrough to the modern era of total joint replacement. The utility of PMMA has been borne out by its continued use for nearly four decades and remains the gold standard to which other methods of fixation must be compared.

PMMA is manufactured as a powdered polymer and a liquid monomer. Once they are mixed, a polymerization process takes place, producing an exothermic reaction. When the PMMA is putty-like, it is packed into the bone by one of a several techniques (see Table 66-2). The prosthetic component is then rigidly held in place while the PMMA hardens, which takes approximately 15 minutes. The majority of the polymerization process occurs within this time. By 24 hours the process is completed, at which time the PMMA is mechanically strongest. The PMMA, which is also called bone cement, acts as a grouting agent, interdigitating with the endosteal surface of the bone to provide a mechanical lock. It has no adhesive properties and is therefore not a glue. Its purpose is to distribute stresses from the prosthesis to the bone. The PMMA itself has poor mechanical properties compared to metal and bone. It demonstrates fatigue failure at relatively low strain rates, particularly in tension (46,47), which may be one of the factors leading to loosening. Despite these concerns, PMMA has demonstrated its clinical effectiveness over time.

Porous Coated—Bony Ingrowth

For many years, it was felt that the PMMA was the primary factor leading to aseptic loosening. Not only could PMMA fail under cyclic loading, but barium granules, which are normally distributed in the powdered polymer to make the material radiopaque (Fig. 66-1), were found in the interface tissues removed from areas of loosening, leading to the concept of cement disease (48). This, in turn, led to the development of systems to produce a biological fixation of the prosthesis to the bone.

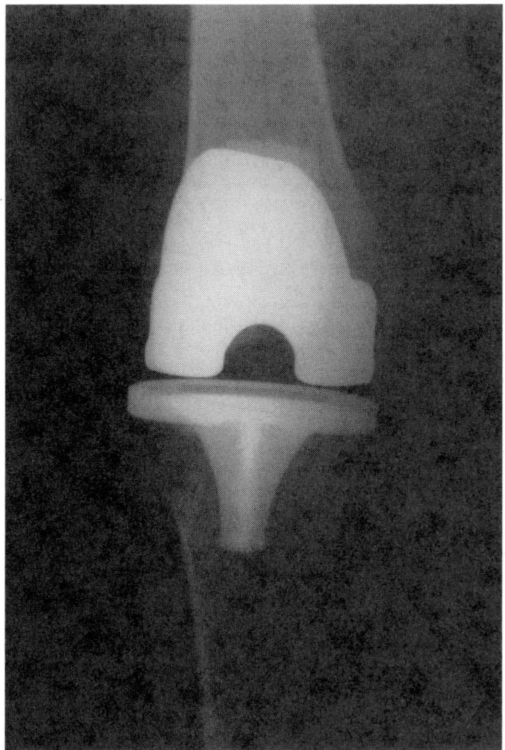
A

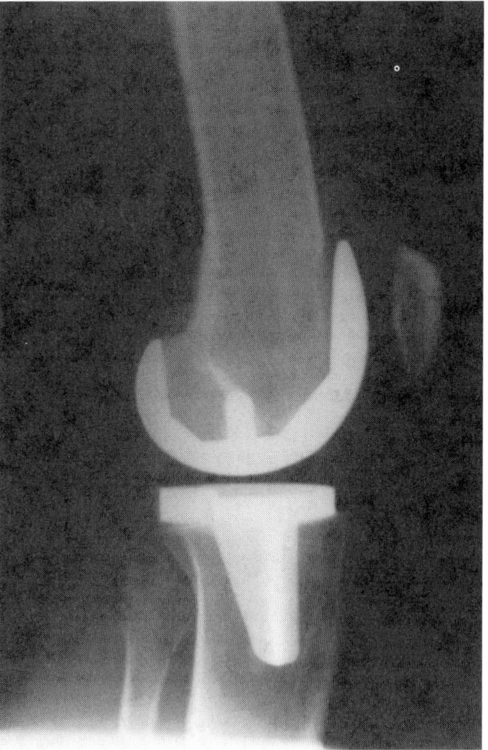
B

FIG. 66-2. A: Anteroposterior radiograph of a noncemented total knee replacement. There is a metal femoral component and a metal tibial tray which holds a radiolucent tibial component made of ultra high molecular weight polyethylene. There is no cement between the components and the bone. **B:** Lateral radiograph of a noncemented total knee replacement. In addition to the components noted in **A,** there is a plastic patellar button articulating with the femoral component.

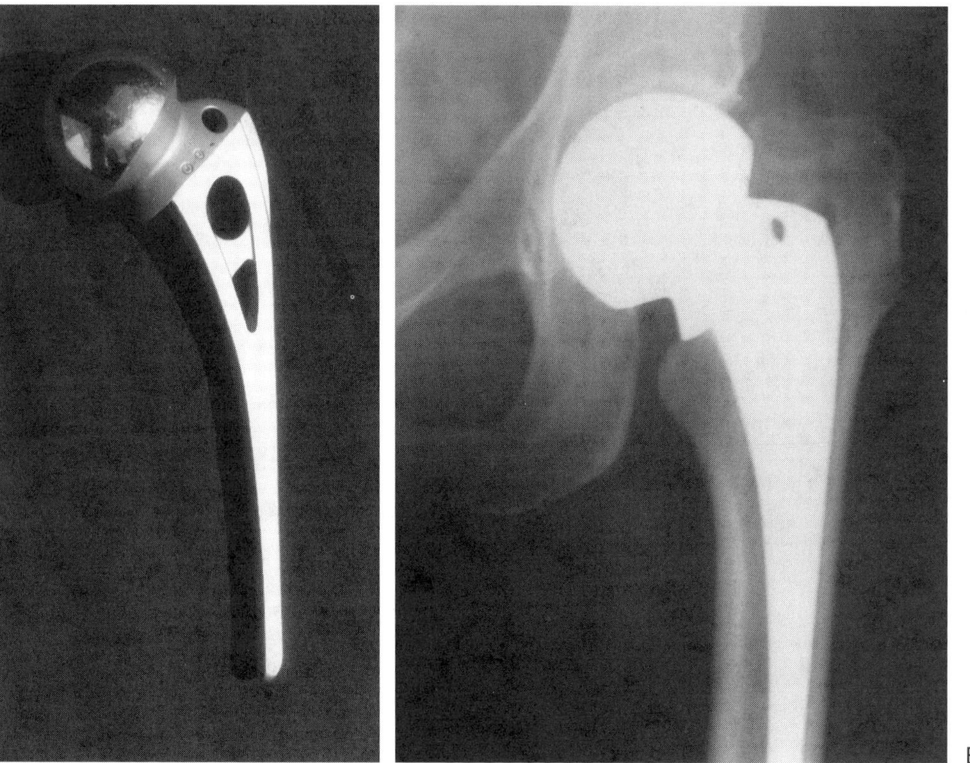

FIG. 66-3. A: An Austin Moore or unipolar hemiarthroplasty. **B:** Radiographic appearance of an Austin Moore hemiarthroplasty. The acetabular cartilage is seen as clear space between the metal head and the superior roof of the acetabulum. This shows that there is no acetabular component, which is the definition of a hemiarthroplasty of the hip.

To manufacture a bony ingrowth surface, a porous metal matrix is bonded onto a metal core. At the time of surgery, a hematoma develops, which will trigger a fracture-healing response, with the eventual development of mature bone in the pores of the matrix (49–51). Motion at the bone–prosthesis interface needs to be minimized as much as possible in the first 6 weeks of this process (52–54), although exactly how much motion can be tolerated remains controversial (55). Initial press-fit stability, as described below, is necessary. All of these studies, however, have been performed on animal models, so that recommendations for optimizing the local macro- and microenvironments in humans are by inference only. Retrieval studies have shown that bone does not grow over the entire porous coated surface, with fibrous tissue often being more abundant than bone. However, extensive bone growth does not appear to be necessary for satisfactory clinical outcomes (46,50,51).

Hydroxyapatite Coating

Calcium hydroxyapatite (HA) and tricalcium phosphate (TCP) are bioactive ceramics that resemble biological apatite. They are capable of producing new bone growth (osteoconduction), to which they directly bond, without intervening soft tissue. This property may allow osseointegration with smooth metal as well as improved bone growth into porous coated prostheses. In animal studies, new bone growth and enhanced fixation are seen with both smooth (56) and porous coated implants (57,58).

Hydroxyapatite is now being used in clinical trials of both smooth and porous coated components. Initial stable fixation, as with noncoated porous implants, is necessary to ensure bony apposition (46). In dogs, micromotion of as little as 100 μm has been shown to impede new bone growth (59). Although early clinical results are encouraging (60–64), long-term follow-up will be necessary to monitor the status of the HA coating (delamination may occur at the HA–prosthesis interface) (65,66) and to determine if functional outcomes differ from other methods of fixation.

Press-Fit Stabilization

Press-fit stabilization implies a tight, stable fit between the implant and the bone after insertion of the component. The surface being prepared must be exactly the same size

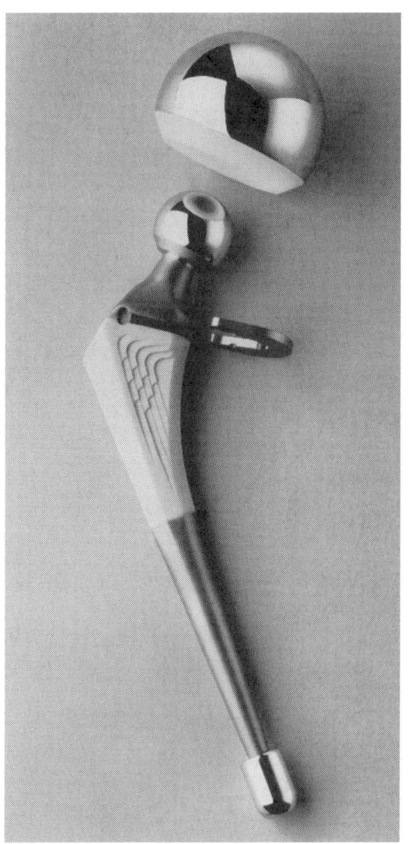
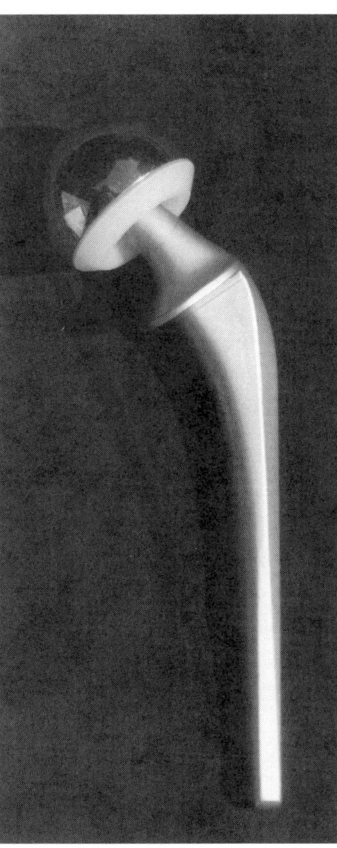
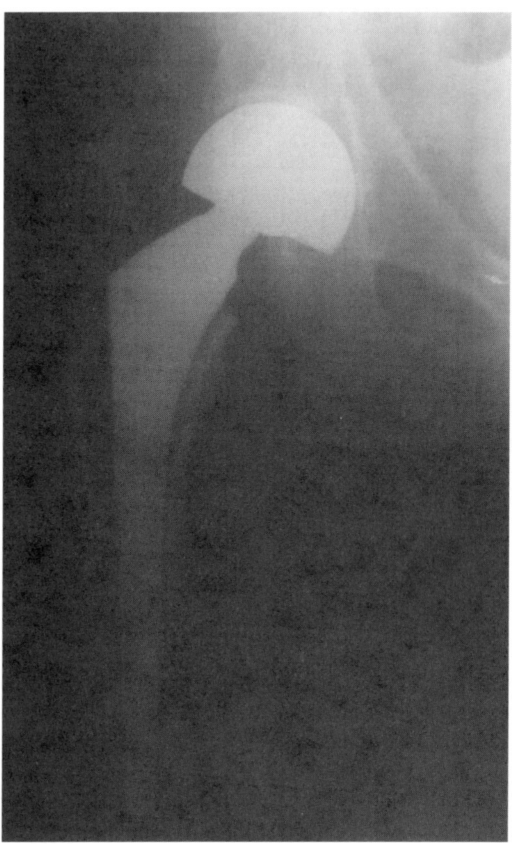

A,B C

FIG. 66-4. A: An expanded view of a bipolar hemiarthroplasty. The femoral component is identical to those used for a total hip arthroplasty. **B:** A fully constructed bipolar hemiarthroplasty. **C:** Radiographic appearance of a bipolar hemiarthroplasty. As in Figure 66-3*B*, the acetabular cartilage is seen superiorly.

as or slightly smaller than the component being inserted. A fracture may occur when the component is hammered into place if the prepared area is too small. The ability to produce a stable press-fit component depends on the geometry of the component, the geometry of the bone, and the skill of the surgeon. With a satisfactory press fit, the macrolock between the component and the bone provides the necessary initial stability for devices with porous or HA coating while minimizing micromotion. Smooth-stem devices, such as the Austin Moore hemiarthroplasty, rely on the press fit to provide long-term stability, as the metal itself has no osteoconductive properties. The usefulness of press-fit stabilization has been demonstrated by over 40 years of clinical use.

COMPLICATIONS OF TOTAL JOINT REPLACEMENTS

Since the modern era of joint replacements began in the early 1960s, a number of postoperative complications have

TABLE 66-1. *Methods of prosthetic fixation*

Polymethylmethacrylate (bone cement)
Porous coated—bony ingrowth
Hydroxyapatite coating
Press-fit stabilization

TABLE 66-2. *Current cementing techniques*

First generation
Removal of loose cancellous fragments
Hand mixing of cement
Finger-packing of cement into the acetabulum and femoral canal
Second generation
Removal of loose cancellous fragments
Sponge drying of prepared surfaces
Hand mixing of cement
Intramedullary femoral canal plug (to restrict cement movement)
Cement gun for retrograde filling of the femoral canal (to improve filling of the canal and reduce voids and laminations in the cement mantle)
Third generation
Intramedullary canal plug
Pulsatile lavage (to remove debris)
Adrenaline-soaked sponges (to reduce bleeding)
Centrifugation or vacuum mixing of the cement (to reduce cement porosity)
Cement gun for retrograde filling of the femoral canal
Pressurization of the cement before insertion of the components (to enhance penetration and interdigitation of the cement at the bone–cement interface)
Precoating the proximal portion of the femoral stem with a very thin layer of polymethylmethacrylate (to enhance bonding to the cement)

been identified. A current knowledge of the concepts, etiology, and treatment paradigms for these complications will help ensure both the short- and long-term health of patients as well as maximize the long-term viability of the implants.

Aseptic Loosening

Charnley's first long-term series reported an infection rate of 4.3% as the most common postoperative complication (13). As perioperative antibiotics and laminar air exchange in the operating room significantly lowered infection rates, aseptic loosening emerged as the major problem following THA (42) and remains so today for both THA (67–69) and TKA (70).

Patients with a loose prosthesis complain of pain in the groin or buttocks after THA or about the knee after TKA, especially with weight bearing. There should be radiographic confirmation of loosening, consisting of movement or fracture of the component or the presence of a continuous radiolucent line around the entire prosthesis (Fig. 66-5). However, patients may have radiographic findings compatible with a loose device without any complaints of pain. This is called radiographic loosening. Clinical series usually report both clinically loose and radiographically loose components as a composite total; those patients with only radiographic loosening are not considered clinical failures but do require further observation.

The earliest clinical series of THA reported rates of loosening of up to 40% for femoral components and 30% for acetabular components, as determined by the need for revision or by radiographic evidence of loosening (71,72). The introduction of newer cementing techniques (see Table 66-2) (73,74) led to significant reductions in the rate of femoral component loosening to less than 3% (73,74). These results are superior to those reported with porous coated stems (75,76). However, the need for the new cementing techniques may be controversial, as there have been several recent long-term series of femoral components inserted with the original techniques that have showed results similar to the newer techniques (77,78).

Loosening of the acetabular component remains a significant long-term problem no matter which fixation technique is used, with loosening rates reported in recent long-term studies as high as 40% (77,79). The concern about long-

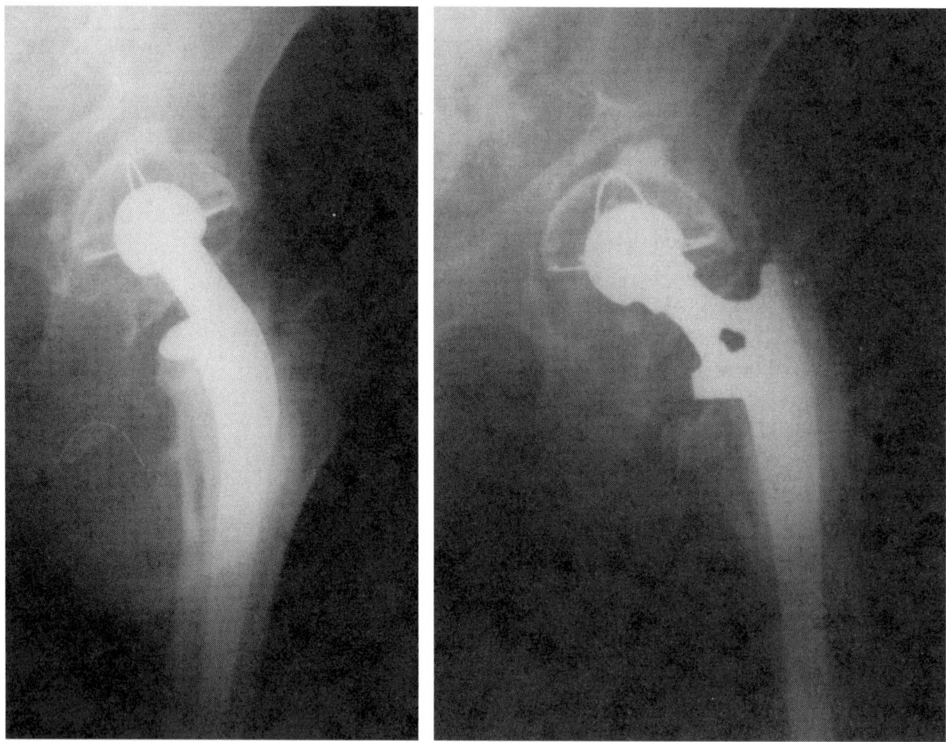

FIG. 66-5. A: A total hip arthroplasty after insertion. There is no complete cement mantle about either the femoral or the acetabular component. There is also a radiolucent line laterally between the acetabular component and the bone. **B:** The same hip after revision of the femoral component for aseptic loosening. Osteolysis in the femur can be seen as an irregular thinning of the cortex (there is extravasation of cement distally) as well as a loss of bone in the region of the calcar (just above the lesser trochanter). A specially designed femoral component must be used to replace this lost proximal bone. About the acetabular component, osteolysis presents as a radiolucent space between the component/cement and the bone, with possible movement of the component. This is a marked change from the initial radiograph. Despite the osteolysis, the acetabular component was well fixed at the time of surgery, so that its revision was not indicated.

term loosening of cemented acetabular components has led to the "hybrid" concept of total hip replacement, in which the femoral component is cemented while a porous coated acetabular component is used. There are similar or improved clinical results using this approach when compared to other combinations of fixation techniques (75,80,81).

Revision rates after hip hemiarthroplasty had been reported to be between 10% and 20% (82), with radiographic signs of loosening in up to 37% (83). Although revision surgery is prompted by pain, it cannot usually be determined whether the pain is caused by femoral loosening or wear of the acetabular cartilage (33). A meta-analysis of outcomes after displaced femoral neck fractures showed that the rates of reoperation were lower with bipolar hemiarthroplasties than with unipolar devices (10% versus 20%) (84).

Aseptic loosening after TKA is seen almost exclusively with the tibial and patellar components (70,85). With improvements in component design and cementing techniques, rates of revision are now less than 3% for the tibia (44,86–88) and 1% for the patella (70). Cemented components showed better long-term survivorship compared to those with bony ingrowth surfaces (86).

Thromboembolic Disease

Although aseptic loosening carries the most significant long-term implications following joint replacement, venous thromboembolic disease (VTED) (e.g., deep venous thrombosis [DVT] and pulmonary embolus [PE]) is the most common and potentially dangerous postoperative complication. Pulmonary embolus is the leading cause of death after total joint replacement (89,90). The incidence of DVT after THA is as high as 70% (91), and 84% after TKA (92). The incidence of nonfatal PE after total joint replacement ranges from 0% to 40%, with fatal PE up to 7% (90). In one survey, 25% of all orthopedic surgeons reported having a patient die of a PE after THA within a 1-year period (93). For these reasons, patients undergoing lower extremity TJR must be considered to be at high risk for PE.

Etiology

The etiology of VTED is multifactoral. Venous stasis and blood pooling may result from intraoperative positioning of the limb (94), immobility (91), local edema, and, for TKA, the use of a tourniquet (95). Direct endothelial damage may occur during manipulation and retraction of the joint (96,97) and from the use of the tourniquet. A hypercoagulable state may develop as a result of activation of tissue and other clotting factors at sites of endothelial injury (98) as well as a reduced level of antithrombin III (99) and inhibition of the fibrinolytic system (100).

Diagnosis of VTED

Most thrombi, both DVT and PE, are small and clinically silent. It is well accepted that the clinical diagnosis of VTED is unreliable (91,92,101). Complete occlusion of the involved vein, which is necessary for the development of most clinical symptoms, occurs no more than 40% of the time (91). Physical examination for DVT, with positive findings such as blanching, pain, edema, and Homan sign, fails to detect 50% to 90% of all DVT and cannot differentiate between proximal and distal DVT (91). Half of all pulmonary emboli are clinically silent, and fewer than 10% of patients with a fatal PE are diagnosed before death (90,102). The clinical and laboratory findings associated with a PE are not only nonspecific but also frequently absent (103).

Because of the unreliability of clinical findings in the diagnosis of VTED, objective screening and diagnostic tests are necessary. Because the primary goal is prevention of PE, any screening test must be able to accurately diagnose the presence of a proximal DVT, which is most often thought to be the primary precursor to a PE (104,105), as well as a distal DVT that could propogate or extend proximally (106,107). Contrast venography, introduced in 1942, has become the gold standard against which other methods are compared (108). However, venography is painful and invasive, can be associated with hypersensitivity reactions, may lead to a secondary thrombosis, and is not a test that can be easily repeated in serial fashion (95,109). Noninvasive screening tests that are now in use include impedance plethysmography (IPG) and compression ultrasonography (US).

IPG has been shown to be less sensitive and to have a lower positive predictive value when compared to US (110,111). Ultrasonography has been compared to venography by a number of investigators and was found to have a sensitivity of 85% to 100% and a specificity of 97% to 100% for the detection of proximal DVT (112–115). Several of these authors also felt that US could be useful for diagnosing distal DVT, but its accuracy was technician dependent (115,116). All of these studies were performed on a relatively small number (approximately 100) of patients. A meta-analysis performed by Wells et al. (117) showed the sensitivity for US to be 62%, specificity 97%, with positive predictive value of 66% when used for detecting proximal DVT. For distal DVT, the meta-analysis showed a sensitivity of only 48% and a positive predictive value of 93%. This analysis demonstrates some of the potential limitations in the use of US as a screening tool.

Prophylaxis for VTED

Because of the possible link between DVT and PE, the presence of a DVT is considered a natural marker for PE (90,118). When the incidence of DVT has been decreased, the incidence of PE and its associated mortality has also been shown to decrease, suggesting that prophylaxis to prevent the development of VTED would be beneficial (89,90,92,95,101,102,118,119). Prevention of VTED through the use of prophylaxis has been shown to be cost effective and preferable to treatment (120,121). Although it does not eliminate the risk of VTED entirely (123–125), prophylaxis has been universally recommended for all patients undergoing THA and TKA (95,102,118,122,126). Prophylaxis, which attempts to alter a part of the pathologic mechanism that leads to the development of VTED, can be either mechanical or chemical.

Mechanical Prophylaxis

Mechanical interventions attempt to decrease venous stasis in the lower extremities. The simplest of these methods, elevation of the limb and early mobilization, are not felt to provide adequate prophylaxis (91), nor do compression stockings (graded or nongraded) significantly reduce the risk of thromboembolism (123). Meta-analysis has confirmed the beneficial effects of intermittent pneumatic stockings after THA (124,125), and they are now used at many institutions. Other mechanical devices that have been tried include a foot pump and, after TKA, the continuous passive motion (CPM) machine. However, there are not enough data to recommend the use of either of these devices for prophylaxis.

Pharmacologic Prophylaxis

Pharmacologic agents attempt to affect various aspects of clot formation. Pharmacologic agents currently in use include aspirin, warfarin, subcutaneous heparin, and low-molecular-weight heparin (LMWH). Two meta-analyses on the formation of DVT after THA (124,125) showed a beneficial effect from all of the agents evaluated except aspirin. The lowest rates of DVT occurred after using LMWH.

There have been no meta-analyses to evaluate prophylactic regimens after TKA or hemiarthroplasty. Thus, recommendation for the use of a specific prophylactic agent is often inferred from THA data. Two studies comparing LMWH and warfarin after TKA showed the LMWH to be the more effective agent (127,128). Both LMWH and warfarin have been shown to be effective prophylactic agents after hip fracture (123), although aspirin may also work in this patient population (129).

Warfarin should be monitored to maintain an anticoagulation effect with an International Normalized Ratio (INR) of 2.0 to 3.0 (130). Prophylactic heparin, given in a 5,000-unit subcutaneous injection 2 to 3 times daily, does not require laboratory monitoring. A LMWH such as enoxaparin is also administered subcutaneously (30 mg every 12 hours) and does not require laboratory monitoring.

Duration of Prophylaxis

There has been only one study to date that has examined in a prospective, randomized fashion, the optimum duration for prophylaxis (131). Most studies examining the various prophylactic regimens chose discharge from the hospital, usually occuring between 7 and 21 days after surgery, as an end point for prophylaxis, unless a DVT has already been diagnosed (127–129). However, it is not known how high the risk is for VTED in the ensuing weeks or months. Seagroatt et al. found DVT to be the most common cause of readmission to the hospital after THA (132). Reports of new, clinically apparent VTED following discharge have ranged from 0 to 2.3% (128,129,133). Bergqvist et al. found an incidence of clinically silent VTED of 39% 1 month after surgery (131).

Currently, there are no standardized regimens or recommendations for how long to continue prophylaxis. Sarasin et al. (134) modeled various treatment options based on current clinical data. They found that oral anticoagulation for 6 weeks, or screening patients with ultrasound at the time of discharge, would be more cost effective than stopping prophylaxis without either of these interventions. The benefit of continued anticoagulation versus ultrasound screening depended on the assumptions made of the rate of major bleeding complications, the cost of the drugs involved, and the sensitivity of the ultrasound test. Bergqvist et al. showed a significant benefit from the continued use of LMWH for 1 month after surgery (131). If patients are not to be monitored by ultrasound during their hospitalization, then consideration should be given for 4 to 6 weeks of anticoagulation with either warfarin or LMWH.

POSTOPERATIVE REHABILITATION PROGRAM

The goal of any rehabilitation program following TJR is not only to maximize the patient's functional status with respect to mobility and activities of daily living (ADL) but also to minimize postoperative complications. In addition, medical and nursing personnel must be vigilant in preventing iatrogenic complications such as sacral and heel decubiti, tape burns, and the adverse effects of drug interactions. Use of narcotic analgesics, parenteral iron, and prolonged bed rest may be the basis on which severe constipation may develop, particularly in the elderly, and it should be guarded against, as should other deleterious effects of prolonged immobilization. Finally, the rehabilitation program, no matter what the setting, should provide the basis for a safe return to the home setting, allow resumption of premorbid activities, and integrate patients back into the social fabric of their communities.

In this section, some general principles regarding the postoperative rehabilitation programs are discussed, followed by specific information necessary for the rehabilitation of both THA and TKA.

General Concepts

In this section, concepts relating to preoperative education, muscle strengthening, range-of-motion exercises, and weight-bearing principles will be discussed. Although most of the literature published on these topics relates to THA, the principles are equally applicable to TKA.

Preoperative Education

Preoperative instructional guides, both written and video, are in common use. In a study of 60 patients undergoing THA, Santavirta et al. (135) found that patients' perceptions of sources of information changed dramatically over time. On admission to the hospital, 35% of patients reported the main source of information as being from their doctors, 20% from other patients, and 17% from a patient guide booklet. Two to three months later, 61% of patients thought they had received most of their information from the physical therapists, 9% from the physician, and 4% from the nursing staff. After surgery was completed, 37% of patients could not name any postoperative complication, and another 37% knew of only one. However, they were better able to choose from a list than to provide answers themselves. Half of these patients had been given an additional intensive educational session before surgery. There was no improvement in the overall level of knowledge with this extra session, except to know when to inform the physician of appropriate symptoms or complications. Overall, patients were satisfied with the booklet but desired as many good illustrations as possible. Patient education must remain an ongoing process throughout the course of the patient's care.

Muscle Strengthening

Many patients will have decreased strength in muscles controlling painful joints (136,137). With relief of pain, muscle strength will improve from increased use of the muscles, accompanied by a return of normal stance and gait patterns. However, studies have shown that weakness can persist for as long as 2 years after surgery. Although this weakness may not interfere with clinical function or gait, the long-term implications remain unknown. Strengthening of muscles about the operated joint, whether isometric, isotonic, or isokinetic, should be continued for a prolonged time (136,137). The effects of specific muscle-strengthening exercises on the stresses in the joint, especially in the immediate postoperative period, remain unknown. Current clinical practices vary widely, without a firm scientific basis for any one regimen. The effects of any exercise on the short- or long-term functioning of the joint also remain unknown.

The only *in vivo* data come from several studies in which an Austin Moore hemiarthroplasty was inserted with transducers placed on the articulating surface of the prosthesis or along the femoral neck of the device (138–141). One month after surgery, Davy and Rydell both showed peak forces during active hip abduction of 1.5 to 2.2 times body weight. Strickland's data showed that the highest peak pressures occurred with active hip flexion and gluteal isometrics during the first two postoperative weeks.

Over the next 2 years, peak pressures during straight-leg raising (SLR) and isometric, side-lying hip abduction exercises stabilized. The stresses generated under these conditions were always less than those seen with full or partial weight bearing (141). Based on this information, these exercises could be performed whenever full or partial weight bearing is allowed. Active supine abduction exercises produced lower peak pressures than the isometric abduction exercises.

Muscle-strengthening exercises, therefore, must be a vital component of any postoperative rehabilitation program. Isometric strengthening of the quadriceps and hip extensor muscles should be started immediately after surgery. Progressive resistive exercises, starting with the weight of the limb itself, may be gradually started for hip flexion (SLR) and knee extension within the first few days of surgery. As long as there is no pain in the joint itself, resistance may be added as tolerated. Initially, active hip abduction should be done in a supine position. For patients who have had a TKA, additional resistance for SLR/knee extension should be avoided until full active extension is achieved. Without full knee extension, the patient may be more susceptible to a rupture of the quadriceps tendon (70,142). Some clinicians will use a knee splint during SLR exercises to maintain the knee in a more extended position, however, there is no evidence that this helps improve quadriceps strength.

In addition to strengthening the muscles directly related to the operated joint, overall muscle strength should be maintained as well. Upper extremity strength is necessary to safely and effectively use assistive devices as well as to perform transfers. Strength must be maintained in the nonoperated limb to allow safe ambulation as well as to perform sit-to-stand transfers and to negotiate elevations. Exercises to strengthen these muscles can be started as a part of the preoperative program and continue immediately after surgery.

Range-of-Motion Exercises

Joint range of motion (ROM) must be maintained to allow patients to perform functional tasks. Full range of motion should be present at all nonoperated joints, including the ankle on the ipsilateral side. This is accomplished by having the patient perform active ROM (AROM) exercises on a daily basis. If AROM exercises cannot be performed for any reason, the joints should be moved passively throughout the full ROM several times a day.

For the patient having a THA or hemiarthroplasty, specific ROM exercises for the involved hip are not indicated. This will be discussed further under the section on total hip precautions. For the patient having a TKA, limitations in both knee flexion and extension may affect function. Knee flexion must be addressed through the use of passive, active assisted, and active ROM exercises and should begin as soon as possible after recovery from surgery. Knee flexion of 83° is needed, under normal functioning conditions, for stair climbing, 70° for normal gait (during swing phase), and 105° for unaided sit-to-stand transfers (143). The role of the continuous passive motion (CPM) machine is discussed below. Although a goal of 90° of flexion on discharge from the hospital may be desirable, the exact relationship between knee ROM and function in the early postoperative period is unknown. A knee extension lag is also present following TKA, the etiology of which may be multifactorial (144). Long-term follow-up studies, though, consistently show maintenance or improvement in knee ROM from preoperative levels, with a mean total arc of motion of 110° to 115°(145).

Total Hip Precautions

After THA or hemiarthroplasty, specific ROM exercises are not performed on the involved hip, thus avoiding an iatrogenic dislocation. A functional ROM is maintained while performing muscle-strengthening exercises (e.g., hip flexion) as well as functional tasks such as sitting, elevations, and transfers. The design of the prosthetic components, combined with the weakened or deficient joint capsule that ensues from surgery, puts the patient at risk for dislocation if the constraints of the prosthesis are exceeded. Thus, total hip precautions are taught to the patient in order to keep the prosthesis within its own constraints. These precautions, which attempt to maintain coverage of the femoral head by the acetabular component and prevent component impingement, include (a) no flexion of the hip past 90°, (b) no adduction of the leg past midline, and (c) no external rotation of the leg (146) (Fig. 66-6). Toward this end, patients must be instructed (a) not to bend forward from the waist more than 90°, (b) not to lift the knee on the side of the surgery higher than the hip, and (c) not to cross the legs, either at the knee or the ankle. To help patients maintain these hip precautions, several pieces of adaptive equipment are necessary. An abduction wedge is most often used while in bed, although a knee immobilizer will restrict hip flexion while the patient is supine (147). Additional equipment, including a reacher, sock-aide, elastic laces, long-handled bath sponge, tub bench, raised toilet seat, and long shoe horn are all necessary to help the patient perform ADLs correctly. The patient must be taught the proper way to transfer, both for bed mobility as well as to standard surfaces, such as a chair and toilet. While in bed, the patient may roll to either side as long as both legs are maintained in an abducted position. Modifications to these hip precautions may be necessary on an individual basis to prevent dislocation (Fig. 66-7).

These precautions are universally accepted and are typically maintained for approximately 3 months, allowing enough time for a pseudocapsule to form. Because the majority of dislocations occur within the first 30 days, (148), there have been no clinical studies to determine the optimum length of time to maintain the hip precautions. If they are maintained too long, contractures may develop that could interfere with future, higher-level activities. Total hip precautions must also be maintained for patients undergoing placement of a hemiarthoplasty, given the risk of dislocation of 1% to 2% (149) and the higher mortality associated with such an occurrence (150).

Continuous Passive Motion Machines

In 1975, Salter et al. (151) first reported on the use of CPM to counteract the detrimental effects of joint immobilization in rabbits. Based on Salter's work, Coutts et al. reported the first prospective study on the use of CPM on patients after TKA (152). Since then, the use of CPM after TKA has been controversial (153,154), although it is used by many surgeons (155,156). Once employed, treatment protocols vary, with total daily usage from 5 hours to 24 hours.

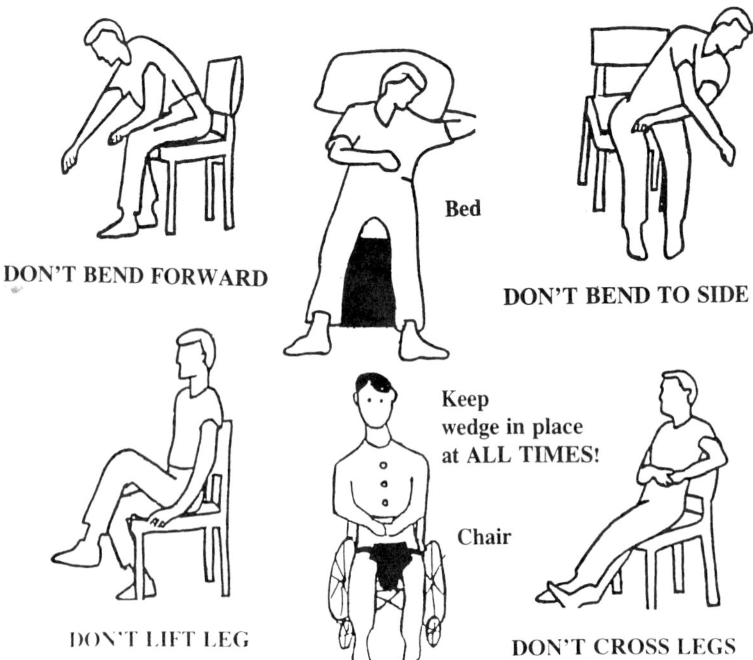

FIG. 66-6. Total hip precautions to prevent dislocation.

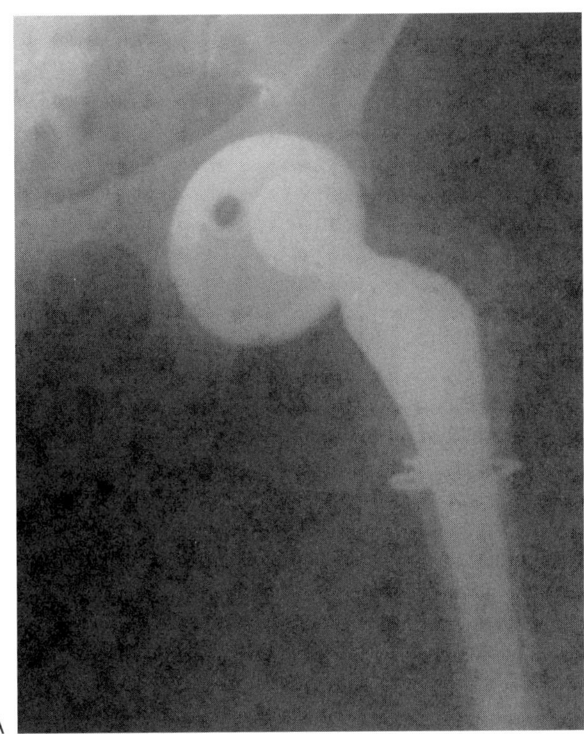

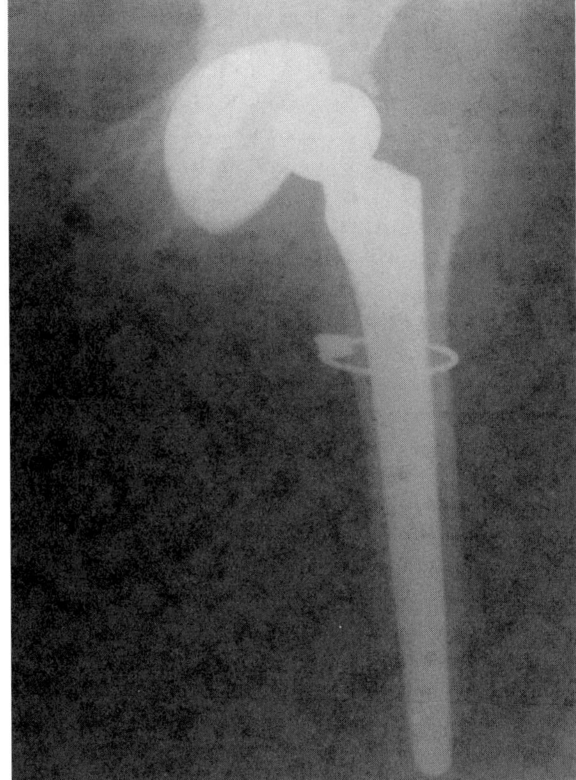

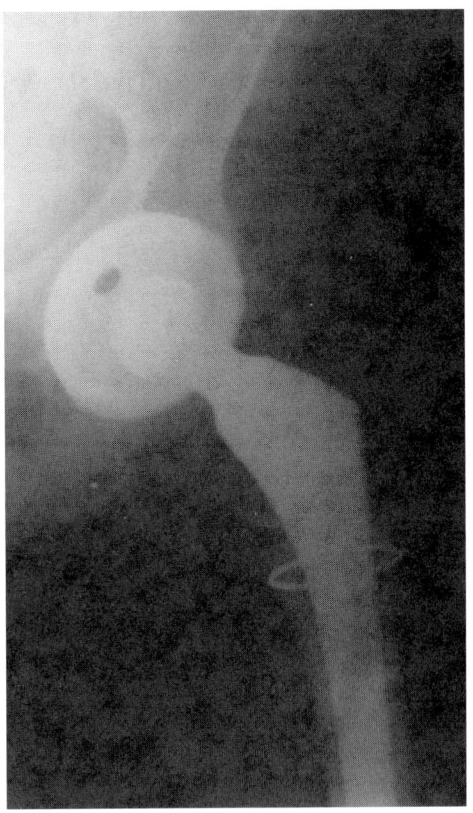

FIG. 66-7. A: Anteroposterior view of a total hip arthroplasty that subluxed/dislocated when the hip was positioned in full extension. This occurred because of the excessive anteversion of the acetabular component. **B:** Lateral view of the same subluxed/dislocated hip. **C:** With slight flexion of the hip, the femoral component is reduced, with the head of the femoral component centered in the acetabulum.

Despite the initial improvements seen with the CPM machine, these authors noted no difference in range of motion or function between groups at 6 weeks after surgery (155,156). Use of CPM has also been reported to reduce knee swelling (155) and has been investigated as a means of DVT prophylaxis after TKA (92,156,157), for which its effectiveness is questionable (157).

The role of CPM for those patients transferred to a rehabilitation facility is unknown. Many times, patients will be continued on the CPM machine if it was used immediately after surgery, with 90° of flexion as an end point to its use. A retrospective study by Nadler et al. on 50 patients admitted to a rehabilitation hospital showed no difference in the final range of motion between CPM and non-CPM groups (158). Presently, there does not appear to be any benefit to using CPM beyond the acute care hospitalization, although this may change as lengths of stay decline.

Weight-Bearing Principles

The effect of weight bearing on the ultimate fixation of the prosthetic components is unknown. Because all of the information regarding the biomechanics of the different fixation methods comes from animal studies, restrictions and recommendations for a particular weight-bearing status after surgery vary widely. In humans, the effectiveness of fixation can be inferred from either radiographic evaluation of the implants or retrieval studies. Although there have been two studies evaluating the degree of subsidence of cemented, bony ingrowth, and HA-coated femoral components over time (159,160), neither used weight-bearing status as an independent variable. In these studies, all of the patients were allowed only toe touch weight bearing for 2 to 3 months, even if the component was cemented, using the theory that early stability of the implant was important to maximize fixation and reduce the risk of later failure. Subsidence of the femoral component of up to 2.7 mm was seen 2 years after surgery, independent of the method of fixation. The greatest rate of subsidence appeared to occur in the first 6 months. With HA-coated prostheses, there was much less subsidence, with occasional proximal migration noted because of early osseointegration. There was no correlation between functional outcome or pain relief and the degree of subsidence or method of fixation. Longer-term data were not available.

Therefore, the optimum weight-bearing status for any method of fixation is unknown, although it is universally agreed that early initial stability is necessary, particularly for noncemented components. This holds true for TKA as well as THA (159). Although the amount of micromotion that can be tolerated and still allow firm fixation is unknown, it is known that excessive motion will interfere with bone ingrowth (54). The study by Givens-Heiss (141), although limited in its scope, showed that peak contact pressures in the acetabulum were highest with full weight bearing (FWB), whereas the lowest stresses were generated with toe-touch weight bearing (TTWB). Intermediate values were generated under partial weight-bearing (PWB) conditions. Contact pressures as high as those seen with partial weight bearing were generated with non–weight-bearing ambulation if the knee was maintained in extension, presumably because of the longer lever arm of the entire leg. With the knee flexed, contact pressures were as low as those seen with TTWB. Based on this information and current clinical practice, patients who have cemented total joints should be allowed to be FWB as soon as they can be mobilized. Patients with bony ingrowth or HA-coated components should have as limited weight bearing as possible, preferably either TTWB or PWB. In clinical practice, though, many of these patients are allowed to be FWB immediately after surgery if good press-fit stability is achieved at the time of surgery. Smooth-surfaced implants that are inserted only by press fit should be allowed FWB immediately after surgery, as there are no osteoconductive properties to the metal, and osseointegration will not take place.

The length of time to allow restricted weight bearing is also not well delineated. Animal models have shown that bone ingrowth can occur within 3 weeks (53), with maximum pullout forces being generated 8 weeks after implantation (161). Although fracture healing in humans often takes 6 weeks, the remodeling process may take a year or more (162). Clinically, weight bearing is most often limited for 6 weeks. Patients are then advanced to a FWB status. However, several authors have suggested that a longer time for restricted weight bearing may be necessary (141,160).

Postoperative Rehabilitation Program

The specific activities that patients must perform as a part of a therapy program after TJR have not changed significantly over the years. Early in the modern era of THA, patients often spent several days or more in balanced suspension before they were allowed to ambulate (77). Patients are now taken out of bed, if possible, on the first day after surgery and begin ambulation training no later than the second postoperative day. Although acute care hospitalizations often lasted up to 2 weeks, 3-day lengths of stay are no longer uncommon. However, the functional needs of the patients have not changed. Postoperative therapy now continues in a variety of settings, depending on the patients' functional and social status. In this section, general guidelines for the rehabilitation programs for THA and TKA are presented. Much of the information needed for the postoperative rehabilitation, i.e., weight-bearing status, ROM exercises, muscle-strengthening exercises, total hip precautions, and CPM machines, have already been presented. In this section, a general time frame for the postoperative rehabilitation program is discussed.

Rehabilitation following a TJR begins on the first postoperative day. The patient can stand at the bedside and, if possible, begin ambulating with an assistive device for upper extremity support. The specific device to be used, whether a standard walker, rolling walker, or axillary crutches, depends on the strength, balance, and endurance of the patient. Patients with severe weakness or deformity of the upper extremities (e.g., rheumatoid arthritis) may benefit from platform extensions to the device. If, on the first day, the patient has only enough endurance to stand, then ambulation must begin by the second postoperative day. At this time, the patient is given further instructions on how to ambulate and perform transfers safely to the bed, chair, and toilet.

Within the first week, the patient should be spending less time in bed, offsetting any deleterious effects from the immobility and bed rest imposed immediately after surgery. Progressive mobilization out of bed will also prevent the development of sacral and heel skin ulcers. The patient should be taught how to perform ADLs with any adaptive equipment, if necessary. Once the patient's endurance and strength are felt to be adequate, elevations should be integrated into the therapy program. By the end of the second week after surgery, most patients should be able to perform mobility tasks at no less than a supervision level. By this time, patients should have been taught how to bathe in the shower or bathtub using appropriate equipment, such as a shower chair. Simple homemaking tasks, such as preparing food and making the bed, should be initiated.

Muscle-strengthening exercises should continue to be performed on a daily basis. The initial ambulatory aid should continue to be used if weight-bearing restrictions exist, although biomechanical analysis shows that the use of cane on the contralateral side will reduce the forces in the joint, especially in the hip (163). Any effect of the type of device on the long-term outcome of the implants is not known. If a patient is allowed full weight bearing, then the use of a cane is indicated if it can be demonstrated that the patient can safely use the device.

By the sixth postoperative week, patients who have been on restricted weight bearing are now allowed to advance to a full weight-bearing status. If a walker or crutches had been used for the first 6 weeks, then advancement to a cane is now indicated. Muscle-strengthening exercises should continue on a long-term basis.

Rehabilitation goals need to be set and reviewed at all stages of the postoperative rehabilitation process. Safety precautions and equipment should be reviewed with the patient on a regular basis. If it appears that a patient will be unable to function safely at home within the first week after surgery, then consideration should be made for a more intensive rehabilitation program.

Although various modalities are used after total joint replacements, there have been very few studies to determine their overall effectiveness or safety. Application of cold after TKA has been shown to be effective in reducing local discomfort associated with an exercise program (164,165). However, neither cryotherapy nor superficial heating modalities have been shown to have any effect on passive range of motion or pain (164). Deep tissue heating using ultrasound over the area of the prosthesis has been shown in several animal models (166–168) to be without adverse local effects. However, the effect of ultrasound on the fixation of the component is unknown. Electrical stimulation of the quadriceps muscle after TKA was shown, in one study, to reduce extension lag, although long-term follow-up was not available (144).

OTHER REHABILITATION ISSUES

Driving

Any procedure performed on the right lower extremity will adversely affect the patient's ability to drive a car safely. After TJR in the right lower extremity, braking reaction time during simulated driving is prolonged (169,170). Return of the braking reaction time to acceptable, safe limits was not seen until 8 weeks after surgery for both THA and TKA. A driving evaluation that would include measurement of the braking reaction time should be considered for any patient for whom driving safety is a concern.

Sexuality

Osteoarthritis of the hip has been shown to have an adverse impact on sexual function (171). Issues of sexuality after total joint replacement have received little attention in the literature and are probably not actively discussed between physician and patient. A questionnaire study by Stern (171) of 100 patients who were satisfied with the overall outcome of their THA showed that, preoperatively, 46% of patients attributed any sexual difficulty to their hip disease, whereas postoperatively only 1% felt this way. Only 7% of all respondents had discussions preoperatively regarding the effect of THA on sexual function. Between 1 and 2 months after surgery, 55% of patients had resumed sexual intercourse. Positions for intercourse were based on comfort. Overall, 89% of patients desired more information in this area, with written material being the most requested. There were no dislocations noted in this group of patients. Although there has been no literature on sexual functioning after TKA, similar considerations are appropriate. Sexual activity can be resumed at the discretion and comfort of the patient and partner. Limitations in the range of motion of the knee may make certain positions more comfortable. A pamphlet presenting this information may be of benefit to any TJR patient.

Sports Activities

Many patients, after successful TJR, would like to resume avocational activities, which may include sports. High-impact sports such as running, singles tennis, racquetball, basketball, and baseball, among others, have been shown to significantly increase the risk of aseptic loosening after THA (172,173) and should be avoided. Patients should be encouraged to participate in low-impact sports such as swimming, cycling, and golf. Similar recommendations exist for total knee arthroplasty (173).

CONCLUSIONS

Total hip and knee arthroplasties are among the most performed and successful of operative procedures, resulting in significant improvements in the patient's quality of life. By alleviating pain, minimizing complications, and maximizing function, patients are often able to resume their desired activities, both vocational and avocational. The postoperative therapy program in which the patient participates can provide the springboard for these positive results. It is essential for any physician working with these patients to understand all the aspects of care that will optimize their outcome.

REFERENCES

1. Graves EJ. *1993 Summary: National hospital discharge survey. Advance data from vital and health statistics; no. 264.* Hyattsville, MD: National Center for Health Statistics, 1995.
2. Charnley J. Arthroplasty of the hip: A new operation. *Lancet* 1961; 1:1129–1132.
3. Yoslow W, Simeone J, Huestis D. Hip replacement rehabilitation. *Arch Phys Med Rehabil* 1976; 57:275–278.
4. Bohannon RW, Cooper J. Total knee arthroplasty: Evaluation of an acute care rehabilitation program. *Arch Phys Med Rehabil* 1993; 74: 1091–1094.
5. Visuri T, Honkanen R. Total hip replacement: Its influence on spontaneous recreation exercise habits. *Arch Phys Med Rehabil* 1980; 61: 325–328.
6. Brander VA, Stulberg SD, Chang RW. Rehabilitation following hip and knee arthroplasty. *Phys Med Rehabil Clin North Am* 1994; 5: 815–836.
7. Total hip replacement. *NIH Consensus Statement* Sept 12–14, 1995; 12(5):1–31.
8. Peterson MG, Hollenberg JP, Szatrowski TP, Johanson NA, Mancuso CA, Charlson ME. Geographic variations in the rates of elective total hip and knee arthroplasties among Medicare beneficiaries in the United States. *J Bone Joint Surg* 1992; 74-A:1530–1539.
9. Stinchfield FE. Total hip replacement: An overview. In: Evarts CM, ed. *Surgery of the musculoskeletal system, vol 6.* New York: Churchill Livingstone, 1983; 157–171.
10. Moore AT. Metal hip joint: A new self-locking vitallium prosthesis. *South Med J* 1952; 11:1015–1019.
11. Swiontkowski MF. Current concepts review. Intracapsular fractures of the hip. *J Bone Joint Surg* 1994; 76-A:129–138.
12. Wiles P. The surgery of the osteo-arthritic hip. *Br J Surg* 1958; 45: 488–497.
13. Charnley J, Cupik K. The nine and ten year results of the low friction arthroplasty of the hip. *Clin Orthop* 1973; 95:9–25.
14. Wallduis B. Arthroplasty of the knee joint using an endoprosthesis. *Acta Orthop Scand [Scand]* 1957; 24:12–26.
15. Gunston FH. Polycentric knee arthroplasty: Prosthetic simulation of normal knee movement. *J Bone Joint Surg* 1971; 53-B:272–277.
16. Rand JA, Ilstrup DM. Suvivorship analysis of total knee arthroplasty. *J Bone Joint Surg* 1991; 73-A:397–409.
17. Harris WH, Sledge CB. Total hip and knee replacement (Part I). *N Engl J Med* 1990; 323:725–731.
18. Harris WH, Sledge CB. Total hip and knee replacement (Part II). *N Engl J Med* 1990; 323:801–807.
19. Scuderi GR, Insall JN, Windsor RE, Moran MC. Suvivorship of cemented knee replacements. *J Bone Joint Surg* 1989; 71-B:798–803.
20. Hori RY, Lewis JL, Zimmerman JR, Compere CL. The number of joint replacements in the United States. *Clin Orthop* 1978; 132:46–52.
21. Overgaard S, Knudsen HM, Hansen LN, Mossing N. Hip arthroplasty in Jutland, Denmark. *Acta Orthop Scand* 1992; 63:536–538.
22. Paavolainen P, Hamalainen M, Mustonen H, Slatis P. Registration of arthroplasties in Finland. *Acta Orthop Scand* 1991; 62(Suppl 24): 27–30.
23. Havelin LI, Espehaug B, Vollset SE, Engesaeter LB, Langeland N. The Norweigian arthroplasty register. *Acta Orthop Scand* 1993; 64: 245–251.
24. Levy RN, Volz RG, Kaufer H, Matthews LS, Capozzi J, Sturm P, et al. Progress in arthritis surgery. *Clin Orthop* 1985; 200:299–321.
25. Madhock R, Lewallen DG, Wallrichs SL, Ilstrup DM, Kurland RL, Melton LJ. Trends in utlilization of primary total hip arthroplasty 1969 through 1990: A population based study in Olmstead County, Minnesota. *Mayo Clin Proc* 1993; 68:11–18.
26. Thomas BJ, Cracchiolo A, Lee YF, Chow GH, Navarro R, Dorey F. Total knee arthroplasty in rheumatoid arthritis. *Clin Orthop* 1991; 265:129–136.
27. Katz RL, Bourne RB, Rorabeck CH, McGee H. Total hip arthroplasty in patients with avascular necrosis of the hip. *Clin Orthop* 1992; 281: 145–151.
28. Jasty M, Anderson MJ, Harris WH. Total hip replacement for developmental dysplasia of the hip. *Clin Orthop* 1995; 311:40–45.
29. Haentjens P, Casteleyn PP, Odecam P. Hip arthroplasty for failed internal fixation of intertrochanteric and subtrochanteric fractures in the elderly patient. *Arch Orthop Trauma Surg* 1994; 113:222–227.
30. Bradley JD, Brandt KD, Katz BP, Kalasinski LA, Ryan SI. Comparison of an anti-inflammatory dose of ibuprofen, an analgesic dose of ibuprofen, and acetominophen in the treatment of patients with osteoarthritis of the knee. *N Engl J Med* 1991; 325:87–91.
31. De Lee JC. Fractures and dislocations of the hip. In: Rockwood CA, Green DP, Bucholz RW, eds. *Fractures in adults, vol 2.* Philadelphia: JB Lippincott, 1991; 1481–1651.
32. Moore AT. Metal hip joint—a new self-locking Vitallium prosthesis. *South Med J* 1952; 45:1015–1019.
33. Gebhard JS, Amstutz HC, Zinar DM, Dorey FJ. A comparison of total hip arthroplasty and hemiarthroplasty for treatment of acute fracture of the femoral neck. *Clin Orthop* 1992; 282:123–131.
34. Taine WH, Armour PC. Primary total hip replacement for displaced subcapital fractures of the femur. *J Bone Joint Surg* 1985; 67-B: 214–217.
35. Sarmiento A, Ebramzadeh E, Gogan WJ, McKellop HA. Total hip arthroplasty with cement. *J Bone Joint Surg* 1990; 72-A:1470–1475.
36. Sullivan PM, MacKenzie JR, Callaghan JJ, Johnston RC. Total hip arthroplasty with cement in patients who are less than fifty years old. *J Bone Joint Surg* 1994; 76-A:863–879.
37. Lehman DE, Capello WN, Feinberg JR. Total hip arthroplasty without cement in obese patients. *J Bone Joint Surg* 1994; 76-A:854–862.
38. Soballe K, Chistensen F, Luxhoj T. Hip replacement in obese patients. *Acta Orthop Scand* 1987; 58:223–225.
39. Stern SH, Insall JN. Total knee arthroplasty in obese patients. *J Bone Joint Surg* 1990; 72-A:1400–1404.
40. Garcia-Ambrelo E, Munvera L. Early and late loosening of the acetabular cup after low friction arthroplasty. *J Bone Joint Surg* 1992; 74-A:1119–1129.
41. Moreland JR. Mechanisms of failure in total knee arthroplasty. *Clin Orthop* 1988; 226:49–64.
42. NIH Consensus Conference: Total hip joint replacement in the United States. *JAMA* 1982; 248:1817–1821.
43. Poss R. Current status of total joint arthroplasty: Observations and projections. *J Rheumatol* 1987; 14(Suppl 15):40–44.
44. Hanssen AD, Rand JA. A comparison of primary and revision total knee arthroplasty using the kinematic stabilizer prosthesis. *J Bone Joint Surg* 1988; 70-A:491–499.
45. Gore DR, Murray MP, Gardner GM, Mollinger LA. Comparison of function two years after revision of failed total hip arthroplasty and primary hip arthroplasty. *Clin Orthop* 1986; 208:168–173.
46. Friedman RJ, Black J, Galente JO, Jacobs JJ, Skinner HB. Current concepts in orthopedic biomaterials and implant fixation. *J Bone Joint Surg* 1993; 75-A:1086–1109.
47. Davies JP, Burke DW, O'Connor DO, Harris WH. Comparison of the fatigue characteristics of centrifuged and uncentrifuged Simplex P bone cement. *J Orthop Res* 1987; 5:366–371.
48. Jones LC, Hungerford DS. Cement disease. *Clin Orthop* 1987; 225: 192–206.
49. Cook SD, Barrack AL, Thomas KA, Haddad RJ. Quantitative analysis of tissue growth into human porous-coated hip components. *J Arthroplasty* 1988; 3:249–262.
50. Collier JP, Bauer TW, Bloebaum RD, Bobyn JD, Cook SD, Galante JO, et al. Results of implant retrieval from post mortem specimens in patients with well functioning, long term total hip replacement. *Clin Orthop* 1992; 274:97–112.
51. Engh CA, Zettl-Schaffer KF, Kukita Y, Sweet D, Jasty M, Bragdon C. Histological and radiographic assessment of well functioning porous-coated acetabular components. *J Bone Joint Surg* 1993; 75-A: 814–824.
52. Cameron H, Pilliar R, McNab I. The effect of movement on the bonding of porous metal to bone. *J Biomed Mater Res* 1973; 7:301–311.
53. Cameron H, Pilliar R, McNab I. The rate of bone growth into porous metal. *J Biomed Mater Res* 1976; 10:295–302.
54. Pilliar RM, Lee JM, Maniatopoulos C. Observations on the effect of movements on bone ingrowth into porous surfaced implants. *Clin Orthop* 1986; 208:108–113.
55. Collier J, Colligan G, Brown S. Bone ingrowth into dynamically

loaded porous coated intramedullary nails. *J Biomed Mater Res* 1976; 10:485–492.
56. Cook S, Thomas K, Kay J, Jarcho M. Hydroxyapatite coated titanium for orthopedic implant application. *Clin Orthop* 1988; 232:225–243.
57. Chae JC, Collier JP, Mayor MB, Surprenant VA, Dauphinaus LA. Enhanced ingrowth of porous-coated CoCr implants plasma-sprayed with tricalcium phosphate. *J Biomed Mater Res* 1992; 26:93–102.
58. Rivero DP, Fox J, Skipor AK, Urban RM, Galante JO. Calcium phosphate coated porous titanium implants for enhanced skeletal fixation. *J Biomed Mater Res* 1988; 22:191–201.
59. Soballe K, Hansen ES, Brockstedt-Rasmussen H, Jorgensen PH, Bunger C. Tissue ingrowth into titanium and hydroxyapatite-coated implants during stable and unstable mechanical conditions. *J Orthop Res* 1992; 10:285–299.
60. Vaughn BK, Lombardi AV, Mallory TH. Clinical and radiographic experience with a hydroxyapatite-coated titanium plasma-sprayed porous implant. *Dent Clin North Am* 1992; 36:263–272.
61. Cook SD, Enis J, Armstrong D, Lisecki E. Early clinical results with the hydroxyapatite coated porous-LSF total hip system. *Dent Clin North Am* 1992; 36:247–255.
62. D'Antonio JA, Capello WN, Crothers OD, Jaffe WL, Manley MT. Early clinical experience with hydroxyapatite-coated femoral implants. *J Bone Joint Surg* 1992; 74-A:995–1008.
63. Moilanen T, Stocks GW, Freeman MAR, Scott G, Goodier WD, Evans SJW. Hydroxyapatite coating of an acetabular prosthesis. *J Bone Joint Surg* 1996; 76-B:200–205.
64. Geesink RGT, Hoefnagels NHM. Six-year results of hydroxyapatiti-coated total hip replacement. *J Bone Joint Surg* 1995; 77-B:534–537.
65. Collier JP, Surprenant VA, Mayor MB, Jensen RE, Surprenant HP. Loss of hydroxyapatite coating on retrieved total hip components. *J Arthroplasty* 1993; 8:389–393.
66. Bauer T, Geesink R, Zimmerman R, McMahon J. Hydroxyapatite coated femoral stems. *J Bone Joint Surg* 1991; 73-A:1439–1452.
67. Goldring SR, Clark CR, Wright TM. The problem in total joint arthroplasty: Aseptic loosening (editorial). *J Bone Joint Surg* 1993; 75-A:799–801.
68. Jasty M, Bragdon C, Jiranek W, Chandler H, Maloney W, Harris WH. Etiology of osteolysis around porous-coated cementless total hip arthroplasty. *Clin Orthop* 1994; 308:111–126.
69. Goetz DD, Smith EJ, Harris WH. The prevalence of femoral osteolysis associated with components inserted with or without cement in total hip replacements. *J Bone Joint Surg* 1994; 76-A:1121–1129.
70. Boyd AD, Ewald FC, Thomas WH, Poss R, Sledge CB. Long term complications after total knee arthroplasty with or without resurfacing of the patella. *J Bone Joint Surg* 1993; 75-A:674–681.
71. Sutherland CJ, Wilde AH, Borden LS, Markes KE. A ten-year follow up of one hundred consecutive Mullen curved-stem total hip arthroplasties. *J Bone Joint Surg* 1982; 64-A:970–982.
72. Stauffer RN. Ten year follow-up study of total hip replacement. *J Bone Joint Surg* 1982; 64-A:983–990.
73. Mulroy RD, Harris WH. The effect of improved cementing techniques on component loosening in total hip replacement: An 11 year radiographic review. *J Bone Joint Surg* 1990; 72-B:757–760.
74. Oishi CS, Walker RH, Colwell CW. The femoral component in total hip arthroplasty: Six to eight year follow up of one hundred consecutive patients after use of a third generation cementing technique. *J Bone Joint Surg* 1994; 76-A:1130–1136.
75. Wixon RL, Stulberg SD, Melhoff M. Total hip replacement with cemented, uncemented, and hybrid prostheses: A comparison of clinical and radiographic results at two to four years. *J Bone Joint Surg* 1991; 73-A:57–70.
76. Evans BG, Salvati EA, Huo MH, Huk OL. The rationale for cemented total hip arthroplasty. *Orthop Clin North Am* 1993; 24:599–610.
77. Schulte KR, Callaghan JJ, Kelley SS, Johnston RC. The outcome of Charnley total hip arthroplasty with cement after a minimum twenty year follow up. *J Bone Joint Surg* 1993; 75-A:961–975.
78. Garellick G, Herberts P, Stromberg C, Malchauh. Long-term results of Charnley arthroplasty: a 12–16 year follow-up study. *J Arthroplasty* 1994; 9:333–340.
79. Garcia-Ambrelo E, Munvera L. Early and late loosening of the acetabular cup after low friction arthroplasty. *J Bone Joint Surg* 1992; 74-A:1119–1129.
80. Schmalzreid TP, Harris WH. Hybrid total hip replacement: A 6.5 year follow-up study. *J Bone Joint Surg* 1993; 75-B:608–615.
81. Mohler CG, Krull LR, Martell JM, Rosenberg AG, Galante JO. Total hip replacement with insertion of an acetabular component without cement and a femoral component with cement: Four to seven year follow up. *J Bone Joint Surg* 1995; 77-A:86–96.
82. Eiskjaer S, Ostgard SE. Survivorship analysis of hemiarthroplasties. *Clin Orthop* 1993; 286:206–211.
83. Lausten GS, Vedel P, Nielsen PM. Fractures of the femoral neck treated wtih a bipolar hemiarthroplasty. *Clin Orthop* 1987; 218:63–67.
84. Lu-Yao, GL, Keller RB, Littenberg B, Wennberg JE. Outcomes after displaced fractures of the femoral neck: A meta-analysis of one hundred and six published reports. *J Bone Joint Surg* 1994; 76-A: 15–25.
85. Moreland JR. Mechanisms of failure in total knee arthroplasty. *Clin Orthop* 1988; 226:49–64.
86. Rand JA, Ilstrup DM. Survivorship anaylsis of total knee arthroplasty: Cumulative rates of survival of 9200 total knee arthroplasties. *J Bone Joint Surg* 1991; 73-A:397–409.
87. Scuderi GR, Insall JN, Windsor RE, Moran MC. Survivorship of cemented knee replacements. *J Bone Joint Surg* 1989; 71-B:798–803.
88. Appel DM, Tozzi JM, Dorr LD. Clinical comparison of all polyethylene and metal backed tibial components in total knee arthroplasty. *Clin Orthop* 1987; 216:151–158.
89. Haake DA, Berkman SA. Venous thromboembolic disease after hip surgery: Risk factors, prophylaxis, and diagnosis. *Clin Orthop* 1989; 242:212–231.
90. Wolfe LD, Hozack WJ, Rothman RH. Pulmonary embolism in total joint arthroplasty. *Clin Orthop* 1993; 288:219–233.
91. Swayze OS, Nasser S, Roberson JR. Deep venous thrombosis in total hip arthroplasty. *Clin Orthop North Am* 1992; 23:359–364.
92. Stulberg BN, Insall JN, Williams GW, Ghelman B. Deep-vein thrombosis following total knee replacement. An analysis of six hundred thirty eight arthroplasties. *J Bone Joint Surg* 1984; 66-A:194–201.
93. Paiement GD, Wessinger SJ, Harris WH. Survey of prophylaxis against venous thromboembolism in adults undergoing hip surgery. *Clin Orthop* 1987; 223:188–193.
94. McNally MA, Mollan RAB. Total hip replacement, lower limb blood flow and venous thrombogenesis. *J Bone Joint Surg* 1993; 75-B: 640–644.
95. Lieberman JR, Geerts WH. Current concepts review. Prevention of venous thromboembolism after total hip and knee arthroplasty. *J Bone Joint Surg* 1994; 76-A:1239–1250.
96. Binns M, Pho R. Femoral vein occlusion during total hip arthroplasty. *Clin Orthop* 1990; 255:168–172.
97. Planes A, Vochelle N, Fagola M. Total hip replacement and deep venous thrombosis. A venographic and necropsy study. *J Bone Joint Surg* 1990; 72-B:9–13.
98. Bredbacka S, Andreen M, Blomback M, Wykkman A. Activation of cascade systems by hip arthroplasty. *Acta Orthop Scand* 1987; 58: 231–235.
99. Gitel SN, Salvati EA, Wessler S, Robinson HJ, Worth MH. The effect of total hip replacement and general surgery on anti-thrombin III in relation to venous thrombosis. *J Bone Joint Surg* 1979; 61-A: 653–656.
100. Erikkson BI, Erikkson E, Gyzander E, Teger-Nillson AC, Risber B. Thrombosis after hip replacement. Relationship to the fibrinolytic system. *Acta Orthop Scand* 1989; 60:159–163.
101. Hull RD, Raskob GE. Current concepts review. Prophylaxis of venous thromboembolic disease following hip and knee surgery. *J Bone Joint Surg* 1986; 68-A:146–150.
102. Thromboembolic Risk Factors (THRIFT) Consensus Group. Risk of and prophylaxis for venous thromboembolism in hospital patients. *Br Med J* 1992; 305:567–574.
103. Fulkerson WJ, Coleman RE, Ravin CE, Saltzman HA. Diagnosis of pulmonary embolism. *Arch Intern Med* 1986; 146:961–967.
104. Kalebo P, Anthmyr BA, Erikkson BI, Zachrisson BE. Phlebographic findings in venous thrombosis following total hip replacement. *Acta Radiol* 1990; 31:259–263.
105. Moser RM, LeMoine JR. Is embolic risk conditioned by location of deep venous thrombosis? *Ann Intern Med* 1987; 94:439–444.
106. Philbrick JT, Becker DM. Calf deep vein thrombosis. A wolf in sheep's clothing? *Arch Intern Med* 1988; 148:2131–2138.
107. Haas SB, Tribus CB, Insall JN, Becker MW, Windsor RE. The significance of calf thrombi after total knee arthroplasty. *J Bone Joint Surg* 1994; 76-A:1649–1657.

108. Lensing AWA, Buller HR, Prandonic P. Contrast venography, the gold standard for the diagnosis of deep vein thrombosis: improvement of observer agreement. *Thromb Haemostas* 1992; 67:8–12.
109. Bettmann MA, Pailin S. Leg phlebography: The incidence, nature, and modification of undesirable side effects. *Radiology* 1977; 122: 101–104.
110. Heijboer H, Buller HR, Lensing AWA, Turpie AGG, Colly LP, Ten Cate WJ. A comparison of real-time compression ultrasonography with impedence plethysmography for the diagnosis of deep vein thrombosis in symptomatic outpatients. *N Engl J Med* 1993; 329: 1365–1369.
111. Katz RL, McCulla MM Sr. Impedance plethysmography as a screening procedure for asymptomatic deep venous thrombosis in a rehabilitation hospital. *Arch Phys Med Rehabil* 1995; 76:833–839.
112. Woolson ST, McCrory DW, Walter JF, Maloney WJ, Watt JM, Cahill PD. B-Mode ultrasound scanning in the detection of proximal venous thrombosis after total hip replacement. *J Bone Joint Surg* 1990; 72-A:983–987.
113. Barnes RW, Nix ML, Barnes CL, Lavender RC, Golden WE, Harmon BH, et al. Perioperative asymptomatic venous thrombosis: Role of duplex scanning versus venography. *J Vasc Surg* 1989; 9:251–260.
114. Froehlich JA, Dorfman GS, Cronan JJ, Urbaneck PJ, Herndon JH, Aaron RK. Compression ultrasonography for the detection of deep venous thrombosis in patients who have a fracture of the hip. *J Bone Joint Surg* 1989; 71-A:245–256.
115. Grady-Benson JC, Oishi CS, Hanson PB, Collwell CW Jr, Otis SM, Walker RH. Routine postoperative duplex ultrasonography screening and monitoring for the detection of deep vein thrombosis. *Clin Orthop* 1994; 307:130–141.
116. Leutz DW, Stauffer ES. Color duplex doppler ultrasound scanning for detection of deep venous thrombosis in total knee and hip arthroplasty patients. *J Arthroplasty* 1994; 9:543–548.
117. Wells PS, Lensing AWA, Davidson BL, Prins MH, Hirsch J. Accuracy of ultrasound for the diagnosis of deep venous thrombosis in asymptomatic patients after orthopedic surgery: A meta-analysis. *Ann Intern Med* 1995; 122:47–53.
118. NIH Consensus Conference. Prevention of venous thrombosis and pulmonary embolism. *JAMA* 1986; 256:744–749.
119. Charnley J. Prophylaxis of postoperative thromboembolism (letter). *Lancet* 1972; 2:134–135.
120. Oster G, Tuden RL, Colditz GA. A cost-effectiveness analysis of prophylaxis against deep-vein thrombosis in major orthpedic surgery. *JAMA* 1987; 257:203–208.
121. Paiement GD, Wessinger SJ, Harris WH. Cost-effectiveness of prophylaxis in total hip replacement. *Am J Surg* 1991; 161:519–524.
122. Hull RD, Raskob GE. Prophylaxis of venous thromboembolic disease following hip and knee surgery. *J Bone Joint Surg* 1986; 68-A: 146–150.
123. Clagett GP, Anderson FA, Hart J, Levine MN, Wheeler HB. Prevention of venous thromboembolism. *Chest* 1995; 108(4 Suppl): 312S–334S.
124. Imperiale TF, Speroff T. A meta-analysis of methods to prevent venous thromboembolism following total hip replacement. *JAMA* 1994; 271:1780–1785.
125. Mohr DN, Silverstein MD, Murtaugh PA, Harrison JM. Prophylactic agents for venous thrombosis in elective hip surgery. Meta-analysis studies using venographic assessment. *Arch Intern Med* 1993; 153: 2221–2228.
126. McNally MA, Mollen RAB. Venous thromboembolism and orthopedic surgery (editorial). *J Bone Joint Surg* 1993; 75-B:517–519.
127. RD Heparin Arthroplasty Group. RD Heparin compared wtih warfarin for prevention of venous thromboembolic disease following total hip or knee arthroplasty. *J Bone Joint Surg* 1994; 76-A:1174–1185.
128. Hull R, Raskob G, Pineo G, Rosenbloom D, Evans W, Mallory T, et al. A comparison of subcutaneous low-molecular-weight heparin with warfarin sodium for prophylaxis against deep vein thrombosis after total hip or knee implantation. *N Engl J Med* 1993; 329:1370–1376.
129. Powers PJ, Gent M, Jay RM, Julian DH, Turpie AGG, Levine M, et al. A randomized trial of less intensive postoperative warfarin or aspirin therapy in the prevention of vneous thromboembolism after surgery for fractured hip. *Arch Intern Med* 1989; 149:771–774.
130. Hirsh J, Dalen JE, Deykin D, Poller L. Oral anticoagulants: Mechanism of action, clinical effectiveness, and optimal therapeutic range. *Chest* 1992; 102(4 Suppl):312S–326S.
131. Bergqvist D, Benoni G, Bjorgell O, Fredin H, Hedlundh U, Nicolas S, et al. Low-molecular-weight heparin (enoxaparin) as prophylaxis against venous thrombosis after total hip replacement. *N Engl J Med* 1996; 335:696–700.
132. Seagroatt V, Tan H, Goldacre M, Bulstrode C, Nugent L, Gill L. Elective total hip replacement: incidence, emergency readmission rate, and postoperative mortality. *Br Med J* 1991; 303:1431–1435.
133. Warwick D, Williams MH, Bannister GC. Death and thromboembolic disease after total hip replacement. *J Bone Joint Surg* 1995; 77-B: 6–10.
134. Sarasin FP, Bounameaux H. Antithrombic strategy after total hip replacement. A cost-effectiveness analysis comparing prolonged oral anticoagulants with screening for deep vein thrombosis. *Arch Intern Med* 1996; 156:1661–1668.
135. Santavirta N, Sarvimaki GLA, Konttinen VHYT, Santavirta S. Teaching of patients undergoing total hip replacement surgery. *Int J Nurs Stud* 1994; 31:135–142.
136. Shih C-H, Du Y-K, Lin Y-H, Wu C-C. Muscular recovery around the hip joint after total hip arthroplasty. *Clin Orthop* 1994; 302:115–120.
137. Long WT, Dorr LD, Healy B, Perry J. Functional recovery of noncemented total hip arthroplasty. *Clin Orthop* 1993; 208:73–77.
138. Davy DT, Kotzar GM, Brown RH, Heysle KG, Goldberg VM, Heysle KG Jr, et al. Telemetric force measurements across the hip after total hip arthroplasty. *J Bone Joint Surg* 1988; 70-A:45–50.
139. Rydell NW. Forces acting on the femoral head prosthesis: a study on strain gauge supplied prostheses in living persons. *Acta Orthop Scand* 1966; 37(88 Suppl):1–132.
140. Strickland EM, Fares M, Krebs DE, Riley PO, Givens-Heiss DL, Hodge WA, et al. *In vivo* acetabular contact pressures during rehabilitation, Part I: Acute phase. *Phys Ther* 1992; 72:691–699.
141. Givens-Heiss DL, Krebs DE, Riley PO, Strickland EM, Fares M, Hodge WA, et al. *In vivo* acetabular contact pressures during rehabilitation, Part II: Postacute phase. *Phys Ther* 1992; 72:700–710.
142. Moreland J. Mechanisms of failure in total knee arthroplasty. *Clin Orthop* 188; 226:49–64.
143. Laubenthal KN, Smidt GL, Kettlekamp DB. A quantitative analysis of knee motion during activities of daily living. *Phys Ther* 1972; 52: 34–42.
144. Gottlin RS, Hershkowitz S, Juris PM, Gonzalez EG, Scott WN, Insall JN. Electrical stimulation effect on extensor lag and length of hospital stay after total knee arthroplasty. *Arch Phys Med Rehabil* 1994; 75: 957–959.
145. Maloney WJ, Schurman DJ. The effects of implant design on range of motion after total knee arthroplasty. *Clin Orthop* 1992; 278:147–152.
146. Seeger MS, Fisher LA. Adaptive equipment used in the rehabilitation of hip arthroplasty patients. *Am J Occup Ther* 1982; 36:503–508.
147. Rao JP, Bronstein R. Dislocations following arthroplasties of the hip. *Orthop Rev* 1991; 20:261–264.
148. Lewinnek GE, Lewis JL, Tarr R, Compere CL, Zimmerman JR. Dislocations after total hip replacement arthroplasties. *J Bone Joint Surg* 1978; 60-A:217–220.
149. Krotenberg R, Stitik T, Johnston MV. Incidence of dislocation following hip arthroplasty for patients in the rehabilitation setting. *Am J Phys Med Rehabil* 1995; 74:444–447.
150. Paton RW, Hirst P. Hemiarthroplasty of the hip and dislocation. *Injury* 1989; 20:167–169.
151. Salter RB, Simmons DF, Malcolm BW. The effects of continuous passive motion on full thickness defects in articular cartilage: An experimental investigation in the rabbit. *J Bone Joint Surg* 1975; 57-A:570–571.
152. Coutts RD, Kaita J, Barr R. The role of continuous passive motion in the postoperative rehabilitation of the total knee patient (abstract). *Orthop Trans* 1982; 6:277.
153. Ritter MA, Grandolf VS, Holston KS. Continuous passive motion versus physical therapy in total knee arthroplasty. *Clin Orthop* 1989; 244:239–243.
154. Gose JC. Continuous passive motion in the postoperative treatment of patients with total knee replacement: a retrospective study. *Phys Ther* 1987; 67:39–42.
155. McInnes J, Larson MG, Daltroy LH, Brown T, Fossel AH, Eaton HM, et al. A controlled evaluation of continuous passive motion in patients undergoing total knee arthroplasty. *JAMA* 1992; 268: 1423–1428.

156. Vince KG, Kelly MA, Beck J, Insall JN. Continuous passive motion after total knee arthroplasty. *J Arthroplasty* 1987; 2:281–284.
157. Lynch AF, Bourne RB, Rorabeck CH, Rankin RN, Donald A. Deep-vein thrombosis and continuous passive motion after total knee arthroplasty. *J Bone Joint Surg* 1988; 70-A:11–14.
158. Nadler SC, Malanga GA, Zimmerman JR. Continuous passive motion in the rehabilitation setting—a retrospective study. *Am J Phys Med Rehabil* 1993; 72:162–165.
159. Karrholm J, Malchau VH, Snorrason F, Herberts P. Micromotion of femoral stems in total hip arthroplasty. A randomized study of cemented, hydroxyapatite-coated, and porous-coated stems with Roentgen stereophotogrammetric analysis. *J Bone Joint Surg* 1994; 76-A(11):1692–1705.
160. Nestor L, Blaha JD, Kjellstrom V, Selvik G. *In vivo* measurements of relative motion between an uncemented femoral total hip component and the femur by roentgen stereophotogrammetric anaylsis. *Clin Orthop* 1991; 269:220–227.
161. Bobyn JD, Pilliar RM, Cameron HU, Weatherly GC. The optimum pore size for the fixation of porous surfaced metal implants by the ingrowth of bone. *Clin Orthop* 1980; 150:263–270.
162. Buckwalter JA, Cruess RL. Healing of the musculoskeletal tissues. In: Rockwood CA, Green DP, Bucholz RW, eds. *Fractures in adults.* Philadelphia: JB Lippincott, 1991; 181–222.
163. Edwards BG. Contralateral and ipsilateral cane usage by patients with total knee or hip replacement. *Arch Phys Med Rehabil* 1986; 67: 734–740.
164. Hecht PJ, Bachmann S, Booth RE, Rothman RH. Effects of thermal therapy on rehabilitation after total knee arthroplasty. *Clin Orthop* 1983; 178:198–201.
165. Ivey M, Johnston RV, Uchida T. Cryotherapy for postoperative pain relief following knee arthroplasty. *J Arthroplasty* 1994; 9:285–290.
166. Lehmann JF, Brunner GD, McMillan J. Influence of surgical metal implants on the temperature distribution in thigh specimens exposed to ultrasound. *Arch Phys Med Rehabil* 1959; 40:483–488.
167. Lehmann JF, Warren CG, Wallace JE, Chan A. Ultrasound: Considerations for use in the presence of prosthetic joints (abstract). *Arch Phys Med Rehabil* 1980; 61:502.
168. Brunner GD Lehmann JF, McMIllan JA, Lane KE, Bell JW. Can ultrasound be used in the presence of surgical metal implants? *Phys Ther* 1958; 38:823–824.
169. MacDonald W, Owen JW. The effect of total hip arthroplasty on driving reactions. *J Bone Joint Surg* 1988; 70-B:202–205.
170. Spalding TJW, Kiss J, Kyberd P, Turner-Smith A, Simpson AH. Driver reaction times after total knee replacement. *J Bone Joint Surg* 1994; 76-B:754–756.
171. Stern SH, Fuchs MD, Ganz SB, Classi P, Sculco TP, Salvate EA. Sexual function after total hip arthroplasty. *Clin Orthop* 1991; 269: 228–235.
172. Kilgus DJ, Dorey FJ, Finerman GA, Amstutz H. Patient activity, sports participation, and impact loading on the durability of cemented total hip replacements. *Clin Orthop* 1991; 269:25–31.
173. McGrory BJ, Stuart MJ, Sim FH. Participation in sports after hip and knee arthroplasty: Review of the literature and survey of surgeon preferences. *Mayo Clin Proc* 1995; 70:342–348.

Rehabilitation Medicine: Principles and Practice, Third Edition,
edited by Joel A. DeLisa and Bruce M. Gans.
Lippincott–Raven Publishers, Philadelphia © 1998.

CHAPTER 67

Health Issues for Women with Disabilities

Kristi L. Kirschner, Carol J. Gill, Judy Panko Reis, and Sandra Welner

BARRIERS: PHYSICAL, ATTITUDINAL, KNOWLEDGE, AND FINANCIAL

"Disabled women . . . are subjected to double discrimination: they are disabled, and they are women." (1)

People with disabilities are no strangers to barriers. The most overt barriers are physical (e.g., stairs, narrow doorways, curbs, inaccessible bathrooms), communication (e.g., lack of sign language interpreters, materials in Braille), and programmatic (e.g., lack of assistants, flexible scheduling, and transportation). The more insidious barriers are erected by ignorance and negative social attitudes about life with disability. Economic barriers also play a significant role in preventing people with disabilities from accessing community services, such as health care. In 1982, Perlman and Arneson (2) described discriminatory practices in employment, education, vocational services, economic programs, access to benefits and services, health care, and parenting activities that disproportionately affect women with disabilities. With the passage of the Americans with Disabilities Act in 1990, and some emerging research and clinical services targeting the needs of women with disabilities, this situation is beginning to improve. We are a long way, though, from full integration, where a woman with a disability can go to a community health center with the expectation that it will be fully accessible with wheelchair-adapted equipment and knowledgeable staff trained to assist women with a variety of disabilities in a manner respectful of their womanhood (Fig. 67-1).

Recent attention has also focused on the unequal representation of women in health care. Historically, women have often been excluded from medical research for a variety of offered reasons—ranging from methodologic concerns about the menstrual cycle to liability concerns related to potential pregnancies (3). As a result, we have little information about the use of medications in women to prevent coronary artery disease, the number one killer for both genders (4). Major causes of morbidity and mortality for women, such as osteoporosis and breast cancer, have only recently received priority funding, as the National Institutes of Health attempts to rectify these neglected areas through the multicenter studies of the Women's Health Initiative. Our data are even more limited in guiding our treatments in women with disabilities. For example, is estrogen a safe and effective treatment in a perimenopausal woman who also has significant immobility osteoporosis as a result of a spinal cord injury 20 years ago? Can combined oral contraceptives be used safely in women with mobility impairments? How soon after the onset of the mobility impairment can they safely be instituted?

This chapter provides an overview of disabled women's health issues with particular attention to the psychosocial concerns that dominate this area. We spend little time in discussing sexuality *per se,* as another chapter in this book (see Chapter 45) is devoted to this topic. Our topics represent issues that women from the disability community have told us are important to them—from their writings, conferences, research, and their collaboration with health care providers. This chapter is meant to highlight principles and provide a guide for comprehensive care for women with disabilities. We have provided a list of resources and model programs in the Appendix for those who wish further information beyond the scope of this chapter.

Just a few words about language: the terms that persons with disabilities use for self-identification are still evolving. In this chapter, the terms "women with disabilities" and "disabled women" are used interchangeably. This usage takes into account recent public statements by prominent

K. L. Kirschner: Department of Physical Medicine and Rehabilitation, Rehabilitation Institute of Chicago, Northwestern University Medical School, Chicago, Illinois 60611.

C. J. Gill: Department of Disability and Human Development, University of Illinois at Chicago, Chicago, Illinois 60608.

J. P. Reis: Health Resource Center for Women with Disabilities, Rehabilitation Institute of Chicago, Chicago, Illinois 60611.

S. Welner: Department of Obstetrics and Gynecology, Sibley Memorial Hospital, Washington, D.C. 20016.

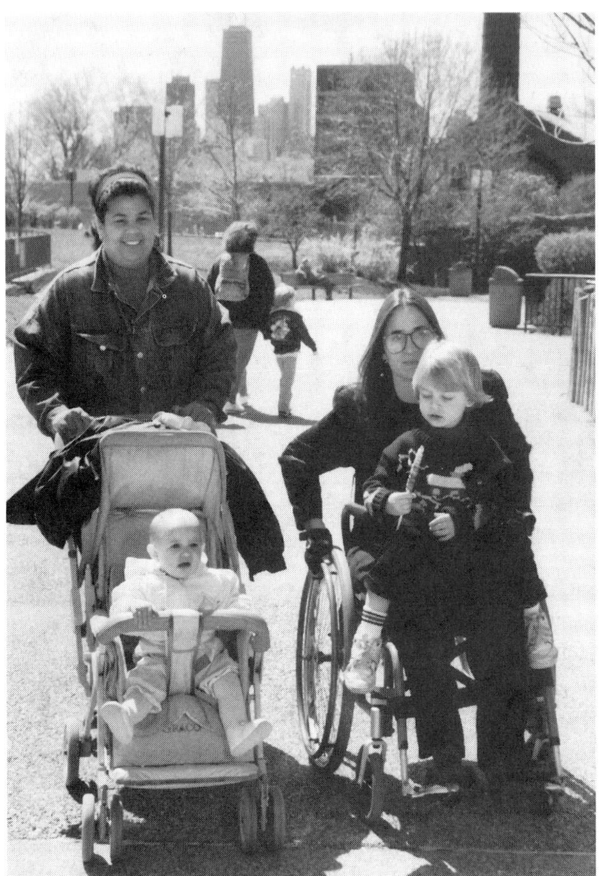

FIG. 67-1. Disabled mother and children and other caregiver.

disability community leaders (e.g., Judith Heumann, University of Minnesota, Minneapolis, MN, August 1, 1994; Barbara Waxman, "Health of Women with Physical Disabilities" conference, National Institutes of Health [NIH], Bethesda, MD, May 10, 1994) suggesting that an insistence on exclusive "person first" terminology might convey disparagement of the disability experience, whereas the term "disabled person" can convey pride in the disability identity. Consistent with this emphasis on disability as a social minority identity rather than purely medically defined deficiency, the authors of this chapter have chosen to use neutral rather than negative terms to describe disabilities, e.g., "extensive disability" rather than "severe disability."

Though this textbook is primarily directed toward the health care services of people with physical disabilities, we have at times used examples of women with sensory and developmental disabilities to illustrate the principle of "inclusiveness" that we believe is central to disabled women's health and to reflect the fact that women with physical disabilities can have other disabilities concurrently. Health care needs to embrace issues of men and women; women's health care needs to embrace nondisabled and disabled; and disabled women's health care needs to embrace physical and nonphysical disabilities. As Gloria Steinem said, in response to an introduction by Marca Bristo, chairperson of the President's Council on Disability and President of Access Living of Chicago, at a political caucus in Chicago:

"We can't go anywhere until you can go everywhere!"

DEMOGRAPHICS

According to current estimates (5), there are approximately 26 million women and girls with disabilities living in the United States, representing about 20% of all female citizens. Their disabilities range from mild (i.e., they report difficulty with one or more functional activities, such as lifting heavy objects) to extensive (in which they report they are unable to manage one or more basic activities of daily living, have one or more specific impairments, or require mobility aids, such as wheelchairs or crutches, to function). Disability types include mobility, sensory, cognitive, mental illness, and disabilities from various chronic disease conditions. Based on respondents' reports of their primary disabling conditions, the three leading causes of disability in women are, in descending order, arthritis, orthopedic impairments, and heart disease (6). Approximately 6.5 million women 15 years and older use a wheelchair, cane, crutches, or walker (7).

The proportion of women and girls with disabilities in the main racial/ethnic/cultural groups is as follows: 20.7% of white women not of Hispanic origin; 21.7% of African-American women; 21.8% of American Indian, Eskimo, or Aleut women; 10.7% of Asian or Pacific Islander women; and 16.2% of women of Hispanic origin (7). Disability, then, is lowest in incidence among Asian-American women and girls. Among working-age women, African-Americans and Native Americans have the highest incidence of extensive disability (7).

Women with disabilities have been described as socially isolated and deprived of the social roles and relationships available to most nondisabled women (8). Demographic data support this characterization. Approximately 18% of all women between the ages of 15 and 64 are women with disabilities. However, approximately 27% of all women in that age group who live alone or have no spouse are disabled. Only 12.7% of women in that age group who are married and have children under age 18 are women with disabilities (7).

In general, women's education level is inversely related to degree of disability. Approximately 20% of all women between 25 and 64 years have disabilities. Of all women in that age group who never completed high school, 36.4% have disabilities. Of those who completed 16 or more years of education, only 10.6% have disabilities, and only 3.7% are women with extensive disabilities (7).

Poverty is a common experience for women with disabilities. Employment rates for disabled women fall behind those of their nondisabled counterparts. For all women between 21 and 64, the employment rate has been reported as 72.6%. For women with disabilities, it is only 45.2% (7). Furthermore, the earning power of women with disabilities who do find employment falls far below that of nondisabled women and even that of men with disabilities. For every dollar earned by nondisabled men, nondisabled women earn 66 cents, men with disabilities earn 88 cents, and women with disabilities earn only 49 cents. If the male experience is extracted from the calculations, and nondisabled women's earnings are used as the standard, women with extensive disabilities earn only 71% of the standard (5). Of all working-age American women receiving means-tested cash assistance, about half are women with disabilities, and 40.5% are women with extensive disabilities (7).

Women with disabilities are as likely as nondisabled women to have healthcare coverage. However, the types of coverage differ significantly between the two groups. Women with disabilities are more likely to have publicly funded coverage (as opposed to private insurance) than nondisabled women. Disabled women report approximately twice the number of annual health service visits as nondisabled women; but given the greater likelihood that their disabling conditions demand more medical attention, it is not yet determined whether this greater number of visits provides adequate service (5).

REPRODUCTIVE HEALTH CARE ISSUES

Women with disabilities have typically not been seen as wives and mothers (9). Dating back to the early 1900s, fears of women with disabilities producing children with disabilities led to some social policies encouraging sterilization and criminalization of marriage (10). Other fears have checkered the reproductive history of disabled women, including the perceived inability of women with disabilities to be ''good'' mothers and exaggeration of health risks for women with disabilities who choose to bear children (11,12).

Improved research and education have helped to break down these stereotypes and oppressive policies, though much work remains to be done. Women with disabilities overwhelmingly report difficulties obtaining balanced information about reproductive healthcare issues—techniques for managing menstruation, birth control, risks associated with pregnancy, techniques for labor and delivery, information about sexual functioning, dating, gender identity, etc. (13–16). This section provides a brief overview of reproductive health care issues for women with disabilities with an emphasis on further resources for providing more detailed information. Consistent with the rehabilitation model, it is our recommendation that the physiatrist work with a team of health care professionals—in particular an obstetrician/gynecologist who has an interest in reproductive health care issues for women with disabilities—to deliver knowledgeable, respectful reproductive health care.

Menstruation and Fertility

Management of Menstruation

Menarche is a symbolic moment in most women's lives, marking the transition from ''girlhood'' to ''womanhood,'' with the attendant procreative possibilities. Though management of the menstrual flow is an issue for all women, it can be particularly cumbersome for women with physical impairments. For girls growing up with disabilities, options for managing menstrual flow should be explored, if possible, before the onset of menstruation. Such discussions offer opportunities for girls with disabilities to develop a sense of control over their emerging sexuality and evolving images of themselves as women. For women with acquired disabilities who are still menstruating, management of menstrual flow should be addressed shortly after the onset of disability, preferably as a part of a rehabilitation program.

Some women may be able to work with a nurse or occupational therapist to develop a system for managing menstrual hygiene. Other women may find that switching to sanitary pads if they had previously used tampons may be all that is needed. Still other women may elect to work with a personal assistant to manage their menstrual hygiene. Some women, particularly those with more extensive physical disabilities, may find these options impractical and choose to look for options to regulate or curtail the menstrual flow if it is safe to do so. Unfortunately, some physical disabilities and chronic disease states are inherently associated with menstrual irregularities, leading exactly to the unpredictable flow that is so unwelcome.

Menstrual Irregularity and Fertility in Women with Physical Disabilities

For most women with physical disabilities, fertility potential is preserved, and menses resemble the patterns of women without disabilities. In some cases, though, menstrual irregularity and fertility problems can occur. The most common hormonal imbalances found in women in general are disorders of prolactin secretion or thyroid function. Women, after traumatic brain injury (TBI) and spinal cord injury (SCI), occasionally exhibit elevated levels of prolactin, with or without galactorrhea (17,18). This hyperprolactinemia interferes with the normal functioning of the hypothalamic–pituitary–ovarian axis, causing menstrual irregularity. This is usually in the form of oligo- or amenorrhea but can manifest in irregular menstrual patterns as well. Galactorrhea, a result of hyperprolactinemia, has been reported in women after SCI. This hyperprolactinemia develops within 3 to 6 months after SCI and can persist up to 24 months (17). Prolactin levels can become markedly elevated immediately postinjury, although this elevation does tend to return to normal within 1 year (19). Almost all women after SCI will resume their normal menses within the first 9 to 12 months postinjury (20).

Occasionally medications can also result in menstrual irregularities. Phenytoin (Dilantin) and corticosteroids may affect thyroid function and ovulation; tricyclic antidepressants and some antihypertensives may also cause menstrual irregularities by affecting prolactin levels (21,22).

Treatment of menstrual irregularities varies with age and

medical condition. Such irregularities are often seen in young girls who have immature hypothalmic–pituitary–ovarian axes and may be producing unbalanced amounts of estrogen and progestin. Treatments need to be individualized. Pregnancy should always be considered and ruled out in evaluating menstrual irregularity. A short course of high-dose estrogen with progestin withdrawal is often helpful in curtailing menorrhagia in young girls (23). Combination oral contraceptives are the standard regimen as a follow-up, but in women with disabilities, in whom these may be contraindicated because of concerns about thrombotic complications, cyclic progestin regimens may also be effective (23).

Thyroid function tests and prolactin levels can be helpful in evaluating women with irregular menstrual periods (23,24). If significant hyperprolactinemia is detected, pituitary studies should be performed to rule out adenoma before consideration is given to bromocriptine treatment. Treatment of thyroid function irregularities should be instituted if abnormalities are detected. Correcting hormonal causes of menstrual irregularities can often regulate the menstrual cycle successfully and reverse subfertility if desired.

Other possible sources of abnormal bleeding include uterine or endocervical polyps, fibroids, cervical pathology, and vulvovaginal lesions (25). Careful gynecologic evaluation is required to determine an appropriate course of treatment. Menstrual irregularities become more common as women reach the climacteric years.

Women with disordered menstrual cycles often have fertility difficulties. Regular menstrual cycles and ovulation are critical components in achieving conception. Although many women with physical disabilities have unaltered fertility potential, some women may have subfertility problems related to hormonal irregularities. If these women desire conception, they need to undergo workups identical to those that would be given to nondisabled women, which includes several months of basal body temperature charting, evaluation of Fallopian tube pathology with hysterosalpingography, and postcoital testing (26). Blood work and biopsies may also be needed. The male partner needs to be involved in the process by providing a semen specimen for analysis, as almost half of all couples in general who present with infertility problems will have a male factor contribution (27).

Contraception

The history of contraception for women with disabilities has at times been coercive and oppressive. Compulsory sterilization, particularly for people with psychiatric and cognitive disabilities, took root in the United States in the early 1900s and in some venues persisted until the 1960s as part of the general eugenics movement (10,12). Concerns about ''physician-controlled'' contraceptives, such as Depo-Provera (Upjohn, Kalamazoo, MI), still percolate in segments of the disability community as a result of this history and the fear that a woman's reproductive choices might be curtailed by physicians, parents, or guardians who make decisions on her behalf (28).

Sensitivity to this history is essential in establishing patient-centered, trusting relationships between health care providers and women with disabilities. Women with disabilities have a right to knowledgeable information about contraception, similar to nondisabled women, and should participate in their reproductive health care decision making to the fullest extent possible. Contraceptive choices may be colored, though, by the nature of the woman's physical impairment or chronic disease condition (29). For example, a woman with impaired hand function may have difficulty using barrier methods such as the diaphragm, sponge, or spermicidal product. Problem solving with an occupational therapist, or working with the woman's partner, may result in an adequate solution for the use of barrier methods. Condoms, of course, always remain an effective method if the male partner is in agreement and provide the dual benefits of contraception and protection from sexually transmitted diseases.

For women who desire hormonal methods of contraception, information about the risks and benefits of various hormonal contraceptive options in women with disabilities is limited. For example, some women with mobility limitations (such as women with spina bifida, SCI, and multiple sclerosis) might have an increased risk for developing thrombotic events when using combination oral contraceptives, but definite statistics are not available (30). Therefore, in this group, alternative options that do not contain estrogen may be considered. Some women who are not candidates for the combination pill may do well with progestin-only contraceptive minipills, Depo-Provera (methoxyprogesterone acetate), or Norplant (subdermal levonorgesterel [Wyeth-Ayerst, Philadelphia, PA]).

These options, however, also have limitations (see Table 67-1). The progestin-only contraceptive pills are associated with an increased risk of abnormal uterine bleeding and are less effective than the combination pills (31). Depo-Provera, an injectable form of progesterone that is effective for at least 10 to 12 weeks, is highly effective, and patients are often pleased with the decreased menstrual flow or amenorrhea that additionally result from this method if taken long enough (32,33). This method is also efficacious and convenient to use. Unfortunately, many women experience some weight gain and reduced estrogen levels, which can lead to osteoporosis (34,35).

Norplant is another option for a progestin-only contraceptive. It is an implantable contraceptive requiring a minor surgical procedure to place and remove and is again associated with menstrual irregularities and amenorrhea (33). Estrogen levels are normal, however, with this method, and therefore, osteoporosis risk is not increased with use of Norplant. This method is again highly efficacious and is effective for about 5 years after placement. Over the last several years sporadic reports of difficulty removing the implants has moderated enthusiasm about using the implants. Inser-

TABLE 67-1. *Common contraception options: efficacy and side effects*[a]

Type of contraception	Failure rate (%)	Reported side effects
Combination oral contraceptives (OC)	3.0	Spotting; up to four times risk of thromboembolic phenomenon compared to nonusers
Progestin only (OC)	9.6	Irregular menses; spotting
Depo-Provera	0.3	Irregular bleeding; hypoestrogenism; osteoporosis
Norplant	0.2	Irregular spotting or amenorrhea, insertion/removal difficulties; ? immunologic-thrombotic concerns under study
Copper IUD	<1	Heavy-flow menses with increased cramping; increased risk of STD
Cervical Cap/ Diaphragm	Up to 18	Manual dexterity required for proper use
Condom	Up to 12	Latex allergies

[a] The pearl index is defined as the number of failures per 100 woman-years of exposure.

Some information taken from Speroff L, Darner P. *A clinical guide for contraception.* Baltimore: Williams & Wilkins, 1992; 3.

tion and removal difficulties may be especially problematic in some women with upper extremity limitations, though these difficulties can be minimized by using an experienced Norplant provider to perform this service.

Intrauterine devices (IUD) are another potential choice when estrogens are contraindicated. Patients with impaired pelvic sensation who desire to use IUDs should be cautioned about the risk of underdiagnosis of infections with this method. Occasional heavier menses with the IUD might also be seen as undesirable, though progestin-containing IUDs might be an option to lessen this effect. This method is also not recommended for women who are nulliparous or who have multiple partners (36).

Pregnancy and Prenatal Preparation

When possible, as with any nondisabled woman, it is best to discuss issues and concerns about pregnancy and motherhood *before* becoming pregnant (37–39). Counselling about health behaviors that can maximize the woman's and fetus's well-being during pregnancy is just one potential benefit. Information about diet, medication use, and potential adverse effects on the fetus of smoking, alcohol, and illicit drug use and the benefits of various vitamin supplementations may maximize the woman's ability to make choices and be an active participant in managing her pregnancy.

For some women, information about their health risks with pregnancy may be useful in facilitating a decision to pursue biological motherhood. A few disabilities may progress with pregnancy, perhaps irreversibly, or require higher-risk interventions and support (40). For example, a woman with multiple sclerosis may expect that her MS could worsen postpartum, or a woman with spinal muscular atrophy may need ventilatory assistance as the gravid uterus pushes up on her diaphragm and impedes ventilatory excursion (41–44).

Other women could expect a temporary decrement in their functional abilities, necessitating more physical assistance as pregnancy progresses (39,45–47). Most women with mobility impairments will be affected to some degree by changes in their center of gravity with increasing weight gain. Women who had previously managed their mobility with braces or assistive devices may find their stamina and balance affected as the pregnancy progresses and elect to temporarily use a manual wheelchair. Women who had previously been independent with manual wheelchairs may notice that they fatigue much more quickly and are unable to navigate the environment independently; these women may choose to use an electric wheelchair for the last trimester. Anticipating these changes will allow the woman and her healthcare provider to anticipate needs that might arise during the pregnancy and proactive interventions (such as referrals to physical therapy in the second trimester) that can be instituted to lessen the impact of some of these changes.

Information about other potential risks associated with pregnancy may assist in a plan of care to obviate or lessen these risks (19,48,49). For example, for women who use indwelling catheters and are chronically colonized with bacteria, the risk of recurrent pyelonephritis may be heightened as the growing uterus causes pressure on the ureters (50,51). Prompt recognition and prevention of UTIs is extremely important in preventing preterm labor (19,49,52). Women who have been accustomed to intermittent catheterization may find their bladder capacitance to be significantly decreased and opt to use an indwelling catheter to maintain continence for the latter part of their pregnancies. For any woman who has a neurogenic bladder and requires regular radiographic procedures to monitor her genitourinary system, these studies are best undertaken before pregnancy before of the risk to the fetus of radiographic exposure during pregnancy.

Excellent skin care and vigilance are extremely important in preventing decubitus ulcers during pregnancy for any woman with a mobility impairment and areas of insensate skin (19,49,51). A pressure-relief program that had previously been adequate in preventing decubiti may no longer be adequate with the increasing weight gain of pregnancy, coupled with hormonal changes that may predispose the skin to break down more easily. Counseling about more frequent pressure reliefs, changing wheelchair cushions, and frequent skin checks can go a long way in preventing this problematic complication. Counseling about padding and positioning is also crucial in preventing this complication with the labor and delivery staff as well.

Constipation and hemorrhoids are potential problems in any pregnancy with changes in diet, hormonal influences on the intestinal tract, iron supplementation, and the gravid uterus pushing on pelvic veins, but these potential complications can be particularly difficult for a woman with a neurogenic bowel who must use a bowel program (53). Vigilance, modifications in diet and the bowel program, and proactive bowel hygiene can again go a long way in preventing potential bowel impaction and hemorrhoidal complications.

Again, pressure on the pelvic veins, hormonal changes in pregnancy, and immobility may predispose a woman to deep venous thromboses, a potential complication of any pregnancy but especially for a woman with paralysis (54). Frequent examinations and counseling about signs and symptoms of deep vein thrombosis (DVT) are extremely important in helping women and care providers quickly recognize and seek assistance in managing this potentially life-threatening complication. Elevation of the legs, minimization of salt, range of motion, and the use of compression stockings may help minimize dependent edema.

For women with respiratory impairments from SCI, neuromuscular disorders such as spinal muscular atrophy, or extensive scoliosis with restrictive lung disease, respiratory function may also be affected with lowering of the functional residual capacity as the uterus grows (54). Pregnant women frequently hyperventilate and develop a mild degree of respiratory alkalosis, believed to be an effect of progesterone (49,54). Women with limited respiratory reserve may be particularly affected by these changes and require some modification in their activities, sleeping positions, and occasionally ventilatory assistance to manage the later stages of pregnancy, labor, and delivery.

A few potential complications of pregnancy can be life-threatening for a woman with disability. One of the best-recognized and frequently written-about complications is autonomic hyperreflexia in a woman with quadriplegia or high paraplegia (usually T6 or above) (55–69). Not only can hyperreflexia signal an issue requiring attention such as bladder distention or infection, bowel impaction, or labor, but the signs and symptoms can be misinterpreted as preeclampsia and lead health care providers down an incorrect path of diagnosis and treatment, with potentially disastrous results including intracerebral hemorrhage and even death. For women who are at risk for hyperreflexia, consultation with an anesthesiologist well before delivery may be prudent (67,70–74). A team approach to pregnancy, with a specialist in SCI working closely with the obstetric staff, can facilitate prevention and management of these potential complications (19,39,45,49,62,75).

Though preventive health care is a major focus for any woman with a disability going through pregnancy, this period also offers an excellent opportunity to help the woman prepare for her future role as a mother (47,76–78). If a woman has an extensive mobility impairment, referrals to an experienced occupational therapist and physical therapist may help her to develop a variety of anticipated skills to maximize her ability to parent (79–82). For example, how will she carry the baby? How will she feed the baby? If she plans to breastfeed, what positioning techniques will work best for her? What about diapering, dressing, and bathing? A home visit may be helpful in setting up the environment with adaptive equipment to facilitate her functional abilities. If the woman will require or chooses to use assistance in managing some of the care tasks required, working out a plan before the baby is born is important.

Many women with disabilities also yearn to talk to other women with similar disabilities about their experiences as mothers. Peer support and referrals can be extremely helpful in facilitating successful adjustment for both mother and baby and in anticipating the needs of each subsequent developmental stage (47,83,84). If a woman uses a wheelchair, how will she manage her toddler and maintain safety and discipline? How will she work with her child around the child's growing perception of her disability (85–87)? Women also report that continued contact with child care specialists from occupational therapy and psychology can be extremely important in adapting to each new developmental stage. More detailed information and resources on mothering with a disability is presented later in the chapter.

Labor and Delivery

Preparation for labor and delivery is an important consideration for the woman with a disability, though, depending on her disability, the traditional Lamaze classes (or variations thereof) may not make sense for her and her partner (47). Information to assist the woman in proper recognition of labor involves understanding expected signs and symptoms in the context of her particular disability (19,49,51). For example, a woman with extensive sensory impairments may not be able to sense pain from uterine contractions but have to rely on manual or electronic detection of the contractions. If she has high paraplegia or quadriplegia, periodic headaches from recurring autonomic hyperreflexia (occurring with each contraction of the uterus) may be the first symptom she recognizes. Recognition of her amniotic fluid breaking and knowing when to seek a checkup with her care provider are important information to discuss. Of course, frequent regular checkups with her obstetrician will also be helpful in predicting impending labor.

As previously mentioned, a discussion of anesthesia before labor and delivery is important in establishing a care plan. For example, a woman with an SCI who develops autonomic hyperreflexia with labor may do well with an epidural catheter, not to manage pain but to block the afferent signal from the uterus to the spinal cord triggering the sympathetic response (36,49,57). For a woman with respiratory compromise, a plan for providing ventilatory support should be discussed if this becomes necessary. If general anesthesia is needed for any reason, pertinent knowledge about disability-related issues that could influence the safety of general anesthesia should be considered. For example, a woman with a spinal cord injury should not receive succinylcholine as a depolarizing agent secondary to the risk of hyperkalemia (70). If a woman has had a cervical fusion of her neck, intubation may be more difficult with traditional methods.

Working with the labor and delivery staff may also be important in anticipating the needs of a woman with disability. If she is at risk for skin breakdown, proper padding and frequent position changes are important. If she has significant contractures and spasticity, tips for managing these issues with range of motion, positioning, and occasionally medication may be advisable (49,53,88). It is always optimal if the woman (and her partner) has an opportunity to tour the facility where she will deliver and to discuss her wishes for her peripartum care with her obstetrician and the nursing staff.

Preventive Healthcare Services

Pap Smears and Gynecologic Examinations

Basic preventive health and gynecologic screening for women with disabilities is often overshadowed by more obvious physical or neurologic problems, which may require more immediate focus. Thus, screening for diabetes, hypertension, hyperlipidemia, and thyroid imbalance, all of which are common concerns for women, may be neglected in women with disabilities. Many women avoid gynecologic care because of difficulty in obtaining an accessible, comfortable, and dignified examination (15,16,89). As a consequence, treatable early-stage problems may escalate and become much more difficult to manage. These concerns include Pap smear screening as well as breast evaluation.

Performance of the pelvic examination must be tailored to a woman's physical impairments (89,90). An accessible examination table that lowers to wheelchair height and has security features such as hand rails, boots, and straps can be indispensable (90a). Leg adjustments should be performed slowly and gradually to minimize pain and spasticity. Liberal application of lidocaine gel to the perineal area can be helpful in minimizing spasticity or in preventing episodes of autonomic hyperreflexia in some spinal-cord-injured women with high lesions (above T6) (49,91).

Breast Self-Exam and Mammograms

National Cancer Institute statistics report that breast cancer is the most prevalent gynecologic cancer occurring in women, with approximately 1¾ million women affected in 1995 (92) (Fig. 67-2). Currently, it is estimated that one in eight women will develop breast cancer. A family history of breast cancer, early menarche, and late menopause are factors that have been linked to an increased risk of breast cancer. It is generally recommended that women learn their breast anatomy and examine themselves on a regular basis to detect changes or abnormalities that may signal breast cancer (93,94). Training can improve the detection rate from 25% to 55% accuracy during breast self-exam, although this is less accurate than physician detection, 85% to 90% (95).

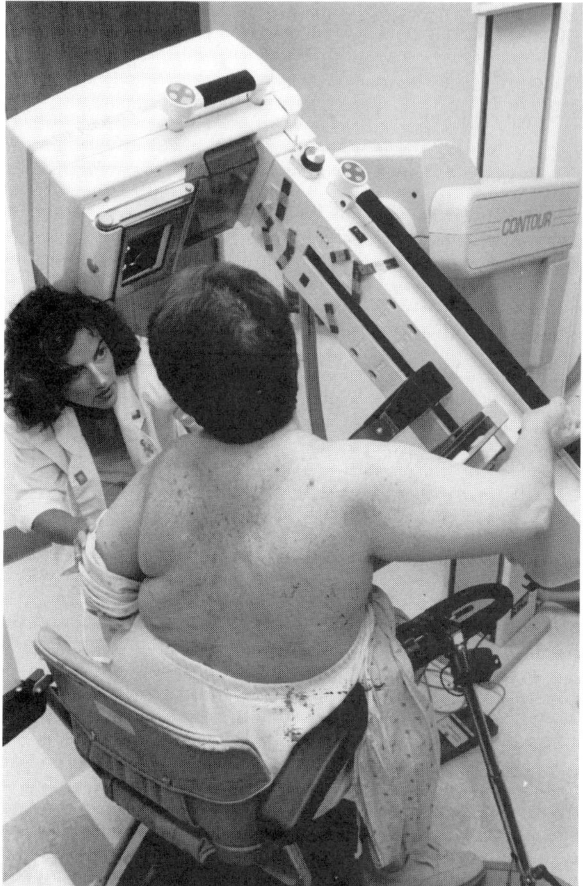

FIG. 67-2. Patient who uses a wheelchair receiving a mammogram.

If a woman with a disability is unable to perform breast self-exam, she may want to work out a system with her physician, personal care assistant, partner, or other available person to assist in breast exam techniques. It is recommended that manual breast exams be done regularly after the menstrual cycle in premenopausal women and on a monthly basis in menopausal women. The technique is simple to learn as long as a systematic approach is used. Up-and-down, side-to-side techniques and spiral techniques are equally effective in detecting abnormalities if done consistently (96).

Menopause and Aging with a Disability

Menopause is the "cessation of menstruation for a year or more. It is caused by ovarian failure and is frequently preceded by anovulatory bleeding" (54). Menopause usually occurs in women between 45 and 55 years of age with a mean age of 51 and is suspected after 6 months of amenorrhea (97). Diagnosis can be confirmed by findings of low estradiol and high follicle stimulating hormone (FSH). These tests can be performed if the diagnosis is in question. The age of onset of menopause can occur earlier in women with chronic disease states such as thyroid disease, diabetes, and in disabilities such as MS (98,99). It is important to properly diagnose the onset of menopause because early intervention can prevent some of the major sequelae of estrogen deficiency such as osteoporosis and cardiovascular disease (100). Symptomatology may also vary in its manifestation and effects on women with disabilities. For example, women with neurologic conditions that are particularly heat sensitive, such as multiple sclerosis, may have difficulty with the "hot flashes" and vasomotor instability of menopause (101).

Some menopausal women with physical impairments who have baseline micturition dysfunction may note a change in their usual pattern. A woman with stroke or multiple sclerosis who was previously continent, for example, may note some difficulties with leakage or frank incontinence. Three main structural components that are important for the control of micturition include the vascularity of urethral structures, soft tissue supports to these structures, and muscular control mechanisms (102). Estrogen deficiency can result in reduced vascularity and tissue turgor in the periurethral area, although muscular function or dysfunction is usually constant. Hormone replacement therapy can improve the variables that respond to estrogen supplementation and may result in improved continence (103).

Some subtle cognitive, sensory, and coordination difficulties have been linked to menopause as well. Estrogen replacement therapy (ERT) has been shown to modestly improve cognitive abilities, such as memory, concentration, and attention, documented by neuropsychological testing (104). In other studies motor control and coordination have also demonstrated some improvement in women taking ERT. Estrogen deficiency states have also been linked to problems with dexterity and two-point discrimination (105).

Women with physical disabilities may be at higher risk than their nondisabled counterparts for the consequences of estrogen deprivation, including osteoporosis, difficulties with skin integrity, and perhaps even cardiovascular morbidity. For example, a woman with weakness or paralysis from a neurologic disability may have extensive immobilization osteoporosis that occurred around the time of onset of the disability. She is still at risk for age-related and menopause-related osteoporosis but will be entering these phases with a lower bone mass to begin with. If she is at increased risk for pressure sores from immobility or loss of sensation, she may note increasing difficulty with maintenance of her skin integrity and turgor around menopause with the loss of estrogen. Aerobic exercise has a recognized benefit in the prevention and management of coronary artery disease, perhaps by affecting the level of high density lipoprotein (HDL)-cholesterol, weight management, and blood pressure (4). For women with extensive mobility impairments, endurance exercise may be difficult, if not impossible. Hormone replacement therapy has been shown to have beneficial effects in forestalling postmenopausal osteoporosis and coronary artery disease and in the maintenance of skin turgor in women in general (4,106,107). The mechanisms for cardioprotective effect of estrogen may be twofold. First, by a direct vasodilatory effect on blood vessels, peripherally and in coronary arteries, as well as by a beneficial alteration of the lipid profile, increasing HDL and decreasing low density lipoprotein (LDL).

Estrogen replacement therapy has been linked to a significant decrease in cardiovascular morbidity in women (108). Women with disabilities resulting from cerebrovascular disease, history of transient ischemic attacks, or vascular occlusive disease may be at a higher risk for developing further cardiovascular morbidity. Though hormone replacement therapy may offer some benefit, the risk of blood clotting is unclear. To minimize this risk in women considering the use of ERT, screening for hypercoagulability before initiation of hormone replacement therapy may be appropriate (109). Hypercoagulability markers should be reviewed, and transdermal estrogen therapy, possibly with the addition of low-dose aspirin therapy every 2 to 3 days, may offer safe treatment and permit the protective effects of hormone replacement therapy on osteoporosis as well as on cardiovascular disease (110).

Women with strong family histories of breast cancer and certain types of breast pathology should carefully weigh estrogen replacement (111). Without this predisposing history, the risk of morbidity and mortality from cardiovascular events is ten times higher than that from breast cancer in women after menopause (108). Women who elect not to use ERT or who have contraindications to being treated with estrogen replacement therapy may still be treated with antiresorptive agents such as calcitonin and alendronate to protect bone structures, although these do not provide the cardioprotective effects of ERT. Detailed discussion of osteoporosis diagnosis and treatment is found elsewhere in the text (Chapter 58).

SEXUALITY

Definition

The World Health Organization definition of sexual health (1975) is "the integration of the somatic, emotional, mental, and social aspects of being sexual beings, in ways that are positively enriching and that include personality and love."

Body image (112) is "an image of self and includes physical appearance, inner feelings, how other people act or react (or one's interpretation of how they react or do not react) and identification."

Sexuality is much more than penile–vaginal intercourse, though prior research has focused heavily on this area to describe sexuality after disability (113–129). Although a broader definition of sexuality is important for all, people with disabilities have been especially helpful in expanding our concepts of human sexuality to include the quality of relationships, imagery, sensuality, self-image, creativity, and emotional connectedness (130–135).

Access to knowledgeable health care professionals can be extremely important in facilitating successful sexual adjustment after disability and problem-solving issues that may arise (136–148,150,151). For example, sexual desire may be suppressed in women who experience significant fatigue or discomfort from a chronic disease or disability. In such cases, analgesics can be considered and timing centered around peak energy level periods. Communication between members of the couple about individual needs can help transcend barriers to desire. For women with sensory impairments, exploration of nontraditional erogenous zones as well as traditional areas may help her to discover pleasurable touching. Discussions about bowel programs, the management of catheters, spasticity, hyperreflexia, contractures, and positioning may all help alleviate anxiety about resuming intimate relationships. Of course, it is important to remember that not all women with disabilities are heterosexual, and their lives may include lesbian relationships. The need to have access to knowledgeable, caring, and open health care professionals is the same.

Self-Esteem/Self-Image and Gender Issues

The development of positive identity is a challenge for any member of a socially devalued community (152). It is especially difficult for an individual to sustain positive identity and self-esteem when surrounded by messages that she or he fails to measure up to culturally prescribed norms. For that reason, scholars specializing in women's issues have denounced the unforgiving standards of physical and functional perfection imposed on all young girls as they mature into womanhood. Heterosexual attractiveness and social success, in particular, are still highly associated with self-esteem in young women (149).

Those standards are exceptionally harsh for women with disabilities. Girls who grow up with visible impairments learn early in life that they are not expected to succeed at womanhood, either esthetically or functionally. In research interviews and their own written accounts of growing up with disabilities (8,153,154), they frequently report that their parents carefully avoided discussions of romance or, worse, explicitly predicted that the daughters would never attract or please a mate. Instead of offering tips on dating, mothers might urge them to hide their limbs or cover up disabled body features with clothing to prevent social rejection. Fathers often encouraged them to study hard and prepare for a good job in lieu of a husband. Nondisabled classmates sometimes openly ridiculed their sexual appeal. The consequences for many adolescent girls with disabilities have been alienation and shame.

Some young women with disabilities, however, including those with extensive physical limitations, have demonstrated amazing resilience in the face of invalidating messages. They have developed positive self-concepts as women and have established enduring intimate relationships. Many give credit to unusually perceptive family members who affirmed their gender roles and who facilitated their social contacts. Others, surrounded by discouragement, refused to internalize it. Seeking strong disabled women role models for support or simply finding validation from within, they have integrated their disabilities into strong and positive identities (149). Accepting disability as a familiar and "normal" part of their lives, they seem to set their own standards for what is valuable, sexually appealing, and womanly.

Women who acquire their disabilities after adolescence may be spared the unique barriers to self-esteem development and sex-role definition experienced by women with early-onset disabilities. However, they frequently report feeling shaken by a change in others' regard for them as women immediately following disability (155), and others have referred to this phenomenon as "degenderization"—being treated as asexual and as no longer female. Divested of the qualities and roles that define women in our society, women with late-onset disabilities may feel a profound loss of identity and meaningful place in their social network (156).

In addition to invalidating messages about their womanliness from family, friends, and greater society, women with disabilities experience degenderization and patronizing attitudes from professionals in medical settings. "Public stripping" is an experience so pervasive and distressing to women with disabilities that they have written about it extensively and given it a name (157). They use this term to refer to the practice of requiring children and adults with disabilities to disrobe for medical educational display and/or clinical photographs, sometimes without adequate preparation or request for permission. Women with disabilities report enduring psychological trauma from their perceived violation of body space and privacy in medical settings, describing such events as assaultive, objectifying or dehumanizing, and dismissive of their gender roles. Many women and girls with disabilities struggle to be respected as valid women with genuine women's health issues, including contraception, fertility, and sexually transmitted disease. When a health care provider expresses undue curiosity or overriding concern regarding aspects of their disability rather than gynecologic health, they may feel "treated like a disability instead of a woman."

In addition to adopting a responsive and respectful clinical approach that acknowledges women with disabilities as women in every way, physicians can help link their patients to community resources for peer support and opportunities for self-expression. Physicians can acquaint themselves with independent living centers—a national network comprising hundreds of centers run by people with disabilities to provide disability-related information, services, and advocacy to others with disabilities and deafness. Most cities have one or more such centers, and many offer peer support groups and domestic violence programs as well as information on housing, health services, transportation, and in-home personal assistance services. Additionally, in many cities there are disability rights and consumer organizations that can be contacted for resources helpful to women with disabilities. State, county, and municipal government offices routinely have departments addressing the needs of citizens with disabilities. By contacting these organizations and programs, physicians and the women with disabilities they serve can inquire about local recreational, artistic, employment, and peer support programs that welcome women with disabilities and encourage their development of positive identity.

Recently, the national disability community has developed a multitude of projects to celebrate the history, culture, and group identity of people with disabilities. Women with disabilities have figured prominently in this movement. As poets, playwrights, scholars, and performers, they have asserted the importance of disabled women's perspective on the world (158). In the past two decades, women with disabilities across the country have established programs to encourage networking for support and mentoring. For example, the Networking Project for Disabled Women and Girls was established in New York by Harilyn Rousso in 1984 to promote connections between girls with disabilities and disabled women who have achieved career and relationship goals. The Project on Women and Disability in Boston under the leadership of Marsha Saxton has developed a variety of projects to encourage women with disabilities to exchange information about their experiences and to learn useful skills such as assertiveness and strategies for effective communication and partnership building with health service providers. The motto of that organization aptly expresses the philosophy underpinning these efforts: ''Female, Disabled, and Proud!'' (Fig. 67-3).

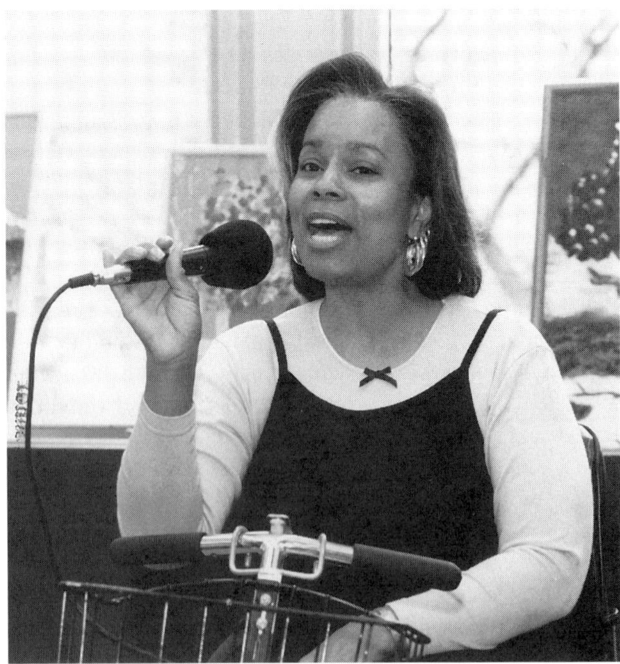

FIG. 67-3. Disabled actress participating in a "coffee-shop" celebrating the arts and talents of disabled women.

Access to Information

Lack of access to information can prevent women with disabilities from achieving self-determination in health and other aspects of life. Their exclusion from sources of information about sexuality and reproductive health options has been caused by inadequate disability accommodations, negative disability attitudes, or a combination of both types of barriers (159).

Many girls with disabilities grow up outside the usual channels for learning about sexuality. For example, they may be denied admission to their neighborhood schools and recreation programs because of access barriers and discriminatory enrollment practices. Consequently, they are denied important informal opportunities to exchange information and experiences regarding sexuality with their peers. Instead, they might be placed in a sheltered and closely supervised ''special education'' school where even formal sex education may not be offered. Their parents are less likely to talk to them about sexuality and reproduction than to their nondisabled sisters (149). Girls and young women who are blind are rarely given tactile anatomic models so they can safely explore and understand the form and function of human body parts. Those who are deaf or hard of hearing may miss conversations about ''the facts of life'' whispered between hearing friends. Girls and women with cognitive disabilities may not fully understand spoken and written information about sexuality and health matters unless it is presented in an illustrated, uncomplicated manner.

In adulthood, information barriers interfere with health maintenance for women with disabilities. Blind women and those with low vision confront clinic signs, instructions, release forms, and educational materials that have not been translated into accessible formats such as Braille, audiotapes, or computer disk versions. Deaf women are not offered interpreters to insure accurate doctor–patient communication. Women with cognitive disabilities are not allowed adequate time and explanation to ensure comprehension and informed consent.

Provider attitudes affect the amount and quality of information offered to women patients with disabilities. Negative disability attitudes in physicians have not only been associated with their lack of complete knowledge about health options for persons with disabilities but also with an inclination to withhold options that are known (160). There is some empirical evidence to confirm that disabled women garner negative judgments from health professionals. In their survey of allied health professionals' knowledge of men and women with disabilities, for example, Westbrook and Adamson (161) found that men generally were perceived by the professionals as better at coping with their disabilities than women. There is also evidence that physician's perceptions of a woman's disability may result in the withholding of information about her health options. One of the first systematic studies to document disabled womens' health service experiences (16) revealed that physicians' inclination to offer disabled women patients information regarding sexuality and contraception was mediated by such factors as the age of onset or extent of a woman's disability.

A useful rule of thumb in working clinically with any woman with a disability, particularly early-onset disability, is to ask if she would like information or guidance about sexuality, reproductive health options, or any other aspect of health. Some women with disabilities are extraordinarily sophisticated about their health options and the workings of their bodies; others lack basic information about anatomy and human sexuality. Many are experts regarding their particular disability but have gaps in general health maintenance knowledge as a result of the information barriers discussed above. It is useful to explore each woman's level of knowledge and desire for more information before concluding any health service contact.

MOTHERING WITH A DISABILITY

Women with disabilities increasingly have been choosing to become mothers, shattering stereotypes of asexuality and maternal incompetency historically ascribed to them by a society that stigmatizes disability. They and mothers who later acquired disabilities are seeking recognition and support for their capabilities. This surge was spurred in the 1970s by the independent living movement and in the 1990s by the passage of the Americans with Disabilities Act and is forcing health care providers to take a closer look at ways to assist mothers with disabilities to achieve self-determination over their parenting activities. Although mothers with disabilities share the same basic needs and concerns as nondisabled mothers, their capabilities to function aptly in a parenting role are greatly enhanced with the use of adaptive equipment, adequate personal assistance, regular access to peer support, and knowledgeable health care providers who understand the concept of self-determination, as well as the sociopolitical barriers confronting women with disabilities (162).

Research

Researchers have found that nature, too, can play a significant role in helping mothers with disabilities become self-determining. Studies conducted by researchers at a California-based agency, Through the Looking Glass (TLG), a pioneer in training, services, and research for parents with disabilities, determined that infants adapt early to their visually impaired parents through a process facilitated by a maternal cuing of sorts, where the sound of the mother's voice may serve as a signal for the child's adaptive behavior (165).

Consistent with these findings, women with spinal cord injuries have observed that weeks after birth, their children began helping their mothers lift them by "balling up" their head and legs as the mothers approached the children and that infants remained in that configuration until the lift occurred. Anecdotal evidence also suggests that adaptations can continue as the child develops. For example, mothers with hemiplegia report that their children knew at an early age always to approach the mother on her stronger side and to refrain from extending arms to be picked up when their mother was standing or not in a more stable, seated position (163,164).

Against a background of scant high-quality research on mothering with a disability and prevalence of early literature condemning the activity of parenting with a disability as a source of potential damage to the children (165–167), Through the Looking Glass continues to spearhead research that helps improve the quality of family life for individuals parenting with a disability. Their Rehabilitation Research and Training Center (RRTC) on Families of Adults with Disabilities is a clearinghouse for parents with disabilities that offers a consultation service, training modules, catalogues of adaptive equipment, and a newsletter (168). In 1993 to 1997, it has undertaken several key research and training projects:

1. Needs assessment: assessing the incidence of different subpopulations of families with parents who have disabilities and the types of supports needed by these families.
2. Family case studies: an in-depth study documenting strategies in successful family formation of families in which at least one parent has a disability.
3. State of the nation: identifying and analyzing federal and state policy barriers to successful family life for parents with disabilities.
4. Parents with deafness: documenting the effectiveness of interventions that integrate infant mental health work, peer teaching, and support for parents who are deaf.
5. Mothers with visual disabilities: exploring the psychological adjustment of new mothers with visual disabilities.
6. A longitudinal study of children of parents with physical disabilities: examining the interactions between parents and their children at two developmental points.
7. Pregnancy and birthing: designing a training module to address the issues described by women with physical disabilities during pregnancy, labor, and delivery.
8. Family support model: developing a model that will respond to the needs of family members experiencing acute onset of disabling conditions.
9. Determining the cost of living for adults with disabilities: determining a living wage for individuals with disabilities to become self-supporting.
10. Increasing access to Head Start for parents with disabilities: exploring the degree to which parents with disabilities have access to Head Start for their children and how the program could improve access.
11. Assistive technology and parenting: developing parenting equipment, and disseminating a national survey and local survey regarding the impact of assistive technology for parents with physical disabilities (165).

Facilitating Self-Determination

Although the introduction of adaptive equipment and parenting resources early in the mothering experience can minimize problems and significantly improve a disabled mother's capacity to provide "totally independent care" for her baby, this is not feasible for all mothers. Financial constraints, scarcity of customized equipment, and physical limitations may still prevent many women from becoming fully self-sufficient in managing the care of a child.

It is thus essential for mothers and health care providers alike to recognize that a disabled woman's lack of independence does not diminish her mothering skill. Rather, it shifts the focus to the value of facilitating self-determination instead of self-sufficiency in the parenting role. This distinction is a crucial one. It suggests that parents with disabilities should be (a) the primary decision makers in the care of their children, (b) encouraged to personally perform as many parenting tasks as they can carry out safely, (c) supported with a caregiver when they cannot or choose not to perform an activity independently.

A caregiver can be a family member, spouse, friend, or hired personal assistant. Caregivers are most beneficial when they enhance the special bond between a parent and child (169). Health professionals and occupational therapists can help maximize the value of hired caregivers by facilitating childcare training to teach the caregiver how to assist the disabled mother ''without taking over the role of the parent'' (82).

Occupational therapists at the Rehabilitation Institute of Chicago have made great strides in developing a protocol and activity analysis to assess child care and parenting skills that facilitate self-determination in mothers with cognitive as well as physical disabilities (Figs. 67-4 and 67-5) (82). This approach identifies a disabled mother's abilities regard-

Item Name: Care of Others (Child Care)

Definitions:

a. **Physical daily care**--Selects proper equipment, uses correct positioning, and performs the following:

- Feeding--breastfeeding, bottle feeding (includes set-up and clean-up), spoon feeding (includes opening jars)
- Changing a diaper--donning and removal (specify type: cloth with pins or diaper cover or plastic with tape) and managing hygiene
- Dressing/undressing--Donning and removal (specify type: one-piece jumpsuit, t-shirt, plastic pants, dress with snaps or buttons, socks, shoes, booties)
- Bathing--Holding, washing, drying off (indicate location: tub, sink, positioning device)
- Preparing for bed--Changing clothes, lifting and lowering side of crib, moving child from crib to lap or wheelchair, covering child with blanket
- Carrying/lifting--Lifting to and from floor and transporting 50 feet

b. **Playing/nurturing**--Selects appropriate toys/activities, uses age-appropriate interaction, and is aware of various intervention strategies for behavior management and facilitation emotional growth

c. **Illness/first aid**--Takes temperature, uses nasal aspirator, manages suppositories, and gives medication. Is aware of symptoms and is able to perform minor emergency procedures (cuts choking, CPR, poisoning), "baby-proofing" of home, and seeking assist in an emergency

d. **Community access/resourcing**--is able to select and access day care/preschool, child supplies, physician, babysitter. Is able to instruct babysitter. Is able to manage stroller and car seat (includes placement and removal from car, placing child in/out of devices), diaper bag, back pack.

Note: Select and note activities appropriate to the patient's lifestyle/abilities.

SCALE POINTS

NO CAREGIVER REQUIREMENT:

7. Complete independence: Patient can perform task safely and consistently within a functional amount of time in any environment without specialized equipment, modifications, or verbal/physical assist.
6. Modified independence: Patient can perform task safely and consistently without caregiver assistance but requires specialized equipment, an adapted environment, and/or excessive time to complete task.

REQUIRES CAREGIVER ASSISTANCE

5. Set-up/infrequent assistance: Patient consistently requires caregiver presence to initiate and/or complete task (e.g., with set-up and/or clean-up), but patient safely and consistently completes interim components independently, *or* patient requires caregiver's assistance for unpredictable occurrences only.
4. Minimal assistance: Patient performs more than three quarters of the task safely and consistently. Because of physical or cognitive impairment, patient requires caregiver to provide physical or verbal assist to complete one quarter of the task.
3. Moderate assistance: Patient performs half to three quarters of the task safely and consistently. Because of physical or cognitive impairment, patient requires caregiver to provide physical or verbal assist to complete on quarter to half the task.
2. Maximal assistance: Patient performs one quarter to half of the task safely and consistently, or may be physically unable to perform any part of the activity but can accurately direct the caregiver. Patient requires caregiver to provide physical or verbal assist to complete the remainder of the task.
1. Dependent: Patient performs less than one quarter of the task consistently. Patient is unable to direct the caregiver and is dependent of the caregiver's physical or verbal assistance for completing more than three quarters of the task.

FIG. 67-4. Rehabilitation Institute of Chicago (RIC) Functional Assessment Scale. The occupational therapy department would like to recognize the contribution made by Sharon Gartland, OTR/L, and Sheila Gupta, OTR/L, in the development of the definition for child care. (Used by permission of the Rehabilitation Institute of Chicago.)

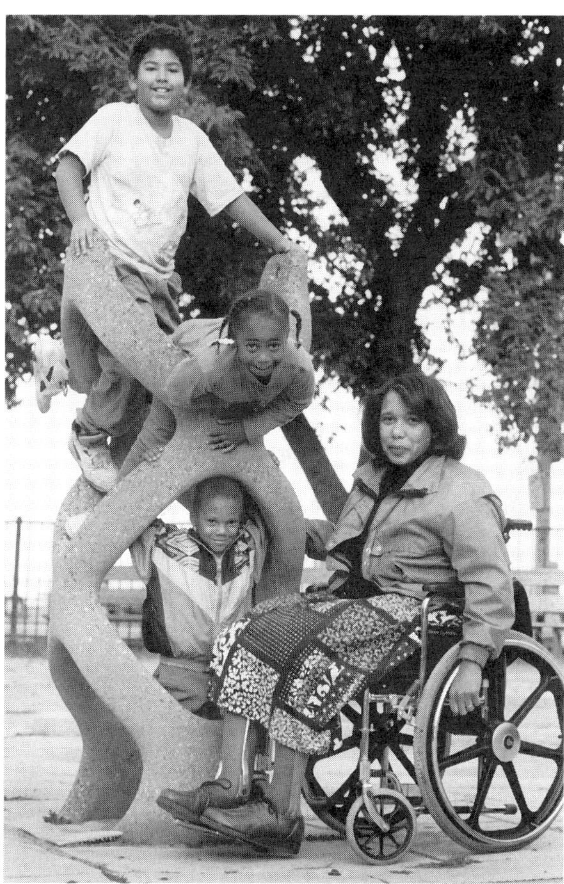

FIG. 67-5. Disabled mother.

ing selective child care tasks and gives her final say in parenting decisions. On the basis of the assessment therapist, mother and spouse or caregiver collaborate to determine the tasks the disabled mother needs simplified, is comfortable performing independently, or will delegate to helpers.

Despite the growing numbers of mothers with disabilities and the positive impact of support resources, the lack of disability-aware social institutions and services can pose real threats to their self-determination. A profound problem related to personal assistance stems from the fact that some states exclude child care as an activity of daily living for which a disabled person can get personal assistant support. Tasks involving dinner preparation for a child or assistance in positioning for breastfeeding or bathing are not considered viable activities for state-funded assistance. Note that this issue is relevant only in cases when the parents are disabled and have nondisabled children. When the child is also disabled, funds for personal assistance are common (170).

Unfortunately, women with disabilities who have a low income and are unable to afford private child care have lost custody of their children because the state refused them assistant services and then deemed them incompetent in parental functioning (11,171). Full knowledge of relevant state policies on the provisions of personal assistants will create realistic expectations on the part of prospective parents and better aid practitioners in educating their clients and peers about ways to reduce the risk for unnecessary removal of children from their disabled parents.

Stereotypes depicting women with disabilities as having to be ''cared for'' rather than as caregivers presents ongoing challenges to those women wishing to adopt children. Other barriers to adoptive services may include the lack of universal definitions for good parenting, permitting agency staff to impose arbitrary standards onto disabled individuals applying for adoptive services (172,173). This point is captured best in the story of a man using a wheelchair who was told that his problems ''playing baseball'' could diminish his capacity to be a fit father for an adoptive son (174). Advocates in the disability community increasingly are inviting health care providers to join them in the quest for creating a level playing field, given the strong competition for adoptable infants (173). Physicians can play a major role in this regard simply by educating other physicians, policymakers, and allied health professionals, such as social workers, about the parenting capabilities of individuals and their countless successes achieving self-determination in parenting activities.

Peer Support

Facing the onslaught of negative messages concerning one's reproductive and parenting capacities can reinforce self-doubts in even the most confident of disabled women. Advocates and experts around the world are finding that a disability consciousness and culture emerging from the power of peer-to-peer contact is the tried-and-true remedy for counteracting the isolation and devaluation women experience when parenting with a disability (162,175). From each other, many women are hearing for the first time that their decision to become mothers is a valid one—a cause for celebration. They rely on one another for a wholeness and strength that come not from independence and self-sufficiency but from interdependence and self-determination.

Violence and Abuse

Unlike many traditional health concerns, domestic violence is a complex social problem rather than a biomedical one (176). It is a crime of power that utilizes fear to control a victim and is an everyday reality in the United States. Above all, domestic violence is an insidious process frequently invisible to the public and most health practitioners. Moreover, disability has long been linked to violence, both as an outcome and as a means for establishing societal perceptions of women's vulnerability. This association creates a cycle of disability and violence, begetting more disability and violence, that easily entraps but proves difficult for a woman to escape (see Fig. 67-6) (177). For the past two decades women with disabilities have been calling attention to the prevalence of violence and abuse in their lives as well

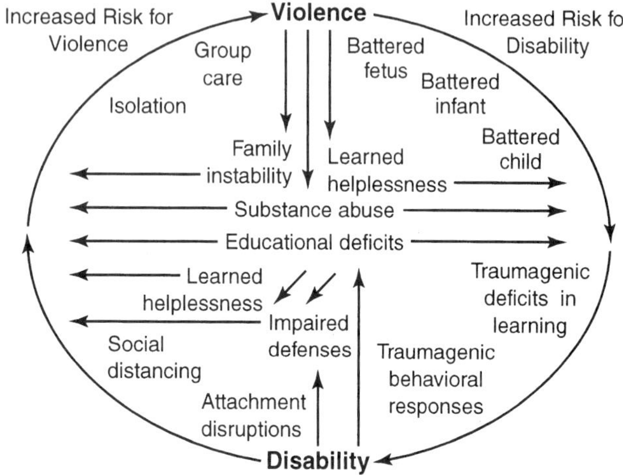

FIG. 67-6. Mechanisms that contribute to the abuse and disability cycle. (From Sobsey D. *Violence and abuse in the lives of people with disabilities: The end of silent acceptance?* Baltimore: Paul H Brookes, 1994; 47, with permission.)

as advocating for disability-inclusive research and support services (178,179).

The abuse experience of women with disabilities is often not reported to law officers (180). They are rarely documented in the media or in studies and given scant attention by providers (181). However, a growing number of experts agree that violence and abuse against women with disabilities are the rule rather than the exception (171,177,180,182). Sobsey states that:

> The risk of only a single incident of abuse for people with disabilities appears to be at least one and a half times as great as the risk for other people of similar age or gender. Because people with disabilities are often repeatedly or chronically abused, the risk becomes even greater when multiple victimizations are considered (177).

Social isolation, lack of sex education, low self-esteem, and dependence on caregivers are frequently cited as contributing factors to the high rate of violence against women and girls with disabilities (177,185). Although physical limitations may be associated with an increased risk and incidence of violence and abuse among women with disabilities, the primacy of cultural factors cannot be ignored. Negative societal perceptions that characterize disabled women as dependent, asexual, and passive greatly heighten the risk for abuse (177,183,185).

Offenders include family members, personal assistants, service providers, institutional staff, spouses, dates, and strangers (182,183,185). Women with disabilities living in institutions are especially vulnerable to violence (184) and run the risk of having their reports of violence discredited when offenders are institutional employees protected by the administrative staff of the institution. The isolation of institutional living can also prevent disabled women who are abused from gaining the support services they require. Reports of neglect, mistreatment, and abuse perpetrated by health care providers are also not uncommon and occur to disabled women living both in institutions and in the community (The Center for Research on Women with Disabilities, Baylor College of Medicine, unpublished fact sheet, 1995). However, most sexual abuse is commonly committed by caregivers, and vulnerability to sexual assault increases when disabled women are involved with multiple caregivers (183).

Anecdotal evidence suggests that, like other abused women, those who are disabled tend to resist reporting their experiences because of denial, guilt, self-contempt, and fear of loss of financial security. However, some experts believe that disabled women are often discouraged from disclosure because they are commonly regarded as less credible and easily discredited as witnesses by virtue of having a disability (186). Threats from abusers to withdraw assistive devices, such as wheelchairs and respirators, as well as personal assistant services add to the fears of disabled women and further inhibit their disclosure of violent incidents. These threats and fears also serve as disincentives to leave abusive relationships with caregivers and family members and reinforce the cycle of violence.

Health care providers are cautioned to discriminate between the signs of sexual abuse and those of disability. Frequently, symptoms of abuse are confused with the sequelae of a woman's disability, or they may be overlooked completely. Common symptoms of sexual abuse include pain, bruises, and bleeding in the genital area, behavioral disturbances, loss of weight, fear of sexual intimacy, and fear of intervention (15,180). Practitioners are also urged to be mindful in recognizing and treating the symptoms of posttraumatic stress syndrome (PTSD), which can manifest in survivors of violence. When she has had previous brain trauma or head injuries acquired through violence, the compounded effects may overwhelm the woman with head trauma and require physicians to invoke the expertise of mental health workers familiar with such cases. Because PTSD can occasionally be a more problematic workplace disability than more visible disabilities such as limited mobility, clinicians treating women with PTSD are urged to link them with appropriate resources to ensure workplace accommodations for the effects of PTSD (187).

Moreover, physicians must take a supportive and facilitative role in identifying and treating violence and abuse. Domestic violence requires practitioners to move beyond the biomedical model and collaborate with advocacy groups committed to ending violence against women (176). They can assist by working to facilitate access to high-quality personal assistants (180) and to prevent the placement of women into nursing homes and other institutions. Healthcare providers can help prevent sexual abuse in women with disabilities by collaborating with other social services to develop comprehensive outreach strategies that are accessible to women with physical, cognitive, sensory, and communication disabilities including those living in institutions.

Offering high-quality health services to disabled women obliges providers to make their services welcoming with accessible equipment, signers, and TTYs (teletype writers). It also dictates that they become knowledgeable about local accessible shelters and their policies regarding personal assistants and children. Shelters and support services are accessible only if they can be accessed by a woman at any time regardless of her physical, sensory, or communication disabilities.

Physicians should be aware of their role in breaking the cycle of violence and disability. They are encouraged to work with social services to prevent isolation to the fullest degree by involving the expertise of disabled women in the design and execution of outreach and education strategies. For example, transportation is a key component in any emergency. It should be factored into any protocol developed in response to abuse encounters.

Most important, health providers can assist in breaking the cycle of violence and disability by implementing a system of detection, reporting, and prosecution for cases of assault. Assaults will continue unless practitioners are willing and able to implement a comprehensive protocol (188).

DEPRESSION/SUICIDAL TENDENCIES AND MENTAL HEALTH SERVICES

It has been well established that women are troubled by significant depression at a rate approximately twice that of men (189). Among the causes hypothesized to explain this disparity have been physiology, social oppression including restricted choices and narrow standards for appearance and behavior, and socially imposed powerlessness. Although little research has specifically addressed depression in women with disabilities, there is no reason to believe this population would be immune from the dynamics of depression affecting all women.

The multiminority status of women with disabilities can, in fact, elevate their risk for stress disorder. The complexities and pressures of daily living with a disability command a balancing act of finding transportation, making appointments, filling out forms, negotiating with service agencies, managing personal assistants, worrying about equipment breakdown, and coping with discrimination. For women, who are more likely than men with disabilities to confront poverty and social isolation, the lack of adequate resources can compound the routine pressures of disability, leading to depression and feelings of hopelessness.

Rintala, Hart, and Fuhrer (190) found that women with spinal cord injuries reported significantly higher levels of perceived stress and scored higher in depression than either men with the same disability or women in the general population. A recent survey study of women with disabilities in Canada found a significant association among suicide, depression, and abuse (191). Of 371 women with a variety of disabilities, over 60% had contemplated suicide, and over 45% of the contemplators had attempted suicide at least once. Approximately half had experienced physical abuse or sexual abuse, and two-thirds had experienced emotional abuse. The more types of abuse a woman had experienced, the more likely she was to have considered suicide. Aside from abuse, the two factors mentioned most by the women as contributing to their suicidal tendencies were poverty and isolation.

The social role loss that all too often accompanies disablement in our society may be a significant risk factor for depression and suicide in elderly women. Osgood and Eisenhandler (192) have found that women who enter nursing homes because of age-related disability often respond to their powerlessness, loss of control over life, and cessation of meaningful social involvement by passively foregoing life-sustaining behaviors, e.g., stopping their medications. The authors refer to this phenomenon as ''acquiescent suicide.''

Treatable depression in disabled women remains undiagnosed when health service providers incorrectly assume that depression is a natural concomitant of disability. Although depression is an expected feature of the initial disability adjustment process, it should be noted and addressed with support, counseling, and other interventions appropriate to situational distress. Beyond the adjustment phase, depression in women with disabilities calls for a thorough exploration of specific causes (whether directly related to the woman's disability or not) and a review of potentially effective interventions by professionals knowledgeable about disability issues. Peer support can be a powerful adjunct to professional treatment.

Unfortunately, many women's clinics and community mental health centers are inaccessible to women with disabilities because of physical, economic, and communication barriers. Residential treatment programs for substance abuse and psychiatric disorders commonly refuse to admit women who use equipment or need physical assistance with activities of daily living. Sexual counseling, psychotherapy, and suicide intervention are rarely available from therapists who are adequately informed about the stressors and options resulting from the interaction of being a woman and being disabled. A concerned physician can be an important ally in a disabled woman's journey through depression, from identification of the problem to support in surmounting the barriers to adequate mental health services. The management of depression can be a critical facet of disabled women's health care, as we are reminded by the disproportionate number of women in the news who have succumbed to assisted suicide.

MODEL HEALTH SERVICES: THE ROLE OF COMMUNITY

A list of health service organizations focused on disabled women's issues is given in the Appendix.

In 1988, Amy Jackson, M.D., Director of the Spain Rehabilitation Center at the University of Alabama in Birmingham, inaugurated the first clinic in the United States offering reproductive health services specifically for women with disabilities (The Women's Clinic for the Disabled). The treatment center is fully wheelchair accessible and has a flexible examining table that facilitates unassisted transfers and eases the examination process. Working closely with an obstetrician/gynecologist, Dr. Jackson offers disabled women the benefit of "combined expertise" (193).

After a long history of neglect by both the medical and women's communities, disabled women are currently finding a voice in both planned and existing health services. Gaining increased respect as the experts in their own lives, they are acquiring decision-making authority and local ownership in programs designed to serve their needs (170). Although the manifestations of these efforts are varied in health service delivery throughout North America, the community-driven perspective emerges as a common theme in several prominent programs addressing disabled women's health concerns. This is illustrated in three programs that developed their community orientation in different ways in Los Angeles, Chicago, and Houston.

The California Family Planning Council initiated a federally funded Americans with Disabilities Act and Reproductive Health Project in 1993 under the direction of Barbara F. Waxman Fiduccia, a disabled woman and certified sex educator expert in disabled women's reproductive concerns. The project, originating in Los Angeles, aims to enable federally funded family planning clinics in the United States to provide accessible medical, educational, and counseling services to individuals with a wide variety of disabilities: mobility, hearing, visual, and cognitive. An important goal of this project is building significant relationships between the council's clinics and women from local disability communities (15). Currently the project is expanding its efforts to include federally funded victim services such as domestic violence shelters.

Programs like this are predicated on a community organization approach to health that encourages community participation rather than institutional dependency (194). This concept stresses that the role of health clinicians is to facilitate community health programs. Successful implementation of a community empowerment model obliges physicians to work collaboratively with members from the local disabled women's community in shaping the delivery of medical services, conducting research, and developing educational resources.

The Health Resource Center for Women with Disabilities (HRCWD) at the Rehabilitation Institute of Chicago brings to life the vision of a balanced partnership between local disabled women activists and the staff of a rehabilitation hospital (see Appendix). The center started in 1991 as a clinic offering accessible, collaborative reproductive health care services. Its goal is to assist disabled women to become self-determining in achieving physical and emotional wellness.

The backbone of the center from its inception has been a community board of 20 women of diverse backgrounds and disabilities who work with medical and rehabilitation staff to find solutions to the access problems preventing women from obtaining reproductive health care services. As members of its community board, they have expanded services to include the center's research component and an educational mission emphasizing psychosocial resources, such as parenting, aging, and antiviolence support. The lifeblood of the center, the community board, sets research and training priorities and provides ongoing feedback to the center's medical director, a woman physiatrist, and the administrative director, a disabled woman professional.

HRCWD is committed to its investment in the leadership abilities of its disabled women professionals who conduct research, ongoing peer support groups, and periodic conferences, seminars, and in-services targeting physicians, clinicians, and consumers. They have also created a resource library that handles information and referrals and collaborates in producing educational videos and an international newsletter published three times a year. Hospital medical and administrative staff assist with fundraising and program development as needed (Fig. 67-7).

The Center for Research on Women with Disabilities at Baylor Medical College in Houston was founded in 1993 by Margaret Nosek, Ph.D. When Nosek, a researcher with a disability, received a grant from the National Institutes of Health to study the psychosocial concerns of women with disabilities, including sexuality, domestic violence, and self-esteem, she was besieged with nationwide requests from disabled women asking to participate in the study. The grant and ensuing outcry from community women moved Nosek to start the center.

In contrast to other community health initiatives, the center offers no treatment services. Instead, Nosek, as the center's director, works with a team of other researchers with disabilities toward the end of improving reproductive health services for disabled women. Nosek supports mainstreaming services for disabled women into community health centers as opposed to offering services solely in specialty clinics (193). To meet this goal, Nosek and her team are committed to dismantling attitudinal and knowledge barriers preventing disabled women from receiving quality care by developing research and training materials for primary care physicians and ob/gyn providers.

This raises a crucial question: Are reproductive health services for disabled women more viable when they reside in specialty clinics or when they are mainstreamed into community health settings? Advocates favoring equal access to neighborhood health centers caution that, taken to the extreme, specialty clinics reinforce negative stereotypes, emphasizing the disability over the woman and suggesting that the disabled woman is without legitimate women's concerns. But others, preferring treatments from physicians who understand their disabilities, warn that traditional community clinics are often staffed with disability-unaware physicians whose practices can unwittingly cause them harm or humiliation. This structure also guarantees outreach to larger numbers of disabled women using the rehabilitation center for other services.

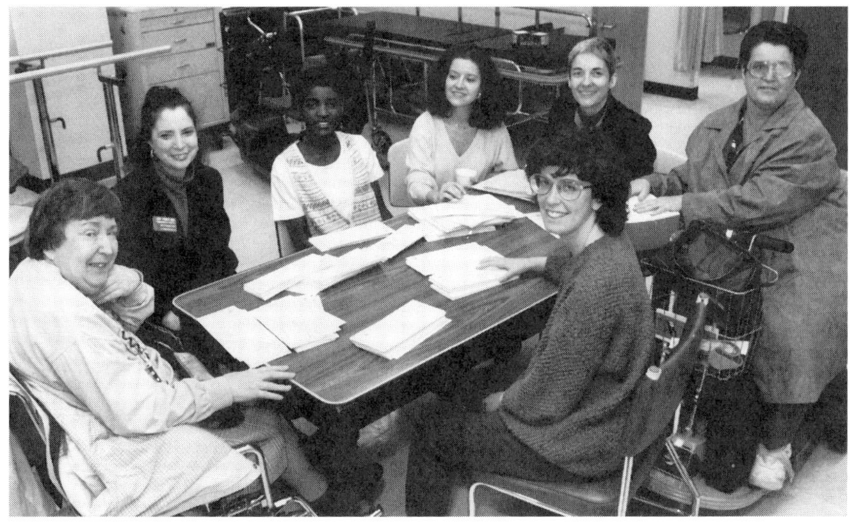

FIG. 67-7. Seminar. Community disabled women and healthcare providers collaborating on an educational seminar.

Mindful of the merits inherent in each model, many professionals and advocates agree that creating a full spectrum of health services available to disabled women is an ideal worth striving for and one that gives women the choices they need to become truly self-determining.

APPENDIX: SOME MODEL PROGRAMS AND RESOURCES FOR WOMEN WITH DISABILITIES

Networking Project for Young People with Disabilities (formerly the Networking Project for Women and Girls with Disabilities)
610 Lexington Avenue
New York, NY 10022
(212) 735-9767 (V)
Founded by Harilyn Rousso, this trailblazing program links disabled young women (and now young men, too) with experienced adult peer mentors who are active in the community.

Domestic Violence Initiative for Women with Disabilities
P.O. Box 300535
Denver, CO 80203
(303) 839-5510 (V)
Directed by Sharon Hickman, this is a nationally respected center of information and support for women with disabilities experiencing domestic violence and for their allies and health professionals.

National Clearinghouse for Women and Girls with Disabilities
114 East 32nd Street
New York, NY 10016
(212) 725-1803 (V)
This is a national repository of information on organizations and services for women with disabilities that publishes and disseminates the publication, Bridging the Gap: A Directory of Services for Women and Girls with Disabilities.

Berkeley Planning Associates (BPA)
440 Grand Avenue, Suite 500
Oakland, CA 94610
(510) 465-7884 (V)
(510) 465-4493 (TTY)
After researching and identifying access barriers to mainstream services for women with disabilities nationally, this organization has prepared materials addressing nine service systems, e.g., adoption, aging services, reproductive health, etc.

Domestic Violence Program
Access Living
310 South Peoria
Chicago, IL 60607
(312) 226-5900 (V)
(312) 226-1687 (TTY)
This program offers support groups for survivors; advocacy for women, children, and family members within the disabled community; appropriate information and referral services to victims of domestic violence who have disabilities.

Americans with Disabilities Act and Reproductive Health Project
Los Angeles Family Planning Council
Satellite Office
19907 Beekman Place
Cupertino, CA 94014-2452
(408)-996-9005
Barbara Waxman Fiduccia, Director
Project works to enable federally funded family planning clinics and victim services centers in United States to provide

accessible medical, educational, and counseling services to individuals with a wide variety of disabilities.

Center on Research on Women with Disabilities
Department of Physical Medicine and Rehabilitation
Baylor Medical College
3440 Richmond, Suite B
Houston, TX 77046
(713) 960-0505 (V and TTY)
(713) 961-3555 (FAX)
e-mail: mnosek@bcm.tmc.edu
Margaret Nosek: Director
The Center works to develop research and training materials for primary care physicians and ob/gyn providers.

Disability, Pregnancy, and Parenthood International
1 Chiswick Staithe
London W4 3TP
England
e-mail: fad36@dial.pipex.com
Mukti Jain Campion: Director
Periodic newsletter by subscription for professionals and parents to exchange information and experience.

Health Resource Center for Women with Disabilities
Rehabilitation Institute of Chicago
345 East Superior Street
Chicago, IL 60611
(312) 908-7997 (V)
Judy Panko Reis: Administrative Director
Kristi L. Kirschner, M.D.: Medical Director
Newsletter Resourceful Woman *written by, about, and for women with disabilities, is published three times a year, available at no charge.*

Mariposa Ministry
905 Encinitas Avenue
Calexico, CA 92231
e-mail KMTD@aol.com
(619)357-4768 or (619)768-0598
Ken Tittle, M.D.: Director
Lupita Redondo: Co-Director
Peer counseling ministry for disabled youth and young adults, with Spanish/English library of commentaries by and about young disabled women.

Through the Looking Glass
P.O. Box 8226
Berkley, CA 94707-8138
(510) 525-8138 (V)
(800) 644-2666
(510) 527-8137 (TTY)
National research and training center on families of adults with disabilities offering free periodic publication, Parenting with a Disability.

Disabled Women's Health Center
Spain Rehabilitation Hospital
1717 6th Avenue South
Birmingham, AL 35233
(205) 934-3330 (V)
Aimee Jackson, M.D.: Director
First collaborative clinic designed to meet the reproductive health care issues of women with disabilities.

Sandra Welner, M.D.
8484 16th Street
Suite 707
Silver Spring, MD 20910
(301) 587-6396 (V)
(301) 585-5467
In 1993, Sandra Welner, M.D., a disabled gynecologist, was recruited to start a new program as the Clinical Director of primary care programs for women with special needs, serving the Washington, D.C. metropolitan area. The center is primarily oriented around service delivery, using accessible facilities and women professionals trained in disability issues working with Dr. Welner. A unique feature of this clinic is a universally accessible examination table designed and patented by Dr. Welner. Research initiatives are also explored regarding contraceptive options for women with disabilities.

ACKNOWLEDGMENT

The authors would like to thank Dr. Raymond Curry and Dr. Eileen Murphy for their critical review of the manuscript.

REFERENCES

1. Sawin KJ. *Physical disability. Contemporary women's health.* Merlo Park, CA: Wesley, 1986.
2. Perlman L, Arneson D. *Women and rehabilitation of disabled persons. A report of the sixth annual Mary E. Switzer Memorial Seminar.* Washington, D.C.: National Rehabilitation Association, 1982.
3. Bulger RE. Special reports: inclusion of women in clinical trials—policies for population subgroups. *N Engl J Med* 1993; 329:288–296.
4. Wenger NK, Speroff L, Packard B. Cardiovascular health and disease in women. *N Engl J Med* 1993; 329:247–272.
5. Altman BM. Causes, risks, and consequences of disability among women with physical disabilities. In: Krotoski DM, Nosek MA, Turk MA, eds. *Achieving and maintaining health and well-being.* Baltimore: Paul H. Brookes, 1996;35–56.
6. LaPlante MP. *Disability risks of chronic illnesses and impairments.* Washington, D.C.: National Institute on Disability and Rehabilitation Research, US Department of Education, Office of Special Education and Rehabilitative Services, 1991.
7. McNeil JM. *Americans with disabilities: 1991–1992.* Washington, D.C.: US Bureau of the Census current population reports, P70-33, US Government Printing Office, 1993.
8. Fine M, Asch A, eds. *Introduction: Beyond pedestals. Women with disabilities: essays in psychology, culture, and politics.* Philadelphia: Temple University Press, 1988.
9. Tilley CM. Sexuality in women with physical disabilities: A social justice or health issue? *Sexuality Dis* 1996; 14:139–151.
10. Larson EJ. *Sex, race, and science: eugenics in the deep South.* Baltimore: John Hopkins University Press, 1995.
11. Mathews J. *A mother's touch: the Tiffany Callo story.* New York: Henry Holt, 1992.

12. Shapiro JP. *No pity: people with disabilities forging a new civil rights movement.* New York: Times Books, 1981.
13. Jackson AB. Pregnancy and delivery. In: Krotoski DM, Nosek MA, Turk MA, eds. Women with physical disabilities: achieving and maintaining health and well-being. Baltimore: Paul H. Brookes, 1996; 91–99.
14. Waxman BF. It's time to politicize our sexual oppression. *Disability Rag* 1991; March/April:23–26.
15. Nosek MA, Rintala DH, Young ME et al. Sexual functioning among women with physical disabilities. *Arch Phys Med Rehabil* 1996; 77: 107–115.
16. Beckmann CRB, Gittler M, Barzansky BM, Beckmann CA. Gynecologic health care of women with disabilities. *Obstet Gynecol* 1989; 74:75–79.
17. Yarkony GM, Novick AK, Roth EJ, Kirschner KL, Rayner S, Betts HB. Galactorrhea: a complication of spinal cord injury. *Arch Phys Med Rehabil* 1991; 73(9):878–880.
18. De Leo R, Petruk KC, Crockford P. Galactorrhea after prolonged traumatic coma: A case report. *Neurosurgery* 1981; 9:177–178.
19. Yarkony GM. Spinal cord injured women: sexuality, fertility and pregnancy. In: Goldstein PJ, Stern BJ, eds. *Neurologic disorders of pregnancy.* Mt Kisco, NY: Futura, 1992; 203–222.
20. Reame NE. A prospective study of the menstrual cycle and spinal cord injury. *Am J Phys Med Rehabil* 1992; 71:15–21.
21. Smith PJ, Surks MI. Multiple effects of 5,5′-diphenylhydantonin on the thyroid hormone systems. *Endocr Rev* 1984; 5:514–524.
22. Kletzky OA, Davajan V. Hyperprolactinemia. In: Mishell DR, Davajan V, Lobo RA, eds. *Infertility, contraception, and reproductive endocrinology.* Boston: Blackwell Scientific Publications, 1991; 809–851.
23. Wathen PI, Hendersen MC, Witz CA. Abnormal uterine bleeding. *Med Clin North Am* 1995; 2:329–344.
24. Ratchev E, Dokumov S. Premenopausal bleeding associated with hyperprolactinaemia. *Maturitas* 1995; 3:197–200.
25. Severino M. Endocrinology, infertility, and genetics. *Gynecol Obstet* 1995; 5:2.
26. Sauer MV. Investigation of the female pelvis. *J Reprod Med* 1993; 38:270.
27. Mosher WD, Pratt WF. *Fecundity and infertility in the United States, 1965–1988. Advance data from vital and health statistics, no. 192.* Hyattsville, MD: National Center for Health Statistics, 1990.
28. Gill CJ. Cultivating common ground: women with disabilities. *Health/PAC Bull* 1992; 22:32–37.
29. Hakim-Elahi E. Contraception for the disabled. *Female Patient* 1991; 16:19–27.
30. Effect of different progestagens in low estrogen oral contraceptives on venous thromboembolic disease. World Health Organization. Collaborative study of cardiovascular disease and steroid hormone contraception. *Lancet* 1995; 346:1582–1588.
31. Speroff L, Glass RH, Kase NG. *Clinical gynecologic endocrinology and infertility, 5th ed.* Baltimore: Williams & Wilkins, 1994.
32. East Tennessee State University James H Quillen College of Medicine, Johnson City. Depo-Provera: an injectable contraceptive. *Am Fam Physician* 1994; 49:891–894, 897–898.
33. Datey S, Gaur LN, Saxena BN. Vaginal bleeding patterns of women using different contraceptive methods (implants, injectables, IUDs, oral pills). *Contraception* 1995; 51:155–165.
34. Mainwaring R, Hales HA, Stevenson K, et al. Metabolic parameter, bleeding, and weight changes in U.S. women using progestin only contraceptives. *Contraception* 1995;51:149–153.
35. Cundy T, Evans M, Roberts H, et al. Bone density in women receiving depot medroxyprogesterone acetate for contraception. *Br Med J* 1991; 303:13–16.
36. ACOG technical bulletin. The intrauterine device. *Int J Gynaecol Obstet* 1993; 41:189–193.
37. DisAbled Women's Network (DAWN). *I want to be a mother I have a disability: What are my choices?* Available from DAWN, Toronto, Ontario M4A 1Z3, 1993.
38. Pischke ME. Parenting with a disability. Special issue: reproductive issues for persons with physical disabilities. *Sexuality Dis* 1993; 11:3.
39. Asrael W. An approach to motherhood for disabled women. *Rehab Literature* 1982; 43:214–218.
40. Rudnik-Schoneborn S, Rohrig D, Nicholson G, Zerres K. Pregnancy and delivery in Charcot-Marie-Tooth disease type 1. *Neurology* 1993; 43:2011–2016.
41. Abramsky O. Pregnancy and multiple sclerosis. *Ann Neurol [Suppl]* 1994; 36:S38–S41.
42. Birk K, Ford C, Smeltzer S, et al. The clinical course of multiple sclerosis during pregnancy and the puerperium. *Arch Neurol* 1990; 47:738–742.
43. Carter GT, Bonekat HW, Milio L. Successful pregnancies in the presence of spinal muscular atrophy: two case reports. *Arch Phys Med Rehabil* 1994; 75:229–231.
44. Sadovnick AD, Eisen K, Hashimoto SA et al. Pregnancy and multiple sclerosis. A prospective study. *Arch Neurol* 1994; 51:1120–1124.
45. Asrael W. The rehabilitation team's role during the childbearing year for disabled women. *Sexuality Dis* 1987; 8:47–62.
46. Guthrie M. Bringing up baby: products for parents with disabilities. *Team Rehab Report* 1997; June:17–19.
47. Rogers J, Matsumura M. *Mother to be, a guide to pregnancy and birth for women with disabilities.* New York: Demos Publications, 1991.
48. Cohen BS, Hilton EB. Spinal cord disorders and pregnancy. In: Goldstein PJ, ed. *Neurological disorders of pregnancy.* Mt Kisco, NY: Futura, 1986; 139–152.
49. Baker ER, Cardenas DD. Pregnancy in spinal cord injured women. *Arch Phys Med Rehabil* 1996; 77:501–507.
50. Bradley WS, Walker WW, Searight MW. Pregnancy in paraplegia. A case report with urologic complication. *Obstet Gynecol* 1957; 10: 573–575.
51. Young BK, Katz M, Klein SA. Pregnancy after spinal cord injury: altered maternal and fetal response to labor. *Obstet Gynecol* 1983; 62:59–63.
52. Daw E. Pregnancy problems in a paraplegic patient with an ileal conduit bladder. *Practitioner* 1973; 211:781–784.
53. Craig DI. The adaptation to pregnancy of spinal cord injured women. *Rehabil Nurs* 1990; 15:6–9.
54. Wynn RM. *Obstetrics and gynecology: The clinical core.* Philadelphia: Lea & Febiger, 1983.
55. Abouleish E. Hypertension in a paraplegic parturient. *Anesthesiology* 1980; 3:348–349.
56. Gimovsky ML, Ojeda A, Ozaki R, Zerne S. Management of autonomic hyperreflexia associated with a low thoracic spinal cord lesion. *Am J Obstet Gynecol* 1985; 153:223–224.
57. Greenspoon JS, Paul RH. Paraplegia and quadriplegia: Special considerations during pregnancy and labor and delivery. *Am J Obstet Gynecol* 1986; 155:738–741.
58. Hardy AG, Warrell DW. Pregnancy and labour in complete tetraplegia. *Paraplegia.* 1965; 3:182–188.
59. Committee on Obstetrics. Maternal-fetal medicince. Management of labor and delivery for patients with spinal cord injury. *ACOG Comm Opin* 1993; 121:1–2.
60. McGregor JA, Meeuwsen J. Autonomic hyperreflexia: A mortal danger for spinal cord-damaged women in labor. *Am J Obstet Gynecol* 1985; 151:330–333.
61. Nath M, Vivian JM, Cherny WB. Autonomic hyperreflexia in pregnancy and labor: A case report. *Am J Obstet Gynecol* 1979; 134: 390–392.
62. Ohry A, Peleg D,Goldman J, David A, Rozin R. Sexual function, pregnancy and delivery in spinal cord injured women. *Gynecol Obstet Invest* 1978; 9:281–291.
63. Ravindran RS, Cummins DF, Smith IE. Experience with the use of nitroprusside and subsequent epidural analgesia in a pregnant quadriplegic patient. *Anesth Analg* 1981; 60:61–63.
64. Robertson DNS. Pregnancy and labour in the paraplegic. *Paraplegia* 1972; 10:209–212.
65. Robertson DNS, Guttmann I. The paraplegic patient in pregnancy and labour. *Proc R Soc Med* 1963; 561:381–387.
66. Saunders D, Yeo J. Pregnancy and quadriplegia—the problem of autonomic dysreflexia. *Aust NZ J Obstet Gynaecol* 1968; 8:152–154.
67. Stirt JA, Marco A, Conklin KA. Obstetric anesthesia for a quadriplegic patient with autonomic hyperreflexia. *Anesthesiology* 1979; 51: 560–562.
68. Verduyn WH. Spinal cord injured women, pregnancy and delivery. *Paraplegia* 1986; 24:231–240.
69. Wanner MB, Rageth CJ, Zach GA. Pregnancy and autonomic hyperre-

flexia in patients with spinal cord lesions. *Paraplegia* 1987; 25: 482–490.

70. Brooke MM, Dononvon WH, Stolov WC. Paraplegia: succinylcholine-induced hyperkalemia and cardiac arrest. *Arch Phys Med Rehabil* 1978; 59:306–308.
71. Schonwald G, Fish KJ, Perkash I. Cardiovascular complications during anesthesia in chronic spinal cord injured patients. *Anesthesiology* 1981; 55:550–558.
72. Snyder SW, Wheeler AS, James FM III. The use of nitroglycerin to control severe hypertension of pregnancy during cesarean section. *Anesthesiology* 1979; 51:563–564.
73. Tabsh KMA, Brinkman CR III, Reff RA. Autonomic dysreflexia in pregnancy. *Obstet Gynecol* 1982; 60:119–121.
74. Thorn-Alquist AM. Prevention of hypertensive crises in patients with high spinal lesions during cystoscopy and lithotripsy. *Acta Anaesth Scand [Suppl]* 1975; 57:79–82.
75. Letcher JC, Goldfine LJ. Management of a pregnant paraplegic patient in a rehabilitation center. *Arch Phys Med Rehabil* 1986; 67:477–478.
76. Saxton M, ed. Special issue: Women with disabilities: Reproduction and motherhood. *Sexuality Dis* 1994; 12.
77. Garee B, ed. *Parenting: Tips from parents (who happen to have a disability) on raising children. An accent guide.* Bloomington, IL: Cheever, 1989.
78. Westgren N, Levi R. Motherhood after traumatic spinal cord injury. *Paraplegia* 1994; 32:517–523.
79. Campion MJ, ed. Who's carrying the baby? *Dis Pregnancy Parent Int* 1993; 3.
80. Freda M, Cioschi HM, Nilson C. Childbearing issues for women with physical disabilities. *Am Occup Ther Assoc* 1989; 12:1–4.
81. Stewart C. Raising children from a wheelchair. *Am Occup Ther Assoc Spec Int Sect Newslett* 1989; 12:5–8.
82. Culler KH, Jasch C, Scanlon S. Childcare and parenting issues for the young stroke survivor. *Top Stroke Rehabil* 1994; 1:48–64.
83. Hughes HE, ed. *The creative woman, swimming upstream: Managing disabilities.* University Park, IL: Governors State University, 1991.
84. Finger A. *Past due: a story of disability, pregnancy and birth.* Seattle: Seal Press, 1990.
85. Beck V, Beck K. Who'll teach Michael to play baseball? *Spinal Network Extra* 1991; Spring:26–28.
86. Buck FM, Hohmann GW. Parental disability and children's adjustment. *Annu Rev Rehabil* 1983; 3:203–241.
87. Crown-Fletcher J. *Mama zooms.* New York: Scholastic, 1993.
88. Delhaas EM, Verhagen J. Pregnancy in a quadriplegic patient treated with continuous intrathecal baclofen infusion to manage her severe spasticity. Case report. *Paraplegia* 1992; 30:527–528.
89. Welner SL. Compassion and comprehension key to care of the disabled woman. *Focus* 1992; 5:1–6.
90. Ferreyra S, Hughes K. *Table manners: A guide to the pelvic examination for disabled women and health care providers.* San Francisco: Planned Parenthood Alameda/San Francisco, 1984.

90a. Waller L, Reader G, Etingen O, et al, eds. *Textbook of women's health—caring for the woman with a disability.* Boston: Little, Brown, 1998.

91. Colachis SC III. Autonomic hyperreflexia with spinal cord injury. *J Am Paraplegia Soc* 1992; 15:171–186.
92. *National Cancer Institute fact book.* Bethesda: National Cancer Institute, 1992.
93. American College of Obstetrics and Gynecology. *Committee opinion 140, Role of ob-gyns in diagnosis and treatment of breast disease.* Washington, D.C.: ACOG, June 1994.
94. American College of Obstetrics and Gynecology. *Publication AP26: Detecting and treatment of breast disease.* Washington, D.C.: ACOG, March 1993.
95. Prout MN. *Breast cancer: epidemiology, screening, and prevention. The medical care of women.* Philadelphia: WB Saunders, 1995.
96. Prout MN. Breast cancer: epidemiology, screening, and prevention. In Carr EP, Freund S, Somani S, eds. *The medical care of women.* Philadelphia: WB Saunders 1995; 153–160.
97. Coney P, Cefalo RC. *Menopause: Acceptance and understanding of its impact. Women's primary health care—office practice and procedures.* New York: McGraw-Hill, 1995.
98. Grinsted L, Heltberg A, Hagen C, Djursing H. Serum sex hormone and gonadotropin concentrations in premenopausal women with multiple sclerosis. *Intern Med* 1989; 226:241–244.
99. Hoek A, Van Kasteren Y, De Haan-Meulman M, Schoemaker J, Drexhage HA. Dysfunction of monocytes and dendritic cells in patients with premature ovarian failure. *Am J Reprod Immunol* 1993; 30: 207–217.
100. Schwartz J, Freeman R, Frishman W. Clinical pharmacology of estrogens: cardiovascular actions and cardioprotective benefits of replacement therapy in postmenopausal women. *J Clin Pharmacol* 1995; 35: 314–319.
101. Smith R, Studd JWW. A pilot study of the effect upon multiple sclerosis of the menopause, hormone replacement therapy, and the menstrual cycle. *J R Soc Med* 1992; 85:612–613.
102. Elbadawi A. Functional anatomy of the organs of micturition. *Urol Clin North Am* 1996; 23:177–210.
103. Cardozo LD, Kelleher CJ. Sex hormones, the menopause and urinary problems. *Gynecol Endocrinol* 1995; 9:75–84.
104. Backstrom T. Symptoms related to the menopause and sex steroid treatments. *Ciba Found Symp* 1995; 191:171–180.
105. Varney NR, Syrop C, Kubu SC, Struchen M, Hahn S, Franzen K. Neuropsychologic dysfunction in women following leuprolide acetate induction of hypoestrogenism. *J Assist Reprod Genet* 1993; 10:53–57.
106. Vickers MR, Meade TW, Wilkes HC. Hormone replacement therapy and cardiovascular disease: the case for a randomized controlled trial. *Ciba Found Symp* 1995; 191:150–160.
107. Most W, Schot L, Ederveen A, Van der Wee-Pals L, Papapoulous S, Lowik C. *In vitro* and *ex vivo* evidence that estrogens suppress increased bone resorption induced by ovariectomy or PTH stimulation through an effect on osteoclastogenesis. *J Bone Miner Res* 1995; 10: 1523–1530.
108. Khaw KT. Women, hormones and blood pressure. *Can J Cardiol* 1996; 12(Suppl D):9D–12D.
109. Kroon UB, Silfverstolpe G, Tengborn L. The effects of transdermal estradiol and oral conjugated estrogens on haemostasis variables. *Thromb Hemostas* 1994; 71:420–423.
110. Vermylen J. Clinical trials of primary and secondary prevention of thrombosis and restenosis. *Thromb Hemostas* 1995; 74:377–381.
111. Bosze P. Should estrogen replacement therapy be applied in women with genital and breast cancer? *Orv Hetil* 1995; 136(8 Suppl 1): 465–472.
112. Griggs W. Sexuality. In: Martin N, Holt NB, Hick D, eds. *Comprehensive rehabilitation nursing.* New York: McGraw-Hill, 1980.
113. Aloni R, Schwartz J, Ring H. Sexual function in post-stroke female patients. *Sexuality Dis* 1994; 12:191–199.
114. Berard JJ. The sexuality of spinal cord injured women: physiology and pathophysiology. A review. *Paraplegia* 1989; 27:99–112.
115. Boldrini P, Basaglia N, Calanca MC. Sexual changes in hemiparetic patients. *Arch Phys Med Rehabil* 1991; 72:202–207.
116. Charlifue SW, Gerhart KA, Menter RR, Whiteneck GG, Manley MS. Sexual issues of women with spinal cord injuries. *Paraplegia* 1992; 30:192–199.
117. Donohue J, Gebhard P, eds. Special issue: The Kinsey/Indiana University report on sexuality and spinal cord injury. *Sexuality Dis* 1995; 13:7–85.
118. Finger WW. Prevention, assessment and treatment of sexual dysfunction following stroke. *Sexuality Dis* 1995; 11:39–56.
119. Freda M, Rubinsky H. Sexual function in the stroke survivor. *Phys Med Rehabil Clin North Am* 1991; 2:643–658.
120. Garden FH, Bontke CF, Hoffman M. Sexual functioning and Marital adjustment after traumatic brain injury. *J Head Trauma Rehabil* 1990; 5:52–55.
121. Geiger RC. Neurophysiology of female sexual response in spinal cord injury. *Sexuality Dis* 1979; 2(4):257–266.
122. Kettl P, Zarefoss S, Jacoby K, Garman C. Female sexuality after spinal cord injury. *Sexuality Dis* 1991; 9:287–295.
123. Kreuter M, Sullivan M, Siosteen A. Sexual adjustment and quality of relationships in spinal paraplegia: A controlled study. *Arch Phys Med Rehabil* 1996; 77:541–547.
124. Lundberg PO, Hulter B. Female sexual dysfunction in multiple sclerosis: A review. *Sexuality Dis* 1996; 14:65–72.
125. Monga TN, Lawson JS, Inglis J. Sexual dysfunction in stroke patients. *Arch Phys Med Rehabil* 1986; 67:19–22.
126. Monga TN. Sexuality post stroke. *Phys Med Rehabil State Art Rev* 1993; 7:225–236.
127. Sipski ML. Spinal cord injury: What is the effect on sexual response? *J Am Paraplegia Soc* 1991; 14:40–43.

128. Szasz G, Paty D, Maurice WL. Sexual dysfunction in multiple sclerosis. *Ann NY Acad Sci* 1984; 436:443–452.
129. Hulter BM, Lundberg PO. Sexual function in women with advanced multiple sclerosis. *J Neurol Neurosurg Psychiatry* 1995; 59:83–86.
130. Badeau D. Illness, disability and sex in aging. *Sexuality Dis* 1995; 13:219–237.
131. Anderson BL, Cyranowski JM. Women's sexuality: behaviors, responses, and individual differences. *J Consult Clin Psychol* 1995; 63: 891–906.
132. Cole SS, Cole TM. Sexuality, disability, and reproductive issues through the lifespan. *Sexuality Dis* 1993; 11:189–205.
133. Gregory MF. *Sexual adjustment: A guide for the spinal cord injured.* Bloomington, IL: Accent, 1986.
134. Holland NJ, Cavallo PF. Sexuality and multiple sclerosis. *Neurorehabilitation* 1993; 3:48–56.
135. Kroll K, Klein EL. *Enabling romance.* New York: Harmony Books, 1992.
136. Bullard DG, Knight SE, eds. *Sexuality and physical disability: Personal perspectives.* St Louis: CV Mosby, 1981.
137. Leyson JFJ, ed. *Sexual rehabilitation of the spinal cord injured patient.* Clifton, NJ: Humana Press, 1991.
138. O'Carroll RE, Woodrow J, Maroun F. Psychosexual and psychosocial sequelae of closed head injury. *Brain Injury* 1991; 5:303–313.
139. The Boston Women's Health Book Collective. *The new our bodies, ourselves.* New York: Touchstone, 1992.
140. Medlar TM. Sexual counseling and traumatic brain injury. *Sexuality Dis* 1993; 11:57–71.
141. McCormick GP, Riffer DJ, Thompson McDougall M. Coital positioning for stroke afflicted couples. *Rehabil Nurs* 1986; 11:17–19.
142. Perduta-Fulginiti PS. Sexual functioning of women with complete spinal cord injury: Nursing implications. *Sexuality Dis* 1992; 10: 115–118.
143. Price JR. Promoting sexual wellness in head-injured patients. *Rehabil Nurs* 1985; Nov/Dec:12–13.
144. Rousso H. Special considerations in counseling clients with cerebral palsy. *Sexuality Dis* 1993; 11:99–108.
145. Vermote R, Peuskens J. Sexual and micturition problems in multiple sclerosis patients: Psychological issues. *Sexuality Dis* 1996; 14: 73–82.
146. Hatzichristou DG. Preface to the special issue: management of voiding, bowel and sexual dysfunction in multiple sclerosis: towards a holistic approach. *Sexuality Dis* 1996; 14:3–6.
147. Finger WW, ed. Special issue: Sexual counseling for people with disabilities. *Sexuality Dis* 1993; 11:1.
148. Hanson EI, Brouse SH. Assessing sexual implication of functional impairments associated with chronic illness. *Jrnl of Sex Education and Therapy* 1983; 9:39–45.
149. Rousso H. Sexuality and a positive sense of self. In: Krotoski DM, Nosek MA, Turk MA, eds. *Women with physical disabilities: Achieving and maintaining health and well-being.* Baltimore: Paul H Brookes, 1996; 109–116.
150. Haseltine F, Cole S, Gray D, eds. *Reproductive issues for persons with physical disabilities.* Baltimore: Paul H Brookes, 1993.
151. Lemon MA. Sexual counseling and spinal cord injury. *Sexuality Dis* 1993; 11:73–97.
152. Mona LR, Gardos PS, Brown RC. Sexual self views of women with disabilities: The relationship among age-of-onset, nature of disability and sexual self-esteem. *Sexuality Dis* 1994; 12:261–277.
153. Gill CJ, Voss LA. *Inclusion beyond the classroom: Asking persons with disabilities about education.* Paper presented at the annual meeting of the Society for Disability Studies, Rockville, MD, June 1994.
154. Rousso H. Daughters with disabilities: defective women or minority women? In: Fine M, Asch A, eds. *Women with disabilities: Essays in psychology, culture, and politics.* Philadelphia: Temple University Press, 1988; 139–171.
155. Hannaford S. *Living outside inside.* Berkeley, CA: Canterbury Press, 1985.
156. Klein BS. We are who you are: Feminism and disability. *Ms* 1992; : 70–74.
157. Blumberg L. Public stripping. *Disability Rag* 1990; 11:18–20.
158. Saxton M, Howe F, eds. *With wings: An anthology of literature by and about women with disabilities.* New York: Feminist Press, 1987.
159. Task Force on Concerns of Physically Disabled Women. *Toward intimacy: Family Planning and sexuality concerns of physically disabled women.* New York: Human Sciences Press, 1978.
160. Paris MJ. Attitudes of medical students and health-care professionals toward people with disabilities. *Arch Phys Med Rehabil* 1993; 74: 818–825.
161. Westbrook MT, Adamson BJ. Gender differences in allied health students' knowledge of disabled women and men. *Women Health* 1989; 15:93–110.
162. Loyola University of Chicago. *Mothers with disabilities: An introduction to issues.* Chicago: Author, Video, 1992.
163. Kirshbaum M. Parents with physical disabilities and their babies. *Zero to Three* 1988; 8:8–15.
164. Brentan A. *The creative woman 1991: Acts of creativity, acts of love: mothering with disabilities.* University Park, IL: Governors State University, 1991.
165. Kirshbaum M. Mothers with physical disabilities. In: Kratoski DM, Nosek MA, Turk MA, eds. *Women with physical disabilities: Achieving and maintaining health and well-being.* Baltimore: Paul H Brookes, 1996; 125–133.
166. Graves WH. Future directions in research and training in reproductive issues for persons with physical disabilites. In: Haseltine FB, Cole SS, Gray DB, eds. *Reproductive issues for persons with disabilities.* Baltimore: Paul H Brookes, 1993; 333–338.
167. Thurman SK. *Children of handicapped parents: Research and clinical perspectives.* New York: Academic Press, 1985.
168. DeMoss A, Rogers J, Tuleja C, Kirshbaum M. Adaptive parenting equipment idea book I. Berkeley, CA: Through the Looking Glass, 1995.
169. Panko Reis J. Parenting with a disability: How different is it really? Resourceful Woman 1992; 1:1–4.
170. Gill CJ, Kirschner KL, Panko Reis J. Women with disabilities: Barriers and portals. In: Dan A, ed. *Reframing women's health.* San Francisco: Sage Publications, 1994; 257–266.
171. Gill CJ. A grieving mother shares her story. *Resourceful Woman.* 1992; 1:2.
172. DeAngelis T. Custody battles challenging for parents with disabilities. *APA Monitor* 1995; 26:39.
173. Cupolo A, Srong M, Barker LT, Haight S. *Meeting the needs of women with disabilities: A blueprint for change. Preliminary summary of key issues.* Berkeley, CA: Berkeley Planning Associates.
174. Starkloff C. The adoption option. In: Haseltine FH, Cole SS, Gray DB, eds. *Reproductive issues for persons with disabilities.* Baltimore: Paul H Brookes, 1993; 103–105.
175. Kirshbaum M. Family context and disability culture reframing: Through the looking glass. *Family Psychologist* 1994; 10:8–12.
176. Warshaw C. *Violence against women with disabilities: Responding to partner abuse, April 22–23, 1996, monograph of conference proceedings, "We've come a long way, but can we survive managed care?" Chicago, IL:* Rehabilitation Institute of Chicago, 1996; 39–42.
177. Sobsey D. *Violence and abuse in the lives of people with disabilities: The end of silence and acceptance?* Baltimore: Paul H Brookes, 1994.
178. Cole SS, ed. Special issue: Sexual exploitation of people with disabilities. *Sexuality Dis* 1991:9; 3:177–279.
179. McCabe MP, Cummins RA, Reid SB. An empirical study of the sexual abuse of people with intellectual disability. *Sexuality Dis* 1994; 12: 297–306.
180. Cole SS. Facing the challenges of sexual abuse in persons with disabilities. *Sexuality Dis* 1984–1986; 7:71–88.
181. Brick A. Addressing domestic violence against women with disabilities. *Resourceful Woman* 1995; 4:1–3.
182. Doucett J. *Violent acts against disabled women.* Toronto: Disabled Women's Network, 1986.
183. Sobsey D, Doe T. Patterns of sexual abuse and assault. *Sexuality Dis* 1991; 9:243–259.
184. Sobsey D. Research on sexual abuse: Are we asking the right questions? *Am Assoc Ment Retard Newslett* 1988; 1:2,8.
185. Nosek MA. Sexual abuse of women with disabilities. In: Krotoski DM, Nosek MA, Turk MA, eds. *Women with physical disabilities: Achieving and maintaining health and well-being.* Baltimore: Paul H Brookes, 1996; 153–173.
186. Cusitar L. Strengthening the links—stopping the violence. Toronto: DisAbled Women's Network (DAWN), 1989.
187. Murphy P. *Making the connections: Women, work and abuse.* Orlando, FL: Paul M Deutsch, 1993.

188. Bacon J. *Violence against women with disabilities: Practical considerations for health care professionals.* Toronto: DisAbled Women's Network (DAWN), 1994.
189. Angold A, Worthman CW. Puberty onset of gender differences in rates of depression: A developmental, epidemiologic and neuroendocrine perspective. J Affect Dis 1993; 29:145–158.
190. Rintala DH, Hart KA, Fuhrer MJ. Perceived stress in individuals with spinal cord injury. In: Krotoski DM, Nosek MA, Turk MA, eds. *Women with physical disabilities: Achieving and maintaining health and well-being.* Baltimore: Paul H Brookes, 1996.
191. Madusa S. *Research summary. SAFETY NET/WORK Community kit: From abuse to suicide prevention and women with disabilities.* Toronto: DisAbled Women's Network of Canada, 1996.
192. Osgood NJ, Eisenhandler SA. Gender and assisted and acquiescent suicide: A suicidologist's perspective. *Issues Law Med* 1994; 9: 361–374.
193. Reichley M. Women with disabilities resource centers. *Adv Phys Ther* 1995; May 8:8–10.
194. McKnight JL. Services are bad for people. *Organizing* 1991; Spring/Summer:41–44.

Rehabilitation Medicine: Principles and Practice, Third Edition,
edited by Joel A. DeLisa and Bruce M. Gans.
Lippincott–Raven Publishers, Philadelphia © 1998.

CHAPTER 68

Hand Rehabilitation[1]

Ann H. Schutt and Keith A. Bengtson

The purpose of hand rehabilitation is to maximize the residual function of a patient who has had surgery to, or an injury or disease of, the hand or upper extremity. Hand rehabilitation is a team effort. The hand physiatrist's role in the rehabilitation team is to evaluate the patient's condition and then prescribe and coordinate the physical therapy, occupational therapy, hand therapy, and psychosocial intervention. Specially trained physical therapists, occupational therapists, hand therapists, and orthotists can provide the physical measures required in hand therapy. The rehabilitation team also may include social workers, psychologists, vocational counselors, and the qualified rehabilitation counselors of an insurance company or an employer. These team members provide emotional, social, and vocational support to the patient (1). Good coordination of this team is essential for efficient and effective rehabilitation (2).

Most injuries to the upper extremity require hand therapy. These may include fractures, tendon injuries, crush injuries, and amputation. Patients with arthritis frequently need hand rehabilitation. Rehabilitation of the hand and upper extremity is essential after such surgical procedures as carpal tunnel release, arthroplasty, tendon transfer or repair, tumor excision, and reconstruction of congenital defects (1). Hand therapy also is essential to patients who have overuse syndromes and work-related injuries, such as epicondylitis, tendinitis, and myofascial pain syndromes (3). Therapy should begin shortly after completion of hand surgery and should be considered essential postsurgical care, even while the patient's limbs are in bulky dressings or casts (1). Hand rehabilitation also may be required for conditions such as congenital deformity, neuropathologic lesion, diabetic neuropathy, traumatic brachial plexopathy, primary myopathy, and muscular dystrophy (4).

[1] This chapter does not imply that Mayo Foundation endorses any of the products mentioned.

A.H. Schutt and K.A. Bengtson: Department of Physical Medicine and Rehabilitation, Mayo Medical Center, Rochester, Minnesota 55905.

EVALUATION OF THE HAND

Precise knowledge of the anatomy, kinesiology, and physiology of the muscles, tendons, nerves, and joints of the upper extremity is essential in evaluating the functional status of the upper extremity and hand. Measurements must be well defined and precisely executed in a standard manner so that they can be reproduced by other evaluators (5–12). If edema is present, a volumeter and specially devised measuring tapes are very helpful to determine the volume and circumference of the digits (5). Small rulers and small, specially adapted goniometers are used to measure the active and passive ranges of motion. More recently, computerized goniometers have been developed for measuring pinch, grip, and vibration.[2] Such instruments are very helpful in recording standard data (Fig. 68-1), although simpler tools can yield the same data without the added costs. It is important that the data gathered be recorded accurately. Special forms and graphs are available to record the patient's progress in such abilities as range of motion and grip strength. Patients should be reevaluated and measured at least weekly during initial treatment and more often if necessary.

Specific techniques are used to measure range of motion of the digits, digital flexion and extension lags, thumb flexion and extension reposition, palmar abduction and opposition, wrist flexion and extension, and forearm pronation and supination. Flexion and extension lags are composite measurements of digital range of motion. The flexion lag of the thumb is defined as the distance between the tip of the thumb and the base of the small finger in full opposition and flexion of the thumb. Flexion lags of the second through fifth digits are the distances between the fingertips and the distal palmar crease with the fingers in full flexion. Extension lags are distances between the thumb or fingernails and a line extending distally from the dorsum of the corresponding metacarpal

[2] Computerized goniometers are manufactured by Loredan Biomedical, Davis, CA; NK Biotechnical Engineering, Minneapolis, MN; BTE, Hanover, MD; and Cybex, Ronkonkoma, NY.

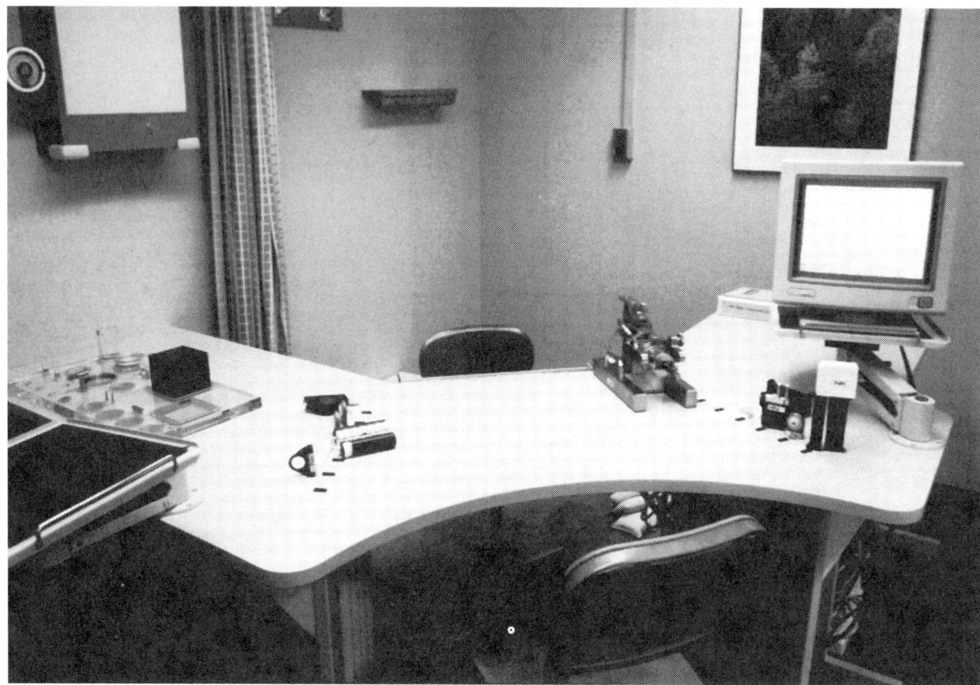

FIG. 68-1. An examining station is equipped with computerized goniometer (NK Biotechnical Engineering, Minneapolis, MN) for measuring pinch, grip, and vibration.

with the digit in full extension. In addition, range of motion of the shoulder (i.e., flexion, abduction, internal rotation, and external rotation) and elbow flexion and extension should be noted (5–11). Details of these measurements are given in Chapter 5. Strength is measured with a dynamometer. Measurements are taken for opposition (i.e., tip pinch), apposition (i.e., lateral pinch), and grip in several positions. Touch, moving touch, two-point discrimination, proprioception, temperature perception, and vibration are important sensations to measure (13,14). Nylon filaments of various diameters, two-point calipers, needles, tuning forks, vibrometers, test tubes of various temperatures, and objects of various sizes, shapes, and weights are used to test sensation and functional discrimination of the hand and upper extremity (15–20).

For preoperative carpal tunnel release and for postoperative follow-up, measurement of range of motion of the wrist and digits is essential. The strength of all muscles supplied by the median nerve should be tested manually and with a dynamometer. The Tinel sign should be noted at the wrist and forearm. The Phalen test is performed by holding the patient's wrists in a fully flexed position with the digits extended. The patient may perform this test alone by pressing the dorsum of one hand against that of the other. A carpal tunnel compression test is performed by applying firm but nonpainful pressure directly over the carpal tunnel. Phalen and carpal tunnel compression tests should be done for at least 60 seconds or until the patient's symptoms are reproduced. The time at which the patient first senses paresthesias should be noted. Two-point discrimination of the digits is also helpful. This is more sensitive than testing simple light touch or pinprick. However, it is thought to be less sensitive than more expensive and time-consuming tests such as vibrometry.

The most common complication following arthroplastic surgery is joint stiffness; therefore, the most important measurement after arthroplastic surgery is that of range of motion. These recordings should be followed serially as recovery and rehabilitation are taking place. Recording of grip and pinch strength is typically deferred for 3 months to allow the arthroplasty to heal sufficiently.

Each evaluation should include the anatomic, kinesiologic, and physiological evaluations necessary for appropriate diagnosis and formulation of a treatment plan. Kinesiologic and physiological evaluations are necessary to afford diagnosis, to allow formulation of the proper treatment plans and goals, to evaluate the outcome of the rehabilitation, and to allow change of the treatment goals and plans as rehabilitation progresses.

Many functional evaluations for upper extremity activities of daily living are available. Some of these are the Jebsen Hand Function Test, the Purdue Pegboard, the Minnesota Rate of Manipulation Test, the Crawford Small Parts Dexterity Test, and the Bennot Hand Tool (9,21–23). Standard vocational assessments applicable to the hand and upper extremity are used by occupational therapists and vocational rehabilitation counselors (10,24,25). Work simulators with various tool attachments, some of which are computerized, have been developed for testing in vocational evaluations, treatments, and work-hardening programs for the patient with an upper extremity impairment (24,26). Work-capacity evaluations simulate the patient's job requirements and measure capabilities and limitations related to return to work (27,28). For development of a workable treatment program, a thorough evaluation of the upper extremity and hand function is imperative (1). Observations are assessed during initial treatment and follow-up examinations. Serial evaluations are valuable in quantifying the outcome of hand therapy.

TREATMENT GOALS

Treatment goals should be prioritized to prevent frustration of the patient and rehabilitation team and to prevent the patient from being overwhelmed, reactions that may lead to ineffective therapy (1). Treatments and priorities should be updated frequently so that both the patient and the rehabilitation team will continue to understand the plan.

Specific goals for hand therapy may include the following (1):

- Prevent and decrease edema
- Assist in tissue healing
- Relieve pain
- Allow relaxation
- Prevent misuse, disuse, and overuse of the muscles
- Avoid joint jamming or injury
- Desensitize areas of hypersensitivity
- Reeducate sensation
- Redevelop motor and sensory functions

The first steps in treatment are to develop comfort, normal motor patterns, good posture, and comfortable functional residual capacities of the hand and upper extremity. Once these are accomplished, increasing the range of motion and redeveloping functional use of the extremity are critical. There must be acceptable motor patterns without muscle substitution, joint jamming, guarding, or overprotection of the extremity at this stage. Once light functional activities can be performed smoothly, consistently, and without discomfort, resistive strengthening exercises for the upper extremity may be introduced. Patients may resume work activities or work hardening once reconditioning, pain-free use, and coordinated motor patterns are established (1).

It is important to maintain and increase range of motion at the proper time, improve independence and endurance in daily functional activities, preserve mechanical alignment, and maintain strength. The hand and upper extremity must be protected from deforming forces, overuse, repetitive stresses, thermal injuries, and other injuries to which insensate hands and upper limbs are particularly susceptible.

Complications of the injury can be prevented by early evaluation and treatment. Some of the complications that can arise include:

- Edema
- Pain
- Loss of range of motion
- Loss of strength
- Adhesions
- Hypersensitivity
- Misuse, disuse, and overuse of the extremity

Overuse of the upper extremity during rehabilitation is harmful and counterproductive. If work hardening or endurance training is begun too quickly, complications such as increased pain and edema can ensue that will prolong the rehabilitation process. Work hardening and endurance training should not be undertaken until the patient is relatively free of pain when using the upper extremity (1).

EDEMA CONTROL

Edema often occurs after injury or surgical procedures, and its prevention and treatment are important components of effective hand rehabilitation. Chronic edema from reduced lymphatic and venous drainage is often caused by immobilization of the upper extremity and loss of the pumping action that moves lymph out of the hand (29–32). When a tourniquet used in surgery is released, the lymphatic channels, particularly in the dorsum of the hand, may be overwhelmed by the rapid return of circulation and by the results of secondary hyperemia (29,32–34). Postfracture edema often occurs after protective casting is removed. Edema that becomes chronic may cause fibrosis of the joints, muscles, fascial planes, vessels, and nerves, leading to stiffness. Chronic edema also promotes infection.

Initially, one may prevent postoperative edema by bulky dressings for gentle, even compression while the hand or extremity is splinted (35,36). The hand usually is splinted in a position of rest, with the wrist midway between pronation and supination and in 12° to 20° of wrist extension and the phalanges slightly flexed. In this position, there is good balance and control between the intrinsic and extrinsic muscles of the hand. The fingers are separated by layers of fluffy gauze. An exception to this positioning is to splint the hand in the intrinsic-plus position (i.e., the metacarpal joints in 90° of flexion and the proximal and distal interphalangeal joints in extension) to protect intrinsic muscle repairs. In instances of tendon transfer, tendon repair, or nerve repair, one may position the hand in a way that protects the tendon or nerve from traction at the site of anastomosis (37).

If postoperative edema is present, the extremity is usually elevated for 3 to 5 days. Elevation and early range of motion are effective preventive measures for edema control. In joints that can be moved, range of motion should be started as soon as possible after surgery, trauma, or fracture. Even the smallest movements of the muscle can assist in removing lymph from the hand and upper extremity. If possible, the extremity should be elevated with the elbow above the level of the shoulder and the hand above the level of the elbow. The elbow should be relatively extended if possible. This position allows two-thirds more circulation than if the elbow and upper extremity are held at the level of the waist (35,36).

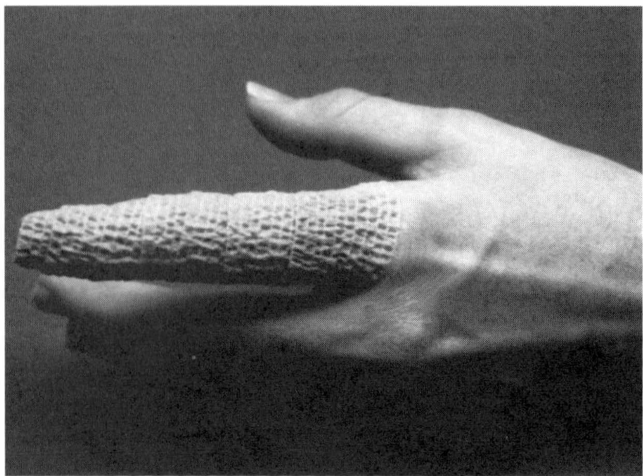

FIG. 68-2. Coban elastic wrap (3-M, Minneapolis, MN) around finger.

The patient should be instructed to keep the hand and upper extremity elevated whenever possible (10).

Decongestive massage is also helpful in the treatment of edema (38). The upper extremity is massaged in the distal-to-proximal direction to facilitate movement of the edema fluid. An elastic wrap, such as Coban (3-M, Minneapolis, MN; Figs. 68-2 and 68-3), Cowrap (Conco Medical, Bridgeport, CT), dental rubber dam, or a thick string finger wrap is wrapped around the fingers from distal to proximal (1,35,39). Elastic wraps or dressings also are helpful. These materials are inexpensive and effective for reducing edema. The wrapping is applied slowly, distally to proximally, in immediately adjacent loops that overlap at each turn by one-half the width of the wrap. The distal portion should be wrapped more tightly than the proximal portion to prevent a blockage in lymph flow. The wrap can be left in place for 5 to 15 minutes, depending on the circulation of the digits and the type of wrap used, and can be applied several times daily. Finger elastic dressings can be left on safely for 6 to 8 hours (39). Active range-of-motion exercises performed during and after wrapping of the hand help reduce swelling through the pumping action of active muscle contractions.

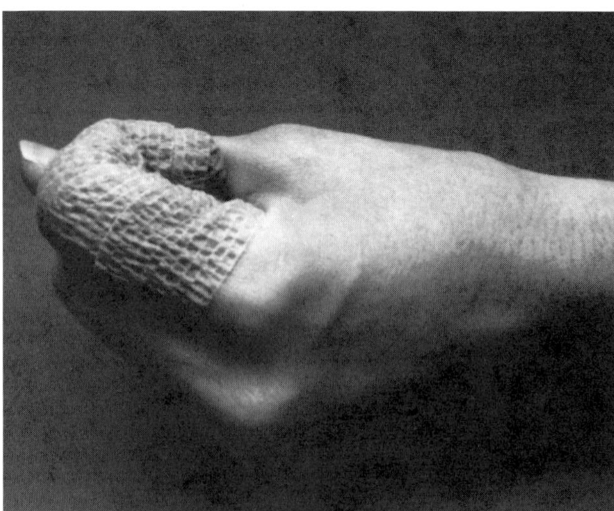

FIG. 68-3. Movement of finger with Coban wrap (3-M, Minneapolis, MN).

Elastic gloves, such as Aris-Isotoner (Aris Gloves, New York, NY), and elastic sleeves with graded pressure, distal to proximal, also help reduce edema (35). These garments are available from the Jobst Institute[3] or the Barton-Carey Company.[4] The elastic garments help reinforce the normal fluid dynamics of the upper extremity and can be worn during activities of daily living (1,30,32,35).

Intermittent pneumatic compression pumps are useful for edema caused by soft tissue injury or reflex sympathetic dystrophy, but they should be used only if the extremity is fairly pain-free (1,40). In dependent or chronic edema (e.g., postmastectomy lymphedema), elastic gloves and sleeves, and wrapping with rubber or elastic after pneumatic pumping, have proved helpful in maintaining edema reduction (35,41). Intermittent pneumatic compression devices can apply even pressure if the upper extremity or hand is placed in a plastic bag of polystyrene beads and then inserted into the pneumatic sleeve of the pump (1,35,41). The sleeve is intermittently inflated to about 50 mm Hg for 30 to 60 minutes at a time, as tolerated.

TISSUE HEALING

Direct pressure over scars can help to realign connective tissue and, therefore, soften scars and inhibit their formation. This can be accomplished by placing elastomer pads over scars and applying even pressure with an elastic glove or pressure garment. Hydrotherapy such as whirlpools or contrast baths may promote tissue healing. The whirlpool can be used to remove dried secretions and superficial necrotic debris and to clean open wounds. A moderate temperature (34° to 36°C) helps minimize formation of edema. Contrast baths are relaxing and cleansing, and they tend to cause less edema than whirlpools (1,42). Because dependency of the extremity in water may cause edema, it should be elevated during submersion if possible. Likewise, active motion assists in counteracting edema, as does minimizing the duration of hydrotherapy treatment. Careful manual debridement in the water, with special attention to blood vessels and nerves, promotes healing. Active motion during secondary healing is extremely important for optimal scar formation and function, particularly in burns, postoperative infections, and release of Dupuytren contracture (1).

PAIN MANAGEMENT

Pain is a common problem in hand rehabilitation. It can occur for short periods after surgery, in neuropathies and

[3] 635 Miami Street, Toledo, OH 43605.

[4] P.O. Box 421, Perrysburg, OH 43552; 1-800-421-0444 or 419-874-0555.

arthritis, and after injury. Pain can cause overprotection and motor pattern incoordination.

Many types of heat modalities are used to relieve pain, but it is important not to increase edema by inappropriate use of heat (43). Contrast baths can be performed in cycles of 10 minutes in warm water, 1 minute in cold water, 4 minutes in warm water, and 1 minute in cold water for about 30 minutes. The temperature of the water may be adjusted downward to prevent edema. Usually, the warm water is 43.7°C, and the cold water is 18.3°C. Occasionally, the temperature of the contrast baths can be modified to 40.6°C for the warm water and up to 21°C for the cold. Raynaud phenomenon may be precipitated by a lower temperature; therefore, lower-temperature water baths are not recommended for patients with this problem (44). Whirlpool baths at a temperature of 35° to 37°C (i.e., skin temperature) can prevent or minimize the formation of edema while relieving pain.

Thermal therapies, such as radiant heat, hot packs, ultrasound, paraffin, and fluidotherapy, have been used to decrease pain and promote relaxation before massage (45,46). Whenever possible, it is helpful to have the extremity elevated during heat therapy. The tissue temperature of the hand is increased most effectively by paraffin or fluidotherapy (45). Again, in many cases heat can promote edema and is therefore contraindicated. Ice massage or cooling methods can be used for acute strains or sprains and for relief of pain.

Transcutaneous electrical stimulation before or during active exercise should be considered for prevention of pain. This treatment is especially helpful in patients with pain and hypersensitivity (47–50) or with sympathetically mediated pain (51,52). Relief of pain by transcutaneous electrical nerve stimulation depends on the shape, duration, and frequency of the pulse wave (48).

MUSCLE REEDUCATION

Abnormal motor patterns can interfere with and limit range of motion. Therefore, voluntary, acceptable motor patterns must be established. Sister Elizabeth Kenny described the classic methods of muscle reeducation for the treatment of poliomyelitis (53). These techniques often are employed before beginning therapy to establish range of motion. Proper motor skills must be redeveloped before therapeutic exercise can begin. Neuromuscular reeducation allows the patient to perform therapeutic exercises in an acceptable manner. The patient must be aware of the desired action of the muscle, feel the muscle or tendon or both, and concentrate on using this muscle for the desired motion (1). The patient often can be helped in this training by observing movement and muscle action in the contralateral hand (1).

Proprioceptive feedback often is used to train and enhance motor control. The patient applies slight pressure with the contralateral (i.e., uninvolved) hand along the muscle or tendon to learn proper muscle control. In training for active movement, auditory or visual feedback from a contracting muscle also may be used for instruction in active, prolonged stretching. Relaxation muscle reeducation and biofeedback techniques are very helpful, particularly if abnormal motor contraction, voluntary or involuntary, and poor relaxation of the muscle are present. These techniques are learned not only for using but also for relaxing the muscle. Gentle bipolar electrical stimulation of the prime movers also may help in reeducation of the muscle. Electrical stimulation and electromyographic biofeedback enhance awareness of muscular action (1).

It is extremely important for patient, therapist, and physician to be aware of and try to prevent misuse, disuse, overuse, and abnormal jamming of the affected muscles and the other muscles of the extremity. With muscle reeducation, abnormal use of the muscles of the extremity can be prevented. "Misuse" is a term that describes an abnormal motor pattern, such as substitution, inappropriate cocontraction, or guarding. Abnormal motor patterns imply dysfunctional use of stabilizing or antagonistic muscle groups, or both. There can be a lack of spontaneous relaxation and coordination after a task is completed and a protective quivering, shaking, trembling, guarding, or tightening of the muscles or parts of the extremity during the motion. Misuse leads to tension myalgia, myofascial pain syndromes, muscle attachment pains, unnecessary compression or jamming of the joints, and unnecessary traction of the soft tissues during motion. The result can be pain and swelling in the joints, pain at the attachment of the muscles, and swelling within the muscles, which then become fatigued and painful. Misuse makes range-of-motion exercises or use of the muscle irritating, inefficient, and extremely painful. Compulsive people who practice exercise despite persistent misuse are prone to the development of increasing pain syndromes (1).

Insufficient use of the extremity can result in disuse of the muscles. This leads to atrophy of the tissues and inefficient muscular performance. Functional hand activities in a supervised treatment plan can avoid muscle disuse. The muscles must be used in a proper, smooth, functional pattern. Early incorporation of proper functional hand activities and activities of daily living in use of the involved extremity can help prevent muscle disuse (1). Increasing use of the hand within a comfortable and safe limit is helpful. Observing the extremity during activities of daily living can determine the patient's muscle habit patterns, which can then be modified (1).

In overuse of muscles, excessive activity is too fast or too forceful (11,54). Overuse often is associated with misuse. Intensive misuse, swelling, pain, hypersensitivity, guarding, limited range of motion, and, eventually, severe deconditioning of the extremity can occur when patients overuse muscles. These effects also occur with repetitive activities or during attempts to return to normal preinjury levels too quickly (1).

Careful monitoring and guidance in progressing from light to moderate to heavy activities are important in hand rehabilitation. To maintain motion without damaging the joints, they should be moved through a full, pain-free range of motion. It is important to differentiate general discomfort, as in a patient with arthritic joints, from the pain caused by overuse of a joint or muscle. The activity should be adjusted so that the level or method of performing a task avoids excessive pain. Pain lasting longer than 12 to 24 hours after activity indicates that the particular activity is too stressful. Arthritic joints and joints that have been operated on are more likely to be damaged when they are painful and swollen. The patient should avoid using the hand in ways that increase the potential for deformities. Tight fists, tight pinching of objects, pushing the fingers toward the little finger, or power gripping may accelerate ulnar deviation of the fingers. Motion of the fingers should be in the direction of the thumb whenever possible to avoid ulnar drifting of the digits. For holding objects, an open hand is preferable to a pinch grip. When a person pushes up on the edge of a table or arms of a chair, the forearms and palms are preferred to the fingers.

The level of coordination achieved by the injured or rehabilitated extremity should determine the speed of use of the muscles. Adequate time must be allowed to teach intermittent relaxation and proper use of the extremity before the patient can be allowed to return to preinjury levels of activity. It is extremely important that the extremity be kept relaxed when not in use. Static splinting can be used at night, and part-time during the day, to promote rest and relaxation of the extremity. If there is extreme overuse of the extremity, static splinting often is helpful for total rest. Once the overused muscles are no longer painful with range of motion, neuromuscular reeducation and strengthening can begin.

RANGE OF MOTION

Hand trauma, arthritic conditions, neuropathies, operations, and severe repetitive overuse of muscles frequently result in loss of range of motion (ROM) (55). Early rehabilitation of the hand is imperative. Edema interferes with mechanical function of the fingers, joints, and muscles of the hand and progresses to fibrosis (1). This, in turn, causes swelling and stiffness to persist and eventually become permanent. Immobilization of the joints results in capsular and ligamentous tightness, which causes loss of ROM. Bones and soft tissue structures that have been repaired require immobilization for healing. For any joint that does not require immobilization, however, ROM exercises should begin as soon as the involved structures can safely be moved (16,56,57).

In active-assistive ROM, the patient moves the part as far as possible before an external force completes the movement through the available range. These exercises are done without stretching. Active-assistive exercises imply that the patient can coordinate and produce muscle contraction through the available range. When the purpose is to increase the arc of motion, active-assistive or active ROM with prolonged stretch is used. This stretching and active force help mobilize adhesions of the tendon, particularly those adhesions proximal to the affected joint. Often, gentle and prolonged contraction of the muscle is the only force that can move the adherent tendon. Thus, active ROM can effectively mobilize and maintain the motion of the adherent tendons after stretching.

Gentle active-assistive ROM exercises should be done without forcing. Tightness and contractures may result from prolonged immobilization. Immobilization also decreases muscle power. Loss of muscle power or innervation of muscle can lead to reduced range of motion, tightness, and contractures. Shoulders can become stiff and painful when a hand or forearm is immobilized and the extremity is not used in a normal manner. Therefore, specific exercises are needed to help the patient maintain shoulder and elbow ROM even if the hand is immobilized (1). These exercises can be done with the patient in the supine, sitting, or standing position. The patient often is more comfortable in the supine position and can relax to avoid guarding, misuse, and overuse.

Active-assistive or passive-relaxed exercises are important for the shoulder in these cases. These exercises should be assisted until the patient can do the shoulder motions actively and correctly. Elbow, forearm, and wrist ROM exercises should be begun when appropriate according to the guidelines above. The surgeon must specify the degrees of permissible ROM on the basis of the operative procedure (58–60). It is important to know the goals to be achieved and the degrees of protection needed for the structures after surgery. The operative reports are essential in understanding and initiating hand rehabilitation. Tendon repairs, ligament or capsular repairs, and stability of joint fractures (61) should be clarified by the surgeon before hand rehabilitation is attempted.

Passive ROM is external force applied to produce motion. Passive ranging may be used after surgery in patients with paralysis, muscle weakness, or neurologic lesions. Continuous passive ROM machines, dynamic splinting, the therapist, and the patient's contralateral hand can be used to perform the required motion (61,62). With this technique, however, muscles must be fully relaxed to prevent harm and undesired force. Passive ROM is not stretching and must be done without muscle contraction. These exercises are done slowly to increase available range during full relaxation of the muscle. More aggressive short-arc ROM has been advocated for operations or injuries of the proximal interphalangeal joints (63).

Gentle and prolonged passive stretching by an external force can be prescribed. These stretches can be as short as 1 minute and as long as 20 minutes. Postoperatively, connective tissue needs about 6 weeks to regain adequate tensile strength, and stretching should be delayed until then. Gentle, prolonged stretch force is much more effective and safe than high deforming force for short periods. Repetitions with rest intervals can be increased as recovery progresses. The patient should tolerate these procedures without pain, swelling, or fatigue.

Finger trapping, web strapping, flexion gloves, and rubber

band strapping also afford prolonged passive stretching. Joint jacks, knuckle benders, and reverse knuckle benders, when used without compromising circulation or injuring the skin, can effectively stretch joint contractures and direct joint motion (1). The arc of motion must be in the proper plane. These devices, however, have to be fit properly and worn effectively to avoid soft tissue damage and increased pain. One must use the longest possible lever arms to prevent compromise of adjacent joint circulation (1).

Various continuous passive ROM devices are on the market.[5] The clinical use of these machines requires careful monitoring. When used properly, they are well tolerated and can aid healing of the cartilage, tendons, and ligaments and can prevent adhesions and joint stiffness without interfering with the healing process. Specific guidelines must be given for use of passive ROM machines, such as when and at what speed to use the machine and at what angle and force to move the joints. These machines can never take the place of active motion, which always is preferable. When newly healed tissues are stressed, however, the movement must be carefully controlled and repetitive. The fatigue of skeletal muscles during active movement and the lack of external control over active movement make passive motion a better choice in properly selected cases (28). The device must be carefully adjusted to ensure proper joint alignment and motion while avoiding the extremes of motion. Often, the patient becomes overly reliant on the devices to the exclusion of other important hand rehabilitation measures. In addition, cost is a factor, because the machines are expensive to rent, and the time needed to initiate treatment, to educate the patient, and to fit the extremity may be excessive. The final result, however, may be found to be cost-effective (28).

Joint mobilization techniques performed properly by the therapist can help to gain capsular motion and full joint movement. With proper technique, overstretching or injury to the joint capsule will not occur.

Friction massage can help improve ROM if the skin is tight over the area or scar tissue is present. This massage can soften scar tissue to allow better ROM. Lubriderm lotion, Eucerin cream, Alpha Keri lotion, white Vaseline Intensive Care lotion (Cheesebrough Ponds, Greenwich, CT), lanolin creams, Vanicream, or cocoa butter can be used during the massage. Elastomer pads, iodoform pads, elastic wrap, or elastic garments can be used to apply constant, firm pressure to help soften scars.

Once an injured worker is back at work, gradually increasing activities at the workplace can be helpful. Increasing work time by 1 hour every 2 to 3 weeks until the worker is able to tolerate a full day of work has been effective in assisting return to work. Activities and exercises for strengthening and endurance must not cause pain, but usual muscle discomfort is acceptable. No signs of overuse or muscle misuse should appear when activities are increased and strengthening exercises are done. Assistive devices may be prescribed and provided for the patient so that activities of daily living can be done or the ability to perform work can be improved. Techniques to train the nondominant hand to take over activities from the dominant hand have been helpful in patients with permanent disability of the dominant hand. Long-term follow-up, especially for the patient with severe injuries, is vital. When the patient is first injured, it often is not known what will be needed in the way of assistance during different stages of recovery.

[5] Danninger Medical, Columbus, OH; Richards Medical, Memphis, TN; Toronto Medical, Pickering, Ontario; Sutter, San Diego, CA.

HEAT MODALITIES

Whirlpool baths, contrast baths, hot packs, radiant heat, fluidotherapy, paraffin baths, and ultrasound heating before or during treatment may allow freer, more relaxed movements (42). Joint mobilization techniques in conjunction with heat modalities can be extremely useful in gaining capsular motion and full joint movement. Overstretching and injury to important capsular structures, however, should be avoided with this joint mobilization.

Ultrasound heating with passive and active gentle, prolonged stretching can be applied across restrictive parts to enhance the process (42,64). Ultrasound heating therapy can be applied under water, around restricted joints for adhesions of the skin, to deeper structures, and for adhesions between movable planes. Postoperative ultrasound treatment can be given once the stitches have been removed. It can be used approximately 6 weeks after arthroplasty, tendon repair, tendon transfer, or wound and fracture healing. Ultrasound wattage should be set to cause periosteal pain within 5 minutes of use. The sound head should be moving at all times to prevent overheating. Severe periosteal pain should be avoided. Periosteal discomfort indicates that the tissues being treated have reached a temperature of 45°C, at which soft tissues are more stretchable. The wattage can then be slightly reduced while the sound head continues to be moved. The prolonged stretching is continued for 5 to 10 minutes. Ultrasound treatment usually is given for only 5 minutes, and the prolonged stretch continues until the tissues are cool (42,64). Ultrasound heating and phonophoresis with 10% hydrocortisone in Aquasonic, Aquaphor, or plastibase can be helpful for tendinitis, epicondylitis, and myofascial pain syndromes. Iontophoresis can be used to infiltrate local areas with hydrocortisone or other drugs (65). Care must be taken, however, not to increase skin irritation under the iontophoretic area.

ORTHOTICS

The use of orthoses is an integral part of hand rehabilitation. Orthoses can be made for individual joints, for an entire region such as elbow–hand–wrist, or for portions of the upper extremity (66,67). Thermoplastic, metal, or light casting material is used for fabrication of the orthosis. Many prefabricated splints of plastic, thermoplastic, canvas, and elastic materials are available, but often they do not fit as well as custom-made orthoses (66,67).

The specific problems for which the orthosis is prescribed determine the duration of wear. If the orthosis is to be worn constantly, it should be fabricated to avoid damage to underlying parts, avoid pressure areas or insensate skin areas, and avoid compression of digital arteries and nerves (57,66,67). Precise fitting of any orthosis is necessary to avoid damage, as these devices often are worn constantly to protect healing tendons or fractures. The physiatrist should determine the schedule for wearing an orthosis. The orthosis should be tolerated well by the patient, and, as needed, the duration and frequency of wear may be decreased gradually.

An orthosis may be either static or dynamic. A static orthosis has no hinges, joints, or movement. The static orthosis is prescribed to support digits that recently have been surgically repaired, to prevent overstretching, to prevent contractures, to facilitate healing of soft tissue or fractures, to prevent movement, and to retain movement gained through mobilization techniques (37,66,67). The static orthosis may need to be serially adjusted when used to maintain increased achieved range of motion or to prevent deformities. Static orthoses provide rest in overuse syndromes and promote healing of fractures and soft-tissue injuries.

Static orthoses are prescribed for the following conditions:

- Posttraumatic tendon injury and repair
- Hyperesthetic or anesthetic fingers
- Swan neck deformities
- Boutonniere deformities
- Ulnar deviation deformities of the wrist
- Claw deformities of the hands from burns, scars, and nerve injuries
- Healing fractures

Static splints can be used to maintain a motion that has been achieved in range of motion. Often, a large C-bar splint holds the thumb in abduction and opposition to obtain web space between the thumb and the index finger and to allow for aid in pinching. Static wrist splints provide support and may be used in conjunction with splinting of the metacarpophalangeal and proximal phalangeal joints or to allow freedom of the fingers and thumb while the wrist is stabilized (68). Wrist splints with the wrist in neutral position and the palm cupped can be quite helpful in the conservative treatment of carpal tunnel syndrome and tendinitis of the wrist muscles at their insertions (66,67). Static splinting with the wrist in a position of function can be used to support a hand with paralysis or weakened wrist extensor muscles. Assistive devices for writing, eating, and other activities can be attached to the static splint.

After nerve repair and tendon repair, the extremity is splinted to prevent traction of the repaired nerves (55). The Kleinert type of splint, which looks like a shepherd's crook, is used after nerve and flexor tendon repairs of the wrist and hand. All splints must be well molded around bony prominences and padded as needed to prevent areas of pressure and sensitivity. For tendon repairs, hooks can be added to the fingers to hold rubber bands attached to the wrist for dynamic-passive flexion of the fingers and for static extension to promote tendon gliding without traction on the repaired flexor tendon (69,70). This splint protects the repaired median and ulnar nerves yet leaves the fingers free for massage, sensory stimulation, and observation. After digital flexor tendon repair, the Kleinert splint is often used in conjunction with the Durand method of tendon rehabilitation, which involves gentle passive range of motion of the digits by the therapist or patient with subsequent placement and holding of the digits in full flexion. This method allows tendon gliding while protecting the tendon repair (69–71).

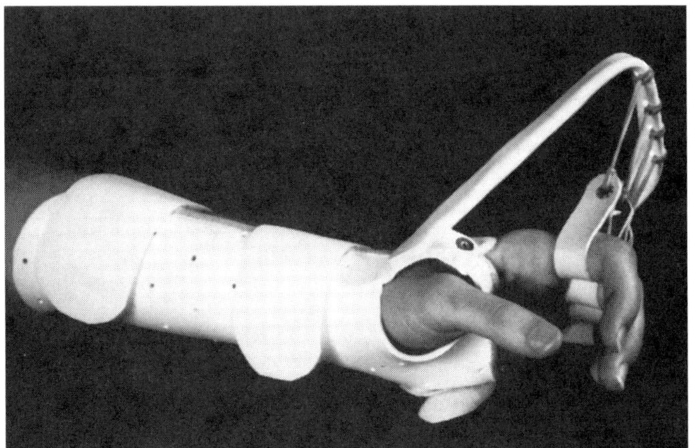

FIG. 68-4. High-profile dynamic orthosis (Johnson & Johnson, New Brunswick, NJ) for metacarpal extension.

When movement is desired but protection of the extremity is needed, dynamic orthoses are prescribed (Figs. 68-4 and 68-5) (37,66,67). Dynamic orthoses are made with hinges or external joints and have a source of power, such as rubber bands, electric motors, other muscles, springs, or compressed gas, to provide the movement. Dynamic orthoses are used to align, resist, assist, and simulate movement. The

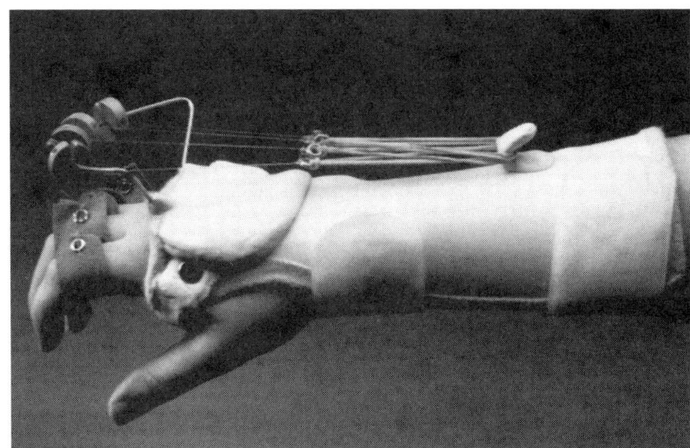

FIG. 68-5. Low-profile dynamic orthosis (Phoenix, Smith & Nephew Rolyan, Menomonee Falls, WI) for metacarpal extension.

dynamic power sources can provide a specific directional control yet allow for mobility of the joint and often substitute for weak or absent muscle power. They can be used to assist movement of the interphalangeal joints, metacarpophalangeal joints, and first metacarpophalangeal joint of the thumb when joint arthroplasty has been performed. While being protected, these joints may be assisted in flexion and extension by outrigger supports, hooks applied to the nails, rubber band sling devices, or springs with slings. These dynamic pulls should be gentle and not cause pain or swelling. Dynamic orthoses are made to assist wrist flexion and extension and elbow flexion, extension, pronation, and supination. They may be used to increase range of motion through the prolonged, gentle stretching that can be accomplished. The physiatrist should prescribe the duration of use of a dynamic orthosis, such as 30 minutes four times a day or 20 minutes with 5 minutes of rest during the waking hours.

In a dynamic orthosis, alignment is important, particularly in arthritic patients and in patients with tendon repairs and periarticular structures requiring protection. Dynamic orthoses can be used to resist abnormal or undesired movements. When protecting a newly repaired tendon from tension, the orthosis must allow gliding of the tendon or, after replacement arthroplasty, protect capsular structures.

Functional movement can be simulated in specially made dynamic orthoses that are activated by the patient's own muscles, as in the shoulder-operated hand orthosis, or by an external power source, as in myoelectric orthoses (37,66,67).

MUSCLE STRENGTHENING AND ENDURANCE

Muscle strength and endurance should be increased gradually. The patient must have nearly full range of motion and be relatively pain-free before beginning a strengthening program. Manual resistance exercises are important in early strengthening. The patient uses the contralateral hand as a resistive force and is able to monitor that force. Progressive resistive exercises (i.e., isotonic, isometric, and isokinetic) with gradually increasing weight and resistance by the unaffected extremity are helpful later (1). A hand helper, hand exerciser, various spring and weight devices, therapeutic putty, elastic strapping, and functional activities gradually increasing in difficulty also are used in a graded program of exercise (Fig. 68-6) (24,72). Devices such as the Cybex isokinetic machine and the Baltimore therapeutic exercise machine assist strengthening and endurance training (24,26,73).[6] Many of these machines are helpful in comparing the affected side with the nonaffected side and for providing permanent records.

Gradually increasing numbers of repetitions of the exercise increase endurance; likewise, slow increases in force can increase strength. The patient may do activities of daily

[6] Computerized goniometers are manufactured by Loredan Biomedical, Davis, CA; NK Biotechnical Engineering, Minneapolis, MN; BTE, Hanover, MD; and Cybex, Ronkonkoma, NY.

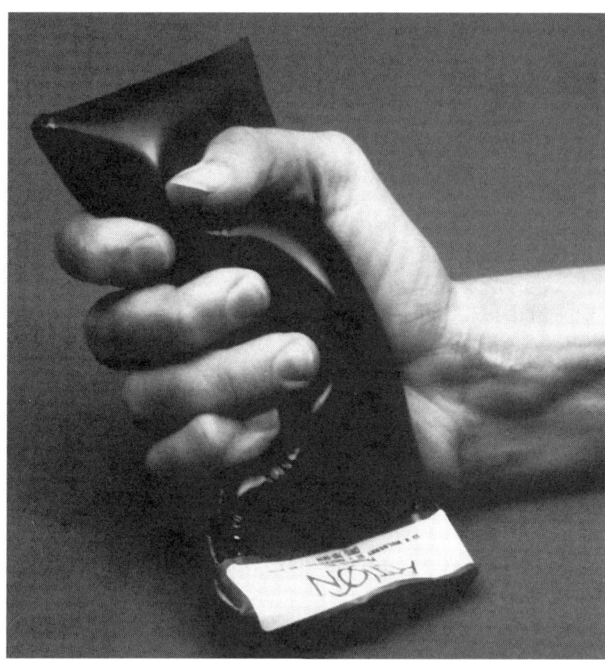

FIG. 68-6. Action hand exerciser (P Products, Hagerstown, MD).

living or special functional activities, gradually increasing the time spent on them; however, activity or exercise must not cause pain, unusual muscular discomfort, or signs of overuse. Assistive devices may be prescribed to improve the patient's performance of activities of daily living (1).

HAND PROTECTION

Conditions such as rheumatoid arthritis, psoriatic arthritis, systemic sclerosis, arteriosclerosis, carpal tunnel syndrome, degenerative joint disease, and overuse syndromes of the hands all require special care of the hands to prevent further damage or aggravation of the existing problem. The Arthritis Foundation provides instructional materials on joint protection and equipment for these conditions (45,74,75).[7] Special joint protection techniques, training, and practice in using the equipment are important.

A patient with scleroderma needs special care. The hands require lubrication with cream or oil to assist in retaining moisture, balance, and suppleness of the skin and to prevent drying, chapping, and cracking of the skin. These lotions, oils, and creams include cocoa butter, Lubriderm lotion, mineral oil, Alpha Keri, Vaseline (Cheesebrough Ponds, Greenwich, CT), Eucerin, and petroleum jelly (1). It is suggested that one of these lubricants be applied three or four times a day, especially after hand washing or exposure to sun, wind, and cold. The hands should be patted almost dry after washing and the lotion applied to slightly damp skin.

[7] National Arthritis Foundation, 3400 Peachtree Road Northeast, Atlanta, GA 30326.

Friction massage to the skin helps to maintain elasticity and reduce swelling and may be easier to perform after cream is applied. If dry skin, particularly on the hands, is a problem, the patient should wear loose white gloves and flannel pajamas to bed after applying the cream. For bathing, Basis soap (Beiersdorf, Norwalk, CT) or superfatty soap is suggested. The hands should be protected from cuts, scratches, and bruises; the cuticles should be cared for to prevent hangnails. They can be softened by applying cream or using a cotton swab soaked in cuticle remover. Sharp objects should not be used to push cuticles back. If a hangnail develops, it should be carefully cut, not pulled, off. The nails should be cut in a rounded shape to the tip of the fingers, with care being taken not to cut the skin during clipping and filing (1).

Patients with scleroderma often have Raynaud's disease and should protect their skin from cold by wearing insulated gloves or mittens. Mittens are preferred and should be down-filled or extra large and fur-lined and always worn in cold weather. Electrically warmed mittens and socks, available from hunting and athletic supply stores, are suggested for patients with scleroderma and severe Raynaud's disease of the extremities. Excessive heat and sunburn should be avoided. When handling frozed foods or removing items from the refrigerator, the patient should wear insulated mittens. Ice cubes should not be touched with bare hands, and cold water should not contact the skin. Drinking water should be tepid or at room temperature. The patient should use insulated cups when drinking hot or cold beverages. In cold weather, preheating the car before traveling helps to avoid acrocyanosis. Large fur- or pile-lined boots and warm socks made of wool should be worn. Tight shoes or boots should be avoided.

To protect the hands while washing dishes, the patient should wear large rubber gloves. These gloves insulate the hands from extremes of water temperature and help the patient avoid accidental cuts from sharp utensils. Nondetergent dishwashing soap, such as Ivory (Procter & Gamble, Cincinnati, OH), should be used. The patient should avoid bumping the arms, legs, hands, and feet against low furniture and counters. While handling hot foods, working around the stove, or ironing, the patient should take care to prevent burns to the skin. The patient should be cautioned about protecting the skin when working near hot motors. Small objects should not be tightly grasped, and the patient with scleroderma should avoid hand sewing, crochet hooks, knitting needles, and coarse yarns and threads. Extreme care should be taken not to stick the fingers with pins or needles. To avoid trauma to the fingertips, the patient should not type on a manual typewriter or play a piano or guitar (40).

Carpal tunnel syndrome results from compression and irritation of the median nerve at the wrist. A common tunnel at the wrist is shared by the median nerve and the nine extrinsic flexor tendons of the digits. Processes that decrease the tunnel space at the wrist may result in symptoms associated with median nerve compression. There are many ways to decrease stress and pressure within the carpal tunnel. The patient should avoid flexing and extending the wrist. A wrist splint may be used during sleep to prevent such flexion and extension (67). The wrist should be held in as much of a neutral position as possible. Because flattening the palm increases symptoms, the patient should keep the hand and palm in a cupped position whenever possible. Hard grasp should be avoided during scrubbing, driving, carrying, and holding. Prolonged gripping of an object, such as a steering wheel, paintbrush, pen, rake, newspaper, or book, should be avoided; the grip should be relaxed frequently when items are held. Pinching activities, such as needlework and writing, should be avoided, done only for short periods, or adapted to decrease stress. For writing, felt- or nylon-tipped pens can be substituted to increase the size of the object held. Repetitive activities should be avoided or performed in short periods. Relaxation of the hand for several minutes before repetitive activities are resumed can be helpful. The patient should avoid repetitive pounding actions, such as stapling, hammering, and keyboarding (1).

The joints affected by rheumatoid arthritis can not tolerate much stress. Pushing, pulling, and twisting activities can contribute to weakness, deformities, and joint pain. The patient with rheumatoid arthritis needs specific suggestions on joint protection techniques and equipment to help with daily activities. For maintaining range of motion without damaging joints, each joint should be moved through its full range of motion at least once a day. The patient with arthritis should avoid overuse of the joints and try to incorporate tasks of daily living into the exercise program. The joints are more likely to be damaged when they are painful or swollen. Tight fists or tight pinching of objects should be avoided. The motion of the digits should be in the direction of the thumb whenever possible. Built-up handles make it easier to grasp objects. The proper height for work surfaces when the patient is sitting is 2 inches below the bent elbow. In the standing position, the work surface should be high enough to avoid stooping over (76).

The person with rheumatoid arthritis should avoid keeping the joints in the same position for prolonged periods. During writing, driving, or handwork, the grip should be released and the hands rested every 10 to 15 minutes. Rest and activities should be balanced during the day. Chores should be spread throughout the entire week. The work should be done at a steady, moderate pace without rushing. Rest is necessary before fatigue and joint and muscle soreness occur. Velcro can substitute for buttons, and large tabs on zippers are suggested. Extra time should be allowed for dressing, grooming, and bathing.

Work areas should be organized so that the items are easy to reach. Energy should be conserved, and the joints protected. Sponges used with an open hand and pressed out with the open hand are preferable to the wringing of dishcloths and washcloths. Larger or built-up pens, lever-arm door handles, and lightweight luggage carts with wheels are suggested. Electric appliances and tools such as food processors, blenders, knives, can openers, drills, power saws, and automatic door openers should be used when feasible. Single-lever faucets are recommended. The principle of joint protection should be applied to hobbies, leisure activities, and recreational activities. More infomation can be obtained from the national or local chapters of the Arthritis Foundation.[8]

HYPERSENSITIVITY

Heightened responses to painful or sensory stimulation often complicate neurologic problems or injuries. The responses and sensations may be bizarre. Hypersensitivity that occurs after nerve injury may precede sensory reeducation (14,22,25,77–81). After nerve injuries, various degrees of dysesthesia and hypersensitivity often occur. Early desensitization is important but is contraindicated if the patient has open wounds or infection in the affected area.

One technique of desensitization is massage applied alternately with smooth, coarse, and rough material. The material is rubbed gently over the area for 1 to 2 minutes, rubbed more vigorously for another 1 to 2 minutes, and rubbed softly again for a final 1 to 2 minutes. This massage, based on the concept of increasing the pain threshold of the nerve, can be repeated as often as necessary. Treatment begins with soft, less irritating material at the patient's level of tolerance (1). Force, duration, and frequency are increased, and more irritating material is added as desensitization occurs.

Sensation also can be decreased by light or heavy tapping over the area (82). Patients must not be bruised on the parts being desensitized. Use of mechanical vibrators or tappers for percussion 10 to 30 munites once or twice a day has been suggested. In another approach to desensitization, the hands are immersed in such material as soft Styrofoam balls, rice, beads, or popcorn. Any stimulus to desensitize the area should be repetitive and be performed constantly for 20 to 30 minutes two or three times a day. Desensitization is started in the least sensitive regions and progresses to the more hypersensitive areas. It is important that the patient remain relaxed at all times during the treatment.

Pain in the hypersensitive hand can be relieved by transcutaneous electrical stimulation, contrast baths, whirlpool baths, and fluidotherapy (50). Applying oil or cream helps retain moisture in the skin of the hypersensitive hand to prevent scaling and cracking. Massaging the cream or oil into the hand can assist in desensitization and simultaneously promote awareness and reeducation of the altered sensation patterns.

SENSORY REEDUCATION

Sensory reeducation is a technique used to develop conscious preception and proper interpretation of distorted or insufficient sensation (22,25,77–81). The goal of sensory reeducation is to teach the patient to distinguish the following:

- Pain (e.g., sharp, dull)
- Temperature (e.g., hot, cold)
- Shape (e.g., sphere, cube)
- Size (e.g., large, small)
- Length (e.g., long, short)
- Texture (e.g., rough, smooth)
- Consistency (e.g., hard, soft)
- Material (e.g., wood, cotton, nylon)
- Weight (e.g., heavy, light)

Sensory reeducation has several training prerequisites (18,25,77,79). The training area should be free of distraction, and the extremity should be free of pain. Adequate time should be allowed for treatment. The patient and therapist should have good rapport. Education of the patient is essential for treatment; the patient should understand the objectives of treatment and the requirements of participation in the training. In addition, the patient must be able to comprehend the instructions, participate actively in the program, and interpret the different sensations. Learning involved in sensory retraining requires perception, recognition, retention, and recall.

The patient is educated to prevent further injuries to areas of absent to decreased sensation. Injuries occur when actvities are done by rote. The patient should be warned to protect the insensate hand when holding a cigarette, grabbing a frying pan or cooking utensil, working near a hot stove or in a freezer, or working around a hot motor. The hand should not be placed in hot water and should be protected in cold weather. The patient should avoid removing toast from a toaster and touching or bumping a hot pan, stove, or popcorn popper. The insensate hand should not be placed over a steaming pot or a hot automobile motor.

Wynn Parry (83,84) with Salter (85) proposed a sensory reeducation program based on a pattern theory. The three main concepts are that the skin is innervated at random, and the patient must learn new patterns of sensation; the more skilled the patient and the more the limb is used, the more likely the patient is to maintain the improvement gained with training; and sensory exercises should begin after protective sensation is recovered, that is, when the patient can recognize pain and temperature.

In the first part of the program, the patient is given several wooden blocks of various shapes, sizes, and weights but is not allowed to see them; a box obstructs that patient's view (Fig. 68-7). The patient moves a block slowly around in the hand to sense the corners and different surfaces. If the object is not recognized within 60 seconds, the patient is told to look at the object and move it in the hand at the same time. In this way, the patient builds up a tactile visual image by relating what is felt with what is seen. The time intervals until recognition are noted for later comparison. As progress is made, the shapes are changed to avoid a training effect.

[8] National Arthritis Foundation, 3400 Peachtree Road Northeast, Atlanta, GA 30326.

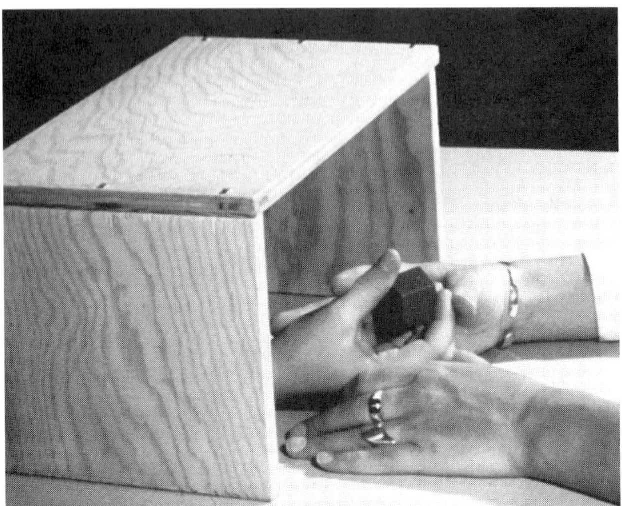

FIG. 68-7. Box occludes the patient's view while she identifies objects held in her hand.

Also in this technique, the examiner uses point localization by touching the hand and asking where the hand has been touched.

The second part of training involves recognition of textures. Again, times are recorded and textures are changed as recognition is mastered. For training in localization of touch, the patient is blindfolded, and the hand is touched in various places. The patient is asked to point to the spot touched. If not able to identify the spot within 60 seconds, the patient fails. The process is repeated with the blindfold off, and the patient begins to learn to localize the areas of the extremity.

The final stage of training requires recognition of everyday objects—from large (e.g., tennis ball, matchbox, peg) to small (e.g., paper clip, safety pin, key, match, domino). The patient slowly explores each object, assessing size, weight, density, texture, and temperature and assembling clues for identification. The affected hand does in slow motion what the normal hand does automatically and quickly. Training sessions are as short as 10 to 15 minutes and should be held several times a day.

Sensory retraining methods seen to be based not only on the pattern theory of sensation but also on the belief that most external stimuli require motor participation. If the median nerve is involved, a thick leather glove covering the portions of the fingers and palm innervated by the ulnar nerve allows the areas innervated by the injured median nerve to relearn the meaning of stimuli and not rely on the ulnar nerve.

External stimuli can be divided into two types: those passively impressed and those requiring active movement for sensation or discrimination. Passive stimuli, rarely encountered in normal life, include the sensation of wind blowing on the skin and the sensation of the ambient temperature. Active sensations are typically those of grasping and manipulating. After sensory retraining, the patient can achieve good sensory function despite a lack of two-point discrimination because movable sensation is often retained. This is the ability to discriminate between one and two points when they are stroked across the palm or digit. Sensory reeducation by the Dellon and Curtis program is based on neurophysiological division of large, myelinated sensory fibers (i.e., group A-beta fibers) into those that adapt quickly and those that adapt slowly to mechanical stimuli (13,14,25,77). This is the specificity theory of sensory reeducation. Quickly adapting fibers can in turn be subdivided into a group maximally responsive to 256 cycles/sec of vibration stimuli and a group maximally responsive to 30 cycles/sec. Slowly adapting fibers mediate the perception not only of vibration by also of moving touch. These investigators stated that the time to begin the reeducation program is determined by the pattern of recovery of sensation. The typical pattern of sensation recovery would be perception of pain (i.e., pinprick), 30 cycles/sec of vibration, moving touch, constant touch, and, finally, 256 cycles/sec of vibration.

During recovery, if a stimulus of 30 cycles/sec is perceived only in a proximal part of the hand, the patient should begin sensory exercises specific for moving touch in that area only. Exercises should be simple, repetitive, and manageable for the patient at home. In the early phase, when the patient can perceive 30 cycles/sec at the fingertips but not moving touch or constant touch, the patient is asked to touch any blunt object, such as another finger or a pencil, within the given area of the fingertips and to vary the pressure. The quickly adapting fibers are reeducated by moving the blunt object across that area. In the later phase, when the perception of constant or moving touch has been recovered, different shapes of nuts and bolts are used for the fingertip exercises.

For reeducation of constant touch, that patient is asked to discriminate between large and small nuts. As discrimination improves, smaller objects are used to increase the difficulty. For reeducation of moving touch, the patient is asked to discriminate between a square nut and a hexagonal one, each of which is rolled across that finger. The patient is asked first to make the distinction with eyes open, observing the stimulus, and then to close the eyes and concentrate on the stimulus involved (14,25,77).

Callahan (59) added to these exercises a program of sensory bombardment and the differentiation of objects from a background medium such as sand, rice, or beans. With special boxes or boards for sensory reeducation of the hands, the patient can screw nuts and bolts while vision is blocked. In addition, various black boxes and screens can obstruct vision while that patient attempts to use the hand to distinguish objects.

COORDINATION

Coordination is the ability to control movement correctly and readily. Coordination involves gross motor movements, such as moving the shoulder, elbow, wrist, and hand, and fine motor movements, such as moving the hand and fingers. Coordination exercises are used to improve upper limb function through gross and fine motor coordination activities. The key to improving coordination is proper performance of many repetitions of an appropriate activity. The movements should be smooth and relaxed. These activities should not be continued to the point of fatigue or pain. If the speed and accuracy of the motion decrease, the exercises should be discontinued. When performing coordination exercises, the patient should rest frequently to relax the joints and the muscles. The coordination exercises should begin at a tolerable level and then be increased as the difficulty of the coordination tasks increases (59,72). The coordination exercises may be enhanced by increasing the speed, changing the size of the objects used, or incorporating tools into the activities. Coordination exercises and activities should not be performed if the quality of the motion is compromised. Coordination can be improved only with practice.

Gross motor coordination exercises often are begun first. Examples of these are raising the arms over the head and then down to a resting position, throwing a ball, washing a wall or window, picking up and placing objects on a shelf, and folding clothes. Examples of fine motor coordination exercises are touching the fingertips, picking up different-sized objects and placing them in a container, and tying knots. Manipulating coins in the hand, opening and closing safety pins, and using a typewriter also can increase coordination, particularly if speed and accuracy are gradually increased. Woodworking, needlework, and knitting, when performed in relatively short periods, can increase coordination. The use of tools such as screwdrivers, hammers, and wrenches also can increase coordination (59,73).

OVERUSE SYNDROME

Overuse syndrome is a term applied when pain develops because of muscle overuse or abuse. This condition should not be confused with one that represents a specific tendinitis, tensynovitis, or nerve entrapment syndrome. Pain frequently develops in muscles used for long periods without adequate rest. Pain may intensify muscle tightness and cause swelling at the tendinous insertion onto bone, at the tendinous attachments to muscle, or in the muscles themselves. It is important to try frequent rest periods to relax muscles during the day. Relaxation of the shoulder and neck muscles allows the arms to relax and dangle. Work positions should be changed frequently, and work surfaces and positions may have to be adapted or changed. Equipment may be needed to modify the way a person grasps or uses the extremity in a work situation (86).

If the overuse syndrome is severe, the patient may need to resume activities only for short periods with frequent breaks for relaxation. Once the symptoms have subsided, a gradual general conditioning program and strengthening program may be helpful (73). Often, the affected area of overuse requires splinting for rest or special devices to decrease the swelling or the pull on the tendon. Rubber tubing or elastic sleeves can be used to decrease the swelling in the muscle. Strapping may be necessary to decrease the tension on the tendon or epicondylar areas while healing takes place.

Adaptations for the work environment may be necessary to prevent further overuse or cumulative trauma. Vocational specialists may be quite helpful in adapting and changing the place of employment to allow better ergonomic positioning of upper limbs. The adaptations to the work area help promote good posture and proper positioning of the limbs to reduce or eliminate neck, shoulder, and upper limb discomfort and stress. Good body posture is important at all times. Excessive reaching, excessive vibration without protection, excessive pinching, and tight grip should be avoided. Excessive bending of the wrist into ulnar or radial deviation can lead to overuse. Relaxation exercises should be performed regularly. Prolonged and repetitive bending of the wrist and frequent continuous stretching and grip shoud be avoided. Hand tools and gloves should be of the proper size at work. Frequent short breaks are helpful. Relaxation exercises in short periods of time can ease stress and fatigue.

Regular physical examinations, updating of the home exercise program, and practicing updated home programs before dismissal from therapy are essential.

AFTER RECONSTRUCTIVE SURGERY

After operative reconstruction of the hand, there may be skeletal, neurovascular, and soft-tissue problems. These may include amputation, crushes, lacerations, or avulsions. The challenge of hand rehabilitation is to obtain an acceptable esthetic and functional extremity through coordinated treatment of the various systems and tissues that are injured. The time to begin treatment varies among the tissue types. There are stages of healing, with different therapeutic goals for each stage. The inflammatory phase lasts about 2 days, and hand rehabilitation is directed toward minimizing pain and edema and promoting healing without complications (28). The fibroplastic or collagen deposition phase extends from about 3 days to 3 weeks after reconstruction. The tensile strength of the wound is very low, and excessive tension can rupture the fragile tissues. Treatment goals are to minimize edema, avoid undue stress, and prevent inflammatory responses. Depending on the type of operation or injury, controlled stress can be initiated to decrease edema and increase or maintain joint and soft tissue mobility. The scar maturation or remodeling phase spans about 3 weeks to 6 to 9 weeks, although the process may continue through 1 year. Therapy goals in this phase are mobility of the scar, soft tissues, and joints and advancement to strengthening, dexterity, and functional use (28).

Skin wounds heal quickly, and sutures can be removed in 7 to 10 days. Grafts and flaps need more protection, with the type of coverage and the size of the graft or wound dictating the length of healing.

Scar adhesions between the skin or superficial tissue and

deep structures can severely limit motion. This is especially true on the dorsum of the hand. This area should be mobilized by gentle massage as soon as healing allows. Further injury may be prevented by proper wound care, edema control, positioning, and gentle pressure dressings (28).

Blood vessel repair requires at least 2 weeks of protection. Arterial and venous insufficiencies should be prevented. Bandages should not be constricting. Positioning of the extremity depends on the microsurgical procedures in instances of reimplantation, free flaps, or revascularization. Elevation may not be indicated in these cases, as it may stress the arterial anastomosis.

Nerve repair requires 3 to 4 weeks of protection from stresses that increase scar formation, such as direct compression on the nerve, positioning in excessive stretch, intermittent stretching, and compression by too-early mobilization of the part injured or operated on. Gentle mobilization after nerve healing avoids nerve stretch, and a desensitization program may forestall severe hypersensitivity. Sensory reeducation must be an integral part of the hand rehabilitation program after nerve repair (59).

A tendon repair or graft generally has sufficient tensile strength to withstand gentle active motion at 3 to 4 weeks and light resistance at 6 to 8 weeks postoperatively. Gentle passive motion is initiated within the first 2 to 3 days to prevent adhesions of the newly repaired tendon. These are general guidelines, and the vascularity of the tendon and the gliding ability of the tendon or surrounding scar will determine the specific timing of mobilization.

Hand fractures may be considered healed as early as 2 to 5 weeks. The type of fracture, fixation, and radiographic evidence of healing determine the course of treatment.

In reimplanted extremities, rigid skeletal stabilization allows therapy to begin early. The level of injury determines the bony fixation.

Patient education is essential. The patient should avoid extreme temperatures and restrictive clothing. An insensate hand should be kept within sight to prevent injury. Articular cartilage heals by fibrocartilage formation and tends to be less elastic. In ligament injuries, scar, by contraction, can limit motion of the joint, and the injured hand should not be immobilized for long periods of time with the ligaments in the shortened position.

ARTHROPLASTY

Flexible implant prostheses of the digits are used most commonly in arthroplasty. There have been experimental prostheses of hinged metal and plastic implants; press fitted, noncemented surface replacement of joints; and rigid, hinged, cemented prostheses. The usual indications are joint pain resulting from rheumatoid or degenerative arthritis or trauma. In addition, decreased range of motion can be an indication for joint arthroplasty. Two orthoses are fabricated about 3 to 7 days after arthroplasty. One is made for night wear, to prevent deformities and allow the joint to rest. In this resting splint, the wrist is placed in slight ulnar deviation of 15° of extension, avoiding supination. The metacarpophalangeal joint is in extension, and the interphalangeal joints are comfortably flexed with the thumb supported. Dividers or elastomer pads are placed in the splint to prevent ulnar deviation of the digits, particularly at the metacarpophalangeal joints. The second orthosis, a dynamic extension splint to hold the metacarpophalangeal joints, is fabricated for daytime wear.

In the first 3 to 4 weeks after arthroplasty, the digits are flexed and extended actively in the dynamic orthosis. From 4 to 6 weeks, the hand is exercised out of the splint. Each joint is moved separately by blocking of the other digital joints. Gentle resistive exercises and gentle stretching can begin approximately 2 months after arthroplasty. The rehabilitation techniques are highly individualized, depending on the type of arthroplasty, the surgical techniques, preferences of the surgeon, and the underlying impairment.

CONCLUSION

Rehabilitation of hand disabilities is time-consuming but, when accomplished correctly, quite rewarding. Delay in starting hand rehabilitation may result in slow and suboptimal recovery, often with permanent contractures or other impairments developing. Cooperation and communication among patient, hand surgeon, physiatrist, hand therapist, and other health care professionals must be fully developed and maintained in practice. These relationships lead to maximum benefit and recovery for the patient.

REFERENCES

1. Goodgold J. *Rehabilitation medicine.* St Louis: CV Mosby, 1988.
2. Wynn Parry CB. The Ruscoe Clarke Memorial Lecture, 1979: the management of traction lesions of the brachial plexus and peripheral nerve injuries of the upper limb: a study in teamwork. *Injury* 1980; 11: 265–285.
3. Grunert BK, Devine CA, Matloub HS, Sanger JR, Yousif NJ. Flashbacks after traumatic hand injuries: prognostic indicators. *J Hand Surg [Am]* 1988; 13:125–127.
4. Hardy MA, Moran CA, Merritt WH. Desensitization of the traumatized hand. *Virginia Med* 1982; 109:134–137.
5. Fess EE. Documentation: essential elements of an upper extremity assessment battery. In: Hunter JM, Schneider LH, Mackin EJ, Callahan AD, eds. *Rehabilitation of the hand: surgery and therapy.* St Louis: CV Mosby, 1990; 53–81.
6. Heck CV, Hendryson IE, Rowe CR. *Measuring and recording of joint motion.* Park Ridge, FL: Committee for the Study of Joint Motion, American Academy of Orthopedic Surgeons, 1965.
7. Jones JM, Schneck RR, Chesney RB. Digital replantation and amputation: comparison of function. *J Hand Surg [Am]* 1982; 7:183–189.
8. Kellor M, Frost J, Silberberg N, Iverson I, Cummings R. Hand strength and dexterity. *Am J Occup Ther* 1971; 25:77–83.
9. Kellor M, Krondrosuk R, Iverson I. *Technical manual: hand strength and dexterity test.* Minneapolis, MN: Kenny Rehabilitation Institute, Research Division, 1971.
10. Mathiowetz V, Kashman N, Volland G, Weber K, Dowe M, Rogers S. Grip and pinch strength: normative data for adults. *Arch Phys Med Rehabil* 1985; 66:69–74.
11. Opitz JL. Reconstructive surgery of the extremities. In: Kottke FJ, Stillwell GK, Lehmann JF, eds. *Krusen's handbook of physical medi-*

cine and rehabilitation, 3rd ed. Philadelphia: WB Saunders, 1982; 851–839.
12. Parkes A. Some thoughts on examination of the hand. *Hand* 1975; 7: 427–431.
13. Dellon AL. The moving two-point discrimination test: clinical evaluation of the quickly adapting fiber/receptor system. *J Hand Surg [Am]* 1978; 3:474–481.
14. Dellon AL. *Evaluation of sensibility and re-education of sensation in the hand.* Baltimore: Williams & Wilkins, 1981.
15. Dellon AL. The vibrometer. *Plast Reconstruct Surg* 1983; 71:427–431.
16. Edinburg M, Widgerow AD, Biddulph SL. Early postoperative mobilization of flexor tendon injuries using a modification of the Kleinert technique. *J Hand Surg [Am]* 1987; 12:34–38.
17. Frohring WO, Kohn PM, Bosma JF, Toomey JA. Changes in the vibratory sense of patients with poliomyelitis as measured by the pall esthesiometer. *Am J Dis Child* 1945; 69:89–91.
18. Frykman GK, Waylett J. Rehabilitation of peripheral nerve injuries. *Orthop Clin North Am* 1981; 12:361–379.
19. Markley JM Jr. The preservation of close two-point discriminination in the interdigital transfer of neurovascular island flaps. *Plast Reconstruct Surg* 1977; 59:812–816.
20. Terzis JK. Sensory mapping. *Clin Plast Surg* 1976; 3:59–64.
21. Jebsen RH, Taylor N, Trieschmann RB, Trotter MJ, Howard LA. An objective and standardized test of hand function. *Arch Phys Med Rehabil* 1969; 50:311–319.
22. Moberg E. Objective methods for determining the functional value of sensibility in the hand. *J Bone Joint Surg Br* 1958; 40-B:454–476.
23. Tiffin J, Asher EJ. The Purdue pegboard; norms and studies of reliability and validity. *J Psychol* 1948; 32:234–237.
24. Curtis RM, Engalitcheff J Jr. A work simulator for rehabilitating the upper extremity: preliminary report. *J Hand Surg [Am]* 1981; 6: 499–501.
25. Dellon AL, Curtis RM, Edgerton MT. Reeducation of sensation in the hand after nerve injury and repair. *Plast Reconstruct Surg* 1974; 53: 297–305.
26. Anderson PA, Chanoski CE, Devan DL, McMahon BL, Whelan EP. Normative study of grip and wrist flexion strength employing a BTE Work Simulator. *J Hand Surg [Am]* 1990; 15:420–425.
27. Ballard M, Baxter P, Brueling L, Fried S. Work therapy and return to work. *Hand Clin* 1986; 2:247–258.
28. Herbin ML. Work capacity evaluation for occupational hand injuries. *J Hand Surg [Am]* 1987; 12:958–961.
29. Casley-Smith JR. The structural basis for the conservative treatment of lymphedema. In: Closius L, ed. *Lymphedema.* Stuttgart: Georg Thieme Verlag, 1977; 13–25.
30. Foldi M. Physiology and pathophysioloy of lymph flow. In: Closius L, ed. *Lymphedema.* Stuttgart: Georg Thieme Verlag, 1977; 1–11.
31. Guyton AC, Granger HJ, Taylor AE. Interstitial fluid pressure. *Physiol Rev* 1971; 51:527–563.
32. Olszewski WL, Engeset A. Intrinsic contractility of prenodal lymph vessels and lymph flow in human leg. *Am J Physiol* 1980; 239: H775–H783.
33. Olszewski W. Pathophysiological and clinical observations of obstructive lymphedema of the limbs. In: Closius L, ed. *Lymphedema.* Stuttgart: Georg Thieme Verlag, 1977; 79–102.
34. Olszewski WL, Engeset A. Intrinsic contractility of leg lymphatics in man: preliminary communication. *Lymphology* 1979; 12:81–84.
35. Stillwell GK. Treatment of postmastectomy lymphedema. *Mod Treat* 1969; 6:396–412.
36. Stillwell GK. The Law of Laplace: some clinical applications. *Mayo Clin Proc* 1973; 48:863–869.
37. Long C, Schutt AH. Upper limbs orthotics. In: Redford JB, ed. *Orthotics etcetera, 3rd ed.* Baltimore: Williams & Wilkins, 1986; 198–277.
38. Knapp ME. Massage. In: Krusen FH, ed. *Handbook of physical medicine and rehabilitation, 2nd ed.* Philadelphia: WB Saunders, 1971; 382–384.
39. Flowers KR. String wrapping versus massage for reducing digital volume. *Phys Ther* 1988; 68:57–59.
40. Griffin JW, Newsome LS, Stralka SW, Wright PE. Reduction of chronic posttraumatic hand edema: a comparison of high voltage pulsed current, intermittent pneumatic compression, and placebo treatments. *Phys Ther* 1990; 70:279–286.
41. Tinkham RG, Stillwell GK. The role of pneumatic pumping devices in the treatment of postmastectomy lymphedema. *Arch Phys Med Reahbil* 1965; 46:193–197.
42. Stillwell GK. Therapeutic hot and cold. In: Krusen FH, ed. *Hnadbook of physical medicine and rehabilitation, 2nd ed.* Philadelphia: WB Saunders, 1971; 264.
43. Wynn Parry CB. *Rehabilitation of the hand, 4th ed.* London: Butterworth, 1981.
44. Delp HL, Newton RA. Effects of brief cold exposure on finger dexterity and sensibility in subjects with Rauynaud's phenomenon. *Phys Ther* 1986; 66:503–507.
45. Borrell RM, Henley EJ, Ho P, Hubbel MK. Fluidotherapy: evaluation of a new heat modality. *Arch Phys Med Rehabil* 1977; 58:69–71.
46. Borrell RM, Parker R, Henley EJ, Masley D, Repinecz M. Comparison of *in vivo* temperatures produced by hydrotherapy, paraffin wax treatment, and fluidotherapy. *Phys Ther* 1980; 60:1273–1276.
47. Fried T, Johnson R, McCracken W. Transcutaneous electrical nerve stimulation: its role in the control of chronic pain. *Arch Phys Med Rehabil* 1984; 65:228–231.
48. Mannheimer JS, Lampe GN. *Clinical transcutaneous electrical nerve stimulation.* Philadelphia: FA Davis, 1984.
49. Sensory rehabilitation of the hand (editorial). *Lancet* 1981; 1:135–136.
50. Thorsteinsson G, Stonnington HH, Stillwell GK, Elveback LR. Transcutaneous electrical stimulation: a double-blind trial of its efficacy for pain. *Arch Phys Med Rehabil* 1977; 58:8–13.
51. Lunter MH, Van Albada-Kuipers GA, Heggelman BGF. Reflex sympathetic dystrophy syndrome of one finger. *Clin Rheumatol* 1990; 9: 542–544.
52. Omer GE Jr, Thomas ST. The management of chronic pain syndromes in the upper extremity. *Clin Orthop* 1974; 104:37–45.
53. Knapp ME. The contribution of Sister Elizabeth Kenny to the treatment of poliomyelitis. *Arch Phys Med Rehabil* 1955; 36:510–517.
54. Opitz JL, Linschied RL. Hand function after metacarpophalangeal joint replacement in rheumatoid arthritis. *Arch Phys Med Rehabil* 1978; 59: 160–165.
55. Weeks PM, Wray RC. *Management of acute hand injuries: a biological approach, 2nd ed.* St Louis: CV Mosby, 1978.
56. Evans RB. Clinical application of controlled stress to the healing extensor tendon: a review of 112 cases. *Phys Ther* 1989; 69:1041–1049.
57. Knapp ME. Aftercare fractures. In: Krusen FH, ed. *Handbook of physical medicine and rehabilitation, 2nd ed.* Philadelphia: WB Saunders, 1971; 579–582.
58. Hung LK, Chan J, Tsang A, Leung PC. Early controlled active mobilization with dynamic spinting for treatment of extensor tendon injuries. *J Hand Surg [Am]* 1990; 15:251–257.
59. Callahan AD. Methods of compensation and reeducation for sensory dysfunction. In: Hunter JM, Mackin EJ, Callahan AD, eds. *Rehabilitation of the hand: surgery and therapy, 4th ed.* St Louis: CV Mosby, 1995; 701–714.
60. Jones RF. The rehabilitation of surgical patients with particular reference to traumatic upper limb disability. *Aust NZ J Surg* 1977; 47: 402–407.
61. Bunker TD, Potter B, Barton NJ. Continuous passive motion following flexor tendon repair. *J Hand Surg [Br]* 1989; 14:406–411.
62. Giudice ML. Effects of continuous passive motion and elevation on hand edema. *Am J Occup Ther* 1990; 44:914–921.
63. Evans RB. Early active short arc motion for the repaired central slip. *J Hand Surg [Am]* 1994; 19:991–997.
64. Lehmann JF. Diathermy. In: Krusen FH, ed. *Handbook of physical medicine and rehabilitation, 2nd ed.* Philadelphia: WB Saunders, 1971; 316–321.
65. Gangarosa LP, Park NH, Fond BC, Scott DF, Hill JM. Conductivity of drugs used for iontophoresis. *J Pharmacol Sci* 1978; 67:1439–1443.
66. Meier RH III, Danek JC, Friedmann LW, Leonard JA. *Prosthetics, orthotics, and assistive devices (syllabus), 2nd ed.* Chicago: American Academy of Physical Medicine and Rehabilitation, Self-Directed Medical Knowledge Program, 1984.
67. Schutt AH. Upper extremity and hand orthotics. *Phys Med Rehabil Clin North Am* 1992; 3:223–241.
68. Prokop LL. Upper extremity rehabilitation: conditioning and orthotics for the athlete and performing artist. *Hand Clin* 1990; 6:517–524.
69. Saldana MJ, Chow JA, Gerbino P II, Westerbeck P, Schacherer TG. Further experience in rehabilitation of zone II flexor tendon repair with dynamic traction splinting. *Plast Reconstruct Surg* 1991; 87:543–546.

70. Stewart KM. Review and comparison of current trends in the postoperative management of tendon repair. *Hand Clin* 1991; 7:447–460.
71. Dovelle S, Heeter PK. The Washington regimen: rehabilitation of the hand following flexor tendon injuries. *Phys Ther* 1989; 69:1034–1040.
72. Krusen FH. *Handbook of physical medicine and rehabilitation, 2nd ed.* Philadelphia: WB Saunders, 1971.
73. Schultz-Johnson K. Work hardening: a mandate for hand therapy. *Hand Clin* 1991; 7:597–610.
74. Bosarge J. Finger replant patient undergoing rehabilitation. *J Rehabil* 1976; 42(6):29–30.
75. Mayo Clinic Occupational Therapy Department. *Joint protection for the arthritic person.* Rochester MN: Mayo Foundation, 1985.
76. Bengston KA, Schutt AH. Rehabilitation of the rheumatoid hand. *Phys Med Rehabil Clin North Am* 1994; 5:729–745.
77. Dellon AL, Jabaley ME. Reeducation of sensation in the hand following nerve suture. *Clin Orthop* 1982; 163:75–79.
78. Dykes RW, Terzis JK. Reinnervation of glabrous skin in baboons: properties of cutaneous mechanoreceptors subsequent to nerve crush. *J Neurophysiol* 1979; 42:1461–1478.
79. Gelberman RH, Urbaniak JR, Bright DS, Levin LS. Digital sensibility following replantation. *J Hand Surg [Am]* 1978; 3:313–319.
80. McQuillen MP. Practical approaches to managing peripheral neuropathies. *Geriatrics* 1975; 30:109–116.
81. Yerxa EJ, Barber LM, Diaz O, Black W, Azen SP. Development of a hand sensitivity test for the hypersensitive hand. *Am J Occup Ther* 1983; 37:176–181.
82. Russel WR. Percussion and vibration. In: Licht SH, ed. *Massage, manipulation and traction.* New Haven: E Licht, 1960; 113–121.
83. Wynn Parry CB. Sensory rehabilitation of the hand. *Aust NZ J Surg* 1980; 50:233–236.
84. Wynn Parry CB. Painful conditions of peripheral nerves. *Aust NZ J Surg* 1980; 50:233–236.
85. Wynn Parry CB, Salter M. Sensory re-education after median nerve lesions. *Hand* 1976; 8:250–257.
86. Lane C. Therapy for the occupationally injured hand. *Hand Clin* 1986; 2:593–602.

Rehabilitation Medicine: Principles and Practice, Third Edition,
edited by Joel A. DeLisa and Bruce M. Gans.
Lippincott–Raven Publishers, Philadelphia © 1998.

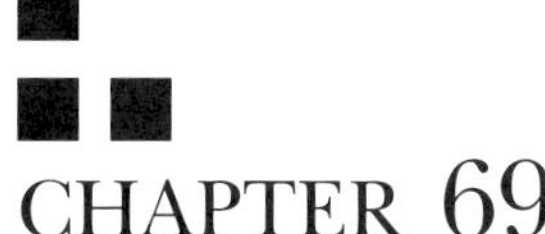

CHAPTER 69

Rehabilitation of the Patient with Visual Impairment

Stanley F. Wainapel and Marla Bernbaum

Visual impairment and blindness have been notably overlooked in the rehabilitation medicine literature (1,2), and only once previously has a chapter in a rehabilitation medicine textbook dealt with this topic (3). The relative neglect of vision rehabilitation by physiatrists is both surprising and unjustified in the context of historical associations and epidemiologic trends, both of which suggest the need for a greater degree of involvement.

THE HISTORICAL CONTEXT

World War II was a turning point in human history as well as a turning point in the development of both vision and medical rehabilitation. The extensive and severe casualties from battle occurred at a time when antibiotics and other medical and surgical techniques saved the lives of many soldiers who would otherwise have succumbed to their injuries. Society was then faced with a tremendous challenge as veterans with limb amputations, traumatic brain injuries, and traumatic spinal cord injuries attempted to take up their social roles as workers and family members. The response by the health care system was the creation of a multidisciplinary and functionally oriented approach that emphasized psychosocial and vocational goals compatible with the needs of these young and predominantly male veterans. Adding life to years rather than years to life (4) became the motto of the physicians who pioneered this approach, and by 1947 the American Board of Physical Medicine and Rehabilitation had been established.

At the same time and under the same circumstances, a large number of blinded veterans entered society with equally urgent needs for retraining and social reintegration. The response of the vision care system was the development of a multidisciplinary and functionally oriented approach that emphasized psychosocial and vocational goals. By 1948 the first civilian vision rehabilitation program had been established at the Veterans Administration Hospital in Hines, Illinois. That program was located within the Department of Rehabilitation Medicine (5).

The parallels between vision rehabilitation and medical rehabilitation are obvious from their shared roots, but the similarities go deeper. The professionals who comprise the rehabilitation team (physical therapist, occupational therapist, etc.) have their counterparts within the vision rehabilitation team, and physiatric areas of expertise such as orthotics and prosthetics have clear homologs for visually impaired patients (Table 69-1). There are notable differences between the two systems, however, and they explain why the systems have tended to diverge from their conjoint origins into parallel but distinct paths over the last 50 years. When vision loss is an isolated sensory deficit affecting a single organ and unassociated with other medical problems, the major focus tends to be on social and vocational issues rather than comprehensive medical management. When vision loss is part of multiple traumatic events or a part of a medical problem (e.g., diabetes mellitus), the approach needs to be comprehensive. Because vision loss is often the only problem, vision rehabilitation services have tended to be funded under social service and vocational sources, and the agencies providing vision rehabilitation have remained separate from the medical mainstream. To some extent this was not a problem when the patient was an otherwise healthy young person such as the blind veteran around whose needs the programs were developed. But this paradigm is increasingly inadequate for the new generation of individuals with visual impairments, whose care will make it essential that medical

S. F. Wainapel: Department of Rehabilitation Medicine, Montefiore Hospital, Albert Einstein College of Medicine, Bronx, New York 10467.

M. Bernbaum: Department of Internal Medicine, Division of Endocrinology, St. Louis University Health Sciences Center, St. Louis, Missouri 63104.

TABLE 69-1. *Comparisons between medical and vision rehabilitation*

Rehabilitation medicine	Vision rehabilitation
Physical therapy	Orientation and mobility
Occupational therapy	Rehabilitation teaching
Social work	Social work
Rehabilitation counseling	Rehabilitation counseling
Orthotics	Vision enhancement
Prosthetics	Vision substitution

and vision rehabilitation systems join forces after a half-century of relative insularity. The new challenge does not come from the ravages of war but from the ravages of age.

THE EPIDEMIOLOGIC CONTEXT

In 1900 only 4% of the American population was aged 65 or older; by 1980 that number had nearly tripled (6), and it will continue to increase as the "baby boom" generation ages during the early 21st century. The physiological changes of aging are protean and affect all body systems or organs (7), and the visual system is no exception. Thus, the new "epidemic" of visual impairment will occur among the geriatric population. Epidemiologic surveys confirm this conclusion. Nelson and Dimitrova (8) have analyzed data from the 1990 Health Interview Survey: 4.3 million Americans had difficulty reading ordinary newspaper print (the equivalent of less than 20/70 corrected visual acuity) even when using reading glasses, and about two-thirds of these were 65 or older (Table 69-2). It is worth noting that this prevalence of visual impairment is greater than that for stroke and lower limb amputation combined. Because both of the latter conditions are frequent diagnoses among the elderly, it is not surprising to find them associated with vision problems, producing the blind amputee (9,10) or the blind stroke patient (11). The prevalence of visual impairment among rehabilitation medicine inpatients has been reported to be about 7% in a retrospective survey of 191 consecutive admissions to an inpatient unit (12). These patients were older than the average but had a length of stay (LOS) that was actually shorter than that for the entire unit's mean LOS (Table 69-3). Vision loss was a comorbidity that did not adversely affect outcome, probably because these patients had lost vision a number of years before this admission and had adjusted to their impairment.

TABLE 69-2. *Prevalence of severe visual impairment in the United States, 1990*

Age	Number with visual impairment	Prevalence
0–17	95,410	1.5/1,000
18–44	349,350	3.2/1,000
45–54	340,510	13.5/1,000
55–64	600,600	28.4/1,000
65–74	1,068,290	59.0/1,000
75–85	1,190,520	118.4/1,000
85 +	648,680	210.6/1,000
Total	4,293,360	17.3/1,000

Adapted from Nelson KA, Dimitrova E. Severe visual impairment in the United States and in each state, 1990. *J Vis Impairment Blind* 1993; 87:80–86; reprinted by permission of the American Foundation of the Blind.

THE FUNCTIONAL CONTEXT

It is not sufficient for visual impairment to be prevalent for it to warrant closer attention from the physiatrist. It must also result in significant functional disability and/or handicap. A number of studies have documented that vision loss has adverse effects on mobility, self-care, and social function.

Vision is one of the three essential components for normal upright stance; vestibular function and proprioception are the other two (13). Loss of this stabilizing influence has been implicated in falls by several authors (14–16), and Felson (17) has graphically demonstrated a greater than twofold increased risk of hip fractures among members of the Framingham Eye Study cohort.

Deficits in basic and/or instrumental activities of daily living (ADL) have been documented in persons with isolated visual impairment in a number of settings in the United States as well as Europe. Carabellese and co-workers (18) studied a large urban Italian community sample of persons aged 70 or older, measuring their self-care status and dividing the sample into groups based on the presence or absence of visual or hearing impairments. Visual impairment alone produced statistically significant losses in ADL and IADL function. Branch and co-workers (19) found IADL deficits in a more heterogeneous sample of older residents of Massachusetts but failed to find statistically significant basic ADL losses. Others (20) have documented that visually impaired persons have lower perceived health status and suffer from a sense of social isolation.

The rationale for physiatrists' increased awareness of and attention to vision-related issues is clear. Visual impairment is a frequent concomitant of the aging process, producing significant disability in its own right. It occurs with some frequency among patients seen by the physiatrist. It affects balance, gait, and self-care activities. It can also occur as part of the syndromes produced by three common rehabilitation medicine diagnoses: stroke, traumatic brain injury, and multiple sclerosis.

VISION PROBLEMS ASSOCIATED WITH AGING

As the eye ages, it undergoes many physiological and morphologic changes, which are summarized in Table 69-4. Familiar changes include the arcus senilis, the loss of accommodation after age 40, which produces the need for reading glasses, and the development of clouding of the crystalline lens, which can lead to full-blown cataract formation.

TABLE 69-3. *Length of stay in rehabilitation facility for patients with visual impairment*

Sex	Age	Rehabilitation diagnosis	Vision diagnosis	Length of stay (days)	Discharge status
F	78	CVA, R hemi	Cataracts	56	Home
F	82	Pelvic fracture	Macular degeneration	17	Home
F	81	Back pain	Macular degeneration	50	Home
F	81	Back pain	Macular degeneration	28	Home
F	82	Gait disorder	Cataracts, macular degeneration	15	Surgery
F	82	S/P VP shunt	Cataracts, macular degeneration	17	Medicine
M	79	Bilateral BKA	Cataracts, glaucoma	24	Home
M	89	CVA, R hemi	Glaucoma	25	Home
M	84	CVA, R hemi	Glaucoma	30	Home
F	69	L BKA	Diabetic retinopathy	30	Home
F	70	CVA, L hemi	Diabetic retinopathy	72	Skilled nursing facility

BKA, below-knee amputation; CVA, cerebrovascular accident; L hemi, left hemiparesis; R hemi, right hemiparesis; VP, ventriculo-peritoneal.

From Wainapel S, Kwon YS, Fazzari PJ. Severe visual impairment on a rehabilitation unit: incidence and implications. *Arch Phys Med Rehabil* 1989; 70:439–441; reprinted by permission of WB Saunders, Co.

Other changes are often quite significant. The pupil becomes smaller with age and limits the amount of light reaching the retina. By age 60, the retina receives less than one-third the light it did at age 20 (7). Ptosis of the upper eyelid can produce a reduction of the upper visual field. Nuclear sclerosis produces heightened glare sensitivity, and yellowing of the lens leads to color distortions.

The great majority of visual impairments in the elderly are caused by one of four diagnoses: cataract, age-related macular degeneration (AMD), glaucoma, and diabetic retinopathy (21). A detailed discussion of their etiology, pathophysiology, and medical/surgical management is beyond the scope of this chapter, but a brief summary of their characteristics is included since the physiatrist will be likely to see many patients with these disorders. An excellent concise guide to the aging eye and its management has been published by the New York Lighthouse and is highly recommended as a reference (22). Figures 69-1 through 69-4 present visual simulations of the identical objects as they would appear to a person with these disorders.

TABLE 69-4. *Changes in the eye associated with aging*

Functional change	Physiological change
Visual acuity	Morphologic change in choroid, pigment epithelium, or retina
	Decreased function of rods, cones, or other neural elements
Extraocular motion	Difficulty in gazing upward and maintaining convergence
Intraocular pressure	Increased pressure
Refractive power	Increased hyperopia and myopia
	Presbyopia
	Increased lens size
	Nuclear sclerosis (lens)
	Ciliary muscle atrophy
Tear secretion	Decreased tearing
	Decreased lacrimal gland function
	Decreased goblet cell secretion
Corneal function	Loss of endothelial integrity
	Posterior surface pigmentation

From Kane RL, Ouslander JG, Abrass IB. Sensory impairment. In: *Essentials of clinical geriatrics, 2nd ed.;* reprinted by permission of McGraw-Hill, Inc.

Cataract is an opacification of the normally clear crystalline lens. It is extremely common with advancing age but may not require specific treatment unless it produces symptoms that impact on the patient's life style and normal activities. Three major types of cataract are distinguished: (a) central (nuclear) cataract, the most common variety; (b) peripheral (cortical) cataract, which is associated with increased age; and (c) posterior (subcapsular) cataract, which occurs most commonly in diabetics or patients receiving corticosteroids (23). Common symptoms include blurred vision, glare sensitivity, and yellow vision. Treatment is surgical and usually takes the form of extracapsular lens extraction or phacoemulsification of the lens, both of which leave the capsule intact and permit the implantation of an intraocular lens (23). The intraocular lens produces much less magnification or distortion than the older techniques of cataract glasses or contact lenses. The surgery is performed on an ambulatory basis and has an extremely high success rate that approaches 90% in patients without comorbid conditions. Follow-up studies have documented that elderly patients experience improved self-care status and even improvement of mental status following intraocular lens implant surgery (24,25).

The most frequent cause of blindness among the elderly is AMD, especially among those aged 75 or older. In this condition the macula suffers damage with a resulting loss of central visual field but preservation of peripheral vision (Fig. 69-2). Detail vision for facial recognition, reading, and close-up observation is severely affected, but mobility is relatively preserved because peripheral vision remains intact. Two types of AMD have been delineated: (a) nonexudative (''dry'') AMD, which may be relatively benign and nonprogressive; and (b) exudative (''wet'') AMD, which

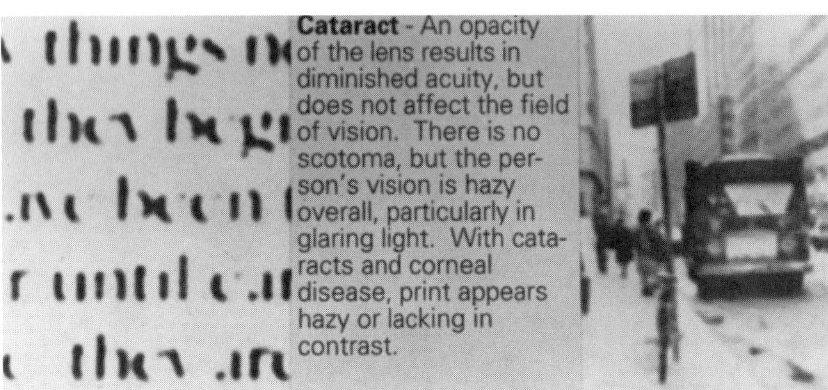

FIG. 69-1. Simulation of visual consequences of cataract. (From Faye EE, Stuen CS. *The aging eye and low vision.* New York: The Lighthouse, 1992; reprinted by permission of The Lighthouse, Inc.)

frequently progresses to total loss of macular function. Although laser photocoagulation surgery has been of some benefit in selected cases of exudative AMD, most patients have no surgical or medical option at the present time. Fortunately, the disease is self-limited, and the patient can be reassured that he or she will not become totally blind, nor will his or her mobility be impaired.

The visual deficit of glaucoma results from damage to the optic nerve from increased intraocular pressure related to abnormal mechanisms of fluid flow between the anterior and posterior chambers of the eye. It presents in one of two ways: (a) a rapidly progressive vision loss with pain from acute angle closure, a true ophthalmologic emergency; or (b) an insidious and silently progressive disease that gradually constricts the peripheral visual fields with resulting ''tunnel vision'' (Fig. 69-3) and, if unrecognized, ultimate total vision loss. Early detection is essential for the second type, which is called open-angle glaucoma; intraocular pressure should be regularly measured in every elderly patient to facilitate early detection and treatment. The management of glaucoma can be purely medical, using various eye drops, but sometimes requires a surgical procedure, usually a laser iridotomy, that reestablishes normal drainage of the aqueous humor.

Diabetic retinopathy is an important cause of blindness in young and middle-aged patients as well as the elderly. Its clinical manifestations can be more variable than the preceding three disorders, but they usually produce central deficits that affect visual acuity (Fig. 69-4). It is discussed in more detail in the following section.

VISION PROBLEMS IN THE YOUNG AND MIDDLE-AGED

As shown in Table 69-2, visual impairment is relatively uncommon below age 55, but when it does occur, its effects can be particularly devastating, interfering with a person's ability to complete educational studies, obtain employment, or continue in the usual social role. Causes of vision loss are more variable than among the elderly, with diabetic retinopathy being by far the most prevalent. Retinopathy of prematurity (ROP), which was formerly called retrolental fibroplasia, is occurring more frequently in recent years because of the improved care of premature infants who would have previously died . Other causes of blindness or visual impairment in infants and children include congenital cataracts, rubella syndrome, and anoxic brain damage with cerebral palsy. Tapetoretinal degenerative disorders, of which retinitis pigmentosa (RP) is the most prevalent, characteristically manifest themselves in childhood or early adulthood with symptoms of night blindness and ''tunnel vision'' from loss of peripheral visual fields with preservation of central vision, similar to the effects of open-angle glaucoma (Fig. 69-3). This type of vision loss produces significant difficulty

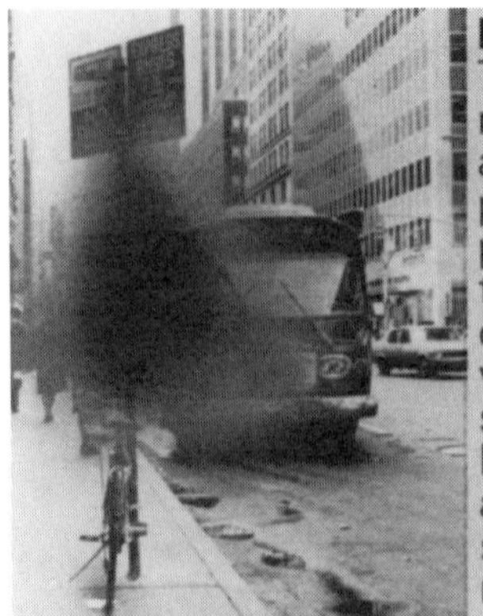

FIG. 69-2. Simulation of visual consequences of macular degeneration. (From Faye EE, Stuen CS. *The aging eye and low vision.* New York: The Lighthouse, 1992; reprinted by permission of The Lighthouse, Inc.)

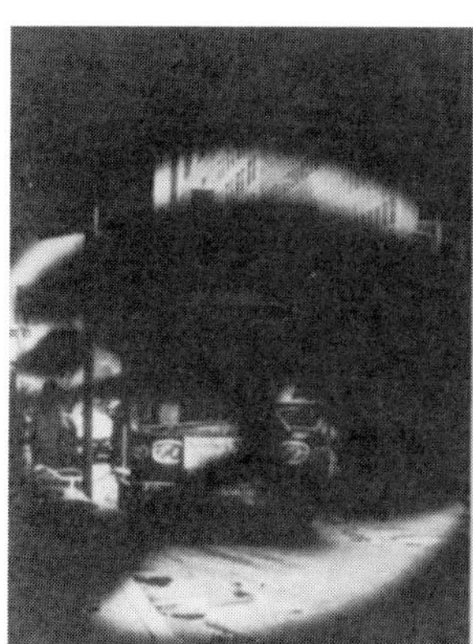

Glaucoma - Chronic elevated eye pressure in susceptible individuals may cause optic nerve atrophy and loss of peripheral vision. Early detection and close medical monitoring can help reduce complications. In advanced glaucoma, print may appear faded and words may be difficult to read.

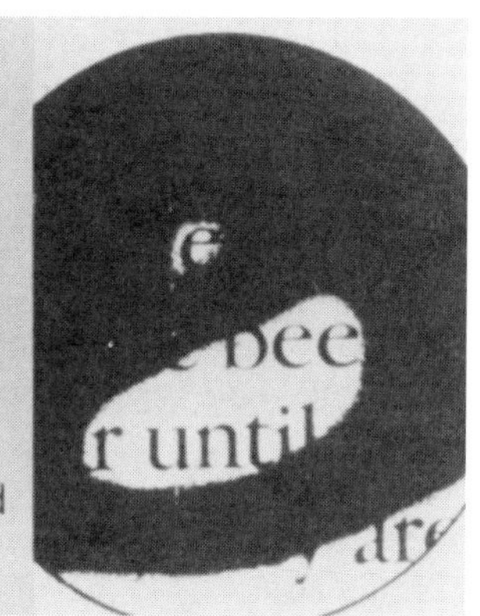

FIG. 69-3. Simulation of visual consequences of glaucoma. (From Faye EE, Stuen CS. *The aging eye and low vision.* New York: The Lighthouse, 1992; reprinted by permission of The Lighthouse, Inc.)

in mobility while leaving reading and detail vision unimpaired. The course of RP is dependent on the particular variant of the disease, but in general there is progressive narrowing of visual field that may progress to total blindness by middle age. Cataract formation may also contribute to the loss of residual central vision in RP.

A relatively new cause of vision loss in the young adult is that associated with cytomegalovirus (CMV) retinitis in patients with acquired immunodeficiency syndrome (AIDS). This infection has been a relatively late manifestation of the disease and has carried a grave prognosis for prolonged survival, but recent advances in treatment using intraocular gancyclovir have extended survival in these patients. Other opportunistic infections of the central nervous system such as cryptococcal meningitis and toxoplasmosis may also produce visual sequelae.

Diabetes mellitus is the leading cause of visual impairment in American adults between the ages of 20 and 74 years and, overall, accounts for 12% of new cases of blindness (26). Development of diabetic retinopathy correlates with disease duration as well as with the degree of blood glucose control (27). After 15 years, background retinopathy is present in 97% of individuals with insulin-dependent diabetes mellitus (IDDM), 80% of individuals with non-insulin-dependent diabetes mellitus (NIDDM) who are insulin treated, and 55% of individuals with NIDDM who are not insulin requiring (26). Small hemorrhages, microaneurysms, and lipid exudates are visible within the retina, although vision is usually unaffected. However, in 8% of individuals, the macula is involved, resulting in moderate to severe visual impairment (28). Early laser photocoagulation can reduce vision loss by 60% (29–31).

Within 15 years of diagnosis, proliferative retinopathy occurs in 30% of individuals with IDDM, 10% to 15% of those with insulin-requiring NIDDM, and 5% of non-insulin-requiring individuals (26). Proliferative retinopathy involves blockages of the microvascular circulation nourishing the retina, leading to the formation of new and abnormal (neovascular) vessels (28). These fragile vessels rupture and hemorrhage easily; they may also grow out of the retina into the vitreous humor, with subsequent traction tears, detachments, and scarring of the retina. Optimal control of the blood glucose can prevent or delay the progression of retinopathy (27). Early intervention with laser photocoagulation can reduce the incidence of serious vision loss (29–31). Individuals who already have severe visual impairment with extensive hemorrhages, fibrosis, or retinal detachments are treated with surgical vitrectomy to remove vitreous hemorrhage and opacities and to release mechanical traction on the retina. Vitrectomy can be very effective in restoring visual

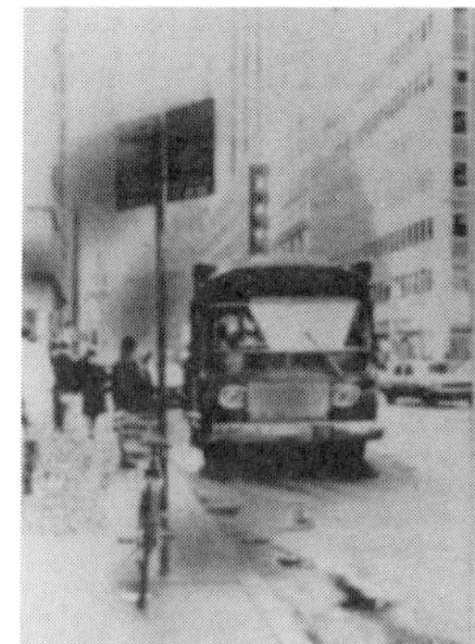

Diabetic Retinopathy - The leaking of retinal blood vessels may occur in advanced or long-term diabetes and affect the macula or the entire retina and vitreous. Not all diabetics develop retinal changes, but the likelihood of retinopathy and cataracts increases with the length of time a person has diabetes.

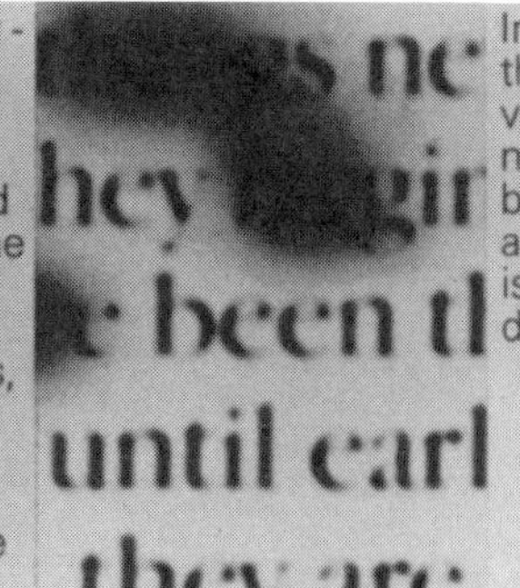

In diabetic retinopathy, reading vision is variable and print may be distorted or blurred. If cataracts are also present, print is hazy as well as distorted.

FIG. 69-4. Simulation of visual consequences of diabetic retinopathy. (From Faye EE, Stuen CS. *The aging eye and low vision.* New York: The Lighthouse, 1992; reprinted by permission of The Lighthouse, Inc.)

acuity, but there is a 25% complication rate, which may lead to further compromise of vision (31,32).

The patient with diabetic retinopathy is a classic example in which the medical and vision rehabilitation systems must interface for optimal outcome. The many medical complications associated with diabetes mellitus—peripheral neuropathy, autonomic neuropathy, peripheral vascular disease, and nephropathy, among others—demand close medical attention, while the physical disabilities that can accompany these conditions—lower limb amputations, weakness, and/or sensory disturbances—warrant the participation of the physiatrist. When one adds the presence of severe visual impairment to the above scenario, it becomes quite evident that vision rehabilitation personnel need to become more familiar with medical rehabilitation issues while physiatrists need to understand the basic principles of vision rehabilitation in order to adequately serve such a patient.

AN OVERVIEW OF VISION REHABILITATION PRINCIPLES AND PRACTICE

As has already been illustrated (Table 69-1), vision rehabilitation has many similarities to the medical rehabilitation model. In the case of the individual with visual impairment or blindness, the process can be divided into the following components:

1. Assessment and classification of the degree and type of visual impairment.
2. Referral to vision rehabilitation system and providers.
3. Devices and techniques to enhance residual vision.
4. Devices and techniques that substitute for lost vision.

Assessment and Classification

Vision assessment should be as routine a part of the physiatrist's evaluation as the peripheral sensory examination. The thoroughness of this assessment cannot be expected to equal that of the ophthalmologist or optometrist (33), but it is essential to rule out this important sensory disability in all rehabilitation medicine patients. A high index of suspicion should be present when examining patients with stroke, multiple sclerosis, traumatic brain injury, or underlying diabetes mellitus. The high prevalence of visual impairment among the elderly, which reaches 27% in those aged 85 or older (34), should be recalled. History taking should include functionally oriented questions about vision: difficulty in reading, night vision problems, glare sensitivity in sunlight, mobility problems related to narrow visual fields, or difficulty in ADL related to vision loss (for example, diabetics unable to draw up or self-administer insulin). The physical examination should include evaluation of extraocular movements, which can be affected in brainstem stroke or multiple sclerosis. Visual acuity can be measured using a portable Snellen eye chart, and even without one it is possible to use a newspaper as a rough screening tool: inability to read the latter corresponds to a visual acuity of less than 20/70. Visual field testing with confrontation at the bedside is a useful method to determine the presence of hemianopia, but more accurate formal perimetry testing is often indicated when subtler deficits are present or suspected. A full ophthalmologic consultation should be requested when any of the above screening tests reveals vision deficits.

Classification of visual impairment is of more than academic significance; it determines the patient's eligibility for state-funded vision rehabilitation services. Two main levels of impairment are usually recognized for classification, based on corrected visual acuity and extent of visual fields. *Legal blindness* is defined as corrected acuity less than 20/200 or visual field of less than 20° in the better eye. *Low vision* is defined as corrected acuity between 20/70 and 20/200 or visual field deficit with residual field of greater than 20° in the better eye. These definitions clearly have major limitations because they exclude patients with significant vision problems who would not meet their criteria. For example, a diabetic who is totally blind in one eye and has 20/60 corrected acuity in the remaining eye would not be considered legally blind. Nevertheless, such a patient would require extensive vision rehabilitation.

Visual impairments can also be classified into central (acuity) or peripheral (field) deficits. The former can be subdivided into discrete deficits such as scotomas or diffuse deficits such as are produced by cataract. The latter can be subdivided into central deficits such as those resulting from AMD or concentric deficits such as those produced by glaucoma or RP.

Referral for Vision Rehabilitation

The vision rehabilitation system varies from state to state, but in general it is administered by the Department of Social Services or a similar agency. Funding for treatment comes from this source rather than from third-party insurance carriers as is the case with most medical care. This distinction is extremely important in light of the previously discussed overlaps between visual and medical disabilities. Certification of legal blindness by an ophthalmologist or optometrist is sent to the appropriate state agency, which then institutes an evaluation by a social worker or rehabilitation counselor, who then determines which rehabilitation services should be provided. This case-management model provides the following major treatment options (see Table 69-1):

1. Orientation and mobility (O&M) instructor: The equivalent of a physical therapist for the visually impaired or blind patient, the O&M instructor (formerly referred to as a peripatologist) teaches ambulation and navigation techniques that allow the patient to safely negotiate indoor and outdoor environments using a variety of assistive devices.
2. Rehabilitation teacher: The equivalent of an occupational therapist, this professional teaches special ADL

and IADL techniques that enable the visually impaired person to function independently. In addition to prescribing self-help devices, the rehabilitation teacher may also instruct the patient in reading and writing Braille.

3. Low-vision specialist: An optometrist is usually consulted for formal low-vision evaluation and prescription of devices that enhance or substitute for vision.
4. Communication/computer specialist: This individual concentrates on skills that will improve reading and writing, such as Braille and computer adaptations.
5. Social worker: As with their medical rehabilitation counterpart, the social worker assists the patient and family with psychosocial issues.
6. Rehabilitation counselor: As with their counterpart in medical rehabilitation, the rehabilitation counselor assists the patient in the areas of education and employment.

This multidisciplinary team provides input as well as specific services for the patient. Treatments are usually given at a specialized nonresidential facility, although in some cases they may be performed in the patient's own home.

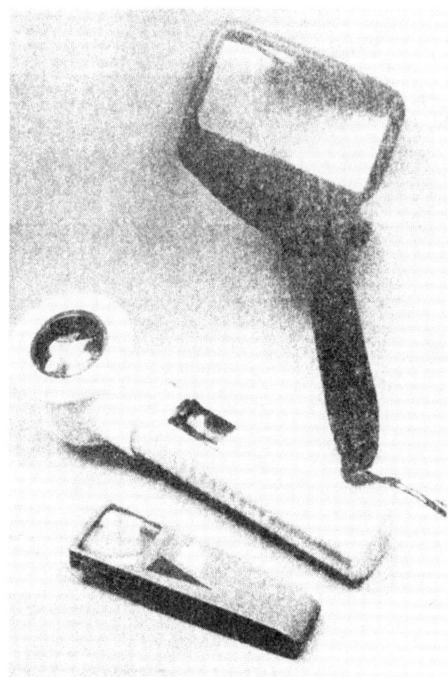

FIG. 69-5. Hand-held magnifiers. (Photograph by permission of Resources for Rehabilitation, Lexington, MA.)

Enhancement of Residual Vision

Vision enhancement, often referred to as low-vision rehabilitation, is a complex subject that is exhaustively discussed in books by Faye (35) and by Cole and Rosenthal (36). In general, there are two basic components: (a) optical devices or techniques that provide magnification of the image or alter the visual field; (b) nonoptical aids that modify environmental factors such as glare, lighting, and contrast.

Ordinary spectacles and contact lenses are the most ubiquitous magnification devices, although their range of enlargement is relatively narrow. Magnifiers come in many shapes and sizes, but they share the advantage of being portable and relatively inexpensive. Hand-held devices (Fig. 69-5) require functional use of the upper extremities (a potential problem for arthritics, hemiplegics, or parkinsonian patients) and must have their focal length adjusted for maximal effect. Stand magnifiers eliminate these difficulties (Fig. 69-6). Adding built-in halogen illumination to a stand magnifier provides even greater visibility (Fig. 69-7). Monocular or binocular spectacle-mounted telescopic lenses are prescribed for patients to facilitate reading (Fig. 69-8) or even for driving. Hand-held monocular telescopes can assist with distance vision, as in the case of patients having difficulty reading street signs. Visual fatigue and a limited field of vision are shared disadvantages of magnifiers and telescopes. The closed-circuit television videomagnifier (CCTV) offers a wide range of magnification from 3 to 60 times normal while minimizing reading fatigue and maximizing the field of view (Fig. 69-9). The reversal of image that gives a black background with white foreground increases contrast and further heightens visibility. The main problem with the CCTV is its relatively high cost and its size, although portable models are now available. Enlarged print books, magazines, and computer output are another magnification option for patients with low vision.

Expansion or shifting of the visual field is the second treatment option for enhancing vision. Reversing a pair of binoculars or opera glasses is a simple expedient to increase the narrow visual fields produced by RP or glaucoma. Prisms or minification lenses are also used for this purpose. Fresnell prisms can divert vision from impaired areas to intact ones, as in the case of stroke or head injury with homonymous hemianopia. A mirror mounted on a pair of glasses (Fig. 69-10) is an alternative option that can be made more cosmetic by mounting it behind the lenses. Central visual field defects produced by AMD may be compensated for by learning the technique of eccentric viewing, in which a new fixation point is trained to substitute for the macula (36).

Modification of external factors within the environment can markedly improve visual function, and conversely, a lack of attention to them can cause great difficulty despite adequate magnification. The nonoptical aids that are used to reduce glare, heighten contrast, and optimize illumination are often simple and quite inexpensive. Glare can be reduced by sunglasses, especially those whose tinting blocks the passage of the blue part of the visible spectrum (orange and yellow tints are particularly effective); a hat or cap with a brim or a simple visor can also decrease glare from light coming from above the viewer. Indirect lighting is also indicated. The amount of illumination that suffices for each patient will vary with age and underlying condition, but it is essential to have an adjustable lighting source for any near-vision activities such as reading, writing, or sewing. Im-

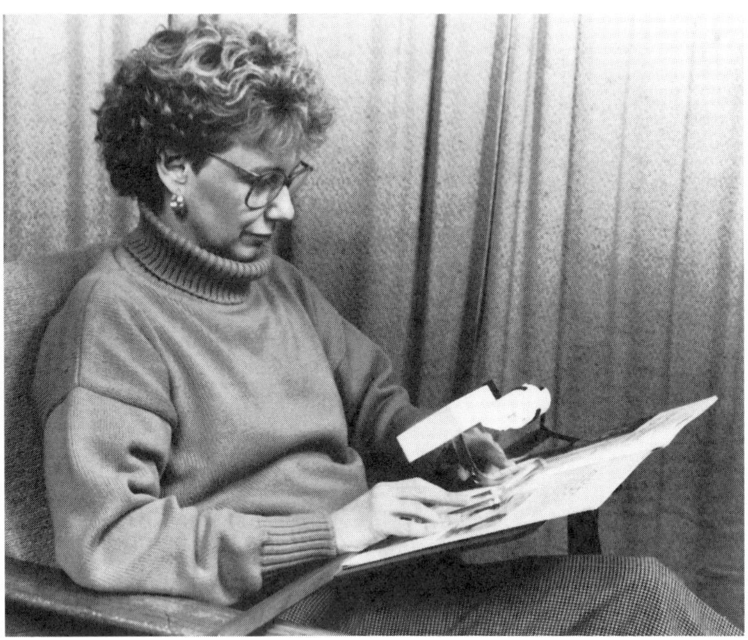

FIG. 69-6. Stand magnifier.

paired night vision can be enhanced by the use of illumination devices originally developed for underwater or wartime activities. Contrast-enhancing devices include sharply contrasting colors on adjacent surfaces, paper with thick and dark lines, felt-tipped or boldly writing pens, and tinted glasses. Typoscopes are made from dark colored material into which a series of apertures are cut, which guide the user to the right position for signing their name, writing a check, or addressing an envelope. They can also be extremely helpful for visual tracking while reading (Fig. 69-11).

Substitution for Lost Vision

Vision enhancement is useful only when there is sufficient residual vision to be enhanced. Often, however, so little remains that it only provides cues about light, shapes, and

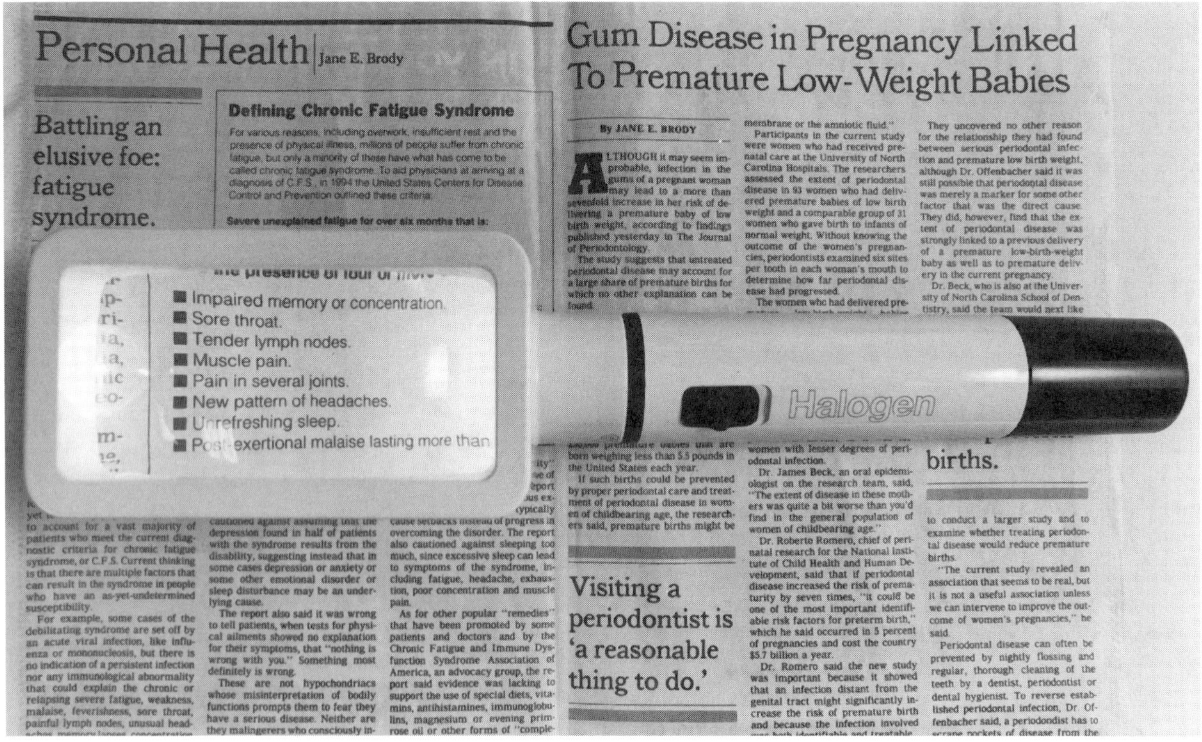

FIG. 69-7. Halogen-illuminated stand magnifier.

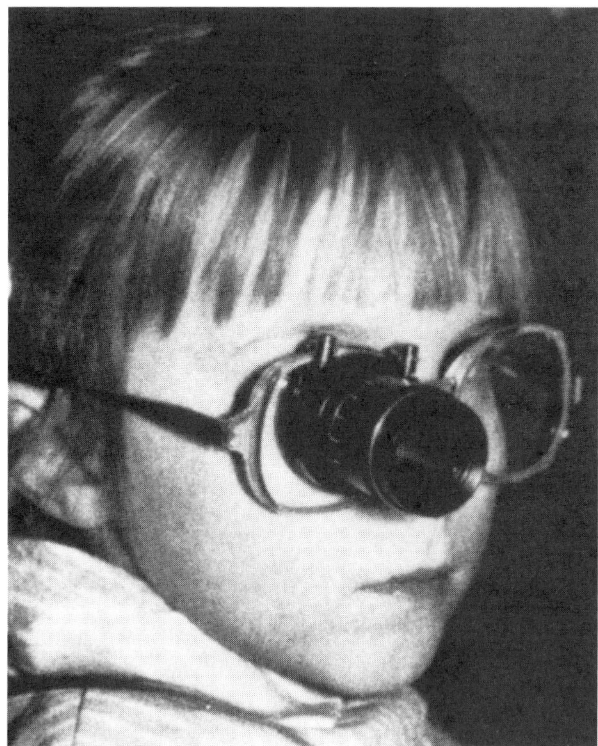

FIG. 69-8. Monocular telescope for reading. (Reprinted by permission of Resources for Rehabilitation, Lexington, MA.)

movement. Although only 12% of the visually impaired population have no light perception (8), a larger proportion have nonfunctional vision, and for these individuals it is necessary to resort to substitutes for vision. New techniques need to be learned for mobility, self-care, and reading/writing. The O&M instructor and the rehabilitation teacher now assume a

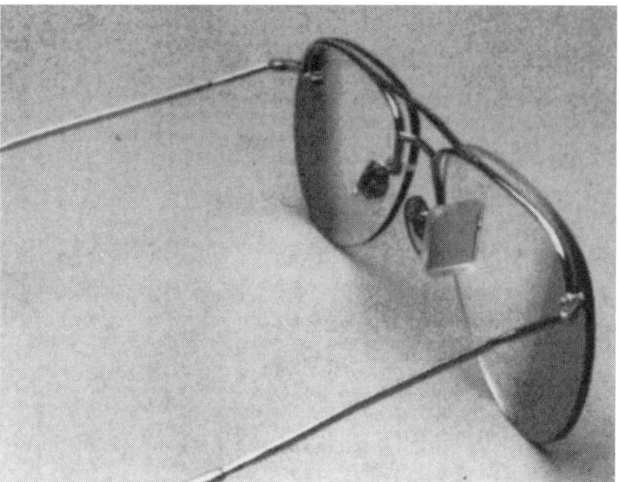

FIG. 69-10. Spectacle-mounted mirror for homonymous hemianopia. (From Cole RG, Rosenthal BP. *Remediation and management of low vision.* St Louis: CV Mosby, 1996; reprinted by permission of Mosby–Year Book Publishers.)

major role in the rehabilitation process. Mobility techniques, tactile substitution, vocal substitution, and specialized ADL techniques are used by these professionals to foster an independent life style.

There are many options available for improving the mobility of a blind person (37,38). The most frequently used techniques are a sighted guide, the long white cane, the guide dog, and various electronic or sonic navigation aids. Sighted guide technique is the correct way for a sighted person to assist one who is blind: the blind person places his or her hand just above the guide's elbow and then walks a step behind, allowing the guide's body movements to be communicated before turning, ascending/descending stairs, or nego-

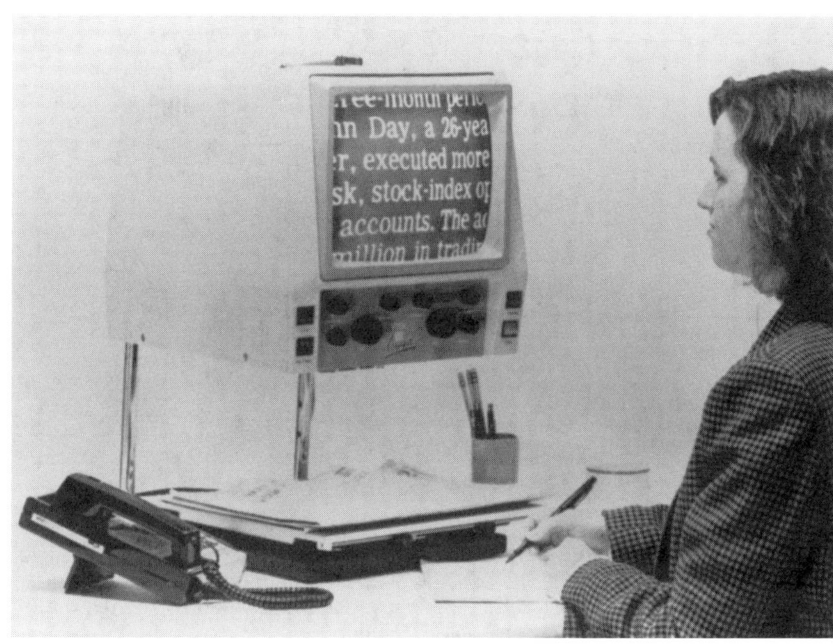

FIG. 69-9. Closed-circuit television video magnifier (CCTV). (Reprinted by permission of VTek, Santa Monica, CA.)

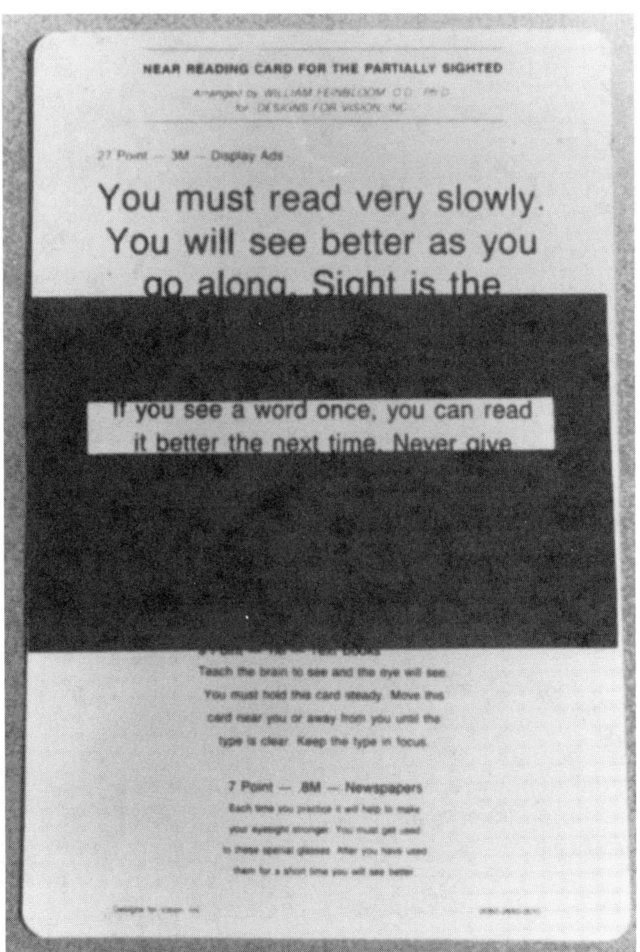

FIG. 69-11. Typoscope for enhanced contrast for reading. (From Cole RG, Rosenthal BP. *Remediation and management of low vision.* St Louis: CV Mosby, 1996; reprinted by permission of Mosby–Year Book Publishers.)

tiating curbs. The long white cane serves as an extension of the sense of touch, warning the blind traveler of upcoming obstacles or terrain changes as it is tapped about two paces in front of the user (the cane is usually 4 to 5 feet long). When used correctly, it allows movement in potentially hazardous circumstances such as descending stairs (Fig. 69-12). The laser cane, though more expensive and difficult to master, provides increased feedback about distant drop-offs and obstacles at head level by sending out three separate light beams, which trigger vibratory signals on the cane when such obstacles are detected (Fig. 69-13). The guide dog allows a greater degree of freedom of movement than the cane as well as a sense of companionship and security, but it requires intensive training of both dog and user, entails extra responsibility for the animal's care, and may be too strenuous for older or frailer individuals. Ultrasonic navigation aids can be worn over the chest by wheelchair users, mounted on walkerettes or wheelchairs, held in the hand, or mounted on a pair of glasses (38). The most recent advance in electronic navigation entails satellite tracking and computer localization with synthetic speech output.

Tactile substitution is used in a wide variety of ways by blind persons. The best known is Braille, a tactile language system developed in France and based on permutations of a series of six small raised dots, which have the form seen on an ordinary domino. With practice it is possible to detect the more than 250 variations that are the basis of grade 2 Braille, which makes fluent reading possible. However, the majority of blind people, particularly those whose vision loss was acquired in later life, will find it difficult to master, although a simpler form (grade 1) can be used for writing labels or brief notes. Written Braille and Braille output from computers are important communication tools, especially in persons with early-onset vision loss. Other tactile techniques include raised-line diagrams (for reading maps or illustrations); raised-dot marking of kitchen utensils to facilitate such activities as weighing, measuring, and using oven or toaster; watches with covers that can be swung away to permit the hands to be felt for keeping time; and raised letters or numbers for use by those unable to learn Braille.

Vocal substitution covers a wide range of techniques and resources in which any type of sound provides feedback or information for the blind individual. Recorded books and magazines are an invaluable source of pleasure and informa-

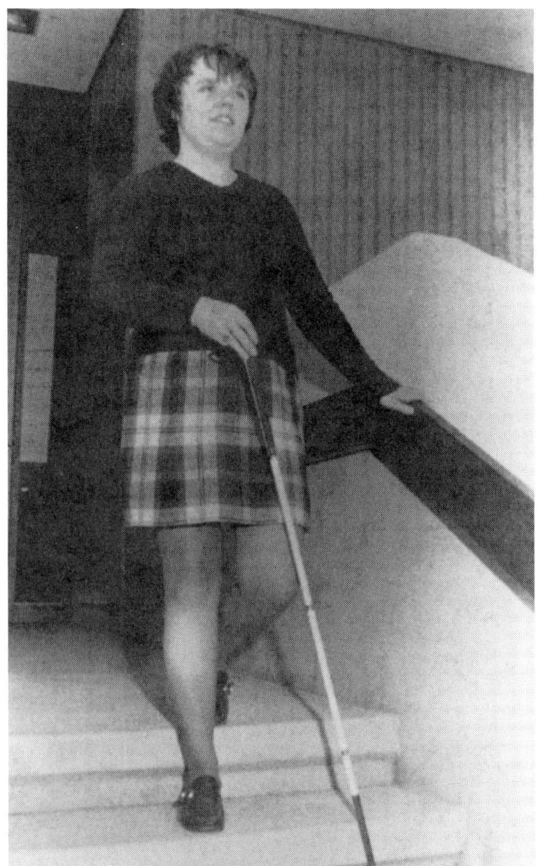

FIG. 69-12. Stair climbing with long white cane. (From Cole RG, Rosenthal BP. *Remediation and management of low vision.* St Louis: CV Mosby, 1996; reprinted by permission of Mosby–Year Book Publishers.)

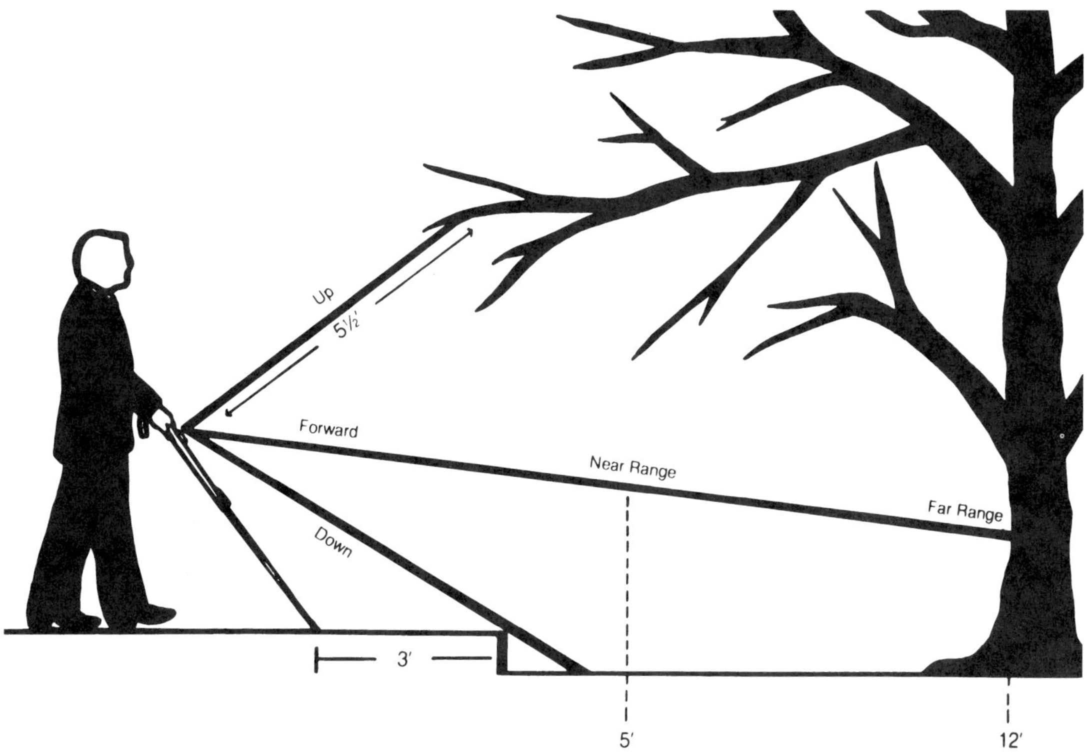

The above distances have been achieved in the laboratory using a neutral test material of tan corrugated cardboard. Distances may vary according to the reflective quality of individual objects in the user's traveling environment.

FIG. 69-13. Laser cane. (Reprinted with permission of Nurion Industries, Inc., Paoli, PA.)

tion for thousands of visually impaired persons who do not have access to Braille. The Talking Book Program of the Library of Congress has recorded versions of most fiction and many nonfiction books in a convenient four-track cassette format recorded at half speed, which allows 6 hours of material on each cassette. Cassettes are sent to participants in plastic containers, and these are returned to the local library distributor free of charge via the mail. A modified cassette recorder is required to play these tapes; a large one is provided to users of the program, and smaller, more portable ones can be purchased for $150 to $250. A physician, optometrist, or vision rehabilitation professional can certify that a patient has a print disability; legal blindness is not a requirement, and the program is also available to those with dyslexia or neuromuscular problems that interfere with normal reading. Recordings for the Blind and Dyslexic of Princeton, New Jersey supplements the Talking Books program with more than 75,000 recorded books, many of which are textbooks that can be used by students with print disabilities. Synthetic speech technology is another form of vocal substitution that has greatly facilitated the lives of visually impaired people, spawning a host of devices that announce their data in clearly audible form: watches, calculators, weight scales, thermometers, glucometers, and even sphygmomanometers. The synthetic speech, screen-reading, and optical character recognition (OCR) software that have been developed in recent years are revolutionizing the field of computer technology for blind individuals, and it is now possible for such a person to read documents using a scanner and to perform other computer activities such as word processing (Fig. 69-14).

Other ADL techniques for the blind combine tactile and vocal substitution strategies. For example, a liquid level indicator emits a tone when a cup of tea or coffee is filled to near the top; coins are identified by touch; dollar bill denominations are made identifiable by folding specific denominations in different patterns; clothing is color-coded using Braille labeling; and food preparation is simplified by using a measuring cup, weight scale, and timer that are marked with raised dots to indicate divisions of volume, weight, and time.

TREATING COMBINED VISUAL AND NEUROMUSCULAR DISABILITIES

The need for closer coordination between vision and medical rehabilitation systems is exemplified in a number of instances in which a neuromuscular impairment coexists with or includes a visual impairment. In some cases the two developed separately, as in the blind person who subsequently suffers an amputation of the lower extremity or a cerebrovascular accident (CVA). Altner, Rusin, and DeBoer

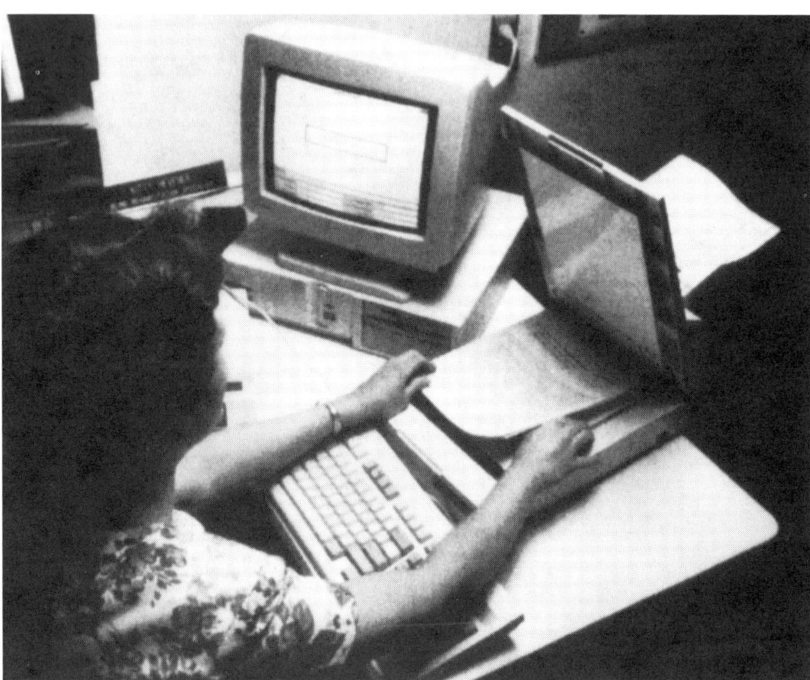

FIG. 69-14. Computer and scanner for the visually impaired individual. (From Cole RG, Rosenthal BP. *Remediation and management of low vision.* St Louis: CV Mosby, 1996; reprinted by permission of Mosby–Year Book Publishers.)

(9) have demonstrated that blind amputees generally become prosthetic users and noted a 66% success rate among 12 such patients. Fisher (10) has added two more cases, both of which had positive outcomes. Wainapel (11) reviewed 220 consecutive stroke admissions to a general rehabilitation medicine unit, seven of whom had preexisting blindness. Although these patients were older and had a more lengthy hospital course, most of them became ambulatory, and four were discharged to their homes. These articles emphasize that blindness plus a second disability is no contraindication to rehabilitation; in fact, it is possible that the prior experience of a disability and its successful rehabilitation might be beneficial in terms of adaptation to a second disability.

Stroke is also associated with its own types of visual impairment, including perceptual–motor problems caused by right-sided brain damage and homonymous hemianopia from damage to the optic radiation on either side. The latter condition may severely interfere with mobility, self-care, and safety. The patient needs to be aware of the presence of this field deficit and to compensate for it by turning the head toward the affected side. Prisms or a spectacle-mounted mirror (Fig. 69-10) can deflect vision from the impaired to the normal portions of the visual field. More recently, it has been suggested that monocular eye patching combined with computer-generated stimulation of the affected visual field may produce beneficial results (39).

Traumatic brain injury (TBI) is also associated with visual disturbances, some of which are similar to those seen with CVA. However, the greater degree of cognitive impairment with TBI makes diagnosis of these problems more difficult. Gianutsos, Ramsey, and Perlin (40) performed visual screening on 55 severely brain-injured patients in a long-term care facility and found that more than half of them had visual impairments. Of the 26 sent to a rehabilitative optometrist, all but two were benefited by this intervention, and many patients showed increased participation in their rehabilitation program following treatment. The optometric examination in such patients is quite difficult and often time-consuming; the participation of a cognitive therapist can be of great help during this exam. This kind of cooperation between the vision and medical rehabilitation systems is precisely what is needed for these complex clinical challenges.

The visual consequences of multiple sclerosis include diplopia, blurred vision, nystagmus, and even monocular or binocular blindness as a result of optic neuritis. Vision enhancement and substitution techniques for such patients may be difficult or impossible because of associated weakness, spasticity, and ataxia of the upper extremities; standing magnifiers are preferable to hand-held ones, and recorded material is definitely more accessible than Braille. Computers may have to be voice-activated because of loss of finger dexterity and coordination. Similar obstacles face the diabetic patient whose retinopathy is combined with peripheral neuropathy. Additionally, diabetics develop autonomic dysfunction that can impact negatively on exercise programs and therapy in the rehabilitation setting. In one study of 29 visually impaired diabetics, 28 had parasympathetic neuropathy manifested by abnormal heart rate changes with respiration, 23 had sympathetic neuropathy manifested by abnormal cardiovascular responses to tilting, and nine developed frank orthostatic hypotension (41). In some of these patients it is advisable to perform physical therapy and occupational therapy as well as general exercise programs in the seated or recumbent position.

ADAPTATIONS FOR THERAPEUTIC AND RECREATIONAL EXERCISE

It is imperative that visually impaired individuals have the same opportunity for physical activity as their sighted counterparts. Although a physical fitness program is recognized as an important component of the education curriculum for visually impaired children, many progress to adolescence and adulthood without the opportunity to develop healthy exercise habits (42). Adults with acquired visual deficits often withdraw from previous activities and are apprehensive to undertake new forms of exercise. Because of social isolation, lack of access, or discomfort with unfamiliar settings, they do not join exercise classes or utilize community exercise facilities. A complete rehabilitation program for visually impaired individuals should encourage lifelong exercise habits and should offer instruction in adaptive exercise training. A comprehensive exercise program design must address (a) modifications of the exercise environment and equipment, (b) safety precautions for unstable eye disease, and (c) accommodations for special problems imposed by concurrent disease and disability.

Environmental Modifications

Visually impaired individuals are more apt to have a positive experience on initiation of an exercise program if they are comfortable with the program personnel and the physical setting. The exercise instructor and support staff should receive sensitivity training and should learn sighted guide techniques. Visually impaired participants should receive hands-on orientation to the exercise facility and equipment. Location of exercise stations, locker rooms, and rest rooms must be included in the orientation.

During warm-up and cool-down exercises, persons with severe visual impairments need to be stationed near a wall, chair, or other solid object, which can be used as a center for spatial orientation and support. Exercise routines should be described verbally, and movements should be demonstrated individually until the routines are mastered. Participants can select from multiple aerobic options such as walking, running, stationary bicycling, and swimming. Visually impaired persons can participate in dance aerobics when time is allowed for proper demonstration of movements (42). Existing indoor and outdoor tracks for walking and running can be modified by installing a guide rope along the perimeter of the track. A single-lane track can be improvised by stringing a guide rope along the length of the exercise room or designating an area adjacent to a long straight segment of wall. By maintaining hand contact with the rope or wall, even a totally blind individual will feel more confident and safe and will be able to focus efforts more effectively on the exercise activity. At home, one may establish a guide rope to walk repetitive laps along a driveway or yard or designate an indoor walking lane along an uncluttered hallway or other wall space. Persons who have honed cane-travel skills can select safe low-traffic walking routes. Those who prefer other forms of indoor exercise, at home or at a public facility, can choose from a variety of aerobic exercise equipment including treadmills, step trainers, stationary bicycles, cross-country ski synthesizers, rowing machines, and exercise gliders. Before using equipment, the visually impaired person should have an opportunity to manually explore all moving parts and controls. Dial settings and touch panels can be marked with Braille or raised dots. Swimming is another excellent aerobic option. Blind swimmers may have difficulty maintaining orientation and staying within the boundaries of designated lap lanes. To overcome this problem, they can align themselves with conventional floating lane markers and periodically brush a hand against the lane marker to maintain a straight course (43–47).

Precautions for Unstable Eye Conditions

Individuals who have had recent eye surgery or those with unstable eye conditions may be advised to curtail physical activities. However, in diseases such as proliferative diabetic retinopathy, the condition may be chronic. Prolonged inactivity will lead to severe cardiovascular and musculoskeletal deconditioning (44,48). If appropriate precautions are taken, an exercise training program can be designed to promote cardiovascular and general fitness without aggravating the pathologic eye condition (43,44). The role of exercise in inducing retinal hemorrhage is uncertain. However, abnormalities in systemic blood pressure and local blood flow to the eye have been observed in patients with proliferative diabetic retinopathy (49). Hence, it seems wise to limit blood pressure excursions during exercise. In one exercise program, involving 29 participants with proliferative diabetic retinopathy, no visual deterioration was noted when systolic blood pressures were maintained below 200 mm Hg and were not allowed to exceed the baseline by an increment greater than 50 mm Hg (44,48).

There are no definitive studies, but cautious recommendations for persons with active diabetic retinopathy and other unstable eye conditions are (a) to keep the head elevated (avoid forward bending from the waist), (b) to avoid the supine or prone position, (c) to avoid contact sports, (d) to avoid vigorous bouncing exercises (e.g., jumping, jogging), and (e) to avoid isometric exercises and heavy weight lifting with the associated Valsalva maneuver.

To adhere to these recommendations, an exercise program can be developed in which warm-up and cool-down exercises are performed from an erect sitting or standing position. Preferred aerobic selections would include low-impact activities such as walking, stationary bicycling, and rowing (43,44).

Special Considerations for Diabetes Mellitus

Diabetes is the leading cause of blindness for middle-aged and older adults in the United States. Rehabilitation specialists involved in designing exercise programs and mobility training for persons with diabetes and visual impairment will need to consider other concurrent complications of the disease. Even when precautions are taken to minimize deterioration of the eye disease, there will be concerns about blood glucose excursions during exercise as well as cardiac, renal, and neurologic dysfunction.

Exercise can induce low blood sugar in persons receiving insulin or oral antiglycemic medications. Previously inactive individuals may experience low blood sugar even with low to moderate levels of activity (41). Because insulin and other medications are planned to match food ingestion, exercise and mobility training sessions should be planned to avoid delays or omissions of meals. The instructor or the participant should carry a source of carbohydrate such as fruit juice, hard candy, or glucose tablets. These items should be ingested if the individual develops symptoms of low blood sugar (weakness, shaking, sweating, palpitations, headaches, confusion), and the training session should be discontinued until these symptoms completely resolve. Some persons with a very high blood sugar will experience fatigue or have difficulty concentrating, necessitating postponement of the training session. Others will have no obvious symptoms and will have no difficulty in continuing with the planned session.

Manifestations of diabetic neuropathy may include diminished sensations in the hands and feet as well as loss of muscle strength and balance. Autonomic nervous system dysfunction may result in orthostatic hypotension and poor exercise tolerance, related to abnormal cardiac and circulatory responses. Persons with these problems may need to perform all exercises stationed near a wall or solid piece of furniture or may need to carry out exercise routines from a seated position. Those with orthostatic hypotension, who are unable to remain standing for sustained periods, may select aerobic activities such as rowing or bicycling from a semirecumbent position. The latter can be achieved by seating the individual in an arm chair placed behind the seat of a conventional stationary bicycle, or through the use of a semirecumbent bicycle (41,44).

Sensory loss to the feet combined with circulatory problems places the individual at high risk for foot injury, which may lead to infection or amputation. Persons with severe neuropathy or existing foot injuries should avoid weight-bearing exercise, although light cycling, rowing, and upper body activities may be appropriate. In all cases, it is essential that footwear be comfortable, properly fitted, and adequately protective. The feet should be inspected before and after each exercise session for signs of pressure and friction injury. Abrasions and blisters should receive appropriate medical attention and should be observed until completely healed (50,51).

Participation in exercise and mobility training may be limited by heart and kidney disease, which frequently accompany failing vision. Individuals should be evaluated by a physician before initiating an exercise program. Aerobic activity should be selected according to the individual's abilities and needs. The heart rate and blood pressure should be monitored throughout the exercise session. Individuals should be taught how to measure their own pulse rates, and they should be given guidelines to curtail exercise if the heart rate or blood pressure exceeds preset limits. Aerobic programs should begin at low levels, and the length and level of the exercise should be gradually incremented as the individual develops improved strength and cardiovascular conditioning. Once individuals have learned the principles of safe exercise and appropriate goals have been determined, they may continue to exercise independently using home equipment or walking in safe environments.

A model 12-week program, including three exercise sessions per week, was designed specifically to meet the needs of visually impaired individuals with diabetes mellitus (43,44). All of the precautions and principles discussed were incorporated into the exercise program. There were moderate improvements in diabetes control with decreased insulin requirements. There were moderate improvements in exercise tolerance, opening the potential for other work and leisure activities. Patients with the poorest baseline conditioning derived the most cardiovascular benefit (48). Improvements in psychosocial function were also observed, which may have been related to enhanced self-confidence, better balance and coordination, and the facilitation of social interactions (43,44,47,52). Other exercise programs have been described for patients with diabetes and visual impairment, although outcome data have not been reported (45,46).

Persons with other neuromuscular problems and systemic disease in conjunction with visual impairment may benefit from similar adaptations to exercise. Specific needs should be analyzed so that individualized exercise programs can be developed. The final objective of every exercise training program should be to teach the participants safe and practical exercise routines that can be maintained in the home environment and that will enhance general health and the ability to undertake occupational and leisure activities.

CONCLUSIONS: BRIDGING TWO WORLDS

The worlds of rehabilitation medicine and vision rehabilitation, which commingled their expertise in the postwar years, have since then gone their separate ways. Both have produced their own specialists and unique therapeutic approaches to the disabilities and handicaps of their target populations. Both continue to have distinct scholarly journals *(Journal of Vision Impairment and Blindness, Journal of Vision Rehabilitation).* And both have established distinct roles as advocates for their patients. But the commonalities are stronger than the distinctions, and contemporary trends favor a return to the earlier intimacy between these worlds. The aging population guarantees an ever-increasing supply of patients with combinations of visual and superimposed medical disabilities; in such cases, a more eclectic treatment approach is necessary to address the multiple functional losses that ensue. Neither system can adequately address this challenge on its own. Similarly, the visual impairments produced by such common rehabilitation diagnoses as CVA, TBI, MS, and IDDM demand greater knowledge of vision rehabilitation options by physiatrists. Finally, the increasing role of managed care in medical decision making and service reimbursement encourages the concept of the physiatrist as primary care physician for people with physical disabilities. Such a conceptual model would be unthinkable if the practitioner were to remain ignorant of the rehabilitation methods appropriate for a group of over 4,000,000 individuals.

A provocative recent article by Massof and co-workers (53) demonstrates that the rehabilitation paradigm can be applied to the vision care system and can be used to justify reimbursement of vision rehabilitation services by third-party payers such as Medicare or Medicaid. Physiatrists are ideally suited for the role of medical coordinator of these patients by virtue of their training, their patient-centered and functionally oriented approach, and their traditional role as advocates for persons with disabilities. This is a wonderful opportunity to expand physiatric involvement into an area with which it has long historical associations. A half-century after the global conflict that spurred their simultaneous evolution into modern specialties, the two worlds need to commingle their respective identities once again, and both of them ought to be the stronger and more effective from their association.

APPENDIX: INFORMATION SOURCES FOR PHYSICIANS AND/OR CONSUMERS

American Council of the Blind (ACB)
1155 15th Street, NW, Suite 720
Washington, D.C. 20005
800-424-8666 (3 p.m. to 5:30 p.m.)
202-467-5081

American Foundation for the Blind (AFB)
11 Penn Plaza, Suite 300
New York, NY 10001
800-232-5463
212-502-7600
212-947-1060

American Printing House for the Blind (APH)
1839 Frankfort Avenue
Louisville, KY 40206
800-223-1839
502-895-2405

Blinded Veterans Association
477 H Street, Northwest
Washington, D.C. 20001-2694
800-699-7079
202-371-8880

Council of Citizens with Low Vision International (CCLVI)
6511 26th Street, West
Bradenton, FL 34207
800-733-2258
941-755-9721

Library of Congress
National Library Service for the Blind
and Physically Handicapped
1291 Taylor Street, Northwest
Washington, D.C. 20542
800-424-8567
202-707-5100

The Lighthouse, Inc.
111 East 59th Street
New York, NY 10022
800-334-5497
212-821-9200

National Association for Visually Handicapped
22 West 21st Street
New York, NY 10010
212-889-3141

National Federation of the Blind (NFB)
1800 Johnson Street
Baltimore, MD 21230
410-659-9314

Recordings for the Blind and Dyslexic
The Anne T. MacDonald Center
20 Roszel Road
Princeton, NJ 08540
800-221-4792
609-452-0606

REFERENCES

1. Wainapel SF. Vision rehabilitation: an overlooked subject in physiatric training and practice. *Am J Phys Med Rehabil* 1995; 74:313–314.
2. Lupinacci M. Physiatric management of the visually impaired disabled patient. *Curr Concepts Rehabil Med* 1990; 5:6–13.
3. Goodpasture RC. Rehabilitation of the blind. In: Krusen FH, Kottke FJ, Ellwood PM, eds. *Handbook of physical medicine and rehabilitation, 2nd ed.* Philadelphia: WB Saunders, 1971.
4. Rusk HA. *A world to care for.* New York: Random House, 1977.
5. Koestler FA. *The unseen minority: A history of the blind in America.* New York: American Foundation for the Blind, 1976.
6. Rabin DL, Stockton P. *Long-term care for the elderly.* New York: Oxford University Press, 1987.
7. Kenney RA. *Physiology of aging, 2nd ed.* Chicago: Year Book Medical Publishers, 1989.
8. Nelson KA, Dimitrova E. Severe visual impairment in the United States and in each state, 1990. *J Vis Impairment Blind* 1993; 87:80–86.
9. Altner PE, Rusin JJ, DeBoer A. Rehabilitation of blind patients with lower extremity amputations. *Arch Phys Med Rehabil* 1980; 61:82–85.
10. Fisher R. Rehabilitation of the blind amputee: a rewarding experience. *Arch Phys Med Rehabil* 1987; 68:382–383.
11. Wainapel SF. Rehabilitation of the blind stroke patient. *Arch Phys Med Rehabil* 1984; 65:487–489.

12. Wainapel SF, Kwon YS, Fazzari PJ. Severe visual impairment on a rehabilitation unit: incidence and implications. *Arch Phys Med Rehabil* 1989; 70:439–441.
13. Tobis JS, Block M, Steinhaus-Donham C, Reinsch S, Tamaru K, Weil D. Falling among the sensorially impaired elderly. *Arch Phys Med Rehabil* 1990; 71:144–147.
14. Tinetti M, Inouye S, Gill T, Doucette J. Shared risk factors for falls, incontinence, and functional dependence. *JAMA* 1995; 273: 1348–1353.
15. Stones MV, Kozma A. Balance and age in the sighted and blind. *Arch Phys Med Rehabil* 1987; 68:85–89.
16. Cohn TE, Lasley DJ. Visual depth illusion and falls in the elderly. *Clin Geriatr Med* 1985; 1:601–620.
17. Felson D, Anderson JJ, Hannan MT, Milton RC, Wilson PWF, Kiel DP. Impaired vision and hip fracture: the Framingham Study. *J Am Geriatr Soc* 1989; 37:495–500.
18. Carabellese C, Appollonio I, Rozzini R, Bianchetti A, Frisoni G, Frattola L, Trabucchi M. Sensory Impairment and Quality of Life in Community Elderly Population. *J Am Geriatr Soc* 1993; 41:401–407.
19. Branch LG, Horowitz A, Carr C. The implications for everyday life of incident self-reported visual decline among people over age 65 living in the community. *Gerontologist* 1989; 29:359–365.
20. Gillman AE, Simmel A, Simon EP. Visual handicap in the aged: Self-reported visual disability and the quality of life of residents of public housing for the elderly. *J Vis Impairment Blind* 1986; 80:588–590.
21. Kahn HA, Liebowitz HM, Ganley JP. The Framingham Eye Study: outline and major prevalence findings. *Am J Epidemiol* 1977; 106: 17–32.
22. Faye EE, Stuen CS. *The aging eye and low vision.* New York: The Lighthouse, 1992.
23. Obstbaum SA. Clinical crossroads: an 82 year old woman with cataracts. *JAMA* 1996; 275:1675–1680.
24. Steinberg EP, Tielsch JM, Schein OD. National study of cataract surgery outcomes: variations in four month postoperative outcomes as reflected in multiple outcome measures. *Ophthalmology* 1994; 101: 1142–1152.
25. Applegate WB, Miller ST, Elam JT, Freeman JM, Wood TO, Gettlefinger TC. Impact of cataract surgery with lens implantation on vision and physical function in elderly patients. *JAMA* 1987; 257:1064–1066.
26. Klein R, Klein BEK. Vision disorders in diabetes. In: National Diabetes Data Group, eds. *Diabetes in America, 2nd ed.* Bethesda: National Institutes of Health, 1995; 293–337.
27. Diabetes Control and Complications Trial Research Group. The effect of intensive treatment of diabetes on the development and progression of long-term complications in insulin-dependent diabetes mellitus. *N Eng J Med* 1993; 329:977–986.
28. Ferris FL 3rd. Diabetic retinopathy. *Diabetes Care* 1993; 16:322–325.
29. Diabetic Retinopathy Study Research Group. Preliminary report on effects of photocoagulation therapy. *Am J Ophthalmol* 1976; 81: 383–396.
30. Early Treatment Diabetic Retinopathy Study Research Group. Photocoagulation for diabetic macular edema. Early Treatment Diabetic Retinopathy Study report number 1. *Arch Ophthalmol* 1985; 103: 1796–1806.
31. Raskin P, Arauz-Pacheco C. The treatment of diabetic retinopathy: a view for the internist. *Ann Intern Med* 1992; 117:226–233.
32. Kohner EM. Diabetic retinopathy. *Br Med J* 1993; 307:1195–1199.
33. Rosenthal BP, Cole RG. *Functional assessment of low vision.* St Louis: CV Mosby, 1996.
34. Havlik RJ. *Aging in the eighties. Impaired senses for sound and light in persons aged 65 years and over. Preliminary data from the Supplement on Aging to the National Health Interview Survey; United States, Jan–June, 1984. Advanced Data from Vital and Health Statistics. DHHS Publication # (PHS) 86-1250.* Hyattsville, MD: United States Department of Health and Human Services, 1986.
35. Faye EE. *Clinical low vision.* Boston: Little, Brown, 1984.
36. Cole RG, Rosenthal BP. *Remediation and management of low vision.* St Louis: CV Mosby, 1996.
37. Walsh R, Blasch BB. *Foundations of orientation and mobility.* New York: American Foundation for the Blind, 1983.
38. Coleman CL, Weinstock RF. Physically handicapped blind people: adaptive mobility techniques. *J Vis Impairment Blind* 1984; 78: 113–117.
39. Butter C, Kirsch N. Combined and separate effects of eye patching and visual stimulation on unilateral neglect following stroke. *Arch Phys Med Rehabil* 1992; 73:133–1139.
40. Gianutsos R, Ramsey G, Perlin R. Rehabilitative optometric services for survivors of acquired brain injury. *Arch Phys Med Rehabil* 1988; 69:573–578.
41. Bernbaum M, Albert SG, Cohen JD. Exercise training in individuals with diabetic retinopathy and blindness. *Arch Phys Med Rehabil* 1989; 70:605–611.
42. Ponchillia SV, Powell LL, Felski KA, Nichlawski MT. The effectiveness of aerobic exercise instruction for totally blind women. *J Vis Impairment Blind* 1992; 86:174–177.
43. Bernbaum M, Albert SG, Brusca SR, Drimmer A, Duckro PN. A team approach. Promoting diabetes self-management and independence in the visually impaired: A model clinical program. *Diabetes Educ* 1988; 14:51–54.
44. Bernbaum M, Albert SG, Brusca SR, et al. A model clinical program for patients with diabetes and vision impairment. *Diabetes Educ* 1989; 15:325–330.
45. Dods J. Two exercise programs for people with diabetes and visual impairment. *J Vis Impairment Blind* 1993; 87:365–367.
46. Weitzman DM. Promoting healthful exercise for visually impaired persons with diabetes. *J Vis Impairment Blind* 1993; 87:361–364.
47. Albert SG, Bernbaum M. Exercise for patients with diabetic retinopathy. *Diabetes Care* 1995; 18:130–132.
48. Bernbaum M, Albert SG, Cohen JD, Drimmer A. Cardiovascular conditioning in individuals with diabetic retinopathy. *Diabetes Care* 1989; 12:740–742.
49. Albert SG, Gomez CR, Russell S, Chaitman BR, Bernbaum M, Kong B. Cerebral and ophthalmic artery hemodynamic responses in diabetes mellitus. *Diabetes Care* 1993; 16:476–482.
50. Caputo GM, Cavanagh PR, Ulbrecht JS, Gibbons GW, Karchmer AW. Assessment and management of foot disease in patients with diabetes. *N Engl J Med* 1994; 331:854–860.
51. Plummer ES, Albert SG. Foot care assessment in patients with diabetes mellitus: A screening algorithm for patient education and referral. *Diabetes Educ* 1995; 21:47–51.
52. Bernbaum M, Albert SG, Duckro PN. Psychosocial profiles in patients with visual impairment due to diabetic retinopathy. *Diabetes Care* 1988; 11:551–557.
53. Massof RW, Dagnelie G, Deremeik JT, DeRose JL, Alibhai SS, Glasner NM. Low vision rehabilitation in the US health care system. *J Vis Rehabil* 1995; 9:3–31.

Rehabilitation Medicine: Principles and Practice, Third Edition,
edited by Joel A. DeLisa and Bruce M. Gans.
Lippincott–Raven Publishers, Philadelphia © 1998.

CHAPTER 70

Rehabilitation of the Hearing Impaired

Paul R. Kileny and Teresa A. Zwolan

HEARING IMPAIRMENT IN ADULTS AND CHILDREN

Hearing loss is the second most common cause of disability in the United States (1). Of the approximately 20 million Americans with impaired hearing, over 2 million are profoundly deaf. The prevalence of hearing impairment increases with age. For instance, for individuals 85 years and older, the prevalence of hearing impairment reaches 48%. Hearing impairment impacts negatively on communication ability, socioeconomic status, reading skills, and cognitive function (2–5).

Accurate diagnosis of hearing loss is an important requirement for the achievement of appropriate treatment and rehabilitation. Often, however, the diagnosis may be delayed or incorrect. In the pediatric age group, diagnosis of hearing loss in the United States does not occur until the age of 2½ on the average (6). This leads to delayed language skills and delayed psychological and cognitive development in congenitally hearing-impaired children (7). Accurate and early detection of hearing loss in infants is readily available, however, through screening programs. These programs may focus on all newborns (i.e., universal hearing screening) or just on those with risk factors for hearing impairment (8). At the University of Michigan Medical Center, for example, screening of high-risk newborns has reduced the average age of diagnosis to below 6 months, making earlier intervention possible and effective. Prompt and accurate diagnosis of hearing impairment in the older patient population may also improve patient outcome. For instance, accurate diagnosis of hearing loss may reduce the occurrence of attributing the behavior associated with hearing loss to dementia (9). Fitting older patients with appropriate amplification and providing them with a rehabilitation program will avoid the isolation associated with hearing impairment and inappropriate institutional placements.

P. R. Kileny: Department of Otolaryngology—Head and Neck Surgery, University of Michigan Medical Center, Ann Arbor, Michigan 48109.

T. A. Zwolan: Department of Otolaryngology, University of Michigan, Ann Arbor, Michigan 48108.

THE AUDITORY SYSTEM: PATHOPHYSIOLOGY AND CLINICAL CORRELATES

The special sense of hearing is supported by a complex sensory system that deals with a variety of acoustic signals originating from a variety of sources. It combines finely tuned biomechanical components (the external and middle ear) and intricate neural receptors (hair cells of the organ of Corti). The auditory signal is further processed along a central nervous system pathway including the cochlear nuclei, superior olivary complex, lateral lemniscus, inferior colliculus, medial geniculate, and auditory cortex.

When dealing with the auditory system for diagnostic or therapeutic purposes, there is a tendency to divide it into four anatomic regions: the external ear, including the auricle and ear canal; the middle ear, including the tympanic membrane and ossicular chain; the inner ear, communicating with the middle ear through the round and oval windows and containing the cochlear receptors or hair cells; and the central auditory pathways, beginning with the neurons of the spiral ganglion and ending up at the auditory cortex. The auricle and the ear canal contribute to sound localization and funnel sound waves to the tympanic membrane. The ear canal resonates at approximately 3,800 Hz and, as a result, modifies incoming sounds. The eardrum and the ossicular chain together constitute a compensatory mechanism for the inherent loss of acoustic energy that occurs at the interface of a low-density gaseous medium and the much-higher-impedance medium of the fluid-filled cochlea. Much of this energy loss is compensated for through two primary mechanisms: the lever advantage of the ossicular chain assembly (malleus, incus, stapes) and the advantage of the area of the eardrum–oval window ratio. Thus, a disorder affecting this transmission or conductive mechanism will result in less energy being transmitted to the inner ear or, in other words, will contribute to the attenuation of the acoustic energy.

Causes for conductive hearing loss may include congenital malformations of the external ear, middle-ear effusion, Eustachian tube dysfunction, fixation of the stapes footplate as a sequel of otosclerosis, and fracture of the ossicular chain resulting from a traumatic head injury. Disorders secondary to middle-ear pathology that may present as neurologic disease include lateral sinus thrombosis, cholesteatoma, glomus jugulare tumor, and mastoiditis (10,11).

Patients with a conductive hearing loss typically report that all types of sounds (speech, music, etc.) are softer; however, they rarely exhibit reduced speech recognition if loudness is sufficiently increased to compensate for the conductive loss. Audiograms of patients with conductive hearing loss are characterized by an air–bone gap, simply indicating that thresholds by air conduction (i.e., sounds delivered by means of an earphone) exceed thresholds obtained by bone conduction (sounds delivered to the ear by means of a bone vibrator coupled to the mastoid process), as illustrated in Figure 70-1.

An additional tool useful in the diagnosis of conductive hearing loss is the acoustic immittance battery. Acoustic immittance instrumentation includes a probe introduced into the external ear canal to form an airtight seal. Testing consists of the delivery of a probe tone to the ear and the measurement of the magnitude of the reflected acoustic energy from the eardrum. The magnitude of the reflected acoustic energy changes as a function of middle-ear and eardrum status: the less compliant the system, the higher the intensity of the reflected tone. Tympanometry, which measures the compliance of the eardrum as a function of changes in air pressure (also varied through the probe) in the ear canal, provides information regarding middle-ear pressure, tympanic membrane mobility, Eustachian tube function, and continuity and mobility of the middle-ear ossicles. Examples of tympanograms showing (a) normal middle-ear pressure and normal mobility and (b) normal mobility with abnormal (negative) middle-ear pressure are presented in Figure 70-2.

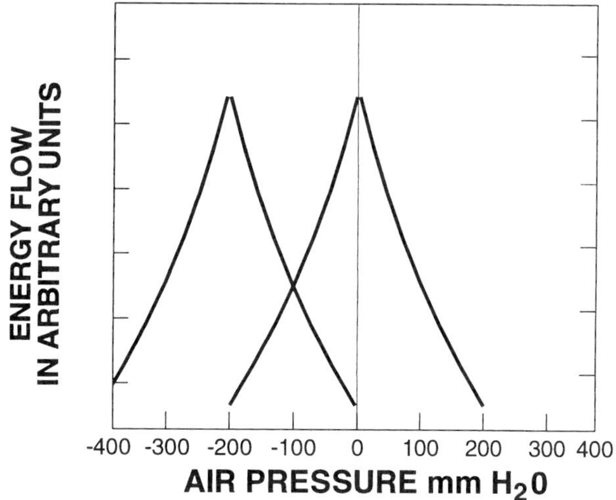

FIG. 70-2. Normal tympanogram with negative-pressure tympanogram (−250 mm H_2O) superimposed.

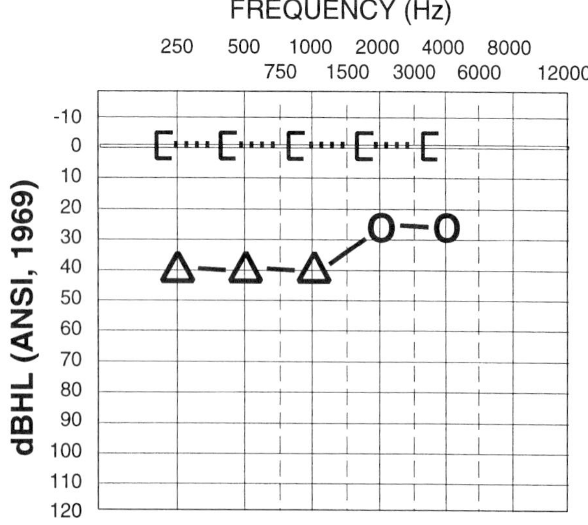

FIG. 70-1. Audiogram indicating a conductive hearing loss.

Acoustic reflex tests, which measure changes in tympanic membrane compliance caused by contraction of the stapedius muscle, are particularly useful for differentiation of cochlear and retrocochlear sites of lesion. The acoustic reflex threshold test determines the softest level of sound that will elicit stapedius muscle contraction, which normally occurs bilaterally following either ipsilateral or contralateral stimulation with pure tones or noise ranging in intensity from 70 to 95 dB sound pressure level (SPL). The stapedius reflex arc includes the ventral cochlear nucleus, the medial superior olive, the motor nucleus of the seventh cranial nerve, and the seventh cranial nerve, which innervates the stapedius (12). Acoustic reflex decay measures the ability of the stapedius muscle to sustain contraction. During this test, a signal is presented 10 dB above the acoustic reflex threshold for a period of 10 seconds. A response is considered abnormal if the amplitude of the reflex response decreases to one-half or less amplitude within 5 seconds. Persons with a conductive hearing loss characteristically demonstrate abnormal tympanograms, elevated or absent acoustic reflex thresholds, and, when measurable, negative acoustic reflex decay.

Conductive hearing losses are potentially amenable to surgical correction. Although there are no firmly established practices, in most cases, otologists will not consider surgical correction of a conductive component that is less than 20 dB. For instance, a conductive hearing loss resulting from a large tympanic membrane perforation may be corrected by a tympanoplasty procedure. This technique involves the use of a temporalis fascia graft to repair the tympanic membrane perforation. An ossicular problem may be reconstructed by means of a variety of implantable prostheses. The most common surgical procedure for the correction of conductive hearing loss is the myringotomy and the insertion of ventilation tubes into the tympanic membrane for the treatment of chronic otitis media. This procedure is most commonly done in younger patients (aged ≤6 years) in whom there is a high prevalence of otitis media.

A conductive pathology may occur simultaneously with a cochlear or retrocochlear problem. Therefore, knowledge regarding outer- and middle-ear function is needed for accurate interpretation of audiologic measures used to evaluate the central auditory system.

The cochlea may be considered to serve a dual role. First, the highly specialized sensory receptors, the hair cells, transduce the mechanical stage of audition to a neurochemical message, the onset of synaptic transmission. Second, the mechanical tuning characteristics of the basilar membrane, which supports the hair cells of the organ of Corti, constitute the earliest and perhaps the most important stage of frequency analysis. Thus, specific regions along the basilar membrane are primarily displaced by certain frequencies, activating segments of the hair-cell populations corresponding to specific frequencies. For instance, the basal end of the basilar membrane (that which is closest to the stapes footplate) is primarily activated by high-frequency sounds, and therefore, a loss of the hair-cell population in that region coincides with a high-frequency hearing loss. Audiograms of patients with cochlear sensorineural hearing loss are characterized by an equal elevation of both air-conduction and bone-conduction thresholds, as shown in Figure 70-3.

The phenomenon of loudness recruitment (an abnormal growth of loudness), which causes reduced dynamic range, has in the past been exploited to differentially diagnose between cochlear and eighth cranial nerve hearing impairment because purely eighth cranial nerve lesions are not characterized by this phenomenon. Two of the best known tests of recruitment are the Alternate Binaural Loudness Balance Test (ABLB) (13) and the Short Increment Sensitivity Index (SISI) (14). The ABLB compares the loudness of a tone in the impaired ear to the same or a different tone in the unaffected ear. In cases of recruitment, tones of equal intensity will be judged equally loud in the impaired and unimpaired ear despite elevated thresholds in the impaired ear. Therefore, the range between threshold and equal loudness sensation is reduced in the impaired ear. The SISI assesses the percentage of 1-dB intensity increments distinguished when superimposed on a continuous tone. The ability to perceive these small increment changes (high percentage SISI scores) is associated with cochlear involvement, whereas low scores are associated with eighth nerve pathology (15).

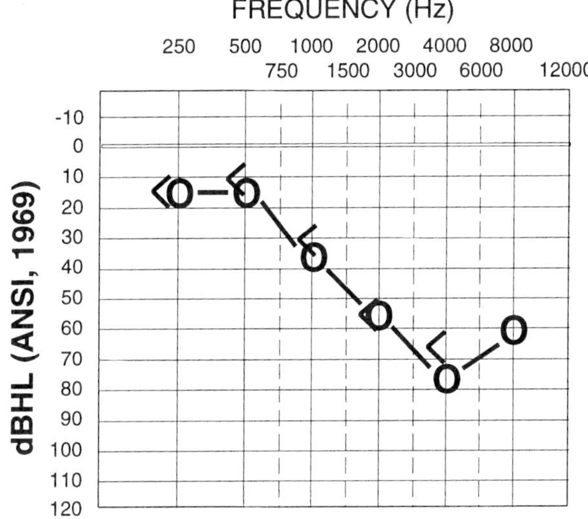

FIG. 70-3. Audiogram indicating high-frequency sensorineural hearing loss.

Another phenomenon associated with a cochlear site of lesion is a reduction in speech recognition, which is usually tested using standardized monosyllabic word lists presented either live voice or, preferably, using taped material (for instance, NU-6 Word List, Auditec, St. Louis, MO). Because a cochlear site of lesion reduces or subtracts neural elements, patients with a sensorineural hearing loss (both cochlear and retrocochlear) typically have reduced speech-recognition scores, even when materials are presented well within their audible range. Therefore, one might consider a cochlear site of lesion as a subtractive lesion, whereas a conductive loss may be considered as an attenuating-type lesion. Patients with lesions of the eighth cranial nerve or beyond tend to have lower speech-recognition scores than those with a cochlear site of lesion. The extreme of this phenomenon is in patients with cortical lesions, who may be entirely unable to understand speech or recognize other complex auditory signals.

Two immittance measures useful for differentiating cochlear and retrocochlear lesions include acoustic reflex threshold and acoustic reflex decay. In patients with a cochlear loss, acoustic reflexes may be present at reduced sensation levels, indicating recruitment. More frequently, however, the acoustic reflex thresholds may be elevated or absent, depending on the severity of the hearing loss. Acoustic reflex decay testing often reveals that patients with a cochlear hearing loss are able to sustain contraction of the stapedius muscle for more than 10 seconds, whereas patients with a retrocochlear loss often demonstrate marked decay in the amplitude of the reflex response.

The most effective audiologic tool for differentiation of cochlear and retrocochlear sites of lesion is the auditory brainstem response (ABR). The ABR is the averaged surface-recorded manifestation of the neuroelectric activation of auditory neural generators extending from the cochlea to upper brainstem or lower midbrain (Fig. 70-4) (16). It is generally agreed that the ABR provides little or no diagnostic information for cochlear hearing impairment (17,18). However, the overall configuration and latency of the ABR are, in general, affected by hearing loss, including cochlear hearing loss. For instance, a 75-dB normal hearing level (nHL) click delivered to a normal-hearing ear in a neurologically normal patient will evoke a well-defined ABR consisting of waves I through V, but the same stimulus delivered to an ear with

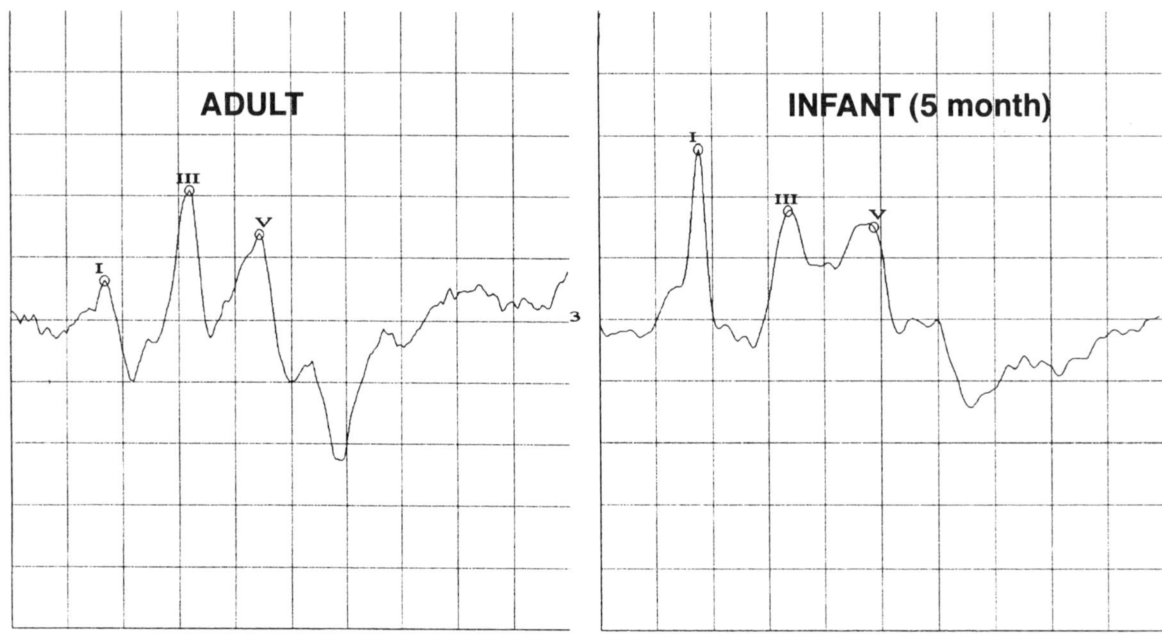

FIG. 70-4. Auditory brainstem responses (ABRs) from normal-hearing and neurologically normal adult **(left)** and 4-month-old infant **(right).** Note similar response morphologies but longer response latency of infant ABR peaks. (Calibration: 1.5 msec/division; 0.15 μV/division.)

a high-frequency cochlear hearing loss will result in an ABR with a poorly defined or absent wave I and a delayed wave V. These changes result from the loss of neural receptor elements in the basal, high-frequency region of the cochlea, which, under normal circumstances, dominate the click-evoked ABR. A delayed wave V in high-frequency cochlear hearing loss is the result of the predominant activation of the more apical regions of the cochlea, and this is associated with an appropriate time delay. In some cases of cochlear hearing loss, an increase in stimulus intensity will compensate the poor morphology of the response, resulting in well-defined waves I through V and normal interpeak latencies but a delay in the overall absolute latency of the ABR (19).

REHABILITATION OF HEARING IMPAIRMENT

In addition to the medical and audiologic components of the diagnosis, management of sensorineural hearing impairment also involves the assessment of the extent to which hearing loss affects communication. If medical or surgical treatment is not considered or is inappropriate, the patient needs to be informed about the availability of appropriate assistive devices to maximize residual hearing. This, of course, includes determination of the best amplification system for the patient. Additionally, information regarding community resources and support networks for hearing-impaired persons is also important.

Hearing Aids

A hearing aid is an electronic prosthetic device that amplifies and shapes acoustic signals delivered to the external auditory canal. There have been significant esthetic and electronic advances in hearing aids since the first bulky electric hearing aids became available 40 to 50 years ago. These first electric hearing aids were not highly effective for sensorineural hearing loss, but marked improvements in technology have made it possible for hearing aids to be effective today in patients with sensorineural hearing losses with a variety of configurations. Although hearing aids are used in patients as young as 6 months of age, the average age of Americans utilizing a hearing aid ranges from 55 to 70 years (20). This average age is the result of the disproportionately large number of elderly hearing-impaired persons using hearing aids.

In 1977, the U.S. Food and Drug Administration (FDA) issued regulations (currently under revision) setting standards to be followed by dispensers of hearing aids. These regulations required that hearing aid candidates receive a medical evaluation within 6 months before the purchase of a hearing aid. This examination may be waived by adults after receiving proper informed consent notification that such an evaluation may be in their best interest. Patients under the age of 18 years must be evaluated by an audiologist (21). Additionally, the FDA regulations further require that a medical consultation be obtained by a hearing aid recipient with any of the following present: visible congenital or traumatic deformity of the ear; active drainage from the ear; sudden or rapidly progressive hearing loss; acute or chronic dizziness; an air–bone gap of 15 dB or greater at 500, 1,000, and 2,000 Hz; evidence of excessive cerumen or foreign body in the ear canal; and/or pain or discomfort in the ear. Most states also require a license or registration for those who sell hearing aids.

In addition to its diagnostic significance, speech recognition testing is an integral component of a hearing aid evaluation. This measure may be used to determine the relative effectiveness of the hearing aid and may provide a basis for comparison of different hearing aids or different settings of the hearing aid. This test can also be performed with background noise to reproduce real-life situations. Patients with very low speech recognition scores may not experience an improvement in speech recognition even with substantial amplification. Hearing aids may not be effective and may be contraindicated in such cases. In addition to auditory factors, nonauditory factors also play an important role in the decision to use amplification (22). Such factors may include the patient's overall communication handicap, ability to tolerate amplification, motivation, and listening requirement. Bess and his colleagues (23) showed that 21% of elderly individuals who met at least one of four expected criteria for significant hearing loss experienced little communication or global dysfunction as a result of the hearing impairment. Children who lose their hearing before they have acquired language often suffer severe limitations in communication and usually benefit from amplification regardless of age. A hearing aid rehabilitation and training program significantly increases the benefit of the device (24).

Based on their physical characteristics, hearing aids may be divided into four basic types: body-aid, eyeglass, behind-the-ear (BTE), and in-the-ear or in-the-canal (ITE or ITC) (Fig. 70-5). Today, the most common types of hearing aids used by patients in the United States are the BTE and ITE/ITC types. A BTE hearing aid fits behind the auricle and has a hook-shaped rigid tube that fits over the ear. To this, a soft polyethylene tube is attached, ending with the custom-made ear mold that couples the hearing aid to the patient's ear canal. The ITE/ITC-type hearing aid consists of a single piece. Its shell is custom molded for each patient's ear canal. Depending on the specific type, this hearing aid may protrude slightly from the ear canal or be completely hidden inside the ear canal.

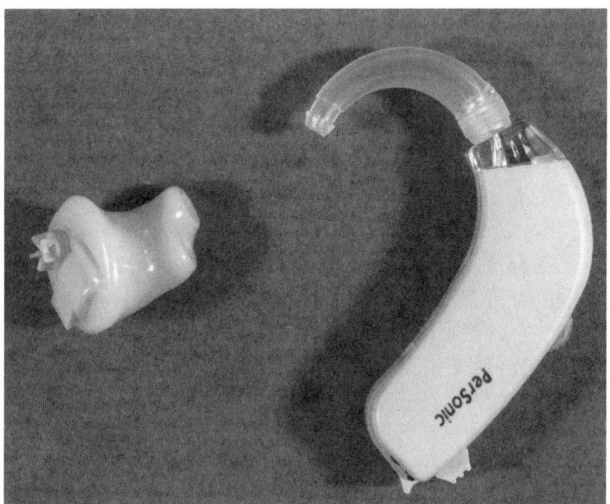

FIG. 70-5. Photographs of an in-the-canal (ITC) and a behind-the-ear (BTE) hearing aid.

Electronically, hearing aids may be divided into analog, hybrid, and digital hearing aids. The analog hearing aids function by converting acoustic energy to an electric signal that can be modified by the electronic components of the hearing aid. This modified electric waveform is then delivered to the speaker transducer of the hearing aid and converted back to acoustic energy, which is delivered to the ear canal through the ear mold of the BTE or through the ITE/ITC-type hearing aid. Hybrid hearing aids function somewhat similarly to analog hearing aids except that digital components are used to control or modify the operation of the analog components in the signal-processing stage. The advantage of the hybrid hearing aids is that they may have more flexibility than a standard analog hearing aid. Digital hearing aids use a different approach. With these, the electric signal is further modified to a digital signal composed of discrete signals coded by binary numbers. As a result, the waveform may be modified in multiple manners through changes in software. Inherent to digital circuitry, these hearing aids may have a higher-fidelity signal because of the absence of limitations imposed by standard analog circuit components that make up analog hearing aids. In theory, digital hearing aids may be programmed for individual specific needs. The disadvantage is that they command a substantially higher price ($2,000 to $3,000 each as opposed to $500 to $1,000 each) than analog hearing aids. Additionally, they also have increased power requirements. Currently, more patients are being fitted with analog and hybrid hearing aids than with digital hearing aids.

The ear mold of the BTE hearing aid and the molded shell of the ITE/ITC hearing aid are important and integral components of a hearing aid. Their shape, canal length, bore size, and vent size may be used judiciously to alter the acoustic output of any type of hearing aid. For instance, a relatively large vent will contribute to the attenuation of low-frequency sounds that is necessary for patients with high-frequency hearing loss and normal low-frequency thresholds (25). In spite of the fact that hearing aids have the potential to enhance communication in many individuals with hearing loss, there are a disproportionate number of hearing aid candidates who do not obtain hearing aids or who obtain them and do not use them. Cost is a major factor, as 59% of hearing aids are dispensed to the elderly, many of whom have limited financial resources (26). Medicare does not cover the cost of hearing aids, and Medicaid coverage varies by state. Franks et al. (27) investigated the use of hearing aids in an elderly population and found that the principal reason for not using hearing aids was high cost. Other reasons included the impression that use of hearing aids may call attention to their handicap, hearing aid dispenser sales techniques, concerns about the nature of the amplified sound, problems with manual dexterity in manipulating hearing aid controls, and lack of knowledge regarding sources for hearing aids. Another study (28) reported that 32% of hearing aid users had a variety of difficulties with their devices. Problems with ear mold fit, annoying acoustic feedback, the amplification of background noise, and distortion were factors most often mentioned in this study.

A knowledgeable and helpful audiologist can offer substantial assistance to patients with hearing aids. Several visits may be necessary before complete satisfaction with the hearing aid is achieved. It is important to note that most hearing aid dispensers provide patients with a 30-day free trial before requiring a final financial commitment. The choice of the specific type of hearing aid depends on several factors. The ITE/ITC-type aids are preferred by most because of their cosmetic appearance. However, as a result of their relatively small size and the difficulty in accessing their controls, patients need to have good vision and manual dexterity to manipulate them. This may be a problem for older patients.

Cochlear Implants (see Chapters 12 and 29)

Often, patients with a severe to profound sensorineural hearing loss are unable to receive benefit from a hearing aid because of an inability to detect the signal and/or inability to recognize speech, even when amplified into a detectable range. Recent surgical and technological advancements have provided such patients with an ability to hear with a cochlear implant.

A cochlear implant is an electronic device that provides useful hearing and improved communication ability for persons who have a severe to profound sensorineural hearing loss and who receive minimal benefit from conventional hearing aids. The technology of cochlear implantation has evolved from a device using a single channel to stimulate the ear to current devices that transmit sound information through multiple electrodes. Cochlear implants have been used with more than 15,000 adults and children worldwide. Cochlear implants are designed to provide useful sound information by directly stimulating surviving auditory nerve fibers. In order to obtain a cochlear implant, patients must have a bilateral severe to profound sensorineural hearing loss, demonstrate minimal benefit from traditional hearing aids, and demonstrate no medical or radiologic contraindications to surgery.

Cochlear implants consist of both internal and external components that work together in order for the patient to hear (Fig. 70-6). The implant works in the following manner: (a) sounds from the environment are picked up by the microphone, which is located on the patient's headset; (b) the sound travels from the microphone to the speech processor via a cable; (c) the speech processor filters, analyzes, and digitizes sound into coded signals; (d) the coded signals are sent from the speech processor to the transmitting coil via the cable (the transmitting coil is housed on the patient's headset); (e) the transmitting coil sends the signal across the patient's skin to the implanted receiver/stimulator via an FM radio signal; (f) the receiver/stimulator delivers the correct amount of electrical stimulation to the appropriate electrodes on the array. The electrodes stimulate the remaining auditory neural elements in the cochlea.

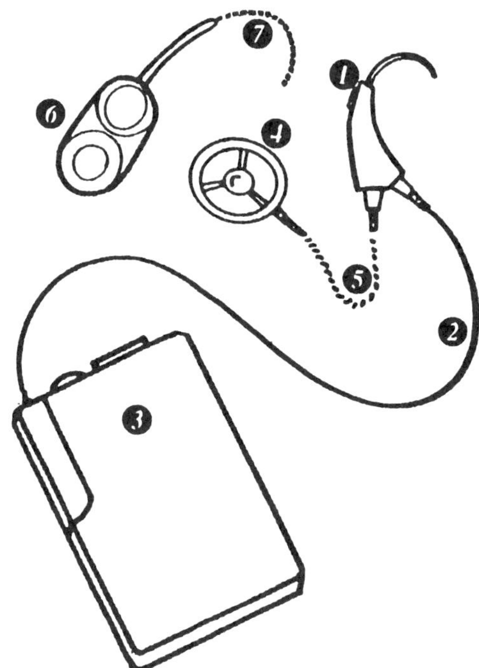

FIG. 70-6. Diagram indicating how a cochlear implant works. **1:** Sounds in the environment are picked up by a small microphone. **2:** The long cable sends the sound from the microphone to the speech processor, a powerful miniaturized computer. **3:** The speech processor filters, analyzes, and digitizes sound into coded signals. **4:** The coded signals are sent from the speech processor to the transmitting coil via the cables. **5:** The transmitting coil sends the signals across the skin to the implanted receiver/stimulator via an FM radio signal. **6:** The receiver/stimulator delivers the correct amount of electrical stimulation to the appropriate electrodes on the array. **7:** The electrodes along the array stimulate the remaining auditory nerve fibers in the cochlea. (Courtesy of Cochlear Corp.)

During cochlear implant surgery, the internal electrode array/receiver/stimulator is placed inside the cochlea. A postauricular incision is made, and a deep well is created in the mastoid bone so the receiver/stimulator will sit flush with the skull. The mastoid bone is drilled out, and the facial recess is opened to access the cochlea. The electrode array is then inserted into the cochlea via a cochleostomy drilled anterior to the round window. Typically, the surgery lasts 3 to 5 hours, and the length of hospital stay is usually limited to 24 hours. Patients who demonstrate cochlear ossification or cochlear malformations are still considered to be candidates for a cochlear implant, although such conditions may limit the amount of speech recognition they receive with their device. Surgery for such patients may be more complex and involve additional risks.

Approximately 4 weeks after surgery, patients return to the clinic for activation of their device. During this visit, the audiologist determines the appropriate levels of "first hearing" (threshold) and "loud but comfortable" for each electrode in the array. Following this programming, the patient is introduced to speech and to how it will sound with the cochlear implant.

The amount of rehabilitation following cochlear implantation varies from patient to patient and is affected by such variables as adjustment to the cochlear implant, frequency of need for reprogramming of the speech processor, rehabilitative services available near home or at school, and geographic location. In general, most adults are seen approximately 8 times during the first year and then annually thereafter. Children require more appointments for programming of their device and are seen approximately 12 times during the first year and, at a minimum, two times per year thereafter. Auditory training and speech and language therapy services are primarily delivered by the child's school. The clinic where the cochlear implant was performed works closely with the child's school to ensure that appropriate rehabilitation services are delivered.

There are several commercially available cochlear implant devices. These devices have received FDA approval for implantation in children (ages 2 to 17), prelingually deafened adults, and postlingually deafened adults with severe to profound sensorineural hearing losses. Additionally, clinical trials are currently under way to evaluate newer devices in both children and adults. Great variability is seen in the results being obtained by patients with cochlear implants in terms of their ability to recognize speech. However, in general, children who receive cochlear implants at a young age demonstrate speech recognition and speech production skills that are better than those being obtained by children with similar hearing losses who continue to use powerful hearing aids (29). Almost all postlingually deafened adults who receive multichannel cochlear implants demonstrate enhanced lip-reading ability when using their device, and most demonstrate enhanced speech recognition ability that enables them to understand some speech when using hearing alone (30). Additionally, many adult cochlear implant users are able to use the telephone. Although improvements in speech recognition skills of prelingually deafened adults are minimal, several of these patients report that they are satisfied with their device and that using the cochlear implant enhances their overall communication ability (31).

ASSISTIVE LISTENING DEVICES

Hearing-impaired patients may require instruction regarding devices (other than hearing aids or cochlear implants) that will enhance their overall communication ability. This includes assistive listening device counseling, fitting, and instruction.

Several types of assistive listening devices are available for persons with hearing impairment. Some of these devices are designed for use in conjunction with a hearing aid or cochlear implant, whereas others are designed to be used alone. The most commonly used types of assistive devices include alerting/warning systems, telephone devices, and devices to improve comprehension of speech.

Alerting/Warning Systems

Assistive alerting/warning systems are vital for many hearing-impaired persons, as they are unable to rely on their sense of hearing for notification that a particular event has occurred. Some of these devices are essential for safety purposes. For example, persons with a severe to profound hearing loss will be unable to hear a smoke alarm if it is activated during the night when they are not wearing their hearing aid or cochlear implant. Activation of a vibrator on the bed or illumination of an extremely bright light may save a life. Other devices may be used to alert them to environmental sounds, such as the telephone and/or doorbell ringing.

Alerting/warning devices may be electronic, visual, or kinesthetic. Alerting devices utilize a microphone to pick up sound in the environment. The information is then transmitted to a receiver, using either hard-wired or wireless technology. The receiver then activates a system that warns the listener about the presence of a particular sound. An auditory device may include a buzz or alarm that is loud and low-pitched and is more likely to be heard by the hearing-impaired person. Visual devices are available that activate a flashing, bright, or incandescent light, and kinesthetic devices may send the information to objects such as a fan, bed shaker, or vibrotactile pager.

One type of assistive listening tool that is becoming increasingly popular is the hearing ear dog. These animals serve as "substitute ears" for the hearing-impaired person and are professionally trained to alert their owners when certain sounds occur.

Telephone Devices

Several types of devices are available to assist hearing-impaired persons with communication over the phone. Most standard telephones employ a high-pitched ring that may be undetectable by a hearing-impaired listener. Therefore, several different devices are available that alert the user of an incoming call. Such devices use various procedures to alert the listener, such as illumination of a steady light or strobe light, activation of a ring that is louder and/or lower-pitched than available with standard telephones, and stimulation of a remote receiver that causes stimulation of a body-worn vibrotactile device.

Auditory telephone devices are available that increase the intensity of the signal delivered to the listener. These devices may be designed for use with or without a prosthetic device and primarily consist of amplifier handsets, in-line amplifiers, and portable amplifiers (32).

Nonauditory telephone devices are available for persons who are unable to understand speech over the telephone. These devices are referred to as telecommunication devices for the deaf (TDDs). The TDDs are based on teletypewriter technology and transmit information over standard phone lines. When using a TDD, both the sender and the receiver must have access to a TDD. The speaker uses the TDD to type his or her end of the conversation. The typed words are then transmitted to the other party, who receives an ongoing printout of the message being sent and may respond by typing on his or her TDD.

Until recently, both parties involved in the conversation needed access to a TDD in order for such a conversation to take place. The development of deaf relay services, however, has greatly increased the accessibility of who may be reached with a TDD call. Such relays provide access to an operator who has a TDD. The operator receives and interprets the typed TDD message and conveys the message to someone who does not have a TDD via spoken voice. The Americans with Disabilities Act (ADA), which was signed into law in 1990, mandates that deaf relay services be available to hearing- and speech-impaired persons in the United States.

Increased utilization of home computers and facsimile (fax) machines has resulted in a large increase in the number of hearing-impaired persons who communicate via electronic mail or by fax. The costs associated with owning either a home computer or a fax machine have dropped recently, making these forms of technology increasingly popular among hearing-impaired persons.

Devices to Improve Comprehension of Speech

There are three primary types of devices designed to improve comprehension of speech: hard-wired systems, wireless, systems and visual devices. When using a hardwired system, the listener is physically connected to the sound source. The sound is picked up by a microphone and delivered to the listener. There are several ways the sound may be received by the listener, including via a headset or via his or her personal hearing aid (direct audio input or inductive coupling). The primary limitation of hard-wired systems is that separation from the sound source is limited by the length of the cord. Wireless systems, on the other hand, are more mobile and are more versatile than hard-wired systems. These devices, which consist of a transmitter that sends a radio signal to a receiver, do not require a direct connection between the listener and the sound source. Wireless systems are often available in large concert halls, classrooms, theaters, museums, and churches and can be easily adapted for use at home. Like hard-wired systems, wireless systems may be used in conjunction with a hearing aid or may deliver the signal to an alternative receiver, such as headphones. Some of the wireless systems available include induction loop, frequency modulation (FM), and infrared.

There are several types of visual devices available to enhance a hearing-impaired person's ability to perceive speech. One of the most popular, closed captioning, refers to a television decoder that provides a printed display of what is being said. Such decoders are used regularly by persons with a severe to profound hearing loss as their primary means for understanding what is being said on the television. The Television Decoder Circuitry Act of 1990 (PL 101-431) greatly increased the accessibility to closed-caption television, as it requires that all televisions with screens 13 inches and larger contain decoder circuitry.

Real-time captioning, like closed captioning, presents the listener with a printed display of the spoken word. A trained court reporter uses a specialized computer system that enables him or her to transcribe what is being said. The computer system then projects the transcribed copy to a projection screen, where persons may read what is being said (with only minimal time delays). Unlike closed captioning, which may or may not be performed live, real-time captioning is almost always performed live.

Provision of Rehabilitation Services Beyond the Fitting of a Prosthetic Device

Most patients' rehabilitative needs related to their hearing loss consist of audiologic evaluation, medical evaluation, and fitting of a prosthetic device. Some patients, however, have rehabilitative needs that require further intervention. Specifically, some patients may require basic instruction regarding hearing loss and its effect on communication ability (including enrollment in individual or group therapy); instruction regarding ways to enhance communication ability, including assistive listening device counseling, fitting, and instruction; and/or formalized instruction aimed at improving their ability to perceive speech.

Basic Instruction Regarding Hearing Loss and Its Impact on Communication

One of the most basic aspects of audiologic rehabilitation entails educating the patient about his or her hearing loss. This includes a review of the patient's audiogram and provision of information regarding the type and severity of the loss. Patients should be able to describe their own hearing loss (type, degree, and severity) and understand the effect the hearing loss has on their ability to recognize speech. They should have information regarding the amount of help that is provided by their prosthetic device and understand its limitations. They need to be aware that hearing aids and cochlear implants do not restore normal hearing. They need to be informed that they will experience difficulty understanding speech in certain situations, such as in the presence of background noise.

Patients should be provided with simple information that will enhance their communication ability. For example, it is inevitable that they will not be able to hear each word that is said. Therefore, they should try to focus on what they do understand rather than on the information they did not understand. They should be taught to follow the overall flow of conversation rather than trying to comprehend each and every word.

Often, patients need to be taught how to educate others

about their hearing loss and about their limitations in understanding speech. They should be able to instruct others regarding how to speak so they will be optimally understood by the hearing-impaired person (e.g., slow down speaking rate, refrain from placing objects in front of the mouth). They should learn to develop a buddy system in which a friend or colleague assists them in communication by keeping them informed of quick changes in the topic of conversation. These factors are important, as they teach the hearing-impaired person to be an assertive listener and to participate actively in conversations. It additionally teaches them to take control of as many factors as possible in order to enhance their communication ability.

Occasionally, clinics may offer patients the ability to enroll in formal auditory rehabilitation classes. These classes may be held individually or in a group setting. Topics covered in such sessions may include the following: maximizing auditory and visual input; improving auditory–visual integration, discrimination, and memory; familiarization with the linguistic aspects of speech, such as vocabulary and context awareness; training in assertive listening and conversation repair; and improving the patient's ability to interact effectively with family and friends (32). Enrollment in a group program is advantageous for many patients, as it provides them with the opportunity to share their feelings and experiences related to their hearing loss with other hearing-impaired persons. Group members frequently provide each other with emotional support as well as with new ideas regarding ways to enhance communication.

Formal Instruction Aimed at Improving Ability to Understand Speech

When faced with dealing with a hearing loss, many patients express interest in enrolling in lip-reading classes in hopes that such instruction will greatly improve their communication ability. These patients need to be informed that lip-reading instruction may provide only limited help. Lip reading is extremely complex and difficult; only about one-third of the spoken message can be understood when one uses lip reading alone. This is because many of the sounds of speech that sound different look identical when produced. Although some patients become very adept lip readers, others experience difficulty even after years of formal instruction.

There are several topics, however, that could be covered in such classes that will facilitate improved communication. For example, formal instruction regarding lip shape and position will help the patient learn to recognize certain categories of speech sounds. This will also foster an understanding that the amount of information that can be derived from lip reading is limited, as many speech sounds are indistinguishable when using lip reading alone. Importantly, patients should be taught that lip reading is most effective when used in conjunction with the auditory signal, even if the auditory signal they receive is limited.

Frequently, patients need to be taught basic strategies for improving their communication ability. For example, they should be instructed regarding ways to make the speaker's face more visible, such as by placing themselves in an optimal location for visualization of the speaker's lip movements. Doing so will enhance the availability of lip-reading cues and may serve to enhance the quality of the auditory signal that is received as well. They often need to be encouraged to use aggressive strategies to optimize their perception. For example, if they will be attending a conference in a large auditorium, they could incorporate any or all of the following: check with the auditorium personnel before attendance to ascertain the availability of assistive listening devices; arrange for preferential seating (up close to the stage where visualization of the speaker's face is optimal); and request that the speaker provide a written copy of his or her speech before its presentation in order to have a visual tool that will aid in overall comprehension.

SUMMARY

There are several options available for rehabilitative treatment of hearing loss. The particular type of treatment suitable for a specific patient will depend on several factors, such as type and severity of the hearing loss and its impact on the affected individual's ability to communicate. It is well documented, however, that early intervention, fitting of an appropriate prosthetic device, and the provision of rehabilitative services are important factors that will optimize a patient's communication ability when faced with the diagnosis of hearing loss.

REFERENCES

1. Current estimates from National Health Interview Survey, 1988. *Vital Health Stat* 1989; 173:1–250.
2. Michigan Commission on Handicapper Concerns, Division of Deafness. *The hearing impaired population of Michigan.* Lansing: Michigan Department of Labor, 1989.
3. Schein JD, Delk MT Jr. *The deaf population of the United States.* Silver Spring, MD: National Association of Deaf, 1974.
4. Uhlmann RF, Larson EB, Rees TS, Koepsell TD, Duckert LG. Relationship of hearing impairment to dementia and cognitive dysfunction in older adults. *JAMA* 1989; 261:1916–1919.
5. Bess FH, Lichtenstein MJ, Logan SA, Burger MC, Nelson E. Hearing impairment as a determinant of function in the elderly. *J Am Geriatr Soc* 1989; 37:123–128.
6. Epstein S, Reilly JS. Sensorineural hearing loss. *Pediatr Clin North Am* 1989; 36:1501–1520.
7. Parving A. Hearing disorders in childhood: Some procedure for detection, identification and diagnostic evaluation. *Int J Pediatr Otorhinolaryngol* 1985; 9:31–57.
8. Joint Committee on Infant Hearing Position Statement. *ASHA* 1982; 24:1017–1018.
9. Weinstein BE. Geriatric hearing loss: Myths, realities, resources for physicians. *Geriatrics* 1989; 44(4):42–48.
10. Hecox K, Hogan K. Neuro-otologic disorders. Part 2: The auditory system. In: Rosenberg R, ed. *The clinical neurosciences.* New York: Churchill Livingstone, 1983; 858–875.
11. Hall JW, Ghorayeb BY. Diagnosis of middle ear pathology and evaluation of conductive hearing loss. In: Jacobson JT, Northern JL, eds. *Diagnostic audiology.* Austin, TX: PRO-ED, 1990; 161–198.
12. Borg E. Dynamic characteristics of the intra-aural muscle reflex. In:

Feldman AS, Wilber LA, eds. *Acoustic impedance and admittance. The measurement of middle ear function.* Baltimore: Williams & Wilkins, 1976; 236–299.

13. Fowler PE. The diagnosis of disease of the neural mechanism of hearing by the aid of sounds well above threshold. *Trans Am Otolaryngol Soc* 1937; 27:207–219.
14. Jerger J, Shedd J, Harford E. On the detection of extremely small changes in sound intensity. *Arch Otolarynogol* 1959; 69:200–211.
15. Olsen WO. Special auditory tests: a historical perspective. In: Jacobson JT, Northern, JL, eds. *Diagnostic audiology.* Austin, TX: PRO-ED, 1990; 19–52.
16. Moller AR, Jannetta PJ. Neural generators of the auditory brainstem response. In: Jacobson JT, ed. *The auditory brainstem response.* Boston: College-Hill Press, 1985; 13–31.
17. Hyde ML. The effect of cochlear lesion on the ABR. In: Jacobson JT, ed. *The auditory brainstem response.* Boston: College-Hill Press, 1985; 33–48.
18. Ruth RA, Lambert PR. Evaluation and diagnosis of cochlear disorders. In: Jacobson JT, Northern JL, eds. *Diagnostic audiology.* Austin, TX: PRO-ED, 1990; 199–215.
19. Schwartz DM, Morris MD. Strategies for optimizing the detection of neuropathology from the auditory brainstem response. In: Jacobson JT, Northern JL, eds. *Diagnostic audiology.* Austin, TX: PRO-ED, 1990; 141–160.
20. Bess FH, Crandell CC. An update on amplification: Some changing directions. *Am J Otol* 1986; 7:470–475.
21. Hearing aid devices—Professional and patient labeling and conditions for sale. *Fed Register* 1977; 42:9286–9296.
22. Golabek W, Nowakowska M, Siwiec H, Stephens SD. Self-reported benefits of hearing aids by the hearing impaired. *Br J Audiol* 1988; 22:183–186.
23. Bess FH, Lichtenstein MJ, Logan SA, Burger MC, Nelson E. Hearing impairment as a determinant of function in the elderly. *J Am Geriatr Soc* 1989; 37:123–128.
24. Stewart IF. After early identification—What follows? *Laryngoscope* 1984; 94:784–799.
25. Bess FH, Crandell CC. An update on amplification: Some changing directions. *Am J Otol* 1986; 7:470–475.
26. Pappas JJ, Bailey HA Jr, Graham SS. Clinical hearing aid dispensing: A five year review. *Laryngoscope* 1980; 90:1475–1480.
27. Franks JR, Beckmann MJ. Rejection of hearing aids: Attitudes of a geriatric sample. *Ear Hearing* 1985; 6:161–166.
28. Tyler RS, Baker LJ, Armstrong-Bednall G. Difficulties experienced by hearing aid candidates and hearing aid users. *Br J Audiol* 1983; 17: 191–201.
29. Miyamoto RT, Osberger MJ, Todd SL, Robbins AM, Stroer BS, Zimmerman-Phillips S, Carney AE. Variables affecting implant performance in children. *Laryngoscope* 1994; 104:1120–1124.
30. NIH consensus statement: Cochlear implants in adults and children. 1995; 13(2):15–17.
31. Zwolan TA, Kileny PR, Telian SA. Self-report of cochlear implant use and satisfaction by prelingually deafened adults. *Ear Hearing* 1996; 17(3):198–210.
32. Montgomery AA. Management of the hearing-impaired adult. In: Alpiner J, McCarthy PA, eds. *Rehabilitative audiology in children and adults.* Baltimore: Williams & Wilkins, 1993; 311–330.

Rehabilitation Medicine: Principles and Practice, Third Edition,
edited by Joel A. DeLisa and Bruce M. Gans.
Lippincott–Raven Publishers, Philadelphia © 1998.

CHAPTER 71

Vestibular Rehabilitation

Shailesh S. Parikh and Champa V. Bid

Dizziness, vertigo, and disruptions of balance have a negative impact on one's ability to perform routines of daily life and to live independently. Normally, maintenance of balance and upright posture does not require conscious effort. The sense of orientation permits individuals to perform normal tasks and to participate in multiple and complex tasks ranging from ice skating and mechanical repair to skyscraper construction.

Visual, vestibular, and somatosensory systems play a role in providing accurate and very rapid information, which is integrated at the cortical level with input from the cerebellum (1). The brain must ignore erroneous information and select information that may be relied on to execute coordinated motor activity for postural control (2,3).

External disturbance to posture and balance control comes from mechanical or informational sources. External mechanical disturbance to balance can come from forces acting on the body that displace the body's center of gravity (COG) beyond the base of support (e.g., a push) or prevent the base of support from being positioned beneath the COG (e.g., tripping). External informational disturbances provide inaccurate orientational information from the environment, creating temporary conflict among visual, vestibular, and somatosensory inputs (e.g., looking at a moving train while standing on the platform creates the illusion of self-motion) (2).

Internal physiological disturbances may affect balance either by disruption of the sensory-motor system (e.g., dizziness or vertigo creating a sense of spinning) or by momentary interference with perfusion of the cerebrum, brainstem, or cerebellum (e.g., postural hypotension, cardiac arrhythmia, or vertebral basilary insufficiency).

Problems with balance are very common in the elderly population. It is estimated that almost 7% of primary care patients over age 85 present with dizziness (4), the most frequent symptom associated with vestibular dysfunction.

FUNCTIONAL ANATOMY AND APPLIED PHYSIOLOGY OF THE VESTIBULAR SYSTEM

Among the three components of the peripheral balance mechanism, visual, vestibular, and somatosensory, the vestibular is the most specialized and complex.

The vestibular system has a peripheral and a central component. Balance and postural control depend on sensory information from various peripheral receptors including the vestibular apparatus reaching the sensory cortex and integration centers in the brainstem and cerebellum. This is the afferent loop of the balance mechanism. Signals then are transmitted via the corticospinal tract and brainstem pathways to the peripheral and extraocular muscles. This is the efferent loop of the balance mechanism.

The vestibular apparatus is a receptor composed of a membranous labyrinth within a bony labyrinth located in the temporal bone. The membranous labyrinth is the functional part of the apparatus, which consists of the cochlea (major sensory area for hearing) and semicircular ducts with utricle and saccule (sensory area of balance). Semicircular ducts, which are responsible for dynamic orientation, have an enlarged portion called an ampulla that contains the crista ampullaris with sensory neuroepithelium including hair cells, on top of which is the gelatinous mass called the cupula. Hundreds of cilia from hair cells located along the ampullary crest are projected into the cupula. The kinocilium of each of these hair cells is always directed toward the same side of the cupula. Bending the cupula in that direction causes depolarization of hair cells, whereas bending toward the opposite side will hyperpolarize the hair cells (5–7). The signals from the hair cells are sent through the vestibular nerve to the central nervous system, indicating a change in the rate and direction of head rotation in three different spatial

S. S. Parikh and C. V. Bid: Department of Physical Medicine and Rehabilitation, University of Medicine and Dentistry of New Jersey, New Jersey Medical School; and Kessler Institute for Rehabilitation, Saddle Brook, New Jersey 07663.

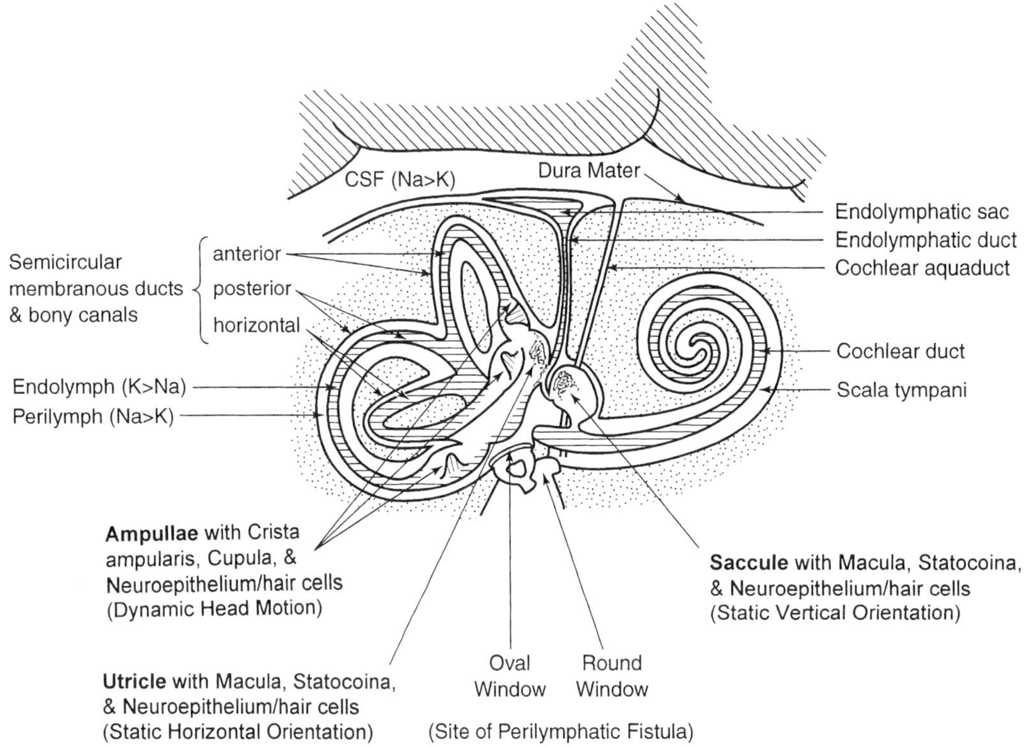

FIG. 71-1. Diagrammatic cross section of the inner ear.

planes. The otolithic organs are the utricle (responsible for static horizontal orientation) and saccule (responsible for static vertical orientation). Each contains a macula and statoconia with sensory neuroepithelium including hair cells. The membranous labyrinth includes two compartments known as the perilymphatic and endolymphatic chambers. The perilymphatic chamber surrounds the endolymphatic chamber within the bony canal and plays a significant role only in the hearing function of the cochlear part of the membranous labyrinth. The endolymphatic chamber contains the sensory neuroepithelium receptors, which are most important for vestibular function (5–7) (Fig. 71-1).

The three semicircular ducts are oriented at right angles to each other and are known as the anterior, posterior, and horizontal ducts. The flow of endolymphatic fluid in the semicircular duct and ampulla excites the sensory organ. The function of the semicircular duct is to measure the angular acceleration in any direction. When the head is tilted forward by 30°, the horizontal duct is parallel to the surface of the earth. The anterior duct then becomes more vertical and projects 45° anterior and lateral to the sagittal plane, and the posterior duct also becomes more vertical and projects 45° posterior and lateral. The anterior duct on one side is parallel to the posterior duct on the opposite side, and they function physiologically as one unit. Horizontal ducts on both sides remain approximately in the same plane.

Vision is an important cue for maintenance of balance and postural stability. Eye and head movements provide information in order to pursue visual targets. The vestibulo-ocular reflex (VOR) drives the eyes with signals from the semicircular duct, thus stabilizing the direction of gaze. It is a well-known fact that postural sway increases when an individual stands in the dark or with his or her eyes closed or covered. Visual depth illusion, decreased occulomotility and accommodation, fixation inaccuracy, decreased contrast sensitivity, and decreased visual and stereo acuity can affect balance, especially in the elderly population when compensation by other sensory modalities is also deficient. Both VOR and the optokinetic system work to smoothe the disrupted visual gaze and dampen nystagmus.

Abnormal visual stimulation alone can create an illusion of self-movement and balance disruption. This abnormal input must be suppressed by noncorresponding vestibular and somatosensory input in normal subjects in order to allow the head to remain fixed in relation to the body.

Peripheral sensory receptors, proprioceptive joint receptors (especially upper cervical facet joints and ankle joint), stretch receptors of the muscles, and vibratory receptors provide information concerning surface, position, motion of muscle and joints, as well as gravitational information. This must respond quickly to perturbational forces and work against external loads. This input correlates with vestibular gravitational information and also provides feedback for the spinal and vestibulospinal reflexes. The upper cervical facet joint proprioceptive receptors play a role in balance through the cervico-ocular reflex (1).

The central nervous system (CNS) also plays an important role in balance. The primary pathway for the maintenance of equilibrium travels along the vestibular nerve to the vestibular nuclei and cerebellum. Signals are also sent to the oculomotor and reticular nuclei of the brainstem as well as to the thalamus and the cortex via vestibulothalamocortical projections and to the spinal cord via vestibulospinal and reticulospinal tracts. These connections facilitate the VOR and vestibulospinal reflex (VSR).

The cerebellum is important in gaze control, postural stability, and gait. Communication between the visual and vestibular systems occurs via the cerebellum. In conditions affecting vestibular nuclear function, the CNS compensation to suppress nystagmus occurs through visual fixation, and the cerebellum is critical for this form of learning (6,7). The cerebellum also helps to time and sequence motor activity, monitors this activity, and facilitates instantaneous corrective adjustment of agonist and antagonist muscles through signaling an increase or decrease in the level of activation of specific muscles.

The cerebral cortex contributes to balance by a process of selection and suppression of sensory references in an altered sensory environment. This probably is accomplished through a vestibulothalamocortical projection (8). Primarily, this process occurs involuntarily, but there may be voluntary control in certain situations. Disturbance of this function may be the reason for imbalance in mild brain injury, or it may be caused by alcohol or medications affecting cognition.

SYMPTOMS AND CAUSES OF VESTIBULAR AND BALANCE DYSFUNCTION

Dizziness is a sense of a disturbed relationship between oneself and one's environment. Words often used to describe changes in balance or dizziness include clumsiness, disequilibrium, drifting, fainting, floating, fuzzy-headedness, giddiness, leaning, lightheadedness, listing, being off balance, reeling, instability, unsteadiness, swaying, swimmy-headed, spinning, wooziness, and being wobbly (1,9). It is important to ask the patient to clarify how he or she is using the term. Dizziness may be caused by vestibular or nonvestibular system disorders (Table 71-1).

The causes of vestibular system dysfunction may be peripheral or central. True vertigo is described as a false sense of unidirectional movement related to one's surroundings. It is more a sense of spinning or rotation. Vertigo is a strong indicator of vestibular system dysfunction. The clinical examination coupled with the history helps differentiate among causes of vertigo (Table 71-2).

Vestibular neuronitis and *acute viral labyrinthitis* are the most common self-limited inner ear conditions. They are usually preceded by viral infection of the upper respiratory or gastrointestinal tract. Initial symptoms are true vertigo, which may be associated with nausea, ataxia, and nystagmus. Most patients have nystagmus toward the normal ear and decreased or absent caloric response in the affected ear. Hearing loss, tinnitus, and increased aural pressure are not

TABLE 71-1. *Causes of dizziness*

Vestibular system disorder (VSD)
- **Peripheral vestibular system disorders** (labyrinth and vestibular nerve)
  - Acute viral labyrinthitis
  - Vestibular neuronitis
  - Recurrent labyrinthitis
  - Autoimmune vestibulopathy
  - Benign paroxysmal positional vertigo (BPPV)
  - Meniere's disease (endolymphatic hydrops, ELH)
  - Perilymphatic fistula (PLF) from barotrauma, cholesteatoma, stapes surgery, Mondini malformation, or syphilis
  - Acoustic neuroma, herpes zoster oticus (Ramsey Hunt syndrome)
  - Ototoxic drugs
  - Traumatic labyrinthine injury, e.g., temporal bone fracture, inner ear concussion, hemorrhage
  - Infection, e.g., herpes zoster, Lyme's disease
  - Other sources of endolymphatic pressure sensitivity
    - Hypermobile stapes foot plate
    - Vestibular fibrosis
    - Vestibular atelectasis
    - Alternobaric vertigo
  - Middle ear disturbances causing vertigo
- **Central vestibular system disorders**
  - Vascular disease, e.g., transient ischemic attack (TIA) of vertebrobasilar system, stroke of posterior circulation, cerebellar hemorrhage, cerebellar infarction, subclavian steal syndrome, cerebral vasculitis
  - Posterior fossa lesion/tumors, vestibular schwannoma
  - Basilar artery migraine
  - Traumatic brain injury (TBI)
  - Demyelinating central nervous system (CNS) disease, e.g., multiple sclerosis
  - Degenerative CNS disease
  - Temporal lobe epilepsy (with vestibular aura)
  - Infection, e.g., meningitis, abscess
  - Drugs (centrally acting)

Nonvestibular system disorders (NVSD)
- **Cardiovascular lightheadedness** (presyncopal type)
  - Anemia
  - Hyperviscosity
  - Hypotension (postprandial syncope, postural hypotension)
  - Carotid sinus hypersensitivity
  - Cardiac arrhythmia
  - Cardiac valvular disease
  - Heart failure
  - Vertebral artery dissection.
- **Cervical dizziness**, e.g., whiplash injury, cervical osteoarthritis
- **Dizziness of unknown causes**: "functional dizziness/vertigo/lightheadedness"
  - Dizziness/ vertigo without objective findings, "nonspecific dizziness"
  - Hyperventilation syndrome
  - Psychiatric disturbances, e.g., psychogenic dizziness/vertigo, phobic postural dizziness/vertigo, agoraphobia, anxiety and panic disorder, major depression, somatization disorder, malingering
- **Endocrine dysfunction**, including diabetes, hypo/hyperglycemia, hypo/hyperthyroidism

TABLE 71-2. *Characteristics of peripheral and central vertigo*

	Peripheral	Central
History		
1. Vertigo severity	Severe	Mild to moderate
2. Frequency	Often intermittent	Often constant
3. Onset	Abrupt, sudden onset	Slow, gradual onset
4. Effect of change of position	More common	Less common
5. Nausea and vomiting	More common	Less common
6. Cochlear symptoms	Common	Uncommon
7. Imbalance	Mild	Severe
8. Oscillopsia	Mild	Severe
Physical examination		
1. Focal neurologic sign	Absent	Present
2. Mental status alteration	None or sometimes	Often present
3. Nystagmus	Always present	May be absent
	Unidirectional	Uni- or bidirectional
	Oblique rotatory or horizontal	
	Never vertical	May be absent
	Inhibited by fixation	Usually little effect of fixation
4. Hearing loss or tinnitus	Often present	Rarely present
Nystagmography		
1. Caloric test	Abnormal	Normal
2. Positional nystagmus	Abnormal	Abnormal
	15 to 30 seconds latency	Almost immediate
	Fatigable	Not fatigable
	<30 seconds duration	>30 seconds duration
3. Optokinetic pursuit	Normal	Abnormal
Compensation	Rapid	Slow

present (10). If hearing loss is present, then the diagnosis of suppurative or serous labyrinthitis, Meniere's disease, neurosyphilis, herpes zoster, acoustic neuroma, and CNS pathology should be considered (11).

Severe distressing symptoms last for 2 to 3 days, and less intense symptoms persist for 1 to 2 weeks. Approximately 10% of patients may take as long as 2 months to improve. Elderly patients and patients with cerebellar degeneration recover much more slowly.

Antiemetic and vestibular suppressants should be used initially (Table 71-3). Patients are instructed to restrict activities during the first 3 days of illness. By the fourth day, vestibular suppressants should be reduced, and the patient is advised to increase activity as tolerated. Vestibular rehabilitation exercise, described below, can be initiated as an outpatient or home exercise program.

Benign paroxysmal positional vertigo (BPPV) is a self-limited condition characterized by episodic vertigo and nystagmus of brief duration. It is provoked by assuming very specific head positions that probably cause movement of debris from the otolithic organ within the semicircular duct. It may be associated with head trauma, infection, or degeneration but can occur spontaneously in the elderly (12–14). The most common precipitating movements are head extension with rotation of the neck or rolling in bed from side to side. The vertigo disappears in 1 to 2 minutes when the precipitating position is maintained. The patient typically does not complain of hearing loss, tinnitus, or aural fullness.

The diagnosis of BPPV can be made when positional vertigo is present and when positional testing using the Dix–Hallpike maneuver (Fig. 71-2) precipitates a burst of upbeating torsional nystagmus (15). This maneuver can be done by positioning the head to orient the posterior canal vertically downward. It can also be diagnosed by using a pair of Fresnel lenses, which brings on rotatory nystagmus toward the dependent ear. In chronic, persistent cases refractory to treatment, magnetic resonance imaging (MRI) is ordered to rule out acoustic neuroma or fourth ventricle tumor.

BPPV is a self-limited disorder that commonly resolves spontaneously, or by a canalith-repositioning maneuver, e.g., the Epley maneuver. The Brandt–Daroff exercise, which involves compensation and habituation, is very effective in most patients (12,16,17). Vestibular suppressants may slow down CNS compensation. They are used only if vertiginous spells are followed by nausea, in which case, mild antihistaminic and anticholinergic medications such as meclizine can be helpful. This approach is often required for elderly patients, whose symptoms can persist because CNS compensation and adaptation are reduced. Surgical options can be considered for severe BPPV unresponsive to exercise and medical management and when symptoms persist for more than 1 year. Posterior canal plugging is presently the procedure of choice (18).

Meniere's disease (endolymphatic hydrops, ELH) is a common disorder of the inner ear characterized by episodic true vertigo. It is preceded by an increasing sensation of aural fullness or aching in the affected ear, by tinnitus, and by fluctuating hearing loss. Nausea and vomiting can occur

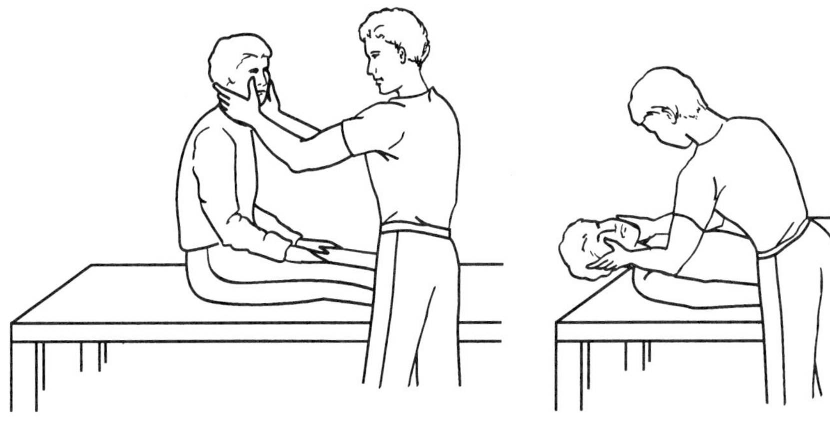

FIG. 71-2. Dix–Hallpike maneuver test. Positional nystagmus is evoked using the Dix–Hallpike maneuvers, which can be accomplished by positioning the head to orient the posterior canal vertically downward.

at the time of the vertiginous spell (19). According to the Vestibular Disorders Association, Meniere's disease affects 2 to 5 million Americans with onset during the third or fourth decade. Approximately 75% of those affected have unilateral and 25% have bilateral ear involvement.

Normal endolymphatic system function requires equal pressure of endolymphatic and perilymphatic fluid. Pressure imbalance can lead to dilation of the endolymphatic system over time. Current theory suggests that endolymphatic hydrops develops because of a mild dysfunction of the resorptive mechanism in the endolymphatic sac. Overproduction of endolymph may also lead to this condition.

Other types of Meniere's disease are known as "cochlear Meniere's disease/hydrops" and "vestibular Meniere's disease/hydrops." In vestibular hydrops, there is episodic vertigo without hearing loss and tinnitus. Cochlear hydrops is characterized by fluctuating hearing loss, tinnitus, and ear pressure without vertigo (18).

TABLE 71-3. *Vestibular suppressants and antiemetics used for treating acute vertigo*[a]

Pharmacologic class	Drug	Adult dose	Precautions and side effects
Vestibular suppressants			
First line of treatment: antihistamine and anticholinergic	Meclizine (Antivert, Roerig Division, New York, NY)	25–50 mg bid	Prostatic enlargement; sedation can worsen dizziness of nonlabyrinthine causes
Second-line treatment	Lorazepam (Ativan, Wyeth-Ayerst, Philadelphia, PA)	0.5 mg bid	Sedation, drug dependency
	Clonazepam (Klonopin, Roche Laboratories, Nutley NJ)	0.5 mg bid	
	Diazepam (Valium, Roche Products, Manati Puerto Rico)	2 to 10 mg (1 dose given acutely PO, IM, or IV)	
Third-line in-hospital treatment, only with close supervision	Diphenidol (Vontrol, SmithKline Beecham Pharmaceuticals, Philadelphia, PA)	Refer to *Physicians' Desk Reference* for details	Hallucinations, disorientation, confusion
Antiemetics			
Phenothiazine	Prochlorperazine (Compazine, SmithKline Beecham Pharmaceuticals, Philadelphia, PA)	5 to 10 mg IM or PO or prn q6–12h; or 25 mg supp q12h	Sedation, extrapyramidal
	Promethazine (Phenergan, Wyeth-Ayerst, Philadelphia, PA)	25 mg PO q6–8h; 25 mg rectal q12h; or 12.5 mg IM q6–8h	
	Thiethylperazine (Torecan, Roxane Laboratories, Columbus, OH)	10 mg PO prn tid; or 2 ml IM prn tid	
	Trimethobenzamide (Tigan, Roberts Pharmaceutical Corp., Eatontown, NJ)	250 mg PO prn tid; or 200 mg IM tid	

IM, intramuscularly; IV, intravenously; PO, orally; prn, as needed.
[a] Refer to current *Physicians' Desk Reference* (PDR) for update.

Low-frequency sensorineural hearing loss with moderate impairment of speech discrimination are classic features of Meniere's disease. Auditory brainstem response (ABR) or MRI with gadolinium enhancement can be done to exclude acoustic neuroma or other tumors (20). Electronystagmography can show normal or a moderately reduced vestibular response.

Elimination of episodic vertigo and prevention of sensorineural hearing impairment are the main goals of treatment. Management of the acute attack in early stages includes bed rest and a vestibular suppressant, e.g., meclizine (Antivert, Roerig Division, New York, NY), 25 mg every 4 hours. If the patient is vomiting, then a 25-mg prochlorperazine (Compazine, SmithKline Beecham Pharmaceuticals, Philadelphia, PA) suppository can be used. Vertigo usually lasts for 2 to 3 hours, and after a severe attack, most people are extremely exhausted and sleep for several hours. If an attack is prolonged and is associated with nausea and vomiting, then intravenous fluid therapy can be initiated to maintain hydration, and 5 to 10 mg intravenous diazepam (Valium, Roche Products, Manati, Puerto Rico) titrated slowly may also be beneficial (21).

In chronic cases a trial of medical management should include a low-salt diet; avoidance of caffeine, alcohol, and tobacco; meclizine, 12.5 to 25 mg three times a day; hydrochlorothiazide, 50 mg each morning, to reduce endolymphatic pressure; and use of a vasodilator such as papaverine hydrochloride (Pavabid, Marion Merrell Dow, Inc., Kansas City, MO), 150 mg twice daily (21,22). Vestibular rehabilitation exercise and counseling can be helpful and are an important part of management in these patients. Surgery should be considered if medical therapy and rehabilitation are deemed inadequate. Should Meniere's disease recur in the unoperated ear after vestibular ablation has been done, streptomycin injection therapy for ablation of vestibular function can be considered. Twenty grams of streptomycin sulfate is given intravenously over a 2-week period with careful monitoring of auditory and vestibular function. The streptomycin dose can be increased to the point of vestibular ablation with preservation of hearing function (19,21,23). A summary of pharmacologic treatment is presented in Table 71-3.

A *perilymphatic fistula* (PLF) is defined as an abnormal communication through which perilymph passes from inner ear to middle ear. The most common causes of PLF are complications from ear surgery, head trauma such as basilar skull fracture, whiplash injury from a motor vehicle accident, barotrauma (e.g., a rupture of the round window during scuba diving), puncturing injury through the tympanic membrane, coughing, straining, nose blowing, and other such maneuvers that increase intrathoracic and cerebrospinal fluid (CSF) pressures and rupture the labyrinthine window. Other rare causes are congenital anomalies of the inner ear that result in spontaneous fistulization (6,24).

Symptoms associated with PLF result from an imbalance in pressure of endolymphatic and perilymphatic fluid (25). Prognosis of PLF is uncertain, and satisfactory diagnostic testing and criteria for surgical candidacy are often unclear. A presumptive diagnosis is based on a high degree of clinical suspicion, history, physical findings, and a positive fistula test.

Auditory symptoms (e.g., sudden onset of mild or profound hearing loss and tinnitus), vestibular symptoms including true vertigo, lightheadedness, dizziness, and vertigo worsened by Valsalva maneuver and low-frequency loud noise (Tullio phenomenon) suggest PLF (25,26). The Romberg test, Fukuda stepping test, and Singleton test are often positive but not specific for PLF. The presence of a few beats of nystagmus or a sensation of dizziness when negative pressure is applied to the affected ear suggests a PLF. High-resolution computed tomography (CT) scan of the temporal bone can be helpful to rule out temporal bone fracture, which may cause PLF. Standard air and bone conduction testing can indicate unilateral sensorineural hearing loss. Electrocochleography (ECOG) can be used for identifying and monitoring PLF (27,28). A most consistent finding for PLF is an abnormal positional test during electronystagmography (ENG) (26,27).

Surgery is indicated for chronic severely disabling symptomatic PLF. The operative procedure consists of packing the oval and round windows with a small soft tissue graft whether or not a clear-cut fistula is demonstrated. The success rate of this treatment is variable.

If the fistula test is negative, the patient should be treated conservatively for 6 months. If there is persistent dizziness, then PLF treatment is reconsidered.

Acoustic neuroma may present as Meniere's disease except that attacks are usually not followed by asymptomatic periods. Vertigo is usually associated with hearing loss and tinnitus. Onset occurs in the fifth and sixth decades, and both sexes are equally affected (29).

Acoustic neuroma originates in the vestibular division of the eighth nerve just within the internal auditory canal. As it grows, it occupies the posterior fossa at the cerebellopontine angle. Facial weakness, facial sensory loss, unilateral ataxia of limbs, and gait abnormality may be present. Audiologic and vestibular evaluation, brainstem evoked responses, and MRI of the internal auditory meatus can be helpful in making the diagnosis. Treatment is surgical excision by a subcapital approach. Occasionally, Von Recklinghausen neurofibromatosis is associated with acoustic neuroma.

Herpes zoster oticus is a viral syndrome involving the eighth nerve and is also known as the Ramsey Hunt syndrome (30). In this syndrome, zoster virus remains dormant in the seventh and eighth nerve ganglia and is reactivated during periods of lower immunity. Patients can develop hearing loss, vertigo, and facial weakness before or after developing vesicular eruption or burning pain in the ear. Herpes external otitis is a self-limited condition; however, eighth and seventh nerve damage can be irreversible. Corticosteroids and antiviral drugs such as acyclovir should be tried.

Aminoglycosides such as streptomycin, gentamycin, and tobramycin can cause vestibular ototoxicity (31). Kanamycin and amikacin primarily cause auditory ototoxicity. "Loop" diuretics, e.g., furosemide and ethacrynic acid, have ototoxic effects in approximately 6% of patients. High doses of salicylate therapy can cause hearing loss, tinnitus, dizziness, loss of balance, and occasionally vertigo in some patients. *Cis*-platinum is associated with both auditory and vestibular ototoxicity in about 60% of patients. Major risk factors for ototoxicity are impaired renal function, high serum level of the drug, a course of more than 14 days, prior use of ototoxic drugs, preexisting sensorineural hearing loss, and age over 65 (5). Preventive methods include periodic auditory and vestibular testing while taking known ototoxic medications. A wide variety of medications prescribed for cardiac conditions, and some antihypertensive medication, can cause dizziness. Psychotropic medications, muscle relaxants, and anticonvulsants can also cause dizziness (32,33). It is important to inquire about alcohol and caffeine intake and any use of over-the-counter medications such as cold preparations and sleeping medication.

Middle ear conditions that can be associated with vertigo include cerumen impaction or its removal, eustachian tube dysfunction, and temporomandibular joint dysfunction. Patients with unilateral wax impaction can develop an "alternobaric vertigo" related to pressure difference between the ears. Vertigo after wax removal may be caused by caloric effect of syringing of the ear or manipulation of the tympanic membrane or mobilizing the stapes foot plate during syringing. Eustachian tube malfunction can be associated with mild vague dizziness, aural fullness, otalgia, and popping/clicking in the ear. Decongestants and intranasal steroid therapy can be used in this situation.

CNS vertigo is much less common than that caused by peripheral vestibular dysfunction. Stroke and transient ischemic attacks account for about 35% of cases. Vertigo from vertebrobasilary migraine accounts for another 15% of cases. In the remaining 50% of patients, neurologic disorders such as multiple sclerosis, postinfectious demyelination, temporal lobe seizure, Arnold Chiari malformation, tumors of brainstem and cerebellum, and cerebellar degeneration are associated with vertigo (18).

Many vertebrobasilar ischemia and stroke syndromes present with vertigo. Lateral medullary syndrome with infarction of the dorsal lateral medulla as a result of occlusion of the vertebral artery or posterior inferior cerebellar artery leads to vertigo, nausea, ipsilateral facial numbness, Horner syndrome, and contralateral loss of body pain and temperature (34,35). Lateral pontomedullary syndrome from occlusion of the anterior inferior cerebellar artery results in infarction of the labyrinth, part of the pontomedullary region, and inferior lateral cerebellum. This can cause severe vertigo, nausea, vomiting, unilateral hearing loss, tinnitus, facial paralysis, and asymmetric signs of cerebellar dysfunction (4,35). Cerebellar infarction can also cause severe vertigo, vomiting, and ataxia. This can be mistaken for labyrinthitis if brainstem signs are absent. Lacunar infarction of the cerebellum, which may be unrecognized on MRI, can cause balance dysfunction (36,37).

In hemispheric stroke, abnormal postural reaction cannot be attributed solely to unilateral sensory-motor impairment. It has been hypothesized that hemispheric stroke may impair vestibular function and that this can affect the postural reaction on both sides of the body by impairment of VOR suppression (24,38). In a stroke patient with weakness, impaired ability of weight transfer, swing phase impairment, difficulty in maintaining stance phase on the paretic side, difficulty in coordinating muscle control, and difficulty in responding to proprioceptive feedback all provide further challenges to the balance mechanism. Balance in stroke patients can be further impaired by postural hypotension, drug side effects, psychological disturbances, altered vision, and other associated conditions such as neuropathy, arthritis, and altered cognitive status.

Most patients with multiple sclerosis experience difficulties with balance during the course of their disease, and about 20% of patients are noted to have true vertigo. The most proximal few millimeters of the vestibular cochlear nerve as well as its entire course within the brainstem are myelinated by CNS myelin (oligodendrocytes) and are, therefore, susceptible to CNS demyelination. Symptoms of diplopia, blurred vision, hearing loss, numbness, paresthesias, weakness, and spasms as well as balance dysfunction can be important neurologic signs in patients with MS.

Vestibular system dysfunction occurs in 30% to 60% of traumatic brain injury patients during the course of their recovery (39–42). Many present with a variety of symptoms related to vestibular pathology, including vertigo, decreased gaze stability and ocular control, disequilibrium, and gait ataxia. The intensity of these symptoms depends on the site and severity of brain injury and associated cognitive and sensory-motor deficits. Fracture of the temporal bone is often associated with injury or concussion of the vestibular apparatus, producing loss of vestibular function on the side of injury. Positional nystagmus, vertigo, and high-frequency sensorineural hearing loss are commonly seen in inner ear concussion injury.

Head trauma can result in displacement of otoconia to cupula or the posterior semicircular canal, possibly causing BPPV or rupture of the round or oval window and resulting in a traumatic perilymphatic fistula (34,43). Injury to the central vestibular system (brainstem and cerebellum) in the form of multiple petechial hemorrhages in mild and moderate cases of head injury has been reported, and outcomes in these patients are worse than for those with peripheral vestibular injury (37). Management includes the treatment of underlying pathology along with a vestibular rehabilitation program, as described below (44).

Nonvestibular System Disorder and Dizziness

Types of dizziness caused by nonvestibular system disorders are presyncopal lightheadedness, disequilibrium, psy-

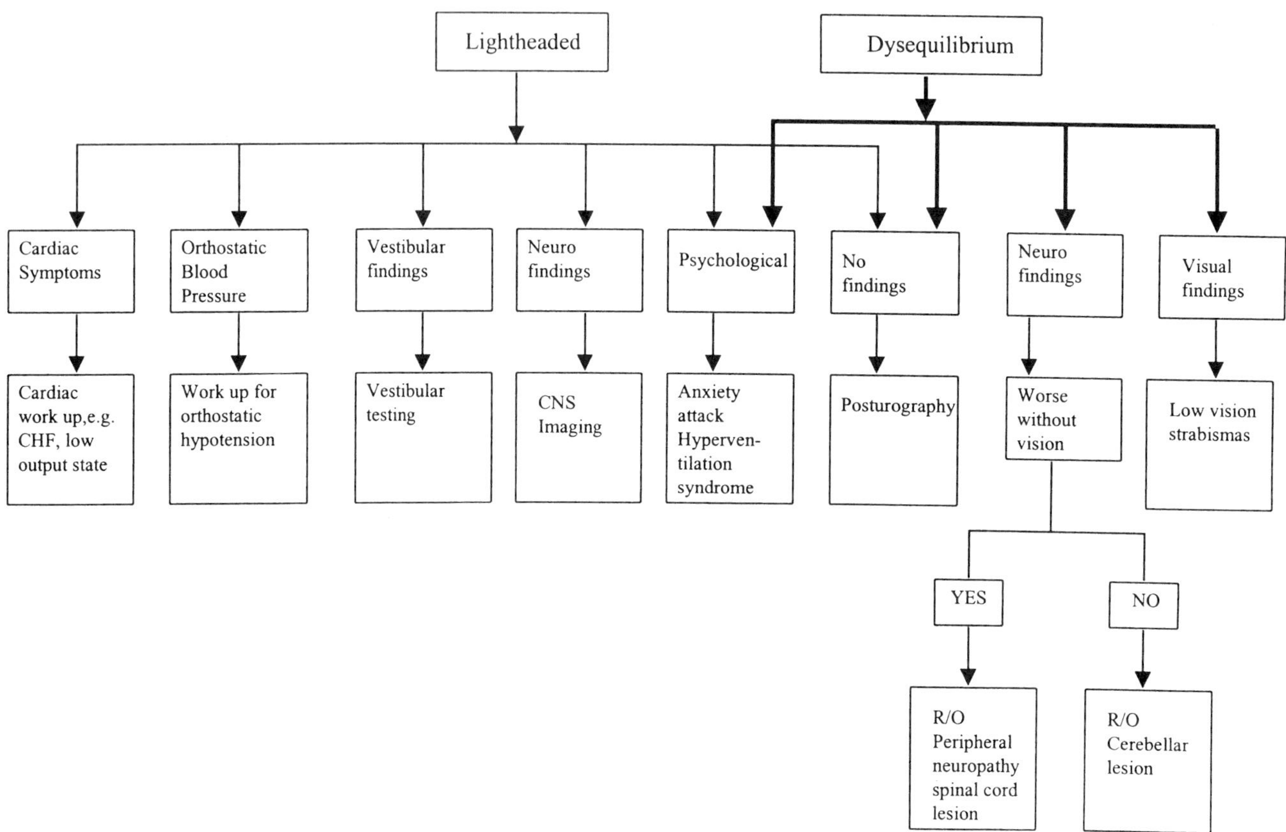

FIG. 71-3. Differential diagnosis for symptoms of lightheadness.

chogenic dizziness, and dizziness as a result of metabolic or endocrine disease. Symptoms of lightheadedness require a differential diagnosis as suggested in Figure 71-3.

Presyncopal lightheadedness is a sensation of impending fainting associated with dimming of vision, feeling cold and clammy, and anxiety that lasts for only a few seconds. It is perceived as a head rather than a body sensation. Possible etiologies are noted in Table 71-1.

Disequilibrium, or a sensation of unsteadiness and being off balance, is perceived as a body sensation. Any disturbance in visual, vestibulospinal, proprioceptive/somatosensory, cerebellar, or motor function can lead to disequilibrium. Common causes of disequilibrium are stroke, medications, multiple neurosensory deficit, peripheral neuropathy, or cerebellar disease.

Psychogenic dizziness is dizziness without objective findings and is associated with psychiatric disturbances. It is described as functional or psychogenic dizziness or lightheadedness.

Imbalance is a condition in which an individual is unable to maintain his or her COG over the base of support. This may present as frequent falls, stumbling, or a change in body posture to bring the COG back to over the base of support. It is usually caused by weakness secondary to sensory or motor dysfunction, which can result from traumatic or degenerative musculoskeletal abnormalities. This is often seen in amputees.

Cervical dizziness usually occurs in older persons with osteoarthritic changes of the cervical spine. It is caused either by temporary disruption of vertebral artery blood flow while turning the head and looking up or by overstimulation of proprioceptive receptors in cervical facet joints (4,45). This presents with episodic vertigo provoked by the assumption of certain neck positions. Cervical dizziness can be differentiated from BPPV by the absence of symptoms when the positions of the head and neck are changed together, e.g., bending forward or turning in bed without movement of the cervical spine facet joints (4). Use of a cervical collar and cervical traction during acute episodes and neck retraction exercises for chronic symptoms may be helpful.

Criteria for postural (orthostatic) hypotension is a 20 mm Hg drop in systolic pressure and/or a 10 mm Hg drop in diastolic pressure within 2 minutes of standing up from a recumbent position (4). Many elderly patients complain of dizziness during this position change; however, they rarely meet the criteria for orthostatic hypotension (4,46,47). Some older patients pool enough blood in their lower extremities to impair cerebral perfusion without lowering their blood pressure enough to have orthostatic hypotension (48,49). In some cases, blood pressure drop occurs 10 to 20 minutes after the change to upright posture, suggesting delayed orthostatic intolerance (4,9). Management can include compressive stockings, lower extremity exercises, maintenance of optimal hydration, and cardioselective beta-blocking medications.

Older patients sometimes present with dizziness from impaired physiological function of multiple systems, e.g., visual impairment from cataracts, physical deconditioning with poor postural control, cervical spondylosis, mild peripheral neuropathy, medications, and unilateral or bilateral vestibular hypofunction as a result of age-related degeneration of otoconia and loss of hair cells (50,51). Treatment can include correction of visual acuity and other reversible factors as well as conditioning exercises to improve strength and coordination, adjustment of medication, and assistive devices (52).

Vestibular symptoms and signs are often associated with diabetes mellitus, chronic renal disease, hypothyroidism, thiamine deficiency, and alcohol intoxication. Diabetes mellitus can lead to cranial neuropathy or atherosclerosis of the vertebrobasilar artery, leading to hearing loss and vertigo. Ototoxic effect of medication, immunosuppressive treatment in transplant patients, and hyponatremia in patients undergoing dialysis are believed to be causes of vestibular symptoms in patients with chronic renal failure and uremia (53,54). Acute alcohol intoxication causes positional vertigo and nystagmus (55). Long-term excessive use of alcohol may cause cerebellar degeneration and atrophy, most likely from malnutrition rather than from any direct effect of alcohol. Thiamine deficiency is the most common cause of Wernicke's encephalopathy, a condition that is also associated with vestibular dysfunction.

Vertigo or dizziness without apparent organic pathology is common and often labeled as "vertigo of unknown etiology," "nonspecific vertigo," "psychogenic vertigo," or "hyperventilation syndrome." Diagnostic workup includes otoneurologic and audiometric evaluations. Patients with position-provoked symptoms should be given a trial of vestibular rehabilitation exercise. If this is not effective, then electronystagmography and MRI studies of the brain may assist in establishing a diagnosis. If a complete diagnostic workup is unrevealing, consultation with a psychiatrist or psychologist is recommended.

Vestibular suppressants, diuretics, migraine prophylaxis, and/or long acting antihistamines can also be tried (Table 71-3). If all measures fail to resolve the symptoms, the patient is nevertheless followed every 6 months, and yearly audiometric screening is performed to screen for acoustic neuroma, BPPV, or very early Meniere's disease.

VESTIBULAR AND BALANCE ASSESSMENT AND REHABILITATION

The goals of rehabilitation are to resolve acute or reversible deficits, compensate for irreversible deficits, minimize the burden of chronic deficits, and minimize danger from falls to restore safe, upright mobility and promote independence.

A comprehensive evaluation of dizziness may require multiple system assessments. A differential diagnosis of vertigo and dizziness assessment are shown in Figures 71-3 and 71-4. It must begin with a history that should include specific questions relevant to the vestibular system and a detailed physical examination (Appendix I; specialized testing is detailed in Appendix II).

With a clear understanding of the balance mechanism, it would be easier to correlate patients' symptoms, examination findings, and specialized testing results to diagnose and plan medical rehabilitation and surgical management.

Physiatric management of patients with vestibular and balance disorders requires a coordinated multidisciplinary program that includes therapeutic exercises and training in compensation (56). Adaptation and habituation to motion-provoked symptoms are believed to occur by readjustment and recalibration of the vestibulo-ocular reflex, visuo-ocular reflex, cervico-ocular reflex, vestibulospinal reflex, and other reflexes. Compensation by substitution is accomplished by effective use of other sensory modalities for input.

Spontaneous resolution occurs in a majority of patients with dizziness and vertigo caused by peripheral vestibular disorders. Failure to resolve spontaneously may result from the severity of the disorder and impaired CNS capacity for spontaneous compensation (57). Central nervous system plasticity is the essential characteristic for the basis of recovery in balance dysfunction (58). Improvements occur by adaptation, habituation, and substitution resulting in compensation. Home visits are essential to prescribe potentially beneficial alterations as well as for caregivers' education. A coordinated multidisciplinary team approach is the most successful and should include psychological counseling for associated neurobehavioral symptoms.

Patients with reproducible symptoms on examination are likely to benefit from rehabilitation. Exercises are presented (Table 71-4), and the regimen is increased gradually while avoiding intolerable symptoms. Motions or positions that mildly provoke or increase vertigo are selected as the starting point for exercise. The most effective exercises are those that provide visual stimuli by movement of the head at different frequencies in various positions. Adaptation response to the exercise program may require 2 weeks to 2 months in unilateral peripheral vestibular lesions and up to 2 years in bilateral lesions. Influencing factors such as diagnosis, age, and conditions affecting the central and peripheral nervous systems as well as the patient's compliance with the exercise program may compromise the process of adaptation and substitution. It is important to grade the degree of intensity of symptoms initially and periodically to determine the efficacy of the exercise program. If there is no progress by 4 weeks, the existing exercise program is reviewed and modified. Lack of progress may indicate that the exercise program is either too vigorous or not sufficiently challenging.

Once symptoms are found to improve with exercise, the program can be modified to incorporate challenges in visual and somatosensory input to facilitate substitution, e.g., standing on foam with eyes open and closed. Habituation

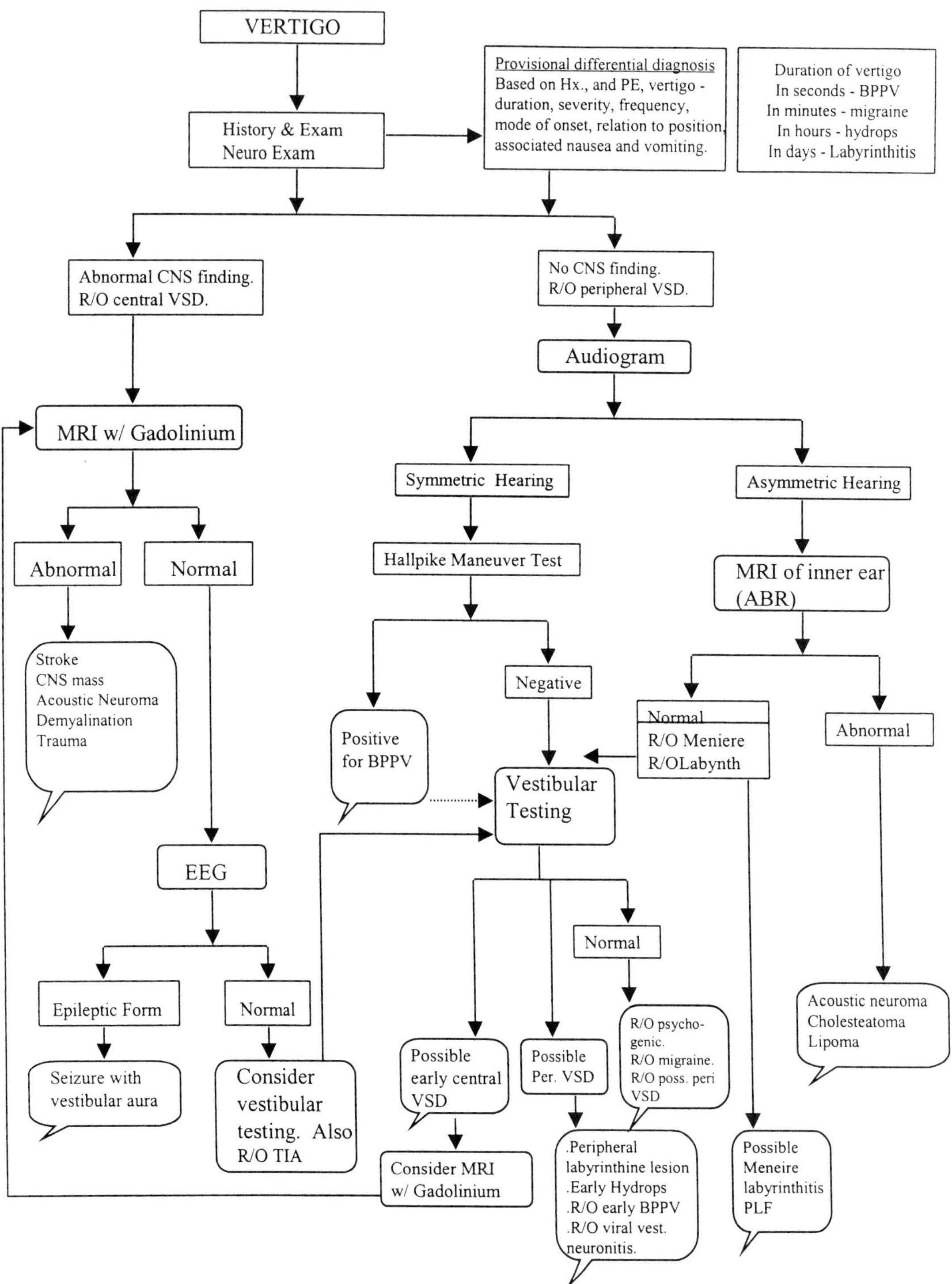

FIG. 71-4. Guidelines to a possible pathway for diagnostic workup in vertigo.

exercises can cause fear, anxiety, or panic in some patients. Habituation exercise involving extreme head and neck movement of extension and rotation are contraindicated in patients with severe cervical spondylosis, stenosis, fusion, or instability, vertebral basilar insufficiency, or other cerebral vascular disease. Reassurance to the patient and proper education are very important for development of trust and compliance. Psychological counseling and support groups may be helpful. Central nervous system adaptation and habituation with therapeutic exercise are least effective if the patient is on vestibular suppressant medication. Adaptive and substitutive capability of the vestibular system is reduced in older persons because of age-related changes in the CNS as well as visual and somatosensory receptors. When indicated, therapeutic exercise programs should also include exercise to improve flexibility, general conditioning in respect to strength and endurance, training with task-oriented functional activities, education and safety awareness, training with appropriate orthotic and assistive devices, mental exercise to improve concentration and attention, and psychological counseling. The results of vestibular rehabilitation are not favorable in sedentary patients, the elderly, patients with bilateral lesions or fluctuating deficits, and the neurologically impaired with multiple sensory deficits.

In 1944, Cawthorne explained the physiological basis of head exercise, and in 1946 Cawthorne and Cooksey presented a concept of vestibular exercise for the rehabilitation of patients with vestibular injuries (59,60). These exercises have been used since then for patients with dizziness along with medical and surgical treatment. McCabe in 1970 described the physiological basis for the methodology of labyrinthine exercise (61). Hecker in 1974 and Norre in 1980 published their experience with Cawthorne–Cooksey exercise and habituation therapy, respectively (62,63). In 1985, Zee suggested a set of exercise protocols for vertigo patients (64).

TABLE 71-4. *Example of vestibular and balance rehabilitation exercise program*[a]

Head–eye coordination exercise (Fig. 71-5)
1. While seated, hold a target at arm's length in front of you, and move your head first side to side, then up and down, while keeping target in focus all the time, gradually increasing velocity and repetitions to tolerance.
2. Focus on a hand-held moving target and move the target in the opposite direction of head movement in horizontal and vertical directions.

Visual–ocular control exercise (Fig. 71-5)
1. While seated in front of wall, holding head still, jump-move your eyes to extreme established target points on the wall in horizontal and vertical planes within your visual field.

Adaptation/habituation exercise for motion-provoked symptoms (Table 71-5)
1. Lie flat on your back with eyes open, then quickly come to a sitting position, wait for 10 seconds, back to supine with head turned to right, wait for 10 seconds. Repeat the same maneuver with head turned to the opposite side.

Sensory substitution-promoting exercise (Table 71-6)
1. Stand on one leg with support and eyes open for 30 seconds, then with eyes closed. Progressively increase challenges by standing on foam or with head movement.

Postural strategy practicing exercise (Fig. 71-6)
1. Standing on flat surface, rock back and forth about the ankle without bending at the hip first with eyes open and then with eyes closed for 30 seconds.
2. Repeat the above standing on foam surface.

General conditioning exercise
1. Self-performed exercise program to improve flexibility and strength if deficit is identified.

Functional activity training
1. Walking program: start with 5 minutes and progress 2 minutes each week until you can walk for 30 minutes.

Exercise for improving attention, concentration, and psychological counseling

Patient/family education support group

[a] Instructions: (a) follow-up visit in 2 to 4 weeks; (b) use Tables 71-5 and 71-6 and Figs. 71-5 and 71-6 to write appropriate detailed exercises in each category. Prescribe and specify number of repetitions and duration of each exercise when applicable.

The most effective approach for rehabilitation of patients with vestibular problems is to devise an individualized program (Table 71-4). This must address deficits in (a) gaze stability and ocular control (Fig. 71-5), (b) adaptation and habituation to motion-provoked symptoms (Table 71-5), (c) postural stability by substitution with unaffected sensory modalities (Table 71-6), (d) postural response strategies (Fig. 71-6), (e) attention, concentration, and psychological adjustment, (f) patient and family education, (g) general conditioning and flexibility contributing to balance dysfunction, (h) functional activities, and (i) adaptation and habituation to positional vertigo (specific exercises for BPPV).

Each individual can have a different degree of impairment responsible for balance dysfunction in each category, so each patient's exercise program should prioritize the category found to be most responsible for his or her balance dysfunction, and the program should be periodically revised to a higher level of challenges in each category as improvement occurs.

Exercise for gaze stability is begun as soon as possible after onset of vestibular dysfunction (Fig. 71-5). Exercise should initially be performed for 1 minute at slow speed, followed by a period of rest. Exercise duration and speed of head movements are gradually increased. When head–eye coordination exercise with a fixed target is well tolerated, exercise progresses to using a moving target. The patient should be warned that the exercise may make him or her dizzy or nauseated, but it should be continued for 1 to 2 minutes, followed by a period of rest, unless vomiting occurs.

For exercise to improve visual ocular control, the head is held in one position, and a moving target is kept in focus all the time. The target moves slowly and smoothly in vertical, horizontal, and circular fashion (smooth pursuit eye movement) and also toward and away from the nose.

Exercise using saccadic eye movement can be done by keeping the head still and jump-looking up and down or side to side to the extreme points. This will accomplish conditioning of extraocular muscles for saccadic ocular control as well as habituation to symptoms provoked by rapidly changing visual images.

CNS compensation by adaptation and habituation can be achieved effectively by gradually progressive symptom-provoking exercises (Table 71-5). Compensation occurs at the level of the vestibular nuclei and cerebellum (integration level) by rebalancing tonic activity at vestibular nuclei as well as modulation by the cerebral cortex (perception level) if resolution of the pathology at the peripheral receptor level does not occur.

Each exercise is done twice a day with increasing repetitions, velocity and range of motion as tolerated. (5 repetitions increasing to 10 repetitions). They may start for a duration of one minute and then increase slowly utilizing rest periods.

I. Progressive head eye coordination exercise:

1. Focus on **fixed target** in front of eyes while sitting then
   a. Move your head side to side.
   b. Move your head up and down.
   c. Move your head in circular fashion.
   Repeat above in different head and neck position in relation to the body, e.g., fixed target on floor or ceiling while seated.

2. Focus on a hand held **moving target** and move the target in an opposite direction of head movement in horizontal and vertical direction.

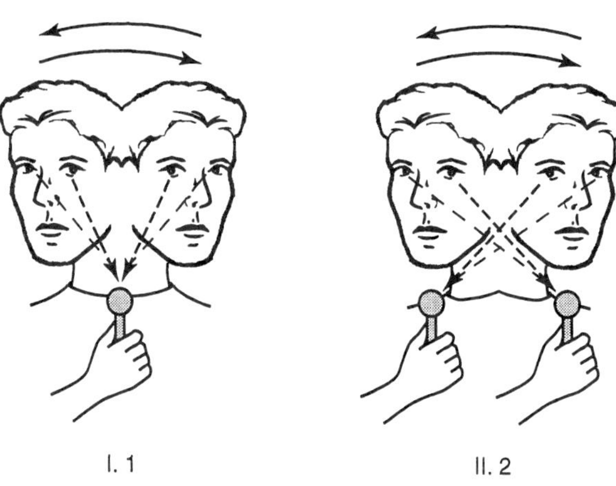

II. Visual-ocular control exercise:

Exercise with **smooth pursuit** eye movement:

1. Keep your **head still** while focusing on a motorized or hand held **smooth moving target** and move the target in horizontal, vertical and circular clockwise and anticlockwise fashion.

Exercise with **saccadic eye** movement:

2. Hold **head still** and jump-move eyes to the extreme points (dot or light) in front in horizontal and vertical fashion.

PRECAUTIONS: The patient may develop nausea and dizziness during exercises. These exercises should begin as soon as vestibular dysfunction is detected.

FIG. 71-5. Gaze stability and ocular control exercises.

An abnormally responding vestibular system is desensitized by repetition of dizziness-provoking rapid movement. This desensitization and habituation effect occurs by physiological CNS compensation as well as by behavioral adjustment to abnormal responses (64,65).

The movements listed in Table 71-5 can be used initially to identify the position changes that provoke the symptoms. These same movements then can be used for exercises with a gradual increase in movement speeds and frequency as habituation develops.

Compensation by substitution with visual or somatosensory information occurs at the CNS level in cases in which vestibular input is deficient, especially in bilateral peripheral vestibular lesions (Table 71-6). The exercise program for postural stability is developed by gradually increasing challenges using various positions and postures for maintenance of the center of gravity over the base of support through musculoskeletal control. While performing this exercise program, the patient is instructed in techniques to prevent falls.

Exercise to improve postural response strategies is used to facilitate the patient's ability to use corrective and protective postural responses. Corrective posture responses improve stability and refer to ankle, hip, and body stiffening and counterbalance responses. Protective posture responses include stepping, grabbing of external support, and rescue responses with support by outstretched arm to minimize the impact of a fall when challenges to the base of support are severe (Fig. 71-6).

Fatigue, irritability, frustration, sleep disturbances, depression, anxiety, and panic are some of the neurobehavioral symptoms associated with vertigo due to peripheral vestibular disorders. Patient education and psychological counseling along with strategies to improve attention and concentration are the most crucial aspects of vestibular rehabilitation. These improve patient compliance with the exercise program, which is essential for habituation and adaptation. The patient may benefit from enrollment in a vestibular support group. The Vestibular Disorder Association (P.O. Box 4467, Portland, OR 97208-4467) can provide patients with a newsletter and information concerning support networks.

The patient also needs to be instructed about precautions if the therapy program is performed on a home basis. Modification of the home environment may be necessary to prevent injury from falls. Good lighting and avoiding the use of throw rugs may prevent potential falls. Medication interactions may be responsible for the patient's falls and should also be addressed.

Balance can be compromised, especially in elderly people, by a decrease in lower extremity range of motion, muscle flexibility, strength, endurance, and general deconditioning. Poor or abnormal posture can also contribute to balance impairment. Strengthening of trunk, hip girdle, and other lower extremity muscles may increase stability and reduce falls.

Training in safety awareness during functional activity and assessment of need for adaptive equipment, orthoses, and assistive devices are considered. A progressive ambulation program can be developed, beginning with 5 minutes and incorporating sensory challenges, e.g., shaking, turning or tilting the head, or quickly pivoting to the right or left. Walking duration can be increased to 30 minutes over a period of several weeks. Rehabilitation of hearing loss, when present, is addressed with auditory training and a hearing aid.

TABLE 71-5. *Adaptation and habituation exercise training for motion-provoked symptoms*

Exercise/motion	Intensity (1, 2, 3)	Duration (1, 2, 3)	Nystagmus (0, +2)	Score
Bed rolling				
Supine to right lateral				
Supine to left lateral				
Supine to sitting				
Supine to sit straight				
Sit to left Hallpike				
Left Hallpike to sit				
Sit to right Hallpike				
Right Hallpike to sit				
Sitting with head movement				
Side to side				
Up and down				
Circular fashion clockwise				
Circular fashion counterclockwise				
Sit to bend forward				
Sit → touch nose to right knee				
Sit → touch nose to left knee				
Sit to stand				
Stand → sudden turn to right				
Stand → sudden turn to left				
Stand → bend forward and up				

Instructions: (a) Document intensity (1, mild; 2, moderate; 3, severe) and duration (1, 0–15 seconds; 2, 15–30 seconds; 3, >30 seconds) of symptoms with each exercise, and +2 for presence of nystagmus. (b) Total score (intensity + duration + nystagmus) denotes severity.

Precautions: These exercises may provoke symptoms. Total score denotes severity. Compensation occurs at the level of vestibular nuclei and cerebellum by rebalancing tonic activity at the vestibular and modulation by cerebral cortex.

TABLE 71-6. *Postural stability exercises*[a]

Motor challenges		Visual challenges		Visual + Vestibular Challenges (head movement, HM)		Visual + Vestibular + Somatosensory Challenges (standing on foam, SOF)			
		Eyes open (EO) (a)	Eyes closed (EC) (b)	HM/EO (c)	HM/EC (d)	SOF/EO (e)	SOF/EC (f)	SOF/ HM/EO (g)	SOF/ HM/EC (h)
Standing Feet apart	Contact support								
	Unsupported								
Feet together	Contact support								
	Unsupported								
In tandem	Contact support								
	Unsupported								
On one leg	Contact support								
	Unsupported								
Walking Normal gait	Contact support								
	Unsupported								
Tandem walk	Contact support								
	Unsupported								
Stairs, up and down	Contact support								
	Unsupported								
Bending	Contact support								
	Unsupported								

[a] These exercises facilitate postural stability by substitution with visual or somatosensory input when vestibular input is deficient. The exercise is to improve compensation by substitution.

Specific Exercise for BPPV: Canalith Repositioning/ Restoration

Benign paroxysmal positional vertigo can be treated by many approaches, including Epley's canalith-repositioning maneuver (for canalithiasis), the Brandt–Daroff exercise (for cupulolithiasis), and the Semont maneuver.

The Epley canalith-repositioning maneuver is also known as the canalith-repositioning procedure (CRP). It is the first line of treatment for BPPV (Fig. 71-7). It can be performed in the office on an adjustable examination table with side rails or on a hospital bed with the patient lying across the bed. Patients who become nauseous during the Hallpike testing are premedicated with antiemetics or any of the vestibular suppressants (17,57).

1. The procedure is started with the patient sitting in head-upright position (position A, Fig. 71-7).
2. Then, the Dix–Hallpike provoking position is assumed (position B, Fig. 71-7). The examiner observes for nystagmus until it stops. A massager is held to the mastoid region of the downward ear to facilitate ampullofugal flow of endolymph. The examiner then waits another 30 seconds to watch again for nystagmus. This entire process takes about 3 to 4 minutes.
3. Then the examiner turns the patient's head to the opposite side while keeping the head extended (Dix–Hallpike) (position C, Fig. 71-7) and waits an additional 30 seconds after nystagmus stops. The massager is used again on the mastoid bone of the downward ear, and the process is repeated. In Dix–Hallpike positions B and C, one normally sees a nystagmus beating toward the upward ear.
4. The head and trunk positions are maintained, and the patient rolls into the right lateral position. In this position, D, the head is 180° opposite to that with respect to position B. Apply the hand-held massager to the mastoid and wait for 30 seconds. Nystagmus will be seen beating toward the upward ear in this position.
5. Maintaining the head position, bring the patient rapidly to the sitting position, rotate the head forward, and wait for 1 minute (position E).
6. This procedure may be stopped after two cycles if nystagmus or dizziness stops. Otherwise, repeat to a maximum

of six cycles. Each cycle takes approximately 3 minutes, and the whole process can be completed in about 20 to 30 minutes. After the test, the patient rests in a semirecumbent position at a 45° angle for 2 days without movement of the head up or down. The patient is also advised to sleep with the affected side up, using two pillows, and to avoid symptom-provoking positions for 1 week. This evaluation and treatment can be repeated in 1 week. Some practitioners do not use the vibrator out of concern that additional debris may break off from the utricle. Occasionally, after the Epley maneuver, debris can move from the posterior canal to the lateral canal and change the nystagmus type from horizontal nystagmus to one in which nystagmus beats downward with respect to the dependent ear. This change of "posterior canal BPPV" to "lateral canal BPPV" is called "canal conversion" (18).

In case of recurrence of symptoms after treatment with the Epley maneuver, or if the maneuver fails to improve

A. **Corrective response exercise**:	Mode of Action:
1. Ankle response: Stand on solid platform longer than size of feet and rock back and forth about ankle without bending hip joint for 30 seconds with eyes open and closed.	This strategy rotates the body about the ankle joint. Effective when COG moves slowly and is well within the limits of stability.
2. Hip response: Stand on compressible surface or surface which is shorter than the size of feet (e.g., round pipe) and rock back and forth bending at hip for 30 seconds.	Hip strategy is effective when the support surface is short or compressible or when COG moves rapidly approaching the limits of stability.
3. Stiffening response: Contract all the agonist and antagonist muscles of the ankle, knee, hip joints, lumbosacral spine and neck muscles (vibrating surface).	Effective when support surface is vibrating and all agonist and antagonist muscles are contracting.
4. Counterbalance response: Counterbalancing movement of the arm to maintain COG over the BOS.	Movement of the arm in front of the body minimizes COG shift from the center to the limits of the stability.
B. **Protective response exercise:** 5. Stepping response. 6. Grabbing of external support response. 7. Rescue response with support by outstretched arm to minimize impact of fall and break the fall.	Train the patient how to prevent fall or how to break fall in cases where challenges of base support are catastrophic.
Precautions: Learn techniques to prevent falls	

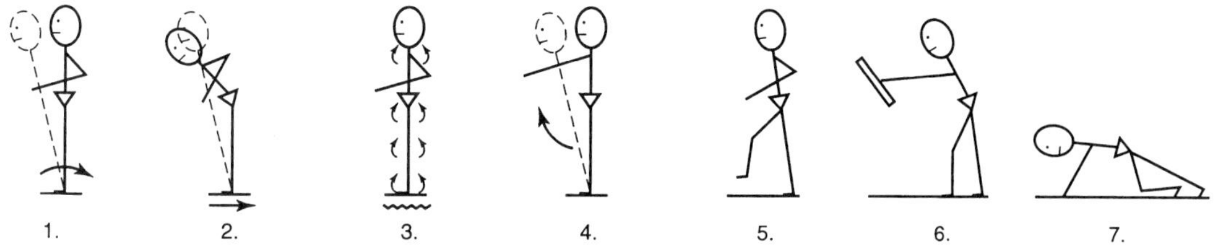

1. 2. 3. 4. 5. 6. 7.

FIG. 71-6. Exercise to improve postural response strategies. These exercises facilitate stability through corrective and protective postural responses.

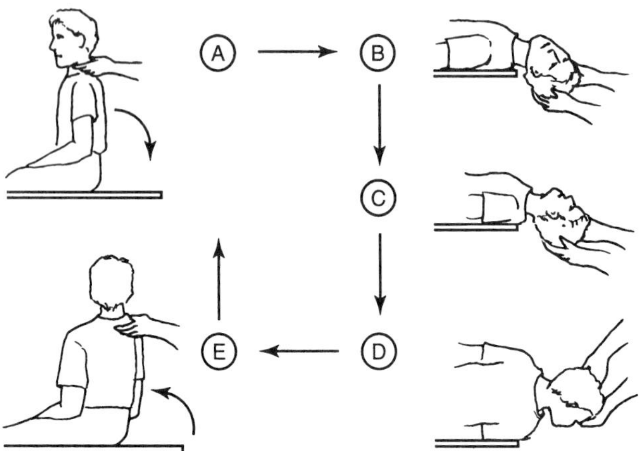

FIG. 71-7. Epley canalith-repositioning procedure for treatment of benign paroxysmal positional vertigo (BPPV).

symptoms, one may proceed with the Brandt–Daroff exercise (Fig. 71-8).

The Brandt–Daroff exercise is used for a home exercise treatment program for BPPV. This exercise approach is based on the following principles: otoconial material in the cupula of the posterior semicircular canal (cupulolithiasis) can be dislodged by frequently moving the patient into a vertigo-provoking position. This subjects the patient repeatedly to a position that brings on the symptom, which fatigues the response and stimulates the CNS to compensate by habituation and adaptation (16,57).

In this exercise (Fig. 71-8), the patient is instructed to sit on the edge of the bed (posterior canal facing posterolaterally at 45°) and quickly move to the right-side lying position with the head rotated 45° facing up (posterior canal oriented vertically downward). This brings on vertigo. The patient then stays in that position for 30 seconds after vertigo stops and then moves rapidly to the left side lying position with the head rotated 45° facing upward for approximately 30 seconds until vertigo stops (right nondependent side posterior canal is oriented horizontally, and left dependent side posterior canal is oriented vertically).

This exercise is repeated five to ten times per session and three times per day (depending on the severity of the

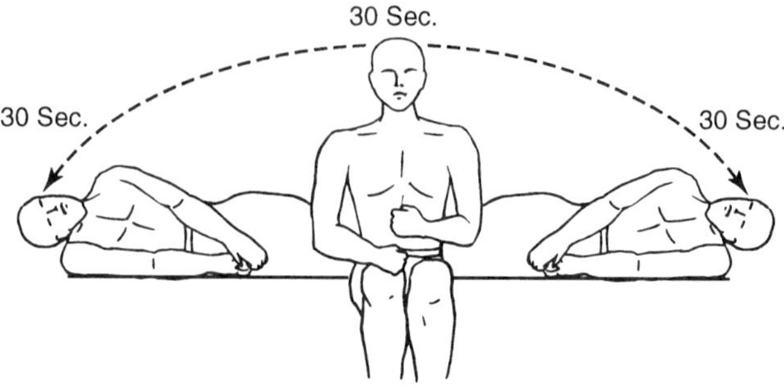

FIG. 71-8. Brandt–Daroff exercise.

provoked vertigo) for several weeks. This procedure is effective in more than 90% of patients with BPPV. If the symptom persists for more than 1 year, surgery can be considered.

The Semont maneuver is used when the affected side is clearly known (60,61). The patient sits with head turned 45° opposite to the involved side. This orients the posterior canal from the posterolateral to the lateral direction. The patient is then moved to side-lying on the affected side while maintaining the head at 45°. This provokes vertigo, as the posterior canal faces vertically down and induces gravity-dependent motion. This position is maintained for 2 to 3 minutes, and then the patient is brought rapidly to the opposite side-lying position and maintains a 45° head rotation toward the unaffected side, with the head facing downward and the posterior canal oriented vertically upward.

If the patient does not experience vertigo in the second position, the head is shaken once or twice in an attempt to free the otolithic debris. The patient stays in this position for 5 minutes and then is slowly brought to sitting. Following this exercise, the patient remains vertical for 48 hours and avoids symptom-provoking positions for 1 week.

CONCLUSION

Recently, newer strategies for evaluation and treatment of balance disorders have become available. Advanced computerized diagnostic and therapeutic equipment is available for vestibular testing and posturography. Physiatric practice should include these techniques and treatments to help reduce balance and mobility dysfunction.

APPENDIX I: CASE EVALUATION

History and Physical Examination

Chief complaint
Dizziness

Onset of symptom
Date of onset
Description
Sudden versus gradual
Frequency
Associated symptoms of nausea/vomiting

Characteristic feature (vertigo, lightheadedness, disequilibrium, imbalance; episodic versus continuous)

1. Symptoms increase with loud noise? (Tullio phenomenon, PLF)
2. Symptoms increase with Valsalva maneuver? (cough and sneeze, PLF)
3. Symptoms occur only in certain position? (BPPV)
4. Associated symptoms of nausea and vomiting? (peripheral VSD)
5. Symptoms increase with rise of temperature? (demyelinating disease)

6. Symptoms ease when eyes open and worsen when eyes close? (visual compensation)
7. Symptoms increase with exercise? (cardiac/pulmonary)
8. Symptoms increase after meals? (postprandial hypotension or syncope)
9. Symptoms while fasting? (hypoglycemia)
10. Symptoms decrease with exercise or distraction? Presence of anxiety and panic? (psychogenic dizziness)

Hearing loss (Right or left)
Duration, progressive, fluctuation?
Tinnitus, fullness?

Past medical history
History of head and neck injury?
Unusual activity, e.g., scuba diving, mountain hiking?
Stress events in life, ear infection, migraine headache, ototoxic medication, diabetes, hypertension, heart disease, CVA, Parkinson's disease, visual problem?

Personal history
Self anxiety rating 0 to 10
General activity level (describe)
Employment status
Smoking history
Alcohol history

Current medication and allergies

Functional history

Describe specific activity that can not be performed as a result of symptoms (self-care, home management, community activity, vocational, leisure activity)

Disability scale by history (Circle one)

0. No disability
1. Bothersome symptoms
2. Mild disability, performs usual duties, symptoms interfere with social activity
3. Moderate disability, disrupts usual duties
4. Recent severe disability, on medical leave, or had to change job
5. Long-term disability, unable to work for extended period

Physical Examination

Blood pressure (sitting, standing), pulse, respiration rate

Examination of heart

Examination of lungs

Vision examination: Snellen chart rating, visual field (full/limited, left, right, upper, lower), extraocular muscles, nystagmus

Ear exam: Otoscopic examination: cerumen impaction, osteoma, malformation, canal obstruction, tympanic membrane, serous otitis media, perforation, evidence of cholesteatoma, hemotympanum (suggestive of bone trauma), painful vesicular eruption (herpes zoster)

Rinne's test: bone conduction (BC) versus air conduction (AC)
BC > AC: negative Rinne test (conductive hearing loss of at least 25 dB)
AC > BC: positive Rinne test (possible normal hearing, sensory-neural hearing loss or conductive loss smaller than 25 dB)

Weber test: Tuning fork on glabella
Sound lateralized to the ear with conductive hearing loss or away from sensorineural hearing loss
Unilateral hearing loss: sound lateralizing to better ear suggests a contralateral sensorineural hearing loss; sound lateralizing to the worse ear is characteristic of conductive hearing loss

Examination of nose, oral cavity, and throat

Examination of neck and cervical spine: carotid bruit, thyromegaly, lymphadenopathy, cervical range of motion

Neurologic exam: cranial nerves

Test for coordination and motor control
Finger to nose, heel to shin, diadochokinesis, finger opposition, rhythmic tapping, pronator drift
Sensation: light touch, pinprick, sharp/dull discrimination, proprioception, vibration
Reflexes: Babinski (up/down)
Muscle tone: hyper, hypo, normal, clonus (+/−)
Muscle strength

Neurologic assessment (circle)
Pyramidal: spasticity, clasp knife, poor distal control, + clonus, +Babinski, hyperreflexia, spastic gait, pronator drift
Extrapyramidal: rigidity (cogwheel, lead pipe), dysrhythmia, dysdiadochokinesis, bradykinesis, shuffle gait
Cerebellar: hypertonia, intention tremor, dysmetria, ataxic gait

Musculoskeletal examination
Head and neck: forward head posture, loss of cervical lordosis, torticollis
Trunk postural deviation: protracted shoulder, kyphosis, scoliosis, excessive lordosis
Range of motion and strength: shoulder, elbow, wrist, hand, hip joint, knee, and ankle
Comments

Stance and gait: short distance walk in straight line with eyes open, then eyes closed

Gait analysis
Standard: normal, unsteady (mild, moderate, severe)
Tandem gait: number of steps on line/20
Head turn/tilt: normal, unsteady (mild, moderate, severe)
Turn (right/left): normal, unsteady (mild, moderate, severe)
Comments

Static postural stability test

Sitting balance; *standing* balance, eyes open; *standing* balance, eyes closed (Rhomberg)

Tandem stance, eyes open; tandem stance, eyes closed

Standing on foam, both legs, eyes open; standing on foam, both legs, eyes closed; *tandem stance on foam*, eyes open; tandem stance on foam, eyes closed

Stance on one leg, eyes open; stance on one leg, eyes closed; stance on one leg, head turning; stance on one leg on foam

Dynamic postural stability test

Walking 25 steps eyes open, document number of fall reactions; walking 25 steps eyes closed, document number of fall reactions

Walking on foam mat 25 steps, eyes open, document number of fall reactions; walking 25 steps on foam mat, eyes closed, document number of fall reactions

Stepping up and down on step stool, 10 times with each leg

Functional postural stability test

Stepping test of Fukuda (65)

Test of ability to make stable turn on command while walking (Singleton test) (66)

Test for limits of stability (standing reach test) (67)

Specialized Testing

Test for motion-provoked symptoms

Dix–Hallpike maneuver test

Fistula tests (with pneumatoscope)

Dynamic posturography: clinical test for sensory interaction on balance (CTSIB) control

Dynamic posturography conditions (68) (Fig. 71-9):

1. Eyes open, support surface stable, visual field stable
2. Eyes closed, support surface stable (Rhomberg test)
3. Eyes open, support surface, visual field swayed
4. Eyes open, support surface swayed, visual field stable
5. Eyes closed, support surface swayed
6. Eyes open, support surface swayed, visual field swayed

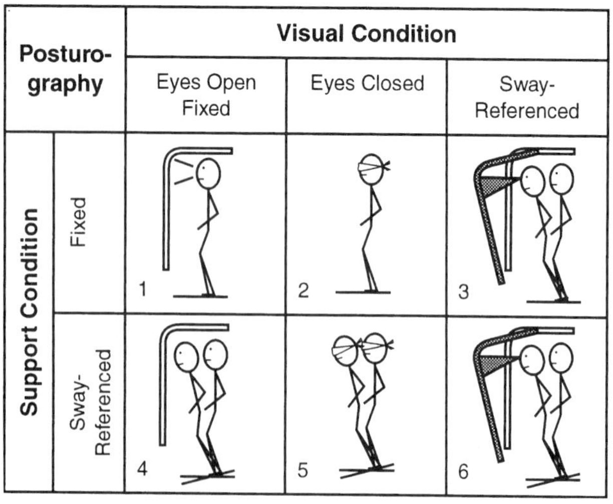

Posturography		Visual Condition		
		Eyes Open Fixed	Eyes Closed	Sway-Referenced
Support Condition	Fixed	1	2	3
	Sway-Referenced	4	5	6

FIG. 71-9. Dynamic posturography.

Document number of falls and increased sway in 30-second trial; common patterns of performance:

i. Normal (no problem in any position)

ii. Vestibular dysfunction (problem with 5,6)

iii. Visual vestibular dysfunction, support-surface-dependent pattern (4,5,6)

iv. Visual preference (problem with 3,4)

v. Somatosensory–vestibular dysfunction, visual dependent pattern (problem with 2,3,5,6)

vi. Severe (combination other than those above)

vii. Inconsistent (e.g., performance on 1 worse than others, 2 worse than 5, 3 worse than 6, 4 worse than 5 and 6)

Vestibular testing

Audiometric studies: audiogram, speech reception threshold (SRT), speech discrimination test (SDT), impedance audiometry, tympanometry, stapedial–acoustic reflex (69,70) test, electrocochleography (EcoG) (28,71,72)

Auditory brainstem response (ABR)

Electronystagmography (ENG)

Spontaneous, gaze evoked, positional nystagmus (73)

EMG test of visual-ocular control with saccadic, smooth pursuit, and optokinetic stimulus (71,74)

Caloric test (bithermal) (75–77): caloric stimuli and ENG for evaluation of horizontal canal vestibulo-ocular reflex

Rotational chair test (78–81), vestibular autorotational test (82–84): rotational stimuli and ENG for evaluation of horizontal canal vestibulo-ocular reflex

Radiographic examination

CT scan with contrast

MRI with gadolinium

Blood test

CBC, blood glucose

Thyroid function test

Cholesterol, triglycerides

Autoimmune test: sedimentation rate, antinuclear antibody, rheumatoid arthritis factor, lupus erythematosus preparation, lymphocyte transformation test, fluorescent treponemal antibody with absorption

APPENDIX II: SPECIALIZED TESTING

Dix–Hallpike Maneuver Test

The Dix–Hallpike test is used primarily to test for BPPV (15,85). In this test (Fig. 71-2), the patient sits on the examination table in a way that, when lying down, his or her head would be hanging off the edge of the table. Throughout this test, the head is supported by the examiner's hand. The patient is first placed in a sitting position with the head facing straight ahead. In the initial maneuver, the patient is brought to supine with the head hanging off the examination table. In about 60 seconds, the patient is brought back to sitting position. The patient is instructed to keep eyes open, looking ahead all the time. During the second maneuver, the patient's head is rotated to one side, and the patient is brought to supine with the head hanging and rotated. Again, 60 seconds later, the patient is brought back to upright. This maneuver is again repeated a third time in the same manner with head turned to the other side.

Rapid change in position results in reorientation of the posterior semicircular canal and ampulla, producing gravity-dependent endolymph and cupula motion. The presence of an otolithic lesion increases the sensitivity of the canal to the above movement and induces the nystagmus. The examiner observes the patient's eyes for nystagmus.

Dynamic Posturography

Dynamic (Fig. 71-9) posturography is a test of a person's ability to maintain balance by effectively using visual, vestibular, and somatosensory inputs separately as well as suppressing or compensating for inaccurate or challenging sensory information. Postural balance requires that the center of gravity (COG) be over the base of support within limits of stability in a given sensory environmental condition. This requires integration of accurate sensory input and proper execution of motor control. The immediate motor control of balance when the body is displaced occurs by automatic postural responses that are not under volitional control. These postural responses are ankle, hip, stiffening, counterbalance, step, and grab responses (3,86,87) (Fig. 71-6).

The dynamic posturography test consists of two components. The first assesses sensory interaction on balance or sensory organization. The second component evaluates automatic postural response and movement coordination. Sensory interaction or organization can be evaluated by systematically altering mechanical somatosensory input and informational visual input and assessing the body's ability to maintain balance (80). Vestibular information cannot be altered by noninvasive methods (51). The method of altering (sway referencing) somatosensory and visual information involves tilting the support surface and visual surround (86). Six combinations of altered visual and support conditions are used to assess sensory interaction and organization as well as the ability to control balance and posture.

Vestibular Testing

The functional integrity of the labyrinthine and cochlear parts of the vestibular apparatus, eighth nerve, and brainstem pathways are tested. In addition, ocular motility is evaluated to screen peripheral and central components of vestibulo-ocular system and for loss of VOR suppression. Tests include audiometric studies (to determine symmetric versus asymmetric), electro-oculography, positional electronystagmography, caloric stimuli with electronystagmography (to help differentiate unilateral from bilateral loss), and rotation stimuli with electronystagmography (to identify reduced gain of vestibular system). Audiologic testing is considered an extension of the clinical examination and is done even if there is no subjective hearing loss.

REFERENCES

1. Brown JJ. A systematic approach to the dizzy patient. *Neurol Clin* 1990; 8:209–224.
2. Maki BE, McIlroy WE. Postural control in the older adult. *Clin Geriatr Med* 1996; 12:635–658.
3. Nashner LM, Peters JF. Dynamic posturography in the diagnosis and management of dizziness and balance disorders. *Neurol Clin* 1990; 8: 331–349.
4. Sloane PD. Evaluation and management of dizziness in the older patient. *Clin Geriatr Med* 1996; 12:785–801.
5. Baloh RW, Honrubia V. *Clinical neurophysiology of the vestibular system.* Philadelphia: FA Davis, 1990.
6. Guyton AC. Cortical and brain stem control of motor function. In: *Textbook of medical physiology, 8th ed.* Philadelphia: WB Saunders, 1991; 602–616.
7. Livingston RB, ed. Vestibular function. In: West JB, ed. *Best and Taylor's physiological basis of medical practice, 11th ed.* Baltimore: Williams & Wilkins, 1985; 1022–1048.
8. Walzl EM, Mountcastle V. Projection of vestibular nerve to the cerebral cortex of the cat. *Am J Physiol* 1949; 159:594–595.
9. Streeten D, Anderson GH. Delayed orthostatic interolance. *Arch Intern Med* 1992; 152:1066–1072.
10. Schuknecht HF, Kitamura K. Vestibular neuritis. *Ann Otol Rhinol Laryngol* 1981; 90(Suppl):1–19.
11. Dawes JDK. Complications of infections of the middle ear. In: Scott-Brown WG, Ballantyne J, Groves J, eds. *Diseases of the ear, nose and throat, 2nd ed.* London: Butterworth, 1965; 475–554.
12. Epley JM. New dimensions of benign paroxysmal positional vertigo. *Otolaryngol Head Neck Surg* 1980; 88:599–605.
13. Hall SF, Ruby RR, McClure JA. The mechanisms of benign paroxysmal vertigo. *J Otolaryngol* 1979; 8:151–158.
14. Schuknecht HF. Cupulolithiasis. *Arch Otolaryngol* 1969; 90:765–778.
15. Dix MR, Hallpike CS. Pathology, symptomatology and diagnosis of certain common disorders of the vestibular system. *Proc R Soc Med* 1952; 45:341–354.
16. Brandt T, Daraff RB. Physical therapy for benign paroxysmal vertigo. *Arch Otolaryngol* 1980; 106:484.
17. Epley JM. The canalith repositioning procedure: for treatment of benign paroxysmal positional vertigo. *Otolaryngol Head Neck Surg* 1992; 107: 399–404.
18. Hain TC. Episodic vertigo. In: Conn H, ed. *Conn's current therapy; latest approved methods of treatment for the practicing physician.* Philadelphia: WB Saunders, 1996; 869–875.
19. Paparella MM, Kimberly BP. Pathogenesis of Meniere's disease. *J Vestib Res* 1990; 1:3–7.
20. Coats AC. The summating potential and Meniere's disease. *Arch Otolaryngol* 1981; 107:199.
21. Brackman DE. Meniere's disease. In: Conn H, ed. *Conn's current therapy; latest approved methods of treatment for the practicing physician.* Philadelphia: WB Saunders, 1996.
22. Baloh RW, Langhofer L, Honrubia V, Yee RD. On-line analysis of eye movements using a digital computer. *Aviat Space Environ Med* 1980; 51:563–567.
23. Balkany TJ, Sires B, Arenberg IK. Bilateral aspects of Meniere's disease: An underestimated clinical entity. *Otolaryngol Clin North Am* 1980; 13:603–609.
24. Fitzgerald DC. Persistent dizziness following head trauma and perilymphatic fistula. *Arch Phys Med Rehabil* 1995; 76:1017–1020.
25. Ackley RS, Ferraro J, Arenberg IK. Diagnosis of patients with perilymphatic fistula. *Semin Hear* 1994; 15:37–41, 63–64.
26. Gulya AJ. Diagnostic testing and perilymphatic fistulas: Critical review. *Semin Hear* 1994; 15:31–36, 63–64.
27. Ferraro JA, Arenberg IK, Hassanein RS. Electrocochleography and symptoms of inner ear dysfunction. *Arch Otolaryngol* 1985; 3:71–74.

28. Arenberg IK, Ackley RS, Ferraro J, Muchnik C. ECoG results in perilymphatic fistula. Clinical and experimental studies. *Otolaryngol Head Neck Surg* 1988; 99:435–443.
29. Adams RD, Victor M, Ropper AH. *Principles of neurology, 6th ed.* New York: McGraw-Hill, 1977; 284–310.
30. Robillard RB, Hilsinger RL Jr, Adour KK. Ramsey Hunt facial paralysis: clinical analysis of 185 patients. *Otolaryngol Head Neck Surg* 1986; 95:292–297.
31. Meyers RM. Ototoxic effects of gentamycin. *Arch Otolaryngol* 1970; 92:160–162.
32. Fisher CM. Lacunar strokes and infarcts: A review. *Neurology* 1985; 32:871–876.
33. Amarenco P, Kase CS, Rosengart A, Pessins MS, Bousser MG, Caplan LR. Very small (border zone) cerebellar infarcts. Distribution, causes, mechanisms and clinical features. *Brain* 1993; 116:161–186.
34. Hollander J. Dizziness. *Semin Neurol* 1987; 7:317–335.
35. Baloh RW. Dizziness in older people. *J Am Geriatr Soc* 1992; 40: 713–721.
36. Catz A, Ron S, Solzi P, Kooczyn A. The vestibuo-ocular reflex and disequilibrium after hemispheric stroke. *Am J Phys Med Rehabil* 1994; 73:36–39.
37. Berman J, Fredrickson J. Vertigo after head injury—a five year follow-up. *J Otolaryngol* 1978; 7:237.
38. Griffith MV. The incidence of auditory and vestibular concussion following minor head injury. *J Laryngol Otol* 1979; 93:253.
39. Nelson JR. Neuro-otologic aspect of head injury. *Adv Neurol* 1979; 2: 107–128.
40. Shumway-Cook A. Rehabilitation of vestibular dysfunction in traumatic brain injury. *Phys Med Rehabil Clin North Am* 1992; 3:355–369.
41. Schuknecht HF. Mechanism of inner ear injury from blows to the head. *Ann Otol Rhinol Laryngol* 1969; 78:253–262.
42. Lehrer JF, Rubin RC, Poole DC, Hubbard JH, Wille R, Jacobs GB. Perilymphatic fistula—a definitive and curable cause of vertigo following head trauma. *West J Med* 1984; 141:57–60.
43. Weiner H. What's causing the dizziness? *Diagnosis* 1980; 2:38–49.
44. Wennmo K, Wennmo C. Drug-related dizziness. *Acta Otolaryngol [Suppl]* 1988; 455:11–13.
45. McClure JA. Vertigo and imbalance in the elderly. *J Otolaryngol* 1986; 15:248–252.
46. Baloh RW, Konrad HR, Dirks D, Honrobia V. Cerebellar-pontine angle tumors. Results of quantitative vestibulo-ocular testing. *Arch Neurol* 1976; 33:507–512.
47. Rutan GH, Hermanson B, Bild DE, Kittner SJ, LaBaw F, Rell GS. Orthostatic hypotension in older adults. The Cardiovascular Health Study. *Hypertension* 1992; 19:508–519.
48. Hackel A, Linzer M, Anderson N, Williams R. Cardiovascular and catecholamine responses to head-up tilt in the diagnosis of recurrent unexplained syncope in elderly patients. *J Am Geriatr Soc* 1991; 39: 663–668.
49. Hargreaves AD, Muir AL. Lack of variation in venous tone potentiates vasovagal syncope. *Br Heart J* 1992; 67:486–490.
50. Bclal A, Glorig A. Disequilibrium of aging (presbyastasis). *J Laryngol Otol* 1986; 100:1037–1041.
51. Norre ME. Sensory interaction posturography in patients with peripheral vestibular disorders. *Otolaryngol Head Neck Surg* 1994; 110: 281–287.
52. Jenkins HA, Furman J, Gulya A, et al. Disequilibrium of aging. *Otolaryngol Head Neck Surg* 1989; 100:272–282.
53. Makishima K, Tanaka K. Pathological changes of the inner ear and central auditory pathways in diabetics. *Ann Otol Rhinol Laryngol* 1971; 80:218–228.
54. Bergstrom L, Jenkins P, Sando I, English GM. Hearing loss in renal disease: Clinical and pathological studies. *Ann Otorhinol Laryngol* 1973; 82:555.
55. Baloh RW, Honrubia V. Clinical neurophysiology of the vestibular system. Philadelphia: FA Davis, 1990; 253–254.
56. Cohen H, Rubin AM, Gombash L. The team approach to treatment of the dizzy patient. *Arch Phys Med Rehabil* 1992; 73:703–708.
57. Igarashi M. Vestibular compensation: an overview. *Acta Otolaryngol* 1984; 406:78–82.
58. Jones GM. Vestibular plasticity. *Otolaryngol Head Neck Surg* 1983; 91:72–75.
59. Cawthorne T. The physiological basis for head exercises. *J Chart Soc Physiother* 1944; 30:106.
60. Cooksey FS. Rehabilitation in vestibular injuries. *Proc R Soc Med* 1946; 39:273–275.
61. McCabe BF. Labyrinthine exercises in the treatment of diseases, characterized by vertigo; their physiologic basis and methodology. *Laryngoscope* 1970; 80:1429–1433.
62. Hecker HC, Haug CO, Herndon JW. Treatment of the vertiginous patient using Cawthorne's vestibular exercises. *Laryngoscope* 1974; 84: 2065–2072.
63. Norre ME, De Weerdt W. Treatment of vertigo based on habituation. Technique and results of habituation training. *J Laryngol Otol* 1980; 94:971–977.
64. Zee DS. Treatment of vertigo. In: Johnson RT, ed. *Current therapy in neurologic diseases.* Philadelphia: BC Decker, 1985; 8–13.
65. Fukuda T. *Statokinetic reflexes in equilibrium and movement.* Tokyo: Tokyo University Press, 1983.
66. Borello-France DF, Whitney SL, Herdman SJ. *Assessment of vestibular hypofunction; vestibular rehabilitation.* Philadelphia: FA Davis, 1994; 247–286.
67. Duncan PW, Weiner DK, Chandler J, Studenski S. Functional reach: A new clinical measure of balance. *J Gerontol* 1990; 45:M192–M197.
68. Horak FB, Nashner LM. Central programming of postural movements: Adaptation to altered support surface confirguration. *J Neurophysiol* 1986; 554:1369–1381.
69. Sheehy JL, Inzer BE. Acoustic reflex test in neuro-otologic diagnosis. A review of 24 cases of acoustic tumors. *Arch Otolaryngol* 1976; 102: 647–653.
70. Silman S, Gelfand SA, Piper N, Silverman CA, Van Frank L. Prediction of hearing loss from the acoustic reflex threshold. In: Silman S, ed. *The acoustic reflex. Basic principles and clinical application.* New York: Academic Press, 1984; 187–223.
71. Dauman R, Aran JM, Charlet de Sauvage R, Portmann M. Clinical significance of the summating potential in Meniere's s disease. *Am J Otol* 1988; 9:31–38.
72. Gibson WP, Prasher DK. Electrocochleography and its role in the diagnosis and understanding of Meniere's disease. *Otolaryngol Clin North Am* 1983; 16:59–68.
73. Gizzi M, Liveson J. Electronystegmography. In: Liveson JA, Ma DM, eds. *Laboratory reference for clinical neurophysiology.* Philadelphia: FA Davis, 1992; 384–394.
74. Baloh RW, Yee RD, Honrubia V. Clinical abnormalities of optokinetic nystagmus. In: Lennerstrand G, Zee D, Keller EL, eds. *Functional basis of ocular motility disorders.* New York: Pergamon Press, 1982; 311–324.
75. Karlson EA, Mikhail HH, Norris CW, Hassanein RS. Comparison of responses to air, water, and closed loop caloric irrigators. *J Speech Hear Res* 1992; 35:186–191.
76. O'Neil G. The caloric stimulus. Temperature generation within the temporal bone. *Acta Otolaryngol* 1987; 103:266–272.
77. Torok N. Differential caloric stimulations in vestibular diagnosis. *Arch Otolaryngol* 1969; 90:52–57.
78. Saadat D, O'Leary DP, Pulec JL, Kitano H. Comparison of vestibular autorotation and caloric testing. *Otolaryngol Head Neck Surg* 1995; 113:215–222.
79. Tabak S, Collewijn H. Human vestibulo-ocular responses to rapid, helmet-driven head movements. *Exp Brain Res* 1994; 102:367–378.
80. Baloh RW, Honrubia V, Yee RD, Hess K. Changes in the human vestibulo-ocular reflex after loss of peripheral sensitivity. *Ann Neurol* 1984; 16:222–228.
81. Honrubia V, Marco J, Andrews J, Minser K, Yee RD, Baloh RW. Vestibulo-ocular reflexes in peripheral labyrinthine lesions III. Bilateral dysfunction. *Am J Otolaryngol* 1985; 6:342–352.
82. Baloh RW, Sakala SM, Yee RD, Langhofer L, Honrubia V. Quantitative vestibular testing. *Otolaryngol Head Neck Surg* 1984; 92:145–150.
83. Houston HG, Watson DR. A review of computerized electronystagmography technology. *Br J Audiol* 1994; 28:41–46.
84. Jenkins HA, Honrubia V, Baloh RH. Evaluation of multiple frequency rotatory testing in patients with peripheral labyrinthine weakness. *Am J Otolaryngol* 1982; 3:182–188.
85. Herdman SJ. Treatment of benign paroxysmal positional vertigo. *Phys Ther* 1990; 70:381–388.
86. Voorhees RL. The role of dynamic posturography in neurotologic diagnosis. *Laryngoscope* 1989; 99:995–1001.
87. Mirka A, Black FO. Clinical application of dynamic posturography for evaluating sensory integration and vestibular dysfunction. *Neurol Clin* 1990; 8:351–359.

Subject Index

Numbers followed by f indicate figures and numbers followed by t indicate tables.

G

J

O

T